EQUINE SURGERY

Equine Surgery

Jörg A. Auer, Dr Med Vet, MS
Dipolmate, ACVS, ECVS
Professor of Surgery
Director, Equine Hospital
Vetsuisse Faculty Zurich
University of Zurich
Zurich, Switzerland

John A. Stick, DVM
Diplomate, ACVS
Professor
Department of Large Animal Clinical Sciences
College of Veterinary Medicine
Chief of Staff
Veterinary Teaching Hospital
Michigan State University
East Lansing, Michigan

With illustrations by
Mathias Haab

Third Edition

SAUNDERS

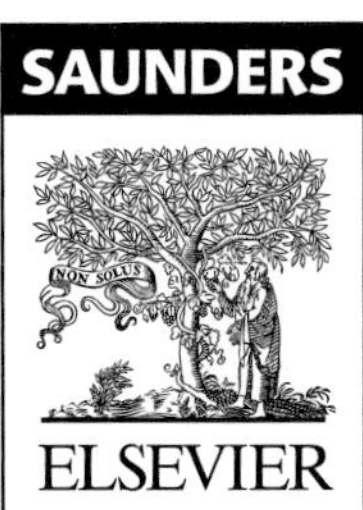

ELSEVIER

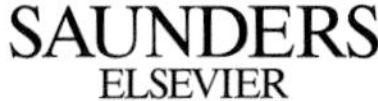

SAUNDERS
ELSEVIER

11830 Westline Industrial Drive
St. Louis, Missouri 63146

EQUINE SURGERY, ed 3

ISBN 13: 978-1-4160-0123-2
ISBN 10: 1-4160-0123-9

Notice

Knowledge and best practice in this field are constantly changing. As new research and experience broaden our knowledge, changes in practice, treatment and drug therapy may become necessary or appropriate. Readers are advised to check the most current information provided (i) on procedures featured or (ii) by the manufacturer of each product to be administered, to verify the recommended dose or formula, the method and duration of administration, and contraindications. It is the responsibility of the practitioner, relying on their own experience and knowledge of the patient, to make diagnoses, to determine dosages and the best treatment for each individual patient, and to take all appropriate safety precautions. To the fullest extent of the law, neither the Publisher nor the Editors assumes any liability for any injury and/or damage to persons or property arising out or related to any use of the material contained in this book.

ISBN 13: 978-1-4160-0123-2
ISBN 10: 1-4160-0123-9

Publishing Director: Linda Duncan
Senior Editor: Liz Fathman
Senior Developmental Editor: Jolynn Gower
Publishing Services Manager: Patricia Tannian
Project Manager: John Casey
Senior Book Design Manager: Julia Dummitt

Printed in United States of America

Last digit is the print number: 9 8 7 6 5 4 3 2 1

DEDICATED TO

Anita and Claudette

our lifelong confidantes,
who keep us focused on the true importance of our existence

and

Ellen and John Stick

my parents (JAS),
for their unconditional encouragement to achieve
and –vibrant as ever in their mid-eighties- for setting an example
of how we should live through their zest for life

and

Renato, Meghan and Mary Katherine

our grown children, for making it all worthwhile

Contributors

Jörg A. Auer, Dr Med Vet, MS, Diplomate, ACVS, ECVS
Professor of Surgery and Director, Veterinary Surgery Clinic, University of Zurich, Zurich, Switzerland
Surgical Instruments
Surgical Techniques
Minimally Invasive Surgical Techniques
Drains, Bandages, and External Coaptation
Principles of Fracture Treatment
Bone Grafts and Bone Replacements
Arthrodesis Techniques
Angular Limb Deformities
Flexural Limb Deformities
Subchondral Cystic Lesions
Tarsus
Craniomaxillofacial Disorders

George W. Bagby, MD, MS (Orthopedics)
Assistant Professor (retired), Washington State University, Pullman, Washington,
Sacred Heart Hospital and Deaconess Hospital (retired), Spokane, Washington, Nalta Hospital (co-founder), Nalta, Bangladesh, Board Member, Prosthetic Outreach Foundation, Seattle, Washington
Surgical Treatment of Developmental Diseases of the Spinal Column

Jeremy V. Bailey, BVSc, MVetSc, Diplomate, ACVS
Professor, Large Animal Surgery, Department of Large Animal Clinical Sciences, Western College of Veterinary Medicine, University of Saskatchewan, Saskatoon, Saskatchewan, Canada
Principles of Reconstructive and Plastic Surgery

Regula Bettschart-Wolfensberger, Dr Med Vet, PhD, Diplomate, ECVA
Equine Hospital Vetsuisse Faculty, University of Zurich, Zurich, Switzerland
Modern Injection Anesthesia for Horses
Recovery from Anesthesia

James T. Blackford, DVM, MS, Diplomate, ACVS
Professor, Department of Large Animal Clinical Sciences, University of Tennessee,
College of Veterinary Medicine, Knoxville, Tennessee
Biomaterials, Surgical Implants, and Instruments
Suture Materials and Patterns

LeeAnn W. Blackford, DVM, Diplomate, ACVS
Blackford Veterinary Surgery Referral, Knoxville, Tennessee
Biomaterials, Surgical Implants, and Instruments
Suture Materials and Patterns

Anthony T. Blikslager, DVM, PhD, Diplomate, ACVS
Assistant Professor, Equine Surgery and Gastrointestinal Biology, College of Veterinary Medicine, North Carolina State University, Raleigh, North Carolina
Stomach and Spleen
Principles of Intestinal Surgery and Determination of Intestinal Viability

Marc Bohner, PhD (Sc Tech)
Dr. Robert Mathys Foundation, Bettlach, Switzerland
Biomaterials, Surgical Implants, and Instruments

Larry R. Bramlage, DVM, MS, Diplomate, ACVS
Rood & Riddle Equine Hospital, Lexington, Kentucky
Tibia

Dennis E. Brooks, DVM, PhD, Diplomate, ACVO
Professor of Ophthalmology, University of Florida, College of Veterinary Medicine,
Gainesville, Florida
Cornea and Sclera
Orbit
Ocular Emergencies and Trauma

H. H. Florian Buchner, Dr Med Vet, PhD
Assistant Professor, Department for Small Animal and Horses, University of Veterinary Medicine, Vienna, Austria
Gait Analysis

Daniel J. Burba, DVM, Diplomate, ACVS
Professor of Equine Surgery, Veterinary Clinical Sciences, Equine Health Studies, School of Veterinary Medicine, Louisiana State University, Baton Rouge, Louisiana
Surgical Site Infection and the Use of Antimicrobials

Shauna L. Cantwell, DVM, MVSc, Diplomate, ACVA
Clinical Assistant Professor, Large Animal Clinical Sciences, College of Veterinary Medicine, University of Florida, Gainesville, Florida
Equine Pain Management

Elizabeth A. Carr, DVM, PhD, Diplomate, ACVIM
Associate Professor, Department of Large Animal Clinical Sciences,
College of Veterinary Medicine, Michigan State University, East Lansing, Michigan
Metabolism and Nutritional Support of the Surgical Patient
Skin Conditions Amenable to Surgery
Pleuropneumonia

Barbara L. Dallap Schaer, VMD, Diplomate, ACVS, ACVECC
Assistant Professor, Department of Clinical Studies, Section of Emergency/Critical Care, New Bolton Center, Kennett Square, Pennsylvania
Hemostasis, Surgical Bleeding, and Transfusion

Charlotte S. Davis, Cert EP, BVSc, MRCVS
Senior Clinical Training Scholar in Equine Orthopaedics, Sefton Equine Referral Hospital, Royal Veterinary College, University of London, London, United Kingdom
Diagnosis and Management of Tendon and Ligament Disorders

Richard M. DeBowes, DVM, MS, Diplomate, ACVS
Professor of Surgery and Chair, Veterinary Clinical Sciences, College of Veterinary Medicine, Washington State University, Pullman, Washington
Principles of Urinary Tract Surgery
Kidneys and Ureters
Bladder
Urethra

Frederick J. Derksen, DVM, PhD, Diplomate, ACVIM
Professor, Department of Large Animal Clinical Sciences, College of Veterinary Medicine, Michigan State University, East Lansing, Michigan
Overview of Upper Airway Function
Diagnostic Techniques in Equine Upper Respiratory Tract Disease

John Disegi, BS, Chemistry
Group Manager, Materials, Chairman AO Materials Expert Group, Product Development, Synthes Technical Center, West Chester, Pennsylvania
Biomaterials, Surgical Implants, and Instruments

Padraic M. Dixon, MVB, PhD, MRCVS
Professor of Equine Surgery, Division of Veterinary Clinical Studies, The University of Edinburgh, Easter Bush Veterinary Centre, Midlothian, Scotland
Oral Cavity and Salivary Glands

Norman G. Ducharme, DVM, MSc, Diplomate ACVS
Medical Director of Equine and Farm Animal Hospitals, Professor of Surgery, College of Veterinary Medicine, Cornell University, Ithaca, New York
Pharynx

Joan Dziezyc, DVM, Diplomate, ACVO
Associate Professor, Texas A & M University, College of Veterinary Medicine, Department of Large Animal Medicine & Science, College Station, Texas
Nasolacrimal System
Intraocular Surgery

Susan C. Eades, DVM, PhD, Diplomate, ACVIM
Professor, Equine Medicine, Department of Veterinary Clinical Sciences, School of Veterinary Medicine, Louisiana State University, Baton Rouge, Louisiana
Sepsis and Endotoxemia

Rolf M. Embertson, DVM, Diplomate, ACVS
Rood & Riddle Equine Hospital, Lexington, Kentucky
Ovaries and Uterus

Andrew T. Fischer, Jr., DVM, Diplomate, ACVS
Chino Valley Equine Hospital, Chino, California
Minimally Invasive Surgical Techniques
Colic: Diagnosis, Preoperative Management, and Surgical Approaches
Kidneys and Ureters
Bladder

Lisa A. Fortier, DVM, PhD, Diplomate, ACVS
Assistant Professor, Department of Clinical Sciences, College of Veterinary Medicine, Cornell University, Ithaca, New York
Shoulder

David E. Freeman, MVB, PhD, Diplomate, ACVS
Professor and Associate Chief of Staff, Large Animal Clinical Sciences, College of Veterinary Medicine, University of Florida, Gainesville, Florida
Sterilization and Antiseptics
Small Intestine
Rectum and Anus
Guttural Pouch

David D. Frisbie, DVM, PhD, Diplomate, ACVS
Assistant Professor, Senior Scientist and Manager of the Orthopaedic Research Center, Clinical Sciences, Colorado State University, Veterinary Teaching Hospital, Fort Collins, Colorado
Synovial Joint Biology and Pathobiology
Principles of Treatment of Joint Disease

Anton E. Fürst, Dr Med Vet, Diplomate, ECVS
Equine Hospital Vetsuisse Faculty, University of Zurich, Zurich, Switzerland
Diagnostic Anesthesia
Emergency Treatment and Transportation of Equine Fracture Patients
Foot

Mathew P. Gerard, BVSc, PhD, DACVS
Assistant Professor of Large Animal Surgery, Department of Clinical Sciences, College of Veterinary Medicine, North Carolina State University, Raleigh, North Carolina
Oral Cavity and Salivary Glands

Brian C. Gilger, DVM, MS, Diplomate, ACVO
Professor of Ophthalmology, Department of Clinical Sciences, North Carolina State University, Raleigh, North Carolina
Surgical Management of Equine Recurrent Uveitis

Barrie D. Grant, DVM, MS, Diplomate, ACVS
San Luis Rey Equine Clinic, Bonsall, California
Surgical Treatment of Developmental Diseases of the Spinal Column

Joanne Hardy, DVM, PhD, Diplomate, ACVS, ACVECC
Clinical Associate Professor, Department of Large Animal Medicine and Surgery, Texas A & M University, College Station, Texas
Fluids, Electrolytes, and Acid-Base Therapy
Minimally Invasive Surgical Techniques
Large Intestine
Postoperative Care and Complications Associated with Abdominal Surgery
Guttural Pouch

Dean A. Hendrickson, DVM, MS, Diplomate, ACVS
Associate Professor of Surgery, James L. Voss Veterinary Teaching Hospital, Colorado State University, Fort Collins, Colorado
Management of Superficial Wounds
Management of Deep and Chronic Wounds

Susan J. Holcombe, VMD, MS, PhD, Diplomate, ACVS, ACVECC
Associate Professor, Department of Large Animal Clinical Sciences, College of Veterinary Medicine, Michigan State University, East Lansing, Michigan
Shock: Pathophysiology, Diagnosis, and Treatment
Physiologic Response to Trauma: Evaluating the Trauma Patient

Michael O. Hottiger, DVM, PhD
Institute of Veterinary Biochemistry and Molecular Biology, University of Zurich, Zurich, Switzerland
Molecular Biology Techniques in Musculoskeletal Research

Vivian E. Jamieson, DVM, Diplomate, ACVO
Veterinary Eye Care, Mount Pleasant, South Carolina
Cornea and Sclera

Barbara Kaser-Hotz, Dr Med Vet, Diplomate, ACVR, ECVDI
Professor Diagnostic Imaging, Vetsuisse Faculty, University of Zurich, Zurich, Switzerland
Diagnostic Medical Imaging

Renée Léveillé, DVM, Diplomate, ACVR
Imaging Center for Animals, Veterinary Specialty Center, Buffalo Grove, Illinois
Minimally Invasive Surgical Techniques

James D. Lillich, DVM, MS, Diplomate, ACVS
Associate Professor of Equine Surgery, Department of Clinical Sciences, Kansas State University, Manhattan, Kansas
Principles of Urinary Tract Surgery
Kidneys and Ureters
Bladder
Urethra

Christophorus J. Lischer, PD, Dr Vet Med, Diplomate, ECVS
Equine Clinic, Vetsuisse Faculty, University of Zurich, Zurich, Switzerland
Foot

Mandi J. Lopez, DVM, PhD, Diplomate, ACVS
Assistant Professor, Veterinary Clinical Sciences, Louisiana State University, Baton Rouge, Louisiana
Bone Biology and Fracture Healing

Joel Lugo, DVM, MS, Diplomate, ACVS
Assistant Professor, Department of Clinical Sciences, College of Veterinary Medicine, Auburn University, Auburn, Alabama
Thoracic Disorders
Pleuropneumonia

Robert J. MacKay, BVSc, PhD, Diplomate, ACVIM
Professor, Large Animal Clinical Sciences, University of Florida, Gainesville, Florida
Anatomy and Physiology of the Nervous System
Diagnostic Procedures
Peripheral Nerve Injury

Mark D. Markel, DVM, PhD, Diplomate, ACVS
Professor and Chair, Department of Medical Sciences, School of Veterinary Medicine, University of Wisconsin, Madison, Wisconsin
Bone Biology and Fracture Healing

Thomas R. Miller, DVM, Diplomate, ACVO
Tampa Bay Veterinary Specialists, Largo, Florida
Eyelids

Nicholas J. Millichamp, BVet Med, PhD, MRCVS, Diplomate, ACVO
Professor of Ophthalmology, Texas A&M University, College of Veterinary Medicine, Veterinary Teaching Hospital, College Station, Texas
Principles of Ophthalmic Surgery
Conjunctiva
Third Eyelid

Rustin M. Moore, DVM, PhD, Diplomate, ACVS
Professor of Equine Surgery, Department of Veterinary Clinical Sciences, School of Veterinary Medicine, Louisiana State University, Baton Rouge, Louisiana
Sepsis and Endotoxemia
Surgical Site Infection and the Use of Antimicrobials

Mark P. Nasisse, DVM
Carolina Veterinary Specialists, Greensboro, North Carolina
Cornea and Sclera

Frank A. Nickels, DVM, MS, Diplomate, ACVS
Professor, Department of Large Animal Clinical Sciences, Michigan State University, College of Veterinary Medicine, East Lansing, Michigan
Nasal Passages and Paranasal Sinuses

Alan J. Nixon, BVSc, MS, Diplomate, ACVS
Professor of Orthopedic Surgery, Cornell University, College of Veterinary Medicine, Ithaca, New York
Phalanges and the Metacarpophalangeal and Metatarsophalangeal Joints

Eric J. Parente, DVM, Diplomate, ACVS
Associate Professor of Surgery, Department of Clinical Sciences, University of Pennsylvania, New Bolton Center, Kennett Square, Pennsylvania
Diagnostic Techniques in Equine Upper Respiratory Tract Disease

John G. Peloso, DVM, MS, Diplomate, ACVS
Surgeon, Equine Medical Center of Ocala, Ocala, Florida
Biology and Management of Muscle Disorders and Diseases

Peter C. Rakestraw, MA, VMD, Diplomate, ACVS
Clinical Assistant Professor, Department of Large Animal Medicine and Surgery, College of Veterinary Medicine, Texas A&M University, College Station, Texas
Large Intestine
Postoperative Care and Complications Associated with Abdominal Surgery

Dean W. Richardson, DVM, Diplomate, ACVS
Charles W. Raker Professor of Surgery, New Bolton Center, Department of Clinical Studies, University of Pennsylvania, Kennett Square, Pennsylvania
The Metacarpal and Metatarsal Bones
Femur and Pelvis

Astrid B. M. Rijkenhuizen, DVM, PhD, RNVA, Diplomate, ECVS
Faculty of Veterinary Medicine, Department of Equine Sciences, University of Utrecht, Utrecht, Netherlands
Minimally Invasive Surgical Techniques

James T. Robertson, DVM, Diplomate, ACVS
Associate Professor Equine Surgery, The Ohio State University, College of Veterinary Medicine, Columbus, Ohio
Traumatic Disorders of the Spinal Column

Sheilah A. Robertson, BVMS, PhD, DACVA, DECVA
Professor, Department of Large Animal Clinical Sciences, College of Veterinary Medicine, University of Florida, Gainesville, Florida
Anesthesia and Analgesia for Foals
Equine Pain Management

Alan J. Ruggles, DVM, Diplomate, ACVS
Rood & Riddle Equine Hospital, Lexington, Kentucky
Carpus

Bonnie R. Rush, DVM, MS, Diplomate, ACVIM
Professor, Equine Internal Medicine, Department of Clinical Sciences, College of Veterinary Medicine, Kansas State University, Manhattan, Kansas
Developmental Vertebral Anomalies

Valerie F. Samii, DVM, Diplomate, ACVR
Associate Professor, Veterinary Clinical Sciences, The Ohio State University, Columbus, Ohio
Traumatic Disorders of the Spinal Column

Sarah N. Sampson, BSc, DVM
Resident, Equine Surgery & Orthopedic Sports Medicine Resident, Department of Equine Surgery, College of Veterinary Medicine, Washington State University, Pullman, Washington
Magnetic Resonance Imaging of the Equine Distal Limb

Robert K. Schneider, DVM, MS, Diplomate, ACVS
Professor and Chief Department of Equine Surgery, Washington State University, College of Veterinary Medicine, Pullman, Washington
Magnetic Resonance Imaging of the Equine Distal Limb
Synovial and Osseous Infections

James Schumacher, DVM, MS, MRCVS, Diplomate, ACVS
Department of Large Animal Clinical Sciences, University of Tennessee, Knoxville, Tennessee
Skin Grafting
Testis
Penis and Prepuce

Anja C. Schütte, Dr Med Vet, PhD
Pferdeklinik Aschheim (Private Equine Hospital), Munich, Bavaria, Germany
Surgical Treatment of Developmental Diseases of the Spinal Column

Roger K. W. Smith, MA VetMB, CertEO, MRCVS, PhD, Diplomate, ECVS
Department of Farm Animal & Equine Medicine /Surgery, The Royal Veterinary College, North Mymms, Hatfield, Great Britain
Diagnosis and Management of Tendon and Ligament Disorders

Bernhard M. Spiess, DVM, Dr Med Vet, Diplomate, ACVO, Diplomate, ECVO
Professor, Veterinary Ophthalmology, Department of Small Animal Medicine, University of Zurich, Zurich, Switzerland
Surgical Management of Equine Recurrent Uveitis

John A. Stick., DVM, Diplomate, ACVS
Professor and Chief of Staff, Department of Large Animal Clinical Sciences, College of Veterinary Medicine, Michigan State University, East Lansing, Michigan
Preparation of the Surgical Patient, the Surgery Facility, and the Operating Team
Cryosurgery
Management of Sinus Tracts and Fistulas
Esophagus
Abdominal Hernias
Larynx
Trachea
Stifle

Lloyd P. Tate, Jr., VMD, Diplomate, ACVS
Professor of Surgery, North Carolina State University, College of Veterinary Medicine, Raleigh, North Carolina
Lasers in Veterinary Surgery

Christine L. Theoret, DVM, PhD, Diplomate, ACVS
Associate Professor, Department of Biomédecine Vétérinaire, Université de Montréal, St-Hyacinthe, Québec, Canada
Wound Repair

Russell L. Tucker, DVM, Diplomate, ACVR
Radiology Director, Veterinary Clinical Sciences, Washington State University, Pullman, Washington
Magnetic Resonance Imaging of the Equine Distal Limb

Gottlieb Ueltschi
Professor of Equine Medicine and Veterinary Radiology, Department of Clinical Medicine, Equine Clinic and Large Animal Radiology, Vetsuisse Faculty, University of Bern, Bern, Switzerland
Diagnostic Medical Imaging

Alexander Valverde, DVM, DVSc, Diplomate, ACVA
Assistant Professor, Department of Large Animal Clinical Sciences, College of Veterinary Medicine, University of Florida, Gainesville, Florida
Advances in Inhalation Anesthesia

P. René van Weeren, DVM, PhD, Diplomate, ECVS
Associate Professor, Equine Surgery, Department of Equine Sciences, Faculty of Veterinary Medicine, Utrecht University, Utrecht, The Netherlands
Osteochondrosis

Brigitte von Rechenberg, Dr Med Vet, PD, Diplomate, ECVS
Musculoskeletal Research Unit, Equine Hospital Vetsuisse Faculty, University of Zurich, Zurich, Switzerland
Saddle Evaluation: Poor Fit Contributing to Back Problems in Horses
Molecular Biology Techniques in Musculoskeletal Research
Bone Grafts and Bone Replacements
Subchondral Cystic Lesions

R. Wayne Waguespack, DVM, MS, Diplomate, ACVS
Assistant Professor of Equine Surgery, Department of Veterinary Clinical Sciences, School of Veterinary Medicine, Louisiana State University, Baton Rouge, Louisiana
Surgical Site Infection and the Use of Antimicrobials

Jeffrey P. Watkins, DVM, MS, Diplomate, ACVS
Professor and Chief of Surgery, Large Animal Medicine and Surgery, College of Veterinary Medicine, Texas A & M University, College Station, Texas
Radius and Ulna

Michael A. Weishaupt, Dr Med Vet, PhD
Equine Hospital, Vetsuisse Faculty, University of Zurich, Zurich, Switzerland
Gait Analysis

David A. Wilson, DVM, MS, Diplomate, ACVS
Associate Professor, Equine Surgery, Section Head, Department of Equine Surgery & Medicine, Associate Chair for Clinical Affairs, College of Veterinary Medicine, University of Missouri, Columbia, Missouri
Stomach and Spleen

Brett Woodie, DVM, MS, Diplomate, ACVS
Rood & Riddle Equine Hospital, Lexington, Kentucky
Vulva, Vestibule, Vagina and Cervix

PREFACE

Since the publication of the first edition in 1992, *Equine Surgery* has been accepted as a definitive clinical reference and teaching text. Like the first two editions, the third edition of the book has been prepared as a foundation text for the art and science of modern equine surgery. Our intent was to produce a comprehensive textbook that would be of practical help to general practitioners, as well as provide specialists and surgeons in training with a single reference source on equine surgery. Accordingly, this third edition of the book has been significantly enlarged and includes new information, new authors, additional illustrations, and many more line drawings and tables.

The task of reviewing the ever expanding literature into concise chapters was considerable. As the editors, we divided the responsibility for organizing the sections and inviting authors between the two of us; and, we believe that the outcome is consistency of content and presentation in the final text. Additionally, we deliberately avoided omitting well-known material and concentrating only on state of the art techniques and procedures. We felt it was important that students, practitioners, and clinicians have a comprehensive textbook, discussing all aspects of this exciting field in-depth, while staying current with new developments.

All chapters in the third edition have been completely revised and updated. Many new chapters were added in areas of this discipline that are rapidly expanding. While many authors remained the same, many new authors have been added to this text, and we are indebted to all contributing authors who helped us produce this book in a timely fashion. We especially would like to thank David Freeman, Anton Fürst, Susan Holcombe, Pete Knox, Wayne McIlwraith and Rolfe M. Radcliff who provided a critical review of the second edition, making suggestions for revision and improvement of the third edition of this text. We are also indebted to the staff of Elsevier, including Elizabeth Fathman, Jolynn Gower (our most pleasant and constant contact), John Dedeke, and especially John Casey (for his tireless quest to keep the project on time and the editors happy). Personal thanks to our administrative assistants, Monika Gutscher (Zurich) and Martha Devlin (East Lansing), without whom our lives would have been much more complicated during the compilation of this book. A special thank you goes to Mathias Haab of Zurich, Switzerland, who did an excellent job in preparing all new art work and in a most efficient manner. Finally, our most sincere thanks to all the specialists who contributed to this textbook, but most especially to the Diplomates in the American and European Colleges of Veterinary Surgery for their outstanding educational contributions.

Jörg Auer and
John Stick, Editors

Contents

Section V Alimentary System

John A. Stick

Section VI Respiratory System

John A. Stick

Section VII Nervous System

John A. Stick

Section VIII Eye and Adnexa

Jörg A. Auer

SECTION I

Surgical Biology

John A. Stick

CHAPTER 1

Shock: Pathophysiology, Diagnosis, and Treatment

Susan J. Holcombe

We commonly think of shock as an event that follows severe hemorrhage or endotoxemia and causes tachycardia, tachypnea, hypotension, depression, and abnormal mucous membranes. The clinical signs of shock reflect hemodynamic responses that are the result of exquisitely controlled neurohumoral mechanisms triggered by depletion of effective circulating volume. Shock results from any inciting event that causes blood flow and oxygen delivery to be insufficient to meet the oxygen demands of the tissues. Decreased blood flow can occur because of inadequate cardiac function, decreased total blood volume, inappropriate distribution of blood volume, or obstruction of cardiac output, all of which result in decreased cardiac output and poor tissue perfusion. Because oxygen is not stored in tissues, the rate of oxygen uptake from the capillaries must match the metabolic requirements of the tissues for aerobic metabolism to continue.[1] When metabolic demand for oxygen exceeds the rate of oxygen uptake by the tissues, anaerobic metabolism ensues, resulting in decreased energy production. When cell dysoxia (the condition in which energy production is limited by the supply of oxygen) produces a measurable change in organ function, the condition is commonly known as shock.[2] If left untreated, progressive tissue hypoxia leads to altered cellular metabolism, cell death, organ failure, and, ultimately, the death of the animal.

Understanding the pathophysiology of shock is essential for developing appropriate treatment strategies and monitoring techniques for the shock patient. As well, several aspects of the patient's response to treatment are relevant to predicting outcome. These topics are addressed here.

CLASSIFICATION OF SHOCK

Historically, shock has been classified on the basis of the *cause* of the impaired circulating blood volume.[3] These causative categories include cardiogenic (caused by primary cardiac dysfunction), hypovolemic or hemorrhagic (due to severe blood or volume loss), distributive (resulting from maldistribution of blood flow caused by sepsis, endotoxemia, or trauma), and anaphylactic or neurogenic shock. Each of these categories ultimately results in insufficient cardiac output and impaired tissue perfusion. Shock may also be classified by *functional* categories that describe the type of effective blood volume depletion responsible for circulatory failure.[4] These functional categories include cardiogenic, hypovolemic, and maldistribution shock. Finally, a third classification encompasses *vasogenic* and *obstructive* forms of shock. Hypovolemia can result from whole blood loss, fluid loss because of severe dehydration, or intestinal hypersecretion. Sepsis, endotoxemia, and anaphylaxis are causes of vasogenic shock, as they lead to maldistribution of blood flow as a result of vasoactive substances that cause extensive vasodilation and impair appropriate venous or arterial constriction. Anaphylactic shock occurs because of an IgE-mediated release of vasoactive substances that produce massive vasodilation and pooling of as much as 60% to 80% of circulating volume.[5] Obstructive shock is caused by something that impedes cardiac output, such as cardiac tamponade. Frequently, disease processes cause more than one type of shock to develop in a patient. For example, a horse may lose 30% of its blood volume and develop hypovolemic shock. Because of hypoperfusion of the gastrointestinal tract and the resultant mucosal ischemia, bacterial translocation and absorption of endotoxin may occur, causing the horse to develop signs of endotoxemia. On the other hand, a horse with acute large colon volvulus may become endotoxemic but also hypovolemic as a result of *hypersecretion* into the gastrointestinal tract.

The depletion of circulating blood volume caused by primary blood loss can be understood intuitively. Hypovolemia caused by gastrointestinal diseases and endotoxemia is more complex. Major fluid shifts with abdominal disease occur because of hypersecretion into the bowel lumen or peritoneal cavity as a result of bacterial toxins, or because of primary endotoxemia. Frequently, both occur. These fluid shifts occur at the expense of the plasma volume, resulting in hemoconcentration and decreased circulating volume. Endotoxins have profound effects on the distribution of fluid and can cause redistribution of up to 20% of the plasma volume into the splanchnic capillary beds. In addition to sodium-rich fluid losses, increased capillary permeability leads to loss of albumin and water into the interstitium, further depleting the plasma volume and reducing the intravascular oncotic pressure. Therefore, although plasma volume is retained within the horse, it is distributed into the interstitium and the gastrointestinal tract, and pooled in the venous circulation.

Classifications of shock are useful for understanding the pathophysiology of shock. They may help direct treatment strategies, but shock is a dynamic process and several causes of shock may develop in one patient. The result is a hypoperfused patient with inappropriate oxygen delivery to and uptake by the tissues.

PATHOPHYSIOLOGY

The initial response to depletion of the effective circulating volume is the movement of fluid from the interstitium into the capillaries. This transcapillary refill helps maintain blood volume but leaves an interstitial fluid deficit. This may be the only response to mild acute hemorrhage (i.e., less than 15% blood volume loss) or volume loss. The interstitial volume is then replaced by increased oral intake of water, stimulated by increased plasma osmolarity.[6]

Clinical signs of volume depletion occur when 15% to 20% of the circulating blood volume is lost acutely.[6] This degree of blood loss causes decreased cardiac output and arterial pressure because of the relationship described in the following equation:

$$\text{Mean arterial pressure} = \text{cardiac output} \times \text{systemic vascular resistance.}$$

Therefore, the reduction in cardiac output lowers the systemic blood pressure. Decreased systemic blood pressure causes decreased tension in the vascular walls, initiating neurohumoral responses in an attempt to increase intravascular volume and cardiac output.[7] Baroreceptors in the aorta and carotid arteries sense decreased stretch of the vascular walls, resulting in a change in baroreceptor afferent discharge to the vasomotor centers in the brain stem (Fig. 1-1). This signal is sent via branches of the glossopharyngeal and vagus nerves (cranial nerves IX and X) to the medulla oblongata, which induces sympathetic inhibition of parasympathetic stimulation.[7] The catecholamines epinephrine and norepinephrine are then released from the adrenal medulla, leading to arterial and venous constriction in an attempt to improve cardiac preload. Direct arteriolar constriction increases systemic vascular resistance, thereby elevating the systemic blood pressure toward normal. Venous constriction increases blood delivery to the heart, because about 70% of the vascular volume is normally contained within the venous system.[7] Myocardial contractility and heart rate are increased, which, in combination with the enhanced venous return, raises the cardiac output. Effective circulating volume depletion sensed at the carotid sinus baroreceptors also stimulates release of antidiuretic hormone from the paraventricular nuclei of the hypothalamus and ultimately from the pituitary gland, leading to increased water reabsorption at the collecting tubules of the kidney in an attempt to preserve circulating volume.[7]

The kidney also has an intrinsic set of mechanisms to monitor and affect blood pressure. Reduction in circulating volume is sensed by baroreceptors in the wall of the afferent arteriole and the cells of the macula densa in the early distal tubule of the kidney.[8] The afferent arteriole of each glomerulus contains specialized cells—the juxtaglomerular cells—that synthesize the precursor prorenin, which is cleaved to the active proteolytic enzyme renin. Active renin is then stored in and released from secretory granules.[8,9] Renal hypoperfusion (resulting from hypotension or volume

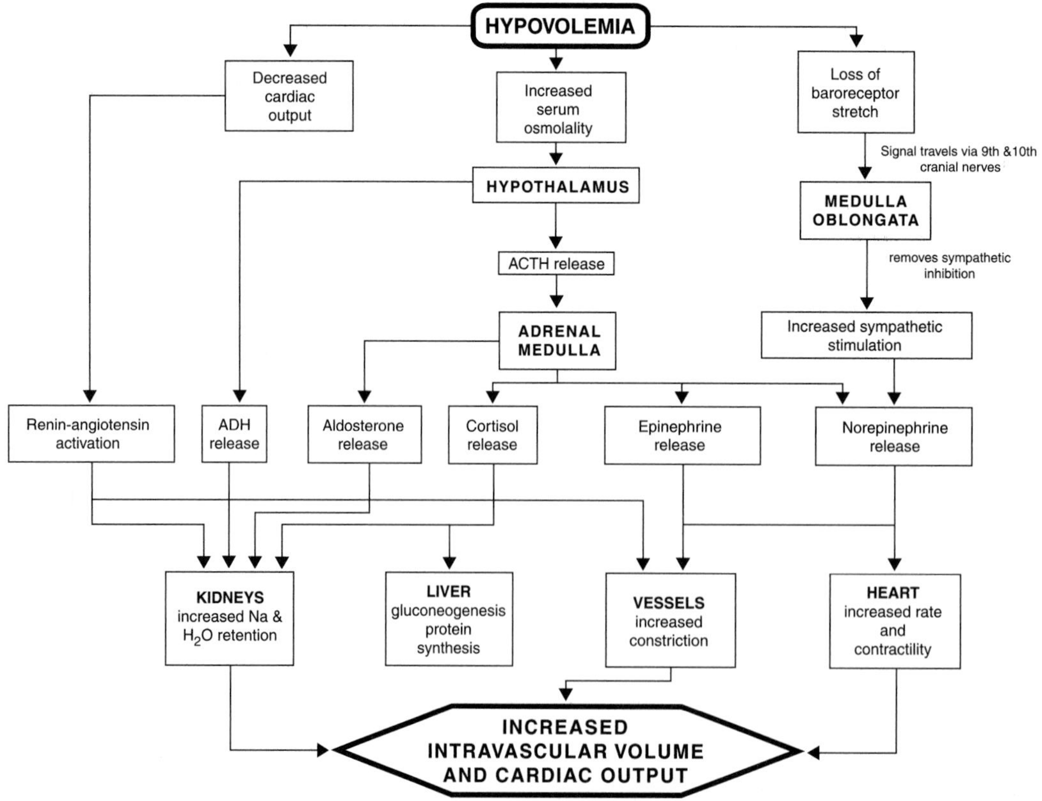

Figure 1-1. Sympathetic response to hypotension. (From Rudloff E, Kirby R: Vet Clin North Am Small Anim Pract 24:1016, 1994.)

depletion), increased sympathetic activity, and release of catecholamines are the major physiologic stimuli to renin secretion. Renin initiates a sequence of steps that begins with cleavage of angiotensin I from angiotensinogen produced in the liver and other organs including the kidney. Angiotensin I is then converted into angiotensin II, catalyzed by angiotensin-converting enzyme, which is located principally in the lung. Most angiotensin II formation takes place in the pulmonary circulation.[9] Angiotensin II promotes renal sodium and water retention and therefore expansion of the plasma volume and ultimately the interstitium. This occurs by at least two mechanisms[10]:

1. Direct stimulation of sodium reabsorption in the early proximal tubule
2. Increased secretion of aldosterone from the adrenal medulla, which also enhances sodium and water conservation by the kidney

Angiotensin II also stimulates systemic vasoconstriction.

In addition to using multiorgan signals to maintain circulating volume, the animal also responds to shock by mobilizing body reserves for increased metabolic demand. Increased circulating catecholamines and adrenocorticotropic hormone released from the hypothalamus in response to hypovolemia and hyperosmolarity result in cortisol secretion from the adrenal glands. Cortisol mobilizes substrates for energy production by stimulating gluconeogenesis and protein synthesis by the liver in an attempt to meet the increased energy demands of the system during the early shock state.[11]

These neurohumoral responses result in a hyperdynamic state that attempts to restore circulating volume and cardiac output.[11] Although these adaptive effects are beneficial, especially in minor insults, peripheral vasoconstriction leads to maldistributed microcirculatory flow with localized areas of hypoperfusion and tissue hypoxemia.[12] During early shock, blood flow is maintained to the heart and brain at the expense of the intestinal tract, skeletal muscle, and other organs. Indeed, normal arterial blood pressure is maintained even when there is observed blood loss, meaning that some organ somewhere is underperfused because of vasoconstriction of its vascular bed.[12] Without aggressive therapy, the patient in a hyperdynamic, compensatory phase of shock begins to decompensate. When tissue oxygen consumption becomes supply dependent, anaerobic metabolism ensues, resulting ultimately in lactic acidosis, cell death, and organ failure. Decreased gastrointestinal perfusion causes decreased mucosal integrity and increased absorption of bacteria and endotoxin, overwhelming the liver's capacity to detoxify the blood. The pancreas releases myocardial depressant factor, which decreases heart rate and contractility, depresses the reticular endothelial system, and decreases the afferent arteriole and glomerular filtration rate, leading to decreased urine production and ultimately to anuria.[13] Ultimately, autoregulatory escape occurs, which is an overriding of sympathetic vasoconstriction resulting in organ vasodilation.[12] This occurs because precapillary constriction leads to decreased tissue perfusion, resulting in a change from aerobic to anaerobic metabolism.[12] As anaerobic metabolism continues, the neuroendocrine sympathetic response becomes ineffective, and dilation of precapillary sphincters with continued constriction of postcapillary sphincters occurs, leading to pooling of blood in the venules.[12] Such secondary sequestration of blood volume in the tissues contributes to maldistribution of blood volume, but it also causes increased capillary hydrostatic pressure, leading to extravasation of water and salt and small amounts of albumin into the interstitium, further depleting the vascular volume. These changes at the capillary level contribute to the maldistribution of blood flow, or the distributive component of shock.[12] As the decompensated phase of shock continues, the hypoxic, acidotic endothelium and poorly perfused capillaries activate macrophages and leucocytes and produce cytokines, including interleukin-1, interleukin-6, tumor necrosis factor, platelet activating factor, eicosanoids, and other immunochemical cascades, which may initiate intravascular coagulation, a state of systemic inflammation, organ failure, and death.[4,12]

The common denominator in early shock is inadequate oxygen delivery. Oxygen is needed to meet normal or increased metabolic activity as measured by oxygen consumption.[12] Two variables describe oxygen transport: the rate of oxygen delivery (DO_2) and the rate of oxygen uptake or consumption (VO_2) (Table 1-1). Delivery of oxygen to the tissues depends on cardiac output and the oxygen content of the arterial blood. Cardiac output depends on heart rate and stroke volume, which are affected by preload, afterload, myocardial contractility, and rhythm.[12] The oxygen content of the arterial blood (Cao_2) is determined by the formula

$$Cao_2 = (1.34 \times Hb \times Sao_2) + (0.003 \times Pao_2)$$

and is thus dependent on the amount of hemoglobin (Hb) and the oxygen saturation of the hemoglobin in the arterial blood (Sao_2). Note that the dissolved oxygen, or partial

TABLE 1-1. Hemodynamic Values

Term	Abbreviation	Formula
Cardiac output	CO	CO = MAP/SVR
Oxygen content of arterial blood	Cao_2	$Cao_2 = (Hb \times 1.34 \times Sao_2) + (Pao_2 \times 0.003)$
Blood volume	—	Blood volume = $0.08 \times$ kg body weight
Oxygen content of mixed venous blood	Cvo_2	$Cvo_2 = (Hb \times 1.34 \times Svo_2) + (Pvo_2 \times 0.003)$
Oxygen extraction, or difference between oxygen contents of arterial blood and venous blood	vO_2	$vO_2 = CO \times (Cao_2 - Cvo_2)$
Oxygen delivery	DO_2	$DO_2 = CO \times Cao_2$

Hb, hemoglobin; MAP, mean arterial pressure; Pao_2, partial pressure of oxygen in arterial blood; Pvo_2, partial pressure of oxygen in venous blood; Sao_2, oxygen saturation in arterial blood; Svo_2, oxygen saturation in venous blood; SVR, systemic vascular resistance.

pressure of oxygen, in the arterial blood (Pa_{O_2}) contributes very little to the oxygen content of the blood. An oxygen debt occurs when the oxygen consumption permitted by delivery is less than that needed. DO_2, the amount of oxygen delivered to the tissues per minute, is described by the formula

$$DO_2 = CO \times Ca_{O_2},$$

where CO is cardiac output. The amount of oxygen consumed by the tissues (V_{O_2}) is equal to the difference between the amount of oxygen in the blood delivered *to* the tissues and the amount of oxygen in the blood returning *from* the tissues:

$$V_{O_2} = CO \times (Ca_{O_2} - Cv_{O_2}),$$

where Cv_{O_2} is the oxygen content of the venous blood (see Table 1-1).

Therefore, measures of oxygen supply to the tissues, such as heart rate, cardiac output, mean arterial pressure, hemoglobin concentration, and arterial oxygen saturation, provide information on oxygen supply but not about adequacy of tissue oxygenation. If a decrease in oxygen uptake is not accompanied by a decrease in metabolic rate, oxygen supply cannot support aerobic metabolism, and anaerobic metabolism ensues. In the aerobic state, glucose is completely oxidized, yielding 36 moles of adenosine triphosphate per mole of glucose.[1] However, when the metabolic demand for oxygen exceeds the rate of oxygen uptake by the tissues, a portion of the glucose metabolism is diverted to the production of lactate, with an energy yield of only 2 moles of ATP per mole of glucose.[1] Therefore, blood lactate levels can help to predict tissue oxygen deficit and, combined with other evidence of inadequate oxygen consumption, can support a diagnosis of hypoperfusion, oxygen debt, and shock.

CLINICAL SIGNS

The clinical stages of shock include (1) the compensatory phase, sometimes referred to as the hyperdynamic phase, (2) the early decompensatory or hypodynamic phase, and (3) the terminal decompensatory phase.[1] These phases of shock follow the depletion of effective circulating volume, neuroadrenal responses to the depletion, and the amount of oxygen debt that is accrued. The American College of Surgeons identifies four categories of acute blood loss based on the percentage loss of blood volume.[4]

- Class I: Loss of 15% or less of the total blood volume. This degree of blood loss is usually fully compensated by transcapillary refill. Because blood volume is maintained, clinical manifestations of hypovolemia are minimal or absent.
- Class II: Loss of 15% to 30% of the total blood volume. The clinical findings at this stage may include resting tachycardia, orthostatic changes in heart rate and blood pressure, decreased urine output, and agitated mental state.
- Class III: Loss of 30% to 40% of the blood volume. This usually marks the onset of hypovolemic shock, with a decrease in blood pressure and continued decreased urine output, possibly to an anuric state. There is evidence that the tachycardia-vasoconstrictor response to hemorrhage can be lost at this stage of blood loss.
- Class IV: Loss of more than 40% of the blood volume. This is a harbinger of circulatory collapse.

The hyperdynamic or compensated phase of shock correlates with early class II blood loss, and clinical signs of compensation begin when the blood volume is acutely depleted by greater than 15%. The initiating event is abnormal tissue perfusion followed by compensatory neurohumoral responses, which cause clinical signs such as tachycardia, tachypnea, hyperemic mucous membranes, fast capillary refill time, and bounding pulse pressure. This high-energy state is achieved by increasing the metabolic rate. If the compensatory response is unsuccessful, because of either the severity of the insult or lack of appropriate treatment, early decompensation ensues.

Early decompensation correlates with late class II and class III blood loss and begins when oxygen delivery does not meet consumptive needs, initiating anaerobic metabolism and lactic acidosis. Clinical signs of early decompensation include progressive tachycardia, tachypnea, prolonged capillary refill time, cold peripheral appendages such as ears, muzzle, and limbs, poor pulse pressure, decreased urine production, and abnormal mentation exhibited as depression or lack of responsiveness.

Late decompensation correlates with class IV blood loss and is associated with marked hypotension, bradycardia, circulatory collapse, pale to gray mucous membranes, progressive abnormal mentation or somnolence, anuria, and other evidence of organ failure. Late decompensation is a nearly lethal stage of shock, and many patients are no longer able to respond to even very aggressive therapy.

TREATMENT

Prompt, aggressive fluid therapy (see Chapter 3) is the hallmark of shock treatment, with the goals of resuscitation being reestablishment of oxygen uptake into the vital organs and sustained aerobic metabolism. Fluid therapy is used to restore intravascular volume, improve tissue perfusion, and overcome regional circulatory deficiencies caused by uneven, maldistributed vasoconstriction. The most commonly used fluids for volume resuscitation are balanced polyionic crystalloids, which are isotonic relative to plasma and have a similar electrolyte composition. They contain water, sodium or glucose, other electrolytes, and, in some instances, a buffer. The principal electrolyte in crystalloid fluids is sodium, which is also the main electrolyte in the extracellular fluid.

Extracellular fluid is distributed between the interstitial and intravascular fluid compartments, with the majority (75%) being in the interstitium.[14] Therefore, within 1 hour of intravenous administration, crystalloids are distributed evenly throughout the extracellular fluid, primarily expanding the interstitial fluid space. For example, administration of 10 L of polyionic crystalloids results in an expansion of approximately 2.5 L or less in blood volume and 7.5 L of interstitial volume. A significant amount may be lost in the urine, depending on the rate of delivery.

Examples of isotonic crystalloid solutions are 0.9% NaCl, lactated Ringer's solution, Plasma-Lyte A, and Normosol-R.

If the horse is sodium or chloride deficient, 0.9% NaCl is a good choice. Lactated Ringer's solution contains potassium, calcium, and lactate as a buffer. Lactated Ringer's—or any solution containing calcium—is incompatible with blood products because the calcium will bind with the citrated anticoagulant, and therefore it should be discontinued during whole blood or plasma transfusions. Normosol-R and Plasma-Lyte A are pH balanced and contain some magnesium. For resuscitation purposes, any isotonic crystalloid solution is appropriate.

To determine the volume of crystalloid fluids to administer to a patient in shock, estimate the blood volume lost; then give four times that volume because the principal distribution of crystalloids is into the interstitial space. Or, as a "shock dose," administer 90 mL/kg at a rate of 6 mL/kg per minute while monitoring the patient closely. The horse's total blood volume is estimated to be 0.08 to 0.09 times its lean body mass in kilograms. Therefore, a shock dose of fluids amounts to the administration of one volume of circulating blood. This is estimated to be 40 to 50 L of fluid for a 500-kg horse. Pulmonary edema from volume overload is unlikely to occur in an adult horse, but it may occur if the horse is in anuric renal failure or has pulmonary contusions or inflammation or cardiac dysfunction.[7]

Achieving a fluid rate of 6 mL/kg per minute in an adult 500 kg horse is difficult without using automated fluid pumps, which can cause endothelial damage and vascular thrombosis. Determinants of flow through a rigid tube are based on the Hagen-Poiseuille equation: the rate of laminar or streamlined flow will vary directly with the fourth power of the inner radius of the catheter (bigger is better) and proportionally with the length (shorter is better).[14] The rate of resuscitation can be improved by using large-bore, short catheters and large-bore extension sets and lines. Crystalloid fluids can be given at 1 L/min, or faster, through a 12- or 10-gauge catheter (Mila International, Inc., Florence, Ky.; 12-gauge, 13-cm Teflon IV catheters) using large-bore extension sets (International WIN, Ltd., Kennett Square, Pa.) with fluids elevated at least 1 m above the horse's withers. Although the most commonly used resuscitative fluids in human and veterinary medicine are the polyionic crystalloids, hypertonic saline may be used if more rapid effective circulating volume expansion is required.

Hypertonic saline (7.5% NaCl) is given at a maximal dosage of 4 mL/kg and will increase the circulating blood volume by two to four times the volume given.[15] Exceeding this dosage puts the patient at risk for a hyperosmolar state. Hypertonic saline is useful in severe life-threatening cases or for patients that have very painful acute abdomen and cannot be resuscitated prior to anesthetic induction. It works by shifting water into the plasma, first from red blood cells and endothelium and then from the interstitial space and tissue cells, so that, ultimately, expansion of the plasma volume occurs as a result of depletion of the intracellular volume.[16] Advantages of hypertonic saline are that it produces (1) a rapid but transient increase in blood volume to support and improve hemodynamics and (2) hemodilution and endothelial cell shrinkage, which decrease capillary hydraulic pressure and improve tissue perfusion.[16] Hypertonic saline is effective at expanding plasma volume, raising blood pressure, improving cardiac output, lowering systemic and pulmonary vascular resistance, and improving oxygen delivery.[15,16] Improved regional tissue perfusion, decreased leucocyte-endothelial cell interaction, and decreased stickiness of leucocytes point to a potential decrease in ischemia/reperfusion injury and subsequent multiple organ failures.[12,17] Because it is the osmolality and not the oncotic pressure that affects water movement in the brain, and because the blood-brain barrier is essentially impervious to sodium, hypertonic saline is an appropriate fluid to use in patients with central nervous system trauma or head injury.[12] After initial hypertonic saline therapy, it is important to administer 10 L of balanced polyionic solution for each liter of hypertonic saline given, to reestablish the intracellular fluid deficit.

If the principal goal of fluid therapy is to restore effective circulating volume, or if oncotic pressure support is required, colloid therapy is warranted. *Colloids,* the principal source of oncotic pressure in the blood, are large molecules that do not pass across diffusion barriers as readily as crystalloids, if at all. Therefore, they stay in the vascular space and enhance effective circulating volume expansion, which is very useful when resuscitating the hypovolemic patient[18] and is critical when resuscitating the hypoproteinemic patient.[19] Oncotic pressure, or colloid osmotic pressure (COP), opposes hydrostatic pressure that favors the movement of water out of capillaries into the interstitium.[18,19] Therefore, the ability of colloids to expand plasma volume is directly related to COP. Albumin is responsible for 75% of the oncotic pressure of the plasma, with other contributions from globulins and fibrinogen.[14] *Plasma* has a COP equal to 20 mm Hg.[14] It is an excellent source of albumin and clotting factors. As a rule of thumb, administration of 10 L of plasma to a 450-kg horse will increase its total protein by 1.0 g/dL, if there are no ongoing losses.

Hetastarch (hydroxyethyl starch), the major synthetic colloid fluid used in large-animal practice, is available as a 6% solution in isotonic saline.[18] It contains amylopectin molecules with atomic mass units of from hundreds to millions of daltons. Colloid osmotic pressure of hetastarch is 30 mm Hg. The dosage is 10 to 20 mL/kg in horses, and it increases the vascular space by 141% of the volume administered.[18] Hetastarch has a half-life of 25.5 hours, so the duration of volume expansion is 12 to 48 hours. Hetastarch increases the COP but not the total protein, and in fact, because of dilution, it may decrease the measured total protein. Advantages of using hetastarch to support COP are its cost (lower than that of plasma) and the lack of risk of adverse anaphylactic reactions. An additional advantage is its ability to reduce the development of multisystem organ failure in patients with shock. The iron chelator deferoxamine combines with hetastarch and attenuates the iron-dependent generation of toxic oxygen-derived radicals during reperfusion of ischemic tissue.[20,21] Hetastarch can also minimize signs of reperfusion injury by decreasing the oxidant-generating enzyme xanthine oxidase.[22] Disadvantages of its use include increased serum amylase and bleeding times. The amylopectin molecules are cleared by amylase enzymes in the bloodstream before they are cleared by the kidney. Therefore, elevations in serum amylase are common. There is a prolongation of partial thromboplastin time when hetastarch is given at 20 mL/kg, because of the interaction with factor VIII, but there are no reports of bleeding after its administration.[14,18] However, in patients with bleeding tendencies, such as uncontrolled hemorrhage from middle uterine artery rupture, thrombocytopenia, or coagulopathy, plasma would be a better choice for volume expansion and to support or restore oncotic pressure. Frequently, both hetastarch and plasma are used in the same patient, because hetastarch can be given quickly and provides excellent oncotic pressure support and vascular volume expansion, while plasma provides albumin, clotting factors, and complement and can be administered in addition to other resuscitative therapy, after the plasma has thawed.

Because oxygen delivery is proportional to cardiac output, hemoglobin level, and oxygen saturation, it is reasonable to first increase oxygen delivery by increasing the blood volume with crystalloids and colloids. If tissue oxygenation is still insufficient, especially if substantial blood loss occurred, or if the packed cell volume drops acutely to below 20% (or chronically to below 12% to 14%) after crystalloid resuscitation, blood transfusion (see Chapter 4) is warranted. The amount of blood required can be calculated by first estimating the amount of blood lost, using the class system proposed by the American College of Surgeons discussed earlier. Practically, if the horse is tachycardic with poor pulse pressures, increased capillary refill time, cold peripheral appendages, and an elevated blood lactate concentration, but it is still standing, it has most likely lost between 25% and 35% of its blood volume, or 0.25 to 0.35 times its body weight in kilograms, or 12 to 17 L for a 500-kg horse. Only a portion of the lost blood volume needs to be replaced with whole blood, and a good estimate is between 15 and 20 mL/kg. The following formula can be used to determine the transfusion volume:

$$\text{Blood (L)} = 0.08 \times \text{body weight (kg)} \times [(PCV_{desired} - PCV_{actual})/PCV_{donor}],$$

where PCV is packed cell volume.

Up to 20% of the blood donor's volume can be collected from an acceptable 450-kg donor, or about 9 L. The donor should test negative for equine infectious anemia and Aa Qa alloantibody. Prior to transfusion, the horse may be treated with flunixin meglumine (1.1 mg/kg, IV) or dexamethasone (0.04 to 0.08 mg/kg) to reduce the chance of an allergic reaction. Blood should be administered slowly for the first 10 to 15 minutes, while the horse is monitored for signs of adverse reactions. Temperature, heart rate, and respiratory rate should be measured every 1 to 2 minutes during this period. Elevations in these parameters, hives, or sweating may indicate that the horse is reacting to the blood transfusion, and the transfusion should be stopped. If no signs of such reactions are seen for 10 to 15 minutes, the rate of administration can be increased to 15 to 25 mL/kg per hour and the horse monitored every 15 to 30 minutes.

Concerns with blood transfusion include adverse reactions, disease, and immunosuppression. Whole blood transfusion causes immunosuppression, has been shown to be positively correlated with the development of postoperative infection, and is an independent risk factor for the development of multisystem organ dysfunction, as blood leads to an imbalance between proinflammatory and anti-inflammatory mediators in people.[12,23] Despite the fact that the marrow begins to increase production of erythrocytes within a few hours of the onset of hemorrhage, complete replacement of erythrocytes can take up to 2 months. Therefore, whole blood transfusion should be given at an appropriate dosage when systemic signs of decreased oxygen delivery are present, but overzealous use of transfusion to maintain packed cell volume is not warranted.

Vasopressor or positive inotropic drugs are rarely used in awake, adult horses, but if, after appropriate volume resuscitation, the patient shows no clinical signs of improved perfusion, these drugs may be used. Dobutamine, a β_1-receptor agonist, stimulates myocardial contraction and, because of mild β_2 effects, causes mild vasodilation, increasing cardiac output without increased mean arterial pressure.[24] It is administered as a continuous intravenous infusion (2 to 15 µg/kg per minute). At a dosage 1 to 3 µg/kg per minute, dopamine, a precursor of norepinephrine, stimulates dopaminergic receptors of the renal, coronary, and cerebral arteries, causing dilation.[24] Higher dosages, 3 to 7.5 µg/kg per minute, produce sympathomimetic effects specifically at β_1 adrenergic receptors of the sinus node and myocardium. At this dosage, dopamine is a positive chronotropic and inotropic agent.[24] In a prospective crossover clinical trial of human patients with shock, dobutamine (compared with dopamine) improved tissue perfusion as reflected by greater increases in VO_2 and greater reductions in pulmonary and systemic vascular resistance.[25] These data are unavailable for horses with shock. It is of paramount importance to be certain that appropriate volume resuscitation precedes therapy with vasoactive drugs, because these drugs may exacerbate peripheral vasoconstriction and poor perfusion at the expense of improved cardiac output.

Injury to organs can continue after apparently successful resuscitation of hypovolemic shock. With resuscitation and reperfusion of hypoxic capillaries, activated cellular and immunochemical cascades are washed into the venous circulation, leading to reperfusion injury of tissues such as the kidney, gastrointestinal tract, and lamina.[3,12] Two potential sources of enhanced oxidant production are activated neutrophils and generation of superoxide radicals.

Lidocaine infusion has been shown in other species to inhibit oxygen radical formation and lipid peroxidation in ischemia and reperfusion injury by inhibition of Na^+/Ca^{2+} exchange and Ca^{2+} accumulation during ischemia, scavenging of hydroxyl radicals, decreased release of superoxides from granulocytes, decreased polymorphonuclear activation and migration, and subsequent endothelial dysfunction.[26] Therefore, lidocaine infusion may help ameliorate the pathologic changes associated with ischemia and reperfusion injury, preventing cell death, tissue injury, and organ failure. Lidocaine is used as a continuous intravenous infusion (0.05 mg/kg per minute) following a bolus (1.3 mg/kg, IV). This infusion can be started intraoperatively if ischemia and reperfusion injury is a concern. According to anecdotal reports, this has been useful in cases of large colon volvulus and incarcerated small intestine.

Monitoring

To determine the effectiveness of the fluid therapy on oxygen delivery and the end point of resuscitation, cardiac output and perfusion are monitored. Signs of improvement include increased heart rate, increased pulse pressure (i.e., the difference between systolic and diastolic pressures), increased arterial pressure, improved mentation, warming of the extremities, decreased capillary refill time, and increased urine production with decreased specific gravity. Trends in packed cell volume and total solids can be useful, especially if hemorrhage occurred or whole blood transfusion was given.

Central venous pressure (CVP) can be measured easily and provides an indication of the venous return to the heart. It is measured at the level of the right atrium by placing sterile polypropylene tubing through a 12-gauge catheter located in the right jugular vein.[27] A three-way stopcock is attached to the tubing and to a manometer primed with heparinized saline. The manometer is zeroed by placing it at the point of the horse's shoulder. Mean CVP in a standing adult horse is 12 cm H_2O.[28] In hypovolemic animals or those with vasodilation, the venous return to the heart is reduced and the CVP is low and will increase with intravenous fluid therapy.[27] The CVP is also very useful in identifying volume overload in a horse with anuric renal failure or cardiac compromise, which can result in pulmonary edema.

The mean arterial blood pressure can be monitored in standing adult horses. It is usually measured indirectly from the middle coccygeal artery, using a manometer or an electronic transducer (Dinamap Pro Series monitor, GE Medical Systems, Milwaukee, Wis.). Normal coccygeal uncorrected systolic blood pressure should be 80 to 144 mm Hg, and the diastolic should be 49 to 105 mm Hg.[27] However, in hypovolemic patients, indirect measurements tend to be spuriously low or at times undetectable, presumably because of peripheral vasoconstriction, and therefore indirect blood pressure monitoring in the adult horse with shock is rarely performed.[14]

Cardiac output can be measured using indicator dilution techniques, with indocyanine green, cold (thermodilution), or lithium as the marker. Lithium dilution is the easiest and most accurate method, requiring only catheterization of a peripheral artery and a jugular vein. It has recently been validated in anesthetized adult horses and neonatal foals.[29] Cardiac output can also be measured using Doppler echocardiography, which is a noninvasive ultrasound-based technique.[29] Serial measurements of cardiac output provide useful information about the patient's response to volume resuscitation and improvement in oxygen delivery. However, hemodynamic measurements such as central venous pressure, mean arterial pressure, and cardiac output can all be improved in horses, especially after application of positive inotropic drugs, while the horse continues to suffer from hypoperfusion and remains in an anaerobic state. This is because these measurements reflect oxygen delivery to part of the horse and not oxygen consumption by the tissues.

A good method for monitoring oxygen consumption by the tissues is the measurement of blood or serum lactate.[1] Blood lactate levels are a good indicator of perfusion; as perfusion and oxygen delivery to the tissues and oxygen utilization improve, serum lactate levels normalize. The serum lactate level may initially increase as "lactic acid washout" occurs, but with restoration of aerobic metabolism in the peripheral tissues, it should return to normal within 2 hours. Blood and plasma lactate levels are equivalent, and these values are useful in predicting outcome in patients treated for shock.[30,31] Anaerobic metabolism is not the only source of lactate. Other causes of hyperlactatemia include hepatic insufficiency and impaired clearance of lactate by the liver, thiamine deficiency as a result of blocked pyruvate entry into mitochondria, alkalosis (which stimulates glycolysis), intense muscular activity, and production by enteric microbes.[1] In sepsis, part of the cause of lactate elevation is attributed to endotoxin. Endotoxins block the actions of the enzyme pyruvate dehydrogenase, which is responsible for the movement of pyruvate into the mitochondria. Subsequently, pyruvate accumulates in the cell cytoplasm, where it is converted to lactate.[1] Once tissue oxygenation is restored, lactate can be used as a fuel source by tissues such as heart, brain, liver, and skeletal muscle.[1] Other measures indicative of improved oxygen transport (in addition to normalization of blood lactate) include increased venous oxygen saturation (greater than 50%), and normalization of base excess and pH.[1,30,31] When venous blood gases are used to measure venous oxygen saturation, the blood gas must be collected anaerobically, stored on ice, and processed quickly to minimize errors. Pulse oximetry may be used to estimate arterial oxygen saturation and calculate oxygen extraction. However, pulse oximetry is unreliable in the underperfused, hypotensive patient and must be applied to a nonkeratinized appendage, such as the tongue, which is difficult in the awake horse.

Controlled Hypotension

Although the goal of therapy is to restore oxygen delivery and effective circulating volume with prompt, aggressive therapy, this resuscitative strategy can be deleterious to the patient if hemorrhage is not controlled.[21,32] Active bleeding from an injured large vessel may be uncontrollable without surgical hemostasis, or it may stop spontaneously by vessel retraction, vasoconstriction, tamponade, or intraluminal or extraluminal thrombus formation.[12] The hemostatic plug, which forms over several minutes, consists of platelet aggregates and fibrin mesh containing blood cells and other plasma components. Increased circulating volume and blood pressure, vasodilation, and decreased blood viscosity secondary to hemodilution—all factors associated with fluid resuscitation—can act to dislodge the hemostatic plug, precipitating continued hemorrhage.[12,33] Evidence suggests that patients with uncontrolled hemorrhage have improved survival rates with controlled hypotension and mild to moderate fluid resuscitation compared with patients that received aggressive fluid resuscitation.[12,33] It was proposed that in a model of vascular injury and uncontrolled hemorrhage, the hemostatic plug could be rendered ineffective because of decreased blood viscosity, dilutional coagulopathy, and "blowout" of the fibrin plug, with accentuation of ongoing hemorrhage or reestablishment of hemorrhage.[32] Therefore, in horses with uncontrolled hemorrhage (e.g., from middle uterine artery rupture), slower, less aggressive methods of fluid therapy may be best. There is evidence to suggest that in patients with continued hemorrhage, the best resuscitative fluid may be whole blood in addition to smaller volumes of polyionic crystalloids, because whole blood provides clotting factors, does not contribute as much to dilutional coagulopathy, and does not decrease blood viscosity. The concern with the controlled hypotensive state is, of course, underperfusion of the tissues, oxygen debt, and organ damage.

PREDICTING OUTCOME

Many human trials have shown improved survival rates, fewer occurrences of organ failure, and lower costs when cardiac output, oxygen delivery, and oxygen consumption by the tissues were promptly restored.[12] A 92% survival rate was reached when the optimal goals were achieved within 24 hours of admission to an intensive care unit, but the mortality rate was 93% when achievement of the goals was delayed, or not reached at all, and lactate levels did not return to satisfactory levels.[12,33] In patients with septic shock, blood lactate levels are closely related to survival, and decreases in blood lactate levels during the course of treatment are indicative of a favorable outcome.[30] Base excess combined with blood lactate has been used to calculate oxygen debt and predict survival.[31]

Unfortunately, such data are not available for the horse. Lack of appropriate response to aggressive resuscitative therapy is considered a poor prognostic indicator in horses. Development of organ dysfunction, such as renal failure or laminitis, after an appropriate response to aggressive resuscitative therapy is also a poor prognostic sign.

ON THE HORIZON

The rate of survival from shock will improve as detection and monitoring techniques advance, alternative crystalloids and colloids become available at reasonable cost, and hemostatic agents are developed to treat uncontrolled hemorrhage. Hetastarch has a limited role in massive resuscitation in bleeding patients because it can prolong bleeding times. A new synthetic colloid, Hextend, produces blood volume expansion without altering coagulation.[34,35] Additionally, alternative crystalloid solutions, such as Ringer's ethyl pyruvate, are being developed that expand the intravascular space and replete the extracellular fluid, but they also have anti-inflammatory properties.[36,37] Coagulation factor replacement, such as recombinant activated factor VII (rFVIIa), are likely to improve survival from recalcitrant coagulopathy. After administration, rFVIIa binds only to exposed subendothelial tissue factor, activating the extrinsic clotting system at the site of injury without causing systemic hypercoagulability.[38,39] Finally, noninvasive monitoring techniques that would allow the clinician to better assess oxygen delivery and consumption, such as transthoracic electrical bioimpedance and transesophageal echocardiography, would be valuable tools in shock management.[40] As an example, near-infrared spectroscopy, which can be used to quantitatively monitor the oxygen saturation of hemoglobin in skeletal muscle and subcutaneous tissue while simultaneously monitoring the cytochrome aa_3 redox state (which reflects mitochondrial oxygen consumption), may become a clinical tool for use in the horse in the future.

REFERENCES

1. Marino PL: Tissue oxygenation. In Marino PL: The ICU Book, ed 2, Baltimore, 1997, Williams and Wilkins.
2. Connett RJ, Honig CR, Gayeski TEJ, et al: Defining hypoxia: A systems view of V_{O_2}, glycolysis, energetics, and intracellular P_{O_2}, J Appl Physiol 1990;68:833-842.
3. Shoemaker WC: Diagnosis and treatment of shock and circulatory dysfunction. In Textbook of Critical Care, ed 4, Philadelphia, 2000, WB Saunders.
4. Rivers E, Nguyen B, Havstad S, et al: Early goal-directed therapy in the treatment of severe sepsis and septic shock, N Engl J Med 2001;345:1368-1377.
5. Barsan WG, Hedges JR, Syverud SA, et al: A hemodynamic model for anaphylactic shock, Ann Emerg Med 1985;14:834-839.
6. Shires GT, Coln D, Carrico J, et al: Fluid therapy in hemorrhagic shock, Arch Surg 1964;88:688-693.
7. Rose BD: Regulation of the effective circulating volume. In Rose BD, Post TW, editors: Clinical Physiology of Acid-Base and Electrolyte Disorders, ed 5, New York, 2001, McGraw-Hill.
8. Rose BD: Renal circulation and glomerular filtration rate. In Rose BD, Post TW, editors: Clinical Physiology of Acid-Base and Electrolyte Disorders, ed 5, New York, 2001, McGraw-Hill.
9. Wagner C, Jensen BL, Kramer BK, et al: Control of the renal renin system by local factors, Kidney Int Suppl 1998;67:S78.
10. Cogan MG: Angiotensin II: A potent controller of sodium transport in the early proximal tubule, Hypertension 1990;15:451.
11. Shoemaker WC, Appell PL, Kram HB, et al: Prospective trial of supranormal values of survivors as therapeutic goals in high-risk surgical patients, Chest 1988;94:1176-1186.
12. Orlinsky M, Shoemaker WC, Reis ED, et al: Current controversies in shock and resuscitation: Vascular trauma—Complex and challenging injuries, Part I, Surg Clin North Am 2001;81:1217-1262.
13. Kawabata H, Yahagi M, Mizumachi K, et al: Evaluation of shock-related cardiotoxic peptide, J Anesth 1989;3:155-165.
14. Marino PL: Colloid and crystalloid resuscitation. In The ICU Book, ed 2, Baltimore, 1997, Williams and Wilkins.
15. Bertone JJ, Shoemaker KE: Effect of hypertonic and isotonic saline solutions on plasma constituents of conscious horses, Am J Vet Res 1992;53:1844-1849.
16. Mazzoni MC, Borgstrom P, Arfors KET, et al: Dynamic fluid redistribution in hyperosmotic resuscitation of hypovolemic hemorrhage, Am J Physiol 1988;255:H629-H637.
17. Corso CO, Okamoto, S, Ruttinger D, et al: Hypertonic saline dextran attenuates leukocyte accumulation in the liver after hemorrhagic shock and resuscitation, J Trauma 1999;46:417-423.
18. Jones PA, Bain FT, Byars DT, et al: Effect of hydroxyethyl starch infusion on colloid oncotic pressure in hypoproteinemic horses, J Am Vet Med Assoc 2001;218:1428.
19. Chiara O, Pelosi P, Brazzi L, et al: Resuscitation from hemorrhagic shock: Experimental model comparing normal saline, dextran, and hypertonic saline solutions, Crit Care Med 2003;31:1915-1920.
20. Bauer C, Walcher F, Holanda M, et al: Deferoxamine-conjugated hydroxyethyl starch reduces reperfusion injury to the liver following hemorrhagic shock, Anaesthetist 1997;46:53-56.
21. Bauer C, Walcher F, Holanda M, et al: Antioxidative resuscitation solution presents leucocyte adhesion in the liver after hemorrhagic shock, J Trauma 1999;46:886-893.
22. Nielsen VG, Tan S, Brix AE, et al: Hextend (hetastarch solution) decreases multiple organ injury and xanthine oxidase release after hepatoenteric ischemia-reperfusion in rabbits, Crit Care Med 1997;25:1565-1574.
23. Jensen LS, Hokland M, Nielsen HJ: A randomized controlled study of the effect of bedside leucocyte depletion on the immunosuppressive effect of whole blood transfusions in patients undergoing elective colorectal surgery, Br J Surg 1996;83:973-977.
24. Marino PL: Hemodynamic drugs. In The ICU Book, ed 2, Baltimore, 1997, Williams and Wilkins.
25. Shoemaker WC, Kram HB, Appel PL: Therapy of shock based on pathophysiology, monitoring, and outcome prediction, Crit Care Med 1990;18:S19-S25.
26. Cassutto BH, Gfeller RW: Use of intravenous lidocaine to prevent reperfusion injury and subsequent multiorgan dysfunction syndrome, J Vet Emerg Crit Care 2003;13:137-148.

27. Cook VL, Bain FT: Volume (crystalloid) replacement in the ICU patient, Clin Tech Equine Pract 2003;2:122-129.
28. Hall LW, Nigam JM: Measurement of central venous pressure in horses, Vet Rec 1975;97:66-69.
29. Corley KT, Donaldson LL, Durando MM, et al: Cardiac output technologies with special reference to the horse, J Vet Intern Med 2003;17:262-272.
30. Backer J, Coffernils M, Leon M, et al: Blood lactate levels are superior to oxygen-derived variables in predicting outcome in human septic shock, Chest 1991;99:956-962.
31. Dunham MC, Siegel JH, Weireter L, et al: Oxygen debt and metabolic acidemia as quantitative predictors of mortality and the severity of the ischemic insult in hemorrhagic shock, Crit Care Med 1991;19:231-243.
32. Stern S: Low-volume fluid resuscitation for presumed hemorrhagic shock: Helpful or harmful? Curr Opin Crit Care 2001;7:422-430.
33. Bishop MW, Shoemaker WC, Kram HB, et al: Prospective randomized trial of survivor values of cardiac output, oxygen delivery, and oxygen consumption as resuscitation endpoints in severe trauma, J Trauma 1995;38:780-787.
34. Moore FA, McKinley BA, Moore EE: The next generation in shock resuscitation, Lancet 2004;363:1988-1996.
35. Gan TJ, Bennett-Guerrero E, Phillips-Bute B, et al: Hextend, a physiologically balanced plasma expander for large volume use in major surgery: A randomized phase III clinical trial, Anesth Analg 1999;88:992-998.
36. Sims CA, Wattanasirichaigoon S, Menconi MH, et al: Ringer's ethyl pyruvate solution ameliorates ischemia/reperfusion-induced intestinal mucosal injury in rats, Crit Care Med 2001;29:1513-1518.
37. Yang R, Uchiyama T, Alber SM, et al: Ethyl pyruvate ameliorates distant organ injury in a murine model of acute necrotizing pancreatitis, Crit Care Med 2004;32:1453-1459.
38. Martinowitz U, Kenet G, Segal E, et al: Recombinant activated factor VII for adjunctive hemorrhage in trauma, J Trauma 2001;51:431-439.
39. O'Neill PA, Bluth M, Gloster ES, et al: Successful use of recombinant activated factor VII for trauma-associated hemorrhage in a patient without pre-existing coagulopathy, J Trauma 2002;52:400-405.
40. McKinley BA, Marvin RG, Cocanour CS, et al: Tissue hemoglobin O_2 saturation during resuscitation of traumatic shock monitored using near infrared spectrometry, J Trauma 2000;48:637-642.

CHAPTER 2

Sepsis and Endotoxemia

Susan C. Eades
Rustin M. Moore

SEPTIC AND ENDOTOXIC SHOCK IN THE HORSE

Pathogenesis

Sepsis refers to the systemic (and commonly overshooting) inflammatory reaction to infection, and endotoxemia refers to the presence of endotoxin in the bloodstream. The general term used to describe these systemic sequelae to inflammatory mediators is *systemic inflammatory response syndrome* (SIRS). During severe infection or after absorption of large amounts of endotoxin, as during acute diarrheal disease, SIRS often occurs. Septic or endotoxic shock develops when the systemic derangements compromise circulatory function.

Septic or endotoxic shock, with its serious life-threatening complications, occurs during numerous diseases in horses. Septic inflammation generally causes a local inflammatory process that compromises the function of the tissues and organs involved. However, a systemic inflammatory response occurs when the infection is local and severe (especially in adult pleuropneumonia, endometritis, peritonitis, or infectious colitis), when more than one organ is infected, or when the infection enters the systemic circulation (especially in neonatal sepsis). Infection with gram-negative baceria is more likely to initiate SIRS because the gram-negative bacterial cell wall contains an endotoxin molecule that is a potent stimulus of equine monocytes and macrophages, resulting in synthesis and release of numerous inflammatory mediators.

The endotoxin of gram-negative enteric bacteria is a lipopolysaccharide (LPS) that is a structural component of the outer cell membrane. It is composed of three parts, each with important biologic characteristics. The inner component, the lipid-A portion, is well conserved among different species of gram-negative bacteria and imparts the toxic qualities to the endotoxin molecule. The middle region of endotoxin is the core oligosaccharide, which links the lipid-A with the outer polysaccharide portion. This core region is also well conserved in gram-negative bacteria. The outermost component is composed of repeating polysaccharides. The composition of this portion differs among bacterial species and accounts for their serologic differentiation.[1]

Because endotoxin is an integral component of the outer cell wall of gram-negative bacteria, it is liberated when the bacterium dies or undergoes periods of rapid proliferation. The gastrointestinal tract lumen harbors large quantities of gram-negative bacteria and free endotoxin.[2] To prevent the development of endotoxemia, the horse has evolved several efficient mechanisms to restrict transmural movement of endotoxin across the bowel wall and to remove endotoxin from the portal blood.[1] The mucosal epithelial cells of the intestine function as a physical barrier against transmural movement and are the first line of the innate immune response.[3] These mucosal epithelial cells also secrete substances such as lysozymes, enzymes, and antibodies, which limit the ability of enteric bacteria to invade the mucosal lining. Endotoxin can traverse compromised intestinal mucosal epithelium either via transepithelial movement (transcellular) or across the intercellular tight junctions (paracellular).[3] If a small quantity of endotoxin traverses the intestinal mucosal barrier and gains access into the portal circulation, Kupffer cells (hepatic macrophages) are effective scavengers of endotoxin. Additionally, many horses have small quantities of circulating antiendotoxin antibodies directed against the core region, which can bind endotoxin and facilitate its removal from the circulation.

If the integrity of the intestinal mucosal barrier is disrupted sufficiently, the quantity of endotoxin traversing the barrier may exceed the ability of these protective mechanisms to remove it from the circulation. Additionally, endotoxin can also traverse full-thickness bowel, enter the peritoneal cavity and lymphatics, and reach the systemic circulation via the thoracic duct.[4] The permeability of the intestinal mucosal barrier is frequently increased in cases of acute equine gastrointestinal tract disease. Plasma tests positive for endotoxin in 10% to 40% of horses with colic.[5,6] Increases in mucosal permeability are most often associated with ischemia/reperfusion injury caused by intestinal strangulation, severe colitis and enteritis, or gastrointestinal rupture.[1] However, because the rate of plasma endotoxin detection is not greater in horses with these diagnoses than in horses with other causes of colic, it is concluded that endotoxemia may accompany all types of gastrointestinal tract disease in horses.[5,7] Endotoxin is three times more likely to be detected in the peritoneal fluid than in the plasma of horses with gastrointestinal tract disease, emphasizing that either endotoxin enters the intestinal lymphatics or it crosses the full-thickness of the bowel wall.[5]

Once endotoxin gains access to the systemic circulation, it may become associated with high-density lipoproteins or lipopolysaccharide-binding protein (LBP), which has a strong avidity for the lipid-A region of endotoxin.[8,9] This protein acts as a shuttle to transfer endotoxin monomers from the endotoxin aggregates to the surface of effector cells that subsequently respond to endotoxin. Although mononuclear phagocytes are capable of responding to endotoxin without LBP, the presence of LBP increases the sensitivity of the response for protection against gram-negative infection. The endotoxin-LBP complex transfers endotoxin monomers to a cell surface receptor antigen, known as CD14, which exists both as a membrane-bound receptor and as a soluble form in biologic fluids.[9,10] The membrane-bound form is present principally on mononuclear cells, but it also exists on other cell types. The soluble form of the receptor may interact with endotoxin and LPB as well as with cells lacking membrane CD14, such as endothelial cells. The CD14 receptor plays a central role in the inflammatory cascade initiated by endotoxin. However, binding of endotoxin to this receptor alone does not result in transmission of the endotoxin signal to the interior of the cell. Thus, because the CD14 is a cell surface receptor that does not cross the cell membrane, binding of endotoxin to it does not directly initiate stimulation of second messenger systems or signal transduction pathways.

Toll-like receptors, originally identified from *Drosophila*, have been shown to have both transmembrane and intracellular components, which permits communication between the interior and exterior of cells.[11] Toll-like receptor 4 (TLR4) has been shown to be responsible for delivery of the endotoxin signal from the cell surface to the interior of the cell.[11-13] Stimulation of theTLR4 causes phosphorylation and subsequent degradation of the intracellular inhibitory protein IκB, resulting in the liberation of nuclear factor κB (NF-κB). This factor subsequently enters the nucleus and binds to the promoter region of genes that encode for the synthesis of inflammatory cytokines (Fig. 2-1). It has been shown that MD-2, a secreted protein that physically associates with TLR4, is required for the responsiveness of TLR4 to LPS.[14,15] Additionally, MD-2 has been shown to enhance the synthesis of cytokines secondary to LPS by activating alternative pathways resulting in increased NF-κB activity.[15]

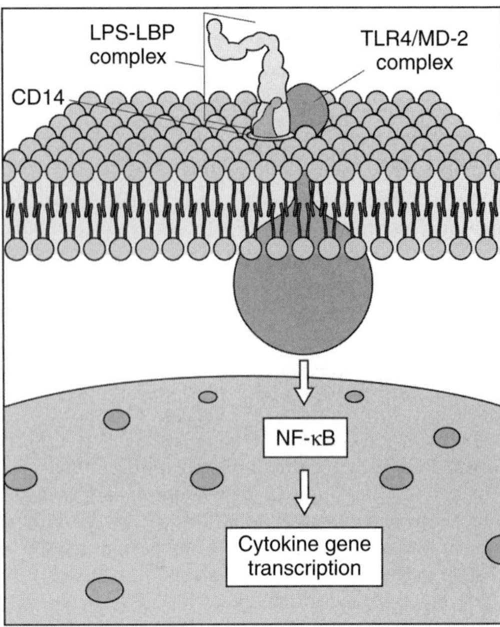

Figure 2-1. Lipopolysaccharide-binding protein (LBP) complexes with lipopolysaccharide (LPS) within the circulation and transports it to the CD14 receptor on effector cells such as mononuclear cells. Because CD14 receptors do not traverse from the cell surface to the cell's interior, Toll-like receptor 4 (TLR4), which is composed of a transmembrane domain, serves to transfer the signal to the interior of the cell. Once the signal enters the interior of the cell, it activates nuclear factor kappa-B (NF-κB), which stimulates cytokine gene transcription. A secreted protein known as MD-2 physically associates with TLR4 and is required for its responsiveness to LPS, and it enhances the synthesis of cytokines secondary to LPS.

Cytokine Activation

Cytokines (which include tumor necrosis factor-alpha [TNF-α], interleukins [IL], chemokines, and growth factors) are glycoprotein molecules that regulate inflammatory and immune responses by acting as a signal between cells (Table 2-1). TNF-α is referred to as the proximal mediator of the response to endotoxin.[1] Administration of TNF-α causes many of the same clinical effects that endotoxin causes. Increased plasma activity of TNF-α has been associated with increased mortality in colic and neonatal sepsis.[5] IL-1 and IL-6 are also major proinflammatory cytokines. The following events result from endotoxin-induced cytokine synthesis:

TABLE 2-1. Mediators Involved in Sepsis and Endotoxemia

Mediator	Source	Vasodilators (+) Vasoconstrictors (–)	Vascular Leakage	Chemotaxis	Leukocyte Adhesion	Other
Complement C3a	Plasma protein (liver)	NA	+	–	–	Opsonin
Complement C5a	Macrophages	NA	+	+	+	NA
Bradykinin	Plasma	+	+	–	–	Pain
Histamine	Mast cells, platelets	+	+	–	–	Pain
Serotonin	Mast cells, platelets	+,–	+	–	–	NA
Prostaglandins (PGE_2 and PGI_2)	Leukocytes, endothelium, epithelium, fibroblasts	+,–	+	–	–	Pain, fever
Thromboxane	Platelets	–	NA	NA	NA	Platelet aggregation
Leukotriene B_4	Leukocytes	NA	–	+	+	NA
Leukotriene C_4, D_4, E_4	Leukocytes	+	+	–	–	Bronchoconstriction
Oxygen metabolites	Leukocytes	+	+	+	+	Endothelial and tissue damage
Platelet activating factor	Leukocytes	+	+	+	+	Bronchoconstriction
Interleukin-1	Macrophages	NA	–	+	+	Acute phase reaction
Tumor necrosis factor-α	Macrophages	+	–	+	+	Acute phase reaction
Chemokines	Leukocytes	NA	–	+	+	NA
Endothelin-1	Endothelium	–	NA	NA	NA	Bronchoconstriction Intestinal motility
Nitric oxide	Macrophages, endothelium	–	+	+	+	Cytotoxicity

- TNF-α and IL-1 stimulate neutrophil adhesion to endothelium and activation of neutrophils.[16]
- TNF-α causes a spectrum of changes in endothelial cells because of increased gene transcription, referred to as endothelial cell activation. In the presence of TNF-α, endothelial cells express procoagulant activity (thromboplastin or tissue factor).[7,17] These responses favor hemostasis and potentiate the coagulopathy present in the systemic inflammatory response syndrome. The coagulopathy may lead to microthrombi, thereby resulting in alterations in tissue perfusion.
- Activated endothelial cells also synthesize nitric oxide (NO) and eicosanoids, thereby altering blood pressure, tissue perfusion, and venous return of blood for cardiac output.
- TNF-α stimulates effector cells (monocytes, macrophages, and endothelial cells) to synthesize cytokines to perpetuate the cycle of the inflammatory response.[18]
- TNF-α, IL-1, and IL-6 stimulate prostaglandin E_2 synthesis in the hypothalamus, thereby increasing the set point for body temperature, resulting in fever. These cytokines are also responsible for the altered mentation and loss of appetite that accompany the systemic responses to inflammation. Central nervous system effects of TNF-α and IL-1 result in increased release of adrenocorticotropic hormone, thereby increasing circulating corticosteroid concentrations.[18]
- IL-1 and IL-6 induce hepatic acute-phase protein synthesis. The proteins include fibrinogen, ceruloplasmin, and α globulins and β globulins produced nonspecifically by the liver during inflammation. Although many of these are synthesized with no specific function, α_1-antitrypsin and α_2-macroglobulin are major inhibitors of leukocyte lysosomal enzymes, which help to keep in check the tissue destruction caused by enzymes released during leukocyte death.[18]

In addition to cytokines, other inflammatory mediators released in response to the action of endotoxin on effector cells include arachidonic acid metabolites, platelet-activating factor (PAF), oxygen-derived free radicals, NO, histamine, kinins, and complement components. The generation of eicosanoids (cyclooxygenase enzymes), leukotrienes (lipoxygenase enzymes), and lipoxins from arachidonic acid in the cellular membrane can mediate virtually every step of inflammation. These steps involve the following agents and processes:

- Thromboxane A_2 is a potent platelet-aggregating agent and vasoconstrictor.[19]
- Increased hypothalamic synthesis of prostaglandin E_2 raises the set point for body temperature.[18]
- Leukotriene B_4 (LTB_4) is a potent chemotactic agent and activator of neutrophils; it causes increased aggregation and adhesion, generation of oxygen radicals, and release of lysosomal enzymes.[20]
- Leukotrienes C_4, D_4, E_4 (LTC_4, LTD_4, LTE_4) cause intense vasoconstriction, bronchospasm, and increased vascular permeability (of venules).[20]
- Lipoxin A_4 stimulates vasodilation.[21]
- Other lipoxins are potent anti-inflammatory substances.[22]

PAF is another phospholipid-derived mediator, synthesized in platelets, basophils, neutrophils, monocytes, macrophages, and endothelial cells.[18,23] Its effects are mediated via a single G protein–coupled receptor and are regulated by a family of inactivating PAF acetylhydrolases. PAF elicits most of the cardinal features of inflammation, including the following:

- At low concentrations, PAF causes vasodilation and increased venular permeability.
- At higher concentrations, PAF causes vasoconstriction, bronchoconstriction, platelet aggregation, and leukocyte chemotaxis and activation.
- PAF boosts the synthesis of eicosanoids.

Oxygen Metabolites

Oxygen-derived free radicals are generated in activated leukocytes through the nicotinamide-adenine dinucleotide phosphate (NADP) oxidative system, and in endothelial cells during reperfusion after ischemia via the xanthine oxidase pathway.[24] Superoxide anion, hydrogen peroxide, hydroxyl radical, and hypochlorous acid are the major radicals released extracellularly from leukocytes where these metabolites can combine with NO to form other reactive nitrogen intermediates (peroxynitrite) responsible for bacterial killing. Activated neutrophils adherent to endothelial cells stimulate xanthine oxidase in endothelial cells, thus causing elaboration of more superoxide. These oxygen metabolites are responsible for much of the host tissue destruction that accompanies endotoxin-induced inflammation. Oxygen metabolites also have proinflammatory functions, including the following:

- Extracellular release of low levels of oxygen metabolites can increase leukocyte adhesion and expression of cytokines to amplify the cascade of the inflammatory response.[25]
- Endothelial cells are damaged by increasing concentrations of oxygen-derived free radicals, resulting in increased vascular permeability.[18]
- Oxygen-derived free radicals inactivate antiproteases, enzymes that degrade the proteases released from activated neutrophils, leading to unopposed protease activity that causes destruction of the extracellular matrix.[18]
- In high concentration, oxygen-derived free radicals lead to injury to other cell types (tumor cells, red cells, and parenchymal cells).

Nitric oxide functions not only as a mediator of inflammatory processes but also as a regulator of local blood flow and tissue perfusion. NO is synthesized by endothelial cells, macrophages, and specific neurons in the brain[26] from L-arginine, molecular oxygen, the reduced form of NADP (NADPH), and other cofactors by the enzyme nitric oxide synthase (NOS). There are three different types of NOS: endothelial (eNOS), neuronal (nNOS), and cytokine inducible (iNOS).[27] These types exhibit two different patterns of expression. The eNOS and nNOS isoforms are constitutively expressed, resulting in low concentrations requiring increased cytoplasmic calcium ions in the presence of calmodulin. On the other hand, when macrophages are activated by cytokines via expression of iNOS, changes in cytosolic calcium are not required. NO acts on target cells through induction of cyclic guanosine monophosphate (cGMP), thereby leading to vasodilation. The in vivo half-life of NO is only a matter of seconds; therefore, the gas acts only on cells in close proximity to the site of its synthesis.

Reactive oxygen species derived from NO synthase possess antimicrobial activity.[28] Reactions between NO and reactive oxygen species lead to the formation of antimicrobial metabolites (e.g., peroxynitrite). However, high concentrations of NO may also damage host cells. The overproduction of NO is responsible for the hypotension noted in many models of septic shock. However, endogenous control mechanisms exist for synthesis of NO in inflammatory conditions. The iNOS response does not appear to be the same in horses as in laboratory animals and humans. Plasma and urine NO concentrations do not increase significantly in horses during the 24 hours after a low dosage (35 ng/kg, IV over 30 minutes) of endotoxin is administered intravenously.[29]

Complement System

The complement system consists of 20 plasma-derived proteins that modulate the systemic response to endotoxin and are directly activated by the presence of endotoxin alone and gram-negative bacteria.[18] The result of activation of the complement system is formation of the membrane attack complex that functions in lysis of bacteria. Concurrently, the activated complement components cause increased vascular permeability, chemotaxis, and opsonization.

Histamine

Histamine is widely distributed in tissues throughout the body. It is preformed and stored in mast cell granules, which are normally present in the connective tissue adjacent to blood vessels. It is released during mast cell degranulation in response to activation of complement fragments (C3a and C5a) and cytokines.[18] Histamine acts on the circulation predominantly through H1 receptors, thereby causing dilation of arterioles and constriction of large arteries. It is the principal mediator of the immediate phase of increased vascular permeability and acts by constricting venular endothelium, causing gaps in the venular wall.

Anti-Inflammatory Response

Concurrent with the synthesis and release of a multitude of inflammatory mediators, sepsis and endotoxemia elicit an anti-inflammatory response designed to hold the inflammatory response in check. The LBP can serve to transfer endotoxin molecules to high-density lipoproteins, thereby decreasing the interaction of endotoxin with CD14 on inflammatory cells. Cytokine-induced endogenous glucocorticoid synthesis may inhibit further synthesis of cytokines.[30] Interleukin-10 is an anti-inflammatory cytokine released in response to endotoxin, and its principal effect is deactivation of mononuclear phagocytes and inhibition of proinflammatory cytokine synthesis.[31] Lipoxins generated during metabolism of arachidonic acid are potent inhibitors of the inflammatory response.[22]

Host Responses

The clinical response to endotoxin may diminish with repeated exposures, a phenomenon known as endotoxin tolerance.[7] Tolerance can also be demonstrated experimentally in vivo and in vitro with decreased synthesis of cytokines (especially TNF-α) in humans, laboratory animals, and horses. Receptor downregulation and inhibition of intracellular signaling pathways are likely mechanisms.

The host response to sepsis and endotoxemia involves defense mechanisms resulting from synthesis of inflammatory mediators and anti-inflammatory mechanisms designed to modulate the inflammatory events. Detrimental consequences occur if excessive and uncontrolled responses culminate in cardiovascular dysfunction, resulting in shock, impaired hemostasis, and organ failure. These pathophysiologic events caused by the cascade of inflammatory mediators result from leukocyte activation, endothelial dysfunction and damage, hemodynamic changes, and coagulopathy.

During sepsis and endotoxemia, cytokines activate integrins (e.g., CD11/CD18) on the surface of neutrophils, causing firm adhesion to the endothelium and leading to transmigration of neutrophils.[32] Leukotriene B4, activated complement components, and antigen-antibody complexes stimulate activation of the neutrophil oxidative burst for bacterial killing.[33] Xanthine oxidase–derived hydrogen peroxide reacts with large quantities of NO (generated via iNOS in neutrophils) to form peroxynitrite, a potent oxidant. Hydrogen peroxide generated in neutrophils also reacts with chloride anions, a reaction catalyzed by myeloperoxidase, resulting in the formation of hypochlorous acid, another potent oxidant. These oxidants are capable of killing bacteria and degrading endotoxin, but they are also powerful mediators of host endothelial and tissue injury.[18]

Normal endothelium functions in the regulation of local perfusion and blood pressure, neutrophil adhesion and activation, transvascular fluid movement, and anticoagulation. Endothelial dysfunction results in a decreased responsiveness to vasoactive (vasodilating and vasoconstricting) agents, increased vascular permeability and edema, and coagulopathy. Cytokines increase expression of intercellular adhesion molecules (ICAM-1) on endothelial cells, which bind to the CD11/CD18 receptors on neutrophils, leading to neutrophil adhesion and activation.[33] Cytokines also stimulate arachidonic acid metabolism, leading to generation of leukotrienes that alter endothelial permeability (LTC_4, LTD_4, LTE_4).[20] Additionally, activated neutrophils release matrix metalloproteinases, which contribute to the tissue injury via breakdown of components of the basement membrane.[30] In horses suffering from endotoxemia, extensive endothelial damage has been documented.[19,34] The end result is poor tissue perfusion and edema, leading to cardiovascular shock.

In addition to the effects of endothelial dysfunction, the inflammatory mediators generated during sepsis and endotoxemia adversely affect vascular and cardiac function, leading to loss of homeostatic control mechanisms. The breakdown of hemodynamic control decreases cardiac output, venous return, and perfusion of vital organs, leading to shock.[34] Normal blood pressure is maintained by vascular smooth muscle tone regulated by endothelial release of endothelin-1 (ET-1) (vasoconstriction), NO (vasodilation), and prostacyclin (PGI_2) (vasodilation). Horses with gastrointestinal tract disease commonly have accompanying endotoxemia and increased venous plasma concentrations of ET-1, which could reduce peripheral perfusion by vasoconstriction.[35] Endotoxemia in horses is accompanied by increases in circulating concentrations of thromboxane, which causes pulmonary hypertension and decreased peripheral perfusion.[1] Endothelial damage during endotoxemia impairs endothelial synthesis of PGI_2 and NO, thereby reducing local perfusion. Very high concentrations of NO generated by iNOS in macrophages lead to vascular blood pooling, and to decreased venous return and cardiac output.[27] Sympathetic nervous system activity increases to compensate for the decreased cardiac output, resulting in tachycardia, increased stroke volume, and increased peripheral vascular resistance. Concurrent with increased ET-1, thromboxane, serotonin, angiotensin, and increased peripheral neurotransmission from sympathetic compensatory reflexes may further impair peripheral perfusion. With progression of sepsis and endotoxemia, decompensated shock results in progressive systemic hypotension caused by synthesis of excessive quantities of prostacyclin, prostaglandin E_2, and NO.[1,7,30] Ultimately, direct myocardial suppression by NO, increased vascular permeability, impaired tissue oxygen extraction, and vascular pooling resulting from the systemic hypotension cause failure of tissue oxygen delivery and progressive metabolic acidosis.

Prevalence and Clinical Impact

Most respondents (73%) to a survey of diplomates of the American College of Veterinary Internal Medicine (ACVIM) and the American College of Veterinary Surgeons (ACVS) indicated that less than 25% of the horses in their practice in the year preceding the survey had evidence of endotoxemia, whereas 26% believed the prevalence was between

25% and 50%.[36] Over 90% of the respondents indicated they believed that enteritis/colitis, intestinal strangulation obstruction, and retained placenta/metritis were commonly associated with endotoxemia in horses, whereas between 75% and 90% of respondents believed that in their practice and in their experience, grain overload, pleuropneumonia, and laminitis were associated with endotoxemia. As many as 30% to 40% of horses admitted to university teaching hospitals for acute gastrointestinal tract disease show detectable endotoxin in the plasma and/or peritoneal fluid, and up to 50% of foals with presumed sepsis have measurable amounts of plasma endotoxin.[6,37,38] Because the half-life of circulating endotoxin in plasma is less than 2 minutes,[39] these results suggest that there is constant movement of endotoxin from the intestinal lumen into the circulation in horses with a compromised mucosal barrier. Most horses with gastrointestinal tract disease and endotoxemia have ischemic or inflammatory bowel disease. Therefore, the prevalence of endotoxemia is greatest for horses with intestinal strangulation obstruction (e.g., small intestinal or large colon volvulus, incarceration), enteritis (colitis, proximal enteritis), and septic peritonitis. Entrance of endotoxin into the systemic circulation results in a complex pathophysiologic cascade of events that frequently leads to morbidity and mortality despite aggressive treatment.

CLINICAL ENDOTOXEMIA AND SHOCK IN THE HORSE

Clinical Findings

Clinical signs associated with early hyperdynamic response to endotoxin include anorexia, yawning, sweating, depression, mild colic, muscle fasciculation, recumbency, increased heart and respiratory rates, mucous membrane hyperemia, decreased borborygmi, and accelerated capillary refill time. Clinical signs observed during the later hypodynamic phase of endotoxemia include brick-red to purple mucous membranes, development of a "toxic ring" around the gum line of the oral mucous membranes, prolonged capillary refill time, decreased arterial pulse strength, tachycardia, tachypnea, hypothermia, decreased venous filling, and scleral reddening (Box 2-1). More subtle signs may occur in horses in which a relatively low level of endotoxin gains access to the systemic circulation, or early in the disease process; these include mild or moderate abdominal pain, anorexia, and depression.

BOX 2-1. Diagnostic Findings for Horses with Sepsis or Endotoxemia

PHYSICAL EXAMINATION

Early Hyperdynamic Phase

- Anorexia
- Yawning
- Depression
- Sweating
- Mild colic
- Muscle fasciculation
- Recumbency
- Tachycardia
- Tachypnea
- Fever
- Mucous membrane hyperemia
- Decreased gastrointestinal borborygmi
- Accelerated capillary refill time

Later Hypodynamic Phase

- Tachycardia
- Tachypnea
- Discolored mucous membranes
  - Brick red to purple color
  - Development of a toxic ring around gum line
- Prolonged capillary refill time
- Decreased arterial pulse strength
- Hypothermia
- Decreased venous filling
- Scleral reddening

COMPLETE BLOOD COUNT

Early Leukopenia

- Neutropenia
- Left shift

Later Leukocytosis

- Neutrophilia

ARTERIAL BLOOD GAS ANALYSIS

- Early arterial hypoxemia
- Hypocapnia due to tachypnea
- Later metabolic acidosis

SERUM ENDOTOXIN OR INFLAMMATORY MEDIATOR CONCENTRATIONS

- Lipopolysaccharide (endotoxin)
- Tumor necrosis factor-α
- Interleukin-1
- Interleukin-6

Assessment and Diagnostic Approach

The diagnostic approach to endotoxemia in horses includes performing a thorough physical examination, complete blood count, and arterial blood gas analysis. Complete blood count often reveals leukopenia, neutropenia, and a left shift, which often is followed by leukocytosis and neutrophilia if the horse survives. An arterial blood gas usually reveals arterial hypoxemia. Horses often develop an early hyperdynamic (systemic arterial hypertension) followed by a more prolonged hypodynamic (hypotension) phase. Horses often develop pulmonary arterial hypertension. A tentative diagnosis of endotoxemia is usually made based upon the clinical signs, clinicopathologic data and the most likely primary disease process. Treatment is often necessary and should be instituted without a definitive diagnosis. Regarding the diagnosis of endotoxemia, most respondents to a survey indicated that neutropenia (94%), oral mucous membrane hyperemia (89%), leukopenia (89%), the appearance of toxic neutrophils and a left shift on the differential white blood cell count (86%), tachycardia (77%) and fever (76%) were clinical indicators of endotoxemia. Other clinical or laboratory findings listed by respondents as indicators of endotoxemia included prolonged capillary refill time (61%), coagulation abnormalities (60%), bacterial growth on blood culture (39%), any other mucous membrane abnormality (32%), increased blood lactate or anion gap concentration (33%) and endotoxin detected on an endotoxin blood assay (21%).[36]

Clinical Management

Treatment

The principal treatments for horses suffering from endotoxemia include (1) prevention of movement of endotoxin into the systemic circulation by the treatment or resolution of the primary disease process, (2) advanced medical and supportive care, (3) neutralization of endotoxin before it interacts with effector cells, (4) prevention of the synthesis, release, or effects of proinflammatory mediators, and (5) prevention of endotoxin-induced cellular activation (Box 2-2).

To a survey about treatment of horses with endotoxemia, respondents indicated that they administer intravenous fluids (100%), low-dose flunixin meglumine (86%), broad-spectrum antimicrobials (85%), hyperimmune antiendotoxic plasma or serum (64%), high-dose flunixin meglumine (60%), dimethyl sulfoxide (41%), hypertonic saline solution (38%), heparin (31%), normal equine plasma (29%), phenylbutazone (23%), aspirin (14%), pentoxifylline (12%), ketoprofen (8%), and corticosteroids (8%).[36]

BOX 2-2. Principles of Treatment for Horses with Sepsis or Endotoxemia

CONTROL PRIMARY DISEASE
- Administer laxatives or emollients
  - Mineral oil
  - Activated charcoal
  - Di-tri-octahedral smectite
- Surgical resection of compromised bowel
- Resect or drain localized areas of infection (umbilicus, pleural/peritoneal cavity)
- Antibiotic treatment

ADVANCED MEDICAL AND SUPPORTIVE CARE
- Intravenous fluid therapy
  - Crystalloids
  - Colloids
- Acid-base and electrolyte correction
- Broad-spectrum antibiotics
- Plasma

NEUTRALIZE CIRCULATING ENDOTOXIN
- Hyperimmune serum or plasma
- Polymyxin B
- Phospholipid emulsion

INHIBIT INFLAMMATORY MEDIATOR SYNTHESIS
- Nonsteroidal anti-inflammatory drugs
- Pentoxifylline
- Dimethyl sulfoxide
- Corticosteroids?

INTERFERENCE WITH CELLULAR ACTIVATION
- Nontoxic lipopolysaccharide or lipid-A compounds

CONTROLLING THE PRIMARY DISEASE

Addressing and resolving the primary disease is one of the most important initial aspects of treatment or prevention of endotoxemia in horses. When the primary disease is of the gastrointestinal tract, this often involves administering mineral oil, activated charcoal, or DTO (di-tri-octahedral) smectite[40] to horses with grain overload or enterocolitis, surgically resecting ischemic bowel, or providing supportive care to horses with inflammatory bowel disease. When it is bacteremia or septicemia or localized areas of infection (e.g., pleuropneumonia, umbilical abscess), treatment involves removal of the source (pleural drainage, omphalophlebectomy) and antibiotic treatment. In mares with retained placenta and metritis, facilitating passage of the placenta, uterine lavage, and antibiotic treatment are indicated.

ADVANCED MEDICAL AND SUPPORTIVE CARE

Supportive care involves administration of IV fluids (crystalloids and colloids) to correct dehydration and volume depletion, and to keep up with ongoing losses (diarrhea, reflux, pleural or peritoneal fluid accumulation). Correction and maintenance of electrolytes and acid-base balance is also important (see Chapter 3). Administering broad-spectrum antibiotics is important in treating horses with septic processes; however, rapid death of gram-negative bacteria could theoretically lead to increased release of endotoxin from their cell walls. It has been shown in an in vitro model of septicemia in foals that amikacin or amikacin combined with ampicillin is less likely to induce endotoxemia and TNF-α synthesis during bactericidal treatment for *Escherichia coli* septicemia, compared with β-lactam antibiotics such as ampicillin, imipenem, and ceftiofur.[41] Administration of plasma is useful to help replenish plasma proteins, especially albumin, which helps maintain the necessary oncotic pressure to keep fluids in the intravascular compartment. Neonatal foals with failure of passive transfer should be administered regular plasma to increase circulating immunoglobulin levels.

NEUTRALIZING CIRCULATING ENDOTOXIN

Hyperimmune serum or plasma can be administered intravenously to horses with endotoxemia and to those predisposed to developing endotoxemia. These products are most likely to be beneficial if administered before the endotoxin gains access to the circulation, because these antiendotoxin antibodies presumably exert a protective effect by forming complexes with endotoxin before they interact with inflammatory cells. The proposed protective mechanisms of action associated with binding of the antibodies with LPS include steric blockage of interaction between lipid-A and cellular receptors, and enhanced bacterial clearance via opsonization. Although there are controversial and contradictory results using these hyperimmune plasma or serum products in experimental and naturally acquired endotoxemia, there may be a place for them in the therapeutic regimen of horses with, or predisposed to develop, endotoxemia.

There are anecdotal reports that administration of 0.5 to 1.0 L of hyperimmune serum or plasma raised against a rough mutant of *E. coli* (J5) or *Salmonella typhimurium* may have fairly profound protective effects in individual horses, depending on the timing of administration and the magnitude of endotoxemia. In a double-blind clinical study performed on horses with clinicopathologic evidence of endotoxemia, treatment with J5 hyperimmune plasma was associated with an increased survival rate (87% versus 53%), improved clinical appearance, and a shorter hospitalization period compared with horses treated with nonspecific hyperimmune plasma.[42] However, in another study of sublethal experimental endotoxemia, J5 hyperimmune serum administration did not improve clinical or clinicopathologic variables.[43] Additionally, pretreatment with 1.5 mL/kg of *Salmonella typhimurium* antiserum administered IV to 3- to 5-month-old foals before challenge with 0.25 μg/kg *E. coli* LPS had no positive protective effect. It was suggested that under certain circumstances, this antiserum could exacerbate the actions of endotoxin.[43]

Forty-five percent of respondents to the previously mentioned ACVIM and ACVS survey answered that they believed administration of hyperimmune antiendotoxic plasma or serum was effective in decreasing the signs of endotoxemia, 45% were uncertain whether there was any beneficial effect, and 10% indicated they believed these products were not useful and could possibly be the cause of subsequent development of laminitis. Most respondents reported that if they used these products, they usually administered 1 to 2 L per horse.[36] The variable effects of administration of hyperimmune plasma or serum to horses with endotoxemia explain the diverse opinions of clinicians regarding the clinical efficacy of these solutions. These products probably have the best chance of having a beneficial effect if administered before or during the early stages of endotoxin absorption. If used, these products should be administered slowly initially and diluted in polyionic fluids to minimize any untoward effects. Anecdotal reports suggest a high rate of untoward reactions to hyperimmune plasma and serum in foals.

Polymyxin B is a cationic polypeptide antibiotic that has been shown to bind lipid A and to neutralize the actions of endotoxin in vitro. Polymyxin B is a broad-spectrum antibiotic, however, and because of a high potential for nephrotoxicity and neurotoxicity, it is not administered systemically to horses. Because polymyxin B exerts antiendotoxic activity at serum concentrations substantially lower than that required for its antimicrobial effects, it has been used in clinical trials for prevention and treatment of endotoxemia in human patients. In some studies, patients given polymyxin B have been shown to have improved immunologic function, decreased plasma endotoxin concentrations, and decreased mortality, compared with patients not given polymyxin B.[44] There were also no adverse effects of polymyxin B observed. Pretreatment with 6000 IU/kg polymyxin B administered IV before 0.25 μg/kg *E. coli* LPS to 3- to 5-month-old foals caused significantly lower maximal TNF-α and IL-6 activities and significantly lower rectal temperature and respiratory rate, compared with foals given endotoxin but no polymyxin B.[43] A study evaluating the effect of polymyxin B conjugated to dextran was performed to evaluate this combination for retaining the polymyxin B within the circulation (and thus preventing extravasation into tissues and toxic interaction with cell membranes, and decreasing the risk for development of adverse effects such as nephrotoxicity).[45] A combination of a 5-mg/kg dose of polymyxin B and 6.6 g/kg of dextran was given to horses 15 minutes before experimental administration of endotoxin. Treatment with this combination prevented the tachycardia, tachypnea, fever, neutropenia, and the increased serum levels of TNF-α, IL-6, thromboxane B_2, and the metabolite of PGI_2 associated with endotoxin administration. This conjugated combination of polymyxin B and dextran is not currently available commercially.

Clinically, polymyxin B is administered to horses at a dosage of 1000 to 5000 IU/kg every 8 to 12 hours diluted in approximately 1 L of polyionic fluid.[46] This therapy is typically continued for approximately 2 to 3 days, or until the signs of endotoxemia subside. Caution should be used in horses that are obviously dehydrated, hypovolemic, or azotemic, and until these abnormalities are corrected. Polymyxin B might have the best chance of providing protection to horses as a preventative measure, if it is possible to administer it before clinical signs develop; administration should probably be considered in horses predisposed to endotoxin absorption, such as horses with ischemic or inflammatory bowel disease.

Treatment of horses with a phospholipid emulsion at a dosage of 200 mg/kg was shown to delay and diminish the effects of low-dose (30 ng/kg, IV) endotoxin administration.[47] Specifically, administration of phospholipid emulsion resulted in significantly decreased rectal temperature, heart rate, cardiac output, right atrial pressure and pulmonary artery pressure, and a higher total leukocyte count. There were also significant differences between treated and control horses for TNF-α, thromboxane B_2, and the PGI_2 metabolite.

INTERFERING WITH SYNTHESIS OR ACTIVITY OF INFLAMMATORY MEDIATORS

Nonsteroidal anti-inflammatory drugs (NSAIDs) are the mainstay of treatment of horses with endotoxemia. Flunixin meglumine and phenylbutazone are the two most commonly used NSAIDs in these horses. In general, flunixin meglumine seems to be more effective at attenuating the cardiovascular effects of endotoxin, whereas phenylbutazone appears to offset the inhibitory effects of endotoxin on bowel motility. Administration of flunixin meglumine at 0.25 mg/kg IV every 8 hours has been shown to decrease eicosanoid concentrations, attenuate hemodynamic effects, and reduce lactic acidemia associated with experimental endotoxemia if administered before endotoxin infusion.[48] Although one study showed that phenylbutazone seems to be more effective for ameliorating the effects of endotoxin on bowel motility in horse, flunixin meglumine is also efficacious.[49] Phenylbutazone can be administered at a dosage of 2.2 mg/kg IV every 12 hours to inhibit the effects of endotoxin on intestinal motility. Although we do not advocate it, some clinicians recommend the combined use of flunixin meglumine (0.25 mg/kg IV three times a day) and phenylbutazone (2.2 mg/kg IV twice a day) to minimize the effects of endotoxin on hemodynamics and intestinal motility *provided the horse is well hydrated*.[49] In a study comparing ketoprofen and flunixin meglumine on the in vitro response of equine peripheral blood mononuclear cells to bacterial endotoxin, they both significantly decreased serum thromboxane B_2, prostaglandin E_2, 12-hydroxy-eicosatetraenoic acid, TNF-α, and tissue factor, suggesting that there does not appear to be any difference in the effects of these two NSAIDs in inhibiting synthesis of inflammatory mediators associated with endotoxemia.[50] It seems that most people continue to use flunixin meglumine to inhibit the effects of endotoxin on the cardiovascular system. Perhaps horses with azotemia or dehydration that may be more predisposed to the toxic effect of NSAIDs would be good candidates for administration of ketoprofen because of its less toxic effects on the gastrointestinal mucosa and renal papilla.[51] Combination NSAID therapy must be administered with extreme caution because of the risk of potentiating the toxic effects on the intestinal mucosa and renal papillae; the drugs should be administered at the lowest possible dosages and for the shortest duration in well-hydrated horses. Because horses with illnesses commonly associated with endotoxemia develop or are predisposed to laminitis, NSAIDs are often the mainstay for prevention and treatment. Phenylbutazone appears to be more effective for musculoskeletal inflammatory conditions and pain, and it is commonly administered for prevention and treatment of laminitis.

Dimethyl sulfoxide (DMSO) is often administered to horses for its putative anti-inflammatory effects, which are related to its ability to scavenge oxygen-derived free radicals. Experimental evidence for the use of DMSO in horses with endotoxemia is lacking, but it has been shown to attenuate endothelial damage, hypoglycemia, hypotension, and lactic acidemia in endotoxic shock in other species.[52] If used, DMSO should be administered at a dosage of 0.1 g/kg to 1 g/kg, and in solution at a concentration no greater than a 10% to 20%. Although it has been demonstrated to decrease ischemia/reperfusion injury of the intestinal mucosa in laboratory animals, no beneficial effects have been reported for ischemia/reperfusion injury in horses. Beneficial effects in laboratory animals have been demonstrated when DMSO is given as a pretreatment and at a dosage of 1 g/kg in these laboratory animals.[53] Pretreatment is not practical in horses with colic, and the dosage that is often used in horses is much greater (100 mg to 1 g/kg). One study reported a potentially deleterious effect of DMSO on the large colon mucosa when administered after ischemia but before the reperfusion period.[54]

Other antioxidants such as allopurinol, a competitive antagonist of xanthine oxidase, and 21-aminosteroids (which inhibit lipid peroxidation) have been shown to be protective against endotoxemia in other species. Allopurinol has been shown to exert some beneficial effect when administered to horses at 5 mg/kg 12 hours before endotoxin challenge.[55] However, again, pretreatment is not particularly practical in the clinical situation,[55] and thus allopurinol is not commonly used in horses.

Pentoxifylline (PTX) is a methylxanthine derivative that has been used for several years to treat intermittent claudication in people. Pentoxifylline is a rheologic agent that improves capillary blood flow by reducing blood viscosity and increased red blood cell deformability. More recently, PTX has been shown to exert pharmacologic effects in vivo and in vitro that may be beneficial in the treatment of endotoxemia, such as inhibition of TNF-α synthesis, decreased thromboxane B_2 concentrations and tissue thromboplastin activity, and increased PGI_2 concentrations. However, PTX has not been shown to attenuate the clinical signs of endotoxemia in human patients, and it does not exert any antipyretic or analgesic effects. Intravenous administration of 8 mg/kg of PTX 15 minutes before and 8 hours after IV administration of 30 ng/kg *E. coli* LPS resulted in a significantly greater PGI_2 concentration at 1.5 hours and lower plasminogen activator inhibitor activity at 12 hours, but TNF-α and IL-6 activities were not different from those in untreated horses.[56] Administration of flunixin meglumine alone (1.1 mg/kg IV) 15 minutes before and again 8 hours after endotoxin administration resulted in a decrease in rectal temperature, total leukocyte count, and thromboxane B_2 concentration. Administration of a combination of flunixin meglumine (1.1 mg/kg IV) and PTX (8 mg/kg IV) did not cause an appreciable difference in the measured variables of this study, compared with administration of flunixin meglumine alone. Because this study did not assess survival as an outcome but rather only clinical signs and clinicopathologic variables, it is difficult to determine if administration of PTX would improve survival of horses with endotoxemia. Treatment with a combination of flunixin meglumine and PTX may be beneficial in horses and deserves further study.

Bolus administration of 7.5 mg/kg PTX immediately after IV administration of 20 ng/kg *E. coli* LPS and followed by an infusion of 3 mg/kg per hour over 3 hours resulted in significant differences in some measured variables compared with horses receiving only endotoxin.[57] Although heart rate, rectal temperature, mean blood pressure, total leukocyte count, whole blood recalcification time, plasminogen activator inhibitor activity, TNF-α and IL-6 activities, and plasma thromboxane B_2 concentrations were significantly changed across time in horses receiving endotoxin and PTX and endotoxin alone, those receiving PTX had lower rectal temperature and respiratory rate and longer whole blood recalcification time than horses that did not receive PTX. Although it appeared that administration of PTX to horses as a bolus followed by a constant infusion caused significant changes in some measured variables, there appear to be minimal beneficial effects of PTX when administered IV using this regimen in this nonlethal equine model of endotoxemia.

Corticosteroids exert a number of beneficial effects that render them potentially useful in the treatment of endotoxemia, including inhibition of phospholipase A_2 and subsequent release of arachidonic acid from cell membranes, and a decreased synthesis of TNF-α, IL-1, and IL-6. However, there are also a number of potentially detrimental effects, including disruption of physiologic processes, inhibition of neutrophil migration, decreased bactericidal activity of neutrophils, increased susceptibility to bacterial and viral infections, and the apparent predisposition of horses to develop laminitis. Although one dose of corticosteroids probably does not put horses at great risk of complications, some clinicians are concerned about the potential for the development of laminitis. The dosage of dexamethasone required to inhibit TNF-α synthesis by equine peritoneal macrophages equates to a systemic dosage of approximately 3 mg/kg, which exceeds the currently recommended dosage that has been shown to have beneficial effects in experimental equine endotoxemia.[58] However, many of the potentially beneficial effects of corticosteroids can be achieved with NSAIDs, and these effects do not outweigh the potential deleterious effects. Therefore, corticosteroids should not be used in the prevention or treatment of endotoxemia in horses.

INTERFERING WITH CELLULAR ACTIVATION

It has been shown that nontoxic LPS or nontoxic lipid-A substances can serve as endotoxin antagonists by competitively inhibiting binding to either LBP or cellular receptors. Because of these effects, numerous attempts to interfere with the interaction of cells and LPS and to halt intracellular signal pathways have been studied in laboratory animals and people.[59,60] Of these substances, LPS and lipid A originating from the phototrophic bacterium *Rhodobacter sphaeroides*, and a synthetic substance with a structure similar to the *R. sphaeroides* LPS, are the most promising. However, unlike in other species, these substances act as potent stimulants of cytokine expression in equine cells.[61] It is believed that this species difference may be associated with TLR4, which indicates that further studies are needed to clarify the potential role of these substances and their mechanism of action in horses.

A typical horse with signs of endotoxemia secondary to gastrointestinal tract disease would most likely be treated for the primary disease (e.g., mineral oil for grain overload, mucosal protectant for inflammatory bowel disease, surgical resection of ischemic-injured bowel), advanced medical and supportive care (e.g., IV crystalloids or colloids, antibiotics), NSAIDs (flunixin meglumine and/or phenylbutazone), neutralizing endotoxin (antiendotoxin serum, polymyxin B), or ancillary anti-inflammatory drugs (dimethyl sulfoxide, pentoxifylline).

Prevention

Maintenance and restoration of the intestinal mucosal barrier is an important factor in the prevention of endotoxemia and sepsis.[4] Conditions favoring intestinal and colonic overgrowth favor development of sepsis and endotoxemia. Administration of antacids in critically ill patients may lead to proximal gut colonization by virulent bacteria because of increased gastric pH. Caution in administering antacids should be exercised, especially in critically ill neonates. Impaired intestinal motility associated with ileus and obstruction often leads to bacterial overgrowth. Therefore, prevention or rapid resolution of ileus should be a goal of management of these horses. Regarding prophylaxis, 77% of respondents to a survey indicated that they treat horses they consider at risk for developing endotoxemia even when the horses do not show clinical signs of endotoxemia. These prophylactic measures include administration of intravenous fluids (92%), low-dose flunixin meglumine (86%), antimicrobials (73%), hyperimmune antiendotoxic plasma or serum (65%), high-dose (1.1 mg/kg) flunixin meglumine (50%), ketoprofen (50%), heparin (35%), aspirin (17%), and/or corticosteroids (7%).[36]

Prognosis

It is difficult to accurately determine the likelihood of survival of horses with endotoxemia, because this condition typically occurs subsequent to a variety of other diseases, each with its own severity, and because of the variation in the rapidity and amount of endotoxin gaining access to the circulation. However, the prognosis for horses with endotoxemia should be guarded because of the severity of the primary disease and the rapidly progressing pathophysiologic processes that are initiated when appreciable quantities of endotoxin gain access to the systemic circulation. Horses that develop endotoxemia secondary to gastrointestinal tract ischemia or inflammation (enteritis, colitis) are often so severely ill that they succumb to the effects of either the primary disease or the inflammatory cascade initiated by the interaction of endotoxin with the host's inflammatory cells. Early, aggressive treatment of the primary disease process along with a combination of the previously mentioned medications could improve the outcome in some horses, if the quantity of endotoxin reaching the systemic circulation is not overwhelming.

ON THE HORIZON

Future therapeutic regimens will probably be developed on the basis of temporal changes in gene expression that are identified through the use of modern molecular biology techniques. These treatments will most likely be geared toward modulation of the proinflammatory and anti-inflammatory cascades that are initiated by the systemic exposure of horses to endotoxin.

Monoclonal antibodies against specific mediators of the inflammatory process have been developed and administered to human patients to modulate the tissue damage in inflammatory diseases. For example, administration of monoclonal antibody directed against TNF-α (infliximab) has successfully suppressed tissue damage in patients with ulcerative colitis and Crohn's disease. New insights into cell-based and gene-based treatments against inflammatory disease in veterinary medicine are needed to apply these therapies to domestic animals.

Leukotriene inhibitors and antagonists have been used with success in a number of human diseases. Although these drugs have not yet been applied to veterinary medicine, research data have shown their effects to be promising. Medications currently available for human use include the following:

- Drugs (e.g., Zileuton and 5-aminosalicylic acid) that inhibit 5-lipoxygenase, thereby preventing metabolism of arachidonic acid to leukotrienes
- Drugs that block 5-lipoxygenase activating protein, preventing the action of 5-lipoxygenase
- Drugs that block the *cys*-leukotriene-1 receptor, which is responsible for the bronchoconstrictor effects of leukotrienes. LTC_4, LTD_4, and LTE_4 cause bronchoconstriction through effects on this receptor. Zafirlukast and montelukast are selective, competitive antagonists of this receptor that are approved for clinical use in people.

Because of species differences, mechanisms identified in humans and laboratory animals and subsequent treatments directed against these pathways or mediators cannot automatically be assumed (or extrapolated) to be effective, safe, and useful in horses. Controlled research studies and case-control clinical trials are needed to accurately determine the efficacy of new treatments in the clinical management of endotoxemia in horses.

REFERENCES

1. Morris DD: Endotoxemia in horses: A review of cellular and humoral mediators involved in its pathogenesis, J Vet Intern Med 1991;5:167.
2. Moore JN, Garner HE, Berg JN, et al: Intracecal endotoxin and lactate during the onset of equine laminitis: A preliminary report, Am J Vet Res 1979;40:722-723.
3. Tomlinson JE, Blikslager AT: Interactions between lipopolysaccharide and the intestinal epithelium, J Am Vet Med Assoc 2004;224:1446-1452.
4. Bellhorn T, Macintire DK: Bacterial translocation, Compend Contin Educ Pract Vet 2004;26:229-236.
5. Barton MH, Collatos C: Tumor necrosis factor and interleukin-6 activity and endotoxin concentration in peritoneal fluid and blood of horses with acute abdominal disease, J Vet Intern Med 1999;13:457-464.
6. Steverink PJGM, Sturk A, Rutten VPMG, et al: Endotoxin, interleukin-6 and tumor necrosis factor concentrations in equine acute abdominal disease: Relation to clinical outcome, J Endotoxin Res 1995;2:289-299.
7. Lohmann KL, Barton MH: Endotoxemia. In Reed SM, Bayly WM, Sellon DC, editors: Equine Internal Medicine, ed 2, St Louis, 2004, WB Saunders.
8. Tobias PS: Lipopolysaccharide-binding protein. In Brade H, Opal SM, Vogel SN, et al, editors: Endotoxin in Health and Disease, New York, 1999, Marcel Dekker.
9. Schuman RR, Leong SR, Flaggs GW, et al: Structure and function of lipopolysaccharide-binding protein, Science 1990;249:1429-1431.
10. Wright SD, Ramos RA, Tobias PS, et al: CD14, a receptor for complexes of lipopolysaccharide (LPS) and LPS binding protein, Science 1990;249:1431-1433.
11. Wurfel MM, Hailman E, Wright SD: Soluble CD14 acts as a shuttle in the neutralization of lipopolysaccharide (LPS) by LPS-binding protein and reconstituted high density lipoprotein, J Exp Med 1995;181:1743-1754.
12. Lien E, Means TK, Heine H, et al: Toll-like receptor 4 imparts ligand-specific recognition of bacterial lipopolysaccharide, J Clin Invest 2000;105:497-504.
13. Chow JC, Young DW, Golenbock DT, et al: Toll-like receptor-4 mediates lipopolysaccharide-induced signal transduction, J Biol Chem 1999;274:10689-10692.
14. Brightbill HD, Modlin RL: Toll-like receptors: Molecular mechanisms of the mammalian immune response, Immunology 2000;101:1-10.
15. Yang H, Young DW, Gusovsky F, et al: Cellular events mediated by lipopolysaccharide-stimulated Toll-like receptor 4: MD-2 is required for activation of mitogen-activated protein kinases and Elk-1, J Biol Chem 2000;275:20861-20866.
16. Le J, Vilcek J: Biology of disease: Tumor necrosis factor and interleukin-1: Cytokines with multiple and overlapping biologic activities, Lab Invest 1987;61:588-602.
17. Barton MH, Collatos C, Moore JN: Endotoxin induced expression of tumour necrosis factor, tissue factor and plasminogen activator inhibitor activity by peritoneal macrophages, Equine Vet J 28:382-389, 1996.
18. Collins T: Acute and chronic inflammation. In Cotran RS, Kumar V, Collins T, editors: Pathologic Basis of Disease, Philadelphia, 1999, WB Saunders.
19. Moore JN, Morris DD: Endotoxemia and septicemia in horses: Experimental and clinical correlates, J Am Vet Med Assoc 1992;200:1903-1914.
20. Henderson WR: The role of leukotrienes in inflammation, Ann Intern Med 1994;121:684-697.
21. Brady HR: Potential vascular roles for lipoxins in "stop programs" of host defense and inflammation, Trends Cardiovasc Med 1995;5:186-192.
22. Maddox JF: Lipoxin B4 regulates human monocyte/neutrophil adherence and motility. FASEB 1998;12:487.
23. Carrick JB, Morris DD, Moore JN: Administration of a receptor antagonist for platelet activating factor during equine endotoxemia, Equine Vet J 1993;25:152-157.
24. Ward PA: Oxygen radicals, inflammation and tissue injury, Free Radic Biol Med 5:403, 1988.
25. Remick DG, Villarete L: Regulation of cytokine gene expression by reactive oxygen and reactive nitrogen intermediates, J Leukocyte Biol 1996;59:471-475.
26. Furchgott RF, Zawadzki JV: The obligatory role of endothelial cells in the relaxation of arterial smooth muscle by acetylcholine, Nature 1980;288:373-376.
27. Nathan C: Inducible nitric oxide synthase: What difference does it make? J Clin Invest 1997;100:2417-2423.
28. Fang FC: Mechanisms of nitric oxide-related antimicrobial activity, J Clin Invest 1997;99:2818-2825.
29. Bueno AC, Seahorn TL, Cornick-Seahorn J, et al: Plasma and urine nitric oxide concentrations in horses given a low dose of endotoxin, Am J Vet Res 1999;60:969-976.
30. Mackay RJ: Treatment of endotoxemia and SIRS. In Proceedings of the Annual American College of Veterinary Internal Medicine Forum, 2001.
31. Hawkins DL, Mackay RJ, MacKay SL, et al: Human interleukin 10 suppresses production of inflammatory mediators by LPS-stimulated equine peritoneal macrophages, Vet Immunol Immunopathol 1998;66:1-10.
32. Lipowsky HH: Leukocyte margination and deformation in post-capillary venules. In Granger DN, Schmid-Schönbein G, editors: Physiology and Pathophysiology of Leukocyte Adhesion, New York, 1996, Oxford Press.
33. Carlos TM, Harlan JM: Leukocyte-endothelial adhesion molecules, Blood 1994;84:2068-2101.
34. Moore JN: Pathophysiology of circulatory shock. In White NA, editor: The Equine Acute Abdomen, Philadelphia, 1990, Lea & Febiger.
35. Ramaswamy CM, Eades SC, Venugopal CS, et al: Plasma concentrations of endothelin-like immunoreactivity in healthy horses and horses with naturally acquired gastrointestinal tract disorders, Am J Vet Res 2002;63:454-458.
36. Shuster R, Traub-Dargatz J, Baxter G: Survey of diplomates of the American College of Veterinary Internal Medicine and the American College of Veterinary Surgeons regarding clinical aspects and treatment of endotoxemia in horses, Am J Vet Res 1997;210:87-92.
37. King JN: Detection of endotoxin in cases of equine colic, Vet Rec 1988;123:269-271.
38. Barton MH, Morris DD, Norton NN, et al: Hemostatic and fibrinolytic indices in neonatal foals with presumed septicemia, J Vet Intern Med 1998;12:26-35.
39. Bottoms GD, Fessler JF, Gimarc S, et al: Plasma concentrations of endotoxin (LPS) following jugular or portal injections of LPS, GI strangulating-obstructions and after colon rupture, Circ Shock 1987;21:335-340.
40. Weese JS, Cote NM, deGannes RVG: Evaluation of in vitro properties of di-tri-octahedral smectite on clostridial toxins and growth, Equine Vet J 2003;35:638-641.
41. Bentley AP, Barton MH, Lee MD, et al: Antimicrobial-induced endotoxin and cytokine activity in an in vitro model of septicemia in foals, Am J Vet Res 2002;63:660-668.
42. Spier SJ, Lavoie JP, Cullor JS, et al: Protection against clinical endotoxemia in horses by using plasma containing antibody to an Rc mutant *E. coli* (J5), Circ Shock 1989;28:235-248.
43. Durando MM, Mackay RJ, Linda S, et al: Effects of polymyxin B and *Salmonella typhimurium* antiserum on horses given endotoxin intravenously, Am J Vet Res 1994;55:921-927.
44. Endo S, Indad K, Kikuchi M, et al: Clinical effects of intramuscular administration of a small dose of polymyxin B to patients with endotoxemia, Res Commun Chem Pathol Pharmacol 1994;83:223-235.

45. MacKay RJ, Clark CK, Logdberg L, et al: Effect of a conjugate of polymyxin B-dextran 70 in horses with experimentally induced endotoxemia, Am J Vet Res 1999;60:68-75.
46. Barton MH: Use of polymyxin B for treatment of endotoxemia in horses, Compend Contin Educ Pract Vet 2000;11:1056-1059.
47. Winchell WW, Hardy J, Levine DM, et al: Effect of administration of a phospholipid emulsion on the initial response of horses administered endotoxin, Am J Vet Res 2002;63:1370-1378.
48. Semrad SD, Hardee GE, Hardee MM, et al: Low dose flunixin meglumine: Effects on eicosanoid production and clinical signs induced by experimental endotoxaemia in horses, Equine Vet J 1987;19:201-206.
49. King JN, Gerring EL: Antagonism of endotoxin-induced disruption of equine bowel motility by flunixin and phenylbutazone, Equine Vet J 1989;7:38-42.
50. Jackman BR, Moore JN, Barton MH, et al: Comparison of the effects of ketoprofen and flunixin meglumine on the in vitro response of equine peripheral blood monocytes to bacterial endotoxin, Can J Vet Res 1994;58:138-143.
51. McAllister CG, Morgan SJ, Borne AT, et al: Comparison of adverse effects of phenylbutazone, flunixin meglumine, and ketoprofen in horses, J Am Vet Med Assoc 1993;202:71-77.
52. Brackett DJ, Lerner MR, Wilson MF: Dimethyl sulfoxide antagonizes hypotensive, metabolic, and pathologic responses induced by endotoxin, Circ Shock 1991;33:156-163.
53. Matsuda T, Eccleston CA, Rubinstein I, et al: Antioxidants attenuate endotoxin-induced microvascular leakage of macromolecules in vivo, J Appl Physiol 1991;70:1483-1489.
54. Moore RM, Muir WW, Berton AL, et al: Effects of dimethyl sulfoxide, allopurinol, 21-aminosteroid U-74389G, and manganese chloride on low-flow ischemia and reperfusion of the large colon in horses, Am J Vet Res 1995;56:671-687.
55. Lochner F, Sangiah S, Burrows G, et al: Effects of allopurinol in experimental endotoxin shock in horses, Res Vet Sci 1989;47:178-184.
56. Baskett A, Barton MH, Norton N, et al: Effects of pentoxifylline, flunixin meglumine, and their combination on a model of endotoxemia in horses, Am J Vet Res 1997;58:1291-1299.
57. Barton MH, Moore JN, Norton N: Effects of pentoxifylline infusion on response of horses to in vivo challenge exposure with endotoxin, Am J Vet Res 1997;58:1300-1307.
58. Frauenfelder HC, Fessler JF, Moore AB, et al: Effects of dexamethasone on endotoxin shock in the anesthetized pony: Hematologic, blood gas, and coagulation changes, Am J Vet Res 1982;43:405-411.
59. Lei MG, Qureshi N, Morrison DC: Lipopolysaccharide (LPS) binding to 73-kDa and 38-kDa surface proteins on lymphoreticular cells: Preferential inhibition of LPS binding to the former by *Rhodopseudomonas sphaeroides* lipid A, Immunol Lett 1993;36:245-250.
60. Bunnell E, Lynn M, Habet K, et al: A lipid A analog, E5531, blocks the endotoxin response in human volunteers with experimental endotoxemia, Crit Care Med 2000;28:2713-2720.
61. Lohmann KL: Lipopolysaccharide from *Rhodobacter sphaeroides* is an endotoxin agonist in equine cells. Presented at the 24th Conference on Shock, Shock Society, June 2001.

CHAPTER 3

Fluids, Electrolytes, and Acid–Base Therapy

Joanne Hardy

Fluid administration for maintenance or replacement purposes is one of the mainstays of equine critical care, and the technology should be readily accessible in any equine hospital. The availability of commercial materials and fluids for use in large animals makes fluid administration easy and cost effective in most situations. This chapter reviews fluid and electrolyte balance, materials needed, and principles to follow when planning fluid administration.

NORMAL FLUID AND ELECTROLYTE BALANCE

Distribution of Fluids

Fluids in the body are distributed in two compartments: the intracellular fluid (ICF) volume and the extracellular fluid (ECF) volume. The ECF is composed of interstitial fluid, plasma, lymph, and transcellular fluids such as synovial, pleural, abdominal, and cerebrospinal fluids. The transcellular fluids do not normally contribute to significant fluid losses, but they may, in disease states such as pleuropneumonia or peritonitis, contribute significantly to volume deficits. For example, it is not unusual to drain 10 to 20 L of fluid from the pleural cavity of horses with severe pleuropneumonia. Additionally, the volume of gastrointestinal secretions in horses plays an important role in fluid distribution. The normal volume of gastrointestinal secretion in horses is approximately equivalent to the extracellular fluid volume, representing approximately 100 L every 24 hours in a 500-kg horse.[1] Therefore, significant fluid sequestration and loss can occur with intestinal obstruction or colitis.

The volume of total body water (TBW) represents 60% of body weight in adults and up to 80% in neonates. The ECF volume represents 20% (in adults) to 40% (in neonates) of total body water, and the ICF volume, approximately 40%. Recent estimates of fluid distribution in horses report values of 0.67 L/kg (67%) for TBW, 0.21 L/kg (21%) for ECF, and 0.46 L/kg (46%) for ICF.[2,3] In neonates, the ECF is approximately 40% of the TBW, and it decreases to approximately 30% by 24 weeks of age.[4] For calculation purposes on substances distributed across the ECF, a factor of 0.3 is used for adults, and 0.4 for young animals. Blood volume in sedentary horses represents approximately 8% of body weight (see Chapter 4).[5] In fit horses, this value can reach 14% of body weight.[6] In neonates, blood volume represents 15% of body weight and decreases to adult values by 12 weeks of age.[4]

Body solutes are not distributed equally through TBW. In plasma, sodium is the main cation, and bicarbonate and chloride are the main anions. Proteins contribute to the negative charges, and they also provide oncotic pressure. Albumin or molecules of similar size are the main contributors to oncotic pressure. The interstitial fluid comprises about 75% of the ECF, and it is composed mainly of sodium, bicarbonate, and chloride, but the concentration of protein there is lower. The slightly increased concentration of anions and decreased concentration of cations in interstitial fluids occurs because of the greater concentration of protein in plasma (according to the Gibbs-Donnan equilibrium). In clinical practice, this difference is small, so that the measured concentration of solutes in plasma is thought to reflect the concentration of solutes throughout the ECF. Table 3-1 lists normal plasma concentrations of electrolytes in adult horses. The composition of the intracellular fluid compartment is different: the important cations are potassium and magnesium, and the important anions are phosphates and proteins (Fig. 3-1).

Transfer of fluid between compartments is an important consideration when planning fluid administration. Some important concepts govern these mechanisms. Osmolality is defined as the concentration of osmotically active particles in solution per kilogram of solvent (mOsm/kg), whereas osmolarity is the number of particles of solute per liter of solvent (mOsm/L). In biologic fluids, the difference between the two concentrations is negligible, and the two terms are often used interchangeably. Normal plasma osmolality in adult horses ranges from 275 to 312 mOsm/kg,[7] and it varies slightly between breeds. Lower values are reported for normal foals.[8] The effective osmolality, or *tonicity*, is the osmotic pressure generated by the difference in osmolality between two compartments. Colloid oncotic pressure is the osmotic pressure generated by proteins, mainly albumin, and is measured using a colloid osmometer (Wescor, Logan, Utah).

TABLE 3-1. Normal Hematologic Values in Adult Horses

Plasma Parameter (Units)	Normal Concentration Range
CATIONS	
Sodium (mmol/L or mEq/L)	132-146
Potassium (mmol/L or mEq/L)	2.4-4.7
Calcium (mmol/L)	2.8-3.4
Ionized calcium (mmol/L)	1.0-1.3
Magnesium (mmol/L)	0.9-1.15
Ionized magnesium (mmol/L)	0.4-0.55
ANIONS	
Chloride (mmol/L or mEq/L)	99-109
Total CO_2 (mmol/L or mEq/L)	24-32
VENOUS BLOOD GAS	
pH	7.32-7.44
PCO_2 (mm Hg)	38-46
PO_2 (mm Hg)	37-56 (arterial, 80-100)
HCO_3^- (mmol/L or mEq/L)	20-28
Base excess (mmol/L or mEq/L)	−2 to +2
OTHER	
Creatinine (mg/dL)	0.9-1.9
Plasma protein (g/dL)	5.8-8.7
Albumin (mg/dL)	2.9-3.8
Plasma lactate (mmol/L)	1.11-1.78

Data from Kaneko JJ, Bruss ML: Clinical Biochemistry of Domestic Animals, 5th ed. San Diego, Calif, Academic Press, 1997.

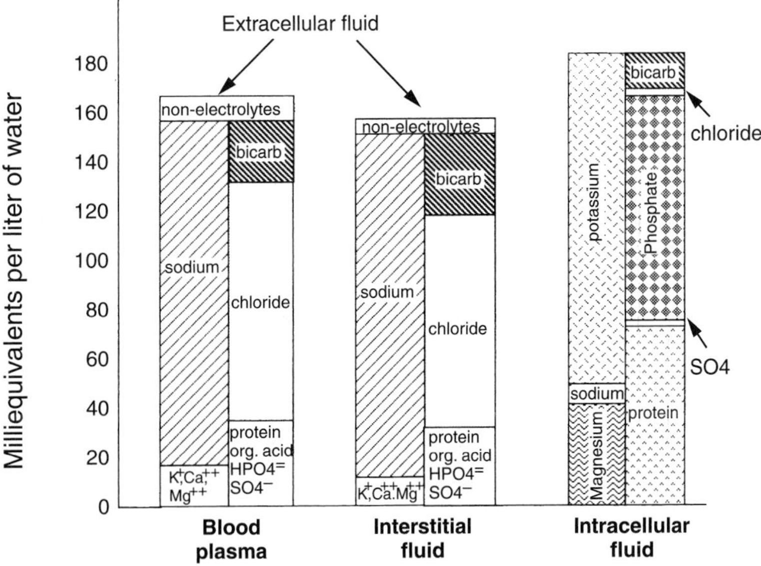

Figure 3-1. The compositions of plasma, interstitial fluid, and intracellular fluid. (Adapted from Guyton AC: Textbook of Medical Physiology, 7th ed. Philadelphia, WB Saunders 1986, p 386; originally modified and reprinted by permission of the publisher from Gamble JL: Chemical Anatomy, Physiology and Pathology of Extracellular Fluid: A Lecture Syllabus. Cambridge, Mass, Harvard University Press, 1954; Copyright 1942 by JL Gamble.)

Normal values of 15.0 to 22.6 mm Hg for foals and 19.2 to 31.3 mm Hg for adult horses have been reported.[9,10] *Water and ionic solute exchange between the vascular and interstitial compartments occurs at the capillary level and is rapid; equilibrium is reached within 30 to 60 minutes.* The rate of exchange or net filtration that occurs between these compartments is controlled by a balance between the forces that favor filtration (capillary hydrostatic pressure and tissue oncotic pressure) and the forces that tend to retain fluid within the vascular space (plasma oncotic pressure and tissue hydrostatic pressure). These relationships are described by Starling's law:

$$\text{Net filtration} = K_f\,[(P_{cap} - P_{int}) - \sigma\,(\pi_p - \pi_{int})],$$

where K_f is the filtration coefficient, which varies depending on the surface available for filtration and the permeability of the capillary wall; P_{cap} and P_{int} are the hydrostatic pressure in the capillary or in the interstitium; π_p and π_{int} are the oncotic pressures in the plasma or interstitial fluid; and σ is the reflection coefficient of proteins across the capillary wall.

Exchanges between the interstitial and the intracellular compartment are governed by the number of osmotically active particles within each space. Sodium is the most abundant cation in the ECF. Consequently, sodium accounts for most of the osmotically active particles in the ECF. Other osmotically active compounds that make a significant contribution to ECF osmolarity are glucose and urea. The most commonly used formula for estimation of serum osmolarity is as follows[11]:

$$\text{ECF osmolality} = 2[\text{Na}^+] + \frac{\text{glucose}}{18} + \frac{\text{urea}}{2.8}.$$

Cells membranes are permeable to urea and K^+. Therefore, the effective osmolarity is calculated as follows:

$$\text{ECF osmolality} = 2[\text{Na}^+] + \frac{\text{glucose}}{18}.$$

The *osmolar gap* is the difference between measured osmolarity and calculated osmolarity; an increased osmolar gap can exist when unmeasured solutes, such as mannitol, are present.[12]

Exchanges between the extracellular and intracellular compartments are comparatively slow, taking up to 24 hours to reach equilibrium.

Acid–Base Balance

The concentration of hydrogen ions, and therefore the pH, is closely regulated in the body to vary between 7.35 and 7.45. This narrow range is maintained by the presence of buffers within different body compartments; a buffer is a compound that can accept or donate protons to maintain the pH within a narrow range. In the body, bicarbonate is the primary buffer system of the extracellular fluid, whereas protein and inorganic and organic phosphates are the principal intracellular buffer system.

The importance of bicarbonate as a buffer in the ECF stems from the fact that it is an open system. The dissociation of carbonic acid is expressed by the law of mass action:

$$H^+ + HCO_3^- \cdot H_2CO_3 \cdot CO_2 + H_2O$$

In the body, this system is open, and carbonic acid, in the presence of carbonic anhydrase, forms CO_2, which is eliminated entirely from the system by alveolar ventilation.

The relationship between pH, bicarbonate, and carbonic acid is expressed in the Henderson-Hasselbach equation:

$$\text{pH} = 6.1 + \log \frac{[HCO_3^-]}{0.03\ \text{P}CO_2},$$

where $\text{P}CO_2$ is the partial pressure of carbon dioxide. This is the clinically relevant form of the equation, which shows that in body fluids, pH is a function of the ratio of HCO_3^- to $\text{P}CO_2$; this ratio is normally approximately 20:1.

The responses to acid or base alterations in the body all combine to normalize pH. For example, an acute increase in hydrogen ions from a fixed acid load is immediately buffered by bicarbonate and intracellular buffers. This is the acute physiochemical response. Alveolar ventilation is subsequently modified, and this is complete within hours to further minimize changes in pH by normalizing the ratio of HCO_3^- to $\text{P}CO_2$. Finally, renal responses result in regeneration of HCO_3^-, resulting in a long-term response. The renal response begins within hours and is complete within 2 to 5 days. An acute increase in volatile CO_2, in contrast, cannot be buffered by HCO_3^-; therefore, the hydrogen ions generated from the dissociation of carbonic acid must be buffered by intracellular buffers. Renal adaptation, characterized by increased HCO_3^- reabsorption and net acid secretion, takes 2 to 5 days to achieve maximal effectiveness.

ACID–BASE DISORDERS

Terminology

Acidosis and alkalosis refer to the processes that cause net accumulation of acid or alkali in the body, respectively. Acidemia and alkalemia refer to the pH of the ECF: in acidemia, the pH of the ECF is lower than normal, and in alkalemia the pH of the ECF is higher than normal. The distinction between these terms is important; for example a horse with chronic reactive airway disease may have a normal blood pH because of effective renal compensation, but in this setting the patient will have increased bicarbonate. This patient has alkalosis but does not have alkalemia.

Primary Acid–Base Disorders

There are four primary acid–base disorders: metabolic acidosis, metabolic alkalosis, respiratory acidosis, and respiratory alkalosis. The metabolic disorders refer to the net excess or deficit of nonvolatile or fixed acid, whereas the respiratory disturbances refer to a net deficit or excess of volatile acid (dissolved CO_2).

Metabolic acidosis is present when there is a decrease in HCO_3^- caused by either loss or buffering of nonvolatile acids. Common causes of metabolic acidosis in horses include accumulation of lactic acid as a result of poor perfusion, and HCO_3^- losses in the gastrointestinal tract resulting from diarrhea. *Metabolic alkalosis* is present when there is an increased concentration of HCO_3^-. Metabolic alkalosis is commonly associated with a disproportionate loss of

TABLE 3-2. Traditional Approach* to Simple Acid–Base Disorders in Adult Horses

Parameter	Metabolic Acidosis	Metabolic Alkalosis	Respiratory Acidosis	Respiratory Alkalosis (Arterial Sample)
pH	7.390	7.49	7.30	7.50
P_{CO_2} (mm Hg)	28.4	49	60	32
P_{O_2} (mm Hg)	42	43	38	55
HCO_3^- (mEq/L)	16.5	34	28	22
Base excess (BE) (mEq/L)	−5.8	+9	−1	−2
Comments	There is a secondary increase in P_{CO_2} to compensate for the primary disorder.	There is a secondary decrease in P_{CO_2} in an attempt at compensation.	This is an acute disorder with increased bicarbonate of 1-2 mEq/L per 10 mm Hg increase in P_{CO_2}. Note that the BE is normal, indicating no metabolic disturbance.	Increased ventilation in response to hypoxemia is the cause of this disorder.

*This traditional approach to the diagnosis of simple acid–base disorders depends on interpretation of the clinical parameters in the left-hand column, without examining the contribution of electrolytes, unmeasured anions, or protein concentrations.

TABLE 3-3. Secondary (Adaptive) Responses to Primary Acid–Base Abnormalities

Disorder	Primary Change	Secondary Response
Metabolic acidosis	↓ HCO_3^-	P_{CO_2} decreases by 1.2 mm Hg for every 1 mEq/L decrease in bicarbonate
Metabolic alkalosis	↑ HCO_3^-	P_{CO_2} increases by 0.6 to 1 mm Hg for every 1 mEq/L increase in bicarbonate
Acute respiratory acidosis	↑ P_{CO_2}	$[HCO_3^-]$ increases by 1 mEq/L for every 10 mm Hg increase in PCO_2
Chronic respiratory acidosis	↑ P_{CO_2}	$[HCO_3^-]$ increases by 3-4 mEq/L for every 10 mm Hg increase in PCO_2
Acute respiratory alkalosis	↓ P_{CO_2}	$[HCO_3^-]$ decreases by 1-3 mEq/L for every 10 mm Hg decrease in P_{CO_2}
Chronic respiratory alkalosis	↓ P_{CO_2}	$[HCO_3^-]$ decreases by 5 mEq/L for every 10 mm Hg decrease in P_{CO_2}

From Brobst D: J Am Vet Med Assoc 1983;183:773-780.

chloride ions. *Respiratory acidosis* is present when the partial pressure of carbon dioxide (P_{CO_2}) is increased in response to alveolar hypoventilation. *Respiratory alkalosis* is present when the P_{CO_2} is decreased. Table 3-2 lists examples of primary acid–base disorders in horses.

For each primary acid–base disturbance, there is a secondary or adaptive response that involves the component opposite the primary disturbance, in an attempt to return the pH toward normal. The secondary response never restores the pH completely to normal. For metabolic disorders, the secondary or adaptive respiratory response begins immediately and is complete within hours. In respiratory disorders, the adaptive response begins with an acute, immediate titration by nonbicarbonate buffers that results in an initial change in plasma HCO_3^- concentration. This is followed by a chronic response mediated by the kidney that involves net acid secretion and bicarbonate resorption. This response begins within hours and takes 2 to 5 days to be complete. Table 3-3 lists expected adaptive responses to acid–base disorders. These expected responses vary slightly across species.[13]

Mixed Acid–Base Disorders

When a primary disorder occurs with the expected secondary response, it is considered a *simple acid–base disorder*. A *mixed disorder* means that two separate primary disorders are present in the same patient. A mixed disorder is suspected when the adaptive response is lower or higher than the expected response from the primary disorder.

MEASUREMENT AND INTERPRETATION OF BLOOD GASES

Measurement

For accurate blood gas analysis, appropriate sampling methods should be followed. Blood (arterial or venous) is collected anaerobically from the puncture site using a syringe that contains the appropriate anticoagulant for the analyzer, usually lithium heparin, taking care to not dilute the sample with excess heparin. Introduction of room air into the sample will falsely increase the partial pressure of oxygen and decrease the partial pressure of carbon dioxide. If a delay in analysis is anticipated, the blood should be placed on ice to decrease cell metabolism. Most blood gas analyzers perform their analysis at 37° C. At extremes of body temperature, a patient's actual value may differ from expected according to the gas law: with increases in temperature, gas is less soluble and therefore its partial pressure in the solution increases; this will increase the Po_2 and Pco_2 of a solution. Similarly, with extreme hypothermia, gas is more soluble, resulting in decreases in Po_2 and Pco_2. Although available in many blood gas analyzers, temperature correction is usually not performed for several reasons: (1) the small changes in body temperature usually do not affect blood gas analyses significantly, (2) the patient's temperature, if extreme, will usually be corrected shortly, and (3) there are no established normal values for extremes in body temperature.

Routine blood gas analyzers provide three measured values, pH, Pco_2, and Po_2, and three calculated values, total CO_2 (TCO_2), HCO_3^-, and base excess (BE). Measured values that are outside of physiologic ranges should be considered a malfunction of the analyzer.

- pH is the negative base 10 logarithm of hydrogen concentration and is a measured value.
- Pco_2 (mm Hg) is the measured partial pressure of dissolved carbon dioxide in the sample. A venous sample will have a slightly higher (5 mm Hg) value than an arterial sample. An increase in Pco_2 is termed *hypercapnia* or *hypercarbia,* and it usually reflects alveolar hypoventilation. However, an increase in venous Pco_2 may also reflect poor tissue perfusion.
- Po_2 (mm Hg) is the measured partial pressure of dissolved oxygen in blood. This is different than oxygen content, which is the total concentration of oxygen carried by blood and includes the portion carried by hemoglobin.
- TCO_2 (mEq/L) is the concentration of total CO_2 in the sample, obtained by adding a strong acid to the sample and measuring the amount of CO_2 produced, and it includes both dissolved CO_2 and HCO_3^-. As HCO_3^- represents 95% of total CO_2, this measurement is indirectly a measurement of HCO_3^-, and it is 1 to 2 mEq/L higher than the concentration of HCO_3^-.
- HCO_3^- (mEq/L) is reported as actual bicarbonate, which is the calculated concentration of bicarbonate in the sample, and standard bicarbonate, which is the calculated concentration of HCO_3^- after the sample has been equilibrated to a Pco_2 of 40 mm Hg.
- BE (mEq/L) is the amount of strong acid or base required to titrate 1 L of blood to a pH of 7.40 at 37° C with the Pco_2 held constant at 40 mm Hg. Because the base excess is changed only by nonvolatile fixed acids, it is considered to reflect *metabolic* acid–base disturbances.

Normal values for the horse are presented in Table 3-1.

Interpretation

To interpret blood gases, a practiced method should be followed. First the pH is measured, and if it is outside the normal range, an acid–base disorder is present. The clinician examines next the HCO_3^- and Pco_2 and determines if an abnormality is present that could explain the abnormal pH. An acidemia is caused by an increase in Pco_2 or a decrease in HCO_3^-, whereas an alkalemia is caused by a decrease in Pco_2 or an increase in HCO_3^-. Once the primary disorder has been characterized, the clinician determines whether a secondary response is present. The absence of a secondary response, or a change in the direction opposite the expected response, is an indication of a mixed disorder. The clinician then determines whether the acid–base disturbance is consistent with the patient's history and clinical findings. Table 3-2 lists examples of simple acid–base disorders in horses.

Another important component of blood gas interpretation is the partial pressure of oxygen (Po_2). The normal Po_2 of arterial blood (Pao_2) is approximately 5 times the fraction of inspired oxygen (Fio_2), or 80 to 100 mm Hg in room air at sea level (Fio_2, 21%). *Hypoxemia* refers to a decreased Pao_2; common causes include a decreased Fio_2 (an example is a decreased barometric pressure associated with high altitude), hypoventilation, ventilation/perfusion mismatch, shunt, or diffusion impairment. The normal Po_2 of venous blood is 40 mm Hg. A low mixed Pvo_2 (*mixed* refers to a sample collected centrally, ideally from the pulmonary artery) in the presence of normal Pao_2 should alert to poor tissue perfusion.

Anion Gap

The anion gap (AG) is the difference between the sum of the commonly measured cations and the sum of the commonly measured anions in serum, calculated as follows:

$$AG = (Na^+ + K^+) - (Cl^- + HCO_3^-).$$

The sum of cations always exceeds the sum of anions, and the difference is an attempt to estimate the concentration of unmeasured anions—for example, lactate. A normal anion gap of 10.4 ± 1.2 mEq/L has been reported in adult horses.[14] Neonates have a slightly higher anion gap because of their increased levels of phosphates and globulins.[14] In exercising horses, the anion gap is useful to estimate plasma lactate concentrations in the presence of relatively normal plasma protein concentrations.[15] In horses with abdominal pain, the correlation between lactate concentration and the AG is excellent, but the presence of other strong ions results in a higher AG than would be expected from lactate measurement.[16] The anion gap is considered a good prognostic indicator of survival in horses with abdominal disorders: a value of greater than 25 mEq/L is associated with a significantly lower survival rate.[17,18]

Lactate

Measurement of lactate is now a routine part of the assessment of perfusion in equine patients, and it is available in most chemistry and point-of-care analyzers.[19] Samples should be analyzed immediately to avoid in vitro lactate production by erythrocytes; alternatively, collection in fluoride-containing tubes, storage on ice, and plasma separation can help minimize this problem. Lactate is the end product of anaerobic glycolysis, and its concentration is another indicator of tissue perfusion and oxygen delivery; an increased blood lactate concentration is most often a result of tissue hypoxia. Although inadequate oxygen delivery to tissues as a result of hypovolemia, decreased oxygen content or impaired myocardial function (absolute hypoxia) is the most common cause of hyperlactatemia, hypermetabolic states or impaired oxygen utilization as a result of mitochondrial dysfunction (relative hypoxia) can also increase blood lactate concentration. Less commonly, increased lactate may result from impaired clearance because of hepatic dysfunction, thiamine deficiency, or increased catecholamine production.[20] Normal blood lactate concentrations in resting adult horses are less than 2 mmol/L; concentrations higher than this in the adult are an indication of inadequate oxygen delivery. Neonates have higher blood lactate concentrations that decrease to adult values by 24 hours of age.[21] Serial measurement of lactate is a useful tool to monitor the adequacy of fluid therapy (see Chapter 1).

Nontraditional Approach to Acid–Base Evaluation

In the traditional approach, the relationship between PCO_2, HCO_3^-, and pH is explained by the Henderson-Hasselbalch equation and appears to stand alone as an explanation for acid–base derangements. This is still the approach most commonly used by clinicians, and it serves to initiate and target therapeutic intervention. However, what this approach fails to do is provide explanations for the influence of other electrolytes, weak acids, and plasma protein on acid–base balance.

The nontraditional approach (or Stewart's approach) to acid–base balance is based on three physical laws: maintenance of electroneutrality, satisfaction of dissociation equilibrium for solutes that are incompletely dissociated, and conservation of mass. In this approach, independent variables are variables that can be changed externally; dependent variables are ones that change only when a change in independent variables occurs. Independent variables include the strong ion difference (SID), PCO_2, and the total concentration of weak acids, or A_{tot}. The SID is the difference between the concentration of strong cations and the concentration of strong anions. The most important cation is sodium; chloride and other unmeasured anions make up the strong anions. Because many strong anions are not routinely measured, the normal strong ion difference accounts for the presence of these anions. An increase in SID indirectly indicates an accumulation of unmeasured anions. The concentration of weak acids in plasma mostly derives from protein and phosphates. Bicarbonate is a dependent variable that changes in response to a change in independent variables. Hypoproteinemia (a decrease in weak acid) results in alkalosis (an increase in HCO_3^-); conversely, an increase in phosphates, as may occur in acute renal failure, causes an acidosis.

In Stewart's approach, the primary disturbance is therefore defined as a change in one or more of the independent variables: [SID], PCO_2, or $[A_{tot}]$. To calculate the contribution of these variables to an acid–base disturbance, determination of the total concentration of nonvolatile weak acids and the effective dissociation constant for weak acids is required, which is impractical in most clinical situations. A simplified version of Stewart's approach, proposed and validated for equine plasma, allows the determination of A_{tot} and K_a and accurately predicts pH.[22]

Another approach to Stewart's concepts involves the characterization of four components of base excess: changes in free water reflected by changes in sodium, changes in chloride, changes in serum albumin concentration, and changes in unmeasured anions. This method has also been used successfully in horses to better characterize acid–base disorders.[23] The example in Table 3-4 illustrates the contributions of protein, chloride, and unmeasured anions to acid–base balance, and it shows how the traditional approach to acid–base balance can sometimes fail to recognize abnormalities when complex disorders are present.

The preceding discussion emphasizes the complexity of interactions between solutes in body fluids, and the importance of recognizing the traditional approach to acid–base interpretation. Although the traditional approach provides a working method for identification of problems, it falls short

TABLE 3-4. Example of Acid–Base Measurements in a Horse with Intestinal Strangulating Obstruction

pH	7.49
PCO_2 (mm Hg)	37
Base excess (BE) (mEq/L)	4.6
Na^+ (mEq/L)	137
Cl^- (mEq/L)	93
HCO_3^- (mEq/L)	32.7
K^+ (mEq/L)	2.7
Total protein (g/dL)	4.4
Packed cell volume (%)	58
Anion gap (mEq/L)	25
BE_{fw} (mEq/L)	0.9
BE_{Cl} (mEq/L)	9
BE_{tp} (mEq/L)	7.5
BE_{ua} (mEq/L)	−12.8

From Whitehair KJ, Haskins SC, Whitehair JG, et al: J Vet Intern Med 1995; 9:1-11.

Using the traditional approach to diagnosing acid-base disorders, the interpretation of blood gas analyses on this horse would indicate a metabolic alkalosis with no secondary or adaptive response (PCO_2 is normal). Further examination reveals hypochloremia and hypoproteinemia, which are responsible for the alkalosis (as indicated by the calculation of their respective base excesses [BE_{Cl} and BE_{tp}]). However, examination of the anion gap and calculation of the BE contributed by unmeasured anions (BE_{ua}) reveal an underlying acidosis that was masked by the hypoproteinemia and hypochloremia. Measurement of lactate would be indicated in this case to further characterize the disorder. Most likely, lactic acidosis is present as a result of poor perfusion (indicated by the marked increase in packed cell volume). BE_{fw}, BE contributed by free water.

in complex mixed acid–base disorders and does not provide a satisfactory explanation when electrolyte, colloidal, and unmeasured anion disorders coexist.

DESIGNING A FLUID THERAPY REGIMEN

Volumes of Fluid to Administer

Fluids can be administered for the purpose of maintenance or replacement. *Maintenance regimens* are often provided via the oral route in equine patients, and oral electrolyte formulations are available for this purpose (see Chapter 5). Intravenous maintenance fluids are lower in sodium and higher in calcium, potassium, and magnesium than replacement fluids. An appropriate maintenance fluid is 0.45% saline to which potassium, magnesium, and calcium were added.

More commonly, a *replacement fluid therapy regimen* is given to equine patients to replace fluids lost through dehydration and ongoing losses. When designing a replacement fluid therapy regimen, three questions must be answered:

1. What volume of fluid must be given?
2. What type of fluid will be given?
3. What will be the rate of administration?

Furthermore, the volume of fluids given must equal the *maintenance requirements* plus the volume needed to *correct hypovolemia* plus that needed to compensate for *ongoing losses*.

Maintenance

In adult horses, maintenance fluid requirements have been estimated at 60 mL/kg per day. This figure probably overestimates the actual needs of a resting, fasted animal in a normothermic environment, but it appears to be safe in most situations. In horses with renal failure, when elimination of excess fluids is difficult, monitoring of body weight and central venous pressures is indicated to help avoid fluid overload. If weight gain, edema, or increased central venous pressures are noted, the fluid rate should be decreased.

Dehydration

Dehydration is the general term used to indicate loss of total body water; *hypovolemia* is a form of dehydration resulting from loss of effective circulating volume. This distinction is important; for example, when the lack of water intake is prolonged, heart rate and parameters of perfusion remain within normal limits, as fluid shifts from the intracellular space to maintain normal circulating volume. In this case, replenishment of intracellular fluid volume should be performed relatively slowly, to allow time for fluid shifts to occur. In contrast, acute intestinal obstruction results in loss of circulating blood volume manifested by altered cardiovascular parameters such as increased heart rate, poor perfusion, and decreased pulse quality. Rapid restitution of effective circulating blood volume is important in this situation. Parameters that may be used for estimation of dehydration include serial body weights, heart rate, mucous membrane color, capillary refill time, skin elasticity (skin tenting), palpation of extremities, and urine output. Useful laboratory parameters include packed cell volume (PCV), total protein, creatinine and lactate concentrations, and urine specific gravity. Table 3-5 lists parameters useful for estimating hypovolemia (loss of effective circulating volume) in the horse.

Once an estimate of hypovolemia has been obtained, the amount of fluids to give is calculated as follows:

$$\text{Correction of hypovolemia} = \text{estimate of loss (\%)} \times \text{body weight (kg)}.$$

Ongoing Losses

Ongoing losses can sometimes be measured and recorded—for example, when nasogastric reflux is present—but usually they must be estimated. Therefore, patient monitoring is used to determine if the calculated fluid volume is meeting the ongoing losses. Monitoring, which may include serial measurements of cardiovascular parameters, PCV and total protein, lactate concentration, and blood gas analyses, is done at least twice a day when patients are on intravenous fluids, but it should be done more frequently (every 2, 4, or 6 hours) depending on the severity of cardiovascular compromise. Creatinine concentration should also be monitored at least once daily when initially elevated, to ensure adequate return to normal. Additional means of monitoring adequate fluid delivery include measurement of central venous pressure, arterial blood pressure, and urine output.

Type of Fluid

The type of fluid chosen depends on the evaluation of the chemistry profile and on the disease state. The first step is to choose a baseline fluid (saline or balanced electrolyte

TABLE 3-5. Parameters to Estimate Degree of Hypovolemia in Adult Horses

% Loss of Effective Circulating Volume	Heart Rate (bpm)	Capillary Refill Time (sec)	PCV/TP (%, g/L)	Creatinine (mg/dL)
6%	40-60	2	40/7	1.5-2
8%	61-80	3	45/7.5	2-3
10%	81-100	4	50/8	3-4
12%	>100	>4	>50/>8	>4

These parameters are useful to estimate the degree of hypovolemia in adult horses, assuming a normal packed cell volume (PCV) of 35% and total protein (TP) of 6.5 g/dL.

solution), and the second is to decide which additives to add to the baseline fluid. The choice of additives depends on the specific deficits or excesses, such as hypo- or hypernatremia, hypo- or hyperkalemia, hypo- or hypercalcemia, hypo- or hypermagnesemia, hypoglycemia, or acid–base disorders.

The two categories of crystalloids commonly used for fluid replacement are 0.09% saline and balanced electrolyte solutions (BESs). Table 3-6 lists the compositions of various commercially available fluids. In general, BESs are chosen when serum electrolytes are close to normal. The BES provides a bicarbonate precursor, which is either lactate, or acetate plus gluconate. Lactate requires hepatic metabolism for conversion to bicarbonate, whereas acetate and gluconate are metabolized by other tissues. All BESs contain some potassium. As noted in Table 3-6, calcium or magnesium is present in different types of BES. Saline (0.09%) is higher in sodium and much higher in chloride than serum concentrations and is used when [Na^+] is lower than 125 mEq/L. Saline is also used in disease processes associated with high [K^+], such as hyperkalemic periodic paralysis or renal failure, where a potassium-free solution is preferred. In cases of long-term maintenance fluid therapy (greater than 4 to 5 days), if the oral route is not available, half-strength basic fluids, to which potassium, calcium, and magnesium are added, should be considered. Long-term fluid therapy solely with a BES will result in hypernatremia, hypokalemia, hypomagnesemia, and hypocalcemia.

In horses, routine fluid replacement also includes *calcium, potassium, and magnesium supplementation,* particularly when there is no oral intake because of gastrointestinal disease. Low concentrations of serum ionized calcium (iCa) and magnesium (iMg) are more prevalent in horses with surgical gastrointestinal disease, particularly in those with small intestinal or large and small colon nonstrangulating infarction or strangulation and in horses with postoperative ileus.[24-26] Horses with enterocolitis also have low iCa and iMg and a decreased fractional clearance of calcium.[27] Total magnesium and calcium concentrations are less reliable for identification of calcium and magnesium status—it is preferable to determine ionized concentrations.[24-26] Measurement of total calcium can be misleading if total protein is low (ionized calcium may still be normal) or if the horse is alkalotic (total calcium may be normal, with a low ionized fraction). Recently, fractional excretion of magnesium has been suggested as a diagnostic tool for assessment of magnesium status in horses.[28] Based on this information, supplemental calcium and magnesium appears beneficial for fluid therapy in horses.

Administration of 50 to 100 mL of 23% calcium gluconate in every 5 L of fluid is usually sufficient to maintain normocalcemia. In the presence of severe hypocalcemia (iCa less than 4.0 mg/dL), administration of 500 mL of calcium gluconate in 5 L of BES is indicated. Hypocalcemia that is refractory to calcium therapy may indicate hypomagnesemia, and concurrent magnesium replacement is required. The maintenance requirement of magnesium in horses is estimated at 13 mg/kg per day of elemental Mg, which is provided by 31 mg/kg per day of MgO, 64 mg/kg per day of $MgCO_3$, or 93 mg/kg per day of $MgSO_4$.[29] In critically ill patients, the requirement may be increased, as indicated by the high prevalence of hypomagnesemia in hospitalized patients.[26] When considering magnesium supplementation, the concentration of elemental magnesium in the compound should be considered. Some crystalloid fluids such as Plasma-Lyte A and Normosol-R contain 3 mEq/L of elemental Mg. This amount may be insufficient to account for the increased losses in sick horses. Administration of 150 mg/kg per day of $MgSO_4$ (0.3 mL/kg of a 50% solution), equivalent to 14.5 mg/kg per day or 1.22 mEq/kg per day of elemental magnesium, administered in saline, dextrose, or polyionic fluids, would provide the daily requirement for the horse.[29]

Hypokalemia may develop because of lack of intake, diuresis, and gastrointestinal loss through diarrhea. Horses with a metabolic acidosis can become hyperkalemic, and potassium excretion can occur after correction of the acidemia. Measurement of serum potassium as an estimate of total body potassium can be misleading, because most of the potassium ion is intracellular. Routine potassium supplementation is indicated if lack of intake and fluid therapy are continued for more than 24 hours. To avoid any complication, it is recommended that animals not receive more potassium than 0.5 mEq/kg per hour. Most horses will benefit from the addition of 12 mEq of potassium chloride per liter of fluids (80 mEq per 5-L bag).

TABLE 3-6. Composition of Commonly Used Intravenous Solutions

Fluid	Na (mEq/L)	K (mEq/L)	Ca (mEq/L)	Mg (mEq/L)	Cl (mEq/L)	Buffer Source (mEq/L)	Osmolality (mOsm/L)
Plasma	132-146	2.8-5.1	9.0-13	1.8-3	99-110	(TCO_2) 20-36	285 ± 10
Lactated Ringer's	130	4	3	0	109	(lactate) 28	274
Normosol-R*	140	5	0	3	98	(acetate, gluconate) 50	295
0.9% NaCl	154	0	0	0	154		308
5% Dextrose	0	0	0	0	0		253
2.5% Dextrose in 0.45% NaCl	77	0	0	0	77		280
1.25% $NaHCO_3$	149	0	0	0	0	149	298

Adapted from Morris DD: Vet Med 34:164, 1987.

*Manufactured by Ceva Laboratories, 10560 Barkley Street, Overland Park, KS 66121.

Bicarbonate supplementation may also be required in horses with *metabolic acidosis*. Because the most common cause of nonrespiratory acidosis is lactic acidemia resulting from poor perfusion, providing fluid replacement should be the first and principal means of correcting this problem. The following are rules of thumb for bicarbonate supplementation in *acute* metabolic acidosis:

- The horse should have normal respiratory function. If it is unable to exhale the generated CO_2 because of a respiratory problem, worsening of the acidosis will result.
- The blood pH should be less than 7.2. In acute acidosis associated with dehydration, fluid replacement will result in restoration of urine output, and renal compensation will follow and usually be complete if the pH is greater than 7.2
- Half of the calculated amount should be administered rapidly, followed by the rest over 12 to 24 hours.
- IV bicarbonate should not be given with calcium-containing solutions.

In chronic metabolic acidosis, particularly when there are ongoing losses of bicarbonate (e.g., when there is diarrhea), the full calculated amount is usually required, partially because the bicarbonate loss is distributed over all fluid compartments, not just the extracellular fluid. Oral is a good means of dealing with ongoing losses in horses with diarrhea. Bicarbonate can be given orally as a powder (1 g $NaHCO_3$ = 12 mEq HCO_3^-).

Administration of *dextrose* is indicated for the treatment of *hypertonic dehydration*, for animals susceptible to or diagnosed with hyperlipemia (miniature horses and donkeys, adult horses with azotemia), and for pregnant mares as a source of energy for the fetoplacental unit.[30,31] As glucose is metabolized rapidly, administration of dextrose in water results in the administration of free water, which is useful for the correction of intracellular dehydration. As a source of energy, 5% dextrose can be administered at a rate of 1 to 2 mg/kg per minute.

Administration of *colloids* is indicated when the total protein concentration is less than 4 mg/dL, the albumin concentration is less than 2.0 mg/dL, or the colloid oncotic pressure is less than 12 mm Hg. Plasma and hetastarch are commonly used colloids in horses (see Chapter 1). Plasma administration is indicated when administration of other plasma products such as coagulation factors or antithrombin III is desired in addition to administration of colloids. The amount of plasma to be administered can be calculated as follows:

$$\text{Plasma to be administered(L)} = \frac{(TP_{des} - TP_{pt}) \times 0.5\ \text{BW (kg)}}{TP_{don}},$$

where TP_{des} is the desired protein concentration, TP_{pt} is the total protein concentration of the patient, and TP_{don} is the total protein concentration of the donor plasma. If the goal of colloid therapy is to restore oncotic pressure, then synthetic colloids can be used. Before the advent of hetastarch, dextran was commonly used, but its administration was associated with more anaphylactic reactions, and because of its lower molecular weight average, it had a shorter duration of effect.[5] Hetastarch is preferred and is used at a dosage of 10 mL/kg. Higher dosages (20 mL/kg) were associated with increased coagulation times caused by a decrease in von Willebrand factor antigen (vWf:Ag) activity and factor VIII coagulant (FVIII:C),[10] and should probably not be used in sick animals with increased susceptibility to coagulopathies. Hetastarch registers at a lower value than protein on a refractometer and can therefore decrease the value of the total protein concentration that is measured. To accurately monitor hetastarch therapy, use of a colloid osmometer is indicated.

Administration of blood or blood substitutes (see Chapter 4) is indicated when loss of oxygen-carrying capacity has occurred through red blood cell loss. Ideally, fresh whole blood collected in a plastic container (to preserve platelet function) from a donor that is negative for the red blood cell antigens A and Q and with an appropriate anticoagulant should be given. Commercially available kits (Dynavet, Veterinary Dynamics, Templeton, Calif.) consist of 2-L collection bags, collection and administration sets, and anticoagulant. Blood stored for greater than 10 days has a decreased concentration of 2,3-diphosphoglycerate, resulting in decreased oxygen release into tissues, increased red blood cell fragility, and increased potassium concentration. For prolonged storage of equine blood, the use of citrate-phosphate-dextrose with supplemental adenine has recently been recommended.[32] In cases of chronic blood loss, the amount of blood required can be calculated as follows:

$$\text{Amount required (L)} = \frac{(PCV_{des} - PCV_{pt}) \times 0.8\ \text{BW (kg)}}{PCV_{don}},$$

where PCV_{des} is the target packed cell volume, PCV_{pt} is the patient's packed cell volume, PCV_{don} is the PCV of the donor, and BW is body weight. When the blood loss is acute, the packed cell volume does not reflect the amount of blood lost for up to 24 hours. If blood loss is considered severe, 10 to 20 mL/kg of whole blood can be administered. When a large volume of anticoagulated whole blood is administered, the patient should be monitored for anaphylactic reaction and hypocalcemia.

Oxyglobin, a hemoglobin-based oxygen carrier, is a glutaraldehyde-polymerized bovine hemoglobin solution that has been administered safely to horses for restoration of oxygen-carrying capacity.[33-35] After administration, volume expansion also occurs because of the colloidal nature of the solution. In one study performed in ponies with experimentally-induced normovolemic anemia, administration of 15 mL/kg given at the rate of 10 mL/kg per hour improved hemodynamics and oxygen transport parameters without adverse renal or coagulation effects; however, one pony suffered an anaphylactoid reaction during infusion.[35] The half-life of Oxyglobin is relatively short; therefore, the patient should be monitored if the need for another transfusion may arise.[32] Expense may limit its use in adult horses.

Rate of Administration

In severe shock, a shock dose of fluids (60 to 90 mL/kg) should be given in the first hour. This can be done only with pressurized bags or a pump. In other situations, the rate of administration is calculated on the basis of 24-hour requirements and estimated as a volume per hour. It is important to keep a tally of the fluids given to ensure that the correct amount is reached.

Oral Fluids

Although the oral route of fluid administration has been neglected with the advent of commercially available intravenous fluids for horses, interest is being revived, particularly in the treatment of impaction colic. Oral fluids should be considered when the gastrointestinal tract is functional and maintenance requirements are needed—for example, in a dysphagic horse and as a principal means of treatment of impaction colic. Enteral fluid therapy may complement and even supplement intravenous fluids. Advantages of enteral fluid therapy include administration of fluid directly into the gastrointestinal tract, stimulation of colonic motility through the gastrocolic reflex, decreased expense, and decreased need for precise adjustment of fluid composition.[36] Enteral fluids may be administered by intermittent nasogastric intubation, or by placement of an indwelling feeding tube (18-French equine enteral feeding tube, Mila International, Florence, Ky.), allowing continuous fluid administration.

An isotonic electrolyte solution can be made by mixing 5.27 g of NaCl, 0.37 g of KCl, and 3.78 g of $NaHCO_3$ per liter of tap water.[36] This solution results in the following electrolyte concentrations: 135 mEq/L of Na^+, 95 mEq/L of Cl^-, 5 mEq/L of K^+, and 45 mEq/L of HCO_3^-, with a measured osmolarity of approximately 255 mOsm/L, representing a balanced, slightly hypotonic electrolyte solution compared with plasma. Plasma electrolyte concentrations remain within normal range with this solution compared with the marked hypernatremia and hyperchloremia observed when 0.9% saline is administered enterally.[37]

Although normal horses can tolerate up to 10 L hourly,[38] it is usually not possible to administer more than 5 L every 2 hours to horses with impactions, as they start to reflux when more fluid is given. Thus, intermittent intubation allows administration of approximately 60 L of fluids per day. When continuous enteral fluids are given, a greater rate of administration is tolerated, and horses can be given between 4 and 10 L/h. At the higher rate of 10 L/h, mild signs of abdominal pain were observed in normal horses,[36] and in horses with large colon impaction, a rate of 5 L/h is better tolerated. In one study, right dorsal colon ingesta hydration was significantly increased after enteral fluid therapy compared with intravenous fluid therapy combined with enteral administration of magnesium sulfate.[39]

FLUIDS USED FOR RESUSCITATION

Isotonic Crystalloids

Isotonic crystalloid fluids are administered intravenously and immediately reconstitute the circulating volume. However, because they are crystalloids, they are distributed to the entire extracellular compartment within a matter of minutes. Because the ECF compartment is approximately 3 times the volume of blood, 3 times as much isotonic crystalloid must be administered to gain the desired amount of circulating volume expansion. As an example, if blood loss is estimated at 30% of blood volume, representing 12 L for a 500-kg horse, then 36 L of a crystalloid fluid is required. An estimated shock dose for crystalloids is therefore 60 to 90 mL/kg per hour.

Hypertonic Crystalloids (7.2% NaCl)

Hypertonic crystalloid fluids (7.2% NaCl) have approximately 8 times the tonicity of plasma and ECF (composition: Na^+, 1200 mOsm/L; Cl^-, 1200 mOsm/L). Their immediate effect is to expand the vascular volume by redistribution of fluid from the interstitial and intracellular spaces. Each liter of hypertonic saline will expand blood volume by approximately 4.5 L. However, this effect is short-lived. As the electrolytes redistribute across the ECF, fluids shift back and the patient once again becomes hypovolemic. Because the principal effect of hypertonic saline is fluid redistribution, there still exists a total body deficit, which must be replaced. The duration of effect of hypertonic solutions is directly proportional to the distribution constant, which is the indexed cardiac output. In horses, the duration of effect is estimated at approximately 45 minutes. The recommended dosage is 4 mL/kg, administered as rapidly as possible. Because of its short duration of effect, hypertonic saline administration must be followed with isotonic volume replacement at shock doses (see earlier).

Colloids

Colloids are fluids that contain a molecule that can exert oncotic pressure. These molecules do redistribute to the ECF, but at a much slower rate than crystalloids, so that the duration of effect is prolonged compared with crystalloids. Hetastarch, because of its long duration of effect, is the most commonly used fluid for volume expansion in horses. Each liter of administered colloid will further expand the circulating blood volume by approximately 1 L, resulting in a total fluid expansion of 2 L. If hetastarch is used at a dosage of 10 mL/kg, the resulting increased colloid pressure will be significant for up to 120 hours in horses.[10] For shock therapy, the combination of hypertonic saline at 4 mL/kg and hetastarch at 4 mL/kg will prolong the resuscitation efforts and be more beneficial than either fluid alone.[40,41]

MATERIALS FOR FLUID ADMINISTRATION

Intravenous Catheters

Intravenous catheters are available in varying materials, construct, length, and diameter (Tables 3-7 and 3-8). In choosing a catheter, the desired fluid rate, the fluid viscosity, the length of time the catheter will remain in the vein, the severity of the systemic illness, and the size of the animal should be considered. The rate of fluid flow is proportional to the diameter of the catheter and inversely proportional to the length of the catheter and the viscosity of the fluid. Standard adult horse catheter sizes are usually 14 ga in diameter and 13 cm (5.25 inches) in length. For more rapid administration rates (shock), a 12 ga or 10 ga should be used. Plasma and blood products flow more slowly because of their increased viscosity, so if volume replacement is also needed, administration of these fluids can be combined with a balanced electrolyte solution. Teflon catheters should be changed every 3 days, whereas polyurethane catheters may remain in the vein for up to 2 weeks. Horses that are

TABLE 3-7. List of Commercially Available Catheter Materials

Material	Manufacturer	Comment
Polypropylene, polyethylene tubing	Medicut	Highly thrombogenic
Teflon	Angiocath	Less thrombogenic
Polyurethane	Mila International, Arrow Medical	Much less thrombogenic
Silastic	Centrasil	Least thrombogenic

very ill (bacteremic, septicemic, endotoxic) are more likely to encounter catheter problems and benefit from polyurethane or silicone catheters.

The catheter construction needs also to be considered (see Table 3-8). Through-the-needle catheters are most common for standard-size adult horses. An over-the-wire catheter is best for foals and miniature horses, or when the lateral thoracic vein is catheterized. Short and long extension sets are available, as well as small- and large-bore diameters. It is best to use an extension that screws into the hub of the catheter, to avoid dislodgement. In horses with low central venous pressures, disconnection of the line may result in significant aspiration of air and cardiovascular collapse. Double extensions are also available when other medications need to be administered with the fluids.

Catheter Maintenance

In adults, catheters are usually not covered with a bandage but rather are sutured in place, so that any problem is quickly identified. Bandages may need to be applied in foals if they are tampering with the catheter. A triple antibiotic ointment may be applied at the insertion site on the skin to decrease the risk of infection. Catheters should be flushed with heparinized saline (10 IU/mL) four times a day if they are not used for fluid administration. When administering a medication, the injection cap should be wiped with alcohol prior to insertion of the needle. The injection cap should be changed daily. All infected catheters should be cultured for identification of the causative organism and for possible nosocomial infection.

Coil Sets and Administration Sets

Coil sets are used for in-stall fluid administration. They are essential as they allow the horse to move around, lie down, and eat without restraint. An overhead pulley system with a rotating hook prevents fluid lines from getting tangled.

Administration sets are used for short-term fluid or drug administration and are available at 10 drops/mL and 60 drops/mL. When using a calibrated fluid pump, care should be taken to use the appropriate set calibrated for the brand of pump. Long coiled extension sets may then be used to connect fluids to the horse. Foal coil sets (18 French equine enteral feeding tube, Mila International, Florence, Ky.) are also available that deliver 15 drops/mL.

Pump Delivery

Calibrated pumps are available that allow delivery at various rates. These pumps have alarms that signal air in the line, empty fluid bags, or catheter problems. The maximal fluid rate these pumps can deliver is 999 mL/hour, which is usually not rapid enough to provide fluid replacement in adult horses, but they are useful for foals or for constant rate infusions. For large-volume fluid delivery, peristaltic pumps are available that can deliver up to 40 L/h. These must be under constant supervision when in use, as the pumps will continue to run even if fluids run out. Large-bore catheters should be used to avoid trauma from the jet effect on the endothelium of the vein.

Sites for Intravenous Catheterization in Horses

Common sites for insertion of intravenous catheters in horses include the jugular, lateral thoracic, cephalic, and saphenous veins. The lateral thoracic vein makes an acute

TABLE 3-8. Catheter Constructs Commercially Available

Type	Description	Advantage	Disadvantage
Butterfly	Needle attached to tubing	Ease of use	Laceration of vessel Vessel puncture Extravascular administration
Over-the-needle	Stylet inside catheter for venipuncture	Available in large diameter	Limited length of catheter Insertion more difficult Break at junction of catheter and hub
Through-the-needle	Short needle is inserted, catheter is threaded through needle	All lengths available	Trocar must be removed or protected
Over-the-wire	Needle serves as guide to insert wire, which serves as guide for catheter	Trocar is removed after catheter insertion Long catheters available Ensures proper catheter placement	More technical expertise required Expensive

angle as it enters the chest at the fifth intercostal space. Therefore, a short (7.5-cm) or an over-the-wire catheter is best used when catheterizing this vein. When catheters are placed in any location other than the jugular vein, more frequent flushings (every 4 hours) are required, as these catheters tend to clot more easily. Leg catheters are usually bandaged, because they are more prone to dislodgment than jugular catheters.

Oral Feeding Tubes

Oral fluid administration offers a good alternative to intravenous fluid therapy in animals that require maintenance fluids because of an inability to swallow, or in horses with impaction colic. Enteral nutrition (see Chapter 6) can also be administered for complete or partial enteral nutrition in foals and adults. Commercially available feeding tubes* for foals, weanlings, and adults enable fluid or liquid diet supplementation while allowing the horse to continue to nurse or eat.

REFERENCES

1. Sellers AF, Lowe JE, Rendano VT, et al: The reservoir function of the equine cecum and ventral large colon: Its relation to chronic non-surgical obstructive disease with colic, Cornell Vet 1982;72:233.
2. Fielding CL, Magdesian KG, Elliott DA, et al: Use of multifrequency bioelectrical impedance analysis for estimation of total body water and extracellular and intracellular fluid volumes in horses, Am J Vet Res 2004;65:320-326.
3. Fielding CL, Magdesian KG, Elliott DA, et al: Pharmacokinetics and clinical utility of sodium bromide (NaBr) as an estimator of extracellular fluid volume in horses, J Vet Intern Med 2003;17:213-217.
4. Spensley MS, Carlson GP, Harrold D: Plasma, red blood cell, total blood, and extracellular fluid volumes in healthy horse foals during growth, Am J Vet Res 1987;48:1703-1707.
5. MacKay RJ, Clark CK, Logdberg L, et al: Effect of a conjugate of polymyxin B-dextran 70 in horses with experimentally induced endotoxemia, Am J Vet Res 1999;60:68-75.
6. Persson SG, Funkquist P, Nyman G: Total blood volume in the normally performing Standardbred trotter: Age and sex variations. Zentralbl Veterinarmed A 1996;43:57-64.
7. Brownlow MA, Hutchins DR: The concept of osmolality: Its use in the evaluation of "dehydration" in the horse, Equine Vet J 1982;14:106-110.
8. Edwards D, Brownlow M, Hutchins D: Indices of renal function: Value in eight normal foals from birth to 56 days, Aust Vet J 1990;67:251-254.
9. Runk DT, Madigan JE, Rahal CJ, et al: Measurement of plasma colloid osmotic pressure in normal thoroughbred neonatal foals, J Vet Intern Med 2000;14:475-478.
10. Jones PA, Tomasic M, Gentry PA: Oncotic, hemodilutional, and hemostatic effects of isotonic saline and hydroxyethyl starch solutions in clinically normal ponies, Am J Vet Res 1997;58:541-548.
11. Rose B, Post T: The total body water and the plasma sodium concentration. In Rose B, Post T, editors: Clinical Physiology of Acid-Base and Electrolyte Disorders, ed 5, New York, 2001, McGraw-Hill.
12. Guglielminotti J, Pernet P, Maury E, et al: Osmolar gap hyponatremia in critically ill patients: Evidence for the sick cell syndrome? Crit Care Med 2002;30:1051-1055.
13. DiBartola S: Introduction to acid-base disorders In DiBartola S, editor: Fluid Therapy in Small Animal Practice, ed 2, Philadelphia, 2000, WB Saunders.
14. Gossett KA, French DD: Effect of age on anion gap in clinically normal Quarter Horses, Am J Vet Res 1983;44:1744-1745.
15. Constable PD, Hinchcliff KW, Muir WW 3rd: Comparison of anion gap and strong ion gap as predictors of unmeasured strong ion concentration in plasma and serum from horses, Am J Vet Res 1998;59:881-887.
16. Gossett KA, Cleghorn B, Adams R, et al: Contribution of whole blood L-lactate, pyruvate, D-lactate, acetoacetate, and 3-hydroxybutyrate concentrations to the plasma anion gap in horses with intestinal disorders, Am J Vet Res 1987;48:72-75.
17. Gossett KA, Cleghorn B, Martin GS, et al: Correlation between anion gap, blood L-lactate concentration and survival in horses, Equine Vet J 1987;19:29-30.
18. Bristol DG: The anion gap as a prognostic indicator in horses with abdominal pain, J Am Vet Med Assoc 1982;181:63-65.
19. Evans D, Golland L: Accuracy of Accusport for measurement of lactate concentrations in equine blood and plasma, Equine Vet J 1996;28:398-402.
20. Friedrich C: Lactic acidosis update for critical care clinicians, J Am Soc Nephrol 2001;12:S15-S19.
21. Silver M, Fowden A, Knox J: Sympathoadrenal and other responses to hypoglycemia in the young foal, J Reprod Fertil 1987; 35(Suppl):607-614.
22. Constable PD: A simplified strong ion model for acid-base equilibria: Application to horse plasma, J Appl Physiol 1997; 83:297-311.
23. Whitehair KJ, Haskins SC, Whitehair JG, et al: Clinical applications of quantitative acid-base chemistry, J Vet Intern Med 1995;9:1-11.
24. Dart A, Snyder J, Spier S, et al: Ionized concentration in horses with surgically managed gastrointestinal disease: 147 cases (1988-1990), J Am Vet Med Assoc 1992;201:1244-1248.
25. Garcia-Lopez J, Provost P, Rush JE, et al: Prevalence and prognostic importance of hypomagnesemia and hypocalcemia in horses that have colic surgery, Am J Vet Res 2001;62:7-12.
26. Johansson A, Gardner S, Jones S, et al: Hypomagnesemia in hospitalized horses, J Vet Intern Med 2003;17:860-867.
27. Toribio RE, Kohn CW, Chew DJ, et al: Comparison of serum parathyroid hormone and ionized calcium and magnesium concentrations and fractional urinary clearance of calcium and phosphorus in healthy horses and horses with enterocolitis, Am J Vet Res 2001;62:938-947.
28. Stewart AJ, Hardy J, Kohn CW, et al: Validation of diagnostic tests for determination of magnesium status in horses with reduced magnesium intake, Am J Vet Res 2004;65:422-430.
29. Stewart A: Magnesium disorders. In Reed S, Bayly W, Sellon D, editors: Equine Internal Medicine, St Louis, 2004, WB Saunders.
30. Fowden AL, Taylor PM, White KL, et al: Ontogenic and nutritionally induced changes in fetal metabolism in the horse, J Physiol 2000;528:209-219.
31. Hughes KJ, Hodgson DR, Dart AJ: Equine hyperlipaemia: A review, Aust Vet J 2004;82:136-142.
32. Mudge MC, Macdonald MH, Owens SD, et al: Comparison of 4 blood storage methods in a protocol for equine pre-operative autologous donation, Vet Surg 2004;33:475-486.
33. Perkins G, Divers T: Polymerized hemoglobin therapy in a foal with neonatal isoerythrolysis, J Vet Emerg Crit Care 2001;11:141-143.
34. Maxson AD, Giger U, Sweeney CR, et al: Use of a bovine hemoglobin preparation in the treatment of cyclic ovarian hemorrhage in a miniature horse, J Am Vet Med Assoc 1993;203:1308-1311.
35. Belgrave R: Effects of a polymerized bovine hemoglobin blood substitute administered to ponies with normovolemic anemia, J Vet Intern Med 2002;16:396-403.
36. Lopes MA, Walker BL, White NA 2nd, et al: Treatments to promote colonic hydration: enteral fluid therapy versus intravenous fluid therapy and magnesium sulphate, Equine Vet J 2002;34:505-509.

*Mila International, Florence, Ky; see www.milaint.com.

37. Lopes MA, Hepburn R, McKenzie H, et al: Enteral fluid therapy for horses, Compend Contin Educ Pract Vet 2003;25:390-397.
38. Lopes MA, Johnson S, White NA, et al: Enteral fluid therapy: Slow infusion versus boluses. In Proceedings of the 11th Annual American College of Veterinary Surgeons Veterinary Symposium, 2001.
39. Lopes MA, White NA: Hydration of colonic ingesta in fistulated horses fed hay and hay and grain. In Proceedings of the 12th Annual American College of Veterinary Surgeons Veterinary Symposium, 2002.
40. Prough DS, Whitley JM, Olympio MA, et al: Hypertonic/hyperoncotic fluid resuscitation after hemorrhagic shock in dogs, Anesth Analg 1991;73:738-744.
41. Vollmar B, Lang G, Menger MD, et al: Hypertonic hydroxyethyl starch restores hepatic microvascular perfusion in hemorrhagic shock, Am J Physiol 1994;266:H1927-1934.

CHAPTER 4

Hemostasis, Surgical Bleeding, and Transfusion

Barbara L. Dallap Schaer

PHYSIOLOGY OF HEMOSTASIS

Physiologic hemostasis is critical in preoperative, intraoperative, and postoperative surgical management. A complete understanding of the physiology of hemostasis, the ability to identify patients at risk for development of hemostatic dysfunction, and knowledge of appropriate and timely therapeutic intervention are essential for any successful surgical outcome. Hemostasis is a balancing act between the ability to rapidly form clots to prevent excessive hemorrhage (coagulation), and the necessary clot dissolution to restore nutrient blood flow to vital tissues and end organs (fibrinolysis). Trauma (surgical or other), endotoxemia, sepsis, and neoplasia are just a few of the possible inciting events that disrupt the delicate balance of physiologic hemostasis. Blood vessels, platelets, coagulation factors, anticoagulants, and fibrinolysis are the pillars of hemostasis and will be discussed individually.

Blood Vessels and the Role of the Vascular Endothelium

Intact blood vessels resist clot formation through a number of mechanisms. The vascular endothelium is responsible for maintaining a nonthrombogenic environment to provide passage for the flow of nutrient blood and the thrombogenic platelet. Vasodilation helps to resist clot or fibrin formation by promoting low-turbulence blood flow in the absence of vascular damage or injury.

The metabolic activities of the vascular endothelium play a large role in maintaining a nonthrombogenic environment. Through the action of prostacyclin synthetase within the endothelial cell, arachidonic acid is converted to prostacyclin, a potent inhibitor of platelet aggregation.[1] Thrombomodulin is also produced by the endothelial cell, which serves to inhibit thrombin and promote the activity of protein C (anticoagulant).[2] The activity of antithrombin, the most potent natural anticoagulant, is enhanced by the production of specific glycosaminoglycans produced within the endothelium.[3]

These mechanisms are kept in careful balance with the *procoagulant* properties of the vascular endothelium, which are activated when there is vascular disruption or denuding of the endothelium. The immediate response of the blood vessel to injury is vasoconstriction. This is mediated through local signaling from damaged endothelial cells, perhaps through interruption of the release of endothelial-derived relaxation factors. Prompt vasoconstriction prevents unnecessary blood loss and promotes rapid fibrin formation. Alternatively, inappropriate or excessive activation of these procoagulant properties may play a role in the hemodynamic instability and end-organ failure often observed in severe endotoxemia or sepsis.[4]

The subendothelium of the blood vessels provides the primary surface on which passing platelets and coagulation factors are activated, and it is traditionally thought to be the primary contributor of the vascular endothelium for the promotion of clot formation. A number of coagulation-promoting proteins are produced, but they are not necessarily exposed on the endothelial surface until activated by inflammatory mediators.[5] Von Willebrand factor (vWF), factor V, platelet activating factor (PAF), and tissue factor are all procoagulant proteins produced in the endothelial cell. It has been proposed that in the presence of inflammatory mediators, the endothelial cell may undergo a monocyte-like phenotype change, resulting in a reduction in the production of endothelium-derived relaxation factors and other antithrombogenic properties.[5] The effect of endotoxin on vessel dysfunction and activation of a procoagulant state has been reported (see Chapter 2).[6,7] A recent study revealed that vascular endothelial damage was the primary cause of multiorgan failure in thrombocytopenic patients, and the damage was most likely linked to the effects of specific inflammatory mediators.[8] Because of the vital role blood vessels and vascular endothelium play in the maintenance of hemostasis, therapeutics aimed at the prevention of endothelial damage in the presence of inflammatory mediators are likely to be a focus of future critical care research. Given the extreme sensitivity of the horse to endotoxin, control of vascular endothelial damage in the horse undergoing surgical treatment of gastrointestinal disease may be quite relevant.

Platelets

In many ways, platelets are the workhorse of a balanced hemostatic system. The interaction of the activated platelet with exposed subendothelium of blood vessels is the basis of primary hemostasis. Platelets also play a key role in secondary hemostasis: once activated, they undergo conformational changes exposing binding sites (platelet factor 3) for specific coagulation factors. Additionally, even though platelets have a relatively simple anuclear structure, they release ADP and a number of regulatory proteins from complex storage granules that are critical in initiating fibrin formation.

Platelet Physiology and Anatomy

Platelets originate from a process of megakaryocytopoiesis, which produces a membrane-encased cytoplasmic fragment of the original megakaryocyte. Megakaryocytes originate primarily in bone marrow. The specific signals responsible for the upregulation of platelet production are not entirely defined, but it is likely that specific hematopoietic growth factors are necessary for platelet growth and development.[9] These anucleate, disc-shaped cells do not have the ability to synthesize proteins, but they are capable of specific metabolic activities such as arachidonate and phospholipid metabolism.[1] The human platelet is approximately 2 to 3 μm in its unactivated state, but its complex cytoskeleton infrastructure and associated microtubules allow it to change shape dramatically once activated, exposing critical binding sites for coagulation factors and cofactors. The platelet plasma membrane is also quite sophisticated, consisting of an open canalicular system that facilitates secretion of essential platelet products.

Dense granules, α-granules, and lysosomes store the majority of platelet proteins needed for the initiation of coagulation. Dense granules store calcium, a common cofactor in platelet–phospholipid interactions, as well as ADP, ATP, and serotonin. Thrombin is the strongest stimulant for the release of the contents of the dense granules, but other agonists for release have also been reported. The α-granules are the largest and most prevalent storage granule, comprising the majority of the storage capacity of the platelet. They contain a number of proteins involved in platelet aggregation and cohesion, including fibrinogen, fibronectin, vWF, platelet-derived growth factor (PDGF), and platelet factor 4. Platelet lysosomes contain predominantly acid hydrolases, responsible for degradation of unwanted cellular debris after complete activation of fibrin formation.

Role of the Platelet in Hemostasis and Clot Formation

The platelet is the initial responder to vascular damage and subsequent endothelial exposure. Platelets rush to cover denuded endothelium, rapidly changing shape and providing an effective monolayer in what is known as the *adhesion* phase. This results in a primary platelet plug (primary hemostasis) that is responsible for preventing leakage of blood from the minute vessel defects that occur daily. If blood flow in this area remains nonturbulent, further platelet aggregation does not occur, and the monolayer generally suffices to plug the small defects or the area of vascular attenuation.[9]

With large vessel disruption, blood flow becomes quite turbulent, resulting in large platelet aggregates coating the exposed endothelium. With the conversion of membrane-derived arachidonic acid to thromboxane A_2, activated platelets release significant amounts of ADP.[10] As an increasing number of platelets adhere and undergo conformational change, ADP levels in the local area increase *(release reaction)*, strongly stimulating further platelet *aggregation*. Other agonists such as thrombin and epinephrine can also stimulate platelet aggregation. Prostacyclin, produced by neighboring healthy endothelial cells, prevents unwanted expansion of platelet aggregates by decreasing further ADP release. Platelet aggregation results in exposure of platelet factor 3, a platelet phospholipid, which serves as a congregation site for the coagulation factors.

The end result of coagulation-factor binding is the production of fibrin, which ultimately stabilizes the platelet plug (secondary hemostasis). In addition to platelet factor 3, platelets express receptors for factors Xa and Va, and for calcium, which is responsible for the conversion of prothrombin to thrombin. Platelets also contain many membrane glycoproteins (GPs) including GP IIb-IIIa, which is a receptor for vWF, and $\alpha_{IIb}\beta_3$, a fibrinogen receptor important for proper platelet aggregation. Manipulation of the glycoprotein receptors has become a focus of much research in an attempt to control the contribution of the platelet in thrombogenic disease processes. Platelets also play a critical role in the activation of the intrinsic coagulation pathway by providing binding sites for factors XIIa and XIa.

Platelets have critical roles in both primary and secondary hemostasis through the processes of *adhesion*, *release reaction*, *aggregation*, and *activation of coagulation*. As mentioned before, platelets have the ability to rapidly change shape and produce metabolic bursts that are responsible for the modulation of coagulation. From preventing leakage from minute vessel defects to initiation of thrombus formation, an appropriate number of properly functioning platelets is essential to the regulation of hemostasis.

Coagulation Factors

Coagulation factors are predominantly serine proteases (except factor XIII) that circulate in an inactive form throughout blood plasma. All coagulation factors, except for factor VIII, are produced in the liver. Factor VIII is produced by megakaryocytes. Activation of each coagulation factor is achieved through cleavage of a portion of the serine protease to reveal an active serine site. This results in the formation of macromolecular aggregates, the net result of which is fibrin formation. In physiologic activation of coagulation, the fibrin is cross-linked by factor XIII, resulting in stable clot formation at the site of a wound or an area of vascular injury. Properly coordinated fibrinolysis is responsible for clot removal and restoration of nutrient blood flow. The following discussion focuses on the characteristics of specific coagulation factors and the traditionally proposed pathways of the coagulation cascade.

It is useful to consider the coagulation factors as members of groups of proteins that share common characteristics or play a role in specific portions of clot formation.[11] Most veterinarians are familiar with the vitamin K–dependent serine proteases, factors II, VII, IX, and X.[12] Proteins C and

S, two anticoagulants, are also vitamin K dependent.[10] All of these factors together are referred to as the *prothrombin complex*. Vitamin K is necessary for the carboxylation of glutamic acid, present on the serine protease, to λ-carboxyglutamic acid. This results in a double negative charge on the surface of the serine protease. This double negative charge facilitates an electrostatic bond with calcium (Ca^{2+}), which is essential for the binding of these molecules to platelet phospholipids.[13]

A second family of proteins characteristically act as substrates for thrombin, or are principally involved in the final phase of clot formation. These are factors I (fibrinogen), V, VIII, and XIII. Activated factors V and VIII serve as cofactors for factors X and IX, respectively, and are essential in the amplification and acceleration of the coagulation cascade. Factor XIII, known as the fibrin-stabilizing factor,[10,11] is responsible for cross-linking fibrin monomer strands and facilitating clot contraction. It is important to note that factors V, VIII, and XIII are extremely labile and are therefore commonly not present (or are present at very low levels) in stored blood products.

The remaining group of coagulation factors are those traditionally involved in the *contact pathway* of coagulation activation. This group consists of high-molecular-weight kininogen (HMWK), prekallikrein, and kallikrein, as well as factors XII and XI.[14] Factor XII is a circulating single-chain glycoprotein that becomes activated through contact with collagen or a negatively charged surface. The activation of factor XII initiates the *intrinsic pathway* of coagulation. Prekallikrein is activated to kallikrein by activated factor XII. Kallikrein can have a significant amplification effect, activating factor XII as well as cleaving HMWK. These proteins form a complex that activates factor XI in the presence of calcium, ensuring continuation of the propagation of the intrinsic pathway. The complex may also be responsible for cross-activation of factor VII in the extrinsic pathway.

Intrinsic Pathway

As mentioned earlier, the intrinsic pathway is initiated by the activation of factor XII and subsequently factor XI through the exposure of blood to a negatively charged surface. Contact proteins such as HMWK and prekallikrein may also be involved in the amplification of the intrinsic pathway through activation of factors XII and XI, by appropriately positioning HMWK, prekallikrein, and factor XI close to surface-bound factor XII.[10] Factor XIa (activated factor XI) in turn activates factor IX in the presence of calcium, presumably in the presence of the activated platelet membrane. Factor VIII, produced by megakaryocytes, becomes bound to vWF, but it circulates in an inactive complex VIIIa:vWF. Cleavage of this complex by thrombin results in the procoagulant activity of factor VIIIa. Factor IXa then binds to procoagulant VIIIa, in the presence of calcium. It is this complex that activates the common coagulation pathway, marked by the activation of factor X (Fig. 4-1).

Common Pathway

The common pathway is initiated by the activation of factor X, which, in the presence of factor Va, calcium, and a platelet phospholipid, converts prothrombin (factor II) to thrombin

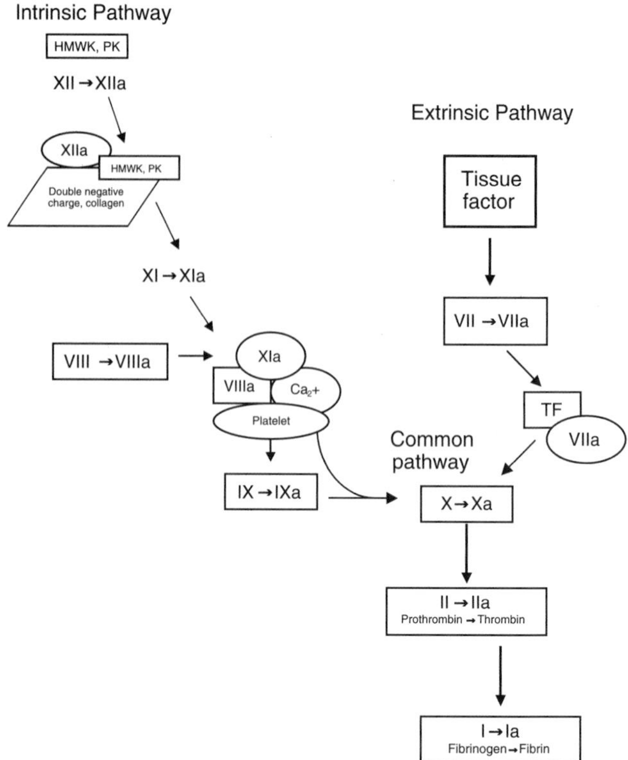

Figure 4-1. Coagulation cascade: intrinsic, extrinsic, and common pathways.

(IIa). In the final step of clot formation, factor IIa converts fibrinogen to fibrin. As mentioned earlier, factor XIII stabilizes the fibrin clot by cross-linking strands of fibrin monomer in the presence of calcium. Thrombin is capable of greatly amplifying the coagulation cascade by activating factors V, VII, and XIII, as well as by stimulating platelet activation.[11]

Extrinsic Pathway

The extrinsic pathway is initiated by the activation of factor VII by tissue factor (TF). TF is present in vascular endothelium and a number of tissues, and it was initially thought to be exposed only secondary to damage or trauma. This explains the early hypotheses that the extrinsic pathway was less significant in physiologic hemostasis, as well as in the development of many types of hemostatic dysfunction. The role of TF was redefined after it was discovered that it commonly activates factor VII in the presence of endotoxin, trauma, and inflammatory mediators.[15] It has been shown that TF levels are increased in disease states such as sepsis, diabetes, and atherosclerosis.[16-18] Studies have shown that inhibition of TF in models of sepsis may improve the outcome and attenuate coagulopathies.[19,20] It was recently demonstrated that protease-activated receptors (PARs) are the mediator between TF, factor VIIa, factor Xa complex, and the proinflammatory, procoagulant effects observed in endotoxemia.[21] The results of this research have placed what is now commonly termed the tissue factor pathway (TFP) into a very prominent position in the study of hemostatic dysfunction in a number of disease processes. In fact, this pathway is now also considered most important as the primary cellular initiation of coagulation.[22]

Fibrinolysis

Simultaneous activation of the fibrinolytic system occurs with activation of coagulation. This is the primary mechanism of clot dissolution and is responsible for prevention of excessive fibrin deposition and restoration of nutrient blood flow to affected tissues. Fibrinolysis, in conjunction with prostacyclin released by surrounding healthy endothelial cells, inhibits unwanted expansion of the fibrin clot.

Plasminogen, an inactive zymogen produced primarily in the kidney and liver, is the principal component of the fibrinolytic system. Plasminogen activators such as tissue plasminogen activator (tPA) and urokinase plasminogen activator (uPA) convert plasminogen to plasmin. Plasmin degrades fibrinogen and fibrin into soluble fibrin(ogen) degradation products (FDPs).[24] The activation of the intrinsic pathway also activates plasminogen conversion to plasmin, through the action of kallikrein. Plasmin also serves to inactivate other members of the coagulation cascade, such as factors V and VIII, and actively degrades prekallikrein and HMWK. Through these mechanisms, plasmin serves not only to degrade fibrin(ogen) but also to downregulate the intrinsic pathway.

The products of fibrinogen or fibrin degradation are the FDPs designated fragment X, fragment Y, and fragments D and E.[11] Fragments D and E have the ability to inhibit platelet aggregation and fibrin formation. Accumulation of these fragments in the blood represents an overwhelming of the mononuclear phagocytic system of the liver, the usual route by which these fragments are removed, either through increased fibrin production (and degradation) or liver dysfunction. Plasmin degradation of fibrin results in the formation of a neoantigen on the D fragment, which subsequently cross-links and is present in the circulation as a dimer (D-dimer). During the maintenance of physiologic hemostasis, a critical balance between fibrin formation and degradation exists. Proper functioning of the fibrinolytic system controls unwanted clot expansion, prevents premature fibrin lysis, and provides appropriately timed restoration of nutrient blood flow to tissues. Increased levels of FDPs, D-dimers, or soluble fibrin monomer in the circulation lead to increased fibrinolysis. This can be interpreted either as being the result of a thrombogenic disease process, or as the patient being in a hypercoagulable state.

Inhibitors of Coagulation and Fibrinolysis

Inhibitors of Coagulation

Inhibitors of coagulation are composed of a family of proteins that enzymatically bind with coagulation factors to form inactive complexes. In some instances, coagulation cofactors or surface receptors are destroyed to downregulate clot formation. The principal inhibitors of coagulation are antithrombin, heparin, protein C, protein S, and tissue factor pathway inhibitor (TFPI).

Antithrombin (AT) is responsible for 70% to 80% of thrombin inhibition in the coagulation system.[10,24] It is the key player in a family of serine protease inhibitors responsible for modulation of clot formation. Antithrombin is a glycoprotein produced in the liver and in endothelial cells that binds aggressively to thrombin through an arginine–serine interaction.[25] A stable thrombin–antithrombin (TAT) complex is the result of this reaction. The cofactor heparin alters the arginine site of AT and dramatically increases its ability to interact with thrombin. AT is also capable of neutralizing other serine proteases, such as factors XIIa, XIa, Xa, and IXa. The AT–heparin complex also slowly inactivates factor VII.[24] The horse appears to have higher concentrations of AT than some other species, such as dogs and humans.[26] Currently, AT is commonly measured in horses suspected of having hemostatic dysfunction. AT loss may occur through consumption via increased thrombin formation, through protein loss, such as nephropathies or enteropathies, or via failure of adequate production.

Heparin is a highly sulfated glycosaminoglycan, ranging in molecular weight from 3 to 30 kDa.[27] It is produced primarily in mast cells located in the lung, liver, kidney, heart, and gastrointestinal tract.[26] In terms of physiologic anticoagulation, heparin's most significant role is its ability to convert the interaction between antithrombin and thrombin from a slow reaction to a very rapid one. Its presence in an area of coagulation activation decreases thrombin-generated fibrin formation significantly. Heparin also releases TFPI from endothelial cells, thereby liberating one of the most effective inhibitors of the factor VIIa-TF complex.[26,27] An additional proposed mechanism of heparin's action may be the synergistic action of protein C, resulting in decreased production of thrombin through inhibition of thrombinase. The hemostatic relationship between vWF and the platelet is also affected by the presence of heparin, resulting in an additional antithrombogenic property. As a result of its many potential effects on coagulation, exogenous heparin administration has been a highly debated topic in the treatment of human and animal coagulopathies. Alterations of its chemical composition to enhance specific anticoagulant properties have been explored, resulting in the marketing of high- and low-molecular-weight heparins.[27]

The thrombomodulin–protein C–protein S pathway has received a lot of attention in recent years. Protein C is a vitamin K–dependent zymogen with primary inhibitory action on factors Va and VIIIa.[10,26] For inhibition to occur, the reaction must take place in the presence of calcium, protein S, and phospholipid. Because these tend to be rate-limiting steps in clot formation, the end result of protein C is to limit thrombus size. In yet another negative-feedback mechanism, thrombin, in the presence of the endothelial cell cofactor thrombomodulin, is responsible for protein C activation.[25] Deficits in this system may lead to hypercoagulability; for example, downregulation of the protein C pathway has been demonstrated in sepsis and the systemic inflammatory response syndrome (SIRS: see later and Chapter 2).

Tissue factor pathway inhibitor is a group of lipoprotein-bound proteins present in platelets and endothelial cells. As mentioned earlier, heparin enhances the release of TFPI into the circulation. In the presence of calcium, TFPI inhibits the factor VIIa-TF activation of factor X, thereby dramatically decreasing the primary cellular initiator of coagulation. Further exploration of TFPI and its activity in veterinary critical care patients is warranted.

Inhibitors of Fibrinolysis

Plasminogen activator inhibitor (PAI) is the principal regulator of plasminogen, through inhibitory effects on tPA.[28] PAI is present in endothelial cells and is stored in α-granules of platelets.[29] The main physiologic inhibitor of plasmin is α-2-antiplasmin, through an almost instantaneous interaction.[10] An alternative inhibitor of plasmin, α-2-macroglobulin, may inhibit plasmin in a limited fashion, particularly if α-2-antiplasmin is overwhelmed. Prevention of premature fibrinolysis and clot dissolution is mediated principally through these inhibitors of plasminogen and plasmin.

HEMOSTATIC DYSFUNCTION

Hemostatic dysfunction is a clinicopathologic syndrome resulting from a multitude of underlying causes that clinically manifests as hypercoagulability, subclinical disseminated intravascular coagulopathy (DIC), or clinical DIC. There has always been a struggle to define the various stages of hemostatic dysfunction; specific definitions of DIC vary from report to report. Scoring systems for DIC have been proposed[30,31] but have not gained widespread use, and they would have to be modified for use in veterinary medicine.

It is perhaps best to consider hemostatic dysfunction as a progressive failure of various arms of the hemostatic system. Clinical (or overt, noncompensated or fulminant) DIC may start as multiple microvascular or large-vessel thromboses, possibly a result of hypercoagulability and decreased fibrinolytic activity, which progress to body cavity hemorrhage and complete failure of primary and/or secondary hemostasis. To help distinguish these phases of dysfunction, hypercoagulability is now commonly described as a specific clinical entity, and a distinction exists between subclinical DIC (compensated, non-overt) and clinical DIC (overt, noncompensated).[32] (On the other hand, hypocoagulability is often *not* described as a specific clinical entity but is instead a feature of progression into stages of pathologic coagulopathy.)

Clearer definitions of the phases of hemostatic dysfunction have led to attempts to identify DIC in its earlier stages in hopes that prompt intervention will improve the outcome.[33] That hemostatic dysfunction increases morbidity and mortality in critically ill human and animal patients is well established, but the exact mechanism of what specifically occurs on a microvascular level is still debated. Most investigators now agree that hemostatic dysfunction and its subsequent clinical syndromes are a component of SIRS, and that ensuing organ failure is the most common cause of death in affected patients.[34] For equine veterinarians struggling with patients that are extremely endotoxin sensitive, the challenges continue to be early detection of patients at risk and the search for effective anticoagulant or component therapy to restore physiologic anticoagulant pathways.

Hypercoagulability

Hypercoagulability, commonly defined as thrombosis formation in inappropriate locations, can be primary or secondary.[35] In humans, the primary causes of hypercoagulability often include specific deficits in anticoagulants, such as antithrombin, protein C, and protein S, or dysfunction of the fibrinolytic system.[35,36] Primary causes of hypercoagulability in veterinary patients are certainly not prevalent in the literature. Secondary causes of hypercoagulability in human patients include diseases or conditions such as malignancy, pregnancy, nephrotic syndrome, platelet abnormalities, or abnormalities of blood vessels and rheology.[37] Again, these secondary causes of hypercoagulability are not commonly reported in veterinary patients. Typically, hypercoagulability observed by veterinarians relates to an early procoagulant phase of hemostatic dysfunction, which may or may not progress to DIC. In this sense, the recognition of hypercoagulability is critical in the prevention of significant thrombotic disease, or in the development of organ dysfunction.

Hypercoagulability is a response to inflammation initiated by a primary disease process (Fig. 4-2). An endotoxin challenge increases cytokines such as interleukin-6 and interleukin-8, which may be responsible for the initiation of a procoagulant state through the activation of the tissue factor pathway.[38] The activation of the hypercoagulable state can be triggered by endothelial damage or TF activation, and, depending on the cross-reactivity of activated serine proteases, inhibition of the fibrinolytic system may occur simultaneously. Although there is not a readily agreed-on set of tests for the diagnosis of hypercoagulability, alterations in certain parameters may identify hypercoagulation as a component of early DIC. In a study evaluating hemostatic markers prior to the onset of DIC, increases in soluble fibrin monomer, D-dimer, and thrombin–antithrombin (TAT) were useful indicators of the onset of coagulopathy,[39] and their presence seemed to indicate an ongoing increase in clot formation. Viscoelastic measures of clot formation, such as thromboelastography (TEG) or the Sonoclot Platelet Function Analyzer (Sonoclot Coagulation and Platelet Function Analyzer, Sienco, Wheat Ridge, Colo.) could be used clinically for early identification of a hypercoagulable state. Otto and colleagues successfully used TEG to demonstrate hypercoagulability in dogs with parvoviral enteritis.[40] Trials using viscoelastic techniques are ongoing in both small- and large-animal applications for identification of hypercoagulability and earlier recognition of hemostatic dysfunction.

Disseminated Intravascular Coagulation: Identification of Patients at Risk

Hemostatic dysfunction may progress to DIC in the equine patient as a result of severe endotoxemia, neoplasia, sepsis, acute trauma or hemorrhage, or possibly the syndrome of hypoxia-ischemia encephalopathy observed in neonates. Reports of DIC in the equine veterinary literature most commonly describe the process as occurring secondary to a primary gastrointestinal disorder.[41] As mentioned earlier, the definition of DIC varies significantly in the human critical care literature. Most reports in the veterinary literature describe clinical DIC, in which the horse had overt clinical signs, or subclinical DIC, in conjunction with an abnormal coagulation profile but lacking signs of a thrombohemorrhagic crisis.

Reports of horses with clinically overt DIC describe the process as occurring secondary to neoplasia, sepsis, or severe

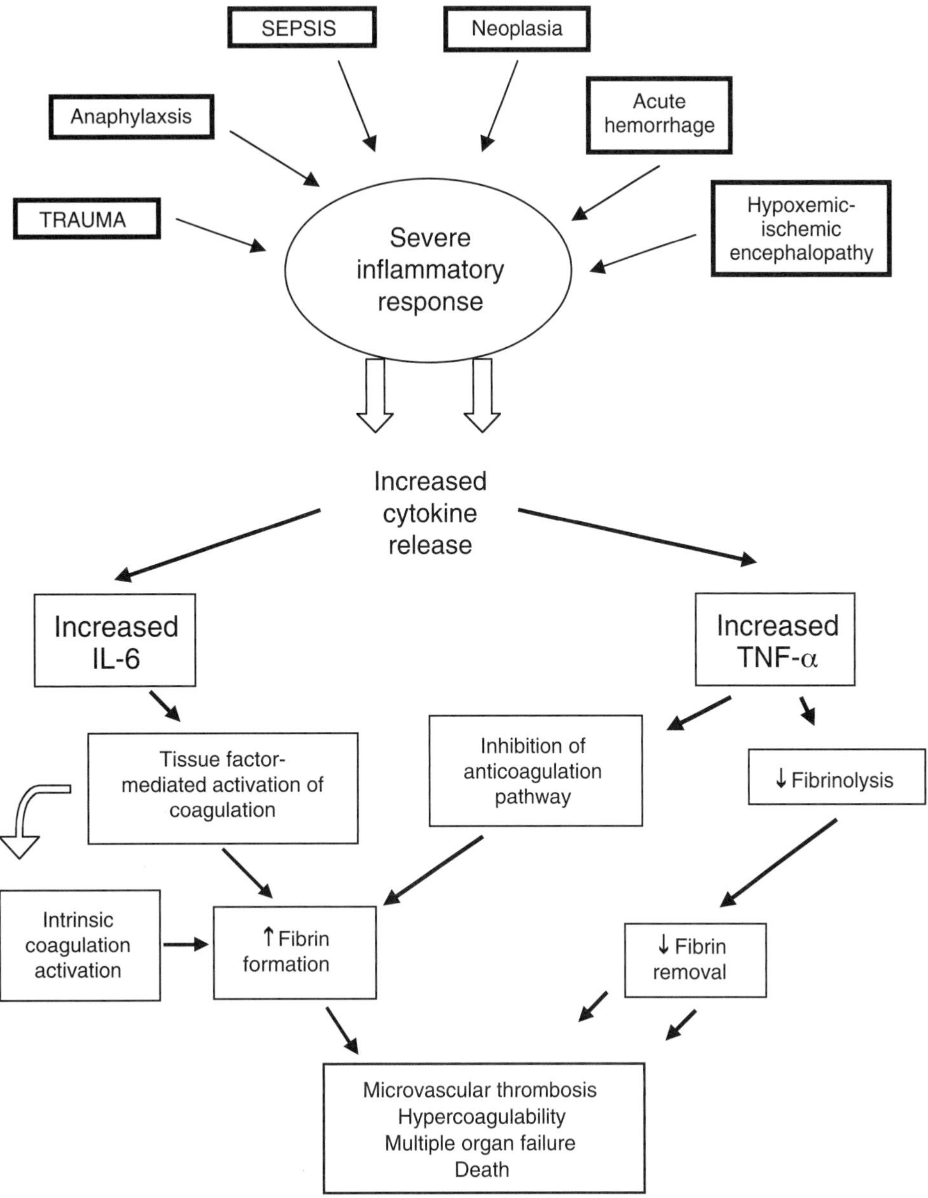

Figure 4-2. Relationships between inciting inflammatory events and the development of systemic inflammatory reaction syndrome (SIRS), hypercoagulability, multiple organ failure, and death.

gastrointestinal disease. Clinical signs in these patients included excessive hemorrhage during surgery, bleeding from venipuncture sites, venous thrombosis, and petechiae. Survival rates for horses with clinical DIC secondary to gastrointestinal disorders range from 34% to 67%,[42] with outcomes worse for horses with severe ischemic bowel disease. There appears to be an association between the development of a coagulopathy and a devitalized small intestine in the horse.[42-44] Large-colon torsion has also been associated with hemostatic dysfunction and poor outcome.[45]

A larger prospective study (*N* = 233) evaluated eight parameters of hemostasis.[46] Parameters associated with increased coagulation and fibrinolysis were observed (decreased AT, protein C, and plasminogen; increased prothrombin time (PT), activated partial thromboplastin time (PTT), and fibrin degradation products). Because this study was designed prospectively, all initial hemostatic parameters were observed to be abnormal in patients that had *not* received a clinical diagnosis of DIC. Failure of parameters to return to normal was associated with the development of overt DIC. This study demonstrated early evidence of subclinical DIC in horses with gastrointestinal disease, suggesting coagulation testing should be performed in these at-risk patients.

Documentation of subclinical DIC in horses with colitis has been reported.[47,48] Approximately one third of horses with colitis presenting to a veterinary teaching hospital were diagnosed with subclinical DIC. Horses were eight times more likely to die if identified as having subclinical DIC. In one study, 70% of horses with surgical treatment of large-colon volvulus had subclinical DIC.[45,49] None of the horses had a coagulation profile ordered as part of perioperative management. Horses were more likely (odds ratio, 47:1) to be euthanized if four to six hemostatic parameters were abnormal in the postoperative period.

Young foals (less than 1 week of age) have also been reported to have alterations in hemostatic indices.[50] Foals with presumed septicemia are even more likely to develop a coagulopathy.[51] In our hospital, foals with severe hypoxic-ischemic encephalopathy undergoing a systemic inflammatory response have had abnormal hemostatic parameters.

The surgeon needs to be aware that very young or sick neonates, and horses with neoplasia, sepsis, or severe gastrointestinal disease, are at risk for development of DIC. Perhaps more critically, many at-risk patients develop *subclinical* DIC, the presence of which may not be obvious but could definitely affect surgical outcome. Identification of subclinical DIC through perioperative coagulation testing in patients at risk could allow appropriate surgical planning and postoperative management.

Coagulation Testing

A standard coagulation profile in our hospital consists of platelet count, PT, PTT, AT, FDPs, and fibrinogen. However, coagulation profiles vary from hospital to hospital, as do normal values established by each laboratory.

Platelet Count

Horses tend to have lower platelet counts than other species, typically in the 150,000 to 250,000/μL range. A platelet count of less than 100,000/μL is considered abnormal. In the literature on humans, thrombocytopenia is a consistent feature of acute coagulopathy, but it may not be present in chronic or compensated DIC. Thrombocytopenia was reported in ponies in a model of severe intestinal strangulation,[43] and it was also a feature of almost half of horses with colitis that developed subclinical DIC.[47] In horses surgically treated for large-colon volvulus, development of thrombocytopenia was significantly associated with poor outcome.[45]

Given the integral role of the platelet in hemostasis, it is understandable that severe thrombocytopenia has an effect on a number of different portions of the coagulation cascade. Not only should a patient have adequate platelet numbers but proper function of the platelets is also critical. Viscoelastic analyzers of clot formation may provide more sensitive information about platelet function, although studies are needed to further evaluate these methods in the equine patient. Petechiae or hemorrhagic oozing of mucosal surfaces are clinical signs of thrombocytopenia.

Prothrombin Time

Prothrombin time is used to evaluate the extrinsic and common pathways of the coagulation cascade. Typically, an increase in time by 20% indicates an abnormal test result. In DIC in humans, PT may not be a particularly useful indicator,[52] perhaps because of a lack of sensitivity when there is significant clinical decline, or perhaps because more sophisticated molecular markers, not commonly available in the veterinary clinical setting, are relied on. In human patients, PT becomes prolonged when fibrinogen is less than 100 mg/dL, prothrombin is less than 30% of its normal plasma concentration, or factors VII, V, and X are decreased to 50% of their normal concentrations.[53]

Prolonged PT was observed only in a portion of horses presenting for colic, but it appeared to be a good predictor of outcome.[42,43] Prolongation of PT was associated with horses that had strangulating gastrointestinal lesions in another study.[46] In horses with surgical treatment of large-colon volvulus, prolonged PT was associated with poor outcome.[45]

Activated Partial Prothrombin Time

A prolonged PTT indicates dysfunction of the intrinsic coagulation pathway. An increase in time by 20% is usually considered abnormal, as seen with PT. PTT is not a particularly useful indicator of DIC in human patients, and it often becomes abnormal when factor VIII or IX is decreased by at least 20%. PT and PTT are also prolonged in people with a fibrinogen level of less than 100 mg/dL,[52] but this would be an uncommon cause of prolongation in the equine patient.

In reports of hemostatic analysis of horses with colic, PTT prolongation was one of the most common findings,[42,44,46] but it was not predictive of patient outcome. Similarly, horses with colitis that developed subclinical DIC often had prolonged PTT, but there was no association with patient outcome.[47]

Both PT and PTT serve as parameters to evaluate the coagulation cascade portion of the hemostatic system. Although PT and PTT are certainly useful indications of significant problems with the coagulation cascade, they may not be sensitive enough to adequately identify early stages of hypercoagulability or DIC. Prolonged PT or PTT may be associated with body cavity bleeding, significant hematuria, or hematochezia. Perhaps wider availability of more specific molecular markers of coagulation will provide the veterinary clinician with earlier clinical data for the diagnosis of hemostatic dysfunction.

Antithrombin

As discussed earlier, AT is one of the most significant and effective serine protease inhibitors in the anticoagulative armamentarium. Much attention has been given to measuring levels (reported as percentage activity) of AT in the human critical care literature, and a poor outcome is expected when AT drops to 60% to 70%. In human cases of DIC or sepsis, AT drops as a result of consumption, or because of destruction by elastase produced by activated neutrophils.[54] Other possible causes for decreased AT activity are protein loss (enteropathy or nephrotic syndrome) and failure of production. AT activity appears to be a more sensitive indicator of an ongoing coagulopathic problem, and many animal studies have reported improvement with the administration of AT concentrate in models of endotoxemia and sepsis.

In the equine patient with acute gastrointestinal disease, AT has been shown to be a useful predictor of outcome.[44,46]

In one study of horses with large-colon torsion, the patients had a significant decrease in AT, and failure for AT to return to normal activity was associated with nonsurvival.[55] AT was significantly greater in the peritoneal fluid of nonsurvivors presenting with acute gastrointestinal disease,[48] indicating a dramatic AT response to intraperitoneal inflammation and a possible decrease in systemic AT circulation. Horses with colitis developed AT deficiency approximately 48 hours after admission, in association with hypoproteinemia.[47] AT levels in the horse are normally greater than in some other species, and it appears that a significant decrease in AT can reliably predict hemostatic dysfunction.

Fibrin(ogen) Degradation Products

FDPs are produced by the proteolytic degradation of fibrin(ogen) by plasmin. They are routinely cleared by the mononuclear phagocytic system (MPS), and an accumulation of FDPs indicates a failure of the MPS to adequately remove them from the circulation. This can be the result of local or systemic hyperfibrinolysis, and it may be indicative of a dramatic increase in clot formation. FDP evaluation is usually performed as a semiquantitative test, resulting in the following possible ranges for FDPs: 0 to 10 μg/mL, 10 to 20 μg/mL, 20 to 40 μg/mL, or greater than 40 μg/mL. In our clinical laboratory, FDPs greater than 10 μg/mL are considered abnormal.

In reports evaluating the predictive value of hemostatic parameters in the equine patient, FDPs were often increased but poorly predictive of development of DIC or patient outcome.[42-47] It is possible that in an animal that produces rather large amounts of fibrinogen in response to inflammation, FDPs are not particularly useful indicators of development of a coagulopathy or of poor outcome.

Fibrinogen

The measurement of fibrinogen as part of a standard coagulation profile is an attempt to document hypofibrinogenemia, which is a somewhat consistent feature of overt DIC in humans. It is not unusual for human patients with significant hemostatic dysfunction to develop a fibrinogen level of less than 100 mg/dL. This does not seem to be a consistent feature of DIC in the horse, however.[42-44,46] Increased fibrinogen levels were present in the intraperitoneal fluid of horses with colic but were not associated with the presence of endotoxin.[48] In the evaluation of fibrinogen in the horse with DIC, it may be possible that the wrong question is being asked. In horses with colitis that developed subclinical DIC, hypofibrinogenemia was not a consistent finding; however, there was a difference in the fibrinogen levels between the DIC and non-DIC groups.[47] Similarly, horses surgically treated for large-colon volvulus and horses suffering from DIC associated with a poor outcome demonstrated lower fibrinogen levels than their surviving counterparts with better hemostatic function. In the horse, perhaps it is the failure of expected fibrinogen increase, rather than the development of hypofibrinogenemia, that could be significant. Further studies are needed to validate this hypothesis.

For both human and veterinary patients, the problem continues to be achieving *prompt* and accurate identification of hemostatic dysfunction early enough to intervene successfully. By the time many of the standard coagulation tests, such those discussed earlier, are significantly abnormal, the therapeutic window of opportunity has often narrowed. It is possible that additional tests of hemostatic dysfunction could provide earlier detection and subsequent intervention.

There is no one specific test that best identifies DIC in the horse. In patients at risk for development of a coagulopathy, a standard coagulation profile should be performed. The parameters that are abnormal relate to both the primary disease and the specific host response to the insult. Although variations in the coagulation profile abnormalities may exist, the profile may point to the component of hemostasis that is most affected, and this could be used to guide therapy. Increased FDPs, decreased fibrinogen, and decreased AT may indicate hypercoagulability. These three abnormal hemostatic parameters indicate subclinical DIC, and they should direct the clinician to take action. Earlier intervention, prior to the onset of clinical DIC, may improve outcome.[31]

Currently, no prospective study is available that compares treatment options for DIC and outcome. Therapy should be aimed at restoration of physiologic hemostasis. Administration of fresh frozen plasma, with or without the addition of heparin, can replace depleted coagulation factors and potentiate the action of AT. Heparin therapy alone may decrease hypercoagulability, although side effects such as thrombocytopenia and anemia are common in the horse treated with repeated doses of unfractionated heparin. Platelet-rich plasma could be used in patients with thrombocytopenia caused by consumption. Hemostatic tests available for veterinarians in a clinical setting are somewhat limited, and debates over proper therapy are common. Performing a standard coagulation profile provides the clinician with the opportunity to attempt to restore physiologic hemostasis, prepare for possible overt DIC and organ dysfunction, and inform the client about a possible poor outcome.

Additional Tests of Hemostatic Dysfunction

Measuring D-dimer is not a particularly new hemostatic test, but it is often not included in coagulation profiles performed in the equine surgical setting. D-dimer is an epitope resulting from the plasmin degradation of fibrin. It is a cross-linked dimer of the two smallest fibrin degradation products, fragment D-D. D-dimer can be measured semiquantitatively by latex agglutination, or by using a latex-enhanced turbidimetric immunoassay performed on a standard coagulation analyzer. Increased D-dimer levels indicate increased fibrinolysis or inability to clear the products from the circulation. In critically ill patients, D-dimer has been used to better characterize acute pulmonary thromboembolism, and to diagnose deep vein thrombosis.

D-dimer concentrations were evaluated in healthy dogs and dogs with DIC.[56] D-dimer was found to be a sensitive and specific test for the identification of dogs with DIC. In this study, DIC was defined as thrombocytopenia in combination with two additional abnormal hemostatic parameters and bleeding from at least two unrelated sites. D-dimer has also been reported to improve the prognostic value of clinical and laboratory data in horses with acute colic.[57] It is possible that the predictive value may be linked to the prognosis of specific types of gastrointestinal lesions. In a study evaluating D-dimer in horses surgically treated for large-colon volvulus, D-dimer was significantly increased in all patients.[45] D-dimer could not be used to distinguish survivors from nonsurvivors, nor was it useful in predicting which horses had abnormal coagulation profiles. It can be stated that D-dimer must be evaluated while considering the primary cause of the inflammatory process. If the primary lesion involves ischemic or strangulating circumstances, D-dimer may be reflective of the inciting event rather than predictive of the development of DIC or mortality.

Thrombin-antithrombin is an irreversible inactive complex between thrombin and antithrombin. TATs are rapidly taken up by a serpin-1 receptor and quickly degraded by the liver, resulting in a short half-life of 5 minutes. TAT levels can be measured using a sandwich enzyme-linked immunosorbent assay (Enzygnost, Dade-Behring, Inc., Wilmington, Del.), which has been evaluated and validated for use in the horse.[58]

TAT complexes have been measured in horses with colic[59] and reveal a significant increase in TAT in nonsurvivors. The most significant increase in TAT level between nonsurvivors and survivors was observed on the admission sample. Horses with strangulating obstructions had significantly higher TATs than horses with nonstrangulating lesions over time. In a study evaluating TAT complexes in horses with surgical treatment of large-colon volvulus, increased TATs were associated with the development of DIC and poor outcome.[45] A statistically significant difference was observed at all three time points between survivors and nonsurvivors. Although measuring TAT complexes seems quite promising for predicting both the development of DIC and poor outcome in horses with acute colic, the test (a 72-well enzyme-linked immunosorbent assay [ELISA]) currently remains difficult to use in a clinical setting. Hopefully, a snap ELISA TAT kit will be developed in the near future, increasing the applicability in the clinical situation.

Viscoelastic analyzers may hold some promise for evaluation of coagulation in the veterinary surgical patient in the future. Thromboelastography and the Sonoclot analyzer are two currently available analyzers that use viscosity and/or elasticity to evaluate clot formation in whole or citrated blood samples. Both analyzers evaluate all phases of clot formation and retraction from a single, small-volume (i.e., 330 μL) sample of blood. A tracing or signature is provided from which values can be derived to assess platelet or coagulation function. Software is provided with each analyzer, resulting in a user-friendly interface and easy storage of data.

In human surgical patients, viscoelastic analyzers are most commonly used to monitor coagulation inhibition during cardiopulmonary bypass procedures and liver transplantations, and to evaluate perioperative hemorrhage. TEG has been used to identify a hypercoagulability state in dogs with parvoviral enteritis.[40] In our clinic, we are using the Sonoclot analyzer for hemostatic evaluation of septic foals, and we are initiating a study to use the analyzer to assess coagulopathy in horses with surgical treatment of acute colic.

SURGICAL BLEEDING

An increased risk for surgical bleeding may be related to an inherited condition in the patient or to an acquired coagulopathy or thrombocytopathy, or it may be a consequence of the procedure being performed. In equine surgery, it is probably most commonly related to an acquired hemostatic dysfunction or the nature of the surgical procedure.

Predisposing Factors

Inherited conditions that result in coagulopathy or thrombocytopathy are relatively uncommon in the horse and much more common in the dog, cat, and human. These conditions include von Willebrand disease, thrombasthenia, hemophilias, and specific coagulation factor deficits. In horses, deficits of prekallikrein[60,61] and of factors VIII, IX, and XI[62] have been reported. These may be difficult to detect preoperatively; a thorough history obtained from the client or observation of clinical signs may indicate a need for specific coagulation testing. If a specific deficit is identified, adequate preparation for surgery is critical, possibly consisting of pretreatment with component therapy or anticoagulants.

Acquired conditions resulting in hemostatic dysfunction may present clinically as DIC, or perhaps as a specific coagulopathy or thrombocytopathy. Primary diseases that could result in DIC (see earlier) and that may be encountered by a surgeon include neoplasia, sepsis, trauma, severe acute hemorrhage, clostridial myositis, and severe endotoxemia associated with acute gastrointestinal disease. Hemostatic dysfunction could also be the result of inappropriate use of heparin (particularly unfractionated), aspirin, or other anticoagulants. The administration of certain drugs such as sulfonamides, penicillin, phenylbutazone, ibuprofen, estrogens, antihistamines, and cardiovascular drugs has been associated with thrombocytopenia in humans and animals. Other diseases associated with hemostatic dysfunction in the horse are severe liver disease, equine infectious anemia, *Anaplasma phagocytophila*, and equine viral arteritis. In general, if any acquired condition that could result in a coagulopathy is noted in the history or detected in the clinical progression of a surgical candidate, appropriate and complete evaluation of the hemostatic system must be performed. If the surgeon is presented with an emergent situation, arrangements should be made for the availability of a blood donor or possible component therapy to attenuate the situation.

Certain surgical procedures, particularly in large-animal surgery, are associated with a significant risk for intraoperative and postoperative hemorrhage. Surgery involving the sinuses or ethmoid area, the cranial reproductive tract, the spleen, or certain neoplasias may result in significant intraoperative hemorrhagic challenges. Because many of these surgeries can be performed electively, careful preoperative planning may alleviate many of the complications of perioperative hemorrhage. Options could include planned autologous transfusion and normovolemic or isovolemic hemodilution, preoperative crossmatch and subsequent whole blood transfusion (see later), or availability of stored blood products and components. Autologous transfusion and normovolemic hemodilution involve collection of the patient's blood in the weeks before surgery (banking) or in the immediate preoperative period, followed by administration of crystalloids prior to induction. Recombinant human factor VII has been used in human surgeries both in trauma situations to decrease life-threatening hemorrhage and as a preoperative procoagulant treatment. Throughout any surgical procedure, it is critical to employ proper hemostatic techniques.

BLOOD TRANSFUSION

The need for blood transfusion in the horse is usually a result of acute blood loss, secondary to either trauma or surgical intervention, or of severe hemolytic anemia, possibly caused by neonatal isoerythrolysis, red maple leaf toxicosis, or immune-mediated thrombocytopenia. Acute blood loss is the situation the surgeon most commonly faces.

Deciding when to transfuse is not easy, and the issue has been debated in both human and veterinary medicine. Transfusions are not without risk, and their pros and cons must be carefully considered. Guidelines regarding this decision fall roughly into three categories: physiologic indicators, indices of red cell mass, and clinical observations. Ultimately, the attending clinician decides when a transfusion is best for the patient, and the clinical situation often plays a large role in the decision. The veterinary surgeon may ask the following questions: Is the patient still bleeding? What is the duration of the blood loss? What are the wishes of the owner? What is the animal's overall prognosis with regard to the primary lesion? Are there reasonable alternatives to transfusion in this patient? Good clinical judgment is just as critical as any single measure to determine the need for perioperative transfusion.

Acute blood loss in the horse can be the result of splenic trauma, uterine artery bleeding, guttural pouch mycosis, or a surgical procedure associated with high risk for hemorrhage. In the event of acute blood loss, the goal is to maintain appropriate oxygen delivery (DO_2) to the tissues. Tissue oxygen delivery is controlled by cardiac output, which affects the volume of blood reaching the tissue, and the oxygen content of the blood reaching that tissue (Cao_2). The first challenge of acute blood loss is the decline in intravascular blood volume, which results in decreased stroke volume and subsequent decrease in cardiac output. As the body loses red cell mass, the oxygen-carrying capacity of the intravascular blood volume decreases. This means tissue oxygen delivery takes a second hit, decreased Cao_2 combined with poor perfusion. The results of inappropriate tissue oxygenation are anaerobic cellular metabolism, increased lactate production, subsequent cellular dysfunction, and probable organ dysfunction and death.

The physiologic response to acute blood loss is immediate redirection of blood flow to essential organs, such as brain, heart, kidneys, and lung (see Chapter 1). The initial drop in intravascular blood volume triggers arterial baroceptors to increase heart rate and respiratory rate, and vasoconstriction of peripheral vessels. Vasoconstriction is rather profound in splanchnic beds, which results in a significant recruitment of blood volume. In the horse, the spleen may contain up to 30% of the circulating red cell mass, and splenic contraction is triggered within minutes of an acute hemorrhagic episode. Other compensatory mechanisms include fluid shift from interstitial to intravascular spaces, a shift of the oxyhemoglobin curve to the right, increased levels of 2,3-diphosphoglycerate, antidiuretic hormone increase, and activation of the renin-angiotensin-aldosterone system.

Indications

Determining when to transfuse is difficult because tissue oxygenation cannot be easily monitored in veterinary patients. Clinicians would welcome a specific guideline that tells when to give a transfusion. However, the degree of acute anemia cannot be appropriately assessed by the PCV, hematocrit, or hemoglobin concentrations and will be normal until fluid shifts occur.[63] These hematologic values reflect only a *relative concentration* of the entire intravascular volume. A number of circumstances, such as crystalloid fluid volume resuscitation or rate of hemorrhage, could make these values difficult to interpret.

Physiologic monitoring of the human patient with acute hemorrhage often involves pulmonary artery catheter placement and measurements of systemic oxygenation saturations and oxygen extraction ratios. The oxygen extraction ratio (O_2 ER) is the ratio of oxygen uptake to oxygen delivery, and it represents the utilization of oxygen by the tissues. Normal O_2 ER is approximately 0.2 to 0.3, or 20% to 30%. As the value for O_2 ER increases, tissues extract a larger portion of the oxygen supplied by the afferent vasculature. Because mixed venous oxygen saturation returning to the pulmonary artery contributes to the systemic arterial concentration, a high O_2 ER represents a continual decline in tissue oxygenation. The O_2 ER may adjust to physiologic circumstances. In trained athletes, it may be up to four times the normal value as the metabolic demands for oxygen dramatically increase. Generally, once the O_2 ER reaches 0.5 in a patient with hemorrhage, tissue oxygenation is impaired,[63] and transfusion is indicated.

In most veterinary clinics, a pulmonary artery catheter is not an option, but O_2 ER can be estimated using pulse oximetry to determine arterial oxygen saturation (Sao_2), and a central venous pressure catheter to estimate mixed venous oxygen saturation (Svo_2), and by calculating as follows:

$$O_2\ ER = \sim Sao_2 - Svo_2$$

Using O_2 ER as an assessment of tissue oxygenation is a more accurate method than relying solely on a specific red cell index such as PCV or hemoglobin. Currently, there are no guidelines for use in the horse, but pulse oximetry and a central venous pressure catheter can be used to estimate O_2 ER. The red cell index that indicates transfusion in humans is hemoglobin below 6 or 7 g/dL, which corresponds to a hematocrit of less than 18% to 21%.[64] A number of additional patient considerations are recommended for use with that numerical cutoff, such as rate of hemorrhage, illness of patient, clinical signs, increased lactate, additional evidence of organ dysfunction, and the O_2 ER.[64]

Recommendations for transfusion in the equine patient are a PCV of less than 20% in an acute bleeding episode, or less than 12% to 14% in a situation of chronic blood loss.

However, during acute bleeding, the PCV will be normal. Therefore, clinical signs associated with acute hemorrhage that may indicate evidence of hypovolemic shock include tachycardia, tachypnea, poor pulse quality, poor perfusion to extremities, poor jugular fill, and pale mucous membranes (see Chapter 1). Indirect blood pressure measurements can be taken, but they have been inaccurate in human patients with hypovolemic shock. Direct blood pressure measurements through an arterial line may be useful in determining the need for transfusion and for measuring the response to fluid volume resuscitation, but blood pressure may remain normal as it is the last parameter to alter before death. Integrating all the available information (clinical signs, red cell indices, and physiologic parameters) is the best approach to determining the need for transfusion.

Donor Selection and Management

Unfortunately, a universal equine donor does not exist. Horses have seven blood categories: A, C, D, K, P, Q, and U, with alloantigen subdivisions. It is desirable for a blood donor to be Aa and Qa alloantigen negative, as these types are the most immunogenic of the identified red cell antigens.[65] It is also helpful if a donor is negative for Aa alloantibodies, given the prevalence of the Aa type. If the blood type is unknown, and a crossmatch is unavailable, a Standardbred or Quarter Horse gelding may be the best option for a donor, as either is less likely to have Aa and Qa alloantigens. Donors should weigh at least 450 kg and be in good health. Mares that have foaled are a poor selection as donors, because they may have developed specific blood type alloantibodies during pregnancy. The donor should be negative for transmissible bloodborne diseases, such as equine infectious anemia, and should not have received any transfusions.

In a veterinary teaching hospital or a large practice setting, blood typing of a group of available donors can be very helpful. Where available, a crossmatch providing evaluation of agglutinins and hemolysins significantly minimizes the risk of transfusion reactions. Alloantibodies in the horses often act as hemolysins. This means lysis studies using rabbit complement are very helpful in determining the compatibility of a donor.[66] The major portion of the agglutination phase of the crossmatch involves washing the donor's red blood cells with the recipient's serum. The minor portion consists of washing the recipient's red cells with the donor's serum. Optimal compatibility is determined by selecting the donor with the least reactivity in all three categories, with the minor being of the least significance.

The amount of blood being collected from the donor is determined by the needs at the time of donation and the physiologic limitations of the donor. Recommendations for volume collected from the donor vary from 16% to 30% of total blood volume, but recent studies favor 25%.[67] In a typical-size donor, 25% of blood volume usually results in about 10 L, which can reasonably provide the recipient with improved tissue oxygenation in most situations. The long- and short-term effects of collecting 25% of a horse's blood volume were recently evaluated, and it was found to be quite safe.[67] Cardiovascular and physiologic parameters were rarely outside the normal range, and they returned to precollection values within 24 to 48 hours. This volume can be safely collected from a donor every 30 days.

To determine an approximate volume of blood needed for transfusion, the following formula is often used:

$$\frac{\text{desired PCV} - \text{recipient PCV} \times (0.8 \times \text{body weight [kg]})}{\text{PCV of donor}}$$

This formula assumes that the recipient has approximately 80 mL of blood volume per kilogram of body weight (thus the 0.8 value). A higher value may be used if a larger blood volume per kilogram is suspected—for example, in a neonatal patient requiring transfusion.

Blood Collection and Administration

Blood is most effectively collected in 3-L plastic bags using an intravenous transfer set. Glass bottles are easily broken, and they may stimulate contact coagulation or platelet dysfunction during collection. The vacuum on many glass collection sets may also damage the red cells. The most commonly available anticoagulants are acid-citrate-dextrose (ACD) and citrate-phosphate-dextrose (CPD). The anticoagulant-to-blood ratio should be 1:9.

Blood is usually administered through an aseptically placed jugular catheter. A blood administration set with filter is recommended for transfusion. Whole-blood administration should be started at a slow drip, and temperature, heart rate, and respiratory rate should be monitored for 15 minutes. If no adverse reactions are observed, the transfusion can proceed at a target rate of 10 to 20 mL/kg.

Complications of Transfusion

Tachycardia, tachypnea, sweating, signs of distress or discomfort, urticaria, and sudden collapse are all signs of a transfusion reaction. If any of these signs occur, transfusion should be stopped immediately and an anti-inflammatory dose of flunixin meglumine or steroids administered. If signs of anaphylaxis are evident, 0.01 to 0.02 mL/kg of a 1:1000 concentration of epinephrine[65] should be administered.

Risks of transfusion include hemolytic reactions and hypersensitivities, acute lung injury, and immunosuppression.[64] Recent reports indicate that transfusions may result in an immunomodulatory response that could affect the surgical outcome. An increase in nosocomial infections has been observed in critically ill patients that have received transfusions.[68] In small-animal surgical patients, transfusion was identified as a risk factor in the development of aspiration pneumonia and acute respiratory distress.[68] The immunomodulatory effects of transfusion are not completely understood, but evidence exists that an impaired immune system is a possible complication.

PLASMA TRANSFUSION

Plasma is administered in the horse in hyperimmunized forms for specific diseases or endotoxemia, or for replacement of clotting factors. It is also used in cases of hypoalbuminemia, but this is not always a cost-efficient method of increasing colloid oncotic pressure in the horse. Plasma hyperimmunized against *Rhodococcus equi* and the *Escherichia coli* mutant J5 portion of endotoxin is available commercially. For the equine surgeon, the most common uses of plasma transfusion are to treat acute endotoxemia and to replace clotting factors in cases of DIC or acute hemorrhage. The dose of plasma administration in these applications is 4 to 5 mL/kg, but if restoration of physiologic anticoagulants is a goal of such an administration, hemostatic monitoring should follow plasma therapy. Administration of plasma should be through a blood administration set, and horses should be monitored for any signs of reaction, although hypersensitivity reactions to plasma are uncommon. Fresh frozen plasma may be obtained via immediate plasmapheresis from individual units of whole blood, and it can be stored for approximately 1 year if frozen properly. Fresh frozen plasma contains the most viable clotting factors, and it is the plasma product of choice when there is any coagulopathy or specific factor deficit.

Platelet-rich plasma (PRP) can be produced by centrifugation of whole blood at a rate of 250 × g,[62] or by more sophisticated methods of thrombocytapheresis available at human hospitals or blood banking facilities. PRP administration may be quite useful in cases of immune-mediated thrombocytopenia or thrombocytopathia, or in cases of dilutional coagulopathy secondary to acute hemorrhage.

REFERENCES

1. Kunicki TJ: Role of platelets in hemostasis. In Rossi EC, Sion TL, Moss GS, Gould SA, editors: Principles of Transfusion Medicine, Baltimore, 1996, Williams and Wilkins.
2. Rosenberg RD, Rosenberg JS: Natural anticoagulant mechanisms, J Clin Invest 1984;74:1-6.
3. Vasiliev JM, Gelfand IM: Mechanisms of non-adhesiveness of endothelial and epithelial surfaces, Nature 1978;274:710-711.
4. Vallet B, Wiel E: Endothelial cell dysfunction and coagulation, Crit Care Med 2001;29:S36-S41.
5. Naworth PP, Worth DM: Endothelial cells as active participants in procoagulant reactions. In Gimbrone MA, editor: Vascular Endothelium in Hemostasis and Thrombosis, Edinburgh, 1986, Churchill Livingstone.
6. Lee M, Schuessler G, Chien S: Time dependent effects of endotoxin on the ultrastructure of the aortic endothelium, Artery 1988;15:71-89.
7. Leclerc J, Pu Q, Corseaux D, et al: A single endotoxin ejection in the rabbit causes prolonged vessel dysfunction and a procoagulant state, Crit Care Med 2000;28:3672-3678.
8. Ueno H, Hirasawa H, Oda S, et al: Coagulation/fibrinolysis abnormality and vascular endothelial damage in the pathogenesis of thrombocytopenic multiple organ failure, Crit Care Med 2002;30:2242-2248.
9. Tomer A, Harker LA: Megakaryocytopoiesis and platelet kinetics. In Rossi EC, Sion TL, Moss GS, Gould SA, editors: Principles of Transfusion Medicine, Baltimore, 1996, Williams and Wilkins.
10. Morris DD: Recognition and management of disseminated intravascular coagulation in horses, Vet Clin North Am Equine Pract 1988;4:115-143.
11. Troy GC: An overview of hemostasis, Vet Clin North Am Small Anim Pract 1988;18:5-20.
12. Mosher DF: Coagulation and fibrinolysis. In MacKinney AA, editor: Pathophysiology of Blood, New York, 1984, John Wiley and Sons.
13. Stenflo JA: A new vitamin K dependent protein: Purification from bovine plasma and preliminary characterization, J Biol Chem 1976;251:355-363.
14. Roncales FJ, Sancho JM: Coagulation activators. In Feldman BF, Zinkl JG, Jain NC, editors: Schalm's Veterinary Hematology, Baltimore, 2000, Lippincott Williams and Wilkins.
15. Nemerson Y, Bach R: Tissue factor revisited, Prog Hemost Thromb 1982;6:237-261.
16. Nieuwland R, Berckmans RJ, McGregor S, et al: Cellular origin and procoagulant properties of microparticles in meningococcal sepsis, Blood 2000;95:930-935.
17. Diament M, Nieuwland R, Pablo RF, et al: Elevated numbers of tissue-factor exposing microparticles correlate with components of the metabolic syndrome in uncomplicated type 2 diabetes mellitus, Circulation 2002;106:2442-2447.
18. Bonderman D, Teml A, Jakowitsch J, et al: Coronary no-reflow is caused by shedding of active tissue factor from dissected atherosclerotic plaque, Blood 2002;99:2794-2800.
19. Dackiw AP, McGilvray ID, Woodsie M, et al: Prevention of endotoxin-induced mortality by antitissue factor immunization, Arch Surg 1996;131:1273-1279.
20. Creasey AA, Chang AC, Feigen L, et al: Tissue factor pathway inhibitor reduces mortality from *E. coli* septic shock, J Clin Invest 1993;91:2850-2856.
21. Pawlinski R, Mackman N: Tissue factor, coagulation protease, and protease-activated receptors in endotoxemia and sepsis, Crit Care Med 2004;32:S293-S297.
22. Mackman N: Role of tissue factor in hemostasis, thrombosis, and vascular development, Arterioscler Thromb Vasc Biol 2004; 24:1015-1022.
23. Darien BJ: Fibrinolytic system. In Feldman BF, Zinkl JG, Jain NC, editors: Schalm's Veterinary Hematology, Baltimore, 2000, Lippincott Williams and Wilkins.
24. Johnstone IB: Coagulation inhibitors. In Feldman BF, Zinkl JG, Jain NC, editors: Schalm's Veterinary Hematology, Baltimore, 2000, Lippincott Williams and Wilkins.
25. Rosenberg RD: The molecular basis of blood diseases. In Stamatoyannopoulos G, Nienhuis AW, Leder P, et al, editors: Regulation of the Hemostatic Mechanism, Philadelphia, 1987, WB Saunders.
26. Johnstone IB, Petersen D, Crane S: Antithrombin III (ATIII) activity in plasmas from normal and diseased horses, and in normal canine, bovine and human plasmas, Vet Clin Pathol 1987;16:14-18.
27. Hirsh J, Warkentin TE, Shaughnessy SG, et al: Heparin and low-molecular-weight heparin: mechanisms of action, pharmacokinetics, dosing, monitoring, efficacy, and safety, Chest 2001; 119:64S-94S.
28. Lawrence DA, Ginsburg D: Plasminogen activator inhibitors. In High KA, Roberts HR, editors: Molecular Basis of Thrombosis and Hemostasis, New York, 1995, Marcel Dekker.
29. Spengers ED, Kluft C: Plasminogen activator inhibitors, Blood 1987;69:381-387.
30. Bick RL: Disseminated intravascular coagulation and related syndromes: A clinical review, Semin Thromb Hemost 1988;14:299-338.
31. Wada H, Gabazza EC, Asakura H, et al: Comparison of diagnostic criteria for disseminated intravascular coagulation (DIC): Diagnostic criteria of the International Society of Thrombosis and Hemostasis and of the Japanese Ministry of Health and Welfare for overt DIC, Am J Hematol 2003;74:17-22.
32. Taylor FB, Wada H, Kinasewitz G: Description of compensated and uncompensated disseminated intravascular coagulation (DIC) responses (non-overt and overt DIC) in baboon models of intravenous and intraperitoneal *Escherichia coli* sepsis and in the human model of endotoxemia: Toward a better definition of DIC, Crit Care Med 2000;28:S12-S19.
33. Wada H, Wakita Y, Nakase T, et al: Outcome of disseminated intravascular coagulation in relation to the score when treatment was begun, Thromb Haemost 1995;74:848-852.
34. Marshall JC: Inflammation, coagulopathy, and the pathogenesis of multiple organ dysfunction syndrome, Crit Care Med 2001;29:S99-S105.
35. Schafer AI: The hypercoagulable states, Ann Intern Med 1985; 102:814-828.

36. Thomas RH: Hypercoagulability syndromes, Arch Intern Med 2001;161:2433-2439.
37. Bick RL: Syndromes of hypercoagulability and thrombosis: A review, Semin Thromb Hemost 1994;20:109-132.
38. Taylor FB: Response of anticoagulant pathways in disseminated intravascular coagulation, Semin Thromb Hemost 2001;27:619-630.
39. Wada H, Sakuragawa N, Mori Y, et al: Hemostatic molecular markers before the onset of disseminated intravascular coagulation, Am J Hematol 1999;60:273-278.
40. Otto CM, Rieser TM, Brooks MB, et al: Evidence of hypercoagulability in dogs with parvoviral enteritis, J Am Vet Med Assoc 2000;217:1500-1504.
41. Morris DD, Beech J: Disseminated intravascular coagulation in six horses, J Am Vet Med Assoc 1983;10:1067-1072.
42. Welch RD, Watkins JP, Taylor TS, et al: Disseminated intravascular coagulation associated with colic in 23 horses (1984-1989), J Vet Intern Med 1992;6:29-35.
43. Pablo LS, Purohit RC, Teer PA, et al: Disseminated intravascular coagulation in experimental intestinal strangulation obstruction in ponies, Am J Vet Res 1983;44:2115-2122.
44. Johnston IB, Crane S: Haemostatic abnormalities in horses with colic: Their prognostic value, Equine Vet J 1986;18:271-274.
45. Dallap BL, Dolente B, Boston R: Coagulation profiles in 27 horses with large colon volvulus, J Vet Emerg Crit Care 2003;13:215-225.
46. Prasse KW, Topper MJ, Moore JN, Welles EG: Analysis of hemostasis in horses with colic, J Am Vet Med Assoc 1993;203:685-693.
47. Dolente BA, Wilkins PA, Boston RC: Clinicopathologic evidence of disseminated intravascular coagulation in horses with acute colitis, J Am Vet Med Assoc 2002;220:1034-1038.
48. Collatos C, Barton MH, Prasse KW, Moore JN: Intravascular and peritoneal coagulation and fibrinolysis in horses with acute gastrointestinal tract diseases, J Am Vet Med Assoc 1995;207:465-470.
49. Feige K, Kaestner SB, Dempfle CE, et al: Changes in coagulation and markers of fibrinolysis in horses undergoing colic surgery, J Vet Med 2003;50:30-36.
50. Barton MH, Morris DD, Crow N, et al: Hemostatic indices in healthy foals from birth to one month of age, J Vet Diagn Invest 1995;7:380-385.
51. Barton MH, Morris DD, Norton N, Prasse KW: Hemostatic and fibrinolytic indices in neonatal foals with presumed septicemia, J Vet Intern Med 1998;12:26-35.
52. Bick RL: Disseminated intravascular coagulation: Objective criteria for diagnosis and management. Med Clin North Am 1994;78:511-543.
53. Colman RW, Marder VJ, Salzman EW, Hirsh J: Hemostasis and thrombosis. In Colman RW, Hirsh J, Marder VJ, et al, editors: Hemostasis and Thrombosis: Basic Principles and Clinical Practice, Philadelphia, 1982, JB Lippincott.
54. de Jonge E, van der Poll T, Kesecioglu J, Levi M: Anticoagulant factor concentrates in disseminated intravascular coagulation: Rationale for use and clinical experience, Semin Thromb Hemost 2001; 27:667-673.
55. Holland M, Kelly AB, Snyder JR, et al: Antithrombin III activity in horses with large colon torsion, Am J Vet Res 1986;47:897-900.
56. Stokol T, Brooks MB, Erb HN, et al: D-dimer concentrations in healthy dogs and dogs with disseminated intravascular coagulation, J Am Vet Med Assoc 2000;61:393-398.
57. Sandholm M, Vidovic A, Puotunen-Reinert A, et al: D-dimer improves the prognostic value of combined clinical and laboratory data in equine gastrointestinal colic, Acta Vet Scand 1995;36:255-272.
58. Topper MJ, Prasse KW, Morris MJ, et al: Enzyme-linked immunosorbent assay for thrombin-antithrombin III complexes in horses, Am J Vet Res 1996;4:427-431.
59. Topper MJ, Prasse KW: Use of enzyme-linked immunosorbent assay to measure thrombin-antithrombin III complexes in horses with colic, Am J Vet Res 1996;57:456-462.
60. Geor RJ, Jakson ML, Lewis KD, et al: Prekallikrein deficiency in a family of Belgian horses, J Am Vet Med Assoc 1990;197:741-745.
61. Turrentine MA, Sculley PW, Green EM, et al: Prekallikrein deficiency in a family of miniature horses, Am J Vet Res 1986; 47:2464-2467.
62. Morris DD: Diseases associated with blood loss or hemostatic dysfunction. In Smith BP, editor: Large Animal Internal Medicine, St Louis, 1990, Mosby.
63. Marino P: Erythrocyte transfusions. In Marino P, editor: The ICU Book, ed 2, Baltimore, 1998, Williams and Wilkins.
64. Jutkowitz LA: Blood transfusion in the perioperative period, Clin Tech Small Anim Pract 2004;19:75-82.
65. Morris DD: Physiology of hemostasis and blood transfusion. In Auer JA, Stick JA, editors: Equine Surgery, ed 2, Philadelphia, 1999, WB Saunders.
66. Malikides N, Hodgson JL, Rose RJ, Hodgson DR: Cardiovascular, haemotological and biochemical responses after large volume blood collection in horses, Vet J 2001;162:44.
67. Taylor RW, Manganaro L, O'Brien J, et al: Impact of allogenic packed red blood cell transfusion on nosocomial infection rates in the critically ill patient, Crit Care Med 2002;30:2249.
68. Alwood AJ, Lafond E, Brainard B, et al: Postoperative pulmonary complications in dogs undergoing laparotomy [abstract], J Vet Emerg Crit Care 2003;13:159.

CHAPTER 5

Wound Repair

Christine L. Theoret

A critical trait of living organisms continually subjected to insults from the environment is their capacity for self-repair. Whether the injury is a deliberate act of surgery or accidental, it generates an attempt by the host to restore tissue continuity. Two processes are involved in healing: repair and regeneration. Regeneration entails the replacement of damaged tissue with normal cells of the type lost, and this is possible only in tissues with a sustained population of cells capable of mitosis, such as epithelium, bone, and liver. Repair is a stopgap reaction designed to reestablish the continuity of interrupted tissues. Tissue forms between the severed parts, without differentiating totally new elements, and ultimately results in scar tissue.[1] Repair is therefore the second-best method of healing, producing a result that is usually less biologically useful than the tissue it replaced and that may adversely affect adjacent normal tissues.

Traumatic wounds occur commonly in horses and often demand labor-intensive and costly treatments. The objective of repair is reestablishment of an epithelial cover and recovery of tissue integrity, strength, and function. Partial-thickness wounds (e.g., abrasions and erosions) heal primarily by migration and proliferation of epidermal cells from the remaining underlying epithelium as well as the adnexal structures (hair follicles, sweat and sebaceous glands), with little participation of inflammatory or mesenchymal cells. In contrast, repair of full-thickness wounds relies principally on three coordinated phases: acute inflammation, cellular proliferation, and, finally, matrix synthesis and remodeling with scar formation (Fig. 5-1). Many traumatic wounds in horses, whether partial- or full-thickness, cannot be sutured because of massive tissue loss, extreme contamination, continuous movement, and skin tension, as well as a long interval since the time of injury. A further number dehisced after attempted primary closure, for similar reasons. A large retrospective study revealed that primary closure was successful in only 24% of horse wounds and 39% of pony wounds, more than half of which were located on the limb.[2] Thus, a significant number of wounds must heal by second intention. Unfortunately, this type of repair leads to formation of a much larger scar tissue than that formed after successful primary closure, and function and appearance may be adversely affected.

PHASES OF WOUND REPAIR

Acute Inflammation

Inflammation prepares the wound for the subsequent reparative phases. It purges the body of alien substances and disposes of dead tissue, while the participating cellular populations liberate mediators to amplify and sustain the events that will follow. Inflammation encompasses vascular and cellular responses whose intensity is strongly correlated to the severity of trauma. The injured endothelial cell membrane releases phospholipids that are transformed into arachidonic acid and its metabolites, which mediate vascular tone and permeability as well as platelet aggregation. The first response of the damaged blood vessel is vasoconstriction, lasting 5 to 10 minutes, after which vasodilation ensues and promotes diapedesis of cells, fluid, and protein across the vessel wall into the extravascular space. Coagulated blood and aggregated platelets together form a clot within the defect that, despite providing limited strength to the wound, seals off the injury and prevents further bleeding. The clot also functions as a scaffold through the presence of a large number of binding sites on blood proteins that are recognized by special surface receptors

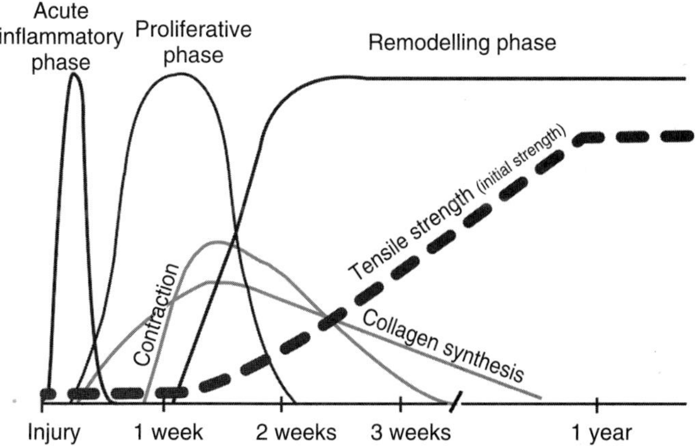

Figure 5-1. Temporal profile of various processes and gain in tensile strength occurring during normal cutaneous wound repair.

(integrins) found on migratory inflammatory and mesenchymal cells. Activated platelets are among the earliest promoters of inflammation, via the release of potent chemoattractants and mitogens from their storage granules. These serve as signals to initiate and amplify the reparative phases of healing and are detailed later. Over time, the surface clot desiccates to form a scab that protects the wound from infection. This scab is in turn lysed by plasmin and sloughs along with dead inflammatory cells and bacteria as healing proceeds underneath. The provisional extracellular matrix (ECM) will be replaced by granulation tissue in the next phase of repair.

Leukocytes are recruited from the circulating blood pool to the site of injury by the numerous vasoactive mediators and chemoattractants supplied by the coagulation and activated complement pathways, by platelets, by mast cells, and by injured or activated mesenchymal cells.[3] These signals initiate the processes of rolling, activation, tight adhesion, and finally transmigration of inflammatory cells through the microvascular endothelium. Chemoattractants additionally stimulate the release of enzymes by the activated neutrophils; these enzymes facilitate the penetration of the inflammatory cells as they migrate through vascular basement membranes. Neutrophil diapedesis is further facilitated by increased capillary permeability after the release of a spectrum of vasodilatory agents. Cellular influx begins early, and neutrophil numbers progressively increase to reach a peak 1 to 2 days after the injury. The neutrophils act as a first line of defense in contaminated wounds by destroying debris and bacteria through phagocytosis and subsequent enzymatic and oxygen-radical mechanisms. The principal degradative proteinases released by the neutrophils to rid the site of denatured ECM components are neutrophil-specific interstitial collagenase, neutrophil elastase, and cathepsin G. Neutrophil migration and phagocytosis cease when contaminating particles are cleared from the site of injury. Most cells then become entrapped within the clot, which is sloughed during later phases of repair. The neutrophils remaining within viable tissue die in a few days and are phagocytosed by the tissue macrophages or the modified wound fibroblasts. This marks the termination of the early inflammatory phase of repair. Although the neutrophils help create a favorable wound environment and serve as a source of proinflammatory cytokines, they are not essential to repair in uninfected wounds.[4]

The rapid increase in macrophage numbers under inflammatory conditions is predominantly caused by the emigration of monocytes from the vasculature, which then differentiate into macrophages to assist resident tissue macrophages at the wound site for a period lasting from days to weeks. In this manner, the responsive and adaptable pluripotent monocytes can differentiate into macrophages, whose functional properties are determined by the conditions they encounter at the site of mobilization. Like the neutrophils, the macrophages are phagocytes and thus carry out débridement and microbial killing. Unlike the neutrophils, the wound macrophages play a key role in the reparative phases of healing. Indeed, adherence to the ECM (which consists of a cross-linked supporting framework of collagen fibrils and elastin fibers, which is saturated with proteoglycans and other glycoproteins) stimulates monocytes to transform into phenotypes that have the ability to

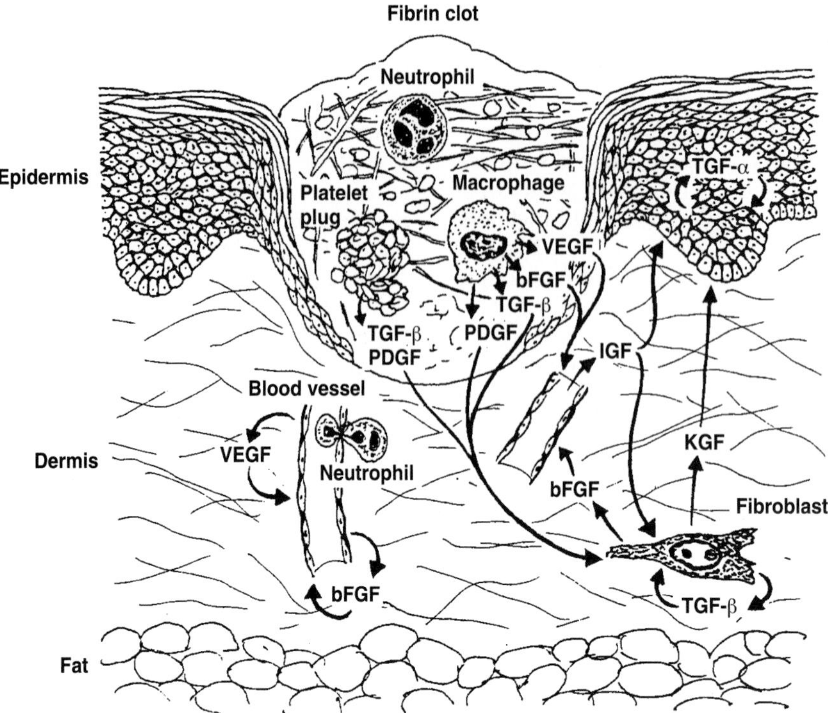

Figure 5-2. Cutaneous wound 3 days after injury. bFGF, basic fibroblast growth factor; IGF, insulin-like growth factor; KGF, keratinocyte growth factor; PDGF, platelet-derived growth factor; TGF, transforming growth factor; VEGF, vascular endothelial growth factor. (Modified from Singer AJ, Clark RAF: N Engl J Med 341:738-746, 1999.)

continually synthesize and express the various cytokines necessary for their survival, as well as for the initiation and propagation of new tissue formation in wounds (Fig. 5-2). A classic series of experiments in the 1970s determined that wounds depleted of both circulating blood monocytes and tissue macrophages exhibited not only severe retardation of tissue débridement but also a marked delay in fibroblast proliferation and subsequent wound fibrosis.[5] Although it has long been considered that the inflammatory response is instrumental in supplying cytokine and growth factor signals that orchestrate the cell and tissue movements necessary for repair, it has recently been shown that mice genetically lacking macrophages and functioning neutrophils are able to repair skin wounds within a time frame similar to that seen in their wild-type siblings, and these repairs appear scar free, possibly in response to an altered local cytokine and growth factor profile.[6]

On arrival at the site of inflammation, macrophages participate in bacterial killing via mechanisms that parallel those of the neutrophils. Three inducible, secreted, neutral proteinases have been identified in macrophages: elastase, collagenase, and plasminogen activator (PA). These proteinases aid in degradation of damaged tissue and debris, which must be cleared before repair can proceed. Despite the new data gleaned from the study on mice without macrophages,[6] acute inflammation is still considered crucial to the normal outcome of wound repair. Indeed, macrophages are regarded as the major inflammatory cell responsible not only for débridement but also for recruitment of other inflammatory and mesenchymal cells, and for subsequent induction of angiogenesis, fibroplasia, and epithelialization. Thus, a general approach for improving wound repair may be to recruit or possibly activate monocytes. For example, it has recently been shown that priming a planned incision site with recombinant proinflammatory cytokines nearly doubles the breaking strength of an acute wound.[7] Likewise, honey and sugar (Intracell, Macleod Pharmaceutical, Ft. Collins, Colo.) applied to open wounds have been shown to enhance fibroplasia and epithelialization, possibly via their chemoattractant and stimulatory activity on the tissue macrophages.[8,9] A β-(1-4)-acetylated mannan, available as a topical hydrogel (Carravet, Veterinary Products Laboratories, Phoenix, Ariz.; Carrasorb, Carrington Laboratories, Irving, Tex.), likewise enhances the early stages of wound repair by stimulating macrophages to produce proinflammatory cytokines.[9]

Paradoxically, prolonged inflammation retards healing and encourages the development of chronic proliferation of fibroblastic granulation. This is thought to contribute to the pathogenesis of a number of diseases characterized by disproportionate scarring, such as pulmonary fibrosis, hepatic cirrhosis, glomerulonephritis, and dermal keloids in humans. Extensive scarring or fibrosis of any organ may cause catastrophic loss of function of that organ. In the horse, a comparable condition is the development of exuberant granulation tissue in skin wounds (Fig. 5-3). Wilmink and colleagues believe this is related to a deficient but protracted inflammatory response in the horse when compared with ponies, especially when wounds are located at the distal aspect of the limb.[10] They found that the number of polymorphonuclear leukocytes (PMNs) was high in ponies during the first 3 weeks after experimental full-

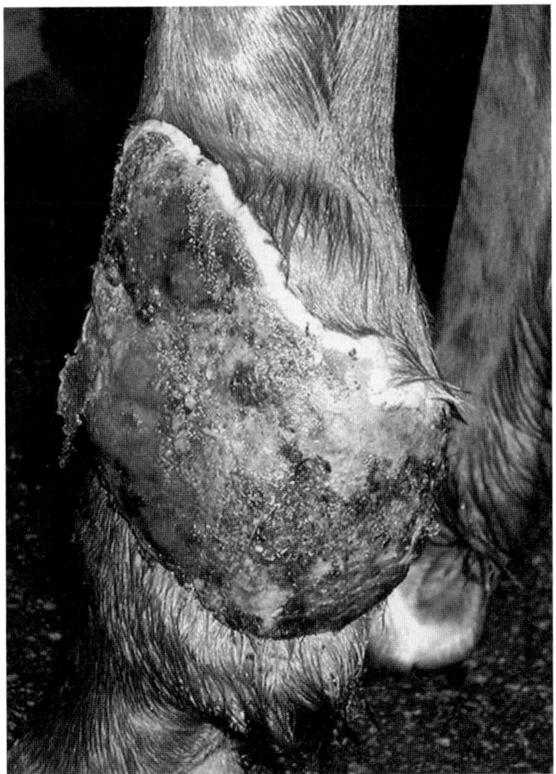

Figure 5-3. Exuberant granulation tissue demonstrating chronic inflammation. (Photo courtesy of FMV, Université de Montréal.)

thickness wounding, but it subsequently decreased rapidly, whereas in the horse the initial number of PMNs was lower, but it remained persistently elevated during the entire 6-week study.[10] Furthermore, peripheral blood leukocytes from ponies produce more reactive oxygen species essential to bacterial killing than do those of horses,[11] which corresponds to the more pronounced initial inflammatory response and to the better local defense against wound infection clinically apparent in the pony.[2]

A handful of equine studies have been undertaken with the intent of encouraging a powerful yet brief acute inflammatory response and thus limiting the subsequent fibrosis that appears in response to injury to the distal portion of the limb in horses. Wilson and colleagues found that although an activated macrophage supernate effectively restrained proliferation of equine fibroblasts in vitro, no significant in vivo effects were found on distal limb wounds.[12] Another study found that a protein-free dialysate of calf blood (Solcoseryl, Solco Basle Ltd., Birsfelden, Switzerland) provoked a greater inflammatory response, with faster formation and contraction of granulation tissue within deep wounds.[13] Subsequently, it inhibited repair by causing protracted inflammation and delaying epithelialization. Finally, a field study was recently performed to determine the efficacy of Vulketan gel (Janssen Animal Health, Beerse, Belgium) in preventing exuberant formation of granulation tissue in equine lower limb wounds.[14] The active ingredient appears to antagonize serotonin-induced suppression of wound macrophages, thus allowing a strong, effective inflammatory response to occur. Vulketan was two to five times more likely to result in successful closure by reducing infection and proud flesh formation, than an antiseptic or a dislodging agent.

Inflammation is a sequence of events: production of mediators; rolling, tethering, and adhesion of neutrophils to vascular endothelium, with subsequent migration through endothelium and basement membranes; altered vascular permeability with passage of fluid into tissues; neutrophil phagocytosis of invading organisms, and release of biologically active materials; emigration of monocytes from the local vasculature; and maturation of monocytes into inflammatory macrophages with subsequent removal of the components of inflammation. Resolution of inflammation should therefore address each one of these events and halt or potentially reverse it. However, despite the importance of the processes by which inflammation normally resolves, little research has been done in this area.

Apoptosis, or programmed cell death, is the universal pathway for the elimination of unneeded cells and tissues in a phagocytic process that does not elicit additional inflammation.[15] This mechanism is prevalent during all phases of wound repair, as each phase relies on rapid increases in specific cell populations that either prepare the wound for repair (inflammatory cells) or deposit new matrices and mature the wound (mesenchymal cells), but the cell populations must then be eliminated prior to progression to the next phase. Indeed, a mature wound is typically acellular.

In conclusion, the termination of inflammation is a complex but closely regulated sequence of events. There are several steps at which the resolution process could go astray, leading to suppuration, chronic inflammation, and/or excessive fibrosis.

Cellular Proliferation

Fibroplasia

The proliferative phase of repair comes about as inflammation subsides and is characterized by the eventual appearance of red, fleshy granulation tissue, which ultimately fills the defect. Although the earliest part of this phase is very active at the cellular level, this does not immediately translate into a gain in wound strength. Indeed, during the first 3 to 5 days after injury, mesenchymal cells such as fibroblasts and endothelial and epithelial cells are rapidly invading the wound in preparation for matrix synthesis and maturation; however, these latter reinforcing mechanisms lag somewhat. Granulation tissue is formed by three elements that move into the wound space simultaneously: macrophages débride and produce cytokines and growth factors, which stimulate angiogenesis and fibroplasia (see Fig. 5-2); fibroblasts proliferate and synthesize new ECM components; and new blood vessels carry oxygen and nutrients necessary for the metabolism and growth of mesenchymal cells, and confer to the granulation tissue its characteristic appearance.[3] This stroma, of which fibronectin and hyaluronan are major components, replaces the fibrin-containing clot to provide a physical barrier to infection and, importantly, to proffer a surface across which mesenchymal cells can then migrate. A number of matrix molecules, as well as chemoattractants, cytokines, and growth factors released by inflammatory cells, are believed to stimulate fibroblasts from adjacent uninjured skin to proliferate and express integrin receptors to assist migration into the wound space. Integrins are transmembrane proteins that act as the major cell-surface receptors for ECM molecules and thus mediate interactions and transduce signals between cells and their environment. They are particularly critical to the migratory movements exhibited by wound-healing cells. Migration immediately precedes advancing capillary endothelial buds but follows macrophages, which have cleared a path by phagocytosing debris. Fibroblasts themselves also possess an active proteolytic system to aid migration into the cross-linked fibrin blood clot; proteinases include PA, various collagenases, gelatinase, and stromelysin.[16]

Once fibroblasts have arrived within the wound space, they proliferate and then switch their major function to protein synthesis and commence the gradual replacement of provisional matrix by a collagenous one, probably under the influence of various cytokines and growth factors. As the wound matures, there is a marked increase in the ratio of type I (mature) to type III (immature) collagen; proteoglycans also become abundant within the mature matrix. The greatest rate of connective tissue accumulation within the wound occurs 7 to 14 days after injury, and thus this is the period with most rapid gain in tensile strength (see Fig. 5-1). Thereafter, collagen content levels off as fibroblasts retract their synthetic machinery; this corresponds to a much slower gain in wound strength, which occurs as the wound remodels. The fibroblast-rich granulation tissue is then replaced by a relatively avascular and acellular scar as the capillary content regresses and fibroblasts either undergo apoptosis[17] or acquire smooth-muscle characteristics and transform into myofibroblasts that participate in wound contraction. The latter phenomena are regulated by the physiologic needs and/or the microenvironmental stimuli present at the wound site. It appears that if the signal to downregulate fibroblast activity is delayed beyond a specific time point, apoptosis is permanently impaired, which ultimately leads to an imbalance between collagen synthesis and degradation[17] and the formation of excessive scar tissue, such as that seen in human keloids.[18]

Following this logic, and since the horse activates wound collagen formation to a greater extent and at an earlier time during repair than do other species,[19] it is hypothesized that excessive fibrosis in the horse may relate to an imbalance between collagen synthesis and lysis in favor of the former, possibly as a result of deficient fibroblast apoptosis. Undeniably, repair of full-thickness wounds in the horse is subject to excessive formation of granulation tissue, with subsequent delays in epithelialization and contraction, especially when wounds are located at the distal aspect of the limb.[20] Predilection for this site remains unexplained, but it may result from a population of dermal fibroblasts possessing particular morphologic and functional characteristics, or it may relate to the local environment of the wound. Surprisingly, in vitro fibroblast growth from tissues isolated from the horse limb is significantly less rapid than growth of fibroblasts from the horse trunk.[21] In vivo, an elevated and persistent mitotic activity exists in distal metatarsal wounds of horses, compared with the activity present in wounds healing normally on the hindquarters.[10] This resembles the different mitotic activities of fibroblasts from various sites in the rat where regional differences in granulation tissue formation also exist,[22] and it may indicate deficient cell death, which could result from downregulation of apoptosis-related genes, as occurs in humans.[23] We recently investigated this hypothesis in the horse and found that the balance of apoptotic signals was altered against apoptosis in limb versus body wounds.[24]

Silicone dressings are used for the prevention of excessive fibroplasia and scarring in man. It appears that this type of synthetic, nonadherent, and fully occlusive dressing surpasses other modalities for decreasing the amount of scar tissue while exerting no negative side effects. In a recent study performed in wounds of the distal limbs of horses, we found that the silicone dressing surpassed a conventional permeable, nonadherent dressing for preventing the formation of exuberant granulation tissue and improving tissue quality.[25]

Angiogenesis

Besides initiating the inflammatory response through interaction with leukocytes, microvascular endothelial cells play a key role in the proliferative phase of repair. The formation of new capillary blood vessels from preexisting ones (angiogenesis) is necessary to sustain the granulation tissue newly formed within the wound bed. Angiogenesis, in response to tissue injury and hypoxia, is a complex and dynamic process mediated by diverse soluble factors from both serum and the surrounding ECM environment—in particular, angiogenic inducers including growth factors, chemokines, angiogenic enzymes, endothelial cell–specific receptors, and adhesion molecules[26] (see Fig. 5-2), many of which are released during the previous inflammatory phase of repair.

Construction of a vascular network requires sequential steps that include augmented microvascular permeability, the release of proteinases from activated endothelial cells with subsequent local degradation of the basement membrane surrounding the existing vessel, migration and sprouting of endothelial cells into the interstitial space, endothelial cell proliferation and formation of granulation tissue, differentiation into mature blood vessels, and stabilization, eventually followed by regression and involution of the newly formed vasculature as the tissue remodels.[27] Angiogenesis depends not only on the cells and cytokines present but also on the production and organization of ECM components, which act both as scaffold support through which endothelial cells may migrate, and as reservoir and modulator for growth factors. Thus, endothelial cells at the tips of capillaries begin their migration into the wound in response to angiogenic stimuli and absence of neighboring cells, on the second day following injury. Cytoplasmic pseudopodia extend through fragmented basement membranes; subsequently, the entire cell migrates into the perivascular space. Cells remaining in the parent vessel near the tip of the angiogenic sprouts begin to proliferate, providing a continuous source of microvascular endothelial cells for angiogenesis. When a new capillary sprout first develops, it is solid; after it fuses with a neighboring sprout to form an arcade it becomes canalized and erythrocytes pass into and through it. Lumen formation probably involves the joining of plasma membranes of individual or adjacent cells, as well as extensive intracellular vacuolization followed by fusion of the vacuoles to form ring cells, which ultimately fuse to form seamless capillaries. Capillaries are then stabilized by endothelial cells and interact with the new basement membrane within 24 hours of new vessel formation. Once the reconstitution of parenchyma is complete, there is no longer the need for a rich vascular supply. Angiogenic stimuli are downregulated or the local concentration of inhibitors increases and most of the recently formed capillary network quickly involutes through the activity of matrix metalloproteinases (MMPs)[28] and apoptosis of endothelial cells. The wound color becomes correspondingly paler as the rich capillary bed disappears from the granulation tissue.

Exuberant granulation tissue that develops in wounds of the lower limbs of horses is characterized microscopically by a great number of microvessels. Although the reason angiogenesis is more prominent in this location remains obscure, it is tempting to speculate that the regional paucity of blood supply may impart an effect via upregulation of various angiogenic factors. Indeed, hypoxia is known to stimulate proliferation and synthetic activity of fibroblasts.[29] In support of this hypothesis, we have recently shown that although a greater number of microvessels are microscopically apparent within the granulation tissue of limb wounds in horses, their lumens are occluded significantly more often than the lumens of microvessels within thoracic wounds, which may corroborate the existence of a hypoxic environment in wounds of the lower limb.[24] Thus, via upregulation of various angiogenic factors, hypoxia may lead to excessive fibrosis. Alternatively, deficient apoptotic signals may lead to persistence of microcapillary endothelial cells and subsequent angiogenic activity.

Epithelialization

All body surfaces are covered by epithelium, which acts as a selective barrier to the environment. Epithelium provides the primary defense against hostile surroundings and is a major factor in maintaining internal homeostasis by limiting fluid and electrolyte loss. The outer region of skin, a multilayered stratified squamous epithelium (the epidermis), interfaces with the musculoskeletal framework by means of a connective tissue layer (the dermis) and a fibrofatty layer (the subcutis). Epidermis is attached to the dermis at the level of the basement membrane, a thin, glycoprotein-rich layer composed primarily of laminin and type IV collagen. This attachment is mediated by hemidesmosomes, which physically attach the basal cells of the epidermis to the underlying dermis, as well as by vertically oriented type VII collagen anchoring fibrils, which bind the cytoskeleton.[30]

It is critical to survival that an epidermal wound be covered without delay. In addition to the aforementioned hemostatic activities, which establish a temporary barrier, centripetal movement of the residual epithelium below the clot participates in wound closure. Although epithelial migration commences 24 to 48 hours after wounding, the characteristic pink rim of new epithelium is not macroscopically visible until 4 to 6 days later, although this is variable because the rate of wound closure depends on the animal species as well as on the wound site, substrate, and size. For example, epithelialization is accelerated in a partial-thickness wound, because migrating cells arise not only from the residual epithelium at the wound periphery but also from remaining epidermal appendages. Furthermore, the basement membrane is intact in this type of injury, precluding its lengthy regeneration. On the other hand, during second-intention healing of a full-thickness wound, epithelialization must await the formation of a bed of granulation tissue to proceed. Wounds in the flank area of a horse epithelialize at a rate of 0.2 mm per day, compared with a rate as slow as 0.09 mm per day for wounds in the distal portion of limbs.[31]

In preparation for migration, basal epidermal cells at the wound margin undergo phenotypic alterations that favor mobility and phagocytic activity. Additionally, various degradative enzymes necessary for the proteolysis of ECM components are upregulated within cells at the leading edge, facilitating ingestion of the clot and debris found along the migratory route. The migratory route is determined by the array of integrin receptors expressed on the surface of migrating epithelial cells, for various ECM proteins. Indeed, a fundamental reason why migrating epidermis dissects the fibrin eschar from wounds is that normal epithelial cells cannot interact with the fibrinogen and its derivatives found within the clot because they lack the appropriate integrin.[32] Once the wound surface is covered by epithelial cells that contact one another, further migration from the margin of the wound inward is inhibited by the expression within the ECM of laminin, a major cell adhesion factor for epithelial cells.

Although initial migration does not require an increase in cellular multiplication, epidermal cells at the wound margin do begin to proliferate 1 to 2 days after injury to replenish the migratory front. This corresponds histologically to epithelial hyperplasia (Fig. 5-4), as cellular mitosis increases 17-fold within 48 to 72 hours. The new cells leapfrog over those at the wound margin to adhere to the substratum, only to be replaced in turn by other cells coming from above

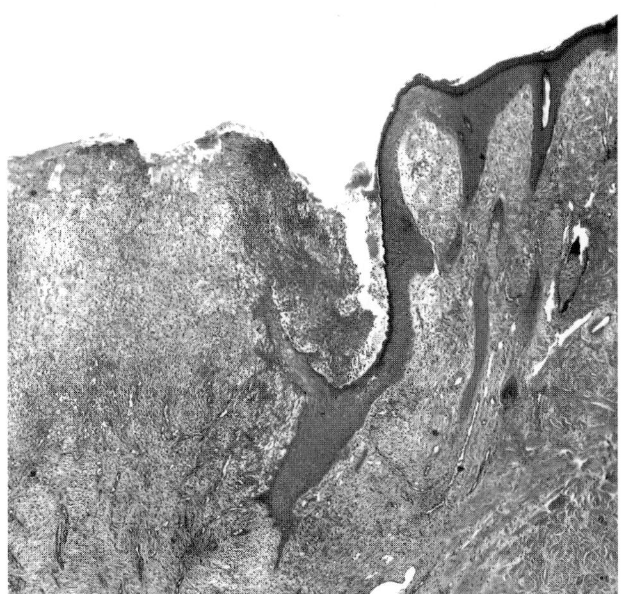

Figure 5-4. Photomicrograph of wound edge biopsy taken 7 days after wounding. Normal unwounded skin to the right; granulation tissue to the left; hyperplastic epithelium in the center.

and behind. The newly adherent monolayer subsequently restratifies in an attempt to restore the original multilayered epidermis.

In full-thickness wounds healing by second intention, such as those commonly managed in equine practice, provisional matrix is eventually replaced by a mature basement membrane zone. Repairing epidermis reassembles its constituents from the margin of the wound inward, in a zipper-like fashion.[3] Epidermal cells then revert to a quiescent phenotype and become attached to this new basement membrane through hemidesmosomes and to the underlying dermis through type VII collagen fibrils. This particular aspect of epithelialization is time consuming, occurring long after total wound coverage is apparent, which may explain the continued fragility of neoepidermis for extended periods after macroscopically complete repair. This is particularly evident in large wounds of the limb, where epidermis at the center is often thin and easily traumatized.

Wounds in horses commonly fail to epithelialize altogether. This occurs in two distinct types of wounds: those in which fibroplasia is excessive and those of an indolent nature. In the former, protruding granulation tissue may act as a physical impediment to epithelial migration and it may inhibit epithelial cell mitosis. The relative absence of epithelial cells could in turn lead to persistent synthesis of fibrogenic growth factors by fibroblasts[33] and defective apoptosis signaling,[15] thus establishing a vicious cycle culminating in proud flesh formation. Conversely, indolent wounds possess a granulation bed of deficient quantity and quality, thus hindering migratory efforts by epithelial cells. In this case, it is critical to encourage the formation of a healthy granulation bed. Although hydrogel dressings have been advocated for this purpose,[34] a recent study is not supportive.[35]

In the case of limb wounds presenting delays in epithelialization but possessing a healthy bed of granulation tissue, the value of skin grafting is undisputed (see Chapter 25). Grafting exerts a significant inhibitory effect on both endothelial cell and fibroblast growth while enhancing proliferation and migration of epithelial cells. It is, however, critical that the graft be obtained from a site that normally heals well and in which contraction is a prominent feature (e.g., from the lateral cervical, abdominal, or pectoral regions). The inhibitory effect of grafts on fibroblast proliferation and collagen synthesis may be regulated by a soluble epithelial cell–derived product,[33] possibly a cytokine or a growth factor such as epidermal growth factor (EGF), which enhances epithelialization via positive effects on epithelial cell migration, proliferation, and differentiation. Following this premise, EGF was recently applied to experimentally induced corneal wounds of horses in hopes of accelerating epithelialization. Unfortunately, it was found that beneficial effects were outweighed by the intensity of the associated inflammatory response, at least in the eye.[36]

To encourage ingrowth of mesenchymal cells in indolent wounds during the proliferative phase, biomaterials such as collagen membranes and sponges have been developed and are appraised as improving rate and quality of repair. Collagen may function as a substrate for hemostasis; as a template for cellular attachment, migration, and proliferation; and as a scaffold for more rapid transition to mature collagen. A porous bovine collagen membrane was shown to generate a strong inflammatory response in full-thickness limb wounds of horses, which may augment the cytokine or growth factor content of wound tissues, although it did not significantly alter the total wound, or the epithelialization or contraction process.[37] A commercially available collagen matrix derived from porcine small intestinal submucosa (Vet BioSISt, Cook Veterinary Products, Inc, Spencer, Ind.) and containing a plethora of proteins and growth factors, has been designed as a scaffold for tissue ingrowth and is promoted as reducing scarring. Regrettably, a recent study determined that it offers no apparent advantage over a nonbiologic, nonadherent synthetic dressing for treatment of small, granulating wounds of the distal limb of horses.[38]

Matrix Synthesis and Remodeling

In addition to epithelialization, contraction contributes to the successful closure of full-thickness wounds. Contraction is defined as a process whereby both dermis and epidermis bordering a full-thickness skin deficit are drawn from all sides centripetally over the exposed wound bed.[39] This occurs usually during the second week after injury. Wound contraction not only accelerates closure but also enhances the cosmetic appearance and strength of the scar, because proportionally less wound area must be covered by newly formed, inferior quality epithelium, which is fragile and lacks normal nervous, glandular, follicular, and vascular components. For this reason, a high degree of wound contraction is a desired feature of wound repair, at least in the horse.

A number of theories have been proposed to explain wound contraction, but most authorities agree that it involves a finely orchestrated interaction of ECM, cytokines or growth factors, and cells—in particular, a specialized fibroblast phenotype, the myofibroblast (Fig. 5-5). Myofibroblasts

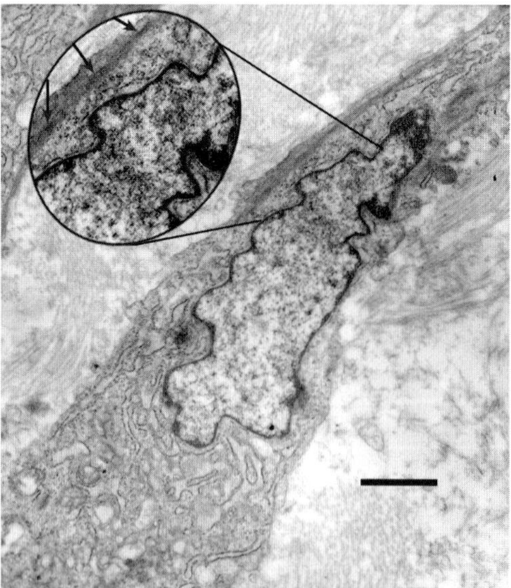

Figure 5-5. Transmission electron micrograph showing a typical myofibroblast with microfilament bundles illustrated in the inset *(arrows)*. Bar = 1 μm.

are the most abundant cellular elements of healthy granulation tissue and are aligned within the wound along the lines of contraction, in contrast to capillaries and macrophages. The most striking feature of the myofibroblasts is a well-developed alpha smooth muscle actin (α-SMA) microfilamentous system, arranged parallel to the cell's long axis and in continuity with ECM components via various integrins. In addition to these cell–substratum links, intercellular connections such as gap junctions and hemidesmosomes ensure that neighboring cells exert tension on one another. Factors producing and regulating contraction are presently unknown, but they appear to include various cytokines and growth factors.

Wound contraction is divided into three phases. An initial *lag phase* (wherein skin edges retract and the wound area increases temporarily for 5 to 10 days) occurs because significant fibroblastic invasion into the wound is a prerequisite for contraction. Subsequently, a period of *rapid contraction* is followed by a period of *slow contraction* as the wound approaches complete closure. The number of myofibroblasts found in a wound appears to be proportional to the need for contraction; thus, as repair progresses and the rate of contraction slows, this number decreases. During wound contraction, the surrounding skin stretches by intussusceptive growth, and the wound takes on a stellate appearance. Contraction ceases in response to one of three events: the wound edges meet and contact inhibition halts the processes of both epithelialization and contraction; tension in the surrounding skin becomes equal to or greater than the contractile force generated by the α-SMA of the myofibroblasts; or, in the case of chronic wounds, a low myofibroblast count in the granulation tissue may result in failure of wound contraction despite laxity in the surrounding skin. In this case, the granulation tissue is pale and consists primarily of collagen and ground substance. Wound contraction is greater in regions of the body with loose skin than in regions where skin is under tension, such as the distal aspect of the limb in the horse. Although it has been speculated that the shape of the wound may influence the process of contraction, this does not appear relevant in wounds at the distal extremities of horse limbs where skin is tightly stretched and not easily moved.[40] Skin grafts have been reported to inhibit contraction by preventing formation of myofibroblasts or by accelerating the myofibroblast life cycle, although this is questionable in the horse.[34,41]

As contraction concludes, myofibroblasts disappear, either by reverting to a quiescent fibroblast phenotype or by apoptosis,[17] primarily in response to reduced tension within the ECM.[42] The myofibroblast persists in fibrotic lesions, where it may be involved in further ECM accumulation and pathologic contracture, a condition rarely encountered in the horse, but leading to significant morbidity particularly when it involves joints or body orifices.

Significant differences exist with regard to contraction between horses and ponies and between distinct areas of the body. Wound contraction is clearly more pronounced in ponies than in horses,[43] and the rate of contraction of limb wounds is at best 25% that of flank wounds.[31] A study reported no difference in the amount of α-SMA in distal metatarsal versus buttocks wounds in horses, but it described a disorganized arrangement of myofibroblasts in chronic wounds of the distal limb.[10] This particular arrangement may be related to fibronexin being scarce between myofibroblasts of the granulation tissue, and it could be responsible for deficient contractile activity within the wounds. Contrary to expectations, it was shown that fibroblasts harvested from the limb do not display a slower rate of contraction than do those harvested from the body, at least in vitro.[44,45] Rather, it appears that tissue environmental factors emanating from the inflammatory response to injury, such as cytokine or growth factor profiles, are instrumental in causing this difference.

The conversion of ECM from granulation to scar tissue constitutes the final phase of wound repair and consists of connective tissue synthesis, lysis, and remodeling, also referred to as maturation. Proteoglycans replace hyaluronan during the second week of repair, support the deposition and aggregation of collagen fibers, and provide the mature matrix with better resilience. Collagen macromolecules provide the wound tissue with tensile strength as their deposition peaks within the first week in primary wound repair, and between 7 and 14 days in second-intention healing. Although this corresponds to the period of most rapid gain in strength, only 20% of the final strength of the wound is achieved in the first 3 weeks of repair. At this time, collagen synthesis is balanced by collagenolysis, which normally prevents accretion of excessive amounts of collagen and formation of pathologic scars. It appears that during the development of exuberant granulation tissue in horses, collagen synthesis continues unabated.[46] The balance between synthesis and degradation determines the overall strength of a healing wound at a particular time. The first newly deposited collagen tends to be oriented randomly and therefore provides little tensile strength, whereas during remodeling the fibers re-form along lines of stress and therefore resist dehiscence more effectively. Crosslinking in the later-formed collagen is also more effective, although never to the same extent as in the original tissue. A recent study has shown that newly accumulated collagen fibrils are disorganized in wounds at the distal aspect of the forelimb of horses but more normally organized in thoracic wounds.[46] The new collagen weaves into the collagen that preexisted and also appears to bond to the ends of old collagen fibers. These welds are points of weakness that may rupture under stress.

Because the ultimate tensile strength of a wound is related to collagen content, therapies that favor its synthesis and deposition are continuously sought. Growth hormone is postulated to stimulate collagen synthesis through fibroblasts and accelerate its maturation, resulting in enhanced wound strength, effects that are probably mediated through various growth factors. Regrettably, a study investigating the effect of intramuscular injections of recombinant equine growth hormone on maturation of limb wounds in horses found that the wounds contracted at a faster rate only after treatment ended.[47]

Collagen degradation within a wound depends on the presence of various proteolytic enzymes released from inflammatory and mesenchymal cells. Most are of the MMP family of zinc-dependent endopeptidases that are collectively capable of degrading virtually all ECM components. Although MMPs are not constitutively expressed in skin, upregulation occurs whenever proteolysis is required, such as during cell migration and matrix remodeling. Inactive precursors (zymogens) of the MMPs are cleaved in the extracellular space by proteinases such as plasmin and trypsin (left over from the inflammatory and proliferative phases) and also by other MMPs. To date, a dozen different MMPs, all distinct gene products, have been characterized (Table 5-1).[16] The best-known subgroup of MMPs are the collagenases (MMP-1, 8, and 13), which possess the unique ability to cleave the triple helix of native types I, II, and III collagens, the rate-limiting step of collagen degradation. The fragments generated are thermally unstable and denature into their constitutive polypeptide chains, forming gelatin peptides. Basal epithelial cells at the migratory front of epithelialization are the predominant source of collagenase during active wound repair,[16] whereas the resolution of granulation tissue also depends on the activity of collagenase, in this case expressed by dermal fibroblasts. Another subgroup of MMPs, the stromelysins, possess a broad substrate specificity. Stromelysin-1 and -2 are strong proteoglycanases and can also degrade basement membranes, laminin, and fibronectin, whereas stromelysin-3 is only weakly proteolytic. Although stromelysin-2 expression is strictly confined to the epidermis, stromelysin-1 is also abundantly expressed by dermal fibroblasts in the granulation tissue associated with wounds, and because of its broad substrate specificity, it may be important in remodeling the matrix—in particular, the newly formed basement membrane—during repair.[16] There are two metallogelatinases: the 72-kDa gelatinase (gelatinase A), which, unlike other MMPs, is produced constitutively by most cells types, and the 92-kDa gelatinase (gelatinase B), produced by most inflammatory cells as well as by epithelial cells. Both types efficiently degrade denatured collagens (gelatins) and also attack basement membranes, fibronectin, and insoluble elastin. Matrilysin is the smallest MMP (28 kDa), but it is a stronger proteoglycanase than stromelysin and also degrades basement membranes, insoluble elastin, laminin, fibronectin, and gelatin.

Homeostasis between collagen synthesis and degradation during the remodeling phase depends on the simultaneous presence of MMPs and nonspecific inhibitors such as α_2-macroglobulin and α_1-antiprotease, as well as the natural specific inhibitors of MMPs, the TIMPs. TIMPs are a gene family of four structurally related members, TIMP-1 through -4, that inhibit conversion of MMPs from a zymogen to an activated state and that irreversibly bind to the catalytic site of active MMPs. The role of TIMPs in wound repair is not limited to remodeling, as they also promote growth in a wide range of cell types, and they are thought to stabilize the basement membrane of regenerating epidermis and to inhibit angiogenesis and induce apoptosis.

Inhibition of MMP activity during the acute inflammatory phase of repair enhances wound strength despite accompanying decreases in the inflammatory response and new collagen synthesis. This is thought to result from decreased collagen turnover or increased collagen maturation and crosslinking, or both.[48] However, under most circumstances, an imbalance between MMPs and TIMPs leads to abnormal resolution and delayed repair. Indeed,

TABLE 5-1. Major Matrix Metalloproteinases (MMP) Involved in Wound Repair

MMP Name	MMP #	Substrates	Source
COLLAGENASES			
Interstitial collagenase	MMP-1	Collagen (I, II, III, VII, IX)	Epithelial cell, fibroblast
Neutrophil collagenase	MMP-8	Collagen (I, II, III)	PMNs
Collagenase 3	MMP-13	Collagen (I, II, III)	—
STROMELYSINS			
Stromelysin 1	MMP-3	PGs, laminin, fibronectin	Epithelial cell
Stromelysin 2	MMP-10	Collagen (III, IV, IX, X)	Epithelial cell, fibroblast
Stromelysin 3	MMP-11	Collagen IV, fibronectin, gelatin, laminin	—
GELATINASES			
Gelatinase A (72 kDa)	MMP-2	Gelatin, collagen (I, IV), elastin	Most cells
Gelatinase B (92 kDa)	MMP-9	Gelatin, collagen (IV, V), elastin	Inflammatory cell, epithelial cell, fibroblast
Matrilysin	MMP-7	PGs, elastin, fibronectin, laminin, gelatin, collagen IV	Epithelial cell
MEMBRANE-TYPE (MT) MMPS			
MT1-MMP	MMP-14	Collagen (I, III), fibronectin	Membrane bound
MT2-MMP	MMP-15	Vitronectin, pro-MMPs	—
MT3-MMP	MMP-16	—	—
MT4-MMP	MMP-17	—	—
MT5-MMP	MMP-20	—	—

PG, proteoglycan; PMN, polymorphonuclear granulocyte.

although the presence of MMPs is essential for normal wound maturation, it may also be responsible for the inability of chronic wounds to heal. For example, chronic wound fluid is characterized by elevated levels of proteinases, particularly MMP-9 and serine proteinases, which lead to excessive protein degradation and the inactivation of critical growth factors. Chronic wounds also contain reduced levels of TIMPs—in particular, TIMP-1.[49] It is interesting that as epithelialization progresses, the production of MMPs by epithelial cells is turned off, allowing the formation of hemidesmosomal adhesions between cells and the basement membrane.

Schwartz and coworkers recently documented greater collagen synthesis in metacarpal than thoracic wounds of horses and attributed this to an imbalance between collagen synthesis and degradation.[46] Although TIMP-1 expression was significantly higher in forelimb than in thoracic wounds at 1 week after the wounding, which may imply that collagen degradation is inhibited at this time, the relationship between concentrations of MMP-1 and TIMP-1 throughout the course of the study was unclear.[46]

Wound remodeling continues for up to 2 years, during which time there is no net increase in collagen content—rather, a rearrangement of collagen fibers into a more organized lattice structure, under the influence of local mechanical factors, progressively increasing the tensile strength of scar tissue. The majority of type III collagen fibers laid down early in the healing process are replaced by collagen type I, the fibers become increasingly cross-linked, and the normal skin ratio of 4:1 type I to type III collagen is achieved. Glycosaminoglycans are steadily degraded until they reach concentrations found in normal dermis. The duration of the maturation phase depends on a variety of factors including the patient's genetic makeup, age, location of the wound on the body, type of injury, and duration of inflammation. At maximum strength, cutaneous wounds remain 15% to 20% weaker than the normal surrounding tissue, although this varies markedly among species[50] (see Fig. 5-1).

MEDIATORS OF WOUND REPAIR: CYTOKINES AND GROWTH FACTORS

Wound repair relies on a complex amalgamation of interactive processes involving formed blood elements, ECM, and mesenchymal cells. Although histologic and morphometric observations have permitted a detailed description of the kinetics of cellular and macromolecular components involved in repair, much remains to be learned about the regulation of such activities. Restoration of structural integrity and partial functional properties appear to rely on soluble mediators synthesized by cells, present in the wound or in the surrounding tissue, that form a dense communication network that coordinates migration, proliferation, and protein synthesis by the various cell populations involved in the repair process.

Cytokines, defined as 4- to 60-kDa signaling glycoproteins released by most nucleated cells, are among the most important soluble mediators regulating wound repair. They act in concentrations of 10^9 to 10^{12} M in an autocrine (same-cell), paracrine (adjacent-cell), or endocrine (distant-cell) fashion. For cytokines to exert an effect, the target cell must express a surface receptor to the specific mediator. Receptors are proteins with an extracellular site to bind the cytokine and a transmembrane site to transmit the signal to the intracellular site, where it must reach nuclear DNA for a specific response to occur. Cells may have different numbers of receptors for different factors; the concentration of factors in the area and the number of receptors that are bound determine the response generated. Growth factors are cytokines, which exert primarily mitogenic influences. The cytokines that play a significant role in cutaneous wound repair are summarized in Table 5-2.

Colony-Stimulating Factors

Four cytokines classified as colony-stimulating factors (CSFs) have been identified: granulocyte (G) CSF, macrophage (M) CSF, granulocyte-macrophage (GM) CSF, and multilineage (ML) CSF.[51] Many cells involved in repair, including macrophages, lymphocytes, fibroblasts, and endothelial cells, synthesize CSFs or are targets of this cytokine.[52] Indeed, the way in which CSFs influence repair is by promoting the differentiation and maturation of hematopoietic stem cells to progenitor cells and, finally, to granulocytes, monocytes, macrophages, and lymphocytes. These mature cells can, in turn, secrete or produce secondary cytokines with subsequent effects on inflammation, angiogenesis, epithelialization, and fibroplasia. Cloning of equine GM-CSF has recently been achieved.[53]

Interferons

Interferons (IFNs) represent a family of cytokines originally discovered because of their antiviral activity, but they also influence general immunity, activating and modulating lymphocytes, macrophages, and natural killer and dendritic cells.[54] Type I IFNs share the same ubiquitously expressed receptor, and they include IFN-α, produced by dendritic cells and monocytes/macrophages, and IFN-β, produced by several mesenchymal cell types. Interferon-γ is a type II IFN with its own distinct and more specifically expressed receptor. In horses, IFN-α1, -β, and -γ were cloned and sequenced earlier,[55] but recombinant proteins allowing the analysis of protein, antibodies, and biologic activity became available only recently.[56] Interestingly, it was revealed that although recombinant equine IFN-γ does not display substantial antiviral activity, it does show immunomodulatory effects on monocytes, at least in vitro. This indicates that IFN-γ may stimulate the inflammatory phase of repair, via release by activated monocytes and macrophages of a plethora of additional cytokines, in particular interleukins (ILs) and growth factors. Interestingly, IFN-γ is thought to prevent excessive fibrosis from occurring in the later stages of repair, which may be of particular significance to wound healing in the horse.[57]

Interleukins

Interleukins are produced by virtually every nucleated cell (in particular, macrophages and lymphocytes) and most cells express IL surface receptors through which the cytokine mediates cell-to-cell and cell-to-matrix interactions. Two different IL-1 peptides with diverging isoelectric focusing points exist: IL-1α and IL-1β. There is very close homology

TABLE 5-2. Cytokines Involved in Wound Repair

Name	Abbreviation	Source	Major Function
Colony-stimulating factor	CSF	Macrophage, lymphocyte, fibroblast, endothelial cell	Differentiation and maturation of hematopoietic stem cells
Interferon	IFN	Monocyte and macrophage, lymphocyte, mesenchymal cell	Proinflammatory; release of other cytokines; inhibit fibrosis
Interleukin	IL	All nucleated cells, in particular macrophage and lymphocyte	Proinflammatory; enhance epithelialization, angiogenesis, and remodeling
Tumor necrosis factor	TNF	Macrophage, lymphocyte, mast cell	Proinflammatory; enhance angiogenesis, epithelialization, and remodeling
Connective tissue growth factor	CTGF	Fibroblast	Mediator of TGF-β activity (cell proliferation and ECM accumulation)
Epidermal growth factor	EGF	Platelet, saliva	Epithelialization; chemotactic and mitogenic to fibroblast; protein and MMP synthesis (remodeling); angiogenesis (TGF-α)
Transforming growth factor-α	TGF-α	Macrophage, epithelial cell	
Fibroblast growth factor	FGF	Inflammatory cell, fibroblast, endothelial cell	Chemotactic and mitogenic to fibroblast and epithelial cell; protein synthesis; angiogenesis
Insulin-like growth factor	IGF	Liver, platelet	Chemotactic and mitogenic to endothelial cell; migration of epithelial cell; fibroblast proliferation, protein and GAG synthesis
Keratinocyte growth factor	KGF	Fibroblast	Chemotactic and mitogenic to epithelial cell
Platelet-derived growth factor	PDGF	Platelet	Chemotactic to inflammatory cell and fibroblast; mitogenic to mesenchymal cell; protein synthesis; contraction?
Transforming growth factor-β	TGF-β	Platelet, lymphocyte, mast cell, monocyte and macrophage, endothelial cell, epithelial cell, fibroblast	Chemotactic to inflammatory and mesenchymal cell; fibroblast proliferation; protein synthesis; ECM deposition (inhibition of MMP; induction of TIMP); wound contraction
Vascular endothelial growth factor	VEGF	Macrophage; fibroblast; endothelial cell; epithelial cell	Angiogenesis

ECM, extracellular matrix; GAG, glycosaminoglycan; MMP, matrix metalloproteinase; TIMP, tissue inhibitor of metalloproteinase.

between the two, and both activate cells and stimulate their proliferation. Interleukin-1 has a wide range of biologic activities, many of which are proinflammatory, but it also aids in the later phases of repair. Notably, IL-1 is synthesized by epithelial cells in response to injury and favors epithelialization by directly stimulating chemoattraction of epithelial cells, and by indirectly enhancing their proliferation by upregulating keratinocyte growth factor (KGF) production by wound fibroblasts. The autocrine nature of epithelial cell–derived IL-1 is emphasized by the fact that it additionally induces the cell to synthesize IL-1, transforming growth factor (TGF)-α, and KGF. Interleukin-1 also influences matrix synthesis and remodeling via stimulation of fibroblast proliferation and enhancement of collagenase production. Circular DNAs (cDNAs) for equine IL-1α and IL-1β,[58] as well as for their natural inhibitor, IL-1 receptor antagonist (IL-1ra), have been cloned, sequenced, and expressed.[59]

Other ILs have also been attributed a role in wound repair. For example, it has been shown, with the help of IL-6–deficient mice, that repair of excisional wounds requires this particular IL to proceed normally via gene expression of IL-1, chemokines, adhesion molecules, TGF-β_1, and vascular endothelial growth factor (VEGF).[60,61] Interleukin-8 appears to accelerate maturation of granulation tissue, encouraging the formation of thicker, more mature collagen fibers.[62] On the other hand, IL-10 seems inhibitory to ECM remodeling during wound repair, reducing tumor necrosis factor (TNF)-α–induced fibroblast proliferation, decreasing concentrations of TGF-β_1, and inhibiting collagen type I protein synthesis by dermal fibroblasts, at least in vitro.[63]

Tumor Necrosis Factor-α

TNF-α is produced by a variety of cell types, including macrophages, T cells, mast cells, and epithelial cells, and exerts principally inflammatory effects. TNF-α may favor angiogenesis through chemoattraction and proliferation of endothelial cells, and it is also thought to enhance remodeling through fibroblast proliferation and upregulation of collagenase as well as TIMP-1 levels.[61] Finally, TNF-α has also been shown to stimulate epithelial cell migration. The gene encoding equine TNF-α has been cloned and characterized.[64]

Growth Factors

Connective Tissue Growth Factor

Connective tissue growth factor (CTGF) is a heparin-binding peptide whose secretion by fibroblasts is selectively induced by TGF-ββ and whose biologic activities resemble those of platelet-derived growth factor (PDGF).[65] CTGF acts in an autocrine and paracrine fashion on connective tissue cells, in particular the fibroblast, in which it mediates TGF-β activity as a downstream effector and thus indirectly stimulates cell proliferation and ECM accumulation.[66] Connective tissue growth factor expression in blood vessels suggests that this growth factor is also involved in angiogenesis. Thus, CTGF is an interesting target for future antifibrotic therapies, as it is conceivable that its inhibition may block the profibrotic effects of TGF-β without affecting the antiproliferative and immunosuppressive effects of TGF-β.[67] Although equine CTGF has not been cloned, an antigenic similarity between human and horse CTGF was recently established in a bioequivalence assay.[68] Interestingly, this same study demonstrated that fibrogenic CTGF is present in horse lacrimal fluid and derives, at least partly, from the lacrimal gland. This may explain why repair of corneal ulcers in horses is often associated with profound corneal stromal fibrosis and scar formation.

Epidermal Growth Factor and Transforming Growth Factor-α

Although plasma levels of EGF are undetectable, platelets release substantial amounts on aggregation. This growth factor is also abundant in saliva, which may represent the physiologic basis for wound licking. As its name would imply, EGF enhances epithelialization through various mechanisms: accrued contractility of epithelial cells allows more efficient migration,[69] and both proliferation and differentiation are favored. Furthermore, EGF exerts positive effects on the wound fibroblast, including chemoattraction, mitogenesis, and upregulation of protein and MMP synthesis, important to the remodeling phase of repair.[32] The coding sequence for equine EGF has been identified and it shows 60% to 70% amino acid identity with EGF sequences of other species.[70]

TGF-α, which has no amino acid homology with TGF-β, is synthesized by activated macrophages and epithelial cells, and although it is distinct from EGF, it binds to the same cell-surface receptor and exhibits similar biologic activities. Like EGF, it is a chemoattractant and mitogen for epithelial cells and fibroblasts; however, it is considered a more potent inducer of angiogenesis, in particular via initiation of tube formation by microvascular endothelial cells.[71] Interestingly, TGF-α has also been attributed a role in host defense during wound repair, by inducing the expression of antimicrobial peptides in proliferating epithelial cells, which complement the physical barrier against microorganisms formed by new epithelium.[72]

Fibroblast Growth Factor

Basic fibroblast growth factor (bFGF), also called heparin-binding growth factor-2, is the most extensively studied member of a growing group of structurally related proteins having high affinity for heparin, and it was one of the first angiogenic factors to be characterized.[73] It is synthesized by a number of major cell types involved in angiogenesis and wound repair, and it is found in the ECM bound to heparin. Although the exact mechanism involved in its cellular release remains unknown, it is postulated to occur upon damage to the synthesizing cell. Dermal wounding could thus trigger the release of bFGF protein preexisting in cells in the wound area, allowing active FGF to exert its mitogenic and chemotactic effects on virtually all cells.

Fibroblast growth factors are mitogenic to mesenchymal cells, whereby they influence many of the processes taking place during the proliferative phase of repair. Notably, bFGF promotes endothelial cell migration during granulation tissue formation by induction of cell surface integrins that mediate the binding of endothelial cells to ECM,[27] and it is thus considered a potent angiogenic factor, particularly in response to the hypoxic wound environment. Additionally, bFGF can augment epithelialization and may stimulate wound contraction via the enhancement of TGF-β_1 activity. Finally, bFGF exerts effects on matrix synthesis and remodeling by reversing the induction of collagen type I production while simultaneously encouraging collagenase production by fibroblasts.[74]

Insulin-like Growth Factor

The insulin-like growth factors (IGFs) are structurally similar to proinsulin and, as their name implies, have insulin-like activity. There are two forms, having separate receptors: IGF-1 and IGF-2. Production of IGF-1 by the liver and other tissues is in part regulated by insulin, estrogen, and growth hormone (GH). Indeed, cell proliferation, tissue differentiation, and protein synthesis engendered by GH are mediated, indirectly, through the production of IGFs.

Unlike other growth factors whose primary source during wound repair is the inflammatory cell, substantial levels of inactive IGF, reversibly bound by high-affinity IGF-binding proteins, are present in blood. Once cleaved, the free IGF can exert its autocrine, paracrine, and endocrine actions. Until recently, IGFs were primarily considered mediators of the growth-promoting effects of GH. Lately, it has been shown that IGF-1, released by platelets during clotting and activated by enzymatic activity, low pH, and decreased oxygen tension present in the wound environment, is a potent chemoattractant and mitogen for vascular endothelial cells,[75] it enhances epithelial cell proliferation in vitro,[76] and it stimulates collagen synthesis by fibroblasts.[77] In addition, IGF-1 stimulates epithelial cell membrane protrusion and facilitates cell spreading, which influences the speed of wound epithelialization.[69] Interestingly, IGF-1 induces TGF-β_1 mRNA and protein expression,[78] which implies that it may, indirectly, influence even more aspects of repair.

As mentioned earlier, the impact of intramuscular injections of equine recombinant GH on maturation of limb wounds in horses was initial further wound retraction followed by contraction at a faster rate only after treatment ended.[47]

Equine IGF-1 cDNA has been cloned and sequenced.[79]

Keratinocyte Growth Factor

Keratinocyte growth factor (KGF)-1 is a member of the rapidly growing FGF family; it is sometimes referred to as FGF-7, and it resembles bFGF (FGF-2). Whereas most FGFs influence proliferation or differentiation of numerous cell types, KGF, weakly expressed in skin but strongly upregulated in dermal fibroblasts after wounding,[80] acts specifically on epithelial cells, in a paracrine fashion.[81] It stimulates migration and proliferation of these cells, but it also affects differentiation of early progenitor cells within dermal appendages in the wound bed and adjacent dermis. Both KGF-1 and -2 have recently been found to enhance granulation tissue formation during wound repair, by increasing angiogenesis and collagen deposition. Indeed, a recent multicenter clinical trial found that recombinant human KGF-2 (repifermin) accelerated repair of chronic venous ulcers.[82]

A partial coding sequence for horse KGF-1 (FGF-7) gene is known.[83]

Platelet-Derived Growth Factor

PDGF is a family of isoforms consisting of homo- or heterodimers of products of two genes, the PDGF A-chain gene and the PDGF B-chain gene. Three isoforms of PDGF exist, depending on the bonds formed between the A- and B-chains: AA, AB, and BB.[84] Although the predominant isoform in human platelets is PDGF-AB, this is species variable and currently unknown in the horse.

The platelet, the first cell to invade the site of trauma, is the largest source of PDGF, although a number of connective tissue cell types are also triggered by wounding to express PDGF-like molecules and receptors. Thus, throughout the normal repair process, wound tissues are continuously bathed in PDGF. PDGF acts initially as a chemoattractant for inflammatory cells and fibroblasts, which it activates in an autocrine fashion. Subsequently it becomes mitogenic for mesenchymal cells through the release of other growth factors—namely, TGF-β, from activated macrophages.[85] In this manner, PDGF may participate in angiogenesis and accelerate epithelialization in normal and pathologic wounds, including those of the horse cornea.[86] Furthermore, it stimulates the production of ECM components and increases collagenase activity by the wound fibroblast, in this manner enhancing remodeling. Finally, the role of PDGF in contraction remains unclear, although it does not appear to be direct.[87] To date, PDGF in its recombinant form is the only growth factor commercially available for use as a wound healing stimulant, in particular for the treatment of diabetic foot ulcers.[88]

Transforming Growth Factor-β

Transforming growth factor-β is widely acknowledged as the growth factor with the broadest range of activities in repair, on the basis of both the variety of cell types that produce or respond to it and the spectrum of its cellular responses.[89] It is an extensively investigated mediator: as of 2004, there were over 20,000 publications on TGF-β, and over 2000 articles have been published annually for the past 5 years.[90] In mammals, three isoforms of TGF-β are currently identified (TGF-β_1 to β_3), whose spatial and temporal distributions are specific. TGF-β_1 is the most abundant in the majority of tissues, and in platelets it is the only isoform.[89] The cDNA for equine TGF-β_1 has been cloned and sequenced; it exhibits 99% identity to mature human TGF-β_1.[91]

TGF-β can be synthesized and released from virtually all cell types participating in the repair process. A unique feature of this peptide is that it can regulate its own production by monocytes and activated macrophages in an autocrine manner.[89] This autoinduction results in a sustained expression at the wound site and extends the effectiveness of both the initial burst of endogenous TGF-β released upon injury and exogenous TGF-β that may be applied to a wound. Thus, this particular growth factor is ubiquitous during repair, when its major effects are to enhance chemoattraction of inflammatory and mesenchymal cells—in particular, fibroblasts—and to modulate the accumulation of ECM. In the former capacity, the effects of TGF-β are exacerbated by its influence on activated macrophages to secrete more TGF-β as well as other angiogenic and fibrogenic mediators. The effects of TGF-β on ECM are more complex and profound than those of any other cytokine, and they are central to increasing the maturation and strength of wounds. In addition to enhancing fibroblast migration to the site of repair, TGF-β regulates the transcription of a wide variety of ECM proteins.[89] Furthermore, it concurrently inhibits ECM turnover by inducing TIMPs and reducing MMP expression. These particular activities have earned TGF-β the nickname "fibrogenic" cytokine. Indeed, a cause-and-effect relationship has been established between TGF-β_1/β_2 and fibrosis, in various tissues.[92] TGF-β has also been found to promote angiogenesis by stimulating endothelial cell migration, differentiation, and tubule formation, as well as by upregulating their integrin receptors. The impact of TGF-β on epithelialization has not been completely elucidated, but it appears to favor epithelial cell migration. Finally, TGF-β_1 enhances wound contraction by inducing α-SMA expression in granulation tissue myofibroblasts.[93]

Because of the importance of cytokines in the repair process, we and others have recently examined their contribution to wound repair in the horse, particularly in relation to the development of proud flesh. It is now apparent that local concentrations of fibrogenic TGF-β_1 remain elevated throughout the proliferative phase of healing in limb wounds whereas they quickly return to baseline values in body wounds after resolution of acute inflammation.[46,94,95] Not surprisingly, we found that wound macrophages and fibroblasts seem responsible for this augmented synthesis.[96] Correspondingly, TGF-β receptors are abundant in limb wounds, particularly those developing proud flesh, which suggests that the signaling machinery for ECM synthesis is in place to contribute to fibrosis.[97] Finally, preliminary studies suggest that natural surgical and traumatic[98]—as well as experimental[99]—wounds healing with exuberant granulation tissue overexpress fibrogenic TGF-β_1 and underexpress antifibrogenic TGF-β_3.

Vascular Endothelial Growth Factor

Vascular endothelial growth factor, also known as vascular permeability factor, is a heparin-binding glycoprotein with potent and selective mitogenic, angiogenic, and permeability-enhancing effects on endothelial cells.[100] VEGF is expressed in a range of cells, predominantly macrophages, in response to soluble mediators, cell-bound stimuli, and environmental factors, and it binds to two endothelial cell-specific receptors. Expression is upregulated during early wound repair, in response to tissue hypoxia, and correlates with the density of granulation tissue developing within the wound. Although VEGF activity is considered essential to optimal wound angiogenesis via stimulation of ECM degradation, and via proliferation of, migration of, and tube formation by endothelial cells,[101] it is not critical to wound closure. Cloning of equine VEGF cDNA has been achieved.[102]

Cytokine Therapy

As mentioned several times, horses commonly manifest difficulty with the repair of wounds of the distal extremities; chronic wounds of either the exuberant or indolent type are particularly frustrating. Evidence supporting the role of an abnormal cytokine profile in the pathogenesis of these conditions is mounting,[46,94,95,98,99] and this has led investigators to manipulate the balance of these mediators in hopes of ameliorating the quality of repair. Although topical application of TGF-β_1 has proven valuable in rodent models of chronic, impaired wound healing, there were no beneficial effects on total amount of granulation tissue formation or the area of epithelialization when it was applied to full-thickness wounds of the distal limb in horses.[103] Promising, though preliminary, results have been obtained with the use of the antifibrogenic isoform, TGF-β_3, in a similar model, where healthy granulation tissue did not become exuberant despite the use of bandages.[104]

Because repair results from complex interactions among blood constituents, soluble mediators, cells, and ECM components, application of a single cytokine is unlikely to mimic natural processes and enhance repair unless impairment was caused by the relative lack of that specific mediator. In particular, timing and mode of application are important factors in clinical applications and remain ill-defined. A rich source of the complex group of growth factors essential to natural wound repair is the platelet α-granule.[105] Numerous studies have shown that platelet releasate substantially improves repair, probably through mediator synergism. A recent study suggests that this form of topical therapy may be beneficial in horse wounds as well.[106]

ELEMENTS INFLUENCING WOUND REPAIR

Endogenous

General Health Status

Wound healing is part of normal body maintenance and depends on the patient's general state of health. A debilitated horse heals more slowly than a healthy one, but the equine species is less commonly affected by diseases exerting a negative impact on repair (e.g., diabetes, hyperadrenocorticism, liver disease or uremia) than companion animals. Although protein intake is important in the recovery from severe injury, in particular burn wounds, nutrition is critical only at extremes. Indeed, serum protein must be less than 2 g/dL before wound repair is impeded in the form of slow gain in tensile strength.[107]

Blood Supply/Anemia/Local Oxygen Gradient

There is a strong correlation between the extent of wound repair and regional blood supply. A healing wound depends on local microcirculation to furnish necessary oxygen and other nutrients; therefore, anything that interferes with it inhibits wound repair. Although the normal microcirculation of equine skin is poorly described, it is common knowledge that wound repair is impaired in the distal limb where there is little tissue cover and a relatively poor vascular bed.[34] Interestingly, it has been determined by laser Doppler velocimetry that cutaneous blood flow and volume in the dorsal metacarpal area exceed those of skin at the thoracolumbar junction.[108] This apparent contradiction supports the notion that dermal repair is contingent on more than strictly cutaneous vasculature.

Hypovolemia is the major deterrent to wound repair in anemia, hemorrhage, and shock. Anemia itself does not delay wound repair if blood volume is normal, because low hemoglobin levels are compatible with normal healing. It is tissue oxygen tension, rather than content, that is critical. Oxygen is necessary for tissue metabolism, and, after trauma, for collagen synthesis. An oxygen gradient exists between the nearest functioning capillary and the wound edge. The oxygen tension near a wound capillary is between 60 and 90 mm Hg; however, near the advancing edge of granulation tissue, the oxygen tension approaches 0 mm Hg. This decrease is caused by the diffusion gradient and the consumption of oxygen by cells at the wound margin. Thus, the activities of the new fibroblasts (migration, proliferation, protein synthesis) depend on the rate at which new capillaries are formed, and thus wound tensile strength is limited by perfusion and tissue oxygen tension. Indeed, perfusion during the first postoperative days seems crucial to the outcome of repair, and it is probable that the difference in the accumulation of collagen on day 7 is already established during the early postoperative period.[109]

Although the normal wound environment is characterized by low levels of oxygen tension, hypoxia can be detrimental. On the one hand, cellular synthetic activity is increased by hypoxia, with preferential production of direct angiogenic substances such as VEGF and bFGF as well as indirect mediators such as PDGF and TGF-β. These favor further production of collagen and possibly excessive fibrosis as seen in the horse. On the other hand, hypoxia may be responsible for delayed wound repair by inducing an increase in MMP-1 synthesis, with subsequent excessive degradation of newly formed collagen. Although controversy surrounds the impact of hypoxia, it is certain that ischemic tissues heal poorly and are easily infected. It is thus advisable to select regional anesthesia over local injection of anesthetic agents, particularly those containing epinephrine, to avoid local vasoconstriction when exploring limb wounds during the initial management. Reflex vasoconstriction subsequent to low environmental temperatures is also blamed for delayed and weak repair. The temperature of the limb of the horse is noticeably less than that of the trunk, and this may have a role in the failure of limb wounds to heal as well as those on the trunk.[34]

Location

Horses frequently experience pronounced difficulty in repairing wounds on the lower extremities, whereas even extensive wounds of the trunk and head heal remarkably well. Specifically, delays in epithelialization and contraction, as well as the exuberant development of granulation tissue, commonly afflict full-thickness wounds of the distal limbs.[21,43] Mechanisms that cause problematic wound repair in the horse limb have yet to be elucidated, although several have been proposed. Better blood supply, a greater amount of adnexal structures, and the thinner epidermis covering the head and neck contribute to the more rapid and cosmetic repair occurring in these areas.[110] Furthermore, wounds to the extremities may be near bony prominences and highly mobile joints, and they have an absence of underlying musculature and more contamination compared with body wounds.[34,45]

Interestingly, a craniocaudal variation in granulation tissue formation has been reported in the rat and is attributed to differing mitotic activity of fibroblasts related to differences in availability of nutrients, hormones, growth factors, or mitotic inhibitors, or to variation in local temperaure.[22] Although an inherent difference between growth characteristics of trunk and limb fibroblasts was similarly believed to contribute to the development of exuberant granulation tissue in the horse, a study showed that fibroblasts isolated from the horse limb grow significantly more slowly than those of the trunk.[21]

Prompt repair relies profoundly on the acute inflammatory response to trauma, as any chronicity in this response retards repair and encourages the development of wounds of either an exuberant or an indolent nature, such as those afflicting extremities. The horse displays a deficient yet protracted inflammatory response compared with the pony, especially when wounds are located at the distal aspect of the limb.[10] Furthermore, leukocytes from ponies are better equipped to kill bacteria than are those of horses.[11] Several studies suggest that an imbalance between collagen synthesis and lysis causes the excessive fibrosis exhibited by limb wounds, and they show that the local cytokine profile is skewed in favor of fibrogenic mediators.[46,94,95,98] Deficient contraction has also been blamed for poor repair of limb wounds in horses, particularly in comparison with body wounds.[43] Although the innate contraction capacities of myofibroblasts from body and from limbs are similar, these cells are poorly arranged in chronic wounds of the limb, which may preclude efficient contractile activity.[43] Furthermore, environmental factors emanating from the inflammatory response to injury, such as cytokine profiles, may negatively affect contractility.[44]

Exogenous

Vitamins (A, E, and C) and Minerals (Zinc)

Vitamin A promotes a healthy integument and enhances immune function through beneficial actions on epithelium. With regard to wound repair, vitamin A exerts positive effects on epithelialization by facilitating cell migration and indirectly controlling cellular growth and differentiation. It also regulates expression of α-SMA in wound myofibroblasts, which may aid wound contraction.[111] Vitamin A deficiency is known to negatively influence neutrophil and macrophage maturation and function, which diminishes their migration from local capillaries into the wound bed, as well as phagocytosis and oxidative metabolism. These adverse effects may impair the inflammatory phase of repair. Furthermore, vitamin A deficiency is associated with production of immature fibroblasts, leading to faulty collagen synthesis and deposition.[112] Both oral and topical vitamin A supplementations mitigate compromised wound repair in animal models, but there is no evidence that administration of vitamin A alters the rate of normal repair.[113]

The physiologic effects of *vitamin E* are hypothesized to include antioxidant activity, promotion of optimal immune system function, protection of skin from radiation and excessive sunlight, and acceleration of repair of specific types of wounds. The beneficial effects of vitamin E on wounds (including direct effects on tissue repair and regeneration and indirect effects on immune function) may go beyond the effects of a simple antioxidant.

Physiologic functions associated with *vitamin C* arise from its ability to act as a reducing agent that balances the potentially harmful byproducts released in oxidative reactions in the body. Vitamin C influences tissue repair and regeneration, in particular with respect to the synthesis of connective tissue. Along with iron it acts as a cofactor for enzymes involved during hydroxylation of proline and lysine in the production of collagen and also during cross-linking of mature collagen. Both of these are critical to the proliferative and remodeling phases of repair. Vitamin C also promotes fibroblast formation, upregulates collagen gene expression, and enhances the biosynthesis of other substances important to wound repair and regeneration, including fibronectin and proteoglycans. Finally, the level of vitamin C in leukocytes is important for phagocytic functions relevant to control of bacteria in wounds.

Zinc is involved in the synthesis or activation of numerous enzymes—in particular, metalloenzymes. It is critical to DNA and RNA synthesis and consequently plays a significant role in wound repair, particularly in the later phases when fibroblast proliferation and collagen synthesis are required.[114] During the initial inflammatory phase of repair, zinc concentrations transiently fall; in contrast, the amount of bioavailable zinc in the blood and wound bed rises during the later phases of repair, when concentrations are 15% to 20% higher than those found in intact skin. Although the precise task of zinc in tissue repair and regeneration is not yet known, it is hypothesized to play a significant role in the synthesis of granulation and scar tissue, as well as in epithelialization. Zinc also exerts an anti-inflammatory effect on phagocytic cells, important to late repair and closure. On the other hand, high concentrations of zinc may be detrimental to repair for the same reason. Zinc deficiency adversely affects inflammatory cells. Studies in both animal models and humans demonstrate that zinc deficiency is associated with an increased risk for chronic wounds.[115]

Nonsteroidal Anti-inflammatory Drugs

Selective inhibition of either cyclooxygenase (COX)-1 (constitutive) or COX-2 (induced by lipopolysaccharide, nitric oxide, and various cytokines) is the basis for the mechanism of action of nonsteroidal anti-inflammatory drugs (NSAIDs). The activity of these rate-limiting enzymes on membrane-derived arachidonic acid generates various eicosanoids, which mediate inflammation and induce fibroblast proliferation and collagen production. COX-2 is the predominant isoform in all stages of the inflammatory response, and its upregulation is accountable for persistent inflammation because the reaction products are responsible for many of the cytotoxic effects of inflammation.[116]

Inflammation protects against infection and is a precursor to the subsequent proliferative phase of repair through the action of macrophage-generated mediators that initiate migration and proliferation of the mesenchymal cells involved in angiogenesis, fibroplasia, and epithelialization. Consequently, controversy surrounds the use of NSAIDs in the early period after trauma, when the normal inflammatory response should not be inhibited. For example, high doses of NSAIDs administered immediately after creation of linea alba incisions in ponies delayed repair,[117] and suppression of inflammation by COX-2 inhibition reduced the extent of granulation/scar tissue without compromising tensile properties of mouse wounds.[118] Although NSAIDs appear to have little effect on the ultimate course or quality of repair when dispensed in pharmacologic doses, selective anti-inflammatory agents, such as COX-2 inhibitors, can be fine-tuned to suppress the imbalances of inflammation, thus leading to a more ideal healing response.

In contrast, chronic inflammation is characterized by excess and persistent neutrophil and macrophage activity and may forestall the normal repair sequence, leading to a number of diseases typified by disproportionate scarring. In these cases, NSAIDs, especially COX-2 selective inhibitors, may be effective in the prevention of excessive scarring.

Corticosteroids

Regardless of the tissue implicated, topical and systemic administration of corticosteroids appears to retard wound repair, depending on the specific glucocorticoid involved and the timing, concentration, and duration of therapy.[119] Cortisone stabilizes lysosomal membranes and consequently inhibits the normal inflammatory response to trauma. This leads to a delay in repair, although ultimate wound strength does not seem affected. Other mechanisms whereby glucocorticoids may alter various phases of repair include angiostasis,[120] decreased rate of fibroblast proliferation with consequent inhibition of protein synthesis, possibly through downregulation of fibrogenic TGF-β[121] and inhibition of KGF production in fibroblasts, which may impair epithelialization.[122]

Traumatic wounds in the distal extremities of horses appear predisposed to an excessive fibroblastic response, leading to the development of proud flesh. Because corticosteroids limit proliferation of both fibroblasts and endothelial cells, topical application may be beneficial in this particular situation. Indeed, glucocorticoids are used extensively by equine practitioners in the treatment of wounds, with mostly favorable results.[123] However, one application at the first sign of excessive fibroplasia is all that is needed—continued application may exert negative effects on wound contraction and epithelialization.

Bandages

Second-intention wound repair depends on contraction and epithelialization. Any therapy that accelerates either of these mechanisms would be a desirable adjunct to the management of wounds in the horse, particularly those located at the distal aspect of the limb and complicated by excessive fibroplasia and subsequent poor strength and cosmetic appearance. Although moist wound healing, such as that occurring under semiocclusive and fully occlusive synthetic dressings, favors rapid epithelialization and cosmetic repair in other species, it has been shown to encourage excessive growth of granulation tissue and delay subsequent repair when applied to wounds located on the distal limb in the horse.[99,124,125] An exception is the nonadherent and fully occlusive silicone dressing that we have recently shown to prevent the formation of exuberant granulation tissue and improve tissue quality in repairing limb wounds of horses.[25] Various semiocclusive biologic dressings are available for use in the horse, such as amnion, allogeneic skin, peritoneal grafts, and porcine small intestinal or urinary bladder submucosa.[38] To date, the only one of these showing beneficial effects when used on granulating limb wounds or grafts sites is species-specific amnion dressing.[126,127] For more details on bandaging and wound management see Chapter 26.

REFERENCES

1. Lipowitz AJ: Tissue regeneration. In Slatter DH, editor: Textbook of Small Animal Surgery, vol 1, Philadelphia, 1985, WB Saunders.
2. Wilmink JM, van Herten J, van Weeren PR, et al: Retrospective study of primary intention healing and sequestrum formation in horses compared to ponies under clinical circumstances, Equine Vet J 2002;34:270.
3. Singer AJ, Clark RAF: Cutaneous wound healing, N Engl J Med 1999;341:738-746.
4. Simpson DM, Ross R: The neutrophilic leukocyte in wound repair: A study with antineutrophil serum, J Clin Invest 1972;51:2009.
5. Leibovitch SJ, Ross R: The role of the macrophage in wound repair: A study with hydrocortisone and antimacrophage serum, Am J Pathol 1975;78:71.
6. Martin P, D'Souza D, Martin J, et al: Wound healing in the PU.1 null mouse: Tissue repair is not dependent on inflammatory cells, Curr Biol 2003;13:1122.
7. Smith PD, Kuhn MA, Franz MG, et al: Initiating the inflammatory phase of incisional healing prior to tissue injury, J Surg Res 2000;92:11.
8. Molan PC: The role of honey in the management of wounds, J Wound Care 1999;8:415.
9. Swaim SF, Bohling MW: Mise au point sur les récents développements en gestion de plaies chez les animaux de compagnie. Med Vet QC 2003;33:99.
10. Wilmink JM, van Weeren PR, Stolk PW, et al: Differences in second-intention wound healing between horses and ponies: Histological aspects, Equine Vet J 1999;31:61.
11. Wilmink JM, Veenman JN, van den Boom R, et al: Differences in polymorphonucleocyte function and local inflammatory response between horses and ponies, Equine Vet J 2003;35:561.

12. Wilson DA, Adelstein EH, Keegan KG, et al: In vitro and in vivo effects of activated macrophage supernatant on distal limb wounds of ponies, Am J Vet Res 1996;57:1220.
13. Wilmink JM, Stolk PW, van Weeren PR, et al: The effectiveness of the haemodialysate Solcoseryl for second-intention wound healing in horses and ponies, J Vet Med A Physiol Pathol Clin Med 2000;47:311.
14. Engelen M, Besche B, Lefay MP, et al: Effects of ketanserin on hypergranulation tissue formation, infection, and healing of equine lower limb wounds, Can Vet J 2004;45:144.
15. Greenhalgh DG: The role of apoptosis in wound healing, Int J Biochem Cell Biol 1998;30:1019.
16. Mignatti P, Rifkin DB, Welgus HG, et al: Proteinases and tissue remodeling. In Clark RAF, editor: The Molecular and Cellular Biology of Wound Repair, ed 2, New York, 1996, Plenum Press.
17. Desmoulière A, Redard M, Darby I, et al: Apoptosis mediates the decrease in cellularity during the transition between granulation tissue and scar, Am J Pathol 1995;146:56.
18. Luo S, Benathan M, Raffoul W, et al: Abnormal balance between proliferation and apoptotic cell death in fibroblasts derived from keloid lesions. Plast Reconstr Surg 2001;107:87.
19. Chvapil M, Pfister T, Escalada S, et al: Dynamics of the healing of skin wounds in the horse as compared with the rat, Exp Mol Pathol 1979;30:349.
20. Jacobs KA, Leach DH, Fretz PB, et al: Comparative aspects of the healing of excisional wounds on the leg and body of horses, Vet Surg 1984;13:83.
21. Bacon Miller C, Wilson DA, Keegan KG, et al: Growth characteristics of fibroblasts isolated from the trunk and distal aspect of the limb of horses and ponies, Vet Surg 2000;29:1.
22. Martson M, Viljanto J, Laippala P, et al: Cranio-caudal differences in granulation tissue formation: An experimental study in the rat, Wound Repair Regen 1999;7:119.
23. Sayah DN, Soo C, Shaw WW, et al: Downregulation of apoptosis-related genes in keloid tissues, J Surg Res 1999;87:209.
24. Lepault É, Céleste CJ, Doré M, et al: Comparative study on microvascular occlusion and apoptosis in normal and pathologic wounds in the horse, Wound Repair Regen 2004 [submitted].
25. Ducharme-Desjarlais M, Céleste CJ, Lepault É et al: Effect of a silicone-containing dressing on exuberant granulation tissue formation and wound repair in the horse, Am J Vet Res 2005 [in press].
26. Liekens S, De Clerq E, Neyts J: Angiogenesis: Regulators and clinical applications, Biochem Pharmacol 2001;61:253.
27. Li J, Zhang YP, Kirsner RS: Angiogenesis in wound repair: Angiogenic growth factors and the extracellular matrix, Microsc Res Tech 2003;60:107.
28. Zhu WH, Guo X, Villaschi S, et al: Regulation of vascular growth and regression by matrix metalloproteinases in the rat aorta model of angiogenesis, Lab Invest 2000;80:545.
29. Falanga V: Chronic wounds: Pathophysiologic and experimental considerations, J Invest Dermatol 1993;100:721.
30. Stenn KS, Malhotra R: Epithelialization. In Cohen IK, Diegelmann RF, Lindblad WJ, editors: Wound Healing: Biochemical and Clinical Aspects, Philadelphia, 1992, WB Saunders.
31. Stashak TS: Chapter 1. In Stashak TS, editor: Equine Wound Management, Philadelphia, 1991, Lea & Febiger.
32. Nanney LB, King LE: Epidermal growth factor and transforming growth factor-α. In Clark RAF, editor: The Molecular and Cellular Biology of Wound Repair, ed 2, New York, 1996, Plenum Press.
33. LePoole IC, Boyce ST: Keratinocytes suppress TGF-β1 expression by fibroblasts in cultured skin substitutes, Br J Dermatol 1999;140:409.
34. Knottenbelt DC: Equine wound management: Are there significant differences in healing at different sites on the body? Vet Dermatol 1997;8:273.
35. Dart AJ, Cries L, Jeffcott LB, et al: Effects of 25% propylene glycol hydrogel (Solugel) on second intention wound healing in horses, Vet Surg 2002;31:309.
36. Burling K, Seguin MA, Marsh P, et al: Effect of topical administration of epidermal growth factor on healing of corneal epithelial defects in horses, Am J Vet Res 2000;61:1150.
37. Yvorchuk-St. Jean K, Gaughan E, St. Jean G, et al: Evaluation of a porous bovine collagen membrane bandage for management of wounds in horses, Am J Vet Res 1995;56:1663.
38. Gomez JH, Schumacher J, Lauten SD, et al: Effects of 3 biologic dressings on healing of cutaneous wounds on the limbs of horses, Can J Vet Res 2004;68:49.
39. Desmoulière A, Gabbiani G: The role of the myofibroblast in wound healing and fibrocontractive diseases. In Clark RAF, editor: The Molecular and Cellular Biology of Wound Repair, ed 2, New York, 1996, Plenum Press.
40. Madison JB, Gronwall RR: Influence of wound shape on wound contraction in horses, Am J Vet Res 1992;53:1575.
41. Ford TS, Schumacher J, Brumbaugh GW, et al: Effects of split-thickness and full-thickness grafts on secondary graft contraction in horses, Am J Vet Res 1992;53:1572.
42. Grinnell F, Zhu M, Carlson MA, et al: Release of mechanical tension triggers apoptosis of human fibroblasts in a model of regressing granulation tissue, Exp Cell Res 1999;248:608.
43. Wilmink JM, Stolk PW, Van Weeren PR, et al: Differences in second-intention wound healing between horses and ponies: Macroscopic aspects, Equine Vet J 1999;31:53.
44. Wilmink JM, Nederbragt H, van Weeren PR, et al: Differences in wound contraction between horses and ponies: The in vitro contraction capacity of fibroblasts, Equine Vet J 2001;33:499.
45. Cochrane CA, Pain R, Knottenbelt DC: In vitro wound contraction in the horse: Differences between body and limb wounds, Wounds 2003;15:175.
46. Schwartz AJ, Wilson DA, Keegan KG, et al: Factors regulating collagen synthesis and degradation during second-intention healing of wounds in the thoracic region and the distal aspect of the forelimb of horses, Am J Vet Res 2002;63:1564.
47. Dart AJ, Cries L, Jeffcott LB, et al: The effect of equine recombinant growth hormone on second intention wound healing in horses, Vet Surg 2002;31:314.
48. Witte MB, Thornton FJ, Kiyama T, et al: Metalloproteinase inhibitors and wound healing: A novel enhancer of wound strength, Surgery 1998;124:464.
49. Yager DR, Chen SM, Ward SI, et al: Ability of chronic wound fluids to degrade peptide growth factors is associated with increased levels of elastase activity and diminished levels of proteinase inhibitors, Wound Repair Regen 1997;5:23.
50. Levenson SM, Geever EF, Crowley LV, et al: The healing of rat skin wounds, Ann Surg 1965;161:293.
51. Metcalf D: The granulocyte-macrophage colony stimulating factors, Science 1985;229:16.
52. Mann A, Breuhahn K, Schirmacher P, et al: Keratinocyte-derived granulocyte-macrophage colony stimulating factor accelerates wound healing: Stimulation of keratinocyte proliferation, granulation tissue formation, and vascularization, J Invest Dermatol 2001;117:1382.
53. Mauel S, Commandeur U, Steinbach F: Cloning of equine granulocyte-macrophage colony-stimulating-factor (eq. GM-CSF), Direct submission to GenBank (AAK72108).
54. Leonard WJ: Type I cytokines and interferons and their receptors. In Paul WE, editor: Fundamental Immunology, ed 4, New York, 1999, Lippincott-Raven Press.
55. Curran JA, Argyle DJ, Cox P, et al: Nucleotide sequence of the equine interferon gamma cDNA, DNA Seq 1994;4:405.
56. Steinbach F, Mauel S, Beier I: Recombinant equine interferons: Expression cloning and biological activity, Vet Immunol Immunopathol 2002;84:83.
57. Ishida Y, Kondo T, Takayasu T, et al: The essential involvement of cross-talk between IFN-gamma and TGF-beta in the skin wound-healing process, J Immunol 2004;172:1848.
58. Howard RD, McIlwraith CW, Trotter GW, Nyborg JK: Cloning of

equine interleukin 1 alpha and equine interleukin 1 beta and determination of their full-length cDNA sequences, Am J Vet Res 1998;59:704.
59. Howard RD, McIlwraith CW, Trotter GW, Nyborg JK: Cloning of equine interleukin 1 receptor antagonist and determination of its full-length cDNA sequence, Am J Vet Res 1998;59:712.
60. Lin ZQ, Kondo T, Ishida Y, et al: Essential involvement of IL-6 in the skin wound-healing process as evidenced by delayed wound healing in IL-6-deficient mice, J Leukoc Biol 2003;73:713,
61. Mori R, Kondo T, Ohshima T, et al: MMP-1 and TIMP-1 mRNA expression were markedly increased with IL-6 and TNF-alpha treatment and remains unchanged with IL-1 beta, Burns 2003;29:527.
62. Moyer KE, Saggers GC, Allison GM, et al: Effects of interleukin-8 on granulation tissue maturation, J Cell Physiol 2002;193:173.
63. Moroguchi A, Ishimura K, Okano K, et al: Interleukin-10 suppresses proliferation and remodeling of extracellular matrix of cultured human skin fibroblasts, Eur Surg Res 2004;36:39.
64. Su X, Deem Morris D, McGraw RA: Cloning and characterization of gene TNFα encoding equine tumor necrosis factor alpha, Gene 1991;107:319.
65. Igarashi A, Okochi H, Bradham DM, et al: Regulation of connective tissue growth factor gene expression in human skin fibroblasts and during wound repair, Mol Biol Cell 1993;4:637.
66. Grotendorst GR: Connective tissue growth factor: A mediator of TGF-β action on fibroblasts, Cytokine Growth Factor Rev 1997;8:171.
67. Blom IE, Goldschmeding R, Leask A: Gene regulation of connective tissue growth factor: new targets for antifibrotic therapy? Matrix Biol 2002;21:473.
68. Ollivier FJ, Brooks DE, Schultz GS, et al: Connective tissue growth factor in tear film of the horse: Detection, identification and origin, Graefes Arch Clin Exp Ophthalmol 2004;242:165, Epub Nov 28, 2003.
69. Haase I, Evans R, Pofahl R, et al: Regulation of keratinocyte shape, migration and wound epithelialization by IGF-1- and EGF-dependent signalling pathways, J Cell Sci 2003;116:3227.
70. Stewart F, Power CA, Lennard SN, et al: Identification of the horse epidermal growth factor (EGF) coding sequence and its use in monitoring EGF gene expression in the endometrium of the pregnant mare, J Mol Endocrinol 1994;12:341.
71. Ono M, Okamuro K, Nakayama Y, et al: Induction of human microvascular endothelial tubular morphogenesis by human keratinocytes: Involvement of transforming growth factor-alpha, Biochem Biophys Res Commun 1992;189:601.
72. Sorensen OE, Cowland JB, Theilgaard-Monch K, et al: Wound healing and expression of antimicrobial peptides/polypeptides in human keratinocytes: A consequence of common growth factors, J Immunol 2003;170:5583.
73. Abraham JA, Klagsbrun M: Modulation of wound repair by members of the fibroblast growth factor family. In Clark RAF, editor: The Molecular and Cellular Biology of Wound Repair, ed 2, New York, 1996, Plenum Press.
74. Kuwabara K, Ogawa S, Matsumoto M, et al: Hypoxia-mediated induction of acidic/basic fibroblast growth factor and platelet-derived growth factor in mononuclear phagocytes stimulates growth of hypoxic endothelial cells, Proc Natl Acad Sci U S A 1995;92:4606.
75. Taylor WR, Alexander RW: Autocrine control of wound repair by insulin-like growth factor 1 in cultured endothelial cells, Am J Physiol 1993;265:C801.
76. Ando H, Jensen PJ: EGF and IGF-1 enhance keratinocyte migration, J Invest Dermatol 1993;100:633.
77. Dunaiski V, Belford DA: Contribution of circulating IGF-I to wound repair in GH-treated rats, Growth Horm IGF Res 2002;12:381.
78. Ghahary A, Shen Q, Shen YJ, et al: Induction of transforming growth factor beta 1 by insulin-like growth factor-1 in dermal fibroblasts, J Cell Physiol 1998;174:301.
79. Otte K, Rozell B, Gessbo A, Engstrom W: Cloning and sequencing of an equine insulin-like growth factor I cDNA and its expression in fetal and adult tissues, Gen Comp Endocrinol 1996;102:11.
80. Beer HD, Gassmann MG, Munz B, et al: Expression and function of keratinocyte growth factor and activin in skin morphogenesis and cutaneous wound repair, J Invest Dermatol Symp Proc 2000;5:34.
81. Werner S: Keratinocyte growth factor: A unique player in epithelial repair processes, Cytokine Growth Factor Rev 1998;9:153.
82. Robson MC, Phillips TJ, Falanga V, et al: Randomized trial of topically applied repifermin (recombinant human keratinocyte growth factor-2) to accelerate wound healing in venous ulcers, Wound Repair Regen 2001;9:347.
83. Welter H., Bollwein H, Einspanier R: Direct submission to GenBank (AJ439891) for *Equus caballus* FGF-7, 2002.
84. Heldin CH, Westermark B: Role of platelet-derived growth factor in vivo. In Clark RAF, editor: The Molecular and Cellular Biology of Wound Repair, ed 2, New York, 1996, Plenum Press.
85. Pierce GF, Vande Berg J, Rudolph R, et al: Platelet-derived growth factor-BB and transforming growth factor beta 1 selectively modulate glycosaminoglycans, collagen, and myofibroblasts in excisional wounds, Am J Pathol 1991;138:629.
86. Haber M, Cao Z, Panjwani N, et al: Effects of growth factors (EGF, PDGF-BB and TGF-beta 1) on cultured equine epithelial cells and keratocytes: implications for wound healing, Vet Ophthalmol 2003;6:211.
87. Saba AA, Freedman BM, Gaffield JW, et al: Topical platelet-derived growth factor enhances wound closure in the absence of wound contraction: An experimental and clinical study, Ann Plast Surg 2002;49:62.
88. Wieman TJ, Smiell JM, Su Y: Efficacy and safety of a topical gel formulation of recombinant human platelet-derived growth factor-BB (becaplermin) in patients with nonhealing diabetic ulcers: A phase III randomised, placebo-controlled, double-blind study, Diabetes Care 1998;21:822.
89. Roberts AB, Sporn MB: Transforming growth factor-β. In Clark RAF, editor: The Molecular and Cellular Biology of Wound Repair, ed 2, New York, 1996, Plenum Press.
90. Chin D, Boyle GM, Parsons PG, et al: What is transforming growth factor-beta (TGF-beta)? Br J Plast Surg 2004;57:215.
91. Penha-Goncalves MN, Onions DE, Nicolson L: Cloning and sequencing of equine transforming growth factor-beta 1 (TGF beta-1) cDNA, DNA Seq 1997;7:375.
92. Shah M, Foreman DM, Ferguson MWJ: Neutralization of TGF-β1 and TGF-β2 or exogenous addition of TGF-β3 to cutaneous rat wounds reduces scarring, J Cell Sci 1995;108:985.
93. Desmoulière A, Geinoz A, Gabbiani F, et al: Transforming growth factor β1 induces α-smooth muscle actin expression in granulation tissue myofibroblasts in quiescent and growing cultured fibroblasts, J Cell Biol 1993;122:103.
94. Theoret CL, Barber SM, Moyana TN, et al: Expression of transforming growth factor β1, β3, and basic fibroblast growth factor in full-thickness skin wounds of equine limbs and thorax, Vet Surg 2001;30:269.
95. van den Boom R, Wilmink JM, O'Kane S, et al: Transforming growth factor-beta levels during second-intention healing are related to the different course of wound contraction in horses and ponies, Wound Repair Regen 2002;10:188.
96. Theoret CL, Barber SM, Gordon JR: Temporal localization of immunoreactive transforming growth factor β1 in normal equine skin and in full-thickness dermal wounds, Vet Surg 2002;31:274.
97. De Martin I, Theoret CL: Spatial and temporal expression of types I and II receptors for transforming growth factor β in normal equine skin and dermal wounds, Vet Surg 2004;33:70.
98. Cochrane CA: Models in vivo of wound healing in the horse and the role of growth factors, Vet Dermatol 1997;8:259.
99. Theoret CL, Barber SM, Moyana TN, et al: Preliminary observations on expression of transforming growth factor β1, β3, and basic fibroblast growth factor in equine limb wounds healing normally or with proud flesh, Vet Surg 2002;31:266.

100. Dvorak HF, Brown LF, Betmar M, et al: Vascular permeability factor/vascular endothelial growth factor, microvascular hyperpermeability, and angiogenesis, Am J Pathol 1995;146:1029.
101. Howdieshell TR, Callaway D, Webb WL, et al: Antibody neutralization of vascular endothelial growth factor inhibits wound granulation tissue formation, J Surg Res 2001;96:173.
102. Miura N, Misumi K, Kawahara K, et al: Cloning of cDNA and high-level expression of equine vascular endothelial growth factor, Direct submission to GenBank (BAB20890).
103. Steel CM, Robertson ID, Thomas J, et al: Effect of topical rh-TGF-β1 on second intention wound healing in horses, Austr Vet J 1999;77:734.
104. Ohnemusl P, von Rechenberg BV, Arvinte T, et al: Application of TGF-β3 on experimentally created circular wounds in horses. In Proceedings of the 8th Annual Scientific Meeting of the European Congress of Veterinary Surgeons, 1999;28:216.
105. Crovetti G, Martinelli G, Issi M, et al: Platelet gel for healing cutaneous chronic wounds, Transfus Apheresis Sci 2004;30:145.
106. Carter CA, Jolly DG, Worden CE, et al: Platelet-rich plasma gel promotes differentiation and regeneration during equine wound healing, Exp Mol Pathol 2003;74:244.
107. Peacock EE: Wound Repair, ed 3, Philadelphia, 1984, WB Saunders.
108. Manning TO, Monteiro-Riviere NA, Bristol DG, et al: Cutaneous laser-Doppler velocimetry in nine animal species, Am J Vet Res 1991;52:1960.
109. Hartmann M, Jonsson K, Zederfeldt B: Effect of tissue perfusion and oxygenation on accumulation of collagen in healing wounds, Eur J Surg 1992;158:521.
110. Moy LS: Management of acute wounds, Dermatol Clin 1993;11:759.
111. Xu G, Bochaton-Piallat ML, Andreutti D, et al: Regulation of alpha-smooth muscle actin and CRBP-1 expression by retinoic acid and TGF-beta in cultured fibroblasts, J Cell Physiol 2001;187:315.
112. Varani J, Warner RL, Gharaee-Kermani M, et al: Vitamin A antagonizes decreased cell growth and elevated collagen-degrading matrix metalloproteinases and stimulates collagen accumulation in naturally aged human skin, J Invest Dermatol 2000;114:480.
113. Gray M: Evidence-based report card from the Center for Clinical Investigation: Does oral supplementation with vitamins A or E promote healing of chronic wounds? J Wound Ostomy Continence Nurs 2003;30:290.
114. Lansdown AB: Zinc in the healing wound, Lancet 1996;347:706.
115. Gray M: Evidence-Based Report Card from the Center for Clinical Investigation: Does oral zinc supplementation promote healing of chronic wounds? J Wound Ostomy Continence Nurs 2003;30:295.
116. Abd-El-Aleem SA, Ferguson MWJ, Appleton I, et al: Expression of cyclooxygenase isoforms in normal human skin and chronic venous ulcers, J Pathol 2001;195:616.
117. Schneiter HL, McClure JR, Cho DY, et al: The effects of flunixin meglumine on early wound healing of abdominal incisions in ponies, Vet Surg 16:101 (abstr).
118. Wilgus TA, Vodovotz Y, Vittadini E, et al: Reduction of scar formation in full-thickness wounds with topical celecoxib treatment, Wound Repair Regen 2003;11:25.
119. Marks JG Jr, Cano C, Leitzel K, et al: Inhibition of wound healing by topical steroids, Dermatol Surg Oncol 1983;9:819.
120. Hashimoto I, Nakanishi H, Shono Y, et al: Angiostatic effects of corticosteroid on wound healing of the rabbit ear, J Med Invest 2002;49:61.
121. Beck LS, Deguzman L, Lee WP, et al: TGF-beta 1 accelerates wound healing: Reversal of steroid-impaired healing in rats and rabbits, Growth Factors 1991;5:295.
122. Chedid M, Hoyle JR, Csaky KG, et al: Glucocorticoids inhibit keratinocyte growth factor production in primary dermal fibroblasts, Endocrinology 1996;137:2232.
123. Barber SM: Second intention wound healing in the horse: the effect of bandages and topical corticosteroids, Proc Am Assoc Equine Pract 1990;35:107.
124. Howard RD, Stashak TS, Baxter GM: Evaluation of occlusive dressings for management of full-thickness excisional wounds on the distal portion of the limbs of horses, Am J Vet Res 1993;54:2150.
125. Berry DB, Sullins KE: Effects of topical application of antimicrobials and bandaging on healing and granulation tissue formation in wounds of the distal aspect of the limbs in horses, Am J Vet Res 2003;64:88.
126. Bigbie RB, Schumacher J, Swaim SF, et al: Effects of amnion and live yeast cell derivative on second-intention healing in horses, Am J Vet Res 1991;52:1376.
127. Goodrich LR, Moll HD, Crisman MV, et al: Comparison of equine amnion and a nonadherent wound dressing material for bandaging pinch-grafted wounds in ponies, Am J Vet Res 2000;61:326.

CHAPTER 6

Metabolism and Nutritional Support of the Surgical Patient

Elizabeth A. Carr

In the last two decades, a tremendous advancement in the care and treatment of the critically ill equine patient has taken place. Survival rates from colic surgery have increased, and large-animal intensive care units are found in most, if not all, major university hospitals and referral practices across the United States and most of Europe. Critical to this success is presurgical evaluation and patient triage. The physical examination data as well as laboratory and diagnostic information are carefully collected and analyzed to determine the severity of the disease process. Any underlying abnormalities and any metabolic derangements that may affect the outcome negatively are carefully determined. Patients may receive fluids, anti-inflammatories, colloids, oxygen insufflation, and other medications prior to anesthesia to ensure that a hemodynamically and metabolically stable patient is taken to the induction stall. The surgical technique is designed to minimize trauma, resolve the underlying problem, and keep postoperative complications at a minimum. After recovery, the patient may be continued on intravenous fluids to maintain hydration, as well as other therapeutics to minimize or prevent postoperative complications, including ileus, pain, and infection, and to maximize the chance of recovery. Despite this proactive approach to treatment and support of adult equine patients, rarely is their nutritional status considered in the initial therapeutic plan. Preoperative and postoperative nutritional status and nutritional support are clearly linked to morbidity and mortality in humans.[1,2] Malnutrition has been shown to negatively impact survival, immune function, wound healing, and gastrointestinal function, and it probably negatively affects numerous other processes.[2-6]

This chapter will discuss the metabolic consequences of food deprivation, the pathologic metabolic responses to illness, nutritional requirements in health and disease, and the indications for and types of nutritional supplementation.

INDICATIONS FOR NUTRITIONAL SUPPORT

The need for interventional nutritional support depends on a number of factors. The healthy adult horse that is undergoing elective surgery and has a body condition score of 4 or 5 (out of 9) rarely requires nutritional supplementation (Box 6-1). These individuals can easily tolerate food deprivation for 48 hours. The majority of healthy adult horses undergoing elective surgery have food withheld for a period of 6 to 12 hours preoperatively, and it is reintroduced after recovery when the animal is deemed capable of eating and swallowing effectively. During this period of starvation, energy demands are met by glycogen reserves, with little effect on overall metabolism.

Regardless of the type and complexity of the surgical procedure, nutritional support should be considered in patients with an increased metabolic rate (e.g., young growing animals), individuals presenting with a prior history of malnutrition or hypophagia, patients with underlying metabolic abnormalities that could worsen with food deprivation, and individuals with disorders such as severe trauma, sepsis, or strangulating bowel obstruction that result in an increased energy demand. Underweight horses require nutritional support earlier. Obese or overconditioned individuals, particularly pony breeds, miniature horses, and donkeys, as well as lactating mares are at risk for developing hyperlipemia and should receive nutritional support if their serum triglycerides are higher than normal values. Older horses, or individuals diagnosed with equine Cushing's syndrome and the more recently described peripheral Cushing's syndrome, are insulin resistant and at greater risk for developing hyperlipemia and fatty infiltration of the liver. If food deprivation is prolonged or there is a concern regarding the individual's desire or ability to eat, early intervention is indicated to prevent more severe malnutrition.

BOX 6-1. Body Condition Score

1. Poor: Animal extremely emaciated. Spinous processes, ribs, tailhead, hooks, and pins projecting prominently. Bone structure of withers, shoulders, and neck easily noticeable. No fatty tissue can be felt.
2. Very thin: Animal emaciated. Slight fat covering over base of spinous processes, transverse processes of lumbar vertebrae feel rounded. Spinous processes, ribs, tailhead, and hooks and pins prominent. Withers, shoulders, and neck structures faintly discernible.
3. Thin: Fat buildup about half way on spinous processes, transverse processes cannot be felt. Slight fat cover over ribs. Spinous processes and ribs easily discernible. Tailhead prominent, but individual vertebrae cannot be visually identified. Hook bones appear rounded but easily discernible. Pin bones not distinguishable. Withers, shoulder, and neck accentuated.
4. Moderately thin: Negative crease along back. Faint outline of ribs discernible. Tailhead prominence depends on conformation; fat can be felt around it. Hook bones not discernible. Withers, shoulders, and neck not obviously thin.
5. Moderate: Back level. Ribs cannot be visually distinguished but can be easily felt. Fat around tailhead beginning to feel spongy. Withers appear rounded over spinous processes. Shoulders and neck blend smoothly into body.
6. Moderate to fleshy: May have slight crease down back. Fat over ribs feels spongy. Fat around tailhead feels soft. Fat beginning to be deposited along the sides of withers, behind the shoulders, and along the sides of the neck.
7. Fleshy: May have crease down back. Individual ribs can be felt, noticeable filling between ribs with fat. Fat around tailhead is soft. Fat deposited along withers, behind shoulders, and along the neck.
8. Fat: Crease down back. Difficult to feel ribs. Fat around tailhead very soft. Area along withers filled with fat. Area behind shoulder filled in flush. Noticeable thickening of neck. Fat deposited along inner buttocks.
9. Extremely fat: Obvious crease down back. Patch fat appearing over ribs. Bulging fat around tailhead along withers, behind shoulders, and along neck. Fat along inner buttocks may rub together. Flank filled in flush.

Scoring is based on visual appraisal and handling (particularly in scoring horses with long hair).

PURE PROTEIN/CALORIE MALNUTRITION

The average, healthy adult horse can easily tolerate food deprivation (pure protein/calorie malnutrition [PPCM] or simple starvation) for 24 to 72 hours with little systemic effect. A decline in blood glucose concentration occurs with food deprivation, insulin levels fall, and energy demands are initially met via glycogenolysis, resulting in an increase in the breakdown of liver glycogen stores. As starvation progresses, glycogen is mobilized from other tissues, including muscle. Lipid mobilization is triggered by alterations in insulin or glucagon levels and the activity of hormone-sensitive lipase. As glucose becomes limited, many body tissues begin to rely on fatty acid oxidation and the production of ketone bodies as energy sources. Glycerol produced from lipid degradation, lactate from the Krebs cycle, and amino acids from muscle tissue breakdown continue to be utilized for gluconeogenesis to provide energy to glucose-dependent tissues (central nervous system and red blood cells). This response to starvation correlates with an increase in circulating levels of growth hormone, glucagon, epinephrine, leptin, and cortisol and a decrease in insulin and thyroid hormones. These hormone fluxes are an afferent stimulus for the hypothalamic response to starvation resulting in an increased drive to eat and a decrease in energy expenditure. Metabolism slows in an effort to conserve body fuels, and the body survives primarily on fat stores, sparing lean tissue.

Individuals with preexisting PPCM are at a disadvantage when intake is restricted because of surgery or illness. In the malnourished or cachectic human patient, presurgical nutritional supplementation has been shown to positively influence both survival and morbidity. Early nutritional supplementation should be strongly considered in animals presenting with preexisting PPCM.

METABOLIC RESPONSE TO INJURY

The metabolic response to injury (e.g., surgical manipulation, critical illness, sepsis, trauma), unlike the response to PPCM, is characterized by an increased metabolism and the onset of a catabolic process leading to excessive breakdown of tissue proteins. This metabolic state is the result of a complex interaction of inflammatory cytokines (interleukin [IL]-1, IL-2, IL-6, tumor necrosis factor [TNF]-α, and γ-interferon; see Chapter 2) released at the site of injury or inflammation, circulating hormones released in response to stress and injury (hypothalamic-pituitary-adrenal axis), and neurotransmitters (sympathoadrenal axis).[7] Infusion of cytokines including IL-6 and TNF-α results in stimulation of corticotrophin, cortisol, epinephrine, and glucagon, leading to an increase in the resting metabolic rate and lipolysis.[8,9] TNF-α activation of nuclear factor kappa (NFκ)-β results in stimulation of proteolytic pathways.[10] In response to injury, there is an increased metabolic activity of the brain. Afferent nerve activity and brain stimulation may result in autonomic nerve stimulation with direct effects on hormone secretion; for example, splanchnic nerve stimulation as a result of injury results in increased glucagon secretion and hyperglycemia.[11] Afferent nerve activity from the injured site also results in hypothalamic-pituitary activation, increasing activity of cortisol, catecholamines, growth hormone, aldosterone, and antidiuretic hormone.[7] In fact, in humans, prolonged infusions of glucagon, cortisol, and epinephrine result in increased protein breakdown and elevated resting metabolic rate.[12] Prolonged elevation of cortisol is associated with onset of insulin resistance. In addition, peripheral nerve endings have been shown to exist on adipocytes, and the stimulation of adipocytes results in increased lipolysis.

During illness or after trauma, food intake frequently falls. However, despite this decline, the adaptive responses to starvation do not occur. Hepatic gluconeogenesis continues and rapid protein catabolism develops. There is an increased mobilization of stored fuels and metabolic cycling, resulting in heat production and energy loss. Insulin resistance develops and hyperglycemia may occur despite the absence of food intake. In severe metabolic stress, the body appears to preferentially utilize skeletal muscle as a metabolic fuel (as opposed to the situation in PPCM, when fat metabolism is the principal source of energy). The adaptive switch to fat utilization is limited, in part because of increased levels of circulating insulin. The result is an increase in lean tissue breakdown, visceral organ dysfunction, impaired wound healing, and immunosuppression.[7,13] Nitrogen losses during this catabolic response may be as high as 20 to 30 g/day versus 4 to 5 g/day in a human experiencing PPCM. Excess protein breakdown and muscle disuse because of inactivity result in muscle weakness and increased morbidity. Because sodium and water retention are a component of this response, weight loss frequently goes unnoticed. Cytokine production results in behavioral changes, including anorexia and decreased activity. Food deprivation during this hypermetabolic/catabolic state results in a much greater loss of lean muscle mass and visceral protein than would be expected during simple starvation. A healthy human allowed access to water can survive approximately 3 months with food deprivation or PPCM. In contrast, the same individual with a critical illness would survive approximately 1 month, and those with preexisting malnutrition, less than 2 weeks.

Although nutritional supplementation will reverse the catabolic processes occurring during simple starvation, it will not completely reverse those occurring during metabolic stress, because as long as tissue injury persists, catabolic processes are maintained. In the critically ill patient, protein catabolism continues despite protein supplementation in the diet. However, nutritional supplementation does have benefits in minimizing the severity of protein loss, providing both essential and conditionally essential amino acids, vitamins, and minerals, and in decreasing morbidity associated with illness.

Although the metabolic response to surgical injury is not likely to be as severe as that expected with sepsis, severe trauma, or other critical illnesses, an increase in metabolic rate is seen postoperatively in humans undergoing simple elective surgery. The combination of an increased energy demand and the metabolic processes already discussed can result in significant loss of lean body mass. These changes may not affect survival, but they can significantly impact the return to performance of a competitive athlete. In equine patients with severe surgical trauma, prolonged recoveries, or complications such as infection and laminitis, food deprivation almost certainly affects overall recovery.

METABOLIC REQUIREMENTS

The total energy of a feedstuff is divided into the digestible energy (DE) and the nondisgestible energy. Digestible energy is further divided into metabolic energy (which is used to provide energy) and that which is lost or nonmetabolizable, such as gases produced and urea excreted in the urine. By convention, energy requirements are calculated in terms of digestible energy.

Adults

The amount of DE needed to meet the maintenance energy requirements (DE_m) of the normally active, non-working horse can be estimated using the following formulas:

- For horses weighing less than 600 kg,

$$DE_m \text{ (Mcal/day)} = 1.4 + (BW \times 0.03).$$

- For horses weighing greater than 600 kg,

$$DE_m \text{ (Mcal/day)} = 1.82 + (BW \times 0.0383) - (BW \times 0.000015).$$

where BW is body weight in kilograms, and 1 Mcal equals 1000 kcal. Alternatively, these requirements can be estimated to be approximately 33 kcal/kg per day.

The resting energy requirement (DE_r) is the amount of energy required for maintenance (neither weight gain nor weight loss) of the completely inactive animal and is determined using a metabolism stall in a thermoneutral environment. The result is approximately 70% of the maintenance energy, and it can be calculated using the following formula:

$$DE_r \text{ (Mcal/day)} = (BW \times 0.021) + 0.975.$$

The maintenance energy requirements of a horse can be affected by several factors, including its age, size, and physical condition; the amount and type of activity; and environmental factors. Even when all these factors are controlled, individual variation occurs.

Increased Energy Demand

Energy requirements in the pregnant mare do not significantly increase until late gestation and are estimated to be 1.1, 1.13, and 1.2 times the DE_m, respectively, in the last 3 months of gestation. During lactation, energy demands peak over the first 3 months and then decline toward weaning and can be calculated using the following equations:

- In the first 3 months of lactation,
  - for 300- to 900-kg mares,

$$DE \text{ (Mcal/day)} = DE_m + (0.03 \times BW \times 0.792),$$

  - for 200- to 299-kg mares,

$$DE \text{ (Mcal/day)} = DE_m + (0.04 \times BW \times 0.792).$$

- After 3 months of lactation,
  - for 300- to 900-kg mares,

$$DE \text{ (Mcal/kg)} = DE_m + (0.02 \times BW \times 0.792),$$

  - for 200- to 299-kg mares,

$$DE \text{ (Mcal/day)} = DE_m + (0.03 \times BW \times 0.792).$$

The energy and protein requirements for the hospitalized surgical patient are not known and probably vary depending on disease state, environment, and level of fitness of the individual. However, they are likely to be close to the resting or maintenance energy requirements. In humans, multipliers have been used to estimate the energy requirements in certain conditions, including severe sepsis, trauma, and burn injuries. However, the increased metabolic demands of illness or surgical trauma and recovery are likely to be balanced by the inactivity of the patient during hospitalization. Consequently, these multipliers may overestimate the caloric requirement of certain illnesses. The exceptions to this are individuals with extreme trauma, burns, or severe sepsis; surgical conditions that require intestinal resection; and patients with large areas of devitalized tissue (e.g., patients with clostridial myositis undergoing multiple fasciotomies). When estimating the energy requirements of the majority of surgical patients, resting energy requirements are an acceptable target. If the patient tolerates nutritional supplementation at this rate, the amount can be gradually increased to meet maintenance needs.

Foals and Weanlings

Foals and young horses that are growing have the highest energy demands. Mare's milk has been reported to provide between 500 and 600 kcal of energy per liter. A healthy neonatal foal drinks between 20% and 30% of its body weight in milk a day, which means that a 45-kg foal drinking 9 to 13.5 L of mare's milk consumes between 4500 kcal (4.5 Mcal) to 7800 kcal per day. This equates to a metabolic rate of between 100 and 173 kcal/kg per day. The resting metabolic rate in the healthy sedated foal has been calculated to be between 45 and 50 kcal/kg per day. As previously discussed, it is unclear whether a sick individual truly has a higher metabolic rate than a healthy individual. A recumbent sick foal is expending significantly less energy than its healthy counterpart in terms of activity level, but disease and its effect on metabolic rate and catabolism must be considered. As with adults, it is probably best to start nutritional supplementation at approximately the DE_r, particularly if starting with the enteral route. If tolerated, it is recommended that this be gradually increased toward growth requirements over a shorter period of time than might be used to increase the adult animal's caloric intake. If using mare's milk or a milk replacement of similar caloric content, DE_r would equate to feeding the equivalent of 10% of the foal's body weight per day. Clinical experience suggests that this would be sufficient in the initial 12 to 24 hours, but additional nutritional support would be required to ensure adequate intake for healing and growth.

The largest growth rate occurs during the first month of life.[14] The following formula can be used to estimate and adjust the energy requirement, in Mcal DE per day, for growth of weanlings and young growing horses:

$$DE_m + \{[4.81 + (1.17 \times M) - (0.023 \times M^2)] \times ADG\},$$

where M is months of age, ADG is average daily weight gain in kilograms, and BW is body weight.

More comprehensive reviews related to the metabolic needs of active and young growing horses are available for readers who need them.[15-17]

PROTEIN REQUIREMENTS

Protein intake must be adequate not only for energy requirements but also to ensure that protein catabolism is minimized. Maintenance requirements for crude protein (CP) in the adult horse can be estimated using the following equation:

$$CP \text{ (in grams)} = 40 \times DE_m \text{ (in Mcal/day)}$$

For example, a 500-kg horse with a DE_m of 16.5 Mcal/day would require 660 g of protein per day. Alternatively, protein requirements can be estimated as 0.5 to 1.5 g protein per kilogram of the horse's body weight per day, or 250 to

750 g/day for a 500-kg horse. The higher end of this estimate should be used when calculating protein needs in a sick patient.

VITAMIN REQUIREMENTS

Vitamins are organic compounds that are important in many enzymatic functions and metabolic pathways. Fat-soluble vitamins include vitamins A, K, D, and E. Water-soluble vitamins include the B vitamins and vitamin C. Vitamin K and all the B vitamins with the exception of niacin are synthesized by the microbial population in the horse's large colon and cecum. Vitamin D, vitamin C, and niacin are produced by the horse, whereas the precursors to vitamin A, beta-carotene, and vitamin E must be ingested. The need for supplemental vitamins and minerals depends on the type and duration of supplementation. Fat-soluble vitamins are stored in body tissues and generally do not require supplementation for short periods of anorexia. Complete pelleted diets have vitamins and minerals added to meet the requirements set by the National Research Council. When feeding a component diet or a parenteral diet, vitamin and mineral supplementation is necessary to ensure adequate intake.

ASSESSMENT OF NUTRITIONAL SUPPORT

Body weight should be measured daily to determine if nutritional support is adequate to maintain body weight. The most accurate method is to use a walk-on floor scale. A weight tape is a useful alternative when a scale is not available. Weight tapes are used to measure the girth just behind the elbow; the circumference correlates with pounds or kilograms. Weight tapes are relatively accurate in predicting the weight of small horses (less than 350 kg) and large ponies (350 to 450 kg). Weight tapes have been shown to be less accurate in estimating weight in heavy stock breeds and Thoroughbred horses.[18] However, in the hospital setting, their value lies in determining the overall trend of body weight, not the actual number.

Body condition scores are used to subjectively determine the animal's body fat stores and are useful to evaluate the long-term nutritional status of the animal (see Box 6-1). Body condition scores are less useful than a scale for determining smaller weight gains and losses in a hospital situation, but they are more accurate for predicting fat stores.

Diet and hydration status can alter body weight by as much as 5% to 10%. For example, a 500-kg horse that presents with colic may be 7% dehydrated at admission. At the time of exploratory celiotomy, the large colon may be emptied to facilitate correction of a surgical lesion. Rehydration of this animal would result in a weight increase of 35 kg. The large colon and cecum can hold between 75 and 90 L of ingesta; removal of a portion of the contents could result in a weight loss of 50 kg or more. Consequently, weight changes need to be considered in light of hydration status, feed intake, and any procedures that have occurred.

ENTERAL NUTRITION

In the critically ill patient with poor perfusion and decreased oxygen delivery to the tissues, the gastrointestinal tract is frequently the most vulnerable organ. Decreased oxygen delivery has been shown to increase mucosal permeability, resulting in increased translocation of bacteria and absorption of bacterial toxins.[19,20] Inflammatory mediators, produced in the gut as a result of ischemia, are absorbed across the damaged mucosa and enter the portal and systemic circulations; this absorption has been implicated in the onset of septic shock or multiorgan failure.[21] Enteral nutrition increases total hepatosplanchnic blood flow in healthy patients, resulting in greater oxygen delivery to the mucosa. In a rat model of *Escherichia coli* sepsis, enteral feeding of glucose resulted in improved intestinal perfusion rates.[22] Enteral nutrition maintains functional and structural integrity of the gut; the absence of enteral nutrition results in mucosal atrophy, increased gut permeability, and enzymatic dysfunction in critically ill human patients.[23]

Enteral nutrition is a trophic stimulus for the gastrointestinal tract both directly via the presence of nutrients and indirectly via stimulation of trophic hormones such as enteroglucagon. Early enteral nutrition (EEN) is the initiation of enteral feeding within 48 hours after surgery. In a large clinical study of surgical and trauma patients, EEN significantly decreased morbidity and length of stay when compared with delayed enteral nutrition and parenteral nutrition.[21] Enteral nutrition has a protective effect against bacterial translocation across the ischemic intestinal wall. In addition, EEN has been shown to blunt the hypermetabolic/catabolic response to injury in several human and animal models.[2] During the hypermetabolic, catabolic state seen with injury or illness, many amino acids, such as glutamine, become conditionally essential. Glutamine is an important fuel for lymphocytes, hepatocytes, and mucosal cells of the gut. During catabolism, glutamine levels may become insufficient to meet these energy demands. The addition of glutamine to both enteral and parenteral diets may improve gastrointestinal function and mucosal cell healing.[24]

Although the decision to supply supplemental nutrition may be clear, the route of supplementation must be considered in light of the original insult, surgical manipulations, and postoperative status of the patient. The enteral route is always preferred when the gastrointestinal tract can be used. Patients with overwhelming bowel ischemia, intestinal resection, and anastomosis or postoperative ileus may not be the best candidates for EEN. However, concerns about the strength and diameter of anastomotic sites after surgical resection and about the risk of obstruction or leakage if enteral feeding is introduced prematurely are not valid. Enterally fed dogs had higher bursting pressures at colonic anastomotic sites and better wound collagen synthesis than unfed controls.[25] Because horses are commonly fed high-fiber diets, the risk of obstruction at the anastomotic site is a valid concern; consequently, when enteral feeding is to be instituted, the type of diet should be carefully considered. Patients with a high risk of postoperative ileus or with a narrow anastomotic site may be better off started on parenteral nutrition and then gradually reintroduced to enteral nutrition. Alternatively, a liquid enteral diet may be instituted until healing is sufficient to allow introduction of roughage.

Types of enteral nutrition can vary from normal feedstuffs (i.e., grains, hay, and complete pelleted diets), slurry diets composed primarily of normal feedstuffs (Table 6-1), and

TABLE 6-1. Nutritional Contents of Selected Horse Feeds

	Equine Senior	Strategy	Purina Horse Chow
Crude Protein	14%	14%	10%
Fat	4%	6%	2%
Fiber	16%	8%	30%
Kcal/kg feed	2695	3300	—

TABLE 6-2. Nutritional Content of Selected Liquid Diets

	Vital HN	Osmolite	Critical Care Meals/Packet
Cal/L	1000	1008	1066
Protein	41.7 g/dL	40 g/dL	12%
Fat	10.8 g/dL	34 g/dL	1%
Carbohydrate	185 g/L	135.6 g/L	73%

liquid diets containing component requirements (Table 6-2). In horses with decreased appetite or complete anorexia, the choices are limited to those diets that can be administered through a nasogastric tube. Complete pelleted diets offer several advantages: they are relatively inexpensive, they are well balanced for the maintenance requirements of the adult horse, and they contain fiber. Fiber is beneficial in increasing colonic blood flow, enzymatic activity, and colonic mucosal cell growth and absorption.[26] The major disadvantage of pelleted diets is the difficulty of giving them via nasogastric intubation. Both human and equine liquid formulations are available and have been used as enteral nutrition support in horses.[27-30]

Alternatively, diets prepared using specific components have been described.[31] Corn oil may be added to the diet to increase the caloric content. The use of human products for the full-size horse can be very expensive, and these products have been associated with diarrhea. Liquid diets may be given via continuous flow using a small nasogastric tube or via periodic intubation and larger meals. When using pelleted diets, approximately 1 kg of a pelleted complete feed is soaked in approximately 4 L of water. Once dissolved, an additional 2 L of water is added and the slurry is administered via a large-bore nasogastric tube. Slurry diets made from complete pelleted feeds will not pass through a nasogastric tube using gravity alone and must be pumped in using a marine-supply bilge pump. If a bilge pump is not available or a large-bore tube cannot be passed, pulverizing the pellets prior to adding water may improve flow. The horse should be checked for the presence of gastric reflux prior to administration, and the slurry should be pumped slowly with attention paid to the horse's attitude and reaction.

The stomach volume of an adult, 450-kg horse is approximately 9 to 12 L, and a feeding should not exceed 6 to 8 L. This volume should be adjusted for smaller horses. Long-term placement of nasogastric tubes is not without the risk of complications.[32] Small-bore, softer (polyurethane) tubes are recommended if intubation is prolonged, but these generally preclude the use of slurry diets. Alternatively, intermittent placement of a nasogastric tube is effective in decreasing complications, but this can be difficult and at times traumatic to the patient. When instituting enteral feeding, particularly in a patient with prolonged anorexia, it is best to start gradually, increasing the amount fed over several days. A maximum of 50% of the calculated requirements should be fed in the first 24 hours. If the patient tolerates the supplementation, it can be increased over the next few days until full supplementation is achieved. Rapid changes in intake, particularly with component feeding or high-fat diets, may be associated with colic or diarrhea.

PARENTERAL NUTRITION

Parenteral nutrition (PN) is used to supply nutrition when the enteral route is unavailable. Parenteral nutrition can provide partial nutritional support (PPN) or total nutritional support (TPN). In the adult horse, it is most commonly used to supply partial nutrition when oral intake is insufficient or inappropriate. Horses with proximal enteritis, colitis, postoperative ileus, esophageal lacerations, or obstructions can receive nutritional support until resolution of the underlying problem allows reinstitution of enteral feeding. Recumbent or dysphagic animals at risk for aspiration pneumonia, individuals with preexisting protein calorie malnutrition or increased energy demands (late gestation, early lactation, and young, growing animals), and those with decreased feed consumption should also be considered as candidates for partial or total parenteral nutrition.

Depending on the desired goals and duration of supplementation, solutions containing various amounts of carbohydrate, amino acids, lipids, vitamins, electrolytes, and minerals may be formulated. Carbohydrate is commonly provided using 50% dextrose solutions (2525 mOsm/L) that contain 1.7 Kcal/mL. Isotonic lipid emulsions contain principally safflower and soybean oil, egg yolk phospholipids, and glycerin and come in 10% and 20% solutions. Amino acid preparations are available in several concentrations: 8.5% and 10% solutions are most commonly used in veterinary medicine. Solutions containing both essential and conditionally essential amino acids are preferable.

Components that may be added to parenteral nutrition include electrolyte solutions and vitamin and mineral supplements. Multivitamin supplements for humans are available and may be added directly to PN solutions. Some vitamins can be given orally (vitamins C and E) or added to crystalloid solutions (B vitamins). Fat-soluble vitamins are stored in body tissues and rarely need to be supplemented unless prolonged periods (weeks) of anorexia occur. Macrominerals, if required, are best supplemented in separate crystalloid solutions, because divalent cations may destabilize lipid emulsions. Although sick animals require trace minerals, such supplementation is rarely given except to patients receiving parenteral nutrition as their sole nutritional source for prolonged periods (greater than 7 days).

Resting energy requirements should be used when calculating PN volumes for adult animals, but protein requirements should be determined using maintenance requirements (see Box 6-1) or estimated using the following formula (as described under "Protein Requirements," earlier):

0.5 to 1.5 g protein per kilogram BW per day.

The higher end of this formula is recommended in sick, compromised patients. The ratio of nonprotein calories to nitrogen should be at least 100:1 in the final solution. Lipids should provide approximately 30% to 40% of the nonprotein calories whenever possible. The addition of lipids to PN is beneficial in patients with persistent hyperglycemia or hypercapnia, as this reduces the dependency on glucose as the principal energy source. The amount of fat utilization will depend on the amount of carbohydrate provided, with fat storage occurring in the presence of excess carbohydrate calories.

The preparation of PN should be performed under a laminar flow hood using aseptic techniques. Lipids should be added last to prevent destabilization of the emulsion in acidic dextrose solutions. Parenteral solutions are an excellent medium for growth of bacteria and should be used within 24 hours of preparation. Prior to use, they should be kept in a dark, cool area to minimize degradation and loss of vitamins. Because these solutions are hyperosmolar, delivery through a central venous catheter is recommended. Ideally, a separate catheter or portal is designated for parenteral nutrition only. Catheter placement and line maintenance should be performed using strict aseptic technique and all lines changed daily. We generally place a 14-gauge double-lumen catheter (Arrow catheter, Arrow International, Reading, Pa.) and designate one port for parenteral nutrition. Gradual introduction of parenteral nutrition is recommended to decrease risk of complications. Initial infusion rates should provide approximately 25% to 50% of the calculated requirement over the first 24 hours. If tolerated, the rate of infusion can gradually be increased over the next few days to provide 100% of the calculated requirement.

Complications of parenteral nutrition include hyperglycemia, hyperammonemia, hyperlipemia, elevation of serum urea nitrogen, thrombophlebitis, and sepsis.[13,33-36] Lipid infusions have been associated with allergic reactions, hyperlipemia, alterations in liver function, and fat embolism. Insulin resistance seen with systemic inflammatory response syndrome can result in hyperglycemia and rebound hypoglycemia when rates are altered too rapidly. Although solutions containing lipids are very useful in providing additional calories, their use should be determined on a case-by-case basis. Lipids should be avoided in patients with a predisposition to or a preexisting hyperlipemia or an underlying liver dysfunction. Thrombocytopenia, coagulopathy, fat embolization, coagulopathies, and alterations in cellular immunity are reported with lipid infusions. Triglyceride levels and platelet counts should be monitored regularly when lipids are added to PN solutions.

Monitoring should include daily assessment of serum electrolytes, blood urea nitrogen, triglycerides, and ammonia and liver function during the acclimation period. Blood glucose should be monitored every 4 to 6 hours and the rate adjusted to maintain blood glucose within the established normal range. If costs are a concern, blood values may be monitored less frequently once a steady state has been achieved.

BOX 6-2. Sample Calculations for Feed Supplementation

- Daily nutritional requirements of a 450-kg horse:

DE_r = (450 kg × 0.021 Mcal/kg) + 0.975 = 10.4 Mcal
DE_m = (450 kg × 0.03 Mcal/kg) + 1.4 = 14.9 Mcal
Crude protein requirements = 40 g/Mcal × 14.9 Mcal = 596 g protein
Alternatively, 0.5 to 1.5 g protein/kg × 450 kg = 225 to 675 g protein

ENTERAL FORMULATION

Equine Senior (horse feed) = 2695 kcal/kg
Corn oil = 1.6 Mcal/cup

- To meet daily DE_r requirements:

10.4 Mcal/2.7 Mcal/kg = 3.8 kg Equine Senior

- Daily protein requirements (maintenance):

12% protein = 120 g/kg feed
3.8 kg × 120 g = 456 g crude protein

- To meet daily DE_m requirements:

4.9 kg Equine Senior (2.7 Mcal/kg × 5.0 kg) = 13.3 Mcal
plus 1 cup corn oil = 1.6 Mcal = 14.9 Mcal
4.9 kg × 120 g protein/kg = 588 g protein

PARENTERAL FORMULATION

1 L of 50% dextrose = 1.7 Mcal
1.5 L of 10% amino acids = 0. 57 Mcal and 150 g of protein
0.5 L of 20% lipids = 1.0 Mcal
Total = 3.27 Mcal/3 L or 1.09 Mcal/L
DE_r = 10.4 Mcal/day
10.4 Mcal/day ÷ 1.09 Mcal/L = 10 L/24 hours = 416 mL/hour
500 g protein/day
Ratio of nonprotein calories to nitrogen = 117:1

DE_m, maintenance energy requirement for active horse; DE_r, resting energy requirement.

The same approach should be used when discontinuing parenteral nutrition. A gradual decrease in the infusion rate should be performed over at least 24 hours. Frequent monitoring of blood glucose during withdrawal is warranted because of the risk of transient hypoglycemia. For examples on how to calculate parenteral nutrition requirements, see Box 6-2.

REFERENCES

1. Ward N: Nutrition support to patients undergoing gastrointestinal surgery, Nutr J 2003;2:18.
2. Robert PR, Zaloga GP: Enteral nutrition. In Shoemaker WC, Ayres SM, Grenvick A, et al, editors: Textbook of Critical Care, ed 4, Philadelphia, 2000, WB Saunders.
3. Studley HO: Percentage weight loss: A basic indicator of surgical risk in patients with chronic peptic ulcer, JAMA 1936;106:458-460.

4. Windsor JA, Hill GL: Risk factors for post operative pneumonia: The importance of protein depletion, Ann Surg 1988;208:209-214.
5. Schroeder D, Gillanders L, Mahr K, et al: Effects of immediate postoperative enteral nutrition on body composition, muscle function and wound healing, JPEN J Parenter Enteral Nutr 1991;15:376-383.
6. Keusch GT: The history of nutrition: Malnutrition, infection and immunity, J Nutr 2003;133:336S-340S.
7. Romijn JA: Substrate metabolism in the metabolic response to injury, Proc Nutr Soc 2000;59:447-449.
8. Stouthard JML, Romijn JA, Van der Poll T, et al: Endocrine and metabolic effects of interleukin-6 in humans, Am J Phys 1995;268:E813-819.
9. Van der Poll T, Romijn JA, Endert E, et al: Tumor necrosis factor mimics the metabolic response to acute infection in healthy humans, Am J Phys 1991;261:E457-465.
10. Langhans W: Peripheral mechanisms involved with catabolism, Curr Opin Clin Nutr Metab Care 2002;5:419-426.
11. Bloom SR, Edwards AV: The release of pancreatic glucagons and inhibition of insulin in response to stimulation of sympathetic innervation, J Phys 1975;253:157-173.
12. Bessey PQ, Watters JM, Aoki TT, et al: Combined hormonal infusion simulates the metabolic response to injury, Ann Surg 1984;200:264-281.
13. Sternberg JA, Rohovsky SA, Blackburn GL, et al: Total parenteral nutrition for the critically ill patient. In Shoemaker WC, Ayres SM, Grenvick A, et al, editors: Textbook of Critical Care, ed 4, Philadelphia, 2000, WB Saunders.
14. Persson SGB, Ullberg LE: Blood volume and rate of growth in Standardbred foals, Equine Vet J 1981;13:254-258.
15. Paradis MR: Nutritional support: Enteral and parenteral, Clin Tech Equine Pract 2003;2:87-95.
16. Lewis L: Growing horse feeding and care. In Lewis L, editor: Equine Clinical Nutrition Feeding and Care. Media, Pa, 1995, Wilkins and Wilkins.
17. Pugh DG, Williams MA: Feeding foals from birth to weaning, Cont Ed Vet Pract 1992;14:526-532.
18. Reavell DG: Measuring and estimating the weight of horses with tapes, formulae and by visual assessment, Equine Vet Ed 1999;1:188-193.
19. Luyer MD, Jacobs JA, Vreugdenhil AC, et al: Enteral administration of high fat nutrition before and directly after hemorrhagic shock reduces endotoxemia and bacterial translocation, Ann Surg 2004;239:257-264.
20. Saito H, Trocki O, Alexander JW, et al: The effect of route of nutrient administration on the nutritional state, catabolic hormone secretion, and gut mucosal integrity after burn injury, JPEN J Parenter Enteral Nutr 1987;11:1-7.
21. Rokyta R, Matejovic M, Krouzecky A, et al: Enteral nutrition and hepatosplanchnic region in critically ill patients: Friends or foes? Phys Res 2003;52:31-37.
22. Gosche JR, Garrison RN, Harris PD, et al: Absorptive hyperaemia restores intestinal blood flow during *Escherichia coli* sepsis in the rat, Arch Surg 1990;125:1573-1576.
23. Hernandez G, Velasco N, Wainstein C, et al: Gut mucosal atrophy after a short enteral fasting period in critically ill patients, J Crit Care 1999;14:73-77.
24. Buchman AL: Glutamine commercially essential or conditionally essential? A critical appraisal of the human data, Am J Clin Nutr 2001;74:25-32.
25. Moss G, Greenstein A, Levy S, et al: Maintenance of GI function after bowel surgery and immediate enteral full nutrition: I. Doubling of canine colorectal anastomotic bursting pressure and intestinal wound mature collagen content, JPEN J Parenter Enteral Nutr 1980;4:535-538.
26. Scheppach W: Effects of short chain fatty acids on gut morphology and function, Gut 1994;35:S35-38.
27. Golenz MR, Knight DA, Yvorchuk-St Jean KE: Use of a human enteral feeding preparation for treatment of hyperlipemia and nutritional support during healing of an esophageal laceration in a miniature horse, J Am Vet Med Assoc 1992;200:951-953.
28. Hallebeek JM, Beynen AC: A preliminary report on a fat-free diet formula for nasogastric enteral administration as treatment for hyperlipaemia in ponies, Vet Q 2001;23:201-205.
29. Sweeney RW, Hansen TO: Use of a liquid diet as the sole source of nutrition in six dysphagic horses and as a dietary supplement in seven hypophagic horses, J Am Vet Med Assoc 1990;197:1030-1032.
30. MD's Choice Critical Care Meals: Available at www.vetsupplements.com.
31. Naylor JM, Freeman DE, Kronfeld DS: Alimentation of hypophagic horses, Comp Cont Ed Pract Vet 1984;6:S93-99.
32. Hardy J, Stewart RH, Beard WL, et al: Complications of nasogastric intubation in horses: Nine cases (1987-1989), J Am Vet Med Assoc 1992;201:483-486.
33. Lopes MAF, White NA: Parenteral nutrition for horses with gastrointestinal disease: a retrospective study of 79 cases, Equine Vet J 2002;34:250-257.
34. Durham AE, Phillips TJ, Walmsley JP, et al: Study of the clinical effects of postoperative parenteral nutrition in 15 horses, Vet Rec 2003;153:493-498.
35. Durham AE, Phillips TJ, Walmsley JP, et al: Nutritional and clinicopathological effects of post operative parenteral nutrition following small intestinal resection and anastomosis in the mature horse, Equine Vet J 2004;36:390-396.
36. Jeejeebhoy KN: Total parenteral nutrition: Potion or poison? Am J Clin Nutr 2001;74:160-163.

CHAPTER 7

Surgical Site Infection and the Use of Antimicrobials

R. Wayne Waguespack
Daniel J. Burba
Rustin M. Moore

One of the most serious complications associated with surgery is the development of infection after an operation. Postoperative surgical site infections (SSIs) are a major source of morbidity and even mortality. The risk of SSI in horses varies greatly depending on interactions between factors that can be categorized as attributable to host, microorganisms, and surgery. Numerous discoveries have contributed to the advancement of modern surgery, such as Semmelweiss's recognition of a surgeon's hands as a source of contagion, Lister's use of antiseptics to reduce the risk for mortality among newborn babies and their mothers, the discovery of penicillin and the resultant antimicrobial era, and the importance of the timing of antibiotic prophylaxis as demonstrated by Burke.[1] These discoveries have been adapted to modern veterinary surgery. However, despite advances in surgical techniques, infection control, and antibiotic prophylaxis, postsurgical infections remain a problem in the equine patient.

WOUND CLASSIFICATION

The presence of purulent drainage from the incision site has typically been the clinical definition of an SSI. However, infection may be present in or around a site that communicates with the incision, complicating the definition of SSI. Therefore, to create a uniform classification of SSI, the Centers for Disease Control and Prevention (CDC) established definitions for surveillance and epidemiologic purposes.[2] In 1992, the CDC redefined surgical wound infections as SSIs to include the incision, regional extension, and organ or visceral infection, but not more-distant infections (e.g., postoperative pneumonia). Distant infections are considered complications and are not classified as SSIs because they are not directly associated with the surgical incision.[3] For surveillance and classification purposes, SSIs are placed into three categories: superficial incisional SSI (involving skin and subcutaneous tissues), deep incisional SSI (involving the fascial and muscle layers), and organ or space SSI (involving any part of the anatomy other than the incision that is opened or manipulated during the surgical procedure)[4] (Table 7-1).

Veterinary medicine has used the wound classification system developed by the National Academy of Sciences and the National Research Council (Table 7-2). This classification system is based on intrinsic intraoperative microbial contamination. Originally, it was believed that as the degree of microbial contamination increased, so did the overall incidence of SSI; however, this may be misleading in equine surgery. In clinical studies in the horse, the correlation between wound classification and surgical infection has been shown to vary greatly between soft tissue and orthopedic procedures.[5-7] In equine abdominal surgery, the performance of enterotomy or resection did not influence the incidence of SSI.[5,7-9] Preexisting dermatitis, poor intraoperative drape adherence, high number of bacterial colony-forming units (CFU) obtained from the celiotomy incision site immediately after recovery from anesthesia, and high number of CFU obtained from the surgery room environment are risk factors associated with abdominal SSI.[10] In contrast, there is a strong association between the risk of postoperative infection and surgical wound classification for equine orthopedic procedures, where surgical wound classification has the strongest association.[6] Clean-contaminated surgeries are approximately 24 times more likely to develop a postoperative SSI than are clean surgeries.[6] For example, long-bone surgeries have a 5.1-fold greater risk of surgical infection than do procedures involving the articular surface.[6]

INFECTION AND SOURCES OF MICROORGANISMS

A variety of microorganisms are capable of causing SSIs in horses, but the most common agents are bacteria. In horses, coagulase-positive and coagulase-negative staphylococci, followed by members of the family Enterobacteriaceae, species of *Streptococcus* and *Pseudomonas,* and anaerobes, were the most common pathogens isolated from infections after joint surgery.[11,12] Postoperative infections after fracture repair were most often caused by Enterobacteriaceae, followed closely by streptococci[6,13] (Table 7-3). In horses with peritonitis after abdominal surgery, streptococci, Enterobacteriaceae, *Actinobacillus* species, and anaerobes, including species of *Fusobacterium, Peptostreptococcus, Clostridium,* and *Prevotella,* and *Bacteroides fragilis* were found.[14,15]

Infection often results from microorganisms introduced into the surgical site at the time of surgery. It is believed that within 24 hours of a surgical procedure, a surgical site is sufficiently sealed to be resistant to microorganism entry.[16] Sources of microorganisms that infect surgical sites include endogenous sources (the patient's flora), remote infections in the surgical patient, and exogenous sources such as operating room personnel, the environment, and the air. Most SSIs are believed to originate from *direct inoculation* of the patient's endogenous flora at or near the surgical site during surgery.[3,12,17,18] For example, contamination during ventral median celiotomies in horses was caused by streptococci, staphylococci, and *Escherichia coli,* which are representative of the horse's endogenous flora.[7]

Endogenous microorganisms located at a distance from the surgical site may also be a source of infection. It was shown that human albumin microspheres applied as tracer particles on a patient's skin remote to the incision site can be recovered from the surgical site, implying that microorganisms located at distant sites could gain entrance to the

TABLE 7-1. Classification of Surgical Site Infections

Surgical Site Infection	Qualifications	Includes One of the Following
Superficial incisional	Infection occurs within 30 days after surgical procedure. Infection involves only the skin or subcutaneous tissue of the incision.	• Purulent drainage from the superficial incision • Organisms isolated from an aseptically obtained culture of fluid or tissue from the superficial incision • At least one of the following signs or symptoms of infection: pain or tenderness, localized swelling, redness or heat • Superficial incision deliberately opened by a surgeon (unless culture of the incision is negative) • Diagnosis of superficial incisional surgical site infection by the surgeon or attending physician
Deep incisional	Infection occurs within 30 days after surgical procedure if no implant was left in place. Infection occurs within 1 year if an implant is in place. Infection appears to be related to the surgical procedure. Infection involves the deep tissues (i.e., fascial and muscle layers) of the incision.	• Purulent drainage from the deep incision but not from an organ space component of the surgical site • A deep incision spontaneously dehisces or is deliberately opened by a surgeon when the patient has at least one of the following signs: fever, localized pain, or tenderness (unless culture of the incision is negative) • An abscess or other evidence of infection involving the deep incision is found on direct examination during reoperation, or by histopathologic or radiologic examination • Diagnosis of deep incisional surgical site infection by the surgeon or attending physician
Organ/space	Infection involves any part of the anatomy, other than the incision, opened or manipulated during the surgical procedure. Infection occurs within 30 days after surgical procedure if no implant was left in place. Infection occurs within 1 year if an implant is in place. The infection appears to be related to the surgical procedure.	• Purulent drainage from a drain placed through a stab incision into an organ/space • Organisms isolated from an aseptically obtained culture of fluid or tissue in the organ/space • An abscess or other evidence of infection involving the organ/space on direct examination, during reoperation, or by histopathologic or radiologic examination • Diagnosis of organ/space surgical site infection by the surgeon or attending physician

surgical site.[19] Microorganisms located at remote sites may infect surgical sites via hematogenous or lymphogenous spread—a likely route of transmission in the neonate but an uncommon route in the adult horse.[12]

Exogenous microorganisms originate from operating room personnel, contaminated equipment, fluids, the inanimate environment, and the air. The hands of operating personnel contain numerous microorganisms and may be a source of contamination of the surgical site through glove perforations. Therefore, preoperative scrubbing is performed to decrease the number of microorganisms on the hands (see Chapter 11) so that glove perforations do not result in an increased incidence of SSI.[17]

Other body sites of the surgical team, including the hair, scalp, nares, and oropharynx, are colonized by microorganisms and may serve as a source of SSI. When human albumin microspheres were applied to the head, neck, and inner surface of surgical face masks, they were recovered from the surgical site.[19] Methicillin-resistant *Staphylococcus aureus* (MRSA), a serious SSI problem in humans, though not considered a very common problem in horses, has been reported to be transmitted from veterinary hospital personnel to equine patients.[20,21] In humans, MRSA colonization precedes infection, and a major site of human colonization is the anterior nares.[20]

Microorganisms associated with the inanimate environment of the operating room, including the air, are rarely associated with SSI.[22] The environment is a potential source of infection when equipment or devices that come into close contact with the surgical site are not adequately disinfected or when there are breaks in aseptic technique.

Microorganisms in the air arise from the patient, the surgical team, and, to a small extent, the inanimate environment. Numerous investigators have studied the effect of airborne transmission in the operating room and the incidence of SSI in human surgical patients. Systems that decrease bacterial counts in the operating room air, including air filtration systems that provide 20 air changes each hour, ultraviolet-irradiated rooms, laminar-flow systems, and surgical team exhaust suits, have not been definitively proven to decrease SSI rates, except in clean orthopedic surgeries such as total hip and knee procedures.[23-25]

TABLE 7-2. National Research Council Operative Wound Classification

Wound Category	Characteristics of the Wound
Clean	Elective, primarily closed, and undrained Nontraumatic, uninfected No inflammation encountered No break in aseptic technique
Clean-contaminated	Gastrointestinal, respiratory, and urogenital tracts entered under controlled conditions and with usual contamination Minor break in aseptic technique
Contaminated	Open fresh traumatic wound Gross spillage of the gastrointestinal tract Entrance into the urogenital or biliary tracts in the presence of infected urine or bile Incisions in which acute nonpurulent inflammation is encountered Major break in aseptic technique
Dirty and infected	Traumatic wound with retained devitalized tissue and foreign bodies, fecal contamination, or delayed treatment or from a dirty source Perforated viscus encountered Acute bacterial inflammation with purulent exudate encountered during the operation

TABLE 7-3. Bacterial Infections in the Horse

Disease Process	Bacterial Isolates
Surgical incisions in general	β-Hemolytic streptococci, staphylococci, Enterobacteriaceae, *Pseudomonas*
Iatrogenic septic arthritis	*Staphylococcus aureus*
Hematogenous septic arthritis	*Escherichia coli, Klebsiella, Actinobacillus equuli, Streptococcus, Salmonella, Rhodococcus equi*
Traumatic septic arthritis, tenosynovitis, bursitis	β-Hemolytic streptococci, staphylococci, Enterobacteriaceae, *Pseudomonas*
Osteomyelitis, infection after orthopedic surgery	Enterobacteriaceae, β-hemolytic streptococci, staphylococci, *Pseudomonas*
Peritonitis after abdominal surgery	*Streptococcus,* Enterobacteriaceae, *Actinobacillus,* anaerobes
Enterocolitis	*Salmonella, Clostridium*
Cellulitis	*Staphylococcus aureus, Clostridium*

RISK FACTORS FOR SURGICAL SITE INFECTION

Many factors influence the development of SSIs. The development of infection is a function of the interaction between the nature and degree of microbial contamination, the microorganism, local and systemic host defenses, and technical factors that relate to the surgery itself.

Microbe-Related Factors

The isolation of a microorganism from a surgical site may indicate that there is an infection, or the surgical site may be colonized by microorganisms without evidence of infection.[26] Whether particular microorganisms cause infection depends on the interplay among the number of infecting microorganisms, their virulence, and the host's local and systemic defenses.

The critical infective dose of a pure culture of obligate aerobic and facultative anaerobic bacteria has been demonstrated to be 10^5 bacteria per gram of tissue or greater; below this concentration, soft tissue wounds heal without evidence of infection.[27,28] However, 10^5 organisms per gram of tissue is a relative number, because SSIs can result from a smaller inoculum if the host's immune response is impaired, a virulent microorganism is involved, or a foreign body is present.[17,29] Joints are particularly vulnerable to infection, and studies have revealed that only 100 CFU of *S. aureus* need be present for a predictable infection of a synovial joint.[30] Although numerous microorganisms may be introduced into the surgical field at the time of surgery, not all microorganisms are equally capable of causing infection. Established infection depends on an agent's intrinsic capabilities (virulence) to infect and cause disease. The agent must be able to attach to eukaryotic cell surfaces, adapt to its current nutritional environment, multiply sufficiently, and evade the host immune system. Attachment to eukaryotic cell surfaces is mediated by bacterial cell surface adhesions that react with host cell receptors. Some staphylococci, for example, produce a large number of cell-associated and extracellular proteins, including various cytolytic toxins and enzymes such as proteases, lipases, and hyaluronidase that are important for colonization and growth in various body tissues.[31] Microorganisms can evade the host immune response by several means, including possession of an antiphagocytic capsule that prevents complement deposition on the bacterial cell surface; antigenic variation of cell surface antigens; secretion of IgA proteases at mucosal sites; possession of O-antigen polysaccharide, which resists complement lysis; and being sequestered as an intracellular pathogen.[32]

Microorganisms can evade host defenses and cause infection by adhering to biomaterials such as sutures, prosthetic devices, or bone, resulting in biofilm formation.[33] Biofilms are often polymicrobial in nature but can be caused by a single microorganism. Gram-positive bacteria such as staphylococci produce an extracellular glycocalyx, or mucin, that promotes adherence to biomaterials in greater numbers than gram-negative bacteria. Adherent bacteria form microcolonies that aggregate and produce exopolysaccharides, thus forming an extensive fibrous matrix that mediates their adhesion to each other and to the substrate. The biofilm is resistant to both local and systemic host defenses and antimicrobial agents.

Some microorganisms cause an infection only if another microorganism is present, a phenomenon known as bacterial synergism. Mixed and synergistic surgical infections often contain aerobic and anaerobic bacteria. Interactions among these bacteria may facilitate colonization, lower host resistance, provide nutritional factors, and enhance virulence of one microorganism by another.[3] Some strains of *S. aureus* and *Fusobacterium necrophorum* secrete leukocidins that are cytocidal to phagocytes and protect a mixed inoculum from phagocytosis.[34] Bacteria that synthesize β-lactamases or other extracellular enzymes that inactivate antimicrobials can protect otherwise sensitive co-pathogens from these antimicrobials.

Host-Related Factors

The quantitative relationship between a host's resistance to infection and the number of bacteria can be altered by both local and systemic factors, including age, weight, metabolic status (see Chapter 5), and presence of remote or distant infections.

Systemic Risk Factors

In humans, advancing age is the most important systemic risk factor associated with increasing infection rates. This correlation has not been reported in horses but may become noticeable as treatment of more geriatric equine patients develops. As an example, complication rates of ventral midline incision were lower in horses less than 1 year of age (15%) than in older horses (43%).[35]

Human patients in shock or severe metabolic derangement are at a greater risk of SSI. Scoring systems are used to index disease severity, and as severity increases, the risk of SSI increases.[36] Such scoring systems do not exist in equine surgery, so retrospective studies are confined to comparing surgery performed electively with surgery performed on an emergency basis. The incidence of incisional complication rate for horses undergoing surgery for acute abdominal disease (39%) was significantly greater than that for those undergoing elective surgical procedures of the abdominal cavity (7%).[35]

Weight and obesity are two important host-related risk factors in humans, where increased weight is often associated with obesity.[36] This is not necessarily true in horses because of the differences in weight variations with breed. However, ventral midline incisional complications in horses weighing less than 300 kg (8%) were fewer than those in horses weighing more than 300 kg (43%).[35] Remote trauma and distant infections have been reported to increase the incidence of SSI by twofold to threefold in humans.[17] Local dermatitis or remote infections, such as pneumonia, are always a concern in horses and should be eliminated or controlled to reduce the risk of SSI. Elective procedures should generally be delayed until the infection has resolved. If a remote infection is not controlled, it may develop into a systemic infection. This is usually a greater concern in neonates than in adult horses. At least four mechanisms exist whereby microorganisms may have an effect elsewhere in the body:

1. Bacteremia or septic emboli may result in deposition of organisms in distant tissues.
2. Bacterial toxins can produce cell damage; this is particularly true in hepatocytes.
3. Local necrosis at the site of infection may allow the release of proteolytic enzymes, which facilitate invasion into adjacent regions. Endotoxins and peptidases from injured tissues can activate vasoactive peptides and the clotting and fibrinolytic cascades, cause platelet aggregation, and alter systemic and pulmonary vascular resistance, membrane function, and energy metabolism.
4. Disseminated intravascular coagulation may occur after activation of the clotting cascades, with subsequent platelet consumption, consumption coagulopathy, and accumulation of fibrin-split products (see Chapter 4).

Local Risk Factors

Local factors are important when determining the outcome of the interaction between the host and the microorganism. Any foreign body, whether accidental or intentional, inhibits the host's local tissue defenses. The magnitude of this damage appears to be related to the chemical activity of the foreign body. Large numbers of *S. aureus* can be applied to intact skin without resulting in a clinical infection, but if these microbes are injected in the presence of a foreign body such as a suture, only 100 bacteria are needed to cause an infection.[29] Soil and dirt are frequent contaminants in traumatic wounds. Specific infection-potentiating factors have been identified in soil, including organic components and inorganic clay fractions.[37] Wounds that contain these fractions require only 100 bacteria per gram of tissue to elicit infection. The ability of these fractions to enhance the incidence of infection appears to be related to their damage of host defenses. In the presence of these fractions, leukocytes are not capable of phagocytizing bacteria because of the interaction between the highly charged soil particles and the white blood cells. In contrast, sand grains are relatively innocuous, presumably because of their large particle size and low chemical activity.

Surgery-Related Risk Factors

Many factors related to surgery itself have been implicated in increasing the likelihood of SSI. As surgery-related factors can be controlled by the surgeon, this is a method of decreasing the risk of SSI.

Duration of Surgery

Longer surgical times are generally associated with a more serious disease or procedure difficulty.[35,38,39] Longer procedures require longer anesthesia times, potentially resulting in decreased tissue perfusion, hypoxemia, and hypovolemia as complicating factors that increase the risk of SSI.[17] Research has demonstrated clinically and experimentally that the infection rate of clean wounds roughly doubles with every hour of surgery.[40] Equine orthopedic procedures taking longer than 90 minutes are 3.6 times more likely to develop SSI than procedures taking less than 90 minutes.[39] The number of incisional complications after ventral midline celiotomy is twice as great in operations lasting longer than 2 hours (47%) than in those lasting less than 2 hours (24%).[35]

The exact mechanism by which prolonged surgical time increases the risk for SSI is unclear. Four possible explanations have been considered[37]:

1. An increase in contamination of the wound
2. An increase in tissue damage because of drying, prolonged retraction, and manipulations
3. An increase in the amount of suture and of electrocoagulation, which may reduce local resistance
4. Greater host defense suppression because of blood loss and shock

To avoid prolongation of operating time, the surgeon should have a working knowledge of the local anatomy and, when possible, should practice on a cadaver specimen prior to operating on a patient.

Patient and Surgeon Preparation

Studies that have evaluated the effects of various equine patient preparation techniques on SSI are lacking. However, the use of antiseptics to prepare the skin of horses significantly decreases the number of skin bacteria.[41] The use of antiseptics in preparing both patient and surgeon decreases the incidence of infection (see Chapters 10 and 11). In people, there is a marked increase in SSI after shaving compared with the use of clipping or depilatories, especially when shaving was done the night before the surgical procedure.[36] Shaving disrupts the skin barrier through microtrauma or lacerations of the surgical site, thus predisposing the patient to SSI. If shaving is performed, it should be completed just before surgery to prevent microbial colonization.

There are several time-honored practices in surgeon preparation, including hand hygiene and the wearing of masks, caps, gowns, and gloves. Many of these practices have been traditionally believed to decrease the incidence of SSI and are considered a gold standard in today's veterinary hospital, even if few are supported by well-designed clinical studies. Even simple procedures such as the use of double gloves can decrease the incidence of infection. Double gloving should be employed in all orthopedic operations involving fracture manipulation because of the high risk of perforation. We do not advocate double gloving for all surgical procedures, but we routinely double glove during the draping procedure because this is commonly where a break in asepsis occurs. The outer gloves are shed prior to the skin incision, or if double gloving will be used throughout the operation, the outer gloves are then changed. Studies show that frequently changing outer gloves during surgery is an effective method of minimizing contamination.[42]

Surgical Technique

The surgeon's skill has a central role in SSI. The risk of infection is decreased by adhering to Halsted's principles of minimizing hemorrhage and tissue trauma; using correct instrumentation, suture materials, and implants; débriding devitalized tissue; and eradicating dead space.[17] Débridement is the most important factor in the management of a contaminated or infected wound.[43] Débridement removes tissue heavily contaminated by soil, infection-potentiating factors, and microorganisms. It also removes devitalized soft tissues that would alter host defenses and encourage the development of infection. Devitalized tissue enhances infection by acting as a culture medium for bacterial growth, inhibiting leukocyte phagocytic activity, and creating an anaerobic environment.

INCISION

The skin incision can be made by three techniques: (1) stainless steel scalpel, (2) electrosurgery, or (3) laser. It is reported that skin incisions made by either electrosurgery or laser have a threefold to 10-fold greater incidence of susceptibility to infection than those made by a stainless steel scalpel.[43] This is probably because of the increase in lateral thermal necrosis observed when using electrosurgery and lasers. However, in cases requiring massive excision, the risk of blood loss frequently outweighs the potential problem of subsequent infection. In addition, equine abdominal surgery that requires approaches through the muscular body wall (flank incisions) have a greater incidence of SSI than those through the ventral midline (88% versus 29%, respectively).[35] The increased incidence of infection after flank incisions is believed to be caused by an increase in dead space and muscle necrosis from excessively tight sutures or muscle trauma during surgery.[10]

SUTURE MATERIALS AND SURGICAL IMPLANTS

Devices placed in or under the skin through surgical intervention may also increase the incidence of surgical infection by acting as a foreign body and altering local tissue defense mechanisms. Bacteria adhere to these devices and proliferate to form a biofilm. Typically, in equine surgery, these are orthopedic devices (screws, wires, plates) or mesh implants. Sutures, particularly nonabsorbable suture materials, should also be considered as a potential source of infection or sinus tract formation.[44] The use of polyglactin 910 to close the linea alba in horses was significantly associated with increased risk of postoperative wound infection, compared with the use of polydioxanone and polyglycolic acid.[45]

Length of Hospitalization

In humans, a prolonged preoperative hospital stay is highly associated with incisional infection. A prolonged stay can promote the proliferation of endogenous or hospital-acquired microorganisms.[17] Hospitalization length is often not reported in equine studies on SSI, but it should be considered as advanced procedures and hospitalized recuperation become more common.

NOSOCOMIAL INFECTION IN THE SURGICAL PATIENT

Hospital-acquired or nosocomial infections are defined as infections acquired within a hospital or clinic that were not present or incubating at the time of admission. The majority of nosocomial infections become clinically apparent while patients are still hospitalized, often after 48 hours of hospitalization. Infections that develop after hospital discharge are also considered nosocomial if there is a direct link between the infection and the hospitalization.

It has been estimated that 5.7% of human patients admitted to acute care hospitals in the United States develop nosocomial infections. Furthermore, approximately 24% of these nosocomial infections are SSIs.[46] This percentage may actually underestimate the true occurrence of SSIs, because 20% to 80% of postoperative infections become clinically apparent only after hospital discharge,[47] and studies often do not include surveillance after hospital discharge.

Published surveillance studies of nosocomial infection rates in veterinary medicine are limited.[48] However, one report determined that 21.9% of 105 hospitalized horses developed nosocomial gram-negative aerobic infections by other than *Salmonella* species, and of these infections, 48% were postoperative SSIs.[49] *Salmonella* appear to be one of the most common causes of nosocomial infections in horses.[49-51] *Salmonella* species have been reported to cause hospital outbreaks of infection in horses, with surgery and antimicrobial therapy being important risk factors.[52-54] Horses may be asymptomatic carriers and shed the organism for weeks or months and serve as a significant reservoir of infection for both patients and personnel. However, determining whether an infection caused by *Salmonella* is nosocomial or the result of a preexisting latent infection may be difficult. Other gram-negative rods, such as *E. coli* and species of *Pseudomonas, Enterobacter, Citrobacter, Proteus,* and *Klebsiella,* have been reported to cause nosocomial infections in horses.[49] Gram-negative rods colonize patients and survive well in the hospital environment, thriving in minute traces of moisture with minimal nourishment, and in the presence of proteinaceous material, they resist desiccation. Other bacteria reported in equine nosocomial infections include gram-positive bacteria and anaerobes such as *Clostridium difficile*.[20,55,56] Bacterial organisms are the most frequently involved in nosocomial infections, but other microorganisms, including viruses, *Chlamydia, Mycoplasma,* fungi, and protozoa, can also cause nosocomial infections.[57]

Nosocomial infections contribute to increased morbidity, prolonged hospitalization, adverse patient outcome, and increased patient care cost. Approximately 2.5 million human nosocomial infections occur each year, costing the U.S. healthcare system over $10 million.[2] Although hospital epidemics or outbreaks are frequently reported in the literature, the majority of nosocomial infections are endemic. Nosocomial infections are frequently caused by the normal microorganisms colonizing the patient at the time of admission or by exogenous, hospital-associated microorganisms that are acquired and subsequently colonize the patient after admission. Colonization of the skin, mucosal membranes, or any other site is an important step before infection; however, whether infection and disease occur depends on interactions between the infecting organism and the host.

Surgical patients are at risk for the development of nosocomial infections. Surgical procedures, surgical implants, and invasive devices such as intravascular catheters, indwelling urinary catheters, and nasogastric and endotracheal tubes compromise the host's normal anatomic epithelial and mucosal antibacterial barriers. Surgical patients receiving antibiotic therapy risk nosocomial infections because the antibiotics alter the normal microbial ecology of the patient's skin; upper respiratory, gastrointestinal, and urogenital tracts; and any other site typically colonized by microorganisms.[51,56] Maintenance of the patient's normal microbial ecology is a potent deterrent to colonization by nosocomial pathogens.

Common types of nosocomial infections that occur in surgical patients include urinary, lower respiratory tract, and hematogenous infections, but SSI is the most common.[4] Nosocomial SSIs are usually the result of the patient's endogenous or hospital-acquired flora.[3] Infections caused by exogenous sources of microorganisms are a result of direct or indirect contamination of the surgical site by operating room personnel, contaminated devices or fluids, and, occasionally, airborne transmission of microorganisms from members of the operating room team. *Outbreaks resulting from nosocomial pathogens occur principally via transmission from colonized or infected patients to other patients via the transiently colonized hands of personnel, who acquire the microorganisms after direct patient contact* or after handling contaminated materials.[58] Transmissions via contaminated equipment, devices, solutions, air, or the inanimate environment occasionally occur.

Increasingly, more nosocomial pathogens cultured from patients postoperatively and from the hospital environment are resistant to antibiotics. Antibiotic resistance is a consequence of selective pressure from their use. Antibiotic pressure can cause susceptible strains to become resistant through mutation or through the acquisition of resistance genes, or it can provide a selective advantage for the emergence of resistant bacterial strains already present but in small quantities. Patients colonized by drug-resistant bacteria serve as a reservoir of these microorganisms and of transferable antibiotic resistance determinants that can be further transferred to susceptible bacteria.

Prevention and control of nosocomial infections are directed at elimination or containment of reservoirs, interruption of infection transmission, and protection of patients, personnel, and visitors from nosocomial infection and disease. A nosocomial infection control program that includes barrier precautions, isolation precautions, disinfection, and sterilization protocols is important in veterinary medicine for the control of nosocomial infections.[59,60] *Hand disinfecting is the most effective method of preventing nosocomial infections.* Monitoring of antibiotic resistance patterns and programs directed at controlling antibiotic use are also important in veterinary medicine if the emergence of antibiotic resistance is to be controlled. Surveillance of surgical patients for nosocomial infections using standard definitions is important to determine endemic rates of infection, to aid in identification of outbreaks, to identify new nosocomial pathogens, and to recognize and alter hospital practices that may contribute to nosocomial infections.

PREVENTION AND MANAGEMENT OF SURGICAL SITE INFECTIONS

Most publications dealing with postoperative infection rates of equine patients contain data on specific conditions rather than being overall reviews* (Table 7-4). Two trends appear from examining these studies. Infection is uncommon in elective general surgery and rarely results in mortality, whereas orthopedic procedures, particularly those

*References 5, 8, 11, 35, 39, 45, 61-83.

TABLE 7-4. Summary of the Incidence of Equine Surgical Site Infection by Procedure

Procedure	Horses (*N*)	Infection Rate	Risk Factors	Mortality from Infection
GENERAL SURGERY				
Emergency Celiotomy	78-274	10%-37%	Enterotomy, use of Vicryl, reoperation	0%
Ovariectomy	77	5%	—	0%
Open joint injuries	58	56%	Inadequate drainage and lavage	67%
Castration				
Routine	23,229	3.2%	—	0%
Cryptorchid	107	0.9%	Lack of drainage; lack of antibiotic prophylaxis	0%
Laryngoplasty	153	3.3%	—	0%
ORTHOPEDIC PROCEDURES				
General orthopedic	452	10%	—	—
Clean	433	8.1%	Procedure classification, long bone affected, surgery duration > 90 min, female patients	—
Clean-contaminated	19	52.6%	—	—
Arthroscopy	591	0.5%	—	0%
Humeral fractures	13	38%	Age++	—
Pins and wires	6	17%	—	0%
Plated	5	80%	—	100%
Intramedullary nail	10	0%	—	NA
Radial fractures	24	29%	Open fractures (age, fracture configuration)++	57%
Olecranon fracture				
Simple	29	13%	—	0%
Comminuted	17	53%	Open wounds (age, weight)	56%
Pins and wires	22	24^	—	60%
Condylar fracture	60	0%	—	NA
Metacarpal/metatarsal III fractures	11	46%	Open fractures, excessive trauma, instability, surgical duration, poor soft tissue coverage (age)++	100%
Open splint bone fractures				
Internal fixation	2	100%	—	0%
Without internal fixation	24	8%	Use of implant	—
Sesamoid fracture (lag screw)	25	8%	Suture sinus	50%
First phalanx fracture				
Simple	65	2%	—	100%
Comminuted	20	55%	—	100%
Secondary phalanx fracture (comminuted)	10	10%	Invasive surgical approach	0%
Femoral fractures	18	38%	Configuration of incision in extensor tendon	88%
Tibial fractures (foals)	9	22%	Seroma formation (age, weight, implant size)++	0%
Arthrodesis				
Fetlock joint	17	8%	Stability, plate luting, closed configuration, age	100%
Pastern joint	21	0%	Extension of preexisting infection Repair of open luxation	NA

++, factor thought to affect overall success; NA, not applicable.
See references 5, 8, 11, 35, 39, 46, 62-84.

involving fracture fixations, have greater rates of infection and mortality. The seriousness of orthopedic infection in the horse is emphasized by a retrospective study that demonstrated a 36% rate of euthanasia because of uncontrolled orthopedic infection, and a resolution of infection in only 48% of horses treated, even after implant removal.[84]

The cost of SSI in horses has not been calculated. However, the mean duration of hospitalization of 25 horses with postoperative septic arthritis was 39 days (range, 6 to 125 days).[85] Therefore, even conservative daily costs would result in a high total treatment cost. Additionally, treatment of infection after internal fixation can be devastatingly expensive,[86] and treatment of many other SSIs in the horse can be similarly costly.

Evaluation of large numbers of human patients has allowed physicians to determine infection rates after surgery and establish risk factors.[40,87-89] This information can be combined with equine postoperative infection rates to propose guidelines for the reduction of postoperative infection in horses; however, not all information from human studies is applicable. The reasons for different infection rates and outcomes after infection in horses compared with humans have yet to be entirely identified. However, equine surgeons encounter challenges that are not present in surgery on humans, and they affect equine postsurgical infection rates. Some disparities most likely result from environmental differences—for example, horses are "hospitalized" in a barn stall, not in a hospital bed. The amount of contamination to a traumatic wound or open fracture is likely to be more significant in horses because of these environmental conditions, which increase the likelihood of developing an SSI.

Diagnosis of Surgical Site Infections

Clinical Signs

Clinical diagnosis of SSI can be challenging. Uninfected and grossly infected wounds are easily identified, but mild to moderate infections may be more difficult to identify.[90] Postoperative fever is one of the earliest and consistent signs of an orthopedic SSI,[91] but it can be the result of other sources of inflammation, such as respiratory or gastrointestinal tract conditions. Superficial and deep incisional wounds are considered infected when one or more of the following is present: (1) discharge of purulent material, (2) spontaneous dehiscence of one or more wound layers, accompanied by serous drainage, (3) organisms isolated from an aseptically obtained culture of the area, or (4) excessive erythema, pain, or swelling in the immediate postoperative period.[90-92] The most common superficial SSI in the horse is infection of the ventral midline incision after an emergency celiotomy. The first clinical signs of infection are excessive edema, pain elicited with digital palpation, and an accumulation of serous or exudative fluid revealed by palpation of the incision.

Recognition of organ or space infections can be more difficult. The first clinical signs often seen in horses with osteomyelitis and septic arthritis are excess fluid accumulation in the surgical site.[92] Lameness is another early clinical signs of an orthopedic SSI. However, if lameness was present before surgery, it can be difficult to differentiate a lameness caused by infection from the preexisting lameness. Because of their remote locations, organ or space infections often require laboratory evaluations of fluid or tissue, or diagnostic imaging, for confirmation.

Laboratory Evaluations

The goal of a laboratory evaluation is to distinguish between posttraumatic or postsurgical inflammation and postsurgical infection. Complete blood counts may be useful but can be within normal limits in the presence of infection. Wound fluid can be obtained from superficial and deep incisional infections after surgical drainage or spontaneous dehiscence. Although cytologic examination of incisional fluid is not commonly performed, it should be cultured to help direct antimicrobial therapy.

Cytologic examination of fluid obtained from a potential infection of an organ or space is valuable in determining if infection is present. Normal postoperative values for peritoneal fluid after laparotomy are available,[93] but similar values are not available for joints. However, laboratory findings on examination of space fluids that indicate infection include increases in both number and concentration of polymorphonuclear leukocytes, an increase in the total protein concentration, and evidence of bacteriophagia by inflammatory cells. Correct interpretation of the results requires knowledge of the cytologic changes that result from surgery alone. Even with this information, these values may be confusing after abdominal surgery when the results are equivocal and the results of bacterial culture of peritoneal fluid are pending. Recently, a study indicated that peritoneal fluid pH and glucose concentration can be used to assist in the identification of horses with postoperative septic peritonitis. The finding that the difference between the glucose concentration in serum and that in peritoneal fluid was greater than 50 mg/dL had the greatest diagnostic value for detection of septic peritonitis. A peritoneal fluid pH of less than 7.3, a glucose concentration of less than 30 mg/dL, and a fibrinogen concentration of greater than 200 mg/dL were also highly indicative of septic peritonitis after an exploratory celiotomy.[94] Nonetheless, clinical evaluation is often the best early indicator of SSI, and treatment should begin when clinical signs are noted. Animals with acute peritonitis are characterized by shock, ileus, abdominal distention, and nasogastric reflux. The animal may be febrile, have a slow capillary refill time, and show evidence of hemoconcentration and leukopenia on a complete blood count. Plasma protein may decline because of its effective loss from the circulation into the peritoneal cavity. Therapy should not be delayed until "conclusive" evidence of infection, such as positive cultures or evidence of degenerative neutrophils in surgical site fluid, is identified.

Osteomyelitis is a serious organ infection in equine surgery because of the fatality rate associated with this infection. Osteomyelitis can (1) be hematogenous in origin, which is common in foals but rare in adults, (2) spread from an adjacent infected soft tissue focus, (3) occur as the result of a penetrating wound, or (4) occur secondary to surgery for fracture repair. Postoperative osteomyelitis may be difficult to diagnose if no accumulation of fluid is apparent. However, if it is present, fluid accumulation should be sampled percutaneously after sterile preparation of the skin, and a finding of greater than 90% neutrophils in the fluid suggests that infection is present.[92] If spontaneous drainage occurs, culture of the draining tract may be useful to identify the pathogen.[92] Enrichment media (blood culture, thioglycolate broth) are generally not recommended, as contaminants or other local nonprincipal pathogenic organisms may have their growth enhanced as well, to the exclusion of the principal pathogen.

Imaging Techniques

Radiography of the surgical site is the most commonly used tool for the diagnosis of osteomyelitis, but it is not particularly sensitive, especially for early diagnosis. Initial radiographic changes result from hyperemia and bone demineralization, but 50% to 75% of bone mineral must be lost before this change can be seen on plain radiographs. Therefore, radiographic signs of infection in bone are not usually apparent for at least 7 to 10 days after the onset of symptoms and can take as long as 3 weeks.[95,96] With chronic infection, radiographic lucencies associated with areas of bone lysis predominate, and radiodense bone sequestra can form. These sequestra may become surrounded by an envelope of proliferative periosteal new bone growth, known as an involucrum.

Alternatively, ultrasonography has been used to diagnose osteomyelitis in human patients[97,98] and osteitis in equine patients.[99] Further work is needed regarding the use of ultrasonography in the early diagnosis of bone or implant infection in horses. However, this technique is invaluable in the evaluation of equine ventral midline incisions.[100] Nuclear scintigraphy using technetium-99m diphosphonate is a very sensitive indicator of bone turnover and can yield positive signs of osteomyelitis 10 to 14 days before radiographic signs are observed.[95] However, a positive bone scan is not specific for infection, and scintigraphy is nonspecific in cases of recent wounding and fracture development, or when recent surgery has occurred. Computed tomography and magnetic resonance imaging have certain specific indications in the diagnosis of osteomyelitis in human patients. As these imaging modalities, especially magnetic resonance imaging, become more available in veterinary hospitals, their role in diagnosing soft tissue infections and osteomyelitis should become more significant.

Prevention of Surgical Site Infections

The identification of preoperative, intraoperative, and postoperative factors that contribute to SSI pathogenesis has led to several interventions that may be applied to decrease the risk of SSI. These interventions include practices that have been scientifically proven in the horse to decrease the risk of SSI as well as those that may theoretically decrease the risk of infection (Table 7-5). The three main components to the prevention of surgical site infections are (1) reduction of bacterial numbers in the surgical site, (2) promotion of clearance of bacteria from the surgical site, and (3) administration of prophylactic antimicrobials. Surgical technique is the most important factor in the prevention of SSI, as it addresses the first of these components.[101] Additionally, to decrease equine SSI, the bacteria most commonly isolated from equine surgical infections must be identified, and therefore hospital surveillance programs should be implemented.

TABLE 7-5. Interventions to Decrease Incidence of Surgical Site Infection in the Horse

Timing	Interventions
Preoperative	Minimize surgical time by preoperative planning. Delay hair removal until just before surgery. Perform emergency surgery only when absolutely necessary. Establish good metabolic status and a positive nutritional plane. Treat remote or distant sites of infection before surgery. Minimize length of preoperative hospitalization. Consider preoperative bathing of patient.
Intraoperative	Prepare the patient's and surgeon's skin with antiseptics such as chlorhexidine or povidone-iodine solutions. Administer perioperative antimicrobial agents when appropriate. Use aseptic technique and barriers such as surgical caps, masks, shoe covers, gowns, gloves, and incisive drapes. Use good surgical judgment when closing contaminated or infected wounds. Use surgical techniques that minimize tissue trauma, hemorrhage, and dead space. Débride infected or devitalized tissue. Minimize use of foreign materials, including suture, drains, and orthopedic and prosthetic devices.
Postoperative	Administer therapeutic antimicrobials when appropriate. Minimize the length of postoperative hospitalization. Cover or bandage wounds for a minimum of 24 to 48 h.

Surveillance

An essential part of an effective infection control program is SSI surveillance, which entails the ongoing systematic collection, analysis, and interpretation of data relating to the frequency and distribution of SSI and the conditions that increase or decrease its risk of occurrence. Programs for surveillance of SSIs in human patients that include feedback of SSI rates to surgeons have been reported to decrease the incidence of infections.[102,103] Surveillance identifies endemic rates of infection and, once established, can result in a more rapid recognition of an outbreak. Identifying risk factors that contribute to SSI allows the institution of appropriate intervention measures and the evaluation of their efficacy. Essential components of a surveillance program include established criteria for the definition of SSI, critical evaluation of data from surveillance activities, involvement of representatives from the surgical and attending staff in the data analysis, and a method for surveillance after discharge.[17,104] Initiation of SSI surveillance programs in veterinary medicine may aid in the development of more effective control and treatment strategies.

Pathogenic Bacteria Associated with Equine SSI

The organisms most commonly associated with equine orthopedic SSI are Enterobacteriaceae, *Pseudomonas, Streptococcus, Staphylococcus*, and anaerobes. Two studies on orthopedic SSI reported 60% and 19% polymicrobial infections, respectively.[105,106] The second striking difference is the 18% incidence of staphylococcal isolations in the first study,[105] whereas in the second study, 52% of the isolates were staphylococcal.[106] The differences between these studies were probably caused by the different sites of infection surveyed. The first study examined only orthopedic procedures, whereas the second study examined cases with septic arthritis and tenosynovitis. Fractures tend to become infected with multiple gram-negative bacteria, whereas septic arthritis is often the result of an iatrogenic inoculation with *Staphylococcus* species. These two studies show that gram-negative and gram-positive aerobic bacteria and anaerobic bacteria all have the potential to cause an equine orthopedic SSI. It is also suggested that nonarticular orthopedic infections should be considered polymicrobial until proven otherwise, and that postoperative septic arthritis is often caused by *Staphylococcus* species. Both studies note that not all patients were cultured for anaerobes, and therefore the incidence of anaerobic infection may be underrepresented.

Reduction of Bacterial Numbers in the Surgical Site

Proper design and maintenance of the surgical suite is important in the reduction of overall bacterial numbers, as is appropriate antiseptic preparation of the surgical site, including the clipping of hair. Removal of devitalized tissue, removal of foreign substances, and wound lavage decreases the number of bacteria in contaminated surgical sites and also reduces SSIs.[107,108] Postoperative wound contamination can also be reduced by keeping a sterile dressing on the surgical site until healing has occurred.

Antibiotic Prophylaxis against Surgical Site Infections

PERIOPERATIVE ANTIBIOTIC THERAPY IN HORSES

Antibiotic therapy constitutes a major component of SSI prophylactic regimens for horses undergoing elective and emergency surgical procedures. Development of an effective and safe antibiotic regimen requires knowledge of their mechanism of action, their toxic side effects, their pharmacokinetics, and other important principles regarding prophylaxis.

ANTIBIOTIC CLASSIFICATION

Antibiotics can be classified as bactericidal versus bacteriostatic, as broad-spectrum versus narrow-spectrum, and by their mechanism of action.[70,109,110] Mechanisms of action include inhibition of cell wall synthesis, reversible or irreversible inhibition of protein synthesis, inhibition of plasma membrane function, inhibition of nucleic acid synthesis, and inhibition of intermediary metabolism (Table 7-6). Classifying antibiotics according to their mechanism of action is useful because the mechanism does not change from patient to patient, concurrent use of more than one

TABLE 7-6. Characteristics of Antibiotics Used for Perioperative Prophylaxis in the Horse

Antibiotic	Classification	Mechanism of Action	Adverse Effects	Mechanism of Resistance
Penicillins Potassium penicillin G Procaine penicillin G	Bactericidal	Inhibits cell wall synthesis	Autoimmune hemolytic anemia Anaphylaxis Transient hypotension Increased large intestinal motility	β-Lactamases Plasmids Chromosomal Failure to penetrate outer cell wall Alteration of penicillin-binding proteins
Cephalosporins Cefazolin Ceftiofur	Bactericidal	Inhibits cell wall synthesis	Enterocolitis	β-Lactamases
Aminoglycosides Gentamicin Amikacin	Bactericidal	Protein synthesis inhibitor via 30S ribosomal subunit	Nephrotoxicity Neuromuscular blockade Ototoxicity	Plasmid-encoded enzymes
Trimethoprim-Sulfonamides TMP-sulfamethoxazole TMP-sulfadiazine	Bactericidal	Inhibition of successive steps in folate synthesis	Enterocolitis Anemia Congenital defects Immune hemolytic anemia	TMP Plasmids Sulfonamides: Chromosomal mutations Plasmids

TMP, trimethoprim.

drug can be rationally formulated, the mechanisms of bacterial resistance are easily understood, and it helps predict or explain toxic or adverse effects.[109]

PROPHYLACTIC VERSUS THERAPEUTIC ANTIBIOTICS

Antibiotics administered for prophylaxis differ from those administered for therapeutic purposes. Antibiotics are administered therapeutically when an infectious process is already present. Prophylactic antibiotics are typically administered perioperatively in horses undergoing surgical procedures. The principles of these two uses differ. Antibiotics used for prophylaxis should always be *bactericidal* and must be administered so that they reach the surgical site in sufficient concentrations at or before the time of the procedure to prevent establishment of infection. Moreover, to decrease the development of bacterial resistance to the antibiotics necessary to treat serious, life-threatening infections, prophylactic antibiotics should not be the same ones typically used to treat established infections. Because there have been limited reports of controlled studies regarding the efficacy of prophylactic antibiotics in horses,[111] most recommendations are based on extrapolations from human studies. The risk of SSI must outweigh the potential adverse effects to warrant the use of prophylactic antibiotics. Most of the risk of SSI in veterinary medicine is related to the skill of the surgeon and thus the duration of the surgery, as well as to the management practices of the hospital.[112] Antibiotic prophylaxis is most effective when administered within 1 hour of bacterial inoculation, and it is ineffective when administered 3 to 4 hours after bacteria inoculate the wound.[70,113]

Guidelines have been established for the use of antibiotic prophylaxis.[70,113] Antibiotics should be used only for procedures with a high likelihood of postoperative infection. Peak serum concentrations of the antibiotics should reach 4 to 8 times the minimum inhibitory concentration (MIC) for bacteria being treated. The antibiotics should achieve adequate tissue levels throughout the duration of the procedure. Effective antibiotics that are least cytotoxic and least costly should be used. Timing of antibiotic administration should permit absorption and distribution to the target tissue, without promoting bacterial resistance. This usually means intramuscular administration of antibiotics 1 to 2 hours before surgery or intravenous administration immediately prior to the time of induction of general anesthesia (approximately 30 to 60 minutes prior to surgery). Recent trials in humans have suggested that a single dose of an appropriate antibiotic regimen 30 to 60 minutes before surgery provides adequate prophylaxis; a second dose is given for procedures lasting longer than 3 hours.[101] There is no apparent benefit to continuing antibiotic prophylaxis for more than 24 hours postoperatively. Therefore, prophylactic antibiotics should generally not be administered for more than 24 hours and definitely no longer than 72 hours.[113] In veterinary medicine, a single preoperative dose is usually sufficient and is more cost effective.[114] If infection develops despite prophylactic antibiotics, the bacteria should be considered resistant. Prolonged administration of prophylactic antibiotics could contribute to the occurrence of adverse effects and might promote the development of resistance.

Prophylactic systemic administration of antibiotics is indicated for all clean-contaminated and contaminated surgical wounds, for clean surgical wounds involving an implant or prosthesis, and for any situation in which development of an infection is considered life threatening.[70,113] Systemic prophylactic antibiotics are also indicated for high-risk patients, animals suffering from a concurrent disease process, animals appreciably underweight or malnourished, animals advanced in age, and possibly animals receiving corticosteroids. Because the infection rate for clean surgical wounds is quite low, systemic antibiotic prophylaxis is generally not needed and may be contraindicated in these procedures. There is much disagreement about indications for systemic prophylactic antibiotic treatment of clean-contaminated surgical procedures.[70,113] Because all procedures involving entry into the upper respiratory, urogenital, and gastrointestinal tracts carry an increased risk of infection, many clinicians recommend the use of prophylactic antibiotics. The decision to administer prophylactic antibiotics should be made individually, taking into account the probable magnitude of contamination, the patient's immune status, and the length of the procedure. If major spillage or contamination is possible, then prophylactic antibiotics are indicated. Systemic antibiotics are mandatory for contaminated and dirty procedures.[70,113] It must also be remembered that antibiotics are often administered prophylactically to horses undergoing general anesthesia and surgery, to prevent pneumonia and pleuropneumonia. The most commonly used antibiotics for systemic prophylaxis in horses includes a combination of penicillin and gentamicin, penicillin alone, trimethoprim-sulfonamides, or ceftiofur.

Topical antibiotics can also be used prophylactically.[70] Some studies have shown that topical antibiotics have a significant advantage over placebo administration. When systemic antibiotic prophylaxis is compared with topical antibiotics, there is no appreciable difference in the rate of SSI. Concurrent use of systemic and topical prophylactic antibiotics has no greater efficacy in preventing infection over either one alone. When topical antibiotics are used, results are optimal when the antibiotic is administered immediately after opening each tissue plane; this prevents bacterial adherence to tissue. Irrigation of the tissues with the antibiotic should continue throughout the surgical procedure, not simply prior to closure. The antibiotics that have been used for topical wound irrigation include penicillin, kanamycin, lincomycin, cephalothin, ampicillin, and a combination of neomycin, bacitracin, and polymyxin B.[70]

SELECTION OF PROPHYLACTIC ANTIBIOTICS

Selecting an antibiotic is an important decision for the prophylaxis of SSI in horses. Knowledge of the most common bacteria isolated from horses with infections involving different sites and their probable antibiotic susceptibility patterns is necessary. Clinical experience and the results of retrospective studies evaluating antibiotic susceptibility patterns of equine bacterial pathogens should assist clinicians in making rational choices regarding antibiotic treatment, both for established infections and for prophylactic use during surgical procedures.[70,109,110,113,115] As an example, Enterobacteriaceae, staphylococci, streptococci, and *Pseudomonas* species represent 69% to 77% of the organisms isolated from infected orthopedic procedures.[13,78] Currently, there are no published data regarding the most common bacteria isolated from surgical sites after general soft tissue surgery. Surgeons should be familiar with the most likely bacteria involved in SSI and the likely antibiotic susceptibility patterns in their own hospitals or practices.

Numerous factors should be considered when selecting an antibiotic regimen in horses.[70,109,110,113] These include the presence or likelihood of an infectious process, the type of infectious process, the most likely bacteria to be isolated, the age and immune status of the animal, the cost of antibiotics, the ease of administration, and potential toxic side effects. The type of established or likely infectious process is important when selecting an antibiotic regimen. Some infections such as septicemia require immediate, aggressive treatment because the infection may be life threatening. On the other hand, a chronic infectious process is usually not immediately life threatening, and therefore a more thorough diagnostic evaluation can be performed prior to initiating antibiotic therapy. Selection of an appropriate antibiotic regimen in these cases usually necessitates knowledge of the most likely organisms to be involved in the infection and the probable susceptibility patterns of these isolates; this is often based on practical experience or retrospective studies. Infectious processes unresponsive to initial antibiotic treatment or complicated infections necessitate identification of the offending bacteria and determining their antibiotic susceptibility pattern. Undoubtedly, refinement of bacterial isolation and identification techniques and antibiotic susceptibility testing has dramatically improved the ability of clinicians to select appropriate antibiotics.

It is generally believed that prophylactic antibiotics are not necessary for horses undergoing routine arthroscopic procedures that do not involve the use of implants. This is because of the extremely low infection rate reported following these procedures, which probably results from the minimally invasive surgery, the relatively short duration of surgery, and the continuous lavage of the joint with a large volume of fluid. However, certain factors may necessitate the need for prophylactic antibiotics, such as the intra-articular administration of corticosteroids in the recent past. Similarly, antibiotics are probably not necessary for routine laparoscopic procedures such an ovariectomy and cryptorchidectomy. Prophylactic antibiotics are often indicated in horses undergoing other types of articular surgery because of the potentially devastating consequences of septic arthritis. When a synovial structure becomes infected postoperatively, staphylococci are commonly isolated, which suggests that an antibiotic effective against staphylococcal species should be chosen.[78] Depending on the results of antibiotic susceptibility testing of bacteria isolated from horses with postoperative orthopedic infections, an aminoglycoside, a cephalosporin, or both have been recommended.[113] Although it has been reported that amikacin is the most effective antibiotic presently available to treat orthopedic infections in horses, it should probably not be used for routine prophylaxis because of the possibility of promotion of antibiotic-resistant strains. Rather, gentamicin is probably more appropriate in this situation, depending on other factors including whether or not implants are involved and the nature of the fracture (open versus closed) or injury.

The risk of potential side effects of an antibiotic must be considered when selecting a prophylactic antibiotic regimen. Horses appear to be susceptible to antibiotic-associated diarrhea, apparently secondary to disruption of the gastrointestinal tract microflora.[116] Antibiotics have been shown to promote the overgrowth of opportunistic bacteria, select for resistant strains, and disrupt bacteria that contain toxins.[117] Although the causal relationship between the administration of antibiotics and diarrhea in horses is poorly understood, anecdotal experience suggests that caution is warranted when selecting prophylactic antibiotics. For example, orally administered antibiotics and administration of antibiotics to highly stressed or anorexic horses should be carefully considered.

ANTIBIOTICS USED FOR PROPHYLAXIS IN HORSES

Penicillin G remains one of the most effective antibiotics for prevention and treatment of certain bacterial infections in horses.[118] The mechanism of action involves interference with synthesis of the bacterial cell wall peptidoglycans, resulting in cell lysis in a hypoosmotic or isoosmotic environment. Penicillin is effective against most β-hemolytic streptococci, β-lactamase-negative staphylococci, and obligate anaerobes other than *Bacteroides* species. Penicillin G is easily inactivated by β-lactamases and has little efficacy against bacteria that can produce these enzymes. It is most useful for the prevention or treatment of β-hemolytic streptococci and anaerobes. Penicillin G is administered either via the intramuscular route as procaine penicillin G or intravenously as the potassium or sodium salt.

Aminoglycosides, particularly gentamicin, are commonly administered for antibiotic prophylaxis. Aminoglycosides are actively pumped into the interior of bacterial cells, where the drug binds to the 30S ribosomal subunit and causes a misreading of the genetic code, interrupting normal bacterial protein synthesis.[118] This interruption in protein synthesis leads to alterations in cell membrane permeability, additional aminoglycoside uptake, additional bacterial cell disruption, and ultimately cell bacterial death. Aminoglycosides exert an effect even after administration has ceased. They are effective against most gram-negative bacteria, including *Pseudomonas,* and they are somewhat effective against staphylococci. Streptococci are often resistant, and because aminoglycosides move into bacterial cells via an oxygen-dependent pump, these drugs are not effective against anaerobic bacteria. Gentamicin and amikacin are the most commonly used aminoglycosides. Gentamicin should probably be used for short-term prophylaxis and amikacin reserved for longer-duration therapeutic use. Amikacin is effective against bacteria that are often resistant to other aminoglycosides, because it is more resistant to bacterial enzymatic inactivation.

Cephalosporins, which inhibit bacterial cell wall synthesis, are sometimes used for prophylaxis, particularly in horses undergoing orthopedic procedures. Ceftiofur, a new-generation cephalosporin, is used in some hospitals for routine antibiotic prophylaxis. It is active against many bacterial pathogens commonly isolated from horses, including streptococci, *Pasteurella* species, obligate anaerobes, and some staphylococci and Enterobacteriaceae. *Pseudomonas* species are usually resistant.[118] Ceftiofur is rapidly metabolized to the active metabolite desfuroylceftiofur; however, the metabolite is less effective against *S. aureus* and *Proteus* species. It is important to know whether the microbiology laboratory uses ceftiofur or desfuroylceftiofur discs for susceptibility testing, as desfuroylceftiofur results for staphylococci and *Proteus* may not be reliable for predicting efficacy of ceftiofur against these bacteria. Cephalosporins should probably be administered intramuscularly because of their rapid elimination after intravenous injection.

Potentiated sulfonamides are usually formulated at a ratio of 1:5 with trimethoprim. Sulfonamides inhibit the bacterial dihydropteroate synthetase in the folic acid pathway, thereby blocking bacterial nucleic acid synthesis.[118] Sulfonamides substitute for para-aminobenzoic acid (PABA), which prevents its conversion to dihydrofolic acid. When used alone, sulfonamides are bacteriostatic. However, in combination with trimethoprim, they inhibit successive steps in the folic acid pathway, so the combination is bactericidal. Trimethoprim inhibits bacterial folic acid synthesis at the next step in the folic acid pathway, inhibiting the conversion of dihydrofolic acid to tetrahydrofolic acid by inhibiting dihydrofolic acid reductase. Sulfonamides have a relatively broad spectrum of activity and are typically effective against streptococci, *Proteus, E. coli, Pasteurella,* and *Salmonella*. Staphylococci, obligate anaerobes, *Klebsiella*, and *Enterobacter* are usually susceptible, but they may develop resistance. On the other hand, *Pseudomonas* species are usually resistant.

TIMING AND DURATION OF ANTIBIOTIC ADMINISTRATION

Prophylactic antibiotics should be administered before the surgical procedure to exert their maximal effect. Although a transient decrease in arterial blood pressure has been reported after the IV administration of sodium penicillin in horses,[119] we believe that penicillin can be used safely in horses when given shortly before anesthetic induction. Evaluation of the horse's heart rate after IV penicillin administration prior to anesthetic induction is recommended. Depending on the length of the surgical procedure and the pharmacokinetics of the given antibiotic, intraoperative redosing may be necessary to maintain high circulating and tissue concentrations of antibiotic.

Much controversy exists over the appropriate duration of prophylactic antibiotic administration. In humans, there is probably no additional benefit after 24 hours of prophylactic antibiotics.[120-122] Furthermore, it has been demonstrated that a single prophylactic dose of antibiotic(s) results in wound infection rates that are similar to the rates obtained with multiple dosing regimens.[123] Despite this finding, antibiotics are often administered prophylactically for extended periods. There is substantial variability in the duration of prophylactic antibiotic administration used by different equine surgeons. Generally, the duration of administration for antibiotic prophylaxis should not exceed 24 hours in horses; however, antibiotics are often administered for up to 24 hours after removal of a surgical drain.[116] This is important because surgical drains are often used with orthopedic procedures, and orthopedic infections are often polymicrobial in nature, which suggests that environmental contamination contributes to these orthopedic infections. Because of the devastating effects of implant-associated infection in orthopedic procedures, many equine surgeons administer prophylactic antibiotics for several days after fracture fixation. The duration of antibiotic administration often depends on the nature of the injury or wound; the length of the surgery; the health of the overlying soft tissues; other factors related to the bacteria, host, and surgery; and the surgeon's preference.

The optimal duration of antibiotic prophylaxis for emergency gastrointestinal tract surgery has not been determined in horses. Because there is a relatively high prevalence of SSI in horses after emergency abdominal surgery,[45] surgeons often choose to administer antibiotics for a longer duration than for many other surgical procedures. However, as there have been relatively high rates of infection in horses receiving prophylactic antibiotics, they may not be particularly efficacious. The duration of antibiotic administration in these horses depends in large part on the diagnosis, and on the presence and magnitude of contamination. Horses with gastrointestinal tract ischemia and those requiring an enterotomy or resection and anastomosis may need to have prophylactic antibiotics administered for a longer period of time. The surgeon determines when to discontinue antibiotic administration in these horses, and the decision should be based on rectal temperature, appearance of the surgical site, and the complete blood count and fibrinogen concentration.

SPECIAL ROUTES OF ADMINISTRATION AND DOSAGES

Topical administration of antibiotics is useful prophylactically to prevent intraoperative wound infections, and it is used in irrigation fluids during surgical débridement and repair of contaminated wounds. The triple antibiotic combination of neomycin, bacitracin, and polymyxin B is recommended. Silver sulfadiazine is a useful topical antibiotic for the treatment of wound infections caused by *Pseudomonas.* The addition of Tris-EDTA to an aminoglycoside such as gentamicin for topical administration increases its effectiveness against *Pseudomonas* by altering the cell membrane and making it more permeable to the aminoglycoside.[125]

Intrathecal administration of gentamicin (150 mg per joint) or amikacin (250 to 500 mg) have been shown to result in synovial fluid concentrations that remain above the MIC of most pathogenic bacteria for 24 hours or greater.[126,127] The advantages of intra-articular antibiotics are that a lower total dose of antibiotic can be used (thus less expensive), and a greater concentration of antibiotic will be maintained in the synovial fluid for a longer period of time than with parenteral administration. Although used most frequently to treat infected joints and tendon sheaths, antibiotics can be injected into synovial structures to prevent perioperative infection at the conclusion of joint or tendon sheath surgery.

Regional limb perfusion with antibiotics has been used experimentally and clinically in horses.[11,128] This method involves the delivery of antibiotic under pressure to a selected region of the limb through the bone or venous system. This is an effective method of delivering high concentrations of antibiotics to bones, joints, and tendon sheaths. Although this route is often used therapeutically to treat orthopedic infections, it can be used intraoperatively or perioperatively to prevent infection. The antibiotic can be delivered via an intravenous catheter or a butterfly catheter placed in a superficial vein, or through a catheter adapter placed in a 4.5-mm hole drilled in the bone. The limbs are usually wrapped tightly with an Esmarch bandage distal to the entrance of the venous system and proximal to the site of infection to occlude the superficial venous system and open the collateral osseous venous circulation. Perfusions are usually administered over a period of approximately 30 minutes at a maximal perfusion pressure of 450 psi. Once the infusion is completed, the Esmarch bandage and catheter are removed (see Chapter 88).

Antibiotic-impregnated plaster of Paris (POP) or polymethylmethacrylate (PMMA) has been used successfully in horses for prophylaxis and treatment of musculoskeletal infections.[78,129] Eighty percent of gentamicin is eluted from POP beads within the first 48 hours after implantation, but it continues to be eluted at concentrations deemed bactericidal for 14 days.[129] The gentamicin also retains its bactericidal activity after ethylene oxide sterilization and storage at room temperature for up to 5 months. PMMA is a high-density plastic formed by combining a fluid monomer and a powdered polymer; the antibiotics are added to the PMMA as it is being mixed, and they become suspended in the PMMA. During the hardening process, the PMMA is molded into round beads or cylinder-shaped implants, which are then placed in the surgical wound. Antibiotics are released from the antibiotic-impregnated PMMA by diffusion; tissue fluids surrounding the PMMA implant create a concentration gradient for elution of the antibiotic from the implant into the fluids. Placement of PMMA in a surgically created wound or at the site of infection provides a prolonged high local tissue concentration of the drug during the first few days after insertion, and the concentration decreases with time.[130] Although it is variable with the antibiotic used, there is sustained release of antibiotic from the implant. Gentamicin- and amikacin-impregnated PMMA release bactericidal concentrations of the antibiotic for at least 30 days, whereas ceftiofur-impregnated PMMA is unlikely to provide long-term bactericidal concentrations.[131] Antibiotic concentrations have been detected more than 2 years after implantation, but elution usually decreases below bacteriostatic level after a few weeks or months. Antibiotics can be added to PMMA used for plate luting in the repair of long-bone fractures or used as implants alongside the repaired fracture in horses.[78] This allows high concentrations to be maintained at the site of repair to help prevent infection involving the bone and implants. Because a combination of cefazolin and amikacin provides the best coverage against the most common bacteria isolated from horses with orthopedic infection,[11,113] the use of these two antibiotics in PMMA implants allows greater concentrations of antibiotics to be achieved locally at much lower cost than with parenteral administration.

LATER ANTIBIOTIC EFFECTS

Some antibiotics continue to exert a deleterious effect on susceptible bacteria after drug concentrations have decreased below the MIC.[132] These postantibiotic effects are believed to occur because of (1) decreased ability of bacteria to grow and reproduce, (2) increased phagocytosis by inflammatory cells as a result of increased opsonization of the bacteria, (3) increased autolytic bacterial enzyme production, and (4) diminished ability of bacteria to adhere to tissues. There is some evidence to suggest that it may in fact be advantageous for the antibiotic concentration to decrease below the MIC for part of the dosing interval to ensure maximal effectiveness. Aminoglycosides, penicillins, cephalosporins, and fluoroquinolones demonstrate an in vitro postantibiotic effect. It is now believed that high peak serum concentrations of aminoglycosides may be more efficacious than prolonged serum concentrations above the MIC.

TOXIC SIDE EFFECTS OF ANTIBIOTICS

Adverse or toxic side effects of antibiotics are not commonly encountered, but when present they can be life threatening (see Table 7-6). Enterocolitis/diarrhea is a relatively common side effect of antibiotic treatment of horses, and it is often associated with *C. difficile* or *Salmonella*.[133,134] Antibiotic-associated diarrhea appears to be most common after oral administration, but it may also occur with parenteral administration. Although objective data are not available, anecdotal reports suggest that ampicillin, trimethoprim-sulfonamides, oxytetracycline, and erythromycin are frequently associated with diarrhea. Some of these reports also report diarrhea with ceftiofur when administered IV more frequently than twice daily.

Neuromuscular blockade is a potential side effect of aminoglycoside therapy.[135] It is recognized infrequently in horses, but it may be more common when used concurrently with anesthetic agents. Although caution is advised regarding the use of a single daily dose of aminoglycosides preoperatively because of the potential for neuromuscular weakness associated with the use of aminoglycosides when combined with inhalant anesthetics,[136] a more recent study has shown that a single high dose of gentamicin does not cause appreciable neuromuscular blockade when administered alone to healthy horses anesthetized with halothane.[137] We have used a 6.6-mg/kg dose of gentamicin preoperatively in horses undergoing elective and emergency surgical procedures with no apparent abnormalities. Ototoxicity is also a potential side effect of aminoglycoside therapy.[135]

Nephrotoxicity is the most common toxic side effect associated with aminoglycoside therapy; it appears to be correlated with a high trough level, which is associated with the accumulation of drug in renal tubules.[135,138] Aminoglycosides are resorbed on the brush border of the proximal tubular cells, and this cortical uptake is saturable. Sustained high serum trough concentrations result in greater nephrotoxicosis. Therefore, single high-dose gentamicin administration avoids the likelihood of this complication.

There are reported deleterious effects of fluoroquinolones (enrofloxacin) on bone, tendon, and cartilage in horses[139-141]; however, the clinical importance of these effects has not been thoroughly documented. These drugs should be used cautiously in foals. They are not, and should not be, used for routine antibiotic prophylaxis.

Anorexia is not uncommon in horses given metronidazole; approximately 2% of horses administered metronidazole per os develop anorexia.[142] Because metronidazole is rarely used prophylactically and because this effect usually develops over time, it is not usually considered a problem in horses undergoing surgery.

EMERGENCE OF BACTERIAL RESISTANCE TO ANTIBIOTICS

The emergence of resistant bacteria has been reported in equine hospitals as it has in human hospitals. The reasons are probably multifactorial, but most likely they are related to the application, perhaps indiscriminate at times, of antibiotics for prophylactic and therapeutic uses. Because penicillins and aminoglycosides are the most commonly used antibiotics for SSI prophylaxis, the mechanisms for development of resistance to these antibiotics will be briefly discussed.

Methicillin-resistant staphylococci have been isolated from normal healthy horses, horses with SSI or other infections, and horses that were involved in outbreaks on farms and in hospitals.[21,143-145] These findings demonstrate the need for even more stringent guidelines for the appropriate use of antibiotics in horses. These bacteria not only pose a risk for horses but also threaten people working with or around them. It is imperative that clinicians be aware of the risk of antibiotic-resistant bacteria, including MRSA, in their hospital or practice.

Resistance to penicillins or other β-lactam antibiotics such as cephalosporins can result from failure of the antibiotic to penetrate the outer bacterial cell layers and from alteration of penicillin-binding proteins, which decreases the affinity of these proteins for the antibiotic.[146] This is the mechanism that occurs in MRSA. Bacteria can also synthesize β-lactamase enzymes, which hydrolyze the cyclic amide bond of the β-lactam ring and inactivate the antibiotic.[147] Bacteria synthesize as many as 50 β-lactamase enzymes, depending on the bacterial species.[148] Most of these enzymes do not inactivate cephalosporins or anti-staphylococcal penicillins. The gram-negative β-lactamase enzymes are a diverse group that can be encoded by either chromosomes or plasmids.[148] *E. coli* also produces a plasmid-derived lactamase that can inactivate penicillins and cephalosporins.

Aminoglycoside resistance is caused principally by enzymes encoded by genes located on bacterial plasmids, which act internally to alter the aminoglycoside and prevent it from binding to ribosomes.[149] Amikacin is the least susceptible of the aminoglycosides to enzymatic inactivation. This plasmid-mediated resistance to aminoglycosides can be transferred between bacteria, so a single type of plasmid may confer cross-resistance to multiple aminoglycosides and to other unrelated antibiotics. Bacteria have developed additional mechanisms to decrease the efficacy of aminoglycosides. For example, some bacteria are less permeable to aminoglycosides, so greater concentrations are required to kill them. Subinhibitory and inhibitory aminoglycoside concentrations lead to resistance in bacterial cells that survive the initial ionic binding.[150] This adaptive resistance is caused by decreased aminoglycoside transport into the bacteria.[149] Exposure to a single dose of an aminoglycoside is sufficient to cause resistant strains of bacteria with altered metabolism and impaired aminoglycoside uptake. Resistance has been shown to occur within 1 to 2 hours after the first dose of an aminoglycoside.

Bacterial resistance to trimethoprim is typically slow to develop, but it is relatively common in bacteria isolated from horses. Bacterial resistance to sulfonamides occurs via chromosomal mutations or via plasmids. Chromosomal alterations may cause increased bacterial synthesis of PABA, which overcomes competitive substitution of the sulfonamides.[118] Cross resistance occurs among sulfonamides.

SUMMARY OF ANTIBIOTIC PROPHYLAXIS

Although antibiotics are an important component of SSI prophylaxis, it is imperative that they be used discriminately. Appropriate principles and guidelines must be followed to decrease the chances of SSI and other complicating infections while minimizing the risk of toxicity, adverse effects, and the emergence of resistant bacterial strains.

REFERENCES

1. Burke JF: Effective period of preventive antibiotic action in experimental incisions and dermal lesions, Surgery 1961;50:161.
2. Perl TM, Golub JE: New approaches to reduce *Staphylococcus aureus* nosocomial infection rates: Treating *S. aureus* nasal carriage, Ann Pharmacother 1998;32:S7-16.
3. Ahrenholz DH, Simmons RL: Mixed and synergistic infections. In Howard RJ, Simmons RL, editors: Surgical Infectious Diseases, ed 3, Norwalk, Conn, 1994, Appleton & Lange.
4. Horan TC, Culver DH, Gaynes RP, et al: Nosocomial infections in surgical patients in the United States, January 1986-June 1992. National Nosocomial Infections Surveillance (NNIS) System, Infect Control Hosp Epidemiol 1993;14:73-80.
5. Kobluk CN, Ducharme NG, Lumsden JH, et al: Factors affecting incisional complication rates associated with colic surgery in horses: 78 cases (1983-1985), J Am Vet Med Assoc 1989;195:639-642.
6. MacDonald DG, Morley PS, Bailey JV, et al: An examination of occurrence of surgical wound infection following equine orthopedic surgery (1981-1990), Equine Vet J 1994;26:323.
7. Ingle-Fehr JE Baxter GM, Howard RD, et al: Bacterial culturing of ventral median celiotomies for prediction of postoperative incisional complications in horses, Vet Surg 1997;26:7-13.
8. Gibson KT, Curtis CR, Turner AS, et al: Incisional hernias in the horse: Incidence and predisposing factors, Vet Surg 1989;18:360-366.
9. Phillips TJ, Walmsley JP: Retrospective analysis of the results of 151 exploratory laparotomies in horses with gastrointestinal disease, Equine Vet J 1993;25:427-431.
10. Galuppo LD, Pascoe JR, Jang SS, et al: Evaluation of iodophor skin preparation techniques and factors influencing drainage from ventral midline incisions in horses, J Am Vet Med Assoc 1999; 215:963-969.
11. Hance SR, Bramlage LR, Schneider RK, et al: Retrospective study of 38 cases of femur fractures in horses less than one year of age, Equine Vet J 1992;24:357-363.
12. Baxter GM: Instrumentation and techniques for treating orthopedic infections in horses, Vet Clin North Am Equine Pract 1996;12:303-335.
13. Snyder J, Pascoe J, Hirsh D: Antimicrobial susceptibility of microorganisms isolated from equine orthopedic patients, Vet Surg 1987;16:197.
14. Moore RM: Antimicrobial therapy in horses. In Colahan P, Mayhew IG, Merritt AM, Moore JN, editors: Equine Medicine and Surgery, ed 5, St Louis, 1999, Mosby.
15. Brown M: Selection and use of antibiotics for equine surgery. In Proceedings of Annual Surgical Forum, American College of Veterinary Surgeons, 1989;17:5.
16. Altemeier W, Culbertson W, Hummel RP: Surgical considerations of endogenous infections: Sources, types, methods of control, Surg Clin North Am 1968;48:277.
17. Wong E: Surgical site infections. In Mayhall C, editor: Hospital Epidemiology and Infection Control, Baltimore, 1996, Williams & Wilkins.
18. Whyte W, Hambraeus A, Laurell G, et al: The relative importance of routes and sources of wound contamination during general surgery: I. Non-airborne, J Hosp Infect 1991;18:93.

19. Wiley AM, Ha'eri GB: Routes of infection: A study of using tracer particles in the orthopedic operating room, Clin Orthop 1979;139:150.
20. Seguin JC, Walker RD, Caron JP, et al: Methicillin-resistant *Staphylococcus aureus* outbreak in a veterinary teaching hospital: Potential human-to-animal transmission, J Clin Microbiol 1999;37:1459-1463.
21. Hartmann FA, Trostle SS, Klohnen AA: Isolation of methicillin-resistant *Staphylococcus aureus* from a postoperative wound infection in a horse, J Am Vet Med Assoc 1997;211:590-592.
22. Ayliffe GA: Role of the environment of the operating suite in surgical wound infection, Rev Infect Dis 1991;13(Suppl 10):S800-804.
23. Kimouth JB, Hare R, Tracy GD: Studies of theater ventilation and wound infection, Br Med J 1958;2:407.
24. Council NR: Postoperative wound infection: The influence of ultraviolet irradiation of the operating room and various other factors, Ann Surg 1964;160(Suppl):1.
25. Altemeier WA, Burke JF, Pruitt BA, et al: Manual on Control of Infection in Surgical Patients, Philadelphia, 1984, JB Lippincott.
26. Hierholzer W: Principles of infectious disease epidemiology. In Mayhall C, editor: Hospital Epidemiology and Infection Control, Baltimore, 1996, Williams & Wilkins.
27. Roettinger W, Edgerton MT, Kurtz LD, et al: Role of inoculation site as a determinant of infection in soft tissue wounds, Am J Surg 1973;126:354-358.
28. Hackett RP, Dimock BA, Bentinck-Smith J: Quantitative bacteriology of experimentally incised skin wounds in horses, Equine Vet J 1983;15:37-39.
29. Elek SD, Conen PE: The virulence of *Staphylococcus pyogenes* for man: A study of the problems of wound infection, Br J Exp Pathol 1957;38:573-586.
30. Gustafson SB, McIlwraith CW, Jones R: Comparison of the effect of polysulfated glycosaminoglycans, corticosteroids and sodium hyaluronate in the potentiation of a subinfective dose of *Staphylococcus aureus* in the midcarpal joint of horses, Am J Vet Res 1989;50:2014-2017.
31. Wolff MA, Ramphal R, Peterson P: The pyogenic cocci. In Howard RJ, Simmons RL, editors: Surgical Infectious Diseases, ed 3, Norwalk, Conn, 1994, Appleton & Lange.
32. Finlay BB, Falkow S: Common themes in microbial pathogenicity, Microbiol Rev 1989;53:210-230.
33. Gristina AG, Oga M, Webb LX, et al: Adherent bacterial colonization in the pathogenesis of osteomyelitis, Science 1985; 228:990-993.
34. Fales WH, Warner JF, Teresa GW: Effects of *Fusobacterium necrophorum* leukotoxin on rabbit peritoneal macrophages in vitro, Am J Vet Res 1977;38:491-495.
35. Wilson DA, Baker GJ, Boero MJ: Complications of celiotomy incisions in horses, Vet Surg 1995;24:506-514.
36. Howard RJ: Surgical Infections, ed 7, New York, 1999, McGraw-Hill.
37. Swaim SF: Surgery of traumatized skin: Management and reconstruction in the dog and cat, Philadelphia, 1980, WB Saunders.
38. Phillips TJ, Walmsley JP: Retrospective analysis of the results of 151 exploratory laparotomies in horses with gastrointestinal disease, Equine Vet J 1993;25:427-431.
39. MacDonald DG, Morley PS, Bailey JV, et al: An examination of the occurrence of surgical wound infection following equine orthopaedic surgery (1981-1990), Equine Vet J 1994;26:323-326.
40. Cruse PJ, Foord R: The epidemiology of wound infection: A 10-year prospective study of 62,939 wounds, Surg Clin North Am 1980;60:27-40.
41. Klohnen AA, Wilson DG, MacWilliams PS, et al: Comparison of three preoperative skin preparation techniques in ponies, Vet Surg 1997;26:419.
42. McCue SF, Berg EW, Saunders EA: Efficacy of double-gloving as a barrier to microbial contamination during total joint arthroplasty, J Bone Joint Surg 1981;63:811-813.
43. Edlich RF, Rodeheaver GT, Thacker JG: Technical factors in the prevention of wound infection. In Howard RJ, Simmons RL, editors: Surgical Infectious Diseases, ed 3, Norwalk, Conn, 1994, Appleton & Lange.
44. Trostle SS, Hendrickson DA: Suture sinus formation following closure of ventral midline incisions with polypropylene in three horses, J Am Vet Med Assoc 1995;207:742-745.
45. Honnas CM, Cohen ND: Risk factors for wound infection following celiotomy in horses, J Am Vet Med Assoc 1997;210:78-81.
46. Haley RW, Culver DH, White JW, et al: The nationwide nosocomial infection rate: A new need for vital statistics, Am J Epidemiol 1985;121:159-167.
47. Holtz TH, Wenzel RP: Postdischarge surveillance for nosocomial wound infection: A brief review and commentary, Am J Infect Control 1992;120:206.
48. Sage R: Nosocomial infections: Listening to human experience may help the horse, Equine Vet J 1998;30:450-451.
49. Koterba A, Torchia J, Silverthorne C, et al: Nosocomial infections and bacterial antibiotic resistance in a university hospital, J Am Vet Med Assoc 1986;189:185.
50. Schott HC, Ewart SL, Walker RD, et al: An outbreak of salmonellosis among horses at a veterinary teaching hospital, J Am Vet Med Assoc 2001;218:1152-1159.
51. House JK, Mainar-Jaime RC, Smith BP, et al: Risk factors for nosocomial *Salmonella* infection among hospitalized horses, J Am Vet Med Assoc 1999;214:1511-1516.
52. Hird DW, Pappaioanou M, Smith BP: Case-control study of risk factors associated with isolation of *Salmonella saintpaul* in hospitalized horses, Am J Epidemiol 1984;120:852-864.
53. Rumschlag ES, Boyce JR: Plasmid profile analysis of salmonellae in a large animal hospital, Vet Microb 1987;13:301.
54. Owen RR, Fullerton J, Barnum DA: Effects of transportation, surgery, and antibiotic therapy in ponies infected with *Salmonella*, Am J Vet Res 1983;44:46.
55. Weese JS, Staempfli HR, Prescott JF: Isolation of environmental *Clostridium difficile* from a veterinary teaching hospital, J Vet Diagn Invest 2000;12:449-452.
56. Jones RL: Clostridial enterocolitis, Vet Clin North Am Equine Pract 2000;16:471-485.
57. Jarvis WR: Nosocomial outbreaks: The Centers for Disease Control's Hospital Infections Program experience, 1980-1990. Epidemiology Branch, Hospital Infections Program, Am J Med 1991;91:101S-106S.
58. Patterson JE, Vecchio J, Pantelick EL, et al: Association of contaminated gloves with transmission of *Acinetobacter calcoaceticus* var. anitratus in an intensive care unit, Am J Med 1991;91:479-483.
59. Centers for Disease Control: Guidelines for the Prevention and Control of Nosocomial Infections. Atlanta, 1981, Public Health Services, Centers for Disease Control.
60. Pugliese G, Kroc KA: Development and implementation of infection control policies and procedures. In Mayhall C, editor: Hospital Epidemiology and Infection Control, Baltimore, 1996, Williams & Wilkins.
61. Wilson DG, Reinertson EL: A modified parainguinal approach for cryptorchidectomy in horses: An evaluation in 107 horses, Vet Surg 1987;16:1-4.
62. Gibson KT, McIlwraith CW, Turner AS, et al: Open joint injuries in horses: 58 cases (1980-1986), J Am Vet Med Assoc 1989;194:398-404.
63. Meagher DM, Wheat JD, Hughes JP, et al: Granulosa cell tumors in mares: A review of 78 cases. Proc Am Assoc Equine Practit 1977;23:133-143.
64. Moll HD, Pelzer KD, Pleasant RS, et al: A survey of equine castration complications, J Equine Vet Sci 1995;15:522.

65. McIlwraith CW, Yovich JV, Martin GS: Arthroscopic surgery for the treatment of osteochondral chip fractures in the equine carpus, J Am Vet Med Assoc 1987;191:531-540.
66. Carter BG, Schneider RK, Hardy J, et al: Assessment and treatment of equine humeral fractures: Retrospective study of 54 cases (1972-1990), Equine Vet J 1993;25:203-207.
67. Watkins JP: Intramedullary interlocking nail fixation of humeral fractures: Results of ten foals. Proc Am Assoc Equine Practit 1996:172.
68. Sanders-Shamis M, Bramlage LR, Gable AA: Radius fractures in the horse: A retrospective study of 47 cases, Equine Vet J 1986;18:432-437.
69. Donecker JM, Bramlage LR, Gabel AA: Retrospective analysis of 29 fractures of the olecranon process of the equine ulna, J Am Vet Med Assoc 1984;185:15.
70. Martin F, Richardson DW, Nunamaker DM, et al: Use of tension band wires in horses with fractures of the ulna: 22 cases (1980-1992), J Am Vet Med Assoc 1995;207:1085-1089.
71. Rick MC, O'Brien TR, Pool RR, et al: Condylar fractures of the third metacarpal bone and third metatarsal bone in 75 horses: Radiographic features, treatments, and outcome, J Am Vet Med Assoc 1983;183:287-296.
72. Denny HR: Diaphyseal fractures of the third metacarpus and third metatarsus bones (cannon bones). In Denny HR, editor: Treatment of Equine Fractures, London, 1989, Wright (Butterworth Scientific).
73. Bramlage LR: Long bone fractures, Vet Clin North Am Equine Pract 1983;5:285.
74. Harrison LJ, May SA, Edwards GB: Surgical treatment of open splint bone fractures in 26 horses, Vet Rec 1991;128:606-610.
75. Henninger RW, Bramlage LR, Schneider RK, et al: Lag screw and cancellous bone graft fixation of transverse proximal sesamoid bone fractures in horses: 25 cases (1983-1989), J Am Vet Med Assoc 1991;199:606-612.
76. Markel MD, Richardson DW: Noncomminuted fractures of the proximal phalanx in 69 horses, J Am Vet Med Assoc 1985;186:573-579.
77. Markel MD, Richardson DW, Nunamaker DM: Comminuted first phalanx fractures in 30 horses, Vet Surg 1985;14:135-140.
78. Crabill MR, Watkins JP, Schneider RK, et al: Double-plate fixation of comminuted fractures of the second phalanx in horses: 10 cases (1985-1993), J Am Vet Med Assoc 1995;207:1458-1461.
79. Young DR, Richardson DW, Nunamaker DM, et al: Use of dynamic compression plates for treatment of tibial diaphyseal fractures in foals: Nine cases (1980-1987), J Am Vet Med Assoc 1989;194:1755-1760.
80. Bramlage L: An initial report on a surgical technique for arthrodesis of the metacarpophalangeal joint in the horse. Proc Am Assoc Equine Practit 1981:257.
81. Martin GS, McIlwraith CW, Turner AS, et al: Long-term results and complications of proximal interphalangeal arthrodesis in horses, J Am Vet Med Assoc 1984;184:1136-1140.
82. Speirs VC, Bourke JM, Anderson GA: Assessment of the efficacy of an abductor muscle prosthesis for treatment of laryngeal hemiplegia in the horse, Aust Vet J 1983;60:294.
83. Anderson DE, Allen D, DeBowes RM: Comminuted, articular fractures of the olecranon process in horses: 17 cases (1980-1992), J Am Vet Med Assoc 1995;207:1085.
84. Snyder JR, Pascoe JR, Hirsh DC: Antimicrobial susceptibility of microorganisms isolated from equine orthopedic patients, Vet Surg 1987;16:197-201.
85. Schneider RK, Bramlage LR, Moore RM, et al: A retrospective study of 192 horses affected with septic arthritis/tenosynovitis, Equine Vet J 1992;24:436-442.
86. Richardson DW: Long bone fractures: Evolving solutions, Equine Vet J 1992;24:333-334.
87. Haley RW, Culver DH, Morgan WM, et al: Identifying patients at high risk of surgical wound infection: A simple multivariate index of patient susceptibility and wound contamination, Am J Epidemiol 1985;121:206-215.
88. Culver DH, Horan TC, Gaynes RP, et al: Surgical wound infection rates by wound class, operative procedure, and patient risk index. National Nosocomial Infections Surveillance System, Am J Med 1991;16:152S-157S.
89. Howard JM, Barker WF, Culbertson WR, et al: Postoperative wound infections: The influence of ultraviolet irradiation of the operating room and of various other factors, Ann Surg 1964;160(Suppl):1.
90. Sawyer RG, Pruett TL: Wound infections, Surg Clin North Am 1994;74:519-536.
91. Schneider RK: Management of implant infection and open fractures. In Proceedings of American College of Veterinary Surgeons, 23rd Annual Surgical Forum, Chicago, Oct 29-Nov 1, 1995, p 56.
92. Horan TC, Gaynes RP, Martone WJ, et al: CDC definitions of nosocomial surgical site infections, 1992: A modification of CDC definitions of surgical wound infections, Am J Infect Control 1992;20:271-274.
93. Santschi EM, Grindem CB, Tate LPJ, et al: Peritoneal fluid analysis in ponies after abdominal surgery, Vet Surg 1988;17:6-9.
94. Van Hoogmoed L, Rodger LD, Speir SJ, et al: Evaluation of peritoneal fluid pH, glucose concentration, and lactate dehydrogenase activity for detection of septic peritonitis in horses, J Am Vet Med Assoc 1999;214:1032-1036.
95. Schauwecker DS, Braunstein EM, Wheat LJ: Diagnostic imaging of osteomyelitis, Infect Dis Clin North Am 1990;4:441-463.
96. Wegener WA, Alavi A: Diagnostic imaging of musculoskeletal infection, Orthop Clin North Am 1991;22:401.
97. Abiri MM: The society for computer applications in radiology: Has DICOM become a victim of its own success? J Digit Imaging 2001;14:163-164.
98. Glasier CM, Seibert JJ, Williamson SL, et al: High resolution ultrasound characterization of soft tissue masses in children, Pediatr Radiol 1987;17:233.
99. Bohn A, Papageorges M, Grant BD: Ultrasonographic evaluation and surgical treatment of humeral osteitis and bicipital tenosynovitis in a horse, J Am Vet Med Assoc 1992;201:305-306.
100. Wilson DA, Badertscher RR, Boero MJ, et al: Ultrasonographic evaluation of the healing of ventral midline abdominal incisions in the horse, Equine Vet J Suppl 1989:107-110.
101. Nichols RL: Surgical wound infection, Am J Med 1991;91:54S-64S.
102. Haley RW, Culver DH, White JW, et al: The efficacy of infection surveillance and control programs in preventing nosocomial infections in US hospitals, Am J Epidemiol 1985;121:182-205.
103. Olson MM, Lee JT: Continuous, 10-year wound infection surveillance: Results, advantages, and unanswered questions, Arch Surg 1990;125:794-803.
104. Howard R: Hospital acquired infections in surgical patients. In Howard RJ, Simmons RL, editors: Surgical Infectious Diseases, ed 3, Norwalk, Conn, 1994, Appleton & Lange.
105. Snyder JR, Pascoe JR, Hirsh DC: Antimicrobial susceptibility of microorganisms isolated from equine orthopedic patients, Vet Surg 1987;16:197-201.
106. Schneider RK, Bramlage LR, Moore RM, et al: A retrospective study of 192 horses affected with septic arthritis/tenosynovitis, Equine Vet J 1992;24:436-442.
107. Merritt K: Factors increasing the risk of infection in patients with open fractures, J Trauma 1988;28:823-827.
108. Stevenson S, Olmstead ML, Kowalski J: Bacterial culturing for prediction of postoperative complications following open fracture repair in small animals, Vet Surg 1986;15:99.
109. Brumbaugh GW: Rational selection of antimicrobial drugs for treatment of infections in horses, Vet Clin North Am Equine Pract 1987;3:191-220.
110. Folz SD, Hanson BJ, Griffin AK, et al: Treatment of respiratory infections in horses with ceftiofur sodium, Equine Vet J 1992;24:300-304.

111. Raidal SL, Taplin RH, Bailey GD, et al: Antibiotic prophylaxis of lower respiratory tract contamination in horses confined with head elevation for 24 or 48 hours, Aust Vet J 1997;75:126-131.
112. Whittem TL, Johnson AL, Smith CW, et al: Effect of perioperative prophylactic antimicrobial treatment in dogs undergoing elective orthopedic surgery, J Am Vet Med Assoc 1999;215:212-216.
113. Brown MP: Principles of antibiotic prophylaxis. In White NA, Moore JN, editors: Current Practice of Equine Surgery, ed 1, Philadelphia, 1992, JB Lippincott.
114. Haven ML, Wichtel JJ, Bristol DG, et al: Effects of antibiotic prophylaxis on postoperative complications after rumenotomy in cattle, J Am Vet Med Assoc 1992;200:1332-1335.
115. Hirsh DC, Jang SS: Antimicrobial susceptibility of bacterial pathogens from horses, Vet Clin North Am Equine Pract 1987;3:181-190.
116. Santschi EM: Diagnosis and management of surgical site infection and antimicrobial prophylaxis. In Auer JA, Stick JA, editors: Equine Surgery, ed 2, Philadelphia, 1992, WB Saunders.
117. Saadia R, Lipman J: Duration of antibiotic treatment in surgical infections of the abdomen: Antibiotics and the gut, Eur J Surg 1996;576(Suppl):39-41.
118. Dowling PA: Antimicrobial therapy. In Reed SM, Bayly WM, Sellon DC, editors: Equine Internal Medicine, ed 2, St Louis, 2004, Saunders.
119. Hubbell JAE, Muir WW, Robertson JT, et al: Cardiovascular effects of intravenous sodium penicillin, sodium cefazolin, and sodium citrate in awake and anesthetized horses, Vet Surg 1987;16:245-250.
120. Classen DC, Evans RS, Pestotnik SL, et al: The timing of prophylactic administration of antibiotics and the risk of surgical-wound infection, N Engl J Med 1992;326:281-286.
121. Mauerhan DR, Nelson CL, Smith DL, et al: Prophylaxis against infection in total joint arthroplasty: One day of cefuroxime compared with three days of cefazolin, J Bone Joint Surg 1994;76:39-45.
122. Righi M, Manfredi R, Farneti G, et al: Short-term versus long-term antimicrobial prophylaxis in oncologic head and neck surgery, Head Neck 1996;18:399-404.
123. DiPiro JT, Cheung RP, Bowden TAJ, et al: Single dose systemic antibiotic prophylaxis of surgical wound infections, Am J Surg 1986;152:552-559.
124. Garber JL, Brown MP, Gronwall RR, et al: Pharmacokinetics of metronidazole after rectal administration in horses, Am J Vet Res 1993;54:2060-2063.
125. Wooley RE, Jones MS: Action of EDTA-Tris and antimicrobial agent combinations on selected pathogenic bacteria, Vet Microbiol 1983;8:271-280.
126. Lloyd KCK, Stover SM, Pascoe JR, et al: Plasma and synovial fluid concentrations of gentamicin in horses after intra-articular administration of buffered and unbuffered gentamicin, Am J Vet Res 1988;49:644-649.
127. Sedrish SA, Moore RM, Barker SM, et al: Synovial fluid concentrations of amikacin after a single intra-articular injection in radiocarpal joints of normal horses, Am J Vet Res 1997 [submitted].
128. Whitehair KJ, Adams SB, Parker JE, et al: Regional limb perfusion with antibiotics in three horses, Vet Surg 1992;21:286-292.
129. Santschi EM, McGarvey L: In vitro elution of gentamicin from plaster of Paris beads, Vet Surg 2003;32:128-133.
130. Holcombe SJ, Schneider RK, Bramlage LR, et al: Use of antibiotic-impregnated polymethylmethacrylate in horses with open or infected fractures or joints: 19 cases (1987-1995), J Am Vet Med Assoc 1997;211:889-893.
131. Ethell MT, Bennett RA, Brown MP, et al: In vitro elution of gentamicin, amikacin, and ceftiofur from polymethylmethacrylate and hydroxyapatite cement, Vet Surg 2000;29:375-382.
132. Brown SA: Minimum inhibitory concentrations and postantimicrobial effects as factors in dosage of antimicrobial drugs, J Am Vet Med Assoc 1987;191:871-872.
133. Baverud V, Gustafsson A, Franklin A, et al: *Clostridium difficile:* Prevalence in horses and environment, and antimicrobial susceptibility, Equine Vet J 2003;35:465-471.
134. Hird DW, Casebolt DB, Carter JD, et al: Risk factors for salmonellosis in hospitalized horses, J Am Vet Med Assoc 1986;188:173-177.
135. Riviere JE, Spoo JW: Aminoglycoside antibiotics. In Adams HR, editor: Veterinary Pharmacology and Therapeutics, ed 7, Philadelphia, 1995, WB Saunders.
136. Brown MP: Antimicrobial selection and advances. Fifth American College of Veterinary Surgeons, Veterinary Symposium, 1995:40-42.
137. Hague BA, Martinez EA, Hartsfield SM: Effects of high-dose gentamicin sulfate on neuromuscular blockade in halothane-anesthetized horses, Am J Vet Res 1997;58:1324-1326.
138. Edens LM: Clinical application of aminoglycoside pharmacokinetics, American College of Veterinary Internal Medicine Forum, 1995:579-581.
139. Bertone AL, Tremaine WH, Macoris DG, et al: Effect of long-term administration of an injectable enrofloxacin solution on physical and musculoskeletal variables in adult horses, J Am Vet Med Assoc 2000;217:1514-1521.
140. Yoon JH, Brooks RLJ, Khan A, et al: The effect of enrofloxacin on cell proliferation and proteoglycans in horse tendon cells, Cell Biol Toxicol 2004;20:41-54.
141. Egerbacher M, Edinger J, Tschylenk W: Effects of enrofloxacin and ciprofloxacin hydrochloride on canine and equine chondrocytes in culture, Am J Vet Res 2001;62:704-708.
142. Sweeney R, Sweeney C, Weiher J: Clinical use of metronidazole in horses: 200 cases (1984-1989), J Am Vet Med Assoc 1991; 198:1045-1048.
143. Yasuda R, Kawano J, Onda H, et al: Methicillin-resistant coagulase-negative staphylococci isolated from healthy horses in Japan, Am J Vet Res 2000;61:1451-1455.
144. Trostle SS, Peavey CL, King DS, et al: Treatment of methicillin-resistant *Staphylococcus epidermidis* infection following repair of an ulnar fracture and humeroradial joint luxation in a horse, J Am Vet Med Assoc 2001;218:554-559.
145. O'Rourke K: Methicillin-resistant *Staphylococcus aureus:* An emerging problem in horses? J Am Vet Med Assoc 2003;223:1399-1400.
146. Dever LA, Dermody TS: Mechanisms of bacterial resistance to antibiotics, Arch Intern Med 1991;151:886.
147. Gold HS, Moellering RC: Antimicrobial-drug resistance, N Engl J Med 1996;335:1445-1453.
148. Smith JT, Lewin CS: Mechanisms of antimicrobial resistance and implications for epidemiology, Vet Microbiol 1993;35:233-242.
149. Prescott JF: Aminoglycosides and aminocyclitols. In Prescott JF, Baggott JD, editors: Antimicrobial Therapy in Veterinary Medicine, ed 3, Ames, 2000, Iowa State University Press.
150. Barclay ML, Begg EJ: Aminoglycoside adaptive resistance: Importance for effective dosage regimens, Drugs 1994;61:713-721.

CHAPTER 8

Physiologic Response to Trauma: Evaluating the Trauma Patient

Susan J. Holcombe

Traumatic injury in horses is common but usually limited to limb or trunk wounds. Less frequently, horses experience more severe trauma resulting in a substantial systemic response. This acute response to trauma is initiated by pain, blood loss and concomitant hypovolemia, hypoxia, acidosis, and sometimes hypothermia, and it is regulated by neurohumoral, immunologic, and inflammatory mediators. The response to trauma is meant to promote homeostatic mechanisms essential to survival and ultimately healing, but the response can be deleterious, leading to systemic inflammatory response (SIRS) (see Chapter 2), coagulopathy (see Chapter 4), remote organ failure, and death. When the tightly regulated equilibrium of proinflammatory and anti-inflammatory cytokines that controls and coordinates the body's response to injury becomes unbalanced, it causes either a hyperinflammatory or a severe immunosuppressive state, neither of which is conducive to longevity.[1]

Classically, the metabolic response to trauma has been described by two phases: ebb (shock phase) and flow (catabolic, followed by an anabolic phase).[2,3] The ebb or *shock* phase occurs during the first several hours after injury and is characterized by the compensatory physiologic responses to shock (see Chapter 1), as well as by acute inflammation. Next, the patient enters the flow phase, which is initiated by a *catabolic* state meant to promote tissue healing.[2,4] This second phase is an intense metabolic state, characterized by a hyperdynamic stress response, fluid retention and edema, and hypermetabolism, which is propagated by cytokines, reactive oxygen metabolites, nitric oxide, and arachidonic acid derivatives.[5] This phase may last for days to weeks. Once volume deficits have been eliminated, wounds have closed, and infection has been controlled, the anabolic stage begins, and this represents the end of the flow phase.[5] It is characterized by a return to normal hemodynamics, diuresis, the reaccumulation of protein and body fat, restoration of body function, and weight gain.[2] This chapter summarizes the acute systemic traumatic responses and then briefly reviews the diagnostic steps for evaluation of thoracic, abdominal, and cranial trauma.

EBB—THE SHOCK PHASE

Components of severe trauma include pain, tissue injury, hypovolemic shock, and, at times, hypothermia. Each of these events contributes to the stress response that results from trauma and is a potent initiator of the sympatho-adrenal axis and secretion of catecholamines and cortisol.[2] Blood loss and resulting hypovolemia cause subsequent release of catecholamines and antidiuretic hormone and activation of the rennin-angiotensin-aldosterone system in an attempt to restore vascular volume.[6] Epinephrine and norepinephrine cause vasoconstriction and increase heart rate and stroke volume to restore perfusion and oxygen delivery to the tissues. Adrenal secretion of cortisol is mediated by the hypothalamic-pituitary-adrenal axis. Stimuli for cortisol release trigger neural afferent signals that stimulate corticotrophin-releasing factor from the hypothalamus, signaling secretion of adrenocorticotropic hormone (ACTH) from the anterior lobe of the pituitary gland.[2] The target organ for ACTH is the adrenal cortex, which stimulates synthesis and release of cortisol. The amount of cortisol released is relative to the degree of injury. Glucocorticoids cause sodium retention, stimulate insulin resistance, and help to fuel a high-energy state by stimulating gluconeogenesis, lipolysis, and protein catabolism.[2] Increased circulating levels of cortisol also enhance the catabolic effects of tumor necrosis factor (TNF) and interleukin (IL)-1 and IL-6, inflammatory cytokines found in high circulating levels in trauma patients.[7,8]

Pain

Pain results from the initial traumatic injury and may persist throughout the healing process. Pain produces a strong sympathetic response and contributes to the stimulus for cortisol secretion. The fact that pain is not experienced during anesthesia may be an important reason that extensive trauma of major surgery is often well tolerated, whereas similar amounts of tissue injury, incurred during accidental trauma, cause more severe metabolic responses.[2,9,10] Such evidence strongly suggests that preemptive and continued analgesic therapy is essential in patients with traumatic injury to minimize the stress response and improve immunologic function and tissue healing[11-16] (Table 8-1). The importance of neural afferents from the site of tissue injury is confirmed in paraplegic humans, in whom the usual perioperative rise in cortisol levels is not seen if the operation is performed below the level of spinal cord damage.[2,17] Pain, as well as other events that stimulate a sympathetic response, enhance endorphin release from the adrenal glands, which functions in part to decrease the sensation of pain. Endogenous opioids also act as regulators of the stress response by modulating the release of catecholamines from the adrenal medulla, exerting inhibitory feedback on pituitary activation and decreasing ACTH release.

Tissue Injury

The response to tissue injury is an essential component of the acute response to trauma. Localized inflammation and coagulation may lead to systemic inflammatory and deranged coagulation events. Endothelial disruption at sites of injury and tissue ischemia initiate the release of inflammatory mediators and coagulation factors. Exposure of the subendothelial collagen and basement membrane activates circulating Hageman factor (factor XII), which initiates the intrinsic coagulation pathway, and the complement cascade,

TABLE 8-1. Analgesic Therapy

Drug	Reference Number	Continuous Rate Infusion	Comments
Lidocaine (2%)	11	1.3 mg/kg, IV bolus 0.05 mg/kg/min, infusion	Repeat bolus if infusion is discontinued for longer than 20 min.
Butorphanol	12	23.7 μg/kg/h	Epidural
Morphine	13	0.1 mg/kg in sufficient saline, 20 mL per 450 kg	—
Morphine, detomidine	14	0.1 mg/kg morphine + 30 to 60 μg/kg detomidine	—
Xylazine	15	0.17 mg/kg in sufficient saline, 20 mL per 450 kg	Transdermal therapeutic system
Fentanyl	16	One 10-mg patch per 200 kg	—

which also incites an inflammatory response.[2,18] Impaired coagulation may be caused by hypothermia as well as by aggressive fluid resuscitation, resulting in dilutional coagulopathy. Another important set of processes activated by injury, ischemia, and endothelial disruption is stimulation of arachidonic acid metabolism, releasing prostaglandins and leukotrienes, which are potent mediators of vascular tone and cause inflammation, cellular activation and cytokine production, and coagulation. The role of cytokines in the pathophysiologic alteration of trauma is not completely understood. There is strong evidence, however, suggesting that one of the important initiating events in posttraumatic inflammation is the overproduction of the proinflammatory cytokines TNF-α, IL-1, and IL-6.[19]

Edema

A vital component of the initial responses to trauma is the restoration of tissue perfusion and maintenance of body fluids. This occurs by a combination of vascular constriction and fluid preservation. Vasoconstriction occurs in an attempt to stop blood loss from the wound and to preferentially perfuse vital organs. Catecholamines, cortisol, aldosterone, and angiotensin II promote sodium and water retention to facilitate the preservation of the blood, interstitial, and intracellular volumes after mild to moderate trauma.[2] The same events that attempt to preserve total body water can result in both local and systemic edema formation. Edema at the site of injury occurs because of loss of capillary integrity and inflammation. Systemic edema occurs because capillary physiology is altered, leading to salt and water loss from the vascular space into the interstitium. This occurs because of the presence of circulating and local vasoactive mediators and increased sympathetic tone, which cause postcapillary vasoconstriction and subsequent increase in intraluminal capillary pressure.

Hypoproteinemia from blood loss and crystalloid resuscitation decreases intravascular oncotic pressure. Increased capillary interstitial pressure and decreased oncotic pressure, in addition to inflammation, which may increase the "leakiness" of capillaries, lead to the egress of salt and water from the capillaries, producing systemic edema formation distant from the original site of injury. The magnitude of edema formation tends to be proportional to the severity of the injury and is progressive as long as the stress state persists.[2] Edema impairs wound healing at the site of injury but also contributes to impaired microcirculatory blood flow, decreased oxygen delivery, and consumption by the tissues, systemically.

Hypothermia

Hypothermia, defined as a core body temperature below 35° C (95° F), may develop in trauma patients as a response to cold exposure, especially if the horse is wet, or as a response to failure of normal physiologic homeothermic mechanisms, which can be a complication of shock.[20] Clinical hypothermia is uncommon in adult horses but common in foals with severe trauma because they have a higher body surface area–to–body mass ratio. Hypothermia may lead to coagulopathies, cardiac arrhythmia, and impaired immune function.[20]

Homeothermia describes the maintenance of constant internal temperature despite changing environmental temperature. This is accomplished by matching metabolic thermogenesis and heat loss. Heat loss occurs by four mechanisms: convection, conduction, radiation, and evaporation.[20] *Convective heat loss* occurs when heat is transferred to the air in contact with the body. It is dependent on air velocity. Therefore, it is important to move injured horses into an enclosed area for evaluation and treatment. *Conductive heat loss* occurs by transfer of heat to an object directly contacting the body. Placing foals on heated water blankets versus cold stainless steel tables minimizes conductive heat loss. *Radiation* is defined as heat loss to the environment based on a gradient of temperature and is minimized by placing blankets on the patient and maintaining a warm ambient temperature. *Evaporation* occurs by conversion of water to the gaseous phase, making it important to keep injured patients dry.[20]

The hypothalamus regulates body temperature and responds to thermoreceptors located along the internal carotid artery, the reticular area of the midbrain, and the preoptic and posterior hypothalamus as well as peripheral receptors in the skin.[20] The normal response to cold includes increased muscular activity or shivering and increased thermogenesis. Increased levels of epinephrine and norepinephrine with a subsequent rise in metabolic rate cause increased metabolic thermogenesis.[20] These processes may be impaired in trauma patients. Three basic mechanisms contribute to hypothermia:

1. Traumatic injury can alter normal central thermoregulation at the hypothalamus and block the shivering response.[21]
2. If the trauma patient experiences hypovolemic shock, thermogenesis decreases because of impaired oxygen delivery to the tissues.
3. Although it is an infrequent cause, infusion of large volumes of cold fluids may contribute to hypothermia.

Hypothermia is a concern because it can lead to coagulopathies that result from impaired platelet function and altered enzymatic kinetics in the coagulation cascade. Severe hypothermia has been shown to impair cardiovascular status by decreasing cardiac output, and by causing hypotension and fatal arrhythmias. Finally, hypothermia causes the oxyhemoglobin dissociation curve to shift to the left, increasing the affinity of hemoglobin for oxygen.[20,22,23]

FLOW—THE CATABOLIC PHASE

After trauma, energy demands increase dramatically because basal metabolic rate can more than double in these patients.[1-3] This hypermetabolic state is directly related to a prolonged stress response, which supports a hyperdynamic circulatory state and increased oxygen consumption as well as generalized inflammation. Cytokines, specifically TNF, formerly known as cachectin, are important mediators of the posttraumatic hypermetabolic state. In research animals, the complete manifestation of the stress response is seen when cortisol, glucagons, and epinephrine were infused into the patient in the presence of inflammation, suggesting that the hypermetabolic response is mediated by a combination of central stress responses and tissue inflammation.[2]

This hypermetabolic state must be fueled. After severe trauma, total-body catabolism is increased, particularly within skeletal muscles.[2,24,25] Amino acids are used for energy production via gluconeogenesis, and glycogen is converted to glucose, leaving patients glycogen depleted and in a negative nitrogen balance. Protein breakdown results in a significant loss of muscle mass and may progress to the loss of visceral protein mass as well. The mediators of altered protein metabolism include cortisol and glucagon as well as elevated levels of catecholamines and cytokines, particularly TNF, IL-1, and IL-6,[2] which can impair wound healing. Nutritional support is vital in trauma patients because of increased energy demands, but protein breakdown and gluconeogenesis will continue through the catabolic phase until anabolism begins.

Insulin levels are initially low after injury but subsequently rise to normal or elevated levels. Hyperglycemia may occur as a result of peripheral insulin resistance caused by persistent elevations of glucagon, cortisol, and epinephrine. Two of the major functions of insulin are inhibition of the rate of hepatic glucose production and stimulation of glucose uptake in peripheral tissues. Therefore, the insulin resistance in the stress state may be central to persistent hyperglycemia as well as to breakdown of muscle, fat, and glycogen. After injury, fat is oxidized at an accelerated rate; this effect is mediated by sympathetic stimulation; increases in epinephrine, glucagon, and cortisol; and insulin resistance.[2,26] Fatty acids are released into the circulation and become available as an energy substrate. However, fat mobilization can be limited by lactate and hyperglycemia.[2]

FLOW—THE ANABOLIC PHASE

The anabolic phase of recovery may last for days to weeks.[2,3] During this time, the systemic neurohumoral system returns to normal, edema dissipates, and catecholamine and cortisol levels stabilize, as do the systemic parameters of the patient.[2,3] Visceral and muscle protein is synthesized and organ function improves. Appetite returns and weight gain begins.

There has been increasing interest in the development of effective agents that can be safely used to promote anabolism in recovering trauma patients and others susceptible to chronic cachexia. An anabolic androgenic steroid, oxandrolone, has been effective in treating catabolic disorders in human patients. Administration of oxandrolone has been associated with improvements in body composition and in muscle strength and function. Improved status of underlying disease, improved recovery from acute catabolic injury, and improved nutritional status are significantly better than placebo in the vast majority of oxandrolone trials.[27]

EVALUATING THE TRAUMA PATIENT

Classes of traumatic injury include blunt and penetrating trauma. Blunt trauma is a distributed dissipation of kinetic energy by concussion or by deceleration.[27] Blunt trauma can lead to direct contusive injury, shearing, vascular disruption, and indirect lacerations secondary to skeletal fracture. A horse suffers blunt trauma during a transportation accident, when a trailer is hit or capsizes, if a moving vehicle hits the horse, or if the horse falls. In these instances, it is imperative to examine each body system, because injuries from blunt trauma may not be obvious and may result in thoracic or abdominal bleeding, diaphragmatic hernia, or cranial injury. Unlike blunt trauma, penetrating trauma is a more focal dissipation of a projectile's kinetic energy, and it leads to direct-impact lacerations and fractures.[27] Examples of penetrating trauma in horses include gunshot injuries and impalement on fenceposts. Although thorough examination of the horse is exigent, injury from penetrating trauma is more obvious as long as an entry wound is found. Blunt or penetrating trauma can result in respiratory, cardiovascular, neurologic, gastrointestinal, or musculoskeletal system injury, and therefore each body system must be assessed during evaluation of the patient.

Thoracic Trauma

Thoracic trauma may result from blunt or penetrating injury. Broadly categorized disorders of thoracic trauma include pneumothorax, hemothorax, thoracic wounds, and fractured ribs. Pulmonary contusions and rib fractures frequently occur with blunt trauma, whereas cardiac tamponade and pneumothorax are more common after penetrating trauma.[28] Injuries that cause blunt trauma may ultimately result in penetrating trauma, because fractured ribs may lacerate pulmonary parenchyma or perforate the heart or cardiac vessels. Blunt thoracic trauma is more common in neonatal foals and may be caused by compression in the pelvic cavity during parturition.[29] In the evaluation and treatment of thoracic wall injury, the principal concerns are cardiovascular embarrassment, pain management, and pulmonary compromise. On an emergency basis, respiratory insufficiency is one of the most serious physiologic consequences of thoracic trauma, and early respiratory support for the injured horse is concerned primarily with restoration and maintenance of adequate ventilation and oxygenation.

The basic principles of treatment of thoracic injury include rapid restoration of the airway, supplemental oxygen, decompression of pneumothorax, and covering open thoracic wounds. Subjectively, horses with thoracic injury may seem anxious because of respiratory distress, or in pain as a result of wounds or fractures. Signs of respiratory distress include excessive respiratory efforts, tachypnea, nostril flaring, audible inspiratory and expiratory sounds, accentuated thoracic and abdominal excursions, and cyanotic mucous membranes.[30] The respiratory rate, pattern, and depth of breathing are evaluated because alterations in the respiratory pattern may be suggestive of specific lesions. For example, a horse with fractured ribs may breathe with a shallow respiratory pattern and decreased tidal volume as a result of thoracic splinting that is caused by pain. Horses with pneumothorax or hemothorax may have a rapid, shallow respiratory pattern, as well. Auscultation of the entire lung fields identifies pneumothorax or hemothorax. With pneumothorax, lung sounds are absent dorsally.[30] With hemothorax, lung sounds are absent or diminished ventrally, but the heart sounds resonate over a large area of the ventral thorax.[30]

Arterial blood gas measurements provide important information on the horse's ability to ventilate and maintain normoxia. Serial samples help determine if the horse is deteriorating or responding favorably to therapy. Palpation of the thoracic cage for swelling, subcutaneous emphysema, and crepitus will help identify injuries such as rib fractures and chest wounds. Thoracic radiographs allow detection of rib fractures, pneumothorax (Fig. 8-1), hemothorax, and thoracic foreign bodies. Thoracic ultrasonography may establish the diagnosis of pneumothorax or the degree of hemothorax present, and it provides guidance for pleurocentesis or placing chest tubes, which are indicated if fluid or air needs to be removed from the pleural space. Thoracoscopy may be performed in the standing and hemodynamically stable horse to assess structures within the chest after thoracic trauma.[31,32] Indications for exploratory thoracoscopy include ongoing hemorrhage, retained hemothorax, suspected diaphragmatic injuries, suspected cardiac injury, intrathoracic foreign body or contamination, and persistent bronchopleurofistula.[33,34] Exploration of each hemithorax can be performed, if warranted, from the caudal dorsal quadrant and continuing cranially. The collapsed lung, diaphragm, aorta, and esophagus can be assessed.[31,32] On the right side, the azygos vein, thoracic duct, and pulmonary veins may be viewed.[31,32]

Cardiovascular assessment of horses with thoracic trauma is important because of the risk of damage to the heart, great vessels, and intercostal and pulmonary parenchymal vasculature. Tachycardia, palpably weak peripheral pulses, and pale mucous membranes may indicate severe, ongoing hemorrhage. Serial arterial blood gases, packed cell volume, and total protein will help assess blood loss and hypoxemia. (For additional details on diagnosis and treatment of thoracic trauma, see Chapter 47).

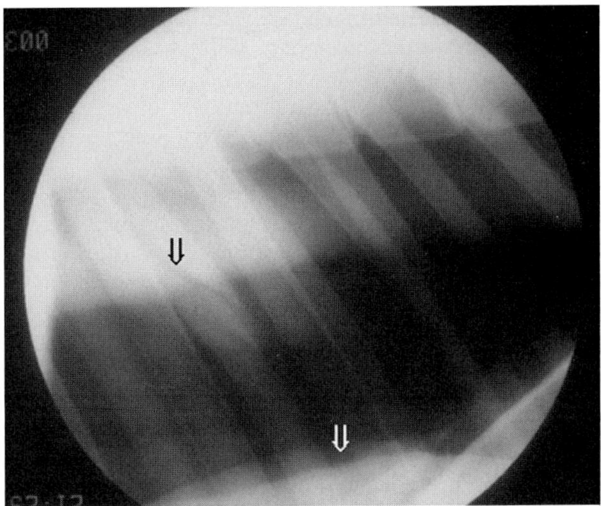

Figure 8-1. Thoracic radiograph of a horse with a rib fracture *(black arrow)* that resulted in pneumothorax, seen as air within the chest *(appears black)*: atelectatic lung *(white arrow)*.

Pneumothorax

Ventilatory embarrassment associated with pneumothorax is believed to be the result of equilibration of atmospheric and intrapleural pressures through a defect in the chest wall or lung. This allows atmospheric air to enter the pleural space, which causes the intrapleural pressure to rise toward atmospheric pressure and produces pneumothorax and collapse of the lung.[35] Bilateral pneumothorax may develop in horses because they have an incomplete mediastinum.[36] Pneumothorax can be categorized as open, closed, or tension pneumothorax. Open pneumothorax results from penetrating, open chest wounds, through which air is drawn into the pleural space during inspiration.[28] Closed pneumothorax is caused by air entering the pleural space from the lung, resulting from a ruptured bulla or closed rib fracture where the rib fragment has lacerated the lung parenchyma.

Tension pneumothorax is present when intrapleural pressure exceeds the atmospheric pressure throughout expiration and often during inspiration as well.[37] Tension pneumothorax usually occurs because of a pleurocutaneous fistula, such as a sucking chest wound, that acts like a one-way valve. During inspiration, when the pleural pressure is negative, air moves into the pleural space while the opening is patent. During expiration, the communication is partially or totally occluded by a flap or valve-like opening, and air accumulates in the pleural space under positive pressure. The development of tension pneumothorax is exceptionally dangerous because of the severe deterioration in the cardiopulmonary status of the horse. This deterioration is the result of severe hypoxemia, and the partial pressure of arterial oxygen (Pa_{O_2}) may fall to 22 to 28 mm Hg.[37]

Diminished venous return to the heart has been implicated as the cause of cardiopulmonary collapse; however, when tension pneumothorax was created experimentally in monkeys and goats, cardiac output was unchanged. The genesis of the distress was related to precipitous decreases in PaO_2, which fell from 90 to 22 mm Hg.[37]

Pneumothorax may be treated after the wounds have been sealed by carefully inserting a large-gauge needle, teat cannula, or thoracostomy tube into the dorsal thoracic cavity just in front of the 12th to 15th rib, avoiding the vessels running on the caudal surfaces of the ribs. The air may be evacuated with a 60-mL syringe and a three-way stopcock or suction apparatus. Reexpansion pulmonary edema is a complication of rapidly reinflating a lung after a period of collapse secondary to pneumothorax, hemothorax, or pleural effusion. Horses with reexpansion pulmonary edema may develop varying degrees of hypoxemia and hypotension. Reexpansion pulmonary edema is likely caused by increased permeability of the pulmonary vasculature.[38] The edema fluid has a high protein content, suggesting that it is leakiness of the capillaries rather than an increased hydrostatic pressure that is responsible for the formation of the edema.[38] Capillary damage may be caused by mechanical trauma associated with lung reexpansion or reperfusion injury.[38] To minimize the risks of reexpansion pulmonary edema, a pressure of −20 cm H_2O or less should be used, and the air should be removed from the thorax slowly.[39] Evacuation may need to be repeated or continuous because of continuing air leaks from the wound.

Hemothorax

Generally, a horse with a massive hemothorax caused by a penetrating wound to the heart succumbs soon after the injury. However, if hemothorax is suspected, restoring circulating blood volume prior to draining the chest cavity is suggested. Evacuating the hemothorax from the pleural cavity will aid in ventilation because the fluid displaces the functional lung, compromising alveolar ventilation. Removing the hemothorax also decreases the risk of developing septic pleural effusion and pleural adhesions.

Thoracentesis is an emergency procedure for hemothorax in which alveolar ventilation is impaired because of decreased lung expansion. Radiography or ultrasonographic examination is used to determine the level and amount of fluid to be removed. A 7-cm area is clipped and surgically prepared, ventrally, at the seventh intercostal space. The skin, subcutaneous tissue, cranial aspect of the rib, and parietal pleura are infiltrated with local anesthetic. A stab incision is made through the skin over the cranial aspect of the rib and then a teat cannula, a catheter, or a chest tube is advanced through the skin incision, intercostal muscles, and parietal pleural lining until a distinct popping sensation is felt. The catheter can be redirected if neither fluid nor air is aspirated. The caudal aspect of the rib's intercostal vessels and nerves and sites more cranial than the seventh intercostal space should be avoided. In cases of hemothorax, a large-bore catheter or chest tube with a trocar may be used to rapidly drain large volumes or thickened fluid with blood clots. A one-way valve, such as a Heimlich valve, can be attached to the tube for continuous one-way flow (see Chapter 18).

Because of the proximity of the abdomen to the thorax, evaluating the horse for signs of acute abdominal crisis is important, especially if penetrating trauma to the thorax invaded the abdomen. Because the dome of the diaphragm extends to the sixth rib on expiration, horses with wounds caudal to this or with deep penetration warrant peritoneal paracentesis to detect potential visceral damage or rupture.[40]

Abdominal Trauma

Abdominal injury can occur with blunt or penetrating trauma and result in hemorrhage, contamination, gastrointestinal viscus rupture, or eventration. Thorough physical examination is indicated because these patients may be cardiovascularly unstable with injuries to other body systems. Penetrating wounds that enter the abdomen causing eventration of intestines require immediate attention. The exposed intestine should be thoroughly lavaged with sterile balanced polyionic solution and replaced within the abdomen. The abdominal wall defect should be closed, if possible, and a large bandage applied to the abdomen to support the wound and keep the abdomen closed. Broad-spectrum antimicrobials and nonsteroidal anti-inflammatory medication should be instituted prior to referral to a surgical facility. Abdominal exploratory surgery is frequently warranted after eventration to assess bowel viability, resect damaged intestine, lavage the abdomen, and properly close the abdominal wound. Penetrating abdominal injury, such as a gunshot wound or an impalement on a fencepost, may cause parenchymal damage to the spleen, liver, or kidneys, resulting in hemorrhage, major vessel injury, or gastrointestinal viscus damage, including serosal tears, mural hematomas, mesenteric avulsion, and intestinal perforation.[41]

Diagnostic techniques used to assess the abdomen after trauma include peritoneal paracentesis, rectal palpation, abdominal ultrasonography, abdominal radiographs, and laparoscopy. The diagnosis of *hemoabdomen* is based on peritoneal fluid evaluation and abdominal ultrasonography. Ultrasonic examination shows free abdominal fluid with a swirling pattern (Fig. 8-2). The presence of blood in the abdomen is confirmed with peritoneal paracentesis and assessment of the packed cell volume and total solids of the fluid. Gastrointestinal *viscus rupture* can also be diagnosed with abdominal ultrasound and peritoneal paracentesis. Free abdominal fluid is detected ultrasonographically and the presence of gastrointestinal contents confirmed with peritoneal fluid evaluation. The fluid is frequently serosanguineous, with a foul odor, and grossly contaminated with feed. Cytologically, multiple populations of bacteria and degenerative neutrophils confirms the diagnosis. If gastrointestinal rupture is suspected but the peritoneal fluid does not appear grossly contaminated, measurements of pH, glucose, and lactate may be helpful, in addition to cytology. Horses with *septic peritonitis* have significantly lower peritoneal fluid pH and glucose concentrations than horses with nonseptic peritonitis and healthy horses. Serum-to-peritoneal fluid glucose concentration differences greater than 50 mg/dL, peritoneal fluid glucose concentration less than 30 mg/dL, peritoneal fluid pH less than 7.3, and fibrinogen concentration greater than 200 mg/dL are also highly indicative of septic peritonitis.[42] Exploratory laparoscopy can be performed in the standing horse after abdominal

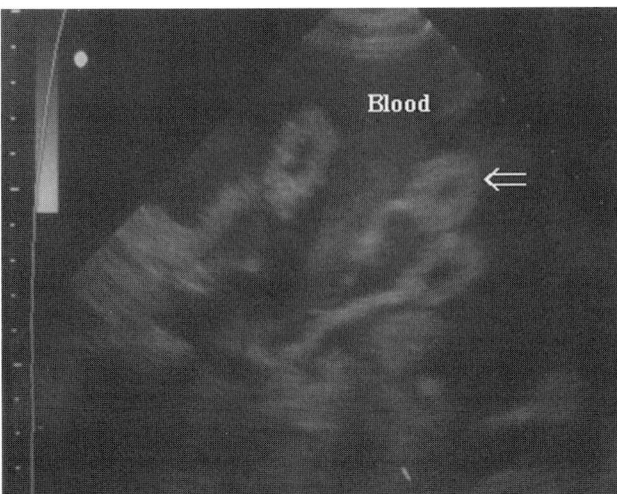

Figure 8-2. Image from an abdominal ultrasonographic examination of a horse with hemoabdomen. Small intestinal loops *(arrow)* "float" in the abdominal hemorrhage.

TABLE 8-2. Modified Glasgow Coma Scale

Modality	Horse's Best Response	Score
Eye opening	Spontaneous	4
	To voice	3
	To painful stimuli	2
	None	1
Response to verbal command	Oriented	5
	Disoriented but responsive	4
	Poor response	3
	None	1
Motor	Obedient	6
	Partially obedient	5
	Withdraws from pain	4
	Abnormal flexion	3
	Abnormal extension	2
	Flaccid/unresponsive	1

Total score = Eye + Verbal + Motor = 3 to 15

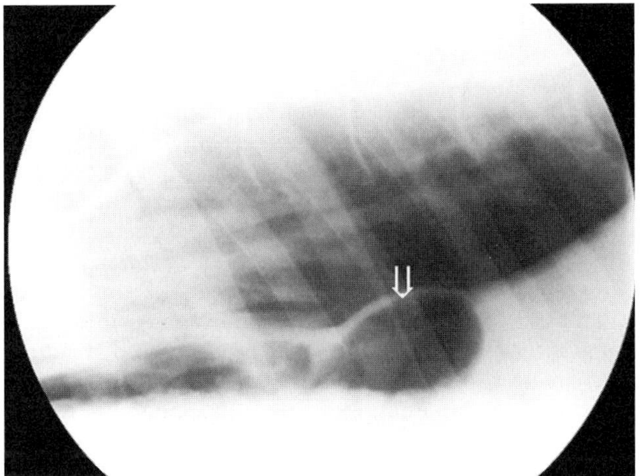

Figure 8-3. Lateral radiograph of the caudodorsal thorax of a horse with a diaphragmatic hernia. Note the gas-filled viscus *(arrow)* within the thoracic cavity.

trauma.[43] Splenic hematoma, mesenteric avulsion, diaphragmatic hernia, and viscus rupture with gross peritoneal contamination have been diagnosed.[43,44] Thoracic radiographs are indicated if diaphragmatic hernia is suspected (Fig. 8-3).

Cranial Trauma

Cranial injuries vary in severity and range from subtle alterations in mentation to unresponsive coma. Physical examination and neurologic evaluation should be performed, and a modified Glasgow Coma Scale can be used to assess mentation[45] (Table 8-2). In human patients, a score of 13 to 15 indicates mild brain injury, 9 to 12 moderate injury, and 3 to 8 severe brain injury. The score is established by adding the horse's best responses in the three categories listed in Table 8-2.

Any portion of the calvaria can be fractured, although certain injuries are more common. Most cranial injuries occur because the horse falls over backwards, striking the poll, or because the horse runs into something or is kicked, injuring the frontal bones. Severe brain injury may occur with or without skull fractures because the brain recoils within the cranial vault, resulting in contusion, vascular injury, and axonal disruption.[46] When horses fall over backwards, striking the poll, portions of the nuchal crest, paramastoid processes, and occipital condyles can fracture.[46] More serious injuries result from the actions of the rectus capitis ventralis muscles on the basisphenoid and basioccipital bones. These muscles originate on the ventral surface of the cervical vertebrae and insert on the ventral aspect of the basisphenoid and basioccipital bones. Contraction of these muscles flexes the head, but when the horse falls and the head is extended, the action of these muscles can result in avulsion fractures of the junction of the basisphenoid and basioccipital bones (more common in young horses) (Fig. 8-4), or in complete avulsion of a portion of the basilar bones[46] (Fig. 8-5). These injuries may lead to fatal hemorrhage if the occipital arteries or their branches are lacerated. Hemorrhage into the cervical tissue planes and between the guttural pouches may occur (Fig. 8-6).

Fracture of the basilar bones can cause injury to cranial nerves V, IX, and X, exhibited by loose jaw tone, decreased facial sensation, dyspnea, and dysphagia. Injury to the petrous temporal bone area may cause vestibular signs and facial nerve paresis because of injury to cranial nerves VII and VIII.[46] Therefore, horses with poll trauma may have evidence of vestibular syndrome and exhibit a head tilt, leaning, or circling toward the side of the lesion. The vestibular signs worsen if the horse is blindfolded. Also, horizontal or rotary nystagmus may be detected. These horses may have a hypometric or spastic gait because of cerebellar injury. If the optic nerves have been stretched or torn, these horses will be blind with absent papillary light response and dilated pupils.[46,47] Examination of the size, symmetry, and response to light of the pupils is critical. A change in pupil size from bilaterally constricted to bilaterally dilated, with lack of response to light, is indicative of progressive brain injury. Asymmetric or bilaterally miotic pupils indicate serious injury, and the prognosis for recovery is poor.[48]

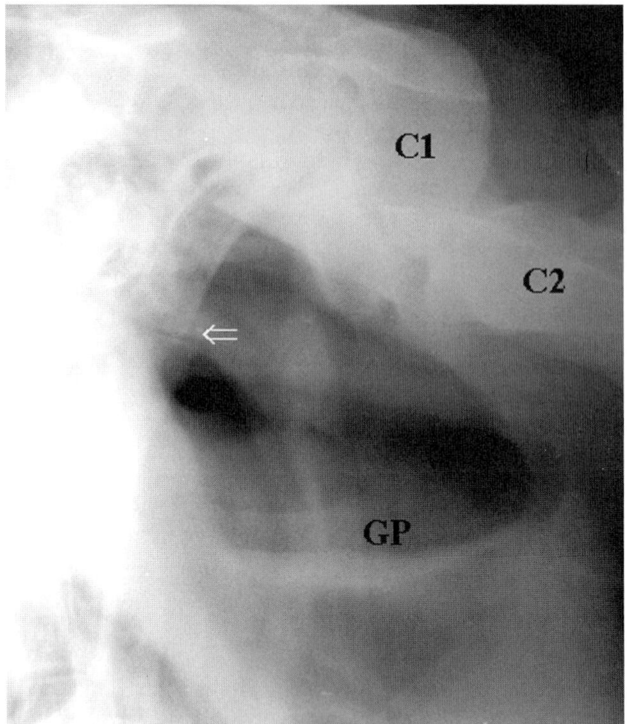

Figure 8-4. Lateral skull radiograph of a 3-month-old foal that flipped over backward, landing on its poll. Notice the bony fragment and step at the junction of the basisphenoid and basioccipital bones *(arrow)*. C1, first cervical vertebrae; C2, second cervical vertebrae; GP, guttural pouch.

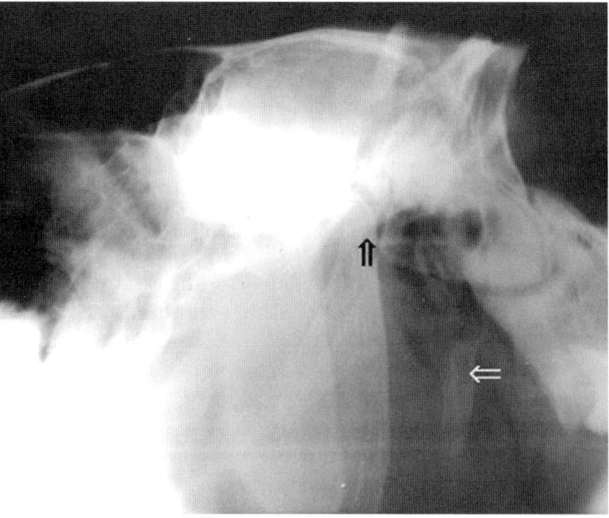

Figure 8-5. Lateral skull radiograph of a 14-year-old horse that flipped over backward and fell. Note the bone fragment *(white arrow)*, which at postmortem examination was determined to be the basisphenoid bone completely avulsed from its normal position at the base of the skull *(black arrow)*.

Horses with frontal or parietal bone trauma frequently have epistaxis from sinus or ethmoid injury. These horses may be depressed, unresponsive, or demented, or they may exhibit compulsive walking or head pressing. If the occipital cortex is injured, vision and the menace response are impaired in the eye contralateral to the lesion. The pupillary light response should be intact.[46]

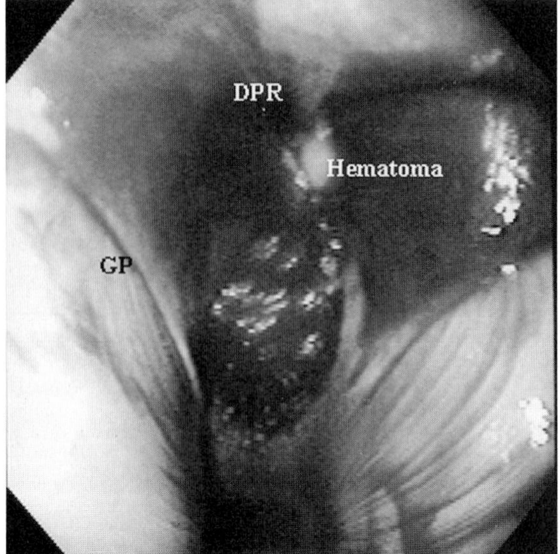

Figure 8-6. Endoscopic image of the dorsal nasopharynx showing hematoma formation within the dorsal nasopharynx and guttural pouch region after fracture of the basisphenoid bone. DPR, dorsal pharyngeal recess; GP, guttural pouch.

Diagnostic modalities for cranial trauma include plain radiographs, computed tomography (CT), CT with contrast enhancement, endoscopy, cerebral spinal fluid evaluation, and magnetic resonance imaging.[49] Because of the complex nature of the anatomy of the equine head, superimposition of numerous structures, and poor soft tissue differentiation, radiography may be of limited value in the diagnosis of basilar skull fractures. However, in many horses, radiographic changes such as soft tissue opacification of the guttural pouch region, irregular bone margination at the spheno-occipital line, attenuation of the nasopharynx, ventral displacement of the dorsal pharyngeal wall, and the presence of irregularly shaped bone fragments in the region of the guttural pouches are suggestive of a fracture of the skull base.[50] CT with or without contrast enhancement is a sensitive diagnostic modality for detecting skull fractures or brain trauma such as focal parenchymal hemorrhage or subdural hemorrhage.[51]

Emergency therapy for horses with head trauma and brain injury includes establishing an airway if needed and oxygen insufflation if the horse is hypoxemic (15 L/min), anti-inflammatory and analgesic medications. Hypertonic saline (7.5%; 4 mL/kg) has been demonstrated to exert neuroprotective properties after traumatic brain injury by osmotic mobilization of parenchymal water and improvement of microcirculation, as well as its having anti-inflammatory properties. When administered with dextran, hypertonic saline resulted in lower intracranial pressure, improved neurologic recovery, and less morphologic damage after subarachnoid hemorrhage in rats.[52,53] Posttrauma administration of magnesium sulfate (100 mg/kg) has been shown to decrease cerebral edema, attenuate defects in the blood-brain barrier, and attenuate long-term motor and cognitive deficits after traumatic brain injury.[54-56] In addition, administration of magnesium sulfate supports endogenous antioxidant function within the brain after injury.[54-56]

REFERENCES

1. DeLong WG, Born CT: Cytokines in patients with polytrauma, Clin Orthop 2004;422:57-65.
2. Waxman K: Physiologic response to injury. In Shoemaker WC, editor: Textbook of Critical Care, ed 4, Philadelphia, 2000, WB Saunders.
3. Cathbertson DP: Post-shock metabolic responses, Lancet 1942;I:433.
4. Wilmore DW: Homeostasis: Bodily changes in trauma and surgery. In Sabiston DC, editor: Textbook of Surgery, ed 13, Philadelphia, 1986, WB Saunders.
5. Hill AG, Siegel J, Rounds J, Wilmore DW: Metabolic responses to interleukin-1: Centrally and peripherally mediated, Ann Surg 1997;225:246-251.
6. Rose BD: Regulation of the effective circulating volume. In Rose BD, Post TW, editors: Clinical Physiology of Acid-Base and Electrolyte Disorders, ed 5, New York, 2001, McGraw-Hill.
7. Ferguson KL, Taheri P, Rodriguez J, et al: Tumor necrosis factor activity increases in the early response to trauma, Acad Emerg Med 1997;4:1035-1040.
8. Perl M, Gebhard F, Knoterl MW, et al: The pattern of preformed cytokines in tissues frequently affected by blunt trauma, Shock 2003;19:299-304.
9. Zaloga GP: Catecholamines in anesthetic and surgical stress, Int Anesthesiol Clin 1988;26:187-198.
10. Kehlet H, Brandt MR, Rem J: Role of neurogenic stimuli in mediating the endocrine-metabolic response to surgery, J Parenter Enteral Nutr 1980;4:152-156.
11. Brianceau P, Chevalier H, Karas A, et al: Intravenous lidocaine and small-intestinal size, abdominal fluid, and outcome after colic surgery in horses, J Vet Intern Med 2002;16:736-741.
12. Sellon DC, Monroe VL, Roberts MC, et al: Pharmacokinetics and adverse effects of butorphanol administered by single intravenous injection or continuous intravenous infusion in horses, Am J Vet Res 2001;62:183-189.
13. Natalini CC, Robinson EP: Evaluation of the analgesic effects of epidurally administered morphine, alfentanil, butorphanol, tramadol, and U50488H in horses, Am J Vet Res 2000;61:1579-1586.
14. Goodrich LR, Nixon AJ, Fubinin SL, et al: Epidural morphine and detomidine decreases postoperative hindlimb lameness in horses after bilateral stifle arthroscopy, Vet Surg 2002;31:232-239.
15. LeBlanc PH, Caron JP, Patterson JS, et al: Epidural injection of xylazine for perineal analgesia in horses, J Am Vet Med Assoc 1988;193:1405-1408.
16. Maxwell LK, Thomasy SM, Slovic N, et al: Pharmacokinetics of fentanyl following intravenous and transdermal administration in horses, Equine Vet J 2003;35:484-490.
17. Hume DM, Egdahl RH: The importance of the brain in the endocrine response to injury, Ann Surg 1959;150:697-712.
18. Fosse E, Mollnes TE, Aasen AO, et al: Complement activation following multiple injuries, Acta Chir Scand 1987;153:325-330.
19. Sherry RM, Cue JI, Goddard JK, et al: Interleukin-10 is associated with the development of sepsis in trauma patients, J Trauma 1996;40:613-616.
20. Peng RY, Bongard FS: Hypothermia in trauma patients, J Am Col Surg 1999;188:685-696.
21. Stoner HB: Thermoregulation after injury, Adv Exp Med Biol 1972;33:495-499.
22. Reuler JB. Hypothermia: Pathophysiology, clinical settings, and management, Ann Intern Med 1978;89:519-527.
23. Flynn P, Hughes R, Walton B: Use of atracurium in cardiac surgery involving cardiopulmonary bypass with induced hypothermia, Br J Anaesth 1984;56:967-972.
24. Cipolle MD, Pasquale MD, Cerra FB: Secondary organ dysfunction: From clinical perspectives to molecular mediators, Crit Care Clin 1993;9:261-298.
25. Ressey PQ, Jian ZM, Johnson DJ, et al: Post-traumatic skeletal muscle proteolysis: The role of the hormonal environment, World J Surg 1989;13:465-470.
26. Long CL, Nelson KM, Atkin JM, et al: A physiologic basis for the provision of fuel mixtures in normal and stressed patients, J Trauma 1990;30:1077-1085.
27. Traks AL. Epidemiology of trauma: In Shoemaker WC, editor: Textbook of Critical Care, ed 4, Philadelphia, 2000, WB Saunders.
28. Pate JW: Chest wall injuries, Surg Clin North Am 1989;69:59-70.
29. Jean D, Laverty S, Halley J, et al: Thoracic trauma in newborn foals. Proceedings of the 14th Annual Veterinary Medical Forum, 1996:735.
30. Mason DE, Ainsworth DM, Robertson JT: Respiratory emergencies in the adult horse, Vet Clin North Am Equine Pract 1994;10:685-701.
31. Vachon AM, Fischer AT: Thoracoscopy in the horse: Diagnostic and therapeutic indications in 28 cases, Equine Vet J 1998;30:467-475.
32. Peroni JF, Horner NT, Robinson NE, et al: Equine thoracoscopy: normal anatomy and surgical technique, Equine Vet J 2001;33:231-237.
33. Manlulu AV, Lee TW, Thang KH, et al: Current indications and results of VATS in the evaluation and management of hemodynamically stable thoracic injuries, Eur J Cardiothorac Surg 2004;25:1048-1053.
34. Ahmed N, Jones D: Video-assisted thoracic surgery: State of the art in trauma care, Injury 2004;35:479-489.
35. Pepe PE: Acute post-traumatic respiratory physiology and insufficiency, Surg Clin North Am 1989;69:157-172.
36. Hare WC: General respiratory system. In Getty R, editor: Sisson and Grossman's The Anatomy of the Domestic Animals, Philadelphia, 1975, WB Saunders.
37. Rutherford RB, Hurt HH, Brickman RD, et al: The pathophysiology of progressive, tension pneumothorax, J Trauma 1968;8:212-227.
38. Pavlin J, Cheney FW: Unilateral pulmonary edema in rabbits after re-expansion of collapsed lung, J Appl Physiol 1979;46:31-40.
39. Light RW, Jenkinson SG, Minh V, et al: Observations on pleural pressures as fluid is withdrawn during thoracentesis, Am Rev Respir Dis 1980;121:799-804.
40. Laverty S: Respiratory tract trauma. Proceedings of the 25th Annual Veterinary Surgical Forum: Upper Respiratory Surgery, 1997:155-157.
41. Vatistas NJ, Meagher DM, Gillis CL, et al: Gunshot injuries in horses: 22 cases (1971-1993), J Am Vet Med Assoc 1995;207:1198-1200.
42. Van Hoogmoed L, Rodger LD, Psier SJ: Evaluation of peritoneal fluid pH, glucose concentration, and lactate dehydrogenase activity for detection of septic peritonitis in horses, J Am Vet Med Assoc 1999;214:1032-1036.
43. Fischer AT: Laparoscopic evaluation of horses with acute or chronic colic. In Fischer AT, editor: Equine Diagnostic and Surgical Laparoscopy, Philadelphia, 2001, WB Saunders.
44. Mehl ML: Laparoscopic diagnosis of subcapsular hematoma. JAMA 1998;213:1171-1174.
45. Winston SR: Preliminary communication: EMT and the Glasgow Coma Scale, J Iowa Med Soc 1979;69:393-398.
46. MacKay RJ: Brain injury after head trauma: Pathophysiology, diagnosis, and treatment, Vet Clin North Am Equine Pract 2004;20:199-206.
47. van Schaik AM, van der Pol BA, van der Linde-Sipman JS: Acute blindness due to trauma in a Welsh pony-colt, Tijdschr Diergeneeskd 1998;123:142-143.
48. Reed SM: Medical and surgical emergencies of the nervous system of horses: Diagnosis, treatment, and sequelae, Vet Clin North Am Equine Pract 1994;10:703-715.
49. Tucker RL, Farrell E: Computed tomography and magnetic resonance imaging of the equine head, Vet Clin North Am Equine Pract 2001;17:131-144.
50. Ramirez O, Jorgensen JS, Thrall DE: Imaging basilar skull fractures in the horse: A review, Vet Radiol Ultrasound 1998;39:391-395.

51. Gardelle O, Feige K, Geissbuhler U, et al: Possibilities for computer tomography of the equine head based on two cases with fracture of the base of the skull, Schweiz Arch Tierheilkd 1999;141:267-272.
52. Zausinger S, Thal SC, Kreimeier U, et al: Hypertonic fluid resuscitation from subarachnoid hemorrhage in rats, Neurosurgery 2004;55:679-686.
53. Bhardwaj A, Ulatowski JA: Hypertonic saline solutions in brain injury, Curr Opin Crit Care 2004;10:126-131.
54. Esen F, Erdem T, Aktan D: Effects of magnesium administration on brain edema and blood-brain barrier breakdown after experimental traumatic brain injury in rats, J Neurosurg Anesthesiol 2003;15:119-125.
55. Vink R, O'Connor CA, Nimmo AJ, et al: Magnesium attenuates persistent functional deficits following diffuse traumatic brain injury in rates, Neurosci Lett 2004;336:41-44.
56. Ustun ME, Duman A, Ogun CO: Effects of nimodipine and magnesium sulfate on endogenous antioxidant levels in brain tissue after experimental brain trauma, J Neurosurg Anesthesiol 2001;13:227-232.

CHAPTER 9

Biomaterials, Surgical Implants, and Instruments

James T. Blackford
LeeAnn W. Blackford
John Disegi
Marc Bohner

IMPLANT CHARACTERISTICS

Biomaterials of either natural, processed natural, or synthetic origin are used as implants and devices to direct, supplement, and replace or restore tissue function. Metals, polymers, ceramics, and composites of these three are the primary substances used today in manufacturing biomaterials. Design, material selection, and biocompatibility are the critical issues surrounding the manufacture of medical implants and devices. Ideally, materials should be inert, strong enough to allow biomechanical loading, easily handled, noncorrosive, nonallergenic, nontoxic, noncarcinogenic, easily sterilized, inexpensive, and resistant to infection. The ideal biomaterial does not exist; however, the discovery of new materials, alterations in biomaterial composites, and combining metals, ceramics, and polymers have improved product structure, quality, and biocompatibility. Just a few examples of biomaterial applications are intravenous, urinary, and gastric catheters; heart valves and vascular grafts; orthopedic devices such as joint replacement components, pins, screws, plates, rods, tacks, suture anchors, and fixators; dental and ophthalmic implants; tissue adhesives; wound dressings; and suture materials. Initially, readily available substances or materials were used, but today biomaterial science is very sophisticated, with endless possibilities in medical application and construct design.

BIOCOMPATIBILITY

Biocompatibility is a descriptive term pertaining to the ability of a material to elicit an appropriate and predictable host response.[1] The definition extends beyond the chemical composition of the implant to include surface and structural compatibility. Surface compatibility is the chemical, biologic, and physical suitability of the implant surface to interact with host tissues. Structural compatibility is the optimal adaptation to the mechanical behavior of the implant in host tissues. Biocompatibility now emphasizes two areas, biosafety and biofunctionality. Biosafety evaluates the deleterious effects of biomaterial on the host. Biofunctionality deals with the ability of the material to perform with an appropriate host response to a specific application. With pressure to reduce animal testing models, new techniques have evolved, and these trends in biocompatibility testing were recently reviewed.[2] Simple and sophisticated in vitro systems have evolved using human cell line cultures designed to evaluate specific applications of medical devices. These techniques have become the industry standard, because biocompatibility reactions occur at the cellular level and many independent events may occur with interacting stimuli contributing to the overall response.

Host Interactions

When biomaterials interact with a biologic system, the host exhibits a variety of complex reactions. Responses differ depending on whether the material is toxic, inert, resorptive, or bioactive. If the material is toxic, the surrounding tissue dies. Inert materials exhibit minimal chemical reactions with exposed tissue, yet fibrous tissue of varying thicknesses forms at the implant–tissue interface. When biomaterials are almost inert and the interface is not chemically or biologically bonded, there is relative movement, and a nonadherent fibrous capsule is formed progressively in both hard and soft tissues.[3] Bioresorbable materials are slowly dissolved by the surrounding tissue or they are used as drug-delivery systems. Bioactive materials are nontoxic and biologically active, and they form an interfascial bond with surrounding tissues through time-dependent, kinetic modification of their surfaces.

Future biomaterials will be used to incorporate biologic factors. They will recruit cell lines and minimize inflammation and infection while improving bioactivity and compatibility with surrounding tissues. Materials will be designed to provide improved mechanical integrity and corrosion resistance while maintaining improved biocompatibility.

Biomaterial Testing

Testing presently encompasses a number of classical test methods for structural and biologic evaluation of medical devices, under the guidance of the International Standardization Organization (ISO). The ISO presents guidelines for suitable tests and defines important principles of these tests. These include positive and negative controls, extraction conditions, choice of cell lines and cell media, and other important aspects of test procedures. Biocompatibility testing includes in vitro and in vivo evaluations.

Cytotoxicity Testing

Cytotoxicity leads the area of importance in the evaluation process. Cell morphology studies measure cell growth, metabolism, and damage from exposure to new materials. Metabolic studies evaluate impairment to the mitochondrial enzyme succinate dehydrogenase. Exposure of cell cultures to new materials is used to evaluate the effects of DNA synthesis on cell proliferation. Membrane integrity tests evaluate structural and functional membrane changes on exposure to new materials. Blood or hemocompatibility studies measure interactions related to immediate, prolonged, or repeated exposure to the device. These studies evaluate platelet, red blood cell, polymorphonuclear cell, and macrophage function. Clotting time measurements are assessed.

Cell Adhesion Testing

Cell adhesion testing ranks second in importance to cytotoxicity testing of biomaterials. Thrombogenicity is a reflection of plasma protein fibrinogen adherence, platelet adhesion and activation, suppression of protein adsorption, and blood cell adhesion resistance. Products are also evaluated for bacterial adhesion properties. The effects of alkaline and acid fluid media on materials are evaluated. Materials are exposed to physiologic fluids including plasma and serum, as well as to organic chemicals. Electron microscopy evaluates cell spreading in those materials designed for integration into host tissues. Cell proliferation studies are critical in fracture repair devices, especially those that are biodegradable, as they will be replaced by host tissues. Tissue sections are immunohistochemically stained to identify cell types present near the implant.

Mechanical testing has become more refined and includes the study of wear products that are released from devices over time. Materials undergo mechanical testing for stress, strain, compression, and cyclic bending. Spectroscopy is used to evaluate the product's elemental surface composition, its absorption behavior, and its structural surface properties before and after mechanical testing. X-ray diffraction measurements evaluate structural information, viscoelasticity, and tensile (stress/strain) properties. Viscosity, thermal properties, and contact angle are evaluated.

Mutagenesis is evaluated by the detection of mutations, seen as changes in metabolic function in bacteria exposed to new materials, as well as by animal model studies. Carcinogenesis is a critical issue for implants designed for long-term function. These studies are carried out in animal models.

As genetic information emerges and new cytokines and growth factors are discovered, an understanding and insight into fundamental cellular mechanisms and specific actions on biologic structure will continue to unfold. Molecular regulators, signaling receptors, and binding sites will be determined and understood, allowing investigators to use bioactive molecules to turn activities on and off, altering cellular function within microenvironments. For example, transgenic mice developed for the study of specific abnormalities are used to test interactions with biomaterials in bone, muscle, tendon, and connective tissue.

Biomaterial Interactions

All materials elicit a host response, but the degree varies greatly between biomaterials. This can be attributed to the biomaterial's properties. Presently, no material implanted in living tissues is totally inert. *Metals* are selected for their high strength, ductility, and resistance to wear. Disadvantages encountered with metals include corrosion, excess stiffness compared with the surrounding tissue, high density, and release of metal ions that may incite allergic tissue reactions.

Corrosion

Corrosion occurs by ionization, oxidation, or hydroxylation. Electrochemical and pH changes are factors in this process. Physical processes also cause corrosion. Crevice corrosion is the most common; it results from improper component fit or develops in the presence of a defect in the metal surface. Scratches or defects caused by improper handling cause pitting corrosion. Galvanic corrosion occurs when dissimilar metals are in direct contact and are exposed to a conductive medium. Stress corrosion occurs when a metal is subjected to opposing mechanical forces, creating an electrochemical potential leading to corrosion. Fretting corrosion occurs when metal is physically removed as a result of motion between two components. The effect of relative movement plays a role, even with quasi-inert implants.

Movement

Movement eventually leads to deterioration in function of an implant, or of the tissue at the implant–tissue interface. Development of a thick fibrous capsule can rapidly lead to implant loosening and subsequent failure. Small implant particles are phagocytosed and removed from the area. With the death of the cell, particles are deposited in lymphatic tissue, where they can migrate and incite a foreign body reaction.

Metal ion release may stimulate neutrophils to release lysosomal enzymes that may result in implant loosening, patient discomfort, and allergic reactions. Some metal plates provide high axial dynamic compression. However, the stiffness of the implant is complicated by bone atrophy below the plate, secondary to stress shielding, which ultimately weakens the bone. Wear particles that are released from metals, ceramics, and polymers can incite inflammatory conditions that vary in severity.

Bioceramics have excellent tissue biocompatibility, corrosion resistance, high compressive strength, and resistance to wear. They are hydrophobic with low frictional properties. Disadvantages of ceramics include brittleness, low fracture strength, difficulty of fabrication, low mechanical reliability, lack of resiliency, and high density.

Polymers are available in a wide variety of compositions, properties, and forms. Polymer materials are either resorptive or nonresorptive. They can be fabricated into complex shapes and structures, but they tend to be too flexible or too weak to meet mechanical demands of certain applications. Some polymeric devices provide the necessary initial strength for orthopedic applications, and strength reduction during degradation is slow enough to allow tissue healing. Polymers can absorb fluid and swell, with the result that undesirable products are leached into the surrounding tissue. The inflammatory reaction that ensues varies greatly, depending on the polymer. Furthermore, sterilization may affect polymer properties. However, polymer composites alleviate many of these undesirable properties. Polymer resorption generally occurs in two phases. Polymer chains are broken down hydrolytically. As the implant loses form, it physically breaks into particles that are attacked by macrophages. The lungs and kidneys excrete phagocytic byproducts. Among the many factors that affect the degradation of resorbable implants are host reaction, type of implant material, implant geometry, site of implantation, and method of sterilization.[4] Reactions vary in severity from mild fluid accumulation, to formation of discharging sinuses, to severe irreversible tissue damage.

IMPLANT FORMS AND MATERIALS

Available implants and implant forms are listed in Table 9-1.

Solid implants are constructed primarily of ceramics and metal materials. Carbon implants and rods are included in this group. Manufacturing includes casting, machining, and crystalline growth.

Tubular implants are made primarily of synthetic nonabsorbable materials. They are manufactured as extrusions or on tubular mandrels, creating seamless forms. Tubular implants are commonly coated to improve longevity and enhance biocompatibility.

Meshes are used primarily for hernia repair. They are available in absorbable and nonabsorbable woven forms and are therefore porous. Absorbable forms include polyglactin and polyglycolic acid. Nonabsorbable forms are commonly manufactured from polypropylene, polytetrafluroethylene, and polyesters, but carbon fibers and metal meshes (of stainless steel and titanium) have also been used. Products are selected on the basis of the amount of material needed and the filament structure, including strength, pore size, long-term stability, and stiffness.[5] Meshes should be used only in clean wounds because of the risk of chronic infection, fistula formation, and extrusion.

Suture materials are made from natural materials and synthetic polymers. They are manufactured as single-strand monofilaments, twisted or braided multifilaments, and staples. They are available as either absorbable or nonabsorbable products. Sutures are used primarily to appose tissues until the healing process maintains normal structural integrity, and to ligate blood vessels. Knowing the advantages and disadvantages, as well as the biologic and physical properties of each material, allows the surgeon to make knowledgeable choices for selecting the material that suits the intended need.

TABLE 9-1. Available Materials and Implant Forms

Material	Implant Form
Carbon	Fibers, implant coatings, orthopedic rods, meshes
Ceramics	Orthopedic devices, bone lattice, implant coatings
Cobalt-chromium	Prosthetic implants
Collagen	Suture material, hemostatic sponge
Cyanoacrylate	Tissue adhesive
Gelatin	Hemostatic sponge
Latex rubber	Surgical drains
Poliglecaprone	Surgical suture
Polyamide	Surgical suture
Polybutester	Surgical suture
Polydioxanone	Surgical suture, surgical staples, orthopedic pins
Polyester	Surgical suture, surgical mesh, vascular grafts
Polyethylene	Tubing, catheters, joint implants
Polyglactin	Surgical suture, surgical mesh, surgical staples
Polyglycolic acid (isomers)	Surgical suture, surgical mesh, surgical staples, orthopedic implants
Polylactide (isomers)	Orthopedic implants
Polymethylmethacrylate	Tissue cement
Polyoxymethylene	Orthopedic washer
Polypropylene	Surgical suture, surgical mesh
Polytetrafluoroethylene	Surgical mesh, vascular grafts
Polyurethane	Pacemaker leads, vascular grafts
Polyvinyl chloride	Tubing, catheters
Regenerated cellulose	Hemostatic fabric
Silicone rubber	Tubing, pacemaker leads, intraocular prosthesis, catheters
Silk	Surgical suture
Stainless steel	Surgical suture, surgical mesh, surgical staples, intramedullary pins, cerclage wire, bone plates, screws
Small intestine submucosa	Collagen scaffold for tissue regeneration
Surgical gut	Surgical suture
Titanium/alloys	Bone plates, screws, prosthetic implants

Organic Absorbable Materials

Surgical Gut

Surgical gut (the word is derived from *intestine*) is made from the submucosa of sheep or the serosa of cattle. It is a multifilament structure that is machine-ground and polished to resemble a monofilament suture. Chromium salts are used to increase strength and decrease the absorption rate of the material. It is phagocytized by macrophages at a variable rate and incites an inflammatory reaction with increased fibrosis at the site. The material has good handling characteristics, but it has poor knot security and may come untied as it swells with fluid exposure. As a result of the bovine spongiform encephalopathy (BSE) crisis, catgut is no longer used in human surgery and may not be manufactured in the future.

Collagen

Collagen is a multifilament suture processed from bovine flexor tendon and treated with formaldehyde or chromium salts, or both. Its characteristics and properties mirror those of gut, but its source and processing simplicity are advantageous. Collagen is also available as a hemostatic sponge. However, the BSE crisis that affected the use of catgut will certainly affect the use and production of this product.

Small Intestine Submucosa

Small intestine submucosa (SIS) is a denatured product from swine. The denaturing process leaves an extracellular matrix (ECM) that is 90% collagen. The ECM contains selected cytokines and signaling molecules, including fibroblast growth factor, transforming growth factor, and endothelial cell growth factor. The material is paper-like when dry but consists of approximately 90% water when moistened. It acts as a scaffold for regeneration of many body tissues[6] and then is degraded and reabsorbed (see Chapter 26).

Synthetic Absorbable Materials

Polyglactin

Polyglactin is a braided copolymer of glycolic and lactic acid that is coated with calcium stearate, decreasing tissue drag. It is absorbed slowly by hydrolysis over a period of 100 to 120 days. It retains tensile strength for 14 to 28 days. Polyglactin is easy to handle, causes minimal tissue reaction, is stable in contaminated wounds, and has high tensile and knot strength. It is stable in alkaline urine and is safely used in the bladder. It is used in manufacturing suture materials, staples, and surgical mesh implants.

Polyglycolic Acid

Polyglycolic acid is a braided multifilament polymer of glycolic acid. It is absorbed by hydrolysis in 100 to 120 days. Degradation products have some antibacterial effect. Tensile strength is retained for 14 to 21 days. It is easy to handle and has a wide variety of uses in clean and contaminated wounds. To ensure knot security, several throws are placed in each knot. Its major disadvantage is premature absorption in urine. It is used in manufacturing suture materials, staples, and surgical mesh implants.

Polydioxanone

Polydioxanone is a monofilament polymer of paradioxanone. It is absorbed by hydrolysis in 180 days. Tensile strength is maintained for 28 to 56 days. Its strength before implantation exceeds that of nylon or polypropylene and it has good knot security. It has poor handling characteristics when compared with braided absorbable materials, primarily because of its stiffness and memory. Polydioxanone is used in manufacturing suture materials, staples, surgical mesh, implants, and orthopedic pins.

Polyglyconate

Polyglyconate is a monofilament copolymer of glycolic acid and trimethylene. It is absorbed by hydrolysis starting at 60 days and completed by 180 days. Its effective strength after implantation is superior to that of all other absorbable sutures. It has good handling characteristics and the best knot security of the absorbable sutures. Polyglyconate is superior to nylon and polybutester for tendon repair and has a wide spectrum of use in veterinary medicine.

Poliglecaprone

Poliglecaprone is a monofilament absorbable copolymer of glycolide and epsilon-caprolactone. Initially, it is one of the strongest absorbable suture materials available, yet it weakens rapidly, losing all significant strength in 14 days. Poliglecaprone elicits minimal tissue reaction and has good knot security and handling characteristics.

Polylactic Acid

Polylactic acid and its L-isomer are used to form absorbable orthopedic rods and screws. The implants absorb slowly, with appreciable loss of strength in 2 to 3 months. Absorption is initially by hydrolysis, commencing with phagocytosis. Predrilling is required prior to implantation because of the poor torsional strength characteristics of the material.

Organic Nonabsorbable Materials

Silk

Silk is a braided multifilament structure made from raw silk spun by the silkworm. It has excellent handling characteristics and knot security. Although it is classified as a nonabsorbable suture, it loses tensile strength over time and is slowly absorbed over several years. It is used in most body tissues as a ligature, and it is commonly used in plastic, cardiovascular, and ophthalmic surgery. The material does incite an inflammatory condition and may potentiate infection.

Silk-based implants for reconstruction of the Achilles tendon or of the cruciate ligaments were described as early as in the late 19th century,[7] but reports of adverse reactions including inflammation and immune responses terminated their use. Novel purification protocols of the native silk (isolating glycosylated and immunogenic proteins from the silk fibroin), however, have resulted in a very compatible material, with fewer inflammatory and immunogenic reactions both in vitro and in vivo.[8,9] These novel purification protocols may stimulate the use of silk-based biomaterials because of their other advantageous properties—the mechanical properties of silks in fiber form exceed those of all other natural polymers and most synthetic materials, rivaling even high-performance fibers such as Kevlar in terms of energy absorbed before failure.[10] Similarly, porous matrices formed from these proteins exhibit a combination of mechanical properties that exceed other polymeric biomaterials.[11] These impressive mechanical properties, along with established biocompatibility and slow degradability,[9] render silk fibrin an interesting biomaterial for further exploration of orthopedic applications.[12,13]

Cotton

Cotton is a multifilament, nonabsorbable material derived from natural cotton fiber. The material slowly loses tensile strength over a period of 6 months to 2 years. However, the material gains tensile strength and knot security when wet. Cotton has a strong capillary action, is tissue reactive, and may potentiate infection. Today there is little use for cotton in equine practice, except as bandage material.

Synthetic Nonabsorbable Materials

Polyamides

Polyamides are available in two forms as synthetic nonabsorbable surgical implants: nylon and caprolactam. Nylon is a mono- or multifilament fiber that is relatively inert and has no capillary action in its monofilament form. It loses about 30% of its tensile strength over a period of 2 years. As a multifilament suture, it retains no tensile strength after 6 months. Degradation products of the material have potent antimicrobial activity. The incidence of infection in contaminated tissues containing monofilament nylon is very low. Poor handling characteristics and knot security are related to its memory. Sharp suture tags (ends) may be irritating to surrounding tissue. Caprolactam is a coated multifilament suture material with biologic properties similar to nylon. However, caprolactam is enclosed in a smooth sheeth of proteinaceous material and should not be buried under the skin, as the coating degrades and can incite a severe inflammatory reaction with excessive swelling and subsequent sinus tract formation.

Polyester

Polyester (Dacron) is a nonabsorbable, multifilament, synthetic fiber made from polyethylene terephthalate. Polyester is widely used as a woven vascular prosthesis and is available as a braided suture material. The material is strong, loses little strength after implantation, and is useful in slowly healing tissues. It is capable of eliciting more severe tissue reaction than other synthetic nonabsorbable suture materials. A polybuterate coating improves handling characteristics, but it reduces knot security, requiring multiple throws to safely anchor the material. The material should not be used in contaminated wounds, as bacteria incorporated within the braids are isolated from antimicrobial and phagocytic cell activity, leading to chronic drainage and sinus tract formation.

Polybutester

Polybutester is a monofilament synthetic copolymer of polybutylene and polytetramethylene. The material displays good handling characteristics and knot security. Polybutester demonstrates a high degree of elastic stretch under low loads, and it is good for wounds where swelling is anticipated, as the material does not cut through the tissue. It is nonreactive in tissues and is applied in the repair of slowly healing wounds.

Polypropylene

Polypropylene is a nonabsorbable suture made from polyolfin plastic. It has the greatest strength of the synthetic nonabsorbable materials, with no appreciable strength reduction after implantation. Polypropylene is one of the most difficult sutures to handle because of its stiffness, slickness when wet, and material memory. It is one of the most inert and least thrombogenic suture materials available and is therefore used frequently in vascular surgery. Knot quality is marginal unless force is applied to the material, creating interlocking of fibers. Polypropylene is used as implantable mesh and as suture material.

Polyethylene

Polyethylene is a thermoplastic polymer, resistant to inorganic chemicals and to acidic and alkaline environments. The material's low coefficient of friction, its high-density formulation, and its excellent wear resistance make the product suitable as a prosthetic implant. Low-density polyethylene is used for catheters. The material has to be sterilized with ethylene oxide or gas plasma because of its low melting point.

Polytetrafluroethylene

Polytetrafluroethylene (Gore-Tex or Teflon) is a copolymer formed by the reaction between polyethylene and fluorine. It is relatively inert with a low coefficient of friction and has uses as vascular graft material, as a blood vessel replacement device, as implantable mesh material, and as a coating for prosthetic joint implants.

Polyurethane

Polyurethane is used as a polymer coating for implants because of its low thrombogenicity. This coating is fabricated onto implant device housings or into tubular mandrels. Its low melting point restricts it to ethylene oxide or gas plasma sterilization. An adhesive urethane membrane is commercially available for use in wound management.

Polyoxymethylene

Polyoxymethylene is a thermoplastic polymer that was used as a hip joint component. Extremely toxic metabolites leaching from the wear surfaces resulted in severe inflammation and tissue necrosis. Presently, the material is used only as orthopedic washers because of its high creep resistance.

Polyvinyl Chloride

Polyvinyl chloride (PVC) is an organochloride polymer used extensively in cannula and catheter production. A diphthalate compound is added to polyvinyl chloride to increase flexibility. However, body fluid exposure leaches out additives, returning stiffness and rigidity to the material. These products should not be exposed to ethylene oxide sterilization as the gas adheres to the material, causing hemolytic reactions upon tissue exposure.

Silicone

Silicone is an organosilicon polymer that is very biocompatible. Because of their low thrombogenic properties, these products are often placed in contact with blood. It is one of the most widely used implantable materials and is easily fabricated into an assortment of steam-sterilized shapes and sizes. Sustained-release antibiotic coatings, minimizing infection, can be applied to the material for prolonged tissue contact.

Polymethylmethacrylate

Polymethylmethacrylate (PMMA) is formed by mixing powdered methylmethacrylate with the liquid polymer dimethytoluidine. As the mixture polymerizes, an exothermic reaction occurs and forms PMMA. The initial reaction may lead to necrosis of exposed tissues. Although it is described as relatively inert, a fibrous tissue capsule usually forms around the implant. The primary use of PMMA is as cement for implanting metal prosthetics. It has also been used for bone-plate luting, increasing contact between the plate and bone. Antibiotics may be mixed in with the material to provide a sustained antimicrobial action, to decrease the chance of infection.

Stainless Steel Sutures

Stainless steel (SS), titanium, and other metal alloys used as orthopedic implants are discussed in detail later—the description here pertains to SS suture material. Steel is an alloy of iron and is processed as suture in monofilament and multifilament forms. It has the greatest tensile strength and knot security of all sutures, and SS is nearly biologically inert. SS sutures are indicated for tissues that heal slowly. Tissue movement against the suture ends may cause inflammation and tissue necrosis. There is a tendency for SS to cut through tissue under tension, it has poor handling characteristics, and cyclic bending may break the material. Multifilament wire may fragment and migrate in tissues, leading to fistula formation.

METALLIC IMPLANT MATERIALS

Commonly used metallic implant materials for fracture fixation include stainless steel, unalloyed titanium (also known as commercially pure titanium), and titanium alloys. Some cobalt-based alloys are also used for specialty applications. Implant materials standardization is covered by the ISO and the American Society for Testing and Materials (ASTM). Trade names vary with the supplier, but all implant material must meet industry requirements for composition, microstructure, mechanical properties, and corrosion resistance.

Stainless Steel

ISO 5832-1 or ASTM F 138 (bar and wire)/ASTM F 139 (sheet and strip) stainless steel is used extensively in the orthopedic implant industry. The iron-based stainless composition is known as wrought 18% chromium–14% nickel–2.5% molybdenum implant alloy,[14] and it contains minor additions of residual elements. This material is also referred to as implant-quality 316L stainless steel in the United States. The alloy is composed of chromium to provide corrosion resistance, nickel for microstructural stability, and molybdenum for improved resistance to pitting and crevice corrosion. The alloy contains a low carbon content (maximum, 0.030% carbon) for improved resistance to intergranular corrosion.[8] Special melting practices ensure that the implant alloy has a low amount of nonmetallic inclusions, no secondary magnetic phases, and elevated chromium and molybdenum levels. The material must meet a compositional index defined by the equation

$$\%Cr + 3.3 \times \%Mo \geq 26$$

to ensure adequate in vivo pitting and crevice corrosion resistance.[15] For multicomponent devices such as plates and screws, it is not advisable to mix SS and titanium implants, because an accelerated form of corrosion known as galvanic corrosion can occur.[14] Implant SS may be used in the annealed or softest condition for reconstruction plates that are highly contoured or for cerclage wire that may be subjected to a large amount of twisting and torsional deformation. The alloy may also be supplied in the cold-worked or moderate-strength condition to resist the stress loading encountered by bone plates and bone screws. Cold-working is a metalworking operation that permanently deforms the material at room temperature to increase construct strength, usually by reducing the cross-sectional area by drawing or rolling. Small-diameter products such as K-wire, Schanz screws, and Steinmann pins may be fabricated from extra-hard or highly cold-worked material with a very high tensile strength (greater than 1350 MPa) for improved bending resistance.[16] Relative tensile property requirements according to ASTM F 138 specification are shown in Table 9-2.

The excellent corrosion resistance of stainless steel is primarily a result of a chromium oxide film known as the passive layer, which is present on the surface. Chemical passivation in nitric acid is a commonly used method of surface finishing for stainless steel implants.[17] Immersion in 20 to 45 volume-percent nitric acid passivation solution removes surface contaminants such as cutting tool transfer films, heat treat oxide, imbedded particles, and burned-in lubricants. The passivation process restores maximal corrosion resistance but does not affect part dimensions.

Electropolishing is another surface treatment that consists of applying an electric current to an implant immersed in a special formulated chemical solution under specified

TABLE 9-2. Minimum Tensile Properties of Implant Quality 316L Stainless Steel Bar

Condition	Ultimate Tensile Strength* (MPa)	0.2% Yield Strength† (MPa)	Elongation‡ (%)
Annealed	490	190	40
Cold-worked	860	690	12
Extra hard	1350	—	—

*Ultimate tensile strength: failure stress (maximum load ÷ cross-sectional area).
†Yield strength: stress at start of permanent deformation (at 0.2% stress to strain offset deviation).
‡Elongation: a measure of ductility (amount of total extension under load).

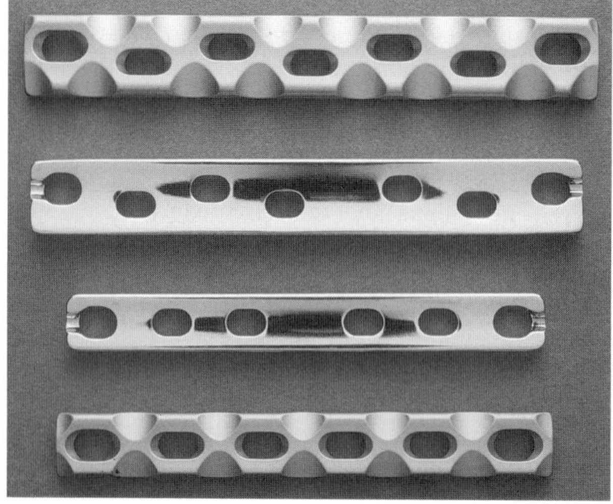

Figure 9-1. Bone plates showing their undersurfaces. The middle two stainless steel plates are electropolished, whereas the top and bottom titanium plates have an anodized surface.

conditions of time and voltage.[18] The treatment removes a microscopic amount of metal, decreases the surface roughness of the implant, provides a low coefficient of friction, improves corrosion resistance, and creates a chemically passivated surface (Fig. 9-1). For certain applications, some implants may be shot-peened before electropolishing. The implant surface is subjected to high-velocity impaction by metallic or ceramic particles under well-defined conditions. Shot peening[19] produces a roughened surface with increased residual compressive stress for enhanced fatigue life.

Implant-quality SS is completely nonmagnetic in all conditions, and implants may be subjected to magnetic resonance imaging (MRI) procedures.[20] AO stainless implants will not exhibit torsional movement, displacement, or heating during MR scans. However, signal artifact may obscure complete MR visualization in the vicinity of the stainless implant because of the high iron content (approximately 62 weight-%). The 15% nickel content may provoke a metal sensitivity reaction and is responsible for about 90% of the metal allergies that are clinically observed in people.[21] Repeated steam autoclaving will not disrupt the passive film or alter the mechanical properties of stainless steel implants.

Titanium

Commercially pure (CP) titanium, also known as unalloyed titanium, is available in five implant compositions designated Ti grade 1 ELI, 1, 2, 3, and 4 according to ISO[22] and ASTM[23] implant industry standards. The extra low interstitial (ELI) composition has the lowest content of nitrogen, carbon, iron, and oxygen. Each grade in the annealed condition has a different combination of tensile strength and ductility. The strength increases and the ductility decreases as the grade changes from the lowest designation (grade 1 ELI) to the highest designation (grade 4). Minimum properties for annealed CP titanium bar according to industry standards are shown in Table 9-3. Cold-working may be used to increase the strength of titanium that is designated grade 4B in ISO 5832-2, but a minimum of 10% elongation must be met. CP titanium has better biocompatibility than stainless steel, typically contains less than 0.05% nickel,[24] and will not cause metal allergy reactions. Unalloyed titanium implants are recommended when metal sensitivity is preoperatively verified or when 316L stainless steel implants have provoked an allergic response.[25]

Titanium also exhibits unique biocompatibility properties, which include soft tissue and bone adhesion to the implant surface.[26] A major advantage of tissue integration at the surface has been the possibility of less bacterial colonization and reduced infection.[27] Tissue adjacent to pure titanium implants becomes well vascularized, with less tendency toward capsule formation. The pitting and crevice corrosion resistance of titanium is superior to that of stainless steel. Titanium implant materials also have a lower density and a lower modulus of elasticity, and they provide

TABLE 9-3. Minimum Tensile Properties of Annealed Implant-Quality CP Titanium Bar

Grade	Ultimate Tensile Strength* (MPa)	0.2% Yield Strength* (MPa)	Elongation* (%)	Reduction of Area† (%)
1 ELI	200	140	30	—
1	240	170	24	30
2	345	275	20	30
3	450	380	18	30
4	550	483	15	25

*See Table 9-2 footnotes.
†Reduction of area: a measure of ductility (the original area minus the area after fracture divided by the original area).

significantly fewer MR artifacts than stainless steel.[28] The density of titanium is 57% of the density of stainless steel and represents a weight reduction of nearly 50% when implants of similar dimensions are compared.

The modulus of elasticity is a constant physical property that describes the stress per unit strain in the elastic region. A material with a high modulus of elasticity transfers less stress from the implant to the bone. This may produce a condition known as stress shielding,[29] which is not ideal because bone must be adequately stressed to consolidate properly during the bone healing stage. The modulus of elasticity of titanium is about 55% of that of stainless steel, and the low modulus is desirable because of increased stress transfer. The modulus consideration is less important for implants with a small cross-sectional area.

Titanium implants may have a special anodized surface finish that increases the thickness of the protective titanium oxide passive film. The titanium implants are immersed in a chemical solution, and a known electrical voltage is applied for a specified time. Visible light diffraction within the oxide film creates a distinct color that depends on the thickness of the oxide film.[30] No pigments or organic coloring agents are present in the anodized titanium film. The titanium anodizing process is capable of producing a variety of colors that permit the design of color-coded implant systems (see Fig. 9-1). Multiple steam sterilization cycles will not significantly change the appearance of anodized titanium implants. However, fingerprint contamination from skin contact should be avoided when handling the implants between autoclave cycles.[24] Gloved handling of anodized titanium implants prevents the discoloration of isolated areas during steam autoclaving.

Titanium Alloys

Titanium–6 aluminum–4 vanadium alloys, which have approximately 6% aluminum and 4% vanadium, are available in two compositions that are identified as Ti-6Al-4V or Ti-6Al-4V ELI. Another titanium alloy widely used as an AO implant material contains titanium, 6% aluminum, and 7% niobium and is identified as Ti-6Al-7Nb. Unique characteristics of titanium alloys include higher tensile strength capability, lower ductility, similar modulus of elasticity, and equivalent density when compared with commercially pure titanium. Important physical properties[25] of CP titanium, titanium alloy, and stainless steel are compiled in Table 9-4. Data on anodic polarization, pitting, and stress corrosion cracking indicate that Ti-6Al-7Nb is an extremely corrosion-resistant alloy.[31] Unalloyed titanium and titanium alloys have well-documented notch sensitivity properties. *Notch sensitivity* is a term that describes the relative effect that local irregularities or stress raisers have on mechanical properties.[32] The notch sensitivity resistance of implant quality stainless steel is similar to that of unalloyed titanium and somewhat better than that of conventional titanium alloys. Titanium-base biomaterials are not classified as notch-sensitive materials on the basis of notch tensile data that has been published.[33] Some newer beta titanium alloys such as Ti-15Mo actually have improved notch sensitivity properties when compared with stainless steel. Implant design and manufacturing methods can influence the notch sensitivity resistance, and clinical factors such as surgical technique and handling must also be considered.

Titanium alloys may be color anodized in the same manner as CP titanium. The major difference is that the anodized film is an oxide mixture composed of thermodynamically stable oxides (i.e., $TiO_2 + Al_2O_3 + Nb_2O_5$).[34]

Retrieval analysis of human hip joint prostheses concluded that the Ti-6Al-7Nb alloy is extremely biocompatible, as evidenced by osseous integration at the implant surface.[35]

Cobalt-Base Alloys

Cobalt-base alloys are used primarily for prosthetic implants such as total hips, total knees, and total disc replacement. Co-26Cr-6Mo is the predominant alloy that is fabricated for total joint applications. The nickel content of this alloy is typically less than 0.5%, and nickel sensitivity reactions have not emerged as a clinical problem. This alloy may be hot forged into complex shapes, the tensile strength can exceed 1170 MPa,[36] and the wear resistance is outstanding. Overall, corrosion resistance is considered to be superior to that of stainless steel but inferior to that of titanium.

Other implantable cobalt alloys have been used for specialty trauma products such as orthopaedic cables, Kirschner wires, and implantable distractor components. Unique properties of cobalt-base alloys include a high modulus of elasticity, which may be 25% greater than stainless steel. Cold-working increases the strength of cobalt-base alloys, and thermal aging heat treatments can significantly increase the yield and ultimate tensile strength. The majority of cobalt-based alloys contain greater than 10% nickel,[37] which may provoke a nickel allergy reaction. The excellent

TABLE 9-4. Physical Properties of Metallic Implant Materials

Material	Specifications ISO ASTM	Density (g/cc)	Modulus of Elasticity (GPa)
316L stainless	F 138 (bar/wire)	7.95	186
	F 139 (sheet/strip)	7.95	186
Ti grade 1 to 4	5832-2 F 67	4.51	103
Ti-6Al-7Nb	5832-11 F 1295	4.52	105
Ti-6Al-4V ELI	5832-3 F 136	4.43	114
Ti-15Mo	F 2066	4.96	78

ASTM, American Society for Testing and Materials; ISO, International Standardization Organization.

corrosion resistance of the cobalt-base alloys is predominately the result of the chromium content, which typically exceeds 18%. Chromium and cobalt are considered metal sensitizing agents, but the clinical incidence of sensitivity reactions is relatively rare when compared with nickel.[21]

METALLIC INSTRUMENT MATERIALS

Stainless Steel

The types of stainless steel that are used for instruments can be classified according to their microstructure, magnetic attraction, corrosion resistance, and hardness. A general comparison of commonly used stainless instrument materials is shown in Table 9-5.[38]

The martensitic (the word describes the type of microstructure associated with 400 series stainless steel, which is magnetic and has moderate corrosion resistance) compositions contain a minimum of 12% to 18% chromium, a medium to high carbon content, and other minor elements. Common types of martensitic alloys of the 400 series of stainless steel include 420A, 431, and 440B, and each grade has an equivalent Deutsches Institut für Normung (DIN) designation. The alloys are fabricated into various instruments in the soft condition and heat-treated to develop full mechanical properties. Heat-treating[39] consists of a hardening process that transforms the microstructure by heat in the range of 930° to 1150° C, followed by a controlled quench in air or a liquid. The hardened structure must be tempered at an intermediate temperature of 150° to 370° C to develop the final optimal properties.[39] For a given alloy, the hardness typically decreases as the tempering temperature increases. Martensitic alloys have high hardness and wear resistance. These alloys are used mainly for cutting instruments such as drills, taps, countersinks, reamers, chisels, and bone-cutting forceps, and for noncutting applications such as screwdriver blades and wrenches.

Precipitation-hardenable (PH) stainless steels contain substantial amounts of chromium, nickel, and copper, plus controlled levels of secondary elements.[39,40] The PH compositions are usually fabricated in the annealed condition, and the heat treatment is finished in a one-step aging treatment that promotes a hardening mechanism as a result of precipitation of a secondary strengthening phase within the martensitic matrix structure. Various age-hardened conditions (e.g., H900 and H950) are available, and the final hardness is inversely related to the age hardening temperature. PH stainless steels are used for a variety of noncutting instruments that require a moderate hardness level. The PH grades do not contain a high carbon content, so edge retention and wear resistance are inferior when compared with the 400 series martensitic compositions. A commonly used alloy contains 17% chromium plus 4% nickel (17-4PH) and is also identified as type 630.

Austenitic (this type of microstructure is nonmagnetic and has high corrosion resistance) stainless steels are known as the 300 series 40 and usually contain 16% to 18% chromium and 8% to 10% nickel. The low carbon grades such as 304L (L indicates low carbon) meet a compositional requirement of a maximum of 0.03% carbon. Other major elements may be added to improve the microstructure stability and corrosion properties. The 300 series stainless steels have excellent corrosion resistance and may be strengthened by cold-working, but they do not have outstanding cutting or wear properties because of the low carbon content. The austenitic alloys, except for 316 and 316L, which contain 2% to 3% molybdenum, also become slightly magnetic as the amount of cold-work increases. Some of the austenitic SSs can be cold-worked to a very high tensile strength and may be used for some noncutting applications including drill guides, clamps, hollow sleeves, springs, and washers. Some typical stainless steel instrument materials[38] are compared in Table 9-6.

TABLE 9-5. Classification of Stainless Steel Instrument Materials

Microstructure	Magnetic Attraction	Corrosion Resistance	Hardness	Common Types
Martensitic	High	Moderate	High	400 series
Precipitation hardenable	High	Moderate	High	PH grades
Austenitic	Low	High	Moderate	300 series

TABLE 9-6. Comparison of Common Stainless Instrument Alloys

Classification	Type (Deutsches Institut für Normung)	Condition	Hardness (HRC)
Martensitic	420A 1.4021	Hardened + tempered	47-50
	431 1.4057	Hardened + tempered	41-46
	440B 1.4112	Hardened + tempered	53-56
PH	630 1.4542	H900	44
	XM-25—	H900	43
Austenitic	302 1.4300	Highly cold-worked	45
	304L 1.4306	Cold-worked 50%	33
	316 1.4401	Cold-worked 50%	37

Aluminum

Aluminum is available in various purities, and a composition frequently used for bone plate or rod templates is known as grade 1100. This grade of aluminum meets a minimum aluminum content of 99.00%, and it is supplied in the soft annealed condition (O temper). Aluminum templates are low in strength, highly ductile, nonmagnetic, and lightweight. They may be color anodized to complement color-coded instrument systems. The anodizing treatment for aluminum is different from the electrolytic anodizing treatment used for titanium. The anodized color produced on aluminum is a result of an organic dye that is infiltrated into the aluminum oxide surface.[41] The surface is then chemically sealed, and other additives may be incorporated into the coating. Additional details regarding surface treatments for aluminum are covered later.

Aluminum Alloys

Aluminum alloys have increased strength and less ductility compared with pure aluminum. The alloys are grouped according to 2xxx through 8xxx identities, depending on the major alloying elements that are present. Aluminum alloy compositions that are frequently used for instruments include 2024, 5052, and 6061. The alloys are usually produced to a designated temper, which covers the heat-treating and/or other finishing operations that define the supplied metallurgical condition. A 5052-H32 designation indicates a 5022 alloy with an H32 temper (strain hardened/stabilized/quarter hard). Another common designation is 6061-T6; the T6 temper refers to solution-heat-treated plus artificially aged condition. Aluminum alloys have been used for depth gauges, IM nail insertion instruments, hollow external fixation rings, graphic case modules, and screw racks. Typical tensile properties for annealed pure aluminum and aluminum alloys with designated tempers are shown in Table 9-7.[42]

Aluminum alloys are nonmagnetic and lightweight. Machined or forged aluminum alloy instruments may be given specialized anodizing treatments to provide modified surface characteristics. The anodizing process for aluminum consists of detergent cleaning, rinsing, electrolytic anodizing, dyeing (optional), rinsing, and sealing. Conventional anodized aluminum films may be clear (nondyed) or may be produced in a variety of colors that meet standardized dye color charts. Conventional anodizing increases the corrosion resistance and surface hardness. Another specialized anodizing treatment is known as hard anodizing or hard coat. Hard anodizing provides an increased surface hardness of around 60 to 65 HRC for improved wear resistance.[41] Hard anodized films may also be produced that contain a polytetrafluroethylene polymer impregnated into the aluminum oxide film or the polymer may be co-deposited during formation of the aluminum oxide coating.[43] In both instances, the polymer plus hard coat provides reduced frictional properties and improved wear and galling resistance (which is a relative measure of the resistance to the adhesive wear that occurs when two metals rub together at high points on their mating surfaces). Chemical cleaning solutions containing chlorine, iodine, or certain metal salts may attack the anodized coating. Aluminum contact with strong alkaline cleaners must be avoided to prevent aggressive chemical attack.

TABLE 9-7. Typical Tensile Properties for Aluminum and Aluminum Alloys

Alloy, Temper	Ultimate Tensile Strength* (MPa)	0.2% Yield Strength* (MPa)	Elongation*† (%)
1100-O	90	35	45
2024-T4	470	325	19
5052-H32	227	193	18
6061-T6	310	276	25

*See Table 9-2 footnotes.
†50-mm-diameter specimens.

Other

Titanium alloys such as Ti-6Al-4V or Ti-6Al-7Nb may occasionally be used for noncutting instrument applications. The nonmagnetic alloys have high strength and low weight, and they may be anodized for color-coded systems. External fixation components have been designed to take advantage of these properties. Cobalt-base alloys have a high modulus of elasticity, which is beneficial for small-diameter guide wires and aiming instruments that require high stiffness.

CERAMICS (M. BOHNER)

There are two main classes of ceramic bone substitutes (CBS): calcium sulfates (CaS) and calcium phosphates (CaP). Both families consist of several chemical compounds representing more than a dozen compositions (Table 9-8).

The first CBS that was used in vivo was β-hemihydrate CaS (β-$CaSO_4 \cdot \frac{1}{2}H_2O$).[44] Addition of water to this material elicits an exothermic reaction, with the end product being a set form of gypsum ($CaSO_4 \cdot 2H_2O$).[45,46] Beside β-$CaSO_4 \cdot \frac{1}{2}H_2O$ and gypsum, there are two other CaS of less clinical importance, which are α-$CaSO_4 \cdot \frac{1}{2}H_2O$ and $CaSO_4$.[46]

Hydroxyapatite [$Ca_5(PO_4)_3OH$], β-tricalcium phosphate [β-$Ca_3(PO_4)_2$], and their composites (commonly called biphasic calcium phosphates) are the most common CaP bone substitutes. However, apatites can be synthesized with various structures and compositions. Additionally, many other calcium phosphates, such as dicalcium phosphate dihydrate and octacalcium phosphate, are available and have been used in vivo.

To simplify matters, there are presently two classes of CaP: low- and high-temperature CaP. Low-temperature CaPs are obtained at room temperature, through either a setting (i.e., hardening; see later) or a conversion reaction. These CaPs can be found in vivo, and they typically have a small average crystal size and a large specific surface area (up to 100 m^2/g for apatites). High-temperature CaPs are obtained by sintering reactions (i.e., heating at temperatures higher than 700° to 800° C). As high-temperature CaPs are easier to synthesize than low-temperature CaPs, most commercial products (e.g., chronOS, the AO standard product) are

TABLE 9-8. Main Ceramic Bone Substitutes

Name	Formula	Ca/P	Mineral Name	Symbol
Monocalcium phosphate monohydrate	$Ca(H_2PO_4)_2 \cdot H_2O$	0.50	—*	MCPM
Dicalcium phosphate	$CaHPO_4$	1.00	Monetite	DCP
Dicalcium phosphate dihydrate	$CaHPO_4 \cdot 2H_2O$	1.00	Brushite	DCPD
Octacalcium phosphate	$Ca_8H_2(PO_4)_6 \cdot 5H_2O$	1.33	—*	OCP
Precipitated hydroxyapatite ("tricalcium phosphate")	$Ca_{10-x}(HPO_4)_x(PO_4)_{6-x}(OH)_{2-x}$	1.50-1.67	—*	PHA
Amorphous calcium phosphate	$Ca_3(PO_4)_2 \cdot nH_2O$ n = 3-4.5; 15-20% $\cdot H_2O$	1.50	—*	ACP
Monocalcium phosphate	$Ca(H_2PO_4)_2$	0.50	—*	MCP
α-Tricalcium phosphate	$\alpha\text{-}Ca_3(PO_4)_2$	1.50	—*	α-TCP
β-Tricalcium phosphate	$\beta\text{-}Ca_3(PO_4)_2$	1.50	—*	β-TCP
Sintered hydroxyapatite	$Ca_5(PO_4)_3OH$	1.67	Hydroxyapatite	HA
Oxyapatite	$Ca_{10}(PO_4)_6O$	1.67	—*	OXA
Tetracalcium phosphate	$Ca_4(PO_4)_2O$	2.00	Hilgenstockite	TetCP
Calcium sulfate	$CaSO_4$	—	—*	CS
Calcium sulfate hemihydrate α	$CaSO_4 \cdot \frac{1}{2}H_2O$	—	—*	α-CSH
Calcium sulfate hemihydrate β	$CaSO_4 \cdot \frac{1}{2}H_2O$	—	Bassanite	β-CSH
Calcium sulfate dihydrate	$CaSO_4 \cdot \frac{1}{2}H_2O$	—	Gypsum	CSD

The first six calcium-phosphate compounds precipitate at room temperature in aqueous systems. The last six calcium-phosphate compounds are obtained by thermal decomposition or thermal synthesis.
*Not known or not indicated.

obtained via sintering reactions. However, low-temperature CaPs, such as dicalcium phosphate dihydrate[47] or precipitated apatite,[48] are likely to become more important in the future, because these compounds are more similar to the CaP present in the body.

Hydraulic cements are obtained via dissolution-precipitation reactions in an aqueous solution. For example, $\beta\text{-}CaSO_4 \cdot \frac{1}{2}H_2O$ dissolves in water and gypsum crystals nucleate and grow. If the powder-to-liquid ratio is large enough (typically greater than 2 g/mL), gypsum crystals grow close enough to entangle and hence provide mechanical stability to the resulting hardened compound. The setting reaction is generally exothermic, but the rate of heat release is too low to cause biocompatibility problems. Hardened cement blocks are nanoporous or microporous, and their porosity is typically in the order of 40% to 50% of the volume.

Whereas plaster of Paris has been known for ages, the discovery of CaP cements is recent.[49] The first products were introduced a decade ago. Many compositions have been proposed, but the end product of the reaction can only be brushite (e.g., chronOS Inject) or an apatite (e.g., Norian SRS). As a result, the terms *brushite cements* and *apatite cements* are used. Because of their higher solubility, brushite cements tend to resorb much faster than apatite cements (see later).

Porosity

The porosity strongly influences the mechanical and biologic properties of CBSs. Generally, there are two types of pores: micropores and macropores (Fig. 9-2). Micropores typically have a diameter in the size range of 1 to 10 μm. Micropores have been considered to promote ceramic resorption,[50-53] but the amount of scientific data is very scarce. It is therefore not possible to define an optimal micropore size or volume fraction. However, micropores are essential to prevent crack propagation[54] and hence should be a standard feature of CBSs. A practical advantage for the clinician is that a microporous CBS can be shaped with a blade. Presently, only few products contain a significant fraction of micropores, one of them being chronOS (Synthes, Inc, Paoli, Pa).

Macropores typically have a diameter in the size range of 50 to 2000 μm. Macropores enable blood vessel and cell ingrowth, hence promoting bone ingrowth and short resorption times.

Mechanical Properties

Compressive strengths as high as 100 MPa (i.e., almost as high as that of bone) have been indicated for some CBSs. Unfortunately, CBSs are ceramics and therefore inherently brittle. As a result, tensile strengths are typically 5 to 20 times lower than compressive strengths, and shear properties are miserable. Therefore, CBSs can break at very small loads (much lower than the indicated average mechanical strength) and hence should be used in combination with an internal or external fixation device.

Many factors, such as porosity, chemistry, and crystal or grain size, influence the mechanical properties of CBS. Typically, an increase in porosity decreases the mechanical properties of a material exponentially. As mentioned before, micropores decrease the brittleness of a CBS.[54] Furthermore, the least soluble CBSs (e.g., hydroxyapatite) tend to have the

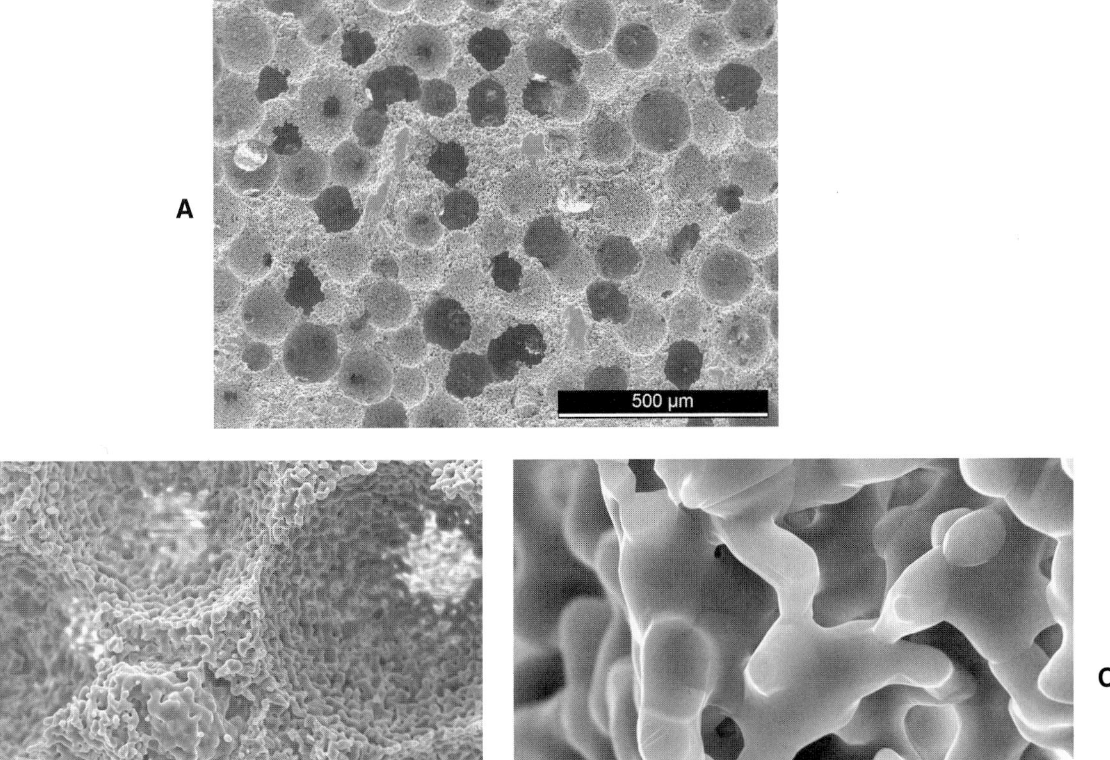

Figure 9-2. Microporosity and macroporosity in a β-tricalcium phosphate bone substitute as seen by scanning electron microscopy. **A,** Overall view of a macroporous bone substitute. **B,** Closer view of the macroporosity. The micropores are visible in the walls of the macropores. **C,** Microporosity. Bar: 500, 100, and 10 µm.

highest mechanical properties. Finally, a small crystal or grain size favors large mechanical properties.

Forms

CBSs are available in various forms: granules, macroporous blocks, hydraulic cements, and putties (paste). Each of these forms has specific advantages and disadvantages. Granules can be filled into any defect, but this procedure is often cumbersome, and granules can migrate. Bone formation and ceramic resorption are both optimal because of the availability of blood vessels and cells, which invade the space between the granules. Blocks, such as cylinders, wedges, and prisms, are difficult to place in complicated defect geometries. However, blocks are mechanically stable and have an optimal porous structure that enables fast blood vessel and cell ingrowth. Hydraulic cements are often injectable. As a result, these cements are easy to apply into any defect and can be shaped. Moreover, cements harden with time, hence providing a stable (but not load-bearing) defect-filling material. However, the cements presently available are not macroporous. Therefore, resorption takes place slowly, layer by layer.

The latest form of CBS is the so-called putty, a term that means that the CBS is a thick paste. The nature of this paste varies from one producer to another. Some putties are also a hydraulic cement and thus behave like a cement. But traditionally, putties consist of a mixture of a gel and granules. The advantage of putties is that they are easier to apply than granules. Moreover, granules do not move out of the defect as easily when accompanied by a gel.

Biologic Behavior

The mechanisms of resorption of CBSs vary widely depending on their solubility. CaS dissolves in vivo because body fluids are undersaturated in CaS. As a result, a change of blood supply or sample volume is expected to modify the dissolution time. A large gap occurs between implant and bone.[55] Typically, the amount and quality of the bone formed in the defect filled with CaS is poor: it consists of very narrow and small trabeculae, which tend to resorb with time. On the other hand, traditional CaPs, such as β-tricalcium phosphate (β-TCP), hydroxyapatite, and their composites, are insoluble in body fluid (e.g., in serum).[56] This low solubility leads to an osteoclast-mediated

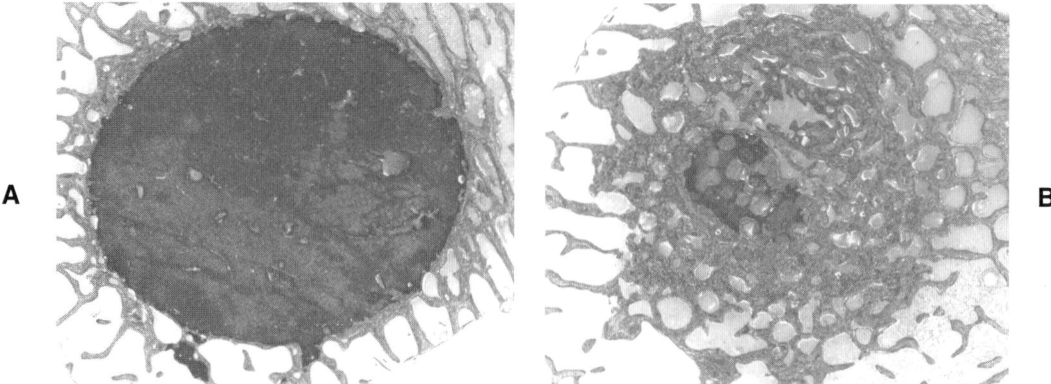

Figure 9-3. General appearance of an 8-mm cylindrical defect filled with apatite (**A**) and brushite (**B**) cement 6 months after implantation in sheep. **A,** Only very small amounts of bone can be seen within the apatite cement (lighter areas within the cement). **B,** Brushite cement is almost completely resorbed and replaced by new bone. (From Disegi JA, Eschbach L: Injury 31[Suppl 4]:2-6, 2000.)

resorption,[57] the rate of which depends on the composition. Whereas β-TCP is typically resorbed within a year,[57] hydroxyapatite is practically nonresorbable[58] (Fig. 9-3). However, for all traditional CaPs, a direct apposition of bone on the ceramic surface is observed. Other calcium phosphates, such as dicalcium phosphate dihydrate (DCPD), have an intermediate solubility and hence an intermediate resorption rate. In that case, resorption occurs primarily via macrophages.[59] Moreover, often a small gap between bone and implant develops. This gap is typically filled with osteoid tissue. Apatite cements are slowly resorbable,[57,59,60] whereas hydroxyapatite is practically nonresorbable.[58] This apparently peculiar difference is caused by a variation in crystal size: apatites obtained from hydraulic cements are nanosized, whereas sintered hydroxyapatite is microsized. Actually, apatite cements are soluble and hence have a resorption rate similar to that of β-TCP.

Many studies have been conducted to determine an optimal pore size for bone ingrowth and resorption rate.[61-69] However, the results are not so conclusive for two main reasons: (1) it is difficult to synthesize ceramics with perfectly controlled geometries, and (2) most in vivo studies have considered only few geometries (e.g., one or two) at few implantation times (e.g., one or two). Nevertheless, it could be shown that a pore diameter in the range of 100 to 1000 μm is adequate,[61-69] the macropores should be interconnected, and the size of the interconnections should be larger than 50 μm.[70] A recent study applied a theoretical approach to determine an adequate pore structure to minimize the resorption time; it revealed that a pore diameter in the range of 200 to 800 μm is optimal, but that this depends on the size of the bone substitute, with larger pieces requiring larger pores.[63]

ADHESIVES

Cyanoacrylate

Cyanoacrylate monomers are clear, colorless liquids with low viscosity and high reactivity. Reactivity is demonstrated by instantaneous polymerization in the presence of moisture, creating a thin, flexible polymer film that adheres to tissue. The film creates a mechanical barrier that is water resistant and resistant to infection, and that maintains a moist wound environment.[71] Two formulations are available for medical application. The butyl formulation is used primarily as a topical bandage, whereas the octyl formula can be used to appose skin edges. Strength of closure is comparable to that of subcuticular skin sutures.[72] Both are useful in controlling subtle hemorrhage. Although the octyl formulation is less cytotoxic than the butyl form, application is for topical use only. Cyanoacrylates are not biodegradable.

Fibrin Glues

Fibrin glues consist primarily of a combination of thrombin and fibrinogen. Autologous glue is composed of fibronectin, thrombin, aprotinin, fibrinogen, factor XIII, and calcium chloride. Autologous fibrin glue can be created by collecting plasma from the patient prior to surgery and then polymerizing an artificial clot. A commercial bovine source is available, but autoimmune reactions are a concern. This compound can be used as a sealant or as a hemostatic agent. Fibrin glues stick to and seal tissue. They have been used to seal leaks in lung, dura, intestine, liver, and spleen.[73] The material is broken down by fibrinolysis.

Glutaraldehyde Glue

Glutaraldehyde glue is a relatively new agent that contains gelatin, resorcinol, formaldehyde, and glutaraldehyde, and it is essentially albumin mixed with adhesion compounds. The glue has a half-life of about 30 days and is used in people as a cardiovascular and pulmonary adhesive. Long-term outcomes are presently unavailable.[73]

Polyethylene Glycol Polymers

Polyethylene glycol polymers are hydrogels that are used for tissue adhesion. This product is a water-soluble agent. It uses light to photopolymerize the substance and activate adhesion. Application is a complicated technique. The compound is degraded over a period of 3 months.[73]

TOPICAL HEMOSTATIC AGENTS

Selected product formulations considered either adhesives or hemostatic agents can perform dual functions. They can be used as adhesive glue or as a hemostatic agent. These products are biocompatible, biodegradable, and easily applied. They incite minimal antigenicity and do not inhibit normal healing.[73,74]

Collagen-Based Adhesive

Collagen-based adhesive is relatively new but demonstrates great potential. The compound is made from a combination of bovine thrombin and freeze-dried bovine collagen powder that is rehydrated, forming a gelatin matrix. On contact with fluids, the gelatin swells, providing a tamponade effect as well as forming a clot matrix, and then delivers fibrinogen to the area. Autologous plasma can be added to the formulation for a better result.

Polysaccharide Powder

Polysaccharide powder is a plant-based microporous derivative. Applied to a bleeding surface, the hydrophilic particles concentrate platelets, red blood cells, thrombin, and fibrinogen, accelerating the natural hemostatic process. Effective hemostasis is rapid.

Purified Gelatin Sponge

A purified gelatin sponge is applied topically to oozing capillaries, achieving hemostasis. On contact with blood, the gelatin absorbs fluid many times its weight, providing a tamponade effect while promoting platelet aggregation. The porosity of the gelatin particles provides a matrix for fibrin deposition and subsequent fibroblast migration. The material is absorbed by phagocytosis over a period of 4 to 6 weeks. Gelatin sponges should not be placed in contaminated wounds as they potentiate infection.

Oxidized Regenerated Cellulose

Controlled oxidization of regenerated cellulose forms a knitted mesh fabric that can be applied to a bleeding surface. Hemostasis is achieved by the formation of an artificial clot, independent of the inherent clotting pathways. The regenerated cellulose also has an affinity for hemoglobin and forms hydrated aggregates that plug exposed vessels. It induces minimal inflammation and fibrosis, and it is known to be bactericidal.

Collagen Absorbable Hemostat

Collagen absorbable hemostat consists of purified and lyophilized bovine collagen containing an abundance of type II collagen, manufactured in a spongelike pad. Subendothelial type II collagen is known to attract platelets, aggregating on the material and releasing coagulation factors that initiate clot formation. Pads are highly cross-linked, pliable, and absorbable. Autoclaving inactivates the product. Absorption occurs by phagocytosis and enzymatic degradation.

Bone Wax

Bone wax consists of a mixture of beeswax, paraffin, and isopropyl palmitate. It controls bleeding from bony surfaces by acting as a mechanical barrier, it can be moderately antigenic, it is nonabsorbable, and it can inhibit orthogenesis, delaying the healing process. Bone wax may cause a mild inflammatory reaction.

REFERENCES

1. Ramakrishna S, Mayer J, Wintermantel E, et al: Biomedical applications of polymer-composite materials: A review, Compo Sci Technol 2001;61:1189.
2. Kirkpatrick CJ, Bittinger F, Wagner M, et al: Current trends in biocompatibility testing, Proc Inst Mech Eng [H] 1998;212:75.
3. Hench LL: Bioceramics, J Am Ceram Soc 1998;81:1705.
4. Ambrose CG, Clanton TO: Bioabsorbable implants: Review of clinical experience in orthopedic surgery, Ann Biomed Eng 2004;32:171.
5. Trostle SS, Rosin E: Selection of prosthetic mesh implants, Compend Cont Educ Pract Vet 1994;16:1147.
6. Badylak SE: The extracellular matrix as a scaffold for tissue reconstruction, Semin Cell Dev Biol 2002;13:377.
7. Lange F: Über die Sehnenplastik, Verh Dtsch Orthop Ges 1903;2:10.
8. Panilaitis B, Altman GH, Chen J, et al: Macrophage response to silk, Biomaterials 2003;24:3079.
9. Meinel L, Hofmann S, Karageorgiou V, et al: The inflammatory responses to silk films in vitro and vivo, Biomaterials 2005;26:147.
10. Altman GH, Diaz F, Jakuba C, et al: Silk-based biomaterials, Biomaterials 2003;24:401.
11. Kim UJ, Park J, Li C, et al: Structure and properties of silk hydrogels, Biomacromolecules 2004;5:786.
12. Meinel L, Hofmann S, Karageorgiou V, et al: Engineering cartilage-like tissue using human mesenchymal stem cells and silk protein scaffolds, Biotechnol Bioeng 2004;88:379.
13. Meinel L, Karageorgiou V, Hofmann S, et al: Engineering bone-like tissue in vitro using human bone marrow stem cells and silk scaffolds, J Biomed Mater Res 2004;71A:25.
14. Disegi JA: AO ASIF wrought 18% chromium-14% nickel-2.5% molybdenum stainless steel implant material, Paoli, Pa, 1998, Synthes.
15. American Society for Testing and Materials: F 138 Standard specification for wrought 18 chromium-14 nickel-2.5 molybdenum stainless steel bar and wire for surgical implants, West Conshohocken, Pa, 2000, ASTM International.
16. Disegi JA, Eschbach L: Stainless steel in bone surgery, Injury 2000;31(Suppl 4):2-6.
17. American Society for Testing and Materials: F 86 Standard practice for surface preparation and marking of metallic surgical implants, West Conshohocken, Pa, 2001, ASTM International.
18. International Standardization Organization: Metallic and other inorganic coatings: Electropolishing as a means of smoothing and passivating stainless steel (15730), Geneva, 2000, ISO.
19. Metal Improvement Company, Inc: Shot peening applications, ed 8, Paramus, NJ, 2001, Metal Improvement Company.
20. Eschbach L: 10 frequently asked questions about magnetic resonance imaging in patients with metal implants, Bettlach, Switzerland, 2003, AO International.
21. Hierholzer S, Hierholzer G: Internal fixation and metal allergy, New York, 1992, Thieme.
22. International Standardization Organization: Implants for surgery: Metallic materials. Part 2: Unalloyed titanium (5832-2), Geneva, 1999, ISO.

23. American Society for Testing and Materials: Standard specification for unalloyed titanium for surgical implant applications (UNS R50250, UNS R50400, UNS 50550, UNS 50700) (F67), West Conshohocken, Pa, 2000, ASTM International.
24. IMI Titanium, Ltd: IMI commercially pure titanium, Birmingham, Ala, IMI Titanium Ltd.
25. Disegi JA: AO ASIF unalloyed titanium implant material, ed 5, Paoli, Pa, 2003, Synthes.
26. Steinemann SG, Eulenberger J, Maeusli PA, et al: Adhesion of bone to titanium. In Christel P, Meunier A, Lee AJC, editors: Biological and Biomechanical Performance of Biomaterials, Amsterdam, 1986, Elsevier.
27. Gristina A: Biomaterials-centered infection: Microbial adhesion versus tissue integration, Science 1987;237:1988.
28. Savolaine ER, Ebraheim NA, Andreshak TG, et al: Anterior and posterior cervical spine fixation using titanium implants to facilitate magnetic resonance imaging evaluation, J Orthop Trauma 1989;3:295.
29. Park JB: Hard tissue replacement implants. In Biomaterials Science and Engineering, New York, 1984, Plenum Press.
30. Disegi JA: Anodizing treatments for titanium implants. In Bumgardner JD, Puckett AD, editors: Proceedings of the 16th Southern Biomedical Engineering Conference, Institute of Electrical & Electronics Engineers (IEEE), 1997.
31. Disegi JA: AO ASIF titanium-6% aluminum-7% niobium alloy, ed 1, Paoli, Pa, 1993, Synthes.
32. Young WC: Roark's formulas for stress and strain, ed 6, New York, 1989, McGraw-Hill.
33. Disegi JA: Titanium alloys for fracture fixation implants, Injury 2000;31(Suppl 4):14-17.
34. Maeusli PA, Bloch PR, Geret V, et al: Surface characterization of titanium and Ti-alloys. In Christel P, Meunier A, Lee AJC, editors: Biological and Biomechanical Performance of Biomaterials, Amsterdam, 1986, Elsevier.
35. Zweymuller KA, Lintner FK, Semlitsch MF: Biologic fixation of a press-fit titanium hip joint endoprosthesis, Clin Orthop 1988;235:195.
36. International Standardization Organization: 5832-12 Implants for surgery: Metallic materials. Part 12: Wrought cobalt-chromium-molybdenum alloy, Geneva, 1996, ISO.
37. Marti A: Cobalt-base alloys used in bone surgery, Injury 2000;31(Suppl 4):18-21.
38. Carpenter Technology Corporation: Carpenter stainless steels, selection, alloy data, fabrication, Reading, Pa, 1999, Carpenter Technology Corp.
39. ASTM F 899 Standard specification for stainless steels for surgical instruments, Conshohocken, Pa, 2002, ASTM International.
40. American Society for Metals: Introduction to stainless steel. In Davis J and Associates, editors: ASM Specialty Handbook, Stainless Steels, Materials Park, Ohio, 1996, ASM International.
41. Military Specification: MIL-A-8625E. Anodic coatings for aluminum and aluminum alloys, Lakehurst, NJ, 1988, Department of Defense.
42. American Society for Metals: Wrought aluminum. In Unterweiser P, editor: Worldwide Guide to Equivalent Nonferrous Metals and Alloys, Metals Park, Ohio, 1990, ASM International.
43. American Society for Metals: 2482C, Hard coating treatment of aluminum alloys Teflon-impregnated or codeposited, Warrendale, Pa, 2000, Society of Automotive Engineers.
44. Dreesman H: Ueber Knochenplombierung, Beitr Klein Chir 1892;9:804.
45. Damien CJ, Parsons JR: Bone graft and bone graft substitutes: A review of current technology and applications, J Appl Biomater 1991;2:187-208.
46. Freyer D, Voigt W: Crystallization and phase stability of $CaSO_4$ and $CaSO_4$-based salts, Monatsheft Chem 2003;134:693-719.
47. Bohner M, Theiss F, Apelt D, et al: Compositional changes of a dicalcium phosphate dihydrate cement after implantation in sheep, Biomaterials 2003;24:3463-3474.
48. Kasten P, Luginbühl R, van Griensven M, et al: A comparison of human bone marrow stromal cells seeded on calcium-deficient hydroxyapatite, β-tricalcium phosphate and demineralized bone matrix, Biomaterials 2003;24:2593-2603.
49. Brown WE, Chow LC: Dental restorative cement pastes, US Patent No 4518430, 1985.
50. de Groot K: Effect of porosity and physicochemical properties on the stability, resorption, and strength of calcium phosphate ceramics, Ann N Y Acad Sci 1988;523:227-233.
51. Koerten HK, van der Meulen J: Degradation of calcium phosphate ceramics, J Biomed Mater Res 1999;44:78-86.
52. Klein CP, Driessen AA, de Groot K: Relationship between the degradation behaviour of calcium phosphate ceramics and their physical-chemical characteristics and ultrastructural geometry, Biomaterials 1984;5:157-160.
53. Klein CP, de Groot K, Driessen AA, van der Lubbe HB: Interaction of biodegradable beta-whitlockite ceramics in bone tissue: An in vivo study, Biomaterials 1985;6:189-192.
54. Morgan JP, Dauskardt RH: Notch insensitivity of self-setting hydroxyapatite bone cements, J Mater Sci Mater Med 2003;14:647-653.
55. Stubbs D, Deakin M, Chapman-Sheath P, et al: In vivo evaluation of resorbable bone graft substitutes in a rabbit tibial defect model, Biomaterials 2004;25:5037-5044.
56. Driessens FC: Physiology of hard tissues in comparison with the solubility of synthetic calcium phosphates, Ann N Y Acad Sci 1988;523:131-136.
57. Steffen T, Stoll T, Arvinte T, Schenk RK: Porous tricalcium phosphate and transforming growth factor used for anterior spine surgery, Eur Spine J 2001;10(Suppl 2):132-140.
58. Linhart W, Briem D, Amling M, et al: Mechanical failure of a porous hydroxyapatite ceramic 7.5 years after treatment of a fracture of the proximal tibia, Unfallchirurg 2004;107:154-157.
59. Apelt D, Theiss F, El-Warrak AO, et al: In vivo behavior of three different injectable hydraulic calcium phosphate cements, Biomaterials 2004;25:1439-1451.
60. Gisep A, Wieling R, Bohner M, et al: Resorption patterns of calcium-phosphate cements in bone, J Biomed Mater Res 2003;66A:532-540.
61. Uchida A, Nade SM, McCartney ER, Ching W: The use of ceramics for bone replacement: A comparative study of three different porous ceramics, J Bone Joint Surg Br 1984;66:269-275.
62. Chang B-S, Lee C-K, Hong K-S, et al: Osteoconduction at porous hydroxyapatite with various pore configurations, Biomaterials 2000;21:1291-1298.
63. Schliephake H, Neukam FW, Klosa D: Influence of pore dimensions on bone ingrowth into porous hydroxyapatite blocks used as bone graft substitutes: A histometric study. Int J Oral Maxillofac Surg 1991;20:53-58.
64. Gauthier O, Bouler J-M, Aguado E, et al: Macroporous biphasic calcium phosphate ceramics: Influence of macropore diameter and macroporosity percentage on bone ingrowth, Biomaterials 1998;19:133-139.
65. Daculsi G, Passuti N: Effect of macroporosity for osseous substitution of calcium phosphate ceramics, Biomaterials 1990;11:86-87.
66. Shimazaki K, Mooney V: Comparative study of porous hydroxyapatite and tricalcium phosphate as bone substitute, J Orthop Res 1985;3:301-310.
67. Chu TM, Orton DG, Hollister SJ, et al: Mechanical and in vivo performance of hydroxyapatite implants with controlled architectures, Biomaterials 2002;23:1283-1293.
68. Lu JX, Flautre B, Anselme K, et al: Role of interconnections in porous bioceramics on bone recolonization in vitro and in vivo, J Mater Sci Mater Med 1999;10:111-120.

69. Eggli PS, Müller W, Schenk RK: Porous hydroxyapatite and tricalcium phosphate cylinders with two different pore size ranges implanted in the cancellous bone of rabbits, Clin Orthop 1988;232:127-138.
70. Bohner M, Baumgart F: Effects of geometrical factors on the resorption of calcium phosphate bone substitutes, Biomaterials 2004;25:3569-3582.
71. Vauthier C, Dubernet C, Fattal E, et al: Poly(alkylcyanoacrylates) as biodegradable materials for biomedical applications, Adv Drug Deliv Rev 2003;55:519.
72. Shapiro AJ, Dinsmore MRC, North JH: Tensile strength of wound closure with cyanoacrylate glue, Am Surg 2001;67:1113.
73. Reece TB, Maxey TS, Kron IL: A prospectus on tissue adhesives, Am J Surg 2001;182:40S.
74. Erne JB, Mann FA: Surgical hemostasis, Compend Cont Educ Pract Vet 2003;25:732.

SECTION II SURGICAL METHODS

Jörg A. Auer

CHAPTER 10

Sterilization and Antiseptics

David E. Freeman

Sterilization refers to the complete destruction or elimination of vegetative bacteria, bacterial spores, viruses, and fungi, by physical or chemical methods.[1] Antisepsis signifies the inhibition of the growth and development of microorganisms without necessarily killing them. Therefore, antiseptics can be applied to living tissues.[1] Physical methods of sterilization include heat (thermal energy), which is the most commonly used type in veterinary hospitals, and filtration and radiation, which are usually applied in the industrial preparation of sterile materials. Ethylene oxide is the most widely used method of chemical sterilization, but physical methods are considered to be more uniformly reliable.

INSTRUMENT PREPARATION AND PACKING

Cleaning

Instruments cannot be sterilized until they are completely clean, because steam cannot penetrate materials such as oil, grease, dried blood, and other organic material.[2-4] Ideally, an assistant should wipe every instrument used during surgery, before it is replaced on the surgery table, to prevent blood drying on the instrument. Once the instruments are returned to the sterilizing room, they are prepared for autoclaving by immediate rinsing in cold water to remove any remaining blood and debris, after which they can be cleaned with a moderately alkaline, low-sudsing detergent, or in an ultrasonic cleaner. Prerinsing in an enzymatic detergent solution is an acceptable alternative to manual cleaning.[5] Enzymatic detergents used for cleaning medical devices (Enzol, Johnson & Johnson, New Brunswick, NJ; Endozyme, Ruhof, Mineola, NY; Sterizyme, Anderson Products, Haw River, NC; and Metrizyme, Metrex Research Division of Sybron Canada, Ltd, Morrisburg, Ontario, Canada) help remove proteins, lipids, and carbohydrates, depending on the formulation.[6] Many of the available enzymatic detergents have a minimum contact time of 2 to 5 minutes (Asepti-zyme, Huntingdon Lab, Ontario, Canada; Gzyme, Germiphene Corp, Brantford, Ontario, Canada; Optim22, Virox Technologies, Mississauga, Ontario, Canada; Adi-Zyme, STERIS Corp, Mentor, Ohio; and Klenzyme, STERIS Corp, Mentor, Ohio) or 10 minutes (Metrizyme, Metrex Research Division of Sybron Canada, Ltd, Morrisburg, Ontario, Canada), and the recommended temperature for most is room temperature.[6] For the majority of them, a maximum soaking time of 30 to 45 minutes is recommended.[7] No commercially available detergents combine cleaning efficiency with microbial killing, with the exception of a newly formulated hydrogen peroxide–based cleaning detergent[6] (Hydrox, Virox Technologies, Mississauga, Ontario, Canada). The advantages of Hydrox are in the realms of protection of healthcare workers from infectious risk and reduced bioburden on instruments before sterilization or disinfection.[6]

Ultrasonic cleaners use high-frequency vibratory waves that clean through cavitation.[7] Minute gas bubbles are produced in this process. The vibratory waves facilitate their touching each other, which results in the formation of bigger bubbles out of many small ones, a process called implosion. The minute vacuum produced by the implosion and then multiplied by their number is responsible for high-pressure waves that radiate and clean all surfaces. Ultrasonic action effectively dislodges impacted debris from holes, jaws, box joints, channels, and complex surfaces, and it disrupts air pockets, ensuring thorough wetting during the cleaning process.[5] The instruments are loosely loaded in wire mesh trays for this process; all box locks are left open; complicated instruments, such as dynamic compression plate (DCP) drill guides, are taken apart; and instruments are thoroughly rinsed afterward to remove detached particles.[7] For ultrasonic cleaning, as used for the manual cleaning step, a nonfoaming enzymatic type of detergent solution is preferable[8] (Asepti-zyme, Huntingdon Lab, Ontario, Canada; Gzyme, Germiphene Corp, Brantford, Ontario, Canada; Sterizyme, Anderson Products, Haw River, NC; Adi-Zyme, STERIS Corp, Mentor, Ohio; Klenzyme, STERIS Corp, Mentor, Ohio; and Metrizyme, Metrex Research Division of Sybron Canada, Ltd, Morrisburg, Ontario, Canada).

After the instruments have been cleaned by these methods, they should be soaked in the oil known as instrument milk, which conditions the instrument surface and lubricates the joints. After an adequate air drying time, they are packed in wrappers that are permeable to steam but not to microorganisms.

Packing

All packs should be marked as to content, date of sterilization, and person responsible for assembling, and the pack should be stored for times appropriate for the material and the method of storage (Table 10-1). For muslin wraps, double layers and two wraps are recommended for each pack. Alternatively, pima cotton can be used, which is a more effective barrier than muslin because of the smaller

TABLE 10-1. Storage Times for Sterilized Packs

	Open Shelf	Closed Cabinet
Single-wrapped muslin (2 layers)	2 days	7 days
Double-wrapped muslin (each 2 layers)	3 weeks	7 weeks
Crepe paper (single-wrapped)	3 weeks	8 weeks
Heat-sealed paper and transparent plastic pouches	At least 1 year	—

From Mitchell SL, Berg J. In Slatter D (ed): Textbook of Small Animal Surgery, vol 1, ed 3, Philadelphia, 2003, WB Saunders.

pore size. Pima cotton wraps can be reused an approximate 75 times, after which so much fabric has been lost that no effective barrier against microorganisms exists.[4] Crepe papers are preferred to noncrepe papers because of their superior durability and handling qualities, and because their safe storage times are longer than that of fabrics.

Instruments can also be sterilized in stackable containers of aluminum composite material (Fig. 10-1) that are dent resistant, available in a variety of sizes, easy to store and transport, and allow safe storage times of up to 1 year (AMSCO Sterilization Container System, STERIS Corporation, Mentor, Ohio). The aluminum composite increases the thermal conductivity of the container during drying to help ensure dry contents. The system is suitable for use in steam, ethylene oxide, and gas plasma sterilization. Three types of filters—cartridge (with internal chemical indicator), disc, or ceramic—are available for this system. The filter is retained in a filter access portal in the lid and base of the units by a retainer ring. Selection of the type of filter is determined by the sterilization cycle to be used, such as prevacuum steam, gravity steam, flash, ethylene oxide, or gas plasma.

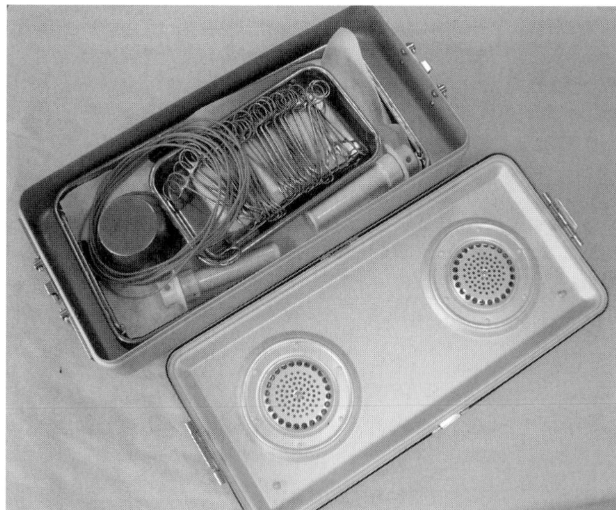

Figure 10-1. Stackable Steriset sterilization container with the lid removed, showing a standard soft tissue instrument set. The instruments located in the bottom of the set are covered by a special paper sheet. On top of it, sponges, towel clamps, the cautery including its electric cord, two sterile light handles, and a sponge forceps are visible. The inside of the lid shows the two valves. In each of the valves, one of three types of filter systems (steam, ethylene oxide, or plasma gas) can be inserted, depending on the type of sterilization being carried out.

Although pima cotton and crepe paper are well suited for instrument packs, these materials are rarely used to wrap single instruments. For this purpose, special sleeves have been developed that are paper on one side and clear cellophane on the other. The sleeves come in different sizes to allow the packing of instruments of different sizes. Also, different sizes are required because the instruments should be double wrapped. The ends of the sleeves are heat sealed. The sharp points of all instruments must be protected by plastic covers. The paper side allows penetration of steam, ethylene oxide, or gas plasma, and the cellophane side provides a view of the contents (Fig. 10-2). These single packs should be identified by date of sterilization and the person who packed it.

Autoclave Indicators

Autoclave indicator systems include chemical indicators that undergo a color change on exposure to sterilizing temperatures, and biologic indicators, such as heat-resistant bacterial spores (e.g., *Bacillus stearothermophilus*).[4,7,9] These spores are extremely resistant to heat, and the indicator systems require a period of incubation after sterilization to ensure the absence of bacterial growth. An indicator tape on the outside of the pack provides no information about the sterility of the pack's contents, so an additional indicator should be placed in the center of the pack. Many of the currently available indicators of sterility are more reliable than simple physical indicators, such as tape, because they indicate that both temperature and time are sufficient for providing sterility (Fig. 10-3), whereas tape merely indicates to the surgeon that the pack was subjected to heat.

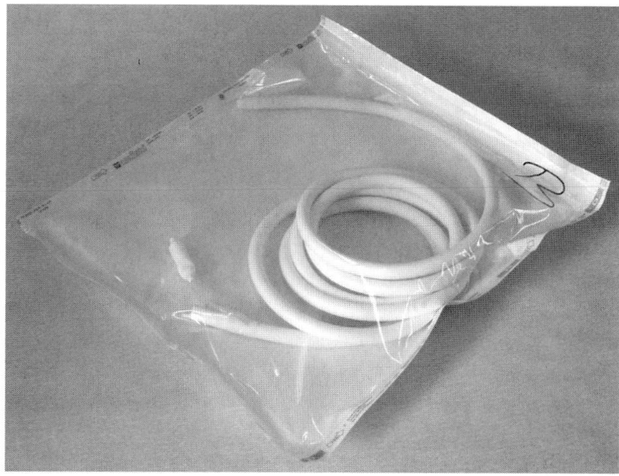

Figure 10-2. A single wrapped catheter in a paper-cellophane sleeve. These wrappers may also be used for single instruments.

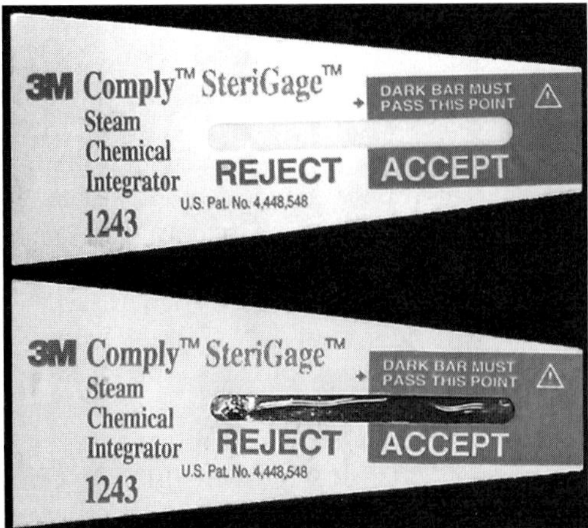

Figure 10-3. Example of a chemical indicator used to confirm that sufficient exposure conditions have been met in the center of the pack. In this 3M Comply (SteriGage) Steam Chemical Integrator, the chemical pellet contained in a paper, film, and foil laminate envelope melts and migrates as a dark color along the paper wick. The distance or extent of migration shown at the *bottom* (compare with unused *top*) depends on exposure to steam, time, and temperature. The dark color should enter the Accept window for an Accept result.

PHYSICAL STERILIZATION

Thermal Energy

Dry heat kills by a combination of oxidation and removal of water, whereas moist heat kills by the coagulation of critical proteins. Moist heat sterilization can coagulate and denature cellular protein at lower temperatures than those required by dry heat and thus can decrease the temperatures and exposure times necessary for sterilization.[2,3]

Exposure time and temperature required to kill microbes are functions of their individual heat sensitivities, which vary with type of organism and the environment to which they are accustomed.[3] For example, bacterial spores are more resistant than the vegetative form of the bacteria.[3] Recommended sterilization times and temperatures are designed to kill all microorganisms, even those that are heat resistant (Table 10-2). Minimum guidelines are an exposure time of 15 minutes at 121° C (249.8° F) and 15 p.s.i. or 2 atmospheres of pressure in a steam autoclave. Because microbial death occurs in a logarithmic fashion, exposure time is as important as temperature. The greater temperatures and water saturation attained by pressurized steam allow for shorter sterilization times. Steam gives up its heat to materials to be sterilized by the process of condensation, and it is able to penetrate porous substances more rapidly than dry heat.[3]

Most autoclaves used in veterinary hospitals use steam pressure to drive air downward and out of the pressure vessel, in a process called gravity displacement[4] (Fig. 10-4). Air displacement by steam is critical to achieve condensation on all surfaces, and air reduces the temperature of steam at any given pressure.[3] Arrangement of trays or bowls within the autoclave must be such that air cannot be trapped by the downward progression of the steam, and bowls should be placed with their openings to the side or facing down.[7,9] Also, packs should be loaded into the autoclave with a loose arrangement to ensure distribution and circulation of steam without the formation of air pockets[9] (Fig. 10-5). Valves in cannulas should be left open to ensure adequate steam penetration.[10] Because air trapped in closed, impervious

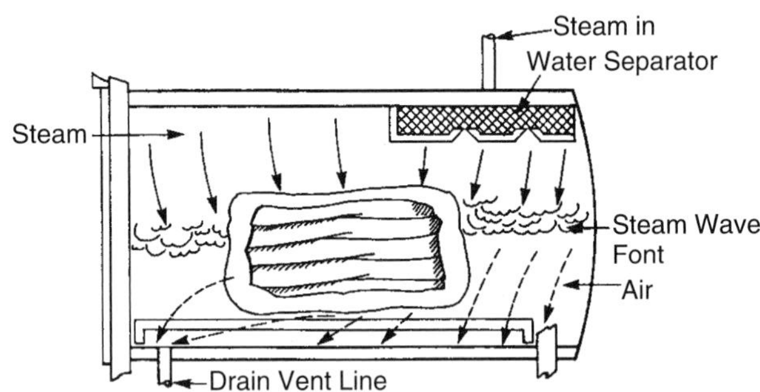

Figure 10-4. Schematic drawing of a gravity displacement autoclave, showing downward displacement of all air by steam in this system. (From Lawrence CA, Block SS: Disinfection, Sterilization, and Preservation. Philadelphia, 1991, Lea & Febiger.)

TABLE 10-2. Exposure Times and Temperatures for Autoclave Sterilization Systems

Procedure and Conditions	Time (min)	Temperature	Comments
Heat-up time (prevacuum and pulse type)	1	Up to 120° C (250° F)	Timing of exposure begins when exhaust line reaches 120 °C.
Minimum standard*	13	120° C	5-10 minutes destroys most resistant microbes; an additional 3-8 minutes provides a safety margin.
Emergency/"flashing" (prevacuum)†	3	131° C (270° F)	Instruments sterilized in perforated metal trays
Large linen packs (gravity-displaced)	30	120° C	—
Large linen packs (prevacuum)	4	131° C	—
Drying period	20	NA	—

*Times are given for gravity displacement autoclaves. Extra time is required for pack contents to reach sterilization temperatures (heat-up time).
†Emergency sterilization is best accomplished in prevacuum autoclaves, which have shorter heat-up times required.
From Southwood LL, Baxter GM: Vet Clin North Am Equine Pract 12:173, 1996 (with permission).

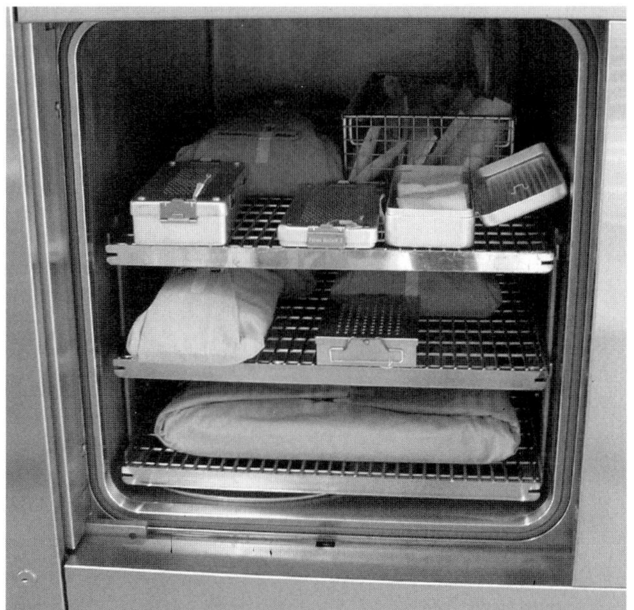

Figure 10-5. A typical sterilization unit in a large hospital, loaded and ready for use. Note that the contents are loosely arranged to facilitate access of steam around each item.

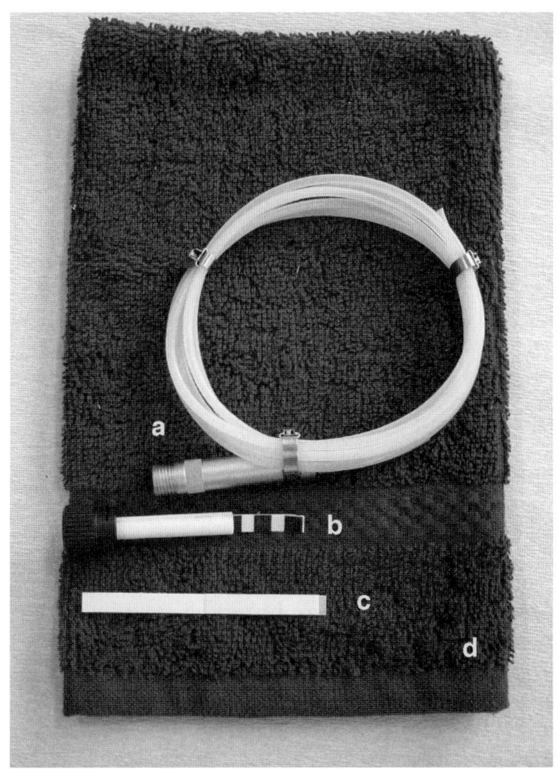

Figure 10-6. The gke Steri-Record Helix Bowie-Dick simulation (BDS) test kit. *a,* Metal test capsule attached to the polytetrafluoroethylene tube. *b,* Lid of the metal capsule holding the integrating indicator (the *dark dots* indicate proper function). *c,* Unused indicator strip. *d,* Cloth container for the BDS kit.

containers can inhibit steam penetration,[2-4] items in glass tubes should be sealed with cotton plugs.[7] Many newer or more sophisticated types of autoclaves use a vacuum to displace air from the materials to be sterilized.[9] This allows shorter sterilization times but adds to the cost of the equipment. Other modifications use pulsed steam pressure and special valve systems to hasten air removal prior to sterilization. Prevacuum steam sterilizers evacuate air from the chamber before steam is admitted, so the time lag for complete air removal is eliminated and the problem of air entrapment is minimized.[3] This system is well suited for "flashing" instruments.[3]

It is also recommended that the steam sterilizer be periodically tested for functionality. The Bowie-Dick test can be used to prove that air removal and steam penetration were complete.[5] The Steri-Record (gke-mbH, Waldems-Esch, Germany) provides two simulation tests for different applications, depending on the sterilization programs used.[11] These Bowie-Dick simulation tests simulate hollow devices, such as trocars, which require more demanding air removal and penetration conditions than porous cotton. The indicator systems consist of a process challenge device (PCD) with an indicator inside. One of the systems is the Helix-PCD, consisting of a polytetrafluoroethylene (PTFE) tube and a metal test capsule holding the integrated indicator (Fig. 10-6). The second system is the Compact-PCD, consisting of an external plastic casing with a stainless steel coil inside that holds the indicator. To ensure proper functioning of the sterilizer, such a kit should be included in each sterilizer charge.

Filtration

Sterilization by filtration is used for air supply to surgery rooms (laminar flow ventilation), in industrial preparation of medications, and for small volumes of solutions in practice settings.[9,12] The laminar air filtering system for surgery suites is discussed in Chapter 11. For fluids, two types of filters are commonly used—depth filters and screen filters.[9,12] Screen filters function like a sieve to remove any microorganisms or particulate matter larger than the pore diameter of the screen.[9,12] Depth filters trap microbes and particles by a combination of random absorption and mechanical entrapment.[12]

Radiation

Sterilization by radiation is used in the industrial preparation of surgical materials that are sensitive to heat or chemical sterilization.[9] The facilities required for ionizing radiation render them unsuitable for use in veterinary hospitals.[9] Although radiation is suitable for items that cannot tolerate heat sterilization, it can change the composition of some plastics and pharmaceuticals.[9,13]

CHEMICAL STERILIZATION

Ethylene Oxide

Ethylene oxide (EO) is the most commonly used agent in chemical sterilization. Because it is a gas, it rapidly penetrates packaging and items to be sterilized at temperatures tolerated by almost all materials. However, its use is limited by the size of the equipment, the time requirement, and concerns about toxicity. It is recommended for use only for items unsuitable for steam sterilization,[14] including laparoscopes, light cables, and camera heads.[10] In fact, because of environmental concerns, ethylene oxide sterilizers are now required by law to be retrofitted with abaters that reduce more of the exhausts to water vapor. Despite the use of abaters, the Environmental Protection Agency has outlawed the use of EO sterilizers altogether in some areas. Gas plasma sterilizers are a logical replacement choice (see later).

Ethylene oxide is an alkylating agent that kills microorganisms by inactivation of proteins, DNA, and RNA, and it is effective against vegetative bacteria, fungi, viruses, and spores.[15] It is supplied as a gas mixed with a carrier agent (Freon or CO_2) to reduce flammability.[4] Mixed with air or oxygen, EO is explosive and flammable.[4] Carbon dioxide is the preferred diluent because of environmental concerns about fluorinated hydrocarbon (Freon) release, although a tendency to stratify from carbon dioxide in storage containers could affect sterilization.[4]

Sterilization by ethylene oxide is influenced by gas concentration, temperature, humidity, and exposure time[16] (Table 10-3). The more sophisticated equipment for EO sterilization includes methods for temperature elevation to shorten sterilization times.[14] Spores require time for humidification to allow optimal killing by ethylene oxide.[9,15,16] The humidity should not be raised by wetting the materials to be sterilized, because ethylene oxide forms condensation products with water that may damage rubber and plastic surfaces. Also, the effectiveness of ethylene oxide sterilization may be reduced below the lethal point by moisture left in needles and tubing.[17] Instruments need to be cleaned as described for steam sterilization.

Because ethylene oxide penetrates materials more readily than steam, a wider variety of materials may be used in packaging items for sterilization and storage. Films of polyethylene, polypropylene, and polyvinyl chloride are commercially available, but nylon should not be used, because it is penetrated poorly by ethylene oxide.[9,15-17] Positioning of packs is less critical than with steam, but overloading and compression in the sterilizer can prevent adequate penetration.[4]

After sterilization by EO, materials must be aerated to allow dissipation of the absorbed chemical (Table 10-4), because residual ethylene oxide can damage tissues.[18,19] For example, inadequate aeration of endotracheal tubes sterilized by EO caused tracheal necrosis and stenosis in horses[20] and dogs.[21] Although some ethylene oxide chambers are equipped with mechanical aeration systems to reduce aeration times (Fig. 10-7), those commonly used in veterinary hospitals use natural aeration in well-ventilated areas.[6] EO sterilization indicator strips should be used on the outside of surgery packs, and chemical or biologic indicators of ethylene oxide exposure are used inside.[17] The 3M (St. Paul, Minn) Comply EO chemical integrators demonstrate a color change and migration on an absorptive strip in response to all the critical aspects of EO sterilization, such as EO concentration, relative humidity, time, and temperature. Safe storage times are 90 to 100 days for plastic wraps sealed with tape, and 1 year for heat-sealed plastic wraps.[17]

Exposure to ethylene oxide can cause skin and mucous membrane irritation, nausea, vomiting, headache,[9] cognitive impairment, sensory loss, reproductive failure, and increased incidence of chromosomal abnormalities.[18] Ability to detect the gas by smell is lost after prolonged exposure.[19] Ethylene chlorohydrin is a highly toxic degradation product of EO that is formed most readily in products that have been previously sterilized by radiation.[9,15,16] This risk is greatest with polyvinyl chloride products.[9]

Gas Plasma

Gas plasma sterilization (Sterrad Sterilization System, Advanced Sterilization Products, a division of Johnson & Johnson Medical, Inc, Irvine, Calif) (Fig.10-8) allows short

TABLE 10-3. Requirements for Ethylene Oxide Sterilization

Variables	Range	Comments
Concentration	450-1500 mg/L	Doubling the concentration approximately halves the sterilization time.
Temperature	21°-60° C	Activity is slightly more than doubled with each 10° C increase.
Exposure time	48 minutes to several hours	Room temperature, 12 h 55° C, 4 h or less "Oversterilization" period allowed
Humidity	40%-60% (Minimum, 33%)	Can be provided by vials of water or sponges

From Southwood LL, Baxter GM: Vet Clin North Am Equine Pract 12:173, 1996.

TABLE 10-4. Average Minimal Aeration Times after Ethylene Oxide Sterilization

Material	Aeration Time*	
	Natural (Days)	Mechanical (Hours)
Rubber products	1-2	46
Latex	7	46
PVC 1/8 inch (thick)	12	46
1/16 inch (thin)	7	46
Polyethylene	2	46
Vinyl	3	32
Plastic wrapped supplies	3	32
Implants	10-15 (recommended)	32

Times are given for natural aeration and, where available, for mechanical aeration. Ethylene oxide sterilizers equipped for mechanical aeration produce significantly shorter aeration times (hours instead of days).

From Clem M: In Auer J (ed): Equine Surgery. Philadelphia, 1992, WB Saunders.

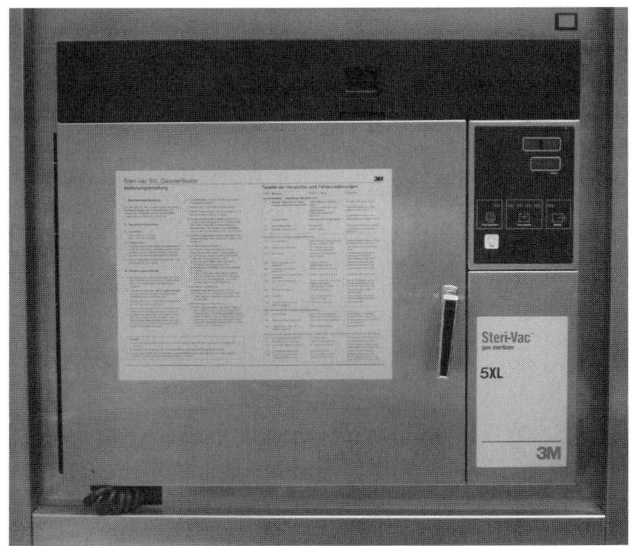

Figure 10-7. A modern ethylene oxide gas sterilizer (3M Health Care, St. Paul, Minn) with aeration capabilities.

instrument turnaround time, has no recognized health hazards, and operates at a low temperature (less than 50° C).[8] An aqueous solution of hydrogen peroxide is injected into the chamber and converted to gas plasma by radio waves that create an electrical field.[4] In this field, hydrogen peroxide vapor is converted to free radicals that collide with and inactivate microorganisms.[7,8] Gas plasma is suitable for heat- and moisture-sensitive instruments (rigid endoscopy lenses and instrument sets, objective lenses for microscopes, nonfabric tourniquets, medication vials, insulated electrosurgery and cautery instruments, and metal instruments).[7,8] Also, the process does not dull the sharpness of delicate microsurgical instruments.[7] Gas plasma is unsuitable for flexible endoscopes, liquids, and items derived from plant fibers (paper products, linens, gauze sponges, Q-tip applicators, cast padding, wooden tongue depressors, gloves, and single-use items), because these materials absorb hydrogen peroxide and inhibit sterilization.[7] Very long narrow lumens, lumens closed at one end, folded plastic bags, and sheeting are unsuitable for sterilization by gas plasma.[8]

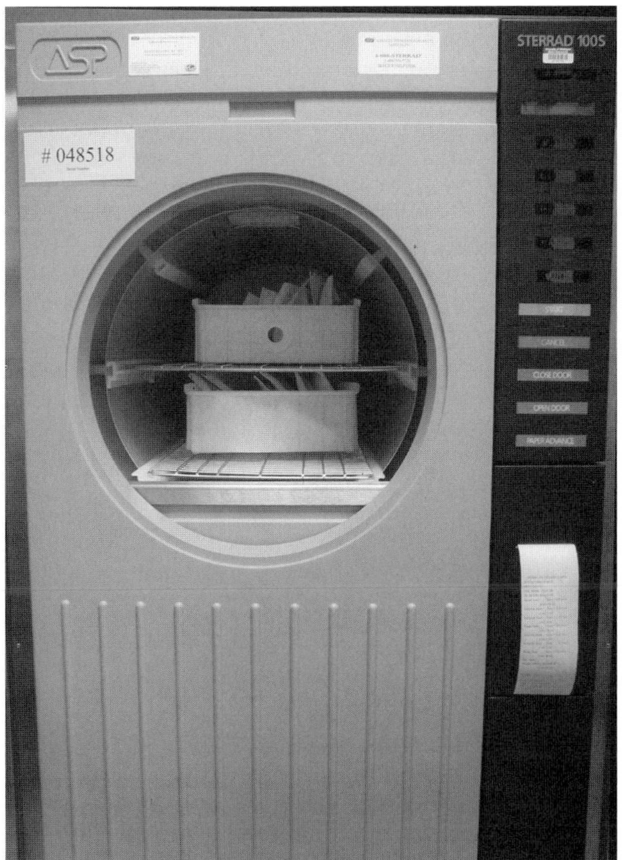

Figure 10-8. Gas plasma sterilization unit (Sterrad) that uses H_2O_2 to generate free radicals, which inactivate microbes.

Peracetic Acid

Peracetic acid (PAA) is available under numerous brand names with different chemical formulations (Nu Cidex 0.35%, Johnson and Johnson; STERIS 0.20%, STERIS Corporation, Mentor, Ohio, and STERIS Limited, STERIS House, Basingstoke, Hampshire, UK; Anioxyde 1000, Clinipak Medical Products, Bourne End, UK; and Sekusept Aktiv, Ecolab Center, St. Paul, Minn). The STERIS Corporation has marketed STERIS 20 Sterilant Concentrate, a 35% peroxyacetic acid concentrate, for use in the STERIS System 1[8] (Fig. 10-9). An arthroscopic camera and telescope can be processed, rinsed, and dried in this system in a 20-minute cycle. It is routinely used to sterilize flexible endoscopes as well. A contact time of 10 or 15 minutes and a concentration of greater than 0.09% PAA are recommended for destruction of bacteria, fungi, viruses, and spores, if used manually.[8] Compared with glutaraldehyde, PAA has a similar or even a better biocidal efficacy and is claimed to be less irritating for staff and safer for the environment. PAA does not fix proteins and therefore does not create a biofilm. It has the ability to remove glutaraldehyde-hardened material from biopsy channels, and its activity is not adversely affected by organic matter. Potential adverse effects are strongly linked to the pH value of the application solution, with minimal effects in a pH range of 7.5 or higher. PAA is less stable than glutaraldehyde, can be corrosive, and has a strong,

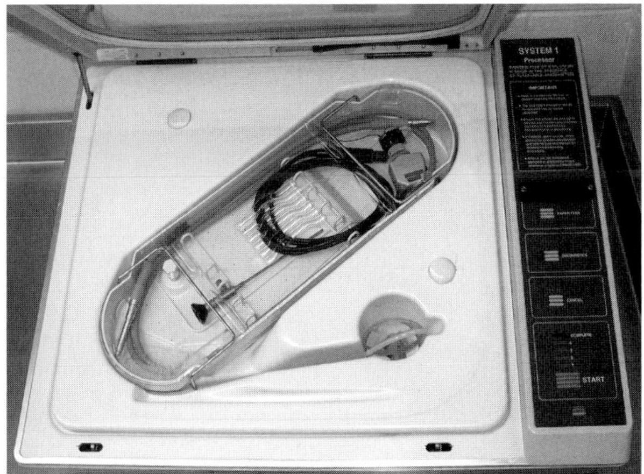

Figure 10-9. Peracetic acid sterilizer (Steris System 1), which is used to sterilize endoscopes, arthroscopes, and other equipment.

vinegar-like odor. Therefore, when using manual immersion methods, PAA should be used with adequate ventilation and personal protective measures. PAA also causes cosmetic discoloration of endoscopes, but without any functional damage if used manually; the STERIS System 1 sterilizer does not have this problem, however, as adequate rinsing is automatic. PAA is also expensive.[8]

Electrolyzed Acid Water

At present, two types of electrolyzed acid water (EAW) are available—electrolyzed strong acid water with a pH of less than 3 (e.g., CleantopWM-S, CBC Medical Device Group, Duesseldorf, Germany) and electrolyzed weak acid water, with a pH of between 6 and 7 (e.g., Sterilox Technologies, Inc, Radnor, Pa).[8] EAW is produced by using water and salt under electrolysis with membrane separation. The process generates hydroxy radicals that have a rapid and potent bactericidal effect. Additionally, the low pH (pH 2.7) and high oxidation-reduction potential (1100 mV) are toxic to microorganisms.[8] EAW breaks the bacterial cell wall and degenerates various inner components of the bacterium (including chromosomal DNA). EAW is nonirritating, has minimal toxicity, and is safe and inexpensive, but the bacterial effect is drastically decreased in the presence of organic matter or biofilm. Also, EAW is unstable, and the full disinfecting potential of EAW and its long-term compatibility for endoscopes remain to be examined.[8]

Sterilox, often referred to as superoxidized water, is a dilute mixture of mild oxidants at neutral pH derived from salt by electrolysis in a proprietary electrochemical cell.[8] The primary active species is hypochlorous acid, an extremely powerful disinfectant completely nontoxic in the low, clinically effective small concentrations produced in Sterilox. Sterilox is generated on site, as needed, and stored no longer than 24 hours. The active agents decompose slowly to harmless species.[8]

Chlorine Dioxide

Chlorine dioxide (e.g., Tristel, Tristel Co, Ltd, Snailwell, UK; Dexit; and Medicide) is a powerful oxidizing agent and is active against nonsporing bacteria, including mycobacteria and viruses, in less than 5 minutes, and is rapidly sporicidal (10 minutes).[8] Chlorine dioxide is more damaging to instruments and components than glutaraldehyde.[8] Experience with chlorine dioxide has demonstrated discoloration of the black plastic casing of flexible endoscopes, and irritation of skin, eyes, and respiratory tract.[8] It emits a strong odor of chlorine and should be stored in sealed containers and handled in well-ventilated areas.[8]

DISINFECTANTS

Antiseptics are intended for use on living tissue, whereas disinfectants are intended for use on inanimate objects and can harm tissue[9] (Table 10-5). An agent can be an antiseptic at low concentrations and a disinfectant at higher concentrations.[9]

Aldehydes

Because heat and moisture are damaging to certain instruments, such as endoscopes, arthroscopes, and laparoscopes, cold disinfection with glutaraldehyde, a dialdehyde (Cidex, Johnson and Johnson Medical, Inc, Arlington, Tex; Omnicide 28, Baxter Healthcare Corp, Deerfield, Ill; Abcocide, Abco Dealers, Inc, LaVergne, Tenn), can be used for these items.[7] Olympus, Pentax, and Fujinon list glutaraldehyde as compatible with their endoscopes,[8] but manufacturer recommendations need to be closely followed for all such instruments. Although glutaraldehyde is effective against a wide range of susceptible organisms (see Table 10-5),[22] Cidex is now classified as a disinfectant by the manufacturer, rather than as a sterilant, and therefore its use on arthroscopic and laparoscopy instruments is questionable.

TABLE 10-5. Characteristics of Selected Antiseptics and Disinfectants

Agent	Trade Name	Action	Effects	Disadvantages
Isopropyl alcohol	Propanol	Protein denaturation	Bactericidal, effective against vegetative bacteria only	Poor against spores, fungi, viruses Cytotoxic in tissue
Glutaraldehyde	Cidex Omnicide Abcocide	Protein and nucleic acid denaturation	Bactericidal, fungicidal, viricidal, sporicidal	Long (10-h) exposure time required for sporicidal effect Limited shelf life once activated Tissue irritant/toxicity
Chlorhexidine	Nolvasan	Cell membrane disruption and cellular protein precipitation	Bactericidal, fungicidal; variable activity against viruses	Not sporicidal
Povidone-iodine	Betadine	Metabolic interference	Bactericidal, viricidal, fungicidal	Poorly sporicidal Some inactivation by organic debris

From Clem M: In Auer J (ed): Equine Surgery. Philadelphia, 1992, WB Saunders.

PAA sterilization would be the best choice to sterilize these items, as discussed earlier. The antimicrobial activity of glutaraldehyde is greatly enhanced in alkaline solutions, although high pH hastens its polymerization and therefore limits its shelf life. To overcome this problem, glutaraldehyde is supplied as an acidic colorless solution that is activated at the time of use by adding an "activator" that converts it to a green (Cidex, Abcocide) or blue (Omnicide) alkaline solution with a sharp odor.[8,22]

Repeated use of an activated solution or placing damp instruments into the solution can dilute it to less than the effective concentration. Solutions should be reused only when the minimum effective concentration, as determined by the appropriate test strip, is assured, and when the pH and temperature are correct (Table 10-6). Solutions should be discarded after the specified reuse period has elapsed, even if the appropriate conditions have been met.

Antimicrobial activity of Cidex increases with increased temperature and decreases with organic matter.[22] Therefore, presterilization cleaning and drying are important, and an enzyme-based presoak detergent can be used.[7] Instruments soaked in glutaraldehyde must be thoroughly rinsed with sterile water before they touch tissue, and gloves must always be worn when removing items from glutaraldehyde baths.

The potential hazards of glutaraldehyde for staff are considerable. Toxicity has been suspected in 35% of endoscopy units, with harmful or potentially harmful problems in 63% of these.[8] Direct contact with glutaraldehyde is irritating to skin and other tissues, and repeated exposure can result in sensitization and allergic contact dermatitis. Vapor may cause stinging sensations in the eye, excess tear production, redness of the conjunctiva, a stinging sensation in the nose and throat, nasal discharge, coughing, symptoms of bronchitis, and headache.[8] Glutaraldehyde is not ideal for chemical disinfection of instruments that are hinged, corroded, or have deep or narrow crevices[23] and it should not be used for critical, single-use devices, such as catheters. Prolonged use of glutaraldehyde can corrode metals and some plastics.[24] As with all aldehydes, glutaraldehyde can fix proteins by denaturing and coagulating them, and this creates a biofilm on instruments.[8]

Orthophthalaldehyde (OPA; Cidex OPA, Johnson & Johnson's Advanced Sterilization Products) is a high-level disinfectant that contains 0.55% 1,2-benzenedicarboxaldehyde. OPA completely destroys all common bacteria in 5 minutes of exposure, does not produce noxious fumes, does not require activation, and is stable at a wide pH range (3 to 9).[8] Exposure to OPA vapors may be irritating to the respiratory tract and eyes, and it can stain linens, clothing, skin, instruments, and automatic cleaning devices.[8]

Succindialdehyde with dimethoxytetrahydrofuran and anticorrosion components (Gigasept FF, Schülke & Mayr UK, Ltd, Meadowhall, Sheffield, UK) is recommended for flexible endoscopes and ultrasonic probes by well-known manufacturers (e.g., Fujinon, Olympus, Hewlett Packard, Acuson, Toshiba). It is a broad-spectrum cold-sterilizing or disinfecting solution with excellent material compatibility and a pH of approximately 6.5. It does not require activation additives and might be preferable when avoiding formaldehyde or glutaraldehyde products is desired.

ANTISEPTICS

Alcohols

Alcohols are commonly used in veterinary medicine, but they are effective only against vegetative bacteria[25] (see Table 10-5). They have a mild defatting effect but they are inactivated by a variety of organic debris and have no residual activity after evaporation.[4,25] Alcohols have higher and more rapid kill rate than chlorhexidine, and third best is povidone-iodine.[26] The bactericidal efficacy of 1-propanol

TABLE 10-6. Recommended Conditions for Use of Three Glutaraldehyde Preparations

	Cidex (Activated)	Cidex 7 (Long-Life Activated)	Cidexplus (28-Day Solution)
Concentration (%)	2.4	2.5	3.4
Maximal reuse period	14 d	28 d	28 d
AS A STERILANT			
Temperature (°C)	25	20-25	20-25
Minimal immersion time	10 h	10 h	10 h
AS A HIGH-LEVEL DISINFECTANT			
Temperature (°C)	25	25	25
Minimal immersion time	45 min	90 min	20 min
AS AN INTERMEDIATE-LEVEL DISINFECTANT			
Temperature (°C)	20-25	20-25	20-25
Minimal immersion time	10 min	10 min	10 min

Sterilant conditions apply to surgical instruments and devices that penetrate skin or are used in sterile tissues; the longer times are required for spores. High-level disinfectants are used for semicritical devices that do not penetrate sterile tissues (endoscopes, anesthesia equipment). Intermediate-level disinfectants are used for noncritical devices that contact skin surface only. Recommendations for other glutaraldehyde preparations may vary—the manufacturer's advice should be followed.
From Southwood LL, Baxter GM: Vet Clin North Am Equine Pract 12:173, 1996, with permission.

can be regarded as superior to that of 2-propanol, and third best is ethanol.[27]

Either alcohol or sterile saline can be used to rinse the surgical scrub solution from the surgery site. Alcohol does not inactivate chlorhexidine gluconate in vitro and has no significant effect on its protein-binding property in vivo.[26] However, isopropyl alcohol rinse can reduce the residual antimicrobial activity of chlorhexidine[28,29] and can inactivate hexachlorophene-based preparations (e.g., PHisoHex).[9] Isopropyl alcohol potentiates the antimicrobial efficacy of povidone-iodine by increasing the release of free iodine, so it should be used as a rinse after this surgical scrub.[30,31]

Chlorhexidine

Chlorhexidine diacetate (2%; Nolvasan Solution and Surgical Scrub, Fort Dodge Laboratories, Inc, Fort Dodge, Iowa) and chlorhexidine gluconate (4%; Hibiclens, Stuart Pharmaceuticals, Division of ICI America, Inc, Wilmington, Del) have a rapid onset of action and a persistent effect[32] but variable and inconsistent activity against viruses and fungi[7] (see Table 10-5). Chlorhexidine binds to protein of the stratum corneum, forming a persistent residue that can kill bacteria emerging from sebaceous glands, sweat glands, and hair follicles during surgery.[33] A recently approved antiseptic for preoperative skin preparation, 2% chlorhexidine gluconate plus 70% isopropyl alcohol (ChloraPrep, Medi-Flex, Inc, Leawood, Kan), provided significantly more persistent antimicrobial activity on abdominal sites at 24 hours than either of the components used separately.[34]

Chlorhexidine has low toxicity as a skin scrub or as an aqueous solution for wound disinfection, oral lavage, and mucous membranes of the urinary tract.[32] Although it can be toxic to fibroblasts in vitro, in vivo lavage with dilute chlorhexidine (0.05%) is not harmful to wound healing.[31] However, the least known bactericidal concentration (0.05%) of chlorhexidine diacetate causes synovial ulceration, inflammation, and fibrin accumulation in the tarsocrural joints of horses.[35] Chlorhexidine (0.0005%) potentiated with 3.2 mM EDTA and 0.05 mM Tris buffer (hydroxymethylaminomethylamine) is 90% lethal to *Escherichia coli*, *Staphylococcus aureus*, and *Streptococcus zooepidemicus* and is not harmful to the synovium or articular cartilage of the tarsocrural joints of ponies.[36] Chlorhexidine (0.02%), like 1% povidone-iodine, promotes intra-abdominal adhesion formation and therefore should not be used for peritoneal lavage.[37]

Iodine Compounds

Inorganic or elemental iodine has a very broad antimicrobial spectrum compared with other agents (see Table 10-5) and a very short kill time at low concentrations, and organisms do not develop resistance to it.[38] Its undesirable characteristics are odor, tissue irritation, staining, radiopacity, and corrosiveness.[38] Iodophors are complexes of elemental iodine with a carrier, such as polyvinylpyrrolidone (PVP), which forms povidone-iodine (PVP-I_2; Betadine surgical scrub, Purdue Frederick Co, Norwalk, Conn). The complex retains the bactericidal activity of iodine, while reducing tissue irritation and staining. Povidone-iodine is usually supplied as a 10% solution with approximately 1% available iodine, which is not equivalent to free iodine but must be converted to free iodine to become bactericidal.[38] However, iodine is so tightly bound to PVP that the standard 10% solution contains as little as 0.8 part per million of free iodine.[38] This concentration may not be sufficient to kill bacteria, especially as some free iodine is readily neutralized by protein and by conversion to iodide in vivo.[38] However, dilution of the 10% solution of povidone-iodine liberates more free iodine than is present in the undiluted solution—thus the diluted solution is more bactericidal.[38] Contamination of 10% povidone-iodine solution by bacteria has been reported, apparently because it liberates an insufficient amount of free iodine at this concentration.[38] At least 2 minutes of scrubbing is required to release free iodine from povidone-iodine.[26] Addition of detergents, as in surgical scrubs, further reduces the release of iodine.[39]

Before application of iodophor compounds, hair should be removed and the skin well cleaned to remove organic debris that can reduce the bactericidal activity of the iodophor. However, when arthrocentesis sites in the midcarpal joint and the distal interphalangeal joint region of horses were not clipped of hair, a 5-minute surgical scrub with povidone-iodine followed by a rinse with 70% alcohol was as effective as the same regimen on corresponding clipped sites.[40] Although a scrub with povidone-iodine, followed by a 24-hour soak in povidone-iodine solution, could reduce bacterial numbers on the surface of the equine hoof, especially if the superficial layer of the hoof capsule was removed, bacterial populations capable of inducing wound infection still remained.[41]

The toxicity of iodine-releasing compounds is low, although individual sensitivities can occur and some horses may develop skin wheals about the head and neck (e.g., at the laryngoplasty site). Undiluted povidone-iodine solutions have no effect on numbers of viable bacteria in wounds, and povidone-iodine surgical scrub can potentiate infection and inflammation.[39] The practice of lavaging the peritoneal cavity with povidone-iodine has been abandoned because of evidence that even dilute solutions can cause a sterile peritonitis in ponies[42] and induce metabolic acidosis.[38] Although 0.1% povidone-iodine has been reported to be bactericidal and to have minimal deleterious effects on the equine tarsocrural joint,[43] it was ineffective in the treatment of experimental infectious arthritis in horses.[44] Concentrations greater than 0.05% in vitro can disrupt neutrophil viability and migration.[45]

A one-step surgical preparation technique using Dura-Prep Surgical Solution (3M Health Care, St. Paul, Minn) is as effective as a two-step povidone-iodine preparation.[30] The antimicrobial properties of the solution are the result of 70% isopropyl alcohol in an iodophor-polymer complex that forms a water-insoluble film with sustained chemical and physical barrier properties on skin.[30] In a study on skin preparation for ventral midline incisions in horses undergoing celiotomy, Dura-Prep was as effective as povidone-iodine and alcohol in reducing colony-forming units up to the time of skin closure, and both methods had comparable rates of incisional drainage.[46] However, preparation time was significantly shorter for Dura-Prep than with the routine skin preparation technique.[46]

Antimicrobial film drapes with adhesive backing (Ioban 2, 3M Animal Care Products, St. Paul, Minn) contain an iodophor and come in different sizes that make them suitable for equine surgery. After the skin has been prepared with an accepted surgical scrub, it is rinsed with isopropyl alcohol and may need to be dried with a sterile towel to improve adherence.[46] In some clinics, the proposed surgery site is shaved with a size 40 blade to improve adherence beyond that achieved by clipping.[46] A medical grade adhesive spray can also be used (Medical Adhesive, Hollister, Inc, Libertyville, Ill; EZ Drape Adhesive, Clinipad Corp, Rocky Hill, Conn), but this is not essential. Adherence to smooth flat surfaces, such as the ventral abdomen, may be better than to the irregular contour of a joint. A tight adherence of the drape in areas of complicated contours can be achieved by applying the adhesive drape circumferentially while pressing the excess edges of the drape tightly together behind the limb on the side opposite the surgical site. Care should be taken that small pieces of the drape not be torn off and dragged into joints by arthroscopic instruments, to end up as free-floating objects in the joint cavity.

The value of antimicrobial adhesive drapes is questionable.[26] In a study on human patients undergoing hip surgery, bacterial contamination of the wound at the end of surgery was reduced from 15% with conventional preparation to 1.6% by use of an iodophor-impregnated plastic adhesive drape (Ioban).[47] In a prospective randomized clinical trial on 1102 patients, isolates of normal skin organisms were less frequent when an iodophor-impregnated plastic incise drape was used in clean and clean contaminated abdominal procedures than when the drape was not used.[48] However, no difference was found between wound infection rates for patients on whom the iodophor drape was used compared with those patients on whom it was not used.[48,49] Although iodophor skin preparations do not produce a radiopaque artifact on intraoperative radiographs, folds in iodophor-impregnated plastic drapes can produce confusing radiographic images.

Chlorhexidine versus Povidone-Iodine

In tests with *E. coli* and *S. aureus* on canine skin, 2% chlorhexidine diacetate was superior to hexachlorophene and povidone-iodine in rapid removal of bacteria and in residual activity.[50] In another study, chlorhexidine and povidone-iodine were effective in reducing bacteria from surgeon's hands, but the apparently greater residual effect of chlorhexidine (120 minutes) was not statistically significant.[51] Such a residual effect could be of value during long surgical procedures, in which rates of glove puncture could be as high as 17% and many perforations are unnoticed by the surgeon.[52] In one study, 4% chlorhexidine gluconate was found to be superior, on the basis of efficacy and prolonged effects, to 7.5% povidone-iodine throughout a 3-hour period after hand antisepsis.[53] Compared with iodine preparations, chlorhexidine preparations are less susceptible to inactivation by organic debris.[32]

Although chlorhexidine's wider range of antimicrobial activity, longer residual action, minimal inhibition by organic material, and greater tolerance by skin would render it superior to povidone-iodine, both agents perform comparably in the surgical setting.[26] In a prospective randomized study of 886 patients, there were significantly fewer wound infections with chlorhexidine preparations for surgical hand washing and patient skin preparation than with povidone-iodine (hand washing and skin preparation) in operations on the biliary tract and in "clean" nonabdominal operations; however, there were no significant differences in a number of other types of surgery.[54] The authors concluded that "on the evidence of this study, there is no overwhelming case for using one compound rather than the other as an all-purpose preparation and scrub."[54]

Povidone-iodine and 4% chlorhexidine gluconate scrubs rinsed with 70% isopropyl alcohol decreased skin microflora in cattle and had similar frequencies of surgical wound infection.[55] Colony-forming unit counts were lower with chlorhexidine and alcohol immediately after scrubbing, but there was no difference in residual effect between the two scrubs.[54] Povidone-iodine solutions are inferior to chlorhexidine for wound lavage.[56] However, chlorhexidine is more expensive than povidone-iodine.[7] Because of concerns about inadequate release of free iodine from povidone-iodine, some consider it to be inferior for skin preparation.[38]

Phenols

Phenol, cresol, and other coal tar derivates, such as hexachlorophene (PHisoHex; see Table 10-5), are generally considered to be inferior to chlorhexidine and povidone-iodine.[9,26] Hexachlorophene has a relatively slow onset of action but a prolonged residual activity, and it is not adversely affected by organic materials. Hexachlorophene-based preparations are inactivated by alcohol.[9,26] Use was largely curtailed after hexachlorophene was shown to be neurotoxic at levels obtained with dermal exposure.[57]

Quaternary Ammonium Compounds

Quaternary ammonium compounds, such as benzalkonium chloride, are cationic surfactants that dissolve lipids in bacterial cell walls and membranes.[58] Drawbacks to the group are ineffectiveness against viruses, spores, and fungi, formation of residue layers, and inactivation by common organic debris and soaps.[8]

Miscellaneous

Hydrogen peroxide is used to clean severely contaminated wounds, but it is a poor antiseptic and is mainly effective against spores, and concentrations lower than 3% are damaging to tissues.[59] Chloroxylenol, or parachlorometaxylenol, a synthetic halogen-substituted phenol derivative, and triclosan, a diphenyl ether, do not appear to offer any advantages over the more commonly used antiseptics in veterinary medicine.[26,52,60]

Current trends in surgical hand disinfection have evolved very rapidly in the last several years and now include alcohol-based and quaternary ammonium compounds using brushless techniques. For a complete discussion on these newer products and techniques, see under "Surgeon's Skin" in Chapter 11.

REFERENCES

1. Dorland's Illustrated Medical Dictionary, ed 30, Philadelphia, 2003, Elsevier.

2. Alder V, Simpson RA: Heat sterilization: Sterilization and disinfection by heat methods. In Russell AD, Hugo WB, Ayliffe GAJ, editors: Principles and Practice of Disinfection, Preservation and Sterilization, Oxford, 1982, Blackwell Scientific.
3. Perkins JJ: Principles and Methods of Sterilization in Health Sciences, Springfield, 1969, Charles C. Thomas.
4. Mitchell SL, Berg RJ: Sterilization. In Slatter DH, editor: Textbook of Small Animal Surgery, ed 3, Philadelphia, 2003, WB Saunders.
5. Association of Perioperative Registered Nurses: Standards, Recommended Practices and Guidelines, Denver, 2001, AORN.
6. Alfa MJ, Jackson M: A new hydrogen peroxide–based medical-device detergent with germicidal properties: Comparison with enzymatic cleaners, Am J Infect Control 2001;29:168.
7. Southwood LL, Baxter GM: Instrument sterilization, skin preparation, and wound management, Vet Clin North Am Equine Pract 1996;12:173.
8. Rey J-F, Kruse A, Neumann C: ESGE/ESGENA technical note on cleaning and disinfection, Endoscopy 2003;35:869.
9. Clem MF: Sterilization and antiseptics. In Auer JA, editor: Equine Surgery, Philadelphia, 1992, WB Saunders.
10. Chamness CJ: Nondisposable instrumentation for equine laparoscopy. In Fischer AT, editor: Equine Diagnostic and Surgical Laparoscopy, Philadelphia, 2002, WB Saunders.
11. Gömann J, Kaiser U, Menzel R: Air removal from porous and hollow goods using different steam sterilization processes, Zentr Steril 2001;9:182.
12. Fifield CW, Leahy TJ: Sterilization filtration. In Block SS, editor: Disinfection, Sterilization and Preservation, Philadelphia, 1983, Lea & Febiger.
13. Silverman GJ: Sterilization by ionizing radiation. In Block SS, editor: Disinfection, Sterilization and Preservation, Philadelphia, 1983, Lea & Febiger.
14. Altenmeier WA, Burke JF, Pruitt BA, Sandusky WR: Manual on Control of Infection in Surgical Patients, Philadelphia, 1984, JB Lippincott.
15. Christensen EA, Kristensen H: Gaseous sterilization. In Russell AD, Hugo WB, Ayliffe GAJ, editors: Principles and Practice of Disinfection, Preservation and Sterilization, Oxford, 1982, Blackwell Scientific.
16. Caputo RA, Odlaug TE: Sterilization with ethylene oxide and other gases. In Block SS, editor: Disinfection, Sterilization and Preservation, Philadelphia, 1983, Lea & Febiger.
17. ATI Company: Principles and Practice of Ethylene Oxide Sterilization, North Hollywood, Calif, 1982, ATI Company.
18. Estrin WJ, Cavalieri SA, Wald P, et al: Evidence of neurologic dysfunction related to long-term ethylene oxide exposure, Arch Neurol 1987;44:1283.
19. American Sterilization Company: Gas Sterilization/Aeration Systems, Erie, Pa, 1982, American Sterilization Company.
20. Schatzmann U, Lang J, Ueltschi G, et al: Tracheal necrosis following intubation in the horse, Dtsch Tierärztl Wochenschr 1981;88:102.
21. Trim CM, Simpson ST: Complications following ethylene oxide sterilization: A case report, J Am Anim Hosp Assoc 1982;18:507.
22. Russell AD: Glutaraldehyde: Current status and uses. Infect Control Hosp Epidemiol 1994;15:724.
23. Sebben JE: Sterilization and care of surgical instruments and supplies, J Am Acad Dermatol 1984;11:381.
24. Geiss HK: New sterilization technologies: Are they applicable for endoscopic surgical instruments? Endosc Surg Allied Technol 1994;2:276.
25. Morton HE: Alcohols. In Block SS, editor: Disinfection, Sterilization and Preservation, Philadelphia, 1983, Lea & Febiger.
26. Schmon C: Assessment and preparation of the surgical patient and the operating team. In Slatter DH, editor: Textbook of Small Animal Surgery, ed 3, Philadelphia, 2003, WB Saunders.
27. Rotter ML: Hand washing and hand disinfection. In Mayhall CG, editor: Hospital Epidemiology and Infection Control, ed 2, Philadelphia, 1999, Lippincott Williams & Wilkins.
28. Osuna DJ, DeYoung DJ, Walker RL: Comparison of three skin preparation techniques in the dog: Part 1. Experimental trial, Vet Surg 1990;19:14.
29. Osuna DJ, DeYoung DJ, Walker RL: Comparison of three skin preparation techniques: Part 2. Clinical trial in 100 dogs, Vet Surg 1990;19:20.
30. Rochat MC, Mann FA, Berg JN: Evaluation of a one-step surgical preparation technique in dogs, J Am Vet Med Assoc 1993;203:392.
31. Lemarie RJ, Hosgood G: Antiseptics and disinfectants in small animal practice, Comp Cont Educ Pract Vet 1995;17:1339.
32. Desrochers A, St-Jean G, Anderson DA, et al: Comparison of povidone iodine and chlorhexidine gluconate for operative-site preparation in cattle, Vet Surg 1994;23:400.
33. Swaim SF, Riddell KP, Geiger DL, et al: Evaluation of surgical scrub and antiseptic solutions for surgical preparation of canine paws, J Am Vet Med Assoc 1991;198:1941.
34. Hibbard JS, Mulberry GK, Brady AR: A clinical study comparing the skin antisepsis and safety of ChloraPrep, 70% isopropyl alcohol, and 2% aqueous chlorhexidine, J Infus Nurs 2002;25:244.
35. Wilson DG, Cooley AJ, MacWilliams PS, et al: Effects of 0.05% chlorhexidine lavage on the tarsocrural joints of horses, Vet Surg 1994;23:442.
36. Klohnen A, Wilson DG, Hendrickson DA, et al: Effects of potentiated chlorhexidine on bacteria and tarsocrural joints in ponies, J Am Vet Med Assoc 1996;57:756.
37. van Westreenen M, van den Tol PM, Pronk A, et al: Perioperative lavage promotes intraperitoneal adhesion in the rat, Eur Surg Res 1999;31:196.
38. LeVeen HH, LeVeen RF, LeVeen EG: The mythology of povidone-iodine and the development of self-sterilizing plastic, Surg Gynecol Obstet 1993;176:183.
39. Rodeheaver G, Bellamy W, Kody M, et al: Bactericidal activity and toxicity of iodine-containing solutions in wounds, Arch Surg 1982;117:181.
40. Hague BA, Honnas CM, Simpson RB, et al: Evaluation of skin bacterial flora before and after aseptic preparation of clipped and nonclipped arthrocentesis sites in horses, Vet Surg 1997;26:121.
41. Hennig GE, Kraus BH, Fister R, et al: Comparison of two methods for presurgical disinfection of the equine hoof, Vet Surg 2001;30:366.
42. Schneider RK, Meyer DJ, Embertson RM, et al: Response of pony peritoneum to four peritoneal lavage solutions, Am J Vet Res 1988;49:889.
43. Bertone AL, McIlwraith CW, Powers BE, et al: Effect of four antimicrobial lavage solutions on the tarsocrural joint of horses, Vet Surg 1986;15:305.
44. Bertone AL, McIlwraith CW, Jones RL, et al: Povidone-iodine lavage treatment of experimentally induced equine infectious arthritis, Am J Vet Res 1987;48:712.
45. Tvedten HW, Till GO: Effect of povidone, povidone-iodine, and iodine on locomotion (in vitro) of neutrophils from people, rats, dogs, and rabbits, Am J Vet Res 1985;46:1797.
46. Gallupo LD, Pascoe JR, Jang SS, et al: Evaluation of iodophor skin preparation techniques and factors influencing drainage from ventral midline incisions in horses, J Am Vet Med Assoc 215:963, 1999.
47. Fairclough JA, Johnson D, Mackie I: The prevention of wound contamination by skin organisms by the pre-operative application of an iodophor impregnated plastic adhesive drape, J Int Med Res 1986;14:105.
48. Dewan PA, Van Rij AM, Robinson RG, et al: The use of an iodophor-impregnated plastic incise drape in abdominal surgery: A controlled clinical trial, Aust N Z J Surg 1987;57:859.
49. Lewis DA, Leaper DJ, Speller DC: Prevention of bacterial colonization of wounds at operation: Comparison of iodine-impregnated ("Ioban") drapes with conventional methods, J Hosp Infect 1984;5:431.
50. Paul JW, Gordon MA: Efficacy of a chlorhexidine surgical scrub

compared to that of hexachlorophene and povidone-iodine, Vet Med Small Anim Clin 1978;73:573.
51. Wan PY, Blackford JT, Bemis DA, et al: Evaluation of surgical scrub methods for large animal surgeons, Vet Surg 1997;26:382.
52. Marchetti MG, Kampf G, Finzi G, et al: Evaluation of the bactericidal effect of five products for surgical hand disinfection according to prEN 12054 and prEN 12791, J Hosp Infect 2003;54:63.
53. Furukawa K, Ogawa R, Norose Y, et al: A new surgical handwashing and hand antisepsis from scrubbing to rubbing, J Nippon Med Sch 2004;71:19.
54. Berry AR, Watt B, Goldacre MJ, et al: A comparison of the use of povidone-iodine and chlorhexidine in the prophylaxis of postoperative wound infection, J Hosp Infect 1982;3:55.
55. Desrochers A, St-Jean G, Anderson DA, et al: Comparative evaluation of two surgical scrub preparations in cattle, Vet Surg 1996;25:336.
56. Sanchez IR, Swaim SF, Nusbaum KE, et al: Effects of chlorhexidine diacetate and povidone-iodine on wound healing in dogs, Vet Surg 1988;17:291.
57. Polk HC, Simpson CJ, Simmons BP, et al: Guidelines for prevention of surgical wound infection, Arch Surg 1983;118:1213.
58. Tracy DL, Warren RG: Small Animal Surgical Nursing. St Louis, 1983, CV Mosby.
59. Swaim SF, Lee AH. Topical wound medications: A review, J Am Vet Med Assoc 1987;190:1588.
60. Faoagali J, Fong J, George N, et al: Comparison of the immediate, residual, and cumulative antibacterial effects of Novaderm R, Novascrub R, Betadine Surgical Scrub, Hibiclens, and liquid soap, Am J Infect Control 1995;23:337.

CHAPTER 11

Preparation of the Surgical Patient, the Surgery Facility, and the Operating Team

John A. Stick

Having the capacity for sound clinical judgment is the ultimate characteristic of the mature veterinary surgeon. To attain this capacity, the surgeon needs to be able to provide an accurate assessment of operative risk. This can be done only if there is thorough preparation of the surgical patient combined with knowledge of the primary problem, experience, and an open mind.

ASSESSMENT OF OPERATIVE RISK

When determining operative risk, each surgeon must consider the relative rewards and risks in treating a specific illness.[1] The surgical risks encompass not only the odds of surviving surgery but also the long-term prognosis, the potential for complications, and the patient's use and quality of life.[2] Basic factors affecting operative risk include age, overall physical status, elective versus emergency operation, physiologic extent of the procedure, number of associated illnesses, and projected surgery time. Although the surgeon can informally consider all this information and make a guess as to the surgical risks based on experience in similar cases, formal assessment schemes are useful. The formal determination of surgical risk can be considered to have two main components: the primary disorder and the general health of the patient.

Primary Disease

Primary diseases with a tendency to progress rapidly and involve other body systems are associated with more risks than those that progress slowly and do not affect the patient's systemic health. The procedure's invasiveness and potential for complications are also considered in risk assessment.

Complications and the risk of death increase with the duration of surgery. The risk of surgery also varies with the system involved. For example, diseases involving the gastrointestinal tract have a tendency to cause shock and sepsis early in their course. Elective orthopedic surgery has a much lower associated risk than nonelective general surgeries and major trauma. When emergency surgery is necessary, the surgical risk increases. When a disorder is fatal without surgery but has the potential for a surgical cure, surgery is likely to be recommended despite a high surgical risk.

General Health Assessment

Surgery and anesthesia are never without risks, and unexpected complications can occur even in the healthiest patient undergoing a minor procedure. However, the risks are increased by a variety of conditions. Risk is increased in the very young and the very old. Neonatal animals are predisposed to hypothermia, hypoglycemia, and infection. Morbidity and mortality increase with age in human and veterinary surgical patients.[2]

The effects of concurrent disease on an animal's general health are important determinants of surgical risk. Animals with normal physical findings and no history of cardiovascular, respiratory, renal, or liver disorders have a relatively low surgical risk. Additionally, the preoperative nutritional status is an important determinant of surgical risk (see Chapter 6). Cachectic animals may have delayed wound healing and a higher incidence of postsurgical wound infection and susceptibility to multiple organ disorders.

The importance of establishing the physical status cannot be overstated. The American Society of Anesthesiologists has created a classification system for human patients based on evaluation of their physical status, and the rankings can be used to determine surgical risk (Table 11-1). In humans, physical status was second only to albumin level in its

TABLE 11-1. American Society of Anesthesiologists Classification System for Physical Status and Recommended Tests for Each Class

Physical Status	Definition	Examples	Recommended Laboratory Tests: Minor*	Recommended Laboratory Tests: Major†	Prognosis
I	Healthy with no organic disease	Elective procedures not necessary for health (ovariohysterectomy)	PCV, TP, urine specific gravity	CBC, U/A, surgical panel‡	Excellent
II	Local disease with no systemic signs	Healthy nonelective surgery (skin laceration, simple fracture)	PCV, TP, urine specific gravity	CBC, U/A, surgical panel‡	Good
III	Disease causes moderate systemic signs that limit function	Heart murmur, anemia, pneumonia, mild chest trauma, moderate dehydration	CBC, U/A, surgical panel‡	CBC, U/A, biochemical panel§	Fair
IV	Disease causes severe systemic signs and threatens life	Gastric torsion, diaphragmatic hernia, severe chest trauma, severe anemia, or dehydration	CBC, U/A, biochemical panel§	CBC, U/A, biochemical panel§	Guarded
V	Moribund, not expected to live for more than 24 hours with or without surgery	Endotoxic shock, severe trauma, multiorgan failure	CBC, U/A, biochemical panel§	CBC, U/A, biochemical panel§	Grave
E	Emergency	Qualifier of above classes	PCV, TP, urine specific gravity	Depends on facilities available	Variable

* Duration less than 60 minutes.
† Duration longer than 60 minutes or patients older than 7 years.
‡ Surgical panel: urea, creatinine, alkaline phosphatase, alanine aminotransferase, glucose, sodium, potassium, chloride, total protein.
§ Biochemical panel: the full panel is the surgical panel tests plus bicarbonate, anion gap, calcium, phosphorus, cholesterol, total bilirubin, γ-glutamyltransferase, albumin.
CBC, complete blood cell count; PCV, packed cell volume; TP, total protein; U/A, urinalysis.

accuracy in predicting survival and postoperative complications.[3,4] Similar findings were observed in high-risk canine surgical patients: 92% of canine patients assigned to American Society of Anesthesiologists class II survived, compared with 73% in class III and 38% in class IV.[5]

Personal Relationships

A bond of communication, cemented with personal responsibility, is established between the surgeon and the client (usually the animal owner), whenever a surgical procedure is being considered. The confidence of the well-informed client is based on a true understanding of the situation, which allows the client to participate in judgments regarding operative risks, outcomes, the process of postoperative recovery, and financial implications. Legal action is rare when a careful effort has been made by the veterinarian to achieve such understanding before an operation.

Veterinary surgeons should also appreciate the importance of an effective relationship with the referring veterinarian. In many situations, patients are referred to surgeons by veterinarians with valuable skills and expertise. It is important to understand the wishes and views of the referring veterinarian. Differences in judgment must be discussed. Both the surgeon and the referring veterinarian should be aware of the expected course of treatment and the extent of the referring veterinarian's participation in postoperative care. This avoids communication errors and contradictory efforts.

True informed consent is attained when there is a full and frank discussion with the client in the presence of an appropriate professional witness.[1] The surgeon should record a summary of this encounter in the hospital chart. The surgeon should also record why the operation is needed, the operative risks, and the problems anticipated intraoperatively and postoperatively. When a condition is expected to have a clinically significant course beyond the duration of the early follow-up period, the client should be told how much continuing commitment will be needed.

PREPARATION OF THE SURGICAL PATIENT

History

The first step in assessment of the patient is interviewing the owner to determine the animal's medical history, its overall health, and the impact of the presenting complaint.[2] At this time, the surgeon should determine the owner's wishes and expectations.

The patient's signalment should be reviewed to determine the potential for problems related to age, breed, and sex.

Questions about the animal's general health and environment can contribute to making the diagnosis. The animal's intended use and the owner's expectations of its future performance are explored to gauge the future satisfaction of the owner with the proposed procedure. Past medical problems should be discussed, because they may influence the outcome.

Physical Examination

Despite a surgeon's natural tendency to focus on the presenting problem, a thorough physical examination should include an assessment of each system. A general physical examination determines the need for in-depth assessment and preoperative stabilization. It is this examination that is most likely to identify risk factors affecting surgical outcome.[2] The animal should first be examined for general demeanor, nutritional status, and gait. Temperature, pulse, and respiration rate are noted as the respiratory and cardiovascular systems are emphasized.

Finally, the affected area and related systems are evaluated. A physical status ranking, based on the American Society of Anesthesiologists classification system (see Table 11-1), should be assigned. This will allow a more accurate determination of what supplemental testing should be performed.

Supplemental Testing

Laboratory testing is not a substitute for the thorough examination, and all abnormal findings in the laboratory data should be interpreted in light of the initial physical findings. When abnormalities in the function of organs (e.g., the heart, kidneys, and respiratory system) are detected, testing may be expanded to include chest radiography, urinalysis, and biochemical profile. However, although preoperative tests that screen for clinically silent disease will not replace the physical examination, some basic laboratory data are recommended for use with the American Society of Anesthesiologists classification system for physical status (see Table 11-1).

Physiologic Preparation

In preparation for elective surgery, steps should be taken to correct physiologic deprivations. Procedures in chronically anemic patients should be delayed until the anemia can be corrected. If fluid deficits exist, plasma or fluids should be administered in appropriate volume, concentration, and composition (see Chapter 3). Although not all volume and concentration deficits need to be corrected before the surgery, a significant fraction of the total deficit should be replaced to enhance the safety of the anesthesia, even in emergency patients. Nutritional replenishment supplementation should be provided for a patient that awaits an elective operation if deficits are obvious.

Infection is a major source of morbidity and a disconcerting source of mortality in some surgical patients. Badly injured or traumatized horses, and those that undergo an operation and survive despite the development of secondary shock and electrolyte disturbances, are at a very high risk for serious infection.

Infection rates of surgical wounds in horses are higher than those seen in people and dogs. Overall infection rates for equine orthopedic surgeries has been reported to be 10%, compared with 4.7% in people, and 5.1% in dogs and cats.[6-9] Infection rates for abdominal surgery in horses have been reported to be 25.4% and 30%.[7,8] Therefore, a primary consideration in preparing the patient is antibiotic prophylaxis. Because equine patients do not live in particularly clean environments, antimicrobial drugs are frequently administered prophylactically even for elective orthopedic surgeries. For additional information on surgical infections and management of sepsis, see Chapters 7, 10, and 88.

Skin Preparation

The patient is the primary source of pathogens involved in surgical wound infections and, therefore, should be groomed before surgery, or even bathed if the hair coat contains a lot of organic material, and the tail should be wrapped.[9] Preparation of the surgical site should include hair removal and cleansing to remove dirt and oil and to reduce resident skin flora. It has been suggested that using a no. 40 clipper blade to clip over the entire surgical area, followed by scrubbing, applying antiseptic solution, and wrapping the limb with a sterile bandage overnight, reduces the chance of contamination in orthopedic cases. However, clipper blades used repeatedly without sterilization have high levels of bacterial contamination and, therefore, are a potential source of infection.[10] Sterilization of clipper blades between uses has been shown to decrease bacterial counts. A study in humans revealed that using razors for the close removal of hair caused significant injury to the skin and increased bacterial colonization by altering wound defense mechanisms and delaying healing.[11] Therefore, if the surgical site is to be shaved, it should be done immediately before surgery and not the night before.

Clipping should be performed whenever possible outside of the surgical theatre, as should the initial skin preparations. The limb from the elbow and stifle distad should be clipped circumferentially in the region of the surgery site. Additionally, the hair should be clipped 10 cm further proximad and distad relative to the intended surgery site to facilitate appropriate skin preparation and draping. If possible, only the final skin preparation should be performed in the surgical theatre to avoid dust, dander, and exfoliated skin cells from contaminating the environment.

The optimal scrub time for maximal reduction of skin flora and lowest wound infection rates has not been determined for the horse. A 5% povidone-iodine solution or 4% chlorhexidine diacetate used for 10 minutes, alternating with an alcohol rinse, is currently recommended, and other scrub solutions are available (see Chapter 10).

Surgical scrubs are applied to an area starting at the expected surgical incision and moving outward in expanding concentric circles, extending the outer margins of the clipped area (Fig. 11-1). This maneuver is repeated, alternating rinse solutions with the antiseptic until the sponges are free of visible soiling. Then a final application of the disinfectant is applied and left in place (Fig. 11-2). When distal limbs are scrubbed, the entire circumference of the limb is prepared, applying the scrub at the proposed surgical site and expanding distad and proximad, as just described.

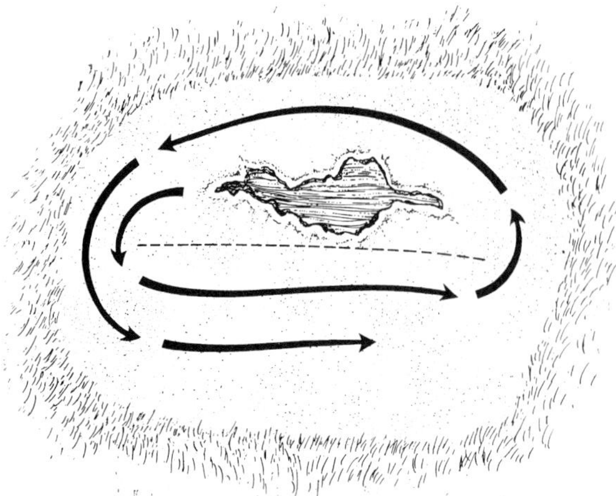

Figure 11-1. Proper method of skin preparation. In the initial preparation, the scrub begins at the anticipated incision site *(dotted line)* and moves outward in expanding concentric circles. The process is repeated until the sponges are free of visible soiling.

Draping the Surgical Field

Ideally, barrier materials prevent the movement of debris and bacteria from nonsterile areas onto the surgical field for the duration of surgery. They should be easy to sterilize and economical, and they should retain their barrier properties if they are washed, sterilized, and reused. Woven fabrics that are intended for reuse consist of interlacing fibers that cross at right angles. The number of threads per square inch reflects the tightness of the weave, and the higher the number is, the tighter the weave and the more effective the barrier.

Reusable woven fabrics fall into two categories: cotton muslin with 140 threads per square inch, and pima cotton with tightly twisted fibers woven into 270 threads per square inch.[2] The cotton muslin is not a good barrier. It instantly allows passage of bacteria when wet (termed strikethrough), and dry penetration of bacteria may also occur because its pore size is 50 to 100 µm, which is large enough to allow bacteria (5 to 12 µm) to pass through.[12] On the other hand, pima cotton has a weave tight enough to prevent penetration by skin squames, but it readily allows penetration of bacteria when wet. A chemical treatment process, Quarpel, makes cotton fabric water resistant by providing a fluorochemical finish in combination with pyridinium or a melamine hydrophobe. This process renders pima cotton an effective barrier for up to 75 washings.[13] It is necessary to record the number of washings each piece of fabric undergoes to ensure that it is replaced before the barrier properties become ineffective.

A disadvantage of reusable woven fabrics is that they can sustain tears or punctures from towel clamps (therefore, only nonpenetrating clamps should be used at the surgical site) and needles, which destroy their barrier function. Although holes can be repaired with vulcanized fabric patches, these patches generally resist autoclave steam penetration, so this material becomes less than an ideal barrier.

Disposable materials are made from cellulose, wood pulp, polyesters, or synthetic polymer fibers, formed into sheets and bonded together. The barrier properties of the various nonwoven materials differ a great deal. Polymeric ingredients in these barriers tend to be more impermeable, but only those with a reinforced polyethylene or plastic film prevent moist and dry penetration at pressure points.[2] Although disposable drapes result in lower particle counts in the operating room (because of the lack of lint from cotton), the air bacterial counts are similar to those of reusable drapes. However, they are reported to decrease the number of bacteria isolated from the surgical wound by up to 90% compared with the cloth draping systems, and surgical wound infection rates decrease by a factor of up to 2½.[14,15] Because the difference between the two materials appears to be small, the choice is often based on economics and convenience; however, when large volumes of liquids are

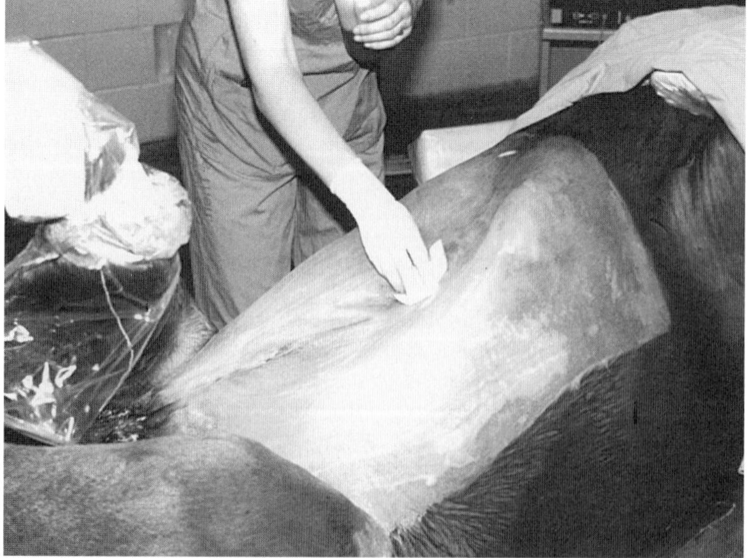

Figure 11-2. After the initial preparation, a sterile preparation is applied using the same methods, with sterile materials, in the operating room.

expected in the surgery (e.g., in colic and arthroscopic surgery), nonwoven disposable materials appear to be the material of choice for barrier drapes.

Before moving the patient into the operating theatre, the patient should be covered with a clean drape and its feet should be covered with plastic bags or other water-impervious coverings to prevent contamination from the foot and distal limbs. After the patient is positioned in the room and the final preparation of the surgery site is completed, draping begins at the surgical site and moves outward.

Drapes are applied to all visible surfaces of the patient, providing a barrier to aerosolization of debris from non-surgically prepared portions of the animal's skin. When applying drapes, the surgeon's gloved hands are positioned on the side of the drape away from the animal's skin and are protected by curling the outer surface of the drape over the hands (Fig. 11-3). The portion of the drape that is to be adjacent to the incision is positioned first and then moved peripherally to the desired location, never the reverse. It is desirable to drape closely, leaving no unnecessary skin exposed. Drapes are generally positioned in a four-quadrant method, with separate drapes in each quadrant, leaving a rectangular area of the surgical field exposed. It is recommended that this process be repeated to double drape the area immediately adjacent to the surgical site.

Self-adhering drapes are helpful when larger areas need to be exposed for topographic orientation and palpation. The goal of multiple layers of draping is to build a waterproof barrier that extends to cover the entire patient. When the distal limb is draped, the quadrant method may be used. However, providing access to the entire circumference of the limb is often preferred, especially during orthopedic procedures. In such a case, the foot is often covered with a rubber glove, and circumferential draping is applied, first by wrapping around the foot and then around the proximal limb. Next, a self-adhering sterile drape (Ioban 2, 3M Health Care, St. Paul, Minn) is applied over the foot and the half-sheet that has been applied to the proximal limb. Then an extremity sheet with a fenestration is passed over the foot and secured around the limb proximal to the surgery site (Fig. 11-4).

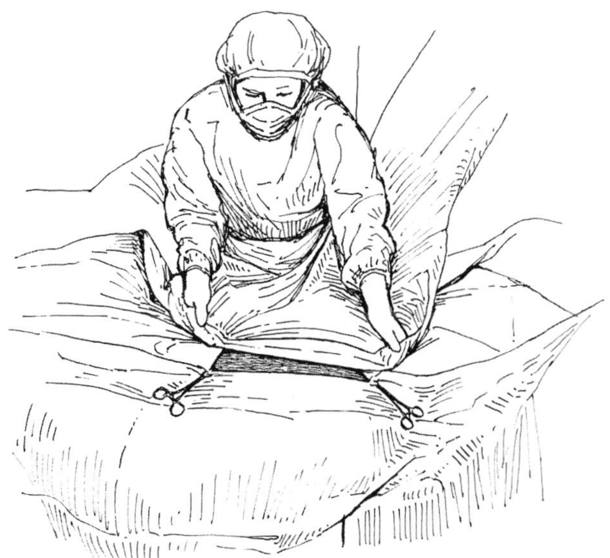

Figure 11-3. Four quadrant draping method with separate drapes in each quadrant, leaving a rectangular area of the surgical field exposed. Note how the surgeon's hands are protected by the drape.

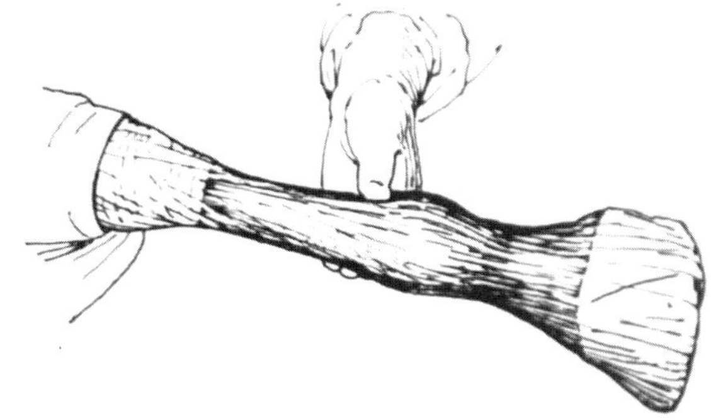

Figure 11-4. After drapes are applied circumferentially above and below the surgery site, they are covered with a self-adhering drape. An extremity sheet for fenestration can be passed over the foot to complete the draping.

Because there is a risk of contamination during draping, it is best to practice double gloving for the act of draping, removing the outer gloves immediately thereafter.

The surgical field is defined by areas above and level with the surgical wound (Fig. 11-5). Even if draped, areas below the level of the wound should be considered contaminated and not part of the surgical field.

THE SURGICAL FACILITY

With the increasing sophistication of surgical techniques and instrumentation available today, surgeries outside a proper surgical facility are becoming less common. If the procedure to be performed is expected to be lengthy, complicated, or sophisticated, use of a designated operating

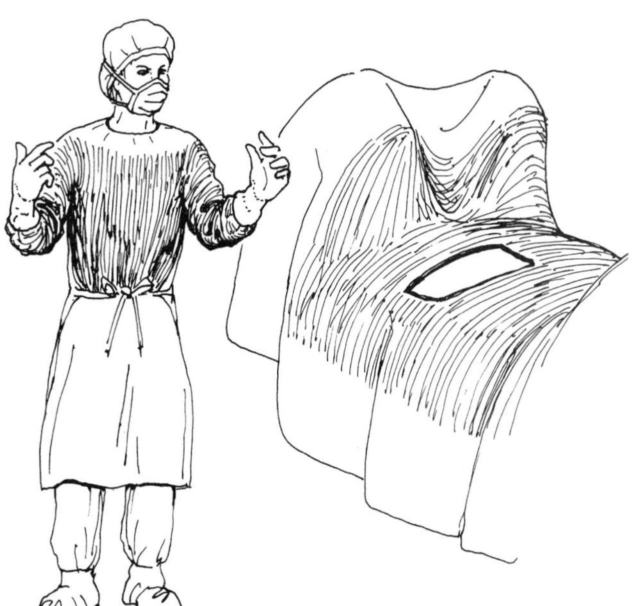

Figure 11-5. The surgical field is defined by the areas above and level with the surgical wound *(shaded area)*. It is extended to include the front of the surgical gown from below the surgeon's shoulders to the waist *(shaded area)*. Areas that are not shaded should be considered to be outside the surgical field.

room is the standard of care. Surgical operating facilities should allow for separate induction, preparation, and recovery rooms and for a minimum of two surgical suites so that clean procedures can be performed in one surgical suite dedicated to strict aseptic surgical procedures, and the other suite can be used for contaminated or infected procedures (Fig. 11-6). The surgery suite should be convenient to the work and have adequate room for the patient, people, and equipment. The average size of an equine operating room should measure 8 m^2 (25 square feet). Separate induction and recovery rooms should be available for each surgical suite. Floors and walls should be surfaced so that cleaning is efficient, and drains should be placed so that water does not pool anywhere in the surgical suite after cleaning. Drains should be of sufficient diameter to remove the material and should contain a flushing system so that they do not harbor potentially dangerous mixtures of blood, feces, and bacteria. One-way traffic should be maintained from patient preparation area to the operating suite and then to the recovery room. After induction of anesthesia, the patient should be properly positioned on the surgery table and prepared for aseptic surgery, and then the table with the horse should be transported into the surgery suite. The suite should not be a high-traffic area, and proper surgical attire, including caps, boots, mask, and surgical caps, should be worn when in the operating theater.

A room temperature of approximately 20° C (70° F) with a relative humidity of 50% provides a comfortable environment.[16] Air within the operating room should be under mild positive pressure, so that when the doors open, air flows out of the room rather than into it. A minimum of 25 air exchanges per hour is recommended if the air is recirculated, and 15 air changes per hour if the air is exhausted to the outside. In selected human surgery suites, especially those used for joint replacement, laminar air filtering system are installed to reduce the number of airborne microorganisms in the surgery suite. The filtering system measures about 3×3 m (Fig. 11-7). The air is directed in a vertical flow of 0.5 m/sec initially through a rough, then through a fine, and ultimately through a high-efficiency particulate air (HEPA) filter. The ultra-clean air reaches the surgical field and is directed around the patient to the floor. From there it is aspirated into exhaust outlets located all around the walls at the ceiling. The air is recirculated through the filtering system. Ideally, the outline of the filtering system is marked on the surgery room floor, which facilitates the positioning of the surgery site, the instrument tables, and surgeons within the field (Fig. 11-8). Such ultra-clean filtering systems

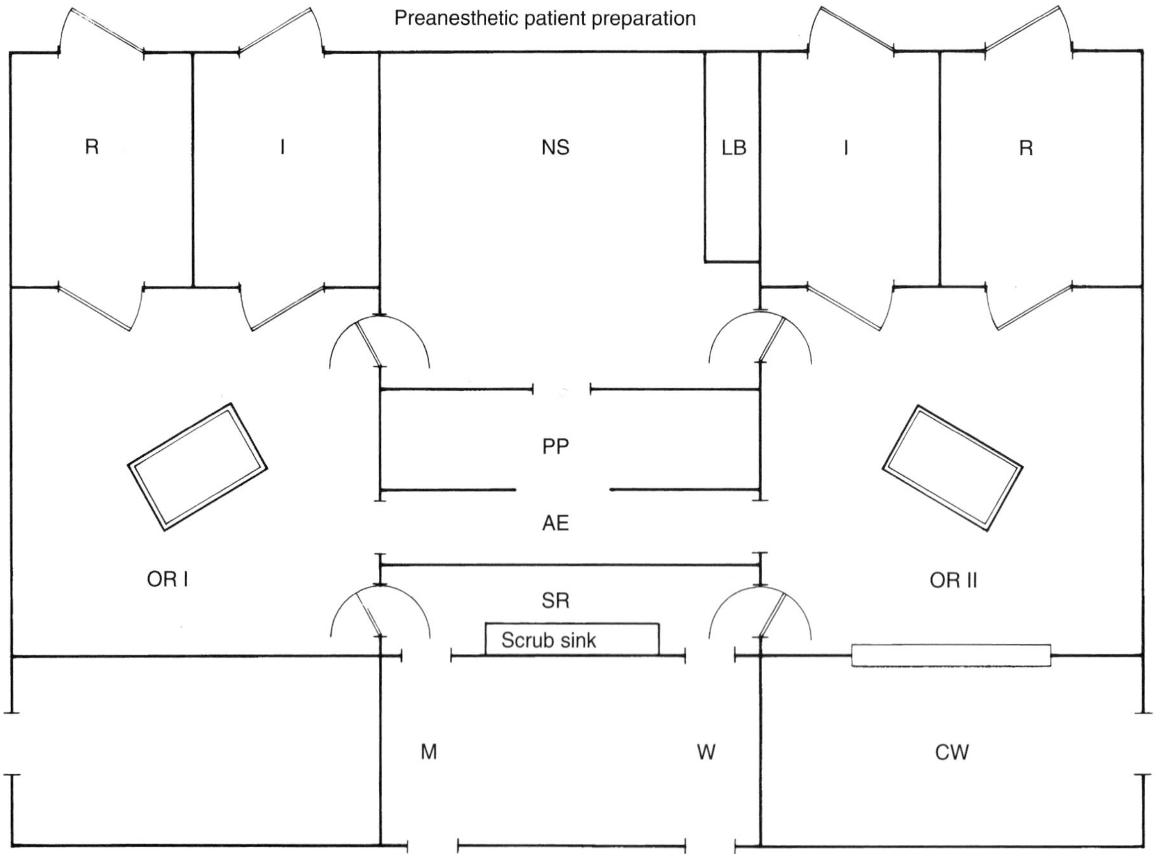

Figure 11-6. Suggested layout for an equine surgical facility. Separate rooms are provided for clean procedures and for contaminated or infected procedures, and a central station supplies both suites. AE, anesthesia equipment; CW, client waiting room; I, induction stalls; LB, laboratory bench; M, men's dressing area; NS, nurse's station; OR, operating rooms; PP, pack preparation and storage; R, recovery stalls; SR, scrub room; W, women's dressing area.

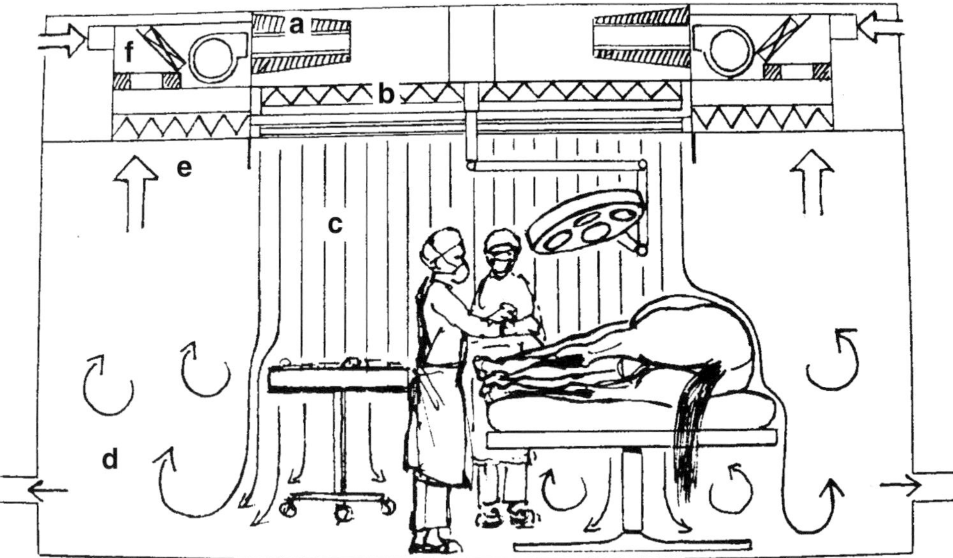

Figure 11-7. Schematic drawing of a laminar air filter system. The surgical site, the surgeons, and the instrument tables must be situated in the field of filtration. *a:* Blower to force filtered air through the pores in ceiling. *b:* Laminar air filter in the ceiling (frequently illuminated). *c:* Laminar air stream gently falling towards the floor. All objects within the field are surrounded by this air. *d:* Once at or near the floor, the air is directed toward the periphery and some of it is lost through doors and other openings. The rest is gently pulled up toward a filter system mounted along the walls in the ceiling. *e:* After being extensively filtered and mixed with clean air from outside, the air is directed through the blower (f) again and reentered into the cycle.

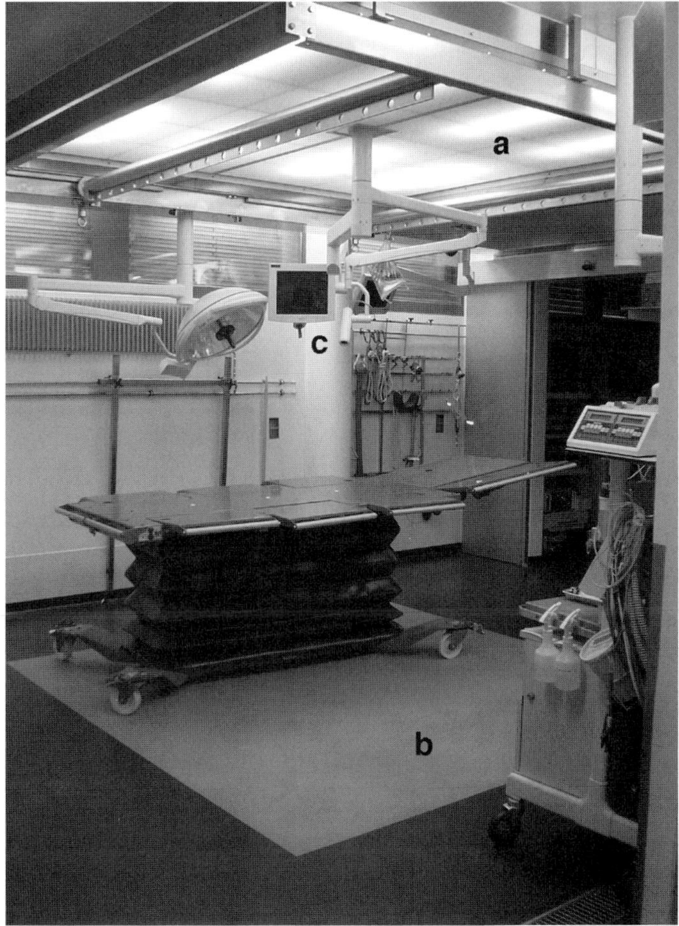

Figure 11-8. View into the aseptic surgery suite of the Equine Hospital, University of Zurich. *a:* The laminar air filter is illuminated. *b:* The grey area marked on the floor delineates the extent of the filter field. The surgery site, the surgeons, and the instrument tables need to be located within this field during surgery. (A mobile Haico Surgery table is shown in the room). *c:* A movable video camera *(left)* is mounted on the ceiling together with a video screen.

are rarely found in equine hospitals and may not be necessary.

The door should be wide enough to allow the surgery table with the horse and other large equipment such as the digital-capture C-arm and radiography machines to pass through easily. Electrical outlets should be located waist high or suspended from the ceiling so they do not become wet during cleaning of the room. Ideally, several locations for hooking up the anesthetic gases and the exhaust pipes of the anesthetic machine should be available. Also, devices should be placed in the wall to allow the application of traction pulleys for the reduction of fractures. Some provision should be made for emergency lighting, either by battery units or with an emergency generator that starts automatically when needed. At least one surgery light in each room should be wired to the emergency system. All cabinets should be recessed into the wall so that the floor can be adequately cleaned after each surgery. Viewing windows are desirable in operating rooms. This is done not only for direct viewing from a doctor or nurse's station but also so the public can view surgeries from an outside hall. Another option is the installation of a closed-circuit video camera system, which can be operated by the owners or students from an observation room distant from the surgery facility.

THE OPERATING TEAM

Scrub Attire

The operating team consists of the people performing the surgery and administering the anesthesia, nonscrubbed assistants, and observers within the operating room. All individuals, regardless of their role in the surgery, contribute to operating room contamination and potential infection of the wound. Therefore, scrub suits, caps, masks, sweat bands, shoe covers, gowns, and gloves are worn to prevent shed particulates and microorganisms from reaching the surgery site.

Scrub suits usually consist of separate pants and shirts and should be clean, comfortable, and dedicated to the operating room (Fig. 11-9) Many blended cotton materials are available for this purpose. Although the design is relatively standard, sizing should accomplish covering the surgeon effectively from neck to ankle while leaving the arms exposed. The bottom of the scrub shirt should be tucked into the pants to prevent shedding of hair, skin cells, and bacteria between the top and the pants. Long-sleeved cuffed jumpsuits for those not needing to gown and glove for the procedure are also quite useful, as they provide a barrier against shedding of skin debris and microorganisms. The scrub suit should not be worn outside the surgery without being covered by a clean laboratory coat, and it should be laundered after each case or at least daily. This scrub clothing should be steam sterilized weekly to ensure removal of the microorganisms that can remain after routine laundry cleaning. Alternatively, bleach can be added to the laundry cycle to reduce the number of bacteria.

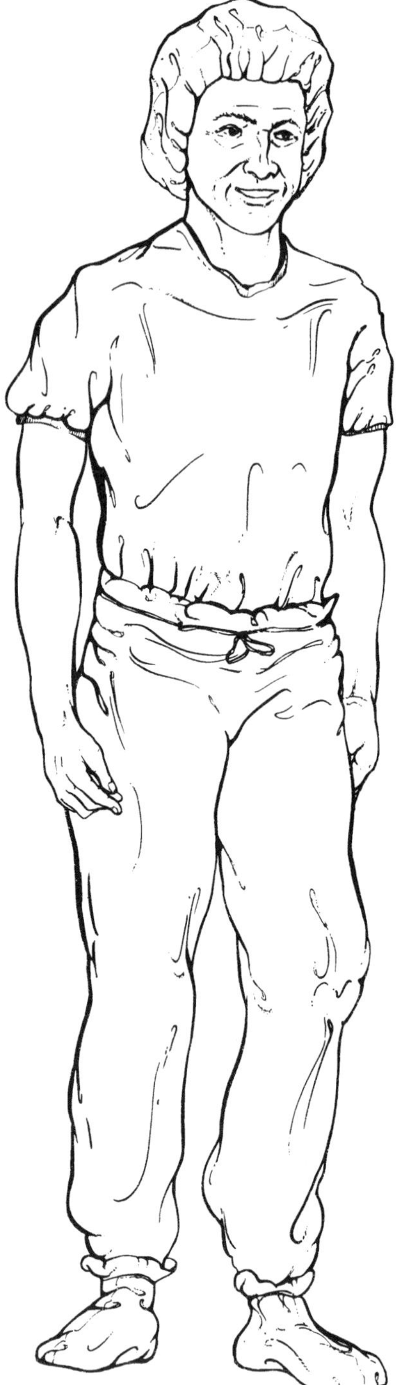

Figure 11-9. Scrub suit recommendations. The scrub shirt should be tucked into the pants. Although not always practical, the pant legs may be tucked into boots or shoecovers. Peripheral personnel may wear long-sleeved tops with elastic cuffs to further limit transmission of skin debris.

Air in an operating room contains approximately 250,000 particles (bacteria, lint, and skin squames) and 11 to 13 bacteria per cubic foot.[17,18] These particles and bacteria increase with the number of people and level of activity in the room, the amount of uncovered skin area, and the amount of talking. Bacterial levels in excess of 400 per cubic foot may be seen in a busy operating theatre. Therefore, barrier apparel is worn to minimize these numbers and their effect on surgical wound rate.

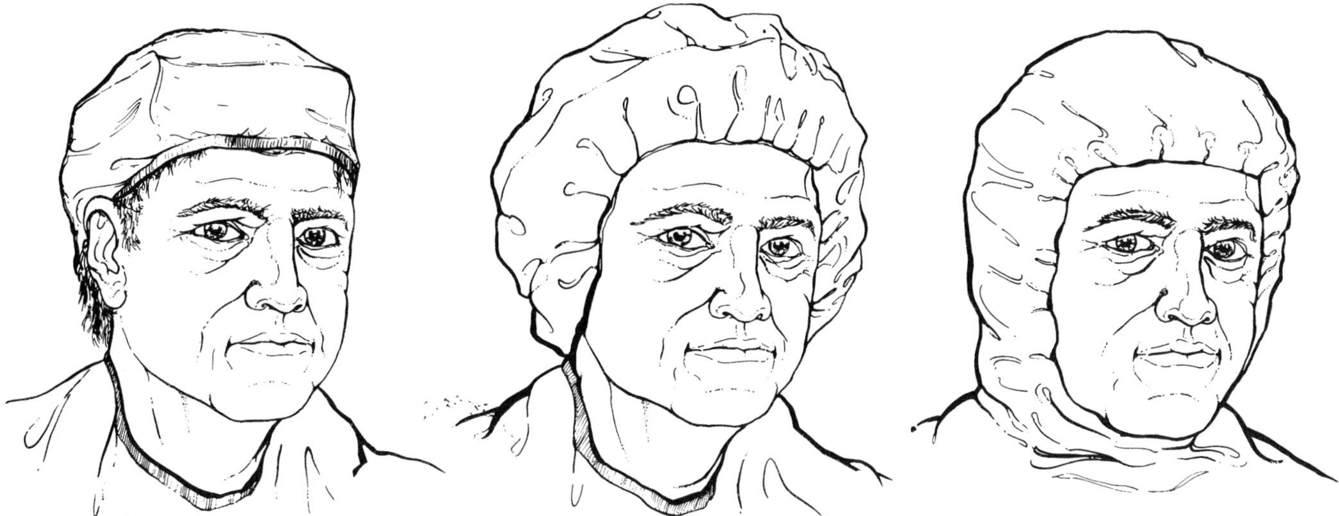

Figure 11-10. Headcover styles are show in order of increasing barrier capability, from left to right. Surgeon's caps, bouffant caps, and hoods offer protection against shedding hair and debris into the surgical wound. Coverage by the old-style surgeon's cap is obviously limited compared with the other types.

Head Covers

Human hair is a major source of bacteria. Because the uncovered hair of the surgeon, who stands over the incision, is frequently a major source of surgical wound contamination, head covers are worn to reduce the shedding of hair and bacteria. All people in the operating room should wear head covers—caps, hoods, or bouffants (Fig. 11-10). These are available in reusable cloth and disposable nonwoven material. The covers should cover all the hair on the head. The reusable head covers should be washed after every procedure (up to a total of 75 times and then, like the reusable drapes, discarded).

Gowns

Gowns provide an aseptic barrier between the skin of the operating team and the patient. The gown should be water resistant as well as comfortable and breathable. It should not produce lint. Gowns are packaged individually and folded so the interior back region is outermost, allowing this area to be handled without contaminating the gown's exterior surface. Once donned, the sterile surgical field extends only above the waist (see Fig. 11-5).

Gowns, like the draping materials, can be made of either reusable woven fabric or nonwoven disposable material. The most effective barrier gown contains some type of polyester or plastic film over a breathable material. Preventing strikethrough when becoming wet is an attribute that is almost mandatory for surgical gowns. Gortex gowns with double-layered barriers in the elbows, chest, and abdominal areas have become popular because they are comfortable and meet the necessary criteria. Gortex is a barrier material consisting of an expanded film of polytetrafluroethylene between two layers of fabric with a maximal pore size of 0.2 mm, which resists strikethrough by water, and bacteria.[19] It allows evaporation of perspiration, which increases comfort for the surgeon. Gortex fabrics are more durable than Quarpel-treated pima cotton and will retain barrier quality characteristics for up to 100 washings.

Gloves

Surgical gloves are made of natural rubber latex and are provided in a sterile, single-use package. Gloves should fit tightly, because gloves that are loose will impair dexterity, but they should not be so tight that the surgeon's fingers lose sensitivity. Modified cornstarch is preapplied to most gloves for easier application, and therefore the outside of the gloves should be rinsed before patient contact.[20] Cornstarch is referred to as "absorbable powder." Magnesium silicate (talcum) powder is no longer used in powdered gloves because it potentiates latex allergies and causes granulomas in patients even when gloves are thoroughly rinsed. However, even absorbable powdered gloves contribute to natural rubber latex allergies (which cause contact dermatitis), and the powder acts as an airborne carrier of natural latex proteins (which can cause respiratory allergies). Therefore, most surgical gloves are treated with multiple washings to reduce the latex proteins. If allergies develop to latex, powderless latex gloves are available, which are chlorinated during manufacturing to decrease their tackiness. (However, these gloves do not store well, and inventory should be monitored to avoid use of these gloves beyond the expiration dates as failure becomes common.) Alternatively, vinyl gloves are available to eliminate this problem, although their performance is less desirable (i.e., dexterity is reduced).

The accepted industry standard for surgical gloves is that 1.5% contain punctures before use.[21] One study found that 2.7% of latex and 4.1% of vinyl gloves leak when filled with water. By the end of surgery, up to 31% of gloves have perforations, and when double gloves are worn, 16% to 67% of the outer gloves and 8% to 30% of the inner gloves contain perforations. Holes are most common on the thumb and index finger of the nondominant hand. Although gloves can be applied using closed or open gloving technique, closed gloving techniques are preferred because the surgeon's skin will not make contact with the outside of the gown cuff. If soiling of the gloves is expected or extra protection is needed during a surgical procedure (i.e., during most orthopedic procedures), many surgeons elect to apply and wear a second pair of gloves. Cuffs of the surgeon's gown should be completely covered, because cuff material is not impervious to water penetration. The use of plastic safety sleeves often helps when the surgeon's hands and arms may be submerged, such as at a colic surgery. Extra-thick gloves are available for orthopedic surgeries, where there is an increased risk of puncturing the gloves from sharp bone spikes and implant materials.

Face Masks

Facial coverings are not effective bacterial filters. When properly fitted, they redirect airflow away from the surgical wound and in doing so reduce the potential for surgical wound infection (Fig. 11-11). Despite clinical reports that facial coverings do not reduce surgical site infections, the use of a face mask is considered mandatory during surgery. Tie-on face masks are tied over the head first, the wire on the top of the mask is fitted over the surgeon's nose, and the lower ties are pulled around and tied behind the neck.[2] The mask should fit tightly around the sides of the face and over the tip of the chin. Cup masks with elastic bands provide a better fit and offer less chance of bacterial contamination.

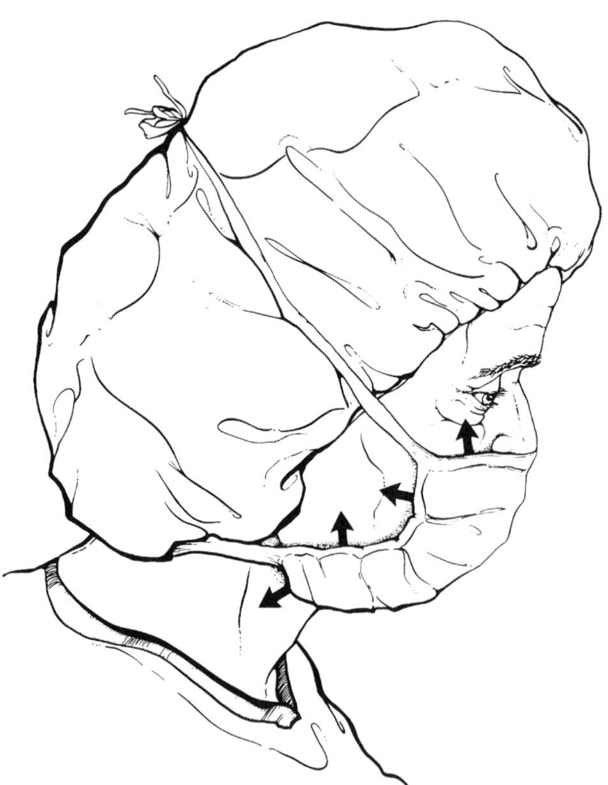

Figure 11-11. Potential leakage sites of the standard surgical mask *(arrows)*. Transmission of contaminants around the edges of the mask can be limited by properly conforming the nosepiece to the nose and tying the mask snugly.

Disposable surgical face masks are recommended over washable gauze because of improved efficiency and comfort. Masks should be worn by all personnel entering the surgery room at any time. Failure to wear masks even when surgery is not in progress promotes contamination of the surgical area. Masks should not be removed and replaced, pushed on the top of head, dangled from the chin, or tucked in a pocket. Each of these common practices risks contamination of scrub clothing with bacteria from inside the mask, which may be transmitted to the patient. The effectiveness of masks and other barriers in a surgery room should probably not be relied on for more than 2 hours.[2] A frequent change of masks, caps, and other apparel is warranted when this time period is exceeded. Bearded surgeons should wear a hood that covers all facial hair in addition to a face mask, which alone is insufficient.

Foot Covers

Disposable shoe covers are usually made of light, nonwoven material fabric and sometimes have polypropylene coatings to avoid strikethrough. Shoe covers help keep the surgeon's feet dry and thus more comfortable during surgical procedures, but they are not believed to be useful in reducing the soil brought to the operating room floor in an equine surgery suite, because of the obvious soiling that occurs with this type of patient. Therefore, shoes dedicated to the operating room are a better option for reducing environment contamination; these shoes should never be worn outside the surgery area without shoe covers, which are then removed prior to reentering the surgery suite.

Surgeon's Skin

Surgeon's hands have higher bacterial counts and more pathogenic organisms than the hands of other medical personnel because of increased exposure to scrub solutions (which irritate the skin) and contaminated wounds.[22] The objective of a surgical hand scrub is to remove gross dirt and oil and decrease bacterial counts, and just as importantly to have a prolonged depressant effect on transient and resident microflora of the hands and forearms. Surgical scrub protocols are based either on scrubbing time or on stroke counting. Principles of the scrub procedure are standard. Fingernails are kept short, clean, and free of polish and artificial nails (chipped nail polish and polish worn for more than 4 days foster an increased number of bacteria on the fingernails, even after a surgical hand scrub).[23] All surfaces of the hands and forearms below the elbow are exposed to antiseptic scrub. Special attention is paid to the area under the nails. The ideal scrub time is controversial, but 2 to 5 minutes seems to be safe and effective, depending on the agent used. Ten-minute scrubs are no longer used because they do not result in additional reductions in bacterial counts (and in one study, counts were increased) and are more irritating to the skin,[24] and 2-minute scrubs result in bacterial count reductions similar to those of longer scrub times. It is currently recommended that brushes or sponges be used for the first scrub of the day, but subsequent scrubs can be brushless.

The residual activity of antisepsis is widely accepted as being useful in the preoperative disinfection of the surgeon's hands. The residual activity of either chlorhexidine gluconate or alcohol chlorhexidine is reported to be superior to that of povidone-iodine against resistant bacteria. Therefore, for procedures lasting less than 1 hour, povidone-iodine is acceptable, but if the procedure is going to exceed 1 hour, alcohol chlorhexidine or chlorhexidine gluconate is the antiseptic of choice.[9]

The primary objective of surgical hand disinfection is destruction or maximal reduction of the resident flora; the secondary objective is elimination of the transient flora. Surgical hand disinfection with alcohol-based hand rubs, many of which contain emollients, is growing in popularity over surgical hand washes made of an antiseptic-based liquid soap, because the rubs have a rapid and immediate action, do not require water or a scrub brush, are considerably faster than the traditional hand scrubs, and cause less skin damage after repeated use.

One large veterinary clinic in Europe (University of Zurich) uses a combination of three products in sequence. A disinfectant solution, Bactolin (Bode Chemie, Hamburg, Germany), is applied with a soft brush or foam pad as the initial wash. Then the hands are dried, and 10 mL of Sterillium (Bode Chemie) is applied for 3 minutes. Postoperatively, Baktolin Balm (Bode Chemie) is applied for rehydration. Sterillium contains 2-propanol (45%) and 1-propanol (30%), and mecetronium ethyl sulfate (MES), a nonvolatile quaternary ammonium compound with skin-soothing and mild antiperspirant effects. Manufacturer's claims are exceptionally good skin protection and skin care, even with long-term use, efficacy against a broad range of microorganisms and viruses (bactericidal, fungicidal, tuberculocidal, virus inactivating), and excellent residual effect. The manufacturer also claims that this preparation permits penetration deep into the stratum corneum of the skin, where it forms a defensive barrier against organisms that emerge with perspiration.

Bacterial examination after disinfection was conducted in two ways. The volunteer rubbed the distal phalanges of one hand (randomly selected) for 1 minute in a Petri dish containing 10 mL of tryptic soy broth (TBS) supplemented with neutralizers (immediate effect). The other hand was gloved for 3 hours for the assessment of the sustained effect. After removal of the glove, sampling was done as for the immediate effect. From the sampling fluid, two 1 mL and two 0.1 mL aliquots were seeded, each in two Petri dishes with solidified TSA. A 1:10 dilution of the sampling fluid in TSB was prepared, and two 0.1 mL aliquots of this were seeded as above. Dishes were incubated at 37° C for 24 to 48 hours. For each dilution the mean number of colony-forming units scored in duplicate dishes was calculated. This was multiplied by the dilution factor to obtain the number of colony-forming units per milliliter of sampling liquid.[25] The examination technique described above has confirmed that rubbing the hands with an antiseptic is significantly more effective than scrubbing with brushes.[25] Hand rubbing with 0.2% chlorhexidine and 83% ethanol (Hibisoft, Sumitomo Pharmaceutical Co, Osaka, Japan) suppressed the number of bacteria and prolonged sterilization for more than 3 hours. In a study conducted according to two European standards for bactericidal efficacy, all alcohol-based surgical hand rubs (Sterillium and Softa Man) and the hand washes, chlorhexidine (Hibiscrub), and povidone-iodine (Betadine) fulfilled the requirements of a bacterial suspension test.[26] However, only the hand rubs met the requirements of the in vivo test of efficacy on resident skin flora, and chlorhexidine failed that test. In another study on surgical hand scrubs, Sterillium was superior to Hibiscrub and alcoholic gels in terms of skin tolerance and microbicidal efficacy.

A 1% chlorhexidine gluconate solution and 61% ethyl alcohol with moisturizers (Avagard, 3M Animal Care Products, St. Paul, Minn) is currently in use as a hand cleaner in the United States. Advantages claimed are greater preservation of the skin's own moisture, pliability and integrity, rapid microbial kill, and activity against a wide range of organisms, including methicillin-resistant *Staphylococcus aureus*. It has been shown to have residual activity comparable to that of chlorhexidine gluconate alone and greater than that of povidone-iodine. A similar product, 0.5% chlorhexidine gluconate plus 70% isopropanol (Hibisol, Promed, Killorglin, Ireland) has greater residual activity against clinically significant test organisms than chlorhexidine digluconate skin cleanser (Hibiscrub), povidone-iodine surgical scrub (Betadine), or 60% isopropanol.

Despite growing evidence in favor of alcohol-based hand rubs for preoperative preparation, many surgeons remain reluctant to switch from an antiseptic soap to an alcohol-based hand rub. Large-animal surgeons pose a considerable challenge to methods employed in human hospitals, because they so often handle heavily contaminated areas on their patients before surgery. Therefore, thorough prewashing is strongly encouraged before using alcohol-based hand rubs.

Additionally, recently developed microbicide products containing substituted phenolic and quaternary phospholipids have 30-second kill times and are used in 2-minute brushless scrubs (Techni-care, Care-Tech Laboratories, Inc., OTC Pharmaceuticals, St. Louis, Mo). These products are less irritating to the skin and are being used in several hospital applications, even including the direct applications to infected and open wounds. All of these products are recommended to be used with a skin balm after surgery to prevent the surgeon's skin from drying with multiple uses.

Staffing the Surgery Area

A minimum of three persons is recommended to perform equine surgery. A surgeon, an anesthetist, and a dedicated surgical technician form the minimal operating team for most efficient operation and least risk to the patient. The properly trained anesthetist allows the surgeon to concentrate entirely on the surgical procedure and must be able to restrain patients effectively and place catheters, calculate drug doses, and be familiar with various sedative and anesthetic agents and regimens. The surgical technician becomes an extension of the veterinary surgeon and usually is more adept than the surgeon in the support areas.

An operating room supervisor is important regardless of the size of the facility. The supervisor is responsible for ordering and stocking all supplies, maintaining a surgery log, and recording all controlled substances and their use. The dedicated surgical technician can fill this role. Additionally, a surgical assistant is invaluable, and technicians with the proper basic training skills and attitude can be acceptably competent in a relatively short time with minimal training, rounding out the team to a perfect four.

REFERENCES

1. Polk HC, Cheadle WG: Principles of pre-operative preparation of the surgical patient. In Sabiston DC, editor: Textbook of Surgery: The Biological Basis of Modern Surgical Practice, ed 15, Philadelphia, 1997, WB Saunders.
2. Shmon C: Assessment and preparation of the surgical patient and the operating team. In Slatter D, editor: Textbook of Small Animal Surgery, ed 3, Philadelphia, 2003, Elsevier.
3. Wolters U, Wolf T, Stutzer H, et al: ASA classification in perioperative variables as predictors of postoperative outcome, Br J Anaesth 1996;77:217.
4. Wolters U, Wolf T, Stutzer H, et al: Risk factors, complication, and outcome in surgery: A multivariate analysis, Eur J Surg 1997; 163:563.
5. Hardy EM, Jayawickrama J, Duff LC, et al: Prognostic indicators of survival in high risk canine surgery patients, J Vet Emerg Crit Care 1995;5:42.
6. MacDonald DG, Morley PS, Bailey JV, et al: An examination of the occurrence of surgical wound infection following equine orthopaedic surgery (1981-1990), Equine Vet J 1994;26:323.
7. Honnas CM, Cohen ND: Analysis of risk factors for postoperative wound infection following celiotomy in horses, J Am Vet Med Assoc 1997;210:78-81.
8. Wilson DA, Baker GJ, Boero MJ: Complications of celiotomy incisions in horses, Vet Surg 1995;24:506.
9. Ingle-Fehr J, Baxter GM: Skin preparation and surgical scrub techniques. In White NA, Moore JN, editors: Current Techniques in Equine Surgery and Lameness, ed 2, Philadelphia, 1998, WB Saunders.
10. Masterson TM, Rodeheaver GT, Morgan RF, et al: Bacteriologic evaluation of electrical clippers for surgical hair removal, Am J Surg 1984;148:301-302.
11. Howard RJ: Surgical Infections, ed 7, New York, 1999, McGraw-Hill.
12. Beck WC: Aseptic barriers in surgery: Their present status, Arch Surg 1981;116:240.
13. Polk HC, Simpson CJ, Simmons BP, et al: Guidelines for prevention of surgical wound infections, Arch Surg 1983;118:1213.
14. Dineen P: Role of impervious drapes and gowns in preventing surgical infection, Clin Orthop 1973;96:210.
15. Moylan JA, Fitzpatrick KT, Davenport KE: Reducing wound infections: Improved gown and drape barrier performance, Arch Surg 1987;122:152.
16. Hobson HP: Surgical facilities and equipment. In Slatter D, editor: Textbook of Small Animal Surgery, ed 3, Philadelphia, 2003, Elsevier.
17. Moylan JA, Kennedy BV: The importance of gown and drape barriers in the prevention of wound infection, Surg Gynecol Obstet 1980;151:465.
18. Sawyer RG, Pruett TL: Wound infections, Surg Clin North Am 1994;74:5-19.
19. Stone WC: Preparation for surgery. In Auer JA, Stick JA, editors: Equine Surgery, ed 2, Philadelphia, 1999, WB Saunders.
20. US Food and Drug Administration—Center for Devices and Radiological Health: Medical Glove Powder Report, Sept 1997.
21. Fog DM: Bacterial barrier of latex and vinyl gloves, AORN J 1989;49:1101.
22. Coelho JC, Lerner H, Murad I: The influence of the surgical scrub on hand bacterial flora, Int Surg 69:305, 1984.
23. Wynd CA, Samstag DE, Lapp AM: Bacterial carriage on the fingernails of OR nurses, AORN J 1994;60:796.
24. O'Farrell DA, O'Sullivan JKM, Nicholson P, et al: Evaluation of the optimal hand scrub duration prior to total hip arthroplasty, J Hosp Infect 1994;26:93.
25. Girou E, Loyeau S, Legrand P: Efficacy of handrubbing with alcohol-based solution versus standard handwashing with antiseptic soap randomised clinical trial, BMJ 2002;325:362.
26. Marchetti MG, Kampf G, Finzi G, et al: Evaluation of the bactericidal effect of five products for surgical hand disinfection according to prEN and prEN 12791, J Hosp Infect 2003;54:63.

CHAPTER 12

Surgical Instruments

Jörg A. Auer

Veterinary surgeons have access to all the instruments used by surgeons who operate on humans, and to an increasing number of instruments specially designed for veterinary applications. However, the instruments actually used by a surgeon are determined by a combination of economics, predicted use, specialty considerations, and personal preference. The costs involved in the purchase of instruments are substantial and demand a clear understanding of manufacturing procedures, maintenance, and potential applications during surgery.[1-4]

Surgical instruments are offered by a large number of manufacturers. As they all compete for the same customers, advertisements usually include an attractive purchase price, which can be the result of compromised quality standards during manufacturing. Unfortunately, there are no international standards for instrument quality. As a result, caution must be exercised before purchasing instruments at bargain prices. When costs for replacement of prematurely worn-out instruments are combined with the frustrations encountered during surgery because of poorly functioning equipment, the higher costs of high-quality instruments are justified. On the other hand, some disposable instruments intended for human surgery can be used repeatedly by veterinary surgeons, which reduces costs considerably.

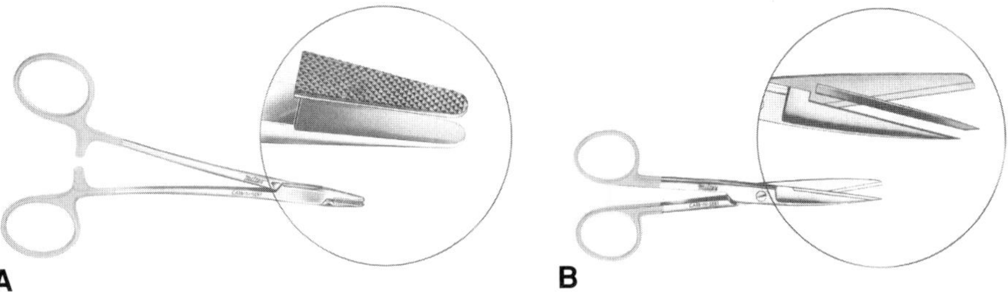

Figure 12-1. **A,** Mayo-Hegar needle holder with tungsten carbide inserts. **B,** Metzenbaum surgical scissors with tungsten carbide inserts. (Reprinted with permission from Miltex Instrument Company, Bethpage, NY, 2004.)

MATERIALS

A description of the different compositions of stainless steels used for manufacturing instruments is found in Chapter 9. Here, only some general comments referring to instrument materials are made.

High-quality stainless steel has become the material of choice for most surgical instruments. In its various forms, stainless steel exhibits a number of desirable instrument characteristics, such as hardness, ability to hold an edge, and resistance to wear and corrosion. Variation in the carbon content of the steel results in changes in the handling characteristics of the material to meet special needs. Currently, most stainless steels used for instrument manufacturing contain a high content of carbon. Although high-carbon stainless steel is resistant to wear and allows the instrument to hold its sharp edge, tungsten carbide inserts have been introduced to replace stainless steel cutting and gripping surfaces[5] (Fig. 12-1). These inserts are even harder and more resistant to wear, prolonging the life of the instrument considerably. The bond between these inserts and the body of the instrument represents a potential problem area, because these bonds may loosen through frequent use and sterilization.[6]

The fine edges and working surfaces required for microsurgery have led to the use of titanium alloys for this specialty instrumentation. Titanium alloys can be produced with excellent corrosion resistance and temperature strength. The brittleness of such alloys complicates the manufacturing process and dictates particular care during use and maintenance. Manufacturers' recommendations for cleaning and sterilization of titanium alloy instruments should be closely followed.

Before the wide availability of low-cost stainless steel, many instruments were manufactured from chrome-plated carbon steel. The chrome plating provided corrosion resistance unavailable with carbon steel alone. Unfortunately, the chrome plating itself is susceptible to early deterioration from frequent rough use and exposure to acidic solutions. Failure of the chrome coating exposes the underlying carbon steel, allowing oxidation and rust formation. Although deteriorated instruments can be refurbished and replated, replacement with higher-quality, longer-lasting stainless steel instruments is more cost effective and is strongly encouraged.

Corrosion resistance can also be improved by the process of passivation. This process uses nitric acid to remove foreign materials from the stainless steel surface, while covering it with a thin coat of chromium oxide. Both actions contribute to corrosion resistance of surgical stainless steel. Polishing the instrument provides a very fine instrument surface, further increasing corrosion resistance.

One popular surface finish for increased corrosion resistance is a dull satin finish. Created by abrasion or sandblasting techniques, the satin finish reduces light reflection and thus eyestrain. A black finish, which serves a similar purpose, is also available. Gold electroplating of instrument handles does little to improve working surfaces but is generally recognized as a symbol of high-quality instrumentation.

GENERAL SURGERY INSTRUMENTS

Hundreds of different instruments are available today, and it is impossible to know them all by name, function, and design. Frequently, similar instruments are modified and manufactured under different names. In this chapter, instruments are discussed in groups according to function, and differences within the groups are mentioned when needed. All basic instruments should be known to all surgeons, which will aid in the selection of the appropriate instrument for a specific procedure and expedite communication during surgery. The parts of a typical surgical instrument are identified in Figure 12-2. Specialty instruments will be covered in subsequent chapters where applicable.

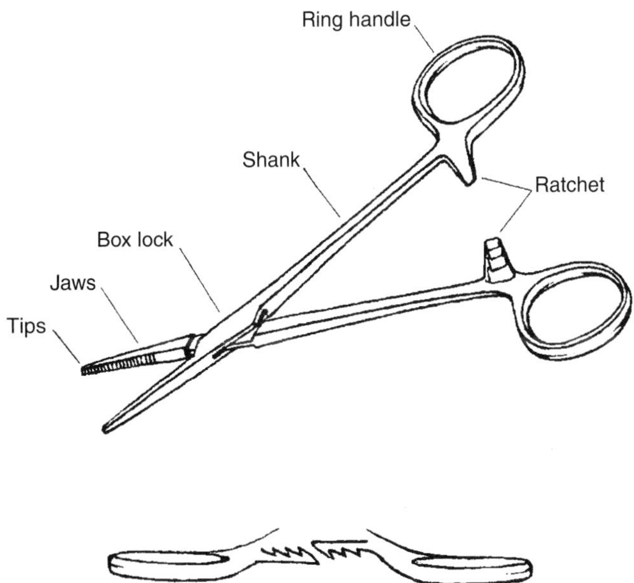

Figure 12-2. *Top:* Labeled parts of a typical surgical instrument. *Bottom:* End-on view of the ratchet mechanism. The ratchets should be slightly separate when the jaws are closed.

Instruments that fall into more than one category are described only once.

Scalpels

Steel Scalpels

Scalpels are available with detachable blades, as disposable units with blades attached, and as reusable units with blades attached. In most clinics, the *Bard-Parker* scalpel handles with different detachable disposable blades are used (Fig. 12-3). The Bard-Parker no. 3 scalpel handle is the most frequently used. Most surgeons prefer the no. 10 blade; the no. 15 blade is a smaller version in a similar shape. The no. 11 blade is frequently used for stab incisions during arthroscopic surgery, and the no. 12 blade is used for periosteal stripping. Two narrow blade handles, Bard-Parker no. 7 and no. 9 (see Fig. 12-3, *C*, and *D*), receive the same blades and are more appropriate for delicate work. The Bard-Parker no. 4 handle accepts larger blades (see Fig. 12-3, *F*). A detachable blade should not be used in joints or deep within heavy connective tissues, where they could break off and be lost from view. The primary advantage of disposable blades is that replacement blades are consistently sharp.

The reusable scalpel with attached blade has a single advantage over the disposable units: the blade will not detach when used in heavy connective tissue, within joints, or in deep tissue planes, where visibility and access for removal are poor. Ethylene oxide or gas plasma sterilization (see Chapter 10) is recommended, as heat and chemicals will dull the blade. Disposable scalpels with nondetachable blades are occasionally used in the field or for bandage removal. In a surgical procedure that requires no other instruments, such a scalpel may be used instead of opening an entire set of instruments.

High-Energy Scalpels

High-energy cutting instruments include the electrosurgical scalpel, the plasma scalpel, the water scalpel, and various forms of lasers. Although their energy sources differ, they share a common cutting mechanism. Energy is focally transmitted to tissue, and the effect depends on the water content of the tissue. The result is vaporization of cells along the line of energy application, a variable degree of thermal necrosis of the wound edges, and a relatively bloodless incision. Electrosurgical incisions are by far the most frequent applications of high-energy cutting.

Electrosurgery uses radiofrequency current to produce one or more of the following effects: incision, coagulation, desiccation, or fulguration of tissues. Most modern electrosurgery units use controlled high-frequency electrical currents ranging between 1.5 and 7.5 mHz.[6] The predominant effect depends on the waveform of the current. Continuous undamped (fully rectified, fully filtered) sine waves provide

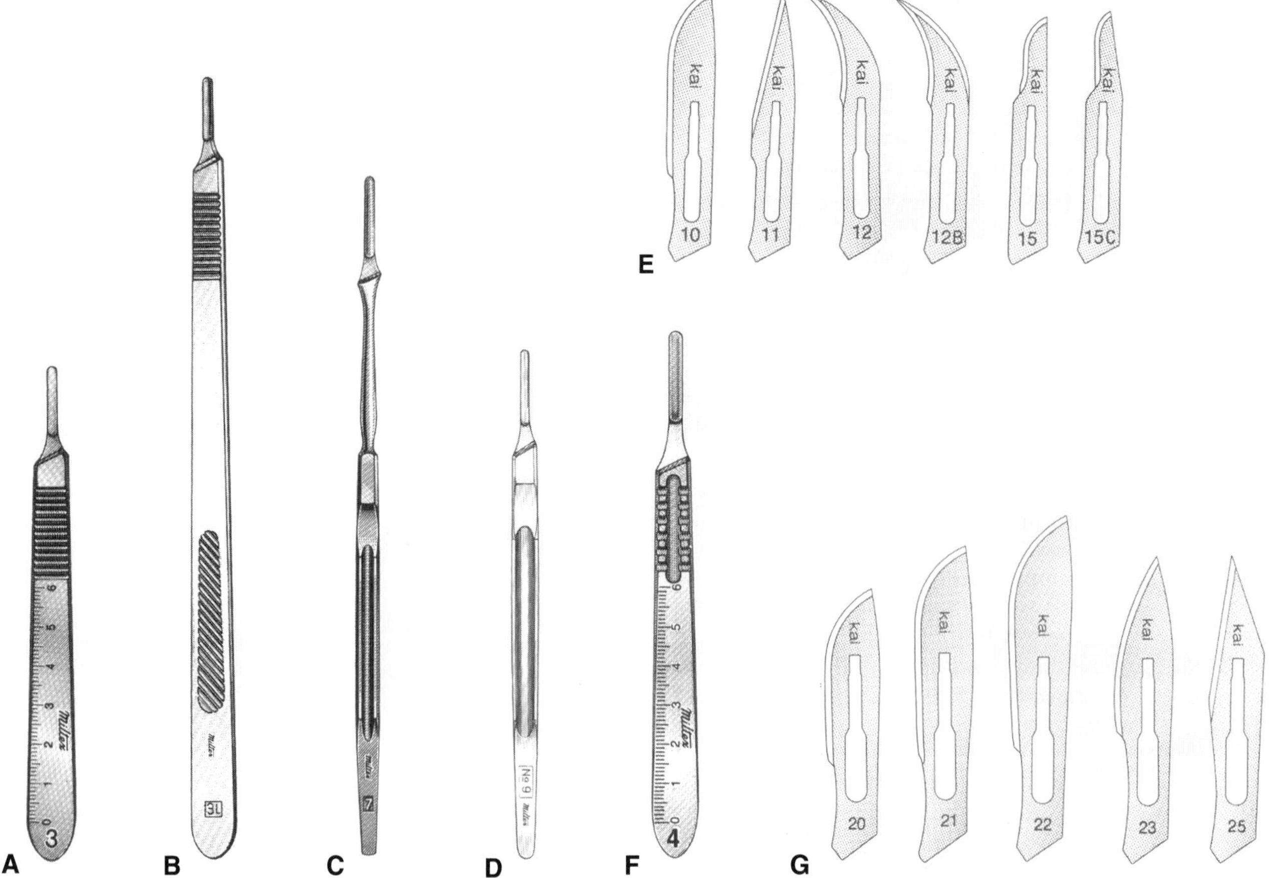

Figure 12-3. Scalpels. **A,** Bard-Parker no. 3 handle. **B,** Bard-Parker no. 3 handle, long. **C,** Bard-Parker no. 7 handle. **D,** Bard-Parker no. 9 handle. **E,** Various shapes of scalpel blades that fit the no. 3, no. 7, and no. 9 scalpel handles. **F,** Bard-Parker no. 4 handle. **G,** Various shapes of scalpel blades that fit the no. 4 scalpel handle. (Reprinted with permission from Miltex Instrument Company, Bethpage, NY, 2004.)

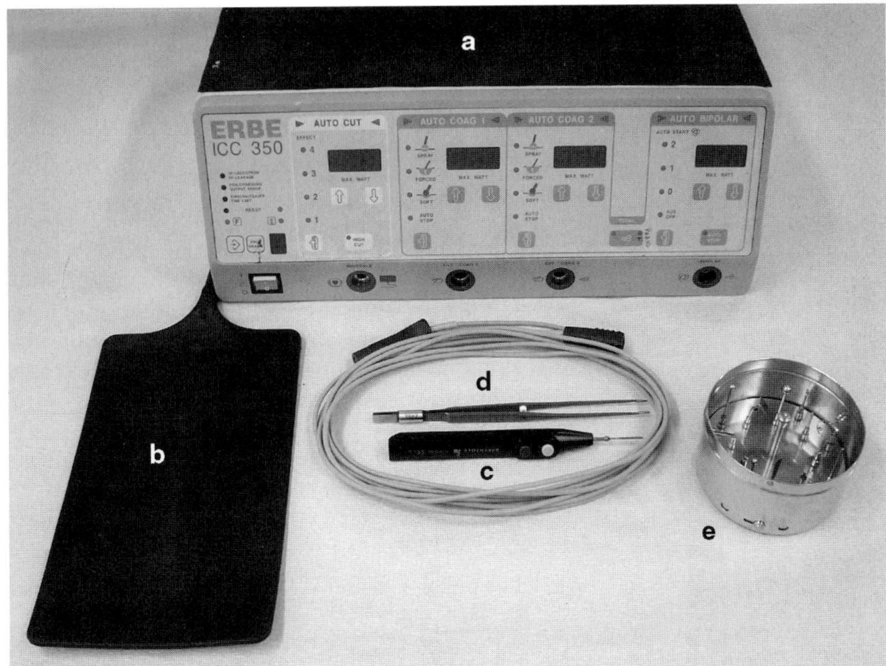

Figure 12-4. Electrosurgical instrumentation. *a,* Electrocautery unit with capacity for monopolar modes of cutting and coagulation, and for bipolar coagulation mode. *b,* Patient grounding plate. *c,* Monopolar handpiece with thin knife. *d,* Bipolar electrode forceps with connection cable. *e,* Exchangeable electrodes for the monopolar handpiece.

maximal cutting and minimal coagulation, and they produce the least amount of lateral heat and tissue destruction.[6] On the other hand, interrupted damped (partially rectified) sine waves maximize coagulation and minimize cutting capabilities. Modulated, pulsed (fully rectified, nonfiltered) sine waves allow simultaneous cutting and coagulation, or "blended" function. The magnitude of the selected effect is directly proportional to the duration and power (in watts) of the applied current.[6]

Because most modern units can be used with unipolar and bipolar instruments, adequate electrical grounding of the patient is required for the unit to function properly in the monopolar mode (Fig. 12-4). The desired function (cutting or coagulation) can be selected by activating a button on the handle. Cutting and coagulation tips are available and can be exchanged as desired. Frequently, needles are used for cutting tissue because of their limited contact area with the tissue, which reduces the amount of tissue necrosis. Correct technique dictates that the tissue be placed under tension and that the contact area of the point be minimized to prevent adjacent tissue destruction. Skin and fascia incise easily, whereas muscle and fat are more easily incised using a cold scalpel. Units can also be used to coagulate vessels less than 1 mm in diameter (see Chapter 13). Coagulation time should be minimized to limit the amount of tissue destruction. The bipolar forceps for direct coagulation of smaller vessels speed up hemostasis, because the initial placement of a hemostatic forceps can be bypassed.

Scissors

Surgical scissors are available in various lengths, weights, blade types (curved or straight), cutting edge types (plain or serrated), and tip types (sharp-sharp, sharp-blunt, and blunt-blunt). The two most commonly used operating scissors for tissue dissection are the *Mayo* and the *Metzenbaum* scissors (Fig. 12-5). The sturdier Mayo scissors, available in 14- to 22.5-cm (5½- to 9-inch) lengths, should be used for cutting connective tissue. Metzenbaum scissors are reserved

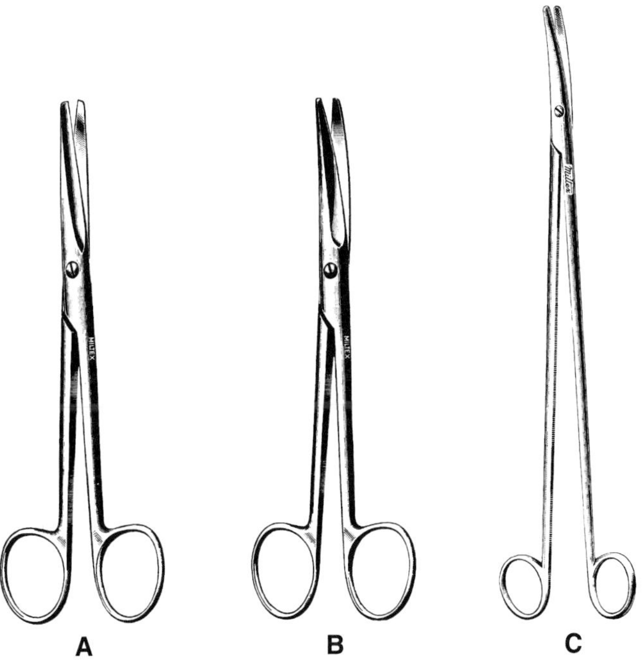

Figure 12-5. Operating scissors. **A,** Straight Mayo scissors. **B,** Curved Mayo scissors. **C,** Metzenbaum scissors. (Reprinted with permission from Miltex Instrument Company, Bethpage, NY, 2004.)

for delicate soft tissue dissection and should not be used for dense tissue dissection. They are available in 12.5- to 34-cm (5- to $14\frac{1}{2}$-inch) lengths.

Specially designated and marked suture scissors are used during surgery to cut the sutures. It is important to use only the suture scissors for cutting sutures, because this job rapidly dulls the blades, making them less effective for soft tissue dissection. The *Olsen-Hegar* needle holders are equipped with cutting edges (see later) to cut sutures, which obviates the need for a special set of suture scissors. Suture removal scissors (Fig. 12-6, *A*) are lighter in weight, and they have a sharp, thin point and a concave lower blade that facilitates blade placement underneath the suture, which reduces suture tension as it cuts. Wire-cutting scissors (see Fig. 12-6, *B*) have been designed specifically for wire suture removal and are typically short and heavy and have serrated blades.

Of the bandage scissors, the *Lister* and the *all-purpose* utility scissors are the best known (see Fig. 12-6, *C*). The lower blade of these scissors has a blunt tip that allows it to be inserted underneath the bandage without damaging the patient's skin. The all-purpose scissor comes with a needle destroyer and a serrated blade (see Fig. 12-6, *D*). The serrated blade reduces bandage material slippage during cutting. Both scissors can be autoclaved.

As a general rule, scissors should be used only as intended by their design. Misuse dulls the edges and causes blades to

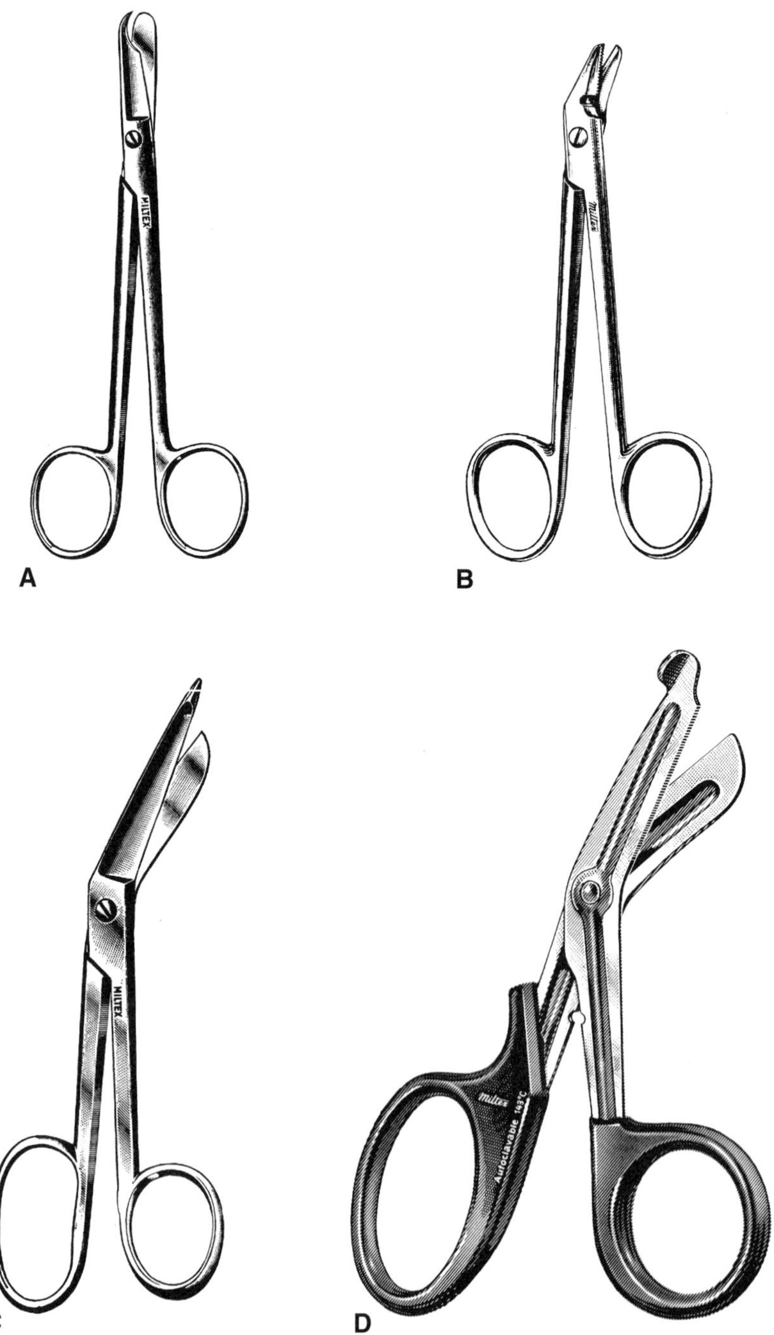

Figure 12-6. A, Littauer stitch scissors. **B,** Wire cutting scissors. **C,** Lister bandage scissors. **D,** All-purpose bandage scissors. (Reprinted with permission from Miltex Instrument Company, Bethpage, NY, 2004.)

separate, rendering them ineffective. Properly functioning scissors should open and close with a smooth, gliding action, and their tips should meet when closed. Scissors should be sharpened only by a qualified person. Incorrect blade sharpening causes the metal to overheat and lose temper, and the cutting edges to become soft, resulting in loss of a sharp edge. Scissors with tungsten carbide inserts maintain sharpness longer. The insert can be replaced when dull.

Needle Holders

A needle holder is selected on the basis of the type of tissue to be sutured, the needle and suture material used, and personal preference. The grasping surfaces of the needle holders are crosshatched with a central longitudinal groove that facilitates the holding of curved suture needles. The two most commonly used needle holders are the *Mayo-Hegar* and the *Olsen-Hegar* (Fig. 12-7). The Olsen-Hegar is a combination of needle holder and scissors. It allows the surgeon working without an assistant to place, tie, and cut suture material swiftly. Its major disadvantage is the occasional inadvertent and premature cutting of suture material, which occurs usually from inexperience with the instrument. Both needle holders are available in various lengths and jaw widths. The choice of jaw width is based on the size of the needle. Narrow jaw widths are recommended for small needles to prevent needle flattening as the ratchet is tightened, whereas wider jaws prevent larger needles from rotating as they pass through dense tissue.

The *Mathieu* needle holder is also popular in equine surgery. It lacks finger holes and has an open box lock that is released by further closing of the handles. Unfortunately, this can occur when a firm grip is applied to the instrument while passing a needle through resistant tissue, making its use somewhat restricted. The efficient use of this needle holder requires practice.

The needle holder is the instrument that receives the most use, and through its constant metal-on-metal action, the most wear. It is advisable to purchase good-quality needle holders with tungsten carbide inserts that facilitate needle grip and instrument durability. The inserts lack a longitudinal groove and are designed with pyramidal teeth to provide a nonslip grip on needles. Instrument life can be prolonged by choosing the appropriate needle for the size of the needle holder. The lock box will be damaged if the instrument is used to grasp too large a needle. Repair is necessary if the needle can be rotated by hand when the instrument is locked at the second ratchet position. New needle holders will hold an appropriate-size needle securely when locked in the first ratchet tooth.[1]

Forceps

Forceps are available in many designs, each intended to perform specific functions or tissue manipulations. They range from simple thumb forceps to instruments containing various hinge configurations and ratchet locks. Selection of appropriate forceps for inclusion in surgical packs can greatly facilitate some maneuvers. Improper use can compound tissue trauma during surgery, increasing inflammation and delaying healing. Also, improper use may alter the shape of the jaws, rendering them useless for the intended application.

Thumb Forceps

Thumb forceps (Fig. 12-8) are designed to grasp and hold tissues and small objects, such as suture needles, and thus

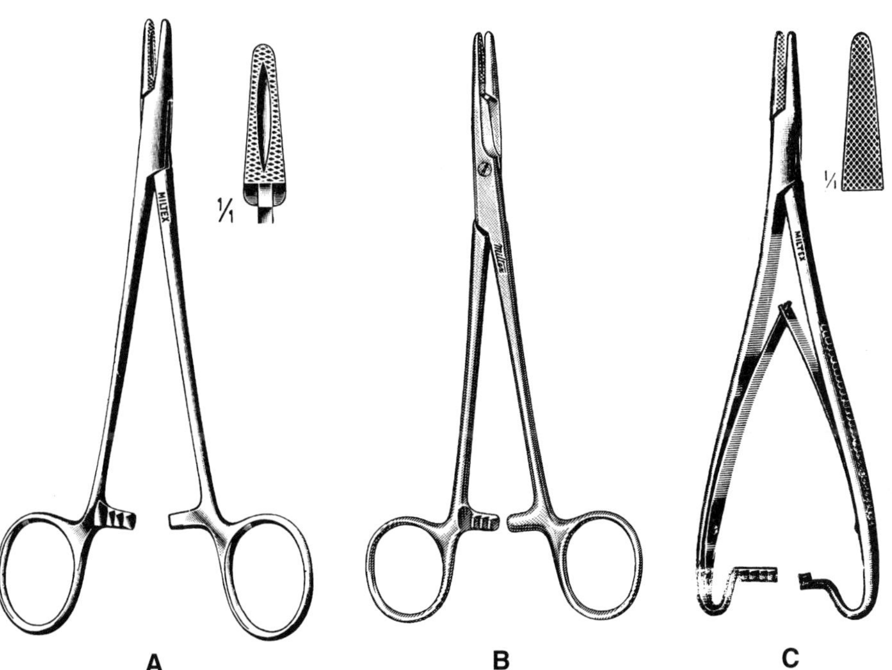

Figure 12-7. Needle holders. **A,** Mayo-Hegar needle holder. **B,** Olsen-Hegar needle holder. **C,** Mathieu needle holder. (Reprinted with permission from Miltex Instrument Company, Bethpage, NY, 2004.)

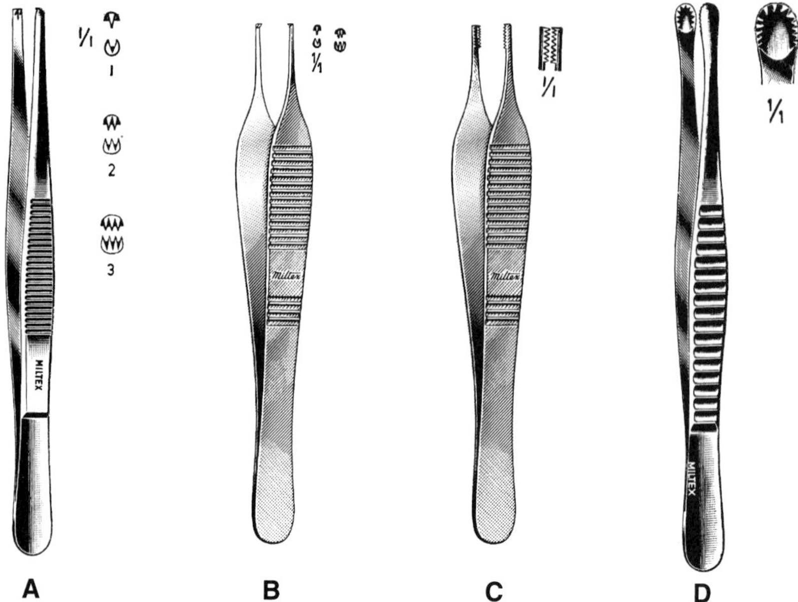

Figure 12-8. Thumb forceps. **A,** Rat-toothed forceps. **B,** Adson forceps. **C,** Brown-Adson forceps. **D,** Russian forceps. (Reprinted with permission from Miltex Instrument Company, Bethpage, NY, 2004.)

they serve as an extension of the surgeon's fingers. They consist of two blades attached at the proximal end, and the tips come together to hold tissue as finger pressure is applied on the blades. The outer surfaces of the blades are grooved to increase digital purchase. Thumb forceps are distinguished by the configuration of the tips. Forceps with smooth tips (without grooves or teeth) crush tissues because a considerable amount of force is necessary to gain purchase on the tissues. These smooth-tipped forceps are called traumatic (or anatomic) thumb forceps and should not be used for surgery.

A variety of serrated and toothed (or surgical) thumb forceps are available. The serrations and teeth allow a secure hold on tissues with minimal digital crushing pressure. The most aggressive of the thumb forceps is the *rat tooth* forceps (see Fig. 12-8, *A*), which is available with 1-to-2 to 4-to-5 interlocking tooth patterns. They are used primarily for manipulating skin and tough connective tissue. The *Adson* forceps has a 1-to-2 toothed tip but affords precise control of instrument pressure (see Fig. 12-8, *B*). The *Adson* forceps is used to grasp thin skin and light fascial planes. The *Brown-Adson* forceps has two longitudinal rows of small, fine, intermeshing teeth (see Fig. 12-8, *C*). The tooth configuration provides a broad but delicate tissue grip and facilitates grasping of the suture needle. The *Russian* forceps, which is not so frequently used, is very sturdy (see Fig. 12-8, *D*). It has a broad, round tip with a grooved perimeter and a concave center. This thumb forceps has a grip that is considered less traumatic than the Adson and Brown-Adson forceps, because pressure on the tissues is spread out over a larger area and it lacks teeth, making it less likely to tear or puncture tissue. The *DeBakey* and *Cooley* forceps lack teeth but are still considered atraumatic forceps because of the serrations in the tips (Fig. 12-9). These forceps are designed with longitudinal grooves and fine, horizontal striations that grip tissue without injury. They are considered ideal for vascular, thoracic, and intestinal surgeries. The DeBakey and Cooley serrated groove patterns are also available on hemostatic forceps.

Hemostatic Forceps

Hemostatic forceps are crushing instruments, designed to collapse vessels until hemostasis occurs or until electrocoagulation or ligation is accomplished (Fig. 12-10). Most of these forceps have transverse grooves on the inner jaw surface that increase tissue purchase. The *Halstead mosquito* forceps (see Fig. 12-10, *A*) are the smallest and most frequently used of these. They are available in 9- and 12.5-cm (3½- and 5-inch) lengths, with thin or standard-width, curved or straight jaws. They should be used only on small vessels. The *Kelly* and *Crile* forceps (see Fig. 12-10, *B* and *C*) are sturdier hemostatic forceps. These instruments are available in a standard 14-cm (5½-inch) length, with curved or straight jaws. The two differ in that the Kelly's transverse grooves are restricted to the distal half of the jaw, whereas the Crile's entire surface is grooved. Both are used for manipulating larger vessels.

To clamp large tissue bundles and vessels, *Rochester-Pean* forceps (see Fig. 12-10, *D*) are recommended. They have deep transverse grooves over the entire jaw surface, are available in 14- to 30-cm (5½- to 12-inch) lengths, and come with straight or curved jaws. *Rochester-Carmalt* forceps (see Fig. 12-10, *E*) are made to assist in pedicle ligation. Their jaw grooves run longitudinally with a few horizontal cross-striations at the tips. The groove design facilitates removal during ligation. *Rochester-Ochsner* forceps (see Fig. 12-10, *F*), available in 18.5- to 25-cm (6¼- to 10-inch) lengths and with curved or straight jaws, are similar in design to the Rochester-Pean, but they differ by having 1-to-2 interdigitating teeth located at the jaw tip to help prevent tissue slippage. *Ochsner* forceps are considered traumatic

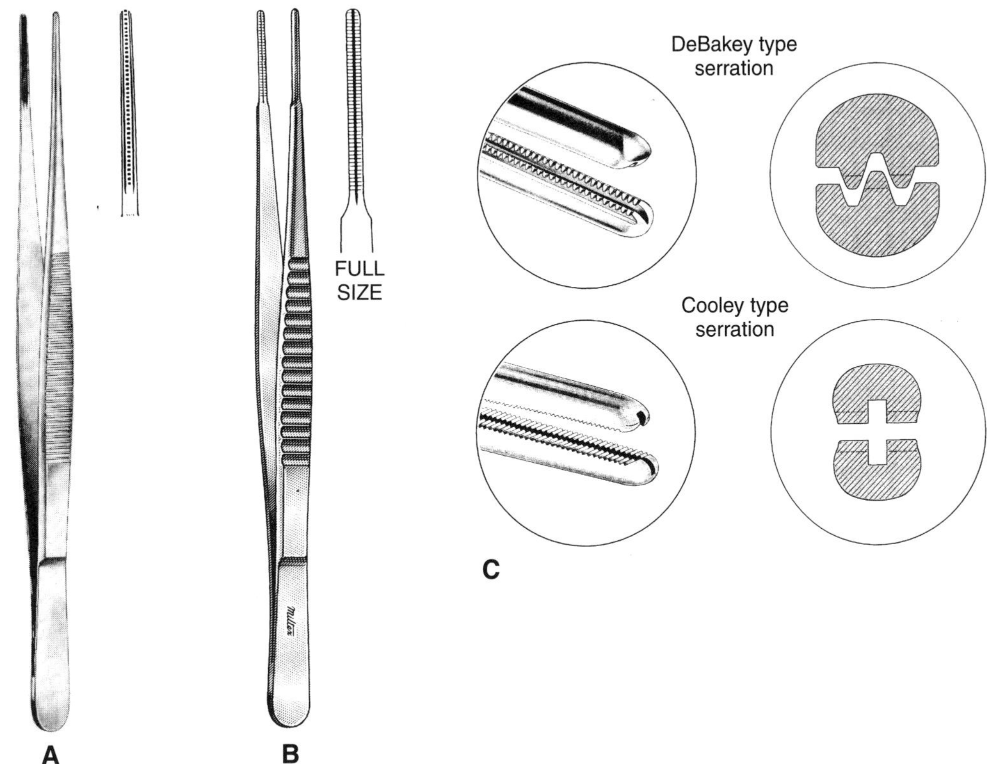

Figure 12-9. A, DeBakey forceps. **B,** Cooley forceps. **C,** Serration patterns. (Reprinted with permission from Miltex Instrument Company, Bethpage, NY, 2004.)

and should be reserved for use on tissue that is to be removed.

Tissue Forceps

Tissue forceps (Fig. 12-11) are available in many shapes and sizes, and for a variety of uses. *Doyen* intestinal forceps, when properly used, are the least traumatic to tissue (see Fig. 12-11, *A*). They are manufactured with slightly bowed, flexible jaws with longitudinal serrations. The longitudinal serrations allow easy removal from the intestine. The instrument is available in 16.5- to 22.5-cm (6½- and 9-inch) lengths with straight or curved jaws, and it can be obtained with a wing nut to secure the tips in a clamping position, which is especially useful for longer forceps. The tips of the jaws should just meet when the ratchet's first tooth is engaged. The instrument will traumatize tissue if the ratchet is closed too tightly.

Allis tissue forceps vary in length between 12.5 and 19 cm (5 and 7¼ inches) and in the number of teeth (4-to-5 and 5-to-6) (see Fig. 12-11, *B*). Designed to grip tissue, the teeth are oriented perpendicular to the direction of pull. The teeth can be traumatic, especially when excessive compression is applied to the handles, and his forceps should be used only on heavy tissue planes or on tissue that is to be excised.

Babcock intestinal forceps, like the Allis tissue forceps, pull in a direction that is perpendicular to the tissue, but the *Babcock* forceps are considered less traumatic (see Fig. 12-11, *C*). The instrument is available in lengths from 13 to 24 cm (5¼ to 9½ inches) and jaw widths of 6 to 10 mm. *Lahey* right-angled forceps (see Fig. 12-11, *D*), *Vulsellum* uterine forceps (see Fig. 12-11, *E*), and *Noyes alligator* forceps (see Fig. 12-11, *F*) are infrequently used, but their unique designs make them useful in a variety of surgical applications.

Hemostatic and tissue forceps should regularly be inspected for instrument wear and damage. When the instrument is closed, the jaws should align perfectly and the teeth, if present, should interdigitate. When clamped on tissue, the instrument should not spring open.

Retractors

Soft tissue retractors are designed to spread the wound edges to facilitate exposure of the surgical field. A classification used by many manufacturers includes the finger-held, the hand-held, and the self-retaining retractors. All three types require an adequate length of incision to prevent tissue tearing when retraction is used. The finger-held and hand-held retractors require a surgical assistant.

Finger-Held Retractors

Senn, Mathieu, Meyerding, Farabeuf, and *Parker* retractors are typical representatives of this group (Fig. 12-12). Senn and Mathieu retractors are similar (see Fig. 12-12, *A* and *B*). Both are available with either blunt or sharp retractor prongs at one end and a right-angled fingerplate on the other. These retract skin and superficial muscle layers but are less useful for retracting a large muscle mass. Meyerding finger retractors (see Fig. 12-12, *C*) have an assortment of gripping blades available and a single-ring handle. Farabeuf and Parker retractors (see Fig. 12-12, *D* and *E*) are larger, with deeper, flat blades on both ends that allow the retraction of more tissue.

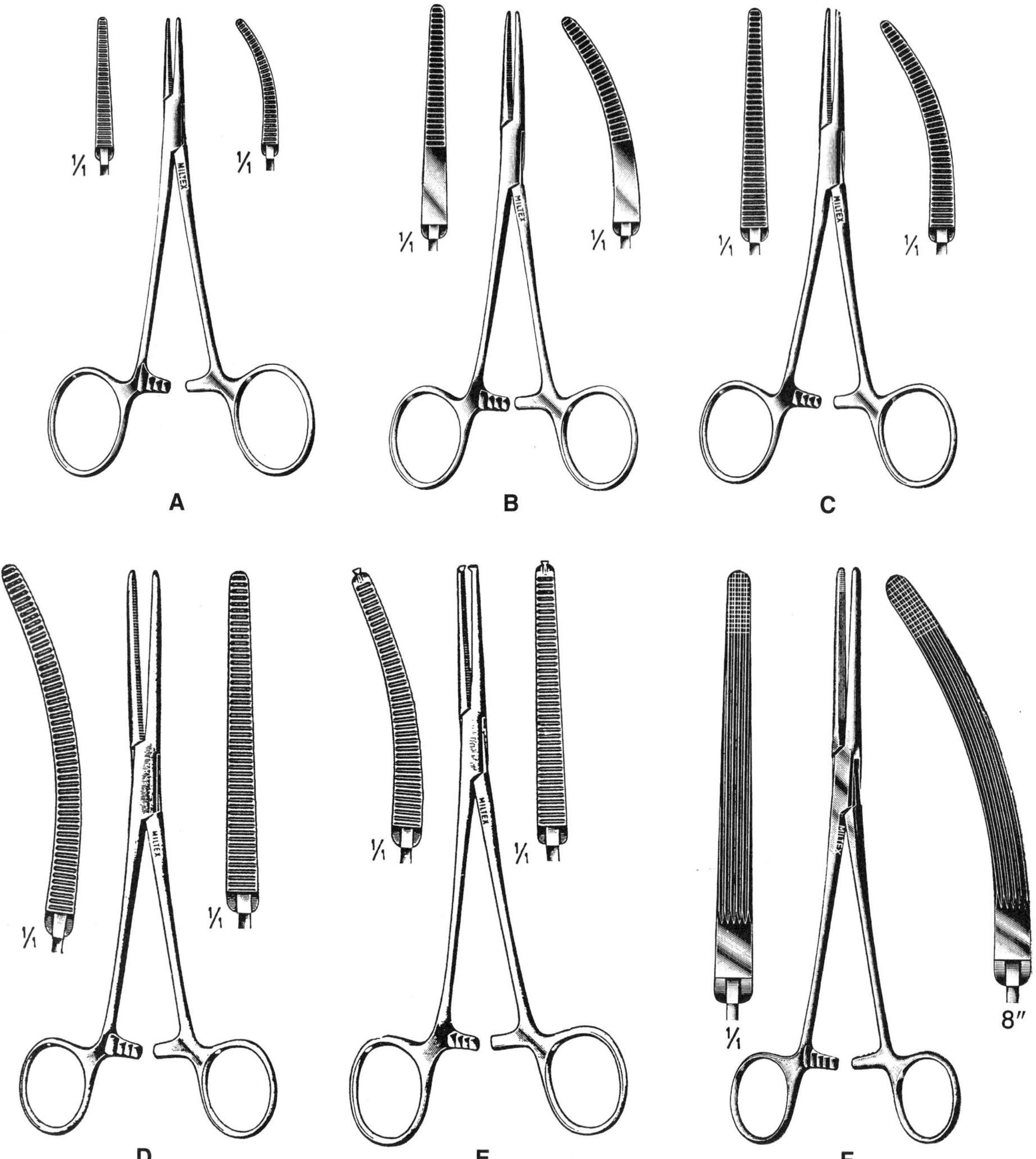

Figure 12-10. Hemostatic forceps. **A,** Halstead mosquito forceps. **B,** Kelly forceps. **C,** Crile forceps. **D,** Rochester-Pean forceps. **E,** Rochester-Carmalt forceps. **F,** Rochester-Oschner forceps. (Reprinted with permission from Miltex Instrument Company, Bethpage, NY, 2004.)

Hand-Held Retractors

Common hand held retractors are the *Army-Navy, Hohmann, Meyerding,* and *Ribbon* retractors (Fig. 12-13). Army-Navy retractors are available in a standard 21.5-cm (8½-inch) length (see Fig. 12-13, *A*). They have double-ended retracting blades of two different lengths, which allow the surgeon to select a blade according to tissue depth. Hohmann retractors are available in 16.5- to 24.5-cm (6¼- to 9¾-inch) lengths, and with blade widths from 6 to 70 mm (see Fig. 12-13, *B*). The blade has a blunt projection that is useful in exposing bone while retracting the muscle in orthopedic and reconstructive procedures. Meyerding retractors are available with three different blade widths and depths (see Fig. 12-13, *C*). The largest blade is 9 cm (3½ inches) wide and 5 cm (2 inches) in depth. *Ribbon* malleable retractors are 32.5 cm (13 inches) in length and available in 2- to 5-cm (¾- to 2-inch) widths (see Fig. 12-13, *D*). The malleable blade can be bent repeatedly, making it a favorite of some surgeons. After prolonged use, it becomes an unaesthetic surgical instrument, although its effectiveness is not altered.

Self-Retaining Retractors

The *Gelpi, Weitlaner, Balfour,* and *Finochietto* retractors (Fig. 12-14) are representatives of the available self-retaining retractors. The Gelpi retractor has a grip-lock mechanism

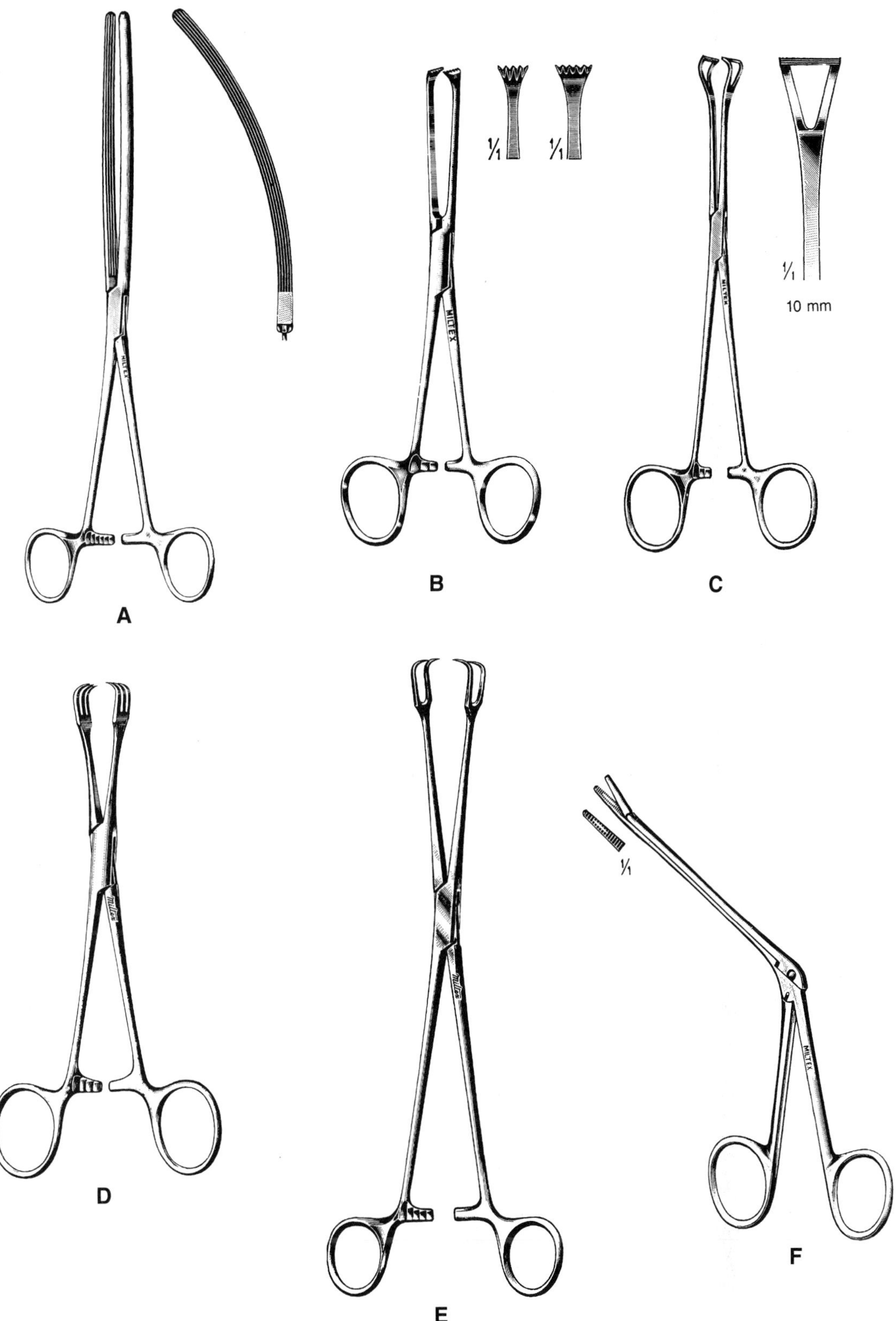

Figure 12-11. Tissue forceps. **A,** Doyen intestinal forceps. **B,** Allis forceps. **C,** Babcock forceps. **D,** Lahey forceps. **E,** Vulsellum forceps. **F,** Noyes forceps. (Reprinted with permission from Miltex Instrument Company, Bethpage, NY, 2004.)

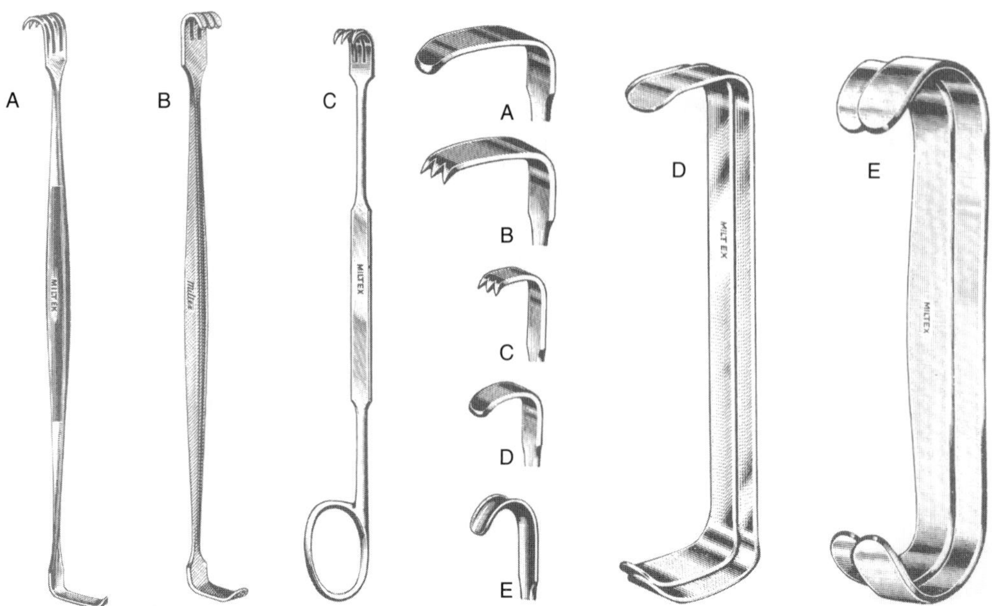

Figure 12-12. Finger-held retractors. **A,** Senn retractor. **B,** Mathieu retractor. **C,** Meyerding finger retractor with various blades for gripping (*A-E,* vertically). **D,** Farabeuf retractor. **E,** Parker retractor. (Reprinted with permission from Miltex Instrument Company, Bethpage, NY, 2004.)

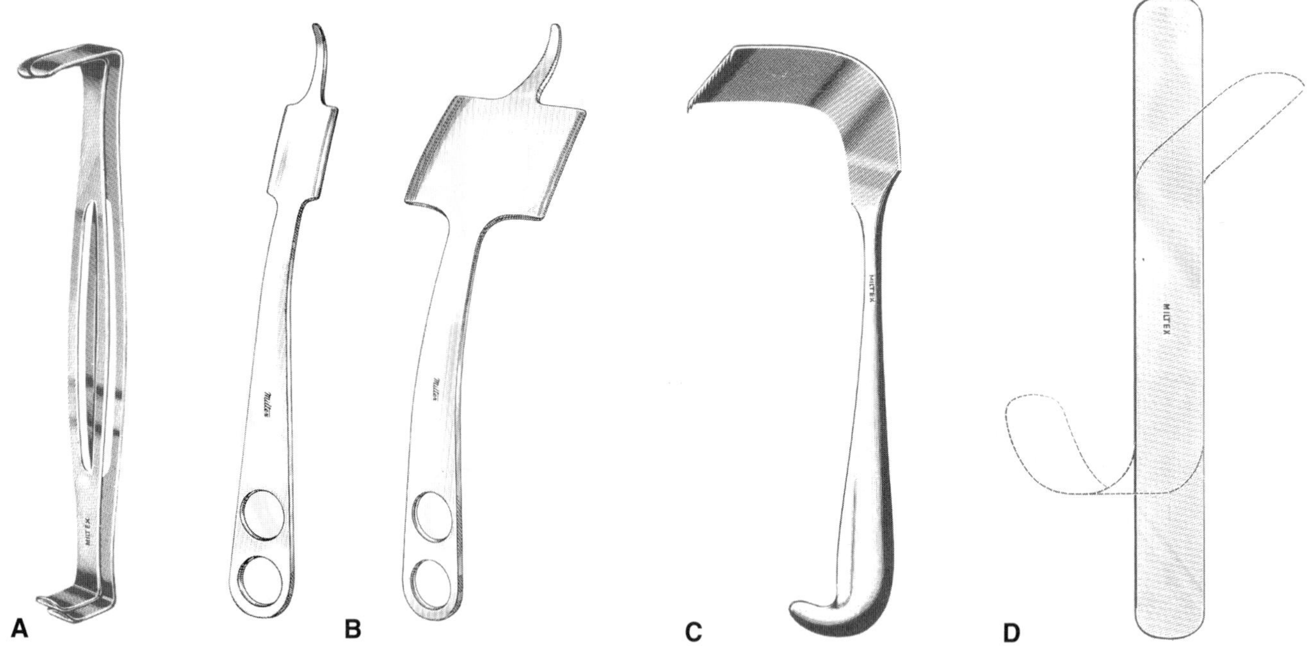

Figure 12-13. Hand-held retractors. **A,** Army-Navy retractor. **B,** Hohmann retractor with two different blades. **C,** Meyerding retractor. **D,** Ribbon malleable retractor. (Reprinted with permission from Miltex Instrument Company, Bethpage, NY, 2004.)

that maintains tension on its two outwardly pointed tips (see Fig. 12-14, *A*). The instrument is available in a 14-cm (5½-inch) pediatric size and a 17-cm (6¾-inch) standard size. The larger version is available with ball stops to prevent excess tissue penetration. Weitlaner retractors range in size from 10 to 23.5 cm (4 to 9½ inches) and are available with 2-to-3 or 3-to-4 outwardly pointed blunt or sharp teeth (see Fig. 12-14, *B*). A 14-cm (5½-inch) Weitlaner is also available with solid blades (see Fig. 12-14, *C*). The *Beckman-Weitlaner* hybrid has blunt or sharp 3-to-4 teeth and hinged jaws (see Fig. 12-14, *D*). The hinge facilitates seating the instrument deep in the incision. The Balfour self-retaining abdominal retractor is available in 17.5- or 25-cm (7- or 10-inch) spreads and with 6.5- to 10-cm (2½- to 4-inch) deep, solid or fenestrated side blades (see Fig. 12-14, *E*). Finochietto rib spreaders have two bladed arms that are spread apart by a strong ratchet system (see Fig. 12-14, *F*). The blunt-ended blades are a standard 48 mm deep by 65 mm wide. The

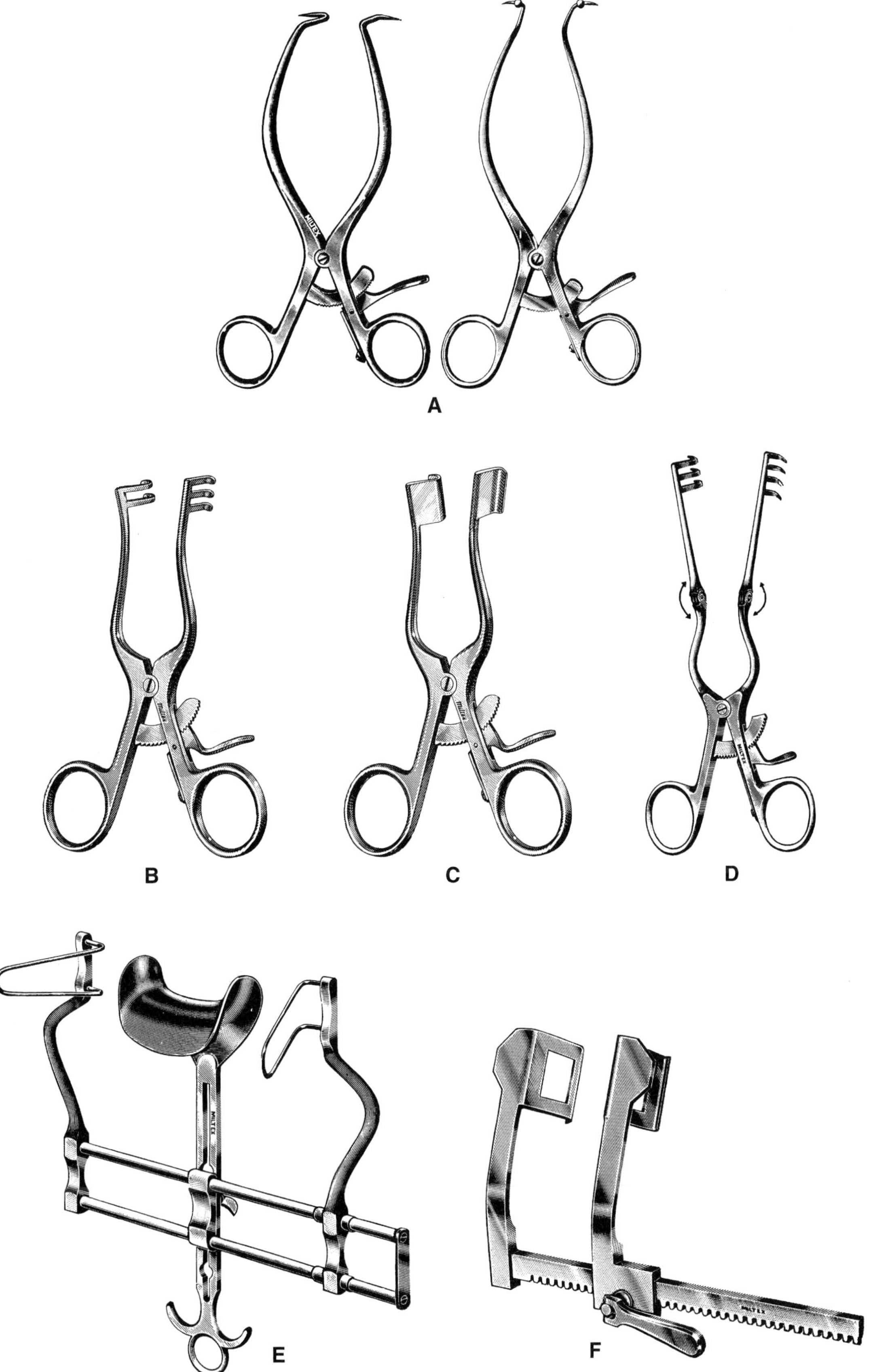

Figure 12-14. Self-retaining retractors. **A,** Gelpi retractor, with and without ball stops. **B,** Weitlaner retractor, 2-to-3 blade. **C,** Weitlaner retractor, solid blade. **D,** Beckman-Weitlaner retractor. **E,** Balfour retractor, open blades. **F,** Finochietto retractor. (Reprinted with permission from Miltex Instrument Company, Bethpage, NY, 2004.)

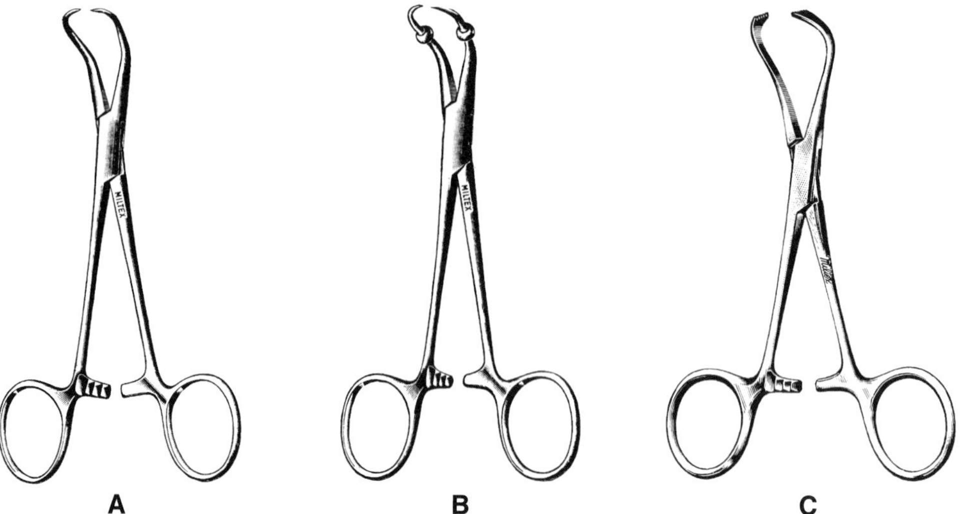

Figure 12-15. Towel clamps. **A,** Backhaus towel clamp. **B,** Roeder towel clamp. **C,** Lorna towel clamp. (Reprinted with permission from Miltex Instrument Company, Bethpage, NY, 2004.)

instrument is available with maximum spreads of 20, 25, or 30 cm (8, 10, or 12 inches).

Towel Clamps

Several types of towel clamps are available (Fig. 12-15). *Backhaus* and *Roeder* towel clamps are the most commonly used (see Fig. 12-15, *A* and *B*). The Roeder clamps have ball stops to prevent deep tissue penetration and minimize towel slippage. The Backhaus clamp is available in 9- and 13-cm (3½- and 5¼-inch) sizes, whereas the Roeder is available only in the larger size. The *Lorna* towel clamps are nonpenetrating and therefore ideal for securing suction lines and cables to drapes (see Fig. 12-15, *C*). Penetrating towel clamp tips should meet when closed, and they should be sharp and free of burrs.

Suction Tips

There are three basic types of suction tips available (Fig. 12-16). The *Yankauer* tip is relatively large, allowing the removal of large volumes of blood or fluid from the surgical site (see Fig. 12-16, *A*). The *Frazier-Ferguson* tip has the smallest diameter and is useful when working in confined areas (see Fig. 12-16, *B*). The suction intensity of these tips can be varied by placing the index finger over the hole located on the handle. Both models are available in stainless steel and in disposable plastic. The *Poole* suction tip has multiple ports along the tube, making it ideal for use within the abdomen, where single-orifice tubes are easily plugged by omentum (see Fig. 12-16, *C*).

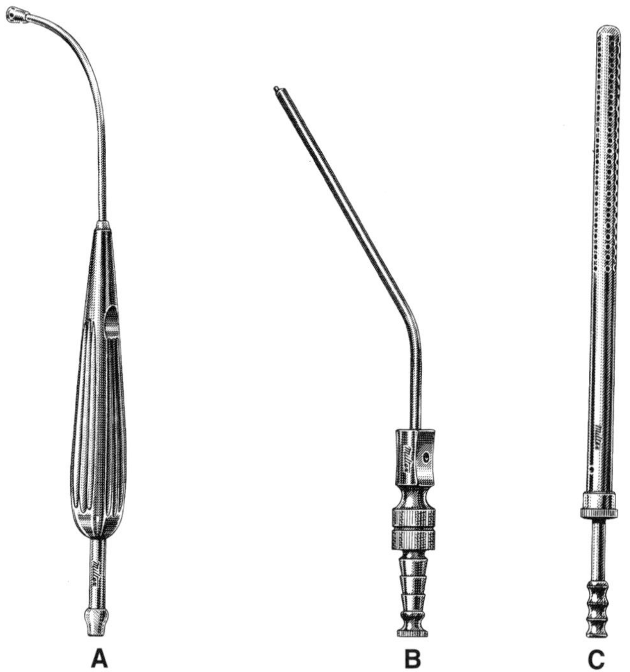

Figure 12-16. Suction tips. **A,** Yankauer suction tip. **B,** Frazier-Ferguson suction tip. **C,** Poole suction tip. (Reprinted with permission from Miltex Instrument Company, Bethpage, NY, 2004.)

ORTHOPEDIC INSTRUMENTS

A wide variety of instruments are associated with orthopedic surgery. Those presented here are used outside the realm of fracture repair. For information regarding instruments used for reconstruction and fracture treatment, the reader is referred to Chapter 81.

Rongeurs

Rongeurs have opposed cutting jaws that allow precise removal of bone, cartilage, and fibrous tissue (Fig. 12-17). Of the several types, most contain either a single- or a double-action mechanism and curved or straight jaws. The double-action rongeurs are stronger and have a smoother action. *Ruskin* rongeurs are available with 3-, 5-, or 7-mm bites. The slightly larger *Stille-Luer* rongeurs are available with 6×12- and 9×15-mm jaws.

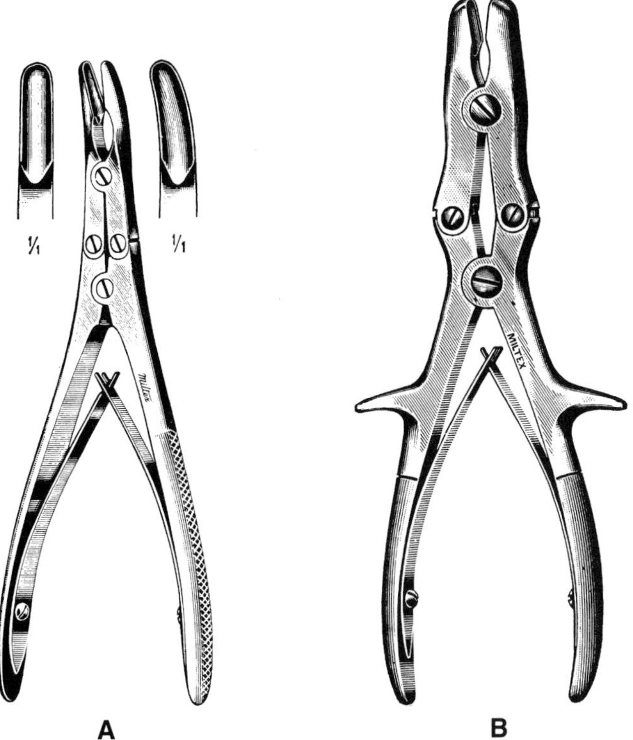

Figure 12-17. Rongeurs. **A,** Ruskin rongeur. **B,** Stille-Luer rongeur. (Reprinted with permission from Miltex Instrument Company, Bethpage, NY, 2004.)

Curets

Curets are easily recognized by their cuplike structure (Fig. 12-18). The sharp, oval or round edges are useful for removing diseased bone, debris, and damaged tissue from dense tissue surfaces. Their shape also makes them ideal for harvesting cancellous bone grafts. Several sizes of curets are available. The *Spratt* curets have a single oval cup at the end of a grooved handle, whereas the *Volkman* curets are double ended, having an oval cup on one end and a round cup on the other.

Periosteal Elevators

As their name suggests, periosteal elevators are designed to elevate periosteum and muscle attachments away from bone. Common elevators include the single-ended *Langenbeck* and *Key* elevators and the double-ended *Sayre* and *Freer* elevators (Fig. 12-19). The Langenbeck elevator is available with either a blunt or a sharp tip, whereas the Key elevator has only a blunt tip, but it comes in widths of up to 2.5 cm (1 inch). The double-ended elevators are narrow and have one end that is blunt and one that is sharp.

Bone-Cutting Instruments

Osteotomes, chisels, and gouges are all hand-held instruments that are used in combination with a mallet (Fig. 12-20). Gouges are easily distinguished by their concave shape. They are available in 4- to 38-mm widths. Osteotomes

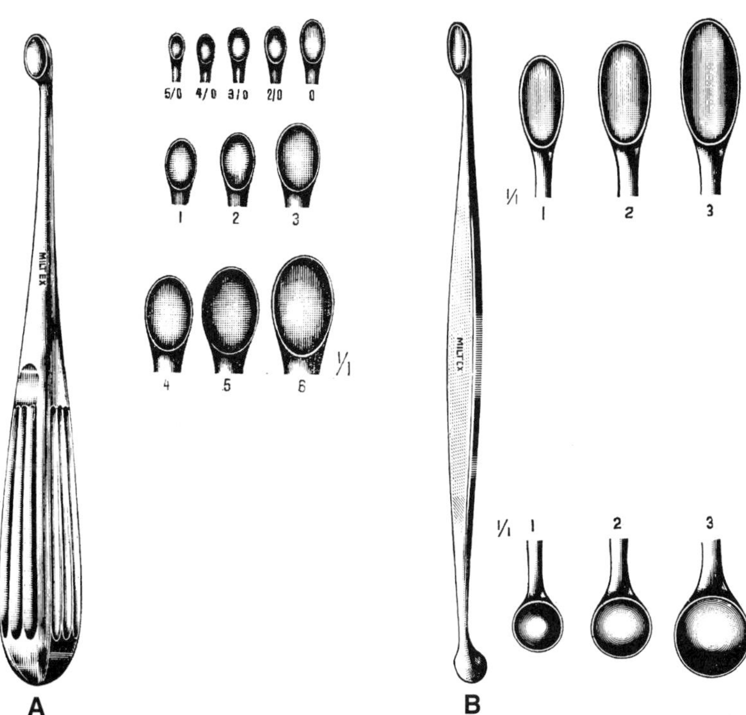

Figure 12-18. Curets. **A,** Spratt curet, with available cup sizes. **B,** Volkman curet, with available cup sizes. (Reprinted with permission from Miltex Instrument Company, Bethpage, NY, 2004.)

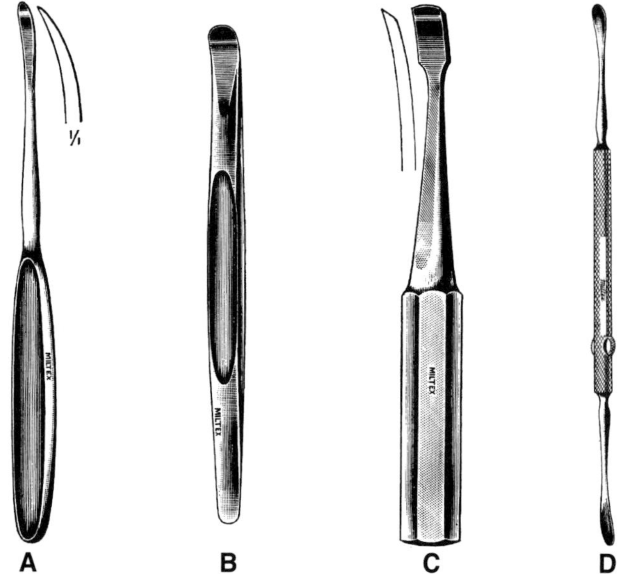

Figure 12-19. Periosteal elevators. **A,** Langenbeck periosteal elevator. **B,** Sayre periosteal elevator. **C,** Key periosteal elevator. **D,** Freer periosteal elevator. (Reprinted with permission from Miltex Instrument Company, Bethpage, NY, 2004.)

are double-beveled at their cutting tip, and chisels are single beveled. The cutting widths vary from 4 to 38 mm. The chisel tends to move in a direction away from the beveled edge. Therefore, it needs to be applied at a somewhat steeper angle relative to its axis. This allows the chisel to move along the bone surface on its beveled edge. If the chisel is reversed, it tends to dive into the bone, leaving sharp edges on the surface. The chisel is the preferred instrument to remove exostoses, but when the direction of bone cutting needs to be more precise, it is better controlled with an osteotome. Common types for these three cutting instruments are *Army-Navy, Hibbs,* and *Smith-Peterson.*

The mallet can be solid stainless steel or have an aluminum handle and a stainless steel head. Polyethylene-capped stainless steel heads are quieter and prevent the production of metal particle flake.

Bone-cutting forceps can be of the single- or double-action type, straight or angled. The *Liston* forceps are representatives of the single-action type, and *Ruskin* and *Stille-Liston* are double-action bone-cutting forceps (Fig. 12-21).

Trephines

Two types of trephines are available, *Michele* and *Galt* (Fig. 12-22). Both are T-shaped and capable of drilling a cylinder of bone. The Michele trephine is available in graduated inner diameters of 0.6 to 3.1 cm (¼ to 1¼ inch). It contains a graduated scale along its shaft, allowing the penetration depth to be measured. It cuts through bone on the end of the shaft only. The Galt trephine can cut bone at the end of the shaft and along the outside perimeter of the shaft. It is available in graduated sizes from 1.25 to 2.5 cm (½ to 1 inch) in diameter and has an adjustable central trocar. The trocar centers the trephine and stabilizes it until a circular trough is cut in the bone.

MICROSURGICAL INSTRUMENTS

Presently, reconstructive vascular and neural surgery is rarely performed in equine patients. The exceptions are thrombectomies, which may be performed with the help of catheters (see Chapter 14). Because horses are rarely used as research animals, microsurgical techniques play a minor role in these aspects. The microsurgical instruments used for ocular surgery can be found in Chapter 55.

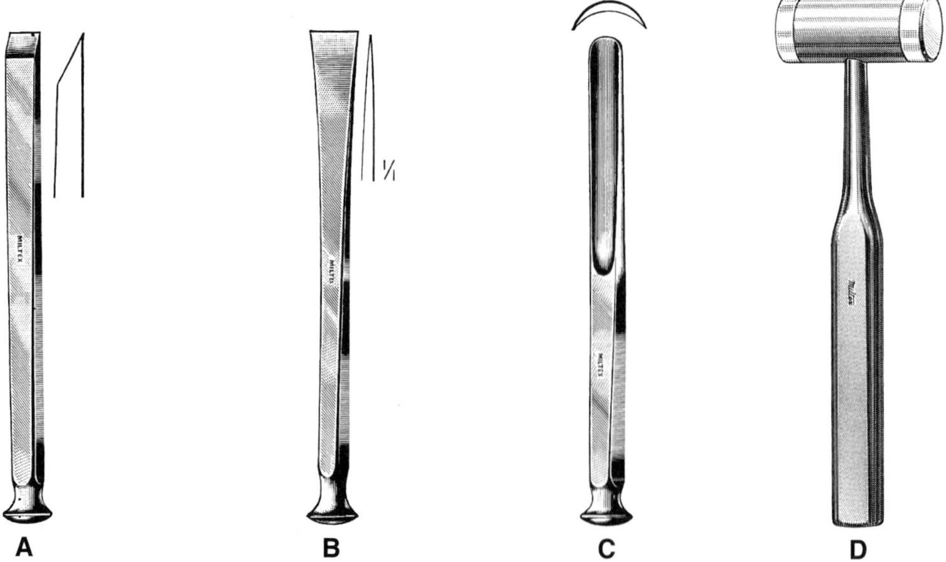

Figure 12-20. A, U.S. Army chisel. **B,** U.S. Army osteotome. **C,** U.S. Army gouge. **D,** Miltex mallet, with caps. (Reprinted with permission from Miltex Instrument Company, Bethpage, NY.)

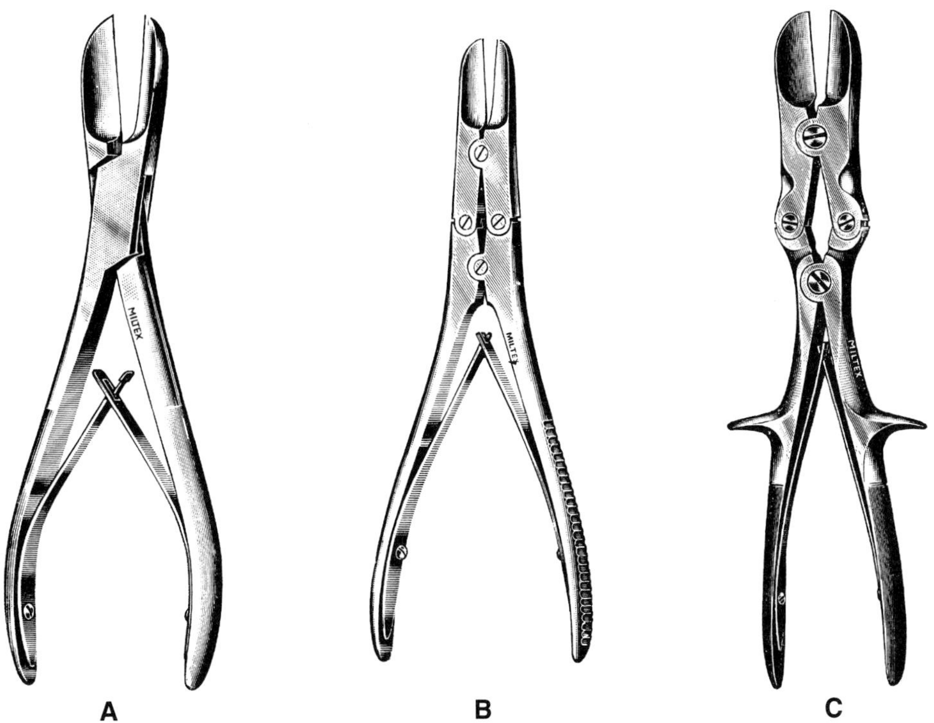

Figure 12-21. Bone cutting forceps. **A,** Liston forceps. B, Ruskin forceps. C, Stille-Liston forceps. (Reprinted with permission from Miltex Instrument Company, Bethpage, NY, 2004.)

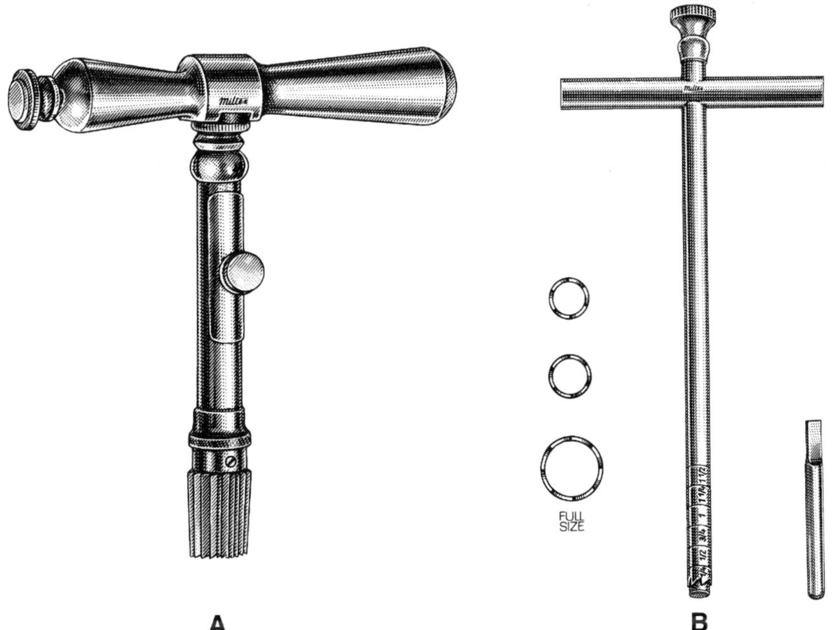

Figure 12-22. Trephines. **A,** Galt trephine. **B,** Michele trephine. (Reprinted with permission from Miltex Instrument Company, Bethpage, NY, 2004.)

INSTRUMENT MAINTENANCE

Proper care maintains long-term instrument serviceability. Instruments should be cleaned immediately after use. Care should be taken to separate sharp and delicate instruments from other instruments that may damage them. When washing them by hand, it is best to use warm water, a neutral-pH detergent, and a soft bristle brush. Ultrasonic cleaners are more effective than hand washing; however, the manufacturer's recommendations for type of water, such as deionized or distilled, and detergent used should be followed (see "Cleaning" in Chapter 10). If cleaning cannot be done immediately, instruments should be submerged, in the open position, in a solution of water and neutral-pH detergent. Hard water, saline solution, and non-neutral-pH detergents (dish washing liquids) should be avoided, because surface discoloration, corrosion, and poor mechanics of the joints may result.[7] Once cleaned, instruments should be rinsed with de-ionized or distilled water. Instruments with a working action should then be treated with an instrument lubricant (instrument milk). The lubricant, which often includes a rust inhibitor, should not be rinsed off. Instruments are then dried and stored or resterilized.

Instrument refurbishing programs are available through most instrument manufacturers. In addition to resharpening cutting edges and replacing tungsten carbide inserts, instruments are cleaned, polished, and refinished to retard corrosion. Refurbishing generally costs less than replacement.

IDENTIFICATION

Instruments are frequently marked to identify their owner or their belonging to an instrument set. Various identification methods are available. Commercially available engravers should be avoided, as should any other method that damages the surface of the instrument. Surface damage, with removal of the corrosion-resistant coating, will shorten instrument life. Electrochemical etching units are acceptable as long as they are properly used. After etching, the instrument must be thoroughly rinsed to neutralize the acid etching fluid.

Autoclavable plastic tapes for instrument identification are available in different colors and are easy to apply. Color coding with tape does not harm the instrument surface. All instruments belonging to a specific set can be marked with the same color. This is helpful in large clinics, where different surgical teams work parallel to each other with different instrument sets. During cleaning and resterilization, instruments belonging to different sets may be mingled. The color coding allows easy and efficient separation. Poorly applied tape, however, may begin to peel off, creating crevices that could harbor debris and microorganisms. Proper selection of a tape marking system should include considerations of color, durability, and adhesive properties to ensure a long life once applied to the instrument. Higher-quality marking systems are frequently marketed through instrument manufacturing companies.

PACK PREPARATION AND STORAGE

Tightly woven linen drapes have long been used to package instrument sets. Their disadvantages include short shelf-life and the cost of laundering for reuse. Because microorganisms can fairly rapidly penetrate linen wrappers, it is prudent to double-wrap the sets with linens. Safe storage times have been established[8] (see Table 10-1).

A variety of paper-type products have been developed to replace linen wrappers. Although these products share some of the disadvantages of linen, they offer longer safe storage times, because the sterilization process closes the pores within the sheet. As a result, these paper-type products cannot be reused and are therefore disposable, so laundry expenses are avoided. On the other hand, disposal costs and the burden on the environment through exhaust gases (e.g., CO_2) from incinerators rise. Many of the newer paper-type wrappers handle like linen.

Both paper and linen prevent visualization of the instruments within the pack. In the case of sets, this is not a problem because the contents are known. However, if instruments are separately wrapped, visualization is important. Therefore, special wraps that consist of a sheet of paper on one side and a clear plastic sheet on the other have become popular. The plastic side allows the instrument to be seen inside, and the paper side allows steam or ethylene oxide to penetrate the package. Sharp points of instruments have to be covered by plastic caps to prevent inadvertent damage to the paper layer. These wrappers are available in tube rolls in several sizes, and most of them contain sterilization indicators (see Chapter 10). The ends are heat sealed. Safe storage time is extended with this type of wrapping, but the paper side is still susceptible to microorganism penetration when wet.

Regardless of the type of wrapping chosen, the instruments should be loosely packed with the jaws slightly opened to allow circulation of steam, ethylene oxide, or gas

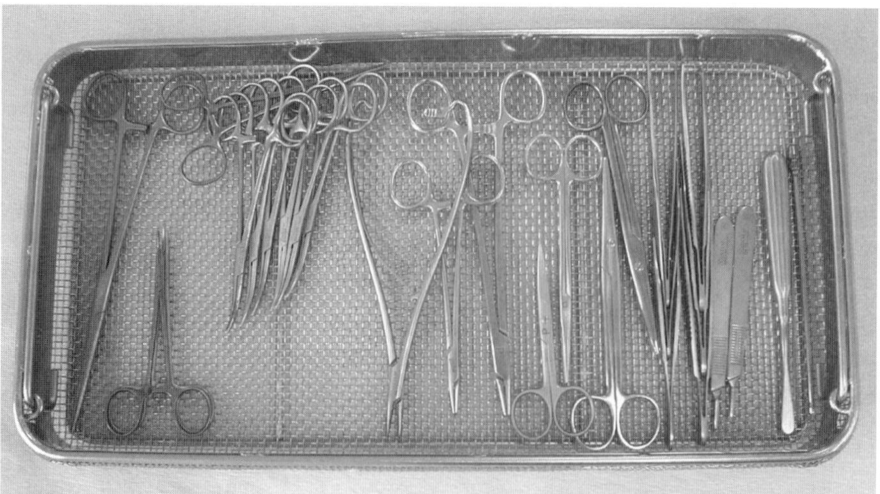

Figure 12-23. Example of a standard soft tissue set. The instruments are neatly arranged in a logical sequence.

plasma[9] (Fig.12-23). All instrument packs should be dated and labeled for easy identification, and for resterilization if they are not used within the safe storage timeframe. For prolonged storage life, the packs may be placed within a plastic envelope or into a glass closet.

Lately, reusable metal sterilization containers enjoy renewed popularity, after having almost disappeared in the late 1980s (Steriset Containers, Wagner GmbH, Munich, Germany) (see Fig. 10-1). These containers are used for holding surgical instrument sets or textiles during vacuum-steam sterilization procedures, and for maintaining sterility of the contents during storage and transport under hospital conditions. They operate with either filters or valves. The filter units are single-use filters, or reusable textile filters with known service life spans. SteriSet valve containers have a closed base and permanent stainless steel pressure-sensitive valves in the inner lid. The sterilization valves react to the change in pressure during the sterilization process. During the vacuum phase, the valves open upward, and the air/steam mixture can escape from the container. During the pressurization phase, the valves open inwardly and allow steam to enter the container. The system is automatically flushed and sterilized by the hot steam rushing through the valve with every sterilization cycle. Outside the sterilizer (i.e., during storage or transport), the valve is closed and serves as a barrier to microorganisms.

REFERENCES

1. Hurov L et al: Handbook of Veterinary Surgical Instruments and Glossary of Surgical Terms, Philadelphia, 1978, WB Saunders.
2. Clem M: Surgical instruments. In Auer JA, editor: Equine Surgery, Philadelphia, 1992, WB Saunders.
3. Provost PJ: Surgical instruments. In Auer JA, Stick JA, editors: Equine Surgery, ed 2, Philadelphia, 1999, WB Saunders.
4. Nieves MA, Merkley DF, Wagner SD: Surgical instruments. In Slatter DH, editor: Textbook of Small Animal Surgery, ed 3, Philadelphia, 2003, WB Saunders.
5. Miltex Instrument Company: Miltex Surgical Instruments, Lake Success, NY, 2003, Miltex Instrument Company, Inc
6. Fucci V, Elkins AD: Electrosurgery: Principles and guidelines in veterinary medicine, Comp Contin Educ Pract Vet 1991;13:407.
7. Patterson CJW, Mackay AM: The effect of ultrasonic cleaning and autoclaving on tungsten carbide burs, Br Dent J 1988;164:113.
8. Selwyn S: Aseptic rituals unmasked, Br Med J 1984;289:1642.
9. Ritter MA, Eitzen H, French MLV, et al: Operating room environment as affected by people and the surgical face mask, Clin Orthop Rel Res 1975;111:147.

CHAPTER 13

Surgical Techniques

Jörg A. Auer

Surgery can be defined as goal-oriented violence to tissue and, therefore, considerations related to minimizing tissue damage are an important part of adequate preoperative planning and proper surgical technique.[1] Adequate preparation for each surgery is the best prevention of unnecessary delays that prolong surgery. Before embarking on an unfamiliar or complicated surgical task, the operator should plan the procedure in a step-by-step manner from skin incision to closure. This chapter describes those aspects of surgical manipulations that are basic to the performance of any procedure—namely, the different techniques of incision, excision, and dissection of tissue, in addition to the methods of surgical hemostasis, tissue retraction and handling, and surgical irrigation and suction. Adherence to the basic principles of state-of-the-art surgical technique, described by Halsted, minimizes tissue trauma, blood loss, and wound dehiscence, resulting in a better surgical result.[2]

BASIC MANIPULATIONS OF SURGICAL INSTRUMENTS

Incising or cutting into tissue represents the initial step of every surgical intervention. The instruments used for this procedure and the manner in which they are applied provide the surgeon with the means to vary the type of incision and its effects on the surrounding tissue. The scalpel and scissors are the basic instruments for incising or excising tissues. Separation along tissue planes is usually accomplished through blunt dissection. Electrosurgery and laser surgery complement the instruments used for incisions and excisions.

Scalpels

Steel Scalpel

The steel scalpel with disposable blades is the instrument most frequently used to incise skin and other soft tissues. It is prudent to apply the blade to the scalpel handle with the help of a needle holder or similar instrument to prevent inadvertent puncture of the surgery gloves, or even worse, cutting of the surgeon's fingers.

There are three ways to hold the blade handle: the pencil grip, the fingertip grip, and the palm grip.[3] With the pencil grip, very precise cuts can be performed. The distal end of the scalpel handle is grasped between the thumb and index finger and rests on the middle finger, while the tip of the middle finger contacts the patient (Fig. 13-1). The surgeon's hand also rests lightly on the patient and the fingers are moved rather than the entire arm, which allows better control of the blade. This grip works best for short incisions where precision is important.[4] Contact with the patient controls precisely the depth of penetration. The disadvantage of this grip compared with the others is the relatively steep angle with which the scalpel is held, thereby decreasing cutting edge contact with the skin.

For the fingertip grip, the tips of the third, fourth, and fifth fingers are placed underneath the handle, while the tip of the thumb is placed on the other side. The index finger

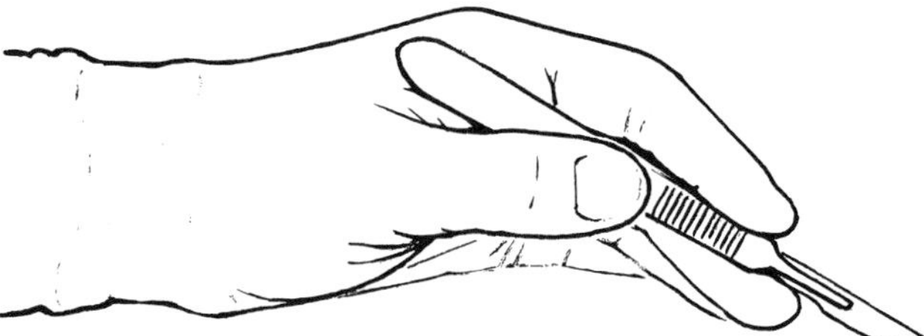

Figure 13-1. The pencil grip for holding a surgical scalpel.

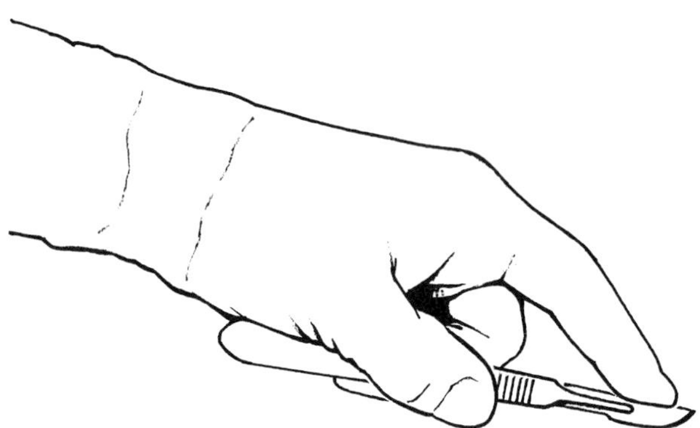

Figure 13-2. The fingertip grip for holding a surgical scalpel.

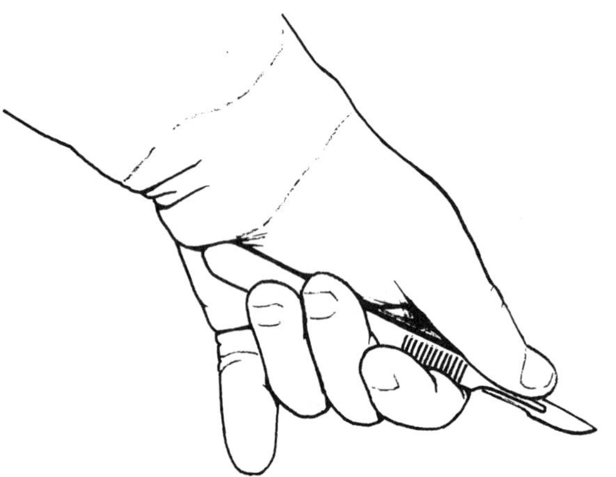

Figure 13-3. The palm grip for holding a surgical scalpel.

rests on the top surface of the blade to create controlled, downward pressure (Fig. 13-2). This grip is useful for long straight, curved, or sigmoidal incisions, because it places the long surface of the blade against the tissue, providing greater cutting surface, better control of the blade angle, and optimal control of incision depth. The blade movement originates in the shoulder, with the entire arm participating in directing the incision.[5]

The palm grip is not commonly used. Some surgeons prefer it for standing flank incisions. It provides the strongest grasp of the scalpel. The scalpel is grasped with the fingers and palm wrapped around the handle, while the thumb is placed on the top edge of the blade to create downward pressure (Fig. 13-3). The small finger is resting on the patient to steady the hand.

Electro Scalpel

Proper cutting technique with the electro scalpel (see Fig. 12-4) differs markedly from that with the steel scalpel. A modified pencil grip is used to hold the instrument almost perpendicular to the tissue surface to be cut, to minimize the area of energy contact at the point of incision. The use of a needle scalpel further minimizes the contact area. The hand piece is held between the thumb and the middle finger tips, leaving the index finger free to activate the trigger button of the hand piece.

Scissors

Operating scissors cut tissues by moving edge contact between two blades that are set slightly toward one another.[6] This action is most effective near the tips of the instrument, dictating their use for precise tissue cutting. Tissues that are too thick or too dense to be cut with the tips of the scissors should be separated with either a larger pair of scissors or a scalpel blade. The blade near the hinge should not be used for cutting, because the tissues are crushed more than cut, resulting in devitalization.

As shown in Chapter 12, many scissors are available with straight and slightly curved blades. The mechanical aspect of scissor cutting is best achieved with straight blades, so straight-bladed scissors should be used in dense tissues. Curved scissors provide a more comfortable positioning of the surgeon's hand and better visualization of the tips in deeper planes, but these instruments are less efficient in cutting tissues.

The classic tripod grip provides the best functional result. The tip of the thumb and last digit of the third finger are placed in the rings of the scissors, while the index finger stabilizes the instrument along the shaft toward the tip of the blades (Fig. 13-4). The tripod formed by the thumb, third finger, and index finger creates a stable and powerful base for cutting.

Suture scissors are usually held in the classic tripod grip to cut the sutures at the designated spot. Because it is the surgeon who is responsible for the lengths of the suture ends, an adequate length must be presented to the assistant so that the scissors can be applied at the desired spot.

A surgeon working without an assistant may use a pair of *Olsen-Hegar* needle holders with the built-in suture scissors, or the suture scissors can be held in the same hand as the needle holders in the manner described for handling multiple hemostats (see later).

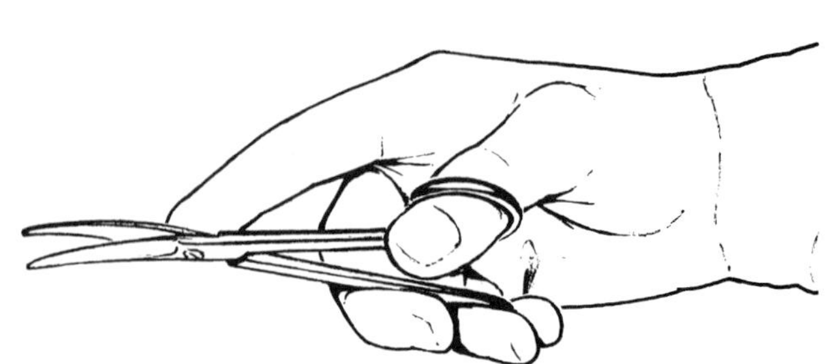

Figure 13-4. The tripod grip for holding surgical scissors.

Needle Holders

There are two methods for holding needle holders. One is the classic tripod grip just described for scissors. This method works best when precise suture placement is indicated. The other is the palm grip, which is useful for rapid instrument manipulation in closure of tissue when precision is not essential; however, the palm grip is not universally accepted as proper technique.[3] With the palm grip, also referred to as the modified thenar eminence grip, the surgeon places the instrument in the palm of the hand with the one ring resting against the thenar eminence of the thumb. The index finger stabilizes the instrument along the shaft. The lock mechanism is disengaged by lateral pressure applied to the instrument using the thenar eminence. The tips of the instrument may be opened and closed by adduction and abduction movements of the thumb. This method of manipulation is useful for rapid closure, because it allows the needle to be more easily grasped, extracted, and readied for the next pass.[7]

A needle holder grips the suture needle along its shaft so that the needle is perpendicular to and near the tip of the instrument. The needle is usually grasped mid-shaft, but it can be grasped closer to the needle tip for greater precision.[7] The needle is passed through tissue by rotation of the surgeon's hand, always following the curve of the needle. Care should be taken to advance the needle so that it protrudes out of the tissue enough to allow the needle holder or tissue forceps to grasp it far enough behind the tip to prevent dulling or bending of the needle. When using the needle holder, the surgeon may pronate the hand for greater precision or supinate the hand for greater speed.[7]

Forceps

Thumb Forceps

Thumb tissue forceps are used to manipulate and stabilize tissue during incising and closing. Thumb forceps are usually held in the nondominant hand using a pencil grip. When not in use, they may rest in the palm.[7] If the surgeon's hand becomes fatigued, the natural tendency is to switch to a palm grip. This grip is less precise and more likely to incite unnecessary tissue trauma.

When closing deep tissue layers, thumb forceps are useful for retracting superficial layers during needle placement, starting on the far side of the incision (Fig. 13-5). As the needle is passed, the forceps moves to the layer being closed, exposing the exit point. The process continues with the tissue forceps being used to grasp tissue layers in opposite order on the near and far side of the incision.[5]

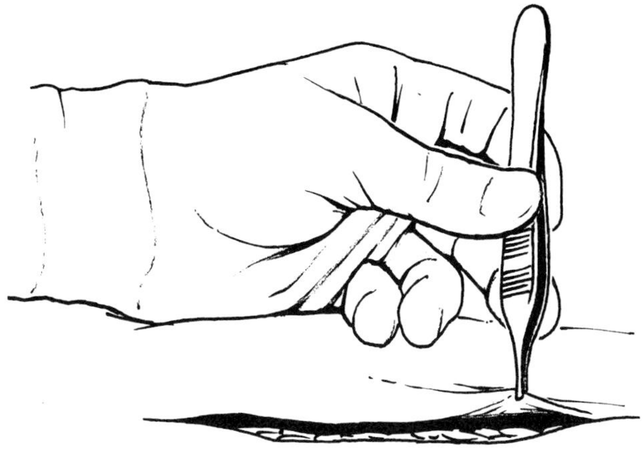

Figure 13-5. Proper technique for holding and using thumb forceps.

Hemostat Forceps

Mosquito and other tissue forceps used for hemostasis are held in the classic tripod grip to grasp the vessel to be ligated. When a surgical assistant is not available and several hemostats have to be applied, time can be saved by introducing the ring finger through the left ring of several such instruments and holding them in the palm of the right hand, while applying a hemostat to a vessel in the tripod grip with the same hand (Fig. 13-6). By arranging the hemostats so that the tips point toward the thumb, the instruments can one by one be rotated into the tripod grip and applied to a bleeding vessel.

Tissue Forceps

The most commonly used tissue forceps in equine surgery are towel clamps, mosquito forceps, Allis tissue forceps, Ochsner forceps, and Carmalt forceps. All these forceps are applied to tissues with the tripod grip. Towel clamps are useful during some procedures for tissue manipulation even though their primary purpose is to secure drapes on the patient. Towel clamps attached to skin edges provide an atraumatic method of retraction for exposing deeper tissues. Because Allis tissue forceps and Ochsner forceps are traumatic and crush the tissue, they are best reserved for securing tissue that can be excised.

TISSUE INCISION AND EXCISION

Slide Cutting

The skin is usually incised with a scalpel because this is the method that is least traumatic and most conducive to primary healing. The incision should be made in one smooth pass of the scalpel through the skin, using the slide-cutting technique, transecting the dermis without cutting deep

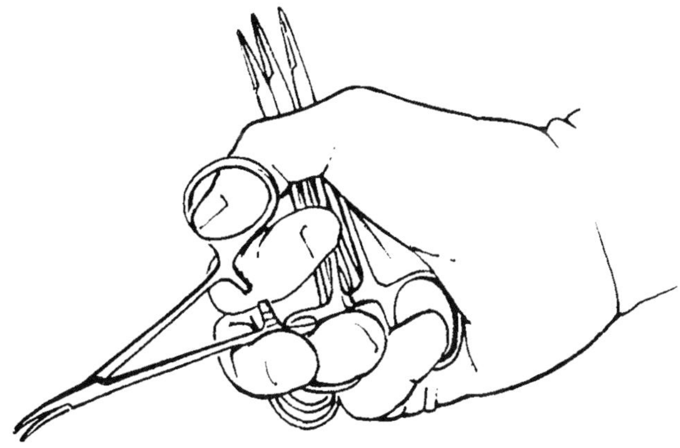

Figure 13-6. Several mosquito forceps are held in the surgeon's palm, allowing effective application to a number of vessels, one after the other.

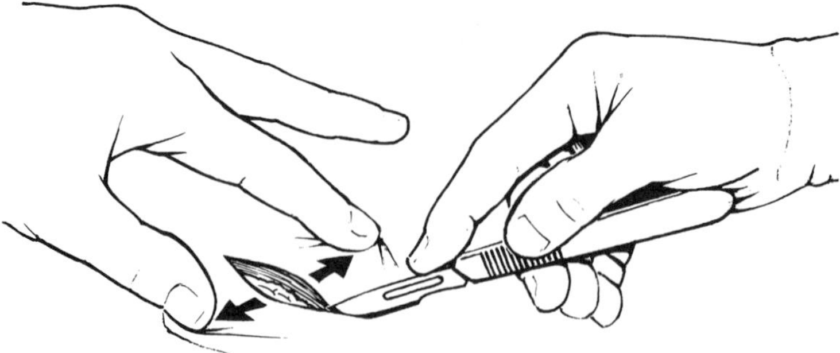

Figure 13-7. Stabilizing and stretching the skin between the thumb and index finger facilitates the incising of the skin.

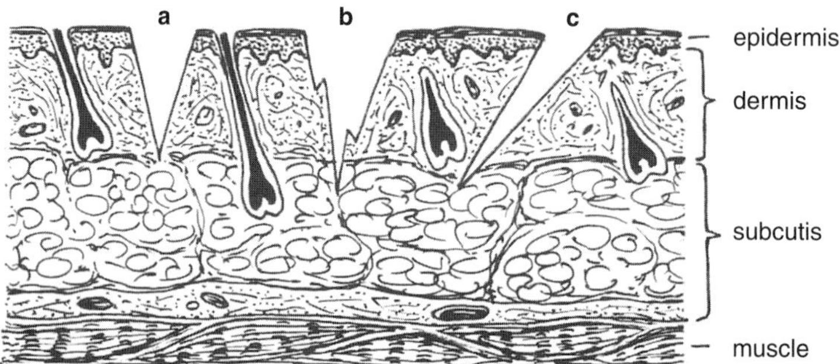

Figure 13-8. Skin incisions. *a,* Correctly performed incision. *b,* Timid slide-cutting resulted in jagged incision edges. *c,* Slide cutting with a sideways-angled blade resulted in an obliquely angled skin incision.

fascial tissue. The surgeon's free hand should stabilize and stretch the skin being incised (Fig. 13-7). When properly transected, skin edges will retract. In a longer incision, it may be necessary to reposition the free hand to put tension on the skin along the entire incision. During this repositioning, the scalpel should not be lifted from the tissues. Each time the scalpel leaves and returns to the tissue, a jagged edge is created that will adversely affect healing[8] (Fig. 13-8).

Stab or Press-Cutting Incision

Stab or press-cutting incisions are generally performed with the scalpel held in the pencil grip in a vertical position (Fig. 13-9). A stab incision results when the bursting threshold of the tissue being incised is exceeded. Press cutting is applied to initiate incisions into hollow, fluid-filled structures, such as the bladder. For this technique to be effective, the tissue to be entered should be under tension. Press-cutting incisions are also used frequently during screw fixation of an anatomically reduced condylar fracture of MCIII/MTIII or of the proximal phalanx. The scalpel is held in a pencil or palm grip, perpendicular to the surface of the tissue. The tissue is entered with a slight thrust, and the incision is extended carefully by pushing the cutting edge of the scalpel through the tissue. With this technique, depth control is poor, but it can be improved by using the index finger as a bumper (Fig. 13-10), effectively limiting penetration of the blade to a predetermined depth.[7] Press cutting with an inverted blade

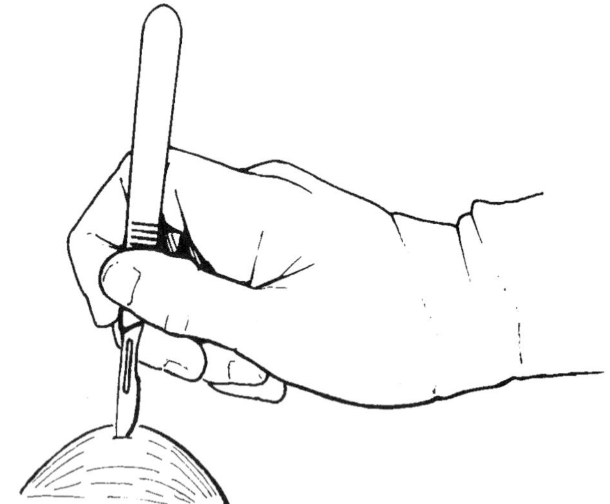

Figure 13-9. Stab or press cutting into a hollow organ.

(Fig. 13-11) elevates the tissues to be transected and provides more safety for the deeper- laying structures, while preventing fluid from exiting a fluid-filled structure or organ.

Two rarely applied techniques are the sawing (or push-pull slide cutting) and the scalpel scraping technique, the latter of which is used to separate fascial planes or for subperiosteal dissection and elevation of muscles.[7]

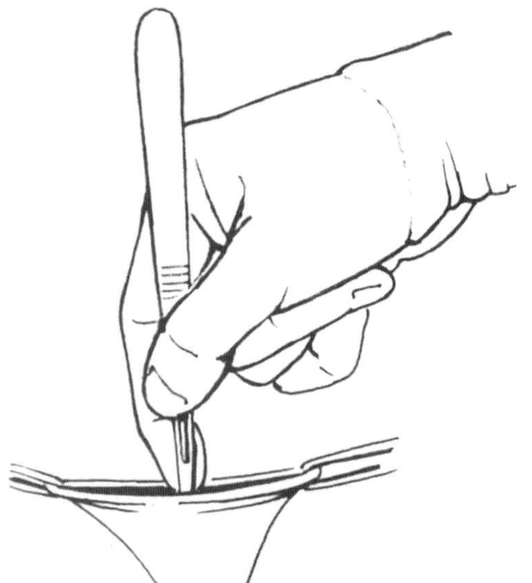

Figure 13-10. Bumper-cutting into a structure elevated and stretched between two Allis forceps.

Scissor Incisions

The scissor tips are often used to transect tissues. Before this technique is used, the tissue to be incised must be isolated from underlying tissues using blunt scissor dissection (see later). This isolates the tissue structures to be cut. Some tissues can be effectively transected by partially opening the scissors, holding the blades motionless relative to each other, and pushing them through the tissue. Allowing the scissors to slide through the tissue creates a clean, atraumatic incision. This method is appropriate for opening fascial planes over muscles or subcutis, or for opening tissue planes in which the start and finish points of the incision are well defined.

Electroincision

Because lateral heat production during electroincision increases with the duration of trigger activation and tissue contact time, the blade is moved at a speed of about 7 mm/s.[7] Only one tissue plane is cut at a time, using only the tip of the blade. Depth control with the electro scalpel is less precise than with the cold scalpel. Because the electrode cuts all tissue it contacts, visual control is of paramount importance. Electrosurgical incision should not be used in areas with ill-defined anatomic planes. Thermal necrosis at the wound edges can be reduced and depth control can be improved by using the lowest setting on the controls that allows clean cutting.

The electrode should be cleaned frequently to ensure proper function. Charred tissue that accumulates at the tip of the electrode acts as an insulator and decreases effective cutting. Three undesirable effects are associated with a charred electrode: (1) higher power is required to incise tissues, (2) current is dispersed to a larger area of tissue, diminishing control, and (3) thermal necrosis of the wound edges is increased.[2] If the buildup of charred material at the tip is rapid or excessive, the power setting may be too high or the cutting speed may be too slow.[9]

Advantages reported for electrosurgical incisions over those made with a steel scalpel are (1) reduction in total blood loss, (2) decreased need for ligatures, and thus reduction in the amount of foreign material left in the wound, and (3) reduced operating time.[10,11] These advantages come at the expense of delayed wound healing and decreased resistance of wounds to infection. Controlled experiments revealed that there is no overall difference in epithelial healing between incisions made with the electro scalpel and those made with the steel scalpel. However, a difference in the initial response of the connective tissue was recorded.[5] Electro incisions of the skin heal primarily, but there is a definite lag time in reaching maximal strength. Because of this delay, skin sutures or staples should remain in place an additional 2 to 3 days if the incision was made with an electro scalpel. Electrosurgical incisions should be avoided in the presence of cyclopropane, ether, alcohol, and certain bowel gases because of the risks of ignition and explosion.[7]

Tissue Excision

Most tissues are excised primarily by scalpels or scissors. Skin, hollow organs, contaminated subcutaneous tissues, and neoplastic tissues are best excised with a scalpel. This is performed by a single passage of the scalpel along or around the periphery of the tissue to be removed. However, repeated passes or a sawing action with the scalpel may be necessary to complete excision of the tissue. This is especially true for thick, dense tissue or en bloc excision. Precise excision of

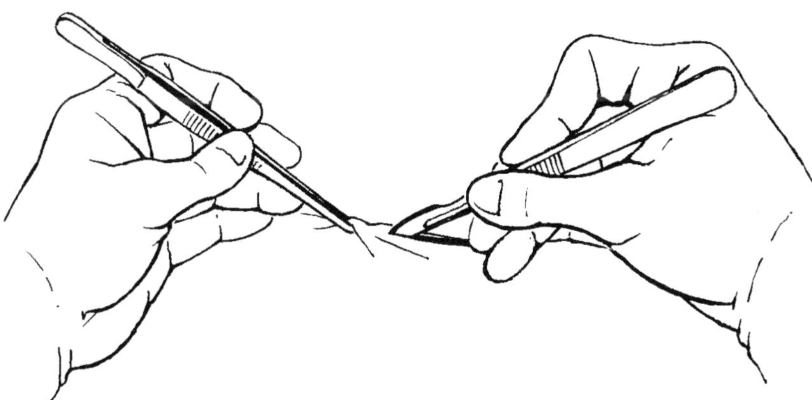

Figure 13-11. The technique of inverted-blade press cutting facilitates blade control.

tissue deep within surgical wounds or body cavities is best performed with scissors.

BLUNT DISSECTION

Blunt dissection is used to reduce or prevent the risk of damaging deeper vital structures during a surgical approach. The technique is performed digitally or with surgical scissors. Blunt dissection is generally carried out along natural tissue planes or parallel to tissue fibers. Excessive dissection and undermining should be avoided, because creation of dead space impedes wound healing and potentiates infection. If scissors are used, the tips are placed in a closed position into the tissue, and the jaws are opened parallel to the tissue fibers or along natural tissue planes (Fig. 13-12). Forceps can be used to stabilize the tissue during dissection. When digital dissection is applied, the gloved index finger of each hand is placed side by side in the same tissue plane and pulled in opposite directions to stretch and separate the tissue, thus increasing surgical wound exposure.

Scissors are useful for dissecting tissues, especially the subcutaneous tissue. The plane of dissection is parallel with the skin, along the incision edges. Limited dissection underneath the skin allows further retraction of the skin away from the center of the incision and facilitates visualization of deeper tissues. Scissor dissection is less useful, and potentially dangerous, in deeper dissections, where vessels or nerves could be severed before they are seen.

SURGICAL HEMOSTASIS

Proper hemostasis prevents the surgical field from being obscured by blood, and it decreases the potential for infection. Hemostasis minimizes blood loss and postoperative hematoma or seroma formation, which may delay healing or potentiate wound dehiscence. Additionally, excessive or uncontrolled hemorrhage can lead to anemia or hypovolemic shock.[7] Therefore, the goal of hemostasis is to prevent blood flow from incised or transected vessels. This is accomplished primarily by interruption of blood flow to the involved area or by direct closure of the vessel walls.[12] There are mechanical, thermal, and chemical techniques to achieve hemostasis.

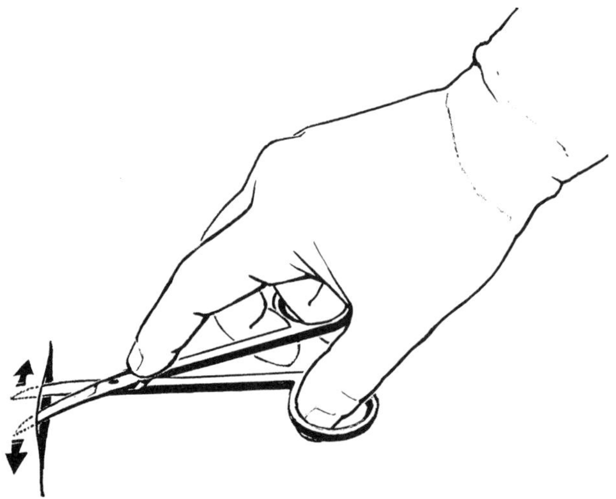

Figure 13-12. Blunt dissection of subcutaneous tissue can be performed by spreading the jaws of the scissors in the tissues.

Mechanical Hemostasis

Pressure

Pressure can be applied directly over the site of a major vessel, or over a major vessel at a site remote from the wound, using the fingers or the hand. Oozing from small vessels is best controlled by direct pressure using sterile gauze. Although this is the least traumatic means of vascular hemostasis, it is not adequate for medium-size and larger vessels, which require some other means of hemostasis.

Gauze packing is used to control hemorrhage from open body cavities (such as the nasal cavity, paranasal sinuses, urogenital tract, and defects created in the hoof wall or sole) and from large body wounds. Hemorrhage is controlled through pressure, allowing time for clot formation. The gauze can be soaked in iced or chilled saline solution, or diluted epinephrine can be added to the saline solution to help control the bleeding. Several gauze rolls tied together may need to be used to effectively pack large defects. The end of the packing is best secured to the body to ensure its presence at the time of removal.

Ligatures

Hemostats can be applied to small, noncritical vessels and held there for a few minutes. The vessel tissue trapped in the jaws is crushed, effectively occluding the vessel.[12] A combination of vasospasms and intravascular coagulation maintains hemostasis when the clamp is released. To facilitate these events, the vessel can be stretched or twisted before the instrument is released. If bleeding control from a critical vessel is necessary, atraumatic hemostatic clamps can be used to limit damage and allow repair.

Suture ligation is commonly used to control bleeding from larger vessels. Absorbable suture material is preferred over nonabsorbable material, as the latter can result in extrusion or sinus tract formation.[12] The number of ligatures required to maintain occlusion depends on vessel size and the material used. A simple circumferential ligature is generally used for small vessels (Fig. 13-13, *A*), whereas pulsating or large vessels, such as arteries, should be ligated with two ligatures, a circumferential followed by a transfixation ligature placed more distally (Fig. 13-13, *B*). This will prevent the circumferential ligature from slipping.

In most situations, a hemostatic clamp is applied to the vessel prior to ligation. The clamp's crushing effect facilitates ligature placement and vessel occlusion. The following steps for proper use of hemostatic forceps should be kept in mind[4]:

1. The smallest forceps that will accomplish the needed hemostasis should be used.
2. Only as much tissue is clamped as is necessary.
3. The tip of the instrument should be used rather than the middle or the base.
4. The mosquito forceps should be applied to small bleeding vessels perpendicular to the cut surface.

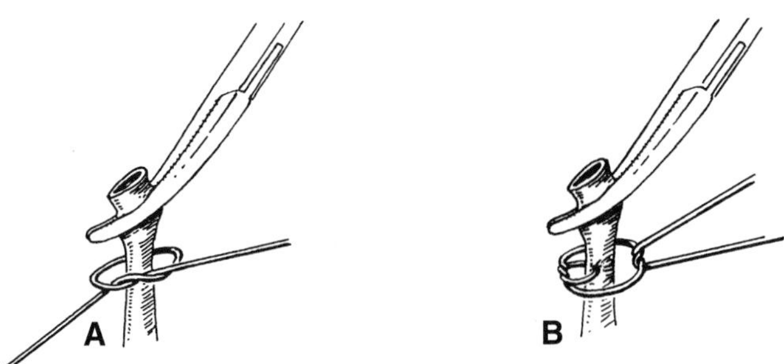

Figure 13-13. Circumferential (**A**) and transfixation (**B**) ligatures.

5. Other forceps should be applied perpendicular to the long axis of the vessel to be ligated.
6. The mosquito forceps should be applied to surface bleeders so that they come to rest lateral to the incision, with the concave part of the curved blades pointing down. In deeper locations, such as in the abdominal cavity, the forceps should be placed such that the tips point upward.
7. The assistant should pick up the hemostat and direct it with the tip pointing toward the surgeon.
8. The hemostat should be held in the nondominant hand. One ring is held between the index finger and the thumb, and the other ring rests on the middle and ring fingers (Fig. 13-14).
9. At the time of the final tightening of the first half hitch around the vessel, the surgeon should give the assistant the sign to release the hemostat.
10. The assistant releases the hemostat by pushing up with the middle and ring fingers while pressing down with the thumb, carefully releasing the ratchet mechanism of the hemostat.
11. Before releasing the hemostat, the instrument should be directed into the incision to release tension on the vessel and prevent it from slipping out of the ligature before the ligature is completely tightened.
12. The surgeon should apply a second half-hitch over the first one, forming a square knot.
13. Then, the assistant should cut the suture ends at the level indicated by the surgeon, with the suture scissors held in the dominant hand. If double ligation is indicated, clamps are placed at each ligature site, approximately 2 to 3 mm apart. Once the vessel is clamped, a circumferential ligature is placed around the vessel adjacent to the proximal hemostat. As the ligature is tightened, the clamp is released. The ligature should fall into the area of the vessel crushed by the clamp. The distal clamp is released and replaced with a transfixation ligature.

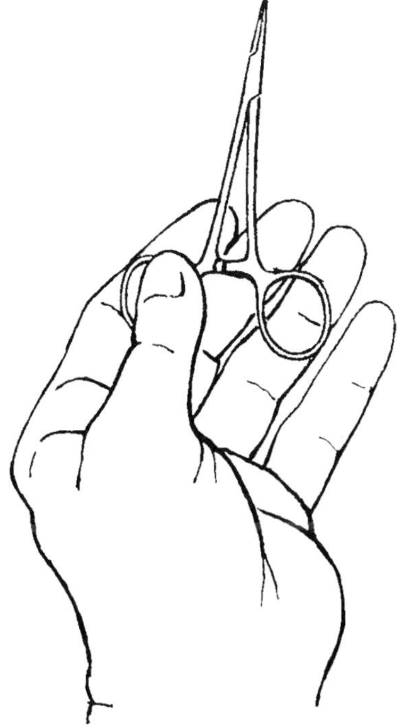

Figure 13-14. The hemostat is held in the nondominant hand. One ring is held between the index finger and the thumb, and the other ring rests on the middle and ring fingers. Pressing the rings toward one another releases the hemostat handle lock.

Large pedicles are preferably divided into smaller units, and each is separately ligated. After ligating the last unit, a suture is placed around the combined units and tied as one pedicle ligation. This is called the "divide and conquer" method.[7] The three-forceps method involves initial clamping of the pedicle with three parallel forceps 1 to 1.5 cm apart, incorporating the entire pedicle. The pedicle is transected between two such forceps, leaving one side with one forceps and the other with two forceps. A loose ligature is applied around the entire pedicle with the two forceps between the base of the pedicle and the first forceps. This forceps is then partially taken off, leaving a strand of crushed tissue behind. The ligature is now solidly tightened, making sure that it comes to lie over the crushed line of tissue. While the surgeon tightens the ligature, the assistant carefully removes the forceps completely. If the pedicle is too large, insufficient hemostasis is often achieved with this technique.[7] In such cases, the "divide and conquer" technique should be used.

Ligation of vessels obscured by perivascular fat accumulation, such as occurs in the omentum, may be a challenge because occasionally the vessel is traumatized by trying to blindly pass a needle around the vessel. In these cases, the blunt end of the needle can be used to place the suture around the vessel. This part of the needle pushes the vessel aside if it is in its path rather than penetrating it. Subsequent ligation of the vessel is routine.

Staples

Vascular staples, which can be used to occlude vessels up to 7 mm in diameter, are an alternative to suture ligation. They offer the advantage of speed and precision in placement. A specially designed instrument (1) applies two vascular staples that are crimped around the vessel simultaneously and (2) divides the vessel between the staples (the ligate-and-divide stapler [LDS] is described in Chapter 17). In cases of extensive intestinal resection with multiple mesenteric arcades, time is saved using this instrument. Disadvantages of staples are potential failure when used on large vessels, and expense.

Surgical Repair

Management of lateral wall defects in vital vessels can be very difficult. Suturing the defect is recommended,[5] incorporating the tunic, adventitia, and media—the major holding layers within the walls of large vessels.[10] Fine suture material (4-0 to 6-0) is recommended, using a continuous pattern with bites placed close together.

Esmarch System

The Esmarch and pneumatic tourniquet systems are excellent methods of temporarily occluding blood flow to a distal extremity (Fig. 13-15). They are used to maintain a bloodless operative field. An inflatable pneumatic cuff is placed around the limb, 10 to 15 cm proximal to the surgical site, prior to preparing and draping the surgical site. If the cuff is applied proximal to the carpus or the tarsus, a gauze roll is placed on the medial and lateral sides of the limb over large vessels underneath the tourniquet to facilitate blood flow occlusion. A long latex rubber bandage is tightly wrapped around the limb to force the blood from the limb, starting over the hoof and proceeding in a proximal direction. Once the Esmarch bandage reaches the pneumatic tourniquet, the cuff is inflated above systolic pressure to occlude blood flow into the limb (approximately 600 mm Hg) (see Fig. 13-15). Subsequently, the Esmarch is removed. Nonpigmented skin will appear blanched. The tourniquet is generally left on the limb for no longer than 2 hours.

Thermal Hemostasis

Electrocoagulation is a commonly used method of hemostasis. Heat generated from high-frequency alternating electrical current traveling between two electrodes causes protein denaturation inside tissue cells.[10] Tissue damage from heat production occurs between 3000 and 4000 Hz. Electrosurgical units can generate currents ranging between 1.5 and 7.5 MHz, and if too high a current is applied, the intracellular fluid boils instantly, potentially causing the vessel to explode without achieving coagulation.[11]

Electrosurgical units can produce different types of currents. A partially rectified waveform achieves the most effective hemostasis.[10] Vessels up to 2 mm in diameter can be coagulated in two ways. Obliterative coagulation is performed by direct contact between the hand-held electrode and the vessel. This causes the vessel wall to shrink, occluding the lumen by thrombosis and coagulum formation.[10,13] Alternatively, hemostasis can be achieved by coaptive coagulation. In this method, the vessel is initially occluded by a hemostatic forceps. The electrode of the electrosurgical unit then contacts an instrument that conducts the energy to the vessel, inducing permanent occlusion of the vessel. This technique allows precise electrocoagulation of a vessel.

Cryogenic hemostasis, as the name implies, is the rapid freezing of vessels to cause coagulation. The technique of cryosurgery is discussed in detail in Chapter 15.

Chemical Hemostasis

Occasionally, epinephrine is used to control hemorrhage. Epinephrine is a potent α-adrenergic agonist that causes peripheral vasoconstriction.[14] A solution of 1:100,000 to 1:20,000 is used to control superficial bleeding of mucosal and subcutaneous tissues.[12] Gauze packing soaked with a dilute epinephrine solution is an effective way to control bleeding.

Intravenous injection of 10% buffered formalin at a dosage of 0.02 to 0.06 mL/kg body weight diluted 1:9 in physiologic saline solution has been shown to be effective in controlling diffuse bleeding.[15] The exact mechanism of action is unknown, but it may be the result of induction of coagulation on the endothelial cell surface. Close monitoring of the patient during application is recommended. This technique is applied to stop bleeding after castrations, colic surgeries, and surgical interventions of the upper airways.

Physical Hemostasis

Soluble sponge-type materials control hemorrhagic oozing by promoting clot formation. Various types of hemostatic materials include gelatin foam, oxidized cellulose, oxidized regenerated cellulose, and micronized collagen. While these materials transmit pressure against the wound surface, the material's interstices provide a scaffold on which a clot can organize.[5] These materials are most beneficial for low-pressure bleeding and in friable organs that cannot be readily sutured.[7] The materials are nontoxic, but they will delay wound healing and can potentiate infection[2] because they are absorbed by phagocytosis.

A
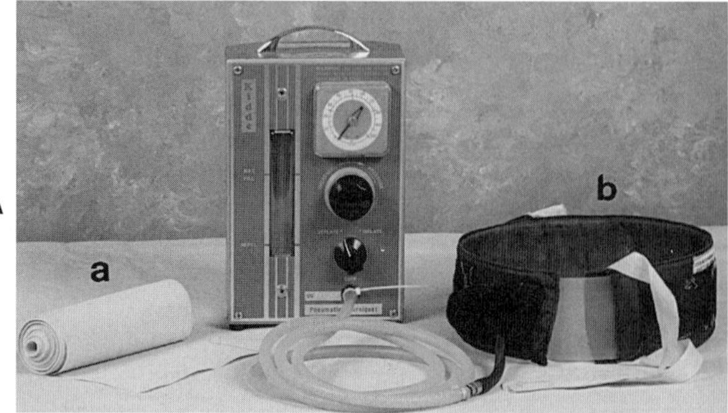

B
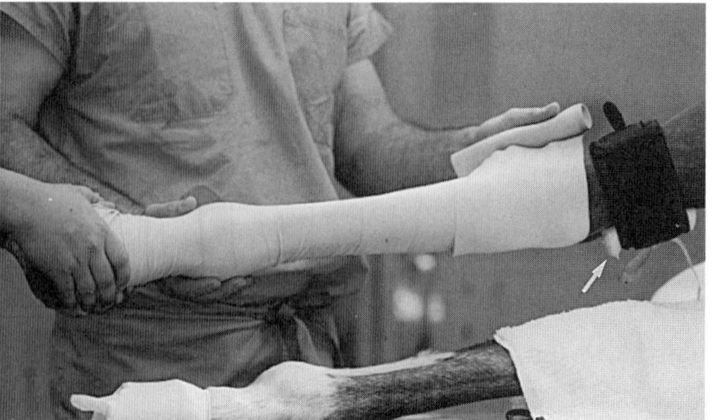

Figure 13-15. A, An Esmarch bandage *(a)* and pneumatic tourniquet *(b)* used for occluding blood flow in a limb. **B,** Application of an Esmarch bandage and a pneumatic tourniquet. Gauze rolls are placed over vascular pressure points under the tourniquet *(arrow)*.

Bleeding from the bone can be controlled with the help of bone wax, which consists of purified and sterilized beeswax. The wax is physically packed onto the bone to block oozing of blood from cut cortical and cancellous bone. The material is relatively nonirritating, but it will remain in contact with the bone for years.[7]

TISSUE RETRACTION AND HANDLING

Retraction

Unnecessary tissue trauma induces inflammation, which can delay healing. Therefore, incisions should be made only as long as necessary to allow adequate exposure. Gentle manipulation of tissue with respect to blood supply, innervation, and hydration is essential for atraumatic surgical technique. To achieve this, instrument retraction may be preferred over direct hand retraction in selected situations.

Hand-held retractors are designed with a single handle and blade, to be used as an extension of the assistant's hand. Alternatively, self-retaining retractors are designed with a locking mechanism on the handles to keep the blades in an open position. The blades of the retractor are placed within the incision and opened until the tissues on each side of the incision are spread maximally. Occasional repositioning or relaxation of the instrument blades, in conjunction with padding (i.e., moist gauze sponges placed between the blades of the retractor and tissue), minimizes tissue damage.

Careful retraction and stabilization of nerves and neurovascular bundles with Penrose drains or umbilical tape should always be considered in place of metallic retractors.[12]

Careful and atraumatic tissue handling is as important as applying aseptic technique during surgery. Rough handling of the tissues may induce inflammation and subsequent delayed wound healing.

Tissue Handling

An incision heals from side to side, not from end to end. Therefore, the incisions should be long enough to facilitate a clear view of the surgical site. Inadequate exposure may lead to increased tension on the tissues through overzealous retraction, jeopardize hemostasis, and increase the risk of traumatizing a nerve or vessel.

Sharp dissection should be carried out with sharp instruments. The use of dull scalpel blades, and dull and worn-out scissors only increases tissue trauma. Whenever possible, natural tissue cleavage planes should be followed during dissection; this prevents inadvertent transection of or tearing of fibrous tissues that heal poorly, if at all. Excessive undermining of tissues should be avoided, because it leads to the formation of dead spaces, which allow hematoma and seroma formation.

Most tissues should be handled with appropriate instruments; fingers should not be used. In small wounds, the introduction of a surgeon's finger prevents adequate evaluation of the deeper structures. Probing with a thin instrument allows simultaneous observation and manipulation. Tissue forceps are available for just about any manipulation necessary. Applying hemostatic forceps to tissues not intended to be excised should be avoided, because the tissues are crushed and devitalized. Allis forceps are designed to hold tissues. However, excessive compression of the tissues in the clamp should be avoided. Stabilization and retraction of tissue may be accomplished in a variety of ways besides by using tissue forceps. In selected situations, the assistant's fingers may accomplish effective atraumatic temporary occlusion of bowel to facilitate an enterotomy. Alternatively, a pair of self-retaining Doyen clamps may serve the same purpose.

Stay sutures can be used in a variety of situations—for example, to stabilize vessels and bowel. These sutures can be placed through very small amounts of tissue and still allow manipulations without pulling out. Hand-held and self-retaining retractors can be used in many surgical procedures to help facilitate certain manipulations.

Nerves and vital vessels should be spared whenever possible. Once they are isolated, they should be manipulated with great care. The identification of these structures with the help of a Penrose drain is atraumatic and effective.

SURGICAL IRRIGATION AND SUCTION

Surgical Irrigation

Operative wound lavage has been associated with reduced rates of postoperative infection for both clean and contaminated wounds in direct proportion to the volume of irrigation solution used.[16,17] This phenomenon has been attributed to the removal of surface bacteria and debris from contaminated wounds, dislodgement and removal of bacteria and exudate from infected wounds, and dilution and removal of toxins associated with infection.[17] An additional benefit of wound lavage and suction is the moistening of tissues to counteract the dehydrating effects of air and surgical lights. Wound lavage removes blood from the surgical site, which also improves visibility. Various types of lavage solutions, delivery systems, and suction devices have been developed, depending on where they are applied (e.g., body cavity, skin), the type of wound (e.g., traumatic, surgical), and the presence or absence of contamination or infection.

The ideal lavage solution is sterile, nontoxic, isoosmotic, and normothermic.[18] Sterile 0.9% physiologic saline, lactated Ringer's solution, and Plasmalyte are examples of available solutions that approach these criteria. Antibiotics are often added to a lavage solution as prophylaxis against possible infection, or if contamination has occurred. Even though some effect has been reported,[19] conclusive evidence that this technique is superior to saline lavage alone is lacking.[7] Infection implies bacterial penetration of tissues, and adequate blood and tissue concentrations of antibiotics via systemic administration are required for effective bacterial destruction.[7] Some antibiotics, such as tetracycline, are irritating when applied to exposed tissue or peritoneal surfaces and should be avoided.[19] Antiseptics such as povidone-iodine and chlorhexidine may be added to lavage solutions.

Fluid delivery systems used for irrigation vary depending on the area being irrigated and the presence or absence of contamination or infection. Lavage of body cavities is accomplished by flooding the cavity with large volumes of sterile solution, followed by suctioning to remove the fluid. This is usually performed by pouring the sterile solution from the bottle or a bowl into the cavity, or with a system capable of delivering large volumes of fluid at low pressure (referred to as diuresis).

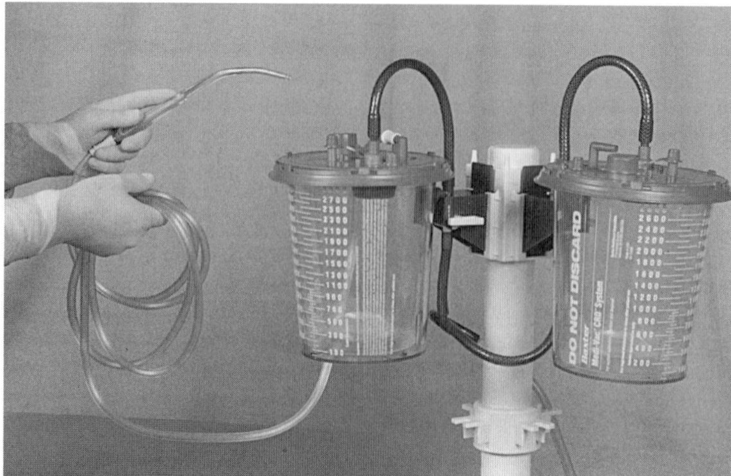

Figure 13-16. A suction tip is connected to sterile tubing to evacuate fluid from the surgical site into a reservoir.

Alternatively, traumatic and surgical wounds of the limbs are usually lavaged with the solutions under pressure. This is especially important if contamination or infection is present, because it dislodges bacteria or debris.[7] A bulb syringe or a 60-cc dose syringe is adequate for keeping tissues moist and removing débrided tissue particles in some circumstances, but automated systems that deliver a high volume of lavage solution at pressures not exceeding 10 to 15 pounds per square inch should be used on heavily contaminated tissues (additional information on wound lavage techniques can be found in Chapter 26).

Suction

Suctioning efficiently removes blood and fluid from the surgical site. A suction tip attached to sterile tubing connected to a suction pump that delivers a vacuum of 80 to 120 mm Hg is recommended[2] (Fig. 13-16). When gentle suction is indicated, such as in deep incisions where exposure is limited, a Frazier tip is used. This tip has a side-hole port near the handle, which can be used to vary the amount of suction force by either leaving the port uncovered or covering it with the index finger. When suctioning a large volume of fluid a Yankauer suction tip with a single port tip can be used. The multifenestrated sump-type design of the Poole tip makes it ideal for use in body cavities, where a single-port tip will plug or injure viscera.[7] Figure 12-16 in the preceding chapter shows these special tips.

CURETTAGE

Curettage refers to the removal of a growth or other tissue from the wall of a cavity or other surface with a curet.[20] Curettage can be used in all types of surgical interventions, but it is mainly applied in orthopedic procedures. Débridement of sequestra, excess bone production such as periosteal exostoses, damaged or diseased articular cartilage, and subchondral bone during an articular procedure (arthroscopy or arthrotomy) represent some surgical procedures that may involve curettage. It can also be used to remove necrotic soft tissue and debris from wounds, such as the tissue covering the bone after removal of a bone plate. The curet is used in an axial rotational motion (utilizing its cuplike design at the instrument tip) to scoop out tissue, or with a pulling motion to scrape tissue from the surgical site. The handle of the instrument is grasped in the palm of the dominant hand and the index finger is placed on the shaft of the instrument to help stabilize the tip against the tissue (Fig. 13-17).

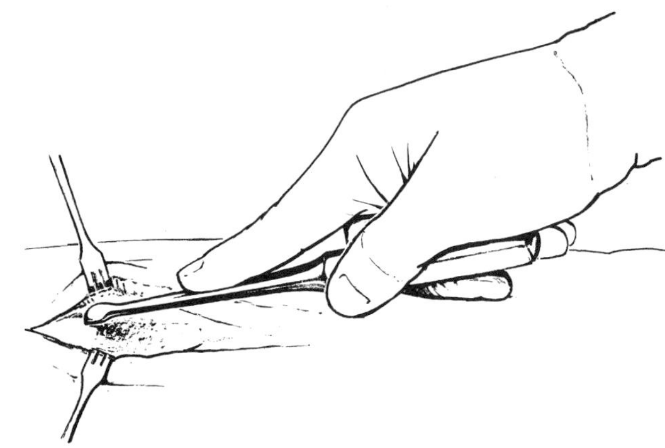

Figure 13-17. Proper technique for holding a curet.

REFERENCES

1. Burba JD, Martin GS: Surgical techniques. In Auer JA, Stick JA, editors: Equine Surgery, ed 2, Philadelphia, 1999, WB Saunders.
2. Wong E: Surgical site infections. In Mayhall CG, editor: Hospital Epidemiology and Infection Control, Baltimore, 1996, Williams & Wilkins.
3. Anderson RM, Romfh RF: Technique in the Use of Surgical Tools, New York, 1980, Appleton-Century-Crofts.
4. Knecht CD, Allen AR, Williams DJ, et al: Surgical instrumentation. In Knecht CD, editor: Fundamental Techniques in Veterinary Surgery, ed 2, Philadelphia, 1981, WB Saunders.
5. Clem MF: Surgical techniques. In Auer JA, editor: Equine Surgery, Philadelphia, 1992, WB Saunders.

6. Kirk RM: Basic Surgical Techniques, ed 2, New York, 1978, Churchill-Livingstone.
7. Toombs JP, Clarke KM: Basic operative techniques. In Slatter D, editor: Textbook of Small Animal Surgery, ed 2, Philadelphia, 2003, WB Saunders.
8. Burba DJ, Martin GS: Surgical techniques. In Auer JA, Stick JA, editors: Equine Surgery, ed 2, Philadelphia, 1999, WB Saunders.
9. Toombs JP, Crowe DT: Operative techniques. In Slatter D, editor: Textbook of Small Animal Surgery, Philadelphia, 1985, WB Saunders.
10. Fucci V, Elkins AD: Electro surgery: Principles and guidelines in veterinary medicine, Comp Cont Educ Pract Vet 1991;13:407.
11. Greene JA, Knecht CD: Electro surgery: A review, Vet Surg 1980;9:27.
12. Schwartz SI: Hemostasis, surgical bleeding, and transfusion. In Schwartz SI, Shires GT, Spencer FC, editors: Principles of Surgery, ed 6, New York, 1994, McGraw-Hill.
13. Kelly HA, Ward GE: Electro surgery. In Green JA, Knecht CD, editors: Electro Surgery: A Review, Philadelphia, 1980, WB Saunders.
14. Adams HR: Adrenergic and antiadrenergic drugs. In Booth NH, McDonald LE, editors: Veterinary Pharmacology and Therapeutics, ed 5, Ames, 1982, Iowa State University Press.
15. Edens LM: Abdominal hemorrhage. In Robinson NE, editor: Current Therapy in Equine Medicine, ed 4, Philadelphia, 1997, WB Saunders.
16. Singleton AO, Julian I: An experimental evaluation of methods used to prevent infection in wounds which have been contaminated with feces, Ann Surg 1960;151:912.
17. Swaim SF: Management of contaminated and infected wounds. In Swaim SF, editor: Surgery of Traumatized Skin: Management and Reconstruction in the Dog and Cat, Philadelphia, 1980, WB Saunders.
18. Daily WR: Wound infection. In Slatter SH, editor: Textbook of Small Animal Surgery, Philadelphia, 1985, WB Saunders.
19. Leff A, Hopewell PC, Costello J: Pleural effusion from malignancy, Ann Intern Med 1978;88:532.
20. Dorland's Illustrated Medical Dictionary, ed 30, Philadelphia, 2003, WB Saunders.

CHAPTER 14

Minimally Invasive Surgical Techniques

Andrew T. Fischer, Jr.
Joanne Hardy
Renée Léveillé
Astrid B.M. Rijkenhuizen
Jörg A. Auer

The evolution of minimally invasive human surgery that peaked in the 1980s has been matched by a parallel development in minimally invasive surgical techniques in the horse. The evaluation of joints by arthrotomy, which was common until the mid 1980s, has been replaced by arthroscopy for almost all indications. Laparoscopic surgical techniques have continued to replace previous open techniques such as cryptorchidectomy, ovariectomy, and inguinal hernia repair. In some cases, new techniques have been developed that were not previously available in the horse (e.g., testicle-sparing mesh repair of the inguinal ring). Thoracoscopic techniques are also continuing to evolve but at a slower pace because of the infrequency of surgical disease of the equine thorax. The three major applications of rigid endoscopy (laparoscopy, arthroscopy, and thoracoscopy) share common surgical techniques and basic equipment. This chapter describes specialized equipment unique to each application.

Embolization and thrombectomy techniques can be conducted through catheters introduced into vessels. These procedures are effective techniques for treating disorders that a few years ago could be attempted only with great risk to the patient.

Computer-assisted surgery has only recently been introduced into equine surgery and may play a major role in orthopedic surgery of the future.

In addition to smaller surgical incisions, minimally invasive surgical techniques are characterized by vastly improved visualization. This has led to improved surgical outcomes and better overall understanding of regional anatomy. Minimally invasive techniques continue to evolve and replace previous open techniques as more surgeons become comfortable with them and as more thought is devoted to their development.

ENDOSCOPY

Equipment

Illumination

Most minimally invasive procedures require a means of getting illumination into the body cavity and a telescope with which to view the target organs. The supply of light into the patient's body cavity was a limiting factor until the development of cold light sources, which allowed high-intensity illumination of the cavity without danger to the patient or surgeon from excessive heat. The next major limitation of early arthroscopy and laparoscopy was the lack of video imaging equipment, which prevented an assistant from participating in the surgery. The inability to be aided by an assistant limited the procedures to those that could be accomplished with one hand. Beam splitters were developed to share the image on the surgical telescope, but they were unwieldy and they markedly decreased the amount of light, resulting in a poor image. As video cameras were developed and refined, arthroscopy, laparoscopy, and thoracoscopy became popular. With time, the complexity of procedures markedly increased, as did the number of surgeons performing them.

Currently, light sources are capable of providing intense illumination to the selected cavity (Fig. 14-1). Most manufacturers produce light sources with 300 watts of output from xenon bulbs. Xenon light sources are preferred, as they offer more lumens per watt than halogen light sources, and the light is whiter, offering more accurate reproduction of colors. A flexible fiberoptic or liquid light cable is needed to transmit the light from the light source to the telescope. Light cables are available in many lengths, but a 10-foot-long cable is generally preferred for equine endoscopy. A fiberoptic light cable must be checked regularly for broken fibers and must be well maintained by thorough cleaning. Poor illumination of the cavity can frequently be traced to a light cable with many broken bundles. However, a liquid light cable does not have this problem. Although a bit more expensive, they are quite durable and not subject to fiber bundle breakage.

When the light source is on and the light cable is connected to the light source, it is important that the distal end of the light cable or the telescope not be left in contact with the patient, drapes, or any other combustible material, as burns may occur or fires may start as a result of the heat produced at the tip.

The three areas of rigid endoscopy all use a trocar and cannula assembly to first enter the body cavity (Fig. 14-2). The cannula protects the telescope after insertion and has stopcocks allowing fluid infusion or gas insufflation for distending the cavity. The cannula has seals to prevent leakage of fluid or gas through it.

Telescopes

A high-quality surgical telescope is very important for all endoscopic procedures (Fig. 14-3). The Hopkins rod lens system provides more light transmission for illumination of the cavity and a wider field of view than traditional optical systems. Light is provided by optical fibers that surround the lens system. Telescopes of 5 mm or less in diameter provide adequate light and visualization for arthroscopy but not for laparoscopy or thoracoscopy. The reasons for this are that the cartilage covering the articular surfaces of the bones in the joints is bright and reflective, and the cavity is smaller. The most common telescope size used in equine laparoscopy and thoracoscopy has a 10-mm outside diameter. The large size allows adequate light transmission with good visualization. The standard length for arthroscopes is 15 to 25 cm with an extra-long 4-mm diameter arthroscope of 35 cm. The standard length for human laparoscopes is approximately 30 cm, but a specially designed 57-cm laparoscope is available for equine use. The distal ends of endoscopes are designed with different lens angles. The most commonly available distal angles are 0, 25, or 30 degrees of visualization. The zero-degree telescope allows more light transmission into the body cavity but does not offer the panoramic view that the 30-degree telescope provides. The 30-degree telescope allows panoramic visualization (which facilitates triangulation techniques), accomplished by rotating the scope (not possible with the zero-degree telescope). For special procedures, a 70-degree arthroscope is available, but it is rarely used.

Video Equipment

A video camera that connects to the telescope is necessary to ensure aseptic surgical technique and allow assistance during surgery. Most cameras contain either one chip or three chips—the charged capacitance devices (CCDs) used in the camera. Three-chip cameras have one chip for each of the primary colors (red, green, and blue) and generally offer better resolution than single-chip cameras. Newer video cameras have an increased light sensitivity, which is very helpful for laparoscopy and thoracoscopy in horses. Zoom features, gain changes, and multimedia image capture may also be offered as options on the various cameras. The video camera should be connected to a good-quality monitor in

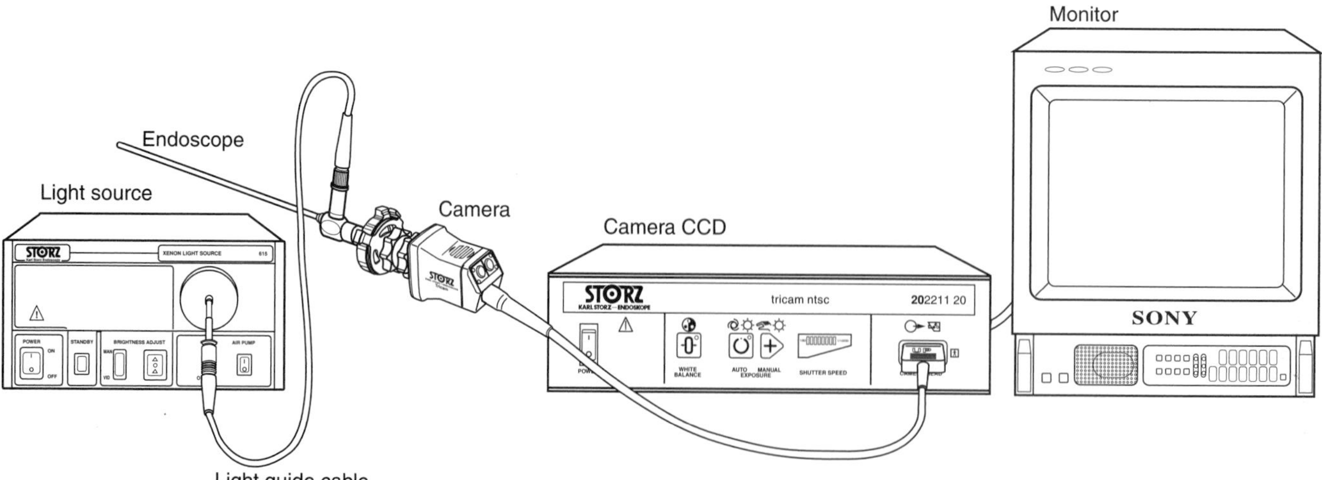

Figure 14-1. Basic equipment set up for minimally invasive surgery consisting of light source, light cable, video camera with camera processor, and monitor.

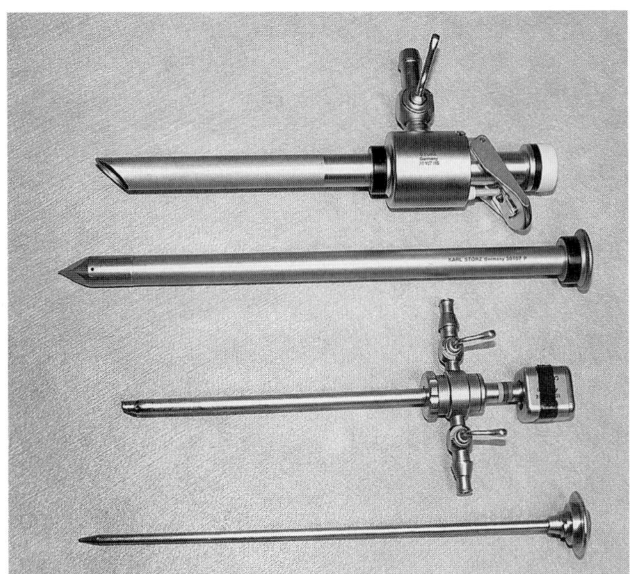

Figure 14-2. Laparoscopic and arthroscopic trocar/cannula assemblies. Note the pyramidal tip of the laparoscopic trocar and the conical tip of the arthroscopic obturator.

the direct line of sight of the surgeon. In some cases, it is helpful to have multiple monitors for the benefit of the assistant surgeon. The choice of cable connections affects monitor image—S-video cables offer the highest resolution. Multimedia digital capture of video-assisted surgery is becoming standard procedure and can be accomplished through the use of personal computers, stand-alone video documentation systems, or video recorders incorporating hard disk storage and DVD burners.

Fluids and Gases

Arthroscopic, laparoscopic, and thoracoscopic procedures all require the creation of an optical cavity. The optical cavity allows separation of the joint capsule or body wall from the contents of the cavity, which facilitates a thorough visual exploration.

Adequate visualization during arthroscopy is accomplished by the use of fluid or gas distention of the joint. Fluids used for joint distention are pH-balanced polyionic solutions such as lactated Ringer's solution. If electrosurgical instrumentation within the joint is going to be used, specially devised fluids suitable for this are needed. Fluid distention is usually obtained by the use of pressure or manually controlled pumps, but it can also be achieved by gravity. Excessive fluid pressure is associated with extravasation of the fluid, resulting in marked subcutaneous edema and poor visualization because pressure on the skin and subcutaneous tissues compresses the joint capsule. Arthroscopy using gas insufflation may be used when the joint surfaces must remain dry (e.g., in insertion of cartilage grafts). The pictures obtained with gas insufflation are clearer and truer to actual intra-articular colors. The insufflation technique is identical to the one described later for laparoscopy.

The abdominal cavity requires insufflation for optimal viewing. Insufflation is accomplished by insufflators that provide a controlled flow of gas into the patient's cavity. Settings on the insufflator should be available that limit flow rate and pressure in the cavity to be examined. Insufflators for equine use should have flow rates that can

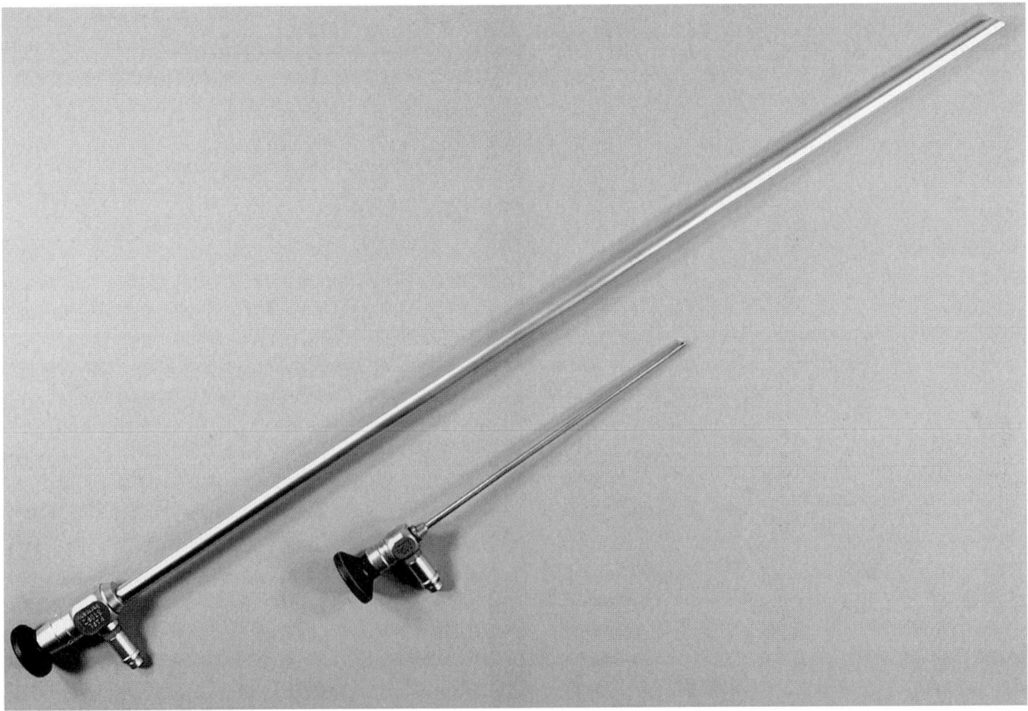

Figure 14-3. Laparoscopic and arthroscopic telescopes.

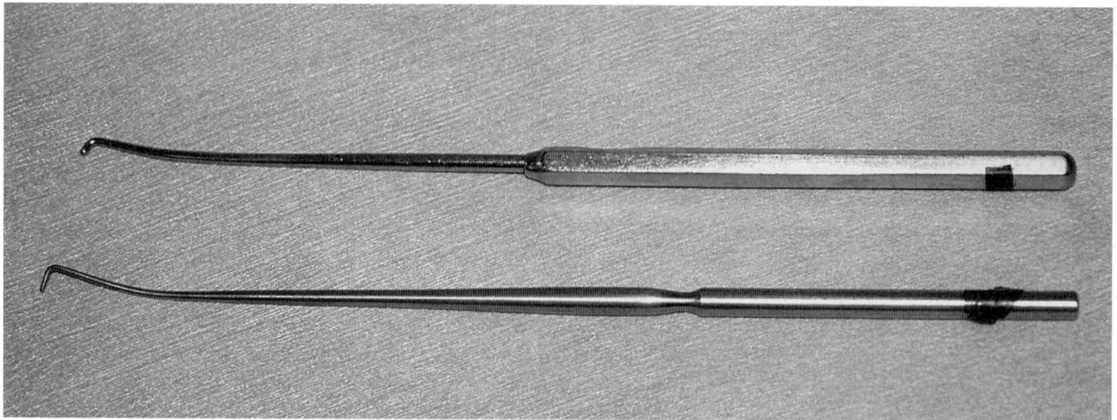

Figure 14-4. Arthroscopic probes.

exceed 10 L/min, and 20 L/min is desirable. Slower-rate insufflators require too long a time for adequate insufflation to occur or for the cavity to be reinflated if it becomes deflated. Initially, the rate of flow of gas into the patient is limited by the smallest diameter in the circuit, which is typically the insufflation needle. Needles such as the Verres needle have flow rates of less than 3 L/min, whereas teat cannulas can accomplish flows of 6 to 7 L/min. Once the laparoscopic trocar is inserted, the limit on flow rate is usually the insufflator.

The most commonly used gas for insufflation is carbon dioxide. Other inert gases have also been used in human medicine. The patient's abdominal pressure is usually 15 mm Hg or less. Higher pressures are associated with increased patient discomfort and respiratory compromise and are not necessary for visualization. Insufflation is less commonly used in thoracoscopy because of the tendency for the lung to collapse when air is allowed to enter the thorax passively. When insufflation is necessary during thoracoscopy, 5 mm Hg is usually adequate. The use of high intrapleural pressures is unnecessary; high pressure decreases cardiac return and interferes with ventilation. Selective bronchial intubation may be performed for thoracoscopy in cases requiring general anesthesia.

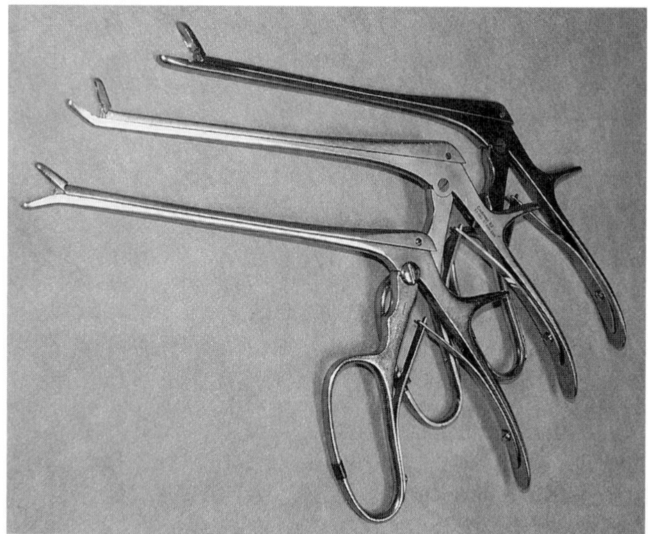

Figure 14-5. Ferris-Smith rongeurs with different cups.

Surgical Instruments

The basic instruments necessary for arthroscopy include probes, rongeurs, grasping forceps, chisels, mallet, curets, periosteal elevator, flush cannula, and a bone awl. Probes are used to evaluate looseness of fragments, determine stability of cartilage, and manipulate structures, testing their integrity or improving visualization (Fig. 14-4). Multiple rongeurs may be used in a single surgery, and the choice is dictated by the operative target. Ferris-Smith rongeurs are available in different sizes and with different jaw angles (straight, angled up, and angled down), and an assortment should be available in each surgical pack (Fig. 14-5). Grasping forceps are used to remove fragments from the joint (Fig. 14-6). Grasping forceps with small teeth in the jaws are better at grasping than rongeurs. Chisels, osteotomes, and

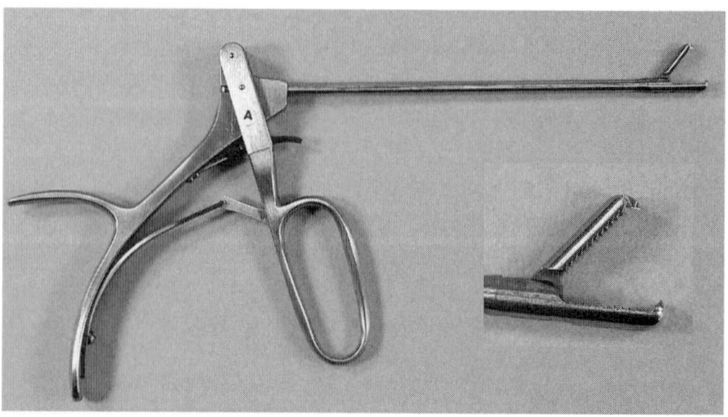

Figure 14-6. Grasping forceps.

periosteal elevators are used to elevate osteochondral fragments with or without the use of a mallet. Curets are used to débride cartilage edges and remove devitalized bone. Several different sizes and angles should be available to maximize access to the base of the defect. Bone awls are used to produce microfractures in the subchondral bone plate, which are thought to improve cartilage adhesion after bone débridement of the articular surface (see Chapter 84). Flush cannulas are useful for lavaging the joint and removing any remaining bits of cartilage or bony debris (Fig. 14-7). Motorized equipment is useful for synovectomy, meniscectomy, tendon débridement, and removal of cartilage flaps. Different blades are used according to the structure being débrided.

The basic instruments used for laparoscopy include probes, Semm claw forceps, scissors, Babcock forceps, and biopsy forceps. Probes are used to probe organs and provide tactile feedback regarding the consistency of the target, and to evaluate organ attachments. Semm claw forceps provide good security when grasping tissue that is to be removed from the patient (Fig. 14-8). Atraumatic forceps such as Babcock forceps allow tissue manipulation without injury and are useful in exploratory laparoscopy or thoracoscopy (Fig. 14-9). Endoscopic scissors are used for dividing tissue after adequate hemostasis has been obtained (Fig. 14-10). Biopsy forceps are used for visceral biopsy (spleen, kidney, liver, and other solid organs) or tumors. Hemostatic devices such as endoscopic staplers, electrosurgical units, ultrasonic scalpels, and different types of lasers are routinely used and will be discussed in appropriate chapters.

Triangulation Technique

Arthroscopic, laparoscopic, and thoracoscopic surgical procedures all share the common technique of triangulation. Triangulation refers to the placing of telescope and instruments through separate portals so that they converge on the operative target. Mastering the technique of triangulation is essential to becoming competent in minimally invasive endoscopic techniques. The visual target should be in front of the surgeon, with the monitor directly behind the visual target. The camera must be kept in an orientation that maintains the true vertical and horizontal axes to facilitate proper movement of the surgical instruments toward the

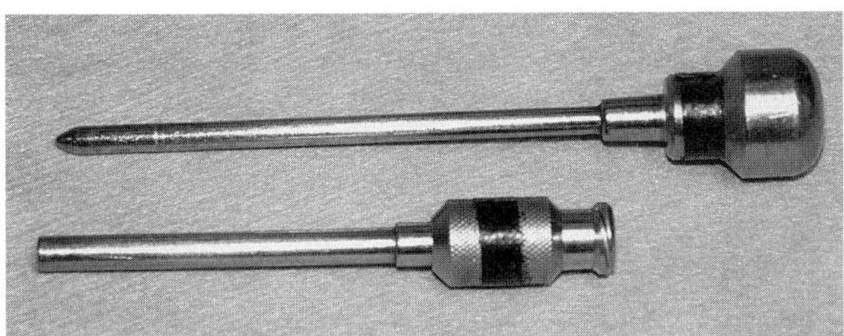

Figure 14-7. Arthroscopic flush cannula.

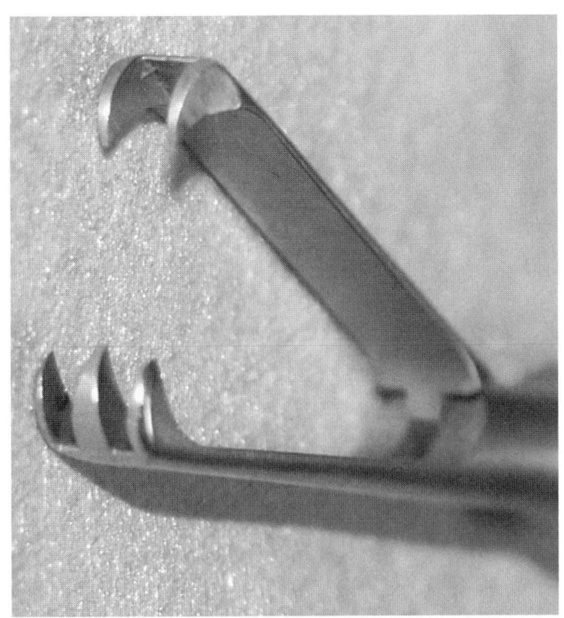

Figure 14-8. Semm claw forceps used for tissue removal.

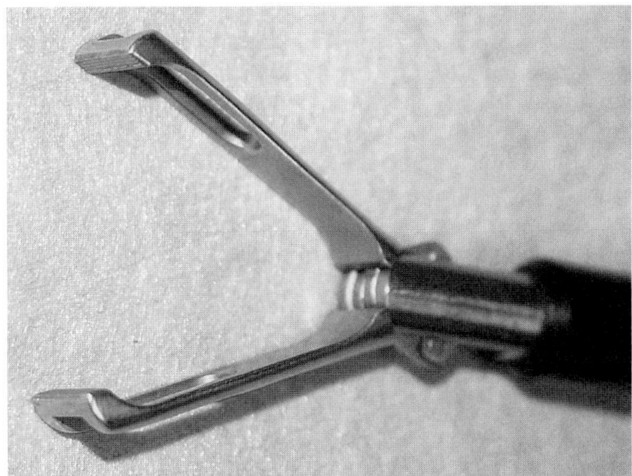

Figure 14-9. Babcock forceps used for atraumatic tissue manipulation.

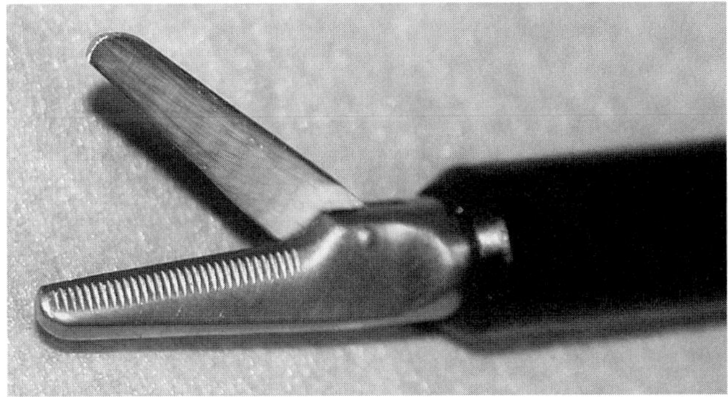

Figure 14-10. Scissors used for laparoscopic surgery. Note the increased length and size needed for efficient cutting.

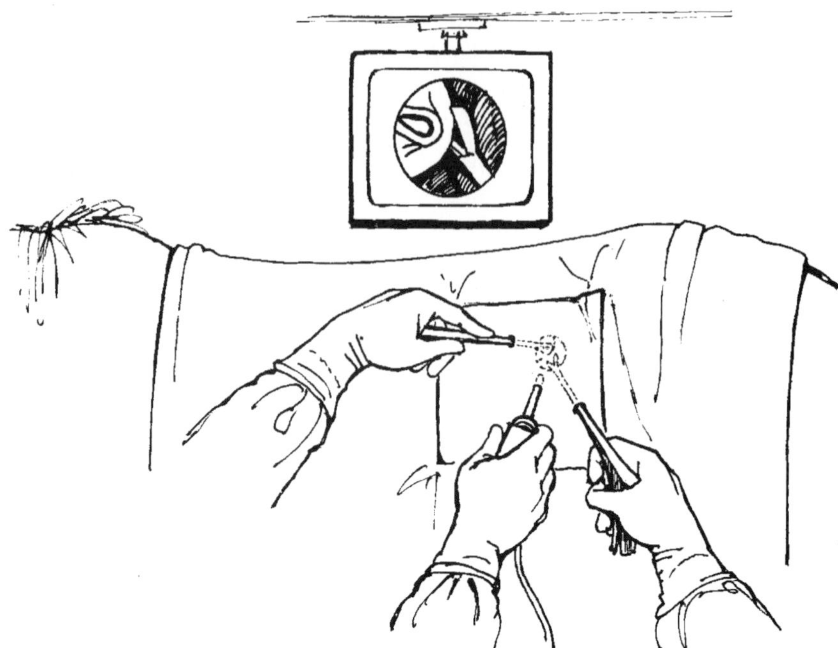

Figure 14-11. The proper use of the triangulation technique.

surgical target (Fig. 14-11). Triangulation techniques should be learned with training boxes before surgery is attempted on clinical cases. In general, the diagnostic evaluation in all minimally invasive surgeries should be performed before instrument portals are established, as they can collapse the optical cavity and interfere with visualization. An exception to this occurs when instrumentation must be introduced to manipulate viscera to facilitate exploration. Once the diagnostic exploration has been accomplished, additional instrument portals are established for the surgical procedure. The details for specific procedures are found in subsequent chapters and specialized texts.[1-3]

EMBOLIZATION

Arterial embolization refers to catheter-directed delivery of particulate material for the purpose of embolizing selected arteries. Currently, microcoils are the most popular embolization material. They have been used for occlusion of normal and abnormal vasculature, and for creating ischemia of neoplastic tissue (Fig. 14-12). In dogs, coil embolization has been used for vascular occlusion of patent ductus arteriosus,[4-8] occlusion of portosystemic shunts,[9-14] treatment of epistaxis,[15] and experimental treatment of cerebral aneurysms.[16] In horses, coil embolization has been used to occlude branches of the common carotid artery usually involved in guttural pouch mycosis.[17-20] The use of emulsions for embolization of tumors for the purpose of creating ischemia and reducing tumor size has also been described.[21] Chemoembolization refers to selective intra-arterial delivery of chemotherapeutic agents in conjunction with particulate material for the purpose of embolizing arteries supplying blood to a tumor.[22] Numerous studies describe its use in humans and dogs, using various chemotherapeutic agents.[23-27]

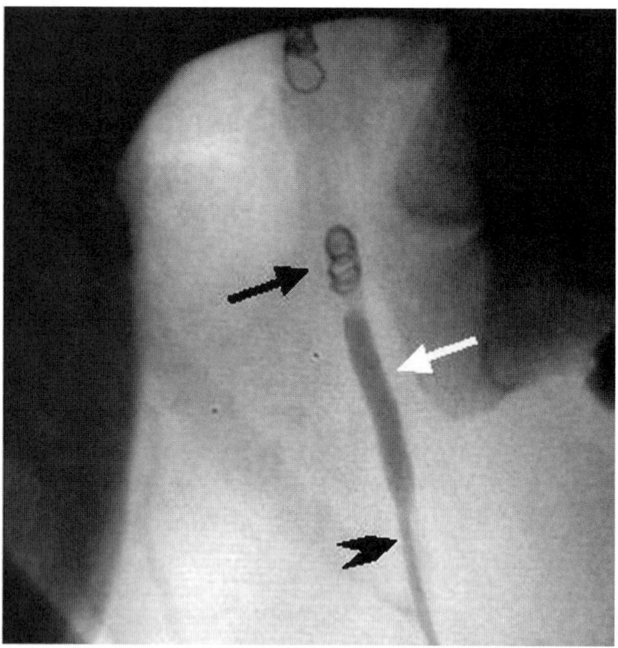

Figure 14-12. Fluoroscopic image of embolization coils *(black arrow)* occluding the internal carotid artery of a horse affected with guttural pouch mycosis. Note the position of the catheter *(white arrow)* within the artery, and injection of contrast material demonstrating arterial occlusion *(arrowhead)*.

Surgical Technique

Catheter-directed embolization involves accessing a peripheral artery, where an introducer is inserted. A catheter is then directed, under fluoroscopic guidance, within the artery until the tip of the catheter is located at the desired site of embolization. Accessing the proper site requires knowledge of local vascular anatomy and variances within individuals. Navigation through the arterial tree is facilitated by using a gliding guide wire inserted within the catheter. Once the site of embolization is reached, the embolization material is delivered. The catheter and introducer are removed, and hemostasis at the arterial puncture site is achieved by direct pressure or suturing.

The sizes and materials used for embolization techniques are very specific, and correct selection of product characteristic for the desired purpose is essential. For example, catheters made of polyvinylchloride (PVC) or vinyl do not allow the coils to glide within the catheter, resulting in occlusion of the catheter. Similarly, selection of too small a coil diameter allows the coil to travel farther into the arterial vasculature, where it might embolize an undesired vessel. For details on use of this technique to control bleeding from guttural pouch mycosis, see Chapter 45.

THROMBECTOMY

Aortic-iliac thrombosis (TAI) in the horse is an unusual cause of hind limb lameness.[28,29] Diagnosis is often difficult, and conservative treatment is usually unrewarding.[28,29] Therefore, a surgical treatment has been explored. Thrombectomy via minimally invasive surgery has been used successfully for chronic arterial occlusive disease of the aorta and its caudal arteries.

The most common manifestation of TAI is a predictable exercise-induced lameness that ceases with a resting period of 5 to 10 minutes. Horses that are forced to train despite the lameness exhibit a more severe lameness and may require significantly more time for the symptoms to resolve. More severely affected horses take longer to recover. After physical activity, there is an absence of sweating, retarded venous vein filling, and hypothermia of the distal extremity of the affected limb. Initially, symptoms are exhibited only after exercise. As the disease progresses, clinical signs are also present at rest, because of ischemia in the hind limb.

TAI is progressive with a gradual onset. The clinical signs are determined by the degree of vascular occlusion, the presence of collateral circulation, and the speed of the onset of the occlusion.[28-30]Affected horses can be asymptomatic or show only vague performance deficits. Occasionally, part of a thrombus dislodges from a proximal location and acutely occludes a distal peripheral artery. After training, acute colic-like signs may occur (pawing, straining, sweating, lying down and rolling), mostly combined with a severe lameness.

Diagnosis is based on history, clinical presentation, and rectal palpation, in combination with ultrasonography, thermography (if available), and scintigraphy.[31-38] Information on the onset of ischemic symptoms, the duration of symptoms, the characteristics of pain, and any alleviating factors is helpful. The absence of a pulse in an extremity is probably the most common physical finding. Rectal ultrasonography is used to recognize the thrombus in the aorta and the internal and external iliac artery. Doppler ultrasonography renders both an anatomic and a functional assessment of the femoral artery in the inguinal region. This technique is also used to estimate the degree of arterial occlusion.[39] The femoral artery is visualized in the femoral triangle (trigonum femorale), which is bordered caudally by the pectineus and cranially by the sartorius muscles, over a distance of approximately 15 cm. In unilateral cases, the unaffected hind limb can be used as a reference.

To monitor the development of hypoxemia in the affected hind limb, the oxygen pressure in venous blood samples before and after a workload can be measured.[33] The samples are taken from the right and left saphenous veins as far proximally as possible—that is, at the level of the stifle joint. Samples are collected anaerobically in heparinized 2-mL syringes, which are immediately sealed so that they are airtight, and then immersed in ice. Within 15 minutes after the first sample is taken, they are tested in a blood gas analyzer.

Conservative treatment with exercise programs and pharmacologic therapy with sodium gluconate, with or without fibrinolytic enzymes, anticoagulants, and vasodilators, has thus far been unsatisfactory.* Promising results were seen in unilaterally affected horses by restoring blood supply to the ischemic regions through thrombectomy with the use of a Fogarty graft thrombectomy catheter.[33]

Surgical Technique

The horse is anesthetized and positioned on the surgery table in lateral recumbency with the affected limb down. The upper hind limb is secured in flexion and abduction. An approximately 10-cm-long incision is made medially over the saphenous vein where its course changes from superficial to deep (Fig. 14-13). Dissection of the vein is continued as it courses proximally, until the femoral artery is identified. The femoral artery is carefully isolated and stabilized with two large sutures, and two vascular clamps (aortic forceps, DeBakey-Morris) are placed proximally and distally to prevent excessive blood loss during surgery. Small arterial branches of the femoral artery are ligated if this is necessary to gain exposure.

A transverse arteriotomy is performed and the blood flow is observed by loosening the clamp and removing the proximal suture. Visible thrombi are loosened from the arterial

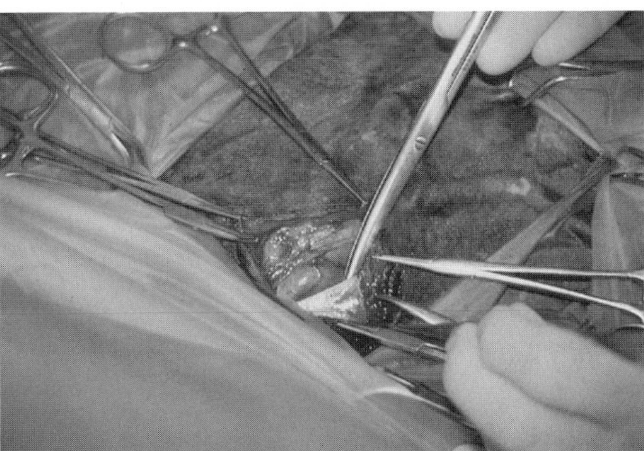

Figure 14-13. Intraoperative view of the saphenous vein. The femoral artery is located by following the saphenous vein proximally.

*References 29, 30, 34, 35, 37, 40.

wall and removed with forceps (Fig. 14-14). Subsequently, the Fogarty catheter (50 cm long, with a closed diameter of 4 mm and an expanded diameter of 16 mm) is inserted in collapsed form into the femoral artery, directed proximally, and positioned beyond the saddle thrombus. The catheter has a flexible wire coil at the distal end that expands when retracted to form a double-helix ring (Fig. 14-15). The sliding knob on the handle of the catheter is retracted slowly, which causes the wire loops to partially expand and move the thrombi distally as the catheter is withdrawn. This procedure is repeated with the diameter of the coil more expanded until no resistance is felt during withdrawal of the catheter, and no more thrombi are retrieved (Fig. 14-16). By removing this blockage, blood flow is restored from the proximal side. When indicated, additional thrombectomies are performed distal to the incision. Before closure of the artery, blood is allowed to flow freely with the distal clamp closed for a short period to remove any detached thrombi and air. Prior to reclamping the artery for closure, 20 mL of a heparin solution (250 IU heparin/mL physiologic saline solution) is injected into the femoral artery, in both a distal and a proximal direction. The incision in the femoral artery is sutured using a simple continuous suture pattern of monofilament polypropylene (5-0). Fascia and subcutis are closed with a simple continuous suture pattern, followed by skin closure using an intradermal continuous suture.

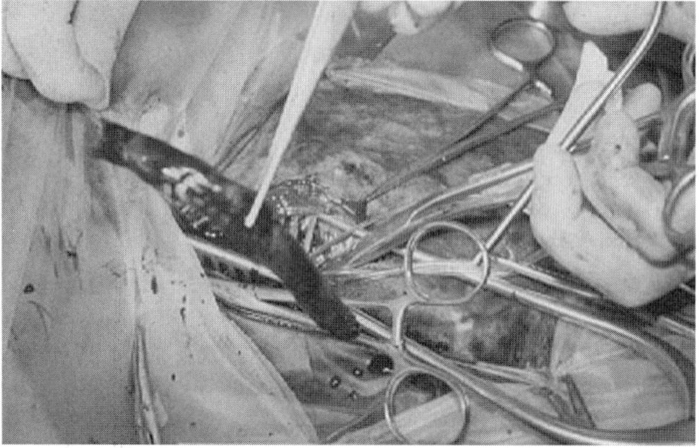

Figure 14-14. A thrombus is removed with the help of a forceps.

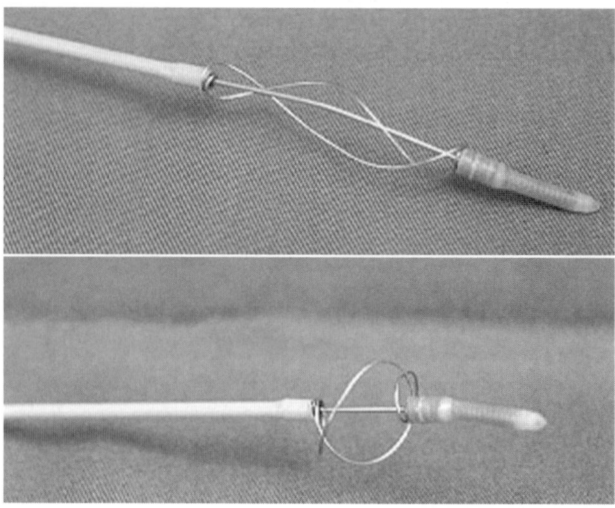

Figure 14-15. Fogarty catheter in closed *(top)* and expanded *(bottom)* position

Anticoagulation is obtained intra-operatively just before arteriotomy by the intravenous administration of 100 IU heparin/kg. This is followed postoperatively by the subcutaneous administration of 50 IU heparin/kg twice daily for 2 days, and carbasalatum calcium 5 mg/kg (Ascal, Dagra Pharma) orally once daily for at least 3 months.

Hand walking is advised immediately after surgery, after which light exercise can begin.

A severe complication is the appearance of TAI in the contralateral limb after surgery because of thromboembolization caused by dislodged clot fragments. Postanesthetic myopathy is seen in 60% of the cases and assumed to be caused by local hypoxemia of various muscle groups.[40] Horses with TAI that have preexisting hypoxemia before surgery are therefore at high risk for this complication. Adequate padding, correct positioning, prevention of intra-operative hypotension, and keeping surgery time as short as possible are important considerations.[40]

The prognosis after surgical intervention is reasonable, with a 50% return to athletic function.

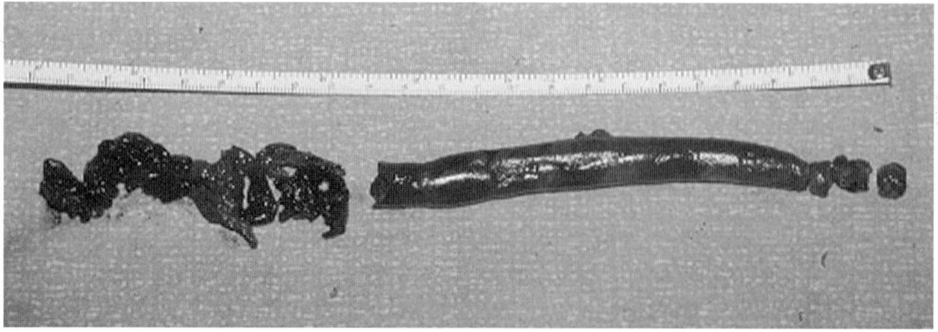

Figure 14-16. Removed thrombi.

COMPUTER-ASSISTED SURGERY

Internal fixation of fractures is usually planned on the basis of a radiographic study. Occasionally, computed tomography (CT) is used to determine the exact course of the fracture line as it courses along the bone. Such a study allows the surgeon to determine exactly where to implant screws. Nevertheless, the actual result depends greatly on the surgeon's skill to insert the implants according to the preoperative plan. Computer-assisted surgery (CAS) allows the surgeon to accurately implement the preoperative plan and to implant screws at the desired location and at the correct angle relative to the fracture plane.[41]

Surgical Technique

The equipment used at the Equine Hospital of the University of Zurich, Switzerland, is composed of instruments equipped with infrared light-emitting diodes (LEDs), the Medivision SurgiGate (Praxim-Medivision, Inc, Grenoble, France) navigation system, and the Siemens Siremobil Iso 3D C-arm (Siemens AG, Munich, Germany) (Fig. 14-17). These instruments together define the fractured bone in three dimensions and allow real-time observation of the actual implantation of the screw in three planes simultaneously.[41]

First, the dynamic reference base (DRB) is securely attached to a Schanz screw, which was previously attached to the fractured bone. Subsequently, the fractured bone is isocentrically positioned between the two components of the C-arm. Positioning is assisted by two laser beams positioned at 90 degrees relative to each other. Special attention is given to allow movement of the C-arm over a 190-degree arc without interfering with any object (e.g., the surgery table). The C-arm and the DRB must be located in the identifiable view of the navigation camera. Over a 2-minute period, the C-arm takes 100 still radiographs over an arc of 190 degrees, which are processed into 256 single pictures and sent to the SurgiGate computer. The radiographic images can be viewed in three planes that are oriented at right angles to each other (in the horizontal, parasagittal, and frontal planes).

The SurgiGate system consists of a navigation camera, a computer unit with sophisticated 3-dimensional software, the instruments (e.g., a power drill and an awl), and a virtual keyboard that allows the surgeon to navigate within the system and calibrate the instruments under aseptic conditions during surgery (Figs. 14-17 and 14-18). The data collected with the Siremobil Iso 3D is subsequently transferred to the SurgiGate computer, where the future location of each screw is planned on the screen and marked. The SurgiGate system is then changed to real time to guide the surgeon during the actual implantation. This is carried out by observation of the computer screen and matching the drill and subsequently needed instruments with the planned image in three planes, similar to an arthroscopic technique (Fig. 14-19). Once the location is matched, drilling is initiated. As soon as the drill bit crosses the fracture plane, which can be seen on the screen, the drill bit is changed to prepare the thread hole (Fig. 14-20). Insertion is then routine.

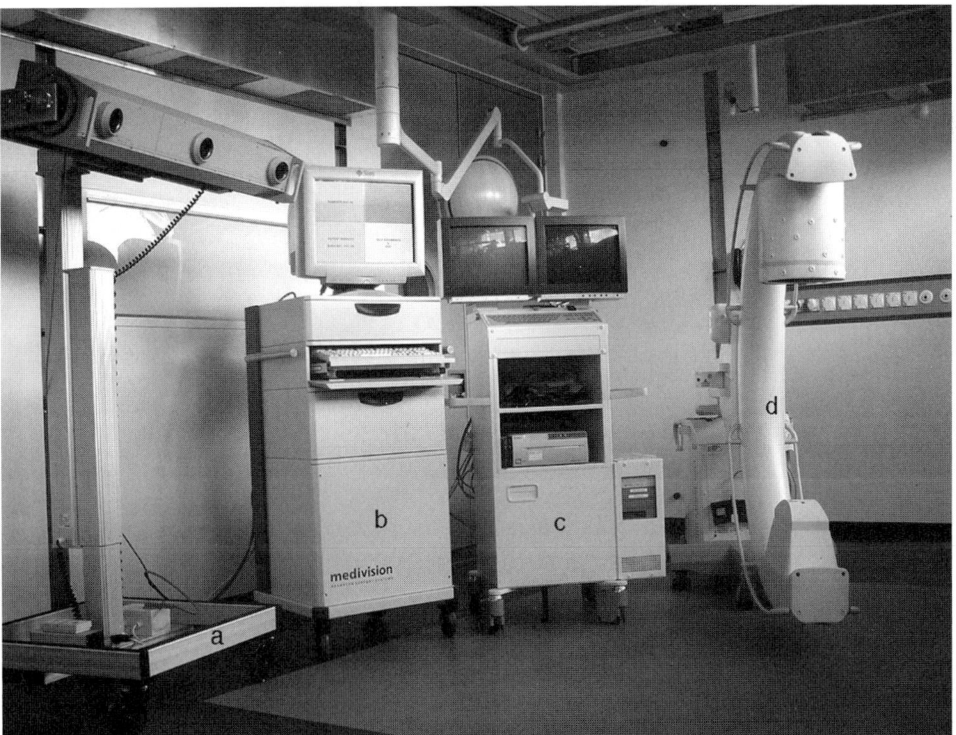

Figure 14-17. *a,* The navigation camera with the three lenses, which converge toward the surgical object. *b,* The corresponding computer with monitor, on which the preoperative planning is performed and subsequent surgical guidance is viewed. *c,* Siremobil Iso 3D with computer screens. *d,* Its corresponding C-arm.

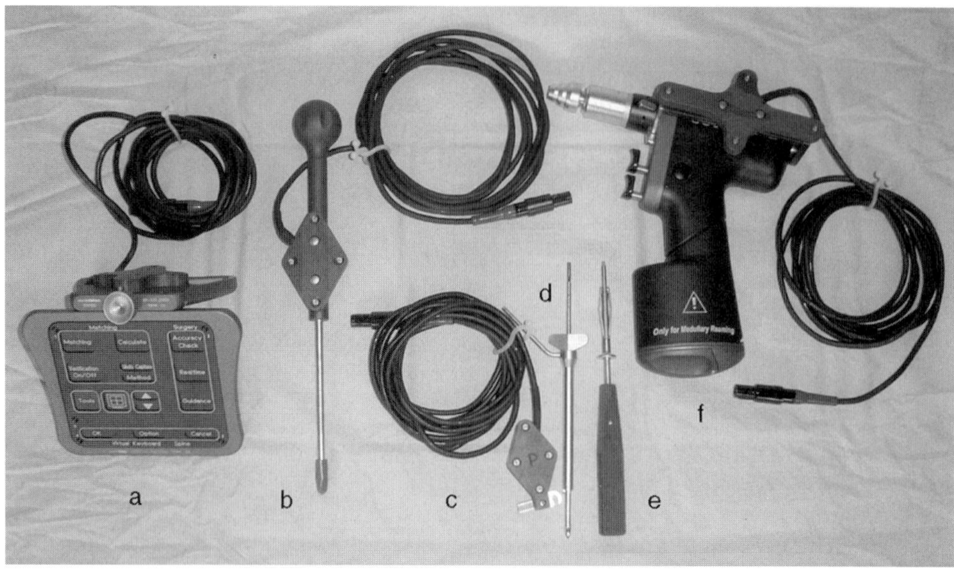

Figure 14-18. The instruments used for navigation. *a,* The virtual keyboard, on which most manipulations can be carried out. *b,* Awl with protection cap. *c,* Dynamic reference base (DRB). *d,* Drill sleeve with the handle on which the DRB is firmly placed over the Schanz screw. The wing nut can be tightened on the drill sleeve to form a solid unit. *e,* 3.5-mm screwdriver for the attachment of the DRB. *f,* Battery-powered Colibri drill (Synthes, West Chester, Pa) with the light-emitting diodes on top, turned toward the viewer.

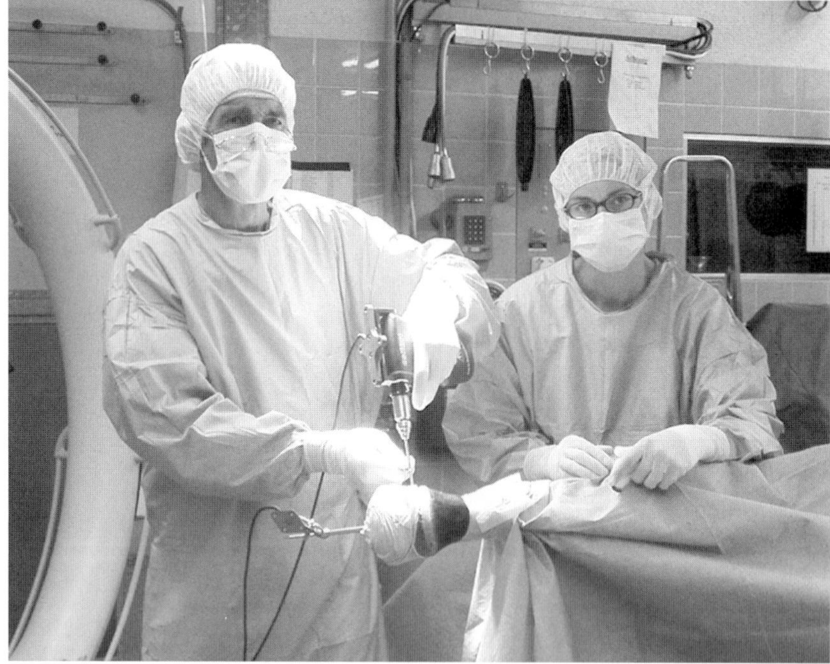

Figure 14-19. Drilling is performed while constantly observing the monitor screen. The dynamic reference base (DRB) can be seen mounted to the hoof.

Three-dimensional navigation systems such as the Medivision SurgiGate in combination with the Siremobil Iso 3D has great potential to be a real advantage for the precise and accurate implantation of lag screws in fractures in the horse. It has been used successfully in a limited number of clinical cases. A controlled study on cadaveric limbs is underway to evaluate the value of the system.[42] Potential future indications for CAS include fractures of the distal, middle, and proximal phalanx, condylar and saucer fractures of MCIII and MTIII, and cystic lesions of the various bones. A study is presently being conducted on the use of CAS in the management of navicular bone fractures.

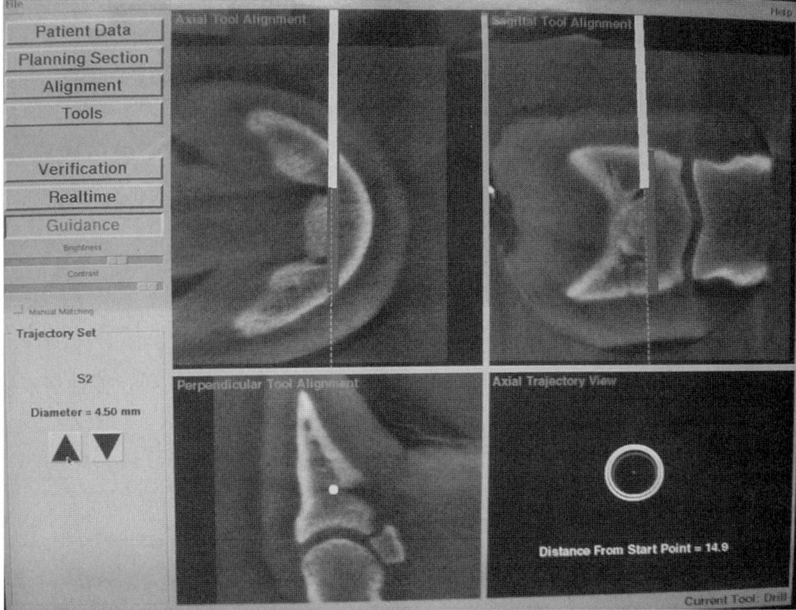

Figure 14-20. The computer screen during the insertion of a 4.5-mm screw into the coffin bone. *Top left:* The *darker line* crossing the birds-eye view of P3 represents the intended location of the screw within the bone. The *light line* represents the drill bit and shows how much of the bone is penetrated. *Top right:* Again, the *darker bar* represents the planned screw location in the frontal plane, whereas the *white line* shows the drill bit. There is more discrepancy between planned and actual location than in the view to the left. *Bottom left:* The *white dot* in the sagittal plane, representing the drill bit, coincides with the darker planned screw location. *Bottom right:* The three *circles* shown on the screen represent the axial trajectory view. Ideally, the circles should be concentrically arranged. The inner circle represents the planned screw location, the one in the middle the tip of the drill bit, and the outer circle the LED marker of the drill. The tip of the drill bit is 14.9 mm inside the bone.

REFERENCES

1. Fischer AT: Equine Diagnostic and Surgical Laparoscopy, Philadelphia, 2002, WB Saunders.
2. Freeman LJ: Veterinary Endosurgery, St Louis, 1999, Mosby.
3. McIlwraith CW: Diagnostic and Surgical Arthroscopy in the Horse, ed 2, Philadelphia, 1990, Lea & Febiger.
4. Fellows CG, Lerche P, King G, et al: Treatment of patent ductus arteriosus by placement of two intravascular embolisation coils in a puppy, J Small Anim Pract 1998;39:196.
5. Hogan DF, Green HW 3rd, Gordon S, et al: Transarterial coil embolization of patent ductus arteriosus in small dogs with 0.025-inch vascular occlusion coils: 10 cases, J Vet Intern Med 2004; 18:325.
6. Schneider M, Hildebrandt N, Schweigl T, et al: Transvenous embolization of small patent ductus arteriosus with single detachable coils in dogs, J Vet Intern Med 2001;15:222.
7. Stokhof AA, Sreeram N, Wolvekamp WT: Transcatheter closure of patent ductus arteriosus using occluding spring coils, J Vet Intern Med 2000;14:452.
8. Tanaka R, Nagashima Y, Hoshi K, et al: Supplemental embolization coil implantation for closure of patent ductus arteriosus in a beagle dog, J Vet Med Sci 2001;63:557.
9. Asano K, Watari T, Kuwabara M, et al: Successful treatment by percutaneous transvenous coil embolization in a small-breed dog with intrahepatic portosystemic shunt, J Vet Med Sci 2003;65:1269.
10. Gonzalo-Orden JM, Altonaga JR, Costilla S, et al: Transvenous coil embolization of an intrahepatic portosystemic shunt in a dog, Vet Radiol Ultrasound 2000;41:516.
11. Leveille R, Pibarot P, Soulez G, et al: Transvenous coil embolization of an extrahepatic portosystemic shunt in a dog: A naturally occurring model of portosystemic malformations in humans, Pediatr Radiol 2000;30:607.
12. Leveille R, Johnson SE, Birchard SJ: Transvenous coil embolization of portosystemic shunt in dogs, Vet Radiol Ultrasound 2003;44:32.
13. Yamakado K, Takeda K, Nishide Y, et al: Portal vein embolization with steel coils and absolute ethanol: A comparative experimental study with canine liver, Hepatology 1995;22:1812.
14. Partington BP, Partington CR, Biller DS: Transvenous coil embolization for treatment of patent ductus venosus in a dog, J Am Vet Med Assoc 1993;202:281.
15. Weisse C, Nicholson ME, Rollings C, et al: Use of percutaneous arterial embolization for treatment of intractable epistaxis in three dogs, J Am Vet Med Assoc 2004;224:1307.
16. Huang Z, Dai Q, Jiang T, Li J: Endovascular embolization of intracranial aneurysms with self-made tungsten coils in a dog model, Chin Med J (Engl) 1996;109:626.
17. Leveille R, Hardy J, Robertson JT, et al: Transarterial occlusion of the internal and external carotid, and maxillary arteries using embolization coils in normal horses, Proc Eur Coll Vet Surg 1999;8:173.
18. Leveille R, Hardy J, Robertson JT, et al: Transarterial coil embolization of the internal and external carotid and maxillary arteries for prevention of hemorrhage from guttural pouch mycosis in horses, Vet Surg 2000;29:389.

19. Matsuda Y, Nakanishi Y, Mizuno Y: Occlusion of the internal carotid artery by means of microcoils for preventing epistaxis caused by guttural pouch mycosis in horses, J Vet Med Sci 1999;61:221.
20. Ragle C, Wooten T, Howlett M: Microcoil embolization of the rostral portion of the internal carotid artery in the horse. In Proceedings of the 7th Annual Symposium of the American College of Veterinary Surgeons, 1997.
21. Sun F, Hernandez J, Ezquerra J, et al: Angiographic study and therapeutic embolization of soft-tissue fibrosarcoma in a dog: Case report and literature, J Am Anim Hosp Assoc 2002;38:452.
22. Weisse C, Clifford CA, Holt D, et al: Percutaneous arterial embolization and chemoembolization for treatment of benign and malignant tumors in three dogs and a goat, J Am Vet Med Assoc 2002;221:1430.
23. Yi SW, Kim YH, Kwon IC, et al: Stable lipiodolized emulsions for hepatoma targeting and treatment by transcatheter arterial chemoembolization, J Control Release 1998;50:135.
24. Ding JW, Wu ZD, Andersson R, et al: Pharmacokinetics of mitomycin C following hepatic arterial chemoembolization with Gelfoam, HPB Surg 1992;5:161-167; discussion, 167-169.
25. Nishioka Y, Kyotani S, Okamura M, et al: A study of embolizing materials for chemo-embolization therapy of hepatocellular carcinoma: Embolic effect of cisplatin albumin microspheres using chitin and chitosan in dogs, and changes of cisplatin content in blood and tissue, Chem Pharm Bull (Tokyo) 1992;40:267.
26. Cho KJ, Williams DM, Brady TM, et al: Transcatheter embolization with sodium tetradecyl sulfate: Experimental and clinical results, Radiology 1984;153:95.
27. Li X, Hu G, Liu P: Segmental embolization by ethanol iodized oil emulsion for hepatocellular carcinoma, J Tongji Med Univ 1999;19:135.
28. Crawford WH: Aortic-iliac thrombosis in a horse, Can Vet J 1982;23:59.
29. Gerhards H, Rosenbruch M: Intermittierendes Hinken beim Pferd: Diskussion ätiologischer und therapeutischer Aspekte an Hand eines Fallberichtes, Prakt Tierarzt 1984;8:645.
30. Maxie MG, Physick-Sheard PW: Aortic-iliac thrombosis in horses, Vet Pathol 1985;22:238.
31. Azzie MAJ: Aortic/iliac thrombosis of thoroughbred horses, Equine Vet J 1969;1:113.
32. Boswell JC, Marr CM, Cauvin ER, et al: The use of scintigraphy in the diagnosis of aortic-iliac thrombosis in a horse, Equine Vet J 1999;31:537.
33. Brama PA, Rijkenhuizen AB, van Swieten HA, et al: Thrombosis of the aorta and the caudal arteries in the horse: Additional diagnostics and a new surgical treatment, Vet Quart 1996;18(Suppl 2):S85.
34. Branscomb BL: Treatment of arterial thrombosis in a horse with sodium gluconate, J Am Vet Med Assoc 1968;152:1643.
35. Moffett FS, Vaden P: Diagnosis and treatment of thrombosis of the posterior aorta or iliac arteries in the horse, Vet Med Small Anim Clin 1978;73:184.
36. Reef VB, Roby KAW, Richardson DW, et al: Use of ultrasonography for the detection of aortic-iliac thrombosis in horses, J Am Vet Med Assoc 1987;190:286.
37. Tillotsen PJ, Kopper PH: Treatment of aortic thrombosis in a horse, J Am Vet Med Assoc 1966;149:766.
38. Tithof PK, Rebhun WC, Dietze AE: Ultrasonographic diagnosis of aorto-iliac thrombosis, Cornell Vet 1985;75:540.
39. Warmerdam EP: Ultrasonography of the femoral artery in six normal horses and three horses with thrombosis, Vet Radiol Ultrasound 1998;39:137.
40. Stashak TS: Adams' Lameness in Horses, ed 4, Philadelphia, 1987, Lea & Febiger.
41. Auer JA: Computer assisted orthopedic surgery (CAOS) in equine fracture treatment, Proc Eur Coll Vet Surg 2003;12:70.
42 Andritzky J, Rossol M, Lischer CJ, Auer JA: Comparison of computer assisted osteosynthesis to conventional technique for the treatment of axial distal phalanx fractures in horses: An experimental study, Vet Surg 2005;34:120.

CHAPTER 15

Cryosurgery

John A. Stick

PRINCIPLES OF CRYOBIOLOGY

Mammalian cells are destroyed when cooled to a temperature of −20° C (−4° F).[1] Primary injury begins with the formation of ice crystals, both intracellular and extracellular. The cell's outer membrane becomes ruptured by intracellular crystals, and ice formation outside the cell dehydrates the cellular environment, resulting in lethal electrolyte concentrations and pH changes. When organelles are damaged, the cell loses its ability to regulate ion permeability, and cell death ensues. Secondary injury from freezing occurs from vascular stasis. As the permeability of vessels is increased, loss of plasma causes local hemoconcentration. Damaged endothelium in arterioles and venules induces thrombus formation of the vessels, and infarction of frozen tissue occurs within hours of freezing.

Rapid freezing results in the greatest intracellular concentration of ice. Thereafter, slow thawing of the tissue results in recrystallization, during which small crystals enlarge, producing more cell damage. To ensure that all target tissue receives a lethal dose of cold, a second freeze/thaw cycle is used. Because precooled tissue freezes faster than normal tissue, repeating this cycle causes necrosis of the target tissue more consistently.

Variations in vascularity, noncellular structure, and water content cause tissues to respond differently to cryonecrosis. Dry tissues (e.g., the cornea) do not readily form ice crystals and therefore do not respond to cryotherapy very well. The cellular components of peripheral nerves are destroyed by freezing, but because the fiber scaffolding of the epineurium is not damaged, regeneration is possible.[2] Tissues near major blood vessels or in highly vascular areas are difficult to freeze rapidly and tend to thaw quickly without loss of function.[3] The use of epinephrine or temporary regional vessel occlusion may be necessary to ensure proper treatment in those tissues.

Although immune responses directed against tumor cells have been documented after cryosurgery, this has not been proven clinically in horses.[4] However, numerous case reports

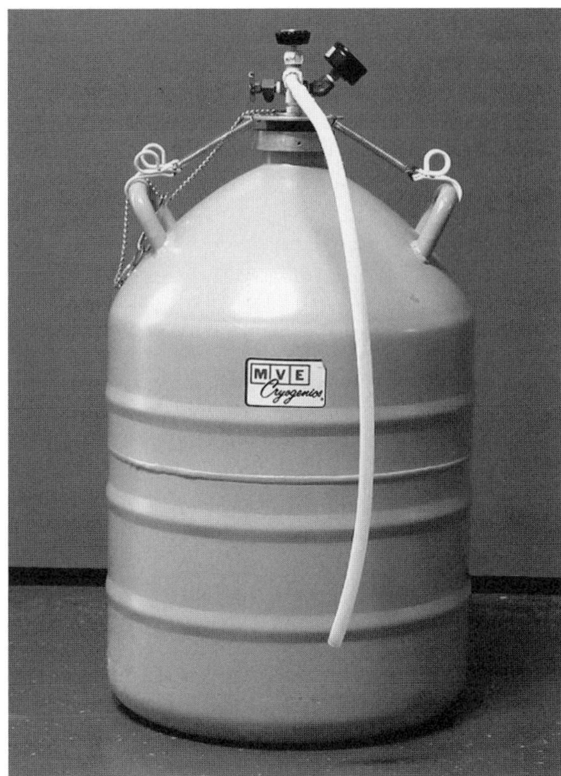

Figure 15-1. Insulated Dewar flasks are used to store liquid nitrogen. This tank is fitted with a special adaptor lid and spray gun attachment. Note the pressure gauges used to regulate the liquid nitrogen.

suggest secondary tumor regression does occur as a result of cryosurgical treatment of a primary tumor.[5,6]

Although liquid nitrogen, nitrous oxide, and carbon dioxide are all cryogens used in veterinary medicine, liquid nitrogen is the most versatile and therefore the most commonly used. Liquid nitrogen has a boiling point of −195.8° C (−320.4° F). Cryogens, usually stored in liquid form in Dewar flasks (Fig. 15-1), can be delivered as a spray or used by super-chilling a probe. Two types of probes are used: hollow probes and solid probes. When hollow probes are used, liquid is circulated through the probe and exits under pressure through a small opening. When solid probes are used, they are chilled by immersion into the liquid cryogen.

Indications

Cryosurgery does not require a sterile field. Therefore, it is a good choice for the treatment of benign and neoplastic cutaneous lesions. It can also be used in the mouth and in ocular surgery. By far the most common tumor that is treated with cryotherapy is the equine sarcoid. However, a plethora of skin conditions amenable to surgery can be treated by cryotherapy (see Chapter 29). Because there is frequently no need for general anesthesia of horses afflicted with skin lesions, cryosurgery has an advantage over other types of surgical extirpations—it frequently can be done on an outpatient basis.

INSTRUMENTATION

Sprays

Self-pressurizing spray guns (Fig. 15-2) deliver a combination of vapor and droplets of liquid cryogen and are a most effective method of cryogen delivery. As liquid nitrogen contacts the tissue, it evaporates, or changes from the liquid to the gas phase. This has been shown to remove a greater amount of heat from treated tissue than is achieved with probes. The volume and size of the spray droplet are controlled by the diameter of the needle orifice (Fig. 15-3) and the trigger in the pressurizing gun. The surgeon can gauge the volume of the cryogen so that the wetting conforms to the shape of the tumor's surface. However, care must be taken to prevent excess liquid cryogen from running off onto surrounding skin. It is common to pack the surrounding area with Vaseline-impregnated sponges to prevent this runoff. Alternatively, a spray cup (Fig. 15-4) can be used that has the advantage of controlling runoff. A cup size (Fig. 15-5) is chosen that fits over the tumor, and as the spray is applied, droplets form a liquid pool over the tumor.

Probes

Hollow probes are cooled by circulating a liquid cryogen through them. Hollow probe freezing is easiest to control, but the rate it cools an area is slow compared with the rate achieved by spray and solid probes. Hollow probes can be

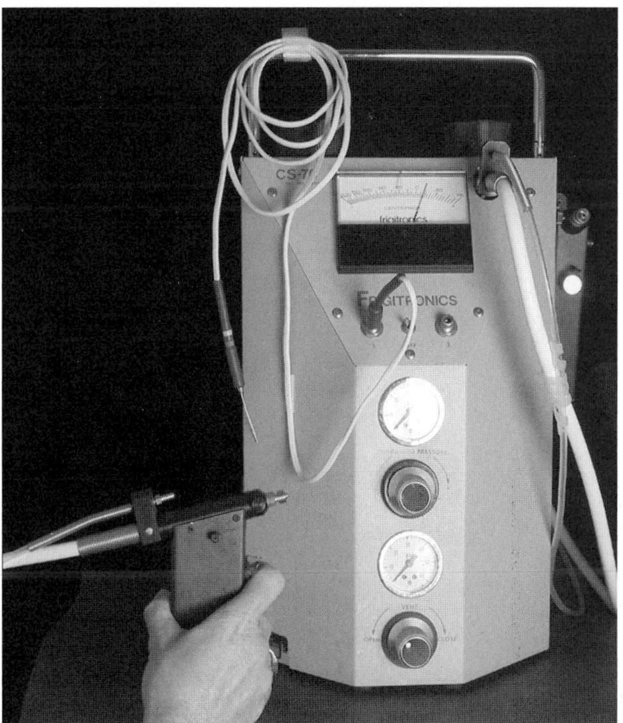

Figure 15-2. Special container used to deliver liquid nitrogen through a self-pressurizing spray gun. A thermocouple needle is to the left of the pyrometer, which is used to measure the temperature achieved beyond the limits of the targeted tissue. This single-channel monitor allows the needle to be placed into the tissue adjacent to the deepest portion of the target. When the temperature reaches −20° C, all unwanted tissue is destroyed.

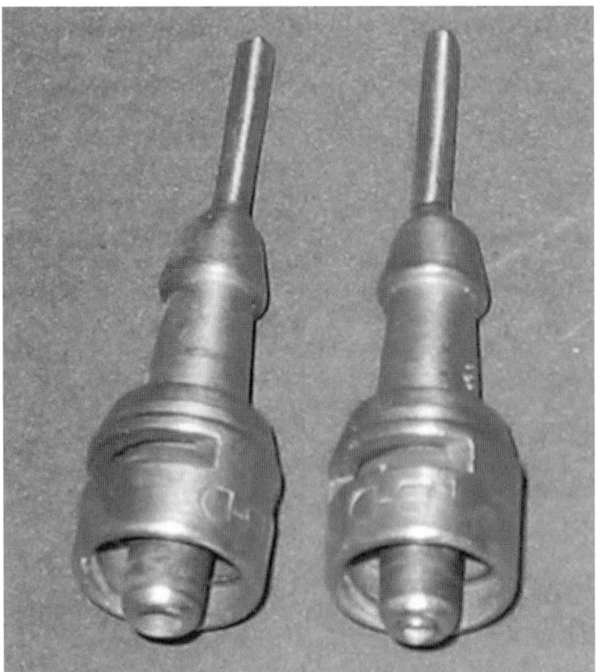

Figure 15-3. Two examples of needles that attach to the spray gun to deliver liquid nitrogen sprays directly onto the tissue to be frozen. The volume and size of the spray drop is determined by the diameter of the needle orifice.

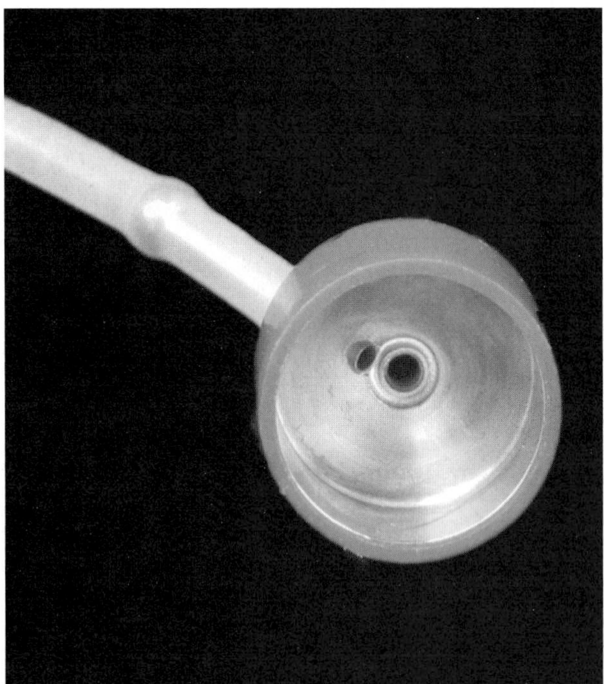

Figure 15-4. View of the inside of the spray cup, which is attached to the self-pressurizing spray gun.

used for either contact or penetration freezing, depending on the configuration of the probe (Fig. 15-6). During freezing, traction can be used to lift the tumor away from underlying structures as an ice ball is extended to the monitored limits.[7] Penetration freezing can be performed in larger lesions where a core biopsy specimen is removed from the

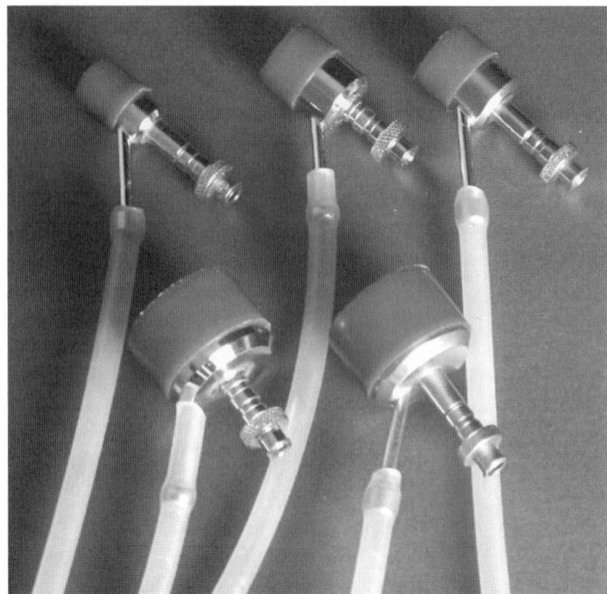

Figure 15-5. Spray cups come in a variety of sizes, so the cup can be fitted over a tumor, and as the spray is applied, droplets form a liquid pool contained by the cup. This prevents runoff generated by the spray method.

center of the tumor (Fig. 15-7) and the cryoprobe is placed within the mass. Contact freezing with solid probes is a very efficient manner of delivering cryotherapy to variously sized tumors, based on the size of the probe (Fig. 15-8). As multiple probes are placed within the liquid nitrogen (Fig. 15-9), they can be removed and used to freeze tumors quite rapidly—a large advantage when multiple tumors need to be frozen in the same patient.

CRYOSURGERY TECHNIQUES

Using either contact or penetration cryotherapy, monitoring the depth of freezing can be done either by subjective inspection or by objective measurement of temperature changes. Subjective assessment is made by visual inspection or palpation of the ice ball. The outer edge of the ice ball is about 0° C (32° F), which is inadequate for tissue destruction. Seventy-five percent of the tissue within an ice ball is destroyed by freezing. The depth of contact freezing is estimated to be slightly less than the radius of the ice ball. Pyrometers are used to measure the temperature achieved beyond the limits of the target tissue. Single- or multiple-channel monitors are available (see Fig. 15-2). Needle probes are placed into the tissue adjacent to the deepest portion of the target. When temperatures of −20° C (−4° F) are recorded, all unwanted tissue is destroyed.

COMPLICATIONS

Normal biologic reactions to freezing include swelling, bleeding, necrosis, depigmentation, and odor of varying degrees. Swelling occurs within hours of freezing because of increased vascular permeability and vasodilation. This is usually self-limiting and resolves in 48 hours. When lesions are biopsied or ulcerated and undergo cryotherapy,

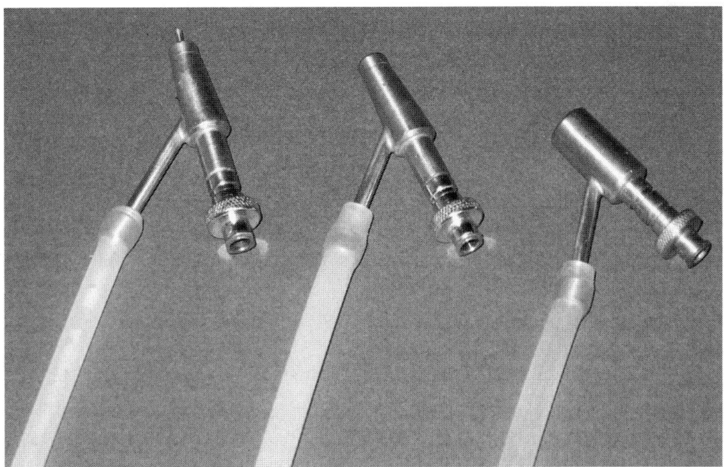

Figure 15-6. Hollow probes come in a variety of shapes and can be used for either contact or penetration freezing.

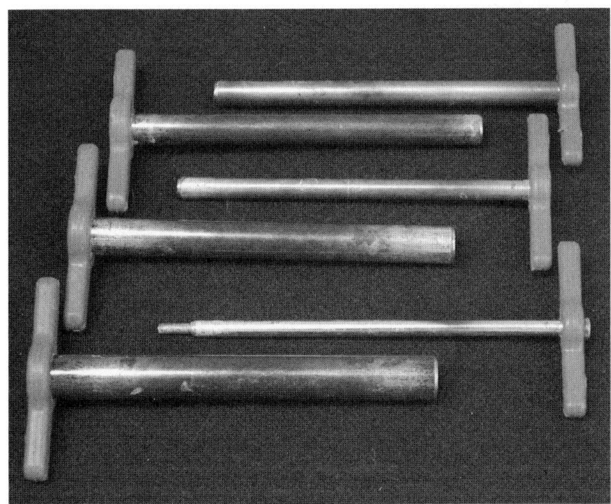

Figure 15-7. Core biopsy instruments used to remove the center of a tumor so that the same size of hollow spray probe can be inserted into the center of the tumor to perform penetration freezing.

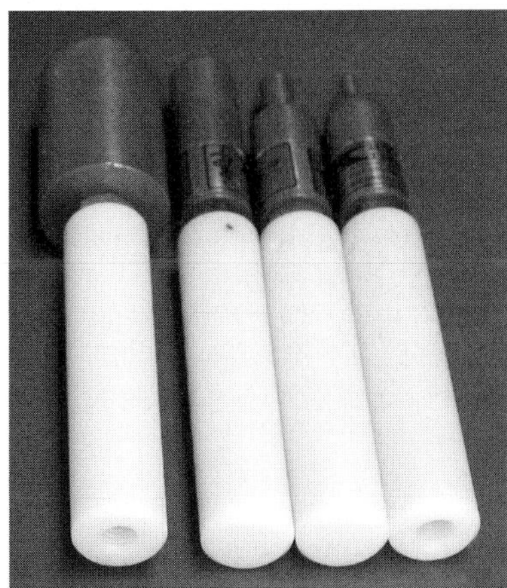

Figure 15-8. Solid probes come in a variety of sizes, each fitted with a separate plastic handle that does not become chilled as the probe is immersed in liquid nitrogen. Various sizes and shapes allow these probes to become a heat sink when pressed onto the surface of the tumor.

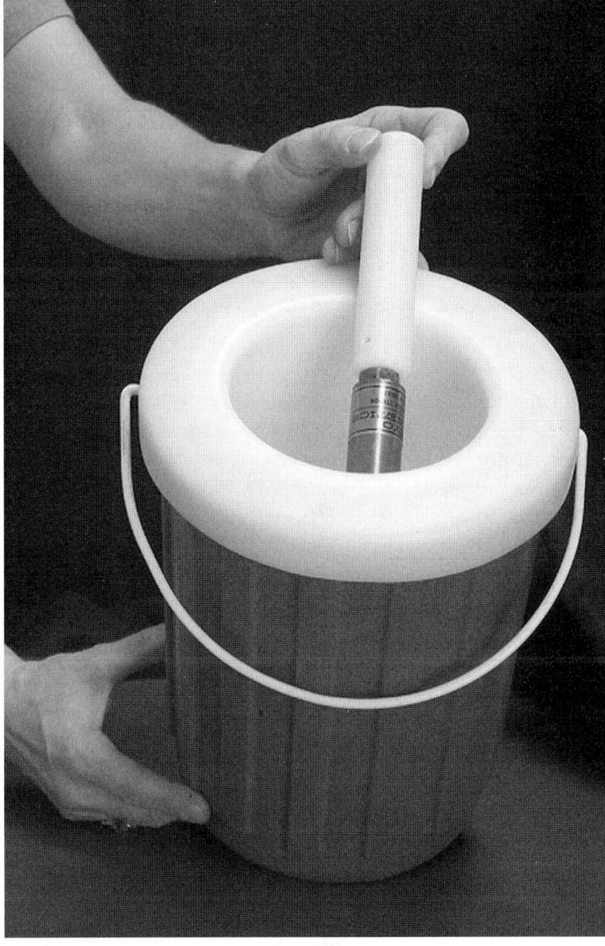

Figure 15-9. A special container is used into which liquid nitrogen is poured and the contact probe is submersed to attain the proper temperature before applying to a tumor.

vasodilation after freezing can cause hemorrhage to become more obvious and may become cosmetically objectionable to an owner. Therefore, some form of hemostasis should be used during the biopsy procedure and on ulcerated lesions.

Necrosis occurs in 14 to 21 days. The wound contracts and epithelializes under a dry eschar that forms over the necrotic tissue. When the eschar sloughs, it usually reveals healthy granulation tissue or recurrence of the tumor. Because melanocytes and hair follicles are destroyed by freezing, the skin will show depigmentation and will not regrow hair. Owners need to be advised of this prior to treatment.

Offensive odors accompany necrosis of large tumors, and cleansing of the area daily and excision of the necrotic tissue may be necessary to ameliorate this problem. Freezing cortical bone causes cell destruction and reduces the strength of the bone by 70%. Spontaneous fractures have been reported months after cryotherapy treatment. Additionally, bone tumors do not respond well to cryotherapy. Auricular cartilage does not respond well to cryotherapy either and can result in shortening or deformity of an ear. Therefore, cryotherapy should be used on skin tumors in the ears with caution.

REFERENCES

1. Wolstenholme GWE, O'Connor M, editors: The frozen cell. A Ciba Foundation Symposium. London, 1970, J & A Churchill.
2. Beazley RM, Bagley DH, Ketcham AS: The effect of cryosurgery on peripheral nerves, J Surg Res 1974;16:231.
3. Gage AM, Montes M, Gage AA: Freezing the canine aorta in situ, J Surg Res 1979;27:331.
4. Neel HB: Immunotherapeutic effect of cryosurgical tumor necrosis, Vet Clin North Am 1980;10:763.
5. Martens A, DeMoor A, Vlaminck J, et al: Evaluation of excision, cryosurgery and local BCG vaccination for the treatment of equine sarcoids, Vet Rec 2001;149:665.
6. Klein WR, Bras GE, Misdorp W, et al: Equine sarcoid: BCG immunotherapy compared to cryosurgery in a prospective randomized clinical trial, Cancer Immunol Immunother 1986;21:133.
7. Holmberg DL: Cryosurgery. In Slatter D, editor: Textbook of Small Animal Surgery, ed 3, Philadelphia, 2003, Elsevier.

CHAPTER 16

Lasers in Veterinary Surgery

Lloyd P. Tate, Jr.

As technology and specialized instrumentation have expanded the realm of minimally invasive surgeries, public and veterinary awareness has greatly increased. Surgeries using lasers are minimally invasive in that they often do not require general anesthesia or an external incision, and they can be performed transendoscopically. The word *laser* is an acronym for *light amplification by stimulated emission of radiation*. Surgical lasers offer veterinarians the potential for expanding their surgical capability, decreasing complications, and improving patient care. To meet these goals and to avoid foreseeable complications, surgeons should understand laser–tissue interactions and the requirements for safe operation of surgical lasers.

FUNCTION OF THE LASER

Laser Physics

Energy is emitted by a laser in the form of light, called a photon. Understanding the emission process is an important first step toward applying the laser surgically. Light is characterized or defined by its frequency, wavelength, amplitude, and velocity. Numeric values given to these characteristics depend on the source from which the light is generated. A large number of medical lasers use the near-infrared spectrum. Examples of laser *sources* include carbon dioxide, argon, neodymium, gallium, and holmium. Each source is referred to as a laser medium (Table 16-1). All photons produced by a given medium have identical wavelengths and frequencies (*frequency* here is called coherence). The medium may exist in one of three forms: as a gas, a crystal, or a liquid. The medium requires an external energy source to produce the photon cascade that results in a laser beam.

The process of energizing a medium involves stimulating electrons and is referred to as pumping. Pumping may occur in several forms, such as heat, light, electricity, or even another laser beam. The pumping process does not determine the characteristics of photons produced by the medium; it is only a method of energizing the medium.

The medium and pumping source are two primary components of the laser. A third component is composed of two reflecting surfaces, one containing a shutter or semitransparent area. The reflecting surfaces are mirrors placed at either end of the medium. The mirrors and medium are contained within a resonating chamber (Fig. 16-1). Photons initially emitted by the medium are continually reflected back into the medium. As pumping continues, electrons from the medium are raised to a highly excited state. The electrons eventually gain sufficient energy to penetrate the semitransparent reflective mirror surface and exit as a laser beam.

Diode lasers do not require a resonating chamber, as they are fashioned from semiconductors and are referred to as solid-state lasers. Diode laser semiconductors are fashioned from gallium salts or more complex compounds. Functionally, semiconductors are made of two materials that vary in their ability to allow electrons to pass through them.[1] At the interface or junction between two types of semiconductors,

TABLE 16-1. Commonly Available Surgical Lasers

Laser Type	Wavelength	Light Spectrum (nm)
Carbon dioxide*	Infrared	10,600
	Blue	488
Argon	Green	515
	Infrared	1064
Nd:YAG*	Infrared	1318
Frequency-doubled Nd:YAG	Green	532
	Red	647
	Yellow	568
Krypton	Green	531
Ruby		
Helium neon	Deep red	694
Gold vapor	Red	632
Copper vapor	Red	632
	Variable with dyes	
	Red	632
Dye laser	Yellow/green	577
Erbium	Infrared	
Excimers		
ArF		193
KrCl		222
KrF		248
XeCl		308
XeF	Ultraviolet	351

*The carbon dioxide and Nd:YAG lasers are popular for photoincision and ablation.
Nd:YAG, neodymium:yttrium aluminum garnet.

an electronic phenomenon occurs. When voltage is applied, electrons flow through the junction, causing a buildup of excited electrons on one side. When the system relaxes or current decreases, the electrons seek equilibrium by de-excitation, which causes an energy release in the form of an emitted photon (Fig. 16-2). The reason for the photon release is that pores present at the junction between the two semiconductors allow the electrons to travel through only when they are in a relaxed state. To return to a relaxed state, the energized electrons must release a photon. By channeling the photons from a series of diodes, the laser beam is produced. The materials used to construct semiconductors, the number of semiconductors used, and the voltage, current, and heat produced determine the frequency and power output of each laser. Large lasers using resonating chambers are being replaced by diode lasers, which have more efficient semiconductor cooling, allowing an increase in power output.

The laser beam is electromagnetic radiation or irradiation produced by stimulated emission from an excited medium or semiconductor.[2] A unique characteristic of the laser beam is that it is spatially and temporally in phase, meaning that the photons are all of the same wavelength and traveling in parallel fashion. This characteristic of the beam is described as being collimated and monochromic. Coherence, collimation, and monochromic light are important parameters for transmission and focusing of laser irradiation. Lenses placed in the system control the beams, the focal length, and focal spot size. Focal spot size is referred to as the focal point, and its size determines the amount of energy delivered to an area of tissue. When laser energy is concentrated into a small focal point, it is used for cutting and vaporizing tissue.[3,4] Divergence means that the focal point is either above or below the tissue surface. Thus, irradiation is less concentrated and requires more time at the same energy level to produce the same thermal effect. Divergent laser beams are often used for vessel coagulation.

Laser output power is expressed as watts, where delivered laser energy over time is expressed as watts per second (W/sec) or joules (J). Energy that is concentrated in a known area is called the power density and is expressed as a watt per square centimeter (W/cm^2).[5] Power density determines the type of biologic change that will be seen in tissue (Fig. 16-3). Laser energy applied over a large area of tissue has a diffuse thermal effect. A small focal spot concentrates the energy, producing deeper tissue penetration, which is preferred for making an incision. Thermal damage to tissue that is not immediately apparent is referred to as latent thermal necrosis. In resecting a tumor, it may be desirable to have latent thermal damage to achieve as much marginal destruction as possible. Latent thermal damage is best appreciated lateral to an incision line (Fig. 16-4). The type of laser, its medium, and how its irradiation is delivered and interacts with tissue influence the laser's effectiveness as a surgical tool.

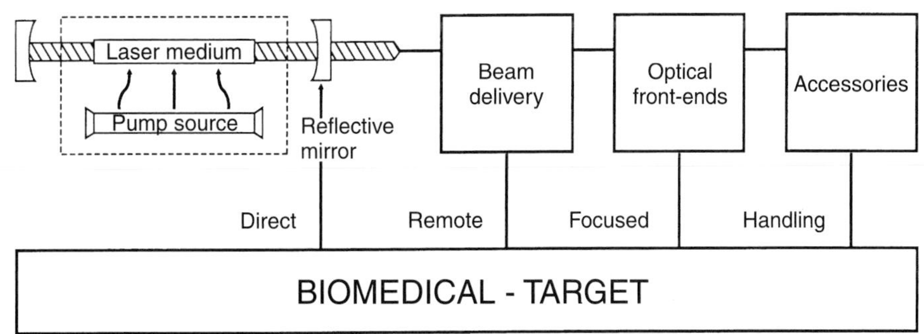

Figure 16-1. Schematic drawing of a laser and its available delivery systems. Structures within *dotted lines* represent resonating chamber.

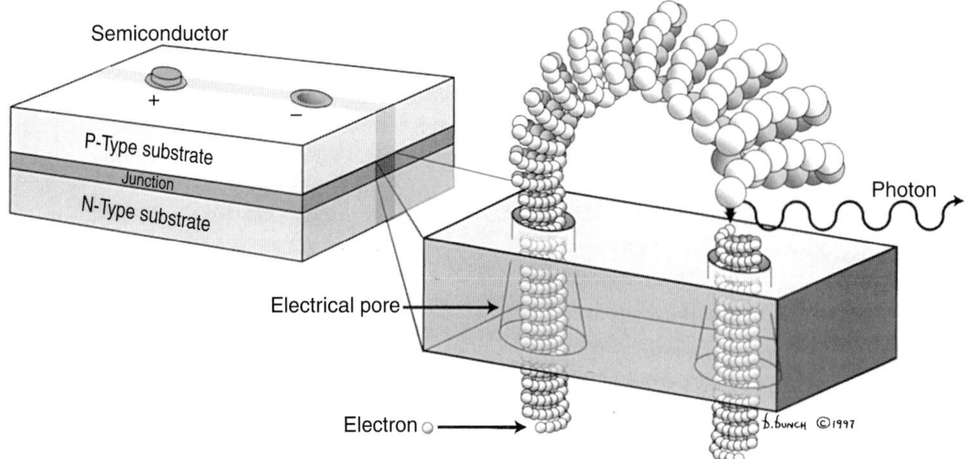

Figure 16-2. Schematic diagram of a semiconductor. A photon is emitted from a semiconductor when electrons return across the junction of the two different substrates, resulting from a change in voltage flux.

Range of Power (in watts/cm^2)	Density Result	Spot Size
1 - 10	Coagulation	mm
10 - 100	Coagulation and vaporization	
100 - 1000	Hemostasis of small vessels	
1000 - 10,000	Rapid cutting or vaporization	
10,000 - 100,000 or higher	Ultra-rapid cutting	
		0.1 mm

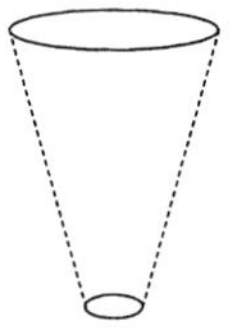

Figure 16-3. Delivery of irradiation to tissue is controlled by power or spot size to produce a biologic change.

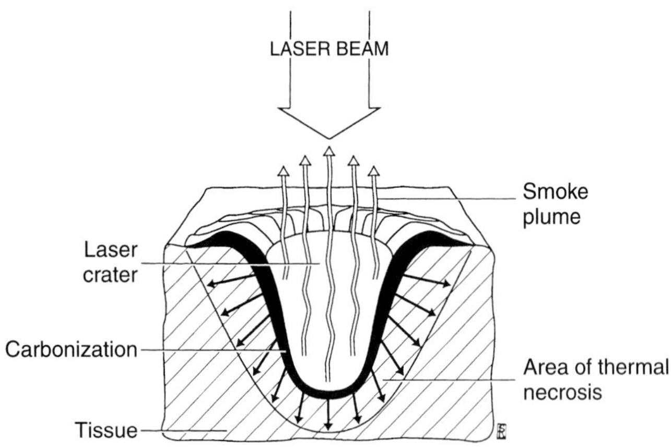

Figure 16-4. Physical changes that occur in tissue from laser beam irradiation.

How a laser is used is influenced by how the beam and energy are delivered. A lens is often used at the delivery point to concentrate the laser beam, but with it, irradiation can be applied only in the direct line of sight. Attaching a transmitting fiber permits the beam to be directed in different directions and allows endoscopic application. The mode and how the laser beam is configured also determine depth of penetration and the amount of latent thermal damage. There are three modes used in delivering laser beams: continuous mode, chopped mode, and superpulse mode.[3] The advantages of the chopped and superpulse modes over the continuous mode are energy efficiency, a decrease in lateral thermal damage, and greater tissue penetration. The continuous mode does not allow marginal tissue cooling during cutting. In the chopped and superpulse modes, cycles of energy are delivered to tissue, which allows cooling between cycles. The faster the laser beam is pulsed, the greater is the amount of energy delivered to the tissue and the deeper the penetration. Choice of which surgical laser to use depends on the method of irradiation delivery, power output, cost, size, and laser–tissue interaction.

Tissue Interaction

The laser's wavelength and frequency determine how it will interact with tissue. Tissue reacts to lasers in one of four ways, or in a combination of any of the four: (1) absorption, (2) reflection, (3) transmission, and (4) scatter (Fig. 16-5).

Absorption represents conversion of laser irradiation into heat, resulting in an incision or tissue vaporization. Denaturation of protein occurs when tissue is heated

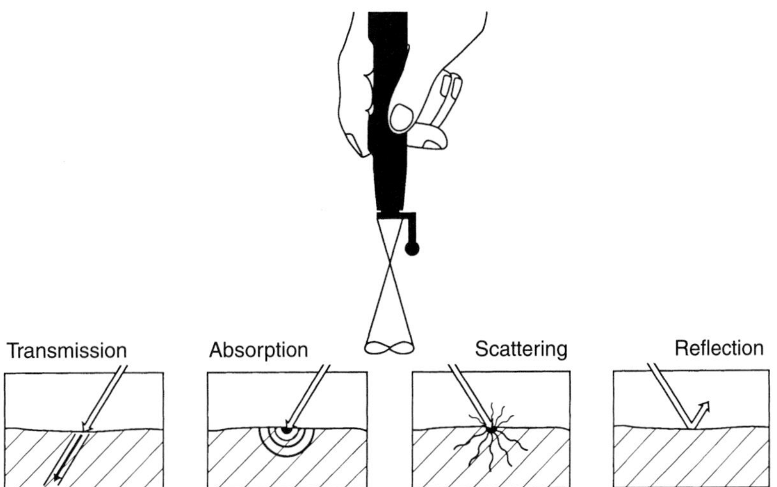

Figure 16-5. Four possible laser tissue interactions. Dominance is determined by laser beam wavelength.

TABLE 16-2. Changes Resulting from Interaction between Laser Beam and Tissue

Temperature (C)	Visual Change	Biologic Change
100°	Smoke plume	Vaporization, carbonization
90°-100°	Puckering	Drying
65°-90°	White/gray	Protein denaturation
60°-65°	Blanching	Blanching
37°-60°	None	Warming, welding

between 60° and 70° C and causes coagulation necrosis[6] (Table 16-2). Tissue vaporization occurs at 100° C, resulting in cellular explosion.[6]

Scattering and reflection cause additional tissue loss.[6] Scattering depends on both the frequency of the energy delivered and the tissue absorption characteristics. Cellular constituents do not equally absorb laser irradiation. Transmission through tissue or fluids surrounding tissue occurs when the absorption curve of pigments, proteins, or fluids does not match the wavelength of the laser beam. The eye is a good example of this laser energy–tissue interaction, because laser irradiation in the visible and near-infrared spectrum are transmitted easily through the clear cornea and lens to be absorbed by the pigmented retina. Water, as an example, absorbs light in the far end of the light spectrum, whereas melanin and hemoglobin absorb light in the near-infrared end of the spectrum. Therefore, the cornea, which contains water, absorbs laser irradiation from the far-infrared spectrum, preventing deeper transmission.

Laser Safety

Laser safety is important because a collimated laser beam can be emitted over a great distance without attenuation. Lasers have been classified for safety by the Bureau of Radiological Health and the Food and Drug Administration.[5] These agencies classify lasers on the basis of energy output and accessibility to the irradiation emitted. Surgical lasers emit high energy levels and belong to class IV lasers, which are considered the most hazardous because burns can result from direct application or from deflected or reflected beams of irradiation. All personnel within an area where surgical lasers are operated need to be aware of the potential damage that can be caused by the apparatus. The patient, operator, and other personnel should be protected.[2-5] All users should understand the safety standards required for each laser they intend to use. For example, the beam of the CO_2 laser is attenuated by water; therefore, drapes should be covered with sterile, moistened towels to avoid fires in the surgical area.[7] The endotracheal tubes used should be resistant to the laser beam or encased in a crinkled aluminum foil.[8] Protection of endotracheal tubes is of the greatest importance, because they carry high concentrations of oxygen; and airway fires are fatal.

Although instruments with a reflective surface can be used with lasers, it is best to use anodized instruments, decreasing the potential of reflected or scattered beams onto adjacent tissues or toward people in the area. Eye damage caused by reflection is a major safety concern. Specifically designed glasses or goggles should be used to filter out the damaging irradiation.[5-8] The CO_2 laser has a high propensity for damaging the cornea and requires the operator to wear simple plastic goggles. The argon, potassium titanyl phosphate (KTP), diode, or various yttrium aluminum garnet (YAG) lasers require specific filtered lenses to prohibit the beam from causing retinal damage. Endoscopic application of lasers should also include protective eyewear or should be performed with the assistance of a video camera attached to the endoscope.[5,9,10] This negates the possibility of infrared irradiation being reflected back through a fiberoptic channel and directly into the eye of the operator. Signs for laser dangers should be posted immediately outside the operating room, and the doors of the room should be locked during laser surgery. Glass windows in operating room doors and walls should be covered with protective shades, and equipment to extinguish a fire should be immediately available.

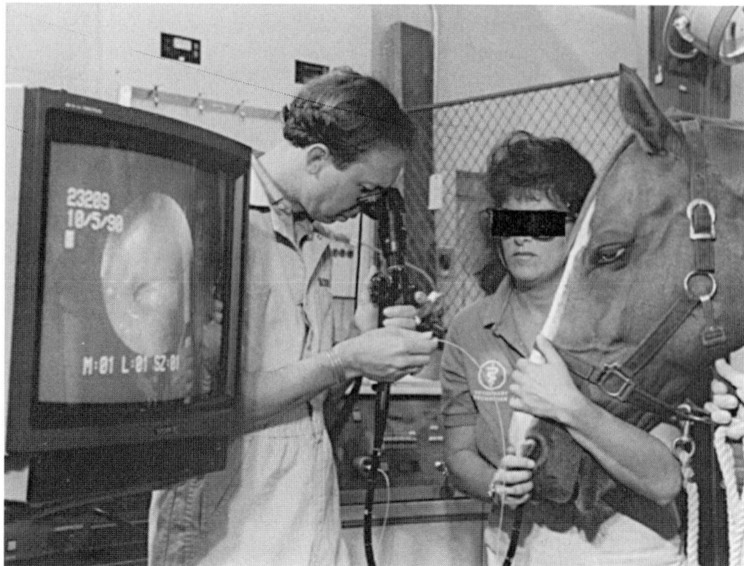

Figure 16-6. Transendoscopic laser surgery being performed. The laser fiber is directed through the biopsy channel of the endoscope. The assistant is wearing protective eyeglasses, and the surgeon views the procedure directly through a lens cap or video monitor.

Video viewing is also preferred because magnification of the target tissue improves the precision of directing the laser beam (Fig. 16-6). Endoscopes constructed with a built-in video chip camera should be certified as laser protected by the manufacturer. Video endoscopes that are not certified will produce a "whiteout" when the laser is activated, preventing observation of laser tissue interaction. Most endoscope manufacturers provide protection for neodymium (Nd):YAG laser irradiation. Diode lasers at a slightly different wavelength can cause a whiteout when the laser is activated. It is important to specify which laser wavelengths will be used when questioning the endoscope manufacturer or representative.

The laser fiber used for transendoscopic application should protrude at least 1 cm out of the distal biopsy port to prevent heat or hot debris from damaging the endoscope. Endoscopes that have a darkened surface at the distal end are more susceptible to damage than a metal or a lighter-colored material, because dark materials absorb infrared irradiation. After finishing a laser procedure, the laser fiber should be examined to ensure that there is no debris attached that could lacerate the inner channel of the endoscope when the fiber is retracted. The fiber should be allowed to cool before pulling it into the biopsy channel.

SUPPORT EQUIPMENT

Support equipment is considered essential for transendoscopic laser application. Commercially available broncho-esophageal grasping forceps, endoscopic snares, and polyethylene tubing are used to irrigate tissue or apply local anesthetics or medications through the biopsy channel.[11,12] Transendoscopic surgery for horses requires a flexible endoscope of at least 60 cm in length, preferably equipped with a video system.[11]

Some newer endoscopes contain a second channel, which may have several advantages for laser surgery, as it provides a route for the removal of smoke, the introduction of additional instruments, and direct irrigation. Endoscopic irrigation is advantageous for two reasons: it provides cool water to the tissues surrounding the target and, when applied in a pulsating mode, it can be used to flush carbonized debris from the tissue. It is crucial that the endoscope have at least a 2.7-mm biopsy channel to allow the passage of the laser fiber. Evacuation of smoke is important, because smoke irritates mucous membranes and obscures vision.[7,13] When a second biopsy channel is not available, smoke is removed by suction or by mechanical filtration attached to a flexible tube passed through the patient's opposite nostril. If standard suction is chosen, an in-line filter is necessary to prevent smoke particles and debris from soiling and obstructing the equipment.[8] The smoke produced during cell vaporization is referred to as *laser plume*. When a laser is used in general surgery, an air filtration device should also be employed to remove smoke from the surgical area.

RESTRAINT

Horses should be placed in stocks and heavily sedated for standing transendoscopic laser surgery. Xylazine (0.3 to 0.5 mg/kg) and butorphanol tartrate (0.025 mg/kg), in combination, provide sedation and analgesia.[8,11,14] Two alternative drug combinations that can be used for restraint are acepromazine maleate (0.033 mg/kg IV), followed by detomidine hydrochloride (0.011 mg/kg IV), or a combination of xylazine (0.4 to 0.6 mg/kg IV) and acepromazine maleate (0.02 to 0.04 mg/kg IV).[15] Topical anesthesia of mucosal surfaces can be provided by either local irrigation or infiltration. For upper respiratory work, the horse's head should be cross-tied in a position that prevents tracheal compression and at a level suitable for endoscope placement.

SURGICAL LASERS

CO_2 Laser

Of all the surgical lasers, the CO_2 laser has received more recognition and is used the most in general surgery. The CO_2 laser, which produces a beam of irradiation in the far-infrared range (10,600 nm), and was the first to be applied surgically, is considered excellent for incising tissue. Because its beam is absorbed rapidly, it produces little latent thermal damage. Its success as a hemostatic device is generally considered poor because it coagulates vessels only up to a diameter of 0.5 mm.[3,4] Its physical appearance is easily recognized; its beam is routinely transmitted through an articulating arm to the target tissue (Fig. 16-7). A series of mirrors and focusing lenses are incorporated into the articulating arm. The mirrors carry the laser beam and the lenses form a small focal spot. This articulating arm restricts the laser's use to lesions within the line of sight. By connecting it to operating microscopes, bronchoscopes, or laparoscopes, applications within certain hollow organs or passageways are possible.[7] Even when coupled to these devices, its application is still restricted to lesions within a straight line or lesions that can be visualized by reflection in mirrors.

Newer CO_2 lasers producing up to 20 W can use a hollow light guide to transmit the irradiation (see Fig. 16-7). Hollow light guides are small flexible metal tubes (4 to 5 mm in diameter) with highly polished or reflective coated inner linings. The hollow light guide is less cumbersome to use in surgery than the articulating arm. At the distal end is a hand piece in which a small tip or nozzle is inserted to focus the irradiation. The smaller the tip, the smaller is the focal point, and thus a greater concentration of irradiation is emitted. In general surgery, the wave-guide hand piece can easily be covered with a sterile barrier.

For endoscopic application, small (1.5 to 2 mm) metal hollow light guides were manufactured that were up to 1 m in length. The metal construction significantly retarded flexibility of the endoscope and easily damaged its biopsy channel. In 2004, a very flexible laminated plastic wave-guide, the OmniGuide, was constructed for CO_2 laser transmission.[16] The wave-guide is over 1 m in length, and its distal tip is under 2.7mm in diameter, allowing it to be passed through the biopsy channel of most endoscopes.

The infrared beam of the CO_2 laser is primarily absorbed by water, raising its temperature to a superheated steam within the cells and causing their membranes to explode. Adjacent tissue and water may serve as heat sinks, producing latent thermal damage. Studies have demonstrated that there is a delay in healing, similar to that produced by electrosurgery, when the CO_2 laser is used for skin incisions.[6,14] For this reason, many surgeons prefer to perform the initial skin incision with a scalpel rather than with the CO_2 laser. Debulking of neoplastic masses with the CO_2 laser is beneficial because it seals small vessels and lymphatics, which could disseminate tumor cells. Sealing of lymphatics and small vessels is also advantageous because it decreases postoperative edema, and pain is mitigated through transection and sealing of small nerves.[4] The surgeon can employ a "no touch" technique with this laser (i.e., tip of the laser never touches the tissue) and tissue separation and penetration depth is visualized as it occurs. In veterinary surgery, the CO_2 laser is generally used for removal of skin masses, general cutting, sterilization of an infected area, or sealing of small vessels and lymphatics. It may also be used in the defocus pattern to produce photovaporization for removal of small tumors, for sterilization of infected wounds, or for shaving away several layers of surface cells.

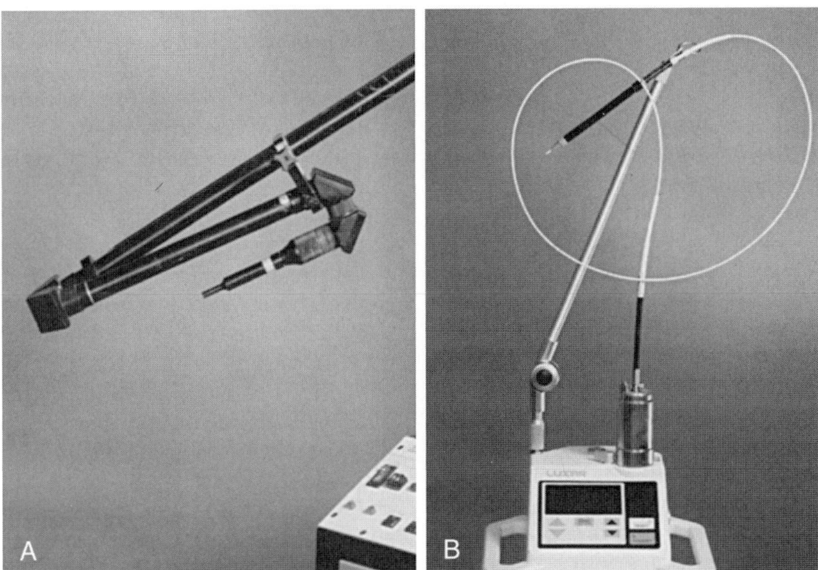

Figure 16-7. CO_2 laser delivery systems. **A,** Articulating arm containing a series of mirrors and focusing lenses used to deliver irradiation to the target tissue. **B,** A hollow flexible light guide is used in conjunction with a focusing hand piece as a substitute for an articulating arm.

The destructive potential of the CO_2 laser is directly proportional to its power output. Because its absorption coefficient in water is very high, the surgeon should use the laser at its highest power in a motion that is as swift as possible. Irradiation is significantly attenuated as it passes through hollow light guides. The smaller and longer the wave-guide, the greater the loss of power at the emitting end. Therefore, the light guides constructed for endoscopic use need to be coupled to a CO_2 laser that produces 20 W or greater to perform transendoscopic surgical procedures. Transendoscopic application of CO_2 laser irradiation through the hollow OmniGuide broadens the versatility of the CO_2 laser. Laser tissue interactions at this wavelength produce less latent thermal necrosis than any other laser, which should improve the surgeon's accuracy and decrease healing time. In the future, these two factors will play an important role in the selection of a laser for endoscopic application in the veterinary field.

Nd:YAG Laser

In large animals, the Nd:YAG laser was the most popular laser applied endoscopically from 1984 to the mid 1990s.* The medium of this laser produces a wavelength of 1064 nm, which allows transmission through quartz fibers. The photons produced by this laser are not absorbed by water. This laser's beam is in the near-infrared portion of the light spectrum; it exhibits stronger tissue absorption than the CO_2 laser. The Nd:YAG laser is better suited than the CO_2 laser for volumetric heating of large tissue masses. The two primary agents that give living tissue its color, melanin and hemoglobin, absorb this laser's wavelength equally. It is the characteristic of scatter and absorptive heating that gives the Nd:YAG laser the unwanted quality of producing substantial latent thermal tissue necrosis compared with the CO_2. This laser does, however, have the advantage of coagulating substantially larger vessels than the CO_2 laser. It is reported to provide good hemostasis in vessels up to 4 mm in diameter.[6] This characteristic is enhanced by its lack of absorption by water, which allows its beam to pass through many body fluids. With proper training, the surgeon can anticipate the amount of latent thermal necrosis that will occur. The Nd:YAG laser has been widely used in the upper respiratory area because of its ability to transmit its energy through fiberoptic cables, provide coagulation, and efficiently photovaporize tissue transendoscopically.

Diode Laser

Diode lasers are advantageous because of their semiconductor construction. They are generally small and portable and require less current than lasers using a medium. The efficiency of the diode laser exceeds that of most other lasers: 20% to 80% of input power is converted to laser energy. Diode lasers manufactured for veterinary surgery produce wavelengths of 810, 980, and 10,600 nm. The lower-wavelength lasers use inexpensive flexible quartz fibers to transmit their irradiation in the free-fiber or contact configuration. For contact application, fibers with a sculptured tip in the form of a cone, wedge, or ball are available.[8,17] The area where diode lasers differ from larger resonating chamber lasers is in power output. Most diode lasers are rated with power outputs up to 25 W; a few diode lasers have a power rating in the 50- to 60-W range. The decreased power output may increase the time that it takes to perform a procedure, because tissue penetration is decreased. Cooling of the internal diode array is critical to their stability and longevity. Therefore, to maintain a small size, manufacturers limit the power output to prevent overheating. However, the diode lasers have gained popularity because they can be manufactured at selective wavelengths and, in many cases, have replaced larger, more cumbersome lasers such as the Nd:YAG and argon lasers. User-friendly characteristics include a high electrical-to-optical efficiency, light weight, compact size, air cooling, and operation from a standard 110 variable AC electrical outlet. In large animal surgery, they can be used transendoscopically to treat many of the upper respiratory diseases.

Argon, KTP, and Holmium Lasers

In veterinary medicine, the argon laser (488 and 515 nm) has been used as the pump source for the dye laser. In the dye laser, a liquid phase moves through the medium and is excited by the argon laser. Therefore, wavelength selection is possible by changing the dye exposure. Because diode lasers can be manufactured at any wavelength, they have been also produced to mimic the dye pump laser. Tunable selection of wavelength is important for the excitation of hematoporphyrin derivatives, referred to as photodynamic therapy.[18] Photodynamic therapy is based on the principle that abnormal tissues, primarily cancer cells, selectively retain compounds on the basis of hematoporphyrin derivatives. Once the body's normal tissues have excreted the hematoporphyrin, tumorous tissue may be exposed to a set wavelength of light, causing an internal reaction and the release of superoxide radicals. This selectively kills tumor cells without destroying normal tissue.

A flash lamp–pulsed dye laser (504 nm) has been used to fragment uroliths in horses.[19,20] The laser fiber is applied transendoscopically, with the endoscope passed up the urethra or through a subischial urethrostomy incision. The procedure can be performed on the standing horse, but best results are achieved with general anesthesia and the horse placed in lateral recumbency. The laser fiber must make contact with the solid calculus for the pulses to properly fragment it. Complete fragmentation of a calculus of 4 to 6 cm in diameter requires thousands of laser pulses over several hours, and debris is removed by periodically replacing the endoscope with a lavage system.[20] For more information on this technique, see Chapter 71.

The KTP laser (532 nm) has been used in general surgery and is excellent for incising tissues. Its irradiation beam is transmitted through fiberoptic cables, which influences its popularity.

The holmium laser (2100 nm) uses fiberoptic transmission for its irradiation beam. It is very effective in liquid media such as joint fluid. Therefore, this device has become popular in upper respiratory, arthroscopic, urogenital, and ocular surgery. In arthroscopy, this device is applied to shrink periarticular tissues,[21] transect ligaments, ablate syn-

*References 6, 8-12, 14, 17, 26, 29-38.

ovial membrane and villi proliferations, and shave off cartilage and meniscal lesions. Arthroscopic removal of plantar or palmar chips of the proximal phalanx is greatly assisted by the use of the holmium laser to ablate the proliferative synovial membrane in the region, thus facilitating better visual perception of the surgical field and ensuring that the entire chip has been removed.[22] Application of the holmium laser in upper respiratory surgery is limited because of the need for contact application of the laser fiber tip for tissue removal. Smaller diode lasers have primarily replaced it in this field of surgery. The holmium laser has been applied to perform lithotripsy, but it has not been as beneficial or as popular as other lasers for this procedure.

DELIVERY SYSTEMS

For the Nd:YAG, holmium, KTP, argon, diode, and several other lasers, energy can be transmitted through small quartz fibers. These fibers are constructed in two forms, solid and coaxial, and they are between 3 and 4 m long (Fig. 16-8, *E* and *F*). Most outside diameters are less than 2.7 mm, allowing the fibers to pass through the biopsy channel of an endoscope.[8,11,12] Initially, devices such as sapphire crystals were connected to the ends of the solid quartz fibers, which, upon absorbing energy, produced a high temperature at the tip and were used for cutting and ablating tissue.

This form of delivery is referred to as contact delivery, in that the device or the end of the quartz fiber has to remain in contact with tissue to transmit the laser's thermal energy.[8,12] Currently, contact delivery systems do not require the sapphire end piece for the fiber to be used either endoscopically or hand held in general surgery. Fibers are now manufactured so that the ends can be either polished or cleaved for multiple uses for contact cutting. These fibers are particularly amenable for use with diode lasers that produce 15 to 25 W. A large-animal veterinarian using this system with one of the diode lasers can easily perform surgical procedures that simply require an incision to relieve the animal of an upper respiratory disorder.

Fiber longevity is increased by cycling the laser's irradiation when activated. For example, using a diode laser set at 18 W with a 600-nm fiber and cycle settings for 0.8 seconds on and 0.2 second off allows cooling of the fiber's cutting end. This could double the fiber's usable application time before it has to be replaced or cleaved. With the older Nd:YAG laser and high-power output diode lasers producing between 50 and 60 W, a second option, referred to as noncontact delivery, is available for delivery of laser irradiation. In this form of delivery system, the quartz fiber is further enclosed by a polyethylene casing, which carries cooling inert gas such as nitrogen or carbon diode, and internally, the laser contains aiming beams whose wavelength is within the visible range[8,11,23] (see Fig. 16-8, *F*). With the contact form of cutting, the incision that is produced is similar to that made with a scalpel.[12] The disadvantage is that the incision must be made before the surgeon can visualize the depth of the tissue that has been disrupted. With noncontact cutting, the fiber is several millimeters away from the tissue, and the surgeon has the advantage of visualizing the depth of the cut as it occurs. Noncontact cutting is also performed using hollow light guides. Those produced for transendoscopic application are smaller than those used in general surgery, which are hand held (see Fig. 16-8, *C* and *D*).

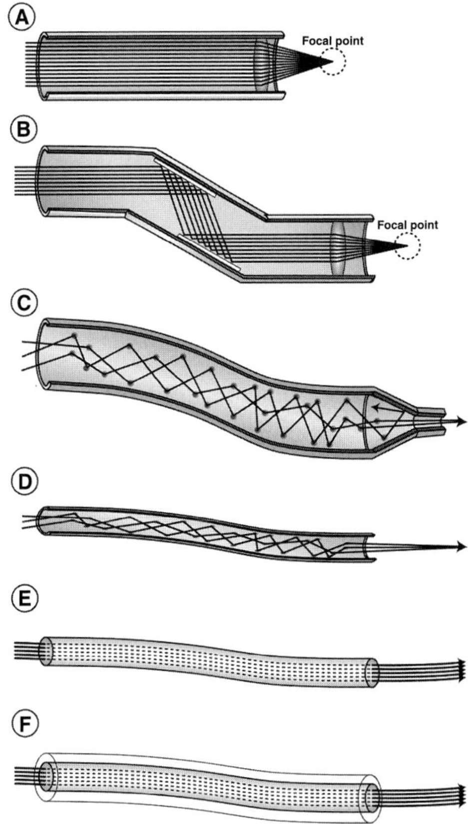

Figure 16-8. Delivery system for CO_2 laser irradiation (A-D). **A,** Lens-focused beam. **B,** Articulating arm (mirrors and lenses). **C,** Hollow light guide with beam-funneling aperture. **D,** Endoscopic light guide. Delivery system for Nd:YAG, holmium, KTP, argon, dye pump, and diode lasers (E-F). **E,** Contact endoscopic or hand-held solid fiber. **F,** Coaxial endoscopic fiber.

APPLICATION OF LASERS

CO_2 Laser

Skin tumors, such as sarcoids or squamous cell carcinoma, are easily ablated with the CO_2 laser.[7,8,24] When the animal is not placed under general anesthesia, it is sedated and local anesthetic is infused sublesionally. In certain cases, the CO_2 laser is used as a scalpel for tissue resection. However, skin tumors that are sufficiently raised above the base of the skin are best removed through sharp scalpel dissection at or below the skin surface. The laser is then applied in the defocused pattern, and all remaining tumorous tissue is removed. Wounds are generally left to heal by second intention. If wounds are closed, skin sutures should be left in place long enough to ensure that complete wound healing occurs prior to their removal. Laser ablation of sarcoids, particularly in the auricular region, is favored over freezing. The defocused beam allows tissue to be shaved away with great precision, avoiding injury to the ear cartilage, which might otherwise be damaged by freezing techniques (see Chapter 15).

Periocular squamous cell carcinomas are excellent indications for CO_2 laser application. Advantages over freezing techniques include better control and significantly less swelling and pain after tumor removal, because the lymphatics, veins, and nerves are sealed. Tumors of the eyelids or nictitating membrane can be removed without general anesthesia, although it is required for ablation of squamous cell carcinomas of the cornea. The laser is usually applied at a setting between 10 and 20 W for ablation of tissue around the cornea, and between 3 and 8 W for vaporizing a tumor off the cornea. Practice and precision are required when working around the eye, especially when the cornea is involved.

The CO_2 laser may be used to prepare granulation beds for skin grafting. An output of between 15 and 25 W is selected, and the laser is applied in a defocused pattern to remove exuberant granulation tissue to a level below the skin surface. Periodically, the area should be flushed with normal saline or daubed with moistened, sterile gauze sponges to remove carbonized tissue debris. The CO_2 laser is superior to the steel scalpel for the preparation of a graft bed, because it seals the small vessels, thus reducing hemorrhage and providing better visualization of the tissue surface. The CO_2 laser sterilizes the tissue surface, and repeated applications produce a healthy-appearing granulation bed. The accuracy of tissue removal is greatly improved by directing the laser's irradiation through a mechanical scanner, which controls the speed and sweep of the beam over the lesion area.

The CO_2 laser can be used to create recipient pockets for pinch grafts. The power setting for this purpose is 7 to 15 W in the focus mode. The pockets are created at a 45- to 60-degree angle to the tissue surface in a downward direction. The dimensions of the pockets should be between 2 and 4 mm in diameter and from 3 to 4 mm in depth. The advantage of using the CO_2 laser is the no-touch technique of tissue sterilization, combined with decreased hemorrhage. Minimal additional damage occurs if the laser is used in a chopped or superpulse mode. Flushing of the pockets is necessary to remove the carbonized tissue debris. Best results are obtained by bandaging the wound for 12 to 24 hours before skin grafting. After that, bandages are removed, the area is flushed, and a skin graft (pinch grafts) is placed into each of the previously created pockets. The rationale for the delay between pocket creation and graft placement is improved capillary growth and graft survival. For additional information on skin grafting, see Chapter 25.

In the urogenital system, the CO_2 laser has advantages over freezing or steel scalpel surgery. For example, in a patient with penile carcinoma, removal can be performed under local anesthesia. Pedunculated masses are resected using the CO_2 laser in a focused pattern, and the edges are further treated in the defocused pattern.[24] Healing occurs by second intention.

Laser palmar digital neurectomy was first performed using the CO_2 laser. Horses are placed under general anesthesia, and after the pastern is prepared for aseptic surgery, the nerve is isolated through a small incision. Laser irradiation is used to transect and remove a segment of the nerve. The thermal effect of the laser's irradiation causes coagulation at the point of transection, which reduces the possibility of axonal reconnection or neuroma formation.[25] Several other lasers, including the Nd:YAG and diode lasers, have been applied in a similar fashion with good results.[25]

Transendoscopic Application: Nd:YAG, Diode Lasers, and CO_2 Wave-Guide

Entrapment of the Epiglottis

Correction of the entrapment by the aryepiglottic fold is achieved by transendoscopic axial division using contact or noncontact delivery fibers in conjunction with the Nd:YAG and diode laser, or OmniGuide, coupled to the CO_2 laser. The Nd:YAG is applied at 100 W using a noncontact fiber or at 15 to 20 W using a contact fiber.[17,23] The diode laser can also be used at the same low wattage setting using the contact fiber.[26] In performing a release of the aryepiglottic fold, care should be taken to avoid secondary thermal damage to the epiglottis, particularly at its tip. It is helpful to make an initial 1- to 1.5-cm horizontal incision just underneath the tip of the epiglottis to assist in providing a complete release of the aryepiglottic fold and decrease the possibility of reentrapment.[27] The laser energy is then applied in a straight line beginning at the caudal border of the aryepiglottic fold and ending at the tip of the epiglottis. Initially, the incision is shallow and provides a path for the laser to track. This path is then deepened with each passage of the laser fiber until release is achieved. As the incision is deepened, inherent tension causes the edges to retract laterally, exposing fresh tissue for the next laser pass. In some instances, premature release of the entrapment may occur before the mucosa is entirely divided, or, if a thickened entrapment is present, it may fail to completely retract beneath the epiglottis. The bronchoesophageal grasping forceps should be employed to elevate the tissue to facilitate completion of the incision. On occasion, when the surgeon is unable to elevate the tissue, laser blanching may be performed to produce delayed necrosis, which results in further tissue separation. Post-treatment evaluation should be performed 14 days after the release of epiglottic entrapment and again at 30 days.

Dorsal Displacement of the Soft Palate

Under general anesthesia, the CO_2 laser can assist in performing a myectomy, in which a portion of the muscle bellies of the sternothyroideus, sternohyoideus, and omohyoideus muscles are incised and resected[7] (see Chapter 43). Transendoscopic application of a diode laser has been used in contact mode to blanch focal points along the caudal border of the soft palate in combination with the myectomy procedure.[15] The premise behind this form of treatment is that the thermal energy will produce scar tissue formation, thus stiffening the soft palate and preventing it from dorsally displacing above the epiglottis. No more than 1000 J should be applied to the soft palate. Applying too much energy to the soft palate can result in complete necrosis of the laser treated area.

Respiratory Masses (Pharynx, Larynx, and Trachea)

Tracheal, pharyngeal, and laryngeal masses including lymphoid hyperplasia, granulomas, and cancer can easily be removed using any of the lasers in either the contact or noncontact delivery configurations.[11,28-31] Large masses can be separated off the pharynx and retrieved using a grasping forceps or an endoscopic snare. Similarly, granulating masses on the surface of the arytenoid cartilage can be cauterized in a similar fashion. Infected fistulas within the arytenoid cartilage can be cauterized with laser irradiation. The laser fiber is inserted into the fistula, either transendoscopically or through a laryngotomy incision performed on the standing sedated horse.[32,33] Transendoscopic drainage or vaporization of respiratory abscesses can be performed using the Nd:YAG or diode laser.[30]

Vocal Cordectomy and Ventriculectomy

Ventriculectomy or vocal cordectomy can be performed transendoscopically. For laser ventriculectomy, a high-powered laser Nd:YAG or diode laser (50 to 100 W) is required to achieve vaporization of the ventricle's mucosal lining.[8,11,34,35] The lining of the ventricle is blanched using a coaxial laser fiber in a noncontact configuration, totaling up to 3500 J of energy.[34]

Swelling of the mucosa develops very rapidly, so the initial irradiation should be directed deep into the sack with the fiber and then drawn toward the opening as the mucosal surface swells and is coagulated. An alternative method is a vocal cordectomy, in which the vocal fold is incised by using a contact fiber and bronchoesophageal forceps.[36,37] The bronchoesophageal forceps are passed through the opposite nostril to grasp the fold and provide traction as the laser fiber is gently drawn along the edges of the vocal fold to separate it from the laryngeal wall. For more details on these surgeries, see Chapter 44.

Progressive Ethmoid Hematoma

Because definitive treatment of a progressive ethmoid hematoma remains controversial, lasers have been employed over the last 20 years to treat primary lesions and ablate early recurrence. It appears that the most effective laser treatment is reserved for those lesions that appear to originate under the middle nasal conchae, or for recurrences that appear after sinus surgery is performed.[38]

For masses appearing to arise from the ethmoid turbinate area and not originating in the paranasal sinuses, initial direct injection of 10% formalin may be considered prior to transendoscopic laser ablation.[39] Two weeks after injection of formalin, a small residual portion of the ethmoid hematoma may remain in the lower ethmoid turbinate areas. The remaining lesion can be approached transendoscopically and irradiated using either noncontact 100-W Nd:YAG laser, 50-W or greater diode laser, or CO_2 laser coupled with the OmniGuide.

An alternative to formalin injection is direct laser irradiation. This requires a high-wattage laser in which the laser energy is directed to the center of the mass protruding into the nasal pharynx.[38] Substantial energy (30,000 to 40,000 J) is used to thermally debulk the mass.[29] In this procedure, laser energy is directed into the center of the lesion, thermal necrosis produces shrinkage within several days, and an endoscopic snare can be used to remove necrotic tissue. Fewer laser applications are required to treat a small mass or early recurrence. Capsular excision followed by evacuation of the contents and dissection of the origin of the ethmoid hematoma has been described using contact laser scalpel technique.[40] The procedure is performed through a sinusotomy approach, with the horse placed under general anesthesia. Application of the laser provides better visibility within the sinus compartment by decreasing hemorrhage.[40] Recurrence of this lesion is common, and repeated laser ablation via endoscopy is a viable method of controlling tumor regrowth.

Guttural Pouch Tympany

Before standing laser surgery is performed, foals should be evaluated for aspiration pneumonia, and if it is present, appropriate systemic antibiotics should be administrated. A Chamber's catheter is inserted into the larger of the two distended guttural pouches. At this time, deflation of both guttural pouches signifies to the surgeon that the guttural pouch that initiated the distention has been identified if the tympany is not bilateral. Bilateral cases do occur, although they are rarer than unilateral cases. The Chamber's catheter in the guttural pouch is rotated so that an endoscope passed up the opposite nostril can identify tented mucosa just inside the guttural pouch. The laser of choice is the Nd:YAG, or a high-powered diode laser using noncontact delivery fiber, or the OmniGuide CO_2 fiber directed at the tented mucosa. Laser irradiation is stopped when a 5- to 10-mm hole has been created between the pharynx and the guttural pouch, and when the ball on the end of the Chamber's catheter can be identified.[41] A no. 24 French catheter is then inserted through the hole and allowed to remain in place for at least 14 days so that a permanent fistula is formed between the guttural pouch and the pharynx.

Removal of a portion of the median septum separating the two guttural pouches can be performed using contact or noncontact transendoscopic laser technique. Creation of a fenestration is technically more difficult than creating a fistula between the guttural pouch and the pharynx and has a greater potential risk of causing thermal damage to the vessels and nerve located within.[8,42]

Cysts: Subepiglottal, Dorsal Pharyngeal, and Intrauterine

Subepiglottal, dorsal pharyngeal, and nasal cysts can be diagnosed by either radiographic means or endoscopic visualization.[8,11] Standing laser ablation requires a high-powered Nd:YAG, diode, or CO_2 OmniGuide laser. Initially, the surface of the cyst is blanched while applying the laser energy in a sweeping motion across the visible surface.[8,43] The purpose is to cause latent thermal necrosis, so that after the cyst is evacuated additional tissue will slough, preventing premature closure of the incision, and recurrence. The laser is then aimed at the most dependent portion of the cyst, and it is irradiated until fluid drains through the incision. Once the cyst is completely drained of fluid, all portions of the cyst still visible are irradiated. Sometimes, subepiglottal cysts prematurely disappear from view below the soft palate. An endoscopic snare or bronchoesophageal grasping forceps can be used to reposition the cyst for completion of the procedure.[44] A post-treatment examination should be made approximately 14 days after surgery and again at 1 month.

Ablation of an intrauterine cyst requires an endoscopic fiber that provides a high-volume flow of inert gases such as

CO_2 or nitrogen to maintain insufflation of the uterus. Laser application mimics the technique used with respiratory cysts, except that care should be taken to not irradiate the base of the cyst, as this could result in either immediate or latent penetration of the uterine wall.[32,43,45] Assessment after the ablation is performed by transrectal ultrasonography, and a small uterine scar can be expected to remain at the surgical site after 30 days.

COMPLICATIONS

Although it is frequently successful, standing transendoscopic laser correction of respiratory disorders has the potential for incomplete correction and recurrence. The anatomic location of the lesion and the movement of surrounding structures contribute significantly. For example, complete photoablation of an ethmoid hematoma with its origin located deep within the ethmoid turbinate is difficult to achieve. Similarly, dorsal displacement of the soft palate may visually obscure an epiglottic entrapment or subepiglottal cyst during the treatment procedure, resulting in incomplete correction. Clients should be made aware that such circumstances may require repeated attempts at correction over several days, or eventually surgery under general anesthesia. Before the initiation of any procedure, proper laser function and beam alignment should be confirmed.

Large-vessel laceration is a potential complication, particularly when the laser is applied within the guttural pouch. Additionally, the nerves traversing the guttural pouch may be damaged by direct laser application or by general heating of the surrounding tissues. Allowing periodic cooling or evacuation of heated air can minimize this. This is of concern when applying any laser within hollow organs or enclosed spaces such as the uterus, trachea, urethra, and bladder. Hemorrhage that cannot be immediately stopped by laser irradiation will obscure the target tissue. Blood also absorbs various laser wavelengths, which will decrease the cutting efficiency of the laser's irradiation. Continuation of the laser procedure then becomes dependent on when hemostasis occurs.

The Nd:YAG laser and those lasers close to its wavelength tend to produce latent necrosis secondary to scatter irradiation.[14] Conservative application is indicated when there is a potential to destroy more tissue than is desired or to inadvertently puncture a hollow organ.

Damage to endoscopic equipment from irradiation backscatter or direct irradiation when the distal scope end is folded back 180 degrees should be avoided. Intraendoscopic damage can occur if hot tips or fibers are pulled through the instrument. Laser fibers coated with debris can lacerate fragile biopsy channels. If an abnormality is observed in the laser fiber, the laser should be inactivated, the endoscope removed from the patient, and the fiber inspected prior to pulling it through the biopsy channel.

REFERENCES

1. Melles JA: Optics Guide IV, Cambridge, UK, 1990, Melles Griot.
2. Wolbarsh ML: Laser Applications in Medicine and Biology, New York, 1971, Plenum Press.
3. Kaplan I: Laser Surgery I and II, Jerusalem, Israel, 1976, Jerusalem Academic Press.
4. Kaplan I: Laser Surgery III, Jerusalem, Israel, 1979, Jerusalem Academic Press.
5. Goldman L: The Biomedical Laser Technology and Clinical Applications, New York, 1981, Springer-Verlag.
6. Joffe SN: Neodymium: YAG Laser in Medicine and Surgery, New York, 1983, Elsevier.
7. Palmer SE: Instrumentation and techniques for carbon-dioxide lasers in equine general surgery, Vet Clin North Am Equine Pract 1996;12:397.
8. Tate LP: Application of lasers in equine upper respiratory surgery, Vet Clin North Am Equine Pract 1991;7:165.
9. Joffe SN: Contact neodymium:YAG laser surgery in gastroenterology: A preliminary report, Lasers Surg Med 1986;6:135.
10. Tate LP, Newman HC, Sweeny CL, et al: An overview of endoscopic laser surgery: Three clinical cases in the standing animal, Proc Am Assoc Equine Pract 1986;32:385.
11. Blikslager AT, Tate LP: History, instrumentation, and techniques of flexible endoscopic laser surgery in horses, Clin North Am Equine Pract 2000;15:251.
12. Tulleners E: Instrumentation and techniques in transendoscopic upper respiratory tract laser surgery, Vet Clin North Am Equine Pract 1996;12:373.
13. Engelbert TA, Tate LP, Malone D, et al: Influence of inhaled smoke from upper respiratory laser surgery, Vet Radiol Ultrasound 1994;35:319.
14. Tate LP, Sweeny CL, Cullen J, et al: An investigation into transendoscopic Nd:YAG laser irradiation in the horse, Am J Vet Res 1989;50:780.
15. Hogan PM, Palmer SE, Congelosi M: Transendoscopic laser cauterization of the soft palate as an adjunctive treatment for dorsal displacement in the racehorse, Proc Am Assoc Eq Pract 2002; 48:228.
16. Tate LP: Why lasers in the airway, Proc Symp Am Coll Vet Surg, 2004.
17. Tulleners E: Transendoscopic contact neodymium:yttrium aluminum garnet laser correction of epiglottic entrapment in standing horses, J Am Vet Med Assoc 1990;196:12.
18. Manyak MJ, Russo A, Smith PD, et al: Photodynamic therapy, J Clin Oncol 1998;6:2.
19. Sullins KE: Noninvasive removal of equine uroliths: Laser lithotripsy, Clin Techn Equine Pract 2002;1:36.
20. Howard RD, Pleasant RS, May KA: Pulsed dye laser lithotripsy for treatment of urolithiasis in two geldings, J Am Vet Med Assoc 1998;212:10.
21. Schaefer SL, Ciarelli MJ, Arnoczky SP, et al: Tissue shrinkage using a holmium:YAG laser: A postoperative assessment of tissue length, stiffness, and morphology, Trans Orthop Res Soc 1997; 43:480.
22. Auer JA: Personal communication, 1998.
23. Tate LP, Sweeny CL, Bowman KF, et al: Transendoscopic Nd:YAG laser surgery for treatment of epiglottal entrapment and dorsal displacement of the soft palate in the horse, Vet Surg 1990;19:356.
24. Palmer SE: Treatment of common cutaneous tumors using the carbon dioxide laser, Clin Techn Equine Pract 2002;1:43.
25. Palmer SE: Palmar digital neurectomy using the GaA1As diode laser, Clin Techn Equine Pract 2002;1:39.
26. Tate LP, Tudor RA: Clinical update: Transendoscopic laser surgery for treatment of epiglottic entrapment, Nd:YAG and 808-nm diode laser applied individually or in combination, Proc Soc Photo-Opt Engin 1999;3590:350.
27. Sullins KE: Personal communication, 2002.
28. Tate LP, Weddle DL, Correa MT: In vitro evaluation of three lasers for the potential treatment of equine pharyngeal lymphoid hyperplasia, Proc Soc Photo-Opt Engin 1993;1880:56.
29. Tate LP, Little ED: A review of treatment of upper airway obstruction caused by various masses both malignant and nonmalignant in the horse using transendoscopic Nd: YAG laser application for treatment, Proc Soc Photo-Opt Engin 1996;2671:67.

30. Tulleners EP: Use of transendoscopic contact neodymium:yttrium aluminum garnet laser to drain dorsal epiglottic abscesses in tow horses, J Am Vet Med Assoc 1991;198:10.
31. Hay WP, Tulleners E: Excision of intralaryngeal granulation tissue in 25 horses using a neodymium: YAG laser (1986 to 1991), Vet Surg 1993;22:129.
32. Sullins KE: Minimally invasive laser treatment of arytenoid chondritis in five horses, Proc Am Assoc Equine Pract 2001;47:120.
33. Sullins KE: Minimally invasive laser treatment of arytenoid chondritis in horses, Clin Techn Equine Pract 2002;1:13.
34. Tate LP, Little ED, Bishop BJ: Experimental and clinical evaluation of Nd:YAG ablation of the laryngeal ventricle and laryngoplasty in horses with left laryngeal hemiplegia, J Clin Laser Med Surg 1993;11:139.
35. Bristol DG, Palmer SE, Tate LP, et al: Complications of Nd: YAG laser ventriculectomy in the horse: A review of 106 consecutive cases, J Clin Laser Med Surg 1995;13:377.
36. Hawkins JF, Andrews-Jones L: Neodymium:yttrium aluminum garnet laser ventriculocordectomy in standing horses, Am J Vet Res 2001;62:4.
37. Ducharme NG, Goodrich L, Woodie B: Vocal cordectomy as an aid in the management of horses with laryngeal hemiparesis/hemiplegia, Clin Techn Equine Pract 2002;1:17.
38. Tate LP, Blikslager A: New perspectives on diagnosis and treatment of progressive ethmoid hematomas, Proc Am Assoc Equine Pract 2002;48:233.
39. Schumacher J, Yarbrough T, Pascoe J, et al: Transendoscopic chemical ablation of progressive ethmoidal hematomas in standing horses, Vet Surg 1998;27:175.
40. Rothaug PG, Tulleners EP: Neodymium:yttrium-aluminum-garnet laser-assisted excision of progressive ethmoid hematomas in horses: 20 cases (1986-1996), J Am Vet Med Assoc 1999;214:7.
41. Tate LP, Blikslager AT, Little ED: Transendoscopic laser treatment of guttural pouch tympanites in eight foals, Proc Am Coll Vet Surg 1995;24:367.
42. Tetens J, Tulleners EP, Ross MW, et al: Transendoscopic contact neodymium: yttrium aluminum garnet laser treatment of tympany of the auditory tube diverticulum in two foals, J Am Vet Med Assoc 1994;204:12.
43. Tate LP: Transendoscopic Nd: YAG ablation of cystic lesions in 27 large animals: 1986-1995, Proc Soc Photo-Opt Engin 1997; 2970:215.
44. Tulleners EP: Evaluation of peroral transendoscopic contact neodymium: yttrium aluminum garnet laser and snare excision of subepiglottic cysts in horses, J Am Vet Med Assoc 1991;198:1631.
45. Blikslager AT, Tate LP, Weinstock D: Effects of neodymium: yttrium aluminum garnet laser irradiation of endometrium and on endometrial cysts in six mares, Vet Surg 1993;22:351.

CHAPTER 17

Suture Materials and Patterns

LeeAnn W. Blackford
James T. Blackford

SUTURE MATERIALS

Sutures serve an important function in wound repair. They are necessary to ligate blood vessels and to hold tissues in apposition as they heal. Suture materials should be selected with regard to their physical and chemical characteristics and the biologic response they elicit from the host. The ideal suture material should have the following properties[1]:

- It should be suitable for any operation.
- It should be easy to handle.
- It should elicit minimal tissue reaction without inducing an environment favorable to bacterial growth.
- It should have high tensile strength and a small diameter.
- It should provide good knot security.
- It should be nonelectrolytic, nonwicking, nonallergenic, and noncarcinogenic.
- It should be easy to sterilize and economical to use.
- Once it has served its purpose, it should be absorbed with minimal tissue reaction.

The ideal suture material does not presently exist, but many of the available materials possess a majority of the ideal properties. Knowledge of the advantages and disadvantages of each suture material allows the surgeon to make an informed choice. The type of tissue involved, the reason for suture application, the patient, and the location and condition of the wound should be considered when choosing a suture material. Although knowledge of the properties of the suture materials is important, more vital is the surgeon's technique in closing the wound. A good surgeon can usually achieve satisfactory results with any type of suture material.[2]

Biologic Properties

Sutures are classified as absorbable or nonabsorbable. Absorbable sutures undergo degradation and rapid loss of tensile strength within 60 days.[2,3] Absorption occurs either by enzymatic degradation and subsequent phagocytosis (e.g., surgical gut) or by hydrolysis, a process in which the suture is broken down by the addition of water and then metabolized. Nonabsorbable sutures retain tensile strength for more than 60 days.[3] Absorption must be distinguished from loss of tensile strength, which has greater significance. Tensile strength is a measure of how much pull a suture can withstand before it breaks. Suture strength is essential for the early healing of wounds, and tensile strength retention is critical in delayed wound healing or when permanent retention of a prosthesis (e.g., a laryngeal prosthesis) is required.[3] Characteristics of the most commonly used absorbable and nonabsorbable suture materials are found in Tables 17-1 and 17-2. Additional information on the physical characteristics and composition of suture materials is found in Chapter 9.

TABLE 17-1. Characteristics of Absorbable Suture Materials

Suture Type	Raw Material	Biologic Properties	Advantages and Uses	Disadvantages
Surgical catgut (plain), multifilament	Submucosa of ovine intestine or serosa of bovine intestine	Absorbed relatively quickly by cellular and tissue proteases	Rarely used	Inflammatory reaction, maintains tensile strength for a relatively short period of time
Surgical catgut (chromic), multifilament	Same as plain. Treated with chromium salts, which increases molecular bonding and improves tensile strength with less tissue reactivity	Absorbed more slowly owing to chemical treatment (90+ days). Retains tensile strength for 14 to 28 days	Good handling characteristics. Used for subcutaneous and other tissues that heal rapidly. May be used in infected wounds. Inflammatory reaction causes an increase in fibrosis that may be desirable in some instances (herniorrhaphies)	Inflammatory reaction; poor knot security; variability in rate of absorption and loss of tensile strength; capillarity; occasional sensitivity reaction
Polyglactin 910 (Vicryl), coated Vicryl, braided, multifilament	Copolymer of glycolic and lactic acid. Coating: calcium stearate	Absorbed by slow hydrolysis in 40 to 90 days. Retains tensile strength for 14 to 21 days	Coated Vicryl easier to handle; less tissue drag. Minimal tissue reaction. Stable in contaminated wounds. Higher tensile and knot strength	Noncoated Vicryl has significant tissue drag
Polyglycolic acid (Dexon), braided, multifilament	Polymer of glycolic acid	Absorbed by hydrolysis in 100 to 120 days. Degradation products have antibacterial effect. Loses tensile strength in 7 to 14 days	Wide variety of uses in clean and contaminated surgical procedures. Easy to handle	Prematurely absorbed in urine. Tends to drag through tissues and may cut friable tissues. Less knot security than surgical gut
Polydioxanone (PDS) monofilament	Polymer of polydioxanone	Absorbed by hydrolysis in 180 days. Retains tensile strength for 28 to 56 days	Good knot security Strength exceeds nylon and polypropylene Low tissue drag	Poor handling characteristics because of stiffness and memory
Polyglyconate (Maxon), monofilament	Copolymer of glycolic acid and trimethylene	Absorbed by hydrolysis starting at day 60 and is complete by 6 mos. Retains tensile strength for more than 21 days	Three times stronger than Vicryl at day 21 of wound healing	—
Poliglecaprone 25 (Monocryl), monofilament	Copolymer of caprolactone and glycolide	Absorbed by hydrolysis in 90 to 120 days	Easy to handle with decreased flexibility; good knot security with minimal memory	Loses 50% of tensile strength in 7 days, should not be used in areas of delayed healing
Glycomer 631 (Biosyn), monofilament	Combined polymer of glycolide, dioxanone and trimethylene carbonate	Absorbed by hydrolysis in 90 to 110 days. Minimal tissue reaction	Excellent initial strength and knot security. Easy to handle with minimal memory	—

TABLE 17-2. Characteristics of Nonabsorbable Suture Materials

Suture Type	Raw Material	Biologic Properties	Advantages and Uses	Disadvantages
Silk, multifilament	Raw silk, spun by silkworm	Loses 80% of tensile strength within 8 days. May be slowly absorbed or persist for several years	Excellent handling characteristics. Used in most body tissues for ligatures. Ophthalmology and plastic surgery. Inexpensive	Inferior to other suture materials in terms of strength. Incites some reaction and may potentiate infection. Should not be used in hollow viscera; capillarity
Cotton, multifilament	Natural cotton fibers	Slowly loses tensile strength in 6 months to 2 years. Is not absorbed	Gains tensile strength and knot security when wet	May potentiate infection; capillarity, tissue reactivity, and inferior handling ability
Surgical steel, monofilament or multifilament	Alloy of iron	Biologically inert	Nonwicking as a monofilalment; greatest tensile strength of all sutures and maintains strength when implanted. Also has greatest knot security. No inflammatory reaction. Good for tissues that heal slowly	Tissue movement against the inflexible ends of suture may cause inflammation and tissue necrosis. Tends to cut tissues; poor handling; cannot withstand repeated bending without breaking. Multifilament wire may fragment and migrate, leading to sinus formation
Nylon (Ethilon), monofilament or multifilament	Polyamide polymer	Biologically inert and nonwicking as a monofilament. Monofilament nylon loses about 30% of tensile strength over 2 years. Multifilament nylon retains no tensile strength after 6 months	Incidence of infection in contaminated tissues containing monofilament nylon is very low. Used effectively as a skin suture. Degradation products are potent antibacterial agents. Good for use in contaminated wounds	Poor handling characteristics and knot security. Not recommended for use within a serous or synovial cavity. The buried sharp ends may cause frictional irritation
Polymerized caprolactam (Supramid or Braunamid), multifilament	Polyamide polymer	Same as multifilament nylon	Available in reels or dispensers. Must be autoclaved before use as a buried suture; however, it may cause excessive swelling and sinus tract formation when used in this fashion	Difficult to handle. Poor knot security. Intermediate tissue reactivity
Polyester fiber (Mersilene), coated polyester (Ethibond), multifilament	Synthetic material made from chemicals. Coating: polybutilate	Has a high initial tensile strength with little or no loss after implantation	One of the strongest nonmetallic suture materials available. Offers prolonged support for slow-healing tissues. Nonwicking. Good handling characteristics	Noncoated polyester has a high coefficient of friction. Coating reduces knot security. Causes the most tissue reaction of the synthetic suture materials. Should not be used in contaminated wounds. Can form sinus tracts

Continued

TABLE 17-2. Characteristics of Nonabsorbable Suture Materials—cont'd

Suture Type	Raw Material	Biologic Properties	Advantages and Uses	Disadvantages
Polypropylene (Prolene), monofilament	Polydelfin plastic	Retains strength after implantation. Inert	Has relatively low tensile strength but greater knot security than all other monofilament, nonmetallic synthetic materials. Least likely to potentiate infection. Best suture material available for skin. Frequently used in vascular surgery	Slippery quality results in difficulty handling and tying
Polybutester (Novafil) monofilament	Copolymer of polybutylene and polytetramethylene	Elicits minimal tissue reaction	Strong, with good handling characteristics and knot security. Provides prolonged support for slow-healing tissues	—

Physical Properties

Sutures are made from naturally occurring substances (e.g., surgical gut, silk), synthetic polymers, or metallic fibers. Sutures are formed as a single strand (monofilament) or multiple strands (multifilament) that are either braided or twisted together. Most surgical staples used in equine surgery are manufactured from stainless steel.

Selecting the Appropriate Suture Material

The selection of suture material should be based on the known biologic and physical properties of the suture, the wound environment, and the response of tissue to the suture. More than 10 suture varieties are available, and some are superior to others in different wound environments.

The suture selected should be as strong as the normal tissue through which it is placed. Skin and fascia are the strongest tissues, stomach and small intestine are much weaker, and the urinary bladder is even weaker.[2] For the first 3 to 4 days, the strength of the sutured wound depends on the suture material. The relative rates at which a wound gains strength and the suture loses strength is important. For example, visceral wounds heal rapidly, gaining strength in 14 to 21 days; therefore, absorbable sutures are adequate for these tissues. However, because fascia heals slowly, attaining only 50% of maximal strength at day 50, nonabsorbable sutures are more suitable for its closure.

When the wounds being sutured are contaminated or infected, the biologic effect of the suture on the healing process is especially important. Most sutures are known to potentiate the development of wound infection. Monofilament sutures are not as likely as multifilament sutures to exhibit capillarity (a wicking action that allows infection to travel along the suture strand), and therefore they withstand contamination better.[4] Sutures with the lowest reported incidence of infection when used in contaminated tissues include polyglycolic acid, polyglactin 910, monofilament nylon, and polypropylene.[5,6] The amount of suture material used in contaminated wounds should be minimized, because even the least reactive suture impairs the ability of the wound to resist infection.[6]

Selecting the Appropriate Suture for a Specific Tissue

The sutures recommended for specific tissues are the following:

- Skin. Monofilament nylon, polypropylene, and polybutester are preferred for skin sutures.[2] Sutures that exhibit capillarity or are reactive should be avoided.
- Subcutis. Synthetic absorbable sutures are preferred.
- Fascia. Synthetic nonabsorbable sutures are recommended if prolonged strength is required, although synthetic absorbable sutures have been effective.
- Muscle. Synthetic absorbable or nonabsorbable sutures may be used effectively in muscle. Nylon and polypropylene are recommended for use in cardiac muscle because of their superior mechanical properties.
- Hollow viscus. Surgical gut, polyglycolic acid, polyglactin 910, poliglecaprone 25, glycomer 631, and monofilament nonabsorbable sutures may be used in viscera. Polyglycolic acid has been observed to absorb prematurely in urine. Multifilament, nonabsorbable sutures should be avoided because they serve as a nidus of calculus formation.
- Tendon. Nylon and stainless steel are commonly recommended for tendon repair. Polydioxanone and polybutester have been suggested for equine flexor tendon repair because they may decrease adhesion formation associated with the prolonged presence of suture.[7] The newly available polyglyconate suture may also be effective as a tendon suture.
- Blood vessel. Polypropylene is the least thrombogenic suture and is the material of choice in vascular repair. Nylon and coated polyester have also been used.
- Nerve. Nylon and polypropylene are recommended for peripheral nerve repair because tissue reactivity is the most important consideration.

Selecting the Appropriate Suture Size

When selecting the proper diameter of suture, the following principles should be considered:

- The strength of a wound is more dependent on the involved tissue's ability to hold a suture than the strength of the suture material itself.[1]
- Use of an oversized suture material may weaken the repaired wound by causing excessive tissue reaction.
- A suture's function is to hold the wound edges together under minimal tension.
- For a wound under tension, increasing suture numbers is better than increasing material size. In general, skin and fascia have the greatest suture-holding power, and fat has the least.

Guidelines for the size of ligature and suture to use for various tissues have not been officially specified for large animal surgery. Table 17-3 reflects the author's preference in suture sizes for various tissues.

TABLE 17-3. Guidelines for Suture Selection in Large Animal Surgery

Tissue Type	Suture Size	Suture Type*
Skin	2-0 to 2	Nonabsorbable monofilament
Subcutis	3-0 to 0	Absorbable monofilament or multifilament
Fascia	0 to 2	Absorbable monofilament or multifilament
Muscle	2-0 to 0	Absorbable monofilament or multifilament
Hollow viscus	3-0 to 0	Absorbable monofilament or multifilament
Tendon	2	Nonabsorbable monofilament
Vessel (ligatures)	3-0 to 2-0	Absorbable multifilament
Vessel (sutures)	6-0 to 5-0	Nonabsorbable monofilament
Nerve	7-0 to 5-0	Nonabsorbable monofilament

* Absorbable or monofilament nonabsorbable sutures should be used in contaminated or infected wounds.

SURGICAL NEEDLES

The appropriate suture needle to be used is based on the type of tissue to be sutured, the location and accessibility of the tissue, and the size of the suture material. Suture needles are manufactured from stainless steel and are available as eyed needles, where the suture has to be threaded, or swaged needles with the suture attached to their ends. Swaged needles are less traumatic to tissues, easier to handle, and always sharp because they are used only once and then discarded. Eyed needles are reusable and less expensive than swaged needles, but they cause greater trauma during suture placement because of the bigger diameter of the end and because a double strand of suture is pulled through the tissue, and they become dull with reuse.[1]

Surgical needles vary in size, shape, and type of needle point. The important aspects of needle size are the length and diameter (Fig. 17-1). The needle should be long enough to penetrate both sides of the incision. To avoid excessive trauma, the diameter should be the smallest that will penetrate the tissue without bending.[1]

The ability of the needle to penetrate tissue depends on the shape of the point and body (Fig. 17-2). Taper-point

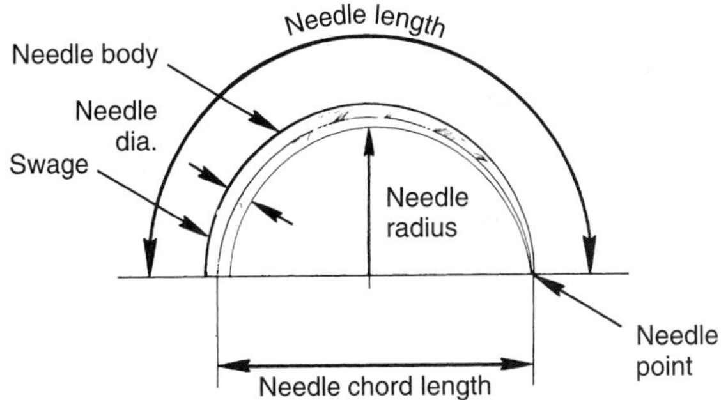

Figure 17-1. Anatomy of a surgical needle. (Redrawn with permission from Ethicon, Inc, Somerville, NJ, 1999.)

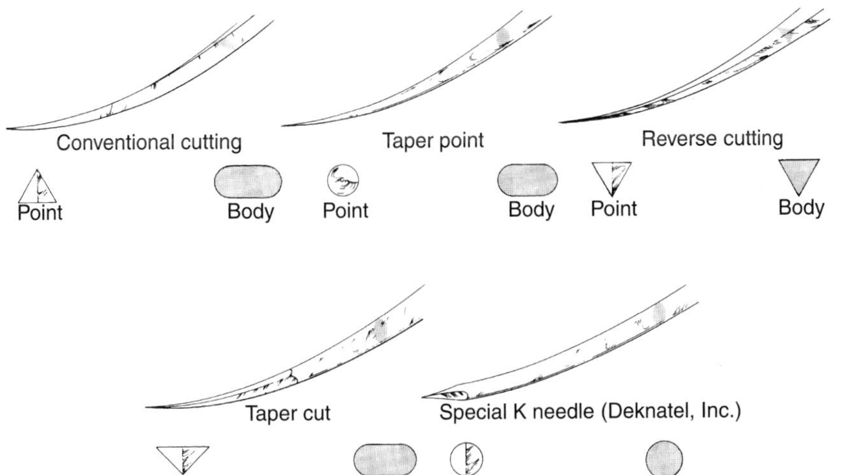

Figure 17-2. Various points and shaft designs of suture needles. (Redrawn with permission from Turner AS, McIlwraith CW: Techniques in Large Animal Surgery. Oxford, UK, 1989, Blackwell.)

needles have a sharp point and cylindric body, and they can be used on nonfibrous soft tissues (such as abdominal viscera) with minimal risk to adjacent vessels and nerves. Cutting needles are used to penetrate dense tissues such as fascia and skin. Cutting needles may be conventional (side cutting) or reverse cutting, in which the cutting edge is located on the convex side of the needle. The inner, flat concave surface of the reverse-cutting needle prevents excessive cutting of tissues when the needle passes through them. The design also improves needle strength.[2] The taper-cut needle combines the reverse-cutting point with a round shaft that is useful in delicate fibrous tissue. The special K needle (Deknatel, Inc, Fall River, Mass) is similar to the taper-cut needle and is useful in tough, dense tissues such as the cartilage of the equine larynx.[8] Additional information is found in Chapter 44.

Needles come in various shapes: straight, half-curved, or with a variable curvature[8] (Fig. 17-3). Wound depth, size, and accessibility to suturing are the factors considered when choosing the needle shape. Straight needles are used in accessible sites (e.g., when performing an anastomosis of exteriorized bowel). When suturing within a deep wound, a half-circle or five-eighths-circle needle is more suitable.[8] Long-stemmed needles are used for placing heavy suture materials (e.g., vaginal prolapse). In most other instances, the 3/8 needle is preferred because it requires the least rotational movement of the hand to traverse the tissue.

When choosing a needle, the following factors should be considered:

- The hole made by the needle should be only large enough to permit suture passage, so that the needle does not weaken the tissue.
- The design and diameter of the needle should result in minimal tissue damage and needle breakage.
- The needle should have the appropriate size, shape, and diameter to permit rapid, accurate, and precise suturing.[9]

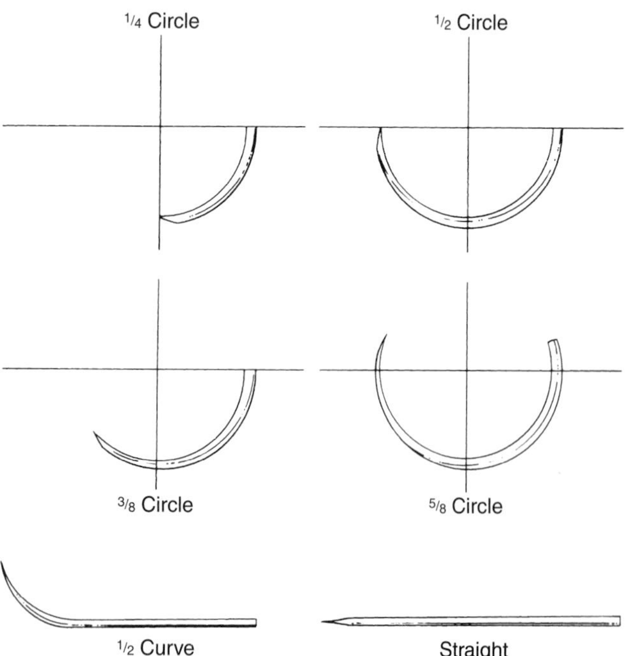

Figure 17-3. Various needle shapes. (Redrawn with permission from Turner AS, McIlwraith CW: Techniques in Large Animal Surgery. Oxford, UK, 1989, Blackwell.)

SUTURE CONFIGURATIONS

Knots and Ligatures

Tying knots rapidly and efficiently is an integral part of any surgical procedure. Types of surgical knots are demonstrated in Figure 17-4. In general, sutures and ligatures (sutures used for occluding blood vessels) are tied in square knots because these are the most secure. The half-hitch is the basic component of three types of knots. Two consecutive half-hitch knots can result in a square knot, a granny knot, or a half-hitch knot. Square knots are made by reversing direction on consecutive half-hitches. Each half-hitch is ideally tightened with even tension on both strands in the same plane as the suture, perpendicular to the incision line. Failure to reverse direction on consecutive throws results in a granny knot. Failure to maintain even tension on the strands or pulling the strands away from the plane of the knot may result in a half-hitch or an asymmetric square knot.[10] Granny and half-hitch knots are prone to slip and generally are not recommended. However, these knots may be used to overcome tissue tension when applying deep sutures or ligatures, because they can be slipped under tension to tighten the suture. When used in this manner, several square knots should be applied on top to prevent slippage.

When the first throw of a square knot does not hold the wound in apposition, a surgeon's knot may be tied by applying a double twist to the first throw. The surgeon's knot should be avoided when not needed, however, because it takes longer to tie and places more suture material into the wound. When using chromic gut, a surgeon's knot is contraindicated. The increased friction weakens the suture by fraying the material at the knot.

During closure of deep layers, tightening the sutures at a 90-degree angle to the suture loop plane or parallel to the

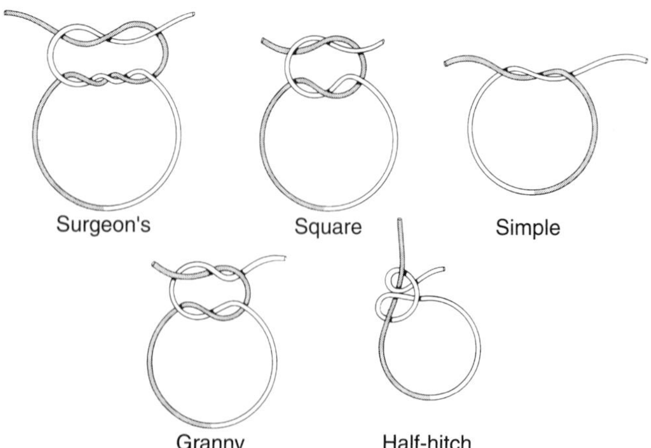

Figure 17-4. Surgical knots. (Redrawn with permission from Toombs JP, Crowe DT: Textbook of Small Animal Surgery. Philadelphia, 1993, WB Saunders.)

incision direction facilitates tissue closure, prevents excessive force, and reduces the risk of suture breakage. Attempting to close deep tissue layers by tightening sutures at a 90-degree angle to the incisional plane distracts the superficial layers while deep tissue layers are apposed, which is counter-productive.

Knot-tying techniques and physical characteristics of suture materials influence knot security. In one study, the minimal number of throws needed (including the first) for a secure square knot were determined to be three for catgut, polyglycolic acid, polyglactin 910, and polypropylene and four for nylon and polydioxanone.[11] However, when beginning a continuous suture pattern with square knots, one additional throw was required with surgical gut, polydioxanone, and nylon. Two or three additional throws were required for knot security when using square knots, to end a continuous pattern with all suture materials tested.[11] In this study, the newer suture materials were clearly not included.

Three methods for tying knots are the one-handed, two-handed, and instrument ties. These techniques[12,13] and other methods of applying ligatures[10,12] are discussed in depth in the literature. The ability to use all of these techniques gives the surgeon versatility in applying secure ligatures and sutures in every situation.

Suture Patterns

A wide variety of suture patterns are available for use in animals. The surgeon should be familiar with the advantages and disadvantages of each and choose one that provides maximal security with minimal alteration of wound healing. The general features and common uses of selected suture patterns are summarized in Tables 17-4 to 17-6. Corresponding illustrations are provided in Figures 17-5 to 17-7.

Interrupted Versus Continuous Patterns

Sutures may be placed in an interrupted or a continuous pattern. Interrupted patterns provide more security because failure of one suture does not jeopardize the entire closure. Suture failure in any portion of a continuous pattern may lead to dehiscence of the entire suture line. Interrupted sutures have the disadvantages of leaving a greater volume of suture material in the tissue (in the form of knots), increased surgery time (to tie multiple knots and cut the suture ends), and lower holding power against stress. Continuous suture patterns result in less suture material in the wound and reduced operative time. In terms of wound-bursting strength, a simple continuous pattern is superior to simple interrupted patterns when used in abdominal fascial closure. The continuous suture tends to distribute tension along the entire length of an incision, instead of isolating tension to each individual suture.[14]

Everting versus Inverting Patterns

Suture patterns that cause slight eversion are useful for skin closure because skin edges tend to invert during healing. To prevent leakage, inverting patterns are desirable for closure of hollow viscera; however, excessive inversion compromises lumen size.[15,16]

TABLE 17-4. Appositional Sutures

Suture Type	General Features	Common Uses
Simple interrupted (SI)	Provides secure, anatomic closure. Precise suture tension possible. Easily applied. Excessive tension may cause wound inversion	Skin, subcutis, fascia, blood vessels, nerves, gastrointestinal tract
Gambee	Modified simple interrupted suture. Less susceptible to wicking of bowel contents than SI. Prevents mucosal eversion, unlike SI. Tied tightly so that suture impresses itself on the bowel	Intestinal anastomosis
Interrupted intradermal or subcuticular	Upside down SI suture placed in dermis and subcutis	Intradermal skin closure
Interrupted cruciate or cross mattress	Provides stronger closure than SI. Resists tension and prevents eversion. Easiest of all mattress sutures to apply	Skin
Simple continuous (Sc)	Saves time and promotes suture economy. Provides good apposition and an airtight or watertight seal. Good for layers under low tension. Provides less strength than SI. Excessive tension causes puckering and strangulation of skin	Skin, subcutis, fascia, blood vessels, gastrointestinal tract
Continuous intradermal or subcuticular	Modified horizontal mattress suture. Saves time and promotes suture economy	Intradermal skin closure
Continuous lock or Ford interlocking	Similar to Sc except that it provides greater security if broken	Skin, diaphragm

From Toombs JP, Crowe DT: Textbook of Small Animal Surgery, Philadelphia, 1985, WB Saunders.

TABLE 17-5. Inverting Sutures

Suture Type	General Features	Common Uses
Lembert (Le)	A variation of the vertical mattress suture. Can be used as interrupted or continuous pattern. Penetrates the submucosa but not the lumen of the bowel	Fascial imbrication or plication; closure of hollow viscera
Halsted (Ha)	A variation of Le	Second layer of closure for viscera
Cushing (Cu)	Penetrates the submucosa but not the lumen of the bowel. Provides less inversion than Le	Closure of hollow viscera
Connell (Co)	Similar to Cu except penetrates bowel lumen. Subject to wicking of bowel contents, unlike Le, Ha, and Cu	First layer of closure for hollow viscera
Parker-Kerr (Pa)	A single layer of Cu sewn over a clamp, pulled tight as a clamp, is removed, and is oversewn with a continuous layer of Le	Closure of hollow visceral stumps
Pursestring (Pu)	A circular variation of Le. Stump must be held inverted as suture is tightened	Inversion of visceral stumps, securing of ostomy tubes and lavage catheters

From Toombs JP, Crowe DT: Textbook of Small Animal Surgery, Philadelphia, 1985, WB Saunders.

TABLE 17-6. Tension Sutures

Suture Type	General Features	Common Uses
Interrupted vertical mattress	Appositional to everting. Stronger in tissues under tension than interrupted horizontal mattress sutures. A single layer can be used for concurrent closure of skin and subcutis to eliminate dead space	Skin, subcutis, fascia
Interrupted horizontal mattress	Appositional to everting suture depending on suture tension and whether suture penetrates tissue full or split thickness. Potential for tissue strangulation can be reduced with stents	Skin, subcutis, fascia, muscle, tendon
Quilled	A variation of interrupted vertical mattress sutures that loops over a stent on either side of the incision. Everting	Combined with appositional suture for skin in areas of extreme stress
Continuous horizontal mattress	A variation of interrupted vertical mattress sutures. Provides necessary tension for wound edge approximation without applying tension to the wound edge itself. Excessive tightening causes inversion	Skin, subcutis, fascia
Near and far	Modified simple interrupted suture passed through skin, subcutis, and fascia, and tied over a gauze roll. Effective obliteration of dead space	Used in combination with appositional closure of skin and subcutis in layers
Stent	Appositional to everting suture depending on suture tension. Facilitates rapid closure	Skin, subcutis, fascia
Locking loop or modified Kessler	Provides superior apposition and equal holding strength compared with other tendon sutures	Tendons
Intraneural	Centrally placed neurorrhaphy suture anchored externally with silicone buttons.	Nerves

From Toombs JP, Crowe DT: Textbook of Small Animal Surgery, Philadelphia, 1985, WB Saunders.

Continuous Intradermal Patterns

Skin closure using a continuous intradermal pattern is popular, especially in conjunction with periosteal stripping.[17] In addition to the technique depicted in Figure 17-5, *F,* application of the pattern in Figure 17-5, *C* in a continuous fashion results in secure closure of the skin. The latter technique has better cosmetic properties. Care is taken not to include the epidermis because of the potential development of suture fistulas. Ideally, a 2-0 or 3-0 absorbable monofilament suture material (polydioxanone [PDS] or polyglyconate [Maxon]) with a reverse-cutting or taper-cut needle is used.[17]

Tension Sutures

Wounds with large defects or tissue loss are difficult to close without tension on the sutures. Tension may cut through or strangulate the tissue, resulting in wound dehiscence. The purpose of tension sutures is to redistribute the tension across the wound edges, minimizing marginal strangulation and necrosis. In horses, tension sutures are frequently indicated for closing traumatic lacerations and surgical wounds over bone plates.

Interrupted vertical mattress, horizontal mattress, quilted, and stent sutures are placed well away from the skin edges to prevent strangulation. These sutures are used to draw the

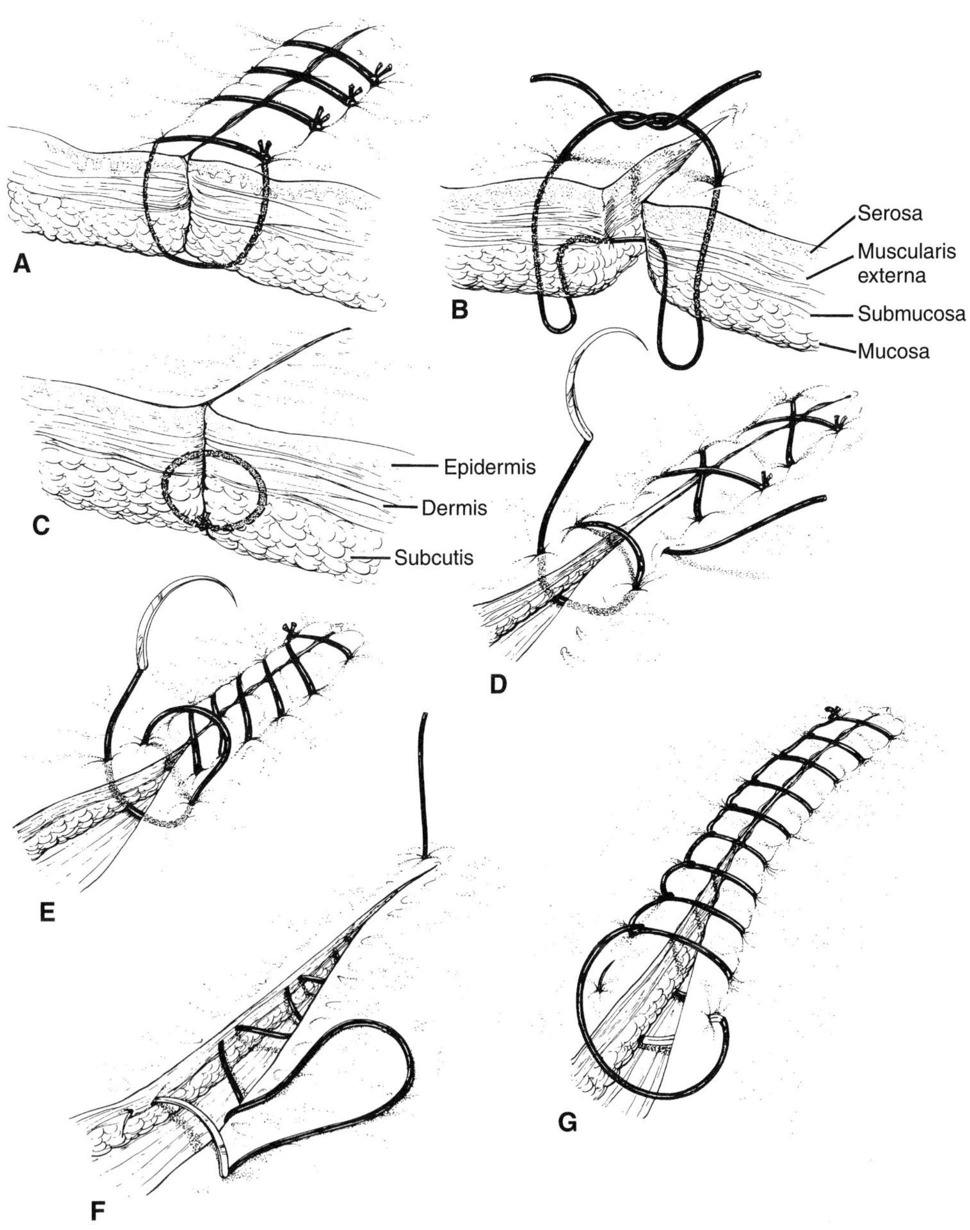

Figure 17-5. Appositional sutures. Refer to Table 17-4 for descriptions. (Redrawn with permission from Toombs JP, Crowe DT: Textbook of Small Animal Surgery. Philadelphia, 1993, WB Saunders.)

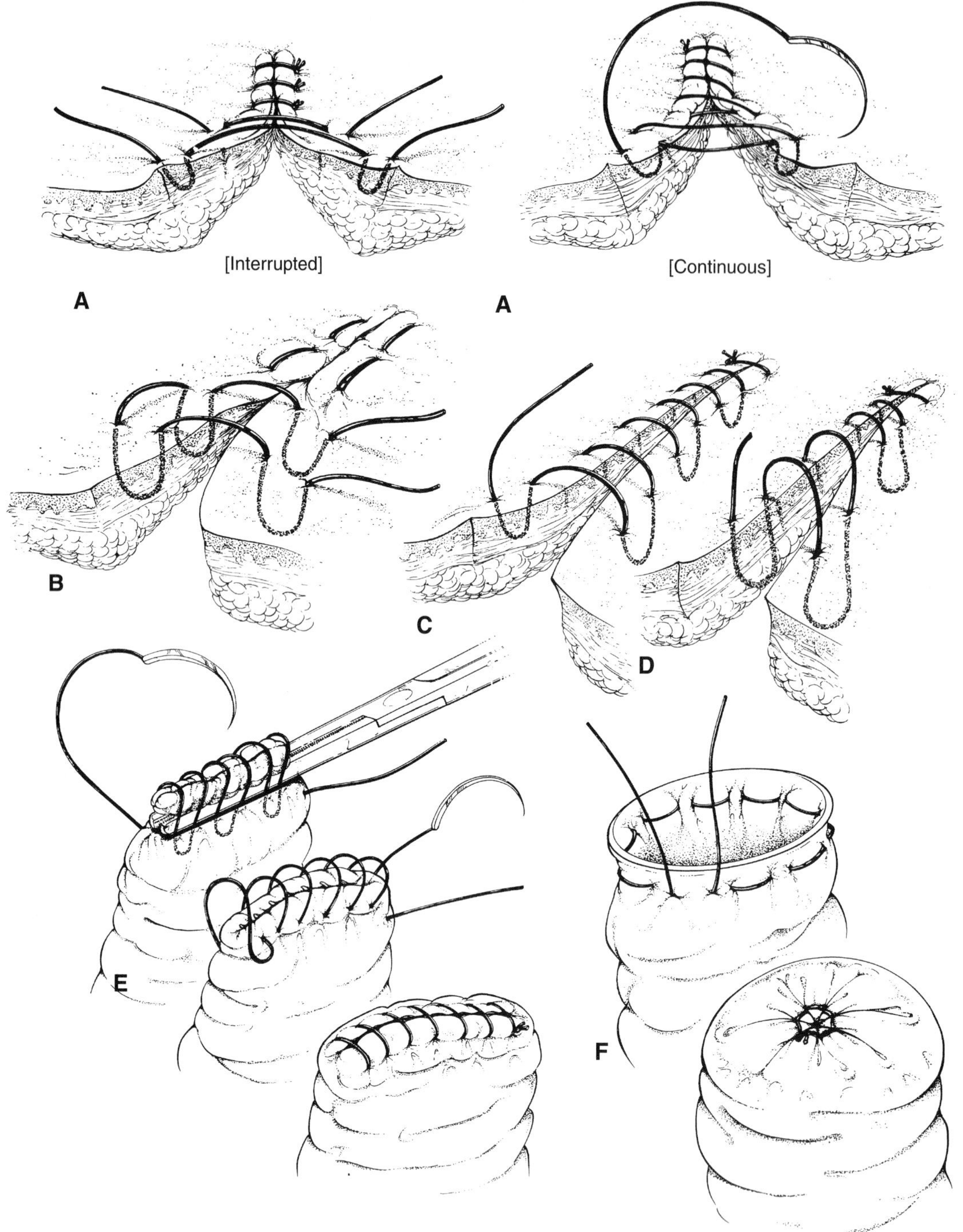

Figure 17-6. Inverting sutures. See Table 17-5 for description. (Redrawn with permission from Toombs JP, Crowe DT: Textbook of Small Animal Surgery. Philadelphia, 1993, WB Saunders.)

wound edges closer together so interrupted sutures can complete the closure without placing excessive tension on the wound margins. Subcuticular sutures are a form of tension suture because they help appose the skin edges, but they also prevent widening of the scar once the skin sutures are removed.[1]

Walking Sutures

"Walking" sutures are buried tension sutures that move skin progressively toward the center or the opposite wound margin (Fig. 17-8). They evenly distribute tension and obliterate dead space. The skin around the wound is undermined, and, using absorbable suture material, the first bite

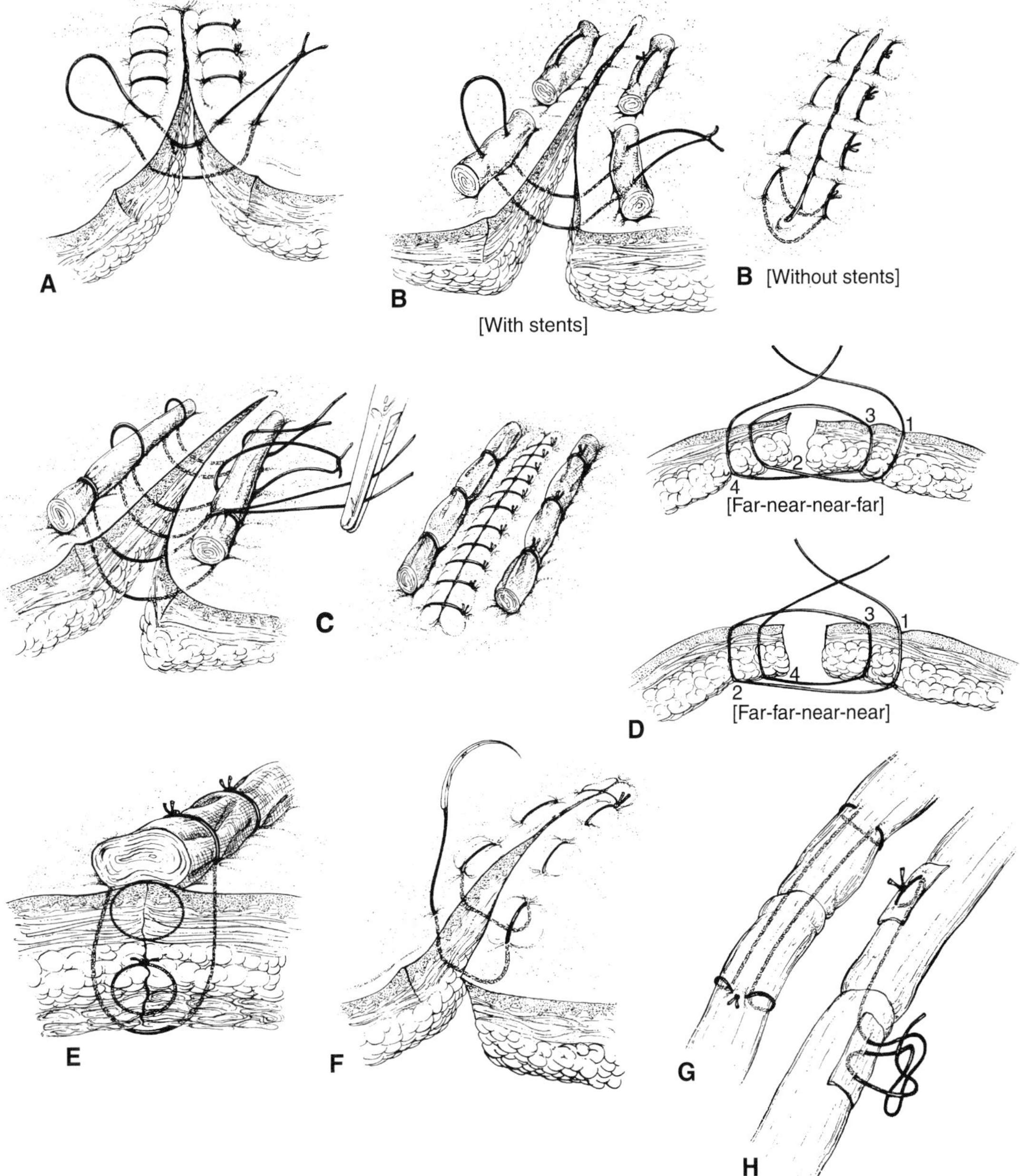

Figure 17-7. Tension sutures. Refer to Table 17-6 for descriptions. (Redrawn with permission from Toombs JP, Crowe DT: Textbook of Small Animal Surgery. Philadelphia, 1993, WB Saunders.)

is taken deep within the dermis without penetrating the full thickness of the skin. The second bite is taken in the underlying fascia toward the center of the wound. As the suture is tied, the skin is advanced toward the center of the wound. The walking sutures are placed on each side of the wound until the skin edges meet and allow closure with simple interrupted skin sutures, placed without tension. With a skin flap, walking sutures are used to advance the flap into place.[18] This technique prevents the formation of serum pockets subcutaneously and facilitates rapid healing and good cosmetic results in large wounds that would otherwise be managed by second-intention healing.

STAPLES

Advances in the development of stapling devices provide the surgeon with an alternative to hand-sutured anastomoses, ligations, and skin closures. Stapling instruments reduce tissue handling, decrease surgery time, minimize contamination, and provide secure visceral, vascular, and dermal closures when used correctly.

Properties

With the exception of fascia and skin staples, wound closure created by a staple instrument consists of inverted or everted

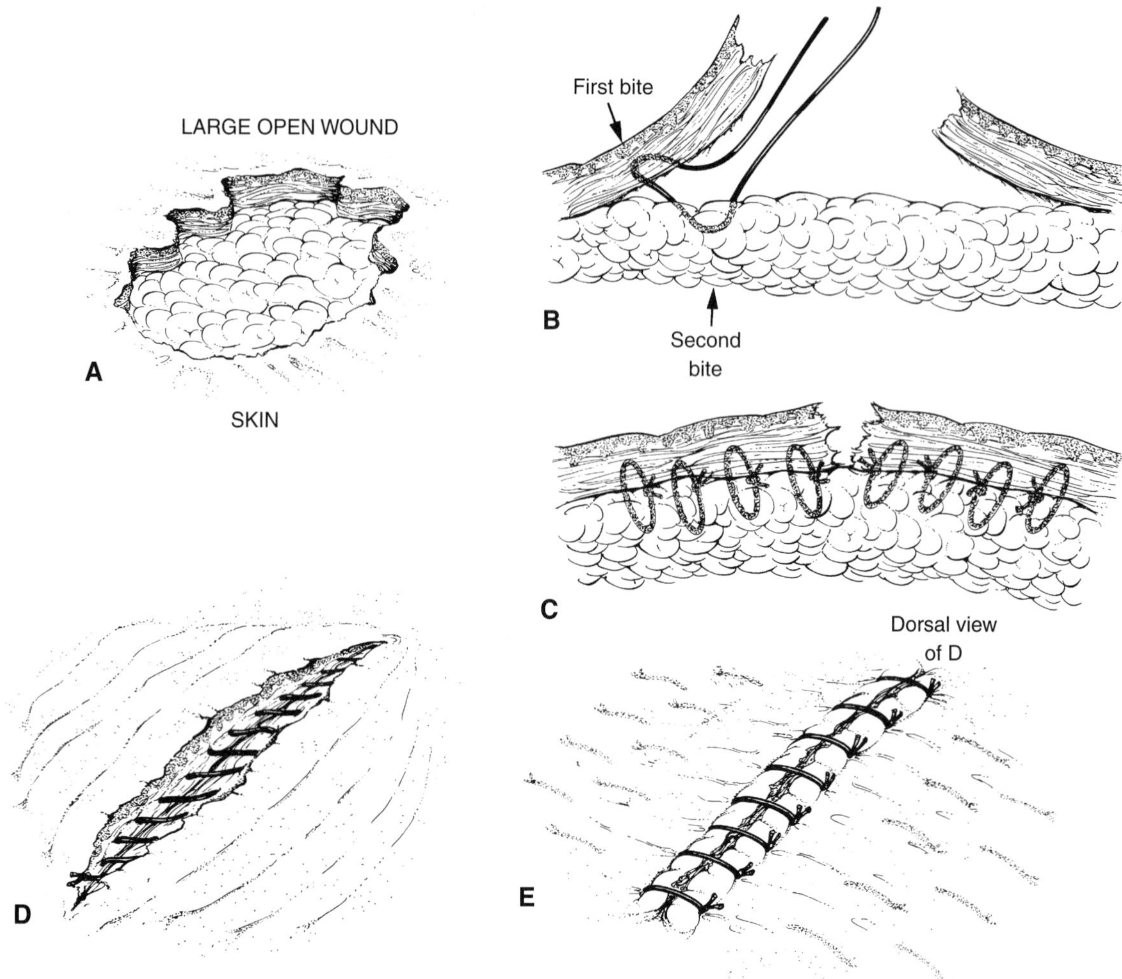

Figure 17-8. A, Closure of a large open wound. **B,** Placement of a walking suture in the deep layer of the dermis and underlying fascia. The first bite of the suture does not penetrate the full thickness of the skin. **C,** Slight advancement of the skin over the wound as the suture is tied. **D,** Almost complete closure of the wound after placement of walking sutures. *Broken lines* indicate sutures are under the skin and are not seen. **E,** Placement of a simple continuous intradermal suture and simple interrupted skin sutures. (Redrawn with permission from Swaim SF: Surgery of Traumatized Skin. Philadelphia, 1980, WB Saunders.)

layers of tissue secured by staggered double rows of B-shaped stainless steel wire staples. The staples are essentially inert and nonreactive, and they reduce the occurrence of tissue inflammation and infection.[19] The B-shaped staple is noncrushing; however, it does compress tissue, providing some hemostasis, yet it permits nutrition of the cut edge, thereby avoiding necrosis. United States Surgical Corporation (Norwalk, Conn) and Ethicon (Summerville, NJ) developed a line of disposable instruments, making their system more convenient with reduced risk of malfunction or misuse.

Stapling Devices

Skin

Skin staples provide a rapid, precise, slightly everted skin closure, which is easily applied and more convenient than conventional suturing (Fig. 17-9, *A*). Each time the trigger is pressed, the instrument discharges a single rectangular staple into the skin (see Fig. 17-9, *B*). When the wound is healed, the clips are opened and removed with the use of a special instrument (see Fig. 17-9, *C*).

Ligatures

Instruments for vascular ligation are designed for application to vascular bundles that can be compressed to the dimension of 0.75×5 or 7 mm.[20] The LDS-2 (ligate and divide stapler, United States Surgical Corporation) is clinically applicable for the rapid ligation of mesenteric vessels (Fig. 17-10, *A*). The instrument is pistol shaped and uses two sizes of disposable staple cartridges. When the trigger is activated, two wire ligatures are placed 1 cm apart, and a knife blade cuts between them (see Fig. 17-10, *B*). The instrument is used after the vessels have been isolated from their connective tissue attachments. Postoperative hemor-

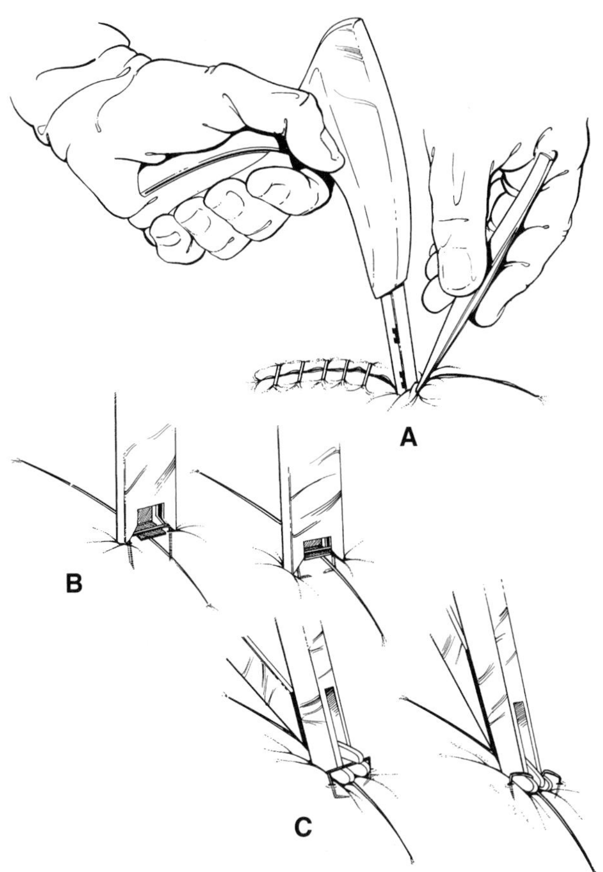

Figure 17-9. Skin-stapling instrument and technique. **A,** The skin edges are apposed with a forceps and stapled. **B,** As the staple penetrates the tissues, it is forced into a rectangular configuration apposing the cut edges. **C,** The staple remover opens the staple for easy removal from the tissues. (Copyright 1974, 1980, 1988, 1998, 2005 United States Surgical, a division of Tyco Healthcare Group LP. All rights reserved. Reprinted with Permission of United States Surgical, a division of Tyco Healthcare Group LP.)

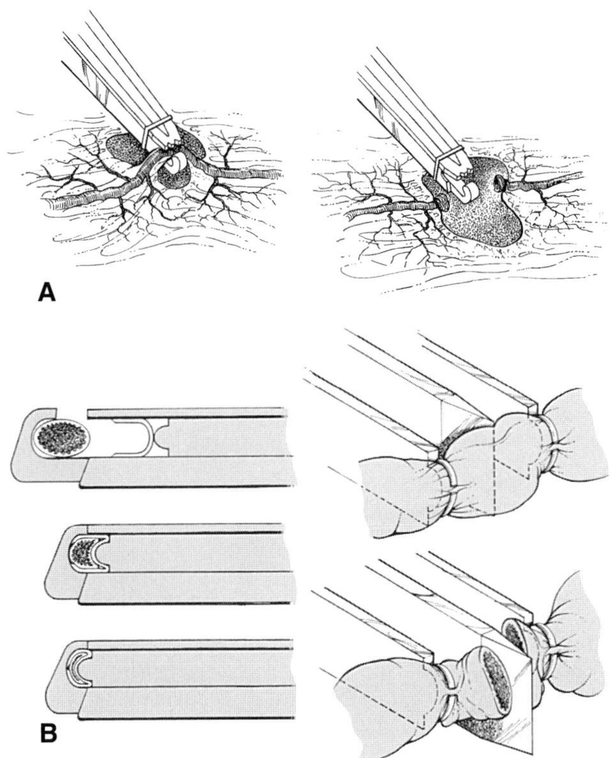

Figure 17-10. Vessel ligation and transection. **A,** The vessel is isolated from its mesenteric attachments and the jaws of the LDS (ligate and divide stapler) are slipped around the vessels. Two staples ligate the vessel simultaneously, and a knife divides the vessel between the staples. **B,** Vascular ligation with the LDS. (Copyright 1974, 1980, 1988, 1998, 2005 United States Surgical, a division of Tyco Healthcare Group LP. All rights reserved. Reprinted with Permission of United States Surgical, a division of Tyco Healthcare Group LP.)

rhage may occur if the diameter restrictions recommended by the manufacturer are not followed; one author even suggests that the vascular staple should not be relied on in adult horses.[21]

Abdominal and Thoracic Surgery

Surgical stapling devices are commonly used in equine abdominal surgery because shortened anesthesia and surgery time and reduced abdominal contamination are critically important. The instruments are either disposable or reusable. Stainless steel and titanium staples are used in most procedures, but absorbable staples are also available. Absorbable staples and specially designed equipment is used primarily in minimally invasive surgery.

The GIA 50 Premium (gastrointestinal anastomosis, United States Surgical Corporation) is the most commonly used stapling instrument in equine abdominal surgery. It consists of two parts and uses disposable staple cartridges (Fig. 17-11, *A*). The cartridge fires two double, staggered rows of stainless steel staples.[21] The two sets of staple lines are positioned 3.5 mm apart, and a knife blade cuts between them (see Fig. 17-11, *B*). One application of this instrument results in an inverting side-to-side anastomosis with a 5-cm-long stoma. It can be used for small-intestinal resection, leaving two secure blind ends that decrease the possibility of contamination by intestinal contents. The GIA is most commonly used to create an inverted side-to-side anastomosis of two hollow organs. Each fork of the GIA is inserted into the bowel lumen where it has been resected or through stab incisions. For a longer anastomosis, the GIA 80 or the ILA 100 (also by United States Surgical Corporation) may be used, providing a stoma approximately double in size. Double application of the GIA 50 in opposite directions will also accomplish this task. The stab incisions should be closed with inverting sutures. The GIA has been used successfully in the horse to perform jejunocecostomies, ileocolostomies, anastomoses of the dorsal and ventral colons, gastrojejunostomies, small-intestinal resections with side-to-side jejunojejunostomy, and functional end-to-end anastomoses.[21] For a secure closure, an additional layer of sutures is often applied using a hand technique. (For details on application of these stapling devices, see Chapters 35 and 36.)

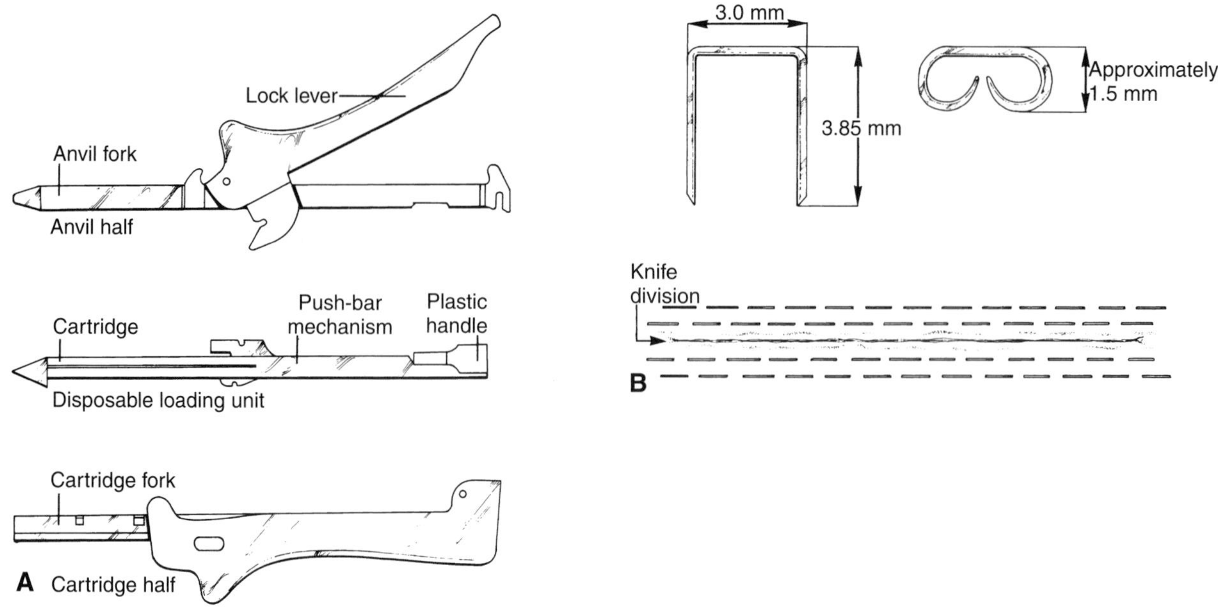

Figure 17-11. A, GIA 50 Premium stapler with disposable cartridge schematic view and nomenclature. **B,** The GIA 50 Premium staple cartridge contains 52 staples arranged in two double-staggered rows. The instrument's knife blade cuts between the two sets of staple lines, ending approximately 5 mm short of the last staple in the distal end. (Copyright 1974, 1980, 1988, 1998, 2005 United States Surgical, a division of Tyco Healthcare Group LP. All rights reserved. Reprinted with Permission of United States Surgical, a division of Tyco Healthcare Group LP.)

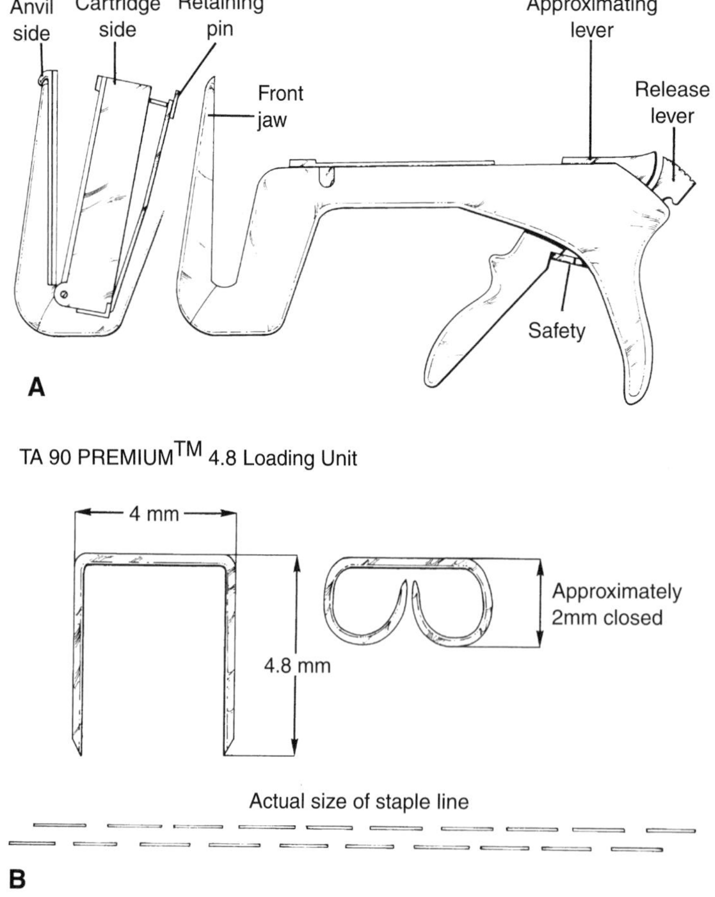

Figure 17-12. A, TA-90 Premium stapler with a disposable cartridge. **B,** TA-90 Premium 4.8 loading stapler contains 33 staples arranged in a double-staggered row 91.5 mm long. (Copyright 1974, 1980, 1988, 1998, 2005 United States Surgical, a division of Tyco Healthcare Group LP. All rights reserved. Reprinted with Permission of United States Surgical, a division of Tyco Healthcare Group LP.)

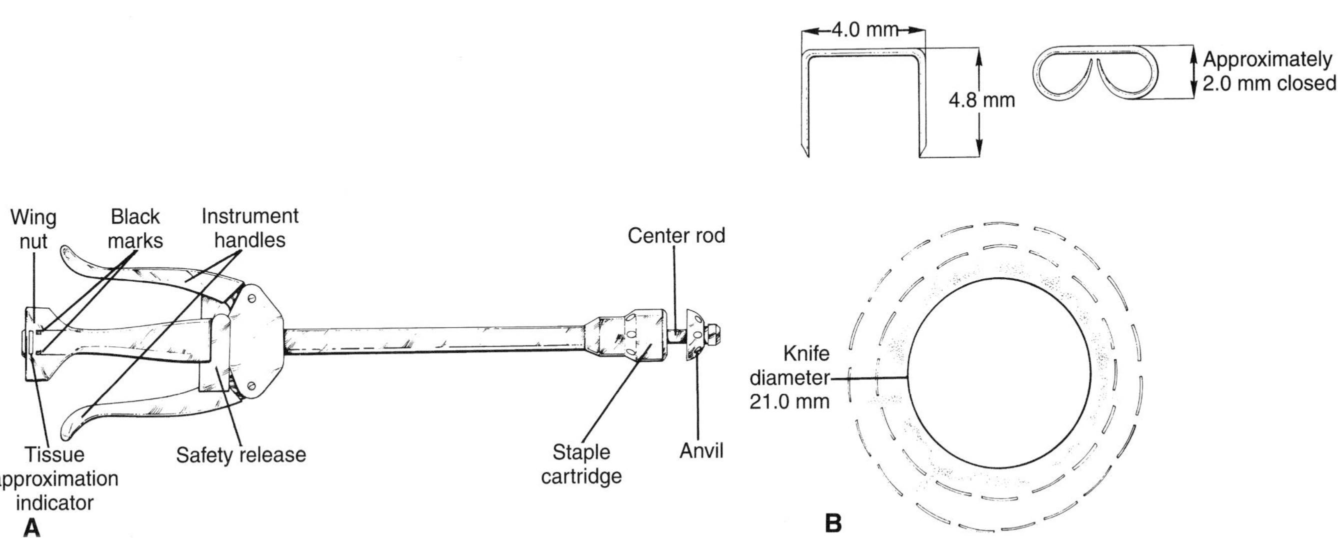

Figure 17-13. A, The EEA surgical stapling instrument. **B,** The disposable EEA 31 staple cartridge contains 35 staples in a staggered fashion, with a knife blade that cuts a stoma within the staple line. (Copyright 1974, 1980, 1988, 1998, 2005 United States Surgical, a division of Tyco Healthcare Group LP. All rights reserved. Reprinted with Permission of United States Surgical, a division of Tyco Healthcare Group LP.)

The TA-90 Premium (tissue anastomosis, United States Surgical Corporation) is pistol shaped and uses disposable cartridges that come in two staple sizes: 3.5 and 4.8 mm (Fig. 17-12, *A*). The instrument places one double, staggered row of staples 91.5 mm long[21] (see Fig. 17-12, *B*). The 4.8-mm staple cartridges are commonly used because of the longer staple leg. The longer staples are more applicable in the thick-walled large colon of the horse. The TA-90 has been used in the horse for large colon resections[22] and may be used for resections of thickened or edematous small intestine. The TA-90 is also useful for partial lung lobe resection in the horse.[23] The TA-35 and TA-55 were designed for tissues of smaller dimensions. For a secure closure, frequently an additional layer of sutures is applied using a hand technique.

The EEA (end-to-end anastomosis, United States Surgical Corporation) uses disposable staple cartridges in a circular design to create an inverting end-to-end or end-to-side anastomosis (Fig. 17-13, *A*). The lumen of each end of the intestine to be anastomosed is tightened to the center rod of the instrument using purse-string sutures. When the intestine is properly aligned, the instrument is fired, producing a circular, double, staggered row of staples, whereas a knife blade cuts a circular stoma within the stapled ring (see Fig. 17-13, *B*). The EEA has limited value in equine surgery because the diameter of the stoma created by the largest EEA is not compatible with the luminal diameter of the adult equine small intestine, but it may be applicable in foals.[20]

TISSUE ADHESIVES

The medical use of cyanoacrylate monomers as tissue adhesives is broadening. The older, short-chain cyanoacrylates were cytotoxic; however, newer relatively nontoxic formulations are used on organ tissues. New interest in the tissue adhesives has occurred because of the formulation of the *N*-butyl groups. Some of the investigational uses include plastic, ophthalmic, orthopedic, vascular, otolaryngeal, and oral surgery, as well as dermal healing. Cyanoacrylates also exhibit some hemostatic and bacteriostatic properties. For example, a 2-octyl cyanoacrylate formula is available as a dermal suture replacement. It has also been used to secure mesh grafts to limb wounds with excellent results (see Chapter 25).

The use of *N*-butyl cyanoacrylate as a topical bandage for horses has been described.[24] These cyanoacrylate bandages were functionally similar to an occlusive bandage: exuberant granulation tissue was inhibited, and the rate and type of healing on distal extremity wounds of horses were no different from conventionally pressure-bandaged limbs.

For a wound to be covered with a cyanoacrylate bandage, it must have a mature granulation bed with a smooth, dry surface. Fluid collecting beneath the bandage will disrupt a portion or all of it. Therefore, corticosteroid-based ointment or cream is applied to the mature wound surface to smooth the wound surface and decrease fluid production.[25]

A host of new adhesives are presently being evaluated for use on tissues (see Chapter 9). They have not been evaluated in the horse.

REFERENCES

1. Swaim SF: General principles of delayed wound excision and closure. In Swaim SF, editor: Surgery of Traumatized Skin, Philadelphia, 1980, WB Saunders.
2. Boothe HW: Suture materials and tissue adhesives. In Slatter DH, editor: Textbook of Small Animal Surgery, Philadelphia, 1985, WB Saunders.

3. Vasseur PB: Principles of operative surgery. In Gourley IM, Vasseur PB, editors: General Small Animal Surgery, Philadelphia, 1985, JB Lippincott.
4. Smeak DD, Wendlelburg KL: Choosing suture materials for use in contaminated or infected wounds, Comp Cont Educ Pract Vet 1989;11:467.
5. Bellenger CR: Sutures: Part II. The use of sutures and alternative methods of closure, Comp Cont Educ Pract Vet 1982;4:587.
6. Edlich RF, Panek PH, Rodeheaver GT, et al: Physical and chemical configuration of sutures in the development of surgical infection, Ann Surg 1973;177:679.
7. Adair HS, Goble DO, Rohrbach BW: In vitro comparison of the locking loop and the three loop pulley suture techniques in the repair of equine flexor tendons, Equine Vet Sci 1989;9:186.
8. Turner AS, McIlwraith CW: Suture materials and needles. In Turner AS, McIlwraith CW, editors: Large Animal Surgery, ed 2, Philadelphia, 1989, Lea & Febiger.
9. Trier WC: Considerations in the choice of surgical needles, Surg Gynecol Obstet 1979;149:84.
10. Toombs JP, Crowe DT: Operative techniques. In Slatter DH, editor: Textbook of Small Animal Surgery, Philadelphia, 1985, WB Saunders.
11. Rosin E, Robinson GM: Knot security of suture materials, Vet Surg 1989;18:269.
12. Turner AS, McIlwraith CW: Knots and ligatures. In Turner AS, McIlwraith CW, editors: Techniques in Large Animal Surgery, ed 2, Philadelphia, 1989, Lea & Febiger.
13. Knecht CD, Allen AR, Williams DJ, Johnson JH: Fundamental Techniques in Veterinary Surgery, ed 3, Philadelphia, 1987, WB Saunders.
14. Pode GV, Meredith JW, Kon ND, et al: Suture technique and wound-bursting strength, Am Surg 1984;50:569.
15. Reinertson EL: Comparison of three techniques for intestinal anastomosis in Equidae, J Am Vet Med Assoc 1976;169:208.
16. Dean PW, Robertson JT, Jacobs RM: Comparison of suture materials and suture patterns for inverting intestinal anastomosis of the jejunum in the horse, Am J Vet Res 1985;46:2072.
17. Auer JA: Periosteal transection for correction of angular limb deformities, Proc Am Assoc Equine Pract 1982;28:232.
18. Swaim SF: Moving local tissues to close surface defects. In Swaim SF, editor: Surgery of Traumatized Skin, Philadelphia, 1980, WB Saunders.
19. Pascoe JR, Peterson PR: Intestinal healing and methods of anastomosis, Vet Clin North Am Equine Pract 1989;5:309.
20. United States Surgical Corporation: Information Manual for Auto Suture Model LDS-2, Norwalk, Conn, 1985, United States Surgical Corporation.
21. Doran RE, Allen D: The use of stapling devices in equine gastro-intestinal surgery, Comp Cont Educ Pract Vet 1987;9:854.
22. Bertone AL, Stashak TS, Sullins KE, Ralston SL: Experimental large colon resection at the cecocolic ligament in the horse, Vet Surg 1987;16:5.
23. Boulton CH, Modransky PD, Grant BD, et al: Partial equine lung resection using a stapling instrument, Vet Surg 1986;15:93.
24. Blackford JT, Shires M, Goble D, et al: The use of *N*-butyl cyanoacrylate in the treatment of open leg wounds in the horse, Proc Am Assoc Equine Pract 1986;32:349.
25. Blackford JT: The effects of an antimicrobial glucocorticosteroid ointment on granulating lower leg wounds in the horse, Vet Surg 1990;19:59.

CHAPTER 18

Drains, Bandages, and External Coaptation

Jörg A. Auer

The application of drains, bandages, and external coaptation is an important step in state-of-the-art wound management. The different dressings used in association with bandages are discussed in Chapter 26.

DRAINS AND DRAINAGE

History

Hippocrates, in the 4th century BC, was the first to use drains, in the form of hollow tubes, to treat empyemas. In the 2nd century AD, Celsus and Galen used conical tubes of brass and lead to drain ascites, and these devices were used for 1500 years. In 1719, Heisler introduced capillary drainage via a gauze wick inside a metal tube.[1,2] In 1859, Penrose used soft rubber tubing as a drain, known today as the Penrose drain. Kehrer modified this technique in 1882 by placing gauze inside the Penrose drain to facilitate drainage, thus creating the "cigarette drain." Today's version of the cigarette drain consists of semirigid vinyl or polyvinyl tubing inserted into a Penrose drain to prevent soft tissue obstruction and increase capillary action.[3,4] All of these drains were applied in a passive system, allowing gravity, capillary action, natural pressure gradients, or overflow to control fluid and gas flow. Negative pressure was subsequently applied to the semirigid tubes to provide an active system, and finally Raffle developed the technique of continuous suction in 1952.[5]

Purposes

Drains are implants designed to channel unwanted fluids such as wound secretions, purulent material, bile, urine, blood, or gases out of the body.[6] Proper use of drains generally speeds up healing time, whereas inappropriate use usually delays healing, occasionally even increasing morbidity and mortality. There are three reasons to place a drain: (1) to facilitate elimination of dead space, (2) to evacuate existing fluid and gas accumulations, and (3) to prevent anticipated formation of fluid collections.[7] Understanding the principles of drain selection, placement, and management minimizes the risks associated with these implants.

Materials

The ideal drain is inert, soft, nonreactive, and radio-opaque. Table 18-1 lists common drain types and materials. Soft latex is frequently used in drains; it allows excellent passive drainage of wound fluids. Because it is pliant and does not maintain a rigid lumen, it fits comfortably within the wound. Polyvinylchloride (PVC) drain tubes provide excellent wound fluid evacuation, especially from body cavities and deep surgical wounds. They are less flexible than latex and have a rigid lumen, allowing them to be used for passive or active systems. Frequently, PVC drains are multifenestrated to permit fluids to exit the wound or body. Other drains are manufactured out of silicone, an organic compound in which all or part of the carbon has been replaced by silicon (a nonmetallic element occurring in nature as silica)[8]. Silastic is the trade name for polymeric silicone substances having the properties of rubber; it is biologically inert and frequently used in applications other than drains.[8] It is softer than PVC, but at some diameters it maintains a rigid lumen. Therefore, Silastic can be used for active or passive drainage systems. The compliance of the material increases the animal's comfort and makes this type of drain ideal for placement in sensitive areas and within small spaces.[9,10]

Placement

The basic principles of wound management, such as clipping of the hair, aseptic preparation of the implantation site, and possibly local anesthesia, are considerations when placing a drain. In sterile wounds, the drain should be applied under aseptic conditions. Additionally, this sterile environment should be maintained as long as possible through covering of the wound and frequent bandage changes. Passive drains should exit below the most ventral aspect of the wound or dead space.

The drains should be placed into the space requiring the most drainage. Occasionally, several drains are needed to evacuate a large area or several different tissue layers. The shortest and most direct avenue for evacuation of secretions should be selected. Drains cause some mechanical injury and therefore should not be placed in the immediate vicinity of blood vessels, nerves, and suture lines. To reduce the risk of suture dehiscence, drains should exit through separate incisions, away from the suture line (Fig. 18-1, *A*). It is important to secure the drains with individual sutures to prevent their loss into or out of the wound. A suture is placed from the skin into the wound, through the drain, and back through the skin, where it is tied (see Fig. 18-1, *B*). The suture used for securing the drain should be easily distinguishable from the skin sutures to avoid inadvertent premature removal of a suture securing the incision. If a drain is placed into a wound that is to be closed, care should be taken to avoid inadvertent incorporation of the drain into the suture line, because drains are usually removed before incisional sutures (see later). The drain end should be long enough to prevent its disappearance into the wound and to evacuate drainage fluids. It is also important to protect the drains from attempts by the patient to remove them. Large openings provide better and longer-lasting drainage. Small exit incisions frequently plug up, even with a drain in place, preventing evacuation of drainage material.

Management

The amount of drainage and its consistency dictate the frequency that bandages need to be changed or vacuum containers emptied. The exit site should be cleaned with antiseptic solutions at every bandage change. If a passive drain is used, it is advisable to protect the adjacent skin from irritation by covering it with a thin layer of Vaseline. Passive drains should seldom if ever be back-flushed, and active drains should not be back-flushed unless obstructed because of the risk of transporting microorganisms into the wound. Additionally, healing may be interrupted by the mechanical disturbance of flushing.

Re-establishing drainage in an obstructed drain exit wound should be performed carefully. If the drain exit site is obstructed, it should be reopened. First the site is prepared for aseptic surgery, followed by insertion of a sterile hemostatic forceps into the opening and gentle spreading of its jaws to separate the wound ends.

Removal

As a general rule, drains should be removed as quickly as possible. An average time for maintaining drains is 2 to 4 days, the duration of the débridement period of wound healing. However, there are exceptions to this rule:

1. When evacuating blood from small cavities, the drain may be removed after approximately 24 hours.
2. When treating bacterial infections, the drain should be maintained for 48 to 72 hours.
3. If large dead spaces remain, as after tumor removal, the presence of a drain may be necessary for as long as 2 weeks.

The best indicator for drain removal is an abrupt decrease in the drainage volume and a change in its characteristics to a serous, non-odiferous, slightly turbid fluid. Because drains are foreign material, they induce the production of secretions. At the time of drain removal, exit sites are prepared for aseptic surgery. While the proximal end is held in place, the distal securing suture is removed, followed by application of slight tension to the distal end of the drain, before it is cut off at skin level. This ensures that the contaminated external part of the drain is not pulled through the wound bed, possibly recontaminating it. The proximal suture is removed, and the rest of the drain is pulled out of the wound bed. The two incisions are left to heal by secondary intention. In case of only one exit portal present, the securing suture(s) is (are) cut and the drain is removed through the distal portal.

If gauze packs are used as tamponade in a bleeding wound, they are removed in stages, with a portion withdrawn and cut off daily, each time leaving a protruding stump to facilitate removal of the next portion.

TABLE 18-1. Drains

	Material	Mechanism of Action; Function	Advantages	Disadvantages
PASSIVE DRAINS				
Gauze drains[1]	Fine mesh gauze	Gravity Capillary action	Economical	Adherence of fibrin clots to gauze
Penrose drain[2]	Soft, pliable latex available in various sizes Hollow tube	Gravity Capillary action Mostly drainage around periphery	Economical Many applications	May easily kink Not applicable in body cavities No suction possible May facilitate ascending infection
Silicone Penrose drain[3,4]	Soft, pliable, nonreactive silicone	As Penrose drain	Less irritating Use in latex-sensitive patients Contains radiodense marker	Not applicable in body cavities No suction possible
Rubber tube drains	Red rubber Smooth surface	Gravity Capillary action	Because of relative stiffness, rarely compressed or occluded Suction may be applied	Increased foreign body reaction
Well drain[5] (German for "waved drain")	Waved sheet of red rubber, stiff, can be cut to size	Gravity Capillary action	Because of relative stiffness, rarely compressed or occluded	Increased foreign body reaction
Flexi-Drain[4]	12 silicone tubes, 3 mm in diameter, joined together parallel to each other	Gravity Capillary action Good drainage along the tubes where they join	Contains radiodense marker Can be split longitudinally to adjust size of drain Suction may be applied	Main drainage externally
ACTIVE DRAINS				
Redon drain[6]	Round, multifenestrated PVC tube with nonfenestrated extension	Closed or open drainage system	Can be used as closed or open drainage system Excellent for evacuation of fluids from body cavities	Depending on location, attaching the container may be difficult. Tube cannot be used universally.
Jackson-Pratt drain[5]	Flat Silastic, multifenestrated drain with nonfenestrated extension	Closed or open drainage system	Can be used as closed or open drainage system Excellent for evacuation of fluids from body cavities Less reactive	Depending on location, attaching the container may be difficult.
Blake drain[1]	Round pliable Silastic drains with slits at the end	Closed and open drainage system	Multifaceted slits reduce the risk of clogging up Minimal tissue irritation	Relatively voluminous Suction function possible only when skin suture is tight
Trocar catheter[7]	Round, multifenestrated tube Inserted with blunt trocar into the chest	Drainage of thoracic cavity	Minimal reaction and irritation Effective fluid drainage from thorax	Relatively easily dislodged, interrupting effective drainage

1. Johnson & Johnson, New Brunswick, NJ; Triclosan-Gauze IVF Hartmann, Neuhausen, Switzerland.
2. Sherwood Medical, St. Louis, Mo.
3. Easy-Flow drain, Degania Silicone LTD, Degania Bet, Israel.
4. Cook Veterinary Products, Eight Mile Plains, Queensland, Australia.
5. Nelaton, Ruesch, Belp, Switzerland.
6. Zimmer, Inc, Dover, Ohio.
7. Mallinckrodt Medical, Athlone, Ireland.

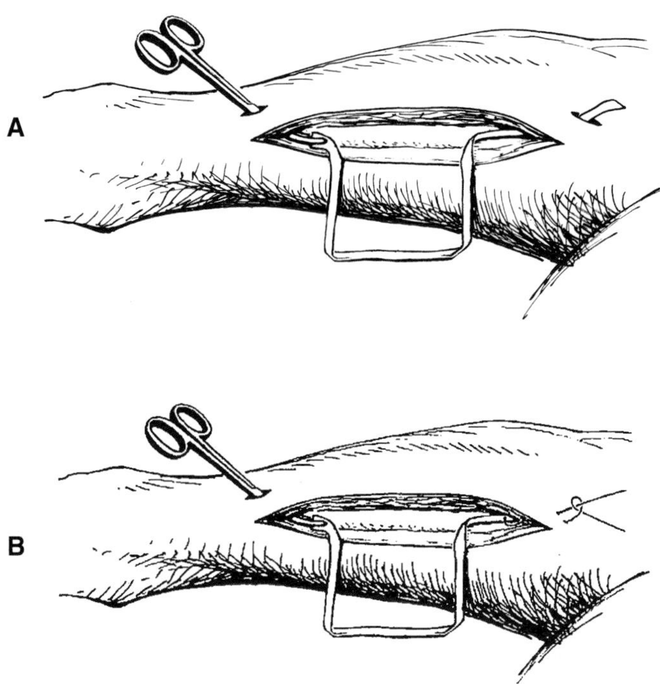

Figure 18-1. Proper placement of a Penrose drain for passive postoperative drainage. **A,** The two exit portals for the drain are placed distant from the primary incision. The ends of the drain are secured with a suture each (using sutures of a different type from the skin sutures for easy recognition). **B,** Only the distal exit portal is made, and the proximal-most aspect of the drain is secured within the wound with a suture that enters proximal to the wound through the skin, passes through the drain, and exits the skin again, where it is tied. The wound is subsequently closed.

Complications

Foreign body response and ascending infection are the most common complications associated with drain use. Because drains are foreign bodies, an adverse response to the drain cannot be avoided. If a portion of the drain is accidentally left in the wound, wound drainage will persist until it is removed. Therefore, the removed drain should be carefully examined to verify complete removal. Ascending infection may aggravate an already existing infection, and the microorganisms in the wound may be resistant to previously used antibiotics. Cultures should be obtained if the character of the wound fluid changes or the volume increases while a drain is in place.

Loss of function may be encountered, especially if the distal exiting portal is too small. It is therefore advisable to initially remove a triangle of skin and subcutaneous tissues at the exiting portal. Another cause of loss of function is the kinking of a tube drain, effectively obliterating the drain lumen. Repositioning of the drain and gentle traction frequently restores function.

Suture dehiscence is an occasional complication that may be attributed to the placement of a drain. Also, vessels and nerves may be damaged during drain placement through stab incisions and blind implantation. Rigid drain tubes may cause pain if they are located near osseous protuberances.

Types of Drains

Drain selection depends on the wound and on expected activity level of the patient. Additionally, the preferences of the surgeon, based on experience, play an important role in the selection of a drain.

Passive Drains

GAUZE DRAINS

Gauze drains are prepared from gauze rolls or gauze sponges. They may be soaked with an antibiotic or even with an antiseptic. The antibiotic may be added at the time of drain placement, or the gauze may come commercially prepared (Fig. 18-2, and see Table 18-1). If a large amount of gauze is used to pack a cavity, several rolls are tied together securely to ensure that eventually they are completely removed. Drainage occurs by gravity and capillary action.

Gauze drains are applied as packing in profusely bleeding cavities (e.g., after nasal septum removal) or in abscesses that cannot be drained at the lowest point. They can be used to evacuate a hematoma (after closed castration). In Europe, gauze drains are frequently attached to the stump of the spermatic cord after castration to facilitate drainage and prevent fluid accumulation in the scrotum. The advantages of gauze drains include cost effectiveness and ease of removal in stages. The adherence of fibrin clots to the gauze is a disadvantage, as it may result in bleeding after removal.

PENROSE DRAINS

Penrose drains are the most commonly used drains because they are soft, pliable, easily sterilized, readily available, and economical, and they cause little foreign body reaction[4] (see Table 18-1). They are available in lengths from 30 to 45 cm (12 to 18 inches) and in widths from 6 to 25 mm ($\frac{1}{4}$ to 1 inch) (see Fig. 18-2). Most drainage occurs extraluminally and is driven by gravity and capillary action. To facilitate intraluminal drainage, the drain may be installed inside the body at its most proximal aspect or fenestrated. However,

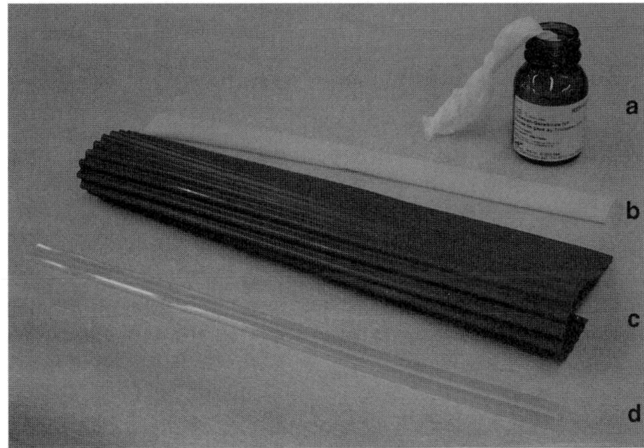

Figure 18-2. Materials frequently used as drains. *a,* Gauze drain soaked with Triclosan (antibiotic) (IVF Hartmann, Neuhausen, Switzerland). *b,* Latex Penrose drains (Sherwood Medical; St. Louis, Mo). *c,* Sheet drain of waved red rubber (Ruesch, Belp, Switzerland). The sheet is folded over. *d,* Easy-Flow silicone drain (Degania Silicone LTD, Degania Bet, Israel).

despite providing access of drainage to the inside of drain, fenestrations reduce the surface area, which decreases their efficacy.[4] Also, the fenestrations weaken the drain and may result in breakage and the risk of subsequent incomplete removal if adhesions between the drain and the soft tissues develop.

Penrose drains can be successfully used in wounds that cannot be completely débrided and in the presence of residual foreign material, massively contaminated tissue, questionably viable tissue, and fluid-filled dead spaces.[3,5,7] Additionally, these drains have been applied with good results underneath skin grafts, in open wounds left to heal by secondary intention, and even in septic joints and tendon sheaths left open for lavage.[11-14] Penrose drains are not suitable for use with suction (because they collapse under a vacuum), in the abdominal cavity (because they are walled off within a short time in the abdomen), or in the thoracic cavity (because they allow air to pass into the thorax).[7]

SHEET DRAINS

Frequently, large wounds over muscular areas have to be drained. In these instances, several drains are needed to effectively drain the entire wound. An alternative is the sheet drain (see Fig. 18-2 and Table 18-1), which is made of red rubber and has a cross-section shaped like a sine wave. The sheet can be trimmed to the desired size. To facilitate additional space in the field to be drained, the sheet can be folded over. Because of its inherent stiffness, there is a gap between the two layers of drain when folded, which resists obstruction. These drains are left in place only a couple of days, but they work efficiently during that time. Red rubber generally induces a significant foreign body reaction.

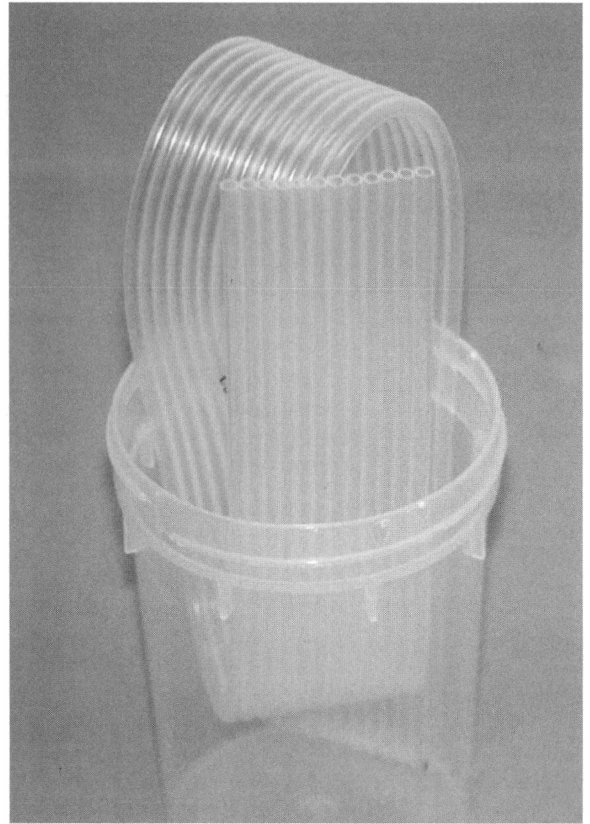

Figure 18-3. A Flexi-drain (Cook Veterinary Products, Eight Mile Plains, Queensland, Australia) folded up in a plastic cup. The 12 single tubes joined to a single drain system is shown.

TUBE DRAINS

Tube drains differ in form and material. They can be relatively stiff, single tubes of red rubber, contain a cross-sectional wave pattern, be of soft, pliable, ribbed, flat Silastic, or they can be tubular silicone drains that consist of 12 single tubes joined together, each with a diameter of 3 mm (Fig. 18-3, and see Table 18-1). These drains function by extraluminal and intraluminal flow and have been successfully applied for draining fluid from wounds as well as from the abdomen and thorax. The more rigid drains have a tendency to induce a greater tissue irritation than Penrose-type drains. Simple tube drains provide only weak capillary action but they are effective for gravity drainage.[4,7] the outer and inner surfaces of the tubes should exhibit a low coefficient of friction to facilitate evacuation of blood clots as well as their own removal. Some of the drains can be connected to a suction apparatus to evacuate fluids without collapsing and to allow irrigation. These drains are inexpensive and readily available, and they cause less interference with tissue healing than Penrose drains.[4]

One disadvantage of tube drains in a passive system is that they are easily obstructed by debris, so that they become ineffective until they are back-flushed to make them patent again, and this may occur frequently. Therefore, their use is limited to grossly contaminated areas where bacterial contamination by back-flushing is not too worrisome. Some materials (such as red rubber) induce greater inflammatory reactions than others (such as PVC or Silastic). Polyethylene contains certain impurities that support bacterial growth.[3,7] When used intra-abdominally, omentum can easily obstruct tube drains.

Active Drains

CLOSED SUCTION SYSTEMS

In equine practice, simple tube drains attached to a suction apparatus providing either intermittent or continuous suction are frequently used in infected joints; in large, deep wounds; to evacuate the pleural space; and under full-thickness skin grafts. Blake and fenestrated tube drains are often used in these situations (Fig. 18-4), and occasionally Snyder Hemovac drains are used (Fig. 18-5, see Table 18-1). Either the end of the drain is multifenestrated or the cross-section consists of a modified cloverleaf pattern with four slits and protected spaces (as in the Blake drain). The external end is made of smooth tubing and is connected through a three-way stopcock, most frequently to a syringe; the plunger of the syringe is withdrawn to achieve the desired negative pressure, and it can be held in that position by introducing a large needle or a small pin across the plunger and resting it on the syringe end (see Fig. 18-5). This provides the most economical suction apparatus. The three-way stopcock allows interruption of the suction action prior to removing the syringe for emptying. This is also an effective means to fight against ascending infection. A study comparing Penrose drains to closed suction drains showed that at 24 hours, 34% of the Penrose drains were contam-

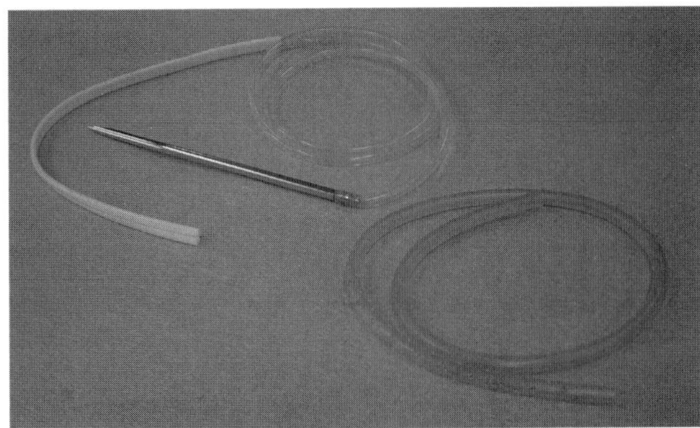

Figure 18-4. A Blake drain (Johnson & Johnson, New Brunswick, NJ) and a multifenestrated Snyder-type tube drain (Zimmer, Inc, Dover, Ohio). The *insert* represents the cross-section of the Blake drain. The trocar at the other end is used to place the drain through the skin.

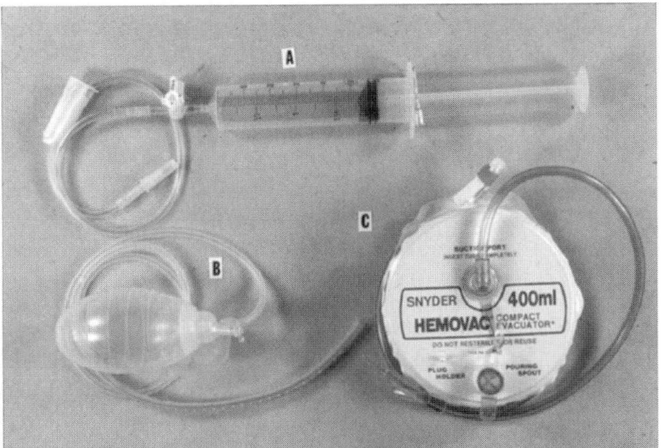

Figure 18-5. Devices used as active drainage systems. A, Syringe-adapted closed-suction device made from a 60-mL syringe by drilling a hole in the shaft, near the plunger. A three-way stopcock and extension set is attached to the syringe and fixed to the drain. The syringe is held open by a 14-gauge needle whose tip is ground flat, placed across the syringe shaft. B, Snyder Hemovac–100 mL (Zimmer, Inc, Dover, Ohio) with a flat silicone fenestrated drain. C, Snyder Hemovac–400 mL (Zimmer, Inc).

inated compared with none of the closed suction drains.[2,4,7] If suction is applied in a continuous manner, soft tissues can rapidly occlude the drain. High negative pressure may cause injury to tissues, and if the system is suddenly disrupted, reflux of evacuated fluid may occur, increasing the risk of infection. The installation of a Heimlich valve into a suction system can prevent reflux of fluid (Fig. 18-6).

A special closed suction system has been used in humans to promote granulation tissue production in large open wounds, especially when there is bone involvement. This device has been successfully applied in horses. The wound to be treated by suction is prepared for aseptic surgery and the wound edges are clipped and trimmed. A sponge is cut to slightly overlap the wound size. The continuous suction device is installed into the sponge. The entire sponge and the suction device are covered by a special adhesive tape, which provides an airtight seal between the wound and the

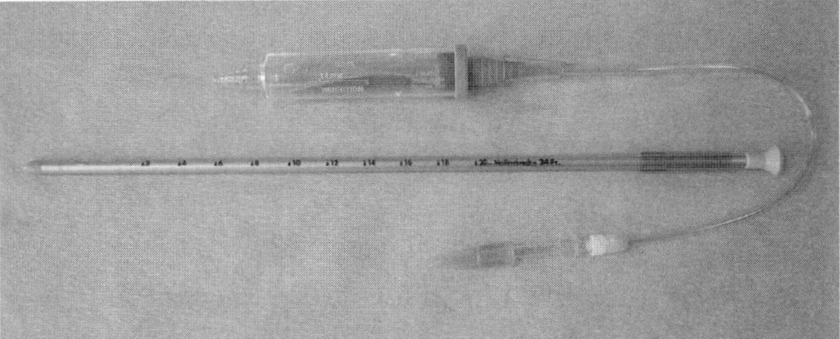

Figure 18-6. *Top:* A spontaneous pneumothorax aspiration system (Heimlich valve) (Cook Veterinary Products, Eight Mile Plains, Queensland, Australia) used to prevent access of ascending air and microorganisms into the cavity to be drained. *Bottom:* A PVC thorax drain (Trocar Catheter, Mallinckrodt Medical, Athlone, Ireland).

normal skin (Fig. 18-7). A bandage is applied to protect the device and maintain external pressure. When suction is applied, the evacuated fluid accumulates in a container. Movements of the horse must be restricted to ensure continuous suction. This method of wound treatment can change an infected, odiferous wound into one covered with healthy granulation tissue within 4 days (Fig. 18-8).

OPEN SUCTION SYSTEMS

Open suction is infrequently applied in equine medicine. One system involves a sump drain, which is a large drain tube with a second, smaller tube in the wall or within the lumen of the larger tube. This "vented" suction apparatus allows the entrance of air to the wound through the narrow lumen tube while debris and fluid are evacuated through the larger tube. Suction may be applied in continuous or intermittent form.[4,7] The airflow improves drainage and decreases the risk of occlusion. However, sump drains do not adapt well to many veterinary hospital situations. Large, portable, or built-in wall units are needed. Also, the large

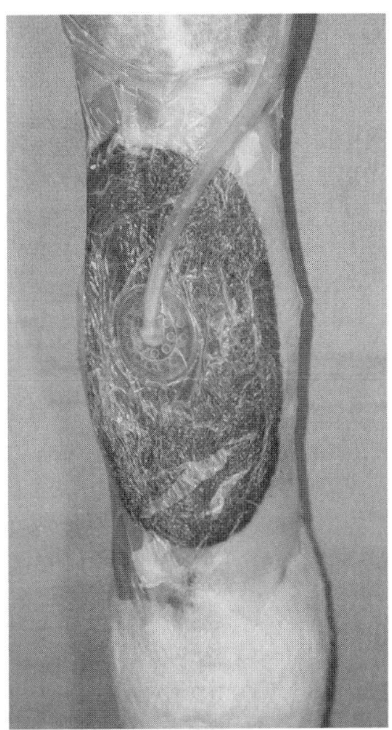

Figure 18-7. The wound in Figure 18-8 was covered with a suction device and sealed under a plastic bandage.

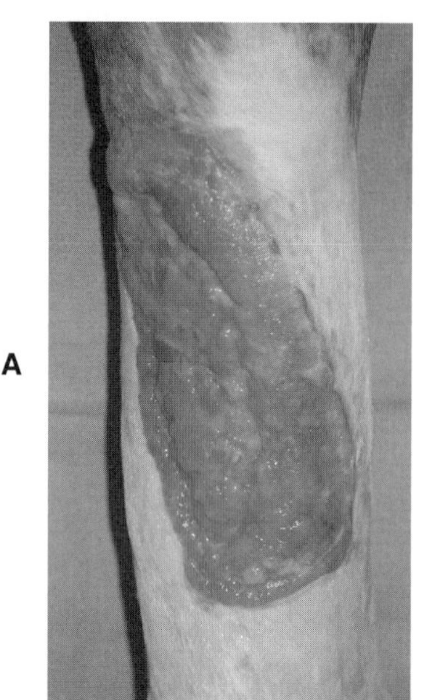

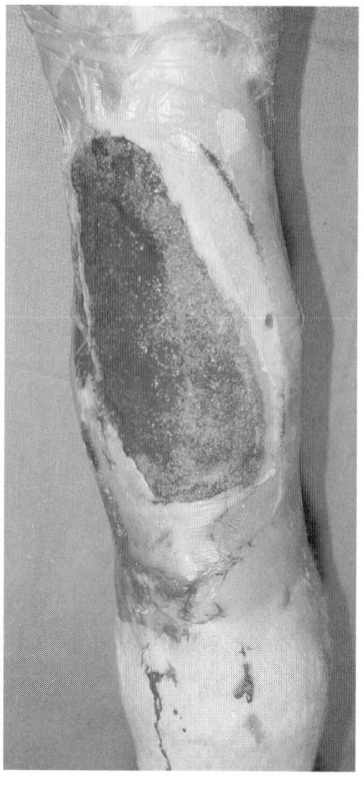

Figure 18-8. A, An old, infected, nonhealing wound over the dorsomedial aspect of third metatarsal bone. The granulation tissue is unhealthy looking and nonresponsive to treatment. **B,** The same wound 4 days later, after removal of the suction device. Healthy granulation tissue covers the wound. The size of the wound is significantly reduced.

quantities of air needed to keep the suction end open may increase the risk of infection and tissue irritation. Bacterial filters over the air inlets have been shown to effectively reduce infection rates.[2]

The application of a Heimlich valve provides an effective barrier to ascending infection in open drainage of body cavities. This device prevents inflow of air but facilitates drainage of fluid and debris (see Fig. 18-6).

Drainage of Body Spaces

Drains in Synovial Spaces

Removal of purulent debris from synovial spaces is facilitated by drain placement. Passive or active drainage systems can be employed for this purpose, but the passive Penrose drains are best. It is important that they be placed in the distal dependent aspect of the synovial space and maintained beneath a sterile bandage. Conversely, active drainage systems can be uncomfortable and abrasive to articular cartilage and tendons because of the rigidity of the material. However, Jackson-Pratt drains, made from Silastic, are multifenestrated and can be placed in these small spaces to provide efficient active drainage.[8]

Drains in Body Cavities

ABDOMEN

Passive drainage of the abdominal cavity requires dependent placement of a rigid-lumen drain tube.[7] PVC and Silastic drains can be used effectively for this purpose. (Penrose drains are not functional for this purpose, and should not be used.) Intraoperative placement of multifenestrated drains should be considered after abdominal lavage, or when large volumes of exudate or transudate are expected. The drain is placed in a dependent position away from the abdominal incision and sutured to the skin to prevent dislodgement. A sharp trocar with a threaded end is provided to place the drain (see Fig. 18-4). It is important to use the trocar to prepare the drain exit portal so that it is just large enough to allow drainage to occur through the drain lumen but not around it. An exit wound that is too large may allow eventration of omentum through it. Bandage placement over abdominal drains is impractical because of the drainage volume obtained. The drain should be removed as soon as drainage slows or ceases. Protecting the drain end is important to prevent ascending infection. A simple method to reduce this risk is to cut off the end of a latex condom, or a finger from a surgical glove, and to place it over the drain, where it acts as a one-way valve. Such valves are commercially available under the name of Heimlich valves (see Fig. 18-6).

Thoracic trocars made from PVC and Silastic can be placed percutaneously for drainage of air, urine, exudates, or lavage fluid from the abdominal cavity. Functional time may be limited by the number of fenestrations in the commercial products, so it is helpful to provide additional fenestrations. Squares holes in the drain may provide better drainage than round holes.[4] To place the drain, a dependent position is identified. If a longstanding peritonitis is present, or if there has been previous surgery, ultrasonographic guidance may be indicated to identify bowel adhered to the body wall. The site is prepared for aseptic surgery, and local anesthetic is infiltrated. A 1-cm incision is made through the skin and the external rectus sheath. An appropriate-diameter thoracic trocar is selected (16-30 Fr), and carefully inserted through the rectus abdominis muscle, internal rectus sheath, and peritoneum. When the abdominal cavity is penetrated, the obturator is removed, minimizing the risk of inadvertent bowel puncture. The drain is subsequently positioned properly and secured. Drains can be sutured to the skin in a variety of patterns. Two useful patterns are the "Chinese finger trap" suture and the "double clove hitch" pattern[9] (Fig. 18-9). If the drain is left in place, the drain end is protected as previously described, or a Heimlich valve may be added.

In cases that benefit from open peritoneal drainage, polypropylene mesh can be used to provide drainage over several days.[7] After correction of the primary problem, the mesh is secured into the abdominal closure with sutures, leaving a gap for fluids to escape. The mesh is left in place until drainage subsides, and it is removed during a second surgical procedure (Fig. 18-10).

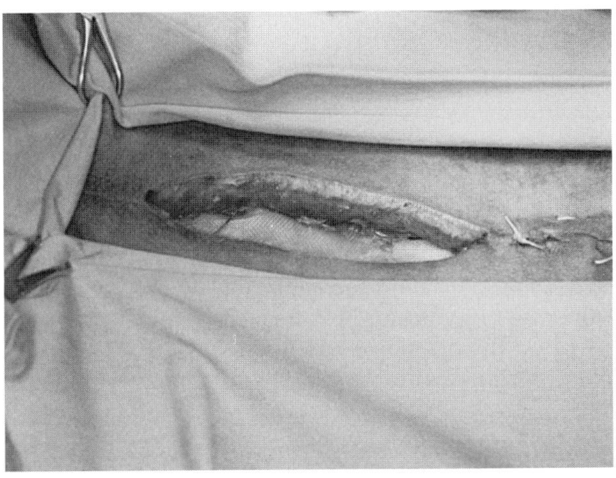

Figure 18-10. Polypropylene mesh used for open peritoneal drainage. The mesh, seen interposed between the wound edges, is ready for removal.

THORAX

Thoracic drainage presents special problems because negative pressure needs to be maintained in the chest despite the frequent presence of air. The use of a rigid drain tube is necessary. Removal of air can be achieved through active or passive mechanisms. To place a drain for removal of air, a dorsal site is selected and prepared for aseptic surgery. Local anesthetic is infiltrated prior to establishing a 1-cm stab incision through the skin. A thoracic trocar is inserted and tunneled cranially for one or two rib spaces and inserted into the thorax along the cranial edge of the rib, avoiding the intercostal vessels located on the caudal border of the rib (Fig. 18-11). Once the thorax has been penetrated, a Heimlich valve is placed on the drain end. The Heimlich valve has a rubber liner, which allows air to exit during expiration, and it collapses on inspiration, restricting backflow of air (see Fig. 18-6). If a large volume of air is present, suction can be applied to the open end of the Heimlich valve, rapidly removing air and reestablishing negative pressure. The drain is secured by one of the means previously described. If the primary problem is corrected, the drain can usually be removed in 24 hours.

Removal of fluid from the thorax is best achieved using an active drainage system. Multifenestrated PVC drains surgically placed, or thoracic trocars percutaneously placed, are suitable for this purpose. A closed suction device is applied to the catheter and maintained until drainage subsides. It is

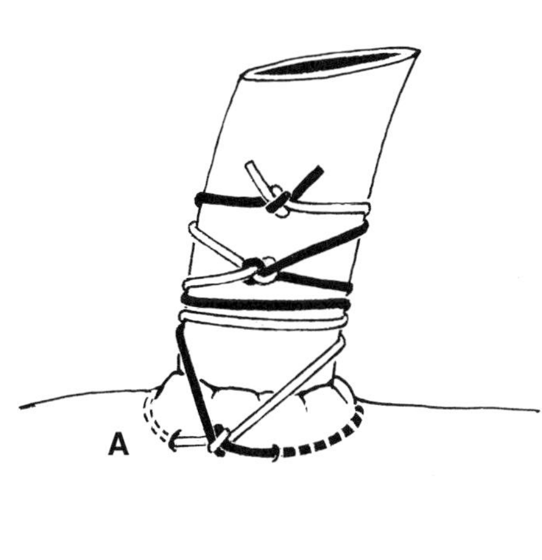

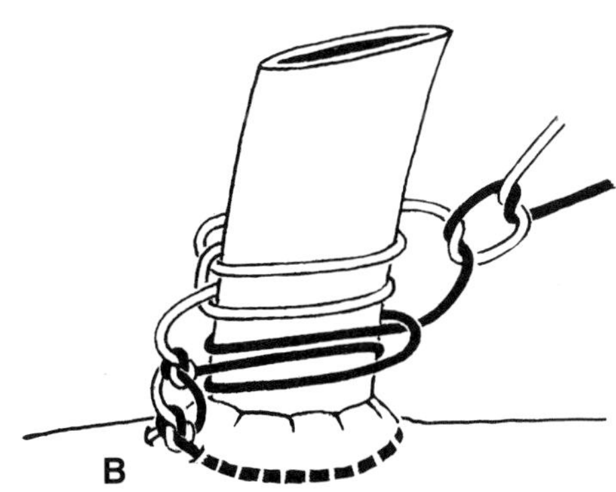

Figure 18-9. Suture patterns used to secure a drain to the body wall. **A,** The "Chinese finger trap" suture pattern. **B,** The "double clove hitch" pattern.

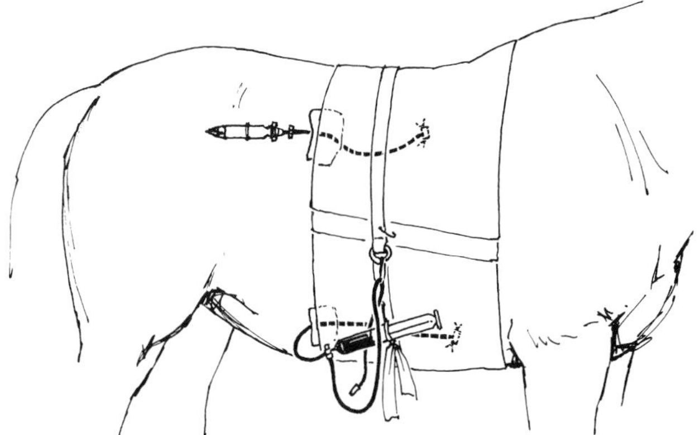

Figure 18-11. Proper placement of thoracic drains. A drain in the dorsal thorax is placed with a Heimlich valve (Heimlich chest drain valve, Bard Parker, Becton Dickinson, Inc, Lincoln Park, NJ) to prevent the backflow of air. A ventral drain uses a syringe-adapted closed-suction device to provide safe removal of fluid accumulating in the ventral thoracic cavity.

important that the closed suction device not become dislodged from the drain, as this would cause a rapid loss of negative pressure and introduce environmental contaminants into the thorax (see Fig. 18-11).

BANDAGES

Bandages are applied to cover wounds protected by dressings, to prevent edema formation after injuries of the limb, and to support the limb in conjunction with an added splint in the case of a fracture of a bone. The type of bandage is chosen on the basis of the location and the nature of the injury.

Foot Bandage

Foot bandages are applied to manage a variety of problems. Part of a roll of cotton is placed over a primary wound dressing (Fig. 18-12). The padding is secured with gauze, and it can be held in place with either cohesive or adhesive bandaging tape. Duct tape placed over the bottom of the bandage will render the bandage more durable and less permeable to urine and water (see Fig. 18-12). Moisture can be controlled from entering the bandage by placing plastic over the foot. An empty 5-L fluid-bag can be opened with a pair of scissors and placed over the hoof capsule and fastened with adhesive tape, attaching it effectively to the foot. This type of bandage is useful if it is desirable to exclude water from the wound environment, when a poultice or soak is applied to the foot, or when preparing a foot or pastern for any type of surgery.

Lower Limb Bandage

A lower limb bandage is applied from the bulbs of the heel up to just below the carpus or tarsus. It usually consists of a roll of cotton, applied in the standard clockwise fashion (pulling the tendons to the inside) (Fig. 18-13). The thickness, or number of layers, of the bandage is dictated by the underlying medical problem. Each layer is secured with conforming roll gauze, wrapped snugly in a spiral pattern, overlapping half the tape width, to prevent the padding from slipping or bunching. The gauze is overlaid with either adhesive or cohesive bandaging tape securing the bandage in position. A single wrap of adhesive tape around the bottom of the hoof and the top of the bandage prevents

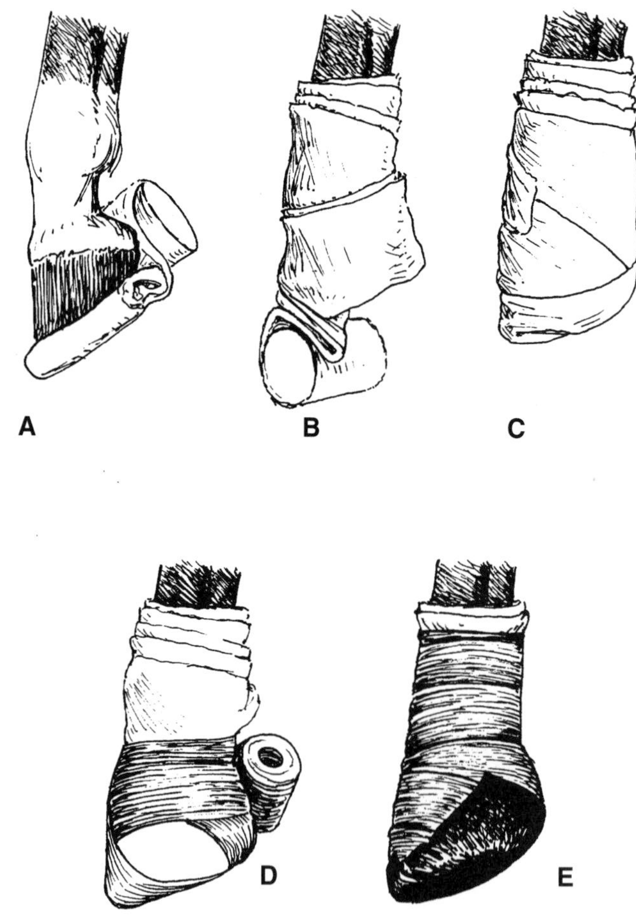

Figure 18-12. A, Several layers of folded-up cotton are placed over the sole of the foot. **B** and **C,** The roll of cotton is subsequently applied in several layers over the foot and fetlock area. **D,** A roll of elastic adhesive tape, tightly applied, finishes the bandage. **E,** Some protection may be applied to the sole to prevent wearing of the bandage. If deemed necessary, the bandage may also be covered with several layers of casting tape to further reduce motion in this region and to stabilize an injury of the bulbs of the heel.

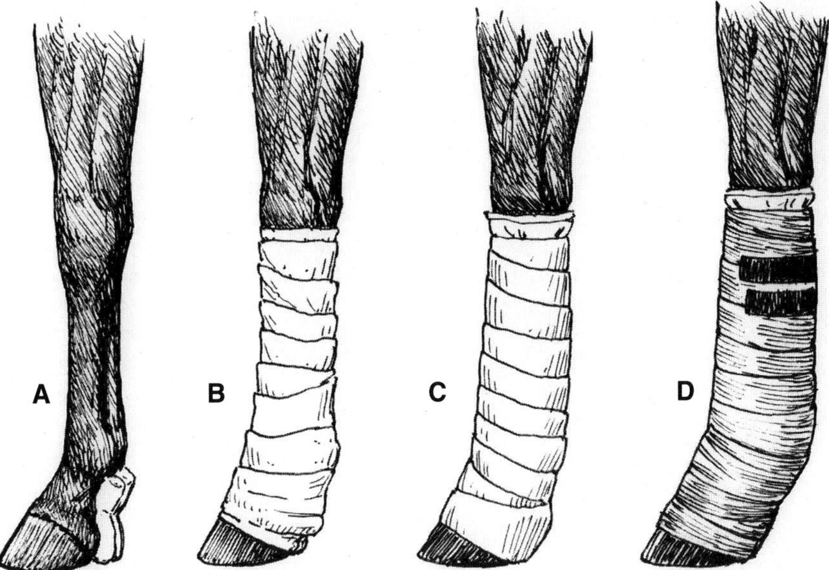

Figure 18-13. **A,** The heel area is first padded with some cotton. **B,** The first layer of the lower limb bandage is placed on the hind limb. **C,** After tightening it with gauze, a second layer is applied. **D,** The bandage is covered with elastic adhesive tape and secured with two pieces of duct tape. To finish the bandage, adhesive tape will be applied to its top and bottom to prevent bedding and dirt from gaining access to the wound (not shown).

bedding materials from gaining access to the underlying skin or wound respectively. Care should be taken to extend the bandage to the level of the carpometacarpal or tarsometatarsal joint, to prevent inadvertent tendon damage if a considerable amount of tension is applied to the elastic bandage tape. At the level of those joints, the tendons are lodged between the vestigial metacarpal bones, which provide protection. Additionally, the coronary band should be included in the bandage so that tape can be applied directly to the hoof capsule.

Full Limb Bandage—Forelimb

A full limb bandage is applied from the bulbs of the heel up to the elbow region (Fig. 18-14). When applying a full limb bandage, movement of the carpus requires that special

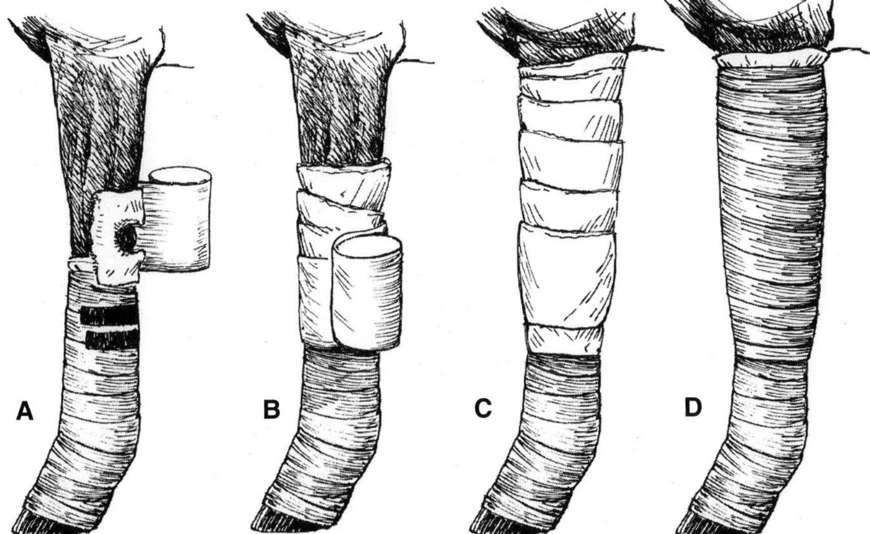

Figure 18-14. A full limb bandage applied to the hind limb. **A,** The distal part of the bandage (shown in Fig. 18-13) is first applied. Cotton arranged in a doughnut shape or a piece of felt with a central hole is placed over the accessory carpal bone before roll cotton is applied to the proximal aspect of the limb. **B,** The carpal area is covered with roll cotton in figure-eight fashion. **C,** The proximal limb is evenly covered with cotton layers, each separately tightened with heavy gauze. **D,** The bandage is covered with tightly applied elastic adhesive tape, and the top and bottom are sealed to prevent access of bedding and dirt.

attention be given to this area to prevent decubital ulcers. The bandage is usually "stacked" to prevent slippage and subsequent irritation over bony prominences. Padding materials are the same as for the lower limb bandage and therefore require placement in two stages. The distal bandage is initially applied as previously described. The proximal part is subsequently added on top of the lower limb bandage, overlapping it for 5 to 10 cm. Applying a doughnut-shaped cotton ring or incising the gauze over the accessory carpal bone helps prevent skin irritation over that area and potential development of skin ulcers. Tightening of the bandage in layers provides more stability and increases the support. If the bandage becomes displaced distally, it is imperative that it be changed at once to prevent skin ulcers from developing over bony prominences.

Full Limb Bandage—Hindlimb

Motion of the tarsus requires special attention when applying a bandage to that region. Primary wound dressings are held in place using gauze applied in a figure-eight (Fig. 18-15). The crossing of the "8" occurs over the dorsal aspect of the tarsus, with the loops applied around the proximal metatarsus and the distal tibia of the limb, leaving the point of the hock open. Caution should be used in applying tension over the gastrocnemius tendon. The bandage is also applied in two steps, as described for the forelimb. The proximal part of the bandage overlaps the distal bandage. Applying soft cotton patches medially and laterally between the tibia and the gastrocnemius tendon provides support and reduces the pressure of the latter, thereby serving as protection against tendon damage that could result from excessive tension. Each layer of padding material is first secured with gauze, applied at a right angle to the limb, as opposed to the figure-eight for the primary dressing. Application of cohesive or adhesive tape completes the bandage (see Fig. 18-15). The bandage is finished by applying elastic adhesive tape around the hoof capsule below, and to the skin on top of the proximal end of the bandage to prevent access of bedding to the skin underneath the bandage.

The application of a full limb bandage to the hind limb decreases the movement of all joints in the limb because of the reciprocal apparatus. Some horses have more problems coping with this situation, especially when gaining or rising from recumbency. Therefore, the patient will need to be observed after such a bandage is applied.

Splints

A special type of full limb bandage is the Robert Jones dressing (RJD), for which several layers of cotton are evenly applied over the entire limb, each layer tightened separately with elastic nonadhesive tape. The final cover of the RJD consists of a layer of tightly applied elastic adhesive tape. The size of the RJD should be approximately double the size of the limb and produce a dampened "ping" when snapped with the finger on the outside. This type of bandage provides good support to a severely injured or fractured extremity, because it adds rigidity, especially if a splint of some kind is incorporated into the bandage. An RJD with an incorporated splint allows weight bearing on a fractured limb.

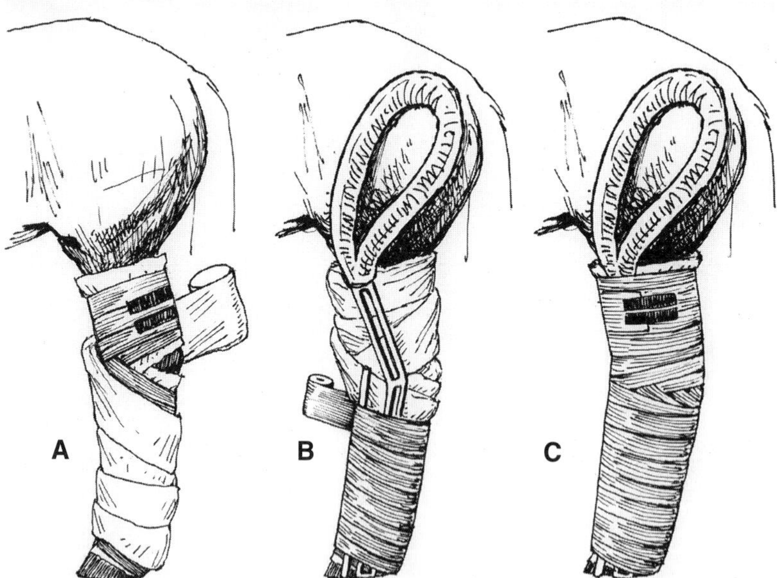

Figure 18-15. A Robert Jones bandage with a lateral splint applied to immobilize a distal tibial fracture prior to surgery. **A,** First, a multilayered full limb bandage is applied to the limb using a technique similar to that described in Figure 18-14. The tarsus is covered with a figure-eight bandage. **B,** The proximally padded commercial metallic splint is applied to the lateral aspect of the limb and attached to the bandage with broad nonelastic tape. **C,** The bandage is tightly applied up to the stifle. The padded loop in the hip area provides counter-pressure and resists the development of a valgus deformity during weight bearing. It is prudent to surgically prepare the skin and use a sterile dressing in the first layer in the event the fracture becomes open after the bandage is applied or during the transport.

Splints must be applied carefully to prevent decubitus ulcers. Splints are commonly made from wood, PVC pipe, or metal, or they can be assembled from cast material incorporated into the bandage. Wood splints are not ideal because they lack strength in small conforming widths, and larger boards do not conform well to the limb. This limitation is overcome by incorporating several small-width slats into the bandage. The sum of the slats used increases the bandage rigidity and achieves the desired result. With adequate padding in place, 1×4-inch (2.5×10-cm) boards can be incorporated into a bandage and arranged in at least two right-angle planes. Board splints should extend from the hoof to the joint proximal to the affected area in at least one plane. If the radius or tibia is to be immobilized, a padded lateral splint extending beyond the top of the bandage should be incorporated to prevent adduction of the limb (see Fig. 18-15).

Excellent rigidity can be achieved by using PVC pipe as splints. The diameter of the schedule 40 PVC pipe selected depends on the size and location of the limb to which it is applied. The material should be cut longitudinally in two or three sections. The splint may be modified by removing half-moon–shaped portions at strategic locations to allow access to regions with a wider diameter, such as the carpus. A good compromise has to be found between the PVC pipe diameter and the diameter of the widest part of the limb to be incorporated into the splint.

Neither PVC pipe nor wood conforms well to the limb, however. Casting tape, on the other hand, conforms well to the bandaged limb, but it does not provide the bandage rigidity that can be achieved with wood or PVC pipe. Splints may be made from casting tape rolls, or purchased in that configuration as a *longuette*. Addition of a casting tape splint reduces the amount of padding needed while providing suitable immobilization in most circumstances. Casting tape splints cannot be applied to extend to the shoulder or hip to prevent adduction of the limb for immobilization of the antebrachium or crus, respectively.

Stainless steel splints are commercially available for temporary immobilization of the distal limb, including the metacarpus in the forelimb. These splints are used as emergency fixation for breakdown injuries of the suspensory apparatus, for flexor tendon injuries, for fractures of the metacarpal condyle, and for phalangeal fractures when a strut of bone remains to support the limb. They are especially useful for transport of horses with such injuries (see Chapter 78).

EXTERNAL COAPTATION (CASTS)

Cast Application

Materials

Historically, plaster of Paris casts have been popular for external coaptation. Plaster is still a viable casting material, because it is easy to apply, has good molding capability, and is inexpensive. Unfortunately, plaster casts also are heavy, disintegrate when wet, and do not allow exchange of air, which makes this type of cast uncomfortable when worn for a prolonged period.[15] Furthermore, plaster is not as strong as fiberglass and thus requires more material to prevent breakage. This results in a heavier cast.

The shortcomings of early fiberglass casts were corrected and they are now made with materials of superior quality; they are lightweight, strong, and radiolucent, and they have excellent molding capability. Additionally, the porosity of the material allows exchange of air across the cast. Although these types of casts are more expensive than plaster casts, they are more durable and require less material for adequate strength. A variety of fiberglass casting materials are presently available on the market. Twenty years ago, the mechanical properties of several of these materials were compared, and differences were seen.[16] However, since then major improvements in handling ability and strength were implemented. For practical purposes today, there are no significant differences between the products on the market.

The strength of a cast is determined mainly through bonding between the tape layers, so swift cast application is of great importance for a strong cast. Fiberglass casts are about 20 times stronger and 4 times lighter than plaster casts. All cast materials exhibit an exothermic reaction (i.e., they release heat) during setting; the more layers applied, the greater the reaction. Immersion in water hotter than 27° C (80.6° F) immediately before application also results in heat production. However, warm water reduces the curing time considerably. Therefore, veterinarians inexperienced in the application of casts should use cool water, which permits a longer application time but ensures that all tape layers will bond together as the cast hardens. Unlike in the procedure for application of plaster casts, water should not be expressed from the fiberglass material before application, because the cooling effect of the water is lost. Also, freshly applied casts should not be covered with bandage materials before they have set. The casts usually set within 4 to 5 minutes and allow weight bearing within 20 to 30 minutes.

Indications

External coaptation by casting is indicated in selected fractures of the phalanges, as adjunct treatment to internal fixation of fractures, for immobilization after tendon repair, and to stabilize wound healing in regions of continuous motion, such as heel lacerations (see Chapter 93). Casts are also applied to protect a limb during recovery from anesthesia—for example, after repair of a condylar fracture of the distal MCIII/MTIII. Tube casts may be applied to foals with incomplete ossification of the cuboidal carpal and tarsal bones to facilitate ossification while weight is distributed evenly across the joints (see Chapter 89).

Technique

Most casts are applied with the horse under general anesthesia. This prevents the animal from moving during the application and setting of the cast, which may weaken the cast or cause pressure points, with subsequent development of decubitus ulcers. However, with adequate sedation, casts can also be successfully applied in standing horses.

Before starting, all materials should be laid out for efficient and swift cast application. The entire portion of the limb to be covered with a cast should be cleaned and dried. It is not advisable to clip the hair unless that is required for a surgical procedure. Special attention should be given to the hoof. It should be trimmed and all excessive sole and frog material removed. It is advisable to paint the sole and frog with a solution containing iodine. Any lacerations or wounds should be débrided, sutured if necessary, and covered with a sterile nonadhering dressing. This dressing should be secured by a gauze or elastic bandage. It is advisable to apply boric acid to the portion of the limb that will be covered with a cast. Boric acid is a drying agent with antibacterial properties. A zinc-containing soft gauze is an alternative, providing protective properties to the skin. A piece of stockinette somewhat longer than twice the proposed length of the cast is prepared by rolling it from each end toward its center. One side is rolled outward and the other side inward (Fig. 18-16). For foals, a 5.0-cm (2-inch)-diameter stockinette should be selected. A 7.5- or 10.0-cm (3- to 4-inch) stockinette is adequate for adult horses. The stockinette should be neither too loose nor too light.

The stockinette is applied to the limb by an outward unrolling of the previously rolled portion (see Fig. 18-16). Once the first layer of stockinette is applied, it should be pulled distally for about 2 cm (¾ inch) to ensure normal alignment of the hair on the limb. The other half of the stockinette is then twisted at the sole region and unrolled like the first half. At this stage, the stockinette should extend about 5 to 10 cm (2 to 4 inches) past the proximal end of the cast. Generally, a ring of orthopedic felt, about 7 cm (3 inches) wide, is applied to the most proximal aspect of the cast between the two layers of the stockinette (see Fig. 18-16). This ring of felt should not be overlapped but should be adjusted to the correct length to perfectly appose both ends. The ends are held in place temporarily by nonelastic adhesive tape.

For plaster casts, a cotton stockinette usually is used, whereas synthetic stockinettes are preferred for fiberglass casts. Because synthetic stockinette is manufactured from acrylic fiber that has little capacity to hold moisture, moisture is transferred away from the body. Also, synthetic stockinette maintains greater bulk, adding to the padding. Some clinicians prefer to add a thin layer of synthetic cast padding between the two layers of stockinette. Additional attention should be given to potential pressure points, such as over the accessory carpal bone, ergot, or calcaneus regions. Extra padding, consisting of a silicone doughnut or orthopedic felt with an elliptic hole, should be applied to these areas. After the stockinette and padding have been applied, the limb should be positioned for application of the cast. In most cases, the limb should be extended with the metacarpal and phalangeal regions in the same frontal plane. In special cases, it may be preferable to cast the limb in a normal weight-bearing position. For this purpose, the carpus is flexed and slight pressure is applied either to the dorsum at the fetlock region or to the sole in a dorsal direction (Fig. 18-17). An assistant must hold the limb in the desired position. The palm of the hand, not the fingertips, should be used to apply pressure to a specific region and thereby help prevent pressure point development.

The polyurethane, resin-impregnated foam introduced in the early 1990s[17] is an efficient means to reduce cast sores. This material is immersed in warm water for about 1 minute. After minimal squeezing, the soft foam is applied evenly over the stockinette. Care is taken to overlap each turn-half of the width, with the result that a double layer of foam is applied over the part of the limb being covered with a cast. Minimal tension is applied. Wearing gloves during application of the foam is strongly encouraged.

To facilitate cast removal under practice conditions, a Gigli wire attached to a long felt strip (Fig. 18-18, *A*) may be placed medially and laterally over the padded limb[18] (see Fig. 18-18, *B*). The wire should be long enough that some excess wire protrudes proximally and distally. Once the cast is finished, the excess wire is rolled up and placed underneath the elastic tape applied to this region (see Fig. 18-18, *C*).

Latex gloves must be worn for application of a fiberglass cast. The airtight packages of the fiberglass tape are opened immediately before application. The fiberglass tape is held with both hands, separating the free end from the rest of the material, before submerging it in the water.[19] The fiberglass tape is held in water at about 21° to 27° C (70° to 80° F) for 5 seconds. During this time, the tape is squeezed four or five times to encourage complete penetration by water. The fiberglass tape is removed from the water dripping wet and immediately applied to the limb. Cast application is started at the foot and progresses in a proximal direction, overlapping at least half the width of the roll until the most proximal aspect is reached. After applying two layers at the

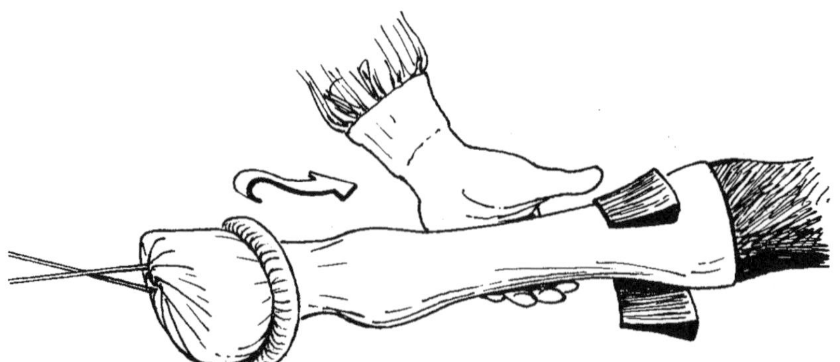

Figure 18-16. The limb is placed in traction and the inner layer of stockinette is rolled up along the limb. The outer layer of stockinette, which was initially rolled up in an inward direction, is twisted axially 360 degrees at the bottom of the foot and rolled up along the limb as well. At the proximal aspect of the cast, a wedge-shaped piece of thick felt is fitted to the limb, secured with tape, and covered with the outer layer of stockinette.

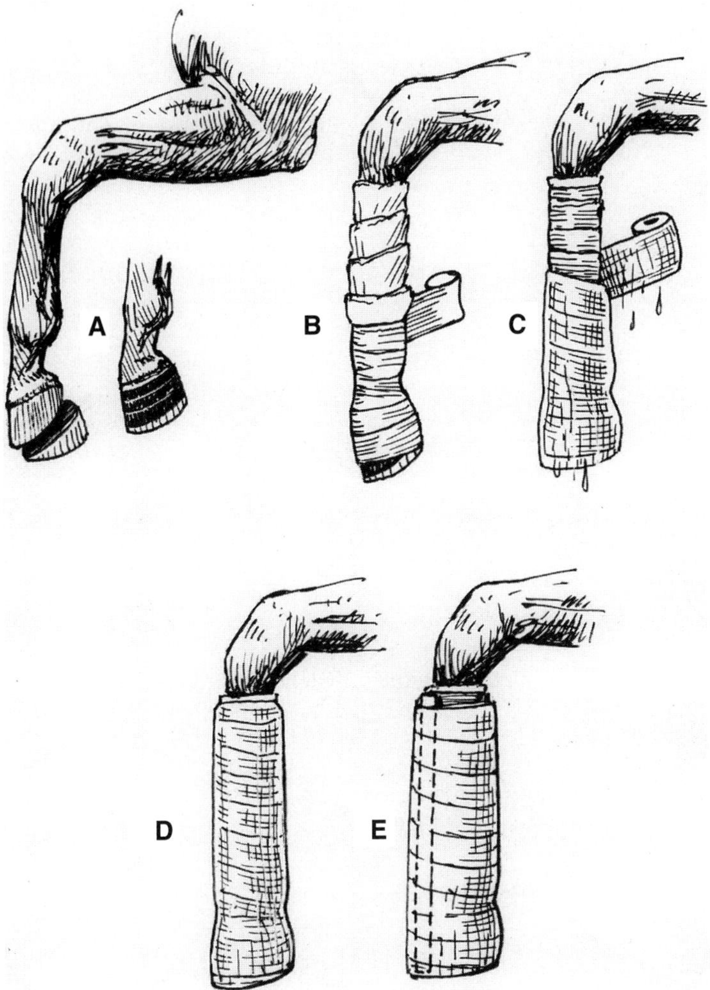

Figure 18-17. A short limb cast applied to the forelimb. The phalanges and MCIII are aligned in the same plane. **A,** A wooden wedge is applied to the foot with adhesive tape. **B** to **D,** The cast material is evenly applied over the synthetic foam in several layers. **E,** If deemed necessary, a straight dorsal splint may be incorporated into the cast.

top, the cast material is directed distally and applied evenly over the limb. As a rule, the cast bandages are applied in progression by continuing with the next bandage where the previous one ended. Changing direction during cast application is done by folding the cast material at one place and smoothing out the fold with the flattened hand. The newer materials adapt so well that in most cases directional changes can be carried out without folding the material over. Care should be taken to follow the contours of the limb and not to apply too much tension to the tape, which could interfere with circulation.

After the first few layers of cast material are applied, the extra stockinette extending on top of the cast is folded distally and covered by the following layers (see Fig. 18-17). Fiberglass cast material is applied until the cast reaches a thickness of 7 to 8 mm (¼ to ½ inch) throughout the total length of the cast. This requires four to six rolls of 12.7-cm (5-inch) fiberglass casting tape for a half-length cast and 10 to 12 rolls for a full-length cast.

If deemed necessary, a straight splint in the shape of an old hoof rasp or any similar type of material may be incorporated into the cast on its dorsal aspect (see Fig. 18-17). This splint should be covered with cast material to prevent accidental trauma to another limb. Such a splint would reduce the amount of cast material needed for a weight-bearing cast.

Once sufficient cast material is applied, the cast is molded over its total length and the surface smoothed out. It is important not to flex the joints under the cast from the time cast application begins until the cast has set. Most casts harden within 5 to 7 minutes after the final roll is applied.

If the limb is cast in an extended position, a wedge should be incorporated in the cast under the heel (see Fig. 18-17). The wedge permits weight to be applied over a greater surface than just at the toe. It is advisable to protect the sole with a layer of hoof acrylic, a piece of old inner tube, or the bottom of a gallon plastic bottle, taped to the foot with nonelastic tape.

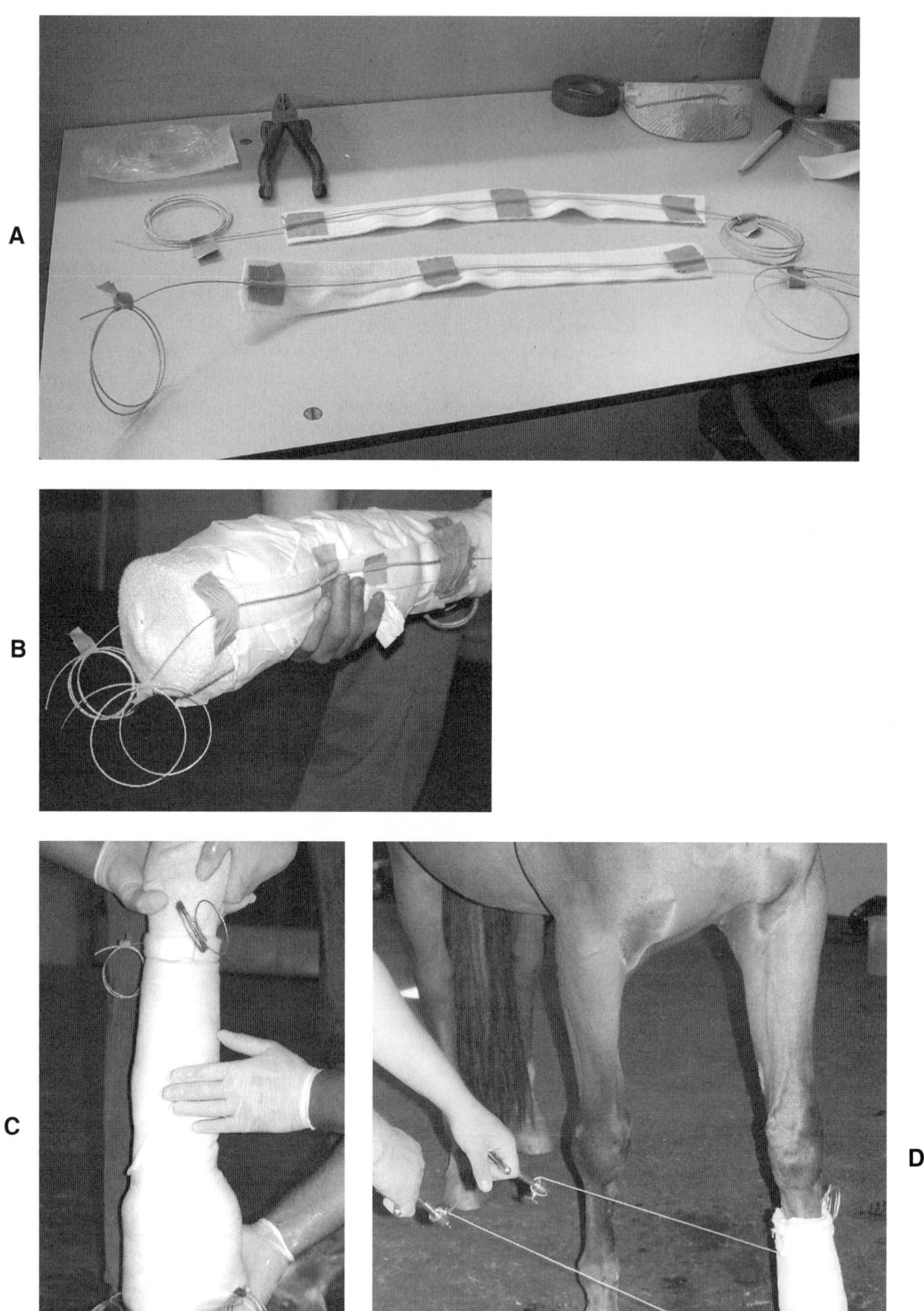

Figure 18-18. A, Two pieces of Gigli wire are attached to felt strips. The two ends are rolled up. **B,** The felt strips with the wire are applied medially and laterally to the padded limb. **C,** The cast is applied in routine fashion. The rolled-up ends of the wire are covered with tape at the end of cast application. **D,** At the time of cast removal, the ends of the wire are attached to the handles, and by slow sawing movements, the medial and lateral sides of the cast are severed apart. Finally, the two shells still connected at the sole are split dorsally and palmarly, allowing the limb to be removed from the cast. (Photos courtesy C. Lischer, Zurich.)

To prevent foreign material, such as wood shavings or straw, from entering at the top of the cast and causing irritation, a collar of adhesive elastic tape should be placed around the top of the cast and continued about 6 cm (2¼ inches) proximally up the limb.

Casts applied with the limb in extension result in a longer limb than the ipsilateral counterpart. Therefore, the cast limb is usually held in an extended or non–weight-bearing position. This may lead to continuous overload of the good limb, which increases the risk of foundering. It is advisable to tape a rubber pad to the ipsilateral foot and in so doing to lengthen it as well, preferably to the same extent as the cast limb. This comforts the patient and facilitates even weight bearing.

Generally, hindlimb casts are applied in the same way as casts for the forelimb. The most likely areas for pressure sore development are the Achilles tendon and the dorsal aspect of the tarsus. The tarsal region presents an additional problem in a full-leg hind limb cast because of the reciprocal apparatus. Attempts of the horse to flex the hind limb in a full limb cast may cause the peroneus tertius tendon to avulse from its attachment or rupture in the tarsal region, allowing flexion of the stifle without flexion of the tarsus. Treatment of this problem is discussed in Chapter 99.

Exercise should be limited for a horse with a cast. It is preferable to keep the horse in a cool environment to prevent excessive sweating under the cast. In this respect, fiberglass casts are superior to plaster casts because fiberglass casts are porous and dissipate heat from the body.

It is advisable to palpate the cast every day, especially over possible pressure points. A localized area of increased heat, palpable through the cast, is an early sign of a developing skin ulcer. Sudden decreased use of the limb under a cast or increased lameness of the affected limb are signs of irritation under the cast. Another sign of such a problem is cast abuse through chewing, stomping, or rubbing. Swelling above the cast usually signifies a far more serious problem under the cast. Should any of these signs be noted, the cast should be changed or removed to alleviate the problem. Repairing a cast or making adjustments is not very often successful and is therefore not recommended.

Cast Removal

Removal of the cast with the horse under general anesthesia is usually uneventful. Removal of the cast while the horse is standing may be more complicated. In most cases, some degree of chemical or physical restraint is necessary to permit safe removal of the cast. If Gigli wires were incorporated into the cast, the ends can be freed up, connected to their handles, and with slow sawing motions the cast can be split in half (see Fig. 18-18, *D*). If cast cutters are used, the cast should be grooved medially and laterally along its entire length to ensure the correct location of the cut. Then, the proximal aspect of the cast is cut completely through, down to the foam or orthopedic felt. This allows assessment of the thickness of the cast and gives the person removing the cast an indication of how deep to cut. Using excessive force may result in perforation of the underlying skin. Once the proximal area of the cast is cut through, the rest of the cast should be cut by maintaining the blade at the same location until the cast is cut through completely before moving distally. Dragging the cast cutter parallel to the limb will promote skin lacerations. After the entire thickness of the cast has been cut through, the two portions of the cast tend to separate somewhat.

The cast covering the foot should be split carefully, because the density of the hoof is similar to that of the cast, and it is often difficult to differentiate between them, resulting in inadvertent penetration of the hoof wall by the saw blade. Although a standing horse may object to such treatment, there will be no reaction to this in the anesthetized animal.

Once the cast is split into two half shells, a cast spreader is applied to widen the gap and allow transection of the cast padding with scissors. The cast is removed and the limb washed thoroughly. If radiographs are made after cast removal, it is advisable not to wash the limb with soap containing iodine. After cast removal, the limb should be covered with a pressure bandage for some time to allow gradual relief of external pressure. Any sores that developed under the cast should be treated immediately using routine wound management.

In selected cases, a bivalve cast is applied to the limb. This can be carried out on the standing and sedated horse or with the horse under general anesthesia. In either case, the padding of the cast is made somewhat thicker and usually consists of a thin bandage, which can later be changed at regular intervals. The cast is subsequently applied using routine technique. It is advisable to let it set for about a day before splitting it into two half-shells. After the bandage is changed, the two shells are reapplied and maintained in apposition by tightly wrapping the two half-shells with nonadhesive tape.

Complications

Cast complications may develop from an overly tight application, resulting in dermal pressure necrosis (that will damage deeper structures if undetected) or in an overly loose application. If the cast is too loose, the limb can shift in the cast, which may result in the development of skin pressure in areas not anticipated. Cast loosening may result from a decrease in the limb swelling, from muscle atrophy, or from compacting of cast padding materials. Application of too-short a half-cast may result in severe tendon injury, because the limb may be partially flexed, causing the top end of the cast to apply a considerable amount of linear pressure on the unprotected tendons. In a properly applied cast, the tendons are protected by the proximal ends of the vestigial metacarpal or metatarsal bones. Wear on the bottom of the cast will also cause the limb to shift within the cast, resulting in serious dermal pressure necrosis.

REFERENCES

1. Arighi M: Drains, dressings, and external coaptation devices. In Auer JA, editor: Equine Surgery, Philadelphia, 1999, WB Saunders.
2. Donner GS, Ellison GW: The use and misuse of abdominal drains in small animals, Comp Cont Educ Pract Vet 1986;8:705.
3. Presnell KR: Drains, dressings and other surgical materials. In Slatter DH, editor: Textbook of Small Animal Surgery, vol 1, Philadelphia, 1985, WB Saunders.
4. Lee AH, Swaim SF, Henderson RA: Surgical drainage, Comp Cont Educ Pract Vet 1986;8:94.

5. Robinson OJ: Surgical drainage: A historical perspective. Br J Surg 1986;73:422.
6. Miller CW: Bandages and drains. In Slatter DH, editor: Textbook of Small Animal Surgery, ed 3, Philadelphia, 2003, WB Saunders.
7. Hampel HL, Johnson RG: Principles of surgical drains and drainage, J Am Anim Hosp Assoc 1985;21:21.
8. Ross MW, Orsini JA, Richardson DW, Martin BB: Closed suction drainage in the treatment of infectious arthritis of the equine tarsocrural joint, Vet Surg 1991;20:21.
9. Chase JP, Beard WL, Bertone AL, et al: Open perineal drainage in horses with experimentally induced peritonitis, Vet Surg 1996; 25:189.
10. Dorland's Illustrated Medical Dictionary, ed 30, Philadelphia, 2003, WB Saunders.
11. Day TG: Drainage in gynecological surgery, Clin Obstet Gynecol 1988;31:744.
12. Diehl M, Ersek RA: Porcine xenografts for treatment of skin defects in horses, J Am Vet Med Assoc 1980;177:625.
13. Hackett RP: Management of traumatic wounds, Proc Am Assoc Equine Pract 1978;24:363.
14. Baxter GM: Retrospective study of lower limb wounds involving tendons, tendon sheaths, or joints in horses, Proc Am Assoc Equine Pract 1987;33:715.
15. Stone WC: Drains, dressings, and external coaptation. In Auer JA, Stick JA, editors: Equine Surgery, ed 2, Philadelphia, 1999, WB Saunders.
16. Bramlage LR: Current concepts of emergency first aid treatment and transportation of equine fracture patients, Comp Cont Educ Pract Vet 1983;5:S564.
17. Wilson DG, Vanderby R: An evaluation of fiberglass cast application techniques, Vet Surg 1995;24:118.
18. Bramlage LR, Embertson RM, Libbey CJ: Resin impregnated foam as a cast liner on the equine limb, Proc Am Assoc Equine Pract 1991;37:481.
19. Murray RC, DeBowes RM: Casting techniques. In Nixon AJ, editor: Equine Fracture Repair, Philadelphia, 1995, WB Saunders.

SECTION III RECENT ADVANCES IN ANESTHESIA

Jörg A. Auer

CHAPTER 19

Advances in Inhalation Anesthesia

Alexander Valverde

Inhalation anesthesia is a versatile technique that facilitates many different types of surgical and diagnostic procedures in the equine patient, ranging from short to long, from elective to emergency, and from routine to complicated.

Halothane and methoxyflurane were introduced into clinical anesthetic practice in the early 1960s and their use became widespread in veterinary medicine. Methoxyflurane is no longer available because of the advent of novel inhalation anesthetics such as isoflurane (in the late 1970s) and more recently, sevoflurane and desflurane (in the 1990s). Halothane is also slowly disappearing from daily use in North America, although it continues to be widely used in Europe.

Novel drugs should provide significant advantages over previously used drugs if they are to replace them. Advantages of novel inhalation anesthetics should include less morbidity and mortality, better and more rapid control of anesthetic depth, less cardiorespiratory depression, and less biotransformation.

ANESTHETIC RISK

"A chance to cut is a chance to kill."
G. Mark Johnson[1]

Complications arising from general anesthesia are common. Not all recognized complications reflect an immediate danger to the patient; however, identifying their significance and addressing them promptly may reduce their impact. Because most surgery is performed under general anesthesia, deaths during that time have been coined "anesthetic deaths." Some deaths can be considered as inevitable—for example, after rupture of major vessels. In addition, cardiac arrest can be a nonanesthetic event related to direct surgical complications, or it could be part of an anaphylactic reaction. Thus, not all causes of death are directly related to anesthesia. The most common causes of cardiac arrest associated with anesthesia include hypoxia because of ventilatory problems, drug overdose, and perioperative hypotension.

The anesthetic death rate in humans has decreased from 1 death per 2700 anesthesias in the 1950s,[2] to 1 in 4761 in the 1970s, and to 1 in 10,000 in the 1980s.[3] Anesthetic deaths have decreased over the years probably as a result of safer anesthetic drugs, better techniques, and more sophisticated monitoring and support equipment that allow early detection of problems and intervention. On the other hand, for these same reasons, it is now common to perform surgery or diagnostic procedures on critically ill patients, which contribute to the overall mortality rate despite recent anesthetic advances.

Equine studies have reported a death rate of 1 per 1250 anesthesias for elective procedures when only anesthetic causes are considered. Mortality increases to 1 in 158 cases when anesthetic and surgical causes, such as bleeding in the immediate postoperative period, fractured limbs during recovery, and shock, are included.[4] If the entire hospitalization period from the time of anesthesia until the final outcome of the case is taken into account, then the overall death rate may be as high as 1 in 28.[4]

Emergency cases had a higher overall death rate of 1 in 3.2 cases (1 in 2.8 for colic and 1 in 6.5 for noncolic cases) than elective cases when the entire hospitalization period is taken into account.[5] Surgical and/or anesthetic deaths represented 1 in 23 cases in the colic group and 1 in 50 cases in the noncolic group if only the immediate postoperative period is considered.[5] From these two studies,[4,5] risk of death is 4.25 times more likely for emergency procedures not associated with colic than for similar procedures carried out electively. Emergency general anesthesia for colic carries an increased risk of death 9.86 times that of elective cases.[5] These numbers are worrisome, but they include death by euthanasia, and that decision is influenced by many factors, including financial and prognosis for athletic future.

Morbidity and mortality studies are necessary to determine if one anesthetic drug or technique can positively influence outcome. However, these studies are difficult to design and execute because of the multiple factors involved. In an effort to identify drugs and techniques that may be linked to anesthetic death in horses, a confidential enquiry into perioperative equine fatalities (CEPEF) analyzed data from over 40,000 anesthetic records.[6]

Findings from the CEPEF study identified an increased risk of death associated with techniques that involved an inhalation anesthetic only as part of the induction technique, a common practice in neonatal foals.[6] Tachypnea and release of catecholamines have been suggested as possible causes that predispose to anesthetic overdose in foals, as well as increased overall requirement for the inhalation anesthetic because premedicant and induction agents are not used.[6] Age was also linked to anesthetic death rate, which was highest in the very young, followed by the older horse, and lowest in young adults.[6]

Maintenance of anesthesia with inhalation anesthetics carried a threefold higher risk of death than injectable anesthetics.[6] Improved outcome with injectable anesthetics may reflect their use for shorter anesthetic procedures, as risk of death also increases with duration of anesthesia and surgery time, a situation in which injectable techniques are less likely to be used.[6,7] In addition, intravenous anesthetics cause less cardiovascular depression than inhalation anesthetics.[8] Most of the anesthetic deaths were related to cardiac arrest (33%),[6] which explains the association between inhalation anesthetics and mortality. Of all anesthetic drugs and protocols used in over 35,400 cases, inhalation anesthetics were used as the maintenance agent in 87%, and injectables or no additional anesthetic were used for the remaining 13%.[6] Despite the higher risk involved with inhalation anesthetics, the ease of administration with appropriate equipment and the ability to alter anesthetic depth makes them the most common method of maintaining anesthesia in equine patients at this time.

In the study by Johnston and colleagues,[6] most of the horses under inhalation anesthesia received halothane (98%) versus isoflurane (2%), and it is unclear whether overall mortality from inhalation anesthetics can be generalized to both drugs. The death rate for halothane was 1 death per 101 cases and 1 in 78 cases for isoflurane, whereas for injectable agents it was 1 in 321 cases.[6]

In a randomized prospective study that included elective and emergency cases from several equine clinics around the world, and with approximately 4100 horses receiving halothane and a similar number isoflurane, comparisons of mortality were similar; 1.7% versus 1.6%, respectively.[9] The only difference between the two inhalants was demonstrated in horses 2 to 5 years of age, where the use of isoflurane reduced the death rate fivefold.[9] The main causes of death in this study were cardiac arrest (32%) and fractures (23%).[9] Isoflurane use was associated with less risk of cardiac-related mortality than halothane (30% versus 70% of cardiac deaths, respectively).[9] Fractures may be related to poor perfusion to muscle groups secondary to cardiovascular depression and the subsequent myopathy that manifests in the recovery period. However, there were no significant differences between isoflurane and halothane in respect to myopathy.[9] Duration of anesthesia (over 90 minutes) and lateral recumbency were the two factors that carried an increased risk of myopathy in this study.[9] Despite the lack of evidence for advantages of isoflurane over halothane, it is generally agreed that isoflurane and novel inhalant anesthetics (sevoflurane and desflurane) depress myocardial function and cardiac output less than halothane[10-15] and should be selected in more critical cases when perfusion and oxygenation may be impaired.

ANESTHETIC DEPTH

The novel inhalation anesthetics such as isoflurane, sevoflurane, and desflurane are less potent and less soluble than older agents such as halothane (Table 19-1). Potency is indicated by the minimum alveolar concentration (MAC), defined as the alveolar concentration of inhalation anesthetic that prevents movement in 50% of subjects in response to a noxious stimulus. Thus, the MAC of novel drugs is higher than that of the older drugs.

TABLE 19-1. Minimum Alveolar Concentration (MAC) and Blood/Gas Partition Coefficient Values of Inhalant Anesthetics in the Horse

		Blood/Gas*	
	MAC (%)	Humans	Horse[35]
Halothane	0.82-0.95[36-39]	2.4	1.66
Isoflurane	1.31[39]	1.4	0.92
Sevoflurane	2.31[40]	0.6	0.47
Desflurane	7.6[41]	0.42	ND

*These values are significantly lower in horses than for people.

The low lipid solubility (expressed as the blood/gas partition coefficient) of novel anesthetics is responsible for their lower potency because a higher concentration is required to achieve equilibrium between the two compartments (blood and alveoli) (see Table 19-1). The concentration of anesthetic in the alveoli is a reflection of the brain concentration for that particular drug. By controlling the concentration in the alveoli, with minimal impact from the lipid solubility of the drug in other tissues, changes in anesthetic plane can be achieved more readily and result in faster onset or disappearance of clinical effects.

In horses, a faster recovery is advantageous only if the animal has fully regained mental and motor function. The unique behavior of the horse compels it to assume a standing position early in the recovery period, and premature attempts to stand may result in a stormy recovery and major injuries. In the recovery period, horses attempt to move and change body position even when end-tidal anesthetic concentrations sufficient for clinical planes of anesthesia are still measurable.[16] The administration of sedative drugs, including alpha-2 agonists, during this time has been advocated to prevent early movement attempts and improve the quality of recovery.[17]

Duration of anesthesia also influences the quality of recovery. Isoflurane results in faster, but often less controlled, recoveries than halothane in horses anesthetized for periods of less than 2 hours.[11,13,18] In horses anesthetized for periods of 3 hours or longer, the recoveries were better with isoflurane, as horses appeared more alert and less ataxic than after halothane.[16] The solubility of halothane may account for more accumulation after a prolonged anesthetic delivery. In contrast, horses recovering from 1 hour of halothane anesthesia tended to have more ideal recoveries than horses recovering from 3 hours of halothane or isoflurane anesthesia.[16]

Sevoflurane results in more controlled recoveries than isoflurane, although no differences in times to standing were demonstrated between the two drugs. The better recoveries after sevoflurane may be the result of its lower solubility.[11] In foals less than 3 months of age, no differences were detected in the induction or recovery times and quality scores between sevoflurane and isoflurane; however, these foals were assisted during recovery.[13]

CARDIORESPIRATORY EFFECTS

In general, cardiovascular depression from inhalant anesthetics is dose dependent. Normally expressed as MAC multiples for the specific inhalant, the higher the MAC multiple delivered to the patient, the more pronounced was the cardiovascular depression. Using MAC multiples allows comparison of different inhalant anesthetics, based on the principle that there is equipotency between them at the same MAC level.

The cardiovascular effects of inhalant anesthetics can be divided into those that occur under mechanical ventilation and those under spontaneous ventilation. Dose-dependent decreases in cardiac output, stroke volume, and blood pressure are common with all inhalant anesthetics. However, these parameters are better maintained during spontaneous than during controlled ventilation because of the stimulatory effects of arterial CO_2, which is higher during spontaneous breathing.[10,19,20] In addition, changes in intrathoracic pressure that occur in ventilated horses have a negative effect on venous return that further depresses cardiac function.[10,20]

Cardiac output, blood pressure, and systemic vascular resistance increased significantly from baseline in horses anesthetized with isoflurane during volume-controlled ventilation that allowed arterial CO_2 tensions to increase to moderate levels ($PaCO_2$ of 75 to 85 mm Hg) from normal values (35 to 45 mm Hg). In this same study, mild hypercapnia (55 to 65 mm Hg) caused only a minor decrease in cardiac output and an increase in vascular resistance.[19]

In horses breathing spontaneously, cardiovascular variables were similar between isoflurane and halothane MAC multiples in one study,[10] and they were less depressed by isoflurane and sevoflurane than halothane in another.[11] Under controlled ventilation, isoflurane caused less depression of cardiac output and stroke volume than halothane, and similar changes in blood pressure, but vascular peripheral resistance was decreased with isoflurane more than with halothane.[10] Similar findings of better cardiovascular function with isoflurane compared with halothane have been described in horses anesthetized under hypoxemic conditions (PaO_2 of 50 mm Hg) for 3 hours.[15]

Changes in cardiac output, blood pressure, and peripheral vascular resistance are similar with isoflurane and with sevoflurane at 1.5 MAC, which represents a moderate plane of surgical anesthesia.[11] Similarly, in foals anesthetized for approximately 1 hour, no differences between sevoflurane and isoflurane were detected in cardiovascular effects.[13] Desflurane causes cardiovascular changes similar to those caused by isoflurane and sevoflurane; it decreases vascular resistance and blood pressure, whereas cardiac output and heart rate remained unchanged at 1 MAC.[14]

Halothane causes a decrease in blood pressure that is more related to a decrease in myocardial contractility and cardiac output than to a decrease in peripheral resistance. On the other hand, isoflurane, sevoflurane, and desflurane lower blood pressure as a result of decreased peripheral resistance and tend to cause less depression of cardiac output and contractility. Based on these findings, isoflurane, sevoflurane, and probably desflurane provide *better tissue flow* both in foals and adult horses and therefore *may be safer*, especially in the critically ill patient.

No major differences in heart rate are observed between isoflurane, sevoflurane, and halothane.[11] The arrhythmogenicity of halothane in response to doses of epinephrine is also higher than for isoflurane, sevoflurane, or desflurane.[21-23]

Halothane-anesthetized horses breathe at a faster rate than horses on isoflurane. Respiratory rate also decreases progressively with increasing doses of isoflurane or sevoflurane but not with halothane.[10,11] Despite these differences, $PaCO_2$ tends to be similar with all inhalant anesthetics, indicating similar minute-ventilation with all of them, most probably as a result of an increased tidal volume in horses receiving isoflurane or sevoflurane, to compensate for the slower respiratory rate and a smaller tidal volume in horses receiving halothane.

In spontaneously breathing anesthetized horses, respiratory rate is decreased to a similar extent by isoflurane, sevoflurane, and desflurane and less by halothane.[11,14] The decrease in rate was accompanied by concomitant increases in $PaCO_2$.[11]

BIOTRANSFORMATION

Respiration is responsible for eliminating most inhalation anesthetics. Liver metabolism is responsible for almost all degradation of inhalation anesthetics that remain in the body, although the lungs, kidneys, and other organs may contribute to overall elimination.

Halothane is the only currently used inhalant anesthetic that undergoes extensive metabolism (up to 20%) by the liver. In comparison, isoflurane, sevoflurane, and desflurane are metabolized to a much lesser extent (0.2%, 3% to 5%, and 0.02%, respectively).[24]

The effects of inhalant anesthetics on hepatic blood flow and metabolism should be minimal so that hepatic function is sustained and toxicity problems are avoided. In animal studies that have included dogs, rats, and pigs, the novel inhalant anesthetics including isoflurane, sevoflurane, and desflurane preserve hepatic metabolism and splanchnic blood flow better than halothane.[25-28] Similarly, in humans, all three of the novel anesthetics are preferred over halothane in patients with liver disease.[29]

Research horses anesthetized for up to 5 hours with only halothane and maintained at 1 to 2 MAC during this time exhibited a significant increase from baseline in aspartate aminotransferase, lactate dehydrogenase, creatinine phosphokinase, and total bilirubin for up to 4 days after anesthesia.[30] Similar changes are observed, although significantly less pronounced, when anesthesia time with halothane is less than 2 hours in clinical cases.[30] In contrast, horses exposed to isoflurane for 5 hours at 1 to 2 MAC did not exhibit significant changes in their serum chemistry values.[31] In a subsequent study, the same authors demonstrated that increasing anesthetic time with halothane beyond 5 hours increases the magnitude and duration of these changes, suggesting liver dysfunction.[32] Hepatic dysfunction in horses has been associated with halothane anesthesia combined with hypoxemia, but not with isoflurane and hypoxemia.[15]

Halothane has been implicated in cases of hepatic dysfunction in other species. Hepatic hypoxia with halothane is reported to be a major cause of such changes because greater reductions in hepatic blood flow occur with halothane than with other inhalation anesthetics. In addition, the increased biotransformation (20%) in the presence of reduced blood flow and oxygenation will promote a reduction of metabolism. As mentioned before, only halothane undergoes this type of metabolism. However, a reduction of metabolism is not always linked directly to hepatotoxicity, as hepatic damage also occurs with other anesthetics.[33]

GENERAL RECOMMENDATIONS

The transition from induction of anesthesia with injectable agents to inhalation anesthesia, and then to emergence from inhalation anesthesia, should be smooth. The use of injectable drugs with sedative or anesthetic properties is advised, especially in the neonate, as shown by mortality studies.

High oxygen flows should be used in the first 10 to 15 minutes of anesthesia to carry the inhalation anesthetic into the circuit and overcome the dilution effects of the anesthetic equipment (canister, reservoir bag, and breathing circuit), the horse's tidal volume and concentration gradients. In the adult horse, oxygen flows of 20 mL/kg per minute are normally used during the first part of anesthesia and then lowered to 10 mL/kg per minute for the remainder of the anesthetic period. In foals, flows of 40 to 60 mL/kg per minute are adequate, and this has less impact on cost and allows the use of small animal anesthetic machines.

Carbon dioxide absorbers should be monitored and changed regularly, usually after 5 to 7 hours of use at the oxygen flow rates just described. This also prevents accumulation of carbon monoxide, which may occur especially with desflurane, isoflurane, and halothane when low oxygen flows are used and soda lime is the choice of carbon dioxide absorbent. Production of compound A from sevoflurane in the presence of barium lime, and to a lesser degree with soda lime, can occur when low oxygen flows are used. This compound is reported to be nephrotoxic in rats,[34] and although similar data are not available in horses, caution is advised.

In conclusion, novel inhalation anesthetics with lower blood/gas partition coefficients have been introduced over the last 40 years. The advantages of these drugs are less biotransformation, less cardiovascular depression, and more rapid changes in anesthetic depth. Isoflurane, sevoflurane, and desflurane are drugs with similar anesthetic effects in the horse and the choice of agent depends on personal preference, available vaporizers, and financial considerations. Whether the novel agents will result in lower fatality rates remains to be seen.

REFERENCES

1. Johnston GM: Equine anaesthesia: A chance to cut is a chance to kill, Proc Assoc Vet Anaesth 2000:1-2.
2. Beecher HK, Todd DP: A study of the deaths associated with anesthesia and surgery: Based on a study of 599,548 anesthesias in ten institutions 1948-1952, inclusive, Ann Surg 1954;140:2.
3. Keenan RL, Boyan CP: Decreasing frequency of anesthetic cardiac arrests, Clin Anesth 1991;3:354.
4. Mee AM, Cripps PJ, Jones RS: A retrospective study of mortality associated with general anaesthesia in horses: Elective procedures, Vet Rec 1998;142:275.
5. Mee AM, Cripps PJ, Jones RS: A retrospective study of mortality associated with general anaesthesia in horses: Emergency procedures, Vet Rec 1998;142:307.
6. Johnston GM, Eastment JK, Wood JLN, et al: The confidential enquiry into perioperative equine fatalities (CEPEF): mortality results of Phases 1 and 2, Vet Anaesth Analg 2002;29:159.
7. Johnston GM, Taylor PM, Holmes MA, et al: Confidential enquiry of perioperative equine fatalities (CEPEF-1): Preliminary results, Equine Vet J 1995;27:193.
8. Taylor PM, Kirby JJ, Shrimpton DJ, et al: Cardiovascular effects of surgical castration during anesthesia maintained with halothane or infusion of detomidine, ketamine and guaiphenesin in ponies, Equine Vet J 1998;30:304.
9. Johnston GM, Eastment JK, Taylor PM, et al: Is isoflurane safer than halothane in equine anaesthesia? Results from a prospective multicentre randomized controlled trial, Equine Vet J 2004;36:64.
10. Steffey EP, Howland D Jr: Comparison of circulatory and respiratory effects of isoflurane and halothane anesthesia in horses, Am J Vet Res 1980;41:821.
11. Grosenbaugh DA, Muir WW: Cardiorespiratory effects of sevoflurane, isoflurane, and halothane anesthesia in horses, Am J Vet Res 1998;59:101.
12. Raisis AL, Young LE, Blissitt KJ, et al: A comparison of the haemodynamic effects of isoflurane and halothane anaesthesia in horses, Equine Vet J 2000;32:318.
13. Read MR, Read EK, Duke T, et al: Cardiopulmonary effects and induction and recovery characteristics of isoflurane and sevoflurane in foals, J Am Vet Med Assoc 2002;221:393.
14. Clarke KW, Song DY, Alibhai HI, et al: Cardiopulmonary effects of desflurane in ponies, after induction of anaesthesia with xylazine and ketamine, Vet Rec 1996;139:180.
15. Whitehair KJ, Steffey EP, Woliner MJ, et al: Effects of inhalation anesthetic agents on response of horses to three hours of hypoxemia, Am J Vet Res 1996;57:351.
16. Whitehair KJ, Steffey EP, Willits NH, et al: Recovery of horses from inhalation anesthesia, Am J Vet Res 1993;54:1693.
17. Santos M, Fuente M, Garcia-Iturralde P, et al: Effects of alpha-2 adrenoceptor agonists during recovery from isoflurane anaesthesia in horses, Equine Vet J 2003;35:170.
18. Donaldson LL, Dunlop GS, Holland MS, et al: The recovery of horses from inhalant anesthesia: A comparison of halothane and isoflurane, Vet Surg 2000;29:92.
19. Khanna AK, McDonell WN, Dyson DH, et al: Cardiopulmonary effects of hypercapnia during controlled intermittent positive pressure ventilation in the horse, Can J Vet Res 1995;59:213.
20. Hodgson DS, Steffey EP, Grandy JL, et al: Effects of spontaneous, assisted and controlled ventilatory modes in halothane-anesthetized geldings, Am J Vet Res 1986;47:992.
21. Pettifer G, Dyson D, McDonell W: The arrhythmogenic dose of epinephrine in halothane and isoflurane anesthetized dogs: An assessment of repeatability, Can J Vet Res 1997;61:221.
22. Hikasa Y, Okabe C, Takase K, et al: Ventricular arrhythmogenic dose of adrenaline during sevoflurane, isoflurane, and halothane anaesthesia either with or without ketamine or thiopentone in cats, Res Vet Sci 1996;60:134.
23. Moore MA, Weiskopf RB, Eger EI 2nd, et al: Arrhythmogenic doses of epinephrine are similar during desflurane or isoflurane anesthesia in humans, Anesthesiology 1993;79:943.
24. Stoelting R: Pharmacology and Physiology in Anesthetic Practice, ed 3, Philadelphia, 1999, Lippincott-Raven.
25. Debaene B, Goldfarb G, Braillon T, et al: Effects of ketamine, halothane, enflurane and isoflurane on systemic and splanchnic hemodynamics in normovolemic and hypovolemic cirrhotic rats, Anesthesiology 1990;73:118.
26. Sugai M: Comparison of the effect of isoflurane and that of sevoflurane on hepatic circulation and oxygen metabolism during acute hypoxia in dogs, Masui 1996;45:608.
27. Bernard JM, Doursout MF, Wouters P, et al: Effects of sevoflurane and isoflurane on hepatic circulation in the chronically instrumented dog, Anesthesiology 1992;77:541.
28. Armbruster K, Noldge-Schomburg GF, Dressler IM, et al: The effects of desflurane on splanchnic hemodynamics and oxygenation in the anesthetized pig, Anesth Analg 1997;84:271.
29. Green DW, Ashley EMC: The choice of inhalation anaesthetic for

major abdominal surgery in children with liver disease, Paed Anaesth 2002;12:665.
30. Steffey EP, Farver T, Zinkl J, et al: Alterations in horse blood cell count and biochemical values after halothane anesthesia, Am J Vet Res 1980;41:934.
31. Steffey EP, Zinkl J, Howland D Jr: Minimal changes in blood cell counts and biochemical values associated with prolonged isoflurane anesthesia of horses, Am J Vet Res 1979;40:1646.
32. Steffey EP, Giri SN, Dunlop CI, et al: Biochemical and haematological changes following prolonged halothane anaesthesia in horses, Res Vet Sci 1993;55:338.
33. Shingu K, Eger EI, Johnson BH, et al: Hepatic injury induced by anesthetic agents in rats, Anesth Analg 1983;62:10.
34. Keller K, Callan C, Prokocimer P, et al: Inhalation toxicology study of a haloalkene degradant of sevoflurane, compound A (PIFE), in Sprague Dawley rats, Anesthesiology 1995;83:1220.
35. Bergadano A, Lauber R, Zbinden A, et al: Blood/gas partition coefficient of halothane, isoflurane and sevoflurane in horse blood, Br J Anesth 2003;91:276.
36. Doherty TJ, Frazier DL: Effect of intravenous lidocaine on halothane minimum alveolar concentration in ponies, Equine Vet J 1998;30:300.
37. Doherty TJ, Geiser DR, Rohrbach BW: Effect of acepromazine and butorphanol on halothane minimum alveolar concentration in ponies, Equine Vet J 1997;29:374.
38. Doherty TJ, Geiser DR, Rohrbach BW: Effect of high volume epidural morphine, ketamine and butorphanol on halothane minimum alveolar concentration in ponies, Equine Vet J 1997;29:370.
39. Steffey EP, Howland D Jr, Giri S, et al: Enflurane, halothane, and isoflurane potency in horses, Am J Vet Res 1977;38:1037.
40. Aida H, Mizuno Y, Hobo S, et al: Determination of the minimum alveolar concentration (MAC) and physical response to sevoflurane inhalation in horses, J Vet Med Sci 1994;56:1161.
41. Tendillo FJ, Mascias A, Santos M, et al: Anesthetic potency of desflurane in the horse: Determination of the minimum alveolar concentration, Vet Surg 1997;26:354.

CHAPTER 20

Modern Injection Anesthesia for Horses

Regula Bettschart-Wolfensberger

The use of inhalational anesthesia is generally limited to larger clinics because of equipment costs, the requirement for an oxygen source, and the need for a scavenging system for waste gases. There is also strong evidence that inhalant techniques are associated with a higher mortality rate in horses (see Chapter 19). Therefore, the use of safe intravenous anesthesia techniques in practice is both desirable and advantageous. The most important features of intravenous protocols are a smooth, excitement-free induction phase with a slow lowering of the body into sternal and lateral recumbency, minimal cardiopulmonary depression, and a calm recovery with a single attempt to stand and minimal ataxia. Other factors include good muscle relaxation and analgesia, as well as the possibility to assess depth of anesthesia and modify depth and duration of anesthesia in a quick and predictable manner.

Injectable anesthetic combinations are presently used for anesthesia induction and for short (up to 30 minutes), minor surgical procedures. Longer surgeries are performed with intravenous anesthesia induction followed by inhalation, or less commonly by total intravenous anesthesia (TIVA). Features of short-duration injection anesthesia are discussed separately from long-duration (anesthetic duration over 30 minutes) TIVA. Anesthetics discussed in this chapter include ketamine and propofol and useful combinations of these two drugs. Older agents such as barbiturates, chloral hydrate, and drugs suitable for the anesthesia of wild Equidae, such as Immobilon (etorphine-acepromazine), will not be discussed.

SHORT-DURATION INJECTION ANESTHESIA

For anesthesia induction, ketamine, tiletamine/zolazepam, or propofol can be used. Adult horses must be adequately sedated before anesthesia induction with a calculated dosage of the selected drug. Only in very young foals and in recumbent, severely compromised horses can anesthesia be induced with administration of an anesthetic to effect. For compromised horses, a mixture of equal volumes of diazepam (5 mg/mL) and ketamine (100 mg/mL) is a safe method for anesthesia induction and usually requires 1 mL/25 kg of the mixture (0.1 mg/kg diazepam + 2 mg/kg ketamine). This protocol avoids the cardiovascular-compromising side effects of α_2-agonists. In foals, the administration of propofol to effect is an alternative (see Chapter 21).

Ketamine

Ketamine is the most widely used drug for anesthesia induction in horses. It provides good, mainly somatic analgesia without inducing hypnosis. However, it is not suitable as a sole agent, as it may cause seizure-like activity and muscle rigidity. Appropriate sedation with α_2-agonists or acepromazine prior to induction is very important.[1-14] The additional use of drugs such as guaifenesin or benzodiazepines (diazepam or midazolam) will further improve muscle relaxation.[15-20] Guaifenesin is a safe drug with minimal side effects at clinical dosages. It should be used as a 5% (50 mg/mL) solution, because higher concentrations are associated with significant irritation of the veins[21] and intravenous hemolysis.

Guaifenesin is administered to the sedated horse to effect (preferably under pressure, as effective dosages are large—often 50 mg/kg, or 500 mL for a 500-kg horse). When the horse begins to buckle at the knees, the induction drug, most commonly ketamine (2 mg/kg), should be given.

Benzodiazepines can be used instead of guaifenesin and can be given mixed with ketamine without causing irritation of the vein. Depending on the dosage used, these drugs may increase the respiratory depression caused by ketamine. To reduce the risk of apnea in the field when respiratory support is not available, low dosages of benzodiazepines (0.02 mg/kg diazepam or midazolam IV) are advocated. For anesthesia induction followed by inhalation anesthesia, higher dosages (up to 0.2 mg/kg IV) can be used and will facilitate intubation. Mechanical ventilation will counteract respiratory depression. To guarantee adequate muscle relaxation in the field where low dosages of benzodiazepines should be used, very deep sedation with relatively high dosages of α_2-adrenoceptor agonists is recommended.

Ketamine is a safe anesthetic for horses. Properly sedated, undisturbed horses will slowly sink into sternal and then lateral recumbency. Recovery at the end of anesthesia is usually quick and coordinated.[1-14] Respiratory depression is minimal. Ketamine's sympathomimetic action[22] is ideal to counteract the bradycardia and hypotensive effects of the drugs used as sedatives. For example, xylazine has been shown to have only minimal influence on cardiovascular function in combination with ketamine in the horse.[7] The judgment of depth of anesthesia can be difficult until one is familiar with these techniques, because the eyes remain open and the reflexes are only minimally depressed. Movements as a result of awakening may occur very suddenly and may be of a strong nature. In healthy horses, I prefer the administration of ketamine according to a fixed time scheme rather than to effect (Table 20-1).

Tiletamine

Tiletamine is a drug similar to ketamine, and both are classified as dissociative agents. It is commercially available as a powder in a fixed (1:1) combination with zolazepam, a benzodiazepine, and it is reconstituted with sterile water immediately before use. It has been used in horses and other Equidae[23-27] at dosage ranges of 1.1 to 1.65 mg/kg IV after sedation with α_2-adrenoceptor agonists. Depending on the dosage selected, the recumbency time was considerably longer than with ketamine combinations, and respiratory depression was more pronounced. Ataxia during recovery was more accentuated than with ketamine, with horses making several attempts to stand up. This feature makes this combination less desirable than xylazine-ketamine.

Propofol

Propofol is a short-acting anesthetic that provides very good hypnosis and muscle relaxation but poor analgesia. It is not suitable as a sole agent in adult horses because anesthesia inductions are unpredictable, and the large volumes required make it impractical and prohibitively expensive.[28] Propofol has been used mainly after sedation with α_2-adrenoceptor agonists under experimental conditions.[29-32] Only a few investigations have looked at propofol in clinical patients.[33] Some authors were happy with propofol as an induction agent. Others reported that the quality of anesthesia induction in individual horses was "not ideal" or "unacceptable."[34,35] It was questioned whether slow administration of propofol would smooth anesthesia induction,[34] but other factors, such as respiratory depression and lack of inherent analgesia in addition to cost, have prevented widespread use of propofol for anesthesia induction and maintenance of anesthesia during short surgical procedures.

In the neonatal foal, the use of propofol, administered to effect, for anesthesia induction (approximate dosage, 2 mg/kg IV) is, however, a good alternative to ketamine, as the duration of action of propofol is short and not dependent

TABLE 20-1. Protocols for Use of Ketamine for Short Surgical Procedures

Sedation		Anesthesia Induction		Duration of Anesthesia	Prolongation
		Muscle relaxant *And*	**Anesthetic**		
Alpha$_2$-agonist: Administer slowly to effect; wait 5 (xylazine)-10 (others) min	Xylazine (0.5)-1 mg/kg IV	*Either* guaifenesin 25-50 mg/kg IV Administer under pressure before ketamine to effect (until horse starts to become wobbly)	Ketamine 2 g/kg IV	10-25 min Duration of anesthesia tends to be longer with detomidine or romifindine sedation	Xylazine-ketamine: half the initial dose of each drug every 10 min
Combine with butorphanol (0.02 mg/kg) *or* methadone (0.1 mg/kg) to increase sedation	*or* detomidine 20-(40) mcg/kg IV *or* romifidine (80)-100 mcg/kg IV	*or* benzodiazepine 0.02-(0.2) mg/kg IV (diazepam, midazolam, climazolam) administered together with ketamine	Ketamine 2 mg/kg IV	Shorter duration in stressed, nervous animals	Ketamine: 0.5-1 mg/kg every 10 min following detomidine or romifidine sedation
Administer (IM) detomidine or romifidine to uncooperative horses					Triple drip (see Table 20-2)

TABLE 20-2. Dosage Regimens for Maintenance of Ketamine-Based TIVA in Horses

Technique	Drugs	Approximate Dosage	Comments
Triple drip	500 mL guaifenesin 10% + 1 g ketamine + 10 mg detomidine	1 mL/kg/h	Even higher dosage during initial 10-15 min; try to reduce dosage rate after 1 h of infusion
	500 mL guaifenesin 5% + 650 mg ketamine + 325 mg xylazine	2 mL/kg/h	
	500 mL guaifenesin 5% + 500 mg ketamine + 250 mg xylazine	2.75 mL/kg	Better relaxation than with preceding mixes (as guaifenesin dose is higher); more ataxia during recovery
Ketamine-climazolam	Ketamine + climazolam	6 mg/kg/h + 0.4 mg/kg/h	20 minutes after the end of infusion, sarmazenil 0.04 mg/kg must be given IV to prevent ataxia

on liver function. Relaxation is better and thus endotracheal intubation easier than with ketamine. Propofol is contraindicated in hypotensive foals, because it will further compromise these patients (see Chapter 21).

TOTAL INTRAVENOUS ANESTHESIA OF GREATER THAN 30 MINUTES' DURATION

Drugs and dosages suggested for maintenance of anesthesia with TIVA in horses are summarized in Table 20-2.

In modern equine practice, TIVA of longer duration is commonly maintained with constant infusions of the so-called triple drip (guaifenesin + α_2-agonist + ketamine), ketamine-climazolam, or propofol in combination with various drugs.

Ketamine combinations can be safely used for up to 1.5 hours to perform minor surgeries in the field. A recumbent horse breathing air will, however, become hypoxic. To prevent complications associated with hypoxia during field procedures of 30 minutes or longer, inspired air should be supplemented with oxygen (15 L/min, via a nasal or endotracheal tube). If the duration of anesthesia exceeds 2 hours, ketamine should not be used, because it produces active metabolites[36,37] that are eliminated very slowly and thus negatively influence the recovery period.

Ketamine-Guaifenesin-α_2-Adrenoceptor Agonist

The triple-drip drug combinations are the most widely used for TIVA. The most commonly used combination is ketamine, guaifenesin, and xylazine. Cardiovascular and respiratory depressions are minimal,[38,39] and these combinations have been successfully used to perform major surgical procedures as well as to prolong field anesthesia in a relatively controlled manner.[40,41] The use of this combination should be restricted to procedures of up to 2 hours' duration, not only because of the cumulative effects of metabolites of ketamine but also because large doses of guaifenesin may result in severe ataxia during recovery. Anesthetic induction performed prior to triple-drip anesthesia should not include guaifenesin, so that the total amount of guaifenesin given to the individual is as low as possible. A suitable induction technique is xylazine followed by ketamine. Because guaifenesin is a centrally acting muscle relaxant, the lack of movements during anesthesia is no guarantee of adequate analgesia. During painful procedures, analgesia should be provided with local anesthesia or the inclusion of opioids such as butorphanol or morphine.

Ketamine-Climazolam

The infusion of climazolam (a long acting benzodiazepine) together with ketamine causes less cardiovascular depression than triple-drip techniques.[17,42] Because climazolam causes severe ataxia, its action has to be reversed with sarmazenil for recovery. Analgesia is sufficient to perform superficial surgeries causing somatic pain. To provide sufficient analgesia for visceral procedures, local anesthesia or additional analgesia (opioids, α_2-agonsits) must be administered.

Propofol

In contrast to ketamine, propofol is an ideal anesthetic for prolonged TIVA. It possesses a short context-sensitive half-life,[36] permitting rapid recovery. It has been used in combination with different α_2-adrenoceptor agonists, guaifenesin, ketamine, and opioids.[34,35,43-46] In combination with medetomidine, anesthesia was maintained for up to 4 hours, and major surgeries were successfully performed. Although recovery was uneventful and relatively quick in all reports, problems, mainly of a respiratory nature (apnea and severe respiratory acidosis), and the relatively high cost of propofol have prevented its widespread use in clinical practice. Also, it offers no major advantages over commonly used inhalation anesthetic protocols—an additional reason for its limited use.

REFERENCES

1. Wright M: Pharmacologic effects of ketamine and its use in veterinary medicine, J Am Vet Med Assoc 1982;180:1462.
2. Crispin SM: Methods of equine general anesthesia in clinical practice, Equine Vet J 1981;13:19.
3. Ellis RG, Lowe JE, Schwark WS, et al: Intravenously administered xylazine and ketamine HCl for anesthesia in horses, J Equine Med Surg 1977;1:259.
4. Fisher RJ: A field trial of ketamine anesthesia in the horse, Equine Vet J 1984;16:176.

5. Hall LW, Taylor PM: Clinical trial of xylazine with ketamine in equine anaesthesia, Vet Rec 1981;108:489.
6. Kaegi B, Pabst B, Bucher R: Xylazin-Ketamin-Narkose beim Pferd, Pferdeheilkunde 1988;4:203.
7. Muir WW, Skarda RT, Milne DW: Evaluation of xylazine and ketamine hydrochloride for anesthesia in horses, Am J Vet Res 1977;38:195.
8. Muir WW, Scicluna C: Anesthesia and anesthetic techniques in horses, Equine Vet Educ 1998;10:33.
9. Parsons LE, Walmsley JP: Field use of an acetylpromazine/methadone/ketamine combination for anesthesia in the horse and donkey, Vet Rec 1982;111:395.
10. Schmidt-Oechtering GU, Alef M, Roecken M: Ein Beitrag zur Anästhesie des Pferdes mit Xylazin und Ketamin: Teil 2. Die Anästhesie des adulten Pferdes, Tierärztl Prax 1990;18:47.
11. Taylor P: Field anesthesia in the horse, In Pract 1983;5:112.
12. Thurmon JC, Benson GJ, Tranquilli WJ: Injectable anesthesia for horses, Mod Vet Pract 1985;66:745.
13. Watkins SB, Watney GC, Hall LW, Houlton JE: A clinical trial of three anesthetic regimens for the castration of ponies, Vet Rec 1987;120:274.
14. Clarke KW, Taylor PM, Watkins SB: Detomidine/ketamine anesthesia in the horse, Acta Vet Scand 1986;82:167.
15. Butera TS, Moore JN, Garner HE, et al: Diazepam/xylazine/ketamine combination for short-term anesthesia in the horse, Vet Med Small Anim Clin 1978;73:490.
16. Cronau PF, Zebisch P, Tilkorn P: Kurznarkose beim Pferd mit Diazepam-Xylazin-Ketamin, Tierärztl, Umsch 1980;35:393.
17. Kaegi B: Injektionsanästhesie mit Xylazin, Ketamin und dem Benhodiazepinderivat Climazolam sowie Anwendung des Benzodiazepinantagonisten Ro 15-3505, Schweiz Arch Tierheilk 1990;132:251.
18. Kerr CL, McDonell WN, Young SS: A comparison of romifidine and xylazine when used with diazepam/ketamine for short duration anesthesia in the horse, Can Vet J 1996;37:601.
19. Muir WW, Skarda RT, Sheenan W: Evaluation of xylazine, guaifenesin, and ketamine hydrochloride for restraint in horses, Am J Vet Res 1978;39:1274.
20. Marnell S, Nyman G: Effects of additional premedication on romifidine and ketamine anesthesia in horses, Acta Vet Scand 1996;37:315.
21. Herschl MA, Trim CM, Mahaffey EA: Effects of 5% and 10% guaifenesin infusion on equine vascular endothelium, Vet Surg 1992;21:494.
22. Ivankovitch AD, Miletich DJ, Reinmann C, et al: Cardiovascular effects of centrally administered ketamine in goats, Anesth Analg 1974;53:924.
23. Matthews NS, Dollars NS, Young DB, et al: Prolongation of xylazine/ketamine induced recumbency time with temazepam in horses, Equine Vet J 1991;23:8.
24. Matthews NS, Hartsfield SM, Cornick, JL, et al: A comparison of injectable anesthetic combinations in horses, Vet Surg 1991;20:268.
25. Matthews NS, Taylor TS, Skrobarcek CL, et al: A comparison of injectable anesthetic regimens in mules, Equine Vet J Suppl 1992;11:34.
26. Matthews NS, Taylor TS, Hartsfield SM, et al: A comparison of injectable anesthetic regimens in mammoth asses, Equine Vet J Suppl 1992;11:37.
27. Muir WW, Gadawski JE, Grosenbaugh DA: Cardiorespiratory effects of a tiletamine/zolazepam-ketamine-detomidine combination in horses, Am J Vet Res 1999;60:770.
28. Mama KR, Steffey EP, Pascoe PJ: Evaluation of propofol as a general anesthetic for horses, Vet Surg 1995;24:188.
29. Mama KR, Steffey EP, Pascoe PJ: Evaluation of propofol for general anesthesia in premedicated horses, Am J Vet Res 1996;57:512.
30. Nolan AM: The use of propofol as an induction agent after detomidine premedication in ponies, J Assoc Vet Anaesth 1989;16:30.
31. Nolan AM, Hall LW: Total intravenous anesthesia in the horse with propofol, Equine Vet J 1985;17:394.
32. Taylor PM: Adrenocortical response to propofol infusion in ponies: A preliminary report, J Assoc Vet Anaesth 1989;16:12.
33. Aguiar A, Hussni CA, Luna St P, et al: Propofol compared with propofol/guaifenesin after detomidine premedication for equine surgery, J Vet Anaesth 1993;20:26.
34. Matthews NS, Hartsfield SM, Hague B, et al: Detomidine-propofol anesthesia for abdominal surgery in horses, Vet Surg 1999;28:196.
35. Bettschart-Wolfensberger R, Freeman S, Bettschart RW, et al: Assessment of a medetomidine/propofol total intravenous anesthesia (TIVA) for clinical anesthesia in Equidae, Pferdeheilkunde 2002;18:39.
36. Nolan A, Reid J, Welsh E, et al: Simultaneous infusions of propofol and ketamine in ponies premedicated with detomidine: A pharmacokinetic study, Res Vet Sci 1996;60:262.
37. Delatour P, Jaussaud P, Courtot D, et al: Enantioselective *N*-demethylation of ketamine in the horse, J Vet Pharmacol Therap 1991;14:209.
38. Greene SA, Thurmon JC, Tranquilli WJ, et al: Cardiopulmonary effects of continuous intravenous infusion of guaifenesin, ketamine, and xylazine in ponies, Am J Vet Res 1986;47:2364.
39. Luna SPL, Taylor PM, Wheeler MJ: Cardiorespiratory, endocrine and metabolic changes in ponies undergoing intravenous or inhalation anesthesia, J Vet Pharmacol Therap 1996;19:251.
40. Young LE, Bartram DH, Diamond MJ, et al: Clinical evaluation of an infusion of xylazine, guaifenesin and ketamine for maintenance of anesthesia in horses, Equine Vet J 1993;25:115.
41. McCarty JE, Trim CM, Ferguson D: Prolongation of anesthesia with xylazine, ketamine, and guaifenesin in horses: 64 cases (1986-1989), J Am Vet Med Assoc 1990;197:1646.
42. Bettschart-Wolfensberger R, Taylor PM, Sear JW, et al: Physiologic effects of anesthesia induced and maintained by intravenous administration of a climazolam-ketamine combination in ponies premedicated with acepromazine and xylazine, Am J Vet Res 1996;57:1472.
43. Bettschart-Wolfensberger R, Bowen MI, Freeman SL, et al: Prolonged anesthesia with propofol-medetomidine infusion in Ponies: Cardiopulmonary function and other observations, Am J Vet Res 2001;62:1428.
44. Bettschart-Wolfensberger R, Freemann SL, Jäggin-Schmucker N, et al: Infusion of a combination of propofol and medetomidine for long-term anesthesia in ponies, Am J Vet Res 2001;62:500.
45. Mama KR, Pascoe PJ, Steffey EP, et al: Comparison of two techniques for total intravenous anesthesia in horses, Am J Vet Res 1998;59:1292.
46. Flaherty D, Reid J, Welsh E, et al: A pharmacodynamic study of propofol or propofol and ketamine in ponies undergoing surgery, Res Vet Sci 1997;62:179.

CHAPTER 21

Anesthesia and Analgesia for Foals

Sheilah A. Robertson

Foals undergo a rapid physiologic transition during the first year of life. Many changes involving the respiratory, cardiovascular, central nervous, and renal systems are unique to foals, and they have a major impact on their anesthetic management. Foals require sedation or general anesthesia for a variety of reasons, but the most common procedures are orthopedic and urogenital. The overall perioperative mortality rate for equine patients under 1 year of age is 1.9%, which is higher than the rate reported for the general horse population.[1,2] Foals between birth and 4 weeks of age pose the greatest risk associated with anesthesia, and within this group abdominal surgery has the highest mortality rate. Data show that the choice of anesthetic technique has a significant impact on outcome.

Despite the risks, the demand for anesthesia in critically ill foals sent to referral centers is greater than ever. Newer surgical and imaging techniques that require general anesthesia, such as laparoscopy[3] and magnetic resonance imaging (MRI),[4] are becoming popular. Importantly, pain management is an integral component of perioperative care, and techniques that are appropriate for foals must be included in the anesthetic plan.

RISKS ASSOCIATED WITH ANESTHESIA IN FOALS

Although outcomes have been reported for surgical treatment of colic[5] and uroperitoneum[6] in foals, it has been difficult to differentiate between mortality associated with anesthesia itself and the surgical procedure. The Confidential Enquiry into Perioperative Equine Fatalities (CEPEF) is an observational multi-institutional prospective study of recovery outcome at 7 days postoperatively, which was initiated by Johnston and others in 1991 to provide evidence-based data on risk factors associated with equine anesthesia.[1] This study is the basis for the following discussion on anesthetic risk in foals.

The most common procedures performed in foals include orthopedic surgery (correction of angular limb deformities and joint flushes) and urogenital surgery (Table 21-1). The greatest risk associated with anesthesia and surgery occurs in foals between birth and 4 weeks of age (Table 21-2), and abdominal surgery is the procedure that carries the highest mortality rate (Table 21-3).

Inhalant agents are associated with more deaths than injectable anesthetic protocols (Table 21-4). If only inhalant agents are used, the fatality rate is 4.4%, compared with 0.8% for total intravenous anesthetic (TIVA) techniques. In the past, inhalant agents were used primarily because of the belief that neonates, including foals, could not effectively metabolize injectable drugs. Future studies on foal anesthesia should focus on total intravenous techniques such as those discussed for adults in Chapter 20.

PHYSIOLOGY OF NORMAL FOALS

The anesthetist must be aware of the normal physiologic values in healthy foals to avoid misinterpretation of data.[7-10] For example, murmurs may be "normal" and arterial oxygen values low in the first week of life.

Cardiovascular System

Heart rates are approximately 100 beats per minute during the first month of life, decreasing to an average of 77 at 2 months and 60 at 3 months of age[7,10] (Table 21-5). These changes most likely reflect a transition from sympathetic dominance to increased vagal influence as the cardiovascular system matures.

Echocardiographic evidence indicates that left ventricular function (as measured by the shortening fraction) is similar in foals and adults,[10] but cardiac output is primarily rate dependent. If cardiac indices are adjusted for metabolic size, foals have a cardiac index (mL/min per kilogram)[7] at least

TABLE 21-1. Reasons for Anesthesia in Foals

Age of Foal (mo)	Colic *N* (%)	Abdominal, Not Colic *N* (%)	Fracture *N* (%)	Orthopedic, Not Fracture *N* (%)	Urogenital *N* (%)	ENT *N* (%)	Other *N* (%)	Total in Group (N)
<1	53 (8)	41 (6)	19 (3)	322 (47)	178 (26)	30 (4)	37 (5)	680
1-2	55 (5)	21 (2)	23 (2)	774 (68)	137 (12)	49 (4)	72 (6)	1131
3-5	54 (5)	23 (2)	23 (2)	474 (41)	438 (38)	51 (4)	96 (8)	1159
6-11	84 (6)	20 (1)	19 (1)	477 (32)	674 (45)	70 (5)	148 (10)	1492
Total for each procedure	246 (6)	105 (2)	84 (2)	2047 (46)	1427 (32)	200 (4)	353 (8)	4462

ENT, ear, nose, or throat surgery.
Data from the Confidential Enquiry into Perioperative Equine Fatalities (Johnston GM, Taylor PM, Holmes MA, et al: Equine Vet J 1995,27:193).

TABLE 21-2. Perioperative Fatality Rate in Foals

Age of Foals (mo)	Animals in Group (*N*)	Fatality Rate (%)
<1	680	4.26
1-2	1131	1.50
2-5	1159	1.38
6-11	1492	1.54
All (0-11 months)	4462	1.9

Data from the Confidential Enquiry into Perioperative Equine Fatalities (Johnston GM, Taylor PM, Holmes MA, et al: Equine Vet J 1995,27:193).

TABLE 21-3. Risk from Surgical Procedures in Foals Aged <12 Months

Surgical Procedure	Foals (*N*)	Deaths (*N*)	Fatality Rate (%)
Abdominal	311	40	12.9
Ear, nose, or throat	197	3	1.5
Fracture	77	7	9.1
Orthopedic (not fracture)	2031	16	0.8
Urogenital	1411	16	1.1
Other	350	3	0.9

Data from the Confidential Enquiry into Perioperative Equine Fatalities (Johnston GM, Taylor PM, Holmes MA, et al: Equine Vet J 1995;27:193).

twice that of adults,[11,12] yet their stroke volume is lower (see Table 21-5). Therefore, any decrease in a foal's heart rate has a significant impact on cardiac output.

Mean arterial blood pressure (MAP) values vary with the measurement technique employed. If indirect techniques such as Doppler ultrasound or electronic sphygmomanometry are used, the MAP may be as low as 50 mm Hg in normal 1-day-old foals, rising to 60 to 70 mm Hg at 2 to 3 weeks of age.[10] More recently, indirect oscillometric techniques have been validated against direct arterial blood pressure measurement, and true blood pressure readings are higher than those reported from Doppler studies.[13] MAP dictates organ perfusion; therefore, this is the most valuable blood pressure variable to obtain. In conscious 30- to 46-hour-old foals, direct MAP ranged from 59 to 113 mm Hg[13] and from 69 to 111 mm Hg using oscillometric techniques.[14]

TABLE 21-4. Anesthesia Technique and Perioperative Fatality Rate in Foals Aged <12 Months

Anesthesia Technique	Anesthesias (*N*)	Deaths (*N*)	Fatality Rate (%)
IV induction + maintenance with inhalant	3258	56	1.7
Single IV bolus only	378	2	0.5
IV induction and IV maintenance	259	2	0.8
Inhalant agent for induction and maintenance	567	25	4.4
Total number of anesthesias	4462	85	1.9

Data from the Confidential Enquiry into Perioperative Equine Fatalities (Johnston GM, Taylor PM, Holmes MA, et al: Equine Vet J 1995;27:193).

Respiratory System

Respiratory rate is high at birth,[15,16] and it declines over the first 6 months of life. At 1 week of age, the respiratory rate (43 ± 8 breaths/min),[15] is four times that of adult horses.[17]

TABLE 21-5. Cardiovascular Variables in Normal Foals and Adults

Variable	AGE								
	12 h	24 h	6-8 d	14 d	21 d	30 d	60 d	4-6 wk	Adult
Heart rate (beats/min)	89 ± 4*	106 ± 17†	114 ± 9* 111 ± 18†	95 ± 5* 100 ± 11†	110 ± 11†	103 ± 14†	77 ± 9†	84 ± 16‡	37 ± 2§
Cardiac index (mL/kg/min)	180 ± 10*	197 ± 12*	—	222 ± 21*	—	—	—	167 ± 16‡	68.9 ± 3.1§ 72.2 to 99#
Stroke volume (mL)	90.4 ± 5.7*	—	—	164 ± 25.9*	—	—	—	151 ± 25‡	889 ± 55§
Total peripheral resistance (dynes•sec•cm^{-5})	858 ± 70*	—	—	497 ± 87*	—	—	—	—	333 ± 18§
Mean arterial pressure (mm Hg)	88 ± 2*	59-113¶	97 ± 5*	100 ± 3*	—	—	—	115 ± 6‡	133 ± 4§

*Thomas WP, Madigan JE, Backus KQ, et al: J Reprod Fertil Suppl 1987;35:623.
†Lombard CW, Evans M, Martin L, et al: Equine Vet J 1984;16:342.
‡ Dunlop CI: Vet Clin North Am Equine Pract 1994;10:67.
§Steffey EP, Dunlop CI, Farver TB, et al: Am J Vet Res 1987;48:7.
#Bonagura JD, Muir WW: In Muir WW, Hubbell JAE (eds): Equine Anesthesia: Monitoring and Emergency Therapy, St Louis, 1991, Mosby.
¶Nout YS, Corley KT, Donaldson LL, et al: J Vet Emerg Crit Care 2002;12:75.

Minute ventilation also declines over this age range,[15] with the high values early in life being necessary to meet the high metabolic rate of foals.[16] Oxygen consumption in 1- to 7-day-old foals is 6 to 8 mL/kg per minute, which is two to three times that of adults,[16] and this must be taken into account when low-flow anesthetic techniques are used. Tidal volume in foals is similar to that in adults, as are values for arterial partial pressure of carbon dioxide. Some of these variables are shown in Table 21-6.

Newborn foals are hypoxic.[16,18] At 1 hour of age, values are 60.9 ± 2.7 (mean ± standard error of the mean) mm Hg and gradually increase to 86.9 ± 2.2 mm Hg by day 7, which is still below adult values of 104 ± 5 mm Hg.[19] Body position influences arterial oxygenation,[9,16] with values up to 14 mm Hg lower in foals that are laterally recumbent than in foals in the upright position.[16] The anesthetist should also be aware of the age-related responses to oxygen administration.[18,20] Although the rise in arterial oxygen pressure (Pa_{O_2}) with oxygen therapy in normal foals is significant, the response is much less in the first 2 days of life compared with day 7 and is not influenced by duration of oxygen therapy (2 minutes versus 20 minutes) or method of administration (face mask versus nasal insufflation).[20] The changes in response to oxygen may be a result of ductal closure or differences in ventilation and perfusion. Premature foals failed to show a response to oxygen therapy,[18] and this should be borne in mind when emergency anesthesia is performed in these patients.

Renal Function

Renal function is an important determinant of the excretion of many drugs. Studies show that although foal kidneys may be structurally immature, they are functionally mature. The glomerular filtration rate and effective renal plasma flow from 1 to 10 days of age are not significantly different from those of adults.[21,22] Blood urea nitrogen values of less than 2 mmol/L are normal up to 3 months of age,[21] whereas the mean adult value is 3.5 mmol/L. Rapid incorporation of amino acids into proteins is thought to be the cause of the low value in foals. Urine production in 4-day-old foals was 148 ± 20 mL/kg per day and had a low specific gravity (less than 1.008).[21] Iohexol clearance may offer a clinically useful method for assessing renal function in neonatal foals.[23] In normal 1- to 10-day-old foals, the pharmacokinetics of amikacin, a renally excreted antibiotic, suggest maturation of kidney function during this time.[24] Hypoxemia and azotemia can markedly alter excretion of amikacin,[25] and the dosage and dosing interval of renally excreted drugs may require adjustment in compromised foals.

Central Nervous System

Changes in drug disposition in growing foals may be explained by alterations in body composition, hepatic metabolism, and renal excretion. An additional factor to consider, especially in regard to anesthetic agents, whose site of action is the central nervous system (CNS), is the permeability of the blood-brain barrier, which separates cerebral spinal fluid (CSF) and nervous tissue from the intravascular compartment.[26,27] Age-related changes in permeability have been reported in some species,[27] but much less is known about the foal. The buffering ability of the CSF is also important to consider, as changes in CNS pH may directly affect brain function and may also alter drug dissociation and action.

Geiser and colleagues studied the CSF buffering capacity of foals less than 12 days of age by measuring the pH and P_{CO_2} of arterial and venous blood and the CSF during normocapnia and hypercapnia.[26] As in other neonates, the CSF of foals was more acidic than blood during normocapnia (Pa_{CO_2}, 35 to 40 mm Hg).[26] Hypercapnia (Pa_{CO_2} greater than 45 mm Hg) produced a rapid increase in CSF P_{CO_2} and a drop in pH. In contrast with blood, the buffering capacity of the CSF was poor and can be explained by the lack of protein, a major buffering system in blood, and the low permeability of the blood–CSF interface to bicarbonate ions compared with highly soluble CO_2. Acute increases in Pa_{CO_2} that may occur in sick, sedated, or anesthetized neonatal foals may have far-reaching effects not only because of their poor CSF buffering capacity but also as a result of vasodilation of cerebral vessels, which results in increased cerebral blood flow and intracranial pressure.[26]

TABLE 21-6. Respiratory and Pa_{O_2} Values in Normal Foals and Adults

Variable	AGE						
	24 h	48 h	7 d	14 d	1 mo	2 mo	Adult
Respiratory rate (breaths/min)	42 ± 4*	54 ± 10† 44 ± 7*	43 ± 8† 42 ± 5*	38 ± 11†	34 ± 11†	32 ± 8†	11 ± 4‡ 16 ± 2§
Tidal volume (mL/kg)	6.4 ± 0.5*	15.8 ± 2.5† 6 ± 0.5*	17.4 ± 2.9† 8 ± 1.2*	14.3 ± 1.9†	13.1 ± 1.6†	9.8 ± 2.6†	14.3 ± 2.3‡
Minute ventilation (mL/min/kg)	—	848 ± 231†	744 ± 169†	523 ± 126†	436 ± 116†	300 ± 42†	162 ± 45‡
Pa_{O_2} (mm Hg)	68 ± 4*	75 ± 3*	87 ± 2*	—	—	—	104 ± 4§

*Stewart JH, Rose RJ, Barko AM: Equine Vet J 1984;16:323.
†Koterba AM, Wozniak JA, Kosch PC: Equine Vet J 1995;27:257.
‡Koterba AM, Kosch PC, Beech J, et al: J Appl Physiol 1988;64:337.
§Wagner AE, Muir WW 3rd, Hinchcliff KW: Am J Vet Res 1991;52:651.

Clinical Chemistry

Bauer and coworkers[28] monitored serum chemistry values in several equine breeds during the first year of life and reported significant changes for alkaline phosphatase, aspartate transaminase, urea nitrogen, and total, direct, and indirect bilirubin, but not for electrolytes or glucose, emphasizing the need to consult age-specific reference values when interpreting this information in a clinical situation.

Mean serum glucose values ranged from 8.0 to 9.3 mmol/L during the first 3 months, with foals less than 12 hours of age having values of 8.0 ± 1.6 mmol/L.[28] Smyth and colleagues reported that 1-day-old foals that had been fasted for 2 hours had serum glucose values of 6.0 ± 0.7 mmol/L.[29] Full-term foals were able to maintain plasma glucose values for 2 hours after birth without suckling, but premature foals had mean values of only 2.31 mmol/L.[30]

Blood lactate is a useful indicator of tissue perfusion, but reference values may vary with age and source of the sample. In Thoroughbred foals aged 1 to 6 months, jugular blood values ranged from 0.9 to 1.65 mmol/L,[31] whereas arterial blood lactate values in 2-day-old foals were 2.17 ± 0.49 mmol/L.[32]

Hematology

Hematologic values change during a foal's first 12 months.[33] Hemoglobin and packed cell volume (PCV) fell during the first 2 weeks of life and then remained in the low normal range reported for adults, with no differences noted between Thoroughbred and Quarter Horse foals.[33] PCV was 0.43 ± 0.03, 0.40 ± 0.03, 0.38 ± 0.03 L/L at birth, 1 and 3 days respectively and progressively fell to 0.34 ± 0.04 L/L at 1 month of age. Hemoglobin and PCV values lower than those reported for healthy foals may result in decreased oxygen delivery to tissues. Total plasma proteins values were 60 ± 8 g/L at day 1 and did not vary more than 10% during the first year.[33]

PHARMACOKINETICS

The disposition of many drugs in foals is different from that in adults, and appropriate changes in both dosage and dose interval may be needed to avoid subtherapeutic or toxic concentrations. Pharmacokinetics may be influenced by both body composition and organ maturation, especially hepatic and renal function. For several drugs, marked pharmacokinetic differences have been noted between newborns, 1-week-old foals, 1-month-old foals, and foals older than 1 month. As a percentage of their body weight, foals have greater total body water, blood plasma, and extracellular fluid (ECF) volumes than adults[34,35] (see Chapter 3). In foals up to 1 month of age, the ECF accounts for 35% to 40% of body weight, compared with 25% in adult horses,[34] and this may influence the uptake and distribution of anesthetic drugs.

Hepatic Metabolism

The liver is the main site of drug metabolism, and it is important to have data on age-related hepatic function so that the anesthetist can make appropriate drug choices. The pharmacokinetics of chloramphenicol during the first week of life suggest that glucuronide synthesis matures rapidly[36] in normal foals, but the longer half-life in one premature foal indicates that their livers are less mature. Elevated bilirubin values in the first week of life may be a result of low glucuronyl transferase activity in foals.[28]

SEDATION

Foals require sedation for a variety of reasons, including radiography, bandage and cast changes, intravenous catheter placement, intensive care procedures, and arthrocentesis, and they should be sedated prior to general anesthesia. Information on the effects of the commonly used sedatives (xylazine, detomidine, diazepam, acepromazine) on foals is available.

There are no significant differences in the cardiopulmonary responses to high dosages (1.1 mg/kg IV) of the alpha$_2$-agonist xylazine in healthy 10- and 28-day-old foals.[37] Unlike adults given a similar dosage, most foals become recumbent. Foals' heart rates fell by about 20% to 30% without the second-degree atrioventricular block that is typically seen in adults. A biphasic (initial increase followed by a decrease) change in blood pressure, similar to that in adult horses, occurred, but the MAP did not fall below 60 mm Hg.[37]

Respiratory rhythm is markedly disrupted after xylazine administration in foals. Frequent upper airway noise indicative of respiratory obstruction lasted for 20 minutes, after which time respiration became slow and regular.[37] The noise is thought to result from upper airway collapse secondary to muscle weakness. Despite this response, healthy foals showed no changes in Pa_{O_2} or Pa_{CO_2}. Foals with respiratory disease, including those with preexisting upper airway obstructions such as guttural pouch tympany or strangles, may not compensate for these respiratory insults and should not be given xylazine. Alternatively, it can be given after establishing an airway by nasotracheal intubation.[38] Lower dosages (0.2 to 0.3 mg/kg IV) provide adequate sedation in a clinical setting and are associated with fewer cardiovascular changes.[39]

Rectal temperature fell significantly after xylazine administration in foals and remained low for more than 2 hours, by which time the sedative effects had worn off.[40] Body temperature should be monitored in all foals given xylazine, and extremes of environmental temperature are best avoided. Unlike in adult horses, xylazine did not produce hypoinsulinemia and hyperglycemia in 10- and 28-day-old foals, suggesting differences in pancreatic response to α_2-adrenergic agonists in neonates.[40] Increased urination occurs after xylazine administration,[40] and this should be considered when it is used to sedate hypovolemic foals.

Detomidine has been studied in foals between 2 weeks and 3 months of age.[41] Increasing the IV dosage from 10 to 40 μg/kg did not provide a greater degree of sedation, but it did prolong the duration of action: sedation lasted 28 ± 4 minutes after 10 μg/kg, and 73 ± 7 minutes after 40 μg/kg. Analgesia as assessed by skin prick was noted only at the 40-μg/kg dosage, but this was inconsistent and present in less than 50% of foals. As in xylazine-treated foals, respiratory stridor and increased urine production were observed. Unlike in foals given xylazine, recumbency did not occur even after high dosages of detomidine. This agent is less desirable than xylazine for sedation and analgesia of young foals, as even low dosages (10 μg/kg) are associated with a 60% incidence of arrhythmias.[41]

Diazepam is widely used in foals as a tranquilizer, muscle relaxant, and anticonvulsant. The pharmacokinetics of diazepam at a commonly used clinical dosage (0.25 mg/kg IV) have been studied in foals at 4, 21, 42, and 84 days of age.[42] Several pharmacokinetic variables were different when the 4-day-old foals were compared with foals of the other ages; the most clinically significant difference was the lower clearance in the 4-day-old age group, because this determines whether or not diazepam could accumulate if repeated doses or constant-rate infusions are used. In foals 21 days and older, pharmacokinetic data were similar to those reported for adult horses.[42,43] Compared with the values seen in other adult species, the free fraction of diazepam was much higher, and this could result in a greater clinical effect.[42] Lower binding ability of fetal albumin or competition for binding sites by elevated bilirubin levels in foals may explain this relatively high free fraction. The active metabolite desmethyldiazepam was measurable in all foals between 4 and 84 days of age[42] but was not detected in adult horses after administration of diazepam.[43] These data suggest a difference between foals and adults in hepatic biotransformation and elimination of drugs. The cardiopulmonary effects of diazepam have not been reported in foals, but dosages of up to 0.4 mg/kg produced no changes in cardiac output, blood pressure, or blood gas values in adult horses.[43]

Clinical effects of diazepam in foals are not widely documented. One study comparing xylazine to diazepam plus butorphanol as a premedicant for foals undergoing periosteal stripping concluded that xylazine provided better muscle relaxation.[44] When diazepam (0.1 to 0.2 mg/kg IV) is administered to foals less than 2 months of age, the usual response is profound sedation, muscle relaxation, and recumbency, whereas in older foals (2 to 4 months old), sedation and muscle relaxation are less pronounced and not always accompanied by recumbency (in my personal experience). These observations correlate with the research studies described earlier. These age-related responses may occur because of differences in permeability of the blood-brain barrier in younger foals.

Acepromazine can be used in foals, and commonly used dosages are 0.03 to 0.05 mg/kg (IM or IV). In adult horses, acepromazine decreases the fatality rate associated with general anesthesia,[1] which may be a reflection of its antiarrhythmic properties. Hypotension secondary to vasodilation is not observed unless foals are hypovolemic. Vasodilation and sedation may enhance heat loss, but there are no reported studies confirming this.

THE PREANESTHETIC PERIOD

The preoperative workup varies depending on the physical status of the foal and the intended surgical procedure. Blood work and physical examination results must be correlated with the distinct age-related changes described earlier. Electrolytes should be measured in foals with uroperitoneum; in one study, 48% of foals had abnormalities, which included hyponatremia, hypochloremia, and hyperkalemia accompanied by a metabolic acidosis.[6,45] Hyperkalemia may be associated with cardiac arrhythmias, which increases the anesthetic risk and must be corrected before surgery. Serum potassium can be decreased by draining the abdomen, by administering intravenous fluids (0.9% NaCl or 5% dextrose), and by correcting the metabolic acidosis with sodium bicarbonate. Insulin is only rarely required.

Although the focus of attention is the foal, the mare must not be forgotten. Allowing the dam to be present at induction of anesthesia is extremely valuable, because this ensures a calm foal. Suckling prior to anesthesia ensures adequate blood glucose levels, and regurgitation or vomiting is not a problem. After the foal has lost consciousness, the mare can be housed nearby but must be sedated, as most mares become agitated when separated from their foals. Xylazine (0.3 to 0.5 mg/kg IV) or detomidine (0.01 mg/kg IV) produces rapid and profound sedation in mares that can be extended by the addition of acepromazine (0.04 mg/kg IM).

GENERAL ANESTHESIA

Injectable Agents

Matthews and coworkers reported their experiences with propofol in healthy foals.[46] Their protocol was 0.5 mg/kg of xylazine IV followed 5 minutes later by a bolus of propofol (2 to 3 mg/kg) given over 45 to 60 seconds. As in other species, propofol must be given slowly to prevent apnea. Immediately after induction, foals were intubated, they were given 100% oxygen, and an infusion of propofol was started (approximately 0.3 mg/kg per minute). After infusions of up to 2 hours, foals had smooth and rapid recoveries. Cardiopulmonary variables were generally well maintained even when foals were placed in dorsal recumbency. A mild respiratory acidosis (Pa_{CO_2} of 60 mm Hg or less) was documented but considered clinically acceptable in healthy foals. It must be emphasized that these foals were all given oxygen supplementation, as hemoglobin saturation declines significantly if foals are allowed to breathe room air during propofol anesthesia (my personal experience).

Foals may react to surgical stimuli when anesthesia is maintained with propofol alone. Therefore, this technique is more suited for short, nonpainful procedures such as cast changes and radiography, when a rapid smooth recovery is desirable. Alternatively, propofol anesthesia could be combined with a local anesthetic in some situations, or sedatives, analgesics, or dissociative agents such as xylazine, butorphanol, or ketamine (respectively) could be added to the protocol. Propofol used alone without premedication provides approximately 5 minutes of general anesthesia. In dogs, propofol is an appropriate agent for patients with neurologic disease.[47,48] In foals, a single bolus should be adequate for collection of CSF samples. For MRI studies in foals suffering from neurologic disorders, propofol could be administered as a continuous infusion, and in these patients, Pa_{CO_2} should be closely monitored and hypercapnia avoided.

The pharmacokinetics of ketamine have not been described for the foal, but in adult horses recovery after a bolus results from redistribution.[49] Ketamine at a dosage of 2.2 mg/kg IV is recommended for foals and is usually given after premedication with xylazine or diazepam, or after administration of the centrally acting muscle relaxant guaifenesin.[39]

Total Intravenous Anesthesia

TIVA is associated with a lower mortality rate in both adults and foals. The so-called triple drip is widely used in foals,[39] but oxygen supplementation is required to prevent hypoxemia. Dunlop[39] recommends making a triple-drip mixture using a 1-L bag of 5% guaifenesin and adding 250 mg of xylazine and 1000 mg of ketamine. Induction can be achieved with 1 to 2 mL/kg of this mixture. Anesthesia is maintained using a rate of 2 to 3 mL/kg per hour, with the infusion rate adjusted on the basis of the clinical signs of depth of anesthesia. TIVA techniques are discussed fully in Chapter 20.

Inhalant Agents

The CEPEF data strongly suggest using TIVA techniques, or to induce the patient with injectable agents followed by maintenance with inhalant agents rather than relying totally on inhalant agents. For the foreseeable future, inhalant agents will continue to be used in foals, so the advantages and disadvantages of each should be well understood.

The time from induction to lateral recumbency was the same for halothane and isoflurane (approximately 4½ minutes) when administered by mask to unmedicated foals up to 2 months of age,[50] and induction was smooth in both groups. After 80 to 90 minutes of anesthesia, time to sternal recumbency was significantly faster in the isoflurane group (8.03 ± 0.93 minutes) than in the halothane group (13.6 ± 1.5 minutes); however, time to suckling was not different. Both agents were associated with a similar increase in $Pa{CO_2}$ values despite the lower respiratory rate in isoflurane-anesthetized foals. In adult horses, there is no difference in overall mortality between halothane and isoflurane,[2] but such data are not yet available for neonatal foals.

Sevoflurane is the most recent inhalant agent to be introduced to the veterinary market. In adult horses, its cardiopulmonary effects are similar to those of isoflurane[51] but recovery is more rapid because of its low solubility.[52] Read and coworkers compared isoflurane and sevoflurane as sole agents for anesthesia in six 1- to 3-month-old foals and noted no differences between the two agents in induction and recovery characteristics or times.[53] Direct MAPs were low in both groups for the first 30 minutes after induction, with a mean of only 44 ± 7 mm Hg and 46 ± 8 mm Hg for sevoflurane and isoflurane, respectively, at 10 minutes.[53] Although MAP improved between 30 and 60 minutes, the cardiac index remained low. The latter varied between 93 and 117 mL/kg per minute in both isoflurane- and sevoflurane-anesthetized foals, which represents approximately a 50% decrease compared with the mean values reported for conscious foals.[7,39] The respiratory depressive effects of sevoflurane could not be assessed because intermittent positive pressure was used.[53]

Inhalant agents seem suitable for maintenance of anesthesia, and using sedatives, tranquillizers, or analgesic agents decreases the minimum alveolar concentration, which may offset the cardiorespiratory depressant effects of the volatile agents. On the basis of the information available, all currently available inhalant agents are suitable for use in foals.

ANALGESIA

Pain has negative physiologic and psychological effects in all species and should be treated. There are very few studies on pain assessment in foals and few on the efficacy of analgesic agents. Traditionally, analgesia is provided by nonsteroidal anti-inflammatory agents (NSAIDs), opioids, α_2-agonists, and local anesthetics. A detailed review of analgesic drugs and techniques of pain management used in horses can be found in Chapter 23.

It is not unusual for foals to respond to pain more abruptly and profoundly than adults—for example, during the initial incision at the start of a surgical procedure—even when the anesthetic depth appears adequate. Dunlop remarked during a study that evaluated the anesthetic potency of isoflurane that foals were hyperresponsive to the initial noxious stimulus.[39] To block the initial response to surgery, local infiltration of the surgical site with lidocaine or bupivacaine is a simple and effective technique, as these agents also provide some analgesia in the early postoperative period.

The agonist-antagonist opioid butorphanol has been used safely in foals and is given IV or IM (0.1 to 0.2 mg/kg). Morphine and fentanyl at dosages similar to those used in adults have been used, but there are no reports on the pharmacokinetics or pharmacodynamics of these drugs in foals.

Several pharmacokinetic studies of NSAIDs (including phenylbutazone,[54] ibuprofen,[55] ketoprofen,[56] and flunixin meglumine[57,58]) in foals have been published. Many of these were primarily aimed at the use of these drugs for their antiendotoxin effect rather than as analgesics. There are differences in volume of distribution, half-life, and clearance for phenylbutazone (2.2 mg/kg IV) between foals and adults, with foals less than 24 hours old showing a reduced ability for drug elimination.[54]

Potential side effects of these drugs include gastrointestinal ulceration, nephrotoxicity, and platelet dysfunction. High dosages (5 mg/kg twice daily for 7 days) of phenylbutazone did not produce clinical signs of renal or gastrointestinal disease, or changes in complete blood counts or clinical chemistries in healthy 7- to 10-day-old foals, but renal changes could be detected through premortem ultrasonic examination, and gastric ulcers and histologic changes in the kidneys were found at necropsy.[59] In healthy 5- to 10-week-old foals, ibuprofen at dosages up to 25 mg/kg three times daily for 6 days produced no unwanted side effects, but the authors cautioned that this may not be true in foals with compromised renal function.[55] In healthy 1-day-old foals, dosages of ketoprofen must be increased to 1.5 times the adult dosage of 2.2 mg/kg to achieve therapeutic plasma concentrations, but because of reduced elimination, dosing intervals may need to be lengthened.[56] It is also suggested that the dosage of flunixin meglumine, like that of ketoprofen, be increased in 1-day-old foals but that the dosing interval be extended.[57] However, when treating septic or dehydrated foals, further adjustments must be made. The pharmacokinetics of flunixin meglumine (1.1 mg/kg IV) are different in foals at 1 day of age, 10 to 11 days, and 27 to 28 days of age.[58] Drug elimination was significantly decreased in the youngest foals, most likely because of decreased hepatic metabolism and renal clearance. Despite these differences, dosages of up to 2.2 mg/kg given over 5 days in 2-day-old foals caused no clinical, complete blood count, clinical chemistry, or pathologic changes.[60] Doses of 6.6 mg/kg did result in gastrointestinal ulceration.[60] These studies suggest that the use of NSAIDs to treat acute perioperative pain in young foals should be safe and effective, but care should be taken in compromised foals.

MONITORING AND INTRAOPERATIVE CARE

Monitor is derived from the Latin word *monere,* which means "one that warns." Monitoring vital functions in anesthetized foals is essential for a successful outcome, but monitoring equipment displays only numbers, and the anesthetist must know what values are normal and how to intervene if aberrations occur. For these reasons, it is important to be familiar with the physiologic data of neonatal foals described earlier. In addition, the anesthetist's physical senses, skill, and experience play a vital role in determining anesthetic depth.

Many of the techniques described for monitoring critically ill neonatal foals, reviewed in depth by Corley,[32,61] apply to anesthetized foals. During anesthesia, ventilation and oxygenation must be maintained, and therefore these variables must be monitored. Optimizing organ perfusion is a primary goal of the anesthetist, but perfusion per se is difficult to measure. Indirect markers of perfusion include cardiac output, blood pressure, urine output, and blood lactate values. Hypothermia has far-reaching deleterious effects, so body temperature should be closely monitored and active warming techniques employed. Foals may be susceptible to hypoglycemia, so blood glucose should be monitored.

Cardiovascular Monitoring

Cardiac output is the parameter that most accurately assesses cardiovascular function, but its measurement has until now been restricted to the research arena because of the technical challenges and dangers associated with cardiac catheterization, which include endocardial damage. New, less invasive technology that requires only a venous and a peripheral arterial catheter and lithium as a marker has revolutionized cardiovascular monitoring, making it the only validated technique currently suitable for clinical use.[32,62] This technique, termed lithium dilution (LiDCO Ltd, Cambridge, United Kingdom), is commercially available. Even more recently, a noninvasive cardiac output technique (NICO, Novametrix, Wallingford, Conn) based on the Fick principle and partial rebreathing of CO_2 has performed well when compared with the lithium dilution technique in dogs,[63] and it is being evaluated in neonatal foals (personal communication, A. Valverde, 2004). This technology can be used only in intubated animals, but because nasotracheal intubation is easily performed,[38] it may be adaptable to conscious foals.

Cardiac output monitoring is invaluable in critically ill foals in the perioperative period. It allows the anesthetists to make prompt and appropriate treatment decisions and to monitor the response to fluid therapy, inotropes, or vasopressors. Normal values were discussed earlier in this chapter.

Blood pressure can be measured directly or indirectly and provides useful information on cardiovascular status, provided the clinician understands the correlation of cardiac output, systemic vascular resistance, and blood pressure, and is aware of the age-related changes in blood pressure. Direct measurement requires insertion of an arterial catheter (with all the associated problems discussed later in this chapter), and for this reason indirect methods are often used. The ultrasonic Doppler technique using a tail cuff as described by Lombard and coworkers[10] was not validated against a direct blood pressure measurement and may have underestimated the blood pressure of neonatal foals. An electronic sphygmomanometer gave consistently lower readings than directly measured blood pressure in anesthetized pony foals,[14] but the authors felt it was sufficiently accurate if a correction factor was used.

More recently, the accuracy of an indirect oscillometric monitor (ProPaq Encore 206EL, Protocol Systems, Inc, Beaverton, Ore) has been reported in both awake and anesthetized foals.[13] There was good agreement between this technique (cuff placed around the tail) and direct measurement (greater metatarsal artery) for mean and diastolic blood pressure, but agreement was less satisfactory for systolic blood pressure. MAP is more clinically relevant, as this is a better predictor of organ perfusion. The authors recommended a ratio of cuff bladder width to tail girth of between 1:1.9 and 1:2.8, and in practical terms, a 52-mm bladder was suitable for foals aged 1 to 2 days and weighing 44 to 68 kg.

On the basis of published results,[13,14] a MAP of 60 mm Hg or below should prompt the clinician to intervene. Corley suggests that supportive therapy be initiated at an MAP of 69 mm Hg and published data indicating that MAPs less than 60 mm Hg in foals less than 1 week old are associated with a higher mortality rate.[32] Foals with low blood pressure may require fluid therapy or inotropic support (see Chapter 1).

Urine output in foals is approximately 6 mL/kg per hour.[21] Urine production reflects adequacy of perfusion, cardiovascular and hydration status, and renal function.[32] Urine production can be measured after placing a urinary catheter using a sterile technique and attaching it to a closed collection system.[32] Less than expected urine production should prompt the anesthetist to review the hydration and cardiovascular status of the foal.

Respiratory Monitoring

Arterial oxygen values in foals change with age and are lower than in adults. However, hypoxemia is a potential problem in awake and anesthetized neonatal foals but frequently goes unnoticed because clinical signs are nonspecific; therefore, reliable monitoring techniques are required. The gold standard is arterial blood gas measurement, but obtaining a sample by direct needle puncture may be technically difficult, maintaining an arterial catheter is challenging, and the site is a potential access for infection.[64] In addition, only periodic information can be obtained. For these reasons, pulse oximetry has been evaluated in foals.[32,64] Pulse oximetry is a continuous, noninvasive technique for estimating arterial oxygen saturation (SaO_2). Commercially available monitors are inexpensive, but clinicians must be aware of their limitations. In anesthetized foals, the accuracy of one pulse oximeter (Nellcor N-200, Nellcor Puritan Bennett, Inc, Pleasanton, Calif) with three different transducers (fingertip, adhesive, and forehead reflectance types) placed at several sites (ear, lip, tongue, and ventral tail base) was evaluated.[64] Pulse oximetry is a valuable technique, but the transducer type, placement site, and range of Sao_2 values have a significant effect on reliability, so pulse oximetry should not totally replace arterial blood gas analysis. A fingertip-type transducer placed on the ear or tongue is the most clinically useful technique.

Carbon dioxide values reflect the balance between production (metabolic rate), cardiovascular function (transport of CO_2 from tissues to the lungs), and elimination (ventilation). As previously discussed, increases in $Paco_2$ may have deleterious effects on CNS function. Elevated CO_2 values may occur in weak and compromised foals, and most sedatives and general anesthetic agents produce respiratory depression and hypercapnia.

The partial pressure of arterial CO_2 ($Paco_2$) is the most reliable indicator of pulmonary ventilation, but because of the difficulty in obtaining arterial blood samples, venous[9] and end-tidal CO_2[65] values have been studied in foals. End-tidal or end-expired CO_2 ($ETCO_2$) reflects alveolar CO_2 tension, which in turn is closely related to arterial CO_2, and is widely used as a noninvasive method for monitoring ventilation in anesthetized and intubated animals.[66] Capnography refers to the graphic display of CO_2 concentration over time and is preferred over capnometry, which provides the anesthetist with only a numerical display of CO_2 concentrations. The attraction of capnography is the continuous display of information compared with intermittent blood gas analysis. Interpretation of the waveform not only provides information on patient factors but also alerts the anesthetist to equipment malfunction, such as kinked endotracheal tubes, airway obstruction, exhausted carbon dioxide absorbent, and incompetent one-way valves. Currently, there are two main types of capnograph available—the mainstream and the sidestream—and in dogs, the former was considered more accurate.[67] However, the authors warned that under hypercapnic conditions (i.e., $Paco_2$ greater than 60 mm Hg), $ETCO_2$ values do not accurately reflect the severity of hypoventilation, as determined by the gold standard of arterial CO_2 measurement.[67] The reliability of $ETCO_2$ measurement in spontaneously breathing, isoflurane-anesthetized foals has been reported.[65] A gradual increase in both $Paco_2$ and $ETCO_2$ occurred over a 90-minute period, with arterial CO_2 always greater than $ETCO_2$.[65] During the first 60 minutes, $ETCO_2$ was a useful indicator. After 60 minutes, $ETCO_2$ was not predictive and greatly underestimated arterial CO_2 values—for example, at 90 minutes, the mean $ETCO_2$ value was 63 mm Hg and $Paco_2$ was 78 mm Hg. The widening of the arterial to end-tidal gradient could be explained by hypoventilation and decreased pulmonary capillary perfusion of alveoli.[65] As in other species,[66] the limitations of capnography must be understood. Capnography may be useful for short anesthetic procedures, but it cannot totally replace blood gas analyses. This technology is primarily thought of as a respiratory monitor, but because carbon dioxide must be transported in blood from tissues to the lungs to be eliminated, sudden decreases in $ETCO_2$ can reflect a cardiovascular crisis.

Blood Glucose

Both hypoglycemia and hyperglycemia are undesirable in anesthetized patients. In a conscious animal, hypoglycemia may result in seizure activity, coma, and CNS damage, all of which are masked by general anesthesia. In the past, the detrimental effects of hyperglycemia were underestimated, but human data strongly implicate elevated blood glucose values as a cause of increased postoperative infection and mortality.[68-70]

Problems associated with interpreting glucose results in foals include the analytical technique, sample site (venous, arterial, or capillary), and which references are used as normal values. The anesthetists must know whether the analytical technique they use measures plasma, serum, or whole blood glucose so that the correct reference data are used. For convenience, bed-side analyzers are commonly used in the operating room. In dogs[71] and foals,[72] there are wide variations in the accuracy of commercially available portable blood glucose monitors. Cohn and coworkers[71] concluded that up to 67% of clinical treatment decisions would have been erroneously altered had the clinician relied on results obtained from some portable blood glucose meters and, according to their study, a point-of-care analyzer (i-STAT portable clinical analyzer, Heska Corporation, Fort Collins, Colo) was the only acceptable portable method.[71] To track trends accurately, blood samples should be collected from the same site and analyzed using the same technique. Healthy foals scheduled for short procedures are unlikely to have problems associated with blood glucose, but premature foals and sick foals, especially those that may be septic and those undergoing surgery lasting several hours, should be monitored. To preserve normoglycemia, foals should be allowed to suckle up until the time of anesthesia and allowed access to their mare's milk as soon as possible after recovery.

Body Temperature

Foals are susceptible to heat loss because of their high ratio of surface area to body weight, and their lack of subcutaneous fat. Hypothermia decreases metabolism of anesthetic drugs, delays recovery, and results in postanesthetic shivering, which increases oxygen requirements. Very low heart rates (less than 60 beats per minute) associated with rectal temperatures less than 36° C (less than 97° F)[32] are detrimental to foals because their cardiac output is more dependent on heart rate than that of adults. Shivering is unpleasant and may increase postoperative pain because of involuntary muscle activity around surgical wounds. Although not well documented in the veterinary literature, intraoperative hypothermia interferes with clotting enzymes, causing increased blood loss in humans.[73,74] Postoperative infections are increased and wound healing is delayed by hypothermia, because cold-induced vasoconstriction results in decreased wound perfusion and oxygen delivery. In addition, antibody and cell-mediated immune systems are depressed by low body temperatures.[68,74,75] Core temperature (at the esophagus, tympanic membrane, or pulmonary artery) is considered the most critical value, but in a clinical setting and in awake foals, it is impractical to obtain. For these reasons, peripheral or shell temperature, usually a rectal temperature, is measured. The relationship between core and peripheral temperature is not well documented in foals, but in anesthetized adult horses, rectal temperatures did accurately reflect core temperature.[76]

Preventing hypothermia is important and can be done using simple and relatively inexpensive techniques such as dry, light-weight blankets, circulating warm water blankets, and forced warm air devices (Bair Hugger Therapy, Arizant, Inc, Eden Prairie, Minn). Additionally, cold operating rooms and excessive use of cold evaporative skin preparation solutions such as alcohol should be avoided.

Fluid Therapy

The fluid intake (milk plus water) of foals is high, with animals aged 11 to 18 days drinking 246 g/kg and those aged 30 to 44 days consuming 202 g/kg.[77] Maintenance fluid rates in neonatal foals are variable but higher than in adults,[78] and as much as 120 mL/kg per day is required in foals up to 1 month of age. Neonates are less tolerant of blood loss and dehydration because of their cardiovascular physiology,[39] so fluid status must be closely monitored and promptly treated. Foals that are septic, have diarrhea, or have lost blood but require surgery should be rehydrated before they are anesthetized. Hypovolemia is best treated with balanced ionic crystalloid solutions such as Normosol-R, Plasmalyte, or lactated Ringer's solution.[78] Large volumes of saline should be avoided, as this can promote acidosis.[78] The response to therapy can be assessed by measuring blood pressure, urine output, and, if the technology is available, blood lactate. During surgery, similar fluids should be administered to replace respiratory and evaporative losses as well as blood loss, although the actual fluid administration rate will vary with each individual case. For a healthy foal undergoing an elective procedure, 10 mL/kg per hour should be adequate. Foals with uroperitoneum and hyperkalemia require specific fluid therapy (see Chapter 3). If blood glucose monitoring indicates it, dextrose may be added to the intravenous fluids.

Colloids, including dextrans and hetastarch, may be required if total protein and albumin are low or if there is a poor response to crystalloid therapy. Hetastarch is readily available and frequently used in neonatal resuscitation[61] at a dosage of 3 mL/kg body weight infused at a rate of 10 mL/kg per hour. Blood loss or anemia can be treated with cross-matched whole blood, but the use of polymerized bovine hemoglobin (Oxyglobin solution, Biopure Corporation, Cambridge, Mass) has been reported in adult horses[79] and could be used in foals. In addition to providing hemoglobin for oxygen carriage, this product is a potent colloid (see Chapter 4).

Blood Pressure Support

During anesthesia, blood pressure can easily be measured. It is recommended that a mean arterial blood pressure of greater than 70 mm Hg be maintained at all times to ensure adequate organ perfusion. If hypotension occurs, the cause must be identified, and it may be hypovolemia, hemorrhage, decreased cardiac output, or vasodilation, or a combination of any of these. If fluid losses are thought to be the problem, they can be addressed as discussed earlier.

Bradycardia has a marked effect on cardiac output and blood pressure in foals because of their high heart rate and fixed stroke volume. One of the main causes of bradycardia is hypothermia, and this must be prevented or treated, because heart rate does not respond to anticholinergic therapy in this situation. Bradycardia may result from vagal stimulation such as bladder manipulation. Such stimuli should be stopped and anticholinergics (atropine or glycopyrrolate) may be required. Anesthetic agents, in particular the inhalant agents discussed previously, are potent cardiovascular depressants. For these reasons, the depth of anesthesia should be closely assessed and, if possible, the vaporizer setting decreased. In addition, the use of an anesthetic-sparing drug such as xylazine, acepromazine, and lidocaine (as an infusion) is recommended to reduce the requirement for inhalant agents.

Although inotropes and vasopressors may be used to increase blood pressure, the goal is to improve organ perfusion, so increasing cardiac output and blood flow should be the first line of treatment.[61] Monitoring cardiac output is the ideal and, as described previously, clinically acceptable techniques are now available. Dobutamine is a widely used inotrope in equine anesthesia and effectively increases cardiac output.[80,81] In 1-month-old isoflurane-anesthetized foals, 3 µg/kg per minute of dobutamine doubled the cardiac output by increasing both heart rate and stroke volume,[39] whereas in adult horses the increase is primarily related to stroke volume. These differences between adults and foals are a result of the changing sympathetic and vagal control of the heart with age. Despite the increased cardiac output, mean blood pressure in dobutamine-treated foals increased only from 60 to 70 mm Hg because of a significant decrease in peripheral vascular resistance.[39] Therefore, blood pressure readings may not reflect the benefits of dobutamine, and monitoring increases in heart rate and urine output may be useful when cardiac output cannot be measured.

Vasopressor agents such as epinephrine (adrenaline) and phenylephrine should be used with caution because they increase cardiac afterload, their effects may vary in different organs, and despite an increase in systemic blood pressure, perfusion of the gastrointestinal tract and kidneys can be severely compromised.[61] Vasopressin is receiving a lot of attention as a therapeutic agent in nonresponsive vasodilatory shock,[82] and it has been used in foals,[83] but its place in treatment of the critically ill and anesthetized foal will not be clear until further studies are conducted. Vasopressors should be used only when the blood pressure has not responded to other therapies. A comprehensive discussion of inotropes and vasopressors is outside the scope of this chapter and the reader is directed to the reviews by Corley.[61,83]

RECOVERY

Foals should be allowed to recover in a dry, warm environment, and they should be propped up in sternal recumbency to optimize their Pa_{O_2}. If they shiver, supplemental oxygen should be provided to prevent hypoxemia. When they can be assisted to stand, foals should be reunited with their dam and allowed to suckle to maintain their fluid and caloric intake and to reestablish maternal bonding.

NEW TECHNIQUES AND CHALLENGES

Two techniques that require new anesthetic skills and knowledge are MRI and laparoscopic surgery. Neurologic disorders are common in foals, but until recently diagnosis has been hampered by the inability to image the brain.[4] MRI is considered the diagnostic technique of choice for many CNS disorders and has become increasingly accessible to veterinarians over the past few years. The challenges of anesthesia in an MRI unit include working in a confined space with limited access to the patient and the incompatibility of conventional anesthetic equipment with the magnetic field and radiofrequency pulses.[84] If inhalant anesthesia is used, the ferrous material in anesthesia machines must be replaced or the equipment adapted so that the machine remains outside the critical Gauss line (magnetic flux density). Alternatively, special MRI-compatible equipment must be purchased, and this option may not be practical for veterinary clinics. However, a more practical alternative is TIVA.[4,46] In both situations, monitoring equipment must be chosen and used carefully to prevent patient burns[85] and interference with the image. Excellent guidelines for anesthesia and monitoring in an MRI unit can be found at the website of the Anesthesia Patient Safety Foundation (www.apsf.org/index.php).

Chaffin and colleagues described an anesthetic technique suitable for MRI in neonatal (3-6 days of age) foals.[4] Xylazine (0.5 mg/kg IV) was followed 5 minutes later by a bolus of propofol (0.2 to 0.4 mg/kg IV). After endotracheal intubation, a constant rate infusion of propofol (0.2 to 0.4 mg/kg) was started, and the rate was adjusted up or down depending on the depth of anesthesia. Oxygen was insufflated through the endotracheal tube using a long nonrebreathing (Bain) circuit attached to an oxygen supply outside the MRI chamber. For reasons previously discussed, $Paco_2$ should be monitored in compromised foals, and controlled ventilation is required to avoid the hypercapnia that occurs in spontaneously breathing foals during propofol anesthesia. Ventilation can be assisted in an MRI unit using an Ambu bag attached to the endotracheal tube, or manual ventilation with a bag attached to the breathing circuit. An oscillometric blood pressure monitor can be placed outside the magnetic field and attached by a long cable.

Laparoscopic surgery under general anesthesia has been reported for resection of umbilical structures[3] and ruptured bladder repair in foals[86] (see Chapter 71). Advantages may include better visibility of intra-abdominal structures and less postoperative soft tissue swelling and discomfort.[3] However, the effects of insufflation with carbon dioxide, abdominal distention, the Trendelenburg position, and longer anesthesia time must also be considered.[3] In adult horses, CO_2 insufflation produced hypercapnia, acidosis, and an increase in cardiac work.[87] In foals, no anesthetic-related complications were noted during or after laparoscopy,[3] but the cardiopulmonary changes associated with this technique have not been critically evaluated in this patient population. It would be prudent to monitor $Paco_2$ and cardiovascular function closely during this procedure.

In conclusion, anesthetizing foals can be a challenge. However, it should be possible to decrease the currently unacceptable fatality rate in this group of patients. The clinician should have knowledge of foals' unique physiology, age-specific pharmacologic data, evidence-based studies of anesthetic risk factors, and emerging technology (in particular, measurement of cardiac output).

REFERENCES

1. Johnston GM, Taylor PM, Holmes MA, et al: Confidential Enquiry of Perioperative Equine Fatalities (CEPEF-1): Preliminary results, Equine Vet J 1995;27:193.
2. Johnston GM, Eastment JK, Taylor PM, et al: Is isoflurane safer than halothane in equine anaesthesia? Results from a prospective multicentre randomised controlled trial, Equine Vet J 2004;36:64.
3. Fischer AT Jr: Laparoscopically assisted resection of umbilical structures in foals, J Am Vet Med Assoc 1998;214:1813.
4. Chaffin MK, Walker MA, McArthur NH, et al: Magnetic resonance imaging of the brain of normal neonatal foals, Vet Radiol Ultrasound 1997;38:102.
5. Vatistas NJ, Snyder JR, Wilson WD, et al: Surgical treatment for colic in the foal (67 cases): 1980-1992, Equine Vet J 1996;28:139.
6. Kablack KA, Embertson RM, Bernard WV, et al: Uroperitoneum in the hospitalised equine neonate: Retrospective study of 31 cases, 1988-1997, Equine Vet J 2000;32:505.
7. Thomas WP, Madigan JE, Backus KQ, et al: Systemic and pulmonary haemodynamics in normal neonatal foals, J Reprod Fertil Suppl 1987;35:623.
8. Machida N, Yasuda J, Too K, et al: A morphological study on the obliteration processes of the ductus arteriosus in the horse, Equine Vet J 1988;20:249.
9. Madigan JE, Thomas WP, Backus KQ, et al: Mixed venous blood gases in recumbent and upright positions in foals from birth to 14 days of age, Equine Vet J 1992;24:399.
10. Lombard CW, Evans M, Martin L, et al: Blood pressure, electrocardiogram and echocardiogram measurements in the growing pony foal, Equine Vet J 1984;16:342.
11. Steffey EP, Dunlop CI, Farver TB, et al: Cardiovascular and respiratory measurements in awake and isoflurane-anesthetized horses, Am J Vet Res 1987;48:7.
12. Bonagura JD, Muir WW: The cardiovascular system. In Muir WW, Hubbell JAE, editors: Equine Anesthesia: Monitoring and Emergency Therapy, St Louis, 1991, Mosby.
13. Nout YS, Corley KT, Donaldson LL, et al: Indirect oscillometric and direct blood pressure measurements in anesthetized and conscious neonatal foals, J Vet Emerg Crit Care 2002;12:75.
14. Franco RM, Ousey JC, Cash RS, et al: Study of arterial blood pressure in newborn foals using an electronic sphygmomanometer, Equine Vet J 1986;18:475.
15. Koterba AM, Wozniak JA, Kosch PC: Ventilatory and timing parameters in normal horses at rest up to age one year, Equine Vet J 1995;27:257.
16. Stewart JH, Rose RJ, Barko AM: Respiratory studies in foals from birth to seven days old, Equine Vet J 1984;16:323.
17. Koterba AM, Kosch PC, Beech J, et al: Breathing strategy of the adult horse *(Equus caballus)* at rest, J Appl Physiol 1988;64:337.
18. Rose RJ, Hodgson DR, Leadon DP, et al: Effect of intranasal oxygen administration on arterial blood gas and acid base parameters in spontaneously delivered, term induced and induced premature foals, Res Vet Sci 1983;34:159.
19. Wagner AE, Muir WW 3rd, Hinchcliff KW: Cardiovascular effects of xylazine and detomidine in horses, Am J Vet Res 1991;52:651.
20. Stewart JH, Rose RJ, Barko AM: Response to oxygen administration

in foals: Effect of age, duration and method of administration on arterial blood gas values, Equine Vet J 1984;16:329.
21. Brewer BD, Clement SF, Lotz WS, et al: Renal clearance, urinary excretion of endogenous substances, and urinary diagnostic indices in healthy neonatal foals, J Vet Intern Med 1991;5:28.
22. Holdstock NB, Ousey JC, Rossdale PD: Glomerular filtration rate, effective renal plasma flow, blood pressure and pulse rate in the equine neonate during the first 10 days post partum, Equine Vet J 1998;30:335.
23. Gonda KC, Wilcke JR, Crisman MV, et al: Evaluation of iohexol clearance used to estimate glomerular filtration rate in clinically normal foals, Am J Vet Res 2003;64:1486.
24. Magdesian KG, Wilson WD, Mihalyi J: Pharmacokinetics of a high dose of amikacin administered at extended intervals to neonatal foals, Am J Vet Res 2004;65:473.
25. Green SL, Conlon PD, Mama K, et al: Effects of hypoxia and azotaemia on the pharmacokinetics of amikacin in neonatal foals, Equine Vet J 1992;24:475.
26. Geiser DR, Andrews FM, Rohrbach BW, et al: Cerebrospinal fluid acid-base status during normocapnia and acute hypercapnia in equine neonates, Am J Vet Res 1996;57:1483.
27. Saunders NR, Knott GW, Dziegielewska KM: Barriers in the immature brain, Cell Mol Neurobiol 2000;20:29.
28. Bauer JE, Harvey JW, Asquith RL, et al: Clinical chemistry reference values of foals during the first year of life, Equine Vet J 1984;16:361.
29. Smyth GB, Young DW, Duran SH: Maturation of insulin and glucose responses to normal feeding in foals. Aust Vet J 1993; 70:129.
30. Fowden AL, Silver M, Ellis L, et al: Studies on equine prematurity: 3. Insulin secretion in the foal during the perinatal period, Equine Vet J 1984;16:286.
31. Lumsden JH, Rowe R, Mullen K: Hematology and biochemistry reference values for the light horse, Can J Comp Med 1980;44:32.
32. Corley KT: Monitoring and treating haemodynamic disturbances in critically ill neonatal foals: Part 1. Haemodynamic monitoring, Equine Vet Educ 2002;14:270.
33. Harvey JW, Asquith RL, McNulty PK, et al: Haematology of foals up to one year old, Equine Vet J 1984;16:347.
34. Kami G, Merritt AM, Duelly P: Preliminary studies of plasma and extracellular fluid volume in neonatal ponies, Equine Vet J 1984;16:356.
35. Spensley MS, Carlson GP, Harrold D: Plasma, red blood cell, total blood, and extracellular fluid volumes in healthy horse foals during growth, Am J Vet Res 1987;48:1703.
36. Adamson PJ, Wilson WD, Baggot JD, et al: Influence of age on the disposition kinetics of chloramphenicol in equine neonates, Am J Vet Res 1991;52:426.
37. Carter SW, Robertson SA, Steel CJ, et al: Cardiopulmonary effects of xylazine sedation in the foal, Equine Vet J 1990;22:384.
38. Webb AI: Nasal intubation in the foal, J Am Vet Med Assoc 1984;185:48.
39. Dunlop CI: Anesthesia and sedation of foals, Vet Clin North Am Equine Pract 1994;10:67.
40. Robertson SA, Carter SW, Donovan M, et al: Effects of intravenous xylazine hydrochloride on blood glucose, plasma insulin and rectal temperature in neonatal foals, Equine Vet J 1990;22:43.
41. Oijala M, Katila T: Detomidine (Domosedan) in foals: Sedative and analgesic effects, Equine Vet J 1988;20:327.
42. Norman WM, Court MH, Greenblatt DJ: Age-related changes in the pharmacokinetic disposition of diazepam in foals, Am J Vet Res 1997;58:878.
43. Muir WW, Sams RA, Huffman RH, et al: Pharmacodynamic and pharmacokinetic properties of diazepam in horses, Am J Vet Res 1982;43:1756.
44. Robertson SA, Holcombe SJ, Colon J, et al: Comparison of xylazine or diazepam/butorphanol followed by ketamine and diazepam for induction of foals undergoing periosteal stripping. In Proceedings of the American College of Veterinary Anesthesiologists Annual Meeting, San Diego, Calif, 1997.
45. Richardson DW, Kohn CW: Uroperitoneum in the foal, J Am Vet Med Assoc 1983;182:267.
46. Matthews NS, Chaffin MK, Erickson SW, et al: Propofol anesthesia for non-surgical procedures of neonatal foals, Equine Pract 1995;17:15.
47. Wooten TL, Lowrie CT: Comparison of cerebrospinal fluid pressure in propofol- and thiopental-anesthetized eucapnic dogs, Vet Surg 1993;22:148.
48. Steffen F, Grasmueck S: Propofol for treatment of refractory seizures in dogs and a cat with intracranial disorders, J Small Anim Pract 2000;41:496.
49. Waterman AE, Robertson SA, Lane JG: Pharmacokinetics of intravenously administered ketamine in the horse, Res Vet Sci 1987;42:162.
50. Steffey EP, Willits N, Wong P, et al: Clinical investigations of halothane and isoflurane for induction and maintenance of foal anesthesia, J Vet Pharmacol Ther 1991;14:300.
51. Grosenbaugh DA, Muir WW: Cardiorespiratory effects of sevoflurane, isoflurane, and halothane anesthesia in horses, Am J Vet Res 1998;59:101.
52. Matthews NS, Hartsfield SM, Mercer D, et al: Recovery from sevoflurane anesthesia in horses: Comparison to isoflurane and effect of postmedication with xylazine, Vet Surg 1998;27:480.
53. Read MR, Read EK, Duke T, et al: Cardiopulmonary effects and induction and recovery characteristics of isoflurane and sevoflurane in foals, J Am Vet Med Assoc 2002;221:393.
54. Wilcke JR, Crisman MV, Sams RA, et al: Pharmacokinetics of phenylbutazone in neonatal foals, Am J Vet Res 1993;54:2064.
55. Breuhaus BA, DeGraves FJ, Honore EK, et al: Pharmacokinetics of ibuprofen after intravenous and oral administration and assessment of safety of administration to healthy foals, Am J Vet Res 1999;60:1066.
56. Wilcke JR, Crisman MV, Scarratt WK, et al: Pharmacokinetics of ketoprofen in healthy foals less than twenty-four hours old, Am J Vet Res 1998;59:290.
57. Crisman MV, Wilcke JR, Sams RA: Pharmacokinetics of flunixin meglumine in healthy foals less than twenty-four hours old, Am J Vet Res 1996;57:1759.
58. Semrad SD, Sams RA, Ashcraft SM: Pharmacokinetics of and serum thromboxane suppression by flunixin meglumine in healthy foals during the first month of life, Am J Vet Res 1993;54:2083.
59. Leveille R, Miyabayashi T, Weisbrode SE, et al: Ultrasonographic renal changes associated with phenylbutazone administration in three foals, Can Vet J 1996;37:235.
60. Carrick JB, Papich MG, Middleton DM, et al: Clinical and pathological effects of flunixin meglumine administration to neonatal foals, Can J Vet Res 1989;53:195.
61. Corley KT: Monitoring and treating haemodynamic disturbances in critically ill neonatal foals: Part 2. Assessment and treatment, Equine Vet Educ 2002;14:328.
62. Corley KT, Donaldson LL, Furr MO: Comparison of lithium dilution and thermodilution cardiac output measurements in anaesthetised neonatal foals, Equine Vet J 2002;34:598.
63. Gunkel CI, Valverde A, Morey TE, et al: Comparison of non-invasive cardiac output measurement by partial carbon dioxide rebreathing with the lithium dilution method in anesthetized dogs, J Vet Emerg Crit Care 2004;14:1.
64. Chaffin MK, Matthews NS, Cohen ND, et al: Evaluation of pulse oximetry in anaesthetised foals using multiple combinations of transducer type and transducer attachment site, Equine Vet J 1996;28:437.
65. Geiser DR, Rohrbach BW: Use of end-tidal CO_2 tension to predict arterial CO_2 values in isoflurane-anesthetized equine neonates, Am J Vet Res 1992;53:1617.
66. Hackett TB: Pulse oximetry and end tidal carbon dioxide monitoring, Vet Clin North Am Small Anim Pract 2002;32:1021.
67. Teixeira Neto FJ, Carregaro AB, Mannarino R, et al: Comparison of

a sidestream capnograph and a mainstream capnograph in mechanically ventilated dogs, J Am Vet Med Assoc 2002;221:1582.
68. Hunt TK, Hopf HW: Wound healing and wound infection: What surgeons and anesthesiologists can do, Surg Clin North Am 1997;77:587.
69. Gore DC, Chinkes D, Heggers J, et al: Association of hyperglycemia with increased mortality after severe burn injury, J Trauma 2001;51:540.
70. DiNardo MM, Korytkowski MT, Siminerio LS: The importance of normoglycemia in critically ill patients, Crit Care Nurs Q 2004;27:126.
71. Cohn LA, McCaw DL, Tate DJ, et al: Assessment of five portable blood glucose meters, a point-of-care analyzer, and color test strips for measuring blood glucose concentration in dogs, J Am Vet Med Assoc 2000;216:198.
72. Magdesian KG: Monitoring the critically ill equine patient, Vet Clin North Am Equine Pract 2004;20:11.
73. Schmied H, Kurz A, Sessler DI, et al: Mild hypothermia increases blood loss and transfusion requirements during total hip arthroplasty, Lancet 1996;347:289.
74. Doufas AG: Consequences of inadvertent perioperative hypothermia, Best Pract Res Clin Anaesthesiol 2003;17:535.
75. Kurz A, Sessler DI, Lenhardt R: Perioperative normothermia to reduce the incidence of surgical-wound infection and shorten hospitalization. Study of Wound Infection and Temperature Group, N Engl J Med 1996;334:1209.
76. Tomasic M, Nann LE: Comparison of peripheral and core temperatures in anesthetized horses, Am J Vet Res 1999;60:648.
77. Martin RG, McMeniman NP, Dowsett KF: Milk and water intakes of foals sucking grazing mares, Equine Vet J 1992;24:295.
78. Palmer JE: Fluid therapy in the neonate: not your mother's fluid space, Vet Clin North Am Equine Pract 2004;20:63.
79. Belgrave RL, Hines MT, Keegan RD, et al: Effects of a polymerized ultrapurified bovine hemoglobin blood substitute administered to ponies with normovolemic anemia, J Vet Intern Med 2002;16:396.
80. Young LE, Blissitt KJ, Clutton RE, et al: Temporal effects of an infusion of dobutamine hydrochloride in horses anesthetized with halothane, Am J Vet Res 1998;59:1027.
81. Swanson CR, Muir WW 3rd, Bednarski RM, et al: Hemodynamic responses in halothane-anesthetized horses given infusions of dopamine or dobutamine, Am J Vet Res 1985;46:365.
82. Holmes CL, Landry DW, Granton JT: Science review: Vasopressin and the cardiovascular system: Part 2. Clinical physiology, Crit Care 2004;8:15.
83. Corley KT: Inotropes and vasopressors in adults and foals, Vet Clin North Am Equine Pract 2004;20:77.
84. Peden CJ, Menon DK, Hall AS, et al: Magnetic resonance for the anaesthetist: Part II. Anaesthesia and monitoring in MR units, Anaesthesia 1992;47:508.
85. Dempsey MF, Condon B: Thermal injuries associated with MRI, Clin Radiol 2001;56:457.
86. Edwards RB, Ducharme NG, Hackett RP: Laparoscopic repair of a bladder rupture in a foal, Vet Surg 1995;24:60.
87. Donaldson LL, Trostle SS, White NA: Cardiopulmonary changes associated with abdominal insufflation of carbon dioxide in mechanically ventilated, dorsally recumbent, halothane anaesthetised horses, Equine Vet J 1988;30:144.

CHAPTER 22

Recovery from Anesthesia

Regula Bettschart-Wolfensberger

Recovery is one of the most critical phases of equine anesthesia. Recent results from a multicenter prospective study of equine anesthetic fatalities reported that 23% of all nonsurvivors sustained inoperable orthopedic lesions during recovery.[1] Because of the size and temperament of the horse, it is not possible to continue full monitoring, and mechanical ventilation during recovery and even fluid administration are discontinued in most cases. Significant problems such as hypoxemia or hypotension that may develop can be recognized only in severe cases. Once the horse starts to wake up, intervention is dangerous for personnel and, depending on the size of the horse and its temperament, often simply impossible. This chapter describes all aspects of recovery from anesthesia in horses.

MANAGEMENT OF HORSES DURING RECOVERY

General Aspects

During recovery, external stimuli (noise, bright light, physical stimuli) should be minimized. The horse's head should be protected by a padded head cover. The recovery box should have a padded floor and walls. Ideally, the box would have an octagonal shape to prevent horses from being trapped in the corners. In some clinics, horses are placed on heavy foam pads for the recovery. These pads prevent the patients from making premature attempts to rise, because it takes a controlled and coordinated effort to "get out" of them and attain sternal recumbency. Frequently, human assistance is necessary to roll them from the mattress onto the recovery box floor. Because the patients cannot leave the mattress too early, there is additional time for inhalant anesthetic to be exhaled, which eventually results in a smoother recovery. Soft mattresses may also prevent nerve damage in cases of prolonged recovery. Depending on the nature of the surgery, the premises, and the personal preferences of anesthetists and surgeons involved, assistance during recovery (ropes, slings, hoists) may be desirable.[2] Sling assistance is sometimes (6%) not well tolerated, and to prevent self-inflicted injury, the patients may have to be reanesthetized. Fracture patients are most successfully recovered in a hydro pool (my personal experience).

In the early stages of recovery, an anesthetist should stay with the horse. Thereafter, continuous observation of the horse will reveal problems at an early stage, allowing immediate intervention. Ideally, horses remain recumbent for at least 20 minutes and then roll into sternal recumbency for another 10 to 20 minutes. The attainment of sternal recumbency is associated with the restoration of more normal breathing patterns, and it reduces ventilation-perfusion mismatching in the lung, which should improve oxygenation.[3] Horses that rest in sternal recumbency prior to attempting to stand usually then stand without complication. They recover best if they are allowed to exhale all of the volatile anesthetic agent before trying to stand and thus should not be stimulated to get up too soon. If a horse has not attempted to stand within 60 minutes after the end of anesthesia and is still in lateral recumbency, stimulation may be appropriate. If it is reluctant to get up, its status must be reevaluated and any problems treated.

For any surgery longer than 1 hour, the use of a urinary catheter is recommended, as it prevents overdistention of the bladder, which is uncomfortable for the horse. Without a urinary catheter, a horse often tries to get up before it is ready to do so. As soon as it is standing, despite being ataxic, it will try to urinate. This can represent a considerable risk, as the floor can become slippery and the horse may lose its balance and injure itself.

Maintenance of Adequate Respiration during Recovery

Insufflation of oxygen (15 L/min per 500 kg), first via the endotracheal tube and after extubation via nasal tubes or directly into the nasal cavity, helps to reduce the development of hypoxemia.[4] If apnea is present, the use of a demand valve helps to ventilate the horse until spontaneous respiration resumes.[5] Short periods of apnea (3 to 5 minutes)—for example, during transport from the surgery suite to the recovery stall—are not harmful. One study demonstrated that mechanically ventilated, anesthetized horses maintain higher values for partial pressure of arterial oxygen (Pa_{O_2}) postoperatively during a brief period of apnea than horses weaned from the ventilator prior to disconnection.[6]

Controversy exists as to the optimal point during recovery for removal of the endotracheal tube. Most anesthetists advocate the removal of the endotracheal tube once the horse is actively swallowing. The presence of an active swallowing reflex helps to ensure that fluid or gastric reflux is not aspirated and that the horse replaces its soft palate into the normal position. Others believe that the tube should be removed only once the horse is standing. Extubation while the horse is in lateral recumbency allows earlier identification of potential respiratory obstruction. The endotracheal tube is then easily reintroduced, and if necessary a tracheostomy can be performed, which would be very difficult in a standing horse with acute dyspnea.

Another reason to remove the endotracheal tube as soon as the horse is swallowing is that some horses will object to this foreign body once they regain consciousness. This negatively influences recovery because the animal may try to get up too early. Therefore, I prefer to remove the endotracheal tube prior to the horse's regaining a standing position. An alternative to this approach is to remove the endotracheal tube once the swallowing reflex is regained, and to place a small endotracheal tube via the nares for recovery. This technique avoids the inadvertent damage to the endotracheal tube from the teeth and still maintains a patent airway (see later).

Most recumbent horses develop nasal edema, and because horses are obligate nasal breathers, this swelling will impair breathing after removal of the endotracheal tube. In severe cases, significant airway obstruction may occur. Transient airway obstruction during recovery can also be caused by a variety of other problems, such as laryngospasm, laryngeal hemiplegia,[7] dorsal displacement of the soft palate, kinking of the head in a corner of the recovery box, or obstructing foreign bodies in the upper airways. Regardless of the cause, any airway obstruction may lead to pulmonary edema or pulmonary hemorrhage, resulting in cardiovascular collapse and death.[7-10]

Phenylephrine (0.15%) can be instilled into the nares to decrease nasal congestion and help prevent obstruction after extubation. An alternative is to insert nasal tubes approximately 20 cm long into one or both nasal cavities. It is necessary to have various diameters available to fit a wide range of horses. Fractious animals find this tube in their nares uncomfortable, however, and I prefer the use of an anticongestant. To achieve optimal effect, the drops are instilled 10 minutes before extubation. If, despite the use of nasal drops, labored breathing or snoring occurs after extubation, nasal tubes should be inserted and the head extended with the tongue pulled out. Should this not result in normal regular breathing, other causes of airway obstruction should be investigated. Orotracheal intubation or a temporary tracheostomy may become inevitable in these cases.

Management of Cardiovascular Function

Administration of fluids, dobutamine, or other vasopressive agents is usually discontinued before recovery. All inhalation anesthetics and total intravenous anesthesia regimens depress cardiovascular function in a dose dependent manner.[11] At the end of anesthesia, the administration of these agents is stopped. Modern anesthetics are relatively quickly exhaled or redistributed, and thus cardiovascular function improves rapidly during recovery, and it is usually not necessary to administer fluids in the recovery period. If horses suffer from severe blood loss or hypotension (possibly as a result of endotoxemia) during anesthesia, continuing fluid administration and inotropic support during recovery is advocated. Depending on the severity of the condition, such horses continue to lose fluid from their circulating volume and thus have problems in maintaining adequate cardiovascular function despite waning of the depressive effect of anesthetic agents. Such horses, especially if they are large, have great difficulty in getting up.

FACTORS INFLUENCING RECOVERY

Severity of Surgery, Temperament of the Horse

Under clinical circumstances, the quality of recovery and ultimate outcome correlate negatively with duration of anesthesia and severity of surgery.[1,12] On the other hand, under experimental conditions, when horses were anesthetized with isoflurane or halothane but did not undergo surgery, the temperament of the individual was the major factor determining the quality of recovery.[13] Therefore, it follows that recovery after surgery in some horses will correlate well with their temperaments.

Inhalation Anesthetic

Different inhalation anesthetics possess different physical properties (see Chapter 19). Blood gas solubility is the major determinant of the speed of action of an anesthetic and thus duration of recovery. With halothane, the relatively high rate of metabolism (about 20%), in comparison to isoflurane (about 0.2%) or sevoflurane (2% to 3%), may have an influence on the quality of recovery in compromised patients. An early report that investigated duration and quality of recovery after 2 hours of anesthesia showed that recovery after isoflurane anesthesia is quicker and of a better quality than after halothane anesthesia.[14] After 3 hours of anesthesia,[13] no difference in duration or quality of recovery was detected between isoflurane and halothane. In another report,[15] the recoveries of horses with or without surgery with isoflurane or halothane were compared. These authors found no difference in the quality of recovery but reported shorter recoveries following isoflurane. This is in contrast to clinical studies that showed that recoveries with halothane are of better quality.[16-18] Another experimental study compared halothane, isoflurane, and sevoflurane and found that recovery quality was better with sevoflurane and halothane, and duration was shorter with sevoflurane and isoflurane.[11] Comparison of recovery after just 90 minutes of isoflurane or sevoflurane anesthesia showed that horses recovered significantly quicker and better with sevoflurane than with isoflurane.[19] To date, there are no reports that compare the quality of recovery of desflurane (the least soluble and therefore fastest-acting inhalant agent presently available) with other inhalant anesthetics. In one report investigating desflurane in ponies,[20] it was stated that "recovery from anesthesia was very rapid, although the quality in the unrestrained ponies was unacceptable."

Sedation, Analgesia

Pain has a negative influence on recovery in horses. To prevent central and peripheral sensitization, analgesia should be addressed before and during the anesthetic period. To provide maximal analgesia for recovery, especially after long, major surgical procedures, some additional analgesia, preferably using a multimodal approach, should be provided (see Chapter 23) (Table 22-1). In a clinical study of 25 horses undergoing arthroscopy, the preoperative use of phenylbu-

TABLE 22-1. Dosages of Drug Used during Recovery in Horses

Drug	Dose/Administration	Indication, Effects	Untoward Effects
Acepromazine	0.03 mg/kg IM (very slowly IV)	Sedation, improvement of perfusion	Hypotension
Xylazine	0.1-0.2 mg/kg slowly IV	Sedation, analgesia	Cardiovascular depression
Medetomidine	2 μg/kg slowly IV	Sedation, analgesia	Cardiovascular depression
Detomidine	1-5 μg/kg slowly IV	Sedation, analgesia	Cardiovascular depression
Romifidine	5-20 μg/kg slowly IV	Sedation, analgesia	Cardiovascular depression
Morphine	0.1-0.2 mg/kg IM (IV)	Analgesia	Minimal after single application
Methadone	0.1-0.2 mg/kg IV (IM)	Analgesia	Minimal after single application
Pethidine	1-2 mg/kg IM	Analgesia	Minimal after single application
Butorphanol	0.02-0.04 mg/kg IV (IM)	Analgesia	Minimal after single application
Dobutamine	Up to 1.25 μg/kg/min IV	Cardiovascular depression, hypotension	Untoward effects at recommended dose rare, tachyarrhythmias with higher doses
Hypertonic saline (7%)	2-6 mL/kg IV over 10-20 min, followed by isotonic electrolyte solutions	Shock, hypovolemia	Bradycardia, hypotension after rapid infusion
Hetastarch/pentastarch	5-10 mL/kg IV together with Ringer's lactate (1:2)	Shock, fatigue	—
Dimethyl sulfoxide	0.5-1 g/kg IV, dilute to conc. <20%, administer slowly (over several hours together with Ringer's lactate)	Myopathy, neuropathy	Hemolysis if administered undiluted
Dexamethasone	2 mg/kg IV	Myopathy, neuropathy	Laminitis
Methylprednisolone	2-8 mg/kg IV	Myopathy, neuropathy	Laminitis
Calcium	0.1-0.2 mEq/kg very slowly IV (over 30 min)	Hypocalcemia, Hyperkalemia	Bradyarrhythmias or tachyarrhythmias

tazone did not alter recovery time but did slightly improve recovery score compared with patients not receiving this nonsteroidal anti-inflammatory drug (NSAID).[21] These results are somewhat in contrast to the previous statements, which advocated continuous administration of analgesics during anesthesia.

The use of opioids in horses is controversial because of the fear of excitement and because of the effect of the opioids on the gastrointestinal tract. Some authors have tried to show the benefit of using opioids for recovery[22,23] but have failed to do so, probably because too many other factors also influence this period. They were, however, able to show that opioids do not negatively influence and prolong recovery or result in an elevated $Pa{CO_2}$ level compared with that in untreated horses. In my experience, every horse benefits from the administration of morphine (0.1 mg/kg IM) 10 minutes before disconnection from the inhalation anesthetic.

α_2-Adrenoceptor agonists such as xylazine slightly prolong the recovery period.[19,24] In clinical cases, this usually results in superior recoveries. The fact that α_2-adrenoceptor agonists act not only as sedatives but also as analgesics certainly adds positively to the calming effect. Most authors advocate the use of 0.1 to 0.2 mg/kg xylazine IV; others use low doses of detomidine, romifidine, or medetomidine.[25] Because α_2-adrenoceptor agonists negatively influence cardiovascular function, the use of low doses of xylazine (especially in compromised patients) is probably safest, as its side effects are less severe and of shorter duration. The α_2-adrenoceptor agonists should be administered only once brisk palpebral reflexes or even nystagmus is present. This guarantees that levels of inhalation anesthetics are lower than during maintenance of anesthesia and that overdose is prevented. Slow administration of the sedative (the full dose over 1 minute or slower) reduces the risk of profound side effects and thus probably increases safety.

Recovery Stall Design and Construction

Although there is no literature comparing the influence of different types of recovery stalls on fatality rates, most anesthetists agree on a number of important design features for recovery stalls. First of all, the recovery box should not be too large; this allows the horses to lean against the walls during their arousal or as soon as they are standing, because most horses show some degree of ataxia immediately after recovery. Ideally, the angles between walls are greater than 90 degrees (Fig. 22-1) to prevent horses getting trapped in a corner with their head in a kinked position. Padding of walls and floor is most important. Floors should provide secure footing with a surface that is not slippery, even when wet (urine, blood, excessive sweating, obstetrical lubricant). On the other hand, the surface must be soft enough to prevent abrasion injuries if horses fall during recovery. Last but not least, the padding should be easy to clean. Linatex (Four D Rubber Co, Ltd, Heanor, Derbyshire, UK) is a commercially available surface providing these qualities.

A recovery stall should also have metal rings (for attaching ropes), an oxygen supply, heating, air conditioning, lights that can be dimmed, a hoist, and easy access for recovery personnel in case of an emergency. Figure 22-2 shows a design for a recovery stall that allows intervention and help

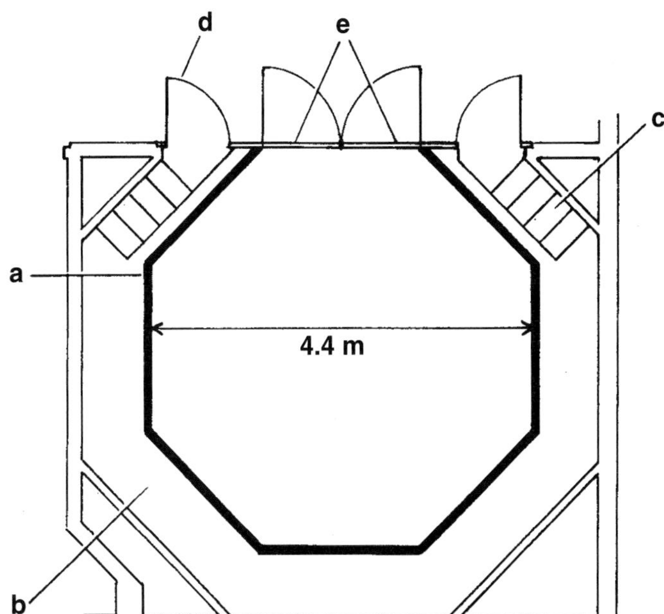

Figure 22-1. Birds-eye view of recovery box, including walkway around the box with access to the horse from above. *a,* Recovery stall wall; *b,* the walkway, the floor of which is elevated relative to the recovery box floor, provides ideal, safe position to assist horse's recovery; *c,* staircase to walkway; *d,* doors to walkway; *e,* doors to recovery box.

for the horse from outside the box, thereby minimizing the risk of injury to people. The ideal size of a recovery box depends on the horse's size. The best option is to have several of different sizes. The size of the box in Figures 22-1 and 22-2 has proved optimal for horses ranging in size from 400 to 800 kg.

Pool Recovery

The major benefit of recovery in a hydro pool is that self-inflicted trauma is minimized because the partially submerged horse struggles against the resistance of the water until it is fully capable of standing. For the people involved in recovery, there is minimal danger while the horse is inside the pool. The critical phase is the removal of the horse from the pool. There are two different systems. At the University of Pennsylvania's New Bolton Center, the horses are secured in a raft inside a round pool. The raft contains a sleeve for each leg and a flotation ring that has supports for the head. With this design, the horse has only minimal contact with the water. However, the stabilization of the horse inside such a pool can be difficult and requires several people during the entire recovery period. Removing the horses from this pool requires them to be lifted out of the raft by a sling attached to an overhead hoist (Fig. 22-3). In this critical phase, if horses do not cooperate, injuries might occur. It may be necessary to implement short-term sedation or anesthesia until the horse is safely in a stall.

Another hydro pool system has been designed to facilitate the process of getting the horse out of the water.[26] The pool has a rectangular shape with the following measurements: 3.5 m long, 1.2 m wide, 2.5 m deep. The water is heated to 38° C and continuously filtered to remove dirt.

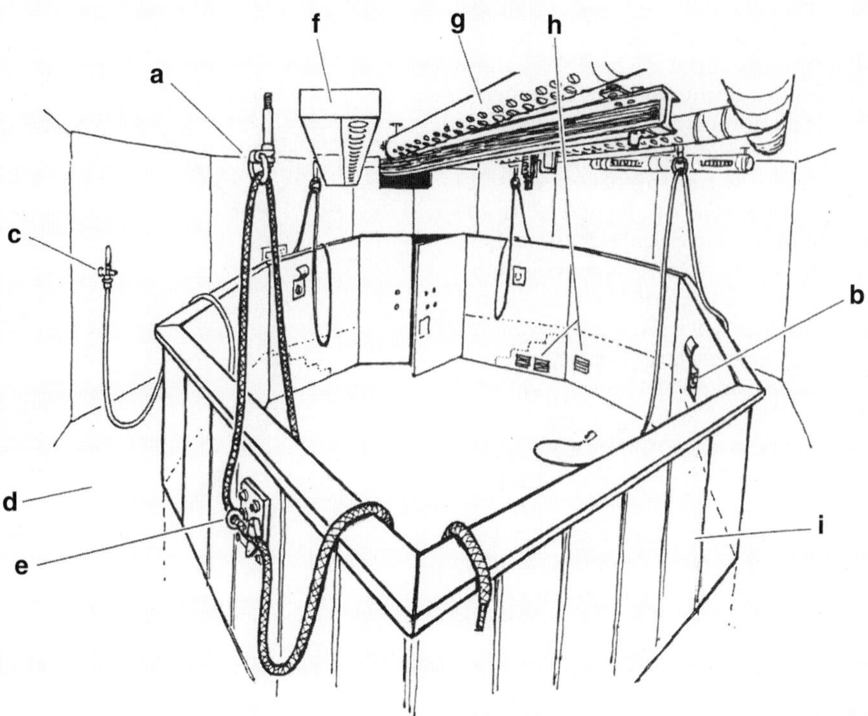

Figure 22-2. Lateral view from the walkway around the recovery box. *a,* Metal rings attached to the ceiling and *b,* metal rings in the recovery box wall to engage ropes for assisted recovery; *c,* oxygen supply; *d,* walkway; *e,* quick-release devices for attaching ropes firmly; *f,* row of infrared lamps; *g,* air conditioning; *h,* fresh air supply *(left),* air removal-suction *(right)*; i, recovery box wall.

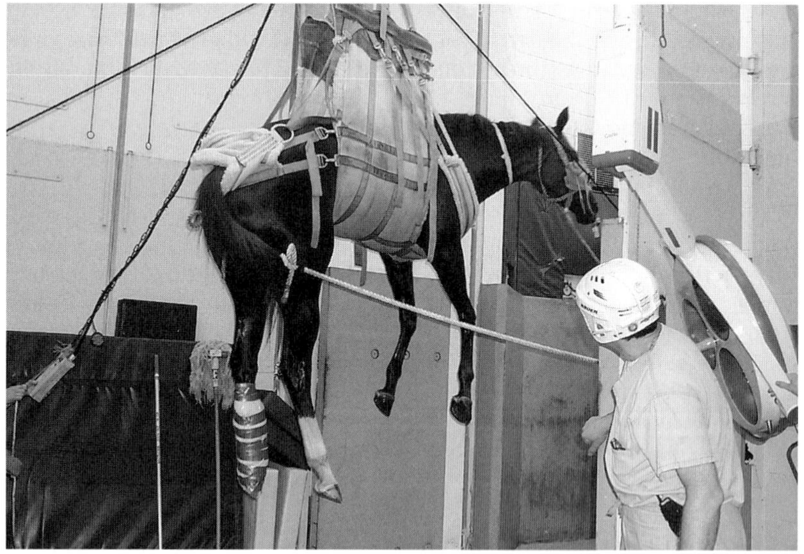

Figure 22-3. Lifting of a horse out of the pool with a Liftex-sling at the New Bolton Centre. (Photograph courtesy of Larry Nann.)

Additionally, bacterial contamination is minimized by passing the water through an ultraviolet filter. Because the horse is immersed in the water, it is impossible to totally prevent exposure of the surgical site to water, so application of a routine bandage for recovery is contraindicated. The wound is covered with an Ioban bandage (Ioban 2, 3M Health Care, St. Paul, Minn) and additional linear application of cyanoacrylate (superglue) around the entire incision. The Ioban sheet is further protected by an elastic adhesive tape.

The horse is placed inside the pool restrained by a sling or a net designed for the helicopter rescue of horses (Fig. 22-4). At that time, the scissor table installed within the pool is collapsed all the way to the bottom of the tank. While the horse is unconscious, its head is supported by a floating mattress. The horse is maintained in a sternal position in the

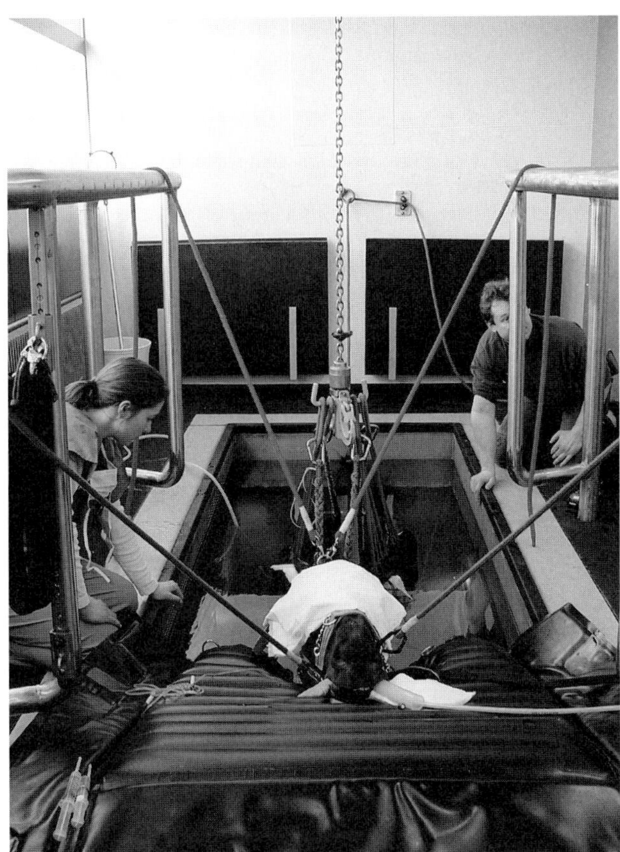

Figure 22-4. A horse recovering from anesthesia in the pool at the University of Zurich. The head is fixed with four ropes on the side bars, the head rests on an air mattress, and the body is secured in the water with a custom recovery net. The eyes are covered and ear-plugs are in place.

water. The head is secured in a vertical position by several ropes attached to metal bars on the sides of the pool (see Fig. 22-4). Once the horse starts to move, the table is elevated by a hydraulic system and the horse allowed to "feel" the table underneath its feet. After the patient has stood securely on all four feet in the water for some time, the table is elevated, pushing the horse up to the level of the room floor (Fig. 22-5). The sling is subsequently removed, the bandage removed, the surgical site prepared aseptically, a bandage reapplied, and once ready, the horse is walked into the recovery box, where it is allowed to dry under an infrared solarium.

This type of hydro pool was originally designed in California[26] and has since been used regularly at Washington State University, Del Mar Race Track, and at the Vetsuisse Faculty University of Zurich, Switzerland. A report on the use of this type of recovery pool on 60 horses documented the following[27]: mean anesthesia time, 182 minutes; mean time in the pool, 108 minutes (range 20 to 270 minutes). Furthermore, three horses showed severe lung edema (one of them died), two horses showed multiple skin abrasions from violent attempts to leave the pool during recovery, two horses showed incisional infections, and one horse developed septic arthritis following stifle joint surgery. These results demonstrate that hydro pool recovery is not risk free, but that it is a relatively safe option when a difficult recovery is anticipated.

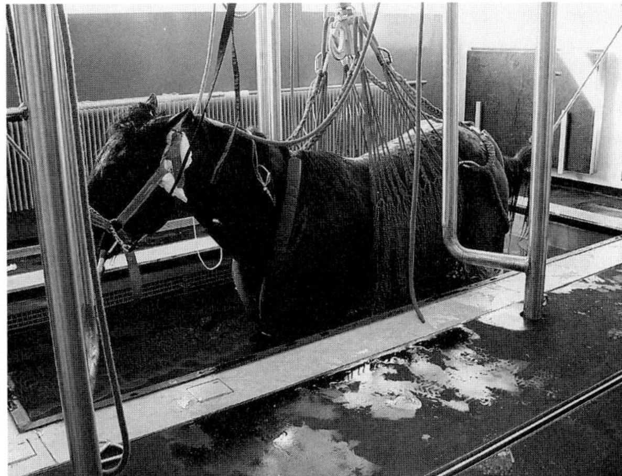

Figure 22-5. A patient quietly standing on the scissor table with the feet still in the water. The recovery net is still in place.

During hydro pool recovery, extrathoracic and pulmonary pressures are increased,[28] which may contribute to an increased incidence of pulmonary edema during anesthetic recovery. To minimize the likelihood of edema formation, all anesthetized horses in Zurich are treated with hetastarch (10%, 4 L/500 kg IV, in addition to Ringer's lactate) to maintain plasma oncotic pressure during hydro pool recovery. Furthermore, acepromazine (0.03 mg/kg) is administered (IM) to produce peripheral vasodilatation and improve perfusion. The administration of acepromazine also provides some calming effect during recovery, without causing ataxia. Supplemental oxygen has decreased the incidence of edema at Washington State.[29] As with any surgery, it is very important to provide multimodal analgesia to optimize recovery quality before hydro pool recovery. For any orthopedic surgery, I advocate the presurgical administration of phenylbutazone, α_2-agonists, and possibly opioids (e.g., morphine 0.1 to 0.2 mg/kg IM); the intraoperative use of a balanced anesthesia regimen (e.g., isoflurane in oxygen + 3.5 mcg/kg per hour medetomidine IV); plus additional analgesia for recovery (e.g., 2 mcg/kg medetomidine IV + 0.1 mg/kg morphine IM). The use of an α_2-agonist such as medetomidine for recovery is advantageous because it provides analgesia as well as sedation. Using this management protocol, lung edema has not occurred in 19 consecutive pool recoveries.

PROBLEMS ENCOUNTERED DURING RECOVERY

Reluctance or Inability to Stand

Most problems that become evident during recovery have developed during anesthesia. Hypotension (resulting in poor muscle perfusion), hypoxemia, and malpositioning on the surgery table are the major factors that result in the problems encountered during recovery in horses.[30-37] Possible causes of prolonged recoveries follow.

Myopathies

Myopathies may affect single groups of muscles or they can occur in a generalized form. Myopathies occur most frequently if hypotension (blood pressure less than

70 mm Hg) is present for more than 15 minutes or anesthesia time exceeds 3 hours.[38,39] Affected muscles are swollen to different degrees and are very painful. Depending on the severity of the myopathy, horses may be unable to stand. Therapy of the acute phase is supportive and symptomatic and should aim at reducing pain, swelling, and anxiety. NSAIDs, opioids, α_2-agonists, and, in severe cases, dimethyl sulfoxide (DMSO), dantrolene sodium, and corticosteroids should be administered. A small dose of acepromazine (0.02 to 0.03 mg/kg IM) may help to calm the horse and to improve peripheral perfusion, but this should be administered only if no major cardiovascular disturbances are present. As long as the horses are recumbent, oxygen should be administered via nasal tubes or directly into the nasal cavity. Ringer's lactate solution or other balanced electrolyte solutions should be infused to help maintain cardiovascular function. In excited horses, the most important factor is to calm them, as repeated attempts to stand up exhaust the horse and the likelihood of a catastrophic injury increases. Head and tail ropes help the horse to lift its weight when getting up and provide some stability, because most affected horses show some degree of ataxia. Be aware that some horses resent the pull on the tail and abandon attempts to get on their feet.

Once the horse is standing, the major life-threatening problem is myoglobinuria resulting in kidney dysfunction. Appropriate fluid administration (to ensure maintenance of urine output) and monitoring of urine production are mandatory. Physiotherapy and infrared light may help the horse to relax its muscles and thus will reduce suffering.

Neuropathies

Neuropathies that impair recovery include femoral nerve paralysis, radial or brachial nerve paralysis, peroneal nerve paralysis, and hemorrhagic myelopathy. Neuropathies can also be accompanied by myopathies, and vice versa. Horses suffering from neuropathies of single nerves are not at as high risk as horses suffering from severe myopathies, but the risk of fractures during recovery is relatively high in all horses with neurologic weakness. Horses are often unable to cope with paralyzed extremities: they get excited and injure themselves before intervention becomes possible. Therapy during recovery is symptomatic and supportive, as for myopathies.

Other, less common causes of reluctance, difficulty, or inability to stand after general anesthesia are hyperkalemic periodic paralysis (HYPP), hypocalcemia, glycogen disease of draft horses, fractures or luxations, severe hypothermia or blood loss, generalized fatigue as a result of underlying disease, and pulmonary embolism.[40]

REFERENCES

1. Johnston GM, Eastment JK, Taylor PM, et al: Is isoflurane safer than halothane in equine anesthesia? Results from a prospective multicentre randomised controlled trial, Equine Vet J 2004;36:64.
2. Liechti J, Pauli H, Jäggin N, et al: Untersuchungen zum assistierten Aufstehen von Pferden während der Aufwachphase nach einer Inhalationsanästhesie, Pferdeheilkunde 2003;19:271.
3. Gasthuys F, DeMoor A, Parmentier D: Haemodynamic effects of change in position and respiration mode during a standard halothane anesthesia in ponies, Schweiz Arch Tierheilk 1991;38:203.
4. Duckert J, Schatzmann U, Ammann E: Die postnarkotische Hypoxämie und ihre Therapie beim Pferd, Pferdeheilkunde 1985;1:95.
5. Waterman AE, Jones RS, Richards DLS: Use of a demand valve for postoperative administration of oxygen to horses, Equine Vet J 1982;14:290.
6. Wright B, Hildebrand S: An evaluation of apnea or spontaneous ventilation in early recovery following mechanical ventilation in the anesthetized horse, J Vet Anaesth Analg 2001;28:26-33.
7. Abrahamsen EJ, Bohanon TC, Bedmarski RM, et al: Bilateral arytenoid cartilage paralysis after inhalation anesthesia in a horse, J Am Vet Med Assoc 1990;10:1363-1365.
8. Kollias-Baker CA, Pipers FS, Heard D, et al: Pulmonary edema associated with transient airway obstruction in three horses, J Am Vet Med Assoc 1993;202:1116-1118.
9. Ball MA, Trim CM: Post anesthetic pulmonary oedema in two horses, Equine Vet Educ 1996;8:13-16.
10. Tute AS, Wilkins PA, Gleed RD: Negative pressure pulmonary edema as a postanesthetic complication associated with upper airway obstruction in a horse, Vet Surg 1996;25:519-523.
11. Grosenbaugh DA, Muir WW: Cardiorespiratory effects of sevoflurane, isoflurane, and halothane anesthesia in horses, Am J Vet Res 1998;59:101-106.
12. Young SS, Taylor PM: Factors influencing the outcome of equine anesthesia: A review of 1314 cases, Equine Vet J 1993;25:147-151.
13. Whitehair KJ, Steffey EP, Willits NH, et al: Recovery of horses from inhalation anesthesia, Am J Vet Res 1993;54:1693-1702.
14. Auer JA, Garner HE, Amend JF, et al: Recovery from anesthesia in ponies: A comparative study of the effects of isoflurane, enflurane, methoxyflurane and halothane, Equine Vet J 1978;10:18-23.
15. Matthews NS, Miller SM, Hartsfield SM, et al: Comparison of recoveries from halothane vs isoflurane anesthesia in horses, J Am Vet Med Assoc 1992;201:559-563.
16. Taylor PM, Watkins SB: Isoflurane in the horse, J Assoc Vet Anaest 1984;12:191-194.
17. Rose JA, Rose EM, Robin P: Clinical experience with isoflurane anesthesia in foals and adult horses, Proc Am Assoc Equine Pract 1989;34:555-561.
18. Donaldson LL, Dunlop GS, Holland MS, et al: The recovery of horses from inhalant anaesthesia: A comparison of halothane and isoflurane, Vet Surg 2000;29:92-101.
19. Matthews NS, Hartsfield SM, Mercer D, et al: Recovery from sevoflurane anesthesia in horses: comparison to isoflurane and effect of postmedication with xylazine, Vet Surg 1998;27:480-485.
20. Jones N, Clarke KW, Clegg P: Desflurane in equine anaesthesia: A preliminary trial, Vet Rec 1995;137:618-620.
21. Raekallio M, Taylor PM, Bennett RC: Preliminary investigation of pain and analgesia assessment in horses administered phenylbutazone or placebo after arthroscopic surgery, Vet Surg 1997;26:150-155.
22. Taylor PM: Effect of postoperative pethidine on the anaesthetic recovery period in the horse, Equine Vet J 1986;18:70-72.
23. Mircica E, Clutton RE, Kyles KW: Problems associated with perioperative morphine in horses: A retrospective case analysis, J Vet Anaesth Analg 2003;30:147-155.
24. Santos M, Fuente M, Garcia-Iturralde P, et al: Effects of alpha-2 adrenoceptor agonists during recovery from isoflurane anaesthesia in horses, Equine Vet J 2003;35:170-175.
25. Taylor PM: Equine anesthesia, Equine Vet Data 1992;13:274-275.
26. Herthel DJ: Systems for recovery from anesthesia. In Nixon AJ, editor: Equine Fracture Repair, Philadelphia, 1996, WB Saunders.
27. Tidwell SA, Schneider RK, Ragle CA: Use of a hydro-pool system to recover horses after general anesthesia: 60 cases, Vet Surg 2002;31:455-461.
28. Richter MC, Bayly WM, Keegan RD, et al: Cardiopulmonary function in horses during anesthetic recovery in a hydro pool, Am J Vet Res 2001;62:1903-1910.
29. Schneider RK: Personal communication, 2004.

30. Trim CM, Mason J: Post anaesthetic forelimb lameness in horses, Equine Vet J 1974;5:71.
31. Friend SCE: Postanesthetic myonecrosis in horses, Can Vet J 1981;22:367-371.
32. Lindsay WA, Pascoe PJ, McDonell WN, et al: Effect of protective padding on forelimb intracompartmental muscle pressures in anesthetized horses, Am J Vet Res 1985;46:688-691.
33. Lindsay WA, Robinson GM, Brunson DB, et al: Induction of equine postanesthetic myositis after halothane induced hypotension, Am J Vet Res 1989;50:404-410.
34. Brearley JC, Jones RS, Kelly DF, et al: Spinal cord degeneration following general anesthesia in a shire horse, Equine Vet J 1986;18:222-224.
35. Dodman NH, Williams R, Court MH, et al: Postanesthetic hind limb adductor myopathy in five horses, J Am Vet Med Assoc 1988;193:83-86.
36. Taylor PM: Risks of recumbency in the anaesthetized horse, Equine Vet J 1984;16:77-80.
37. Dyson S, Taylor PM, Whitwell K: Femoral nerve paralyses after general anaesthesia, Equine Vet J 1988;20:376-380.
38. Grandy JL, Steffey EP, Hodgson DS, et al: Arterial hypotension and the development of postanesthetic myopathy in halothane-anesthetized horses, Am J Vet Res 1987;48:192-197.
39. Richey MT, Holland MS, McGrath CJ, et al: Equine post-anesthetic lameness: A retrospective study, Vet Surg 1990;19:392-397.
40. Jones RS, Payne-Johnson CE, Seymour CJ: Pulmonary micro-embolism following orthopaedic surgery in a Thoroughbred gelding, Equine Vet J 1988;20:382-384.

CHAPTER 23

Equine Pain Management

Shauna L. Cantwell
Sheilah A. Robertson

A discussion of equine pain and its relief must encompass the underlying neurophysiology of each type of pain; the mode of action of, indications for, and side effects of available drugs and analgesic techniques; and the current and rapidly expanding amount of evidence-based information.

PHYSIOLOGIC CONSEQUENCES OF PAIN

Pain occurs in a conscious state and is an unpleasant sensory or emotional experience associated with actual or potential tissue damage. It is a consequence of ascending impulses mediated by nociceptive fibers. Physiologic responses occur at the level of the spinal cord and include increased sympathetic tone, vasoconstriction, and increased myocardial work, which may lead to oxygen debt and arrhythmias. Increased blood pressure can compromise delicate tissues and surgical procedures in areas such as the eye. Decreased gastrointestinal motility is a common complication of untreated pain in horses. Increased skeletal muscle tone occurs on a segmental level and can potentiate oxygen demand, metabolic acidosis, and muscle spasms, which can augment pain. Muscle tension can also lead to abdominal splinting, reluctance to cough, hypoventilation, atelectasis, and hypoxemia.

The stress response or neuroendocrine response to pain can be dramatic, as is well documented in horses.[1] Nociception stimulates adrenocorticotropic hormone (ACTH), cortisol, and renin/angiotensin II; it decreases insulin and testosterone; and it can interfere with osteoblastic and fibroblastic activity and subsequent healing. Metabolic responses include sodium and water retention, hyperglycemia, lipolysis, and catabolism. Central responses such as fear and anxiety can promote further sympathetic responses, resulting in a vicious cycle.

The historic argument against analgesic intervention is the loss of guarding behavior that protects the injured or surgical site. However, in addition to delaying healing, pain may cause anxiety and panic, leading to sudden and unbalanced movement, further harming an already injured animal. For example, horses with a closed fracture may panic, move frantically, and develop a catastrophic comminuted open fracture. A pain-free state is not necessarily ideal, but an acceptable level of comfort is the goal. Allowing pain to persist is no longer acceptable or necessary with the drugs and methods available to veterinarians today.

PAIN ASSESSMENT

Analgesia should be provided to reach a desired effect, but recognizing pain in horses is not always easy, especially in chronic pain states where signs may be subtle and their onset insidious. Electroencephalograms (EEG tracings) have been analyzed in horses under general anesthesia and correlated with a noxious stimulus.[2] Pain-associated behaviors have been studied,[3,4] but they are not the same in all horses because of differences in temperament, environment, and individual responses to drugs. Pain is not directly related to heart and respiratory rate, but these variables may be useful in an overall assessment of a patient.

Behaviors that strongly indicate pain include lip-curling, inappetence, sham eating, lowered head, disinterest in surroundings, and staying at the back of the stall. In addition to these, the more overt behaviors of guarding the painful site, unusual postures, and aggression or complacency should be noted. Catecholamines and corticosteroids are indicators of stress, which is frequently a component of pain. Their measurement is not practical in a clinical setting, but they have been used as objective markers in research studies. Palpation and gait analysis are evaluation methods that are suitable in a clinical setting. To develop a treatment plan, the patient should be assessed and reassessed at regular intervals after initiating treatment. Assessment methods should be consistent. Using an objective scoring system to record the patient's response is perhaps most practical.

Characterization of Pain States

Acute Pain

Tissue damage and inflammation cause acute pain. This is perceived as sharp, shooting pain mediated by large, myelinated A-δ fibers. Local anesthetics block these fibers by inhibiting propagation of action potentials. The slower onset of deep aching pain is mediated by C-fibers, which are also stimulated by inflammation, and this type of pain is opioid responsive. Continued stimulation of the C-fibers causes central changes, loss of central inhibition, *N*-methyl-D-aspartate (NMDA) receptor stimulation (or "wind-up") and self-perpetuated nervous discharge. This is the basis of pain sensitization and of phantom pain.[5]

Central Sensitization

Acute pain and inflammation lead to upregulation of nociceptive pathways, often within minutes of the inciting cause. Various types of pain states arise as a result of the plasticity of the nervous system. These pain states look different, require diverse treatment regimens, and represent central sensitization.[5] Nociceptive input to the nervous system, because it is so plastic, results in rewiring of pathways and creates upregulated pain states. *Hyperalgesia* occurs when the magnitude of pain is greater than that expected from a nociceptive stimulus. Examples include pharyngitis causing pain when swallowing, or urinary tract inflammation causing pain during micturition. Hyperalgesia in the surrounding noninjured area is termed secondary hyperalgesia. Here, light touch stimulates low-threshold mechanoreceptors, which elicit a nociceptive stimulus. This *allodynia* occurs when an animal exhibits an exaggerated reaction after being touched in an area removed from the injury. *Sympathetically maintained pain,* which is not commonly acknowledged in veterinary medicine, is pain that depends on activity in the sympathetic nervous system. It can manifest in a variety of situations, such as chronic arthritis, soft tissue trauma, or neuropathies. Sympathetic pain is a subset of neuropathic pain. Persistent, spontaneous, phantom pain is pain perception resulting from central nociceptive activity without actual peripheral tissue damage. Chronic pain can include any one or a combination of these, and it may also have an acute component.

Pain Modulation

The body has protective mechanisms against pain that are centrally mediated, and we veterinarians try to emulate this endogenous network pharmacologically. Melzack and Wall first described the "gate theory" in 1965, in which ascending nociceptive transmission stimulates negative-feedback neurotransmission loops to inhibit the transmission and hence pain awareness.[6] Centrally located endogenous opioids, norepinephrine, serotonin, and nicotinic cholinergic neurons, among many other neurotransmitters, contribute to pain inhibition.

PRINCIPLES OF PAIN MANAGEMENT

Diagnosis

Acute pain is often characterized by overt signs of pain, obvious tissue damage, response to palpation, and the horse's history. Inflammation is usually obvious, or it occurs soon after the injury. If tissue damage, inflammation, or pain behavior is present, then pain sensitization should be assessed. Primary hyperalgesia may be tested by palpation over the area in question. Secondary hyperalgesia, or allodynia, can be tested by innocuous touch outside the region of the obvious cause of pain. The history of pain behavior or duration of the lesion may help define whether the pain is acute, or chronic with a superimposed acute component. Cause, severity, and duration should be documented.

Preemptive Analgesia and Continuous Treatment

Treatment of postoperative pain is facilitated by preventing the establishment of central pain sensitization. This is accomplished by administering analgesics before nociception occurs (i.e., prior to the start of a surgical procedure), and by treating continuously and not allowing pain breakthrough.[7] Fewer analgesic drugs are needed with this approach, and the benefit is fewer side effects. Put in practical terms, pain is easier to prevent than treat.

Multimodal and Synergistic Approach

A balanced and layered approach to pain management is optimal (Box 23-1). To achieve synergism, prevention of nociceptive transmission at as many steps in the ascending pathway as possible should be attempted. Local anesthetics, opioids, anti-inflammatory agents, epidural drugs, and anxiolytics or sedatives should all be considered, depending on the type of pain already present or anticipated.

Ancillary Pain Management

Many factors other than simple tissue damage potentiate pain. The treatment of para-pain factors is important. Surgical methods may aid management—for example, reduction of impinging dorsal spinous processes causing back pain, arthrodesis for chronic osteoarthritis, and laparoscopic surgery to shorten postoperative recovery and healing time. Contact lenses may confer corneal ulcer pro-

BOX 23-1. Strategies for Treatment of Pain

- Nerve blocks, including ganglionic blocks
- Intra-articular local and opioid blocks
- Epidural local, opioid, α_2-agonist, or other analgesics
- Segmental thoracolumbar local analgesia
- Topical capsaicin
- Lidocaine patch
- Fentanyl patch
- Infusions: α_2-agonists, lidocaine, butorphanol, ketamine, other opioids
- Central sensitization drugs
- Complementary therapy

tection, speed healing, and lessen the duration of pain. Sedation or tranquilization or improving the environment may decrease the anxiety that potentiates acute pain. Nutritional needs increase with pain, especially if the patient is in a catabolic state (up to two times the basal metabolic rate; see Chapter 6). Antiendotoxins, antithrombotic agents, special shoeing techniques, bandaging, and tissue support are methods that increase comfort and decrease pain. For chronic disorders, exercise regimens, saddle fit, and training techniques should be addressed.

Continuous Reevaluation

The analgesic treatment is only as good as the effect it produces. Because all animals respond differently (probably as a result of genetic variability) and because the neurophysiologic state is in flux, response to therapy must be carefully evaluated. Breakthrough pain and side effects of treatment must be monitored. A scoring system is recommended so that the horse's comfort can be tracked as objectively as possible and to keep therapeutic goals in sight.

ANALGESIC DRUGS AND MODES OF ACTION

Nonsteroidal Anti-Inflammatory Drugs

Many painful conditions have an inflammatory component, and nonsteroidal anti-inflammatory drugs (NSAIDs) have historically been the foundation of equine pain management. NSAIDs inhibit the cyclooxygenase (COX) enzymes and decrease the release of prostaglandins and thromboxane, thereby interfering with the inflammatory cascade.[8,9] Until recently, it was thought that a distinct delineation between the functions of the COX-1 and COX-2 enzymes existed. COX-1 was considered constitutive and responsible for gastrointestinal protection, renal arteriodilation, and platelet function, whereas COX-2 was thought to be responsible for the prostaglandins that mediate inflammation and pain.

Phenylbutazone and flunixin meglumine are potent COX-1 inhibitors, whereas carprofen is a weak COX-1 inhibitor[10] that does not inhibit COX-2 in equine blood.[11] Phenylbutazone is more effective for acute synovitis than ketoprofen at clinically relevant dosages[12] and is still the most commonly used NSAID. Vedaprofen is licensed for use in horses in the United Kingdom and is more COX-1 selective than COX-2.[10] In addition to the traditionally used drugs (phenylbutazone, flunixin meglumine, and ketoprofen), the newer NSAIDs carprofen, meloxicam, and etodolac are now available and have been used in horses, although pharmacokinetic and clinical data are lacking. Meloxicam has partial selectivity for COX-2.[10] It is now known, however, that COX-2 is not only inducible but constitutive in some tissues, including the kidney, central nervous system, and stomach.[8] This may be the reason that newer-generation COX-2 specific antagonists have not been devoid of deleterious side effects.

The actions of NSAIDs are complex and the therapeutic and toxic actions may also be in part caused by centrally mediated COX actions or COX-independent actions. Contraindications for any of the NSAIDs are preexisting bleeding disorders, renal or hepatic disease, and gastrointestinal ulceration. For a comprehensive review, see Moses and colleagues (2002).[9]

Opioids

Opioids other than butorphanol are not commonly used in horses, most likely because of the perceived side effects of excitatory behavior (rather than sedation) and decreased gastrointestinal motility. Excitatory effects of morphine and butorphanol at high dosages include restlessness, shivering, dangerously increased motor activity, ataxia, and sedation.[13,14] These effects are uncommon when α_2-agonists or acepromazine is concurrently administered, or when the drugs are given to a horse in pain. Sellon and coworkers reported adverse gastrointestinal effects after a bolus injection of butorphanol.[15] However, butorphanol can be given alone as an infusion for at least 24 hours with few side effects[15] (Box 23-2). Opioid antagonists are being investigated for their usefulness in diminishing the gastrointestinal effects of many agonists without affecting analgesia.[16]

Opioids have a definite place in analgesia protocols and can be administered as boluses, as infusions, epidurally, intra-articularly, and transdermally. Not only do opioids produce an antinociceptive effect by inhibiting C-fiber transmission but they also decrease inflammatory pain by inhibiting substance P release from peptidergic neurons.[17] Opioid receptors are present in the brain and spinal cord.[18] When administered under general anesthesia, opioids produce analgesia and possible central nervous system stimulation at the same time, but they do not necessarily decrease the amount of inhalant necessary. In my (SC) personal experience, morphine (0.1 mg/kg intravenously) maintained a lighter anesthetic depth with less response to surgical stimulation and smoother recoveries but with arousal tendencies; also, in some horses, euphoria occurred. Mircica and colleagues reported that in a large clinical retrospective study, morphine given intraoperatively (0.1 to 0.17 mg/kg) did not result in more complications than if it were not given,[19] demonstrating a lack of undesirable clinical side effects. However, another multicenter retrospective study showed that the postoperative incidence of colic was positively associated with morphine given at 0.1 mg/kg compared with either butorphanol or no opioid.[20] Intramuscular morphine (0.66 mg/kg, higher than used clinically) produced effective analgesia for experimental superficial pain in ponies, whereas butorphanol intramuscularly (0.22 mg/kg) had little effect.[13] Xylazine administered

BOX 23-2. Infusion Dosages

Medetomidine	7 μg/kg intravenously, followed by 3.5 μg/kg/h
Butorphanol	17.8 μg/kg intravenously, followed by 23.7 μg/kg/h
Detomidine infusion	7.5 μg/kg loading dosage, then 0.6 μg/kg/min, halved every 15 min
Lidocaine	1-2 mg/kg intravenously, followed by 20-75 μg/kg/min
Ketamine	0.5 mg/kg intravenously, followed by 3-10 μg/kg/min

intramuscularly (2.2 mg/kg) was more effective than either opioid.[13] In a similar study, intravenous butorphanol (0.01 to 0.04 mg/kg) produced dosage-related superficial analgesia for 15 to 30 minutes.[14] Butorphanol given intravenously (0.22 mg/kg) provided visceral analgesia for 60 minutes and was associated with ataxia but no excitement.[21] At this dosage, the dysphoric effects are minimized when the opioid is given to a patient already in pain. Butorphanol given during surgery also reduces the need for additional doses of NSAIDS.[22]

Peripheral opioid receptors are present in equine synovial tissue,[23] which supports the practice of intra-articular opioid administration. In humans, intra-articular opioids decrease the need for systemic administration of postoperative analgesics,[24] and perioperative analgesia shortens the time of return to mobility and normal range of motion.[25] The small space and minimal vascularization of the joint prevents rapid uptake of opioid and allows a much longer duration of effect without systemic signs of sedation, or decreased gastrointestinal motility. A common clinical practice is to inject 0.1 mg/kg of morphine, diluted with saline or local anesthetic, into the joint at the end of surgery.

Transdermal fentanyl patches are useful as an adjunct in acute pain management, or as primary management of some pain states such as burns, laminitis, and pleuritis. Two or three patches (10 mg each) placed on a shaved area over the neck, antebrachium, or gaskin may confer 48 to 72 hours of continuous analgesia. Uptake occurs within 1 hour of application, and plasma levels decrease rapidly once the patches are removed.[26] Replacement of the patches at the end of their life span should allow a constant systemic level to be maintained.

Alpha-2 Agonists

Xylazine (0.2 to 2.2 mg/kg), romifidine (80 to 120 μg/kg), detomidine (10 to 20 μg/kg), and medetomidine (4 to 7 μg/kg) are α_2-agonists commonly used for sedation and analgesia.[27-29] Medetomidine infusions (see Box 23-2) have been used during general anesthesia[30] and significantly decrease inhalant agent requirements, and recoveries are generally excellent (see Chapter 20). With α_2-agonists, sedation outlasts analgesia and one must be cognizant of this during invasive procedures or when treating pain.[31] The cardiovascular side effects of bradycardia, bradyarrhythmias, increased vascular resistance, and decreased cardiac output[32,33] seem to be well tolerated in healthy horses, but the impact of these have not been well studied in hypotensive, hypovolemic, or sick horses. The historical use and pharmacology of α_2-agonists were recently reviewed.[34]

Local Anesthetics

Local anesthetics can be utilized topically, as specific nerve blocks, and by infiltration, either regionally or systemically. Sites for common perineural infiltration have been described in detail[35] (see Chapter 74). In addition to being used for lameness evaluation, local anesthetic blocks can be used during standing surgery, to diminish postsurgical pain, to decrease the amount of inhalant agent needed during general anesthesia, and to comfort the horse during anesthetic recovery. The authors find that when proprioceptive deficits are prevented, perioperative local anesthesia of limbs results in a smoother recovery. Local anesthesia of nerves lacking a sensory component (e.g., the auriculopalpebral nerve) may facilitate pain management as well as diagnosis by decreasing muscle tone and blepharospasm. Paravertebral thoracolumbar anesthesia can be performed to allow a surgical approach to the flank.[36] Deeper nerve anesthesia is not commonly performed, but a sacroiliac joint block can be an effective management strategy for back pain,[37] and cervical stellate ganglion blocks have been described for sympathetic pain disorders.[38] Intrapleural, intercostal, dental, and pudendal local anesthetic blocks should also be considered when appropriate.

Systemic Lidocaine Administration

Intravenous lidocaine is used to treat ileus after abdominal surgery in horses.[39] It significantly decreases the requirement for inhalant agents.[40] Intravenous lidocaine can be a useful adjunct to other analgesic protocols. At clinically recommended dosages, it does not have the associated excitatory and gastrointestinal side effects of opioids or the profound sedating and cardiovascular depressant effects of α_2-antagonists, and it is inexpensive. Infusions can be administered to both awake and anesthetized horses (see Box 23-2). Toxicity is easily recognized and managed. Sedation, muscle tremors, and progression to severe ataxia and collapse occur if the plasma concentrations are too high.[41] If the infusion is discontinued, lidocaine is rapidly cleared and the effects quickly abate. Lidocaine has been used in conscious horses at a loading dosage of 1 to 5 mg/kg given over 10 to 20 minutes, followed by an infusion rate of 15 to 75 μg/kg per minute. Robertson and colleagues[42] have shown that in normal horses, lidocaine increased the thermal threshold of skin, suggesting somatic analgesia, but it did not have an effect on visceral pain as measured by duodenal or rectal balloon distention. Further research on pharmacokinetics and dynamics in horses is ongoing, and more investigation is needed to clarify the role of lidocaine in equine analgesia.

Drugs for the Treatment of Central Sensitization

Once a sensitized state is suspected or diagnosed, therapy is aimed toward reducing the sensitization. Some examples of pain states that are related to sensitization include the chronic pain of osteoarthritis or laminitis, chronic wounds, and healing after orthopedic surgery.

NMDA antagonists, monoamine reuptake inhibitors, and anticonvulsants are the classes of drugs currently used to treat upregulated pain states. These drugs do not treat acute or ongoing pain but act to diminish sensitization and the abnormal neurologic states that cause hyperalgesia, referred pain, increased receptive fields, and allodynia. They are used as adjuncts to acute pain management. For many years, ketamine has been used as a component of anesthetic induction protocols and may have provided analgesia and prevented wind-up in addition to inducing dissociative anesthesia. As an NMDA receptor antagonist, ketamine can prevent or diminish central wind-up and self-propagation of nociceptive impulses. In humans, small subanesthetic dosages have been used in conjunction with opioids for management of chronic ongoing pain such as burns.

Ketamine infusions at dosages of 3 to 40 μg/kg per minute are used in small animals for treatment of pain sensitization and for intraoperative and postoperative pain management[43] (see Box 23-2). Amantadine is an NMDA receptor antagonist that has been used in small animals, and it may have a role in equine pain management. Anticonvulsants such as gabapentin may have a future in equine analgesia, although phenytoin has been used in the past and may be much more economical.

Monoamine reuptake inhibitors such as the tricyclic antidepressants are used in human and small animal medicine for chronic pain at dosages that are less than those used for their antidepressant effects. There may also be a role in horses for these drugs. Tramadol, a weak opioid with nonopioid action, has been placed in the epidural space of horses.[44] Its activity is in part from monoaminergic reuptake inhibition, which prevents ascending nociception. Reuptake inhibition allows an increase in central levels of catecholamines, which aid in negative feedback to nociception transmission. Many of the discussed drugs are not labeled for use in the horse, and species-specific pharmacokinetic data for them are not available.

INTRA-ARTICULAR ANALGESIA

As previously discussed, intra-articular opioids such as morphine can provide relief for up to 24 hours. Corticosteroids are primarily indicated for treatment of acute synovitis, although these drugs are also used for treatment of chronic lameness and osteoarthritis. Triamcinolone acetonide, methylprednisolone acetate, and betamethasone are frequently used intra-articularly for nonseptic joint disease, but the deleterious effects of intra-articular steroids must be considered.[45] Hyaluronic acid and polysulfated glycosaminoglycan are used to promote joint health when the joints are the source of pain and lameness (see Chapter 84). Polysulfated glycosaminoglycan stimulates proteoglycan synthesis in chondrocyte monolayers, whereas betamethasone suppresses synthesis at high concentrations.[46] Phenylbutazone increases sulfate uptake in chondrocyte cultures at low concentrations.[47] Intra-articular local anesthetics such as lidocaine or bupivacaine can be administered for short-term relief.

EPIDURAL ANALGESIA

Epidural analgesia is used to produce local anesthesia in the perineal and tail regions or in the hindlimbs. Local anesthetic drugs such as lidocaine, mepivacaine, and ropivacaine are commonly used for this purpose. Opioids, including morphine and fentanyl, are also used. α_2-Agonists such as xylazine and detomidine can be used in conjunction with opioids. Ketamine and tramadol have also been reported, alone or in combination with other more traditional analgesics.[44,47]

The goal of using epidural analgesia differs from the goal of using anesthesia. Anesthesia is utilized with local anesthetics administered in such a volume that they inactivate action potentials in the spinal cord caudal to the branching of the sciatic and femoral nerves. Local anesthesia allows surgical incision to the perineal and tail area by blocking nociceptive, sensory, and motor transmission. Most anesthetics cause severe ataxia if the nerve blockade extends too far cranially, and this limits their use to perineal anesthesia. Analgesia, on the other hand, may include local anesthesia, but it has a much broader range of application. Indications include hindlimb, abdominal, thoracic, and sometimes front limb pain. Opioids, α_2-antagonists, ketamine, and tramadol[44,47] have been used clinically with minimal motor impairment. Systemic absorption and side effects vary depending on the solubility and other physical properties of the drug administered.

Drug combinations are most effective in the epidural space to provide analgesia. Local anesthetics are often combined with opioids or α_2-agonists. Ropivacaine is a local anesthetic shown to block A-δ and C-fibers of nociception before compromising larger motor fibers; this results in less ataxia. Ropivacaine used together with fentanyl has been described.[48]

For a surgical flank approach or for abdominal analgesia, subarachnoid analgesia can be performed. Segmental thoracolumbar analgesia with local anesthetic administered through a catheter has been well described[49] in standing horses. Subarachnoid mepivacaine would facilitate standing surgical procedures such as ovariectomy, laparoscopic cryptorchidectomy, and flank laparotomy, with onset of analgesia at 10 minutes and lasting 23 to 68 minutes. Epidural morphine (0.1 mg/kg)[50] and epidural methadone (0.1 mg/kg)[51] do not cause excitement, ataxia, or a decrease in defecation. Morphine may be absorbed systemically and may cause mild sedation.[52] Both of these drugs migrate cranially and cause ascending analgesia. However, methadone has a quicker onset and shorter duration, most likely because of its greater lipophilicity. Morphine could be used with local anesthetics, α_2-agonists, or ketamine to create synergistic and longer-lasting analgesia. Butorphanol does not create significant epidural analgesia.[44] Tramadol (1 mg/ kg) can produce relatively long lasting ascending analgesia (up to 6½ hours)[52] and can be combined with fentanyl to manage horses with severe intractable pain (of 12 to 24 hours' duration). Ketamine has commonly been used in human medicine both systemically and epidurally to decrease pain sensitization.[53,54] In horses, epidural ketamine alone lasts only 30 to 90 minutes and may not confer surgical analgesia,[47,55] but it is suitable when combined with morphine or xylazine to treat chronic or severe pain associated with laminitis and other painful orthopedic conditions. Surgical pain can be interrupted for a short duration by ketamine.[56] Ketamine may also have local anesthetic properties[57] and can be used for palmar digital nerve blocks in horses.[58]

Placing an epidural catheter (Fig. 23-1) allows repeated dosing of analgesics for days to weeks. The drugs used for epidural analgesia and anesthesia are summarized in Table 23-1.

Complications

Injections into the epidural space should not be performed at a rate faster than 1 mL per 10 to 20 seconds, because rapid injections can cause ataxia and recumbency. Sedation can occur from systemic uptake of drugs. Morphine may cause other side effects, such as pruritus,[59] and incorrectly placed epidural catheters may become knotted or contaminate the epidural space. Bleeding disorders, infection at the

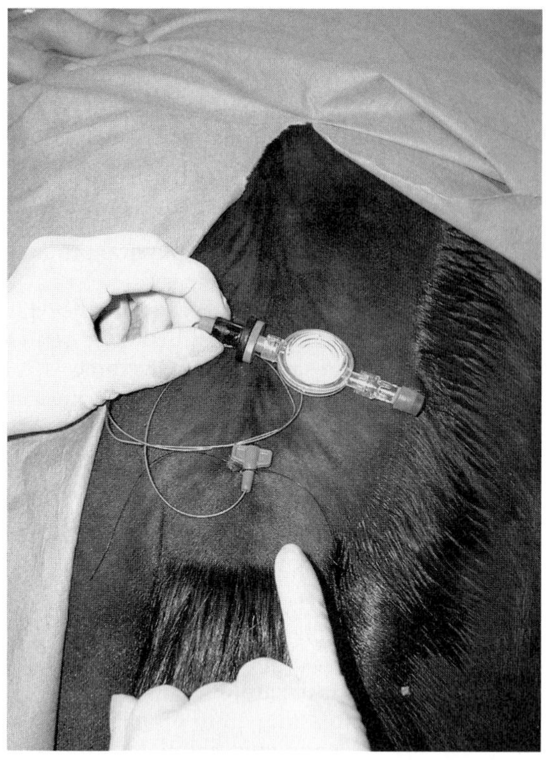

Figure 23-1. Epidural catheter being placed for long-term use.

placement site, and septicemia are contraindications for epidural catheter use.

COMPLEMENTARY THERAPY

Acupuncture

Acupuncture is becoming a respected and widely used form of therapy, especially for pain management in both human and veterinary medicine. In conjunction with electrical stimuli (electroacupuncture), it produces analgesia via nonopioid means as well as through release of β-endorphin into the cerebrospinal fluid.[60] The effects are varied, and studies support endorphin release because the effects can be reversed with naloxone.[61] Differences in response between sexes has been shown.[62] Navicular pain has resolved and laminitis has been treated successfully.[63] The International Veterinary Acupuncture Society (IVAS) and the Chi Institute are two well-respected veterinary training organizations for those interested in learning more about this treatment modality.

Other Treatment Modalities

Manual therapy, such as chiropractic manipulations, physical therapy, osteopathy, and massage, can facilitate a return to normal function. In chronic pain states when tissue damage has healed or scarred, tissue hypersensitivity and locomotion restriction may still exist. In addition to drugs

TABLE 23-1. Epidural Drugs

Drug	Dosage	Volume	Onset	Duration	Comments
Morphine	0.1 mg/kg	20 mL (saline)	45 min to 1 h	6 to 24 h	Longer onset and shorter duration cranially
Methadone	0.1 mg/kg	20 mL (saline)	15 min to 2 h	3 to 7 h	Longer onset and shorter duration more cranially
Lidocaine	2%	5 to 7 mL	7 to 10 min	1 to 3 h	Perineal anesthesia only at this volume
Ropivacaine	0.5%	8 mL	11 min	3 h	Less motor loss
Detomidine	5-60 μg/kg	—	10 to 15 min	2.5 h	Much is absorbed systemically
Xylazine	0.17-0.22 mg/kg	—	15 min	3 h (perineal)	Much is absorbed systemically
Ketamine	0.8-1.2 mg/kg	—	5 to 10 min	30 to 90 min	Decreases sensitization, used in combination for chronic, severe pain
Tramadol	1.0 mg/kg	—	30 min	12 to 18 h	—
Tramadol + fentanyl	1.0 mg/kg 100 μg total	—	30 to 60 min	18 to 24 h	For intractable pain
Ropivacaine + fentanyl	0.5% 100 μg total	8 mL	11 min 3.5 h	3^+ h	No sedation due to fentanyl, better analgesia than ropivacaine alone
Morphine + detomidine	0.1 mg/kg 5-60 μg/kg	Sufficient quantity (20 mL) saline	15 min	20 to 24 h 2.5 h	Detomidine causes sedation
Lidocaine + xylazine	2% 0.17-0.22 mg/kg	5 to 7 mL	7 to 10 min 15 min	5.5 h	Xylazine potentiates and prolongs the lidocaine block

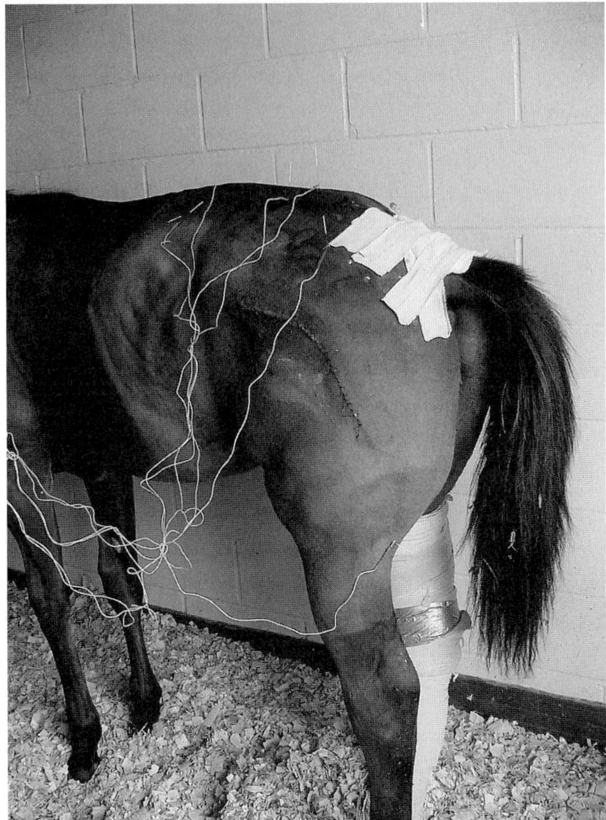

Figure 23-2. The filly shown here has chronic pain from a previous trauma and femoral head excision. She has mixed acute ongoing and chronic pain from developing laminitis as well as allodynia. She is shown with an epidural catheter and electroacupuncture. Therapy included phenylbutazone, xylazine, and morphine, and ketamine and lidocaine for surgery. Postoperative management included detomidine and morphine epidurally, acupuncture, ketamine boluses, anti-inflammatories, and massage and physiotherapy. The filly might have benefited from phenytoin or gabapentin in addition to unweighting the other limbs. The animal was eventually euthanized because of progressive laminitis.

directed toward alleviating neuropathic pain, joint and muscle manipulation can restore proprioceptive and mechanoreceptor input to normalize segmental and suprasegmental reflexes and decrease sensitized nociceptive input.[64]

Therapeutic ultrasound for soft tissue injuries has been shown to increase blood flow and decrease pain.[65] These therapies have a place in intensive pain management situations as well as sports medicine. Magnetic, extracorporeal shockwave, and laser therapy are also management modalities of interest, and controlled studies in these fields are ongoing. Herbal therapy is backed by extensive clinical experience but not by widely published controlled studies.[66] Good reviews of herbs used in equine pain management have been published.[67,68]

Figure 23-2 shows a comprehensive approach to pain management.

NOVEL THERAPIES

Capsaicin ointment has local analgesic effects and can be considered for perineural treatment of laminitis, osteoarthritis, and any other painful situation that is amenable to topical analgesics. Use of capsaicin is not a new idea, as it was used in ancient times in the original form of hot chili peppers. Capsaicin is used to deplete substance P and decrease A-δ and C-fiber nociceptive transmission.[69] In palmar digital skin application, it causes dramatic analgesia of the foot for up to 4 hours.[70]

Transdermal delivery of analgesics to localized areas presents an interesting form of directed analgesia. Lidocaine (5%) patches (Lidoderm, Endo Pharmaceuticals, Chadds Ford, Pa) have provided promising results.[71] Cathodic iontophoresis has the potential to deliver anionic anti-inflammatory drugs to superficial sites, although intra-articular sites may be too deep, as evidenced by work with ketoprofen by Eastman and coworkers.[72] Other constant-rate drug delivery systems are being developed. Surpass (IDEXX Laboratories, Greensboro, NC) is a topical formulation of 1% diclofenac applied to joints for isolated anti-inflammatory effects.[73] Nanotechnologic techniques are being used in the investigation and development of drug delivery methods.[74,75]

FUTURE DEVELOPMENTS

Immune-modulating drugs such as rubeola virus immunomodulator for chronic myofascial pain have been described and utilized in veterinary clinical practice, although this has not been published in a peer-reviewed journal.[76] Central nervous system immunomodulation holds promise as a therapeutic target for chronic pain and opioid tolerance.[77]

The vanilloid receptor VR-1 is a peripheral component of the nociceptive pathway, and it can be targeted to permanently remove pain but not sensation. Perhaps there will be a role in such conditions as laminitis or navicular disease. Controlled studies are ongoing.[78]

REFERENCES

1. Robertson SA: Some metabolic and hormonal changes associated with general anesthesia and surgery in the horse, Equine Vet J 1987;19:288-294.
2. Murrell JC, Johnson CB, White KL, et al: Changes in the EEG during castration in horses and ponies anaesthetized with halothane, Vet Anaesth Analg 2003;30:138-146.
3. Price J, Catriona S, Welsh EM, et al: Preliminary evaluation of a behavior-based system for assessment of post-operative pain in horses following arthroscopic surgery, Vet Anaesth Analg 2003; 30:124-137.
4. Raekallio M, Taylor PM, Blomfield M: A comparison of methods for evaluation of pain and distress after orthopaedic surgery in horses, J Vet Anaesth 1997;24:17-20.
5. Raja SN, Meyer RA, Ringkamp M, et al: Peripheral neural mechanisms of nociception. In Wall PD, Melzack R, editors: Textbook of Pain, Philadelphia, 1999, Churchill Livingstone.
6. Melzack R, Wall PD: Pain mechanisms: A new theory, Science 1965;150:971-999.
7. Woolf CJ, Chong MS: Preemptive analgesia: Treating postoperative pain by preventing the establishment of central sensitization, Anesth Analg 1993;77:362-379.
8. Nolan A: Pharmacology of analgesic drugs. In Flecknell PA, Waterman-Pearson AE, editors: Pain Management in Animals, London, 2000, WB Saunders.
9. Moses VS, Bertone AL: Nonsteroidal anti-inflammatory drugs, Vet Clin North Am Equine Pract 2002;18:21-37.
10. Lees P, May SA, Coert A, et al: A pharmacodynamic and pharmacokinetic study with vedaprofen in an equine model of

acute nonimmune inflammation, J Vet Pharmacol Ther 1999; 22:96-106.
11. Brideau C, Van Staden C, Chan CC: In vitro effects of cyclooxygenase inhibitors in whole blood of horses, dogs, and cats, Am J Vet Res 2001;62:1755-1760.
12. Owens JG, Kamerling SG, Stanton SR, et al: Effects of pretreatment with ketoprofen and phenylbutazone on experimentally induced synovitis in horses, Am J Vet Res 1996;57:866-874.
13. Kalpravidh M, Lumb WV, Wright M, Heath RB: Effects of butorphanol, flunixin, levorphanol, morphine, and xylazine in ponies, Am J Vet Res 1984;45:217-223.
14. Kalpravidh M, Lumb WV, Wright M, Heath RB: Analgesic effects of butorphanol in horses: Dose-response studies, Am J Vet Res 1984; 45:211-216.
15. Sellon DC, Monroe VL, Roberts MC, Papich MG: Pharmacokinetics and adverse effects of butorphanol administered by single intravenous injection or continuous intravenous infusion in horses, Am J Vet Res 2001;62:183-189.
16. Liu SS, Hodgson PS, Carpenter RI, et al: ADL 8-2698, a trans-3,4-dimethyl-4-(3-hydroxyphenyl) piperidine, prevents gastrointestinal effects of intravenous morphine without affecting analgesia, Clin Pharmacol Ther 2001;17:66-71.
17. Yaksh TL: Pharmacology and mechanisms of opioid analgesic activity, Acta Anaesthesiol Scand 1997;41:94-111.
18. Tobin T, Combie J, Miller JR, et al: The pharmacology of narcotic analgesics in the horse: II. Studies on the detection, pharmacokinetics, urinary clearance times and behavioral effects of pentazocine and fentanyl in the horse, Irish Vet J 1979;33:169-176.
19. Mircica E, Clutton RE, Kyles KW, et al: Problems associated with perioperative morphine in horses: A retrospective case analysis, Vet Anaesth Anal 2003;30:147-155.
20. Senior JM, Pinchbeck GL, Dugdale AHA, et al: Retrospective study of the risk factors and prevalence of colic in horses after orthopedic surgery, Vet Rec 2004;155:321-325.
21. Muir WW, Robertson JT. Visceral analgesia: Effects of xylazine, butorphanol, meperidine, and pentazocine in horses, Am J Vet Res 1985;46:2081-2084.
22. Johnson CB, Taylor PM, Young SS, et al: Postoperative analgesia using phenylbutazone, flunixin, or carprofen in horses, Vet Rec 1993;133:336-338.
23. Sheehy JG, Hellyer PW, Sammonds GE, et al: Evaluation of opioid receptors in synovial membranes of horses, Am J Vet Res 2001;62:1408-1412.
24. Joshi GP, McCarroll SM, Obrien TM, et al: Intraarticular analgesia following knee arthroscopy, Anesth Analg 1993;76:333-336.
25. Capdevila X, Barthelet Y, Biboulet P, et al: Effects of perioperative analgesic technique on the surgical outcome and duration of rehabilitation after major knee surgery, Anesthesiology 1999;91:8-15.
26. Maxwell LK, Thomasy SM, Lovis N, et al: Pharmacokinetics of fentanyl following intravenous and transdermal administration in horses, Equine Vet J 2003;35:484-490.
27. Freeman SL, England GCW: Investigation of romifidine and detomidine for the clinical sedation of the horse, Vet Rec 2000;147:507-511.
28. Wilson DV, Bohart GV, Evans AT, et al: Retrospective analysis of detomidine infusion for standing chemical restraint in 51 horses, Vet Anaesth Analg 2002;29:54-57.
29. Ramsay EC, Geiser D, Carter W, et al: Serum concentrations and effects of detomidine delivered orally to horses in three different mediums, Vet Anaesth Analg 2002;29:219-222.
30. Bettschart-Wolfensberger R, Clarke KW, Vainio O, et al: Pharmacokinetics of medetomidine in ponies and elaboration of a medetomidine infusion regime which provides a constant level of sedation, Res Vet Sci 1999;67:41-46.
31. Kamerling SG, Cravens WM, Baywell CA: Objective assessment of detomidine induced analgesia and sedation in the horse, Eur J Pharm 1988;151:1-8.
32. Bueno AC, Cornick-Seahorn J, Seahorn TL, et al: Cardiopulmonary and sedative effects of intravenous administration of low doses of medetomidine and xylazine to adult horses, Am J Vet Res 1999;60:1371-1376.
33. Singh S, Young SS, McDonell WN, et al: Modification of pulmonary and intestinal motility effects of xylazine with glycopyrrolate in horses, Can J Vet Res 1997;61:99-107.
34. Daunt DA, Steffey EP: Alpha-2 adrenergic agonists as analgesics in horses, Vet Clin North Am Equine Pract 2002;18:39-46.
35. Schmotzer WB, Timm KIJ: Local anesthetic techniques for diagnosis of lameness, Vet Clin North Am Equine Pract 1990;6:705-728.
36. Moon PF, Suter CM: Paravertebral thoracolumbar anaesthesia in 10 horses, Equine Vet J 1993;25:304-308.
37. Dyson S, Murray R: Pain associated with the sacroiliac joint region: A clinical study of 74 horses, Equine Vet J 2003;35:240-245.
38. Skarda RT, Muir WW, Swanson CR, et al: Cervicothoracic (stellate) ganglion block in conscious horses, Am J Vet Res 1986;47:21-26.
39. Brianceau P, Chevalier H, Karas A, et al: Intravenous lidocaine and small-intestinal size, abdominal fluid, and outcome after colic surgery in horses, J Vet Intern Med 2002;16:736-741.
40. Doherty TJ, Frazier DL: Effect of intravenous lidocaine on halothane minimum alveolar concentration in ponies, Equine Vet J 1998;30:300-303.
41. Meyer GA, Lin HC, Hansons RR, et al: Effects of intravenous lidocaine overdose on cardiac electrical activity and blood pressure in the horse, Equine Vet J 2001;33:434-437.
42. Robertson S, Sanchez C, Merritt A, et al: Effect of systemic lidocaine on visceral and somatic nociception on conscious horses, Equine Vet J 2005;37:122.
43. Wagner AE, Walton JA, Hellyer PW, et al: Use of low doses of ketamine administered by constant rate infusion as an adjunct for postoperative analgesia in dogs, J Am Vet Med Assoc 2002; 221:72-75.
44. Natalini CC, Robinson B: Evaluation of the analgesic effects of epidurally administered morphine, alfentanil, butorphanol, tramadol, and U50488H in horses, Am J Vet Res 2000;61:1579-1586.
45. Frisbie DD, Kawcak CE, Baxter GM, et al: Effects of 6alpha-methylprednisolone acetate on an equine osteochondral fragment exercise model, Am J Vet Res 1998;59:1619-1628.
46. Frean SP, Cambridge H, Lees P: Effects of anti-arthritic drugs on proteoglycan synthesis by equine cartilage, J Vet Pharmacol Ther 2002;25:289-298.
47. Robinson EP, Natalini CC: Epidural anesthesia and analgesia in horses, Vet Clin Equine 2002;18:61-82.
48. Ganidagli S, Cetin H, Biricik HS, et al: Comparison of ropivacaine with a combination of ropivacaine and fentanyl for the caudal epidural anesthesia of mares, Vet Rec 2004;154:329-332.
49. Skarda RT, Muir WW: Segmental thoracolumbar spinal (subarachnoid) analgesia in conscious horses, Am J Vet Res 1982; 43:2121-2128.
50. Valverde A, Little CB, Dyson DH, et al: Use of epidural morphine to relieve pain in a horse, Can Vet J 1990;31:211-212.
51. Olbrich VH, Mosing M: A comparison of the analgesic effects of caudal epidural methadone and lidocaine in the horse, Vet Anaesth Analg 2003;30:156-154.
52. Natalini CC, Robinson EP: Effects of epidural opioid analgesics on heart rate, arterial blood pressure, respiratory rate, body temperature, and behavior in horses, Vet Ther 2004;4:364-375.
53. Persson J, Axelsson G, Hallin RG, et al: Beneficial effects of ketamine in a chronic pain state with allodynia, possibly due to central sensitization, Pain 1995;60:217-222.
54. Yang C, Wong C, Chang J, et al: Intrathecal ketamine reduces morphine requirements in patients with terminal cancer pain, Can J Anesth 1996;43:379-383.
55. Doherty TJ, Geiser DR, Rohrback BW: Effect of epidural morphine, butorphanol, and ketamine on halothane MAC in ponies, Equine Vet J 1997;29:30-373.
56. Redua MA, Valadao CAA, Duque JC, et al: The pre-emptive effect of epidural ketamine on wound sensitivity in horses tested by using

von Frey filaments, Vet Anaesth Analg 2002;29:200-206.
57. Dowdy EG, Kaya K, Gocho Y: Some pharmacologic similarities of ketamine, lidocaine, and procaine, Anesth Analg 1973;52:839-842.
58. Lopez-Sanroman FJ, Cruz JM, Santos M, et al: Evaluation of the local analgesic effect of ketamine in the palmar digital nerve block at the base of the proximal sesamoid (abaxial sesamoid block) in horses, Am J Vet Res 2003;64:475-478.
59. Haitjema H, Gibson KT: Severe pruritus associated with epidural morphine and detomidine in a horse, Aust Vet J 2001;79:248-250.
60. Skarda RT, Tejwani GA, Muir WW: Cutaneous analgesia, hemodynamic and respiratory effects, and β-endorphin concentration in spinal fluid and plasma of horses after acupuncture and electroacupuncture, Am J Vet Res 2002;63:1435-1442.
61. Chu TC, Potter DE: Ocular hypotension induced by electroacupuncture, J Ocul Pharmacol Ther 2002;18:293-305.
62. Bossut DFB, Page EH, Stromberg MW: Production of cutaneous analgesia by electroacupuncture in horses: Variations dependent on sex of subject and locus of stimulation, Am J Vet Res 1984;45:620-625.
63. Xie H: Personal communication, 2004.
64. Pickar J: Neurophysiological effects of spinal manipulation. Spine J 2002;2:357-371.
65. Millis DL, Levine D: The role of exercise and physical modalities in the treatment of osteoarthritis, Vet Clin North Am Small Anim Pract 1997;27:913-930.
66. Chen J: Herbal alternative to drugs: pain management. Presented at the 8th Annual Conference of the Acupuncture and Oriental Medicine Alliance, Safety Harbor, Fla, May 2001.
67. Fleming P: Nontraditional approaches to pain management, Vet Clin North Am Equine Pract 2002;18:83-101.
68. Xie H, Preast V: Traditional Chinese Veterinary Medicine: Vol 1. Fundamental Principles, Reddick, Fla, Jing Tang, 2002.
69. Winter J, Bevan S, Campbell EA: Capsaicin and pain mechanisms, Br J Anaesth 1995;75:157-168.
70. Seino KK, Foreman JH, Greene SA, et al: Effects of topical perineural capsaicin in a reversible model of equine foot lameness, J Vet Intern Med 2003;17:563-566.
71. Bidwell LA, Wilson DV, Caron JP: Systemic lidocaine absorption after placement of Lidoderm patches on horses: Preliminary findings. Presented at the Veterinary Midwest Anesthesia and Analgesia Conference, Indianapolis, Ind, 2004.
72. Eastman T, Panus PC, Honnas CM, et al: Cathodic iontophoresis of ketoprofen over the equine middle carpal joint, Equine Vet J 2001;33:614-616.
73. Caldwell FJ, Nueller POE, Lynn RC, et al: Effect of topical application of diclofenac liposomal suspension on experimentally induced subcutaneous inflammation in horses, Am J Vet Res 2004; 65:271-276.
74. Neuberger T, Schöpf B, Hofmann H, et al: Superparamagnetic nanoparticles for biomedical applications: Possibilities and limitations of a new drug delivery system, J Magnetism Magn Mater 2005;293:483-496.
75. Schulze K, Koch A, Schöpf B, et al: Intraarticular application of superparamagnetic nanoparticles and their uptake by synovial membrane: An experimental study in sheep, J Magnetism Magn Mater 2005;293:419-432.
76. Vasko KA, McMichael J: Use of an immuno-modulating agent in the treatment of myofascial pain, J Equine Vet Sci 1998;8:399.
77. DeLeo JA, Tanga FY, Tawfik VL: Neuroimmune activation and neuroinflammation in chronic pain and opioid tolerance/hyperalgesia, Neuroscientist 2004;10:40-52.
78. Karai L, Brown DC, Mannes AJ, et al: Deletion of vanilloid receptor 1-expressing primary afferent neurons for pain control, J Clin Invest 2004;113:1344-1352.

SECTION IV INTEGUMENTARY SYSTEM

John A. Stick

CHAPTER 24

Principles of Reconstructive and Plastic Surgery

Jeremy V. Bailey

Skin lacerations and other traumatic injuries of the integument are frequently seen in equine practices and range from relatively minor cuts to severe, potentially debilitating injuries. The challenges facing the practitioner managing these injuries are numerous, and treatment is dictated by the nature and size of the wound, the area of the body on which the wound occurs, and several aspects of wound healing unique to horses. The age of the wound, integrity of the local blood supply, degree of contamination, location of the injury, skin loss, and local tissue damage must all be considered when deciding on the most appropriate method for managing a particular wound. In addition to biologic factors, the physical size of equine patients and the environment in which they are kept present unique management challenges not encountered in the treatment of soft tissue injuries in other species.

Primary, or even delayed primary, closure may not be a viable option, and many wounds are best treated by secondary closure or as open wounds. To get the best cosmetic and functional results, open granulating wounds should be managed in such a way as to allow maximal contraction and optimal epithelialization. Carefully planned reconstructive and skin mobilizing techniques can be used in conjunction with primary, delayed primary, or secondary wound closure, and as part of an overall strategy of open wound management to minimize the potential cosmetic and functional shortcomings of excessive epithelialization (scarring). Besides traumatic wounds, there are other clinical situations, such as the planned excision of skin lesions, in which reconstructive procedures can be used to facilitate closure of surgical incisions.

The overall objective in the management of any wound is to achieve a result that is as functional and as cosmetically appealing as possible. The benefits of successfully using reconstructive procedures in wound management include an increased percentage of the wound covered with full-thickness skin, improved cosmetic appearance and function, and a reduction of overall healing time.

The combination of skin loss and the amount of redundant or loose skin surrounding a wound has an obvious influence on the clinician's ability to close a wound and the extent to which wound contraction will contribute to the final result. The effects of the location of the wound on the body as well as breed differences on wound healing in horses are well recognized,[1,2] as is the influence of surrounding skin tension on wound contraction.[3] Similarly, the extent to which some reconstructive and skin mobilization techniques can be used depends on the presence of adequate tissue surrounding the wound.

Financial and time constraints are often imposed on the practitioner, and it is advisable to spend time discussing the owner's expectations, the possible complications, and the costs associated with these procedures before beginning. When these techniques are used, particularly in elective, cosmetic procedures, failures can result in significant client dissatisfaction. The application of reconstructive and mobilization techniques has not been studied in horses to the same extent as in other species.

Understanding the principles and limitations of reconstructive procedures, adhering to the basic principles of equine wound management, and providing appropriate postoperative care all contribute to a successful outcome.

CUTANEOUS BLOOD SUPPLY

Detailed descriptions of the vascular supply to the skin in humans and dogs have been the basis for significant advancement of cutaneous reconstructive procedures. A full appreciation of the normal anatomy and function of the cutaneous vascular supply, particularly as it pertains to the healing process, contributes to sound clinical judgment, allows the selection of appropriate surgical techniques, and provides an insight into the possible reasons for surgical failures. Two types of vessels supply the skin—musculocutaneous vessels, which are perforator vessels that pass through the body of underlying muscle, and direct cutaneous arteries, which reach the skin by passing through the fascial septa between muscle bodies. Direct cutaneous vessels run subdermally and supply a larger area of skin than do musculocutaneous vessels.

In most animals with loose-fitting skin, the skin is supplied by direct cutaneous vasculature. These cutaneous vessels run parallel to the skin surface and are closely associated with the panniculus muscle in areas where this structure is present. In the distal extremities, where no panniculus muscle exists, the direct cutaneous arteries run beneath and parallel to the dermis.

The term *angiosome* has been applied to an area that is supplied by a single artery. A total of 374 such angiosomes have been plotted in humans.[4] In a similar study in other mammals and vertebrates, the cutaneous perforator vessels were found to be larger and sparser in areas where skin was very mobile but smaller in diameter and more densely packed in areas where skin was less mobile.[5] This finding was consistent in the species studied and, although horses were not included in the study, it seems reasonable to assume that a similar pattern exists in equine skin.

Smaller vessels branch off these cutaneous arteries and arborize in the dermis, forming three closely interconnecting plexuses—the deep subcutaneous plexus, the middle cutaneous plexus, and the superficial subpapillary plexus—which together supply the dermis and adnexal structures of the skin.[6] The superficial plexus is an important component of the thermoregulatory system, and all three are crucial in maintaining the integrity of the blood supply and are thus of importance when manipulating skin in reconstructive procedures.

A number of skin flaps based on the major cutaneous arteries of the trunk are commonly used in dogs.[7] These include axial pattern flaps, island arterial flaps, and vascularized free flaps. A skin flap based on the cutaneous portion of the caudal branch of the deep circumflex iliac artery has been described and used in experimental studies for a vascularized free tissue transfer in the horse.[8] Although regional differences in blood supply and the influence this has on wound healing in horses is well recognized,[1] more detailed descriptions of the vascular supply to the equine skin are required to expand our understanding and use of reconstructive procedures.

PHYSICAL AND BIOMECHANICAL PROPERTIES OF SKIN

The physical and biomechanical properties of skin are the focus of increasing attention in reconstructive surgery, and application of these characteristics is an integral part of many procedures in reconstructive surgery. Although many of the techniques have not been tested in horses, they provide some interesting potential opportunities in equine reconstructive surgery.

The biomechanical properties of skin are the product of three structural components: collagen fibers that impart strength, elastic fibers, and the ground substance (predominantly proteoglycans). Interactions between these components give skin its viscoelastic properties. It is important to note that these components vary considerably between individuals and between different sites of the body. In humans, they are known to be affected by aging, solar radiation, disease, and chemical and physical trauma.[9] The effect of superficial hydration of the skin on its mechanical properties has potential benefits in reconstructive surgery. Twenty minutes after the application of wet paper towels, covered by a plastic wrap, a significant increase in the distensibility was seen, but the skin became more plastic in its behavior.[10] This study concluded that the deep structures of the skin were unlikely to be affected by the short-term hydration and postulated that the contribution of the epidermis to the mechanical properties of skin may explain the mechanical differences seen between a pure collagen model and skin. The positive benefits of superficial hydration of the skin in a limited number of clinical cases supported the experimental observations.[10]

Tension

The normal tension that exists in skin is a result of the elastic fibers in the dermis and is the reason skin edges retract when incised. In 1861, Professor Langer expanded on previous work and mapped out the so-called Langer's lines of tension (cleavage lines, or "splittability" lines) over the surface of the human body. This work followed the unexpected observation that when skin was punctured by a conical instrument, an elliptical, not a circular, defect resulted. Langer's lines were established in cadaveric studies and were referred to as lines of maximal tension, but Langer's studies did not take into account body or limb position or movement. However; since skin is anisotropic, these tension lines are influenced by muscle contraction, movement of joints, and other external forces, and thus Langer's lines are more accurately referred to as relaxed skin tension lines.[11] Relaxed skin tension lines were thought to result from the overall orientation of connective tissue strands within the dermis, but histology and scanning electron microscopy have not confirmed this theory.[11,12] Nonetheless, it is these tensile forces that result in the retraction of skin edges after an incision. Incisions made parallel to lines of maximal tension will gap to a lesser extent and heal with a finer scar than incisions made at right angles to them. Incisions made at right angles to lines of tension will heal with scars that, over time, become stretched and less cosmetically acceptable.

Skin extensibility is another important physical property of the dermis that is used to advantage in reconstructive surgery. Lines of maximal extensibility have been shown to run at right angles to Langer's lines, which logically could also be referred to as lines of minimal extensibility.[12] Pinching skin into folds at the site of a proposed reconstructive procedure can be used to roughly determine the extent of orientation of skin extensibility and to assess whether or not the edges of the remaining defect can be brought into apposition after excision of a lesion or the revision of a scar.[12] When excising an elliptical piece of skin, closure is facilitated by ensuring that the long axis of the ellipse is aligned to Langer's lines. Because the lines of maximal extensibility are at right angles to Langer's lines, the width of the ellipse can be wider if the long axis is parallel rather than perpendicular to Langer's lines. Tension lines and lines of extensibility in the human skin are well documented, and diagrams showing their locations can be found in most plastic and reconstructive surgery texts.

Tension lines have been described in dogs, but they have been investigated to only a very limited extent in the horse[13,14] (Fig. 24-1). Lines of maximal extensibility have been mapped for the equine carpus, which has given credence to the clinical practice of making longitudinal incisions over the dorsal aspect of the carpus.[15] Diagrams showing the orientation of tension lines in the dog resemble the color patterns seen on the tiger and zebra, and it has been suggested that the lines of the skin color pattern in these animals closely mimic lines of tension.[11] In the absence of detailed information, these generalities can be used to advantage in planning reconstructive procedures in

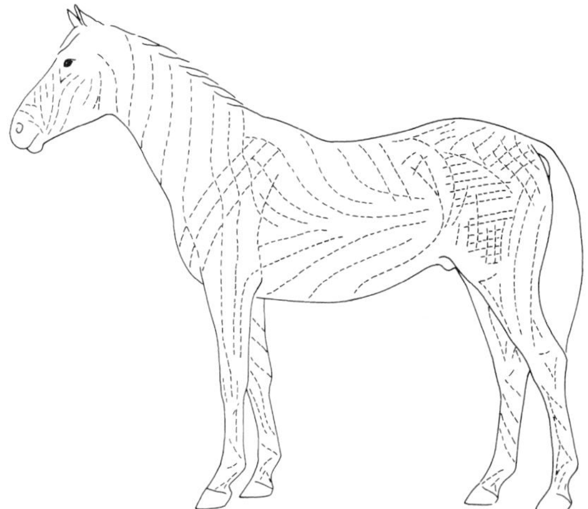

Figure 24-1. Cleavage lines of equine skin. (Redrawn from Hrudka F, Popesko P, Komarek V: Principal Morphology of Domestic Animals, Bratislava, Czechoslovakia, 1962, Slovak Publishing House of Agricultural Literature, based on work by Najbrt.)

horses. However, to make full use of such surgical procedures as Z- and W-plasties in the horse, a much greater understanding of the physical properties of the equine skin is required.

Creep and Stress Relaxation

As a result of its viscoelastic properties, skin demonstrates two related, time-dependent biomechanical properties referred to as creep and stress relaxation. Creep is the increase in length (strain) that occurs when a constant force (stress) is exerted on a piece of skin. Creep results from the normally convoluted collagen fibers becoming straightened and aligned in a parallel fashion. Water is displaced from the collagen network, and disruption of elastic fibers occurs. Stress relaxation, on the other hand, is the decrease in the stress that occurs when the strain imposed on a piece of skin is kept constant, which explains why the tension on a suture line decreases to some extent a few minutes to hours after surgery.

Mechanical creep must be differentiated from biologic creep, which is the generation of new tissue in response to chronic tension. Biologic creep occurs during pregnancy, as a result of obesity, or in association with clinical situations such as hernias and large skin tumors.

A number of surgical techniques in reconstructive surgery utilize these viscoelastic properties of skin; however, there are only limited documented accounts of the application of these procedures in horses. Used alone or in combination with the other techniques described in the following paragraphs, they provide interesting possibilities for the management and reconstruction of skin wounds in horses.

SKIN EXPANSION AND STRETCHING TECHNIQUES

Presuturing

Presuturing is a preoperative suturing technique to plicate skin over an area of proposed excision.[16] The technique utilizes the mechanical creep properties of skin and in a pig model has been shown to decrease the tension required to close a standardized wound by 40%. When compared with simply undermining the surrounding skin, presuturing did result in some tissue gain and an initial decrease on closing tension, although this advantage diminished over time.[17] In this study, it was concluded that the demonstrated progressive increase in water content of the tissue resulted in the skin's becoming stiffer and thus harder to close. The duration of presuturing is thus important, and clinical observations in the horse support this. Where the preplaced sutures were left in place for 24 to 30 hours, moderate edema resulted that was not seen when the sutures were removed after 4 to 8 hours.[18,19] Periods as short as 2½ hours have been shown to be beneficial.[16] Placement of the plicating sutures can be carried out under local anesthesia. Optimally, the sutures should be placed in the direction that will take greatest advantage of the inherent extensible nature of the skin. As discussed previously, although the lines of maximal extensibility have not been mapped out for the horse, sound clinical observation and assessing extensibility by pinching the skin into folds over the proposed area will provide useful information.

The original description of this procedure suggests that presuturing avoids the potential complications that can be associated with undermining.[16] However, the combination of presuturing and undermining may provide additional advantages.

Intraoperative Tissue Expansion

Intraoperative tissue expansion has been advocated as a means of decreasing incision closure tension, and, since the original description of intraoperative sustained limited expansion,[20] a number of synonyms for this strategy have developed, all of which imply a single-stage procedure involving the rapid expansion of the surrounding skin. The techniques for achieving this have varied from the manual application of traction using towel clamps applied to the skin edges, to the use of Foley catheters and the short-term subcutaneous implantation of other inflatable balloon devices.[21] Variations in technique have been described ranging from tension being applied in three or four cycles of 3 to 5 minutes, to a single loading cycle applied for 20 minutes. The original explanation that this technique utilized the creep phenomenon has been challenged, and it has been suggested that this technique utilizes only the normal elastic properties of skin.[22,23] Histologic studies support this, as none of the changes in the dermis associated with mechanical creep are seen with acute intraoperative tissue expansion.[24] There is considerable controversy regarding the benefits of intraoperative tissue expansion, and although several studies have been designed to demonstrate the benefits of intraoperative expansion,[25-27] other studies have concluded that it is in fact the undermining of the surrounding skin required for the placement of the inflatable balloons that accounts for the decrease in closing tensions.[22,28]

Intraoperative skin expansion relies on the inherent extensibility of the skin and, as previously mentioned, these properties vary at different locations on the body. Although there are no published reports of using this technique in equine reconstructive surgery, there are sufficient reports of the potential benefits in other species to justify considering this procedure as part of a strategy to manage tension across a wound closure.

External Skin-Stretching Devices

Externally applied devices designed to recruit skin from the surrounding area have been described.[29,30] The successful use of a relatively simple system using adherent skin pads and elastic connecting cables has been described in dogs.[30] The placement of the adherent pads relative to the skin edge can be varied according to the amount of skin recruitment required. By subjective assessment, a moderate amount of tension is applied on the cables and is increased every 6 to 8 hours. The greatest gains in recruitment of surrounding skin appeared to be achieved 48 to 72 hours after application. The technique was reported as being well tolerated, and no biologic complications were encountered with separation of the adhesive pads associated with excessive tension being the most common technical complication.

The suture tension adjustment reel (STAR) is an externally applied device that allows tension on a preplaced horizontal mattress suture to be adjusted after the knot has been tied.[31] This device can be used preoperatively as an adjunct to the presuturing technique and has been advocated as a means of achieving intraoperative tissue expansion.

Elastomers

Studies in other species have shown encouraging results with the use of silicone elastomer tissue expanders in reconstructive procedures, but descriptions of the use of this technique in horses are limited.[32] This procedure entails placing a silicone pouch under the intact skin immediately adjacent to the scar that is to be repaired. After the implant incision is healed, the pouch is expanded over a period of 4 to 7 days by the injection of small amounts of saline through an injection port, thereby stretching the overlying skin. The elastomers are available in various sizes and shapes to allow flexibility in the amount of tissue expansion. Once sufficient skin expansion has been achieved, the elastomer is removed and the expanded tissue is used to form a skin flap to cover the defect. This procedure takes advantage of both mechanical and biologic creep, and the microscopic changes seen in the skin are consistent with mechanical creep. In addition, new tissue is generated in response to the chronic forces.[24]

The use of expanders may be of substantial benefit where limited skin is available for reconstructive procedures. Canine studies have recorded increases of 35.9% and 37.3% in the surface areas of skin on the antebrachium and crus following controlled expansion.[33] Other studies in dogs have shown that these are well tolerated and provided sufficient additional skin for the development of pedicle flaps to cover defects on the tarsus.[34]

Other advantages include similarity of the color and hair coverage of the donor skin to the surrounding area, the absence of a donor site defect, and the quality of the skin that is generated. The optimal inflation pressure of the elastomer has not been determined in large animals. In a canine study, 20 to 40 mm Hg was initially used, but pressures approaching capillary pressure have been shown to be safe.[34] Excessive pressure can lead to ischemia and necrosis of the overlying skin. Skin color and transcutaneous partial pressure of oxygen have been used in human patients to monitor the integrity of the blood supply to the expanding skin.

In cattle, where the skin is thicker and stiffer, the increased pressure required resulted in rupture of the elastomer, suggesting that a more resilient device may be required for use in large animals.[32] Random pattern flaps created from expanded skin have a longer survival rate than those raised from nonexpanded skin. When compared with controls, the survival length of delayed random pattern flaps and similar flaps raised from expanded skin was increased 73% and 117%, respectively. This increased viability is attributed to similar effects seen in the delay phenomenon.[35,36]

Histologic changes seen in expanded skin are consistent with mild inflammation that includes edema and the formation of a fibrous capsule around the expander.[33,36] The initial thickening of the epidermis and thinning of the dermis seen immediately after expansion has been shown to return to normal 24 weeks after transfer of expanded skin in dogs, and similarly the capsule that forms around the expander disappears.[37] However, this fibrous capsule results in an overall thickening of the raised flap and loss of elasticity of the expanded skin.[34] This increased stiffness may compromise the surgeon's ability to manipulate the flap in the reconstructive procedure. Removing this fibrous capsule may resolve this problem to some extent, and the effect of capsulectomy on the blood supply to the expanded skin has been investigated.[38] Although some controversy surrounds this issue, it appears that removing or incising the capsule to facilitate advancement of the flap does not critically affect the survival of the expanded tissue.[38]

Complications include implant failure, wound dehiscence, and premature exposure of the expander necessitating its removal before adequate expansion had been achieved. Although more experience is required with the use of tissue expanders, they add an exciting new dimension to the treatment and repair of skin defects in horses.

SUTURES AND PATTERNS

The proper placement and use of appropriate suture patterns are important technical considerations in reconstructive surgery. The selection of a suture pattern is often based on personal preference; however, in some instances, there are definite advantages and disadvantages associated with particular patterns that should be taken into consideration. The choice of suture material is of less importance.[7,11] Manipulation of the tissue when placing sutures should be performed as atraumatically as possible. If instruments are used to stabilize or manipulate the skin edges, crushing and abrading tissue, which is detrimental to future healing, should be avoided; using one's gloved fingers is probably the least traumatic method. Most reconstructive procedures can be performed using a standard instrument set; however, the addition of a limited number of instruments will greatly assist the surgeon. The addition of sharp skin hooks or Lahey traction forceps aids in minimizing trauma when stabilizing tissue. Sterile Backhaus towel clamps are an acceptable alternative. Stabilization of the skin using an instrument that penetrates the tissue is less damaging to the skin and its microvasculature than using an instrument that has a crushing action.

To facilitate optimal healing, accurate apposition of the skin edges with minimal interference to the blood supply should be the goal when suturing wounds. The pattern and technique of suture placement, the number of sutures, and suture line support all play an important role in ensuring an optimal outcome.

The spacing of sutures plays an important role in maintaining optimal apposition of the skin edges. As a rule sutures should be placed at a distance from the skin edge equal to the thickness of the skin itself.[39] However, other factors, such as the tension on the wound edges and the thickness and stiffness of the skin, must also be taken into consideration. The collagenolytic and inflammatory processes that take place during early wound healing serve to weaken the suture-holding ability of skin, and as a result, sutures should be placed at a distance of at least 0.5 cm from the skin edge for improved security.[40] Clinical experience with equine wounds treated by secondary closure shows that wound edges where newly epithelialized tissue exists have little or no holding strength, making it important to place the sutures well back from the skin edge to ensure optimal holding strength. In laboratory animals, the levels of matrix metalloproteinases (MMP) have been shown to be higher in keratinocytes during reepithelialization,[41] and in a porcine model, the levels of these collagenolytic enzymes have also been shown to be higher and to persist longer in granulating wounds than in sutured wounds.[42] Neutrophil-derived MMP has been associated with nonhealing wounds in human patients, and overexpression of this particular collagenase may be part of the pathogenesis of chronic ulcers.[43] A sound working knowledge of the biology of wound healing improves clinical judgment and reduces the risk of failure of repair (see Chapter 5).

Sutures should be placed as close together as is necessary to achieve good approximation of skin edges. In human surgery, placing interrupted sutures 0.5 cm apart has been shown to give good tissue apposition and to minimize tension on individual sutures.[40] The suggestion that the distance between individual sutures should be twice the thickness of the skin may apply, although in some instances, this procedure may result in an excessive number of sutures being used, leading to impaired healing as a result of excessive tissue reaction.[39]

The tension applied when placing and tying skin sutures should be sufficient to appose the skin edges, but overtightening of sutures can result in failure of the suture line. The overall tension on a suture is a combination of intrinsic and extrinsic tension. Intrinsic tension is the constricting effect within the suture loop, which, if excessive as a result of the suture being tied too tightly, causes strangulation of the blood supply to tissue within the loop of the suture. A higher degree of intrinsic tension can be generated with heavier suture material, and any postoperative swelling will increase the intrinsic tension of a suture. Extrinsic tension results from opposing forces exerted by the surrounding skin on the suture when drawing the skin edges together. Extrinsic tension is related to the size of the defect being sutured and to the amount of redundant or loose skin in the area.[44] Tension on sutures can lead to tissue necrosis by interfering with local blood supply, increasing edema, and decreasing the oxygen supply to the skin. The clinical result of this can include wound dehiscence, sloughing of tissue, and delayed healing which, depending on the location of the suture line, may have catastrophic consequences.

Basic Suture Patterns

Simple Interrupted Sutures

Simple interrupted sutures are commonly used and give good tissue apposition, provided they are not placed too far back from the skin edge or pulled too tightly, which will cause inversion of the skin edges. Placement with slight eversion is preferred to inversion.[45] A simple interrupted pattern also allows adjustments for good alignment of skin edges in irregularly shaped defects. If placed correctly, this pattern results in minimal interference with the blood supply, and skin wounds closed with interrupted patterns have been shown to have greater tensile strength and less compromise of the microvasculature than those closed with simple continuous sutures.[46,47] If tension exists across the suture line, the attributes of simple interrupted sutures can be combined with other tension suture patterns.

Simple Continuous Sutures

As with any continuous pattern, knot failure or suture breakage results in breakdown of a large part or all of the incision line. Continuous patterns are quickly placed, but it is not possible to vary the tension on the suture line to the same degree as with an interrupted pattern. Continuous patterns have been shown to result in increased edema and compromised circulation, and to have a prolonging effect on the inflammatory phase of wound healing.[46,47] Although a simple continuous pattern has some advantages, the lack of precise skin apposition probably makes it inappropriate for use in plastic or reconstructive procedures.

Corner Suture

Also called a three-point or half-buried mattress suture, the corner suture is used to secure the sharp intersecting point of a Y-shaped incision[39] (Fig. 24-2). The intersecting apex of a Y-incision is predisposed to ischemia, and the design of this suture pattern is such that it will not further compromise the blood flow. The three-point suture can also be used in other situations in which a piece of skin has a similar acute angle that is in danger of being underperfused. The corner suture pattern begins like a routine horizontal mattress suture, but instead of penetrating the full thickness, only a partial-thickness bite is taken. The suture is then passed horizontally through the dermis at the point of the V and completed as it was started with a partial-thickness bite.

Tension Sutures

Tension along suture lines can result from attempting to close wounds where there has been loss of skin, swelling in the area, or loss of elasticity in the surrounding tissue of more chronic wounds.[48] Closing wounds under tension should always be performed with caution, but the relationship between the tension on sutures and the incidence of necrosis of skin flaps has been challenged in a study that concluded the vascular damage resulted primarily from the process of undermining the tissue, and that skin with a good

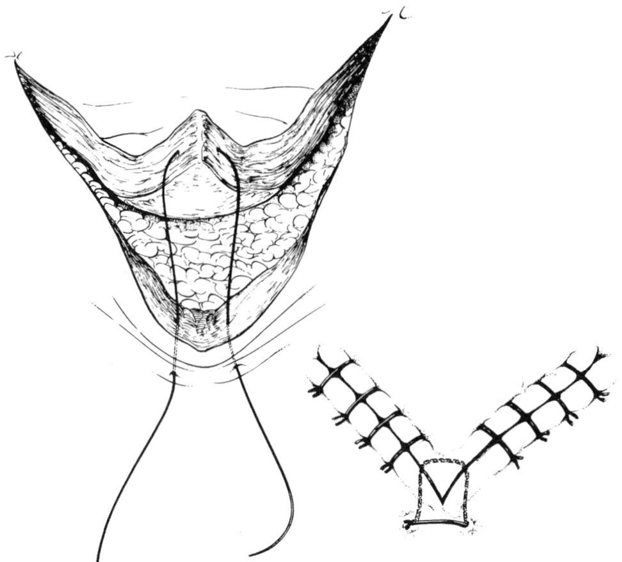

Figure 24-2. Corner suture used to minimize vascular compromise to the tip of the flap.

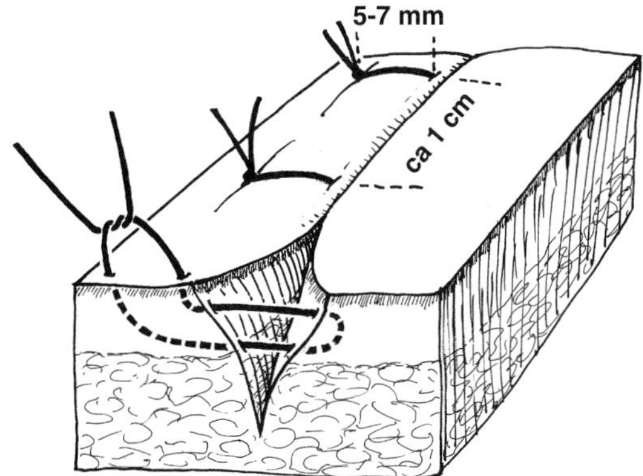

Figure 24-3. The Allgöwer corium vertical mattress suture pattern allows good apposition with minimal or no eversion of the skin edges.

blood supply could be closed under considerable tension without fear of necrosis.[49] Careful judgment is required when increasing stress on suture lines; however, clinical experience suggests that equine wounds can be closed under a reasonable amount of tension and, provided there is a good blood supply and the suture line is well supported by bandages, healing is not delayed. If the force required on individual sutures to appose the skin edges increases to the point where vascular compromise is becoming a threat, tension sutures can be used to minimize the risk. Tension sutures can be used either alone or in combination with appositional patterns such as simple interrupted sutures.

Mattress Sutures

Mattress sutures are described as vertical or horizontal, depending on their orientation to the skin edge. These patterns can be used when there is mild-to-moderate tension, and both provide reasonable apposition but have a tendency to evert the skin edges. The vertical pattern is stronger under tension than the horizontal pattern and, as with a simple interrupted suture, results in little if any compromise to the microcirculation.[50] The configuration of the horizontal pattern is such that, if ischemic necrosis results from tissue strangulation, all the tissue within the loop of the suture will be lost, which may compromise subsequent efforts to reconstruct the defect. Mattress sutures can be used together with simple interrupted sutures, and buttons, tubing (rubber, plastic), or gauze can be incorporated into mattress sutures to form a quilled or stented suture to further disperse the pressure forces on the skin.[50] Although quilled sutures are particularly useful on the body where pressure bandages cannot be used to support the suture line, they should be avoided if pressure wraps or casts are to be used.[51]

The corium vertical mattress pattern results in minimal trauma (Fig. 24-3). The suture penetrates the skin and exits at the wound level through the corium (dermis). On the opposite side of the skin defect to be closed, the suture is placed entirely in the corium, where it exits intradermally at the skin edges, penetrates the dermis again at the other side of the defect, and exits near the initial penetrating suture, where the knot is tied. This results in a cosmetically superior closure because the sutures exit on only one side of the defect, which ensures perfect alignment of the skin edges without inversion or eversion.[52]

Far-Near-Near-Far Suture

The far-near-near-far suture pattern (or its modified form, the near-far-far-near pattern) combines a tension suture, the *far* portion, and an appositional suture, the *near* portion, with the name denoting the order and relative distance the sequential suture bites are taken from the skin edge (Fig. 24-4). This pattern has a higher tensile strength than either a simple interrupted or a mattress pattern, but it has the disadvantage of requiring that a large amount of suture material be placed in the wound.[50,52]

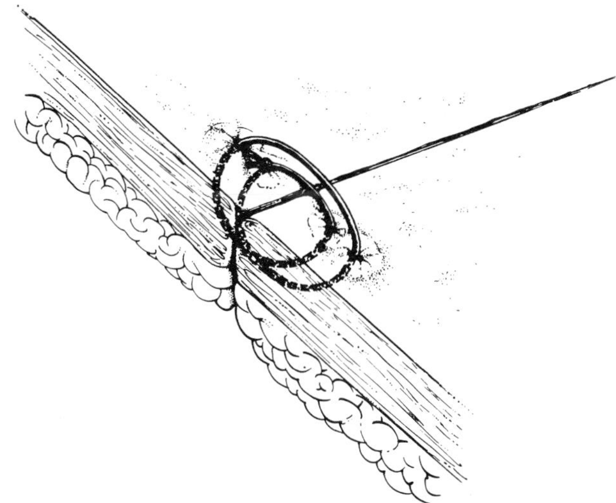

Figure 24-4. Near-far-far-near suture pattern. This serves as an excellent tension suture while also providing good tissue apposition.

Walking Suture

Walking sutures have been described for closing skin defects in small animals, particularly in areas where the skin fits loosely, such as the trunk.[52,53] (For additional information on this technique see Chapter 17.)

Support for Suture Lines

Supplying adequate support for sutured wounds can make the difference between success and failure in reconstructive procedures. The method of choice is determined to some extent by the location of the lesion and the amount of tension on the suture line. In many areas, bandages may be used to support a suture line, immobilize adjacent skin and joints, minimize edema formation, and obliterate dead space.[54] Pressure bandages are frequently used to support suture lines; however, a subtle balance exists between providing adequate support of the suture line and causing interference with regional blood flow. As a result of absorption of moisture and compression of the material, pressure bandages constructed from cotton or linen materials soon lose their compressive effect and hence their support.[54] To maintain effectiveness, it is necessary either to change these bandages at frequent intervals or to apply tension with an elastic bandage. (A more in-depth discussion on this topic can be found in Chapter 18.)

When dealing with repairs on the upper limb or body, the clinician is often limited to the use of stent bandages (tie-over bandages). Stent bandages can provide effective support of suture lines, but they are less effective in preventing or minimizing edema formation. Careful monitoring of these sites is important.

COSMETIC CLOSURE OF SKIN DEFECTS OF VARIOUS SHAPES

When undertaking scar revisions or the closure of traumatic wounds, the size of the lesion, the amount of redundant skin in the area, the elasticity of the surrounding skin, and the inherent lines of extensibility are all factors that must be considered during the planning process, and sound clinical judgment remains the cornerstone of making the required surgical decisions. Complex mathematical analyses have been developed to assess the optimal closure patterns of wounds with complex shapes,[55] and these analyses may provide helpful information in the future. The amount of skin that can be excised, the extent of undermining of the surrounding skin, the type of tension-relieving techniques used, the type of suture patterns to be applied, and postoperative support of the repair are other details that should be carefully contemplated when reconstructive or skin mobilization procedures are undertaken.

Fusiform Defects

Fusiform defects have sometimes been incorrectly referred to as elliptical defects; the latter do not have the tapered or spindle-shaped appearance of a fusiform excision and do not close as well.[11,52] Fusiform excisions can be used for elective scar revision, with the long axis of the defect being oriented parallel to the lines of skin tension. A 3:1 or 4:1 length-to-width ratio will allow closure of the defect with a fairly even distribution of tension along the length of the suture line.[44,52] Shorter, broader defects result in uneven tension and in the formation of dog-ears at the end of the suture line.[56] In fusiform incisions, dog ears can be prevented by tapering the ends of the excised portion of skin. Dog-ears may flatten out over time, but there are methods to surgically manage these irregularities (described later). As with any reconstructive procedure, careful marking of the proposed incision facilitates excision of a piece of skin that has the optimal orientation and length-to-width ratio.

Triangular, Square, and Rectangular Defects

Where sufficient movable skin is present to permit closure, triangular defects should be closed from the points of the triangle toward the center, which will result in the formation of a Y-shaped suture line. There is a tendency for the skin at the center of the Y to develop ischemic necrosis. A half-buried horizontal mattress suture in a three-point closure (see Fig. 24-2) can be used to secure this central point with minimal interference with the blood supply.[45,52]

Square and rectangular defects can also be closed by beginning to suture at the corners of the defect and closing toward the center.

V-Shaped Defects

V-shaped defects are fairly commonly encountered in veterinary medicine, and often part of the V-flap is lost or requires débridement prior to closure. After débridement, the resulting chevron-shaped defect can be closed with a Y-pattern in a similar fashion as that described for triangular defects. If the chevron-shaped defect is long and narrow, provided there is sufficient movable skin in the surrounding area, a fusiform incision could be made around it, which is then closed like a linear defect.

Circular Defects

Closure of circular defects commonly results in the formation of dog-ears, and several techniques have been described to prevent their occurrence. It is possible to close the defect without modifying its circular appearance by orienting the suture line along the relaxed skin lines of tension, followed by removal of any dog-ear as described later. A circle can be converted into either an X- or a Y-shape by tightening sutures placed at three or four points equidistant to each other around the circumference of the defect. The closure can then be completed, although this method also results in the formation of dog-ears.

The simplest method of facilitating closure of a circular defect is to excise two triangles on opposite sides of the circle, thereby creating a fusiform defect. From a geometric point of view, the height of each triangle should be at least equal to the diameter of the circle; this will result in the removal of normal skin equivalent to 1.5 times the area of the original defect.[57] The implications of removing this amount of normal skin must be carefully evaluated.

The double S-shaped incision with a bi-winged excision, the bow tie, and the combined V-incision are alternative methods of modifying circular defects that have been well described.[58] These methods are all designed to minimize scarring and dog-ear formation in human cosmetic surgery and are best applied to small circular defects.

Management of Skin Puckers (Dog-Ears)

Skin puckers or dog-ears often develop at the end of the suture line when closing oval or irregularly shaped defects or when using skin flaps as part of a reconstructive procedure. These dog-ears, if ignored, will flatten out to some extent over time and may be of little consequence. If the pucker is small and the cosmetic appearance of limited importance, they can be managed by placing small sutures through half the thickness of the skin. In some locations, however, this conservative approach may result in an unsightly blemish. Because correction of dog-ears requires lengthening of the incision, it is worthwhile to assess the extent to which the cosmetic result will be compromised if the pucker is left alone.

To remove the puckered skin, the dog-ear can be stabilized with an appropriate instrument and removed by incising around the base, which results in a lengthening of the incision line (Fig. 24-5, *A*). An alternative method is to close the incision until the dog-ear becomes well defined, and then to extend the initial incision through the middle of the dog-ear. This converts the pucker into two small triangular flaps of skin (Burow's triangles), which can be excised at their base (see Fig. 24-5, *B*).

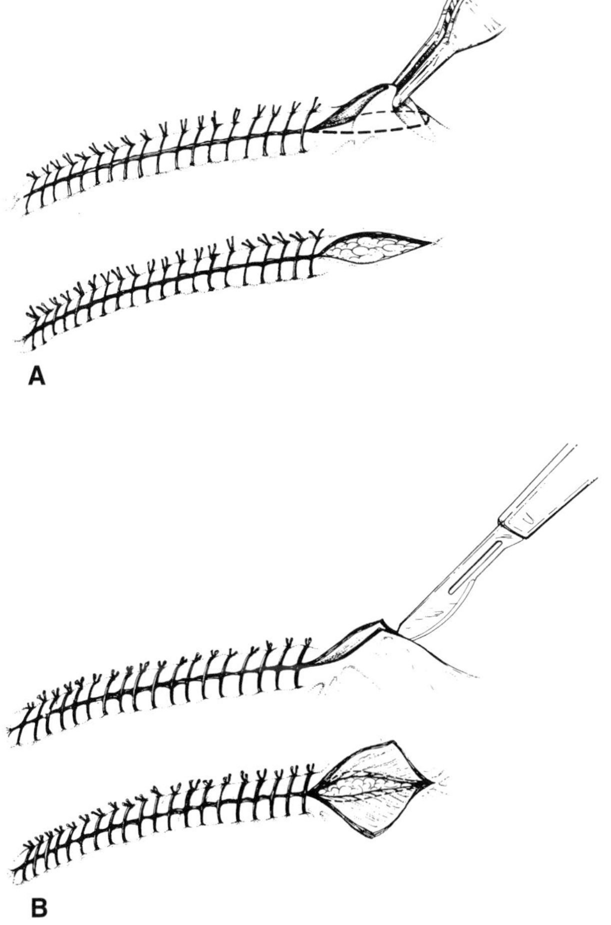

Figure 24-5. Methods for removal of dog-ears. **A,** The dog-ear is held securely, elevated, and excised level with the surrounding skin, leaving a small fusiform defect to close. **B,** The dog-ear is bisected to form two small triangular flaps, which are resected level with the skin surface.

TENSION-RELIEVING AND SKIN-MOBILIZATION PROCEDURES

Tension on suture lines can result in discomfort for the animal, increased scarring, ischemia of the skin margin, and suture line breakdown with partial or complete wound dehiscence. Allowing for some species variation in the amount of redundant skin, the hair coverage, the vascular supply, and tension on skin, suture lines present less of a problem in animals than in humans. Because of these basic differences, skin wounds in dogs can be closed under moderate tension without deleterious effects provided there is an adequate blood supply to the area.[48,52] The effect of suture line tension is also influenced by the anatomic location of the lesion. On the lower limb, where there is essentially no redundant skin, excessive tension on suture lines may create a tourniquet effect around the limb, leading to vascular compromise.[53]

The consequences of tension across suture lines can be attenuated by undermining the surrounding skin, by using tension sutures, or by using tension-relieving incisions or skin-mobilization techniques. These techniques may be used alone or in combination.

Surgical procedures in plastic and reconstructive surgery can vary from simple tension-relieving incisions to complex, vascularized, free tissue transplants. Although skin wounds should be closed using the simplest possible technique, despite the paucity of redundant skin, the use of skin-advancement techniques or skin flaps to cover defects is often overlooked by equine practitioners. By successfully using skin-mobilization techniques, the potentially deleterious effects associated with contraction and epithelialization can be overcome; these include excessive scarring, fragile epithelial coverage, and impaired function. Early wound coverage results in a reduced healing time and a more rapid return to function.

Although many of the reconstructive techniques that have been described for both humans and small animals have obvious practical limitations in horses, certain techniques are applicable.

Undermining Skin

Simple undermining can be used alone or in conjunction with other reconstructive procedures, and it is a time-honored method of reducing tension on a suture line when closing a skin defect. As with any surgical procedure, the skin should be handled as gently as possible, with every effort being made to protect the integrity of the blood supply and health of the tissue. Undermining the skin entails separating it from its underlying subcutaneous attachments by dissecting along fascial planes.

Skin can be undermined through either sharp or blunt dissection using scissors or a scalpel (Fig. 24-6). Opening the blades of scissors that have been inserted closed into fascial planes or using the handle of a scalpel in a back-and-forth motion are both accepted methods for bluntly

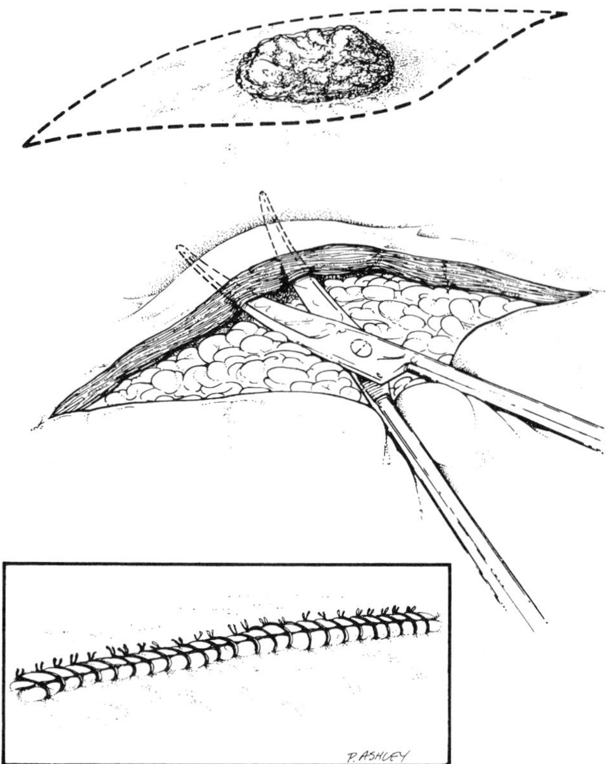

Figure 24-6. Fusiform excision. After excision, the skin is undermined to facilitate closure of the defect. Optimal length-to-width ratio of the fusiform defect should be 4:1.

undermining skin. Blunt dissection has the advantage of minimizing damage to the blood vessels in the area. In chronic, fibrotic wounds, blunt dissection may be difficult to perform, making it necessary to use careful sharp dissection with either a scalpel or scissors; this, however, results in the severance of small subcutaneous blood vessels, increasing both the amount of intraoperative hemorrhage and the chances of hematoma formation after closure. Hematomas have several detrimental effects. They may increase the tension on the suture line, they provide an excellent medium for bacterial growth, and they can interfere with revascularization of transferred flaps.[45,52] If clinical assessment indicates the possibility of subcutaneous hematoma formation, the surgeon should consider preventive measures such as the use of drains or carefully applied pressure bandages.[45,52]

The depth at which skin is undermined depends on the vascular supply to the skin and the presence of superficial nerves in the particular area. To prevent damage to these structures, the regional anatomy should be reviewed. Skin on the trunk should be elevated below the level of the panniculus muscle to preserve the small direct cutaneous vessels. On the distal limbs, where no panniculus muscle exists, the dissection plane should be as deep as possible between the subcutaneous tissue and the deep fascia.[44,52]

Fascial planes are quite easy to identify where an elective incision has been made and primary closure is being used. In older wounds, however, because of scar tissue that develops as a result of the inflammatory process, these planes are not as readily identified until the dissection has been continued some distance from the skin edge. In these situations, it seems appropriate, from a clinical perspective, to begin the dissection at a level that approximates the original thickness of the skin.

The degree to which skin needs to be undermined can be estimated by drawing the skin edges together with towel forceps. As a rule, in a fresh wound, a distance equal to the width of the defect itself should be elevated on each side of the wound. If this is not sufficient, undermining can be extended half as much again. Given the potential to disrupt cutaneous blood supply, the cost-to-benefit ratio of expanding the area of undermining requires careful clinical judgment. The extent to which skin can be undermined without significantly damaging the blood supply and causing necrosis has not been objectively studied in either small animals or horses. In small animals, it is thought that undermining can be quite extensive without causing necrosis, provided there is limited interference with the blood supply. Clinical experience suggests the same is true for horses.[52,53,59] Used in conjunction with a mesh-expansion technique to repair large defects on the limbs of dogs, 360-degree undermining was not associated with any major complications.[60]

The benefits derived from undermining skin are the result of freeing the skin from its underlying subcutaneous attachments, which allows the surrounding skin to be drawn toward the defect and makes use of the elastic properties of the surrounding skin. The baseline closing tension on standard-size wounds varies significantly in different locations and is related to the amount of loose-fitting skin in the area.[22,28] Studies in pigs have shown an incremental decrease in wound closure tension associated with increasing the extent of undermining, but the benefits diminished as the extent of the undermining increased.[22]

The physical properties of skin vary at different sites on the body, and thus the benefits of undermining are affected by the location of the wound and any other factors that alter the biomechanical properties of skin. In chronic wounds, as the process of wound healing proceeds, first the inflammatory edema and later the development of fibrous tissue will both lead to a loss of skin elasticity, which may necessitate undermining the adjacent skin more extensively to achieve the desired effect. Having an appreciation of the concept of lines of maximal tension and extensibility in different regions of the body will allow the surgeon to take full advantage of the gains made by undermining.

Tension-Release Incisions

A tension-release incision may be thought of as a bipedicle advancement flap, which is described in more detail later. This technique is used to allow the movement of a limited amount of skin in those areas where simple undermining alone does not result in adequate tension relief, yet the size of the defect to be closed does not justify the use of more elaborate procedures. The secondary defect created by the relief incision should be closed, but when planning relief incisions, efforts should be made to create the secondary defect over healthy tissue, thereby minimizing problems associated with second-intention healing should closure not be feasible.

Mesh Expansion

A combination of tension-relieving incisions, mesh expansion, and tissue mobilization has been used successfully to facilitate primary, delayed primary, or secondary closure of wounds in a variety of locations.[59] When compared with open treatment of wounds in horses, the mesh expansion method has been shown, in both experimental and clinical cases, to facilitate closure, to greatly reduce the overall healing time, and to markedly improve the end result.[61] This technique has the advantage of increasing the percentage of the wound that is eventually covered by full-thickness skin, thus providing a better cosmetic and functional result. Technically, the procedure is simple, does not require any special instruments, and could be performed in most general practices, provided anesthetic facilities are available.

After the surrounding skin is undermined, small stab incisions are made in the undermined skin to permit expansion of this tissue, as is done for a meshed skin graft. The stab incisions are made in staggered rows, parallel to the wound edge (Fig. 24-7). Applying traction to the skin edges provides a good indication for the optimal location and orientation of the stab incisions to gain maximal relief of tension.[61] As a guideline, in fresh wounds, the distance between the individual stab incisions and between the adjacent rows should measure approximately 1 cm.[59] Placing either the rows or the incisions too closely should be avoided so as to prevent the possibility of the adjacent stab incisions becoming confluent or causing focal vascular compromise. The appropriate length of the stab incisions varies depending on the degree of elasticity and pliability of the undermined skin. In fresh wounds, more expansion can be obtained with smaller incisions, whereas for those wounds where the surrounding skin is thickened and fibrotic, longer incisions are required to achieve the same result.

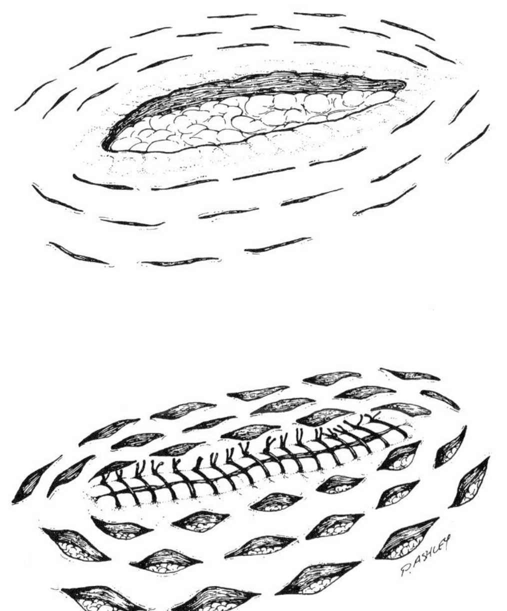

Figure 24-7. The mesh expansion method of closure. After undermining of the skin around the defect, two or three staggered rows of stab incisions are made parallel to the skin edges. After closure of the defect, the stab incisions gape open to provide both tension relief and drainage.

In some older wounds, the stab incisions do not readily open at the time of suturing, but clinical experience has shown that expansion does occur within a few hours postoperatively as a result of the viscoelastic nature of skin. Stress relaxation results in the undermined skin's becoming fatigued over time and in the stab incision's opening, which together result in reduced tension on the suture line.

When this technique is used in conjunction with delayed closure in clinical cases, careful excision of excessive granulation tissue from the wound bed to a level slightly below the skin surface has been beneficial. Excising granulation tissue does result in some hemorrhage, which can be controlled by pressure. Hematoma formation is seldom a problem because the presence of the stab incisions allows drainage. A simple interrupted suture pattern, a far-near-near-far tension suture, or a combination of the two is the preferred method of skin closure.

Postoperative support of the closure is extremely important and, depending on the location of the repair, strong consideration should be given to the use of cast immobilization for 10 to 14 days. Experimental evidence revealed that the use of padded cast bandages did not provide the required support.[59] This was assumed to be caused by compression of the padding, and therefore; if padded bandages are used, they should be changed daily.

As mentioned, wounds on the limbs of horses are often not suited to the use of rotating skin flaps, but the mesh expansion technique has been used on these wounds and to wounds on the head with a very good cosmetic and functional result.

V-to-Y-Plasty and Y-to-V-Plasty

The V-to-Y-plasty technique for relieving tension requires a V-shaped incision with the point of the V directed away from the defect to be closed. Once closure of the original defect has been accomplished, closure of the V incision is done by converting it to a Y (Fig. 24-8). The longer the legs of the V, the greater will be the degree of tension relief; however, this method provides only a limited amount of skin movement. This technique has been advocated for scar revision of the eyelid (see Chapter 56) and for relieving tension when closing elliptical defects.[51,52] It is less useful for management of large defects.

Conversely the Y-to-V-plasty may be used if additional tension is required, as in the surgical correction of an entropion.

Z-Plasty

Z-plasties can be used to relieve tension along a linear scar, to change the orientation of an incision line or a scar, or to relieve tension when closing a large defect.[12,52,58] These effects are achieved by recruiting loose tissue from the sides of the surgical site,[46,52] and the success of the procedure depends on the presence of sufficient loose skin in the area to permit mobilization of tissue. If this situation does not exist, as in the lower limb of the horse, other procedures may be more suitable.

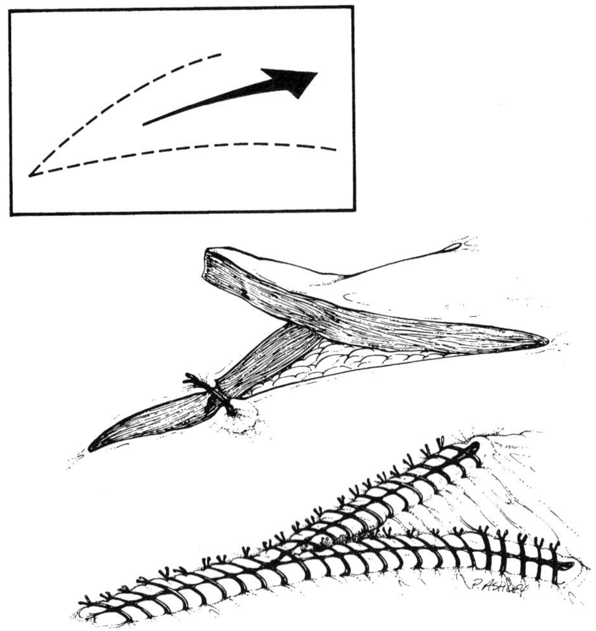

Figure 24-8. V-to-Y-plasty for tension relief. With this technique, tissue is mobilized in the direction of the arrow.

A Z-plasty represents a modification of a transposition flap. The basic Z-plasty is performed by making a Z-shaped incision with subsequent undermining and transposition of the two triangular portions of skin formed by the dissection (Fig. 24-9). This technique results in a change in the orientation of the central limb of the Z and a gain in its length. The gain in length achieved by this procedure is in the direction of the original central limb—that is, before transposition occurs. Commonly, the Z is symmetric, with the three limbs of equal length and the same angle between the two arms and the central limb. An angle of 60 degrees is most frequently used, which results in a 75% gain in length. Varying the angles of the Z and the length of the arms influences the amount of elongation, and decreasing the angles results in a decreased gain in length. Maintaining a 60-degree angle and lengthening the limbs of the Z can achieve an increased gain in length; however, the greater the increase in length, the greater will be the resultant tension in the surrounding tissue. Using multiple small Z-plasties in the place of a single large procedure can minimize this problem.[44,52] Although the biomechanics and mathematics of Z-plasties have been examined extensively,[62] this has been done using laboratory models, which are not influenced by the same forces as those found in living tissue.

When Z-plasties are used to realign scars in humans, the limbs of the Z are oriented to follow the lines of minimal tension in the area, and the angles between the limbs of the Z vary according to the obliquity of the scar in relation to the lines of tension. If the procedure is to be used successfully for scar revision in horses, more information on the lines of tension and extensibility in the equine integument is needed.

In the horse, Z-plasties have been recommended as a relaxation procedure for closing elliptical defects and for revision of scars involving the eyelids that have resulted in an acquired entropion.[63] Although other uses undoubtedly exist, the procedure does have some limitations and potential complications. The most common complication encountered with the use of a Z-plasty is ischemia and necrosis of the tips of the triangular skin flaps. The risk of this problem occurring can be reduced by making the base of the flap as broad as possible, and by minimizing tension on the suture line.

W-Plasty

W-plasties are designed to improve the cosmetic appearance of a scar. Scars that are at right angles to lines of maximal tension tend, over time, to widen and become cosmetically less acceptable. By using a W-plasty, such a scar is excised by making a series of opposing zigzag incisions in such a way that, when sutured, the incisions will interdigitate, with the result that the final suture line resembles a series of Ws. In using this technique, the orientation of the single scar is changed from being at right angles to the lines of maximal tension, to a series of connected smaller scars that are better aligned with the force of maximal tension and are thus not inclined to widen. Because this procedure involves the removal of tissue, with a subsequent increase in tension on

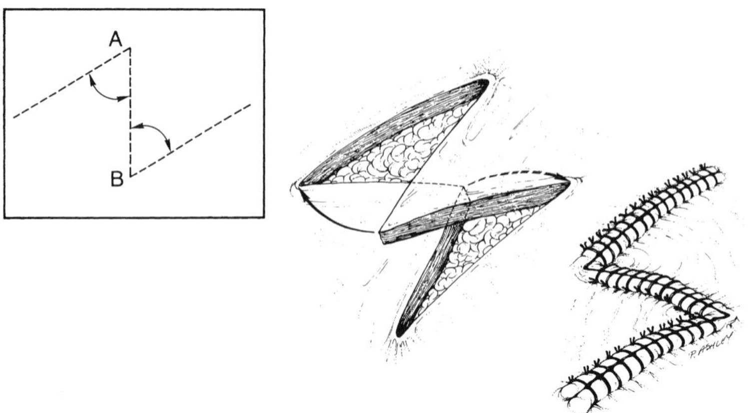

Figure 24-9. Z-plasty. The length of the central limb (*A* to *B*) is equal to the length of the two arms, and tissue movement occurs along the plane of the central limb. After closure, the orientation of the Z incision changes.

the surrounding skin, and because it is primarily aimed at cosmetic improvement, careful consideration should be given to the need to undertake the surgery in the first place. If the technique is to be used, a template should be fashioned and the incision lines drawn carefully on the skin to ensure that the two opposing incisions are adequately aligned.

SKIN FLAPS

A skin flap or pedicle graft is a portion (or flap) of skin that, once created, can be moved from its original location to a second location on the body while, by virtue of its attachment (or pedicle), it maintains its vascular supply.[56] The survival of these grafts, unlike that of free skin grafts, is not dependent on successful revascularization from the recipient site. Because they are fully vascularized, pedicle grafts can be used to cover areas that, because of an inadequate blood supply, would be unsuitable for free skin grafts. When successful, pedicle grafts reduce healing time, minimize wound contraction and epithelialization, and provide a more acceptable cosmetic result with better-quality skin coverage and more hair growth.[64] In contemplating the use of a skin flap, the clinician should evaluate the amount of loose skin in the area. It is preferable to be able to close the secondary defect that is created when the flap is raised, so sufficient skin must be available to be moved without producing excessive tension, either on the donor site or on the suture line at the new location. For this reason, large wounds on the distal limb may not be suitable candidates for a local skin flap, although some success with the use of both advancement flaps and rotating flaps has been reported in treating wounds on the dorsal aspect of the tarsus and in the area of the metacarpophalangeal joint.[32,65,66] Pinching the adjacent skin into folds or pushing it toward the center of the primary defect can be used to assess availability of surrounding skin.

Flaps can be classified as local or distant, depending on the relationship of the donor site to the recipient site. Distant flaps usually involve either multiple surgical procedures or a degree of postoperative immobilization and patient compliance that makes them impractical in equine surgery. Local flaps (including rotation flaps, transposition flaps and interpolating flaps) are usually one-stage procedures and can be simple advancement or rotating flaps. These types of flaps have been used successfully in the horse (discussed in more detail later).

Skin flaps can also be categorized as random or axial pattern flaps according to the nature of their vascular supply. Random pattern flaps, which do not have a defined vascular pattern, depend on the subdermal plexus for their survival and have been referred to as subdermal plexus flaps.[7,52] Axial pattern flaps, on the other hand, contain at least one major direct afferent and efferent cutaneous vessel and are usually named in accordance with that vessel. In the dog, the omocervical, thoracodorsal, and caudal superficial epigastric flaps are well recognized and established axial pattern flaps. In horses, local random pattern flaps have greater potential use than axial pattern flaps.

Flap survival depends on the survival of its intrinsic vasculature. Random pattern flaps have traditionally been defined by the length-to-width ratio. Although the detailed differences in regional blood supply to the skin have not been studied in the horse, differences have been reported in other species, and those studies show that the optimal ratio for a flap varies with the location on the body. Length-to-width ratios from 1:1 to 3:1 for single-pedicle and 1.5:1 to 3:1 for bipedicle flaps have been reported in the veterinary literature. However, studies in dogs and pigs have shown that flaps of a standard length with similar vascularity survive regardless of the flap width.[67] In horses, a correlation of flap width to viable length in random-pattern pedicle flaps of the trunk has been shown.[64] Length-to-width ratios of 1.5:1 and 3:1 have been used successfully on the limb and head, respectively.[32] The narrower the pedicle of the flap, the more maneuverable it will be, but the greater will be the chances of compromising its blood supply. On the other hand, a wide-based flap will have a good vascularity, but mobility, particularly rotational, is limited.

The delay phenomenon has been used to enhance the blood supply to the skin to increase the chances of flap survival. This two-stage technique involves incising and undermining the skin and subcutaneous tissue of the proposed flap and then leaving it sutured in its original location for a period of time. The incision may be on three adjacent sides of the flap or on two opposite sides, and undermining may extend to involve all or part of the flap. The most appropriate period of delay varies between species[56]: in rabbits and pigs, 8 to 10 days is adequate, whereas circulation in single-pedicle flaps in dogs rose to 150% of normal in 3 weeks.[68] Although the mechanism by which flap survival improves using this technique is not well understood, both denervation and ischemia have been shown to play a role. Both contribute, with a resultant increase in the number and diameter of the vessels as well as an increase in blood flow into the flap through its primary attachments.[56] Although this technique is not commonly used in equine reconstructive surgery, as the horizons of plastic surgery in the horse are advanced, specific studies are required to determine the most appropriate method and optimal time delay.

Tension applied to pedicle grafts has been shown to decrease blood supply and thus increase flap necrosis in pigs.[69] However, a study assessing the effect of tension on perfusion of axial and random pattern flaps in foals concluded that adequate perfusion was maintained in equine axial pattern flaps even when subjected to high tension.[70] Assessment of flap viability based on clinical criteria, such as temperature and color, is probably adequate. Other, more sophisticated techniques, such as radioisotope tests, histamine wheal, and fluorescein tests, have been described[44,52] but are not routinely used. It is debatable whether venous compromise or arterial compromise, or a combination of both, is of prime importance in flap necrosis; however, tension on the pedicle from stretching or over-rotating should be avoided to help prevent flap necrosis. Several methods for improving flap survival, in addition to the delay phenomenon, have been suggested; these include the use of vasodilators, massage, dimethyl sulfoxide, and hyperbaric oxygen, but all are of questionable clinical value and require further investigation before they can be recommended.[44,52]

Attention to the specific anatomy of local cutaneous vasculature is important in flap elevation. Flaps raised on the trunk should be elevated beneath the cutaneous musculature, whereas on the limb, dissection should be performed deep in the subcutaneous tissue. Careful design of the flap and good postoperative care greatly improve the success rate achieved. Planning should include determining which type of skin flap is to be used as well as mapping and marking the borders of the piece of skin to be elevated. This can be done using a paper towel or a cloth template of the defect to be covered. The flap should be slightly larger than the defect. Sharp corners, which may be prone to ischemia, should be avoided.

Advancement Flaps

Advancement flaps are random pattern flaps that can be of either the single or the bipedicle type. They have also been referred to as sliding flaps because there is no rotation of the elevated skin. A V-Y-plasty is an example of an advancement flap.

Simple bipedicle advancement flaps are performed either by making a single longitudinal incision on one side of the wound or by incising on each side of the defect. These incisions are made parallel to the wound edge to create skin flaps that are approximately the same width as the original defect. The bipedicle nature of this flap (Fig. 24-10) provides two sources of blood supply to ensure survival of the mobilized portion of skin. The flaps and surrounding skin can be undermined and the initial defect closed. Depending on the nature of the surrounding skin, the new defects can be either closed or left to heal by contraction and epithelialization. As with many types of flaps, moving a single or bipedicle advancement flap may create some laxity in the adjacent skin. This can be managed by removing small triangular portions of skin called Burow's triangles, thereby preventing the formation of a dog-ear at the end of the suture line.

An H-plasty is a modification of a single-pedicle flap and is used to mobilize tissue during closure of a rectangular defect. Two single-pedicle flaps are used on opposite sides of the defect to advance the skin, and Burow's triangles are excised at the base of both pedicles to avoid dog-ear formation (Fig. 24-11).

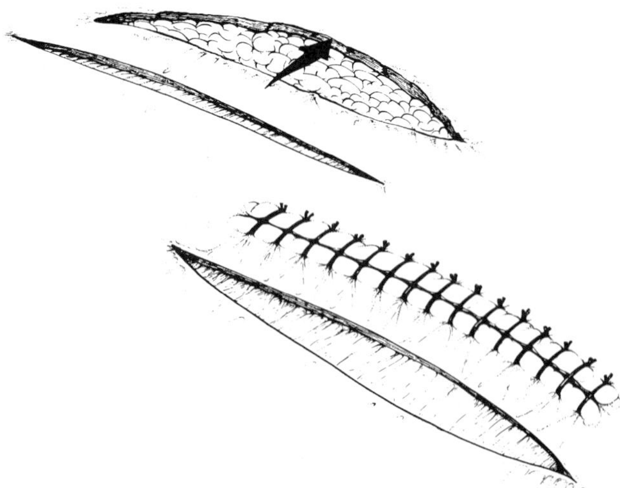

Figure 24-10. Simple bipedicle flap. This can be used with a single incision as depicted here, or a second incision can be made on the opposite side of the primary defect. By using two relaxing incisions, it may be possible to close the secondary defects.

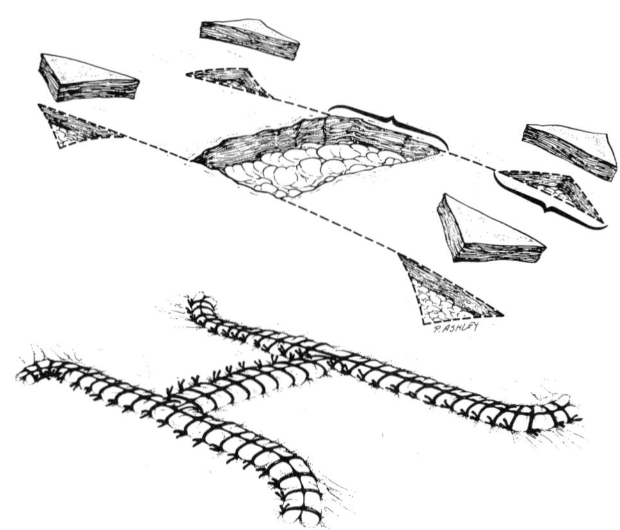

Figure 24-11. Sliding H-plasty. Burow's triangles are created and excised to prevent dog-ear formation after mobilization of the skin.

Rotating Flaps

Rotating flaps can be one of three types: rotation, transposition, or interpolating flap. A rotation flap requires making a semicircular incision and moving the tissue laterally to cover the defect (Fig. 24-12). A rectangular, single-pedicle flap that is created adjacent to a defect and subsequently rotated on its pedicle is called a transposition flap (Fig. 24-13). These can be rotated up to 180 degrees, but increasing the amount of rotation has the effect of shortening the flap, which must be considered when planning the surgery. Moving a similar rectangular flap onto an immediately adjacent defect (i.e., the pedicle bridges an intact portion of the skin) creates an interpolating flap (Fig. 24-14). The successful use of a rotating flap has been described in the management of a lesion on the craniolateral aspect of the tarsus of a horse.[65]

VASCULARIZED FREE TISSUE TRANSFERS

Vascularized free tissue transfers, based on axial pattern flaps and using microvascular surgical techniques, have gained popularity and are now commonly used in many small animal surgical practices. Attempts have been made to adapt this technology for use in repairing skin defects in horses. In the horse, a large axial pattern flap has been described using the deep circumflex iliac artery and vein,[8] and a smaller one is based on the saphenous artery and the medial saphenous

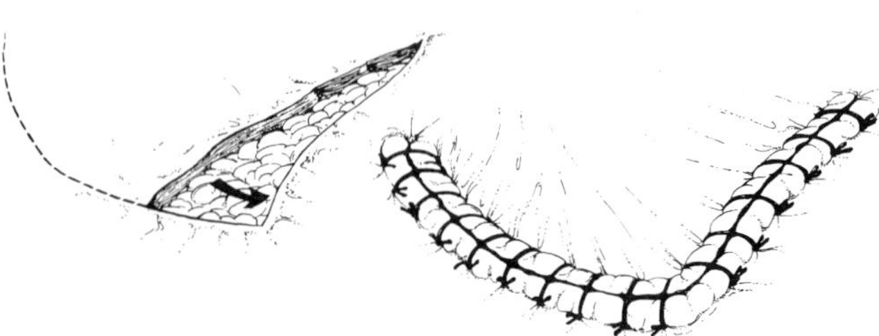

Figure 24-12. Rotation flap. This pedicle flap is semicircular and can be used to cover small defects.

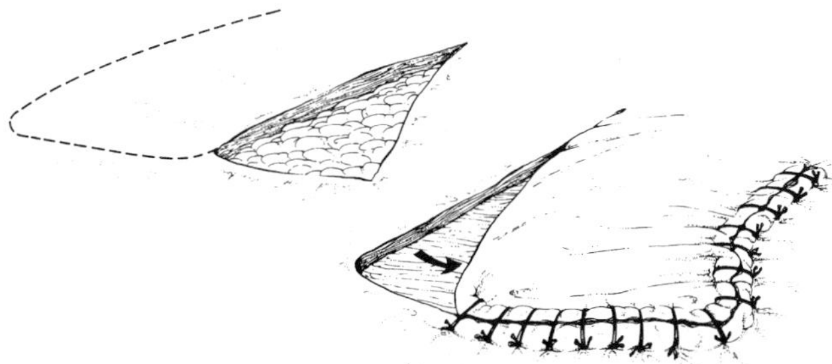

Figure 24-13. Transposition flap. This rectangular pedicle flap can be rotated up to 180 degrees to cover a defect.

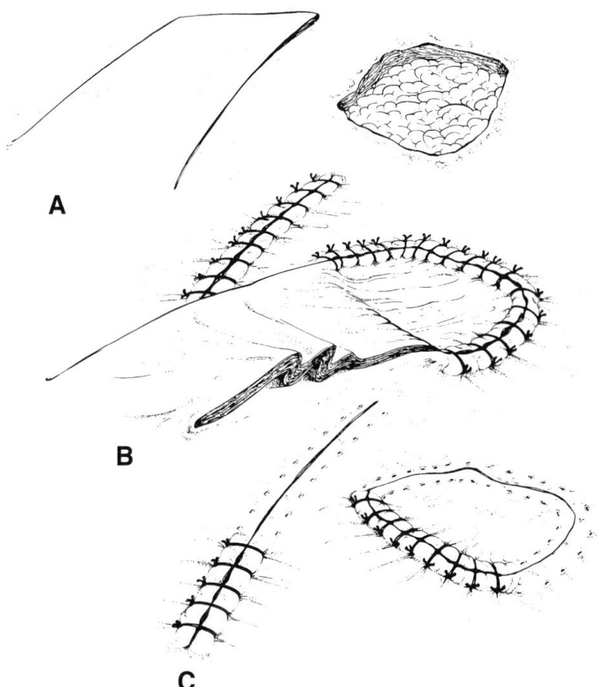

Figure 24-14. Interpolating flap. **A,** A pedicle flap is lifted from the skin adjacent to the defect. **B,** The flap bridges normal tissue to cover the defect. **C,** After the defect has healed, the pedicle is resected and the incised edges are sutured.

vein.[71] Attempts to use these flaps to cover distant defects in experimental models have been unsuccessful. In two separate studies, none of the heterotopically transferred flaps survived for longer than 4 to 6 days. The reasons for failure are not fully understood but may include poor perfusion as a result of vasospasm, a species tendency toward vascular thrombosis, or ischemia-reperfusion (IR) injury. Neutrophils are a significant source of the oxygen free radials that mediate IR injury. A study to assess the role that IR injury plays in the failure of vascularized free tissue transfer in the horses showed no difference in neutrophil accumulation between control myocutaneous flaps and those subjected to a period of ischemia and reperfusion.[72]

Although the initial results are disappointing, further studies may resolve the difficulties encountered and make this technique a viable option in the future.

REFERENCES

1. Jacobs KA, Leach DH, Fretz PB, et al: Comparative aspects of the healing of excisional wounds on the leg and body of horses, Vet Surg 1984;13:83.
2. Wilmink JM, Stolk PW, Van Weeren PR, et al: Differences in second-intention wound healing between horses and ponies: Macroscopic aspects, Equine Vet J 1999;31:53.
3. Walton GS, Neal PA: Observations on wound healing in the horse, Equine Vet J 1972;4:93.
4. Taylor GI, Palmer JH: The vascular territories (angiosomes) of the body: Experimental study and clinical applications, Br J Plast Surg 1987;40:113.
5. Taylor GI, Minabe T: The angiosomes of the mammals and other vertebrates, Plast Reconstr Surg 1992;89:181.
6. Pavletic MM: Vascular supply to the skin of the dog: A review, Vet Surg 1980;9:77.
7. Palvetic MM: Canine axial pattern flaps using the omocervical, thoracodorsal, and deep circumflex iliac direct cutaneous arteries, Am J Vet Res 1981;42:391.
8. Lees MJ, Bowen CV, Fretz PB, et al: Transfer of deep circumflex iliac flaps to the tarsus by microvascular anastomosis in the horse, Vet Surg 1989;18:292.
9. Edwards C, Marks R: Evaluation of biomechanical properties of human skin, Clin Dermatol 1995;13:375.
10. Jemec GBE, Jemec B, Jemec BIE, et al: The effect of superficial hydration on the mechanical properties of human skin in vivo: Implications for plastic surgery, Plast Reconstr Surg 1990;85:100.
11. Borges AF: Elective Incisions and Scar Revision, Boston, 1973, Little, Brown.
12. Converse JM: Reconstructive Plastic Surgery, Philadelphia, 1978, WB Saunders.
13. Irwin DHG: Tension lines in the skin of the dog, J Small Anim Pract 1966;7:593.
14. Hrudka F, Popesko P, Komarek V: Principal Morphology of Domestic Animals, Bratislava, Slovakia, 1962, Slovak Publishing House of Agricultural Literature.
15. Cartee RE, Cowles WR: Surgical implications of extensibility of the skin of the equine carpus, Am J Vet Res 1978;39:387.
16. Liang MD, Briggs P, Heckler FR, et al: Presuturing: A new technique for closing large skin defects: Clinical and experimental studies, Plast Reconstr Surg 1988;81:694.
17. Neves RI, Saggers GC, Mackay DR, et al: Assessing the role of presuturing on wound closure, Plast Reconstr Surg 1998;97:807.
18. Bigbie R, Shealy P, Moll D, et al: Presuturing as an aid in the closure of skin defects created by surgical excision, Proc Am Assoc Equine Pract 1990;36:613.
19. Harrison IW: Presuturing as a means of reducing skin tension in excisional biopsy wounds in four horses, Cornell Vet 1991; 81:351.
20. Sasaki GH: Intraoperative expansion as an immediate reconstructive technique. Facial Plast Surg 1988;5:362.
21. Johnson TM, Brown MD, Sullivan MJ, et al: Immediate intraoperative tissue expansion, J Am Acad Dermatol 1990;22:283.
22. Mckay DR, Saggers GC, Kotwal N, et al: Stretching skin: Undermining is more important that intraoperative expansion, Plast Reconstr Surg 1990;86:722.
23. Siegert R, Weerda H, Hoffman S, et al: Clinical and experimental evaluation of intermittent intraoperative short-term expansion, Plast Reconstr Surg 1993;92:248.
24. Johnson TM, Lowe L, Brown MD, et al: Histology and physiology of tissue expansion, J Dermatol Surg 1993;19:1074.
25. Shapiro AL, Hochman M, Thomas JR, et al: Effects of intraoperative tissue expansion and skin flaps on wound closing tensions, Arch Otolaryngol Head Neck Surg 1996;122:1107.
26. Wee SS, Logan SE, Mustoe TA: Continuous versus intraoperative expansion in the pig model, Plast Reconstr Surg 1992;90:808.
27. Chandawarkar RY, Cervino AL, Pennington GA: Intraoperative

acute tissue expansion revisited: A valuable tool for challenging skin defects, Dermatol Surg 2003;29:834.
28. Hochman M, Branham G, Thomas RJ: Relative effects of intraoperative tissue expansion and undermining on wound closing tensions, Arch Otolaryngol Head Neck Surg 1992;118:1185.
29. Hirshowitz B, Lindenbaum E, Har-Shai Y: A skin-stretching device for the harnessing of the viscoelastic properties of skin, Plast Reconstr Surg 1993;92:260.
30. Pavletic MM: Use of an external skin-stretching device of wound closure in dogs and cats, J Am Vet Assoc 2000;217:350.
31. Cohen BH, Cosmetto AJ: The suture tension adjustment reel, J Dermatol Surg Oncol 1992;18:112.
32. Madison JB, Donawick WJ, Johnston DE, et al: The use of skin expansion to repair cosmetic defects in animals, Vet Surg 1989;18:15.
33. Spodnick GJ, Pavletic MM, Clark NC, et al: Controlled tissue expansion in the distal extremities of dogs, Vet Surg 1993;22:436.
34. Keller WG, Aron DN, Rakich PM, et al: Rapid tissue expansion for the development of rotational skin flaps in the distal portion of the hindlimb of dogs: An experimental study, Vet Surg 1994;23:31.
35 Cherry GW, Austad E, Pasyk K, et al: Increased survival and vascularity of random-pattern skin flaps elevated in controlled, expanded skin, Plast Reconstr Surg 1983;72:680.
36. Madison JB: Tissue expansion, Vet Clin North Am Equine Pract 1989;5:633.
37. Zeng Y, Huang K, Zhang J, et al: Biorheolgical characteristics of skin after expansion, Biorheology 2001;38:367.
38. Morris SF, Pang CY, Mahoney J, et al: Effect of capsulectomy on the hemodynamics and viability of random-pattern skin flaps raised on expanded skin in pigs, Plast Reconstr Surg 1989;84:314.
39. Swaim SF: Surgery of traumatized skin. In Swaim SF, editor: Management and Reconstruction in the Dog and Cat, Philadelphia, 1980, WB Saunders.
40. Forrester JC: Suture materials and their uses, Nurs Mirror 1975;140:48.
41. Madlener M, Parks WC, Werner S: Matrix metalloproteinases (MMPs) and their physiological inhibitors (TIMPs) are differently expressed during excisional skin wound repair, Exp Cell Res 1998;242:201.
42. Agren MS, Taplin CJ, Woessner JF, et al: Collagenase in wound healing: Effect of wound age and type, J Invest Dermatol 1992;99:709.
43. Nwomeh BC, Liang HX, Cohen IK, et al: MMP-8 is the predominant collagenase in healing and non-healing ulcers, J Surg Res 1999;81:189.
44. Swaim SF: Principles of plastic and reconstructive surgery. In Slatter DH, editor: Textbook of Small Animal Surgery, Philadelphia, 1985, WB Saunders.
45. McGregor IA: Fundamental Techniques of Plastic Surgery and Their Surgical Application, Edinburgh, 1980, Churchill Livingston.
46. Cocke WM, McShaw RH, Silverton JS: Essentials of Plastic Surgery, Boston, 1980, Little, Brown.
47. Speer DP: The influence of suture technique on early wound healing, J Surg Res 1979;27:385.
48. Dixon AC: The secondary closure of wounds, Vet Rec 1963;75:1133.
49. Myers MB, Combs B, Cohen G: Wound tension and wound sloughs: A negative correlation, Am J Surg 1965;109:711.
50. Knecht CO, Algernon RA, Williams AA, et al: Fundamental Techniques in Veterinary Surgery, Philadelphia, 1987, WB Saunders.
51. Stashak TS: Reconstructive surgery in the horse, J Am Vet Med Assoc 1977;170:143.
52. Allgöwer M, Liebermann-Meffert D: Wundheiling. In Allgöwer M, Siewert D, editors: Chirurgie, ed 5, Berlin/New York, 1992, Springer-Verlag.
53. Swaim SF: Management of skin tension in dermal surgery, Comp Cont Educ Pract Vet 1980;11:758.
54. Swaim SF: The physics, physiology and chemistry of bandaging open wounds, Comp Cont Educ Pract Vet 1985;7:146.
55. Lott-Crumpler DA, Chaudhry HR: Optimal patterns for suturing wounds of complex shapes to foster healing, J Biomech 2001;34:51.
56. Kernahan DA, Vistnes LM: Biological Aspects of Reconstructive Surgery, Boston, 1977, Little, Brown.
57. Pavletic MM: Pedicle grafts. In Slatter DH, editor: Textbook of Small Animal Surgery, Philadelphia, 1985, WB Saunders.
58. Swaim SF, Lee AH, McGuire JA: Techniques for reconstructing circular defects in dogs, Vet Surg 1984;13:18.
59. Bailey JV, Jacobs KA: The mesh expansion method of suturing wounds on the legs of horses, Vet Surg 1983;12:78.
60. Vig MM: Management of integumentary wounds of extremities in dogs: An experimental study, J Am Anim Hosp Assoc 1985;21:187.
61. Beard WL, Wilkie DA: Partial orbital rim resection, mesh skin expansion, and second intention healing combined with enucleation or exenteration for extensive periocular tumors in horses, Vet Ophthalmol 2002;5:23.
62. Furnas DW, Fisher GW: The Z-plasty: Biomechanics and mathematics, Br J Plastic Surg 1971;24:144.
63. Turner AS, McIlwraith CW: Techniques in Large Animal Surgery, Philadelphia, 1982, Lea & Febiger.
64. Hinchcliff KW, MacDonald DR, Lindsay WA: Pedicle skin flaps in ponies: Viable length is related to width, Equine Vet J 1992;24:26.
65. Peyton LC, Campbell ML, Wolf GA, et al: The use of random skin flaps in equine reconstructive surgery, J Equine Vet Sci 1983;3:80.
66. Peyton LC: Reconstructive surgical techniques in the horse, J Am Vet Med Assoc 1981;179:260.
67. Pavletic MM: Caudal superficial epigastric arterial pedicle grafts in the dog, Vet Surg 1980;9:103.
68. Hoffmeister FS: Studies on timing of tissue transfer in reconstructive surgery: 1. Effect of delay on circulation in flaps, Plast Reconstr Surg 1957;19:283.
69. Larrabee WF, Holloway GA, Sutton D: Wound tension and blood flow in skin flaps, Ann Otol Rhinol Laryngol 1984;93:112.
70. Bristol D: The effect of tension on perfusion of axial and random pattern flaps in foals, Vet Surg 1992;21:223.
71. Miller CW, Hurtig M: Identification and transfer of free cutaneous flaps by microvascular anastomosis in the pony, Vet Comp Orthop Traumatol 1989;1:21.
72. Scott MW, Fowler D, Matte G, et al: Effect of ischemia and reperfusion on neutrophil accumulation on equine microvascular tissue flaps, Vet Surg 1999;28:180.

CHAPTER 25

Skin Grafting

James Schumacher

INDICATIONS FOR GRAFTING

The most common indication for applying a skin graft to a horse is a wound so large that it cannot heal by any other means, but the presence of any open wound that cannot be sutured is an invitation for grafting (Fig. 25-1). The rapid healing achieved with a skin graft may make grafting the most economical choice for managing some wounds that cannot be sutured. A healed skin graft contains some epidermis, dermis, and some adnexa, including hair follicles, so it is likely to be more cosmetic and resilient than a wound healed primarily by epithelialization. Skin grafting should not be regarded as an option of last resort and should not be avoided because of fear of failure. Many techniques of skin grafting require little experience and only basic surgical equipment.

GRAFT CLASSIFICATION

The two basic types of skin grafts are the pedicle graft and the free graft.[1-3] A *pedicle* graft remains connected to the donor site, at least temporarily, by a vascular pedicle that sustains the graft, ensuring its viability. A pedicle graft is useful for covering a poorly vascularized wound, because the graft does not depend on the vascularity of the recipient site. The cosmetic appearance of wounds healed by application of a pedicle graft is good, because all components of skin are transferred. Cutaneous wounds of horses are rarely covered with a pedicle graft because the inelastic nature of equine skin makes mobilizing an adequate amount of skin for advancement difficult.[4] In humans and dogs, skin flaps that incorporate a direct cutaneous artery and vein (i.e., axial-pattern flaps) can be transferred to adjacent sites, or even to remote sites, by using microsurgical techniques to anastomose the flap's vessels to local recipient vessels.[5] Similar transfers in horses are unsuccessful, apparently because of reperfusion injury to the graft.[6,7]

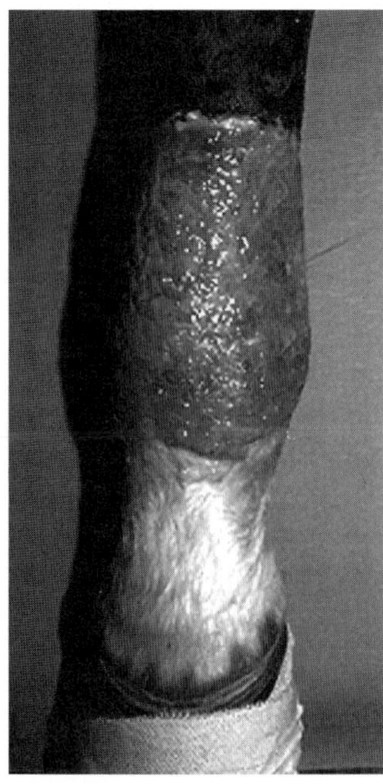

Figure 25-1. A granulating wound on the fetlock of a horse. This wound is so extensive that it cannot heal by any means other than skin grafting.

A *free* skin graft is a piece of skin that has been completely separated from its local blood supply and transferred to a wound at another site, where it must establish new vascular connections to survive.[8,9] Free grafts can be categorized in several different ways, one of which is by their source. Most skin grafts applied to wounds of horses are *autografts* (or isografts), which are grafts transferred from one site to another on the same individual[10] (Table 25-1). The recipient of an autograft mounts no detrimental immune response against the graft because the recipient and donor are one and the same. Autografting is the most common and practical type of grafting of wounds of horses.

A graft transferred between different members of the same species is an *allograft* (or homograft), and a graft transferred from one species to another is a *xenograft* (or heterograft). The recipient of an allograft or xenograft mounts an immune response against the graft, causing the graft to be eventually rejected.[8,11] A second allograft from the same donor applied to the wound survives only a few days, but an allograft from a different donor survives for about the same time as the first allograft.[8] Because the immune mechanism is highly specific, an allograft from a different donor is not affected by circulating lymphocytes sensitized against the first allograft. Although allografts and xenografts are rarely applied to wounds of horses, these grafts are occasionally useful as a biologic bandage.[12-14]

Free skin grafts can be categorized according to their thickness. Full-thickness grafts are composed of epidermis

TABLE 25-1. Graft Terminology*

Greek	Latin	Definition
Autograft	Isograft	A graft transferred from one site to another on the same individual
Allograft	Homograft	A graft transferred between different members of the same species
Xenograft	Heterograft	A graft transferred from a member of one species to a member of another species

Adapted from Boykin JV, Molnar JA: Burn scar and skin equivalents. In Cohen IK, Diegelmann RF, Linblad WJ, editors: Wound Healing, Philadelphia, 1992, WB Saunders.

*To avoid confusion, Greek and Latin prefixes that identify the source of the graft should not be used interchangeably in discussions.

and the entire dermis; split-thickness (or partial-thickness) grafts are composed of epidermis and only a portion of the dermis. The percentage of dermis within the graft influences the graft's acceptance, durability, and cosmesis at the recipient site. The thickness of dermis within the graft is directly proportional to the graft's durability and cosmesis but inversely proportional to the ability of the graft to survive.

Full- or split-thickness free skin grafts can be applied to the surface of wounds as solid or meshed sheets, or they can be embedded in granulation tissue as pinch, punch, or tunnel grafts. Each method of free grafting has its merits and drawbacks, and the method selected depends on circumstances, such as the size and location of the wound, the necessity for cosmesis, the financial constraints imposed by the owner, the equipment available, and the expertise of the surgeon.

PHYSIOLOGY OF GRAFT ACCEPTANCE

Recipient Bed Characteristics

A prime requisite for free grafting is a recipient bed that is vascular and free of infection and devitalized tissue. A free graft cannot be expected to survive if placed on bone denuded of periosteum, tendon denuded of paratenon, or cartilage denuded of perichondrium, but practically any other tissue is capable of supporting a free graft.[15-18] Fresh, surgically created wounds or fresh, clean wounds caused by accident are vascular and free of infection and so readily accept a graft.[15,19] Granulating tissue is also capable of accepting a graft, although not as readily as is fresh tissue.[2,19,20] Granulation tissue healthy enough to allow epithelium to proliferate at its margin is generally healthy enough to accept a skin graft[15] (Fig. 25-2).

Adherence

The graft is initially adhered to the recipient site by fibrin, which binds to collagen within the graft.[9,17,21,22] Vessels and fibroblasts invade the fibrin matrix by the 4th or 5th day, and the graft becomes firmly united to the recipient bed by around the 10th day.

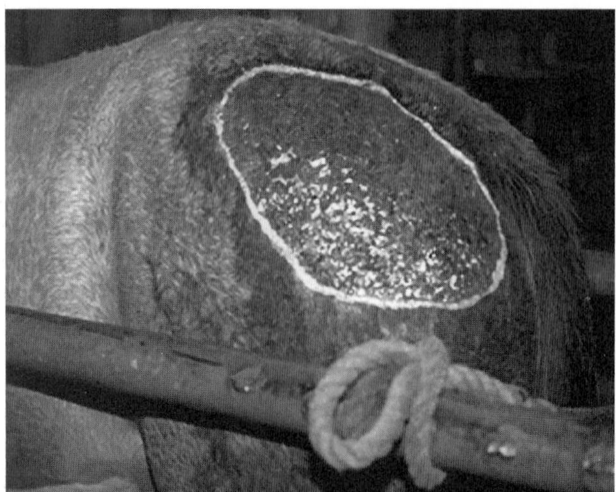

Figure 25-2. Proliferating epithelium at the margin of a wound on the hip of a horse. Proliferating epithelium, represented by the pale ring around the edge of the wound, indicates that the wound is healthy enough to accept a skin graft.

Serum Imbibition (Plasmatic Circulation)

The newly applied graft is nourished by plasma-like fluid that it passively imbibes, by capillary action, into its open vessels, a process referred to as plasmatic imbibition or plasmatic circulation.[9,17,23] Oscillating movement of fluid into the vessels keeps the vessels open for revascularization. The graft becomes edematous and remains so until vascular connections to the graft are restored.

Revascularization

After about 48 hours, new capillaries generated in the recipient bed traverse the fibrin layer to anastomose with those in the graft, a process called *inosculation*.[9,17,23,24] Simultaneously, new capillaries from the recipient bed invade preexisting vessels within the graft, and others cut new vascular channels into the dermis (called *neovascularization*). The graft revascularizes between the 4th and 5th day after grafting, and reestablishment of circulation and lymphatic drainage brings about resolution of edema.[24]

Vascular bridging is a phenomenon that may enable a portion of the graft overlying a relatively avascular portion of the wound to revascularize.[16,25] With vascular bridging, capillaries enter the portion of the graft overlying the avascular portion of the wound from the relatively highly vascular aspects of the surrounding recipient bed to create a vascular bridge across the avascular portion of the wound. For vascular bridging to occur, the avascular area of the wound must be small, and the surrounding area must be highly vascular. Full-thickness grafts bridge avascular areas better than split-thickness grafts, because collateral circulation within the dermis of a full-thickness graft is less interrupted than that within the dermis of a split-thickness graft.[25]

Organization (Organic Union)

The epidermis of the graft becomes hyperplastic after grafting and can double in thickness during the first 2 weeks.[18,26] The epidermis, especially that of a full-thickness graft, may die and slough in some areas, exposing pale dermis beneath it[26] (Fig. 25-3). The exposed dermis may closely resemble granulation tissue, so a surgeon may remove the upper layer of the wound in preparation for a second graft, not realizing that a portion of the dermis has been accepted. Dermis can be differentiated from granulation tissue by its paler color. Exposed dermis becomes covered with epithelial cells that migrate from the hair follicles and the eccrine glands within the dermis.

Split-thickness skin grafts of humans usually begin to develop pigment about 4 weeks after grafting,[2,17,18] and the same is true of split-thickness grafts of horses.[26] Split-thickness grafts often remain scaly for several months, until the eccrine glands regenerate.[2,19,26] Split-thickness grafts of horses, no matter the thickness at which the grafts are harvested, are likely to be devoid of sweat glands,[27,28] and even full-thickness grafts of horses may be devoid of sweat glands.[28] Hair begins to appear in split-thickness grafts at

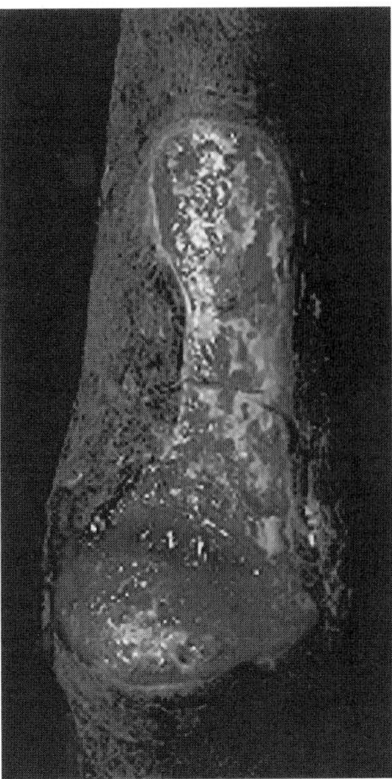

Figure 25-3. Grafted wound of a horse. The epidermis has sloughed in some areas of the graft, exposing pale dermis beneath it. This wound contained enough dermis to allow rapid healing.

between 4 and 6 weeks[26] and often grows to a greater than normal length.[29]

Re-innervation returns more rapidly, but to a lesser extent, in split-thickness grafts than in full-thickness grafts.[17,30] Sensation in split-thickness grafts of humans usually first appears between the 7th and 9th weeks but can occasionally be present as early as the 10th day.[31] Sensation in split-thickness grafts remains incomplete and patchy. Regional nerves enter the base and margins of the graft and, by following vacated neurilemmal sheaths, reconstruct the innervation pattern of the grafted skin.[30] Humans sometimes suffer from hyperesthesia of the grafted wound,[18,30] and this may occur in horses also.

Graft Contraction

After being harvested, grafts immediately shrink because of recoil of the elastic fibers within the deep, dermal layers.[15] This shrinkage is referred to as *primary contraction*. Primary contraction is greatest in full-thickness grafts and decreases as grafts become thinner. Full-thickness grafts from humans contract to close to half their original size after being harvested. Split-thickness grafts that are about half the thickness of the whole skin contract to about three-quarters of their original size, and grafts composed solely of epidermis do not shrink at all. The consequences of primary contraction are minor, because it is reversed when the graft is stretched and sutured or stapled to the recipient site.

Although grafts appear to contract after being accepted, this contraction is probably caused by contraction of the recipient bed, not by the graft itself.[15] Open wounds heal, at least in part, by contraction, which is brought about by the action of contractile fibroblasts, or myofibroblasts, within the wound.[15,32] Skin grafts inhibit wound contraction, to various extents, by accelerating the life cycle of the myofibroblasts within the wound.

The extent to which a skin graft is capable of inhibiting wound contraction is influenced by the relative thickness of the graft's dermis and the stage of healing of the recipient bed at the time of grafting.[15,32,33] The total percentage of the dermis grafted is more important than the absolute thickness of the skin graft in preventing wound contraction. Fresh or granulating wounds of humans and rats receiving a full-thickness graft tend to contract less than wounds receiving a split-thickness graft, even when the full-thickness graft is thinner than a split-thickness graft, indicating that physical or biochemical differences between the upper and lower portions of the dermis may strongly influence the effect of the skin graft on wound contraction.[32-34]

In a study on the effects of grafts on wound contraction in horses, fresh or granulating wounds to which a split-thickness graft was applied contracted at the same fractional rate as fresh or granulating wounds to which a full-thickness graft was applied.[35] The fractional rate of contraction of grafted fresh wounds, however, was less than that of grafted, granulating wounds.

Contraction of wounds of humans can sometimes lead to considerable cosmetic defects and to *contracture*, which is deformity of one or more joints caused by contraction of the wound.[8] Contraction of wounds of humans is sometimes intentionally inhibited by autografting or allografting to prevent cosmetic and functional defects caused by contracture.[2] Skin of horses is more mobile than that of humans and so is more capable of healing by contraction. Contraction of wounds of horses rarely, if ever, causes contracture of joints, so contraction of wounds of horses, before or after grafting, should be considered beneficial. If applied to a wound after contraction has commenced, skin grafts, regardless of whether they are full-thickness or split-thickness, appear to have little effect on inhibiting contraction in horses.[36]

GRAFT FAILURE

Reasons for graft failure include fluid accumulation beneath the graft, movement, and infection.[15,18,22,23,29] Grafts applied to horses fail most frequently because of infection.[37]

Fluid Accumulation

The graft must contact the wound intimately to prevent fluid from becoming interposed between the graft and the wound.[23] A hematoma, seroma, or exudate beneath the graft prevents fibrin from attaching the graft to the wound and acts as a barrier to the ingrowth of new vessels.[16,23] A graft can survive for only several days by imbibing nutrients from the hematoma or seroma, and if budding capillaries from the recipient bed are unable to traverse this barrier within this time, the graft expires. To avoid formation of a hematoma or seroma beneath a graft, grafting of a hemorrhagic wound should be delayed until hemorrhage has ceased.

Infection

Granulation tissue always has resident bacteria at its surface, but it contains abundant blood vessels and phagocytic cells that act as a partial barrier to bacterial invasion.* The wound becomes infected when the concentration of bacteria in the tissue exceeds the ability of humoral and cellular defenses to destroy the bacteria, and for most types of bacteria, this concentration seems to be about 10^5 organisms per gram of tissue. Survival of a skin graft is better correlated to the concentration of bacteria in the recipient bed than to any other single factor.[40,41] If a wound is found, by quantitative bacterial analysis, to contain more than 10^5 bacteria per gram of tissue, the wound should not be grafted.

Because quantifying the concentration of bacteria in a wound is time-consuming and often impractical, at least for most veterinary surgeons, and because the concentration of bacteria in the wound is sometimes not as important as the *type* of bacteria,[22] the bacterial status of a wound to be grafted is usually assessed qualitatively. A wound that shows signs of inflammation, such as redness, swelling of the surrounding area, and formation of exudate, should be assumed to be infected. Bacteriologic culture of a wound that appears to be infected should precede grafting, and isolates should be tested for antimicrobial susceptibility. Unfortunately, even a wound that has no signs of inflammation and appears to be healthy may have more than 10^5 bacteria per gram of tissue.[41]

The concentration of some bacteria, most notably β-hemolytic streptococci, required to infect a wound is much less than 10^5 per gram of tissue.[22,38] β-Hemolytic streptococci produce proteolytic enzymes, including streptokinase and staphylokinase, that are destructive to both the graft and its recipient bed. These bacterial enzymes, and others, destabilize the fibrin network between the graft and the recipient wound by catalyzing the conversion of plasminogen to plasmin, which digests fibrin.[22,42] *Pseudomonas* species also critically weaken a graft's fibrinous attachment by producing elastase, which specifically degrades elastin in the dermis of the graft to which fibrin attaches.[22]

Motion

The graft must remain immobilized long enough to become vascularized. Shearing forces between the graft and the underlying recipient bed dislodge the fibrin seal, impairing plasmatic imbibition, inosculation, and capillary ingrowth. Shearing forces occur when the recipient wound is located in a highly mobile area, such as over a joint, or when the grafted area is inadequately immobilized.

GRAFTING TECHNIQUES

Preparation of the Recipient Site

Preparation of the recipient site is the most important contributor to survival of a free graft.[4] Factors to consider when determining if a wound is prepared sufficiently to accept a graft are the wound's vascularity and whether the wound appears to be infected.[17] Grafting should be delayed if the wound appears to have inadequate vascularity to support a free graft or if it appears to be infected or to have a higher than ordinary vulnerability for developing infection.

*References 8, 16, 17, 22, 38, 39.

Highly vascular granulation tissue readily accepts a graft, but as the granulation tissue matures, its vascularity and ability to accept a graft diminish[38] (Fig. 25-4). Fibrous, poorly vascularized granulation tissue, or granulation tissue plagued by unremitting infection, should be excised to a level below the margin of the wound to allow the wound to form fresh, vascular granulation tissue free of infection before a graft is applied.[29] Granulation tissue can usually be excised with the horse standing, because granulation tissue has no innervation.

Delaying grafting of a fresh wound for several days may decrease the time required for the graft to revascularize.[43] Sprouting capillaries capable of rapidly revascularizing the graft develop in the wound within 48 hours, so, by delaying grafting for 2 days after wounding, the time before the graft begins to revascularize (i.e., the phase of plasmatic imbibition) can be reduced by about one half. Wounds that are allowed several days to develop sprouting capillaries before being grafted are referred to as prepared wounds.

Although eliminating all bacteria from a wound is difficult, removing streptococci is relatively easy, because streptococci are nearly always susceptible to penicillin.[38,44,45] Occasionally, penicillin or other β-lactam antibiotics are ineffective in resolving a streptococcal infection, because other resident bacteria, particularly staphylococci and gram-negative bacteria, produce β-lactamase, an enzyme that inactivates β-lactam antibiotics.[44] The efficacy of the β-lactam antibiotic against streptococci can be preserved if

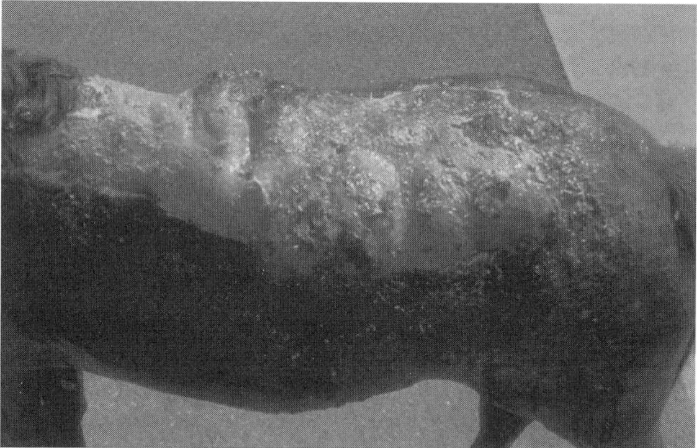

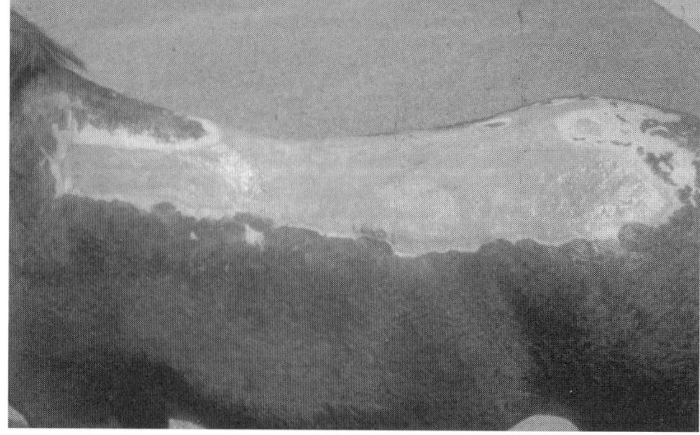

Figure 25-4. Burn wound on the back of a horse. The wound contained exuberant, relatively avascular granulation tissue that was excised to skin level, with the horse standing, in preparation for grafting. The fresh tissue accepted a split-thickness skin graft.

the β-lactam antibiotic administered is effective against β-lactamase–producing bacteria as well as streptococci. The activity of the β-lactam antibiotics can also be preserved by administering clavulanic acid, a potent inhibitor of β-lactamase, in conjunction with the β-lactam antibiotic.[44] Clavulanic acid has no therapeutic value when administered alone. Pseudomonads are usually sensitive to topically applied mafenide acetate, aminoglycosides, or polymyxin-B sulfate.[15,46]

Topical application of an antimicrobial drug to an infected, granulating wound is often more effective for eliminating infection than is systemic administration of the same antimicrobial drug, because systemically administered antimicrobial drugs often fail to reach therapeutic concentrations within granulation tissue.[17,47] Fibrin within granulation tissue appears to prevent adequate penetration of the antimicrobial drug.

Before a wound is grafted, it should be evaluated thoroughly for evidence of damage to synovial structures, ligamentous or tendinous tissue, or bone. Bone beneath slowly healing wounds or beneath wounds with draining tracts should be examined radiographically for evidence of a foreign body and for evidence of infection or sequestration of bone (Fig. 25-5). Granulation tissue within chronic, slowly healing wounds, particularly those wounds that appear to be pruritic, should be examined histologically for the presence of larvae of the equine stomach worm *Habronema*. Some neoplasms, such as sarcoids or carcinomas, sometimes resemble granulation tissue.

Preparation of the recipient bed immediately before grafting should include clipping or shaving the skin around the wound. A surgical scrub solution can be used to cleanse the skin around the wound, but the wound itself should be cleansed by rinsing it with physiologic saline solution or a balanced electrolyte solution. Contact between the wound and the detergent found in surgical scrub solutions increases the wound's susceptibility to infection.[48]

Preparation of the Donor Site

The area selected as the donor site depends on the technique of grafting selected, and on whether the graft is to be harvested with the horse anesthetized or standing. Because harvesting skin creates a wound, the donor site, especially the donor site of a split-thickness graft, should be at an inconspicuous location.

Hair is removed from the donor site by clipping with a no. 40 clipper blade, by shaving, or by applying a chemical depilatory agent. Although chemical depilatory agents may irritate the donor skin, they have no clinically apparent detrimental effect on acceptance of grafts (my observation). When hair is removed completely from the surface of the donor site by shaving or by depilation, the graft should be marked in such a way that ensures that when the graft is applied, the direction of its hair growth matches that of the skin surrounding the recipient site. The direction of hair growth on the graft remains visible when the donor site is clipped. After the donor site is scrubbed, it should be rinsed thoroughly with water or physiologic saline solution so that no residue detrimental to the graft, such as isopropyl alcohol, remains.

Full-Thickness Sheet Grafting

The site most suitable for procuring a full-thickness graft is the cranial pectoral region, where the skin is relatively mobile (Fig. 25-6).[49,50] The graft can be removed, and the donor site sutured, with the horse anesthetized or with the

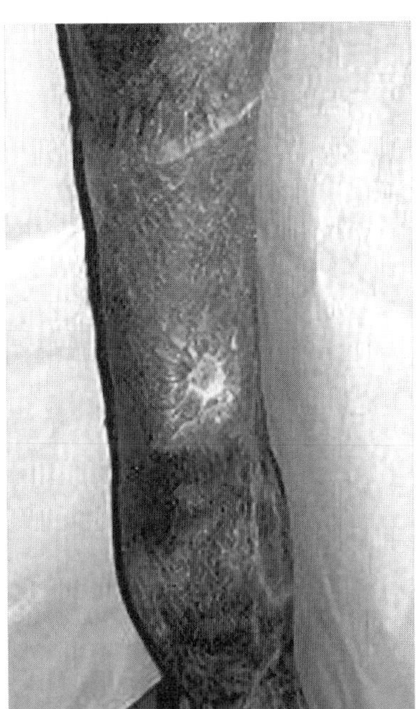

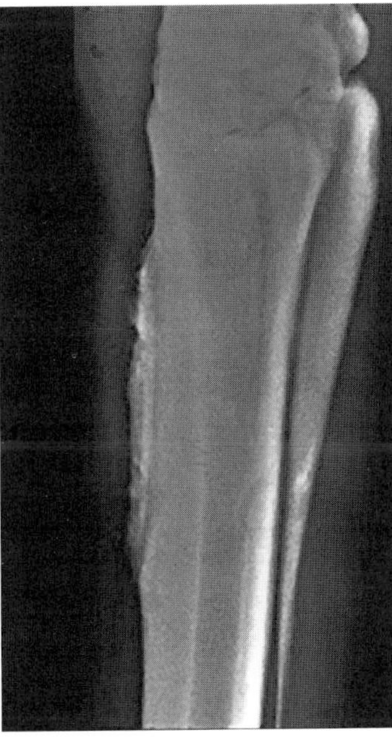

Figure 25-5. A graft applied to a healthy-appearing, granulating wound on the dorsal aspect of a metacarpus was completely accepted, but a draining tract soon appeared in the healed wound. Drainage was caused by infection of bone beneath the wound.

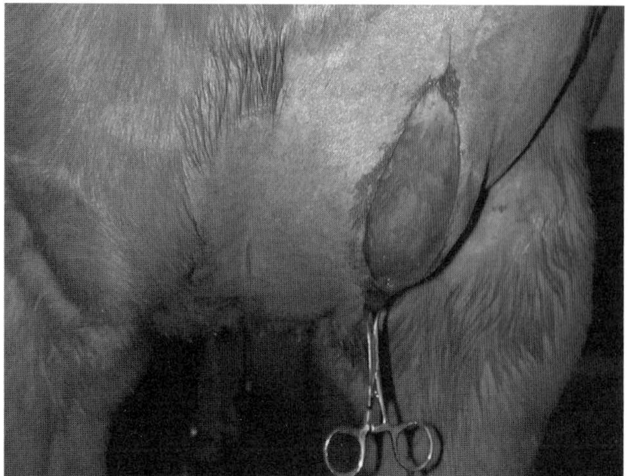

Figure 25-6. Cranial pectoral area from which a full-thickness graft was obtained. The graft was obtained with the horse standing. The incision was closed with skin staples.

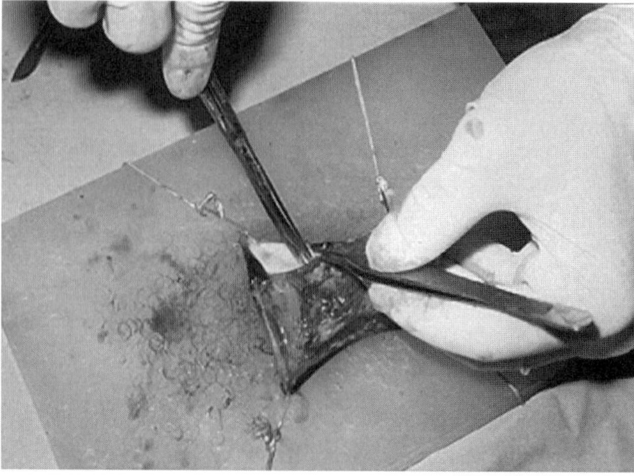

Figure 25-7. Removing fascia and fat from a full-thickness graft using sharp dissection. A scalpel blade can also be used.

horse standing and sedated after desensitizing the donor site with local anesthetic solution. If a sutured wound in this region should dehisce, healing occurs rapidly by contraction with little or no scarring (my observation). The graft should be cut slightly larger than the recipient site, even though the shrinkage caused by recoil of elastic fibers is largely reversed when the graft is stretched and fixed to the margin of the wound.[3,15]

Subcutaneous tissue attached to the undersurface of the graft acts as a barrier to plasmatic imbibition and ingrowth of new vessels, so it must be removed to expose the dermis and its vasculature.[1,3,23] Fascia and fat should be removed by sharp dissection, because scraping the subcutaneous tissue from the graft can injure the dermis and its vasculature (Fig. 25-7). The graft should be attached to the recipient site with slight tension to keep the small dermal vessels open for inosculation.[51]

Full-thickness sheet grafting requires no sophisticated equipment for harvesting and can be performed with the horse standing. Full-thickness skin grafts resist trauma better than split-thickness skin grafts, and because they contain all the properties of the surrounding skin, full-thickness skin grafts provide the best cosmetic appearance and function of any type of free graft.[2,3,8,37,52]

Full-thickness grafts are not accepted as readily as split-thickness grafts, because they have fewer exposed blood vessels than split-thickness grafts, and because their requirement for nourishment is greater.[8,23,52,53] Circumstances for full-thickness grafting must be ideal, because blood vessels in a full-thickness graft that are available for diffusion of nutrients or for inosculation by vessels in the recipient wound are few in number and large in diameter. Although healthy, highly vascular granulation tissue is capable of accepting a full-thickness skin graft,[35] full-thickness grafting is usually reserved for fresh, uncontaminated wounds.[2,8,17,26,38]

A considerable disadvantage of full-thickness grafting of wounds of horses is the horse's lack of redundant donor skin. This disadvantage makes full-thickness grafting practical for covering only relatively small wounds, provided that the surgeon intends to suture the donor site after the graft is harvested. A full-thickness graft can be used to cover a wound larger than the graft itself by meshing and expanding the graft, but full-thickness skin of horses is too thick to be easily meshed using some commercial meshgraft dermatomes, such as the Zimmer mechanical skin mesher (see "Meshing Sheet Grafts," later).

Split-Thickness Sheet Grafting

A split-thickness graft is composed of epidermis and a portion of the dermis. The thickness of a split-thickness graft is determined by the relative amount, rather than the absolute amount, of dermis included in the graft, because the thickness of the dermis varies between individuals and between regions.[2,28,29] To obtain a split-thickness graft, a portion of the dermis with its overlying epidermis is harvested with a free-hand knife, a drum dermatome, or a power-driven dermatome. Relatively inconspicuous donor sites for obtaining a split-thickness graft from horses are the ventral portion of the abdomen and the ventrolateral aspect of the thorax, caudal to the elbow.[49,54-56]

Hand Instruments

Scalpel blades, double edged razor blades, and surgical straight razors are sometimes used to harvest small, split-thickness grafts from humans, but these types of dermatomes are of little use for harvesting skin grafts from horses, because they can be used to harvest only relatively small grafts, and because their use requires considerable technical expertise to obtain a graft of consistent thickness.

Large grafts necessary to cover wounds of horses can be cut with a variety of knives designed specifically for harvesting skin. The Watson skin grafting knife (Padgett Instruments, Inc, 1520 Grand, Kansas City, Mo), a modification of the Braithwaite knife, can harvest a graft 100 mm (4 inches) wide, uses disposable blades, and is fitted with an adjustable roller in front of the blade to control the depth of the cut (Fig. 25-8). Because the thickness of the graft is controlled by the adjustable roller, only a moderate amount of practice is required to develop the expertise necessary to achieve a uniform, split-thickness graft of the desired thick-

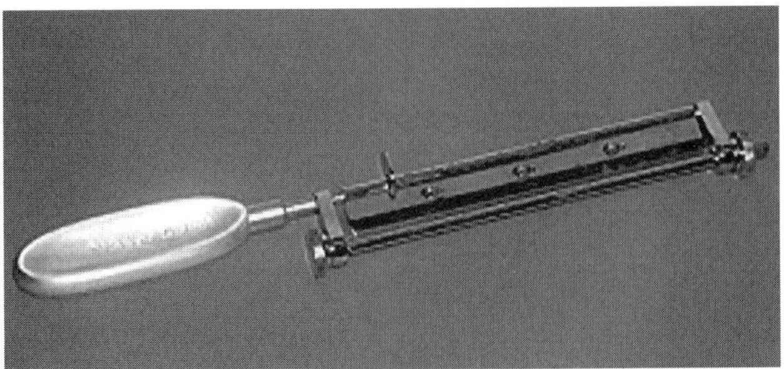

Figure 25-8. The Watson skin grafting knife. Using this dermatome, a surgeon can harvest a graft 100 mm (4 inches) wide. The knife uses disposable blades and is fitted with an adjustable roller in front of the blade to control the depth of cut.

ness. The position of the adjustable roller is controlled by a screw marked with calibrations at one end and a lock at the other. The thickness of graft represented by each calibration is learned by experience. The thickness of the graft depends not only on the position of the roller but also on the angle of incidence at which the skin is cut, and on the pressure applied to the knife while cutting.[38] The heavier the pressure and the greater the angle of incidence, the thicker is the harvested skin.

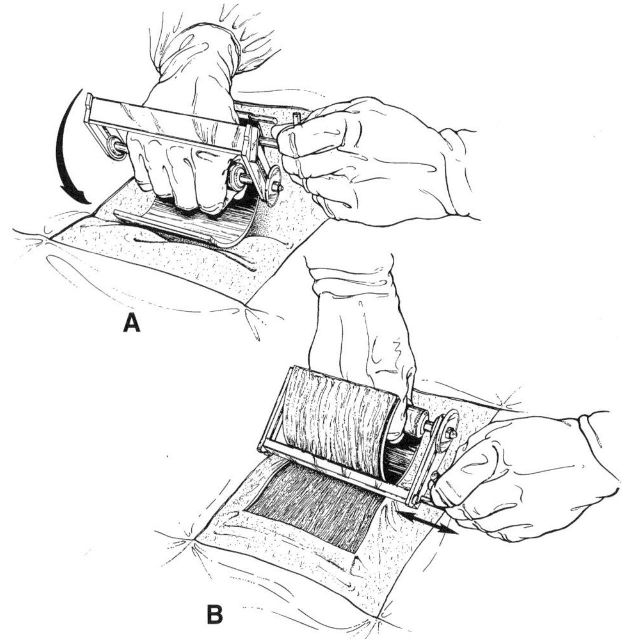

Figure 25-9. Harvesting a skin graft with a drum dermatome. **A,** Rotating the drum of a drum dermatome elevates skin to which it has been glued. **B,** The skin attached to the drum is cut at a precise depth with a knife that oscillates back and forth on a piston.

Drum Dermatomes

A clinician with only minimal training can harvest a uniform section of skin with a drum dermatome.[2,17,23] The drum dermatome uses a knife that oscillates back and forth on a piston to precisely split the dermis of a section of skin that has been glued to the drum of the dermatome (Fig. 25-9). The depth of cut is predetermined by the caliber of shims placed next to the blade.

The drum dermatome allows the surgeon to harvest a graft of the exact dimensions to fit the wound for which the graft is intended.[17] Using a template from the recipient site, glue is applied only to a similar area on the drum, so that as the drum is rotated, only that portion of skin that adheres to the drum is cut. The drum dermatome requires no external power source. It is considerably more expensive than a free-hand knife but not as expensive as power-driven dermatomes.[8] A major drawback to the use of the drum dermatome to harvest grafts for wounds of horses is that the length of the graft is limited by the circumference of the drum. An example of a drum dermatome is the Padgett Manual Dermatome (Z-PD-100R, Padgett Instruments, Inc, Kansas City, Mo).

Power-Driven Dermatomes

Power-driven dermatomes use a rapidly oscillating blade, driven by an electric motor or gas turbine to harvest a split-thickness skin graft with predictable precision. The depth and width of cut can be adjusted precisely. Commonly used power-driven dermatomes are the Stryker electric dermatome (Stryker Electro-Surgical Unit, Kalamazoo, Mich) and the Brown pneumatic or electric dermatome (Zimmer, Warsaw, Ind) (Fig. 25-10). The cutting head of a pneumatic dermatome oscillates more rapidly than that of an electric dermatome, making harvesting smoother.[23]

The Davol-Simon skin graft dermatome (Davol Inc, Cranston, RI) is a relatively inexpensive dermatome powered by a rechargeable handle, similar to the handle of an electric toothbrush.[15,16] A disposable, nonadjustable cutting

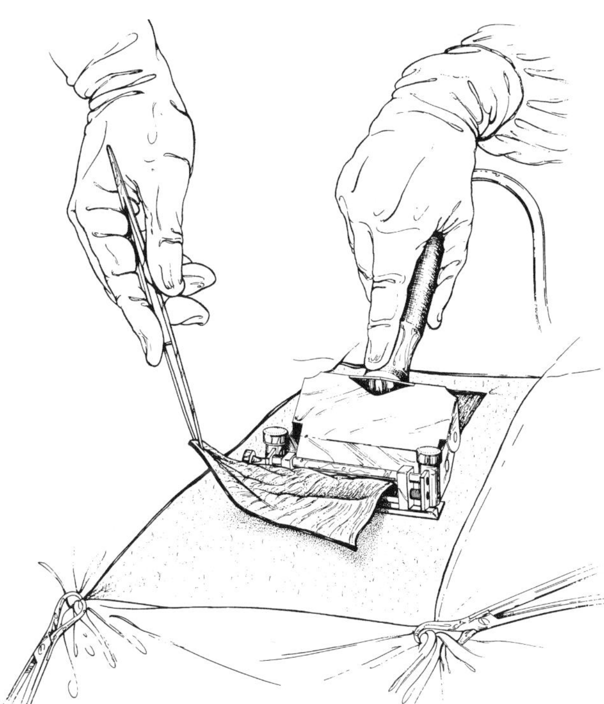

Figure 25-10. Harvesting a split-thickness skin graft with a pneumatic dermatome. Although they are expensive, power-driven dermatomes allow the cutting of very uniform grafts by minimally experienced operators.

head harvests a split-thickness skin graft 33 mm (1½ inches) wide and 0.38 mm (0.015 inch) thick. Grafts obtained with this skin graft dermatome are too thin to impart a cosmetic appearance to wounds of horses, but they may be useful for covering relatively small wounds when cosmetic appearance is not important.

Although a power-driven dermatome provides precision harvesting, the widest graft that can be harvested with many power dermatomes is only 76 mm (3 inches). A surface firmer than the ventral aspect of the abdomen, the least conspicuous donor site on the horse, is often necessary when harvesting with a power-driven dermatome. Although operating a power-driven dermatome requires only a minimum of experience, a power-driven dermatome requires skilled maintenance.[8] Because of their expense, power-driven dermatomes are found primarily only at large equine surgical referral centers.

An advantage of the free-hand knife over the power-driven dermatome is that consistently uniform grafts more than 100 mm wide (4 inches or greater) can be harvested using a free-hand knife. Grafts can be harvested from the ventral aspect of the abdomen with a free-hand knife, which is a difficult feat for a power-driven dermatome. A free-hand knife is far less expensive than a power-driven dermatome, requires less maintenance, has fewer parts to malfunction, and is easier to sterilize and to transport.

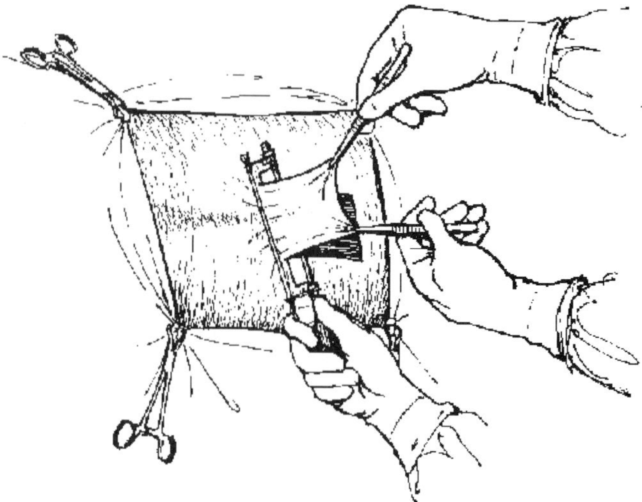

Figure 25-11. Harvesting split-thickness skin from the ventral aspect of the abdomen using a free-hand knife. The ventral portion of the abdomen must protrude over the edge of the table to accommodate the handle of the hand-held knife.

Technique of Harvesting a Split-Thickness Graft

A split-thickness skin graft can be harvested from any convex surface of the body, but the cosmetic appearance of the horse should be considered when selecting a donor site, because a split-thickness graft of acceptable durability and hair-coverage cannot be obtained without creating a large epithelial scar at the donor site. Harvesting a split-thickness skin graft is painful to the horse and can be accomplished only when the horse is anesthetized.

To harvest skin from the ventral aspect of the horse's abdomen using a free-hand knife, the horse is positioned in lateral recumbency with its abdomen protruding beyond the edge of the table. The ventral portion of the abdomen must protrude over the edge of the table to accommodate the handle of the hand-held knife. The donor site is prepared for aseptic surgery, but draping is not necessary. Harvesting usually begins at the umbilicus and extends cranially. The donor site can be stabilized, if necessary, by assistants stretching the skin with towel clamps. The knife is applied to the skin at an acute angle of about 5 to 10 degrees, and the skin is cut using a regular sawing motion, concentrating on moving the blade back and forth, rather than pushing it forward (Fig. 25-11). Lubricating the donor site with physiologic saline solution and the blade with a light coating of mineral oil reduces friction. Mineral oil does not adversely affect acceptance of the graft.[8,15] Slight, uniform tension should be applied to the cut end of the graft as the graft is harvested.

After several centimeters of graft have been cut, the graft and donor site should be inspected to ensure that the graft is the desired thickness before harvesting is continued. The thickness of the graft can be assessed subjectively by examining the graft for translucency and the donor site for the pattern of bleeding.[15,16] A shallow cut through the dermis produces a translucent graft and exposes many small bleeding vessels, whereas a deep cut produces a more opaque graft and exposes fewer but larger bleeding vessels. If subcutaneous fat is exposed, the graft is full thickness and therefore much too thick. The depth of cut can be changed by repositioning the adjustable roller, by changing the pressure applied to the knife, or by raising or lowering the knife's angle of incidence. When the desired length of graft has been cut, the knife is tilted upward to sever the graft. If the graft is to be meshed and fully expanded, the length of graft should be considerably longer than the wound to which it is applied, because expanding the graft's width also shortens the graft's length.

The split-thickness graft is the most useful type of graft, because it can be used to cover defects too large to be covered by a full-thickness graft, and because it survives more readily than does the full-thickness graft.[8,20,38,53] The cosmetic appearance of a wound healed by split-thickness skin grafting is inferior to that of a wound healed by full-thickness skin grafting, but it is superior to that of a wound healed by island grafting (see "Island Grafts," later). A split-thickness graft is less conveniently procured than a full-thickness graft, because to obtain a split-thickness graft, the horse must be anesthetized.

Meshing Sheet Grafts

A split-thickness or full-thickness sheet graft can be applied to a recipient bed as a solid or as a meshed sheet. A graft is meshed by uniformly fenestrating it manually with a scalpel blade or mechanically with a meshgraft dermatome. The primary reason for meshing a sheet graft is to allow the graft to uniformly cover a wound larger than the graft itself.* Grafts are also meshed to prevent serum, blood, or exudate from mechanically disrupting a newly applied graft from its delicate fibrinous and vascular attachments to the recipient

*References 2, 16, 17, 23, 29, 49, 54-59.

bed. Fenestrations also enable a topically applied antimicrobial agent to contact a large portion of the recipient wound. A meshed graft conforms to an irregular surface better than does a nonmeshed graft, and its ability to expand allows it to better tolerate motion. Fenestrations in the graft fill with fibrin, which increases the graft's stability on the recipient bed.[37]

An example of a meshgraft dermatome is the Padgett mechanical skin mesher (Mesh Skin Graft Expander, No. Z-PD-170, Padgett Instruments, Kansas City, Mo). This instrument consists of an aluminum block with staggered, parallel rows of blades and a Teflon rolling pin. The graft is positioned on the block, dermal side down, and pressed into the cutting blades, in the direction of the blades, with the rolling pin (Fig. 25-12). The rolling pin should first be rolled lightly across the graft to secure the graft to the blades of the mesher and then firmly so that the blades pierce the graft. The staggered cuts produce a meshed pattern that allows the graft to be expanded to three times its original width.

The Zimmer mechanical skin mesher (Zimmer Meshgraft Dermatome, Zimmer, Warsaw, Ind) is a more elaborate and expensive meshing instrument, capable of expanding the graft to one and one-half, three, six, or nine times its original area. The graft is positioned dermal side down on a specially grooved plastic carrier selected according to the degree of expansion desired, and the graft and carrier are fed through the mesh cutter by turning a hand-crank (Fig. 25-13). The pattern engraved onto the plastic carrier determines the distance between cuts. The graft must be placed on the ridged surface of the carrier, because placing the graft on the smooth side of the carrier causes the graft to be shredded into spaghetti-like strips.

An important consideration when purchasing a meshgraft dermatome is the width of grafts routinely harvested with the skin graft dermatome. Grafts up to 100 mm wide are harvested routinely with a free-hand skin graft knife, but a graft wider than 76 mm is difficult to mesh with a Zimmer mechanical skin mesher. Grafts up to about 110 mm wide can be fitted onto the cutting surface of the Padgett mechanical skin mesher. Although the Padgett mechanical skin mesher accommodates a graft only 13.5 cm (5.3 inches) long, a longer graft can be meshed in sections.

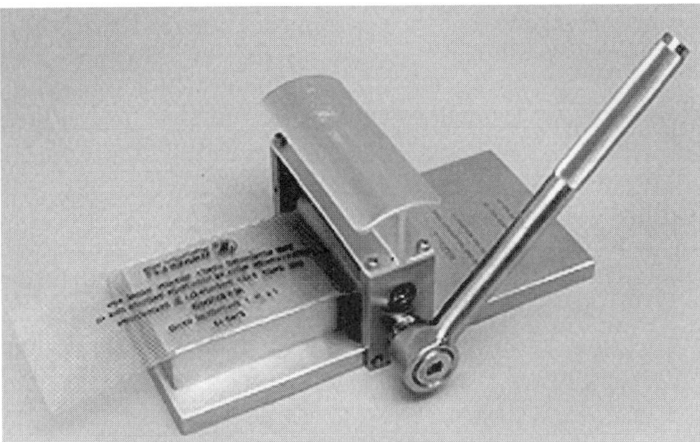

Figure 25-13. A Zimmer mechanical skin mesher. The mesher is capable of expanding the graft to many times its original area. The graft is positioned on a specially grooved plastic carrier, and the graft and carrier are fed through the mesh cutter by turning a hand-crank.

Full-thickness sheet grafts of horses are difficult to mesh on commercial meshing instruments and often must be meshed manually. Meshing a graft manually is tedious, especially if the graft is large or if it must be greatly expanded. The skin is fixed to a cutting board, such as sterile sheet of cardboard or Styrofoam, with the dermal side up, and after removing the subcutaneous fascia, staggered, parallel rows of incisions are created using a scalpel blade. The longer and the more numerous are the incisions, the greater is the expansion.

An expanded, meshed graft has the appearance of chicken wire or chain-link fencing and uniformly exposes portions of the wound within the fenestrations (Fig. 25-14). The amount of wound exposed within the fenestrations depends on the degree to which the graft is expanded. Portions of the wound covered by the graft heal primarily, but each portion of the wound exposed within the fenestrations must heal by contraction and epithelialization. The exposed portions of the wound epithelialize rapidly because of the

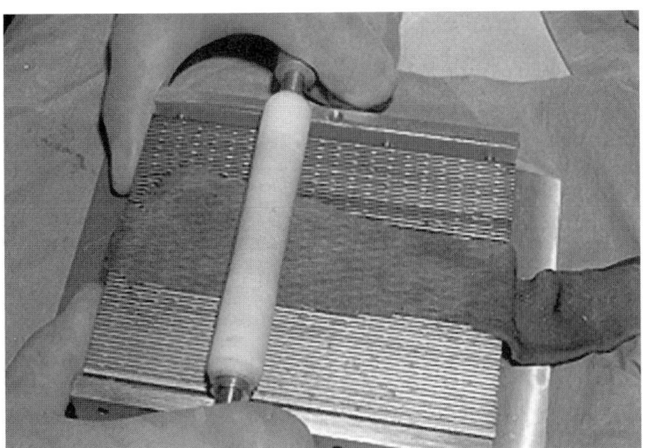

Figure 25-12. A Padgett mechanical skin mesher. The mesher consists of an aluminum block with staggered, parallel rows of blades and a Teflon rolling pin. The graft is positioned on the block, dermal side down, and pressed into the cutting blades with the rolling pin.

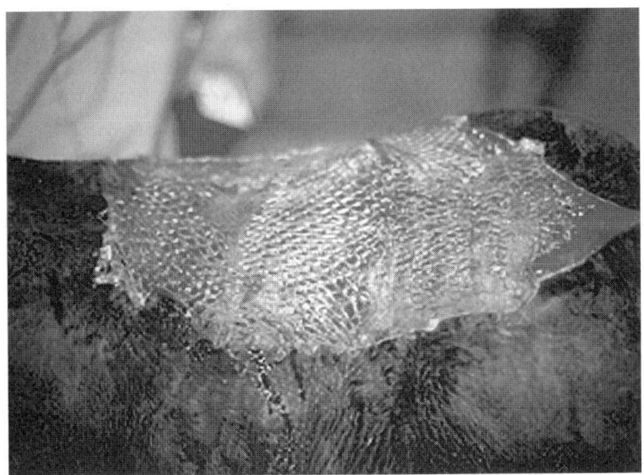

Figure 25-14. An expanded, meshed graft on the back of a foal. The graft has the appearance of chain-link fencing and uniformly exposes portions of the wound within the fenestrations. These exposed portions of the wound must heal by contraction and epithelialization.

enormous increase in the border of the graft from which epithelial cells migrate.[54,56] The epithelium that eventually covers the expanded fenestrations has no adnexa, causing the wound to heal with abundant, diamond-shaped epithelial scars. The more a graft is expanded at application, the more apparent are the diamond-shaped scars.[2,38,54,56] The size of the epithelial scars can be reduced by attaching the graft to the wound so that the fenestrations within the graft are parallel with the skin lines (i.e., parallel to the long axis of the limb).[55] The diamond-shaped epithelial scars within the grafted wound diminish in size as the grafted wound contracts.

Applying Sheet Grafts

Excess granulation tissue should be excised before the graft is harvested, to allow time for hemorrhage to stop before the graft is applied. Excising exuberant granulation tissue 24 hours in advance of grafting ensures hemostasis and provides time for budding capillaries to develop at the surface of the wound for rapid vascularization of the graft[43] (see "Preparation of the Recipient Site," earlier). If granulation tissue is not exuberant, the surface of the wound should be rubbed with a gauze sponge or gently scraped with a scalpel blade held 90 degrees to the wound, until serum exudes from the wound's surface.

The graft should be situated on the wound so that the direction of its hair growth conforms to that of the surrounding skin. A graft harvested with the horse anesthetized can be sutured or stapled to the wound's margin before the horse is allowed to recover from anesthesia. To avoid constant disturbance of the fibrin seal at the edge of the graft when securing the graft with sutures, the suture needle should pass from the graft to the surrounding skin, rather than from the surrounding skin to the graft.[23] To suture or staple the graft to the wound's margin with the horse standing, the margin of the wound must first be desensitized using local or regional anesthesia. The graft can be fixed to the margin of the wound, with the horse standing, without using local or regional anesthesia, by overlapping and gluing the margin of the graft to the margin of the wound with cyanoacrylate glue (Superglue, Loctite Co, Cleveland, Ohio), provided that sufficient skin has been harvested to allow overlap of the graft (Fig. 25-15). Applying the graft with the horse standing reduces the time of general anesthesia and eliminates the possibility of damage to the graft that may occur while the horse recovers from general anesthesia.

A graft need only be fixed to the wound's margin, because fibrin produced by the wound fixes the graft to the wound's surface within minutes after the graft is applied.[2,26] If the wound is large or is in an area that is difficult to immobilize, however, such as the dorsum of a fetlock, the graft can be further secured, with simple interrupted sutures placed through the fenestrations in the meshed graft. To suture a graft to the bed of a fresh wound, with the horse standing, the wound must first be desensitized with regional or local anesthesia. A graft can be sutured to granulation tissue, with the horse standing, without anesthesia, because granulation tissue has no innervation (Fig. 25-16). Sutures can be removed in 6 or 7 days when acceptance of the graft is ensured. Catgut is convenient to use as a suture because it

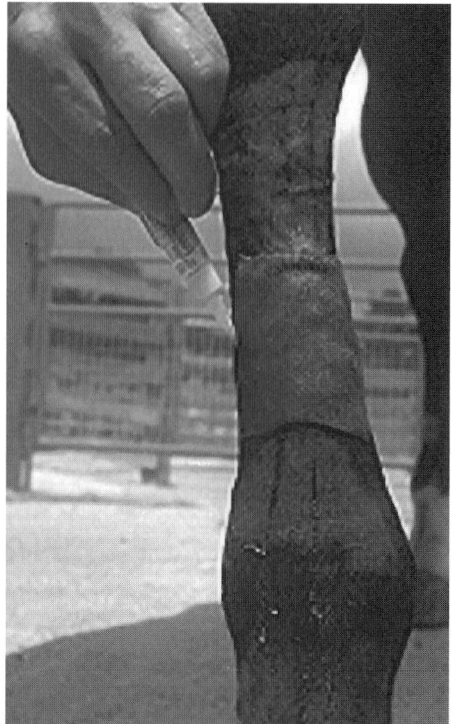

Figure 25-15. Attaching a graft to the margin of a wound, with the horse standing. The graft is attached by overlapping and attaching the margin of the graft to the margin of the wound with cyanoacrylate glue.

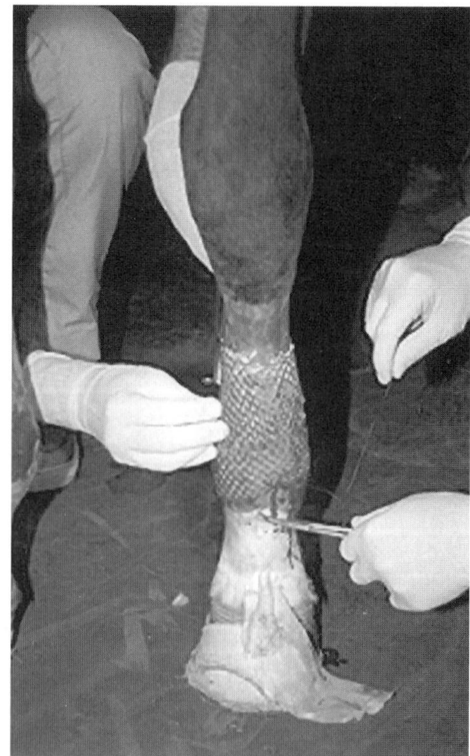

Figure 25-16. Suturing a graft to granulation tissue with the horse standing Anesthesia is not necessary because granulation tissue has no innervation.

swells, causing the knot to loosen. If tied with a square knot, the suture can usually be removed by applying gentle traction to one end of the suture with a hemostat. Removing sutures in this fashion is easier than cutting the sutures.

Acceptance and Cosmesis

The thickness of a graft greatly influences its acceptance at the recipient wound.* The thinner the graft, the less are its metabolic demands, and the less are its demands for vascularity at the recipient bed. Blood vessels branch as they ascend the dermis, so the thinner the graft is, the greater the number of exposed vessels. The greater the number of exposed vessels, the better is the absorption of nutrients from the recipient wound, and the more rapid is revascularization from inosculation. The thinner the graft, the poorer is its durability and cosmetic appearance.

Split-thickness grafts obtained from the hip, gaskin, or ventral aspect of the abdomen of horses that are 0.5 mm (0.020 inch) or less thick lack durability and have sparse or no hair coverage.[20] Split-thickness grafts harvested from these areas and from the ventrolateral aspect of the thorax that are between 0.63 mm (0.025 inch) and 0.76 mm (0.030 inch) thick have moderate to good piliation and good durability.[20,29] The thickness to which the graft should be harvested is a matter of judgment, because the thickness of the dermis varies between horses and between donor sites.[29] Although one of the aims of split-thickness grafting is to provide adequate piliation at both the donor and recipient sites, occasionally piliation is inadequate at either site.[52]

Island Grafts

An island graft is a small piece of full-thickness or split-thickness skin, placed either into or onto a granulating wound.[60-62] Other names for this type of graft include implantation graft and seed graft.[3,4] Implanting island grafts into granulation tissue of horses, rather than applying them to the surface of the wound, avoids shearing forces between the graft and the bandage. The purpose of island grafting is to increase the area of epidermis from which epithelialization can proceed; consequently, wounds that receive island grafts heal primarily by epithelialization. Types of island grafts used to graft wounds of horses are the punch graft, the pinch graft, and the tunnel graft.

Punch Grafts

Punch grafts are small, full-thickness plugs of skin that are harvested and implanted into granulation tissue using skin biopsy punches. Punch grafts can be taken directly from the horse or from an excised, full-thickness sheet of skin.

Common donor sites for obtaining punch grafts directly from the horse are the ventrolateral aspect of the abdomen, the perineum, and the portion of the neck that lies beneath the mane. The donor site is clipped, scrubbed, and desensitized with a local anesthetic agent. The perineal area can be desensitized using caudal epidural anesthesia. Removing punch grafts directly from the horse with a skin biopsy punch creates small blemishes at the donor site (Fig. 25-17). Therefore, the grafts should be harvested in a symmetrical pattern about 1 cm apart to improve cosmesis.[37] The small wounds created by the biopsy punch need not be closed, but suturing or stapling each wound may produce less obvious blemishes.

Subcutaneous fascia and fat should be sharply excised from each individual graft before it is implanted to facilitate plasmatic imbibition and revascularization.[63] Removing subcutaneous tissue from each small plug of skin is a tedious process. One method is to stretch the subcutaneous tissue between one thumb forceps grasping the top of the plug and another thumb forceps grasping the subcutaneous tissue. A second person excises the taut subcutaneous tissue from the dermis with a scalpel blade.

Punch grafts can also be harvested from an elliptical, full-thickness sheet of skin, which is usually harvested from the cranial pectoral area, where the skin is relatively mobile.[1] A 10-cm-long by 4-cm-wide section of skin provides enough punch grafts to cover most wounds and allows easy primary closure of the donor site.[50] The section of skin is stretched and secured, epidermal side down, to a sterile piece of cardboard or Styrofoam or to a sterile polypropylene block. After all subcutaneous tissue is sharply excised from the section of skin, full-thickness plugs are cut from the skin using a 6- to 7-mm-diameter skin biopsy punch (Fig. 25-18). The grafts are stored on a gauze sponge moistened with physiologic saline solution until they are implanted, and the wound created at the donor site is closed in one or two layers. Applying a stent to the sutured wound decreases tension on the suture line.

Exuberant granulation tissue at the recipient site should be excised to the level of the margin of the wound 24 to 48 hours prior to grafting. The recipient holes in the granulation tissue should be created before the grafts are harvested to allow hemostasis to occur prior to implantation. The depth of the recipient holes should correspond to the thickness of the grafts to be inserted.[1] To avoid obscuring the wound with hemorrhage that occurs when the recipient

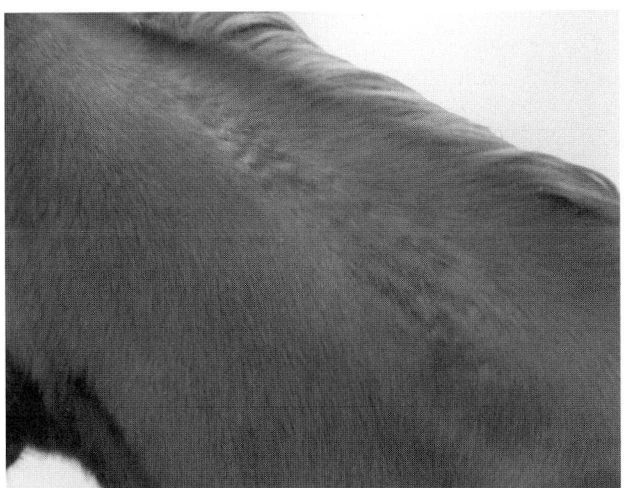

Figure 25-17. Blemishes on a horse's neck created with a skin biopsy punch.

*References 8, 15, 20, 23, 27, 38, 53.

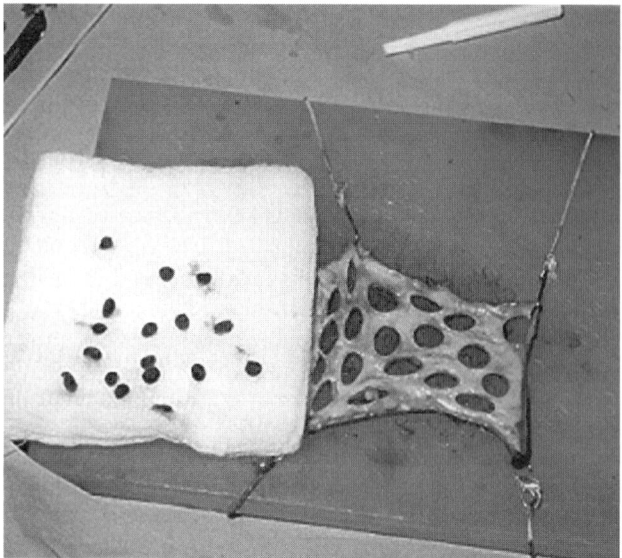

Figure 25-18. Punch grafts harvested from a full-thickness section of skin. The section of skin was obtained from the pectoral region. Full-thickness plugs are cut from the skin using a skin biopsy punch.

holes are created, creation of the recipient holes should begin distally and proceed in a proximal direction.[63] A cotton-tipped applicator inserted into the recipient holes enables each hole to be located easily for insertion of a graft and prevents a blood clot from forming in the hole (Fig. 25-19). Spraying the wound with phenylephrine before creating the recipient holes may improve visibility by decreasing hemorrhage. Creating the recipient holes hours in advance of implantation ensures a hemorrhage-free wound for grafting.[50] The holes should be placed about 6 mm (about ¼ inch) apart in a symmetrical pattern.[1]

The recipient holes are created with a slightly smaller biopsy punch than that used to harvest the grafts, to allow for contraction of the graft. For example, if the grafts are harvested with a 7-mm-diameter biopsy punch, the recipient holes should be created with a 5-mm biopsy punch (Fig. 25-20). The grafts are inserted into recipient holes, and the grafted wound is covered with a nonadherent dressing and a bandage. Consideration can be given to the direction of the hair growth on the graft when the graft is inserted, but the cosmetic outcome is little affected by properly orienting the direction of the hair.

The pigmented, superficial portions of the grafts frequently slough, exposing nonpigmented deeper layers. By 3 weeks, each plug of skin is surrounded by a red ring, which represents migrating epithelium.[1] Acceptance of the grafts is ensured if the grafts remain within the recipient hole,[37] but survival of 60% to 75% of the grafts is a realistic expectation.[50] The time required for the wound to completely epithelialize is inversely proportional to the amount of wound covered by viable plugs. Punch grafting requires no expensive or sophisticated equipment and little expertise, and the grafts are accepted into recipient beds that are unsuitable for sheet grafting.[1] Punch grafting can be performed with the horse standing, making this an inexpensive method of grafting wounds. Punch grafting is usually reserved for small wounds where cosmesis is not important. Wounds healed by punch grafting are covered primarily by an epithelial scar from which grow sparse tufts of divergent hair (Fig. 25-21).

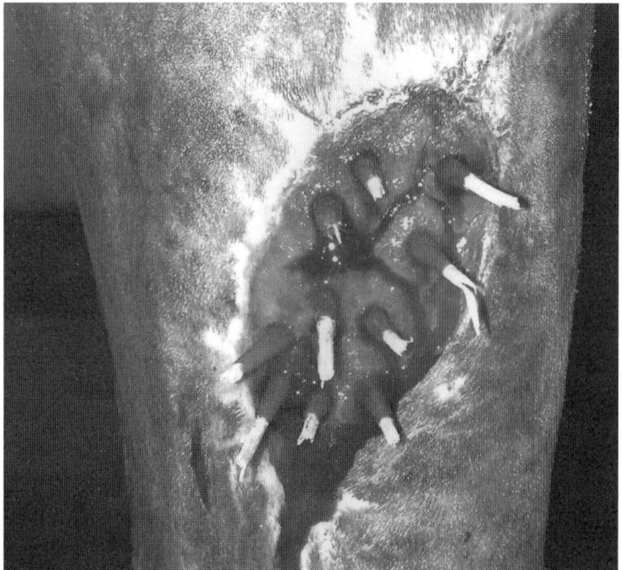

Figure 25-19. Cotton-tipped applicators inserted into recipient holes in a granulating wound. An applicator enables a hole to be located easily and prevents a blood clot from forming in the hole.

Pinch Grafts

Pinch grafts are small discs of skin, harvested by excising an elevated cone of skin, that are laid onto or implanted into granulation tissue.[26,45,51,60-62] The pinch graft is sometime referred to as a Reverdin graft.[62] The donor sites for obtaining pinch grafts from the horse are the same as described for punch grafts; small blemishes created at these donor sites are relatively inconspicuous. A disc of optimal size is approximately 3 mm in diameter, which approaches full thickness toward its center, but its thickness diminishes toward its periphery.[60]

Preparation of the donor site is identical to that described for punch grafts. A cone of skin is elevated using a tissue forceps, a suture needle, or a hypodermic needle with a bent point, and it is excised with a scalpel blade (Fig. 25-22).[45,51,60-62] A no. 11 scalpel blade is most suited for

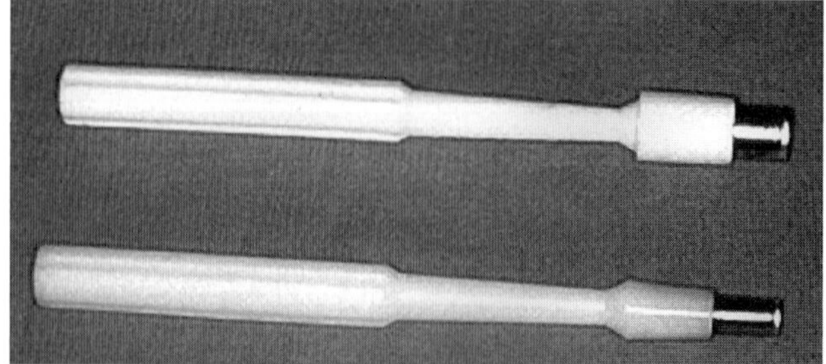

Figure 25-20. Skin biopsy punches used for harvesting punch grafts and for creating recipient holes. The recipient holes for punch grafts are created with a slightly smaller skin biopsy punch than that used to harvest the grafts. The larger punch is used to harvest punch grafts, and the smaller biopsy punch is used to create recipient holes.

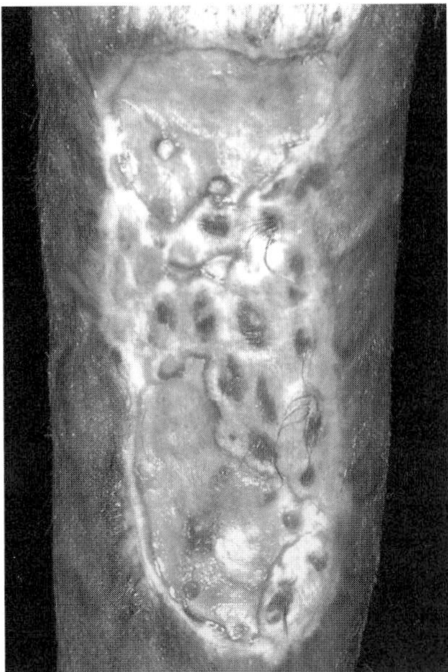

Figure 25-21. A nearly healed, punch-grafted wound. The non-pigmented tissue between the pigmented punch grafts is epithelium. This epithelium will eventually become pigmented.

excising the cone of skin. The grafts are stored on a gauze sponge moistened with physiologic saline solution until they are implanted.

The recipient site is prepared in the same way as for punch grafts. The recipient pockets can be created hours in advance of implantation to ensure a hemorrhage-free wound for grafting, but locating the pockets after hemorrhage has ceased may be difficult.

To implant a graft, a no. 15 scalpel blade is stabbed into the granulation tissue of the recipient bed at an acute angle to create a shallow pocket into which the graft is inserted. Implantation should begin distally and proceed proximally, because the pockets are obscured by hemorrhage after they are created. The grafts should be implanted about 3 to 5 mm apart.[60] Each graft is laid onto the wound, epidermal side up, proximal to the pocket and slid into the pocket using a hypodermic needle, a straight suture needle, or the scalpel blade used to create the pocket. Consideration can be given to the direction of the hair growth on the graft when the graft is inserted, but the cosmetic outcome is little affected by properly orienting the direction of the hair. To speed implantation, three or more grafts can be laid onto the granulation tissue at once, each 15 to 20 mm proximal to its proposed site of implantation. Hydrostatic pressure prevents the grafts from falling from the wound. The surgeon creates a pocket distal to a graft and inserts the graft into the pocket using the same scalpel blade that was used to create the pocket. The surgeon can create and implant the pockets in rapid succession without looking away from the wound.

Wounds created at the donor site are left to heal by second intention or closed with a single suture or staple. The grafted wound is covered with a nonadherent dressing and a bandage.

The thin layer of granulation tissue covering each pinch graft usually sloughs between the first and second week after grafting.[60] Grafts initially appear as dark spots on the wound's surface (Fig. 25-23), but frequently the superficial, pigmented portion of the graft sloughs, causing the graft to appear as a white spot surrounded by pink granulation tissue. Within 3 weeks, each disc of skin is surrounded by a red ring, which represents migrating epithelium. Epithelium migrates from the margin of the wound, as well as from the margin of each graft, so that eventually the entire wound is

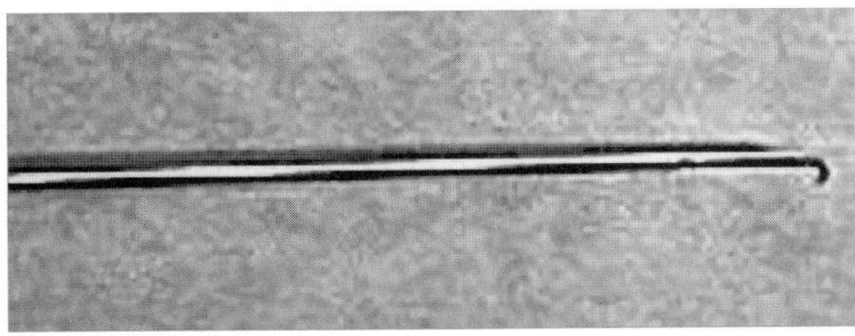

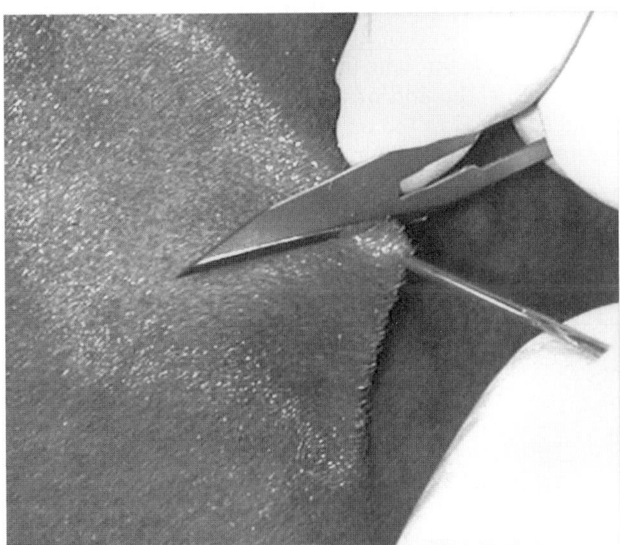

Figure 25-22. Harvesting a pinch graft. A cone of skin is elevated using a hypodermic needle with a bent point, and the elevated cone of skin is excised with a scalpel blade.

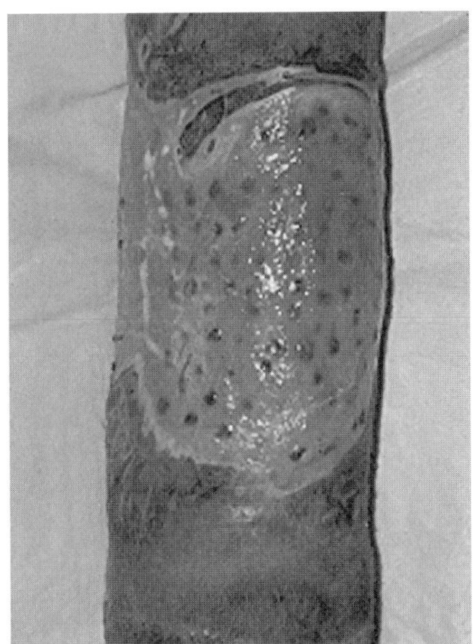

Figure 25-23. A wound covered with pinch grafts.

covered with epithelium. Even under adverse conditions, one can expect at least 50% to 75% of the grafts to survive.[60]

Pinch grafting, like punch grafting, is a relatively inexpensive technique of grafting, because the procedure can be performed with the horse standing, and because only basic instruments are required. Little expertise is necessary, and the grafts can survive in a granulation bed that is less than ideal.[3,61] Pinch grafting is tedious, however, and imparts a poor cosmetic appearance, because the wound is left covered by an epithelial scar from which grow sparse tufts of divergent hair.

Tunnel Grafts

Tunnel grafts are strips of split-thickness or full-thickness skin implanted into tunnels created in granulation tissue.[4,64,65] The grafts are exposed days later, when they have revascularized, by excising the overlying granulation tissue that forms the roof of the tunnel. Donor skin can be harvested from various sites on the horse, using various techniques, and implanted with the horse anesthetized or standing and sedated.

Split-thickness or full-thickness strips of skin can be harvested conveniently from the portion of the neck that lies beneath the mane or the ventral aspect of the flank.[4,64,65] In preparation for harvesting strips of skin, linear wheals, 2 to 3 cm wide and slightly longer than the wound to be grafted, are created along the longitudinal axis of the donor site by subcutaneously injecting local anesthetic solution (or physiologic saline solution, if the graft is to be harvested with the horse anesthetized).

A straight intestinal forceps is applied to the base of each wheal so that skin protrudes slightly above the jaws of the forceps.[4,64,65] If a strip of skin longer than the jaws of the forceps is required, two intestinal forceps are applied end-to-end to the base of the wheal. The thickness and width of the graft is determined by the amount of skin that protrudes above the jaws. The protruding skin is severed with a scalpel (Fig. 25-24). If the excised strip of skin is full thickness, subcutaneous tissue should be removed from it to expose the dermis, and the wound at the donor site should be closed with staples or sutures. If the strip of skin is split thickness, the donor site can be closed or left open.

Full-thickness strips of skin can also be harvested from the neck or ventral portion of the abdomen by making a series of parallel incisions 2 mm apart.[65] Strips are excised,

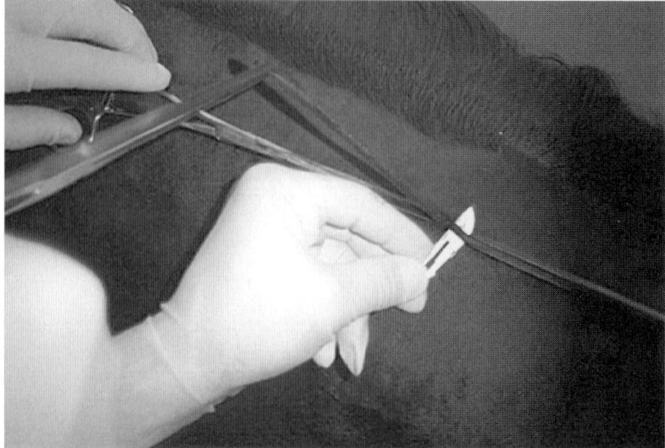

Figure 25-24. Harvesting a tunnel graft. One or two straight intestinal forceps are applied to the skin, so that skin protrudes slightly above the jaws of the forceps. The protruding skin is severed with a scalpel.

and subcutaneous tissue attached to the dermis is sharply excised. The donor sites are closed with sutures or staples.

To implant a strip of skin in the granulation bed, the end of a long, thin, rat-tooth, alligator forceps is inserted into granulation tissue at the edge of the wound and advanced through the granulation tissue at a depth of about 5 or 6 mm until it emerges at the opposite margin of the wound.[4,65] One end of the graft is grasped in the jaws of the forceps, with the epidermis positioned toward the surface of the wound, and pulled through the tunnel. The grafts should be embedded at right angles to the convex surface of the wound to aid entry and exit of the forceps.[65] A wound that is not convex is more easily grafted if granulation tissue is allowed to proliferate so that it protrudes slightly above the margin of the wound.[4] The strips should be embedded about 2 cm apart.[65]

The strip of skin is embedded in two steps if the alligator forceps is not long enough to completely span the wound, or if the wound is too convex for the alligator forceps to completely span it.[4,64,65] In either case, the forceps is advanced through the granulation tissue as far as possible and exited, one end of the graft is grasped, and the forceps is pulled back through the tunnel, with the graft in tow (Fig. 25-25). The end of the forceps is reinserted into the granulation bed at the opposite margin of the wound and advanced beneath the surface of the granulation tissue until

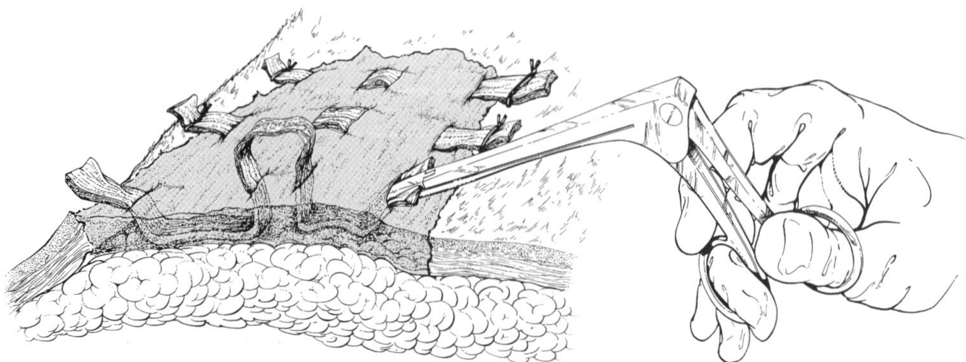

Figure 25-25. Implanting a tunnel graft using an alligator forceps. The strip of skin is embedded in two steps if the forceps is not long enough to completely span the wound.

it emerges at the site of exit of the graft. The end of the graft is grasped in the jaws of the forceps, and the forceps, with graft in tow, is pulled back through the second tunnel.

The graft can also be embedded by positioning the strip of skin onto a strip of adhesive tape, with the epidermis next to the tape.[64] The purpose of the adhesive tape is to prevent the edges of the strip from folding inward and to act as a guide when the grafts are later exposed. The tape should extend 5 cm beyond one end of the strip, and excess tape at this end is folded over the skin so that about 1 cm of the end of the strip is covered by tape. Excess tape along the graft's margin is trimmed with scissors. The tape-covered end of the graft is fitted through the eye of a 10- to 12-cm cutting needle with a flat curve, and the graft–tape composite is implanted by advancing the needle beneath the surface of the granulation bed. If the needle is not long enough to span the wound completely, or if the wound is too convex for the needle to completely span it, the needle is advanced beneath the bed as far as possible, exited, and reentered at the point of exit for a second bite. Another method of creating the strips of graft and tape is to lay a sheet of split- or full-thickness skin, hair side down, onto the sticky side of a similarly sized sheet of adhesive tape; strips of skin and tape are cut from this composite.[50]

The exposed ends of the embedded strips are attached to the margin of the wound with a suture, staple, or cyanoacrylate glue, and the wound is covered with a nonadherent dressing and a pressure wrap. Six to 10 days after grafting, the roof of each tunnel is removed, with the horse sedated or anesthetized, to expose the grafts, and if necessary, to remove adhesive tape.[4,64,65] To remove the roof of a tunnel, a smooth, malleable probe is inserted into the tunnel superficial to the graft, and a V-shaped strip of granulation tissue is carefully excised over the probe with a scalpel blade to expose the graft. The roof of each tunnel can also be sawed off using a twisted, doubled piece of fine wire threaded through the tunnel.[64]

Accidentally removing a graft while attempting to expose it or failure to locate buried grafts can detract from the success of tunnel grafting.[65] These complications can best be avoided by applying a tourniquet proximal to the wound to enhance visibility, or by exposing the grafts with the horse anesthetized. Placing the grafts closer than 2 cm apart may affect the viability of granulation tissue surrounding the grafts. About 60% to 80% acceptance of the strips can be expected.[64,65]

Tunnel grafting is recommended primarily for wounds located in areas where immobilizing other types of grafts would be difficult, such as the dorsal aspect of the hock.[64,65] Tunnel grafts are unaffected by movement in highly mobile areas, because the grafts are circumferentially encompassed and immobilized by granulation tissue. Tunnel grafting does not require expensive equipment and can be performed with the horse standing, but the technique requires the presence of a granulation bed, and aspects of this technique, especially removing the top of the tunnels, make tunnel grafting relatively tedious.

AFTERCARE OF THE DONOR SITE

The donor site of a split-thickness graft retains a portion of the dermis and is comparable to a deep abrasion.[15,17,29] Blood and fibrin form a scab over the abrasion, and beneath this scab, epithelial cells from the wound's edge and epithelial cells produced by adnexa in the remaining dermis migrate to cover the surface of the abrasion. The wound at the donor site is usually covered by epithelium within 1 to 3 weeks, depending on the depth of the cut (Fig. 25-26).[20,54] The new, pink epithelium covering the donor site begins to develop pigment within a month after it forms, causing the epithelial scar to become black. The quantity of adnexa is greatest in the upper layers of the dermis, and consequently, healing of the donor site proceeds more quickly when a thin skin graft is harvested.[17,20] When grafts between 0.63 mm and 0.76 mm thick are harvested from the horse, the donor site heals with a noticeable epithelial scar.[20,56]

Pain caused by exposure of nerves at the donor site of a split-thickness graft can be reduced by bandaging the donor site,[17] but split-thickness grafts of horses are virtually always taken from an area that is difficult to bandage. Pain can be decreased by covering the donor site with fine-mesh gauze or a biologic bandage, such as a stored allograft or xenograft (see "Allografts and Xenografts" and "Storage of Grafts," later). The gauze or biologic bandage falls off when the donor site is completely epithelialized. An uncovered donor site develops a scab, and this scab should not be removed. Any attempt to remove the scab is met with violent resistance from the horse, and its removal interferes with epithelialization that proceeds beneath it. An analgesic drug, such as phenylbutazone, should be administered before the graft is harvested and for several days after surgery.

AFTERCARE OF THE RECIPIENT SITE

The grafted wound should be covered with a sterile, nonadherent dressing, such as cotton nonadherent film dressing (Telfa Sterile Pads, Kendal Co, Hospital Products, Boston, Mass), rayon polyethylene dressing (Release, Johnson & Johnson Products, Inc, New Brunswick, NY), or petrolatum-impregnated gauze dressing (Adaptic, Johnson & Johnson Inc, Fort Dodge, Iowa). Petrolatum-impregnated gauze dressings can be prepared by steam-autoclaving a container filled with gauze sponges topped with a dollop of petrolatum. The petroleum impregnates the gauze as it melts. The

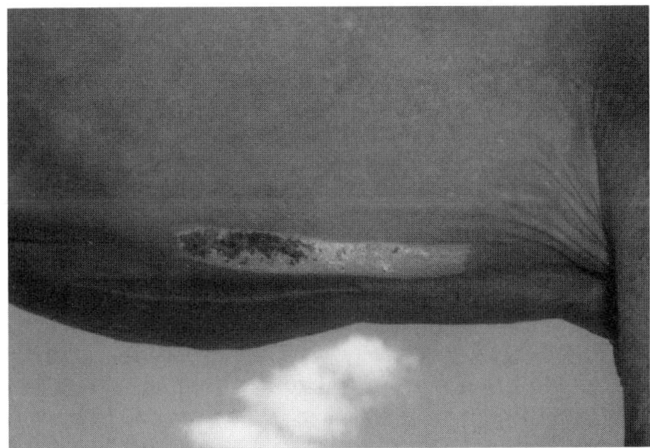

Figure 25-26. The donor site of a split-thickness graft 2 weeks after the graft was harvested. The donor site is nearly covered by epithelium. The new, pink epithelium will begin to develop pigment within a month, causing the epithelial scar to become black.

wide weave of a gauze sponge, however, makes the sponge more likely to adhere to the grafted wound than would a commercially available petrolatum-impregnated gauze dressing with a close weave (my observation).

The primary dressing is secured to the grafted wound with sterile, elastic, conforming, rolled gauze. If the grafted wound is in an area that is difficult to immobilize, such as the dorsal aspect of the hock, securing the primary dressing with staples[37] or with elastic adhesive tape, rather than rolled gauze, may help to decrease shearing forces between the graft and the bandage. The secondary layer of the bandage should be bulky, to decrease motion of the limb, and absorbent, to wick bacteria and destructive enzymes from the grafted wound. Immobilizing the limb with a cast is usually not necessary unless the grafted wound is located in a highly mobile area, such as the dorsum of the fetlock. A splint or a Robert Jones bandage applied to the limb usually immobilizes the grafted wound sufficiently.

The bandage should not be changed for 4 or 5 days after grafting, unless virulent, nosocomial infections are a common problem in the hospital, because changing the bandage may disturb the graft's delicate attachment to the wound. However, if such infections are a common problem in the hospital, the bandage should be changed daily, or even twice daily, for at least 5 days. Changing the bandage daily allows exudate, which contains destructive enzymes, to be removed from the wound, and it allows application of an appropriate antimicrobial drug to the wound. Complete loss of a sheet graft, from infection or motion, later than 5 days after grafting is uncommon.[37] Streptococci or pseudomonads can quickly destroy a recently applied graft (Fig. 25-27), so prompt recognition of infection and application of an appropriate antimicrobial drug to the grafted wound are necessary. Exudate that develops on a grafted wound should be cultured for bacterial growth, and isolates should be tested for antimicrobial susceptibility. Until the results are known, a broad-spectrum antimicrobial agent, effective against both β-hemolytic streptococcus and *Pseudomonas,* such as a combination of ticarcillin disodium and clavulanate potassium, should be applied topically to the wound.[46]

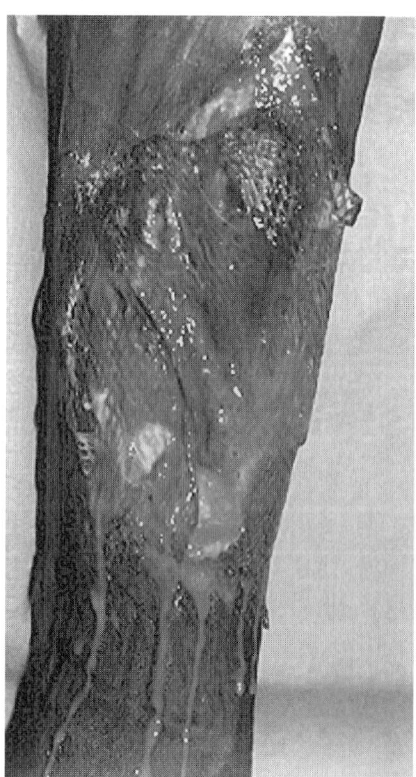

Figure 25-27. A recently applied graft destroyed by streptococcal infection.

If the limb has been immobilized in a cast, and if nosocomial infection from streptococci or pseudomonads is a common problem in the hospital, an antimicrobial drug should be applied periodically to the wound through an infusion tube fixed to the grafted wound and exited through the top of the cast. A good infusion tube can be prepared from silicon tubing by sealing its distal end and perforating it (with a 25-gauge needle) in multiple places along the portion that lies adjacent to the wound.

Even a docile horse should be heavily sedated during the initial bandage changes to help avoid movement that may disturb the delicate, vascular connections forming between the recipient bed and the graft. Adherence of the primary dressing to the grafted wound by fibrin that exudes through a meshed graft usually indicates that the graft is well adhered to the wound by a fibrin seal. Soaking the primary dressing with physiologic saline solution may ease removal of the dressing, but if the primary dressing cannot be removed easily, it should be left in place.

Exuberant granulation tissue that inhibits epithelial migration may grow through the latticework of a meshed graft, especially if the graft was applied to the wound fully expanded. A corticosteroid applied to the grafted wound causes the exuberant granulation tissue within the graft to regress, allowing epithelial migration to proceed, even if at a slower than normal pace.[29,66-68]

Ideally, grafted wounds on limbs should be protected by a bandage until epithelialization is complete. If bandaging becomes impractical before epithelialization is complete, small, nonepithelialized areas within the grafted wound can be allowed to heal beneath a scab, which soon forms when the wound is left exposed.

A grafted wound in an area that is difficult to wrap, such as the abdomen or thorax, can be protected with a "tie-over" bolus dressing, sometimes referred to as a stent.[4,29,63] To apply a stent, the grafted wound is covered with a nonadherent dressing followed by a bolus of gauze. Long ends of interrupted sutures, preplaced around the margin of the grafted wound, are tied tightly over the bolus (Fig. 25-28).

Pressure on a graft from a bandage is not necessary for the graft to be accepted, so, for areas that are difficult to bandage or for wounds that are chronically plagued with infection, the grafted wound can be left uncovered.[2,23] "Open" grafting avoids shearing forces imposed by a bandage and avoids maceration of the graft by allowing constant drainage of exudate. To successfully employ open grafting, precautions, such as tying the horse or applying a neck cradle, must be taken to prevent the horse from disturbing the exposed graft.

Some horses probably suffer from hyperesthesia at the grafted wound, so, when bandaging is discontinued, temporarily applying a neck cradle or tying the horse may be prudent to prevent the horse from mutilating its grafted wound. Drying and scaling of the healed donor and recipient sites of a split-thickness graft, caused by reduced con-

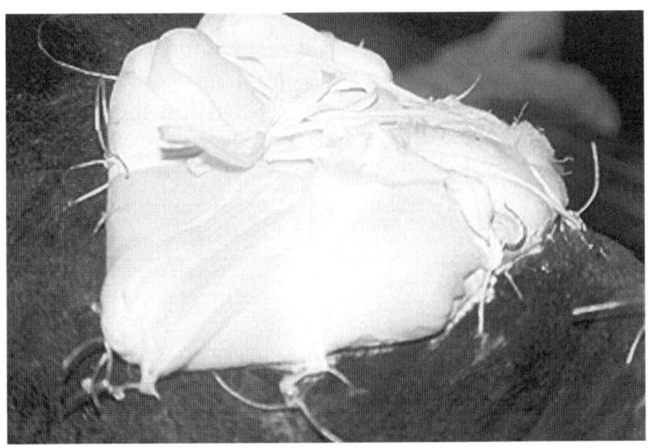

Figure 25-28. A stent bandage applied to a grafted wound on the back of a horse. A grafted wound in an area that is difficult to wrap can be protected with a stent bandage. To apply a stent bandage, the grafted wound is covered with a nonadherent dressing followed by a bolus of gauze. Long ends of interrupted sutures, preplaced around the margin of the grafted wound, are tied tightly over the bolus.

centration of eccrine glands, can be lessened by periodically applying an ointment containing lanolin until enough glands regenerate that scaling is no longer a problem.[8]

ALLOGRAFTS AND XENOGRAFTS

Cutaneous allografts (i.e., skin grafts taken from one animal and transplanted to another of the same species) or cutaneous xenografts (i.e., skin grafts taken from one animal and transplanted to another of a different species) can be used as a biologic dressing on wounds of horses. Cutaneous allografts and xenografts, usually pigskin, have been used extensively since the middle of the 19th century to temporarily dress large wounds on humans. Although xenografts have been used to dress wounds of horses,[12,13,69,70] the use of cadaveric, cutaneous allografts to dress their wounds has only recently been investigated.[14] Viable, cutaneous allografts can be obtained from refrigerated cadavers 24 hours or longer after death.[71] Allografts applied to wounds of horses seem to survive between 2 and 3 weeks, but the length of survival can be difficult to determine, because even when the superficial portion of the graft appears to be desiccated, the deeper portion of the graft may still be viable and attached to the recipient wound by strong vascular connections.

A cutaneous allograft or xenograft can be used to temporarily cover a wound if autografting is physically unfeasible or economically impractical. An allograft or xenograft encourages healing by promoting epithelialization and angiogenesis at the recipient bed.[2,12,13,71,72] The allograft or xenograft also retards formation of exuberant granulation tissue and acts as a bacterial barrier to protect the wound from infection.[12,69,71] A cutaneous allograft or xenograft revascularizes, and this vascularization may explain, at least in part, the ability of the cutaneous allograft or xenograft to resist infection.[11] Acceptance of a graft is not essential for bacterial destruction, however, because bacterial colonization decreases even beneath nonviable grafts, perhaps because the fibrin that forms between the graft and the wound enhances phagocytosis.[12,13,17,39,73] Adherence of an allograft or xenograft to a wound is a useful indicator that the wound is sufficiently healthy to accept an autograft.

The use of cutaneous porcine xenografting in humans arose from the need for a substitute for allografts as a biologic dressing because of the short supply of cadaveric skin, but clinical comparisons in humans have shown that cutaneous porcine xenografts are inferior to cutaneous allografts.[11] Cutaneous porcine xenografts are more poorly adhered than allografts, allow higher bacterial counts in the wound, and cause a more intense immunologic rejection.

STORAGE OF GRAFTS

Autografts or allografts can be applied successfully to wounds after being stored for several weeks at refrigeration temperature, in gauze that has been soaked in either physiologic saline solution or lactated Ringer's solution.[8,16,23] Skin can be stored in a refrigerator, for much longer periods in a nutrient medium, such as McCoy's 5A Medium (Gibco Laboratories, Inc, Grand Island, NY) to which serum has been added.[71,74-76]

McCoy's 5A Medium is a tissue-culture medium composed of a balanced electrolyte solution to which amino acids, vitamins, dextrose, and a pH indicator (phenol red) have been added. Adding vitamins, amino acids, dextrose, and serum to the electrolyte solution greatly extends the time that a graft can be stored. Skin from humans has been stored successfully in refrigerated nutrient media for 6 to 8 weeks.[71,76] Wounds of horses have been grafted using split-thickness skin grafts refrigerated at 4° C in a solution of McCoy's 5A Medium and horse serum for 3 weeks, with consistently successful results,[74] and wounds of some horses have been grafted successfully using skin stored for as long as 12 weeks.

The concentration of serum in the storage medium should be between 10% and 33%.[77] A concentration of serum greater than 33% stimulates the metabolic activity of the graft. Antigenic reaction of the serum to the graft is avoided by using a commercially available antibody-free serum (GG-Free Horse Serum, Gibco Laboratories, Inc, Grand Island, NY), pooled homologous serum, or the horse's own serum.[76] The stored grafts should be allowed access to air.[71]

To prepare a meshed split-thickness skin graft for storage, the graft is laid on a sterile gauze swab or gauze dressing, with the epidermis of the graft next to the gauze. The gauze–graft composite is rolled up, with the gauze to the outside of the roll (Fig. 25-29), and placed in a sterile container containing approximately 1 to 2.5 mL of the storage medium for each square centimeter of stored graft[76,77] (Fig. 25-30). The storage medium should be examined occasionally for a color change brought about by a change in pH. A color change in the McCoy's 5A Medium from cherry-red to orange-yellow indicates excessive accumulation of catabolites and the need for immediate application of the graft or replacement of the medium. Only half of the volume of medium should be replaced, because total replacement affects the graft deleteriously.[76]

A split-thickness skin graft, harvested while the horse is anesthetized for treatment of a wound, such as removal of a bone sequestrum, can be stored until the wound's condition has improved enough to permit grafting.[23,78,79] A graft can be

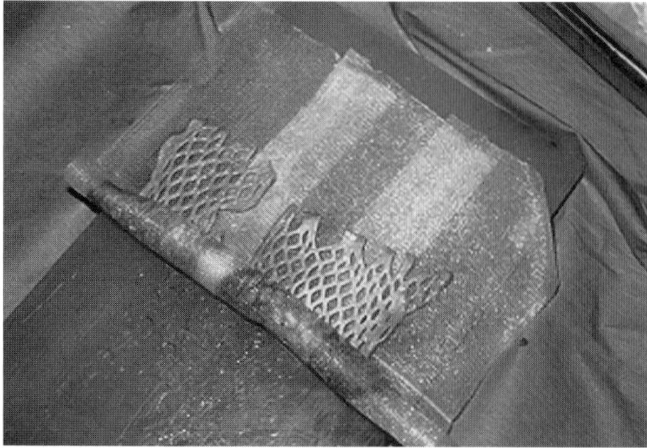

Figure 25-29. Preparing the graft for storage. The gauze–graft composite is rolled up, with the gauze to the outside of the roll.

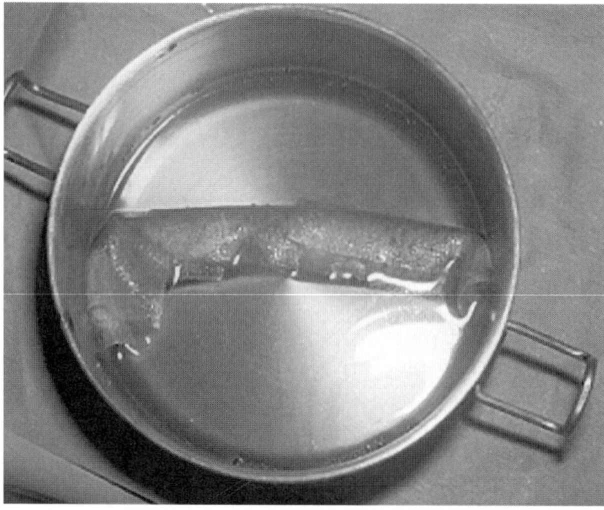

Figure 25-30. Storing the graft. The gauze-graft composite is stored, in a refrigerator, in a sterile container containing McCoy's 5A Medium to which horse serum has been added.

stored for delayed grafting of an excisional defect accompanied by excessive hemorrhage. Storing the graft, so that it can be applied with the horse standing, shortens the anesthetic period and eliminates the risk of the graft's being disturbed during recovery. A stored graft is often more readily accepted than a fresh graft, because grafts stored for 24 hours or more release anaerobic metabolites that stimulate rapid revascularization of the graft.[43,80] For this reason, a stored graft is sometimes referred to as a "prepared graft."

A stored graft is useful for covering a defect created when all or a portion of a primary graft sloughs, and for this reason, harvesting more skin than is required to cover a wound is often prudent, especially when grafting has a greater than usual possibility of failure. A stored graft not required for autografting can be used as a biologic dressing for a wound of another horse, when circumstances permit.

REFERENCES

1. Boyd CL, Hanselka DV: A skin punch technique for equine skin grafting, J Am Vet Med Assoc 1971;158:82.
2. Peacock E: Wound Repair, ed 3, Philadelphia, 1984, WB Saunders.
3. Ross GE: Clinical canine skin grafting, J Am Vet Med Assoc 1968;153:1759.
4. Wilson DG: Applications of skin grafting in large animals, Probl Vet Med 1990;2:442.
5. White R: Reconstruction of skin deficits: Assessing the options, Equine Vet J 1992;24:3.
6. Lees MJ, Fretz P, Bowen CVA, et al: Experimental cutaneous free flap transfers in the horse, Microsurgery 1991;12:130.
7. Lees MJ, Bowen CV, Fretz PB, et al: Transfer of deep circumflex iliac flaps to the tarsus by microvascular anastomosis in the horse, Vet Surg 1989;18:292.
8. Bell R: The Use of Skin Grafts, New York, 1973, Oxford University Press.
9. Mir Y ML: Biology of the skin graft, Plast Reconstr Surg 1951;8:378.
10. Boykin JV, Molnar JA: Burn scar and skin equivalents. In Cohen IK, Diegelmann RF, Lindblad WJ, editors: Wound Healing, Philadelphia, 1992, WB Saunders.
11. May S: The effects of biological wound dressings on the healing process, Clin Mater 1991;8:243.
12. Diehl M, Ersek RA: Porcine xenografts for treatment of skin defects in horses, J Am Vet Med Assoc 1980;177:625.
13. Diehl M, Jeanmonod CA, Muller M, et al: Porcine skin as temporary covering of extensive skin defects in the horse, Schweiz Arch Tierheilk 1979;121:23.
14. Gomez JH, Schumacher J, Swaim SF, et al: Effects of three biological dressings on healing of cutaneous wounds on the limbs of horses, Can J Vet Res 2004;68:49.
15. Rudolph R, Fisher JC, Ninnemann JL: Skin Grafting, Boston, 1979, Little, Brown.
16. Rothstein AS: Skin grafting techniques, J Am Podiatry Assoc 1983;73:79.
17. Argenta LC, Dingman RO: Skin grafting. In Epstein E, editor: Skin Surgery, ed 6, Philadelphia, 1987, WB Saunders.
18. Flowers RS: Unexpected postoperative problems in skin grafting, Surg Clin North Am 1970;50:439.
19. Jensen EC: Canine autogenous skin grafting, Am J Vet Res 1959;20:898.
20. Frankland AL: Autologous, split skin transplantation on the lower limbs of horses, Vet Rec 1979;104:590.
21. Tavis MJ, Thornton JW, Harney JH, et al: Mechanism of skin graft adherence: Collagen, elastin, and fibrin interactions, Surg Forum 1977;28:522.
22. Teh B: Why do skin grafts fail? Plast Reconstr Surg 1979;63:323.
23. Vistnes LM: Grafting of skin, Surg Clin North Am 1977;57:939.
24. Converse JM, Smahel J, Ballantyne DL, et al: Inosculation of vessels of skin graft and host bed: A fortuitous encounter, Br J Plast Surg 1975;28:274.
25. Gringrass PJ, Grabb WC, Gringrass RP: Skin graft survival on avascular defects, Plast Reconstr Surg 1975;55:65.
26. Hogle R, Kingrey BW, Jensen EC: Skin grafting in the horse, J Am Vet Med Assoc 1959;135:165.
27. Frankland AL, Morris PGD, Spreull JSA: Free, autologous, skin transplantation in the horse, Vet Rec 1976;98:105.
28. Boyd CL: Equine skin autotransplants for wound healing, J Am Vet Med Assoc 1967;151:1618.
29. Meagher DM, Adams OR: Split-thickness autologous skin transplantation in horses, J Am Vet Med Assoc 1971;159:55.
30. Fitzgerald MJ, Martin F, Paletta FX: Innervation of skin grafts, Surg Gynecol Obstet 1967;124:808.
31. Kernwein G: Recovery of sensation in split-thickness skin grafts, Arch Surg 1948;56:459.
32. Rudolph R: Inhibition of myofibroblasts by skin grafts, Plast Reconstr Surg 1979;63:473.

33. Corps B: The effect of graft thickness, donor site and graft bed on graft shrinkage in the hooded rat, Br J Plast Surg 1969;22:125.
34. Rudolph R: The effect of skin graft preparation on wound contraction, Surg Gynecol Obstet 1976;142:49.
35. Ford TS, Schumacher J, Brumbaugh GW, et al: Effects of split-thickness and full-thickness skin grafts on secondary graft contraction in horses, Am J Vet Res 1992;53:1572.
36. Schumacher J, Brumbaugh GW, Honnas CM, et al: Kinetics of healing of grafted and nongrafted wounds on the distal portion of the forelimbs of horses, Am J Vet Res 1992;53:1568.
37. Booth L: Equine wound reconstruction using free skin grafting, Calif Vet 1991;45:13.
38. Cason J: Skin grafting and diagnosis of depth of burn. In Cason J, editor: Treatment of Burns, London, 1981, Chapman and Hall.
39. Eade GG: The relationship between granulation tissue, bacteria, and skin grafts in burned patients, Plast Reconstr Surg 1958;22:42.
40. Krizek TJ, Robeson MC, Kho E: Bacterial growth and skin graft survival, Surg Forum 1967;18:518.
41. Robson M, Krizek TJ: Predicting skin graft survival, J Trauma 1973;13:213.
42. Currie LJ, Sharpe JR, Martin R: The use of fibrin glue in skin grafts and tissue-engineered skin replacements: A review, Plast Reconstr Surg 2001;108:1713.
43. Smahel J: Free skin transplantation on a prepared bed, Br J Plast Surg 1971;24:129.
44. Boon RJ, Beale AS: Response of *Streptococcus pyogenes* to therapy with amoxicillin or amoxicillin-clavulanic acid in a mouse model of mixed infection caused by *Staphylococcus aureus* and *Streptococcus pyogenes*, Antimicrob Agents Chemother 1987;31:1204.
45. James J: Skin grafting in difficult situations, Trop Doct 1999;29:41.
46. Moore R: Antimicrobial therapy in horses. In Colahan P, Merritt AM, Moore JN, Mayhew IG, editors: Equine Medicine and Surgery, ed 5, St Louis, Mosby, 1999.
47. Robson MC, Edstom LE, Krizek, TJ: The efficacy of systemic antibiotics in the treatment of granulating wounds, J Surg Res 1974; 16:299.
48. Edlich RF, Schmolka IR, Prusak MP, et al: The molecular basis for toxicity of surfactants in surgical wounds, J Surg Res 1973;14:277.
49. Hanselka DV, Milne FJ: Inexpensive mesh grafting technique in the horse, Proc Am Assoc Equine Pract 1976;21:191.
50. Stashak TS: Skin grafting in horses, Vet Clin North Am 1984;6:215.
51. Davis JS, Trout HF: Origin and development of the blood supply of whole thickness skin grafts: An experimental study, Ann Surg 1925;82:871.
52. French DA, Fretz PB: Treatment of equine leg wounds using skin grafts: Thirty-five cases, 1975-1988, Can Vet J 1990;31:761.
53. Valencia IC, Falabella AF, Eaglestein WH: Skin grafting, Dermatol Clin 2000;18:521.
54. Hanselka DV: Use of autogenous meshgrafts in equine wound management, J Am Vet Med Assoc 1974;164:35.
55. Hanselka DV, Boyd CL: Use of mesh grafts in dogs and horses, J Am Anim Hosp Assoc 1976;12:650.
56. Booth LC: Split-thickness autogenous skin transplantation in the horse, J Am Vet Med 1982;180:754.
57. MacMillan BG: The use of mesh grafting in treating burns, Surg Clin North Am 1970;50:1347.
58. Tobin GR: The compromised bed technique: An improved method for skin grafting problem wounds, Surg Clin North Am 1984; 64:653.
59. Lees ML, Fretz PB, Bailey JV, et al: Principles of grafting, Comp Cont Educ Pract Vet 1989;11:954.
60. Mackay-Smith MP, Marks D: A skin grafting technique for horses, J Am Vet Med Assoc 1968;152:1633.
61. Davis JS: The use of small deep skin grafts, J Am Med Assoc 1914;63:985.
62. Oien RF, Hansen BU, Hakansson A: Pinch graft skin transplantation for leg ulcers in primary care, J Wound Care 2000;9:217.
63. Lindsay WA: Step-by-step instructions for equine skin grafting techniques, Vet Med 1988;83:598.
64. Bjorck GTK: Tunnel skin grafting in the equine species, Proc Am Assoc Equine Pract 1971;17:313.
65. Lees MJ, Andrews GC, Bailey JV, et al: Tunnel grafting of equine wounds, Comp Cont Educ Pract Vet 1989;11:962.
66. Baker BL, Whitaker WL: Interference with wound healing by the local action of adrenocortical steroids, Endocrinology 1950; 46:544.
67. Ehrlich HP, Hunt TK: The effects of cortisone and anabolic steroids on the tensile strength of healing wounds, Ann Surg 1969;170:203.
68. Howes EL, Plotz CM, Blunt JW, et al: Retardation of wound healing by cortisone, Surgery 1950;28:177.
69. Ambler J: Porcine xenografts to facilitate integumental wound healing, Vet Rec 1980;106:437.
70. Marden DT: Use of pigskin to repair leg wounds in the horse, Vet Med Small Anim Clin 1974;69:771.
71. Brown JB, Fryer MP, Zaydon TJ: A skin bank for postmortem homografts, Surg Gynecol Obstet 1955;101:401.
72. O'Donoghue MN, Zarem HA: Stimulation of neovascularization—comparative efficacy of fresh and preserved skin grafts, Plast Reconstr Surg 1971;48:474.
73. Burleson MD, Eiseman B: Mechanism of antibacterial effect of biological dressing, Ann Surg 1973;177:181.
74. Schumacher J, Chambers M, Hanselka DV, et al: Preservation of skin by refrigeration for autogenous grafting in the horse, Vet Surg 1987;16:358.
75. Hurst LN, Brown DH, Murray KA: Prolonged life and improved quality for stored skin grafts, Plast Reconstr Surg 1984;73:105.
76. Gresham RB, Perry VP, Thompson VK: Practical methods of short-term storage of homografts, Arch Surg 1963;87:417.
77. Allgoewer M, Blocker TGJ: Viability of skin in relation to various methods of storage, Texas Rep Bio Med J 1952;10:3.
78. Shephard G: The storage of split skin grafts on their donor sites, Plast Reconstr Surg 1972;49:115.
79. Lehman JA, Saddawi N: Delayed open skin grafting, Br J Plast Surg 1975;28:46.
80. Smahel J: Preparation-phenomenon in a free skin graft, Br J Plast Surg 1971;24:133.

CHAPTER 26

Management of Superficial Wounds

Dean A. Hendrickson

The skin is the largest organ in the body and is very adaptable to the environment. The main functions of the skin are to protect against wear and bacterial invasion, to aid in thermal regulation, and to prevent water loss.[1,2]

The anatomy of the equine skin was first completely described by Talukdar and colleagues in 1972.[3] Using normal horses of ages 2 to 17, they collected skin from 49 different areas. The average skin thickness of the body skin was 3.8 mm, the skin near body openings 3.3 mm, and the skin at the main and tail 6.2 mm. Skin was thicker in older geldings than in younger horses and at the extensor surface of the legs than at the flexor surface of the legs. In general, the skin of the horse is thicker than that of swine, goats, and sheep; thinner than that of beef cattle; and similar in thickness to that of dairy cattle.[3]

The epidermis is composed of four layers: the stratum basale, stratum spinosum, stratum granulosum, and stratum corneum (Fig. 26-1). The stratum corneum slows water loss and functions as a barrier to harmful substances. Other cells found in the epidermis include melanocytes for production of melanin, Merkel cells for mechanoreception of light touch, and Langerhans' cells to help fight infection by engulfing foreign material. The dermis is separated into two layers, the superficial papillary layer and the deep reticular layer, and it provides support for the epidermis. The dermis in the lumbar, sacral, and gluteal regions has a third layer of collagenous fibers. The dermis also contains a rich vascular network that supplies the skin with a continuous blood supply. The vascular system is very important in temperature regulation, access of nutrients to the skin, absorption of topical medications, delivery of systemic medications, and the healing of wounds (see Chapter 5). The main vascular supply comes from the subcutaneous area. In the thinner-skinned areas, the hair angle is more acute. The hair follicles in the general skin areas where the hair length changes with the season are shorter than the hair follicles in the areas of mane and tail. In most cases, two sebaceous glands are associated with each hair follicle. The sweat glands are apocrine.[2,3] The hairs are surrounded by nerves that provide sensation by responding to pressure on the hair shaft. The primary nerve supply comes from the subcutaneous region.

Cleavage lines (Langer's lines of tension:—see Chapter 24) have been described in many species. The pattern is determined by placing an awl through the epidermis into the dermis and observing the orientation of the split or cleavage formed.[4] In a review, Rooney[4] cites the work of Schouppe,[5] who studied cleavage lines. Schouppe found that horses had cleavage lines whose orientation was parallel to the predominant orientation of the collagen fibers. These cleavage lines changed very little between adult horses, and wounds that healed best were parallel to the cleavage lines. In general, the cleavage lines were parallel to the long axis of the legs, head, and torso, and perpendicular to the long axis of the neck and flank. This is different from the cleavage lines found in dogs, which look more like stripes on a tiger.[6] In my opinion, cleavage lines on horses more closely approximate those of dogs than was reported by Schouppe (see Fig. 24-1). When possible, incision lines should be made parallel to the cleavage lines.

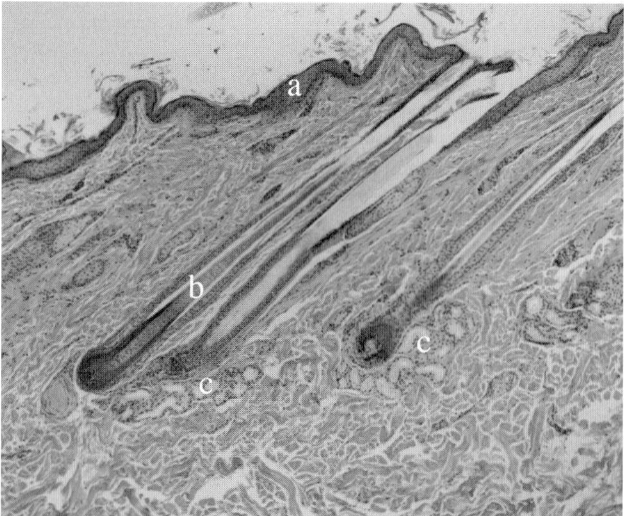

Figure 26-1. Photomicrograph of normal equine skin epidermis *(a)*, hair shaft and follicle *(b)*, and sweat glands *(c)*.

FIRST AID

Appropriate wound care is always a balance between improving the wound environment and harming the cells that are integral to the healing process. Consequently, the veterinarian must carefully weigh the benefits and the detriments of any particular action, not only for the immediate results but also for the long-term healing process.

ASSESSMENT

Wound assessment is one of the most important steps in wound therapy. More repaired wounds fail because of improper preparation and assessment than because of improper therapy. Properly preparing the wound provides an accurate assessment of the wound and deeper structures. Wound preparation begins with placing the animal in a location and environment that will allow the clinician to best determine the status of the wound. If the environment is not adequate to perform all of the tasks in the following paragraphs, it may be a good idea to move the horse to a place where these procedures can be done more efficiently and easily.

INITIAL MANAGEMENT

Restraint and Analgesia

For the horse with a wound, many types of restraint are appropriate, from simply holding its head to general anesthesia. Before using sedation, the horse's systemic status should be determined. It is uncommon for a horse to lose enough blood to cause problems with sedation, but if this is the case, the horse may collapse. Many commonly used sedative agents cause hypotension. Physical examination, blood work including packed cell volume, and skin turgor testing can help determine the systemic status of the horse and allow the clinician to decide if sedation is feasible (see Chapters 1, 4, and 8). Alternatives to systemic sedation include manual restraint such as a twitch, or local anesthesia of the affected area. In many cases, local anesthetic agents provide the best opportunity to prepare and examine the affected area, and to eventually treat the wound.[7]

Initial Preparation

After the horse has been restrained appropriately and the area has been desensitized with local anesthetic, the clinician decides whether to treat the wound with aseptic technique or if a simple clean technique is adequate. If there is a possibility of cross-contaminating a wound while preparing and exploring, aseptic technique should be used. The next step is to clip the hair over and around the wound site. To minimize the amount of clipped hair that gets into the wound, it can be covered with water-soluble, sterile, lubricating gel prior to clipping. It is best to put on a pair of examination or sterile gloves, apply the gel onto the fingers, and rub the gel into place (Fig. 26-2). This technique generally ensures that the gel will remain in contact with the wound bed. As the hair is clipped, it is trapped in the gel. The gel with the trapped hair can simply be rinsed from the wound with water or saline. Only when the entire wound area has been clipped and prepared can the clinician begin to fully appreciate the complexity of the wound. In many cases, seemingly insignificant wounds had invaded synovial structures, and because appropriate aggressive therapy was not instituted, the horse was eventually euthanized.

DÉBRIDEMENT

Débridement is an effective way to reduce the bacterial load within a wound and to minimize necrotic tissue. The benefits of débridement have been widely discussed in the field of human wound care.[8] Necrotic tissue and bacterial infection are major roadblocks to effective and cosmetic wound healing. The presence of foreign material reduces the number of bacteria necessary for infection by a factor of 10 (i.e., from 10^5 to 10^4 bacteria per gram of tissue). Each type of débridement has positive and negative consequences for wound healing, and it is important to select the technique that provides the best benefit-to-detriment ratio. The most common types of débridement are sharp, mechanical, chemical, and autolytic.

Sharp Débridement

Sharp débridement is one of the least traumatic methods available to the equine clinician, yet it is often underutilized. The major drawback to sharp débridement is that once the tissue is removed, it cannot be put back, so it is wise to be conservative in the removal of tissue. If the margin between viable and nonviable tissue is not clear, it is often better to leave some tissue for removal at a later time if necessary. Many skin flaps, especially on the head, retain viability even though they are cool at presentation. Tools for sharp débridement include a scalpel, scissors, and lasers. Scalpel débridement is the least traumatic of these techniques (Fig. 26-3), and it should be used whenever possible in the initial

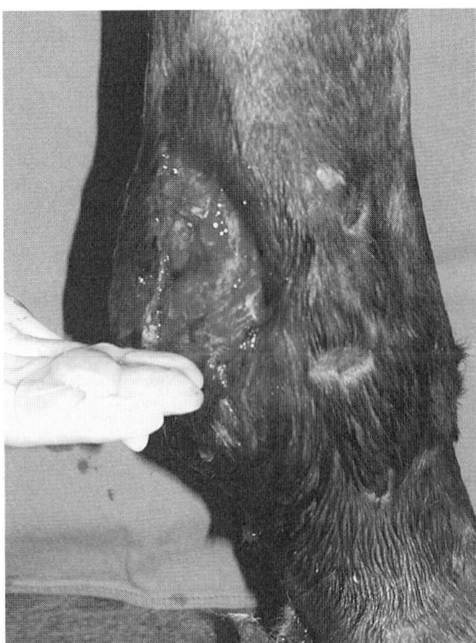

Figure 26-2. Application of sterile water-soluble gel to wound before clipping.

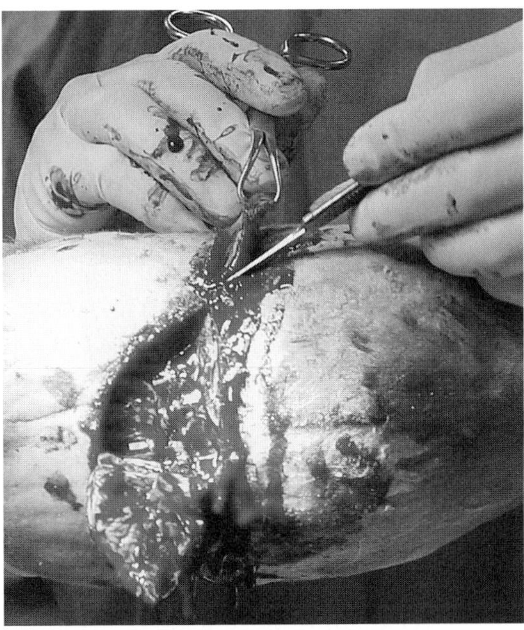

Figure 26-3. Sharp débridement of a wound on the dorsal and lateral aspect of the pastern region.

wound treatment stages. Other types of sharp débridement play a more secondary role.

Mechanical Débridement

Mechanical débridement is more traumatic, and unfortunately it is probably the most commonly used method in the horse. It can be performed using woven gauze (Fig. 26-4), lavage (Fig. 26-5), wet-to-wet, or wet-to-dry dressings. Mechanical débridement can be a useful tool, and it can be beneficial in the healing process, but it can be very traumatic. Often, when using gauze, too much pressure is applied and trauma to the wound bed ensues. Only gentle pressure should be used. If more aggressive débridement is necessary, sharp débridement should be performed. Woven gauze provides mechanical débridement characteristics superior to those of nonwoven gauze (Fig. 26-6).

Lavage can be used successfully for mechanical débridement. It involves two critical components, the selection of a noncytotoxic cleansing solution and the delivery of that solution to the wound surface with appropriate pressure and volume to wash away the necrotic debris without pushing it further into the tissue planes of the wound.[9] The pressure should be between 10 and 15 pounds per square inch (psi). One way to achieve this pressure is to attach a 19-gauge needle or catheter to a 35-mL syringe.[10] Many devices are available. Showerheads are safer and more effective than single-jet lavage systems. Therefore, devices that produce high pressures (e.g., the WaterPik) should not be used. A simple, gentle, low-pressure lavage system can be made by using a 16-gauge needle to punch four to eight holes in the cap of a 1-L bottle and then squeezing saline out (Fig. 26-7, and see Fig. 26-5).

The fluids most commonly used in veterinary medicine are dilute antiseptics. However, there is no evidence that dilute antiseptics successfully kill bacteria when there is

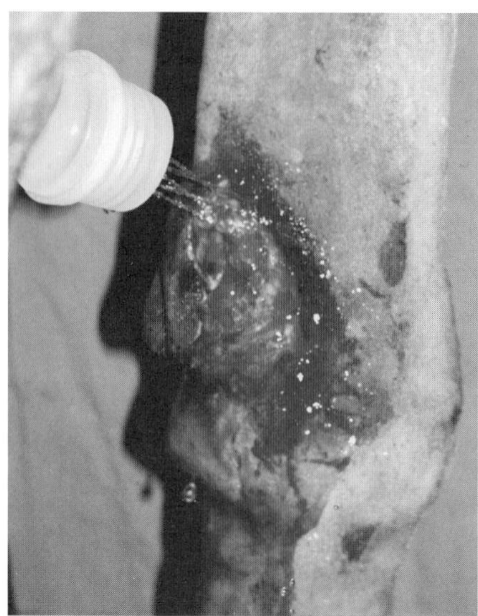

Figure 26-5. Mechanical débridement with sterile saline.

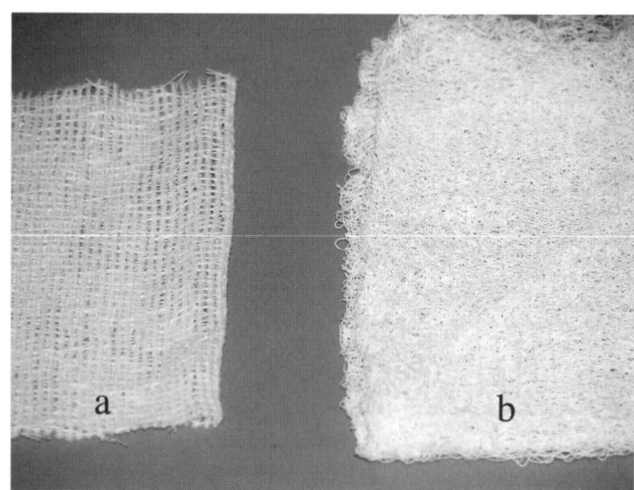

Figure 26-6. Nonwoven (*a*) and woven (*b*) gauze.

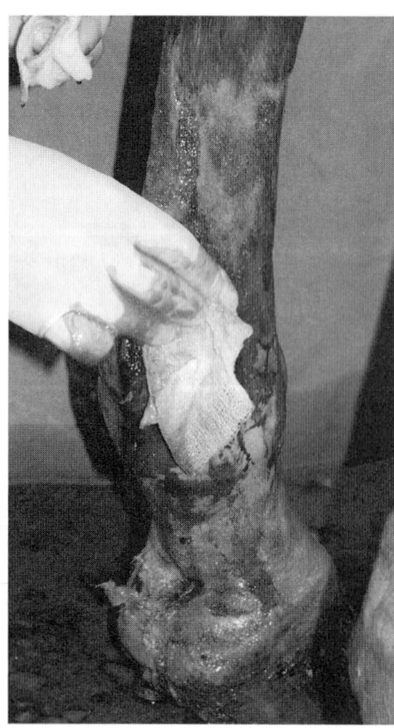

Figure 26-4. Mechanical débridement with woven gauze.

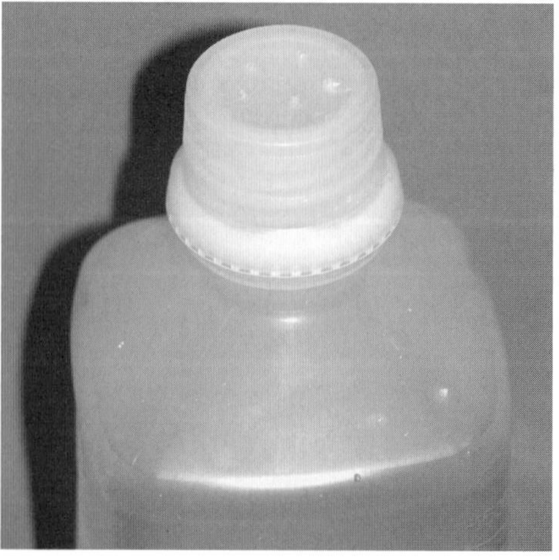

Figure 26-7. Saline bottle, with 16-gauge holes in the cap, used for lavage (see Fig. 26-5).

necrotic tissue in the wound. To achieve bacterial killing in necrotic tissue, high concentrations of antiseptic are necessary, and high concentrations have a negative effect on the cells necessary for wound healing. Antiseptics are best used around the wound, but not in the wound.[11] Saline has been shown to be effective in reducing bacterial counts in an infected wound[12] but to have no effect on wound healing in clean wounds.[13] In one study comparing saline and water in an infected wound in a rat model, saline reduced the bacterial counts by 81.6% whereas tap water reduced bacterial counts by 82%.[14] However, work by Buffa and coworkers suggests that tap water is very toxic to fibroblasts.[15] When exudate is present, surfactant-based wound cleansers are more effective than saline or polyionic fluids (Fig. 26-8).[10,16-18] In summary, the surgeon should avoid putting something in a wound that would not be tolerated in the eye[18] or should not be consumed.[16] If wound infection is present, sharp débridement together with systemic antibiotics is necessary to rid the host of bacteria. Local antibiotics, either by intravenous perfusion or topical, can also be helpful.

Wet-to-wet or wet-to-dry dressings can be used for mechanical débridement. Wet-to-wet dressings are intended to stay wet, whereas the wet-to-dry dressings are intentionally designed to dry out between bandage changes. Wet-to-wet dressing may have to be remoistened up to six times a day. These dressings are much more effective at removing necrotic tissue than is mechanical débridement using gauze, and the fibroblasts and epithelial cells suffer less damage. However, it is very time consuming and is generally available only in an intensive care hospital environment. Wet-to-dry dressings are performed by moistening the primary dressing (the dressing against the wound bed) with saline while leaving the rest of the dressings dry. The concept is that the absorbent secondary dressing will pull the fluid from the primary dressing, pulling the wound exudate into the primary dressing also. Because it is difficult to keep the primary dressing moist unless a large amount of exudate is produced by the wound, the primary dressing often becomes dry between bandage changes. When the dried primary dressing is removed, it effectively débrides the wound bed, and this débridement is very nonselective. Thus the usefulness of a wet-to-dry bandage is questionable. Primary dressings should never be allowed to become dry, as this reduces the effectiveness of autolytic débridement (see later) and leads to indiscriminate removal of epithelial cells and fibroblasts.

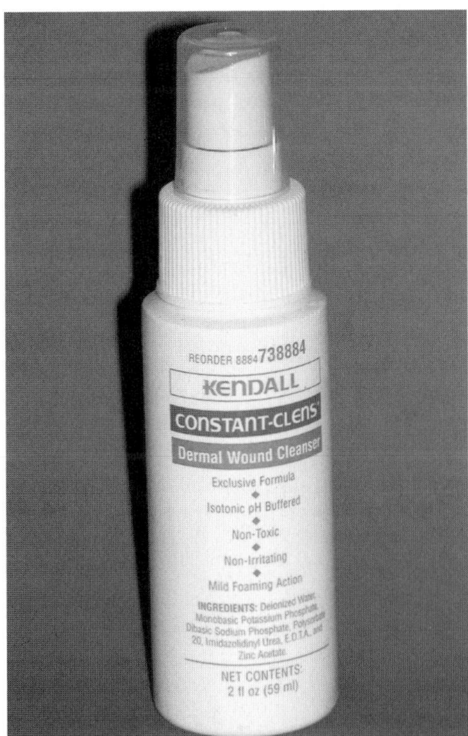

Figure 26-8. Constant-Clens (Kendall/Tyco Healthcare), a surfactant-based wound cleanser.

Chemical and Enzymatic Débridement

Chemical débridement has been used in many different forms in medicine. Dakin's solution, a diluted sodium hypochlorite (bleach) solution, was originally used during World War I. Other chemical agents are hydrogen peroxide, acetic acid, and, more recently, hypertonic saline. Chemical débridement is nonselective and should be reserved for very contaminated wounds. However, although hypertonic saline is good in selected cases, sharp débridement is probably a better technique for removing large amounts of necrotic debris. Hypertonic dressings provide an effective chemical débridement with minimal damage to the wound in the early stages of wound healing (see "Second-Intention Healing," later).

Enzymatic débridement involves placing enzymes directly onto the wound bed. The most commonly used enzymes are streptokinase/streptodornase, collagenase, DNase/fibrinolysin, papain/urea, and trypsin. Enzymatic débridement is limited when large amounts of necrotic tissue have to be removed and should be used only after an initial sharp débridement.

Autolytic Débridement

Autolytic débridement is the least traumatic of these techniques. It is achieved by leaving wound fluid (containing white blood cells and enzymes released from dead white blood cells) in contact with the wound bed. The white blood cells and enzymes affect only the dead and necrotic tissue, leaving healthy cells intact for wound healing. This can occur only in moist wounds (Fig. 26-9). When wounds are allowed to dry, autolytic débridement is slowed significantly. Autolytic débridement reduces the bacterial count by allowing access of white blood cells to the wound bed without causing continued trauma to the wound bed. However, sharp débridement should be performed before using autolytic débridement, as the latter technique is ineffective in the presence of large volumes of necrotic material.

OPTIONS FOR WOUND CLOSURE

The options for wound closure can generally be categorized as *primary closure, delayed primary closure,* and *second-intention healing.* To choose the most appropriate technique, the stages and classification of wounds must be understood.

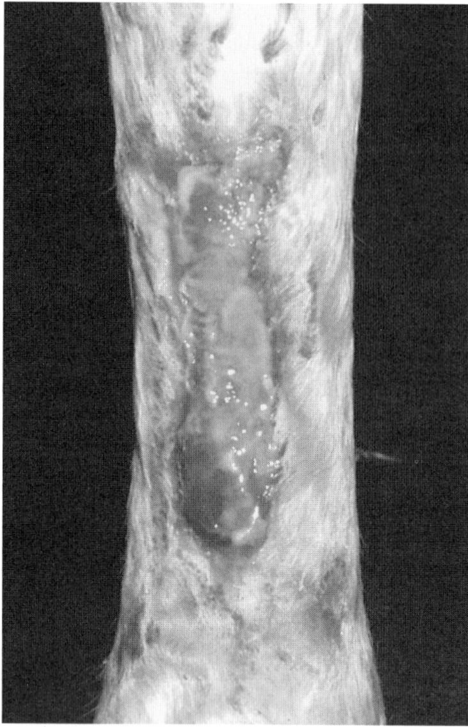

Figure 26-9. Wound undergoing autolytic débridement. This is a normal amount of exudate between bandage changes.

Stages of Wound Healing

There are four stages of wound healing: the inflammatory/cellular reaction stage, the débridement stage, the tissue formation/proliferation stage, and the maturation/remodeling stage. However, these stages overlap during the wound healing process (see Chapter 5). The duration and intensity of the *inflammatory stage* are generally determined by the extent of injury. For example, a surgical wound has a much shorter inflammatory stage than a severe degloving wound. The inflammatory stage is prolonged in the presence of necrotic debris, foreign material, or infection. The inflammatory stage should be reduced to the shortest amount of time possible. Extension of the inflammatory stage results in a delayed repair process.[8]

The *débridement stage* begins early in the inflammatory stage and is marked by migration of neutrophils and macrophages into the wound site. The white blood cells phagocytize bacteria and enzymatically remove necrotic tissue. The length of this stage depends on the size of the wound and the amount of necrotic debris present.

The *tissue formation (or proliferation) stage* involves fibroblast migration and proliferation as well as epithelialization of the wound. The fibroblasts migrate into the wound along the fibrin scaffold. They secrete the ground substance of the wound as well as the collagen that will eventually provide tensile strength in the wound. Granulation tissue, which is highly vascular and important in wound contraction, quickly becomes evident in a noninfected wound. Wound contraction is the process by which full-thickness skin is drawn together by specialized fibroblasts known as myofibroblasts, which are similar to smooth muscle cells. Myofibroblasts cause thinning of the surrounding skin as they pull the wound edges together. Wound contraction, which is most effective in areas with excess skin, stops when cells of the same type are brought together, or when skin tension equals the ability of the myofibroblasts to contract. Epithelialization, which is part of the repair phase of the wound and begins early in the wound healing process, can be stopped with infection, drying of the wound surface, exuberant proliferation of granulation tissue, and repeated dressing changes.

The *maturation stage* of wound healing occurs when there is an equilibrium between collagen production and collagen destruction. It is during this stage that the collagen fibers are realigned along the lines of tension, and when wound tensile strength increases. The number of fibroblasts is also reduced.

Wound Classification

Wounds are typically classified on the basis of degree of contamination. Clean wounds, usually seen only in surgical situations, are not infected and do not involve the respiratory, alimentary, or urogenital tract. Clean contaminated wounds, generally seen in surgical situations, involve the lumen of the respiratory, alimentary, or urogenital tract. Contaminated wounds are generally traumatic in nature and may have gross contamination and necrotic debris. Infected wounds generally involve large numbers of bacteria, inflammation, edema, and suppuration.[19] (For additional details on wounds, see Chapter 7.)

In summary, in the early stages of wound healing (i.e., in the inflammatory or débridement stage), wounds that are clean or clean contaminated are the best candidates for primary or delayed primary closure. Wounds that are in the later stages of healing or are contaminated or infected heal best by second intention.

BACTERIA IN WOUNDS

All wounds contain bacteria, but not all bacteria in wounds are cause for concern. Bacterial *contamination* describes the presence of bacteria in a wound without active multiplication or trauma to the host. Bacterial *colonization* indicates that the bacteria have attached to the tissue and are multiplying but are not necessarily causing trauma to the host. High numbers of bacteria in the absence of a host response may indicate an impaired immune response. Bacterial *infection* occurs when bacteria invade healthy tissue and actively multiply, overwhelming the host's immune response.[20]

Bacteriologic Assessment

One method of bacteriologic assessment used in equine practice is qualitative. Determining the types of bacteria in the wound, coupled with sensitivity testing, can guide the clinician in choosing antibiotics for treatment. The second method is quantitative. Bacterial counts greater than 10^5 per gram of tissue are generally indicative of an active infection. The number of bacteria needed to produce an active infection is reduced if foreign material (e.g., suture, necrotic debris, a foreign body) is present, if the virulence of the bacteria is high, or if host resistance is decreased. Quantitative bacteriology is rarely performed in veterinary medicine, but it should be considered when a wound is not progressing as anticipated or when a skin graft fails. Clinical observation is generally adequate for determining if a wound is infected. Signs such as discolored granulation tissue, edema in and around the wound, purulent exudate, odor, and lameness can indicate an infection. However, a wound can be infected without these overt signs. If infection is suspected, the wound should be cultured.

Technical Considerations in Contaminated Wound Closure

The three main strategies for preventing bacterial infection of wounds are effective wound cleansing and débridement (see "Débridement," earlier), appropriate use of advanced dressings and procedures for dressing changes (see "Second-Intention Healing," later), and appropriate use of topical antimicrobial agents.[9]

Antiseptic agents, in use since the 1800s, are effective against a broad range of gram-positive and gram-negative bacteria. However, they do not penetrate necrotic debris well and are unlikely to reduce bacterial populations deep in a wound bed.[10] Many researchers have looked at the use of antiseptic and antimicrobial agents in the wound.[21-27] In one study, the use of saline in combination with gauze was more effective in reducing bacterial numbers and encouraging wound healing than silver or povidone-iodine.[26] In a review, Rodeheaver noted that the following antiseptics have been used in the false hope of killing bacteria without negatively affecting the wound bed: acetic acid, alcohols, aluminum salts, boric acid, chlorhexidine, formaldehyde, gentian violet, hexachlorophene, hydrogen peroxide, hypochlorite, iodine, povidone-iodine, Merthiolate, permanganate, and silver nitrate.[10] It is clear that antiseptics should be reserved for use on the normal skin surrounding the wound, and not on the wound bed itself.

Unlike antiseptics, topical antimicrobial agents provide efficacy against bacteria within the wound bed, and, depending on the vehicle, they have minimal negative side effects on wound healing. In one study in horses with experimentally created leg wounds, silver sulfadiazine used alone without wound dressings resulted in less formation of granulation tissue than wounds covered with pressure bandages.[28] Antiseptics cannot target specific bacteria, but topical antibiotics can. However, antimicrobial resistance has rendered some antimicrobials ineffective, so the use of systemic antibiotics alone has been advocated to control the appearance of resistant organisms. In some chronic infections, the blood supply to the surface is diminished, and topical antimicrobials are required. Antimicrobials should always be selected on the basis of culture and sensitivity or on the basis of a judgment about the most likely bacteria to be found in the wound. When possible, to reduce concerns about antibiotic resistance, the antimicrobial chosen for topical use should be one that is unlikely to be used systemically. Wound débridement is still the best way to reduce the bacterial count in wounds with necrotic debris, and it should be performed before either an antiseptic or a topical antimicrobial is used.

Systemic antibiotics should be used for chronic or acute wounds that have a large degree of trauma or are close to critical structures such as bones or joints. If possible, cultures and sensitivity test results should be obtained to determine an appropriate antibiotic. Triple antibiotic ointment has been shown to be one of the most effective topical antibiotics in wound healing. Nitrofurazone, at least in current vehicles, is quite toxic to wounds and cannot be recommended.

WOUND CLOSURE TECHNIQUES

After the wound has been successfully débrided, cleaned, and examined, it needs to be closed. The options are suture closure, healing by second intention, skin grafting, or some combination of these to provide a continuous epithelial surface over the wound. The type of closure technique to use depends on what caused the wound, the time from injury, the degree of contamination, the extent of the injury, and potential dead space. That there is a "golden period" of 6 hours from the wounding, after which the wound is considered to be infected, is no longer deemed correct, and it behooves the clinician to examine the wound carefully to determine which of the following techniques to use for wound closure.

Primary Closure

Primary closure is a technique whereby the wound is closed immediately and completely, using strict aseptic technique. This is the technique most likely to provide the best cosmetic result. Unfortunately, primary closure is acceptable only in wounds with minimal tissue loss, minimal bacterial contamination, and minimal tension on the wound edges after closure.

Regardless of whether primary closure or delayed primary closure (see later) is performed, the wound needs to be cleaned and prepared for closure, because excess bacteria in the wound increase the possibility of wound dehiscence. There are many suturing techniques for wound closure (see Chapter 17) and many reviews of suture types for primary closure.[29-33] For areas of tension, complex suture patterns such as the near-far-far-near, vertical mattress, and horizontal mattress patterns provide more tension reduction than simple patterns such as a simple interrupted or simple continuous pattern (see Chapters 17 and 24). The near-far-far-near suture pattern (see Fig. 24-4) is most satisfactory, as it provides apposition of the skin edge at the same time as tension relief. Additionally, the mattress patterns can be used with stents to reduce pull-through at the skin–suture interface. A large-diameter suture material should be used if tension exists. Small-diameter suture can be used between tension-relieving sutures for tissue apposition and cosmetic purposes. The wound edges should be undermined whenever possible, preserving blood supply, to reduce tension on the closed wound.

When closing a wound, the management of dead space is very important. Failure to obliterate dead space can lead to the development of a hematoma or a seroma, providing an excellent medium for bacterial growth. One or a combination of four techniques can be used to manage dead space in a wound: *suture, meshing, passive or active drains,* and *pressure bandages*. Each technique has benefits and risks that need to be weighed. Suture material, although very useful in wound closure, can also act as a foreign body. Excess suture use (too much suture, too large a diameter, or too many knots) can potentiate infection.[34] Consequently, the clinician should use the smallest-diameter suture material possible, use monofilament, absorbable suture material, and use only surgeon's knots (or interrupted sutures if absolutely necessary when the suture material must be buried). Good surgical technique also benefits the patient, as it reduces trauma to the wound site. If dead space cannot be managed by suture placement, meshing (see Chapter 24) or suction drains (passive or closed) should be employed (see Chapter 18). However, drains not only allow evacuation of dead space but can also act as a conduit for bacteria to enter the wound. Drains should be left in place only as long as necessary to reduce the possibility of infection. Pressure bandages can and should be used whenever possible in addition to sutures, meshing, or drains, or sometime in place of them to reduce dead space. A properly applied bandage closes dead space without adding any foreign material. However, if a bandage is too tight, the blood supply to the wound may be compromised, leading to wound failure.

Delayed Primary Closure

In a delayed primary closure, the wound is initially treated as an open wound to allow débridement and reduce bacterial contamination. Next, the wound is closed primarily. In some cases, only a portion of the wound can be completely closed (Fig. 26-10). Delayed primary closure is reserved for wounds that have mild to moderate bacterial contamination, minimal tissue loss, and minimal tension on the wound edges after closure. Drains may be placed to evacuate fluid after closure. Delayed wound closure is very useful in the management of abdominal incisions after colonic rupture in humans.[35-37] These studies showed as much as a twofold increase in incisional infection with primary closure of contaminated abdominal wounds. Delayed primary closure after 3 to 5 days did not result in an increased hospital stay.

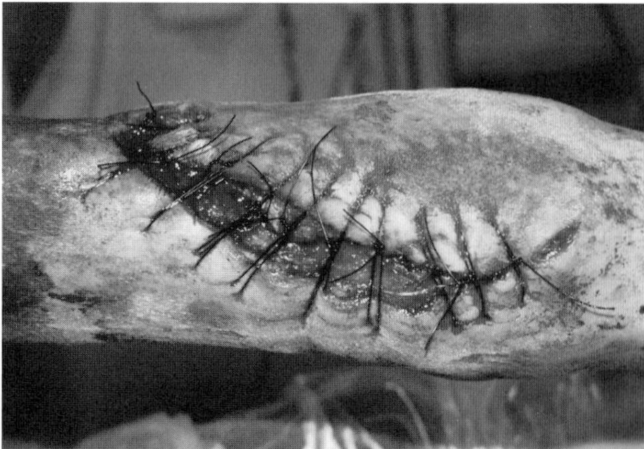

Figure 26-10. A chronic wound that has been débrided and partially closed with near-far-far-near sutures.

Wounds destined for delayed primary closure should be débrided and cleaned to reduce the bacterial burden. Hypertonic saline dressings (see "Second-Intention Healing," next), topical antimicrobials, and systemic antimicrobials can be very useful in treating wounds prior to closure.

Second-Intention Healing

Second-intention healing occurs when primary or delayed primary closure cannot be accomplished. In most cases, these wounds have gross contamination and moderate to severe tissue loss that would make closure difficult. They must heal completely through the process of contraction, granulation, and epithelialization.

A relatively new concept in wound healing is *moist wound healing*, which occurs when the wound exudate is purposefully left in contact with the wound bed. In 1962, George Winter showed that in both swine and humans, full-thickness skin wounds kept in a moist environment reepithelialized in approximately 12 to 15 days, whereas similar wounds exposed to the air took 25 to 30 days to heal.[38,39] Moist wound healing resulted in wounds that were less inflamed, caused less itching, had less eschar formation, and were more likely to heal without scarring. However, the earliest reports of moist wound healing were by Bloom and Bull in the mid 1940s. Bloom, an army surgeon, sterilized cellophane to treat burn wounds at a World War II prisoner of war camp. His primary goal was to reduce the risk of bacteria entering the wound. Although the dressing reduced bacterial infection, unanticipated benefits included movement with less pain, and less plasma loss.[40] Bull and colleagues studied a transparent nylon that stopped bacterial and fluid penetration yet allowed wound exudate to escape from the dressing. Benefits included faster healing and fewer dressing changes.[41]

The concept behind moist wound healing is that the wound exudate provides the necessary cells, and a substrate rich in enzymes, growth factors, and chemotactic factors controls infection and provides the best environment for healing. Enzymes come from the breakdown of white blood cells and metalloproteinases. Occlusive dressings keep the wound fluid in contact with the wound bed to encourage autolytic débridement. This in turn provides a good foundation for the rest of the wound healing process. Local growth factors and cytokines (see Chapter 5) provide a stimulus for the fibroblasts, epithelial cells, and angiogenesis. Chemotactic factors stimulate more neutrophils and macrophages for continued bacterial control and débridement. A moist environment allows better migration of neutrophils and macrophages than a dry wound environment. It has also been shown that wound fluid, even without white blood cells, has some antimicrobial action.[42] Another benefit of occlusion is constant thermal regulation. Concerns with moist healing include bacterial colonization, folliculitis, and the possibility of trauma to periulcer borders. Although bacterial colonization is a concern, a wound that is not infected before occlusion is unlikely to become infected afterward. Another benefit of moist wound healing is that the reduced frequency of dressing changes means that the wound is less exposed to the environment, so it is less likely to become contaminated.

DRESSINGS, GROWTH FACTORS, AND DRUGS

The wound changes as it heals, and different dressings provide better results when used during specific stages of the healing process.[43] Consequently, dressing manufacturers have developed many different dressings. Under the following headings, some of the more common dressings are described, and the wounds for which they are best used are mentioned. The ideal dressing keeps the wound bed moist, but not overly so, and the surrounding skin dry. The clinician needs to learn how to manage the amount of exudate present while making sure the wound does not dry out. Experience will quickly guide the use of the different dressing types. The dressings are described in the order a surgeon might use them when treating a wound.[44]

Hypertonic Saline Dressing

Most wounds have necrotic tissue and need débridement. Hypertonic saline dressings (Curasalt, 20% hypertonic saline on a Kerlix gauze, Tyco Healthcare/Kendall) have been designed for use on necrotic or heavily exuding wounds. They work by osmotic action to remove necrotic tissue and bacteria (Fig. 26-11). They provide a nonselective chemical débridement and consequently need to be monitored carefully. Dressings need to be changed every 24 to 48 hours at the beginning of the treatment period to maintain the hypertonicity and thus the effectiveness. These dressings can be used effectively in most abscess situations. This dressing is available in a 6×6-inch loosely woven gauze with a 6-mm (¼-inch) cotton tape for packing small draining tracts. After the necrotic tissue or bacterial infection has been removed, another dressing type should be used.

Antimicrobial Dressings

Antimicrobial dressings have been designed to stop bacterial penetration. The agents are very effective against bacteria and minimally traumatic to the wound. I use a dressing called Kerlix AMD (Tyco Healthcare/Kendall) (Fig. 26-12). The active agent is polyhexamethylene biguanide (PHMB), and it is available bound to Kerlix Super Sponge, Kerlix roll gauze, and other types of dressings. PHMB belongs to a class of cationic surface-active agents that have been used as preservatives in aqueous solutions and as disinfectants and antiseptics (e.g., in cosmetics, contact lens solutions, baby wipes, and pool sanitizers). Increased concentrations, when impregnated into fabric, have shown the ability to suppress microbial growth and penetration. Microbial death occurs by destabilization and disruption of the cytoplasmic membrane, resulting in leakage of macromolecular components. This response is irreversible, and the microbe cannot adapt or become resistant to the PHMB. These dressings are particularly useful in preventing bacterial infection in surgical incisions or where wounds are close to synovial structures and subsequent deep penetration of bacteria would be catastrophic. Although the dressings have been designed to prevent bacterial penetration, they have also been useful in reducing the bacterial load in the wound (Fig. 26-13). As these dressings are dry, and made with woven gauze, they should be premoistened before being placed in a wound. They can also be used to cover surgically closed incisions. Silver has recently been impregnated into dressings as well, and they can be used in a similar fashion. The dressings should be changed every 3 to 7 days (the shorter times when used for open wounds, and the longer times for surgically closed wounds). After the wound has been cleared of infection, the dressing should be replaced with one of the following dressings.

Hydrogels

Hydrogel dressings were designed to provide moisture in a wound that has dried out. Hydrogels are medical-grade gels composed of water, glycerin, and polymers. They conform to the wound, are nondrying, and provide a bacterial barrier and eventually a moist environment. They are available as amorphous gels, in gel-impregnated gauze, or in a mesh-reinforced pad (Fig. 26-14). They are completely occlusive and provide an excellent environment for autolytic débridement, white blood cell migration, and thermal regulation, and they thus result in improved wound healing. The gel dressing should be changed every 4 to 7 days, depending on

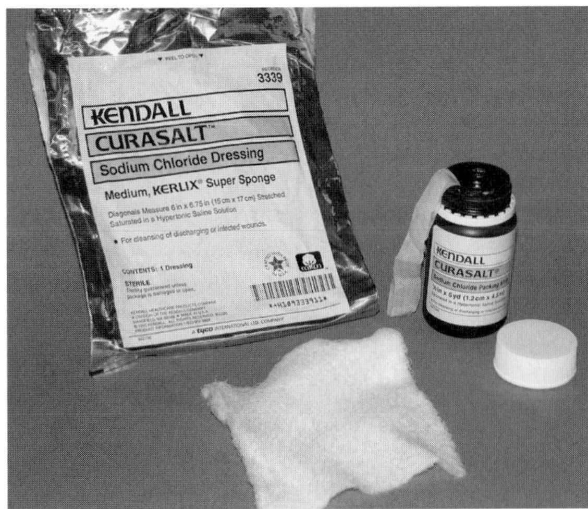

Figure 26-11. Curasalt (Kendall/Tyco Healthcare), a 20% hypertonic saline dressing, 6×6-inch woven gauze, and packing tape.

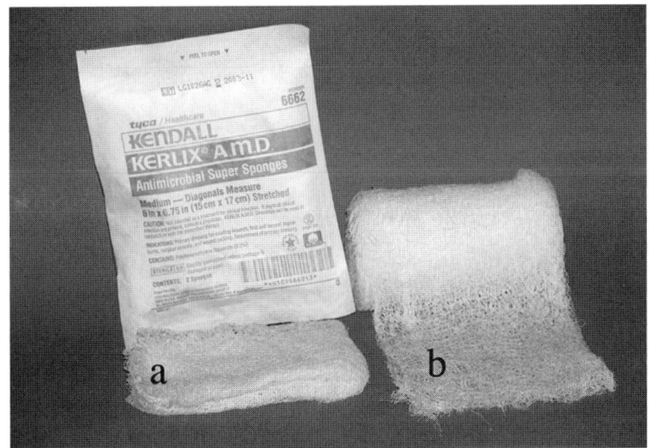

Figure 26-12. Antimicrobial dressing, 6×6-inch woven gauze (*a*), and roll gauze (*b*).

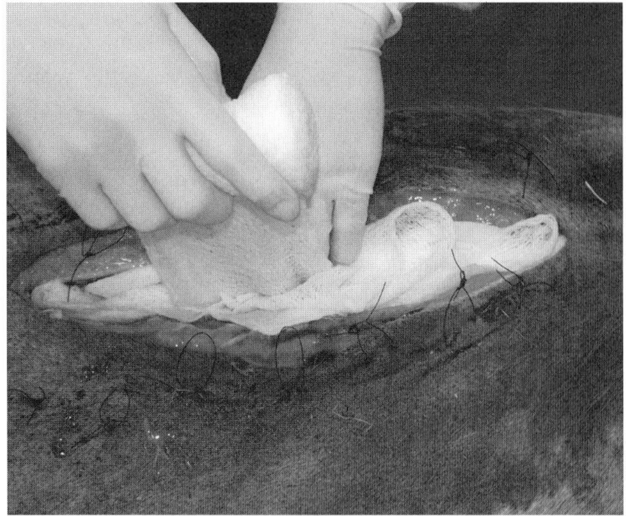

Figure 26-13. Saline-moistened Kerlix AMD antimicrobial dressing roll gauze used for chronic back wound after dorsal spinous process removal (Kendall/Tyco Healthcare).

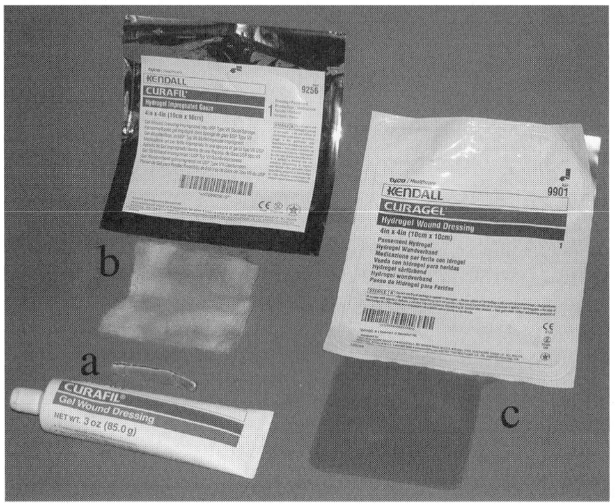

Figure 26-14. Gel dressings (Kendall/Tyco Healthcare). *a,* Curafil as an amorphous gel. *b,* Curafil as a gel-impregnated gauze dressing. *c,* Curagel, a gel pad.

the amount of exudate. Once the wound is moist, a different dressing should be used.

Calcium Alginate Dressings

Calcium alginate dressings are used primarily for the granulating phase of wound repair. They are made from alginate, a derivative of seaweed. The calcium in the dressing interacts with sodium in the wound, providing a wound exudate that stimulates myofibroblasts and epithelial cells and speeds wound homeostasis.[45] The calcium also modulates epithelial cell proliferation and migration. Alginate dressings come in nonwoven pads and rope dressings. They conform well to the wound, have excellent vertical wicking properties, and are designed for moderately to heavily exudative wounds. If a wound has a granulation tissue defect and does not have a moderate amount of exudate, the pad should be premoistened with saline before use. The dressings can be changed every 3 to 7 days, depending on the amount of exudate.

Topical Dressings: Collagens, Maltodextrins

Topical dressings such as collagens and maltodextrins are designed for use in the granulating stage of wound repair. They are both hydrophilic and should maintain a moist wound bed. They are available in powder or gel form. If the wound does not have a lot of exudate, it is probably best to use the gel form to prevent drying out of the wound bed. Maltodextrins may provide nutrition to the wound bed.[46,47] As soon as adequate granulation tissue is present, a semiocclusive foam dressing should be used.

Biologic Dressings

Various substances have been used recently as biologic dressings. These dressings are intended to provide a framework over which other cells migrate, and as a stimulant to those cells to form the tissue that is desired. Some of the more commonly used biologic dressings include porcine small intestinal submucosa (SIS), porcine bladder basement membrane, equine amnion, and various skin products. The porcine small intestinal submucosa and bladder products are not rejected by the host as other xenografts are. From clinical experience, they appear to be best if they are kept moist. In a recent study, SIS dressing was applied to fresh and chronic wounds. Compared with similar wounds treated without SIS, exuberant granulation tissue was reduced and drainage was facilitated, which reduced wound exudation and improved epithelialization. Overall, wound healing was faster and costs for bandages and hospitalization were reduced.[48] Other studies have shown that the use of equine amnion reduces wound retraction and granulation tissue formation while improving epithelialization.[49] Amnion has been shown to be beneficial as a nonadherent dressing in skin grafting.[50]

Growth Factors

Growth factors (see Chapter 5) have become very popular in experimental studies of wound care. The benefit of platelet-derived growth factor (PDGF) in decreasing wound-healing times has been shown.[51,52] It acts as a chemotactic agent and mitogen for fibroblasts, smooth muscle cells, and inflammatory cells. Other growth factors have been studied in horses to determine their effects on granulation tissue formation. In one study, it was determined that transforming growth factor-β (TGF-β) has a profibrotic function in wound healing, in that it seems to encourage formation of granulation tissue. It was also found to be more upregulated in limb wounds than in trunk wounds.[53] A human study has shown the benefit of leaving wound fluid in contact with the wound bed by stimulating fibroblast and endothelial cell growth.[54] Various cytokines have been found useful in treatment of experimentally infected wounds.[55] More studies need to be performed to look at different combinations of growth factors, used sequentially through the wound healing process to determine the true effectiveness of exogenous growth factors. The growth factors may be most useful in the granulating and epithelialization stages of wound healing and may be used in conjunction with other synthetic dressings.

Semiocclusive Foam Dressings

Semiocclusive foam dressings are designed for use on mildly exudative wounds (Fig. 26-15). They are best used after the wound has been cleaned up, necrotic debris has been removed, bacteria are brought to a count below that needed for infectivity, and healthy granulation tissue is present. The dressings should not be used in the presence of infection. Foam dressings provide a moist environment and thermal regulation that will enhance epithelialization while minimizing exuberant granulation tissue. It is best to surgically débride exuberant granulation tissue prior to application of a foam dressing. Foam dressings have also been useful as a nonadherent dressing in skin grafting. They should be changed every 4 to 7 days, depending on the amount of exudate.

Corticosteroids

Corticosteroids are commonly used in equine wound care to reduce the volume of, or to inhibit the formation of, exuberant granulation tissue. However, in vitro studies have shown that hydrocortisone upregulates plasminogen activator inhibitor-1 and downregulates plasminogen activators. The plasminogen activators play an important role in wound homeostasis. This change probably inhibits proteolytic matrix degradation and reepithelialization, which are both necessary for rapid and efficient wound repair.[56] Dexamethasone has been shown to interfere with the synthesis and degradation of types I and III collagen in rats. Type III collagen plays a major role in the induction of wound healing and is affected more dramatically by dexamethazone.[57] Triamcinolone has been shown to decrease vascular growth and consequently granulation tissue formation in rabbits. Topical administration was more severe in reducing angiogenesis than was systemic therapy. Testosterone has been shown to delay wound healing in mice.[58] Based on this information, steroids should not be used to inhibit excess granulation tissue formation. There are better ways to accomplish this, such as effective wound débridement and moist wound healing.

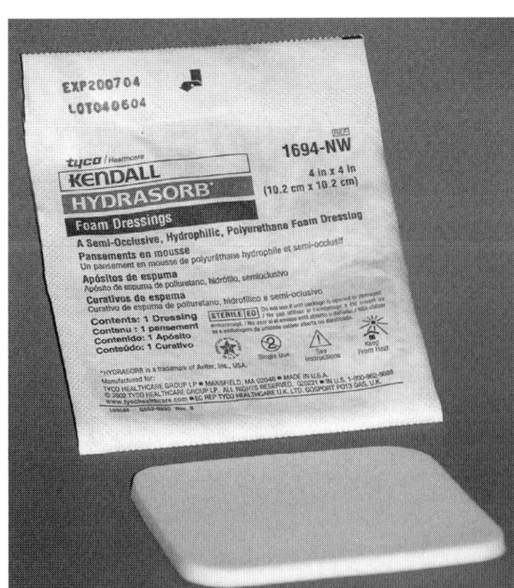

Figure 26-15. Semiocclusive foam dressing (Hydrasorb, Kendall/Tyco Healthcare).

Nonsteroidal Anti-inflammatory Agents

Inflammation is an important part of the wound healing process. However, to achieve the most cosmetic and functional results, the inflammatory stage should be minimized.[8] At therapeutic doses, studies have shown that there are few deleterious effects of using anti-inflammatory drugs during wound healing.[59,60] In time, the selectivity of new antiprostaglandin drugs may provide better efficacy without potential side effects, which will make the use of these drugs even more beneficial.

TETANUS PROPHYLAXIS

Tetanus, caused by *Clostridium tetani,* should be prevented if at all possible. Adequate protection can be achieved by vaccination, but therapy after infection is often unrewarding.[61,62] Although it has been shown that horses given an initial vaccination and a single booster should be protected for 5 years,[63,64] it is probably better to have an annual booster.[62] This is especially true in horses with an uncertain vaccination history. Unvaccinated horses should receive both a tetanus toxoid and a tetanus antitoxin.

REFERENCES

1. Dyce KM, Sack WO, Wensing CJG: The common integument. In Textbook of Veterinary Anatomy, Philadelphia, 1987, WB Saunders.
2. Montes LF, Vaughan JT: Structure and function of the skin. In Atlas of Skin Diseases of the Horse, Copenhagen, 1983, Munksgaard.
3. Talukdar AH, Calhoun ML, Stinson AW: Microscopic anatomy of the skin of the horse, Am J Vet Res 1972;33:2365.
4. Rooney JR: Hair patterns and dermal cleavage lines of the horse, J Equine Vet Sci 2000;20:238.
5. von Schouppe K: Ueber die Spaltbarkeit der Pferdekutis, Arch Wissensch Prakt Tierheilk 1913;39:112.
6. Irwin DHG: Tension lines in the skin of the dog, J Small Anim Pract 1966;7:595.
7. Phillips TJ: Initial management of equine wounds: Part II, Equine Vet Educ 1995;7:193.
8. Rodeheaver GT, Baharestani MM, Brabec ME, et al: Wound healing and wound management: Focus on debridement, Adv Wound Care 1994;7:22.
9. Ovington LG: Battling bacteria in wound care. Home Healthc Nurse 2001;19:622.
10. Rodeheaver GT: Wound cleansing, wound irrigation, wound disinfection. In Kraner D, Rodeheaver GT, Sibbald RG, editors: Chronic Wound Care: A Clinical Source Book for Healthcare Professionals, ed 3, Wayne, Pa, 2001, HM Communications.
11. Booth L: Early wound management in the horse, Equine Pract 1992;14:2.
12. Badia JM, Torres JM, Tur C, et al: Saline wound irrigation reduces the postoperative infection rate in guinea pigs, J Surg Res 1996;63:457.
13. Hollander JE, Richman PB, Werblud M, et al: Irrigation in facial and scalp lacerations: Does it alter outcome? Ann Emerg Med 1998;31:73.
14. Moscati R, Mayrose J, Fincher L, et al: Comparison of normal saline with tap water for wound irrigation, Am J Emerg Med 1998;16:379.

15. Buffa EA, Lubbe AM, Verstraete FJM, et al: The effects of wound lavage solutions on canine fibroblasts: An in vitro study, Vet Surg 1997;26:460.
16. McEwan C: Wound cleansing and dressing, Am J Clin Dermatol 2000;1:57.
17. Witkowski JA, Parish LC: Wound cleansers, Clin Dermatol 1996;14:89.
18. Brown CD, Zitelli JA: A review of topical agents for wounds and methods of wounding, J Dermatol Surg Oncol 1993;19:732.
19. Lindsay W: Wound healing in horses: Guidelines for classification, Vet Med Equine Pract 1988;83:387.
20. Dow G: Infection in chronic wounds. In Kraner D, Rodeheaver GT, Sibbald RG, editors: Chronic Wound Care: A Clinical Source Book for Healthcare Professionals, ed 3, Wayne, Pa, 2001, HM Communications.
21. Booth JH, Benrimoj SI, Nimmo GR: In vitro interactions of neomycin sulfate, bacitracin, and polymyxin B sulfate, Int J Dermatol 1994;33:517.
22. Boyce ST, Warden GD, Holder IA: Cytotoxicity testing of topical antimicrobial agents on human keratinocytes and fibroblasts for cultured skin grafts, J Burn Care Rehabil 1995;16:97.
23. Geronemus RG, Mertz PM, Eaglestein WH: Wound healing: The effects of topical antimicrobial agents, Arch Dermatol 1979; 115:1311.
24. Hansbrough JF, Achauer B, Dawson J, et al: Wound healing in partial thickness burn wounds treated with collagenase ointment versus silver sulfadiazine cream, J Burn Care Rehabil 1995;16:241.
25. Kjolseth D, Frank JM, Barker JH, et al: Comparison of the effects of commonly used wound agents on epithelialization and neovascularization, J Am Coll Surg 1994;179:305.
25. Kucan JO, Robson MC, Heggers JP, et al: Comparison of sliver sulfadiazine, povidone-iodine, and physiologic saline in the treatment of chronic pressure ulcers, J Am Geriatr Soc 1981;29:232.
27. Swaim SF: Bandages and topical agents, Vet Clin North Am Small Anim Pract 1990;20:47.
28. Berry DB, Sullins KE: Effects of topical application of antimicrobials and bandaging on healing and granulation tissue formation in wounds of the distal aspect of the limbs in horses, Am J Vet Res 2003;64:88.
29. Johnston DE: Tension-relieving techniques, Vet Clin North Am Small Anim Pract 1990;20:67.
30. Bailey JV: Repair of large skin defects on the limbs of horses, Wien Tierarztl Mschr 1991;78:277.
31. Gusman D: Wound closure and special suture techniques, J Am Podiatr Med Assoc 1995;85:2.
32. Chaudhry HR, Bukiet B, Siegel M, et al: Optimal patterns for suturing wounds, J Biomech 1998;31:653.
33. Lott-Crumpler DA, Chaudhry HR: Optimal patterns for suturing wounds of complex shapes to foster healing, J Biomech 2001;34:51.
34. DeHoll D, Rodeheaver G, Edgerton MT, et al: Potentiation of infection by suture closure of dead space, Am J Surg 1974;127:716.
35. Velmahos GC, Vassiliu P, Demetriades D, et al: Wound management after colon injury: Open or closed? A prospective randomized trial, Am Surg 2002;68:795.
36. Cohn SM, Giannotti G, Ong AW, et al: Prospective randomized trial of two wound management strategies for dirty abdominal wounds, Ann Surg 2001;233:409.
37. Bender JS: Factors influencing outcome in delayed primary closure of contaminated abdominal wounds: A prospective analysis of 181 consecutive patients, Am Surg 2003;69:252.
38. Winter GD: Formation of the scab and the rate of epithelization of superficial wounds in the skin of the young domestic pig, Nature 1962;193:293.
39. Winter GD: Effect of air exposure and occlusion on experimental human skin wounds, Nature 1963;200:378.
40. Bloom H: Cellophane dressing for second degree burns, Lancet 1945;2:559.
41. Bull JP, Squire JR, Topley E: Experiments with occlusive dressings of a new plastic, Lancet 1948;2:213.
42. Hohn DC, Granelli SG, Burton RW, et al: Antimicrobial systems of the surgical wound: II. Detection of antimicrobial protein in cell free wound fluid, Am J Surg 1977;113:601.
43. Reiter D: Methods and materials for wound management, Otolaryngol Head Neck Surg 1994;110:550.
44. Hendrickson DA: Second intention healing. In Hendrickson DA, editor: Wound Care for the Equine Practitioner Made Easy Series, Jackson Hole, Wyo, 2004, Teton New Media.
45. Lansdown ABG: Calcium: A potential central regulator in wound healing in the skin, Wound Rep Reg 2002;10:271.
46. Purna Sai K, Babu M: Collagen based dressings: A review, Burns 2000;26:54.
47. Swaim SF, Gillette RL, Sartin EA, et al: Effects of a hydrolyzed collagen dressing on the healing of open wounds in dogs, Am J Vet Res 2000;61:1574.
48. Dressel C, Fürst A, Imhof A, et al: Einsatz von Small Intestine Submucosa (SIS) zur Wiundversorgung bei 11 Pferden: Erste Erfahrungen. Wien Tieraerztl Mschr 2004;91:142.
49. Bigbie RB, Schumacher J, Swaim SF, et al: Effects of amnion and live yeast cell derivative on second-intention healing in horses, Am J Vet Res 1991;52:1376.
50. Goodrich LR, Moll HD, Crisman MV, et al: Comparison of equine amnion and a nonadherent wound dressing material for bandaging pinch-grafted wounds in ponies, Am J Vet Res 2000;61:326.
51. Carter CA, Jolly DG, Worden CE, et al: Platelet-rich plasma gel promotes differentiation and regeneration during equine wound healing, Exp Mol Pathol 2003;74:244.
52. Cohen MA, Eaglstein WH: Recombinant human platelet-derived growth factor gel speeds healing of acute full-thickness punch biopsy wounds, J Am Acad Dermatol 2001;45:857.
53. Theoret CL, Barber SM, Moyana TN, et al: Expression of transforming growth factor beta (1), beta (3), basic fibroblast growth factor in full-thickness skin wounds of equine limbs and thorax, Vet Surg 2001;30:269.
54. Katz MH, Alvarez AF, Dirsner RS, et al: Human wound fluid from acute wounds stimulates fibroblast and endothelial cell growth, J Am Acad Dermatol 1991;25:1054.
55. Kovalchuk LV, Gankovskaya LV, Chadaev AP, et al: Cytokine therapy of experimental purulent wounds, Bull Exp Biol Med 1997; 123:590..
56. Hashimoto I, Nakanishi H, Shono Y, et al: Angiostatic effects of corticosteroid on wound healing of the rabbit ear, J Med Invest 2002;49:61.
57. Oishi Y, Fu ZW, Ohnuki Y, et al: Molecular basis of the alteration in skin collagen metabolism in response to in-vivo dexamethasone treatment: Effects on the synthesis of collagen type I and III, collagenase, and tissue inhibitors of metalloproteinases, Br J Dermatol 2002;147:859.
58. Ashcroft GS, Mills SJ: Androgen receptor-mediated inhibition of cutaneous wound healing, J Clin Invest 2002;110:615.
59. Donner GS, Ellison GW, Pwyton LC, et al: Effect of flunixin meglumine on surgical wound strength and healing in the rat, Am J Vet Res 1986;47:2247.
60. Gorman HA, Wolff WA, Frost WW, et al: Effect of oxyphenbutazone on surgical wounds of horses, J Am Vet Med Assoc 1968;152:487.
61. Blood DC, Radostits OM: Veterinary medicine: A textbook of diseases of cattle, sheep, pigs, goats, and horses, ed 7, London, 1989, Bailliere Tindall.
62. Green SL: Equine tetanus: A review of the clinical features and current perspectives on treatment and prophylaxis, Proc Am Assoc Equine Pract 1992;38:299.
63. Liefman CE: Active immunization of horses against tetanus including the booster dose and its application, Aust Vet J 1981;57:57.
64. Scarnell J: Recall of immunity in horses previously immunized with an aluminum-based tetanus toxoid, Vet Rec 1974;95:62.

CHAPTER 27

Management of Deep and Chronic Wounds

Dean A. Hendrickson

DEEP WOUNDS

Wounds in different parts of the body heal at different rates and often produce disparate cosmetic results.[1,2] Wounds on the head, neck, and body often appear to heal better than wounds on the extremities. In a review on the topic, Knottenbelt discussed reduced vascularity in the extremities as a possible cause for prolonged wound healing there.[2] However, increased infection, increased inflammatory response, and reduced regional temperature are all involved in the equation as well.[3-5] The first part of this chapter is devoted to deeper wounds of the head, neck, thorax, abdomen, and extremities, and the second part discusses chronic wounds. Please see Chapters 5 and 26 for more in-depth information on specific wound healing events.

Head and Neck

The head and neck have an extensive vascular supply that provides nutrition, oxygen, and white blood cells to the wound for healing. There is good soft tissue support to most areas of the head and neck, which also provides a good basis for healing.[2,6] Unfortunately, many other important structures, such as the cranium, eyes, ears, sinuses, salivary ducts, and nares, can be involved in lacerations, and exploring them to make sure that nothing is missed requires a thorough knowledge of their anatomy. For example, one horse had hit its head on a feeder, causing a laceration in front of the ear. At the initial presentation, the wound looked very superficial, but a more thorough examination revealed that it involved the cranium and had actually penetrated into the brain (Fig. 27-1). The horse had no obvious neurologic signs indicating the puncture. Thus, a thorough and complete physical examination is necessary to adequately assess wounds to the head and neck. Often, horses with head wounds should be heavily sedated before wound preparation and exploration.

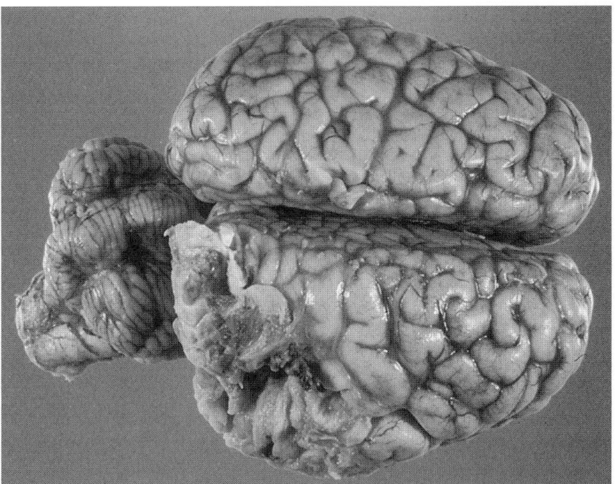

Figure 27-1. The brain of a horse with a penetrating injury to the head.

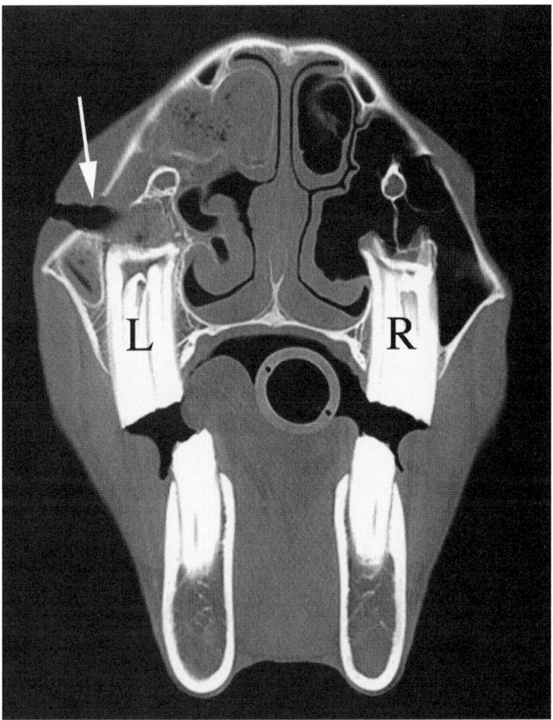

Figure 27-2. Computed tomography scan of a horse with trauma to the left maxillary sinus and subsequent filling of the sinus with blood. *Arrow,* entry wound.

Diagnostic aids for evaluating head and neck wounds include radiographs, ultrasonography, computed tomography (CT), and magnetic resonance imaging (MRI). Radiographs of the head can be difficult to evaluate because of all of the overlapping bones.[8] CT (Fig. 27-2) and MRI provide excellent renderings of abnormalities, but they are expensive and not always available. Fortunately, good wound preparation and digital examination often provide enough information about the amount of bone involvement in a head laceration. Fractures should be considered whenever there is a laceration to the head. When cranial fractures are suspected, a thorough neurologic examination should be performed to help determine the extent of the laceration. If the cranium is involved, aggressive therapy should be instituted to reduce the possibility of bacterial penetration and eventual septic encephalitis.

Lacerations around the orbit should be examined to determine involvement of the bone and the globe of the eye (see Chapter 63). To avoid trauma to the cornea, special care is needed when cleaning around the eye. Chlorhexidine should not be used in this area.[9] If possible, lacerations around the eye should be closed primarily to reduce functional problems of the lids. Lacerations to the lids should be closed using small-diameter, absorbable suture material in many layers (see Chapter 56). Multiple layers of small-diameter suture provide more stability in areas of increased motion yet will not unnecessarily add to the foreign body volume of the wound. Orbit fractures can be treated using bone reconstruction plates (Fig. 27-3).

Repair of ear lacerations can be particularly difficult because ears have considerable mobility. Their range of motion is nearly 270 degrees, and they are supported by cartilage. Ear lacerations, like eyelid lacerations, should be closed primarily whenever possible for the best cosmetic and functional results. Because of the location and blood supply of the ear, lacerations there are rarely too contaminated to close primarily, but sometimes the wounds are too old to hold suture and must heal by second intention, with revision at a later date. General anesthesia should be used to repair ear lacerations for the best cosmetic result. Rolled gauze or radiographic film can be used as a support to minimize ear movement and improve healing.

Lacerations that involve the frontal and maxillary sinuses may lead to bone sequestration and eventual fistula formation.[10] Prompt intervention can make the difference between a wound that can be closed primarily and one that requires multiple surgeries and wound revisions. Stable bone fragments should be elevated back into position, whereas loose fragments devoid of periosteal coverage should be removed. Rotational skin and periosteal flaps may be necessary to close defects in this area. If there is a large bone defect, the addition of a periosteal flap may improve the possibility of bone formation in the area. Other dressings, such as ACell (ACell, Inc, Jessup, Md), have been suggested for use in this type of wound to encourage bone formation.

Mandibular lacerations can involve other structures such as the salivary ducts or even the mandibular incisors. Depending on the cause of the laceration, evaluation of the ducts can be very difficult, especially if extensive trauma has occurred. When possible, the integrity of the duct should be confirmed by feeding the horse and observing salivary fluid loss. If transected ends of the parotid salivary duct can be visualized and anastomosed, the result will be better, but this is rarely achievable. If the ends cannot be anastomosed, the salivary gland may have to be chemically ablated.

Lacerations of the nares are common in equine practice. Successful reconstruction depends on thorough wound débridement, good case selection, and using multiple layers of suture closure to reduce the chance of incisional dehiscence. Fresh wounds are easiest to treat if there is not a large volume of tissue missing. When horses present with wounds that are 7 to 20 days old, the wounds should probably be allowed to heal by second intention and reconstructed at a later date when they are more likely to hold sutures. In all cases of nares lacerations, multiple layers of closure are necessary for a successful closure.[10]

Thorax

Lacerations of the thorax can involve the ribs, which can penetrate the pleural cavity and cause a pneumothorax. Consequently, the wounds must be carefully examined to be absolutely certain of the depth of penetration. The area should be clipped and aseptically prepared to allow a thorough examination of the site (see Chapter 26) Aseptic technique should be used for all thoracic wounds, as involvement of the pleura cannot be ruled out until after the manual examination. If the examination area is quiet, the surgeon may be able to hear air being sucked into the wound during inspiration. Thoracic auscultation should also be performed to help rule out pneumothorax. Radiographs and ultrasonography can be helpful adjuncts to the examination (Fig. 27-4). If the wound has entered the pleural cavity, a chest tube should be placed to evacuate the air from the chest (see Chapter 18). If the surgeon cannot place a chest tube, the wound should be closed in as many layers as possible, bandaged, and then referred (see Chapters 8 and 47). As an alternative to a chest tube, a teat cannula can be attached to a 60-mL syringe with a three-way stopcock to remove air from the chest cavity. With time, it is

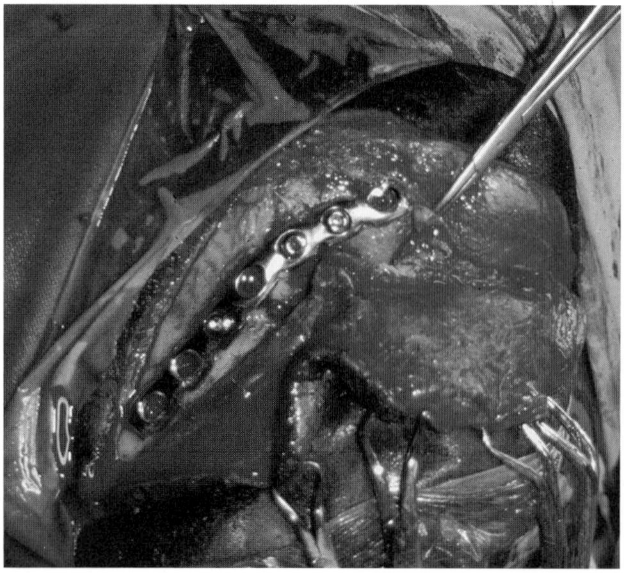

Figure 27-3. Intraoperative photograph of a horse with an orbital fracture repaired with a reconstruction plate.

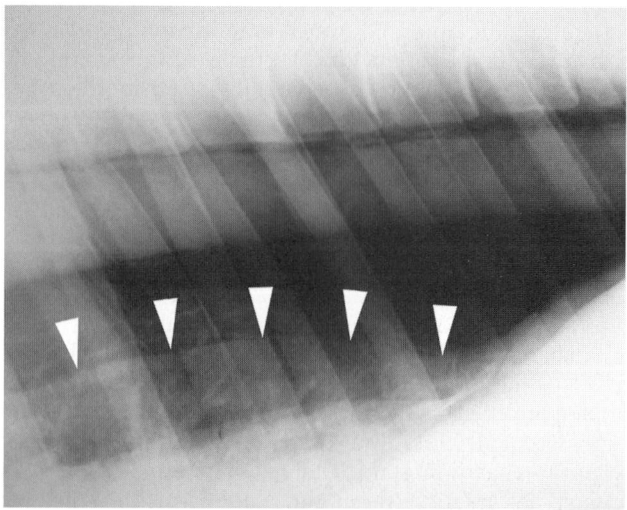

Figure 27-4. Lateral radiographic view of a horse with a thoracic injury and subsequent pneumothorax. Note the dorsal edge of lung outlined by *arrows*.

possible to evacuate most of the air from the pleural cavity with this technique, but a suction pump is more efficient. The chest tube or the teat cannula should be placed in the upper third of the chest to enable removal of the largest volume of air. When there is pleural penetration, broad-spectrum antibiotics should be instituted. The wound care instituted should be appropriate for the stage of healing. Stent bandages can be used to cover the primary dressing.

Abdomen

Lacerations to the abdominal wall offer a diagnostic challenge. The abdominal wall has numerous layers that vary depending on the location. The hair should be clipped, and aseptic technique should always be used on abdominal wounds until peritoneal penetration has been ruled out. If the entry point is small, it may be useful to enlarge the wound to better explore the deeper layers, and the horse may have to be sedated to allow thorough examination. The skin is generally more resistant to tearing than the fascial planes and muscles of the abdominal wall. All tissue planes should be examined for involvement. It is possible for the tissue planes to move, allowing overlap of the layers. An abdominocentesis may help, but in many cases, the cell counts and total protein are not abnormal. Confirmation of abdominal penetration may not be possible, so the veterinarian must carefully monitor the patient for signs of peritonitis after the wounding.

If the wound does not involve the peritoneal space, it should be débrided and closed in multiple layers if at all possible. A drain may be helpful in evacuating dead space. Wounds that have a large amount of tissue loss may be predisposed to herniation. However, it is not advisable to place a mesh in a contaminated wound. Therefore, the wound should be treated until healed, and then a mesh can be placed to reduce the chance of hernia formation. Abdominal bandages can be useful to help support the body wall. The need for abdominal support may be minimal, but the bandage often reduces edema formation at the wound site and encourages more rapid wound healing. Broad-spectrum antibiotics are often indicated in abdominal wounds.

If peritoneal penetration has occurred, an abdominal bandage should be placed on the animal for transport to a surgical facility for an abdominal exploration. Whenever peritoneal penetration has occurred, it is possible that there has been trauma to the viscera. Abdominal lavage using copious amounts of polyionic fluid should be performed, and broad-spectrum antibiotics should be instituted.

Extremities

Axillary Lacerations

Horses that present with lacerations of the axillary region often have subcutaneous emphysema (Fig. 27-5). The emphysema is created when the horse moves its leg forward,

A

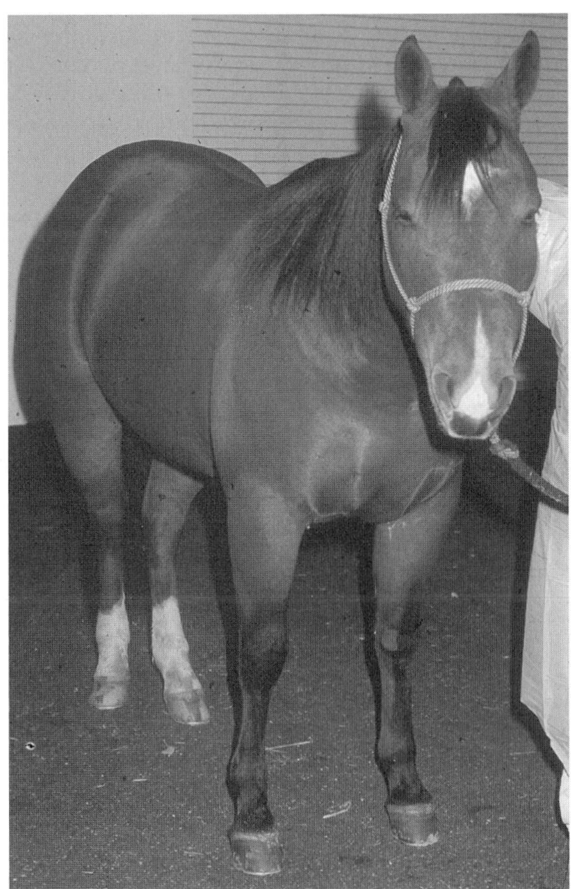

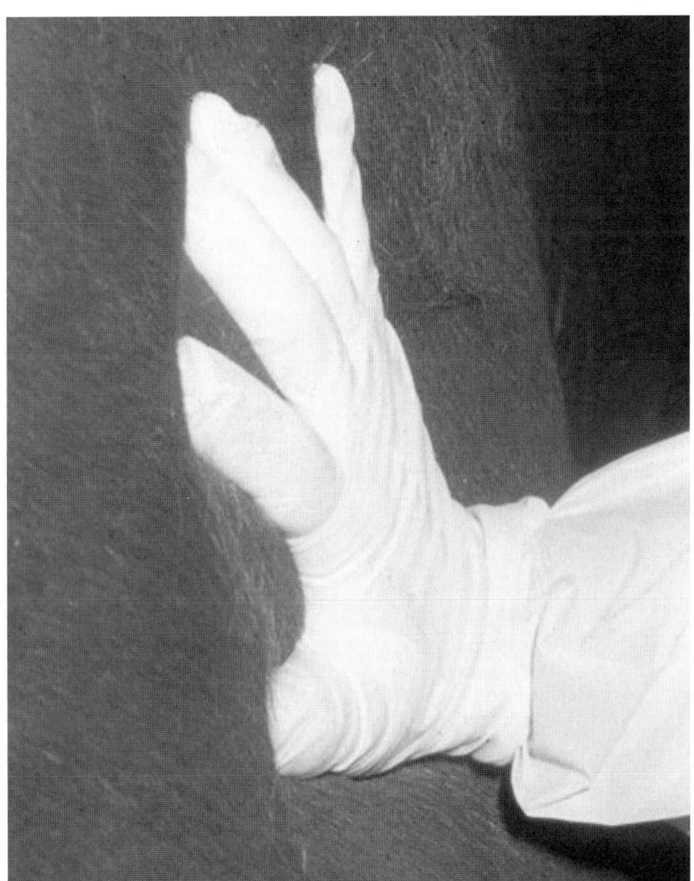

B

Figure 27-5. A, A horse with an axillary wound and subsequent subcutaneous emphysema. **B,** Close-up showing digital indentation over the shoulder.

opening the wound and filling it with air. When the horse moves forward and the leg becomes caudal relative to its forward position, the air is trapped and forced into the surrounding tissues. In some cases, a pneumomediastinum occurs, which can lead to a pneumothorax.[11] The hair over these wounds should be clipped, and they should be cleaned and débrided. Packing the wound is difficult, but it reduces the accumulation of air. The best way to reduce subcutaneous air accumulation is to limit the movement of the horse. Once the air has accumulated, it must be reabsorbed, and there is no efficient way to remove it. Calcium alginate dressings may encourage formation of granulation tissue, speeding the sealing of the wound.

Lacerations Involving Synovial Structures

Lacerations into synovial structures must be identified and aggressively treated as early as possible. The veterinarian must know the locations of the synovial structures—repeated and thorough reviews of equine anatomy are helpful. Whenever a laceration occurs that is close to one of these structures, synovial involvement must be determined. The best way to confirm the involvement of a synovial structure is to place a needle into the structure at a site distant from the wound and distend the structure with sterile saline (Fig. 27-6). Strict aseptic technique is a prerequisite for this injection. If the wound involves a synovial structure, aggressive therapy, including lavage, intravenous antibiotics, local perfusion, and effective wound dressings, should be performed (see Chapters 8 and 88).

Heel Bulb Lacerations

Lacerations to the heel bulb area are common in equine practice and can involve anything from the skin to the coffin joint, so the structures involved must be identified. Synovial involvement of either the digital flexor tendon sheath or the coffin joint should be ruled out before treatment. If there is no synovial involvement, heel bulb lacerations are often best repaired using delayed primary closure. Because the foot is in contact with the ground, most heel bulb lacerations are very contaminated. Effective wound preparation, débridement, and treatment are critical (see Chapter 26). After the wound is cleaned, it can be sutured and a slipper cast applied.[11] The slipper cast reduces movement in the area and allows much more rapid and cosmetic healing (Fig. 27-7). Additional information of the management of heel bulb wounds is found in Chapter 93.

CHRONIC WOUNDS

Chronic wound care can be challenging and demanding. In human medicine, "a chronic wound is a window to underlying disease. Each wound is a symptom of underlying infirmities that undermine the potential for healing."[12] The local wound environment is part of the larger milieu of the body, and chronic, nonhealing wounds can indicate a larger problem in the macroenvironment of the body.[13] Consequently, it is critical to examine the entire animal when a nonhealing or chronic wound is present. Chronic wounds in both people and horses are commonly found on the extremities. In people, they are often secondary to chronic metabolic diseases, whereas horses often have some type of underlying infection.

Much work has been done on the local wound environment of nonhealing wounds in humans. Studies have shown that wound fluid found in chronic wounds inhibits the growth of fibroblasts by affecting the cell cycle.[14,15] The negative effect of the wound fluid can be reversed by high temperatures. Tumor necrosis factor-α (TNF-α) may play a

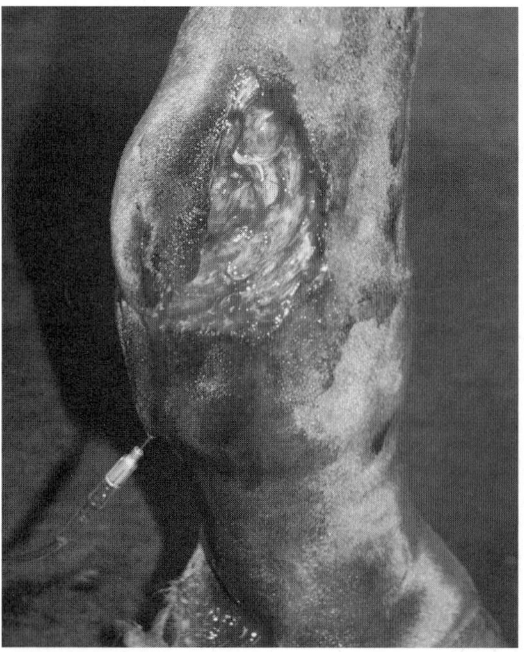

Figure 27-6. The digital tendon sheath is filled with sterile saline solution to determine if communication exists with the laceration on the lateral aspect of the fetlock region.

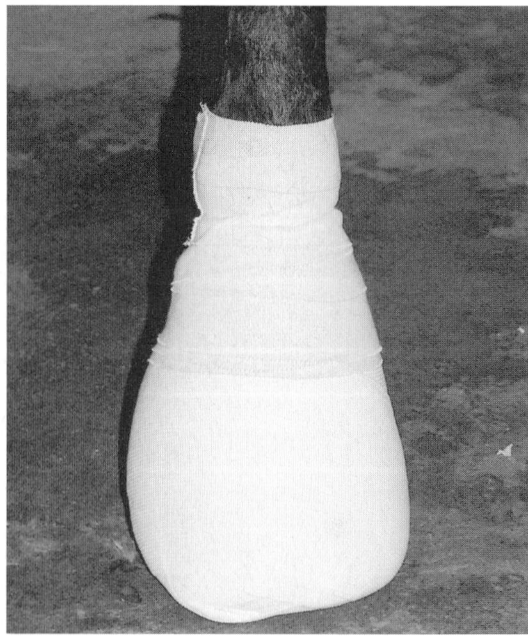

Figure 27-7. A horse in a slipper cast after reconstruction of a coronary band laceration.

role in the reduction of fibroblast growth rates, whereas interleukin-1β (IL-1β) and transforming growth factor-β1 ($TGF\text{-}\beta_1$) did not significantly affect growth rates.[15] Other studies have shown an increase in fibroblast proliferation when these cells are exposed to wound fluid from chronic wounds.[16] Differences in experimental conditions may have caused the difference in results, which underscores the importance of further research into the effects of chronic wound fluid.

Another difference in wound fluid obtained from acute versus chronic wounds is in proteolytic activity. In acute wound fluids, the plasminogen activator system is active, and in chronic wound fluids, the urokinase-type plasminogen activator and urokinase-type plasminogen activator receptors are active.[17] Different proteins are expressed at different levels during the wound healing process. Heat shock protein, platelet-derived growth factor (PDGF), fibroblast growth factor (FGF), vascular endothelial growth factor (VEGF), and their receptors were increased in the wound within 24 hours of skin injury. The levels declined to normal levels by day 7 to day 14, coinciding with healing. The expression of these factors in chronic wounds was delayed or inhibited, suggesting that addition of these agents might improve wound healing in chronic wounds.[18]

Sarcoids are the most common cutaneous tumor in the horse. It is not uncommon for sarcoids to occur at the location of previous wounds.[19] A study designed to look at the response of cells—isolated from sarcoids, granulation tissue, and normal dermal fibroblasts grown from primary cell cultures—to growth factors showed different morphologic features for each cell type. Sarcoid-derived and granulation tissue–derived cells grew more slowly than the normal dermal cells. When growth factors (epidermal growth factor, acidic fibroblast growth factor, and basic fibroblast growth factor) were added, the sarcoid-derived cells and normal cells were stimulated, but the granulation tissue–derived cells were inhibited. However, when TGF-β was added, the granulation tissue–derived cells were not preferentially inhibited.[20] Continued research in wound healing should help to identify ways to change chronic wounds to acute wounds, thereby improving the healing response.

Chronic wounds often heal with a poor functional and cosmetic result. For the most functional and cosmetic healing, the best environment for wound healing should be provided early. The best way to treat a chronic wound is to not allow the wound to become chronic in the first place. As this is not always possible, the surgeon is required to treat horses with chronic, nonhealing wounds.

As with an acute wound, the first step in treating a chronic wound is to prepare the wound for examination (see Chapter 26). The examination generally starts with digital exploration. The wound should be explored for pieces of foreign material (e.g., bone, wood, metal, suture material). In some cases, draining tracts are found that guide the exploration (see Chapter 28). In others, the foreign material is walled off and difficult to palpate. In those cases, ancillary methods such as radiology, ultrasonography, CT, or MRI can be useful. Radiographs are best for bone and other radiodense objects. Ultrasonography can be very useful for radiolucent objects such as wood. CT and MRI may be very useful but are often cost prohibitive.

Infection should be suspected whenever a wound does not heal in the anticipated timeframe. In a review of wound infection, Dow identified studies that show the effect of chronic wound infection on wound healing.[21] He also identified the best ways to diagnose wound infection, the most common being by the clinical appearance of the wound. Inflammation, edematous granulation tissue, discolored granulation tissue, draining tracts in the granulation tissue, and odor are clinical signs that should increase suspicion of infection (Fig. 27-8).

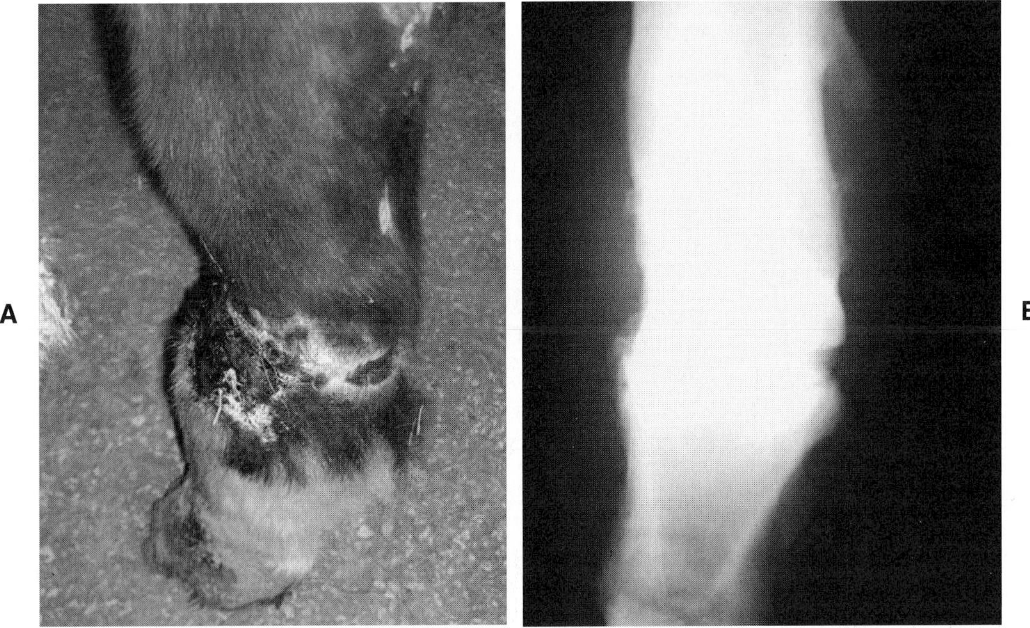

Figure 27-8. A, A chronic wound near the fetlock. **B,** Radiographic evidence of osteomyelitis and new bone production.

A second (and the absolute) way to determine infection in a wound is by bacterial culture. However, all wounds contain bacteria. A wound with a bacterial burden of 10^5 or 10^6 bacteria per gram of tissue is generally considered to be infected.[21] Quantitative bacteriology involves submitting a defined amount of tissue (at least a gram) for bacterial culture and calculating the number of bacteria per gram of tissue. This is rarely done in equine medicine, but it should be considered when wound healing does not progress as expected. Qualitative culture should be done to determine the types of bacteria in the wound, and antibiotic sensitivity testing should be performed to determine the most effective antibiotic. (See Chapter 26 for information on topical antibiotics, antiseptics, and systemic antibiotic therapy.) The most important step in reducing wound infection is adequate débridement and removal of foreign material.

After examining and exploring the wound, the surgeon decides the next step in wound care. In many cases, the wound needs to be "freshened" to stimulate it to heal. Surgical débridement, commonly used to accomplish this (Fig. 27-9), can essentially turn a chronic wound into an acute wound. It generally reduces the bacterial load and removes foreign material. Surgical débridement is a vital adjunct for wound care in humans with diabetic foot ulcers,[22] and it is an important part of chronic wound therapy.[23] Any infected bone or tissue should be removed by the débridement, so that no foreign material is left behind.

As previously described, growth factors hold promise for wound healing. An understanding of the wound environment is necessary before growth factors are routinely used.[24] Purified growth factors may be useful only in combination.

After surgical débridement, wound closure may be attempted (see Chapter 26). A benefit of working with a chronic wound is that the granulation and scar tissue often stretch the skin. After the scar tissue and granulation tissue are removed, there is ample skin to close the defect. In some cases, only a portion of the wound can be closed, and the rest is allowed to heal by second intention or skin grafting (see Fig. 26-10). The skin within approximately 1 cm of the skin edge is usually not healthy enough to hold sutures, and it is often best to remove this tissue during wound débridement.

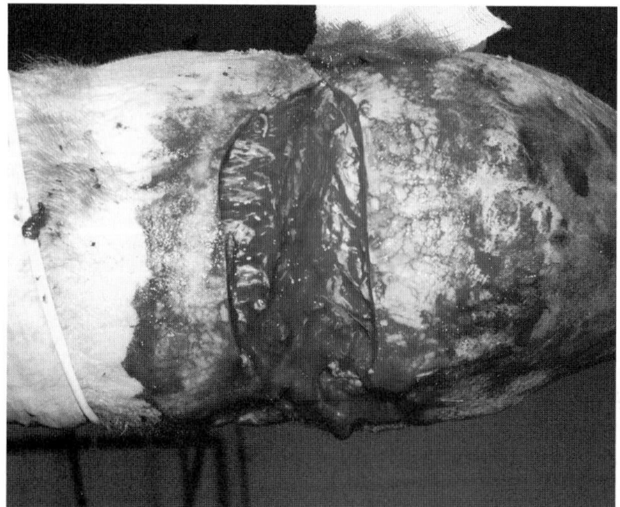

Figure 27-9. A chronic wound after débridement to encourage wound healing.

Sometimes, wounds do not respond in an anticipated fashion, and keloids or excess scar tissue results. Keloids are distinguished from hypertrophic scars in that keloids extend beyond the original wound and rarely regress.[25] The pathogenesis of keloid or hypertrophic scar formation is unknown, but it has been linked to an increased number of epidermal Langerhans' cells.[26] The epidermal immune barrier may play an important role in the development of hypertrophic scars, which have been noted to have increased blood flow in humans evaluated with laser Doppler.[27] In the normal wound healing process, the vasculature diminishes, allowing the completion of healing. Hypertrophic scars may represent an interruption in this healing process. Possibly, vasoconstrictive agents employed in the maturation stage of healing would reduce the proliferation of vasculature, which might inhibit hypertrophic scarring. In humans, there is a familial disposition to keloid formation. Steroid injection, surgical excision, radiation therapy, compression, and tension reduction have been used for treatment of keloids.[28,29] In vitro culturing of fibroblasts from keloids with the dietary compound quercetin (a flavonol) has shown some promise in inhibiting proliferation and contraction of the cells.[30]

REFERENCES

1. Jacobs KA, Leach DH, Fretz PB, Townsend HGG: Comparative aspects of the healing of excisional wounds on the leg and body of horses, Vet Surg 1984;13:83-90.
2. Knottenbelt DC: Equine wound management: Are there significant differences in healing at different sites on the body? Vet Derm 1997;8:273-290.
3. Schwartz AJ, Wilson DA, Keegan KG, et al: Factors regulating collagen synthesis and degradation during second-intention healing of wounds in the thoracic region and the distal aspect of the forelimb of horses, Am J Vet Res 2002;63:1564-1570.
4. Cochrane CA, Pain R, Knottenbelt DC: In vitro wound contraction in the horse: Differences between body and limb wounds, Wounds 2003;15:175-181.
5. Theoret CL, Spencer BM, Terence MN, Gordon JR: Expression of transforming growth factor β_1, β_3, and basic fibroblast growth factor in full-thickness skin wounds of equine limbs and thorax, Vet Surg 2001;30:269-277.
6. Moy LS: Management of acute wounds, Wound Healing 1993; 11:759-765.
7. Sinha AK, Hendrickson DA, Kannegieter NJ: Head trauma in two horses, Vet Rec 1991;128:518-521.
8. Tabor E: Corneal damage due to eye contact with chlorhexidine gluconate, JAMA 1989;261:557-558.
9. Wyn-Jones G: Interpreting radiographs: 6. Radiology of the equine head (Part 2), Equine Vet J 1985;17:417-425.
10. Modransky P, Welker B, Pickett JP: Management of facial injuries, Vet Clin North Am Equine Pract 1989;5:665-682.
11. Hance SR, Robertson JT: Subcutaneous emphysema from an axillary wound that resulted in pneumo-mediastinum and bilateral pneumothorax in a horse, J Am Vet Med Assoc 1992;200:1107-1110.
12. Hendrickson DA: Specific wound considerations. In Hendrickson DA, editor: Wound Care for the Equine Practitioner Made Easy Series, Jackson Hole, Wyo, 2004, Teton New Media.
13. Kane DP: Chronic wound healing and chronic wound management. In Krasner DL, Rodeheaver GT, Sibbald RG, editors: Chronic Wound Care, ed 3, Wayne, Pa, 2001, HMP Communications.
14. Phillips TJ, Al-Amoudi HO, Leverkus M, Park HY: Effect of chronic wound fluid on fibroblasts, J Wound Care 1998;7:527-532.

15. Mendez MV, Raffetto JD, Phillips T, et al: The proliferative capacity of neonatal skin fibroblasts is reduced after exposure to venous ulcer wound fluid: A potential mechanism for senescence in venous ulcers, J Vasc Surg 1999;30:734-742.
16. Chufa HE, Hughes MA, Cherry GW, Arnold F: Effects of chronic wound fluid on the bioactivity of platelet-derived growth factor in serum-free medium and its direct effect on fibroblast growth, Wound Rep Reg 1999;7:97-105.
17. Weckroth M, Vaheri A, Myohanen H, et al: Differential effects of acute and chronic wound fluids on urokinase-type plasminogen activator, urokinase-type plasminogen activator receptor, and tissue-type plasminogen activator in cultured human keratinocytes and fibroblasts, Wound Rep Reg 2001;9:314-322.
18. Shukla A, Dubey MP, Srivastava R, Srivastava BS: Differential expression of proteins during healing of cutaneous wounds in experimental normal and chronic models, Biochem Biophys Res Commun 1998;244:434-439.
19. Knottenbelt DC, Pascoe RR: Color Atlas of Diseases and Disorders of the Horse, Prescott, Ariz, 1994, Wolfe.
20. Cochrane CA, Freeman KL, Knottenbelt DC: Effect of growth factors on the characteristics of cells associated with equine wound healing and sarcoid formation, Wound Rep Reg 1996;4:58-65.
21. Dow G: Infection in chronic wounds. In Krasner DL, Rodeheaver GT, Sibbald RG, editors: Chronic Wound Care, ed 3, Wayne, Pa, 2001, HMP Communications.
22. Steed DL, Donohoe D, Webster MW, Lindsley L: Effect of extensive debridement and treatment on the healing of diabetic foot ulcers, J Am Coll Surg 1996;183:61-64.
23. Shearman CP: The role of surgical intervention in chronic wounds. In Mani R, editor: Chronic Wound Management, Boca Raton, Fla, 2003, Parthenon Group.
24. Falanga V: Growth factors and chronic wounds: The need to understand the microenvironment, J Dermatol 1992;19:667-672.
25. Peacock EE, Madden JW, Trier WC: Biological basis of treatment of keloid and hypertrophic scars. South Med J 1970;63:755-760.
26. Niessen FB, Schalkwijk J, Vos H, Timens T: Hypertrophic scar formation is associated with an increased number of epidermal Langerhans' cells, J Pathol 2004;202:121-129.
27. Ehrlich HP, Kelley SF: Hypertrophic scar: An interruption in the remodeling of repair—A laser Doppler blood flow study, Plast Reconstr Surg 1992;90:993-998.
28. Murray JC: Scars and keloids, Dermatol Clin 1993;11:697-708.
29. Myers BA: Wound healing. In Myers BA, editor: Wound Management: Principles and Practice, Upper Saddle River, NJ, 2004, Prentice Hall.
30. Phan TT, Sun L, Bay BH, et al: Dietary compounds inhibit proliferation and contraction of keloid and hypertrophic scar-derived fibroblasts in vitro: Therapeutic implication for excessive scarring, J Trauma 2003;54:1212-1224.

CHAPTER 28

Management of Sinus Tracts and Fistulas

John A. Stick

Sinus tracts are distinct from fistulas, although the terms are often used interchangeably. A fistula is an abnormal passage or communication, usually between two internal organs or leading from an organ to the surface of the body.[1] Examples include communications between a tendon sheath and a joint (synovial fistula), from the intestine through the abdominal wall (enterocutaneous fistula), and between the mouth or esophagus and the surface of the body (orocutaneous or esophageal fistula).[2,3] A sinus tract, on the other hand, is defined as a cavity or channel, and it may be normal (e.g., a venous sinus), or it may be a pathologic condition (e.g., an abnormal channel or fistula that permits the escape of pus through the skin).[1] In this chapter, the discussion is limited to the management of sinus tracts. Fistulas are described in chapters dealing with the specific affected anatomic organ or space.

ETIOLOGY

Chronic sinus tracts in horses commonly occur secondary to trauma and foreign bodies. Those involving the lower limbs are frequently associated with bone sequestra (Fig. 28-1).

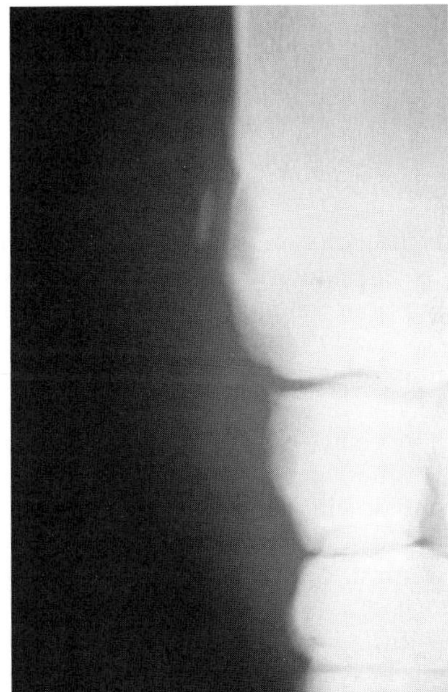

Figure 28-1. Radiograph of the carpal region of a horse that had a draining sinus tract just proximal to the carpus. Note the sequestrum on the distal radius.

Many of these become self-limiting, as the sequestrum undergoes natural débridement or will resolve immediately after sequestrectomy. However, chronic sinus tracts associated with foreign bodies have been described in many areas of the body and are sometimes quite difficult to resolve, especially if the foreign body is inert and not easily degraded by lysosomal enzymes released from white blood cells. Foreign bodies can be wood, metal, and even plastic.[4] Frequently, nonresorbable suture material results in a chronic sinus tract.[5]

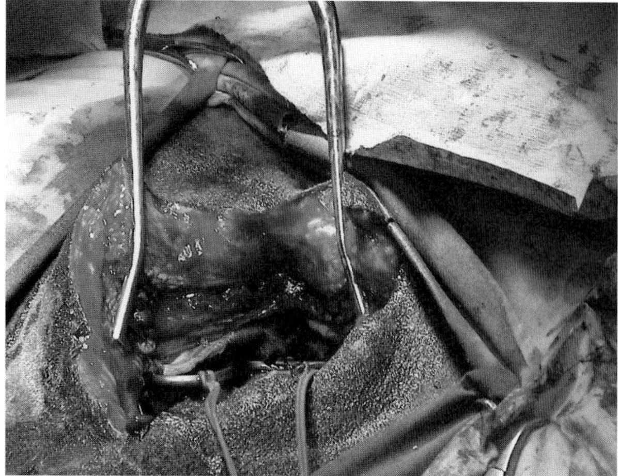

Figure 28-2. These hemostatic forceps are being removed from the thoracic wall of a horse 8 years after surgery, presumably for an umbilical hernia. Umbilical tape sutures are placed through the finger holes to provide traction. The horse had chronic draining tracts over a period of years, and these forceps had traveled approximately 18 inches from the original surgery.

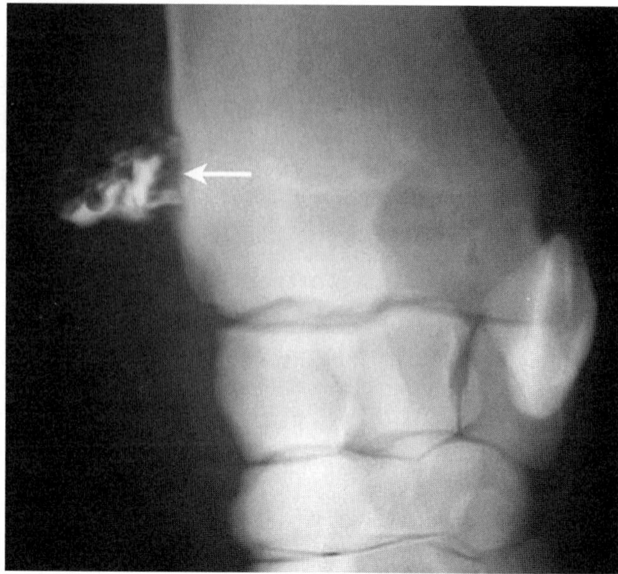

Figure 28-3. Positive-contrast sinography (performed on the horse shown in Fig. 28-1) outlines the extent of a sinus tract. Note that the contrast material outlines the sequestrum.

Sharp foreign bodies have a tendency to travel, especially when one end is blunt and the other is sharp, and can be found at some distance from the original site of entry. Examples of this include wood and metal foreign bodies with one blunt and one pointed end and even surgical instruments (Fig. 28-2).

DIAGNOSIS

Because foreign bodies are suspected at any time a chronic sinus tract is encountered, identification of the type of foreign body prior to surgery is always attempted. Foreign bodies are frequently noted as radiographic abnormalities on survey films, and, therefore, survey films should always be taken. Metallic foreign bodies are easily diagnosed this way. Other abnormalities include soft tissue swelling, thickening, gas densities, and soft tissue and periosteal reactions near bone, any of which may allow the foreign material to be located and identified.

Positive-contrast sinography is easily performed with water-soluble contrast medium (Fig. 28-3). It is particularly useful for identification of radiolucent foreign bodies, which frequently appear as space-occupying lesions in the center of the contrast material. Ultrasonography is also useful in the diagnosis of foreign bodies such as wood, especially those embedded in muscle. Water-bath studies have shown that bone, wood, and large tendons all demonstrated acoustical shadowing in equine muscle.[6] Differences in hyperechogenicity and acoustical shadows help detect and identify a foreign body.

EXPLORATION

Extirpation of the foreign body is the treatment of choice for a chronic sinus tract. Exploration of the sinus is carried out with a malleable probe and a groove director (Fig. 28-4). A malleable probe is used to determine the direction in which the exploration should occur (Fig. 28-5), and a

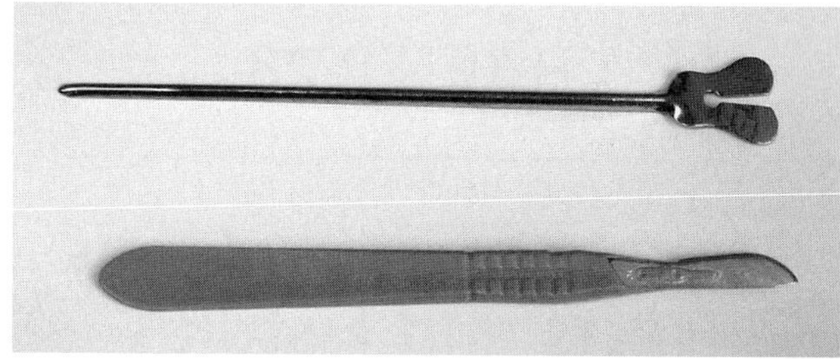

Figure 28-4. A groove director (next to a scalpel blade). When the scalpel blade is placed within the groove director with the point ventrad, the groove director guides the blade into the tract, and the incision can be made from the sinus tract outward. (See Fig. 28-6.)

groove director allows sharp dissection of the superficial portion of the sinus tract, which can be opened rapidly without bypassing the tract. Frequently, sinus tracts travel at varying angles and need to be opened in several directions. Occasionally, they even need to be opened a fair distance from the opening in the skin.

After exploration with a malleable probe, the groove director is inserted through the opening in the skin and guided along the probe. The probe is removed, and with the point of a no. 10 scalpel blade placed in the groove, the tract is opened toward the skin (Fig. 28-6).

This process is repeated if the tracts continue in other directions. When sinus tracts are quite deep, Weitlaner retractors are useful to hold open the incision. The tract itself usually has a dark purple membrane, which allows easy identification. Initial infusion of a vital dye such as Evan's blue further facilitates recognition of the tract during surgery, as it stains the tract lining dark blue.

After the foreign body has been identified and removed, all linings of the sinus tract should be curetted so that most of the bacterial contamination is removed and the sinus

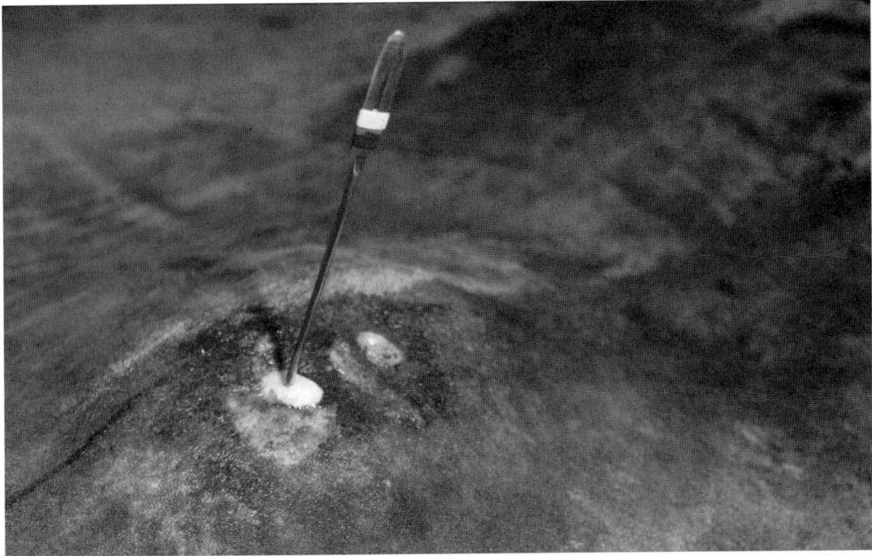

Figure 28-5. A malleable probe is inserted into one of the draining tracts in the ventral abdomen of a horse to localize the foreign body (nonabsorbable suture material in this case).

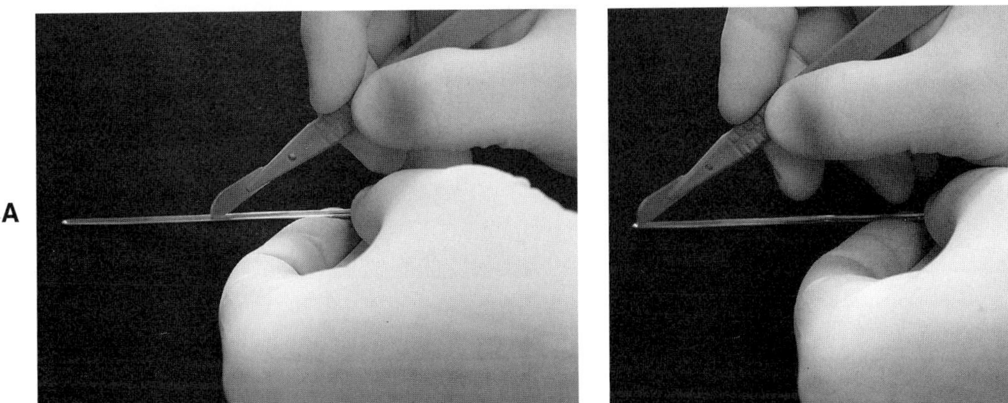

Figure 28-6. The groove director is inserted through the cloaca into the sinus tract. This is followed by sliding a no. 10 scalpel blade point in the groove of the tract (**A**) and opening toward the skin. As the scalpel blade reaches the end of the groove director, it has a stop (**B**); therefore, the incision cannot be made beyond the extent of the end of the groove director.

tract will stop draining. The membrane itself will produce purulent material for some time. The tract should be thoroughly flushed with sterile saline. Although much of the tract may be closed after this procedure, it is usually better to simply débride the cloaca rather than to close it.

SPECIAL CONSIDERATIONS

The location of the sinus tract may be an indication that the tract did not develop secondary to a foreign body. Any time a sinus tract develops on the head, a sinus infection or a dental problem should be suspected, especially if sinography outlines the tract to the apex of a tooth. A sinus tract opening found near the base of the ear is usually the result of a conchal cyst ("ear tooth"). This can easily be diagnosed with radiography (Fig. 28-7). (For details on surgical treatment of this condition, see Chapter 29.) A sinus tract over the pole or the withers region may indicate the development of an infected bursa in this area (Fig. 28-8). The former is called pole evil and the latter is called fistulous withers. If either is the case, a blood sample should be taken to determine a *Brucella* titer, as brucellosis is a human health hazard.

COMPLICATIONS

Lacerations or incisions into large vessels, or even into internal organs, are possible when following a sinus tract. Therefore, caution is necessary when sinus tracts are deeply embedded in and around body cavities. Also, some sinus tracts may contain more than one foreign body, especially if the foreign body is made of wood or nonabsorbable suture material. Owners should be warned that recurrence is a possibility any time this exploration is attempted, and that, in fact, foreign bodies sometimes cannot be found. Another surgery may be necessary when a new cloaca forms from a new sinus tract.

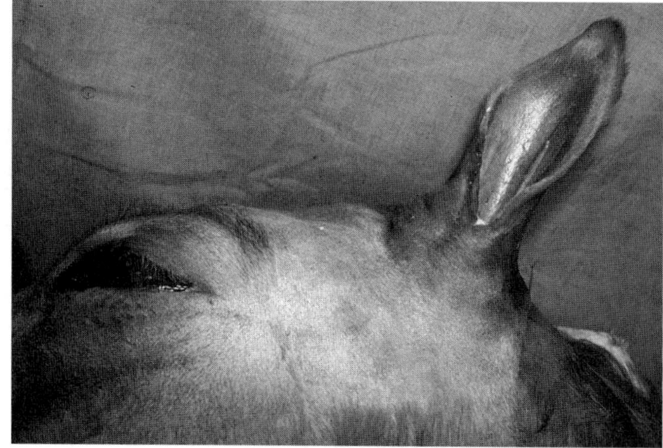

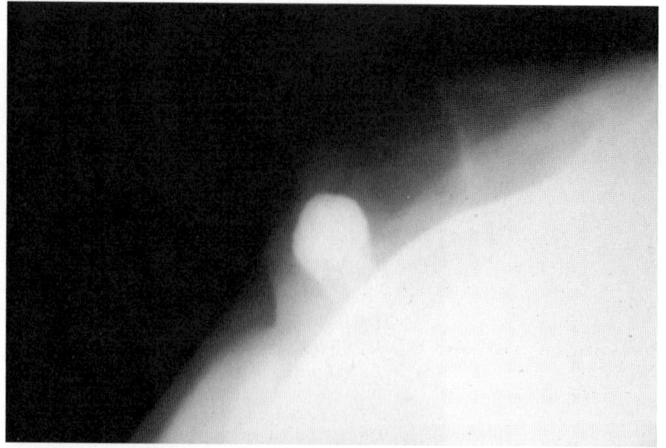

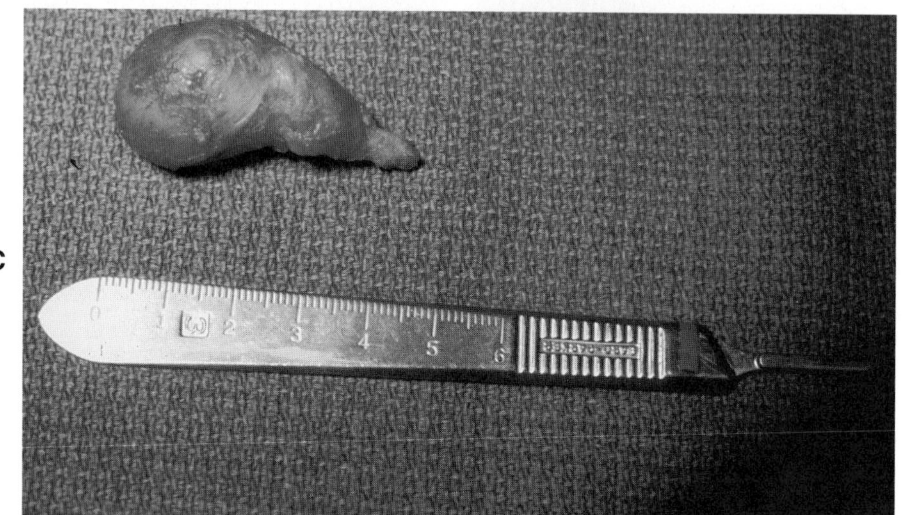

Figure 28-7. Sinus tracts located at the base of the ear usually indicate the presence of a conchal cyst. This can usually be palpated just cranial to the ear as an enlargement (**A**), radiographs confirm that it is a tooth (**B**), and the aberrant tooth with its cyst lining is removed in its entirety (**C**).

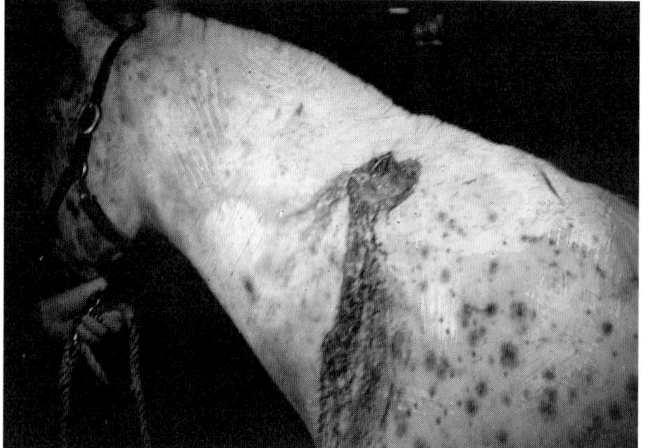

Figure 28-8. Any time a sinus tract develops along the withers, the condition of fistulous withers is suspected, and this can be confirmed with radiographs. However, because this may be a zoonosis involving infection with *Brucella,* cultures and a titer should be obtained prior to further diagnostic workup and treatment.

REFERENCES

1. Dorland's Illustrated Medical Dictionary, ed 30, Philadelphia, 2003, WB Saunders.
2. Johnson JE, Ryan GD: Intersynovial fistula in the carpus of a horse, Cornell Vet 1975;65:84.
3. Bristol DG: Enterocutaneous fistulae in horses: 18 cases (1964 to 1992), Vet Surg 1994;23:534.
4. McEvoy FJ, Lamb CR, White RN: An application of sonography in the small animal practice, Vet Rec 1993;132:183.
5. Hosgood G, Pechman RD, Casey HW: Suture sinus in the linea alba of two dogs, J Small Anim Pract 1992;33:285.
6. Cartee RE, Rumph PF: Ultrasonographic detection of fistulous tracts and foreign object in muscles of horses, J Am Vet Med Assoc 1984;184:1127.

CHAPTER 29

Skin Conditions Amenable to Surgery

Elizabeth A. Carr

The vast majority of equine skin diseases requiring a surgical consultation or surgical intervention are neoplastic in origin. Consequently, the major focus of this chapter is on neoplasms of the skin. The biologic behavior, predisposing factors, diagnosis, prognosis, and treatment options are discussed. When available, comparative reviews of treatment protocols are included. The goal of this chapter is to provide information to assist the clinician in determining the best approach to treatment of a particular neoplastic condition. In addition, a handful of other skin conditions are reviewed. This is not an exhaustive review of all skin conditions but instead a review of the more common diseases, with an emphasis on those that are amenable to surgical resolution.

SARCOIDS

The equine sarcoid was first described by Jackson in 1936.[1] The most common tumor in horses worldwide, sarcoid is a cutaneous, fibroblastic neoplasia with a proliferative epithelial component.[1] Sarcoids are frequently classified histopathologically as benign tumors because of the morphologic characteristics of the fibroblasts and because many sarcoids are slow growing and cause little if any physical problems in the affected animal. This classification is misleading, however, and ignores the large number of tumors whose clinical behavior can only be described as malignant.[2]

Sarcoids are subtyped, on the basis of clinical appearance, into occult, verrucous, nodular fibroblastic, ulcerative fibroblastic, mixed tumors, and malevolent. This classification correlates with their biologic behavior (Fig. 29-1). The most aggressive subtype consists of malevolent sarcoids, which infiltrate locally along fascial planes and vessels; grow rapidly, and have a high recurrence rate after excision.[2]

Sites of predilection vary with geographic location and include the face (muzzle, ears, and periocular region), distal limbs, neck or ventral abdomen, and areas of previous injury and scarring.[3] Location has been reported to affect prognosis, with sarcoids on the distal limb and periorbital region having a worse prognosis for resolution than sarcoids in other locations.

Epidemiology

The relationship between breed and risk for development of sarcoid was evaluated in a large number of horses admitted to the New York State College of Veterinary Medicine between 1975 and 1987.[4] Quarter Horses and related stock breeds were almost twice as likely to develop sarcoid as Thoroughbreds. Standardbred horses were less than half as likely to develop sarcoid as Thoroughbred horses. A direct genetic linkage has been reported between equine leukocyte antigens (ELA) and risk for equine sarcoid. ELA alleles A3 and W13 were strongly associated with risk for sarcoids in Thoroughbreds and Swiss, French, and Irish Warmblood horses.[5-7] The absence of the W13 allele in the Standardbred population may confer relative resistance to sarcoid. Interestingly, a familial predisposition has been reported in a herd in which all five descendants of a sarcoid-affected mare developed sarcoid, whereas none of the unrelated animals on the premises developed these tumors.[8]

Spontaneous malignancies that develop as a result of serial genetic mutations are more common in older animals. Sarcoids generally develop in younger individuals, suggesting a genetic predisposition or an exogenous factor. Individuals with a genetic predisposition have an inherited gene defect that increases their susceptibility to further mutation. Consequently, these individuals develop tumors at a much earlier age. The genetic predisposition for and the age of onset of sarcoids suggest that both genetic factors and exogenous factors may play a role in development. A long-term epidemiologic study of a large herd of donkeys suggests the possibility of transmission of sarcoids between individuals housed in close contact.[9] In addition, an epizootic outbreak was reported in a small herd.[8] Incidence peaked in young horses over a 1-year period. Interestingly, only related, highly inbred animals were affected. A vector such as a fly may explain the predisposition for tumors to develop around the eye, distal limbs, and ventrum (common feeding locations for these insects).

A specific viral etiology was first proposed by Olsen and Cook.[10] While studying the transmissibility of cutaneous papillomas, they noted a striking similarity between equine sarcoid and experimental lesions induced by the injection of bovine wart extracts into the skin of individual horses. Several research groups have since confirmed the presence of bovine papillomavirus (BPV) DNA in nearly all equine sarcoid tissues examined.[11-20] Papillomaviruses play a role in oncogenic transformation in other species, but viral infection alone is not enough to trigger transformation, as BPV DNA can be found in normal skin of sarcoid-affected horses.[20,21] Papillomavirus infection of an abnormal host (such as BPV infection in a horse) generally results in a nonproductive infection; consequently, no viral capsids are produced. Instead, the virus maintains its presence by production of several housekeeping genes, including two, E5 and E6, known to be capable of transforming cells to malignancy. The production of one of these two transforming genes, E5, has been documented in a small number of sarcoids examined.[22] Expression of the viral E5 protein appeared to correlate with the grade of tumor malignancy. Furthermore, although viral DNA was detected in normal skin surrounding sarcoids, E5 protein expression was not. A triggering event such as trauma may be required to activate a latent viral state. This could be one explanation for the tendency for sarcoids to occur at the sites of previous injuries. Experimental inoculation of purified viral DNA has resulted in sarcoid-like tumors, but the majority of these lesions regress spontaneously.[23]

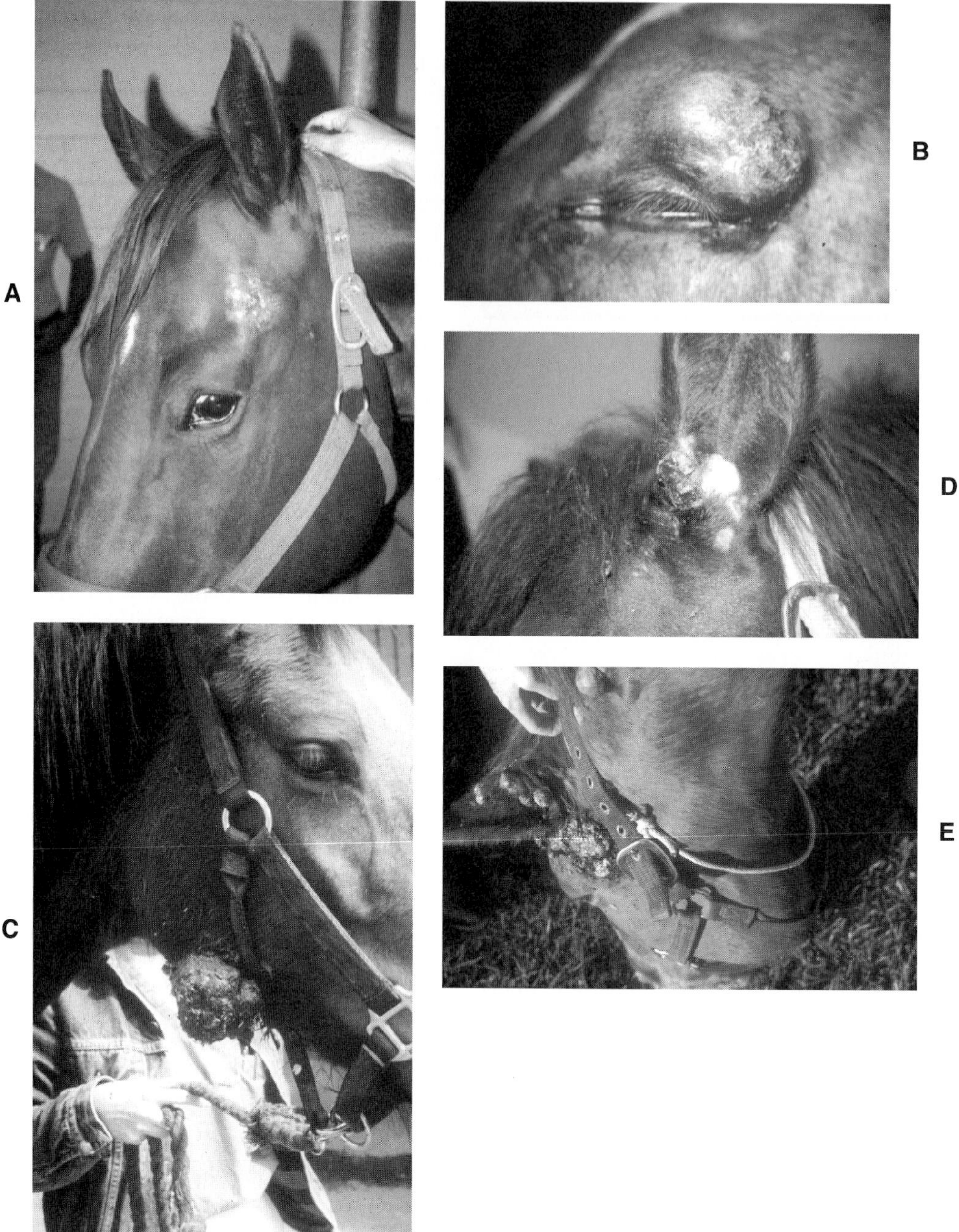

Figure 29-1. Subtypes of sarcoids. **A,** A verrucous sarcoid on the temporal region of the head. **B,** A subcutaneous fibroblastic sarcoid. **C,** An ulcerative fibroblastic sarcoid. **D,** A mixed form consisting of both verrucous and fibroblastic components. **E,** A horse with a malevolent sarcoid. The lesion had spread down the neck along lymphatic chains, and to the retropharyngeal and parotid lymph nodes.

A viral role is strongly suggested by the finding of viral DNA and viral transforming proteins in all sarcoids examined. However, the mechanism of viral transformation is unclear. Given the genetic and breed predispositions, sarcoid occurrence is most likely the result of host, viral, and environmental factors.

Treatment

There are numerous articles regarding treatment of sarcoids. The number of treatment options reflects the variable success as well as the costs of certain treatments. Efficacy is difficult to critically assess; most early studies were not controlled and were based on a subset of cases sent to referral hospitals. Sarcoids commonly referred for treatment are usually more aggressive variants or tumors that have recurred after unsuccessful treatment. Sarcoids can transform to a more aggressive phenotype after incomplete or unsuccessful treatment and are then harder to resolve. In contrast to those tumors typically seen at referral centers, there is anecdotal evidence of a subset of sarcoids that remain quiescent and of others that undergo spontaneous regression.

Surgical Excision

Surgical excision without adjunctive therapy has been reported to be one of the least successful treatment options, having a recurrence rate of 15.8% to 82%.[3,24-26] The reason for this may in part be that tumor projects fronds of malignant cells into the surrounding "normal tissue."[27] Because these projections are infrequent, they are missed on histopathologic review, leading to an incorrect assumption of complete excision. In addition, the possibility exists that a viral agent may remain latent in the surrounding tissue.[20,21] Surgical trauma and the subsequent growth stimulation may trigger viral activation and expression of viral oncogenes. In a recent prospective trial, the detection of viral DNA at the surgical margin of an excised sarcoid correlated with an increased risk of recurrence.[21]

Laser Ablation

Laser ablation of tumors has been used to remove or debulk tumor mass.[24,28-31] Laser ablation causes less damage to the surrounding tissues and less spread of malignant cells to healthy regions than sharp surgical excision with mechanical tools. A large retrospective study evaluating CO_2 laser excision of 60 sarcoids documented an overall recurrence rate of 38%.[29] The use of laser ablation in conjunction with intralesional chemotherapy or other adjunctive therapy may improve overall success rates.

Cryotherapy

Cryotherapy (see Chapter 15) has historically been one of the most commonly used methods for treatment of equine sarcoid.[32-34] Success rates of 60% to 100% have been reported. However, a recent retrospective study evaluating treatment success in a large number of periorbital sarcoids reported a recurrence rate of 91% (9% success rate) in tumors treated by cryotherapy.[26] Longer follow-up time may explain the discrepancy in successful outcome. Cryotherapy has its greatest success with veterinarians who use it frequently and have experience with duration and depth of freeze, which are important for an effective response. Thermocouples can be utilized for more precise measurement of the tissue temperature and depth of freeze. In one report, the use of a three-treatment, −30° C protocol was felt to be more effective than a two-treatment −20° C protocol, with an overall initial success rate of 68%.[32] With multiple repeat treatments, the success rate improved to 85% (85 tumors resolved of 100 retreated). Thirty-three of the 50 horses were cured of their sarcoids using a liquid nitrogen spray apparatus, although many required multiple treatments.[33] Three horses in this study had spontaneous regression of untreated tumors after cryotherapy of another lesion. This seems to indicate that destruction of one tumor can result in an immune response against other, distant sarcoids.

Hyperthermia

Hyperthermia has been reported to be successful in a small number of equine sarcoids, with spontaneous resolution of some of the nontreated tumors.[35] Differences in the metabolic rate of tumor cells compared with normal cells is thought to make the tumor cell more heat sensitive.

Radiotherapy

Radiotherapy using locally implanted iridium-192 has been reported to be successful in the treatment of sarcoids.[26,36,37] The recurrence rate was low, with 1-year tumor-free incidences of 94%, 87.5%, and 100%. Radiotherapy using a linear source of iridium-192 has been reported to have a 100% success rate in a small number of sarcoids.[38] All cases were reported to resolve after a single dose of radiation. Recurrence rate at 1 year was zero for all tumor types, but the number of cases actually followed for a full year was not reported. The 1-year progression-free survival was 86.6% in 62 sarcoids treated with iridium interstitial brachytherapy.[39] Treatment complications included hair and pigment loss as well as fibrosis, cataract formation, and corneal ulceration when treating periocular tumors. Radioactive gold-198 implants have been reported to have a high success rate for treatment of sarcoids—a rate similar to that for the other implant therapies.[40] Although reported success rates using radiation therapy are high, treatment is expensive, requires special equipment and housing, and is potentially hazardous. General anesthesia may be required to implant iridium needles or to deliver a radiation dose via a linear source. These limitations make radiation therapy a difficult and infrequently utilized method of treatment and confine its use to referral centers.

Immunotherapy

Immunotherapy has been used to successfully treat sarcoids in several reports.[26,34,41-43] Several immunostimulants have been utilized, including *Mycobacterium* cell wall extracts, live whole-cell bacille Calmette-Guérin (BCG), and propionibacterial cell wall extracts. These products are thought to stimulate cell-mediated immunity, leading to recognition of tumor cell–specific antigens and subsequently to tumor cell destruction. Most immune stimulants require multiple intralesional injections with or without prior cytoreduction of the tumor mass. Success rates are high for smaller tumors, tumors located periorbitally, and fibroblastic tumors. Knottenbelt and Kelly reported a poorer success rate with occult or verrucous periorbital lesions and hypothesized that this was because of the inability to saturate the tumor bed effectively.[26] Multiple treatments are generally required. Local tissue swelling can be quite severe, and complications include death from anaphylactic shock, particularly after two or more injections.[43] Spontaneous regression of untreated tumors has also been reported with immunotherapy.[34] Recurrence rates vary from 0% to 40%, depending on the study and observation time.[26,34,41-43]

Intralesional Cisplatin

Intralesional cisplatin in an oily emulsion is reported to have an 87% 1-year relapse-free rate for sarcoids.[44] The repositol effect of the oily emulsion prevents significant systemic levels, avoiding systemic toxicity, and maintains effective tissue levels of the chemotherapeutic for prolonged periods of time.[44] Epinephrine can be added to the emulsion (1:1000, diluted 1:10). The resultant vasoconstriction prolongs tumor cell exposure to cisplatin. A dosage of 1 mg cisplatin per cubic centimeter of tumor mass, with a minimum of four treatments, is recommended. Cytoreduction to decrease the mass of the tumor is beneficial when treating large tumors. Intralesional cisplatin instituted at the time of surgical excision or debulking was not shown to affect wound healing.[45] The repositol effect of the oily emulsion is critical for treatment success. A 66% recurrence rate after cisplatin treatment was reported by Knottenbelt.[26] However, the concentration used was lower than that recommended by the original authors.[44]

Intralesional tumor necrosis factor (TNF) combined with a xanthate compound has also been used with success.[46]

Topical Application of Chemotherapeutics

Topical application of chemotherapeutic agents, including 5-fluorouracil (5-FU) and a series of compounded creams, AW3-LUDES and AW4-LUDES, have been reported to be successful in the resolution of sarcoids.[26,47,48] 5-FU had a resolution rate of 66% in nine tumors treated daily for 15 days, but only small occult or verrucous sarcoids were chosen for this treatment protocol.[26] In the same report, the AW4-LUDES cream had a resolution rate of 35% (56 of 146 tumors treated) without complication. The authors reserved this treatment for small, previously untreated verrucous lesions. Six additional tumors resolved with the topical application of AW4-LUDES but had significant scarring after treatment. As with 5-FU, the authors recommend avoiding the use of these creams on tumors in close proximity to the eye. Topical application of a compounded cream containing bloodroot and zinc is anecdotally reported to be extremely effective in the treatment of equine sarcoid, but few controlled studies have been done. I evaluated one sarcoid-affected horse that was treated with this compound; in response to the compound, the tumor became very swollen and ulcerated and began to grow rapidly. More controlled studies evaluating the efficacy of bloodroot and zinc against different types of sarcoid tumors are needed.

Spontaneous regression of untreated tumors suggests that immune recognition plays a role in tumor resolution.[35] Anecdotal reports of successful vaccination therapy exist, but controlled studies are rare. In one report, successful resolution was achieved in 11 of 12 horses treated with an autogenous tumor vaccine.[49] A second vaccination protocol resulted in resolution of the one recurrence. All 12 cases had had no previous tumor treatment. A lower success rate was reported in horses with previously treated, recurrent sarcoids.

With large, aggressive, or multiple tumors, it is recommended that a combination of treatment modalities be employed. At the Veterinary Teaching Hospital at Michigan State University, surgical excision or laser ablation is commonly combined with intralesional chemotherapy or radiation therapy. Unfortunately, these combination treatment regimens are expensive and require a significant time commitment from the owner or caretaker of the patient.

SQUAMOUS CELL CARCINOMA

Epidemiology

Squamous cell carcinoma (SCC), a malignant, locally invasive neoplasia of squamous epithelial cells, is the second most common tumor in horses.[50,51] Although SCC can develop anywhere on the integument, sites of predilection include areas lacking pigmentation, poorly haired regions, and skin near mucocutaneous junctions. SCC is the most common neoplasm of the equine eye, conjunctiva, ocular adnexal structures, and external genitalia.[52] It has also been reported in the nasal cavity, paranasal sinuses, pharynx, larynx, and hoof capsule, and it should be considered in horses with chronic, refractory foot abscesses.[53-56] Ultraviolet light–induced damage is thought to predispose to SCC. Many tumors arise from precancerous lesions, including actinic keratosis, carcinoma in situ, squamous metaplasia of the penile epithelium, and irritant-induced chronic keratitis.[57,58] Proposed irritants include topically applied chemicals, smegma, and flies. SCC has been reported to develop in areas of chronic, poorly healing wounds and at sites of previous burn injury.[52,59,60] Breeds with poorly pigmented, pink-skinned areas including Appaloosas and paint-colored horses are more prone to develop SCC; 69% of all ocular SCC cases occur in individuals lacking periocular pigmentation.[61] It has been suggested that draft breeds have an increased incidence of SCC.[56]

Tumors are classified as ulcerative or proliferative and generally arise as solitary lesions. *Ulcerative SCC* may develop over time, with early lesions appearing as small nodules underlying normal-haired skin. Ulcerative lesions can be mistaken for nonhealing wounds and chronic granulation tissue, resulting in delayed treatment. Ocular lesions can begin as small ulcerative lesions on lid margins, or as keratitic plaques on the cornea, so SCC should be suspected whenever raised red lesions appear on the lid margins, sclera, or conjunctiva, particularly in unpigmented skin (Fig. 29-2). Squamous cell carcinoma of the ocular structures can invade the orbit, calvarium, tear duct, and sinuses if left untreated. *Proliferative* pedunculated lesions on the penis often have a cauliflower-like appearance. SCC typically spreads to surrounding tissues and local lymph nodes, but distant metastasis is rare (see Chapter 66). Tumors with local or distant metastases or large, invasive tumors have a poor prognosis for cure.

Treatment

Surgical excision, radiation therapy, topical application of antimitotics, intralesional chemotherapy, cryotherapy, laser excision, hyperthermia, and immunotherapy have all been successfully used to treat equine SCC.[40,44,62-75] Surgical excision alone should be reserved for small tumors and has a better overall success rate when combined with adjunctive therapies such as chemotherapy, cryotherapy, or radiation therapy.[45,62,63] Keratoplasty with or without adjunctive radiation therapy has been used successfully to treat corneal SCC.[64,65] Cryotherapy is reported to be most useful in small periocular lesions and lesions arising from the external genitalia. Larger lesions may benefit from surgical debulking prior to cryotherapy.[66,67] Frequent reexamination is recommended to monitor regrowth and may be the most important determinant of success. Failure to retreat small recurrences quickly may allow tumor regrowth and failure of the treatment protocol.

Irradiation

Several *radiation* modalities have been used to successfully treat SCC, including external beam radiotherapy, implanted

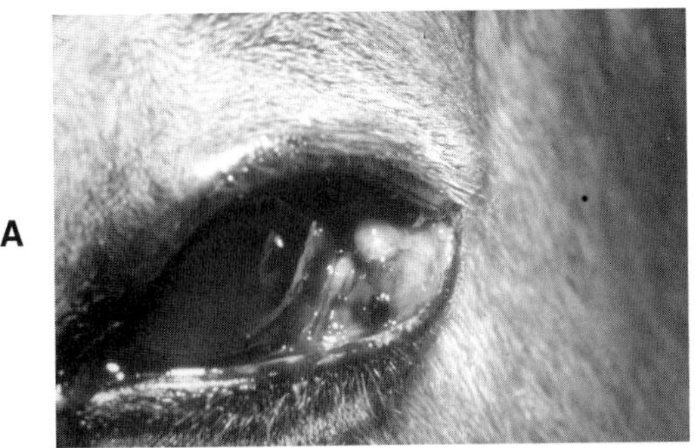

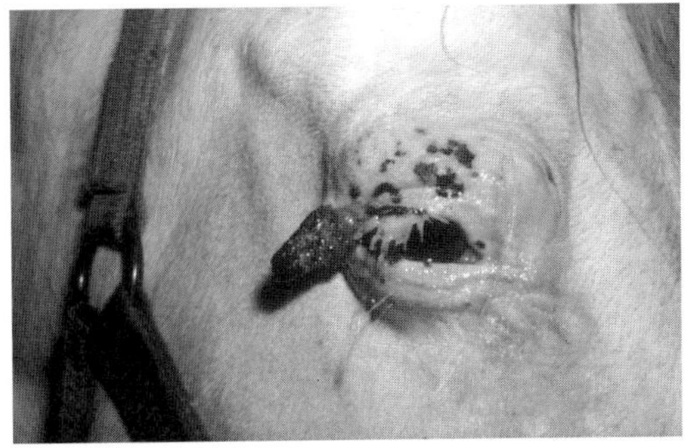

Figure 29-2. Squamous cell carcinoma. **A,** Ulcerative, proliferative lesion involving the conjunctiva of the eye in a bay Quarter Horse mare. **B,** Pedunculated lesion involving the margin of the upper eyelid in an Appaloosa mare.

radiation devices, and β-emitting wands. Strontium wands (β-radiation) can be used to treat small superficial plaques on the cornea, sclera, or conjunctiva.[68-70] Beta irradiation has a very short penetration depth, making it extremely useful for small corneal lesions; an 89% nonrecurrence rate was reported in one study.[69] Both radioactive implants and external beam therapy have been reported as successful in the treatment of SCC.[40,71-73] External beam therapy can be performed on an outpatient basis, whereas radiation implants require hospitalization and special housing during treatment protocols. Radiation therapy is generally limited to referral practices because of the licensure requirement, specialized equipment, and housing requirements.

Intralesional Chemotherapy

Intralesional chemotherapy is very effective in treating SCC, whether as an adjunctive treatment after surgical cytoreduction or as a sole treatment protocol.[44,45] *Cisplatin* binds directly to DNA and inhibits its synthesis in dividing cells. Mixing cisplatin in an oily emulsion creates a repositol effect, maintaining the drug in the local tissues for a prolonged period of time. Intralesional cisplatin in oily emulsion used with or without surgical cytoreduction has a 2-year local control rate of 89% for SCC. Overall success is better with SCC of the external genitalia than with periorbital SCC. Cosmetic results are generally excellent. Drawbacks include the multiple treatments needed, the expense, and potential exposure of the staff, but overall success rates are high.

Topical Chemotherapy

Topical 5-flurouracil, with or without surgical débridement, has a reported success rate of 90% in the treatment of SCC of the male external genitalia.[74] In another small case series, three individuals with superficial SCC were successfully treated with repeated application of topical 5-FU.[75] Topical application was associated with local inflammation and swelling. The use of 5-FU as a sole treatment modality is best reserved for small superficial tumors.

Successful treatment of a recurrent SCC of the lower lip using the nonsteroidal anti-inflammatory *piroxicam* is reported.[76] Nonsteroidal anti-inflammatory drugs inhibit cyclooxygenase (COX) enzymes that catalyze the conversion of arachidonic acid to prostaglandins. Overexpression of the COX-2 enzyme by neoplastic tissue has been reported.[77] Both the lower lip and metastatic lesions resolved with oral piroxicam therapy. No recurrence was reported at the 5-year follow-up. Successful treatment of periocular SCC using immunotherapy has also been reported, but case numbers are small.[78]

In a retrospective study of 43 horses with ocular SCC, nonrecurrence rates were 55.6% for surgical excision, 75% for radiation therapy, and 33.4% for cryotherapy, and combination therapy had a greater success rate than single-modality treatment.[62] In a retrospective study of 147 cases of ocular/adnexal SCC, factors that influenced survival included tumor location and size. Prior treatment modalities, the presence of multiple tumors, and treatment modality used at the time of examination did not influence survival.[79]

MELANOMA

Epidemiology

Equine melanoma is one of the most common skin tumors in horses. Histopathologic surveys report that melanomas comprise 4% to 15% of all skin tumors.[58,80] The vast majority of melanomas occur in gray horses; breed predispositions are most likely caused by the incidence of the color gray within a breed. Virtually all gray horses will develop melanoma over time. In a population study of Lipizzan horses, less than 6% of horses 16 years of age or older were melanoma free.[81] Melanocytic tumors in gray horses are thought to arise because of a disturbance in melanin transfer from dermal melanocytes to follicular cells.[82] Progression from melanocyte accumulation to melanoma formation has been documented in melanoma-prone locations. Interestingly, sites of predilection are the first areas to show depigmentation changes (vitiligo) with aging.[83] There are four types of equine melanomas: melanocytic nevi, dermal melanomas, dermal melanomatosis, and malignant melanomas.[84] *Melanocytic nevi* are composed of larger pleomorphic melanocytes with an increased number of mitotic figures, binucleate cells, and variable cytoplasmic pigmentation. Melanocytic nevi are typically single or multiple discrete nodules and are found in similar frequency in both gray and nongray individuals.[84]

Dermal melanoma and *melanomatosis* appear benign on histopathologic examination and are composed of smaller, homogenous dendritic cells with condensed chromatin, dense pigmentation, and no visible mitosis. Dermal melanomas originate in the deeper dermis and are typically small singular or multiple nodules (Fig. 29-3). *Dermal melanomatosis* is defined as confluent multiple large melanomas. The risk of dermal melanomatosis increases with age and its occurrence is associated with an increased risk of metastases.[81,84] True *malignant melanomas* are rare and are classified on the basis of the presence of both histopathologic and clinical characteristics of malignancy.[84] In one retrospective study, only two of 53 cases were classified as malignant. Both occurred in aged horses (older than 20 years), and both recurred within 10 months after surgical excision.[84] Malignant melanomas are frequently invasive and associated with a poor prognosis for complete resolution.[84-89]

The vast majority of melanomas are located around the perineum and base of the tail, with lesions around the head (lips, eyes, parotid region) and other sites less frequently reported. Melanomas have also been reported in the foot, meninges, thorax, ocular structures, and abdominal cavity. These unusual locations appear to be associated with a poor prognosis.[84-91]

Treatment

Despite their histopathologic differences, dermal melanomas and melanocytic nevi have similar clinical characteristics, and surgical excision is curative in the majority of cases. Smaller lesions can be sharply excised; alternatively, the use of the CO_2 laser has been recommended.[92] The ability to cauterize the wound bed and control hemorrhage makes laser excision particularly useful in sites where primary closure cannot be achieved (e.g., the base of the tail).

Complete excision is difficult with larger lesions such as dermal melanomatosis, but surgical debulking can be palliative.[93] Oral cimetidine has been recommended to treat melanomas, particularly larger lesions and those exhibiting a rapid growth phase.[94-98] Cimetidine has antitumor activity and is a histamine receptor antagonist. Immunomodulation of lymphocyte activity via histamine receptor interaction is postulated to be a mechanism of antitumor activity. Reports of the effectiveness of cimetidine in the treatment of equine melanoma are variable. Response is reported to be the highest in tumors exhibiting a rapid growth phase; successful response was achieved using a dose of 2.5 mg/kg every 8 hours. The frequency of dosing may be the most critical factor in predicting clinical response. Treatment is recommended for 3 months, or for 3 weeks after cessation of tumor growth. Although a complete cure has rarely been reported, cimetidine may have some benefit in halting rapidly growing tumors and returning them to a more quiescent state.[93]

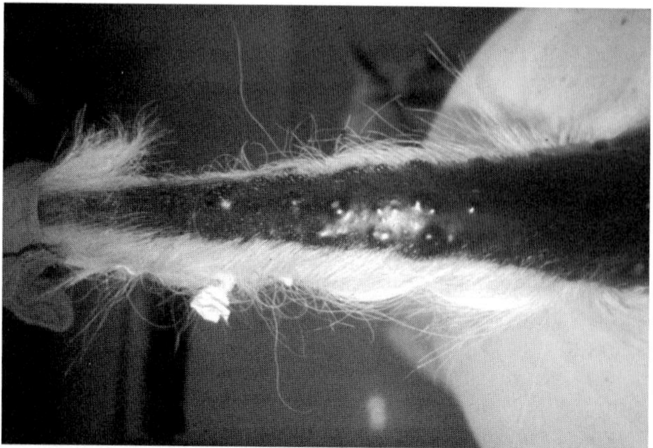

Figure 29-3. Dermal melanomas on the ventral surface of the tail in a gray horse.

Additional treatments for equine melanoma include intralesional chemotherapy and cryotherapy. Successful treatment of smaller nodules has been reported using intralesional cisplatin, and this is beneficial in decreasing the size of larger tumors prior to surgical excision.[98,99]

A melanoma vaccine is available and has been reported to have some success.[100] The successful treatment of equine melanoma using intratumoral injections of human interleukin (IL)-12 has also been reported.[101]

In one study that examined melanomas in a population of gray horses, all patients exhibited normal quality of life regardless of tumor number and type.[81] Consequently, it is frequently suggested that melanomas be treated with benign neglect, as they are rarely the cause of significant disease in affected horses. However, with age, the risk of progression to dermal melanomatosis and metastases increases. Small nodules are easily removed and rarely recur, but owners need to be informed that new tumors will quite likely develop over time. Although conservative management is reasonable in the majority of cases, more aggressive treatment, including early removal of smaller tumors, may decrease the risk of melanomatosis or metastases as the animal ages.

Malignant melanomas have a higher recurrence rate with simple excision. Combination therapy, including surgical debulking and intralesional chemotherapeutic injections, may offer palliation, but the prognosis for cure is poor.[83,87]

MAST CELL TUMORS

Epidemiology

Equine cutaneous mastocytosis (ECM) is less common in horses than in small animals.[102] The benign, solitary, nodular cutaneous form is the most common, although malignant ECM and congenital disseminated forms have been recognized.[103-105] It has been suggested that the benign nodular form is not a true neoplasia and is instead the result of an inflammatory reaction to dysplastic mast cells and recruited eosinophils.[106] The release of inflammatory products from accumulated eosinophils and mast cells results in necrosis, and later a granulomatous reaction develops with fibrosis and subsequent encapsulation of the nodule. The histopathologic findings of a necrotic focus, a granulomatous inflammatory response, and fibrosis surrounding well-differentiated mast cells differentiates equine cutaneous nodular mastocytosis from malignant ECM, which contains abnormal mast cells with increased nuclear-to-cytoplasmic ratios, anisokaryosis, and increased mitotic figures.[104]

Treatment

The majority of cutaneous nodular ECMs are successfully treated with wide surgical excision (margins of 1 cm or greater).[102] Reports of resolution after incomplete resection exist. Intralesional injection of glucocorticoids has also been used to successfully treat cutaneous nodular ECM. Malignant ECM is not responsive to surgical excision and is associated with a poor prognosis for cure.

LIPOMAS

Epidemiology

External lipomas are a relatively uncommon neoplasia in horses. Unlike mesenteric lipomas, they are principally found in young horses.[107-109] Subcutaneous lipomas are generally encapsulated, singular, nonpainful masses that are fluctuant to firm on palpation, although infiltrative lipomas have been reported in the horse.[107-109] Sites of occurrence include the limbs, thorax, abdominal wall, and eyelids. Histopathologic examination reveals encapsulated well-differentiated adipocytes. Infiltrative lipomas consist of similar cell types infiltrating surrounding muscle tissue.[110]

Treatment

Lipomas are generally encapsulated, slow-growing masses, and thus they are benign, clinically insignificant, and typically a cosmetic concern only. Surgical excision is reported to be curative in all cases; recurrence has not been reported even with incomplete excision of infiltrative or large lipomas.

CUTANEOUS HABRONEMIASIS

Epidemiology

Cutaneous habronemiasis is a proliferative ulcerative lesion produced by aberrant migration of the larvae of three endoparasites (*Habronema muscae, Habronema microstoma,* and *Draschia megastoma*) that inhabit the stomach of horses.[111] Eggs, shed in the feces of horses, hatch, and the larvae are ingested by maggots of the house fly, *Musca domestica,* or the stable fly, *Stomoxys calcitrans*. Third-stage infective larvae migrate to the head of the fly and are passed to the horse when the fly feeds on a warm, wet surface. The larvae are then swallowed by the horse and mature to adults in the stomach. The cutaneous form, also called summer sores, develops when larvae are attached to wound beds or aberrant moist surfaces, including the penis, prepuce, and ocular adnexa.[112,113] Lesions are most commonly seen on the penis, in cutaneous wounds, or around the eye. The proliferative, ulcerative, granulomatous lesions are thought to result from a hypersensitivity reaction to the larvae, and mild to severe pruritus may develop.[114]

Ophthalmic habronemiasis can develop in the conjunctiva or nasolacrimal ducts, resulting in third-eyelid granulomas or granulating ulcers below the medial canthus. Clinical signs include epiphora, chemosis, and photophobia. The presence of pale yellow granular material, or the finding of larvae on impression smears, may aid in the diagnosis. Histopathologic examination is recommended, because habronemiasis can develop secondary to an underlying neoplastic or infectious condition. The incidence of disease has declined dramatically since the development of ivermectin anthelmintics. Lesions occur principally in warm months and are associated with increased fly populations and poor manure collection.

Treatment

Lesions have been reported to resolve with onset of cooler weather.[113] Treatment is aimed at reducing the size of the lesions, resolving the inflammatory or allergic component, and preventing reinfestation.[113] Treatment with systemic ivermectin will kill migrating larvae but may not result in resolution of the lesion, because the dead parasite can continue to cause a severe inflammatory reaction. In some cases, oral ivermectin results in an increase in pruritus and self-trauma. Larger masses may require surgical cytoreduction. The intralesional injection of corticosteroid is recommended to decrease the allergic or inflammatory reaction to the larvae. Successful resolution using systemic corticosteroids alone has been reported.[114] Re-infestation can be prevented by application of topical organophosphates or by placing the wound under a bandage. Topical preparations that combine organophosphates, corticosteroids, dimethyl sulfoxide, and nitrofurazone have been used.[102,113] The ophthalmic form of habronemiasis can be treated with oral ivermectin, topical corticosteroid eye drops, and curettage. Careful assessment of the corneal integrity should be made prior to the use of ophthalmic corticosteroids.

PYTHIOSIS

Epidemiology

Pythiosis is a cutaneous disease caused by invasion of the organism *Pythium insidiosum,* a fungus-like oomycete.[115] The disease occurs principally in warm, tropical regions; the organism has an aquatic life cycle and requires relatively warm temperatures for reproduction.[115] Pythiosis is commonly seen in the southern United States during the late summer and early fall. Horses are infected when invasion occurs through small wounds or skin breaks, typically in lakes, swamps, or flooded lands. Zoospores, released during reproduction, are attracted to organic debris and invade open wounds.[115] Characteristic lesions are ulcerative masses of granulation tissue. Rapid enlargement can occur, even within a matter of days. Pythiosis is often pruritic; sinus tracts are visible and often contain gritty, coral-like masses, called "kunker" or "leeches."[116] Kunker are made of necrotic vessels, inflammatory cells, and *Pythium* hyphae. Pythiosis occurs most commonly on the distal extremities and ventral body wall.[117] In chronic, untreated infections, invasion of deeper tissues, including bone, joints, tendons sheaths, and lymph nodes, can occur.[117,119-121] The diagnosis of pythiosis is made on the basis of the history and clinical signs, when the causative organism is found on culture or histopathologic examination.

Treatment

Surgical excision is the treatment of choice for pythiosis. If surgical excision is impossible because of the size or location of the lesion, the prognosis for resolution is poor. Systemic, topical, and intralesional antifungals have been used, but recurrence is common.[121]

Amphotericin B is administered intravenously at a dosage of 0.3 mg/kg diluted in 1 L of 5% dextrose.[122] The dose is increased by 0.1 mg/kg every 3rd day until a maximal dosage of 0.8 to 0.9 mg/kg is achieved. Treatment can be continued daily for 30 days and then every other day until the horse is cured. *Sodium iodide* administered intravenously has been recommended as an adjunctive therapy.[121]

In addition, a topical dressing containing 50 mg amphotericin B, 10 mL sterile water, and 10 mL dimethyl sulfoxide is recommended.[120] Because amphotericin B is nephrotoxic, serum creatinine, urea nitrogen, hydration status, water consumption, and urine output should be closely monitored. Reported side effects of amphotericin B include depression, anorexia, pyrexia, and urticaria.

Immunotherapy using a vaccine made from fungal cultures is reportedly curative if administered early in the course of the disease.[123] In a study of 40 horses with pythiosis, 53% were cured with vaccination alone. Surgical cytoreduction combined with vaccination improved success rates if vaccination was performed within 2 weeks of surgical débridement.[123]

NODULAR NECROBIOSIS

Epidemiology

Nodular necrobiosis, also called collagenolytic granulomas or eosinophilic granulomas with collagen degeneration, is reported to be one of the most common skin diseases in horses.[124] The underlying etiology is unclear; insect hypersensitivity has been proposed, and the propensity for lesions to develop at pressure points (under the saddle region, in particular) suggests trauma may play a role.[125] Diagnosis is based on histopathologic findings of a granulomatous reaction containing eosinophils, lymphocytes, and histiocytes, with collagen degeneration.[126] Typical lesions are 0.5- to 1.0-cm subcutaneous nodules and are most commonly found on the withers and dorsum but can occur anywhere on the body. The differential diagnosis includes equine amyloidosis, foreign body granuloma, dermoid cysts, habronemiasis, equine sarcoid, and other neoplasia.

Treatment

Single asymptomatic lesions that are not a cosmetic concern can be left untreated. Single lesions can be surgically excised. Alternatively, intralesional injection of glucocorticoids such as triamcinolone acetonide (3 to 5 mg per lesion) or methylprednisolone acetate (5 to 10 mg per lesion) can be performed.[124] Lesions that are calcified can be difficult to inject and may require surgical excision.[102] Systemic corticosteroids have been recommended to treat multiple lesions—for example, prednisolone at 1 mg/kg orally, daily for 14 days, followed by 0.5 mg/kg orally for an additional 14 days. Lesions may recur and require multiple retreatments for resolution.

PAPILLOMATOSIS

Epidemiology

Papillomaviruses are very host and tissue specific and are the causative agents of the majority of warts seen in mammals. Equine papillomatosis and aural plaques are caused by equine papillomaviruses (EqPV).[127] Papillomaviruses infect the basal layer of the epidermis, resulting in an abnormal proliferation and hyperkeratosis of the epithelium. Clinical syndromes include aural plaques and juvenile papillomas (juvenile warts). Congenital neonatal papillomatosis was thought to be the result of in utero infection by papillomavirus; however, recent reports suggest that congenital papillomatosis is in reality a hamartomatous lesion and not a virus-induced growth.[128] Affected foals are born with a large wartlike lesion located anywhere on the integument.

Juvenile Papillomatosis

Juvenile papillomatosis most commonly occurs in young horses (6 months to 4 years), but older horses can be affected. Multiple small (5-mm) gray-pink, vegetative, cauliflower-like warts usually develop on the lips, muzzle, face, distal limbs, and external genitalia. Lesions can be spread by direct contact, contamination of the local environment, and vectors. Large numbers of infectious virus are shed in the superficial keratinocytes.

Aural Plaques

Aural plaques are raised, white or tan, smooth plaques arising on the internal surface of the pinnae (Fig. 29-4). Fly irritation may exacerbate these lesions, making them crack and causing the horse discomfort. Equine papillomavirus DNA has been identified in both aural plaques and juvenile papillomas, but different viral subtypes are suspected.

Treatment

Congenital papillomas can be removed surgically or ligated and allowed to undergo necrosis. In the majority of cases, juvenile warts will spontaneously regress once immune recognition occurs. Immunologic compromise may result in failure to regress; in these cases, surgical excision may be necessary. Vaccination using wart tissue has been recommended.[129] Alternative treatments include cryotherapy, intralesional chemotherapy, and radiofrequency hyperthermia.

Historically, treatment protocols for aural plaques have been unrewarding, although successful resolution using laser ablation has recently been reported. The lesions are manually débrided with a dry gauze pad to remove

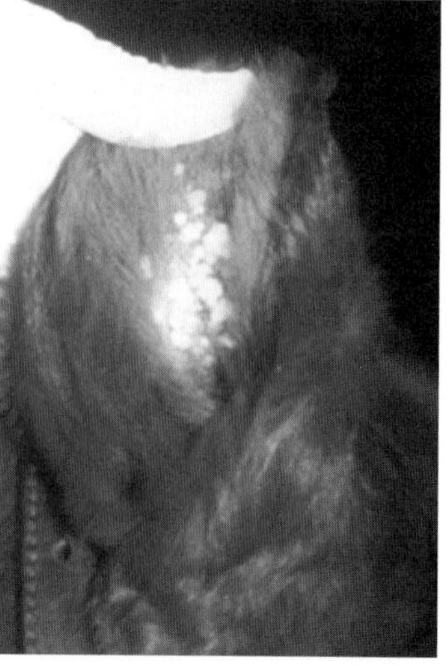

Figure 29-4. Typical appearance of aural plaques in the pinna.

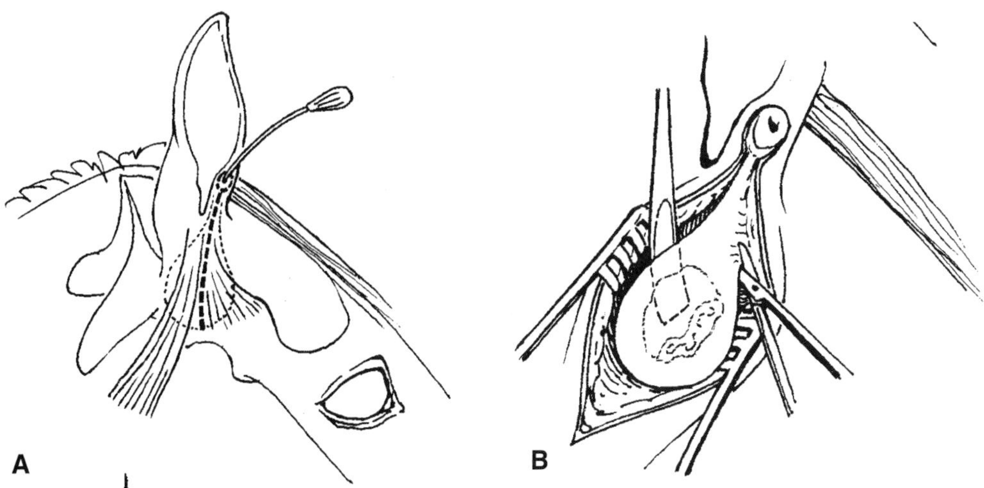

Figure 29-5. Dentigerous cyst. **A,** Identification of the sinus tract is made easier with a malleable probe inserted into the cloaca until it touches the dental material. **B,** After closure of the sinus tract, the cyst is removed intact. The dental material may need to be loosened with an elevator or an osteotome to complete cyst removal.

keratinous debris, and then the lesions are lightly painted with the laser probe. Recurrence has not been reported.[130]

DENTIGEROUS CYSTS

Etiology

A dentigerous cyst is a congenital defect. It arises as a result of incomplete closure of the first branchial cleft during embryologic development. By definition, dentigerous cysts contain dental elements, such as enamel, dentin, and cementum.[131] The epidermal lining differentiates as does normal epidermis, and the cyst becomes nodular as it begins to fill with keratin. Lesions are usually asymptomatic. They may be present from birth, but they remain unnoticed until they enlarge.[131,132] They typically appear as a unilateral swelling at the base of the ear but can occur in other locations on the head and sinuses.[131-134] The secretory, cystic lining produces a mucoid fluid that may drain intermittently from the nodule. Diagnosis is frequently made on the basis of location, clinical history, and the presence of pale yellow, mucoid, cystic fluid.[132] Definitive diagnosis requires surgical excision and histopathologic examination.

Treatment

No treatment is required. However, if desired, surgical excision with complete extirpation of the cyst lining is necessary to prevent recurrence.[135] Preoperative radiographic evaluation is recommended to determine the location of dental material and the number of cysts, and prior to anesthesia, the extent of the cyst should be defined by careful palpation. The preparation and surgical scrub should include the pinnae to allow manipulation during surgery. The sinus tract, which is identified using a malleable probe (Fig. 29-5), is opened and the neck of the cyst sealed with a ligature prior to dissection. The plane of dissection should be as close to the wall of the cyst as possible to prevent damage to the auriculopalpebral nerve and auricular muscles, as well as to minimize hemorrhage. Distention of the cyst aids in its identification and removal. The auricular muscles are small and can be difficult to visualize because of the aberrant connective tissue associated with the dentigerous cyst. Opening the cyst should be avoided at all cost; spillage can result in contamination of the incision site and result in infection, dehiscence, and excessive scarring. The dental tissue can vary in size from a small and easily removable tooth to large areas of enamel-covered bone. Careful excision using a chisel or drill is required in such cases to prevent damage to the cranium and brain.[133] Failure to remove all the dental tissue may result in dehiscence and refistulization. Auricular muscles and fascial layers are apposed with 3-0 polydioxanone, and skin closure is routine. Postoperative antibiotics are not routinely indicated, although anti-inflammatory drugs are recommended, particularly when forceful extraction of dental tissue was required. In one report, an ectopic tooth was found compressing the cerebellum.[133]

REFERENCES

1. Jackson C: The incidence and pathology of tumours of domestic animals in South Africa: A study of the Onderrstepoort collection of neoplasms with special reference to their histopathology, Onderstepoort J Vet Res 1936;6:1.
2. Knottenbelt D, Edwards S, Daniel E: Diagnosis and treatment of equine sarcoid, In Pract 1995;March:123.
3. Marti E, Lazary S, Antczak DF, et al: Report on the first international workshop on equine sarcoid, Equine Vet J 1993;13:235.
4. Angelos J, Oppenheim Y, Rebhun W, et al: Evaluation of breed as a risk factor for sarcoid and uveitis in horses, Anim Genet 1988;19:417.
5. Meredith D, Elser AH, Wolf B, et al: Equine leukocyte antigens: relationship with sarcoid tumors and laminitis in two pure breeds, Immunogen 1986;23:221.
6. Lazary S, Gerber H, Glatt PA, et al: Equine leucocyte antigens in sarcoid-affected horses, Equine Vet J 1985;17:283.
7. Bronstrum H, Fahlbrink E, Dubath ML, et al: Association between equine leucocyte antigens (ELA) and equine sarcoid tumors in the population of Swedish halfbreds and some of their families, Vet Immunol Immunopathol 1988;19:21523.

8. James VS: A family tendency to equine sarcoid, Southw Vet 1968; 21:235.
9. Reid SW, Gettinby G, Fowler JN, et al: Epidemiological observations on sarcoids in a population of donkeys (*Equus asinus*), Vet Rec 1994;134:207.
10. Olsen C, Cook RH: Cutaneous sarcoma-like lesions of the horse caused by the agent bovine papilloma, Proc Soc Exper Biol Med 1951;77:281.
11. Lancaster WD, Olson C, Meinke W: bovine papilloma virus: Presence of virus-specific DNA sequences in naturally occurring equine tumors, Proc Natl Acad Sci U S A 1977;74:524.
12. Lancaster WD, Theilen GHH, Olson C: Hybridization of bovine papilloma virus type 1 and 2 DNA to DNA from virus-induced hamster tumors and naturally occurring equine tumors, Intervirology 1979;11:227.
13. Amtmann E, Muller H, Sauer G: Equine connective tissue tumors contain unintegrated bovine papilloma virus DNA, J Virol 1980;35:962.
14. Lancaster WD: Apparent lack of integration of bovine papillomavirus DNA in virus-induced equine and bovine tumor cells and virus-transformed mouse cells, Virology 1981;108:251.
15. Trenfield K, Spradbrow PB, Vanselow B: Sequences of papillomavirus DNA in equine sarcoids, Equine Vet J 1985;17:449.
16. Angelos JA, Marti E, Lazary S, et al: Characterization of BPV-like DNA in equine sarcoids, Arch Virol 1991;119:95.
17. Lory S, von Tscharner C, Marti E, et al: In situ hybridisation of equine sarcoids with bovine papilloma virus, Vet Rec 1993;132:133.
18. Otten N, von Tscharner C, Lazary S, et al: DNA of bovine papillomavirus type 1 and 2 in equine sarcoids: PCR detection and direct sequencing, Arch Virol 1993;132:121.
19. Teifke JP: [Morphologic and molecular biologic studies of the etiology of equine sarcoid], Tierärztl Prax 1994;22:368.
20. Carr EA, Theon AP, Madewell BR, et al: Presence of bovine papillomavirus DNA in equine sarcoids in horses living in the Western United States, Am J Vet Res 2001;62:741.
21. Martens A, De Moor A, Demeulemeester J, et al: Polymerase chain reaction analysis of the surgical margins of equine sarcoids for bovine papillomaviral DNA, Vet Surg 2001;30:460.
22. Carr EA, Theon AP, Madewell BR, et al: Expression of a transforming gene (E5) of bovine papillomavirus in sarcoids obtained from horses, Am J Vet Res 2001;62:1212.
23. Carr EA: Unpublished data, 1999.
24. Ragland WL, Keown GH, Spencer GR: Equine sarcoid, Equine Vet J 1970;2:2.
25. Diehl M, Vingerhoets M, Stornetta D: Spezifische Methoden zur Entfenung des equinen Sarkoides, Tierärzt Prax 1987;7:14.
26. Knottenbelt DC, Kelly DF: The diagnosis and treatment of periorbital sarcoid in the horse: 445 cases from 1974-1999, Vet Ophthalmol 2000;3:169.
27. Pascoe RR, Knottenbelt DC: Equine sarcoid, In Pascoe RR, Knottenbelt DC, editors: Manual of Equine Dermatology, London, 1999, WB Saunders.
28. McCauley CT, Hawkins JF, Adams SB, et al: Use of a carbon dioxide laser for surgical management of cutaneous masses in horses: 32 cases (1993-2000), J Am Vet Med Assoc 2002;220:1192.
29. Carstanjen B, Jordan P, Lepage OM: Carbon dioxide laser as a surgical instrument for sarcoid therapy: A retrospective study on 60 cases, Can Vet J 1997;38:773.
30. Palmer SE: Carbon dioxide laser removal of a verrucous sarcoid from the ear of a horse, J Am Vet Med Assoc 1989;195:1125.
31. Vingerhoets M, Diehl M, Gerber H, et al: [The treatment of equine sarcoidosis by carbon dioxide laser], Schweiz Arch Tierheilk 1988;130:113.
32. Fretz PB, Barber SM: Prospective analysis of cryosurgery as the sole treatment for equine sarcoids, Vet Clin N Am Sm Anim Prac 1980;10:847.
33. Lane JG: The treatment of equine sarcoids by cryosurgery, Equine Vet J 1977;9:127.
34. Klein WR, Goosen EB, Misdorp W, et al: BCG immunotherapy compared to cryosurgery in a prospective randomized clinical trial, Can Immunol Immunother 1986;21:133.
35. Hoffman KD, Kainer RA, Shideler RK: Radio-frequency current-induced hyperthermia for the treatment of equine sarcoid, Equine Prac 1983;5:24.
36. Walker M, Adams W, Hoskinson J, et al: Iridium-192 brachytherapy for equine sarcoid, one and two year remission rates, Vet Radiol 1991;32:206.
37. Turrel JM, Stover SM, Gyorgyfalvy J: Iridium-192 brachytherapy of equine sarcoid, Vet Radiol 1985;26:20..
38. Wyn-Jones G: Treatment of equine cutaneous neoplasia by radiotherapy using iridium 192 linear sources, Equine Vet J 1983;15:361.
39. Theon AP, Pascoe JP: Iridium-192 brachytherapy for equine periocular tumours: treatment results and prognostic factors in 115 horses, Equine Vet J 1994;27:117.
40. Wyn-Jones G: Treatment of periocular tumours of horses using radioactive gold^{198} grains, Equine Vet J 1979;11:3.
41. Owen R, Jagger DW: Clinical observations on the use of BCG cell wall fraction for treatment of periocular and other equine sarcoids, Vet Rec 1987;120:548.
42. Lavach JD, Sullins KE, Roberts SM, et al: BCG treatment of periocular sarcoid, Equine Vet J 1985;17:445.
43. Vanselow BA, Abetz I: BCG emulsion immunotherapy of equine sarcoid, Equine Vet J 1988;20:444.
44. Theon AP, Pascoe JR, Carelton GP, et al: Intratumoral chemotherapy with cisplatin in oily emulsion in horses, J Am Vet Med 1993;15:261.
45. Theon AP, Pascoe JR, Meagher DM: Perioperative intratumoral administration of cisplatin for treatment of cutaneous tumors in Equidae, J Am Vet Med Assoc 1994;205:1170.
46. Otten N, Marti E, Soderstrom C, et al: Experimental treatment of equine sarcoid using a xanthate compound and recombinant human tumour necrosis factor alpha, J Vet Med 1994;41:757.
47. Knottenbelt DC, Walker JA: Topical treatment of the equine sarcoid, Equine Vet Ed 1994;6:72.
48. Roberts D: Experimental treatment of equine sarcoid, Proc Am Assoc Equine Pract 1969;15:69.
49. Kinnunen RE, Tallberg T, Stenback S: Equine sarcoid tumour treated by autogenous tumour vaccine, Antican Res 1999;19:3367.
50. Baker JR: Histologic survey of tumours of the horse, with particular reference to those of the skin, Vet Rec 1975;96:419.
51. Sundberg JP, Burnstein T, Page EH, et al: Neoplasia of equidae, J Am Vet Med Assoc 1977;170:150.
52. Strafus C: Squamous cell carcinoma in horses, J Am Vet Med Assoc 1976;168:61.
53. Dixon PM, Head KW: Equine nasal and paranasal sinus tumours: Part 2. A contribution of 28 case reports, Vet J 1999;157:279.
54. Jones DL: Squamous cell carcinoma of the larynx and pharynx in horses, Cornell Vet 1994;84:15.
55. Berry CR, O'Brien TR, Pool RR: Squamous cell carcinoma of the hoof wall in a stallion, J Am Vet Med Assoc 1991;199:90.
56. Durham AE, Walmsley JP: Squamous cell carcinoma of the epidermal laminae, Equine Vet Ed 1997;9:30.
57. Hargis AM: A review of solar induced lesions in domestic animals, Comp Cont Educ Pract Vet 1981;3:287.
58. Dugan SJ, Curtis CR, Roberts SM, et al: Epidemiologic study of ocular/adnexal squamous cell carcinoma in horses, J Am Vet Med Assoc 1991;198:251.
59. Fessler JF, Faber NA, Blevins WE, et al: Squamous cell carcinoma associated with a chronic wound in a horse, J AM Vet Med Assoc 1993;202:615.
60. Schumacher J, Watkins JP, Wilson SR, et al: Burn-induced neoplasia in two horses, Equine Vet J 1986;18:410.
61. Madewell BR, Theilen GH: Tumors of the skin and subcutaneous tissues. In Madewell BR, Theilen GH, editors: Veterinary Cancer Medicine, ed 2, Philadelphia, 1987, Lea & Febiger.

62. King TC, Priehs DR, Gum GG, et al: Therapeutic management of ocular squamous cell carcinoma in the horse: 43 cases (1979-1989), Equine Vet J 1991;23:449.
63. Mair TS, Walmsley JP, Phillips TJ: Surgical treatment of 45 horses affected by squamous cell carcinoma of the penis and prepuce, Equine Vet J 2000;32:406.
64. Rebhun WC: Treatment of advanced squamous cell carcinoma involving the equine cornea, Vet Surg 1990;19:297.
65. Van der Woerdt A, Gilger BC, Wilkie DA: Penetrating keratoplasty for treatment of recurrent squamous cell carcinoma of the cornea in a horse, J Am Vet Med Assoc 1996;208:1692.
66. Hilbert BJ, Farrell RK, Grant BD: Cryotherapy of periocular squamous cell carcinoma in the horse, J Am Vet Med Assoc 1977; 170:1305.
67. Joyce JR: Cryosurgical treatment of tumors of horses and cattle, J Am Vet Med Assoc 1976;168:226.
68. Elkon D, Constable WC: The use of strontium-90 in the treatment of carcinoma in situ of the conjunctiva, Am J Ophthalmol 1979; 87:84.
69. Frauenfelder HC, Blevins WE, Page EH: 90Sr for treatment of periocular squamous cell carcinoma in the horse, J Am Vet Med Assoc 1982;180:307.
70. Owen LN, Barnett KC: Treatment of equine squamous cell carcinoma of the conjunctiva using strontium 90 applicator, Equine Vet J 1983;15:125.
71. Gavin PR, Gillette EL: Interstitial radiation therapy of equine squamous cell carcinomas, J Am Radiol Soc 1978;19:138.
72. Theon AP, Pascoe JP: Ir-192 interstitial brachytherapy for equine periocular tumors—treatment results and prognostic factors in 115 horses, Equine Vet J 1995;27:117.
73. Walker MA, Goble D, Geiser D: Two-year non-recurrence rates for equine ocular and periorbittal squamous cell carcinoma following radiotherapy: comparison to previous reports, Vet Radiol 1986; 27:146.
74. Fortier LA, Mac Harg MA: Topical use of 5-fluorouracil for treatment of squamous cell carcinoma of the external genitalia of horses: 11 cases (1988-1992), J Am Vet Med Assoc 1994;205:1183.
75. Paterson S: Treatment of superficial ulcerative squamous cell carcinoma in horses with topical 5-fluorouracil, Vet Rec 1997; 141:626.
76. Moore AS, Beam SL, Rassnick KM, et al: Long-term control of mucocutaneous squamous cell carcinoma and metastases in a horse using piroxicam, Equine Vet J 2003;35:715.
77. McEntee MF, Cates JM, Neilsen N: Cyclooxygenase-2 expression in spontaneous intestinal neoplasia of domestic dogs, Vet Pathol 2002;39:428.
78. McCalla TL, Moore CP, Collier LL: Immunotherapy of periocular squamous cell carcinoma with metastasis in a pony, J Am Vet Med Assoc 1992;200:1678.
79. Dugan SJ, Roberts SM, Curtis CR, et al: Prognostic factors and survival of horses with ocular/adnexal squamous cell carcinoma: 147 cases (1978-1988), J Am Vet Med Assoc 1991;198:298.
80. Johnson PJ: Dermatologic tumors (excluding sarcoids), Vet Clin North Am Equine Pract 1998;14:625.
81. Seltenhammer MH, Simhofer H, Scherzer S: Equine melanoma in a population of 296 grey Lipizzaner horses, Equine Vet J 2003;35:153.
82. Levine A: Equine melanotic disease, Tumori 1971;57:133.
83. Fleury C, Berard F, Balme B, et al: The study of cutaneous melanomas in Camargue-type gray-skinned horses: (1) Clinical-pathological characterization, Pigment Cell Res 2000;13:39.
84. Valentine BA: Equine melanocytic tumors: Retrospective study of 53 horses (1988-1991), J Vet Intern Med 1995;9:291.
85. Honnas CM, Liskey CC, Meagher DM: Malignant melanoma in the foot of a horse, J Am Vet Med Assoc 1990;197:756.
86. Kirker-Head CA, Loeffler D, Held JP, et al: Pelvic limb lameness due to malignant melanoma in a horse, J Am Vet Med Assoc 1985;186:1215.
87. Kunze DJ, Monticello TM, Jakob TP, et al: Malignant melanoma of the coronary band in a horse, J Am Vet Med Assoc 1986;188:297.
88. MacGillivray KC, Sweeney RW, Del Piero F: Metastatic melanoma in horses, J Vet Intern Med 2002;16:452.
89. Murphy J, Young S: Intraocular melanoma in a horse, Vet Pathol 1979;16:539.
90. Schott HC, Major MD, Grant BD, et al: Melanoma as a cause of spinal cord compression in two horses, J Am Vet Med Assoc 1990;11:1820.
91. Giuffre G, Muscarella A, Todaro P, et al: Malignant hypomelanotic melanoma of mules: A histologic, immunohistochemical and ultrastructural study of a case with unknown primary site and widespread metastases, Pathologica 1995;87:100.
92. McCauley CT, Hawkins JF, Adams SB, et al: Use of a carbon dioxide laser for surgical management of cutaneous masses in horses: 32 cases (1993-2000), J Am Vet Med Assoc 2002;220:1192.
93. Goetz TE, Long MT: Treatment of melanomas in horses, Comp Cont Educ Pract Vet 1993;15:608.
94. Warnick LD, Graham ME, Valentine BA: Evaluation of cimetidine treatment for melanomas in seven horses, Equine Pract 1995; 17:16.
95. Bowers JR, Huntington PJ, Slocombe RF: Efficacy of cimetidine for the therapy of skin tumours of horses: 10 cases, Aust Vet J 1994;12:30.
96. Goetz TE, Ogilvie GK, Keegan KG, et al: Cimetidine for the treatment of melanomas in three horses, J Am Vet Med Assoc 1990; 196:449.
97. Goetz TE, Boulton CH, Ogilvie GK: Clinical management of progressive multifocal benign and malignant melanomas of horses with oral cimetidine, Proc Am Assoc Equine Pract 1989;35,431.
98. Hare JE, Staempfli HR: Cimetidine for the treatment of melanomas in horses: Efficacy determined by client questionnaire, Equine Pract 1994;16:18.
99. Theon AP: Cisplatin treatment for cutaneous tumors. In Robinson NE, editor: Current Therapy in Equine Medicine IV, Philadelphia, 1997, Saunders.
100. Jeglum KA: Melanomas. In Robinson NE, editor: Current Therapy in Equine Medicine IV, Philadelphia, 1997, WB Saunders.
101. Heinzerling LM, Feige K, Reider S, et al: Tumor regression induced by intratumoral injection of DNA coding for human interleukin 12 into melanoma metastases in gray horses, J Mol Med 2001; 78:692.
102. Mathison PT: Eosinophilic nodular dermatoses, Vet Clin North Am Equine Pract 1995;11:75.
103. Riley CB, Yovich JV, Howell JM: Malignant mast cell tumours in horses, Aust Vet J 1991;68:346.
104. Malikides N, Reppas G, Hodgson JL, et al: Mast cell tumors in the horse: 4 case reports, Equine Pract 1996;18:12.
105. Prasse KW, Lundvall RL, Cheville NF: Generalized mastocytosis in a foal, resembling urticaria pigmentosa of man, J Am Vet Med Assoc 1975;166:68.
106. McEntee MF: Equine cutaneous mastocytoma: morphology, biological behaviour and evolution of the lesion, J Comp Pathol 1991;104:171.
107. Bristol DG, Fubini SL: External lipomas in three horses, J Am Vet Med Assoc 1984;185:791.
108. Lepage OM, Laverty S, Drolet R, et al: Infiltrative lipoma in a quarter horse, Cornell Vet 1993;83:57.
109. Hammer EJ, Chope K, Lemire TD, et al: A lipoma of the extensor tendon sheaths in a horse, Vet Radiol Ultrasound 2002;43:63.
110. Pulley LT, Stannard AA: Skin and soft tissue. In Moulton JE, editor: Tumors in Domestic Animals, Berkeley, 1990, University of California Press.
111. Georgi JR: Nematodes. In Georgi JR, editor: Parasitology for Veterinarians, ed 4, Philadelphia, 1985, WB Saunders.
112. Pascoe RR, Knottenbelt DC: Metazoan/parasitic diseases. In Pascoe RR, Knottenbelt DC, editors: Manual of Equine Dermatology, London, 1999, WB Saunders.

113. Scott DW: Parasitic diseases. In Scott DW, editor: Large Animal Dermatology, Philadelphia, 1988, WB Saunders.
114. Fadok VA, Mullowney PC: Dermatologic disease of horses: Part I. Parasitic dermatoses of the horse, Comp Cont Educ Pract Vet 1983;5:S615.
115. Scott DW: Fungal disease. In Scott DW, editor: Large Animal Dermatology, Philadelphia, 1988, WB Saunders.
116. Miller RI, Campbell RS: The comparative pathology of equine cutaneous phycomycosis, Vet Pathol 1984;21:325.
117. Miller RI, Campbell RS: Clinical observations on equine phycomycosis, Aust Vet J 1982;58:221.
118. Murray DR, Ladds PW, Johnson RH, et al: Metastatic phycomycosis in a horse, J Am Vet Med Assoc 1978;172:834.
119. Neuwirth L: Radiographic appearance of lesions associated with equine pythiosis, Comp Cont Educ Pract Vet 1993;15:489.
120. Pascoe RR, Knottenbelt DC: Fungal diseases. In Pascoe RR, Knottenbelt DC, editors: Manual of Equine Dermatology, London, 1999, WB Saunders.
121. Miller RI: Equine phycomycosis, Comp Cont Educ Pract Vet 1983;5:S472.
122. Chaffin KM, Schumacher J, McMullan WC: Cutaneous pythiosis in the horse, Vet Clin North Am Equine Pract 1995;11:91.
123. Miller RI: Treatment of equine phycomycosis by immunotherapy and surgery, Aust Vet J 1981;57:377.
124. Pascoe RR, Knottenbelt DC: Immune mediated/allergic diseases. In Pascoe RR, Knottenbelt DC, editors: Manual of Equine Dermatology, London, 1999, WB Saunders.
125. Scott DW: Miscellaneous dermatosis. In Scott DW, editor: Large Animal Dermatology, Philadelphia, 1988, WB Saunders.
126. Yager JA, Scott DW: The skin and appendages. In Jubb KVF, Kennedy PC, Palmer N, editors: Pathology of Domestic Animals, ed 3, London, 1985, Academic Press.
127. Scott DW: Neoplastic diseases. In Scott DW, editor: Large Animal Dermatology, Philadelphia, 1988, WB Saunders.
128. White KS, Fuji RN, Valentine BA, et al: Equine congenital papilloma: pathological findings and results of papillomavirus immunohistochemistry in 5 cases, Vet Dermatol 2004;15:240.
129. Pascoe RR, Knottenbelt DC: Viral diseases. In Pascoe RR, Knottenbelt DC, editors: Manual of Equine Dermatology, London, 1999, WB Saunders.
130. Stick J: Personal communication, 2005.
131. Rashmir-Ravin A, DeBowes RM, Cash WC, et al: Dentigerous cysts, Comp Cont Educ Pract Vet 1990;12:1120.
132. DeBowes RM, Gaughan EM: Congenital dental disease of horses. In Gaughan EM, DeBowes RM, editors: Veterinary Clinics of North America Equine Practice: Dentistry, London, 1998, WB Saunders.
133. Hunt RJ, Allen D, Mueller PO: Intracranial trauma associated with extraction of a temporal ear tooth (dentigerous cyst) in a horse, Cornell Vet 1991;81:103.
134. Fessler JF: Heterotophic polydontia in: Nine cases (1969-1986), J Am Vet Med Assoc 1988;192:535.
135. Adams SB, Fessler JF: Atlas of Equine Surgery, Philadelphia, 2000, WB Saunders.

SECTION **V** ALIMENTARY SYSTEM

John A. Stick

CHAPTER 30

Oral Cavity and Salivary Glands

Padraic M. Dixon
Mathew P. Gerard

DENTISTRY

After almost a century of inactivity, equine dentistry has made rapid progress over the past 10 years, and equine dental disorders are now documented as one of the most common diseases recognized by U.S. practitioners.[1] Additionally, up to 10% of British equine practitioners' time is spent dealing with dental-related disorders.[2] This part of the chapter will concentrate on the many surgical aspects of this expanding field of study. The modified Triadan system of dental nomenclature (Fig. 30-1) is used here.

Examination of the Oral Cavity and Teeth

The equine incisors and canine teeth are readily examined in the unsedated horse. With the mouth closed, the rostral aspect of the mandible should be pushed sideways and the distance of lateral movement of the lower incisors in relation to their upper counterparts (e.g., 1 cm) prior to separation of the incisors (as the angled occlusal surfaces of opposing cheek teeth [CT] come into contact) should be measured. This measurement can be used to assess the angulation of the CT occlusal surfaces and can also detect the presence of major CT overgrowths.[3] This maneuver is easier to perform in sedated horses, as is visual examination of the oral cavity. Because of a combination of factors, including the limited angle of opening of the equine mouth (common to all herbivores), the rostral positioning of the lip commissures, and the length of the equine CT rows, it is very difficult to visually examine the CT, particularly in unsedated horses. Palpation through the cheeks may reveal food pocketing or major dental irregularities (such as a displaced or missing maxillary CT, or a large overgrowth of the rostral CT). Even if no abnormalities are palpable, stimulation of a pain response during this palpation may indicate the presence of sharp overgrowths on the lateral aspect of the upper CT. A useful test for suspected cases of dental disease is to feed the (unsedated) horse a small amount of forage. Affected horses may not make the normal vigorous crunching sounds of mastication, may show restricted mandibular movements that may be confined to one side of the mouth, or may quid (drop boluses of partially masticated forage) if a painful dental disease is present.

A detailed equine oral examination can only be performed using a full mouth speculum (gag), and every equine practitioner should have one (Fig. 30-2). It is possible to perform a safe digital examination of the CT and oral cavity of most unsedated horses, but a more complete visual examination requires sedation, especially with

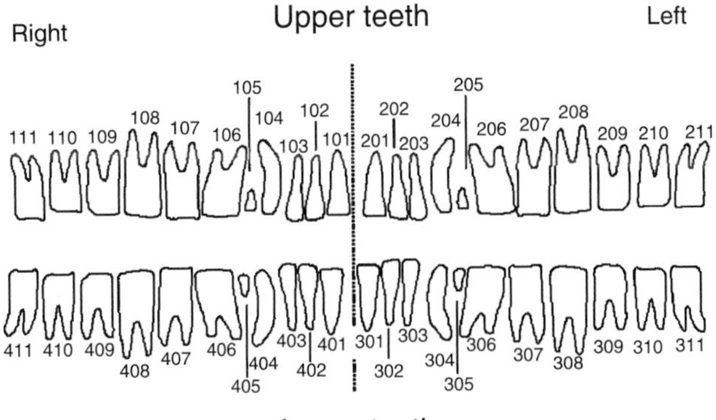

Figure 30-1. The modified Triadan system of equine dental nomenclature. To identify deciduous teeth, add 4 to the first number of its permanent successor. For example, the deciduous incisor 501 is replaced by permanent incisor 101.

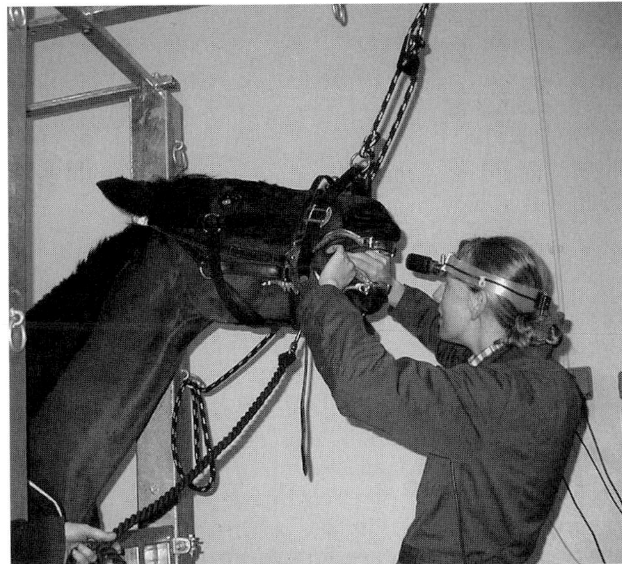

Figure 30-2. This horse is having a dental examination while being restrained in stocks, which has an overhead extension to allow a dental head collar to be attached. Note the use of the Hausmann speculum and headlight for this examination.

painful disorders and in difficult horses. Food retained in the oral cavity should be removed by flushing the mouth using a large dental (dosing) syringe and water or a very dilute chlorhexidine solution. The use of a strong headlight (a hand-held light is much less satisfactory), a dental probe or metal examination "basket" to displace the tongue, and an equine dental mirror (or a rigid dental endoscope, if available) allows full visual examination of the equine oral cavity.

Unless each tooth and the adjacent soft tissues (gums, cheeks, and tongue) are carefully visualized and palpated, major disorders, especially of the caudal CT and of the adjacent periodontal membranes, can readily be missed. A long dental mirror or intraoral endoscope is essential to examine the gingival margins of the CT, especially their buccal aspects, and also to visualize their occlusal surfaces (e.g., to detect pulpar exposure and more fully assess dental fractures and infundibular caries). It is also useful to smell the oral cavity for halitosis, which usually indicates anaerobic infections—most commonly as a result of periodontal food pocketing with infection, but occasionally caused by advanced dental infections (caries) or CT fractures.

A very significant disorder, especially in the younger horse, is CT apical (the roots are often not yet even formed) abscessation. In most cases, little *obvious* change is visible on the clinical crown, except with some maxillary CT apical infections, where gross infundibular caries or sagittal fractures of the clinical crown may be present. However, close examination of the occlusal surface of the suspect CT with a dental mirror or endoscope, and probing the secondary dentine on the occlusal surface with a fine steel probe, will reveal pulpar exposure (i.e., dull, darker areas of the secondary dentine, with pitting and food pocketing into the pulp chamber) in about 25% of infected teeth.[4] This finding can be of enormous value when other clinical findings and radiology are inconclusive in cases of apical infection.

Disorders of the Incisors

Overjet and Overbite ("Parrot Mouth")

Many horses have some degree of what the older textbooks term mandibular brachygnathism ("parrot mouth," "overshot jaw")—that is, a rostral projection of the upper incisors beyond the lower incisors in a horizontal direction, which should be termed "overbite." However, in some of these cases, there may not be shortness of the mandible. Instead, an overlong maxilla (maxillary prognathism) may be present. Both of these conditions induce CT wear disorders.[5] Consequently, a major significance of overjet is that it very commonly occurs with overgrowths of the rostral aspects of 106 and 206 and of the caudal aspects of 311 and 411. In older horses with overjet, the reduced wear on upper incisors 101 and 201, in particular, may cause them to overgrow, and the upper incisors subsequently develop a convex occlusal surface, which has been termed a "smile." In more severe cases, the upper incisors lie rostral to the lower incisors in a vertical direction (i.e., *overbite*), and this may prevent the small, normal amount of rostrocaudal mandibular movement that occurs in horses,[6] and it may even retard mandibular growth, thus exacerbating CT abnormalities.[7] Unless contact between opposing incisors is totally absent, overjet/overbite rarely causes the horse trouble in prehending food, as its mobile lips and tongue can compensate. However, this condition is aesthetically undesirable, especially in show horses.

In affected foals, overjet can be corrected by use of an incisor orthodontic brace—that is, by placing steel wires (a tension band) around the upper incisors and fixing these wires around the 506 and 606, or upper 07s, to retard growth of the premaxilla and maxilla.[7,8] This surgery is best performed at around 3 months of age, but it can be of value in foals up to 8 months old. Under general anesthesia, a 1-cm horizontal stab incision is made in the skin of the cheeks, as dorsal as possible to avoid damaging branches of the dorsal buccal nerve, opposite the interdental spaces between the upper 06s and 07s, or between the 07s and 08s. A short Steinmann pin fitted to a handle (or a bone drill within a guide) can now be pushed through the skin wound to puncture the cheeks and enter the oral cavity (Fig. 30-3). Using a finger in the oral cavity for guidance, the point of the pin is directed into the interdental space, as close to the gingiva as possible, and it is then forcibly pushed (while twisting) through this tight space and directed to exit at the medial (palatal) interdental space, again close to gingiva (at the border of the hard palate). The Steinmann pin is then withdrawn and a 14-gauge needle is inserted along its path, and a 60-cm length of 6 or 7 metric (18 U.S. gauge) stainless steel wire is inserted through the needle into the interdental space and into the oral cavity (Fig. 30-4). Most of the wire is drawn into the oral cavity and pulled rostrally to the incisors, and the needle is withdrawn.

The external free end of the wire is then directed beside the initial part of the wire through the buccal incision into the oral cavity, taking great care not to entrap any soft tissue (possibly the buccal nerve). The second wire end is palpated as it penetrates the buccal mucosa, again as close as possible to the lateral (buccal) gingival margin of the interdental space. This part of the wire is subsequently drawn into the

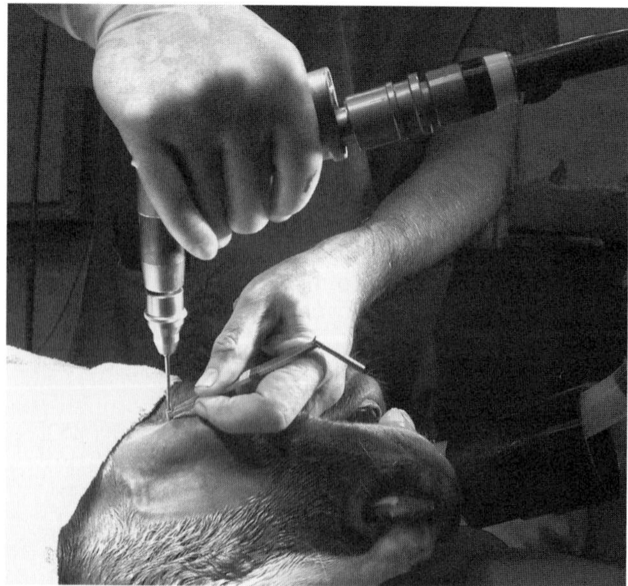

Figure 30-3. A bone drill and drill sleeve have been inserted through a horizontal stab incision in the skin and buccal muscles of this foal with overjet in order to drill between the deciduous cheek teeth for placement of a tension-band prosthesis.

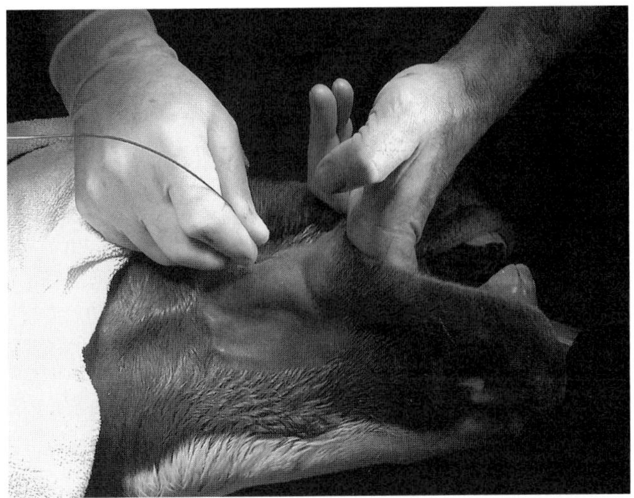

Figure 30-4. A length of 7 metric stainless steel wire is being inserted through the cheek incision into the interdental space between the 1st and 2nd cheek teeth (606 and 607).

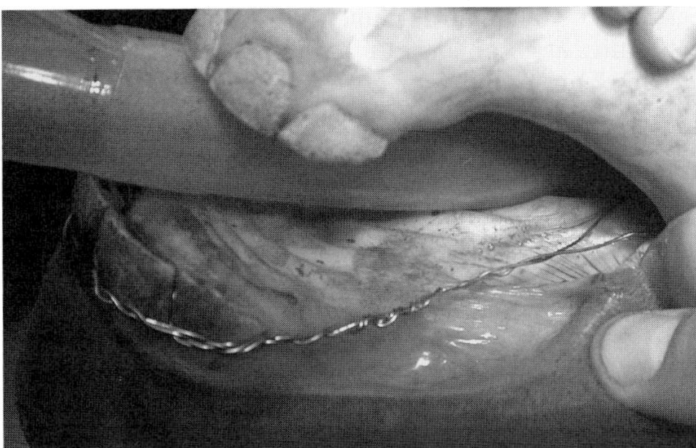

Figure 30-5. The twisted wires that are attached bilaterally to the cheek teeth have been interwoven between some incisors and then tightly joined together in front of the incisors, to retard premaxillary and maxillary growth.

oral cavity along the lateral aspect of the CT. As the last of the wire is pulled through the cheek incision, a kink will occur in it, and this area of weak wire should later be discarded.

The two free ends of the wire are withdrawn from the mouth, on either side of the cheek teeth, while making them even in length. While pulling them rostrally, the free ends are twisted back to the rostral border of the upper 06s, as dorsally as possible. The twisted wires are then placed over the labial (rostral) aspect of the incisors. This procedure is then repeated on the other side of the mouth, and the free ends of the both pairs of wires are twisted tightly together, just below the gingival borders of the upper incisors (or interwoven between some incisors at the gingival level) and their ends are trimmed (Fig. 30-5). The wire knot can be embedded in acrylic to prevent soft tissue trauma.

If overbite is also present in such foals, the tension from this orthodontic brace may well cause further caudoventral deviation of the upper incisors and premaxilla toward the rostral aspect of the lower incisors, and this would simply worsen the overbite, rather than retard premaxillary and maxillary bone growth. In such foals, a "biteplate" can additionally be fitted along with the orthodontic brace to promote indirect occlusion between the upper and lower incisors.[7] The biteplate can be fashioned from a perforated aluminium plate (2 to 4 mm thick) that is cut to fit the shape of the rostral aspect of the hard palate, extending caudally about 4 to 5 cm from the incisors The biteplate should be raised caudally, so that the sloped plate will tend to push the lower incisors more rostrally during prehension.

Having fitted the brace as just described, the underlying hard palate is covered in Vaseline, and the bite plate, covered in wet acrylic, is placed on the hard palate. Additional acrylic is used to join the biteplate to the wires of the brace (Fig. 30-6), ensuring that the acrylic does not extend too high on the gingiva above the incisors, where it can form a sharp rim that can traumatize the lip mucosa. After a biteplate is fitted, foals may have trouble suckling. The biteplate may also hurt the mare's udder during suckling, causing her to temporarily prevent the foal from suckling. In such cases, the mare

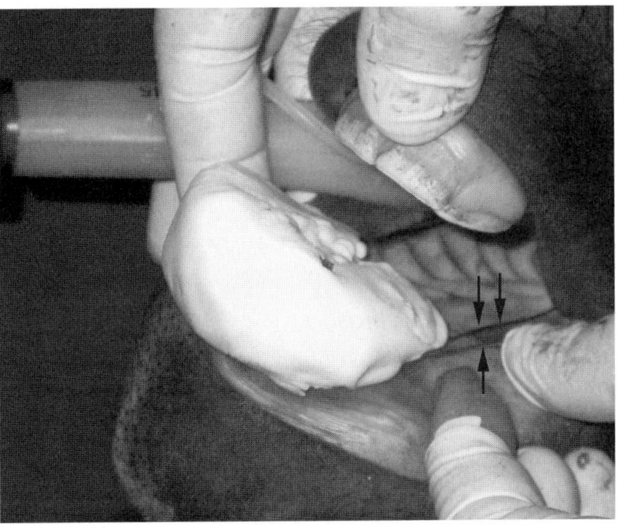

Figure 30-6. This foal had marked overbite as well as overjet, and it has had a perforated aluminium "bite plate" embedded in acrylic, attached to the orthodontic brace. The still soft methylmethacrylate is being moulded around the prosthetic wires *(arrows)* (untwisted in this case).

should be milked for a few days and the foal bottle fed with her milk. If the foal is uncomfortable because of the brace, it should be given low doses of nonsteroidal anti-inflammatory drugs and anti–gastric ulcer medication, such as omeprazole. Some clinicians recommend that foals be weaned before fitting orthodontic braces with biteplates. Any overgrowths on the rostral aspects of the upper 06s and on the caudal aspects of the lower 08s should be rasped off, to promote free rostrocaudal mandibular movement.

Wires may break unilaterally or bilaterally and thus cause the biteplate to loosen. Consequently, the foal's mouth needs to be regularly inspected, and broken wires need to be replaced, usually under general anesthesia. The brace can be removed when the incisors are aligned or nearly so. With severe overjet or overbite, complete resolution may not be possible, but aesthetically pleasing results, and certainly much reduction in the concurrent CT overgrowths, can be achieved. The ethics of these orthodontic procedures, especially in animals that may be used for breeding, are debatable, and some breed societies do not allow registration of horses that have been treated with this technique. This aspect has to be discussed with the owners in detail before orthodontic wires and biteplates are applied.

Orthodontic treatment is not feasible in adult horses. Large overjet/overbite incisor overgrowths in adult horses should be reduced if very overgrown, using power or manual instruments, in stages of about 5 mm, to prevent pulpar exposure. To remove incisor overgrowths, it is best to sedate the horse and use a plastic pipe in the interdental space (circular metal gags, such as Swale's gag, can fracture CT, and rubber wedge gags promote constant chewing). Once the overgrown incisors have been reasonably reduced, they should be rasped level biannually, as should concurrent CT overgrowths (see "Disorders of the Cheek Teeth," p. 327).

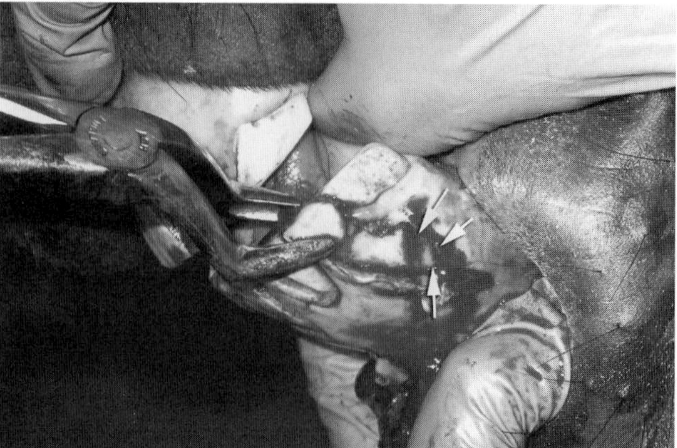

Figure 30-7. This horse has a large retained 702 (deciduous precursor of 302), and minimal resorption of its apex and reserve crown has occurred. A lingual (caudal) deviation of the permanent tooth is now present that would cause a permanent incisor malocclusion. About 5 cm of the rostral aspect of the alveolar wall of 702 was removed *(white arrows)*. The tooth was then loosened with elevators and is now being extracted with incisor forceps.

Underbite ("Sow Mouth")

Prognathism ("undershot jaw," "underbite") is uncommon in the horse, except in miniature horses, and is also usually clinically insignificant unless there is a total lack of occlusion between the upper and lower incisors. Severely affected horses eventually develop a concave upper incisor occlusal surface, which has been termed a "frown" and may develop *lower* 06 and *upper* 11 overgrowths.

Correction may be achieved using the same orthodontic procedures as discussed just previously.

Retained Deciduous Incisors

Deciduous incisors, which normally lie rostral (i.e., labial) to their permanent counterparts, are occasionally retained beyond their normal time of shedding, and they will then cause the permanent incisor to be displaced caudally, and they may even cause permanent changes in the incisor occlusal surface. If retained incisors are very loose, they can be removed using small-animal dental extraction forceps or equine "wolf teeth" forceps. If more firmly attached, they should be extracted under sedation and local anesthesia (by injecting 2 to 5 mL lidocaine, directed 2 to 4 cm caudally, into the ostium of the mental or infraorbital canal) using a small-animal dental elevator. If a permanent incisor does not erupt beneath its deciduous predecessor, little resorption of its reserve crown may occur and up to 6 cm of the deciduous reserve crown may remain in the alveolus. In such cases, some of the rostral aspect of the alveolus will have to be removed with a bone chisel to extract the retained incisor (Fig. 30-7). Occasionally, a permanent incisor will erupt *rostrally* to the deciduous incisor and great care must be taken in removing the deciduous incisor that is now positioned on the caudal (lingual) aspect of the permanent incisor.[9]

Supernumerary Incisors

Supernumerary incisors are permanent teeth that are additional to the normal six permanent incisors on each arcade and must be differentiated from retained incisors. Supernumerary incisors may have long (greater than 7.0 cm) reserve crowns that may be intimately related to the reserve crowns and roots of the normal permanent incisors, and therefore they are usually impossible to differentiate, both clinically and radiographically, from normal incisors.[10] Consequently, extraction of supernumerary incisors is technically very difficult and also risks damaging the normal teeth. If they are grossly displaced rostrally (labially) and thus protrude submucosally, they are amenable to extraction, as described for a large retained deciduous incisor. As most supernumerary incisors cause few clinical problems, they are usually best left alone (except, perhaps, in show horses), with biannual rasping of any incisors that are not in occlusion to prevent overgrowths.

Fractures of the Incisors

Fractures of the incisor teeth, and often of their supporting mandibular or premaxillary bones, can occur because of trauma (usually from kicks) and commonly result in exposure of the pulp (i.e., complicated dental fractures).[10,11] Idiopathic incisor fractures are rare, in contrast to fractures of the CT. All young equine teeth (incisors and CT) have very wide apical foramina (root canal openings), along with a very large, vascular pulp, which can resist the infection, and more so the inflammation, that inevitably develops in orally exposed pulp.[12] Consequently, pulpar exposure, especially in younger horses, does not necessarily lead to the degree of pulpar inflammation that compresses its vascular supply (with subsequent pulpar ischemia and necrosis, and death of the tooth), as usually occurs with pulpar exposure in brachydont (e.g., human or canine) teeth. Cases of incisor fracture should receive tetanus prophylaxis and prolonged (7 to 10 days) antibiotic (e.g., trimethoprim/sulfadiazine) therapy.

Endodontic (root canal) treatment can be performed through the damaged occlusal aspect to help save the tooth. This usually consists of vital pulpotomy—that is, removal of devitalized pulp with a fine-pointed scalpel, control of hemorrhage from the underlying vital pulp with paper "points" or hemostatic agents, followed by sealing the healthy pulp with a calcium hydroxide preparation that promotes reparative tertiary dentine formation at this site. Having sealed off the vital pulp, the remaining open pulp canal should now be prepared for filling by etching it for 1 minute with a phosphoric acid gel (to make the dental surface more porous to bond to dental restorative materials), which is then flushed away with water and air-dried. The pulp canal is then thinly coated with a bonding agent (Fig. 30-8) and sealed with a modern, compound restorative material (Fig. 30-9).

Alternatively, débridement of the exposed pulp and application of calcium hydroxide paste, along with the antibiotic treatment described, could be performed by veterinarians who are not dental specialists. In some young horses, the pulp becomes sealed off at the site of exposure by reparative (tertiary) dentine formation even without treatment, with the tooth remaining vital and continuing to erupt normally.[10] Treatment of premaxillary and mandibular fractures involving the incisors is discussed in Chapter 103.

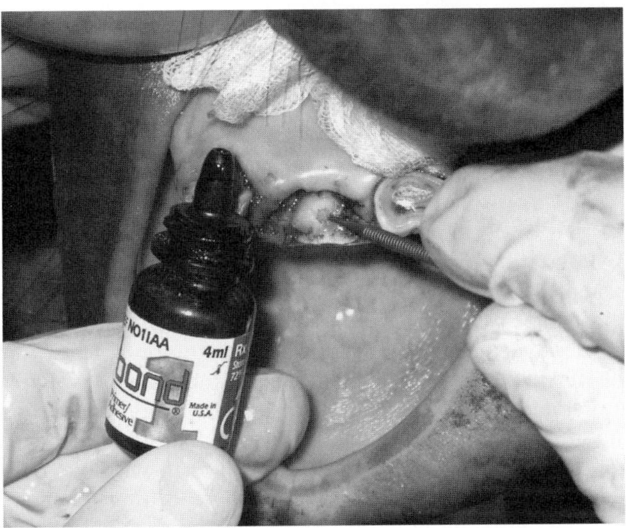

Figure 30-8. This horse is having endodontic treatment of its traumatically damaged incisors (402 and 403). Exposed necrotic pulp in 402 has been removed to the level of healthy pulp, which has then been sealed with calcium hydroxide paste, and the pulp canal above has been acid etched. A bonding agent is now being applied to the sealed pulp canal.

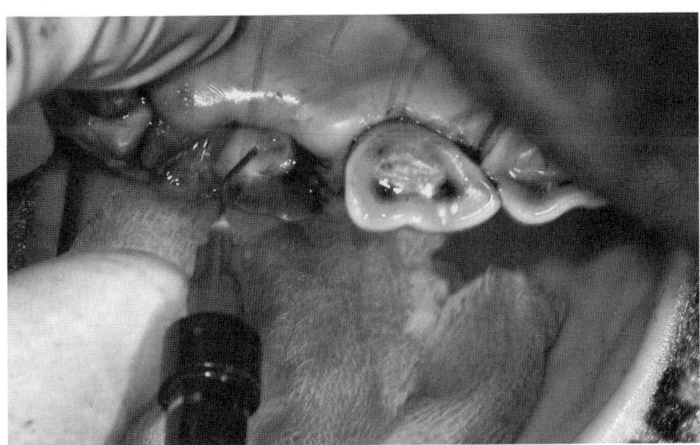

Figure 30-9. A modern, self-curing composite filler is being inserted into the prepared pulp cavity on top of the calcium hydroxide layer to further seal off the underlying vital pulp (same horse seen in Fig. 31-8).

Abnormalities of Incisor Wear

Incisor disorders include rectangular overgrowth of individual incisors ("steps") as a result of traumatic loss, or of maleruption (e.g., delayed eruption or displacement) of the opposing teeth, in addition to the previously noted incisor overgrowths occurring with overjet or underjet. Abnormal wear pattern of the rostral aspect of the 01s and occasionally of the 02s occurs in crib biters. Another common abnormality of incisor wear is a tilted or slanted incisor occlusal surface—that is termed "slope mouth" or "slant mouth." This defect is invariably associated with a major *unilateral* abnormality of the CT that has caused a pronounced unilateral chewing action, which causes uneven wear of the incisors.[10,13] The disorder of "wry nose" can also cause this incisor defect as a result of incisor malocclusion. Such incisor overgrowths should be reduced as previously described. The practice of arbitrarily reducing the height of the incisor, sometimes very extensively, purportedly to allow the CT to develop better occlusal contact ("incisor bite alignment techniques") has little scientific or clinical merit and should be avoided.

Disorders of the Canine Teeth (Triadan 04s)

Occasionally, displaced or grossly enlarged canine teeth interfere with the bit. Such teeth should be ground down, retaining at least 1 cm of crown above the gingiva, to avoid pulpar exposure that may cause pulpitis and possibly death of the tooth, which may not become evident until years later.[14] The sharp tips, or even most of the clinical crown of the canine teeth, are rasped off by some operators to prevent these teeth from causing lacerations of the operator's hands during dental procedures and allegedly to prevent them from interfering with the bits.

Rarely, canines may need to be extracted—for example, as a result of traumatic fracture or infection (Fig. 30-10), possibly associated with long-term calculus formation, or because long-term (greater than 12 months) unerupted canines are causing mucosal ulceration and bitting problems in horses older than 6 or 7 years. Because of the great length

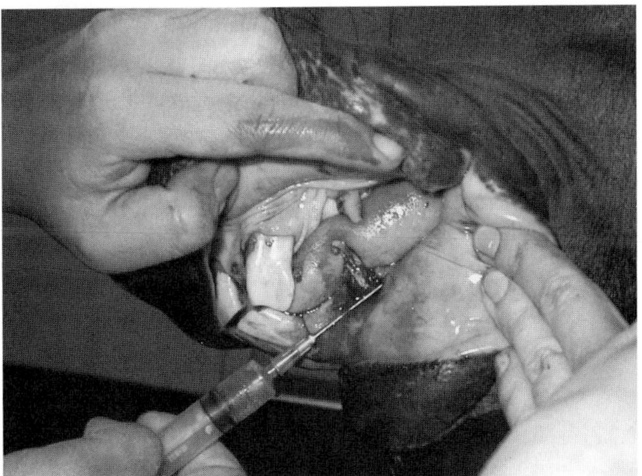

Figure 30-10. In this horse, which has gross caries and secondary periodontal disease of its left mandibular canine (304), a local anesthetic injection is applied into the periodontal membranes to facilitate removal of this tooth.

of their unerupted crown (up to 7 cm long), extraction of uninfected canine teeth is difficult and should never be undertaken without good reason. Extraction is performed by initially removing the vertical aspect of the lateral alveolar wall (Figs. 30-11 and 30-12) of the tooth. A dental elevator is then used to further loosen the canine tooth in the more horizontal, apical aspect of the alveolus, to allow complete extraction (Fig. 30-13). It is a difficult procedure, and firmly attached younger teeth and the apical aspect of the canine tooth may fracture during extraction. In the absence of apical infection, up to one third of the root (canine teeth are brachydont teeth) may be left in the alveolus without causing postoperative problems.

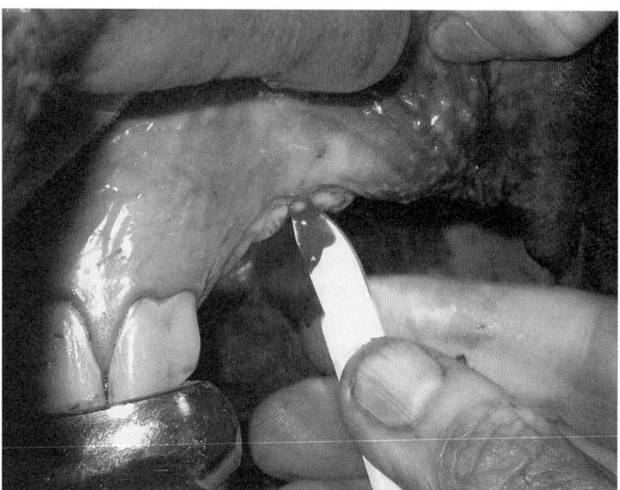

Figure 30-11. This horse had a long-term bitting problem associated with a partially erupted canine tooth (204) that caused chronic painful ulceration of the overlying mucosa. After sedation and infraorbital nerve block, an incision is being made over the ventrolateral aspect of the 204 alveolus.

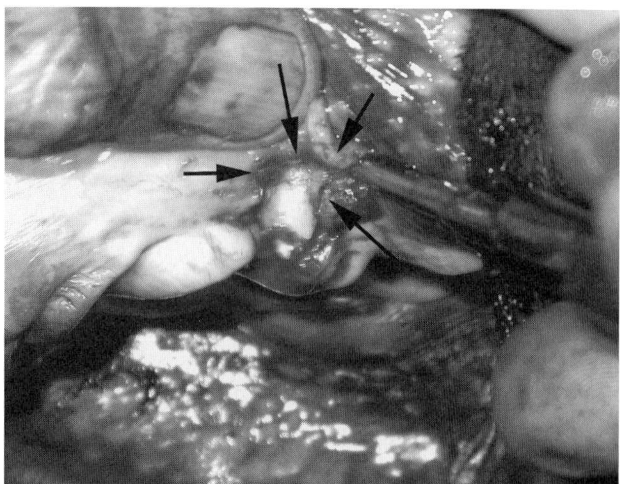

Figure 30-12. After retraction of the incised mucosa, the ventrolateral aspect of the alveolar wall of 204 has been removed with a dental elevator, revealing the vertical aspect of the crown of the problematic canine *(arrows)*.

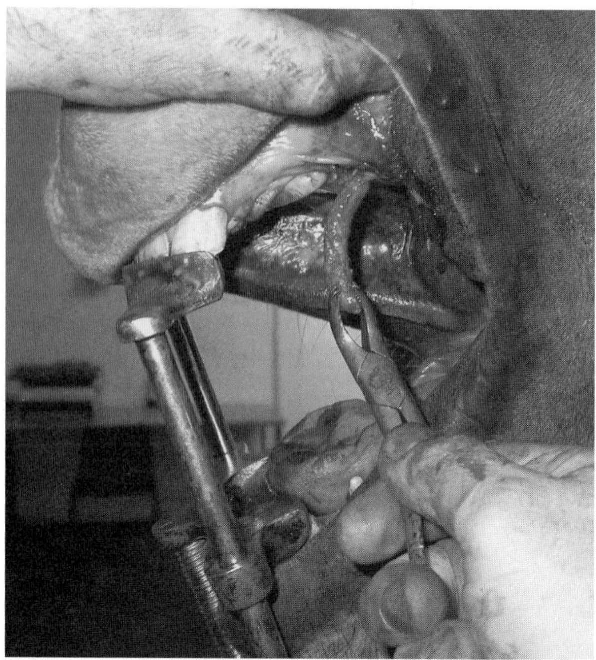

Figure 30-13. Note the great length and the curvature of the canine tooth, which has been extracted intact. A Butler's gag is being used.

Disorders of "Wolf Teeth" (Triadan 05s)

Wolf teeth (Premolar 1, Triadan 05) are small vestigial teeth (usually 1 to 3 cm long) that are blamed for many behavioral and bitting problems in horses and therefore are frequently extracted. Wolf teeth most commonly develop in the maxilla, lying in front of the 06s. If normally positioned and small, it is difficult to envisage how upper wolf teeth can interfere with the bit. However, displaced, enlarged, fractured, or unerupted ("blind") wolf teeth with overlying painful or ulcerated mucosa may cause bitting problems and may also prevent "bit seats" from being made on the rostral aspects of the upper 06s. Such wolf teeth should be extracted, as should all mandibular wolf teeth. Unless digitally loose (mainly in younger horses), wolf teeth should be extracted under sedation using subgingival local anesthesia. When extracting the more deeply embedded wolf teeth commonly found in older horses, it is better to perform infraorbital or mental nerve blocks (as described later) that will anesthetize the more relevant sensory nerves deep in the periodontal ligament.

A variety of specialized instruments (e.g., Burgess or Musgrave elevators) can be used to separate the gingiva around these teeth, and an elevator is subsequently inserted into the periodontal space to loosen the teeth (Fig. 30-14), followed by forceps extraction when adequately loosened. Large (often unerupted) wolf teeth may have to be extracted using a mucosal incision, followed by loosening them from the underlying premaxilla using an osteotome and mallet. In contrast, small mobile wolf teeth in younger horses may be extracted using forceps only. It is imperative to separate firmly attached wolf teeth from the alveolus and, most importantly, not to break them off *above* alveolar level, where the protruding fragment will cause more oral discomfort than was present prior to extraction. If the roots or adjacent apical

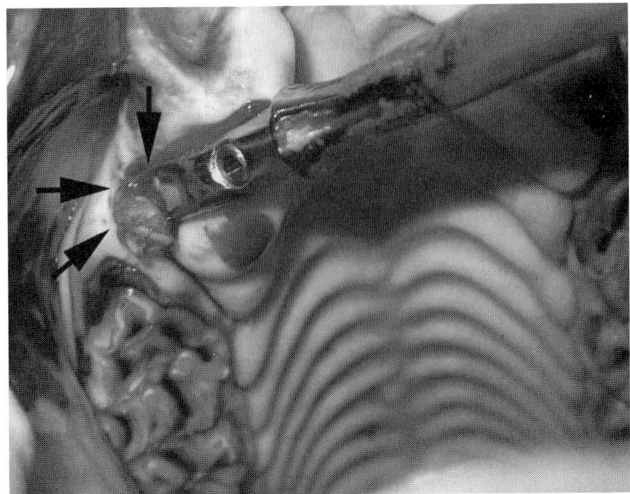

Figure 30-14. This large and rostromedially displaced "wolf tooth" (105) *(arrows)* has been loosened from its periodontal attachments with a Musgrave elevator. The intact, loosened tooth can now be readily extracted with forceps.

parts of wolf teeth fracture below alveolar level during extraction, these alveoli will usually heal over fully and so should be of little concern. The greater palatine artery can be lacerated during wolf tooth extraction, and infection and tetanus can also develop after such procedures.

Disorders of the Cheek Teeth

Developmental Disorders of the Cheek Teeth

RETAINED DECIDUOUS CHEEK TEETH

Retention of the remnants of the deciduous CT ("caps") can occur in horses between 2 and 5 years of age. When loose, and especially when partially retained by their gingival attachments, they may cause oral pain, and affected horses may show quidding, bitting problems, and, occasionally, loss of appetite for a couple of days.[14] Such signs in this age group warrant a careful examination of the rostral three CT for evidence of loose deciduous CT. Loose caps should be removed using specialized cap extractors.

The prolonged retention of caps has been alleged to cause delayed eruption of permanent CT, and the development of large eruption cysts ("bumps" in 3- or 4-year-olds) under the apices of the erupting permanent CT (07s and 08s),[15] but another study found no evidence of this.[16] The presence of very enlarged eruption cysts, especially if unilateral, should prompt a thorough oral and, if necessary, open-mouth radiographic examination for the presence of retained deciduous CT.[17] Additionally, standard radiographic views for evidence of apical infection should also be obtained. However, the practice of methodically removing deciduous teeth at set ages in horses results in the premature removal of some deciduous CT, exposing their underlying permanent counterparts too early. In the upper CT, this leads to loss of blood supply to the still-developing infundibular cementum, possibly leading to infundibular cemental hypoplasia (patent infundibulum) and thus predisposing the tooth to infundibular caries and possible apical infection or CT fracture later in life.

DIASTEMATA

The occlusal surfaces of all six CT are normally compressed closely together, and each CT row should function as a single grinding unit. This compression of the CT together is achieved by the action of the angled rostral and caudal CT compressing together the occlusal aspects of all six CT.[12] Even with age, the progressively smaller reserve crowns usually remain tightly compressed at the occlusal surface (the CT taper in slightly from crown to apex). However, if spaces, or diastemata, develop between the occlusal aspects of adjacent CT, clinical problems will occur.[16,18] Very severe clinical problems occur when these spaces are narrow (often only 2 to 3 mm wide) at the occlusal surface and wider at the gingival margin, a condition known as valve diastemata.[19] In some cases, CT diastemata are caused by lack of sufficient angulation of the rostral and caudal CT to provide enough compression of the occlusal surface of the six CT. In other cases, diastemata occur with apparently normal angulation, suggesting that the dental buds developed too far apart.[16] Individual diastema can also be caused by displaced or supernumerary CT, or it may occur adjacent to overgrown CT (e.g., rostral to an overgrown lower 11 or caudal to an overgrown upper 06 that has been displaced caudally and rostrally, respectively, because of their focal overgrowths).

Food becomes impacted into these abnormal interdental spaces by the prolonged grinding of tough forage (Fig. 30-15), and this leads to progressively deeper and more painful packing of food into the sensitive periodontal spaces, which causes a secondary, malodorous periodontal infection. Diastemata can be recognized by visually (with a dental mirror or intraoral endoscope) or digitally detecting food fibers protruding between these teeth, most commonly at the gingival level. In a longer standing case, this food pocketing and periodontal disease may extend along the full width of affected teeth and extend deep into the mandible or maxilla (including into the maxillary sinuses). Evaluation of the severity and numbers of diastemata can be difficult. Oral endoscopy or intraoral mirrors, or obtaining 10- to 15-degree, latero-oblique radiographs with the horse's mouth open, can be very useful.[20,21]

Treatment of CT diastemata is difficult. Cleaning out the periodontal pockets manually (with dental picks and long

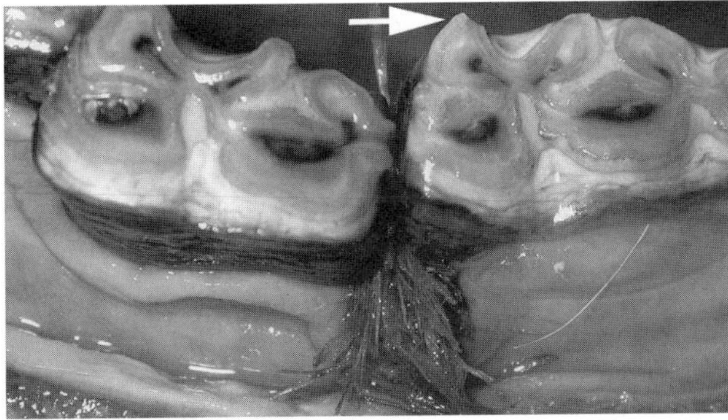

Figure 30-15. A diastema with deep interdental food pocketing is present between this 410 and 411, both of which have slight medial displacement. A slight "steplike" overgrowth is also present on 411 *(arrow)*, which may have caused caudal displacement of this cheek tooth and so predisposed to the diastema.

forceps) or with pneumatic or high-pressure water instruments, and filling the periodontal defects with antibiotics and plastic impression material, gives only temporary relief unless the underlying mechanical predisposition to this food impaction is also treated. Many horses show severe clinical signs when fed hay and then improve greatly when out at grass in the summer. Likewise, feeding only a finely chopped (milled) diet, such as grass or alfalfa cubes (whose fiber length is too short to become entrapped in diastemata), often reduces or fully removes clinical signs.

In younger horses with mild developmental diastemata, provided there is sufficient angulation of their CT (as adjudged radiographically), the abnormal spaces may close when further dental eruption occurs. Such horses should not have their diastemata widened.

Currently, the best treatment for this disorder in mature horses appears to be to widen problematic diastemata—to about 6 to 8 mm wide on the occlusal surface—using a specialized burr (Powerfloat, D&B Enterprises, Inc, Calgary, Alberta, Canada). Cases should be evaluated and selected by clinical examination and possibly by open-mouth radiography. Horses to be treated should be heavily sedated and the periodontal pockets and diastemata cleared of food, the former usually causing much discomfort to the horses. During widening of diastemata, water should be sprayed over the CT being burred to prevent thermal pulpar damage. As much tooth as possible should be removed from the rostral aspect of the tooth positioned *caudal* to the diastema, to help avoid exposing dental pulp (Fig. 30-16). If just a single painful diastema is causing a problem, extraction of a tooth on one side of the diastema may result in complete cessation of quidding, as food will not become trapped in a wider space. Some young horses with severe, multiple diastemata and osteomyelitis of alveoli and supporting bones will be very difficult if not impossible to treat.

ROSTRAL POSITIONING OF THE MAXILLARY CT ROWS

A common dental abnormality in horses is a rostral positioning of the maxillary CT rows relative to their mandibular counterparts, invariably in conjunction with overjet ("parrot mouth"). This disorder eventually leads to the development of focal overgrowths of the rostral aspect of the upper 06s, which may cut the cheeks and interfere with the bit. If small, these overgrowths can be manually rasped level with a solid carbide float, but if they are large, a power tool is best to reduce them, in stages of about 5 mm at a time and a few months apart, to avoid pulpar exposure.

Similar overgrowths on the caudal aspect of 311 and 411 frequently go undetected and can lacerate the tongue and wear down the opposite CT (maxillary 11s) to gum level. There is very little room between the occlusal surfaces of the caudal maxillary and mandibular CT, especially if large overgrowths are present on these teeth. Consequently, these overgrowths are best reduced using power tools, grinding them from their medial aspect if there is not enough room to reduce them from their occlusal surface. Molar cutters and percussion guillotines (which encircle this caudal hook) can fracture these teeth, causing pulpar exposure, especially in smaller breeds (e.g., Arabian and Welsh ponies) that have marked dorsal curvature (curve of Spee) of the caudal occlusal surface of their CT. Such dental fracture and pulpar exposure may lead to life-threatening cellulitis of the mandibular and pharyngeal areas; at the very least, this necessitates CT extraction.

DISPLACEMENTS OF THE CHEEK TEETH

Most severe cases of equine (medial, lateral, rotatory) CT displacements are developmental and appear to be caused by overcrowding of the CT during eruption. This type of displacement is often marked and also may be bilateral.[16] Gross dental overgrowths later develop on areas of the displaced tooth and its occlusal counterparts that are not in contact, causing soft tissue trauma. Additionally, painful food pocketing develops in diastemata that are invariably present on both sides of the displaced CT. This often causes severe and painful periodontal disease (Fig. 30-17) and even osteomyelitis, sinusitis, or oro-sinus fistula formation. *Acquired* CT displacements (usually medial displacements of the lower 10s and 11s) can also develop in older horses and are usually associated with lesser degrees of CT displace-

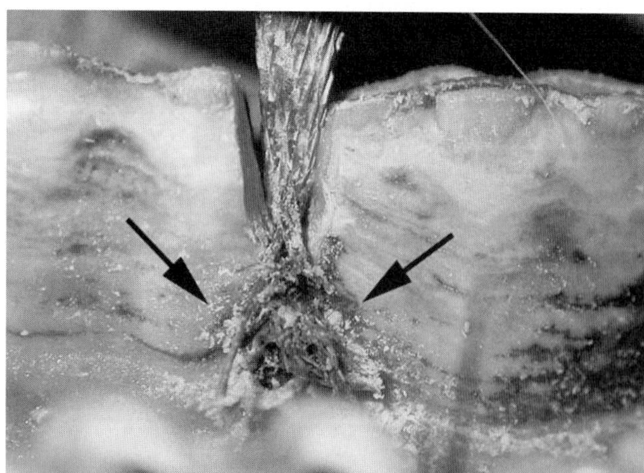

Figure 30-16. A diastema burr (Powerfloat, D&B Enterprises, Inc, Calgary, Alberta, Canada) is being used to widen the occlusal, interdental space in this specimen, which had diastema and food pocketing *(arrows)*. With valvelike diastemata, inserting the burr from the lateral and medial directions into the wider subocclusal space, and then burring occlusally and caudally, is a more effective technique.

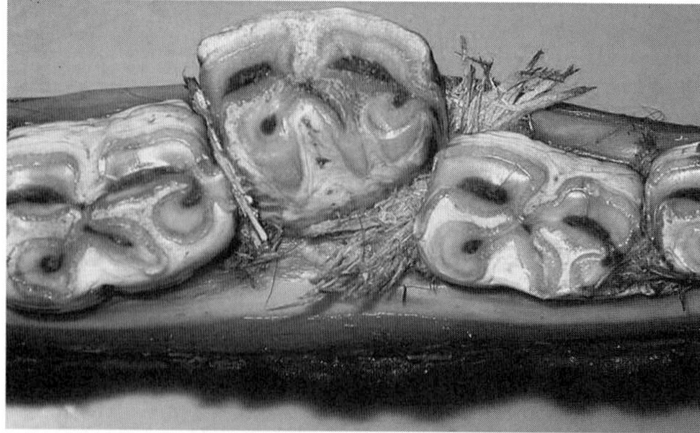

Figure 30-17. This mandible has a grossly, laterally displaced cheek tooth (CT) that is probably developmental in origin. Because of its angulation, the displaced CT *appears* wider than its counterparts. Note the severe periodontal food pocketing in diastemata beside the displaced CT and to a lesser extent between other CT. Oral extraction of this displaced CT is indicated.

ment and overgrowth, but they still may cause painful diastemata.[16]

Abnormal protrusions or overgrowths on displaced CT should be removed, preferably with a power tool. Painful diastemata can be widened with a diastema burr, and this often alleviates periodontal pain and thus quidding. When a cheek tooth is very displaced and has advanced periodontal disease, the displaced tooth should be extracted. This is readily performed per os in the sedated horse using CT extraction forceps (see later), and these horses usually cease quidding immediately. Overgrowths on opposing CT should be reduced at 6-month intervals.

SUPERNUMERARY CHEEK TEETH

Supernumerary CT (i.e., the presence of more than six cheek teeth in a row) are not uncommon in horses, usually occurring at the *caudal* aspect of the maxillary, and less commonly the mandibular, CT rows. These may be large connated structures (i.e., formed from two to three fused, maldeveloped CT). Because they are sometimes large and irregularly shaped, or because of overcrowding of adjacent CT, abnormal spaces and thus periodontal food pocketing occurs between the supernumerary and adjacent teeth, with resultant pain and quidding and occasionally deeper infections.[16] Additionally, if the supernumerary teeth are present in just one row (i.e., are unopposed), they later form large overgrowths. If severe periodontal disease develops, particularly if associated with sinusitis or an oro-sinus fistula, the supernumerary CT should be extracted. Extraction should be performed *per os* if possible, as repulsion of the caudally positioned (usually suborbital) and also caudally angulated reserve crown and apex is technically very difficult. In the absence of periodontal disease, 6-monthly removal of overgrowths on supernumerary CT is required.

Acquired Disorders of the Cheek Teeth

ACQUIRED OVERGROWTHS OF CHEEK TEETH

Feeding concentrates greatly alters the masticatory action of horses, causing them to chew with a more vertical rather than lateral mandibular action, and also for a much shorter time, than a horse that is eating forage. This restricted lateral mandibular movement predisposes horses to develop overgrowths (initially involving primarily enamel) of their CT.[22] If these painful enamel overgrowths are neglected, the sharp enamel points eventually merge into a steeply angulated (e.g., 45 degrees versus the normal 10 to 15 degrees) occlusal surface, termed shearmouth or "scissor mouth". A mechanical obstruction now additionally obstructs the normal side-to-side mandibular masticatory movements, rendering mastication even less efficient. Food stagnation and secondary periodontal disease also commonly develop. In advanced cases of dental overgrowths, undulating irregularities of the occlusal surface of the CT rows in the rostrocaudal plane (i.e., "wavemouth") develop.

Some horses may chew very slowly, make soft slurping sounds (instead of the normal vigorous crunching sounds) when chewing forage. Some affected horses may use just one side of their mouth for chewing rather than alternating sides (and develop a sloping incisor occlusal surface—"slope mouth," "slant mouth"), or they may hold their head in an abnormal position during chewing. Affected horses may also have abnormal head carriage, and bitting problems. The prime role in equine dental care is to prevent these overgrowths from developing by routine oral examinations and effective teeth rasping. Further information on this important area is available in the literature.[23]

TRAUMATIC DISORDERS OF THE CT AND BARS OF THE MOUTH

In young horses, traumatic mandibular fractures inevitably cause damage to the long CT reserve crowns, which occupy much of this bone (see Chapter 103). In most cases of unilateral, nondisplaced mandibular fractures, conservative therapy (1 to 2 weeks of antibiotic therapy and feeding a soft diet, such as soaked grass cubes for 2 to 3 months) is adequate, with the CT at the fracture site helping to stabilize the fracture, and the undamaged hemimandible acting as an effective splint. Traumatic fractures of maxillary CT are less common because of their anatomic position. Even if external sinus tracts develop after fracture of their supporting bones, it is worthwhile persevering with conservative therapy until radiographic changes (including the use of a metallic probe in any sinus tracts present) definitively confirm the presence of dental infection. Extraction of infected CT should be delayed for at least 3 months to allow mandibular or maxillary fracture healing to occur.

Bit-induced injuries to the dorsal aspect of the mandible at the interdental space (bars of mouth) can occur as a result of very excessive bit force.[11,24] In most cases, a superficial periostitis or sequestration of the dorsal mandibular cortex will occur at this site. However, pathologic fractures of the mandible, mandibular osteomyelitis, and lower 06 CT infection can also occur.[11,24,25] These mandibular bone injuries should be assessed radiographically and sequestra removed under sedation. The horses should be ridden with a bitless bridle for 4 to 6 weeks, and thereafter a rubber bit should be used with restraint. Exostoses may develop at the sites of bitting injuries (especially on the caudal aspect of the lower bars of mouth).[26] However, some normal horses have a raised and variably sharp ridge at this site, and some also have some roughening of the mandibular cortex at the insertion of the buccinator muscles. Very large and irregular exostoses at this site may cause damage to the overlying mucosa because of bit contact, and in doing so they cause permanent bitting problems. Such large bony protrusions can be removed under sedation and local anesthesia using an osteotome.[26]

Idiopathic fractures of the CT

Idiopathic CT fractures (i.e., CT fractures in the absence of known trauma) are common in horses.[25] Most commonly, "slab" fractures occur through the two lateral pulp cavities (Fig. 30-18), usually of the upper 09s.[27] Less commonly, lower CT also suffer from such fractures. The fracture site usually becomes filled with fibrous food, thus laterally displacing the smaller lateral CT fragment into the cheeks, causing buccal lacerations with subsequent quidding and bitting problems. Removal of the smaller, loose fragment with CT fragment forceps (Fig. 30-19) usually resolves the clinical signs, even though radiographic and scintigraphic evidence of apical inflammation and alveolar remodeling often occur in these cases. In many cases, the remaining pulps become effectively sealed off from the fracture site

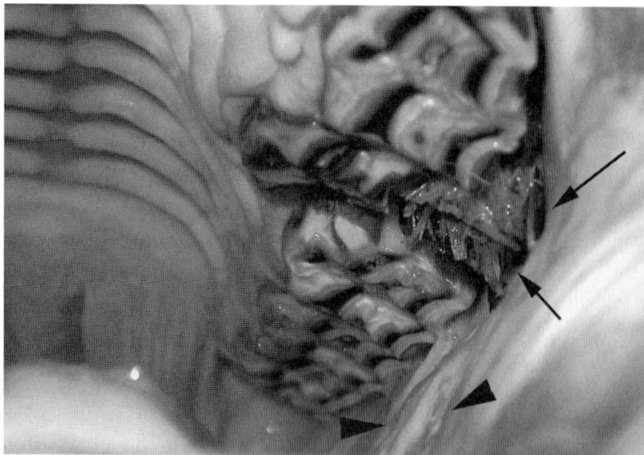

Figure 30-18. Intraoral view of a horse with a lateral "slab" fracture of 208. The fracture site is filled with food that has slightly displaced the larger medial portion into the hard palate and markedly displaced the thin, lateral fragment *(arrows)* into the cheeks, where it has caused buccal ulceration *(arrowheads)*.

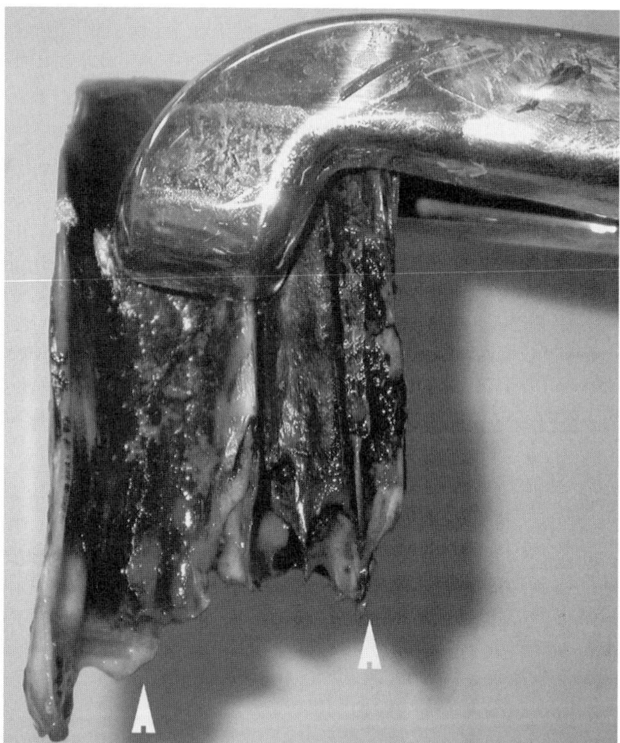

Figure 30-19. A lateral "slab" fracture of a maxillary cheek tooth that was readily removed with forceps. Gross caries on its medial aspect and destruction of its apical area *(arrowheads)* are evident.

with reparative dentine, and the remainder of the CT erupts normally. Less commonly, pulpar exposure is present in the remaining larger (medial) fragment, indicating that pulpar death has occurred, and this remaining fragment is likely to have to be removed within a year or so when it loosens, or if it causes clinical signs of apical infection.

Midline (sagittal) fractures of the maxillary CT occur less commonly than slab fractures, but the 09s are again most commonly affected.[25,27] This type of fracture is believed to be secondary to advanced infundibular caries, with coalescence of two carious infundibula leading to mechanical weakening and fracture of the CT and subsequent infection of the underlying pulp and periapical aspect of the tooth. Maxillary sinusitis sometimes accompanies these types of fractures if the infection spreads *outside* the alveolus. If clinical signs of apical infection occur, the affected tooth should be extracted, per os if possible, even though the clinical crown is weakened.[28] This can best be performed by cleaning out the food in the fracture site and using CT extractors to close the two fragments together, and then gently rocking the combined fragments until loose. Because of concurrent periodontal disease, extraction is usually easy (Fig. 30-20). Sinus lavage is also required if sinusitis is present. In the absence of clinical signs of apical infection, extraction of the looser fracture fragment (usually the lateral) is sufficient. The remaining, stable dental fragment should be reduced in height to prevent medial displacement during mastication. Its retention prevents drifting of adjacent CT into its space, for a few years perhaps, and also partially prevents the development of major overgrowths ("stepmouth") on the opposite CT.

FILLING OF CARIOUS INFUNDIBULA

An endodontic-type treatment has been used for treating deep caries of the infundibulum, to prevent further decay and to structurally strengthen these CT, and so prevent them from fracturing and also to prevent extension of the caries into the pulp, leading to apical infection. After cleaning out food with a dental pick (Fig. 30-21) or high-pressure aerosol or water lavage, the carious cementum in the infundibula is removed using a dental drill (Fig. 30-22) or by high-pressure aerosol abrasion with fine silica or aluminium powder (Fig. 30-23) (Equine Dental System, Pacific Equine Dental Institute, El Dorado Hills, Calif).[29] The cleaned infundibulum is then acid-etched and a bonding agent is applied (Fig. 30-24) before it is filled with a composite restorative material (Fig. 30-25) as previously described (for incisor fractures). As access to these carious infundibula (usually in

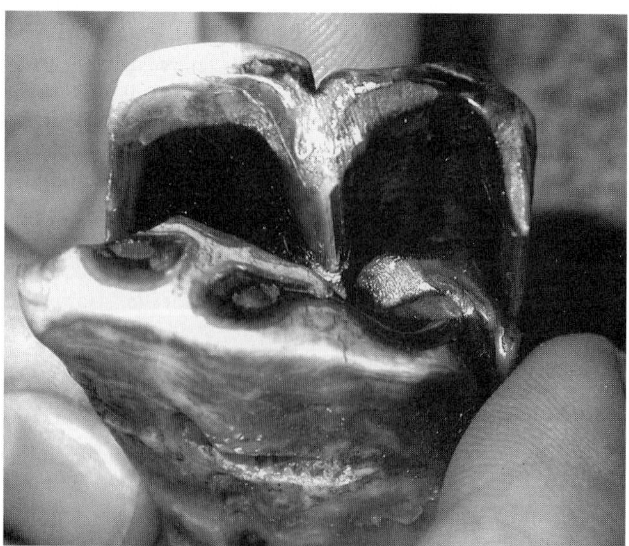

Figure 30-20. This mandibular tooth had a sagittal fracture and subsequent food impaction and displacements. Both parts of the fractured (and now carious) cheek tooth were orally extracted with little difficulty (see extractor forceps marks on tooth).

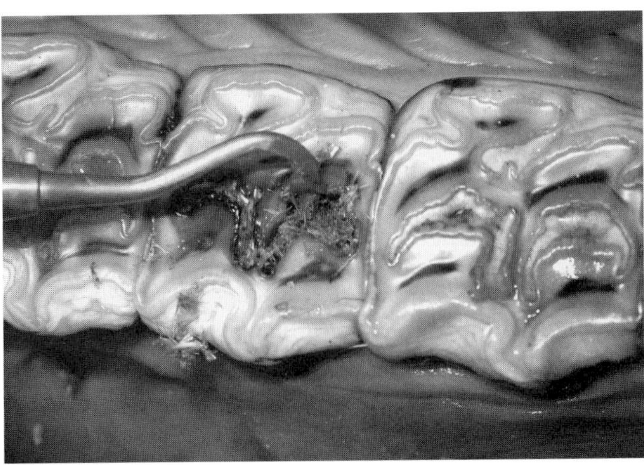

Figure 30-21. This maxillary cheek tooth specimen has impacted food in a carious (note dark infundibular enamel) infundibulum that is being removed with a dental pick.

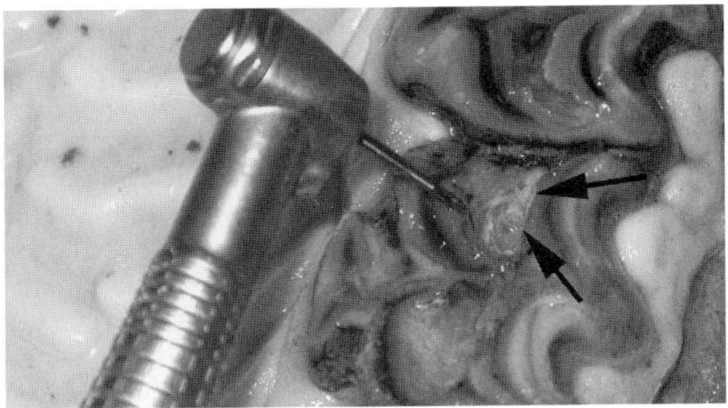

Figure 30-22. The carious infundibulum of Figure 30-21 has had all of the carious cementum and enamel removed with a high-speed dental drill *(arrows)*. The caudal infundibulum is filled with drill coolant water.

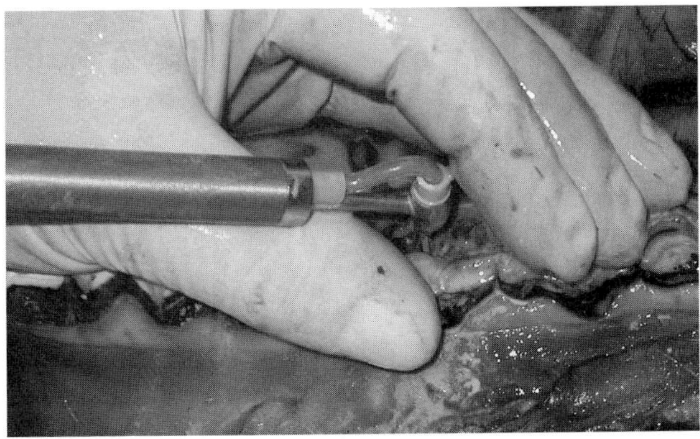

Figure 30-23. A high-pressure aerosol containing microfine aluminium powder (Equine Dental System, Pacific Equine Dental Institute, El Dorado Hills, Calif) is being used to clean out a carious infundibulum in this specimen.

the upper 09s) is difficult, it may not always be possible to fully remove all carious cement (or enamel) deep in the infundibula. Therefore, it is unclear whether this therapy can always prevent progression of caries to involvement of the adjacent pulp or apex, but it should make the affected upper CT more mechanically sound and thus help prevent sagittal fractures.

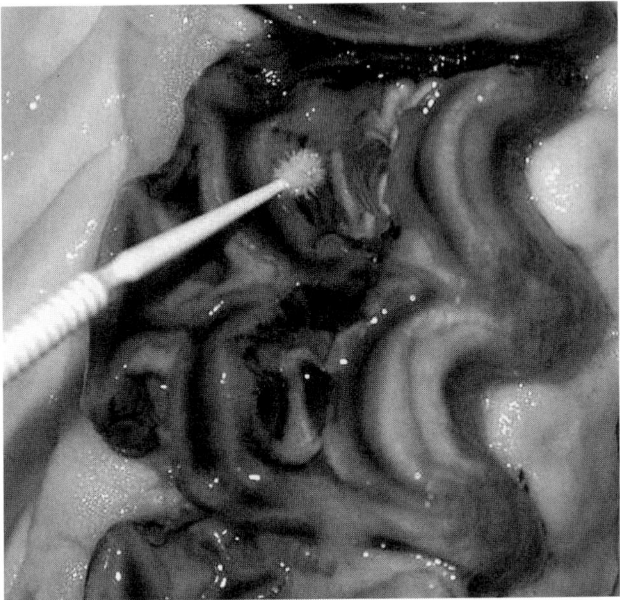

Figure 30-24. The cleaned infundibulum, which has also been acid-etched, washed, and dried, is now having bonding material applied with a flexible brush.

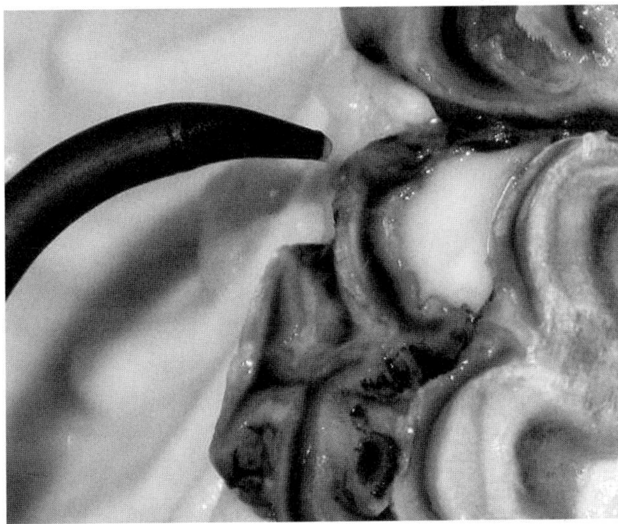

Figure 30-25. The prepared infundibulum has now been filled with a modern, self-curing, composite restorative material.

DENTAL (ODONTOGENIC) TUMORS

Dental tumors are rare in horses, but when present they can mimic apical infections (i.e., with the presence of maxillary and mandibular swellings that later may become much larger than the swellings commonly associated with apical infections). Additionally, these swellings do not usually develop sinus tracts, and they are firm and painless. Dental tumors include ameloblastomas, which are noncalcified epithelial tumors derived from the epithelium that forms enamel. A similar tumor, an ameloblastic odontoma, does induce calcification of adjacent mesenchymal tissues (and reciprocally of enamel epithelium) and so also contains dentine, cementum, and enamel. The appearance of these tumors can therefore vary from a noncalcified, polycystic, fibrous-type tumor to growths containing such tissues along with calcified dental tissues.

Dental tumors also include a variety of calcified tumors from dentinal tissues (odontoma) or cement (cementoma) or more commonly combinations of all three dental components (compound odontoma or ameloblastic odontoma).[30,31] These horses typically present with slowly growing, hard focal mandibular or maxillary masses that are usually very radiodense. The prognosis depends on how well defined they are from the surrounding bones to allow complete surgical excision to be performed.[30-32]

CHEEK TEETH PERIAPICAL INFECTION

Etiology and diagnosis

Apical (true roots may not even be formed at the time of infection) infections of CT may occur secondary to previously discussed abnormalities, including dental fractures or descending periodontal disease (e.g., beside a diastema). However, in most cases, the etiology is not obvious, so they can be termed primary apical infections.[33] The proposed etiologies include bloodborne infection of pulp (or anachoresis), possibly predisposed to by impaction of the rostral CT, which subsequently develop hyperemic, enlarged eruption cysts; deep infundibular caries with extension of infection from the infundibulum into the pulp cavity (maxillary CT only); and exposure of pulp on the occlusal surface (caused by an imbalance between CT wear and the formation of secondary dentine).[33] A recently described equine CT pulp nomenclature (Fig. 30-26) can be used to identify individual pulps in mature CT.[34] Regardless of its etiology, if an apical infection (with death of pulp) has been present for more than 6 to 12 months, the secondary dentine normally worn away on the occlusal surface by mastication is not replaced and therefore pulpar exposure occurs over all pulp horns (Fig. 30-27). Examination for pulpar exposure using a dental mirror or endoscope and a fine steel probe is a simple and valuable clinical test for dental viability that is currently rarely used (Fig. 30-28).

In the early stages, an anachoretic infection may remain confined to the apex, and all the pulp horns (or the common pulp in immature CT) may remain vital. At this early stage of infection, antibiotic treatment (e.g., 2 to 4 weeks of trimethoprim/sulphonamide) may suffice. Surgical curettage of the affected apex has also been utilized with varying success,[33,35] possibly because this procedure may further compromise pulpar blood supply by damaging the apical vasculature. Later, the common pulp or some of the pulp horns may become ischemic, causing pulpar death. At this stage, dental extraction or possibly endodontic therapy is required.

Primary apical infections occur mainly in younger horses, which have long reserve crowns and largely healthy periodontal membranes. Consequently, the infection cannot drain into the oral cavity but instead spreads to the alveolus and its adjacent supporting bones. Mandibular apical infections are invariably accompanied by unilateral, painful, ventral mandibular swellings that often develop external draining tracts. Infections of the upper 06 and 07 (occasionally the 08) CT cause focal swellings of the rostral maxilla (rostrodorsal to the rostral aspect of the facial crest), which are almost pathognomonic for dental infections. Some of these horses also develop an external sinus tract or, less commonly, a tract drains into the nasal cavity. Apical infections of the caudal three maxillary CT (09s to 11s)

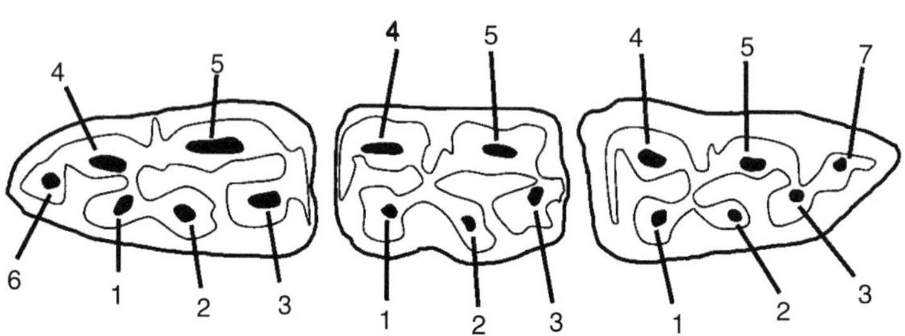

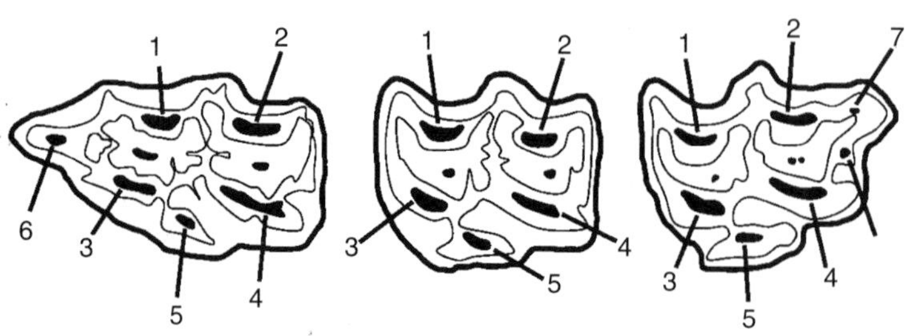

Figure 30-26. Identification of the individual pulp chambers of mature equine cheek teeth according to reference 34. The 06s (left side of figure) have six pulp horns. The 07s-10s (center of figure) have five pulp horns. The 11s (right side of figure) have six or seven horns.

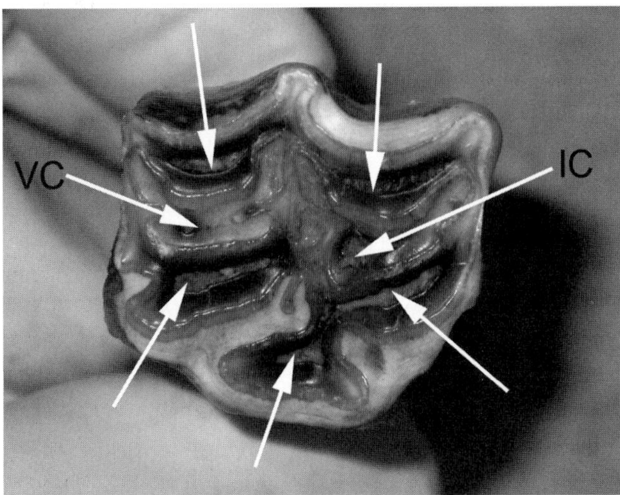

Figure 30-27. The occlusal surface of a cheek tooth extracted because of apical infection shows pulp exposure at all five pulps, all of which contain impacted food material *(arrows)*. One infundibulum contains a distinct vascular channel (VC), but the other has localized infundibular cemental caries (IC), which are not clinically significant in this case.

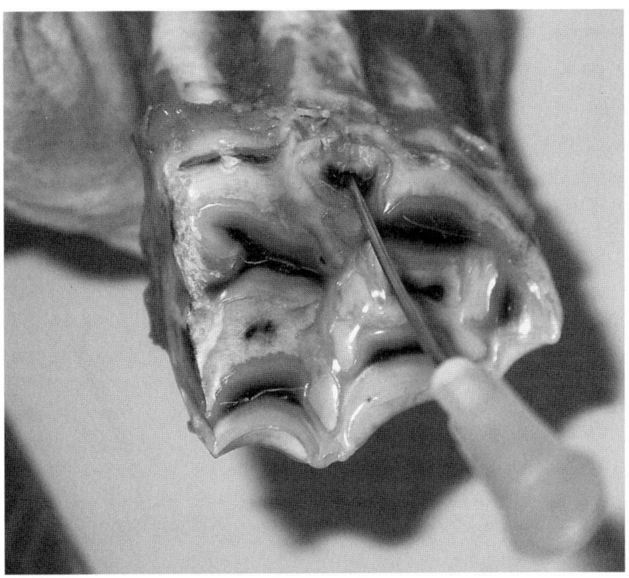

Figure 30-28. The occlusal surface of this cheek tooth (06s have six pulp horns) has intact secondary dentine over five pulp cavities but has a pulp exposure over one (pulp horn five, with needle inserted). Some minor discoloration is present in both infundibula.

usually result in a secondary maxillary sinusitis, with a chronic, malodorous, unilateral nasal discharge, but facial swelling or tracts are uncommon with this type of sinusitis. In older horses, apical infections commonly drain through the shorter periodontal membrane into the mouth, and therefore swellings of the supporting bones and sinus tract formation seldom occur.

A thorough clinical examination should be made, including intraoral examination for evidence of abnormalities, such as CT fractures; gross infundibular caries, or pulpar exposure (see Figs. 30-27 and 30-28). Radiographic evaluation of the horse should include 45-degree ventrolateral-lateral oblique projections for imaging mandibular CT apices and 30-degree dorsolateral-lateral oblique projections for imaging maxillary CT apices. The interpretation of equine dental radiographs is often difficult because of the frequent presence of overlying anatomic structures and because of combinations of lucent areas (from demineralization of apices and adjacent alveoli) and radiodense areas (from apical hypercementosis, alveolar sclerosis, and surrounding soft tissue inflammation). Interpretation is especially problematic in early apical infections in young horses where radiolucent normal eruption cysts have radiographic similarities to apical infections. If a sinus tract is present (e.g., as occurs with mandibular or rostral [06s-09s] maxillary CT infections), it is essential to obtain radiographs with a metallic probe in situ to confirm apical infection (Fig. 30-29). This procedure also provides surgical landmarks (helpful if the infected tooth is to be extracted by repulsion). Similarly, metallic markers should be placed over areas of maximal facial swelling. When available, computed tomography imaging allows these complex three-dimensional structures to be more fully assessed. Endoscopic examination of the sinuses (sinoscopy) may be helpful, as it sometimes demonstrates normal alveoli and indicates that nondental sinusitis is present. These examinations aim to definitively confirm if any of the CT are diseased and need to be extracted.

When doubt exists about whether apical infection is present, scintigraphy may provide additional evidence. If any doubt still remains, conservative therapy should be used—for example, 2 to 4 weeks of oral potentiated sulphonamides (possibly along with oral metronidazole therapy) for suspected mandibular infections and rostral (06 to 08) maxillary CT apical infections, and maxillary sinus lavage and similar antibiotic therapy for suspected caudal (09 to 11) maxillary CT apical infections. Failure to respond to this conservative therapy should prompt a further clinical and radiographic evaluation for apical infection (serial radiographs may detect subtle changes from previous radiographs). Only when *definite* evidence of dental infection is present should dental extraction be considered.[13,33]

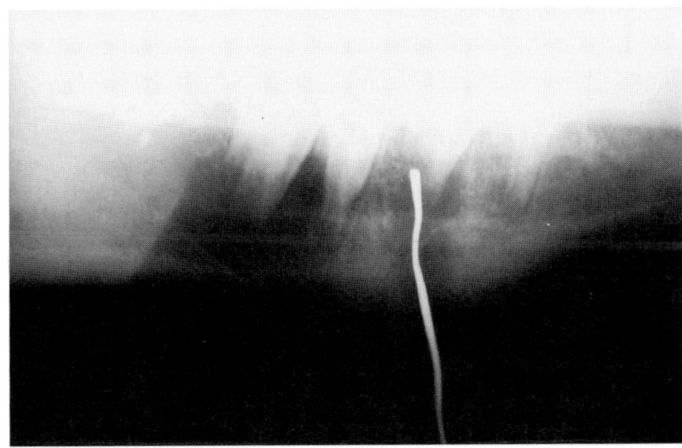

Figure 30-29. This radiograph shows an apically infected mandibular cheek tooth, with thickening of the underlying mandible, that also contains a lytic track leading to its caudal root. The caudal aspect of this root has been destroyed and is thickened more dorsally. The probe inserted up the sinus tract further confirms that infection is present in this CT.

Treatment of Disorders of the Cheek Teeth

EXTRACTION OF CHEEK TEETH

Most CT apical infections occur in younger horses, and in these cases the infection is usually confined locally to the apical area, and great mechanical force is required to break down the remaining extensive healthy periodontal membranes. Consequently, extraction of a long-crowned equine cheek tooth is a major surgical procedure with many possible immediate and delayed sequelae.[28] Oral extraction is the technique of choice for removal of most equine CT, as it can be performed in the standing horse, does not require surgery of the supporting bones, and has greatly reduced postoperative complications compared to the repulsion or buccotomy technique.[28]

Oral extraction of cheek teeth

The availability of today's safe and effective sedatives and analgesics is a major reason for the revival of the oral extraction technique. Most of the instrumentation has remained unchanged for over 100 years.[13,28,36,37]

A prerequisite for oral extraction of equine CT is excellent chemical restraint of the horse. This can be achieved by a combination of an alpha agonist and morphine or butorphanol. A detomidine, continuous-infusion technique has also been used successfully (loading doses of 4 mg IV of detomidine and 10 mg IV of butorphanol are given followed by 2 drops per second of a drip that contains 14 mg of detomidine in 250 mL of saline). *Local anesthesia* of the mental and infraorbital nerves can be used—for example, the upper 06s or 07s can be anesthetized by inserting a 5-cm-long, 21-gauge needle 3 to 4 cm caudally in the infraorbital canal and then slowly injecting 3 to 5 mL of lidocaine. The mental nerve, which is sensory to all mandibular teeth, can be anesthetized as it enters the mandibular canal on the medial aspect of the mandible. The mandibular foramen lies at the intersection of a vertical line at the caudal limit of the orbit, with a line parallel to the occlusal surface of the CT. After subcutaneous local anesthetic infiltration and aseptic skin preparation, a 15-cm long, 18-gauge spinal needle is "walked" up the periosteum of the medial aspect of the mandible and 20 to 30 mL of lidocaine is deposited at, and 1 to 2 cm dorsocaudally to, the site.

With more difficulty, the maxillary branch of the trigeminal nerve can be anesthetized as it enters the caudal aspect of the infraorbital canal. After aseptic skin preparation, a 9-cm spinal needle is inserted caudal to the highest point of the zygomatic arch and is then walked ventro-rostromedially down the orbital aspect of the frontal bone to the caudoventral aspect of the orbit, where 20 to 30 mL of lidocaine is deposited.

For oral CT extraction, the horse should be restrained in stocks with its head on a headstand or suspended in a dental head collar. At least one assistant is needed to stabilize the head and help with the extraction. A good headlight is also required, especially when extracting caudal CT, to absolutely ensure that the correct CT are being separated and that the correct tooth is subsequently removed. In many horses, the medial aspect of the *upper* CT contains very little exposed crown, with the gingival margin in some horses lying just a few millimeters below the occlusal surface. In such cases, a long-handled metal dental pick is used to detach the gingiva around the affected tooth to the level of the alveolar crest on the medial aspect of the tooth. This procedure normally exposes enough of the dental crown to allow CT extractors to be firmly applied on both the lateral and medial aspects of the tooth to be extracted.

A narrow-blade CT separator (molar spreaders) can now be slowly inserted into the interdental space in front of and caudal to the affected tooth (Fig. 30-30). The separator should be kept in place for about 5 minutes to excessively stretch and so damage the periodontal ligaments. A wider-blade CT separator can then be used to further stretch the periodontal ligaments. When extracting an 07, separators should not be used between the 06 and 07, in case the 06 is excessively displaced rostrally and loosened. Separators must also be cautiously used when extracting caudal CT in horses with a marked curve of Spee, because the vertical blades of the separator will not fit the nonvertical interdental spaces of such CT and may instead fracture them.[13,28]

A CT extractor is then firmly attached to the crown of the diseased tooth and the CT is rocked in the horizontal plane (Fig. 30-31). After a variable period, depending on the extent and health of the periodontal membranes, a "squelching" sound is heard. Increased movement of the forceps can now be appreciated and foamy blood can be seen at the gingival margin. After 20 to 120 minutes, the tooth usually becomes digitally loose, and only at this stage should a fulcrum be placed on the occlusal surface of the tooth rostral to the infected tooth. Vertical pressure is now exerted on the forceps, drawing the affected tooth intact from the alveolus. With caudal mandibular CT, it may be safer not to attempt elevation with a fulcrum, in case this *vertical* force fractures the *obliquely* positioned teeth. Instead, the tooth should be made digitally loose and extracted in a rostrodorsal direction using manual force (Fig. 30-32). Unlike repulsed CT, the apexes of extracted CT are virtually always intact (Fig. 30-33).[28]

If no sinus tract or secondary sinusitis is present, the empty alveolus can simply be plugged with one or two swabs (containing metronidazole or iodine) (Fig. 30-34), to prevent fibrous food from being trapped in very deep alveoli

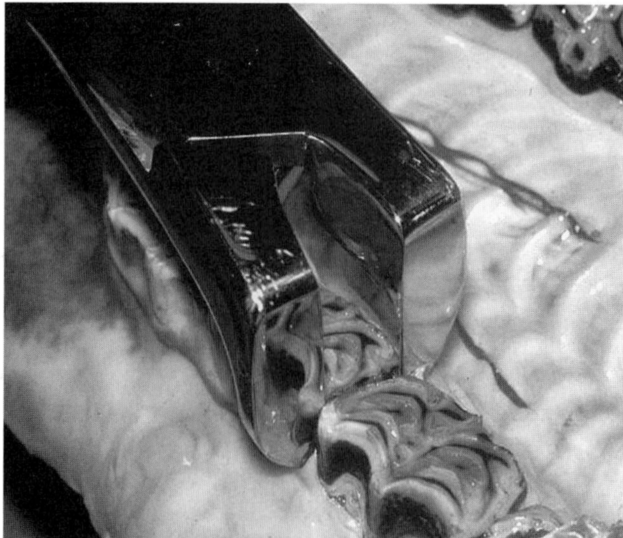

Figure 30-30. A narrow-blade, cheek tooth (CT) separator (CT spreader) is being inserted between two CT in this specimen.

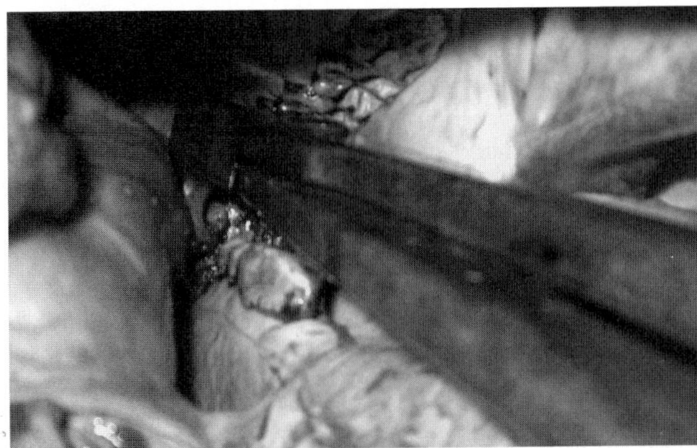

Figure 30-31. A Routeledge-type cheek tooth (CT) extractor applied to a mandibular CT (308), in the latter stages of dental extraction, when this CT has been elevated 2 to 3 cm into the oral cavity.

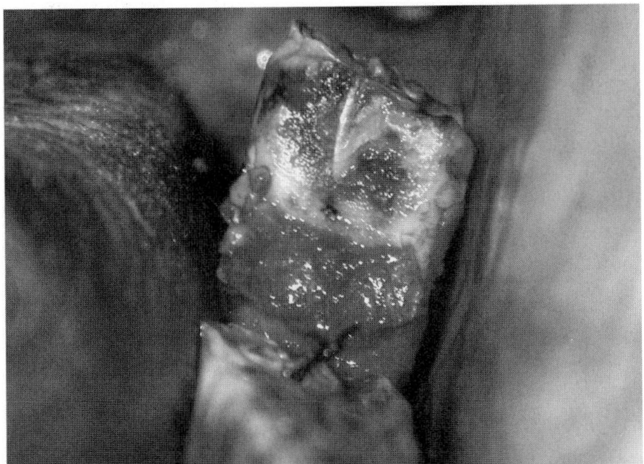

Figure 30-32. The final stages of oral cheek tooth (CT) extraction shows a mandibular CT that has been elevated into the oral cavity. It can be digitally removed at this stage.

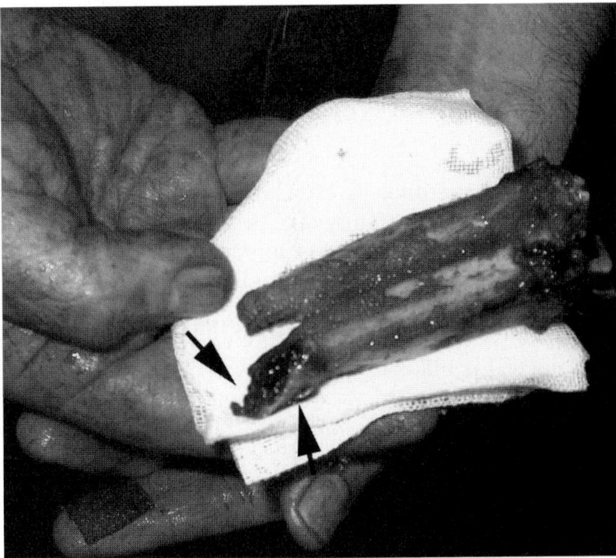

Figure 30-33. The extracted mandibular cheek tooth (shown in Figs. 30-29 to 30-32) has extensive, healthy periodontal covering over all of the reserve crown and apex, except at the tip of the thickened, infected root *(arrows)*.

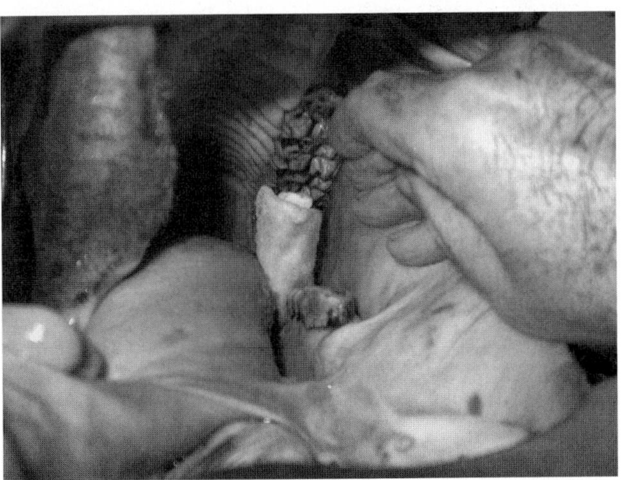

Figure 30-34. Surgical gauze, impregnated with antibiotics, is being inserted into a mandibular cheek tooth alveolus. It will be left in place for a couple of weeks to prevent impaction of food deep within the alveolus.

before it granulates closed. In older horses with shallower alveoli (less than 5 cm deep), no alveolar packing is required. The alveolus should be checked 2 to 4 weeks later and the swab removed if still present. The alveolus should now also be palpated for rough areas, usually caused by sequestration of areas of alveolar cortex. Loose fragments should be digitally removed or curetted, if detected. Specialized, long-handled, right-angled alveolar curettes (Kruuse Worldwide, Marslev, Denmark) are necessary to effectively curette the more caudal alveoli. Alveoli that still have a deep, large lumen may have a swab replaced for a further 2 weeks before being similarly rechecked.

If an external sinus tract was present prior to extraction, the bone at the base of the tract can be gently curetted percutaneously and they will usually spontaneously heal within a few days. In these cases, it is advisable to seal off the oral aspect of the alveolus with dental wax or an acrylic plug and to irrigate the sinus tract with a dilute iodine solution for a couple of days.

Oral extraction of the CT can also be performed on horses with infection of the caudal maxillary CT, which have a secondary sinusitis. If the apical aspect of the alveolus digitally feels intact after CT extraction, it can simply be packed with an antibiotic-impregnated swab, as described earlier. If the alveolus appears disrupted (very rare), an acrylic plug should be inserted to prevent the development of an oromaxillary fistula. In all cases of maxillary sinusitis caused by dental infections, a separate small (e.g., 10-mm diameter) portal should be made in the ipsilateral frontal sinus to allow postoperative lavage of the interconnecting infected maxillary sinus. The affected sinus should be lavaged twice daily, with 5 L of very dilute iodine solution for a week or so, or until the lavage fluid runs clear.

After successful oral extraction of CT by experienced surgeons, postoperative complications are rare (they occur in about 10% of cases) and are usually of a minor nature—

for example, nonhealing alveoli caused by alveolar sequestra, or localized osteitis. Most can be resolved by sequestrum removal, or alveolar curettage, using long-handled equine dental curettes and antibiotic therapy.[28]

Repulsion

The standard method for extracting equine CT in the late 19th and the 20th century has been CT repulsion under general anesthesia.[13] This procedure has the expense and the inherent risks for morbidity and mortality of equine general anesthesia, and it is also associated with a high level of postoperative complications. A surgical window (e.g., 2 cm in diameter) is made using a bone saw, trephine, or chisel, adjacent to the infected apex. For mandibular CT repulsion, this site is beneath the ventral mandible (Figs. 30-35 and 30-36), and for repulsion of maxillary 06, 07, and occasionally 08 CT, it is on the dorsorostral aspect of the rostral maxillary bone. For the latter trephination, care must be taken to avoid the infraorbital canal and nerve. Larger (e.g., 5 to 6 cm square) caudal maxillary bone flaps (hinged in a dorsal direction) can be used to perform a sinusotomy (see Chapter 42), and this is preferable to making a small sinus trephine opening for repulsion of the caudal maxillary CT. Such larger windows allow a visual and digital inspection of the apices of the 09 to 11 CT and then allow their repulsion, *if* apical infection is confirmed. Infected apices lose the smooth, rounded, soft tissue–covered appearance of normal apices; instead, sharp edges of exposed apical enamel or the edges of alveoli are palpable, and local granulation tissue and mucosal inflammation are evident.

Intraoperative radiographs should always be obtained if there is any doubt about the site and the direction of placement of the repulsion punch (Figs. 30-37 and 30-38). Radiographs should also be obtained after the extraction, unless the surgeon is certain that the tooth has been fully repulsed. As wide a punch as possible should be used during repulsion, with offset punches most suitable for upper

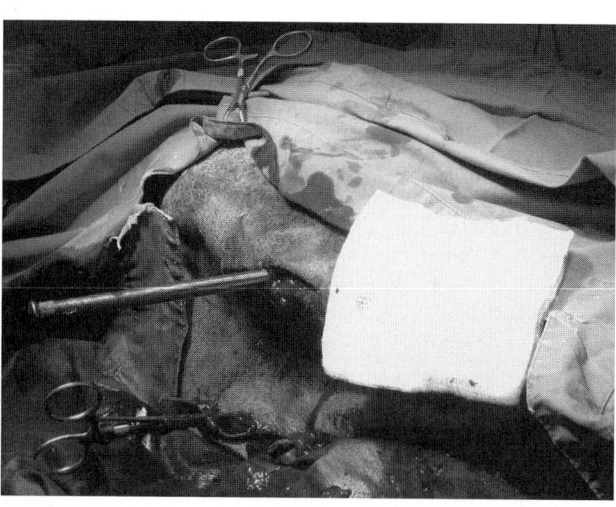

Figure 30-35. This horse is having a mandibular cheek tooth repulsed under general anesthesia. Note the steel punch in a ventral mandibular site.

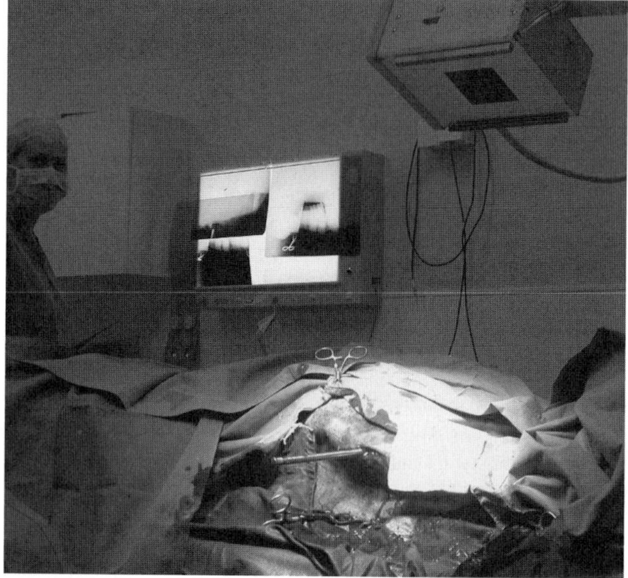

Figure 30-37. Intraoperative radiography of a horse having a mandibular cheek tooth (CT) repulsed. This radiograph is being obtained to confirm punch positioning and angulation to prevent iatrogenic damage to adjacent CT.

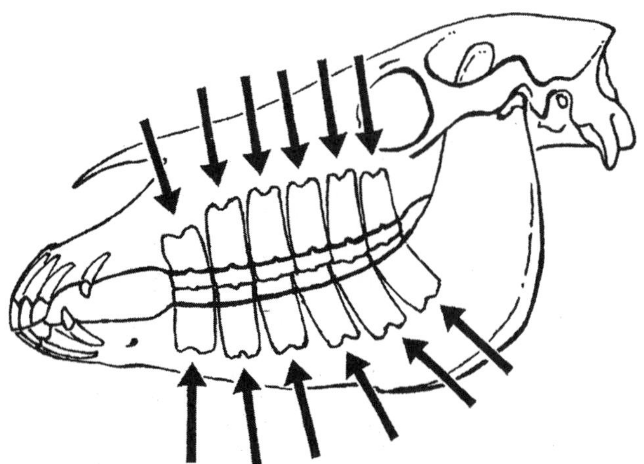

Figure 30-36. The direction of repulsion of the cheek teeth in a young horse.

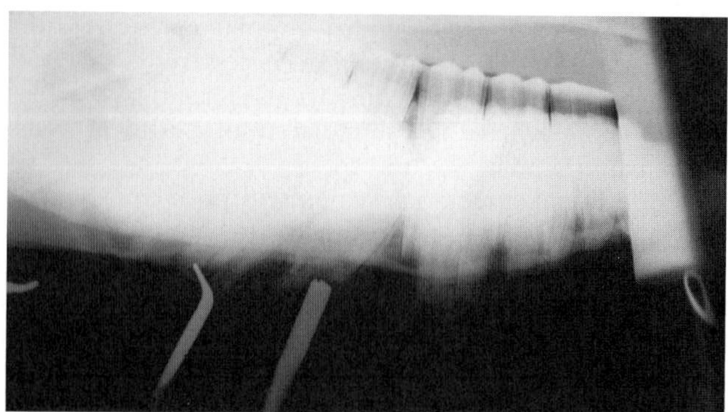

Figure 30-38. This intraoperative radiograph shows the punch correctly positioned over the affected apex and also shows that it is facing in a suitable direction to effectively remove this (09) cheek tooth.

CT repulsion. Hammering a thin metal blade down the periodontal space, especially on the (flat) rostral and caudal CT margins, can greatly decrease the time and trauma necessary to repulse a cheek tooth.

After CT repulsion, it should be determined that the alveolus is free of dental or alveolar remnants by examining the extracted CT and by the use of postoperative radiographs. The oral (occlusal) aspect of the alveolus should now be fully dried and sealed with a dental wax plug (after mandibular or rostral maxillary CT repulsions), or with an acrylic plug attached to the two adjacent CT (for caudal maxillary CT repulsions). The plugs should lie below the occlusal level; otherwise they will loosen quickly with the high, continual forces of mastication. They should also not extend more than 3 to 4 cm into the alveolus, or they will delay alveolar healing. The surgical site used for repulsion of rostral maxillary or mandibular CT should be left open and irrigated (e.g., with a very dilute povidone-iodine solution) for a few days, especially if they remain purulent or malodorous. Broad-spectrum antibiotics should also be administered for at least 3 days after dental repulsions.

Complications very commonly occur after repulsion of apically infected CT from younger horses, because much mechanical damage occurs to the alveolar and supporting mandibular or maxillary bones during the repulsion. These problems include nonhealing alveoli as a result of remaining dental fragments or alveolar sequestra; localized osteomyelitis; oronasal, orofacial, and oromaxillary fistulae; chronically draining facial tracts; damage to adjacent teeth; and chronic sinusitis. A number of studies have shown that between 32% and 70% of cases of equine dental repulsion require additional surgical and nonsurgical treatments, with most complications following maxillary CT repulsions (Fig. 30-39).[33,38-41] Careful radiographic assessment for the presence of dental or bone sequestra, osteomyelitis, adjacent damaged or infected CT, and chronic sinusitis helps (in cases where such problems are detected) in the selection of an appropriate treatment modality, such as replacing loose alveolar plugs, sinus lavage, and antibiotic therapy.

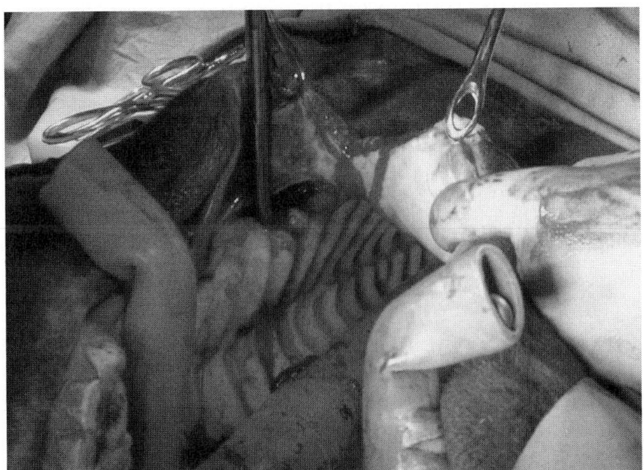

Figure 30-39. This horse had 206 and 207 repulsed some years previously, leaving it with a chronic, nonresponsive oro-nasal-facial fistula. After incision of the lips for access, a sliding hard-palate flap was used to close the large oral defect.

Removal of the lateral alveolar plate (lateral buccotomy technique)

A further technique for equine dental extraction involves the removal of the lateral alveolar plate and has been used for over 100 years. It is most suitable for extraction of the rostral upper three CT,[13] but it has been adapted for extraction of the rostral three mandibular CT by the buccotomy technique[40,42] and also for the more caudal mandibular CT by dissecting through the masseter muscles.[43]

This is the most suitable technique for the rare cases of chronically (sometimes of many years' duration) apically infected CT, where progressive, dense cement deposition has occurred around the infected apex and adjacent reserve crown, making this area and its surrounding alveolus larger than the more occlusal aspect of the alveolus and thus mechanically preventing its oral extraction or repulsion. Under general anesthesia, a surgical approach is made directly through the skin and subcutaneous tissues to the lateral wall of the affected alveolus. A horizontal incision (to reduce the risk of cutting the buccal nerves) is made in the skin and soft tissues overlying the affected mandibular CT. The buccal nerve (and possibly the parotid duct) should be identified and isolated to avoid damage, if they cross the surgical field. A vertical incision is now made in the periosteum over the lateral aspect of the affected CT and the periosteum is reflected. Through use of a bone saw or burr, the lateral wall of the alveolus is removed. The full length of the crown of the exposed diseased tooth is then sectioned longitudinally with a diamond wheel or burr before the CT is extracted in sections.

The occlusal aspect of the alveolus is plugged with dental wax and the remaining alveolus is packed with an iodine-impregnated gauze bandage, which is gradually withdrawn through a small stab incision adjacent to the surgical site. A potential major disadvantage of this technique for extraction of the mandibular CT is that it can cause buccal nerve damage with nasal paralysis and parotid duct rupture.[44] In athletic animals, the former sequela is a disaster, as active dilation of the nostrils cannot occur anymore. Prolonged anesthesia is also required for this technique, which is a further disadvantage.

ENDODONTIC THERAPY

A number of workers have attempted to treat apically infected CT by use of endodontic (pulp canal) therapy. A major advantage of endodontics, if successful, is that the infected tooth is preserved and thus continues to erupt normally (at about 2 to 3 mm per year). This prevents the development of overgrowths ("stepmouth") of the opposing CT and drifting of the adjacent CT into the site of the extracted tooth. This drifting eventually causes focal overgrowths ("hooks") on the caudal and rostral aspects of the opposing CT row.

Equine CT endodontic treatment has been performed mainly through the apex of the affected CT,[45,46] but it is also performed via an occlusal approach (as is used in brachydont teeth endodontics).[47] Endodontic treatment cannot be used in CT with gross sepsis of the apex or where there is extensive periodontal disease (e.g., descending apical infections because of deep periodontal disease at a diastema). Apical endodontic therapy is performed via surgical approaches through the mandibular or maxillary bones. A consequence of this approach is the need for prolonged general anesthesia and surgical exposure of the overlying bone and affected apex for endodontic therapy. The exposed apex is visually assessed, and grossly infected or discolored calcified dental tissue is removed by high-speed, water-cooled burrs.

The large, common pulp (in young horses) or individual pulp horns (five pulp horns in all mature CT, except the 06s have six, and 11s have six or seven—see Fig. 30-26) are then assessed for viability and removed with barbed broaches if found to be nonvital. Any impacted vegetable material (as a result of occlusal pulpar exposure) is removed and the canals are then filed using long endodontic files, until normal-appearing dentine is reached (as adjudged by the color of the filings). The pulp canal can be sterilized by irrigation with 2.5% sodium hypochlorite solution (household bleach) and then lavaged with water and air-dried. The canal lining is then etched with a phosphoric acid preparation and lavaged and dried again. The surface is subsequently coated with a dental bonding agent (some agents need to be cured by UV light) and the pulp canal is then filled, in layers, as completely as possible, with a modern, compound restorative material, some of which also need to be cured by UV light in stages. Air pockets may preclude complete filling of the occlusal aspects of some long, narrow equine CT pulp canals in mature horses.

Baker described an 84% success rate with (apical) endodontic therapy for mandibular 08s and 09s, but poor success with maxillary CT.[45] Other workers have had poor results in trying to treat infected teeth with apical endodontic therapy,[46] with some horses requiring two to three courses of treatment, under general anesthesia, sometimes taking over 2 hours per treatment. Such repeated and prolonged surgery under general anesthesia is costly and has safety considerations for the horse. It is believed that in younger horses, the presence of a very large common pulp cavity is one reason for the failure of this technique in this age group. Consequently, some authors advocate that endodontic treatment should be reserved for more mature teeth (e.g., CT that have been erupted for at least 3 or 4 years). Specialized training and equipment (including long drills and reamers) are required for endodontic therapy of the long equine pulp canals. Additionally, there is still debate over what is the most suitable material (e.g., modern two-part composites, self- or light-cured; amalgam or glass ionomers) for pulp canal filling in horses. Endodontic therapy offers much potential benefit in treating apical infections, but until larger studies have more fully evaluated case selection criteria, long-term efficacy, costs, and the safety of this technique, its wider role in equine dentistry remains unclear.

More recently, endodontic therapy via the oral cavity has been advocated in cases of pulpar exposure on the occlusal surface of CT. However, many such horses have deeply impacted vegetable matter down their pulp canals that may be impossible to fully remove, even with use of high-pressure silicate or aluminium powder aerosols, and after completely drilling out the full occlusal surface of these canals. After cleaning, exposed pulp cavities are sealed with restorative material as previously described. If the affected canal still contains food material or if inaccessible areas of caries have not been removed, it is possible that endodontically sealing off its occlusal drainage may transform a nonclinical apical infection to one with clinical involvement of the supporting bones and sinuses. Notwithstanding these theoretical arguments against occlusal endodontic therapy, some operators have reported success with this therapy.[47]

ORAL CAVITY SOFT TISSUE TRAUMA

The soft tissues of the oral cavity are susceptible to traumatic injuries by harness bits or other oral tack, sharp external objects, blows to the head, injury during recovery from general anesthesia, and iatrogenic damage during intraoral procedures—for example, dental extraction or transoral epiglottic entrapment release.[48-51] The face and oral cavity soft tissues have a tremendous capacity for repair. Minor, superficial lacerations of the mucosa, lips, and tongue can heal effectively by second intention, usually within 2 weeks, without leaving a scar. Management may entail flushing of the oral cavity after meals with an antiseptic solution, warm salt water or clean water, and the use of nonsteroidal anti-inflammatory drugs. Larger wounds should be considered for surgical repair, to maintain tissue function, and for cosmesis. For these repairs, antimicrobial therapy may be needed in selected cases.

Tongue

Lacerations of the tongue are not uncommon and can be severe, with transverse lacerations more frequent than longitudinal ones.[48,52,53] The free portion of the tongue is usually involved because of bit location and because this part has more exposure to the external environment. Clinical signs include oral hemorrhage, ptyalism, inappetence, anorexia, dysphagia, malodorous breath, pyrexia, and tongue protrusion from the mouth. Management of tongue lacerations is guided by the severity, duration, and location of the injury. Partial glossectomy, primary wound closure, or secondary wound healing are approaches to treatment. Surgical procedures are most easily performed on the anesthetized patient; however, the tongue can be operated on in the standing horse with effective sedation and infiltration of local anesthetic. Traction on the tongue for exposure can be achieved by placing towel clamps in the tongue caudal to the laceration or by using a gauze snare at this site, which also serves as a tourniquet.[52,54]

Partial glossectomy is reserved for cases in which the rostral tongue tissue is devitalized and minimal attachment is left between the severed section and the remaining body. Tissue color, temperature, and evidence of bleeding at an incision can be used to assess viability. Observation of fluorescence after intravenous administration of sodium fluorescein allows a more objective assessment of tissue vascularization.[54] After amputation, the remaining stump is meticulously débrided of nonviable tissue. Mucosal-to-mucosal closure of the stump is not imperative[53] but can be performed to aid hemostasis and hasten wound healing. Correct dorsal to ventral apposition is assisted by removing a wedge of intervening musculature and closing the created space with multiple rows of interrupted absorbable 2-0 or 0 sutures. The mucosal edges are subsequently closed with

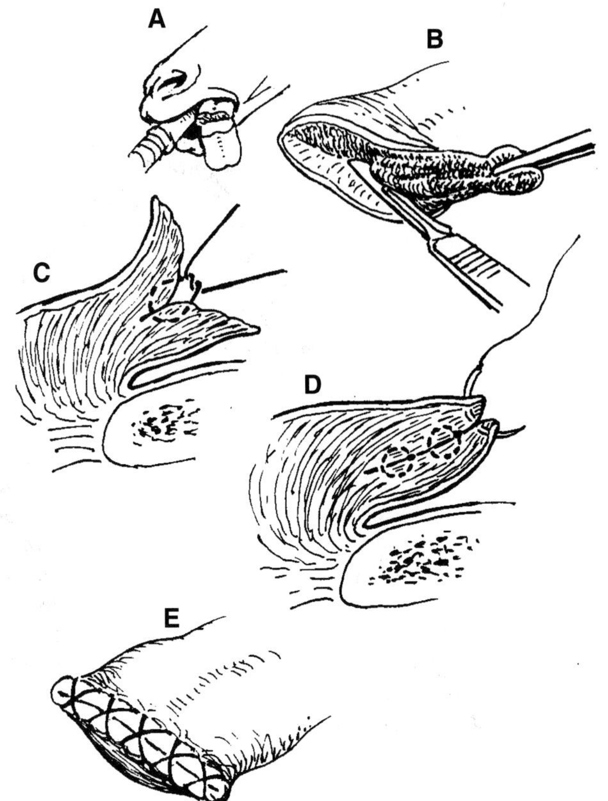

Figure 30-40. Closing the tongue stump after partial glossectomy. After amputation of the severely lacerated tongue (**A**), a wedge of intervening musculature is removed (**B**). The created space is closed with multiple interrupted rows of sutures (**C, D**) before closing the mucosa (**D, E**).

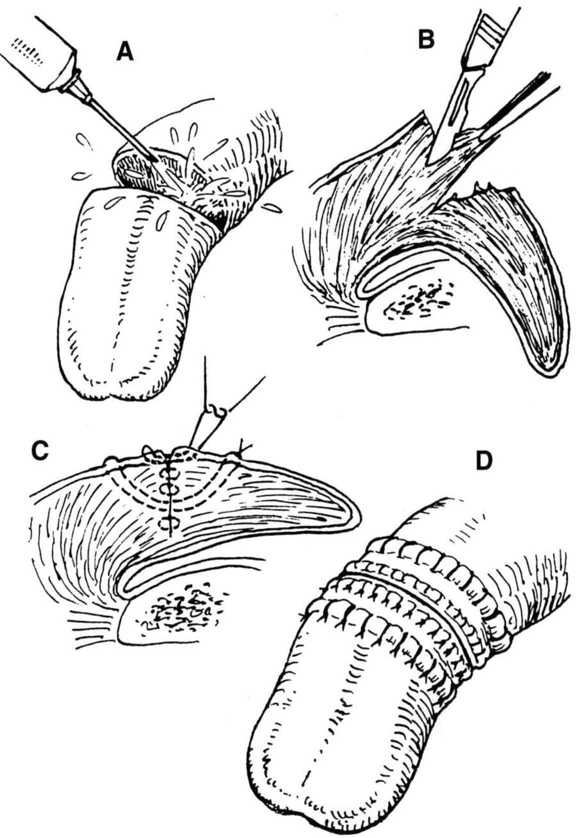

Figure 30-41. Tongue laceration repair. After vigorous lavage of the wound (**A**) and débridement of devitalized tissues (**B**), the laceration is closed with multiple layers of interrupted sutures (**C, D**). The large vertical mattress tension-relieving sutures are placed first, deep in the tongue musculature.

buried sutures of a similar size (Fig. 30-40).[52] Involuntary loss of saliva from the mouth may be observed after amputation of a large part of the free portion of the tongue.[53]

Primary closure of severe tongue lacerations is encouraged whenever possible. The wound edges are débrided of necrotic and contaminated tissue and lavaged vigorously. A multilayer closure to eliminate dead space is recommended.[48,49,52,54] To relieve tension on the closure, vertical mattress sutures are preplaced deep in the muscular body of the tongue with absorbable or nonabsorbable size 0 or 1 monofilament suture. Buried rows of simple interrupted 2-0 to 0 monofilament absorbable sutures are then used to appose the muscles, obliterating dead space. The vertical mattress sutures are tied, and the lingual mucosa is apposed with simple continuous or interrupted vertical mattress sutures (Fig. 30-41).

Second-intention wound healing for management of tongue lacerations is a viable option, particularly when economic constraints preclude surgical repair, and for chronic and less extensive lacerations. Oral lavage with a clean antiseptic solution after meals and careful attention to the horse's ability to eat and drink are indicated. Lacerations that have healed by second intention but result in poor tongue functionality can be reconstructed using primary closure techniques after sharp débridement of scar tissue.[50,52]

After lingual surgery, most horses eat normally, and temporary feeding via a nasogastric tube is rarely required. Gruels of pelleted feeds mixed with water, bran mashes, and wetted hay can be given before introducing drier feeds.[48,52] Nonsteroidal anti-inflammatory drugs are administered, and antimicrobial therapy is used according to the level of tissue devitalization. Nonabsorbable sutures are removed in 2 weeks. Postoperative complications include excessive swelling of the tongue and suture dehiscence. The cosmetic appearance is usually highly acceptable.

Lips

Lip trauma occurs from protruding rigid objects in the horse's environment, such as metal buckets, nails, bolts, and hooks, or from iatrogenic bit damage.[49,50] When there is major disruption, surgery is indicated to preserve lip function and cosmetic appearance. Injuries with extensive tissue contusion and devitalization should be managed by delayed primary closure to optimize the amount of healthy tissue for suturing; otherwise, most lacerations can be repaired at presentation.[49] General anesthesia facilitates a meticulous repair, but standing surgery is possible with regional anesthesia techniques. The wound edges are prepared routinely by sharp débridement and lavage. The lips are highly mobile tissues, and close adherence of the mucosa and skin to underlying musculature results in excessive motion at suture lines during prehension. This leads to a high incidence of dehiscence unless techniques are employed to stabilize the repair.[49,50,54]

To reduce motion on the suture lines, the margins of the skin and oral mucosa are sharply undermined for 1 to 1.5 cm from the edges of the wound. Vertical mattress 0 to 1 nonabsorbable sutures are then preplaced from the extraoral side through the lip musculature and tied over quills of soft rubber tubing[49] or through buttons.[50] The mucous membrane is closed with simple continuous or interrupted 2-0 monofilament absorbable suture. The skin is apposed with simple interrupted or vertical mattress 2-0 to 0 nonabsorbable monofilament sutures. At the mucocutaneous junction, a vertical mattress pattern is recommended for precise apposition.

Chronic lip lacerations are reconstructed using similar principles as for the repair of acute injuries. A three-layer closure is employed, with the layers being created by sharp dissection of the skin and mucous membrane from the intervening lip muscle and granulating scar tissue. When repairing lacerations involving the commissure of the lips, additional vertical mattress tension-relieving sutures are placed rostral to the primary repair for increased support in this highly mobile area[49] (Fig. 30-42). For an extensive lower lip laceration with loss of tissue, a rotational flap may be used.[55] Avulsions of the lower lip should be supported with large mattress sutures passed through the mandibular symphysis. Wire or nonabsorbable suture material is threaded through holes drilled from the outside of the lip and chin to exit caudal to the incisors in the oral cavity, and stents of soft tubing or buttons are placed under the sutures on the oral and external sides.[49,50] Primary closure of the lip and gingival mucosa is performed if practical.

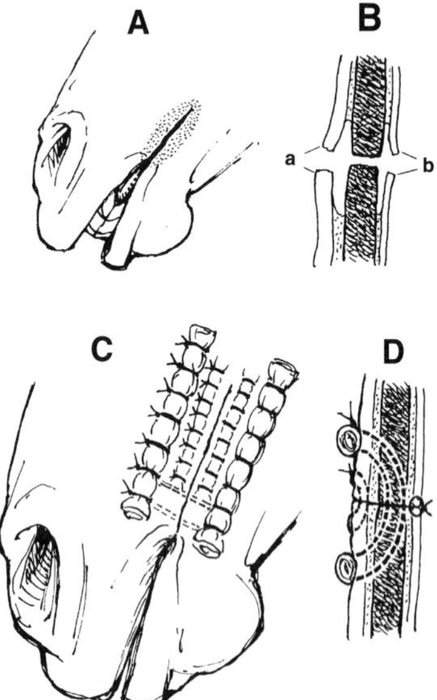

Figure 30-42. Repair of a laceration involving the commissure of the lips. **A** and **B,** After appropriate débridement and lavage of the laceration, the skin and mucous membrane margins of the laceration are undermined 1.0 to 1.5 cm (*stippled area* in **A**). **B** is cross-sectional view with *a,* skin; *b,* mucous membrane. Then vertical mattress sutures tied over stent material are preplaced through the lip musculature before closing the mucous membrane and skin layers to reduce motion at the suture lines (**C, D**). Extra vertical mattress sutures can be placed rostral to the repair to further stabilize the site (**C**).

Nonsteroidal anti-inflammatory drugs are administered, and the oral cavity is lavaged with a dilute antiseptic solution or hose water after meals. Antibiotic administration is not required in most cases. A normal diet can be offered after surgery, and feeding by nasogastric tube or esophagotomy is unnecessary.[49] The stent sutures can be removed after 7 to 10 days and skin sutures after 2 weeks. Mattress sutures used for repair of avulsion injuries are removed 2 to 3 weeks postoperatively. The most common postoperative complication is dehiscence of the repair. Horses have a tendency to rub the repair site, which can be limited by muzzling or cross-tying.[50]

Cheek and Gums

Partial-thickness labial vestibule and buccal cavity lacerations are managed by second-intention wound healing with oral lavaging after meals and nonsteroidal anti-inflammatory drugs. Large, full thickness injuries may be reconstructed to prevent oro-cutaneous fistula development. Repairing the oral aspect of the wound is difficult because of limited space. Suturing the wound from the external side, starting with the mucosal layer, is more practical. Tension-relieving vertical mattress sutures should be used for the musculature.

ORAL CAVITY FOREIGN BODIES

Various types of metallic, usually linear, foreign bodies can penetrate the soft tissues of the oral cavity after inadvertent ingestion.[56,57] Plant matter, such as grass awns or wood splinters, is also a frequent cause of foreign body reaction.[58] External clinical signs include focal or diffuse intermandibular, retropharyngeal, and facial swelling, depending on where the foreign body has lodged or what it is migrating through. Swellings typically have increased heat, and the horse has evidence of pain to palpation of them. Often, antibiotic therapy causes a reduction in the size of the swelling but it recurs when drugs are discontinued. Ptyalism, halitosis, dysphagia, inappetence, and anorexia can be observed. Additionally, there may be a painful response and difficulty when attempts are made to open the jaw. Oral and oropharyngeal examinations (float the teeth before performing the latter) can reveal firm, painful swellings, the end of the foreign body, or ulcerated mucosal surfaces where the foreign body has penetrated the tissue, or where an abscessed site has ruptured spontaneously.

Diagnosis requires a combination of thorough history taking, external and oral examination, and imaging aids. Radiography is indispensable for metallic foreign bodies, but care must be taken not to miss a fine, short structure. Open-mouth head radiographs can prevent tongue soft tissues from being superimposed over radiodense dental elements that may conceal a subtle metallic body (Fig. 30-43). Ultrasonography is very useful to help pinpoint the exact location of a foreign body.[59] Direct tongue ultrasonography may be performed in the standing, sedated horse, with a speculum in place, or when the horse is under general anesthesia. The narrow dimensions for contact of the ultrasound probe limit access to the rostral tongue body via the intermandibular space even when a microconvex head is used.

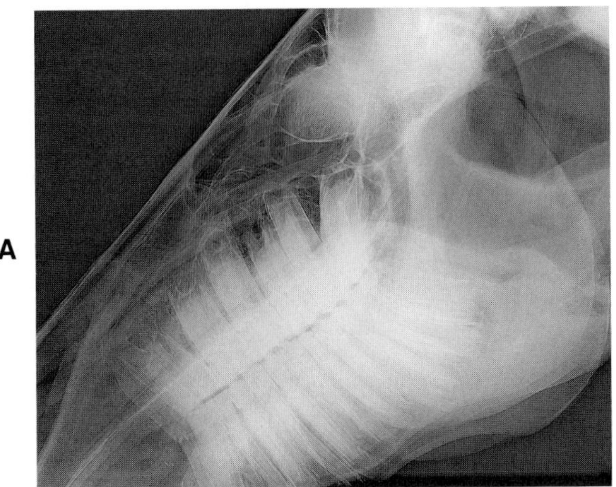

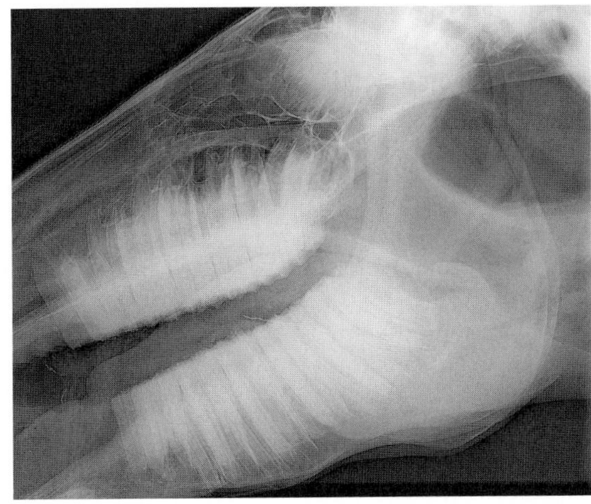

Figure 30-43. A, Closed-jaw, lateral radiographic view of a horse's skull. A barely discernable horizontal, linear opacity is visible superimposed under the mandibular cheek teeth (09s and 10s). **B,** Open jaw, radiographic lateral view of the same horse's skull. Separation of the dental arcades allows easy visualization of the opaque foreign body located in soft tissue (in this case, determined to be the tongue), surrounded by a lucent cavity.

Once a diagnosis is established, the treatment of choice is removal of the foreign body. Surgical approaches may have to be creative. An external approach to a foreign body that has migrated into the deep part of the masseter muscle requires care to avoid trauma to facial nerve branches, parotid duct, and blood vessels in that region. Foreign bodies associated with intraoral swelling may be approached by incising the mass on the oral side and draining exudate into the mouth. Digital or instrumental exploration and débridement of the cavity can then be performed. The cavity is lavaged and allowed to heal by second intention. Lingual foreign bodies can be very awkward to reach when they have implanted or migrated into the caudal body or base of the tongue.[57] Surgery can be associated with significant hemorrhage if large lingual vessels are invaded. An ulcerative defect on the tongue surface provides a useful starting point for exploring the necrotic tract that is associated with the path of the foreign body. A ventral approach between the hemimandibles is necessary in some cases and allows triangulation techniques to narrow down the field of exploration when a second instrument is also passed via the oral cavity into the tongue body. When necessary, the caudal body or base of the tongue can be exposed more effectively after a mandibular symphysiotomy.[57] An oral speculum, an excellent light source, and long-handled instruments are valuable aids. The mouth should not be extended fully open for prolonged periods of time in a speculum (more than 30 to 45 minutes), to prevent muscle and temporomandibular joint soreness postoperatively. Intraoperative ultrasonographic, fluoroscopic, and radiographic guidance may be required to locate the foreign body. Oral endoscopy can aid visualization.

Surgical and necrotic tracts in the tongue are left to heal by second intention. Postoperative care may consist of a combination of oral lavaging, necrotic tract lavaging, and antibiotic and anti-inflammatory therapy. Ptyalism and tongue swelling can be a feature of the early recovery period. Soft feeds and gruels are fed after extensive tongue exploration, until the horse is more comfortable eating. The prognosis is excellent once the foreign body is removed.

PERSISTENT LINGUAL FRENULUM

Ventral ankyloglossia (persistent lingual frenulum) is a very rare congenital condition in foals. The tongue is unable to be protruded as normal because of a mucosal attachment between the ventral rostral free part of the tongue and the floor of the oral cavity. Difficulty with suckling may also occur. The condition is diagnosed by oral examination and is usually noted during the first routine neonatal assessment. Frenuloplasty is the treatment of choice, taking care not to incise the normal lingual frenulum. This may be performed under sedation and local anesthesia or under short-acting general anesthesia. The membrane is sharply transected with scissors. Electrocautery and laser division of the tissue are alternative approaches. With adequate release, the tongue should be easily extended from the mouth.

ORAL CAVITY SOFT TISSUE NEOPLASIA

Neoplasia of the oral cavity soft tissues is infrequently encountered but of considerable clinical significance when identified. The most common primary oral neoplasm is squamous cell carcinoma, affecting any of the mucosal surfaces.[60,61] Other primary or metastatic tumors include melanoma, fibrosarcoma, hemangiosarcoma, lymphosarcoma, rhabdomyoma, and rhabdomyosarcoma of the tongue.[58,60,62-66] Clinical signs include ptyalism, halitosis, quidding, nasal discharge with food material in it, dysphagia, inappetence, anorexia, and weight loss.[58,63,67] Tumor invasion of local bony and soft tissues is often advanced, and regional metastasis may have already occurred before clinical signs become apparent and prompt veterinary attention. Direct visualization of the oral cavity reveals most tumors. Radiography can determine bony involvement, and nasal endoscopy can indicate soft tissue masses on the tongue base displacing the soft palate dorsal to the epiglottis.[63] The definitive diagnosis requires biopsy and histopathologic examination. Often, submandibular lymphadenopathy in horses with oral neoplasia is caused by reactive inflammation rather than metastatic disease, so biopsy of these lymph nodes may be negative in the presence of oral neoplasia.

Successful treatment depends on the type and size of tumor present and its accessibility. Tumors of the lips and rostral tongue are most readily resolved, as they are often noticed early and can be adequately excised or are accessible for intralesional chemotherapy and radiotherapy. Invasive squamous cell carcinomas have a high recurrence rate after surgical excision and have often metastasized by the time they are diagnosed.[58,67]

Complementary radiotherapy after radical surgical excision of squamous cell carcinoma may prevent or prolong time to recurrence.[68] Fibrosarcomas also tend to recur after excision and are less responsive to radiation therapy. The prognosis for resolution of oral squamous cell carcinoma and fibrosarcoma is generally poor.[58] Lingual rhabdomyosarcoma can be managed by surgical excision,[63] but the long-term prognosis is unknown.

Nonneoplastic conditions that should be differentiated from tumors are focal gingival hyperplasia, epulis, and exuberant granulation tissue.[62,66,69,70] These masses can appear neoplastic, but they carry a more favorable prognosis.

SALIVARY GLANDS

Anatomy

The major salivary glands in the horse are the paired parotid, mandibular (submaxillary), and polystomatic sublingual glands. There are also smaller buccal, labial, lingual, and palatine salivary glands.[71] The distribution of serous and mucous cells within the salivary glands determines the nature of the saliva secreted. The parotid salivary gland secretes mainly serous fluid, whereas the mandibular and sublingual glands produce a combination of serous and mucous fluids.

The largest of the salivary glands, the parotid, is located in the retromandibular fossa between the vertical ramus of the mandible and the wing of the atlas. The rostral border reaches and may partially overlap the temporomandibular joint and the masseter muscle along the caudal border of the mandible. The caudal border extends to the wing of the first cervical vertebra. Dorsally, the gland extends to the base of the ear, and ventrally it extends into the intermandibular space. The surfaces of the parotid gland are associated with important vascular and neural structures.[71] Glandular secretions are drained by multiple small ducts that converge at the rostroventral aspect of the gland and exit as the single parotid (Stensen's) duct. The parotid duct initially passes along the medial surface of the mandible in close association with the facial artery and vein. The three structures then travel rostrolaterally around the ventral border of the mandible at the location of the easily palpable facial artery pulse. The duct ascends along the rostral edge of the masseter muscle and opens into the buccal cavity opposite the maxillary 4th premolar tooth (108, 208). A parotid papilla identifies the buccal ostium.

The mandibular salivary gland extends from the atlantal fossa to the basihyoid bone. Most of its lateral surface is covered by the parotid salivary gland and part by the mandible, and its medial surface covers the larynx, common carotid, vagosympathetic trunk, and guttural pouch. Many small radicles unite to form a common duct that travels rostrally, ventral to the tongue. The duct opens a few centimeters rostrolateral to the lingual frenulum, at the sublingual caruncle. The sublingual gland lies beneath the oral mucosa between the body of the tongue and the mandible. It extends from the level of the mandibular symphysis to approximately the first or second mandibular molar (09s and 10s). Sublingual ducts (about 30) open independently at small papillae on the sublingual fold.[71]

Disorders

Trauma

Trauma to the salivary glands is very infrequent, with lacerations or penetrating wounds occasionally occurring. Because of their superficial location, the parotid salivary gland and duct are more subject to traumatic injury than the two other, more deeply located glands.

The hallmark sign of disruption of the gland or duct is the flow of saliva from the wound. This flow is accentuated when the horse is fed, and observation of the wound while offering feed to the horse provides a simple test to confirm that the discharge is saliva.

Diagnosis of duct disruption may be facilitated by catheterizing the duct via the buccal ostium, with the horse under general anesthesia, and seeing the catheter exit the wound. Locating and gaining access to the parotid papilla for retrograde catheterization usually requires a buccotomy incision at the level of the 108 (or 208).[72] A second incision can be made a few centimeters rostral or caudal to the buccotomy to allow tunneling of the tubing subcutaneously to the buccotomy site. Retrograde contrast radiography can also be used to determine communication with a salivary gland in the case of a suspected salivary fistula. If there is no clear indication that a salivary duct or gland has been damaged, it is recommended that parotid wounds be left to heal by second intention.[73] When the duct has been disrupted but this was not recognized at the time of injury, horses may be presented later with a chronically draining tract.[74] Surgical management of salivary gland and duct trauma is fundamentally aimed at repairing the damaged structure or, alternatively, at eliminating saliva secretion. Most salivary fistulas spontaneously close eventually, so deferring treatment for a period of weeks is a worthwhile option.[74]

Fresh wounds of the parotid gland can be débrided and reconstructed with a multilayer closure, starting with the parotid capsule. The potential for suture material that penetrates the glandular tissue to provide a nidus for calculus formation should be considered. Open wound management and healing by second intention is an alternative for older or heavily contaminated wounds and for economic reasons, and this often allows successful healing without the development of a salivary fistula.[58,73,74]

Treatment of lacerated salivary ducts may also be by primary surgical closure or secondary wound healing. Primary closure of an acutely lacerated duct or a nonhealing salivary fistula is facilitated by suturing it over an intraluminal tube[58,72-75] or by placing three sutures to appose the two cut ends as a triangle and suturing between the apices. Cannulation of the parotid papilla may not be practical in some cases.[75] Alternatively, no. 2 nylon suture is threaded normograde through the distal lacerated duct end to the parotid papilla. Tubing is passed via a 14- to 16-gauge needle cannula inserted through the cheek tissue externally to internally to enter the oral cavity just rostral to the parotid papilla. The tubing is then guided over the nylon suture into the duct, and the nylon and needle are removed.[72] When the tip of the tube emerges from the lacerated duct at the wound, it is redirected into the proximal part of the duct and passed to the ventral aspect of the parotid gland. The duct is closed with fine absorbable or nonabsorbable suture (5-0 to 7-0) using a simple interrupted pattern.[72,73,75] The external end of the tube is sutured to the side of the face, allowing for ease of later removal and the ability to check for continued patency of the duct. The need to leave the stent tube in place while the duct is healing after anastomosis, and how long to leave it are unclear.[74-76] The tubing may support the suture line and prevent stricture development while maintaining saliva flow.[72] A gauze mask can be placed over the horse's head to help prevent premature tube removal. If anastomosis of the duct is not possible because of loss of too much intervening tissue, an interposition polytetrafluoroethylene tube graft may be successful in restoring duct continuity.[77] Other options for salvaging salivary secretion capacity are to create a fistula from the duct to the buccal cavity proximal to the injury or alternatively perform duct translocation.[58,73,74,78] These techniques divert saliva from the distal wound site, allowing it to heal, but they are no longer favored because of inconsistent results.

Attempts to reduce salivation after duct or gland repair by withholding feed and water or feeding through a nasogastric tube for a few days have been recommended.[58,76] Others believe this management to be unnecessary and the continued flow of saliva to be important to prevent obstruction.[73-75] Perioperative nonsteroidal anti-inflammatory drugs and antibiotic therapy are administered.

The alternative approach to managing a chronic parotid salivary duct fistula is to attempt to eliminate saliva secretion. Horses can tolerate the loss of one parotid gland.[73,74] This may be performed by surgical removal of the gland, duct ligation, or chemical ablation of the gland. Parotid gland extirpation is difficult, as very careful avoidance of intimately associated large vessels and nerves is required, and removal of all glandular tissue may be impractical because of intervening vital structures.[79,80] Consequently extirpation has been largely replaced by chemical ablation.[74]

Chemical ablation and duct ligation are more economical and easier procedures to perform than major duct reconstruction. For ligation, the parotid duct is readily located where it crosses the tendon of insertion of the sternomandibularis muscle close to its origin from the gland. A catheter is passed retrograde through the duct from the salivary fistula site, toward the gland. The catheter can be palpated in the duct, and this allows definitive isolation of the duct during dissection. Two or three heavy-gauge nonabsorbable sutures should be used for duct ligation and should not be tied too tightly to avoid cutting through the duct wall.[58,81] The distal suture is tied first to distribute resulting back-pressure after ligation.

Successful chemical involution of the parotid gland was first described using Lugol's iodine, with 1 to 2 mL injected transcutaneously into the gland at multiple sites.[81] However, patient discomfort, severe swelling, and the potential for nasopharyngeal collapse and consequent airway obstruction make this method unacceptable today. Other agents that have been examined critically are 10% formalin, 2% chlorhexidine, and 2% and 3% silver nitrate.[82] Of these chemicals, 10% formalin produces the least amount of necrosis and suppurative inflammation, so it is currently recommended.[73,82] Water-soluble iodinated contrast material is also effective in eliminating glandular secretions.[74,82] This must be considered when retrograde sialography is undertaken to investigate a draining fistula or duct atresia. If the contrast material is allowed to drain out and then the duct and gland are lavaged with sterile saline solution, this complication is less likely. When using 10% formalin, the duct is cannulated and a ligature tied to prevent leakage. Thirty-five milliliters of formalin is injected through the cannula into the gland. It is left in for 90 seconds and then allowed to drain out. The cannula is left in place for 36 hours. Cessation of salivary secretions occurs by 3 weeks. Nonsteroidal anti-inflammatory drugs are administered after treatment for pain relief. Postoperative complications after chemical ablation include periocular and facial swelling, transient facial nerve paralysis, anorexia, and dyspnea. Most of these complications have been associated with chlorhexidine and silver nitrate and not with formalin.[73,82]

Sialoliths

Sialoliths are hard concretions composed of calcium carbonate and organic matter that develop within a salivary duct or less commonly a gland.[83-86] Plant material is often found as a nidus of the sialolith formation.[83,84] Sialoliths appear smooth or slightly spiculated, and gray, yellowish, or white.[87] They are rarely recognized but when they occur, they tend to affect older horses and the parotid duct is most commonly involved. Typically, a nonpainful, movable, firm structure is palpable on the lateral aspect of the face near the rostral end of the facial crest (Fig. 30-44). In some cases, the sialolith may be palpable orally.

Obstruction of the duct is often incomplete, and saliva may continue to pass around the sialolith. However, with more severe obstruction, backpressure may cause duct and gland distention, which is noticed as a possibly painful swelling in the intermandibular and retromandibular space.[72,83] Other clinical signs, including the presence of purulent material in the mouth, reddening at the parotid papilla, mild icterus, fever, difficulty masticating, quidding, and decreased appetite, have also been reported in association with sialoliths.[72,83,84] Sialoliths usually occur singularly. If multiple calculi are present in the same duct, a grating sound or sensation may be heard or felt on palpation.[86] Septic sialoadenitis is a rare occurrence in domestic animals but may precede or be a consequence of a developing sialolith.[58] Inflammation and infection of the duct (of ascending, hematogenous, or traumatic origin) results in obstruction by exudates, desquamated cells, and mucus. This material may provide the nidus necessary for a sialolith to form. Partial obstruction of the duct by a sialolith may decrease natural clearance of secretions, resulting in stasis and facilitating proximal movement of bacteria. Diagnosis of sialolithiasis is assisted by radiographs,[83,84] but soft tissue swelling can impede identification of a concretion.[72]

Definitive treatment is by removal of the sialolith. Smaller calculi may be massaged out of the parotid papilla.[58] If this

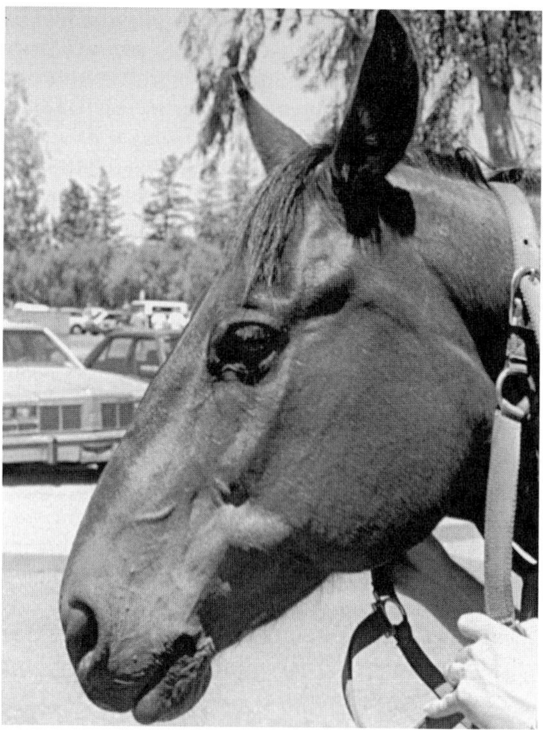

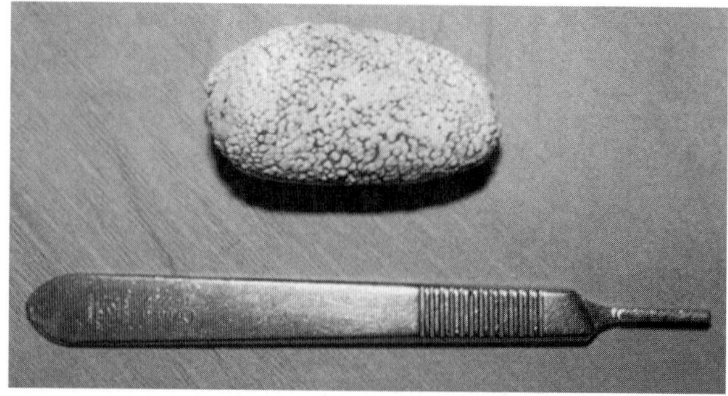

Figure 30-44. A, Photograph of a horse with a sialolith located in the left parotid duct near the rostral edge of the facial crest. **B,** Sialolith removed from a parotid salivary duct. (B, with permission, Equine Veterinary Education 1995;7:315.)

is not possible, and the calculus is near the papilla, direct intraoral incision over the sialolith, leaving the wound to heal by second intention, is preferred.[73,78,81] This approach avoids the risk of external salivary fistula development. Calculi inaccessible by the intraoral route must be removed by external longitudinal incision of the duct. This can be performed as a standing surgery with local anesthesia. Cannulation of the parotid duct via the parotid papilla can be helpful to locate the exact calculus position and then may act as a stent for suturing the duct if primary closure is performed.[83] The entire duct and gland should be lavaged with sterile polyionic solution. Closure of the duct is with a simple interrupted or continuous pattern of fine absorbable suture material. The incision can be left to heal by second intention, and few develop fistulas. Postoperative care is similar to repair of a duct laceration or fistula. Antibiotics and lavage of the duct and gland via catheterization of the oral papilla are recommended in infected cases.[83]

Atresia of the Parotid Salivary Duct

Congenital or acquired functional discontinuity of the parotid salivary duct is very rare in the horse.[79,88,89] Proximal to the obstruction, the dilated duct is characterized by a nonpainful, tortuous, subcutaneous, fluid-filled tube that extends caudally from a point rostral to the masseter (where the obstruction often is located) along the ventral surface of the mandible to the base of the ear on the affected side[74,88,89] (Fig. 30-45). In congenital cases, swelling is present at birth and can increase with time. Swelling may also increase temporarily when the horse is presented with food. Aspirated fluid has the consistency of saliva with an alkaline pH and an acellular, proteinaceous background.[74,89] The swelling recurs after needle drainage, and occasionally saliva continues to drain into subcutaneous tissues after aspiration, setting up a severe inflammatory reaction, followed by persistent sialocele. Diagnosis is based on clinical appearance but can be confirmed with positive-contrast sialography and aspirated fluid analysis. Dilated glandular radicles are seen coalescing into a single grossly distended parotid duct that terminates distally before reaching the buccal cavity.

Treatment options include surgically creating a new buccal ostium, duct excision and proximal ligation, gland extirpation, and chemical ablation of the salivary gland. A buccal fistula is not recommended because of probable spontaneous closure and the potential for ascending contamination of the duct.[74] In one case, removing a large portion of the distended duct and ligating individual radicles was successful.[89] Duct ligation may not be appropriate in a chronic case, as severe dilation may not allow enough back pressure to be generated to cause atrophy of the gland and cessation of secretory activity.[90] Chemical ablation of the gland is an economical, effective, and practical solution and is recommended for most cases. Surgical removal of the duct can be performed for cosmetic reasons after ablation of the gland, but it is a difficult procedure.[74]

Salivary Mucocele and Ranula

Accumulations of saliva can occur in spaces adjacent the local gland or duct, possibly when an external wound has healed but the duct or gland continues to leak. A *mucocele* or *sialocele* refers to a pocket of saliva in a space not lined by epithelium. A *ranula* ("honey cyst") represents a mucocele of one of the sublingual salivary gland ducts and is seen as a bluish-tinged cyst on the floor of the mouth.[87] Fluid aspirated from a sialocele is generally brown and mucinous with a higher concentration of calcium and potassium than is seen in other accumulations of fluid.[76] Salivary fluid also contains amylase. Contrast sialography can determine any

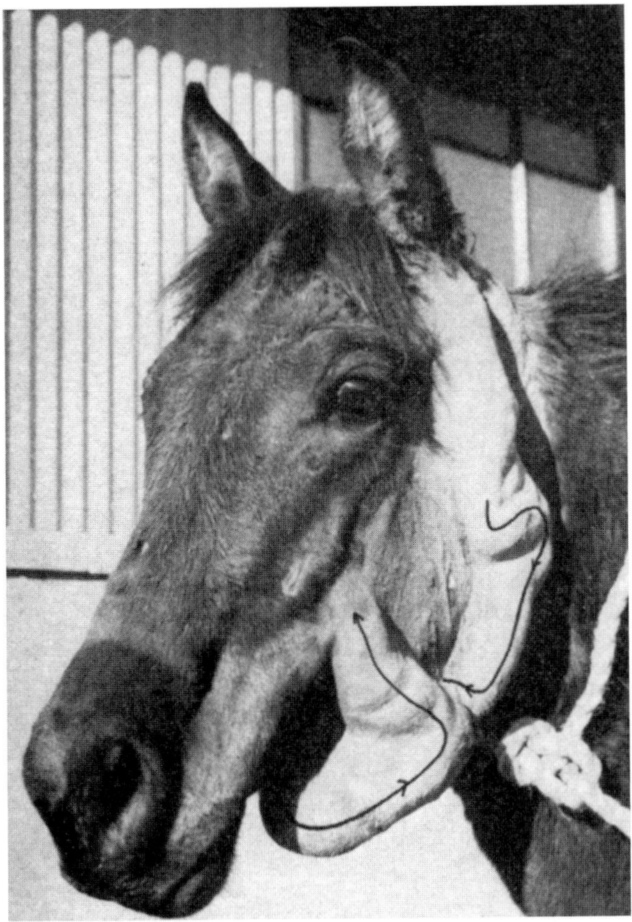

Figure 30-45. Severely dilated parotid salivary duct and gland of a one year old Quarter Horse gelding with congenital atresia of the parotid duct. The duct ended blindly approximately 1.4 cm from the normal site for the buccal ostium. Line arrows mark the course of the duct. (With permission, Journal of the American Veterinary Medical Association 1965;146:1404.)

communication between the cavity and duct or gland. In some cases, complete surgical removal of the structure is appropriate. Ranulas respond well to marsupialization into the oral cavity.[74,76] A catheter can be sutured in place for 2 to 3 weeks to create a permanent fistula. Marsupialization of a mucocele into the buccal cavity is less likely to be successful because of a lack of epithelial lining.[74] Chemical ablation of the parotid gland would be effective and may be the simplest approach if this gland is known to communicate with the mucocele directly or via the duct.[73,74] Later, the mucocele can be drained without expected recurrence.

Heterotopic Salivary Tissue

Salivary tissue found in an abnormal location is a rarely diagnosed disorder and is described as heterotopic salivary tissue. It is possible that this condition goes unrecognized more frequently than it is confirmed; for example, unclassified subclinical lateral nasopharyngeal masses seen endoscopically may be heterotopic salivary tissue.[74] Heterotopic tissue associated with seromucoid draining tracts has been reported in the temporal region and the mid cervical region.[74,91] Drainage of saliva from heterotopic tissue does not increase when the horse is presented with feed. Definitive diagnosis is by histopathology, and complete surgical removal resolves the condition. Chemical ablation of the tissue may also be performed, if the nature of the tissue can be ascertained beforehand.[74]

Idiopathic Parotiditis, "Grass Glands"

Idiopathic parotiditis, or grass glands, refers to a syndrome of recurrent salivary gland swelling that occurs acutely in association with pasture turnout.[92,93] Typically, the parotid salivary glands become swollen during the day while the horse is on pasture, and the swelling resolves overnight when the horse is stalled. The condition is well recognized in Europe and Australia but is uncommon in the United States. Characteristically, there is a rapid development of bilateral swelling of the parotid gland. Glandular swelling is innocuous, firm, and nonpainful, occasionally causes edema at the caudal mandible, and can be mistaken for guttural pouch disease or enlarged lymph nodes (Fig. 30-46). Once the horse is removed from pasture, the glandular swelling resolves. A pasture toxin is suspected but has not been identified. Sporadic or herd outbreaks are possible.

Neoplasia

The salivary glands are a rare site for neoplasia in the horse. Adenocarcinoma, acinar cell tumors, lymphomas, melanomas, and mixed cell tumors have been reported.[87,94,95] Melanomas are commonly seen in the parotid salivary gland of gray horses and may represent a primary or metastatic tumor.[64,95] Tumors in the parotid region can be identified by external swelling and are occasionally painful on palpation. Melanomas typically present as nonpainful, firm, irregular- or smooth-surfaced masses (Fig. 30-47). Diagnosis of neoplasia may require endoscopy, radiology, ultrasonography, and cytology of a fine-needle aspirate. Biopsy and histopathology are indicated for a definitive diagnosis. Treatment is often palliative, as wide surgical margins frequently fail to prevent benign mixed cell tumors, acinar tumors, or

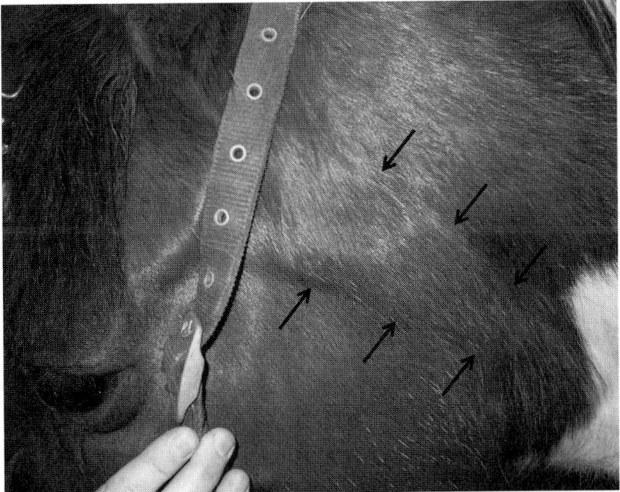

Figure 30-46. Parotid region of a pony showing a nonpainful swelling *(arrows)* that occurred when the pony was at pasture but resolved when it was kept stalled. (Courtesy Dr P. Dixon, Edinburgh University.)

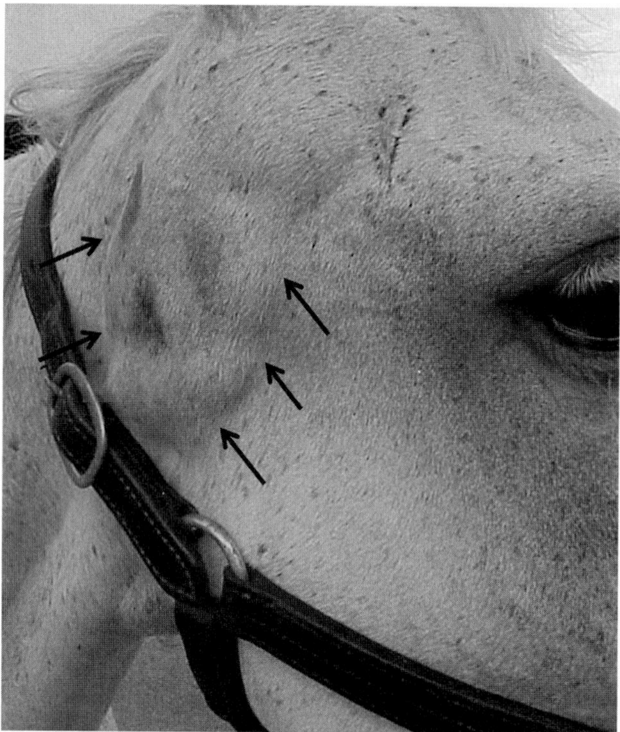

Figure 30-47. Parotid region of an aged Thoroughbred mare showing an irregular-surfaced, firm, nonpainful swelling *(arrows)* caused by melanoma development in the parotid salivary gland. Similar masses were present on the opposite side, and melanomas were visualized in this mare's guttural pouches.

melanomas from recurring. As previously mentioned, total parotidectomy is challenging and generally considered impractical in the horse.[74] Adenocarcinomas often metastasize.[94] Lymphomas can respond to radiation therapy.[96] Cimetidine may help with melanomas,[97-99] but often this treatment is not justified because they are slow growing and most have low malignancy.

TEMPOROMANDIBULAR JOINT

Anatomy

The horse has diarthrodial temporomandibular joints (TMJ) formed by the condylar process of the mandible and the articular tubercle of the temporal bone.[71] Dorsal and ventral compartments are completely[100,101] or incompletely[102] separated by a fibrocartilaginous disc. The large dorsal compartment, referred to as the discotemporal joint, has a prominent caudolateral extension.[102,103] The smaller ventral compartment, the discomandibular joint, has rostrolateral and caudolateral extensions.[101,103] Fibrocartilage, rather than hyaline cartilage, covers the articular surfaces of the joint. The intra-articular disc, shaped like a slightly straightened C, ensures a congruent joint that is essential for mediolateral movement of the mandible in relation to the maxilla to provide effective grinding between the dental arcades.[104] There is a close relationship between the planar angles of the TMJ (15 degrees) and the occlusal surfaces of the CT and the palatine ridges. This angular association is significant for functional mastication and bolus development for deglutition.[104] The caudal margin of the TMJ is closely associated with the rostral border of the parotid salivary gland, and there may be slight dorsal overlap of the gland.[102,105] Caudal and lateral ligaments support the joint but have been difficult to identify in anatomic studies.[101,103]

Disorders affecting the TMJ include luxation, fracture, trauma, and nonseptic and septic arthropathies.[100] Reports of TMJ disorders and treatment are sporadic,[104,106-110] although the literature of the past few years abounds with papers on diagnostic procedures.[101-103,105] The prevalence of disease may be greater than is currently recognized, and it is likely to increase as more methods of TMJ examination are utilized.

Clinical Signs

The clinical signs of TMJ dysfunction are varied and often nonspecific. Dysphagia, quidding, inappetence, chronic weight loss, incisor malocclusion, altered range of motion and pain on manipulation of the mandible, localized pain and heat on palpation of the TMJ, localized swelling over the TMJ, muscle asymmetry, and draining fistulas may be identified (Fig. 30-48). Behavioral manifestations of TMJ pain include signs of depression, head shaking, altered head carriage, altered prehension and mastication, resistance to accepting the bit and other head tack, and abnormalities detected by the rider or driver during exercise. Trauma to the TMJ resulting in fractures or luxations results in acute pain and swelling, impaired prehension, and inability to appose the upper and lower incisors.[100,104,106-109,111]

Diagnosis

The history and clinical examination may raise the level of suspicion for TMJ pathology. However, synovial fluid analysis and effective imaging are important in determining a definitive diagnosis of the condition. TMJ effusion may not be grossly visible, but arthrocentesis of the dorsal joint

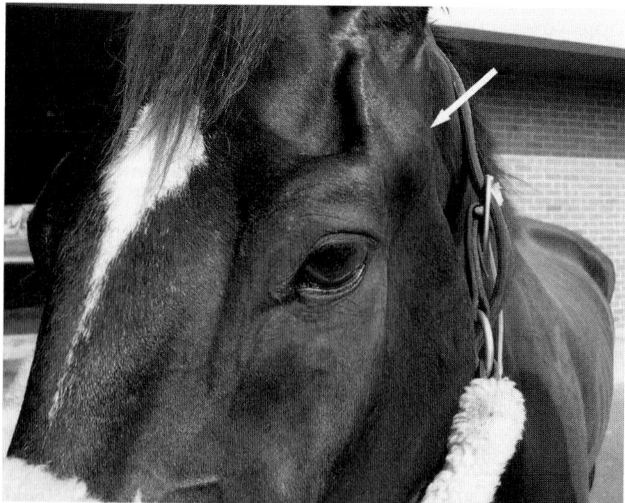

Figure 30-48. A firm enlargement of the left temporomandibular joint *(arrow)* is present in this horse, diagnosed with a septic arthritis. Atrophy of the left masseter muscle is also apparent. The horse exhibited signs of pain when eating and when attempts were made to open its mouth.

compartment is still practical using anatomic landmarks.[102] It is also suggested that the ventral compartment be accessed for synovial fluid collection.[103] Intra-articular anesthesia of the TMJ with 2 to 4 mL of local anesthetic may confirm it as a source of pain; however, it must be determined whether pain alleviation indicates a primary joint condition or TMJ pain secondary to another condition such as dental disease.[100,104]

Radiographs have traditionally been unrewarding in diagnosing TMJ pathology because considerable superimposition of head structures makes interpretation difficult.[100,107] Oblique views provide the most useful of the limited information. Obvious joint disparity (e.g., a luxation or fracture) can be confirmed on radiographs, but bone lysis or proliferation is unlikely to be readily identified (Fig. 30-49).

Ultrasonographic examination of the TMJ provides a noninvasive method of assessing the lateral aspect of the joint capsule, and the articular disc and surfaces.[103] A 7.5-MHz linear array transducer is used in B mode to examine the TMJ in a minimum of three transverse views. The caudolateral space, lateral middle area, and rostrolateral space are imaged. Thin articular cartilage is barely visible in aged horses but is about 3 mm thick in foals. Articular fluid is typically not seen in the normal TMJ. Any changes in the normal ultrasonographic appearance of the TMJ are indicative of pathology.[103] Findings associated with severe degenerative joint disease of the TMJ have included irregular articular surfaces, absence of the intra-articular disc, a narrowed joint space, and a thickened fibrous capsule[107] (Fig. 30-50).

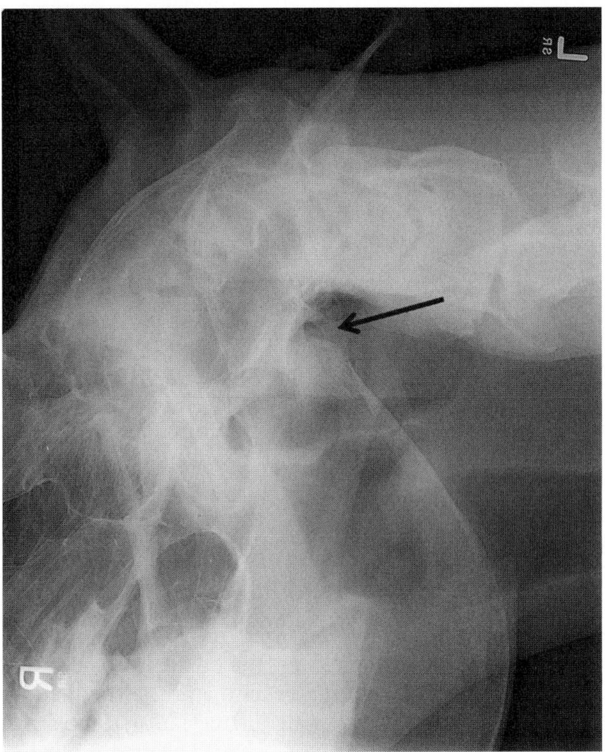

Figure 30-49. Radiographic oblique view of the left temporomandibular joint indicating a widened and incongruent joint space *(arrow)* that was interpreted as evidence of subluxation. This horse is shown in Figure 30-48.

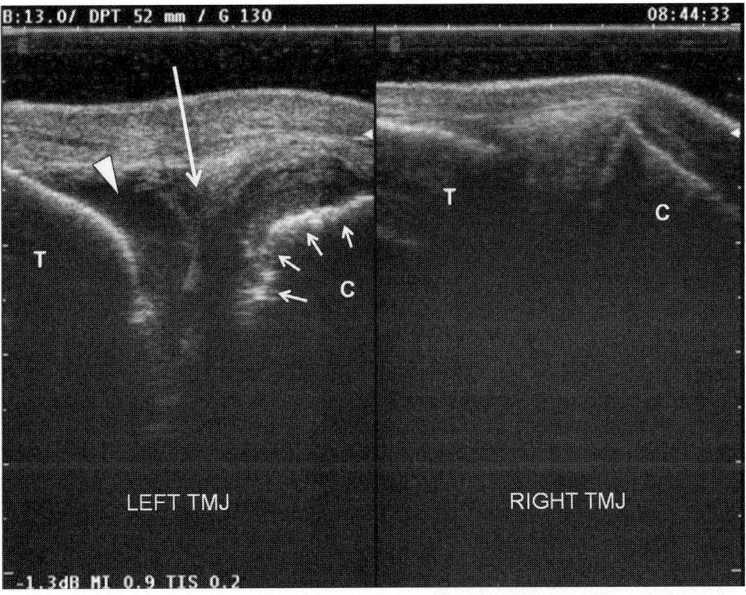

Figure 30-50. Ultrasonographic images obtained in similar planes of the left and right temporomandibular joints of the horse seen in Figure 30-48. Note a widened joint space, irregular bony margins to the mandibular condyle *(short arrows)*, loss of definition of the fibrocartilaginous disc *(long arrow)*, increased synovial fluid *(arrowhead)*, and increased soft tissue thickness at the left temporomandibular joint compared with the normal right temporomandibular joint. C, mandibular condyle; T, temporal articular process; TMJ, temporomandibular joint.

Soft tissue and bone phase nuclear scintigraphy of the head are useful for confirming the TMJ as the location of an active process, but it is not specific for any one type of disorder.[107,112] Computed tomography provides a method to evaluate the TMJ without superimposition of structures, and its usefulness has been reported in clinical cases[106,111] (Fig. 30-51). The disadvantages are cost, limited facilities with tomography for horses, and the need for general anesthesia. Magnetic resonance imaging also provides an excellent means to evaluate the TMJ, but it has similar disadvantages.[113]

Diagnostic arthroscopy of the TMJ has been described using a 4-mm, 30-degree, forward-viewing scope.[101,105] A caudodorsal approach provided the best evaluation of the lateral aspect of the dorsal compartment of the TMJ, including the articular disc. Visualization of the medial aspect of the compartment is very limited. Access to the lateral aspect of the ventral compartment is complicated by the position of the transverse facial artery and vein, but the rostrolateral area can be explored.[101] Synovial villi are seen in both compartments in selected locations. An instrument portal can be created using a triangulation technique, but manipulations are restricted by the small space available, and separating articular surfaces with a probe results in too much iatrogenic damage.[101] Lateral translational movement of the mandibular condyle away from the surgeon improves observation of the dorsal compartment. Fluid flow through the joint may be via an ingress-and-egress cannula or via a hypodermic needle attached to a partially filled syringe, followed by allowing back-and-forth fluid instillation and withdrawal with the syringe. Subcutaneous extravasation of fluids will occur if the joint is overdistended. Use of ultrasonography to determine the safest location of portals to avoid damaging adjacent vital structures is recommended.[101]

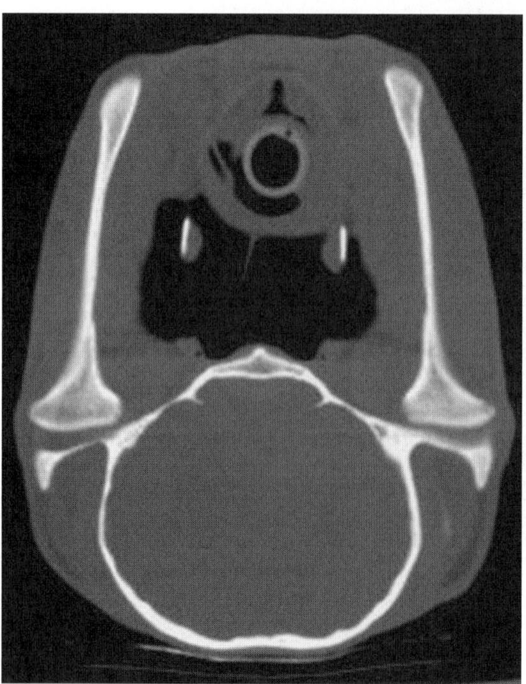

Figure 30-51. Computed tomographic image of a miniature horse in dorsal recumbency, showing the temporomandibular joints. Slight asymmetry from one side to the other is caused by positioning.

Postoperatively, mild pain on palpation of the TMJ can be expected for 1 to 2 days, but eating should be as it was preoperatively.

Treatment

Treatment approaches for TMJ diseases follow the same principles used for other joints. Arthroscopic débridement, joint lavage, systemic and intra-articular antibiotics, and anti-inflammatory drugs are indicated for septic conditions of the TMJ.[106] Nonseptic arthropathies may respond to anti-inflammatory drugs, applied systemically and intra-articularly.[100,107] Conservative treatment of TMJ luxation is possible.[109] Arthroscopic evaluation of a luxated TMJ may provide prognostic information in terms of the degree of damage to articular surfaces and joint soft tissues. Acute luxation of the TMJ can be reduced under general anesthesia, but the long-term prognosis for reduction is not known.[110]

Unilateral or bilateral mandibular condylectomy may be used to treat painful and dysfunctional TMJs that have developed secondary to luxations, condylar fractures, severe arthritis, or ankylosis.[108,114,115] The procedure is performed with the horse under general anesthesia and in lateral recumbency. A 6-cm horizontal skin incision is made, centered on the TMJ. Soft tissues, containing transverse facial neurovascular structures, are reflected ventrally to expose the joint capsule. The capsule is incised horizontally to expose the joint. The periosteum on the mandibular condyle is incised vertically for 2.5 cm and then elevated with a periosteal elevator both rostrally and caudally. An oscillating bone saw is used to make a 2-cm-deep, horizontal cut in the mandibular condyle, about 2.5 cm ventral to the articular margin (Fig. 30-52). An osteotome is inserted into the osteotomy and then lifted dorsally to fracture off the lateral portion of the condyle. Removal of this part of the condyle provides room to continue the osteotomy through the medial aspect of the condyle, using the oscillating bone saw. The condyle is grasped with forceps and freed from medial capsular attachments with scissors before removal. The meniscus is removed by incising its soft tissue attachments

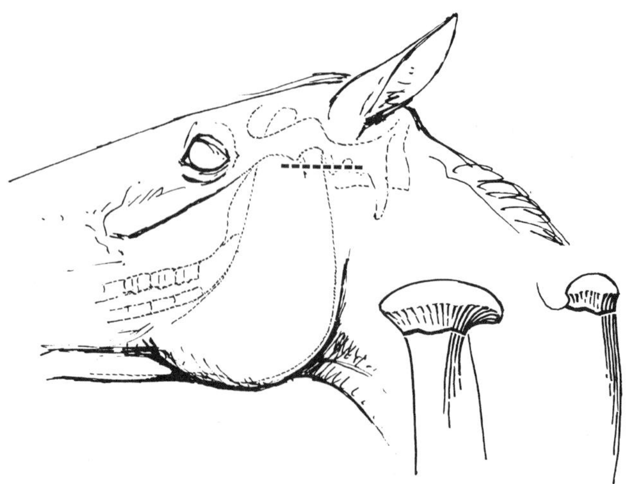

Figure 30-52. Mandibular condylectomy showing the line of incision and the level of resection of the mandibular condyle from two sides

with a scalpel or scissors. A three-layer closure is performed: periosteum and joint capsule combined, the subcutaneous tissue, and the skin.

Close attention to addressing the primary problem is always paramount. Many TMJ disorders may be secondary to dental wear abnormalities, so appropriate dentistry procedures must be performed when indicated.[100,104]

REFERENCES

1. Traub-Dargatz JL, Salman MD, Voss JL: Medical problems of adult horses as ranked by equine practitioners, J Am Vet Med Assoc 1991;198:1745.
2. BEVA: British Equine Veterinary Association survey of equine disease, 1962-63, Vet Rec 1965;77:528.
3. Rucker BA: Equine cheek teeth angle of occlusion: How to calculate and clinical use, Equine Vet Educ 2004;16:137.
4. Dacre IT, Dixon PM: Clinical aspects of the dento-pulpal complex in equine dental disease, Proc 17th Annu Vet Dental Forum, 2003:193.
5. Miles AEW, Grigson C: Colyer's Variations and Diseases of the Teeth of Animals, revised ed, Cambridge, UK, 1990, Cambridge University Press.
6. Carmalt JL, Townsend HGG, Allen AL: Effect of dental floating on the rostro-caudal mobility of the mandible of horses, J Am Vet Med Assoc 2003;223:666.
7. Easley KJ: Basic equine orthodontics. In Baker GJ, Easley KJ, editors: Equine Dentistry, ed 1, London, 1999, WB Saunders.
8. McIlwraith CW: Equine digestive system. In Jennings PB, editor: The Practice of Large Animal Surgery, Philadelphia, 1984, WB Saunders.
9. Alexander K, McMillen RG, Easley J: Incisor extraction in a horse by a longitudinal forage technique, Equine Vet Educ 2001;13:179.
10. Dixon PM, Tremaine WH, Pickles K, et al: Equine dental disease: Part 1. A long-term study of 400 cases—Disorders of incisor, canine and first premolar teeth, Equine Vet J 1999;31:369.
11. Greet TRC: Oral and dental trauma. In Baker GJ, Easley KJ, editors: Equine Dentistry, ed 1, London, 1999, WB Saunders.
12. Dixon PM: The gross, histological, and ultrastructural anatomy of equine teeth and their relationship to disease, Proc Am Assoc Equine Pract 2002;48:421.
13. Easley KJ: Equine tooth removal (exodontia). In Baker GJ, Easley KJ, editors: Equine Dentistry, ed 1, London, 1999, WB Saunders.
14. Scrutchfield WL: Dental prophylaxis. In Baker GJ, Easley KJ, editors: Equine Dentistry, ed 1, London, 1999, WB Saunders.
15. Barrion P, Blin PC, Moliner F: Contribution a l'étude du mecanisme de formation de fistule des premolaires chez de jeune cheval, Bull Acad Vet de France 1980;53:285.
16. Dixon PM, Tremaine WH, McGorum BC, et al: Equine dental disease: Part 2. A long-term study of 400 cases—Disorders of development, eruption and variations in position of the cheek teeth, Equine Vet J 1999;31:519.
17. Dixon PM: Dental anatomy. In Baker GJ, Easley KJ, editors: Equine Dentistry, ed 2, London, 2004, WB Saunders.
18. Wafa NSW: A study of dental disease in the horse. MVM thesis, National University of Ireland, Dublin, 1988:77.
19. Carmalt JL: Understanding the equine diastema, Equine Vet Educ 2003;15:34.
20. Easley J: A new look at dental radiography, Proc Am Assoc Equine Pract 2002;48:412.
21. Barakzai SZ, Dixon PM: A study of open-mouthed oblique radiographic projections for evaluating lesions of the erupted (clinical) crown, Equine Vet Educ 2003;15:143.
22. Leue G (1941), cited by Becker E: Zaehne. In Dobberstein J, Pallaske G, Stuenzi H, editors: Handbuch der Speziellen Pathologischen Anatomie der Haustiere, ed 3, Band V. Berlin, 1962, Verlag Paul Parey.
23. Baker G, Easley J, editors: Equine Dentistry, ed 2, London, WB Saunders, 2004.
24. Smith JC: Osteitis and sequestrum formation of the interdental region of the mandible in 11 polo ponies, Vet Rec 1993;133:188.
25. Dixon PM, Tremaine WH, McGorum BC, et al: Equine dental disease: Part 3. A long term study of 400 cases—Disorders of wear, traumatic damage, other fractures, tumours and miscellaneous disorders of the cheek teeth, Equine Vet J 2000;32:9.
26. Johnson T: Surgical removal of mandibular periostitis (bone spurs) caused by bit damage, Proc Am Assoc Equine Pract 2002;48:458.
27. Dacre IT, Dixon PM: The histopathology of cheek teeth fractures, Proc 17th Annu Vet Dental Forum, 2003:232.
28. Dixon PM, Dacre I, Dacre K, et al: Standing oral extraction of cheek teeth in 100 younger horses (1998-2003), Equine Vet J 2005;37:105.
29. Johnson T, Basil T: Personal communications, 2003.
30. Head KW: Tumours of the alimentary tract. In Moulton JE, editor: Tumours of the domestic animals, Berkeley, 1990, University of California Press.
31. Pirie RS, Dixon PM: Mandibular tumours in the horse: A review of the literature and 7 case reports, Equine Vet Educ 1993;5:287.
32. Knottenbelt DC: Oral and dental tumours. In Baker GJ, Easley KJ, editors: Equine Dentistry, ed 1, London, 1999, WB Saunders.
33. Dixon PM, Tremaine WH, McCann J, et al: Equine dental disease: Part 4. A long term study of 400 cases—Apical infections of cheek teeth, Equine Vet J 2000;32:182.
34. Dacre IT: A pathological, histological and ultrastructural study of diseased equine cheek teeth. PhD Thesis, University of Edinburgh, 2004.
35. Carmalt JL, Barber S: Periapical curettage: An alternative surgical approach to infected mandibular cheek teeth in horses, Vet Surg 2004;33:267.
36. Tremaine WH: Oral extraction of equine cheek teeth, Equine Vet Educ 2004;16:151.
37. Dixon PM: Dental extraction and endodontic techniques in horses, Comp Cont Educ Prac Vet 1997;19:628.
38. Prichard MA, Hackett RP, Erb HN: Long-term outcome of tooth repulsion in horses: A retrospective study of 61 cases, Vet Surg 1992;21:145.
39. Orsini PG, Ross MW, Hamir AN: Levator nasolabialis muscle transposition to prevent an orosinus fistula after tooth extraction in horses, Vet Surg 1992;21:150.
40. Lane JG: Equine dental extraction: Repulsion vs. lateral buccotomy, techniques and results, Proceedings of the 5th World Veterinary Dental Congress, Birmingham, UK, 1997:135.
41. Tremaine WH, Dixon PM: Equine sinonasal disorders: A long-term study of 277 cases. Part II. Treatment and long-term response to treatment, Equine Vet J 2001;33:283.
42. Evans LH, Tate LP, LaDow CS: Extraction of the equine 4th upper premolar and 1st and 2nd molars through a lateral buccotomy, Proc Am Assoc Equine Pract 1981;27:249.
43. Lane JG, Kertesz P: Equine dental surgery. In Kertesz P, editor: A Colour Atlas of Veterinary Dentistry and Oral Surgery, London, 1993, Wolf.
44. Boussauw B: Indications and techniques for buccotomy, Proceedings of 42nd British Equine Veterinary Association Congress, Birmingham, UK, 2003:264.
45. Baker GJ: Endodontic therapy. In Baker GJ, Easley KJ, editors: Equine Dentistry, ed 1, London, 1999, WB Saunders.
46. Schramme M, Robinson J, Boswell J, Butson R: Results of endodontic therapy for periapical infection in nineteen equine CT, Proc Am Assoc Equine Pract 2000;46:119.
47. Tom Johnson: Personal communications, 2004.
48. Adams SB, Becht JL: Surgical repair of a severe laceration in a horse's tongue, Vet Med Small Anim Clin 1978;73:1394.
49. Howard RD, Stashak TS: Reconstructive surgery of selected injuries of the head, Vet Clin North Am Equine Pract 1993;9:185.

50. Hague BA, Honnas CM: Traumatic dental disease and soft tissue injuries of the oral cavity, Vet Clin North Am Equine Pract 1998; 14:333.
51. Ross MW, Gentile DG, Evans LE: Transoral axial division, under endoscopic guidance, for correction of epiglottic entrapment in horses, J Am Vet Med Assoc 1993;203:416.
52. White NA, Hoffman PE: Surgical repair of equine lingual lacerations, Equine Pract 1980;2:37.
53. Mohammed A, Ribadu AY, Hassan SU: Partial glossectomy in a stallion, Vet Rec 1991;128:355.
54. Stashak TS: Wound management and reconstructive surgery of the head region. In Stashak TS, editor: Equine Wound Management, Philadelphia, 1991, Lea & Febiger.
55. Smyth GB, Brown RG, Juzwiak JS, et al: Delayed repair of an extensive lip laceration in a colt using an Estlander flap, Vet Surg 1988;17:350.
56. Kiper ML, Wrigley R, Traub-Dargatz J, Bennett D: Metallic foreign bodies in the mouth or pharynx of horses: seven cases (1983-1989), J Am Vet Med Assoc 1992;200:91.
57. Engelbert TA, Tate LP Jr: Penetrating lingual foreign bodies in three horses, Cornell Vet 1993;83:31.
58. Koch DB: The oral cavity, oropharynx and salivary glands. In Mansmann RA, McAllister ES, editors: Equine Medicine and Surgery, ed 3, Santa Barbara, Calif, 1982, American Veterinary Publications.
59. Rose PL, Penninck D: Use of intraoperative ultrasonography in six horses, Vet Surg 1995;24:396.
60. Dorn CR, Priester WA: Epidemiologic analysis of oral and pharyngeal cancer in dogs, cats, horses, and cattle, J Am Vet Med Assoc 1976;169:1202.
61. Schuh JC: Squamous cell carcinoma of the oral, pharyngeal and nasal mucosa in the horse, Vet Pathol 1986;23:205.
62. Colahan PT: Diseases of the lips, mouth, tongue, and oropharynx. In Colahan PT, Merritt AM, Moore JN, Mayhew IG, editors: Equine Medicine and Surgery, ed 5, St Louis, 1999, Mosby.
63. Hanson PD, Frisbie DD, Dubielzig RR, Markel MD: Rhabdomyosarcoma of the tongue in a horse, J Am Vet Med Assoc 1993;202:1281.
64. MacGillivray KC, Sweeney RW, Del Piero F: Metastatic melanoma in horses, J Vet Intern Med 2002;16:452.
65. Hance SR, Bertone AL: Neoplasia, Vet Clin North Am Equine Pract 1993;9:213.
66. Barker IK, Van Dreumel AA, Palmer N: Tumors of the oral cavity. In Jubb KVF, Kennedy PC, Palmer N, editors: Pathology of Domestic Animals, ed 4, San Diego, 1993, Academic Press.
67. MacFadden KE, Pace LW: Clinical manifestations of squamous cell carcinoma in horses, Comp Cont Educ Pract Vet 1991;13:669.
68. Orsini JA, Nunamaker DM, Jones CJ, Acland HM: Excision of oral squamous cell carcinoma in a horse, Vet Surg 1991;20:264.
69. Handy LH, Peyton LC, Calderwood-Mays MB, Ackerman N: Focal gingival hyperplasia in a horse, J Am Vet Med Assoc 1993; 202:1287.
70. Verstraete FJ, Ligthelm AJ: Excessive granulation tissue of periodontal origin in a horse, Equine Vet J 1988;20:380.
71. The head and ventral neck of the horse. In Dyce KM, Sack WO, Wensing CJG, editors: Textbook of Veterinary Anatomy, Philadelphia, 1987, WB Saunders.
72. Olivier A, Steenkamp G, Petrick SW, Gottschalk RD: Parotid duct laceration repair in two horses. J S Afr Vet Assoc 1998;69:108.
73. Rakestraw PC: Pathology of the salivary glands and esophagus. In 8th Geneva Congress of Equine Medicine and Surgery, Geneva, Switzerland, 2003:38.
74. Schumacher J, Schumacher J: Diseases of the salivary glands and ducts of the horse, Equine Vet Educ 1995;7:313.
75. Newton SA, Knottenbelt DC, Daniel EA: Surgical repair of the parotid gland in a gelding, Vet Rec 1997;140:280.
76. Moore JN: Diseases of the salivary glands. In Colahan PT, Mayhew IG, Merritt AM, Moore JN, editors: Equine Medicine and Surgery, ed 4, Goleta, Calif, 1991, American Veterinary Publications.
77. Kannegieter NJ, Ecke P: Reconstruction of the parotid duct in a horse using an interposition polytetrafluoroethylene tube graft, Aust Vet J 1992;69:62.
78. Pascoe JR: Oral cavity and salivary glands. In Auer JA, Stick JA, editors: Equine Surgery, ed 2, Philadelphia, 1999, WB Saunders.
79. Peddie JF, Tobler EE, Walker EJ: Extirpation of the parotid gland in a mare, Vet Med Small Anim Clin 1971;66:605.
80. Bracegirdle JR: Removal of the parotid and mandibular salivary glands from a pony mare, Vet Rec 1976;98:507.
81. Frank ER: In Veterinary Surgery, 7th ed. Minneapolis, 1964, Burgess.
82. Schmotzer WB, Hultgren BD, Huber MJ, et al: Chemical involution of the equine parotid salivary gland, Vet Surg 1991;20:128.
83. Baskett A, Parks AP, Mahaffey M: Sialolith and sialadenitis associated with a foreign body in a mare, Equine Vet Educ 1995;7:309.
84. Bouayad H, Ouragh L, Johnson DW, et al: Sialoliths in the horse, Equine Pract 1991;13:25.
85. Ramey DW: Sialolith in a horse, Mod Vet Pract 1987:308.
86. Singh AP, Rifat JF, Soliman AS, et al: Sialoliths in a mare, Equine Pract 1987;9:27.
87. Barker IK, Van Dreumel AA, Palmer N: The salivary glands. In Jubb KVF, Kennedy PC, Palmer N, editors: Pathology of Domestic Animals, ed 4, San Diego; 1993, Academic Press.
88. Fowler ME: Congenital atresia of the parotid duct in a horse, J Am Vet Med Assoc 1965;146:1403.
89. Sadler VM, Wisner ER, Robertson JT, Moses VS: Congenital atresia of the parotid duct in a horse, Vet Radiol Ultrasound 1999;40:259.
90. Talley MR, Modransky PD, Welker FH, et al: Congenital atresia of the parotid salivary duct in a 7-month-old Quarter Horse colt, J Am Vet Med Assoc 1990;197:1633.
91. Dahlgren LA, DeBowes RM, Gift LJ, Veatch JK: Heterotopic salivary tissue in a weanling colt, J Am Vet Med Assoc 1992;201:303.
92. Dixon PM: Swellings of the head region in the horse. In Pract 1991;13:257.
93. Knottenbelt DC, Pascoe RR: Color Atlas of Diseases and Disorders of the Horse, London, 1994, Mosby-Wolfe.
94. Stackhouse LL, Moore JJ, Hylton WE: Salivary gland adenocarcinoma in a mare, J Am Vet Med Assoc 1978;172:271.
95. Fintl C, Dixon PM: A review of five cases of parotid melanoma in the horse, Equine Vet Educ 2001;13:17.
96. Coumbe KM: Primary parotid lymphoma in a 10-year-old Hanoverian gelding, Equine Vet Educ 1994;6:91.
97. Goetz TE, Long MT: Treatment of melanomas in horses, Comp Cont Educ Pract Vet 1993;4:608.
98. Hare JE, Staempfli HR: Cimetidine for the treatment of melanomas in horses: Efficacy determined by client questionnaire, Equine Pract 1994;16:18.
99. Warnick LD, Graham ME, Valentine BA: Evaluation of cimetidine treatment for melanomas in seven horses, Equine Pract 1995; 17:16.
100. Moll HD, May KA: A review of conditions of the equine temporomandibular joint, Proc Am Assoc Equine Pract 2002;48:240.
101. Weller R, Maierl J, Bowen IM, et al: The arthroscopic approach and intra-articular anatomy of the equine temporomandibular joint, Equine Vet J 2002;34:421.
102. Rosenstein DS, Bullock MF, Ocello PJ, Clayton HM: Arthrocentesis of the temporomandibular joint in adult horses. Am J Vet Res 2001;62:729.
103. Weller R, Taylor S, Maierl J, Cauvin ER, May SA: Ultrasonographic anatomy of the equine temporomandibular joint, Equine Vet J 1999;31:529.
104. Baker GJ: Equine temporomandibular joints (TMJ): Morphology, function, and clinical disease, Proc Am Assoc Equine Pract 2002;48:442.
105. May KA, Moll HD, Howard RD, et al: Arthroscopic anatomy of the equine temporomandibular joint, Vet Surg 2001;30:564.
106. Warmerdam EP, Klein WR, van Herpen BP: Infectious temporo-

mandibular joint disease in the horse: Computed tomographic diagnosis and treatment of two cases, Vet Rec 1997;141:172.
107. Weller R, Cauvin ER, Bowen IM, May SA: Comparison of radiography, scintigraphy and ultrasonography in the diagnosis of a case of temporomandibular joint arthropathy in a horse, Vet Rec 1999;144:377.
108. Patterson LJ, Shappell KK, Hurtig MB: Mandibular condylectomy in a horse, J Am Vet Med Assoc 1989;195:101.
109. Hurtig MB, Barber SM, Farrow CS: Temporomandibular joint luxation in a horse, J Am Vet Med Assoc 1984;185:78.
110. Hardy J, Shiroma JT: What is your diagnosis? Rostral luxation of the right temporomandibular joint, J Am Vet Med Assoc 1991;198:1663.
111. Tietje S, Becker M, Bockenhoff G: Computed tomographic evaluation of head diseases in the horse: 15 cases, Equine Vet J 1996; 28:98.
112. Metcalf MR, Tate LP, Sellet LC: Clinical use of 99m Tc-MDP scintigraphy in the equine mandible and maxilla, Vet Radiol 1989;30:80.
113. Tucker RL, Farrell E: Computed tomography and magnetic resonance imaging of the equine head, Vet Clin North Am Equine Pract 2001;17:131.
114. Beard W: The skull, maxilla, and mandible. In Auer JA, Stick JA, editors: Equine Surgery, ed 2, Philadelphia, 1999, WB Saunders.
115. Barber SM, Doige CE, Humphreys SG: Mandibular condylectomy: Technique and results in normal horses, Vet Surg 1985;14:79.

CHAPTER 31

Esophagus

John A. Stick

The clinical signs, diagnosis, and therapy of esophageal disease are specific and unlike those of the rest of the alimentary system. Clinical evaluation of the equine patient with esophageal disease includes physical, radiographic, and endoscopic examinations. Early and definitive diagnosis is paramount when dealing with esophageal injury, especially when signs of disease recur after initial treatment. Therapy of esophageal disorders often centers around conservative medical and manipulative management, with dietary alterations being a primary component of therapy. However, surgical management of esophageal disease in the equine patient has become commonplace and necessitates discussion of surgical anatomy, diagnostic and therapeutic considerations, surgical techniques, and complications.[1-3]

SURGICAL ANATOMY

The esophagus of adult horses varies in length from 125 to 200 cm (49 to 78 inches), depending on the size of the animal, and consists of cervical, thoracic, and abdominal parts. As it courses caudally, it deviates from a position dorsal to the trachea in the cranial one third of the neck to the left side of the medial plane in the middle one third of the neck. (In a small percentage of horses, the esophagus courses to the right side of the median plane.) It comes to lie ventral to the trachea at the thoracic inlet.[4] The cervical part of the equine esophagus is most accessible to surgery and makes up over 50% of the total length of the esophagus.

The wall of the esophagus is composed of four layers: a fibrous layer (tunica adventitia), muscular layers (tunicae muscularis), a submucosal layer (tela submucosa), and a mucous membrane (tunica mucosa). The muscular layers are striated from the pharynx to the base of the heart, where they gradually blend into smooth muscle. As the esophagus courses caudally, its muscular layers increase in thickness, whereas the lumen diminishes. Except at the upper esophageal sphincter, the two muscular layers are arranged spirally and elliptically.[5] On surgical incision, the esophageal wall separates easily into two distinct layers. The elastic inner layer, composed of mucosa and submucosa, is freely movable within the relatively inelastic outer muscular layer and adventitia (Fig. 31-1). The mucosa, which provides the greatest tensile strength on closure of an esophageal incision, is covered with stratified squamous epithelium and lies in longitudinal folds that obliterate the lumen except during deglutition. The mucosa is very heavily colonized by bacteria, and therefore surgery on this organ necessitates the use of prophylactic antimicrobial agents (Fig. 31-2).

The arterial supply to the cervical part of the esophagus originates from the carotid arteries. The thoracic and relatively short (2- to 3-cm [¾- to 1¼-inch]) abdominal esophagus is supplied by the bronchoesophageal and gastric arteries. The vascular pattern is arcuate but segmental,

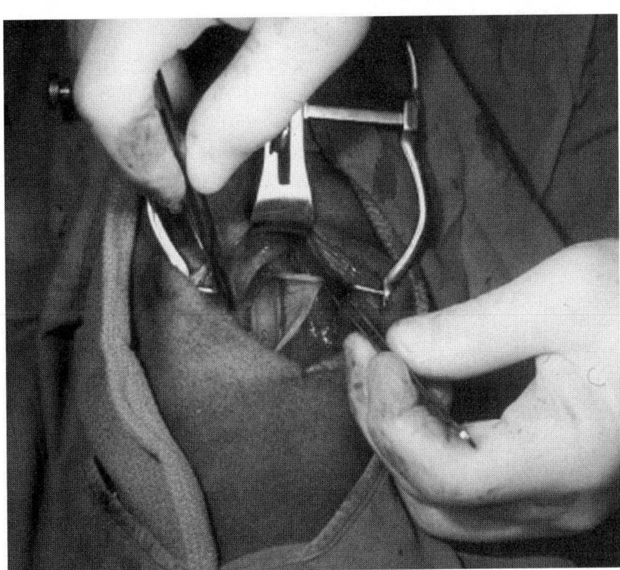

Figure 31-1. Traction on the incised esophagus, with a nasogastric tube in place, shows the elastic properties of the mucosa and submucosa (inner layer).

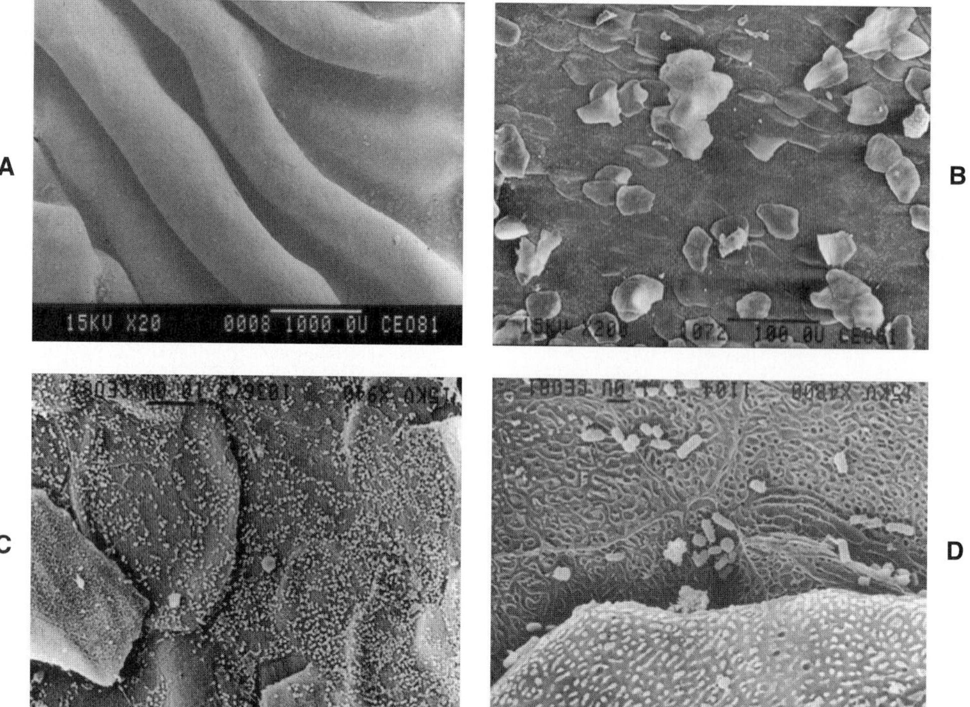

Figure 31-2. Scanning electron micrographic images of the esophageal lumen. **A,** Longitudinal mucosal folds. **B,** At a higher power, squamous epithelial cells. **C,** Colonization of bacteria on squamous cells. **D,** Close-up of squamous cells with mixed populations of bacteria. Because the lumen of the esophagus is heavily colonized under normal circumstances, prophylactic antibiotics are necessary any time this organ is incised.

without generous collateral circulation, necessitating careful preservation of vessels during surgery.

Innervation of the esophagus is derived from the ninth and tenth cranial nerves and the sympathetic trunk, as well as mesenteric ganglion cells within the muscle layers.

CLINICAL MANIFESTATIONS AND EVALUATION OF ESOPHAGEAL DISEASE

The obstructive disease of "choke" may be manifested by ptyalism, dysphagia, coughing, and regurgitation of food, water, and saliva from the mouth and nostrils. Attempts at ingestion are often followed by odynophagia (painful swallowing), repeated extension of the head and neck, and other signs of distress or agitation. The time interval from swallowing until these signs are shown by the patient depends on the location of the lesion within the esophagus. With obstruction of the distal esophagus, odynophagia and retching may occur 10 to 12 seconds after swallowing. With proximal esophageal obstruction, the signs may be evident immediately. This occurs because the propagation speed of the equine esophagus is about 9.4 cm/sec in the proximal two thirds but only 4.6 cm/sec in the distal one third. Therefore, over an average length of 116 cm (45¼ inches), a bolus of food would take about 16 seconds to traverse the body of the esophagus.[6,7] Intermittent signs of choke followed by periods of relief may indicate a disease other than simple feed impaction, and further diagnostic procedures are warranted. Anorexia, electrolyte imbalances, and dehydration accompany cases of long duration (see "Complications of Esophageal Surgery," p. 371). Aspiration pneumonia frequently follows esophageal obstruction, and the clinical signs may be present as early as 1 day after the onset of choke.

Physical Examination

A thorough oral examination should be performed to rule out an oral foreign body, dental disease, cleft palate, or oropharyngeal neoplasms. Observation and palpation of the neck in the area of the jugular furrows may reveal enlargement of the cervical esophagus. Simple food impaction of the cervical esophagus may be localized in this manner. Crepitation of a diffuse, firm enlargement may indicate loss of integrity of the esophageal wall. Passage of the nasogastric tube often confirms luminal obstruction and localizes the site of involvement. Gentle lavage of warm water through the tube may permit material to be flushed free of the obstruction if feed or consumption of bedding is the cause of the problem. At this time, sedation of the animal with xylazine (1.1 mg/kg IV) lowers the horse's head and prevents further aspiration. Lavage may be continued until the obstruction is relieved, and further diagnostic studies may be unnecessary. However, reobstruction indicates that other esophageal disease may be present, and the diagnosis should be pursued.

With any esophageal disease, auscultation and radiography of the thorax are indicated to monitor development of aspiration pneumonia. This complication is common when an esophageal problem is encountered.

Radiographic Evaluation

Esophagography in horses is diagnostic in most instances and should be considered a part of the complete esophageal examination in problems other than simple obstruction. A survey film is necessary to establish radiographic technique and the presence or absence of disease without contrast material (e.g., feed impaction or foreign body) (Fig. 31-3). Barium paste (85% wt/vol with water, 120 mL) given by mouth outlines the longitudinal mucosal folds of the esophagus with the lumen undistended and localizes the obstruction or any disruption of the lumen (Fig. 31-4). A feed impaction becomes coated with the barium, a complete obstruction halts barium flow at the site of the lesion (Fig. 31-5), and rupture of the esophagus permits barium to escape into surrounding soft tissues. If possible, sedation of the patient should be avoided during this procedure because it suppresses the swallowing reflex and causes barium to be held in the mouth, reducing the amount available to coat the esophagus.

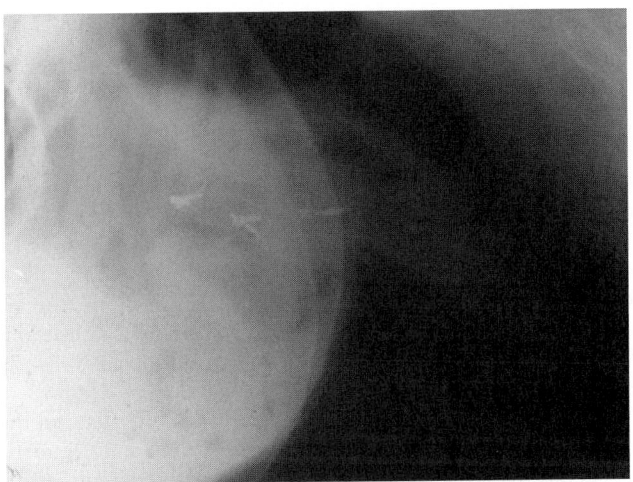

Figure 31-3. Lateral cervical radiograph of a 9-year-old gelding with anorexia and odynophagia. A metallic foreign body (fishing lure) is lodged in the cranial esophageal sphincter.

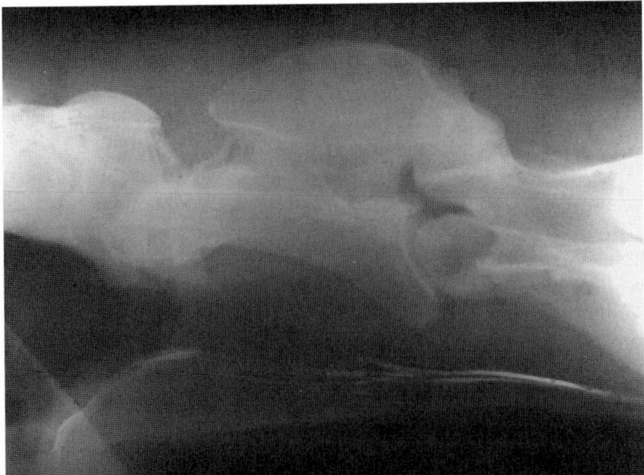

Figure 31-4. Barium paste (120 mL) given by mouth outlines the normal longitudinal folds of the mucosa in the undistended lumen of the esophagus.

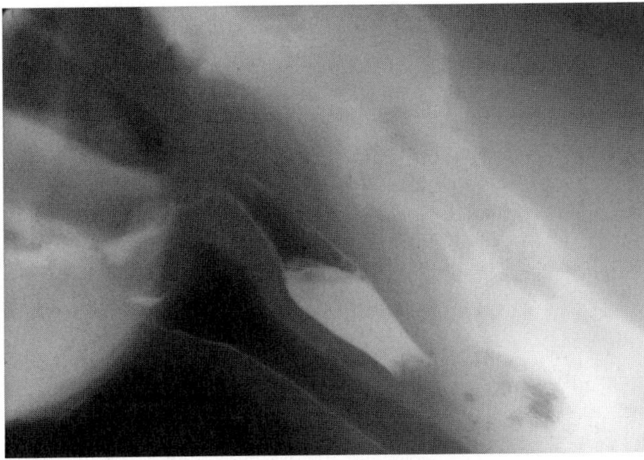

Figure 31-5. Complete obstruction of the esophagus is localized on esophagography after barium paste swallow. This adult horse had an esophageal stricture. Note the prestenotic dilation.

Liquid barium (72% wt/vol with water, 480 mL) may be administered under pressure by a dose syringe through a cuffed nasogastric tube to prevent reflux into the pharynx (Fig. 31-6). This technique demonstrates strictures and associated prestenotic dilation of the esophagus, as well as space-occupying masses that displace the esophagus. Liquid barium (480 mL) followed by air (480 mL), delivered by dose syringe under pressure, provides a double-contrast study (Fig. 31-7), permitting examination of mucosal folds with the esophagus distended. This latter technique gives the best definition of mucosal lesions, such as circumferential mucosal ulcers after feed impaction. Although a diagnosis can often be made without using all three techniques, each technique demonstrates lesions not seen with the other two.

In the cranial cervical area, where the esophagus lies dorsal to the trachea, lesions that restrict distention of the esophageal lumen can be demonstrated with negative-contrast radiography (Fig. 31-8). A flexible endoscope can be

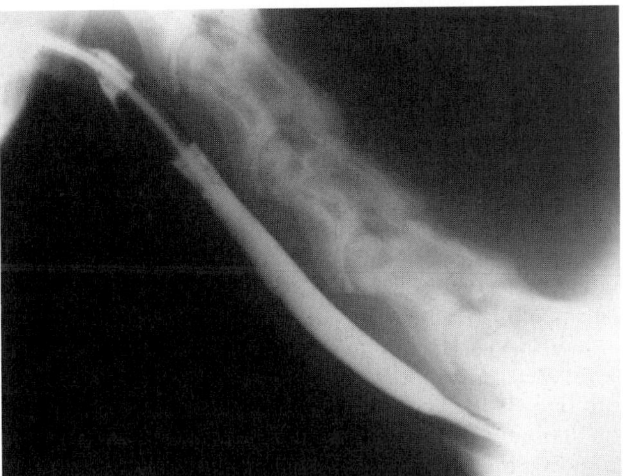

Figure 31-6. Positive-contrast esophagogram (using liquid barium administered under pressure through a nasogastric tube fitted with an inflatable cuff) shows the distended lumen of the normal esophagus. The cuff prevents reflux of barium into the pharynx and aspiration into the trachea.

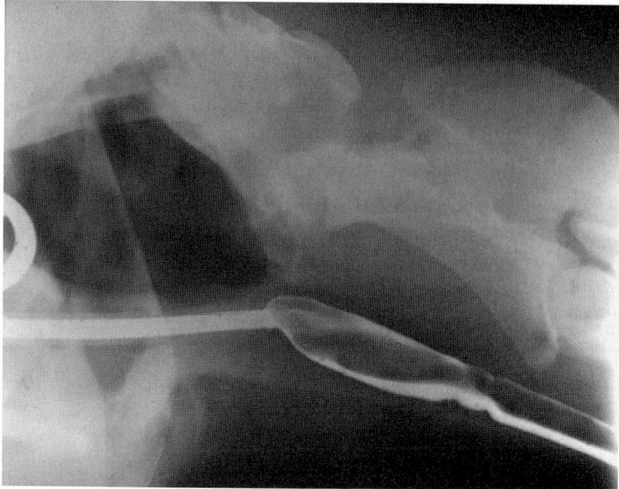

Figure 31-7. Double-contrast esophagogram (using liquid barium followed by a bolus of air) shows the esophagus with the lumen distended. This technique outlines any abnormal transverse mucosal folds and identifies a circumferential ulcer in this horse.

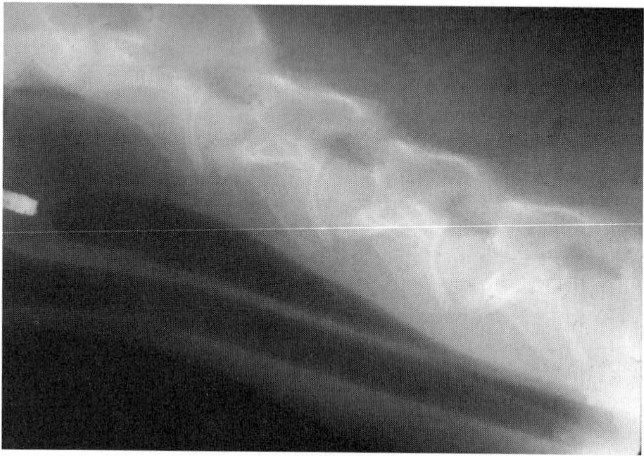

Figure 31-8. Negative-contrast esophagogram (using air insufflation introduced through the flexible endoscope) permits visual localization of the lesion with the endoscope and demonstrates a stricture.

used to localize the lesion and permits insufflation of the esophagus during radiography. Alternatively, air (480 mL) can be delivered by dose syringe under pressure through a cuffed nasogastric tube to achieve the same results. However, negative-contrast radiography alone does not yield much information about the caudal cervical and thoracic portions of the esophagus because of superimposition of the air density of the trachea and lungs.

Swallowing during contrast studies, when the lumen is being distended, produces false signs of esophageal stricture (Fig. 31-9). Xylazine (1.1 mg/kg IV), 5 minutes before the barium-under-pressure, double-contrast, or negative-contrast esophagogram, helps eliminate this swallow artifact by decreasing the reflex "secondary swallows" that follow luminal distention. However, if detomidine is used, false signs of megaesophagus can persist for more than 30 minutes.[8]

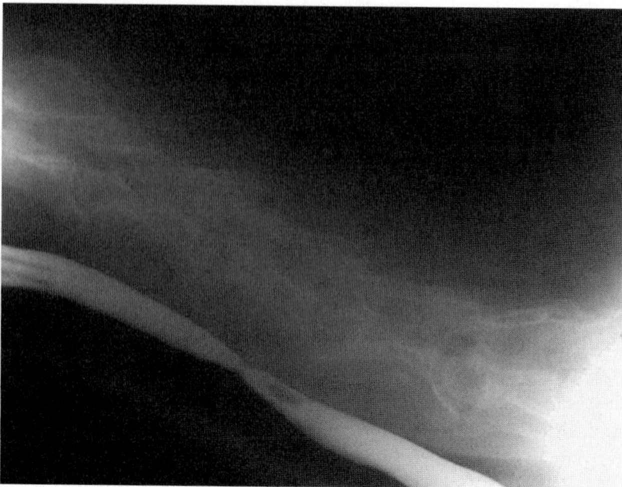

Figure 31-9. Barium esophagogram shows false signs of a stricture when barium is administered under pressure and the radiograph is made during swallowing. This swallow artifact can be avoided if xylazine is administered 5 minutes before the study is begun.

Endoscopic Evaluation

Esophagoscopy may better define the severity and extent of esophageal lesions diagnosed on radiography and can be used as an ancillary diagnostic aid. Additionally, endoscopic examination should always be performed when radiographic findings are not diagnostic. If the endoscope is 200 cm (78 inches) or longer, the entire esophagus may be examined, and esophageal lesions in the thorax of the adult horse undetected on radiographic examination can be diagnosed. A flexible endoscope that allows irrigation and insufflation is necessary to provide good observation of mucosal lesions and changes in luminal size.

Endoscopic examination may be performed safely on the restrained standing animal in most instances. Diagnostic observations are best made by starting with the endoscope fully inserted and the esophageal lumen insufflated, then slowly withdrawing the endoscope tip toward the horse's head. After each swallow, the endoscope should be cleared by irrigation and the esophagus dilated before further withdrawal. Several passes should be made over any area of suspected disease.

Longitudinal mucosal folds in the esophagus are normally seen when the endoscope tip is moved proximad and the esophagus is in the relaxed position (Fig. 31-10). Insufflation flattens these folds and permits observation of luminal size (Fig. 31-11). Inability to insufflate the esophagus and flatten the longitudinal mucosal folds usually indicates disease. This is noted cranial and caudal to a stricture. Transverse folds can be produced iatrogenically by moving the endoscope tip toward the stomach. When the cervical esophagus is insufflated, the outline of the trachea can often be seen through the esophageal wall. Swallowing produces changes in the lumen that give the appearance of diverticula or strictures to the untrained observer. The normal mucosa is white to light pink; reddened discolorations are evidence of mucosal disease.

The cranial aspect of the cervical esophageal sphincter is difficult to examine because the swallowing reflex is stim-

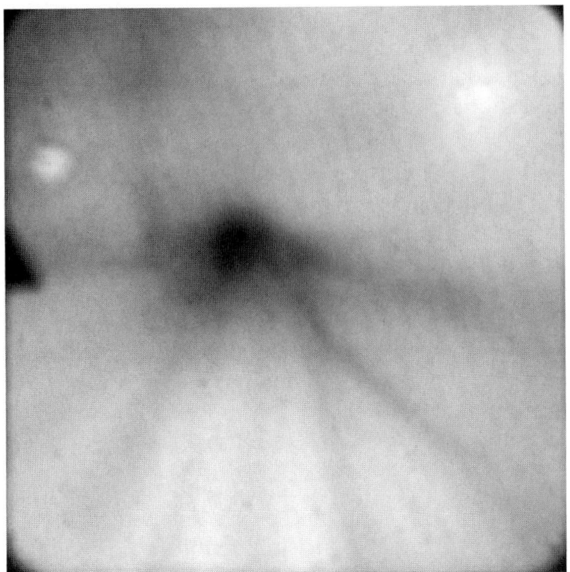

Figure 31-10. Appearance of the normal longitudinal mucosal folds of the undistended esophagus when the endoscope is pulled craniad (toward the head).

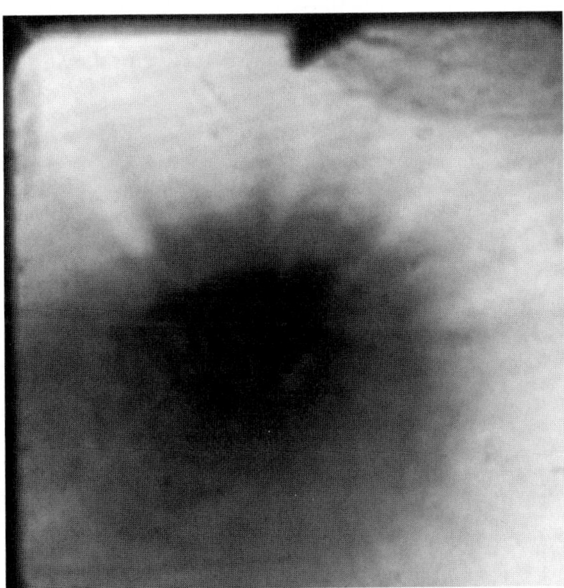

Figure 31-11. Appearance of the normal esophageal lumen when it is insufflated and the endoscope is pulled craniad (toward the head).

ulated repeatedly and the larynx directs the endoscope tip dorsally. Radiographic assessment of this area may be more diagnostic. Additionally, the longitudinal mucosal folds along the rest of the esophagus are absent in this area.

Frequently, the endoscopic appearance of an esophageal obstruction is obscured by saliva mixed with ingesta that collects proximal to the obstruction. This should be removed by suction through a nasogastric tube, and the endoscope should be reinserted immediately to observe the area of obstruction.

Manometric Evaluation

Esophageal dysfunction in humans is routinely evaluated using intraluminal pressure manometry. Manometric techniques have been developed, and reference esophageal pressure profiles have been established in healthy horses. The four functionally distinct regions of the esophagus demonstrated were cranial esophageal sphincter, caudal esophageal sphincter, and "fast" (cranial two thirds) and "slow" (caudal one third) regions in the body of the esophagus (Fig. 31-12). In some physiologic disorders of the equine esophagus, manometry may better define problems in which more conventional methods have not yielded a diagnosis. Manometry has yielded new information on clinical manifestations of esophageal obstruction and the effect of drugs used to treat it. However, the availability and technical

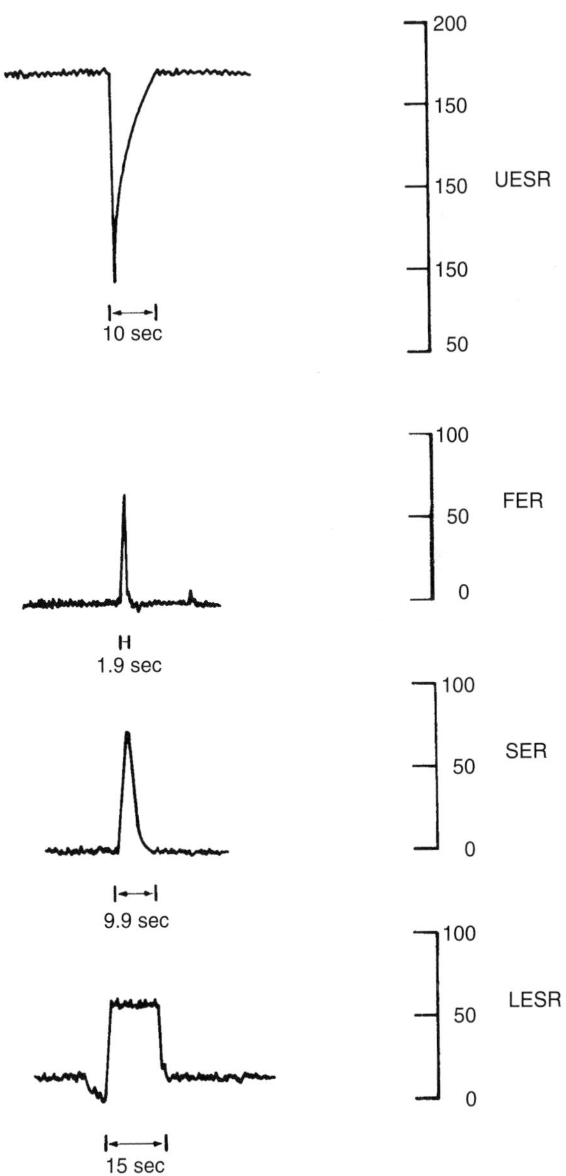

Figure 31-12. Manometric recording of a swallow as it passes through the four functionally distinct regions of the esophagus. FER, fast esophageal region; LESR, caudal, or lower, esophageal sphincter region; SER, slow esophageal region; UESR, cranial, or upper, esophageal sphincter region; units in mm Hg.

difficulty of manometry have limited its use as a diagnostic tool in equine practice.

Figure 31-13 outlines a systematic scheme of examination using physical, radiographic, and endoscopic findings to diagnose esophageal disorders. Alternative pathways may be used, depending on the disease, clinical signs, available diagnostic aids, and experience of the clinician. Physical examination, including passage of a nasogastric tube and esophageal lavage, and radiography yield a diagnosis for most common esophageal problems. Endoscopy allows definitive diagnosis of some anatomic disorders not observed with radiography. Manometry, cineradiography, and electromyography are seldom necessary and have not been commonly used in diagnosis of esophageal diseases.

SURGICAL APPROACHES

Three surgical approaches to the equine esophagus can be used. Each approach is dictated by anatomic location of the lesion and purpose of the surgery. The ventral cervical approach is best used for esophagotomy, esophagomyotomy, and resections involving the proximal third of the cervical esophagus. A ventrolateral approach is recommended for placing a feeding tube in the mid-cervical esophagus (esophagostomy) or for approaching the distal one fourth of the cervical esophagus, especially near the thoracic inlet. Thoracotomy is necessary to approach the distal half of the esophagus; the choice of intercostal space is dictated by the aim of the surgery and location of the lesion.

If the surgeon expects to invade the esophageal lumen, broad-spectrum antibiotics are indicated and should be chosen on the basis of sound surgical principles, expected complications, and recognized bacterial colonization of this organ.[9] Before induction of anesthesia, a nasogastric tube should be passed as far into the esophagus as the surgical site (or beyond if possible) to facilitate identification of the esophagus at surgery. It also is necessary to avoid damage to the recurrent laryngeal nerve and vagosympathetic trunk, which are easily traumatized when retracting the carotid artery away from the esophagus. Owners should be advised that laryngeal hemiplegia is a common complication of esophageal surgery.

Ventral Approach

Surgical procedures are conducted with the animal under general anesthesia and placed in dorsal recumbency. A 10-cm-long (4 inch) skin incision permits exposure of about 6 cm (2½ inches) of the esophagus. The skin and subcutaneous fascia are divided sharply using a scalpel. The paired muscles of the sternothyroid, sternohyoid, and omohyoid are separated along the midline to expose the trachea (Fig. 31-14). Blunt separation of fascia along the left side of the trachea permits identification of the esophagus containing the nasogastric tube. Retraction of the trachea to the right of the median plain and gentle sharp dissection of overlying loose adventitia expose the ventral wall of the esophagus.

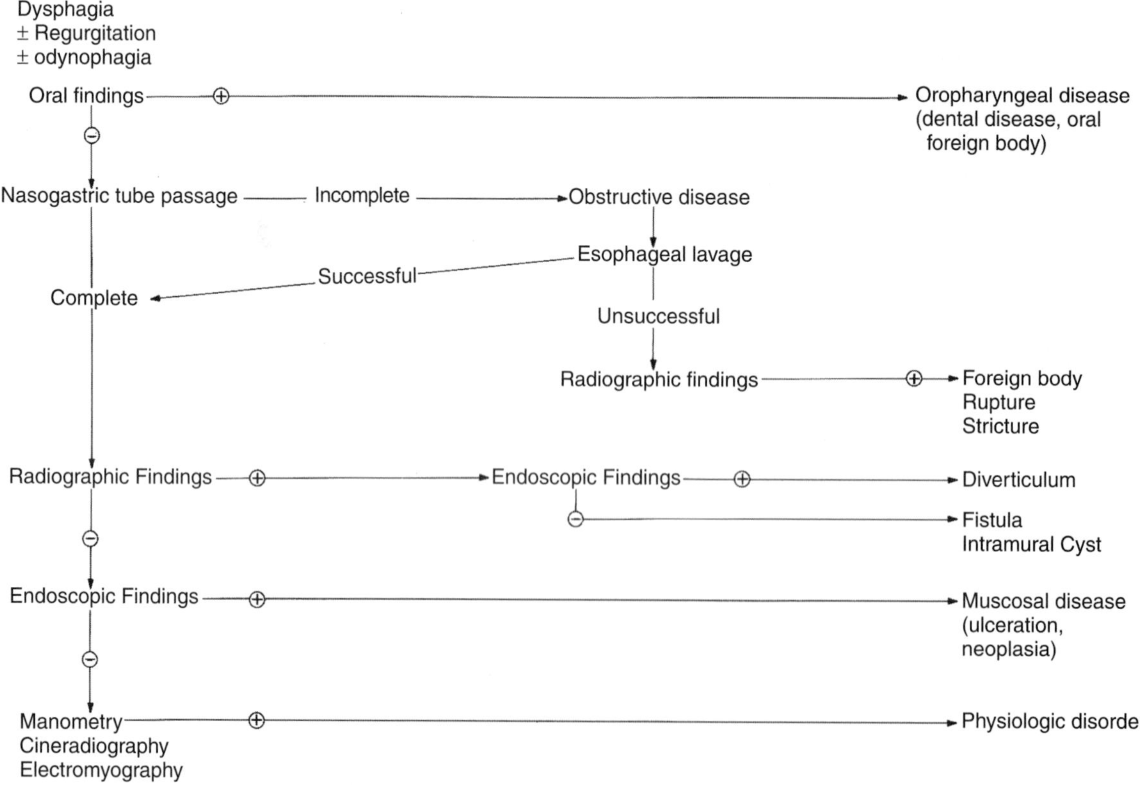

Figure 31-13. Scheme of examination of esophageal disorders. *Arrows* outline pathways that are usually diagnostic for the conditions shown at the right.

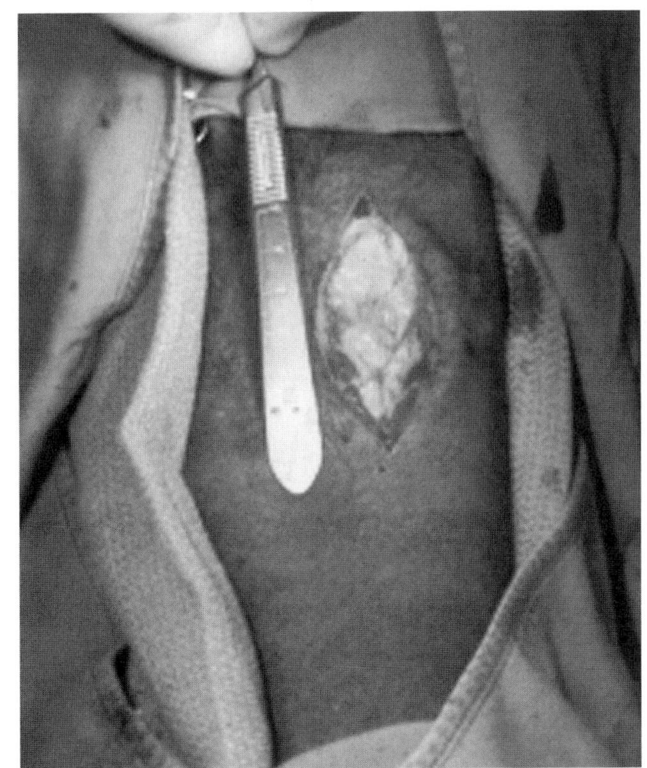

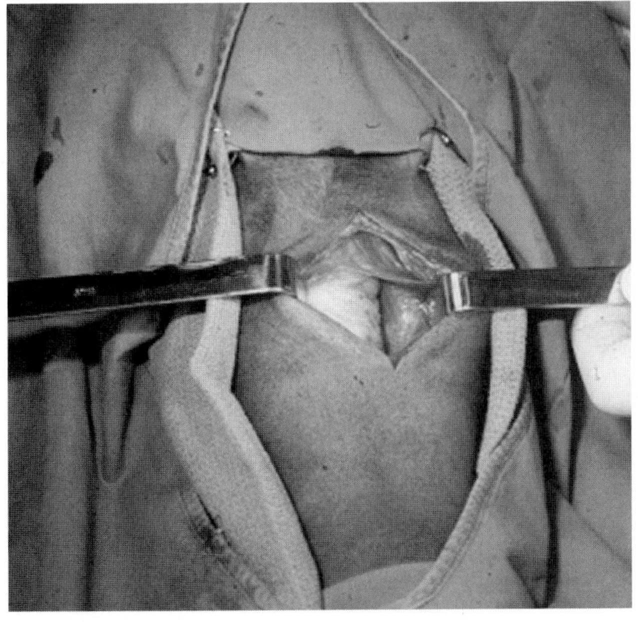

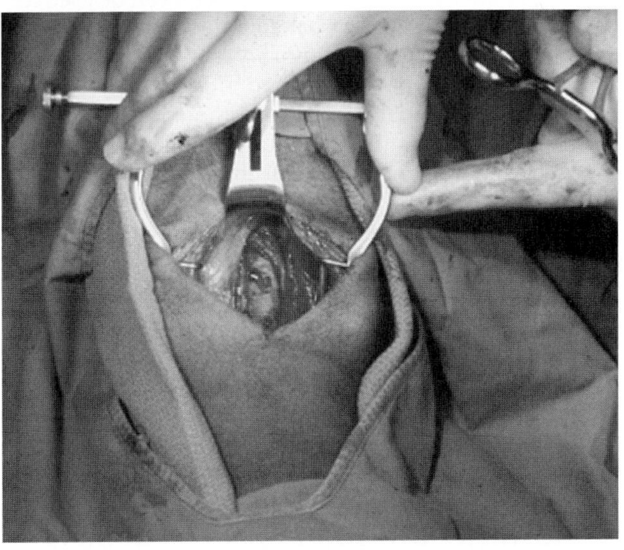

Figure 31-14. **A,** A 10-cm-long incision through the skin and subcutaneous fascia, which is sharply divided using the scalpel. **B,** The paired muscles of the sternothyroid, sternohyoid, and omohyoid are separated along the midline to expose the trachea. **C,** A baby Balfour retractor placed through the incision allows easy access to the esophagus.

Ventrolateral Approach

Placement of a feeding tube using the ventrolateral approach facilitates firm anchorage of the tube to the skin and permits it to lie in a comfortable position on the patient's neck while avoiding impingement of the feeding tube on the trachea (Fig. 31-15). This approach also affords better access to the middle and distal cervical esophagus, where the ventral cervical musculature becomes more heavily developed, making the ventral approach less desirable. This surgical approach may be made with the horse standing, using local anesthesia, or with the horse in dorsal or right lateral recumbency, under general anesthesia.[10]

A 5-cm-long (2 inches) skin incision (for feeding tube placement) is made just ventral to the jugular vein. The sternocephalicus and brachiocephalicus muscles are separated, and the deep cervical fascia is incised to expose the

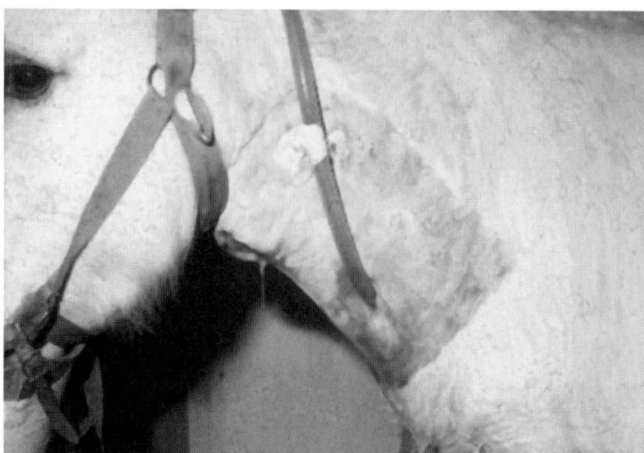

Figure 31-15. Placement of a feeding tube ventral to the jugular vein permits it to lie in a comfortable position on the neck. Note the butterfly tape bandage sutured to the skin to firmly anchor the tube, along with saliva loss around the tube.

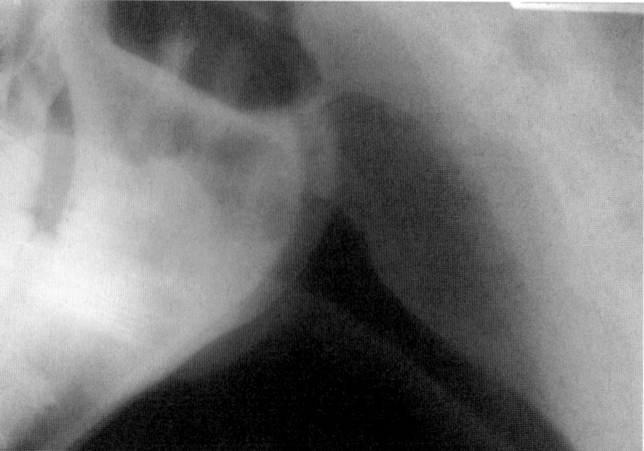

Figure 31-16. Lateral cervical radiograph shows typical appearance of impaction of ingesta in the cranial cervical esophagus.

esophagus. It may be necessary to incise the cutaneous colli muscle in the distal cervical area.

Approach to the Thoracic Esophagus

An approach through the thoracic esophagus can be used for vascular ring anomalies (two patients in my experience, in which the left fourth or right fifth interspace was used) or when the suspected lesion can be resolved surgically without entering the esophageal lumen. A 5-month-old foal was successfully treated for an intrathoracic esophageal stricture with esophagomyotomy through the eighth intercostal space,[11] and an intrathoracic esophageal pulsion diverticulum was resected in a 7-month-old foal by resecting the left eighth rib.[12]

The patient is placed in right lateral recumbency under general anesthesia and positive-pressure ventilation is used. The skin, subcutaneous tissue, cutaneous trunci, serratus ventralis, and latissimus dorsi are sharply divided. A subperiosteal rib resection has been described. However, in my experience, this is not necessary in foals, because rib retractors provide adequate exposure.

MANAGEMENT OF ESOPHAGEAL DISORDERS

Impaction

The most common type of obstructive esophageal disease is impaction with ingesta or bedding. It can occur in the normal esophagus of a gluttonous animal and has a typical radiographic appearance (Fig. 31-16). Nasogastric tube passage and gentle warm water lavage are usually successful in relieving the obstruction. Xylazine sedation to lower the patient's head during this procedure greatly reduces the hazard of aspiration of ingesta that is flushed free and passes up the esophagus into the nasopharynx.

Several alternative techniques may be necessary if gentle lavage meets with failure. A cuffed nasogastric tube may be placed, the animal sedated, and water lavaged under pressure with a dose syringe or stomach pump. The tube helps prevent reflux or ingesta into the pharynx while permitting pressure of the water to push the obstruction distally. External massage and to-and-fro movement of the water resolve most impactions. If this technique is not successful, the animal should be muzzled to prevent food and water intake and left alone for 8 to 12 hours, and the treatment should then be repeated. Frequently, the initial treatment softens the impaction and it becomes dislodged by swallowing or is easily relieved by a second treatment. Some clinicians claim that atropinization (0.02 mg/kg) for a horse with esophageal impaction aids dissolution of the impaction by promoting esophageal relaxation and reduces salivary secretions that might otherwise be inhaled. The effect of acepromazine on esophageal relaxation is supported in one experimental study.[13] However, oxytocin administered intravenously (at 0.11 and 0.2 IU/kg) results in short-term significant relaxation of esophageal musculature in experiments,[14] and it has become popular as an adjunct treatment for esophageal impaction. Because xylazine has similar effects, these drugs could be used together to reduce the tone of the esophageal musculature, allowing passage of the obstructions with reduced risk of esophageal injury.

Refractory cases or intractable horses may benefit from general anesthesia and water lavage under pressure. This method has the advantages of providing some relaxation of the esophageal musculature, reducing the chances of aspiration (because the horse's head is lowered), and decreasing the risk of esophageal perforation with the tube in an intractable horse. Gentle manipulation is mandatory with this technique to avoid rupture of the esophagus. Impactions that do not respond to conservative therapy should be definitively identified by radiographic and endoscopic examination and, if amenable, relieved by longitudinal esophagotomy (see "Foreign Body," next). Surgery is preferable to repeated trauma of the esophagus through attempts to relieve the obstruction with a nasogastric tube. Use of the nasogastric tube as a probang is not recommended and can result in severe trauma to the larynx and esophagus.[15] Cervical esophagotomy can be performed with the horse standing or under general anesthesia, and obstructions can be lavaged through the incision if necessary.

One aftermath of simple impaction is fusiform dilation of the esophagus that predisposes to reobstruction (Fig. 31-17). This condition resolves in 24 to 48 hours, provided the dilation is kept free of ingesta. Food should be withheld

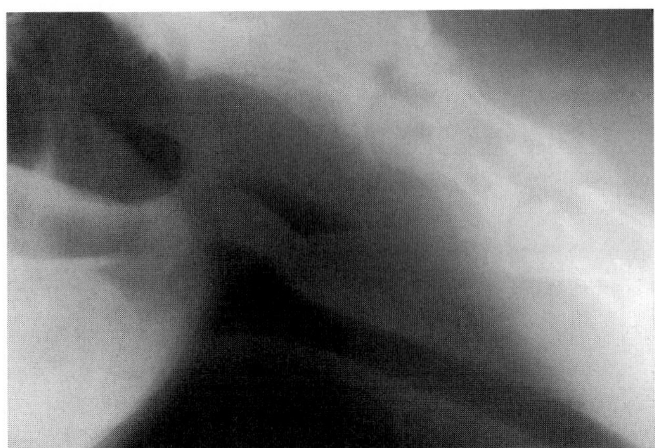

Figure 31-17. Lateral cervical radiograph of a horse after impaction of the esophagus has been relieved shows fluid line in an area of dilation that extends from the distal point of obstruction proximally to the upper esophageal sphincter. The fluid line is produced by saliva that has collected in the dilated area.

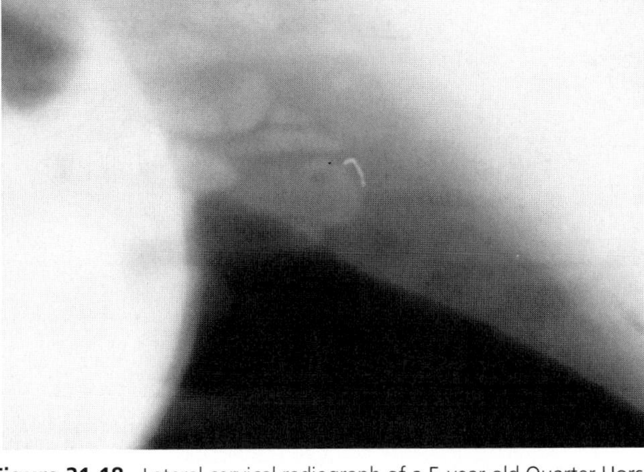

Figure 31-18. Lateral cervical radiograph of a 5-year-old Quarter Horse gelding with cervical swelling, dysphagia, and odynophagia. A metallic foreign body (wire) is lodged in the lateral wall of the cranial esophagus. A nasogastric tube passed easily. Note the gas in the tissues.

or only small quantities of a soft diet fed for 2 days after an episode of choke to permit the lumen to resume its normal diameter. Glucose–electrolyte solutions for drinking should be provided in addition to fresh water so the electrolyte abnormalities secondary to salivary loss can be compensated.

Broad-spectrum antimicrobial therapy is indicated for 5 to 7 days because the risk of aspiration pneumonia is high after choke. If pneumonia is not the major limiting factor in this disease, simple obstruction has a favorable prognosis.

When an obstruction has been present for several days or is refractory to initial treatment, examination using radiography or endoscopy is warranted after the obstruction has been relieved. Circumferential mucosal ulceration is not uncommon in these cases and can result in esophageal stricture.

Foreign Body

Small pieces of wood, wire, fishing tackle, and medication boluses can become esophageal foreign bodies in horses.[16,17] They often perforate the esophageal wall, resulting in phlegmon or abscessation (Fig. 31-18). The swelling that accompanies these conditions usually obstructs the esophageal lumen and results in impaction. Diagnosis is made by radiography or esophagoscopy.

Retrieval of small sharp foreign bodies under endoscopic guidance is possible but difficult; general anesthesia is recommended to prevent the swallowing movements during manipulation that may produce pain and further esophageal trauma. It is necessary to relieve the impaction before attempting this method of treatment. Blunt or round foreign bodies may be treated similar to feed impactions. Although the nasogastric tube may be used as a probe to push the object into the stomach, the risk of perforation is great. Gentle manipulation is mandatory to avoid rupture. Additionally, this technique has the risk of moving the foreign body from the cervical region only to have it lodge in the thorax, a more inaccessible site. Longitudinal esophagotomy with primary closure results in minimal complications when performed in a region of normal esophagus and has become the accepted method of removing a foreign body.[18,19]

Esophagotomy

Surgery is preferred to manipulations that induce further esophageal trauma. Passage of a nasogastric tube as far as the foreign body (or beyond, if possible) facilitates identification of the esophagus during surgery. General anesthesia is preferred if closure is to be attempted. The patient is placed in dorsal recumbency, and the skin of the ventral surface of the neck is prepared and draped for aseptic surgery. A 10-cm (4-inch) skin incision is made. Care should be taken to preserve the small vessels that supply the esophagus. Elevation of the esophagus from its bed of adventitia should be avoided. The left carotid sheath, containing the carotid artery and vagus and recurrent laryngeal nerves, should be retracted laterally. Pediatric-size Balfour abdominal retractors aid exposure to the esophagus, which then can be sharply incised through the muscle, submucosa, and mucosa cranial to, caudal to, or directly over the foreign body (Fig. 31-19). Where the incision is made into the esophagus depends on the mobility of the foreign body within the lumen and the amount of swelling in and compromise to the esophageal wall.

After removal of the foreign body, if the esophagus has a normal appearance in the area of the incision, closure should be completed using a simple-continuous suture of 3-0 polypropylene suture material with the knots tied in the lumen (see Fig. 31-19). Esophageal musculature may be apposed with simple-interrupted sutures of 3-0 absorbable or monofilament nonabsorbable suture material, at the surgeon's preference. Muscular layers, subcutaneous tissue, and skin may be apposed with 0 suture material in a simple-interrupted pattern. A polyethylene drain with an outer diameter of 0.63 cm (¼ inch) is placed beside the esophagus and exits ventral to the skin incision through a small stab wound. This drain is maintained under constant suction for 48 hours to remove serum and blood from the surgical site

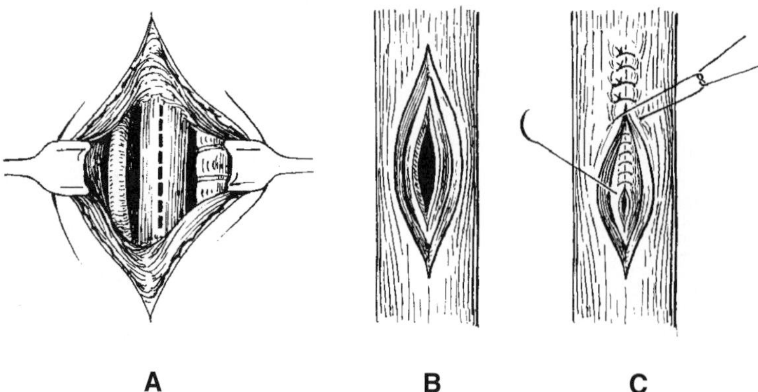

Figure 31-19. **A,** Longitudinal skin incision exposes the carotid artery *(left)*, esophagus *(center)*, and trachea *(right)*. **B,** In this longitudinal esophagotomy, a scalpel is used to incise both the outer layer (muscularis and adventitia) and the inner layer (mucosa and submucosa). **C,** The esophagotomy is closed with simple-continuous sutures in the inner layer (mucosa and submucosa) and simple-interrupted sutures in the outer layer (muscularis and adventitia).

and to provide early detection of salivary leakage should dehiscence occur.

Postoperatively, feed should be withheld for 48 hours. Parenteral administration of electrolyte solution, the composition of which depends on the horse's acid–base and hydration status, may be used to maintain hydration. Small quantities of pelleted feed in a slurry should be fed over the next 8 days before normal feeding can be resumed. Most esophagostomy incisions heal by first intention, and the intraluminal suture will slough into the lumen within 60 days (Fig. 31-20).

If removal of the foreign body is necessary through an obviously diseased segment of the esophagus, the incision may be closed and an esophagostomy tube placed through a separate incision closer to the stomach or directly into the esophagotomy incision (see "Esophagostomy," later).

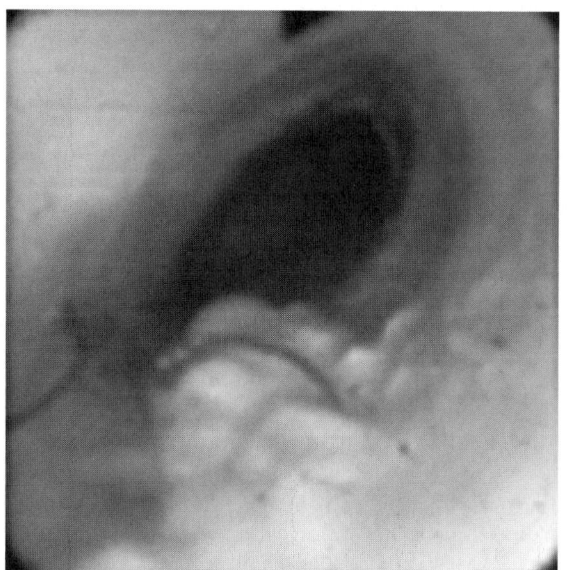

Figure 31-20. Endoscopic appearance of a longitudinal esophagostomy that healed by first intention 48 days after surgery. One loop of the suture remains in the healed esophagotomy site.

Feeding of a complete pelleted diet through the esophagostomy tube can begin immediately after surgery. Particular attention to the patient's water and electrolyte balance is necessary when closure of the esophagus is not possible[20] (see "Acid–Base and Electrolyte Alterations," p. 372).

Ulceration and Esophagitis

Mucosal ulceration and esophagitis commonly occur secondary to longstanding impactions. Longitudinal mucosal ulcers can be produced from impactions; more frequently, circumferential ulcerations occur. Other causes of esophageal ulceration in foals include phenylbutazone toxicity, in which generalized gastrointestinal mucosal disease is a feature, and severe gastroduodenal ulcer disease that produces secondary reflux esophagitis. Diagnosis of esophageal ulceration is best made by endoscopy (Fig. 31-21), although contrast radiography frequently defines the margins of the ulcer (see Fig. 31-7).

Conservative management should be instituted to minimize trauma to the mucosa, reduce inflammation, and control infection. A low-bulk, minimally abrasive diet (mash), nonsteroidal anti-inflammatory drugs (NSAIDs) (only if they are not implicated as causative agents), and broad-spectrum antimicrobial therapy are indicated. Because this diet results in hunger, the patient should be muzzled between feedings, or all bedding should be removed from the stall to avoid ingestion of straw or wood chips. Reexamination is recommended every 10 to 14 days. Stricture (see later) may occur within 30 days of the original insult, when the circumferential ulcer is more than 2.5 cm (1 inch) long.[21] Longitudinal mucosal ulcers (especially if they are not extensive and are localized to one area of the esophagus) and circumferential ulcers less than 2 cm (¾ inch) long usually heal without stricture.

Rupture, Perforations, and Lacerations

Rupture of the esophagus can occur secondary to longstanding obturation, repeated or aggressive nasogastric tube passage, foreign body perforation, external trauma to the

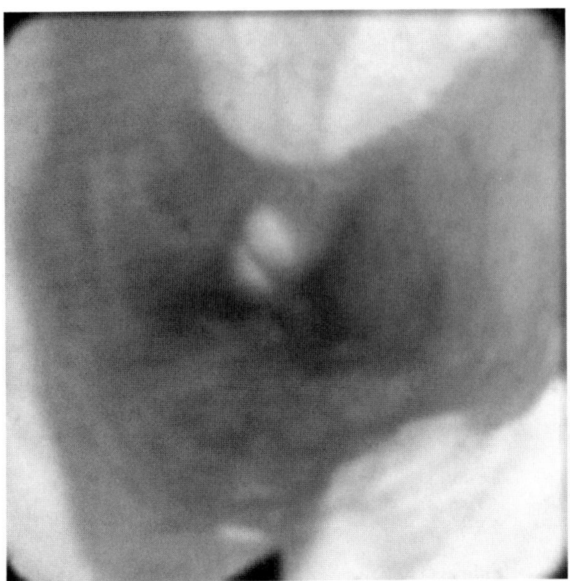

Figure 31-21. Endoscopic appearance of esophagitis with circumferential ulceration 24 hours after feed impaction. A stricture subsequently formed but responded to medical management.

cervical area (usually a kick), or extension of infection from surrounding strictures.[22-26] Cervical swelling usually prevents successful passage of a nasogastric tube, even after irrigation of the esophagus with water. Swallowed air escapes from the rupture and causes subcutaneous emphysema; this can be recognized on radiographs (see Fig. 31-18). Positive-contrast techniques demonstrate escape of barium into surrounding tissues (Fig. 31-22).

Ruptures that cannot drain to the outside result in leakage of saliva and ingesta into tissues of the neck, resulting in severe infection and phlegmon. Ruptures or perforations that allow escape of saliva and ingesta through the skin are less likely to cause systemic illness and extension of infection into the thorax. Early establishment of drainage, preferably on the ventral midline, is necessary with all ruptures of the esophagus to avoid mediastinitis, pleuritis, and even septicemia (Fig. 31-23). This should be followed with daily lavage.

Perforation or lacerations of the esophagus accompanied by minimal escape of saliva and ingesta can be repaired using the technique described for esophagotomy. Drainage and the feeding regimen used after esophagotomy should be employed. Secure closure of a ruptured or perforated defect is usually possible only in patients operated on shortly after the perforation has occurred (within 12 hours). In early cases, when esophageal tissues are too damaged to hold sutures or when infection or contamination with ingesta has already occurred, some means of draining the esophageal contents to the outside must be provided. The patient should receive systemic antibiotics and water; electrolyte and nutritional requirements should be met by tube feeding. In some cases, the feeding tube can be placed through the site of rupture into the stomach (Fig. 31-24). An alternative method of feeding that allows spontaneous healing of the rupture or successful repair of the rupture when edema and infection have been controlled is an esophagostomy performed distal to the rupture (closer to the stomach).

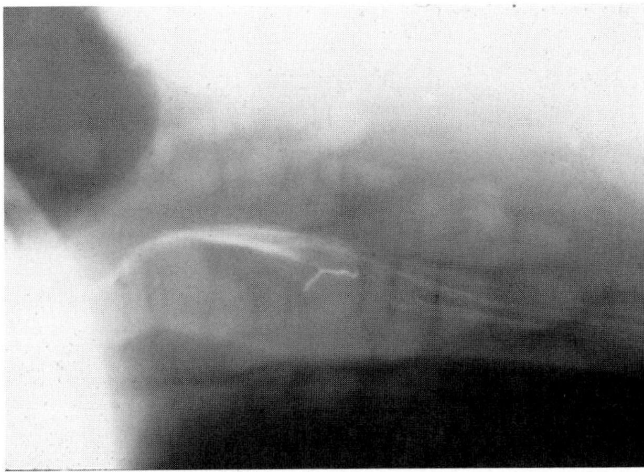

Figure 31-22. Barium swallow in a horse with a penetrating foreign body (wire) shows swallowed air and barium that has escaped into the periesophageal tissue. (Same horse as in Fig. 31-18.)

Esophagostomy

Cervical esophagostomy is an excellent method of extraoral alimentation that avoids the discomfort and irritation of the indwelling nasogastric tube. An additional advantage is avoidance of deleterious influences on healing of an esophageal wound by an intraluminal tube located in the immediate region.[27] To use this advantage, the esophagostomy should be placed distal to the area of esophageal injury. The surgery can be performed with the horse in lateral recumbency under general anesthesia or standing under mild tranquilization and local anesthesia. Passage of a nasogastric tube facilitates identification of the esophagus at surgery.

The skin over the left jugular furrow is prepared for surgery in the desired area. The esophagus is occasionally located on the right side of the trachea and should be approached over the right jugular furrow in those horses. A 5-cm (2-inch) skin incision is made ventral to the vein. The esophagus is sharply incised longitudinally for 3 cm (1¼ inches) down to the indwelling nasogastric tube. The nasogastric tube is removed, and a polyethylene nasogastric tube (with an outer diameter of 14 to 24 mm [½ to 1 inch]) is placed into the stomach through the esophagostomy. Failure to place the tube into the stomach allows easy dislodgement. Care should be taken to ensure that the end of the tube is placed into both the elastic inner layer and the inelastic outer muscle layer of the esophagus. Difficulty in tube placement is usually an indication that the incision in the muscle layer is inadequate to accommodate the diameter of the tube. Sutures can be placed in the mucosa to form a seal around the tube but probably are unnecessary because they do not prevent leakage of saliva. The tube should be secured firmly, first with butterfly tape bandages sutured to the skin (see Fig. 31-15) and then with elastic tape bandages. Tubes of large diameter are preferred to avoid plugging with ingesta during feeding. They should be capped between feedings and flushed with water at the end of each feeding to maintain patency.

Esophagostomy tubes should remain in place for a minimum of 7 to 10 days to permit granulation tissue to form a true stoma (Fig. 31-25). A longer period is necessary

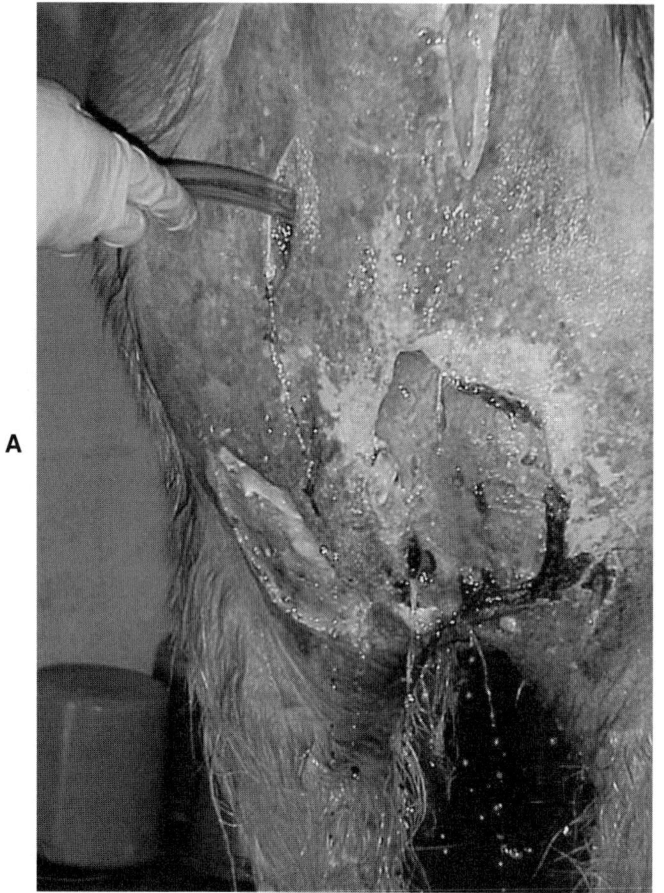

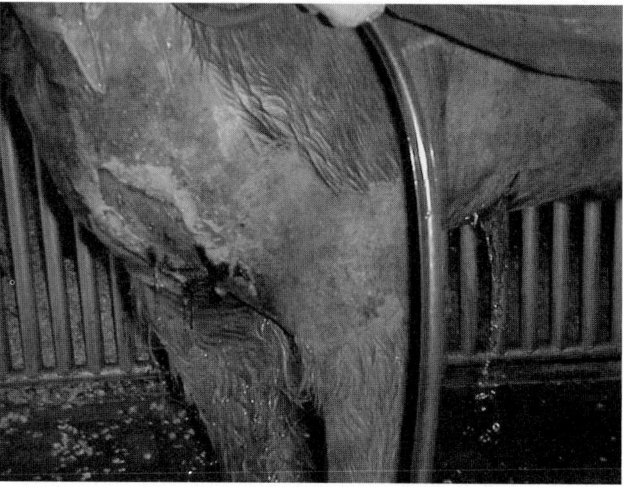

Figure 31-23. A, Establishment of a ventral drainage following esophageal rupture in which multiple incisions needed to be made to drain food material from the cranial pectoral area. **B,** Daily lavage with copious amounts of water through the incisions shows the communication between the caudal cervical esophageal incisions and incisions in the pectoral area and caudal chest area behind the elbow.

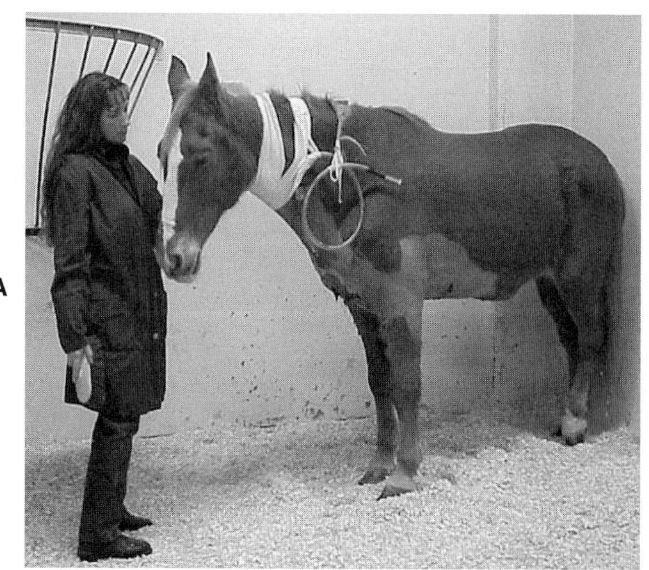

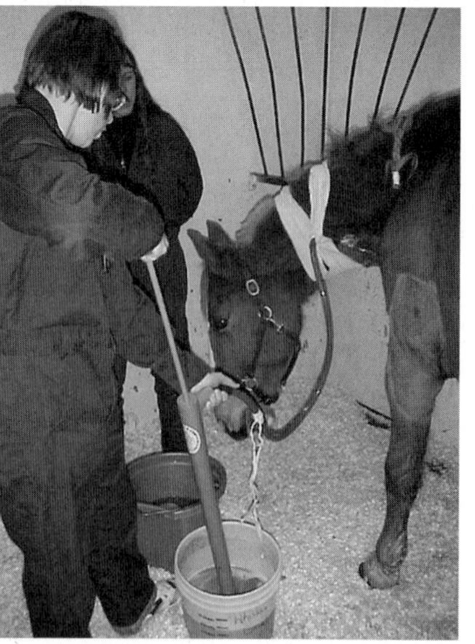

Figure 31-24. A, Electrolyte nutritional requirements can be met by placing the feeding tube through the site of esophageal rupture. **B,** Slurry made of complete pelleted feed is used to meet this requirement.

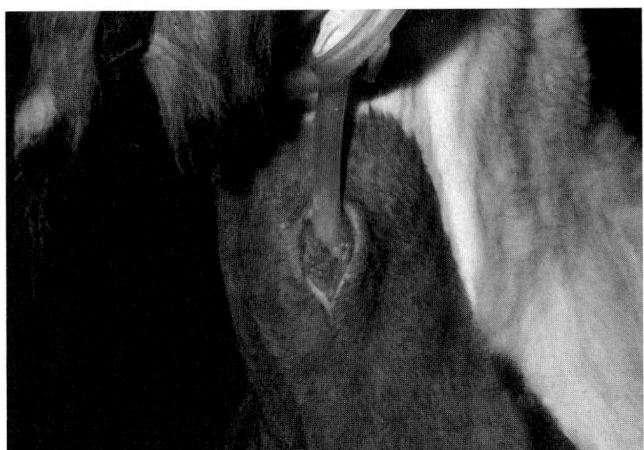

Figure 31-25. Esophagostomy tube should remain in place for a minimum of 7 to 10 days to permit granulation tissue to form a true stoma.

if the tube is placed in the area of a rupture or perforation. When the tube is removed, normal feeding may be resumed. A large portion of swallowed feed may be lost through the stoma when the patient is fed from the ground (Fig. 31-26). When feed is placed at the height of the withers, however, less of the bolus is lost through the stoma with each swallow. The stoma heals spontaneously after the tube is removed, and fistula formation is rare (Fig. 31-27).

However, complications of this form of alimentation are well documented and can result in death. Early detection and ventral drainage of infections that dissect along the trachea and esophagus are vital for a successful outcome. Patients should be maintained on antimicrobial therapy until a mature stoma develops (7 to 10 days).

Resection of the esophagus after rupture is warranted if the muscular layer is obviously necrotic and does not act as a tube along which the mucosa may regenerate, and if the proximal and distal segments of the esophagus can be anastomosed without undue tension (see "Partial Resection" and "Resection and Anastomosis," pp. 365 and 366). Few ruptures of the esophagus requiring resection occur without necrotizing cellulitis. Usually a delay in repair is necessary to permit acute inflammation to subside before surgery. During this period, the patient may be accommodated with a change in diet and tube feeding.

Stricture

Narrowing of the esophageal lumen because of stricture formation is usually an annular lesion and can be classified into the following three types, depending on the anatomic location of induration and fibrosis: (1) mural lesions that involve only the adventitia and muscularis, (2) esophageal rings or webs that involve only the mucosa and submucosa, and (3) annular stenosis that involves all layers of the esophageal wall. Stricture of the esophagus may be acquired as a result of external or internal trauma to the esophageal walls (especially after impactions that produce circumferential ulceration), leakage of saliva or dehiscence after surgery, or external compression by or attachment to adjacent structures. In most instances, strictures are less likely to occur when traumatic insults involve only a portion of the circumference of the esophagus. For this reason, mobiliza-

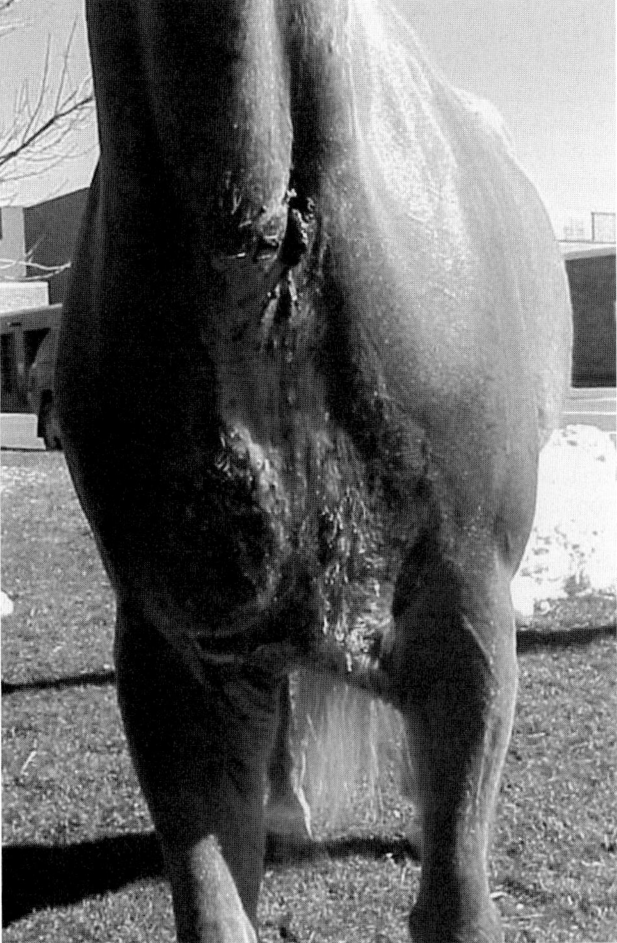

Figure 31-26. After removal of the esophagostomy tube, a large portion of masticated feed and saliva may be lost through the stoma when the patient is fed from the ground. Placing the feed at the height of the withers allows less of the bolus to be lost through the stoma with each swallow. The horse may electively eat the masticated feed, and this should be encouraged because the salt content from the saliva will be reswallowed and eventually ingested.

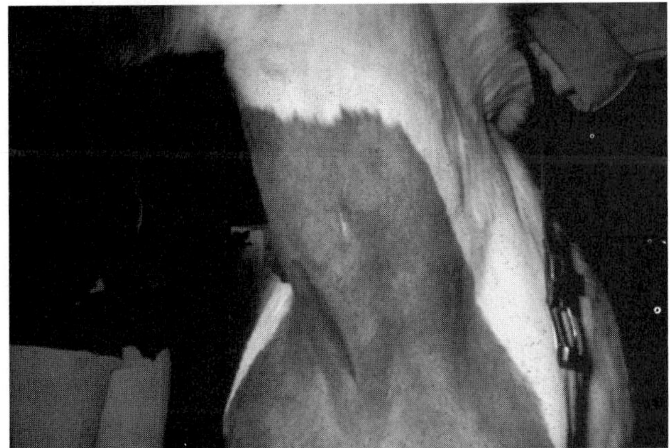

Figure 31-27. The stoma heals spontaneously after the tube is removed, and fistula formation is rare. (Three weeks after tube removal from the animal seen in Fig. 31-25.)

tion of the esophagus from its fascial attachments during surgery should be avoided when possible.

Strictures usually impede complete passage of the nasogastric tube and are best demonstrated by positive-pressure contrast esophagograms (Fig. 31-28). Conservative management of a stricture is aimed at dilation of the stenotic segment. Bougienage or pneumatic or hydrostatic dilators have limited practical value in adult horses because of the inaccessibility of special equipment and the chronicity of the problem. There is a report describing resolution of an esophageal stricture in a 1-month-old colt using a balloon dilation procedure.[28] However, early lesions, such as post-surgical strictures or those following circumferential ulceration, can be dilated with the frequent feeding of small quantities of soft food over a period of several months. In seven horses that developed stricture after esophageal impaction, observation over 2 months revealed that the esophageal lumen was maximally reduced (strictured) 30 days after circumferential ulceration was observed (Fig. 31-29), after which lumen diameter increased to normal by 60 days. This also has been documented after experimental resection and anastomosis and has been observed in a series of cases involving foals.[29] Therefore, a low-bulk diet and anti-inflammatory and antimicrobial therapy should be used, and surgical intervention should be delayed for 60 days after the original insult. It is important to impress on horse owners that several episodes of choke may occur up to 40 days after the original obstruction.

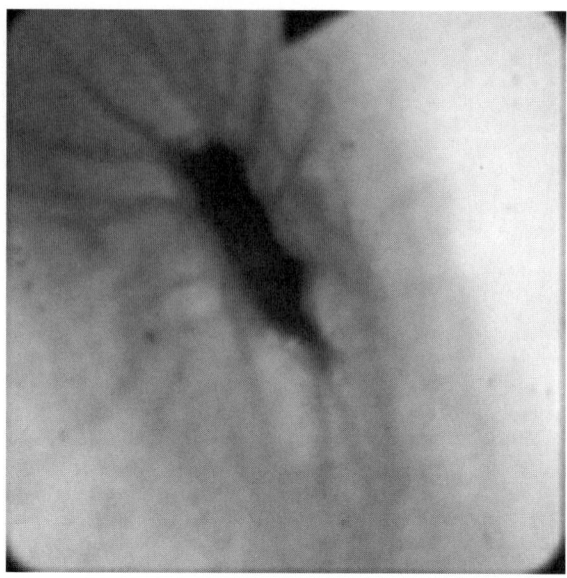

Figure 31-29. Endoscopic appearance of a stricture 30 days after circumferential ulceration.

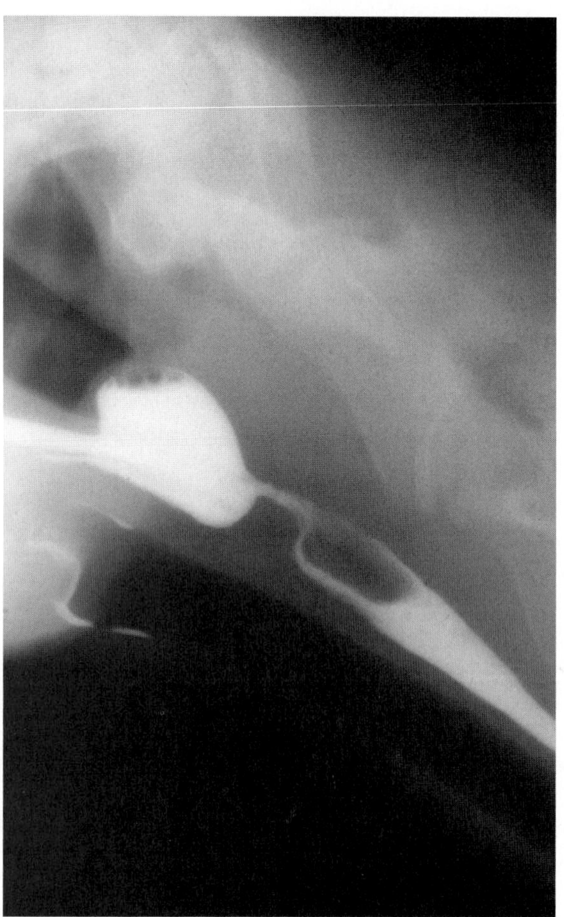

Figure 31-28. Positive-pressure esophagogram showing a stricture in a foal. Note the prestenotic dilation. The lesion was resolved by partial resection and anastomosis.

Strictures more that 60 days old have usually matured to the point where the cicatrix is too firm to yield to dilation by this method and therefore may be classified as chronic (Fig. 31-30). Chronic strictures of the esophagus may be corrected by esophagomyotomy, partial or complete resection and anastomosis, or patch grafting. Complications may occur with any of these surgical treatments, and the surgeon should take care to pick the most conservative therapy that will meet the aim of treatment. Leakage of luminal contents and reformation of the stricture requiring prolonged medical management are to be expected after resection and patch grafting. Strictures that are mural in origin respond to myotomy and have the best prognosis for recovery without

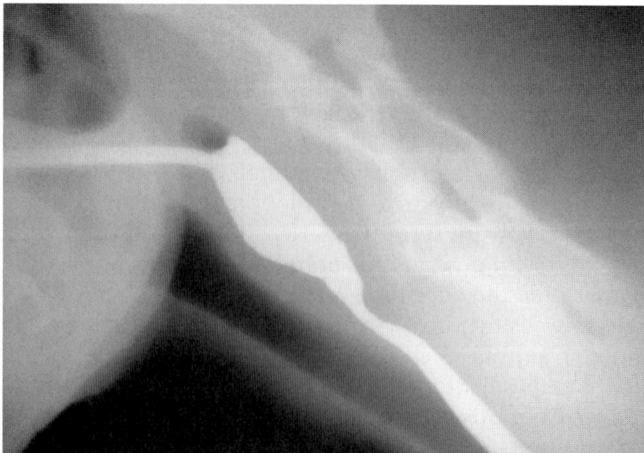

Figure 31-30. Positive-contrast esophagogram using liquid barium administered under pressure through a cuffed nasogastric tube shows stricture with prestenotic dilation. The stenosis was subsequently resolved by esophagomyotomy.

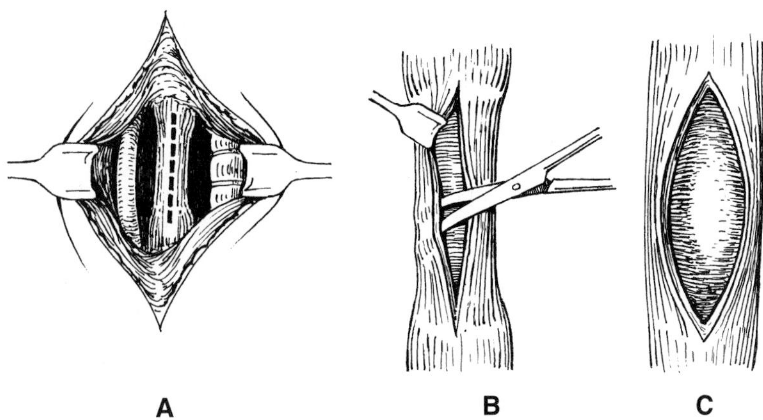

Figure 31-31. A, Esophagomyotomy: longitudinal incision of the outer layer of the esophageal wall. **B,** Elevation and separation of the outer (muscularis and adventitia) and inner (mucosa and submucosa) layers of the esophageal wall to complete the esophagomyotomy. **C,** The muscularis and adventitia are not sutured.

restricture. Three successful reports appear in the literature; I have had similar experience with five other horses.[30,31] The surgery should be performed with the horse under general anesthesia, with a nasogastric tube passed to the level of the stricture to permit easy identification of the involved area.

Esophagomyotomy

The esophagus is incised longitudinally to the level of the mucosa, through the stricture, and 1 cm ($^1/_2$ inch) distal and proximal to it (Fig. 31-31, *A*). The nasogastric tube may be passed through the stenotic area at this point. From this single incision, the muscularis is separated by sharp dissection from the mucosa around the entire circumference of the esophagus (see Fig. 31-31, *B*). When the mucosa is freed in this manner, removal of a portion of the muscularis or multiple myotomy incisions are seldom necessary. The myotomy is not sutured (see Fig. 31-31, *C*), and the approach incision is closed and drained in a routine manner. If the mucosa is opened inadvertently, it should be closed immediately with 3-0 polypropylene sutures in a simple-continuous pattern. Postoperatively, feeding small but frequent quantities of soft feed may be necessary if a prestenotic dilation was present before surgery. When this dilation is no longer evident radiographically, normal feeding may be resumed.

Recurrence of postsurgical cicatricial stricture is slow to develop, with clinical signs occurring weeks or months after the operation. Conservative treatment (changing from hay to a complete pelleted diet) may be all that is necessary to resolve recurrent obstructions. A postsurgical stricture seen long after the original operation usually is the result of a mature nonresilient cicatrix and may not respond to dilation. If surgery is necessary, the surgeon should not hesitate to perform a second esophagomyotomy; however, performing another surgery in a stenotic area of the esophagus before allowing the acute inflammation of the previous surgery to subside greatly increases the propensity for restricture. If such is the case, a more hazardous procedure may have to be selected eventually to correct the problem.

Partial Resection

Longitudinal esophagomyotomy combined with mucosal resection provides relief of stricture caused by esophageal rings or webs or annular stenosis of all muscle layers.[32,33] Performed under general anesthesia, the procedure is indicated when the cicatrix involves the mucosa and prevents passage of a nasogastric tube after myotomy.

The esophagus is exposed and incised as described previously for esophagomyotomy. A longitudinal incision is made through the mucosa long enough to permit identification of the diseased segment (Fig. 31-32, *A*). The mucosal scar is separated by sharp dissection from normal or diseased muscle layer. Circumferential incisions are made at the proximal and distal edges of the mucosal cicatrix and it is removed, leaving the muscular tube intact (see Fig. 31-32, *B*).

If cut edges of the mucosa can be brought into apposition without undue tension, they are apposed by three equally spaced 3-0 polypropylene simple-continuous sutures with the knots tied in the lumen (see Fig. 31-32, *C*). When mucosal rings or webs are the cause of stenosis, the normal esophageal muscle should be apposed over the mucosal anastomosis (see Fig. 31-32, *D*), but in the case of an annular stenosis that involves the entire esophageal wall, the muscularis should not be sutured. A drain is placed next to the esophagus, and the approach incision is closed. If space permits, tube feeding through an esophagostomy placed through a separate incision distal to the stricture is ideal. When this is not possible, frequent feeding of small quantities of soft food may begin 48 hours after surgery and should be continued for 10 days before normal roughage is offered to the patient.

When the stricture is extensive and the mucosa cannot be sutured, regeneration within the muscle tube occurs readily. The muscularis may be sutured if it is healthy, or it may be left open if only scar tissue remains. Spontaneous healing is aided if esophagostomy tube feeding (located closer to the stomach than the operative site) is used. When the stricture is located too close to the thoracic inlet to permit placement of a separate esophagostomy incision, the tube

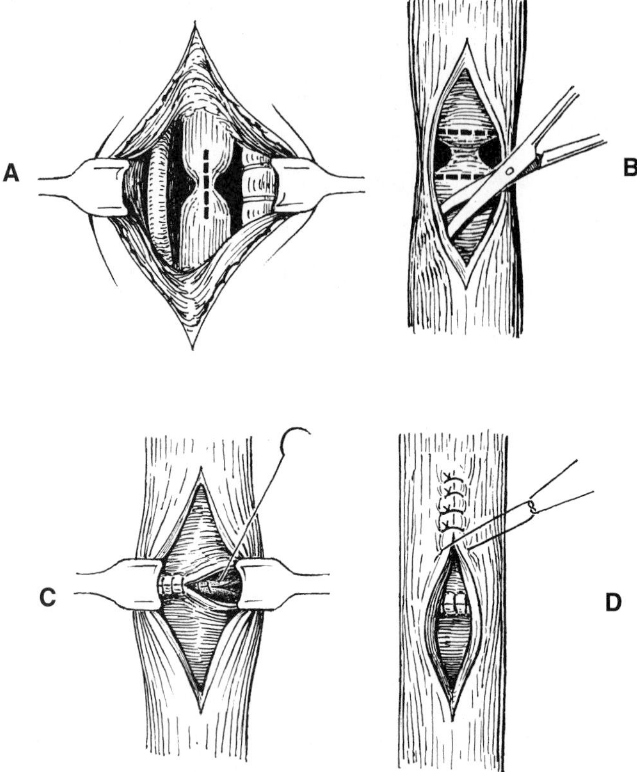

Figure 31-32. Partial resection and anastomosis. After longitudinal incision of the outer layer **(A)**, the inner layer is resected **(B)** and, when possible, closed transversely using several simple-continuous sutures **(C)**. The outer layer is then closed with interrupted sutures **(D)**.

may be inserted directly through the stricture site. Recurrence of stricture after this procedure may be an indication for esophagomyotomy or an esophagostomy tube placed through the stricture.

Resection and Anastomosis

Complete resection and anastomosis should be reserved for rupture of the esophagus in which the muscularis is not viable. The esophagus is exposed as described previously. The area to be resected and several centimeters of normal esophagus distal and proximal to it are mobilized. Umbilical tape or rubber drain tubing (0.63 cm [¼ inch]) is placed around the esophagus and held in place with hemostatic forceps to occlude the lumen a convenient distance from the area to be resected. Crushing clamps of any type should not be used on the esophagus. A point is selected proximal to the diseased segment, where the esophagus is sharply transected, leaving healthy tissue for closure. This procedure is repeated distally and the diseased portion is removed. The mucosal-submucosal layer is apposed with 3-0 simple-interrupted monofilament nonabsorbable polypropylene sutures placed about 3 cm (¼ inch) from the cut edge, 2 to 3 mm ($^1/_{12}$ to ¼ inch) apart, with the knots tied in the lumen. Tension of the sutures is adequate to form a tight seal without interference of the blood supply.

The esophageal muscle is apposed with interrupted horizontal mattress sutures of 2-0 polydioxanone or monofilament nonabsorbable suture material. The muscle layer has limited elasticity and, if necessary, a relief incision in the form of a circular myotomy 4 to 5 cm (1½ to 2 inches) proximal or distal to the anastomosis can decrease tension on the repair. The approach incision is closed as described previously.

Alternative successful methods of closure have been described, but postoperative management is a major determinant of the outcome of this procedure, regardless of closure technique.[34,35] Prevention of undue tension on the anastomosis by use of a standing martingale and special feeding regimen is necessary (Fig. 31-33). If oral alimentation is elected, soft foods should be given only after 48 hours and until endoscopic or radiographic evaluation of the surgery shows primary healing has occurred. Esophagostomy is the preferred method of feeding, if possible. An extensive cervical esophageal stricture produced by annular stenosis of the entire wall may preclude successful repair by techniques described previously. The diameter of the equine esophageal lumen can be increased by using a patch graft of the sternocephalicus muscle.[36]

Patch Grafting

Antibiotics should be given preoperatively and maintained for 6 to 10 days after surgery. With the horse under general anesthesia, a ventral midline or lateral approach to the esophagus is made and, depending on location of the defect and the approach used, the brachiocephalicus and sternocephalicus muscles serve as donors for the graft. With a nasogastric tube passed to the level of the stenosis, a longitudinal incision is made through the muscularis from a point 3 cm (1¼ inch) distal to and extending 3 cm proximal to the stricture. The mucosa and submucosa are sharply incised as the nasogastric tube is passed into the stomach. A caudal portion of the muscle belly of the brachiocephalicus or sternocephalicus is mobilized by blind separation of muscle fibers. The strip of muscle should maintain its proximal and distal attachments and should be freely movable so as not to exert tension on the closure when the patient's head and neck are moved. The graft should be wide enough to appreciably increase the lumen of the esophagus.

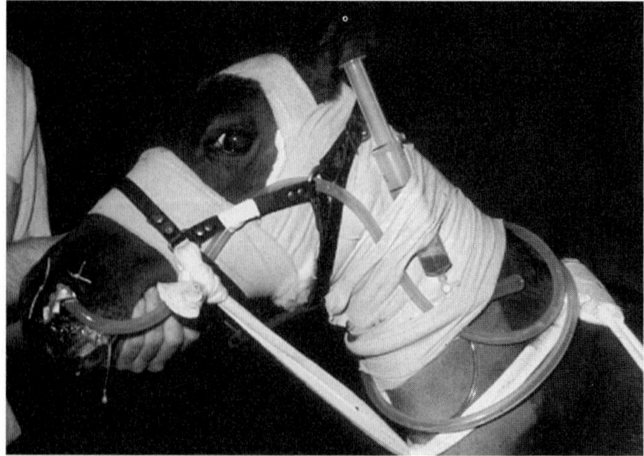

Figure 31-33. When complete resection anastomosis is performed, undue tension frequently results in dehiscence. Undue tension on the anastomosis can be prevented by using a standing Martingale, as shown, which prevents extension of the head and neck.

The edges of the mucosa and submucosa are sutured to the muscle graft using 3-0 polypropylene interrupted through-and-through mattress sutures, and the edges of the muscularis are sutured to the graft with 3-0 simple-interrupted sutures of monofilament polypropylene. Preplacement of mattress sutures and closure of both layers on one side of the esophageal defect at a time facilitate repair. The nasogastric tube should be removed before the second edge is closed. Suction drains are placed next to the esophagus, and the approach incision is closed.

Postoperatively, extraoral alimentation is preferred for 10 days (by esophagostomy, if space allows, or intravenous feeding), but soft foods may be given per os as early as 48 hours if salivary leaking has not occurred. An indwelling nasogastric tube provides a stimulus for salivation and increases the incidence of fistula formation.

Fistula

Fistulae of the esophagus result from causes previously described for ruptures and may be treated similarly. However, small fistulae may be a diagnostic challenge. Occasionally, they may be observed endoscopically (Fig. 31-34). More frequently, findings of endoscopic examinations and barium swallow esophagograms are normal. Esophageal fistulae should be included in the differential diagnosis when cervical swelling, fever, and dysphagia are present; a nasogastric tube can be passed to the stomach; and endoscopic findings are normal. Contrast radiography, using liquid barium administered under pressúre, best demonstrates the lesion (Fig. 31-35). When ventral drainage has been established, fistulae almost always heal spontaneously. During this time, food and water may be expelled through the cloaca (Fig. 31-36). Large fistulas can extrude copious amounts of masticated food and saliva. Elevating the food and water sources will decrease the amount lost. If healing does not occur, resection of the sinus tract and closure of the esophageal stoma may be necessary (Fig. 31-37). Closure of the esophageal defect should be performed as for esophagotomy.

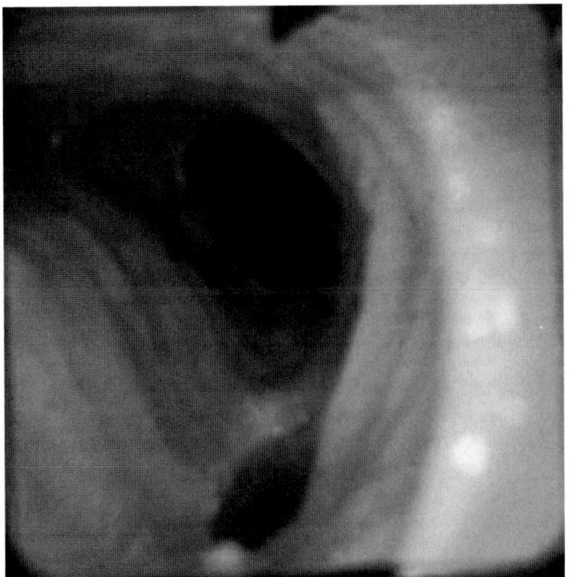

Figure 31-34. Endoscopic appearance of a large esophageal fistula. Smaller fistulae are often difficult to locate endoscopically.

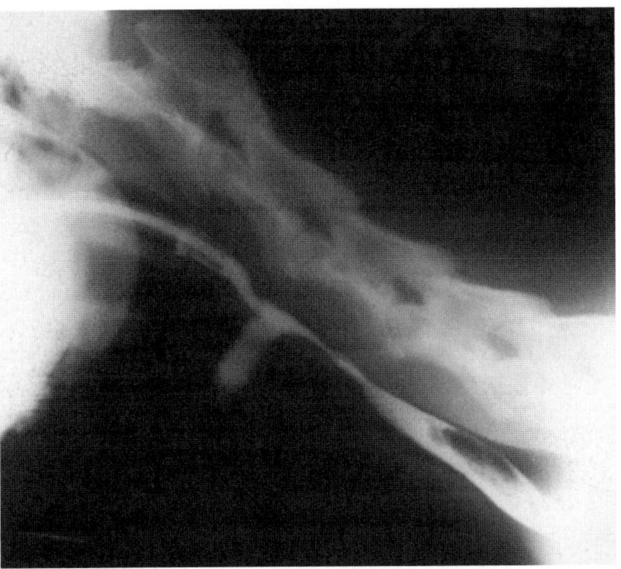

Figure 31-35. Positive-contrast esophagogram shows a large fistula remaining after removal of the esophagotomy tube. The cuff on the nasogastric tube prevents reflux of barium into the pharynx.

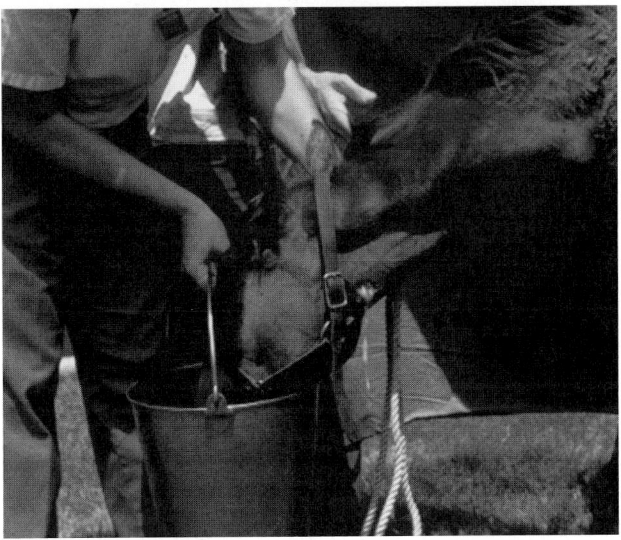

Figure 31-36. A horse drinking, with a large esophageal fistula. When the water source is below the head, almost all of the water is lost. Therefore food and water should be elevated to decrease the amount lost through the fistula.

Diverticulum

In horses, diverticula of the esophagus only occasionally cause esophageal dysfunction. Usually they are acquired lesions that result from contraction of periesophageal fibrous scar tissue, causing outward traction and tenting of all layers of the esophageal wall (traction, or true diverticulum). Or they can occur from protrusion of mucosa and submucosa through a defect in the esophageal muscularis (pulsion, or false diverticulum) (Fig. 31-38).

A traction diverticulum commonly develops at the site of a healed esophagostomy, at the site of a postsurgical or

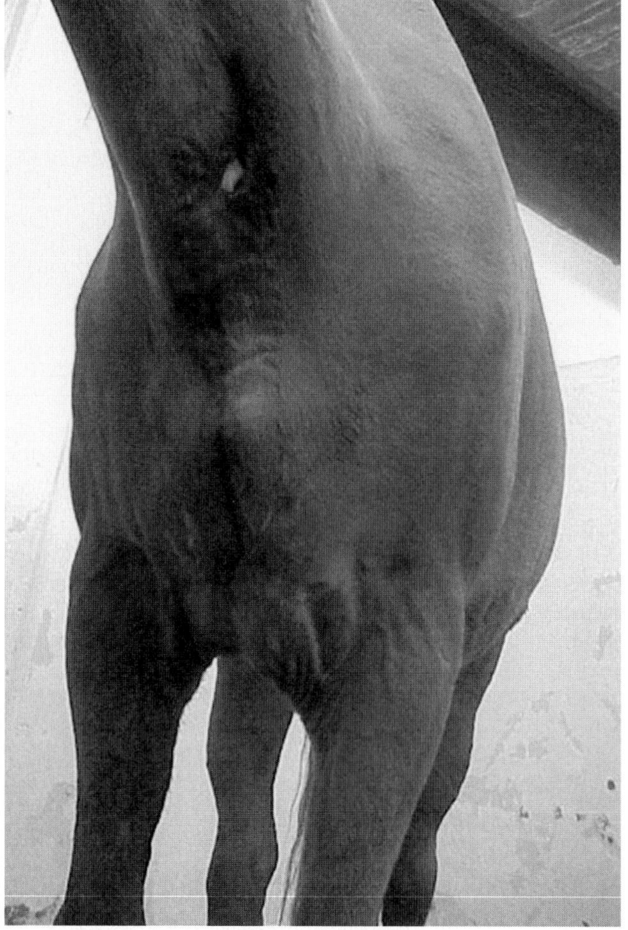

Figure 31-37. An esophageal fistula resulting from placement of the esophagostomy tube through a ruptured esophagus. Redundant mucosa prevented this fistula from healing spontaneously, and it was closed using the techniques described for esophagotomy.

posttraumatic wound of the esophagus that is allowed to heal by second intention as a fistula, or after penetration of the esophageal lumen (traumatic or surgical) in which leakage of saliva has caused inflammation or abscess. Pulsion diverticula are caused by fluctuations in esophageal intraluminal pressure and over-stretch damage to esophageal muscle fibers by impacted feedstuffs. A more probable cause is external trauma to the cervical area.[37-39]

Diverticula in the cervical esophagus should be considered when an enlargement in the neck results in dysphagia and yet a nasogastric tube can be passed. On barium swallow esophagograms, traction diverticula are spherical and have a wide neck (Fig. 31-39), whereas pulsion diverticula are flasklike in configuration, with a narrow neck. Differentiation of these two types of diverticula can be aided by additional contrast techniques that distend the esophageal lumen and outline the opening into the evagination. Esophagoscopy also defines the relative size and configuration of the opening of a diverticulum (Fig. 31-40).

A traction diverticulum, even when quite large, produces few clinical signs and seldom requires treatment. A pulsion diverticulum, however, has a tendency to enlarge progressively so that risk of obstruction and rupture increase with time. Surgical repair is indicated. A pulsion diverticulum can be repaired by diverticulectomy with resection of the mucosal-submucosal sac, followed by reconstruction of the mucosa, submucosa, and muscularis, or by inversion of the mucosal-submucosal sac with reconstruction of the muscular layer. Diverticulectomy should be used when the mucosal sac is very large and the neck of the diverticulum very narrow. There are reports of repair of apparent congenital esophageal diverticula using this technique.[40]

However, mucosal inversion is the preferred technique because it decreases the chance of postoperative leakage, infection, or fistula formation and does not appear to predispose to postoperative obstruction complications.

Mucosal Inversion

The esophagus is exposed, and the diverticulum and defect in the muscularis are identified by careful dissection (Fig. 31-41). Inadvertent perforation of the mucosa and submucosa should be repaired immediately. The edges of the muscular defect should be débrided back to healthy-appearing tissue. The sac is inverted, and the edges of the muscularis are apposed with simple-interrupted sutures of 3-0 polypropylene in a manner to avoid undue tension on the closure and prevent stenosis of the esophageal diameter.

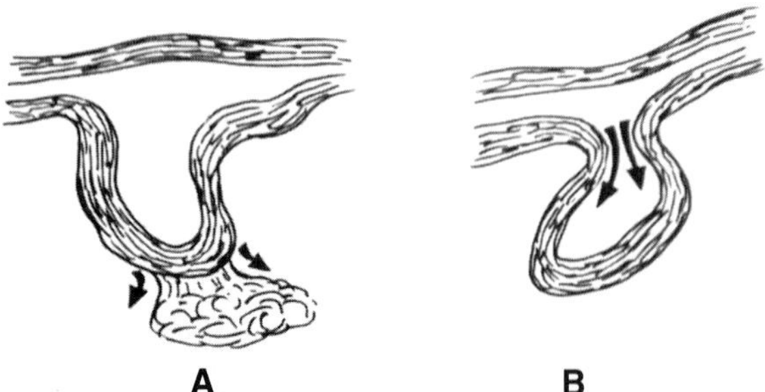

Figure 31-38. A, Traction diverticulum or true diverticulum develops at the site of a postsurgical or posttraumatic wound of the esophagus that is allowed to heal by second intention (e.g., a fistula or penetration of the esophageal wound). This type of diverticulum has a wide neck that seldom needs surgical correction. **B,** Pulsion diverticulum is caused by external trauma to the cervical area that ruptures the muscular layer. This type of diverticulum has a narrow neck and may continue to enlarge or ferment feed within the lumen, requiring surgical correction.

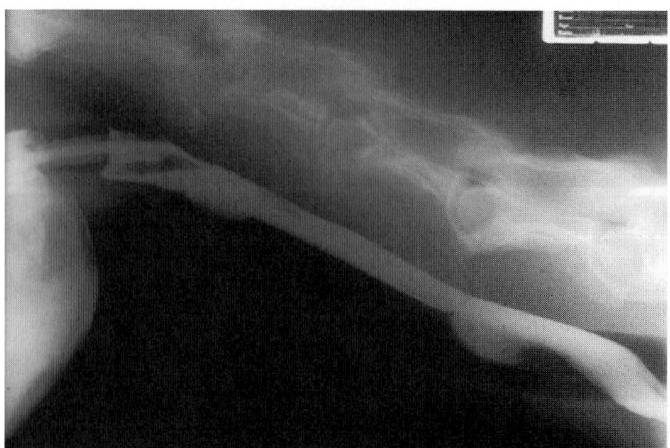

Figure 31-39. Barium swallow procedure in a horse with an esophagotomy that healed by second intention shows a traction diverticulum. Note the wide neck of the diverticulum.

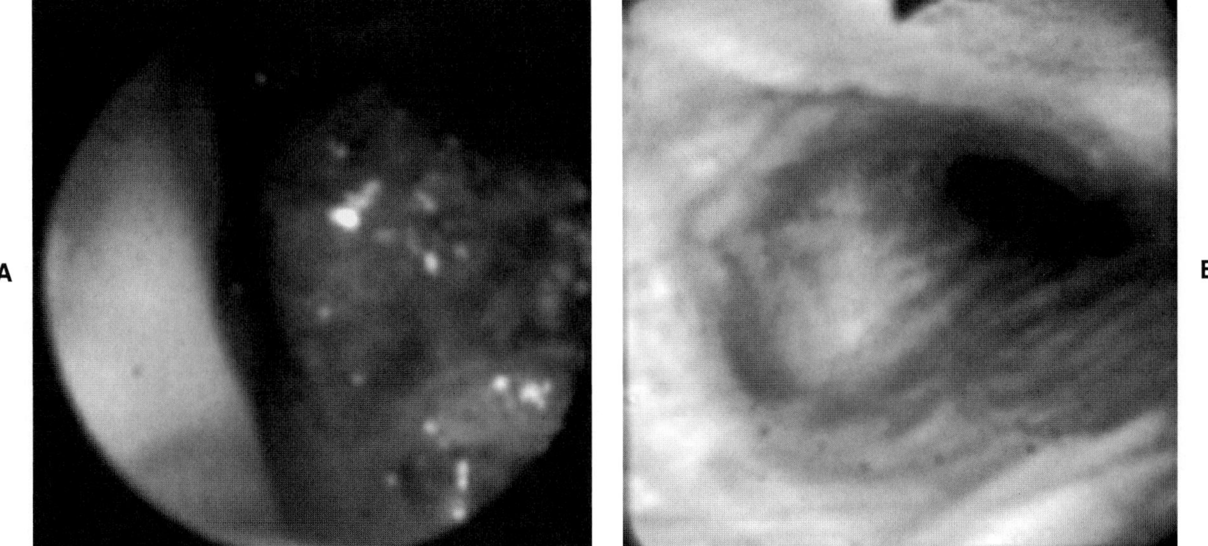

Figure 31-40. Endoscopic appearance of an opening into a traction or true esophageal diverticulum. Note feed in the diverticulum **(A)** and the normal-appearing mucosa **(B)** after lavage via drinking.

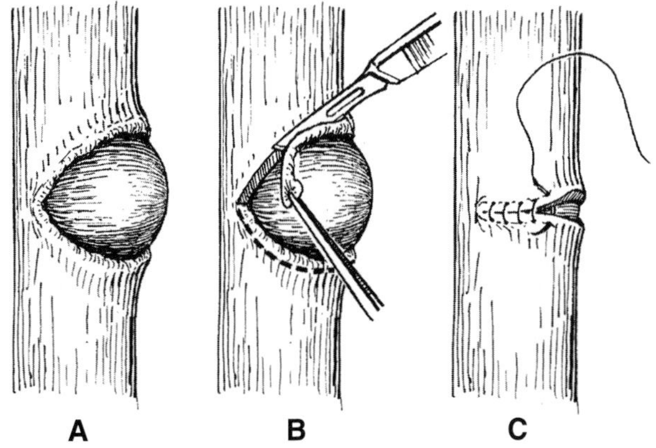

Figure 31-41. A, A pulsion diverticulum repaired by inversion of the mucosal/submucosal sac with reconstruction of the muscular layer. **B,** The edge of the muscular defect should be débrided back to healthy tissue. **C,** The sac is inverted, and the edges of the muscularis are apposed with simple-interrupted sutures of 3-0 polypropylene in a manner that avoids undue tension on the closure and prevents stenosis of the esophageal diameter.

Postoperatively, feeding should consist of soft foods for 4 to 6 weeks.

Intramural Cyst

Esophageal cysts are uncommon in all species, but several equine cases have been documented.[41-43] I have seen three additional horses with esophageal cysts, a 3-year-old Morgan mare, in which the cyst lining had radiographic signs of calcification, and two yearling Quarter Horse colts, both admitted for dysphagia. In all horses, an epithelial inclusion cyst (lined by stratified squamous epithelium and filled with keratinaceous debris) was found in the esophageal wall. Mural cysts are probably a developmental anomaly.

Clinical findings include dysphagia, regurgitation, a palpable soft tissue mass in the neck, and resistance to passage of a nasogastric tube at the site of the cyst. The diagnosis can be made on survey films if the cyst has started to calcify (Fig. 31-42). However, it is better confirmed on contrast radiography by the classic appearance of a filling defect caused by a mural lesion (Fig. 31-43). Endoscopically, the esophageal lumen may appear partially occluded, but significant gross changes are usually not observed because the mucosa appears normal. Intramural esophageal cysts may be removed through enucleation with inversion or resection of redundant mucosa. The esophagus is exposed, and the cyst is identified by manipulation of a nasogastric tube within the esophageal lumen. A longitudinal incision

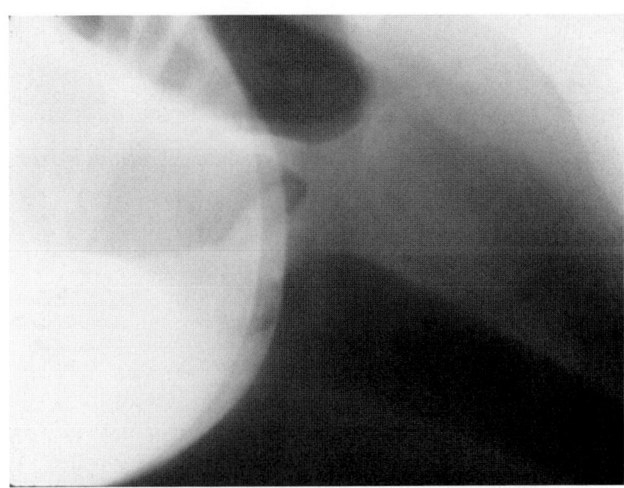

Figure 31-42. Radiographic appearance of an inner mural inclusion cyst of the esophagus in a 3-year-old Morgan mare in which the cyst lining had radiographic signs of calcification. This is an unusual finding, as survey films are usually nondiagnostic.

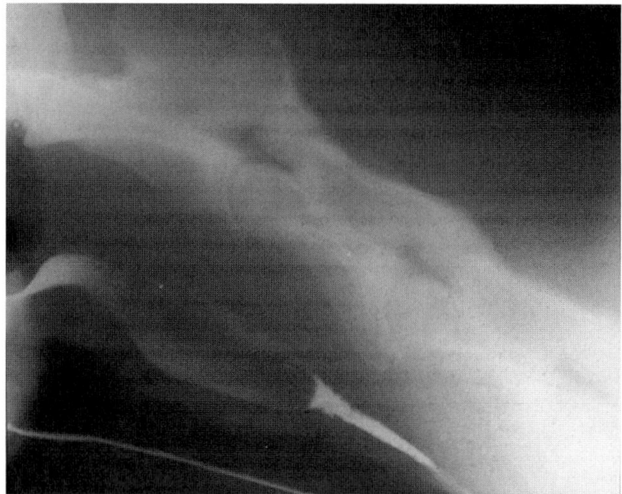

Figure 31-43. Barium esophagogram shows the classic appearance of an intramural lesion of the esophagus—in this case, an epithelial inclusion cyst. The esophageal lumen is narrowed caudally and is dilated but not filled with barium cranially because the mural mass produces a filling defect.

is made through the muscularis over the cyst. By careful dissection, the cyst is separated from its position between the mucosa/submucosa and the muscularis and is removed intact (Fig. 31-44). The cyst can be mistaken for an abscess if it is inadvertently incised by the inexperienced surgeon. Positioning the nasogastric tube caudal to the cyst helps prevent inadvertent perforation of the mucosa. After the cyst is removed, it leaves an area of redundant mucosa, or a sac, which may be treated as a pulsion diverticulum (i.e., by inversion, preferably, or by diverticulectomy). The muscularis is closed with simple-interrupted 3-0 sutures of polydioxanone or polypropylene at the surgeon's preference.

Megaesophagus

Megaesophagus is dilation and muscular hypertrophy of the esophagus oral (proximal) to a constricted distal segment. Although idiopathic muscular hypertrophy does occur in the horse (without dilation), it is an asymptomatic and an incidental finding at necropsy.[44] Therefore, the term *megaesophagus,* as used here, includes congenital ectasia (dilation of unknown origin), achalasia (failure of the distal esophagus to relax because of neural dysfunction, resulting in proximal dilation), and megaesophagus secondary to vascular ring anomalies. One case of vascular ring anomaly causing megaesophagus in a foal has been reported.[45] The anomalous defect was a result of a persistent right aortic arch and was suspected on radiographic examination and confirmed on necropsy. Another case of megaesophagus was reported secondary to chronic gastroesophageal reflux.[46]

Although hypomotility of the esophagus has been documented in one foal and neural defects of the esophagus were found in another, achalasia as defined in dogs and humans has not been reported.[47,48] Treatment of these horses was not successful, even with a modified Heller's myotomy in one foal. I have treated congenital ectasia con-

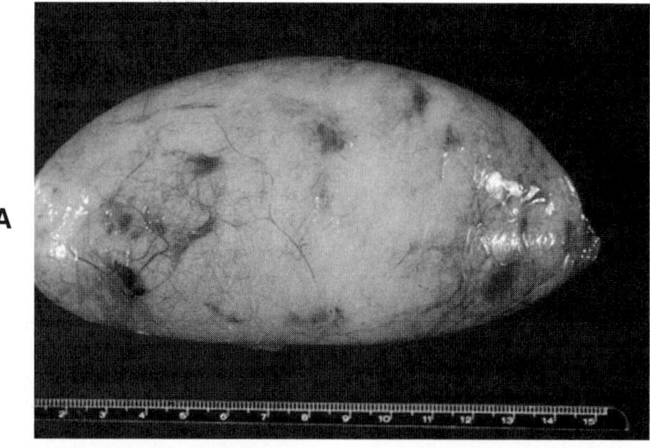

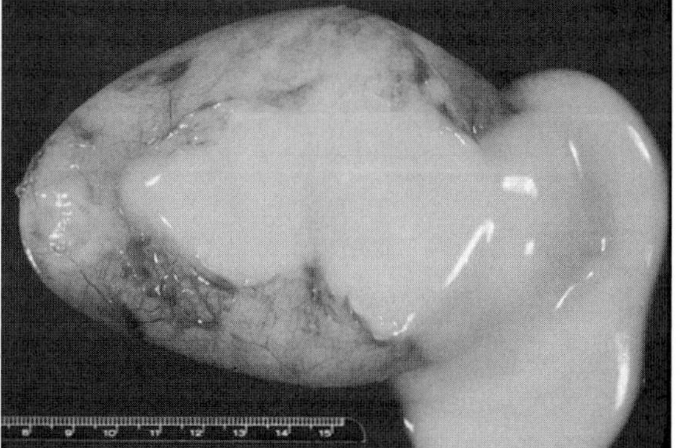

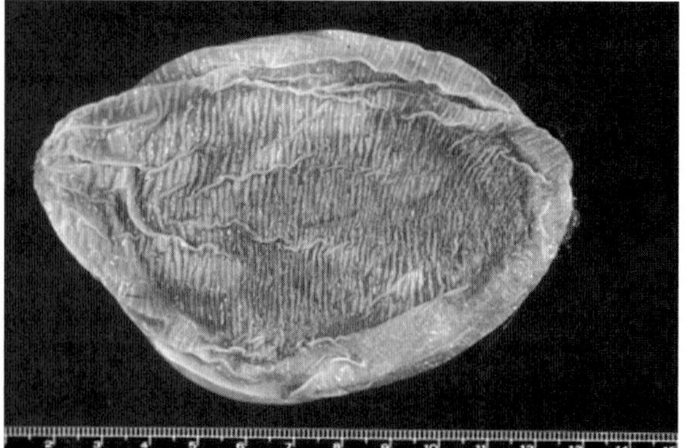

Figure 31-44. An excised intramural inclusion cyst **(A)** following puncture **(B)**. The epithelial cell contents could be mistaken for an abscess ruptured during surgery. The cyst lining is normal esophageal mucosa **(C)**.

servatively with good results. A 5-month-old foal was admitted because of recurrent choke that began at the time of weaning. Esophageal lavage produced 8 L of feed regurgitated through the nasogastric tube. On radiography and endoscopy, generalized ectasia was found from the mid-cervical to the mid-thoracic esophagus (Fig. 31-45), with an annular ring noted at the point where the esophagus passed through the thoracic inlet (Fig. 31-46). The foal was fed a mash diet (pellets mixed with warm water) for 6 months, with the feed trough elevated above the animal's withers. The mash diet was changed to complete pelleted feed for an additional 6 months before the horse was fed normal feed. Although fluid did not pool in the lumen of the esophagus after 6 months of the mash diet and the size of the dilated esophagus did not change over the next 24 months during several radiographic examinations, the horse could eat normally and is being used for show and pleasure riding. Conservative management of this problem should be considered if the owners are willing to provide the extensive nursing care (no access to roughage, including bedding in the stall, and total confinement, with exercise in-hand only)

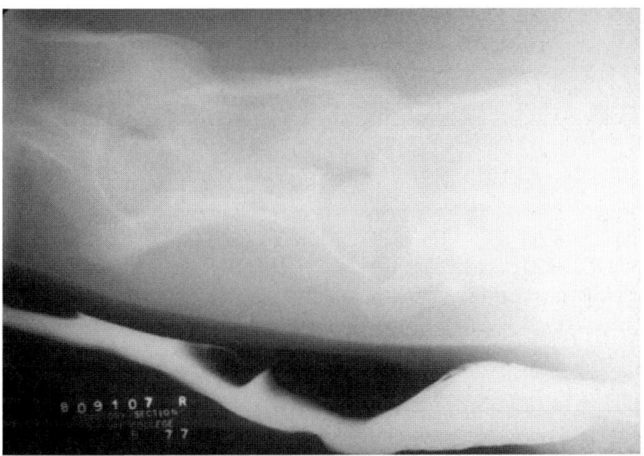

Figure 31-45. Positive-contrast esophagogram shows megaesophagus at the mid-cervical level. The foal was managed with a mash diet and recovered esophageal function over a 1-year period.

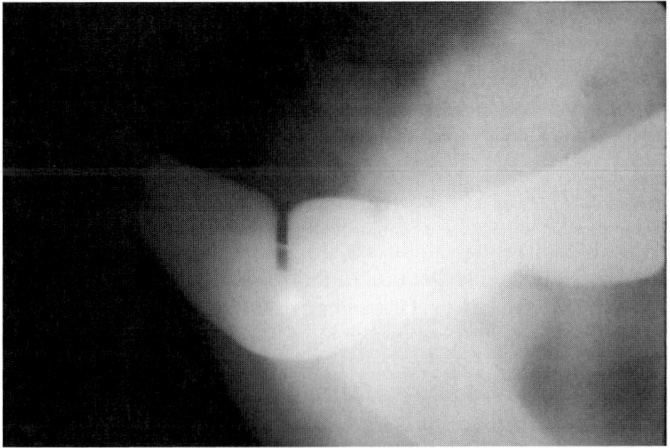

Figure 31-46. Barium pressure esophagogram shows megaesophagus in the foal seen in Figure 31-45. Note the narrowing of the esophageal lumen as it passes through the thoracic inlet.

and are willing to face the possibility of several episodes of "choke" requiring treatment.

Reduplication

It is not clear whether reduplication of the esophagus is a congenital or an acquired condition, but it is included here for the sake of completeness. This condition has been reported twice.[49,50] Clinical signs were similar to those of other forms of esophageal obstruction. Diagnosis may be difficult, but the problem does appear to be amenable to surgery. This condition closely resembles one of the complications of esophagostomy tube feeding, in which a dissecting tract develops parallel to the esophageal wall or within it, causing signs of obstruction.

Neoplasia

Neoplasms causing signs of esophageal obstruction are rare.[1] Squamous cell carcinoma is the most common neoplasm and has been reported in detail in four cases. One was an extension of gastric carcinoma, one was located in the tracheal bifurcation, and two were located in the distal cervical esophagus.[51-54] Biopsy and cytologic examination of brush samples obtained through the endoscope may provide an early diagnosis before stenosis of the esophagus develops, but advanced cases may be detected on radiography. The value of resection is questionable.

COMPLICATIONS OF ESOPHAGEAL SURGERY

The surgeon has the following three clinical objectives: (1) to obtain leak-proof healing of a primary anastomosis or incision, (2) to dilate a restricted aperture, and (3) to return the enlarged or disrupted esophagus to near-normal size and function. Despite meticulous technique, complications can occur. If managed properly, however, they can be resolved with a favorable outcome for the patient.

Dehiscence and Stricture

The keys to handling breakdown of a sutured esophageal incision are early recognition and treatment. For this reason, a suction drain placed next to the esophagus at the time of surgery serves a second function in addition to drainage of the serum and blood from the surgical site. It provides a method to detect salivary leakage. Not all incisions that leak saliva dehisce, especially if the saliva is removed from periesophageal tissues. However, if extreme amounts of saliva are leaking through the incision or complete dehiscence occurs, the original approach incision should be completely opened and lavaged daily to remove any ingesta or saliva. Dissection planes ventrally along the trachea should be drained to the outside to prevent eventual mediastinitis or pleuritis. Dissecting infections can occur after esophagostomy as well, and inadvertent placement of a dislodged feeding tube into a dissection plane or the thorax would clearly have an unfavorable outcome.

The patient may be permitted to drink, which in many cases lavages the wound. Nutritional requirements may be met by oral feeding or placement of a feeding tube into the esophagus at the point of dehiscence or distally through a separate esophagostomy. The outcome of this complication from this point depends on management of water and electrolyte balance. The most common complication after treatment of an annular lesion is stricture (see Fig. 31-30). This complication is the bane of the esophageal surgeon, and its successful treatment is limited by the owner's financial commitment.

Acid–Base and Electrolyte Alterations

In the face of adequate nutrition, daily losses of large amounts of saliva result in hyponatremia, hypochloremia (Fig. 31-47), and transient metabolic acidosis followed by progressive metabolic alkalosis (Fig. 31-48). The alkalosis probably results from renal compensation for electrolyte imbalances. Oral administration of sodium chloride daily reverses the electrolyte imbalance (potassium requirements are adequately met in feed); alkalosis is corrected through renal mechanisms.

Laryngeal Hemiplegia

Manipulative procedures or disease of the esophagus in the cervical area can easily result in laryngeal hemiplegia because of the proximity of the recurrent laryngeal and vagus nerves. The surgeon should be aware that apparently minor manipulations of these nerves can have deleterious effects on their function.

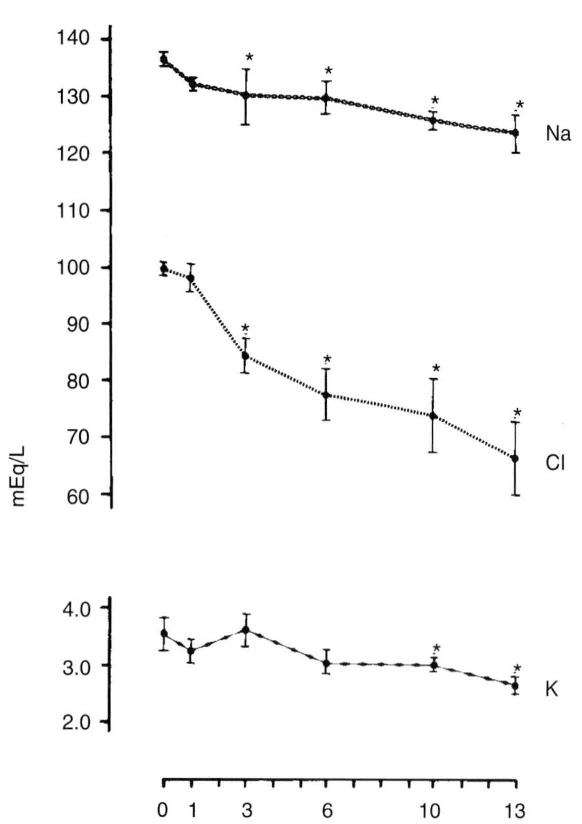

Figure 31-47. Influence of salivary depletion on serum electrolyte levels (Na, K, Cl) before (day 0) and after the esophageal fistulation. Bars indicate ±1 SE (N = 6). Stars indicate days on which serum electrolyte levels were significantly different from baseline values (day 0).

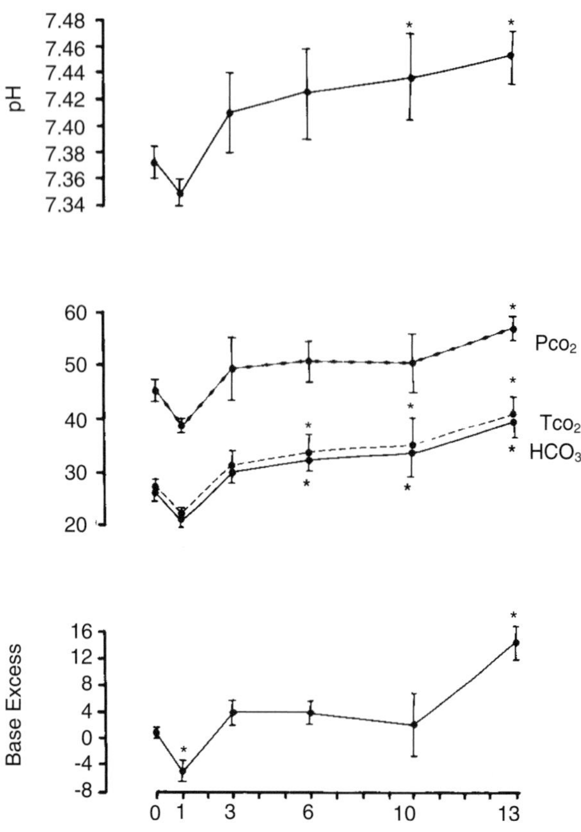

Figure 31-48. Effect of salivary depletion and serum electrolyte alterations on acid–base values (pH, Pco_2 [mm Hg], Tco_2 = total CO_2 [mEq/L], HCO_3^- [mEq/L], and base excess [mEq/L]) before (day 0) and after esophageal fistulation. Bars indicate ±1 SE (N = 6). Stars indicate days on which each value was significantly different from baseline values (day 0).

Carotid Artery Rupture

Chronic feeding tubes placed in the distal third of the cervical esophagus can lead to jugular vein or carotid artery ulceration. Bleeding episodes should be an indication for exploratory and vessel ligation to prevent exsanguination.

REFERENCES

1. Stick JA: Surgery of the esophagus, Vet Clin North Am Large Anim Pract 1982;4:33.
2. Stick JA: Esophageal disease. In Robinson NE, editor: Current Therapy in Equine Medicine 2, Philadelphia, 1987, WB Saunders.
3. Stick JA: Diseases of the esophagus. In Colahan PT, Mayhew IG, Merrett AM, et al, editors: Equine Medicine and Surgery, ed 5, Chicago, 1998, Mosby.
4. Nickel R, Schummer A, Seifferle E, et al: The Viscera of the Domestic Animals, ed 2, New York, 1973, Springer-Verlag.
5. Slocombe RF, Todhunter RJ, Stick JA: Quantitative ultrastructural anatomy of the esophagus in different regions of the horse: Effects on alternate methods of tissue processing, Am J Vet Res 1982;43:1137.

6. Stick JA, Derksen FJ, McNitt DL, et al: Equine esophageal pressure profile, Am J Vet Res 1983;44:272.
7. Clark ES, Deem Morris D, Whitlock RH: Esophageal manometry in horses, cows, and sheep during deglutition, Am J Vet Res 1987; 48:547.
8. Watson TDG, Sullivan M: Effects of detomidine on equine esophageal function as studied by contrast radiography, Vet Res 1991;129:67.
9. Stick JA, Derksen FJ, Scott EA: Equine cervical esophagostomy: Complications associated with durations and locations of feeding tubes, Am J Vet Res 1981;42:727.
10. Freeman DE, Naylor JM: Cervical esophagostomy to permit extraoral feeding of the horse, J Am Vet Med Assoc 1978;172:314.
11. Nixon AJ, Aanes WA, Nelson AW, et al: Esophagomyotomy for relief of an intrathoracic esophageal stricture in a horse, J Am Vet Med Assoc 1983;183:794.
12. Ford TS, Schumacher J, Chaffin MK, et al: Surgical repair of all intrathoracic esophageal diverticula in a horse, Vet Surg 1991; 20:316.
13. Wooldridge AA, Eades SC, Hosgood GL, Moore RM: Effects of treatment with oxytocin, xylazine butorphanol, guaifenesin acepromazine, and detomidine on esophageal manometric pressure in conscious horses, Am J Vet Res 2002;63:1738.
14. Meyer GA, Rashmir-Raven A, Helms RJ, Brashier M: The effect of oxytocin on contractility of the equine oesophagus: A potential treatment for oesophageal obstruction, Equine Vet J 2000;32:151.
15. Hardy J, Stewart RH, Beard WL, et al: Complications of nasogastric intubation in horses: nine cases (1987-1989), J Am Vet Med Assoc 1992;201:483.
16. Lundvall RL, Kingrey BW: Choke in Shetland ponies, caused by boluses, J Am Vet Med Assoc 1958;133:75.
17. DeBowes RM, Grant BD, Sande RD: Esophageal obstruction by antibiotic boluses in a Thoroughbred filly: A case report, J Equine Vet Sci 1982;2:23.
18. Stick JA, Krehbiel JD, Kunze DJ, et al: Esophageal healing in the pony: A comparison of sutured vs non-sutured esophagotomy, Am J Vet Res 1981;42:1506.
19. Stick JA , Slocombe RG, Derksen FJ, et al: Esophagotomy in the pony: Comparison of surgical techniques and form of feed, Am J Vet Res 1983;44:2123.
20. Stick JA, Robinson NE, Krehbiel JD: Acid-base and electrolyte alterations associated with salivary loss in the pony, Am J Vet Res 1981;42:733.
21. Todhunter RJ, Stick JA, Trotter GW, et al: Medical management of esophageal stricture in seven horses, J Am Vet Med Assoc 1984;185:784.
22. Raker CW, Sayers A: Esophageal rupture in a Standardbred mare, J Am Vet Med Assoc 1958;133:371.
23. DeMoor A, Wouters L, Mouens Y, et al: Surgical treatment of a traumatic oesophageal rupture in a foal, Equine Vet J 1979;11:265.
24. Wingfield-Digby NJ, Burguez PN: Traumatic oesophageal rupture in the horse, Equine Vet J 1982;14:169.
25. Peacock EE: Wound Repair, ed 3, Philadelphia, 1984, WB Saunders.
26. Lunn DP, Peel JE: Successful treatment of traumatic oesophageal rupture with severe cellulitis in a mare, Vet Rec 1985;116:544.
27. Todhunter RJ, Stick JA, Slocombe RF: Comparison of three feeding techniques after esophageal mucosal resection and anastomosis in the horse, Cornell Vet 1986;76:16.
28. Tillotson K, Traub-Dargatz JL, Twedt D: Balloon dilation of an oesophageal stricture in a one-month-old Appaloosa colt, Equine Vet Educ 2003;15:67.
29. Knottenbelt DC, Harrison LJ, Peacock PJ: Conservative treatment of oesophageal stricture in 5 foals, Vet Rec 1992;131:27.
30. Wagner PC, Rantanen NW: Myotomy as a treatment for esophageal stricture in a horse, Equine Pract 1980;2:40.
31. Steward KA, Reinertson EL: Congenital esophageal stricture in a pony foal, Mod Vet Pract 1983;64:753.
32. Derksen FJ, Stick JA: Resection and anastomosis of esophageal stricture in a foal, Equine Pract 1983;5:17.
33. Craig D, Todhunter RJ: Surgical repair of an esophageal stricture in a horse, Vet Surg 1987;16:251.
34. Lowe JE: Esophageal anastomosis in the horse, Cornell Vet 1964;54:636.
35. Suann CJ: Oesophageal resection and anastomosis as a treatment for oesophageal stricture in the horse, Equine Vet J 1982;14:163.
36. Hoffer RE, Barber SM, Kallfelz FA, et al: Esophageal patch grafting as a treatment for esophageal stricture in a horse, J Am Vet Med Assoc 1977;171:350.
37. Aanes WA: The diagnosis and surgical repair of diverticulum of the esophagus, Proc Am Assoc Equine Pract 1975;19:211.
38. Hackett RP, Dyer RM, Hoffer RE: Surgical correction of esophageal diverticulum in a horse, J Am Vet Med Assoc 1978;173:998.
39. Harrison IW, Cartel RE: Surgical correction of a traumatic esophageal diverticulum in a horse, Cornell Vet 1990;80:279.
40. Haasjes C: Esophageal diverticulum, J Am Vet Med Assoc 1946; 109:2789.
41. Scott EA, Snoy P, Prasse KW, et al: Intramural esophageal cyst in a horse, J Am Vet Med Assoc 1977;171:652.
42. Stick JA, Boles CL, Scott EA: Esophageal intramural cyst in a horse, J Am Vet Med Assoc 1977;171:1133.
43. Saims AE, Weldon AD, Rakestraw P: Surgical treatment of intramural esophageal inclusion cysts in three horses, Vet Surg 1993;22:135.
44. Benders NA, Veldhuis Kroeze EJB, Van der Kolk JH: Idiopathic muscular hypertrophy of the oesophgus in the horse: A retrospective study of 31 cases, Equine Vet J 2004;36:46.
45. Bartels JE, Vaughan JT: Persistent right aortic arch in the horse, J Am Vet Med Assoc 1969;154:406.
46. Murray MJ, Ball MM, Parker GA: Megaesophagus and aspiration pneumonia secondary to gastric ulceration in a foal, J Am Vet Med Assoc 1988;192:381.
47. Bowman KF, Vaughn JT, Quick CB, et al: Megaesophagus in a colt, J Am Vet Med Assoc 1978;172:334.
48. Rohrback BW, Rooney JR: Congenital esophageal ectasia in a Thoroughbred foal, J Am Vet Med Assoc 1980;177:65.
49. Swanstrom OG, Dade AA: Reduplication of the esophageal lumen in a Quarter Horse filly, Vet Med Small Anim Clin 1979;74:75.
50. Gaughan EM, Gift LJ, Frank RK: Tubular duplication of the cervical portion of the esophagus in a foal, J Am Vet Med Assoc 1992; 201:748.
51. Moore JN, Kintner LD: Recurrent oesophageal obstruction due to squamous cell carcinoma in a horse, Cornel Vet 1976;66:589.
52. Pommer A: Carcinomstenose des Oesophagus beim Pferd, Wien Tieraerztl Monatsschr 1947;34:193.
53. Roberts MC, Kelly WR: Squamous cell carcinoma of the lower cervical oesophagus in a pony, Equine Vet J 1979;11:199.
54. Campbell-Beggs CL, Kiper ML, MacAllister C, et al: Use of esophagoscopy in the diagnosis of esophageal squamous cell carcinoma, J Am Vet Med Assoc 1993;202:617.

CHAPTER 32

Stomach and Spleen

Anthony T. Blikslager
David A. Wilson

STOMACH

Anatomy

The equine stomach is small relative to the body size of the horse, having a capacity of approximately 5 to 15 L.[1] Even when the stomach is filled to capacity, it does not reach the ventral body wall. It is located predominantly on the left side of the abdomen under the cover of the ribs, with only the pyloric aspect of the stomach to the right side of midline. Its most caudal component is the fundus, which lies adjacent to the 14th and 15th rib spaces (Fig. 32-1).[2] The stomach can be divided into several regions, including the cardia at the opening of the esophagus, the fundus (which forms a blind sac), the body, and the pyloric region. The stomach is sharply curved at its lesser curvature so that the cardia and pyloric regions lie adjacent to one another.[2] The cardia is attached to the diaphragm by the gastrophrenic ligament. This ligament is a continuation of the phrenicosplenic ligament and the gastrosplenic ligament on the left side of the abdomen. The greater omentum attaches along the greater curvature of the stomach, and it blends into the gastrophrenic ligament.[1,2] The greater omentum forms a blind, potential space called the omental bursa. The entrance to this bursa is the epiploic foramen, which is located between the caudate process of the liver and the right lobe of the pancreas. The epiploic foramen is also bordered dorsally and ventrally by the caudal vena cava and portal vein, respectively. The lesser omentum, which connects the stomach and duodenum to the liver, consists of the hepatogastric and hepatoduodenal ligaments.[2] The stomach receives its blood supply from the celiac artery. Venous drainage from the stomach is via gastric veins to the portal vein.[1]

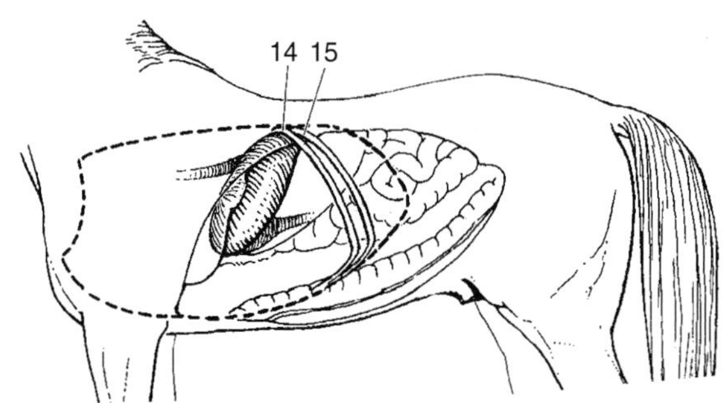

Figure 32-1. Diagram of the anatomic location of the equine stomach in the abdomen.

Physiology

During digestion, the stomach is capable of dramatically lowering the pH of its contents, and of secreting pepsinogen to begin breaking down protein. However, both HCl and pepsinogen (which is converted to pepsin) are inherently damaging to mucosa, which possesses a number of mechanisms to prevent injury, depending on the region of the stomach. There are four regions of the stomach based on the type of mucosal lining (in an orad-to-aborad order): nonglandular stratified squamous epithelium, cardiac epithelium, proper gastric mucosa (glandular mucosa), and pyloric mucosa.[3] The equine stomach has a very extensive region of stratified squamous mucosa that occupies approximately half of the stomach mucosal surface area, and this changes abruptly to cardiac glandular mucosa at a line of demarcation called the margo plicatus.[4] The function of the stratified squamous mucosa in the horse is unknown, since this region of the stomach does not have the ability to secrete ions, although the squamous mucosa may protect underlying tissues from abrasion by roughage.[3] However, the squamous mucosa does not frequently come into contact with stomach contents, as the gastric fill line is typically the margo plicatus. The cardiac epithelium forms a belt of tissue adjacent to the margo plicatus. Relatively little is known about this mucosal region, although it has the ability to secrete bicarbonate in other species and has been shown to contain cells capable of secreting somatostatin in equine mucosa, which serve as a negative feedback mechanism for gastric acid secretion. The proper gastric mucosa contains secretory glands containing HCl-secreting parietal cells and pepsinogen-secreting zymogen cells. In addition, this segment of mucosa contains enterochromaffin-like (ECL) cells that secrete histamine in response to various stimuli, which in turn amplifies HCl secretion by the parietal cells. The pyloric mucosa contains both G-cells, which secrete gastrin, and D-cells, which secrete somatostatin. These hormones enhance or reduce gastric acid secretion, respectively.[4]

Gastric Barrier Function

Mechanisms by which the stratified squamous mucosa resists injury are critical in the horse, where ulceration is prevalent.[5-7] When mounted in Ussing chambers for the purpose of measuring epithelial transport function, equine stratified squamous epithelium has baseline transepithelial resistance measurements of approximately 2000 to 3000 ohms.cm^2, which is an order of magnitude higher than that of the adjacent cardiac mucosa.[5] Since transepithelial resistance is essentially a measure of permeability to ions, the stratified squamous mucosa is exceptionally impermeable. This is the only mechanism of defense against injury present in this type of mucosa. The stratified squamous epithelium consists of four layers: the outer stratum corneum, the stratum transitionale, the stratum spinosum, and the basal stratum germinativum. However, not all of these layers contribute equally to barrier function. Interepithelial tight junctions in the stratum corneum, and muco-substances secreted by the stratum spinosum are mainly responsible for barrier function.[5,8] The stratified squamous mucosa in other species is relatively impermeable to HCl,[9] suggesting that although most of the literature on equine ulceration pertains to the effects of HCl and inhibitors of HCl secretion,[10-13] other factors may be critical to the development of gastric ulcer disease. Nonetheless, exposure of equine stratified mucosa to acid (pH 1.7) results in significant reductions in measurements of transepithelial electrical resistance, regardless of whether other injurious compounds are added, indicating that acid alone can damage the mucosa.[14] What is not clear is whether less acidic solutions can also cause damage alone, or whether other injurious factors, such as bile or pepsin, become important.

The site of HCl secretion (proper gastric mucosa) is protected from so-called back-diffusion of H^+ ions by a relatively high transepithelial electrical resistance (compared to cardiac mucosa), but there is also a number of other critical mechanisms to prevent acid injury. The gastric mucosa secretes both mucus and bicarbonate, which together form an HCO_3–containing gel that titrates acid before it reaches the lumen.[15,16] However, the mucus layer does not form an absolute barrier to back-diffusion of acid. Thus, for acid that does diffuse back into the gastric mucosa, epithelial Na^+/H^+ exchangers are capable of expelling H^+ once the cell reaches a critical pH.[16]

Gastric Mucosal Pathophysiology

Mechanisms of Gastric Ulceration

Ulceration in horses most commonly involves the stratified squamous epithelium and is somewhat analogous to gastroesophageal reflux disease in people.[5] This may occur because the glandular portion of the stomach has a number of protective mechanisms, including mucus and bicarbonate secretion, whereas the squamous mucosa has none of these protective mechanisms and is periodically exposed to acid contents.[4] Although stratified squamous epithelium is relatively impermeable to HCl, a number of factors can dramatically enhance the damaging effects of HCl in this epithelium. In particular, bile salts and short-chain fatty acids are capable of breaking down the squamous epithelial barrier at an acid pH, thereby exposing deep layers to HCl, with subsequent development of ulceration. Relatively high concentrations of short-chain fatty acids normally exist in the equine stomach as a result of microbial fermentation.[5] These weak acids penetrate squamous mucosa, and they appear to damage Na^+ transport activity, principally in the stratum germinativum. Bile salts may also be present in the proximal equine stomach as a result of reflux from the duodenum. Although such reflux has a relatively high pH, it appears that bile salts adhere to stratified squamous epithelium, becoming lipid soluble and triggering damage once the pH falls below 4.[17] Diet and management (e.g., periods of fasting) also play crucial roles in the development of conditions conducive to gastric ulceration. Typically, there is a pH gradation in horses from proximal to distal compartments of the stomach, with the lowest pH values in the distal stomach.[18] However, during periods of fasting, this stratification is disrupted, so that low pH values may be recorded in the proximal stomach.[19] Fasting conditions also increase the concentration of duodenal contents within the proximal stomach, particularly bile.[17] The type of diet also influences the stratification of stomach contents.

Mechanisms inducing injury to proper gastric mucosa may be entirely different from those inducing injury to stratified squamous mucosa. In people, the majority of gastric mucosal ulcers are induced by infection with *Helicobacter pylori,* which has the effect of raising gastric pH because of disruption of gastric glands, but which also induces an inflammatory reaction that causes damage.[20] In particular, *H. pylori* containing the *cagA* gene is most pathogenic. However, there is very little evidence that this organism is involved in gastric ulcers in domestic animal species. In the absence of a known role for infectious agents in equine gastric ulcer disease syndrome, ulceration most likely develops from an imbalance between protective mechanisms and injurious factors, which include gastric acid, bile, and nonsteroidal anti-inflammatory drugs (NSAIDs). However, some factors that are important to induction of squamous epithelial ulceration may not be important in development of proper gastric mucosal ulceration. For example, feed deprivation and intensive training reproducibly induce squamous epithelial ulceration in horses, but they have little effect on proper gastric mucosa in horses.[21] Gastric acid very likely plays a key role, whereas other factors such as NSAIDs serve to reduce gastric defense mechanisms. In particular, inhibition of prostaglandin production reduces mucus and bicarbonate secretion, while also reducing gastric mucosal blood flow, and would be expected to produce ulceration of proper gastric mucosa.[22] In addition, some of the NSAIDs also have a topical irritant effect, but this appears to be of minor significance, since the route of administration (oral or parenteral) seems to have little influence on development of ulceration.[23]

Gastric Reparative Mechanisms

Mechanisms of gastric repair are highly dependent on the extent of injury. For instance, superficial erosions can be rapidly covered by migration of epithelium adjacent to the wound—a process termed epithelial restitution. However, ulceration (full-thickness disruption of mucosa and penetration of the muscularis mucosae) requires repair of submucosal vasculature and matrix. This is initiated by formation of granulation tissue, which supplies connective tissue elements and microvasculature necessary for mucosal reconstruction. Connective tissue elements include proliferating fibroblasts that accompany newly produced capillaries that form from proliferating endothelium. Recent studies indicate that nitric oxide is critical to both of these processes,[24,25] which probably explains the reparative properties of NO in the stomach.[26] Once an adequate granulation bed has been formed, newly proliferated epithelium at the edge of the wound begins to migrate across the wound. In addition, gastric glands at the base of the ulcer begin to bud and migrate across the granulation bed in a tubular fashion.[27] Epidermal growth factor is expressed by repairing epithelium, and it appears to facilitate these processes.[28] In addition, these events are facilitated by a mucoid cap, which retains reparative factors and serum adjacent to the wound bed. Importantly, this cap maintains a neutral pH to facilitate healing.[22] Once the ulcer crater has been filled with granulation tissue and the wound has been reepithelialized, the subepithelial tissue remodels by altering the type and amount of collagen.[29]

Diagnostic Techniques

Endoscopy

Prior to gastric endoscopy, foals up to 20 days of age should be held off feed for 3 hours, whereas older foals require up to 10 hours to sufficiently empty the stomach. Adult horses should be held off feed for 24 hours to allow complete visualization of the stomach.[1] A 3-m endoscope is required to adequately visualize the stomach, including the pylorus, in adult horses, whereas a 1-m endoscope may be sufficient for foals.[1] Although endoscopy is the principal diagnostic aid for detection of gastric ulceration, a recent study comparing endoscopic to histologic scoring of the severity of ulceration indicated that endoscopy tends to underestimate the number and severity of gastric ulcers of the nonglandular equine stomach. Furthermore, endoscopy may not allow detection of glandular gastric ulcers. Therefore, clinicians should realize that ulceration is frequently more severe and extensive than that observed via the endoscope.[30]

Ultrasonography

Ultrasonography can be used to image the wall of the stomach, and it may be particularly useful in foals with suspected gastric outflow obstruction. The stomach is best imaged from the left side of the abdomen between rib spaces 8 and 14. If gastric outflow obstruction is present, a distended stomach with a gas–fluid interface may be detected. The duodenum can also be imaged at this site, and it may show evidence of thickening and reduced motility. The duodenum can additionally be imaged from the right paralumbar fossa, cranial to the right kidney, where there may be additional evidence of thickening or obstruction.[31]

Radiography

Contrast radiography can be performed to allow visualization of the stomach. In a series of foals with gastroduodenal obstruction, barium sulfate solution was administered.[32] In addition, functional gastric emptying can be determined by the administration of barium sulfate after a 12- to 18-hour fasting period. In normal horses, barium appears in the small intestine by 10 minutes, and none remains within the stomach by 35 minutes. With pyloric outflow obstruction, barium may remain in the stomach for up to 8 hours.[1] Barium sulfate solutions should be diluted 1:1 with water, and a volume of approximately 1 L should be administered into the thoracic portion of the esophagus by nasogastric tube.[33] Double-contrast radiography with insufflation of air, followed by administration of a barium sulfate suspension, can enhance visualization of the stomach. This technique has been useful in the diagnosis of gastric outflow obstruction and gastric neoplasia.[1]

Measurement of Gastric Emptying

Assessment of gastric emptying can be performed by nuclear scintigraphy, acetaminophen absorption,[34] or breath testing after the administration of ^{13}C-octanoic acid.[35,36] For scintigraphic determination of gastric emptying, one study involved administration of 370 megabecquerels of 99m-technetium sulfur colloid incorporated into egg albumin (to determine solid phase gastric emptying) and 37 MBq of 111-indium–labeled diethylenetriamine-penta acetic acid (DTPA) in 120 mL of water (to determine liquid phase gastric emptying). These labeled products were administered via a nasogastric tube after a 12-hour fasting period. Scintigraphic images obtained from the left and right flanks were then used to assess gastric emptying. Liquid phase and solid phase 50% gastric emptying times are 30 and 90 minutes, respectively, in normal horses.[37] In experimental trials assessing efficacy of breath testing, ponies were fasted for 14 hours, after which they ingested a test meal with ^{13}C-octanoic acid. Breath samples were then analyzed by mass spectrometry for the appearance of the isotope.[36] This method correlated closely with gastric emptying documented with nuclear scintigraphy after administration of Tc^{99m} sulfur colloid.[35] Similarly, acetaminophen absorption has been shown to closely correlate with scintigraphic measurements of gastric emptying. For example, in one research trial, acetaminophen (20 mg/kg) and Tc^{99m} pentetate (10 mCi) were administered in 200 mL water, and their clearance from the stomach was shown to be similar, based on serum acetaminophen and scintigraphic analyses, respectively.[38]

Disorders

Gastric Ulcer Clinical Syndromes

The clinical syndromes of gastric ulceration are age dependent; the age categories are neonates, weanling foals, and horses older than 1 year.[39] In neonates, ulceration of the glandular mucosa is the most clinically important. Clinical signs include poor appetite, colic, and diarrhea, but foals may have ulcers and not demonstrate overt clinical signs of gastric pain or failure to thrive.[40] The pH of neonatal gastric contents is not typically as low as that of older foals or adults, suggesting that other factors may be important in the pathogenesis of ulceration.[13]

In suckling and weanling foals, ulceration frequently occurs in the squamous mucosa adjacent to the margo plicatus. Severe ulceration of the squamous portion of the stomach in foals of this age group is frequently associated with diarrhea, but foals may also appear unthrifty, with a rough hair coat and a pot-bellied appearance.[39] Diffuse ulceration is also typically associated with teeth grinding and colic. This age group of foals may also be affected with gastroduodenal ulceration, which may result in gastric outflow obstruction (see later).

In yearlings and adult horses, lesions also occur predominantly in the squamous portion of the stomach adjacent to the margo plicatus. These horses may have very subtle signs of disease, such as poor performance, reduced appetite, and failure to thrive, but they do not typically suffer from diarrhea. The diagnosis of gastric ulcers is confirmed with gastroscopy.[7] When evaluating squamous lesions in foals, it is important to differentiate ulceration from desquamation.[8] The latter involves shedding of sheets of epithelium without ulceration, and it is unlikely to be clinically important.[41] Treatment is aimed at elevating the pH of the gastric contents, which may be achieved with a number of histamine receptor (H2) antagonists, such as ranitidine (6.6 mg/kg, PO every 8 hours, or 1.5 to 2 mg/kg IV every 6 to 8 hours) or proton pump inhibitors such as omeprazole (2 to 4 mg/kg PO every 8 hours).[40]

Gastric Impaction

Impaction of the stomach typically consists of excessive dry, fibrous ingesta, but it may also consist of ingested materials that form a mass, such as persimmon seeds or mesquite beans.[42-44] Other feeds that tend to swell after ingestion, including wheat, barley, and sugar beet pulp, may also cause impaction. Furthermore, dental disease may increase the likelihood of gastric impaction because of improper chewing of feed. Clinical signs include colic that ranges from acute and severe to chronic and mild. For example, in one report on four horses with gastric impaction, colic was moderate or severe and of 8 to 12 hours' duration,[45] whereas in another report on a pony with gastric impaction, colic was chronic (7 days' duration) and associated with prolonged recumbency, anorexia, and lethargy.[44] Additional signs may include dysphagia, dropping of feed, and bruxism.[44,46]

The diagnosis is frequently made at the time of surgery, although endoscopy reveals gastric impaction and may provide information on the specific nature of the impaction. Medical treatment includes nasogastric intubation and frequent attempts at softening the ingesta with water, followed by refluxing the fluid contents, or by using back-and-forth agitating movements of water with a 16-ounce dose syringe attached to the nasogastric tube. At surgery, the impaction can be massaged and infused, most commonly via insertion of a needle adjacent to the greater curvature, followed by infusion of a balanced polyionic fluid such as saline. There is also a report including the details of a pony and a horse in which the impacted stomach was packed off from the abdomen with towels, and an incision was made parallel and caudal to the attachment of the omentum on the greater curvature of the stomach. The stomach contents were then evacuated, followed by a double-layer inverting closure. In the horse in this report, the ventral midline incision was extended cranially to the xiphoid process.[46] However, this aggressive approach is seldom necessary, as the impaction can usually be resolved with more conservative management.

Gastric Rupture

Rupture of the stomach appears to have two general causes: primary, where there may be excessive accumulation of ingesta, or no identifiable cause, and secondary, in which another causative condition, such as obstruction of the small intestine, is identified.[47] The site of the rupture is most commonly the greater curvature of the stomach, although other sites of rupture have been identified, including the lesser curvature of the stomach.[48] The condition is almost universally fatal, because the rupture of stomach contents into the abdomen causes septic shock that cannot be adequately reversed with abdominal lavage and repair of the stomach defect. However, there are some case reports of gastric rupture that has been repaired. In one report, subserosal hematoma associated with a focal serosal perforation was repaired by use of a two-layer inverting closure, and the horse survived.[49] In another report, a seromuscular tear with intact mucosa bulging from the tear was noted, and it was oversewn with an inverting suture pattern. However, in neither case was there any evidence of abdominal contamination with gastric contents.[50]

In a report on 54 horses, 11% of deaths in horses with colic taken to surgery were attributable to gastric rupture. Interestingly, at least 6 of the 54 horses had indwelling stomach tubes, indicating that nasogastric intubation does not negate the possibility of gastric rupture.[47] In a separate report on gastric rupture, it was determined that 5.4% of all colic accessions had gastric rupture. One of the striking clinical findings was that the abdominal fluid cell counts were frequently inaccurate, most likely because the acid stomach contents lysed cells infiltrating into the abdomen. However, a number of abdominal fluid samples were not analyzed because they had the appearance of ingesta. This report also determined a number of risk factors for gastric rupture, including the feeding of a diet exclusively of grass hay, or grass and alfalfa hay, and drinking water from a bucket, stream, or pond. Alternatively, horses fed grain had a reduced risk.[48] The cases in this study were principally primary gastric ruptures (60%), and predisposing factors may include the opportunity to consume excessive water or roughage, which may then expand and rupture the stomach.

Gastric Neoplasia

Neoplasia of the stomach is rare. The most common form of gastric neoplasia is squamous cell carcinoma, which typically forms in the cardia of the stomach. In one report, a tumor encircled the esophagus at the cardia of the stomach, where it caused recurrent esophageal obstruction.[51] Clinical signs may include anorexia, weight loss, abdominal distention, abnormal chewing behavior, dysphagia, fever, and ventral abdominal edema.[52-54] The diagnosis can be based antemortem on results of gastric endoscopy and biopsy,[55] or on thoracoscopy and biopsy.[56] In addition, approximately 50% of horses have had neoplastic cells evident in abdominal fluid[53,57] or in thoracic fluid.[58] Other nonspecific laboratory findings have included anemia, neutrophilia, and hypoalbuminemia.[53] Additionally, one horse had a clinical diagnosis of pseudohyperparathyroidism in association with gastric carcinoma, based partially on evidence of hypercalcemia and hypophosphatemia.[58] In a case series on gastric squamous carcinoma, horses have had multiple metastases, including masses throughout the abdomen. Therefore, the prognosis is grave, and the condition has been universally fatal.[53,54,57]

Other neoplasms that have been identified in the stomach include leiomyosarcoma and adenocarcinoma. A leiomyosarcoma was diagnosed in a 12-year-old Thoroughbred gelding that was evaluated because of anorexia, weight loss, and intermittent fever. At surgery, an inoperable mass was discovered in the cranial abdomen, which was found to be a leiomyosarcoma after histopathologic analysis. The mass was associated with the distal portion of the esophagus and the cranial two thirds of the stomach.[59] Adenocarcinoma has been documented in the glandular portion of the equine stomach.[1]

Gastric Outflow Obstruction

Gastric outflow obstruction may be the result of pyloric stenosis, which can be caused by congenital muscular hypertrophy,[60,61] or by development of a mass at the pylorus that reduces gastric outflow. A mass may develop at the pylorus associated with gastroduodenal ulceration or neoplasia.[62-64] Clinical signs include weight loss, reduced appetite, abdominal pain, teeth grinding, and ptyalism. Foals with gastric outflow obstruction are typically 2 to 6 months of age, with signs of gastric ulceration and an unthrifty appearance. However, foals may also have a history of enteritis, and an absence of clinical signs typical of foals with gastric ulcers.[31]

Gastric outflow obstruction can be diagnosed using endoscopy, radiography, ultrasonography, and gastric emptying tests, as described previously. Medical treatment for foals includes decompression of the stomach, antiulcer medications, broad-spectrum antibiotics, prokinetics, and intravenous fluids. However, surgery is indicated if medical treatment does not reverse clinical signs within a short period of time.[31] The principle of surgery for treatment of gastric outflow obstruction is bypass of the pylorus, typically by performing a gastrojejunostomy. Pyloric stenosis has been relieved in a 2-month-old Thoroughbred by a modification of the Heineke-Mikulicz technique, in which a full-thickness longitudinal incision through the pylorus was closed transversely.[61] The pylorus was mobilized by severing the hepatoduodenal ligament.

Alternatively, a series of bypass techniques can be performed, depending on the location of the obstruction.[33] In one series evaluating surgical results in 13 foals with gastroduodenal obstruction, bypass procedures included gastroduodenostomy, duodenojejunostomy, or gastrojejunostomy. A jejunojejunostomy was also performed with the latter two surgical procedures to allow outflow of proximal small intestinal contents.[32] These anastomoses can be hand-sewn or performed with automated stapling equipment (Figs. 32-2 to 32-4). However, hand-sewn anastomoses may be simpler to perform because of the limited space within a foal's abdomen, which reduces maneuverability of larger stapling instruments.[33] Although a three-layer hand-sewn technique has been described (seromuscular, muscular, and mucosal layers), one case report suggested that a two-layer hand-sewn anastomosis (seromuscular and mucosal layers) was sufficient and more rapidly performed in a foal in which a gastroduodenostomy was created.[33]

The prognosis for foals with gastric outflow obstruction is guarded.[31] In one report on results of surgical intervention in foals with gastroduodenal obstruction, 6 of 13 foals (46%) survived.[32] One report indicated that foals with a localized pyloric obstruction should have a more favorable prognosis than foals with pyloric and duodenal obstructions, because the surgery for the former (gastroduodenostomy) is simpler than the surgery for the latter (gastrojejunostomy and jejunojejunostomy).[33]

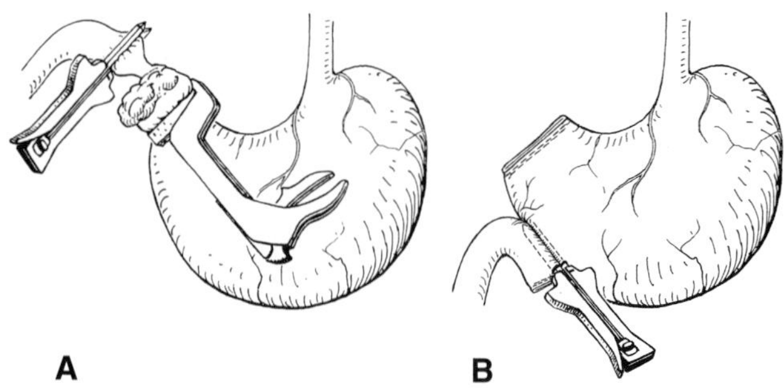

Figure 32-3. Partial gastrectomy (**A**) and gastroduodenostomy (**B**) to relieve pyloric obstruction. Stapling instruments have been applied proximal and distal to the obstruction, allowing resection of the distal stomach. Care is taken to avoid the hepatic duct in the proximal duodenum by stapling proximal to it. The blind-ending duodenum is subsequently anastomosed to the distal stomach using an automated stapling device. (Redrawn from Orsini JA, Donawick WJ: Surgical treatment of gastroduodenal obstruction in foals, Vet Surg 1986;15:205.)

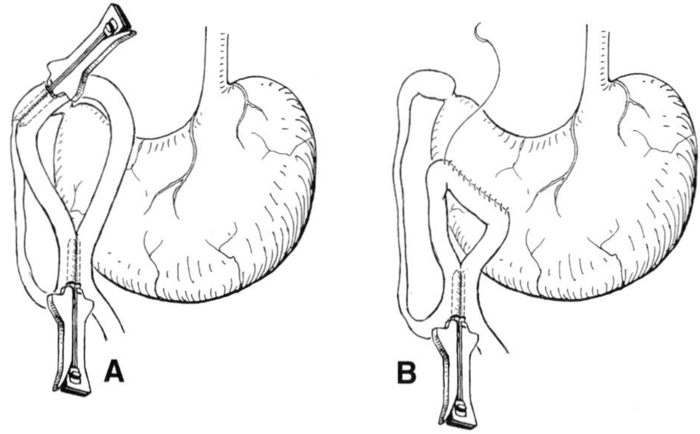

Figure 32-4. Duodenojejunostomy (**A**) or gastrojejunostomy and jejunojejunostomy (**B**) may be performed to bypass the pylorus. The duodenojejunostomy and jejunojejunostomy are performed using an automated stapling device or a three-tiered suturing technique. The duodenojejunostomy is performed with the duodenal component proximal to the hepatic duct, and the jejunojejunostomy is performed with a segment of jejunum distal to the duodenocolic ligament. (Redrawn from Orsini JA, Donawick WJ: Surgical treatment of gastroduodenal obstruction in foals, Vet Surg 1986;15:205.)

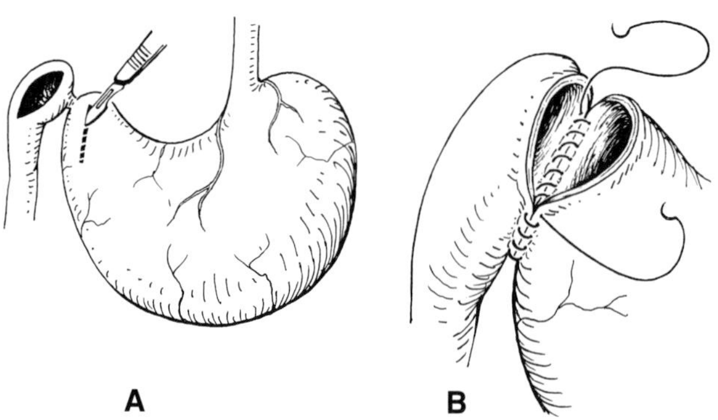

Figure 32-2. A. Locations for incisions for a gastroduodenostomy to bypass a pyloric stenosis. **B.** A 3-tiered hand-sutured anastomosis to complete the gastroduodenostomy. (Redrawn from Orsini JA, Donawick WJ: Surgical treatment of gastroduodenal obstruction in foals, Vet Surg 1986;15:205.)

SPLEEN

Anatomy

The spleen is a falciform or sickle-shaped organ located in the left mid-dorsal part of the peritoneal cavity (Fig. 32-5). The exact position of the spleen varies, depending on, for example, the amount of the stomach filling, intestinal distention or displacement, and splenic disease. The cranial border of the spleen is concave and the caudal border is convex. The parietal or lateral surface is slightly convex and is in intimate contact with the diaphragm.[65] The visceral or

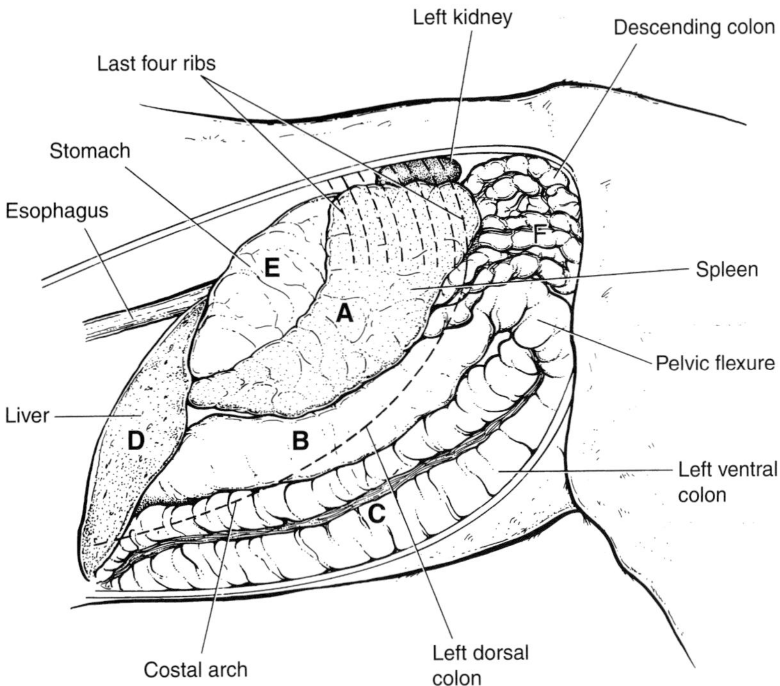

Figure 32-5. Relative topography of the abdominal viscera as viewed from the left side. The lateral and ventral walls are removed. The proximal one third of the last four ribs *(short dotted lines)* shows the relative position of the spleen protected by the rib cage (*long dotted line* defines the ventral and caudal border of the rib cage). A, spleen; B, left dorsal colon; C, left ventral colon; D, liver; E, stomach; F, small bowel.

medial surface is generally concave and contains a longitudinal ridge, the hilus, in which the vessels and nerves are located. The area cranial to the hilus is in contact with the left side of the greater curvature of the stomach. The area caudal to the ridge is more extensive and is variably in contact with the descending colon, and the left parts of the ascending colon and the small intestine. The dorsal extremity or base of the spleen is located between the left crus of the diaphragm and sublumbar muscles dorsally, and on its medial surface by the pancreas and left kidney. The base generally corresponds to the last three or four ribs, exceeding the 18th rib caudally in the paralumbar fossa by 2 to 3 cm. Only the caudodorsal angle (between the base and the caudal border) can be palpated per rectum. The ventral extremity or apex is small and usually found opposite the 9th, 10th, or 11th rib, proximal to the costal arch. The spleen is suspended within the peritoneal cavity by means of the phrenicosplenic and the renosplenic (or nephrosplenic) ligaments, and attached to the stomach by the gastrosplenic ligament. The latter continues with the superficial wall of the greater omentum.[66]

The size and weight of the spleen vary greatly, both among and within animals, depending on the amount of blood it contains. Its weight varies from about 0.5 to 3.5 kg. The spleen is approximately 50 cm long and about 20 to 25 cm wide. It is usually bluish red to purple.[65,67]

The hilus protects the vessels and nerves of the spleen. The splenic artery, a branch of the celiac artery, runs within the groove of the hilus and branches to supply the spleen and short gastric arteries that nourish the greater curvature of the stomach (Fig. 32-6). The splenic vein is an affluent of the portal vein and lies caudal to the artery in the hilus. The splenic lymph nodes are scattered along the splenic artery and drain lymph to the celiac lymphocenter. The splenic plexus, branching from the celiac plexus, supplies the spleen with both sympathetic fibers from the major splanchnic nerve and parasympathetic fibers from the vagus nerve.

The splenic tissue is intimately covered by a fibrous capsule, which sends numerous trabeculae into the substance of the spleen. The capsule consists of collagen and elastin fibers and contains many smooth muscle cells.[66,68] The trabeculae form a spongy framework, which is the support of the splenic pulp. The splenic pulp is mostly red or dark red and is known as the red pulp.[68] The red pulp consists of arterial capillaries, small venules, and a reticulum filled with macrophages and blood. Throughout the red pulp are scattered gray foci just visible to the naked eye,[69] which are known as the white pulp. The white pulp represents the lymphatic tissue of the spleen organized as lymphatic nodules.[67] Lymphocytes and macrophages supported by a scaffolding of branched connective cells called reticular cells make up the lymphatic tissue. The reticulum is made up of a meshwork of supporting cells and extracellular fibers. The white pulp is distributed along the course of the arterial vessels,[70,71] and it is almost as abundant as the red pulp.[67]

Physiology

The spleen has several important functions, including storage of erythrocytes and platelets, removal of aged or damaged erythrocytes and platelets, hematopoiesis during fetal development, iron recycling, and immunologic functions.[70-]

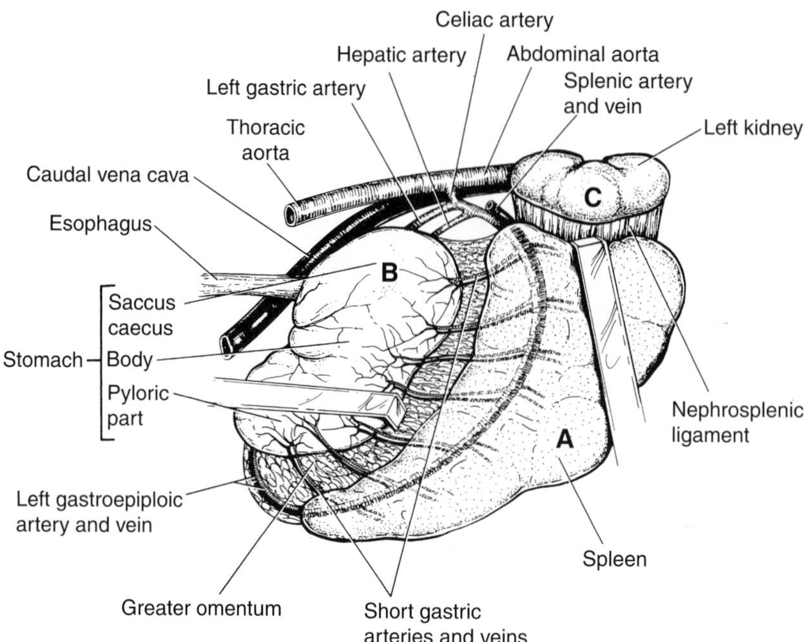

Figure 32-6. Left view of the spleen (A), stomach (B), and left kidney (C) with pertinent vascular supply. Retractors are placed along the greater curvature of the stomach to reveal the short gastric arteries and veins and along the dorsal extremity of the spleen to show the left kidney.

[73] Unlike human spleens, animal spleens have the ability to store red blood cells. The equine spleen is particularly well adapted and can regulate the red cell storage by relaxation and contraction. The equine spleen can store up to 60% of circulating red blood cells.[74] The contractile ability is under sympathetic control and, in times of stress or strenuous exercise, is stimulated to release the stored red blood cells into the circulation, increasing the red cell concentration of the blood. At least one report has questioned the role of splenic emptying in exercise-induced changes in red cell indices.[75] Phenylephrine (an α_1-adrenergic receptor agonist) administration has been reported to cause a transient, dose-dependent splenic contraction of up to 83% of the original splenic mass and may be useful for certain medical or surgical procedures in the horse, such as during splenectomy or as an adjunct to nonsurgical correction of nephrosplenic entrapment of the ascending colon.[76] Epinephrine has also been reported to transiently reduce splenic length approximately 68% when administered as a bolus.[77]

The removal of aged or damaged erythrocytes occurs in the spleen because of its unique structure. Blood is circulated through the splenic red pulp, terminating in small, highly porous capillaries. The blood cells then pass out of the capillaries into the cords of the red pulp and eventually return to circulation through the endothelial wall of the venous sinuses. The red pulp and venous sinuses are loaded with macrophages (reticuloendothelial cells), which phagocytize unwanted debris and old or abnormal red blood cells. Also removed by the phagocytic cells are abnormal platelets, bloodborne parasites, and bacteria.[68]

In addition to its filtering and phagocytic activity, the spleen has another role in the immune-mediated defense against disease. It has a direct effect on the pattern and level of antibody response of the body. The spleen in several species has been determined to be the most important organ in the production of IgM. Decreased levels of IgM occur after splenectomy. The role of IgM occurs in the initial antibody response to disease and, therefore, splenectomized animals may be somewhat compromised.[78]

The resistance of the horse to disease caused by blood protozoa such as *Babesia* species or *Theileria* species is significantly decreased after splenectomy.[79-84] Subclinical infections by protozoa may become patent infections after removal of the spleen.

Diagnostic Procedures

Surgical disorders of the spleen may be relatively difficult to diagnose because of their rare occurrence and nonspecific clinical signs. Rectal palpation usually reveals thickening and rounded margins of an enlarged spleen. Ultrasonography either per rectum or through the left abdominal wall may also reveal an enlarged spleen. A splenic biopsy may be performed for histologic evaluation of splenomegaly. Normal coagulation function should be determined before a percutaneous biopsy is performed. Laparoscopy may also be used to aid in the diagnosis of splenic abnormalities and to help with the decision between medical therapy and splenectomy.[85,86]

To examine the spleen, a long (30 cm) laparoscope is introduced into the dorsal aspect of the left paralumbar fossa facing cranially. The head of the spleen, left kidney, and renosplenic ligament can be readily identified in the left dorsal quadrant of the abdomen. The caudal edge and lateral wall of the spleen can be visualized as the laparoscope is swept down toward the left ventral quadrant, and abnormalities over most of the body of the spleen can be identified. Lesions in this region can be biopsied with additional instruments placed through separate portals in the left paralumbar fossa. Biopsies can be obtained with laparoscopic scissors as wedge biopsies, or with a biopsy instrument similar to a uterine biopsy forceps. Hemorrhage should be expected, and it can be controlled with bipolar cautery forceps.[86] Additional diagnostic procedures used to differentiate disorders of the spleen include a complete history and physical examination, complete blood cell count, including total plasma protein and plasma fibrinogen, coagulation profile, abdominocentesis, the Coggins test (agar gel immunodiffusion test for equine infectious anemia), Coombs' test, and aerobic and anaerobic bacterial cultures.

Indications for Surgery

Splenectomies are performed primarily for research purposes, to aid in the evaluation of the cardiovascular system during exercise[87-92] and to alter the reticuloendothelial system, which controls to a great extent the infections caused by blood protozoa such as *Babesia* or *Theileria*.[79-84] Splenomegaly with or without splenic infarction has been the only reported disease process requiring splenectomy.[93-95] Other possible indications for surgery include neoplasia, trauma, rupture, infarction, and possibly an autoimmune disease in which the spleen would play a role in erythrocyte destruction.[96]

Splenomegaly

Splenomegaly in the horse has been attributed to subcapsular hematoma,[85,97] equine infectious anemia, lymphoma-leukemia (lymphosarcoma), metastatic melanoma, isoimmune hemolytic anemia, salmonellosis, anthrax,[98] and chronic congestion.[93] Infarctions[94,95,99] have also been reported as causes or consequences of splenomegaly. Splenectomy is indicated for splenomegaly for chronic congestion, thrombosis, or primary tumors of the spleen with no evidence of metastases. Clinical signs of horses with splenomegaly include tachycardia, anemia, colic, arching of the back, and standing with the limbs drawn together beneath the body.[94,97,99]

Neoplasia

Lymphosarcoma (malignant lymphoma), metastatic melanoma, and hemangiosarcoma are the only primary neoplastic diseases of the equine spleen.[100-108] Lymphosarcoma is a neoplastic disease of cells of the lymphoid cell series. Splenic lymphosarcoma is classified as an alimentary form of the disease.[103] The cells metastasize via the lymphatics (i.e., in the spleen, the white pulp is first infiltrated). In later stages of the disease, the spleen's architecture may become so distorted that the pathway of spread is not apparent. Leukopenia and anemia are often present.

Melanomas may occur as a primary tumor of the spleen of horses, but the spleen is more likely a site of metastasis.[100,109-111] Hemangiosarcoma or hemangioendothelioma is a frequent primary tumor of other domestic animals and humans but has been only rarely reported as a primary tumor in the horse.[108,112] This tumor is more commonly reported in the spleen of the horse as a site of metastasis.[108,113-117] All of these tumors may cause splenomegaly and may present with clinical signs of an acute abdominal disease because of an increased weight of the spleen and stretching of the splenic ligaments.[102,103,108,109,118]

Splenic Infarction and Splenic Abscesses

Splenic infarction occurs concurrently with splenomegaly.[94,95] Venous thrombosis and infarction may occur any time the spleen is enlarged. Splenic arterial or venous thrombosis, or both, is seen with autoimmune hemolytic anemia, purpura, hemorrhagic pancreatitis, and splenic abscess. Splenic abscesses have been reported to be caused by *Habronema*,[119] *Strongylus*,[98,119] *Bacteroides*, *Clostridium*, and *Streptococcus*.[120]

Splenic Rupture

Splenic rupture is relatively uncommon in horses.[121-125] It may be caused by direct, severe trauma, or it may occur secondary to anthrax, lymphosarcoma, echinococcus infestation, or splenic hematoma or hemorrhage.[100] In all reported cases, horses have been found dead, died during the course of the illness, or were euthanatized shortly thereafter. The cause of rupture is usually unknown, but in one report, it was thought to be as a result of a previous splenomegaly.[124] Most of the ruptures occur on the visceral surface of the spleen. Very few cases of rupture to the parietal surface have been reported.[123,124] Two cases of nonfatal subcapsular hematoma on the parietal surface have been reported.[85,97] The clinical signs include serosanguineous or sanguineous peritoneal fluid, pale mucous membranes, anemia, tachycardia, dyspnea, profuse sweating, anorexia, and colic. Immediate surgery is indicated to control hemorrhage.

Preoperative Considerations

Preoperative considerations for splenectomy include assessment of hydration, acid–base status, and clotting function. The presentation of horses requiring a splenectomy is usually on an emergency basis (i.e., acute abdominal disease, acute blood loss), and therefore the horses may be dehydrated and in shock. Careful assessment should differentiate those with pain because of stretching of the splenic ligaments from those with pain because of acute blood loss from splenic rupture.

Surgical Techniques

Splenectomy

APPROACHES

Several reports have described the technique for splenectomy.[79,93,94,96,126-132] All the methods describe an approach from the left side, with the animal standing or in right lateral recumbency. The variations in the techniques center on the exact position of the skin incision. Originally, the procedure was described as a paralumbar approach (i.e., caudal to the last or 18th rib).[126] Because of the difficulty in accessing the base of the spleen, and therefore its primary vessels, various techniques have been proposed to gain better access. Techniques have been described for access to the spleen between the last two ribs,[129,130] resection of the 18th rib,[128,131] the 17th rib,[79,94,129-132] or the 16th rib.[79,131] One report also describes removal of the distal aspect of the last three ribs.[127] Another report describes removal of the 17th and transecting of the 16th and 18th ribs for removal of an enlarged spleen.[93]

Laparoscopic splenectomy has been reported in humans,[133,134] but its potential use in the horse at this time is only speculative. Hand-assisted techniques may soon be developed similar to those reported for removal of diseased kidneys and ovarian tumors in horses.[135,136] The friability of the diseased spleen and its vascular supply will very likely complicate potential laparoscopic procedures, although the visualization afforded by laparoscopy may well offset the potential complications.[94]

The caudal reflection of the pleural cavity should be considered when determining the technique to be used. The lateral thoracic wall attaches to the diaphragm along a line called the diaphragmatic line of pleural reflection. This line extends from the eighth and ninth costal cartilages dorsocaudally in a gentle, increasing curve, so that its most caudal aspect is at about the middle of the cranial border of the last rib forming the caudal border of the pleural cavity.[137] Therefore, resection of either the 16th or 17th rib is almost always associated with opening the pleural cavity, resulting in a pneumothorax. This is not necessarily a significant problem, because many horses have an intact mediastinum. However, if the mediastinum is incomplete, assisted ventilation is required to maintain respiration.

17TH RIB RESECTION TECHNIQUE

The horse is placed under general anesthesia in right lateral recumbency and prepared for aseptic surgery. A vertical incision is made over the 17th rib from the lumbar muscles (iliocostalis thoracis and longissimus muscles) proximally to the costochondral junction distally. The dissection continues through the subcutaneous tissues, and the cutaneous trunci, serratus dorsalis caudalis, and external abdominal oblique muscles to expose the lateral periosteum of the 17th rib. The periosteum is incised and elevated from the lateral aspect of the rib with a periosteal elevator starting at the costochondral junction and continuing proximally. Circumferential elevation of the periosteum over the full length of the exposed rib is achieved using a large Doyen, Alexander, or other similar periosteal elevator. An obstetrical cable (Gigli wire), bone-cutting forceps, or an oscillating bone saw is used to transect the rib as far proximally as possible. The body of the rib is disarticulated at the costochondral junction through lateral and ventral pull and is removed. The medial periosteum and underlying peritoneum are incised. Proximally, the pleural cavity may be entered. The cavity should be closed by suturing the diaphragm to the intercostal muscles using an absorbable suture in a continuous pattern. While the pleural cavity is open, the horse's respiration may need to be assisted with mechanical ventilation or intermittent manual compression of the rebreathing bag.

The edges of the incision should be draped with saline-moistened laparotomy sponges and separated with a Finochietto rib spreader. The dorsal part of the spleen may be elevated into the incision (Fig. 32-7). The nephrosplenic ligament is transected to expose the splenic vein. The vein is located more superficial or lateral than the artery and may be isolated for separate ligation. Care should be taken not to tear the vein. Intravenous infusion of phenylephrine will result in significant, transient splenic contraction to reduce the weight of the spleen and allow better access to its visceral portion. Some specialists recommend separate ligation of the vessels, with the artery being ligated first and the spleen massaged to remove any excess blood from the organ. A variation is to inject 10 to 15 mL of 1:1000 epinephrine at several sites in the spleen to expedite its contraction. The vessels should be triple-ligated and transected between the distal ligatures, leaving two ligatures on each (if ligated separately) of the vessels. The remainders of the nephrosplenic, phrenicosplenic, and gastrosplenic ligaments are transected near the hilus. Ligatures or stainless steel hemo-

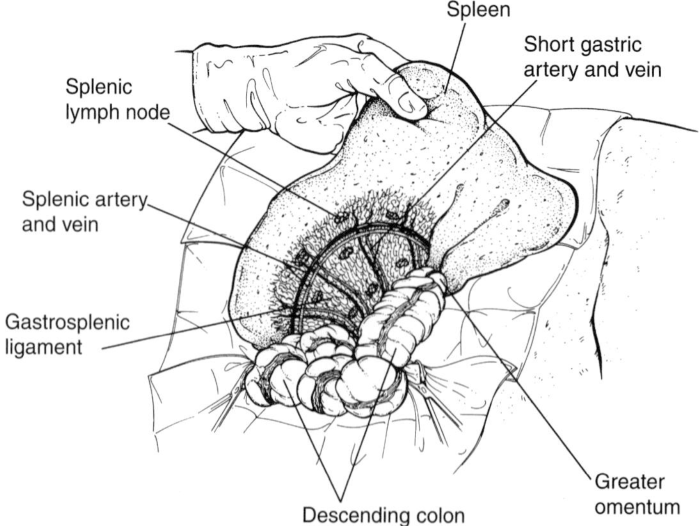

Figure 32-7. Intraoperative view showing elevation of the dorsal part of the spleen into the incision. The renosplenic ligament prohibits complete elevation of the spleen.

static clips are applied to the short gastric vessels as needed. As the spleen is separated from its attachments, the free, cut edge of the greater omentum may be sutured to the free, cut edge of the gastrosplenic ligament. This is most easily performed while the spleen is still attached.

Abdominal wall closure is accomplished in three layers as per the surgeon's preference. The initial layer includes the peritoneum and periosteum, the second layer consists of the subcutaneous tissues, and the skin is the final layer. Either active or passive drains are recommended between muscle layers to minimize serum accumulation and subsequent wound dehiscence.

Splenorrhaphy and Partial Splenectomy

Lacerations of the spleen, such as may occur during abdominocentesis or minor ruptures of the splenic capsule, may be corrected by splenorrhaphy. Absorbable sutures placed across the defect are usually sufficient to control hemorrhage. Large vessels may need to be individually ligated. Partial splenectomy or splenorrhaphy has not been reported in the horse. Various techniques have been described in humans and canines, including the use of mattress sutures,[138-140] stapling devices,[71,141] hemostatic (hemostyptic) agents,[139,140,142] ultrasonic cutting devices,[143] CO_2 lasers,[144] a microwave coagulator,[145] an argon-beam coagulator,[146] and absorbable mesh consisting of polyglycolic acid[147,148] or polyglactin 910.[149] We have applied a TA-90 stapling device, followed by application of an oxidized cellulose hemostatic agent (Surgicel, Ethicon, Somerville, NJ), to accomplish partial splenectomy without complication in a horse with a splenic mass (Fig. 32-8).

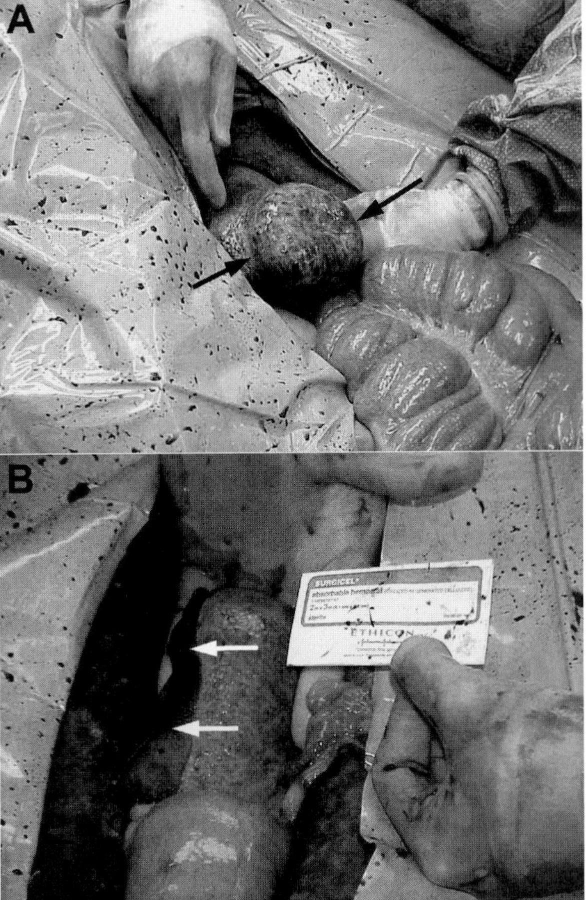

Figure 32-8. Intraoperative view of a partial splenectomy. **A,** A splenic mass confined to the distal third of the spleen was identified via a midline laparotomy. It was associated with a history of chronic colic in a horse. **B,** An automated stapling device has been used to resect the distal third of the spleen. The resection margin has been covered with an oxidized cellulose product to reduce minor hemorrhage from the spleen.

Closure of the Renosplenic Space

Closure of the renosplenic space has been advocated to prevent recurrence of left dorsal displacement of the large colon.[150] More recently, laparoscopic techniques have been described for closing the renosplenic space[151,152] (see Chapter 36). The techniques involve suturing the most dorsal visceral surface of the spleen to the renosplenic ligament to eliminate the area between the spleen and the left kidney to which the large colon frequently becomes displaced.[150-152] There have been no reported cases of left dorsal displacement after closure of the renosplenic space, and there have been no reported complications of the procedure.

Aftercare

After recovery from anesthesia, the animal should be placed in a stall and hand-walked for the first 7 to 10 days. Body temperature, pulse and respiratory rates, and appetite should be monitored regularly. The incision should also be monitored for signs of heat, swelling, drainage, seroma formation, or infection. Antibiotics may be administered as indicated by clinical signs and the results of bacterial culture and sensitivity testing. Analgesics such as flunixin meglumine, ketoprofen, or phenylbutazone should be administered during recovery and for at least 24 hours after surgery to control pain. Drains placed at the time of surgery should be removed after 2 to 3 days. Drainage and lavage of the incision site should occur if evidence of seroma formation or infection is noted.

Complications

The most serious complication after splenectomy is intra-abdominal hemorrhage.[96] Incisional complications include drainage, seroma, edema, infection, and dehiscence.[79,96,127] Additional complications related to the transthoracic approach include pyothorax, pneumothorax, and pleuritis.[96] Complications in humans after splenectomy include atelectasis, pleural effusion, pneumonia, hemorrhage, subphrenic abscess formation, pancreatic fistula and pancreatitis, gastric fistula, thrombocytosis and thrombosis, and sepsis.[153]

REFERENCES

1. Vatistas NJ: The stomach. In Auer JA, Stick JA, editors: Equine Surgery, Philadelphia, 1999, WB Saunders.
2. Schummer A, Nickel R, Sack WO: The Viscera of the Domestic Mammals, ed 2, New York, 1979, Springer Verlag.

3. Stevens CE, Hume ID: Comparative Physiology of the Vertebrate Digestive System, ed 2, New York, 1995, Cambridge University Press.
4. Merritt AM: Normal equine gastroduodenal secretion and motility, Equine Vet J Suppl 1999;29:7.
5. Argenzio RA: Comparative pathophysiology of nonglandular ulcer disease: A review of experimental studies, Equine Vet J Suppl 1999;29:19.
6. Murray MJ: Endoscopic appearance of gastric lesions in foals: 94 cases (1987-1988), J Am Vet Med Assoc 1989;195:1135.
7. Murray MJ, Grodinsky C, Anderson CW, et al: Gastric ulcers in horses: A comparison of endoscopic findings in horses with and without clinical signs, Equine Vet J Suppl 1989;7:68.
8. Murray MJ, Mahaffey EA: Age-related characteristics of gastric squamous epithelial mucosa in foals, Equine Vet J 1993;25:514.
9. Argenzio RA: Mechanisms of acid injury in porcine gastroesophageal mucosa, Am J Vet Res 1996;57:564.
10. Andrews FM, Sifferman RL, Bernard W, et al: Efficacy of omeprazole paste in the treatment and prevention of gastric ulcers in horses, Equine Vet J Suppl 1999;29:81.
11. Vatistas NJ, Snyder JR, Nieto J, et al: Acceptability of a paste formulation and efficacy of high dose omeprazole in healing gastric ulcers in horses maintained in race training, Equine Vet J Suppl 1999;29:71.
12. Murray MJ: Suppression of gastric acidity in horses, J Am Vet Med Assoc 1997;211:37.
13. Campbell-Thompson ML, Merritt AM: Basal and pentagastrin-stimulated gastric secretion in young horses, Am J Physiol 1990;259:R1259-R1266.
14. Widenhouse TV, Lester GD, Merritt AM: Effect of hydrochloric acid, pepsin, or taurocholate on bioelectric properties of gastric squamous mucosa in horses, Am J Vet Res 2002;63:744-749.
15. Schreiber S, Nguyen TH, Stuben M, Scheid P: Demonstration of a pH gradient in the gastric gland of the acid-secreting guinea pig mucosa, Am J Physiol Gastrointest Liver Physiol 2000;279:G597-G604.
16. Flemstrom G: Gastric and duodenal mucosal secretion of bicarbonate. In Johnson LR, editor: Physiology of the Gastrointestinal Tract, New York, 1994, Raven Press.
17. Berschneider HM, Blikslager AT, Roberts MC: Role of duodenal reflux in nonglandular gastric ulcer disease of the mature horse, Equine Vet J Suppl 1999;29:24-29.
18. Baker SJ, Gerring EL: Technique for prolonged, minimally invasive monitoring of intragastric pH in ponies, Am J Vet Res 1993; 54:1725-1734.
19. Murray MJ: Equine model of inducing ulceration in alimentary squamous epithelial mucosa, Dig Dis Sci 1994;39:2530-2535.
20. Peek RM Jr: *Helicobacter pylori* strain-specific activation of signal transduction cascades related to gastric inflammation, Am J Physiol Gastrointest Liver Physiol 2001;280:G525-G530.
21. Murray MJ: Pathophysiology of peptic disorders in foals and horses: A review, Equine Vet J Suppl 1999;29:14-18.
22. Wallace JL: Nonsteroidal anti-inflammatory drugs and gastroenteropathy: The second hundred years. Gastroenterology 1997;112:1000-1016.
23. Henry D, Dobson A, Turner C: Variability in the risk of major gastrointestinal complications from nonaspirin nonsteroidal anti-inflammatory drugs. Gastroenterology 1993;105:1078-1088.
24. Wallace JL, Miller MJ: Nitric oxide in mucosal defense: A little goes a long way. Gastroenterology 2000;119:512-520.
25. Schaffer MR, Efron PA, Thornton FJ, et al: Nitric oxide, an autocrine regulator of wound fibroblast synthetic function, J Immunol 1997;158:2375-2381.
26. Konturek SJ, Brzozowski T, Majka J, et al: Inhibition of nitric oxide synthase delays healing of chronic gastric ulcers, Eur J Pharmacol 1993;239:215-217.
27. Tarnawski A, Tanoue K, Santos AM, Sarfeh IJ: Cellular and molecular mechanisms of gastric ulcer healing. Is the quality of mucosal scar affected by treatment? Scand J Gastroenterol Suppl 1995;210:9-14.
28. Tarnawski A, Stachura J, Durbin T, et al: Increased expression of epidermal growth factor receptor during gastric ulcer healing in rats, Gastroenterology 1992;102:695-698.
29. Podolsky DK: Mucosal immunity and inflammation. V. Innate mechanisms of mucosal defense and repair: The best offense is a good defense, Am J Physiol 1999;277:G495-G499.
30. Andrews FM, Reinemeyer CR, McCracken MD, et al: Comparison of endoscopic, necropsy and histology scoring of equine gastric ulcers, Equine Vet J 2002;34:475-478.
31. Sprayberry KA: Gastric outflow obstruction in young horses. In Robinson NE, editor: Current Therapy in Equine Medicine, Philadelphia, 2003, WB Saunders.
32. Orsini JA, Donawick WJ: Surgical treatment of gastroduodenal obstructions in foals, Vet Surg 2004;15:205-213.
33. Aronoff N, Keegan KG, Johnson PJ, et al: Management of pyloric obstruction in a foal, J Am Vet Med Assoc 1997;210:902-905.
34. Doherty TJ, Andrews FM, Provenza MK, Frazier DL: Acetaminophen as a marker of gastric emptying in ponies, Equine Vet J 1998;30:349-351.
35. Sutton DG, Bahr A, Preston T, et al: Validation of the ^{13}C-octanoic acid breath test for measurement of equine gastric emptying rate of solids using radioscintigraphy, Equine Vet J 2003;35:27-33.
36. Wyse CA, Murphy DM, Preston T, et al: The (13)C-octanoic acid breath test for detection of effects of meal composition on the rate of solid-phase gastric emptying in ponies, Res Vet Sci 2001;71:81-83.
37. Ringger NC, Lester GD, Neuwirth L, et al: Effect of bethanechol or erythromycin on gastric emptying in horses, Am J Vet Res 1996;57:1771-1775.
38. Lohmann KL, Roussel AJ, Cohen ND, et al: Comparison of nuclear scintigraphy and acetaminophen absorption as a means of studying gastric emptying in horses, Am J Vet Res 2000;61:310-315.
39. Andrews FM, Nadeau JA: Clinical syndromes of gastric ulceration in foals and mature horses, Equine Vet J Suppl 1999;29:30-33.
40. Sanchez LC: Diseases of the Stomach. In Reed SM, Bayly WM, Sellon DC, editors: Equine Internal Medicine, Philadelphia, 2004, WB Saunders.
41. Murray MJ, Murray CM, Sweeney HJ, et al: Prevalence of gastric lesions in foals without signs of gastric disease: An endoscopic survey, Equine Vet J 1990;22:6-8.
42. Kellam LL, Johnson PJ, Kramer J, Keegan KG: Gastric impaction and obstruction of the small intestine associated with persimmon phytobezoar in a horse, J Am Vet Med Assoc 2000;216:1279-1281.
43. Cummings CA, Copedge KJ, Confer AW: Equine gastric impaction, ulceration, and perforation due to persimmon *(Diospyros virginiana)* ingestion, J Vet Diagn Invest 9:311-313, 1997.
44. Honnas CM, Schumacher J: Primary gastric impaction in a pony, J Am Vet Med Assoc 1985;187:501-502.
45. Barclay WP, Foerner JJ, Phillips TN, Macharg MA: Primary gastric impaction in the horse, J Am Vet Med Assoc 1982;181:682-683.
46. Owen RA, Jagger DW, Jagger F. Two cases of equine primary gastric impaction, Vet Rec 1987;121:102-105.
47. Todhunter RJ, Erb HN, Roth L: Gastric rupture in horses: A review of 54 cases, Equine Vet J 1986;18:288-293.
48. Kiper ML, Traub-Dargatz J, Curtis CR: Gastric rupture in horses: 50 cases (1979-1987), J Am Vet Med Assoc 1990;196:333-336.
49. Hogan PM, Bramlage LR, Pierce SW: Repair of a full-thickness gastric rupture in a horse, J Am Vet Med Assoc 1995;207:338-340.
50. Steenhaut M, Vlaminck K, Gasthuys F: Surgical repair of a partial gastric rupture in a horse, Equine Vet J 1986;18:331-332.
51. Moore JN, Kintner LD. Recurrent esophageal obstruction due to squamous cell carcinoma in a horse, Cornell Vet 1976;66:590-597.
52. Tennant B, Keirn DR, White KK, et al: Six cases of squamous cell carcinoma of the stomach of the horse, Equine Vet J 1982;14:238-243.

53. Olsen SN. Squamous cell carcinoma of the equine stomach: A report of five cases, Vet Rec 1992;131:170-173.
54. Wester PW, Franken P, Hani HJ: Squamous cell carcinoma of the equine stomach: A report of seven cases, Tijdschr Diergeneeskd 1980;105:103.
55. Keirn JM, White KK, King JM, et al: Endoscopic diagnosis of squamous cell carcinoma of the equine stomach, J Am Vet Med Assoc 1982;180:940-942.
56. Ford TS, Vaala WE, Sweeney CR, et al: Pleuroscopic diagnosis of gastroesophageal squamous cell carcinoma in a horse, J Am Vet Med Assoc 1987;190:1556-1558.
57. McKenzie EC, Mills JN, Bolton JR: Gastric squamous cell carcinoma in three horses, Aust Vet J 1997;75:480-483.
58. Meuten DJ, Price SM, Seiler RM, et al: Gastric carcinoma with pseudohyperparathyroidism in a horse, Cornell Vet 1978;68:179-195.
59. Boy MG, Palmer JE, Heyer G, et al: Gastric leiomyosarcoma in a horse, J Am Vet Med Assoc 1992;200:1363-1364.
60. Munroe GA: Pyloric stenosis in a yearling with an incidental finding of *Capillaria hepatica* in the liver, Equine Vet J 1984;16:221-222.
61. Barth AD, Barber SM, McKenzie NT: Pyloric stenosis in a foal, Can Vet J 1980;21:234-236.
62. Church S, Baker JR, May SA: Gastric retention associated with acquired pyloric stenosis in a gelding, Equine Vet J 1986;18:332-334.
63. Laing JA, Hutchins DR: Acquired pyloric stenosis and gastric retention in a mare, Aust Vet J 1992;69:68-69.
64. McGill CA, Bolton JR: Gastric retention associated with a pyloric mass in two horses, Aust Vet J 1984;61:190-191.
65. Saar LI, Getty R: Equine lymphatic system. In Getty R, editor: Sisson and Grossman's The Anatomy of the Domestic Animal, Philadelphia, 1975, WB Saunders.
66. Schaller O: Illustrated Veterinary Anatomical Nomenclature, Stuttgart, 1992, Ferdinand Enke Verlag.
67. Barone R: Anatomie comparée des mammifères domestiques, tome3, Splanchnologie, Lab d'Anat, École Nat Vét Lyon, 1976:586.
68. Schummer A, Nickel R, Sack WO: Textbook of the Anatomy of the Domestic Animals: The Viscera of the Domestic Mammals, vol II, ed 2 (English edition translated and revised from the 4th German edition), Berlin, 1979, Verlag Paul Parey.
69. Dyce KM, Sack WO, Wensing CJG: Textbook of Veterinary Anatomy, Philadelphia, 1987, WB Saunders.
70. Guyton AC: Textbook of Medical Physiology, ed 7, Philadelphia, 1986, WB Saunders.
71. Lipowitz AJ, Blue J: Spleen. In Slatter D, editor: Textbook of Small Animal Surgery, vol 1, ed 2, Philadelphia, 1993, WB Saunders.
72. Pope ER, Rochat MC: Spleen. In Bojrab MJ, editor: Disease Mechanisms in Small Animal Surgery, Philadelphia, 1993, Lea & Febiger.
73. Wintrobe MM, Lee GR, Boggs DR, et al: Clinical Hematology, ed 8, Philadelphia, 1981, Lea & Febiger.
74. Irvine CHG: The blood picture in the race horse: I. The normal erythrocyte and hemoglobin status—A dynamic concept, J Am Vet Med Assoc 1958;133:97.
75. Masini AP, Baragli P, Tedeschi D, et al: Behaviour of mean erythrocyte volume during submaximal treadmill exercise in the horse, Comp Haematol Int 2000;10:38-42.
76. Hardy J, Bednarski RM, Biller DS: Effect of phenylephrine on hemodynamics and splenic dimensions in horses, Am J Vet Res 1994;55:1570.
77. Venner M, FurkertKorsa B, Deegen E: Influence of different epinephrine applications on the dimensions of the spleen in the horse, Pferdeheilkunde 2001;17:135-140.
78. Lockwood CM: Immunological functions of the spleen, Clin Haem 1983;12:449.
79. Dennig HK, Brocklesby DW: Splenectomy of horses and donkeys, Vet Rec 1965;77:40.
80. Uilenberg G: Notes sur les babesioses et l'anaplasmose des bovins à Madagascar: II. Influence de la splénectomie, Rev Elev Méd Vét Pays Trop 1969;22:237.
81. Mahoney DF, Wright IG, Frerichs WH, et al: The identification of *Babesia equi* in Australia, Aust Vet J 1977;53:461.
82. Knowles DP, Kappmeyer LS, Perryman LE, et al: Specific immune responses are required to control parasitemia in *Babesia-equi* infection. Infect Immun 1994;62:1909.
83. Ambawat HK, Malhotra DV, Kumar S, et al: Erythrocyte associated haemato-biochemical changes in *Babesia equi* infection experimentally produced in donkeys, Vet Parasit 1999;85:319-324.
84. Kumar S, Malhotra DV, Dhar S, et al: Vaccination of donkeys against *Babesia equi* using killed merozoite immunogen, Vet Parasit 2002;106:19-33.
85. Mehl ML, Ragle CA, Mealey RH, et al: Laparoscopic diagnosis of subcapsular splenic hematoma in a horse, J Am Vet Med Assoc 1998;213:1171-1173.
86. Trostle S: Gastrointestinal endoscopic surgery, Vet Clin North Am 2000;16:329-341.
87. Persson SGB, Lydin G: Circulatory effects of splenectomy in the horse: III. Effect on pulse-work relationship, Zbl Vet Med A 1973;7:521.
88. Persson SGB, Bergsten G: Circulatory effects of splenectomy in the horse: IV. Effect on blood flow and blood lactate at rest and during exercise, Zbl Vet Med A 1975;22:801.
89. Davis JL, Manohar M: Effect of splenectomy on exercise-induced pulmonary and systemic hypertension in ponies, Am J Vet Res 1988;49:1169.
90. McKeever KH, Hinchcliff KW, Reed SM, et al: Plasma constituents during incremental treadmill exercise in intact and splenectomized horses, Equine Vet J 1993;25:233.
91. McKeever KH, Hinchcliff KW, Reed SM, et al: Splenectomy alters blood pressure response to incremental treadmill exercise in horses, Am J Physiol 1993;265:R409.
92. Rivas LJ, Hinchcliff KW: Effect of furosemide and subsequent intravenous fluid administration on right atrial pressure of splenectomized horses, Am J Vet Res 1997;58:632.
93. Varra DL, Nelson AW: Primary splenomegaly in a horse, J Am Vet Med Assoc 1976;168:608.
94. Roy MF, Lavoie JP, Deschamps I, et al: Splenic infarction and splenectomy in a jumping horse, Equine Vet J 2000;32:174-176.
95. Westerduin FE, Lankveld DPK, Van der Velden MA, et al: Splenectomy in a dressage pony: End of career? Tijdschr Diergeneeskd 2003;128:406-411.
96. Rigg DL, Reinertson EL, Buttrick ML: A technique for elective splenectomy of Equidae using a transthoracic approach, Vet Surg 1987;16:389.
97. McGorum BC, Young LE, Milne EM: Nonfatal subcapsular splenic hematoma in a horse, Equine Vet J 1996;28:166.
98. Valli VEO: The hematopoietic system. In Jubb KVF, Kennedy PC, Palmer N, editors: Pathology of Domestic Animals, Orlando, Fla, 1985, Academic Press.
99. Scott EA, Trapp AL, Derksen FJ: Splenomegaly and splenic infarction in a Standardbred colt, Vet Med Small Anim Clin 1978; 73:1549.
100. Sudakow NA: Diseases of the cardiovascular system, blood and blood-forming organs. In Dietz O, Wiesner E, editors: Diseases of the Horse (English translation by AS Turner). Basel, 1984, Karger AG.
101. Traub JL, Bayly WM, Reed SM, et al: Intraabdominal neoplasia as a cause of chronic weight loss in the horse, Comp Cont Educ Pract Vet 1983;5:S526.
102. Nyack B, Padmore CL, Dunn D, et al: Splenic lymphosarcoma in a horse, Mod Vet Prac 1984;65:269.
103. Browning AP: Splenic lymphosarcoma in a stallion associated with an acute abdominal crisis, Vet Rec 1986;119:178.
104. Marr CM, Love S, Pirie HM: Clinical ultrasonographic and pathological findings in a horse with splenic lymphosarcoma and pseudohyperparathyroidism, Equine Vet J 1989;21:221.

105. Chaffin MK, Schmitz DG, Brumbaugh GW: Ultrasonographic characteristics of splenic and hepatic lymphosarcoma in three horses, J Am Vet Med Assoc 1992;201:743.
106. Tanimoto T, Yamasaki S, Ohtsuki Y: Primary splenic lymphoma in a horse, J Vet Med Sci 1994;56:767.
107. Ringger NC, Edens L, Bain P, et al: Acute myelogenous leukemia in a mare, Aust Vet J 1997;75:329-331.
108. Southwood LL, Schott HC, Henry CJ, et al: Disseminated hemangiosarcoma in the horse: 35 cases, J Vet Intern Med 2000; 14:105-109.
109. Mostafa MSE: A case of malignant melanoma in a bay horse, Br Vet J 1953;109:201.
110. Patterson Kane JC, Sanchez LC, Uhl EW, et al: Disseminated metastatic intramedullary melanoma in an aged grey horse, J Comp Path 2001;125:204-207.
111. MacGillivray KC, Sweeney RW, DelPiero F: Metastatic melanoma in horses, J Vet Internal Med 2002;16:453-456.
112. Geelen SN, Sloet van Oldruitenborgh-Oosterbaan MM: [A pony with a metastasized hemangiosarcoma] [Dutch]. Tijdschr Diergeneeskd 1996;121:544.
113. Waller T, Rubarth S: Haemangioendothelioma in domestic animals, Acta Vet Scand 1967;8:234.
114. Waugh SL, Long GG, Uriah L, et al: Metastatic hemangiosarcoma in the equine: Report of 2 cases, J Equine Med Surg 1977;1:311.
115. Reinacher M: Hämangioendotheliome in der Skelettmuskulatur eines Pferdes, Berl Munch Tierarztl Wochenschr 1978;91:121.
116. Johnson JE, Beech J, Saik JE: Disseminated hemangiosarcoma in a horse, J Am Vet Med Assoc 1988;193:1429.
117. Katayama Y, Oikawa MA, Yoshihara T, et al: Clinical and immunohistochemical observation of hemangiosarcoma in a racing thoroughbred, Equine Pract 1996;18:24.
118. Rebhun WC, Bertone A: Equine lymphosarcoma, J Am Vet Med Assoc 1984;184:720.
119. Swan RA: Splenitis in horses, Aust Vet J 1968;44:459.
120. Spier S, Carlson GP, Nyland TG, et al: Splenic hematoma and abscess as a cause of chronic weight loss in a horse, J Am Vet Med Assoc 1986;189:557.
121. Finocchio EJ: Splenic rupture in a horse, Vet Med Small Anim Clin 1971;66:223.
122. Steiner JV: Splenic rupture in the horse, Equine Pract 1981;3:37.
123. Zhao Q: A case of hematoma and rupture of the spleen in a mule, Chin J Vet 1982;8:27.
124. Dyke TM, Friend SCE: Ruptured splenic haematoma in a mare, Equine Vet J 1988;20:138.
125. Merkt H: Expert opinions about a case of injury which by a failure of a restraining device caused a life-threatening injury to a breeding stallion, Tierarztl Prax 1996;24:113.
126. Quinlan J, DeKock G, Marais IP: The operation of splenectomy in horses, cattle, sheep, goats, pigs, dogs, and some South African antelopes: A summary of the results of 98 splenectomies, Onderstepoort J Vet Sci Anim Indust 1935;5:273.
127. Witzel DA, Mullenax CH: A simplified approach to splenectomy in the horse, Cornell Vet 1964;S4:628.
128. Alberti CD, Gerosa R, Marenda JL, et al: Esplenectomia en el equino, Rev Med Vet Argent 1974;55:253.
129. Roberts MC, Groenendyk S: Splenectomy in the horse, Aust Vet J 1978;54:196.
130. Brejov GD, Castaguino OM: Esplenectomia en caballos, Rev Militar Vet 1981;26:333.
131. Tantawy M, Bolbol AE, Samy MT: Comparative techniques for splenectomy in donkeys, Assist Vet Med J 1981;8:15.
132. Brunnberg L, Schebitz H, Bohm D: Splenectomy in the horse, Berl Munch Tierarztl Wochenschr 1983;96:75.
133. Tulman S, Holcomb GW III, Karamanoukian HL, et al: Pediatric laparoscopic splenectomy, J Pediatr Surg 1993;28:689.
134. Hashizume M, Sugimachi K, Kitano S, et al: Laparoscopic splenectomy, Am J Surg 1994;167:611.
135. Rodgerson DH, Brown MH, Watt BC, et al: Hand-assisted laparoscopic technique for removal of ovarian tumors in standing mares, J Am Vet Med Assoc 2002;220:1503-1507.
136. Keoughan CG, Rodgerson DH, Brown MP: Hand-assisted laparoscopic left nephrectomy in standing horses, Vet Surg 2003;32:206-212.
137. Hare WCD: Equine respiratory system. In Getty R, editor: Sisson and Grossman's The Anatomy of the Domestic Animal, Philadelphia, 1975, WB Saunders.
138. Furneaux RW: Surgical techniques for the spleen and liver, Vet Clin North Am 1975;5:363.
139. Traub A, Giebink GS, Smith C, et al: Splenic reticuloendothelial function after splenectomy, spleen repair, and spleen autotransplantation, N Engl J Med 1987;317:1559.
140. Beal SL, Spisso JM: The risk of splenorrhaphy, Arch Surg 1988; 123:1158.
141. Uranus S, Kronberger L, Kraft-Kline J: Partial splenic resection using the TA-stapler, Am J Surg 1994;168:49.
142. Schelling G, Block T, Gokel M: Application of a fibrinogen-thrombin-collagen-based hemostyptic agent in experimental injuries of liver and spleen, J Trauma 1988;28:472.
143. Derderian GP, Walshaw R, McGehee J: Ultrasonic surgical dissection in the dog spleen, Am J Surg 1982;143:269.
144. Reynolds M, LoCicero J III, Young S, et al: Partial splenectomy with the CO_2 laser: An alternative technique, J Surg Res 1986; 41:580.
145. Chen HH, Yan NS, Hou KY, et al: Subtotal splenectomy with a microwave coagulator, Br J Surg 1993;80:612.
146. Stylianos S, Hoffman MA, Jacir NN, et al: Sutureless hemisplenectomy, J Pediatr Surg 1991;26:87.
147. Rogers F, Baumgartner N, Nolan P, et al: Repair of traumatic splenic injuries by splenorrhaphy with polyglycolic acid mesh, Curr Surg 1987;44:112.
148. Lange DA, Zaret P, Merlotti GJ, et al: The use of absorbable mesh in splenic trauma, J Trauma 1988;28:269.
149. Tribble CG, Joob AW, Barone GW, et al: A new technique for wrapping the injured spleen with polyglactin mesh, Am Surg 1987;53:661.
150. Zekas LJ, Ramirez, S, Brown MP: Ablation of the nephrosplenic space for treatment of recurring left dorsal displacement of the large colon in a racehorse, J Am Vet Med Assoc 1999;214:1361-1363.
151. Marien T, Adriaenssen A, Hoeck FV, et al: Laparoscopic closure of the renosplenic space in standing horses, Vet Surg 2001;30:559-563.
152. Rocken M, Mosel G: Indications and clinical experiences with laparoscopic closure of the renosplenic space in horses, Pferdeheilkunde 2003;19:451-458.
153. Ellison EC, Fabri PJ: Complications of splenectomy: Etiology, prevention, and management, Surg Clin North Am 1983;63:1313.

CHAPTER 33

Colic: Diagnosis, Preoperative Management, and Surgical Approaches

Andrew T. Fischer, Jr.

THE ACUTE ABDOMEN

Horses presented for colic offer equine clinicians one of the most challenging and interesting problems encountered in practice. Rapid and accurate diagnosis can be life saving and professionally satisfying. A thorough but efficient diagnostic evaluation needs to be performed in the presence of emotionally stressed owners who are watching their horse in discomfort, frequently at a referral hospital that is new to them.

Horses presented for colic to a referral hospital fall into one of several groups: immediate surgical management or euthanasia, medical management with further monitoring and possible surgery, or medical management with no possibility of surgery (usually because of financial constraints). It is the clinician's goal to rapidly and accurately sort the acute abdominal equine patient into the appropriate diagnostic and therapeutic category. A systematic, standardized evaluation facilitates case management.

DIAGNOSIS

History and Signalment

A thorough medical and management history facilitates accurate evaluation of the horse with colic and may serve to guide the selection of additional diagnostic tests specific to the case. The past medical history should be evaluated to see if there are any links to this episode of acute colic. Repetitive bouts of previous colic should make the clinician inquire about previous abdominal surgery, passage of enteroliths, ingestion of sand, or a possible linear foreign body. Management should be examined, with specific attention focused on changes of diet, consumption of water, changes in exercise level, stabling changes, recent dentistry, or other treatments or medications.

The signalment and history may guide the clinician to a presumptive diagnosis and shape the diagnostic workup. The following are some examples of signalment leading to presumptive diagnosis:

- A young racehorse with a recent orthopedic injury should be evaluated for impactions of the large colon or cecum.
- A broodmare that recently foaled and is now presented with acute severe colic should be evaluated for a large colon volvulus.
- Older, obese horses with colic may have a lipoma strangulating the small intestine.
- Adult horses, especially Arabian and Quarter Horses, in the southwestern United States, that have mild recurrent colic and are passing mineral oil and scant feces should be evaluated for enterolithiasis.
- Cribbers should be evaluated for epiploic foramen entrapments.
- Foals with a recent history of deworming may have an ascarid impaction.

The use of signalment and history to form a presumptive diagnosis can improve the efficiency of diagnostic evaluations selected. For example, a geriatric horse presented for a high heart rate would be evaluated with ultrasonography before abdominal radiography, because the most likely diagnosis is a small intestinal strangulation rather than an enterolith.

Clinical Observation

Horses presented for colic should be observed in a box stall to appreciate their true level of discomfort. Many normal horses roll when first placed in a new stall and then stand up and shake the bedding off their hair coat, but horses with colic roll and then stand up *without* shaking off the bedding. The horse should be evaluated for signs of abdominal distention by watching the flank regions. Pain may be exhibited by sweating, muscle fasciculations, and areas of self-inflicted trauma. Evaluation of the facial expression is very important, but this is subjective and not easily described. Flaring of the nostrils, grimacing, and a dull look to the eyes are all indicators of significant pain. It should not be concluded that a horse has no pain after simply observing that it is quiet in standing stocks, because this same horse may roll and exhibit other signs of discomfort once let loose in a box stall.

Signs of Pain

Pain is probably the single most accurate indicator of the need for exploratory surgery in the horse presented for colic, and it must be interpreted with consideration of the horse's temperament. Draft horses and older horses may be very stoic and may not exhibit obvious signs of pain despite having a lesion that requires surgery. The duration and severity of the pain is also important. Acute severe colic may simply be gas related, but if the pain continues and does not respond to analgesic administration, it is an indicator for surgery. Chronic intermittent low-grade colic is typical of partial intraluminal obstructions (enteroliths) or displacements.

The behavioral manifestations of colic include repetitive lying down and getting up (usually without shaking off bedding), rolling, getting cast, straining to defecate, frequent small amounts of urination, pawing, kicking at their abdomen, looking at the flank region, and assuming a "stretched out" posture. Sweating, playing with the water, tail swishing, and depression are other signs of colic that may be seen, although sweating can also be induced with the administration of some analgesics. Horses with small colon obstructions or other large intestinal impactions may be noted backing up into the walls of their box stalls. The owner or handler of the horse can be of valuable help in interpreting an individual horse's expression of pain and should be consulted.

Pain is frequently evaluated by the severity, duration, and quality of response to administered analgesic medications and by the horse's response to environmental factors. *Mild colic pain* may be hidden by handling or hand-walking. Administration of flunixin meglumine will typically keep the horse comfortable for 8 to 12 hours or longer. *Moderate pain* is usually manifested by some of the behavior patterns mentioned previously—it can be temporarily interrupted by hand-walking, but return when the horse is replaced in its box stall. Relief from analgesics may last for several hours but redosing is frequently required and is usually an early indicator of the need for surgical intervention. *Moderate to severe pain* is noted by very short or no response to administered analgesics, and the horse is uncontrollable even with constant walking or handling. Horses with uncontrollable pain are a danger to themselves and to handlers and should be treated as such. Horses with colic that is likely to need surgery, frequently stay comfortable for 1 hour or less after the administration of xylazine (0.2 to 0.5 mg/kg IV).

All horses presented for colic should have a complete physical examination performed. It should include determination of temperature, heart and respiratory rates, pulse quality, mucous membrane assessment with capillary refill time, and auscultation of the thorax and abdominal cavities. An elevated body temperature should be thoroughly evaluated prior to surgery, because few operable lesions are associated with fever. Enteritis, colitis, and respiratory disease need to be ruled out in horses presented for colic and fever. It is important to remember to obtain the temperature prior to rectal examination, as the access to air resulting from the examination will lower the rectal temperature. Subnormal temperatures can be an indicator of severe shock, or they may be merely spurious. Heart rate and respiratory rate frequently increase with pain, but they may remain normal because of analgesic administration. An elevated heart rate often reflects cardiovascular compromise and impending endotoxic shock. Elevated respiratory rates may be seen with colic but also with respiratory disease. Pulse quality and mucous membrane assessment provide further evaluation of the cardiovascular system.

Auscultation

Abdominal auscultation is a part of the examination of the horse with colic. However, normal gastrointestinal sounds may be heard in horses with colic requiring surgery, and borborygmi may be absent in normal horses that have been sedated. It is important to listen for several minutes to allow a full cycle of contractions of the bowel to occur. Increased abdominal sounds may be heard in horses with impending colitis or enteritis. The presence of sand within the gastrointestinal tract may be determined by listening to the ventral abdominal wall caudal to the xiphoid process and are described as being similar to the sounds heard when listening to a seashell. An absence of gastrointestinal sounds may be caused by administration of a sedative, or it may imply that surgery is needed. In general, an *absence* of intestinal noises is more significant than the presence of sounds in evaluating the horse with the acute abdomen, and it usually implies significant disease.

Gas pockets and tympany may be localized by simultaneous auscultation and percussion. Areas of tympany are more reliably located in the right paralumbar fossa, where the cecum and colon are in direct contact with the body wall. Auscultation of the thorax is important to rule out thoracic disease in horses that are exhibiting signs of colic. Colic may be suspected in horses with bronchopneumonia (see Chapter 48). Pleural effusion can be detected by auscultation, but in horses with colic, the heart sounds radiate over a larger area than is typical and decreased lung sounds are heard ventrally.

Rectal Examination

Abdominal palpation per rectum can offer important information to the clinician evaluating the horse presenting with colic. A systematic examination should be performed on each horse. Restraint of the horse in stocks and sedation or the administration of spasmolytic agents may improve the diagnostic yield and the clinician's safety. Abnormalities noted on abdominal palpation per rectum can include distended or edematous small intestine, small intestinal impactions, large colon distention, impaction or edema, displacements of the large colon, space-occupying masses (abscesses, neoplasia), abnormalities of the urogenital tract (uterine torsion or hemorrhage into the broad ligament), inguinal herniation, and free abdominal gas associated with visceral rupture. Enteroliths are rarely felt because of their location in the transverse colon or proximal small colon, but they are occasionally found. (Abdominal palpation during laparoscopic observation is a useful training tool for students and clinicians.)

Nasogastric Intubation

Nasogastric intubation should be performed on all horses presented for colic. When there is gastric dilation (either primary or secondary), it may prevent gastric rupture and save the life of the horse. Large-bore stomach tubes facilitate recovery of gastric fluid because they are less likely to become occluded by gastric contents than are smaller tubes. Stomach tubes are routinely left in place during anesthesia for colic surgery to facilitate gastric decompression and decrease uncontrolled gastric reflux (which can cause pharyngeal burns or pneumonia if aspirated). Flushing of fluid into the nasogastric tube can start a siphoning action to empty the stomach. Effective emptying of the stomach can be verified by ultrasonography or gastroscopy.

Clinical Pathology

Horses presented for colic are frequently operated on despite minimal clinical pathologic data because of the emergency nature of the acute abdominal crisis and the decreased levels of staff available in the middle of the night. Baseline data (packed cell volume [PCV], total protein) are easily obtained to assess the hydration status. Decreased total protein with an elevated PCV indicates protein loss and dehydration, which together indicate a poor prognosis. However, modern laboratory equipment has become simpler to use, and if full electrolyte panels and serum chemistries are available at the time of evaluation, they should be utilized. Electrolyte levels and blood gas status may be assessed to guide fluid replacement prior to and during anesthesia to minimize complications (see Chapters 3 and 8). White blood cell counts are useful if available. Decreased white blood cell values should make the clinician evaluate the horse for the presence of colitis or a possible visceral rupture. Creatinine levels should be evaluated for the possibility of renal disease or dehydration. Elevations of gamma-glutaryl-transferase may indicate liver disease. Horses with colonic displacements may have elevated liver enzymes because of biliary outflow obstruction.

Abdominocentesis

Abdominocentesis is frequently performed in horses presented for colic when a diagnosis has not been reached by other methods. It is not generally necessary when a decision has already been made for surgical intervention, unless the clinician is concerned about visceral rupture. Multiple methods exist for obtaining abdominal fluid. The most dependent part of the abdomen is prepared for the abdominocentesis on the midline by clipping the hair and preparing with antibacterial soap. Local anesthetic is infiltrated into the skin and linea alba. A no. 15 blade is used to make a skin incision and stab into the linea alba. A teat cannula (7.5 cm) or bitch catheter is then forced into the abdominal cavity through the stab incision and punctures the peritoneum. Alternatively, an 18-gauge needle may be used to obtain the abdominal fluid, and only local anesthesia is necessary. The abdominal fluid should be collected into a serum tube without any ethylenediamine-tetra-acetic (EDTA) for total protein (because total protein may be elevated when collected into an EDTA tube) and into an EDTA tube for cytology and cell counts. The needle or cannula may be left in place for several minutes to obtain fluid.

Abdominocentesis carries the risk of bowel laceration or enterocentesis, or amniocentesis in the term mare. Horses with sand accumulations are particularly at risk because the weight of the colon holds it in apposition to the ventral body wall. Abdominal ultrasonography can be used to localize accumulations of abdominal fluid and select alternative abdominocentesis sites. Abdominocentesis can also be dangerous to the collector if the horse decides to kick, so caution is always indicated. Additionally, the needle technique should be used with caution in foals because the distended bowel is easily punctured .

Analysis of abdominal fluid includes cell counts, cytology, total protein, and in some centers biochemical analysis. Normal white blood cell count in abdominal fluid is less than 10,000/μL[1] in adults and less than 1500 cells/μL in foals, but this value varies between clinics. Peritoneal protein collected into serum tubes is usually below 2.0 g/dL. Cytologic evaluation of the abdominal fluid should include examination for degeneration of cells and classification of cell populations, as well as for the presence of bacteria. It is not unusual for a horse to need an exploratory celiotomy despite normal abdominal fluid analysis data, and the reverse can be true (normal horse with abnormal abdominal fluid analysis data). The results of abdominal fluid analysis are less clear in horses that have recently undergone an exploratory celiotomy,[2] castration, or laparoscopy, because they have elevated white blood cell counts and total proteins.[3]

Ultrasonography

Abdominal ultrasonography has become a routine part of the diagnostic evaluation of the horse presented for colic, because it offers information that cannot be obtained with other diagnostic methods. The horse's abdomen is sprayed with alcohol to improve acoustic coupling, and a systematic examination is performed on both sides of the horse from the line of the diaphragmatic reflection down to ventral midline. A lower-frequency probe (2 to 3.5 MHz) is employed in adult horses to allow visualization of deeper structures. Higher-frequency probes may be used in smaller horses and foals for more detail. The stomach can be evaluated for the presence of gastric fluid or squamous cell carcinoma. The small intestine can be assessed for the presence of movement, mural thickness, and dilation. Normal small intestinal wall thickness is 3 mm or less. In horses with enteritis, the small intestinal wall is frequently thickened, motionless, and full of fluid or ingesta (Fig. 33-1). When there is intestinal obstruction, the small intestine is distended, fluid filled, and hypomotile (Fig. 33-2). Ultrasonography has been demonstrated to be more accurate than abdominal palpation per rectum for the identification of small intestinal strangulations.[4] The strangulated intestine is most frequently located in the ventral abdominal cavity. Other small intestinal lesions that are found on ultrasonography include intussusceptions and inguinal herniation. Lesions involving the cecum may be imaged and include cecocolic and cecocecal intussusceptions. Large colon torsions may be diagnosed by imaging the large colon from the ventral abdomen, with a transmural thickness of 9 mm or greater indicating a likely diagnosis (with a sensitivity of 67%).[5] Intra-abdominal fluid accumulations and masses involving intra-abdominal viscera may also be imaged. Ultrasonography is not useful for the detection of enteroliths because of their location and because the acoustic echo from a stone and a gas shadow are similar.

Radiography

Abdominal radiography is very valuable in diagnosing enteroliths and sand accumulations (see Fig. 36-11) in adult horses and is routinely used in areas of the United States where these problems are endemic. However, the failure to image an enterolith does not mean that one is not present, as false negatives do occur.[6] Enteroliths in the small colon are more difficult to image in the horse that is distended. Sand accumulations are easily imaged in most horses in the ventral abdomen, even with low-powered radiograph machines. Calcifications around linear foreign bodies are also occasionally demonstrated on radiographs. Diaphragmatic hernias may be demonstrated on abdominal or thoracic radiographs, but it is more common to discover this defect at surgery.

Abdominal radiography can offer more detail in foals and small horses. Noncontrast radiography is useful in the neonate with colic and should be supplemented by ultrasonography. Gastric dilation and small intestinal and large intestinal distention may all be diagnosed on noncontrast

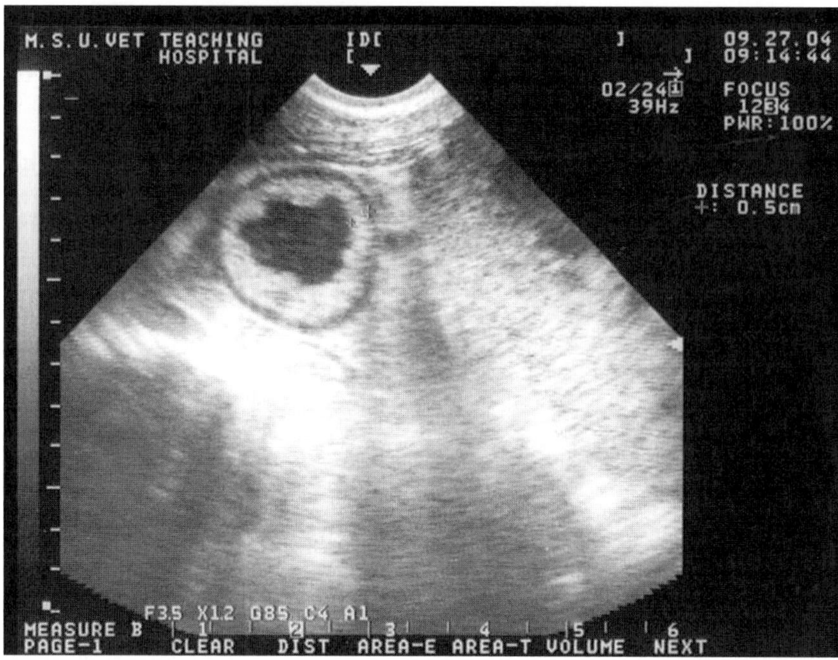

Figure 33-1. Sonogram of the ventral abdomen of a horse with enteritis. The wall of the jejunum is markedly thickened, measuring over 1 cm in some areas. The layers of the bowel wall are easily distinguished because of edema. (Courtesy Dr. Kristin Chaney, Michigan State University.)

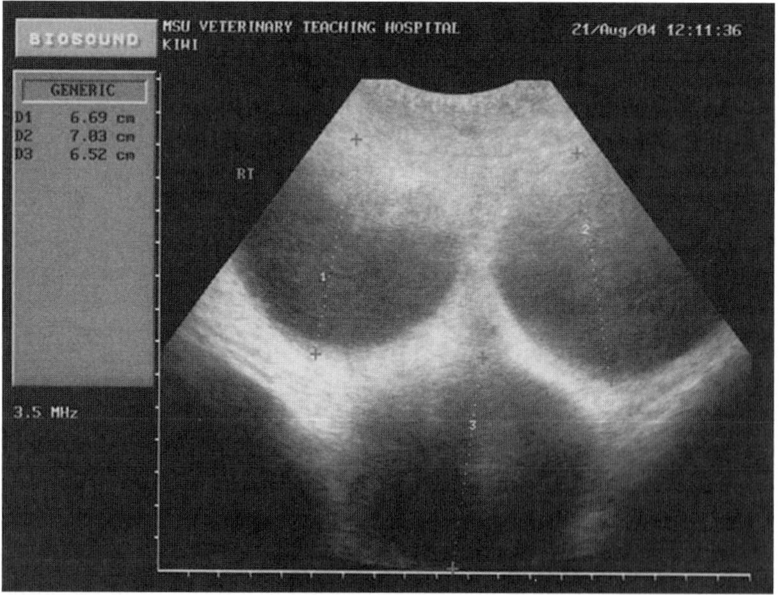

Figure 33-2. Sonogram of the ventral abdomen of a horse with ileus. Many loops of small intestine are fluid distended and hypomotile (in real time). Thickness of the bowel wall is near normal. (Courtesy Dr. Kristin Chaney, Michigan State University.)

abdominal radiography.[7] Contrast media consisting of 30% wt/vol barium sulfate radiography may be administered either orally or rectally and is useful for delineating obstructions or delays in transit. Meconium or other obstructions of the small and large colon, as well as segmental atresias, are readily demonstrated with retrograde contrast radiography.[8]

DECISION FOR SURGERY

The decision to perform an exploratory celiotomy in the horse with colic requires consideration of the diagnostic evaluation and all the other information available to the clinician. In most cases, the decision can be based on the available information and is fairly clear. Horses that are not in pain require further observation and diagnostic evaluation to reach the proper decision. Because of improvements in preoperative stabilization and anesthesia, exploratory celiotomy is less dangerous in terms of morbidity and mortality. Early surgical intervention, even if it is unnecessary (e.g., the lesion found may have been amenable to medical management) is less dangerous to the horse with colic than delayed surgical intervention that results in visceral rupture. Exploratory celiotomy should be strongly considered in horses with colic that have any of the following conditions:

- Persistent or recurrent pain despite the administration of analgesics
- Presence of an enterolith on abdominal radiography
- Presence of distended edematous small intestine without motility on ultrasonography
- Physiologic deterioration despite attempted stabilization with intravenous fluids and other supportive treatments
- Progressive abdominal distention
- Persistent gastric reflux
- Abdominal palpation findings of small intestinal distention, colonic displacement, or very firm intraluminal mass (enterolith or foreign body)
- Serosanguineous abdominal fluid with elevated protein

ANCILLARY DIAGNOSTIC AIDS

Endoscopy

Endoscopic evaluation of the gastrointestinal tract is limited to the esophagus, stomach, duodenum, rectum, and distal small colon by the length of commercially available endoscopes. A 3-m working-length endoscope is commonly used in equine practice. Gastroscopy is useful for the detection of gastric ulcers, gastric impactions, and gastric squamous cell carcinoma. Gastric ulcers are frequently a secondary lesion in horses with colic and indicate the need for further diagnostic workup if antiulcer medication does not alleviate signs of discomfort. Examination of the distal small colon and rectum is most commonly performed in horses with suspected rectal tears or palpable intraluminal masses in these areas.

Laparoscopy

Laparoscopy can be a useful diagnostic tool in horses with both acute and chronic colic. In horses with acute colic, laparoscopy can confirm the need for an exploratory celiotomy or euthanasia. A sensitivity of 82% was found for horses with acute colic, coupled with a specificity of 66%, indicating that if a lesion was found at laparoscopy, it was the likely cause but a significant number of lesions were missed.[9] It is uncommon for a standing laparoscopy to be therapeutic in the horse with acute colic. When performing laparoscopy in the horse with acute colic, it is important to carefully enter the abdominal cavity to avoid penetration of a gas-distended viscus. An open-approach laparoscopy may be performed in horses with abdominal distention. In cases of chronic colic, the horse may be fasted and good visualization of the abdominal cavity may be obtained during diagnostic laparoscopy. The sensitivity for lesion identification in horses with chronic colic declined to 63% with a specificity of 17%. Laparoscopy may be performed in either the standing or the anesthetized horse, depending on where the suspected lesion is located.

Laparoscopy has been used to diagnose trauma after foaling (tears of the small colon mesocolon, uterine rupture, hemorrhage into the broad ligament), abdominal cavity trauma (penetrating wounds), and splenic disease (tumors, hematomas, and ruptures). It also helps identify adhesions (Fig. 33-3), small intestinal strangulations, large colon displacements (Fig. 33-4), visceral rupture, and abdominal neoplasia.[10]

Technique for Diagnostic Standing Laparoscopy

The horse is restrained in standing stocks with the tail secured to prevent contamination of the flank region during surgery. A sedative analgesic combination (e.g., xylazine [0.4

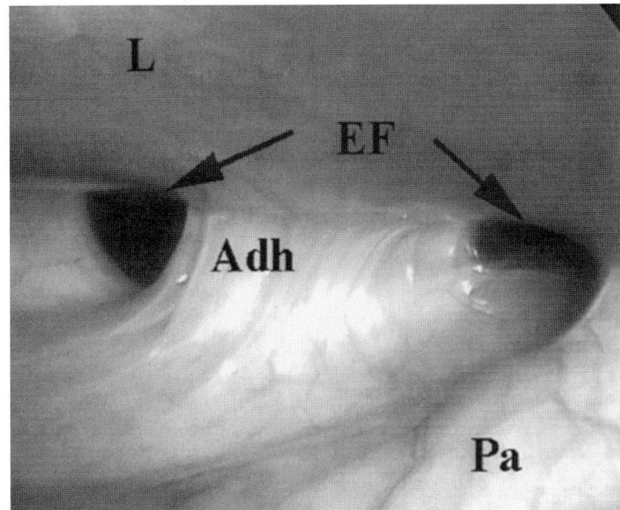

Figure 33-3. An adhesion (Adh) spanning the epiploic foramen (EF) as viewed from the right side. The caudate lobe of the liver (L) and the pancreas (Pa) border the epiploic foramen.

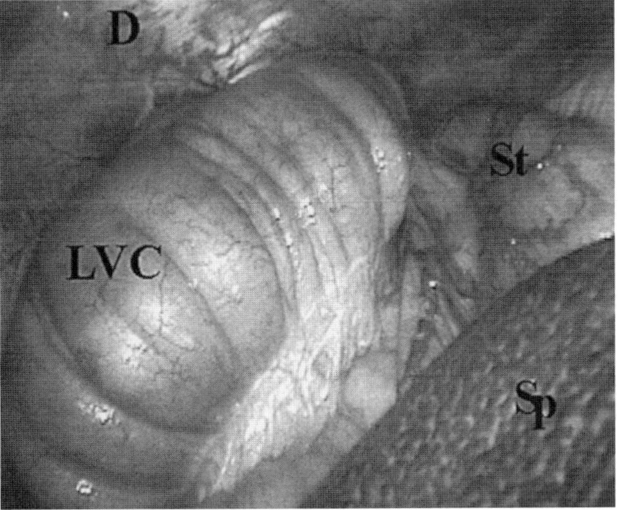

Figure 33-4. Left side laparoscopic view of a large colon displacement (i.e., retroflexion of the pelvic flexure). D, diaphragm; LVC, left ventral colon; St, stomach.

to 0.6 mg/kg IV] and butorphanol tartrate [0.022 mg/kg]) is administered, and both flank regions are prepared for aseptic surgery. Additional analgesics may be administered as needed during the procedure. Local anesthesia (10 to 30 mL) is infiltrated into the sites of trocar introduction both subcutaneously and intramuscularly. The primary site of trocar introduction is usually at the dorsal margin of the internal abdominal oblique muscle midway between the last rib and the tuber coxae. Accessory portals are established above or below this for instrument introduction. The use of adherent drapes is less traumatic to the standing horse than the use of penetrating towel clamps, unless all sites are infiltrated with local anesthesia.

The flank regions should have been previously evaluated for the presence of adherent viscera (via ultrasonography) or other contraindications for laparoscopic portal placement in that region. A 1.5-cm stab incision is made through the skin and underlying fascia to allow introduction of the first laparoscopic trocar or cannula (15 cm in length) assembly. The assembly is inserted aiming at the contralateral coxofemoral joint until resistance decreases. The laparoscopic telescope is then inserted and penetration into the abdominal cavity is confirmed or the laparoscope is found to still be in the retroperitoneal space. If the telescope is in the retroperitoneal space, a quick thrust with the 30-degree telescope will tear the peritoneum. Correct placement into the abdominal cavity is confirmed visually and by being able to freely move the laparoscope without patient discomfort. Insufflation with carbon dioxide to 10 to 15 mm Hg is commenced. Once the abdomen has been insufflated, systematic exploration should occur. Additional portals may be placed to allow introduction of instruments to facilitate manipulation of viscera.

When evaluating the left side of the abdomen, the first structure typically seen is the nephrosplenic ligament with the spleen and associated perirenal fat (Fig 33-5). The mesenteric root is then seen, as are sections of the small intestine and the colon. Passing the laparoscope over the nephrosplenic ligament cranially, the lateral and dorsal surface of the stomach is examined. The diaphragm and left part of the liver are seen further cranially. The evaluation of the caudal abdomen includes visualization of the urogenital organs (the ovary, uterus, and broad ligament in the mare, or the vas deferens and mesorchium in the male, and the urinary bladder). The rectum is noted dorsal to the urinary bladder. The inguinal rings may be evaluated.

The right side of the abdomen is typically evaluated by a separate entry portal in the right paralumbar fossa. The base of the cecum and duodenum are seen when first entering the abdomen. Looking above the duodenum, the right renal outline is seen. The liver is located ventrad and craniad to this, and the epiploic foramen may be entered. Looking caudally, the root of the mesentery is seen, as are sections of the small and large intestine. The right side of the urogenital tract is evaluated similarly to the left side. The use of a biopsy forceps or chambers catheter through a separate portal is helpful to probe organs and move viscera to improve visualization.

At the termination of the laparoscopic evaluation, the valves in the cannula assembly are held open to allow as much of the insufflating gas as possible to leave the abdominal cavity to improve postoperative patient comfort. The skin is sutured and nonsteroidal anti-inflammatory agents are administered if necessary.

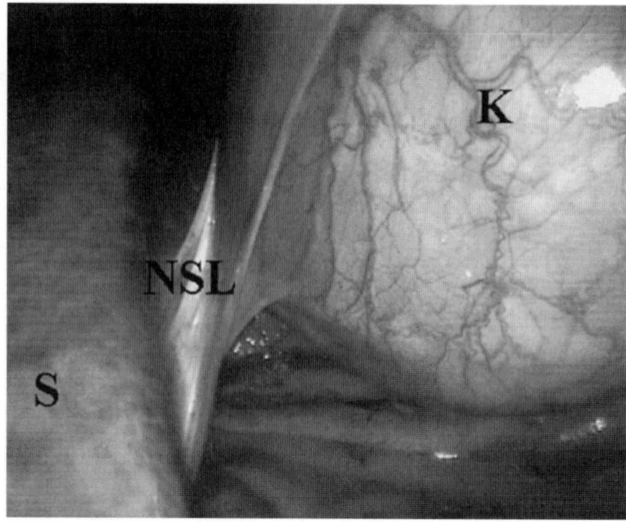

Figure 33-5. The nephrosplenic ligament (NSL) extends from the kidney (K) to the spleen (S).

PREOPERATIVE MANAGEMENT OF THE ACUTE ABDOMEN

Pain Control

Alleviation of pain in the horse with colic is important, but it must be carried out carefully, because if excessive pain relief disguises colic that needs surgery, visceral rupture may occur. Flunixin meglumine (0.5 to 1.1 mg/kg) may be administered as a presurgical anti-inflammatory drug and to help protect against the effects of endotoxemia. Repetitive dosing can mask signs that would otherwise dictate surgical intervention. Most horses that are referred to surgical centers have already been given flunixin meglumine, and more should not be administered in the hospital unless surgery has been performed or no surgical option is available.

Xylazine (0.2 to 0.4 mg/kg IV) is a potent analgesic and may be used to control moderate to severe abdominal discomfort, with a reasonably short duration of action. It is particularly useful during the evaluation period of the horse with colic to allow diagnostic procedures to be performed, because it has a rapid onset of action with a short duration of pain relief. Horses that require exploratory celiotomy typically begin demonstrating signs of colic in 30 to 60 minutes after administration of xylazine. If additional analgesia or duration of sedation is necessary, butorphanol tartrate may be administered (0.011 to 0.022 mg/kg IV). Repetitive dosing of xylazine or other analgesics is rarely indicated in horses that have a surgical option. Use of longer-acting sedatives or analgesics such as detomidine should be reserved for horses without option of surgical intervention.

Preoperative Preparation

Once the decision to perform surgery has been made, induction of anesthesia may occur. An intravenous catheter should be placed to allow high-volume fluid replacement if necessary. The horse's mouth should have been washed out and a nasogastric tube placed that will remain for the duration of surgery. It is important to have stabilized the horse as well as possible preoperatively with intravenous fluids (see Chapter 8). Preoperative antibiotics and tetanus prophylaxis should be provided. The operating room with necessary supplies should be set up in advance to minimize wasted anesthesia time. Preparation of the ventral abdominal wall takes place under general anesthesia and is usually more efficient and safer than attempting to prepare the horse while still standing.

APPROACHES TO THE ABDOMEN

Ventral Midline Celiotomy

Ventral midline celiotomy (VMC) (Fig. 33-6) through the linea alba is the most common approach for equine abdominal surgery because it allows exteriorization of 75% of the intestinal tract (Fig. 33-7). The stomach, duodenum, distal ileum, dorsal body and base of the cecum, distal right dorsal and transverse colon, and terminal descending colon are the only segments that cannot be exteriorized. The VMC creates minimal hemorrhage, is easy to extend, and has strong fibrous tissue for closure.

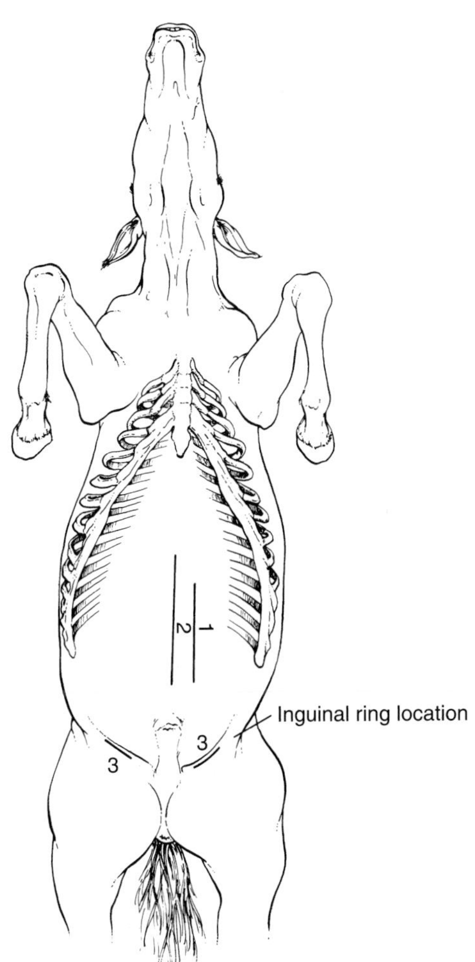

Figure 33-6. Abdominal approaches through the ventral abdominal wall: paramedian (1), ventral midline (2), and inguinal (3). (Redrawn from Adams SB: Surgical approaches to the equine abdomen, Vet Clin North Am Large Anim Pract 1982;4:89.)

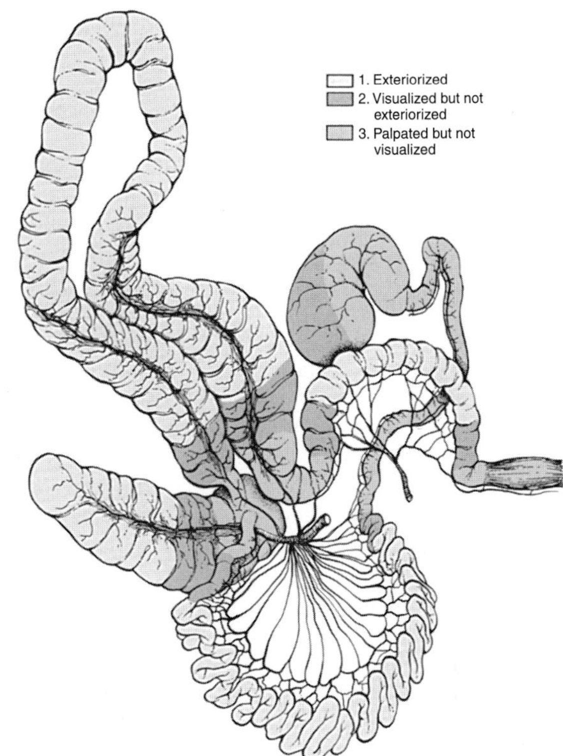

Figure 33-7. Anatomic drawing of the equine intestinal tract. Differential shading (KEY) indicates the portions that may be (1) exteriorized, (2) visualized and palpated but not exteriorized, and (3) palpated only via a standard ventral midline celiotomy approach. (Redrawn from Sack WO: Guide to the Dissection of the Horse, Ann Arbor, 1977, Edwards Brothers.)

The linea alba is a combination of the median fibrous raphe of the aponeuroses of the external abdominal oblique muscle, the internal abdominal oblique muscle, and the transverse abdominal muscle extending from the xiphoid process to the prepubic tendon. Histologically, the linea alba consists of dense connective tissue composed of sheets of collagen bundles and fibroblasts. The fibers of the sheets cross between one another, adding to its mechanical strength.

In horses, the thickness of the cranial part of the linea alba may reach 0.3 mm, whereas the caudal part reaches 1 cm.[11] The midline incision is made as long as necessary to complete the exploratory surgery (averaging about 30 cm in the adult horse). The incision should be large enough to allow exteriorization of necessary viscera and not put excessive pressure on the intestine (which would increase the risk of iatrogenic tears). The time saved in the procedure and the increased safety of a larger incision more than compensate for the extra several minutes spent suturing a longer incision. The incision through the linea should begin at the umbilicus where it is the thickest and continue cranially, avoiding the rectus abdominis muscle.

Closure techniques of the celiotomy incision vary between surgeons and are usually a matter of personal preference. The optimal distance that a suture should be placed from the incisional edge of the linea alba in horses is 1.2 to 1.5 cm.[11] Excessive tension on sutures causes microscopic tissue necrosis and is the most common surgical error made during closure of the linea alba.[11]

Ventral Paramedian Approach

The ventral paramedian incision, the second most common approach used in colic operations, is made 10 cm lateral to the midline (see Fig. 33-6). The incision may be made on either the right or left of midline through the rectus abdominis muscle, which creates a thicker border to the incision than the ventral midline approach but does not significantly limit surgical exposure of the abdominal cavity. The deep and superficial epigastric vessels may be encountered during this incision and should be avoided if possible. The ventral paramedian incision typically hemorrhages more than the linea alba incision, but this does not seem to generate any clinical problems and the wound generally heals well. Some surgeons favor the paramedian incision, particularly if wound healing is thought to be compromised, because fewer hernias are observed to be associated with this incision. Some surgeons prefer to use the paramedian incision when relaparotomy is required. It is better to avoid a previous linea alba incision if there are signs of excessive inflammation, infection, or possible adhesions. Closure of the paramedian incision involves suturing of the external fascia of the rectus abdominis sheath. Suturing of the muscle belly does not appear to contribute to the strength of the closure.

Flank Approach

A standing flank approach to the abdomen is easily performed but less easily applied to the correct clinical situation (Fig. 33-8). The small colon is the most accessible part of the intestinal tract approached from the flank. A nondistended large colon can be exteriorized through a flank incision but not if the viscus is edematous or filled with ingesta. A standing flank approach can also be used for surgical treatment of abdominal pain because of uterine torsion.[12] The flank incision is made on the right side for a clockwise torsion, or vice versa. The exposure offered by a standing flank laparotomy is too limited for it to serve as a routine abdominal exploratory approach.

The most commonly used approach for flank laparotomy is the modified grid approach. The horse is restrained in standing stocks with the tail tied, and the flank region is prepared for aseptic surgery. A sedative-and-analgesic combination is administered, and local anesthesia is infiltrated subcutaneously and intramuscularly at the planned site of incision. The skin is sharply incised in a vertical line midway between the last rib and the tuber coxae, starting dorsal to the palpable dorsal edge of the internal abdominal oblique and continuing ventrally (see Fig. 33-8). The external abdominal oblique muscle is subsequently sharply divided. The internal abdominal oblique and transverse abdominal muscles are bluntly divided parallel to their fiber direction, exposing the peritoneum, which is then punctured, giving access to the abdominal cavity. Closure of the incision is by muscle apposition with absorbable sutures for the deep layers and subsequent closure of the external abdominal oblique muscle layer for a second layer. The subcutaneous tissues may be included in this layer or sutured separately. The skin is sutured or stapled.

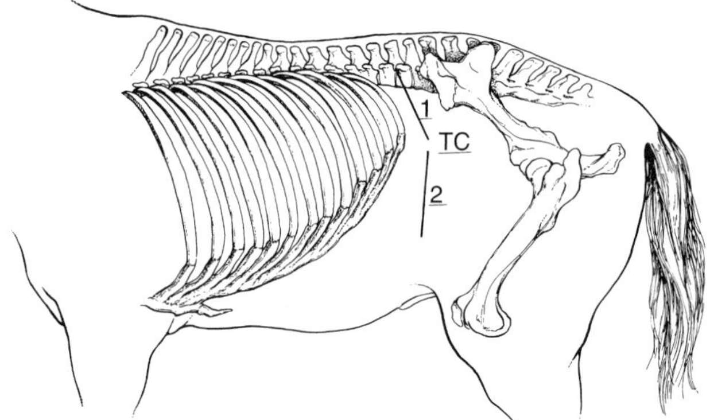

Figure 33-8. Abdominal approaches through the flank: paralumbar incision (1), transverse flank incision (2). TC, tuber coxae.
(Redrawn from Adams SB: Surgical approaches to the equine abdomen, Vet Clin North Am Large Anim Pract 1982;4:103.)

Inguinal Approach

The inguinal approach is used in conjunction with a ventral midline incision when operating on stallions with inguinal or scrotal hernias (see Fig. 33-6). The inguinal approach alone usually does not allow a thorough exploration and decompression of the nonherniated bowel. The inguinal herniorrhaphy often is combined with unilateral castration of the affected testicle. Most hernias are of the indirect type with the vaginal tunic intact. After repair of the intestinal lesion, the tunic can be ligated to bolster the inguinal closure. The external inguinal ring is closed using 2 or 3 polyglactin 910 in a simple-continuous or a simple-interrupted pattern, with sutures placed 1.5 to 2.0 cm apart. The subcutaneous tissues and skin are closed as separate layers. (For more details on anatomy and surgery of the inguinal ring, see Chapters 38 and 65) Alternatively, laparoscopy allows internal repair of the inguinal ring damaged by herniation through mesh secured by staples or laparoscopic suturing techniques.[13]

REFERENCES

1. Grindem CB, Fairley NM, Uhlinger CA, et al: Peritoneal fluid values from healthy foals, Equine Vet J 1990;22:359.
2. Santschi EM, Grindem CB, Tate LP, et al: Fluid analysis in ponies after abdominal surgery, Vet Surg 1988;17:6.
3. Fischer AT, Lloyd KCK, Carlson GP, et al: Diagnostic laparoscopy in the horse, J Am Vet Med Assoc 1986;189:289.
4. Klohnen A, Vachon AM, Fischer AT: Use of diagnostic ultrasonography in horses with signs of acute abdominal pain, J Am Vet Med Assoc 1996;209:1597.
5. Pease AP, Scrivani PV, Erb HN, et al: Accuracy of increased large intestine wall thickness during ultrasonography for diagnosing large colon torsion in 42 horses, Vet Radiol Ultrasound 2004;45:220.
6. Yarbrough TB, Langer DL, Snyder JR, et al: Abdominal radiography for diagnosis of enterolithiasis in horses—141 cases (1990-1992), J Am Vet Med Assoc 1994;205:592.

7. Fischer AT, Kerr LY, O'Brien TR: Radiographic diagnosis of abdominal disorders in the foal, Vet Radiol 1987;28:42.
8. Fischer AT, Yarbrough TY: Retrograde contrast radiography of the distal portions of the intestinal tract in foals, J Am Vet Med Assoc 1995;207:734.
9. Walmsley JP: Review of equine laparoscopy and an analysis of 158 laparoscopies in the horse, Equine Vet J 1999;31:456.
10. Fischer AT: Laparoscopic evaluation of horses with acute or chronic colic. In Fischer AT, editor: Equine Diagnostic and Surgical Laparoscopy, Philadelphia, 2002, WB Saunders.
11. Trostle SS, Wilson DG, Stone W, et al: A study of the biomechanical properties of the adult equine linea alba: Relationship of tissue bite size and suture material to breaking strength, Vet Surg 1994; 23:435.
12. Pascoe JR, Meagher DM, Wheat JD: Surgical management of uterine torsion in the mare: A review of 26 cases, Am Vet Med Assoc 1981;179:351.
13. Fischer AT, Vachon AM, Klein SR: Laparoscopic inguinal herniorrhaphy in two stallions, J Am Vet Med Assoc 1995;207:1599.

CHAPTER 34

Principles of Intestinal Injury and Determination of Intestinal Viability

Anthony T. Blikslager

Intestinal injury, although typically associated with ischemic lesions, occurs during any obstructive intestinal disease to varying degrees depending on the type of obstruction and the extent of vascular compromise. In addition, in some instances, the intestinal lumen is patent, but there is vascular compromise—for example, in nonstrangulating infarctions. Intestinal obstructive lesions are classified as either simple or strangulating obstructions. A great deal of work has been done to assess the level of injury encountered with these lesions at surgery and during the postsurgical phase following correction and reperfusion of these lesions. Although more is known about mucosal injury than about injury encountered in other intestinal layers, it is clear that substantial injury also occurs at the levels of the serosa and the muscularis, which very likely contributes to postoperative complications such as adhesion formation and ileus. Understanding the pathophysiology of these lesions allows the surgeon to more adequately perform surgical and postoperative procedures to optimize patient survival. For example, attention has been focused on the development of intestinal injury during reperfusion, and the possibility of inhibiting these lesions with various treatments. Furthermore, to combat the postoperative complication of serosal inflammation and secondary adhesion formation, surgeons have adopted a number of new treatments.

TYPES OF OBSTRUCTION

Simple Obstruction

Although simple obstruction, most commonly caused by an intraluminal impaction, does not initially result in intestinal injury, studies show that, as distention progresses, mucosal lesions similar to those encountered during ischemic injury occur.[1,2] More specifically, there are critical intraluminal pressure levels beyond which intramural vascular compression takes place, reducing tissue perfusion.[3,4] Furthermore, direct compression of the intestinal wall by obstructive masses may lead to a lesion that has the appearance of an infarction as a result of occlusion of the local arterial supply. Causes of these compressive lesions tend to be hard masses such as enteroliths or fecaliths, which, if not recognized during early lesion formation, may result in intestinal rupture.[5] Injury caused by progressive intestinal distention, particularly in the case of fluid accumulation proximal to a small intestinal obstruction, is more difficult to recognize clinically than compressive infarctions, but nonetheless it is important to be aware of it to minimize postsurgical morbidity.

Strangulating Obstruction

Strangulating obstruction results from simultaneous occlusion of the intestinal lumen and its blood supply. The clearest examples of such lesions include large colon volvulus, and strangulation of the small intestine within an internal hernia or via an abnormal band of tissue such as the stalk of a pedunculated lipoma. The degree of injury attributable to occlusion of the blood supply depends on the nature of vascular occlusion. In most instances, the veins are occluded earlier in the course of strangulating obstruction than the arteries because of their thinner and more compliant walls. This results in a disparity in blood flow during the early phases of strangulating obstruction, with continued pumping of arterial blood into the intestinal wall, which, in the absence of patent outflow, causes a hemorrhagic lesion termed *hemorrhagic strangulating obstruction*. This results in not only ischemic injury but also tremendous congestion of the tissues. Alternatively, the strangulation may exert sufficient pressure on the veins and arterial supply that both are occluded simultaneously, resulting in so-called *ischemic strangulating obstruction*. This results in rapid degeneration of the mucosa.[6]

Clinically, hemorrhagic or ischemic strangulating obstruction may be noted in horses with large colon volvulus. In horses with a 360-degree large colon volvulus, hemorrhagic strangulating obstruction is most frequently noted, particularly if there is ample ingesta within the lumen to reduce how tightly the intestine twists around its mesenteric axis. However, there are also cases of ischemic strangulating obstruction, particularly in horses with a volvulus that exceeds 360 degrees, or in horses with little ingesta in the lumen.[7]

Nonstrangulating Infarction

Nonstrangulating infarction most commonly occurs secondary to cranial mesenteric arteritis caused by migration of *Strongylus vulgaris*,[8] which has become a relatively rare disorder since the advent of broad-spectrum anthelmintics. Although thromboemboli have been implicated in the pathogenesis of this disease, careful dissection of naturally occurring lesions has not revealed the presence of thrombi at the site of intestinal infarctions in most cases. These findings suggest that vasospasm plays an important role in this disease.[8] Any segment of intestine supplied by the cranial mesenteric artery or one of its major branches may be affected, but the distal small intestine and large colon are more commonly involved.[8] These lesions have no obvious cause of obstruction, but they have clearly demarcated regions of degeneration or necrosis, depending on the extent of vascular occlusion.

MECHANISMS OF INJURY

Luminal Distention

Investigators have examined the role of small intestinal intraluminal distention and decompression on the microvasculature. In one study, distention of the jejunum to an intraluminal hydrostatic pressure of 25 cm H_2O for 120 minutes resulted in a significant reduction in the number of perfused vessels in the seromuscular and mucosal layers, and vascular perfusion remained abnormal after decompression.[2] This in turn led to epithelial sloughing, similar to that noted in ischemic lesions.[9] Alternatively, earlier studies indicated that there was no histologic evidence of epithelial sloughing with pressures up to 18 cm H_2O for 4 hours, although the authors did note mucosal and submucosal edema.[3] Thus, it is clear that the nature of mucosal lesions depends on the degree of intraluminal pressure. In experimental studies on the effects of distention, the seromuscular layer appeared to be more severely affected, and it had evidence of mesothelial cell loss, neutrophil infiltration, and edema that progressed after decompression, suggesting reperfusion injury in this tissue.[10]

This type of inflammatory seromuscular lesion has also been noted in studies of the proximal resection margins of naturally occurring small intestinal strangulating obstructions, indicating that distention leads to seromuscular injury proximal to obstructive lesions, despite the fact that this intestine may appear grossly normal.[11] Experimentally, this seromuscular injury and inflammation leads to adhesion formation. Thus, foals subjected to intraluminal distention of a segment of jejunum to 25 cm H_2O for 2 hours in one study developed bowel-to-bowel and bowel-to-mesentery adhesions within 10 days of the surgical procedure.[12] Similar experiments in the large colon have revealed that the colon is far more resistant to seromuscular injury than the small intestine.[10]

Mucosal Ischemic Injury

To understand how the mucosa becomes injured during ischemia, critical anatomic features of the mucosa have to be taken into consideration. In the equine small intestine, the villus tip is the region most susceptible to ischemia, largely because of the countercurrent exchange mechanism of blood flow in the small intestinal villus.[13] This countercurrent exchange mechanism is attributable to the vascular architecture, which consists of a central arteriole that courses up the core of the villus, arborizes at the tip, and is drained by venules coursing down the periphery of the villus.[14] As oxygenated blood enters the central arteriole, oxygen diffuses across the wall of the arteriole, through the interstitial tissues, and into the peripheral venules, which are flowing in the opposite direction. Although this enhances intestinal absorption, it short-circuits the oxygen supply, resulting in a villus tip that is relatively hypoxic even under normal conditions. Countercurrent exchange is exacerbated when the rate of the arterial blood flow is reduced, essentially providing more time for the oxygen to diffuse out of the arteriole across to the venules. When the arterial flow is reduced to a critically low level, the tip of the villus becomes absolutely hypoxic, with attendant epithelial injury.[13,15] This mechanism may explain why the small intestinal mucosa is more susceptible to ischemic injury than the colon, which has no villi. For example, the time required to produce severe morphologic damage to the equine colon is approximately 25% longer than that for the small intestine.[16]

Mucosal epithelium is particularly susceptible to hypoxic injury because of the relatively high level of energy required to fuel the Na^+/K^+–ATPase mechanism that regulates epithelial ion and nutrient transport. The first biochemical event to occur during hypoxia is a loss of oxidative phosphorylation. The resulting diminished ATP concentration causes failure of the energy-dependent Na^+/K^+–ATPase mechanism, resulting in intracellular accumulation of sodium and water. The pH of the cytosol drops as lactic acid and inorganic phosphates accumulate from anaerobic glycolysis, which damages cell membranes and results in their detachment from the basement membrane.[17]

As epithelium separates from the underlying basement membrane in the small intestine, a fluid-filled space termed Grüenhagen's space forms at the tip of the villus.[15] The fluid accumulation exacerbates epithelial separation from the basement membrane. Subsequently, epithelium progressively sloughs from the tip of the villus (Fig. 34-1) toward the crypts, which are the last component of the intestinal mucosa to become injured.[18-20] The relative resistance of the crypts to injury probably relates to their vascular architecture, since crypts receive a blood supply that is separate from the vasculature involved in the villus countercurrent exchange mechanism. The early morphologic changes observed in the equine large colon during ischemia are similar to those described in the equine small intestine, with

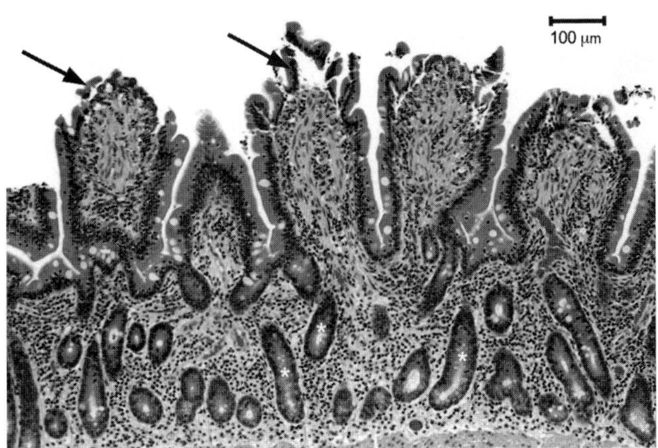

Figure 34-1. Photomicrograph of jejunal mucosa from a horse subjected to complete ischemia, similar to that seen in natural cases of ischemic strangulating obstruction. Note sloughing of epithelium into the lumen *(arrows)*. This sloughing progresses from the tips of the villi toward the crypts *(asterisks)* as the duration of ischemia progresses.

initial loss of the more superficially located surface cells, followed by cellular injury and sloughing within the crypts.[16,21]

Reperfusion Injury

Events that culminate in reperfusion injury in the small intestine are initiated during ischemia when the enzyme xanthine dehydrogenase is converted to xanthine oxidase, and its substrate, hypoxanthine, accumulates as a result of ATP utilization.[22,23] However, there is little xanthine oxidase activity during ischemia, because oxygen is required as an electron acceptor. During reperfusion, xanthine oxidase rapidly degrades hypoxanthine in the presence of oxygen, which acquires a single additional electron, producing superoxide.[22] Superoxide contributes to oxidative tissue damage, but this reactive oxygen metabolite is relatively lipid insoluble, limiting the level of injury.

However, the more important role for superoxide is in the generation of neutrophil chemoattractants.[24,25] Superoxide interacts with lipid membranes, triggering arachidonic acid metabolism and generation of lipid neutrophilic chemoattractants such as leukotriene B_4. Because of the critical role of xanthine oxidase, inhibition of this enzyme in feline studies of intestinal ischemia/reperfusion injury prevented infiltration of neutrophils and subsequent mucosal injury.[25,26] Studies went on to show that reperfusion injury could be inhibited at several levels of the reperfusion cascade, including scavenging superoxide with superoxide dismutase, inhibiting neutrophil infiltration with monoclonal antibodies directed against neutrophil adhesion molecules, and scavenging neutrophil-released reactive oxygen metabolites.[22,25] Researchers were initially optimistic that this would provide practical therapeutic interventions, because many of the treatments tested, including the xanthine oxidase inhibitor allopurinol, could potentially be administered prior to reperfusing an ischemic lesion at surgery (Fig. 34-2).

Unfortunately, treatment of mucosal reperfusion injury has not proven to be highly effective in most cases of strangulating obstruction. One important reason for this is that strangulating obstruction induces maximal mucosal

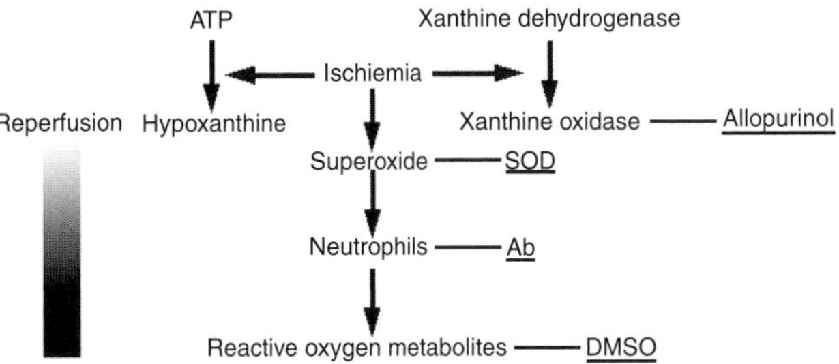

Figure 34-2. Diagram of the events that lead to reperfusion injury. Note that as reperfusion progresses *(shaded bar)*, the concentration of reactive oxygen metabolites amplifies as neutrophils are attracted to the site of injury. Points of experimental therapeutic intervention to block critical stages of reperfusion injury are *underlined*.

injury during the ischemic phase, as compared with studies in laboratory animals in which "low-flow" ischemia was used.[27] The latter involves reduction but not cessation of arterial flow, which induces relatively minor levels of injury, while priming tissues for injury during subsequent reperfusion.[28,29] Studies in horses using low-flow ischemia indicate that equine tissues are susceptible to reperfusion injury after this type of ischemia.[9,30-32] For example, studies of equine jejunum have shown that increased capillary permeability is associated with neutrophil infiltration during reperfusion.[30] Although a direct link to xanthine oxidase has not been shown, equine small intestine expresses substantial levels of xanthine dehydrogenase, which is converted to xanthine oxidase during ischemia.[33] Low-flow ischemia studies in equine colon have shown continued mucosal degeneration during reperfusion associated with marked neutrophil infiltration, despite the fact that equine colon does not express appreciable levels of xanthine oxidase. Alternative oxidant enzyme sources such as aldehyde oxidase have been offered as potential sources of reactive oxygen metabolites.[31]

Once the capacity of equine tissues to develop reperfusion injury was shown, additional studies were performed to determine whether reperfusion injury occurs after clinically applicable models of ischemia that simulate strangulating obstruction. For example, in one study assessing either arteriovenous or venous occlusion in equine jejunum, a small degree of reperfusion injury was documented after 3 hours of ischemia. However, the level of ischemic injury was nearly maximal after 3 hours, and the additional injury that developed during reperfusion was not sensitive to allopurinol, a xanthine oxidase inhibitor, or dimethyl sulfoxide, a reactive oxygen metabolite scavenger.[34] The likely cause of reperfusion injury in this instance was initiation of epithelial injury during ischemia that could not be reversed during reperfusion.[17] More recent studies in equine small intestine,[18] and studies in equine colon[35] using ischemic models relevant to strangulating obstruction have failed to detect any level of reperfusion injury. Studies in laboratory animals on strangulating obstruction have also shown that this type of ischemic insult is less likely to develop into reperfusion injury.[36,37]

In a veterinary review of the pathogenesis of intestinal reperfusion injury in the horse, the concept of a therapeutic window wherein treatment of reperfusion injury would be beneficial was suggested.[22] The basis of this concept is that there are certain conditions under which ischemic injury is minimal, and that tissues are severely damaged during reperfusion.[36] Thus, under conditions of low-flow ischemia, very little injury is demonstrated during 3 hours of ischemia, but remarkable injury occurs during 1 hour of reperfusion.[24-26] However, a very narrow therapeutic window may exist under conditions of strangulating obstruction, where severe injury occurs rapidly during ischemia, leaving relatively little potential for further injury that can be potentially offset with treatments such as antioxidants during reperfusion.

Nonetheless, this does not mean that treatments directed against reperfusion injury have no potential place for treatment of horses with strangulating obstruction, particularly as these treatments become more effective. For example, multimodal therapies involving intravascular or intraluminal infusion of solutions containing antioxidants, intestinal nutrients, and vasodilators have proven very effective in vitro and in vivo, although these treatment modalities have been used predominantly in low-flow ischemia models.[38-41] It is also becoming clear that the consequences of reperfusion injury are widespread and involve tissues other than the intestinal mucosa. For instance, low-flow ischemia models have demonstrated neutrophil infiltration into the seromuscular layers that very likely contributes to important complications such as adhesions and postoperative ileus.[12,42] This neutrophil infiltration appears to be relevant to strangulating obstruction, because similar neutrophil infiltrates were noted in the resection margins of resected strangulated small intestine.[11] Thus, although antioxidant-based therapies may be unable to reduce mucosal injury because of its rapid onset during ischemia, they may be able to reduce neutrophil infiltration in other layers of the intestine.

DETERMINATION OF INTESTINAL VIABILITY

Clinical Assessment of Bowel Viability

The viability of intestinal tissue is most commonly assessed by clinical observation—observing the color of the serosa and assessing the color of the mucosa, which may in some instances be observed prior to resection. For example, when a pelvic flexure enterotomy is performed in horses with large colon volvulus, the mucosa can be directly observed prior to making any decisions on recovering the horse or performing a resection. Changes in coloration are not uniform between the mucosa and the serosa, suggesting that much information can be gained by observing both of these layers of the intestine. For example, in one study on naturally occurring cases of large colon volvulus, the serosa was noted to turn from various shades of purple to pink in some instances as the colon was reperfused, whereas the mucosa consistently remained black. This probably relates to the metabolic demand of mucosa, which requires tremendous energy reserves to fuel the Na^+/K^+-ATPase mechanism that is responsible for driving mucosal transport function. Although there has been some concern about the utility of assessing mucosal color at the pelvic flexure, and about whether this accurately reflects the level of injury in the more proximal regions of the colon, recent studies suggest that injury is uniform throughout the strangulated portion of the large colon.[43]

Clinical determination of viability has the obvious advantage of being noninvasive and rapid to perform, but it has the disadvantage of being inaccurate for fully determining the level of injury. For example, in a study assessing the resection margins after small intestinal resection, it was noted that there was marked serosal inflammation at the proximal resection margin, a region where surgeons would have had the choice to resect additional intestine if needed.[11] In other instances, when the resection margins are forced by anatomic considerations, surgeons can frequently discern substantial intestinal injury, but they have to decide whether the horse can survive if injured intestine is left in place. This is a particular problem with ileal resection and with large colon resection. Generally, if the intestine appears completely nonviable (on the basis of dark coloration, a dull appearance to the serosa, and an inability of the surgeon to rehydrate the surface of the intestine with lavage solutions), owners are advised that euthanasia is the most reasonable option.[7]

However, bowel that appears nonviable sometimes does survive. For example, in a study of ponies subjected to small intestinal venous strangulation obstruction, in which assessment of viability was based on color, wall thickness, peristalsis, and palpable mesenteric arterial pulsation, clinical assessment was only 54% accurate in predicting viability. In particular, clinicians were misled by intramural hemorrhage and edema, which resulted in the faulty judgment of nonviable tissue in some instances.[44] Ultimately, histopathology is the gold standard for determining viability, but when this service is unavailable because the situation is an emergency, any change in coloration during reperfusion, or evidence of bleeding from the vasculature during resection, may be used as evidence that there is some likelihood of survival. On the other hand, hemorrhage and edema within the tissues must be interpreted with caution, because some apparently devitalized bowel may survive.

Ancillary Methods of Determining Intestinal Viability

Fluorescein Dye

Fluorescein dye may be administered intravenously (6.6 to 15 mg/kg), after which it is rapidly distributed throughout the body, including the intestinal tract. Perfusion can be detected by illumination of the bowel with an ultraviolet light within 60 seconds of administration. Although there are distinct patterns of fluorescence in different segments of the intestinal tract, this technique has not gained wide clinical usage, most likely because of inconsistencies of the technique in enhancing accuracy of viability determination. In particular, a complete lack of fluorescence may be noted in clinical cases of ischemic small intestine that has subsequently been documented to survive.[45] This may be caused by the degree of intestinal distention, or by the compromised systemic cardiovascular status, both of which are common problems in horses with colic. One way to overcome this problem is to carefully compare a segment of suspected ischemic intestine with adjacent normal-appearing intestine. A generalized lack of fluorescence over the entire region would indicate that the technique should not be used to make definitive decisions in that particular case, whereas fluorescence in adjacent normal intestine would at least suggest that fluorescein is adequately perfusing the intestinal segment of interest.

In a study comparing the accuracy of fluorescein administration with clinical judgment and Doppler ultrasound in determining viability in strangulated small intestine, fluorescein administration uniformly predicted viability correctly in cases of ischemic strangulating obstruction, but it was very poor in predicting viability in cases of hemorrhagic strangulating obstruction. The latter may result from reduction in fluorescence as a result of the presence of hemorrhage and edema, leading to an overly pessimistic interpretation of viability.[44] As opposed to viability of the small intestine, large intestinal viability may be more adequately assessed using the fluorescein technique. However, great caution has to be exercised when interpreting the results. For example, a patchy pattern of fluorescence is not necessarily an indication of nonviability, but if the fluorescent patches constitute a minor portion of the colonic surface, nonviability is likely. On the other hand, a diffuse granular pattern of fluorescence is usually indicative of tissue that is viable.[45]

Surface Oximetry

An alternative technique for assessing viability is the measurement of intestinal serosal surface oximetry, which is an indirect measure of tissue oxygenation. As with other techniques for assessment of viability, other circulatory factors have to be taken into consideration, including the overall cardiovascular status of the patient. A contact probe may be placed on the intestinal serosal surface, which measures surface oxygen partial pressure (P_{SO_2}). Normal P_{SO_2} values for the jejunum, ileum, and pelvic flexure of healthy anesthetized horses are 71 ± 20, 61 ± 8, and 55 ± 13 mm Hg, respectively.[46] This information has been used to assess the viability of the colon after correction of large colon volvulus. Overall, the accuracy of surface oximetry in predicting colonic viability was 88%, using a set point of 20 mm Hg surface oxygen tension.

Additional analyses revealed that a horse with a P_{SO_2} value of 20 mm Hg or less was 7.4 times more likely to die than a horse with a higher P_{SO_2} value. However, P_{SO_2} values have to be interpreted cautiously. In particular, the sensitivity of the technique was only 53% (calculated as the number of horses with an oximetry value of 20 mm Hg or less divided by the total number of horses that died), whereas the specificity was 100% (calculated as the number of horses that survived with an oximetry value of greater than 20 mm Hg divided by the total number of horses that survived). Thus, the technique is very useful for detecting horses that will survive, but predicting nonsurvival in horses with low P_{SO_2} values is very inaccurate.[47] The other major disadvantage of this technique is that it measures surface oxygen tension in focal areas of application and cannot be used to give an indication as to the viability of an entire region of intestine.[44]

Doppler Ultrasonography

Doppler ultrasonography has been used to discern viability on the basis of detection of flow through the microvasculature. A study described earlier (see "Fluorescein Dye") compared Doppler ultrasonography to use of clinical judgment and intravenous fluorescein.[44] Doppler ultrasonography was shown to be the most accurate technique for detecting viability in poststrangulated small intestine (accuracy values of 88%, 53%, and 53% for Doppler, clinical judgment, and fluorescein, respectively). The increased accuracy for Doppler ultrasonography was particularly evident in horses with experimental small intestinal hemorrhagic strangulating obstruction, in which viability was far more accurately determined with Doppler than other techniques. However, clinical judgment and fluorescein were slightly more accurate than Doppler for determining viability in experimental small intestinal ischemic strangulating obstruction.[44]

Luminal Pressure

Increased intraluminal pressure is correlated with nonsurvival in horses with small intestinal obstruction and is probably related to the degree of mucosal injury generated by compression of the intramural blood supply. For example, in one study, survivors and nonsurvivors with small intestinal lesions had mean pressures of 6 cm H_2O and 15 cm H_2O, respectively.[4] Although 15 cm H_2O is lower than the level that induced epithelial sloughing in experimental studies,[3] the duration of the pressure changes may be far greater in horses with naturally occurring lesions. Thus, a single pressure measurement may not be predictive of the severity of mucosal lesions without factoring in the duration of the disease. In horses with large colon volvulus, an increasing pressure is also correlated with nonsurvival.[48] Using a set value of 38 cm H_2O, survivors were separated from nonsurvivors (with a sensitivity and specificity of 89% and 91%, respectively), indicating that this test is highly accurate for predicting survival of horses with large colon volvulus.

Histopathology

The gross and histopathologic appearances of tissues were carefully evaluated in horses with naturally occurring large colon volvulus,[16] and a number of parameters described in this study were subsequently used to predict survival in horses with large colon volvulus. Biopsies were taken from the pelvic flexure (previously shown to accurately reflect mucosal changes along the length of the colon[43]) and histologically examined.[49] The study used biopsies fixed in 10% neutral buffered formalin or frozen in liquid nitrogen. Although the latter technique resulted in some loss of tissue detail, the authors did not feel that this impaired the use of these biopsies for determination of survival. Furthermore, frozen tissues would be required if this technique were to be used intraoperatively. However, postoperative evaluation of formalin-fixed specimens may provide useful information on horses that have survived surgery but that are experiencing major problems in the postoperative period. Owners may elect euthanasia in some cases, if the lack of postoperative progress is reinforced by histopathology that suggests nonviability of bowel remaining in the horse.

Specific parameters recorded on histologic evaluation in these studies included the percentage loss of surface epithelium, the percentage loss of glandular epithelium, and the width of the crypts and of the interstitial space between the crypts. The latter measurements were expressed as an interstitium-to-crypt width (I:C) ratio. Normal values for this ratio are 1 or less. Additional scored parameters included the degree of hemorrhage and the degree of edema (0, no edema or hemorrhage; 4, marked edema or hemorrhage), but these scores were not used in overall survival analyses. Colonic tissue was considered to be nonviable when the I:C ratio was greater than 3 and the loss of glandular epithelium was greater than 50%. Using these parameters, survival was correctly predicted in 94% of horses.[49]

REFERENCES

1. Dabareiner RM, White NA, Donaldson LL: Effects of intraluminal distention and decompression on microvascular permeability and hemodynamics of the equine jejunum, Am J Vet Res 2001;62:225-236.
2. Dabareiner RM, Sullins KE, Snyder JR, et al: Evaluation of the microcirculation of the equine small intestine after intraluminal distention and subsequent decompression, Am J Vet Res 1993; 54:1673-1682.
3. Allen DJ, White NA, Tyler DE: Morphologic effects of experimental distention of equine small intestine, Vet Surg 1988;17:10-14.
4. Allen DJ, White NA, Tyler DE: Factors for prognostic use in equine obstructive small intestinal disease, J Am Vet Med Assoc 1986; 189:777-780.
5. Hassel DM, Langer DL, Snyder JR, et al: Evaluation of enterolithiasis in equids: 900 cases (1973-1996), J Am Vet Med Assoc 1999; 214:233-237.
6. Meschter CL, Tyler DE, White NA, et al: Histologic findings in the gastrointestinal tract of horses with colic, Am J Vet Res 1986; 47:598-606.
7. Snyder JR, Pascoe JR, Olander HJ, et al: Vascular injury associated with naturally occurring strangulating obstructions of the equine large colon, Vet Surg 1990;19:446-455.
8. White NA: Intestinal infarction associated with mesenteric vascular thrombotic disease in the horse, J Am Vet Med Assoc 1981;178:259-262.
9. Dabareiner RM, Snyder JR, Sullins KE, et al: Evaluation of the microcirculation of the equine jejunum and ascending colon after ischemia and reperfusion, Am J Vet Res 1993;54:1683-1692.
10. Dabareiner RM, Sullins KE, White NA, et al: Serosal injury in the equine jejunum and ascending colon after ischemia-reperfusion or intraluminal distention and decompression, Vet Surg 2001;30:114-125.
11. Gerard MP, Blikslager AT, Roberts MC, et al: The characteristics of intestinal injury peripheral to strangulating obstruction lesions in the equine small intestine, Equine Vet J 1999;31:331-335.
12. Lundin C, Sullins KE, White NA, et al: Induction of peritoneal adhesions with small intestinal ischaemia and distention in the foal, Equine Vet J 1989;21:451-458.
13. Shepherd AP, Granger DN: Metabolic regulation of intestinal circulation. In Shepherd AP, Granger DN, editors: Physiology of Intestinal Circulation, New York, 1983, Raven Press.
14. Dart AJ, Snyder JR, Julian D, et al: Microvascular circulation of the small intestine in horses, Am J Vet Res 1992;53:995-1000.
15. Chiu CJ, McArdle AH, Brown R, et al: Intestinal mucosal lesion in low-flow states: I. A morphological, hemodynamic, and metabolic reappraisal, Arch Surg 1970;101:478-483.
16. Snyder JR, Olander HJ, Pascoe JR, et al: Morphologic alterations observed during experimental ischemia of the equine large colon, Am J Vet Res 1988;49:801-809.
17. McAnulty JF, Stone WC, Darien BJ: The effects of ischemia and reperfusion on mucosal respiratory function, adenosine triphosphate, electrolyte, and water content in the ascending colon of ponies, Vet Surg 1997;26:172-181.
18. Laws EG, Freeman DE: Significance of reperfusion injury after venous strangulation obstruction of equine jejunum, J Invest Surg 1995;8:263-270.
19. Arden WA, Slocombe RF, Stick JA, et al: Morphologic and ultrastructural evaluation of effect of ischemia and dimethyl sulfoxide on equine jejunum, Am J Vet Res 1990;51:1784-1791.
20. Arden WA, Stick JA, Parks AH, et al: Effects of ischemia and dimethyl sulfoxide on equine jejunal vascular resistance, oxygen consumption, intraluminal pressure, and potassium loss, Am J Vet Res 1989;50:380-387.
21. Meschter CL, Craig D, Hackett R: Histopathological and ultrastructural changes in simulated large colonic torsion and reperfusion in ponies, Equine Vet J 1991;23:426-433.
22. Moore RM, Muir WW, Granger DN: Mechanisms of gastrointestinal ischemia-reperfusion injury and potential therapeutic interventions: A review and its implications in the horse, J Vet Intern Med 1995;9:115-132.
23. Parks DA, Williams TK, Beckman JS: Conversion of xanthine dehydrogenase to oxidase in ischemic rat intestine: A reevaluation, Am J Physiol 1988;254:G768-G774.
24. Granger DN: Role of xanthine oxidase and granulocytes in ischemia-reperfusion injury, Am J Physiol 1988;255:H1269-H1275.
25. Grisham MB, Hernandez LA, Granger DN: Xanthine oxidase and neutrophil infiltration in intestinal ischemia, Am J Physiol 1986; 251:G567-G574.
26. Nilsson UA, Schoenberg MH, Aneman A, et al: Free radicals and pathogenesis during ischemia and reperfusion of the cat small intestine, Gastroenterology 1994;106:629-636.
27. Blikslager AT, Roberts MC, Gerard MP, et al: How important is intestinal reperfusion injury in horses? J Am Vet Med Assoc 1997;211:1387-1389.
28. Parks DA, Granger DN: Contributions of ischemia and reperfusion to mucosal lesion formation, Am J Physiol 1986;250:G749-G753.
29. Kubes P, Hunter J, Granger DN: Ischemia/reperfusion-induced feline intestinal dysfunction: Importance of granulocyte recruitment, Gastroenterology 1992;103:807-812.
30. Dabareiner RM, Snyder JR, White NA, et al: Microvascular permeability and endothelial cell morphology associated with low-flow ischemia/reperfusion injury in the equine jejunum, Am J Vet Res 1995;56:639-648.
31. Moore RM, Bertone AL, Bailey MQ, et al: Neutrophil accumulation in the large colon of horses during low-flow ischemia and reperfusion, Am J Vet Res 1994;55:1454-1463.
32. Moore RM, Bertone AL, Muir WW, et al: Histopathologic evidence of reperfusion injury in the large colon of horses after low-flow ischemia, Am J Vet Res 1994;55:1434-1443.
33. Prichard M, Ducharme NG, Wilkins PA, et al: Xanthine oxidase formation during experimental ischemia of the equine small intestine, Can J Vet Res 1991;55:310-314.
34. Horne MM, Pascoe PJ, Ducharme NG, et al: Attempts to modify reperfusion injury of equine jejunal mucosa using dimethylsulfoxide, allopurinol, and intraluminal oxygen, Vet Surg 1994; 23:241-249.
35. Reeves MJ, Vansteenhouse J, Stashak TS, et al: Failure to demonstrate reperfusion injury following ischaemia of the equine large colon using dimethyl sulphoxide, Equine Vet J 1990;22:126-132.
36. Park PO, Haglund U, Bulkley GB, et al: The sequence of development of intestinal tissue injury after strangulation ischemia and reperfusion, Surgery 1990;107:574-580.
37. Haglund U: Gut ischaemia, Gut 1994;35:S73-S76.
38. Dabareiner RM, White NA, Donaldson L: Evaluation of Carolina Rinse solution as a treatment for ischaemia reperfusion of the equine jejunum, Equine Vet J 2003;35:642-646.
39. Young BL, White NA, Donaldson LL, et al: Treatment of ischaemic jejunum with topical and intraluminal Carolina Rinse, Equine Vet J 2002;34:469-474.

40. Van Hoogmoed LM, Nieto JE, Snyder JR, et al: In vitro evaluation of an intraluminal solution to attenuate effects of ischemia and reperfusion in the small intestine of horses, Am J Vet Res 2002; 63:1389-1394.
41. Van Hoogmoed LM, Snyder JR, Nieto J, et al: In vitro evaluation of a customized solution for use in attenuating effects of ischemia and reperfusion in the equine small intestine, Am J Vet Res 2001; 62:1679-1686.
42. Nieto JE, Van Hoogmoed LM, Spier SJ, et al: Use of an extracorporeal circuit to evaluate effects of intraluminal distention and decompression on the equine jejunum, Am J Vet Res 2002;63:267-275.
43. van Hoogmoed L, Snyder JR, Pascoe JR, et al: Evaluation of uniformity of morphological injury of the large colon following severe colonic torsion, Equine Vet J Suppl 2000;32:98-100.
44. Freeman DE, Gentile DG, Richardson DW, et al: Comparison of clinical judgment, Doppler ultrasound, and fluorescein fluorescence as methods for predicting intestinal viability in the pony, Am J Vet Res 1988;49:895-900.
45. Sullins KE: Determination of intestinal viability and the decision to resect. In: White NA, Moore JN, editors: The Equine Acute Abdomen, ed 1, Philadelphia, 1990, WB Saunders.
46. Snyder JR, Pascoe JR, Holland M, et al: Surface oximetry of healthy and ischemic equine intestine, Am J Vet Res 1986;47:2530-2535.
47. Snyder JR, Pascoe JR, Meagher DM, et al: Surface oximetry for intraoperative assessment of colonic viability in horses, J Am Vet Med Assoc 1994;204:1786-1789.
48. Moore RM, Hance SR, Hardy J, et al: Colonic luminal pressure in horses with strangulating and nonstrangulating obstruction of the large colon, Vet Surg 1996;25:134-141.
49. van Hoogmoed L, Snyder JR, Pascoe JR, et al: Use of pelvic flexure biopsies to predict survival after large colon torsion in horses, Vet Surg 2000;29:572-577.

CHAPTER 35

Small Intestine

David E. Freeman

ANATOMY

The equine small intestine varies from 10 to 30 m in length, with an average length of approximately 25 m.[1] The duodenum, with an average length of 1 m, extends from the pylorus to the right of the midline, along the right dorsal abdomen, to a point caudal to the root of the mesentery. The duodenal ampulla and cranial flexure bend the first segment into the S-shaped sigmoid ansa. The major duodenal papilla (opening of the bile and pancreatic duct) and the minor duodenal papilla (opening of the accessory pancreatic duct) are located in the cranial flexure. Caudal to the right kidney, the duodenum is attached to the transverse colon by the duodenocolic fold. It forms the duodenojejunal flexure at its junction with the jejunum.

The jejunum measures 17 to 28 m in adult horses and is situated mainly in the left dorsal quadrant of the abdomen, between loops of small colon. The arterial supply from the cranial mesenteric artery is carried in arcades in the long mesojejunum (40 to 60 cm), which allows the jejunum much mobility. Each vascular arcade is composed of a major jejunal vessel, an arcuate vessel that forms a loop with the next jejunal vessel, and several vasa recta that pass from the arcuate vessels to the intestinal wall. Veins run parallel to the arterial supply and enter the portal vein to provide venous drainage. The ileum is 0.7 m long, and its length is marked by the distinct ileocecal fold that attaches its antimesenteric side to the dorsal band of the cecum.[1] The arterial supply is provided by the ileocecal artery, a branch from the cranial mesenteric artery that travels along the ileum to anastomose with the jejunal arteries.[2]

The terminal ileum forms a papilla that projects into the cecum. The ileal orifice is located in the center of the papilla, surrounded by the cecal musculature,[3] an annular fold of mucous membrane, and a venous network.[2,4] The muscle of the ileocecal papilla is composed of three layers: an inner circular layer, a central longitudinal muscle layer from the ileum, and an outer layer formed from the circular muscle of the cecum and arranged into two semicircular lips.[3,4] The papilla lacks a true sphincter, although the lumen of the ileum appears reduced at the ileocecal junction.[5] The proposal that the venous network and annular fold contribute to the sphincter mechanism[3,4] is rendered less tenable by the observation that the veins are most engorged when the ileum is discharging its contents into the cecum.[4] A functional sphincter does exist and appears to contract in synchrony with contractions of the cecal base.[5,6] Endoscopic studies of the cecal base of the horse have demonstrated that the ileal papilla is very prominent and that it becomes more prominent when the cecum is active.[4]

Digestive Anatomy

Digestion and absorption of nutrients take place predominantly in the upper half of the small intestine.[7] Unique to the small intestine in adults are finger-like projections of the epithelial surface called villi, and each villus is surrounded by approximately six to nine crypts of Lieberkühn.[8] The equine small intestine lacks mucosal folds and/or plicae circulares.[9]

Columnar absorptive cells or enterocytes constitute most of the small intestinal epithelial cells (about 90%), and the remainder are mucous (goblet) cells, enteroendocrine cells, Paneth cells, and undifferentiated columnar cells.[10] After at least two divisions within the crypt, the columnar cells migrate onto the villus as mature absorptive cells, and they are finally extruded at the villous tip, usually with a turnover time of 2 to 3 days.[8,11] Cells in the upper third of the villi are capable of surface digestion of nutrients and active transport of digestion products.

The apical surface of a mature enterocyte is arranged into microvilli that form a brush border membrane. Enterocytes are connected to each other by tight junctions that restrict

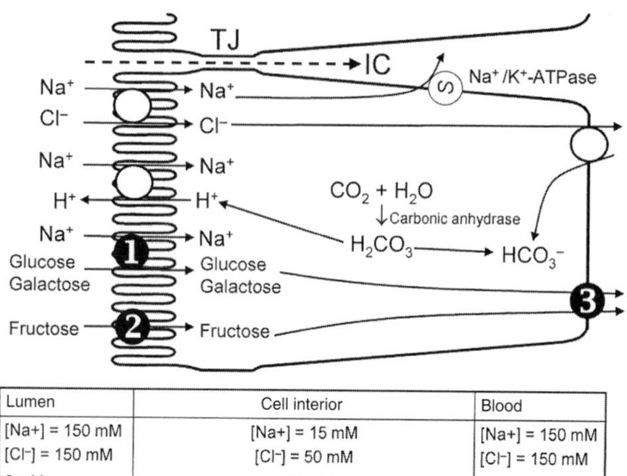

Lumen	Cell interior	Blood
[Na+] = 150 mM	[Na+] = 15 mM	[Na+] = 150 mM
[Cl-] = 150 mM	[Cl-] = 50 mM	[Cl-] = 150 mM
0 mV	– 40 mV	+ 5 mV

Figure 35-1. Role of sodium in providing energy for different transport systems in a surface epithelial cell of the small intestine. Examples are cotransport with chloride and exchange with hydrogen generated within the cell, as well as cotransport with glucose by the SGLT1 transporter *(1)*. Fructose movement from the lumen into the cell by facilitated diffusion through the GLUT5 transport system *(2)* does not require sodium. All absorbed monosaccharides diffuse down their concentration gradient into plasma through a GLUT2 passive transport mechanism *(3)*. The bottom panel gives approximate concentrations of sodium and chloride and potential differences across cell membranes. This illustrates that sodium enters the cell down its electrical gradient (–40 mV) and chemical gradient (15 mM, interior concentration) but exits against its electrochemical gradient, hence the need for the sodium pump, or Na^+/K^+–ATPase. *Arrow with a broken line* designates diffusion through the paracellular route, composed of the tight junction (TJ) and intercellular space (IC).

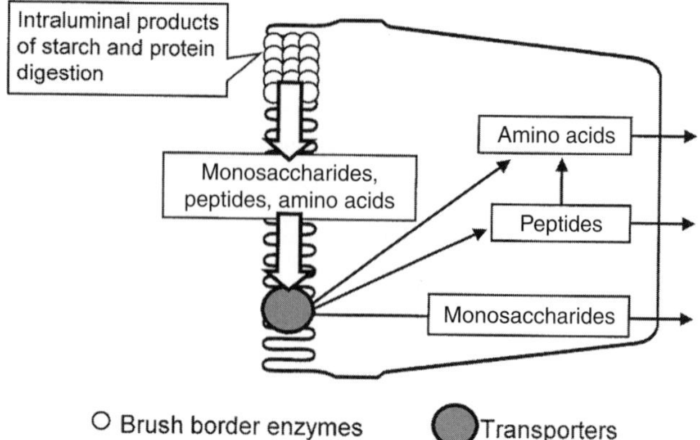

Figure 35-2. Role of brush border membrane in both digestion and absorption of products of intraluminal digestion of carbohydrates and proteins. Enzymes and transporters are simplified, but several oligosaccharidases, disaccharidases, and peptidases exist in the membrane, as well as highly selective carriers for their breakdown products. The largest peptides that can be transported into the cell are tripeptides.

the transmucosal flux of large molecules, although they are permeable to water and many low-molecular-weight substances[12,13] (Fig. 35-1). The intercellular space and the tight junctional complexes form the paracellular channel,[14] and the intercellular space expands during water absorption.[13] Enzymes that complete digestion of carbohydrates (disaccharidases) and proteins (peptidases) as well as various specific transport systems for absorbing digestive end products are located within the microvilli (Fig. 35-2).

PHYSIOLOGY

Intraluminal Digestion

Dietary carbohydrates, fats, and proteins are broken down by pancreatic enzymes in the small intestine, and their breakdown products are hydrolyzed further by brush border enzymes.[8,15] Hydrogen ion in the duodenum causes the release of secretin from S-cells, which stimulates the pancreas and liver to secrete HCO_3^- and water.[11,16] Bicarbonate neutralizes H^+ ions in the proximal small intestine and thereby prevents acid-pepsin damage to duodenal mucosa, provides a functional pH for pancreatic and brush border enzymes, and increases solubility of bile acids and fatty acids.[7] Protein and fat in the duodenum stimulate the release of cholecystokinin (CCK) from I-cells, and CCK causes the pancreas to secrete enzymes for the digestion of carbohydrates (amylase), fat (lipase), and protein (trypsin, chymotrypsin, carboxypeptidase, and elastase), as well as cofactors (colipase) that aid in enzymatic digestion.[7,16]

Trypsinogen, the precursor form (or zymogen) of trypsin, must reach the small intestine to be activated by the brush border enzyme enterokinase.[7] Other enzymes that are secreted as zymogens can be activated only by trypsin.

Resting pancreatic secretions in the horse are profuse, apparently continuous (10 to 12 L/100 kg body weight per day), and increased rapidly by eating.[17] The concentration of HCO_3^- is low, so that Cl^- remains the predominant inorganic anion in the horse's pancreatic secretion at all rates of flow.[17,18] Therefore, the pancreatic secretion may provide a source of anion (Cl^-) for exchange with HCO_3^- in the terminal ileum to buffer products of fermentation in the cecum and colon.[17,18] Although content and output of pancreatic enzymes is small in the horse compared with other animals,[17] digestion and absorption appear to be as efficient.[19]

In the liver, cholic acid and chenodeoxycholic acid[20] combine with glycine and taurine to form conjugated bile salts. Lipolysis in the small intestine requires emulsification of fat by bile salts.[7] Micelles form when the bile salts reach the critical micellar concentration (CMC) in the small intestine to aid in fat absorption (see "Fat Absorption," p. 403). Approximately 94% of bile salts are reabsorbed by the small intestinal mucosa, they pass to the liver, and they are then resecreted, a process called enterohepatic circulation of bile.[7,20] Active transport by a Na^+-dependent process in the ileum and by passive absorption in the jejunum combine to reclaim intraluminal bile. Secondary bile salts are produced from bacterial deconjugation and dehydroxylation of bile salts that are not absorbed in the small intestine and enter the colon. These secondary bile salts are lost in feces and are replaced continually by liver cells.[7,20]

Absorption of Ions and Water

Most water absorption takes place in the distal third of the small intestine, but the bulk of intestinal water is absorbed by the large intestine.[18] However, Na^+ and water absorption in the small intestine is important in absorption of nutrients and other ions.

The routes for transepithelial movement of ions and water (see Fig. 35-1) are through the cells (transcellular) and through the paracellular space (extracellular).[13,14] Transcellular movement of Na^+ involves entry from the lumen into the cell, down an electrochemical gradient. However, exit of Na^+ from the cell is against an electrochemical gradient and is therefore an active process that requires energy from the Na^+ pump (Na^+/K^+–ATPase), located along the basal and lateral membranes.[14,18] The active transport of Na^+ across the cell creates a transmucosal electrical potential difference.

The electrochemical gradient for Na^+ across the apical membrane has sufficient potential energy to move Cl^- into the cell against its electrical gradient. The cotransport of both ions is brought about by a carrier mechanism on the luminal membrane that is specific for Na^+ and Cl^- (see Fig. 35-1). The net movement of Cl^- by this mechanism is called secondary active transport.[21] The Na^+ gradient also energizes uptake of hexoses (glucose), amino acids, and most B vitamins against their chemical gradients into the cell.[21]

Water transport is passive, closely coupled to solute movement, and is primarily paracellular[14] (see Fig. 35-1). As absorbed Na^+ is pumped across the basolateral membrane, it creates an osmotic gradient that draws water into the intercellular space.[14,21] As water accumulates in this space, it increases the hydrostatic pressure, and this pressure forces the water across the basolateral membrane toward the capillary. Although the tight junction restricts backflow of absorbed water and electrolytes into the lumen, paracellular permeability and back-leak through this route is high in the jejunum. Therefore, Starling forces have a considerable influence on ion and fluid transport in the proximal bowel, just as in the proximal tubule of the kidney.[13,18]

Net water movement from lumen to plasma through the paracellular route will "drag" permeant ions and low-molecular-weight substances with it (sugars, amino acids, Ca^{2+}, and Mg^{2+}), and this mechanism is called solvent drag, or convection.[13,18] Fluid absorbed by the epithelium moves into the central lacteal of the villus, from which it moves into the deeper lymphatics.[14] There is little proof that the intestinal villus has a countercurrent multiplier that could enhance water and solute absorption, at least in the dog.[22]

Carbohydrate Absorption

Several brush border oligosaccharidases and disaccharidases hydrolyze initial products of starch digestion by amylase to produce monosaccharides, such as D-glucose, D-fructose, and D-galactose[8] (see Fig. 35-2). In horses on a grass-based diet, sucrase activity in the proximal small intestine is comparable to that reported in other nonruminants.[23] Maltase distribution is constant along the equine small intestine, and its activity is higher than in other species.[23] Lactase activity is higher in equine jejunum than in other parts of the small intestine, and it does decrease with maturity.[23]

D-glucose and D-galactose are transported across the enterocyte membrane by a high-affinity, low-capacity, Na^+-dependent cotransporter *type 1* isoform, SGLT1[8,23] (see Fig. 35-1). The major site of D-glucose uptake by the SGLT1 transporter in horses is the duodenum, followed by the jejunum and then the ileum.[23] Fructose moves from the lumen into the cell by facilitated diffusion through the GLUT5 transport system, which is a high-capacity, low-affinity, Na^+-independent transporter in the equine small intestine.[8,24] The monosaccharides diffuse down their concentration gradient in the absorptive cell into plasma through a GLUT2 passive transport mechanism and then enter the portal venous system.[7,8]

Protein Absorption

Small neutral peptides yielded by pancreatic peptidases are broken down by brush border oligopeptidases (see Fig. 35-2) into dipeptides and tripeptides or amino acids.[7,15] In the enterocyte, the peptides are hydrolyzed by cytoplasmic oligopeptidases into their constituent amino acids, which move passively into portal blood down a concentration gradient. Consequently, many dipeptides and tripeptides are transported into the cell, but mostly free amino acids enter portal circulation.[15] The intestine has several distinct amino acid transport systems, with varying degrees of specificity for amino acids and differences in Na^+ dependence.[15] The transport systems for small peptides are H^+ dependent.[15] Circulating and intraluminal amino acids can also be used by the intestinal epithelial cells as energy sources.[11]

Fat Absorption

Long- and medium-chain triglycerides are split into constituent fatty acids and monoglycerides by pancreatic lipase interacting with colipase.[7] The resulting long-chain fatty acids and 2-monoglycerides, as well as fat-soluble vitamins and cholesterol, must combine with bile acids to form a water-soluble mixed micelle.[25] This micellar solubilization facilitates movement of lipids through the unstirred water layer to the brush border, where the micelles release their components for absorption.[20] Because of their fat solubility, the released long-chain fatty acids and 2-monoglycerides can traverse the membrane down a concentration gradient. Fatty acids and 2-monoglycerides in the mucosal cell undergo reesterification and formation of chylomicrons, and chylomicrons are taken up by the lymphatics.[20]

Absorption of Iron, Calcium, and Magnesium

Iron transport is closely regulated to meet the body's needs. Some absorbed iron combines with an intracellular protein, called apoferritin, to form an iron complex called ferritin.[12,21] If no binding protein is available, absorbed ferrous iron is transported out of the cell through transferrin receptors and is released to the circulation.[21,26] If iron stores are low in the body, crypt cells migrating to the villus tip are low in apoferritin but high in basolateral transferrin receptor.[26] As ferrous iron enters the cell from the lumen, it is not bound and is therefore free to enter the circulation to replenish iron stores. On the other hand, with a large iron store in the body, the crypt cell reaches the villus tip as a mature cell high in apoferritin. As ferrous iron enters the cell from the lumen, it is therefore bound and stored, and this bound iron is lost as the cell exfoliates at the end of its life span.[12,26]

Lumen-to-plasma flux of calcium is highest in the duodenum.[12] A high concentration of dietary magnesium can decrease calcium absorption through competition for the calcium transport site.[12] Absorbed calcium enters the cell down an electrochemical gradient and is transported through the cytoplasm complexed with a specific calcium-binding protein.[12] This protein is regulated by the biologically active form of vitamin D, 1,25-dihydroxycholecalciferol. Extrusion from the cell is against an electrochemical gradient through the Ca^{2+}-ATPase.[12]

Magnesium absorption is of interest because magnesium sulfate is used as a laxative in horses, and the extent of absorption could alter its laxative effects and the risk for magnesium toxicity.[27] Mean magnesium absorption is approximately 40% to 70% in growing foals and mature ponies, and the absorption occurs primarily in the proximal small intestine.[28]

Intestinal Secretion

Crypts of Lieberkühn are located over the mucosal surface of the small intestine and they secrete an almost pure extracellular fluid that maintains chyme in a fluid state, delivers secretory IgAs, and flushes crypts of noxious and infectious agents.[14] Intestinal water and electrolyte secretion is determined primarily by Cl^- secretion by crypt cells, with movement of Na^+ and water following. Intestinal secretion is under a degree of neural and eicosanoid tone.[29]

Protective mucus is secreted by mucous cells located extensively over the surface of the intestinal mucosa, and by Brunner's glands, which are located in the first 9.6 m of the equine duodenum.[9] The function of mucus from Brunner's glands is to protect the duodenal wall from digestion by gastric secretions.

Motility

Small intestine has an outer longitudinal smooth muscle and an inner circular muscle layer, and the latter is divided into a thick outer lamella and a thin inner lamella.[30] Rhythmic segmentation in circular smooth muscle and synchronous shortening of the longitudinal muscle causes aborad transit during peristalsis.[31] The interstitial cells of Cajal are thought to act as pacemakers[32] for the generation of electrical slow waves that propagate into the longitudinal muscle layer.[30]

Two basic components of myoelectrical activity of gastrointestinal smooth muscle are the slow wave (basic electrical rhythm, or electrical control activity) and the action potential ("spike potential"). Slow waves are phasic oscillations of the smooth muscle resting membrane potential that are considered responsible for the rhythmicity and polarity of intestinal contractions.[32,33] In the pony, as in other animals, slow-wave frequency is greater in the duodenum and decreases toward the ileum.[33] This determines the direction and propagation rates of associated motility.[34]

An action potential is generated if something lowers the threshold of the smooth muscle cells, allowing a slow-wave oscillation to reach a threshold and cause a rapid depolarization that triggers intestinal contractions.[34] Mechanical (stretch), neural, and hormonal stimuli determine if that threshold will be reached. Action potentials do not necessarily occur with every slow wave, but slow-wave frequency determines the maximal frequency of action potentials.[34]

These wave forms produce a distinct pattern of myoelectrical activity called the migrating motor complex (MMC).[34] Three phases of activity are recognized. Phase I, or no spiking activity (NSA), has slow waves only and no action potentials (Fig. 35-3). Phase II, or intermittent or irregular spiking activity (ISA), has intermittent action potentials on some slow waves. Phase III, or regular spiking activity (RSA), is evident as an action potential for every slow wave and thus is associated with intense, sustained contractions.[34-36] The MMC is always present during an "interdigestive state" (time between meals when stomach and small intestines are essentially empty) and plays an important role in reducing bacterial colonization in the small intestine.[34] Phases II and III are associated with intestinal contractions, and most of an ingested meal is moved through the small intestine by phase II activity.

Control of Motility

Control of motor events in the small intestine involves myogenic, neural, and hormonal mechanisms. Neural control involves the vagus nerve and components of the sympathetic nervous system, as well as an intrinsic system called the enteric nervous system.[32] The enteric nervous system consists of ganglia in the myenteric (Auerbach's) plexus and the submucosal (Meissner's) plexus, and it mediates reflex behavior independent of input from the brain or spinal cord.[32] Myenteric neurons are the main source of innervation of longitudinal muscle and the outer lamella of circular muscle.[30] Submucosal neurons innervate the inner lamella of circular muscle.[30] Hormonal control of motility involves neurotransmitters and other neural agents that act on intestinal smooth muscle. Motilin, a peptide produced by endocrine cells in the mucosa of the proximal small intestine, is released during fasting, and it regulates the interdigestive migrating motor complex.[37] A coordinated release

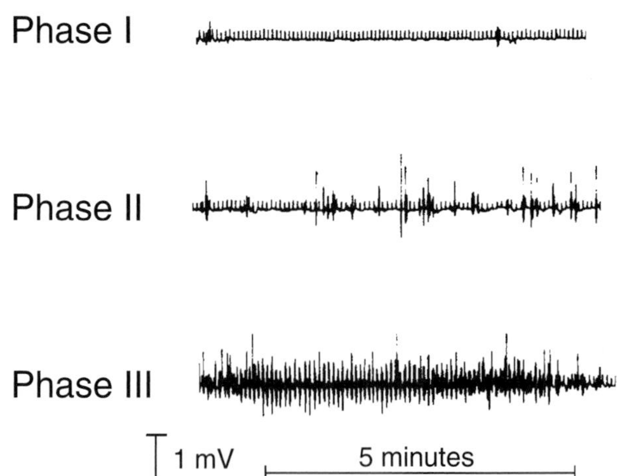

Figure 35-3. Myoelectrical activity of the duodenum of a clinically normal horse, demonstrating all components of the migrating motor complex (phases I through III). The slow wave frequency is about 14 per minute in all segments. (Modified from Merritt AM, Burrow JA, Hartless CS: Effect of xylazine, detomidine, and a combination of xylazine and butorphanol on equine duodenal motility, Am J Vet Res 1998;59:619-623, with permission.)

of excitatory and inhibitory transmitters coordinates the peristaltic reflex responsible for propulsive activity.[30]

Motility of the Ileum

The migrating action potential complex (MAPC) can be recorded in the pony ileum[38] as intense spike bursts of short duration that propagate rapidly aborally,[39] but they are absent in the pony jejunum.[35,40,41] In the ileum of mature ponies, all phases of the MMC can be recorded, but irregular spiking activity (phase II) predominates during the interdigestive period (the period between feeding).[38] Withholding food for 24 hours decreases the frequency of ileal MAPC, but it has no effect on mean slow-wave frequency, MMC phase distribution, MMC phase duration, MAPC conduction velocity, or conduction velocity of spike bursts in RSA.[38] Differences between the ileum and the jejunum in ponies might be related to the unique position of the ileum at the junction of the small and large intestines.

The MAPC is seen directly before retrograde cecal myoelectric activity 73% of the time, indicating a possible myoelectric coupling of the ileum and cecum, and it may be responsible for transit of digesta from the ileum to the cecum.[38] Also, ileal contents are discharged into the cecum at times when the cecum is inactive.[4] Ileal and cecal filling appear to be more important in regulating ileocecal motility events in ponies than stimuli associated with feeding.[38]

Local stimulation of chemoreceptors could be important in the regulation of ileal motility in the horse[5,42] and humans.[6] Also, the human ileum, and possibly the equine ileum, act as reservoirs, discharging contents into the cecum in response to intraluminal stimuli.[6] At neutral pH, tonic activity of the human ileum, but not of the jejunum, is increased by intraluminal short-chain fatty acids, whereas bile acids and lipids can induce ileal relaxation.[6] In the pony, serotonin and luminal fatty acids increase ileal peristalsis.[5] The response to luminal acidification could stimulate ileal emptying of refluxed bacteria and cecal contents[6] and could thereby augment the sphincter function of the ileal papilla.[5,42] Although tone of the ileal papilla increases during contractions of the cecal base in horses, some cecal contents do reflux into the ileum.[5,42]

Sympathetic relaxation of ileal smooth muscle is mediated mainly by activation of β-atypical receptor subtypes,[43] and increased ileal sphincter tone is mediated through α1 receptors.[6] Whereas epinephrine decreases ileal and cecal activity, it increases ileal sphincter tone through α1 receptors.[5,42]

Altered Motility

Xylazine, atropine, meperidine, butorphanol, and pentazocine can increase the mean duration of MMC in pony distal jejunum, whereas flunixin meglumine, dipyrone, metoclopramide, and panthenol have no effect.[35,41] Xylazine and butorphanol (as separate treatments) reset the duodenal MMC in the horse, but without serious disruption of proximal gastrointestinal tract motility.[44,45] However, routine doses of xylazine, detomidine, or a xylazine and butorphanol combination significantly reduce pressure peaks in the duodenum.[46] Common anesthetic regimens decrease myoelectric activity in horse ileum for up to 150 minutes after induction.[36]

After small intestinal resection and anastomosis in the dog, the aboral progression of the MMC stops at the anastomotic site, and alternate pacemakers initiate regular spiking activity distal to the anastomosis.[47] In the distal segment, the number of phases are reduced, disrupted, and delayed, and transit time is delayed also.[47,48] Therefore, timing of the MMC appears to depend on bowel continuity and integrity of intrinsic innervation.[49]

Nonstrangulating obstruction of distal jejunum causes immediate continuous spiking activity proximal to the obstruction.[50] This response is not associated with fluid distention and does not cause signs of colic until accompanied by increased intraluminal pressures.[50] Occlusion of blood supply to the pony ileum decreases motility in the ischemic bowel, increases motility in the more proximal segment, and has no effect on the distal segment.[51] A low dose of endotoxin and intravenous infusion of prostaglandin E_2 alter regular spiking activity in pony jejunum, which suggests a role for endotoxin in postoperative ileus.[52,53] The effects of endotoxin can be partly blocked by pretreatment with phenylbutazone and flunixin meglumine. Increased sympathetic stimulation could decrease intestinal motility in horse jejunum and be relevant to development of ileus.[31] Nitric oxide also appears to act as an inhibitory neurotransmitter to circular smooth muscle of equine jejunum and could be released from invading macrophages in distended or inflamed small intestine.[54]

PATHOPHYSIOLOGY

Small Intestinal Distention

Intestinal obstruction causes prestenotic distention with gas, fluid, and ingesta that can compress intestinal veins.[55] Most of the resulting increase in venous pressure is transmitted to the capillary beds, and consequently capillary pressure increases.[56] The intestinal wall becomes thicker because of edema induced by increased capillary filtration.[56] The resulting filtration of fluid from capillaries into the interstitium is opposed by changes in Starling forces that attempt to maintain the tissues in a more dehydrated state.[56] As these compensatory mechanisms become overwhelmed, continued capillary filtration increases tissue edema and movement of fluid in large volumes into the intestinal lumen, producing a net secretion of fluid into the intestine.[57,58]

An experimentally induced intraluminal pressure of 25 cm H_2O (18.4 mm Hg) for 120 minutes in equine jejunum causes shortening of villi, loss of mesothelial cells, neutrophil infiltration, edema in the seromuscular layer, and a decreased number of perfused vessels in the seromuscular layer as well as in the mucosa.[59] Decompression of distended equine jejunum may not prevent progression of the morphologic lesions, but it permits partial recovery of vascular density.[59] Serosal edema and infiltration with erythrocytes and leukocytes increases significantly after distended equine jejunum is decompressed, and to a greater extent than in reperfused ischemic jejunum.[60] These serosal changes could contribute to complications in distended bowel proximal to an obstructive lesion, such as serosal adhesions.[59,60]

Small Intestinal Ischemia

Venous occlusion occurs rapidly when thin-walled veins are compressed by the edges of a hernial ring or by twisting of mesentery. The increased venous pressure causes edema and net secretion of fluid, as well as a myogenic response (the *Bayliss effect*) that protects the tissues from an increased vascular load.[56] This effect increases vascular resistance to arterial inflow, which combines with the decreased pressure gradient from artery to vein to reduce blood flow.[56] This response, coupled with arterial compression caused by displacement, eventually blocks arterial inflow and causes ischemia. Erythrocytes extravasate through altered capillaries and cause the characteristic intramural hemorrhage, which is known as *hemorrhagic infarction*.[61] Equine jejunum strangulated in a closed space[62] develops tissue changes more slowly than in the open abdomen model[61,63] and therefore might be more representative of a naturally acquired strangulation.

Because ischemia reduces oxygen delivery to the metabolically active mucosa, morphologic changes develop that can be graded in severity from grade I (development of a subepithelial space, called Gruenhagen's space, and slight epithelial lifting at the villus tip) to grade V (complete loss of the villus architecture, with severe mucosal hemorrhage and loss of the lamina propria).[64] The intermediate grades represent a progressive loss of the epithelial layer, starting at the villus tip.[64] As a consequence of this mucosal damage, the important epithelial barrier is lost, and endotoxin can leak across to the peritoneum and be absorbed into the circulation, causing endotoxemia.[65]

In a pattern similar to that seen in other animals, the equine jejunal villus is supplied by an eccentrically placed arteriole that spirals to the villus tip and then "fountains" into a meshlike capillary network that descends along the periphery of the villus to drain into one to three venules.[66] This creates a countercurrent mechanism that allows capillaries near the villus base to "shunt" oxygen from the tip, rendering it more sensitive to hypoxia relative to the rest of the villus.[65] However, this does not appear to be the only or even the most important explanation for the sensitivity of villus cells to anoxia, because anoxic injury to equine jejunum in vitro causes the same progression of epithelial damage.[67] Most likely, cells on the villus tip are the first to succumb to anoxia because they are closer to the end of their life span.

Intestinal smooth muscle is more resistant to hypoxia than mucosa, and crypt cells are more resistant than villus cells—factors that can play a part in recovery from an ischemic insult.[63,64] In the early stages of mucosal repair, viable cells migrate from the crypts to cover the exposed villus stroma, whereas damaged cells are removed by detachment and phagocytosis.[68] This repair process is called *restitution,* and it explains how equine jejunum subjected to a grade IV injury becomes covered with stunted villi, lined with cuboidal epithelium, within 12 hours.[63,68] Normal architecture of the mucosal lining is restored rapidly from this point. Although the intestinal wall can recover from venous strangulating obstruction, mesentery subjected to hemorrhage and edema is prone to fibrosis, shortening,[63] and adhesions.[61] Serosal edema and infiltration with erythrocytes and leukocytes increase significantly after ischemia/reperfusion in equine jejunum to an extent that could predispose to adhesions.[60]

Other factors that can contribute to the mucosal injury in ischemic intestine are those that alter capillary permeability, such as endotoxin, reactive oxygen metabolites, histamine, and activated neutrophils[65] (for an in-depth discussion of intestinal injury, see Chapter 34).

DIAGNOSIS OF SMALL INTESTINAL OBSTRUCTION

Preoperative prediction of a small intestinal versus large intestinal lesion is highly successful,[69] but identification of the specific intestinal lesion is rarely possible, except for strangulation in an external hernia. Clinical findings vary enormously, and small intestinal diseases that require surgery are difficult to distinguish from those that can respond to medical treatment, such as duodenitis–proximal jejunitis and ileal impaction.

Horses with small intestinal strangulating obstruction usually exhibit signs of acute, severe abdominal pain and hypoperfusion, have an elevated heart rate and packed cell volume, and develop acidosis. The signs of distal obstructions develop more slowly, and the electrolyte imbalances and cardiovascular responses are less severe initially than with proximal lesions. Horses with proximal jejunitis may have severe abdominal pain initially; this progresses to depression and less pain than in horses with ileal impaction[70] or strangulating obstruction.[71] After gastric decompression, horses with proximal enteritis usually improve in overall attitude and their heart rate decreases, whereas horses with mechanical obstructions do not improve.

Distended loops of small intestine on rectal palpation indicate small intestinal obstruction from any cause. In studies on horses with small intestinal strangulation, distended loops were palpated in 50% to 98% of horses on which a rectal examination was performed.[72-74] In some horses with small intestinal strangulation, a large colon abnormality can be found on palpation per rectum[72,73] that may not be evident at surgery.[72] Many severely dehydrated horses with small intestinal diseases develop a "vacuum-packed" large colon, evident on rectal palpation as dehydrated colon contents contained within prominent colon haustra. These should not be mistaken for large colon impactions but might be considered as highly suggestive of small intestinal strangulation.[73] The degree of intestinal distention is very variable, with severe distention more likely to be associated with a strangulating lesion than with ileal impaction or proximal enteritis. The amount of gastric reflux varies from none in the early stages of a lesion in the distal part of the small intestine, to several liters with a long-standing lesion or a lesion in the proximal part of the small intestine. Borborygmi are usually diminished or absent in all small intestinal diseases.

Abdominal distention is negligible to moderate in adult horses with small intestinal obstruction but can be pronounced in foals. Abdominal pain can be difficult to assess in foals with small intestinal strangulation because they can alternate between periods of violent colic and periods of depression. The latter can be interpreted erroneously as evidence of improvement. Inability to perform a rectal palpation in foals further complicates their examination, but ultrasonography is very informative in foals.

Peritoneal Fluid Analysis

Analysis of peritoneal fluid is important, but abdominocentesis is not necessary if other clinical findings indicate the need for surgery. Although the complications of enterocentesis are rare, peritonitis and abdominal wall cellulitis may develop after puncture of distended bowel.[75] The risk of enterocentesis is greater in foals than in adult horses, although ultrasonography can identify fluid pockets to be sampled and also gives an impression of the volume and solid contents of the fluid.[76] Omentum can prolapse through the puncture site in a foal if a needle of 18 gauge or larger is used.

The nucleated cell count in peritoneal fluid of normal adult horses ranges from 5000 to 10,000 cells per microliter, but more than 1500 nucleated cells per microliter should be considered elevated in foals.[76,77] Peritoneal fluid protein concentration is within the same range in foals as adults (0.3 to 1.8 g/dL).[76,77] Peritoneal fluid usually becomes serosanguineous with a strangulating lesion, but this is not a consistent finding, especially early in the disease. Accidental blood contamination does not appear to significantly affect nucleated cell count and total protein concentration in a peritoneal fluid sample.[78] Strangulated bowel in an inguinal hernia or intussusception is less likely to alter the peritoneal fluid than an intra-abdominal lesion but can produce serosanguineous fluid with elevated nucleated cell count and total protein.[79-82] Small intestinal rupture or perforation will produce changes in peritoneal fluid suggestive of digesta contamination, such as cloudy or green discoloration, increased protein and cell count, and intracellular bacteria; however, normal cell counts and protein can also be recorded and plant material may not be evident.[83]

Peritoneal fluid from horses with proximal enteritis is rarely serosanguineous, and nucleated cell count and total protein concentration increase to a lesser extent than with a strangulating obstruction.[71,84] Therefore, peritoneal fluid is of some value in distinguishing between these diseases. Total protein can be elevated and eosinophils found in peritoneal fluid from horses with focal eosinophilic enteritis, a cause of small intestinal obstruction in horses.[85] Peritoneal and serum phosphate levels can be used to predict major intestinal injury, although the ranges in horses with surgical and nonsurgical colic can have considerable overlap.[86] (For an in-depth discussion of diagnostic approaches to the horse with colic, see Chapter 33.)

Gastrointestinal Tract Imaging

Ultrasonography is invaluable for examining horses with small intestinal obstruction. Liberal application of alcohol and gel to the horse's hair coat are sufficient to improve acoustic coupling in most horses without clipping, but clipping of long hair coats can improve image quality.[87] Most abnormalities gravitate to the ventral abdomen, where they are accessible for ultrasonography.[87] A lower-frequency ultrasound transducer should be used (2 to 3.5 MHz) to penetrate deeper into the abdomen (approximately 24 cm) and higher-frequency transducers (5.0 or 7.5 MHz) can improve image detail in foals or superficial structures.[87]

Small intestinal strangulating obstruction, peritonitis, peritoneal effusion, bowel rupture, intussusception, inguinal hernia, diaphragmatic hernia, cholelithiasis, abdominal neoplasia, abdominal abscess, and ascarid impactions can be detected by ultrasonography.[76,79,88-90] Transabdominal ultrasonographic findings of small intestine that is edematous (wall thickness greater than 3 mm), distended, and amotile strongly suggest strangulating obstruction[76,88] (see Figs. 33-1 and 33-2). As obstructed small intestine fills with fluid, its contents become more hypoechoic. The five ultrasonographic layers of the intestinal wall are lost in strangulated segments.[91] Ultrasonography may be helpful in assessing gastric distention and in determining the efficacy of gastric decompression. The stomach can be located on the left side of the abdomen between the 11th and 13th intercostal spaces, at the level of the shoulder, dorsal to the splenic hilus and its large splenic vein.[87] The greater curvature of the stomach is seen as a bright gas echo that curves toward the skin surface, deep to the spleen. Distention of the stomach can displace the spleen caudally or obscure it.[87]

Regardless of the motility status, abdominal ultrasonography can provide a sensitivity of 98%, a specificity of 84%, a positive predictive value of 62%, and a negative predictive value of 99% for small intestinal strangulation obstruction from a variety of lesions.[88] Under the same conditions, palpation per rectum can provide a sensitivity of 50% for small intestinal strangulation obstruction, which means that it is considerably inferior to ultrasonography in finding a small intestinal abnormality when one does exist.[88] In horses with small intestine strangulated in the epiploic foramen, ultrasonography could accurately detect small intestinal distention in 94% to 100% of horses, compared with 74% to 78% for palpation per rectum.[73,92] With this lesion, distended or edematous small intestine is found more often in the ventral right paralumbar fossa, caudal ventral abdomen, and middle right paralumbar fossa.[88] For strangulating lipomas, similar intestinal changes are found more often in the caudal ventral abdomen, middle ventral abdomen, and ventral right paralumbar fossa than in other regions[88] (see Chapter 33).

Abdominal radiography is useful in the foal with gastroduodenal obstruction, necrotizing enterocolitis, enteritis, impaction, displacement, intussusception, ruptured viscus, congenital anomalies, and inguinal hernia, and in the adult horse and foal with diaphragmatic hernia.[76] In foals, radiographs can distinguish small intestinal distention from large intestinal distention with gas.[93] Contrast radiography has been used in foals to demonstrate abnormalities of gastrointestinal transit time and gastrointestinal obstruction[94] (see Chapters 32 and 33).

Laparoscopy

Although diagnostic laparoscopy has a sensitivity of 82% and a specificity of 66% for horses with acute abdominal pain, localized lesions or lesions inaccessible to the selected portals cannot be detected, and ileal lesions, such as ileocecal intussusception and ileal hypertrophy, can be missed.[95]

Duodenal lesions can be seen in the standing horse.[95] Care must be taken when inserting the trocar assembly into the abdomen in a horse with colic to avoid damage to distended viscera[76] (for details on this technique, see Chapters 14 and 33).

SURGICAL DISEASES OF THE SMALL INTESTINE

In nine reports from referral institutions, 25% to 64% of all colic cases involved small intestinal diseases (Table 35-1), with a median of 34%.[73,96-103] The proportion was the same in foals as in adults.[102,104] The ileum was involved in 41% to 46% of all small intestinal obstructions.[101,103,105] The majority of small intestinal colics (58% to 85%) are caused by strangulating lesions, and the remainder by nonstrangulating obstruction (simple and functional obstructions).[96,97,100,103,106] Rankings of disease prevalence must consider that the prevalence of different lesions can vary considerably between clinics (see Table 35-1).

Nonstrangulating Obstruction

Ileal Impaction

Impaction of the ileum is usually a primary condition in an apparently normal ileum, but it can occur secondary to other ileal diseases. The impaction forms a doughy-to-solid, tubular mass up to 90 cm long that extends proximally from the ileocecal junction.[70,107-110] The disease has a regional distribution in the United States, with most cases diagnosed in the Southeast, where the high prevalence may be related to feeding coastal Bermuda grass hay.[70] Ileal impaction also occurs in parts of the United States and in Europe where coastal Bermuda grass hay is not fed.[97,105] The disease appears to be more common in the United States from June through November, especially in the fall,[107,110] although a seasonal effect was not found in one study.[111] In that study, the risk for impaction was not reduced by combining coastal Bermuda hay with other hay, it appeared to be increased by recent introduction or feeding poor-quality hay, and it appeared to be lowered by feeding a pelleted-concentrate feed in addition to hay.[111] The disease has been reported in a wide age range,[107,108] including newborn[112] and older foals.[102] In a large series of cases, mares and Arabian Horses were significantly overrepresented.[109]

In the United Kingdom, where coastal Bermuda grass hay is not fed, ileal impaction was strongly associated with both coprologic and serologic evidence of tapeworm infection in horses.[113] This was supported by a study of 78 horses in North Carolina, which showed that feeding coastal Bermuda hay and failure to administer pyrantel pamoate (effective against tapeworms) placed horses at risk for ileal impaction.[111] Mucosal ulceration and submucosal edema caused by tapeworms at the ileocecal valve is proportional to the number of parasites present and could predispose to obstruction at that site.[113] Orbatid mites are the intermediate hosts for *Anoplocephala perfoliata* and their preference for humid regions (southeast)[113] could also contribute to the geographic predisposition to ileal impaction in the United States.

Early pain from ileal impaction is attributed to spasmodic contraction of the bowel around the impaction, but pain becomes more severe and constant as small intestinal dis-

TABLE 35-1. Prevalence of Small Intestinal Diseases That Cause Colic

	% of Total Cases of Colic	% of All Cases of Small Intestinal Colic	Ileum Involved as % of All Ileal Obstructions	References
Volvulus	3.8-7.3	7-28	3	96, 97, 98, 100, 105, 137, 208, 326
Volvulus (foals)	15-19	39-50	—	93, 102
Epiploic foramen	2.1-8.4	5-23	15	73, 74, 92, 96-98, 100, 105, 137, 186, 188, 196, 326
Ileal impaction (United States)	6.5-7.4	2.2-23	—	99, 107, 110, 196
Ileal impaction (Europe)	3.7-11	5.5-17	12-42	96, 97, 100, 103, 105, 326
Proximal enteritis	1.5-7	3-22	—	97, 99, 100, 326
Lipoma	0.3-11	0.5-41	9	96, 97, 98, 100, 105, 137, 188, 196, 200, 202, 208, 326
Intussusception (all types)	0.8-5.2	1.5-29*	13	82, 97, 98, 100, 105, 137
Mesenteric rent	2.4-4.6	4.8-13.4	4	97, 98, 100, 105, 137, 196, 208
Mesenteric bands	1.1-4.6	4.4-13.4	13	96, 97, 98, 105
Inguinal/scrotal hernia	0.08-2.8	2.4-11	4-15	96, 97, 98, 103, 105, 137, 196, 208
Gastrosplenic ligament	1.2-2.5	1.1-7.3	—	97, 98, 196
Thromboembolic disease	1.8-2.6	3.5-6.3	—	98, 100
Ileal muscular hypertrophy	0.14-2	0.6-5.5	12	96, 100, 105, 196
Intussusception (ileocecal)	1.9-3.2	3.3-5	12.5	82, 103, 196
Umbilical hernia	0.4-1.4	1.7-3.7	3	96, 97, 98, 105, 137

Diseases recorded for all ages combined, but prevalence among foal diseases is also given, where available. Not all diseases were listed in all reports.

*This is an unusually high prevalence for this lesion among all small intestinal lesions, but it was the most common small intestinal lesion in this study.[137]

tention progresses.[70] Small intestinal distention is generally a consistent rectal examination finding, and the impacted ileum is more easily palpated early in the disease course before small intestinal distention becomes severe.[70,107,108] Gastric reflux can be obtained in most horses but not all, depending on the duration of obstruction.[107,109,110] Distinction between ileal impactions, strangulating obstructions, and proximal enteritis cases can be difficult (see preceding).

Medical treatment is a viable alternative if surgery is excluded by a lack of finances and can be successful early in the disease, when the impaction can be felt per rectum.[70,108] Medical treatment consists of a balanced electrolyte solution administered intravenously at 5 L every 2 hours and flunixin meglumine at a rate of 0.5 mg/kg three or four times daily.[70] Mineral oil should be administered when gastric reflux has ceased. If surgery is required, the impaction is broken down by manual massage, aided by mixing it with fluid from the proximal bowel or from saline infusion.[110] Although dioctyl sodium sulfosuccinate has been included in the infusion, this is a very irritating drug to mucosal surfaces. Excessive manipulation can cause serosal damage and adhesions, enterotomy is contraindicated in all except rare instances, and jejunocecostomy[109] is not recommended in the absence of a predisposing lesion or severe changes in the muscle wall.[70,110,111]

If treated early, the prognosis is favorable,[108,110] although ileus, gastric rupture, laminitis, mucosal necrosis, and perforation of the ileum are complications when the diagnosis is delayed.[107] Re-impactions are rare.[114] Because tapeworms may play a role in this disease, anthelmintics are recommended, such as pyrantel pamoate at 6.6 mg/kg to 13.2 mg/kg[111] and dewormer combinations approved by the U.S. Food and Drug Administration, with praziquantel as the active ingredient against tapeworms.

Muscular Hypertrophy of the Ileum

Muscular hypertrophy of the ileum can cause ileal impaction, but it is more likely to cause recurrent colic. Unlike the muscular hypertrophy that develops proximal to a chronic obstruction, ileal hypertrophy causes marked luminal constriction (Fig. 35-4). The condition is considered idiopathic.[115] Chronic mucosal inflammation can cause smooth muscle hypertrophy in rats,[116] but mucosal inflammation may[117] or may not[118] be evident in ileal hypertrophy in horses. Ileal hypertrophy and rupture were documented in a pony distal to an ileocecostomy that had been performed 3 years previously to bypass a short, reducible ileocecal intussusception.[119] At the time of the original surgery, that segment of ileum had been judged to be normal.

The affected segment is usually 1 m long, and both the circular and longitudinal layers are increased in thickness[115,120] and diverticula are common (see Fig. 35-4). Full-thickness rupture can occur.[115,120,121] The terminal segment of ileum and the ileocecal junction are spared in some cases.[101,115] The distal jejunum can undergo compensatory hypertrophy in longstanding cases but with an increase in lumen diameter.[120]

The disease has been reported in horses over a wide age range,[115] including foals,[121] but it is most common in mature horses.[101,115,117,118,120] There does not appear to be a breed predilection.[120]

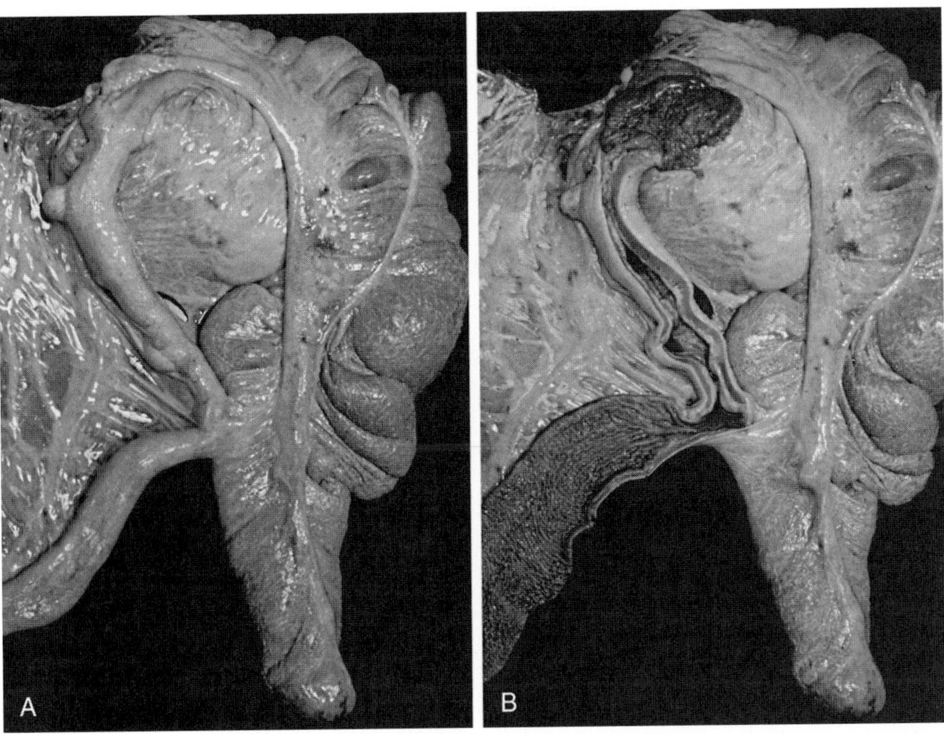

Figure 35-4 A, Ileal muscular hypertrophy treated 1 year previously by side-to-side incomplete bypass. Note the prominent diverticula and tubular appearance of the ileum. Death was from a nonrelated cause. **B,** The horse seen in **A,** with jejunum and ileum opened to demonstrate the thick wall of the ileum and the narrow lumen compared with normal bowel, as well as the diverticula.

Most horses are presented with a history of recurrent, low-grade colic of variable duration, up to 2.4 years in one case.[120] Partial anorexia and weight loss are common. The involved segment was palpated per rectum in 20% of horses in one study.[120] Clinical findings and history are similar to those of horses with chronic ileocecal intussusception, but most cases have been described in older horses (more than 5 years).[101,115,117,118,120]

Side-to-side ileocecostomy or jejunocecostomy with or without transection or removal of part of the ileum (incomplete bypass) is usually successful[101] (see Fig. 35-4). The stoma is made proximal to the constricted segment, and if the space between the ileum and cecum is large, it is not closed.[101]

Ascarid Impactions

Intestinal stages of *Parascaris equorum* can cause small intestinal obstruction, intussusception, abscessation, and rupture in foals and weanlings (median age of 5 months, range of 4 to 24 months).[122] Affected foals usually appear parasitized and unthrifty. Impaction usually (54%) follows shortly after anthelmintic treatment.[122] Ascarids in feces and in gastric reflux are of no diagnostic value because of the high prevalence of this parasite in foals. Ultrasonographic examination can demonstrate ascarids in the small intestine.[89] Recent evidence that *Parascaris equorum* can acquire resistance to ivermectin[123] could mean that foals and young horses are at increased risk for this disease.

Some ascarid impactions can be resolved manually or by typhlotomy, and these cases seem to have the best prognosis, possibly because they have minimal small intestinal damage.[124] Enterotomy is required to evacuate the impaction in more severe cases (Fig. 35-5), although resection is indicated if the bowel is devitalized.[102,122] Not all the worms can be removed at surgery, regardless of method, and anthelmintic treatment after surgery is recommended.[124] Postoperative mortality can be as high as 92%, with focal necrotizing enteritis, peritonitis, abscess formation, and adhesions accounting for most deaths.[122,124] Reasons for such a poor prognosis after surgery include undetected ascarid-induced damage in the intestinal wall, release of toxins from the ascarids, release of antigenic proteins after organophosphate-induced rupture of the cuticle, preexisting debilitation, low-grade liver disease, low-grade pneumonia, and failure to remove all worms at surgery.[124]

Prevention of ascarid impaction requires a sound deworming program, careful environmental management, and fecal egg counts to assess anthelmintic efficacy. Foals should be wormed at 6 weeks of age, and again at 6-week intervals for 6 months.[124] In heavily parasitized foals at high risk for impaction, concurrent administration of mineral oil with an anthelmintic agent is recommended. However, the choice of anthelmintic is controversial, which reflects a lack of information on the role of anthelmintics in the disease process.[124] Some recommend a rapid kill or complete paralysis to prevent impaction from worms undergoing agonal contortion (piperazine, organophosphates).[124] Others recommend a slower kill that would allow gradual elimination of worms in groups too small to induce impaction (fenbendazole, ivermectin, or pyrantel pamoate).[124]

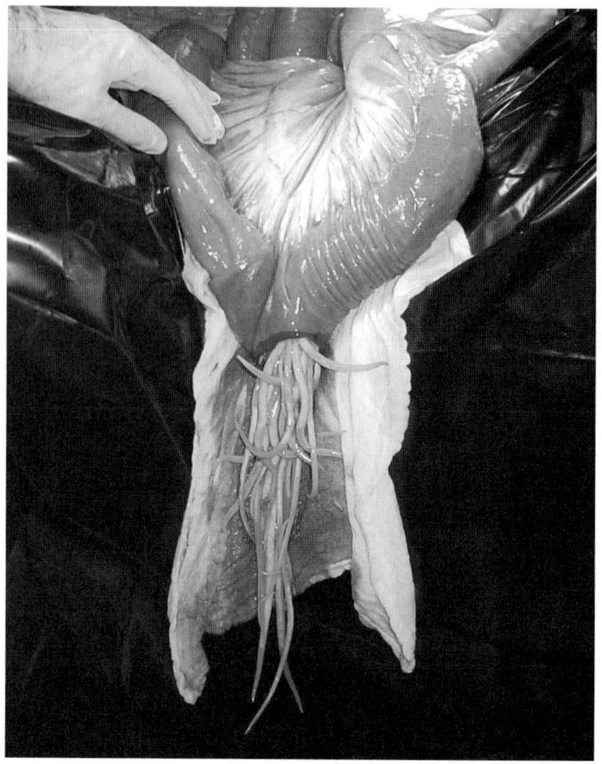

Figure 35-5. Removal of impacted ascarids through an enterotomy in the jejunum. Note that small intestine on the left is dimpled at sites where ascarids remain attached as they are drawn through the incision.

If ivermectin resistance is a problem, fenbendazole at 10 mg/kg PO should be effective.[123]

Duodenitis-Proximal Jejunitis

Duodenitis-proximal jejunitis (DPJ), also called gastroduodenitis-jejunitis, hemorrhagic fibrinonecrotic duodenitis, proximal jejunitis, proximal enteritis, and anterior enteritis, involves inflammation of the proximal part of the small intestine, fluid accumulation in the stomach and small intestine, and endotoxemia. The cause is unknown. Severity of clinical signs varies over a wide range, and age, breed, and sex predispositions have not been established. Although usually diagnosed in horses over 1½ years of age,[71] it does occur in nursing foals. The prevalence of the disease has been reported as 3% to 22% of all small intestinal colics, which is less common in some clinics than volvulus, strangulation in the epiploic foramen, and ileal impaction, and more common than strangulation by lipoma.[96-99] Prevalence in California is lower than in other parts of the United States and Europe, and the disease appears to be more severe in the southeastern United States[84] than in the Northeast.[71]

The clinical hallmark of the disease is nasogastric reflux of a large volume of fluid (usually greater than 48 L in the first 24 hours) in a horse that demonstrates signs of mild to severe pain initially and then depression.[125] Most horses with DPJ have tachycardia, prerenal azotemia, dehydration, hypotension, and electrolyte abnormalities. In contrast to horses with strangulating lesions, horses with DPJ can have a fever, leukocytosis, and a greater volume of gastric reflux.[71,84]

After gastric decompression, a horse with DPJ usually demonstrates relief from pain and becomes quiet, and its heart rate decreases, whereas a horse with mechanical obstruction improves little if at all. On rectal examination, the degree of small intestinal distention with DPJ is subjectively less than with ileal impaction.[70] Peritoneal fluid from horses with DPJ is rarely serosanguineous, and nucleated cell count and total protein concentration increase to a lesser extent than with a strangulating obstruction.[70,71]

The most important goals in treatment of horses with DPJ are frequent gastric decompression, correction of disturbances in water and electrolyte homeostasis, and restoration of normal intestinal function. Horses must be kept off food and water until it is concluded that the condition has resolved, and attention should be paid to calcium and potassium, both of which can become depleted in horses with intestinal injury and decreased food intake. Rate of fluid administration and the types given should be largely determined by clinical and laboratory evidence of hydration status and electrolyte balance.

Flunixin meglumine can attenuate the hemodynamic responses to lipopolysaccharide (endotoxin) and reduce lipopolysaccharide-induced increases in plasma concentrations of thromboxane and prostaglandins.[126] Nonsteroidal anti-inflammatory drugs also could block the effects of lipopolysaccharide on intestinal motility that could exacerbate or sustain ileus in horses with DPJ. Antilipopolysaccharide antibodies in plasma products, such as J5 *Escherichia coli* or Re *Salmonella* mutants could be used; however, there is some controversy regarding efficacy.[126] The amphipathic cyclic polypeptide antimicrobial drug polymyxin B can avidly bind with the lipid A and thereby remove lipopolysaccharide from the circulation,[126] although nephrotoxic side effects in dehydrated horses are valid concerns with use of this drug. Pentoxifylline, a methylxanthine derivative, can reduce lipopolysaccharide-induced production of cytokines and thromboxane in horses.[126] Antibiotic use in DPJ is controversial, but horses in one study received metronidazole (2 g IV, then 1 g IV twice a day) and procaine penicillin (4.5 g IM twice a day), based on a high rate of positive cultures of gastrointestinal contents for *Clostridium perfringens*.[127] Treatment could include prokinetic drugs to improve gastric emptying and small intestinal motility (see paragraphs on postoperative ileus in Chapter 39). Prophylaxis against development of laminitis should be considered, including confinement in a sand stall or on deep wood shavings and application of frog support.

Surgery is performed in at least 6% of cases.[71,125] At surgery, the serosal surface of affected bowel appears smooth, with bright to dark red petechial and ecchymotic hemorrhages and mild edema. Although the prognosis is considered to be reduced by surgery in some areas in the United States, in two studies survival was similar in horses that underwent surgery as in those that did not.[125,128] In a recent report, 40 of 42 horses (95%) recovered rapidly and completely after surgical decompression, suggesting that a prompt recourse to surgery could be indicated for this disease.[127] In addition to a favorable outcome, other advantages of prompt surgical treatment are avoiding delay if a physical cause of obstruction cannot be ruled out and early return of normal circulation and peristalsis to the distended intestine.[127] However, all forms of DPJ might not respond favorably to this treatment, and the longer period of inactivity necessitated by surgery could be a disadvantage.[127] Also, regardless of the procedure used, horses with DPJ that undergo surgery are at risk for obstructive adhesions.

Reported survival rates for DPJ range from 25%[84] to 94%,[71,125] and recurrence is rare.[128] Anion gap, abdominal fluid total protein concentration, and volume of gastric reflux in the first 24 hours were significantly associated with death by univariate analysis.[125] Laminitis is a life-threatening complication of DPJ and the risk is greater in horses with hemorrhagic reflux at the time of admission.[129] The considerable cost of prolonged medical treatment can necessitate euthanasia in protracted cases.

Neoplasia

Obstruction of the gastrointestinal tract by intestinal wall tumors is rare. Lymphosarcoma, adenocarcinoma, ganglioneuroma, intestinal carcinoid, leiomyosarcoma, and leiomyoma have been reported to cause small intestinal obstruction in the horse.[130-137] Horses are presented with a single bout of acute colic or with repeated bouts of mild colic and will respond well to surgical removal of the tumor, if it is discrete, focal, and accessible.[130,132,133,135] Resection of an isolated lymphosarcoma lesion can be curative, but this is generally a multiorgan disease with a grave prognosis.[131]

Gastroduodenal Obstructions

Duodenal inflammation, ulcers, stenosis, and perforation can develop in foals, particularly those treated with phenylbutazone or subjected to stress, surgery, transportation, or illness.[138] Foals younger than 4 months are at greater risk, although duodenal obstruction has been reported in yearlings and in an adult horse.[94,138-140] The incidence of gastroduodenal obstructions has decreased because of increased awareness and earlier treatment with antiulcer medication.[94] Duodenal obstruction can cause reflux of duodenal contents into the bile and pancreatic ducts, inducing diffuse cholangiolitis, perilobar hepatitis, and pancreatitis, with acute erosive and fibrinous inflammation of the large ducts.[138]

Many affected foals are depressed, weak, and anorectic in the days or weeks preceding diagnosis. Clinical signs of duodenal ulcers and obstruction are teeth grinding (odontoprisis), salivation, gastric reflux, fever, diarrhea, and signs of colic (e.g., dorsal recumbency).[94] Abdominal pain may be worse after nursing. Rupture of duodenal ulcers causes signs of peritonitis.[138]

Diagnostic signs on plain radiographs include aspiration pneumonia, dilated fluid-filled esophagus, and gastric distention.[94] Gas may be evident in the hepatic duct.[94] Endoscopy is more sensitive and specific than radiography in diagnosing gastric and duodenal lesions,[76,94] although ultrasonography could be used to demonstrate any abnormalities in duodenal peristalsis, wall thickness, and lumen size.[141,142]

Surgical bypass of the obstruction[94,140] should be followed by medical treatment of gastric ulcers[94] (see Chapter 32). Contrast radiographs are recommended 24 hours after surgery to confirm successful bypass of the obstruction. Barium in dilated bile ducts after surgery is indicative of cholangitis or cholangiohepatitis.[94]

Intestinal Inflammation and Fibrosis

A number of diseases characterized by inflammation or fibrosis in the small intestinal wall have been identified as causes of colic in horses. Intestinal fibrosis has been reported as a cause of weight loss and colic in horses in a small geographic distribution in Colorado,[143] but the disease appears to be more widespread and the signs more variable than originally reported.[144] Equine proliferative enteropathy from *Lawsonia intracellularis* infection in the small intestine causes weight loss, colic, hypoproteinemia, and diarrhea in weanling foals.[145,146] Although erythromycin alone or with rifampin is an effective treatment,[145] resection or bypass of the affected segment may be required.[146]

Eosinophilic gastroenteritis is a well-known but poorly understood cause of colic, diarrhea, and weight loss in horses.[85] In one series of cases, weight loss was not a feature, but affected horses had colic from jejunal obstruction with a red intramural mass or circumferential plaque of fibroplasia and infiltration on the antimesenteric surface.[85] The seasonal distribution of the cases corresponded to the grazing period, suggesting a dietary association.[85] Treatment by complete or wedge resection was successful because of the focal nature of the lesions.[85]

A similar but distinct cause of acute or chronic colic is characterized by small, focal to multifocal, well-demarcated areas of intestinal thickening and fibrosis that form constrictive mural bands in the jejunum and other parts of the intestinal tract.[147] These are free of mucosal ulceration and granulomatous response, but they have histologic evidence of lymphocytic, plasmacytic, and eosinophilic infiltration of all layers, and most lesions are associated with the vasculature.[147] Treatment with surgical resection or medical treatment with corticosteroids can be effective.[147]

Pythiosis caused by *Pythium insidiosum* is a granulomatous disease, typically of skin and subcutis, that is most commonly diagnosed in the Gulf Coast states but also in the Midwest.[148] Jejunal obstruction caused by *P. insidiosum* granuloma can cause weight loss and signs of mild, intermittent abdominal pain.[148] Reported cases have been amenable to resection,[148,149] which can be successful.[149]

Miscellaneous Simple Obstructions

Duodenal obstruction in horses can cause severe pain, gastric reflux is voluminous, and some horses have spontaneous gastric reflux through the nostrils.[70,150] Impactions of the duodenum and jejunum are rare, and causes include impacted feed material,[70,151,152] compressed cracked corn,[153] trichophytobezoar,[154] compacted wood fragments,[155] persimmon fruit,[156,157] molasses-based stable treats,[150] baling twine,[158] and a cholelith.[159] The stomach, duodenum, and jejunum can become impacted intermittently, and weight loss can develop in horses that consume ripe persimmon fruits during fall and winter in the South.[156,157] The ripe persimmons at that time are palatable to animals,[157] and water-soluble tannins in the fruit form a solid phytobezoar when exposed to gastric acid.[156] Diagnosis can be confirmed by identifying persimmon seeds in the gastric impaction on gastroscopy.[156]

Small intestinal perforation by wire,[160,161] a porcupine quill,[162] ulcers,[163] and unidentified causes may lead to diffuse or localized peritonitis, localized intestinal necrosis, and even occlusion of mesenteric vessels.[160] Localized lesions can be resected.[160,162] A recent report describes jejunal perforation in three young horses that were presented with fever, acute colic, depression, and hypovolemic shock.[83] No cause could be identified for the discrete perforations, 1.5 cm or smaller, in an otherwise healthy segment of jejunum.[83]

Congenital segmental aplasia of jejunal lymphatics may cause chyloperitoneum and colic in foals within 12 to 36 hours after birth.[164,165] Resection of the thickened intestine can produce a satisfactory outcome,[165] but mild cases can respond to conservative treatment. Ruptured lymphatics and chyloperitoneum can also develop secondary to tearing of postsurgical mesenteric adhesions and other intestinal lesions.[166] An ileal diverticulum that is not a remnant of the omphalomesenteric structures[167] (see later), other rare forms of intestinal malformation,[168] and congenital jejunal duplications have been described as causes of recurrent small intestinal obstruction in horses.[169] Extraluminal causes of simple obstruction include intra-abdominal abscesses,[100] intramural hematoma[170] (Fig. 35-6), and adhesions.

An idiopathic disease of the duodenum reported in three horses older than 12 years is characterized by mural thickening and marked distention in approximately 30 cm of duodenum.[171] The distention starts 20 cm from the pylorus and ends in a contracted segment with aganglionosis, immediately proximal to the caudal duodenal flexure.[171]

Strangulating Obstruction

Volvulus

Volvulus is defined as a rotation of more than 180 degrees in a segment of jejunum, or in jejunum and ileum, about the mesentery. Most are 360-degree rotations[72] and involve long segments of intestine (Fig. 35-7). Volvulus may develop as a primary displacement or as secondary to preexisting

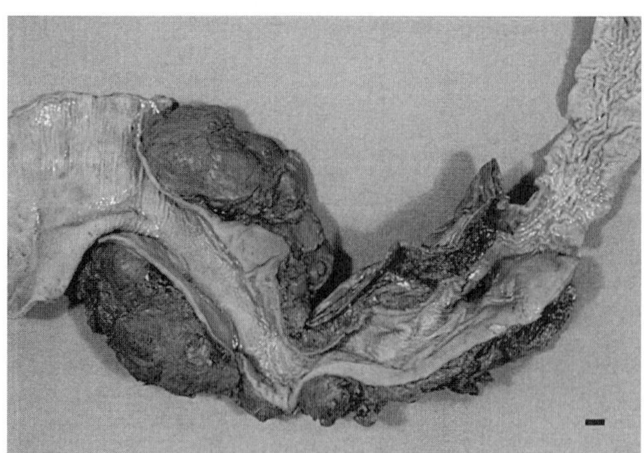

Figure 35-6. Intramural hematoma that caused an obstruction in the jejunum by collapse of the intestinal lumen. Note the healthy mucosa in the affected segment. *Bar,* 1 cm.

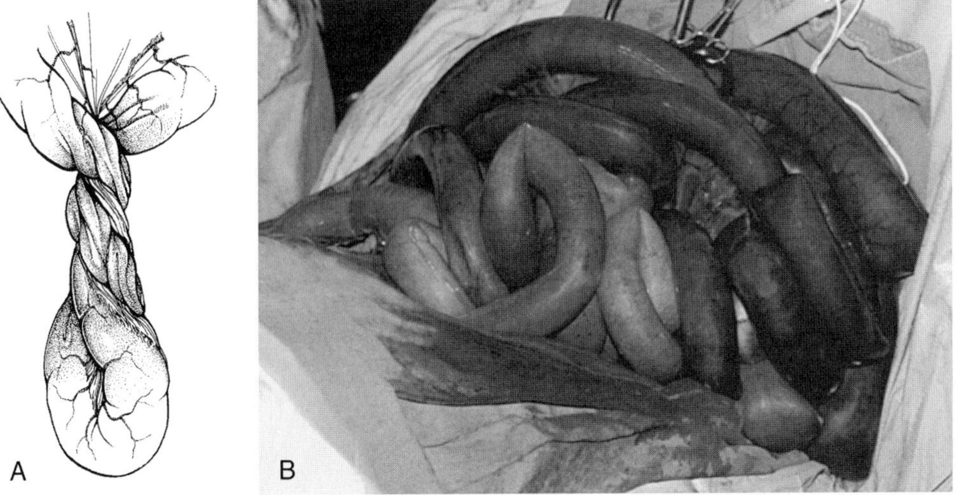

Figure 35-7. Small intestinal volvulus. **A,** Diagram. **B,** Intraoperative presentation. Note typical appearance of numerous coils of distended and ischemic small intestine stacked one on another.

lesions, such as an acquired inguinal hernia,[79,172,173] a mesodiverticular band,[174] a Meckel diverticulum,[175] strangulation in mesenteric rents,[174] distention from any cause, and fixation by vitelloumbilical bands[176] and adhesions.[177] Primary volvulus can affect a horse of any age, but it is the most common indication for intestinal surgery in foals,[102] especially those between 2 and 4 months of age (see Table 35-1). In the most common form of volvulus, the mesentery twists the intestine into distinct spirals. Volvulus nodosus is a less common form of volvulus, formed by the ileum and jejunum undergoing a 360-degree torsion that forms a mesenteric pouch in which prestenotic jejunum becomes entrapped.[178,179] Distention of the entrapped bowel draws the ileum into the mesenteric pouch to form a tight loop that knots the entrapment.[179] Volvulus nodosus is seen typically in foals 2 to 7 months of age,[179] and it can account for 27% of small intestinal lesions that require surgery in foals.[93]

Clinical signs are typical of acute small intestinal strangulating obstruction, and stacks of tightly distended small intestine can be palpated per rectum. In foals, severe pain seems to alternate with periods of depression, and the abdomen becomes markedly distended. Treatment involves correction of the volvulus, followed by resection and anastomosis (see later). Correction can be difficult in foals and adults with volvulus nodosus,[178] but it can be accomplished by massaging the contents of the entrapped loop into the proximal segment, thereby allowing the bowel to be pulled through the ring formed by the ileum.[179] If the bowel involved in a volvulus nodosus is necrotic, time can be saved by resecting the entire lesion without reduction, followed by a jejunocecostomy.[179]

Entrapment in the Epiploic Foramen

The epiploic foramen, or foramen of Winslow, is the 4-cm-wide entry into the vestibule of the omental bursa from the peritoneal cavity. Its dorsal and craniodorsal boundary is the visceral surface of the base of the caudate process of the liver[180] (Fig. 35-8). The portal vein contributes to the

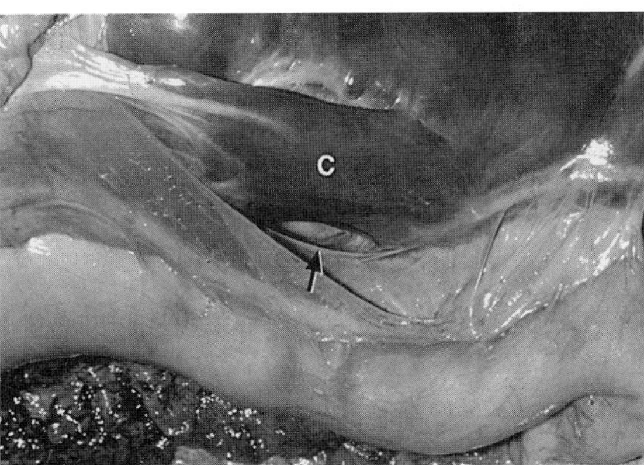

Figure 35-8. Epiploic foramen as viewed from the right side with the duodenum in the foreground, the liver dorsally, and with the cranium to the right. The *arrow* points to the ventral edge of the foramen formed by the gastropancreatic fold. C, caudate lobe.

cranioventral border, and the gastropancreatic fold becomes evident as a band where it forms the ventral border of the foramen.[180] From 8 cm to 18 m of intestine can become incarcerated in this space.[73,74,181,182] Variations include simultaneous strangulation of two loops of small intestine, strangulation of the cecum by the involved small intestine,[173] simultaneous incarceration of the cecum and jejunum, incarceration of a Meckel's diverticulum (Littre's hernia),[74] a parietal (or Richter's) hernia of the ileum,[183] a parietal hernia of the duodenum,[184] and impaction in the incarcerated segment.[185] Entrapment in the epiploic foramen (EFE) can occur from right to left[181]; however, one study reported left-to-right entrapment (Fig. 35-9) in all of 53 horses,[73] another reported it in 138 of 143 horses,[74] and another in 97% of horses.[186] The ileum was involved in 66% to 72% of cases, either alone (12% to 25%) or in combination with the jejunum (41% to 60%), and involvement of the jejunum alone occurred in 28% to 34% of cases.[73,74,92,186] The longer the duration of colic, the more likely that ileum will become involved in the strangulation.[74]

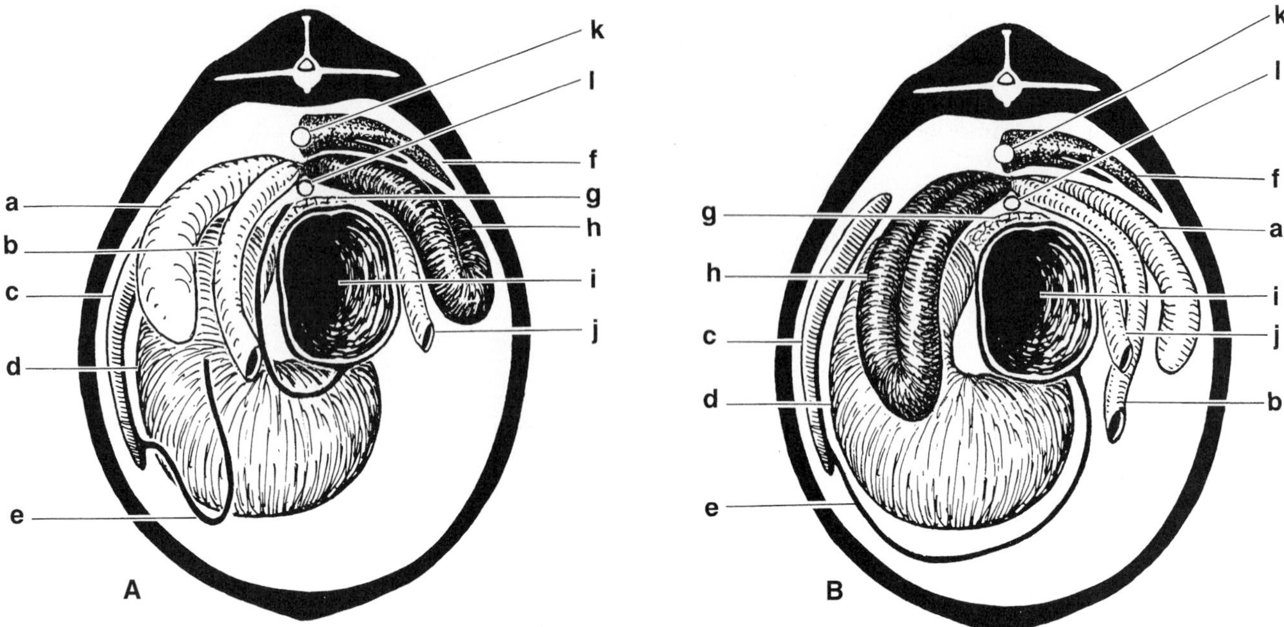

Figure 35-9. Epiploic foramen strangulation. Left to right (**A**) and right to left (**B**) herniation of the small intestine through the epiploic foramen. a, jejunum proximal to strangulation; b, jejunum distal to strangulation; c, spleen; d, stomach; e, greater omentum, torn during strangulation; f, liver; g, pancreas; h, strangulated loop; i, right dorsal colon; j, duodenum; k, vena cava; l, portal vein.

The apparent predisposition to EFE in older horses and the predisposing enlargement of the epiploic foramen with age[187] were not confirmed in recent studies.[180,188] Horses of all ages can be affected, including foals, and horses 11 months to 3 years.[73,74,93,180-182,188-190] In some of the larger studies, 47% to 71.3% of horses were under 11 years old,[74,180,188] and no horse over 20 years was reported with this disease.[73,74,182,188] Some studies found Thoroughbreds and Thoroughbred crosses to be at a higher risk,[73,181,186,191] and males constituted 68.5%[74] and 76%[73] of cases in two studies. In one study from the United Kingdom, 74% of the cases were seen between November and March, mainly in January, suggesting that stabling played a role in cause of this disease.[186] According to data from one U.S. and one U.K. university hospital, up to 68% of horses with EFE were cribbers before surgery, compared with 6% to 10.4% in the control groups, significant evidence that cribbing is associated with this disease.[192]

Clinical findings can be confusing. In one study, 38% of horses with herniation of small intestine through the epiploic foramen did not show signs of abdominal pain at the referral hospital, and in 52% of these horses no gastric reflux was obtained.[73] The signs of abdominal pain were sufficiently mild in one case to cause delay of referral for 2½ days.[193] Changes in the peritoneal fluid do not always represent the extent of intestinal damage.[73,182] Traction on the ventral band of the cecum is reported to induce a painful reaction in horses with the ileum incarcerated in the epiploic foramen[173]; however, this test was not reliable in one report.[182] With transabdominal ultrasonography, distended or edematous small intestine is found more often in the ventral right paralumbar fossa, followed by the caudal ventral abdomen and the middle right paralumbar fossa.[88]

At surgery in most cases, strangulation in the epiploic foramen can be corrected by careful traction combined with pushing of the strangulated bowel in the same direction. Careful milking of fluid into the empty and collapsed distal segment may be necessary to decompress the strangulated bowel. If possible, nonstrangulated bowel can be drawn into the foramen so that distention of the strangulated segment can be reduced by spreading its contents into the nonstrangulated bowel.[73] To avoid tearing the dorsal aspect of the portal vein and causing fatal hemorrhage during traction,[73,181,194] bowel should be drawn in a horizontal direction and not upward to the abdominal incision.[195]

When bowel cannot be drawn back through the epiploic foramen by these methods, jejunum approximately 1 m proximal to the obstruction must be emptied through an enterotomy or by transection.[195] The empty segment of jejunum is subsequently drawn through the foramen. After reduction, abnormal bowel is resected to include the transection or the enterotomy sites.

The short-term survival rate after completed surgery for EFE varies from 63% to 88%,* and the long-term survival rate varies from 35% to 70%.[73,92,182,186] Although these numbers compare favorably with other small intestinal strangulations, an earlier study reported 18% survival[190] and a recent study reported 50% survival[196] after completed surgery. In recent studies on long-term survival after colic surgery, EFE was the only categorical variable associated with decreased survival[197] and horses with this lesion were more than four times as likely to have relaparotomy than horses with other colics.[198] Fatal hypoglycemia, a large thrombus in the portal vein, and areas of ischemic necrosis in the liver have been reported in a horse after treatment of an epiploic entrapment.[199] Rupture of the portal vein is a complication of correction.[73,181,194]

*References 73, 74, 92, 97, 182, 186.

Pedunculated Lipoma

A pedunculated lipoma is a benign, smooth-walled fat tumor that is suspended by a thin mesenteric pedicle of variable length. It can be a solitary tumor, or several of them can be found in the same horse, with 90% found in the small intestine and 9% in the small colon.[200] Some can develop in the omentum. Mesenteric lipomas are usually located close to the root of the mesentery and cause strangulating obstruction when the pedicle wraps around intestine and its mesentery (Fig. 35-10). A large lipoma attached close to the intestine can cause simple, recurrent obstruction, but this is uncommon.[201,202] In general, the length of the stalk rather than the size of the tumor seems to influence the risk for strangulation.

Intestinal strangulation by a mesenteric lipoma is a disease of older horses, with a mean age of 14 to 19.2 years at diagnosis,[98,188,200,202,203] and the youngest reported at 8 years.[203] Incidence of lipomas is five times higher in horses older than 15 years compared with 10- to 15-year-old horses.[180] Ponies, Arabians, and Quarter Horses have been reported to be at a higher risk, whereas Thoroughbreds are at a lower risk for this disease.[180,203] Not all affected horses are overweight.[202] Four studies revealed a significantly higher risk for geldings.[200,202,203]

Pedunculated lipomas should always be suspected in old horses with clinical evidence of strangulating obstruction, although clinical signs can be subtle and not always suggestive of this lesion.[202] In one study, 6 of 17 horses did not show signs of pain at the referral institution.[202] Consequently, this disease can be confused with duodenitis–proximal jejunitis, especially in horses with a large volume of reflux.

At surgery, the lipoma can be found wrapped in the jejunal mesentery, and the involved intestine can be difficult to exteriorize. Blind resection of the pedicle is necessary in many cases but carries the risk of creating a mesenteric rent and mesenteric bleeding.[136] Spontaneous rupture of the lipoma pedicle and correction of the obstruction has been reported, based on surgical findings.[204] Incidental lipomas with distinct pedicles should be removed with the ligate divide stapler (see Fig. 17-10), by ligation and transection. Small, broad-based tumors should not be removed because they are less likely to cause problems and their removal creates a mesenteric defect that should be sutured. A significant association between postoperative ileus and strangulation by lipoma has been reported,[198] and published short-term survival rates for this strangulation range from 48%[203] to 78.6%.[202]

Intussusception

Jejunojejunal, jejunoileal, and ileoileal intussusceptions are reported in the horse.[82] Suspected predisposing factors are segmental motility differences caused by enteritis, heavy ascarid burden, infection with the tapeworm *Anoplocephala perfoliata*, mesenteric arteritis, and abrupt dietary changes.[82,205] A transverse enterotomy,[206] functional side-to-side anastomosis,[207,208] end-to-end anastomosis,[209] and pedunculated mucosal mass, such as a papilloma, leiomyoma, cryptococcal granuloma, granuloma of unknown cause, and carcinoid, can form the leading edge of a jejunojejunal intussusception in horses.[81,82,210,211]

Ileocecal intussusception is the most common type[98] and constituted 74% of all small intestinal intussusceptions in one report, with 27% of these causing chronic, intermittent colic.[80] Chronic ileocecal intussusceptions represented approximately 1% of all surgical colic in one study.[212] Horses with a chronic intussusception usually have a short intussusceptum that is not strangulated but causes an incomplete obstruction. Ileoileal intussusceptions usually form a short, doughnut-like lesion, and most cause chronic recurrent colic.[82,213-215] Jejunojejunal intussusceptions (Fig. 35-11) usually involve long segments of bowel and cause complete obstruction,[81] although short intussusceptions can cause recurrent colic.[81,215]

With chronic intussusceptions, the repeated bouts of obstruction cause compensatory changes in almost half the jejunum proximal to the lesion (Fig. 35-12), including marked jejunal dilation, even when empty; thickening of the muscular coat; and areas of ecchymosis along the

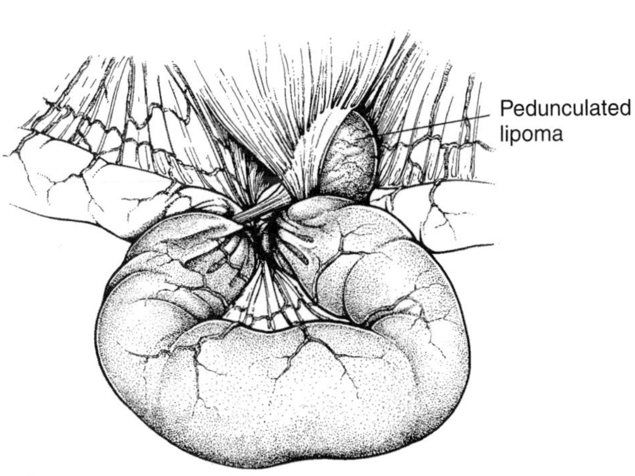

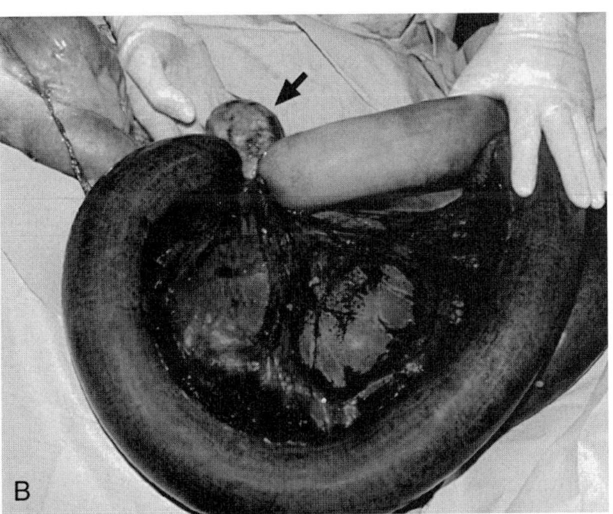

Figure 35-10. A, A pedunculated lipoma causing strangulation obstruction of the small intestine. **B,** Intraoperative presentation (the *arrow* points toward the lipoma). (**A** Redrawn from McIlwraith CW, Robertson JT: Equine Surgery: Advanced Techniques, ed 2, Oxford, UK, 1998, Blackwell.)

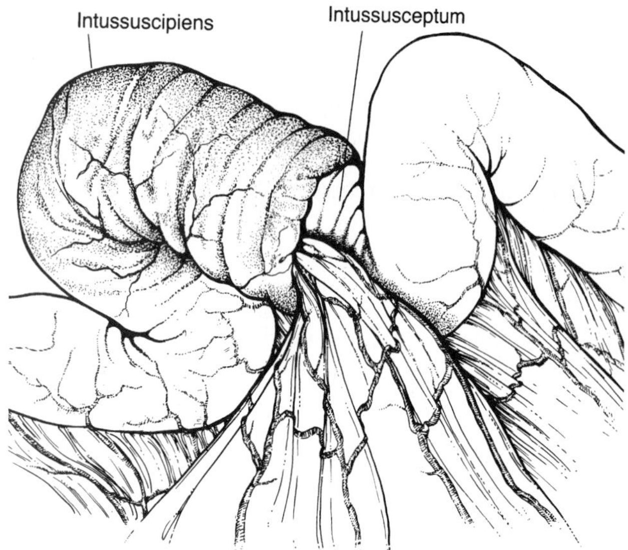

Figure 35-11. Small intestinal intussusception. (Redrawn from McIlwraith CW, Robertson JT: Equine Surgery: Advanced Techniques, ed 2, Oxford, UK, 1998, Blackwell.)

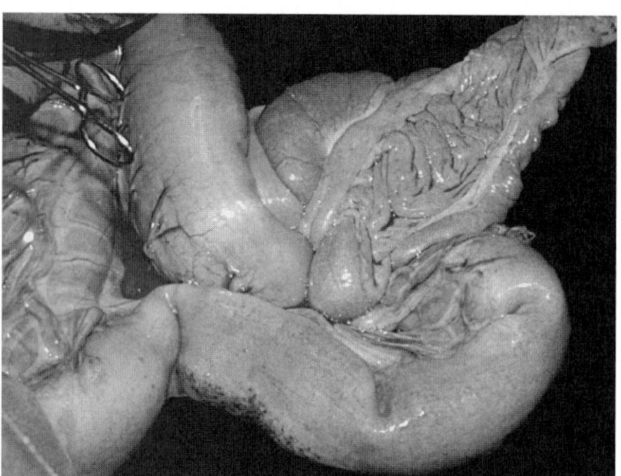

Figure 35-12. Compensatory changes in the jejunum proximal to a chronic ileocecal intussusception. The bowel is dilated but empty; its wall is thick, which is especially evident at the folds; and it has ecchymoses on the antimesenteric surface. (From Ford TS, Freeman DE, Ross MW, et al: Ileocecal intussusception in horses: 26 cases [1981-1988], J Am Vet Med Assoc 1990;196:121.)

antimesenteric surface.[80,212] These changes do not appear to contribute to the obstruction.

Females accounted for six of seven (86%) intussusceptions in one study, and this was significantly different from the sex distribution in the hospital population.[191] The female predisposition was less pronounced in five larger studies, ranging from 45% to 68%.[80,82,205,212,214] One study reported an apparently higher risk for Thoroughbred horses,[214] and another reported a higher risk for ponies.[82]

Although regarded mainly as a disease of foals, intussusceptions have been reported over a wide age range up to 24 years,[80-82] with few reported in young foals.[82,102] Intussusceptions were the most common cause of surgical colic in horses 3 to 12 months of age in one study, particularly ileocecal intussusceptions.[104] In younger foals, intussusceptions were less common and only jejunojejunal intussusceptions were recorded.[104] Ileocecal and ileoileal intussusceptions, both of which are more likely to cause recurrent mild to moderate colic, are more common in horses 3 years of age and younger.[80,82,205,212-215]

Intussusceptions of long segments cause signs of severe small intestinal obstruction.[80-82] Short intussusceptions cause colic that is mild, intermittent, and usually postprandial, and they also cause reduced appetite and feces, elevated temperature, weight loss, and failure to thrive compared with herdmates.[80] An ileal intussusception should be strongly suspected in a horse between weaning and 3 years of age that is unthrifty and has a history of recurrent mild colic.

Rectal examination may reveal distended loops of small intestine, and the intussusception can be palpated as a firm, painful, tubular structure in some cases.[81,82] Ileocecal intussusceptions were palpated in the right dorsal quadrant of the abdomen in 31% of horses in one report[80] and in 50% in another.[82] During an episode of pain in a horse with a chronic intussusception, the hypertrophied small intestine proximal to the obstruction (see Fig. 35-12) can be palpated per rectum as large-diameter, moderately distended loops with thick walls.[80] In young horses and foals too small for rectal palpation, a cross-sectional view of a jejunojejunal or ileocecal intussusception can be seen on ultrasonography as concentric rings with a bull's-eye appearance.[76,90]

White blood cells and protein concentration may be increased in the peritoneal fluid of horses with acute ileocecal intussusceptions[80] and jejunojejunal intussusceptions.[81] Peritoneal fluid protein concentration alone can increase in chronic ileocecal intussusceptions.[80] In one study, 8 of 16 horses with acute ileocecal intussusceptions had serosanguineous fluid.[80]

SURGERY: ILEOCECAL, AND ILEOILEAL INTUSSUSCEPTIONS

In chronic intussusceptions of ileum, short segments (approximately 10 cm) are involved. Reduction is difficult, even in the absence of adhesions, because of chronic folding of the intestinal wall.[80] Reduction was impossible in 11 of 16 ileoileal intussusceptions[214] and in 6 of 7 chronic and 10 of 19 acute ileocecal intussusceptions.[80] Ileocecal and ileoileal intussusceptions have been treated successfully by reduction only[213,214] or by reduction and myotomy.[214,216] Incomplete bypass by ileocecostomy is recommended if there are concerns about permanent ileal changes and the risk of recurrence,[80,212,217] and a hand-sewn technique is recommended over stapling instruments because the ileal wall is so thick. There is no need to resect the involved ileum in chronic cases or the hypertrophied jejunum.

Ileocecostomy for chronic ileocecal intussusception has excellent short-term results,[80] but apparently rare long-term complications include stomal impaction,[80,82] ileal hypertrophy, and rupture distal to the stoma.[119] Also, the size of the stoma can become smaller over time, which could predispose to these complications.[119]

In acute cases, the intussuscepted ileum and jejunum can be too edematous and hemorrhagic to allow reduction. Bypass by a jejunocecostomy without reduction can cause postoperative hemorrhage.[80] Removal of the intussusceptum through a typhlotomy can cause severe contamination,[80] although suturing an impermeable plastic drape around the typhlotomy can contain leakage.[218] In a technique devised to facilitate this surgery,[219] the jejunum proximal to the intussusception is transected with the GIA or the ILA stapler as close to the ileocecal junction as possible.[218] A 10-cm incision is made in the cecum to allow the intussusception to be exteriorized, and another incision is made through the outer wall of the intussusceptum to expose the inner loop (Fig. 35-13). This inner loop then is pulled through the incision in the outer layer until the closed transected end is distal to the selected site for transection.[219] If too much bowel is drawn through this incision, or if the jejunal transection was made far from the ileocecal junction, mesenteric vessels will tear and cause fatal hemorrhage.[218,219] Much of the necrotic bowel is removed by incision along the edge of a TA-90 stapler applied across the inverted ileum within the cecum (see Fig. 35-13).

SURGERY: JEJUNOJEJUNAL INTUSSUSCEPTION

A jejunojejunal intussusception forms a corkscrew configuration because of tension on the mesentery of the intussusceptum, and short to long segments can be involved.[210] Reduction is accomplished by slow traction on the intussusceptum and gentle massage of the distal end of the intussuscipiens.[210] If it is nonreducible, the entire intussusception can be removed by resection only,[81] although this can make ligation of mesenteric vessels difficult.[82]

Prognosis is favorable for all intussusceptions, but the bowel wall and intussuscepted mesenteric vessels can be torn during reduction.[80] Some horses can have a protracted recovery after surgery for a chronic ileocecal intussusception, with slow weight gain and mild episodes of colic.[80] Because *A. perfoliata* may be involved in the pathogenesis of ileocecal intussusceptions in horses, the treatment of affected horses and pasturemates with pyrantel pamoate and praziquantel is recommended.[80,205,220]

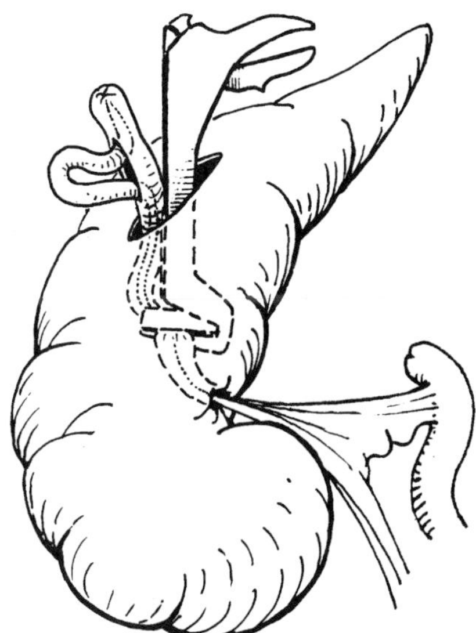

Figure 35-13. Method for resecting the intussusceptum of an acute ileocecal intussusception with the TA-90 stapler applied through a typhlotomy.

Mesenteric Rents

Mesenteric rents can be congenital in origin, secondary to mesodiverticular bands (Fig. 35-14), or may develop as primary lesions of unknown cause. Trauma or mesenteric stretching by another lesion may play a role, and some can develop years after a small intestinal surgery at a site remote to the anastomosis.[73,221] Horses of a wide age range appear to be prone, although females are more likely to be affected, especially in the postpartum period when the tear is possibly induced by vigorous movements of the foal, as has been implicated in tears of the small colon mesentery.[221,222] Such tears in postparturient mares can cause segmental ischemic necrosis of the related segment of jejunum or predispose to later strangulation of a more distant portion of small intestine.[223] The jejunal mesentery is involved in most cases, although tears in the ileal and duodenal mesentery have been reported, as well as tears in multiple sites.[221,223]

Prognosis for surgical treatment appears to be worse than after other strangulating lesions of the small intestine.[221] Possible reasons for this are inability to reduce the hernia, the long segments of bowel involved, hemorrhage from the affected mesentery, and failure to close all of the mesenteric defect.[221] Closure of the entire defect can be difficult or impossible through a ventral midline approach.[224] Elective laparoscopic closure of the full defect can be accomplished as a standing procedure shortly after the ventral midline celiotomy is performed to treat the original strangulation.[224] Both sides of the abdomen may need to be examined to locate the tear.[224]

Inguinal Hernia

An indirect inguinal hernia is the most common form in horses, and it involves small intestine passing through the vaginal ring into the vaginal tunic (see also Chapter 38). In the less common direct inguinal hernia, jejunum and occasionally the testicle escape through a rent in the peritoneum and transverse fascia, adjacent to the vaginal ring, to lie in the subcutaneous space of the scrotum and prepuce[225-228]

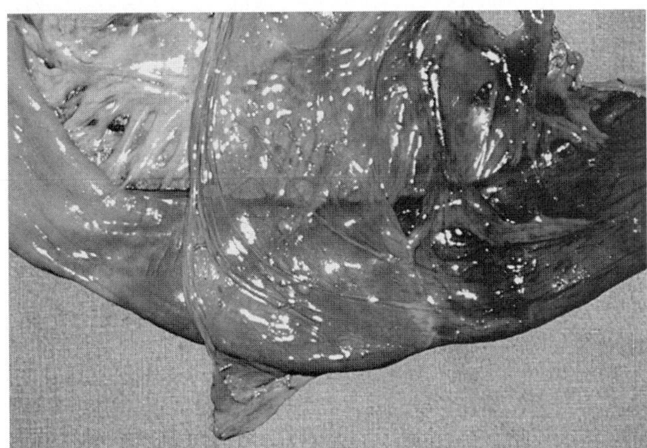

Figure 35-14. The mesodiverticular band is evident as a thin fold extending to the antimesenteric surface of the jejunum. The jejunum was strangulated in a mesenteric rent at the point of attachment of the band and mesentery.

(Fig. 35-15). Direct hernias are more common in foals than in adults,[225-230] but they can involve greater lengths of intestine in adults than are recorded with indirect hernias.[231]

Indirect inguinal hernias in adult horses involve short segments of small intestine (median of 15 cm)[231] and are usually acquired and nonreducible, whereas congenital inguinal or scrotal hernias in foals involve long segments and are reducible. In acquired hernias in adults, the loop of intestine rarely advances to the level of the testicle before it becomes strangulated, whereas a variable length of intestine (approximately 1 m) can reach the fundus of the vaginal tunic in foals and remain viable (Fig. 35-16). This difference can be attributed to the shorter, wider, and more direct configuration of the foal's inguinal canal. Contrary to popular misconception, the size of the external inguinal ring is irrelevant to development of an inguinal hernia, because it is the last structure for the bowel to traverse and is always sufficiently large for intestine to negotiate easily. The vaginal ring is the first structure to be negotiated by herniated intestine,[173] but the intestine is actually strangulated in an adult horse by a ring 2 to 3 cm further distally, formed by merging of the internal spermatic fascia into loose connective tissue in the neck of the vaginal process.[232]

Ileum, alone or with jejunum, was involved in 49% to 53% of adult inguinal hernias in three reports,[79,229,231] but jejunum was involved in eight of eight horses in another.[233] Ileal involvement may be more likely with increased duration of strangulation.[173]

Many breeds can be affected,[233,234] but a higher prevalence of inguinal/scrotal hernia has been reported in Standardbreds[191,234] Tennessee Walking Horses, and American Saddlebreds.[79] Standardbreds also appear to be at a higher risk for intestinal eventration after an open castration.[235] In acquired inguinal hernias, almost all age groups over 1 year are at risk.[180,234] Predisposing factors are not always evident[233] but include a history of recent strenuous exercise, recent breeding,[79,234] and trauma.[79,225] Direct and indirect inguinal hernias are rare in geldings.[230,234,236,237]

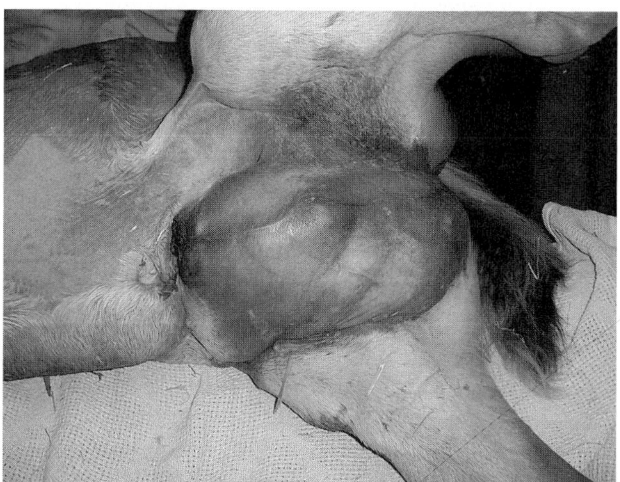

Figure 35-15. Direct inguinal hernia in a foal, with massive preputial and scrotal swelling from loops of small intestine beneath the skin. The tunic ruptured, allowing bowel to escape into a subcutaneous position. (From Bartmann C-P, Glitz F, von Oppen T, et al: Diagnosis and surgical management of colic in the foal, Clin Tech Equine Prac 2003;1:125, with permission.)

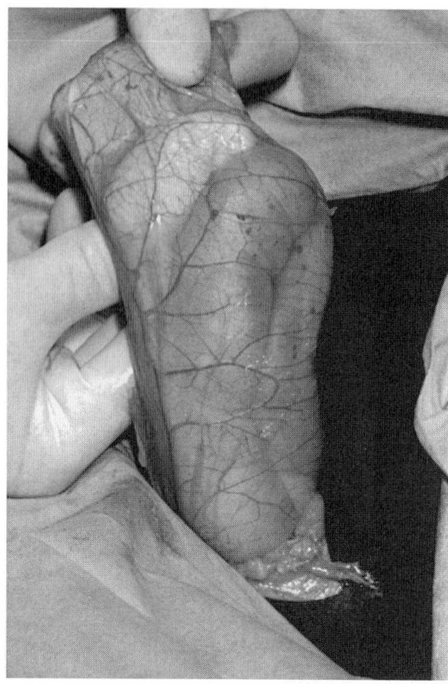

Figure 35-16. Dissected vaginal tunic in a foal with a congenital scrotal hernia, demonstrating the jejunum and the testicle above it and to the left. The cremaster muscle is evident on the left side.

Congenital scrotal hernias are noted shortly after birth, are easily reduced when the foals are rolled onto their backs, and usually resolve spontaneously within 3 to 6 months. Intestinal strangulation is rare. Although the problem is usually unilateral, bilateral cases can occur. Direct or ruptured inguinal hernias in foals are evident within 4 to 48 hours after birth and cause intermittent colic, depression, severe scrotal and preputial swelling (see Fig. 35-15), and edema, with skin excoriation and splitting caused by abrasion against the inside of the thigh.[226,227] These hernias are not reducible and are treated as surgical emergencies, although strangulation is rare.

Acquired inguinal hernias in adult horses cause signs of mild to severe colic.[233] As it becomes strangulated, the intestine compresses the testicular vessels and causes the testicle to become swollen, firm, and cold. Although the strangulated intestine may not be evident on external examination, rectal examination reveals small intestine entering the vaginal ring and distention of the small intestine. Bilateral cases are very rare.[233,238] Ultrasonography can facilitate early diagnosis and is especially useful if rectal palpation is not possible.[79]

SURGERY: CONGENITAL HERNIAS

Surgical correction is indicated if the hernia does not resolve spontaneously, the owner is concerned because of an apparent increase in size of the hernia, or the vaginal tunic ruptures. Surgical correction can be accomplished in foals through an inguinal approach with exposure of the tunic and its contents (see Fig. 35-16), removal of the cremaster muscle, twisting of the testicle and tunic to force the bowel into the abdomen, and then closed castration combined with a transfixation ligature of 0 polydioxanone through the tunic (see Chapter 38). Closure of the external inguinal ring is suggested but not essential[195] and may not prevent reherniation.[227,229] Alternative methods are laparoscopic repair with[239] or without castration,[240] an inguinal approach without castration,[241] or a midline celiotomy with closure of the vaginal ring. The testicle can atrophy after the latter two methods.

For repair of a direct or ruptured inguinal hernia in foals, the torn edges of the common vaginal tunic are identified and drawn upward to create a funnel through which the bowel is returned to the abdomen. The bowel can be directed into the abdomen by careful digital manipulation or by grasping the bowel in unclosed sponge forceps. The torn tunic should be repaired as much as possible to the level of the vaginal ring. Usually, the intestine is viable and does not require resection, although delayed necrosis has been reported.[227] Castration facilitates the repair and closure of the vaginal tunic.

SURGERY: ACQUIRED HERNIAS

In the early stages, a direct hernia in an adult may correct spontaneously after the anesthetized horse is placed in dorsal recumbency[229] or can be corrected by applying gentle traction to the bowel per rectum,[234] with or without external massage of the scrotum.[242] External massage alone may also be effective and can be guided by laparoscopy,[232] which also allows assessment of intestinal viability. In such cases, laparoscopic inguinal herniorrhaphy may be performed 1 week later to prevent recurrence, using either a mesh onlay graft[242] or a cylindrical mesh plug.[243] Spontaneous reduction or reduction by traction does not rule out the possibility of complications from progressive intestinal necrosis.[229]

A nonreducible inguinal hernia is corrected through an inguinal incision directly over the external inguinal ring and along the spermatic cord. The abdomen should be prepared for a ventral midline celiotomy, if needed, to allow intra-abdominal traction on the bowel, to assess viability of the released bowel, to decompress or examine proximal bowel, or for a jejunocecal anastomosis. The tunic is dissected from the surrounding tissues, with care taken to not damage the pudendal vein and branches. A cranial incision is made in the vaginal tunic, which needs to be extended far enough distally to cut the constricting ring formed by the internal spermatic fascia and release the strangulated intestine.[232] The tunic edges should be grasped with hemostats to maintain access for closure. Medial and cranial retraction on the edge of the internal abdominal oblique muscle with a Deaver retractor will improve exposure to the tunic edges, and a finger is used to direct bowel away from the suture line.

Because short segments (less than 25 cm) of intestine are usually involved,[229,231] resection is rarely needed if appearance of the bowel improves markedly after the strangulation has been released. A unilateral castration is recommended to allow more complete closure of the vaginal tunic and abolish the risk of recurrence.[234] In addition, the involved testicle can become cystic or nonfunctional in time, and postoperative swelling could induce degeneration of the other testicle. Techniques to correct the hernia and prevent recurrence have been described.[240-244]

If the vaginal ring can be closed, closure of the external inguinal ring is not essential and does not ensure against evisceration.[229] However, if the vaginal ring closure is not secure, closure of the external inguinal ring is recommended. Closure of the thick subcutaneous fascia and skin incision is accomplished in two layers. After surgery, the scrotum on the castrated side usually lies against the prepuce, and swelling is minimal. Any method of correction that does not involve exploration of the abdomen would fail to detect a concurrent small intestinal volvulus, a rare complication of inguinal hernia that could cause postoperative colic.[79,172,173]

A survival rate of up to 76% has been reported for acquired inguinal hernia.[229,233,234] Adhesions at the vaginal ring are rare causes of later strangulation.[233]

Incarceration through the Gastrosplenic Ligament

The gastrosplenic ligament is a broad but thin attachment between the left part of the greater curvature of the stomach and the hilus of the spleen.[1] Small intestine can pass from caudal to cranial through acute tears in this ligament so that the strangulated loop is lateral to the stomach and craniolateral to the spleen[245] (Fig. 35-17). At surgery, the strangulation is easily corrected by traction, and enlarging the rent does not cause problems or predispose to recurrence. If the most ventral edge of the defect in the ligament is accessible, it can be transected between two ligatures to disrupt continuity of the ring.[246]

Vitelline Anomalies

A mesodiverticular band develops from a vitelline artery and associated mesentery that fail to atrophy during early embryonic development.[174] The band is usually found in the distal jejunum, approximately 1.5 m from the ileocecal junction. It extends from one side of the mesentery, usually the left, to the antimesenteric surface of the small intestine to form a triangular space (see Fig. 35-14). Intestine may

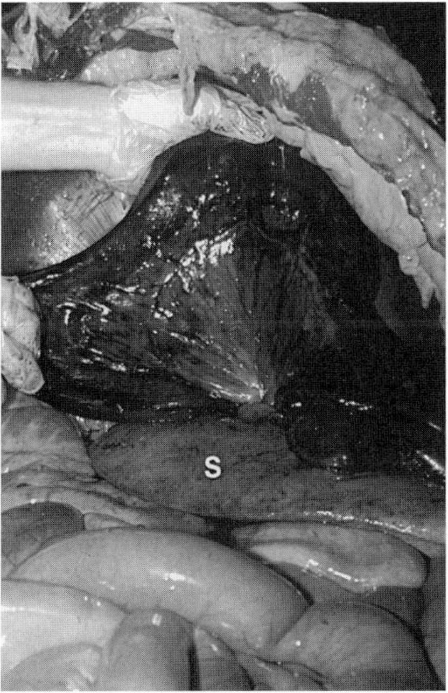

Figure 35-17. The jejunum is strangulated in a rent in the gastrosplenic ligament and lying in the left cranial part of the abdomen. S, spleen.

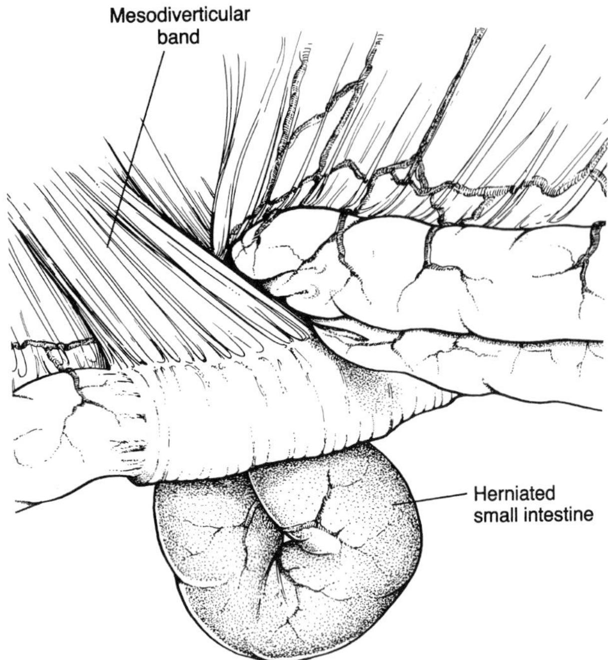

Figure 35-18. A mesodiverticular band and secondary mesenteric rent resulting in incarceration of the small intestine. (Redrawn from McIlwraith CW, Turner AS: Equine Surgery: Advanced Techniques, Oxford, UK, 1987, Blackwell.)

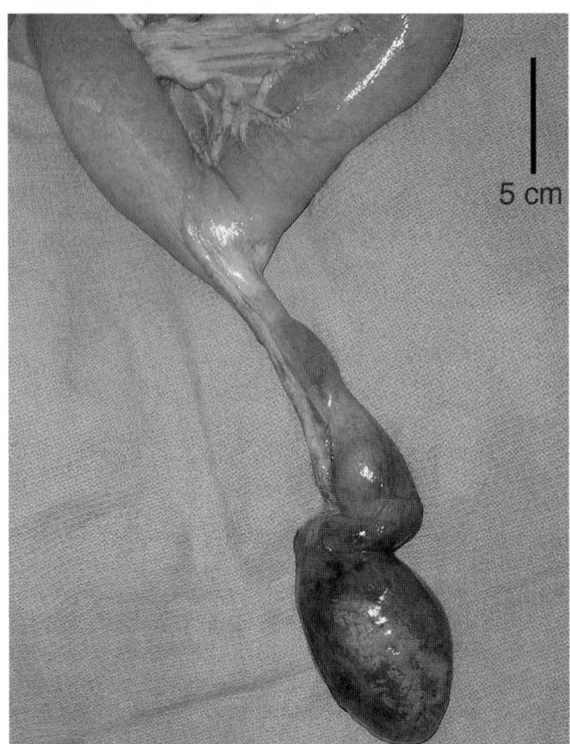

Figure 35-19. Meckel's diverticulum that was knotted around the jejunum in a 5-month-old Clydesdale foal. The diverticulum was resected and the linear defect in the jejunum was oversewn. (From Bartmann C-P, Glitz F, von Oppen T, et al: Diagnosis and surgical management of colic in the foal, Clin Tech Equine Prac 2003;1:125, with permission).

become strangulated in a mesenteric rent that forms in that space (Fig. 35-18), and secondary volvulus of the small intestine follows.[174] A mesodiverticular band alone can also cause a volvulus because the band shortens the mesentery at the point of attachment. Although a mesodiverticular band represents a congenital anomaly, it can cause obstruction in mature horses and may be an incidental finding at necropsy.[174]

Meckel's diverticulum is a remnant of the omphalomesenteric (vitelline) duct that provides a communication between the yolk sac and early embryonic gut. It forms a conical blind extension from the antimesenteric surface of the distal jejunum or ileum, 40 to 120 cm from the ileocecal junction[247,248] (Fig. 35-19). It can be up to 35 cm long, but it is usually 10 to 15 cm long and 5 to 10 cm in diameter.[247] Occasionally, a fibrous band persists from the apex of Meckel's diverticulum to the umbilicus—the vitelloumbilical band—and creates an axis for volvulus of the jejunum and ileum.[176]

In one review of 15,000 necropsies, Meckel's diverticulum was responsible for the death of all five horses (0.03%) in which it was found.[247] Meckel's diverticulum can become impacted[249] and achieve enormous proportions[250] or become necrotic and rupture to cause fatal peritonitis.[247] Meckel's diverticulum can also entangle and strangulate small intestine[248,249,251] or form an axis for volvulus nodosus.[175] In one horse, a Meckel diverticulum was found adhered to and impacted in an umbilical hernia,[252] thereby forming a Littre hernia. Although Meckel's diverticulum represents a congenital anomaly, it can cause colic in horses of a wide age range.[247-251]

Strangulated Umbilical Hernia

Strangulation of a loop of small intestine in an umbilical hernia is rare, and the involved intestine can rupture through the hernial sac and dissect subcutaneously in a caudal direction to cause an inguinal enlargement[253] (see also Chapter 38). More commonly, only a portion of the antimesenteric wall of the ileum is incarcerated, and this is termed a parietal, or Richter's, hernia.[253,254] A parietal hernia should be suspected when an umbilical hernia becomes nonreducible, large, turgid, edematous, and painful to palpation. A parietal hernia can cause umbilical abscessation, which may lead to rupture of the hernia and formation of an enterocutaneous fistula.[253,254] Ultrasonography may be used to evaluate the hernia and its contents.[94] Colic can develop in horses with a parietal hernia, but it is not observed in all cases of an umbilical abscess or enterocutaneous fistula.[253,254] Surgical correction of these umbilical lesions is successfully accomplished by making a 10- to 15-cm celiotomy cranial to the ring, and digitally guiding en bloc removal of the umbilical lesion through this incision. Resection and anastomosis of involved intestine may be required.

Diaphragmatic Hernias

A diaphragmatic defect can be congenital in origin or acquired, although the distinction is difficult. Small intestinal strangulation in diaphragmatic defects has been reported in foals as causes of death at 7 hours to 8 days after birth.[255] A congenital diaphragmatic defect or a diaphragmatic tear inflicted by a rib fracture, usually at or close to the costochondral junction of ribs 3 to 8, are likely causes of diaphragmatic hernia in foals.[255,256] The most common causes of diaphragmatic hernia in adult horses are trauma, parturition (particularly dystocias), and recent strenuous activity.[257] In some horses, the presence of omental adhesions to a callus on fractured ribs on the thoracic side of the defect is suggestive of previous trauma,[258,259] possibly at birth. Although several abdominal organs can enter the diaphragmatic defect, small intestine is the most commonly reported.[260] There does not appear to be an age, breed, or sex predisposition to this disease.

Large defects are more likely to cause dyspnea from pulmonary compression by intrathoracic displacement of the colon, but they do not incarcerate bowel and cause colic.[257,261] Small defects are more likely to strangulate small intestine and manifest as acute and severe colic, clinically indistinguishable from strangulation by any other cause. Abnormalities can be detected on auscultation and percussion of the thorax in some horses.[262]

Both radiography and ultrasonography allow preoperative diagnosis.[263-266] Ultrasonography may be superior to radiography in evaluating diaphragmatic hernias in horses, especially for small tears with little visceral displacement, or when pleural effusion obscures the ventral portion of the diaphragm.[267] The diaphragm can be imaged with 5- or 7.5-MHz transducer adjacent to and parallel with the body wall ventrally, then diverging dorsally and medially to lie behind the echogenic lung.[267] The curved shape of the diaphragm may prevent complete evaluation.[267]

SURGERY

A diaphragmatic hernia can be missed at surgery.[268] If strangulated bowel is found free in the abdomen, a careful search must be conducted to ensure that it did not fall out of a diaphragmatic defect when the horse was placed in dorsal recumbency.[268]

Ideally, a respirator should be used to provide controlled positive-pressure ventilation and correct the diminished pulmonary function. An advantage of preoperative diagnosis is that the abdominal incision can be placed further cranially than the standard approach. Access to ventral defects is not difficult, but access to more dorsal defects can be improved by extending the cranial end of the incision laterally for approximately 12 to 15 cm at an angle of 60 to 90 degrees in a paracostal fashion.[195] The table can be tilted to raise the cranial end of the horse's abdomen so abdominal contents can fall away from the diaphragm.

A small defect may have to be enlarged with scissors[195,258,262] or a curved fetotome[264] to release the bowel. Most defects can be closed with a continuous pattern using heavy absorbable or nonabsorbable material, and the suture line should be completed at full inspiration to reduce the pneumothorax present. Mesh coverage is required for defects that cannot be sutured because of their large size or because the edges are too firm to allow apposition. Successful repair of a dorsal rent that was inaccessible for suture placement was accomplished by blind fixation of a doubled polypropylene mesh (Marlex Mesh #1266, Dowd Inc, Providence, RI) with 4-mm stainless steel staples (Disposable Skin Stapler, Richard-Allen Medical, Richland, Mich).[266] Another inaccessible defect was repaired in the standing horse by suture closure through a thoracic rib resection that was placed by guidance from thoracoscopy and manual direction through a flank incision.[269] Indwelling chest tubes covered by a Heimlich valve (see Chapter 18) can be placed to correct pneumothorax and fluid accumulation in the chest.[195]

Successful repairs of diaphragmatic hernias have been reported in adult horses and foals,* and horses can race, participate successfully in various forms of competition, and deliver foals after repair.[258,264,266] One horse with a small defect that was inaccessible for repair returned to a full athletic career.[264] Unrepaired diaphragmatic defects can partly seal by adhesion of adjacent stomach and liver to the edges,[269] although recurrence of intestinal incarceration immediately after anesthetic recovery is also likely.[266]

Miscellaneous Strangulating/Ischemic Diseases

Small intestine can become strangulated in mesenteric ligamentous bands that cannot be exteriorized at surgery and must be cut blindly with scissors. Small intestine can also become strangulated by uterine torsion[270]; through rents in the mesometrium,[98,271] gastrohepatic ligament,[97] small colon mesentery,[97,173] lateral ligament of the urinary bladder,[272] cecocolic fold,[96,98,173,273] and mesentery of the large colon[98]; by components of the spermatic cord, particularly the mesoductus deferens[274]; and by omental adhesions.[100] Evisceration through a lacerated vaginal fornix, a defect in the bladder and urethra,[275] or a castration wound[235] may cause small intestinal strangulating obstruction. Entrapment of small intestine within the nephrosplenic space has been reported in two horses, with the bowel passing from cranial to caudal.[276] Both horses were presented alert and in stable condition, and the affected segments of bowel did not require resection.[276] Mesenteric hematomas of unknown cause can cause colic and ischemic necrosis of affected intestine.[277] Surgical access to the source of hemorrhage may be difficult.[277] Duodenal torsion has been reported[171] but is rare.

Adhesions after small intestinal surgery or any intra-abdominal procedure can form an axis around which attached small intestine can form a volvulus, or adhesions can form fibrous bands through which small intestinal loops can become strangulated.[177,278] Nonstrangulating infarction and necrotizing enterocolitis in the small intestine are rare and have a poor prognosis.[94,279]

SURGICAL TECHNIQUES

Success of small intestinal surgery in the horse is dependent on (1) identification and correction of the primary problem, (2) intraoperative decompression of distended small intestine, (3) resection of all abnormal intestine, (4) preservation of anatomic and physiologic continuity of the intestine, (5) rapid completion of the surgery with minimal trauma, (6) early return of intestine to normal function, and (7) appropriate postoperative support, including repeat laparotomy when indicated.

---

*References 195, 254, 257, 258, 261, 263, 264.

If the lesion is not revealed quickly by a cursory examination of the abdomen, the cecum should be found and the ileocecal fold traced to the ileum, followed by progressive examination of the jejunum in a cranial direction until the involved segment is found. If several discontinuous loops of small intestine are exteriorized through the incision, they form tight bands of mesentery that can prevent extraction of other distended loops. Rarely, a horse may have two apparently unrelated, strangulating lesions of the small intestine.[173,280] However, it is more common for a horse to have a concurrent large intestinal lesion, such as volvulus, displacement, or impaction.[72,138]

Viability Assessment

Viable small intestine refers to the ability of intestine to survive without developing adhesions (for additional information, see Chapter 34). The observation that increased duration of surgery and length of bowel resected can adversely affect prognosis provides impetus to improve viability assessment and thereby avoid resection whenever possible.[197] Clinical criteria of viability are serosal color, improvement in color after correction of the strangulation, presence or absence of mesenteric arterial pulses, and intestinal motility, spontaneous or evoked (by snapping a finger against the intestinal wall). Clinical judgment tends to be pessimistic. Fluorescein fluorescence offers little improvement over clinical judgment but is accurate when it produces a viable fluorescent pattern.[281]

Intestine can be considered viable if the predominant clinical findings are hemorrhage and edema in the bowel wall, especially if the color improves within approximately 15 minutes after release of the obstruction.[282] Spontaneous or evoked motility appears sluggish in viable strangulated bowel because of "splinting" of the muscle wall by edema and hemorrhage. Enterotomies are not recommended for viability assessment in the small intestine because of the risk for adhesion formation and because mucosal changes are usually sufficiently severe to cause an incorrect prediction in viable bowel. With long segments of questionable viability, the risk for adhesions must be balanced against the risks of additional anesthesia time and the occurrence of adhesions after resection and anastomosis.

Resection

After the lesion has been corrected, the bowel must be arranged in its correct orientation and then decompressed, if necessary. Decompression is accomplished through the strangulated bowel, but only after the bowel has been freed from its mesentery and mobilized from the surgical field. For this purpose, a ligature of 3-0 polydioxanone (PDS) is applied to the first mesenteric vessel in the strangulated bowel, level with the proposed line of mesenteric resection. The mesenteric vessel is then transected distal to the ligature with the ligate divide stapler (LDS) (see Fig. 17-10). The short end of the ligature is secured with a hemostat, and the long end is used to gather the trimmed edge of mesentery as each mesenteric vessel is transected with the LDS instrument (Fig. 35-20). Ideally, the line of mesenteric resection should remain at a constant distance from the bowel, because any deviation toward the mesenteric root will shorten the mesentery and kink the bowel.[195] The two ends of the suture are tied to close the gathered mesentery after the bowel is decompressed, and a gap will remain to be closed between the bowel and the line of mesenteric resection (see Fig. 35-20). With this method, any bleeders can be retained in view outside the abdomen, and a large mesenteric gap is avoided that would allow rotation or entrapment of bowel.[195]

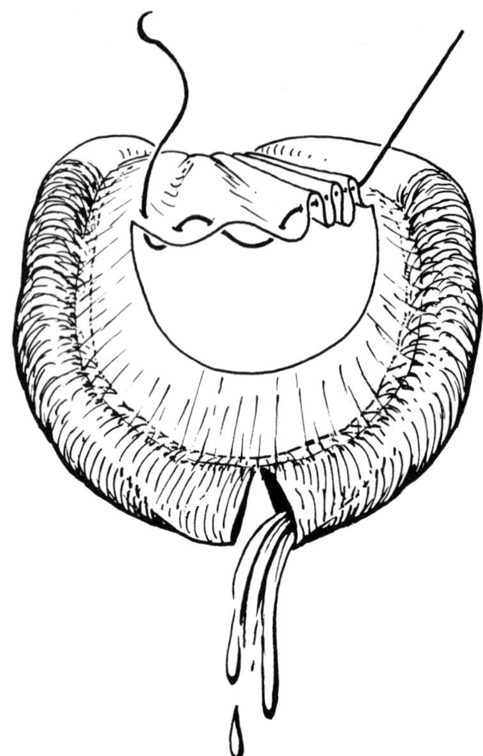

Figure 35-20. Method of resecting and gathering the mesenteric edge and then draining the bowel through the strangulated segment. Note that the line of resection should stay parallel to the bowel. (Redrawn from Freeman DE: Surgery of the small intestine, Vet Clin North Am Equine Pract 1997;13:261.)

The nonviable intestine can now be exteriorized from the abdomen, far from the surgical field, to drain into a container, taking care not to stretch and tear remaining mesenteric attachments. As much intestine as possible proximal to the site of transection is manually stripped of its fluid and gas contents, with care taken not to tear the mesentery (Fig. 35-21). This amount of intestinal handling does not appear to predispose to adhesions, and decompression seems to minimize problems with postoperative ileus. If resection is not needed, small intestinal distention should be relieved through a typhlotomy and not a small intestinal enterotomy, because the latter may lead to adhesion formation and obstruction.

Strangulated bowel is removed along with approximately 30 to 50 cm of contiguous healthy intestine at each end. A large arcuate artery, approximately 10 cm from its origin from the major mesenteric vessel, is left to supply the anastomosed ends. Approximately 2 to 10 cm of mesentery is left beyond the last major vessels and branches to prevent inadvertent vascular occlusion or puncture during closure of the mesenteric gap. After the anastomosis is complete, the

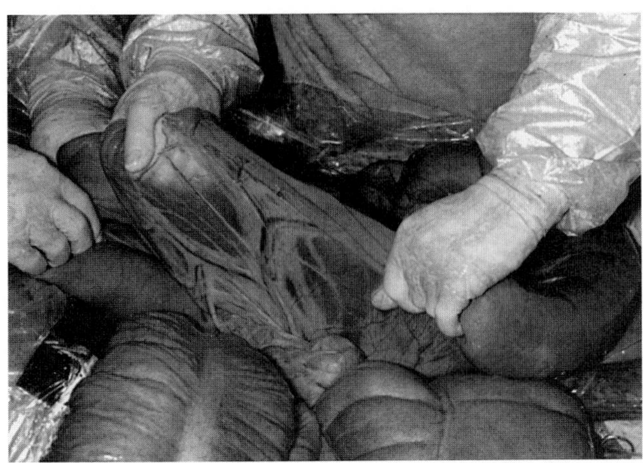

Figure 35-21. A method of stripping the distended bowel to decompress it.

bowel is lavaged. The defect remaining in the mesentery is closed with 2-0 or 3-0 PDS in a simple continuous pattern, with care taken to avoid mesenteric vessels or creating an accordion effect that could kink the bowel.[195] If the mesenteric stump is inflamed and hemorrhagic, adjacent healthy mesentery can be wrapped around it.[97]

Hand-sewn End-to-End Jejunojejunostomy

To prevent leakage into the surgical field, a Penrose drain may be applied at least 15 cm proximal to the anastomosis site to avoid trauma to this critical area (Fig. 35-22). Penrose drains are less traumatic than Doyen clamps and facilitate manipulation and positioning of the bowel. To create a large stoma, the intestine should be transected at approximately 50 to 60 degrees from the mesenteric attachment; an S-shaped line of transection will increase the diameter further without creating sharp angulations in the incision edges. A suture is placed through the mesenteric and antimesenteric edges of both segments to draw them into alignment and to maintain them at similar diameters. With all end-to-end anastomoses, special care must be taken to appose the mesenteric border first, because rapid edema formation at this area can make it difficult to identify the seromuscular layer.

A popular method for end-to-end anastomosis of equine small intestine is a two-layer continuous pattern.[283] This involves a simple continuous pattern of 2-0 or 3-0 absorbable suture for the submucosa/mucosa, followed by a continuous Lembert or Cushing pattern in the seromuscular layer (see Fig. 35-22). The Lembert pattern can be placed so as to produce minimal inversion. Mucosal and seromuscular rows are interrupted at the mesenteric and antimesenteric margins or at thirds of the circumference to prevent a pursestring effect. The Cushing pattern exposes less foreign material to the serosa and therefore poses less risk for adhesion formation than the Lembert pattern, but the Cushing is more likely to pursestring the bowel. The degree of inversion is greater with the Lembert pattern, so special care is needed to minimize this effect (see Fig. 35-22). Combinations of patterns that involve two layers in the seromuscular wall,[209,249] such as continuous appositional, Lembert, Cushing, or Connell oversewn with Lembert or Cushing, produce excess seromuscular inversion, stomal constriction, and a

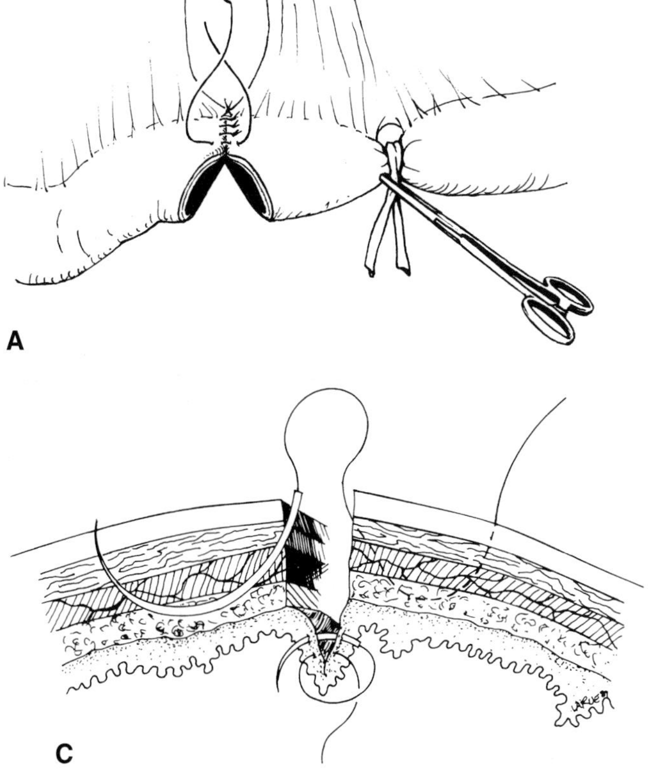

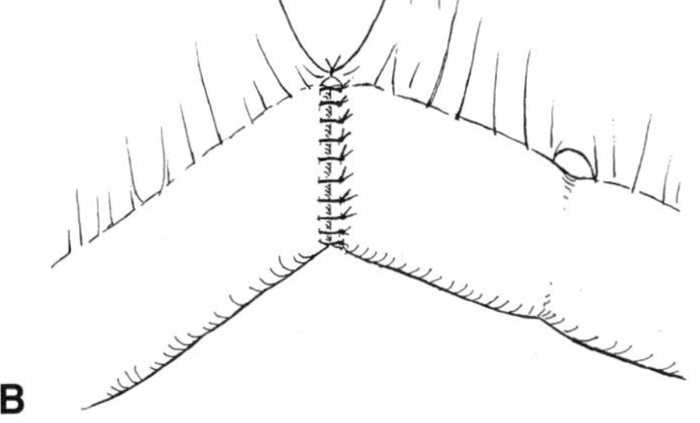

Figure 35-22. A and **B,** The lumen of the small intestine is occluded temporarily with a Penrose drain proximal to the anastomosis site. A one-layer closure consisting of interrupted Lembert sutures is carried out. **C,** Close-up of an alternate (two-layer) anastomosis technique: a simple-continuous apposition of the mucosa over three times a third of the circumference, followed by a minimal inversion pattern of the seromuscular layer.

high risk for postoperative obstruction. There is ample evidence that single-layer anastomoses work well in equine small intestine (for additional details on suture patterns, see Chapter 17).[106,195,283-285]

The Gambee and other interrupted patterns are more likely to cause anastomotic adhesions in the horse than continuous patterns,[283,286] although results of one study did not confirm this.[284] Larger sizes of suture material, such as 0 PDS or polyglactin 910 (Vicryl),[283,286] could predispose to adhesions because they place a greater volume of foreign material along the anastomosis than 3-0 PDS, which is preferred.[195] An interrupted Lembert pattern is used with approximately 6- to 8-mm bites that penetrate within 1 mm from the cut edge of the seromuscular layer and are 6 to 8 mm apart (Fig. 35-23). This pattern may be less likely to induce adhesions than the Gambee method, and it is quicker.[195]

A single-layer anastomosis with 3-0 PDS through the full thickness of the equine jejunum and wrapped with a sodium carboxymethylcellulose and hyaluronate membrane was faster than mucosal closure followed by a Cushing pattern.[285] Also, the single-layer anastomosis reduced lumen diameter from normal adjacent lumen by 35.6%, compared with a 44% reduction for mucosal closure and a Cushing pattern.[285] It also developed significantly fewer peri-anastomotic adhesions than a single-layer anastomosis without the membrane.[285] With this single-layer pattern, care must be taken to minimize mucosal eversion, because mucosa does tend to protrude between the seromuscular edges,[285] which could lead to adhesion formation.

Stapled Jejunojejunostomy

The major advantages of stapling instruments are speed, reduced tissue handling, improved tissue blood flow, and minimal contamination.[287] If the staple line is oversewn, the first two advantages are lost and the prevalence of adhesions becomes comparable to that with hand-sewn anastomoses in horses.[287] The most important disadvantage of staples is expense. The security of the closure with staples can be affected by tissue thickness, and the 4.8-mm staples (green cartridge) are preferable to the 3.8-mm staples (blue cartridge) for equine gastrointestinal surgery.

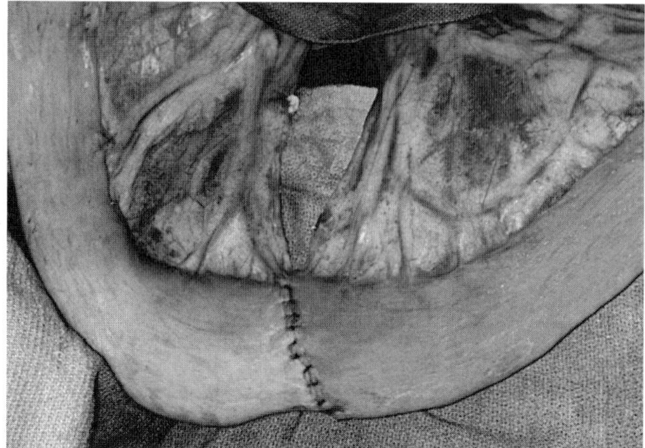

Figure 35-23. End-to-end anastomosis with interrupted Lembert sutures before the mesentery is closed. Note the darker discoloration of the bowel to the right, which is caused by prestenotic distention.

With the exception of the end-to-end anastomosis instrument (see Fig. 17-13), which is too small for adult equine intestine, other available stapling instruments are used in a side-to-side manner. By necessity, side-to-side anastomoses disrupt the normal anatomic and physiologic polarity of the bowel. In canine jejunum, 91% of MMCs can cross an end-to-end anastomosis at 12 weeks after surgery compared with 56% at 2 years after a functional end-to-end anastomosis.[288] Stomal dilation and delayed obstruction have been reported after a stapled side-to-side anastomosis in dogs[288] and after a hand-sewn version of a side-to-side anastomosis in horses[97] and rats.[288] In a study on dogs, the functional end-to-end anastomosis also altered intraluminal flora compared with a hand-sewn end-to-end anastomosis, evidence that it imposed some nonphysiologic changes on intestinal function.[288] In addition, increasing the number of raw edges (although inverted) and the number of suture lines and staple lines increases the number of potential foci of inflammation. In a recent retrospective study in horses, no difference was found between hand-sewn end-to-end anastomoses and stapled side-to-side and stapled functional end-to-end anastomoses with regard to short- and long-term survival, duration of surgery, or prevalence of postoperative ileus.[208] However, the stapled side-to-side anastomoses had a shorter duration of postoperative ileus than the others,[208] a finding weakened because of the wide variety of different types of hand-sewn anastomoses used and because some had two inverting layers.

Side-to-Side Stapled Jejunojejunostomy

The isoperistaltic side-to-side technique involves creating blind stumps of the proximal and distal ends of the jejunum with either a Parker-Kerr technique (see Fig. 17-6) or stapling instruments[195] (see Figs 17-11 and 17-12). The gastrointestinal anastomosis (GIA) instrument is used to create the stoma in the overlapped segments. This places two parallel rows of staggered staples on each side of a stoma cut simultaneously by advancement of the knife blade (Fig. 35-24). If the GIA-50 is used, it is placed proximally and then distally through the same stab incisions on the antimesenteric side, effectively doubling the size of the stoma. Care must be taken to ensure that the staple lines overlap on the far side of the stab incisions[289] or that any defect on that side is oversewn. If the Multifire GIA-80 or ILA-100 (United States Surgical Corp, Norwalk, Conn) is used, a single application is sufficient. The two mesenteric edges are sutured to the adjacent mesenteric surfaces at the points of overlap.

Functional End-to-End Stapled Jejunojejunostomy

With the functional end-to-end anastomosis, the bowel ends are lined up in antiperistaltic fashion, the stoma is created with the GIA instrument along apposing surfaces, and bowel ends are closed.[195,290] A closed, stapled, one-stage, end-to-end jejunojejunostomy realigned itself into an end-to-end configuration as it healed and did not cause adhesions in normal horses.[290] Intussusception of a functional end-to-end anastomosis has been reported in ponies at 2 and 26 days after surgery[207] and in a horse at 8 months after surgery.[208]

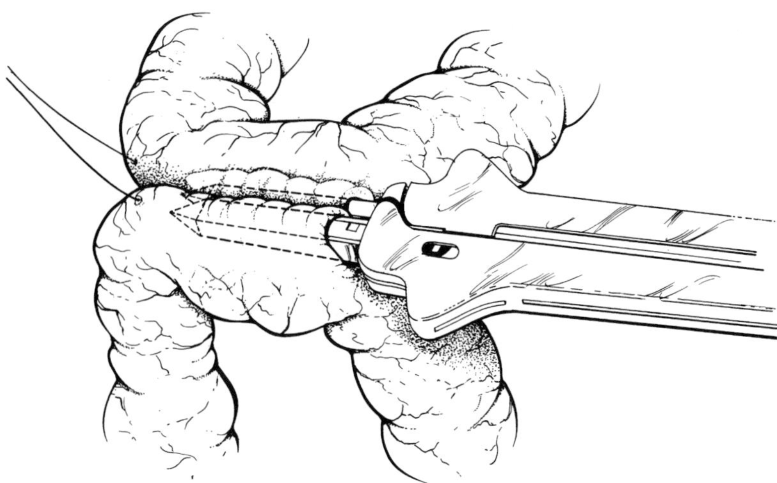

Figure 35-24. GIA-50 Premium stapler with disposable cartridge used for a side-to-side anastomosis. Stay sutures are placed at either end of the proposed anastomotic site to approximate the bowel segments side by side, and a stab is made into both bowel segments large enough to accommodate each fork of the instrument. The instrument forks are inserted fully to maximize stomal size. The stab incisions are apposed with an inverting suture pattern (not shown). (Copyright 1974, 1980, 1988, 1998, 2005 United States Surgical, a division of Tyco Healthcare Group LP. All rights reserved. Reprinted with Permission of United States Surgical, a division of Tyco Healthcare Group LP.)

Jejunocecal and Ileocecal Anastomoses

Jejunocecal and ileocecal anastomoses are indicated when a portion of the ileum is involved in a strangulating lesion. These techniques can constitute 36% to 68% of all small intestinal anastomoses.[74,196,291] Proponents of the side-to-side jejunocecostomy believe that it creates a larger stoma than is possible with the end-to-side technique[97] and that it is associated with fewer postoperative problems from stomal edema.[292] In a study that compared the two techniques in clinical cases, 83% of horses with a side-to-side jejunocecostomy were discharged from the clinic, compared with 37% that had an end-to-side jejunocecostomy.[293] The latter also had more repeat celiotomies, necessitated by such complications as bowel kinking at the anastomosis, adhesion formation, impaction, intussusception of the anastomosis, and volvulus or torsion.[293] An angled line of transection of the jejunum or ileum, with or without a longitudinal incision on the antimesenteric side, allows construction of a stoma of adequate size with the end-to-side technique.[195]

The mesentery and small intestine are prepared as for an end-to-end anastomosis except that the ileum is transected and oversewn using either stapling instruments or a Parker-Kerr technique[195] (see Fig. 17-6). The ileal stump should be as short as possible, because an intussusception can form into the cecum over time,[294] and a long stump can progress into and obstruct the cecocolic orifice.[295,296] The ileal stump remains nonfunctional and therefore can tolerate more severe ischemia than would be acceptable in bowel that is expected to regain normal activity. One method proposed to reduce problems from an ischemic stump is to suture omentum over the suture line.[297]

For extensive ileal necrosis, the TA-90 can be used for a distal transection down to the ileocecal orifice.[298] The 4.8-mm-length staples are recommended for this purpose.[73] An incision is made in the mesentery dorsal to the ileal artery and in the ileocecal fold, and it is continued to the level of ileal transection to create a tract for passage of a loose ligature to that point.[298] This ligature is tied to compress all mesenteric tissues at the level of transection, including the ileal artery and vein. The disadvantage of this and other methods of deep ileal transection is that they create a large mesenteric defect[298] that could entrap bowel. An alternative method is to attach the ileum to a length of stomach tube that can be used to invert the necrotic stump into the cecum.[299]

End-to-Side Anastomosis

The stoma should be created as close to the base of the cecum as possible to reduce the gravitational effects of cecal contents.[195,300] The stoma is made midway between the dorsal band and the medial band, and the small intestine is aligned so that it is directed toward the base of the cecum (Fig. 35-25).

A noncrushing intestinal clamp can be used to clamp off a pouch of the cecum, or upward tension on stay sutures or on Babcock forceps can be used to maintain the cecal opening above the cecal contents. After the mesenteric and antimesenteric ends of jejunum are attached to the selected area on the cecum by simple-interrupted sutures of 3-0 PDS, a Lembert or Cushing pattern apposes the back side of the jejunum to the cecum. An incision is then made in the cecum 5 mm from the suture line that corresponds with the opening in the jejunum. The next row is a simple-continuous, full-thickness pattern, interrupted at the mesenteric and antimesenteric borders before it is continued for 360 degrees. A Cushing or a continuous Lembert pattern on the near side completes the anastomosis. The free edge of mesentery is sewn to the cecum and then to the ileocecal fold, ending at the oversewn end of the ileum and the

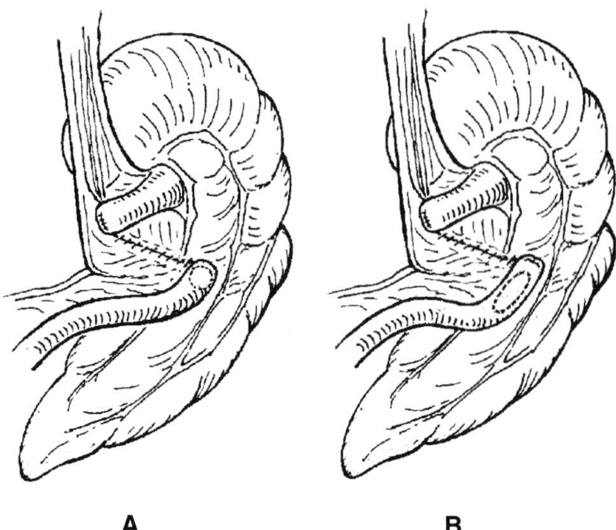

Figure 35-25. Completed end-to-side (**A**) and side-to-side jejunocecal anastomoses (**B**). In both methods, the ileum is oversewn by the Parker-Kerr technique and the mesenteric defects are closed. (From Freeman DE: Surgery of the small intestine, Vet Clin North Am Equine Pract 1997;13:261, with permission.)

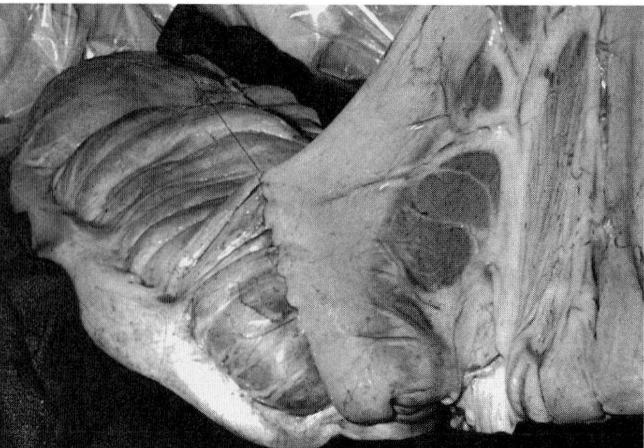

Figure 35-26. Side-to-side jejunocecostomy with the oversewn end of the jejunum in the foreground and facing the cecal base. The apparent divergence of the jejunum toward the medial band of the cecum is not real but the result of close positioning at the edge of the incision.

previously gathered mesenteric stump (see Fig. 35-25). Failure to close this mesenteric defect can lead to subsequent passage of small intestine through it, followed by obstruction and even strangulation.[221,301]

Side-to-Side Anastomosis

After the strangulated segment of small intestine is resected, the jejunum is transected and oversewn as for the ileum. The jejunum is attached to the selected area on the wall of the cecum (see "End-to-Side Anastomosis," just previously) with interrupted sutures of 3-0 PDS at the oversewn end and 10 to 12 cm proximal to this point (see Fig. 35-25). Either a hand-sewn side-to-side method, GIA stapling instruments, or the cutting thread or saw technique[297,302] can be used. A saw technique (with steel wire protected in catheters) can effectively achieve a side-to-side anastomosis and reduces contamination more than the stapling method but without the cost.[302] The oversewn end of the jejunum should not extend beyond the stoma or a stagnant loop will form, and it should be directed toward the cecal base (Fig. 35-26). A stabilizing suture line between cecum and jejunum proximal to the stoma is optional.[195] If the ileum is obstructed by a tumor, muscular hypertrophy, or chronic intussusception, an incomplete bypass can be used.[80]

The colon of horses with small intestinal strangulation is usually tightly contracted around dehydrated contents, although it is not truly impacted. Removal of these contents[303] should eliminate some downstream resistance and provide a more favorable pressure gradient for emptying of the small intestine into the cecum in horses with ileocecal or jejunocecal anastomoses.

Jejunoileal Anastomosis

Jejunoileal anastomosis is an alternative to jejunocecal anastomosis (if sufficient ileum is available) and can be performed more quickly because fewer steps are required. It also eliminates potential problems with jejunocecostomy related to bypassing the ileocecal valve.[300] This anastomosis has a tendency to obstruct and does not function as consistently as a jejunojejunostomy.[195] However, this anastomosis functioned very well in a recent retrospective study.[304] The two-layer anastomosis used, with a simple-continuous pattern in the mucosa and a simple-continuous pattern in the seromuscular layer, eliminated the problem of luminal cuff formation with inverting patterns,[285] and this could explain the lack of obstruction.[304]

Surgery of the Duodenum and Duodenal Bypass

Access to duodenum through a ventral median celiotomy is considerably easier in a foal than in an adult horse.[94,141] The abdominal incision should be extended to the xiphoid cartilage, and a J-shaped incision is required in an adult horse.[141] In addition, the table should be tilted to elevate the front end of an adult horse.[141] Access can be improved by retraction, packing of the abdomen with saline-soaked towels, and suction to remove some unavoidable contamination.[141]

Pyloric stenosis has been successfully corrected by pyloromyotomy, Heineke-Mikulicz pyloroplasty, gastrojejunostomy, or gastroduodenostomy.[94,141,142] For a side-to-side gastroduodenostomy, a hand-sutured anastomosis is preferred over the GIA instrument,[94,140,141] because stapled incision edges can heal together at the commissures of the stoma and cause stomal occlusion.[94] Additionally, stapling instruments are difficult to use in the limited space.[94] In one foal, a focal duodenal stricture was corrected by transverse closure of a full-thickness longitudinal incision that spanned the lesion.[305] Choledochojejunostomy and duodenojejunostomy have been used successfully in foals with obstruction of the common bile duct and duodenum at the level of the hepatopancreatic ampulla.[94]

A duodenojejunostomy can be used to bypass a duodenal stricture beyond the hepaticopancreatic ampulla.[94] A side-to-side gastrojejunostomy is used to bypass an extensive duodenal lesion and has been used in an adult horse with proximal enteritis.[306] A side-to-side jejunojejunostomy is performed distal to bypass procedures to prevent intestinal contents from stagnating in the blind loop between the obstruction and the stoma.[94] The contents of this loop can pass aborally through this stoma, without entering the stomach.

In protracted cases of DPJ that do not respond to appropriate medical therapy, bypass procedures have been developed to drain the affected segment of small intestine into more normal distal segments, so that the large volumes of fluids can be reclaimed by intestinal absorption. In one method, a temporary duodenocecostomy is performed through a 25- to 30-cm-long incision between the 17th and 18th ribs[307] to approach the duodenum before it turns through its caudal flexure behind the base of the cecum. Adjacent portions of duodenum and cecum are joined by the "cutting thread" technique, which creates a stoma 2 cm in diameter. The goal is to allow the distended duodenum to drain into the cecum, with spontaneous closure of the fistula when the condition has resolved. A carbohydrate absorption test can be used during the recovery stage to determine if the stoma has healed spontaneously. For horses with DPJ, a duodenojejunostomy through a ventral midline celiotomy is an alternative procedure that is effective in reducing gastric distention and reflux.[84] An adult horse that had a gastrojejunostomy for DPJ became lethargic for 1 to 2 weeks after a grain diet, suggesting that it had developed the "dumping syndrome," a metabolic consequence of rapid influx of gastric contents into the jejunum.[306] Although this horse did well for a follow-up period of 8 years after gastrojejunostomy, it had trouble maintaining body weight for the first year after surgery.[306]

Duodenal impactions can be treated successfully with massage of the intestinal contents into the stomach for removal by gastrotomy,[154] or into the jejunum for manual disruption or removal by enterotomy.[150,156] Failure of these methods can be followed by enterotomy through an incision in the dorsal paralumbar space, 3 cm caudal to the 18th rib.[152] Location of this incision over the duodenal obstruction could be guided with some precision by ultrasonography.

Small Intestinal Enterotomy

A longitudinal enterotomy on the antimesenteric surface of the small intestine can be required for removal of impactions with food components, foreign material, or ascarids (see Fig. 35-5), or to empty a segment of distended bowel to facilitate reduction of a strangulation in the epiploic foramen.[195] An exception is ileal impaction with digesta, such as coastal Bermuda grass hay, which can be managed by other means (see earlier). Methods to prevent adherence of intestinal contents to the serosa around the incision include constant lavage of the bowel with warm saline or precoating the proposed enterotomy site with sodium carboxymethylcellulose. The enterotomy can be closed with a single layer (Lembert or Cushing pattern) using 2-0 PDS on a taper needle, or in two layers, such as a simple-continuous pattern in the mucosa followed by an inverting pattern. Advantages of the Cushing pattern for the final row are that less suture material is exposed to the peritoneal cavity, and there is minimal inversion. Any closure method should minimize lumen reduction and risk for adhesions.

An enterotomy is indicated to a lesser extent in small intestinal surgery than in colon surgery, and it should be avoided if possible and if other options are available, because the resulting closure could be a focus for adhesion formation. For example, viability can be assessed by seromuscular changes without need for mucosal inspection (see earlier). Extensive strangulating lesions can be corrected without removing fluid contents, although gas can be removed through a 14-gauge needle tunneled beneath the seromuscular layer and connected to a suction device. The tunnel staggers puncture sites in the different layers so suture closure is unnecessary. A focal impaction with dehydrated intestinal contents can be softened by injection of saline through an 18-gauge needle into its substance or by mixing it with more proximal liquid contents. If a resection is not indicated, distended small intestine can be decompressed by massaging contents into the cecum, from which they can be removed by typhlotomy.

AFTERCARE FOR SMALL INTESTINAL SURGERY

Routine use of an indwelling nasogastric tube does not ensure against gastric rupture in horses[79,308] and possibly contributes in some way to the secretory component of postoperative ileus.[195] Therefore, decompression of the stomach is indicated only by clinical findings, such as pain and increased heart rate. I do not use an indwelling tube.

Most horses can be offered a small handful of good-quality hay within 18 to 24 hours after surgery.[195] This can be repeated at 3- to 4-hour intervals and the amount increased slowly to a full ration within 3 to 4 days. The refeeding process requires great care and close observation, but it can stimulate return of intestinal function.[195] Early feeding is very well tolerated in horses with jejunojejunostomy.

Broad-spectrum antibiotics and flunixin meglumine are administered before surgery and continued for 3 days afterward. Intravenous fluids are administered at 2 L/hr to a 450-kg horse for the initial 12 hours after surgery; the rate is subsequently adjusted for changes in packed cell volume and total plasma protein (see Chapters 3 and 39).[303] Prokinetic drugs are used almost routinely by some surgeons[303] or as needed by others.[195]

REPEAT CELIOTOMY

Repeat celiotomy is a life-saving procedure and can be required for 12% to 27% of small intestinal diseases[73,74,106,196,301] and for 4% to 12.5% of all colic surgeries.[100,309-311] The need for repeat celiotomy is far greater after small intestinal surgery than after large intestinal surgery,[311] and it is greater after jejunocecostomy than after jejunojejunostomy.[106,298,312] Although making the distinction between postoperative ileus and mechanical obstruction from anastomotic impaction, ischemia, adhesions, or others can be difficult, horses with mechanical obstruction usually demonstrate a greater degree of pain and have a progressive increase in heart rate.[106,303,311] The median time to relaparotomy in one study was 48 hours, with 67% of horses undergoing surgery within 72 hours of the first procedure.[311]

Two important disadvantages of a second abdominal exploratory intervention are the risk for incisional infection[100,106] and the expense; however, the benefits of this procedure can outweigh the risks and disadvantages in most cases, including prompt termination of hopeless cases and salvage of others with treatable lesions. Survival after a repeat celiotomy ranges from 36% to 56.4%[73,74,106,196,309-311] and can be as low as 20% on a long-term basis.[309] However, in one study, 74% of horses that were recovered after a second celiotomy were alive at 1 year after the second surgery.[311]

COMPLICATIONS AND PITFALLS

The most common complications of small intestinal surgery in the horse are anastomotic obstructions (Fig. 35-27), adhesions, and postoperative ileus (POI). The clinical distinction between these three complications is difficult, and each can contribute to the pathogenesis of the other. The first two cause mechanical obstruction and are associated with greater and more persistent signs of abdominal pain than with POI. Technical errors are not well tolerated in small intestinal surgery in horses and can account for many complications. In a recent study of 74 horses that recovered from general anesthesia after small intestinal surgery, technical errors and errors in judgment were responsible for 8 of 14 repeat celiotomies (57%) and for 7 of 11 deaths during hospitalization (64%).[106]

Anastomotic Obstruction

Mechanical obstruction of the anastomosis can be caused by impaction, hematoma, constriction, excessive shortening of the mesentery, and other errors in technique. Prolonged obstruction of an anastomosis can lead to adhesion formation (see Fig. 35-27). Stomas of marginal size are prone to obstruction because they are further reduced by postanastomotic edema.[313] Thereafter, the stoma reduces in size for up to 3 weeks because of wound contraction. Small intestinal volvulus may develop in distended jejunum and at points of small intestinal fixation, such as at a jejunocecal anastomosis. Risk of this complication is increased in a jejunocecal anastomosis by failure to decompress intestine during surgery and by placement of the jejunum toward the apex of the cecum, which twists the jejunum 180 degees.[106] Intussusception of the anastomosis has been reported in horses and ponies after functional end-to-end anastomosis,[207,208] hand-sewn anastomosis,[209,286,314] and inverting closure of a transverse enterotomy.[206]

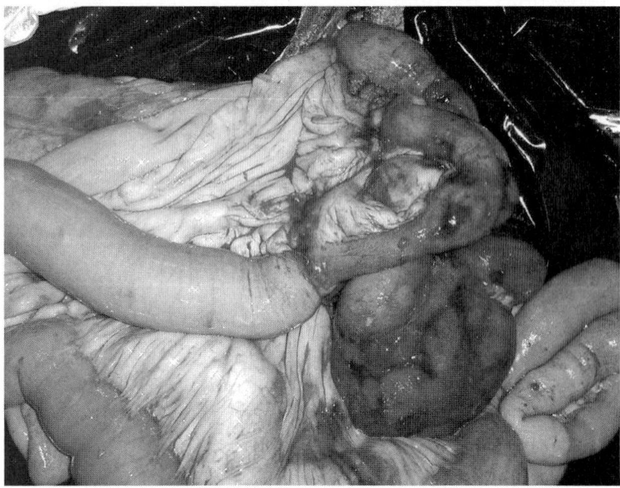

Figure 35-27. Effects of prolonged (5 days) anastomotic obstruction caused by excessive shortening of the mesentery at the anastomosis. Note the hemorrhage in the proximal bowel to the right and the fibrinous adhesions in the loops in the right foreground.

Jejunocecal and ileocecal anastomoses are usually associated with more postoperative complications than jejunojejunostomy.[106,298,312] This difference can be explained by the bypass of the ileocecal valve and by the creation of a sharp transition between intestinal segments of dissimilar functions.[195] The jejunum must overcome intracecal pressure to empty, without the coordinating mechanism of the ileum and ileocecal valve.[4,5,38] Another factor that could contribute to postoperative complications is the presence of adhesions to a devitalized ileal stump and mesentery. In addition, with a jejunocecostomy, all the remaining small intestine was subjected to prestenotic distention that could delay return of function,[59,60] whereas only a portion of the remaining intestine was subjected to distention with jejunojejunostomy.

Postoperative Ileus

Postoperative ileus has a reported prevalence that varies from 10%[106] to 55.6%[315] and a mortality rate of 13% to 86%,[315,316] accounting for 9% to 43% of all deaths after small intestinal surgery.[106,315] In one study on small intestinal surgery, no horse developed POI after jejunojejunostomy, whereas 20% of horses that had had a jejunocecostomy did.[106] Although prokinetic drugs can be used for treatment (see Chapter 39), the role of mechanical obstruction must not be overlooked, because this delays the use of repeat laparotomy. Many horses with postoperative ileus will benefit from decompression at a second surgery.[73] Pelvic flexure enterotomy (see Chapter 36) may reduce the risk for POI, possibly by reducing resistance to ileal emptying and by decreasing compression of hypomotile intestine by a full colon.[317]

Adhesions

Adhesions have been documented in 6% to 26% of horses after small intestinal surgery, with a marked decline in prevalence over time.[73,100,106,278,291] Adhesions usually cause signs of intestinal obstruction in the first 2 months after surgery, but adhesion-related obstruction can arise at any time. Although foals are considered to be especially prone,[318] adhesion formation in juvenile Thoroughbreds after surgery for lesions of all parts of the gastrointestinal tract has been reported at 8%, similar to the percentage reported for adult horses.[319] Foals of 15 days to 6 months seem more likely than weanlings and yearlings to develop adhesions and require multiple surgeries.[319] Factors that could contribute to adhesions are postoperative ileus, ischemia, foreign material, serosal abrasion by towels, excessive handling of bowel, and use of large suture material.

Short Bowel Syndrome

Short bowel syndrome has been documented in horses after extensive small intestinal resection,[73,106,308] although horses can tolerate loss of 10 m to 10.7 m of small intestine.[210,291] According to one study, resection of 60% or more of small intestine can lead to malabsorption.[320] A subsequent study demonstrated that resection of 70% of the small intestine of ponies is well tolerated.[321] Clinical experience supports this conclusion,[106] although the limit for resection can vary among horses, and residual bowel can compensate over time.[210] Mural congestion caused by venous strangulation can increase the length of the affected segment of small intestine by as much as 36%, so some correction for an increase in length after strangulation is needed to avoid an overly pessimistic estimate of the risk for short bowel syndrome.[322] A correction factor that would apply to different severities of strangulation encountered in clinical cases is difficult to establish, and therefore assessment of the remaining length of small intestine could be a more meaningful predictor of postoperative absorptive capacity.[322] A minimal length of 4.5 m (15 feet) of remaining small intestine would be adequate in an adult horse,[73] which approximates what would be left after resection of 75%.[322] Removal of longer segments does not appear to be well tolerated, although one 450-kg horse left with 3.7 m (12.3 feet) did not develop short bowel syndrome, which is evidence of a tremendous individual variation.[106]

Other potential complications of extensive small intestine resection are liver disease[320] and anorexia.[195] Bypass of the ileocecal junction by jejunocecal anastomosis without resection can allow cecal bacteria to seed the small intestine and cause an abnormal xylose absorption test in ponies,[320] which is apparently not the case in horses.[323] Although based on findings from laboratory animals, postoperative dietary recommendations that may apply to horses with short bowel syndrome include complex nutrients as potent stimulants of intestinal adaptation, and fiber to increase colonic production of short-chain fatty acids (see Chapter 6).[322] Carbohydrates should be fed sparingly, as they are more likely than fats and proteins to induce osmotic diarrhea.[322]

Miscellaneous

Anastomotic dehiscence and peritonitis are rare in most studies, but they were a leading cause of death when staples were used for all small intestinal anastomoses in horses.[137] Failure to effectively ligate mesenteric vessels can lead to postoperative hemorrhage. Occlusion or kinking of vessels or postoperative thrombosis of mesenteric vessels for unknown reasons can cause anastomotic necrosis.[106] Mesenteric rents at sites remote to the anastomosis have been described as causes of recurrent small intestinal strangulation and death, years after the original surgery.[73,221] Other complications include pyrexia, jugular vein thrombosis, long-bone fracture, cecal impaction, myositis, endotoxemia, gastric ulceration, recurrent colic, incisional infections, diarrhea,[73,92,196-198,221] and pulmonary aspegillosis.[324] Some horses have concurrent large intestinal displacement[72] or develop large intestinal distention or impaction after surgery.[106]

PROGNOSIS

At least six studies reported survival rates to discharge of 80% to 88% in horses that had surgery of the small intestine and were allowed to recover from anesthesia.* Advances in management and early referral are important determinants of survival, and of the severity of endotoxemia and other complications, such as jugular thrombosis, postoperative ileus, and wound infection.[198] In 115 horses with small intestinal volvulus, nonsurvivors had higher heart rates, longer capillary refill time, greater hemoconcentration, and more exudation of cells and protein into peritoneal fluid at admission than survivors.[325] After small intestinal resection, postoperative factors that were associated with nonsurvival were ileus, heart rate greater than 60 beats per minute at 24 hours, and repeat celiotomy.[196] In 143 horses with entrapment in the epiploic foramen, survival was 75.6% if surgery was performed within 8 hours from the onset of colic, compared with 45.1% survival in horses that underwent surgery 12 hours or more after onset.[74] Multiple logistic analysis demonstrated that duration of surgery was not a factor associated with short-term survival in horses that had small intestinal resection,[196] in contrast to its negative effect on survival when all types of colic are considered.[326] In one study on small intestinal surgery, surgeon experience was the only factor that appeared to influence survival significantly.[106]

In horses with colic from small intestinal disease, survival after simple obstruction is not significantly different from survival after strangulation obstruction.[100,106] Although length of resection does not appear to influence outcome,[291,325] a trend toward lower survival has been reported after resection of greater than 2 m of intestine.[196] Another study found an approximately linear inverse relationship between survival and intestinal resection length.[326] The length of bowel strangulated in the epiploic foramen was longer in nonsurvivors than survivors in another study.[74] Lesions that appear to have an adverse influence on survival are strangulation in the epiploic foramen[197,301] and in mesenteric rents,[221] and ascarid impactions.[122] Prognosis tends to be better after a jejunojejunostomy than after a jejunocecostomy or ileocecostomy,† and jejunocecostomy is associated with increased likelihood of postoperative abdominal pain and repeat celiotomy.[106,312,325] Volvulus at the anastomosis, infarcted jejunum at the anastomosis, and technical errors accounted for most complications from jejunocecostomy in one study,[106] whereas problems with the ileal stump caused 47% of surgery-related complications in another.[312] However, survivals after jejunojejunostomy and jejunocecostomy become similar over the long term.[106] Survival after jejunocecostomy or ileocecostomy without resection is better than after the same procedures with resection.[137] Correction by reduction, bypass, enterotomy, or "kneading" has a better prognosis than after resection and anastomosis.[103,106,137]

In a report on foals with surgical colic, only 10% of those younger than 14 days survived to maturity compared with 45.8% of foals 15 to 150 days old.[102] In one study, 59% of

*References 72, 97, 106, 137, 182, 208.
†References 103, 106, 196, 200, 291, 298, 301.

foals that had surgery for colic survived to discharge, with 25% being euthanized while under anesthesia.[93] The survival for foals that had a small intestinal lesion (46%) was worse than for those with large intestinal lesions (80%).[93] Survival in foals is also greater after nonstrangulating lesions or simple obstruction than after strangulating obstruction.[93,104]

The pattern of survival after surgery for horses with small and large intestinal colics follows a triphasic pattern.[326] Most deaths occur during the first 10 postoperative days, with 69% during the first 100 days after surgery and a slower decline in death rate after that.[326] A study on horses that had small intestinal surgery confirmed this observation and also demonstrated that the risk for death from surgery-related problems diminishes markedly after 12 months.[106]

REFERENCES

1. Schummer A, Nickel R, Sack WO: Viscera of the Domestic Mammal, Berlin, 1979, Springer Verlag.
2. Kotzè SH: Arterial blood supply to the ileocecal junction in the horse, J South Afr Vet Assoc 1990;61:2.
3. Kotzè SH: The arrangement of the muscle layers at the ileocaecal junction, J South Afr Vet Assoc 1988;59:67.
4. Dyce KM, Hartman W: An endoscopic study of the caecal base of the horse, Tijdschr Diergeneesk 1973;98:957.
5. Roger T, Malbert CH: Caractéristique anatomo-fonctionelles de la jonction iléocaecale du poney, Rev Med Vet 140:851, 1989.
6. Coffin B, Lemann M, Flourie B, et al: Local regulation of ileal tone in healthy humans, Am J Physiol 1997;272:G147.
7. Johnson LR: Digestion and absorption. In Johnson LR, editor: Gastrointestinal Physiology, ed 6, St Louis, 2001, CV Mosby.
8. Wright EM, Hirayama BA, Loo DDF, et al: Intestinal sugar transport. In Johnson LR, editor: Physiology of the Gastrointestinal Tract, New York, 1994, Raven Press.
9. Titkemeyer CW, Calhoun ML: A comparative study of the small intestines of domestic animals, Am J Vet Res 1955;16:152.
10. Alpers DH: Digestion and absorption of carbohydrates and proteins. In Johnson LR, editor: Physiology of the Gastrointestinal Tract, New York, 1994, Raven Press.
11. Johnson LR, McCormack SA: Regulation of gastrointestinal mucosal growth. In Johnson LR, editor: Physiology of the Gastrointestinal Tract, New York, 1994, Raven Press.
12. Civitelli R, Avioli LV: Calcium, phosphate, and magnesium absorption. In Johnson LR, editor: Physiology of the Gastrointestinal Tract, New York, 1994, Raven Press.
13. Madara JL, Trier JS: The functional morphology of the mucosa of the small intestine. In Johnson LR, editor: Physiology of the Gastrointestinal Tract, New York, 1994, Raven Press.
14. Chang EB, Rao MC: Intestinal water and electrolyte transport. In Johnson LR, editor: Physiology of the Gastrointestinal Tract, New York, 1994, Raven Press.
15. Ganapathy V, Brandsch M, Leibach FH: Intestinal transport of amino acids and peptides. In Johnson LR, editor: Physiology of the Gastrointestinal Tract, New York, 1994, Raven Press.
16. Walsh JH: Gastrointestinal hormones. In Johnson LR, editor: Physiology of the Gastrointestinal Tract, New York, 1994, Raven Press.
17. Alexander F: The salivary and pancreatic secretions of the horse. In Phillipson TA, editor: Physiology of Digestion and Metabolism in the Ruminant, Newcastle-upon-Tyne, 1969, Oriel Press.
18. Argenzio RA: Physiology of digestive, secretory, and absorptive processes. In White NA, editor: The Equine Acute Abdomen, Philadelphia, 1990, Lea & Febiger.
19. Hintz HF: Digestive physiology of the horse, J South Afr Vet Assoc 1975;46:13.
20. Hofman AF. Intestinal absorption of bile acids and biliary constituents. In Johnson LR, editor: Physiology of the Gastrointestinal Tract, New York, 1994, Raven Press.
21. Johnson LR: Fluid and electrolyte absorption. In Johnson LR, editor: Gastrointestinal Physiology, ed 6, St Louis, 2001, CV Mosby.
22. Eade MN, Pybus J, Ready J: No evidence of a countercurrent multiplier in the intestinal villus of the dog, Gastroenterology 1990;98:3.
23. Dyer J, Fernandez-Castaño M, Salmon KSH, et al: Molecular characterization of carbohydrate digestion and absorption in equine small intestine, Equine Vet J 2002;34:349-358.
24. Fernandez-Castano Merediz E, Dyer J, Salmon KSH, et al: Molecular characterization of fructose transport in equine small intestine, Equine Vet J 2004;36:532.
25. Tso P: Intestinal lipid absorption. In Johnson LR, editor: Physiology of the Gastrointestinal Tract, New York, 1994, Raven Press.
26. Rucker RB, Lönnerdal B, Keen CL: Intestinal absorption of nutritionally important trace elements. In Johnson LR, editor: Physiology of the Gastrointestinal Tract, New York, 1994, Raven Press.
27. Henninger RW, Horst J: Magnesium toxicosis in two horses, J Am Vet Med Assoc 1997;211:82-85.
28. Harrington DD, Walsh JJ: Equine magnesium supplements: Evaluation of magnesium oxide, magnesium sulphate and magnesium carbonate in foals fed purified diets, Equine Vet J 1980;12:32-33.
29. Castro GA: Immunological regulation of epithelial function, Am J Physiol 1982;243:G321.
30. Makhlouf GM: Neuromuscular function of the small intestine. In Johnson LR, editor: Physiology of the Gastrointestinal Tract, New York, 1994, Raven Press.
31. Malone ED, Brown DR, Trent AM, et al: Influence of adrenergic and cholinergic mediators on the equine jejunum in vitro, Am J Vet Res 1996;57:884.
32. Gershon MD, Kirchgessner AL, Wade PR: Functional anatomy of the enteric nervous system. In Johnson LR, editor: Physiology of the Gastrointestinal Tract, New York, 1994, Raven Press.
33. Phaneuf LP, Grivel ML, Ruckebusch Y: Electromyography during normal gastrointestinal activity, painful or non-painful colic and morphine analgesia, in the horse, Can J Comp Med 1972;36:138.
34. Weisbrodt NW: Motility of the small intestine. In Johnson LR, editor: Gastrointestinal Physiology, ed 6, St Louis, 2001, CV Mosby.
35. Adams SB, Lamar CH, Masty J: Motility of the distal portion of the jejunum and pelvic flexure in ponies: Effects of six drugs, Am J Vet Res 1984;45:795.
36. Lester GD, Bolton JR, Cullen LK, et al: Effects of general anesthesia on myoelectric activity of the intestine in horses, Am J Vet Res 1992;53:1553.
37. Walsh JH: Gastrointestinal hormones. In Johnson LR, editor: Physiology of the Gastrointestinal Tract, New York, 1994, Raven Press.
38. Ross MW, Cullen KK, Rutkowski JA: Myoelectric activity of the ileum, cecum, and right ventral colon in ponies during interdigestive, nonfeeding, and digestive periods, Am J Vet Res 1990;51:561.
39. Berry CR, Merritt AM, Burrows CF, et al: Evaluation of the myoelectrical activity of the equine ileum infected with *Strongylus vulgaris* larvae, Am J Vet Res 1986;47:27.
40. Lamar CH, Masty J, Adams SB, et al: Impedance monitoring of equine intestinal motility, Am J Vet Res 1984;45:810.
41. Sojka JE, Adams SB, Lamar CH, et al: Effect of butorphanol, pentazocine, meperidine, or metoclopramide on intestinal motility in female ponies, Am J Vet Res 1988;49:527.
42. Roger T, Malbert CH, Benouali-Pelissier S: Ileo-caecal junction motility disorder in the horse: A hypothesis of the pathogenesis of intussusception of the ileum in this species, Revue Med Vet 1995;146:29.

43. Re G, Belloli C, Badino P, et al: Identification of β-adrenergic receptor subtypes mediating relaxation in isolated equine ileum, Am J Vet Res 1997;58:621.
44. Merritt AM, Campbell-Thompson ML, Lowrey S: Effect of butorphanol on equine antroduodenal motility, Equine Vet J Suppl 1989;7:21-23.
45. Merritt AM, Campbell-Thompson ML, Lowrey S: Effect of xylazine treatment on equine proximal gastrointestinal tract myoelectrical activity, J Am Vet Med Assoc 1989;50:945-949.
46. Merritt AM, Burrow JA, Hartless CS: Effect of xylazine, detomidine, and a combination of xylazine and butorphanol on equine duodenal motility, Am J Vet Res 1998;59:619-623.
47. Bueno L, Praddaude F, Ruckebusch Y: Propagation of electrical spiking activity along the small intestine: intrinsic versus extrinsic neural influences, J Physiol 1979;292:15.
48. Quigley EM, Thompson JS: The motor response to intestinal resection: motor activity in the canine small intestine following distal resection, Gastroenterology 1993;105:791.
49. Pearce AN, Wingate DL: Myoelectric and absorptive activity in the transected canine small bowel, J Physiol 1980;302:11P.
50. MacHarg MA, Adams SB, Lamar, CH, et al: Electromyographic, mechanical, and intraluminal pressure changes associated with acute extraluminal obstruction of the jejunum in conscious ponies, Am J Vet Res 1986;47:7.
51. Davies JV, Gerring EL: Effects of experimental vascular occlusion on small intestinal motility in ponies, Equine Vet J 1985;17:219.
52. King JN, Gerring EL: The action of low dose endotoxin on equine bowel motility, Equine Vet J 1991;23:11.
53. King JN, Gerring EL: Antagonism of endotoxin-induced disruption of equine bowel motility by flunixin and phenylbutazone, Equine Vet J 1989;7(Suppl):38.
54. Rakestraw PC, Snyder JR, Woliner MJ, et al: Involvement of nitric oxide in inhibitory neuromuscular transmission in equine jejunum, Am J Vet Res 1996;57:1206.
55. Shields R: The absorption and secretion of fluid and electrolytes by the obstructed bowel, Br J Surg 1965;52:774.
56. Mortillaro NA, Taylor AE: Interaction of capillary and tissue forces in the cat small intestine, Circ Res 1976;39:348.
57. Swabb EA, Hynes RA, Donowitz M: Elevated intraluminal pressure after rabbit small intestinal transport in vivo, Am J Physiol 1982;242:G58.
58. Lifson N: Fluid secretion and hydrostatic relationships in the small intestine. In Binder HJ, editor: Mechanisms of Secretion, New York, 1979, Alan R. Liss.
59. Dabareiner RM, Sullins KE, Snyder JR, et al: Evaluation of the microcirculation of the equine small intestine after intraluminal distention and subsequent decompression, Am J Vet Res 1993;54:1673.
60. Dabareiner RM, Sullins KE, White NA, et al: Serosal injury in the equine jejunum and ascending colon after ischemia-reperfusion or intraluminal distention and decompression, Vet Surg 2001;30:114.
61. Sullins KE, Stashak TS, Mero KN: Pathologic changes associated with induced small intestinal strangulation obstruction and nonstrangulating infarction in horses, Am J Vet Res 1985;46:913.
62. Ruggles AJ, Freeman DE, Acland HM, et al: Changes in fluid composition on the serosal surface of jejunum and small colon subjected to venous strangulation obstruction in ponies, Am J Vet Res 1993;54:333.
63. Freeman DE, Cimprich RE, Richardson DW, et al: Early mucosal healing and chronic changes in pony jejunum after various types of strangulation obstruction, Am J Vet Res 1988;49:810.
64. Chiu CJ, McArdle AH, Brown R, et al: Intestinal mucosal lesions in low flow states, Arch Surg 1970;191:478.
65. Snyder JR: The pathophysiology of intestinal damage: Effects of luminal distention and ischemia, Vet Clin North Am 1989;5:247.
66. Dart AJ, Snyder JR, Julian D, et al: Microvascular circulation of the small intestine in horses, Am J Vet Res 1992;53:995.
67. Johnston JK, Freeman DE, Gillette D, et al: Effects of superoxide dismutase on injury induced by anoxia and reoxygenation in equine small intestine in vitro, Am J Vet Res 1991;52:2050.
68. Blikslager AT, Roberts MC: Mechanisms of intestinal mucosal repair, J Am Vet Med Assoc 1997;211:1437.
69. Blikslager AT, Roberts MC: Accuracy of clinicians in predicting site and type of lesion as well as outcome in horses with colic, J Am Vet Med Assoc 1995;207:1444.
70. White NA, Dabareiner RM: Treatment of impaction colics, Vet Clin North Am Equine Pract 1997;13:243.
71. Johnston JK, Morris DD: Comparison of duodenitis/proximal jejunitis and small intestinal obstruction in horses: 68 cases (1977-1985), J Am Vet Med Assoc 1987;191:849.
72. Stephen JO, Corley KTT, Johnston JK, et al: Small intestinal volvulus in 115 horses: 1988-2000, Vet Surg 2004;33:333.
73. Vachon AM, Fischer AT: Small-intestinal herniation through the epiploic foramen: 53 cases (1987-1993), Equine Vet J 1995;27:373.
74. Scheidemann W: Beitrag zur Diagnostik und Therapie der Kolik des Pferdes: Die Hernia foraminis omentalis, Doctoral thesis, Ludwig-Maximilians-Universität, Munich, 1989.
75. Tulleners EP: Complications of abdominocentesis in the horse, J Am Vet Med Assoc 1983;182:232.
76. Fischer AT: Advances in diagnostic techniques for horses with colic, Vet Clin North Am Equine Pract 1997;13:203.
77. Grindem CB, Fairley NM, Uhlinger CA, et al: Peritoneal fluid values from healthy foals, Equine Vet J 1990;22:359.
78. Malark JA, Peyton LC, Galvin MJ: Effects of blood contamination in equine peritoneal fluid analysis, J Am Vet Med Assoc 1992;201:1545.
79. Blackford JT, Toal RL, Latimer FG, et al: Percutaneous ultrasonographic diagnosis of suspected acquired inguinal and scrotal herniation in horses, Proc Am Assoc Equine Pract 1992;38:357.
80. Ford TS, Freeman DE, Ross MW, et al: Ileocecal intussusception in horses: 26 cases (1981-1988), J Am Vet Med Assoc 1990;196:121.
81. Gift LJ, Gaughan EM, DeBowes RM, et al: Jejunal intussusception in adult horses: 11 cases (1981-1991), J Am Vet Med Assoc 1993;202:110.
82. Edwards GB: Surgical management of intussusception in the horse, Equine Vet J 1986;18:313.
83. Elce YA, Kraus BM, Habecker PL, et al: Jejunal perforation in three young horses, Equine Vet J 2003;35:720.
84. White NA, Tyler DE, Blackwell RB: Hemorrhagic fibrinonecrotic duodenitis-proximal jejunitis: 20 cases (1977-1984), J Am Vet Med Assoc 1987;190:311.
85. Southwood LL, Kawcak CE, Trotter GW, et al: Idiopathic focal eosinophilic enteritis associated with small intestinal obstruction in 6 horses, Vet Surg 2000;29:415.
86. Arden WA, Stick JA: Serum and peritoneal fluid phosphate concentrations as predictors of major intestinal injury associated with equine colic, J Am Vet Med Assoc 1988;193:927.
87. Scharner D, Rötting A, Gerlach K, et al: Ultrasonography of the abdomen of the horse with colic, Clin Tech Equine Prac 2002;1:118.
88. Klohnen A, Vachon AM, Fischer AT: Use of ultrasonography in horses with signs of acute abdominal pain, J Am Vet Med Assoc 1996;209:1597.
89. Reef VB: Ultrasonographic evaluation and diagnosis of foal diseases. In Robinson NE, editor: Current Therapy in Equine Medicine, ed 3, Philadelphia, 1992, WB Saunders.
90. Bernard WV, Reef VB, Reimer JM, et al: Ultrasonographic diagnosis of small-intestinal intussusception in three foals, J Am Vet Med Assoc 1989;194:395.
91. Freeman S: Diagnostic ultrasonography of the mature equine abdomen, Equine Vet Educ 2003;15:319.
92. Jenei TM, Garcia-Lopez JM, Provost PJ, et al: Surgical management of small intestinal incarceration through the epiploic foramen: 63 cases, Vet Surg 2003;32:489.

93. Bartmann C-P, Glitz F, von Oppen T, et al: Diagnosis and surgical management of colic in the foal, Pferdeheilkunde 2001;17:676.
94. Orsini JA: Abdominal surgery in foals, Vet Clin North Am Equine Pract 1997;13:393.
95. Walmsley JP: Review of equine laparoscopy and an analysis of 158 laparoscopies in the horse, Equine Vet J 1999;31:456.
96. Siebke A-U: Statistische Erhebung über Kurzund Langzeitergebnisse von 718 operativ behandelten Kolikpatienten, Med Vet Thesis, Der Freien Universität, Berlin, 1995.
97. Huskamp B: Diagnosis and treatment of acute abdominal conditions in the horse: Various types and frequency as seen at the animal hospital in Hochmoor, Proc Equine Colic Res Symp 1982;1:261.
98. Tennant B: Intestinal obstruction in the horse: Some aspects of differential diagnosis in equine colic, Proc Am Assoc Equine Pract 1975;21:426.
99. Morris DD, Moore JN: Signalment and management factors of horses presented to the University of Georgia with ileal impaction or proximal enteritis, Proc Equine Colic Res Symp 1988;3:19.
100. Phillips TJ, Walmsley JP: Retrospective analysis of the results of 151 exploratory laparotomies in horses with gastrointestinal disease, Equine Vet J 1993;25:427.
101. Edwards GB: Obstruction of the ileum in the horse: A report of 27 clinical cases, Equine Vet J 1981;13:158.
102. Vatistas, NJ, Snyder JR, Wilson WD, et al: Surgical treatment for colic in the foal (67 cases): 1980-1992, Equine Vet J 1996;28:139.
103. Kersjes AW, Bras GE, Nemeth F, et al: Results of operative treatment of equine colic with special reference to surgery of the ileum, Vet Q 1988;10:17.
104. Cable CS, Fubini SL, Erb HN, et al: Abdominal surgery in foals: A review of 199 cases (1977-1994), Equine Vet J 1997;29:257.
105. Edwards GB: Obstruction of the ileum: A common indication for surgery, Proc Bain-Fallon Memorial Lectures, Sydney, Australia, 1992;14:129.
106. Freeman DE, Hammock P, Baker GJ, et al: Short- and long-term survival and prevalence of postoperative ileus after small intestinal surgery in the horse, Equine Vet J Suppl 2000;32:42.
107. Embertson RM, Colahan PT, Brown MP, et al: Ileal impaction in the horse, J Am Vet Med Assoc 1985;186:570.
108. Hanson RR, Schumacher J, Humburg J, et al: Medical treatment of horses with ileal impactions: 10 cases (1990-1994), J Am Vet Med Assoc 1996;208:898.
109. Parks AH, Doran RE, White NA, et al: Ileal impaction in the horse: 75 cases, Cornell Vet 1989;79:83.
110. Hanson RR, Wright JC, Baird AN, et al: Surgical reduction of ileal impactions in the horse: 28 cases, Vet Surg 1998;27:555.
111. Little D, Blikslager AT: Factors associated with development of ileal impaction in horses with surgical colic: 78 cases (1986-2000), Equine Vet J 2002;34:464.
112. McClure SR, Chaffin MK, Vacek JR, et al: Ileal impactions in two foals, Vet Med 1995;90:1160.
113. Proudman CJ, French NP, Trees AJ: Tapeworm infection is a significant risk factor for spasmodic colic and ileal impaction in the horse, Equine Vet J 30:194,1998.
114. Hanson RR, Baird AN, Pugh DG: Ileal impaction in horses, Comp Cont Educ Pract Vet 1995;17:1287.
115. Lindsay WA, Confer AW, Ochoa R: Ileal smooth muscle hypertrophy and rupture in a horse, Equine Vet J 1981;13:66.
116. Blennerhassett MG, Vignjevic P, Vermillion DL, et al: Inflammation causes hyperplasia and hypertrophy in smooth muscle of rat small intestine, Am J Physiol 1992;262:G1041.
117. Schneider JE, Kennedy GA, Leipold HW: Muscular hypertrophy of the small intestine in a horse, J Equine Med Surg 1979;3:226.
118. Rooney JR, Jeffcott LB: Muscular hypertrophy of the ileum in a horse, Vet Rec 1968;83:217.
119. Mair TS, Lucke VM: Ileal muscular hypertrophy and rupture in a pony three years after surgery for ileocecal intussusception, Vet Rec 2000;146:472.
120. Chaffin MK, Fuenteabla IC, Schumacher J, et al: Idiopathic muscular hypertrophy of the equine small intestine: 11 cases (1980-1991), Equine Vet J 1992;24:372.
121. King JM: Ileal rupture secondary to idiopathic hypertrophy, Vet Med 1994;89:616.
122. Southwood LL, Ragle CA, Snyder JR, et al: Surgical treatment of ascarid impactions in horses and foals, Proc Am Assoc Equine Pract 1996;42:258.
123. Hearn FPD, Peregrine AS: Identification of foals infected with *Parascaris equorum* apparently resistant to ivermectin, J Am Vet Med Assoc 2003;223:482.
124. Southwood LL, Baxter GM, Bennett DG, et al: Ascarid impaction in young horses, Comp Cont Educ Prac Vet 1998;20:100.
125. Seahorn TL, Cornick JL, Cohen ND: Prognostic indicators for horses with duodenitis-proximal jejunitis: 75 horses (1985-1989), J Vet Int Med 1992;6:307.
126. Moore JN, Barton MH: An update on endotoxemia: Part 2. Treatment and the way ahead, Equine Vet Educ 1999;11:30.
127. Edwards GB: Duodenitis-proximal jejunitis (anterior enteritis) as a surgical problem, Equine Vet Educ 2000;12:318.
128. Leeth B, Robertson JT: A retrospective comparison of surgical to medical management of proximal enteritis in the horse, Proc Am Assoc Equine Pract 1989;34:69.
129. Cohen ND, Parson EM, Seahorn TL, et al: Prevalence and factors associated with development of laminitis in horses with duodenitis/proximal jejunitis: 33 cases (1985-1991), J Am Vet Med Assoc 1994;204:250.
130. Allen D, Swayne D, Belknap JK: Ganglioneuroma as a cause of small intestinal obstruction in the horse: A case report, Cornell Vet 1989;79:133.
131. Bertone AL, Yovich HV, McIlwraith CW: Surgical resection of intestinal lymphosarcoma in a mare, Comp Cont Educ Pract Vet 1985;7:506.
132. Livesy MA, Hulland TJ, Yovich JV: Colic in two horses associated with smooth muscle intestinal tumours, Equine Vet J 1986;18:334.
133. Hanes GE, Robertson JT: Leiomyoma of the small intestine in a horse, J Am Vet Med Assoc 1983;182:1398.
134. Orsini JA, Orsini PG, Sepesy L, et al: Intestinal carcinoid in a mare: An etiologic consideration for chronic colic in horses, J Am Vet Med Assoc 1988;193:87.
135. Honnas CM, Snyder JR, Olander HJ, et al: Small intestinal adenocarcinoma in a horse, J Am Vet Med Assoc 1987;191:845.
136. Mair TS, Taylor FGR, Brown PJ: Leiomyosarcoma of the duodenum in two horses, J Comp Path 1990;102:119.
137. Fugaro MN, Coté NM: Survival rates for horses undergoing stapled small intestinal anastomosis: 84 cases (1988-1997), J Am Vet Med Assoc 2001;218:1603.
138. Acland HM, Gunson DE, Gillette DM: Ulcerative duodenitis in foals, Vet Pathol 1983;20:653.
139. Ettlinger JJ, Ford T, Palmer JE: Ulcerative duodenitis with luminal constriction in two horses, J Am Vet Med Assoc 1990;196:1628.
140. Ross MW, Bernard WV, Orsini PG, et al: Surgical management of duodenal obstruction in an adult horse, J Am Vet Med Assoc 1989;194:1312.
141. Aronoff N, Keegan KG, Johnson PJ, et al: Management of pyloric obstruction in a foal, J Am Vet Med Assoc 1997;210:902.
142. Kirberger RM, van den Berg JS, Gottschalk RD, et al: Duodenal ultrasonography in the normal adult horse, Vet Radiol Ultrason 1995;36:50.
143. Traub-Dargatz JL, Schultheiss PC, Kiper ML, et al: Intestinal fibrosis with partial obstruction in five horses and two ponies, J Am Vet Med Assoc 1992;201:603.
144. Johnson PJ, Pace LW, Mrad DR, et al: Small intestinal fibrosis in two horses, J Am Vet Med Assoc 1997;211:1013.
145. Lavoie JP, Drolet R, Parsons D, et al: Equine proliferative enteropathy: A cause of weight loss, colic, diarrhea and hypoproteinaemia in foals on three breeding farms in Canada, Equine Vet J 2000;32:418.

146. Schumacher J, Schumacher J, Rolsma M, et al: Surgical and medical treatment of an Arabian filly with proliferative enteropathy caused by *Lawsonia intracellularis*, J Vet Intern Med 2000;14:630.
147. Scott EA, Heidel JR, Snyder SP, et al: Inflammatory bowel disease in horses: 11 cases (1988-1998), J Am Vet Med Assoc 1999;214:1527.
148. Purcell KL, Johnson PJ, Kreegero JM, et al: Jejunal obstruction caused by a *Pythium insidiosum* granuloma in a mare, J Am Vet Med Assoc 1994;205:337.
149. Allison N, Gillis JP: Enteric pythiosis in a horse, J Am Vet Med Assoc 1990;196:462.
150. Mair TS: Small intestinal obstruction caused by a mass of feedblock containing molasses in 4 horses, Equine Vet J 2002;34:532.
151. Dixon RT: Intestinal obstruction in a gelding, Aust Vet J 1965;41:20.
152. Durham AE: Flank laparotomy for the removal of a duodenal conglobate in a filly, Equine Vet Educ 1998;10:8.
153. Bohanon TC: Duodenal impaction in a horse, J Am Vet Med Assoc 192:365,1988.
154. Turner TA: Trichophytobezoar causing duodenal obstruction in a horse, Comp Cont Educ Pract Vet 1986;8:977.
155. Green P, Tong JMJ: Small intestinal obstruction associated with wood chewing in two horses, Vet Rec 1988;123:196.
156. Kellam LL, Johnson PJ, Kramer J, et al: Gastric impaction and obstruction of the small intestine associated with persimmon phytobezoar in a horse, J Am Vet Med Assoc 2000;216:1279.
157. Wilson RB, Scruggs DW: Duodenal obstruction associated with persimmon fruit ingestion by two horses, Equine Vet Sci 1992;12:26.
158. Baker GJ, Dodman HN, Clayton HM: Foreign body obstruction of the small intestine of a foal, Vet Rec 1974;95:293.
159. Laverty S, Pascoe JR, Williams JW, et al: Cholelith causing duodenal obstruction in a horse, J Am Vet Med Assoc 1992;201:751.
160. Davies JV: Ischaemic necrosis of the jejunum of a horse caused by a penetrating foreign body, Equine Vet J 1983;15:66.
161. Dobson H, Lopez A: Intestinal obstruction and gastric rupture involving a penetrating foreign body, Equine Vet J 1981;13:204.
162. Modransky PD, Traub JL, Krpan MK, et al: Penetration of the small intestine by an unusual foreign body resulting in colic in a horse: A case report, J Equine Vet Sci 1983;3:100.
163. Hunter R: Perforated ulcer in the small intestine of a mare, Vet Med/Small Anim Clin 1975;70:199.
164. Campbell-Beggs CL, Johnson PJ, Wilson DA, et al: Chyloabdomen in a neonatal foal, Vet Rec 1995;137:96.
165. Edwards GB, Scholes SR, Edwards SER, et al: Colic in 4 neonatal foals associated with chyloperitoneum and congenital segmental lymphatic aplasia, Proc Equine Colic Res Symp 1994;5:35.
166. May KA, Cheramie HS, Prater DA: Chyloperitoneum and abdominal adhesions in a miniature horse, J Am Vet Med Assoc 1999;215:676.
167. Madison JB, Dreyfuss DJ, Charlton C: Ileal diverticulum as a cause of chronic colic in a horse, J Am Vet Med Assoc 1991;198:453.
168. Riccaboni P, Tassan S, Mayer P: Rare intestinal malformation (diverticulum confluens) in a horse, Equine Vet J 2000;32:351.
169. Yovich JV, Horney FD: Congenital jejunal diverticulum in a foal, J Am Vet Med Assoc 1983;183:1092.
170. Kobluk CN, Smith DF: Intramural hematoma in the jejunum of a mare, J Am Vet Med Assoc 1988;192:379.
171. Huskamp B, Scheidemann W, Schusser GF: Idiopathic muscular hypertrophy and aganglionosis of the proximal duodenum (pars cranialis et pars descendens duodeni) in colic horses, Proc Equine Colic Res Symp 1998;6:50.
172. Moll HD, Juzwiak JS, Santschi EM, et al: Small intestinal volvulus as a complication of acquired inguinal hernia in two horses, J Am Vet Med Assoc 1991;198:1413.
173. Kopf N: Über die Entstehung der Darmverlagerungen des Pferdes, Pferdeheilkunde 1985;1:131.
174. Freeman DE, Koch DB, Boles CL: Mesodiverticular bands as a cause of small intestinal strangulation and volvulus in the horse, J Am Vet Med Assoc 1979;175:1089.
175. Röcken M, Reckels FJ, Schmidt-Oechtering GU, et al: Eine Sonderform des Meckel-Divertikels am Jejunum eines Pferdes, Pferdeheilkunde 1989;5:49.
176. Grant BD, Tennant BD: Volvulus associated with Meckel's diverticulum in the horse, J Am Vet Med Assoc 1973;165:550.
177. Crouch GM, Snyder J, Harmon BG: Adhesion of the ileum to the inguinal ring in a gelding, Equine Pract 1983;9:32.
178. Crowhurst RC, Simpson DJ, McEnery RJ, et al: Intestinal surgery in the foal, J South Afr Vet Assoc 1975;46:59.
179. Huskamp B, Toth J: The pathogenesis and surgical treatment of nodular volvulus. Magyar Allatorvosok Lapja 1998;120:10.
180. Schmid A: Die Anatomie des Foramen epiploicum und seiner benachbarten Strukturen und die Auswirkungen von Alter, Rasse und Geschlecht auf Darmstrangulation durch das Foramen epiploicum, Inguinalhernie, Lipoma pendulans und Invagination, Med Vet Thesis, Ludwig-Maximilians-Universität, Munich, 1997.
181. Vasey JR: Incarceration of the small intestine by the epiploic foramen in fifteen horses, Can Vet J 1988;29:378.
182. Engelbert TA, Tate LP, Bowman KF, et al: Incarceration of the small intestine in the epiploic foramen: Report of 19 cases (1983-1992), Vet Surg 1993;22:57.
183. Hammock PD, Freeman DE, Magid JH, et al: Parietal hernia of the small intestine into the epiploic foramen of a horse, J Am Vet Med Assoc 1999;214:1354.
184. Edwards GB. Diseases of the equine stomach, In Proc Geneva Congr Equine Med Surg 1997;5:97.
185. Mair TS: Incarceration and impaction of a short segment of ileum into the epiploic foramen in a horse, Equine Vet Educ 2003;15:241.
186. Archer DC, Proudman CJ, Smith J, et al: Epiploic foramen entrapment of the small intestine: A review of 68 cases (1991-2001). In Proceedings of the Equine Colic Research Symposium, Manchester, England, 2002:93.
187. Wheat JD: Diseases of the small intestine: Diagnosis and treatment, Proc Am Assoc Equine Pract 1972;18:265.
188. Freeman DE, Schaeffer DJ: Age distribution of horses with strangulation of the small intestine by a lipoma or in the epiploic foramen: 46 cases (1994-2000), J Am Vet Med Assoc 2001;219:87.
189. Murray RC, Gaughan EM, DeBowes RM, et al: Incarceration of the jejunum in the epiploic foramen of a four month old foal, Cornell Vet 1994;84:47.
190. Turner TA, Adams SB, White NA: Small intestine incarceration through the epiploic foramen of the horse, J Am Vet Med Assoc 1984;184:731.
191. Sembrat RF: The acute abdomen in the horse: Epidemiologic considerations, Arch Am Coll Vet Surg. 1975;4:34.
192. Archer DC, Freeman DE, Doyle AJ, et al: Association between cribbing and entrapment of the small intestine in the epiploic foramen in horses: 68 cases (1991-2002), J Am Vet Med Assoc 2004;224:562.
193. Walmsley JP: Subacute colic caused by epiploic foramen incarceration of the small intestine in a horse, Equine Vet Educ 1991;3:13.
194. Livesey MA, Little CB, Boyd C: Fatal hemorrhage associated with incarceration of small intestine by the epiploic foramen in three horses, Can Vet J 1991;32:434.
195. Freeman DE: Surgery of the small intestine, Vet Clin North Am Equine Pract 1997;13:261.
196. Morton AJ, Blikslager AT: Surgical and postoperative factors influencing short-term survival of horses following small intestinal resection: 92 cases (1994-2001), Equine Vet J 2002;34:450.
197. Proudman CJ, Smith JE, Edwards GB, et al: Long-term survival of equine surgical colic cases: Part 2. modeling postoperative survival, Equine Vet J 2002;34:438.

198. French NP, Smith JE, Edwards GB, et al: Equine surgical colic: risk factors for postoperative complications, Equine Vet J 2002;34:444.
199. Davis DM, McClure JR, Bertone AL, et al: Hypoglycemia and hepatic necrosis after small intestinal incarceration through the epiploic foramen in a horse, Cornell Vet 1992;82:173.
200. Garcia-Seco E, Wilson DA: Intestinal lipoma in the horse: 101 cases (1987-2002), Vet Surg 2003;32:600.
201. Downes EE, Ragle CA, Hines MT: Pedunculated lipoma associated with recurrent colic in a horse, J Am Vet Med Assoc 1994;204:1163.
202. Blikslager AT, Bowman KF, Haven ML, et al: Pedunculated lipomas as a cause of intestinal obstruction in horses: 17 cases (1983-1990), J Am Vet Med Assoc 1992;201:1249.
203. Edwards GB, Proudman CJ: An analysis of 75 cases of intestinal obstruction caused by pedunculated lipomas, Equine Vet J 1994;26:18.
204. Jansson N: Spontaneous correction of a nonstrangulating ileal obstruction caused by a pedunculated lipoma in a 14-year-old pony, Equine Vet Educ 2000;12:183.
205. Barclay WP, Phillips TN, Foerner JJ: Intussusception associated with *Anoplocephala perfoliata* infection in five horses, J Am Vet Med Assoc 1982;180:752.
206. Lowe JE: Intussusception in three ponies following experimental enterotomy, Cornell Vet 1968;58:288.
207. Frankeny R, Wilson D, Messer N, et al: Jejunal intussusception: A complication of functional end to-end stapled anastomosis in two ponies, Vet Surg 1995;24:515.
208. Semevolos SA, Ducharme NG, Hackett RP: Clinical assessment and outcome of three techniques for jejunal resection and anastomosis in horses: 59 cases (1989-2000), J Am Vet Med Assoc 2002;220:215.
209. Boswell JC, Schramme MC, Gains M: Jejunojejunal intussusception after an end-to-end jejunojejunal anastomosis in a horse, Equine Vet Educ 2000;12:303.
210. Collier MA, Trent AM: Jejunal intussusception associated with leiomyoma in an aged horse, J Am Vet Med Assoc 1983;182:819.
211. Boulton CH, Williamson L: Cryptococcal granuloma associated with jejunal intussusception in a horse, Equine Vet J 1984;16:548.
212. Hackett MS, Hackett RP: Chronic ileocecal intussusception in horses, Cornell Vet 1989;79:353.
213. Mason TA, Johnston DE, Wallace CE, et al: Laparotomy in equine colic: A report of thirteen clinical cases, Aust Vet J 1970;46:349.
214. Greet TRC: Ileal intussusception in 16 young Thoroughbreds, Equine Vet J 1992;24:81.
215. Scott EA, Todhunter R: Chronic intestinal intussusception in two horses, J Am Vet Med Assoc 1985;186:383.
216. Horney FD, Funk KA: Ileal myotomy in the horse, Mod Vet Pract 1971;52:49.
217. McLean AA, Church S, Dyke TM, et al: An alternative approach for treatment of irreducible ileocecal intussusception in six horses, Equine Vet Educ 1991;3:10.
218. Beard W: Nonreducible intussusception. In White NA, Moore JN, editors: Current Techniques in Equine Surgery and Lameness, ed 2, Philadelphia, 1998, WB Saunders.
219. Beard W, Byrne BA, Henninger RW: Ileocecal intussusception corrected by resection within the cecum in two horses, J Am Vet Med Assoc 1992;200:1978.
220. Proudman CJ: Intestinal tapeworm infestation. In Robinson NE, editor. Current Therapy in Equine Medicine, ed 5, Philadelphia, 2003, WB Saunders.
221. Gayle JM, Blikslager AT, Bowman KF: Mesenteric rents as a source of small intestinal strangulation in horses: 15 cases (1990-1997), J Am Vet Med Assoc 2000;216:1446.
222. Dart AJ, Pascoe JR: Mesenteric tear of the distal jejunum as a periparturient complication in a mare, Aust Vet J 1994;71:427.
223. Zamos DT, Ford TS, Cohen ND, et al: Segmental ischemic necrosis of the small intestine in two postparturient mares, J Am Vet Med Assoc 1993;202:101.
224. Sutter WW, Hardy J: Laparoscopic repair of a small intestinal mesenteric rent in a broodmare, Vet Surg 2004;33:92.
225. Moore JN, Johnson JH, Garner HE, et al: A case report of inguinal herniorrhaphy in a stallion, J Equine Med Surg 1977;1:391.
226. Spurlock GH, Robertson JT: Congenital inguinal hernias associated with a rent in the common vaginal tunic in five foals, J Am Vet Med Assoc 1988;193:1087.
227. van der Velden MA: Ruptured inguinal hernia in new-born colt foals: A review of 14 cases, Equine Vet J 1988;20:178.
228. Vasey JR: Simultaneous presence of a direct and an indirect inguinal hernia in a stallion, Aust Vet J 1981;57:418.
229. van der Velden MA: Surgical treatment of acquired inguinal hernia in the horse: A review of 51 cases, Equine Vet J 1988;20:173.
230. van der Velden MA, Stolk PWT: Different types of inguinal herniation in two stallions and a gelding, Vet Q 1990;12:46.
231. Mezerová J, Zert Z, Kabes R, et al: Hernia inguinalis incarcerata beim Pferd: 43 Fälle, Pferdeheilkunde 2003;19:263.
232. Huskamp B, Kopf N: Hernia inguinalis incarcerata beim Pferd, Prakt Tierarzt 1997;78:217.
233. Weaver AD: Acquired incarcerated inguinal hernia: A review of 13 horses, Can Vet J 1987;28:195.
234. Schneider RK, Milne DW, Kohn CW: Acquired inguinal hernia in the horse: A review of 27 cases, J Am Vet Med Assoc 1982;180:317.
235. Hutchins DR, Rawlinson RJ: Eventration as a sequel to castration of the horse, Aust Vet J 1972;48:288.
236. Breukink HJ, Nemeth F, Dieten JSMM: Incarcerated scrotal hernia in a gelding, Tijdschr Diergeneeskd 1980;105:242.
237. Bickers RJ, Lewis RD, Hays T, et al: Acquired inguinal hernia in a gelding, Equine Pract 1998;20:28.
238. Alves GES, Santos RL, Henry M, et al: Acquired bilateral inguinal hernia in a stallion, Equine Vet Educ 2000;12:335.
239. Klohnen A, Wilson DG: Laparoscopic repair of scrotal hernia in two foals, Vet Surg 1996;25:414.
240. Marien T, van Hoeck F, Adriaenssen A, et al: Laparoscopic testis-sparing herniorrhaphy: A new approach for congenital inguinal hernia repair in the foal, Equine Vet Educ 2001;13:69.
241. Bignozzi L: Surgical treatment of scrotal hernia in foals and yearlings without orchectomy, Tijdschr Diergeneeskd 1973;98:1025.
242. Fischer AT, Vachon AM, Klein SR: Laparoscopic inguinal herniorrhaphy in two stallions, J Am Vet Med Assoc 1995;207:1599.
243. Marien T: Standing laparoscopic herniorrhaphy in stallions using cylindrical polypropylene mesh prosthesis, Equine Vet J 2001;33:91.
244. Meagher DM: Surgery of the small intestine in the horse, Arch Am Coll Vet Surg 1974;3:3.
245. Yovich JV, Stashak TS, Bertone AL: Incarceration of small intestine through rents in the gastrosplenic ligament in the horse, Vet Surg 1985;14:303.
246. Marien T, Steenhaut M: Incarceration of small intestine through a rent in the gastrosplenic ligament in five horses, Equine Vet Educ 1998;10:187.
247. Sprinkle TP, Swerczek TW, Crowe MW: Meckel's diverticulum in the horse, J Equine Vet Sci 1984;4:175.
248. Hooper RN: Small intestinal strangulation caused by Meckel's diverticulum in a horse, J Am Vet Med Assoc 1989;194:943.
249. Barakzai SZ, Swain JM, Else RW, et al: Two cases of small intestinal strangulation involving Meckel's diverticula, Equine Vet Educ 2003;15:375.
250. Weaver AD: Massive ileal diverticulum: An uncommon anomaly, Vet Med 1987;82:73.
251. Behrens E: Meckel's diverticulum in a horse, Vet Med 1996;83:208.
252. Hilbert BJ, Jacobs KV, Cullen LK: Umbilical hernia of a diverticulum of the vitelline duct in a horse, Aust Vet J 1981;57:190.
253. Freeman DE, Orsini JA, Harrison IW, et al: Complications of umbilical hernias in horses: 13 cases (1972-1986), J Am Vet Med Assoc 1988;192:804.
254. Markel MD, Pascoe R, Sams AE: Strangulation umbilical hernias in horses: 13 cases (1974-1985), J Am Vet Med Assoc 1987;190:692.

255. Collobert C, Gillet J-P, Esling W: A case of congenital diaphragmatic hernia in a foal, Equine Pract 1988;10:43.
256. Schambourg MA, Laverty S, Mullim S, et al: Thoracic trauma in foals: post mortem findings, Equine Vet J 2003;35:78.
257. Bristol DG: Diaphragmatic hernias in horses and cattle, Comp Cont Educ Pract Vet 1986;8:407.
258. Santschi EM, Juzwiak JS, Moll HD, et al: Diaphragmatic hernia repair in three young horses, Vet Surg 1997;26:242.
259. Coffman JR, Kintner LD: Strangulated diaphragmatic hernia in a horse, Vet Med/Small Anim Clin 1972;67:423.
260. Wimberly HC, Andrews EJ, Haschek WM: Diaphragmatic hernias in the horse: A review of the literature and an analysis of six additional cases, J Am Vet Med Assoc 1977;170:1404.
261. Speirs VC, Reynolds WT: Successful repair of a diaphragmatic hernia in a foal, Equine Vet J 1976;8:170.
262. Hill FWG, Knottenbelt DC, van Laeren K: Repair of a diaphragmatic hernia in a horse, Vet Rec 1987;120:127.
263. Verschooten F, Oyaert W, Muylle E, et al: Diaphragmatic hernia in the horse: Four case reports, J Am Vet Radiol Soc 1977;18:45.
264. Edwards GB: Diaphragmatic hernia: A diagnostic and surgical challenge, Equine Vet Educ 1993;5:267.
265. Markel MD, Kerr LY: What is your diagnosis? J Am Vet Med Assoc 1987;190:1599.
266. Dabareiner RM, White NA: Surgical repair of a diaphragmatic hernia in a racehorse, J Am Vet Med Assoc 1999;214:1517.
267. Bryant JE, Sanchez LC, Rameris S, et al: What is your diagnosis? J Am Vet Med Assoc 2002;220:1461.
268. Firth EC: Diaphragmatic herniation in horses, Cornell Vet 1976;66:353.
269. Malone ED, Farnsworth K, Lennox T, et al: Thoracoscopic-assisted diaphragmatic hernia repair using a thoracic rib resection, Vet Surg 2001;30:175.
270. Ruffin DC, Schumacher J, Comer JS: Uterine torsion associated with small intestinal incarceration in a mare at 126 days of gestation, J Am Vet Med Assoc 1995;207:329.
271. Becht JL, McIlwraith CW: Jejunal displacement through the mesometrium in a pregnant mare, J Am Vet Med Assoc 1980;177:436.
272. Hawkins JF, Schumacher JS, McClure SR, et al: Small intestinal incarceration through the lateral ligament of the urinary bladder in a horse, J Am Vet Med Assoc 1993;202:89.
273. Gayle JM, MacHarg MA, Smallwood JE: Strangulating obstruction caused by intestinal herniation through the proximal aspect of the cecocolic fold in 9 horses, Vet Surg 2001;30:40.
274. Moll HD, Howard RD, May KA, et al: Small intestinal strangulation by components of the spermatic cord in two geldings, J Am Vet Med Assoc 1999;215:824.
275. Tulleners EP, Richardson DW, Reid BV: Vaginal evisceration of the small intestine in three mares, J Am Vet Med Assoc 1985;186:385.
276. Goodrich LR, Dabareiner RM, White NA: Entrapment of the small intestine within the nephrosplenic space in two horses, Equine Vet Educ 1997;9:177.
277. Van Hoogmoed L, Snyder JR: Acute small intestinal injury associated with hematomas in the mesentery of four horses, J Am Vet Med Assoc 1996;209:1453.
278. Baxter GM, Broome TE, Moore JN: Abdominal adhesions after small intestinal surgery in the horse, Vet Surg 1989;18:409.
279. White NA: Intestinal infarction associated with mesenteric vascular thrombotic disease in the horse, J Am Vet Med Assoc 1981;178:259.
280. van der Velden MA: Concurrent presence of mesenteric hernia and jejunal intussusception in a horse, Vet Rec 1989;125:605.
281. Freeman DE, Gentile DG, Richardson DW, et al: Comparison of clinical judgment, Doppler ultrasound, and fluorescein fluorescence as methods for predicting intestinal viability in the pony, Am J Vet Res 1988;49:895.
282. Freeman DE, Schaeffer DJ, Baker GJ: A clinical grading system for intraoperative assessment of small intestinal viability, Proc Am Assoc Equine Pract 2001;47:105.
283. Dean PW, Robertson JT: Comparison of three suture techniques for anastomosis of the small intestine in the horse, Am J Vet Res 1985;46:1282.
284. Reinertson EL: Comparison of three techniques for intestinal anastomosis in Equidae, J Am Vet Med Assoc 1976;169:208.
285. Eggleston RB, Mueller POE, Quandt JE, et al: Use of a hyaluronate membrane for jejunal anastomosis in horses, Am J Vet Res 2001;62:1314.
286. Dean PW, Robertson JT, Jacobs RM: Comparison of suture materials and suture patterns for inverting intestinal anastomosis of the jejunum in the horse, Am J Vet Res 1985;46:2072.
287. Baxter G, Hunt R, Tyler D, et al: Sutured end-to-end and stapled side-to-side jejunal anastomosis in the horse, Vet Surg 1992;21:47.
288. Hocking MP, Carlson RG, Courington KR, et al: Altered motility and bacterial flora after functional end-to-end anastomosis, Surgery 1990;108:384.
289. Mackey VS, Pascoe JR, Peterson PR: A potential technique error in stapled side-to-side anastomosis of the small intestine of the horse, Vet Surg 1987;16:189.
290. Latimer FG, Blackford JT, Valk N: Closed one stage end-to-end jejunojejunostomy in horses with use of linear stapling equipment, Vet Surg 1998;27:17.
291. MacDonald M, Pascoe J, Stover S, et al: Survival after small intestine resection and anastomosis in horses, Vet Surg 1989;18:415.
292. Blackwell R: Jejunocecostomy in the horse: A comparison of two techniques, Proc Equine Colic Res Symp 1982;1: 288.
293. Röcken M, Ross MW: Vergleichsstudie über die Jejunocaecostomie als End-zu-Seitanastomose und Seit-zu-Seitanastomose, Pferdheilkunde 1994;10:311.
294. Peterson FB, Stewart JV: Experimental ileocecal anastomosis in the horse, Equine Med Surg 1978;2:461.
295. Schumacher J, Hanrahan L: Ileocecocolic intussusception as a sequel to jejunojejunostomy in a mare, J Am Vet Med Assoc 1987;190:303.
296. Erkert RS, Crowson CL, Moll HD, et al: Obstruction of the cecocolic orifice by ileocecocolic intussusception following jejunocecostomy in a horse, J Am Vet Med Assoc 2003;222:1743.
297. Edwards GB: Resection and anastomosis of the small intestine: Current methods applicable to the horse, Equine Vet J 1986;18:322.
298. Bladon BM, Hillyer MH: Effect of extensive ileal resection with a large resulting mesenteric defect and stapled ileal stump in horses with a jejunocaecostomy: A comparison with other anastomotic techniques, Equine Vet J Suppl 2000;32:52.
299. Vasey JR, Julian RJ: Elective inversion of the distal ileal stump into the caecum of the horse, Equine Vet J 1987;19:223.
300. Huskamp B: Ileum-resektion und Jejunocaecostomie beim Pferd, Berl Münch Tierärztl Wochenschr 1973;86:161.
301. van den Boom R, van der Velden MA: Short- and long-term evaluation of surgical treatment of strangulating obstructions of the small intestine in horses: A review of 244 cases, Vet Q 2001;23:109.
302. Tóth J, Birke H, Huskamp B, et al: Die Ausführung der Jejunozäkostomie beim Pferd mittels einer Sägetechnik, Pferdeheilkunde 1998;14:385.
303. Van Hoogmoed L, Snyder J: Adjunctive methods in equine gastrointestinal surgery, Vet Clin North Am Equine Pract 1997;13:221.
304. Loesch DA, Rodgerson DH, Haines GR, et al: Jejunoileal anastomosis following small intestinal resection in horses: Seven cases (1999-2001), J Am Vet Med Assoc 2002;221:541.
305. McIntosh SC, Shupe JR: Surgical correction of duodenal stenosis in the foal, Equine Pract 1981;3:17.
306. Gillis JP, Taylor TS, Puckett MJ: Gastrojejunostomy for management of acute proximal enteritis in a horse, J Am Vet Med Assoc 1994;204:633.
307. Huskamp, B: Diagnosis of gastroduodenojejunitis and its surgical

treatment by a temporary duodenocaecostomy, Equine Vet J 1985;17:314.
308. Ducharme NG, Hackett RP, Ducharme GR, et al: Surgical treatment of colic: Results in 181 horses, Vet Surg 1983;12:206.
309. Parker J, Fubini S, Todhunter R: Retrospective evaluation of repeat celiotomy in 53 horses with acute gastrointestinal disease, Vet Surg 1989;18:424.
310. Huskamp B, Bonfig H: Relaparotomy as a therapeutic principle in postoperative complications of horses with colic, Proc Equine Colic Res Symp 1985;2:317.
311. Hainisch EK, Proudman CJ, Edwards GB: Indications, surgical intervention and outcome of relaparotomy in 27 cases, Proceedings of the European College of Veterinary Surgeons Annual Symposium, Glasgow, Scotland, 2003:224.
312. Pankowski RL: Small intestinal surgery in the horse: A review of ileo and jejunocecostomy, J Am Vet Med Assoc 1987;190:1608.
313. Chan STF, Kapadia CR, Johnson AW, et al: Extracellular fluid volume expansion and third space sequestration at the site of small bowel anastomoses, Br J Surg 1983;70:36.
314. Rumbaugh ML, Burba DJ, Natalini C, et al: Evaluation of a vessel-sealing device for small intestinal resection and anastomosis in normal horses, Vet Surg 2003;32:574.
315. Hunt JM, Edwards GB, Clarke KW: Incidence, diagnosis and treatment of postoperative complications in colic cases, Equine Vet J 1986;18:264.
316. Blikslager AT, Bowman KF, Levine JF, et al: Evaluation of factors associated with postoperative ileus in horses: 31 cases (1990-1992), J Am Vet Med Assoc 1994;205:1748.
317. Roussel AJ, Cohen ND, Hooper RN, et al: Risk factors associated with development of postoperative ileus in horses, J Am Vet Med Assoc 2001;219:72.
318. Southwood LL, Baxter GM: Current concepts in management of abdominal adhesions, Vet Clin North Am Equine Pract 1997;13:415.
319. Santschi EM, Slone DE, Embertson RM, et al: Colic surgery in 206 juvenile Thoroughbreds: Survival and racing results, Equine Vet J Suppl 2000;32:32.
320. Tate LP, Ralston SL, Koch CM, et al: Effects of extensive resection of the small intestine in the pony, Am J Vet Res 1983;44:1187.
321. Haven ML, Roberts MC, Argenzio RA, et al: Intestinal adaptation following 70% small bowel resection in ponies, Proc Equine Colic Res Symp 1991;4:54.
322. Freeman DE, Laws EG: Effect of venous strangulation obstruction on length of equine jejunum and relevance to small-intestinal resection, Vet Surg 2001;30:218.
323. Bertone AL, Stashak TS, Ralston SL, et al: A preliminary study on the effects of jejunocaecostomy in horses, Equine Vet J Suppl 1992;13:51.
324. Sweeney CR, Habecker PL: Pulmonary aspergillosis in horses: 29 cases (1974-1997), J Am Vet Med Assoc 1999;214:808.
325. Stephen JO, Corley KTT, Johnston JK, et al: Factors associated with mortality and morbidity in small intestinal volvulus in horses: 1988-2000, Vet Surg 2004;33:340.
326. Proudman CJ, Smith JE, Edwards GB, et al: Long-term survival of equine surgical colic cases: Part 1. Patterns of mortality and morbidity, Equine Vet J 2002;34:432.

CHAPTER 36

Large Intestine

Peter C. Rakestraw
Joanne Hardy

CECUM

Anatomy and Physiology

The cecum is positioned between the small intestine and the large colon and located primarily on the right side of the abdomen.[1] It is a large cul-de-sac with an average length of 1.25 m and an average capacity of 30 L.[1] It has a comma-shaped appearance and is divided into three parts—the base, body, and apex (Fig. 36-1). The base, which is the most dorsal part, is positioned in the right iliac and sublumbar region. It has a greater curvature dorsally and lesser curvature ventrally.[2] It extends craniad to the 14th or 15th rib, forming a blind end pointing ventrally. A transverse fold, arising from the floor of the cecal base craniad to the ileocecal junction, divides the base into a cranial and a caudal portion.[3] The cranial part of the base is developmentally part of the ascending colon and is called the cupula.[2] The cranial and caudal parts of the cecal base appear to function separately. The body of the cecum travels cranioventrally from the cecal base. Caudally, it lies against the right flank moving to a slightly more medial position as it extends craniad along the ventral body wall, narrowing toward the cecal apex, which is situated between the right and left ventral colon approximately 20 cm caudal to the xiphoid cartilage.[1,2] The cecal base is attached dorsally to the ventral surface of the right kidney, to the right lobe of the pancreas, and to a part of the abdominal wall caudal to these structures.[1,2] The cecal base is attached medially to the transverse colon and the root of the mesentery from which the vascular supply reaches the cecum.

The body of the cecum has four longitudinal bands (teniae) located on the dorsal, ventral, medial, and lateral surfaces. The dorsal and medial bands end at the cecal apex. The ventral band usually joins the medial band near the cecal apex, and the lateral band may extend to the apex or fade out before reaching the apex.[1] The ileocecal fold runs from the antimesenteric border of the ileum to the dorsal cecal band. The cecocolic fold (ligament) runs from the lateral cecal band to the lateral free band of the right ventral colon.

The cecal blood supply derives from the cecal artery, a branch of the ileocolic artery. The cecal artery divides into the medial and lateral cecal arteries, which run with the corresponding veins in the medial and lateral cecal bands, respectively. The medial cecal artery is the major vascular supply to the cecal apex. The cecum is thought to be at risk for thromboembolic disease, since both cecal arteries arise from a single vessel without collateral circulation, and since the lateral and medial cecal arteries have minimal mixing of

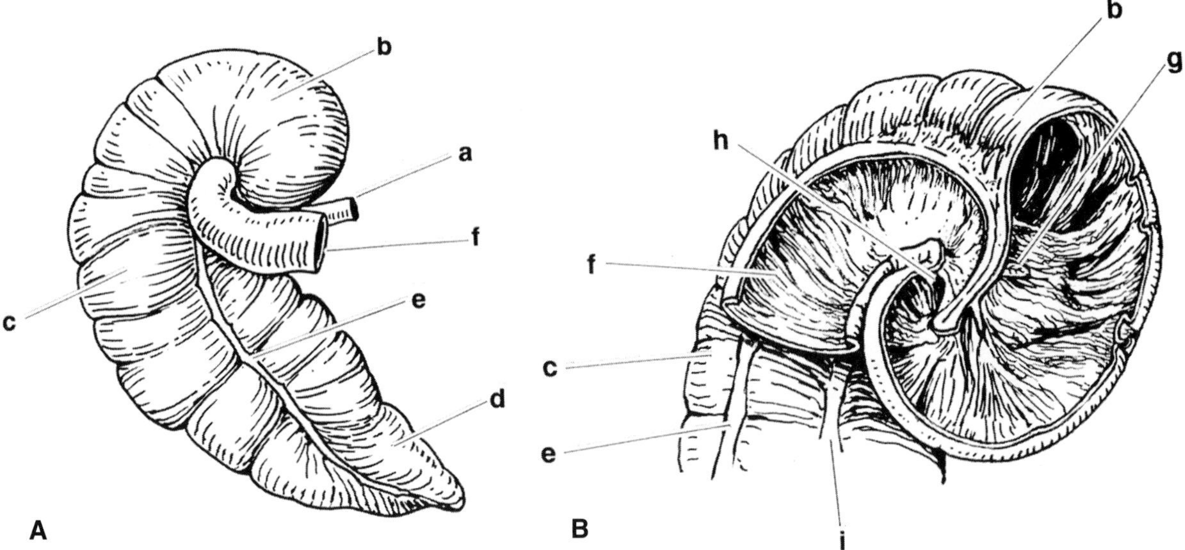

Figure 36-1. A, Cecum of the horse, right lateral aspect. **B,** Base of the cecum and the proximal part of the ascending colon (right ventral colon) of the horse, opened laterally to show the ileal and cecocolic orifices. Fixed in situ. Lateral aspect. a, ileum, elevated; b, base of cecum; c, body of cecum; d, apex of cecum; e, lateral teniae; f, proximal part of right ventral colon; g, ileal orifice on papilla; h, cecocolic orifice; j, dorsal teniae with ileocecal fold.

their two circulations.[4] However, microvascular studies indicate that there is a cecal rete arising from each of the cecal arteries that supplies an extensive submucosal plexus and that may provide an alternative blood supply in the event of a cecal embolus[4] (Fig. 36-2).

The ileocecal orifice is located in the lesser curvature of the cecal base approximately 5 to 7 cm to the right of the median plane and at the level of the first or second lumbar vertebra.[1] The end of the ileum is partly telescoped into the cecum, which positions the ileal orifice in an elevation of an annular fold of mucous membrane. The annular fold contains a network of veins, which can distend the annular fold when engorged.[2] In this way, the ileocecal orifice is narrowed, preventing reflux of cecal contents back into the ileum. The lack of this functional sphincter may contribute to cecal reflux into the small intestine after a jejunocecostomy. The cecocolic orifice is located distal to the ileocecal orifice. Because the cranial cecal base curves ventrally and caudally, the cecocolic orifice is positioned caudal and lateral to the ileocecal orifice (see Fig. 36-1, *B*). It lies between two folds of tissue, which form the cecocolic valve. There is no sphincter at the cecocolic orifice.[2]

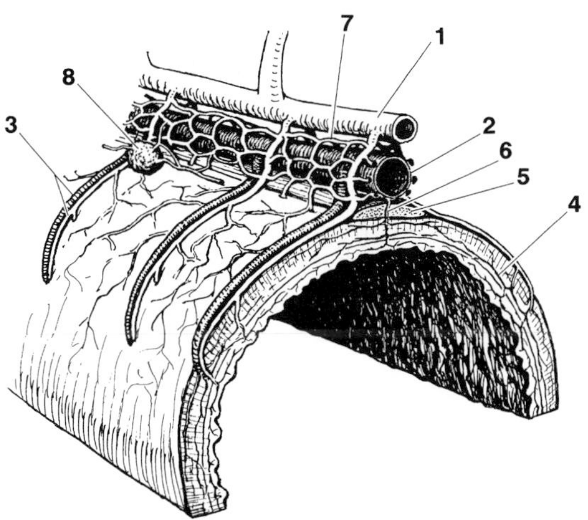

Figure 36-2. Schematic diagram of the cecal arterial rete that forms a meshlike network around the cecal veins before continuing on into the submucosal network plexus. The extensive rete and submucosal network may provide an alternative route for blood flow in the case of an arterial embolus. 1, marginal artery; 2, marginal vein; 3, secondary arcade; 4, long artery and vein; 5, teniae; 6, branch supplying the teniae; 7, vascular rete; 8, lymph node and lymph vessels (shown only at one place).

The two primary physiologic functions of the cecum (as well as of the large colon) are to absorb electrolytes and water and to serve as a site of microbial digestion.[5] The large intestine of a 160-kg pony reabsorbs a total of approximately 30 L of water a day, a volume equivalent to its extracellular space.[5] The cecum appears to be the site of greatest quantitative net water absorption (Fig. 36-3). In an experimental model in ponies, the cecum demonstrated a net transmucosal influx of water during the first 2 hours after a meal, followed by a net absorption of approximately 600 to 800 mL/hr during the next 10 hours between meals.[5] Net increases in daily absorption of water from the ventral and small colon can compensate for decreased cecal water absorption.[5] Microbial digestion is the other important physiologic function of the cecum. A significant amount of soluble and most of the insoluble (e.g., cellulose, hemicellulose) dietary carbohydrate is digested by microbial enzymes in the cecum (and large colon) with production of organic acids (volatile fatty acids).[6] The marked decrease in bicarbonate in the cecum is because of the buffering effect of the organic acids. Although osmotic changes in organic acid (or volatile fatty acid) production has been speculated to control net water movement, sodium transport is probably more important.[5,6]

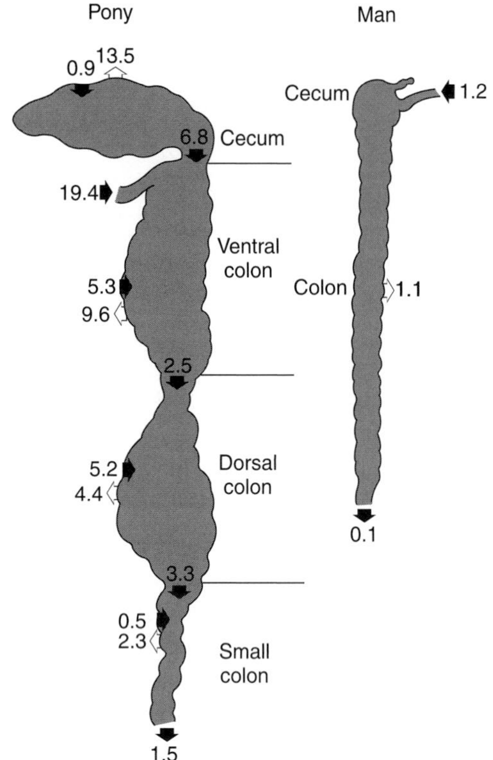

Figure 36-3. Net water movement through the large intestine of a 70-kg man and a 160-kg pony. Both species absorb approximately 90% of ileal outflow, but in a pony, this represents approximately 30 L/day. The volume is roughly equivalent to the animal's extracellular fluid volume. Note that the cecum of the pony has the greatest net water absorption. (Redrawn from Argenzio RA, Lowe JE, Prickard DW, et al: Digesta passage and water exchange in equine large intestine, Am J Physiol 1974;226:1035.)

Cecal Motility

The transit time for liquid and particulate markers through the cecum is relatively rapid compared with that in the large colon.[6] There does not appear to be any retrograde movement of ingesta through either the ileocecal or the cecocolic orifice. Several studies have described normal cecal motility by examining cecal myoelectric activity patterns.[7-9] Ingesta enters the cecum from the ileocecal orifice propelled by the migrating action potential complex, a rapidly progressive electrical event extending from the ileum to the cecum. In the cecum, four different patterns of activity have been characterized. Three are associated with mixing of cecal ingesta: pattern I begins at the cecal apex and is conducted to the cranial base, and patterns II and III begin at the caudal and cranial cecal base, respectively, and are conducted to the cecal apex.

Pattern IV, a progressive pattern, begins at the cecal apex and is conducted through the cecal base and cecocolic orifice and into the right ventral colon (RVC). Pattern IV occurs once every 3 minutes in the fed horse, is associated with a loud distinctive "rush" of digesta (heard on auscultation), and is probably responsible for the transit of digesta from the cecum to the RVC.[8,9] In endoscopic studies of cecal emptying, ingesta was seen to move from the body up to the cranial aspect of the cecal base (cupula), which was separated from the caudal base by a ring of constriction. The cupula then contracted and the cecocolic orifice was elevated and opened, allowing ingesta to flow into the RVC.[10,11] In the RVC, both aborally directed propulsive spike bursts and orally directed retropulsive spike bursts were seen. The orally directed spike bursts may allow the RVC to function as a reservoir. The oral spike bursts were not propagated onto the cecum. An electrical pacemaker region is thought to be located near the cecal apex.[8] There is also indication of possible myoelectric coupling between the ileum, cecum, and RVC.[8,12] Abnormal cecal motility is thought to contribute to several cecal problems, most notably cecal impaction caused by cecal dysfunction.

Cecal motility has been shown to be altered by pharmacologic agents. Xylazine HCl (0.5 mg/kg IV) depresses the progressive motility pattern and mechanical activity for 20 to 30 minutes, and it prolongs cecal emptying.[12-15] Butorphanol tartrate (0.04 mg/kg IV) also depresses the progressive cecal motility pattern for 10 minutes.[14,15] The combination of xylazine and butorphanol prolongs the inhibition of spike bursts.[14,15] Neostigmine methylsulfate (0.025 to 0.033 mg/kg IV or SC) produces a significant increase in the frequency of progressive cecal motility and rate of cecal emptying.[15,16] Bethanechol chloride (0.025 mg/kg IV) increases the rate of cecal emptying.[16] Erythromycin lactobionate (1.0 mg/kg or 0.10 mg/kg) administered as an IV infusion over 60 minutes increases the rate of cecal emptying.[17] All of these studies have been performed in normal horses, so caution should be exercised extrapolating the results to horses with pathology of the cecum.

Cecal Impaction

Pathogenesis

The most common pathologic condition of the cecum is cecal impaction, and it accounts for between 40% and 55% of cecal disease, 5% of all intestinal impactions, and 2% of all referral colics.[18-21] Fatalities as high as 43% have been reported, primarily because of perforation or rupture.[20,21] The etiology of cecal impaction is most likely multifactorial. Suggested predisposing factors include poor dentition, feeding of poor-quality roughage, decreased water intake, parturition, and parasite-induced thromboembolism.[22-27] Tapeworms *(Anoplocephala perfoliata)* located at the cecocolic orifice have been associated with cecal impaction and perforation, possibly as the result of disruption of motility.[28-30] In one study, Arabian, Appaloosa, and Morgan horses, as well as horses older than 15 years, were at an increased risk for developing cecal impactions.[19] In our experience, horses from regions where coastal Bermuda grass hay is the predominant diet are also at an increased risk.

Another predisposing factor for cecal impaction, which may lead to cecal perforation, is hospitalization or prior surgery (within the previous 5 days). Often these horses are hospitalized or have surgery for reasons not related to the gastrointestinal tract, such as elective arthroscopy.[23,31-35] Some of these impactions may be related to a motility dysfunction. During and after general anesthesia, motility of the gastrointestinal tract is disrupted, with the cecum taking the longest time to return to normal function.[36] Use of nonsteroidal anti-inflammatory drugs (NSAIDs) and lack of exercise have also been associated with the development of cecal impaction or rupture in these cases.[19,34,37,38] The association of NSAIDs with cecal rupture has been attributed to masking of gastrointestinal pain associated with cecal impaction, exacerbation of existing ulceration associated with concurrent disease, and primary ulcer development.[3,19,24,39] There is also a group of horses that develop cecal "impactions" that do not appear to have a mechanical obstruction. In these horses, the accumulated ingesta is of normal or often fluid consistency instead of the firm, dry, compacted ingesta typically associated with feed impactions. A functional motility obstruction has been suggested in this group of horses. A disruption in the progressive motility pattern, which starts at the cecal body and propagates aborally to the cecal base and into the right ventral colon, would lead to accumulation of ingesta in the cecum.[7,8] Although altered blood flow secondary to parasite damage, dietary changes, and other clinical conditions have been hypothesized to disrupt the cecal pacemaker located at the cecal apex and to result in interruption of progressive motility, no predisposing cause can be found in many of these cases.

Chronic recurrent cecal impaction has also been associated with hypertrophy of the muscle layers in the cecal base or body.[40] The muscular hypertrophy is thought to result from chronic uncoordinated hypercontractility because of neuronal deficits in the myenteric plexus of the cecal base.[40,41] Ingesta accumulates in the cecum as a result of failure of the motility patterns to move ingesta from the cecum into the RVC. These horses have chronic weight loss with mild signs of colic. To our knowledge, this type of cecal disease has not been recognized in the United States.

Clinical Signs and Diagnosis

Often, horses with cecal impaction show only mild signs of pain, with intermittent periods of increased severity, that may continue for several days to several weeks.[19,23,42-44] The mild signs of colic include lying down, looking at the flank, decreased appetite, and depression. The heart rate is often normal to slightly elevated. Borborygmi are decreased, and feces may be soft with decreased production. Because gas, fluid, and some ingesta may pass through the cecum over the impaction, the small intestine proximal to the cecum is usually not distended. Although some horses may be presented with or may develop moderate to severe pain as the impaction progressively worsens, some affected horses remain relatively comfortable as the cecum becomes tightly distended. Horses with cecal impaction may be presented with cecal rupture with no history of significant abdominal pain.[3,19,34] There are reports of horses with cecal impaction deteriorating so rapidly, even when being monitored in a hospital environment, that surgical intervention before cecal rupture was not possible.[23,24,34] Laboratory evaluation is often normal in horses with cecal impactions. Although changes in peritoneal fluid may help in determining when and if surgical intervention should be performed, they are not always a sensitive predictor of cecal deterioration and may occur too late to be of any value in the decision-making process.[19,23,24]

The diagnosis is confirmed by rectal palpation in most cases.[3,23,38] The first indication of a cecal impaction may be increased tension in the ventral cecal band. As the impaction enlarges, the cecal body begins to fill and the sacculations in the cecal body and a rounded cecal base are palpable. With increasing filling, the sacculations disappear and a large distended structure can be felt filling the right side of the abdomen. Because the cecum is attached dorsally to the body wall, the examiner is not able to pass a hand dorsally over the impaction.[39] This may help differentiate a cecal impaction from a large colon impaction. However, rectal palpation in some cases is not definitive in distinguishing between a distended cecum and a distended colon.[26] Additionally, some horses have cecal impaction involving only the cupula. Since the cupula of the cecum lies more cranial than the body, these can be missed on rectal palpation.[40]

Primarily on the basis of rectal palpation findings, cecal impactions have been divided into two types of obstruction.[21,38] One type has firm, dry, or doughy ingesta at the base or body of the cecum. The mass can be indented with the fingers on rectal palpation, and the cecal wall does not feel thickened. Peritoneal fluid is usually normal in these horses. These cases are thought to include the mechanical obstructions and will be referred to as type 1 cecal impactions. In the other type of cecal impaction, referred to here as type 2 cecal impactions, the cecum is tightly distended with gas and ingesta of normal or fluid consistency. These have been described as cecal dysfunction.[21,38] These horses may have an increased level of pain and an increased heart rate compared with type 1 cecal impactions. They may also show signs of endotoxemia. The cecal wall is usually tightly stretched and may feel thickened. Peritoneal fluid may have elevated protein, and as the disease progresses it becomes serosanguineous. At surgery, the cecal wall appears thickened and hyperemic, and it has decreased motility.[21,38] Although this categorization may be helpful in selecting a treatment modality (see "Treatment," next), it is not without limitations. First, it can be difficult to place a horse accurately into one of the two categories, even with physical, rectal, laboratory, and surgical findings. Second, although the progression of the disease and the response to treatment modalities may be more similar between horses within a group than between horses in different groups, clinically there are significant exceptions.

Treatment

The treatment of cecal impactions is quite controversial. Some reports suggest that cecal impactions can routinely be successfully treated with medical therapy, whereas other reports recommend surgical intervention.* To differentiate horses that will respond to medical therapy from those that will not, attempts have been made to correlate the characteristics of the impaction (the nature of the material in the cecum) with the response to medical therapy. Type 1 cecal impactions, thought to be mechanical obstructions from impacted ingesta, should be more likely to respond to medical therapy.[21,38] Type 2 cecal impactions, thought to be caused by a cecal motility dysfunction, should be less likely to respond to medical therapy and so be more likely to require surgical intervention. Although type 1 cecal impactions can initially be treated with medical therapy, some may not respond. Since these horses may not show

*References 3, 23, 24, 38, 39, 43.

much pain at any stage of the disease, they should be carefully monitored by rectal examination to determine which ones are not responding.

Another area of controversy is associated with the timing of performing a surgical bypass of the cecum. This question arose out of several retrospective studies that identified horses with recurrent cecal tympany or impaction after a prior typhlotomy without bypass had been performed to treat cecal impaction.[45] The nature of the impaction has been used to help with this decision. Type 1 impactions should be more likely to respond to decompression only, whereas cecal dysfunction, the type 2 impactions, should be more likely to require a bypass. However, this has been questioned by some authors.[26] In our opinion, cecal impactions that occur in the postanesthetic period can be treated medically if they are diagnosed prior to the cecum's becoming overdistended. However, it should be stressed that the clinical signs may be mild and their clinical significance underestimated. In a retrospective study of cecal perforation, 13 of 66 horses with cecal disease developed cecal perforation while in a hospital setting without having a prior diagnosis of cecal disease. All of these horses had some sort of painful condition, many related to a musculoskeletal condition. Seven of theses 13 cases had general anesthesia several days prior to cecal perforation. Although these horses exhibited signs such as reduced fecal output and mild abdominal pain, the signs were not recognized as clinically significant prior to cecal perforation or sudden death. These horses were found to have a large and firm cecum filled with ingesta and an empty colon at necropsy.[34] If surgery is required for decompression of postoperative cecal impactions, or if horses develop cecal impaction while hospitalized for other conditions, most cases will not need a bypass. The logic is that the dysfunction is temporary in nature and related to anesthesia (for the horses who had surgery) or to a painful condition, to treatment with NSAIDs, or to a change in management, such as decreased exercise,[36,38] and therefore the patients should respond to a more conservative surgical treatment (i.e., decompression only). These horses should be held off hay for the first 36 to 48 hours postoperatively, exercised with hand-walking and limited grazing to stimulate motility, and slowly reintroduced to a more laxative diet.

MEDICAL THERAPY

The goal of medical therapy in type 1 impactions is to soften the ingesta to allow cecal contractions to empty the cecal contents into the right ventral colon. Feed should be withheld and the horse started on intravenous fluid therapy. Oral laxatives administered by nasogastric tube may assist in softening the impaction. Mineral oil (5 to 10 mL/kg every 12 hours) is commonly used as a lubricant but may have difficulty penetrating the mass. Magnesium sulfate (1 mg/kg) is a saline laxative that exerts an osmotic effect, pulling water into the intestinal lumen. It can be administered once or twice a day for 2 to 3 days if the horse is well hydrated. Magnesium toxicity has been reported after the use of magnesium sulfate in dehydrated horses and in horses that have been treated with a combination magnesium sulfate and dioctyl sodium sulfosuccinate (DSS), which is thought to increase the absorption of magnesium.[46] Psyllium hydrophilic mucilloid (1.0 kg every 6 to 8 hours) has also been recommended for treatment of cecal impactions.[39] Because complete fasting causes cessation of cecal motility, stimulating motility by walking and limited controlled grazing may be beneficial.[3,9]

Analgesics such as flunixin meglumine (0.5 to 1.1 mg/kg IV every 12 hours) can be used if necessary for pain relief in both types of impactions. Caution should be exercised in using xylazine and butorphanol, since both drugs have been shown to decrease cecal contractile activity[13-15] and their analgesic effect may inappropriately delay the decision for surgical intervention. There is no consensus on the use of prokinetics. Erythromycin, bethanechol, and neostigmine have all been shown to increase contractile activity in the normal cecum as stated previously.[15,17] Given the apparent large force of drug-induced activity in the normal cecum, some authors do not recommend the use of neostigmine in horses with cecal impaction.[16] The clinical efficacy and safety of bethanechol and erythromycin for the treatment of cecal impaction are not known.

Although separation into type 1 and type 2 cecal impactions provides some guidance in choosing which cases are more likely to respond to medical therapy, horses undergoing medical therapy for cecal impaction remain at risk for developing cecal rupture.[24,39] Consequently, close monitoring of their physical status, including heart rate and level of pain, as well as transrectal monitoring of the impaction are imperative when treating any cecal impaction medically. Surgery should be considered if there is no improvement on rectal palpation during a 24- to 36-hour period, if there is any sign of systemic deterioration, if there is a significant increase in pain, or if the cecum feels tight enough to rupture.[39]

The prognosis with medical therapy is difficult to assess from previous reports. One study reported a good prognosis for horses with cecal impactions treated with medical therapy when they lived longer than 24 hours after admission.[39] However, horses that may have been treated medically initially and that developed cecal rupture before the 24 hours were not included in the medically treated group. Consequently, it is difficult to interpret the significance of the reported survival rate (89%) of medically treated cecal impactions. Nine of 10 horses (90%) were treated successfully medically in another study, where the majority of cases (21 of 31 treated) were managed surgically. In another study, medical therapy alone was unsuccessful in 12 out of 21 horses with cecal impaction.[23] Poor results with medical therapy have been reported by other authors.[3,24]

SURGICAL THERAPY

The ventral midline celiotomy is the most common approach for surgical access to the cecum. Because the cecal base is firmly attached to the dorsal body wall, only the apex and a portion of the body of the cecum can be exteriorized. The entire base (including the cupula), a portion of the cecal body, and the cecocolic and ileocecal orifices will remain within the abdominal cavity. A right paracostal approach made through an 18th rib resection has been described for complete typhlectomy or enlargement of the cecocolic orifice in horses with cecal impaction associated with cecal hypertrophy.[40,47] In Europe, enlargement of the cecocolic orifice has met with limited (50%) success in treating this particular type of cecal disease.[40]

Surgical options are infusion of fluid with massage of cecal contents, typhlotomy with evacuation of cecal contents, and bypass procedures including cecocolic anastomosis, ileocolostomy, and jejunocolostomy.[23,45,48,49] Poor to good results have been reported with infusion combined with massage.[23,45] This technique has been of limited value in our experience. For type 1 impactions, the mass of ingesta is usually too large and too tightly packed for infusion and massage to be of significant benefit in breaking down the impaction. Type 2 impactions already contain a significant amount of fluid and so are not likely to respond to additional fluid infused to break them down. There is still controversy concerning the criteria to use in deciding when to perform a bypass procedure. As a general rule, horses fitting into the type 2 category should be considered candidates for a cecal bypass. Some authors state that if the cecal wall appears normal and has reflex motility, and if the ventral colon contains a normal amount of ingesta, the cecum is not bypassed, whereas if the cecal wall is thickened and hyperemic and has minimal motility after evacuation, and if the ventral colon is almost empty, suggesting a cecal motility problem, the cecum should be bypassed.[38,50] These are valid guidelines, although there appear to be exceptions.[26]

Typhlotomy: The preferred surgical approach for a typhlotomy is through a ventral midline celiotomy, although the procedure can be performed through a flank laparotomy in the standing animal.[23,24] The cecum is usually quite large and tightly distended, sometimes making it difficult to exteriorize a sufficient portion of the apex to perform the typhlotomy. Extending the celiotomy incision improves the exposure. The cecum should be manipulated carefully with hands and arms placed around the body of the cecum, lifting the cecal body to allow exteriorization of the apex. Tilting the table, or tilting the horse slightly to the right side, can also facilitate exposure of the apex for the typhlotomy procedure.[38] The exteriorized apex should be isolated from the sterile field over the side of the horse. Stay sutures can be placed adjacent to the typhlotomy site to stabilize the cecum and prevent the cecal apex from retracting back into the abdomen.[38] We prefer having an assistant stabilize the cecal apex with their hands, as stay sutures may tear, allowing the cecal apex to retract. An 8- to 12-cm typhlotomy incision is made between the lateral and ventral cecal bands. The size depends on the consistency of the ingesta. The surgeon manipulating the base of the cecum should continue to exteriorize an additional portion of the body of the cecum as the distention is relieved. A sterile tube is placed in the typhlotomy incision, and warm water is infused to aid in flushing out the cecal contents.[23,38,50] The cupula may be difficult to empty since it forms a pouch at the base of the cecum. In the rare case, we have placed a large-bore tube into the cecum through the typhlotomy along with the lavage tube to siphon cecal contents as the lavage loosened the ingesta. By using these lavage techniques, placing an arm into the cecum to remove contents from the caudal cecal base is rarely required as described in some reports.[38] Once the cecal contents have been evacuated, the contaminated region around the typhlotomy incision should be thoroughly rinsed with electrolyte solution. The typhlotomy incision is closed with a double-inverting suture pattern or an appositional followed by an inverting pattern using 2-0 or 0 polyglactin 910. Some surgeons have recommended resecting the apex of the cecum and closing with the TA-90 stapling instrument if the apex becomes excessively contaminated during the typhlotomy.[3,38] With copious lavage, partial typhlectomy of the apex is usually not necessary.

In one case series, seven of eight horses (88%) with cecal impaction treated by typhlotomy and evacuation survived,[23] and in another study, 9 of 10 horses (90%) survived.[26] It is interesting to note that in this second study the impactions were categorized as cecal dysfunction. However, in two other studies, 4 of 14 horses (29%) were euthanized because of recurrence of the impaction after typhlotomy only,[19] and cecal filling continued to occur postoperatively in the other horses, with only one of five surviving.[42]

Cecocolic anastomosis: This procedure was developed because of the poor response seen in horses with cecal impactions managed by typhlotomy only.[45] In this technique, a cecocolic anastomosis (CCA) is performed to create an alternative route for ingesta to pass from the cecum to the right ventral colon. The rationale is that cecal impactions may be caused by a cecal outflow problem, possibly because of motility dysfunction.[45] The cecum is approached by a ventral midline celiotomy. In most cases, a typhlotomy is recommended to evacuate the cecum prior to performing the anastomosis.[45] The CCA is performed between the lateral and dorsal bands of the cecum and between the lateral and medial free bands of the right ventral colon (Fig. 36-4). Although the anastomosis can be hand-sutured with a two-layer side-to-side technique, we recommend that the CCA be performed with intestinal stapling instruments to

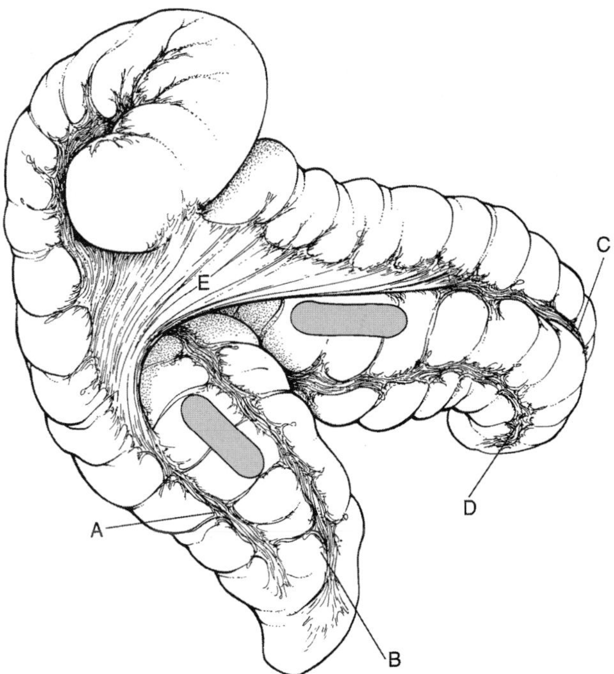

Figure 36-4. The cecum and origin of the right ventral colon (RVC). The marked areas show the location of the cecocolic anastomosis, a surgical procedure useful for horses with recurrent cecal impaction. The anastomosis is performed between the lateral (A) and dorsal (B) cecal bands, and the lateral (C) and medial (D) free bands of the RVC. The cecocolic ligament (E) runs between the lateral cecal band and the lateral free band of the RVC. (Redrawn from Ross MW, Tate LP, Donowick WJ, et al: Cecocolic anastomosis for the surgical management of cecal impaction in horses, Vet Surg 1986;15;85,)

reduce peritoneal and serosal contamination.[45] For the stapling technique, stay sutures attaching the cecum and colon are placed at each end of the selected anastomosis site, approximately 20 cm apart. The seromuscular layer of the cecum and colon are apposed on one side of the intended stoma in a simple-continuous pattern using 2-0 polyglactin 910. Two small stab incisions are made on either side of the midpoint of the 20-cm suture line, one into the cecum and the other into the colon to allow insertion of the stapling instruments. The GIA-90 or ILA-100 stapling instrument is used twice, once orad and once aborad, taking care to overlap the staple lines, which makes a stoma between 15 and 20 cm in length (Fig. 36-5). The stab incisions are closed and the front side of the stapled seromuscular layer is oversewn. To reduce the possibility of internal hernia formation between the cecum and the colon, the seromuscular closures are continued dorsally to the level of the cecocolic ligament.

In one study, three of four horses survived after this technique.[39] In another case series of 14 horses treated by CCA, the long-term survival (12 months) was 71%. However, 4 of the 10 long-term survivors experienced chronic, intermittent, mild abdominal pain thought to be associated with gaseous distention of the cecum.[45] This was considered to be a result of failure of normal gas transit between the two organs, or reflux of gas from the colon into the cecum.[45] Because of the number of horses continuing to experience postoperative problems related to the cecum after the CCA, alternative techniques that bypass the cecum have been recommended in horses with cecal impactions.

Jejunocolostomy or ileocolostomy: For cecal impactions arising from abnormal cecal motility or compromised outflow at the cecocolic orifice, procedures that bypass the cecum entirely have been recommended to prevent cecal tympany or the recurrence of cecal impaction. In these bypass procedures, an anastomosis is made between the ileum or jejunum and the right ventral colon. A partial bypass has been described in which the ileum is not transected.[49] However, in an experimental study comparing a partial to a complete cecal bypass, the partial cecal bypass failed to decrease the size of the cecum or volume of ingesta in the cecum. Consequently, this was thought to be a risk for reimpaction and perforation.[51] Additionally, intermittent colic with cecal distention has been reported after partial cecal bypass.[45] The complete bypass, by taking the cecum out of the flow of ingesta, results in cecal atrophy and prevents postoperative cecal filling and rupture.[51,52] For these reasons, the complete bypass is recommended over the partial bypass.[3,24,51]

The cecum is approached through a ventral midline celiotomy and the cecal impaction evacuated through a typhlotomy. The ileal vascular arcade is double-ligated on both sides of the area of transection. The transection can be completed by hand, with the TA-90 stapling instrument positioned on the distal end and sharply transecting proximal to the instrument, or with a GIA-90 or ILA-100 that will cut between stapled proximal and distal ends.[51,53-55] Doyen intestinal clamps are placed across the ileum oral and aboral to the line of transection for hand-sutured techniques. The proximal and distal ends of the hand-transected ileum are closed with a full-thickness continuous appositional or inverting pattern followed by a partial-thickness

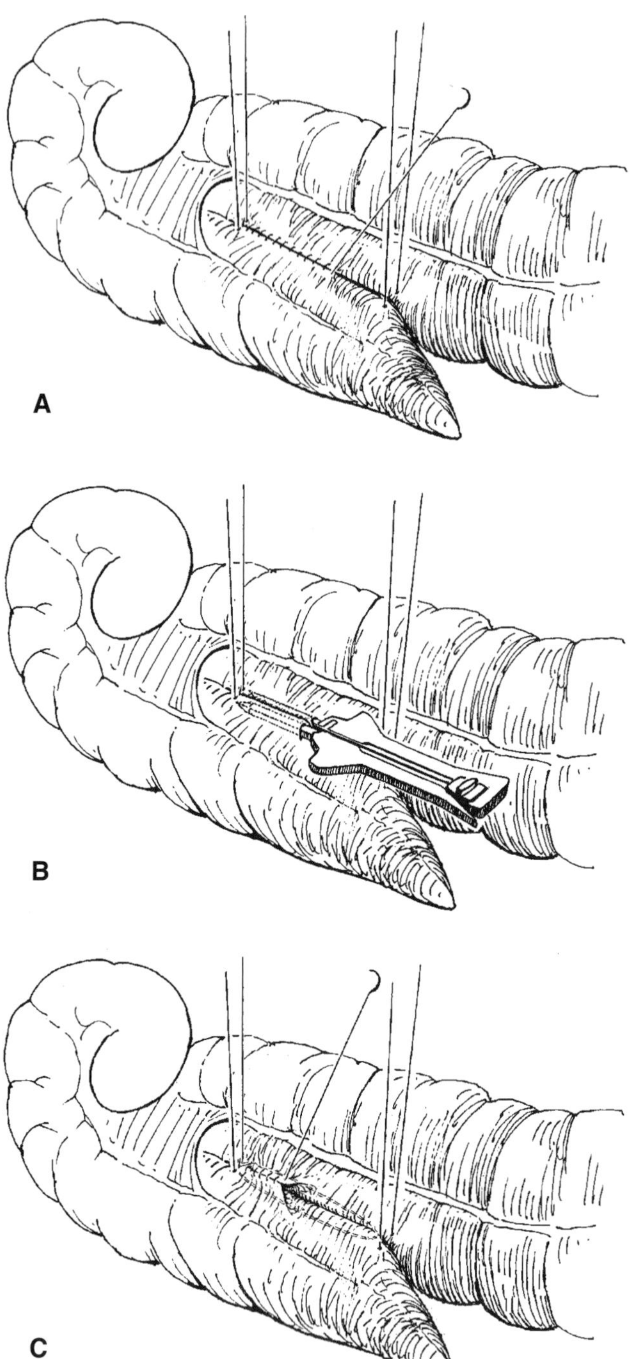

Figure 36-5. The cecum and the origin of the right ventral colon are shown. **A,** Stay sutures attaching the cecum and colon are placed at each end of the selected anastomosis site, approximately 20 cm apart, and the seromuscular layer of the cecum and colon are apposed on one side of the intended stoma in a simple-continuous pattern. **B,** Two small stab incisions are made on either side of the midpoint of the 20-cm suture line, one into the cecum and the other into the colon, to allow insertion of the stapling instruments. The GIA-90 or ILA-100 stapling instrument is used twice, once orad and once aborad, taking care to overlap the staple lines, which creates a stoma between 15 and 20 cm in length. **C,** The stab incisions are closed and the front side of the stapled seromuscular layer is oversewn.

inverting pattern using an absorbable suture. All stapled ends should be oversewn with a partial-thickness inverting pattern. The proximal blind end of the ileum is directed orally, toward the base of the cecum, as it is positioned on the most proximal exteriorized portion of the right ventral colon between the lateral and medial free bands (Fig. 36-6). Stay sutures are placed 15 cm apart to attach the distal end of the ileum to the RVC. A Penrose drain is placed proximal on the ileum, and intestinal clamps placed on the RVC to minimize contamination during the anastomosis. Although a hand-sutured side-to-side anastomosis can be used, we prefer the use of intestinal stapling equipment to shorten surgery time and decrease contamination. Stab incisions are made in adjacent areas of the attached ileum and RVC. The arm of a GIA or ILA stapling instrument is inserted into one stab incision and the anvil inserted into the other stab incision. The stapler is discharged and the blade pushed to form the stoma that is approximately 10 cm in length.[55] The stab incisions are oversewn, followed by a single inverting-suture pattern circumferentially around the entire staple line at a distance of 5 to 8 mm. The ileocecal fold, portions of the cecocolic fold, and the bowel serosa are apposed in a simple-continuous pattern to close the mesenteric defect and eliminate the potential for an internal hernia.[51,55] A variation of this technique describes the resection of a 15- to 30-cm segment of the ileum or ileum and distal jejunum prior to performing the anastomosis. By constructing the distal free end of the small intestine adjacent to a jejunal mesenteric vascular arcade, some surgeons feel the chances of an inadequate blood supply to the anastomosis are decreased.[54]

Several studies have reported on prognosis and complications after cecal bypass.[19,51,54] In one case series, five of six horses (83%) with cecal impaction treated by ileocolostomy returned to their previous activity with a minimal follow-up period of 6 months.[51] Surviving until discharge were six of seven (86%) in another study.[19] In a third study, nine horses that failed to respond to medical therapy received an ileocolostomy or jejunocolostomy.[54] All horses survived until discharge, with all seven horses available for long-term follow-up (range, 7 to 54 months; mean, 1.5 years). Several important observations were made relative to complications in this study. Positioning the small intestine aborally on the RVC makes closure of the mesenteric defect technically difficult, predisposing the horse to entrapment or strangulation of the small intestine in the mesenteric defect. To avoid this problem, the small intestine should always be placed on the RVC facing *orally* and the mesentery closed. Another problem encountered was kinking at the anastomosis. Suturing a 5- to 10-cm segment of the distal small intestine to the colon proximal to the anastomosis is recommended to prevent this problem.[54] A further recommendation was to evacuate the cecum prior to performing the anastomosis to avoid cecal impaction in the postoperative period. The authors emphasized the importance of gradual return to feed, because the most common postoperative complication was mild signs of colic within several days of reintroduction to feed. Although the cecum plays an important role in water absorption and bacterial degradation of dietary fiber,[5,56] no detrimental consequences related to hydration and nutritional states have been observed with the bypass procedure.[51,54]

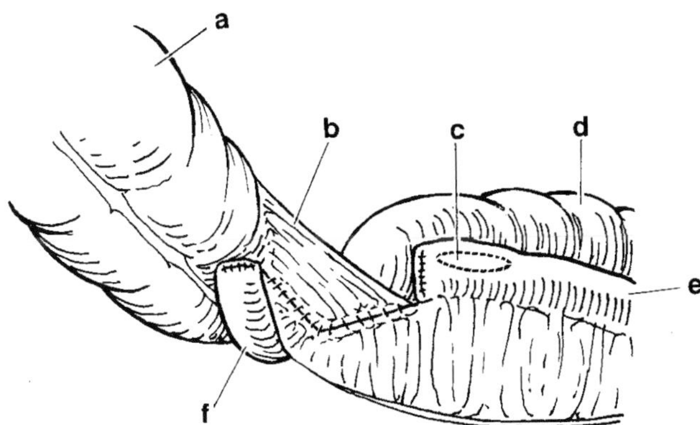

Figure 36-6. Jejunocolic anastomosis. Notice that the blind end of the small intestine is directed orally and the mesenteric defect has been closed. *a*, cecum; *b*, cecocolic ligament; *c*, jejunocolic anastomotic stoma; *d*, right ventral colon; *e*, jejunum, *f*, blind end of the jejunum sutured to the cecum and directed toward the base of the cecum. (Redrawn from McIlwraith CW, Robertson JT, editors: McIlwraith and Turner's Equine Surgery: Advanced Techniques, ed 2, Oxford, UK, 1998, Blackwell.)

Postoperative Care

Horses are treated with broad-spectrum perioperative antibiotics and NSAIDs. The antibiotics may be discontinued 24 hours after surgery or continued for a therapeutic treatment course of 5 to 7 days, depending on the amount of contamination that occurred during the surgical procedure. The NSAIDs are continued for 3 to 5 days. During the initial postoperative period, intravenous fluids should be provided at a slow but constant rate. After 12 to 24 hours, the horse should be offered small amounts of water. Once it has demonstrated a tolerance for oral fluid, the water intake is increased and the intravenous fluids decreased. Postoperative feeding is very important. It has been recommended that feed be withheld for a minimum of 36 to 48 hours, followed by grazing and feeding a bran mash with small quantities of good quality hay at frequent intervals.[54]

Cecocecal or Cecocolic Intussusception

Pathogenesis

Cecocecal and cecocolic intussusception occur when the cecal apex invaginates into the cecal body (cecocecal) or continues through the cecocolic orifice and enters the large colon (cecocolic). Intussusception of the cecum was the most common cause of cecal obstruction in a report from the United Kingdom, whereas it accounted for only 3% to 3.5% of horses with primary cecal disease and for 1.3% of horses undergoing exploratory laparotomy for colic in other reports.[19,31,57-59] The relative frequency of cecocecal compared with cecocolic intussusception varies markedly depending on the study.[32,59-61] The etiology is unknown, but altered motility has been suggested to play a role. Dietary changes, cecal wall abscess, *Salmonella, Eimeria leuckarti, Strongylus vulgaris* arteritis, organophosphates, and administration of parasympathomimetic drugs have all been implicated as potential risk factors.[58,59,62-64] Tapeworm infestation is often encountered in horses with cecal intussusception, leading some to speculate a causative association, possibly from mucosal inflammation initiating the intussusception.[29,58,62,64,65] However, other studies have not found a difference in tapeworm infestation rates between horses with and without cecal intussusception.[19,66,67] Young horses (less than 3 years) and Standardbreds appear to be at increased risk.[32,57,58,62]

Clinical Signs and Diagnosis

Clinical signs may vary considerably depending on the degree of vascular compromise and mechanical obstruction of the ingesta.[19,32,58,60,62] Approximately 55% of horses in one report presented with acute, moderate to severe pain requiring immediate surgical intervention, and 30% presented with a subacute form (3 to 8 days) characterized by intermittent mild to moderate pain with soft feces or diarrhea. A smaller group (13%) presented with a chronic form (6 to 180 days) characterized by weight loss, scant soft feces, and mild abdominal pain.[62] Fever is common in horses suffering from this problem over a longer period of time. Cecocecal intussusceptions are more likely to be nonstrangulating, incomplete obstructions producing mild pain, and they develop into a chronic disease.[62] Cecocolic intussusceptions typically develop ischemic necrosis of the distal end of the intussusceptum, including the cecal apex and part of the body.[63] Rectal examination may be unremarkable in horses with cecocecal intussusception, as the intussuscepted cecal apex may not be palpable and the colon and small intestine are usually not obstructed. In horses with cecocolic intussusception, the cecum may feel malpositioned or may not be palpable at all. A mass or edematous bowel may be palpable in the right caudal abdomen.

Ultrasonography may aid in the making the diagnosis.[57,62,68] Frequently, the compromised portion of the cecum is sequestered within the colon (or cecum), rendering peritoneal fluid analysis an insensitive indicator of pathology.[57] With time and progression of the disease, peritoneal fluid changes may be seen.[58,62,64] Often, the diagnosis is made at surgery after the horse fails to respond to medical therapy.[19,58,62-64]

Treatment

Surgical reduction with partial typhlectomy: The surgical approach is through a ventral midline celiotomy. During the abdominal exploration, the cecal apex is found to be intussuscepted into the body of the cecum in the case of a cecocecal intussusception, whereas the cecum is "absent" from its normal position (with a palpable mass in the right ventral colon) in the case of a cecocolic intussusception. In rare cases, the base of the cecum may be intussuscepted into the colon while the cecal apex remains everted. In these cases, the cecum cannot be exteriorized to the normal extent while the invagination is palpable at the cecal base. Manual reduction is attempted by inserting one hand to grasp and place traction on any portion of the cecum within the intussuscipiens, while the other hand is placed on the colon over the intussuscepted cecum to gently massage the inverted cecum to an everted position. Approximately one third of cecal intussusceptions may be reduced in this manner.[62] The intussusceptum is frequently vascularly compromised, necessitating a partial typhlectomy. To prepare for the partial typhlectomy, the lateral and medial cecal vessels are double-ligated with 0 absorbable suture. Doyen intestinal clamps are placed proximal to the intended amputation site across the cecum to decrease fecal contamination, and the surgical area is draped off. The compromised cecum is often too edematous to allow the use intestinal stapling instruments during the resection. After sharply resecting the compromised cecal apex and body, the cecum is closed using either an inverting or an appositional pattern, followed by an inverting suture pattern with no. 0 absorbable suture.

Cecal amputation through a colotomy: Manual reduction of cecocolic intussusceptions is frequently not successful because of edema and adhesion formation (Fig. 36-7, *A*). In these cases, reduction of the intussusception should be approached through a colotomy.[58,62,69] The large colon should be exteriorized from the abdomen and first evacuated through a pelvic flexure enterotomy if it contains an appreciable amount of ingesta. After closure of the pelvic flexure enterotomy, a second enterotomy is made on the ventral surface of the right ventral colon centered over or immediately distal to the intussusceptum. A sterile plastic bag or a plastic enterotomy drape with a 25-cm-long hole in the center can be sutured to the colon before the enterotomy is made to limit contamination during the colostomy[69] (see Fig. 36-7, *B*). Attempts can be made to manually reduce the intussusception through the colotomy, but this is often unrewarding. In these cases, a partial resection of the invaginated cecum will facilitate reduction of the remaining cecum. The medial and lateral aspects of the inverted cecum are blindly ligated with two parallel transfixation sutures to occlude the cecal vessels. Overlapping mattress sutures, staples, or an encircling ligature with umbilical tape or a natural rubber ligature are placed to occlude the lumen of the cecum[69,70] (see Fig. 36-7, *C*). The invaginated cecum is then transected and the remaining cecal stump reduced using both gentle traction on the cecal body and pushing the remaining inverted cecum out. The colotomy incision is closed with a two-layer inverting pattern using 2-0 or 0 absorbable suture. The now everted cecal stump is subsequently examined for viability. If necessary, further resection of the cecum is performed (see Fig. 36-7, *D*). The cecum is closed with a double-inverting pattern using no. 0 absorbable suture.

If the cecum cannot be reduced after partial resection within the colon, or if the remaining cecal stump is friable and necrotic, the cecal stump is left invaginated within the colon and a cecal bypass procedure is performed.[64,71] In these cases, a partial typhlectomy is performed to remove as much of the necrotic cecum from inside the colon as possible, after which the cecal stump is sutured in a horizontal overlapping mattress pattern followed by a simple-continuous pattern. The colotomy incision is then closed and the surgical area lavaged. To prevent leakage of ingesta, the serosal surface of the cecum at its point of invagination into the colon is oversewn.[64] However, complete oversewing at the point of intussusception may not be possible and may be unnecessary.[71] The ileum is subsequently transected, and an ileocolostomy or jejunocolostomy is performed adjacent to the closed colotomy incision (see "Jejunocolostomy or

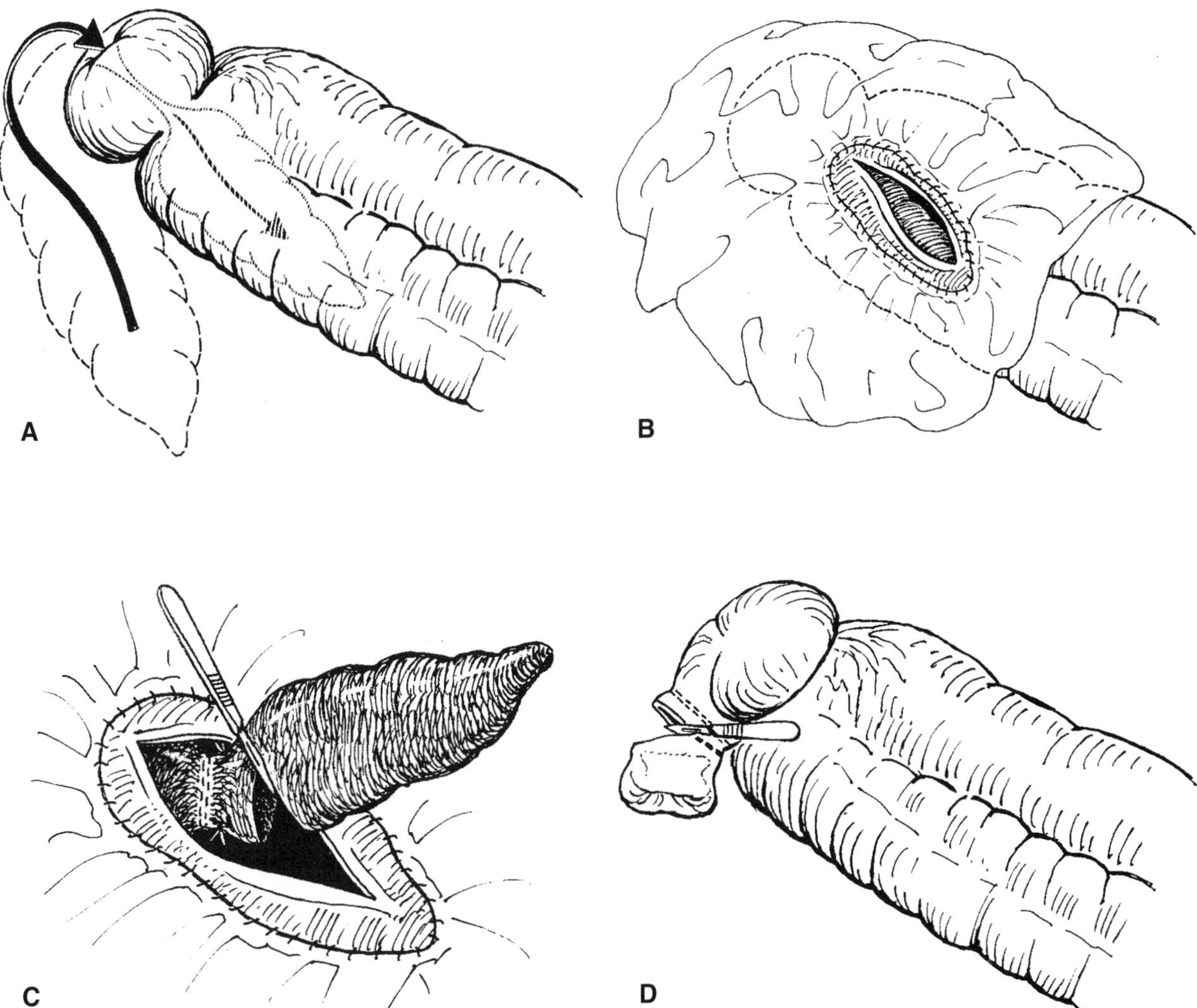

Figure 36-7. Cecal amputation within the right ventral colon (RVC) for nonreducible cecocolic intussusception. **A,** Cecum intussuscepted into the RVC through the CCO. The *dashed lines* represent the outline of the invaginated cecum. **B,** Right ventral colostomy exposing the cecal intussusception. A sterile plastic bag or drape has been sutured to the seromuscular layer of the RVC prior to the colostomy to help contain contamination. **C,** Occluding mattress sutures (or TA staples) have been placed across the inverted cecum to facilitate removal of as much of the cecum as possible, thus enabling reduction of remaining invaginated tissue. The intussusception is then amputated through the RVC. **D,** After eversion of the cecal stump, the remaining compromised part of the remaining cecum is amputated, repeating the technique used for the amputation in the colon.

ileocolostomy" under "Cecal Impaction," p. 442). The devitalized cecal stump is thought by some to slough inside the colon and pass in the feces, whereas others question whether this occurs.[62,64]

Postoperative Care and Prognosis

Horses are treated with intravenous fluids, broad-spectrum antibiotics, and NSAIDs. In cases of cecocecal intussusception with minimal contamination, the antibiotics may be discontinued 24 hours after surgery. Horses with cecocolic intussusceptions requiring cecal amputation within a colostomy are more likely to have been exposed to contamination and consequently require a therapeutic course of antimicrobial therapy. Postoperative abdominal lavage for 2 to 3 days also may aid in reducing the incidence and severity of postoperative peritonitis. The horse can be started back on feed 24 hours after surgery if there is no evidence of pain.

The prognosis is related to the amount of cecum intussuscepted, the ability to manually reduce the intussusception without opening the colon, the amount of contamination at surgery, and the viability of the cecum or the remaining cecal stump.* The prognosis after surgical correction for cecocecal intussusception is good.[60] Although a poor prognosis was associated with partial typhlectomy through a colotomy in one report,[58] other studies revealed a good prognosis associated with this technique.[62,69] Despite some contamination, which is inevitable during reduction through a colostomy, even with careful packing of the abdomen, clinical evidence of postoperative peritonitis is infrequent.[62,69] In one report, four of six horses with irreducible cecocolic intussusception with ileal obstruction survived after a bypass procedure without partial typhlectomy of the invaginated cecum.[57]

*References 3, 24, 32, 58, 60, 62.

However, the complication rate associated with the bypass procedure compared with partial typhlectomy and reduction through a colotomy suggests that the bypass procedure should be reserved for those cases where reduction after partial typhlectomy is not possible.[58,62,69]

Cecal Perforation or Rupture

Cecal perforation has been described in several retrospective studies.[19,31,34,39,72] Cecal perforation secondary to cecal impaction is well recognized.[3,19,39] Primary cecal perforation, unrelated to cecal impaction, has been described to occur in horses during treatment for an unrelated disease. In these horses it appears to be associated with hospitalization, NSAIDs administration, or anesthesia. Primary cecal perforation has also been reported in periparturient mares.[19,24,27,34,73] Dystocia has been observed in approximately 50% of these horses. Horses with cecal perforation typically exhibit signs of pain soon after foaling, presumably as a result of cecal rupture from excessive pressure placed on the cecum during parturition. Primary cecal perforation has also been associated with tapeworm infestation.[28] As discussed previously, some horses with cecal impaction caused by cecal dysfunction may rupture without demonstrating significant clinical signs.[19,34] Consequently, it is not possible to know how many of these cases that have been described as primary cecal perforation have in fact been caused by a cecal dysfunction resulting in cecal distention caused by gas and fluids that went unnoticed prior to cecal perforation.

Cecal Volvulus or Torsion

Cecal volvulus or torsion secondary to large colon volvulus is not uncommon.[3] Because of the substantial dorsal attachments of the cecal base to the body wall and colon, it is not common for the cecum to develop a primary torsion or volvulus. Incidental displacements of the cecum may be encountered at surgery and are sometimes classified as a torsion (usually 90 degrees). These typically are not a pathologic problem.[55] Primary volvulus may be related to anatomic abnormalities such as hypoplasia of the cecocolic fold and the normal cecal attachments to the body wall.[35,74] However, in one report, 9 of 96 horses (9%) with cecal disease were described to have primary cecal torsion with no apparent anatomic abnormalities.[19] Horses with cecal torsion or volvulus are presented with a sudden onset of severe abdominal pain. Rectal palpation is typically not diagnostic. Peritoneal fluid protein and nucleated cell count may be elevated. The diagnosis is made during an exploratory laparotomy. Partial typhlectomy with resection of the compromised cecum is recommended. The prognosis will depend on the viability and amount of compromised cecal tissue remaining after partial typhlectomy. In one report, three of five horses (60%) with cecal torsion treated by partial typhlectomy survived until discharge.[19] If extensive cecal damage extending to the cecal base is found at surgery, complete cecal amputation can be performed through a right flank approach with an 18th rib resection.[47] Cecal amputation leaving part of the cecal cupula to form a conduit between the ileocecal and cecocolic junctions has also been described in a case with extensive cecal ischemia from prolapse through a flank wound.[75] Recurrence has been reported after surgical correction in one horse with abnormal mesenteric attachments.[35]

Cecal Infarction

Cecal infarction has been reported to occur in 10 of 96 (11%) horses with cecal disease.[19] Verminous arteritis from *Strongylus vulgaris* infestation and multifocal infarction from larval cyathostomes are two proposed etiologies.[19,76] Mild abdominal pain increasing in severity over 24 hours is the most common clinical sign. Diarrhea, sudden severe pain, and acute cardiovascular collapse have also been described.[3,19] Peritoneal fluid evaluation reveals changes consistent with intestinal ischemia.[3,19] Rectal palpation may reveal a hard mass in the area where the cecum is located in approximately one third of the cases.[19] Surgical intervention is based on persistent abdominal pain and peritoneal fluid abnormalities, with the diagnosis of cecal infarction made at surgery. Subtotal typhlectomy is the recommended treatment.[19] In one report, seven of eight horses (88%) with cecal infarction treated by subtotal typhlectomy survived to discharge.[19] Although complete typhlectomy requiring an 18th rib resection in left lateral recumbency has been described, the favorable prognosis with partial typhlectomy indicates that the more difficult procedure performed through a right flank approach is usually not necessary.[19,47]

Cecal Tumors

Primary cecal tumors have rarely been reported in horses.[19,77,78] Three of 96 horses (3%) with cecal disease had primary tumors.[19] All three horses were 20 years or older and were presented for chronic weight loss rather than abdominal pain. Histologic diagnoses were leiomyoma, hemangiosarcoma, and papillary adenoma. Treatment should be surgical resection if possible and feasible.

Miscellaneous

Other reported conditions include cecal abscesses that may be associated with adhesions.[19,79] Horses may be presented with mild abdominal pain and peritoneal fluid changes consistent with peritonitis. Transrectal or transabdominal ultrasonography may aid in the diagnosis of cecal abscessation.[19,79] The treatment consists of surgical resection of the abscess and adhesions. Cecocutaneous fistulas have also been described, occurring after repair of body wall hernias with hernia clamps.[80] We have repaired several enterocutaneous fistulas that developed with entrapment of the cecal wall in an umbilical hernia with no history of hernial clamps. The prognosis after surgical repair is good.

LARGE COLON

Anatomy

The equine ascending colon begins at the cecocolic orifice and ends in the transverse colon. It measures approximately 3 to 3.7 m in length and has a capacity of 50 to 60 L. It is composed of the ventral and dorsal areas of the colon, which are connected by a short mesentery. Only rarely does

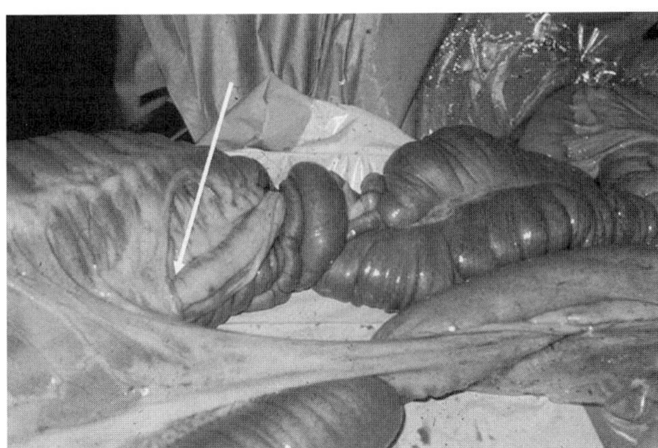

Figure 36-8. Large colon of a horse exteriorized onto a colon tray, showing a defect in the mesentery between the dorsal and ventral colon (*arrow*) that had resulted in a volvulus.

a mesenteric defect occur between the ventral and dorsal colons (Fig. 36-8). In situ, the large colon is further folded such that four segments are designated as the right and left ventral colon and the right and left dorsal colon. The transition from the left and right ventral colons forms the sternal flexure, and the transition from the left and right dorsal colons forms the diaphragmatic flexure. The maximal diameter is seen in the right dorsal colon and can reach 50 cm. The narrowest diameter occurs in the left dorsal colon, which measures about 8 to 9 cm. The bands of the colon (teniae coli) support the colon. The ventral colon has four bands, of which the two ventral ones are free, and the two dorsal ones are associated with the mesentery. The medial dorsal band is associated with the colonic vasculature. The pelvic flexure has one band, which can be palpated on rectal examination. The left dorsal colon has one band, which is joined by two other bands in the right dorsal colon. The roles of the teniae coli are to provide mechanical support to the colon, to maintain orientation of the colon within the abdomen, and to allow distention and contraction of the intestinal segments depending on the degree of ongoing fermentation. The teniae are composed of smooth muscle and collagen in varying proportions, depending on the role of each intestinal segment. In the ventral colon, the site of bacterial fermentation, the teniae have a greater proportion of elastin than in the dorsal colon. In the right dorsal colon, the site of transport and regulation of ingesta through the transverse colon, smooth muscle cells are present in greater proportion.[81]

The blood supply to the ascending colon is derived from the cranial mesenteric artery. The colic branch of the ileocecocolic artery supplies the ventral colon to the pelvic flexure, where it joins the right colic artery, another branch of the cranial mesenteric artery. The middle colic artery, also a branch of the cranial mesenteric artery, provides blood supply to the transverse colon and to the initial part of the small colon. The microvascular circulation of the ascending colon has been well described.[82] The arteries branch from the colonic vessels every 2 cm and anastomose with vessels lying orally and aborally to form a colonic rete before continuing into the colonic tissue. The function of the colonic rete is unclear, but it may provide collateral blood supply, increasing the resistance of the colon to thromboembolic disease.[7] Vessels enter the submucosa through the tunica muscularis to form a complex anastomosing network of submucosal vessels. The extensive collateral supply to the colonic tissue can be expected to enhance healing, particularly where there are areas of devitalized tissue. Arterioles ascend from the submucosal plexus to the mucosa, where an extensive capillary network forms around the colonic glands (Fig. 36-9). This capillary network is drained by more sparsely distributed venules (Fig. 36-10). The submucosal venous plexus is characterized by regular mural helical smooth muscle constrictions that give the veins a sacculated appearance. The venous network is proposed to act as a capacitance system, storing large volumes of blood, which can be actively or passively directed into the systemic circulation as required. Alternatively, because of the large volumes of blood stored within the ascending colon, these smooth muscle constrictions may aid in maintaining blood flow through a low pressure system.[82] The abundant colonic blood supply makes it more susceptible to severe intraluminal hemorrhage after enterotomies.[83]

Physiology

The most critical functions of the equine large colon are storage, microbial digestion, and fluid absorption. In a 24-hour period, the large intestine must recover a quantity of water approximately equivalent to the extracellular fluid volume of the horse (approximately 20% to 30% of body weight, or 90 to 135 L for a 454-kg horse).[6] The storage function of the large colon allows time for microbial digestion and absorption of volatile fatty acids, the main source

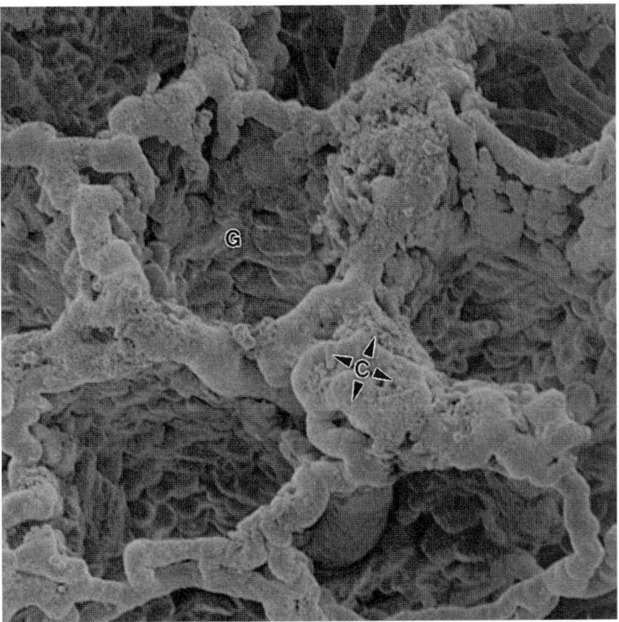

Figure 36-9. Scanning electron micrograph of a vascular replica at the luminal surface of the ascending colon. The capillary network ascends around the colonic glands (G) to the lumen where the capillaries (C) in a network surrounding adjacent glands anastomose and look like a honeycomb.

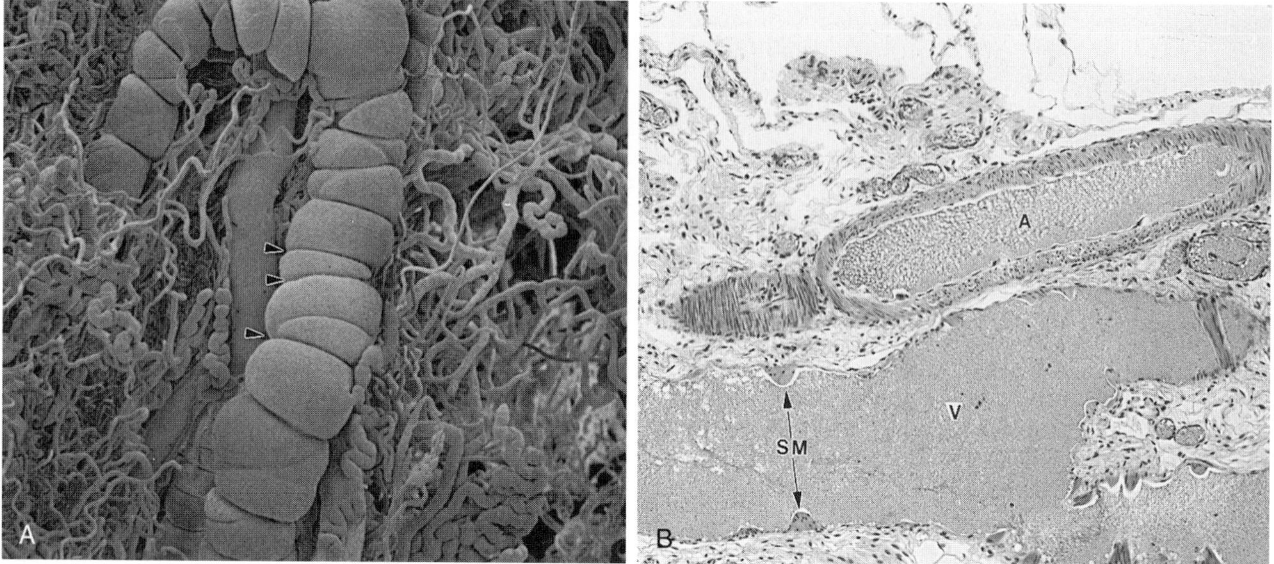

Figure 36-10. A, Scanning electron micrograph of a vascular replica of a colonic submucosal vein. Segmented sacculations are within the vessel wall *(arrowheads)*. **B,** Histologic section of submucosal colonic artery (A) and vein (V). Rings of smooth muscle (SM) are present within the colonic vein, resulting in segmented sacculations identified on the vascular replicas.

of energy in the horse.[84] The principal mechanism for delay in transit is the retropulsive activity initiated in a pacemaker region near the pelvic flexure (approximately 30 cm aboral to the termination of the medial and lateral free teniae of the left ventral colon).[85,86] The coordinated contractions originating at the pelvic flexure pacemaker promote physical separation of small, well-digested particles, which are propelled aborally, and of coarser particles, which are propelled orally for further digestion.[87] This may explain the roles of poor-quality feed and dentition in the development of large colon impaction.

Large Colon Tympany

Large colon tympany (gas colic, spasmodic colic) is the most commonly reported colic in horses.[88-90] It is thought to result from excessive gas fermentation in the colon, resulting in distention and pain. In one study evaluating risk factors for simple colonic obstruction and distention colic in horses (including large colon impaction), an increased risk was associated with crib-biting or windsucking, increasing number of hours spent in a stable, recent change in the regular exercise program, lack of administration of ivermectin or moxidectin anthelmintic in the previous 12 months, and a history of travel in the previous 24 hours.[91] Other factors that increased the risk of simple colonic obstruction and distention included history of previous colic, recent (less than 4 weeks) lameness, and increased time since last dental care.[91] An association between tapeworm infestation and spasmodic colic has been demonstrated.[92] Horses fed a hay and grain diet containing large amounts of soluble carbohydrates and less fiber had decreased water content in ingesta and increased gas, which predispose to gas colic.[93] Although large colon tympany can be self-limiting, it is thought to precede large colon displacements; therefore, identification of risk factors in affected horses may help decrease the risk of future occurrences.

Diagnosis

Horses examined for large colon tympany have acute pain and may show signs of visible external abdominal distention. Although in pain, they are minimally compromised and clinicopathologic parameters including abdominocentesis remain within normal reference range. The challenge for the clinician is to differentiate this type of colic from other, more serious causes of abdominal pain. The differential diagnosis for gas colic resulting in large colon distention includes large colon displacement, large colon torsion, ileus (impending colitis), and aboral obstruction (transverse or small colon obstruction). Rectal palpation reveals moderate to severe gas distention of the large colon.

Treatment

Treatment includes administration of analgesics and withholding feed. The response to medication is favorable and, if the diagnosis is correct, the horse will remain comfortable. Lack of response to analgesics may indicate a more serious problem. If the response to treatment is unsatisfactory, early referral is recommended, considering that large colon volvulus is a differential for this condition.

Large Colon Impaction

Large colon impaction is the second most commonly reported cause of colic in horses, and it is the most frequent type of simple obstruction.[94,95] It represents up to 13.4% of colics examined at referral centers.[37,96] Risk factors identified in one study included crib-biting or windsucking, increasing number of hours spent in a stable, recent change in the regular exercise program, absence of administration of ivermectin or moxidectin anthelmintic in the previous 12 months, and a history of travel in the previous 24 hours.[91] Additional factors identified in that study included history of previous colic, recent (less than 4 weeks) lameness, and increasing time since last dental care. In another study, 79 of 147 horses (53.7%) had a change in routine in the 2 weeks prior to development of a large colon impaction, and 17 of 147 (11.5%) developed the impaction while hospitalized for a reason other than gastrointestinal disease.[37] Decreased water intake and parasites are factors also mentioned although not well documented. High grain diets may predispose to colonic impactions, since grain feeding was shown to be associated with an internal fluid flux and subsequent dehydration of ingesta, setting the stage for impaction.[97] Right colon dry-matter content was higher when grain was part of a free choice hay diet.[98] In another study, water consumption was 40% greater in ponies offered warm drinking water under cold weather conditions, suggesting that cold weather may predispose to colonic impaction.[99] Hospitalization and general anesthesia have been suggested as risk factors for the development of impaction colic.[37,100] In one study, 37 of 85 hospitalized horses (43.6%) developed postoperative reduced fecal output, and 10 horses (12%) developed signs of colic; two of nine horses that had a rectal examination had pelvic flexure impactions. In that study, administration of phenylbutazone decreased the risk of reduced fecal output.[100] In contrast, in vitro studies have shown a negative effect of NSAIDs on large colon intestinal smooth muscle motility.[101,102] The benefits of NSAID administration for pain control, considering their negative effects on intestinal health, remains a matter of debate.[100,103]

Amitraz, an acaricide, has been used to induce experimental large colon impaction in horses.[104] Topical spraying of horses with amitraz was associated with systemic illness and impaction colic in three horses.[105] Amitraz, atropine, glycopyrrolate, and morphine significantly prolonged intestinal transit time in horses.[106] Atropine (0.044 mg/kg and 0.176 mg/kg IV) resulted in decreased intestinal motility and decreased appetite for 2 to 7½ hours after injection; signs of abdominal pain were observed in 3 of 10 ponies after administration.[107] Topical ocular administration of 1 mg of atropine hourly resulted in decreased intestinal motility (as assessed by auscultation for 2 to 18 hours after administration), and signs of abdominal pain were observed in four of six horses.[108] Subconjunctival administration of 3 mg of atropine resulted in decreased intestinal sounds in three of six horses, and signs of abdominal pain in one.[108] Lowering the luminal temperature to 20° C (room temperature) over a 100-cm length of colon cranial and caudal to the pelvic flexure for 2 hours significantly decreased conduction velocity, as well as amplitude and duration of pressure peaks in the intestinal wall. These findings have direct relevance to surgery of the large colon, where the colon is exteriorized from the abdomen, sometimes for prolonged periods of time, and where luminal lavage is performed. Minimizing the time of exteriorization and using warm water for luminal lavage may help the colon recover from the effects of reduced temperature.

The role of intestinal parasites on pelvic flexure motility has been evaluated. In one study, arteritis of the cranial mesenteric artery induced by inoculation of *Strongylus vulgaris* larvae resulted in reduced relative colonic blood flow; but it did not cause altered motility patterns.[109] In another study, increased motility patterns were observed in the cecum and colon at intermittent intervals for several days after infection.[110] Horses with chronic (more than 24 hours) obstructions of the large colon or with previous obstruction had decreased neuron density in the pelvic flexure, which may predispose to future obstructions.[41] Megacolon with myenteric hypoganglionosis has been described in a 6-month-old foal with severe large colon impaction and colic.[111] Recurrent impactions of the large colon were diagnosed in a mare with eosinophilic enterocolitis.[112] In that mare, diarrhea, hypoproteinemia, and weight loss characteristic of the disease were not present, and the intestine appeared grossly normal at surgery and at postmortem examination. These cases support the use of intraoperative intestinal biopsies in horses with unexplained recurrent large colon impaction.

Large colon impactions usually affect horses older than 1 year, although miniature horses may be predisposed to impactions as foals. Historically, horses are presented to referral centers for chronic colic (i.e., of longer than 24 hours' duration).[37]

Diagnosis

The most common location for large colon impaction is the pelvic flexure, followed by the right dorsal and transverse colon. On physical examination, horses typically show mild to moderate abdominal pain, decreased or absent intestinal sounds, decreased or absent fecal production, and occasionally mild to moderate abdominal distention.[37] Nasogastric reflux is rarely present. Rectal palpation is diagnostic in cases of pelvic flexure impaction. However, impactions of the right dorsal and transverse colon can be difficult to palpate in adult horses. When a large colon impaction is suspected on the basis of rectal palpation, it is essential to differentiate that from a large colon displacement with secondary right dorsal colon impaction.[113] Prolonged treatment of a large colon displacement with fluids and cathartics could result in preoperative or intraoperative colonic rupture.

In the case of a large colon displacement, the right dorsal colon may become severely impacted; during rectal palpation, when the hand follows the colon, it travels to the right, and lateral to the cecum. This is in contrast to a pelvic flexure impaction where the end of the pelvic flexure can readily be identified. Another important differential diagnosis of large colon impaction is small intestinal obstruction, which can result in dehydrated dry fecal contents in the large colon as identified by palpation. In contrast to large colon impaction, the teniae and haustra of the ventral colon in such cases become more prominent and distinguishable.[113]

Laboratory data typically observed in horses with large colon impaction show mild to moderate dehydration, a normal leukogram, and normal electrolyte data and blood gas analysis. The abdominocentesis results should be within normal range. Deteriorating cardiovascular status or peritoneal fluid changes are an indication of bowel degeneration.[37]

Treatment

Medical treatment of large colon impaction includes fluid therapy, analgesics, cathartics, and withholding of feed until the impaction is resolved. Intravenous fluids are reserved for impactions of longstanding (more than 24 hours) duration, when dehydration is documented, or when nasogastric reflux is present precluding the use of enteral fluid therapy.

Balanced electrolyte solutions are administered at twice the maintenance rate, or 120 mL/kg per day, both to restore circulating blood volume and to allow secretion of fluid into the large colon in response to cathartics. Overhydration in combination with an oral cathartic such as magnesium sulfate is thought to promote rehydration of ingesta.[114,115] Systemic rehydration should be performed before administration of cathartics.

Enteral fluid therapy can complement and even supplement intravenous fluids. Advantages of enteral fluid therapy include administration of fluid directly in the gastrointestinal tract, stimulation of colonic motility through the gastrocolic reflex, decreased expense, and decreased need for precise adjustment of fluid composition.[115] Enteral fluids can be administered by intermittent nasogastric intubation, or by nasal placement of an indwelling feeding tube (18 French equine enteral feeding tube, Mila International, Florence, Ky), allowing continuous fluid administration. An isotonic electrolyte solution can be made by mixing 5.27 g of NaCl, 0.37 g of KCl, and 3.78 g of $NaHCO_3$ per liter of tap water.[115] This solution results in electrolyte concentration of 135 mEq/L of Na, 95 mEq/L of Cl, 5 mEq/L of K, and 45 mEq/L of HCO_3, with a measured osmolality of approximately 255 mOsm/L, representing a slightly hypotonic electrolyte solution compared with plasma.[115] Plasma electrolyte concentrations remained within normal range with this solution compared with the marked hypernatremia and hyperchloremia observed when 0.9% saline is administered enterally.[115] Despite the fact that normal horses can tolerate up to 10 L hourly through intermittent nasogastric intubation,[116] it is usually not possible to administer more than 5 L every 2 hours in horses with impactions, because these horses start to reflux when more fluid is administered. Therefore, intermittent intubation is used, allowing administration of approximately 60 L of fluids per day. When continuous enteral fluids are given, a greater rate of administration is tolerated, and horses can be given between 4 and 10 L/hour. At the higher rate of 10 L/hour, mild signs of abdominal pain were observed in normal horses,[115] and in horses with large colon impaction, a rate of 5 L/hour is better tolerated. For enteral fluid therapy, the fluid used can be water, or water and electrolytes. In one study, right dorsal colon ingesta hydration was significantly increased after enteral fluid therapy compared with intravenous fluid therapy combined with enteral administration of magnesium sulfate.[115]

Cathartics are useful to increase the amount of water in the large colon or to promote ingesta transit. Mineral oil is a mixture of aliphatic hydrocarbons obtained from petrolatum; it is indigestible and absorbed to a limited extent. It is an intestinal lubricant that can also serve as a marker of intestinal transit. Administration of 5 to 10 mL/kg is usually recommended, and oil should be evident in the feces 12 to 24 hours after administration. Unformed feces were apparent 18 to 24 hours after its administration in normal horses.[117] Administration to normal horses decreased glucose absorption and intestinal transit time.[118,119] Chronic usage can result in a foreign body reaction in the intestinal mucosa.[120] Careful administration is necessary, since inadvertent administration into the lungs results in lipid pneumonitis, which is severe and often fatal.[121,122] Mineral oil is easily confused with propylene glycol, used in the treatment of ketosis in cattle; inadvertent administration of propylene glycol was the cause of death in a horse.[123]

Dioctyl sodium sulfosuccinate is an anionic surface-active agent that by lowering surface tension may facilitate penetration of the fecal mass by water and fats. Effects on motility and secretion are also attributed to this product. The recommended dose range is 16.5 mg/kg to 66 mg/kg, and the maximal recommended dose is 0.2 g/kg. Death because of circulatory shock can occur at doses of 1 g/kg.[124] In one study in normal horses, toxic signs were observed at a dosage of 50 mg/kg.[114] It is important to correctly label the product to avoid overdosing. Its advantage is that it requires a low volume of administration. However, the drug's low margin of safety and lack of efficacy at low dosages make its use questionable. Concurrent absorption with mineral oil may result in emulsification and subsequent systemic absorption of oil. Therefore, the use of the combination is frequently discouraged, although the significance of this finding is unknown.

Osmotic or saline cathartics such as magnesium sulfate or sodium sulfate are the most effective products to increase colonic water content.[114,125] Because of their efficacy, these products should be used after systemic rehydration. Recommended dosages are 0.5 to 1 g/kg. Absorption of magnesium resulting in signs of toxicity was reported in two horses that had received a combination of dioctyl sodium sulfosuccinate and magnesium sulfate.[46] Raw linseed oil produced from flaxseed was a commonly used laxative for the treatment of impactions. The addition of metallic salts and boil oil or boil pure oil enhances its properties as a wood preservative and is highly toxic. Only raw linseed oil should be used. Administration of 2.5 mL/kg to normal horses resulted in watery diarrhea, anorexia, mild signs of colic, and neutropenia.[117] Although raw linseed oil has greater laxative effects than mineral oil, the toxic effects may preclude its use, particularly in horses with compromised intestinal mucosa.[117] Polyethylene glycol 3350 is an effective osmotic laxative that is used in humans for the treatment of constipation or for colonic cleansing.[126,127] This product has not been evaluated rigorously in horses, although we have used it successfully to treat large colon impactions. Its cost is much greater than that of the other cathartics mentioned. Castor oil has been used as a model for experimental colitis in ponies.[128] Its use for the treatment of impaction colic is not recommended.

Analgesics are indicated as part of the management of large colon impaction. NSAIDs are commonly used. Use of low-dose flunixin meglumine may help control pain without affecting large colon motility. In the course of treatment of severe impactions, some horses may require intermittent dosing with xylazine to relieve intestinal spasm.[129] Alternatively, a constant-rate infusion of lidocaine can be used to modulate pain.

Prognosis

Most horses respond well to medical therapy. In one study, only 24 of 147 horses required surgery.[37] Indications for surgery included uncontrollable pain, deteriorating cardiovascular status, or peritoneal fluid changes indicating bowel compromise. Of the horses that went to surgery, five were euthanized after tearing of the colon during exteriorization.[37]

Surgical management of large colon impaction involves evacuation of the colon by pelvic flexure enterotomy. Complications of surgery include intraoperative rupture of the colon, postoperative diarrhea, incisional drainage, and, rarely, septic peritonitis.[37] The prognosis for large colon impaction is excellent, and the majority of horses respond to medical therapy. The prognosis is better for horses treated medically than surgically. In one study, long-term outcome for horses treated medically was 95.1%, compared with 57.8% for horses treated surgically.[37] The most common complication was jugular vein thrombophlebitis, so catheter sites should be monitored carefully. In the management of these horses, it is important to avoid risk factors that predispose to impactions. These horses are at risk for re-impaction if the same conditions remain. A small number of horses require permanent dietary modifications to avoid reimpaction.

Sand Impaction

Accumulation of sand in the equine large colon can result in variable signs, including colic, diarrhea, weight loss, and poor performance. Sand should be considered in the evaluation of chronic diarrhea in foals and adult horses.[130,131] Risk factors for sand impaction include insufficient roughage in the diet, access to sand, and mineral composition of the soil. Sand impaction has been diagnosed in horses that were exposed to sand 3 to 8 weeks before examination.[132] Higher incidences of sand colic are reported in California, Florida, Michigan, and coastal regions. Although most horses with sand impaction are older than 1 year,[132] sand accumulation has been documented in foals.[133,134] Miniature horses may also be predisposed to sand impaction because of environmental and management practices.

Diagnosis

Horses with sand impaction manifest signs similar to those of large colon impaction, unless a concurrent large colon displacement or torsion is present. Large colon displacements or torsion were identified in 10 of 40 (25%) and 26 of 48 (54%) of horses with sand impaction.[132,133] These clinical signs include mild to moderate abdominal pain, reduced fecal production, and decreased intestinal sounds. The sound of sand may be auscultated when the ventral abdomen is auscultated behind the xyphoid. These horses are responsive to analgesics, and signs can be present for several weeks. The cardiovascular status should be normal unless dehydration or intestinal devitalization has occurred. Occasionally, horses with sand impaction show signs of endotoxemia, presumably as a result of mucosal or intestinal damage associated with the weight and abrasiveness of the sand.[134]

Diagnostic procedures that are used to detect the presence of sand include observation of sand in the feces, sand obtained or palpated during abdominocentesis, abdominal auscultation, rectal palpation of a sand-filled viscus, abdominal radiography, and abdominal ultrasonography.[133-135] In one study, 23 of 40 horses (58%) were diagnosed with intestinal sand before surgery by one or more methods.[133] Fecal sedimentation is performed by adding water to six fecal balls in a rectal sleeve, and allowing the sand to settle to the bottom. The presence of more than 1 teaspoonful of sand is considered excessive. The presence of sand on sedimentation, however, may be incidental, and horses with sand impaction may not have sand in their feces at the time of examination. The appearance of sand in the feces during treatment is considered a sign of clearance of the sand.[134]

Abdominocentesis results are often normal, or show an increased total protein. Abdominocentesis is not diagnostic for sand colic but rather indicates the degree of intestinal compromise. However, the weight of the colon makes it easy to perform an unintentional enterocentesis during the procedure, and sand can be palpated with the tip of the needle or cannula.[132] In one study, 13 of 23 horses correctly diagnosed with sand impaction before surgery were identified by the presence of sand obtained or palpated during abdominocentesis.[133] Abdominal auscultation for the detection of sand is performed on the ventral abdomen, with emphasis on the area caudal to the xiphoid process.[136] The sound produced has been described as similar to the sound produced by sand in a partially filled paper bag and slowly rotated.[136] The intensity of sound is loudest with larger accumulations of coarse as opposed to fine sand.[136] In an experimental study of sand impaction in horses, all horses had, at some time, sand sounds that could be auscultated, but in most cases only after receiving several doses of sand, and after several repeated 5-minute auscultation periods.[136] Rectal palpation of horses with sand impaction most commonly reveals distention of the cecum or large colon. The impaction is rarely palpated on rectal examination; however, if coarse sand is present, it may be palpated through the intestinal mucosa.

Abdominal radiography provides the best method to evaluate the amount of sand accumulation, and it serves as a tool for monitoring disappearance of sand with treatment[134] (Fig. 36-11). Imaging of the cranioventral abdomen is the most useful projection.[134] Abdominal ultrasonography can be used to diagnose sand impaction, but it is best used in combination with abdominal radiography to monitor clearance of the sand.[137] Ultrasonographic evidence

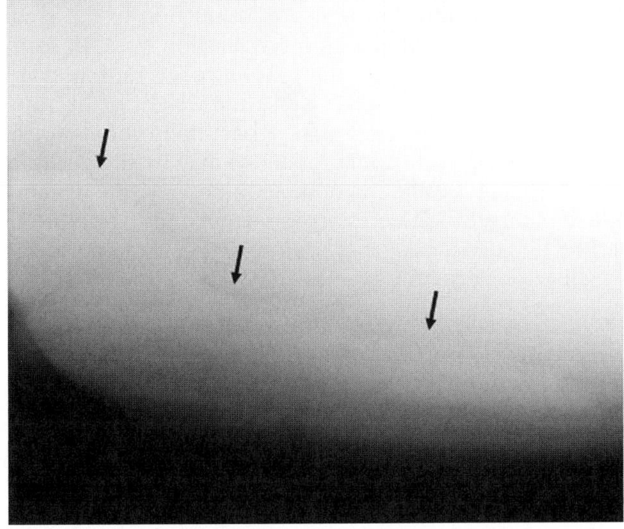

Figure 36-11. Lateral radiographic projection of the ventral abdomen of a horse showing accumulation of sand in the ventral colon *(arrows)*.

of sand accumulation is more subjective and includes close and increased contact of the large colon with the ventral body wall, decreased or absent intestinal motility, and hyperechoic acoustic shadowing. In one study, radiography and ultrasonography outcomes were similar in only 50% of cases.[135] Because ultrasonography is more readily performed and can be easily repeated, it is thought to be a useful tool for monitoring once a diagnosis has been made, although repeated radiographs may be indicated when results of the ultrasonography are equivocal.[135]

Treatment

Medical treatment of sand impaction includes removing the horse from access to sand, rehydration by intravenous or oral methods, and the use of laxatives. Mineral oil is usually not effective, as it will pass around the sand. Magnesium sulfate or psyllium is used to promote evacuation of sand. In one study, psyllium failed to increase evacuation of sand in an experimentally induced model of sand impaction.[138] However, numbers were small and the model may not reflect naturally occurring disease. In a clinical study, horses with sand impaction that were refractory to treatment were responsive to administration of magnesium sulfate and mineral oil.[134]

Monitoring of the resolution of the impaction can be performed using abdominal radiography or ultrasonography.[134,135] Horses with sand impaction can develop abnormal motility patterns and subsequent large colon displacement. These horses are have more pain and develop gas distention of the large colon. Surgical intervention is indicated when a displacement is suspected or diagnosed, when abdominal pain is uncontrolled, in the presence of deteriorating cardiovascular parameters, or when there is evidence of intestinal devitalization.[132,133] Standing flank laparotomy does not allow sufficient access to the large colon for evacuation in the presence of sand, and injection of the impaction is not successful in providing relief.

Therefore, a surgical approach through a ventral midline is recommended. At surgery, the sand is evacuated through a pelvic flexure enterotomy (Fig. 36-12). The most common location for accumulation of sand is the right dorsal colon, but any location, from the ileocecal junction to the small colon, is possible, and multiple impaction sites are commonly encountered. Care must be exercised during exteriorization of the large colon, since the weight of the sand predisposes the colon to rupture, especially in chronic cases. To facilitate exteriorization, the horse may be tilted toward the left side of the abdomen. In addition, only the minimal length of large colon necessary to safely perform a colotomy should be exteriorized; as the colon is evacuated, more of its length can be carefully exteriorized from the abdomen.

Prognosis

Results of surgical treatment of sand impaction report a good long-term survival. The most common complication is postoperative diarrhea, but this complication is commonly noted after surgical evacuation of the large colon for any reason. Other complications include peritonitis associated with intestinal devitalization from pressure necrosis.

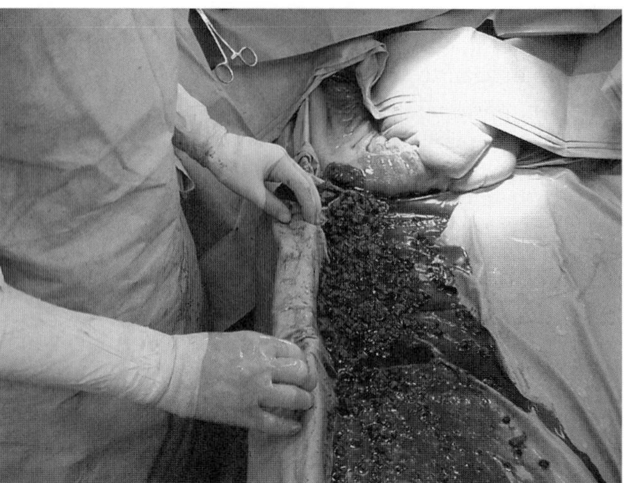

Figure 36-12. Pelvic flexure enterotomy for evacuation of a gravel impaction in the large colon of a horse.

Prevention of sand impaction includes provision of adequate roughage, feeding off the ground, and provision of additional roughage when pastures are insufficient. The use of different formulations of psyllium (pellets or flakes) has been advocated at different dosage regimens (once a day for 3 weeks, then 1 week off, to twice a day for 2 weeks, then 1 week off), but the efficacy of these different dosage regimens in prevention of further sand accumulation has not been documented. There is concern that long-term use of psyllium results in alteration of the colonic microflora with subsequent bacterial digestion of the psyllium and decreased efficacy[138]; this is the rationale behind interrupted administration.

Enterolithiasis

Obstruction of the large or small colon by enteroliths is a well-documented cause of intestinal obstruction in the horse. Risk factors include geographic location (with California and Florida having high prevalence for this cause of colic), breed predisposition (e.g., Arabians and Arabian crosses, Morgans, American Saddlebreds, donkeys, and Miniature Horses), feeding alfalfa hay, and less than 50% of time spent outdoors.[139,140] Other factors to explain why other horses fed the same diet in the same geographic area do not develop enteroliths are as yet unidentified.

Diagnosis

Enterolithiasis can result in acute severe luminal obstruction or cause intermittent mild signs of colic, depending on the location and size of the enterolith. Those in the large colon are usually localized in the right dorsal colon and cause mild signs of intestinal discomfort. Once they migrate into the transverse or small colon, signs of acute luminal obstruction develop, with progressive abdominal distention. Although this condition causes a simple colonic obstruction, transmural pressure necrosis can occur. Critical attention to results of the abdominocentesis helps determine such occurrence. An increase in total protein above the normal range and an increase in white blood cell count can alert the clinician to such occurrence.

Physical examination parameters also vary, depending on the location of the enterolith and whether intestinal devitalization has occurred. Rectal palpation may be normal or may reveal large colon distention. The enterolith can rarely be palpated. Results of the abdominocentesis are often normal, although an increased total protein is an early sign of intestinal devitalization. Radiographs are a useful diagnostic method for the detection of enteroliths, although the sensitivity and specificity vary depending on the location of the enterolith and the prevalence of the disease for the hospital population.[141] In one study performed in a high-prevalence area for enteroliths,[141] the sensitivity of radiographic diagnosis of enterolithiasis was 84.3% for those located in the large colon, compared with 50.0% for those located in the small colon. The mean overall positive predictive value for radiographs was 96.4%, and the negative predictive value was 67.5%.[141]

Surgical removal is indicated. If the enterolith is located in the large colon, the large colon is evacuated via a pelvic flexure enterotomy. A second enterotomy may be required in the right dorsal colon if the enterolith is too large to be evacuated through the pelvic flexure enterotomy. If the enterolith is lodged in the transverse colon, retrograde flushing by enema can facilitate its movement back into the dorsal colon. If the enterolith is in the small colon, it is removed by a small colon enterotomy. A partial-thickness enterotomy can facilitate movement of the enterolith to a more accessible portion of the small colon.[142] If there is significant pressure necrosis of the intestinal wall at the site of the obstruction, a resection may be required.

Prognosis

The prognosis is usually excellent. However, local necrosis of the intestine in an area that cannot be exteriorized, such as the transverse colon, is associated with a grave prognosis. In one study, bypass of the transverse colon by end-to-side anastomosis of the ventral colon to the small colon was successful in a Miniature Horse with intestinal necrosis after obstruction by a fecalith in the transverse colon. The recurrence rate of enteroliths is unknown, but dietary modifications such as avoidance of alfalfa hay are usually recommended. Other recommendations include removing horses from dirt or gravel, which can serve as a nidus, adding psyllium to the diet, and adding cider vinegar (1 cup twice daily) to the diet. In geographic areas where the water has a high mineral concentration, providing an alternate source of water can be useful.[140] Wheat bran should be minimized because of its high phosphorus content. Control of the dietary cation–anion balance (DCAB) has been suggested, although the benefits are unproven.[143] The target DCAB, calculated by the following equation:

$$\text{DCAB} = ([\text{Na}] + [\text{K}] + 0.15\,[\text{Ca}] + 0.15\,[\text{Mg}]) - ([\text{Cl}] + 0.25\,[\text{S}] + 0.5\,[\text{P}]),$$

is +200 to 300 mEq/kg. Grass hays and cereal grains have a DCAB within that range, whereas that of alfalfa is higher.

Large Colon Displacement

The equine large colon, because of its lack of mesenteric attachment to the body wall, is freely mobile and prone to displacement. In addition, normal longitudinal shortening of the left colon, promoted by contractions of the longitudinal layers, move the pelvic flexure toward the diaphragm, followed by backward movement toward the pelvis during relaxation; alterations in this motility pattern, initiated at the pelvic flexure pacemaker, could result in displacements and torsion.[87] The normal equine diet is composed of soluble and insoluble carbohydrates. Insoluble carbohydrates are digested by microbial fermentation, resulting in production of volatile fatty acids that are absorbed for energy production. When excess soluble carbohydrates are fed, alterations in the microbial population of the large colon may result in excessive fermentation, gas distention, and subsequent displacements.

Large colon displacements have been classified into left dorsal displacement of the large colon (also referred to as nephrosplenic entrapment or renosplenic entrapment), right dorsal displacement of the large colon, and nonstrangulating volvulus of the large colon. The large colon may adopt a location intermediate to these displacements, such that the exact description of the displacement can be difficult to describe.

Nephrosplenic Entrapment

Nephrosplenic entrapment (also termed renosplenic entrapment or left dorsal displacement of the large colon) is a form of nonstrangulating large colon displacement in the horse, in which the left dorsal and ventral colons migrate lateral to the spleen in a dorsal direction until entrapped in the nephrosplenic space (Fig. 36-13). It has been reported in horses of any age, and in foals as young as 9 months.[144] Although one report mentions the increased prevalence in male horses, others have not substantiated that finding.[144-146] Miniature horses and pony breeds have not been reported to acquire this problem. It is theorized that excessive gas formation within the left colon, perhaps in association with abnormal motility, causes the left colon to displace lateral to the spleen and dorsally into the nephrosplenic space; alternatively, horses may displace during rolling episodes.[90,147-149] In most cases, there is also ventromedial rotation of the left colon, such that the left dorsal colon is rotated ventral to the left ventral colon. The weight of the colon causes the spleen to displace medially and ventrally, and to become congested. Because of impaired flow of ingesta over time, with duration there is also concurrent impaction of the left dorsal colon. With continued gas formation, the sternal and diaphragmatic flexures can migrate cranial and dorsal to the stomach and become lodged between the stomach and the left lobe of the liver,[150,151] a displacement classified as type II in one report.[150] Nephrosplenic entrapment is a nonstrangulating lesion of the large colon; however, when duration of the condition increases to longer than 24 hours, colonic congestion and edema can develop, and mural damage may follow.[147] Obstruction to gastric outflow occurs because of pressure of the colon on the duodenum, or tension on the mesentery. Entrapment of the small colon or small intestine in the

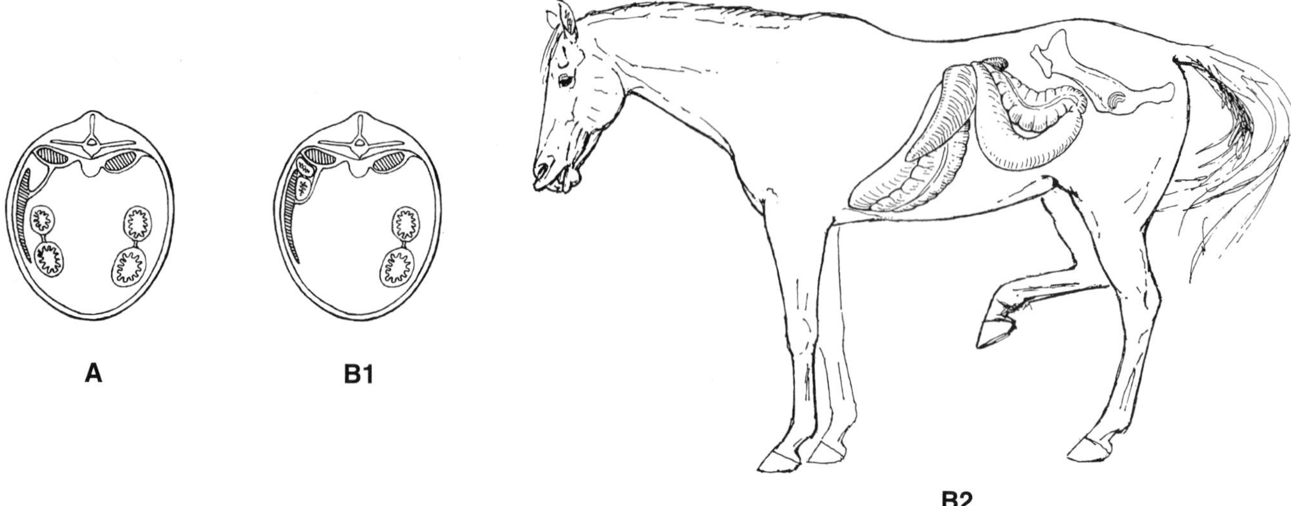

Figure 36-13. **A,** Left dorsal displacement of the ascending colon. The normal anatomic relationships of the colon to the spleen are shown. **B,** The dorsal and ventral colon may displace and become trapped in the nephrosplenic space.

nephrosplenic space have been described, but these conditions are rare.[152,153]

Horses with nephrosplenic entrapment show variable degrees of pain depending on the location of the colon, the amount of gas distention, and the presence of secondary gastric distention. Location of the colon lateral to the spleen is associated with minimal to no discomfort and is found in the resolving stages of the displacement. Entrapment of the colons within the nephrosplenic space with the spleen in a relatively normal position is a very painful condition. Affected horses crouch, want to go down, and often lean to the left. When the spleen is pushed away from the body wall and displaced ventrally by the colons, effectively opening the nephrosplenic space, there is less pressure on the colon, and horses show only mild signs of abdominal pain.

DIAGNOSIS

The diagnosis of nephrosplenic entrapment is based on the presence of abdominal pain (which can be mild to severe, depending on the location of the colon and the degree of gas distention) and relatively normal cardiovascular parameters, consistent with a simple obstruction. The complete blood count and blood chemistry values should be normal or consistent with mild dehydration. A low packed cell volume (PCV) in the face of dehydration has been reported as an indication of red blood cell sequestration in the spleen. The abdominocentesis results should be within normal range, and collection of splenic blood (characterized by a higher PCV than in peripheral blood) is supportive of a diagnosis of nephrosplenic entrapment. In one study, these results were obtained in 25% of horses at admission.[145] Horses with an increased white blood cell count (WBC) in the peritoneal fluid were more likely to suffer from a longer duration of the condition and to be treated surgically.[145] Nasogastric reflux is commonly obtained in horses with nephrosplenic entrapment as a result of pressure on the duodenum or mesenteric tension. Up to 43% of horses with nephrosplenic entrapment were reported to have nasogastric reflux.[144] In one study, resistance to nasogastric intubation was encountered in horses with displacement of the sternal and diaphragmatic flexures dorsal to the stomach.

An ultrasonographic examination of the abdomen may serve as an adjunctive tool in the diagnosis of nephrosplenic entrapment, and it was diagnostic in 88% (36 of 41) horses with nephrosplenic entrapment.[154] A 2.5- or 3.5-MHz ultrasound probe is placed over the 15th to 17th intercostal space in a direction parallel to the ground, and the spleen is imaged. In the normal horse, the left kidney is imaged deep to the spleen. In horses with nephrosplenic entrapment, the presence of gas-filled colon dorsal to the spleen precludes imaging the kidney. Finding ventral displacement of the dorsal aspect of the spleen is also consistent with nephrosplenic entrapment. If the colons are displaced lateral to the spleen, then imaging of the spleen is obscured as well. It is important to direct the probe in a horizontal direction; if the probe is angled in a dorsoventral direction, the kidney can occasionally still be imaged, giving a false-negative diagnosis. The inability to image the left kidney is supportive only of a nephrosplenic entrapment and should be used in conjunction with rectal palpation. Nonspecific large colon distention or the normal presence of small colon in the nephrosplenic space can impair imaging of the left kidney.[155] In addition, if the colon is filled with fluid, imaging of the left kidney is still possible, but the entrapped bowel is also seen.[154]

Rectal palpation remains the mainstay of diagnosis of nephrosplenic entrapment. On palpation, the left colon is most often gas distended, and the ventral colon is located dorsal to the left dorsal colon; often, an impaction of the left dorsal colon is present as well. The colon can be followed up into the nephrosplenic space. It is important for the correct diagnosis to follow the colon into the nephrosplenic space, because in other conditions (ranging from gas colic to large colon torsion), the colon may assume a dorsal position within the abdomen, leading to a false diagnosis of nephrosplenic entrapment.[156] This could be disastrous if nonsurgical management is attempted and the horse effectively has a large colon torsion. Rectal palpation correctly identified left dorsal displacement of the large colon in 61.2%, 68.7%, and 72% of cases in three studies,[144-146] although an early study reported a much lower rate of correct identification (only 18%).[150] Rectal palpation can be impaired by patient size, temperament, or the presence of severe distention.

A thorough physical examination, rectal palpation, and abdominal ultrasonography should be performed in horses diagnosed with nephrosplenic entrapment, because a small number of them will have another primary lesion involving another segment of the gastrointestinal tract. Gastric rupture, small intestinal volvulus, ileal impaction, large colon displacement, large colon volvulus, cecal torsion, and small colon obstruction have been documented in association with nephrosplenic entrapment.[144-146,154,157]

TREATMENT

Once a diagnosis of nephrosplenic entrapment has been made and the clinician is confident that there are no other abnormalities present, options for treatment are evaluated. These include medical therapy with intravenous fluids and withholding of feed; exercise with or without the use of a pressor agent; rolling under general anesthesia, with or without the use of pressor agents; standing flank laparotomy; and ventral midline celiotomy.

Medical treatment

Medical therapy with intravenous fluids supplemented with calcium gluconate is indicated when the colons are located lateral to the spleen. This type of treatment was successful in nine affected horses.[144] When the colons are localized in the nephrosplenic space and the horse is in pain, nonsurgical management can be attempted. In one study, horses that were successfully treated nonsurgically had a shorter duration of clinical signs, a lower peritoneal fluid WBC, and a higher blood lymphocyte count than horses treated surgically.[145] In that study, failure at nonsurgical correction was also felt to be related to severity of gas distention, which would also increase with duration. It is important to emphasize again that the diagnosis must be certain before attempting this option.

With all nonsurgical options, *phenylephrine* is often used to cause splenic contraction and facilitate correction. Bleeding the horse was described in the early literature to reduce splenic size,[158] but this seems unnecessary and possibly detrimental. Phenylephrine (Neo-Synephrine HCl, 10 mg/mL, Winthrop Pharmaceuticals, New York, NY) is an α_1-adrenergic receptor agonist that causes vasoconstriction in most vascular beds, and splenic contraction. In one study, the splenic area was reduced to 28% of baseline and thickness to 48% of baseline after administration of phenylephrine at 3 μg/kg/min over 15 minutes.[159] Side effects were minimal at that dose and included hypertension and reflex bradycardia. We use a total dose of 10 mg for horses with a body weight of 450 kg or less and 20 mg for larger horses, diluted in 50 mL of saline and given slowly intravenously over 5 minutes.

Vigorous exercise is an option for correction of this problem, providing the horse is not lame. This is more successful when performed early in the course of the disease, before large colon distention develops.[144,156] If there is significant distention of the left colons, they can be trocarized before exercise. For trocarization, an area over the left flank is clipped and prepared for aseptic surgery. A 14-gauge angiocatheter with a catheter extension is used to puncture the flank in a perpendicular direction. The end of the catheter extension is placed in a water container to facilitate observation of gas exiting the colons. Once in place, the trocar portion of the catheter is withdrawn for a few millimeters to avoid laceration of the bowel. The catheter may need to be inserted farther as the colon is deflated. When doing so, care must be taken not to lacerate the tip of the catheter with the trocar. Rectal palpation can help manipulate the colon to facilitate gas evacuation. Once done, the trocar portion of the catheter is removed and 1 to 2 mL of gentamicin is injected as the catheter is withdrawn. Once the trocarization is completed, phenylephrine is administered and the horse is exercised either on a lunge line or in a small paddock for approximately 15 to 30 minutes. Rectal palpation is performed to ascertain the position of the colon. Exercise can be repeated if correction is not achieved.

Correction by rolling under general anesthesia is another nonsurgical option for this disorder.[157,158] This has also been reported useful in a small number of horses with other forms of large colon displacements.[160] This option is preferred if the horse is lame, or if there is marked large colon distention. Previous abdominal surgery may preclude it, however, as splenic adhesions may prevent successful correction of the displacement.[161] For this procedure, the colon is not trocarized unless the distention is severe, as gas translocation is used to achieve correction of the displacement. The horse is prepared for short-term intravenous anesthesia. Sedation is given, followed by phenylephrine infusion as described previously. The horse is subsequently anesthetized and dropped into right lateral recumbency. Using a knee or two-handed fist, the clinician then shakes vigorously the abdomen in the region of the right flank, as the horse's hind legs are being hoisted dorsally. If a hoist is not available, the horse is slowly rolled into dorsal recumbency while abdominal compressions are performed. With the hoist, the hind legs are elevated until the horse's body reaches a 60-degree vertical position, while the clinician continues to vigorously shake the abdomen. After 1 or 2 minutes, the horse is replaced in right lateral recumbency. At this stage, some clinicians prefer to place the horse in left lateral recumbency, roll the horse into sternal position, and return it to right lateral recumbency. The procedure is repeated two more times. After the last manipulation, the horse is returned into left lateral recumbency for recovery. Between manipulations, the clinician may check the position of the colon. It is our experience that it is difficult to determine successful correction of the entrapment, either by ultrasonography or palpation, with the horse under general anesthesia. Therefore, we always recover the horse to determine if correction was achieved. Some clinicians prefer to follow immediately with surgical correction without recovery if it is suspected that correction was not achieved.[156]

One author describes manipulation of the colons per rectum. With the horse in right lateral recumbency, the hand lifts the colons off the spleen as the horse is being turned to left lateral recumbency. The use of muscle relaxants is recommended when this procedure is used to relax the rectum. Rectal manipulation must be performed with extreme caution, as rectal tears represent a definitive risk of the procedure.[157]

Rectal palpation after manipulation often reveals that the colon is lateral to the spleen and has not completely resumed its normal position. Administration of fluids and calcium often results in complete correction within a few hours. Some horses may show mild abdominal pain after manipulation even though it is suspected that correction was achieved. This is probably a result of residual large colon distention or impaction, and it is usually responsive to analgesics.

Surgical treatment

If nonsurgical manipulations are unsuccessful, surgical intervention is indicated. Standing flank laparotomy or ventral midline celiotomy are options to consider. The advantages of the standing flank laparotomy are avoidance of general anesthesia, direct access to the problem, access to the nephrosplenic space for closure as an option for prevention of recurrence, and more rapid return to use of the horse. The major disadvantage, as is the case for nonsurgical manipulation, is if an incorrect diagnosis was made, precluding correction by this approach. The advantages of the ventral midline celiotomy are that it ensures successful correction, particularly in cases where the colons are located dorsal and cranial to the stomach, and it allows correction of other undiagnosed problems. The disadvantages include the need for general anesthesia, longer postoperative recovery, and increased cost.

Standing flank laparotomy: The horse is restrained in stocks with the tail bandaged and tied to avoid contamination of the incision. Sedation with xylazine, with or without butorphanol, is sufficient for most horses. After standard preparation of the surgical site, local anesthesia is performed. This can be accomplished with a paravertebral block,[162] an L-block or a line block, taking care to add local anesthesia for placement of towel clamps. In our experience, the paravertebral block often requires additional local anesthetic in the distal aspect of the planned incision. Draping is routine, with the addition of a drape folded to form a pocket for support of the exteriorized bowel. The standard surgical approach for a flank laparotomy is midway between the last rib and the cranial aspect of the tuber coxae, starting approximately 2 cm above the palpable internal oblique muscle. In the standing horse, the modified grid approach is preferred, as the muscles will contain the intestinal contents after surgery. In the modified grid approach, the external oblique muscle is incised in vertical direction but the internal oblique and transverse abdominal muscles are bluntly separated along the course of their muscle fibers by finger traction. Additional topical application of anesthetic may be required before perforating the peritoneum. Once the abdomen is entered, the spleen and large colon are located. In our experience, it is easier to push the spleen down and under the large colon than to lift the large colon over the spleen. Once the colon is lateral to the spleen, it is gently pushed down into the ventral abdomen. Closure is routinely performed.

Ventral midline celiotomy: This approach is recommended for correction of nephrosplenic entrapment if nonsurgical management is unsuccessful and the surgeon is not comfortable with the flank approach or if there are clinical or clinicopathologic findings that indicate either the loss of intestinal integrity or the presence of another lesion. It is also used when a presurgical diagnosis is not possible because the small size of the patient precludes rectal palpation, or because excessive large colon distention is present. A routine ventral midline approach is performed, although to facilitate access to the nephrosplenic space the horse may be slightly rotated to the right. In the presence of excessive splenic congestion, or excessive weight of the colon, phenylephrine may be administered to reduce splenic size and facilitate correction. The base of the spleen is grasped, and the spleen is lifted and pushed medial to the colon, thus freeing it from the nephrosplenic space. The colon is subsequently cradled over the forearm and lifted out of the abdomen. Although there is often feed accumulation in the dorsal colon, evacuation is usually not necessary since the feed redistributes when the displacement is corrected. The colon is assessed for signs of devitalization. Rarely, a large colon resection will have to be performed.

Reported recurrence rates of nephrosplenic entrapment are between 7.5% and 8.5%.[144,145] Considering this relatively low risk of recurrence, surgical intervention procedures for prevention of recurrence are not recommended after a first incidence. However, feeding and management practices should be carefully reviewed to minimize the risk of gas formation in the large colon and subsequent displacement.

PREVENTION OF RECURRENCE

Procedures that have been advocated for prevention of recurrence of left dorsal displacement of the large colon include closure of the nephrosplenic space, large colon colopexy, and large colon resection. The reader is referred to other sections (later) for reference to large colon resection and colopexy procedures.

Closure of the nephrosplenic space does not prevent migration of the large colon lateral to the spleen, or the occurrence of other forms of large colon displacement. The procedure can be performed through a flank laparotomy or though a minimally invasive laparoscopic approach.[118,163,164] The flank approach is performed in the standing or laterally recumbent horse. The abdomen is entered either through a modified grid or laparotomy approach. The spleen and nephrosplenic ligament are identified, and the nephrosplenic space is verified to be free of intestine. Cruciate sutures are then placed between the ligament and the tip of the spleen, using a nonabsorbable suture such as 2-polypropylene in a cruciate pattern. Approximately 6 to 12 sutures are preplaced and tied. The abdomen is closed in a routine fashion. Alternatively, laparoscopic ablation of the renosplenic space can be performed in the standing horse[163]; this has been reported in five experimental animals. The procedure is performed using three laparoscopic portals and polyglactin 910 suture material in a simple-continuous pattern. Two series with small numbers of horses have reported long-term efficacy for this procedure.[163,164]

Right Dorsal Displacement of the Large Colon

This type of displacement is thought to be initiated by retropulsive movement of the pelvic flexure, with subsequent migration of the left colon cranially and then to the right abdominal quadrant, until the right ventral and dorsal colons are located between the cecum and the body wall (Fig. 36-14). The colon can also rotate on its long axis, resulting in variable degree of venous congestion.

DIAGNOSIS

The location of the colon at the time of examination is related to the clinical signs. When the colon is displaced cranially, all parameters are within normal limits, and abdominal pain is mild and intermittent. These horses may be comfortable when held off feed, with abdominal pain recurring when feed is reintroduced. These horses continue to pass small amounts of manure. On rectal palpation, there is no abdominal distention, but the examiner is unable to find the pelvic flexure. As the colon continues to migrate in a clockwise direction, the flow of ingesta is impaired, and a secondary impaction of the right dorsal colon may develop. Gas distention also becomes more significant, as does the associated abdominal pain. When a dorsal colon impaction develops, it is important not to mistake it for a pelvic flexure impaction, as continued medical treatment may result in rupture of the colon. This condition can be differentiated from a pelvic flexure impaction by the fact that the colon travels cranially to the right, and that the pelvic flexure cannot be identified. In right dorsal displacements, the cecum can be enlarged and filled with fluid.

Horses with right dorsal colon displacements are presented with mild to moderate abdominal pain. Depending on the degree of displacement, rectal palpation reveals absence of the pelvic flexure, presence of large colon lateral to the cecum, large colon distention, and right dorsal colon impaction. Nasogastric reflux may be present if there is large colon distention. Laboratory data are usually unremarkable, although a significant number of horses are presented with an elevated gamma-glutamyl-transferase, probably related to partial obstruction of the duodenum.

TREATMENT

When horses are presented early, with normal parameters, mild abdominal pain, and minimal to moderate large colon distention, medical therapy may be attempted. Intravenous fluids are administered and the horse is monitored for resolution of the distention and relocation of the large colon.

When the pain is severe, or there is marked large colon distention or a severe secondary impaction, surgical intervention is recommended. Although in some specific circumstances we have successfully corrected right dorsal colonic displacements via a standing flank laparotomy, a ventral midline celiotomy is preferred because of ease of exposure and correction.

At surgery, the pelvic flexure is identified, the large colon is exteriorized, and the displacement is corrected. When a severe large colon impaction coexists, the large colon is exteriorized at the pelvic flexure, but an attempt to correct the displacement is not made until the large colon has been evacuated, to avoid rupture during colonic manipulations. Although there is one report of successful treatment of a horse after intraoperative rupture during surgery,[165] most of these cases are fatal.

PROGNOSIS

The prognosis for large colon displacement is excellent. Recurrence is possible, and we have had horses redisplace within 48 hours of the first procedure. In our opinion, it is important not to completely evacuate the large colon but to

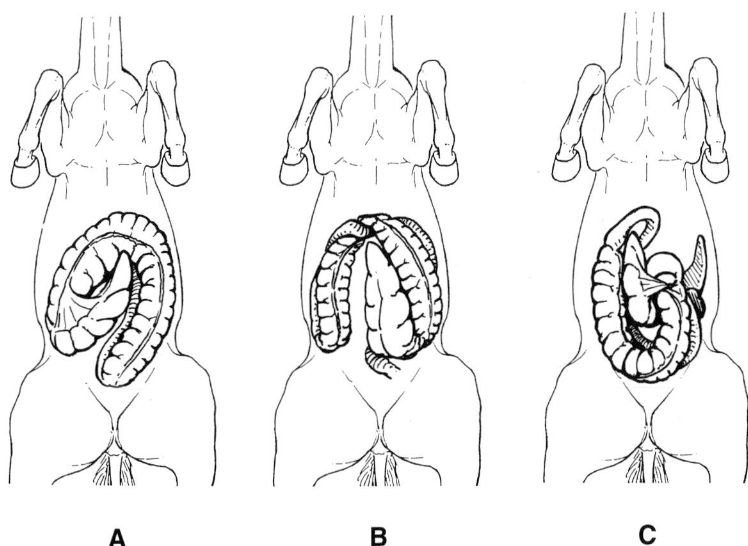

Figure 36-14. Right dorsal displacement of the ascending colon (ventral views). **A,** The normal anatomic relationship of the ascending colon. **B,** The most common direction for a right dorsal displacement is migration of the pelvic flexure in a counterclockwise direction when viewed from the caudal and ventral aspect of the horse at the time of surgery. **C,** Although less common, the ascending colon may develop a right dorsal displacement characterized by a clockwise migration of the pelvic flexure when viewed from the caudal and ventral aspects of the horse at the time of surgery.

leave some ingesta. We also return these horses to feed within 8 hours of surgery, again to try to maintain bulk in the large colon.

Nonstrangulating Volvulus of the Large Colon

Nonstrangulating volvulus of the large colon is identified when the colon is rotated from 90 to 270 degrees along its long axis, a step that precedes the 360-degree large colon volvulus.

DIAGNOSIS

Horses with this type of displacement have a clinical presentation very similar to that of other simple large colon displacements; minimal cardiovascular compromise, mild to moderate abdominal pain, normal abdominocentesis, and mild to moderate large colon distention on rectal palpation. As in other displacements, medical management may be attempted. Horses that remain in pain or that have worsening of abdominal distention are candidates for surgical intervention. At surgery, the colon is replaced in its normal position.

As in all forms of large colon displacements or volvulus, prevention of recurrence should be considered. Colopexy and large colon resection are two procedures that are performed in an attempt to prevent recurrence. Usually these procedures are not recommended on a first time occurrence, but should be considered for horses that have two or more displacements.

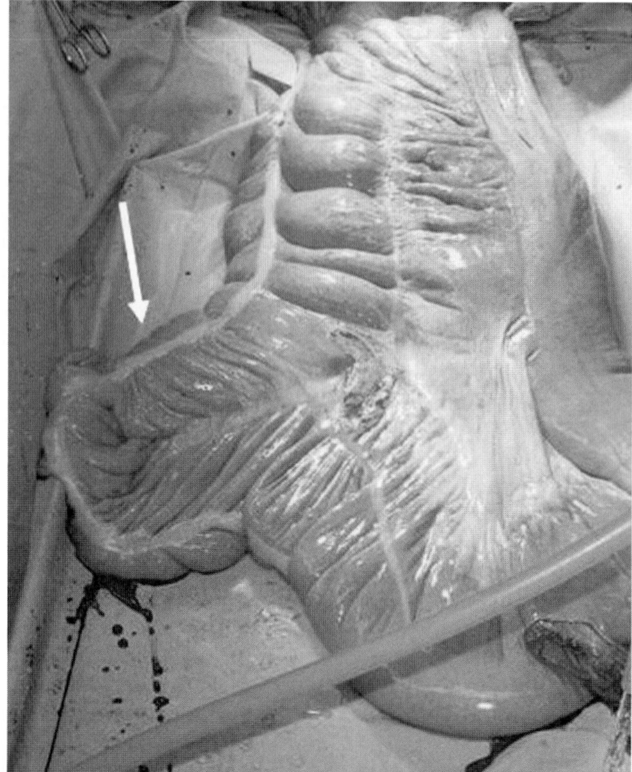

Figure 36-15. Congenital malformation of the large colon in an 8-month-old American Bashkir Curly filly with a history of recurrent colic. The ventral colon has a large diverticulum *(arrow)*. A large colon resection was performed and the filly made an uneventful recovery.

Other Simple Obstructions of the Large Colon

Congenital malformation of the large colon was reported as a cause of recurrent colic in a horse, and we have identified it in several horses[166] (Fig. 36-15). Resection of the colon oral to the malformation and anastomosis successfully resolved the problem.

Fibrosis and stricture of the large colon caused by focal fibrosis at the pelvic flexure was identified in three horses and corrected by transverse closure of a pelvic flexure enterotomy performed at the site of the fibrosis.[167]

Pelvic flexure adhesions resulting in impaction were reported in a filly with peritonitis. Laparoscopic adhesiolysis was successfully performed to allow return of transit.[168]

A massive duplication cyst of the ascending colon was reported in a 27-year-old mare with a history of recurrent colic and a pendulous abdomen. The cyst was successfully removed and the mare made an uneventful recovery.[169]

We have observed defects in the mesentery of the large colon in several horses (see Fig. 36-8). The presence of the defect allows displacement or torsion of the colon upon itself, since it is no longer confined by the mesentery. The problem can be corrected by closure of the defects with the help of sutures.

Large Colon Torsion or Volvulus

Large colon volvulus is one of the most painful and devastating gastrointestinal problems in the horse (Fig. 36-16) Successful management depends on rapid referral and prompt surgical intervention. Without intervention, death occurs in a matter of hours in horses. The prevalence of large colon volvulus is increased in geographic areas with high concentration of brood mares. Risk factors include recent parturition, recent dietary changes, and recent access to a lush pasture.

Diagnosis

The history of horses with large colon volvulus varies depending on the rapidity and totality of the development of a complete volvulus. Some horses are presented with a history of chronic (more than 24 hours) colic that suddenly worsens to intractable pain; others are presented with an acute onset of uncontrollable pain. Initially, despite the severe pain, horses maintain normal cardiovascular parameters, and rectal palpation can be unremarkable. As time elapses, these horses develop progressive large colon distention and accompanying progressive cardiovascular collapse. In mares, the color of the vaginal mucosa changes and reflects the degree of compromise of the large colon. If untreated, horses with large colon torsion die of hypovolemic shock caused by abdominal compartment syndrome associated with the severe distention, by pooling of blood in the strangulated large colon, and by poor pulmonary expansion because of severe distention.

Treatment

The treatment of large colon torsion is surgical. However, during preparation for surgery, resuscitative measures should be initiated to increase circulating blood volume and

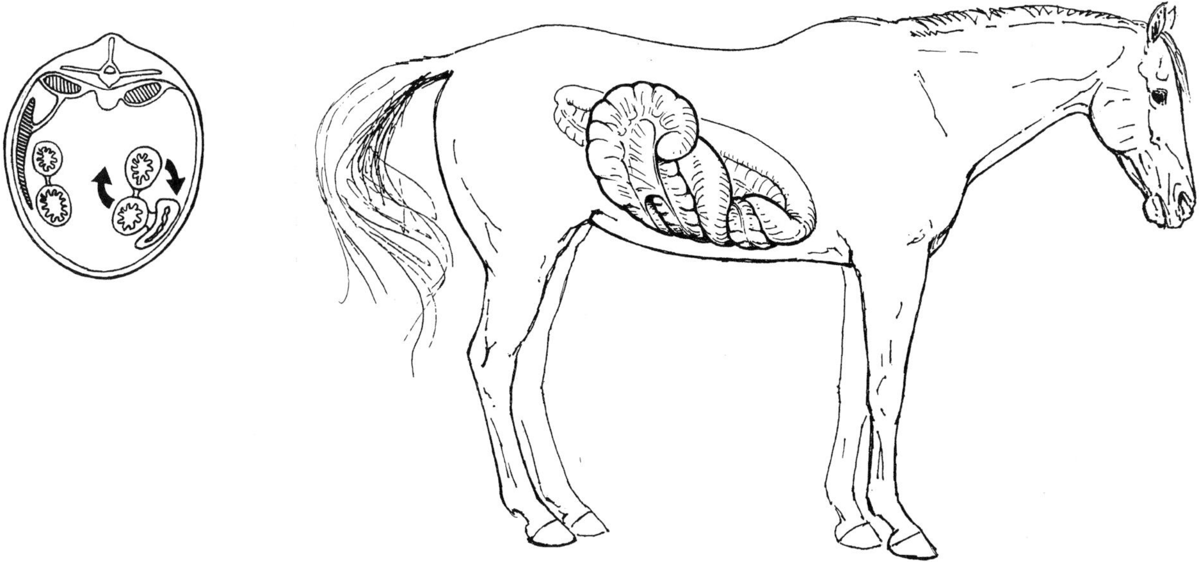

Figure 36-16. A schematic diagram representing the two directions in which the ascending colon may twist during torsion. The *arrows* indicate the more common dorsomedial torsion.

decrease abdominal pressure. Shock fluid therapy, including hypertonic saline, colloids, and crystalloids, needs to be initiated (see Chapter 3). Trocarization to relieve abdominal distention may improve lung expansion and venous return, and it can help support the horse during induction, until the colon can be exteriorized and decompressed.

In preparation for surgery, the horse can be tilted to one side to facilitate exteriorization of the colon and remove pressure on the caudal vena cava. Administration of intravenous lidocaine allows a decrease in the concentration of inhalant agents. A long ventral midline incision is performed to help in exteriorization of the colon. A more cranial approach is preferred, to facilitate exposure of the colonic base.

The direction of the torsion is best described in relationship to the position of the ventral colon, which obviates the need to describe it from the observer's position. Thus, a dorsomedial volvulus indicates rotation of the right ventral colon medially and dorsally.[170] Most are in a dorsomedial direction, and the location of the volvulus is at or proximal to the cecocolic ligament. Occasionally, a volvulus involving the sternal and diaphragmatic flexures is encountered. Volvuli of 270 to 720 degrees have been described.[171] Correction of the volvulus can be difficult, particularly if the colon is full or edematous; this places the colon, particularly the right dorsal colon, at risk for rupture during surgical manipulation. The ascending colon is exteriorized; if the colon is full or edematous and friable, a pelvic flexure enterotomy is performed to empty the colon prior to manipulation. To correct the volvulus, the surgeon, situated on the left side of the horse, places both hands in the abdomen around the base of the colon and gently manipulates the colon in a clockwise direction. The surgical assistant can facilitate manipulation by rotating the exteriorized portion of the colon in the same direction. Gas translocation and return of serosal color are indications that the colon is manipulated correctly. Once a 360-degree rotation has been achieved, the surgeon must ascertain that the volvulus is corrected, and that another rotation of the colon is not needed. This is accomplished by examining the normal position of the cecum and the normal position of the cecocolic ligament, and by ensuring by palpation that the mesenteric attachment of the right dorsal colon to the dorsal body wall is straight. Palpation of the duodenum cranial to the right dorsal colon is possible after the volvulus is completely corrected.

Once the colon has been returned to its normal position, the surgeon must decide between euthanasia, recovery of the horse without further intervention, colopexy for prevention of recurrence, and large colon resection. It is essential to involve the owner in the decision-making process, particularly if the colon is compromised, since the cost of further intervention and postoperative care can be significant. The surgeon must also understand that if the colon is not resected and the horse is recovered, it is unlikely that a second laparotomy will be an option. By the time clinical signs indicate that a second laparotomy with a possible large colon resection is warranted, the horse's condition will have deteriorated to the point that the chances of survival after a resection will be poor. Several factors are useful to help the surgeon reach a decision. A critical one is the horse's systemic condition both preoperatively and intraoperatively. A PCV above 50% (and increasing during surgery) associated with a decreasing total protein is a poor indicator of survival. An inability to maintain mean arterial blood pressure, despite the use of pressor agents, persistent hypoxemia, and persistent tachycardia during surgery, is also associated with poor survival. Examination of the colon can provide some additional information. Return of a normal pink serosal color after volvulus correction is a positive indicator, but it does not relate to mucosal viability; severe postoperative endotoxemia may still occur if the mucosa is devitalized. Visual examination of the mucosa made through a pelvic flexure enterotomy provides additional information.

The presence of dark red or black mucosa with no active bleeding is a poor prognostic indicator. Frozen sections allow calculation of the interstitial-to-crypt (I:C) ratio and percent loss of epithelium, which correlate well with survival. An I:C ratio of 3:1 or greater, or loss of greater than 95% of the epithelium, was associated with 95% death in one study. However, this requires personnel able to obtain and evaluate frozen sections. Other research tools that have been used to evaluate colonic viability include surface oximetry, fluorescein dye, and Doppler flow; none of these tools has gained popularity in a clinical setting (see Chapter 34).

The decision to perform a colon resection should also be based on the location of the volvulus. If the line of devitalized bowel is located distal to the cecocolic ligament, the outcome of a large colon resection is much more favorable, because resection of the affected bowel is possible. However, in most instances, the line of devitalization is located at the base of the colon oral to the cecocolic ligament; resection must be performed in a compromised portion of the bowel, which places the resection site at risk for dehiscence. Surgeons who are advocates of large colon resection for the treatment of large colon volvulus make a case that removing the majority of the diseased colon decreases the endotoxic load and therefore increases the likelihood of survival; in addition, removal of the large colon prevents recurrence of the condition. Surgeons who do not routinely perform large colon resections for large colon volvulus state that the procedure in itself has a high risk of complications, and that in most cases it does not result in removal of the entire diseased colon; in addition, the increased anesthesia time may be detrimental to the animal. These debates emphasize the complexity of the decision-making process in these cases, the importance of experience and familiarity with surgical techniques, and the influence of types of cases on the decision-making process. For example, horses that are referred quickly and have a short duration of illness seldom require a large colon resection.

Prognosis

Preoperative parameters indicative of poor survival include PCV greater than 50%, rectal temperature greater than 39.5° C (102° F), and a heart rate greater than 80 beats per minute.[172] Intraoperative factors associated with a poor survival include black mucosal color, poor return of perfusion after detorsion, and an increasing PCV and decreasing total protein during surgery.[172] Abdominocentesis is usually normal in horses with large colon volvulus; an increase in total protein in the abdominal fluid is associated with decreased survival.[153] Abdominocentesis therefore does not provide information that will alter the decision for surgical treatment, and it has an increased risk of enterocentesis or injury to personnel because these animals are in severe pain.

Reported mortality for large colon volvulus varies from 56% to 65%. However, in one study, the short-term survival rate was 84%; this higher survival rate was thought to be related to a shorter duration of illness and faster intervention time.[173] Although short-term mortality is high after surgical correction of large colon volvulus, a long-term probability of survival of .8 has been reported once discharge from the hospital occurred.[174]

Right Dorsal Colitis

Right dorsal colitis is a specific type of ulcerative colitis observed in the right dorsal colon of the horse, specifically the aboral segment of the dorsal colon as it joins the transverse colon. The condition is recognized in association with administration of NSAIDs, and it has been reproduced experimentally by administration of phenylbutazone. Horses with nervous predisposition seem more prone to the development of the disease despite the administration of appropriate dosages of NSAIDs. Although NSAID administration is commonly associated with this condition, it has also been documented in the absence of NSAID administration.

Diagnosis

Clinical signs of right dorsal colitis can manifest as acute colic, endotoxemia, diarrhea, and even death. The disease is more common in the chronic form, where horses are presented for weight loss, hypoproteinemia, intermittent signs of colic, and intermittent diarrhea.

The diagnosis of right dorsal colitis is based on anamnestic information, particularly related to NSAID administration, and ruling out other causes of weight loss, hypoproteinemia, and diarrhea. Diagnostic ultrasonography of the right dorsal colon may help identify the thickened colon[175] (Fig. 36-17). More recently, scintigraphy with radiolabeled white blood cells has been described to diagnose the condition.[176]

Treatment

Medical management is recommended for the initial treatment of right dorsal colitis. This includes discontinuation of NSAIDs, dietary modifications, anti-inflammatory drugs, intestinal protectants, and metronidazole. Dietary modifications are important to help control the signs of colic.

In cases of protracted colic, or when intermittent colic is so frequent as to prevent the horse from maintaining itself, surgical exploration may be recommended. At surgery, the right dorsal colon feels markedly thickened, and it may be strictured with scar tissue (Fig. 36-18). Once the disease is

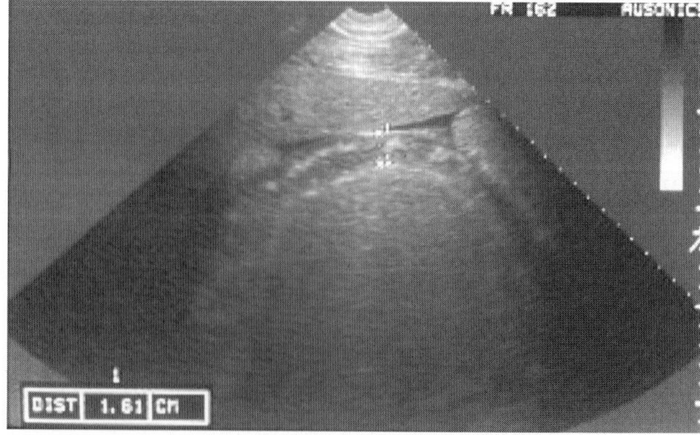

Figure 36-17. Sonographic image of the right dorsal colon showing marked thickening of the colonic wall in a horse with right dorsal ulcerative colitis associated with phenylbutazone toxicity. The image was obtained using a 7.5-MHz probe directed into the 10th right intercostal space.

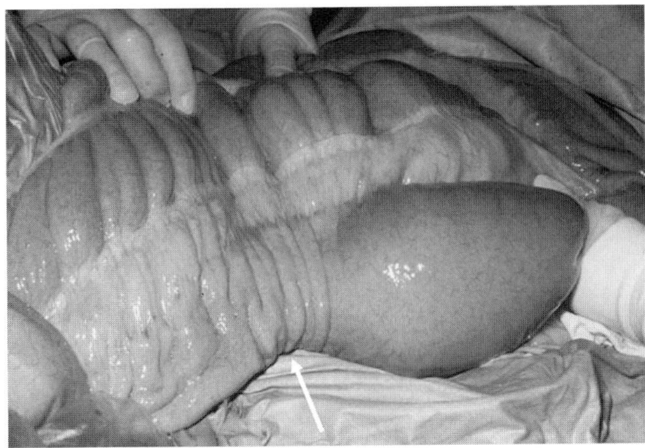

Figure 36-18. Intraoperative image of the right dorsal colon of a horse with right dorsal colitis. Note the markedly thickened colon with stricture at the diseased site *(arrow)*.

identified at surgery, treatment options include right dorsal colon bypass, resection of the affected portion of the colon, large colon resection, or large colon resection and bypass.

Bypass of the affected area of the large colon is performed by exteriorizing the large colon on a colon tray. The small colon is then exteriorized and a 20- to 30-cm side-to-side anastomosis between the right dorsal colon (oral to the lesion) and the small colon approximately 1 m distal to the transverse colon is performed[177] (Fig. 36-19). When this procedure is performed, transient diarrhea has been observed. This procedure does not remove the affected portion of the colon, so the patient can continue to suffer from weight loss and hypoproteinemia until the colitis has resolved. Resection of the affected colon through a 16th rib resection has been reported in one horse.[178] This approach requires either prior knowledge of the disease or a second celiotomy approach once the diagnosis has been made. Resection and end-to-end anastomosis is possible only if the lesion does not extend too far aborally. In cases of severe right dorsal colitis with stricture of the right dorsal colon, large colon resection and anastomosis in a side-to-side fashion can be performed to restore intestinal transit. However, complete removal of the ulcerated area would not be possible with this approach. Another approach, which has not been described for the treatment of this condition, would be to amputate the large colon, particularly the dorsal colon, as far aborally as possible, and to perform an end-to-side anastomosis between the right ventral colon and the small colon. This approach has been reported for the management of nonfunctional dorsal colon lesions in two horses.[179,180]

Mural Infarction (Thromboembolic Colic)

Compromise to the mesenteric vasculature without evidence of strangulation has been described in association with arteritis resulting from *Strongylus vulgaris* larval migration, or in horses with severe colitis and coagulopathies (Fig. 36-20). Cases of larval arteritis can be acute (with signs of ischemic bowel disease and peritonitis) or chronic (with signs of recurrent colic and weight loss). Horses with acute thromboembolic colic demonstrate significant changes in their abdominocentesis, consistent with those seen with peritonitis; horses with recurrent colic often have a normal abdominocentesis.

In acute cases, the decision for surgical intervention is based on the signs of colic and the presence of peritonitis. At surgery, mural infarction is identified, and if possible, resection of the affected segment of intestine is performed. Careful palpation of the cranial mesenteric artery should be performed; identification of severe enlargement, aneurysm, or abscessation is an indication for a guarded to poor prognosis. A regular systemic deworming program should be instituted as part of the postoperative care.

When horses with colitis show acute signs of abdominal pain and abdominal distention, thromboembolic colic and necrotizing colitis should be suspected. Many of these horses have extensive lesions that preclude surgical intervention. In addition, their systemic status, as a result of the primary colitis, makes them poor surgical candidates.

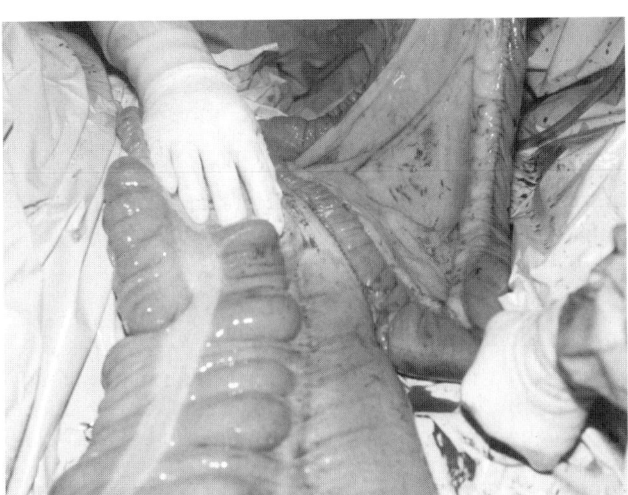

Figure 36-19. Side-to-side anastomosis of the right dorsal colon to the small colon in a horse with right dorsal ulcerative colitis.

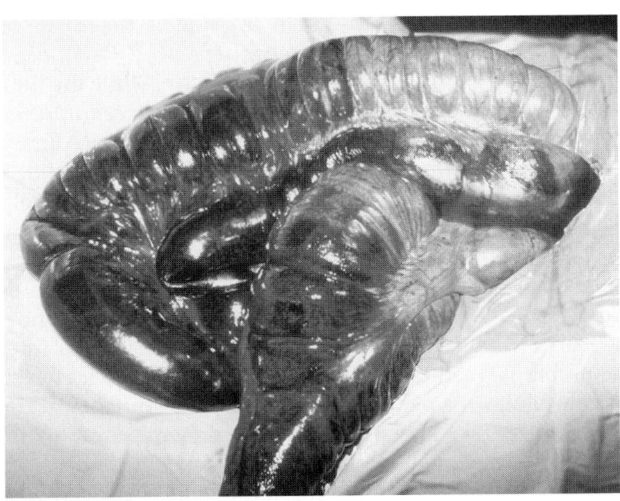

Figure 36-20. Mural infarction in a horse with colitis associated with salmonellosis.

Other Strangulating Lesions of the Large Colon

Other strangulating lesions of the equine large colon that have been reported include incarceration in the epiploic foramen[48] or the gastrosplenic ligament[181]; large colon intussusception[182,183]; and volvulus associated with abnormal mesenteric bands or defects.[35,184] Surgical intervention is dictated in these cases by the increasing degree of abdominal pain, abnormal rectal palpation, and abdominocentesis indicative of intestinal compromise. Resection and anastomosis of the affected colon is required to correct these conditions.

Surgical Procedures

Large Colon Enterotomy

The most commonly performed procedure in the large colon is pelvic flexure enterotomy for evacuation of the large colon. Enterotomy procedures are also performed for removal of foreign bodies, usually in the right dorsal colon. Finally, right ventral colon enterotomy is used to access the cecum in cases of cecocolic intussusceptions.

Pelvic flexure enterotomy and large colon evacuation: For this procedure, the large colon is exteriorized and placed on a colon tray (Enterotomy table, Kimzey Metal Products, Woodland, Calif), either on the left side of the horse or caudally between the horse's hind legs. If a colon tray is not available, the colon is best exteriorized between the hind legs. Some surgeons place the end of the laparotomy drape onto the tray to create a shelf for the colon to rest on. The enterotomy drape is then placed on top of the laparotomy drape and secured with towel clamps. The colon tray is angled at about 20 degrees. A modified trashcan with an ingesta strainer and a liquid outflow hose is used in some clinics to collect and evacuate the contents of the colon[185] (Fig. 36-21). Alternatively, the end of the tray can be positioned over a disposal system built into the surgery room (Fig. 36-22). In anticipation of colonic evacuation, a lavage system should be established. This can be done by using two garden hoses, or one hose with a Y-connection. One hose is used for intraluminal lavage and evacuation of the colon, and the other for extraluminal lavage, using warm water (37° C [98.6° F]).[185] If these are not available, stomach tubes, buckets, and pumps are used.

A full-thickness, 8- to 12-cm incision is made on the antimesenteric border of the pelvic flexure.[186] One hose is inserted and gently advanced into the colon, while the other is used to continuously lavage the serosal surface to prevent fecal contamination. During the evacuation procedure, it is useful to lift the colon and ensure that the underside is lavaged as well. With sterile technique, an assistant helps to feed the hose into the colon and massage its contents. Although a modified colon tray has been described to evacuate the colon, it is not deemed necessary by most surgeons.[187] At this time, if colonic evacuation is performed as part of the correction of a large colon torsion, an intestinal biopsy can be collected. Closure of pelvic flexure enterotomies is performed using 2-0 absorbable suture material in two layers: a simple-continuous seromuscular layer followed by a Lembert or a Cushing pattern.[188] The colon is rinsed thoroughly with sterile saline and replaced in the abdomen.

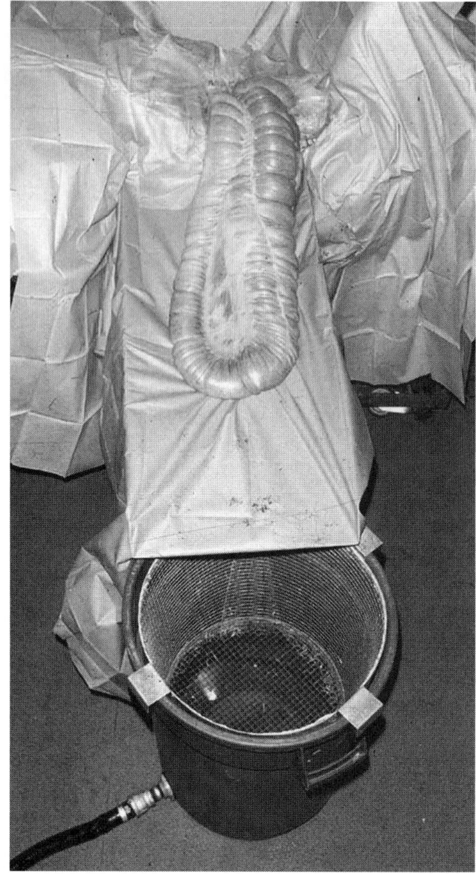

Figure 36-21. Modified colon tray used to evacuate the large colon. In this case, the contents are collected in a modified trash can with a strainer that allows fluids to be evacuated through the drainage system.

Enterotomies in the right dorsal or ventral colon are performed after the colon has been draped off from the main surgical field. In the ventral colon, enterotomies are performed between teniae, since the fibrous nature of the teniae precludes successful inversion during suturing. In the dorsal colon, the location of the enterotomy is not as critical. Enterotomies performed at these sites are more likely to suffer from postoperative luminal hemorrhage; a full-thickness closure (simple-continuous or Connell) is therefore performed on the first layer to achieve better hemostasis.[83] A Lembert or Cushing pattern is used as the second layer.

A modified Heineke-Mikulicz technique for pelvic flexure enterotomy closure has been described in two horses with extensive stricture of the large colon.[167] A longitudinal incision was centered over the stricture and closed using a transverse closure, effectively increasing the diameter of the colon at that site.

Large Colon Resection

Resection of the large colon is performed for removal of full-thickness mural defects in the large colon. Causes include strangulation, infarction, thromboembolic disease, neoplasia, and scar tissue formation.[167,181,189-195]

Removal of 50% to 95% of the large colon has been described.[196-200] Techniques for resection of the large colon

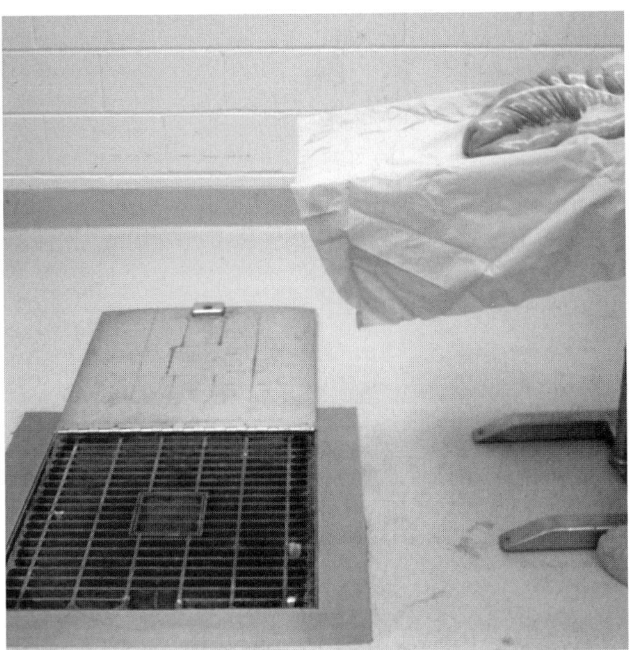

Figure 36-22. Built-in disposal system for collection of fecal material during evacuation of the intestine.

include resection and end-to-end anastomosis, and resection and side-to-side anastomosis. End-to-end procedures are performed for removal of the colon up to 10 to 12 cm from the cecocolic ligament.[172] When resection of the colon closer to or proximal to the cecocolic ligament is required, a side-to-side technique is preferred because the end-to-end technique exerts too much tension on the anastomotic site, placing it at risk for dehiscence. In our experience, it is important to ensure that apposition of the colons in an end-to-end fashion is achieved without tension, and this requires that a substantial amount of colon remain distal to the cecocolic fold.

For a *resection and end-to-end anastomosis,* the colon is exteriorized on a colon tray and draped off; the cecum is replaced in the abdomen. All ingesta are massaged into the segment to be removed. If the colon is full, a pelvic flexure enterotomy is performed to evacuate the colon; care must be taken to remove all ingesta and water from the right dorsal and ventral colons to minimize contamination during the resection. For the resection, a site is chosen that is located in the healthy part of the colon (if possible) and that is easily held by the assistant surgeon without tension on the mesentery.[172] The colon is positioned to expose the right colic artery and the colic branch of the ileocolic artery within the mesocolon; the colonic vessels are isolated by blunt finger dissection and double-ligated using 1 polyglactin 910 (Fig. 36-23). Alternatively, two double rows of staggered staples (TA-90 Premium, United States Surgical Corp, Norwalk, Conn) are applied across the mesocolon, followed by a third double-staggered row 4 cm distal. The mesocolon is transected between the proximal and distal staple lines. Hemostasis is verified and any bleeding vessels are ligated. The right ventral colon is transected in a line transverse to its long axis, whereas the dorsal colon is transected at a 30-degree angle to its long axis, with the antimesenteric border

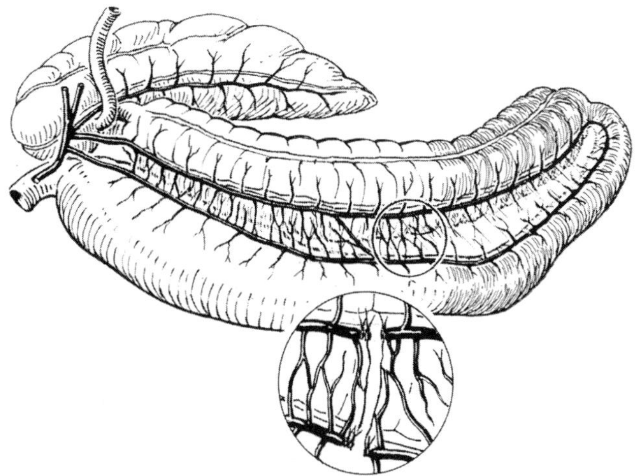

Figure 36-23. The ascending colon is placed on a colon tray with the vessels facing uppermost. The colonic vessels are isolated by blunt finger dissection and double- or triple-ligated before transection *(inset).*

shorter so that the diameters of the colons are similar (Fig. 36-24, *A*). In the original description of the procedure, a V-shaped stoma was then created between the mesenteric border of the dorsal and ventral colons using an inverting linear anastomotic instrument (GIA Premium 55, United States Surgical) reinforced with a double-layer, simple-continuous pattern. This step was omitted in later descriptions of the procedure.[201] Starting at the mesenteric border and suturing from the lumen, the colons are apposed with a double-row, simple-continuous pattern using 0 polydioxanone or Vicryl. The second layer should be full thickness to achieve hemostasis (see Fig. 36-24, *B*). Once the mesenteric portion of the anastomosis is completed, suturing is approached from the serosal side, and the colons are apposed using a double layer, starting with a Connell followed by a Lembert pattern (see Fig. 36-24, *C*). The colon is lavaged and replaced in the abdomen.

For a *side-to-side anastomosis,* the site of resection is usually more proximal, at the cecocolic ligament or oral to it. The colon is exteriorized to the left of the horse on a colon tray and the colonic vasculature is transected as previously described. The stoma is then created *before* the resection, taking advantage of the weight of the colons to facilitate exposure of the anastomotic site. The site for creation of the stoma is identified, taking care to end it just proximal to colonic vessel ligation, so that a blind sac is not formed. A three-tier side-to-side stoma is created; the first layer apposes the seromuscular layers of the colons using 1 polyglactin 910 in a Lembert or Cushing layer for a length of 20 cm (Fig. 36-25, *A*). A full-thickness incision is made in each colon and a full-thickness simple-continuous circumferential closure interrupted at 180 degrees is made to create the stoma (see Fig. 36-25, *B* and *C*). The upper layer is then apposed using a Cushing or Lembert pattern (see Fig. 36-25, *D*). Alternatively, the stoma can be created using stapling instrumentation. This may minimize contamination, but it may not be possible if the colons are too thick and edematous as a result of the underlying disease process. For an adequate-size stoma, the stapling instrument is fired twice if the ILA-100 or the GIA-90 is used, and three times if

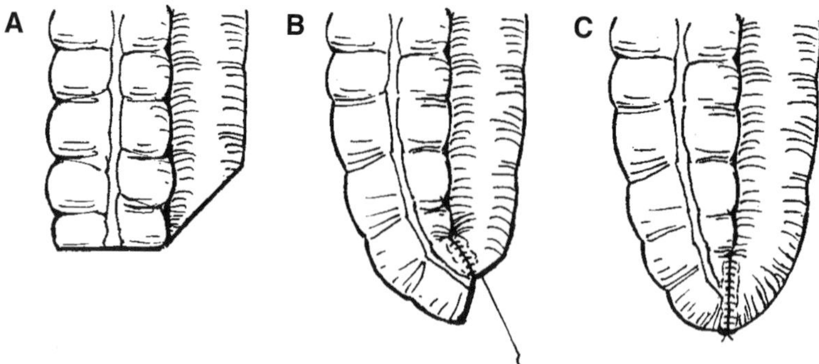

Figure 36-24. Amputation of the large colon. **A,** The right ventral colon is transected in a line transverse to its long axis, whereas the dorsal colon is transected at a 30-degree angle to its long axis. **B,** Starting at the mesenteric border, and suturing from the lumen, the colons are apposed with a double-row simple-continuous pattern using 0 polydioxanone or Vicryl. **C,** Once the mesenteric portion of the anastomosis is completed, suturing is approached from the serosal side, and the colons are apposed using a double-layer pattern, starting with a Connell and followed by a Lembert.

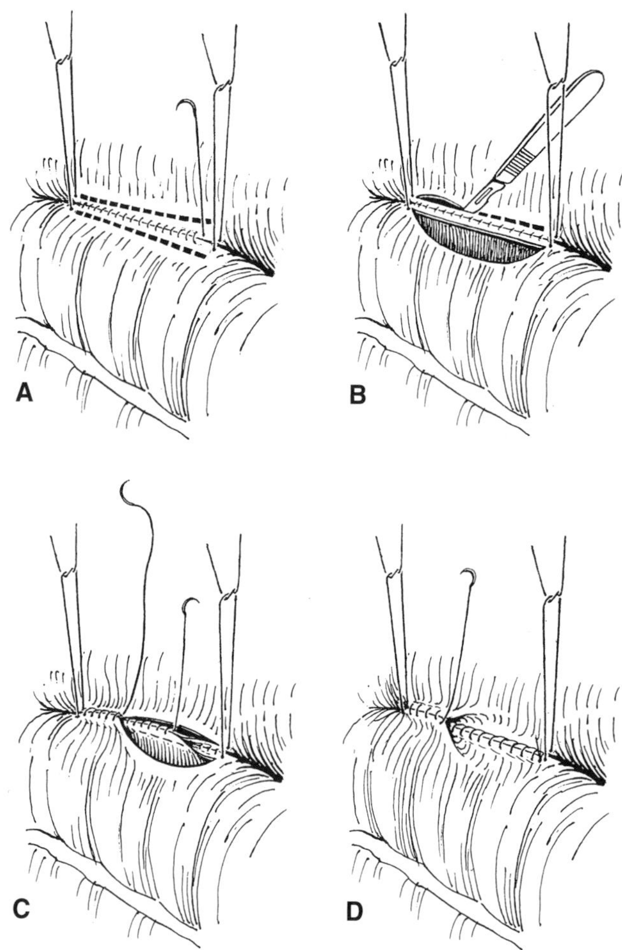

Figure 36-25. A hand-sutured side-to-side anastomosis of the ascending colon. **A,** Placement of stay sutures at either end of the intended stoma. Note that the anastomosis is performed with the diseased part of the colon still in situ. The seromuscular layers of the ventral and dorsal colons are apposed with a Lembert or Cushing pattern, using an absorbable suture material. **B,** A full-thickness incision is made in each colon, and a full-thickness simple-continuous circumferential closure, interrupted at 180 degrees, is made to create the stoma, shown in **(C)**. **D,** The upper layer is then apposed using a Cushing or Lembert pattern.

the GIA-55 is used (the staples for the latter are smaller). Staple lines should be oversewn. Once the staples have been applied, the down layer cannot be approached for oversewing. This layer should therefore be performed first, before application of the stapling instrument. Once the stoma is created, the colons are resected, starting with the ventral colon, taking care to resect them at the site of colonic vessel ligation. The lumens are closed using a full-thickness simple-continuous or Connell pattern, and oversewn with a Lembert or Cushing pattern (Fig. 36-26). The resected colons are lavaged and replaced in the abdomen. Although resection of the large colon has been reported using stapling instrumentation, this is usually not possible after correction of large colon torsion, since the intestinal edema and congestion do not allow proper closure of the instrument and adequate formation of the staples.

An early method of large colon resection has been described that uses a luminal approach to create the side-to-side anastomosis, followed by closing the ends of the colons.[198] The technique described earlier for end-to-end resection represents a modification of this technique.

Successful bypass of the right dorsal colon for the treatment of large colon volvulus has been described in one horse.[180] In that report, the large colon was judged to be nonviable after correction of a large colon volvulus. The right dorsal colon was transected as far distally as possible within the abdomen, using a TA-90 stapling instrument, and the suture line was partially oversewn. The right ventral colon was transected 10 cm from the cecocolic ligament, and an end-to-side anastomosis between the right ventral colon and the descending colon was performed using a double-layer inverting pattern. Two mild episodes of colic and diarrhea for 1 week were the reported complications. In a similar fashion, anastomosis of the right ventral colon to the descending colon to bypass a nonfunctional descending colon anastomosis in a miniature pony was reported.[179] A two-layer hand-sewn end-to side anastomosis was performed between the right ventral colon and the small colon. One episode of colic successfully treated with medical therapy was the only postoperative complication encountered in this case.

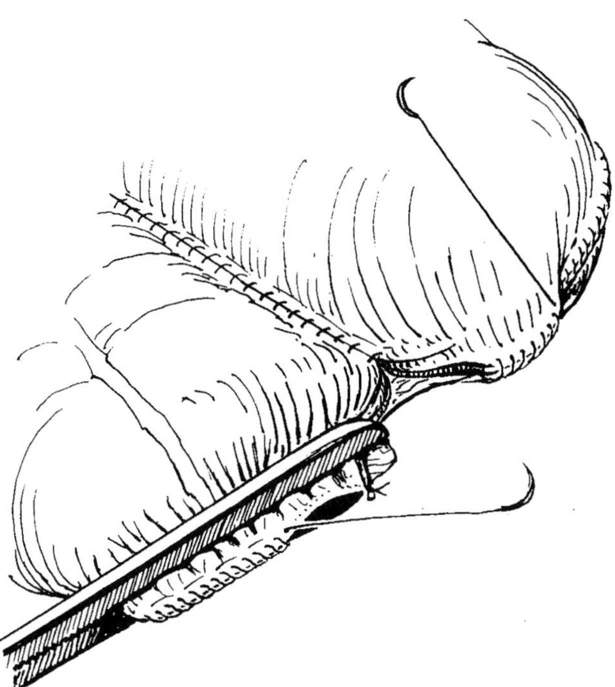

Figure 36-26. The amputated ends of the large colon are closed with a hand suture technique. Note that the amputation of the colon occurred next to the anastomosis site to prevent the formation of a blind end. The lumens are closed using a full-thickness simple-continuous or Connell pattern, oversewn with a Lembert or Cushing pattern.

COMPLICATIONS

Complications from large colon resection are usually a result of the primary disease. They include persistent endotoxemia and peritonitis caused by continued bowel devitalization. This is because the site of torsion is usually at or proximal to the site of resection, so that some portion of compromised large colon cannot be removed. It is therefore essential for the surgeon to remove as much of the devitalized colon as possible. In our experience, this requires a side-to side resection at or proximal to the cecocolic fold. Even then, a segment of devitalized colon may remain in the abdomen, leading to subsequent complications. Most horses that succumb to endotoxemia and peritonitis do so within 3 to 7 days postoperatively after requiring considerable intensive care. In contrast, survivors see an improvement in clinical signs within 24 hours of the procedure.

Postoperative pain is common in horses after large colon resection. It is a painful procedure, even in normal horses. Administration of NSAIDs, lidocaine, and opiates can help alleviate the pain.

Signs of endotoxemia are common after large colon resection for large colon volvulus. Signs include fever, tachycardia, injected mucous membranes, dehydration, and hypoproteinemia. Signs of large colon ileus, such as distention, which can be quite severe, may also occur. Supportive care with fluids, plasma, and antiendotoxin modalities are important (see Chapter 2). Horses should be monitored for signs of postoperative hemorrhage, which is more prevalent with large colon procedures and occasionally requires a blood transfusion.

Postoperative diarrhea is commonly observed after large colon resection, because of mucosal damage or the reduced surface area available for fluid absorption. The diarrhea is usually self-limiting and resolves within a few days if it is not of infectious origin. However, isolation procedures should be followed as dictated by hospital protocol, and infectious diseases should be ruled out.

Horses with successful resection of the large colon usually regain normal fecal consistency within 5 to 7 days. Because of the decreased surface area available for digestion and water absorption, these horses have increased water and phosphorus requirements and require a highly digestible diet.

SMALL COLON

Anatomy

The transverse colon is the continuation of the right dorsal colon. It begins at the level of the 17th or 18th thoracic vertebra where the right dorsal colon narrows significantly in diameter as it turns medially.[1,2] The transverse colon is short and passes from right to left, cranial to the cranial mesenteric artery. It is connected dorsally to the pancreas, to the dorsal aspect of the abdominal cavity, and by a short transverse mesocolon to the root of the mesentery. These attachments prohibit visualization of the transverse colon during a celiotomy. To the left of the root of the mesentery, the transverse colon continues as the descending colon, also known as the small colon. The small colon occupies the left caudodorsal quadrant of the abdominal cavity. The small colon is approximately 3.5 m long and maintains a 7- to 10-cm width throughout its entire length. It is suspended by a long descending mesocolon, which allows good surgical access to all but the most proximal and distal portions of the small colon. The descending mesocolon originates from the left surface of the root of the mesentery and continues caudally attached to the dorsal body wall until it turns into the mesorectum at the pelvic inlet.[1,2] The mesocolon often contains a significant amount of fat. The small colon is attached to the terminal duodenum by the duodenal colic fold, which is an important surgical landmark when exteriorizing the proximal jejunum. The small colon has two longitudinal muscular bands called teniae, one within the mesocolon and the other on the antimesenteric border. Contractile activity of the longitudinal bands and circular muscle produce sacculations in which feces are formed into fecal balls.[202]

The vascular supply to the small colon is derived from the caudal mesenteric artery with anastomoses cranially from the cranial mesenteric artery and caudally from the middle and caudal rectal arteries. The caudal mesenteric artery divides into two major branches, the left colic artery and the cranial rectal artery, with the left colic artery supplying the proximal three fourths of the descending colon and the cranial rectal, the distal one fourth.[203] The left colic artery branches into four to eight arcuate arteries, each dividing into a cranial and caudal branch, which run parallel to the small colon to anastomose to adjacent arcuate arteries (Fig. 36-27). The cranial rectal artery gives off similar arcuate vessels. These anastomosing arcades running parallel to the bowel are called marginal arteries. A secondary anastomosing arcade branching off the marginal arteries runs between the marginal artery and bowel wall, sending off short branches that perforate the mesenteric teniae, and long branches that anastomose in the antimesenteric teniae with

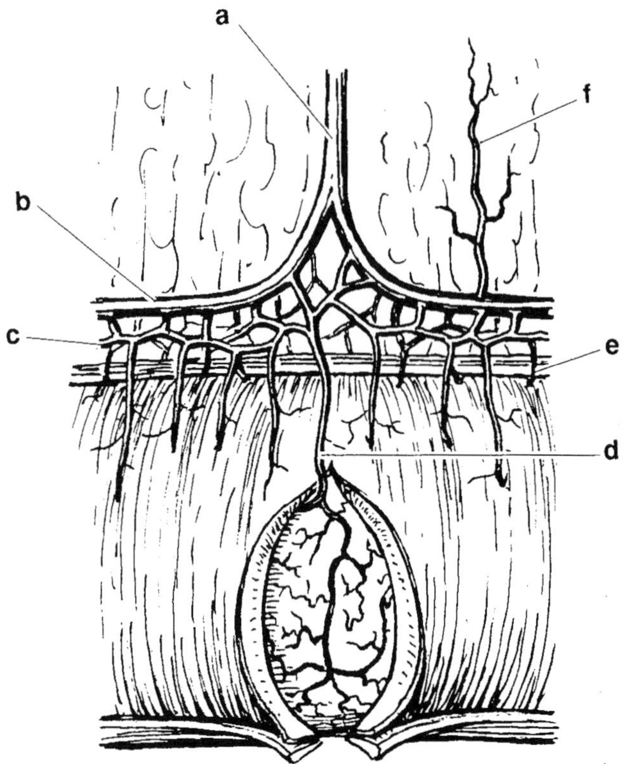

Figure 36-27. Vascular supply of the descending colon, lateral view. a, arcuate artery; b, marginal artery; c, secondary arcade; d, long artery; e, small branch supplying mesenteric teniae; f, small branch to mesocolon.

branches from the other side[203] (see Fig. 36-22). Venous return parallels the arterial supply. The presence of fat in the mesentery makes identification of blood vessels difficult.

Pathology of the Small Colon

Horses with small colon disease make up 1.9% to 18.5% of horses admitted to referral centers with signs of gastrointestinal disease.[96,153,204] The incidence of small colon disease is approximately 4% in horses undergoing surgical treatment for colic.[21,205] Arabian Horses, ponies, and American Miniature Horses are more predisposed to diseases of the small colon.[153] Female horses and horses older than 15 years are more likely to have small colon disease, whereas horses younger than 5 years are less likely to be affected.[153] Diseases may be broken down into congenital abnormalities, such as atresia coli and colonic aganglionosis; simple obstructions, including fecal impaction, fecaliths, phytobezoars, trichobezoars, enteroliths, and retained meconium; vascular lesions, including intramural hematomas and mesocolon tears; strangulating lesions such as lipomas, internal hernias, and volvulus; and neoplasia. (Distal iatrogenic tears, described as rectal tears, although frequently occurring in the small colon, are discussed in Chapter 37.)

Diagnosis

According to one report, 84% of surgical conditions of the small colon were simple obstructions, whereas 16% were vascular or strangulating lesions.[153] Because the obstruction generally affects the distal part of the gastrointestinal tract, horses with small colon disease exhibit slow deterioration of physical status and slow worsening of clinical and laboratory evaluations, making the decision for both referral and surgical intervention more prolonged than is seen with other surgical conditions of the gastrointestinal tract.[153,202,205-207] Early clinical signs are nonspecific and include lethargy, dullness, and inappetence. As the obstruction progresses, signs include abdominal pain, diarrhea, decreased fecal production, tenesmus, and abdominal distention. Strangulating lesions have a more sudden and severe onset of clinical signs. Gastric reflux is rare but may occur as a sequela of the distal obstruction, leading to distention of the ascending colon, which places pressure on the proximal small intestine and obstructs gastric outflow. Changes in the nucleated cell count and the total protein concentration in peritoneal fluid, along with rectal palpation findings, are the key indicators for surgical intervention.[153,202,205] Abdominal ultrasonography may also aid in making a diagnosis.[208] Medical and surgical interventions often carry a good to excellent prognosis.

Simple Obstructions

Fecal Impaction

Horses with small colon fecal impaction represent 1.9% to 2.5% of all those admitted for signs of abdominal pain. Fecal impaction has been reported to be the most common pathologic condition of the small colon except in regions with a high incidence of enterolithiasis.[153,202,204,209] Suggested risk factors are poor dentition, poor-quality hay, lack of water, parasite damage, lack of exercise, submucosal edema, and motility problems.[207,209,210] The fall and winter seasonal predilection observed in some studies may be the result of inadequate water consumption or change of feed.[204,209] Older horses (older than 15 years), American Miniature Horses, and ponies were at an increased risk in several studies, but age and breed were not significant risk factors in other reports.[20,153,204,209]

DIAGNOSIS

The most common clinical signs, in order of decreasing frequency, are abdominal pain, decreased manure production, diarrhea, anorexia, fever, straining to defecate, and depression.[204,209] The colic is initially manifested as mild abdominal pain with a slow progression of signs. The heart rate can be mildly to moderately elevated. Leukopenia with a left shift is not uncommon in horses with small colon feed impactions,[209] whereas serum biochemical and peritoneal fluid values are typically within normal ranges.[204,209] The diagnosis can frequently (i.e., in 75% to 83% of cases) be made by palpation of the impaction per rectum.[204,209] Other palpation findings that have been noted are distention of the large intestine and cecum, edematous or rough rectal mucosa, blood on the rectal sleeve or manure, and unformed feces.[205,207,209] Nasogastric reflux is occasionally obtained. The presence of diarrhea, fever, leukopenia, and irritated rectal mucosa often encountered in a subset of these cases suggests that colitis may predispose some horses to small colon impaction, possibly through motility disturbances. Conversely, the gastrointestinal stasis and inflammation associated with small colon impaction may predispose horses to colitis.[209,211]

MEDICAL TREATMENT

Most fecal impactions are initially managed medically. The goal is to improve hydration, stimulate motility, and soften the impaction. All feed should be withheld and the impaction hydrated. This is accomplished through administration of both intravenous fluids (two to three times the maintenance volume) and oral fluids (2 to 4 L every 4 to 6 hours).[209,211] Oral fluids have the additional benefit of initiating a gastrocolonic reflex, whereby gastric distention stimulates contractile activity of the colon.[114,212] Oral laxatives such as mineral oil, dioctyl sodium sulfosuccinate, or magnesium sulfate administered by nasogastric tube are commonly used to soften the impaction. Mineral oil (5 to 10 mL/kg every 12 hours) is frequently used to lubricate the impaction, and its presence in the perineum is an indication that the obstruction is incomplete. Magnesium sulfate administered to normal horses at 1 g/kg in 6 L of water has been shown to increase total weight of fecal excretion and fecal water excretion compared with administration of a lower dose (0.5 mg/kg), whereas DSS (50 mg/kg in 6 L of water) failed to increase the weight of feces excreted or fecal water excretion.[114] Magnesium sulfate can be administered once daily for 2 to 3 days if the horse is well hydrated. Magnesium toxicity appears more likely to develop in dehydrated horses or in horses treated simultaneously with DSS.[46,213] Flunixin meglumine (0.25 mg/kg three times a day, or 1.1 mg/kg twice a day IV) is administered to treat endotoxemia and to control pain if necessary. Antibiotics may be indicated in horses with signs of septicemia, severe leukopenia, or concurrent diarrhea. Other antiendotoxin therapy such as polymyxin B (2000 to 6000 U/kg IV) or *Salmonella typhimurium* antiserum may also be beneficial.[209] Standing enemas may be used in selected cases to break down impactions in the distal small colon, but extreme caution should be exercised to avoid producing a rectal or small colon tear.[202,207,209] The horse should be adequately sedated and restrained, and epidural anesthesia should be performed. The enema should be administered, without pressure, by gravity flow. Because of the potential for iatrogenic trauma, some authors do not recommend enemas for treatment of small colon impactions.[202,204,209]

SURGICAL TREATMENT

Surgical management is indicated in horses with increasing abdominal pain, increasing abdominal distention, or changes in abdominal fluid indicating deterioration of the bowel. In some horses, large colon displacement or volvulus may occur secondary to gas distention proximal to the impaction. The small colon is exteriorized through a ventral midline celiotomy. The most common technique to relieve the impaction is intraluminal lavage with warm water introduced by stomach tube inserted through the anus by an assistant using aseptic technique. The surgeon manipulates the tube to the distal extent of the impaction and then manually clamps off the small colon lumen anad to the end of the tube to allow water distention around the distal extent of the impaction. Extraluminal massage is used to gently work the fluid into the feces to break up the distal portion of the impaction. These manipulations are repeated working orad until the impaction is relieved. To decrease mechanical damage to the serosa during the massage, sterile carboxymethylcellulose should be placed on the small colon that is being massaged.[209] In some cases, when the small colon impaction cannot be relieved by intraluminal lavage with external massage, a small colon enterotomy is performed in the antimesenteric teniae adjacent to the impacted small colon, and lavage is used to evacuate the impacted fecal material through the enterotomy (see "Small Colon Enterotomy," p. 471). In rare cases, mural ischemia or thrombosis of the mesenteric vessels necessitates resection of a segment of small colon (Fig. 36-28) (see "Small Colon Resection and Anastomosis," p. 472). Ingesta in the large colon should be evacuated through a pelvic flexure enterotomy to prevent postoperative impaction in the edematous and inflamed small colon.

Postoperatively, horses should be started back on feed slowly. Feeding a complete pelleted diet for several weeks may help prevent reimpaction.[207] Extension of perioperative use of antibiotics (24 hours postoperatively) to therapeutic use of antibiotics (5 to 7 days postoperatively) is made on a case-by-case basis, dictated by surgical findings and clinical and laboratory evaluation of the horse. In most cases, antibiotics can be discontinued within 24 hours.

PROGNOSIS

Survival after medical therapy has been reported to be good to excellent (72% to 100%), and survival after surgical therapy has been reported to be fair to good (47% to 75%).[153,204,211] The most common complications after medical or surgical therapy are diarrhea and jugular thrombophlebitis.[153,204,211] Other complications seen are fever, laminitis, peritonitis, incisional infection, incisional hernia, recurrent colic, recurrent impaction, and small colon adhesions.[153,204,211] Surgical cases in which the colon was not evacuated at surgery are more likely to develop postoperative pain.[211] Fecal cultures for *Salmonella* are positive in up to 43% of surgically treated horses.[204,211] Postoperative antibiotic therapy may increase the risk of these horses developing salmonellosis by altering gastrointestinal flora.[202,207]

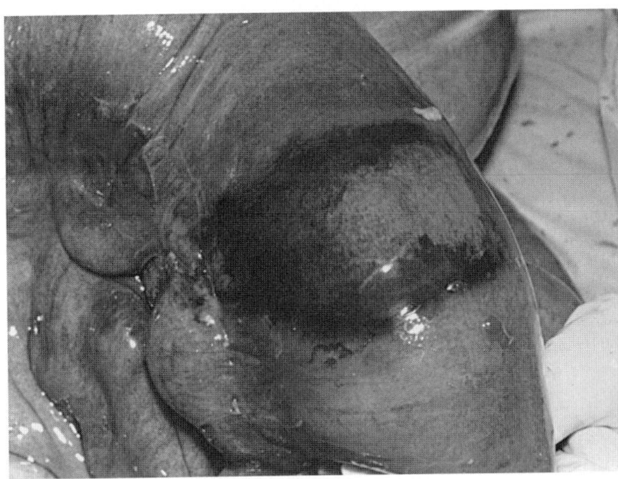

Figure 36-28. An intraoperative photograph of a horse with a descending colon impaction showing an area of compromised tissue.

Intestinal Concretions and Foreign Bodies

Enterolithiasis

The small colon is the site of the obstruction in approximately 45% to 57% of horses with enteroliths, accounting for up to 35% of all small colon diseases in certain geographic regions such as California.[139,140,153,214] The etiology was discussed in the large colon section.

DIAGNOSIS

Horses commonly exhibit multiple episodes of mild colic, most likely from intermittent obstruction in the large colon or proximal transverse colon, before the enterolith enters the small colon. Once the enterolith enters the small colon, the clinical course is determined by the size of the enterolith. Although some are small enough to pass through the small colon without clinical problems, it is not uncommon for the enterolith to become wedged within the lumen of the transverse or small colon, usually in a more proximal segment. Horses typically show signs of increasing abdominal pain, although in some horses rupture occurs with little or no observed abdominal pain. On rectal examination, the large colon may have palpable gaseous distention. Peritoneal fluid analysis should be monitored closely. It is not uncommon for enteroliths wedged in the transverse and small colons to cause pressure necrosis at the area of obstruction. A slight elevation in peritoneal fluid protein may indicate the need for surgical intervention. Radiographs successfully diagnose small colon enteroliths in approximately 40% of horses, as compared with 83% of horses with large colon enteroliths.[141] Surgical exploration is based on signs of increasing pain, increasing abdominal distention, peritoneal fluid changes, and radiographic evaluation.[139-141,214] The most common site of gastrointestinal tract rupture in horses with enteroliths is in the descending colon.[140] Since some horses show little pain prior to rupture, careful monitoring of horses with suspected enterolithiasis is critical to ensure timely surgical intervention.

TREATMENT

Treatment is surgical removal through an antimesenteric small colon enterotomy or retropulsion and removal through an enterotomy in the dorsal colon or pelvic flexure.[140,215] Horses are started on broad-spectrum antibiotics and a ventral midline celiotomy is performed. Retropulsion with lavage can be accomplished by inserting a hose up the rectum. Alternatively, a hose can be inserted through a pelvic flexure enterotomy and advanced to the transverse or small colon obstruction, and lavage can be used to distend the small colon on the oral side with the anal side being clamped off manually. The most important aspect of these techniques is letting the water gradually distend the bowel to aid in dislodging the enterolith. Pressure necrosis can make the bowel wall susceptible to rupture.[216]

When enteroliths are removed by a small colon enterotomy, it is important to ascertain if there are additional enteroliths located proximally. In one study, 45% of horses with enterolithiasis had multiple stones.[140] Particular attention should be paid to the right dorsal and transverse colon, since it may be difficult to palpate a small enterolith if there is an appreciable amount of ingesta in the large colon. Commonly, a pelvic flexure enterotomy is performed prior to the small colon enterotomy to evacuate ingesta from the large colon. This also will decrease the amount of fecal material passing over the small colon enterotomy site in the immediate postoperative period.

PROGNOSIS

Horses recovering from surgery for enteroliths in the small colon have a good to excellent prognosis (up to 92.5%).[139,140] In most cases, antibiotics are discontinued 24 hours after surgery. It is not uncommon for the area where the enterolith was wedged in the small colon to slough some of the mucosa after surgery with absorption of endotoxin. NSAIDs should be continued for 3 to 5 days, depending on the extent of intestinal insult found at surgery. Complications noted after surgery are diarrhea, incisional infection, incisional hernia formation, positive fecal cultures for *Salmonella*, laminitis, septic peritonitis, and adhesions.[139,140,214] Dietary and management changes have been discussed in the large colon section. Recurrence has been identified in 7.7% of cases.[140]

Fecaliths, Phytobezoars, Trichobezoars, Phytotrichobezoars, and Phytoconglobates

Fecaliths are inspissated balls of fecal material that form as a result of poor-quality diet, poor mastication, or reduced water intake.[207,217] They have been reported to occur in approximately 7% of horses with small colon disease, but they probably make up a larger proportion of small colon disorders in regions where enteroliths are not common.[153] Small colon fecaliths have a tendency to occur in young (less than 1 year old) and older (more than 15 years old) horses. Ponies, American Miniature Horses, and mixed-breed horses appear to be at an increased risk.[153,218,219] Phytoconglobates are concretions of matted plant residues formed into balls. Bezoars are combinations of concretions of magnesium ammonium phosphate and plant material (phytobezoars) or hair (trichobezoars). Concretions composed of hair and plant material are called phytotrichobezoars.[206,207,209] Obstruction caused by ingestion of fibrous, nondigestible material occurs most commonly in horses less than 3 years old and in horses with poor dentition.[207] Fecaliths, phytobezoars, trichobezoars, and phytotrichobezoars form in the large colon and become symptomatic as they pass into the small colon and obstruct the lumen. Clinical signs are similar to those of foreign body obstructions. Treatment is surgical removal by small colon enterotomy, or by retropulsion into and removal from the large colon.

Foreign Body Obstructions

Obstruction of the small colon with foreign objects has been reported in several studies.[220-223] The obstructing objects include rubberized fencing and nylon tires, baling twine, rope, disposable plastic sleeves, feed sacks, and cloth material.[220-223] Young horses (less than 3 years of age) with indiscriminate eating habits are thought to be more likely to develop these foreign body impactions. Poor pasture may also contribute to consumption of inappropriate material.[221]

Signs reported are similar to those seen in other small colon obstructions, such as getting up and down, stretching, anorexia, and scant passage of feces.[220-223] Walking backward and dog sitting have also been reported.[221] The heart rate can be normal to markedly elevated. Depending on the configuration of the foreign body, the obstruction may be incomplete, allowing some passage of gas and ingesta, or complete, producing tympany and impaction proximal to the obstruction. With complete obstruction and proximal distention, the abdominal pain becomes more severe. Nasogastric reflux from the distended large intestine compressing the proximal small intestine may occur. In horses with a distal obstruction, tenesmus is common.[207] On rectal palpation, horses frequently exhibit marked abdominal straining, have a large intestine distended with gas and feces, and have no fecal balls in the small colon. In some cases, the obstructing mass is palpable per rectum, although frequently the obstruction is in the proximal small colon out of reach of rectal palpation.[221]

Foreign bodies may produce pressure necrosis of the wall of the small colon where they are lodged. In these cases, peritoneal fluid analysis reveals an elevated protein concentration and sometimes an increase in nucleated cell count. Treatment is surgical removal via a small colon enterotomy in the majority of cases, or through retropulsion into the dorsal colon if the obstruction is at an inaccessible portion of the proximal small colon or transverse colon.

Meconium Impaction

Meconium is a mucilaginous material in the intestine of the fetus, composed of intestinal glandular secretions, bile, epithelial cells, and swallowed amniotic fluid.[202,224] Typically, peristaltic activity moves meconium into the colon or rectum before birth, and it is evacuated between 3 and 24 hours after birth.[202] Meconium is considered retained if the foal makes frequent attempts but fails to produce meconium by 12 hours of age.[225] Retained meconium is the most common cause of colic in the neonate.[96,202,224] Meconium impaction accounted for 0.8% of all cases of equine colic in one study, with a mortality rate of 15.2%.[44] Ingestion of colostrum promotes gastrointestinal activity and may have a laxative effect to aid in expulsion of meconium from higher up in the colon. Delayed ingestion of colostrum, and conditions that compromise the foal such as asphyxia, dystocia, prematurity, low birth weight, and dehydration are thought to be risk factors for meconium impaction.[226] Males are more commonly affected, most likely because of their smaller pelvic size.[227]

DIAGNOSIS

Clinical signs begin with restlessness, tail switching, straining to defecate, and disinterest in nursing.[224] As the condition progresses, foals develop signs of more severe colic, such as lying down and getting up, rolling, lying upside down, and abdominal distention.[225] The diagnosis is based on clinical signs, historical absence of meconium passage, and detection of a firm mass on digital rectal palpation. Plain and retrograde contrast abdominal radiography can show tympanic bowel and often dense meconium.[228,229] Ultrasonography may show a distended large colon. The differential diagnosis is ruptured bladder, atresia coli, ileocolonic aganglionosis, and enteritis.

TREATMENT

The preferred method of treatment is multiple administration of enemas along with intravenous fluids and nasogastric administration of laxatives for more persistent obstructions. Commercially available phosphate enemas (Fleet enemas, CB Fleet Co, Inc, Lynchburg, Va) are frequently used. More recently, 4% acetylcysteine enema solutions have been recommended for treatment of retained meconium.[225,230] The compound cleaves the disulfide bonds in the mucoprotein molecules and decreases the tenacity of the meconium. The 4% solution can be made by mixing 40 mL of a commercial 20% acetylcysteine solution (Ben Venue Inc, Bedford, Ohio) with 160 mL of water. Because the activity of acetylcysteine increases with increasing pH (pH 7 to 9), 20 g (1½ level tablespoons) of $NaHCO_3$ powder (baking soda) is added to the 200 mL of diluted solution. Alternatively, 8 g (1 packed tablespoon) of a powdered form (*N*-acetylcysteine, Sigma Chemical Company, St Louis, Mo) can be mixed with 200 mL of water to which 20 g of $NaHCO_3$ is added. The foals are restrained, sedated with diazepam (0.2 to 0.4 mg/kg IV), and placed in lateral recumbency. A 30-Fr Foley catheter with a 30-mL bulb is inserted about 2.5 to 5 cm into the rectum. The balloon is slowly inflated, using care to not damage the rectum. Between 100 and 200 mL of the 4% solution is administered slowly by gravity flow and retained for 30 to 45 minutes.[225] This can be repeated up to three times over a 24-hour period. The prognosis after acetylcysteine enemas has been reported to be excellent.[225] High meconium retention can be treated with intravenous fluids and mineral oil administered by nasogastric tube.

Surgery should be performed only on foals that have failed to respond to aggressive medical therapy. Postoperative complications involving adhesion formation are not uncommon after gastrointestinal surgery of neonates.[77,231] In one study, 8 of 28 foals with meconium impactions failed to respond to medical therapy and required surgery. Two of seven surgical cases available for follow-up were euthanized as a result of serosal adhesions.[232] These results suggest that if surgical treatment is required, techniques to reduce adhesion formation, such as minimal handling of the bowel and topical carboxymethylcellulose during bowel manipulation, should be practiced.

Vascular Lesions

Intramural Hematoma

The incidence of small colon intramural or submucosal hematoma is very low, less than 1% of surgical colics.[61,233,234] Most often the cause of the lesion is unknown, although focal ulceration with infection and iatrogenic trauma have each been described in one horse.[233,234] Although it has been stated that older horses are at an increased risk, the low number of reported cases makes this difficult to ascertain. Four of seven cases were 10 years old or younger, whereas one of seven was older than 20 years in two case series.[233,234] In another report of six horses, the age range was between 9 and 18 years.[205]

The intramural hematoma causes obstruction of the small colon lumen initially with subsequent ischemic necrosis of the bowel wall leading to septic peritonitis, endotoxemia, circulatory shock, and death if not treated.[205]

Horses are often presented with varying degrees of abdominal pain that may become acutely severe. Heart rate is mildly to markedly elevated. Rectal palpation findings may reveal gas distention of the large intestine, decreased fecal content, and occasionally dark or clotted blood.[205,233,234] In some cases, a solid mass is palpable per rectum.[233,234] During surgical exploration, the lesion is readily identified as a soft, dense, circumscribed mass occupying the bowel lumen and attached to the bowel wall. The lesion has been described as involving between 20 and 55 cm in a series of six cases.[202,205] Treatment is surgical resection and anastomosis. The prognosis can be good if the lesion is located in a region that allows its complete resection, and if surgical intervention occurs before transmural necrosis or bowel rupture leads to bacterial peritonitis.[207,233] Colostomy should be considered if the lesion is too far caudal to allow exteriorization.[207]

Mesocolic Rupture

The incidence of rupture of the mesocolon has been reported to be between 0.4% and 2.5% in horses undergoing exploratory laparotomy for colic.[24,61,235] Rupture of the mesocolon leading to segmental ischemic necrosis of the small colon has been described as a complication of parturition in the mare.[61,236,237] The vigorous reflex kicking and head movement of the foal that allows it to rotate into a dorsal position for delivery is thought to mechanically tear the mesentery that is caught between the uterus and dorsal body wall.[207,236,237] Mesocolon rupture may also occur as a consequence of type III or IV rectal prolapse, often associated with tenesmus after parturition.[31,61,237,238] If more than 30 cm of the rectum prolapses, ischemic necrosis of the rectum and small colon should be expected from disruption of the mesocolon and vascular arcade.[31,61,207,237,238] Mares are typically middle aged and pluriparous. Foaling may have been normal or required assistance.[38,236,237]

Time from foaling to the onset of colic is variable, ranging from 0 to 24 hours, with referral 12 to 48 hours later. The severity of abdominal pain varies greatly from no demonstrable pain to severe pain. The initial mild abdominal discomfort may be incorrectly attributed to uterine involution, delaying the recognition of a surgical problem. There is a consistent lack of feces. Rectal examination findings vary from normal to feed-impacted small colon with gas-distended large intestine. Peritoneal fluid has an elevated protein and nucleated cell concentration, with intra-abdominal hemorrhage seen in some cases.[237] The decision for surgery is often based on duration of pain and peritoneal fluid changes.[236] Laparoscopy can be useful in making the diagnosis and determining the extent of damage.

Treatment consists of surgical resection and anastomosis if viable proximal and distal small colon is accessible for the anastomosis. A temporary colostomy to divert feces away from the compromised bowel has been suggested to facilitate healing if an anastomosis can be performed.[238] In most cases, tears resulting from rectal prolapse do not have sufficient viable distal small colon to allow for an anastomosis. A permanent colostomy is required in these cases. Often the prognosis is poor as a result of the extent of the tear or the delay in surgical intervention.[207,236,237]

Nonstrangulating Infarction

Nonstrangulating infarction of the small colon is uncommon, perhaps because the majority of the blood supply to the small colon is through the caudal mesenteric artery, which is not a common site of occlusive verminous arteritis.[202,205] In a review of 38 cases of small colon obstruction, the three cases with nonstrangulating infarction of the small colon showed no evidence of verminous arteritis.[205] Clinical signs are similar to those described previously for mesocolic rupture, with mild intermittent abdominal pain of 10 to 72 hours' duration. Peritoneal fluid most likely has an elevated protein concentration and nucleated cell counts. Treatment consists of surgical resection and end-to-end anastomosis. Since, in most cases, viable proximal and distal small colon is accessible for the anastomosis, the prognosis should be good as long as surgical intervention occurs before ischemic necrosis of the infarcted segment causes septic peritonitis. When the infarcted segment cannot be exteriorized through a laparotomy, a colostomy or transrectal exteriorization followed by rectocolostomy should be considered.[207]

Strangulating Lesions

Strangulating Lipomas

Strangulating lipomas of the small colon account for approximately 11% of small colon disease.[153] They are most commonly seen in horses older than 15 years and are not reported in horses younger than 8 years.[153,205,239] Geldings may be at an increased risk compared with mares and stallions.[205,240] Ponies have been reported to be at increased risk.[205] It is not uncommon for lipomas to form in the mesentery of the small colon because of the amount of fat it contains. However, unlike in the small intestine, many do not cause clinical problems, as the thickness and diameter of the small colon wall and the fecal balls within its lumen prevent the pedunculated lipoma from encircling and strangulating the bowel. In horses with strangulating pedunculated lipomas, approximately 7% are located in the small colon, whereas 93% are located in the small intestine.[205,240] In some cases, the pedunculated lipoma encircles the small colon, causing obstruction without significant vascular impairment.[205]

Although some horses with small colon strangulating lipomas demonstrate signs of severe colic, others do not show the amount of abdominal pain commonly seen with strangulating lesions involving other areas of the gastrointestinal tract. Peritoneal fluid changes include increased nucleated cell count and protein concentration. The predominant abnormal rectal findings are gas distention of the large colon and cecum with absence of fecal balls in the small colon. In certain cases, the clinician's hand can be advanced to the area of the constriction. A fibrous band encircling the colon may be palpable. Transrectal ultrasonography may indicate increased thickness of the small colon wall with intestinal distention.[208] Treatment consists of surgical removal of the lipoma with resection and anastomosis of any compromised small colon.[153,202,205,207]

Volvulus, Herniation, Intussusception

Volvulus of the small colon is a very rare cause of colic, most likely as a result of its fixed extremities and its relatively short length.[241] The firm fecal balls within the lumen and its fatty mesentery may also prevent the small colon from twisting around its mesentery. Adhesions and abscesses have been associated with small colon volvulus.[25] Herniation of the small colon, which may result in a strangulating obstruction, has been reported to occur with umbilical, inguinal, and body wall hernias, as well as through omental, mesenteric, uterine, vaginal, broad ligament, and gastrosplenic ligament tears.[25,202,242] Intussusception not associated with rectal prolapse has been reported in foals and one broodmare.[60,243,244] If the point of invagination is at the distal end of the small colon, the intussusceptum may protrude from the anus. In this case, a finger can be inserted between the protruding bowel and the anal sphincter and advanced cranially until reaching a blind end.[60]

Clinical signs are similar to those seen with strangulating lipomas of the small colon. There is usually a sudden onset of colic, although the clinical course may be more prolonged than seen with strangulating lesions of the more proximal gastrointestinal tract.[207] Rectal examination reveals lack of feces and gas distention of the large colon. In some cases, the small colon is under considerable tension, limiting the rectal examination.[241,242] Blood staining of feces may be present with an intussusception.[243] Peritoneal fluid is often serosanguineous in color, with increased nucleated cell count and protein concentration.

Treatment involves surgical resection and anastomosis through a ventral midline laparotomy. Rectocolostomy has been described as a treatment for distal intussuscepted small colon protruding through the anus in an 8-week-old foal.[205] In this transrectal procedure, an encircling incision was made in the outer layer of the intussusception 4 cm caudal to the anal sphincter. Ligatures were placed around the mesenteric vessels. Continuity was restored by a colorectostomy using simple-interrupted sutures of 2-0 polyglactin.

Atresia Coli

Atresia coli is a very rare condition in the foal, involving the large, transverse, or small colon. It should not be confused with ileocolonic aganglionosis, seen in the recessive lethal white foal syndrome of the overo white foal. In the lethal white syndrome, which is always fatal, foals are born with no pigment (except for the eyes) and have stenotic colons that have thin muscular walls and few myenteric plexuses, leading to megacolon and death.[206,245] Although the cause of atresia coli remains unknown, it has been proposed that a vascular injury during fetal development leads to focal ischemic necrosis of the intestinal segment.[246-248] Atresia coli does not appear to have a breed or sex predisposition.[249]

Three basic types of intestinal atresia have been recognized. Type 1, membrane atresia, is caused by a membranous diaphragm occluding the lumen of the intestine. Type 2, cord atresia, is characterized by a fibrous band or muscular cordlike remnant of gut connecting the blind ends. Type 3, blind end atresia, is caused by an absence of a segment of intestine, with disconnected ends and a gap in the mesentery. Atresia coli in foals is typically described as type 3.[249-252] Foals with atresia coli develop acute signs of colic within the first 24 hours after birth (mean, 8.2; range, 2 to 26 hours).[249] The most consistent finding on physical examination is absence of meconium staining after repeated enemas. Radiographic examination may indicate gas distention of the gastrointestinal tract proximal to the atretic segment. Radiographic evaluation after a barium enema may indicate a blind end.[249,253]

Surgical repair is often unsuccessful, since the remaining intestine lacks sufficient length or diameter to perform an anastomosis.[249,250,254] If surgical repair is attempted, it is recommended that the severely dilated proximal portion be resected to obtain a normal vascularized segment.[254] Also recommended is an end-to-end or end-to-oblique-end anastomosis to avoid a "blind loop" syndrome. Suggested alternative surgical approaches include colostomy and a pull-through procedure suturing the small colon to the anus.[202] Other congenital abnormalities have been found in some of these foals, such as ventricular septal defect, common truncus arteriosus, hydrocephalus, cerebellar dysplasia, dermal hemangioma, and renal agenesis.[249,254]

Neoplasia

Small colon neoplasia is very rare. Lipomas have been discussed previously. A leiomyoma of the small colon found during exploratory laparotomy for a large colon displacement was successfully treated in a 4-year-old Thoroughbred with resection and anastomosis.[255] Leiomyoma has been reported to cause an intussusception in the small colon,[256] and a lymphoma causing perforation of the small colon has been reported.[257]

Miscellaneous Conditions

Other conditions of the small colon that have been reported are partial obstruction by an abdominal testicular teratoma,[258] obstruction from an ovarian pedicle in a foal,[259] and, in three mares,[205] obstruction from a granulosa cell tumor,[260,261] and secondary chronic idiopathic intestinal pseudo-obstruction (myenteric ganglionitis) in a 4-year-old Standardbred causing recurrent impaction.[262]

Surgical Procedures

Small colon enterotomy: Small colon enterotomy is indicated to remove various types of intraluminal obstruction of the small colon, such as fecal impactions, enteroliths, fecaliths, and foreign bodies.[153,204,209,214,263] In most cases, a ventral midline celiotomy is performed to provide access to the small colon. However, in select cases, such as a fecalith or foreign body, if there are financial constraints, a flank incision may provide adequate access to the lesion. The preferred location for the enterotomy is a longitudinal incision on the antimesenteric teniae. Enterotomies in this location have been found to be stronger, to allow easier apposition, to develop less intraoperative hemorrhage, and to maintain an increased postoperative lumen size compared with enterotomies that do not involve the teniae.[263,264]

The segment of small colon where the enterotomy is to be performed is exteriorized and draped separately from the abdomen and the rest of the gastrointestinal tract. Intestinal clamps or Penrose drains are placed proximal and distal to the enterotomy site to prevent spillage of fecal material during the enterotomy. Stay sutures are placed approximately 1 cm from the ends of the enterotomy incision. The incision is made sharply with a #10 scalpel blade. A two-layer closure is performed using a full-thickness simple-continuous pattern followed by a seromuscular inverting pattern with 2-0 polyglactin 910, taking care to invert a minimal amount of tissue.

In some horses, the intraluminal obstruction, typically an enterolith, is lodged in the proximal small colon where the short mesocolon prevents adequate exteriorization, increasing the risk of peritoneal contamination during the enterotomy. If retropulsion into the right dorsal colon is not feasible, a modified teniotomy can be performed and may facilitate normograde movement of the obstruction to a more accessible location.[142] In this technique, the large colon is first evacuated to decrease fecal material proximal to the obstruction. The site of obstruction is isolated from the rest of the abdominal cavity with sterile moistened drapes. Stay sutures are placed within the antimesenteric tenia proximal to the site of obstruction and 10 to 15 cm distal to the site. Fluid and ingesta are stripped away from the area. Topical 2% lidocaine can first be applied to reduce muscular spasm. A 1-cm longitudinal seromuscular incision is made with a scalpel blade in the antimesenteric tenia 10 to 15 cm aboral to the obstruction. The seromuscular incision is continued orally to the widest part of the obstruction using Metzenbaum scissors. Gentle pressure applied through the wall of the small colon is used to advance the obstruction to a more accessible location, where the mucosa is incised and the obstruction removed. The enterotomy incision is closed as described earlier. This technique is most suitable for obstructions with a smooth surface, such as enteroliths, making them more likely to move distally. In one report, enteroliths were moved distances of 4 to 15 cm.[142]

Small colon resection and anastomosis: Several techniques have been described for small colon anastomosis. These include hand-sutured single-layer end-to-end anastomosis, hand-sutured double-layer end-to-end anastomosis, and triangulated end-to-end everting stapled anastomosis.[265-267] A two-layer technique consisting of a full-thickness appositional pattern oversewn with a partial-thickness continuous inverting layer has less risk for dehiscence, peritonitis, and adhesion formation than the hand-sutured single-layer and stapled closure. As well, it creates less tissue inversion than a double inverting pattern, decreasing the chances of postoperative impaction at the anastomosis site.[265-267]

The vascular arcade supplying the compromised small colon is traced back to normal bowel. The marginal artery at the oral and anal side of the lesion is identified and isolated within the mesenteric fat and is triple-ligated. To prevent inadvertent puncture of a vessel to be ligated with the pointed taper needle, especially if the vessel is partly covered by fat, the needle can be advanced around the vessel with its back first, since this blunt end avoids vessels (Fig. 36-29). Once the suture is placed around the vessel, tightening the loop and the knot results in secure ligation of the vessel, because firm tightening cuts through the fat tissue surrounding the vessel. The vessels are transected with the vessels remaining in situ double-ligated. Vessels supplying the intestine to be removed are triple-ligated and sectioned. The ingesta is milked out of the segment of small colon to be resected and Penrose drains or intestinal clamps are positioned approximately 10 to 20 cm proximal and distal to the resection area to occlude the bowel lumen and decrease contamination from luminal contents during the resection. Doyen intestinal clamps are placed across the descending colon at the oral and anal extent of the resection, angled at approximately 30 degrees from perpendicular so that the length of the small colon at the antimesenteric angle is shorter than the intestine at the mesenteric angle[217] (Fig. 36-30). This should improve blood supply to the antimesenteric border and increase the luminal size of the anastomosis compared with perpendicular transection angles. Moistened sterile drapes are used to isolate this region from the abdomen and adjacent bowel. A scalpel is used to sharply transect the colon, cutting adjacent to the

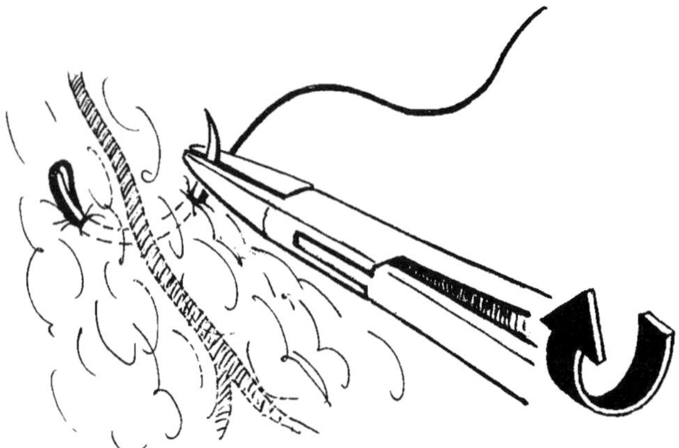

Figure 36-29. Using the blunt back end of a taper-point needle to place a ligature around a semi-hidden (by fat) mesenteric vessel allows safe placement of a ligature around vessels without inadvertent trauma to the vessel.

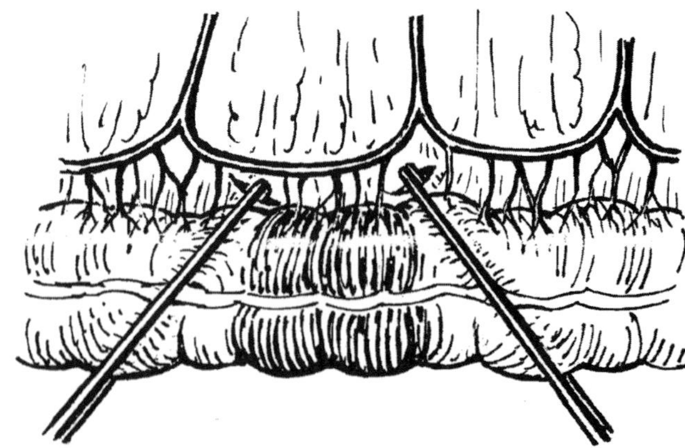

Figure 36-30. Penrose drains or intestinal clamps are positioned approximately 10 to 20 cm proximal and distal to the resection area to occlude the bowel lumen and decrease contamination from luminal contents during the resection (not shown). Doyen intestinal clamps are placed across the descending colon at the oral and anal extent of the resection, angled at approximately 30 degrees from perpendicular so that the length of the small colon at the antimesenteric angle is shorter than the intestine at the mesenteric angle. A scalpel is used to sharply transect the colon, cutting adjacent to the Doyen intestinal clamps and using them to guide a straight transection line.

Doyen intestinal clamps and using them to guide a straight transection line.

The proximal and distal segments are aligned with stay sutures placed at the mesenteric and antimesenteric borders. A slight rotation of the two segments of bowel offsets the mesocolon attachments, allowing a more secure closure at the mesenteric border.[202] The first layer placed is a full-thickness simple-continuous pattern tied at the mesenteric and antimesenteric angles, or a simple-interrupted pattern using no. 0 or 2-0 absorbable suture material. The second layer is a partial-thickness inverting layer using 2-0 absorbable suture interrupted at 180 degrees. The mesentery is closed with a simple-continuous pattern.[202,217,266]

POSTOPERATIVE CARE AND COMPLICATIONS

Because of the high concentration of both aerobic and anaerobic bacteria, broad-spectrum antimicrobial coverage with potassium penicillin (22,000 IU/kg, twice a day IV), gentamicin sulfate (6.6 to 8.8 mg/kg, once a day IV), and metronidazole (15 mg/kg, twice a day IV) is recommended. If the bowel is healthy and the surgical procedure is performed with minimal and contained contamination, perioperative (for 24 hours) use of antibiotics can be appropriate. More extended postoperative administration (therapeutic course) of antibiotics (for 5 to 10 days) should be chosen if the horse has compromised bowel, has any signs of peritonitis, or has acquired abdominal contamination during the surgical procedure. Adjunctive antiendotoxin therapy, such as polymyxin B and hyperimmune serum, should be considered in horses with signs of endotoxemia or septicemia.

Postoperative complications with small colon surgery are dehiscence, stricture and adhesion formation, and impaction at the enterotomy or anastomosis.* Other complications, such as peritonitis, diarrhea, thrombophlebitis, and laminitis, are associated with endotoxemia and septicemia.[204,209] It has been proposed that several factors specifically affect small colon surgery adversely compared with surgery of other areas of the gastrointestinal tract. These are the high concentration of collagenase in the small colon, the high concentration of bacteria (including anaerobic bacteria), the mechanical stress placed on the surgical site by firm fecal balls passing over the incision, and the poor vascular supply.[24,206,268,269] Other authors have questioned some of these assumptions. One study has shown that the small colon vascular arcade system has adequate collateral blood supply. If the lesion is in an area that allows adequate surgical access, the blood supply should not be a limiting factor.[203] The small colon is at risk for postoperative impactions because of the character of the feces and the size of the lumen. Impaction places further stress on an enterotomy or anastomosis site, increasing the risk of dehiscence. Although evacuation of the large colon decreases the risk of this occurring, postoperative feeding should also be carefully controlled to further decrease the risk of impaction at the enterotomy or anastomosis site. Reports suggest that with good surgical technique and attention to postoperative management (such as careful reintroduction to feed), horses have a good prognosis after small colon surgery.[44,153,205,209]

*References 38, 153, 202, 204, 217, 219.

REFERENCES

1. Getty R: Sisson and Grossman's The Anatomy of the Domestic Animal, ed 5, Philadelphia, 1975, WB Saunders.
2. Nickel R, Schumer A, Seiferle E: The Viscera of Domestic Animals, ed 2, New York, 1979, Springer-Verlag.
3. Ross M, Hanson R: The large intestine. In Auer J, editor: Equine Surgery, ed 1, Philadelphia, 1992, WB Saunders.
4. Dart AJ, Snyder JR, Julian D, et al: Microvascular circulation of the cecum in horses, Am J Vet Res 1991;52:1545.
5. Argenzio RA, Lowe JE, Pickard DW, et al: Digesta passage and water exchange in the equine large intestine, Am J Physiol 1974;226:1035.
6. Argenzio R: Functions of the equine large intestine and their interrelationship in disease, Cornell Vet 1975;65:303.
7. Ross MW, Donawick WJ, Sellers AF, et al: Normal motility of the cecum and right ventral colon in ponies, Am J Vet Res 1986;47:1756.
8. Ross MW, Rutkowski JA, Cullen KK: Myoelectric activity of the cecum and right ventral colon in female ponies, Am J Vet Res 1989;50:374.
9. Ross MW, Cullen KK, Rutkowski JA: Myoelectric activity of the ileum, cecum, and right ventral colon in ponies during interdigestive, nonfeeding, and digestive periods, Am J Vet Res 1990;51:561.
10. Dyce KM, Hartman W: An endoscopic study of the caecal base of the horse, Tijdschr Diergeneeskd 1973;98:957.
11. Dyce KM, Hartman W, Aalfs RH: A cinefluoroscopic study of the caecal base of the horse, Res Vet Sci 1976;20:40.
12. Lester GD, Merritt AM, Neuwirth L, et al: Myoelectric activity of the ileum, cecum, and right ventral colon, and cecal emptying of radiolabeled markers in clinically normal ponies, Am J Vet Res 1998;59:313.
13. Clark ES, Thompson SA, Becht JL, et al: Effects of xylazine on cecal mechanical activity and cecal blood flow in healthy horses, Am J Vet Res 1988;49:720.
14. Rutkowski JA, Eades SC, Moore JN: Effects of xylazine butorphanol on cecal arterial blood flow, cecal mechanical activity, and systemic hemodynamics in horses, Am J Vet Res 1991;52:1153.
15. Rutkowski JA, Ross MW, Cullen K: Effects of xylazine and/or butorphanol or neostigmine on myoelectric activity of the cecum and right ventral colon in female ponies, Am J Vet Res 1989;50:1096.
16. Lester GD, Merritt AM, Neuwirth L, et al: Effect of alpha 2-adrenergic, cholinergic, and nonsteroidal anti-inflammatory drugs on myoelectric activity of ileum, cecum, and right ventral colon and on cecal emptying of radiolabeled markers in clinically normal ponies, Am J Vet Res 1998;59:320.
17. Lester GD, Merritt AM, Neuwirth L, et al: Effect of erythromycin lactobionate on myoelectric activity of ileum, cecum, and right ventral colon, and cecal emptying of radiolabeled markers in clinically normal ponies, Am J Vet Res 1998;59:328.
18. Boles C: Surgical techniques in equine colic, J South Afr Vet Assoc 1975;46:115.
19. Dart A, Hodgson D, Snyder J: Caecal disease in equids, Aust Vet J 1997;75:552.
20. Tennant B, Wheat J, Meagher D: Observations on the causes and incidence of acute intestinal obstruction in the horse, Proc Am Assoc Equine Pract 1972;19:251.
21. White N: Epidemiology of colic. In White N, editor: The Equine Acute Abdomen, Philadelphia, 1990, Lea & Febiger.
22. Blood D, Henderson J, Radostitis O: Veterinary Medicine, ed 5, Baltimore, 1979, Lea & Febiger.
23. Campbell ML, Colahan PC, Brown MP, et al: Cecal impaction in the horse, J Am Vet Med Assoc 1984;184:950.
24. Hackett R: Cecal impaction. In White N, Moore J, editors: Current Practice of Equine Surgery, Philadelphia, 1990, JB Lippincott.
25. Meagher D: Obstructive disease in the large intestine of the

horse: Diagnosis and treatment, Proc Am Assoc Equine Pract 1972;18:169.
26. Roberts CT, Slone DE: Cecal impactions surgically managed by typhlotomy, 11 cases (1988-1998), Proceedings, Equine Colic Research Symposium 1998;6:29.
27. Voss JL: Rupture of the cecum and ventral colon of mares during parturition, J Am Vet Med Assoc 1969;155:745.
28. Beroza G, Barclay W, Phillips T, et al: Cecal perforation and peritonitis associated with *Anoplocephala perfoliata* infection in three horses, J Am Vet Med Assoc 1983;183:804.
29. Proudman CJ, Edwards GB: Are tapeworms associated with equine colic? A case control study, Equine Vet J 1993;25:224.
30. Ryu SH, Bak UB, Kim JG, et al: Cecal rupture by *Anoplocephala perfoliata* infection in a Thoroughbred horse in Seoul Race Park, South Korea, J Vet Sci 2001;2:189.
31. Edwards G: The clinical presentation and diagnosis of caecal obstruction in the horse, Equine Vet Educ 1992;4:237.
32. Edwards G: Cecal diseases that can result in colic. In Mair DT, Ducharme N, editors: Manual of Equine Gastroenterology, Philadelphia, 2002, WB Saunders.
33. Hilbert B, Little C, Bolton J, et al: Caecal overload and rupture in the horse, Aust Vet J 1987;64:85.
34. Ross MW, Martin BB, Donawick WJ: Cecal perforation in the horse, J Am Vet Med Assoc 1985;187:249.
35. Ross MW, Bayha R: Volvulus of the cecum and large colon caused by multiple mesenteric defects in a horse, J Am Vet Med Assoc 1992;200:203.
36. Lester GD, Bolton JR, Cullen LK, et al: Effects of general anesthesia on myoelectric activity of the intestine in horses, Am J Vet Res 1992;53:1553.
37. Dabareiner RM, White NA: Large colon impaction in horses: 147 cases (1985-1991), J Am Vet Med Assoc 1995;206:679.
38. Dabareiner R, White NA: Diseases and surgery of the cecum, Vet Clin North Am 1997;13:303.
39. Collatos C, Romano S: Cecal impaction in horses: Causes, diagnosis, and medical treatment, Comp Cont Ed 1993;15:976.
40. Huskamp B, Scheideman W: Diagnosis and treatment of chronic recurrent caecal impaction, Equine Vet J Suppl 2000;32:65.
41. Schusser G, Scheidemann W, Huskamp B: Muscle thickness and neuron density in the caecum of horses with chronic recurrent caecal impaction, Equine Vet J Suppl 2000;32:69.
42. Ross M, Donawick W, Martin B: Cecal impaction and idiopathic cecal perforation in the horse, Vet Surg 1984;13:57.
43. Wheat J: Causes of colic and types requiring surgical intervention, J South Afr Vet Assoc 1975;46:95.
44. White N, Lessard P: Risk factors and clinical signs associated with cases of equine colic, Proc Am Assoc Equine Pract 1986;32:637.
45. Ross MW, Tate LP, Donawick WJ: Cecocolic anastomosis for the surgical management of cecal impaction in horses, Vet Surg 1986;15:85.
46. Henninger RW, Horst J: Magnesium toxicosis in two horses, J Am Vet Med Assoc 1997;211:82.
47. Huskamp B: Diseases of the digestive system and peritoneum. In Dietz O, Wiesner E, editors: Disease of the Horse: A Handbook for Science and Practice, Basel, Switzerland, 1984, Karger.
48. Foerner JJ, Ringle MJ, Junkins DS, et al: Transection of the pelvic flexure to reduce incarceration of the large colon through the epiploic foramen in a horse, J Am Vet Med Assoc 1993;203:1312.
49. Ross M, Orsini J, Ehnen S: Jejunocolic anastomosis for surgical management of recurrent cecal impaction in a horse, Vet Surg 1987;16:265.
50. White N: Diseases of the cecum. In White N, editor: The Equine Acute Abdomen, Philadelphia, 1990, Lea & Febiger.
51. Craig DR, Pankowski RL, Car BD: Ileocolostomy: A technique for surgical management of cecal impaction, Vet Surg 1987;16:451.
52. Kersjes A, Bras G: The surgical treatment of ileus in the horse, Tijdschr Diergeneeskd 1973;98:968.
53. Dart A, Dowling B: Cecal disease, Equine Vet Educ 1999;11:182.
54. Gerard M, Bowman K, Blikslager A, et al: Jejunocolostomy or ileocolostomy for treatment of cecal impaction in horses: Nine cases (1985-1995), J Am Vet Med Assoc 1996;209:1287.
55. McIlwraith C, Robertson J: Advanced Techniques in Equine Surgery, ed 2, Baltimore, 1998, Williams and Wilkins.
56. Hintz H, Schryver H: Digestive physiology of the horse, J Equine Med Surg 1978;2:147.
57. Boussauw BH, Domingo R, Wilderjans H, et al: Treatment of irreducible caecocolic intussusception in horses by jejuno(ileo)-colostomy, Vet Rec 2001;149:16.
58. Gaughan EM, Hackett RP: Cecocolic intussusception in horses: 11 cases (1979-1989), J Am Vet Med Assoc 1990;197:1373.
59. Gaughan EM, van Harreveld P: Cecocecal and cecocolic intussusception in horses, Comp Cont Ed Pract Vet 2000;22:616.
60. Edwards G: Surgical management of intussusception in the horse, Equine Vet J 1986;18:313.
61. Huskamp B: Diagnosis and treatment of acute abdominal conditions in the horse: Various types and frequency as seen at the animal hospital in Hochmoor, Proc Equine Colic Res Symp, University of Georgia, 1982:261.
62. Martin BB, Jr., Freeman DE, Ross MW, et al: Cecocolic and cecocecal intussusception in horses: 30 cases (1976-1996), J Am Vet Med Assoc 214:80,1999.
63. Robertson J: Cecocolic and cecocolic intussusception. In White N, Moore J, editors: Current Practice of Equine Surgery, Philadelphia, 1990, JB Lippincott.
64. Ward JL, Fubini SL: Partial typhlectomy and ileocolostomy for treatment of nonreducible cecocolic intussusception in a horse, J Am Vet Med Assoc 1994;205:325.
65. Barclay WP, Phillips TN, Foerner JJ: Intussusception associated with *Anoplocephala perfoliata* infection in five horses, J Am Vet Med Assoc 1982;180:752.
66. Lyons ET, Tolliver SC, Drudge JH, et al: Parasites in Kentucky Thoroughbreds at necropsy: emphasis on stomach worms and tapeworms, Am J Vet Res 1983;44:839.
67. Owen R, Jaggar D, Quan-Taylor R: Cecal intussusception in horses and the significance of *Anoplocephala perfoliata*, Vet Rec 1989;124:34.
68. McGladdery A: Ultrasonographic diagnosis of intussusception in foals and yearlings, Proc Am Assoc Equine Pract 1996;42:239.
69. Hubert JD, Hardy J, Holcombe SJ, et al: Cecal amputation within the right ventral colon for surgical treatment of nonreducible cecocolic intussusception in 8 horses, Vet Surg 2000;29:317.
70. Wiemer P, van der Veen H: Nonreducible caecocolic intussusception, Equine Vet Educ 1999;11:179.
71. Tyler R: Caecocolic intussusception in a yearling Thoroughbred filly and its surgical management by ileocolostomy, Equine Vet Educ 1992;4:229.
72. Edwards J, Ruoff W: Idiopathic cecal rupture in foals after anesthesia for gastric endoscopy, J Am Vet Med Assoc 1991;198:1421.
73. Littlejohn A, Ritchie J: Rupture of the cecum at parturition, J South Afr Vet Assoc 1975;46:87.
74. Harrison I. Cecal torsion in a horse as a consequence of cecocolic fold hypoplasia, Cornell Vet 1989;79:315.
75. Steyn D: Typhlectomy in a horse, J South Afr Med Assoc 1966;37:440.
76. Mair T, Pearson G: Multifocal non-strangulating intestinal infarction associated with larval cyathostomiasis in a pony, Equine Vet J 1995;27:154.
77. Cable CS, Fubini SL, Erb HN, et al: Abdominal surgery in foals: A review of 119 cases (1977-1994), Equine Vet J 1997;29:257.
78. Cotchin E, Baker-Smith J: Correspondence: Tumours in horses encountered in an abattoir survey, Vet Rec 1975;97:339.
79. Travillian C, Anderson B, Collet M: An unusual paracecal abscess associated with *Fusobacterium necrophorum* in a horse, Aust Vet J 1998;76:659.
80. Brown M, Meagher D: Repair of an equine cecal fistula caused by application of a hernia clamp, Vet Med Small Anim Clin 1978;73:1403.

81. Burns GA: The teniae of the equine intestinal tract, Cornell Vet 1992;82:187.
82. Snyder JR, Tyler WS, Pascoe JR, et al: Microvascular circulation of the ascending colon in horses, Am J Vet Res 1989;50:2075.
83. Doyle AJ, Freeman DE, Rapp H, et al: Life-threatening hemorrhage from enterotomies and anastomoses in 7 horses, Vet Surg 2003;32:553.
84. Lopes MA, Pfeiffer CJ: Functional morphology of the equine pelvic flexure and its role in disease: A review, Histol Histopathol 2000;15:983.
85. Sellers AF, Lowe JE, Brondum J: Motor events in the equine large colon, Am J Physiol 1979;237:E457.
86. Sellers AF, Lowe JE, Rendano VT, et al: The reservoir function of the equine cecum and ventral large colon: Its relation to chronic non-surgical obstructive disease with colic, Cornell Vet 1982;72:233.
87. Sellers AF, Lowe JE: Review of large intestinal motility and mechanism of impaction in the horse, Equine Vet J 1986;18:261.
88. Traub-Dargatz JL, Kopral CA, Seitzinger AH, et al: Estimate of the national incidence of and operation-level risk factors for colic among horses in the United States, spring 1998 to spring 1999, J Am Vet Med Assoc 2001;219:67.
89. Cohen ND, Matejka PL, Honnas CM, et al: Case-control study of the association between various management factors and development of colic in horses, J Am Vet Med Assoc 1995;206:667.
90. Hackett RP: Nonstrangulated colonic displacement in horses, J Am Vet Med Assoc 1983;182:235.
91. Hillyer MH, Taylor FG, Proudman CJ, et al: Case control study to identify risk factors for simple colonic obstruction and distension colic in horses, Equine Vet J 2002;34:455.
92. Proudman CJ, French NP, Trees AJ: Tapeworm infection is a significant risk factor for spasmodic colic and ileal impaction colic in the horse, Equine Vet J 1998;30:194.
93. Lopes MA, White NA: Hydration of colonic ingesta in fistulated horses fed hay and hay and grain. In Proceedings, American College of Veterinary Surgeons 12th Annual Veterinary Symposium, 2002.
94. Cohen ND, Carter GK, Mealey RH, et al: Medical management of right dorsal colitis in 5 horses: A retrospective study (1987-1993), J Vet Intern Med 1995;9:272.
95. Proudman CJ: A two year, prospective survey of equine colic in general practice, Equine Vet J 1991;24:90.
96. White N: Epidemiology and etiology of colic. In White NA, editor: The Equine Acute Abdomen, Philadelphia, 1990, Lea & Febiger.
97. Clarke LL, Roberts MC, Argenzio RA: Feeding and digestive problems in horses. Physiologic responses to a concentrated meal, Vet Clin North Am Equine Pract 1990;6:433.
98. White NA: Enteral fluids for promoting colonic hydration. In Proceedings, American College of Veterinary Surgeons Annual Meeting, 2003.
99. Kristula M, McDonnell S: Effect of drinking water temperature on consumption and preference of water during cold weather in ponies. In Proc Am Assoc Equine Prac 1994:95.
100. Little D, Redding WR, Blikslager AT: Risk factors for reduced postoperative fecal output in horses: 37 cases (1997-1998), J Am Vet Med Assoc 2001;218:414.
101. Van Hoogmoed LM, Snyder JR, Harmon F: In vitro investigation of the effect of prostaglandins and nonsteroidal anti-inflammatory drugs on contractile activity of the equine smooth muscle of the dorsal colon, ventral colon, and pelvic flexure, Am J Vet Res 2000;61:1259.
102. Van Hoogmoed L, Rakestraw PC, Snyder JR, et al: In vitro effects of nonsteroidal anti-inflammatory agents and prostaglandins I2, E2, and F2alpha on contractility of taenia of the large colon of horses, Am J Vet Res 1999;60:1004.
103. Campbell NB, Blikslager AT: The role of cyclooxygenase inhibitors in repair of ischaemic-injured jejunal mucosa in the horse, Equine Vet J Suppl 2000;Jun:59.
104. Roberts MC, Seawright A: Experimental studies of drug induced large colon impaction in the horse, Equine Vet J 1983;15:222.
105. Auer DE, Seawright AA, Pollitt CC, et al: Illness in horses following spraying with amitraz, Aust Vet J 1984;61:257.
106. Roberts MC, Argenzio RA: Effects of amitraz, several opiate derivatives and anticholinergic agents on intestinal transit in ponies, Equine Vet J 1986;18:256.
107. Ducharme NG, Fubini SL: Gastrointestinal complications associated with the use of atropine in horses, J Am Vet Med Assoc 1983;182:229.
108. Williams M, Spiess B, Pascoe P, et al: Systemic effects of topical and subconjunctival ophthalmic atropine in the horse, Vet Ophthalmol 2000;3:193.
109. Sellers AF, Lowe JE, Drost CJ, et al: Retropulsion-propulsion in equine large colon, Am J Vet Res 1982;43:390.
110. Lester GD, Bolton JR, Cambridge H, et al: The effect of *Strongylus vulgaris* larvae on equine intestinal myoelectrical activity, Equine Vet J Suppl 1989;Jun:8.
111. Murray MJ, Parker GA, White NA: Megacolon with myenteric hypoganglionosis in a foal, J Am Vet Med Assoc 1988;192:917.
112. Bassage LH, Johnston JK, Krotec K, et al: Eosinophilic enterocolitis associated with recurrent colonic impactions in a mare, Equine Vet J 1997;29:322.
113. Mueller PO, Moore J: Rectal examination of horses with acute abdominal pain, Comp Cont Educ Pract Vet 2000;22:606.
114. Freeman DE, Ferrante PL, Palmer JE: Comparison of the effects of intragastric infusions of equal volumes of water, dioctyl sodium sulfosuccinate, and magnesium sulfate on fecal composition and output in clinically normal horses, Am J Vet Res 1992;53:1347.
115. Lopes MA, Walker BL, White NA, 2nd, et al: Treatments to promote colonic hydration: Enteral fluid therapy versus intravenous fluid therapy and magnesium sulphate, Equine Vet J 2002;34:505.
116. Lopes MA, Johnson S, White NA, et al: Enteral fluid therapy: Slow infusion versus boluses. In Proceedings, 11th Annual Veterinary Symposium, American College of Veterinary Surgeons, 2001.
117. Schumacher J, DeGraves FJ, Spano JS: Clinical and clinicopathologic effects of large doses of raw linseed oil as compared to mineral oil in healthy horses, J Vet Intern Med 1997;11:296.
118. Macoris DG, Gandolphi W: Intestinal transit in equine: Effect of therapy with flunixin meglumine, combination dipyrone-hioscine, and mineral oil. In Proceedings, 6th Equine Colic Research Symposium, 1998:27.
119. Rodrigues C: Use of markers to study equine gastrointestinal passage after intragastric infusion of mineral oil. In Proceedings, 6th Equine Colic Research Symposium, 1998:28.
120. Brunton L: Agents affecting gastrointestinal water flux and motility: Emesis and antiemetics—Bile acids and pancreatic enzymes. In Hardman J, Limbird L, editors: Goodman and Gilman's Pharmacological Basis of Therapeutics, New York, 1996, McGraw Hill.
121. Bos M, de Bosschere H, Deprez P, et al: Chemical identification of the (causative) lipids in a case of exogenous lipoid pneumonia in a horse, Equine Vet J 2002;34:744.
122. Scarratt WK, Moon ML, Sponenberg DP, et al: Inappropriate administration of mineral oil resulting in lipoid pneumonia in three horses, Equine Vet J 1998;30:85.
123. Dorman DC, Haschek WM: Fatal propylene glycol toxicosis in a horse, J Am Vet Med Assoc 1991;198:1643.
124. Moffat R, Kramer L, Lerner D, et al: Studies on dioctyl sodium sulfosuccinate toxicity: Clinical, gross and microscopic pathology in the horse and guinea pig, Can J Comp Med 1975;39:434.
125. Rowe EL, White NA, Buechner-Maxwell V, et al: Detection of apoptotic cells in intestines from horses with and without gastrointestinal tract disease, Am J Vet Res 2003;64:982.
126. Cleveland MV, Flavin DP, Ruben RA, et al: New polyethylene glycol laxative for treatment of constipation in adults: A randomized, double-blind, placebo-controlled study, South Med J 2001;94:478.

127. Beck DE, Harford FJ, DiPalma JA, et al: Bowel cleansing with polyethylene glycol electrolyte lavage solution, South Med J 1985;78:1414.
128. Roberts MC, Clarke LL, Johnson CM: Castor-oil induced diarrhoea in ponies: A model for acute colitis, Equine Vet J Suppl 1989;Jun:60.
129. Lowe JE, Sellers AF, Brondum J: Equine pelvic flexure impaction: A model used to evaluate motor events and compare drug response, Cornell Vet 1980;70:401.
130. Ramey DW, Reinertson EL: Sand-induced diarrhea in a foal, J Am Vet Med Assoc 1984;185:537.
131. Bertone JJ, Traub-Dargatz JL, Wrigley RW, et al: Diarrhea associated with sand in the gastrointestinal tract of horses, J Am Vet Med Assoc 1988;193:1409.
132. Specht TE, Colahan PT: Surgical treatment of sand colic in equids: 48 cases (1978-1985), J Am Vet Med Assoc 1988;193:1560.
133. Ragle CA, Meagher DM, Lacroix CA, et al: Surgical treatment of sand colic. Results in 40 horses, Vet Surg 1989;18:48.
134. Ruohoniemi M, Kaikkonen R, Raekallio M, et al: Abdominal radiography in monitoring the resolution of sand accumulations from the large colon of horses treated medically, Equine Vet J 2001;33:59.
135. Korolainen R, Kaikkonen R, Ruohoniemi M: Ultrasonography in monitoring the resolution of intestinal sand accumulation in the horse, Equine Vet Educ 2003;5:423.
136. Ragle CA, Meagher DM, Schrader J, et al: Abdominal auscultation in the detection of experimentally induced gastrointestinal sand accumulation, J Vet Intern Med 1988;3:12.
137. Korolainen R, Ruohoniemi M: Reliability of ultrasonography compared to radiography in revealing intestinal sand accumulations in horses, Equine Vet J 2002;34:499.
138. Hammock PD, Freeman DE, Baker GJ: Failure of psyllium mucilloid to hasten evaluation of sand from the equine large intestine, Vet Surg 1998;27:547.
139. Cohen ND, Vontur C, Rakestraw PC: Risk factors for enterolithiasis among horses in Texas, J Am Vet Med Assoc 2000;216:1787.
140. Hassel DM, Langer DL, Snyder JR, et al: Evaluation of enterolithiasis in equids: 900 cases (1973-1996), J Am Vet Med Assoc 1999;214:233.
141. Yarbrough TB, Langer DL, Snyder JR, et al: Abdominal radiography for diagnosis of enterolithiasis in horses: 141 cases (1990-1992), J Am Vet Med Assoc 1994;205:592.
142. Hassel DM, Yarbrough TB: A modified teniotomy technique for facilitated removal of descending colon enteroliths in horses, Vet Surg 1998;27:1.
143. Stratton-Phelps M, Fascetti A: Nutritional therapy in gastrointestinal disease. In Saunders W, editor: Current Therapy in Equine Medicine, ed 5, Philadelphia, 2003, WB Saunders.
144. Hardy J, Minton M, Robertson JT, et al: Nephrosplenic entrapment in the horse: A retrospective study of 174 cases, Equine Vet J Suppl 2000;Jun:95.
145. Baird AN, Cohen ND, Taylor TS, et al: Renosplenic entrapment of the large colon in horses: 57 cases (1983- 1988), J Am Vet Med Assoc 1991;198:1423.
146. Sivula NJ: Renosplenic entrapment of the large colon in horses: 33 cases (1984-1989), J Am Vet Med Assoc 1991;199:244.
147. Testa M, Hilbert BJ: Case report of surgical resection of the pelvic flexure following nephrosplenic ligament entrapment in the horse, Equine Vet Sci 1987;7:35.
148. Markel MD, Orsini JA, Gentile DG, et al: Complications associated with left dorsal displacement of the large colon in the horse, J Am Vet Med Assoc 1985;187:1379.
149. Deen T: Surgical correction of nephrosplenic entrapment of the left colon, Vet Med 1984;79:801.
150. Livesey MA, Arighi M, Ducharme NG, Equine colic: Seventy-six cases resulting from incarceration of the large colon by the suspensory ligament of the spleen, Can Vet J 1988;29:135.
151. Milne D, Tarr M, Lochner F, et al: Left dorsal displacement of the colon in the horse, J Equine Med Surg 1977;1:47.
152. Goodrich LR, Dabareiner RM, White NA: Entrapment of the small intestine within the renosplenic space in two horses, Equine Vet Educ 1997;9:177.
153. Dart AJ, Snyder JR, Pascoe JR, et al: Abnormal conditions of the equine descending (small) colon: 102 cases (1979-1989), J Am Vet Med Assoc 1992;200:971.
154. Santschi EM, Slone DE Jr, Frank WM 2nd: Use of ultrasound in horses for diagnosis of left dorsal displacement of the large colon and monitoring its nonsurgical correction, Vet Surg 1993;22:281.
155. Reef VB: Adult abdominal ultrasonography. In Equine Diagnostic Ultrasound, Philadelphia, 1998, WB Saunders.
156. Johnston JK, Freeman DE: Diseases and surgery of the large colon, Vet Clin North Am Equine Pract 1997;13:317.
157. Kalsbeek HC: Further experiences with non-surgical correction of nephrosplenic entrapment of the left colon in the horse, Equine Vet J 1989;21:442.
158. Boening K, von Saldern F: Nonsurgical treatment of left dorsal displacement of the large colon of horses under general anesthesia. In Proceedings of the Equine Colic Research Symposium, 1986:325.
159. Hardy J, Bednarski RM, Biller DS: Effect of phenylephrine on hemodynamics and splenic dimensions in horses, Am J Vet Res 1994;55:1570.
160. Kobluk CN: Nonsurgical therapeutic procedures for equine colic. In Gordon BJ, Allen D, editors: Field Guide to Colic Management in the Horse, Lenexa, Kan, 1988, Veterinary Medicine.
161. Moll HD, Schumacher J, Dabareiner RM, et al: Left dorsal displacement of the colon with splenic adhesions in three horses, J Am Vet Med Assoc 1993;203:425.
162. Moon PF, Suter CM: Paravertebral thoracolumbar anaesthesia in 10 horses, Equine Vet J 1993;25:304.
163. Marien T, Adriaenssen A, Hoeck FV, et al: Laparoscopic closure of the renosplenic space in standing horses, Vet Surg 2001;30:559.
164. Zekas LJ, Ramirez S, Brown MP: Ablation of the nephrosplenic space for treatment of recurring left dorsal displacement of the large colon in a racehorse, J Am Vet Med Assoc 1999;214:1361.
165. Schumacher J: Treatment of a horse following rupture of the colon during surgery, Equine Vet Educ 2001;3:29.
166. Suann CJ, Livesey MA: Congenital malformation of the large colon causing colic in a horse, Vet Rec 1986;118:230.
167. Rose PL, Schumacher J, Taylor TS: Surgical correction of strictures of the large colon in three horses, Vet Surg 1991;20:260.
168. Boure L, Marcoux M, Lavoie JP, et al: Use of laparoscopic equipment to divide abdominal adhesions in a filly, J Am Vet Med Assoc 1998;212:845.
169. Bassage LH, Habecker PL, Russell EA, et al: Colic in a horse associated with a massive cystic duplication of the ascending colon, Equine Vet J 2000;32:565.
170. Harrison IW: Equine large intestinal volvulus: A review of 124 cases, Vet Surg 1988;17:77.
171. Snyder JR, Pascoe JR, Olander HJ, et al: Strangulating volvulus of the ascending colon in horses, J Am Vet Med Assoc 1989;195:757.
172. Hughes FE, Slone DE: A modified technique for extensive large colon resection and anastomosis in horses, Vet Surg 1998;27:127.
173. Cook G, Embertson RM, Levine J, et al: Early recognition and treatment of large colon volvulus in the horse. In Proceedings, Equine Colic Symposium, 1994:41.
174. Proudman C, Smith J, Edwards G, et al: Long-term survival of equine surgical colic cases: Part 1. Patterns of mortality and morbidity, Equine Vet J 2002;34:432.
175. Jones SL, Davis J, Rowlingson K: Ultrasonographic findings in horses with right dorsal colitis: five cases (2000-2001), J Am Vet Med Assoc 2003;222:1248.
176. East LM, Trumble TN, Steyn PF, et al: The application of technetium-99m hexamethylpropyleneamine oxime (99mTc-

HMPAO) labeled white blood cells for the diagnosis of right dorsal ulcerative colitis in two horses, Vet Radiol Ultrasound 2000;41:360.
177. Andrews FM, Robertson JT: Diagnosis and surgical treatment of functional obstruction of the right dorsal colon in a horse, J Am Vet Med Assoc 1988;193:956.
178. Simmons TR, Gaughan EM, Ducharme NG, et al: Treatment of right dorsal ulcerative colitis in a horse, J Am Vet Med Assoc 1990;196:455.
179. Dowling BA, Dart AJ, McClintock SA, et al: Anastomosis of right ventral colon to descending colon to bypass a non-functional descending colon anastomosis in a miniature pony, Aust Vet J 2000;78:90.
180. Freeman D, Richter RA: Extensive large colon resection with bypass of the right dorsal colon to treat large colon volvulus in a mare. In Proceedings of the 6th Equine Colic Research Symposium, 1998:27.
181. Trostle SS, Markel MD: Incarceration of the large colon in the gastrosplenic ligament of a horse, J Am Vet Med Assoc 1993;202:773.
182. Dyson S, Orsini J: Intussusception of the large colon in a horse, J Am Vet Med Assoc 1983;182:720.
183. Robertson JT, Tate LP Jr: Resection of intussuscepted large colon in a horse, J Am Vet Med Assoc 1982;181:927.
184. Mogg TD, Groenendyk S, Sutton RH: Volvulus of the colon in a horse associated with a mesocolic-umbilical band, Aust Vet J 1992;69:11.
185. Markel M, Stover SM, Pascoe J, et al: Evacuation of the large colon in horses, Comp Cont Educ Pract Vet 1988;10:95.
186. Hardy J, Bertone A: Surgery of the equine large colon, Comp Cont Educ Pract Vet 1992;14:1501.
187. Marien T, Adriaenssen A, Segers L: Design and clinical use of a modified colon tray for large colon evacuation in the horse, Equine Vet J Suppl 2000;Jun:81.
188. Young RL, Snyder JR, Pascoe JR, et al: A comparison of three techniques for closure of pelvic flexure enterotomies in normal equine colon, Vet Surg 1991;20:185.
189. Watt BC, Trostle SS, Cooley AJ: Intraluminal leiomyoma colon polyp in a mare, Equine Vet J 2001;33:326.
190. Dabareiner RM, Sullins KE, Goodrich LR: Large colon resection for treatment of lymphosarcoma in two horses, J Am Vet Med Assoc 1996;208:895.
191. Embertson RM, Schneider RK, Granstedt M: Partial resection and anastomosis of the large colon in a horse, J Am Vet Med Assoc 1982;180:1230.
192. Rottman JB, Roberts MC, Cullen JM: Colonic adenocarcinoma with osseous metaplasia in a horse, J Am Vet Med Assoc 1991;198:657.
193. Steenhaut M, Vandenreyt I, Van Roy M: Incarceration of the large colon through the epiploic foramen in a horse, Equine Vet J 1993;25:550.
194. Wilson DG: Intussusception of the left dorsal colon in a horse, J Am Vet Med Assoc 1983;183:464.
195. Robertson JT, Johnson FM: Surgical correction of cecocolic intussusception in a horse, J Am Vet Med Assoc 1980;176:223.
196. Arighi M, Ducharme NG, Horney FD, et al: Extensive large colon resection in 12 horses, Can Vet J 1987;28:245.
197. Bertone AL, Stashak TS, Sullins KE: Large colon resection and anastomosis in horses, J Am Vet Med Assoc 1986;188:612.
198. Boening K, von Saldern F: Resection of the left large colon in horses. In Proceedings of the Second Colic Research Symposium, 1986:337.
199. Ducharme NG, Burton JH, van Dreumel AA, et al: Extensive large colon resection in the pony. II. Digestibility studies and postmortem findings, Can J Vet Res 1987;51:76.
200. Ducharme NG, Horney FD, Baird JD, et al: Extensive large colon resection in the pony: I. Surgical procedures and clinical results, Can J Vet Res 1987;51:66.
201. Hughes FE, Slone DE Jr: Large colon resection, Vet Clin North Am Equine Pract 1997;13:341.
202. Edwards GB: Diseases and surgery of the small colon, Vet Clin North Am Equine Pract 1997;13:359.
203. Beard WL, Lohse CL, Robertson JT: Vascular anatomy of the descending colon of the horse, Vet Surg 1989;18:130.
204. Ruggles AJ, Ross MW: Medical and surgical management of small-colon impaction in horses: 28 cases (1984-1989), J Am Vet Med Assoc 1991;199:1762.
205. Edwards G: A review of 38 cases of small colon obstruction in the horse, Equine Vet J Suppl 1992;13:42.
206. Keller S, Horney F: Diseases of the equine colon, Comp Cont Ed Pract Vet, 1985;113.
207. Schumacher J, Mair T: Small colon obstruction in the mature horse, Equine Vet Educ 2002;68:27.
208. Freeman SL, Boswell JC, Smith RK: Use of transrectal ultrasonography to aid diagnosis of small colon strangulation in two horses, Vet Rec 2001;148:812.
209. Rhoads W: Small colon impactions in adult horses, Comp Cont Ed Vet Pract 1999;21:770.
210. Livesay M: Small colon obstruction. In White NA, Moore JN, editors: Current Practice of Equine Surgery, Philadelphia, 1990, JB Lippincott.
211. Rhoads WS, Barton MH, Parks AH: Comparison of medical and surgical treatment for impaction of the small colon in horses: 84 cases (1986-1996), J Am Vet Med Assoc 1999;214:1042.
212. Wiley J, Tatum D, Keinath R, et al: Participation of gastric mechanoreceptors and intestinal chemoreceptors in the gastrocolonic response, Gastroenterology 1988;94:1144.
213. Clark ES, Becht JL: Clinical pharmacology of the gastrointestinal tract, Vet Clin North Am Equine Pract 1987;3:101.
214. Blue MG: Enteroliths in horses: A retrospective study of 30 cases, Equine Vet J 1979;11:76.
215. Taylor T, Valdez H, Norwood G: Retrograde flushing for relief of obstructions of the transverse colon in the horse, Equine Pract 1979;2:22.
216. Faleiros RR, Macoris DG, Alessi AC, et al: Effect of intraluminal distention on microvascular perfusion in the equine small colon, Am J Vet Res 2002;63:1292.
217. Dart A, Dowling B, Hodgson DI: The large intestine. In Auer JR, Stick J, editors: Equine Surgery, ed 2, Philadelphia, 1999, WB Saunders.
218. McClure JT, Kobluk C, Voller K, et al: Fecalith impaction in four miniature foals, J Am Vet Med Assoc 1992;200:205.
219. Ragle CA, Snyder JR, Meagher DM, et al: Surgical treatment of colic in American miniature horses: 15 cases (1980-1987), J Am Vet Med Assoc 1992;201:329.
220. Boles CL, Kohn CW: Fibrous foreign body impaction colic in young horses, J Am Vet Med Assoc 1977;171:193.
221. Gay CC, Speirs VC, Christie BA, et al: Foreign body obstruction of the small colon in six horses, Equine Vet J 1979;11:60.
222. Getty S, Ellis D, Krehbiel J, et al: Rubberized fencing as a gastrointestinal obstruction in a young horse, Vet Med 1976;71:221.
223. Meagher D: Impaction of the cecum, Proc Am Assoc Eq Pract 1971;17:174.
224. Madigan J: Meconium retention. In Madigan J, editor: Manual of Neonatal Medicine, Woodland, Calif, 1987, Live Oak.
225. Pusterla N, Magdesian K, Maleski K, et al: Retrospective evaluation of the use of acetylcysteine enemas in the treatment of meconium retention in foals: 44 cases (1987-2002), Equine Vet Educ 2004;27:170.
226. Semrad S, Shaftoe S: Gastrointestinal diseases in the neonatal foal. In Robinson NE, editor: Current Therapy in Equine Medicine, ed 3, Philadelphia, 1992, WB Saunders.
227. Martens R: Pediatrics. In Mannsman RA, McAllister ES, editors: Equine Medicine and Surgery, ed 3, Santa Barbara, Calif, 1982, American Vet.

228. Fisher A, Kerr L, O'Brien T: Radiographic diagnosis of gastrointestinal disorders in the foal, Vet Radiol 1987;28:42.
229. Fischer AT, Yarbrough TY: Retrograde contrast radiography of the distal portions of the intestinal tract in foals, J Am Vet Med Assoc 1995;207:734.
230. Madigan J, Goetzman B: Use of acetylcysteine solution enema for meconium retention in the neonate foal, Proc Am Assoc Eq Pract 1990;36:117.
231. Vatistas NJ, Snyder JR, Wilson WD, et al: Surgical treatment for colic in the foal (67 cases): 1980-1992, Equine Vet J 1996;28:139.
232. Hughs F, Moll H, Slone D: Surgical management of meconium impactions in 8 foals, Proc 5th Equine Colic Res Symposium, Athens, Ga, 1994:32.
233. Pearson H, Waterman AE: Submucosal haematoma as a cause of obstruction of the small colon in the horse: A review of four cases, Equine Vet J 1986;18:340.
234. Speirs VC, van Veenendaal JC, Christie BA, et al: Obstruction of the small colon by intramural haematoma in three horses, Aust Vet J 1981;57:88.
235. Pearson H, Pinsent P, Denny H, et al: The indications for equine laparotomy: An analysis of 140 cases, Equine Vet J 1975;7:131.
236. Dart AJ, Pascoe JR, Snyder JR: Mesenteric tears of the descending (small) colon as a postpartum complication in two mares, J Am Vet Med Assoc 1991;199:1612.
237. Livesey M, Keller S: Segmental ischemic necrosis following mesocolic rupture in postparturient mares, Comp Cont Ed Pract Vet 1986;8:763.
238. Bailey G, Hutchins D: Small colon intussusception in a mare managed with a diverting colostomy, Aust Vet J 1987;64:114.
239. Mason T: Strangulation of the rectum of a horse by a pedicle of a mesenteric lipoma, Equine Vet J 1978;10:269.
240. Blikslager AT, Bowman KF, Haven ML, et al: Pedunculated lipomas as a cause of intestinal obstruction in horses: 17 cases (1983-1990), J Am Vet Med Assoc 1992;201:1249.
241. Kirker-Head C, Steckel R: Volvulus of the small colon in a horse, Mod Vet Pract 1988;69:14.
242. Rhoads WS, Parks AH: Incarceration of the small colon through a rent in the gastrosplenic ligament in a pony, J Am Vet Med Assoc 1999;214:226.
243. McClure S, Faber N, Mealey R: Diagnosing and correcting an intussusception of the small colon in a foal, Vet Med 1995;90:977.
244. Ross MW, Stephens PR, Reimer JM: Small colon intussusception in a broodmare, J Am Vet Med Assoc 1988;192:372.
245. Schneider J, Leipold H: Recessive lethal white in two foals, J Equine Med Surg 1978;2:479.
246. Tsujimoto C, Sherman F, Rovitch M: Experimental intestinal atresia in the rabbit fetus, John Hopkins Med 1972;131:287.
247. Earlam RJ: A study of the aetiology of congenital stenosis of the gut, Ann R Coll Surg Engl 1972;51:126.
248. Barnard C: The genesis of intestinal atresia, Surg Forum 1957;7:393.
249. Young RL, Linford RL, Olander HJ: Atresia coli in the foal: A review of six cases, Equine Vet J 1992;24:60.
250. Cho D, Taylor H: Blind-end atresia coli in two foals, Cornell Vet 1986;76:11.
251. Overboaugh K: Intestinal anomalies in a neonatal foal, Vet Med Small Anim Clin 1983;78:224.
252. Van der Gaag I, Tibboel D: Intestinal atresia and stenosis in animals: A report of 34 cases, Vet Pathol 1980;17:565.
253. Neil N: Foal colic: Practical imaging of the abdomen, Equine Vet Educ 2003;65:335.
254. Schneider J, Leipold H, White S: Repair of congenital atresia of the colon in a foal, J Equine Sci 1981;1:121.
255. Haven ML, Rottman JB, Bowman KF: Leiomyoma of the small colon in a horse, Vet Surg 1991;20:320.
256. Mair TS, Davies EV, Lucke VM: Small colon intussusception associated with an intraluminal leiomyoma in a pony, Vet Rec 1992;130:403.
257. King J: Lymphoma in a horse, Vet Med (Praha) 1993;88:513.
258. Parks A, Wyn-Jones G, Cox J, et al: Partial obstruction of the small colon associated with an abdominal testicular teratoma in a foal, Equine Vet J 1986;18:342.
259. Evard JH, Fischer AT, Greenwood LD: Ovarian strangulation as a cause of small colon obstruction in a foal, Equine Vet J 1988;20:217.
260. Mair T: Small colon impaction associated with a granulosa cell tumor in a pony mare, Equine Vet Educ 2002;14:17.
261. Wilson DA, Foreman JH, Boero MJ, et al: Small-colon rupture attributable to granulosa cell tumor in a mare, J Am Vet Med Assoc 1989;194:681.
262. Burns GA, Karcher LF, Cummings JF: Equine myenteric ganglionitis: A case of chronic intestinal pseudo-obstruction, Cornell Vet 1990;80:53.
263. Beard WL, Robertson JT, Getzy DM: Enterotomy technique in the descending colon of the horse: Effect of location and suture pattern, Vet Surg 1989;18:135.
264. Archer RM, Parsons JC, Lindsay WA, et al: A comparison of enterotomies through the antimesenteric band and the sacculation of the small (descending) colon of ponies, Equine Vet J 1988;20:406.
265. Bristol DG, Cullen J: A comparison of three methods of end-to-end anastomosis in the equine small colon, Cornell Vet 1988;78:325.
266. Hanson RR, Nixon AJ, Calderwood-Mays M, et al: Evaluation of three techniques for end-to end anastomosis of the small colon in horses, Am J Vet Res 1988;49:1613.
267. Hanson RR, Nixon AJ, Calderwood-Mays M, et al: Comparison of staple and suture techniques for end-to-end anastomosis of the small colon in horses, Am J Vet Res 1988;49:1621.
268. Hawley PR, Faulk WP, Hunt TK, et al: Collagenase activity in the gastrointestinal tract, Br J Surg 1970;57:896.
269. Stashak T: Techniques for enterotomy, decompression, and intestinal resection/anastomosis, Vet Clin North Am Large Anim Pract 1982;4:147.

CHAPTER 37

Rectum and Anus

David E. Freeman

The rectum is approximately 30 cm long in an adult horse and extends from the pelvic inlet to the anus.[1] The distance from the anus to the peritoneal reflection is highly variable and is shorter in young horses and in horses with little body fat.[2,3] The peritoneal part of the rectum is attached dorsally by the mesorectum, which is a continuation of the mesocolon.[1] The retroperitoneal part of the rectum forms a dilation called the rectal ampulla, which has thick longitudinal muscle bundles.[1] The anal canal is approximately 5 cm long and is enclosed by the internal anal sphincter, which is a thickening of the circular smooth muscle, and the external anal sphincter, which is composed of striated muscle.[1] The levator ani muscle arises from the ischiatic spine and sacrotuberal ligament and ends under the external anal sphincter.[1] Its action overcomes the tendency of the anus to prolapse during defecation.

RECTAL TEARS

Rectal tears caused by palpation per rectum commonly result in malpractice claims against veterinarians in the United States.[4] However, the standard of care for a horse that has incurred a rectal tear is also subject to claims for negligence,[4] and this is an area in which most veterinarians leave themselves vulnerable to malpractice suits. Copious lubrication of the hand and forearm and adequate restraint of the horse, including sedation if necessary, should be regarded as the minimal measures required to prevent iatrogenic rectal tears. Once a rectal tear is suspected, the veterinarian must assess the tear for severity, inform the owner about the nature of the problem (without making statements that imply admission of guilt or responsibility for payment), and apply appropriate treatment, including referral. Failure to follow these guidelines will weaken a veterinarian's legal defense. The veterinarian should also contact his or her liability insurance company promptly.

Causes

Most rectal tears result from rupture of the rectal wall as it contracts around the examiner's hand or forearm rather than from penetration with the finger tips. To avoid a tear, no attempt should be made to force against straining or a peristaltic wave, and intra-abdominal structures should be palpated only when the hand has been inserted beyond the contraction and then withdrawn to that level. Special precautions should be taken with Arabian horses, ponies, small breeds, horses that have had a previous rectal tear or injury, horses that are unaccustomed to palpation per rectum, fractious horses, and horses with colic.[2,5]

Less common causes of rectal tears are enemas, meconium extraction by forceps, sadism, dystocia, animal bites, chronic impaction at a stricture, misdirection of a stallion's penis,[2,5-7] spontaneous tears,[8] rectal thrombosis,[9] and sand impactions.[3] In one report of five horses with idiopathic tears, four presented with colic, and the tear developed in one horse during a lameness examination.[10] Idiopathic tears tend to be transversely oriented.[10]

Classification and Locations

Rectal tears are divided into four grades based on severity. In grade I tears, only the mucosa and submucosa are torn.[2] In grade II tears, only the muscular layer is disrupted, causing the mucosa and submucosa to prolapse through the defect and create a site for fecal impaction.[2] These are rare (3 of 85 tears in one series), but chronic impactions in the diverticulum may necessitate euthanasia.[11] Grade III tears involve all layers except the serosa (grade IIIa) or mesorectum and retroperitoneal tissues (grade IIIb).[5,12] It is not unusual for grade IIIb tears to pack with feces and produce a large plane of dissection cranially and dorsally, even approaching the left kidney. The feces packed in retroperitoneal spaces can be a source of bacterial contamination of the peritoneal cavity (Fig. 37-1). A grade IV tear involves all layers and is the most serious, since it allows fecal contamination of the peritoneal cavity.[2] Most tears involve the dorsal aspect of the rectum, are located 15 to 55 cm from the anus,[11,12] and occur parallel to the longitudinal axis.[2] Distance from the anus is not a reliable indicator of tear location relative to the retroperitoneal reflection.[1,3,5]

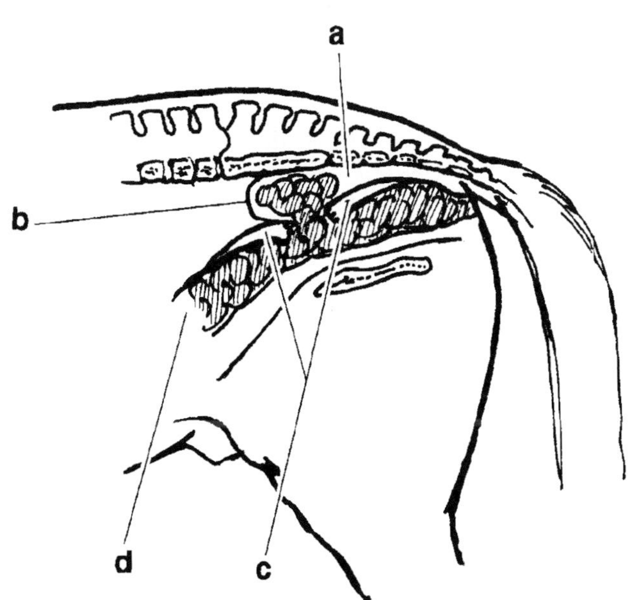

Figure 37-1. Impaction of feces into a grade IIIb rectal tear (a), causing progressive enlargement of the perirectal space and bacterial leakage across the peritoneum (b), swelling of the rectal wall (c), and small colon impaction (d). (From Freeman DE, Richardson DW, Tulleners EP, et al: Loop colostomy for management of rectal tears and small colon injuries in horses: 10 cases [1976-1989], J Am Vet Med Assoc 1992;200:1365, with permission.)

Clinical Signs and Diagnosis

Early diagnosis is essential for successful treatment and to avoid legal repercussions. When a tear occurs, the veterinarian may feel a sudden release of pressure or suddenly be able to directly palpate abdominal organs.[5] Alternatively, the examiner may not sense the torn rectum.[5] A rectal tear should be suspected if a large amount of blood is evident on the rectal sleeve on withdrawal of the hand or if the rectum suddenly relaxes while the horse is straining.[2] Within 2 hours after a rectal tear occurs, the horse usually shows signs of peritonitis and endotoxic shock. Signs of colic are also present initially, but these soon give way to depression.[5] Feces can be hemorrhagic initially and defecation can be accompanied by straining.[13] Idiopathic tears are usually presented as colic of variable duration, and, because there is no reason to suspect a rectal tear, referral can be delayed.[10]

Before examination of the tear, straining and rectal contractions are stopped with epidural anesthesia or xylazine (0.1 to 0.2 mg/kg body weight IV), alone or in combination with butorphanol tartrate (0.1 mg/kg IV).[11-16] Butylscopolamine bromide (Buscopan), 20 mg IV, relaxes the rectum and small colon very well, allowing examination of rectal tears. A lidocaine enema can be given (12 mL of 2% lidocaine in 50 mL of tap water) or lidocaine jelly applied to the rectal mucosa[17] before inspecting the tear digitally or through a tube speculum or endoscope. For digital palpation, the examiner can use the bare hand or wear a surgeon's glove and apply copious lubrication with a water-soluble gel. Because the abundant mucosal folds tend to obscure the rectal tear, more information can be gained from careful palpation than by visual inspection. Failure to accurately grade a tear can cause inappropriate treatment selection. A grade I tear can feel like a flap of mucosa, but a grade III tear can feel as if its edges are rigid and thick and separated, often by packed feces. Abdominocentesis should be performed to assess peritonitis.

Initial Treatment

First aid is applied as soon as the diagnosis is made and includes (1) reduction of activity of the rectum, (2) gentle removal of feces from the tear and rectum, (3) treatment of septic shock and peritonitis, and (4) administration of epidural anesthesia and packing of the rectum.[14,18]

Flunixin meglumine (1.1 mg/kg every 24 hours IV) and antibiotics, such as sodium or potassium penicillin (22,000 IU/kg of body weight every 6 hours IV), gentamicin (6.6 mg/kg every 24 hours IV), and metronidazole (15 mg/kg every 6 hours PO) should be administered and continued as indicated. Intravenous fluids are required to treat shock. Antibiotics and laxatives may be sufficient treatment for grade I and II tears, with daily inspection and careful evacuation of the rectum as needed.[5]

Rectal packing can prevent conversion of a grade III to a grade IV tear and can protect the tear from fecal contamination in the interval before definitive treatment is applied.[5,18] The packing material of choice is a 3-inch stockinette filled with 0.25 kg of moistened rolled cotton, sprayed with povidone-iodine, and lubricated with surgical gel.[18] The packing should fill the rectum without distention to a point 10 cm proximal to the tear, taking care not to pack the tear itself.[18] The anus is subsequently closed with towel clamps or a pursestring suture, and the epidural anesthetic is repeated as necessary to decrease straining.[5,18]

Surgical Management

A temporary indwelling rectal liner[19] and colostomy[20-22] divert feces away from grade III and grade IV rectal tears and thereby prevent contamination and impaction of perirectal tissues, enlargement of the tear, and progression of peritonitis. Each can be combined with direct suture repair and thereby used to protect the suture line during healing.

Temporary Indwelling Rectal Liner

A temporary indwelling rectal liner can be constructed by gluing a palpation sleeve with the hand portion removed, or the plastic cover for an arthroscope camera, to a 5-cm-diameter and 7.5-cm-long rectal prolapse ring with holes through which Dacron loops are laced.[5,19] With the horse anesthetized in dorsal recumbency, an unscrubbed assistant passes the well-lubricated ring and liner through the anus so the surgeon can guide it through a ventral midline celiotomy, cranial to the tear but far enough caudally that the sleeve does not retract into the rectum when the horse stands[5,19] (Fig. 37-2). A circumferential suture of size 3 surgical gut is placed tightly around the small colon over the central groove of the prolapse ring, and four equidistant retention sutures (2-0 polyglycolic acid) are placed to incorporate the circumferential suture, all layers of the rectal wall, and the Dacron loops in the modified prolapse ring.[19] Then, the serosal surface is apposed over the circumferential suture with a Lembert pattern.[19] The large colon is emptied through a pelvic flexure enterotomy, and the small colon is emptied by flushing with a hose directed through the ring and liner from the anus.[5]

The circumferential suture will cut through the rectal wall and allow passage of the ring and liner in feces within approximately 9 to 12 days, by which time the apposed colon walls will have healed.[19] The four retention sutures help maintain the ring in a coaxial relationship with the small colon so that it does not twist and obstruct the lumen.[5,19] Horses are usually cross-tied to prevent them from lying down, which would allow the sleeve to retract forward. Failures have been caused by tearing of the sleeve,

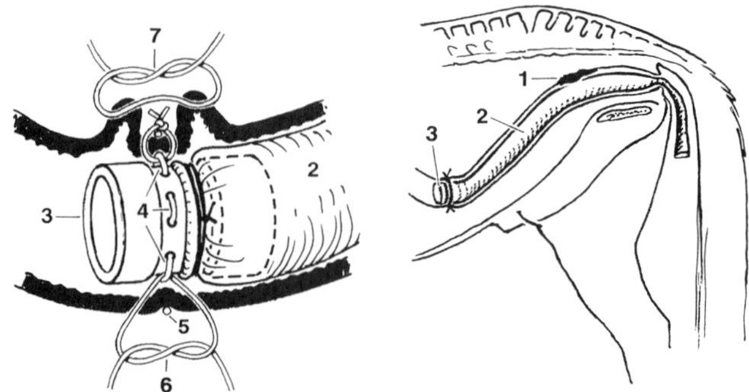

Figure 37-2. Placement of a temporary indwelling rectal liner to divert feces from a rectal tear. The expanded view demonstrates the construction of the liner and the method of securing it in place. 1, Tear; 2, rectal liner; 3, rectal prolapse ring; 4, Dacron anchor suture; 5, circumferential suture; 6, retention suture; 7, interrupted Lembert suture.

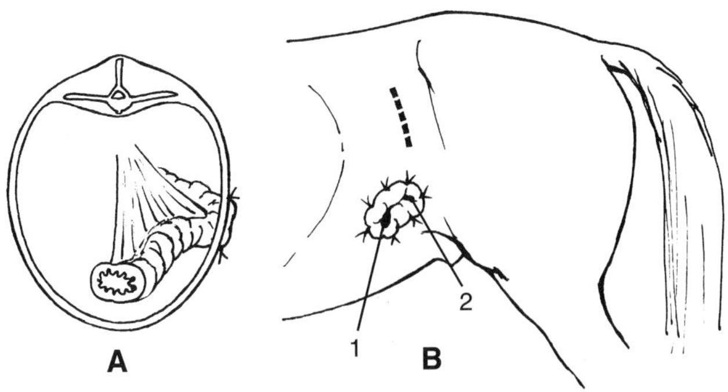

Figure 37-3. **A,** View through the transverse section of the abdomen shows the placement of the loop in the body wall. **B,** Loop colostomy created with a double-incision technique with the high flank approach *(broken lines)* and placement of the stoma in a small low flank incision. The left opening (1) is the proximal opening, and the right opening (2) is the distal opening through which the distal part of the small colon is flushed to prevent atrophy. (Redrawn from Freeman DE, Richardson DW, Tulleners EP, et al: Loop colostomy for management of rectal tears and small colon injuries in horses: 10 cases [1976-1989], J Am Vet Med Assoc 1992;200:1365.)

retraction of the sleeve into the rectum uncovering the tear, and formation of a rectoperitoneal fistula.[5,19]

Colostomy

LOOP COLOSTOMY

The loop-colostomy technique (Fig. 37-3) is preferred over the end-colostomy technique because it is easier and quicker to establish and to reverse later.[20,21] Concerns about incomplete diversion of feces do not apply to a loop colostomy in horses because gravity, combined with correct construction of the stoma, prevents passage of feces into the distal small colon and rectum.[20-22]

A loop colostomy can be created in a left high flank, a left low flank, or a ventral midline incision, and all have advantages and disadvantages (Table 37-1). A single-incision colostomy involves placing the stoma in the same incision used to explore the abdomen and prepare the colon loop, whereas a double-incision colostomy involves a separate flank incision for the stoma.[20] Exploration of the abdomen through the ventral midline is necessary if the horse has a surgical colic that preceded the tear,[21] if intra-abdominal repair of the tear is considered feasible,[14,23] or if the surgeon elects to empty the large and small colons to reduce stress on the colostomy. Colostomy placement in the anesthetized horse has the following *disadvantages:* (1) accurate placement of the stoma is difficult because muscle layers shift and landmarks become distorted in the recumbent horse compared with the standing horse, (2) it is expensive, and (3) dehiscence of the stoma is a risk of rough anesthetic recovery.[20,21] Marking the selected site on the skin with a pen or suture preoperatively while the horse is standing does not obviate the first problem, because the muscle layers disrupt the attachments when the horse stands, even when the skin incision is accurately located. With single-incision colostomies, incorporation of the colostomy in the abdominal closure weakens the body wall repair and makes the ventrally placed stomas, such as the low flank and ventral midline placements, prone to prolapse and herniation.[20] With the double-incision technique, the stoma is placed in a snug low flank incision so that it is surrounded by intact body wall and the risks of prolapse and herniation are reduced.[20]

With the double-incision technique, a high flank incision is used to prepare the colon loop and guide it into a separate low flank incision, midway between the flank fold (just rostral to the stifle) and the costal arch, and at the same level as the fold[20] (Figs. 37-4 and 37-5). The distal incision is approximately 8 cm long and extends through all layers, and deep dissection is guided by a hand through the high flank incision. It is angled dorsally at its caudal end by 20 to 30 degrees. Small transverse incisions are made in muscles and fascia to eliminate constricting bands that could restrict fecal passage. The stoma should not be large and loose fitting, because this would reduce the risk of stomal obstruction but predispose to the more serious complications of prolapse and herniation.[20,21]

If general anesthesia and ventral midline celiotomy are required, this stage of the surgery should be completed as needed to correct the problem. The horse is subsequently placed in lateral recumbency to complete the colostomy in a separate flank incision.[21] This somewhat reduces problems from shifting muscle layers when the horse stands. A heavy retrieval suture (size 2 nylon) is placed on the antimesenteric band of the prepared loop of small colon before closing the midline incision, so that only a small flank incision is

TABLE 37-1. Different Types of Colostomies in Horses

Type of Colostomy*	Abdominal Approach	Stoma Placement	Suitable as Standing Procedure	Suitable for Abdominal Exploration	Suitable for Emptying the Colon	Disadvantages
Single-incision	High flank	High flank	Yes	No	No	Fecal soilage of incision and skin
	Low flank	Low flank	No	No	No	Risk of prolapse and herniation
	Ventral midline	Ventral midline	No	Yes	Yes	Risk of prolapse and herniation
Double-incision	High flank	Low flank	Yes	No	No	Difficult construction
	Ventral midline	Low flank	No	Yes	Yes	Difficult construction

*Information applies to both loop and end colostomies.

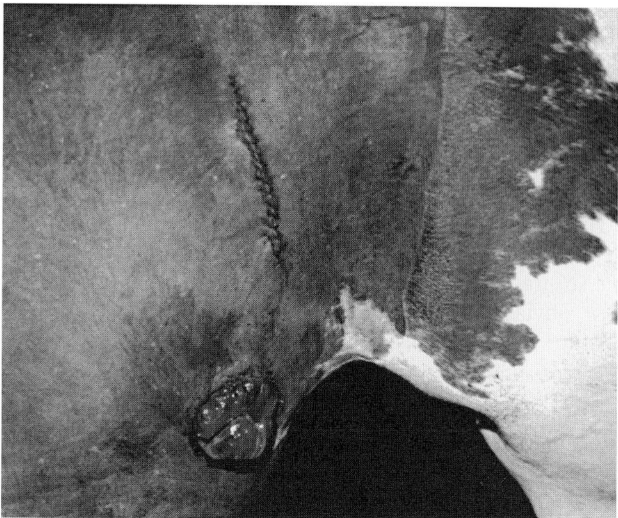

Figure 37-4. Loop colostomy placed in the low flank by a double-incision technique as a standing procedure 2 days earlier. Congestion in the mucosal shelf separating the proximal and distal parts of the small colon is typical for this stage.

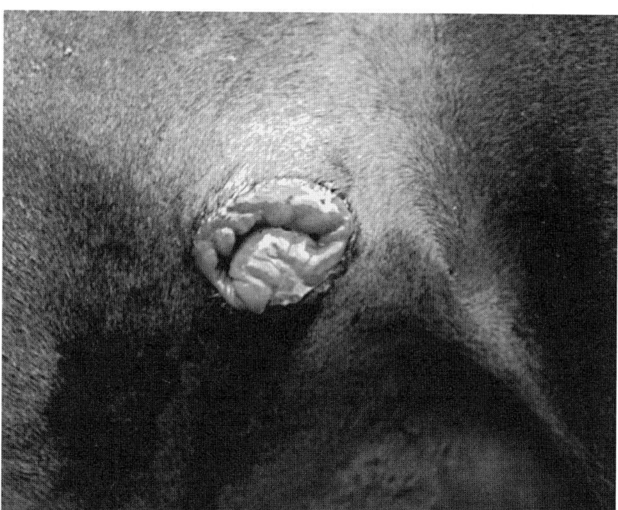

Figure 37-5. Loop colostomy placed in the low flank by a double-incision technique as a standing procedure, 60 days later (horse is not that shown in Fig. 37-4). The stoma is mature and healed to the surrounding skin; the mucosal shelf is evident as a small bulge in its midpoint.

required to form the colostomy.[5,21] The ends of the retrieval suture are placed on a long needle and brought through the body wall at the site marked for the colostomy.[5,21] The midline incision is closed, the horse is placed in lateral recumbency, and the low flank incision for the stoma is made as described earlier for the double-incision technique.[5,21] Unlike with the double-incision technique, the surgeon must bring the prepared loop of small colon through the small incision at the site of the stoma, without being able to direct the loop though a separate larger incision.

Regardless of the approach, the stoma is made in a segment of small colon at least 1 m from the rectum so that the small colon can be easily exteriorized for colostomy reversal. This segment of small colon is folded to form a loop, and the two arms of the loop are sutured together with an absorbable material in a continuous Lembert pattern for 8 to 10 cm, midway between the mesenteric and antimesenteric teniae.[21] This suture line is brought closer to the mesentery at the folded end of colon to turn the antimesenteric tenia along the outer edge of the fold.[20] The adhesion along this suture line creates a more complete mucosal separation between the proximal and distal segments of small colon and thereby enhances complete fecal diversion. The adhesion can also stabilize the loop within the body wall, reducing the risk of prolapse.[20] The prepared loop of small colon is subsequently inserted into the flank incision so that the proximal loop is slightly ventral to the distal loop and the antimesenteric tenia projects beyond the skin by at least 3 cm.[20]

The seromuscular layer of the colon is sutured to the abdominal muscles and fascia using several interrupted sutures of 0 or 2-0 absorbable material, taking care not to puncture or occlude mesenteric vessels.[20] To form the stoma, an 8-cm incision is made along the exposed antimesenteric tenia of the colon, and the cut edges are folded back and sutured to the skin with simple-interrupted sutures of 2-0 nylon or polypropylene[20] (see Fig. 37-3). The opening thus formed is approximately the same size as the small colon lumen[20] (see Fig. 37-5). Because fecal balls are eliminated individually as they pass through the small colon, without being stored to form piles, as in the rectum, the risk of obstruction is low.

An alternative method for loop colostomy is to suture the colon loop to skin only and to detach and oversew the stoma at 14 days.[24] The abdominal muscle layers and skin are then closed.[24] Disadvantages of this method are that such an attachment may allow peristomal herniation and that the rectal tear is unlikely to heal in 14 days.[20-22]

END COLOSTOMY

Some surgeons prefer an end colostomy because of the concern about incomplete fecal diversion with the loop colostomy method,[16,25] a concern most likely carried over from experiences with the supine human patient. However, the loop colostomy method does allow complete fecal diversion, because gravity causes fecal balls to drop away from the stoma rather than turn into the distal segment. For the end colostomy, the colon is transected, the distal segment is closed by the Parker-Kerr method, and the proximal end is incorporated into the body wall as for the loop colostomy.[26] The distal segment tends to atrophy, so its diameter and length may become reduced by 50%.[26] This makes colostomy reversal by future anastomosis difficult and causes anastomotic impactions and dehiscence.

AFTERCARE FOR COLOSTOMY

Antibiotics and laxatives (mineral oil, 2 to 4 L/450 kg, and magnesium sulfate, 1 g/kg) are continued for 3 to 5 days. Horses are held off feed or fed grass and alfalfa hay at half the usual amounts for the first 2 to 3 days after the colostomy is established, and petrolatum-based ointment is applied to the skin around the stoma to protect it from scalding. A cradle is applied because most horses have a tendency to mutilate the colostomy.

When the loop colostomy is created, the mucosal protrusion of the stoma becomes markedly congested over the first 5 to 7 days after surgery (see Fig. 37-4) and slowly sloughs, to be replaced with healthy tissue (see Fig. 37-5). Considerable ventral edema can develop, but it resolves with time.

With the loop colostomy, it is possible to exercise the distal part of the small colon and prevent the atrophy that complicates anastomoses with the end colostomy.[20,21] When the tear has started to granulate, usually after 5 to 7 days, the distal loop of the small colon and the rectum are flushed daily in normograde fashion with approximately 20 L of warm water through a garden hose.[20]

COLOSTOMY REVERSAL

For colostomy reversal, usually 6 weeks or more after the colostomy, the horse is anesthetized in right lateral recumbency, the stoma is resected en bloc, and a colonic anastomosis is performed through the resulting flank incision.[5,20] Even if the colon is not penetrated during dissection, incisional infection is a common complication of stomal resection.[20] Penrose drains should be inserted in deeper tissue layers and left in place for approximately 3 days.

For anastomosis, the distal segment is transected along a more acute mesenteric angle than the proximal segment to correct for a slight reduction in distal diameter. A single layer of interrupted Lembert sutures with 3-0 polydioxanone (PDS) is used for anastomosis[5] (Fig. 37-6), but other methods also are suitable. The stapled side-to-side technique is likely to become impacted despite the large stoma.[22] The postoperative feeding, antibiotic, and laxative regimens are similar to those used after the colostomy procedure.

COMPLICATIONS OF COLOSTOMY

Complications of colostomy are dehiscence, abscessation, peristomal herniation, prolapse, prolapse with rupture of mesenteric vessels, infarction, rupture of the colostomy, spontaneous closure,[6,27] and stomal obstruction, as well as anastomotic impaction and dehiscence after reversal. Herniation and prolapse have been attributed to ventral placement of the stoma and to a stoma that is too large.[20,21] There is a tendency to make the stoma large to prevent stomal obstruction, although stomal obstruction is rare, probably because fecal balls are voided individually.[20]

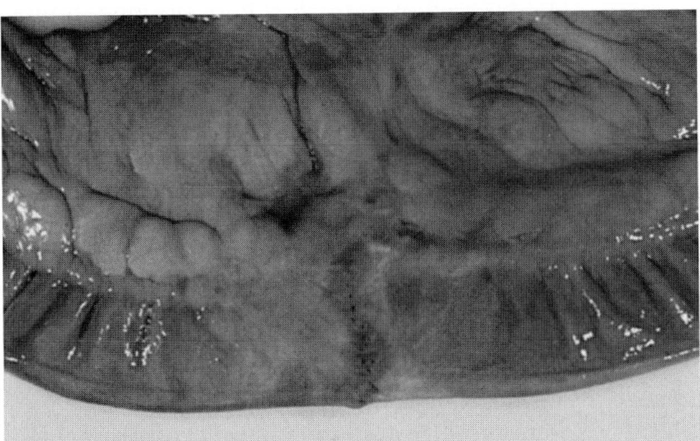

Figure 37-6. End-to-end anastomosis of the small colon with an interrupted Lembert pattern, using a 2-0 silk suture. The colostomy was reversed 21 days earlier, but the horse was euthanized because of laminitis.

CHOICE OF DIVERTING PROCEDURE

The choice between colostomy and temporary indwelling rectal liner for definitive treatment of a rectal tear is influenced largely by cost and by the surgeon's preference, because the two methods have comparable success rates.[12,19-22] The outcome is most likely to be determined by complications of the tear that developed before application of the diverting procedure.[20] Colostomy does have inherent, life-threatening risks and is more expensive because it is a two-stage procedure. A potential advantage of colostomy is that it allows the surgeon more complete control over the duration of fecal diversion,[20,21] which could be important if healing of the tear is delayed.[5] Colostomy is preferred for large tears, small horses, and a tear that is too far proximal to accommodate a rectal liner.[19]

The most difficult decision is whether a fecal diversion procedure is required at all, because some horses with grade III rectal tears can make a full recovery without surgery (see later).[3] Although few criteria can be used to guide treatment selection, the decision to use diverting procedures must be made quickly to derive full benefit, preferably within 12 hours after the tear occurred.[20,21] Because the cost of diverting procedures can be considerable, many owners may opt for less expensive procedures, such as direct suturing or medical treatment combined with repeated manual rectal evacuation.[28-30]

Suture Repair

Suture repair can promote healing and prevent progression of a grade III tear to a grade IV tear.[5,12,19] It should be combined with a diverting procedure if there is any concern about the integrity of the repair, but this is not always necessary and can be precluded for economic reasons. The surgery is easiest to accomplish on a thin horse with a tear that is fresh, clean, and close to the anus.[12,14] Long-handled instruments with pistol grips and a 60-cm-long expandable rectal speculum or "cage" have been developed to facilitate suture repair of rectal tears in horses.[31] The anal sphincter can be incised to improve access to a rectal tear and to ease defecation afterward.[32,33] A large wound of long duration can be partly closed or left open to allow drainage, and the defect can be packed with antiseptic-soaked gauze to prevent fecal impaction and dissection.[12,32] A grade IV tear has been repaired successfully with the TA-90 Premium stapling instrument (United States Surgical Corp, Norwalk, Conn), because the tear created a pneumoperitoneum and equilibration of pressure across the rectal wall that allowed it to be drawn through the anus.[34] If the rectal tear is not accessible through the anus, it can be prolapsed through it from a caudal ventral midline laparotomy[14] or repaired through an antimesenteric enterotomy from a ventral midline approach.[23] Suture repair under laparoscopic control[35] appears to be a promising method for the future, but the instruments may be too short in some cases.

A technique for nonvisual direct suturing has been reported to have favorable results and is a simple and inexpensive standing procedure.[12,28] If the tail is elevated and the anal sphincter relaxed from the caudal epidural anesthesia, the rectum fills with air and the surgeon has more room in which to manipulate the needle.[28] This ballooning effect is poor in rectums with grade IV tears because of the equilibration between intra-abdominal and atmospheric pressure, and it diminishes in grade III tears if surgery is prolonged. Fecal material is digitally removed from the rectum and distal small colon, and the defect and lumen walls are cleaned carefully and thoroughly by wiping with moistened 4×4 gauze sponges. If the tear does not involve the full thickness of the wall, gentle gravity lavage can be used to clean the tear. In a grade IV tear, the severity of peritoneal contamination determines whether a repair should be attempted.

The left hand is used for tears on the right side, and vice versa, and gloves are not worn.[28] The preferred suture is size 5 Dacron (Deknatel Inc, Fall River, Mass), 100 to 150 cm long, with a 6- to 8-cm, half-circle cutting or trocar point needle placed in the middle of the suture.[28] A cruciate or simple-interrupted pattern is used. With both ends of the suture outside the rectum, the needle is manually advanced to the tear. The first bite is placed in the center of the caudal edge of the tear, holding the needle with the thumb and first two fingers. The needle is inserted approximately 1.5 cm from the edge of the wound and guided into the defect subserosally by the second or third finger (Fig. 37-7). The needle is pulled through the tissue, again grasped with the thumb and first two fingers, and then placed in the center of the cranial edge. This bite begins subserosally within the defect and exits 1.5 cm from the edge. The third finger is used to guide the exit point and press the tissue onto the needle. The needle is subsequently brought out the rectum, leaving a single strand of suture in the tear with the other end extending 10 to 15 cm distal to the anal sphincter. The suture is then clamped with a hemostat between the needle and the point of exit from the tear and the needle remains threaded on the proximal half of the suture. An assistant holds the clamped suture to one side to close the defect into a transverse plane, and the needle is carried into the rectum. The suture is then passed through both cranial and caudal edges of the defect in one bite using digital manipulation as before, and finally the needle is brought out the rectum. The hemostat is released and the needle end of the suture is drawn through to form a cruciate suture. The knots are tied outside the rectum and pushed inside with one hand while tension is maintained on the suture with the other hand. Additional throws are placed to secure the knot.

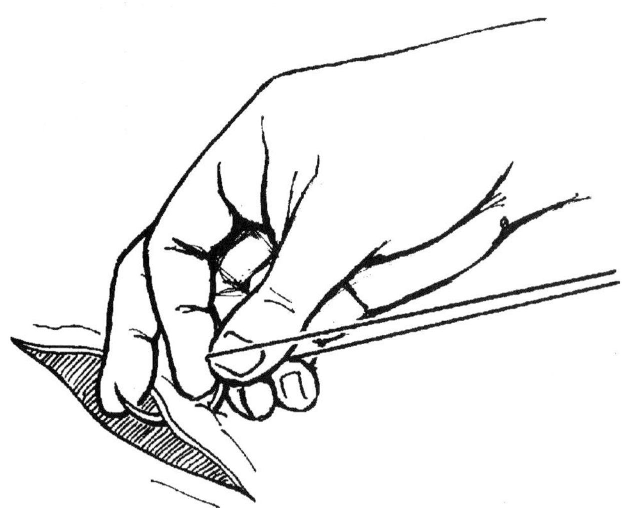

Figure 37-7. Diagram showing the first bite of the nonvisual direct suturing technique being placed in the center of the caudal edge of the tear. The needle, held with the thumb and first two fingers, is inserted approximately 1.5 cm from the edge of the wound and guided into the defect subserosally by the second or third finger. (Drawn from Eastman TG, Taylor TS, Hooper RN, Hague, BA: Treatment of grade 3 rectal tears in horses by direct suturing per rectum, Equine Vet Educ 2000;12:63, with permission.)

Traction on the first suture should convert the tear to a transverse orientation, which facilitates placement of about two or three more sutures on each side of the first.[28] Care must be taken to prevent lumen reduction by the closed defect as its edges turn into the lumen. The suture ends are cut long to facilitate their removal, but if the feces cannot be kept soft, the ends should be cut short so that they do not get pulled out by fecal balls.[28] The sutures are checked at 24- to 48-hour intervals, and any suture that feels slack from loosening or reduction of edema is replaced. The sutures are removed in 12 to 14 days.[28]

Nonvisual direct suturing may not be easily mastered and can require extensive practice.[28] It is a useful technique for tears involving half or less of the rectal circumference, and for tears that have very small perforations of the serosa, but it is recommended as an adjunct and not as a primary treatment for grade IV tears.[28]

The 45-cm-long Deschamps needle (Eickemeyer, Tuttlingen, Germany), which is made in both right- and left-handed configurations (Fig. 37-8), is ideal for one-handed suturing in a deep recess (Fig. 37-9) and has been used successfully for standing repair through the anus.[33] The needle tip should be sharp. Both chromic catgut and polyglycolic acid suture have been used. A right-handed surgeon guides the Deschamps needle rectally to the wound, with the left hand serving as protection and the right hand turning the handle[33] (see Fig. 37-9). The caudal end of the perforation is grasped with the index finger and thumb of the left hand, and the needle is guided through the mucosa, muscularis, and serosa (if present), about 1 cm away from the wound edge.[33] The ventral wound edge is penetrated, the suture is removed from the eye of the needle, and a surgical knot placed outside the rectum is pushed in with the left hand. An assistant pulls the ends of the first knot through the anus to stabilize the repair and bring the wound edges together. Additional single sutures are placed from caudal to cranial, 1 cm apart, so that the wound closes to form a ridge (see Fig. 37-9). If the suture bites exceed 1.5 cm from the wound's edge, the rectum becomes too narrow.[33]

The preferred suture for repair of rectal tears should be long, have low memory, resist stretching, and resist fecal digestion.[28] Small suture tends to cut through the friable tissue edges, and catgut tends to stretch.[28] Continuous suture patterns are not recommended because they reduce the lumen diameter, which predisposes to impaction and dehiscence.[28] A complete pellet ration can be fed after a 2-day fasting period to produce a small fecal bulk, and mineral oil can be used to soften feces.[28] Mineral oil is not used if the repair of a grade IV tear is tenuous, because it could leak into the abdomen.[28]

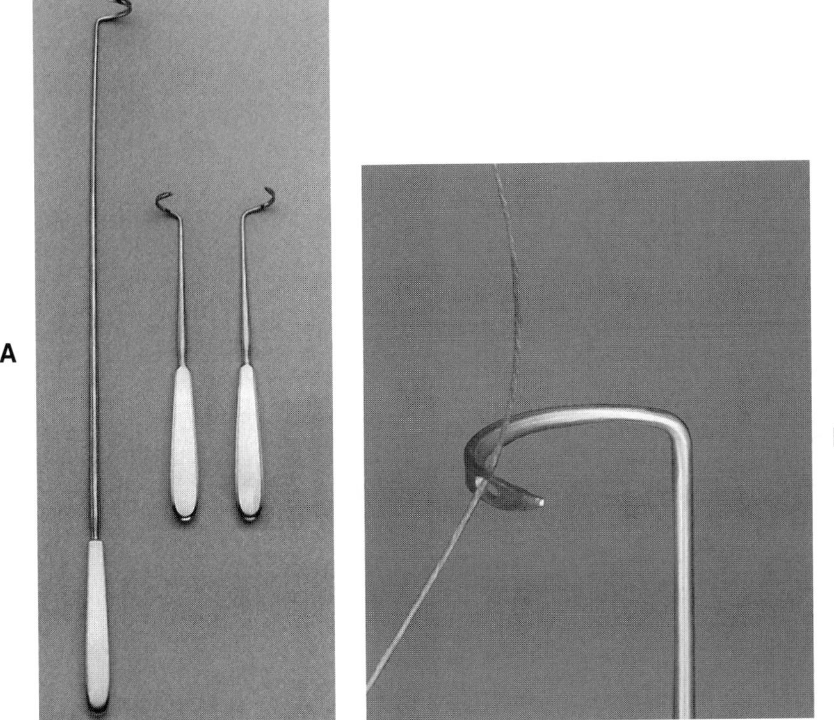

Figure 37-8. A, Deschamps needles, showing the right- and left-handed configurations with 20-cm needles *(right)* and the 45-cm needle that is suitable for rectal tears *(left)*. **B,** Close view of the end of a Deschamps needle. The threaded eye near the pointed tip allows easy retrieval of the suture without the need for complete penetration by the needle. Once the suture is grasped at the tip of the needle, the instrument is rotated backward out of the tissue and can be rethreaded for the next bite.

Nonsurgical Treatment

Grade I and II tears rarely require surgical treatment and grade I tears respond in most cases to antibiotics (e.g., trimethoprim sulfonamide, 20 mg/kg PO every 12 hours), and flunixin meglumine (1.1 mg/kg IV or PO, every 12 hours), mineral oil (1 gallon via nasogastric tube every 24 hours), and dietary changes such as bran mashes, moistened pellets, or grass to reduce fecal volume and soften the consistency. If all or a significant portion of the submucosa layer remains intact, grade I tears should heal with medical management without complications.

Although grade III tears usually require surgical treatment, medical management can be successful and is considerably less expensive than surgical methods.[13,29,30] In one report, six of eight horses with grade IIIb rectal tears were treated successfully with broad-spectrum antibiotics (penicillin, gentamicin, and metronidazole) and nonsteroidal anti-inflammatory agents, maintenance of soft feces with a diet of grass and bran mashes and daily administration of mineral oil by nasogastric tube, and daily manual removal of feces from the rectum after sedation and epidural anesthesia.[30] All horses developed septic peritonitis, and three of the six survivors developed a rectal diverticulum in the tear, without any apparent clinical effects.[30] The authors felt that manual evacuation of feces should be performed only if the tear became impacted, and the procedure should be conducted with extreme care.[30]

In another report on successful medical treatment of four horses with grade IIIb tears, the authors recommended frequent manual evacuation of feces on a daily basis.[29] Frequency of manual evacuation decreased from every 1 to 2 hours to every 6 to 8 hours by the 4th and 5th day, and the evacuations were discontinued between 9 and 21 days.[29] The underlying principle in this approach was to eliminate the storage function of the rectum and thereby eliminate impaction of feces into the tear.[29] Although this treatment is simpler to perform than bypass procedures, it is labor intensive and does require repeated epidurals through an epidural catheter.[29]

Full-thickness tears into the retroperitoneal space may be treated with manual evacuation of feces, antimicrobial therapy, fecal softener, and packing with gauze soaked in antiseptic solution until the defect fills with granulation tissue.[3,14,36] Perirectal abscesses that follow this treatment can be drained into the rectum or perianally with a chest trocar. Ventral tears in mares can be drained through the dorsal vaginal wall.[14] As with any method of treatment, peritonitis from the tear can be treated by peritoneal lavage, although this approach was not used in many cases reported in the literature.

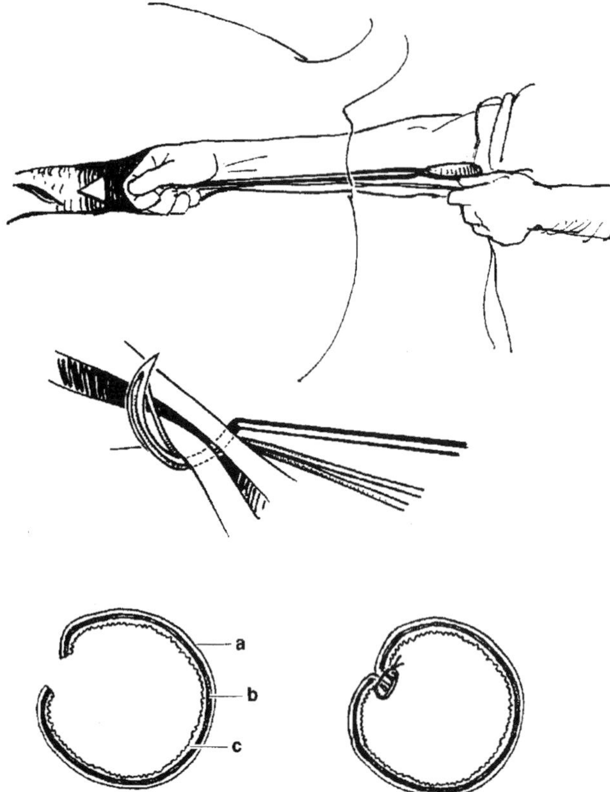

Figure 37-9. Method of inserting the Deschamps needle into the rectum and guiding it to the tear while protecting the tissues with the right hand. The close-up in the *middle* shows how the Deschamps needle grasps both sides of the tear and pulls the suture through it as well. The *lower* diagrams show the suture placement for a grade IV tear. a, serosa; b, muscularis; c, mucosa.

Prognosis for Rectal Tears

Complications of grade III rectal tears are extensive and include cellulitis, abscess formation, severe toxemia, peritonitis, laminitis, and recurrent intestinal obstruction from adhesions.[12,14,19-22] The time required for healing of rectal tears varies from 2 to several weeks.[19-22] Most tears heal with little residual damage, but some can form a stricture,[6] a diverticulum,[30] or perirectal abscessation.[20] Such abscesses must be drained into the rectum by finger puncture and can delay colostomy reversal for up to 60 days.[20,21] Grade III and IV tears can heal to form a mucosal or submucosal hernia that can subsequently become impacted with feces,[14] and a grade IV tear can form a rectoperitoneal fistula.[19]

In one survey of 85 horses, conservative management (medical treatment or no treatment) of 15 horses with grade I tears yielded a 93% survival rate.[11] Grade IIIa rectal tears had a 70% survival rate in this study (16 of 23 horses), and grade IIIb rectal tears had a 69% survival (9 of 13),[11] compared with a 44% survival rate in a previous study.[12] Survival for grade IV tears was 2 of 31 horses.[11]

Nonvisual direct suturing of rectal tears in the horse has a higher success rate than that reported for other techniques.[28] In one study, 75% (15 of 20) of horses treated by this technique survived until discharge. Eighty-one percent of horses (13 of 16) with grade IIIa tears, and 50% of horses (2 of 4) with grade IIIb tears were discharged alive after suture repair.[28] The sutures did not hold in three horses, and the tears converted to grade IV at 1 to 7 days after surgery, and one horse died of peritonitis from an unidentified grade IV tear oral to the sutured grade III tear.[28] Long-term follow-up was available for 10 of 15 survivors (66%), all of which survived at least 6 months. Horses discharged alive were hospitalized an average of 15 days (range, 9 to 24 days).

RECTAL PROLAPSE

Causes of rectal prolapse are straining from diarrhea, dystocia, intestinal parasitism, colic, proctitis, rectal tumor, and rectal foreign body.[16,37,38] In many cases, a cause cannot be identified. The condition is more common in females than in males and may affect any age group.[38]

Classification

In a type I rectal prolapse, only the rectal mucosa and submucosa project through the anus, sometimes more so on one side than on the other.[32,33] A type II lesion represents a complete prolapse of the full thickness of all or part of the rectal ampulla.[39,40] Type I and II prolapses are the most common.[38] In a type III prolapse, a variable amount of small colon intussuscepts into the rectum in addition to a type II prolapse.[39,40] In a type IV prolapse (Fig. 37-10), the peritoneal rectum and a variable length of the small colon form an intussusception through the anus.[39,40] This type of prolapse is seen with dystocia in mares.[16]

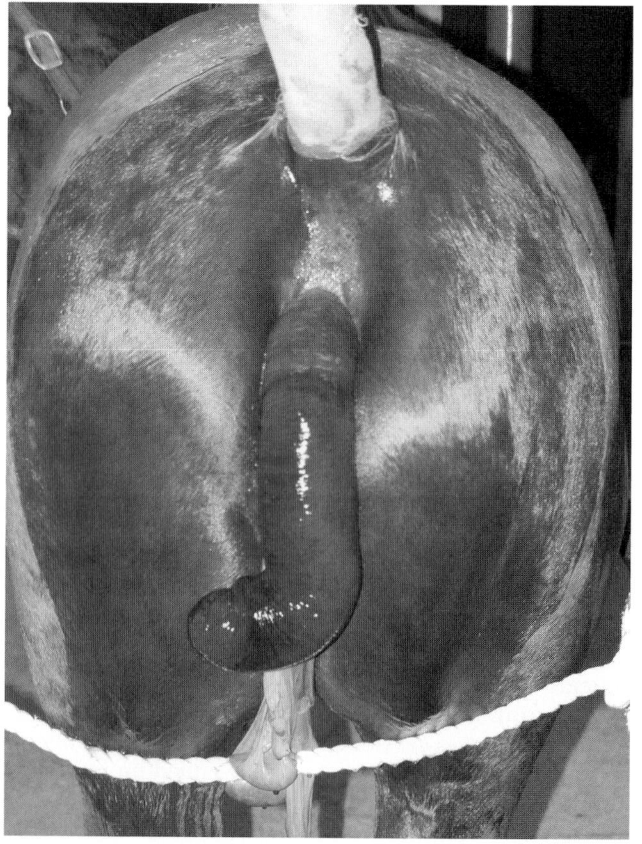

Figure 37-10. Type IV rectal prolapse in a postpartum mare.

Clinical Signs and Diagnosis

The usual presentation of a prolapse is a mucosal mass (types I, II, and III) or tube (type IV) protruding beyond the anus, with a variable amount of inflammation, cyanosis, bruising, or necrosis. Colic and peritonitis develop with types III and IV, and abdominocentesis should be performed in such cases.[41]

Treatment

Most early type I and II prolapses respond to reduction and treatment of the primary problem. In many type I and II prolapses, mucosal edema and irritation can be reduced by topical application of glycerin, sugar, magnesium sulfate, and lidocaine jelly, or lidocaine enemas (12 mL of 2% lidocaine in 50 mL of water).[16,17] Epidural anesthesia may be applied to reduce straining and to facilitate manual correction. To prevent recurrence, doubled 6-mm ($^1/_4$-inch) umbilical tape can be placed with four wide bites in loose pursestring fashion, 1 to 2 cm lateral to the anus. Normal feces cannot pass through the pursestring, so it has to be opened every 2 to 4 hours to allow defecation or manual removal of feces. Mineral oil enemas and intragastric infusions of mineral oil or other laxatives should be given as needed, and the horse should not be fed for 12 to 24 hours. From then on, a laxative diet should be fed for at least 10 days. If it is well tolerated, the pursestring suture can be left in place for 48 hours. If a horse with a type IV prolapse is to be referred to a hospital for definitive treatment and if the prolapsed tissue appears nonviable, it might be better to leave it prolapsed so the surgeons can evaluate and treat it. Reduction of necrotic tissue can lead to peritonitis and complicate treatment, because access through a celiotomy is limited, especially compared with access to the prolapsed tissue.

If type III and IV prolapses are treated by manual reduction alone, serial peritoneal fluid samples should be obtained to monitor changes in bowel wall viability.[38] Frank blood in the rectum after correction of a prolapse may be evidence of bowel necrosis.[42] Laparoscopy can be used to determine whether the mesocolon is ruptured and to assess viability of the involved small colon.[43] Access for resection of the necrotic bowel may be difficult through a celiotomy, and re-creation of the prolapse might be required to allow a submucosal resection outside the anus. A colostomy could be performed,[16,38] but continued necrosis ultimately leads to failure.[20]

Submucosal Resection

A submucosal resection may be indicated if the prolapsed tissues are devitalized, the prolapse recurs after conservative treatment, or the horse continues to strain.[38] The procedure can be performed with epidural or general anesthesia. After preparation for surgery, two 18-gauge, 15.0-cm (6-inch) spinal needles, or 14-gauge, 13-cm (5$^1/_4$ inch)-long Teflon catheters with the stylet in place are inserted at right angles to each other through the external anal sphincter and healthy mucosa to maintain the prolapse during dissection.[38] Starting at the 12 o'clock position, circumferential incisions are made in healthy tissue for one third of the prolapse circumference.[38] These incisions should be combined with deep dissection to elevate a strip of edematous and necrotic mucosa and submucosa. Remaining healthy proximal and distal edges of the mucosa and submucosa are apposed with size 1 or 2 medium chromic gut or PDS in an interrupted, horizontal mattress pattern.[38] These steps are repeated for each of the remaining thirds of the circumference until all necrotic tissue has been removed.[38] Mucosal edges are subsequently apposed with simple-interrupted sutures with buried knots, or preferably with a simple-continuous pattern interrupted at three equidistant points around the circumference.[38] A 2-0 absorbable suture material is used for this layer. The purpose of the mucosal suture is to cover all denuded areas and to prevent extensive granulation, scarring, and stricture formation.[38] Postoperative management includes laxatives, a laxative diet, and, if necessary, careful digital removal of impacted feces from the rectum.

Resection and Anastomosis

Resection and anastomosis may be indicated for type IV prolapse if the prolapsed tissues are devitalized or too much tissue is involved to allow reduction. The procedure can be performed as for submucosal resection, except that full-thickness circumferential incisions are made through the inner and outer walls of the intussusceptum in healthy tissue (Fig. 37-11). The healthy proximal and distal edges are apposed with size 1 or 2 PDS in an interrupted, full-thickness, horizontal mattress pattern (Fig. 37-12). These steps are repeated for each of the remaining thirds of the circumference until all necrotic tissue has been removed. Care must be taken during resection to identify and ligate any mesenteric vessels in the prolapse. Mucosal edges are then apposed in a simple-continuous pattern with 2-0 PDS, interrupted at three equidistant points around the circumference. The transfixing cross-needles and the weight of the necrotic tissue through most of the procedure maintain the line of anastomosis outside the rectum. Postoperative management is the same as for submucosal resection.[38]

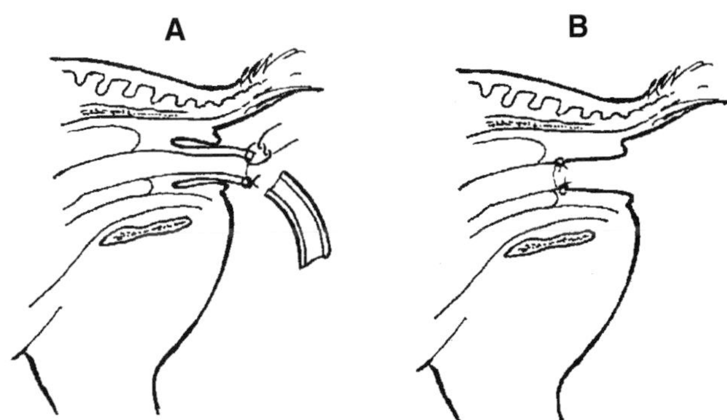

Figure 37-11. Treatment of a type IV rectal prolapse with intussusception of the distal part of the small colon and peritoneal segment of the rectum. **A,** The prolapsed tissues are resected as described and the healthy tissues anastomosed. **B,** When the stabilizing cross-catheters or needles are released, the anastomosis assumes its position in the proximal part of the rectum. (From Edwards GB: Diseases and surgery of the small colon, Vet Clin North Am Equine Pract 1997;13:359, with permission.)

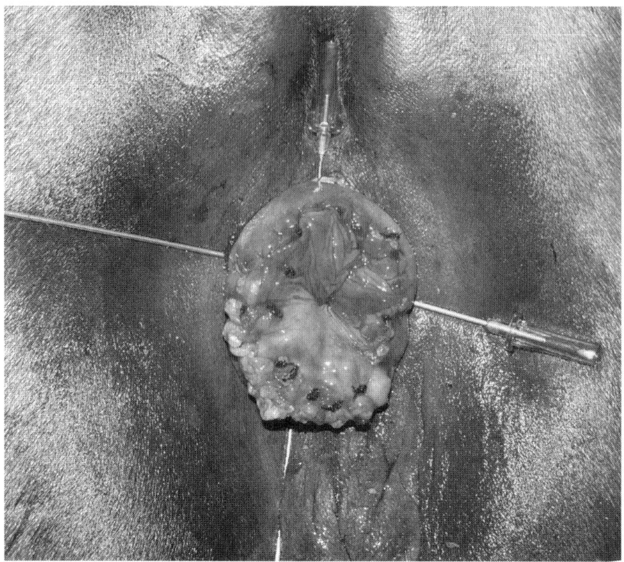

Figure 37-12. Partially completed anastomosis retained in position outside the anus with crossed 14-gauge, 5¼-inch-long Teflon catheters with the stylet in place. The mucosal closure has been completed on top and the visible sutures are full-thickness horizontal mattress sutures. This mare (the same one shown in Fig. 37-10) made a complete recovery.

Prognosis

The prognosis is favorable with types I and II prolapses, but the severity of vascular damage and mesenteric disruption worsens the prognosis for types III and IV prolapses.[39,42,44]

PERIRECTAL ABSCESS

In most cases, the cause of perirectal abscessation is unknown, although possible causes are rectal puncture or tear, rectal inflammation, and gravitation of a gluteal abscess after injection.[45] Enlarged anorectal lymph nodes have been reported as causes of rectal obstruction in young horses (3 to 15 months of age), and such nodes can progress to form abscesses.[46] *Streptococcus zooepidemicus* and *Escherichia coli* have been isolated.[45,46]

Clinical Signs and Diagnosis

The most common signs are low-grade abdominal pain and depression, anorexia, reduced fecal production, dyschezia, tenesmus, and fever.[45,46] Urinary tract dysfunction, manifested as dysuria, may develop from neuritis secondary to regional inflammation.[46] The abscess can be palpated as a firm submucosal mass. Purulent material can be aspirated for culture and sensitivity testing through a needle inserted percutaneously or through the rectal mucosa. Ultrasonographic examination is helpful, especially to monitor the response to treatment, but it cannot always provide a clear distinction between a reactive lymph node and an abscess, a hematoma, or a tumor.[46]

Treatment

Epidural anesthesia or sedation and local anesthesia are used for restraint. A lateral abscess can be drained lateral to the anus, a dorsal abscess can be drained into the rectum, and a ventral abscess can be drained into the vagina in mares or ventral to the anus in males. Postoperatively, the abscess cavity is flushed daily for approximately 6 days with a 10% povidone-iodine solution.[45] A laxative diet is fed, and mineral oil is given as needed by nasogastric tube.

Rarely, the abscess may involve abdominal organs and cause peritonitis.[45] An exploratory celiotomy may be required to drain the intra-abdominal component by marsupialization or to facilitate drainage into the rectum or vagina.[45] In horses without abdominal involvement, the prognosis for recovery is favorable.[45] Surgical drainage does not appear to be necessary in young horses with enlarged or abscessed anorectal lymph nodes, and a successful outcome is possible with treatment by antibiotics, analgesics, laxatives, and diet modification.[46]

ATRESIAS OF THE ANUS AND RECTUM

Atresia ani is rare[47] and may be associated with atresia coli, atresia recti, persistent cloaca, absence of a kidney, renal hypoplasia and dysplasia, absence of the tail, musculoskeletal deformities, micro-ophthalmia, rectourethral fistula, and other urogenital abnormalities.[48-56] Atresia coli is also rare (0.44% to 1.3% of hospitalized foals), and affected foals have a normal anus but may have a blind and empty rectum.[57]

Clinical Signs and Diagnosis

Signs of atresia ani are evident shortly after birth and include straining to defecate, tail flagging, abdominal discomfort, and abdominal distention. The anus is absent, but an anal sphincter may be present (Fig. 37-13). Signs of intestinal obstruction are not seen in foals with atresia and congenital rectovaginal fistula because they can void feces through the vagina. Three of seven foals in one study on atresia coli had atresia of the rectum or a blind-ending

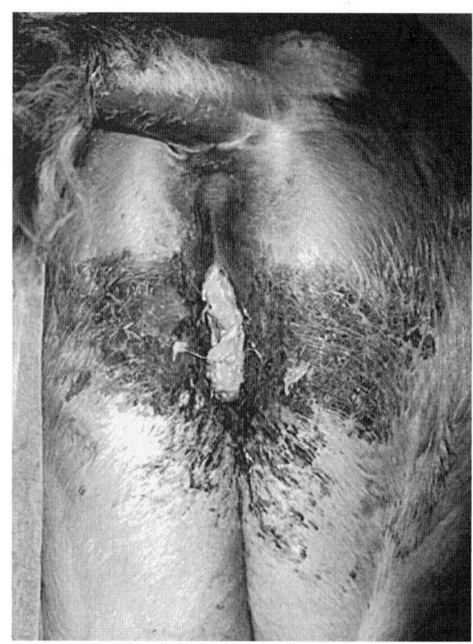

Figure 37-13. Atresia ani in a 5-day-old filly, with meconium staining of the perineum caused by defecation through a rectovaginal fistula.

rectum that could be diagnosed by digital palpation.[57] As with all foals with atresia coli, these foals had a history of failure to pass meconium and a lack of meconium staining of the perineum.[57]

Treatment

In foals with a complete rectal pouch, the persistent anal membrane is incised or a small circular piece of skin is removed, and the anal sphincter is spared, if possible. The rectal wall is subsequently sutured to the skin with simple-interrupted sutures. If the distal rectum is atretic, deeper dissection is needed. Any communication with the urogenital tract should be closed by transection between structures and closure by inverting sutures or by simultaneous closure and transection with autosuture instruments (GIA, United States Surgical Corporation). The prognosis for life is favorable, but normal anal function may not be obtained. The prognosis for atresia coli, with or without rectal involvement, is poor.[57]

POLYPS AND NEOPLASIA

The most common neoplasms of the perineal region and anus of the horse are squamous cell carcinomas and melanomas.[58-62] Squamous cell carcinomas are necrotic, foul smelling, and locally invasive lesions that metastasize slowly.[58] Diagnosis is based on biopsy. Treatments includes surgical excision, cryosurgery, electrosurgery, laser surgery, hyperthermia, radiation therapy, immunotherapy, and combinations of these methods.[58] Colostomy can be used to bypass rectal obstruction by a large tumor.[62]

Approximately 80% of Gray Horses over 15 years of age have melanomas.[59] Melanomas may be solitary or multiple, and they most commonly occur in the perineum and along the ventral surface of the tail[58] (Fig. 37-14). Although most equine melanocytic tumors are benign, dermal melanomatosis can occur on the perineum and have a high metastatic rate[63] (for details, see Chapter 29). Diagnosis is made by clinical features and biopsy.[63] Treatment is indicated if the lesion is large enough to cause clinical problems or is esthetically unacceptable. The treatment of choice is early excision or cryosurgery,[58] although removal of all lesions in a diffuse cluster is not always feasible or necessary. Successful treatment with radiation therapy, cimetidine, and bacillus Calmette-Guérin has been reported.[60]

Rectal polyps,[48] adenocarcinoma,[38] and leiomyosarcoma[64] are rare in horses and can be treated successfully by transection of attachments to the rectal mucosa.[38,64] A hamartomatous polyp (focal disordered growth of mature tissue indigenous to the organ affected) obstructed the distal part of the small colon in a 2-day-old Standardbred foal and caused abdominal pain, tenesmus, and rectal bleeding.[65] The mass could be identified on radiographs after a contrast enema, but it was not readily accessible for removal.[65] Rectal strangulation by a mesenteric lipoma has been treated successfully by twisting the lipoma off its pedicle through a colpotomy.[66]

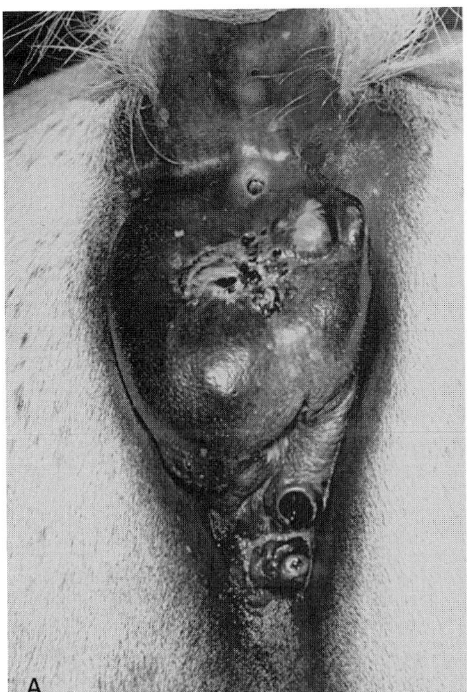

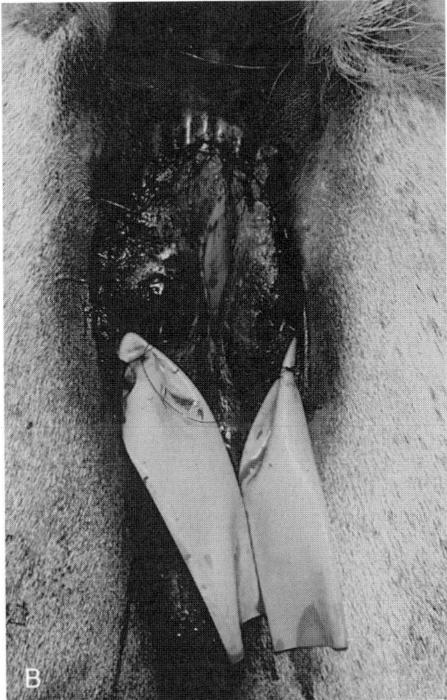

Figure 37-14. A, A large melanoma that deformed the anus and interfered with defecation. **B,** The same horse after excision. Penrose drains are placed in the dead space created by the deep perirectal dissection required to remove the large masses completely. Small tumors were not removed so that sufficient skin remained for closure.

REFERENCES

1. Sisson S: Equine digestive system. In Getty R, editor: Sisson and Grossman's The Anatomy of the Domestic Animals, ed 5, Philadelphia, 1975, WB Saunders.
2. Arnold S, Meagher D, Lohse C: Rectal tears in the horse, J Equine Med Surg 1978;2:55.
3. Mazan MR: Medical management of a full-thickness tear of the retroperitoneal portion of the rectum in a horse with hyperadrenocorticism, J Am Vet Med Assoc 1997;210:665.
4. Wilson JF, Quist CF: Professional liability in equine surgery. In Auer JA, editor: Equine Surgery, Philadelphia, 1992, WB Saunders.
5. Baird AN, Freeman DE: Management of rectal tears, Vet Clin North Am Equine Pract 1997;13:377.
6. Speirs VC, Christie BA, van Veenendaal JC: The management of rectal tears in horses, Aust Vet J 1980;56:313.
7. Reece D: Rectal rupture in a mare, Aust Vet Pract 1981;11:140.
8. Slone DE, Humburg JM, Jagar JE, et al: Noniatrogenic rectal tears in three horses, J Am Vet Med Assoc 1982;180:750.
9. Guglick MA, MacAllister CG, Ewing PJ, et al: Thrombosis resulting in rectal perforation in a horse, J Am Vet Med Assoc 1996;209:1125.
10. Scheidemann W, Huskamp NH, Odenkirchen S: Idiopathische Rektumruptur bei fünf Pferden, Tierärztl Prax 2003;31:1.
11. Eastman TG, Taylor TS, Hooper RN, et al: Treatment of rectal tears in 85 horses presented to the Texas Veterinary Medical Center, Equine Vet Educ 2000;12:342.
12. Watkins JP, Taylor TS, Schumacher J, et al: Rectal tears in the horse: An analysis of 35 cases, Equine Vet J 1989;21:186.
13. Alexander GR, Gibson KT: Non-surgical management of rectal tears in two horses, Aust Vet J 2002;80:137.
14. Arnold J, Meagher D: Management of rectal tears in the horse, J Equine Med Surg 1978;2:64.
15. Richardson D: Rectal tears. In Robinson NE, editor: Current Therapy in Equine Medicine, Philadelphia, 1983, WB Saunders.
16. Rick MC: Management of rectal injuries, Vet Clin North Am Equine Pract 1989;5:407.
17. Brown MP: Conditions of the rectum, Vet Clin North Am Large Anim Pract 1982;4:185.
18. Baird AN, Taylor TS, Watkins JP: Rectal packing as initial management of grade 3 rectal tears, Equine Vet J Suppl1989;7:121.
19. Taylor TS, Watkins JP, Schumacher J: Temporary indwelling rectal liner for use in horses with rectal tears, J Am Vet Med Assoc 1987;191:677.
20. Freeman DE, Richardson DW, Tulleners EP, et al: Loop colostomy for management of rectal tears and small colon injuries in horses: 10 cases (1976-1989), J Am Vet Med Assoc 1992;200:1365.
21. Freeman DE, Robertson JT, Richardson DW, et al: Loop colostomy for management of rectal and small colon injuries in horses, Proc Am Assoc Equine Pract 1992;38:133.
22. Blikslager AT, Bristol DG, Bowman KF, et al: Loop colostomy for treatment of grade-3 rectal tears in horses: Seven cases (1983-1994), J Am Vet Med Assoc 1995;207:1201.
23. Wilson DG, Stone WC: Antimesenteric enterotomy for repair of a dorsal rectal tear in a mare, Can Vet J 1990;31:705.
24. Shires M: The temporary loop colostomy: Another choice. In Byars TD, Moore JN, White NA, editors: Equine Colic Symposium, Athens, Ga, 1982, University of Georgia Press.
25. Stashak TS, Knight AP: Temporary diverting colostomy for management of small colon tears in the horse: A case report, J Equine Med Surg 1978;2:196.
26. Herthel DJ: Colostomy in the mare, Proc Am Assoc Equine Pract 1974;20:187.
27. Azzie MAJ: Temporary colostomy in the management of rectal tears in the horse, J South Afr Vet Assoc 1975;46:121.
28. Eastman TG, Taylor TS, Hooper RN, et al: Treatment of grade 3 rectal tears in horses by direct suturing per rectum, Equine Vet Educ 2000;12:63.
29. Katz LM, Ragle CA: Repeated manual evacuation for treatment of rectal tears in four horses, J Am Vet Med Assoc 1999;215:1473-1477.
30. Mair TS: The medical management of eight horses with grade 3 tears, Equine Vet J Suppl 2000;32:104.
31. Spensley MS, Meagher DM, Hughes JP: Instrumentation to facilitate surgical repair of rectal tears in the horse: A preliminary report. Proc Am Assoc Equine Pract 1985;31:553.
32. Embertson RM, Hodge RJ, Vachon AM: Near circumferential retroperitoneal rectal tear in a pony, J Am Vet Med Assoc 1986;188:738.
33. Huskamp B: Die operative Versorgung von Mastdarmverletzungen, Prakt Tierarzt 1994;11:943.
34. Stewart RH, Robertson JT: Surgical stapling for repair of a rectal tear in a horse, J Am Vet Med Assoc 1990;197:746.
35. Brugmans F, Deegen E: Laparoscopic surgical technique for repair of rectal and colonic tears in horses: An experimental study, Vet Surg 2001;30:409.
36. Schumacher J: Rectal tears of horses, Equine Vet Ed 1999;11:23-28.
37. Levine SB: Surgical treatment of recurrent rectal prolapse in a horse, J Equine Med Surg 1978;2:248.
38. Turner TA, Fessler JF: Rectal prolapse in the horse, J Am Vet Med Assoc 1980;177:1028.
39. Turner TA: Rectal prolapse. In Robinson NE, editor: Current Therapy in Equine Medicine, ed 2, Philadelphia, 1987, WB Saunders.
40. O'Connor JJ: Dollar's Veterinary Surgery, ed 4, Chicago, 1943, Alexander Eger.
41. Ross MW, Stephens PR, Reimer JM: Small colon intussusception in a broodmare, J Am Vet Med Assoc 1988;192:372.
42. Jacobs KA, Barber SM, Leach DH: Disruption of the blood supply to the small colon following rectal prolapse and small colon intussusception in a mare, Can Vet J 1982;23:132.
43. Ragle CA, Southwood LL, Galuppo LD, et al: Laparoscopic diagnosis of ischemic necrosis of the descending colon after rectal prolapse and rupture of the mesocolon in two postpartum mares, J Am Vet Med Assoc 1997;210:1646.
44. Livesey MA, Keller SD: Segmental ischemic necrosis following mesocolic rupture in postparturient mares, Comp Cont Educ Pract Vet 1986;8:763.
45. Sanders-Shamis M: Perirectal abscesses in six horses, J Am Vet Med Assoc 1985;187:499.
46. Magee AA, Ragle CA, Hines MT, et al: Anorectal lymphadenopathy causing colic, perirectal abscesses, or both in five young horses, J Am Vet Med Assoc 1997;210:804.
47. Priester WA, Glass AG, Waggoner NS: Congenital defects in domesticated animals: General considerations, Am J Vet Res 1970;31:1871.
48. Keller SD, Horney FD: Diseases of the small colon, Comp Cont Educ Pract Vet 1985;7:S113.
49. Furie WS: Persistent cloaca and atresia ani in a foal, Equine Pract 1983;5:30.
50. Brown CM, Parks AH, Mullaney TP, et al: Bilateral renal dysplasia and hypoplasia in a foal with an imperforate anus, Vet Rec 1988;116:91.
51. Chaudhry NI, Cheema NI: Atresia ani and rectovaginal fistula in an acaudate filly, Vet Rec 1980;107:95.
52. Kingston RS, Park RD: Atresia ani with an associated urogenital tract anomaly in foals, Equine Pract 1982;4:32.
53. Gideon L: Anal agenesis with rectourethral fistula in a colt, Vet Med Small Anim Clin 1977;72:238.
54. Schneider JE: Agenesis or atresia of the colon in newborn foals, Proc Am Assoc Equine Pract 1981;27:285.
55. Baker GJ: Covered anus with anobulbar fistula in an Arabian foal, Vet Surg 1987;16:82.
56. Fuchslocher D, Rusch K: Atresia recti bei einem Vollblutfohlen, Dtsch Tierärztl Wochenschr 1971;78:519.
57. Nappert G, Laverty S, Drolet R, et al: Atresia coli in 7 foals (1964-1990), Equine Vet J 1992;13:57.

58. Scott DW: Large Animal Dermatology, Philadelphia, 1988, WB Saunders.
59. Stannard AA, Pulley LT: Tumors of the skin and soft tissues. In Moulton JE, editor: Tumors in Domestic Animals: II. Berkeley, 1978, University of California Press.
60. Vaughan JT: Equine urogenital system. In Jennings PB, editor: The Practice of Large Animal Surgery, Philadelphia, 1984, WB Saunders.
61. Madewell BR, Theiler GH: Skin tumors of mesenchymal origin. In Theiler GH, Madewell BR, editors: Veterinary Cancer Medicine, Philadelphia, 1987, Lea & Febiger.
62. Wilson DA: Management of perianal squamous cell carcinoma with permanent colostomy in a mare, J Am Vet Med Assoc 1994;205:1430.
63. Valentine B: Equine melanocytic tumors: A retrospective study of 53 horses (1988 to 1991), J Vet Intern Med 1995;9:291.
64. Clem MF, DeBowes RM, Leipold HW: Rectal leiomyosarcoma in a horse, J Am Vet Med Assoc 1987;191:229.
65. Colbourne CM, Bolton JB, Yovich JV, et al: Hamartomatous polyp causing intestinal obstruction and tenesmus in a neonatal foal, Aust Equine Vet 1996;14:78-80.
66. Mason TA: Strangulation of the rectum of a horse by the pedicle of a mesenteric lipoma, Equine Vet J 1978;10:269.

CHAPTER 38

Abdominal Hernias

John A. Stick

A hernia is a protrusion of an organ or tissue through an abnormal opening.[1] Hernias usually involve protrusion of abdominal contents through part of the abdominal wall, the diaphragm, or the inguinal canal. The defect or opening in the abdominal wall is an important factor in herniation, whether a protrusion through the opening is present or not.[2]

CLASSIFICATION

Various classification schemes are used to characterize hernias. One scheme names the hernia by the type of herniated tissue, such as intestine or omentum. Another classification scheme uses epidemiology of the hernia, wherein they are referred to as either congenital or acquired hernias. A congenital hernia is a defect that is present at birth, although the protrusion may not develop until later. In an acquired hernia, the defect occurs after birth and may be to the result of blunt trauma, surgical trauma (wound disruption), degeneration (prepubic tendon rupture in late pregnancy mares), or because of an increased diameter of a normal body opening (inguinal canal).

A third classification scheme defines a hernia by the opening or defect. In true hernias, the protrusion occurs through a normal aperture in the abdomen and contains a complete peritoneal sac (inguinal or scrotal hernia). These hernias are sometimes referred to as indirect hernias. Conversely, in false hernias, the protrusion does not arise through a normal aperture in the abdomen. False hernias do not initially contain a complete peritoneal sac and are usually created by trauma to the abdomen or develop after breakdown of a surgical entry (incisional hernias). These are also referred to as direct hernias.

Hernias may be further categorized as reducible, incarcerated, or strangulated. A hernia is classified as reducible when the protruding hernial contents are freely movable and can readily be manipulated back into the abdominal cavity. When the hernial contents cannot be reduced, the hernia is classified as incarcerated (or irreducible), and this is frequently the result of adhesions that form between the contents and the surrounding tissue, effectively fixing the contents in an abnormal location. Incarceration frequently causes obstruction of the lumen of a hollow viscus, and either signs of bladder or bowel obstruction may be the presenting complaint. A hernia is classified as strangulated when incarceration obstructs the vascular supply to the herniated tissue, usually at the edge of the defect. Strangulation usually results in tissue necrosis and is the most serious type of hernia.

The anatomic site of herniation is frequently used for classification and allows the best discussion of etiology, clinical signs, and treatment. In this chapter, abdominal hernias are divided into umbilical, ventral midline (incisional), lateral abdominal, diaphragmatic (internal abdominal), and caudal abdominal (inguinal) hernias.

ANATOMY OF A HERNIA

Hernias consist of three portions: the ring, the sac, and the contents.[2] The ring forms the actual defect in the limiting wall and may be small or quite large. Wound healing leads to thickening of the leading edge of the ring through collagen maturation, which usually allows its borders to be identified through digital palpation. If this healing results in contraction of the scar, contents may become strangulated. Inflammation in the sac from trauma to the contents frequently leads to incarceration. Loops of intestine frequently move in and out of the ring of the hernia through peristalsis. Sometimes this leads to strangulation when the contents enter at a rate faster than they leave. Additionally, secretion of fluid into the bowel segment located in the hernial sac may cause distention and may eventually lead to strangulation.

The hernial sac is made up of tissues that cover the contents. This usually includes the mesothelial covering. In the initial stages, peritoneum may not line the sac of the hernia; however, chronic hernias are frequently completely lined with peritoneum. Although the contents of an abdominal hernia are usually parts of the intestine, other structures such as the omentum frequently are involved. The type of bowel in the hernial sac frequently predicts the clinical signs that are seen.

SIGNS OF HERNIATION

Most external abdominal hernias have swelling as a classic sign. However, internal abdominal hernias (diaphragmatic hernias) frequently show signs attributed to intestinal obstruction or respiratory problems. In uncomplicated external hernias, no pain may be elicited on palpation, and the consistency of the swelling depends on the contents. When inflammation or infection or luminal distention of a viscus is present, a definitive diagnosis is difficult to make on palpation alone. Also, the site of the swelling may be some distance from the actual hernial ring, as contents can migrate into the subcutaneous space. However, a tentative diagnosis is frequently made on the basis of clinical signs and location of the swelling. Palpation becomes an important part of the examination to determine if the hernia is reducible, incarcerated, or strangulated. Infrequently, radiography shows luminal gas distention if the hernia contents are bowel in origin. Diagnosis is frequently confirmed by reduction of the hernia and palpation of the hernial ring. The incarcerated hernia presents more of a diagnostic challenge, and ultrasonography is the diagnostic modality of choice in these instances. Fine-needle aspiration to try to rule out hernial contents is contraindicated, as it frequently results in contamination of an otherwise uninfected site.

UMBILICAL HERNIAS

The most common type of hernia in the horse is umbilical in origin and is estimated to occur in 0.5% to 2.0% of foals (Fig. 38-1). Most umbilical hernias are congenital and may have a hereditary component. In a recent study of the closure of a body wall defect at the umbilicus, 19 of 44 foals had a defect in the body wall at the umbilicus with a palpable umbilical ring at birth.[3] This defect closed within 4 days in 18 of these foals. Additionally, in this same study, 12 of 44 foals developed an umbilical hernia between 5 and 8 weeks of age.

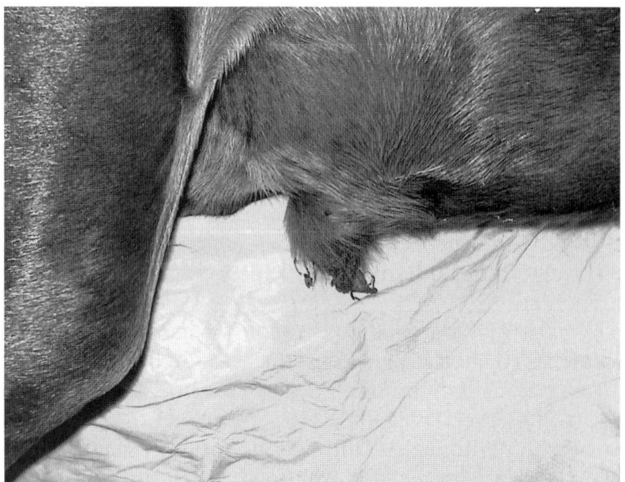

Figure 38-1. Typical appearance of an umbilical hernia in a 3-day-old foal. The majority of umbilical hernias in foals at this age spontaneously regress within the first 3 weeks of life.

Etiology

The development of umbilical hernias has been attributed to trauma to the umbilical cord during birth, excessive straining, and umbilical cord infection.[4] Very rarely, evisceration occurs immediately after the birth as a result of trauma to the umbilical cord. This condition necessitates emergency surgical reconstruction in the abdominal wall. However, in most foals, umbilical hernias are chronic in nature, small, and uncomplicated by underlying organic diseases. They usually represent a cosmetic defect but are a potential site of bowel incarceration. In fact, between 8% and 10% of umbilical hernias referred to tertiary hospitals sustain complications that are life threatening and mandate emergency surgery.[5]

Diagnosis

Digital palpation of the hernia determines the size and shape of the hernia ring, the nature of the contents of the sac, and the reducibility of the hernia. Firm, thickened rings hold sutures quite well during herniorrhaphy, whereas a thin and indistinct ring is an indication that repair may be more difficult. Hernial sacs usually contain subperitoneal fat, omentum, or intestine. These hernias are almost always reducible and are rarely incarcerated. However, when incarceration does occur, strangulation of a portion of the intestinal wall is usually suspected. In some instances, only a portion of the intestinal wall is incarcerated (Richter's hernia or parietal hernia), and luminal wall destruction usually does not occur. When incarceration is present, any increase in hernia size, firmness, edema, or pain on palpation is an indication that surgery should be undertaken as soon as possible. Umbilical hernias need to be differentiated from abscessation and local infection of the umbilical cord and associated structures. Ultrasonographic examination of the hernia and ventral abdominal wall is indicated to determine the nature of the hernial contents in complicated hernias of this type (Fig. 38-2).

Treatment

Reducible umbilical hernias less than 5 cm in diameter frequently close spontaneously as the foals mature. Daily digital reduction of the hernia is indicated to monitor for changes in size or incarceration of hernia contents. Hernias that are not spontaneously regressing by the time the foal is 4 months old should be surgically repaired.

Umbilical hernias greater than 10 cm in diameter are not treated with conservative methods because the risk of strangulating obstruction is so great. Additionally, a hernia of that size very rarely closes on its own. Although most umbilical hernia repairs are elective procedures and are performed on foals for cosmetic reasons, obviously strangulating obstructions of the small intestine necessitate emergency repair.

Two methods have been historically used for repairing hernias. The application of a hernia clamp is one method of management, but this is not commonly practiced and therefore is not part of this discussion. It poses a serious complication if entrapment of the intestine into the hernial clamp occurs, and this has led to intestinal obstruction,

A

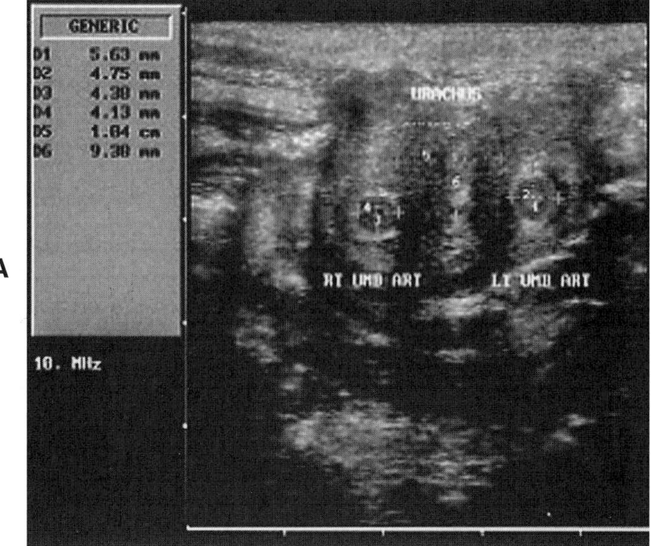

B

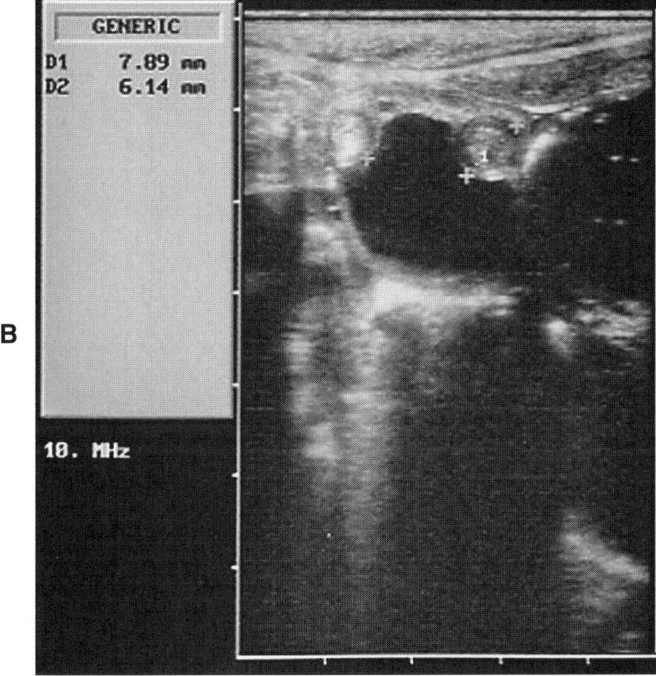

Figure 38-2. A, Sonogram of the urachus and both umbilical arteries obtained from a 1-week-old Thoroughbred foal with an umbilical hernia. The umbilical arteries are normal. **B,** Sonogram of the umbilical arteries obtained from a 12-day-old foal with omphalophlebitis. Notice the thickened left umbilical artery with the swollen hyperechoic vessel wall and hypoechoic fluid center.

peritonitis, or enterocutaneous fistulas. Also, inadvertent dislodging of the clamp has led to eventration. Because of these complications, this technique is strongly discouraged.

Surgical repair of umbilical hernias is accomplished with the horse in dorsal recumbency and under general anesthesia. Careful preparation of the surgical site is especially important in male foals, in which the preputial orifice should be temporarily closed with sutures to reduce contamination during surgery. Surgical repair is initiated by making an elliptical skin incision around the hernia, with the points of the ellipse cranial and caudal (Fig. 38-3). Skin and loose subcutaneous tissue are removed to expose the external sheath of the rectus abdominal muscle. Sharp dissection generally results in less swelling than blunt dissection in this area, and this dissection is continued to about 1 cm peripheral to the hernial ring. The hernial sac can be inverted and the hernia repaired without removal (closed technique). However, the sac is usually removed (open technique). To do this, the hernial sac is incised along the edge of the hernial ring (see Fig. 38-3, *E*). The contents of the sac are examined. It is unusual, but abscesses in the umbilical veins and umbilical remnants can be entered at this point, and care should be taken, especially in the caudal aspect of the incision, to prevent such mishaps. Once the contents have been inspected and appropriately treated, the body wall should be closed. Varying suture materials and patterns can be used; however, a nicer closure without a dog-ear can be achieved if the ventral body wall defect is converted to an ellipse with the point cranial and caudal, similar to the skin incision before closure. A simple-continuous appositional suture pattern is recommended using appropriate-size absorbable suture material. Synthetic monofilament absorbable suture material (1, 2, or 3) is selected on the basis of the body size of the patient. Thereafter, the subcutaneous tissues and skin are closed independently, once again using absorbable suture material in a simple-continuous pattern.

Aftercare

An abdominal support wrap is applied to decrease dead space and reduce edema for about 48 hours. The foal should be confined for 30 to 45 days. Skin sutures do not need to be removed if absorbable suture material has been used. Although laparoscopic surgery is described (see Chapter 71) for disorders of the foal umbilical structures, there are few indications for laparoscopic surgery of umbilical hernias.

VENTRAL MIDLINE HERNIAS

Ventral hernias usually occur as a result of inadequate healing of a previous incision or excessive strain at the site of an abdominal wall scar (Fig. 38-4). Obesity, age, and wound infection are the most common predisposing causes in people,[6] and the incidence is between 1% and 11%. Risk factors for incisional hernias in dogs include intra-abdominal pressure because of pain, entrapped fat between hernia edges, inappropriate suture material use, chronic steroid treatment, and infection.[7] Although sequelae to incisional hernias are often serious and costly, the incidence is much lower in small animals.

In horses, large abdominal wall defects commonly arise from partial incisional dehiscence after ventral midline celiotomy or after failed umbilical herniorrhaphy. Incisional herniation is strongly associated with wound separation. With the proper suture placement, suture selection (in terms of size and material), and soft tissue handling using aseptic technique, primary-intention healing of a ventral midline incision usually occurs. Experimentally, optimal bite size is 15 mm from the incision edge ($\frac{1}{2}$ inch).[8] Ninety-three percent of sutures fail at the knot and suture loops fail

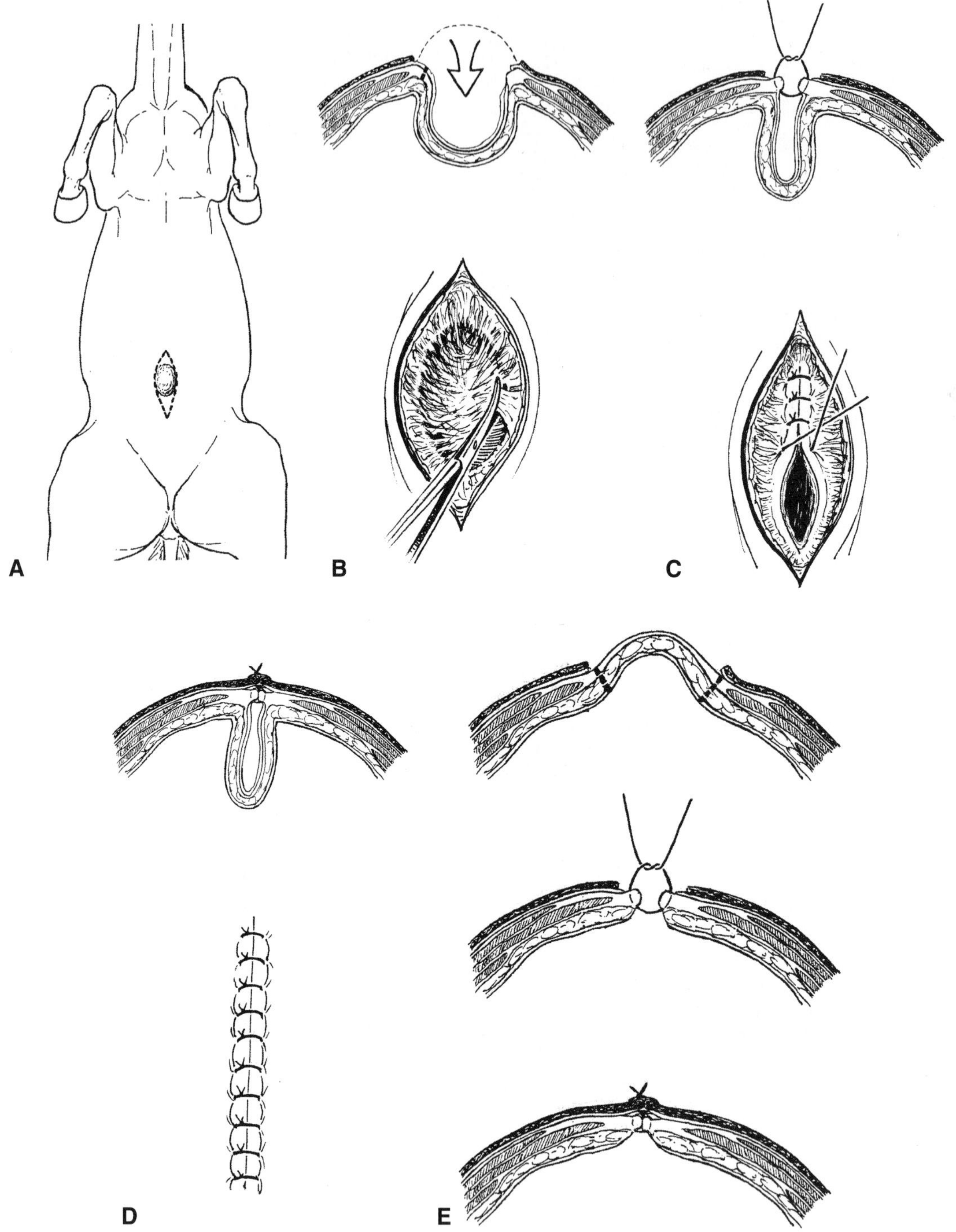

Figure 38-3. Illustrations of umbilical hernia repair. **A,** An elliptical skin incision is made around the hernial sac. The skin is dissected free from the hernial sac and discarded. **B,** The hernial ring is dissected free from the surrounding hernial sac so that the ring can be clearly identified. **C,** The sac can be inverted and the ring prepared for suturing, or the hernial sac can be removed. (The latter technique allows the round hernial ring to be converted into an ellipse for easier closure.) **D,** The ring is closed with a simple-continuous suture of appropriate-size suture material, and the subcutis and skin are closed in separate layers. **E,** In most cases, the open technique is applied: the hernia sac is excised and, after brief inspection of the abdominal cavity, the abdominal wall is closed in three layers.

before complete fascial disruption. The strongest synthetic absorbable suture materials tested were 3 polyglactin 910 and 2 polyglycolic acid. Because the linea alba is thickest near the umbilicus and tends to become thinner cranially, it has been suggested that the cranial portion of the linea alba may be more susceptible to dehiscence. Clinically, the hernias that develop are usually located in the cranial portion of the incision rather than near the umbilicus. In one study of 210 horses undergoing midline celiotomy for abdominal disease, the incisional hernias were as high as 16%, and all hernias were evident within 4 months of surgery.[9]

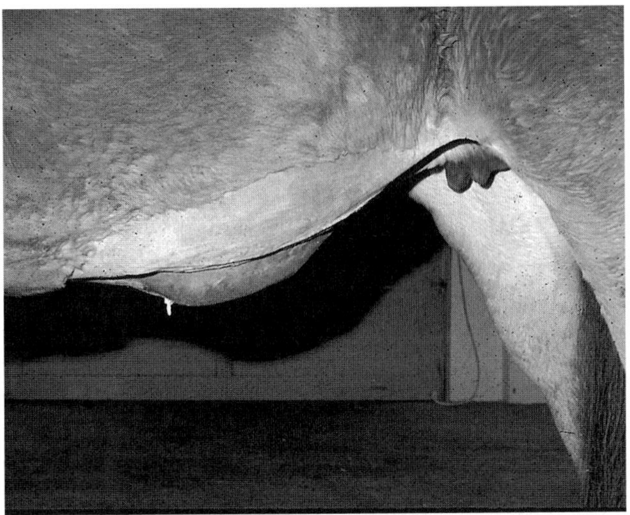

Figure 38-4. Appearance of a ventral abdominal hernia that occurred from dehiscence of a celiotomy incision. Note the purulent material at the cranial aspect of the hernia.

In addition to sepsis, other factors that may affect breakdown of an incision are abdominal distention immediately after recovery, and incisional trauma from excessive struggling during recovery from general anesthesia, or from rolling associated with uncontrolled postoperative pain.[4] For the purposes of treatment, incisional hernias may be broken down into two types: acute total dehiscence and chronic insidious hernia formation.

Acute Total Dehiscence

Disruption of the abdominal incision that occurs within the first 4 to 7 days after surgery constitutes an emergency to prevent eventration. A belly bandage should be applied for support and the horse anesthetized for the repair. Complete acute dehiscence is detected by observing excessive peritoneal fluid leaking from the incision and palpable gaps in the sutured abdominal wall. The horse is placed in dorsal recumbency and all sutures are removed and the site prepared for surgery.

All devitalized tissue is sharply incised and removed. The wound is cultured and thoroughly flushed. The septic surgical closure uses monofilament stainless steel wire to close the abdominal wound. This is a through-and-through interrupted vertical mattress pattern, with sutures placed 2 to 3 cm apart. This suture is passed through skin, fascia, and rectus abdominal muscle about 5 cm from the wound edge (Fig. 38-5). The wire is passed through hard rubber tubing used as stents before the close bites of the vertical mattress pattern are placed. These bites are taken 2.5 cm from the wound edge. The rubber suture is necessary to reduce the tendency of the wire to cut through the skin and underlying tissues. The sutures are pre-placed and the wound is closed by putting tension on all sutures simultaneously. The wires are twisted rather than tied, and the cut ends of the wire are bent back into the lumen of the rubber tubing. If tissues are infected, which is usually the case, the skin edges are left unsutured to facilitate drainage.

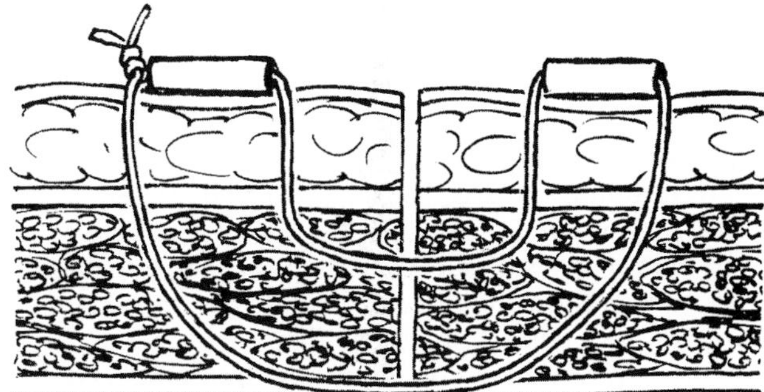

Figure 38-5. Schematic representation of the through-and-through interrupted vertical mattress suture that is used to repair acute total dehiscence of an abdominal incision.

Prior to recovery, a self-adhering drape is placed over the incision, and after recovery, a sterile abdominal compress is secured with Elasticon to form an abdominal bandage. The bandage compress should be changed every 24 hours until the incisions have healed (at about 30 days). Beginning the 14th day after surgery, alternate wire sutures and rubber tubing are removed, and all remaining sutures are removed on day 21. Daily cleaning of the wound is necessary, as well as re-bandaging until the skin is healed.

Chronic Incisional Hernias

The factors responsible for acute total wound disruption usually are the same as the cause of partial dehiscence and eventual hernia formation. Incisional infection is usually part of the medical history preceding hernia formation.[10]

Many hernias can be managed conservatively. If infection is present, the wound should be cultured for bacterial growth and the animal treated with appropriate antimicrobial agents. Sterile abdominal compresses may require daily changing. Flushing is not recommended because of the likelihood of disseminating the infection subcutaneously to other sutured portions of the incision. Chronic abdominal bandaging for 1 to 2 months during treatment of the wound infection reduces the size of the hernia. In some cases, chronic wound bandaging for up to 6 or 8 months will eliminate the necessity for surgical repair of a wall defect. To decrease the amount of disposable bandaging material necessary to accomplish this, commercially available reusable elastic bandages (Surgimed, Hospital Marketing Services, Inc, Naugatuck, Conn) can be purchased and have been used successfully in a number of cases.

When the hernia has failed to heal or enlarges after turnout, surgical repair becomes necessary, especially if the horses are used in an athletic capacity. Large defects in the abdominal wall require prosthetic reconstruction with a synthetic mesh and are preferentially repaired in this manner. Knit polypropylene mesh (Marlex) is strong, elastic, and inert, and it resists infection. Tissue grows through the knit mesh to be incorporated into the healing herniorrhaphy tissue. Failure to use the synthetic mesh in the repair usually results in enough tension to produce a recurrence of the hernia. All infection should be eradicated before prosthetic reconstruction of the defect. This may require surgical removal of infected suture material from sinus tracts (see Chapter 28).

Prophylactic antimicrobial therapy is indicated because most incisional hernias have had some type of infection, and small pockets of bacteria may remain when surgical herniorrhaphy is undertaken. The horse is placed in dorsal recumbency under general inhalation anesthesia and a strict aseptic technique is used. The skin is incised for 180 degrees at the margin of the hernial ring (Fig. 38-6, *A*). Likewise, the fascia and fibrous tissue overlying the hernial ring are incised along the same planes. This fascia is removed using retroperitoneal dissection, leaving the peritoneum intact. The mesh is placed retroperitoneally and subfascially. In some cases, this is not possible, because there is an adhesion between the peritoneum and the fascia, or there is such a thin fascia that it cannot be separated. Then only intraperitoneal and subfascial placement is possible. A single layer of mesh is cut to correspond to the size and contour of the defect, allowing the edges of the mesh to be folded over so the sutures pass through a double layer.

Horizontal mattress sutures are placed about 2.5 cm from the cut edge of the mesh. Each bite is approximately 2.5 cm wide. Sutures are placed 0.5 cm apart (close enough together to prevent the small intestine from becoming incarcerated between the sutures). Number 2 polypropylene suture material is used. The sutures are pre-placed so that when they are tied, the mesh should lie flat and snugly under a moderate amount of tension deep to the hernia ring. The hernial flap then is trimmed and the free edge sutured to the hernial ring for reinforcement of the hernial mesh (see Fig. 38-6, *D*). Simple-continuous synthetic absorbable sutures may be used. Subcutaneous tissues and skin are closed in a routine fashion. All redundant subcutaneous tissues and skin are trimmed so that the skin also is under a moderate amount of tension when closed.

On recovery from surgery, an abdominal bandage is used for 7 to 10 days to prevent edema and seroma formation. Parenteral antibiotics are discontinued on the second or third day after surgery. Horses are confined to a stall for 60 days with hand-walking only.

LATERAL ABDOMINAL HERNIAS

Lateral abdominal hernias are usually the result of blunt trauma injuries from farm machinery, fence posts, or kicks from other horses (Fig. 38-7). Penetrating abdominal wounds may require immediate reconstruction to prevent evisceration, peritonitis, and wound infection. However, more commonly, traumatic wounds are not penetrating, and the horse can be treated with local therapy and abdominal bandaging. After 60 days, small residual defects in the body wall can be treated by direct suture apposition. When they are very large, they can be treated by prosthetic reconstruction with synthetic mesh, as previously described.

Abdominal wall hernias in pregnant mares that do not involve rupture of the prepubic tendon can be similarly repaired. However, it is suggested that the pregnancy be terminated by cesarean section if repair is necessary before parturition.

DIAPHRAGMATIC HERNIAS

Internal abdominal hernias include a multitude of intestinal accidents, including mesenteric hernias, entrapment in the epiploic foramen, and diaphragmatic hernias. Although diaphragmatic hernias are rare, both congenital and acquired hernias have been described.[11-13] Diaphragmatic hernias can be congenital, resulting from failed fusion of many of the four embryonic components of the diaphragm, or acquired from trauma. Diaphragmatic hernias can be classified by anatomic location as peritoneal pericardial or peritoneal pleural, depending on where the tear occurs and into which thoracic compartment bowel enters. Congenital defects usually have smooth round edges, and some hernias can be quite small, only 2.5 cm in diameter. On the other hand, acquired diaphragmatic hernias, because they are associated with some form of violence and increased intra-abdominal pressure, are usually large and frequently originate along the dorsal body wall.

Diaphragmatic hernias result in low-grade, chronic recurrent abdominal pain and sometimes are found incidentally at necropsy. However, this is the exception; more commonly, horses are presented in distress with either a serious abdominal crisis (subsequently found during exploratory celiotomy) or in acute respiratory distress. Diagnosis can be made on physical examination, with borborygmi auscultated during examination of the thorax. However, other signs associated with the acute abdominal crisis may be equivocal, since a rectal examination and abdominocentesis may not be abnormal. Ultrasonography is quite accurate in revealing gas-filled loops of intestine in the thorax (Fig. 38-8). Likewise, radiography may show a loss of the diaphragmatic line at the level of the hernia, or, more commonly, radiopacity in the ventral aspect of the chest. Occasionally, gas-filled loops of large colon can be visualized on thoracic radiographs (Fig. 38-9).

Repair of the diaphragmatic hernia is accomplished with the horse placed in dorsal recumbency and with a ventral midline celiotomy that extends cranially to the xiphoid. Assisted ventilation is necessary during anesthesia. Abdominal viscera should be repositioned into the abdomen, and tilting the horse with front end elevated may aid in reduction of the hernia.

Small defects (less than 5 cm), particularly those ventrally positioned, may be closed by primary apposition using large-gauge suture material in a simple-continuous pattern. Débridement is usually not undertaken, because once the hernial ring is removed, the muscular portion of the diaphragm is less likely to hold sutures as well as the hernial ring. Larger defects require prosthetic reconstruction with a synthetic mesh. The mesh is secured to the perimeter of the defect with simple-interrupted horizontal mattress sutures similar to those used for mesh herniorrhaphy for the ventral midline. Sutures are pre-placed prior to tying to ensure that tension is maintained on the mesh. The mesh is preferentially placed on the abdominal side of the incision.

Traumatic diaphragmatic hernias are quite often associated with very large defects, dorsally positioned, and inaccessible, precluding safe closure. In these instances, thoracotomy is used to gain better access. The diaphragm holds sutures quite well if a linear tear has occurred, and mesh reinforcement may not be necessary. Prior to closing the abdominal incision, the lungs should be maximally inflated to expel as much air as possible from the thorax. A chest tube with a Heimlich valve (see Chapter 18) should be used to manage a pneumothorax.

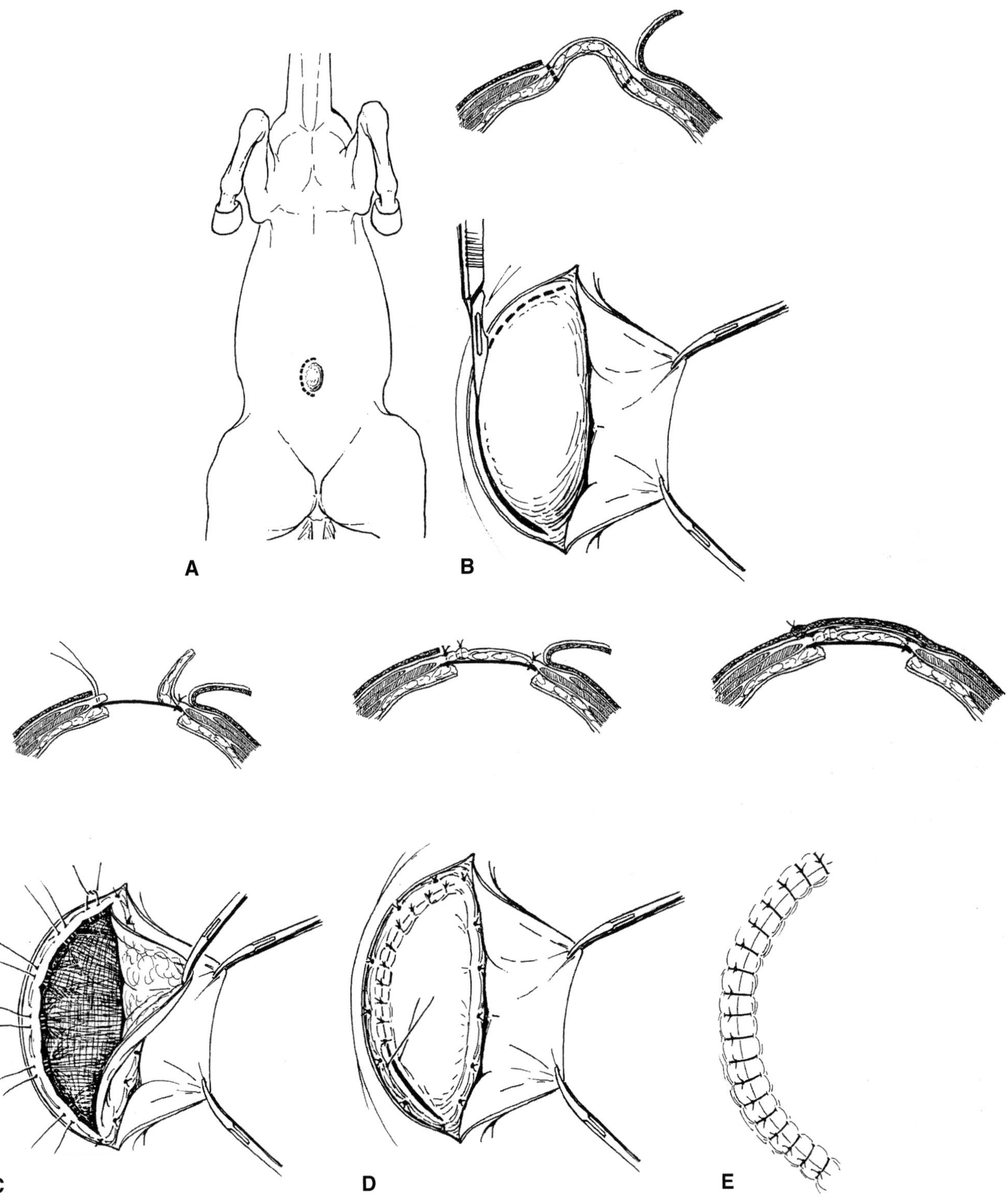

Figure 38-6. Illustrations of herniorrhaphy using a synthetic mesh and fascial overlay. **A,** Semi-elliptical incision extending beyond the cranial and caudal margins of the hernia is made. **B,** The skin flap and subcutaneous tissue are reflected off the hernia and held with towel clamps. The fibrous hernial sac is then reflected toward its attached base, leaving the peritoneum in place if possible. **C,** The mesh is anchored on the inside of the abdominal wall with through-and-through horizontal mattress sutures. Some of these are pre-placed. **D,** The fascial overlay is then sutured back in place using simple interrupted or a simple-continuous suture. **E,** Routine closure of the skin follows.

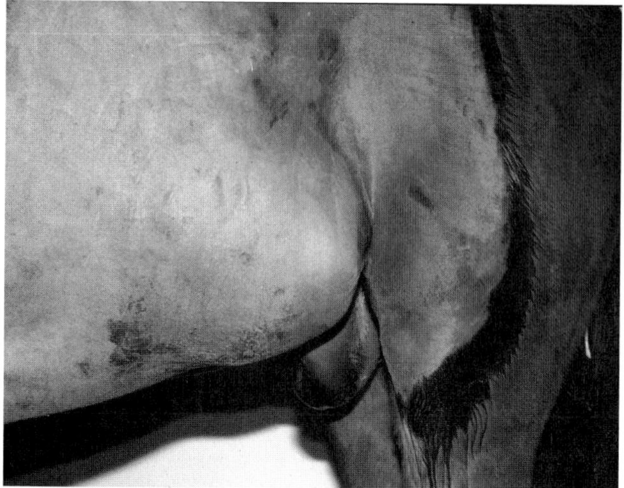

Figure 38-7. A horse that has a traumatic hernia in the lateral body wall as a result of blunt trauma.

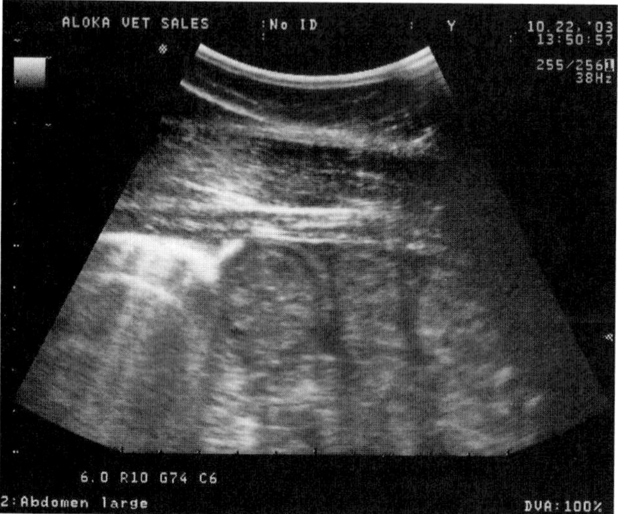

Figure 38-8. Thoracic ultrasonogram in a horse with a diaphragmatic hernia clearly demonstrates a circular viscus (bowel wall) between two ribs.

Dehiscence of the repair is not uncommon, and rupture of the diaphragm in another location has been reported. Prognosis for diaphragmatic hernia repair is guarded.

CAUDAL ABDOMINAL (INGUINAL) HERNIAS

Bilateral congenital inguinal hernias are often encountered in young colts, but they usually resolve without surgery during the first few weeks of life. The colt is confined to a box stall and observed, and the owner is instructed how to manually reduce the hernia several times daily. Larger hernias may benefit from support provided by an inguinal bandage constructed from rolled cotton and gauze. Reduction of the hernia is usually facilitated by casting the animal in lateral recumbency. For surgical descriptions of repair of inguinal hernias including via laparoscopy,[14] please refer to Chapter 65.

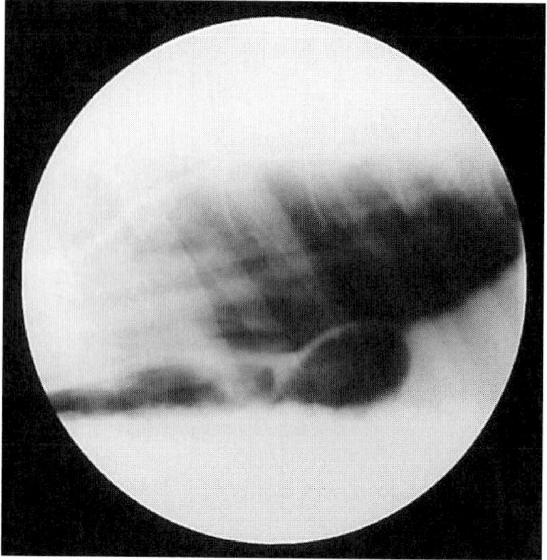

Figure 38-9. Thoracic radiographs of a horse with a diaphragmatic hernia demonstrate a gas-filled loop of bowel in the thorax and loss of diaphragmatic contour. Note fluid in the ventral aspect of the thorax.

By definition, inguinal hernias are present when there are intestinal contents in the inguinal canal. Scrotal hernias occur when the contents continue on into the scrotum. However, the term *inguinal hernia* is usually used to refer to both disorders. Distal jejunum and ileum are the intestinal contents most commonly encountered in inguinal hernias, but omentum and even the small colon are sometimes involved. Equine inguinal hernias usually are indirect (or true) hernias, with the contents passing through the vaginal ring and into the vaginal tunic. In a direct (or false) inguinal hernia, which occurs in humans, the contents do not pass through the ring but protrude through a weakness in the body wall. This occasionally can occur in foals, but it is highly unusual.

The clinical sign of an inguinal hernia is scrotal swelling. The testicle is often cool in the adult horse, probably because of vascular compromise. Frequently, the spermatic cord is enlarged and extremely hard and very painful to the touch. All stallions with colic should be checked for this type of inguinal hernia. Frequently, scrotal herniation in foals occurs without intestinal incarceration and may be the result of abdominal straining. Before repair is undertaken, conservative management may be advisable for several weeks. Diagnosis of inguinal hernias is made on the basis of external palpation, and rectal palpation in adult horses permits further evaluation of the internal inguinal ring. Intestinal incarceration in the ring can be easily palpated. Differential diagnoses include thrombosis of the testicle; testicular artery, seroma, or hematoma of the scrotum; neoplasia; and torsion of the spermatic cord.

REFERENCES

1. Dorland's Illustrated Medical Dictionary, ed 30, Philadelphia, 2003, WB Saunders.
2. Read RA, Bellenger CR: Hernias. In Slatter D, editor: Textbook of Small Animal Surgery, ed 3, Philadelphia, 2003, WB Saunders.
3. Enzerink E, van Weeren PR, van der Velden MA: Closure of the abdominal wall at the umbilicus and the development of umbilical

hernias in a group of foals from birth to 11 months of age, Vet Rec 2000;147:37.
4. Tulleners EP: Diseases of the abdominal wall. In Colahan PT, Merritt AM, Moore JN, Mayhew IG, editors: Equine Medicine and Surgery, ed 5, St Louis, 1999, Mosby.
5. Adams SB, Fessler JF: Abdominal wall surgery: Umbilical herniorrhaphy. In Atlas of Equine Surgery, Philadelphia, 2000, WB Saunders.
6. Mingoli A, Puggioni A, Sgarzini G, et al: Incidence of incisional hernia following emergency abdominal surgery, Ital J Gastroenterol Hepatol 1974;31:449.
7. Smeak DD: Abdominal hernias. In Slatter D, editor: Textbook of Small Animal Surgery, Philadelphia, 2003, WB Saunders.
8. Trostle SS, Wilson DG, Stone WC, et al: A study of the biomechanical properties of the adult equine linea alba: Relationship of tissue bite size and suture material to breaking strength, Vet Surg 1994;23:435.
9. Gibson KT, Curtis CR, Turner AS, et al: Incisional hernias in the horse: Incidence and predisposing factors, Vet Surg 1989;18:360.
10. French NP, Smith J, Edwards GB, et al: Equine surgical colic: Risk factors for postoperative complications, Equine Vet J 2002;34:444.
11. Speirs VC, Reynolds WT: Successful repair of a diaphragmatic hernia in a foal, Equine Vet J 8:170, 1976.
12. Dabareiner RM, White NA: Surgical repair of a diaphragmatic hernia in a racehorse, J Am Vet Med Assoc 1999;214:1517.
13. Santschi EM, Juzwiak JS, Moll HD, et al: Diaphragmatic hernia repair in three young horses, Vet Surg 1997;26:242.
14. Fischer AT Jr, Vachon AM, Klein SR: Laparoscopic inguinal herniorrhaphy in two stallions. J Am Vet Med Assoc 1995;207:1599.

CHAPTER 39

Postoperative Care and Complications Associated with Abdominal Surgery

Joanne Hardy
Peter C. Rakestraw

Postoperative management of horses with abdominal disorders should be targeted toward identification and management of pain, support of the cardiovascular system, treatment of endotoxemia, identification and treatment of surgical infection, restoration of gastrointestinal function, and management of secondary complications (diarrhea, thrombophlebitis, laminitis). Disorders of the gastrointestinal (GI) tract can result in significant systemic derangements in affected horses. Strangulating lesions lead to intestinal distention proximal to the lesion, third-space pooling of fluid in the intestinal tract, and intestinal mucosal damage with subsequent endotoxin absorption. Despite correction of the primary condition, problems encountered in the postoperative period usually represent a natural progression of the events triggered by the primary lesion. This chapter reviews the management of horses after abdominal surgery and addresses complications related to specific surgical procedures.

FLUID THERAPY

Dehydration and electrolyte imbalances are commonly encountered as a result of abdominal disorders. Even though a horse is stabilized in the perioperative period and the primary problem is corrected, continued replacement of previous and ongoing fluid losses is critical to a successful outcome. Knowledge of basic electrolyte and fluid homeostasis is essential to the successful management of these cases (see Chapter 3). The daily maintenance fluid requirement in adult horses is 50 to 60 mL/kg, and in foals, 70 to 80 mL/kg. The volume of GI secretions in adult horses is equivalent to their extracellular fluid volume, approximately 30% of body weight. With ileus or diarrhea, these fluids are not reabsorbed by the large colon, resulting in considerable fluid losses. These losses must be added to the maintenance requirements. Fluids available for replacement therapy in horses include lactated Ringer's solution (Baxter Healthcare Corp, Deerfield, Ill), which contains lactate as a buffer and calcium (4 mEq/L), Plasmalyte A (Baxter Healthcare Corp), and Normosol-R (Abbott Laboratories, North Chicago, Ill), which do not contain calcium but have acetate or gluconate as buffer sources. Intravenous fluid administration systems are commercially available (Baxter Laboratories, Deerfield, Ill) and provide a convenient method of administering large volumes of fluid to horses.

A significant complication of endotoxemia, particularly in postoperative cases of large colon torsion with significant mucosal damage, is increased capillary permeability resulting in fluid and protein loss into the interstitium. Vascular volume can be difficult to maintain in these horses because of the tremendous fluid loss in both the interstitium and the GI tract and the development of hypoproteinemia. The goal of therapy is to maintain enough vascular volume to sustain cardiac output. A reasonable indicator is the ability to maintain the heart rate at less than 80 beats per minute, packed cell volume (PCV, hematocrit) at less than 50%, and total protein at greater than 4.1 g/dL. PCV and total protein should be measured every 6 hours and therapy adjusted accordingly. If plasma protein decreases to less than 4.1 g/dL (corresponding to a plasma oncotic pressure of 12 mm Hg[1]), it may be necessary to administer colloids to prevent severe edema and allow continued administration of fluids. In surviving patients, capillary permeability is restored within 24 to 36 hours. Plasma proteins that were lost into the interstitium are quickly reabsorbed, and plasma protein concentration returns to normal range within a few days. Available colloids for administration to horses include plasma and synthetic colloids such as dextrans and hydroxyethyl starch.

Colloids

Plasma provides a source of protein, coagulation factors, and antithrombin III (AT-III). Plasma should be thawed slowly in a 37° C water bath if preservation of coagulation factors is desired and then used immediately. Storage of frozen plasma for more than 1 year or of thawed plasma for more than 24 hours at 1° to 6° C can result in significant deterioration of coagulation factors, particularly factors V and VIII.[2] Plasma should be administered slowly, using an in-line filter, to avoid adverse reactions. The volume of plasma to be given can be estimated as (PPg − PPr) • (0.05 BWr)/PPd, where PPg is the goal plasma protein concentration, PPr and PPd are the plasma protein of the recipient and donor, respectively, and BWr is the body weight in kilograms of the recipient. Usually, a volume of 2 to 4 mL/kg is sufficient to raise the plasma protein to greater than 4.1 g/dL, but repeated administration may be required.

Dextrans are polysaccharides composed of linear glucose residues.[3] Dextrans are available as dextran 40 or dextran 70, corresponding to a molecular weight of 40,000 or 70,000, respectively. Dextran 70 has a 6-hour and dextran 40 a 2-hour half-life. These colloids are available as a 6% solution and are administered at a rate of 4 mL/kg over 15 to 20 minutes. Dextrans also prolong the effects of hypertonic saline (transient effect in the horse of 30 to 60 minutes) to increase vascular volume.

Hydroxyethyl starch, available as hetastarch or pentastarch, is a substituted amylopectin composed of a heterogeneous group of molecules with a number average molecular weight of 69,000 and a weight average molecular weight of 450,000. Pentastarch is more rapidly degraded than hetastarch (half-life of 2.5 hours versus 25 hours).[3] Hetastarch infusion to clinically normal ponies significantly increased plasma colloid oncotic pressure for 120 hours using a dosage of 10 mL/kg.[4] Hetastarch exerts a dose-dependent effect on hemostasis, which may be significant at higher dosages of 20 mL/kg.[4] Synthetic colloids are not a substitute for plasma or blood products when red blood cells (RBCs), platelets, antithrombin, or coagulation factors are needed.

Electrolyte Replacement

Electrolyte derangements, specifically hypocalcemia, hypokalemia, and hypomagnesemia, can become significant in postoperative patients. Low serum ionized calcium (iCa) and magnesium (iMg) concentrations are more prevalent in horses with surgical GI disease, particularly in those with small intestinal or large and small colon nonstrangulating infarction or strangulation and in horses with postoperative ileus.[5-7] Horses with enterocolitis also have low iCa and iMg, and a decreased fractional clearance of calcium.[8] Total magnesium and calcium concentrations are less reliable for identification of the calcium and magnesium status, and, preferably, ionized concentrations should be determined.[5-7] Measurement of total calcium can be misleading if total protein is low (ionized calcium may still be normal) or if the horse is alkalotic (total calcium may be normal, with a low ionized fraction). Recently, fractional excretion of magnesium has been suggested as a diagnostic tool for assessment of the magnesium status in horses.[9] Based on this information, supplemental calcium and magnesium appears beneficial in the care of horses after abdominal surgery. Administration of 50 to 100 mL of 23% calcium gluconate in every 5 L of fluid is usually sufficient to maintain normocalcemia. In the presence of severe hypocalcemia (iCa less than 4.0 mg/dL), administration of 500 mL of calcium gluconate in 5 L of lactated Ringer's solution is indicated. Hypocalcemia that is refractory to calcium therapy may indicate hypomagnesemia, requiring concurrent magnesium replacement. Maintenance requirements of magnesium in horses are estimated at 13 mg/kg per day of elemental Mg, which is provided by 31 mg/kg per day of MgO, 64 mg/kg per day of $MgCO_3$, or 93 mg/kg per day of $MgSO_4$. In critically ill patients, these requirements may be increased, as indicated by the high prevalence of hypomagnesemia in hospitalized patients.[7] When magnesium supplementation is being considered, the concentration of elemental magnesium in the compound should be considered. Some crystalloid fluids such as Plasmalyte-A and Normosol-R contain 3 mEq/L of elemental Mg. This amount may be insufficient to account for the increased losses in sick horses. Administration of 150 mg/kg per day of $MgSO_4$ (0.3 mL/kg of a 50% solution), equivalent to 14.5 mg/kg per day or 1.22 mEq/kg per day of elemental magnesium, administered in saline, dextrose, or polyionic fluids would provide daily requirements for the horse.

Hypokalemia may develop because of lack of intake, diuresis, and GI loss through diarrhea. Horses with a metabolic acidosis can become hyperkalemic, and potassium excretion can occur after correction of the acidemia. Measurement of serum potassium as an estimate of total body potassium can be misleading, because most of the potassium ion is intracellular. Routine potassium supplementation is indicated if a lack of both intake and fluid therapy is continued for more than 24 hours. It is recommended that, to avoid any complication, animals not receive more potassium than 0.5 mEq/kg per hour. Most horses benefit from the addition of 12 mEq of potassium chloride per liter of fluids (80 mEq per 5-L bag).

Acid–base imbalances are uncommon in horses with acute abdominal disorders unless they are severely dehydrated and compromised, in which case a metabolic acidosis can be present. Rehydration and establishment of renal function often leads to correction of the acidosis. Correction of a metabolic acidosis is not recommended or necessary unless the pH is less than 7.2, blood bicarbonate is less than 15 mEq/L, or base excess deficit is greater than 10 mEq/L. Half the calculated requirement of bicarbonate can be administered over 1 hour, with the remainder administered over 12 to 24 hours. Concurrent rehydration should always be established. Care should be taken to minimize bicarbonate administration in severely distended animals with respiratory impairment until distention is corrected, to avoid accumulation of carbon dioxide.

ENDOTOXEMIA

Endotoxemia in horses causes decreased circulating vascular volume, increased capillary permeability, ileus, and coagulation disorders. It is manifested clinically as pain, tachycardia, edema, hypomotility, intestinal distention, nasogastric reflux, and thrombosis or bleeding tendencies. Hypovolemia results from GI stasis with losses through nasogastric reflux, increased capillary permeability resulting in fluid loss into the interstitium, and maldistribution of fluids with venous pooling. The increased capillary permeability typically observed with endotoxemia also results in protein loss (particularly of albumin) and potential edema formation. Fluid therapy is an important part of the treatment of the hypovolemia associated with endotoxemia and must be carefully adjusted to prevent significant hypoproteinemia. If plasma proteins fall to less than 4.1 g/dL, plasma administration should be considered.

Potential strategies to decrease endotoxin activity include prevention of absorption, chelation and elimination of the endotoxin molecule, and pharmacologic management of the cascade of mediators triggered by endotoxin. Endotoxin absorption can be minimized by restoring and maintaining mesenteric blood flow, which will preserve mucosal integrity, by decreasing luminal contents through emptying of the GI tract, and by luminal binding and inactivation of endotoxin. Luminal lavage, particularly after correction of a large colon volvulus, has been recommended to decrease the luminal endotoxin load. Administration of activated charcoal has also been recommended to bind endotoxin and prevent its absorption. Recently, di-tri-octahedral smectite (Bio-sponge, Platinum Performance, Buellton, Calif) has been shown to actively bind endotoxin and clostridial enterotoxin.[10,11] Its administration has been recommended for use in horses with colitis as well as in horses at risk for the development of postoperative diarrhea. Intraoperative administration through the pelvic flexure enterotomy after the large colon has been lavaged is easily performed. The use of endotoxin adsorbents through hemofiltration has been investigated but has not been attempted in horses. Although oral administration of antibiotics such as neomycin to decrease colonic bacterial content is recommended in other species, this is generally not recommended in horses because of the risk of drug-induced colitis.

Currently, two therapeutic agents are recommended to bind circulating endotoxin; hyperimmune plasma/serum or polymyxin B. Hyperimmune serum is prepared by harvesting serum from horses immunized with the lipid A core of lipopolysaccharide. Two products are currently available: a Re-mutant *Escherichia coli* plasma product (Polymune-J, Veterinary Dynamics, Templeton, Calif), and a Re-mutant *Salmonella typhimurium* serum product (Endoserum, Immvac Inc, Columbia, Mo). These products must be administered diluted. Although they are used in many equine hospitals, documentation of efficacy via randomized clinical trials has not been performed. Recently, four fatal cases of serum hepatitis associated with the administration of commercial plasma to horses have been described.[12] Although uncommon, the potential for complications when administering plasma should be considered. Active immunization through vaccination is also promoted by one company (ENDOVAC-equi, IMMVAC Inc, Columbia, Mo). Although a rapid anamnestic response would theoretically be advantageous in a horse acutely exposed to endotoxin, the benefit of prior immunization has not been demonstrated.

Polymyxin B is a cyclic cationic polypeptide antibiotic that binds lipid A and neutralizes the actions of endotoxin in vitro and has been used to prevent and treat endotoxemia in human patients.[13] In an experimental study performed in foals given low-dose endotoxin, pretreatment with polymyxin B resulted in lower rectal temperature, respiratory rate, and plasma tumor necrosis factor (TNF) and interleukin-6 (IL-6) activities compared with saline pretreatment. Interestingly, in that study, hyperimmune serum worsened the endotoxin response. Polymyxin B was given at a dosage of 6000 IU/kg intravenously (IV). In another study,[14] polymyxin B treatment before or after administration of endotoxin significantly reduced fever, tachycardia, and serum TNF compared with horses receiving saline.

Detergents consisting of a polyethylene oxide polymer of *p*-tert-octophenol,[15] or phospholipids,[16] when administered as a pretreatment to horses given endotoxin, resulted in decreased pulmonary artery hypertension, absence of leukopenia, and absence of fever, suggesting a beneficial effect in attenuating the response to endotoxin. Clinical efficacy or safety of these products has not been determined. Concerns over adverse effects, such as hemolysis, during administration have precluded their use in a clinical setting.[16]

Pharmacologic targeting of inflammatory mediators triggered by endotoxin is an effective modality in the management of endotoxemia. Endotoxin stimulates the release of several mediators, including eicosanoids and cytokines. Nonsteroidal agents, particularly flunixin meglumine, are used routinely to decrease endotoxin-mediated prostaglandin (PG) release. At low doses, flunixin inhibits the PG-mediated vasodilator effects of endotoxin and may minimize the hypotension observed after an acute endotoxic event. Phenylbutazone was more efficacious than flunixin in improving endotoxin-mediated ileus.[17] Ketoprofen can also be administered to mediate the endotoxin-mediated PG release. It has the advantage of being less ulcerogenic than flunixin or phenylbutazone.[18] Claims of ketoprofen's inhibitory effect on the lipoxygenase pathway have not been substantiated. In vitro treatment of ischemia-injured equine jejunum with flunixin meglumine was shown to retard recovery of barrier function.[19] Subsequent in vivo studies confirmed that nonselective inhibition of PG production by flunixin meglumine retarded mucosal recovery and prolonged the increased mucosal permeability induced by ischemia.[20,21] The clinical consequences of these findings are not documented, but the beneficial analgesic, anti-inflammatory, and antiendotoxic effects or these drugs may outweigh the potential deleterious effect on intestinal barrier function.

Endotoxin results in significant macrophage release of TNF and significant increase in pro-coagulant activity. Pentoxifylline, a methylxanthine derivative, is a vasodilator; it improves RBC rheology, decreases platelet aggregation, and may improve microcirculation.[22] In addition, pentoxifylline decreases TNF and IL-6 release by macrophages and thromboxane B_2 by platelets. Currently, only an oral formulation is available, given at a dosage of 8.5 mg/kg every 12 hours.[22] The vasodilatation and decreased thrombin formation may also be beneficial in laminitis prevention.

The coagulation disorders triggered by endotoxemia result in significant thrombotic tendencies or, in the end stages, bleeding tendencies. The increased pro-coagulant activity induced by endotoxemia can result in catheter problems or in intestinal thrombosis. Sodium heparin is used to prevent these complications at a dosage of 20 to

40 IU/kg every 8 hours. Although a higher dosage of sodium heparin (80 IU/kg) was shown to improve hypotension after colonic detorsion, such a dosage should be used with caution in postoperative cases, since significant hemorrhage can result. Calcium heparin may also be administered at a dosage of 150 IU/kg subcutaneously (SC), followed by 125 IU/kg every 12 hours for six doses and then 100 IU/kg every 12 hours after the seventh dose. Aspirin, a thromboxane inhibitor, has been recommended to prevent platelet aggregation and decrease thrombus formation. However, an in vitro study concluded that equine platelet aggregation induced by endotoxin was mediated by platelet-activating factor and therefore not affected by a thromboxane inhibitor.[23]

PAIN

Control of pain is an essential component of the management of postoperative patients. Drugs used for pain management should provide a good clinical response while minimally affecting GI motility.

Postoperative pain can originate from peritoneal inflammation, abdominal incision, or intestinal distention. Flunixin meglumine controls postoperative pain and improves the cardiovascular manifestations of endotoxemia. Flunixin meglumine combined with progesterone supplementation may help maintain pregnancy in mares with endotoxemia in the first trimester of gestation. Flunixin meglumine provides analgesia in a dosage-related manner up to a maximal dosage of 1.1 mg/kg. Smaller dosages (0.25 mg/kg) have been shown to improve cardiovascular parameters after endotoxemia.[24] Butorphanol is an agonist-antagonist narcotic that can be used to control postoperative pain and at low dosages (0.01 mg/kg) does not affect GI motility. Continuous-rate infusion of butorphanol (13 μg/kg per hour) to horses after celiotomy improved behavior scores and recovery characteristics and decreased plasma cortisol concentration.[25] However, time to first passage of feces was delayed significantly in treated horses.[25] Therefore, continuous-rate infusion of butorphanol may be contraindicated for certain GI problems. Horses with ileus occasionally require more potent analgesia. In such cases, administration of xylazine, an α_2-agonist, may be necessary, even though it can negatively affect GI motility. The duration of analgesia may be prolonged by combined intravenous and intramuscular administration.

Intravenous lidocaine has been advocated for the management of visceral pain. In people, lidocaine is used and has synergistic effects with other drugs. In vitro studies have shown a potential benefit of lidocaine on smooth muscle contraction.[26] One clinical study suggested an improvement in small intestinal motility, peritoneal fluid values, and outcome in horses after intestinal surgery; however, the low number of horses with small intestinal lesions makes the value of the results questionable.[27] Lidocaine has also been shown to have anti-inflammatory properties and to reduce reperfusion injury in experimental models of ischemia reperfusion.[28] One publication reported the use of lidocaine for the management of postoperative ileus in horses, using a loading dose of 1.3 mg/kg IV, followed by an infusion rate of 0.05 mg/kg per minute IV.[29] The use of lidocaine is most beneficial with other analgesics and allows the dosage of analgesics to be decreased.

POSTOPERATIVE ILEUS

Adynamic ileus is one of the most commonly encountered complications in horses after GI surgery and is often referred to as postoperative ileus (POI). In horses, POI occurs predominantly after correction of lesions involving the small intestine. Occasionally, POI is seen after correction of large colon problems, primarily large colon volvulus. Intestinal ischemia, distention, peritonitis, electrolyte imbalances, endotoxemia, traumatic handling of the intestine, resection and anastomosis, and anesthesia have all been proposed as potential contributing factors. Risk factors that have been identified for horses developing POI are age greater than 10 years, Arabian breed, PCV greater than 45%, high serum concentrations of protein and albumin, elevated serum glucose, anesthesia for longer than 2.5 hours, surgery longer than 2 hours, resection and anastomosis, lesions in the small intestine, and ischemic small intestine.[30-32] There is some evidence that performing a pelvic flexure enterotomy (bowel decompression) and intraoperative administration of lidocaine may decrease the risk of developing POI.[30,31]

In the current literature, the incidence of POI in horses undergoing surgical treatment of colic has been reported to range from 10% to 21%.[31-33] As expected, the survival rate was lower for horses that developed POI than for those that did not develop POI (87% and 84.1% survival rates in horses with POI, versus 93% and 94.1% survival rates in horses without POI). This is a marked improvement over a previous study, which reported a mortality rate of 86% in horses with POI.[34] Although management and prognosis of these cases has improved, POI is still associated with 38% to 40% of all postoperative deaths in horses treated for colic.[31,32]

Disruption of propulsive motility results in the sequestration of fluid, gas, and ingesta in the segment of the GI tract that is dysfunctional and in the intestine proximal to the dysfunctional area. Since small intestine strangulating lesions are the most common problems leading to POI, the distention occurs primarily in the small intestine and stomach. With colitis, endotoxemia, or ischemia following a large colon volvulus, distention may occur in the cecum and large colon. Signs of ileus are progressive and directly related to the accumulation of gas and fluid within the GI tract. Gastric distention usually occurs within 12 to 48 hours after recovery from anesthesia as fluid and gas back up from the small intestine. With increasing GI distention, the animal becomes more depressed and shows signs of increasing abdominal pain such as pawing, flank watching, lying down, and rolling.[35-37] Borborygmi are usually decreased or absent. The heart rate is usually elevated as a result of pain associated with distention. Hemoconcentration is reflected by increases in the PCV and total protein, as well as in elevated heart rate and increased capillary refill time. Decreases in plasma chloride and potassium are the most commonly observed electrolyte abnormalities, although sodium and calcium may also be low.[34-37] Rectal examination, ultrasonography, and abdominal radiography (in foals) can aid in determining if the small intestine or large intestine is involved. Nasogastric decompression often retrieves from 3 to 10 L of fluid. The response to nasogastric decompression provides an important clue that the problem is functional (i.e., POI). After decompression, the horse should show improvement, with decreased pain and heart rate. If no alleviation of signs is observed after repeated attempts at decompression, careful thought should be given as to the likelihood that the problem may be mechanical, such as a complication with the anastomosis, and not a functional POI.

Supportive Therapy

Because of the therapeutic limitations of available prokinetic agents (discussed later), the hallmark of treatment of POI in the horse is supportive therapy. Included in this supportive therapy are fluid, acid–base, and electrolyte therapies. Antibiotics are also indicated if there is compromised intestine or the possibility of bacterial contamination resulting in peritonitis. Along with fluid therapy, nasogastric decompression remains the primary method to treat POI in the horse. Questions concerning when to place the tube, whether the tube should be left in place, and when to start feeding have not been adequately investigated. A study in normal horses indicated that leaving a nasogastric tube in place increases the rate of gastric emptying over a 24-hour period (T. Lammers, Texas A&M University, unpublished data). The clinical significance of this finding in the postoperative horse is unknown. In humans, eliminating or decreasing routine nasogastric intubation with early return to enteral feeding has been shown to be safe and may actually reduce POI.[38-40] There is some thought among equine surgeons that early removal of the nasogastric tube or passing the tube only when indicated predicated on pain, heart rate, rectal examination, and volume of previous reflux may attenuate the duration and severity of POI in the horse. This has yet to be substantiated.

Prokinetics

It is logical to assume that during POI in the horse, an imbalance of factors controlling excitation and inhibition of GI smooth muscle occurs. Historically, pharmacologic modulation of GI motility in the horse has been directed at increasing excitatory cholinergic activity with administration of parasympathomimetic agents such as bethanechol or neostigmine, or blocking inhibitory sympathetic hyperactivity with α-adrenergic blockers such as yohimbine and acepromazine.[34,41-43] In addition to being affected by sympathetic and parasympathetic input, contractility of gastrointestinal muscle is directly mediated by enteric inhibitory neurotransmitters such as vasoactive intestinal peptide, adenosine triphosphate, and nitric oxide, and enteric excitatory neurotransmitters such as substance P and acetylcholine.[44-47] It is likely that abnormalities involving the enteric nervous system and its neurotransmitters, as well as insult to the enteric smooth muscle cells and interstitial cells of Cajal (astrocytes), which are responsible for generating patterns of electrical activity in the enteric smooth muscle cells that mediate contractile activity, are also involved in the pathophysiology of POI.[48-51] At this time, treatment of POI in the horse is limited to pharmacologic agents that influence only a small number of the mediators of motility. This most likely contributes to the limited response seen.

Prokinetics are used for the treatment of POI in the horse. The following is a summary of some of the more frequently used prokinetics in horses.

Bethanechol

Bethanechol chloride is a muscarinic cholinergic agonist that stimulates acetylcholine receptors (M_2 receptors) on GI smooth muscles or at the level of the myenteric plexus, causing gastrointestinal contractile activity.[47] In an equine POI model, bethanechol (2.5 mg SC at 2 and 5 hours postoperatively in ponies) shortened transit time as measured by the passage of beads, and reduced the time until normal activity levels returned throughout the GI tract when administered in combination with yohimbine, an α-adrenergic receptor blocker.[42] This drug combination, however, was not as effective as metoclopramide in restoring coordinated gastroduodenal motility patterns in these ponies. Although efficacy in treating motility dysfunction has been questioned in the horse and other species, the prokinetic effects in normal horses and the clinical impression of its benefit in treating horses with ileus provides some support for its use in the treatment of certain motility dysfunctions such as POI and gastric and cecal impactions.[43,47,52] The recommended dosage is 0.025 mg/kg IV or SQ, every 4 to 6 hours. The most common side effects of bethanechol are salivation with abdominal cramping and diarrhea.

Neostigmine

Neostigmine methylsulfate is a cholinesterase inhibitor that prolongs the activity of acetylcholine by retarding its breakdown at the synaptic junction. In studies on normal horses, the effects of neostigmine (0.022 mg/kg IV) varied depending on the portion of the gastrointestinal tract examined.[41,52,53] Neostigmine was shown to delay gastric emptying and decrease propulsive motility in the stomach and jejunum but to increase propulsive motility in the pelvic flexure.[41,53] These results suggest that the drug would not be appropriate for gastric and small intestinal problems but may be beneficial for large intestinal motility dysfunction. However, neostigmine increased the amplitude of rhythmic contractions in both the resting and distended jejunum in anesthetized ponies, and it induced contractile activity in the ileum and increased the rate of cecal emptying in other studies, supporting its use for motility dysfunction in both small and large intestine.[52,54] There has been no consensus as to the recommended use of this drug for treatment of motility disorders in horses. It is rarely used as a prokinetic agent in humans.[47] There is anecdotal support that neostigmine can reduce the severity of POI in horses, particularly if the large colon is involved. However, its use for impaction colic or in cases with excess GI distention has not been recommended by some authors because of the apparent force of drug-induced contractions.[52] The dosage used clinically is 0.0044 mg/kg (2 mg per adult horse) SC or IV, repeated in 20 to 60 minutes. If there is no response and the horse is not exhibiting any side effects, the amount can be increased by 2-mg increments to a total of 10 mg per treatment. A side effect commonly seen with this drug is abdominal pain.

Acepromazine and Yohimbine

Acepromazine and yohimbine are both α-adrenergic antagonists. Their use is based on the assumption that sympathetic hyperactivity contributes to POI. Afferent stimulation during surgery is thought to activate inhibitory sympathetic efferents. Norepinephrine released by post-synaptic sympathetic neurons at the enteric ganglia inhibits the release of the excitatory neurotransmitter acetylcholine by stimulating α_2-receptors located presynaptically on cholinergic neurons. Elevated serum catecholamines that can last for the duration of POI have been associated with increased synthesis of norepinephrine in the bowel wall in humans after laparotomy.[45,55]

Acetylpromazine maleate facilitates small intestinal transit in normal ponies.[56] On the basis of clinical impression, acepromazine administered at 0.01 mg/kg intramuscularly (IM) intraoperatively and then every 4 hours is thought to reduce the severity of POI in horses with small intestinal lesions. Because acepromazine is a nonselective α-blocker that can produce hypotension through α_1-receptor antagonism, the animal should be well hydrated before the drug is administered.

Yohimbine hydrochloride is a competitive antagonist that is selective for α_2-adrenergic receptors. When administered at 0.15 mg/kg IV at 1, 4, 7, and 10 hours postoperatively in an experimentally induced POI model, it reduced the severity of POI, especially when combined with bethanechol.[42] Yohimbine administered at 75 μg/kg was demonstrated to attenuate some of the negative effects that endotoxin has on propulsive motility.[57] Since yohimbine is a selective α_2-adrenergic, it should not produce the hypotensive response seen with acepromazine.

Metoclopramide

Metoclopramide is a first-generation substituted benzamide whose prokinetic activity is both through dopamine 1 (DA_1) and 2 (DA_2) receptor antagonism and through 5-hydroxytryptamine 4-receptor (5-HT_4) agonism and 5-HT_3 receptor antagonism.[42,47,58] Stimulation of DA_2 receptors inhibits the release of acetylcholine, whereas stimulation of 5-HT_4 receptors enhances the release of acetylcholine from the myenteric ganglia.[47] Metoclopramide has been shown to stimulate in vitro contractile activity of circular muscle from the stomach and small intestine in the horse.[26] In a POI model in ponies, metoclopramide was more effective in restoring GI coordination than adrenergic antagonists and cholinomimetics used individually or in combination. In horses, metoclopramide is most commonly administered at a dosage of 0.25 mg/kg, diluted in 500 mL of saline, IV over 30 to 60 minutes. In a retrospective study, metoclopramide administered as a continuous infusion (0.04 mg/kg per hour) decreased the total volume, duration, and rate of gastric reflux when used prophylactically after small intestine resection and anastomosis.[59] Metoclopramide may cause extrapyramidal side effects such as excitement, restlessness, sweating, and abdominal cramping.

Cisapride

Cisapride is a second-generation substituted benzamide, which until recently was the most popular and effective prokinetic in human medicine.[47] Although it has been taken off the human market because of its cardiotoxic effects, it is discussed here because it is still available through some compounding agencies, and drugs with similar mechanisms of action will soon be available.[60] Cisapride functions as an indirect cholinergic stimulant by selectively enhancing the release of acetylcholine from postganglionic neurons in the myenteric plexus.[61,62] Unlike that of metoclopramide, the main prokinetic activity of cisapride appears to be mediated through 5-HT_4 receptor agonism and 5-HT_3 receptor antagonism and not through dopamine antagonism.[63] In the horse, cisapride has been shown to act partly through a noncholinergic effect mediated by 5-HT_2 receptors.[26] In experimental studies and in clinical trials in humans, cisapride's prokinetic effects were consistently equal to or superior to those of metoclopramide and of domperidone, a dopamine antagonist used as a prokinetic in humans.[62,64] In normal horses, cisapride augments the amplitude of gastric contractions, stimulates jejunal activity coordinated with gastric contractions, enhances contractile activity of the large and small colon, and stimulates coordinated activity in the ileocecocolonic junction.[6,43,65,66] In a clinical trial in horses, cisapride (0.1 mg/kg IM every 8 hours) significantly decreased the incidence of POI.[67] There are conflicting data on its efficacy for correcting motility dysfunction caused by endotoxin. One study reported no benefit, whereas another suggested that cisapride can attenuate the motility dysfunction induced by endotoxin.[68]

Cisapride suspended in saline and administered per rectum is very poorly absorbed, and suspended in dimethyl sulfoxide (DMSO), it is inconsistently absorbed.[69] Recent work has determined that mixing 400 mg of cisapride with 10 mL of tartaric acid and heating at 50° C for 20 minutes, then adding sterile water to bring the volume to 100 mL and mixing for another 20 minutes at 50° C, followed by sterilizing by filtration, consistently yields a 3-mg/mL solution for IV administration. This should be administered at 0.1 mg/kg every 8 hours.

A recent report has shown that levosulpride, a new substituted benzamide with dopamine (D_2) receptor antagonist activity as well as 5-HT_4 receptor agonist and 5-HT_3 receptor antagonist activity, is as effective as cisapride in treating dysmotility in humans.[70] Prokinetics such as levosulpride, and drugs with similar activity, such as tegaserod and prucalopride, are currently replacing cisapride.[71]

Erythromycin

Erythromycin is a macrolide antibiotic with recognized GI side effects. Erythromycin is a motilin agonist that influences motility partly by acting on motilin receptors on smooth muscles. Motilin is a hormone that is released by enterochromaffin cells and stimulates contractile activity in the stomach and small intestine. Motilin infusion in the horse causes strong contractions in the proximal jejunum in vivo.[66] Erythromycin also acts on enteric cholinergic neurons through motilin and/or 5-HT_3 receptors to stimulate the release of acetylcholine.[47,72] Motilin and erythromycin have been shown to initiate phase III of the migrating motor complex.[73] When administered at subtherapeutic antimicrobial levels, erythromycin has been shown to stimulate gastric emptying, antroduodenal coordination, and phase III activity in the duodenum in humans and laboratory animals.[73]

The dosage that has been used clinically in horses is 1.0 mg/kg in 1 L of saline infused over 60 minutes, every 6 hours. In normal horses, a dosage of 1 mg/kg is effective in stimulating both cecal and small intestinal contractile activity.[74] Dosages higher than 10 mg/kg can potentially disrupt propulsive activity. The prokinetic response may diminish with repeated treatments. Erythromycin can downregulate motilin receptors, which would explain this desensitization. Although the recommended prokinetic dosage is supposed to be below the effective antimicrobial level, there have been some anecdotal reports of severe colitis associated with its use, making many clinicians reluctant to use it. In support of this clinical impression, an association between low-dose erythromycin (1.25 mg/kg PO every 8 hours) and *Clostridium difficile* colitis was demonstrated in one report.[75] Erythromycin has been commonly used to treat gastroparesis in humans, but many of the prokinetic therapeutic benefits that were anticipated have failed to materialize.

Lidocaine

Intravenous lidocaine shortens the duration of paralytic ileus in the colon in humans after abdominal surgery.[76] Sympathetic inhibitory spinal and prevertebral reflexes are involved in the pathogenesis of POI.[45] Lidocaine may act by (1) reducing the level of circulating catecholamines by inhibition of the sympathoadrenal response, (2) suppressing activity in the primary afferent neurons involved in reflex inhibition of gut motility, (3) stimulating smooth muscles directly, and (4) decreasing inflammation in the bowel wall through inhibition of prostaglandin synthesis, inhibition of granulocyte migration and their release of lysosomal enzymes, and inhibition of free radical production.[76] Lidocaine causes an in vitro increase in contractility of the circular muscle from the proximal duodenum of horses.[26] In a clinical trial in horses, lidocaine was effective in decreasing the duration of reflux in horses with POI and in horses with duodenitis–proximal jejunitis.[29] In a retrospective study, intraoperative administration of lidocaine appeared to decrease the risk of POI.[30]

The recommended protocol requires an initial bolus of 1.3 mg/kg IV administered slowly over 5 minutes, followed by 0.05 mg/kg per minute in saline or lactated Ringer's solution over 24 hours.[29] Side effects include muscle fasciculations, trembling, and ataxia.

Anti-Inflammatory and Analgesic Therapy

Recently, a large body of evidence has accumulated to indicate that motility disorders such as POI and ileus associated with enteritis or colitis are, in part, mediated by an inflammatory cell infiltrate into the intestinal wall.[77-79] Intestinal manipulation, lipopolysaccharide administration, and ischemia/reperfusion injury have all been shown to produce significant decreases in in vitro contractile activity of jejunal smooth muscle. In experimental animals, blocking this influx of leukocytes by antiadhesion antibodies eliminates the disruption of motility, supporting a cause-and-effect relationship between intestinal inflammation and POI.[77] Intestinal distention, ischemia, and trauma inflicted during decompression or during resection and anastomosis induce inflammation in the bowel wall, with production of inflammatory mediators such as prostacyclin, PGE_2, and TNF. Endotoxemia, associated with necrotic intestine, also stimulates production of inflammatory mediators. Infusions of endotoxin, PGE_2, and TNF have been shown to disrupt normal motility.[17,57] Both phenylbutazone and flunixin meglumine were shown to significantly attenuate the disruption of gastric, small intestine, and large colon motility elicited by endotoxin infusion.[17,68] Administration of these nonsteroidal drugs decreases the production of inflammatory mediators that directly inhibit smooth muscle contractility, while reducing postoperative pain and thus attenuating potential inhibitory sympathetic reflexes. On the basis of these observations, nonsteroidal anti-inflammatory drugs (NSAIDs) are recommended for prevention and treatment of motility disorders associated with GI inflammation.

Besides NSAIDs, adrenergic agonists and opioids are the other two classes of drugs commonly used in horses to control pain associated with colic. Xylazine and detomidine are α_2-adrenergic agonists that may inhibit presynaptic acetylcholine release in the myenteric plexus, resulting in a decrease in motility.[80] In the horse, xylazine and detomidine have been shown to decrease motility as measured by myoelectrical activity of the distal jejunum, pelvic flexure, cecum, and right ventral colon, and to decrease cecal emptying based on radiolabeled markers.[41,52,81-83] However, in another study, xylazine was not thought to seriously disrupt gastrointestinal motility.[84] Opioid agonists should be avoided if possible, as they have been shown to depress motility in most species studied.[82,85,86] Naloxone, an opioid antagonist, has been suggested by some investigators to be a potentially beneficial drug for treating motility disorders.[65] There is some evidence that naloxone may enhance progressive motility in the horse; however, it has also been shown to cause diarrhea and colic in the horse.[87] Butorphanol tartrate, an opioid agonist-antagonist, has been shown to inhibit myoelectrical activity in the jejunum, whereas it has no effect on pelvic flexure activity.[88] Butorphanol prolonged xylazine-induced inhibition of myoelectrical activity of the cecum and right ventral colon in one study, whereas it produced no undesirable effect on antroduodenal activity in another study.[81,84]

Prognosis

The prognosis for resolution of POI is favorable.[31-33] Although this discussion has been limited to pharmacologic interventions, good surgical technique and appropriate aftercare, including fluid and electrolyte replacement, antibiotic and analgesic therapy, and nasogastric decompression, are critical to the outcome of these cases. Because of the intensive postoperative medical management of these cases, successful treatment is often costly. Frequently, the limiting factor in determining the outcome is the economic constraint imposed by the owner.

ADHESIONS

Peritoneal adhesions are one of the most frequent complications seen after colic surgery in horses. Adhesions occur more frequently after surgery for lesions involving the small intestine, and they cause postoperative signs of pain and intestinal obstruction in as many as 22% of these horses.[89,90] Adhesions are the second most common reason for repeated laparotomy in horses with GI disease.[91] Foals seem to be more predisposed to development of adhesions than adults.[92]

Adhesion formation can be viewed as a variant of the normal physiologic healing process. An intact mesothelial cell layer is critical to the prevention of adhesion formation. Ischemia, distention, drying, or abrasion of the peritoneum during manipulation and decompression of the intestine, as well as hemorrhage, the introduction of foreign material, or infection in the peritoneal cavity, can all result in peritoneal inflammation initiating adhesion formation.[93] Once the mesothelial cells are disrupted, the underlying connective tissue containing blood vessels, collagen, lymphocytes, fibroblasts, mast cells, macrophages, and plasma cells becomes exposed. The release of vasoactive substances such as PGE_2, serotonin, bradykinin, and histamine from the exposed submesothelial tissue mediates increased vascular permeability with extravasation of a fibrinogen-rich inflammatory exudate. The release of thromboplastin (tissue factor) and exposure of subendothelial collagen activate both the intrinsic and the extrinsic clotting cascade, leading ultimately to thrombin-mediated conversion of fibrinogen to fibrin, with the fibrin adhering to sites of injury. In the normal healing process, the fibrin tags are lysed by plasmin, and the peritoneal injury is covered within 2 to 5 days by a single layer of mesothelial cells originating from metaplasia of underlying mesenchymal cells, attachment of free-floating mesothelial cells, or transformation of macrophages.[94] However, if there is inadequate fibrinolysis, fibroblasts migrate over the fibrin scaffold with neovascularization and produce collagen by day 4, initiating the formation of fibrous adhesions.[95]

Tissue plasminogen activators are proteases released by mesothelial and endothelial cells that convert inactive plasminogen to plasmin, an important part of the fibrinolysis pathway. After peritoneal injury from mechanical trauma, ischemia, inflammation, or bacterial infection, plasminogen activator activity is decreased. This was thought to occur because of damage to the cells producing plasminogen activator.[96] A more recent finding suggests that there is an increased production of plasminogen activator inhibitor, which reduces the level of plasminogen activator activity.[93,97,98] Extensive damage to either the parietal or the visceral peritoneal surface tips the balance in favor of adhesion formation, first by increasing the extent of fibrin formation and deposition and second by decreasing fibrinolytic activity.

Several strategies are currently being used to prevent or minimize adhesion formation. The most important one involves minimizing trauma by paying attention to good surgical technique, such as keeping the bowel moist at all times, providing adequate hemostasis, leaving as little suture material as possible exposed, removing as much damaged tissue as possible, and handling the tissue as gently as possible. Trauma is also reduced by making the decision to perform surgery in a timely manner. Both ischemia/reperfusion and intraluminal distention and decompression have been shown to cause severe changes in the seromuscular layer of the small intestine, such as serosal edema, leukocyte infiltration, and erythrocyte leakage with fibrin accumulation, whereas a similar insult to the ascending colon does not result in comparable seromuscular lesions.[90,99] Prophylactic strategies include intervention in the inflammation, coagulation, and fibrinolysis cascades with anti-inflammatory or heparin therapy, and using therapies that provide mechanical separation of the injured areas.

Perioperative NSAIDs and antibiotics are used routinely during GI surgery. Because both inflammation and infection may predispose to adhesion formation, this combination of chemotherapy should curtail the production of adhesions. Broad-spectrum antibiotics should be administered prophylactically or therapeutically, depending on the degree of compromise to the affected segment of bowel. NSAIDs are continued after surgery for 3 to 5 days to reduce the inflammatory response. DMSO (20 mg/kg IV twice a day for 72 hours) may also reduce inflammation. There is experimental evidence that this combination of anti-inflammatory and antimicrobial therapy is effective in reducing adhesion formation in horses.[100,101] In a recent experimental study of ischemia-induced adhesions in foals, administration of flunixin meglumine and antibiotics or administration of DMSO appeared to be more effective than 3% sodium carboxymethylcellulose or heparin in preventing the formation of adhesions.[102] It is interesting to note that a 3% solution was used in this study, compared with the 1% solution in studies discussed later in this chapter.

Heparin is composed of a family of naturally occurring sulfated glycosaminoglycans that are synthesized by connective tissue mast cells.[103,104] By binding to AT-III, a glycoprotein synthesized in the liver and vascular endothelium, heparin markedly enhances the rate of AT-III–mediated inactivation of clotting factors (factors IX, X, XI, and XII and thrombin).[105,106] The AT-III–heparin complex, by neutralizing thrombin, suppresses thrombin-mediated amplification of the coagulation cascade and inhibits thrombin-mediated conversion of fibrinogen to fibrin.[105] Heparin sodium (40 IU/kg IV intraoperatively, followed by 40 IU/kg SC twice a day for 2 days) decreased adhesion formation in ponies after experimentally induced intestinal ischemia.[91] Based on pharmacokinetic studies using calcium heparin instead of sodium heparin, an initial dose of 150 IU/kg SC followed by 125 IU/kg SC twice a day for six doses and then 100 IU/kg SC twice a day is recommended to maintain therapeutic anticoagulant levels.[107] Some evidence suggests that calcium ions inhibit the heparin–AT-III–thrombin reaction. Consequently, a higher dosage of calcium heparin than sodium heparin is required to reach therapeutic levels,[108] although this finding is questioned.[109]

Plasma AT-III levels are reported to be decreased in some horses with abdominal disease.[110,111] Because heparin acts as a cofactor to AT-III, heparin therapy would be of limited value if peritoneal AT-III were depleted significantly. However, changes in plasma AT-III levels do not always correlate with changes in peritoneal levels.[112] Peritoneal AT-III levels have actually been found to be increased in some horses with colic.[113] The most common complication reported with heparin therapy in horses is anemia induced by erythrocyte agglutination.[114]

Intraperitoneal sodium carboxymethylcellulose (SCMC) is effective in preventing adhesions in experimental models using laboratory animals, and there is evidence to support its efficacy in the prevention of experimentally induced adhesions in horses.[115,116] The proposed mechanism of action is the "siliconizing" effect that SCMC has on the bowel. This mechanical lubricating barrier minimizes the duration of direct apposition of traumatized tissue, preventing the establishment of fibrin tags between two surfaces, although the effect is most likely transient, because the SCMC is cleared rapidly from the abdomen. A 1% solution of SCMC (7 mL/kg body weight) is infused into the peritoneal cavity through a sterile stallion catheter before tying the last suture in the linea alba.[115] No adverse effects on abdominal incisional wound healing were observed in horses treated with SCMC.[117] In several experimentally induced adhesion studies, horses treated with 1% SCMC had reduced frequency of intra-abdominal adhesions compared with controls.[118,119]

Sodium hyaluronate (HA) has also been used by itself and in conjunction with SCMC to reduce adhesions. Application of a 0.4% HA solution to the serosal surface of the jejunum significantly decreased the incidence of experimentally induced intra-abdominal adhesion formation in ponies, whereas SCMC did not significantly reduce adhesions.[120] A bio-resorbable hyaluronate-carboxymethylcellulose membrane that is applied over an anastomosis site or an area of localized trauma has also been shown to be beneficial in reducing adhesion formation.[121-123]

Intraperitoneal instillation of crystalloid solutions is often used to prevent adhesion formation, but conflicting results have been reported regarding their efficacy.[95] The proposed mechanism is hydroflotation of the abdominal organs. However, large volumes of fluid in the peritoneal cavity may compromise the host's ability to fight infection by interfering with opsonization and phagocytosis.[124] An alternative approach is the use of peritoneal lavage, which should remove fibrin and other inflammatory mediators while providing mechanical separation of the bowel at the time of lavage. Standing postoperative peritoneal lavage significantly reduced the number of adhesions in horses that received two peritoneal lavages for 2 days postoperatively with 10 L of lactated Ringer's solution delivered through a 32-French chest trocar inserted in the abdomen during surgery.[125] Another technique for abdominal drainage is through the use of a closed suction intra-abdominal drain with intermittent peritoneal lavage. This technique has been associated with a high incidence of minor complications such as partial obstruction of the drain (26%), leakage of fluid around the drain (16%), and subcutaneous fluid accumulation (12%).[126]

SURGICAL COMPLICATIONS

Significant complications, such as hemoperitoneum or peritonitis, may result from surgical procedures. Abdominal surgical procedures must adhere to basic principles of good surgical practice (after Halsted), including accurate homeostasis, gentle tissue handling, approximation of tissue, obliteration of dead space, minimal contamination, accurate ligation, and minimal foreign material. Postoperative hemorrhage can result from ligature slippage or from mucosal hemorrhage following intestinal resection and anastomosis. Fatal hemorrhage resulting from tearing of the portal vein or, less commonly, the caudal vena cava has been reported after manual reduction of epiploic foramen entrapment.[127-129] Therefore, reduction of an epiploic foramen entrapment should be performed with one hand on each side of the foramen and gentle feeding of the entrapped bowel through the foramen in a horizontal direction, because pulling the bowel in an upward direction may lead to tearing of the previously mentioned major vessels. Hemorrhage has also been reported as a complication of enterotomies, particularly those performed in the large colon. Therefore, in these locations, a full-thickness suture pattern may be indicated as a first layer.[130]

Administration of whole blood may be necessary if signs of hemorrhagic shock develop (increased heart rate, pale mucous membranes, weakness, and collapse). Fresh blood collected in plastic bags to preserve platelet activity should be given, as stored blood requires several hours to restore RBC oxygen-carrying capacity. Because signs of hemorrhagic shock develop after loss of 25% to 30% of blood volume, transfusion of 6 to 8 L of whole blood may be required (see Chapter 4).

Complications have been reported that are unique to specific surgical techniques. Small intestinal volvulus may develop after side-to-side anastomosis in ponies. Intussusceptions have been reported after small intestinal surgeries. Jejunojejunal intussusception was reported after a stapled functional end-to-end anastomosis in two pony mares[131] and in two ponies after inverting closure of small intestinal transverse enterotomies,[132] suggesting that excessive cuff formation should be avoided during small intestinal closure. Chronic intermittent colic with small intestinal distention can occur after functional end-to-end jejunojejunostomies. Significantly dilated anastomoses found on re-laparotomy may hinder the passage of the peristaltic wave and are related to excessive length of the anastomosis.

Internal herniation is a possible complication of small intestinal resection, and care should be taken to obliterate all possible internal spaces. Closure of the ileocecal fold after jejunocecostomy, mesenteric closure after small intestinal resection or ileocolostomy, and closure of potential spaces after intestinal bypass are recommended to avoid this problem.[133,134]

Extensive small intestinal resection (greater than 60%) has been associated with malabsorption, diarrhea, weight loss, and liver damage in ponies.[135] In a separate study, a short-interval feeding program (pelleted ration divided into eight feedings per day) prevented the development of a clinical malabsorptive syndrome after 70% of small intestinal resections in ponies.[136]

Jejunocecostomy procedures are reported to have an increased risk for postoperative complications. An ileocecocolic intussusception was reported after jejunocecostomy in one horse.[137] Alterations in calcium absorption and fat absorption and microbial derangements in normal flora have been suggested as potential complications. Attaching the jejunum as close to the base of the cecum as possible decreases backflow pressure, discouraging fluid ingesta in the cecum from traveling orally back into the jejunum.

Ileal impactions may recur in the immediate postoperative period, particularly if a bypass procedure was not performed. Horses need to be fed carefully, using a laxative diet, to avoid this complication.

There is a 15% recurrence rate reported for large colon displacements and torsion. Factors contributing to recurrence have not been thoroughly identified. Recurrence of large colon displacements can be prevented by colopexy and large colon resection. Colopexy of the large colon has been reserved for nonperformance animals because of reported intestinal rupture after colopexy.[138] Extensive large colon resection is associated with short-term decreased absorption of water, decreased absorption of phosphorus, and weight loss.[139] Horses that have undergone large colon resection therefore have increased requirements of water, phosphorus, and better-quality protein.

Recurrence of small colon impaction is also a problem. Surgical evacuation of the large colon is recommended after surgical correction of small colon impactions. These horses should be managed with a laxative diet in the immediate postoperative period.

Management of postoperative complications may require repeat celiotomy. Clinical signs indicating the need for repeat celiotomy include persistent abdominal pain despite successful gastric decompression, marked and progressive intestinal distention, systemic deterioration associated with degenerative changes in the abdominocentesis, and presence of bacteria. In one study, 8.2% of horses (53 of 648) were subjected to repeat celiotomy. The long-term outcome of horses subjected to a second surgery was significantly worse than that of horses undergoing a single surgery.

SEPTIC PERITONITIS

Septic peritonitis is one of the most frequent fatal postoperative complications following exploratory laparotomy in horses (other common fatal complications are adhesions and ileus).[140,141] In one study, 56% of horses with septic postoperative peritonitis did not survive.[142] Postoperative peritonitis may result from necrosis of a segment of the GI tract before or after surgical intervention, contamination occurring at surgery, or leakage from the anastomosis or enterotomy site. In response to bacterial contamination, peritoneal macrophages and mast cells release histamine and prostaglandins, leading to vasodilatation and increased permeability of the peritoneal vessels. The subsequent peritoneal exudate contains fibrin, complement, immunoglobulins, and clotting factors. Chemotaxins such as IL-1, leukotriene B_4, and TNF produced by activated macrophages, mast cells, and neutrophils stimulate a further influx of neutrophils, exacerbating the inflammatory response.[143,144] Bacteria and other particles can be cleared from the peritoneal cavity through the diaphragmatic lymphatics. Movement of the diaphragm during respiration facilitates the uptake of peritoneal fluid into stomata, which are intercellular gaps between mesothelial cells covering the diaphragm. The stomata communicate with lymphatic lacunae, which drain peritoneal fluid into the substernal lymph nodes and subsequently via the thoracic duct into the bloodstream. Systemic effects from peritonitis may be initiated by the entrance of bacteria into the bloodstream, by the action of inflammatory mediators produced by macrophages and neutrophils, or by absorption of endotoxin from the peritoneal cavity into the portal venous system, which then acts on the Kupffer cells of the liver, contributing to the septic response.[145]

Clinical signs commonly associated with peritonitis include mild colic, depression, anorexia, ileus, diarrhea, fever, tachycardia, and tachypnea.[142,144,146] Besides relying on clinical signs, the diagnosis of peritonitis is based on peritoneal fluid analysis. Peritoneal fluid from normal horses has a nucleated cell count of less than 5000 cells/μL and a protein concentration of less than 2.5 g/dL. However, after an exploratory laparotomy, the peritoneal nucleated cell count, percentage of neutrophils, fibrinogen, and protein concentration become markedly elevated.[144,147] The mean nucleated cell count peaks at approximately 200,000/μL at day 4 and remains elevated at 40,000/μL through day 6; the mean protein concentration remains elevated and peaks at 6 g/dL on day 6 after an exploratory laparotomy. Therefore, absolute values and differential counts may not provide sufficient information on which to base a diagnosis of postoperative septic peritonitis. Hence, cytologic evaluation of the peritoneal fluid is crucial for a definitive diagnosis. Toxic or degenerative changes in neutrophils and the presence of intracellular or extracellular bacteria are indicative of septic peritonitis. Peritoneal pH and peripheral and peritoneal glucose may also be evaluated to diagnose septic peritonitis. A serum-peritoneal glucose difference greater than 50 mg/dL or a peritoneal pH less than 7.2 with a peritoneal glucose of less than 30 mg/dL is highly suggestive of septic peritonitis.[148] Peripheral blood values determined by complete blood count and fibrinogen should be compared with peritoneal fluid. A left shift, thrombocytopenia, or hypo-proteinemia is also indicative of septic peritonitis.[147,149] Peritoneal fluid should be submitted for both aerobic and anaerobic cultures and sensitivity.

Treatment should be directed first toward stabilization of the animal and then toward the inciting cause. IV fluids should be administered to correct dehydration and acid-base and electrolyte abnormalities. Patients are often hypoproteinemic (total protein less than 4.4 g/dL) and require plasma. If sepsis is caused by gram-negative bacteria, administration of hyperimmune serum (Polymune, Veterinary Dynamics, San Luis Obispo, Calif; and Endoserum, IMMVAC, Columbia, Mo) may attenuate the degree of endotoxemia. Flunixin meglumine (0.25 mg/kg IV three times a day) attenuates symptoms of endotoxemia. Broad-spectrum IV antibiotics are imperative. The most common organisms isolated from horses with peritonitis include the aerobic bacteria *E. coli, Staphylococcus, Streptococcus,* and *Rhodococcus equi* and the anaerobic bacteria *Bacteroides, Clostridium,* and *Fusobacterium*.[142,145,146] If necrotic intestine or leakage of an anastomosis or enterotomy is considered to be the cause of septic peritonitis, a second exploratory laparotomy is indicated.

Open peritoneal drainage has been described for the treatment of mild inflammatory peritonitis in an experimental model in horses,[150] but the efficacy of this technique in clinical septic peritonitis is not known. However, peritoneal lavage is an important component of the treatment protocol. Placement of an abdominal lavage system in the animal at the time of surgery is indicated if the animal is at risk for developing peritonitis (i.e., with a necrotic intestine or significant contamination at surgery). Enterotomies performed in the large and small colon to remove enteroliths do not significantly increase the risk of the horse's developing septic peritonitis, and a drain is not necessary. A closed fenestrated drain system (International Win Ltd, Kennett Square, Pa) allows infusion of fluid, and the suction drain system (Snyder Hemovac, Zimmer, Dover, Ohio) provides a continuous active evacuation of residual fluid. The drains may also be placed in a standing, sedated animal. Approximately 5 to 10 L of lactated Ringer's is infused every 6 hours. After infusion of the fluid, the horse is walked for 10 minutes to help circulate the fluid before draining the infusate. Heparin is often added to the lavage solution (5000 IU) or administered systemically (20 to 40 IU/kg SC every 8 hours). Heparin decreases peritoneal fibrin formation to give the antimicrobial agents better access to the bacteria.[143] The lavage is maintained until there is a decrease in the nucleated cell count and protein concentration, an increase in pH and glucose of the peritoneal fluid, and improvement in the cytologic appearance of the cells. By evacuating bacteria, cellular debris, fibrinogen, fibrin, and inflammatory mediators, this technique reduces the systemic effects of peritonitis, helps to resolve the infection, and decreases the incidence of adhesion formation, one of the complications of septic peritonitis.[125,151]

The prognosis for horses with septic peritonitis depends on the extent of the insult and how quickly the initiating cause is corrected. Horses that have extensive contamination because of leakage of the anastomosis or necrosis of devitalized bowel that was not removed during the initial surgery are likely to have a guarded prognosis.[141] Horses with less severe contamination often respond favorably to the preceding therapeutic protocol, although the cost of postoperative management is substantially increased.

INCISIONAL COMPLICATIONS

Incisional complications after exploratory celiotomy in horses include infection, dehiscence, suture sinus formation, and herniation. The frequency of incisional infections in horses after colic surgery is 10% to 37%.[141,152,153] A frequency of 28.6% was reported after one colic surgery, and 87.5% after two or more celiotomies.[152] Predisposing factors for incisional complications include repeat celiotomy, increased duration of surgery, use of a near-far-far-near pattern, use of chromic gut, leukopenia, incisional edema, postoperative pain, weight (greater than 300 kg), and older age (older than 1 year).[152,154,155] Incisional hernias are reported in 13% to 16% of horses after celiotomy. The single most important risk factor for herniation is incisional infection, which had a relative risk of 17.8 for causing herniation.[155]

Horses developing incisional infections are initially febrile without any localizing signs. Excessive tenderness and edema are sometimes noted. Most incisional infections develop 3 days or more after surgery, and drainage can sometimes be delayed up to 14 days. Systemic antibiotics delay the onset of drainage. Once drainage is noted, it is important to provide a route for exudation by removing a few staples or sutures at the site of the drainage. Culturing of the drainage identifies potential hospital problems. Horses that are afebrile after drainage has been established and in which excessive edema or cellulitis is not evident do not require systemic antibiotics. However, fever and significant tissue reaction are indications for antibiotic therapy. Flushing of the wound should be performed with caution, because it can propagate the infection along the entire incision line. An abdominal support should be provided, because dehiscence may occur.

Incisional infection rates can be decreased by shortening surgery time, using adequate draping, isolating any enterotomy incision from the clean surgical field, and minimizing trauma to the incision during exploration of the abdomen. A plastic ring drape can be used to protect the incision and is preferred by some surgeons for all exploratory surgeries. Bacterial culturing of the wound does not have predictive value for the incisional infection rate.[156] Closure of the linea alba should be performed with a suture material that is minimally reactive. Chromic gut has been associated with increased incisional drainage in horses, and braided nonabsorbable suture may cause suture sinus formation. Suture patterns do not particularly influence incisional infection rate, although in one study, a near-far-far-near pattern was associated with increased postoperative drainage.[152] Care should be taken, however, not to take overly large bites and to avoid excessive force when tightening sutures, since this can lead to ischemia, predisposing to incisional infection.

If incisional infection is present, or in cases of repeat laparotomy in the presence of an infected incision, the wound can be apposed with large stainless steel tension-releasing sutures, placed distant from the incision, which help support the abdominal wall (see Chapter 38). The linea alba is closed, and the subcutaneous tissues and skin can be left open for drainage.[157]

The reported rate of acute incisional dehiscence is low (2.0% to 2.9%), but this is the most serious acute incisional problem and can be fatal. Violent recovery, severe postoperative abdominal pain, prolonged surgery time, and use of a continuous suture pattern in the linea alba have been associated with early postoperative dehiscence.[152,158] Acute incisional dehiscence is best managed by immediate repair under general anesthesia if the intestine has not been severely traumatized.[159] For details on repair of acute total incisional dehiscence, see Chapter 38.

Incisional herniation is the most significant problem resulting from incisional infection. Incisional hernias do not necessarily require repair if they are small and do not cause deformation in the body wall. Large hernias that protrude from the abdomen require repair for cosmetic reasons but also because they are subject to repeated trauma. Hernias must be repaired only after the incision is healed and free of infection and the hernial ring has gained strength. This usually requires a minimum of 3 months after the original surgery. No skin abrasions, open wound, or drainage should be present at the time of hernia repair, because these may contaminate the surgical site, which could have serious implications, especially if an implant is used to repair the hernia. In preparation for surgery, the horse should be fasted to decrease abdominal weight. If the hernia is large, a complete pelleted feed can be substituted for hay 2 weeks before surgery to further decrease abdominal contents.

The horse is positioned in dorsal recumbency and draped in a routine manner. Three methods of hernia repair are described: primary closure, mesh implantation, and mesh implantation combined with fascial overlay.[160] An elliptic incision is made over the hernial defect, and the excess skin is removed by subcutaneous dissection, leaving the hernia sac intact. At this time, the potential for primary closure of the defect is determined. If this is judged feasible, the hernia sac is removed and the edges of the defect are freshened. A near-far-far-near or cruciate pattern is used to close the defect using a large monofilament nonabsorbable (polypropylene) or slowly absorbable (polydioxanone) suture material.

If excessive tension is of concern with primary closure, a mesh implant can be placed to reinforce closure. The hernia sac is left in place, and the mesh is trimmed to fit the defect. The mesh is inserted over the hernia sac and deep to the abdominal wall (retroperitoneally). Vertical mattress sutures of a large monofilament material (polypropylene or polydioxanone) are used to suture one side of the mesh to the body wall. The same material and patterns are used to pre-place sutures on the other side, estimating the distance needed to completely close the defect. The sutures are pulled tight. The linea is then apposed with a single-interrupted pattern. When the edges of the linea cannot be apposed, the mesh must be pulled tight to avoid sag and maintain a more cosmetic result. In the fascial overlay technique (see Chapter 38 for details), an elliptic incision is made through all layers on one side of the hernial sac, leaving the base attached. The mesh is implanted deep to the abdominal wall but superficial to the peritoneum and retroperitoneal fat. The edges of the mesh are folded toward the outside or laid flat, to avoid intestinal irritation and possible perforation.[161]

Materials used for hernia repair in horses include polypropylene (Marlex, Davol Inc, Cranston, RI) and plastics (Proxplast, Goshen Laboratories, Goshen, NY). The polypropylene is more resilient and may sag more than the plastic implants. Studies in other species indicate

TABLE 39-1. Postoperative Monitoring of Horses After Abdominal Surgery

		Monitoring				
			Hemodynamics			
Surgical Findings	**Possible Problems**	**Exam**	**TPR**	**Lab Work**	**Reflux**	**Fluids**
Small Intestine						
Simple obstruction	Ileus	q 1 hr while on fluids	q 4 hr	PCV/TP q 6 hr until no reflux; monitor electrolyes and creatinine daily until no reflux	q 4 hr	Until no reflux
Anterior enteritis	Ileus, laminitis	q 1 hr while on fluids	q 4 hr	PCV/TP q 6 hr until no reflux; monitor electrolytes and creatinine daily until no reflux	q 4 hr	Until no reflux
Strangulating obstruction	Ileus, endotoxemia, adhesions	q 1 hr	q 2–4 hr	PCV/TP q 6 hr until no reflux; monitor electrolytes and creatinine daily until no reflux	q 2–4 hr	Until cardiovascular status stable and no reflux
Large Intestine						
Simple obstruction	Postoperative diarrhea	q 4 hr	q 4 hr	If febrile: CBC, monitor for leukopenia	No	Correct preoperative dehydration
Strangulating obstruction	Endotoxemia: dehydration, protein loss; diarrhea; laminitis	q 1 hr	q 4 hr	PCV/TP q 6 hr until no reflux; monitor electrolytes and creatinine daily until no reflux; monitor rise in PCV with protein loss	No	Until cardiovascular status stable

*Preoperative antibiotics are broad spectrum: penicillin and gentamincin. Add metronidazole if significant intraoperative contamination.
†2.2 mg/kg IV over 60 min q 6 hr.
‡Loading dose: 1.3 mg/kg IV slowly over 5 min; maintenance: 0.05 mg/kg/min infusion IV.
§0.0044 mg/kg (2 mg per adult horse) SC or IV.

that the inertness of the polyester mesh in the presence of infection enables wound healing without formation of persistent abscesses or sinus tracts,[162] but the cost is much higher. In equine cases of postoperative infection, the implant may have to be removed to resolve persistent drainage.

Postoperative care after hernia repair includes minimizing abdominal weight for 2 weeks, stall rest for 4 weeks, and light exercise for 4 to 6 weeks. An abdominal bandage may help reduce edema in the initial postoperative period. All straining should be avoided in the postoperative period. The most serious complication after mesh repair is infection of the surgical site. Although systemic antibiotics are sometimes successful in treating the infection, in most cases the implant has to be removed to eliminate this complication. When infection develops, recurrence of the hernia may be a problem.

Recently, a postsurgical abdominal wrap has been advocated for the management of incisional hernias (CM Heal, CM Equine Products, Norco, Calif). These abdominal bandages provide firm even abdominal support, with a special pocket designed to apply direct pressure over the hernia site and they are available in different sizes. Anecdotal reports and the authors' experience are favorable for healing of incisional hernias without surgical intervention. An additional benefit is the ability to start the horse in an exercise program while the abdominal support is in place. Additional indications include the need for additional support after surgery in advanced pregnancies, and correction of umbilical hernias in foals.

POSTOPERATIVE MONITORING

Principles of monitoring horses after abdominal surgery are based on restoration of circulating fluid volume, electrolyte and acid–base equilibrium, and GI function. Table 39-1 summarizes the care of horses after abdominal surgery based on surgical findings. However, these are only guide-

TABLE 39-1. Postoperative Monitoring of Horses After Abdominal Surgery—cont'd

Drugs				Feeding		
NSAIDs	Antibiotics*	Pre-motility Agents	Other	Time	Type	Frequency
Flunixin meglumine 0.25 mg/kg IV tid	Perioperative (24 hr)	Erythromycin† Lidocaine‡		After 2 hr no reflux¶	Wet hay or grass	q 4 hr
Flunixin meglumine 0.25 mg/kg IV tid		Erythromycin† Lidocaine‡	Prevention of laminitis; acepromazine, nitroglycerin	After 12 hr no reflux	Wet hay or grass	q 4 hr
Flunixin meglumine 0.25 mg/kg IV tid	Until 24 hr afebrile	Erythromycin† Lidocaine‡	Plasma, hyperimmune serum, polymyxin B Prevention of laminitis: acepromazine, nitroglycerin	After 12 hr no reflux	Wet hay or grass	q 4 hr
Flunixin meglumine 0.25 mg/kg IV tid	Until 24 hr afebrile	Erythromycin† Neostigmine§		At 12 hr**	Grass, hay	q 4 hr
Flunixin meglumine 1.1 mg/kg IV bid, then reduce to 0.25 mg/kg tid	Until 24 hr afebrile	Erythromycin† Neostigmine§	Plasma, hyperimmune serum, polymyxin B Prevention of laminitis: acepromazine, nitroglycerin	When no large colon distention‡	Grass, hay	q 4 hr

¶For ileal impaction, feed a laxative diet and limit intake for 4 to 5 days.
**For cecal or large colon impaction, feed a laxative diet, give mineral oil, and monitor for reimpaction.
††For large colon resection, increase water intake and feed alfalfa hay.
CBC, Complete blood count; *IV*, intravenously; *PCV/TP*, packed cell volume/total protein; *SC*, subcutaneously; *TPR*, temperature, pulse, respiration.

lines, and therapy should be adjusted to individual cases based on physical and laboratory examination.

As a rule, horses on IV fluid therapy should be observed hourly and their hydration status evaluated every 6 hours by PCV and total protein determination. Horses that had significant bowel damage or ileus should be examined (including body temperature, pulse, respiration rate) every 4 hours until they have stabilized. Creatinine should be monitored daily until values are within the normal range. Postoperative fever is common within the first 24 hours of surgery but should resolve thereafter. A persistent fever should be investigated (impending colitis, peritonitis, catheter sepsis). Small intestinal diseases have a high incidence of postoperative ileus, whereas diarrhea more commonly follows large intestinal disorders. Laminitis is a risk for all horses but is more likely to occur if significant bowel damage was present. For all horses that are at risk for the development of endotoxemia, hyperimmune serum or polymyxin B is administered to bind endotoxin. For all horses that are at risk for the development of laminitis, a systemic (acepromazine) or topical (nitroglycerin) vasodilator is indicated, because these drugs are most effective before the onset of clinical signs of laminitis.

Perioperative antimicrobial agents should be of the broad-spectrum type and should have minimal effects on GI flora—for example, penicillin combined with gentamicin or, if significant elevation in creatinine is present, ceftiofur. Perioperative antibiotic therapy is applied in procedures in which the bowel lumen was not entered, and continues until the horse is afebrile for 24 hours and all systemic parameters have improved after enterotomies or resection and anastomosis procedures. Objective criteria that can be used for the discontinuation of systemic antibiotics include a normal white blood cell count without bands, normal temperature, absence of abdominal discomfort, and return of normal appetite.

Analgesic therapy is indicated after celiotomies. Flunixin meglumine is recommended for a minimum of 24 hours and then as needed, depending on the horse's systemic condition and comfort level.

In small intestinal disorders, feeding is resumed in small amounts after 12 hours if the horse has not developed reflux. The horse should first be offered water, followed by small amounts of wet hay or fresh grass. In large colon disorders, feeding can be resumed as early as 8 hours after surgery, provided there is good intestinal health. In cases of large colon torsion, feeding is delayed until there is evidence of mucosal integrity. Ileal, cecal, and large and small colon impactions should be closely monitored when feeding is resumed, because these animals are at risk for reimpaction. The use of laxatives such as mineral oil is recommended in the immediate postoperative period for impactions. For details on nutritional support for the critical surgical patient, see Chapter 6.

REFERENCES

1. Allen DJ, Kvietys PR, Granger N: Crystalloids vs colloids: Implications in fluid therapy in dogs with intestinal obstruction, Am J Vet Res 1986;47:1751.
2. Killingsworth CR: Use of blood and blood components for the feline and canine patient, J Vet Crit Care 1984;7:6.
3. Rudloff E, Kirby R: The critical need for colloids: Selecting the right colloid, Comp Cont Educ 1997;19:811.
4. Jones PA, Tomasic M, Gentry PA: Oncotic, hemodilutional, and hemostatic effects of isotonic saline and hydroxyethyl starch solutions in clinically normal ponies, Am J Vet Res 1997;58:541.
5. Dart AJ, Snyder JR, Spier SJ, et al: Ionized calcium concentration in horses with surgically managed gastrointestinal disease: 147 cases (1988-1990), J Am Vet Med Assoc 1992;201:1244.
6. Garcia-Lopez JM, Provost PJ, Rush JE, et al: Prevalence and prognostic importance of hypomagnesemia and hypocalcemia in horses that have colic surgery, Am J Vet Res 2001;62:7.
7. Johansson A, Gardner S, Jones S, et al: Hypomagnesemia in hospitalized horses, J Vet Intern Med 2003;17:860.
8. Toribio RE, Kohn CW, Chew DJ, et al: Comparison of serum parathyroid hormone and ionized calcium and magnesium concentrations and fractional urinary clearance of calcium and phosphorus in healthy horses and horses with enterocolitis, Am J Vet Res 2001;62:938.
9. Stewart AJ, Hardy J, Kohn CW, et al: Validation of diagnostic tests for determination of magnesium status in horses with reduced magnesium intake, Am J Vet Res 2004;65:422.
10. Herrera P, Burghardt RC, Phillips TD: Adsorption of *Salmonella enteritidis* by cetylpyridinium-exchanged montmorillonite clays, Vet Microbiol 2000;74:259.
11. Weese J, Cote N, deGannes R: Evaluation of the ability of di-tri-octahedral smectite to adhere to *Clostridium difficile* toxins and *Clostridium perfringens* enterotoxin in vitro, Proceedings American Association of Equine Practitioners 2002;48:127.
12. Aleman M, Nieto J, Carr E, et al: Serum hepatitis associated with commercial plasma transfusion in horses, J Vet Intern Med 2005;19:120.
13. Durando MM, MacKay RJ, Linda S, et al: Effects of polymyxin B and *Salmonella typhimurium* antiserum on horses given endotoxin intravenously, Am J Vet Res 1994;55:921.
14. Barton MH, Parviainen A, Norton N: Polymyxin B protects horses against induced endotoxaemia in vivo, Equine Vet J 2004;36:397.
15. Longworth KE, Smith BL, Staub NC, et al: Use of detergent to prevent initial response to endotoxin in horses, Am J Vet Res 1996;57:1063.
16. Winchell WW, Hardy J, Levine DM, et al: Effect of administration of a phospholipid emulsion on the initial response of horses administered endotoxin, Am J Vet Res 2002;63:1370.
17. King JN, Gerring EL: Antagonism of endotoxin-induced disruption of equine gastrointestinal motility with the platelet-activating factor antagonist WEB 2086, J Vet Pharmacol Ther 1990;13:333.
18. MacAllister CG, Morgan SJ, Borne AT, et al: Comparison of adverse effects of phenylbutazone, flunixin meglumine, and ketoprofen in horses, J Am Vet Med Assoc 1993;202:71.
19. Campbell NB, Blikslager AT: The role of cyclooxygenase inhibitors in repair of ischaemic-injured jejunal mucosa in the horse, Equine Vet J Suppl 2000;Jun:59.
20. Tomlinson JE, Blikslager AT: Effects of cyclooxygenase inhibitors flunixin and deracoxib on permeability of ischaemic-injured equine jejunum, Equine Vet J 2005;37:75.
21. Tomlinson JE, Wilder BO, Young KM, et al: Effects of flunixin meglumine or etodolac treatment on mucosal recovery of equine jejunum after ischemia, Am J Vet Res 2004;65:761.
22. Geor RJ, Weiss DJ, Burris SM: Effects of furosemide and pentoxifylline on blood flow properties in horses, Am J Vet Res 1992;53:2043.
23. Jarvis GE, Evans RJ: Platelet-activating factor and not thromboxane A2 is an important mediator of endotoxin-induced platelet aggregation in equine heparinised whole blood in vitro. Blood Coagul Fibrinolysis 1996;7:194.
24. Semrad SD, Hardee GE, Hardee MM, et al: Low dose flunixin meglumine: Effects on eicosanoid production and clinical signs induced by experimental endotoxemia in horses, Equine Vet J 1987;19:201.

25. Sellon D, Roberts M, Blikslager A, et al: Effects of continuous rate intravenous infusion of butorphanol on physiologic and outcome variables in horses after celiotomy, J Vet Intern Med 2004;18:555.
26. Nieto JE, Rakestraw PC, Snyder JR, et al: In vitro effects of erythromycin, lidocaine, and metoclopramide on smooth muscle from the pyloric antrum, proximal portion of the duodenum, and middle portion of the jejunum of horses, Am J Vet Res 2000;61:413.
27. Brianceau P, Chevalier H, Karas A, et al: Intravenous lidocaine and small-intestinal size, abdominal fluid, and outcome after colic surgery in horses, J Vet Intern Med 2002;16:736.
28. Cassuto B, Gfeller R: Use of intravenous lidocaine to prevent reperfusion injury and subsequent multiple organ dysfunction syndrome, J Vet Emerg Crit Care 2003;13:137.
29. Malone ED, Turner TA, Wilson JH: Intravenous lidocaine for the treatment of ileus in the horse. Proc Equine Colic Res Symp 1994;5:39.
30. Cohen ND, Lester GD, Sanchez LC, et al: Evaluation of risk factors associated with development of postoperative ileus in horses, J Am Vet Med Assoc 2004;225:1070.
31. Roussel AJ Jr, Cohen ND, Hooper RN, et al: Risk factors associated with development of postoperative ileus in horses, J Am Vet Med Assoc 2001;219:72.
32. Blikslager AT, Bowman KF, Levine JF, et al: Evaluation of factors associated with postoperative ileus in horses: 31 cases (1990-1992), J Am Vet Med Assoc 1994;205:1748.
33. Freeman DE, Hammock P, Baker GJ, et al: Short- and long-term survival and prevalence of postoperative ileus after small intestinal surgery in the horse, Equine Vet J Suppl 2000;Jun:42.
34. Hunt JM, Edwards GB, Clarke KW: Incidence, diagnosis and treatment of postoperative complications in colic cases, Equine Vet J 1986;18:264.
35. Adams SB: Recognition and management of ileus, Vet Clin North Am Equine Pract 1988;4:91.
36. Becht J, Richardson D: Ileus in the horse: Clinical significance and management. Proceedings American Association of Equine Practitioners 1981;27:291.
37. Gerring E: Management of intestinal ileus in the horse, Comp Cont Educ Pract Vet 1992;14:1102.
38. Ortiz H, Armendariz P, Yarnoz C: Is early postoperative feeding feasible in elective colon and rectal surgery? Int J Colorectal Dis 1996;11:119.
39. Hartsell PA, Frazee RC, Harrison JB, et al: Early postoperative feeding after elective colorectal surgery, Arch Surg 1997;132:518.
40. Cheatham ML, Chapman WC, Key SP, et al: A meta-analysis of selective versus routine nasogastric decompression after elective laparotomy, Ann Surg 1995;221:469.
41. Adams SB, Lamar CH, Masty J: Motility of the distal portion of the jejunum and pelvic flexure in ponies: Effects of six drugs. Am J Vet Res 1984;45:795.
42. Gerring EE, Hunt JM: Pathophysiology of equine postoperative ileus: Effect of adrenergic blockade, parasympathetic stimulation and metoclopramide in an experimental model, Equine Vet J 1986;18:249.
43. Gerring HL: All wind and water: Some progress in the study of equine gut motility, Equine Vet J 1991;23:81.
44. Grider JR: Neurotransmitters mediating the intestinal peristaltic reflex in the mouse, J Pharmacol Exp Ther 2003;307:460.
45. Livingston EH, Passaro EP: Postoperative ileus, Dig Dis Sci 1990;35:121.
46. Sarna SK, Otterman M: Myoelectric and contractile activities In Shuster M, editor: Atlas of gastrointestinal motility in health and disease, Baltimore, 1993, Williams and Wilkins.
47. Reynolds JC, Putman PE: Prokinetic agents, Gastroenterol Clin North Am 1992;21:567.
48. Ward SM, Sanders KM, Hirst GD: Role of interstitial cells of Cajal in neural control of gastrointestinal smooth muscles, Neurogastroenterol Motil 2004;16(Suppl 1):112.
49. Holte K, Kehlet H: Postoperative ileus: A preventable event, Br J Surg 2000;87:1480.
50. Hudson N, Mayhew I, Pearson G: A reduction in interstitial cells of Cajal in horses with equine dysautonomia (grass sickness), Auton Neurosci 2001;92:37.
51. Huizinga JD: Neural injury, repair, and adaptation in the GI tract: IV. Pathophysiology of GI motility related to interstitial cells of Cajal, Am J Physiol 1998;275:G381.
52. Lester GD, Merritt AM, Neuwirth L, et al: Effect of alpha 2-adrenergic, cholinergic, and nonsteroidal anti-inflammatory drugs on myoelectric activity of ileum, cecum, and right ventral colon and on cecal emptying of radiolabeled markers in clinically normal ponies, Am J Vet Res 1998;59:320.
53. Adams SB, MacHarg MA: Neostigmine methylsulfate delays gastric emptying of particulate markers in horses, Am J Vet Res 1985;46:2498.
54. Parks AH, Stick JA, Arden W: Effects of distention and neostigmine on jejunal vascular resistance, oxygen uptake, and intraluminal pressure changes in ponies, Am J Vet Res 1989;50:54.
55. Furness JB, Costa M: Adynamic ileus, its pathogenesis and treatment, Med Biol 1974;52:82.
56. Davies JV, Gerring EL: Effect of spasmolytic analgesic drugs on the motility patterns of the equine small intestine, Res Vet Sci 1983;34:334.
57. Eades SC, Moore JN: Blockade of endotoxin-induced cecal hypoperfusion and ileus with an alpha 2 antagonist in horses, Am J Vet Res 1993;54:586.
58. Fernandez AG, Maasingham R: Peripheral receptor populations involved in the gastrointestinal motility and the pharmacological actions of metoclopramide-like drugs. Life Sci 1985;36:1.
59. Dart AJ, Peauroi JR, Hodgson DR: Efficacy of metoclopramide for the treatment of ileus in horses following small intestinal surgery: 70 cases (1981-1992). Aust Vet J 1996;280:280.
60. Rampe D, Roy ML, Dennis A, et al: A mechanism for the proarrhythmic effects of cisapride (Propulsid): High affinity blockade of the human cardiac potassium channel HERG, FEBS Lett 1997;417:28.
61. Megans A, Awouters F, Niemegeers C: General pharmacology of the four gastrointestinal motility stimulants bethanechol, metoclopramide, trimebutine, and cisapride, Arzeneim-Forsch 1991;41:631.
62. Wiseman L, Fauds D: Cisapride: An updated review of its pharmacology and therapeutic efficacy as a prokinetic agent in gastrointestinal motility disorders, Drugs 1994;47:116.
63. Barone JA, Jessen LM, Colaizzi JL, et al: Cisapride: A gastrointestinal prokinetic drug, Ann Pharmacother 1994;28:488.
64. Orihata M, Sarna SK: Contractile mechanisms of action of gastroprokinetic agents: Cisapride, metoclopramide, and domperidone, Am J Physiol 1994;266:G665.
65. Ruckebusch Y, Roger T: Prokinetic effects of cisapride, naloxone and parasympathetic stimulation at the equine ileo-caeco-colonic junction, J Vet Pharmacol Ther 1988;11:322.
66. Sasaki N, Yoshihara T: The effect of motilin on the regulation mechanism of intestinal motility in conscious horses, J Vet Med Sci 1999;61:167.
67. Gerring EL, King JN, Edwards GB: A multicenter trial of cisapride in the prophylaxis of equine postoperative ileus, Equine Vet Educ 1991;3:143.
68. Valk N, Doherty TJ, Blackford JT, et al: Effect of cisapride on gastric emptying in horses following endotoxin treatment, Equine Vet J 1998;30:344.
69. Cook G, Papich MG, Roberts MS, et al: Cisapride pharmacokinetics in the horse after IV and rectal administration, Proc Am Coll Vet Int Med, Lake Buena Vista, Fla, 1997.
70. Mearin F, Rodrigo L, Perez-Mota A, et al: Levosulpiride and cisapride in the treatment of dysmotility-like functional dyspepsia: A randomized, double-masked trial, Clin Gastroenterol Hepatol 2004;2:301.

71. Pandolfino JE, Howden CW, Kahrilas PJ: Motility-modifying agents and management of disorders of gastrointestinal motility, Gastroenterology 2000;118:S32.
72. Parkman HP, Pagano AP, Vozzelli MA, et al: Gastrokinetic effects of erythromycin: myogenic and neurogenic mechanisms of action in rabbit stomach, Am J Physiol 1995;269:G418.
73. Peeters T: Erythromycin and other macrolides as prokinetic agents, Gastroenterology 1993;105:1886.
74. Lester GD, Merritt AM, Neuwirth L, et al: Effect of erythromycin lactobionate on myoelectric activity of ileum, cecum, and right ventral colon, and cecal emptying of radiolabeled markers in clinically normal ponies, Am J Vet Res 1998;59:328.
75. Gustafsson A, Baverud V, Gunnarsson A, et al: The association of erythromycin ethylsuccinate with acute colitis in horses in Sweden, Equine Vet J 1997;29:314.
76. Rimback G, Cassuto J, Tollesson P: Treatment of postoperative paralytic ileus by intravenous lidocaine infusion, Anesth Analg 1989;70:414.
77. Kalff JC, Carlos TM, Schraut WH, et al: Surgically induced leukocytic infiltrates within the rat intestinal muscularis mediate postoperative ileus, Gastroenterology 1999;117:378.
78. Eskandari MK, Kalff JC, Billiar TR, et al: LPS-induced muscularis macrophage nitric oxide suppresses rat jejunal circular muscle activity, Am J Physiol 1999;277:G478.
79. Kalff JC, Schraut WH, Simmons RL, et al: Surgical manipulation of the gut elicits an intestinal muscularis inflammatory response resulting in postsurgical ileus, Ann Surg 1998;228:652.
80. Hsu WH: Xylazine-induced delay of small intestinal transit in mice, Eur J Pharmacol 1982;83:55.
81. Rutkowski JA, Ross MW, Cullen K: Effects of xylazine and/or butorphanol or neostigmine on myoelectric activity of the cecum and right ventral colon in female ponies, Am J Vet Res 1989;50:1096.
82. Roger T, Bardon T, Ruckebusch Y: Comparative effects of mu and kappa opiate agonists on the cecocolic motility in the pony, Can J Vet Res 1994;58:163.
83. Clark ES, Thompson SA, Becht JL, et al: Effects of xylazine on cecal mechanical activity and cecal blood flow in healthy horses, Am J Vet Res 1988;49:720.
84. Merritt AM, Campbell-Thompson ML, Lowrey S: Effect of xylazine treatment on equine proximal gastrointestinal tract myoelectrical activity, Am J Vet Res 1989;50:945.
85. Pasternak GW: Pharmacological mechanisms of opioid analgesics, Clin Neuropharmacol 1993;16:1.
86. Frantzides CT, Cowles V, Salaymeh B, et al: Morphine effects on human colonic myoelectric activity in the postoperative period, Am J Surg 1992;163:144.
87. Kamerling SG, Hamra JG, Bagwell CA: Naloxone-induced abdominal distress in the horse, Equine Vet J 1990;22:241.
88. Sojka JE, Adams SB, Lamar CH, et al: Effect of butorphanol, pentazocine, meperidine, or metoclopramide on intestinal motility in female ponies, Am J Vet Res 1988;49:527.
89. Baxter GM, Broome TE, Moore JN: Abdominal adhesions after small intestinal surgery in the horse, Vet Surg 1989;18:409.
90. Dabareiner RM, Sullins KE, White NA, et al: Serosal injury in the equine jejunum and ascending colon after ischemia-reperfusion or intraluminal distention and decompression, Vet Surg 2001;30:114.
91. Parker JE, Fubini SL, Car B: Prevention of intraabdominal adhesions in ponies by low-dose heparin therapy, Vet Surg 1987;16:459.
92. Trevor PB, White NA, Sullins KE: Use of sodium hyaluronate to prevent adhesions in the horse and rabbit, Abstract, Equine Colic Research Symposium, 1991.
93. Ryan GB, Grobety J, Majno G: Postoperative peritoneal adhesions: A study of mechanisms, Am J Pathol 1971;65:117.
94. DiZerega GS: Contemporary adhesion prevention, Fertil Steril 1994;61:1219.
95. Gomel V, Urman B, Gurgan T: Pathophysiology of adhesion formation and strategies for prevention, J Reprod Med 1996;41:35.
96. Buckman RF, Buckman P, Hufnagel J: A physiologic basis for the adhesion-free healing on deperitonealized surfaces, J Surg Res 1976;21:67.
97. Thompson JN, Paterson-Brown S, Harbourne T: Plasminogen activating activity: Possible mechanism of adhesion formation, Br J Surg 1989;76:382.
98. Vipond MN, Whawell SA, Thompson JN: Peritoneal fibrinolytic activity and intra-abdominal adhesions, Lancet 1990;335:1120.
99. Dabareiner RM, White NA, Donaldson LL: Effects of intraluminal distention and decompression on microvascular permeability and hemodynamics of the equine jejunum, Am J Vet Res 2001;62:225.
100. Sullins KE, White NA, Lundin CS: Treatment of ischemia induced peritoneal adhesions in foals, Proc Am Coll Vet Surg Veterinary Symposium, 1992.
101. Freeman DE, Cimprich RE, Richardson DW, et al: Early mucosal healing and chronic changes in pony jejunum after various types of strangulation obstruction, Am J Vet Res 1988;49:810.
102. Sullins KE, White NA, Lundin CS, et al: Prevention of ischaemia-induced small intestinal adhesions in foals, Equine Vet J 2004;36:370.
103. Darien BJ: Heparin therapy: rationale and clinical implications, Comp Cont Educ 1993;15:1273.
104. Lam L, Silbert J, Rosenberg R: The separation of active and inactive forms of heparin. Biochem Biophys Res Comm 1976;69:570.
105. Moore BR, Hinchcliff KW: Heparin: A review of its pharmacology and therapeutic use in horses, J Vet Int Med 1994;8:26.
106. Chan T, Chan V: Antithrombin III, the major modulator of intravascular coagulation is synthesized by human endothelial cells, Thromb Haemost 1981;46:504.
107. Gerhards H: Low dose calcium heparin in horses: plasma heparin concentration, effects on red blood cell mass and on coagulation variables, Equine Vet J 1991;23:37.
108. Speight MO, Griffith MJ: Calcium inhibits the heparin-catalyzed antithrombin III/thrombin reaction by decreasing the apparent binding affinity of heparin for thrombin, Arch Biochem Biophys 1983;225:958.
109. Hirsh J: Drug therapy: Heparin, N Engl J Med 1991;324:1565.
110. Darien BJ, Potempa J, Moore JN: Antithrombin III activity in horses with colic: An analysis of 46 cases, Equine Vet J 1991;23:211.
111. Johnstone IB, Crane S: Haemostatic abnormalities in horses with colic: Their prognostic value, Equine Vet J 1986;18:271.
112. Baxter GM, Parks AH, Prasse KW: Effects of exploratory laparotomy on plasma and peritoneal coagulation/fibrinolysis in horses, Am J Vet Res 1991;52:1121.
113. Collatos C, Barton MH, Prasse KW, et al: Intravascular and peritoneal coagulation and fibrinolysis in horses with acute gastrointestinal tract disease, J Am Vet Assoc 1995;207:465.
114. Moore JN, Mahaffey EA, Zboran M: Heparin-induced agglutination of erythrocytes in horses, Am J Vet Res 1987;48:68.
115. Moll HD, Schumacher J, Wright JC, et al: Evaluation of sodium carboxymethylcellulose for prevention of experimentally induced abdominal adhesions in ponies, Am J Vet Res 1991;52:88.
116. Fredericks CM, Kotry DI, Holtz G, et al: Adhesion prevention in the rabbit with sodium carboxymethylcellulose solutions, Am J Obstet Gynecol 1986;155:667.
117. Mueller PO, Hunt RJ, Allen D, et al: Intraperitoneal use of sodium carboxymethylcellulose in horses undergoing exploratory celiotomy, Vet Surg 1995;24:112.
118. Murphy DJ, Peck LS, Detrisac CJ, et al: Use of a high-molecular-weight carboxymethylcellulose in a tissue protective solution for prevention of postoperative abdominal adhesions in ponies, Am J Vet Res 2002;63:1448.
119. Hay WP, Mueller PO, Harmon B, et al: One percent sodium carboxymethylcellulose prevents experimentally induced abdominal adhesions in horses, Vet Surg 2001;30:223.

120. Eggleston RB, Mueller PO, Parviainen AK, et al: Effect of carboxymethylcellulose and hyaluronate solutions on jejunal healing in horses, Am J Vet Res 2004;65:637.
121. Mueller PO, Harmon BG, Hay WP, et al: Effect of carboxymethylcellulose and a hyaluronate-carboxymethylcellulose membrane on healing of intestinal anastomoses in horses, Am J Vet Res 2000;61:369.
122. Mueller PO, Hay WP, Harmon B, et al: Evaluation of a bioresorbable hyaluronate-carboxymethylcellulose membrane for prevention of experimentally induced abdominal adhesions in horses, Vet Surg 2000;29:48.
123. Eggleston RB, Mueller E, Quandt JE, et al: Use of a hyaluronate membrane for jejunal anastomosis in horses, Am J Vet Res 2001;62:1314.
124. Dunn DL, Barke RA, Ahrenholz DH: The adjuvant effect of peritoneal fluid in experimental peritonitis, Ann Surg 1984;199:37.
125. Hague BA, Honnas CM, Berridge BR, et al: Evaluation of standing postoperative peritoneal lavage for prevention of experimentally induced abdominal adhesions in horses, Proc Am Assoc Equine Pract 1996:42.
126. Nieto JE, Snyder JR, Vatistas NJ, et al: Use of an active intra-abdominal drain in 67 horses, Vet Surg 2003;32:1.
127. Livesey MA, Little CB, Boyd C: Fatal hemorrhage associated with incarceration of small intestine by the epiploic foramen in three horses, Can Vet J 1991;32:434.
128. Vachon AM, Fisher AT: Small intestinal herniation through the epiploic foramen: 53 cases (1987-1993), Equine Vet J 1995;27:373.
129. Vasey JR: Incarceration of the small intestine by the epiploic foramen in fifteen horses, Can Vet J 1988;29:378.
130. Doyle AJ, Freeman DE, Rapp H, et al: Life-threatening hemorrhage from enterotomies and anastomoses in 7 horses, Vet Surg 2003;32:553.
131. Frankeny RL, Wilson DA, Messer NT, et al: Jejunal intussusception: A complication of functional end-to-end stapled anastomoses in two ponies, Vet Surg 1995;24:515.
132. Lowe JE: Intussusception in three ponies following experimental enterotomies, Cornell Vet 1968;58:288.
133. Schumacher J, Hanrahan L: Ileocecocolic intussusception as a sequel to jejunocecostomy in a mare, J Am Vet Med Assoc 1987;190:303.
134. Gerard MP, Bowman KF, Blikslager AT, et al: Jejunocolostomy or ileocolostomy for treatment of cecal impaction in horses: nine cases (1985-1995), J Am Vet Med Assoc 1996;209:1287.
135. Taylor TS, Martin MT, McMullan WC: Bypass surgery for intestinal occluding abscesses in the equine: A report of two cases, Vet Surg 1981;10:136.
136. Tate LP, Ralston SL, Koch CM, et al: Effects of extensive resection of the small intestine in the pony, Am J Vet Res 1983;44:1187.
137. Haven ML, Roberts MC, Argenzio RA, et al: Intestinal adaptation following 70% small bowel resection in ponies, Proc Equine Colic Res Symp 1991;4:54.
138. Hance SR, Embertson RM: Colopexy in broodmares: 44 cases (1986-1990), J Am Vet Med Assoc 1992;201:782.
139. Ralston SL, Sullins KE, Stashak TS. Digestion in horses after resection or ischemic insult of the large colon, Am J Vet Res 1986;47:2290.
140. Ducharme N, Hackett RP. Surgical treatment of colic: Results in 181 cases, Vet Surg 1983;12:206.
141. Phillips TJ, Walmsey JP: Retrospective analysis of the results of 151 exploratory laparotomies in horses with gastrointestinal disease, Equine Vet J 1993;25:427.
142. Hawkins JF, Bowman KF, Roberts M: Peritonitis in horses, J Am Vet Med Assoc 1993;203:284.
143. Maddaus M, Ahrenholz D, Simmons RL: The biology of peritonitis and implications for treatment, Surg Clin North Am 1988;68:431.
144. Dabareiner RM: Peritonitis in horses In Smith BP, editor: Large Animal Internal Medicine, St Louis, 1996, Mosby.
145. Mair TS, Hillyer MH, Taylor FGR: Peritonitis in adult horses: A review of 21 cases, Vet Rec 1990;126:567.
146. Dyson S: Review of peritonitis in adult horses, Equine Vet J 1983;15:25.
147. Santshi EM, Grindem CB, Tate LP: Peritoneal fluid analysis in ponies after abdominal surgery, Vet Surg 1988;17:6.
148. Rodgers L: Evaluation of peritoneal pH, glucose, and lactate dehydrogenase levels as an indicator of intra-abdominal sepsis, Proc Am Coll Vet Intern Med 1994;12:173.
149. Kopcha M, Schultze AE: Peritoneal fluid: Part I. Pathophysiology and classification of neoplastic effusions, Comp Cont Educ 1991;13:519.
150. Chase JP, Beard WL, Bertone AL, et al: Open peritoneal drainage in horses with experimentally induced peritonitis, Vet Surg 1996;25:189.
151. Nieto JE, Rakestraw PC, Vatistas NJ: Use of a close intra-abdominal drain in horses: 72 cases, J Am Vet Med Assoc, 1997 (submitted).
152. Kobluk CN, Ducharme NG, Lumsden JH, et al: Factors affecting incisional complication rates associated with colic surgery in horses: 78 cases (1983-1985), J Am Vet Med Assoc 1989;195:639.
153. Honnas CM, Cohen ND: Risk factors for wound infection following celiotomy in horses, J Am Vet Med Assoc 1997;210:78.
154. Wilson DA, Baker GJ, Boero MJ: Complications of celiotomy incisions in horses, Vet Surg 1995; 24:506.
155. Gibson KT, Curtis CR, Turner AS, et al: Incisional hernias in the horse: Incidence and predisposing factors, Vet Surg 1989;18:360.
156. Ingle-Fehr JE, Baxter GM, Howard RD, et al: Bacterial culturing of ventral median celiotomies for prediction of postoperative incisional complications in horses, Vet Surg 1997;26:7.
157. Tulleners EP, Donawick WJ: Secondary closure of infected abdominal incisions in cattle and horses, J Am Vet Med Assoc 1983;182:1377.
158. Stone WC, Lindsay WA, Mason DA, et al: Factors associated with acute wound dehiscence following equine abdominal surgery. Proceedings, Fourth Equine Colic Research Symposium, 1991:52.
159. Curtis MB, Eicker SW, Archer M, et al: Anesthetic management of incisional dehiscence in recovery following exploratory laparotomy in a horse, J Am Vet Med Assoc 1992;200:692.
160. Tulleners EP, Fretz PB: Prosthetic repair of large abdominal wall defects in horses and food animals, J Am Vet Med Assoc 1983;182:258.
161. McIlwraith CW, Turner AS: Surgery of the gastrointestinal tract, In Equine Surgery: Advanced Techniques. Philadelphia, Lea & Febiger, 1987.
162. Fox SM, Bright R, Hammond DL: Reconstruction of tissue deficits with Marlex mesh, Comp Cont Educ 1988;10:897.

SECTION **VI** RESPIRATORY SYSTEM

John A. Stick

CHAPTER 40

Overview of Upper Airway Function

Frederik J. Derksen

The upper airway has complex physiologic functions including olfaction, phonation, deglutition, thermoregulation, filtering and conditioning of the inspired air, and protecting the lower airway from aspiration. Most important, the upper airway also functions as a conduit for airflow to and from the lung, and, because the horse is an obligate nasal breather, a normal upper airway is critical in this species. To accommodate the many diverse demands placed on it, the upper airway was not ideally designed for any one activity. For example, the equine upper airway has a large dead space volume, it has high resistance to airflow, and it tends to collapse in response to negative pressures generated during inspiration.[1-4] Although none of these characteristics is ideal for an airflow conduit, compromises in design are necessary to accommodate the other upper airway functions. For these reasons, the upper airway may well be a limiting factor in the horse's exercise capacity, and tolerances in the upper airway are minimal. Even the smallest lesion before surgery or remaining after completion of a surgical procedure may further limit performance. This makes surgical interventions in the upper airway challenging, and if upper airway function is not fully considered, surgical outcome is often suboptimal. Consequently, surgeons must have a working understanding of upper airway physiology. The purpose of this chapter is to provide the surgeon with information that should be considered when performing upper airway surgery in the horse.

THE UPPER AIRWAY AND PERFORMANCE

The capacity of horses to increase ventilation in response to the demands of exercise is truly enormous. A normal horse at rest breathing 15 times a minute with a tidal volume of 5 L has a minute ventilation of 75 L. During exercise, respiratory rate and tidal volume increase to achieve a minute ventilation of approximately 1500 L.[3] The upper airway must accommodate this 20-fold increase in airflow by undergoing changes in caliber, rigidity, and shape. In spite of these adaptations to exercise, evidence suggests that in exercising horses upper airway resistance becomes a large portion of total respiratory resistance, and this increase in resistance may limit performance.[5] In strenuously exercising horses, the $Pa{O_2}$ decreases and the $Pa{CO_2}$ increases. This perturbation in gas exchange is in part caused by insufficient alveolar ventilation, although diffusion limitation also plays a major role. Substituting a mixture of helium and oxygen for air reduces airway resistance, and blood oxygenation is improved.[5] Taken together, this is strong evidence to suggest that upper airway resistance limits arterial blood oxygenation in exercising horses, thereby limiting oxygen delivery to tissues and performance. Thus, if the function of the upper airway as a conduit for airflow is taxed to the maximum during exercise in normal horses, it is easy to understand that small upper airway lesions can significantly impact upper airway function during exercise and further affect performance.

MECHANICS OF AIR FLOW

The respiratory muscles, primarily the diaphragm, provide the force needed for ventilation. The pumping action of these muscles results in large pressure changes in the airways. On exhalation, pressure in the upper airway becomes positive, driving the air out against the atmospheric pressure, whereas on inhalation, pressures are negative, resulting in movement of air from the outside to inside the lung. The greater the exercise intensity, the greater are the airflow rates and the larger are the pressure changes. During high-intensity exercise, the pressure in the trachea is approximately 15 cm H_2O on exhalation, and it is −30 cm H_2O on inhalation[6] (Fig. 40-1). Positive pressure in the upper airway during exhalation encourages upper airway dilation in this phase of the respiratory cycle. On inhalation, however, the

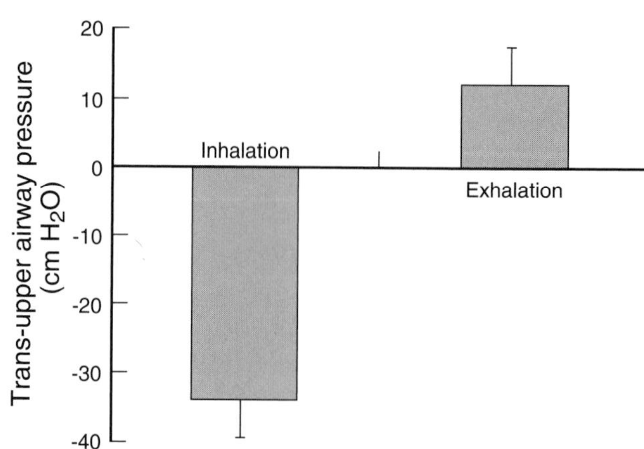

Figure 40-1. Trans-upper airway pressures of normal horses during intense exercise. Note that inspiratory pressures are more than twice as great as expiratory pressures.

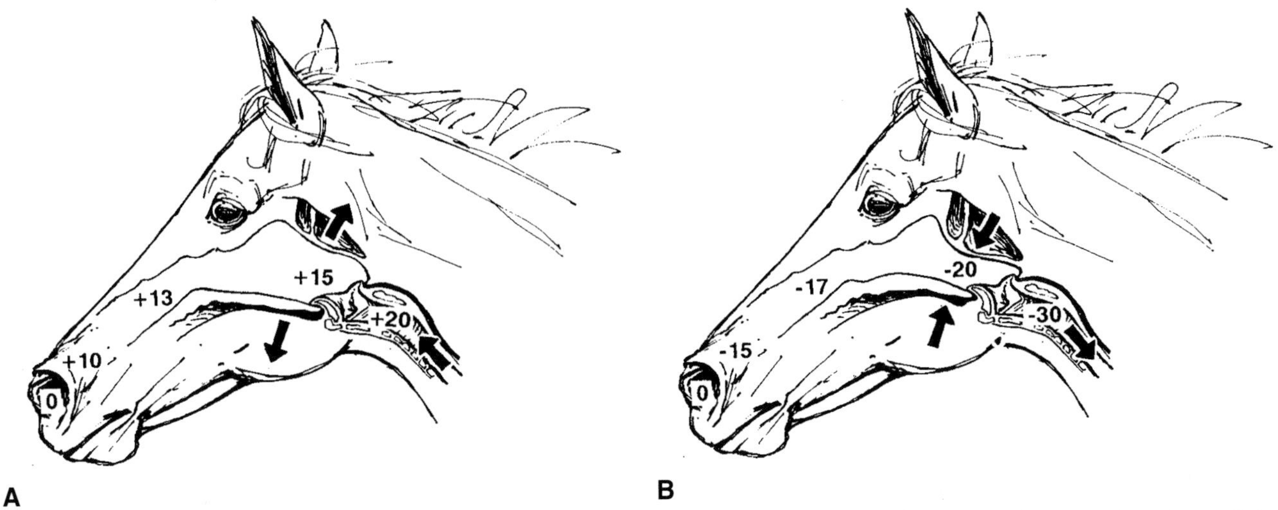

Figure 40-2. **A,** In exercising horses, upper airway pressures are positive relative to the atmosphere during expiration, facilitating airway dilation. **B,** During inspiration, upper airway pressures are negative, narrowing the airway lumen.

negative pressure in the upper airway encourages tissues to collapse, thus narrowing the upper airway (Fig. 40-2).

The ratio of driving pressure and the resulting airflow is called impedance. Impedance is a very useful calculated variable, because it is a measure of how much the airflow is opposed by the respiratory system. One of the most important determinants of impedance is airway resistance. Airway resistance in turn is primarily determined by airway diameter. Many surgically correctable conditions of the upper airway (e.g., recurrent laryngeal neuropathy) narrow the airway lumen, decrease its diameter, and therefore increase impedance.[7] Measurements of upper airway impedance on inhalation and exhalation demonstrate that, even in normal horses, the upper airway is only partially able to withstand these pressure swings, especially during exercise. During inhalation, subatmospheric intraluminal pressures cause the airway to narrow, whereas positive intraluminal pressures enlarge the airway diameter during exhalation. As a consequence, impedance is approximately twice as high on inhalation as it is during exhalation[8] (Fig. 40-3).

At first glance, it may be surprising that upper airway pressure swings are sufficient to cause such large changes in resistance in normal horses. This phenomenon is explained by the observation that small changes in airway caliber cause large changes in resistance. The relationship between resistance (R) of a cylindrical tube with a length (L) and radius (r) is given by the following formula,

$$R = 8 \times u \times L/r^4,$$

where u is the viscosity of the air. This equation demonstrates that the radius is a very important determinant of resistance, and that reducing the radius by half increases resistance 16-fold. Thus, a relatively small decrease in upper airway caliber can significantly increase resistance to flow and limit performance. Once the cross-sectional area of an airway region is decreased, air velocity increases and intraluminal pressure decreases further. This phenomenon, called the Bernoulli effect, reduces airway cross-sectional area even further, setting up a vicious cycle that results in airway collapse (called dynamic collapse).

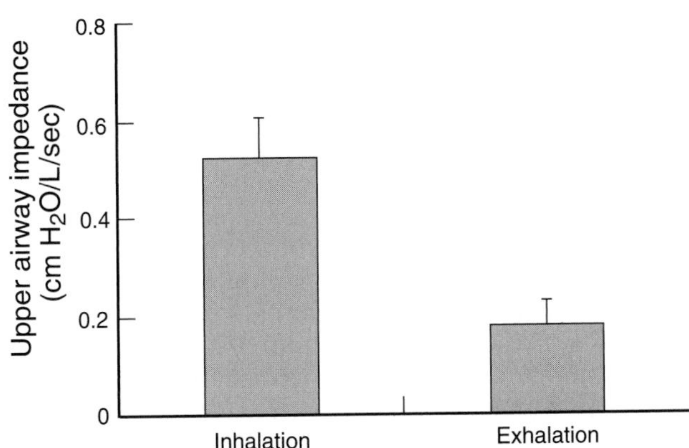

Figure 40-3. Upper airway impedance of normal horses during intense exercise. Note that inspiratory impedance is more than twice as large as expiratory impedance.

DISTRIBUTION OF AIRWAY RESISTANCE

In the horse, as in most mammals, upper airway resistance is a significant proportion of total resistance to flow. In the resting horse, a full two thirds of the total resistance to airflow resides in the upper airway.[2] This portion increases during exercise. Because of this, most animal species switch to mouth breathing during exercise, which provides a low-resistance pathway for the greater airflow required during exercise and minimizes the work of breathing. The horse cannot breathe through its mouth effectively, and the approximately 20-fold increase in airflow that occurs during exercise must be totally accommodated by the upper airway. Obligate nasal breathing is the result of a tight seal between the soft palate and the laryngeal cartilages. When the nasal passages are occluded, this seal may be broken and mouth breathing results. However, in the horse, the resistance to airflow through the mouth is apparently very high.

During exercise, the distribution of airflow resistance changes significantly. In the exercising horse, during inhalation, intrathoracic resistance is less than 25% of total resistance to flow and the remaining resistance is almost evenly divided between nasal and laryngeal resistance. On exhalation, the intrathoracic and extrathoracic resistances are about even.[2]

The upper airway caliber varies with the region. Airway diameters are smallest at the external nares and larynx and largest throughout the nasal turbinate area and pharynx. This observation has practical implications, because it means that lesions in high-resistance areas (external nares and larynx) are more likely to cause clinically significant upper airway obstruction than similar-size lesions in regions such as the pharynx. For example, a small granulomatous lesion located on the axial surface of the arytenoid cartilage is a concern because it reduces the airway caliber in a region of the upper airway that is already narrow. In contrast, pharyngeal lymphoid hyperplasia is not likely to significantly increase total resistance to airflow, because this space-occupying lesion is located in the pharynx, which has a large cross-sectional area, and therefore the lesion contributes less to airflow resistance.

STABILIZING THE UPPER AIRWAY

The upper airway is designed to prevent collapse on inhalation. The simplest way to prevent a tube from collapsing in response to negative intraluminal pressure is to make the wall rigid. Indeed, for some of its length, the upper airway is rigidly supported by bone and cartilage. In other regions of the airway such as the external nares, pharynx, and larynx, rigid support by bone or cartilage is incompatible with other functions such as swallowing and protecting the lower airways. In these regions, the upper airway is supported by muscular activity. Neural reflexes regulate the activity of upper airway dilator muscles.[9-11] On inhalation, these muscles begin to contract just before the diaphragm, and they remain active during inhalation. In this way, the upper airway stiffens before it is exposed to subatmospheric pressures. This phasic activity is finely tuned by pressure- and flow- (temperature-) sensitive receptors in the upper airway that, when stimulated, enhance reflex activation of upper airway dilator muscles. These muscles then provide appropriate tension to prevent dynamic collapse of tissues on inhalation.[12,13]

External Upper Airway Support

Recently, a nasal strip became commercially available as an external nasal dilator. It mechanically supports the soft tissue that forms the lateral wall at the narrowest portion of the nasal cavity (nasal valve), located just rostral to the nasoincisive notch. This region is bound medially by the nasal septum, ventrally by the concha, and dorsolaterally by the skin and dorsal conchal fold. The strip consists of three polyester springs sandwiched between two layers of material, and it adheres to the horse's nose. When the strip is applied, endoscopic examination shows that the strip dilates the nasal valve region.[14] Furthermore, in exercising horses, the nasal strip decreases inspiratory impedance.[14] Interestingly, the nasal strip also decreases the severity of exercise-induced pulmonary hemorrhage (EIPH).[15,16] These findings suggest that in exercising horses, the nasal strip reduces upper airway tissue collapse on inhalation. This would result in decreased inspiratory impedance during exercise, and less negative inspiratory pressures. Less negative inspiratory pressure may reduce the transmural pulmonary capillary pressure. Because excessive transmural pulmonary capillary pressure is responsible for EIPH,[17,18] reduction in this pressure very likely accounts for the observed decrease in the severity of EIPH.

Head Position

Horses are often required to exercise with their heads and necks in unnatural positions. For example, Standardbred horses are raced with an overcheck, which forces the head and neck into extension. Sport horses, such as dressage horses, commonly exercise with head and neck flexed. Head and neck position significantly affects upper airway impedance.[19] In resting horses that are holding their heads in a natural position, the air entering the upper airway turns approximately 90 degrees to flow from the nasal passages into the trachea. This change in direction contributes to the work of breathing. Normally, horses straighten their head and neck during exercise. When the horse's head and neck are flexed, upper airway impedance during exercise is about 50% greater than that of a horse exercising with head and neck in the extended position.[19]

Straightening of the head and neck not only provides a more direct route to the lung, it also tends to stretch upper airway tissues, making them more rigid and resistant to collapse. It stands to reason, therefore, that dynamic upper airway obstructions, especially those involving the pharynx, are often more apparent when affected horses are exercised with a flexed head and neck position.

External Nares

The external nares of the horse are very mobile and can completely close the upper airway (as occurs during swimming) or fully dilate it (e.g., during intense exercise). The external nares and adjacent nasal valve are among the narrowest portions of the upper airway; therefore, lesions in this region significantly affect performance.[20] The dilator muscles of the external nares, such as the dilator naris lateralis, and the transversus nasi are innervated by the facial nerve, and horses with facial nerve dysfunction have marked inspiratory airway obstruction during exercise.

Nasal Turbinate Region

The nasal turbinate region has convoluted conchae that encourage particle deposition and conditioning of the inspired air. This portion of the upper airway is rigidly supported by cartilage and bone. However, marked changes in airway caliber are possible even in this bone- and cartilage-supported region. The upper airway is lined by mucosa that contains vascular sinuses. The purpose of this extensive vasculature is thermoregulation and humidification of inhaled air. These vessels are potentially very large and have the ability to fill with blood, thickening the upper airway mucosa to the point of occlusion. Normally, the size of capacitance vessels is kept small by tonic sympathetic innervation. During exercise, the sympathetic tone increases, capacitance vessels are constricted, and the airway diameter is increased.[21] Injury to the sympathetic trunk innervating this region—for example, in Horner's syndrome—can cause complete nasal occlusion of the affected side. Unilateral airway obstruction is often the longest-lasting condition associated with Horner's syndrome, and it causes significant exercise intolerance. Nasal vascular engorgement also has been identified as a cause of airway obstruction in horses recovering from general anesthesia after removal of the orotracheal tube. This obstruction is sufficiently severe to cause hypoventilation and hypoxemia. Phenylephrine, an α-adrenoceptor, can be used to decrease nasal vascular engorgement after anesthesia to prevent upper airway obstruction in these horses.[22]

Nasopharynx

The nasopharynx participates in swallowing as well as breathing, and it must be able to constrict to propel a bolus of food into the esophagus, and to dilate during exercise to allow unimpeded airflow to and from the lung. These functions are achieved by muscles that are uniquely positioned so that, as a group, they can both constrict and dilate the pharynx.[23-25] In the horse, the exact functions of these muscles are incompletely understood, but from studies in horses and in other species, a general picture is emerging.

The hyoid apparatus is a very important structure that supports the pharynx as well as the root of the tongue and the larynx. The muscles of the hyoid apparatus dilate the pharynx by contracting on inhalation in the following manner. The geniohyoid and genioglossus muscles pull rostrally and ventrally, whereas the sternohyoid and sternothyroid muscles pull in a caudal ventral direction. The net effect is extension of the stylohyoid-ceratohyoid articulation, a ventral movement of the hyoid bone, and nasopharyngeal stabilization or even dilation (Fig. 40-4). One of the recommended surgeries for dorsal displacement of the soft palate is sectioning of the sternohyoid and sternothyroid muscles.[26,27] The objective of this surgery is to move the epiglottis cranially, thereby better engaging the soft palate. From the aforementioned discussion, it is clear that sectioning of the sternohyoid and sternothyroid muscles prevents pharyngeal dilation and may encourage pharyngeal collapse. Indeed, measurements in exercising horses have indicated that sternohyoid and sternothyroid muscle sectioning slightly increases upper airway resistance in exercising horses.[28]

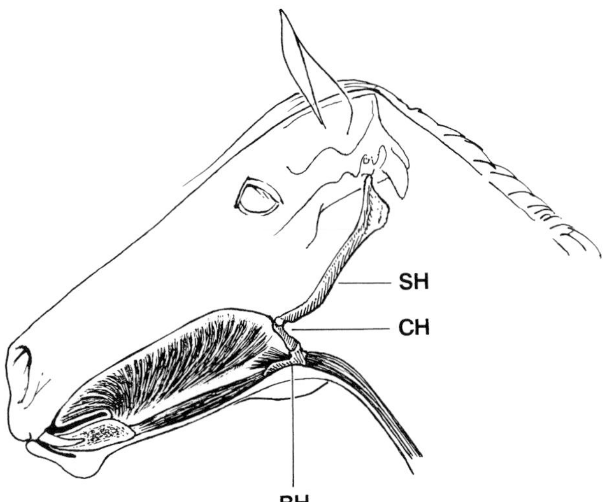

Figure 40-4. The hyoid apparatus and the pharynx. The hyoid apparatus is made up of the stylohyoid (SH), the ceratohyoid (CH), and the basihyoid (BH) bones. Contraction of the geniohyoid and sternohyoid muscles stabilizes the hyoid apparatus and the pharynx.

In racehorses, the tongue is often pulled forward and tied down to the mandible to prevent dorsal displacement of the soft palate. The tongue is attached to the hyoid bone via the genioglossus and hyoglossus muscles. Therefore, it is possible that the tongue-tie could dilate the pharynx. However, recent upper airway flow mechanics and computed tomographic studies have indicated that, in normal horses, the tongue-tie does not pull the hyoid apparatus forward and does not dilate the pharynx.[29,30]

The dorsal pharyngeal wall is supported by the stylopharyngeus muscles. These muscles insert on the dorsal nasopharyngeal wall, perpendicular to it, so that contraction of the stylopharyngeus muscles raises the wall of the dorsal nasopharynx, expanding, supporting, and preventing its collapse as pressures within the airway become more negative during inspiration (Fig. 40-5). Blockade of the ninth cranial nerves, which innervate these muscles, results in dorsal pharyngeal collapse and inspiratory airway obstruction during exercise.[31]

The upper airway is richly endowed with receptors that, when stimulated, activate upper airway dilator muscles, thereby stiffening the upper airway. For example, when the laryngeal mucosa is anesthetized, exercising horses have nasopharyngeal collapse and upper airway obstruction.[32] During nasal occlusion, these horses can also experience dorsal displacement of the soft palate. This demonstrates that, in exercising horses, sensory and motor functions must be fully coordinated to maintain upper airway patency. The message to the surgeon is that the upper airway is a finely tuned instrument that can be easily disturbed by disease or surgical intervention.

The Soft Palate

The soft palate is another upper airway structure with multiple functions. It separates the nasopharynx from the oral pharynx and forms a tight seal around the larynx during breathing. However, during swallowing, the soft palate is elevated and closes the posterior nares, protecting the nasal passages from food and water. The position of the soft palate is determined by four muscles: the tensor veli palatini, levator veli palatini, palatinus, and palatopharyngeus muscles.[33] Dysfunction of the tensor veli palatini destabilizes the cranial portion of the soft palate closest to the hard palate. In affected horses, the cranial portion of the soft palate bulges into the nasopharynx on inhalation.[34] The pharyngeal branch of the vagus nerve innervates all of the muscles controlling the soft palate, except for the tensor veli palatini. Blockade of this nerve with a local anesthetic agent results in dorsal displacement of the soft palate.[35] This demonstrates that coordinated activity of these muscles is necessary to stabilize the soft palate during breathing. The pharyngeal branch of the vagus nerve courses through the guttural pouch and lies in close proximity to the retropharyngeal lymph nodes. It is thought that, in clinical cases, dorsal displacement of the soft palate is the result of injury to this

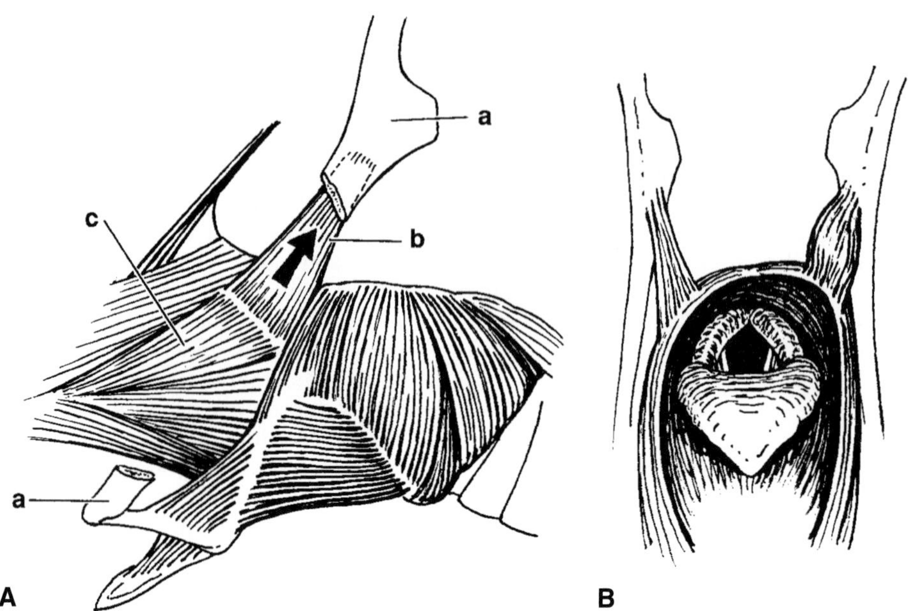

Figure 40-5. A, The stylopharyngeus muscle originates on the stylohyoid bone (a), and broadly inserts on the dorsal pharyngeal wall. Contraction of the stylopharyngeus muscle (b) stabilizes and dilates the dorsal pharynx during exercise. c, palatopharyngeus muscle. **B,** Note the difference in size of the left and right dorsal pharynx when the stylopharyngeus muscle contracts unilaterally.

nerve because of retropharyngeal lymph node or guttural pouch inflammation.

Most upper airway conditions cause inspiratory airway obstruction, and expiratory airflow is unaffected. Dorsal displacement of the soft palate is an exception to this rule, since it is an expiratory obstruction. During exhalation, the paralyzed soft palate billows dorsally into the nasopharynx, markedly obstructing airflow and causing airway obstruction[35] (Fig. 40-6).

The Larynx

The larynx functions as a very important guard, preventing food and water from entering the trachea. During swallowing, the arytenoid cartilages adduct completely, and the epiglottis pivots around its base so that the tip of the epiglottis moves dorsally and caudally. These maneuvers close the rima glottidis and prevent aspiration. Of course, during exercise the larynx must be opened maximally to allow unimpeded airflow. The larynx is one of the narrowest portions of the upper airway, and consequently lesions in this region cause significant airway obstruction. A good example of this is recurrent laryngeal neuropathy, also known as idiopathic laryngeal hemiplegia. In this condition, dysfunction of the left recurrent laryngeal nerve prevents appropriate contraction of the cricoarytenoideus dorsalis muscle, which fails to abduct the arytenoid cartilage during inhalation.[36,37] In resting horses, pressure changes are insufficient to move the affected arytenoid cartilage and vocal fold into the airway lumen. On exhalation, positive pressures in the upper airway move the affected arytenoid cartilage abaxially, increasing airway caliber. However, on inhalation during exercise, luminal pressures are sufficiently negative to move the affected arytenoid cartilage and associated vocal fold into the airway, causing significant obstruction. The objective of surgical intervention in horses with recurrent laryngeal neuropathy is to prevent dynamic collapse of the affected arytenoid cartilage. For example, in these cases, prosthetic laryngoplasty is effective because the procedure stabilizes the affected arytenoid cartilage, preventing dynamic collapse. An example of a surgical procedure that is ineffective because it fails to adhere to this principle is subtotal arytenoidectomy.[38] In this procedure, only the body of the arytenoid cartilage is removed, while the muscular process and the corniculate cartilage are left in place to help prevent postsurgical aspiration. However, during exercise the unsupported cartilage moves axially and obstructs the rima glottidis.[38]

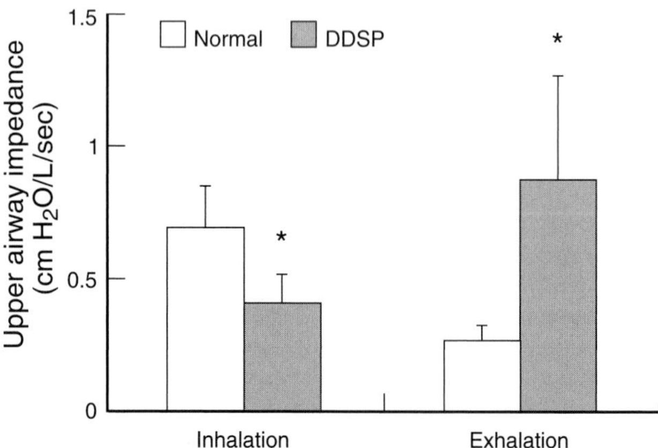

Figure 40-6. Upper airway impedance in intensely exercising horses before and after experimentally induced dorsal displacement of the soft palate. Note that expiratory impedance is increased, whereas inspiratory impedance is decreased.

As mentioned earlier, during swallowing the epiglottis pivots around its base, protecting the trachea. However, during breathing and especially during exercise, the epiglottis must be stabilized. This is the function of the hyoepiglotticus muscle, which originates on the basihyoid bone and inserts on the base of the epiglottis. When the hyoepiglotticus muscle contracts, the epiglottis is pulled ventrally toward the base of the tongue, stabilizing the epiglottis. The hyoepiglotticus muscle is innervated by the hypoglossal nerves, and bilateral blockade of this nerve results in epiglottic retroversion during inhalation in exercising horses.[39,40] Clinical cases of epiglottic retroversion have been described and probably are the result of disease interfering with neuromuscular control of upper airway dilator muscles, specifically the hyoepiglotticus muscle.[41]

MEASUREMENT OF UPPER AIRWAY FUNCTION

Thus it is clear that the upper airway has often-competing functions, that small perturbations in function may cause significant airway obstruction, and that, for the surgeon, tolerance for error is small. Quantitative measurements of upper airway function help determine the effect of a particular condition on upper airway flow mechanics and the efficacy of surgical treatment. The best way to ensure that a surgical procedure is efficacious is to use quantitative methods of evaluation. The simplest method of evaluating upper airway flow mechanics is to measure the pressure needed to move air through the upper airway while the horse is undergoing a standard exercise test. Airway pressures may be measured using a multiple-hole catheter inserted into the trachea via the nostrils or percutaneously.[42] When airway pressures and airflow rates are measured simultaneously, upper airway impedance can be calculated as the ratio of pressure and flow.[7] Measurement of impedance provides a more direct evaluation of changes in airway caliber than pressure measurements alone. Pressure and flow measurements have been used to determine the efficacy of many surgical procedures used in the treatment of upper airway conditions, such as recurrent laryngeal neuropathy and dorsal displacement of the soft palate.[35,43,44]

Quantitative information may also be gained from analysis of airflow rates during the respiratory cycle. Flow-volume loop analysis is a test in which airflow rate is continuously plotted against breath volume. This test is particularly useful when performed in exercising horses, and in some instances it is more sensitive than the measurement of upper airway impedance in the evaluation of upper airway function[8,45] (Fig. 40-7).

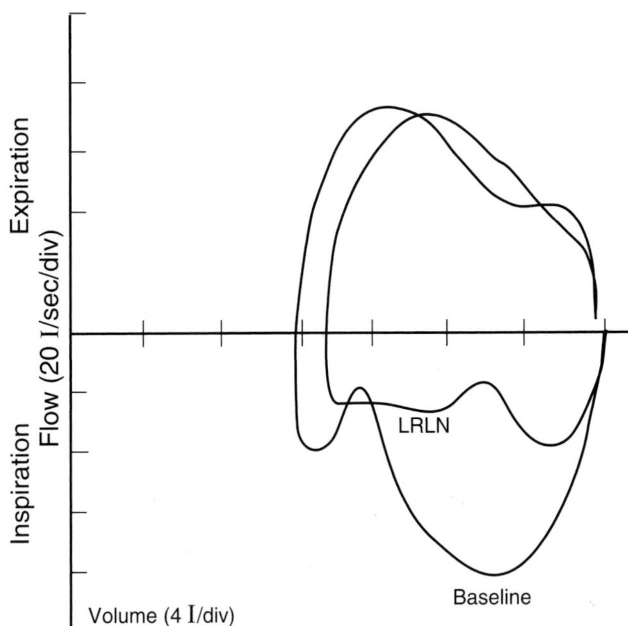

Figure 40-7. Tidal breathing flow-volume loop from a horse exercising at maximal heart rate before (baseline) and after induction of laryngeal hemiplegia (LRLN). Note that expiration is unaffected, but there is severe inspiratory flow limitation with LRLN throughout the inspiratory portion of the tidal volume.

REFERENCES

1. Gallivan GJ, McDonell WN, Forrest JB: Comparative ventilation and gas exchange in the horse and the cow, Res Vet Sci 1989;46:331.
2. Art T, Serteyn D, Lekeux P: Effect of exercise on the partitioning of equine respiratory resistance, Equine Vet J 1988;20:268.
3. Art T, Anderson L, Woakes AJ, et al: Mechanics of breathing during strenuous exercise in Thoroughbred horses, Respir Physiol 1990;82:279.
4. Morris EA, Seeherman HJ: Evaluation of upper respiratory tract function during strenuous exercise in racehorses, J Am Vet Med Assoc 1990;196:431.
5. Erickson BK, Seaman J, Kubo K, et al: Mechanism of reduction in alveolar-arterial P_{O_2} difference by helium breathing in the exercising horse, J Appl Physiol 1994;76:2794.
6. Tetens J, Derksen FJ, Stick JA, et al: Efficacy of prosthetic laryngoplasty with and without bilateral ventriculocordectomy as treatments for laryngeal hemiplegia in horses, Am J Vet Res 1996;57:1668.
7. Derksen FJ, Stick JA, Scott EA, et al: Effect of laryngeal hemiplegia and laryngoplasty on airway flow mechanics in exercising horses, Am J Vet Res 1986;47:16.
8. Lumsden JM, Derksen FJ, Stick JA, et al: Use of flow-volume loops to evaluate upper airway obstruction in exercising Standardbreds, Am J Vet Res 1993;54:766.
9. Mathew OP: Upper airway negative-pressure effects on respiratory activity of upper airway muscles, J Appl Physiol 1984;56:500.
10. Sant'Ambrogio G, Mathew OP, Sant'Ambrogio FB, Fisher JT: Laryngeal receptors responding to respiratory events, Prog Clin Biol Res 1985;176:171.
11. Mathew OP, Sant'Ambrogio G, Fisher JT, et al: Laryngeal pressure receptors, Respir Physiol 1984;57:113.
12. Sant'Ambrogio G, Mathew OP, Fisher JT, et al: Laryngeal receptors responding to transmural pressure, airflow and local muscle activity, Respir Physiol 1983;54:317.
13. Sant'Ambrogio G, Tsubone H, Sant'Ambrogio FB: Sensory information from the upper airway: Role in the control of breathing, Respir Physiol 1995;102:1.
14. Holcombe SJ, Berney C, Cornelisse CJ, et al: Effect of commercially available nasal strips on airway resistance in exercising horses, Am J Vet Res 2002;63:1101.
15. Kindig CA, McDonough P, Fenton G, et al: Efficacy of nasal strip and furosemide in mitigating EIPH in Thoroughbred horses, J Appl Physiol 2001;91:1396.
16. Geor RJ, Ommundson L, Fenton G, et al: Effects of an external nasal strip and frusemide on pulmonary haemorrhage in Thoroughbreds following high-intensity exercise, Equine Vet J 2001;33:577.
17. Birks EK, Durando MM, McBride S: Exercise-induced pulmonary hemorrhage, Vet Clin North Am Equine Pract 2003;19:87.
18. West JB, Mathieu-Costello O, Jones JH, et al: Stress failure of pulmonary capillaries in racehorses with exercise-induced pulmonary hemorrhage, J Appl Physiol 1993;75:1097.

19. Petsche V, Derksen FJ, Berney C, et al: Effect of head position on upper airway function in exercising horses, Equine Vet J Suppl1995;18:18.
20. Robinson NE, Sorenson PR: Pathophysiology of airway obstruction in horses: A review, J Am Vet Med Assoc 1978;172:299.
21. Olson LG, Strohl KP: The response of the nasal airway to exercise, Am Rev Respir Dis 1987;135:356.
22. Lukasik VM, Gleed RD, Scarlett JM, et al: Intranasal phenylephrine reduces post anesthetic upper airway obstruction in horses, Equine Vet J 1997;29:236.
23. Strohl KP, Olson LG: Concerning the importance of pharyngeal muscles in the maintenance of upper airway patency during sleep: An opinion, Chest 1987;92:918.
24. van Lunteren E, Strohl KP: The muscles of the upper airways, Clin Chest Med 1986;7:171.
25. Van de Graff WB, Gottfried SB, Mitra J, et al: Respiratory function of hyoid muscles and hyoid arch, J Appl Physiol 1984;57:197.
26. Hanes PF: Dorsal displacement of the soft palate and epiglottic entrapment: Diagnosis, management and interrelationships, Comp Cont Educ Pract Vet 1983;5:S379.
27. Anderson JD, Tulleners EP, Johnston JK, et al: Sternothyrohyoideus myectomy or staphylectomy for treatment of intermittent dorsal displacement of the soft palate in racehorses: 209 cases (1986-1991), J Am Vet Med Assoc 1995;206:1909.
28. Holcombe SJ, Beard WL, Hinchcliff KW, et al: Effect of sternothyrohyoid myectomy on upper airway mechanics in normal horses, J Appl Physiol 1994;77:2812.
29. Cornelisse CJ, Rosenstein DS, Derksen FJ, et al: Computed tomographic study of the effect of a tongue-tie on hyoid apparatus position and nasopharyngeal dimensions in anesthetized horses, Am J Vet Res 2001;62:1865.
30. Cornelisse CJ, Holcombe SJ, Derksen FJ, et al: Effect of a tongue-tie on upper airway mechanics in horses during exercise, Am J Vet Res 2001;62:775.
31. Tessier C, Holcombe SJ, Derksen FJ, et al: Effects of stylopharyngeus muscle dysfunction on the nasopharynx in exercising horses, Equine Vet J 2004;36:318.
32. Holcombe SJ, Derksen FJ, Berney C, et al: Effect of topical anesthesia of the laryngeal mucosa on upper airway mechanics in exercising horses, Am J Vet Res 2001;62:1706.
33. Holcombe SJ, Derksen FJ, Stick JA, et al: Pathophysiology of dorsal displacement of the soft palate in horses, Equine Vet J Suppl 1999;30:45.
34. Holcombe SJ, Derksen FJ, Stick JA, et al: Effect of bilateral tenectomy of the tensor veli palatini muscle on soft palate function in horses, Am J Vet Res 1997;58:317.
35. Holcombe SJ, Derksen FJ, Stick JA, et al: Effect of bilateral blockade of the pharyngeal branch of the vagus nerve on soft palate function in horses, Am J Vet Res 1998;59:504.
36. Duncan ID, Griffiths IR, McQueen A, et al: The pathology of equine laryngeal hemiplegia, Acta Neuropathol (Berl) 1974;27:337.
37. Duncan ID, Griffiths IR, Madrid RE: A light and electron microscopic study of the neuropathy of equine idiopathic laryngeal hemiplegia, Neuropathol Appl Neurobiol 1978;4:483.
38. Belknap JK, Derksen FJ, Nickels FA, et al: Failure of subtotal arytenoidectomy to improve upper airway flow mechanics in exercising Standardbreds with induced laryngeal hemiplegia, Am J Vet Res 1990;51:1481.
39. Holcombe SJ, Derksen FJ, Stick JA, et al: Effects of bilateral hypoglossal and glossopharyngeal nerve blocks on epiglottic and soft palate position in exercising horses, Am J Vet Res 1997;58:1022.
40. Holcombe SJ, Cornelisse CJ, Berney C, et al: Electromyographic activity of the hyoepiglotticus muscle and control of epiglottis position in horses, Am J Vet Res 2002;63:1617.
41. Parente EJ, Martin BB, Tulleners EP: Epiglottic retroversion as a cause of upper airway obstruction in two horses, Equine Vet J 1998;30:270.
42. Ducharme NG, Hackett RP, Ainsworth DM, et al: Repeatability and normal values for measurement of pharyngeal and tracheal pressures in exercising horses, Am J Vet Res 1994;55:368.
43. Tetens J, Derksen FJ, Stick JA, et al: Efficacy of prosthetic laryngoplasty with and without bilateral ventriculocordectomy as treatments for laryngeal hemiplegia in horses, Am J Vet Res 1996;57:166.
44. Shappell KK, Derksen FJ, Stick JA, et al: Effects of ventriculectomy, prosthetic laryngoplasty, and exercise on upper airway function in horses with induced left laryngeal hemiplegia, Am J Vet Res 1988;49:1760.
45. Lumsden JM, Derksen FJ, Stick JA, et al: Evaluation of partial arytenoidectomy as a treatment for equine laryngeal hemiplegia, Equine Vet J 1994;26:125.

CHAPTER 41

Diagnostic Techniques in Equine Upper Respiratory Tract Disease

Eric J. Parente
Frederik J. Derksen

PHYSICAL EXAMINATION

Although a large portion of the upper respiratory tract is not easily seen or palpated, a thorough physical examination can provide critical details that assist in its overall assessment. A physical examination is an essential part of any evaluation. It not only provides information on present pathology but also reveals clues about previous surgical procedures. Before beginning the examination, a complete history should be obtained. Specific questions should be asked about respiratory noise, dysphagia, exercise intolerance, coughing, nasal discharge, and any previous treatments or surgery. All of this information should be interpreted in conjunction with the physical examination findings and the results of the other diagnostic procedures to establish a diagnosis.

The physical examination begins with visual assessment of any asymmetry of the head and nares, and inspection for the presence of any nasal or ocular discharge. Facial deformity in front of the eye is consistent with either primary or secondary sinus disease. There may be associated nasal discharge via the nasomaxillary opening, or ocular discharge from occlusion of the nasolacrimal duct. Furthermore, chronic sinus disease may result in nasal passage obstruction. Placing a hand in front of each nostril provides a crude indication of airflow from each nostril. Subtle changes are very difficult to detect, but an obstructive lesion in one nasal passage may result in significant asymmetric airflow. Percussion of a normal sinus should result in a hollow sound. The presence of an abnormal structure in the sinus can change the character and intensity of the sound, but this depends on many factors and can often be misinterpreted.

Nostril disease is uncommon, but palpation of each nostril and the alar folds in the dorsal aspect of the nares can often determine if a problem is present. If alar fold redundancy and obstruction during exercise is suspected, the alar folds can be tied with umbilical tape over the bridge of the nostril during an exercise period. Mitigation of noise confirms the diagnosis.

Palpation of the larynx can be a difficult skill to develop, but once mastered it is very helpful in assessing laryngeal function. An assistant should hold the horse's head slightly elevated. The clinician can stabilize the right side of the larynx with one hand and palpate the left side of the larynx with the other hand. By alternating hands, both sides of the larynx can be compared. The muscular processes of the larynx are in a fairly dorsal position and are slightly smaller than a person's knuckle. The caudal border is attached to the cricoarytenoideus dorsalis muscle, and when the muscle is atrophied, the muscular process feels more prominent than on the other side. Mild asymmetry is a common finding in horses with normal laryngeal function, but more overt asymmetry is usually consistent with the horse's inability to maintain abduction of the affected arytenoid cartilage. If the left muscular process cannot be easily palpated, it may be covered by scar tissue from a previous laryngoplasty, or the arytenoid cartilage may be chondritic. A scar from laryngoplasty is not easily palpated at the level of the skin and therefore cannot be used to definitively determine if previous surgery was performed. Clipping the hair ventral to the linguofacial vein makes it easier to detect a scar if surgery was performed. If the right muscular process cannot be palpated easily, the arytenoid may be chondritic, or a fourth branchial arch abnormality may be present.[1] Infrequently, stertorous breathing can be elicited with firm palpation of the larynx, and this may indicate some inability of the horse to maintain an adequate lumen from conditions such as severe arytenoid chondrosis or bilateral arytenoid paresis, or a combination of both.

Other common sites for respiratory surgery should be evaluated during the examination. Previous surgery involving a laryngotomy often leaves a palpable scar. The skin ventral to the larynx should be palpated for a scar by pinching the skin below the larynx. Often, a fibrous band forms between the skin and larynx that can be palpated when drawing the fingers like a rake across the skin in this area. The accessory respiratory muscles (sternothyrohyoideus) should be examined for any sign of a defect secondary to a myectomy, and the tracheal rings should be palpated for any abnormalities associated with trauma or previous surgery.

DIAGNOSTIC IMAGING

Videoendoscopic Examination at Rest

The endoscopic examination of the upper airway is still the primary diagnostic tool. Most diagnoses can be obtained from a complete resting endoscopic examination. Videoendoscopic equipment, commercially available for over 20 years, provides the best method for viewing the upper airway. Several companies produce videoendoscopes with similar specifications, and user preference and cost often determine which system is purchased. The main components of a videoendoscopy system consist of the videoendoscope itself, the video processor, the light source, and the video monitor. A videoendoscope with an outer diameter of less than 9.5 mm can be used easily on all adult horses and on most foals. Smaller videoendoscopes with an outer diameter of less than 8.5 mm are also available for younger foals, but the tradeoff is a smaller biopsy channel (2.2 mm versus 2.8 mm). Most videoendoscopes have a field of view of 120 degrees, and tip deflection angles of 210 to 90 degrees. The working length for most videoendoscopes is approximately 103 cm, which is ample for upper respiratory work. Light sources are fairly standard xenon lamps with illumination of 300 watts. Fiberoptic endoscopes typically have only half the illumination of the videoendoscopes, and a much smaller field of view, which significantly limits the clinician's ability to clearly view all abnormalities.

Image storage is crucial for documentation and reevaluations. It is therefore beneficial to have a recording unit or a printer with any videoendoscopic system. Any VHS tape deck can be used as a recording unit. More recently, advancements have been made that allow digital images to be downloaded directly to a laptop computer or a compact disk.

The clinician should have a plan of how and what to evaluate during the examination. The patient should not be sedated and should be restrained only with a twitch to ensure no interference with any assessments of airway function. It is easiest to have an assistant pass the endoscope down the ventral meatus of one nostril until the tip of the endoscope enters the pharynx. The pharynx and larynx should be evaluated first, and then the nasal passage can be evaluated while backing the endoscope out of the horse's nose. If there is a suspected abnormality in the nasal passage, the normal side should be evaluated first to minimize any trauma to or resentment from the horse before evaluating the abnormal side.

The amount of lymphoid hyperplasia in the pharynx is variable and depends on the horse's age. It is common for the younger horse to have lymphoid hyperplasia, but it has not been correlated with any specific dysfunctions.[2,3] The epiglottis should always be positioned dorsal to the palate and should have a distinct serrated edge with a clear vascular pattern on the dorsal surface. The corniculate processes of the arytenoid cartilages should be evaluated for their overall appearance, relative position, and degree of movement. Thickening, ulcerations, or granulation tissue are probably indicative of chondrosis (Fig. 41-1). Inability to fully abduct relative to the other side is indicative of recurrent laryngeal neuropathy. (*Recurrent laryngeal neuropathy* is the term used to depict the naturally occurring form of laryngeal

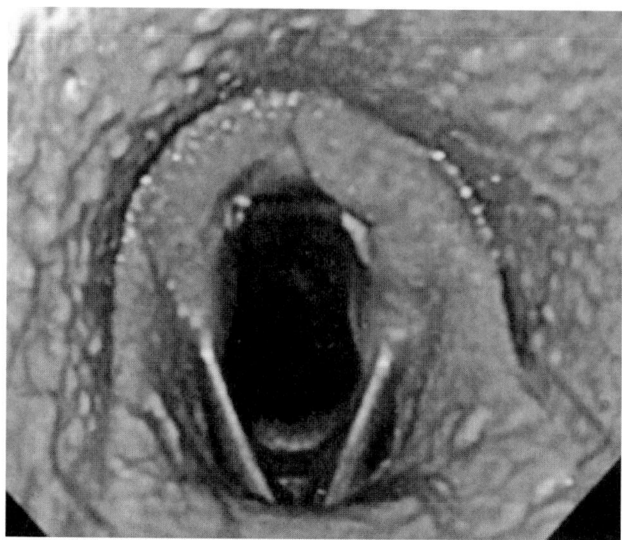

Figure 41-1. Left arytenoid chondritis with a thickened misshapen corniculate process and incomplete abduction.

hemiplegia. In this and subsequent chapters, the two terms are used interchangeably. See Chapter 44 for details.)

A 1 to 4 grading system for assessing arytenoid cartilage movements in horses at rest was developed by Rakestraw and colleagues[4] (Table 41-1). When these assessments are made, abduction of the arytenoids is induced by either swallowing or occlusion. Swallowing yields only a brief period to evaluate full abduction. Nasal occlusion may result in a longer duration of abduction, but it requires a horse to tolerate nasal occlusion for an extended period. Although nasal occlusion may result in negative pharyngeal pressures similar to those experienced by horses during exercise,[5] the degree of abduction after swallowing appears to have a better correlation with the degree of abduction during exercise.[6] Racehorses that are unable to fully abduct one arytenoid (grade 3 or 4) are much more likely to experience dynamic collapse of that arytenoid during high-speed exercise.[7] It may appear to make sense to evaluate the horse's throat from both nares to get a more accurate assessment of arytenoid abduction, but the authors do not think it makes a significant difference.

TABLE 41-1. Subjective Laryngeal Grades for Resting Horses

Grade	Movement
1	Symmetric, synchronous abduction and adduction of the left and right arytenoid cartilages
2	Some asynchronous movement (hesitation, flutter, or abductor weakness) of the left arytenoid cartilage during any phase of respiration. Full abduction of the left arytenoid cartilage can be maintained by swallowing or nasal occlusion.
3	Asynchronous movement (hesitation, flutter, or abductor weakness) of the left arytenoid cartilage during any phase of respiration. Full abduction of the left arytenoid cartilage *cannot* be induced and maintained by swallowing or nasal occlusion.
4	There is no substantial movement of the left arytenoid cartilage during any phase of respiration.

Inability to fully adduct an arytenoid cartilage may be a result of previous laryngoplasty, and palpation of the larynx and assessing the skin for a surgical scar should help determine the diagnosis. The slap test can be used to induce adduction of the arytenoid cartilages, but this is not a valuable test to fully evaluate laryngeal function.[8] The vocal cords and saccules should also be examined for any evidence of previous surgery. Incomplete ablation with the laser may yield scarring and deformation of the vocal cords, or a cord may be absent (Fig. 41-2).

The endoscope should be passed into the trachea to determine the presence of any discharge or feed material, indicative of aspiration. When the endoscope exits the trachea, it is common for the horse to displace its soft palate, but a normal horse should replace it quickly. If the horse does not replace its palate quickly, it can be stimulated to swallow by infusing water into the pharynx or by quickly bumping the pharyngeal wall with the endoscope. If the horse still does not replace the palate below the epiglottis, this may indicate some structural abnormality under the epiglottis, or some pharyngeal dysfunction that may be best observed during high-speed exercise.[9] If a subepiglottic abnormality is suspected, other imaging techniques may be indicated, but the clinician can also spray the epiglottic region with topical anesthetic through the biopsy channel of the videoendoscope, followed by manipulation of the epiglottis with a long bronchoesophageal forceps through the nose to look underneath.

Once the examination of the pharynx and larynx is complete, the remainder of the upper respiratory tract should be examined. The guttural pouch openings should be clear of any discharge. The presence of discharge at the opening of the guttural pouch may be an incidental finding caused by discharge originating from another location and becoming lodged at the opening. Despite this, further endoscopic evaluation of the guttural pouches is always warranted. This is most often done at the end of the examination, and it may require a small dose of intravenous sedation. Temporohyoid disease can often be seen as an enlargement of the stylohyoid bone at the most dorsal aspect of the guttural pouch (Fig. 41-3). The ethmoid recess, turbinates, septum, and region of the nasomaxillary openings (caudal middle meatus) should all be evaluated as the endoscope is slowly withdrawn from the nostril. Discharge running down the ventral turbinate, with material exiting the nasomaxillary opening, is often a sign of sinus disease. Both nasal passages should be evaluated if there is any suspicion of a sinus or nasal passage problem. It is often difficult to discern small deviations in the nasal passage because the endoscopic view provides a very magnified but small field of view. Radiographs are a helpful complementary procedure if septal deviation or some type of sinus disease is suspected.

Videoendoscopic Examination during Exercise

Although a great deal of information can be gained from endoscopy in the resting horse, there are many occasions when a functional abnormality is suspected but no abnor-

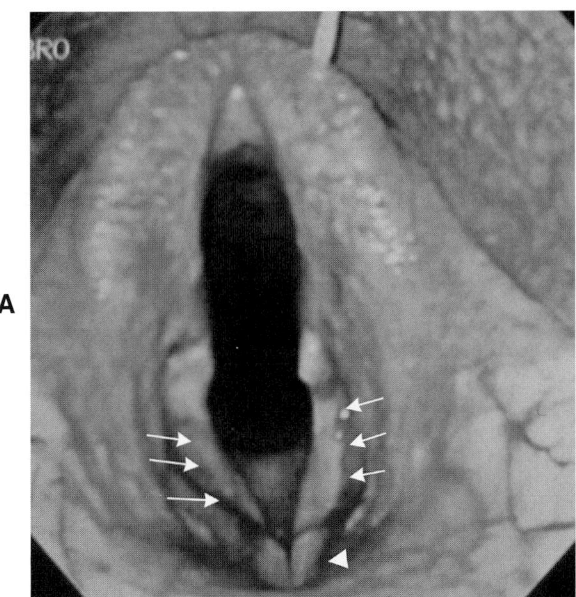

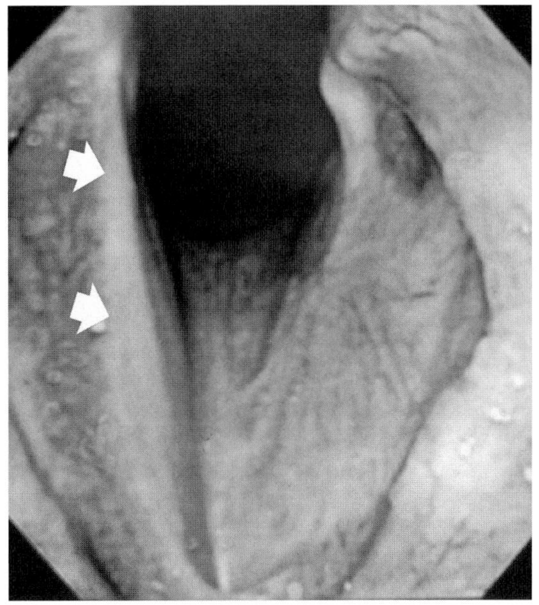

Figure 41-2. A, Scarred vocal cords *(small arrows),* and remaining normal vocal cords ventrally *(arrowhead).* **B,** A close-up videoendoscopic view of the vocal cords. Absent left vocal cord from laser resection. Normal remaining right vocal cord *(arrowheads).*

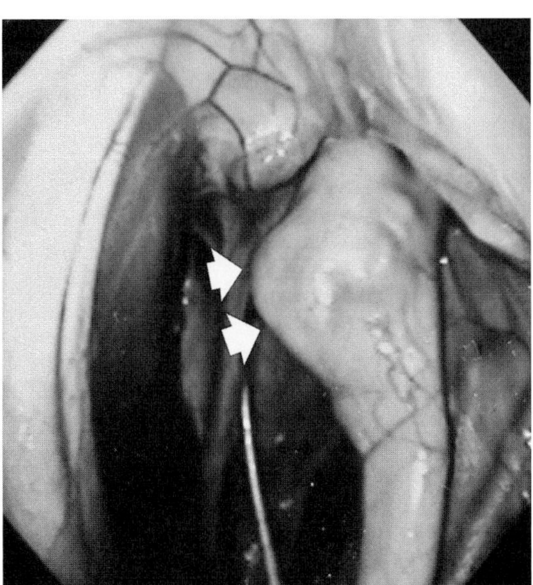

Figure 41-3. Swelling of the stylohyoid bone at the temporohyoid joint within the guttural pouch.

malities are detected during the resting endoscopic examination—for example, when there is exercise intolerance or abnormal respiratory noise during exercise. Conditions that can lead to this scenario include forms of pharyngeal collapse, axial deviation of the aryepiglottic folds, epiglottic retroversion, intermittent epiglottic entrapment, and dorsal displacement of the soft palate. Endoscopic examination immediately after exercise may be valuable in some cases, but it can be misleading. Even normal horses have a much more flaccid-looking upper airway that displaces more easily when first pulling up after exercise. Like all skeletal muscles, the muscles that maintain structural integrity of the upper airway relax at the conclusion of strenuous exercise. Therefore, any conclusion based on an endoscopic examination after exercise, particularly with respect to the functional stability of the pharynx, may be inaccurate.

Treadmill endoscopy may seem to be the easiest and most reliable way to make a diagnosis, but this examination must also be evaluated critically. Accurate conclusions from an endoscopic examination on a high-speed treadmill cannot be drawn from an endoscopy while a horse is running, without specifying the exertional effort. The exercising conditions must simulate the horse's normal working conditions as closely as possible. In the lower respiratory tract, the effects of running a longer distance at a slower speed are not equivalent to the effects of running a shorter distance at a faster speed.[10] This may also be the case in the upper respiratory tract. Furthermore, some of the upper respiratory problems are not only dynamic but also intermittent, and if all the same conditions (e.g., speed, head/neck flexion, fatigue) are not reproduced, a false-negative outcome is likely be obtained (Fig. 41-4). A Holter monitor can be employed to record the horse's heart rate during exercise, and if it is approximately 220 beats per minute or greater, the record will provide evidence that the horse is exercising at or near its maximal heart rate. Of the known upper respiratory abnormalities, dorsal displacement of the soft palate is the most likely not to be reproduced on a high-speed treadmill examination despite circumstantial evidence of the condition under field conditions.

Horses that can be examined by treadmill endoscopy must be as fit as they are for competition. A horse out of work may be too unfit to withstand a maximal exertional effort on the treadmill, and the problem to be diagnosed may not manifest itself. All horses must first be acclimatized to the treadmill before attempting an actual test. This can usually be accomplished with 1 to 2 hours of schooling, taking the horses through the different gaits, and making

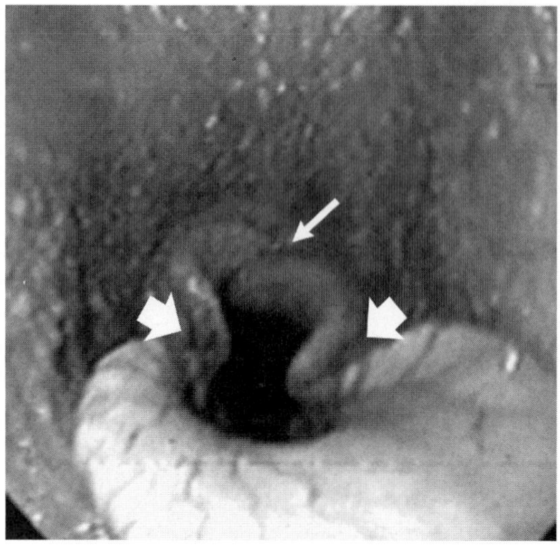

Figure 41-4. Subluxation of the apices of the arytenoid cartilages *(small arrow)* and axial deviation of the aryepiglottic folds *(large arrows)* induced during high-speed treadmill exercise only after increasing head/neck flexion. The larynx was normal without head/neck flexion.

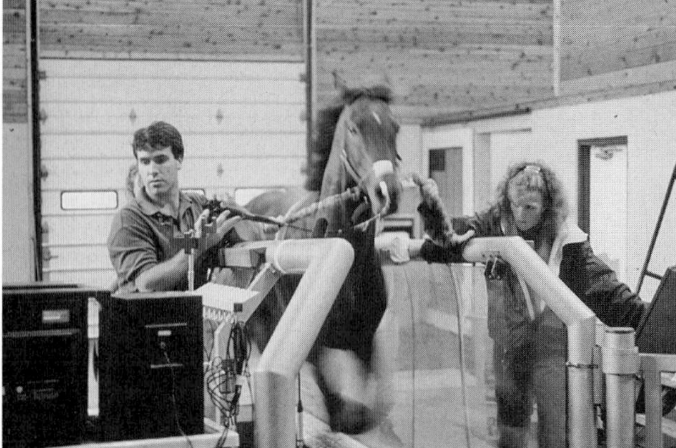

Figure 41-5. Horse during high-speed treadmill endoscopy.

sure they can obtain adequate speed. During the schooling and testing periods, protective boots and leg wraps are recommended. Hobbles and harness are always recommended for pacing Standardbreds and are introduced in the schooling period. The horse must be in condition and should be prepared for the examination as if it were the date of a competition or race.

The treadmill must be capable of obtaining a speed of at least 14 m/s with relatively rapid acceleration and deceleration potential for any racehorse examinations. Padded rails with polycarbonate sides, or an equivalent material, should be present to maintain the animal's position on the belt and protect individuals on either side of the treadmill. Large overhead fans in a temperature-controlled environment are also required. Sweat evaporation is the horse's primary form of body temperature regulation. Under racing conditions, the animal creates its own breeze to enhance evaporation; however, on the treadmill, the horse is stationary, and fans are required to prevent overheating. Two people, holding ropes that are attached to both sides of horse's halter, keep the horse centered on the treadmill. An individual behind the horse encourages the horse forward, and another person closely monitors the horse's gait and controls the treadmill speed, ensuring the horse's position on the treadmill. One final person is needed to guide the endoscope during the examination (Fig. 41-5). For safety reasons, and to ensure a valid test, it is extremely important that the team of individuals carrying out the examination be experienced. The specific protocol used depends on the type of competition the horse is normally engaged in, and it should mimic these circumstances as closely as possible. Generally, after an initial warm-up period, the treadmill is stopped, the endoscope is passed via the right nostril into the pharynx, and its position is maintained by Velcro straps connecting the shaft of the endoscope and the noseband of the horse's halter (Fig. 41-6). A typical exercise protocol for the Thoroughbred racehorse is as follows:

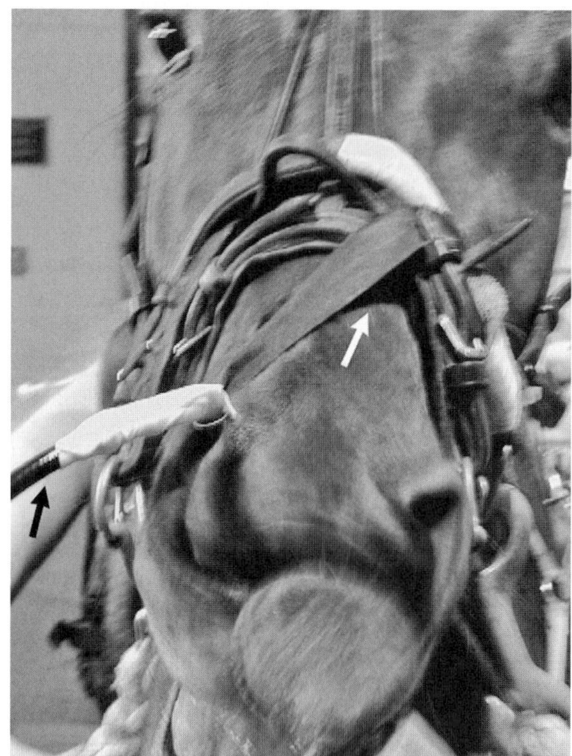

Figure 41-6. The videoendoscope *(dark arrow)* is being held in position up the horse's right nostril by a Velcro strip taped to the scope and then attached to the noseband of the halter *(white arrow)*.

1. Warm up through a combination of walk/trot/canter for 2000 m.
2. Walk again until heart rate is 80 to 90 beats per minute, stop, and pass endoscope.
3. Accelerate to 9 m/s (incline treadmill to 3 degrees for Thoroughbreds).
4. Accelerate to 11 m/s for 400 meters.
5. Accelerate to 12 m/s for 400 meters.
6. Accelerate to 14 m/s for 1600 meters.
7. Decelerate to 12 m/s for 400 meters.

Most horses suffering from a poor performance problem are unable to meet the demands of this protocol. Such horses should be exercised at their own maximal exertional effort. Determination of maximal effort is a subjective assessment by the clinician in conjunction with heart rate evaluation. Recording the entire endoscopic examination, and reviewing it on slow-motion playback, is sometimes necessary, because most abnormalities occur rapidly within the respiratory cycle. Occasionally, stimulating a swallow with water through the endoscope, or altering the speed of the treadmill during the test, will induce the dynamic respiratory problem.

Radiography

Although treadmill endoscopy is invaluable for evaluating the dynamics of the upper respiratory tract during exercise, other imaging techniques, such as radiography and computed tomography, are just as essential in fully evaluating the upper respiratory tract. Radiography and computed tomography are particularly valuable in the assessment of structural abnormalities in areas that are difficult to explore with the endoscope.

The larynx, pharynx, and guttural pouches can be clearly imaged with standard radiographic techniques. Computed radiography and digital radiography provide greater detail and ability to manipulate images. To acquire a lateral image of the laryngeal structures, the x-ray beam should be centered just rostral and dorsal to the angle of the mandible. A dorsoventral projection is usually not of benefit in evaluating these structures.

Air throughout the upper respiratory tract provides good contrast for structures within the pharynx and larynx. Any masses or swelling external to the lumen will lead to obvious compression of the pharyngeal vault. The epiglottis should appear as a thin structure on top of the soft palate. Subepiglottic or palatal lesions may cause dorsal displacement of the soft palate (Fig. 41-7), but heavy sedation of the horse may also precipitate displacement of the palate, and this finding should not be over-interpreted. Measurements have been made of epiglottic length on lateral radiographs and correlated with dynamic upper respiratory dysfunction.[11] Clinicians depend more often on their endoscopic assessment of epiglottic length and apparent stiffness than on radiography. The arytenoids and the remainder of the laryngeal cartilages can be seen dorsal and caudal to the epiglottis. Mineralization of these structures may be associated with normal aging or with an inflammatory process such as arytenoid chondritis.[12,13] Infrequently, abnormal air density may be seen around the larynx and could be consistent with severe laryngeal infection. The saccules should be seen as small air densities between the epiglottis and corniculate processes.

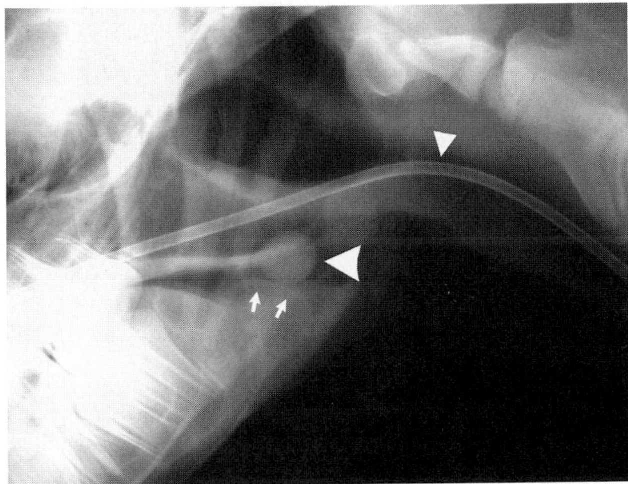

Figure 41-7. Lateral radiograph of a foal with persistent dorsal displacement of the soft palate. The epiglottis *(small arrows)* is unable to assume its normal position because of a large cyst *(large arrowhead)* on the free edge of the palate. A feeding tube is in the esophagus *(small arrowhead)*.

The guttural pouches are thin-walled, air-filled cavities that extend from the pharynx and project dorsal to the larynx. The guttural pouches are outpouchings of the eustachian tubes, and normally the stylohyoid bone is seen traversing through the guttural pouch. Enlarged retropharyngeal lymph nodes may lead to compression of the guttural pouch ventrally. Fluid associated with guttural pouch empyema or hemorrhage can typically be seen as increased soft tissue density or a fluid line. Temporohyoid disease may be seen as enlargement of the stylohyoid bone, but this condition is more reliably detected during the endoscopic examination.[14]

Radiography can be very beneficial in imaging most abnormalities within the sinus, but the technique does have limitations. Dorsoventral, lateral, and oblique projections are the minimum of radiographic views that should be taken to fully evaluate the sinuses. Although air density provides good contrast, superimposition of structures can make interpretation difficult, and familiarity with normal sinus architecture is essential. A fluid line can be seen in the lateral projection in many cases of sinusitis, but if the entire sinus is full, only increased soft tissue density will be seen (Fig. 41-8). Often the borders of the frontal and maxillary sinuses can be discerned easily. The septum between the caudal and rostral maxillary sinuses can be best appreciated on a lateral radiograph, but sinusitis or neoplasia may result in significant distortion of normal anatomy. Contrast sinusography can be used to better help delineate abnormalities. Contrast material can be injected through standard portals for sinus centesis, and filling defects will define the extent of lesions.[15,16]

Sinusitis can be primary, or secondary to another problem such as tooth infection or neoplasia. It can be difficult to make this distinction with standard radiography, but this determination is essential in developing an appropriate treatment plan. If bony lysis is present on standard radiographs, the sinusitis is most likely secondary to some other, primary problem, but the absence of lysis is not definitive for a primary sinusitis. Sinuscopy can be used to visualize the internal aspects of the sinus, but it has limited application.[17] More sensitive imaging techniques are often of greater benefit.

Scintigraphy

Scintigraphy is an extremely sensitive technique for bony remodeling. It can be used to evaluate the equine head reliably for the presence of dental disease, and it can be used to distinguish between dental disease, neoplasia, and

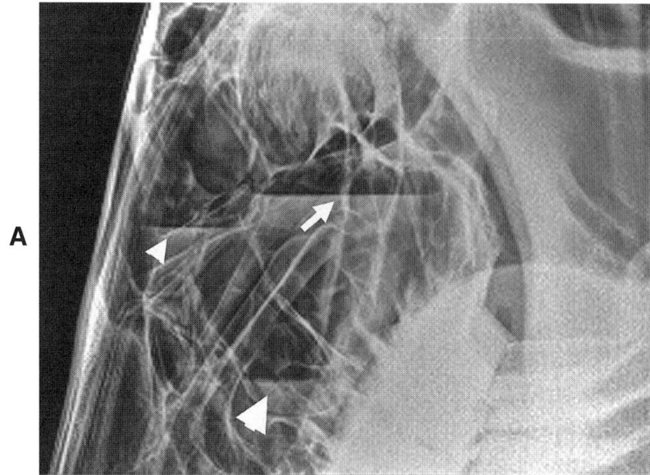

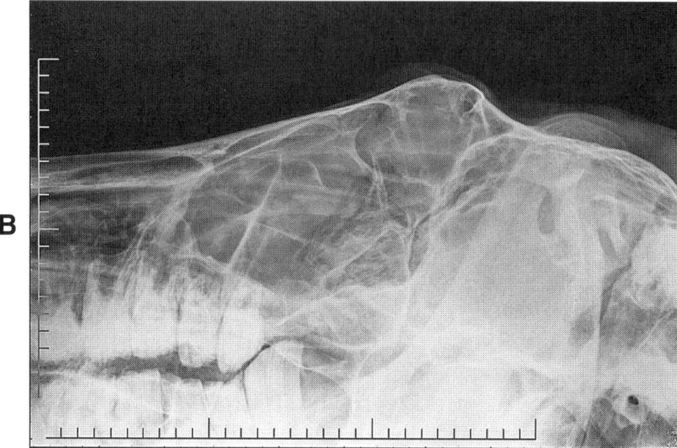

Figure 41-8. A, Lateral skull radiograph with multiple fluid lines. Rostral maxillary sinus *(large arrowhead),* caudal maxillary sinus *(arrow),* dorsal conchal sinus *(small arrowhead).* **B,** Oblique radiograph of the skull with complete opacity of sinus from chronic disease.

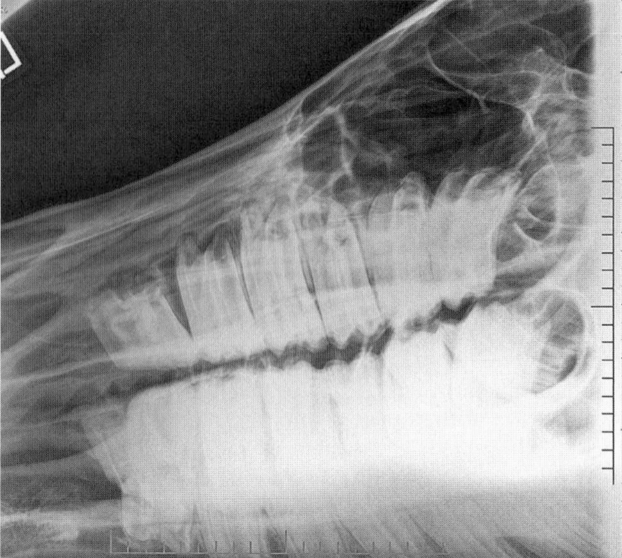

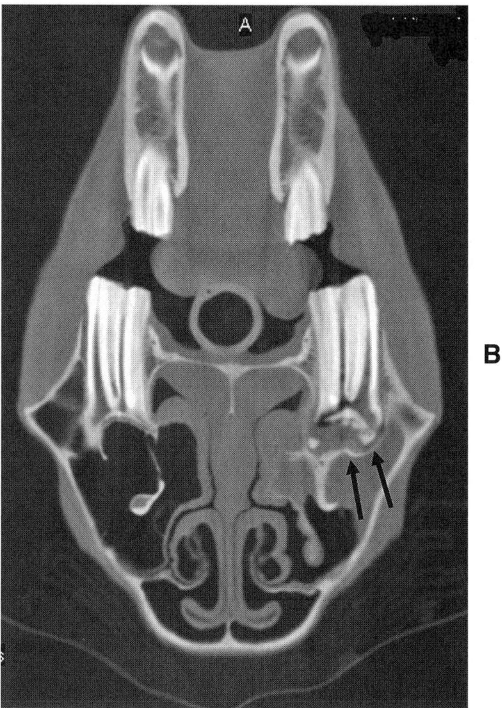

Figure 41-9. A, Lateral radiograph of a horse with purulent drainage from one side of the face and from the ipsilateral nostril. There is no bony lysis around any tooth roots to confirm a suspected diagnosis of tooth root infection. **B,** The CT image at the level of the first molar of the same horse in dorsal recumbency and under general anesthesia. The root structures on the left side are abnormal *(arrows),* and consistent with infection. (Image courtesy Section of Veterinary Imaging, Cornell College of Veterinary Medicine.)

primary sinusitis.[18] Bone phase images are acquired 3 to 4 hours after an intravenous injection of a radioisotope. The images are obtained by a gamma camera, and regions of interest are analyzed. Although scintigraphy can be used to determine the presence of dental disease, it may be difficult to discern the specific tooth that is involved with great certainty. Scintigraphy has a significant advantage over other imaging techniques because general anesthesia is not required. The images are acquired with the standing sedated animal, and multiple views can be taken to help minimize superimposition of structures. Many hospitals now have scintigraphic capability.

Computed Tomography and Magnetic Resonance

Computed tomography (CT) has a distinct advantage over scintigraphy and standard radiography because highly detailed cross-sectional images can be obtained. CT can discriminate tissues with only a 0.5% difference in density, whereas a 10% change in density is necessary to detect a radiographic difference.[19] The images are obtained using x-rays, but the x-ray tube and detectors encircle the patient, acquiring images from many angles. The resulting images are cross-sectional slices of a specified thickness (Fig. 41-9). This eliminates the problem of superimposition encountered with conventional radiography, and it allows precise determination of an abnormality. By knowing in greater detail the extent of a lesion, a more precise surgical plan can be made. Unfortunately, this imaging modality is available only at certain larger hospitals and requires general anesthesia and specially adapted equipment to accommodate large animals.

Magnetic resonance (MR) imaging is another diagnostic modality that can be used to diagnose upper respiratory disease, but it is not as readily available as the other techniques. Furthermore, MR also requires general anesthesia to acquire images of the head. It is generally thought to be a superior imaging technique for soft tissue, but MR can be just as good at discerning bony abnormalities. The normal cross-sectional anatomy of the equine head has been described.[20] A distinct advantage of MR over CT is that MR imaging can be multiplanar without image quality loss. CT slices are always oriented perpendicular to the long axis of the table and body region in the gantry. The CT images can be reconstructed with computer software to provide images in other planes, but there is a significant loss of image quality.

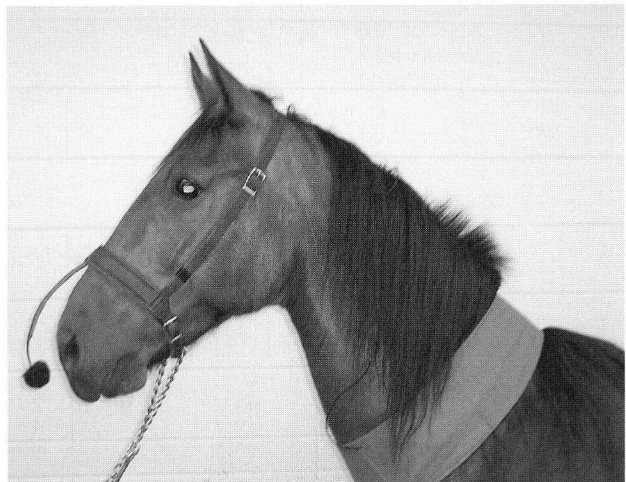

Figure 41-10. Cavison-mounted microphone used to record respiratory sounds in exercising horses.

SOUND ANALYSIS

Horses with upper airway conditions often have exercise intolerance and make a respiratory noise. Although reduced performance may be caused by dysfunction of many body systems, respiratory noise during exercise is a specific indication of upper airway disease. Furthermore, in sport horses, the respiratory noise associated with an upper airway condition is often more worrisome to the owner than reduced performance.

One cannot hear respiratory noises in exercising horses very well. Even the jockey, driver, or rider, who is nearest to the source of the noise most of the time, does not hear respiratory sounds well because the noise is obscured by other sounds associated with exercise such as wind noise and footfall. A listener standing near the track gets "a snapshot" of the noise at best. Also, respiratory sounds do not always occur throughout the exercise period. In some instances, the sounds are more obvious at maximum exercise, but in other cases the sounds are intermittent, or occur as the horse is finishing the exercise. For these reasons, recording of respiratory sounds in exercising horses is advantageous, and it also permits analysis after the recording. Recording of respiratory sounds in exercising horses is simple and inexpensive and requires minimal equipment. The sounds can be recorded throughout the exercise period, in the field, and under conditions in which the horse normally works. This gives the veterinarian complete and verifiable information about the respiratory noise.

Evaluation of respiratory sound during exercise is also useful in the assessment of effectiveness of surgical procedures used in the treatment of upper airway conditions.[21,22] In many horses with upper airway conditions, the primary objective of surgery is to reduce the respiratory noise. In these cases, evaluation of sound production before and after surgery is a good way to determine surgical success.

Methodology

Although several methods are described in the literature, the authors record respiratory sounds in exercising horses in the following manner.[23-26] A unidirectional microphone with a cardioid pickup pattern is attached via a flexible wand to a cavison (Fig. 41-10). This type of microphone centers the sound pickup toward the front of the microphone and helps reduce extraneous sounds such as footfall and track noise that originate behind and to the side of the microphone. The microphone is covered with a windscreen, and it is placed equidistant between the horse's nostrils, approximately 4 cm from the horse's nose. In this way, the microphone is as close to the source of sound to be recorded as possible without being placed in the respiratory air stream. The microphone is attached to an audio recorder with a compression circuit. This kind of recorder automatically adjusts the gain, decreasing the recording of extraneous noises. The advantages of this technique are that it is easily used in the field, and it records respiratory sounds that are also heard by human observers.

Just listening to the audiotape of respiratory sounds made by exercising horses is revealing. The listener can appreciate factors such as respiratory rate and consistency, the number of swallows, the frequency of stride lead changes, and whether abnormal respiratory sounds are present.

Sound can be characterized in terms of time, frequency, and intensity. A sound analysis technique that evaluates these characteristics concurrently is spectrogram analysis. A spectrogram is a three-dimensional plot of frequency on the vertical axis, time along the horizontal axis, and sound intensity in the third dimension. Sound intensity is often plotted in terms of color, or relative darkness. This powerful technique has been used commonly to study human voice or biologic sounds such as bird songs, and also to evaluate upper respiratory sounds made by exercising horses.[25,27-29] Spectrogram analysis requires a personal computer and commercially available software. Listening to the audiotape and viewing the spectrogram at the same time is an effective method of sound evaluation.

Upper Airway Sounds in Exercising Horses

In normal exercising horses, most sounds are heard during exhalation and are present throughout this portion of the respiratory cycle[25,30] (Fig. 41-11). Inspiratory sounds are less than half as loud as sounds made during exhalation.[26] Sound level increases as speed increases. Almost all of the sound intensity occurs at frequencies below 4 kHz, with

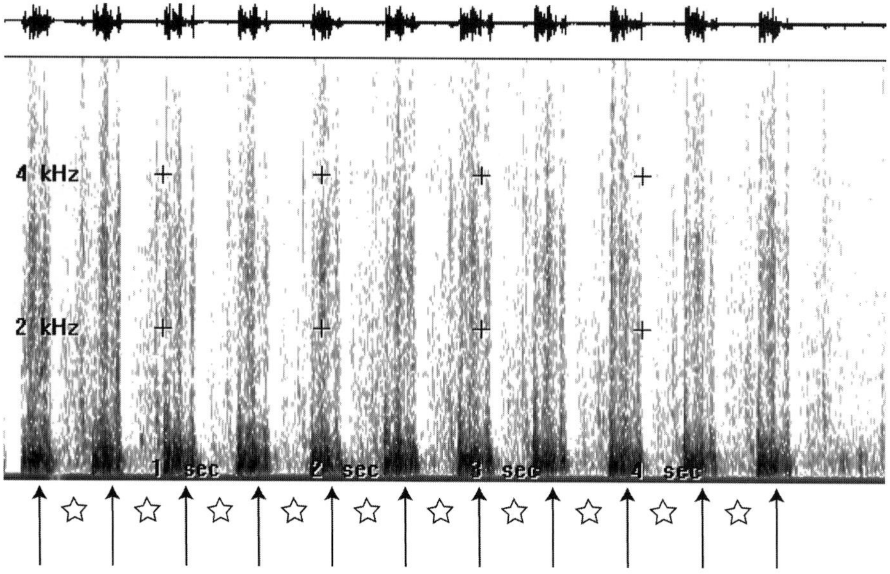

Figure 41-11. Spectrogram of respiratory sounds in a normal galloping horse. Timing is on the abscissa, frequency on the ordinate. The gray scale indicates sound intensity. Inspiration is indicated by a *star,* expiration by an *arrow.*

most of the sound intensity concentrated at frequencies below 800 Hz.[22,26,30]

Recurrent laryngeal neuropathy (RLN) and experimentally induced laryngeal hemiplegia (LH) are characterized by a loud inspiratory noise. This noise contains higher frequencies than normal expiratory sounds and has three bands in the frequency domain called formants. These formants are centered at approximately 300, 1700, and 3700 Hz[22,30] (Fig. 41-12). Human hearing is most acute between 2000 and 4000 Hz. The sound formant centered at about 1700 Hz has significant sound intensity and is in the range of acute human hearing, so this is the one that contributes most to the perception of the high-frequency whistle or roar associated with RLN. The highest-frequency formant has the least sound intensity, and it is not present in all RLN-affected horses. The sound intensity of the formant centered at about 300 Hz is in a region where human hearing is less acute, so this lower-frequency noise does not appear prominent to the human ear. Whether the spectral pattern just described is *unique* for RLN remains to be determined. If this is the case, spectrum analysis of upper airway sounds in exercising horses could be used as a definitive diagnostic tool for RLN.

Dorsal displacement of the soft palate occurs intermittently during exercise; therefore, the abnormal noise associated with this condition is also intermittent.[26] Often, the soft palate displaces near the end of the exercise, or as the horse pulls up. In some horses, the abnormal sound can be heard throughout the exercise period. In affected horses, expiratory sounds are abnormal. The noise is characterized by rattling, which is seen on the spectrogram in the time

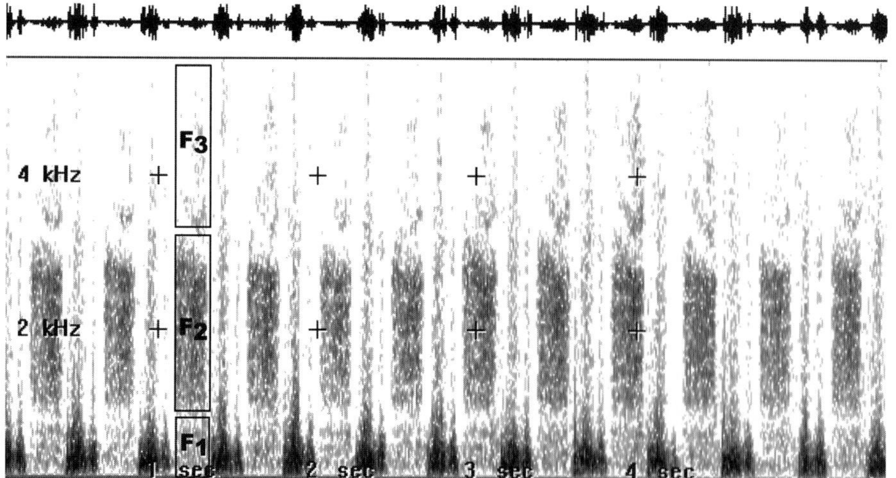

Figure 41-12. Spectrogram of respiratory sounds in a galloping horse with experimentally induced laryngeal hemiplegia. Notice the inspiratory bands of sound (formants) centered at approximately 0.3, 1.7, and 3.7 kHz (F_1, F_2, and F_3, respectively).

domain as bars of sound with a periodicity of about 32 ms (Fig. 41-13). Most of the sound energy is below 4000 Hz, but the range is up to approximately 10,000 Hz.[30] In some horses with dorsal displacement of the soft palate, respiratory sounds are normal, but in others, an inspiratory noise similar to the noise described for exhalation is also heard. In these cases, the inspiratory noise is often less loud than the expiratory noise. During exercise, affected horses often swallow frequently, presumably in an attempt to keep the soft palate in its normal position.

It is likely that vibrations of the dorsally displaced soft palate are the source of the upper airway noise. The rate and amplitude of soft palate vibration are a function of the airflow velocity, the compliance of the dorsally displaced soft palate, and the geometry of the individual horse's upper airway. Combined, these factors explain why some horses with dorsal displacement of the soft palate make no noise, whereas in others the noise is also apparent during inhalation. Listening to the recorded respiratory sounds made by a horse with dorsal displacement of the soft palate while concurrently viewing the spectrogram is an effective way to diagnose the condition.

RLN and dorsal displacement of the soft palate can be experimentally reproduced and are the most common upper airway conditions of horses.[31,32] Consequently, noises associated with these conditions have been studied best. However, upper airway conditions such as pharyngeal collapse, epiglottic entrapment, aryepiglottic fold collapse, and rostral soft palate collapse are also associated with respiratory noise during exercise. Although the associations between specific conditions and their corresponding spectrogram patterns must still be made, in the future it is likely that each upper airway condition associated with noise production will have a well-described "voiceprint," allowing a presumptive spectrogram-based diagnosis of the condition in the field.

Surgical Treatment for Recurrent Laryngeal Neuropathy

Surgical procedures used to treat RLN include prosthetic laryngoplasty, various combinations of laryngeal ventricle and vocal cord excision, often combined with laryngoplasty, and nerve–muscle pedicle grafting.[33-38] The effect of these surgical procedures on upper airway function has been well studied.[31,33,38-40] Fewer studies have investigated the ability of these procedures to reduce respiratory noise.[22,30] In one study, bilateral ventriculocordectomy effectively reduced respiratory noise in horses with experimentally induced laryngeal hemiplegia.[22] Respiratory noises associated with the condition were almost completely eliminated, although spectrum analysis revealed some residual abnormal respiratory sounds (Fig. 41-14). Noise reduction required up to 90 days after the surgery.

The most commonly used surgical technique to treat RLN is prosthetic laryngoplasty.[34-36] The procedure significantly improves upper airway flow mechanics in RLN-affected horses, and many horses have raced successfully after surgery.[35,36] Prosthetic laryngoplasty reduces upper airway noise in horses with laryngeal hemiplegia, but it is not as effective as bilateral ventriculocordectomy in this regard (see Fig. 41-14). Additionally, respiratory noise reduction occurs more rapidly than with bilateral ventriculocordectomy. Residual respiratory noise after surgery is often used to determine the surgical success of prosthetic laryngoplasty.[34] This method of evaluation assumes a tight correlation between respiratory noise and airway obstruction. In fact, in horses with experimentally induced LH, the correlation between residual airway obstruction after prosthetic laryngoplasty and residual noise is weak.[41] Therefore, the residual noise during exercise cannot be used as a predictor of improvement in upper airway function in individual horses after laryngoplasty.

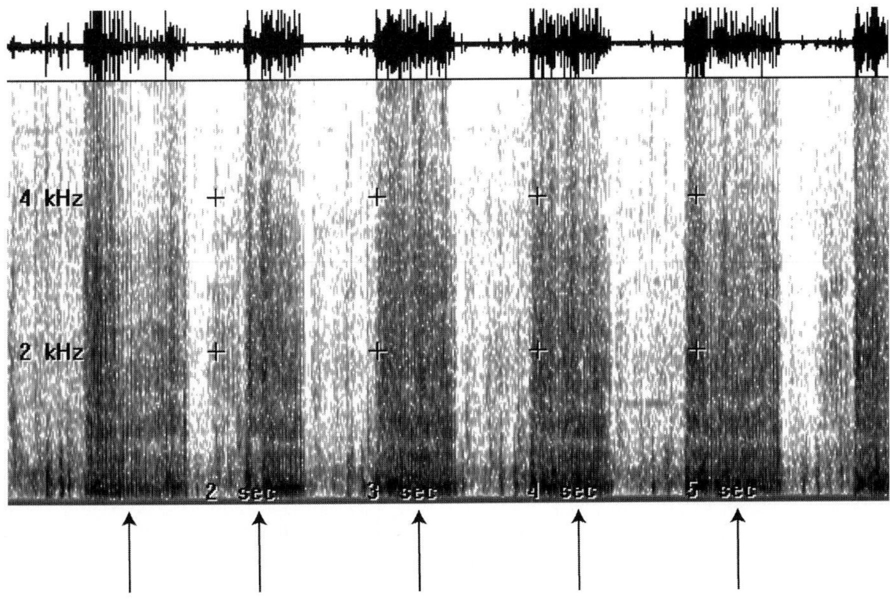

Figure 41-13. Spectrogram of respiratory sounds in a galloping horse with experimentally induced dorsal displacement of the soft palate. Note the "rattling" of the expiratory sound *(arrows)*.

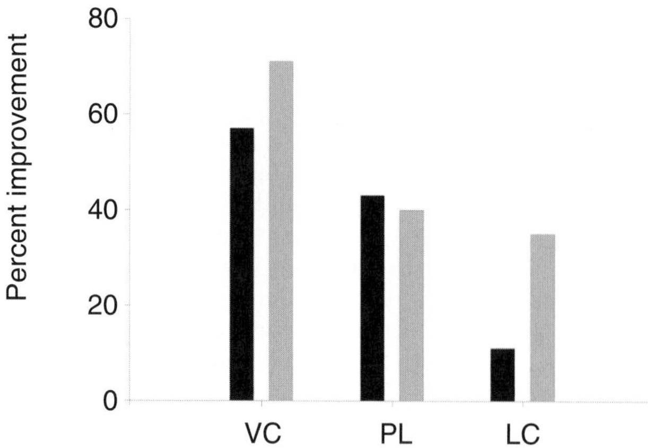

Figure 41-14. Percent improvement of inspiratory sound level *(black bar)* and sound intensity of formant 2 *(gray bar)* in galloping horses with laryngeal hemiplegia 90 days after treatment with bilateral ventriculocordectomy (VC), prosthetic laryngoplasty (PL), and unilateral laser cordectomy (LC). Note that respiratory noise reduction is most effective after VC, and least effective after LC.

Endoscopically guided laser surgery has been used to perform vocal cordectomy in RLN-affected horses.[39,42] In a recent study, the authors evaluated unilateral laser cordectomy and concluded that the procedure does not effectively reduce upper airway noise in horses with experimentally induced laryngeal hemiplegia (see Fig. 41-14). Unilateral laser cordectomy results in removal of the left vocal cord but not of the entire laryngeal ventricle.[42] This study suggests therefore that the laryngeal ventricle rather than the vocal cord may be the primary source of LH-associated noise.

In summary, respiratory sound recording in exercising horses is easy and inexpensive and can be accomplished under field conditions. The sound can be analyzed by simply listening to the recording, and by spectrogram analysis. Just listening to the recording gives the veterinarian insight into breathing patterns and abnormal noises during exercise. Spectrogram analysis provides a voiceprint that in many cases suggests the presence of a specific upper airway condition. Respiratory sound analysis can also be helpful in evaluating surgical procedures aimed at reducing respiratory noise in horses with upper airway disease.

REFERENCES

1. Lane JG: Larynx. In Traub-Dargatz JL, Brown CM, editors: Equine Endoscopy, ed 2, St Louis, 1997, Mosby-Year Book.
2. Parente EJ, Martin BB, Tulleners EP, et al: Dorsal displacement of the soft palate in 92 horses during high speed treadmill examination (1993-1998), Vet Surg 2002;31:507.
3. King C, Evans D, Rose R: Cardiorespiratory and metabolic responses to exercise in horses with various abnormalities of the upper respiratory tract, Equine Vet J 1994;26:220.
4. Rakestraw PC, Hackett RP, Ducharme NG, et al: Arytenoid cartilage movement in resting and exercising horses, Vet Surg 1991;20:122.
5. Holcombe SJ, Derksen FJ, Stick JA, et al: Effect of nasal occlusion on tracheal and pharyngeal pressures in horses, Am J Vet Res 1996;57:1258.
6. Parente EJ: Correlation of resting and treadmill endoscopy, Proceedings Am Coll Vet Surg Ann Surg Symp 1997;7:158.
7. Hammer EJ, Tulleners EP, Parente EJ, et al: Video-endoscopic assessment of dynamic laryngeal function during exercise in horses with grade-III left laryngeal hemiparesis at rest: 26 cases 1992-1995, J Am Vet Med Assoc 1998;212:399.
8. Newton-Clarke MJ, Divers TJ, Valentine B: Evaluation of the thoraco-laryngeal reflex ("slap test") as an indicator of laryngeal adductor myopathy in the horse, Equine Vet J 1994;26:355.
9. Parente EJ, Martin BB: The correlation between standing endoscopic examinations and those made during high-speed exercise in horses: 150 cases, Proc Am Assoc Equine Pract 1995;41:170.
10. Manohar M: Pulmonary vascular pressures of Thoroughbreds increases rapidly and to a higher level with rapid onset of high-intensity exercise than slow onset, Equine Vet J 1994;26:496.
11. Linford RL, O'Brien TR, Wheat JD, et al: Radiographic assessment of epiglottic length and pharyngeal and laryngeal diameters in the Thoroughbred, Am J Vet Res 1983;44:1660.
12. Orsini PG, Raker CW, Reid CF, et al: Xeroradiographic evaluation of the equine larynx, Am J Vet Res 1989;50:845.
13. Tulleners EP, Harrison IW, Raker CW: Management of arytenoid chondropathy and failed laryngoplasty in horses: 75 cases (1979-1985), J Am Vet Med Assoc 1988;192:670.
14. Walker AM, Sellon DC, Cornelisse CJ, et al: Temporohyoid osteoarthropathy in 33 horses (1993-2000), J Vet Intern Med 2002;16:697.
15. Behrens E, Schumacher J, Morris E, et al: Equine paranasal sinusography, Vet Rad 1991;32:98.
16. Behrens E, Schumacher J, Morris E: Contrast paranasal sinusography for evaluation of disease of the paranasal sinuses of five horses, Vet Radiol 1991;32:105.
17. Ruggles AJ, Ross MW, Freeman DE: Endoscopic examination and treatment of paranasal sinus disease in 16 horses, Vet Surg 1993;22:508.
18. Archer DC, Blake CL, Singer JC, et al: Scintigraphic appearance of selected diseases of the equine head, Equine Vet Educ 2003;15:391.
19. Kraft SL, Gavin P: Physical principles and technical considerations for equine computed tomography and magnetic resonance imaging, Vet Clin North Am Equine Pract 2001;17:115.
20. Arencibia A, Vazquez JM, Jaber R, et al: Magnetic resonance imaging and cross sectional anatomy of the normal equine sinuses and nasal passages, Vet Radiol Ultrasound 2000;41:313.
21. Derksen FJ, Holcombe SJ, Hartmann W, et al: Spectrum analysis of respiratory sounds in exercising horses with experimentally induced laryngeal hemiplegia or dorsal displacement of the soft palate, Am J Vet Res 2001;62:659.
22. Brown JA, Derksen FJ, Stick JA, et al: Ventriculocordectomy reduces respiratory noise in horses with laryngeal hemiplegia, Equine Vet J 2003;35:570.
23. Attenburrow DP: Respiratory sounds recorded by radio-stethoscope from normal horses at exercise, Equine Vet J 1978;10:176.
24. Attenburrow DP: The development of a radio-stethoscope for use in the horse at rest and during exercise, Equine Vet J 1978;10:14.
25. Cable CS, Ducharme NG, Hackett RP, et al. Sound signature for identification and quantification of upper airway disease in horses, Am J Vet Res 2002;63:1707.
26. Franklin SH, Usmar SG, Lane JG, et al: Spectral analysis of respiratory noise in horses with upper airway disorders, Equine Vet J 2003;35:264.
27. Heaton JT, Farabaugh SM, Brauth SE: Effect of syringeal denervation in the budgerigar *(Melopsittacus undulatus)*: The role of the syrinx in call production, Neurobiol Learn Mem 1995;64:68-82.
28. Wollemann M, Olaszy G: Spectrogram analysis of different alarm calls in gulls and waders, Agressologie 1977;18:97.
29. Kent RD: Vocal tract acoustics, J Voice 1993;7:97.
30. Derksen FJ, Holcombe SJ, Hartmann W, et al: Spectrum analysis of respiratory sounds in exercising horses with experimentally induced laryngeal hemiplegia or dorsal displacement of the soft palate, Am J Vet Res 2001;62:659.
31. Derksen FJ, Stick JA, Scott EA, et al: Effect of laryngeal hemiplegia and laryngoplasty on airway flow mechanics in exercising horses, Am J Vet Res 1986;47:16.

32. Holcombe SJ, Derksen FJ, Stick JA, et al: Effect of bilateral blockade of the pharyngeal branch of the vagus nerve on soft palate function in horses, Am J Vet Res 1998;59:504.
33. Tetens J, Derksen FJ, Stick JA, et al: Efficacy of prosthetic laryngoplasty with and without bilateral ventriculocordectomy as treatments for laryngeal hemiplegia in horses, Am J Vet Res 1996;57:1668.
34. Marks D, Mackay-Smith MP, Cushing LS, et al: Use of a prosthetic device for surgical correction of laryngeal hemiplegia in horses, J Am Vet Med Assoc 1970;157:157.
35. Hawkins JF, Tulleners EP, Ross MW, et al: Laryngoplasty with or without ventriculectomy for treatment of left laryngeal hemiplegia in 230 racehorses, Vet Surg 1997;26:484.
36. Russell AP, Slone DE: Performance analysis after prosthetic laryngoplasty and bilateral ventriculectomy for laryngeal hemiplegia in horses: 70 cases (1986-1991), J Am Vet Med Assoc 1994;204:1235.
37. Fulton IC, Stick JA, Derksen FJ: Laryngeal reinnervation in the horse, Vet Clin North Am Equine Pract 2003;19:189.
38. Ducharme NF, Hackett RP: The value of surgical treatment of laryngeal hemiplegia in horses, Comp Cont Educ Pract Vet 1991;13:472.
39. Ducharme N, Woody B: Vocal cordectomy as an aid in the management of horses with laryngeal hemiparesis/hemiplegia, Clin Tech Equine Pract 2002;1:17.
40. Shappell KK, Derksen FJ, Stick JA, et al: Effects of ventriculectomy, prosthetic laryngoplasty, and exercise on upper airway function in horses with induced left laryngeal hemiplegia, Am J Vet Res 1988;49:1760.
41. Brown JA, Derksen FJ, Stick JA, et al: Effect of laryngoplasty on respiratory noise reduction in horse with laryngeal hemiplegia, Equine Vet J 2004;36:420-425.
42. Hawkins JF, Andrews-Jones L: Neodymium:yttrium aluminum garnet laser ventriculocordectomy in standing horses, Am J Vet Res 2001;62:531.

CHAPTER 42

Nasal Passages and Paranasal Sinuses

Frank A. Nickels

FUNCTIONAL ANATOMY

External Nares

The external nares or nostrils in the horse are the openings into the nasal passages; they are widely placed and have an unusual shape.[1] The dorsal and lateral margins of the nares, the alae, are supported by the alar cartilages, which are attached to the rostral end of the nasal septum dorsally. The thick alar fold divides each naris into dorsal and ventral parts. The dorsal part leads into a blind sac called the nasal diverticulum, which occupies the nasoincisive notch formed by the incisive bone ventrally and the nasal bone dorsally. The ventral part of the naris leads directly into the nasal cavity.

Nasal Cavity

The nasal cavity is divided into equal halves by the nasal septum and the vomer bone. The reserve crowns of the upper cheek teeth and a portion of the paranasal sinus system occupy this area of the skull. Two major nasal conchae (thin scrolls of cartilage and bone) in each nasal cavity divide the nasal passage into the dorsal, middle, ventral, and common meatus. The dorsal concha extends from the cribriform plate of the ethmoid bone to the level of the 106/206 (2nd premolar in the upper arcade). The ventral concha extends from the level of the 111/211 (3rd molar) to the level of 106/206 (see Chapter 30).[2] Numerous small ethmoturbinates project into the caudal part of the nasal cavity from the lateral mass of the ethmoid bone.

Paranasal Sinuses

The horse's extensive paranasal sinus system consists of six pairs of sinuses: the dorsal (endoturbinate I), middle (endoturbinate II), and ventral nasal conchal sinuses; the sphenopalatine sinus; the frontal sinus; and the maxillary sinus (Fig. 42-1). The major clinically significant sinuses are the frontal and maxillary sinuses. All the sinuses communicate with the nasal cavity directly (maxillary sinus) or indirectly (dorsal, middle, and ventral conchal sinuses; frontal sinus; and sphenopalatine sinuses) through the maxillary sinus. The paranasal sinuses are important clinically because they are susceptible to infections that extend from the nasal cavity or from the alveoli of the caudal upper cheek teeth (see Chapter 30).

Conchal Sinuses

Each conchal sinus is divided into a rostral and a caudal compartment by a septum. The caudal compartment of the dorsal concha forms the dorsal conchal sinus, which communicates with the frontal sinus, forming the conchofrontal sinus. The caudal compartment of the ventral concha forms the ventral conchal sinus, which communicates with the rostral maxillary sinus over the infraorbital canal through the conchomaxillary opening.[2]

Maxillary Sinus

The maxillary sinus is the largest of the sinuses. It is divided into rostral and caudal compartments by an oblique septum. The root of the maxillary 1st molar tooth (109/209) (see Fig. 30-1) usually enters the rostral compartment, and the roots of the 2nd (110/210) and 3rd molars (111/211) usually enter the caudal compartment. The caudal maxillary sinus is partially divided by the infraorbital canal, over which it communicates with the sphenopalatine sinus. It communicates dorsally with the conchofrontal sinus via the

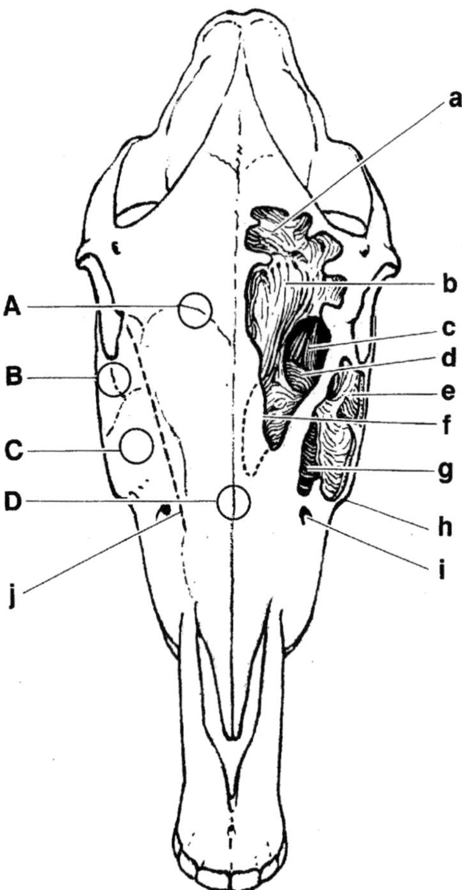

Figure 42-1. Diagram of the skull depicting the location of the equine paranasal sinuses and sites for trephination. A site for entering the frontal sinus is labeled A. The sites for entering the caudal maxillary compartment (B) and the rostral maxillary compartment (C) are above the facial crest and below the nasolacrimal duct (j). The nasal bones start to diverge at (D), which is the site for exposing the nasal septum. (For a detailed description for entering the frontal sinus over the frontomaxillary opening, see Sinoscopy under "Diagnosis" in the text.) The *dotted line* outlines the medial floor of dorsal conchal sinus. a, frontal sinus; b, ethmoid mass; c, frontomaxillary opening; d, dorsal bulla of ventral conchal sinus; e, caudal maxillary sinus; f, dorsal conchal sinus; g, rostral maxillary sinus; h, facial crest; i, infraorbital foramen; j, course of nasolacrimal duct.

frontomaxillary opening at the level of the osseous lacrimal canal and the medial wall of the orbit. It also communicates with the nasal cavity through a compressed nasomaxillary opening into the caudal aspect of the middle meatus. The rostral maxillary sinus is also divided by the infraorbital canal into medial and lateral compartments. The medial compartment of the rostral maxillary sinus communicates with the middle nasal meatus via a narrow slit, the nasomaxillary opening. The rostral compartment communicates with the ventral conchal sinus over the infraorbital canal through the conchomaxillary opening. The volume of the sinus continues to increase from birth through the life of the horse as the teeth continue to erupt and migrate forward. The maxillary sinus is more predisposed to disease than the other sinuses because of direct communication with the nasal cavity and its association with the dental alveoli.

Frontal Sinus

The frontal sinus occupies the dorsal part of the skull. It extends from a point midway between the infraorbital foramen and the medial canthus of the eye to a point midway between the caudal margins of the orbit in the mature horse. An extensive communication exists between the rostromedial aspect of the frontal sinus and the dorsal conchal sinus; together they are referred to as the conchofrontal sinus.

Sphenoid and Palatine Sinuses

The sphenoid and palatine sinuses are usually contiguous in the horse, forming the sphenopalatine sinus. The sphenoid and palatine sinus compartments communicate under the ethmoidal labyrinth. The sphenopalatine sinus communicates freely with the caudal maxillary sinus.

DISEASES OF THE NARES

Diseases of the nares are relatively rare. The most common clinical signs are reduced airflow, nasal stertor, and occasionally facial distortion. The condition of the nares can usually be determined by observation and palpation.

Epidermal Inclusion Cysts (Atheromas)

These cysts, located in the dorsolateral aspects of the nasal diverticulum, were once thought to be sebaceous cysts and were referred to as atheromas.[3,4] A more recent report describing the histologic appearance found no remnants of sebaceous glands or cells in the cyst wall; thus, a more accurate and descriptive name, epidermal inclusion cysts, has been proposed.[5] These cysts are usually single, unilateral, spherical nodules that can vary from 3 to 5 cm in diameter. Epidermal inclusion cysts of the nasal diverticulum are easily identified by visual appearance and location. An accurate diagnosis can be confirmed by cytologic examination of a fine-needle aspirate.[5] Epidermal inclusion cysts are rarely associated with impaired athletic performance and need not be removed unless indicated for cosmetic reasons.

Surgical extirpation can be performed on a standing horse with sedation and local infiltration anesthesia. The skin of the external nares is prepared for aseptic surgery, as is the nasal diverticulum because of the possibility of inadvertent penetration into the diverticulum. The skin and subcutaneous tissue are incised over the lesion, and the cyst is removed by dissection. Care is taken not to rupture the cyst wall. Closure of the incision is routine, and the aftercare is minimal. An alternative method of removal of epidermal inclusion cysts has been described. The cyst is lanced into the nasal diverticulum through a stab incision, and the cyst lining is everted using a roaring burr. The lining is transected using scissors, and the wound is left to heal by second intension. Recurrence has not been reported.[6]

Redundant Alar Folds

The alar fold has been incriminated as a source of respiratory noise in the horse. To determine whether this is the source of abnormal noise or exercise intolerance, a large temporary mattress suture can be placed through the skin of each alar fold and tied over the bridge of the nose. Because the noise is apparent only at exercise, the horse should be exercised after suture placement to determine if the alar fold is the cause of the problem.

Treatment of flaccid or redundant alar folds consists of bilateral resection of the fold. This procedure can be performed either through the external nares[7] or by incising the lateral alae of the external nares. Incising the alae facilitates resection of the alar fold, but the resulting scar may be undesirable in show horses.

The patient is anesthetized and positioned in either dorsal or lateral recumbency. Dorsal recumbency provides adequate access if the procedure is performed through the external nares. Lateral recumbency provides the best exposure to the alar fold if the alae of the external nares are incised. The resection involves incising the alar fold caudal to the alar cartilage on the lateral wall of the nasal cavity to the rostral end of the ventral concha (Fig. 42-2). A second incision is directed caudally along the medial attachment of the alar fold to join the first incision. Approximately 2 cm of the rostral end of the ventral nasal concha is removed with the alar fold. Profuse hemorrhage may occur once the cartilage has been incised. A 22.5-cm curved Rochester-Carmalt forceps can be used as a guide for the incisions and to control hemorrhage (Fig. 42-3). Because ligation of bleeders is almost impossible when the approach through the external nares is used, hemostasis is achieved by closure of the incision using a simple-continuous suture pattern with size 0 absorbable suture material, commencing at the caudal limit. Healing is usually complete within 10 to 12 days, at which time the horse can return to work.

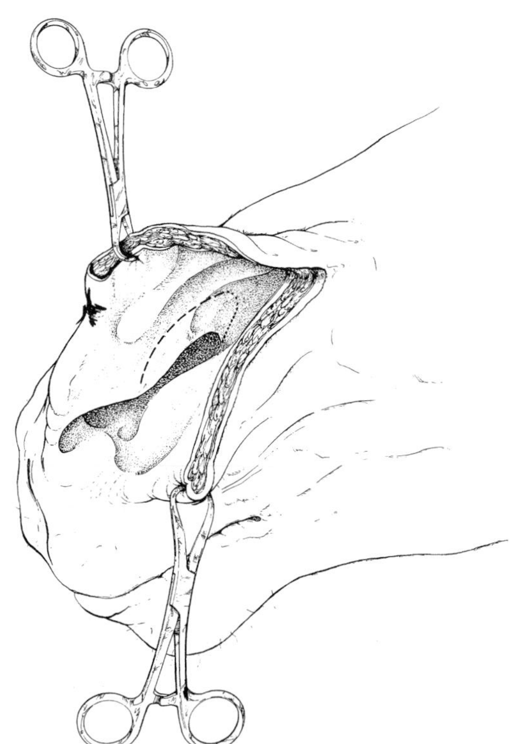

Figure 42-2. Resection of an alar fold. The *dashed line* represents the first incision, which extends caudally from the alar cartilage to the rostral end of the ventral concha. The *dotted line* represents the second incision.

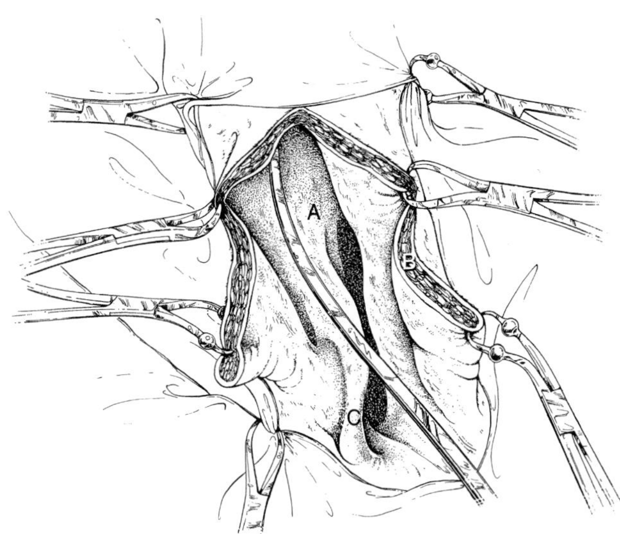

Figure 42-3. Resection of an alar fold. Long, curved forceps are used to control hemorrhage and act as a guide for incisions. A, alar fold; B, incised edges of alae; C, alar cartilage.

DISEASES OF THE NASAL CAVITY

The most common clinical signs of nasal cavity disease are nasal stertor and unilateral nasal discharge and can include a fetid odor and facial distortion. Endoscopy or radiography or both are usually required for diagnosis.

Facial Fractures

Facial fractures involving the paranasal sinuses and nasal cavities are common and result from direct trauma. Fractures of the paranasal sinuses and nasal cavity most commonly involve the nasal and frontal bones but may also involve the maxillae and lacrimal bones.

Diagnosis of fractures of the paranasal sinuses and nasal cavity is based on history, clinical examination, and radiography. Radiographs of the skull should always be taken to assess the severity of the fracture, but the extent and degree of displacement of the fracture fragments may be more readily determined by palpation.

Even though the skin may be intact, these fractures should be considered open, because penetration of the sinus and nasal mucosa usually occurs. Reconstructive surgery should be performed as soon as it is feasible, because primary open reduction provides the best cosmetic results. Some facial fractures of the paranasal sinuses and nasal cavity heal spontaneously; however, failure to treat them may result in chronic sinusitis, bone sequestra, nonhealing wounds, facial deformity, and secondary nasal septal thickening or necrosis.[4,8,9]

Many different reconstructive techniques have been described for facial fractures of the paranasal sinuses and nasal cavity.[9-13] Procedures are performed with the patient anesthetized and positioned in lateral recumbency. Large, slightly curved or S-shaped incisions extending beyond the margins of the fracture are used to expose the traumatized area. Attempts should be made to preserve the periosteal attachments to the fragments. The fracture site is thoroughly débrided and irrigated to remove blood clots and debris.

Detached bone fragments devoid of periosteum can be thoroughly cleansed and replaced, but there is the possibility of eventual sequestration. If a paranasal sinus is involved, it should also be thoroughly lavaged to remove blood clots, small bone fragments, and other debris. Some small fractures may be elevated with a thin osteotome or a narrow periosteal elevator, whereas large fragments require other techniques to elevate them into position. The temporary use of orthopedic screws in the fragment[14] and the use of holes drilled in solid bone adjacent to the fracture for insertion of a Langenbeck elevator[9,15] have been described to assist in elevating the fragments into their normal anatomic position (Fig. 42-4). The use of suture material depends on the stability of the fractured fragments after reduction. Unstable fragments can be held in position using 20- to 22-gauge wire or size 1 monofilament absorbable sutures placed strategically through small holes drilled into the fragment and parent bone.

The incision is closed in two layers. The periosteum is reapposed when possible using an absorbable suture. The use of a simple-continuous intradermal suture pattern to reappose the skin edges has been reported to provide the best cosmetic results, but skin staples are faster and are also very cosmetic.[9] A pressure bandage placed over a nonadherent dressing is recommended for 3 to 4 days to protect the area and minimize postoperative swelling. Systemic antibiotic therapy should be continued for 5 to 6 days.

A serosanguineous nasal discharge may be present for 1 to 2 weeks postoperatively. If this drainage continues, however, it may indicate the presence of a sequestrum or sinusitis.[8] For additional information on facial fractures, see Chapter 103.

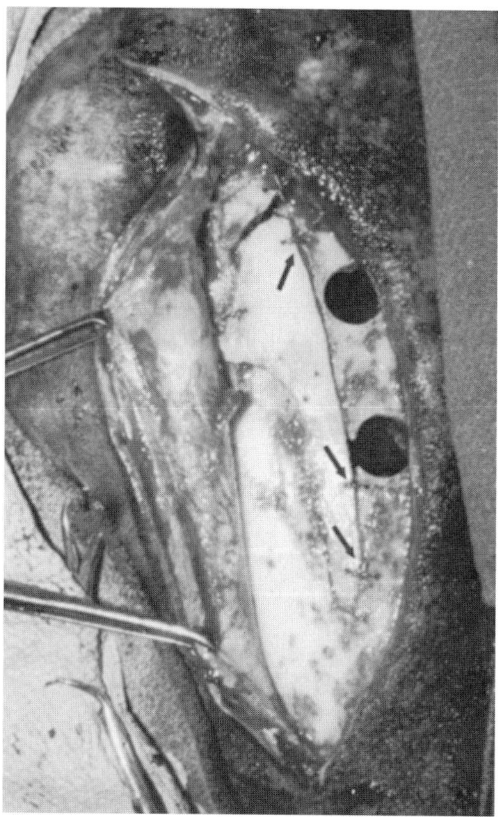

Figure 42-4. Fracture of the nasal and frontal bones. The holes in the parent bone adjacent to the fracture were made to insert a Langenbeck elevator to raise the fragment into its anatomic position. Interrupted stainless steel sutures were used to stabilize the fragment *(black arrows)*.

Nasal Septum Diseases

Diseases of the nasal septum are relatively rare and may cause thickening, malformation, or deviation of the septum. Specific diseases include cystic degeneration,[16] malformation of normal tissue (hamartoma),[17] abscess,[18] traumatic thickening and necrosis secondary to septal fracture,[4] longitudinal deviation of the incisive bones and nasal septum,[19] and neoplasm.[14,20] All of these lesions may produce similar clinical signs, such as decreased airflow or complete obstruction unilaterally, nasal stertor, nasal discharge, and occasionally facial distortion. Endoscopy, radiography, and computed tomography are useful to determine the exact site, extent, and nature of the involvement.

Some of these conditions may improve with removal of the nasal septum. Resection of the nasal septum may involve removal of a small portion or the majority of the septum. Incising the lateral alae of the nostril is the best approach for localized lesions of the rostral aspect of the septum, whereas a subtotal resection of the nasal septum[21,22] or an alternative resection technique is used when the majority of the septum is involved.[16]

Because of the likelihood of profuse hemorrhage during surgery, it is advisable to identify a suitable blood donor and collect 4 to 8 L of blood before surgery in case a blood transfusion becomes necessary. In addition, the administration of large volumes of intravenous fluids during surgery may be necessary to help alleviate hypotension. The most effective method of controlling hemorrhage is to use a nasal tampon after surgery.

The surgery is performed with the horse anesthetized and positioned in lateral recumbency. An airway should be established via a tracheotomy and the anesthetic delivered through it. The surgery for subtotal resection begins by making an 18-mm trephine hole on the bridge of the nose to gain access to the caudal portion of the septum. The center for this opening is located just rostral to the frontal sinuses where the nasal bones begin to diverge (see Fig. 42-1, *D*). A curved incision is made through the skin and periosteum, and the periosteum is reflected to provide exposure for the trephine. The nasal septum is easily identified once the bone plug has been removed and the mucosa has been incised. Doyen intestinal forceps or other suitable straight forceps are placed vertically on the nasal septum down to the floor of the nasal cavity (Fig. 42-5). The forceps act as a stop for the guarded chisel when severing the dorsal and ventral attachments of the nasal septum, and they act as a guide for making the caudal incision in the septum. The rostral division in the nasal septum is performed by making a curved incision with a scalpel, starting from the ventral aspect of the septum and extending in a dorsocaudal direction, leaving at least 4 to 5 cm of the rostral septum to support the alar cartilages and external nares. A guarded chisel is used to incise the dorsal and ventral attachments of the septum caudal to the forceps. The caudal incision is made with a narrow osteotome immediately rostral to the Doyen forceps. The septum is then grasped through the external nares with heavy Vulsellum forceps and removed.

Obstetric wire can be used instead of a guarded chisel to sever the dorsal and ventral attachments of the nasal septum. This causes less trauma and hemorrhage. Another advantage of this technique is removal of more of the ventral aspect of the septum than with the guarded chisel. When using obstetric wire for a subtotal resection, the caudal incision is made before the incisions of the dorsal and ventral attachments. The obstetric wire is threaded through the trephine opening on either side of the septum to the external nares. To incise the ventral attachment, the obstetric wire has to be forced to the most ventral aspect of the caudal septal incision. The septal attachments are severed easily with obstetric wire, so care should be taken not to incise beyond the rostral incision of the septum. Digital palpation or visual inspection using a flexible endoscope can be used to determine if all of the ventral attachment of the nasal septum has been removed. Ferris-Smith rongeurs can be used to remove the remaining portions.

An alternative technique has been described to remove the remainder of the nasal septum (see Fig. 42-5). The differences between this technique and the subtotal resection are as follows: the caudal incision is made at a 60-degree angle to the nasal bones in a dorsocaudoventral direction, the entire ventral septal attachment is incised up to the rostral incision, and the dorsal and ventral incisions are created by using obstetric wire. The obstetric wire is passed through the ventral meatus around the caudal aspect of the nasal septum and back through the opposite nasal passage to incise the ventral attachment. This is accomplished by passing the wire through the ventral nasal meatus into the nasal pharynx, and retrieving the wire through the opposite side using a rat-tooth forceps passed through the biopsy channel in a flexible endoscope. Another instrument that can be used to retrieve the wire is a long flexible grasping forceps (see Chapter 44). For the dorsal incision, the obstetric wire is threaded through the trephine opening on either side of the septum to the external nares. The caudal incision is made at a 60-degree angle to the nasal bones using a long narrow osteotome or a grooved cutting instrument fashioned from a standard wide-tipped screwdriver.[16] The tip of the screwdriver is ground concave and the edges are rounded so that the cutting edge sits better on the septum, reducing trauma to the nasal conchae.

Packing the nasal cavity with sterile cotton roll gauze controls hemorrhage. Excessive packing of the nasal cavity may cause the nasal tampon to extend into the nasopharynx, where it may be inhaled or swallowed. The end of the gauze should be secured to the skin of the nares to prevent inadvertent removal of the pack.

The skin and periosteal incisions are closed in a routine manner. A tracheotomy tube is placed immediately after extubation.

Aftercare includes the use of systemic antibiotic therapy for 5 to 6 days. The nasal packing may be removed after 48 or 72 hours. The nasal cavity should be flushed daily with warm physiologic saline to remove dried blood, debris, and tissue fragments. Complete healing of the septal incisions occurs within approximately 4 to 6 weeks.

The prognosis for restoring normal function is guarded. Complications such as formation of excessive granulation tissue of the caudal septal stump or adhesions to the nasal conchae with subtotal resection may result in a persistent noise or exercise intolerance. Development of the technique that removes additional parts of the caudal septum has minimized these complications. Excellent cosmetic results can be expected except in foals younger than 6 months and in some Standardbreds, in which flattening of the bridge of the nose may occur even when adequate cartilage is left for support.[16]

Ethmoid Hematoma

Ethmoid hematomas are well-encapsulated masses originating in or around the ethmoid labyrinth or occasionally from the paranasal sinuses.[23,24] The cause is unknown, but hemorrhage occurs in the submucosa of an endoturbinate

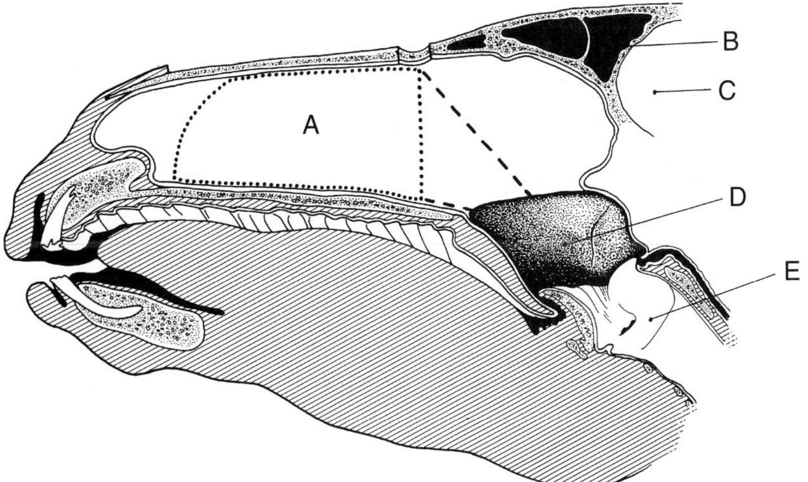

Figure 42-5. Resection of the nasal septum. The *dotted lines* outline the area of the septum removed in the subtotal resection. The *dashed lines* outline the caudal area of the septum removed in addition when a near-total nasal septal resection technique is used. Access to the caudal nasal septum is via a midline trephine opening. *A,* nasal septum; *B,* frontal sinus; *C,* cranial cavity; *D,* nasopharynx; *E,* larynx.

or a sinus, causing the mucosa to stretch and thicken, forming the capsule of the hematoma. An enlarging lesion of the ethmoid labyrinth can extend dorsally into the frontal sinus or ventrally into the sphenopalatine sinus by disrupting the tectorial plate. It may further extend into the maxillary sinus and nasal cavity as it enlarges.[23]

In gross appearance, an ethmoid hematoma has a smooth, glistening surface that may be mottled or green-tinged. Histologically, the lesions are very distinct. The capsule is composed of respiratory epithelium and fibrous tissue. The stroma contains blood, fibrous tissue, macrophages, and giant cells with deposits of hemosiderin and occasionally calcareous deposits.[25] Progressive ethmoid hematomas have been reported in horses ranging from less than 1 year to 20 years of age, with a mean of 9.9 years.[26] Although the condition occurs mostly in middle-aged male horses, it has also been described in young horses and in females; one report found no statistical difference between the occurrence in males and females.[23,26,27] Most cases have been reported in Thoroughbreds, but an ethmoid hematoma also has been described in other breeds.[23,24,27-31]

The most consistent clinical sign is a mild, intermittent, unilateral epistaxis that is usually spontaneous but may occur with exercise.[23,27] An abnormal respiratory noise may be heard when the hematoma extends into the nasal cavity or causes a distortion of the paranasal sinuses. Other possible clinical signs include malodorous breath, facial swelling, head shyness, and head shaking.[23] A tentative diagnosis can be made from the history, clinical signs, and endoscopic and radiographic findings. A definitive diagnosis is made by histologic examination of the tissue. Endoscopic findings early in the development of an ethmoid hematoma can include a trickle of blood from the ethmoidal meatus or middle meatus, and a discoloration or enlargement of the great ethmoturbinate.[23] Hence, small lesions of the sinuses may not be detected endoscopically.[32] However, as the condition progresses, a greenish yellow to purplish red mass may be seen obscuring the fundus of the nasal cavity (Fig. 42-6) or the entire nasal passage.

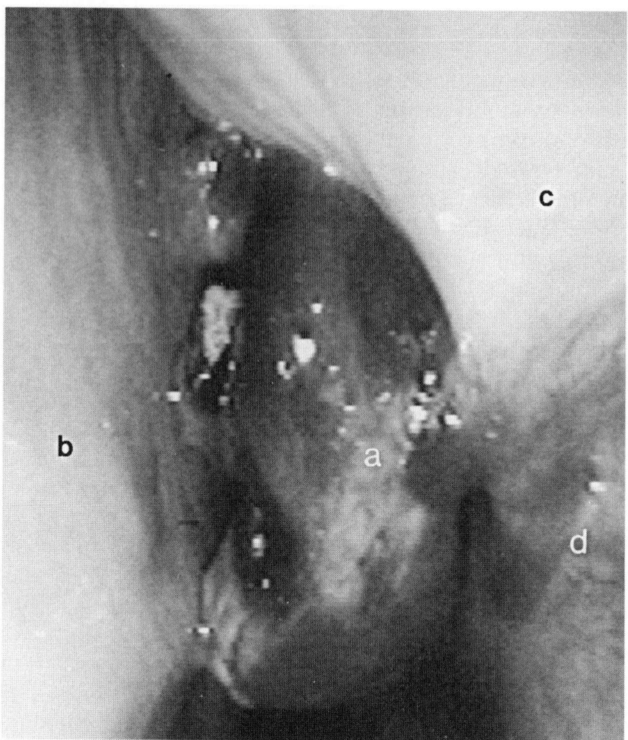

Figure 42-6. Endoscopic appearance of an ethmoid hematoma (a) in the left nasal fundus, located between the nasal septum (b), the dorsal concha (c), and the ventral concha (d).

The most characteristic radiographic abnormality is a smooth, discrete, rounded density in the frontal or maxillary sinus; however, radiographic changes may include fluid lines or diffuse opacities of the sinuses.[23,33] Computed tomography (CT) is useful to determine the exact location and extent of the hematoma involvement (Fig. 42-7), because it provides a cross-sectional view of the skull, which eliminates the superimposition of the paranasal sinuses and nasal cavity that occurs with the lateral radiographic projection.

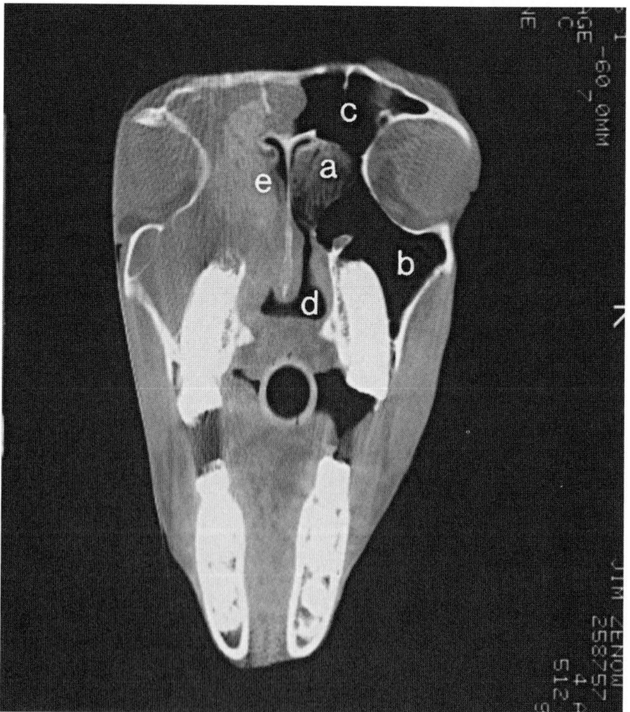

Figure 42-7. A computed tomographic image of a horse's head in a transverse plane at the level of the orbits, demonstrating the right normal ethmoidal labyrinth (a), caudal compartment of the maxillary sinus (b), frontal sinus (c), ventral nasal meatus (d), and a soft tissue density (e) in the frontal and maxillary sinuses on the affected left side. (The asymmetry of the scan is caused by the horse's lateral recumbency during imaging.)

Differential diagnoses include other conditions that may result in persistent or intermittent epistaxis or blood-stained nasal discharge, such as ulcerative or fungal rhinitis; foreign body; ethmoidal neoplasia; mycosis or neoplasia of the guttural pouch; skull fracture; neoplasia, infection, or cyst of the paranasal sinuses; pulmonary abscess or neoplasm; or infectious pleuropneumonia.[33,34]

The goal of surgery is removal of the mass and destruction of its origin. The surgical approach for removal depends on mass size and location. Lesions limited to the fundus of the nasal cavity and less than 5 cm in diameter can be treated transendoscopically using a neodymium:yttrium-aluminum-garnet (Nd:YAG) laser in a standing patient or by intralesional injection of formalin (see later).[32,35,36]

Lesions that are large and extend into the nasal passage or sinuses are best approached via bone flap techniques, gaining access to the origin of the lesion with the horse anesthetized and in lateral recumbency. These techniques can be used to expose the maxillary sinus, frontal sinus, and nasal cavity.[28,30,36-38] One of these techniques, the frontonasal bone flap, gives improved access and has more versatility than other approaches, especially if there is involvement in both the nasal cavity and the frontal sinus.[30] It also allows the creation of a large endoscopic portal to the sinuses, which permits future evaluation for recurrence and treatment with the Nd:YAG laser in a standing patient (Fig. 42-8).

Intraoperative hemorrhage is an expected complication from damage to the normal nasal or sinus mucosa, to the ethmoturbinates, or from the ethmoid hematoma itself. Various techniques have been described to provide hemostasis during surgery, such as bilateral carotid artery ligation, roll gauze packing, epinephrine-soaked gauze packing, vascular clips, lavage with sterile physiologic saline solution (cold or ice slush), and liquid nitrogen spray. Cryosurgical removal of the lesion is reported to lower the incidence of recurrence, but this requires adequate exposure of the base as well as a relatively blood-free surgical field. If the lesion is large, sequentially freezing and removing segments of the mass until the origin is frozen helps to minimize hemorrhage. The use of thermocouples controls the depth of freezing, especially in the ethmoid labyrinth to help protect the cribriform plate. Single freezes of −30° C are suggested to avoid damage to normal structures.[23] The use of the Nd:YAG laser for removal of the lesion has been reported to decrease the amount of hemorrhage and the chance of recurrence.[32,35]

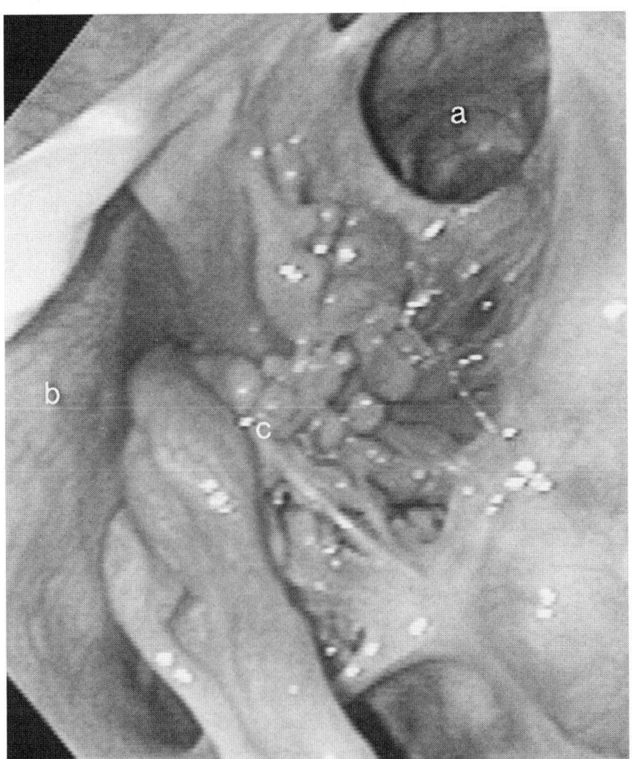

Figure 42-8. Endoscopic appearance of the nasal fundus 4 months after surgery, showing the permanent opening into the frontal sinus (a), the nasal septum (b), and the remains of the endoturbinates (c).

Thorough presurgical planning reduces delays and significant blood loss. In preparation, besides collecting 4 to 8 L of blood for a possible transfusion, it is advisable to administer at least 10 L of intravenous fluids immediately before the induction of anesthesia, and to continue to administer fluids throughout the surgery, thereby alleviating hypotension associated with blood loss. The amount of hemorrhage is usually minimal until disruption of the base of the lesion or other highly vascular structures such as the tectorial plate of the ethmoid labyrinth or the conchal wall of the conchofrontal sinus. Frequently, it is necessary to invade these structures to gain access to the base of the lesion.

Regardless of the removal technique, the most effective method for controlling hemorrhage is firm packing of the sinus or nasal cavity with sterile, cotton roll gauze after surgery. The bone flap is closed in a routine manner. Before closure of the flap, a catheter is placed through the adjacent bone to simplify lavage of the sinus once the pack has been removed. To facilitate removal of the gauze, it can exit either from an aperture on the free edge of the bone flap or through the nasal cavity. The end of the gauze should be secured to the skin of the nares to prevent inadvertent removal of the pack.

Broad-spectrum systemic antibiotics are started before surgery and continued for 3 to 4 days. Administering a sedative and analgesic facilitates removal of the packing 48 to 72 hours after surgery. The use of an indwelling lavage system decreases labor and reduces the horse's resentment of the daily treatment. Lavage of the sinus is helpful in removing exudate, blood clots, and tissue debris, but its effectiveness depends on having adequate drainage through either the nasomaxillary opening or a surgically created opening into the nasal cavity (see later). The horse should be confined to stall rest with only hand-walking for at least 3 weeks. It is common to see fungal and necrotic tissue plaques develop on devitalized mucosal tissues for up to 60 days after surgery, but these usually resolve with no further treatment.

Prognosis is unfavorable without treatment because the lesion is progressive and eventually causes obstruction and dyspnea.[23] The chance of recurrence after routine surgical removal is relatively high (approximately 43%).[23,27] Clients should be advised of the importance of periodic endoscopic examinations after surgery to detect recurrence, so that prompt therapy can be instituted. Because bilateral involvement does occur, endoscopic examination of both nasal passages should always be performed. The use of the Nd:YAG laser on recurrent lesions shows promise in preventing the future recurrence, especially when access to the sinuses via the nasal passage has been provided.

Reported *ablation techniques* for the treatment of progressive ethmoid hematomas in a standing, sedated horse include transendoscopic use of the Nd:YAG laser, intralesional formaldehyde injection, and cryotherapy. The Nd:YAG laser is effective in the standing horse for lesions less than 5 cm in diameter when limited to the nasal fundus only.[35] Therefore, the technique is not applicable for lesions extending into the sinuses. Several laser applications are usually required to ablate the lesion successfully. Lesions are best photo-ablated using noncontact technique at 60 W of power. Once a carbonized surface develops, at least a 7-day delay is recommended before the next treatment, to allow sloughing of the carbonized tissue.

Chemical ablation of ethmoid hematomas has been reported to be effective, inexpensive, and apparently safe.[36] Lesions are injected transendoscopically with a 4% formaldehyde solution. The solution is injected through a commercial polypropylene catheter with a retractable, swedged-on 23-gauge needle (Mill-Rose Laboratories. Inc, Mentor, Ohio) or a polypropylene tube inserted through the biopsy channel of the endoscope. The end of the tube is beveled to permit penetration of the mass. The volume of the injected solution depends on the size of the lesion. The mass is injected until it begins to distend and leakage of solution is noticed around the tube. The treatment is repeated at 3- to 4-week intervals until the lesion is obliterated or too small to inject. A range of 1 to 18 treatments with a mean of five injections has been reported.[36] Complications included laminitis in one horse and the risk of nasal obstruction with treatment of bilateral lesions. In one report, a severe complication occurred using this technique: there was erosion and necrosis of the cribriform plate that may have allowed the formalin to reach the brain.[39]

Transendoscopic use of cryogen for the treatment of progressive ethmoid hematomas cannot be recommended because of potential damage to the endoscope, the lack of control of freezing depth, and damage to surrounding tissues with this direct evaporation technique.

DISEASES OF THE PARANASAL SINUSES

The primary clinical features of paranasal sinus disease are unilateral nasal discharge, facial swelling, and decreased nasal airflow. Occasionally seen are externally draining tracts, malodorous breath, ocular discharge, and stertor. The character of the discharge may be serous, purulent, mucopurulent, or serosanguineous, but hemorrhage usually indicates granulomatous or neoplastic lesions.

Diagnosis

A tentative diagnosis of paranasal sinus disease can be made from the history, clinical signs, and physical examination. The physical examination should include percussion of the paranasal sinuses and an oral examination. *Endoscopy* can be useful for determining the origin of a nasal discharge or evaluating the integrity of the nasal passage of the affected side. *Radiography* is the most useful diagnostic procedure to establish the location and extent of paranasal sinus disease.[8] Abnormal radiographic findings of the paranasal sinus include opacity, free fluid accumulation (see Fig. 41-8, *A*), dental abnormalities, and related bone pathology. Radiography is more reliable in revealing dental disease in the upper premolars rostral to the maxillary sinus than those located within the sinus.[33] Radiographic evidence of free fluid accumulation in the maxillary sinus is similar in frequency and quantity in both dental disease and primary sinusitis, but opacification of both the maxillary and the frontal sinus rarely occurs in dental disease, whereas it is frequent with primary sinusitis.

Sinocentesis is a useful diagnostic or therapeutic procedure for paranasal sinus disease. When it is performed as a diagnostic procedure, both compartments of the maxillary sinus should be sampled. The area is prepared for aseptic surgery. Anesthesia is provided by local infiltration of a 2% solution of lidocaine. The skin, subcutaneous tissue, and periosteum are readily desensitized by a small quantity of local anesthetic. After a stab incision is made through the skin and periosteum, a hole is made in the bone using a Steinmann pin or bone drill of slightly larger diameter than an indwelling plastic catheter or rigid catheter (such as a canine urinary catheter). If no sample is obtained, 20 to 30 mL of warm saline should be infused before subsequent aspiration, or the sinus may be lavaged with 0.5 L of saline and the nasal discharge examined for evidence of purulent exudate.

Sinoscopy of the paranasal sinuses has been reported to be a useful procedure for the diagnosis and treatment of some disorders of the paranasal sinuses.[40] It can be a valuable diagnostic aid when other noninvasive procedures are inconclusive. It can be carried out in a standing, conscious horse or under general anesthesia. The examination is performed with a 4-mm, 30-degree arthroscope using portals created with a 6.25-mm (¼-inch) Steinmann pin. Anatomic locations for these portals are as follows: (1) frontal sinus—60% of the distance in a lateral direction from the midline to the medial canthus and 0.5 cm caudal to the medial canthus, (2) caudal maxillary sinus—2 cm rostral and 2 cm ventral to the medial canthus, (3) rostral maxillary sinus—50% of the distance from the rostral end of the facial crest to the level of the medial canthus and 1 cm ventral to a line joining the infraorbital foramen and the medial canthus.[41] The skin incisions for the portals are closed in a routine manner. A mild, local subcutaneous emphysema occurs at the portal sites but resolves spontaneously within 14 days.[41]

Sinusitis

Sinusitis is the most commonly encountered disease of the paranasal sinuses. It may be classified as either primary or secondary and as either acute or chronic. Empyema refers to purulent exudate within the sinus and is not necessarily synonymous with chronic sinusitis. Primary bacterial sinusitis usually results from previous upper respiratory tract infections. *Streptococcus* species are the most commonly reported organisms of primary sinusitis.[14,42]

The principles of therapy for *primary sinusitis* are to provide adequate drainage and to use the appropriate systemic antimicrobial agents based on antibiotic culture results and sensitivity testing. Drainage may be enhanced by lavaging the sinus once or twice daily. Drainage and lavage are accomplished by either placing an indwelling catheter percutaneously into the maxillary sinus (see the preceding paragraph on sinocentesis for the procedure) or by using a small, sterile, flexible plastic stallion catheter through a trephine opening in the frontoconchal sinus. The skin over the site for entering the frontoconchal sinus is anesthetized with 2% Carbocaine (see later). A small, slightly curved incision is made through all layers of tissue to the bone. The skin incision should be larger than the opening in the sinus to facilitate closure. The tissues are reflected from the bone together, and a circular opening is made using a 19-mm

Gault trephine. The exudate is most efficiently removed from the sinus by inserting a 6.6-mm (OD) sterile, flexible plastic stallion catheter into the frontoconchal sinus and flushing with a mild salt solution (1.2 ounces of salt per gallon of water) via a sterile stomach pump.

Primary paranasal sinusitis usually resolves with systemic antibiotic therapy and lavage, but when the exudate becomes inspissated in the ventral conchal sinus, surgical treatment becomes necessary.[43,44] This condition should be suspected when a primary paranasal sinusitis does not resolve with systemic antibiotics and lavage. Other features of a ventral conchal sinusitis are as follows:

1. The radiographic presence of a soft tissue density over the roots of the superior 4th premolar (108/208), and the 1st (109/209) and 2nd molars (110/210)
2 Distortion of the sinus, seen as a narrowing of the nasal passage caused by an accumulation of inspissated exudate in the ventral conchal sinus

Surgical treatment includes removal of the exudate from the ventral conchal sinus and providing additional drainage if necessary. The ventral conchal sinus can be accessed via a maxillary bone flap or by trephining the frontal sinus in the standing horse (see later).

Secondary sinusitis may be caused by dental disease, facial fractures, granulomatous lesions, or neoplasms. Identifying the cause of sinusitis radiographically can be very difficult with exudate in the sinus. Removal of the exudate via lavage through a trephine opening into the sinus may enhance the radiographic and endoscopic examination of the sinus. After removal of the exudate, the frontoconchal and caudal maxillary sinuses can be reexamined either radiographically or endoscopically. The skin is closed temporarily with skin staples to allow daily flushing. Dental disease is the most common cause of secondary sinusitis[31,45] (see Chapter 30). Secondary sinusitis is generally more difficult to treat and requires surgical intervention to remove the underlying cause (see "Surgical Approaches to the Paranasal Sinuses," later).

Paranasal Sinus Cysts

Occurrence of paranasal sinus cysts is well documented.[46-50] The exact etiology and pathogenesis are unknown, but the cysts are suspected to be of dental origin.[43] There is some evidence that these cysts may have a common origin with ethmoid hematomas.[46] The condition is usually seen in horses ranging in age from nursing foals to young adults, but it is also seen in adult horses. The most common clinical features are dyspnea, facial swelling, and nasal discharge. As the cysts expand, the pressure causes distortion of the ventral nasal concha, the normal internal structures of the sinus, and the maxilla, resulting in obstruction of the common nasal meatus and possibly deviation of the nasal septum and facial deformity. The cysts are typically filled with a yellow, viscous fluid unless they become secondarily infected. There have been no reports of spontaneous regression. Surgical management consists of removing the cysts completely, establishing drainage, and repelling any teeth that may be involved. Complete exposure of the sinus can be provided only via a bone flap technique.[36] Although the prognosis is usually guarded because of the accompanying distortion of the ventral nasal concha and nasal septum, there are reports of regression of the nasal obstruction and facial deformity after surgery in young, growing horses.[48,50]

Neoplasia

The most common tumor of the paranasal sinuses is squamous cell carcinoma. Other invasive tumors reported include spindle-shaped sarcoma[20]; osteogenic sarcoma, lymphosarcoma, and a poorly differentiated carcinoma[50]; ethmoid carcinoma[51]; hemangiosarcoma[52]; and adenocarcinoma.[53] Solid, noninvasive neoplasms such as fibroma,[53] osteoma,[54,55] and ameloblastic odontoma[56] have been reported. Useful clinical signs that may aid in differentiating neoplasia from other sinus diseases are malodorous breath without evidence of dental disease and radiographic evidence of widespread bone destruction. The prognosis is generally unfavorable unless the neoplasm is a solid noninvasive tumor, because the majority are malignant.[53]

SURGICAL APPROACHES TO THE PARANASAL SINUSES

Surgical access to the paranasal sinuses can be obtained by either trephination or bone flap techniques.[30,42] The bone flap techniques are superior to trephination because they provide better exposure, visualization, and access for surgical manipulation within the sinuses, and they eliminate the need for multiple trephine openings. The bone flap technique was first described for exploration of the maxillary sinus,[36] but the technique can be used for the frontal sinus and nasal cavity.

Trephination is the traditional approach for surgical access to the paranasal sinuses. It is useful for diagnostic and therapeutic access to the sinuses. The approximate sites for trephination of the frontal, caudal, and rostral maxillary sinuses are shown in Figure 42-1. The age of the horse should be considered when selecting the site for trephination of the maxillary sinus. The alveoli of the caudal three cheek teeth form the ventrolateral wall of the sinus. In horses 3 years old and younger, the alveoli lie immediately under the osseous infraorbital canal. As the horse ages and the teeth advance, the sinus becomes larger. The trephination sites usually heal within 3 to 4 weeks with minimal blemish.

For the *maxillary bone flap* (Fig. 42-9), the *rostral* margin is a line drawn from the rostral end of the facial crest to the infraorbital foramen; the *dorsal* margin is a line from the infraorbital foramen to the medial canthus of the eye; the *caudal* margin is a line (parallel to the rostral margin) from the medial canthus of the eye to the caudal aspect of the facial crest; and the *ventral* margin is the facial crest. These boundaries provide maximal exposure of the maxillary sinus while protecting the vulnerable infraorbital canal and nasolacrimal duct.

Alternatively, for the *frontonasal bone flap* (Fig. 42-10), the *caudal* margin is a perpendicular line from the dorsal midline to a point midway between the supraorbital foramen and the medial canthus of the eye; the *lateral* margin begins

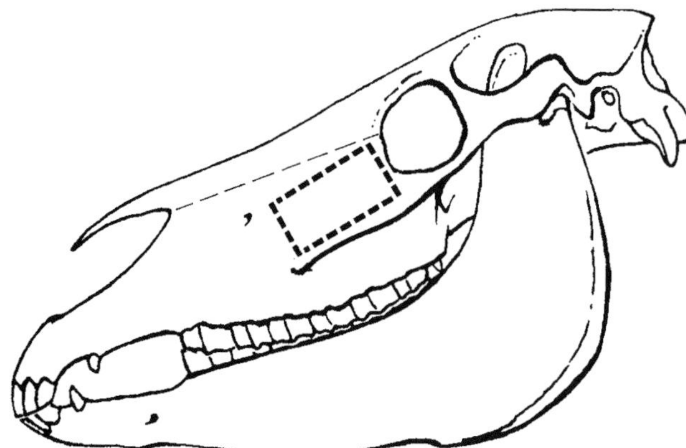

Figure 42-9. Diagram of the skull demonstrating the site for the bone flap technique for exposing the maxillary sinus. The boundaries outlined by *bold dashed lines* provide maximal exposure of the maxillary sinus while protecting the nasolacrimal duct and infraorbital canal. The *long dashed line* from the medial canthus to the incisive notch depicts the approximate course of the nasolacrimal duct. (For a description of the margins of the maxillary bone flap, see "Surgical Approaches to the Paranasal Sinuses" in the text.)

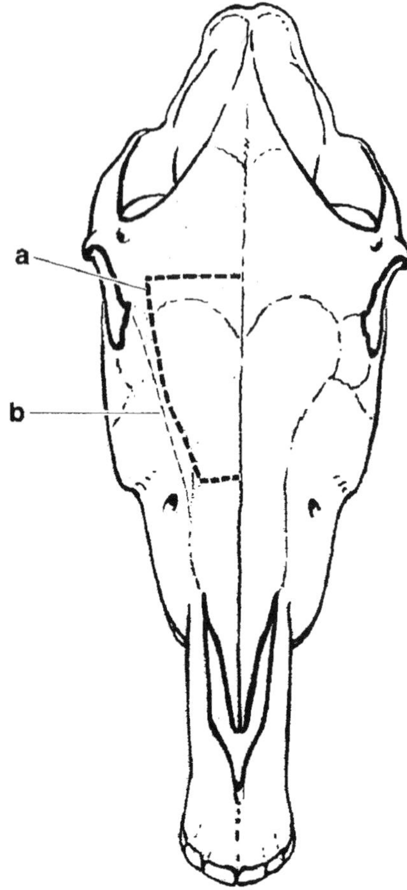

Figure 42-10. Diagram of the skull demonstrating the site for the frontonasal bone flap technique for exposing the caudal aspect of the nasal cavity, dorsal conchal sinus, and frontal sinus. The *long dashed line* from the medial canthus to the incisive notch depicts the approximate course of the nasal lacrimal duct. (For a description of the margins of the frontonasal bone flap, see "Surgical Approaches to the Paranasal Sinuses" in the text.)

at the caudal margin 2 to 2.5 cm medial to the medial canthus of the eye and extends to a point approximately two-thirds the distance from the medial canthus of the eye to the infraorbital foramen; and the *rostral* margin is a perpendicular line from the dorsal midline to the rostral extension of the lateral margin. The estimated course of the nasolacrimal duct is a line from the medial canthus of the eye to the nasoincisive notch. In some horses, the rostral portion of the lateral margin has to be angled toward the midline to avoid the duct (see Fig. 42-10).

Once the boundaries of the area to be explored are determined, a skin incision is made along the rostral, ventral or lateral, and caudal borders. The incision is continued through the subcutaneous tissue to the periosteum, which is exposed and incised. The periosteum is reflected from the site of the proposed osteotomy incision approximately 5 mm.

The osteotomy can be performed using an oscillating bone saw, a pneumatic drill with a tapered burr, or an osteotome and mallet. The osteotomies should be beveled so that when the bone flap is replaced it will provide a more secure closure. Once the osteotomy has been completed on all three sides, the bone flap can be slowly elevated until it fractures along the fourth (or dorsal) side of the rectangle beneath intact tissue. The fracture can be controlled by steady, even pressure and the bone flap completely elevated to expose the area. Before closure, an indwelling lavage system is usually placed through the adjacent bone or a corner of the flap and secured to the skin to facilitate daily lavage. Closure is initiated by pressing the bone flap into its original position and by closure of the periosteum with 2-0 absorbable suture using a simple-continuous pattern. A simple-interrupted stainless steel or monofilament nonabsorbable suture placed at each corner of the flap may occasionally be necessary to secure the flap to the parent bone, but these are frequent sites of fistula formation and should be avoided when possible. The subcutaneous tissue and skin are closed in routine manner. The skin incision usually heals rapidly with minimal scarring.

Frequently, creating a surgical opening into the *nasal cavity* is necessary to improve drainage. Identifying such a site in the conchofrontal sinus (Fig. 42-11) can be aided by passing a mare urinary catheter caudally in the dorsal meatus and feeling the catheter tip through the thin conchal portion of the sinus. The conchal wall is perforated using a curved forceps. The catheter is passed through the opening to aid in the placement of a seton drain threaded through the nasal cavity from the sinus. The site for establishing communication between the rostral maxillary sinus and the nasal cavity is located dorsally over the infraorbital canal in young horses and ventral to the canal in older horses. Caution should be used to prevent damage to the infraorbital canal. The use of a Seton drain helps maintain the patency of the newly created opening to the nasal cavity; a mushroom catheter is usually used instead of gauze or Penrose tubing with the bone flap technique. Once the Seton drain has been removed, the newly created opening may remain permanently open or it may close naturally; therefore, the Seton drain should not be removed until the underlying disease is resolved.

Gaining Surgical Access to the Ventral Conchal Sinuses

The ventral conchal sinus can be entered over the osseous infraorbital canal through the conchomaxillary opening in young horses or by penetrating the thin bony plate (see Fig. 42-11) below the osseous infraorbital canal in older horses. After removing the inspissated exudate, the nasomaxillary opening should be assessed for patency by flushing the sinus with saline and observing for nasal outflow. The medial or ventromedial wall of the sinus can be fenestrated to create an opening into the nasal passage if the nasomaxillary opening is not functional. Removal of inspissated exudate from the ventral conchal sinus has also been reported in the standing horse via a 19-mm trephine opening (a larger trephine opening is better for surgeons with large fingers) into the conchofrontal sinus[43] (see Fig. 42-1). The caudodorsal (bulla) wall of the ventral conchal sinus is identified by palpating ventral and slightly rostral to the trephine opening (see Fig. 42-1). The wall can be perforated with an index finger. The exudate is removed by inserting a 6.6-mm (OD) sterile, flexible plastic stallion catheter into the ventral conchal sinus and flushing with a mild salt solution (1.2 ounces of salt per gallon of water) via a sterile stomach pump.

One of the most important aspects of the treatment of sinusitis is lavage of the sinus to remove exudate, blood, blood clots, or tissue debris. The effectiveness of the lavage depends on adequate drainage, either through a patent nasomaxillary opening or through surgically created openings into the nasal cavity. The frequency and volume are probably more important than the type of lavage solution. Sterile physiologic saline is as effective as antiseptic solutions in most cases and reduces irritation of the mucous membranes. The use of an indwelling lavage system decreases labor and reduces the horse's resentment to daily lavage. Placing a sterile tube through a small trephine opening and pumping a mild salt solution through a sterile pump is a very simple, inexpensive method of flushing the sinuses (see treatment modalities under "Sinusitis," earlier).

The use of systemic antibiotic therapy depends on the primary disease and should be based on bacterial cultures and antibiotic sensitivity results. Feeding the horse on the floor enhances drainage and reduces contamination by hay and dust. Gauze plugs placed in trephine openings or a protective hood made from stockinette also reduces contamination and protects surgical sites in the facial area.

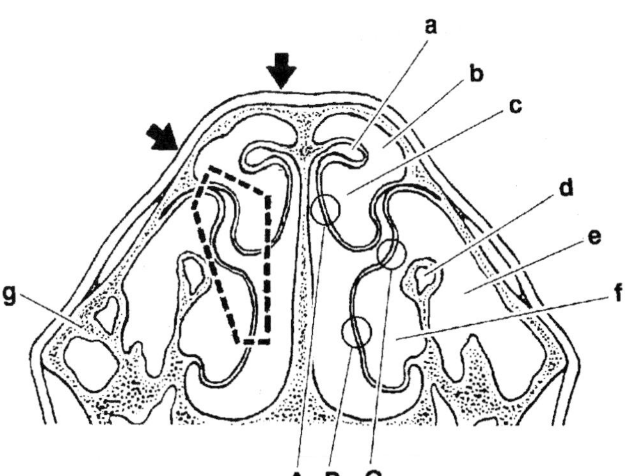

Figure 42-11. Sites for establishing drainage from the paranasal sinuses into the nasal cavity (cross-section of the skull at the level of the 1st molar). The ventral concha may be fenestrated at (A) or (B) to establish drainage into the nasal cavity. Fenestration of the ventromedial wall of the dorsal conchal sinus (C) creates ventral drainage of the conchofrontal sinus into the nasal cavity. This diagram of the skull also demonstrates the medial and lateral edges of the frontonasal bone flap *(arrowheads)* at this level. The structures within the *dashed lines* have to be removed to provide access to the dorsal conchal and maxillary sinuses and the nasal passage. a, dorsal meatus; b, frontal sinus; c, dorsal conchal sinus; d, infraorbital canal; rostral maxillary sinus; f, ventral conchal sinus; g, oblique septum between the rostral and caudal compartments of the maxillary sinus.

REFERENCES

1. Hare WCD: Equine respiratory system. In Getty R, editor: Sisson and Grossman's The Anatomy of the Domestic Animals, ed 5, Philadelphia, 1975, WB Saunders.
2. Hillmann DJ: Skull. In Getty R, editor: Sisson and Grossman's The Anatomy of the Domestic Animals, ed 5, Philadelphia, 1975, WB Saunders.
3. Baker CJ: Surgery of the head and neck. In Catcott EJ, Smithcors JF, editors: Equine Medicine and Surgery, ed 2, Wheaton, Ill, 1972, American Veterinary Publications.
4. Schneider JE: The respiratory system. In Oehme FW, Prier JE, editors: Textbook of Large Animal Surgery, Baltimore, 1974, Williams & Wilkins.
5. Gordon LR: Cytology and histology of epidermal inclusion cysts in the horse, J Equine Med Surg 1978;2:370.
6. Schumacher J, Moll HD, Schumacher J, et al: A simple method to remove an epidermal inclusion cyst from the false nostril of horses, Equine Pract 1997;1:11.
7. Foerner JJ: The diagnosis and correction of false nostrils noises, Proc Am Assoc Equine Pract 1967;13:315.
8. Boulton CH: Equine nasal cavity and paranasal sinus disease: A review of 85 cases, Equine Vet Sci 1985;5:268.
9. Turner AS: Surgical management of depression fractures of the equine skull, Vet Surg 1979;8:29.
10. Levine SB: Depression fractures of the nasal and frontal bones in the horse, J Equine Med Surg 1979;3:186.
11. Stashak TS: Reconstructive surgery in the horse, J Am Vet Med Assoc 1977;170:143.
12. Valdez H: The use of fluorocarbon polymer and carbon fiber for restoration of facial contour in a horse, J Am Vet Med Assoc 1981;178:249.
13. Campbell ML, Peyton LC: Muscle flap closure of a frontocutaneous fistula in a horse, Vet Surg 1984;13:185.
14. Haynes PF: Surgery of the equine respiratory tract. In Jennings PB, editor: Practice of Large Animal Surgery, Philadelphia, 1984, WB Saunders.
15. Wheat JD: Fractures of the head and the mandible, Proc Am Assoc Equine Pract 1975;21:233.
16. Tulleners EP, Raker CW: Nasal septum resection in the horse, Vet Surg 1983;12:41.
17. Servantie D, Sautet JY: Hamartoma of the nasal septum in a yearling, Equine Pract 1986;8:11.
18. McAllister ES: Obstructive upper respiratory disease. In Mansmann RA, McAllister ES, editors: Equine Medicine and Surgery, ed 3, Santa Barbara, Calif, 1982, American Veterinary Publications.
19. Valdez H, McMullan WC, Hobson HP, et al: Surgical correction of deviated nasal septum and premaxilla in a colt, J Am Vet Med Assoc 1978;173:1001.

20. Mason BJE: Spindle-cell sarcoma of the equine paranasal sinuses and nasal chamber, Vet Rec 1975;96:287.
21. Bemis HE: Removal of the nasal septum, J Am Vet Med Assoc 1916;2:397.
22. Frank ER: Veterinary Surgery, ed 7, Minneapolis, 1964, Burgess.
23. Cook WR, Littlewort MCG: Progressive haematoma of the horse, Equine Vet J 1974;6:101.
24. Sullivan M, Burrell MH, McCandlish IAP: Progressive hematoma of the maxillary sinus, Vet Rec 1984;114:191.
25. Platt H: Hemorrhagic nasal polyps of the horse, J Pathol 1975;115:51.
26. Bell BLT, Baker GJ, Foreman JH: Progressive ethmoid hematoma: Background, clinical signs and diagnosis. Comp Cont Educ Pract Vet 1993;15:1101.
27. Specht TE, Colahan PT, Nixon AJ, et al: Ethmoidal hematoma in nine horses, J Am Vet Med Assoc 1990;197:613.
28. Blackford JT, Goble DO, Henry RW, et al: Triangulated flap technique for nasofrontal surgery: Results in five horses, Vet Surg 1985;14:287.
29. Etherington WG, Vasey JR, Horney FD: Ethmoid hematoma in the equine, Can Vet J 1982;23:231.
30. Freeman DE, Orsini PG, Ross MW, et al: A large frontonasal bone flap for sinus surgery in the horse, Vet Surg 1990;19:122.
31. Stickle RL: Nasal polyp in a horse, Vet Med Small Anim Clin 1978;72:911.
32. Tate LP: Application of laser in equine upper respiratory surgery, Vet Clin North Am Equine Pract 1991;7:176.
33. Gibbs C, Lane JG: Radiographic examination of the facial, nasal and paranasal sinus regions of the horse: II. Radiographic findings, Equine Vet J 1987;19:474.
34. O'Callaghan MW: Bleeding from the nose. In Brown CM, editor: Problems in Equine Medicine, Philadelphia, 1989, Lea & Febiger.
35. Tulleners EP: Ethmoid hematoma. In Auer JA, editor: Equine Surgery, Philadelphia, 1992, WB Saunders
36. Schumacher J, Honnas C, Yarbrough T, et al: Treatment of horses with ethmoidal hematoma by intralesional injection of formaldehyde solution, Proc Ann Symp Am Coll Vet Surg 1997;7:150.
37. Haynes PF: Bone flaps. In Jennings PB, editor: The Practice of Large Animal Surgery, Philadelphia, 1984, WB Saunders.
38. Meagher DM: The elevation and surgical treatment of ethmoid hematomas in the horse, Vet Surg 1986;15:128.
39. Frees KE, Gaughan EM, Lillich JD, et al: Severe complications after administration of formalin for treatment of progressive ethmoidal hematoma in a horse, J Am Vet Med Assoc 2001;219:950-952.
40. Wheat JD: Sinus drainage and teeth repulsion in the horse, Proc Am Assoc Equine Pract 1973;19:171.
41. Ruggles AJ, Ross MW, Freeman DE: Endoscopic examination and treatment of paranasal sinus disease in 16 horses, Vet Surg 1993;229:508.
42. Ruggles AJ, Ross MW, Freeman DE: Endoscopic examination of normal paranasal sinuses in horses, Vet Surg 1991;20:418.
43. Schumacher J, Honnas C, Smith B: Paranasal sinusitis complicated by inspissated exudate in ventral conchal sinus, Vet Surg 1987;16:373.
44. Schmacher J, Crossland LE: Removal of inspissated purulent exudate from the ventral conchal sinus of three standing horses, J Am Vet Med Assoc 1994;205:1312.
45. Mason JE: Empyema of the equine paranasal sinuses, J Am Vet Med Assoc 1975;167:727.
46. Cannon JH, Grant BD, Sande RD: Diagnosis and surgical treatment of cyst-like lesions of the equine paranasal sinuses, J Am Vet Med Assoc 1976;169:610.
47. Lane JG, Longstaffe JA, Gibb C: Equine paranasal sinus cyst: A report of 15 cases, Equine Vet J 1987;19:537.
48. Cook WR: Skeletal radiology of the equine head, J Am Vet Radiol Soc 1970;11:33.
49. Leyland A, Baker JR: Lesions of the nasal and paranasal sinuses of the horse causing dyspnea, Br Vet J 1975;131:339.
50. Sanders-Shamis M, Roberston JT: Congenital sinus cyst in a foal, J Am Vet Med Assoc 1987;8:1011.
51. Acland HM, Orsini JA: Congenital ethmoid carcinoma in a foal, J Am Vet Med Assoc 1984;184:979.
52. Stencel E, Grotelueschen D: Hemangiosarcoma involving the frontal sinus of a horse, Equine Pract 1989;11:14.
53. Madewell BR, Priester WA, Gillette KL: Neoplasms of the nasal passages of the paranasal sinuses in domesticated animals as reported by 13 colleges, Am J Vet Res 1976;37:851.
54. Peterson FB, Martens RJ, Montali RJ: Surgical treatment of an osteoma in the paranasal sinuses of a horse, J Equine Med Surg 1978;2:279.
55. Kold SE, Ostblom LC, Philipsen HP: Headshaking caused by a maxillary osteoma in a horse, Equine Vet J 1982;14:169.
56. Roberts MC, Groenendyk S, Kelly WR: Ameloblastic odontoma in a foal, Equine Vet J 1978;10:91.

CHAPTER 43

Pharynx

Norman G. Ducharme

ANATOMY AND PHYSIOLOGY

The pharynx is a musculomembranous tubular structure unsupported by bone or cartilaginous matrix. It has different roles during breathing, deglutition, and vocalization. The pharynx extends from the caudal end of the nasal cavity to the larynx and is equally divided by the soft palate to form the nasopharynx dorsally and the oropharynx ventrally.[1] During normal breathing, the caudal free margin of the soft palate intimately contacts the subepiglottic tissue at the base of the equine larynx (Fig. 43-1) and prevents communication between the oropharynx and nasopharynx. The nasopharynx is attached to the pterygoid, palatine, and hyoid bones and to the laryngeal, cricoid, and thyroid cartilages by muscles, which cause dilation and constriction of the nasopharynx.[2] Although the nasopharynx is not directly supported by cartilage or bone, it must withstand large changes in intraluminal pressures (from 24 to 50 cm water) that occur at varying airflow velocities (up to 90 L/s), with minimal changes in diameter. It does this through muscular contraction.

Several groups of muscles alter the size and configuration of the nasopharynx, including the muscles that move the tongue, insert on the hyoid apparatus and larynx, and regulate soft palate position.[3-9] Some muscle contractions alter the position of the hyoid apparatus. Specifically, ventral displacement of the basihyoid increases nasopharyngeal size and stability by increasing the diameter or decreasing compliance of the nasopharynx.[4,5] The relevant musculature

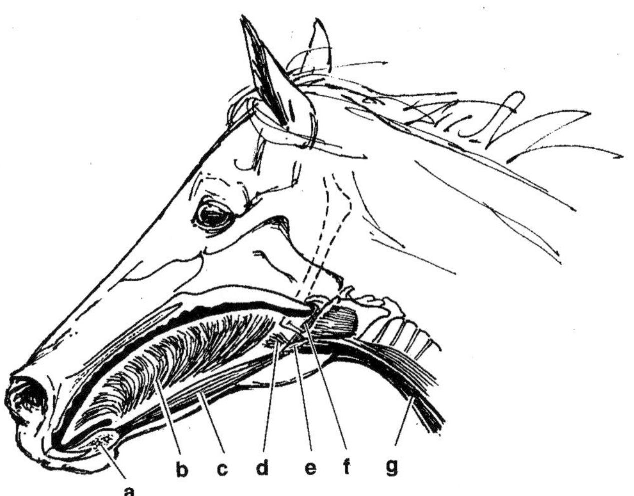

Figure 43-1. Illustration of the extrinsic structures relevant to equine nasopharynx stability, showing the definition of the nasopharynx and relative relationships of the hyoid apparatus, larynx, and extrinsic muscular attachments. a, mandible; b, genioglossus muscle; c, geniohyoideus muscle; d, hyoglossus muscle; e, basihyoid bone; f, hyoepiglotticus muscle; g, sternohyoideus muscle.

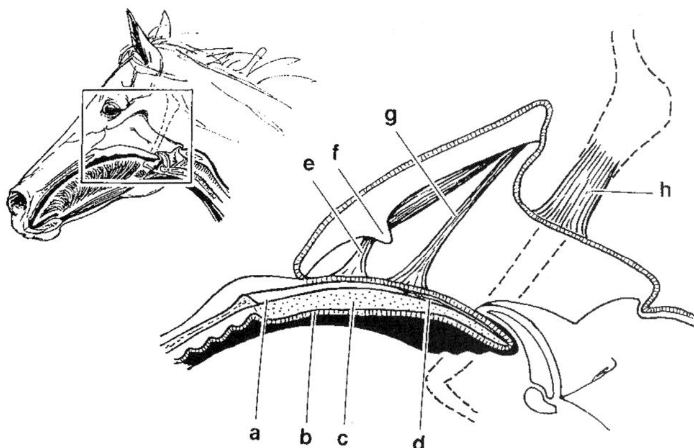

Figure 43-2. Illustration of the intrinsic structures of the nasopharynx. The nasopharynx forms the passageway that transfers airflow from the caudal aspect of the nasal cavity to the larynx. The floor of the nasopharynx is formed by the soft palate and its relevant structures (a, palatine aponeurosis; b, oral mucosa; c, glandular layer; d, palatinus muscle) and is normally in a subepiglottic position during respiration. The hamulus (f) of the pterygoid bone, and the tensor veli palatini (e), levator veli palatini (g), and palatopharyngeus (not shown) muscles are underneath the mucosa of the lateral walls of the nasopharynx. The stylopharyngeus (h) with the palatopharyngeus muscles add to the stability of the roof of the nasopharynx.

can be classified as intrinsic or extrinsic to the nasopharynx.[10] The *intrinsic* muscles, which include those of soft palate and nasopharyngeal musculature, insert on the mucosa or the confined walls and roof of the nasopharynx. The *extrinsic* muscles include those of the larynx and the hyoid apparatus (musculature not part of the nasopharyngeal walls that affect either the position of the basihyoid bone or larynx).

Intrinsic Musculature

The intrinsic musculature contributes to the stability of the nasopharynx mainly by timely muscular contractions that tense and dilate the pharyngeal wall (Fig. 43-2). The floor of the nasopharynx is formed by the soft palate extending caudally from the hard palate to the base of the larynx. The soft palate consists of oral mucous membrane that contains the palatine glands and their ductile openings, palatine aponeurosis, palatinus and palatopharyngeus muscles, and nasopharyngeal mucous membrane.[2] The palatine aponeurosis is formed by expansion of the tendon of the tensor veli palatini muscle.[2,9] This aponeurosis attaches to the caudal margin of the hard palate. It is thick cranially and very thin caudally, where the soft palate is more muscular. The caudal free margin of the soft palate continues dorsally on either side of the larynx, forming the lateral pillars of the soft palate. Muscle fibers of the palatinus muscle course beneath the nasopharyngeal mucosa and extend along the pillars of the soft palate. These pillars unite dorsally, forming the palatopharyngeal arch.[2]

The position of the soft palate is determined by the coordinated function of four muscles (Fig. 43-3, and see Fig. 43-2): the tensor veli palatini, levator veli palatini, palatinus, and palatopharyngeus muscles. The tensor veli palatini muscle is innervated by the mandibular branch of the trigeminal nerve, and the other three are all innervated by the pharyngeal branch of the vagus nerve.[2,6,7,9] The *levator veli palatini* muscle arises from the muscular process of the petrous part

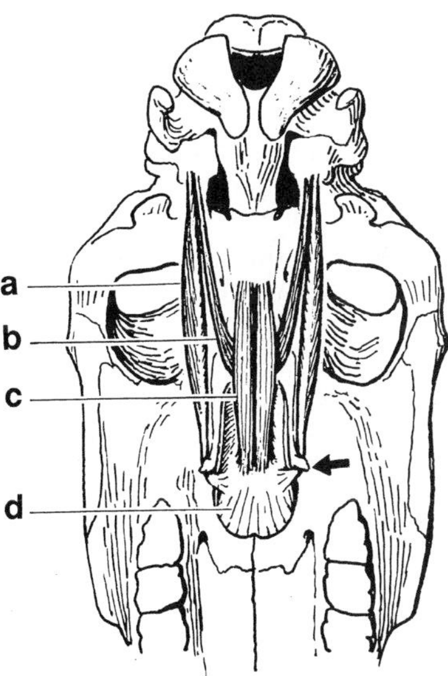

Figure 43-3. Illustration of the intrinsic structures of the nasopharynx viewed from the ventral aspect of the nasopharynx, showing the muscles of the soft palate, the palatine aponeurosis (d), and the hamulus of the pterygoid bone *(arrow)*. a, tensor veli palatini muscle; b, levator veli palatini muscle; c, palatinus muscle.

of the temporal bone and the lateral lamina of the auditory tube and passes along the lateral wall of the nasopharynx to insert within the soft palate dorsal to the glandular layer.[2] This muscle elevates the soft palate during swallowing, closes the nasopharynx, and facilitates oral ventilation in nonobligate nasal breathers. The *palatinus* muscle consists of a paired fusiform muscle that originates at the caudal aspect of the palatine aponeurosis and courses through the middle of the soft palate, just beneath the nasal mucosa, to ramify in the caudal free margin of the soft palate. The *palatopharyngeus* muscle arises from the palatine aponeurosis (lateral to the palatinus muscle attachment) and from the palatine and pterygoid bones.[2] The fibers continue caudally on the lateral wall of the pharynx and partially insert into the upper edge of the thyroid cartilage. The remainder of the muscle continues dorsally and inserts at the median fibrous raphe. The palatinus and palatopharyngeus muscles shorten the soft palate and depress it toward the tongue.[3] The *tensor veli palatini* muscle is a fusiform muscle that originates at the muscular process of the petrous part of the temporal bone, pterygoid bone, and lateral lamina of the auditory tube and travels rostroventrally along the lateral wall of the nasopharynx lateral to the *levator veli palatini*.[2] The tendon courses around the hamulus of the pterygoid bone and ramifies in the palatine aponeurosis. This muscle tenses the rostral aspect of the soft palate by using the hamulus as a pulley and retracts the soft palate away from the dorsal pharyngeal wall,[9] expanding the nasopharynx and slightly depressing it ventrally during inspiration.

The final intrinsic muscle of the nasopharynx is the *stylopharyngeus*, which is divided into two parts.[11] The *stylopharyngeus rostralis* originates from the medial surface of the rostral end of the stylohyoid bone and inserts on the pharyngeal raphe. It is a pharyngeal constrictor that is not stimulated during exercise, so it will not be discussed further. The *stylopharyngeus caudalis* is a pharyngeal dilator muscle that originates from the medial aspect of the caudal third of the stylohyoid bone and courses ventrally and rostrally to attach on the dorsolateral wall of the pharynx[7,11] (see Fig. 40-5, *A*). It is innervated by the glossopharyngeal nerve and is responsible for tension on the roof of the nasopharynx (Fig. 43-4) that helps it resist collapsing with inspiratory pressure.

The blood supply to the soft palate is derived from the linguofacial trunk, and maxillary artery and venous drainage occurs via the accompanying veins.[2] The lymph vessels drain toward the retropharyngeal lymph nodes. The afferent innervation from branches of the trigeminal, glossopharyngeal, and vagus nerves arises from pressure, mechanical, and temperature receptors lining the mucous membrane of the nasopharynx, including the soft palate.

Extrinsic Musculature

The extrinsic muscles contribute to the respiratory patency of the nasopharynx by increasing its diameter or by increasing the stability of the soft palate, or both. In dogs and humans, ventral displacement of the basihyoid bone results in increases in the nasopharynx diameter. The genioglossus muscle is a fan-shaped extrinsic tongue muscle that originates within the median plane of the tongue and attaches to the oral surface of the mandible, caudal to the symphysis[2] (see Fig. 43-1). Contraction of the genioglossus muscle protracts the tongue and pulls the basihyoid bone rostrally. In horses, this activity was once thought to result in an increase in nasopharyngeal diameter and improvement in airway patency. This was the hypothesis behind using a tongue-tie in racing horses, which has been disproved by recent studies. Computed tomographic imaging showed no measurable improvement in nasopharyngeal diameter by using a tongue-tie in normal horses.[12] Likewise, no improvement in airway patency during treadmill exercise was shown by using a tongue-tie in normal horses.[13]

Contraction of muscles that insert on the hyoid arch increases upper airway size and stability by increasing the diameter and stiffness of the nasopharynx.[4,5] The rostrohyoid and caudohyoid muscle groups exert rostral and caudal forces, respectively, on the hyoid apparatus. The geniohyoideus is a rostrohyoid muscle that originates, in conjunction with the genioglossus, on the medial surface of the mandible near the symphysis and inserts on the basihyoid bone. Its action draws the hyoid apparatus rostrally. The sternohyoideus and sternothyroideus muscles are caudohyoid muscles that originate on the sternal manubrium and extend cranially. The sternothyroideus inserts on the caudal abaxial aspect of the thyroid cartilage, and the sternohyoideus muscle inserts on the basihyoid bone and lingual process of the hyoid apparatus. Contraction of these muscles results in caudal traction on the hyoid apparatus and larynx. In dogs and humans, muscles that put rostral traction on the basihyoid bone work in a coordinated fashion with muscles that apply caudal traction, and the sum of these vector forces is a net ventral displacement of the basihyoid bone.[4] This motion increases the angle at the ceratohyoid–stylohyoid joint, increasing the dorsal ventral dimension of the nasopharynx. In doing so, the lateral walls of the nasopharynx expand slightly and become taut.[4] Although this has not been demonstrated conclusively in horses, dysfunction of the strap muscles (*sternohyoideus* and *sternothyroideus*) in horses has been shown experimentally to increase the upper airway pressure at exercise.[14] This suggests that nasopharyngeal impedance is increased by dysfunction of these extrinsic muscles.

Another extrinsic muscle known to increase the patency of the nasopharynx is the hyoepiglotticus muscle (see Fig. 43-1), which attaches to the hyoid bone at the base of the epiglottis and, during its contraction, pulls the epiglottis ventrally toward the base of the tongue, thereby increasing the ventral dimension of the rima glottidis.[2,8] The hyoepiglotticus muscle is the only muscle that inserts on the epiglottis.

Finally, the thyrohyoideus muscle, which extends from the lateral lamina of the thyroid cartilage to the caudal aspect of the thyrohyoid bone (see Figs. 40-5 and 43-4) was thought to move the larynx rostrally only during deglutition.[2] However, resection of this muscle disrupts the normal stability of the nasopharynx during exercise, resulting in dorsal displacement of the soft palate (DDSP).[15] Therefore, the mechanism of action of the thyrohyoideus muscle is to enhance soft palate stability during exercise by moving the larynx rostrally so the thyroid cartilage rests more dorsal and rostral in relation to the basihyoid.[15]

The geniohyoideus, genioglossus, and hyoepiglotticus muscles are all innervated by the hypoglossal nerve,[2] whereas sternohyoideus and sternothyroideus muscles receive motor innervation from branches of the first and second cervical nerves.[2] Although it has been reported that the thyrohyoid branch of the hypoglossal nerve is responsible for innervation of the thyrohyoideus muscle, recent investigations suggest that the pharyngeal branch of the vagus is responsible for this innervation.[16] Arterial blood supply to the pharynx is provided by the common and external carotid arteries and the linguofacial trunk.[2] Venous drainage is provided by the accompanying veins.[2] Lymph vessels drain

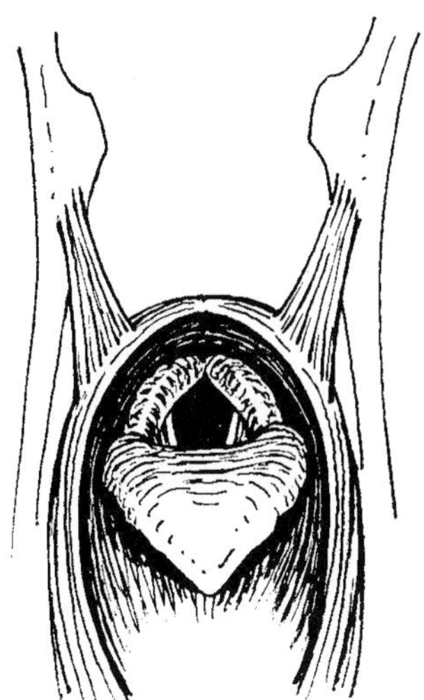

Figure 43-4. Schematic of the intrinsic muscles that form the wall and roof of the nasopharynx. Note that contractions of the *stylopharyngeus caudalis* support the roof of the nasopharynx. Also, compare Fig. 40-5, *A* and *B*. Note the direction of the *stylopharyngeus caudalis* fibers and therefore the direction of its contractions.

toward the retropharyngeal and cranial cervical lymph nodes.[2] The trigeminal, vagus, and glossopharyngeal nerves provide afferent sensory innervation to the nasopharyngeal mucosa.

ANATOMIC DISORDERS OF THE NASOPHARYNX

Nasopharyngeal Cicatrix

Nasopharyngeal cicatrix was a condition first reported as being more commonly seen in aged female horses,[17] but more recent data suggest only a slight predisposition for mares (60% of 87 horses).[18] Affected animals range in age from 5 to 29 years.[17,18] This anomaly is seen almost exclusively in hot climates (mostly in eastern and southern Texas, with occasional reports from Mississippi, Louisiana, Oklahoma, and Florida) in horses kept on pasture. An environmental allergen is thought to lead to nasopharyngeal inflammation and subsequent damage to the nasopharyngeal and laryngeal mucosa and submucosa. Secondary healing results in a web of nasopharyngeal scarring that reduces the diameter of the nasopharynx, or restricts its function when severe[17,18] (Fig. 43-5). In nearly 95% of reported cases, deformed epiglottic, arytenoid, or medial cartilage of the guttural pouch opening is seen[17,18] (Fig. 43-6). Because of the larger cross-sectional area of the nasopharynx in comparison to the rima glottidis and extrathoracic trachea, only severe scarring of the nasopharynx causes functional abnormalities. The degree of involvement of other structures determines clinical signs.

Clinical signs for this condition include upper respiratory noise and exercise intolerance, with dysphagia rarely seen. The airway sounds may be variable, depending on whether nasopharyngeal scarring results in DDSP or arytenoid chondritis. Involvement of one or both of the arytenoid cartilages is the most common reason for exercise intolerance and respiratory noise. The degree of performance interference

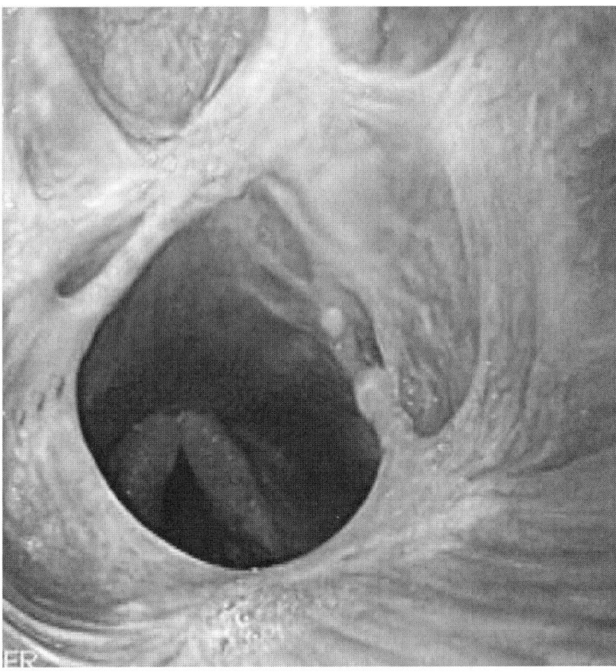

Figure 43-5. Endoscopic photograph of a nasopharyngeal cicatrix in a horse, characterized by scar formation across the floor of the nasopharynx. (Courtesy P. Rakestraw, Texas A&M University.)

depends on the athletic demands and degree of ventilation interference.

The diagnosis is made by endoscopic examination. In the earliest stages, hyperemic mucosa is observed; there may also be yellow or discolored areas (plaques) on the pharyngeal walls, even in areas where a cicatrix does not form

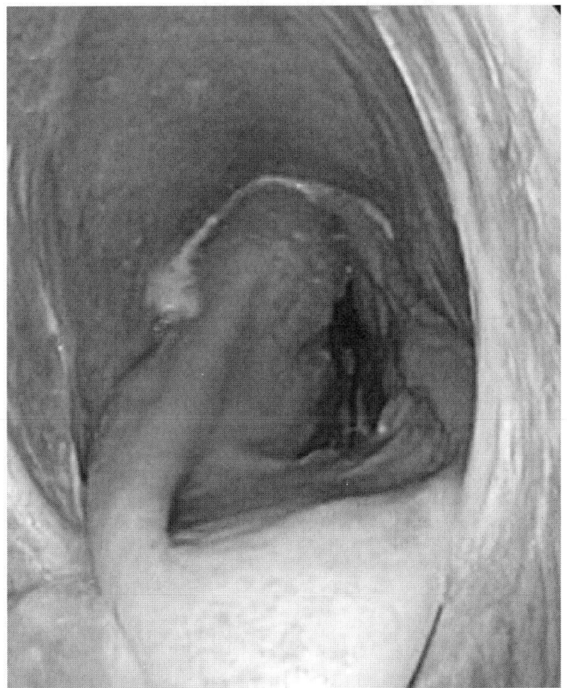

Figure 43-6. Endoscopic photograph of a nasopharyngeal cicatrix affecting the larynx and epiglottic cartilage. Note the deformation of right arytenoid cartilage, as well as scar formation across the floor of the nasopharynx. (Courtesy P. Rakestraw, Texas A&M University.)

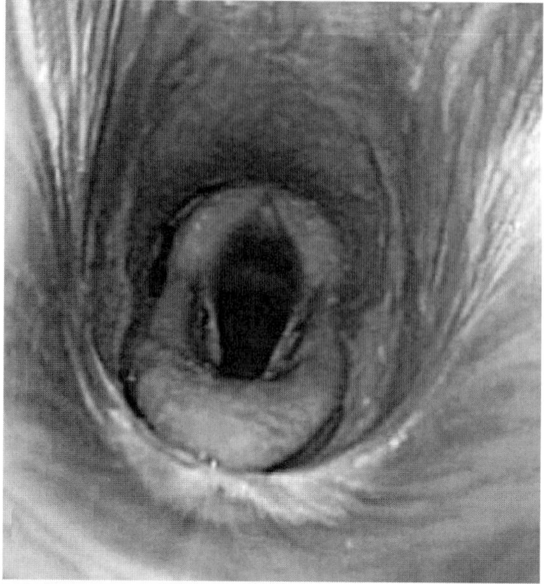

Figure 43-7. Endoscopic view of early nasopharyngeal inflammation, a precursor of nasopharyngeal cicatrix. (Courtesy P. Rakestraw, Texas A&M University.)

(Fig. 43-7). The cicatrix can be limited to a local area or involve the entire circumference of the pharynx, and it usually includes one or more transverse bands of tissue located between the guttural pouch opening and the larynx (see Fig. 43-5). In 20% of the cases reported, one of the guttural pouch openings was involved in the cicatrix.[17] Because this type of cicatrix is generally associated with epiglottic and arytenoid chondropathy (see Fig. 43-6), the anatomic integrity of these structures should be assessed as well as the position of the soft palate.

As soon as the diagnosis is made, the horse should be removed from the pasture and anti-inflammatory therapy initiated.[18] Horses housed in a dry lot or box stall do not seem to be affected by this disease. If the cicatrix causes nasopharyngeal obstruction, it can be transected in two or three places under videoendoscopic guidance with the horse standing, using a diode or other appropriate laser. Although nasopharyngeal stenting has been reported, its use does not seem to have significant value.[18,19] If airway obstruction is associated with chondritis, a permanent tracheostomy (as described in Chapter 46) should be performed. Partial arytenoidectomy in this heavily scarred environment leads to an inappropriate diameter of the rima glottidis during postoperative healing and, therefore, should not be performed.

Nasopharyngeal Masses

Nasopharyngeal masses occur rarely in horses. When masses are present in the nasopharynx, they usually are extensions of paranasal sinus, guttural pouch, or oropharyngeal diseases. However, primary masses involving the nasopharynx can include benign lesions such as fungal granulomas and cysts and neoplastic lesions such as lymphosarcoma and squamous cell carcinoma.[20-22] Depending on the size and location of these masses, they may result in DDSP, dysphagia, or airflow obstruction. Therefore, clinical signs may include exercise intolerance, respiratory noise, nasal drainage, and weight loss. If the mass extends into the rostral nasopharynx or nasal cavity, uneven airflow can be detected at the nostril, and mucopurulent drainage may be present.

The diagnosis of nasopharyngeal masses is made by endoscopic examination on recognition of these clinical signs (Fig. 43-8). A thorough evaluation of adjacent structures (nasal cavity, paranasal sinuses, and guttural pouches) is imperative. Radiography and/or general anesthesia followed by oral manual or oral endoscopic examination may help identify masses extending into the oropharynx. A biopsy sample of the mass can be taken by sedating the horse and using uterine biopsy forceps (Richard Wolf Medical Instruments Corporation, Vernon Hills, Ill). Two or three samples can be taken with a small amount of local hemorrhage. A biopsy of the mass yields the critical information necessary for appropriately managing and treating the lesion.

Treatment is based on the extent of the lesion and the biopsy results. Surgical access to the nasopharynx is limited, and three main options are available: videoendoscopy-assisted laser resection, intralesional injection of a necrosing pharmacologic agent (10% formaldehyde), and surgical attention through an oral approach or pharyngotomy. The author prefers the oral approach.

Videoendoscopy-Assisted Laser Resection

Videoendoscopic-assisted laser resection is performed as follows. The average 450-kg horse is sedated with a solution of detomidine (6 mg) and butorphanol (4 mg). One should err toward a smaller dosage of butorphanol, because some horses experience "head tics" that interfere with the surgical procedure using this medication. The videoendoscope is passed into the right nostril, and the mass is desensitized by applying 50 mL of a topical anesthetic solution (2% lidocaine or mepivacaine hydrochloride) and 10 mL of vasoconstrictive agent (0.15% phenylephrine) through the

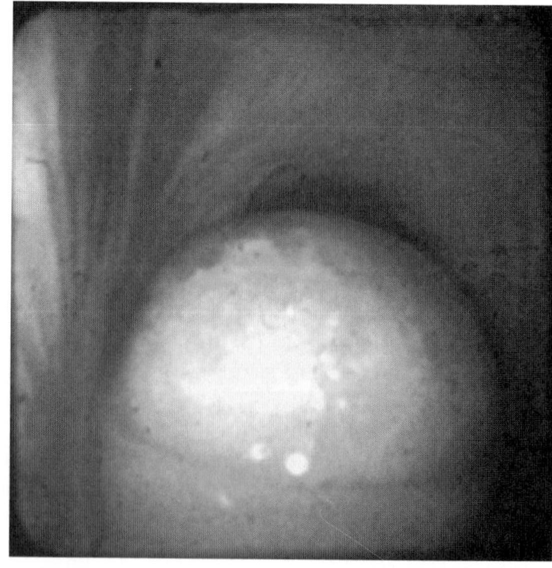

Figure 43-8. Endoscopic view of a pharyngeal mass in a 20-year-old horse. The mass originated at the root of the tongue. (Courtesy J. Stick, Michigan State University.)

biopsy channel of the videoendoscope. The videoendoscope is withdrawn to the nasal cavity near the dorsal meatus, and local anesthetic is applied to desensitize this area and thus facilitate forceps manipulation. The videoendoscope is passed through the left nostril, and the bronchoesophagoscopic forceps are passed into the right nostril to grasp or otherwise facilitate access to the base of the mass. Using a diode (12 to 15 watts) or neodymium:yttrium aluminum garnet (Nd:YAG, 30 to 35 watts) laser, the base of the mass is incised with the laser. A large mass that cannot be removed nasally should be removed in smaller sections. Some masses must be reduced by intralesional injection prior to laser resection.

Intralesional Injection

Treatments by intralesional injection to induce chemical necrosis of the mass, or local treatment with antimicrobials or antifungal agents, can be used if mass resection is not possible. A polyethylene catheter is passed through the endoscope biopsy channel until it emerges from the biopsy port of the endoscope. A 16-gauge needle is attached to the tubing by removing the needle hub and securing the needle 5 to 7 mm into the tubing. The needle should fit tightly so that it will not dislodge during the injection. The horse is sedated before the injection as described earlier for the laser procedure. Fungal granulomas, such as seen in coccidioidomycosis, are treated with weekly intralesional injections of amphotericin B (100 mg of a 100 mg/mL preparation) combined with 3 mL of a 90% solution of medical-grade dimethyl sulfoxide (DMSO). In addition, potassium iodide (125 mL of a 20% sodium iodide solution IV, once a day for 3 days, followed by 30 g PO once a day for 30 days) is given after clinical remission or until signs of iodine toxicity (dry skin) are noted (see Merck Manual).[11] Most masses, other than abscesses and polyps, are treated with repeated intralesional injection of 10% formaldehyde (10 to 20 mL). The masses are reinjected at 3- to 4-week intervals until resolution, or until the size has been reduced. After each treatment, the horse receives a 3- to 5-day course of phenylbutazone (1 mg/lb PO twice a day) or a similar nonsteroidal anti-inflammatory drug (NSAID).

Occasionally, pedunculated cysts or polyps originate near the guttural pouch opening, obstructing the nasopharynx. These masses can be extracted with the horse under general anesthesia using laparoscopic instruments and videoendoscopic guidance.

SURGICAL APPROACHES TO THE NASOPHARYNX OR OROPHARYNX

The nasopharynx is best approached through nasal videoendoscopy, although limited exposure can be obtained by a pharyngotomy with rostral retraction of the caudal free edge of the soft palate. The oropharynx also can be approached orally (see "Tension Palatoplasty" and "Thermal Palatoplasty," later), orally after a mandibular symphysiotomy (see "Surgical Approaches" under "Cleft Palate," later), and through a laryngotomy via incision of the cricothyroid ligament (see "Staphylectomy," later).

Approaches to the oropharynx are performed with the horse under general anesthesia, and the surgical procedures are best performed using long instruments. The pharyngotomy allows access to the caudal third of the soft palate for cleft repair or removal of associated cysts or masses. Likewise, a pharyngotomy provides access to remove a subepiglottic mass or cyst, but a laryngotomy approach has less morbidity, making it preferable. The major disadvantages of the pharyngotomy approach are its limited exposure and the possibility of damaging the hyoepiglotticus muscle (see Fig. 43-1) or its innervation. This can result in significant disability, as epiglottic retroversion during exercise is the consequence of neuromuscular damage to the hyoepiglotticus muscle (see Chapter 44). Therefore, the pharyngotomy approach should be reserved for conditions that cannot be approached through the oral route or a laryngotomy.

With the horse under general anesthesia and in dorsal recumbency, the ventral aspect of the basihyoid bone and thyroid cartilage is palpated on the ventral midline (Fig. 43-9). The skin incision is extended from the rostral aspect of the thyroid cartilage forward toward the basihyoid bone. The *sternohyoideus* muscles are separated bluntly on the ventral midline, and the incision is extended to the loose fascia between the thyroid cartilage and the basihyoid bone (Fig. 43-10). The *hyoepiglotticus* muscle is enclosed in elastic fascia (hyoepiglotticus ligament) deep to the loose fascia. The *hyoepiglotticus* muscle within its fascia is retracted to one side of the incision (Fig. 43-11), and the incision is extended through multiple layers of loose fascia until the oropharyngeal mucosa is reached. The latter is picked up with a rat's tooth forceps and opened with curved scissors. Further exposure is obtained by splitting the basihyoid longitudinally

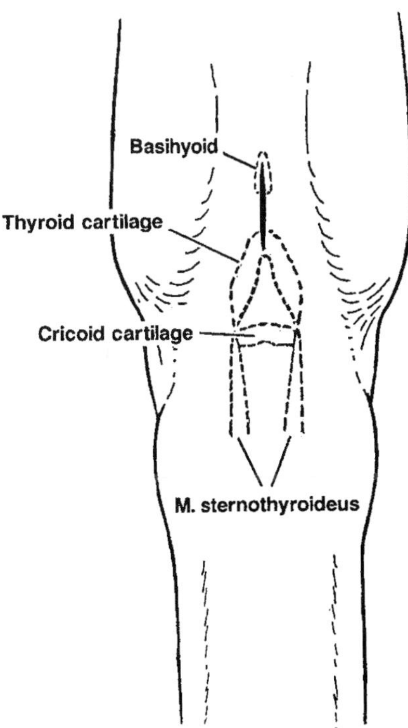

Figure 43-9. Pharyngotomy. Schematic shows the view of the ventral cervical area of a horse in dorsal recumbency and illustrates the landmarks for a pharyngotomy. The *bold line* represents the line of incision extending from the basihyoid to the thyroid cartilage. The incision extends rostrally to the rostral aspect of the basihyoid.

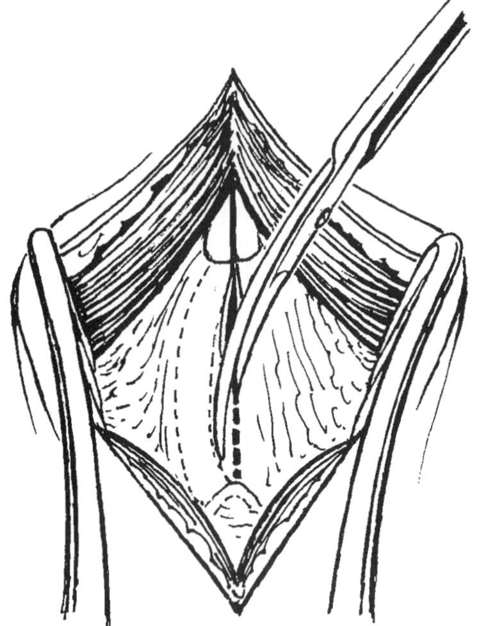

Figure 43-10. Pharyngotomy. The sternohyoideus muscles have been bluntly separated, allowing exposure to the underlying fascia. The basihyoid has been split longitudinally with an osteotome (an optional step), and the superficial fascia is being incised with curved Mayo scissors exposing the underlying hyoepiglotticus muscle.

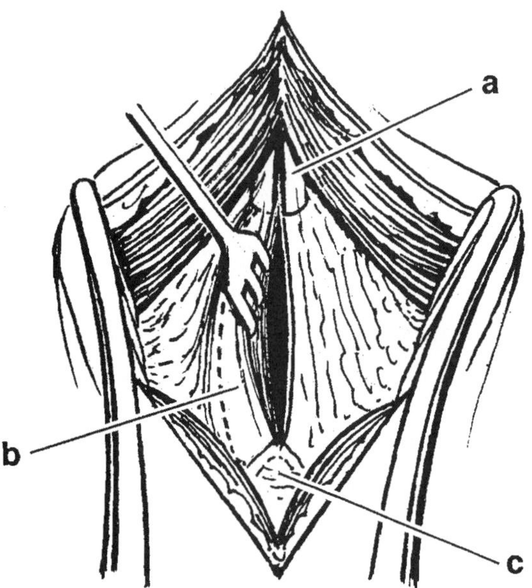

Figure 43-11. Pharyngotomy. The hyoepiglotticus muscle within the hyoepiglotticus ligament is being retracted to one side prior to extending the incision into the oropharynx. a, basihyoid, split longitudinally; b, hyoepiglotticus muscle; c, thyroid cartilage.

with an osteotome. Malleable or Langenbeck retractors are needed to retract each side of the incision laterally and the root of the tongue rostrally.

The incision is closed using no. 0 polyglactin 910 or no. 0 poliglecaprone (Monocryl, Ethicon, Johnson and Johnson) in a simple-interrupted-continuous pattern on the oropharyngeal mucosa. A few simple-interrupted sutures are used to reappose the loose areolar tissue ventral to the oropharyngeal mucosa. The basihyoid (if it was split) is reapposed using a simple size 2 steel suture. The *sternohyoideus* muscle is reapposed using a no. 0 polyglactin 910 or no. 0 Monocryl in a simple-continuous pattern. The subcutaneous tissue and skin are closed only over the split basihyoid bone. Complete closure is not recommended because of the clean-contaminated nature of the incision.

FUNCTIONAL DISORDERS OF THE NASOPHARYNX

Rostral Pharyngeal Collapse

Rostral pharyngeal collapse (i.e., fluttering of the rostral aspect of the soft palate) has been observed during treadmill videoendoscopy and was once thought to be a precursor to DDSP. This condition has been reproduced experimentally by bilateral transection of the tendon of the tensor veli palatini muscle.[9] In this experimental model, rostral instability of the soft palate caused inspiratory obstruction, but DDSP did not occur. The rostral aspect of the soft palate billows dorsally during inspiration, since it is unable to resist nasopharyngeal pressures (Fig. 43-12). It is displaced ventrally during exhalation, so it interferes only with ventilation during inhalation.

Horses with rostral pharyngeal collapse are presented with a history of upper respiratory noise caused by billowing of the rostral soft palate. The diagnosis can be obtained only by videoendoscopic examination of nasopharyngeal function while the horse is exercising on a treadmill. The clinical significance of this condition as it relates to athletic performance is unknown, but it is unlikely to be performance limiting because of the minor obstruction observed. However, rostral soft palate instability may be associated with DDSP; therefore, evaluating the horse for DDSP is required. If billowing of the rostral aspect of the soft palate

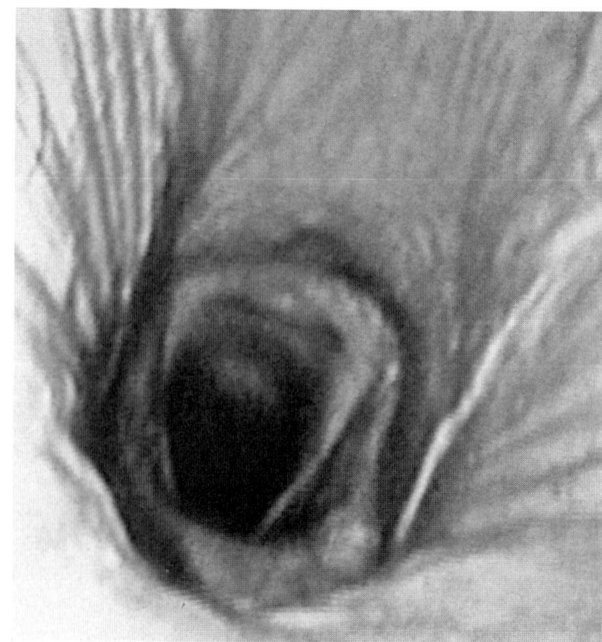

Figure 43-12. Endoscopic photograph of the collapse of the rostral portion of the soft palate in a horse exercising on a treadmill.

is detected, the horse should also be evaluated for any evidence of neuromuscular disorders, such as equine protozoal myelopathy, white muscle disease, or inherited hyperkalemic periodic paralytic episode (HYPP) in Quarter Horses.

If significant nasopharyngeal inflammation is present, the use of local and systemic anti-inflammatory agents is indicated. The author administers 20 mL of a throat spray twice a day (composed of 250 mL of glycerin, 250 mL of 90% DMSO, 500 mL of nitrofurazone, and 50 mL of prednisolone 25 mg/mL) and a course of dexamethasone (30 mg IV or PO once a day for 3 days, followed by 20 mg IV or PO once a day for 3 days, then 10 mg IV or PO once a day for 3 days, and finally 10 mg IV or PO every other day for three treatments). In addition, the author empirically recommends a dropped or figure-eight nose band to maintain airflow into the oropharynx.

There is no proven surgical treatment, but decreasing the compliance of the rostral aspect of the soft palate is logical.[23-25] The author has used *laser thermoplasty,* a diode laser (12 watts) with a contact fiber of 600 μm and pulse duration of 3 seconds (Fig. 43-13) to topically laser the soft palate. In addition, it seems rational to consider two other treatments, tension and thermal palatoplasty, which were designed to decrease compliance of the rostral soft palate because their authors hypothesized that this condition was a precursor to DDSP. These two treatments are both performed through an oral approach.

Thermal Palatoplasty

The horse is placed under general anesthesia using an intravenous agent, and a mouth gag is placed. The tongue is pulled rostrally and the head elevated to facilitate an oral view of the proximal aspect of the ventral soft palate (appropriate lighting is required).[24] A metal instrument is used to protect the tongue during the procedure. Custom-built "irons" made of two 1-cm-diameter, 50-cm-long steel rods, with a 4- to 6-cm length welded on one end to form a T shape. Using a heated T-shaped metal instrument, the ventral surface of the soft palate (oropharynx) is cauterized, from the hard palate extending caudally to beyond the palatoglossal arch (Fig. 43-14, *A* and *B*). Cauterization obliterates the two parasagittal longitudinal folds of the soft palate (see Fig. 43-14, *B*), and this results in a permanent scar (see Fig. 43-14, *C*), which is thought to decrease the compliance of the soft palate.

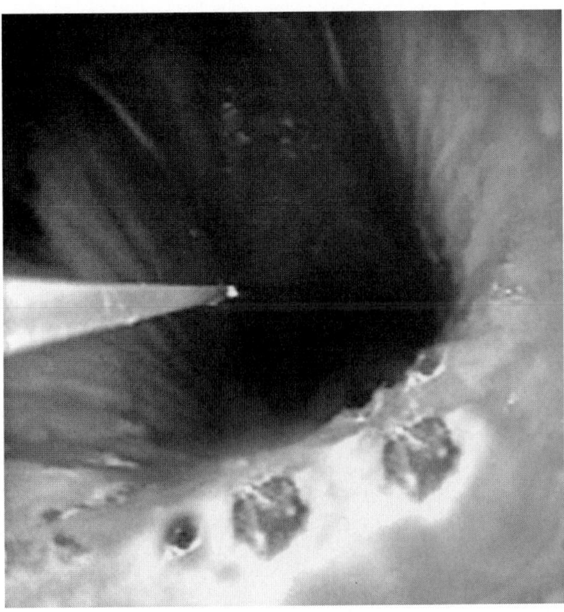

Figure 43-13. The rostral aspect of the soft palate after being treated with a laser to induce local fibrosis. This 3-year-old Standardbred filly had rostral nasopharyngeal collapse during exercise.

A

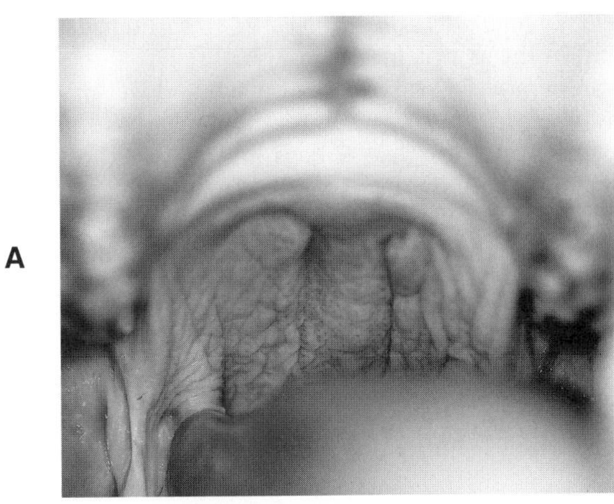

B

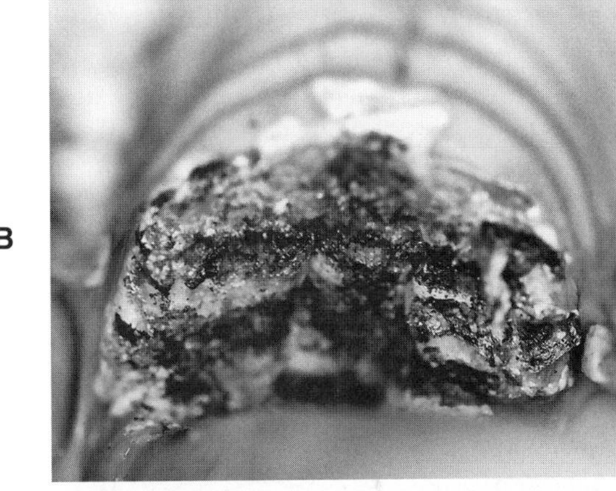

C

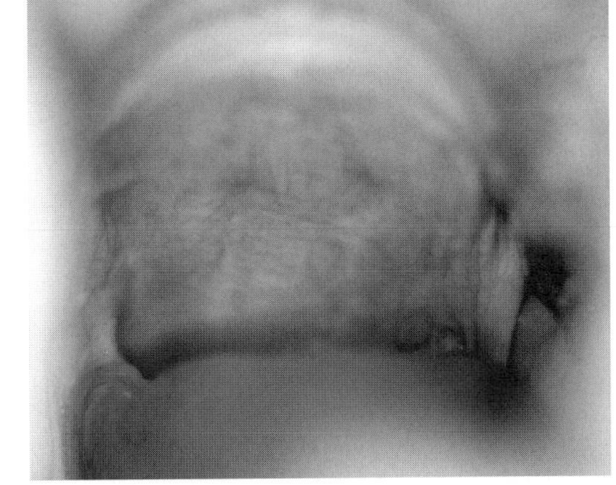

Figure 43-14. Thermal rostral palatoplasty. **A,** Rostral aspect of the soft palate viewed through the oropharynx immediately before surgery. Note parasagittal longitudinal folds on the oropharyngeal mucosa of the rostral aspect of the soft palate. **B,** Appearance of the soft palate immediately after cauterizing. **C,** Appearance of the soft palate 3 months after treatment. (Courtesy R. Ordidge, Rainbow Equine Clinic, UK.)

Tension Palatoplasty

After general anesthesia induction and placement of a mouth gag, an elliptical incision is made through the oral mucosa, starting immediately caudal to the caudal edge of the hard palate. An elliptical section of approximately two thirds of the rostral soft palate mucosa and submucosa is excised (9 to 12 cm long by 1 to 2 cm wide) using long-handled forceps and curved Metzenbaum scissors[25] (Fig. 43-15). The mucosal and submucosal edges are reapposed using 0 Vicryl or Monocryl in a simple-interrupted pattern. The procedure can be repeated in 4 weeks (a procedure termed *maximum tension palatoplasty*) to further increase the tension in the soft palate.

Postoperatively, horses are fed mash and wet hay for 3 to 7 days before returning to work. They are administered phenylbutazone for 3 to 5 days and a trimethoprim and sulfonamide combination for 5 to 7 days. Walking exercise is resumed after 2 days (walking and trotting only), and training can resume in 4 weeks. The degree of postoperative pain is reportedly minimal after thermal palatoplasty (2 to 3 days) compared with tension palatoplasty (up to 7 days in some cases).

Prognosis is related to the degree of collapse. A guarded prognosis should be given, since the current knowledge of this condition is limited.

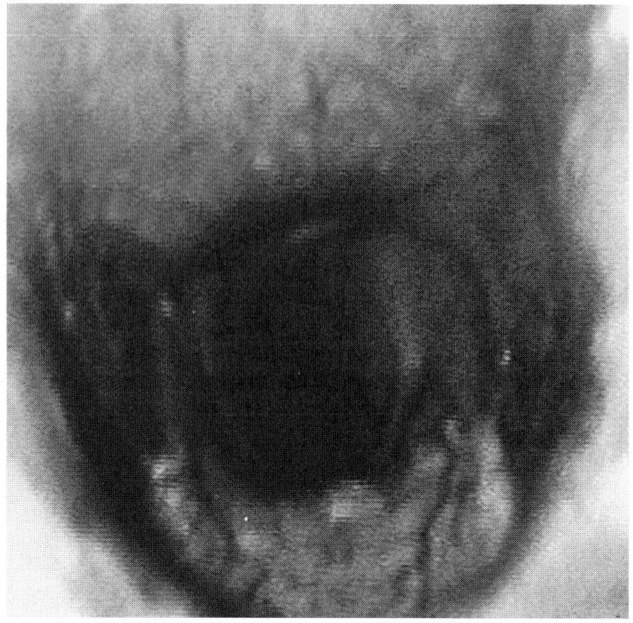

Figure 43-16. Video endoscopic image of the nasopharynx of an exercising horse, demonstrating partial collapse of the dorsal pharyngeal wall. The corniculate processes of the arytenoid cartilages are obstructed from view by the ventral displacement of the roof of the nasopharynx.

Dorsal/Lateral Nasopharyngeal Collapse

Some horses with exercise intolerance and upper respiratory noise are observed to have (1) unilateral or bilateral ventral displacement of the roof of the nasopharynx (Fig. 43-16) or (2) axial displacement of the lateral walls of the nasopharynx, or both[26,27] (Fig. 43-17). A certain degree of collapse is normal in horses during exercise. For instance, the roof of the nasopharynx does normally displace ventrally at the end of expiration during exercise.[28] At rest, the pressure in the guttural pouches, which form the roof of the nasopharynx, is in phase with nasopharyngeal pressure, and the pressure

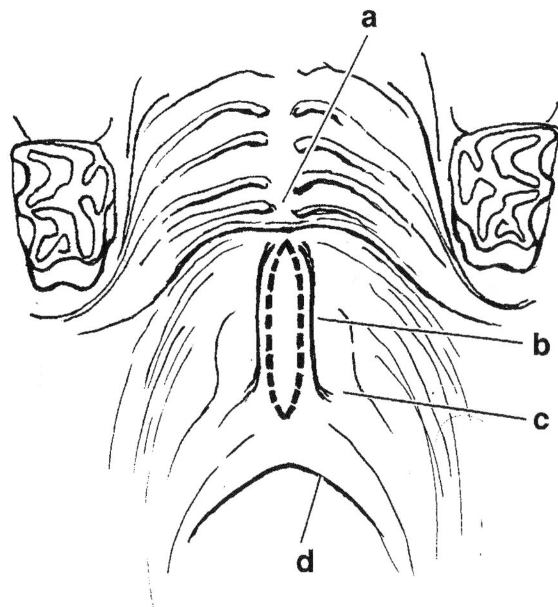

Figure 43-15. Tension rostral palatoplasty. Schematic drawing shows the location of the elliptical incision *(dotted line)* on the ventral and rostral aspect of the soft palate as viewed though the oropharynx. This incision leads to resection of the oropharyngeal mucosa and glandular portion of the soft palate in that specific location. a, Hard palate; b, isthmus faucium; c, sagittal fold; d, caudal border of the soft palate.

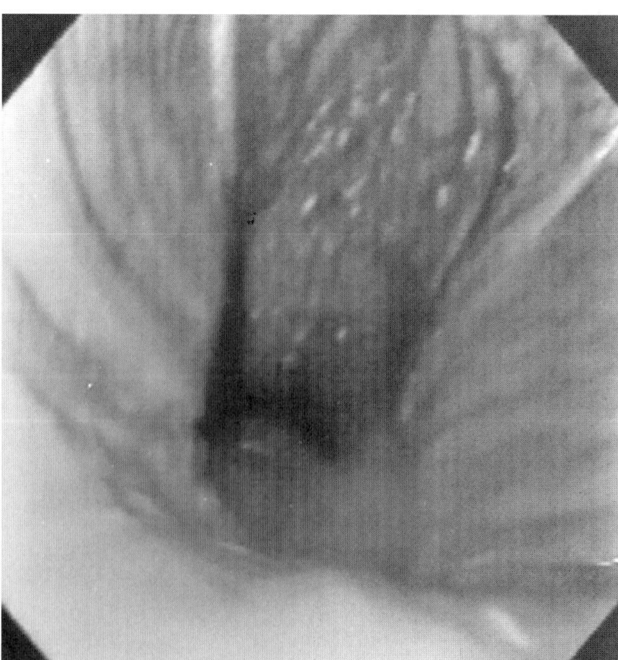

Figure 43-17. Endoscopic photograph of axial collapse of the lateral walls of the nasopharynx during treadmill exercise. Note the lateromedial reduction of the nasopharynx.

in the guttural pouches is subatmospheric when no airflow is present at rest.[28] During exercise, guttural pouch pressure does not stay in phase with nasopharyngeal pressure. Nasopharyngeal peak expiratory pressure is reached earlier than in the guttural pouch during the expiratory cycle, so peak expiratory pressure in the guttural pouch lags behind pressure changes in the nasopharynx.[13] Therefore, the roof of the nasopharynx normally collapses at the end of expiration, but this should not extend beyond the ventral surface of the fully abducted arytenoid cartilages. It is known from experimental studies[7] that dysfunction of the *stylopharyngeus caudalis* muscle (see Fig. 43-4) results in collapse of the roof of the nasopharynx. Presumably, intraluminal collapse of the lateral walls of the nasopharynx occurs because of dysfunction of the *palatopharyngeus* muscles. Dysfunction of these muscles may be associated with severe inflammation or neuritis of the pharyngeal branch of the vagal or glossopharyngeal nerve. Alternatively, dorsal and lateral nasopharyngeal collapse may be the result of a sensory dysfunction that prevents appropriate reflex contraction of the intrinsic musculature of the nasopharynx. Guttural pouch distention leads to ipsilateral nasopharyngeal roof collapse. Other systemic diseases, like an HYPP episode, botulism, or equine protozoal myelitis, could be the cause. Finally, nasal obstruction may lead to more negative inhaling airway pressure, overwhelming the muscular activity of the intrinsic nasopharyngeal musculature.

In the clinical disease, collapse of the nasopharynx occurs during inhalation, causing a greater reduction in the diameter of the lumen of the nasopharynx than in the cross-sectional diameter of the rima glottidis. In the author's experience, this condition is most commonly seen in 2- and 3-year-old racehorses. Clinical signs of dynamic dorsal pharyngeal collapse include inspiratory upper respiratory noise and exercise intolerance.[26,27] Diagnosis can be made by endoscopic examination during nasal occlusion (without sedation) or, more accurately, during treadmill exercise. The guttural pouches and both nasal cavities should also be examined, looking for the primary cause of this disease.

Treatment should be directed toward resolution of the primary condition (e.g., guttural pouch disease, nasal obstruction, systemic disease). In young horses, an anti-inflammatory protocol (as described under "Rostral Pharyngeal Collapse," earlier) should be considered. Affected 2-year-old horses can be allowed to mature until their 3-year season. Some experimental treatments are under investigation, but there is no stabilizing treatment available yet.

Dorsal Displacement of the Soft Palate

Intermittent DDSP is a performance-limiting upper airway condition in horses that was identified in 1.3% of a population of 479 horses examined endoscopically at rest.[29] However, the prevalence of this condition is probably higher, because palate displacement is a dynamic condition that occurs most frequently during intense exercise, making diagnosis at rest difficult. The prevalence of this condition is probably closer to 10% to 20% of 2- to 3-year-old racehorses.

The horse is an obligate nasal breather, perhaps to allow the olfactory senses to function during deglutition. The normal epiglottis is positioned dorsal to the soft palate and contacts the caudal free margin, forming a tight seal around the base of the soft palate. The pillars of the soft palate converge dorsally, forming the palatopharyngeal arch. When the soft palate displaces dorsally, the epiglottis cannot be seen in the nasopharynx and is positioned in the oropharynx (Fig. 43-18). The caudal free margin of the soft palate billows across the rima glottidis during exhalation, creating airway obstruction (see Fig. 43-18). Upper airway pressure measurements made in horses clinically affected with DDSP during treadmill exercise indicate that DDSP is an expiratory obstruction.[30] This observation was confirmed by measuring upper airway mechanics in horses in which DDSP was induced by bilaterally blocking the pharyngeal branch of the vagus nerve. Tracheal expiratory pressure and impedance were increased, minute ventilation was reduced, and horses were more hypoxic and hypercarbic than controls.[31]

DDSP was first reported in 1949,[32] and since then the understanding of the pathophysiology of this disease has increased. DDSP usually interferes only with ventilation during exercise, producing upper respiratory noise. In some cases, there is a digestive disturbance that leads to feed, water, and saliva contamination, predominately of the upper airways. It is important to identify this digestive disturbance for the following reasons. Horses with DDSP are usually presented with a respiratory deficit only, which occurs during intense exercise. This presentation carries a reasonable prognosis, and treatment varies depending on the specific cause. However, DDSP with digestive deficit generally indicates a more advanced deficit of the *palatinus* muscle (or its innervation) or an anatomic deficit (such as cleft palate or an acquired deficit of the caudal free edge of the soft palate—i.e., staphylectomy or loss of epiglottic cartilage secondary to septic epiglottis or surgical resection) that allows feed contamination of the nasopharynx from the oropharynx. In addition, marked tracheal aspiration of feed material into the trachea (generally from laryngeal disease or its treatment) can lead to DDSP (although the pathophysiology of this association is not clear). Equine clinicians should

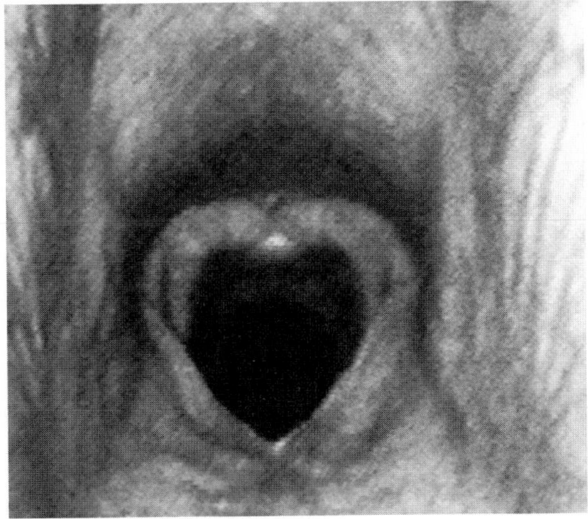

Figure 43-18. Videoendoscopic of the rima glottidis of a horse experiencing dorsal displacement of the soft palate during exercise. The palate collapses into the rima glottidis during inhalation but billows dorsally as air escapes into the oral pharynx during exhalation.

carefully attempt to identify the cause if feed contamination of the upper airway is seen in association with DDSP, and they should be aware that routine treatment of intermittent DDSP may not be successful and could even worsen the condition.

Clinical Study–Based Hypotheses of the Etiology of DDSP

A series of mainly mechanical factors have been implicated in the etiopathogenesis of DDSP, and all are supported only by clinical association and not by experimental investigations. The condition was initially attributed to a paretic or an overly long soft palate.[32] No data support the overly long soft palate hypothesis except perhaps in rare cases in foals.[33] Cysts on the caudal free edge of the soft palate have been observed to interfere with the normal subepiglottic position of the soft palate. This seems to be a mechanical effect, since removing the cyst results in immediate postoperative correction of the DDSP. Other lesions that mechanically interfere with the junction of the caudal free edge of the soft palate and subepiglottic tissue are also believed to result in DDSP. They include subepiglottic or palatal granuloma (Fig. 43-19), masses, and cysts (see Fig. 44-25). The current understanding is that these masses predispose to DDSP, either by mechanically interfering with the seal between the caudal free edge of the soft palate and subepiglottic tissue or by causing irritation or pain that stimulates DDSP.

Epiglottic hypoplasia or deformation has been implicated as a cause of DDSP in horses.[34,35] It was thought that inadequate length or rigidity of an epiglottis might make it unable to "hold" the soft palate in a subepiglottic position.[34,35] Equine practitioners have noted that some horses affected with intermittent DDSP have what appears to be a hypoplastic or flaccid epiglottis. The author has noted that horses experience DDSP at exercise after a progression of morphologic changes prior to DDSP (as observed endoscopically during high-speed exercise). First, caudal retraction of the larynx leads to an increase in "apparent flaccidity" of the epiglottic cartilage and billowing of the soft palate, followed by DDSP. A swallow seems to reset the larynx and the subepiglottic position of the soft palate to the correct rostral position. This progression of events is repeated a few times before persistent DDSP is seen.

Therefore, a flaccid epiglottis is probably a result rather than a cause of the DDSP seen when checking the larynx position or tone of intrinsic/extrinsic musculature. Indeed, the role or importance of an abnormal epiglottis as the initiating factor in DDSP is questionable, because DDSP does not occur despite the fact that epiglottic cartilage is not present to "hold the palate down" when epiglottic retroversion is experimentally induced.[36] Also, there was no statistical correlation between the epiglottic appearance of horses that exhibited DDSP during treadmill examination and those that did not displace their soft palate, suggesting that epiglottic appearance may not directly correlate with the occurrence of DDSP.[30] Therefore, the author no longer believes that epiglottic augmentation[35] should be used routinely to treat horses with intermittent DDSP, but a description of the technique can be found in Chapter 44 for the sake of completeness.

Other factors implicated in the pathogenesis of DDSP include caudal retraction of the tongue, caudal retraction of the larynx because of excitement, and opening of the mouth.[37] If the tongue is retracted, the base of the tongue may "push" the soft palate dorsally, inducing DDSP. In this instance, a tongue-tie pulls the tongue out of the mouth and prevents this occurrence. As mentioned earlier, recent experimental investigations failed to identify a morphologic or physiologic effect from a tongue-tie.[12,13,38] One report showed that DDSP was reversed in two out of six horses by using a tongue-tie.[39] The presence of excessive muscle contractions leading to caudal retraction of the larynx because of a horse's excitement or nervousness during racing or

A 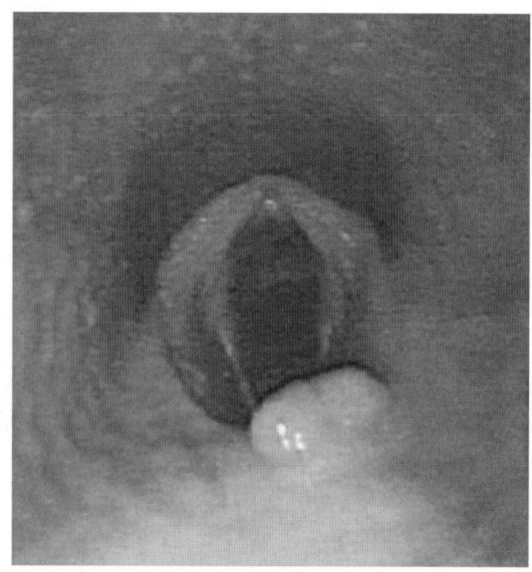

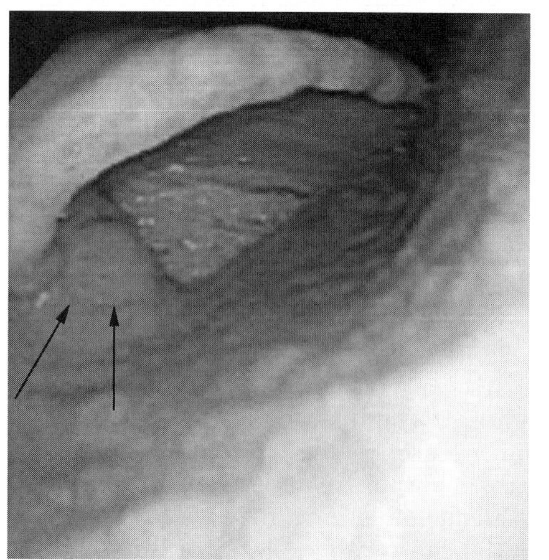 B

Figure 43-19. A, Palatal granuloma in a 2-year-old Thoroughbred with dorsal displacement of the soft palate. **B,** Appearance of the granuloma dorsal to the palate and ventral to the epiglottic cartilage *(arrows)* with the soft palate replaced.

performance has been proposed as another cause of DDSP.[37] This has led to sedation or to surgical transection of the strap muscles to prevent the larynx from retracting.

The clinical association of opening the mouth or swallowing during exercise and the induction of DDSP has led to the following hypothesis. Opening the mouth lets air enter the oropharynx, disturbing the stabilizing effect of the subatmospheric pressure on the ventral surface of the soft palate.[1] This has led to the use of a dropped or figure-eight nose band to prevent DDSP during exercise. There is no experimental data investigating this hypothesis.

Experimental Study–Based Hypotheses of the Etiology of DDSP

Many studies described at the beginning of this chapter have led to the identification of intrinsic and extrinsic factors responsible for the stability of the nasopharynx at exercise. Events that interfere with the neuromuscular control of the nasopharynx, such as a deficit of the pharyngeal branch of the vagus nerve or palatinus or thyrohyoideus muscle function, can lead to DDSP. Deficits of the palatinus muscle function also lead to feed and water contamination of the upper airway.[6]

History and Clinical Signs

Racehorses with intermittent DDSP generally have a history of exercise intolerance and may make a gurgling or vibrating noise during exhalation.[37] These horses may be described as "choking down" or "swallowing their tongue." Concurrent with these signs is open-mouth breathing. Other horses used for show or pleasure riding may exhibit only the respiratory noise described earlier.

Diagnosis

The diagnosis of intermittent DDSP is based on a history of poor performance associated with respiratory noise, observation of the horse competing or racing, physical examination, and endoscopic examination of the upper airway at rest, preferably immediately after strenuous exercise or while the horse is exercising on a treadmill. A complete physical examination is important to rule out other causes of exercise intolerance, such as pulmonary disease, cardiac abnormalities, lameness, and neurologic disease.

Treatment

Neuromuscular pathology has been suggested as a possible etiology of DDSP.[6] Dorsal displacement of the soft palate was historically referred to as soft palate paresis.[32] Recently, persistent DDSP was created by bilaterally blocking the pharyngeal branch of the vagus nerve as it coursed through the guttural pouch.[6] Therefore, dysfunction of the pharyngeal branch of the vagus nerve associated with inflammatory disease in the guttural pouch can interfere with palatinus and palatopharyngeus muscle tone, leading to DDSP. Lending credence to this theory, horses with intermittent DDSP have an elevated prevalence of upper respiratory inflammatory diseases such as pharyngitis that may affect the function of the pharyngeal branch of the vagus nerve.[6,40]

Treatment is initially directed at modifying or eliminating factors associated with DDSP occurrence. Unfit horses should be conditioned and reevaluated before surgical intervention is considered. Tack changes may be suggested to alter the horse's head position, and a figure-eight noseband used to keep the horse from opening its mouth. The bit may be changed, and a bit that secures the tongue (such as a W bit, a spoon bit, or a "Serena song" bit) may be used. These bits are designed to restrict caudal movement of the tongue and are generally used in addition to a tongue-tie.

Tongue-tie use has been popular for many years. Initially the hypothesis was that it prevented "swallowing of the tongue" or, perhaps more medically accurate, prevented the root of the tongue from applying dorsal pressure on the ventral surface of the soft palate.[37] As mentioned earlier, four recent papers looked at the efficacy of the tongue-tie.[12,13,38] In one study, two out of six horses were improved with a tongue-tie, as evidenced by treadmill videoendoscopy.[39] The author has observed two horses exercising on a high-speed treadmill that were normal without a tongue-tie and displaced their palate only when the tongue was tied. The three other papers failed to detect a mechanical effect (a change of nasopharyngeal diameter or upper airway patency) when the tongue-tie was used.[12,13,38] A "bit-less" bridle (see www.bitlessbridle.com) was recommended as a treatment of this condition, on the basis of the belief that a bit in the mouth caused DDSP. More recently, a throat-support device that positions the larynx and basihyoid more rostrally during exercise has been shown to prevent DDSP at exercise in experimentally created DDSP[41] and shows promise as a management tool in clinically affected horses (Throat Support Device,* Vet-Aire, Inc, Ithaca, New York; see www.Vet-Aire.com).

The data are insufficient to draw clear conclusions on these training aids. Using the tongue-tie, removing the tongue-tie, trying different bits, and using a figure-eight nose-band are all valid changes when the diagnosis is first made. If upper respiratory tract inflammation was diagnosed during the examination, treatment should include judicious use of systemic anti-inflammatory medication and topical anti-inflammatory agents such as glycerin, DMSO, and nitrofurazone. Medical treatment should be continued for 30 days, and subsequently the horse should be re-evaluated before training is resumed or surgical intervention is considered. A recent study reported a 60% success rate when these medical treatments were used alone,[42] a figure similar to the outcome seen after many surgeries!

SURGICAL OPTIONS

If medical treatment and tack management fail to correct soft palate displacement at exercise, many surgical options are available. The following is a description of the more commonly used techniques. Tension[25] and thermal palato-

*Conflict-of-interest disclosure: The author and Cornell University both benefit through patent royalties and have equity interest with the company marketing the product.

plasty,[24] described previously, are recommended by some surgeons to treat soft palate displacement as well.

Of all these procedures, which should be used? No double-blind controlled studies have been performed, and experienced surgeons (e.g., H. Lewellyn, P. Hogan, T. Ahern, R. Oldridge, J. Robertson, J. Stick, G. Lane, E. Parente) often disagree on the procedure of choice for treating DDSP. The author believes that morphologic or anatomic abnormalities involving the nasopharynx or subepiglottic and epiglottic cartilage (such as bacterial or viral epiglottitis, cyst, granuloma, aryepiglottic entrapment) should be addressed medically or surgically through a nasal, oral, or laryngotomy approach. Otherwise, the best treatment is a laryngeal tie-forward combined with a partial resection of the thyrohyoideus muscle or tendon.

STAPHYLECTOMY

Staphylectomy, or partial soft palate resection, originally was described as a treatment for an excessively long soft palate.[32] This condition does not exist except perhaps in neonatal foals,[25] so staphylectomy should be discontinued as a routine treatment of DDSP. When more than 0.75 cm of the soft palate is removed, the seal between the oropharynx and the nasopharynx can be disturbed and allow the passage of feed and fluids (water and saliva) into the nasopharynx. Staphylectomy should be reserved to resect a granuloma or cyst from the caudal free edge of the soft palate.

Preoperatively, the horse can be treated with NSAIDs and broad-spectrum antibiotics. Staphylectomy is performed with the horse under general anesthesia and positioned in dorsal recumbency with the head and neck extended and prepared for a *laryngotomy*[43,44] (Fig. 43-20). A 10- to 12-cm skin incision is made along midline, centered over the cricothyroid space. The sternohyoideus muscles are divided bluntly using a curved Mayo or Metzenbaum scissors. A self-retaining retractor, such as a Weitlaner or a Hobday, is placed between the separated sternohyoideus muscles, exposing the cricothyroid membrane. The cricothyroid membrane is sharply incised (along with the underlying laryngeal mucosa) with a scalpel along the midline, from the cricoid cartilage to the junction of the thyroid cartilages (see Fig. 43-20). A small blood vessel is usually also incised at the level of the caudal two thirds of the membrane. The vessel is ligated or cauterized. The self-retaining retractor is subsequently placed within the cricothyroid space. The caudal free margin of the soft palate rostral to the incision is identified. If the horse was not intubated, the soft palate may not displace, and the caudal edge of the soft palate may have to be freed from beneath the epiglottis using a pair of sponge forceps. If the horse was intubated orally, the palate will be displaced and the endotracheal tube should be retracted at this time. The mass or cyst is identified and resected using a curved Satinsky thoracic scissors. If the palate is being trimmed for DDSP, the mucosa of the caudal free margin of the soft palate is grasped with an Allis tissue forceps on the midline, and a second pair of forceps is used to grasp the mucosa 2 to 2.5 cm lateral to the midline. If desired, the caudal free margin of the soft palate is trimmed between the Allis tissue forceps, beginning laterally and ending on the midline. An Allis tissue forceps is placed on the other side of the soft palate, again approximately 2 to

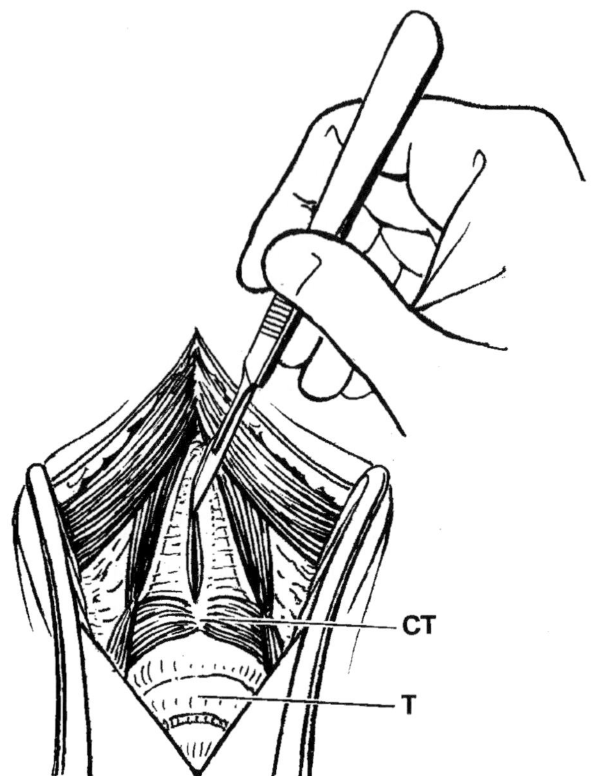

Figure 43-20. Schematic showing view of the ventral cervical area of a horse in dorsal recumbency and illustrating the landmarks for a laryngotomy. The sternohyoideus muscles have been bluntly separated on the ventral midline, and the cricothyroid membrane and underlying laryngeal mucosa is sharply incised from the cricoid rostrally to the thyroid cartilage T, tracheal ring; CT, cricothyroid muscle overlying the ventral aspect of the cricoid cartilage.

2.5 cm from midline, and the caudal margin of the soft palate is trimmed from the lateral forceps toward the midline. A crescent-shaped 4- to 5-cm-long piece of mucosa that is 0.5 cm wide on the midline and tapered toward both ends should be resected.

The laryngotomy incision may be left to heal by second intention, or preferably the cricothyroid membrane is reapposed using no. 0 polyglactin 910 suture material in a simple-continuous pattern. Some surgeons may elect to completely close the laryngotomy incision, but this step increases morbidity unnecessarily. Postoperatively, the horse should wear a muzzle for several hours. Systemic antibiotic therapy is continued for 7 days, and anti-inflammatory medication is continued for 3 days. The laryngotomy incision should be cleaned twice daily until it is healed (approximately 3 weeks). The horse can begin training 2 to 3 weeks later. A success rate of 50% to 60% is reported for treating DDSP after this procedure.

Complications of staphylectomy are uncommon but can occur if too large a section of the soft palate is resected. These horses may be dysphagic, leading to signs of aspiration that include coughing, expulsion of feed material through the nose, and pneumonia. In addition, horses may develop permanent DDSP.

STANDARD MYECTOMY

Standard myectomy (a partial sternohyoideus and sternothyroideus, with or without omohyoideus resection) is performed to reduce caudal retraction of the larynx.[37,43-45] Sections of the sternothyroideus and sternohyoideus muscles are removed with the horse standing as the procedure was first described. If the plan is to also remove a section of omohyoideus muscle, the procedure should be performed under general anesthesia with the horse positioned in dorsal recumbency and the head and neck extended. This is because a more extensive dissection is required when the omohyoideus muscle is resected.

The horse should be treated preoperatively with NSAIDs and broad-spectrum antibiotics. It is restrained in a set of stocks, a stanchion, or a stall doorway. Tranquilization may be necessary or useful. (Alternatively, the horse is anesthetized and placed in dorsal recumbency.) The hair is clipped from the ventral surface of the neck, and the skin is aseptically prepared. Local anesthetic is infiltrated along the midline at the junction of the proximal third and the middle third of the neck.

A 10-cm ventral midline incision is made through the skin, continuing through the cutaneus colli muscles. The paired sternohyoideus muscles are identified. Using curved forceps, the sternohyoideus and sternothyroideus muscles are undermined. The sternothyroideus muscle is positioned caudolateral to the sternohyoideus muscle at this level of the neck. The muscles are elevated through the incision and clamped with a Rochester-Carmalt forceps at the proximal and distal extent of the incision. The muscle bellies are sharply transected between the forceps, and a 6- to 8-cm long section of muscle is removed. The muscle tissue that was removed should be inspected to ensure that sections of both sternohyoid muscles and the smaller sternothyroid muscles were indeed removed. If the omohyoideus muscles are also removed, the dissection (under general anesthesia) must extend laterally up to the ventral border of the left and right jugular veins. More significant dead space is created, so the use of a Penrose drain and application of a postoperative cervical bandage are indicated. The subcutaneous and skin layers are closed routinely. If a Penrose drain is used, it is placed alongside the ventral aspect of the trachea and tunneled through a stab incision distal to the surgical incision. A firm bandage is applied around the neck and may be removed along with the drain 24 hours later.

NSAIDs can be continued for 3 days, and antibiotics should be continued for 5 to 7 days. The horse is kept in a stall with daily hand-walking for 2 weeks. Training can be resumed 2 weeks after surgery, when the sutures are removed. Complications are usually related to the incision and include incisional seromas and infections. No long-term complications are notable except for the cosmetic defect associated with the lack of muscle tissue at the surgical site. Reports indicate a success rate of 58% to 71% for treating DDSP after this procedure.

MINIMALLY INVASIVE MYECTOMY

Minimally invasive myectomy (partial sternothyroidectomy or the Llewellyn procedure) is rapidly performed and has minimal morbidity. Partial sternothyroideus myectomy and tenectomy is performed with the horse under general anesthesia.[46] A 5- to 7-cm ventral midline skin incision is made centered on the cricoid cartilage. The subcutaneous tissue is incised, and the sternohyoideus muscles are divided bluntly using a curved Mayo or Metzenbaum scissors. The blunt dissection is continued dorsal to the sternohyoideus muscle, exposing the caudolateral border of the thyroid cartilage. The tendon of insertion of the sternothyroideus muscle at the thyroid cartilage is identified, undermined, and elevated. The tendon is transected 1 cm caudal to its attachment to avoid the caudal laryngeal artery. Using one index finger, the muscle is freed from the surrounding fascia and transected more proximally, thus removing a 3-cm section of sternothyroideus muscle. This same procedure is performed on the contralateral sternothyroideus tendon. The incision is closed by reapposing the sternohyoideus muscles, and the skin is closed in an acceptable manner.

Postoperatively, NSAIDs are given for 3 to 7 days. Training often is resumed 2 to 3 days postoperatively in Standardbreds and 2 to 3 weeks in Thoroughbreds. The reported success rate for this procedure is 58% to 70%.[44,45]

INDUCTION OF PALATAL FIBROSIS

This procedure is usually performed in combination with the partial sternothyroideus resection.[48] It has been proposed that the compliance of the soft palate can be reduced by induction of fibrosis. This fibrosis was induced in the past by performing a staphylectomy. A laser is used to induce fibrosis on the nasopharyngeal mucosa on the caudal aspect of the soft palate. The stiffening that results is thought to increase the intrinsic strength of the caudal soft palate so that it is able to resist pressure changes during strenuous exercise.

Horses undergoing transendoscopic laser cautery of the soft palate are sedated and restrained in stocks. The endoscope is passed through the nasal passage into the nasopharynx, and a local anesthetic is applied topically. The 600-μm laser fiber is passed through the biopsy channel, and the caudal free margin of the soft palate is lased as follows. The fiber contacts the soft palate for 1 to 2 seconds at 2- to 4-mm intervals along the entire caudal free margin and extending 1.5 cm rostrally (15 watts, 600 to 800 joules) (Fig. 43-21). Routine laser safety precautions must be applied, including protective eyewear appropriate for the laser wave length and laser signs restricting entry into the operating theater to ensure safety of all personnel.

LARYNGEAL TIE-FORWARD

The recently described laryngeal tie-forward is performed with the horse anesthetized and in dorsal recumbency.[49] The ventral cervical and intermandibular areas extending 10 cm rostral to the basihyoid bone are prepared aseptically. A ventral skin incision is made starting 2 cm caudal to the cricoid cartilage and extending 2 cm rostral to the basihyoid bone. The sternohyoideus muscle is separated on the midline and bluntly dissected free of the dorsolateral aspect of the larynx lateral to the thyrohyoideus muscles. Using a 3.2-mm drill bit, a hole is made in the rostral aspect of the basihyoid bone, taking precautions to avoid damage to the vascular structures dorsal to the basihyoid bone (Fig. 43-22). The needle of two nonabsorbable sutures (size 2 or 5 polyblend sutures, Arthrex Inc, Naples, Fla) is placed from

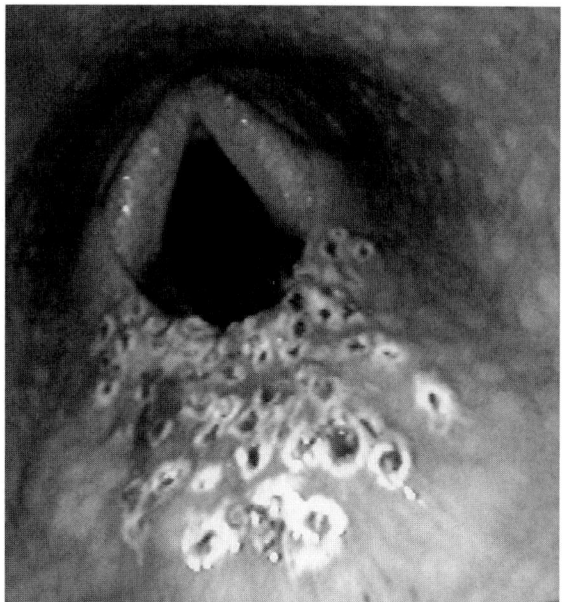

Figure 43-21. Postoperative appearance of the caudal free edge of the soft palate after laser treatment to induce local fibrosis and decrease its compliance. (Courtesy J. Stick, Michigan State University.)

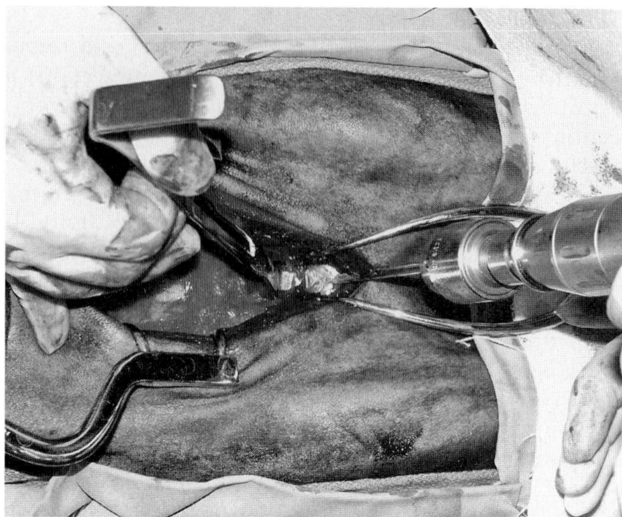

Figure 43-22. Intraoperative view of the laryngeal tie-forward procedure. Surgical view showing a 3.2-mm drill bit making a hole in the rostral aspect of the basihyoid bone. An Army-Navy retractor is placed dorsal to the basihyoid bone to avoid inadvertent damage to adjacent vascular structures.

the ventral to the dorsal aspect of the basihyoid bone. One suture is then passed twice into the right lamina of the thyroid cartilage near the insertion of the tendon of the sternothyroid tendon (Fig. 43-23). The procedure is repeated with the other suture in the left lamina of the thyroid cartilage. A bilateral partial sternothyroidectomy is performed at this time. The sutures are tied so the rostral aspect of the thyroid cartilage is located immediately dorsal and 0.5 to 1 cm rostral to the caudal border of the basihyoid bone (Fig. 43-24). Closure is obtained by reapposing the sternohyoideus muscles with no. 0 poliglecaprone (Monocryl, Ethicon, Johnson and Johnson) in a simple-continuous pattern. To prevent postoperative seromas, the loose fascia overlying the larynx is incorporated into that closure. The subcutaneous tissues and skin are then closed in an acceptable manner. In the first clinical population ($N = 116$) of racehorses where the procedure was performed, an 80% to 82% success rate was obtained after surgery.[49]

NASOPHARYNGEAL DISORDERS OF FOALS

Choanal Atresia

Early in embryonic development, a membrane separates the oral and the nasal cavities.[50] Choanal atresia, a rare upper respiratory malformation in horses,[51-54] is a congenital abnormality associated with failure to resorb this bucco-

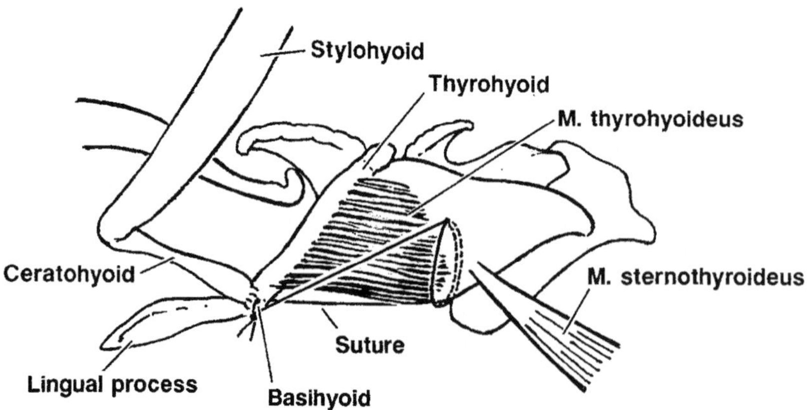

Figure 43-23. Schematic showing the principle of the laryngeal tie-forward procedure. Note that the sutures are placed from the basihyoid into the lateral and caudal aspects of the lamina of the thyroid cartilage. The point where the needle is inserted to place the suture in the thyroid cartilage is immediately ventral to the tendon of the sternothyroid muscle. The suture is passed twice through the thyroid cartilage and tied with a slip knot on the ventral aspect of the basihyoid bone.

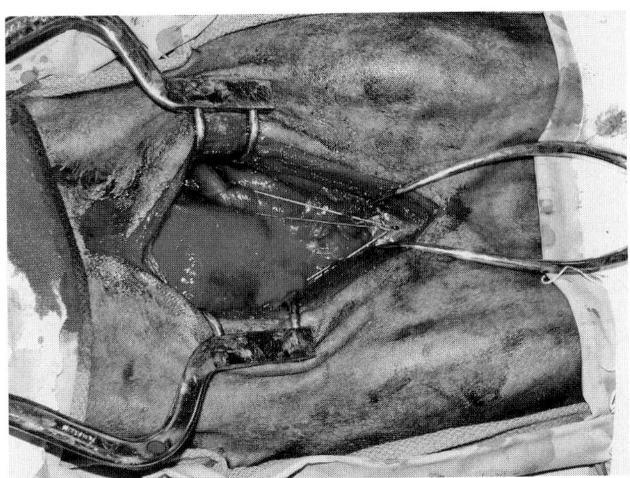

Figure 43-24. Intraoperative view of the laryngeal tie-forward procedure, after the sutures have been tied. The sutures extend from the caudal aspect of the thyroid cartilage to the basihyoid bone.

nasal membrane during embryonic development. Because horses are obligate nasal breathers, bilateral choanal atresia usually results in foal death unless an emergency tracheostomy is performed at birth.[52] When the atresia occurs unilaterally, foals exhibit loud respiratory noise and exercise intolerance, and the nasopharynx can be observed through one nostril, whereas a membrane obstructs the caudal nasal passage of the other nostril. These horses are usually asymptomatic at rest; however, asymmetry of airflow from the nostrils can be detected at rest. The diagnosis is made by endoscopic examination, skull radiography, contrast radiography, and computed tomography.[52-55]

Although the author's experience is very limited, the author believes that foals with unilateral choanal atresia should be allowed to grow untreated until 1 year of age, for three reasons. First, the larger nasal cavity facilitates surgical exposure with less likelihood of postoperative fibrosis, reduced diameter of the choana, or, even worse, complete closure. In addition, the need for a postoperative nasal stent is avoided. Finally, the larger size of the airway allows the procedure to be performed less invasively under videoendoscopic control with the animal standing.

Three treatment approaches have been used to treat this condition. In the first, the yearling is sedated, usually with a combination of detomidine and butorphanol, and topical anesthesia with phenylephrine (2% lidocaine or mepivacaine hydrochloride and 10 mL of 0.15% phenylephrine) is applied to the membrane and nasal cavity. The videoendoscope is placed in the affected nostril and the outline of the choanal membrane is identified using bronchoesophagoscopic forceps. Using a 600-μm laser fiber placed in the biopsy channel of the videoendoscope and a diode laser at 15 watts (pulse duration, 3 seconds), the membrane is incised, creating two lines of incision perpendicular to each other that cross at the center of the choanal membrane. This cross incision is made because the membrane (even though it appears thin) is vascular, and local pressure to stop the bleeding may be needed at times. When excessive bleeding occurs, a nasotracheal tube is passed through the membrane into the nasopharynx, where the cuff is inflated to apply pressure that promotes clotting at the surgical site. After a few minutes, the tube is removed and each flap resected (the aforementioned forceps may be used to apply tension on the flaps as needed). Postoperatively, the animal receives a 5-day course of phenylbutazone (1 mg/lb PO bid) or a similar NSAID.

The second treatment approach is used when the choanal membrane is osseous or the condition is bilateral, and a nasal flap giving access to the caudal aspect of the nasal passage is required. The choanal membrane (bone) is resected, as well as part of the nasal septum using a nasal bone flap. The foal is anesthetized and placed in lateral recumbency, and an endotracheal tube is placed through a tracheostomy. A C-shaped incision (for unilateral lesions) or an S-shaped incision (for bilateral lesions) is made over the nasal bones starting at the level of the medial canthus of the eye and extending rostrally to approximately the middle of the nasal cavity, which is near the level of the infraorbital foramen. The periosteum is incised on the midline extending laterally to an area near the nasomaxillary suture, taking care to stay at least 1 cm axial to the infraorbital canal. A nasal bone flap is created along the line of the periosteal incision by placing an osteotome at a 45-degree angle to create a ridge for the bone flap to rest on at the end of surgery. The nasal bone flap is made in the shape of the periosteal incision. The procedure must be performed bilaterally if the atresia is bilateral. The nasal mucosa is excised, and the choanal membrane is identified and resected, along with the caudal nasal septum if necessary. The area is packed with sterile rolled gauze, which exits the nostril and is sutured to the false nostril.

If necessary to operate on a young foal, the third approach can be used. The membrane is resected through a laryngotomy after placing the endoscope through the nares to illuminate the persistent membrane. The author's preference is to incise the membrane using endoscopic control and to place a stent in the nostril to prevent stricture.[53] In the author's limited experience, Nd:YAG laser dissection of the membrane has been unrewarding because profuse hemorrhage rapidly obscures the endoscopic view, preventing the application of local pressure in a small foal.[53] The membrane is incised best using laparoscopic scissors with unipolar or bipolar cautery under endoscopic control, while the foal is under general anesthesia. A nasotracheal tube is placed through the surgically created fenestration and sutured to the false nostrils. The stents are removed 14 days postoperatively. Appropriate antibiotic therapy is used.

Because of the rarity of this condition, the prognosis is not well known, and persistence of airway obstruction is a possible complication. The heritability of this condition is unknown.

Nasopharyngeal Dysfunction

Nasopharyngeal dysfunction, characterized by respiratory distress, respiratory stridor, and dysphasia, can occur in foals during the first month of life. Endoscopic examination may reveal severe nasopharyngeal edema, laryngeal edema, milk pooling in the nasopharynx, and persistent DDSP.

The etiology of this obstructive syndrome is unknown. However, on the basis of information obtained from neonatal laboratory animals and human infants, nasopharyngeal dysfunction in neonatal foals may be related to immaturity of the neuromuscular reflexes and defense mechanisms that support the nasopharynx and larynx.[56] Specifically, newborns have a smaller number of pressure and flow receptors in the upper airways than adults, and these receptors discharge at a slower rate.[56] Some of the sensory and motor nerves that supply the larynx and nasopharynx are demyelinated at birth, and they change and mature morphologically until 12 months of age.[56] Perhaps this immature neural circuit causes muscular dysfunction and incoordination in the nasopharynx that results in dysphasia and nasopharyngeal collapse, although this is only speculation.

A thorough physical examination, an endoscopic examination, and radiography of the thorax and pharyngeal region should be performed when evaluating a foal with nasopharyngeal dysfunction. While examining the foal, precautions should be taken to provide it with a patent airway if the examination induces respiratory distress. Appropriate blood work, including serum chemistry, complete blood count, serum IgG levels, and an arterial blood gas, should be performed.

Treatment may begin by securing a patent airway for the foal. Respiratory distress may be sufficiently severe that an emergency tracheotomy is performed immediately. If the foal has persistent DDSP, a laryngotomy followed by placement of a tracheostomy tube usually corrects this problem. Rarely, a staphylectomy may be needed to correct this problem.[35] However, surgical intervention is not necessary in many foals. It is best to support the foal medically for 1 month to see if the problem resolves. Clearly, surveillance and prophylaxis for possible aspiration pneumonia should be strongly considered. White muscle disease should be identified and treated, because this may also cause nasopharyngeal dysfunction. If edema is present, anti-inflammatory medication may be useful in improving function. If the foal is dysphagic, enteral feeding can be performed through a nasogastric feeding tube, or parenteral feeding can be initiated.

Most often, these foals recover from nasopharyngeal dysfunction in 10 to 30 days. The nasopharyngeal edema resolves and dysphasia dissipates. Long-term survival rates and effects of this episode on future athletic performance are unknown.

Cleft Palate

Cleft palate (palatoschisis) is a rare congenital defect in foals.[57] The cleft is caused by an interruption in embryologic closure that occurs along the midline in a rostral-to-caudal direction of the palatal folds and may, therefore, involve portions of the soft palate, or of the hard and soft palate.[57] Defects in the lips and maxilla that frequently occur with cleft palate in people have never been reported in horses. The exact etiology of this defect is unknown, but genetics, nutrition, teratogens, and traumatic mechanical factors that could affect palatal fold closure during the 47th day of gestation are possible causes.[57]

Clinical signs of a cleft palate include milk draining from the foal's nose after nursing, coughing, and signs of aspiration.[57-60] The cleft may be observed during an oral examination or diagnosed by digital palpation, or both. Endoscopic examination, using a pediatric endoscope, is helpful in making the definitive diagnosis and assessing the extent of the defect. A careful endoscopic examination is necessary as the field of view with a pediatric endoscope is small. A small but clinically significant cleft may be obscured by epiglottic cartilage or saliva. It is helpful to make the foal swallow a few times to ensure that the palate is intact. The margins of the soft palate will be visible, and the epiglottis will be positioned in the oropharynx. Once a cleft palate has been diagnosed, the foal should be examined for other congenital defects.

If the cleft is small (about one third of the soft palate) and tracheal aspiration is minimal, it may be better to delay surgery while closely monitoring the foal so that aspiration pneumonia does not go undetected. Weaning the foal early seems to decrease tracheal aspiration, as feed reaches the trachea less readily than milk. The advantage of delaying surgery is that a larger oropharynx facilitates surgical manipulation and more precise surgical repair. If the cleft is large or tracheal aspiration of milk is significant, treatment options should be restricted to either surgical repair of the cleft palate or euthanasia. Allowing foals to continue with the cleft palate is a poor choice, because of their resultant poor quality of life and morbidity from chronic aspiration pneumonia. Surgical repair of a cleft palate is considered a salvage procedure, and it is fraught with complications.[58,61] Palatoplasty usually results in some degree of failure because of complete or partial dehiscence of the repair.[61] Reoperation is frequently needed and often unsuccessful.[58] Pneumonia can be a serious, even life-ending, complication despite attempts to repair the cleft, because of the initial aspiration of milk or feed material.

The prognosis is affected by the size of the defect, the length of the soft palate involved, involvement of the hard palate, and pneumonia.[58,61] Repair of asymmetric defects should not be attempted, because there will not be sufficient tissue available for reconstruction.[58] Also, similarly, if more than 20% of the soft palate tissue is missing, repair should not be attempted.[58] Cleft palate defects that occur on the midline with minimal tissue missing have a successful prognosis of 50%.[58] If the hard palate is involved, the chance of success, defined as an animal that can eat and grow normally, drops significantly. Little information is available on whether the respiratory function of the soft palate during strenuous exercise can be restored (i.e., there are no reports about the prognosis for athletic endeavors).

Surgical Approaches

Preoperative care includes broad-spectrum antibiotic coverage and plasma transfusion if the IgG level is inadequate. If the foal already has pneumonia and is aspirating feed material, the surgery should be postponed, systemic antibiotics continued, and the foal fed enterally through a nasogastric feeding tube or parenterally.

Surgical approaches to the palate include a transoral approach, laryngotomy, pharyngotomy, and mandibular symphysiotomy.[59,61-63] Pharyngotomy with a split of the basihyoid bone is used to repair a cleft involving the caudal third of the soft palate[59] (see previous description of pharyngotomy under "Surgical Approaches to the Nasopharynx or Oropharynx," and Figs. 43-9 and 43-10). Mandibular symphysiotomy provides the best exposure to the hard and soft palate[63] (Fig. 43-25). To perform a palatoplasty using the mandibular symphysiotomy approach, the foal is placed under anesthesia and positioned in dorsal recumbency. A tracheotomy is performed, and the endotracheal tube is placed in the trachea (see Fig. 43-25, *A*). Hair is clipped from the lower lip to the proximal trachea, and the skin is prepared for aseptic surgery. A skin incision is made from the hyoid to the lower lip (Fig. 43-25, *B*). The skin and gingiva over the mandibular symphysis are completely incised, and the mandibular symphysis is severed using a scalpel blade (in a neonate), an osteotome, or an oscillating

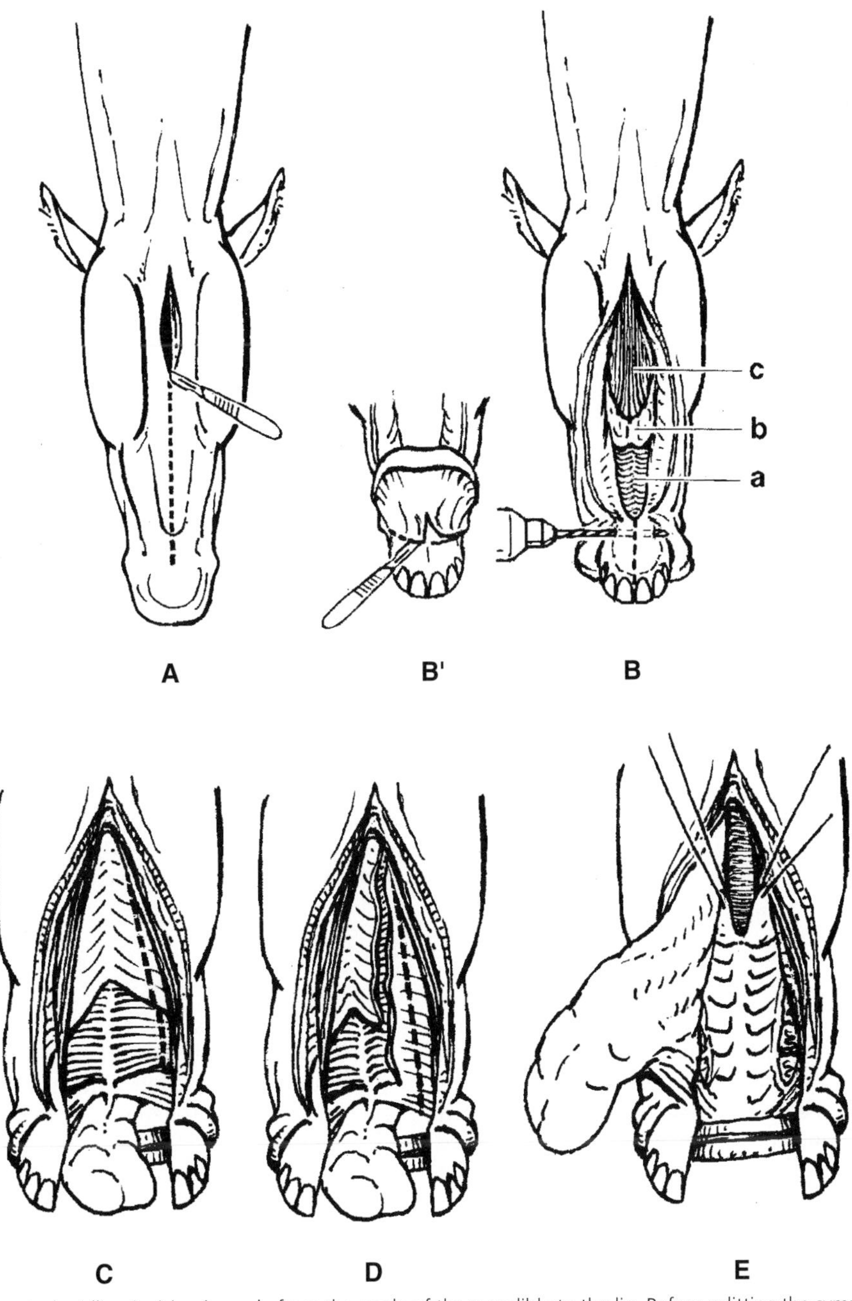

Figure 43-25. A and **B,** A ventral midline incision is made from the angle of the mandible to the lip. Before splitting the symphysis, a hole is prepared to facilitate realignment of the bones during closure. The lip has been moved orally to avoid morbidity associated with incising it. a, mylohyoideus; b, mandibular lymph nodes; c, sternohyoideus and omohyoideus muscles. **C,** The mandibles are spread, and the rostral oral mucosa is incised. The mylohyoid and geniohyoideus muscles are incised near their tendinous origin. They should be cut with enough tissue left to suture them together for closure. **D,** The exposed ventral surface of the oral mucosa is tensed by further spreading of the mandibles. It is incised as far caudally as possible. Care is taken to avoid the sublingual salivary gland near the mandible and the lingual nerve near the tongue. **E,** The edges of the incision are covered with moistened sponges or towels and spread as far as possible. The nasotracheal tube is visible through the cleft. Two stay sutures are placed at the caudal corners of the cleft.

Continued

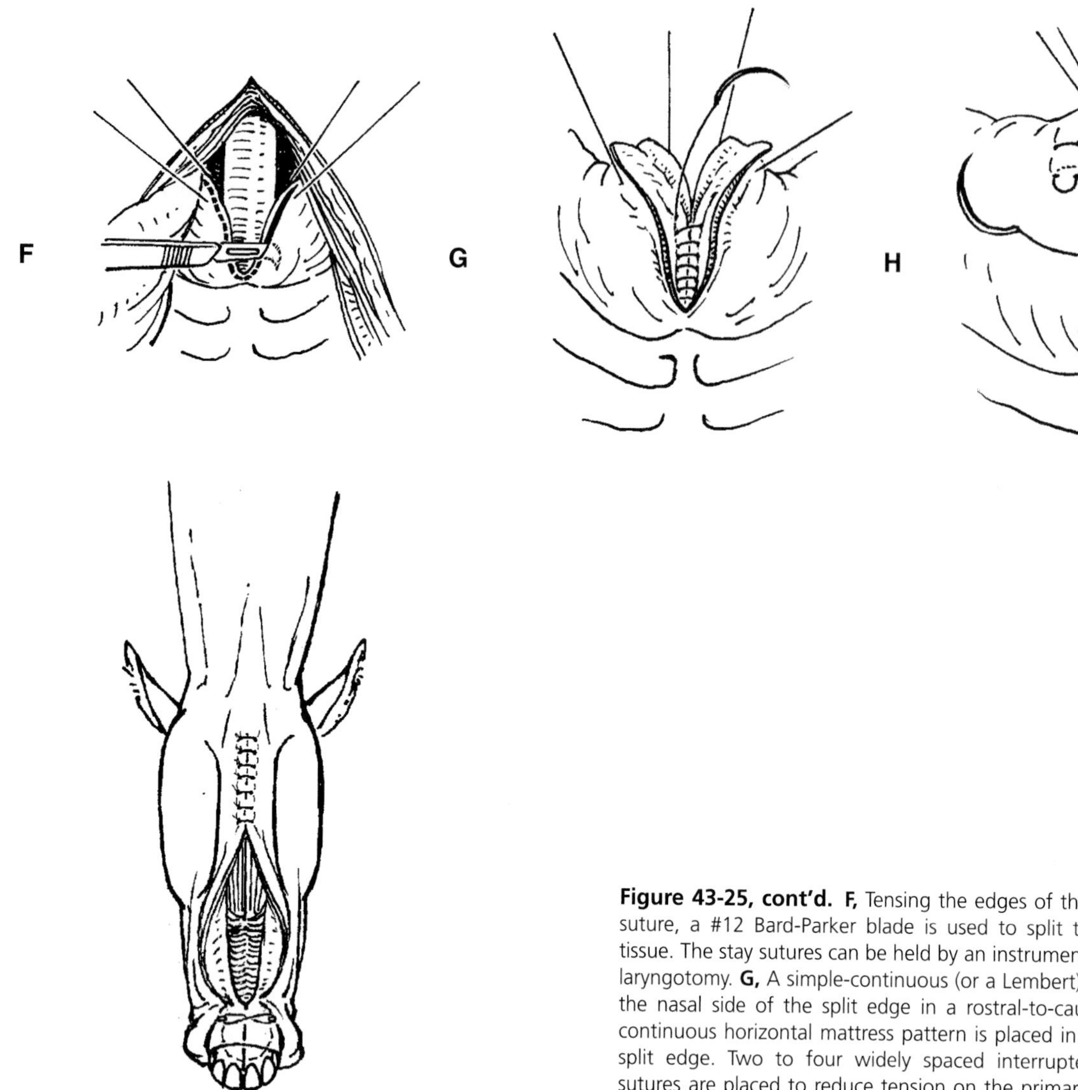

Figure 43-25, cont'd. F, Tensing the edges of the cleft with the stay suture, a #12 Bard-Parker blade is used to split the thickness of the tissue. The stay sutures can be held by an instrument inserted through a laryngotomy. **G,** A simple-continuous (or a Lembert) pattern is placed in the nasal side of the split edge in a rostral-to-caudal direction. **H,** A continuous horizontal mattress pattern is placed in the oral side of the split edge. Two to four widely spaced interrupted vertical mattress sutures are placed to reduce tension on the primary suture line. **I,** Soft tissues are apposed and a lag screw or pin with figure-eight wire is placed using the previously drilled hole. A cerclage wire around the rostral mandible just caudal to the erupted incisors augments stability.

bone saw. It is preferable to avoid incising the lip to minimize postoperative dehiscence[61] and discomfort. This is achieved by making a transverse incision at the base of the lip so the lip can first be moved caudally to give access to the symphysis. After splitting the symphysis, the lip is moved orally. The mandible spread achieved is slightly less after splitting the mandibular symphysis compared with splitting the lower lip, but it reduces morbidity. Surgical dissection subsequently proceeds along the right ramus of the mandible, and the attachments of the mylohyoid, geniohyoid, and genioglossus muscles are transected, exposing the buccal mucosa. The buccal mucosa is sharply incised, allowing the rami of the mandibles to be retracted (Fig. 43-25, *C* and *D*). A thin malleable retractor may be inserted through the laryngotomy incision over the base of the tongue to push the tongue out of the surgical field. Moist towels should be used to retract the mandibles.

After the cleft is repaired, the mandibles are apposed and stabilized with a single ASIF cancellous screw or a Steinmann pin supplemented by a hemi-cerclage, and the central incisors are wired together. The buccal mucosa is closed, and the geniohyoid and mylohyoid muscle layers are apposed and reattached. The lip is reconstructed by closing the gingiva, muscle layer, and skin (Fig. 43-25, *I*). The laryngotomy is left open, and the skin incision from the mandibular symphysis to the laryngotomy incision is closed with sutures interrupted by 2-cm gaps for drainage.[57]

A successful two-step repair of a cleft palate through a purely transoral approach was reported in a 4-week old colt.[64] Because the instruments were too short, the procedure had to be stopped 4 cm short of the caudal rim, and it was completed 4 weeks later, after the initial repair had healed. In this procedure, a special mouth speculum with a long, narrow extension into the mouth was used to elevate the tongue out of the surgical field. Illumination of the surgical field was provided by a pediatric endoscope, which was introduced through one of the nasal passages.[64]

SOFT PALATE REPAIR

Graffe was the first surgeon to attempt surgical closure of cleft palate in humans in 1816, but he reported poor results.[65] Little progress was made until Langenbeck (1961) described a new technique to close a palatal cleft using two bridge flaps. The technique was further modified in 1967, when Kriens suggested that the main surgical problem with palate repair was caused by the misoriented muscles in the soft palate, which, instead of building a velopharyngeal sphincter mechanism, have an insertion in the hard palate[66] (Fig. 43-26). To solve this problem, the faulty origin of the palatopharyngeus and levator veli palatini muscles was resected from the hard palate and subsequently included in the cleft repair, which resulted in a more anatomically correct reconstruction of the soft palate. The interposition of the palatal muscles between the oral and nasal mucosa led to good functional results in humans.[67]

The soft palate is identified, and the cleft is evaluated. A surgical light is directed into the incision. If a pharyngotomy was used for access, the videoendoscope is placed orally. If a mandibular symphysiotomy was chosen, the endoscope can be positioned through a laryngotomy incision to improve visibility at the caudal margin of the soft palate. A stay suture is passed through the soft palate at the caudal extent of the cleft, and these stay sutures are secured at the laryngotomy site to tense the edges of the defect (see Fig. 43-25, *E*). A thin

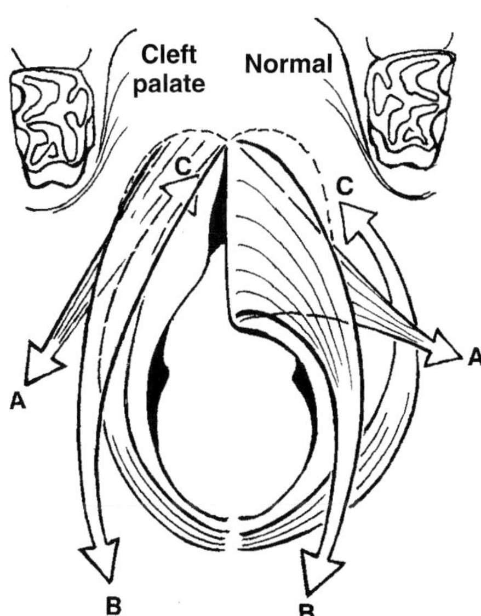

Figure 43-26. Origin and direction of insertion of the three velar muscles—palatopharyngeus (A), levator veli palatini (B), and constrictor pharynges (C)—that form the velopharyngeal sphincter mechanism in the normal horse *(right side)* and in the horse with a cleft palate *(left side)*. In the cleft palate situation, A and B originate from the hard palate, whereas in the normal situation they originate from the median of the soft palate (the muscles of the left and right side have a common origin). C inserts on the median in the normal situation but on the hard palate in the cleft palate situation. (Adapted from the human situation.)

strip of mucosa is excised from each edge of the cleft, and a narrow incision is extended into the palate using a #12 hooked blade (see Fig. 43-25, *F*). The nasal mucosa is closed first, beginning at the caudal free margin of the soft palate, using 2-0 absorbable suture material in a simple-continuous pattern (see Fig. 43-25, *G*). The oral mucosa and muscular layers are closed together using vertical mattress sutures of absorbable material or silk (see Fig. 43-25, *H*). Silk has excellent handling characteristics and good knot security.[58] The oral mucosa is closed with absorbable material in a simple-continuous pattern.

Tension on the repair can lead to dehiscence; therefore, tension-relieving incisions are made parallel to the closure plane in the lateral mucosa axial to the molar teeth. Alternatively, widely spaced interrupted vertical mattress sutures can be placed in the palate to relieve the tension. The tendon of the tensor veli palatini muscle can be transected bilaterally or osteotomy of the hamulus of the pterygoid can be performed to decrease tension applied to the caudal half of the soft palate by the tensor veli palatini muscle. These latter procedures should be used with caution, as they can lead to instability of the rostral aspect of the soft palate and may interfere with respiratory soundness at exercise.

A minimally invasive technique to reconstruct a cleft palate can be achieved with a technique similar to that used for human cleft palate closure.[64] After dividing the oral and nasal mucosa on both sides of the cleft, the muscular layer was exposed. Through two palatal incisions, the hard palate is inspected at its caudal end. The misoriented muscles are detached from their anatomically abnormal insertion on the hard palate and redirected into the correct orientation (see Fig. 43-26). In a first layer, the nasal mucosa is repaired using 2-0 monofilament nylon sutures in an interrupted everting pattern. Subsequently, the previously dissected muscle ends are sutured in the midline to build up a new velar sphincter. Finally, the oral mucosal layer is closed in a pattern identical to that used for the nasal mucosa.

Because it is difficult to repair the caudal end of the soft palate, a combined transoral and laryngotomy approach is an alternative to provide good apposition and reconstruction of the cleft palate.[68] To provide better access to the caudal aspect of the soft palate, the thyroid cartilage may be split sagittally (Fig. 43-27). The surgical repair of the soft palate is identical to the one previously described. At the end of the procedure, the thyroid cartilage is sutured with three single interrupted sutures of no. 2 monofilament nylon.[68] The incision of the cricothyroid membrane is closed in a simple-continuous pattern with 2-0 polyglactin 910 suture material. The subcutaneous tissues and skin are left to heal by second intention.

HARD PALATE REPAIR

Repair of hard palate defects is performed using mucoperiosteal flaps. Hemorrhage can be controlled by injecting small volumes of 2% lidocaine with epinephrine along the incision lines in the hard palate. A mucoperiosteal incision is made parallel to the maxilla from the junction of the hard and soft palate to a few centimeters beyond the defect. The entire width of the mucoperiosteum is elevated to the edge of the defect using a periosteal elevator. Care is taken to preserve the palatine artery, which can be seen as it emerges

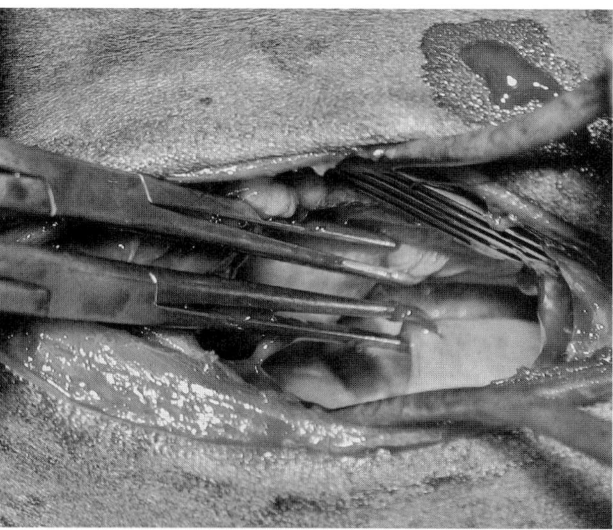

Figure 43-27. Laryngotomy approach for repair of the caudal aspect of a cleft palate. The two parts of the cleft palate are retracted with Allis forceps. Good visibility of the cleft palate was achieved by splitting the thyroid cartilage longitudinally. (Courtesy J. Auer, University of Zurich, Switzerland.)

from the palatine foramina at the caudolateral aspect of the hard palate at the level of the second molar. As the flap is elevated, the palatine artery stretches, and the entire flap is moved axially. The rostral (rostral hard palate) and caudal (junction of the hard and soft palates) attachments of the mucoperiosteal flap are preserved. The nasal mucosa of the flap is closed in a simple-continuous pattern using absorbable suture material, and the mucoperiosteal flaps are sutured together with horizontal mattress sutures. The defects along the lateral aspect of each mucoperiosteal flap heal by second intention.

Postoperative Care

If only the soft palate was repaired, the foal is allowed to nurse. If the soft palate defect was extensive or the hard palate was repaired, or both, the foal should be fed enterally through a nasogastric feeding tube or parenterally for 7 to 10 days. Broad-spectrum antibiotics should be continued for 5 days unless the foal has pneumonia, in which case antibiotics are continued until the pneumonia resolves. The repair may be assessed by careful oral examination (by looking in the mouth, not by digital palpation), but endoscopic examination is not recommended during the early postoperative period.

Dehiscence is the most likely and most severe complication. Generally, dehiscence is apparent within the first 7 to 14 days and is evidenced by nasal reflux of food and coughing. Other complications include pneumonia, osteomyelitis of the mandible, salivary fistulas, and incisional infections.[61]

REFERENCES

1. Odeh M, Schall R, Gavriely N, et al: Effect of upper airway muscle contraction on supraglottic resistance and stability, Respir Physiol 1993;56:139.
2. Hare WCD: Equine respiratory system. In Getty R, editor: Sisson and Grossman's The Anatomy of Domestic Animal, ed 5, Philadelphia, 1975, WB Saunders.
3. Kuehn DP, Folkins JW, Cutting CB: Relationships between muscle activity and velar position, Cleft Palate J 1982;19:25.
4. Van de Graaff WB, Gottfried SB, Mitra J, et al: Respiratory function of hyoid muscle length and upper airway volume, J Appl Physiol 1984;57:197.
5. Van Lunteren E, Haxhiu MA, Cherniak NS: Effects of tracheal airway occlusion on hyoid muscle length and upper airway volume, J Appl Physiol 1989;67:2296.
6. Holcombe SJ, Derksen FJ, Stick JA, et al: Bilateral nerve blockade of the pharyngeal branch of the vagus nerve produces persistent soft palate dysfunction in horses, Am J Vet Res 1998;59:504-508.
7. Tessier C, Holcombe SJ, Derksen FJ, et al: Effects of stylopharyngeus muscle dysfunction on the nasopharynx in exercising horses, Equine Vet J 2004;36:318.
8. Holcombe SJ, Cornelisse CJ, Berney C, et al: Electromyographic activity of the hyoepiglotticus muscle and control of epiglottis position in horses, Am J Vet Res 2002;63:1617-1621.
9. Holcombe SJ, Derksen FJ, Stick JA, et al: Effect of bilateral tenectomy of the tensor veli palatini muscle on soft palate function in horses, Am J Vet Res 1997;58:317-321.
10. Holcombe SJ, Ducharme NG: The function of extrinsic and intrinsic musculature in stabilizing the upper airway. In Proc World Equine Airway Symposium, CD Edinburg, Scotland, 2001.
11. Schummer A, Nickel R, Sack WO: Pharynx. In Schummer A, Nickel R, Sack WO, editors: The viscera of domestic animals, New York, 1979, Springer-Verlag.
12. Cornelisse CJ, Rosenstein DS, Derksen FJ, et al: Computed tomographic study of the effect of a tongue-tie on hyoid apparatus position and nasopharyngeal dimensions in anesthetized horses, Am J Vet Res 2001;62:1865-1869.
13. Cornelisse CJ, Holcombe SJ, Derksen FJ, et al: Effect of a tongue-tie on upper airway mechanics in horses during exercise, Am J Vet Res 2001;62:775-778.
14. Holcombe SJ, Beard WL, Hinchcliff KW, et al: Effect of sterno-thyrohyoid myectomy on upper airway mechanics in normal horses, J Applied Physiol 1994;77:2812-2816.
15. Ducharme NG, Hackett RP, Woodie JB, et al: Investigations into the role of the thyrohyoid muscles in the pathogenesis of dorsal displacement of the soft palate in horses, Equine Vet J 2003;35:258-263.
16. Fukushima S, Shingai T, Kitagawa J, et al: Role of the pharyngeal branch of the vagus nerve in laryngeal elevation and UES pressure during swallowing in rabbits, Dysphagia 2003;18:58-63.
17. Schumacher J: Nasopharyngeal cicatrices in horses: 47 cases (1972-1985), J Am Vet Med Assoc 1987;191:239.
18. Rakestraw P: Equine nasopharyngeal cicatrix syndrome. In Proc Texas Equine Vet Pract Meeting, November, 2003.
19. McClure SR Schumacher J, Snyder JR: Transnasal incision of restricted nasopharyngeal cicatrix in three horses, J Am Vet Med Assoc 1994;205:461.
20. Gaughan EM, Gift LJ, Debowes RM, et al: Squamous cell carcinoma as a sign of dyspnea and blindness, Cornell Vet 1991;81:295.
21. Rastegaev J: The aberrant parasitism of horse botflies *(Diptera gastrophilidae)*, Parazitologiia 1990;24:154.
22. Zamos DT, Schumacher J, Loy JK: Nasopharyngeal conidiobolomycosis in a horse, J Am Vet Med Assoc 1996;208:100.
23. Greet T: Personal communication, 1998.
24. Ordidge RM: Thermal cautery of the equine soft palate as a treatment for displacement of the soft palate during exercise, In Proc 7th World Congress 2001;7:287.
25. Ahern TJ: Oral palatopharyngoplasty: A survey of one hundred post-operative raced horses, Equine Vet Sci 1993;13:670-672.
26. Smith CM, Taylor RJ, Dixon PM: Unilateral ventral displacement of the roof of the nasopharynx as a cause of stridor in a pony, Vet Rec 1994;134:140.

27. Strand E, Staempfli HR: Dynamic collapse of the roof of the nasopharynx as a cause of poor performance in a Standardbred colt, Equine Vet J 1993;25:252-254.
28. Rehder R: Equine upper airway and guttural pouch pressures during exercise. Master's Thesis, Cornell University, 1995.
29. Raphel C: Endoscopic findings in the upper respiratory tract of 479 horses, J Am Vet Med Assoc 1982;181:470.
30. Rehder R, Ducharme NG, Hackett RP, et al: Measurement of upper airway pressures in exercising horses with dorsal displacement of the soft palate, Am J Vet Res 1995;56:269.
31. Holcombe SJ, Derksen FJ, Stick JA, et al: Bilateral nerve blockade of the pharyngeal branch of the vagus nerve produces persistent soft palate dysfunction in horses, Am J Respir Crit Care Med 1997;155:A412.
32. Quinlan J, Van Rensburg SWJ, Starke NC: The soft palate (palatinum molle) as a cause of dyspnoea in two racehorses, J South Afr Vet Assoc 1949;20:125-127.
33. Shappel KK, Caron JP, Stick JA: Staphylectomy for treatment of dorsal displacement of the soft palate in two foals, J Am Vet Med Assoc 1989;195:1395.
34. Linford RL, O'Brien TR, Wheat JD, et al: Radiographic assessment of the epiglottic length and pharyngeal and laryngeal diameters in the Thoroughbred, Am J Vet Res 1983;44:1660.
35. Tulleners EP, Hamir A: Evaluation of epiglottic augmentation by use of polytetrafluoroethylene paste in horses, Am J Vet Res 1991;52:1908.
36. Holcombe SJ, Derksen FJ, Stick JA, et al: Effects of bilateral hypoglossal and glossopharyngeal nerve blocks on epiglottic and soft palate position in exercising horses, Am J Vet Res 1997;58:1.
37. Cook WR: Some observations on form and function of the equine upper airway in health and disease: 1. The pharynx, Proc Am Assoc Equine Pract 1981;27:355.
38. Beard WL, Holcombe SJ, Hinchcliff KW: Effect of a tongue-tie on upper airway mechanics during exercise following sternothyrohyoid myectomy in clinically normal horses, Am J Vet Res 2001;62:779-782.
39. Franklin SH, Naylor JR, Lane JG: The effect of a tongue-tie in horses with dorsal displacement of the soft palate, Equine Vet J Suppl 2002;34:430-433.
40. Hobo S, Matsuda Y, Yoshida K: Prevalence of upper respiratory tract disorders detected with a flexible videoendoscope in Thoroughbred racehorses, J Vet Med Sci 1995;57:409-413.
41. Woodie JB, Ducharme NG, Hackett RP, et al: The effects of a laryngohyoid stabilizer on prevention of experimentally created dorsal displacement of the soft palate in exercising horses, Vet Surg 2003;32:500.
42. Barakzai SZ, Dixon PM: Conservative treatment for Thoroughbred racehorses affected with dorsal displacement of the soft palate, Proc Br Equine Vet Assoc, 2004:98.
43. Anderson JD, Tulleners EP, Johnson JK, et al: Sternothyrohyoideus myectomy or staphylectomy for treatment of intermittent dorsal displacement of the soft palate in racehorses: 209 cases (1986-1991), J Am Vet Med Assoc 1995;206:1909.
44. Carter B, Robertson JT, Beard WL, et al: Sternothyroideus myectomy, tenectomy and staphylectomy for treatment of dorsal displacement of the soft palate in horses, Vet Surg 1993;22:374.
45. Harrison IW, Raker CW: Sternothyrohyoideus myectomy in horses: 17 cases (1984-1985), J Am Vet Med Assoc 1988;193:1299.
46. Llewellyn HR, Petrowitz AB: Sternothyroideus myotomy for the treatment of dorsal displacement of the soft palate, Proc Am Assoc Equine Pract 1997;43:239.
47. Tulleners EP, Stick JA, Leitch M, et al: Epiglottic augmentation for treatment of dorsal displacement of the soft palate in racehorses: 59 cases (1985-1994), J Am Vet Med Assoc 1997;211:1022.
48. Hogan PM, Palmer SE, Congelosi M: Transendoscopic laser cauterization of the soft palate as an adjunctive treatment for dorsal displacement of the soft palate in the racehorse, Proc Am Assoc Equine Pract 2002;48:228-230.
49. Ducharme NG, Woodie JB: Treatment consideration for DDSP, Proc 13th Annual ACVS Symposium CD, 2003.
50. Morgan DW, Baily CM: Current management of choanal atresia, Int J Pediatr Otorhinolaryngol 1990;19:1.
51. Grouch GM, Morgan SJ: Bilateral choanal atresia in a foal, Comp Cont Educ Pract Vet 1983;5:s206.
52. Aylor MK, Campbell ML, Goring RL, et al: Congenital bilateral choanal atresia in a Standardbred foal, Equine Vet J 1984;16:396.
53. Hogan PM, Embertson RM, Hunt RJ: Unilateral choanal atresia in a foal, J Am Vet Med Assoc 1995;207:471.
54. Richardson JD, Lane JG, Day MJ: Congenital choanal restriction in 3 horses, Equine Vet J 1994;26:162-165.
55. Garabedian EN, Ducroz V, Leperchey F, et al: Malformations of the nasal fossa and paramedian clefts: New perspectives, Ann Otolaryngol Chir Cervicofac 1996;113:373.
56. Mortola JP, Fisher JT: Upper airway reflexes in newborns. In Mathew OP, Sant'Ambrogio G, editors: Respiratory Function of the Upper Airway, vol 43, New York, 1988, Marcel Dekker.
57. Mason TA, Speirs VC, Maclean AA, et al: Surgical repair of cleft soft palate in the horse, Vet Rec 1977;100:6.
58. Robertson JT: Pharynx and larynx. In Beech J, editor: Equine Respiratory Disorders, Philadelphia, 1991, Lea & Febiger.
59. Semevolos SA, Ducharme N: Surgical repair of congenital cleft palate in horses: Eight cases (1979-1997), Proc Am Assoc Equine Pract 1998;44:267-268.
60. Jones RS, Maisels DO, DeGeus JJ, et al: Surgical repair of cleft palate in the horse, Equine Vet J 1975;7:86.
61. Bowman KF, Tate LP, Evans LH, et al: Complications of cleft palate repair in large animals, J Am Vet Med Assoc 1982;180:652.
62. Kirkham LE, Vasey JR: Surgical cleft soft palate repair in a foal, Aust Vet J 2002;80:143-146.
63. Nelson AW, Curley BM, Kainer RA: Mandibular symphysiotomy to provide adequate exposure for intraoral surgery in the horse, J Am Vet Med Assoc 1971;159:1025.
64. Sader R, Zeilhofer HF, Fricke R, et al: About the successful intraoral closure of a cleft palate in a foal, Proc Eur Coll Vet Surg 2003;12:154.
65. Sader R: Untersuchungen zur velopharyngealen Funktion bei Patienten mit Lippen-Kiefer-Gaumenspalten und Dysgnathien, Habilitation Thesis, University of Technology, Munich, 1999.
66. Kriens O, Pfeiffer G: On growth disorders following injuries of the mid-face bones in the 1st years of life.
67. Sader R, Zeilhofer HF, Dietz M, et al: Levatorplasty, a new technique to treat hyper nasality: Anatomical investigations and preliminary clinical results, J Craniomaxillofac Surg 2001;29:143.
68. Auer J: Personal communication, 2005.

CHAPTER 44

Larynx

John A. Stick

ANATOMY

The larynx forms the communicating channel between the pharynx and the trachea, and it functions during breathing, vocalization, and deglutition. It is composed of cartilage and muscle and is lined with a mucous membrane composed of stratified squamous and pseudostratified columnar ciliated epithelium.[1]

The cricoid, thyroid, and epiglottic cartilages are unpaired, whereas the arytenoid cartilages are paired. The cricoid cartilage is shaped like a signet ring and is positioned rostral to the first tracheal ring and connected to the trachea by the cricotracheal membrane.[1] The thyroid cartilage is the largest of the laryngeal cartilages and is situated just rostral to the cricoid cartilage. The arytenoid cartilages are positioned on either side of the cricoid cartilage and connected to it by the cricoarytenoid articulations. The articulation is a diarthrodial joint that allows the arytenoid cartilage to rotate dorsolaterally during abduction, and axially during adduction.[1] Each arytenoid cartilage has a corniculate process that forms part of the dorsal border of the rima glottidis, a cuneate process, and a muscular process that serves as origin for the cricoarytenoideus dorsalis muscle. The epiglottis rests on the dorsal surface of the body of the thyroid cartilage and is held there by the thyroepiglottic ligaments. It consists of elastic cartilage and is shaped like an oblanceolate leaf.[1]

Contraction of the intrinsic laryngeal muscles produces changes in caliber of the rima glottidis by abducting and adducting the corniculate processes of the arytenoid cartilages and the vocal folds and therefore altering airway resistance. These muscles include the paired cricoarytenoideus dorsalis, thyroarytenoideus (ventricularis and vocalis muscles), and cricothyroideus and cricoarytenoideus lateralis muscles, plus the unpaired transverse arytenoideus muscle.[2] The cricoarytenoideus dorsalis is the principal abductor muscle that widens the laryngeal aperture by abducting the corniculate process of the arytenoid cartilage and tensing the vocal folds.[2,3] Contraction of the arytenoid transversus muscle also provides arytenoid abduction by drawing the dorsomedial margins of the arytenoid cartilages together.[1] The thyroarytenoideus, arytenoideus transversus, and cricoarytenoideus lateralis muscles adduct the corniculate processes of the arytenoid cartilages, narrowing the rima glottidis and protecting the lower airway during swallowing.[1,3] The cricothyroideus muscle tenses the vocal folds during vocalization but receives efferent motor innervation from the external branch of the superior laryngeal nerve, a branch of the vagus nerve, whereas all other intrinsic laryngeal muscles receive motor innervation from the recurrent laryngeal branch of the vagus nerve.[1,2]

The extrinsic laryngeal muscles of the larynx include the thyrohyoideus, hyoepiglotticus, and sternothyroideus muscles[1] and are involved in stabilization of the larynx and pharynx during exercise.

The mucosa of the larynx is closely adhered to the cartilages and contains many different types of afferent receptors. The mucous membrane covering the epiglottic cartilage reflects off the lateral border of the epiglottis and blends with the mucous membrane covering the corniculate processes of the arytenoid cartilages, forming the aryepiglottic folds.[1] The mucous membrane covers the vocal ligament, forms the vocal folds, and lines the lateral ventricles, forming the laryngeal saccules. These saccules are 2.5 cm deep with a capacity of 5 to 6 mL.[1] They extend between the medial surface of the thyroid cartilage and the ventricularis and vocalis muscles. The laryngeal mucosa contains mechanoreceptors specialized in their sensory modalities for the detection of different stimuli, including transmural pressure changes, airflow, temperature, and laryngeal motion.[4] These receptors receive afferent neural supply from the internal branch of the superior laryngeal nerve, a branch of the vagus nerve.[4] This rich sensory supply is the main source of many respiratory reflexes that influence upper airway patency and breathing patterns.[4,5]

The larynx receives arterial blood supply from the caudal laryngeal and branches of the ascending pharyngeal arteries. Venous drainage is provided by the caudal laryngeal and ascending pharyngeal veins, which flow to the external jugular vein via the thyroid vein. The lymph chains that serve the laryngeal area include the retropharyngeal and the cranial and deep cervical lymph centers.[1]

ARYTENOID CARTILAGES

The paired arytenoids are the most dynamic of the laryngeal cartilages (along with the epiglottis). The articulations with the cricoid cartilage allow complete closure of the glottis during swallowing (adduction) and maximal opening (abduction) during exercise (Fig. 44-1). These dynamics of the arytenoids make them vulnerable to injury, inflammation, and dysfunction and also dictate the impact their dysfunction has on performance. Therefore, the necessity for treatment becomes obvious for athletes.

The body or laminar portion of the arytenoids, like the thyroid and cricoid cartilages, consists of hyaline cartilage, which is subject to ossification with age or trauma. However, the apex of the arytenoids, which curves upward and backward, forms a pitcher-shaped lip (from which the cartilages derive their name) that is readily observed on endoscopic examination.

Laryngeal Hemiplegia (Recurrent Laryngeal Neuropathy)

Etiology and Incidence

Horses can develop unilateral or bilateral paralysis of the arytenoids.[6-9] Unilateral left-sided laryngeal paralysis is most commonly encountered (Fig. 44-2) and results from progressive loss of large myelinated nerve fibers in the left recurrent laryngeal nerve, hence the term *recurrent laryngeal neuropathy* has been suggested as a name for this disease.[6] In

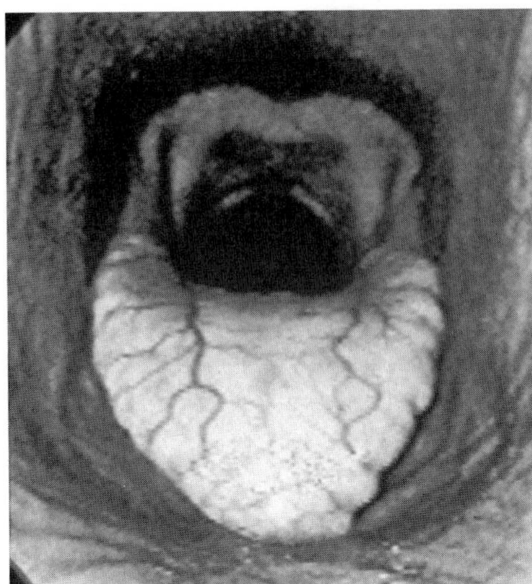

Figure 44-1. Endoscopic appearance of the normal larynx during inhalation, showing maximal abduction of the arytenoid cartilages and a normal-appearing epiglottis.

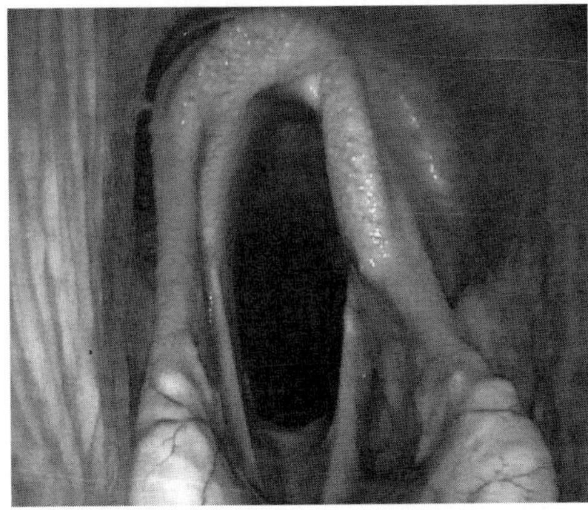

Figure 44-2. Endoscopic appearance of grade 4 laryngeal hemiplegia. (Courtesy M. Weishaupt, Zurich.)

almost all of these horses, no precise cause is evident and the term *idiopathic laryngeal hemiplegia* is applied, although a genetic predisposition is most likely.[9-11] Progressive neurogenic atrophy of the intrinsic laryngeal musculature, most importantly the cricoarytenoideus dorsalis muscle, results in progressive loss of both abductor and adductor arytenoid function.[6] Laryngeal hemiplegia occurs in horses from a few months to 10 years of age and older, with large-breed horses more commonly affected than small-breed horses or ponies.[12,13] Incidence is highest in young horses and commonly discovered in Thoroughbred yearlings that are examined at sale time, before they have started any type of training, or in 2- and 3-year-olds that are racing or are in race training.[13-15] Although the incidence of complete idiopathic laryngeal hemiplegia was 2.75% in a study of Thoroughbred yearling sales, overall incidence in the entire yearling population is likely to be higher.[15,16] In fact, in a recent study of 427 Thoroughbred sale yearlings, 64% had asynchronous/asymmetrical arytenoid cartilage movements and 25% (107) had laryngeal asymmetry that was significantly associated with decreased racing performance.[17]

In a normal horse during sustained exercise, the larynx dilates fully to maximize airflow. Complete arytenoid cartilage abduction is sustained, despite the increased negative inspiratory pressure, throughout the respiratory cycle as exercise intensity increases. In the horse with laryngeal hemiplegia, arytenoid abduction on the affected side cannot be achieved and there is a progressive collapse of the arytenoid cartilage and vocal cord into the airway as negative inspiratory pressures increase[18] (Fig. 44-3). This produces airflow limitations that result in hypoxemia, hypercarbia, and metabolic acidosis, which develop more rapidly than in a normal horse with the same workload,[19,20] causing early fatigue and poor performance.

A specific etiology can be identified in some horses with acquired laryngeal paralysis, unilateral or bilateral. The recurrent laryngeal nerve can be damaged as a result of perivascular injection intended for the jugular vein, guttural pouch mycosis, trauma from injuries or surgical procedures of the neck, strangles abscessation of the head and neck, and impingement by neoplasms of the neck or chest.[9] Organophosphate toxicity, plant poisoning, hepatic encephalopathy, lead toxicity, and central nervous system diseases have also been shown to cause laryngeal paralysis.[21,22] In a recent study of 375 cases of laryngeal hemiplegia in a mixed-breed population of horses, 94% (351) were idiopathic in origin.[23] However, in non-idiopathic cases (6%), over half were bilaterally affected.

Diagnosis

A presumptive diagnosis of laryngeal hemiplegia is made on the basis of history and the findings of a physical examination. Horses with left recurrent laryngeal neuropathy have a history of upper airway obstruction during exercise that includes an abnormal inspiratory respiratory noise, characterized as a whistle or a roar, and exercise intolerance. The noise is the result of air turbulence created as air passes over the affected vocal cord, and over the ventricle, which acts as a resonator.

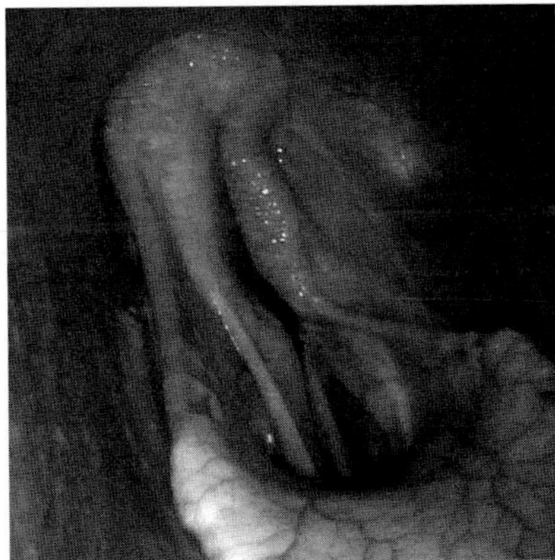

Figure 44-3. A videoendoscopic image of the larynx of a horse with grade 4 laryngeal hemiplegia, showing complete collapse of the larynx and vocal folds during high-speed exercise. (Courtesy M. Weishaupt, Zurich.)

Physical examination should include palpation of the neck and larynx, because horses with complete paralysis of the left arytenoid cartilage will have palpable atrophy of the cricoarytenoideus dorsalis muscle.[16] The larynx should also be palpated for congenital malformation and evidence of arytenoid chondritis.[21,24] If there was previous laryngeal surgery and a laryngotomy was performed, there is usually a linear scar on the ventral aspect of the larynx, over the cricothyroid membrane, which can be palpated. Laryngoplasty and laryngotomy scars can be identified visually after clipping the hair over the incisions.

A definitive diagnosis is made on endoscopic examination when there is a loss of abductor function on the affected side of the larynx (see Fig. 44-2). Because various descriptions of the loss of abductor function (hemiplegia, complete and incomplete paralysis, and paresis) lead to confusion, a four-point laryngeal function grading system has been adopted to more precisely describe arytenoid cartilage activity as assessed on endoscopic examination in resting horses[25] (see Table 41-1). Arytenoid abduction can be stimulated by inducing swallowing or by nasal occlusion in the resting horse. If there is any question as to whether a horse shows complete or incomplete abduction, an exercise test can be carried out and endoscopy performed immediately after cessation of exercise. A more reliable alternative is to perform videoendoscopy during exercise on a treadmill, observing for dynamic collapse of the arytenoid cartilage and the associated vocal cord (see Chapter 41). The video image can be recorded and reexamined in slow motion later.[26]

In the absence of access to a high-speed treadmill, endoscopic examination of the upper airway of horses standing at rest is still commonly performed not only for the diagnosis of suspected upper respiratory obstructive disorders but also as routine surveillance for horses in training and for prepurchase examinations. This has strengthened the recognition that variations in arytenoid cartilage movements of the equine larynx are common. The laryngeal movements in a horse unaffected by clinically significant recurrent laryngeal neuropathy would have complete synchronous and symmetrical abduction maintained during nasal occlusion during a resting endoscopic examination. However, it is recognized that asynchronous and asymmetric arytenoid cartilage movements are common and may or may not indicate failure of arytenoid function during athletic exercise.[17] The clinical significance of these variations in cartilage movement has been controversial. However, it is generally recognized that increasing degrees of laryngeal movement dysfunction result in poor athletic performance and, therefore, it is an undesirable characteristic found during the endoscopic examination of the equine athlete. Furthermore, it is recognized that horses with laryngeal neuropathy, even after treatment with prosthetic laryngoplasty, often have a guarded prognosis for full restoration of athletic performance.[27]

Therefore, interpretation and significance of altered laryngeal cartilage movements during the endoscopic examination falls to the veterinarian, who must make an educated prediction of how these altered movements will affect the horse's performance. To do this, the veterinarian must not only determine how severely affected the larynx is but also answer the question, "Will these altered laryngeal movements progress to complete laryngeal paralysis?" The 1982 literature contained a study in which 168 horses were examined over a period of several years, and there was no apparent progression from asynchronous abductor function to complete paralysis.[28] This led the investigators to conclude that such movement was normal. Subsequently, the four-point classification system for arytenoid cartilage movements was developed to predict present and future arytenoid dysfunction based on resting endoscopic evaluation. Although clinical and experimental studies suggested that the laryngeal neuropathy may have been progressive, no factual evidence was available in the literature.

However, a recent study showed that recurrent laryngeal neuropathy *is* progressive.[29] The long-term histories and clinical findings of 351 horses suffering from recurrent laryngeal neuropathy were examined for evidence of progression of laryngeal asymmetry. Fifty-two out of 351 cases (15%) had evidence of progression of the degree of laryngeal dysfunction over a median period of 12 months. The implication is that today's findings do not apply to the future and, therefore, periodic reexamination is indicated, and prognosis for athletic prowess can change as a direct result.

This study also indicated that many of the adult horses had an *acute* onset of exercise intolerance and inspiratory stertor. If this disease is thought of as progressive, it is assumed to be slow and insidious. However, the clinical signs may, in fact, be caused by a slow progression that finally reaches a threshold, at which point cranial arytenoideus dorsalis muscle fatigue occurs, permitting complete arytenoid collapse during exercise. This manifestation could result in a history of acute onset.

Last, variation in the endoscopic appearance of arytenoid cartilage movements has been reported to be common.[17] It has been suggested that this variation, when it occurs days or even hours later, is often because of intra-assessor variation or laryngeal muscular fatigue from multiple reexaminations. However, differences in clinical and endoscopic findings between veterinarians who perform prepurchase and postpurchase examinations, perhaps just weeks apart, may in some cases simply reflect clinical progression of recurrent laryngeal neuropathy rather than intra-assessor variation.

Treatment

Treatment of laryngeal hemiplegia includes laryngoplasty, ventriculectomy (sacculectomy), ventriculocordectomy, occasionally arytenoidectomy, and neuromuscular-pedicle grafting.[26] However, selection of a particular surgery to treat laryngeal hemiplegia is based on the presenting complaint, use of the horse, and class of arytenoid cartilage movement. When considering this decision, the surgeon should recognize that some horses with laryngeal hemiplegia are able to work to capacity despite the upper airway obstruction. The decision to operate on the upper airway should be based on clear evidence that it is needed, because complications are too frequent to operate on a horse simply because the owners or trainers want to fix all blemishes on their athlete. Some sport horses tolerate upper airway embarrassment quite well when speed is not the issue. Therefore, each of the surgical techniques used to treat laryngeal hemiplegia should target a particular problem.

It is well recognized that horses that work at speed for longer than one-half mile could be greatly affected by obstructions of the upper airway.[27] At these speeds and distances, reduction in the laryngeal aperture by 50% increases the work of breathing 16-fold. Therefore, intervention in the form of a laryngoplasty to eliminate this obstruction is warranted.[28] However, there is evidence that combining ventriculectomy or ventriculocordectomy with this procedure neither prolongs the life of the surgery nor improves upper airway flow mechanics.[30,31]

In the show and performance horse, the respiratory noise caused by laryngeal hemiplegia is an important clinical problem because being "unsound of wind" may result in penalization. Therefore, the primary goal of surgery in the performance and show horse is to eliminate the respiratory noise caused by laryngeal hemiplegia rather than to reduce the airway obstruction. In a recent study, it was shown that bilateral ventriculocordectomy effectively reduces inspiratory noise in laryngeal hemiplegia–affected horses by 90 days after surgery.[32] Conversely, it was shown that laser vocal cordectomy does not effectively reduce the noise associated with laryngeal hemiplegia by 120 days after surgery.[33] Both of these techniques modestly improve airway flow mechanics, but bilateral ventriculocordectomy is the treatment of choice for noise reduction. Clinical experience suggests that bilateral standing ventriculectomy has a very similar result in draft breeds, decreasing airway noise while improving air flow mechanics. Although laryngoplasty reduces respiratory noise in horses with laryngeal hemiplegia, ventriculocordectomy is more efficacious in reducing airway noise in the normal hearing range.[34] A further advantage of ventriculocordectomy over laryngoplasty is that postoperative complications after laryngoplasty are more prevalent and severe and include dysphagia, aspiration pneumonia, chronic cough, wound infection, and prosthetic failure. Furthermore, sound production should not be used as an indicator of surgical success in horses when restoration of upper airway flow mechanics is the primary goal of surgery.[34] There is a poor correlation between the sound indices and degree of airway obstruction as measured by inspiratory pressure. In fact, it has been shown that there was a strong positive correlation in the degree of arytenoid abduction and sound indices. It would have been predicted that a greater abduction would be correlated with less respiratory noise, but the opposite was true.

Occasionally, partial arytenoidectomy is chosen to treat laryngeal hemiplegia when there is a congenital malformation of the cartilages or the laryngoplasty technique has failed because of fractures in the cartilage. Likewise, neuromuscular pedicle grafting is reserved for young horses where return to athletic function is not expected before 4 months after surgery, particularly when laryngeal cartilage movements are still present but are expected to affect performance (grade 3).

Before laryngeal surgery, horses are fasted for 8 to 12 hours. Preoperative and perioperative nonsteroidal anti-inflammatory medication (phenylbutazone) and broad-spectrum antibiotics are indicated for these surgeries for a period of 5 days. The anesthetist should be aware that some horses with a longstanding unilateral arytenoid paralysis can be difficult to intubate with a standard-size tube, and a smaller-diameter tube should be available. The laryngoplasty procedure is performed with the horse in right lateral recumbency. In unique situations, the horse may be first placed in dorsal recumbency to allow for visual and digital inspection of the arytenoid cartilages through a laryngotomy. This approach might be taken when endoscopic observations suggest the presence of subtle arytenoid chondritis or when there has been previous laryngeal surgery. If the cartilage is diseased or has lost flexibility and cannot be pushed into an abducted position, the surgeon may elect to proceed directly to an arytenoidectomy rather than perform a laryngoplasty.

LARYNGOPLASTY

Laryngoplasty is the placement of a prosthesis (suture) between the cricoid and arytenoid cartilages[35,36] (Fig. 44-4). The goal of the laryngoplasty technique (tieback) is to achieve some degree of permanent abduction of the affected arytenoid cartilage. The perfect result for an individual horse is the arytenoid position that achieves a balance between giving the horse enough of a laryngeal opening to perform but not so much abduction as to allow aspiration of saliva, food, and water during swallowing. The art of performing this surgery is finding that balance.

With the affected side uppermost, the head and neck are extended for best surgical exposure. A videoendoscope can be secured in position at this time to allow intraoperative viewing of the larynx by the surgeon. The surgical site is routinely prepared and draped, and a 10- to 12-cm skin incision is made ventral and parallel to the linguofacial vein, extending caudally from a point 4 cm cranial to the ramus of the mandible. This position is the center of the incision over the caudal aspect of the larynx. With Metzenbaum scissors, the linguofacial vein is separated from the omohyoideus muscle along the length of the incision. To maximize exposure, it may be necessary in some horses to ligate and divide the vascular pedicle from the linguofacial vein that enters the omohyoideus muscle. The lateral and dorsal aspects of the larynx are exposed using blunt digital separation of the loose connective tissue, avoiding dissection beyond the dorsal midline of the larynx. A malleable retractor is used in the dorsal portion of the incision to expose the larynx. The muscular process lies beneath the cranial portion of the cricopharyngeus muscle and is exposed by sharply separating the cricopharyngeus and thyropharyngeus muscles along their aponeurosis. The esophagus, thyroid gland, laryngeal and thyroid vessels, and ventral branch of the 1st cervical and cranial laryngeal nerves should be avoided during site preparation and suture placement.[35]

Two sutures of silicone-treated, braided polyester (no. 5 Ticron, Sherwood-Davis & Geck, St. Louis, Mo) or similar large-caliber nonabsorbable suture materials are used for the prosthesis. The large, swaged-on, reverse-cutting needle on the Ticron is used, or the suture can be placed through the eye of a no. 3 Martin uterine reverse-cutting needle and the ends tagged with a small hemostat. (This type of needle is less likely to break off in the laryngeal cartilages than a cutting needle, and it pierces cartilage more easily than a tapered point needle.) Using the left index finger as a guide, the needle is walked off the caudal aspect of the cricoid cartilage just lateral to the dorsal midline until the point slips under the cartilage. (There is a notch in the cricoid at

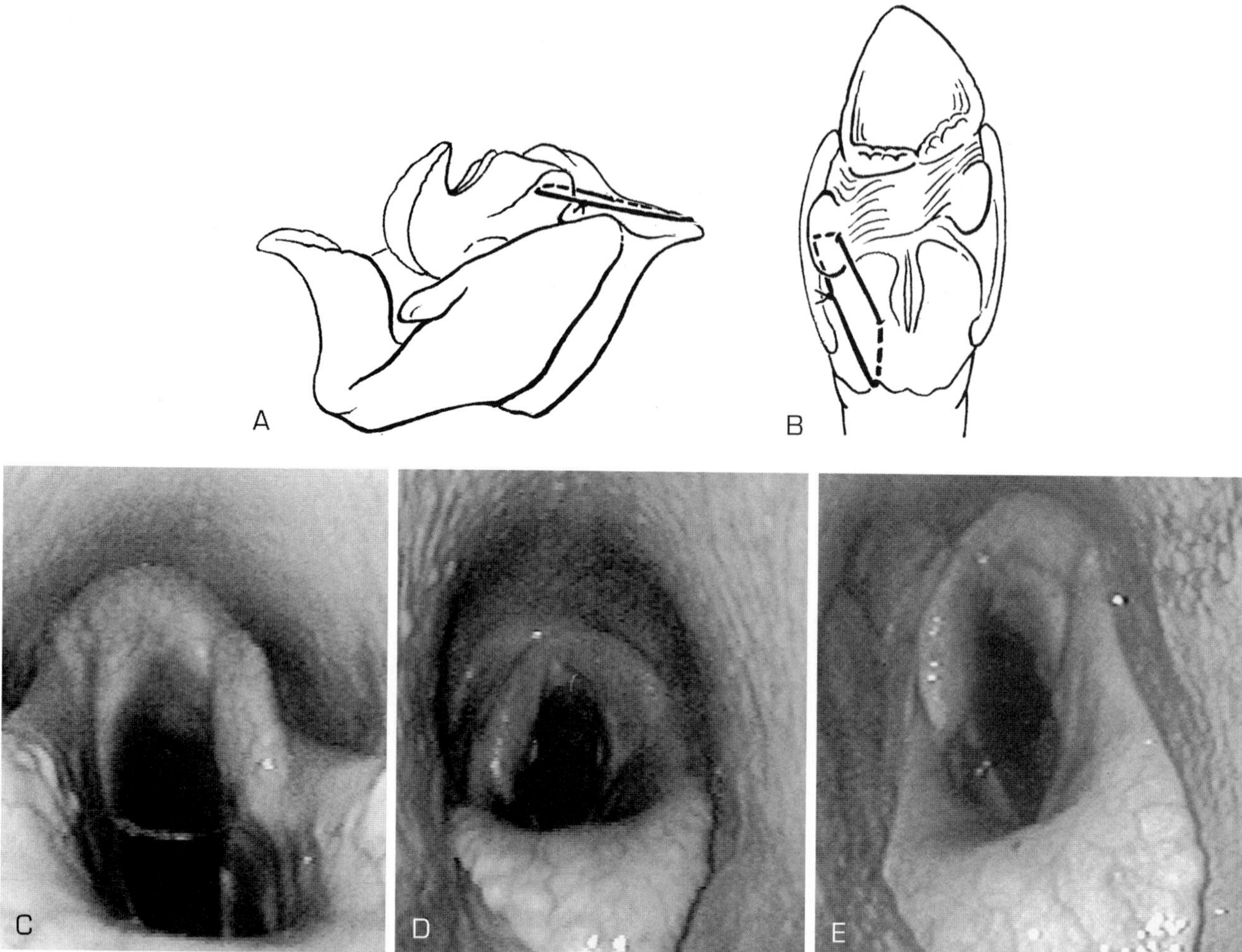

Figure 44-4. Schematic illustration of the correct placement of the laryngoplasty suture and its effects on arytenoid position. **A,** Lateral view of single prosthetic suture in place and tied. **B,** Dorsal view of the larynx, showing configuration of the laryngoplasty suture. **C,** Endoscopic image of a grade 4 laryngeal hemiplegia before laryngoplasty. **D,** Endoscopic appearance of the larynx after laryngoplasty with the left arytenoid cartilage in moderate abduction. **E,** Endoscopic image of an overabduction of the left arytenoid cartilage because of excessive tension of the suture.

this site, but its location can be quite variable.) The needle is advanced in a cranial direction, avoiding the lumen of the larynx. Then the needle is rotated to penetrate the cricoid cartilage 2 to 3 cm cranial to its caudal border and 1 cm lateral to the dorsal ridge (Fig. 44-5, *A*). The left index finger is used to ascertain the site of penetration. The needle is drawn through the cartilage and out of the incision. The needle is cut off and the suture ends are tagged with a small hemostat. A large hemostat is passed under the cranial aspect of the cricopharyngeus muscle, and the points are brought out at the site of penetration of the cranial end of the prosthetic suture. This end is then grasped and drawn under the muscle and brought out of the incision. The lead ends of the prosthetic suture are then placed on a smaller (no. 6 Martin uterine reverse-cutting) needle, which will be used for placing the suture through the muscular process. The needle is positioned on the caudomedial aspect of the muscular process and passed in a craniolateral direction through the muscular process, drawing the prosthetic suture through the muscular process (see Fig. 44-5, *B*). The needle is removed and tension is placed on the cranial and caudal portion of the suture to remove any slack and to be certain that it is tight against the larynx. A second suture is placed in a similar position but 1 cm more caudal in the muscular process. The trailing ends of the prosthetic sutures are then drawn under the cricopharyngeus muscle with a hemostat and the sutures are tied (see Fig. 44-4). Care must be taken to ensure that each trailing suture end is matched to its leading end, and that each suture is placed before one is tied (to avoid cutting the tied suture).

The thyropharyngeus and cricopharyngeus muscles are reapposed with single-interrupted sutures, and the fascia adjacent to the linguofacial vein is apposed to the omohyoideus muscle with simple-interrupted sutures of 2-0 synthetic nonabsorbable suture material. The skin is closed with staples or 2-0 nonabsorbable monofilament suture material.

Variations of the laryngoplasty technique include placement of one prosthetic suture; the use of a crochet hook, rather than a needle, to pull the leading edge of the prosthesis through the muscular process; and the use of tension and crimping devices to adjust and secure the prosthetic

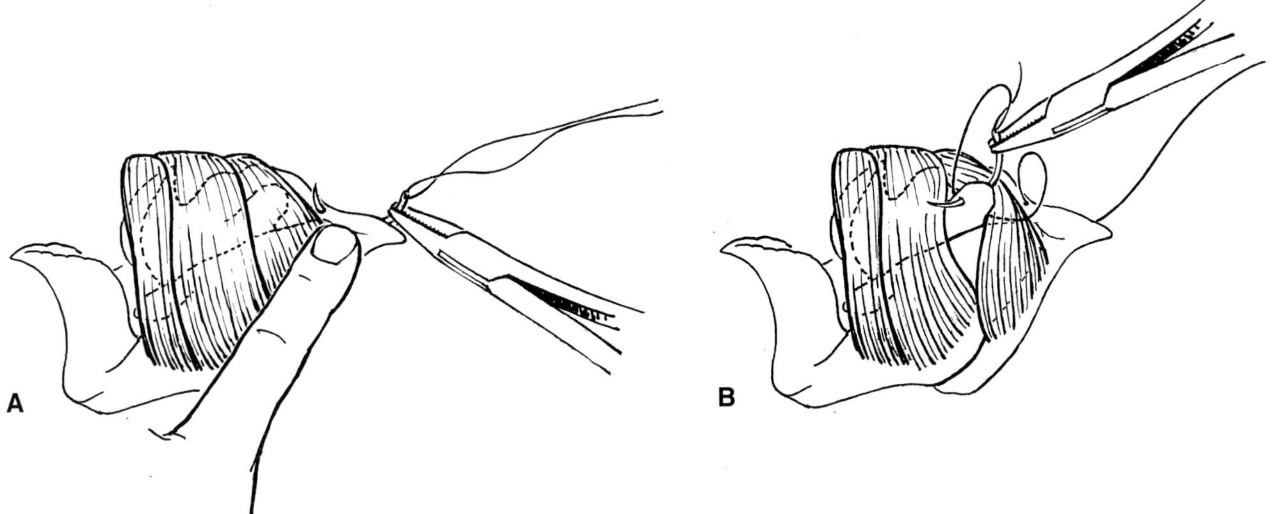

Figure 44-5. Schematic illustration of the laryngoplasty technique. **A,** Placement of the prosthesis in the dorsal, caudal border of the cricoid cartilage. **B,** Placement of the prosthesis in the muscular process of the arytenoid cartilage.

suture (Securos Equine Tie-back System, Chalton, Me).[35,36] Regardless of the technique used, the following principles should be observed:

- Tissue trauma associated with the initial blunt dissection over the larynx should be minimized to prevent damage to adjacent structures (particularly nerves), to reduce the possibility of postoperative dysphagia.[37]
- The prosthetic suture should be seated securely in the cricoid cartilage and the muscular process to minimize cartilage failure.
- Placement of the suture dorsally in the cricoid cartilage, almost on the midline, is important for achieving adequate abduction. Placement of the suture too far laterally results in inadequate abduction.
- The suture must not penetrate the lumen of the larynx. (Placement of the suture in the cricoid cartilage is most likely when the lumen can be penetrated. Therefore, the endotracheal tube should be moved [approximately 4 cm] back and forth before the sutures are tied.)

Following laryngoplasty, stall rest is recommended for 30 days. Hand-walking is allowed for exercise. During the 2nd postoperative week, the swelling in the laryngoplasty incision area subsides. During the 5th and 6th postoperative weeks (30 to 45 days after surgery), the horse is exercised lightly or turned out in a small paddock or round pen. After this, training is resumed. The owner should be advised to feed hay from the ground and that the horse may develop a chronic cough associated with eating.

Complications

Intraoperative complications include bleeding from deep in the surgical site, needle breakage, and prosthetic suture "cut-through" of either the cricoid cartilage or muscular process. Significant hemorrhage can arise from laryngeal vessels that are inadvertently punctured as the needle is passed through the cricoid cartilage. Temporary packing with sponges slows bleeding and allows the placement of the prosthetic suture through the muscular process. The bleeding usually stops when the suture is tightened and tied. Therefore, the surgery should be hastened to accomplish tying of the suture as soon as possible. If the needle breaks, reasonable attempts should be made to retrieve the broken portion, but if it is securely embedded in cartilage or buried in the adjacent soft tissues and has not penetrated the lumen of the larynx, it is not likely to cause a problem. However, it will be clearly visible with radiography of the horse's head or neck.

During the operation, when the prosthetic suture is tightened, having the suture pull through either of the cartilages is a serious problem. The suture must be replaced, avoiding the damaged portion of the cartilage and using less tension. In this instance, a second suture is always used to secure the arytenoid cartilage in an abducted position.

After surgery, large seromas may develop at the laryngoplasty site, and an endoscopic examination may show nasopharyngeal compression on the affected side. If the horse is eating well and remains afebrile (temperature less than 101° F), and if the swollen area is relatively pain free, warm compresses and anti-inflammatory drugs may be used to reduce the size of the seroma. If the horse develops a mild fever, systemic antibiotic treatment is warranted. Drainage of the laryngoplasty incision is indicated if medical treatment fails to resolve the swelling, but rarely does the prosthetic suture become infected. If the suture does become infected, chronic drainage of purulent material may occur for months. Antimicrobial therapy usually resolves the problem, and suture removal is rarely necessary and should be delayed for 4 months, since early removal may result in failure of arytenoid abduction.

Following laryngoplasty, many horses experience some degree of coughing and dysphagia. Initially, pain is associated with swallowing, and the horse may be reluctant to swallow. In the first few days after surgery, saliva, water, and food material may enter the trachea when the horse eats and drinks. This usually resolves within 7 to 10 days. In many cases, the cough persists, particularly when the horse eats.[37-39] The cough is most likely the result of continued aspiration of saliva, water, or food material into the trachea. The cause for this pharyngeal dysfunction resulting in aspiration may be neurologic in origin or related to over-abduction of the arytenoid cartilage.

Chronic aspiration of material causes the chronic cough and, in some horses, repeated episodes of lung infection when they resume training. The diagnosis of aspiration can be made endoscopically by viewing food material in the trachea. Removal of the laryngoplasty suture may resolve the aspiration problem and even the chronic cough in some horses. Time may allow this problem to resolve in others.

Suture pull-out or failure of laryngoplasty seems more likely to occur in yearlings or 2-year-old horses, although experimentally there is no significant effect of age on the in vitro cartilage retention of the prosthesis.[40] In that study, it was also shown that the muscular process is the part of the laryngoplasty fixation that is most likely to fail during progressive tensile loading. It was suggested that partial muscular process cartilage failure is the likely cause of postoperative "relaxation" of the suture, with some loss of abduction.[40] This is a well-recognized phenomenon that occurs during the first 30 days after surgery.[34,41] One retrospective clinical study revealed a much higher rate of successful outcome after prosthetic laryngoplasty in horses that were 2 years old or younger than in horses 3 years old or older.[38] It therefore appears that there is no reason to exclude young horses (younger than 2 years) from laryngoplasty treatment, and that they are at no greater risk for laryngoplasty failure than older horses.[38-40]

The reported success rates for laryngoplasty are variable because of the criteria that are used to measure success, the intended use of the horse, and patient selection. Although reported success rates have ranged from 5% to 90%,* it is realistic to expect that 50% to 70% of racehorses treated with a laryngoplasty will have improved racing performance after surgery.[21,38,39] The outcome is likely to be more successful in horses that are not intended to race after surgery.[38] In a retrospective performance analysis after prosthetic laryngoplasty, the degree of arytenoid abduction achieved did not necessarily correlate to a successful surgical outcome.[38] Likewise, noise production should not be used as a measure of airway obstruction.[34] For the surgery to be successful in racehorses, it appears that the arytenoid cartilage must be positioned at least just beyond an intermediate position and at somewhat less than maximal abduction. However, laryngoplasty should be viewed as a salvage procedure in racehorses, because even the horse with near maximal abduction of the arytenoid cartilage will have some flow limitations at racing speeds.[30]

Reoperation for failed laryngoplasty

During the surgical approach in a horse with a previous laryngoplasty incision, care must be taken not to penetrate the linguofacial vein during the dissection between the vein and the omohyoideus muscle. If the reoperation is within 10 days of the original surgery, a seroma will be encountered in the dead space created at the first surgery, and the local dissection required to expose the dorsal aspect of the cricoid cartilage usually creates a good deal of hemorrhage. In the horse that has a mature surgical area, dense scar tissue makes it difficult to expose the cricoid cartilage and the muscular process of the arytenoid cartilage. Breaking down this scar tissue digitally and with scissors can produce bleeding that will fill the surgical field. Temporary pressure from sponges packed into the incision helps to reduce hemorrhage. Intraoperative suction is necessary in these cases. Usually the object of reoperation is to remove the original laryngoplasty suture and replace it with another suture (or sutures) that pulls the arytenoid cartilage into a more abducted position. If a surgery report describing the original surgery is not available, the surgeon should be aware that there may be more than one prosthetic suture. Although the suture is buried in scar tissue, the knot can usually be found caudal to the muscular process. The suture is cut and removed entirely. The scar tissue along the lateral and caudal surfaces of the muscular process must be incised with scissors to mobilize the arytenoid cartilage. This is accomplished using the points of Metzenbaum scissors with digital guidance. A laryngoplasty suture is then placed and tied as tightly as possible.[44]

Having a videoendoscope in place or having an assistant view the larynx with a fiberoptic endoscope allows the assessment of the position of the arytenoid cartilage after the prosthetic suture is tied[21,26] (Fig. 44-6). It is important to know if the arytenoid cartilage is pulled into a more abducted position. If the cartilage is elevated away from the endotracheal tube, then it is likely that the goal of improving abduction has been achieved. If not, it is likely that the reoperation attempt will fail. With this intraoperative knowledge, the surgeon can decide whether to place another suture to try and achieve greater abduction or whether to proceed with an arytenoidectomy.[21]

Prosthetic suture removal to correct aspiration

If over-abduction after laryngoplasty produces aspiration that necessitates reoperation, the original sutures can be removed. Another suture can be placed that fixes the arytenoid cartilage in a less abducted position after suture removal if the reoperation is performed within 2 weeks of the initial surgery. If the surgical site is mature (greater than 120 days) at the time of reoperation, simple removal of the sutures, without placing another suture, may be all that is necessary. If dissection around the muscular process during

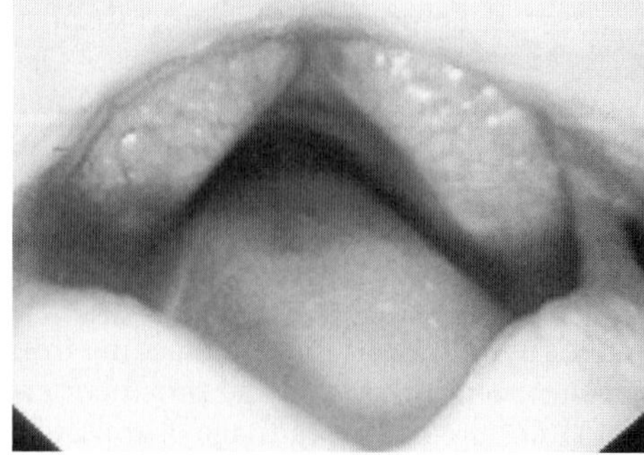

Figure 44-6. Endoscopic appearance of the arytenoid cartilages during laryngoplasty. The tracheal tube has been positioned in the rima glottidis through the mouth, and the displaced palate is seen ventrally. The space between the endotracheal tube and the left arytenoid cartilage indicates that the laryngoplasty position is adequate in the abducted position.

*References 16, 26, 38, 39, 42, 43.

suture removal is minimized, scar tissue around the muscular process usually holds the arytenoid in moderate abduction.

Special Considerations

A number of conditions that appear similar to but are separate entities from idiopathic left-sided laryngeal hemiplegia affect the prognosis for return to athletic activity and deserve discussion. They include vocal fold collapse, bilateral laryngeal hemiplegia, rostral displacement of the palatopharyngeal arch, and right-sided laryngeal hemiplegia.

Vocal Fold Collapse

Vocal fold collapse is a condition observed on videoendoscopy during high-speed exercise. It occasionally occurs in horses with grade 3 laryngeal movements (see Table 41-1). Rarely, it is observed in some horses after laryngoplasty when a concurrent ventriculectomy has not been performed. Clinical signs and history are similar to those of laryngeal hemiplegia. Diagnosis is confirmed on slow-motion playback of an exercising videoendoscopic examination (Fig. 44-7). Treatment for this condition is bilateral ventriculocordectomy (described later).

Bilateral Laryngeal Paralysis

Bilateral laryngeal paralysis has been associated with organophosphate toxicity and with central nervous system diseases such as equine protozoal myeloencephalitis (EPM).[7] Horses with bilateral arytenoid dysfunction usually show severe exercise intolerance with a minimal amount of exercise or stress. Some are in severe distress and make a loud inspiratory noise even at rest. Horses can die of respiratory collapse if a tracheostomy is not performed as an emergency procedure.

On endoscopic examination, there is reduced movement of both arytenoid cartilages. One arytenoid may be more severely affected than the other. Both guttural pouches should be examined endoscopically and, if the horse shows signs of ataxia, a cerebrospinal fluid tap should be performed for EPM testing.

Horses with bilateral laryngeal paralysis that is associated with a diagnosis of EPM can show improved laryngeal function after medical treatment for EPM. In horses that are in danger of asphyxiation, a temporary tracheostomy should be performed (see Chapter 46). In nonresponsive cases, a unilateral laryngoplasty and sacculectomy can be performed on the most severely affected side to salvage the horse for nonperformance activities, but aspiration can be severe because adductor function on the contralateral side may be compromised. Therefore, some estimate of adductor function should be made before unilateral laryngoplasty is undertaken. Bilateral laryngoplasty is not recommended and permanent tracheostomy should be considered.

Rostral Displacement of the Palatopharyngeal Arch

The term *rostral displacement of the palatopharyngeal arch* is used to describe a condition that is part of a complex of congenital pharyngeal and laryngeal abnormalities[45-48] (Fig. 44-8). The caudal margin of the ostium intrapharyngeum is displaced rostral to the corniculate processes of the arytenoid cartilages. It is commonly seen in conjunction with thyroid cartilage abnormalities and an absence of the cricopharyngeus muscles. The laminae of the thyroid cartilages are abnormally shaped and do not articulate normally with the cricoid cartilage. Often, the malformed laminae of the thyroid cartilages limit the normal range of movement of the arytenoid cartilages. Additionally, there can be a variety of intrinsic laryngeal muscle abnormalities. A developmental abnormality of the 4th branchial arch has been proposed as the cause of the anatomic abnormalities of the thyroid cartilage and the affected laryngeal muscles, which can be unilateral or bilateral. *Cricopharyngeal-laryngeal dysplasia* is a more inclusive term that has been proposed to better describe this syndrome.[48] Endoscopically, these horses can appear to have *right* laryngeal hemiplegia.

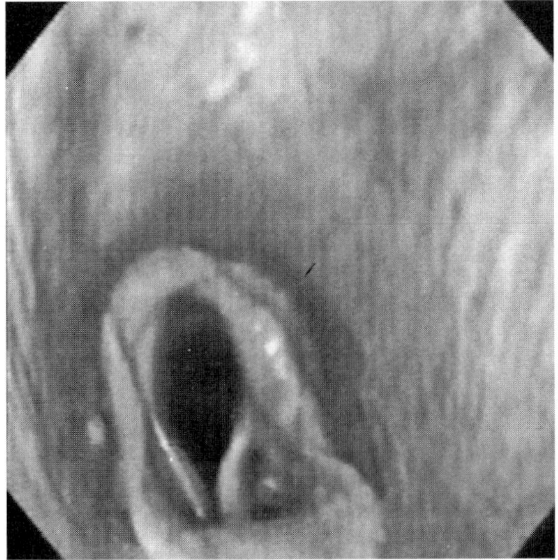

Figure 44-7. Videoendoscopic image (freeze-frame) of the larynx of a horse during exercise, demonstrating vocal fold collapse.

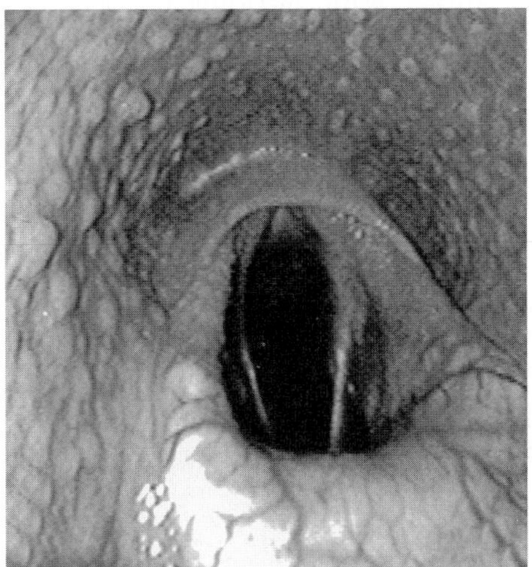

Figure 44-8. Videoendoscopic image of the larynx showing rostral displacement of the palatopharyngeal arch. The palatopharyngeal tissue is covering the apical portions of the corniculate processes, and both arytenoid cartilages show very limited abduction.

The effects of this syndrome are variable, depending on the degree of deformity present. Horses with a severe deformity show signs of respiratory obstruction and dysphagia at rest, whereas less severe deformities produce signs of upper airway obstruction only during exercise. Surgical treatment of this condition is usually unrewarding, but right arytenoidectomy can be considered.

Right-Sided Laryngeal Hemiplegia

Right-sided laryngeal hemiplegia is rare in horses, and an etiology should be sought, because the idiopathic form of laryngeal hemiplegia does not usually affect the right side. If none of the aforementioned causes can be detected, the surgeon should suspect congenital malformation of the laryngeal cartilages in young horses.[24] Palpation of the muscular process of the arytenoid cartilage is an important part of the physical examination. Additionally, endoscopically these horses appear as if the corniculate process of the arytenoid cartilage on the right side is much smaller than on the contralateral side. In a series of horses treated for right-sided laryngeal hemiplegia, 7 of 11 Thoroughbreds had congenital malformation of the laryngeal cartilages. This makes the rate of laryngoplasty failure in this group of horses very high, and partial arytenoidectomy may be selected as a treatment. Although spontaneous recovery from right-sided laryngeal hemiplegia has been reported, it would not be expected to be found in the young yearling to 2-year-old Thoroughbred. A poor prognosis should be given to the owner, and some consideration should be given to performing a neuromuscular pedicle graft. However, the author's personal experience is that right-sided laryngeal hemiplegic horses have a very guarded prognosis for return to athletic activity.

VENTRICULECTOMY (SACCULECTOMY)

Ventriculectomy (unilateral or bilateral) refers to the removal of the mucosal lining of the laryngeal ventricle located caudal to the vocal fold.[26] It is usually performed to eliminate noise and can have some beneficial effects on performance. Because it does not produce abduction of the arytenoid cartilage, ventriculectomy is not recommended as a sole procedure for racing horses affected with laryngeal hemiplegia.[26] However, it reduces soft tissue collapse during exercise and can be quite successful if performed on certain show horses. Because the complication rates of laryngoplasty (e.g., failure, anesthetic problems, coughing) approach 30% in draft horses, the author prefers to perform a bilateral ventriculectomy in the standing horse.[49]

The horse is placed in the stocks and sedated with loading doses of detomidine (4 mg IV) and butorphanol (10 mg IV). After starting a detomidine drip (14 mg added to 250 mL of saline) to effect (approximately 2 drops per second for 15 minutes, 1 drop per second for 15 minutes, and so on, as the effect is highly variable), the horse's head is elevated and the laryngotomy site is prepared. Local anesthetic is injected underneath the skin in the area of the laryngotomy approach (see Chapter 43). After the final preparation, a 10-cm incision is made on the ventral midline, centered over the junction of the horizontal and vertical rami of the mandible. The paired sternothyrohyoideus muscles are separated on the midline and the characteristic V in the thyroid cartilages is palpated. Laryngotomy is performed with a #10 scalpel blade. A burr is introduced into the ventricle to its depth and twisted, engaging the mucosa in the projections on the burr (Fig. 44-9, *A* and *B*). Occasionally, the ventricle is so large that it is necessary for the operator to press on the laminar portion of the arytenoid cartilage to enable the burr to engage the mucosa of these large saccules at their apex. The burr is then withdrawn slowly from the ventricle, everting the attached saccule. Swallowing usually occurs during this procedure and helps evert the saccule. A large hemostat is placed across the everted saccule proximal to the head of the burr (see Fig. 44-9, *C*), and with traction on the clamp, a second clamp is placed behind it. With digital pressure on the opening of the ventricle, the entire saccule is everted and then excised with Metzenbaum scissors (see Fig. 44-9, *D*). The same procedure is repeated on the opposite ventricle, which is allowed to heal along with the laryngotomy incision by second intention. The author now performs this procedure as an outpatient surgery.

Postoperative management

It is important that the horses receive loading doses of antibiotics any time the respiratory tract is invaded. Anti-inflammatory therapy is an important component of mini-

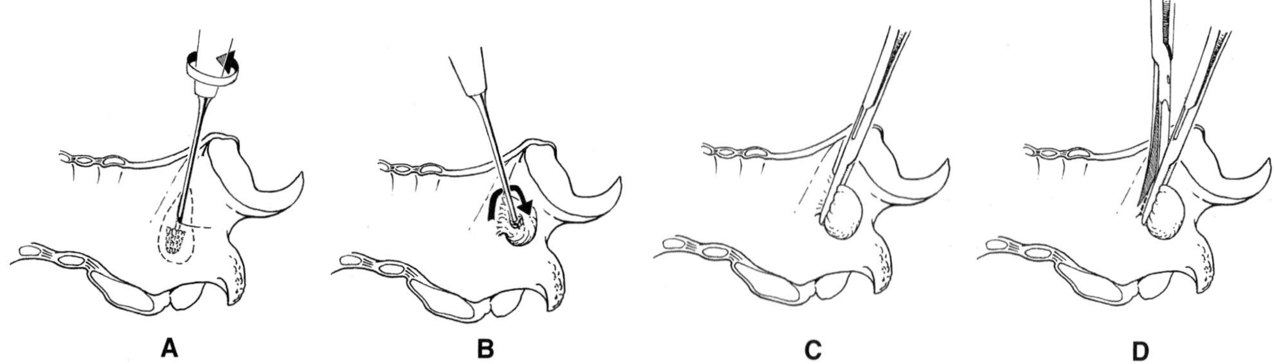

Figure 44-9. Schematic illustration of the ventriculectomy technique with the horse in dorsal recumbency. **A,** The "roaring" burr is placed into the laryngeal ventricle and rotated so that the head of the burr engages the mucosa of the laryngeal saccule. **B,** Once the saccule is firmly engaged, it is everted into the lumen of the larynx by steadily pulling on the burr. **C,** A large hemostat is placed across the saccule immediately adjacent to the vocal fold, and the burr is removed. **D,** The saccule is completely excised using Metzenbaum scissors adjacent to the hemostat.

mally invasive upper respiratory tract surgery. Phenylbutazone (4.4 mg/kg, IV) or flunixin meglumine (1.1 mg/kg, IV) is given immediately before surgery. Horses needing only minimal continued anti-inflammatory support are subsequently given phenylbutazone (2.2 mg/kg PO, twice a day for 7 days); alternatively, dexamethasone powder (0.022 mg/kg) is given orally once daily in the morning feed for 3 consecutive days, day 4 is skipped, and the same dosage is then given on the 5th postoperative day. If a longer course of corticosteroid therapy is deemed necessary, 0.9 mg/kg of prednisone is given orally starting the day after surgery once daily in the morning feed for 7 days. The same dosage is then given every other day for three treatments. The dosage is subsequently reduced to 0.45 mg/kg, given every other day for three treatments.

Topical administration of a pharyngeal medication, a mixture of nitrofurazone (Furacin) or pediatric trimethoprim sulfa (oral preparation), dimethyl sulfoxide, glycerin, and prednisolone also appears to be beneficial. A no. 10 French catheter is advanced along the floor of the nasal passage into the nasal pharynx, and 10 to 15 mL of the solution is sprayed slowly through this catheter at 12-hour intervals for 7 days. The horse is restricted to hand-walking exercise for the 1st week after surgery. After this time, an endoscopic reexamination is performed to assess wound healing and to determine if the horse can return to paddock exercise or if additional rest and anti-inflammatory medication are necessary. The horse should not be returned to training for 90 days.

VENTRICULOCORDECTOMY

Ventriculocordectomy refers to the removal of the mucosal lining of the laryngeal ventricle as described earlier, as well as to removal of a crescent-shaped wedge of tissue from the leading edge of the vocal fold. Again, because this technique does not produce abduction of the arytenoid cartilage, its use as a sole procedure for most racing horses with laryngeal hemiplegia running over long distances is not recommended. However, its use to reduce noise in sport horses has been established.[32] It has also been documented that there is some reduction in airway obstruction using this technique. Therefore, case selection could include the following:

- Sport horses with grade 4 laryngeal movements where the primary complaint is respiratory noise and exercise intolerance is not a feature (hunters and other show horses)
- Race horses with grade 3 laryngeal movements that do not experience arytenoid collapse during high-speed exercise but do experience vocal fold collapse
- Race horses that have had a laryngoplasty and still experience vocal fold collapse during high-speed exercise. (Caution must be used in performing a ventriculocordectomy in racehorses that have had a laryngoplasty where noise is a complaint, because noise cannot be correlated with upper airway obstruction.[34])

The horse is placed in dorsal recumbency with the head and neck extended. A laryngotomy is performed. The endotracheal tube can be removed if necessary to allow easier access to the ventricles, but usually this is not necessary. Ventriculectomy is performed as described earlier. A 2-cm-long and 2-mm-wide, crescent-shaped wedge of tissue is removed from the leading edge of the vocal fold. Using a continuous suture of 2-0 polydioxanone, the outside (abaxial edge of the vocal fold) and inside (axial) border of the ventricle are apposed. Suturing limits hemorrhage at the time of surgery while lessening cicatrix formation and redundant tissue folds as the surgery site heals. Therefore, it leaves a smooth surface over the ventral half of the rima glottidis. This is repeated on the other side. Preoperative and postoperative care is the same as that given for ventriculectomy via laryngotomy.

Complications

Inflammation and infection of the open laryngotomy incision rarely cause a problem that cannot be resolved by establishing good drainage followed by applying a topical antimicrobial ointment. A clostridial infection at the laryngotomy site, however, can be catastrophic or even fatal. Within a 24-hour period after surgery, a clostridial infection can produce tremendous swelling of the head and neck that results in a massive tissue slough. The use of perioperative penicillin may avoid such an infection, and if it does occur, early recognition and prompt treatment with intravenous penicillin is critical.

Rarely, excessive granulation tissue forms in the ventricles after sacculectomy. This problem usually resolves with time and the application of anti-inflammatory sprays.

Special Considerations

Attempts to develop a technique for laser ventriculocordectomy in standing horses have not been successful.[50] When a neodymium:yttrium aluminum garnet (Nd:YAG) laser was used in noncontact fashion via a nasal approach, or in contact fashion via an oral approach, viable mucosa of the ventricle remained after surgery, sometimes resulting in a mucocele. Additionally, although laser vocal cordectomy alone is used clinically, a recent study showed that laser vocal cordectomy does not effectively reduce the noise associated with laryngeal hemiplegia by 120 days after surgery.[33,51]

Therefore, refinements in surgical technique are required before laser ventriculocordectomy can be used with confidence to obviate noise production in horses affected with laryngeal hemiplegia.

NEUROMUSCULAR PEDICLE GRAFT

Young horses affected by laryngeal hemiplegia and horses with grade 3 laryngeal movements are good candidates for laryngeal reinnervation.[52] The technique involves implantation of a nerve–muscle pedicle (NMP) graft into the cricoarytenoideus dorsalis (CAD) muscle. The 1st cervical nerve and omohyoideus muscle are used to make the NMP graft because of their proximity to the larynx. Additionally, the 1st cervical nerve is used because it depolarizes during inspiration and therefore causes abduction of the CAD muscle after reinnervation.

The patient is prepared as if for laryngoplasty, because the surgical approach is very similar. Antimicrobial and anti-inflammatory medications are instituted as for other laryngeal surgeries. Surgical instruments should include small thumb forceps, a spay hook, and small Weitlaner self-retaining retractors in addition to the instruments used for laryngeal surgery.

The horse is placed in right lateral recumbency under general anesthesia, and the head and neck are positioned for an approach for laryngoplasty. A 12-cm linear incision is made along the ventral border of the linguofacial vein that is carefully separated from the omohyoideus muscle. The 1st cervical nerve lies just under a branch of the linguofacial vein that is positioned midway between the rostral and caudal aspects of the incision. The ventral branch of the 1st cervical nerve emerges through the alar foramen of the atlas, and it descends over the cricopharyngeal muscle caudal to the larynx before dividing and entering the omohyoideus muscle (Fig. 44-10, *A*). This nerve is commonly encountered during dissection for laryngoplasty and can be traced from the atlas to the omohyoideus muscle. The main body of the 1st cervical nerve is identified, and ventral retraction of the omohyoideus muscle is achieved with Allis tissue forceps. Insertions of the 1st cervical nerve can be found in the dorsal aspect of the muscle belly (see Fig. 44-10, *B*). Meticulous dissection is necessary to expose several branches of the 1st cervical nerve as they enter the omohyoideus muscle. A middle branch of the 1st cervical nerve often divides into smaller branches and can be traced to a point of muscle entry, allowing creation of the muscle pedicles. The main branch of the 1st cervical nerve is gently retracted using a spay hook and is freed from its fascial attachments on the caudal aspect of the larynx. When harvesting the muscle pedicles, sterile mepivacaine hydrochloride is used to bathe the area so that muscles do not contract during harvesting. Nerve branches that do not end in the omohyoideus muscle are transected and can be used as branches to be directly

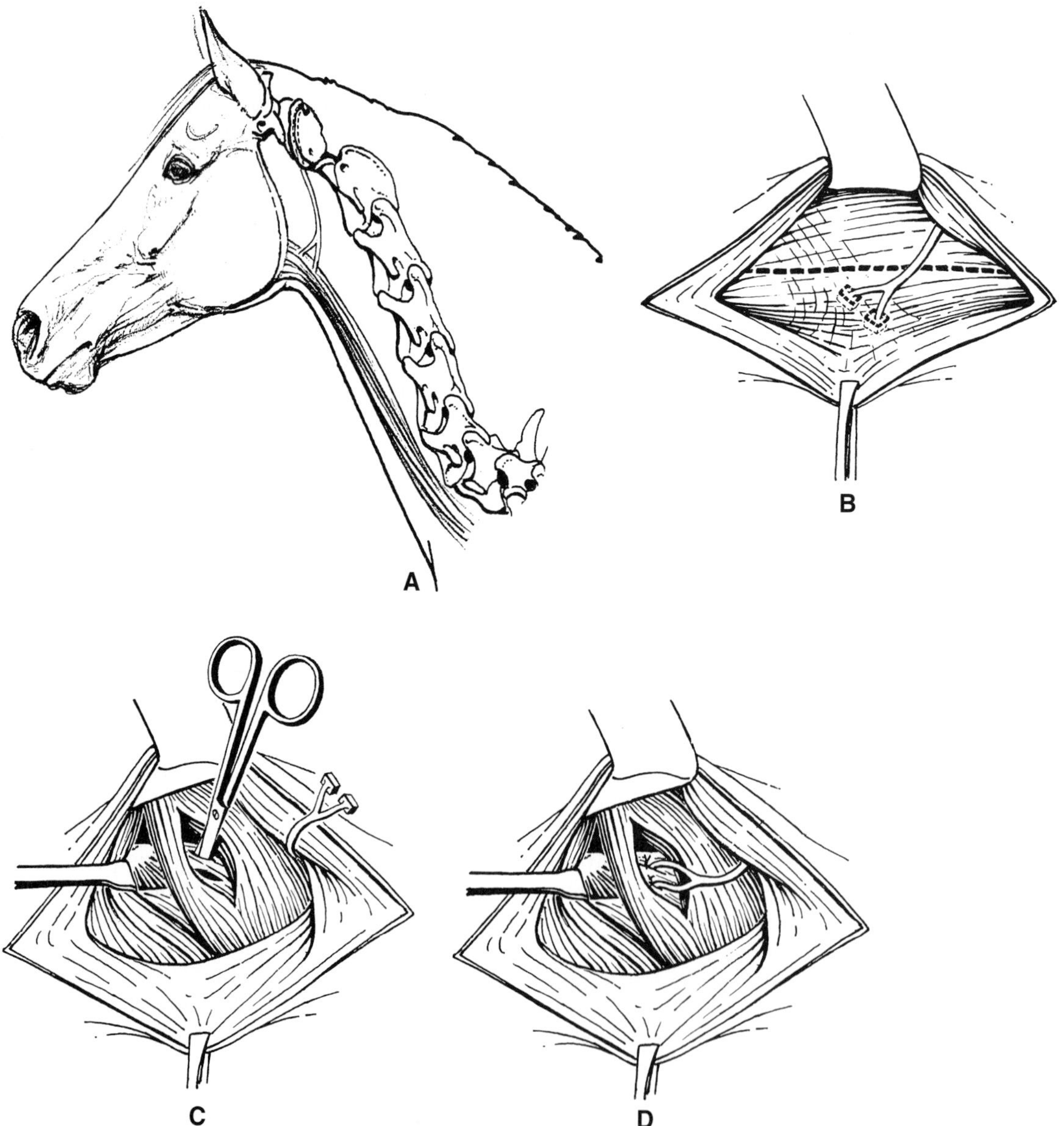

Figure 44-10. Schematic illustration of the neuromuscular pedicle graft technique. **A,** The origin and insertion of the 1st cervical nerve into the omohyoideus muscle is shown. (This nerve and muscle serve as the neuromuscular pedicle graft donors for treatment of laryngeal hemiplegia.) **B,** The 1st cervical nerve and future pedicle grafts of the omohyoideus muscle, which has been retracted with Allis tissue forceps. **C,** The muscular process of the arytenoid cartilage and the exposed cricoarytenoideus dorsalis muscle, and small scissors separating the CAD muscle fibers to create pockets for placement of the muscle pedicle graft. **D,** The nerve muscle pedicle graft implanted into the CAD muscle.

implanted into the CAD muscle. The NMPs are created with fine scissors and are about 3 mm square.

The larynx is then rotated laterally by traction on the wing of the thyroid cartilage. The cricopharyngeus and thyropharyngeus muscles are separated along their aponeurosis. The CAD muscle is bluntly exposed and inspected for donor site access. Then blunt separation of the cricopharyngeus muscle over the area just caudal to the muscular process exposes the CAD muscle. The window over the CAD muscle is maintained using a Weitlaner retractor. By separation of CAD muscle fibers, pockets are created and the pedicles are placed into the CAD muscle (see Fig. 44-10, *C*). Each muscle pedicle or nerve branch is sutured into a pocket using 4-0 polydioxanone (see Fig. 44-10, *D*). Closure of the incision is routine.

Horses are confined to a stall for 2 to 3 weeks after surgery until sutures are removed and inflammation has subsided. Perioperative antibiotic therapy and anti-inflammatory medications are continued for 3 to 4 days after surgery.

After stall confinement, the horse receives paddock turnout for 12 weeks. At this stage (16 weeks after surgery), the horse is put into training. This time frame is based on information from studies on dogs,[53] people,[54] and horses,[55,56] which indicates that the earliest time to see clinical evidence of reinnervation is around 12 weeks after surgery. When the horses are returned to exercise, episodes of fast exercise should be introduced as early and as frequently as possible. Because the omohyoideus muscle is an accessory muscle of respiration, considerable respiratory effort must be undertaken to activate the 1st cervical nerve.

After 6 weeks of training, trainers and owners are requested to present the horse for endoscopic assessment of the larynx. At rest, the left arytenoid cartilage most commonly looks exactly as it did before surgery. This is because the 1st cervical nerve is inactive at rest; thus, there is no depolarization of the nerve and no CAD muscle contraction. Two diagnostic reflexes have been developed to stimulate contraction of the omohyoideus muscle and the newly innervated CAD muscle.[52] The first involves stretching the horse's head and neck upward as high as possible while closely observing the larynx through the endoscope. If reinnervation has occurred, there is often a spontaneous flicker or single abduction of the left arytenoid cartilage. The second reflex involves pulling back rapidly with a finger or thumb on the commissure of the horse's lips. Again, a sudden abduction of the left arytenoid cartilage occurs if reinnervation has been successful. This reflex can be stimulated from the left or right side of the head.

An abductor movement of the left arytenoid cartilage indicates there has been reinnervation of the CAD muscle. Once this has been identified, the recommendation to the trainer is to continue training toward a return to racing. If there is no evidence of movement at the first revisit, the horse is turned out again for another 8 weeks, receives 6 weeks of training, and is reexamined. Horses can take up to 12 months to show evidence of successful reinnervation.[55] Clinical experience suggests that if there is no arytenoid abduction as a result of reinnervation 9 months after surgery, there is only a small chance of improvement from that point. Reinnervation probably occurs in nearly all patients by 4 to 5 months.

The best evidence of successful reinnervation in an individual horse is derived from a treadmill endoscopic or upper airway flow mechanics study. In treadmill studies, the authors have found that those horses with movement of the left arytenoid cartilage visible at rest after NMP graft surgery maintained arytenoid abduction during vigorous exercise.[55] If movement in the affected arytenoid could not be demonstrated in the standing horse, a dynamic collapse occurred during exercise.

Complications

Complications associated with laryngeal reinnervation are few when compared with prosthetic laryngoplasty. The most frequent complication is seroma formation 3 to 5 days after surgery. The large potential dead space that exists after the nerve graft procedure lends itself to the formation of a seroma. In the author's opinion, many of the seromas that form are caused by leaking lymphatic vessels that are inadvertently cut during surgery. Large lymph vessels travel along the lateral border of the omohyoideus muscle and can be transected during the surgical approach. Disruption of the parotid salivary gland has the potential to produce large volumes of fluid continually for a number of days after surgery. Some of these seromas have resolved without intervention. Treatment of other seromas and sialoceles has involved open drainage and daily lavage. The horses have been placed on procaine penicillin therapy until the open tract discontinues draining. Some sinus tracts have become infected, and these have been treated with antibiotics selected from culture and sensitivity results. Because of the ventral position of the incision, once opened, the seroma and sialoceles drain easily and require minimal nursing care apart from daily lavage and attention to the skin around the incision. Horses that have suffered a postoperative incisional infection have gone on to have successful reinnervation; thus, it would seem that this complication does not necessarily compromise success of the NMP graft.[52]

Prognosis

From experimental and clinical work, it is clear that reinnervation of the CAD muscle following an NMP graft varies from 6 to 12 months depending on the amount of CAD muscle atrophy.[55-57] Therefore, horses with grade 3 laryngeal movements will respond sooner (in 4 to 6 months) than those that have grade 4 movements (complete paralysis).[57] Because of the length of this time period, horses that are best suited for the transplantation technique are those whose immediate return to performance is not necessary. Horses that have had previous laryngoplasty for the treatment of laryngeal hemiplegia are not candidates for this surgery because of disruption of the 1st cervical nerve during that surgery. To date, over 140 horses have received NMP grafts for idiopathic laryngeal hemiplegia. Following race records in these Thoroughbreds, 60% have shown improved performance, whereas 80% have been considered a successful reinnervation. NMP grafting has allowed horses to compete successfully, and laryngeal function improves with time. Current success rate is on a parity to that of prosthetic laryngoplasty. For young horses who have never been raced and horses of high value because of their breeding potential, the NMP graft can be offered as a viable treatment for laryngeal hemiplegia. If the result of NMP grafting is unsatisfactory, a laryngoplasty may still be performed.

Arytenoid Chondritis

Arytenoid chondritis is a progressive inflammatory process of the laminar portion of the arytenoid cartilage and results in a space-occupying mass within the larynx that produces respiratory noise and exercise intolerance.[26] Because the history and endoscopic appearance of arytenoid chondritis in the standing horse is similar to that of laryngeal hemiplegia, it should always be considered in the differential diagnosis. Careful endoscopic examination is sometimes necessary to detect the hallmark sign of chondritis: a small sinus tract or granulation tissue that protrudes into the airway from the affected arytenoid (Fig. 44-11). Additionally, the corniculate cartilage is usually distorted and frequently causes mild rostral displacement of the palatopharyngeal arch (Fig. 44-12). Occasionally, palpation of the larynx for thickening around the muscular process is the only diagnostic finding.

In the acute form, horses may be presented in respiratory distress from laryngeal edema. These horses are usually treated with antimicrobials and anti-inflammatories, but occasionally they need a tracheotomy to resolve the acute condition. Medical treatment will resolve the emergency and the condition may not return. In fact, some horses remain with chronic arytenoid chondritis and perform quite well if the abnormal arytenoid cartilage does not result in residual laryngeal obstruction. However, if there is mechanical obstruction to abduction or the laminar portion of the arytenoid cartilage is thickened sufficiently when in the chronic form, surgical removal of the affected arytenoid cartilage is usually necessary. This condition is most often unilateral and therefore treated with unilateral arytenoidectomy.

ARYTENOIDECTOMY

Preparation of the patient should include broad-spectrum antimicrobial therapy and anti-inflammatory medication. The skin should be clipped and prepared for a laryngotomy approach (see Chapter 43) as should the mid-neck region in preparation for placement of a tracheostomy tube. If the horse has bilateral arytenoid chondritis or is dyspneic, the tube can be placed before induction of general anesthesia using local anesthetic under sedation. The author prefers this approach because often the placement of an endotracheal tube through a chondritic larynx is difficult or impossible.

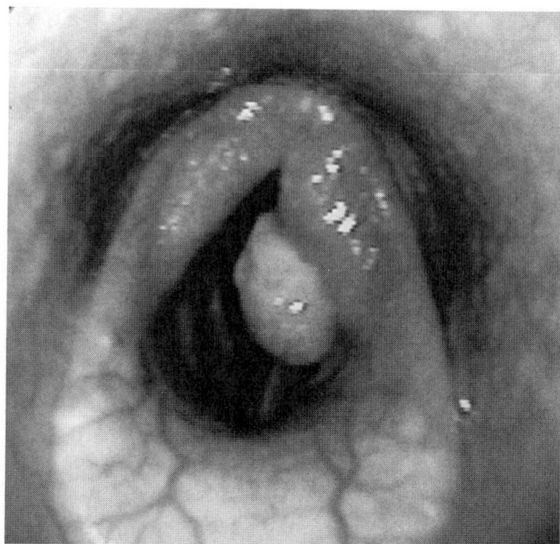

Figure 44-11. Endoscopic appearance of arytenoid chondropathy, showing incomplete abduction on the left side and granulation tissue on the medial surface of the arytenoid at the entrance to a fistula.

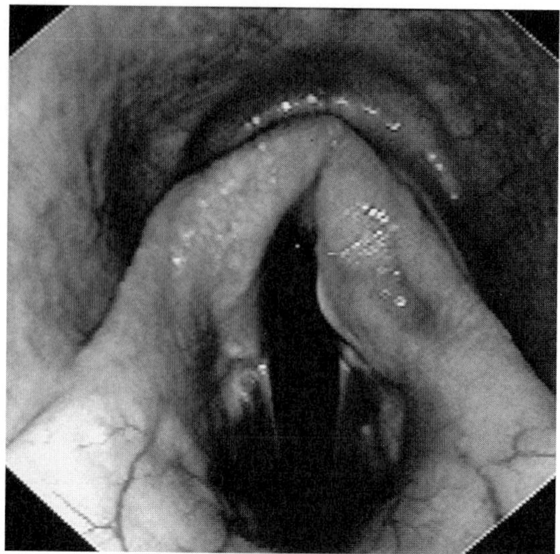

Figure 44-12. Videoendoscopic appearance of the rima glottis of a horse with arytenoid chondritis that shows distortion of the left arytenoid cartilage. The corniculate cartilage is in an abnormally abducted position, often making this condition look like laryngeal hemiplegia or hemiparesis early in the disease process.

Two methods of arytenoidectomy have been described[58,59]: *subtotal*, in which the muscular process and rim of the corniculate process are left intact, and *partial*, in which only the muscular process is left intact (Fig. 44-13). The merits of subtotal and partial arytenoidectomy have been evaluated subjectively on the basis of the assessment of performance and postoperative complications in a series of retrospective studies.[58,60,61] However, in a quantitative evaluation in 1990,[62] it was demonstrated that *subtotal* arytenoidectomy failed to improve upper airway function in horses exercising on a high-speed treadmill with surgically induced left laryngeal hemiplegia. The effect of *partial* arytenoidectomy on upper airway function was evaluated by tidal breathing flow-volume analysis, measurement of upper airway impedance, and videoendoscopic examination of the larynx in strenuously exercising horses with surgically induced left

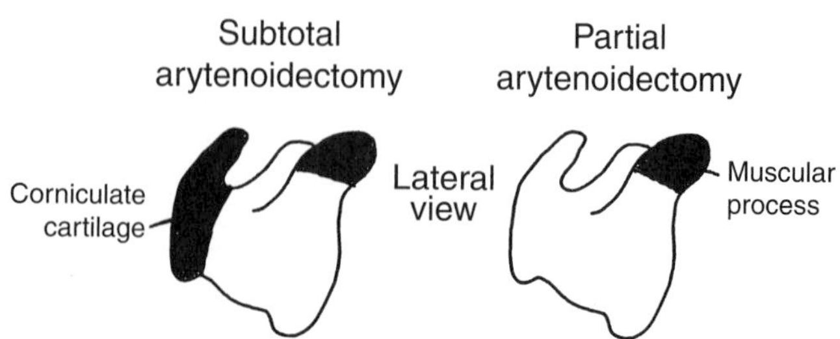

Figure 44-13. Schematic representation of a lateral view of the arytenoid cartilage, demonstrating the portions of the cartilage that are removed *(unshaded)* during subtotal and partial arytenoidectomy.

laryngeal hemiplegia in 1994.[63] This study showed that *partial* arytenoidectomy improved upper airway function in exercising horses with surgically induced left laryngeal hemiplegia and was superior to *subtotal* arytenoidectomy as a treatment for both failed laryngoplasty and arytenoid chondropathy.

The authors recommend combining a partial arytenoidectomy with a ventriculocordectomy and closing the entire incision in such a way that no redundant or loose tissue is left in the airway and all excised mucosal edges are apposed. In the author's experience, any redundant tissue left in the airway creates turbulence and noise and may interfere with airway function. This tissue should be removed at 30 days after surgery via laser ablation before cicatrix formation and mineralization make it impossible. Tidal breathing flow-volume loop analysis shows that partial arytenoidectomy does not completely restore the upper airway to normal,[63] but that the procedure is a viable treatment option for arytenoid cartilage malfunction in the horse. A detailed description of the technique for partial arytenoidectomy follows.

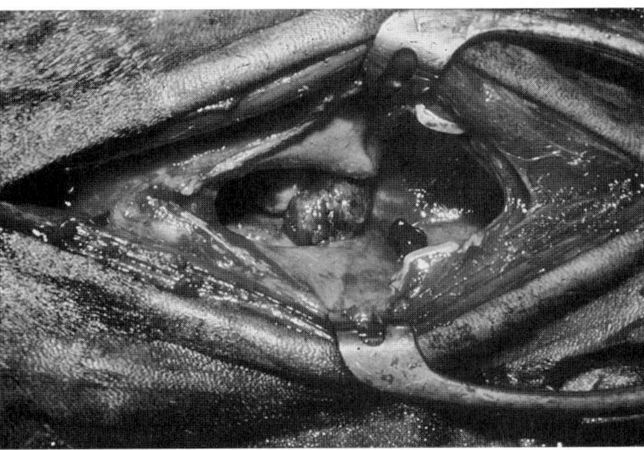

Figure 44-15. After laryngotomy, it is common to find granulomatous masses observed on the affected arytenoid cartilage when a horse is affected with arytenoid chondropathy. Self-retaining retractors provide good access for arytenoidectomy.

PARTIAL ARYTENOIDECTOMY

Horses are placed in dorsal recumbency under general anesthesia with an endotracheal tube placed through a tracheotomy incision (Fig. 44-14). After an approach through a ventral laryngotomy incision, granulomatous masses are often observed on the affected arytenoid cartilage (Fig. 44-15). Self-retaining retractors are used to maintain exposure and allow easy access to the lumen of the larynx. The corniculate cartilage is removed en bloc with its mucosa (Fig. 44-16, *A*). The arytenoid cartilage is exposed by scalpel incision of the overlying mucosa (see Fig. 44-16, *B*). The incision, which extends from the dorsal midline to the vocal process, is made along the caudal border of the laminar portion of the arytenoid cartilage and continued craniad along its ventral border. The mucosa is elevated from the underlying cartilage with a periosteal elevator and reflected cranially and caudally to expose the full medial surface of the arytenoid cartilage. The laminar portion of the arytenoid cartilage is then freed from its deep muscular attachments using a periosteal elevator and Mayo scissors. The remaining arytenoid cartilage is subsequently severed from its muscular process, transected at its articulation with the thyroid cartilage, and removed (see Fig. 44-16, *C*). A ventriculocordectomy is then performed, excess mucosa is excised, and all combined incisions are closed in a simple continuous suture pattern (see Fig. 44-16, *D*). During closure, the surgeon should take care to smooth the airway as much as possible by removing all redundant tissue. The laryngotomy is left unsutured because of the possibility of laryngeal edema and subsequent airway obstruction.

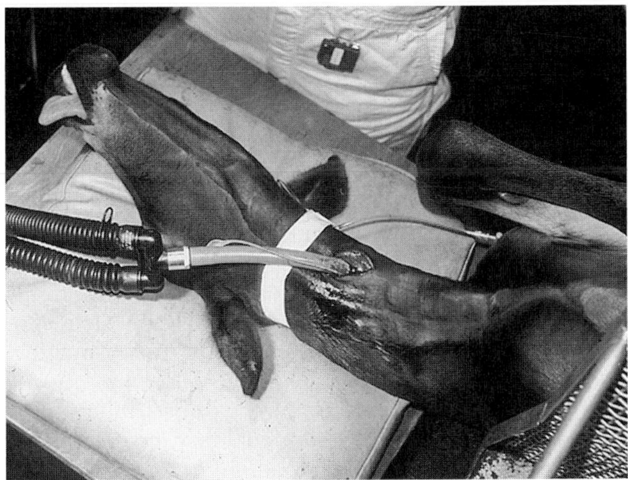

Figure 44-14. Preparation of a foal for arytenoidectomy shows an endotracheal tube placed through a tracheotomy incision located distal to the larynx.

Antimicrobial agents such as penicillin and gentamicin, as well as anti-inflammatory drugs such as phenylbutazone, are administered before surgery and continued for at least 3 days after surgery. A tracheostomy tube should be removed and cleaned twice daily and used until there is endoscopic evidence that the edema in the laryngeal region has subsided. Postoperative endoscopic evaluations should reveal a hemilarynx devoid of vocal folds, ventricle, and corniculate cartilage (Fig. 44-17). Airway patency may also be assessed by plugging the endotracheal tube and listening for respiratory stridor. Horses are reintroduced to food 24 hours after surgery. At that time, wet hay only should be fed until the horses are able to swallow without coughing; then dry feedstuffs can be reintroduced. Horses are stall-rested for 4 to 6 weeks prior to complete healing, which usually occurs within 8 to 10 weeks.

Complications

Dyspnea and dysphagia are the most important complications. Dyspnea frequently occurs as the result of edema or the development of bleeding under the closed mucosa of the larynx. Therefore, the tracheostomy tube should be left in place until airway patency is confirmed. Antimicrobial and anti-inflammatory medications are continued until dyspnea is resolved, and then the tracheostomy tube is removed. Dysphagia may take longer to resolve. Coughing during eating is not uncommon and may continue for some months. Occasionally, large amounts of food and water may be regurgitated through the nose after this procedure. Aspiration is another complication that may occur, and it too may improve with time. Owners are encouraged to feed

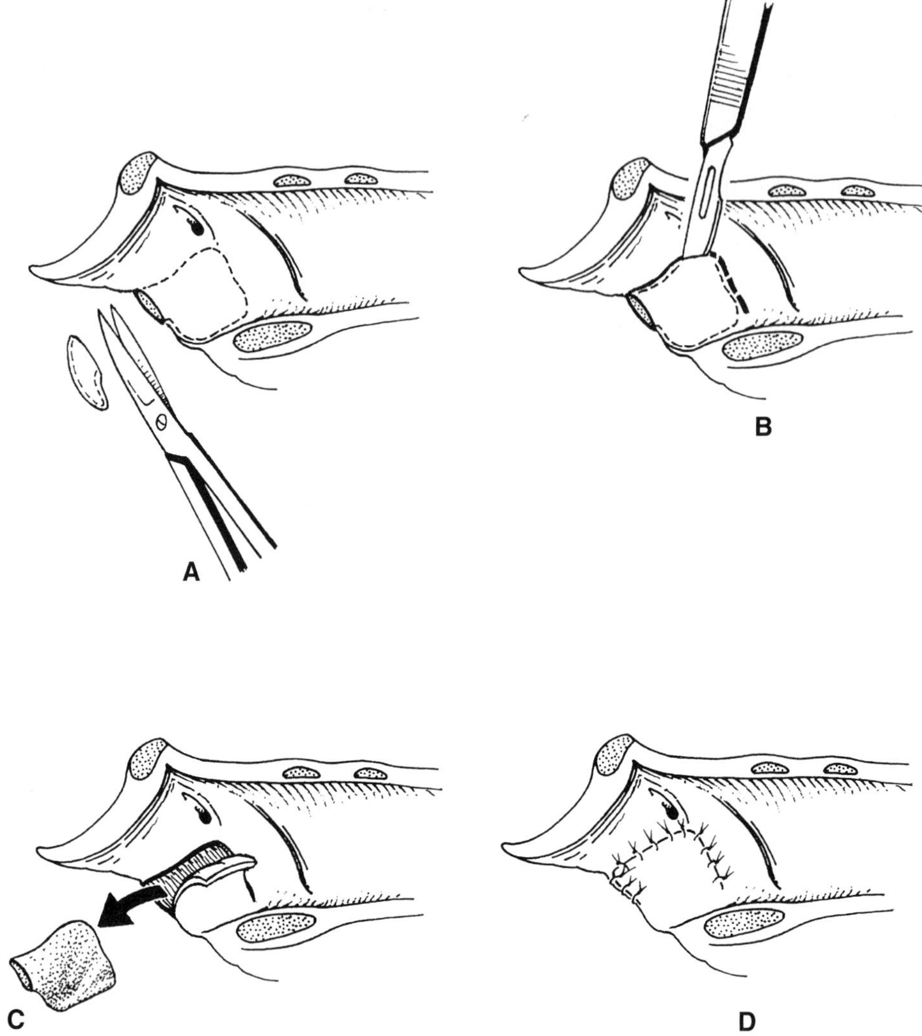

Figure 44-16. Schematic illustration of partial arytenoidectomy technique. **A,** The corniculate cartilage is separated from the arytenoid cartilage with Metzenbaum scissors and removed. (The arytenoid cartilage is outlined by the *dotted line.*) **B,** Beginning at the ventral border of the junction of the corniculate and arytenoid cartilages, an incision is made through the mucosa along the ventral border of the arytenoid cartilage *(heavy dark line)*. The incision is carried dorsally along the caudal border of the laminar portion of the arytenoid. **C,** The mucosa is elevated from the arytenoid cartilage using a periosteal elevator, which exposes the laminar portion of this cartilage. The cartilage is then freed from its deep attachments in a similar fashion. After transection of the muscular process with heavy scissors or a scalpel, the arytenoid cartilage is disarticulated from the thyroid cartilage and removed. Then the ventricle and vocal fold are removed. **D,** The mucosa is completely apposed using a simple continuous or interrupted sutures of 2-0 polydioxanone, taking care to remove any redundant tissue during closure.

the animal on the ground, and pasture feeding may be beneficial.

Granulomas

Occasionally, particularly in Thoroughbred and Standardbred racehorses, a mass projecting from the medial surface of the corniculate process of the arytenoid is seen on endoscopic examination. These lesions are commonly referred to as chondromas; however, histologic examination of the excised tissue invariably reveals granulation tissue.[64] An ulcerated mucosal defect is often seen on the medial surface of the opposing arytenoid where the granulation tissue rubs during laryngeal adduction. However, in a recent survey of 3312 Thoroughbred sale yearlings, the incidence of arytenoid mucosal ulceration was encountered in 21, and only a small percentage progressed to granulomas or chondromas.[65] Ventriculectomy with focal curettage or laser ablation of these lesions has been advocated for some patients to avoid arytenoidectomy.

Transendoscopic laser excision of this granulation tissue without removal of cartilage may be a desirable method of treatment, particularly if the underlying arytenoid cartilage appears grossly normal or is only mildly thickened, and if the arytenoid cartilage has a normal or only mildly affected range of motion.[64] Excision of the granulation tissue does not alter any preexisting underlying cartilage abnormalities, but it is carried out in an attempt to allow the mucosal defect to epithelialize and to prevent contact injury to the opposing arytenoid. This technique may be temporarily successful when combined with antibiotic and anti-inflammatory therapy in some performance horses and many sedentary patients. However, when dealing with an equine athlete, arytenoidectomy is usually required eventually.

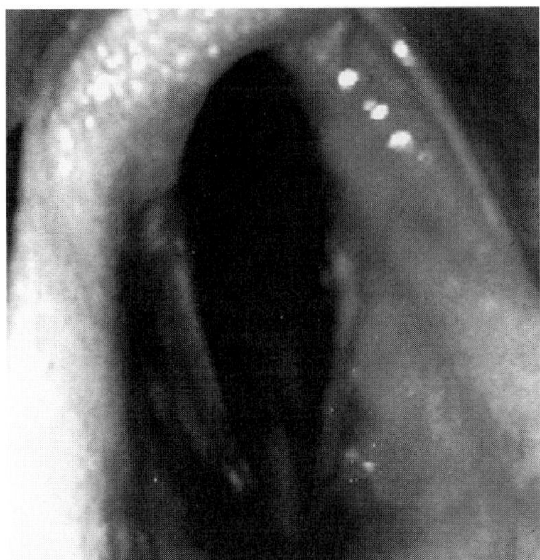

Figure 44-17. Videoendoscopic view of the rima glottidis of a horse 4 weeks after left partial arytenoidectomy and ventriculochordectomy. Note that all redundant tissue has been removed from this airway.

The horse is sedated and the lesion and surrounding tissue are transendoscopically topically anesthetized. Using an Nd:YAG laser, a 2.2-mm-outer-diameter laser fiber with a chisel probe attached or an 800-μm sculpted fiber is introduced through the endoscope biopsy channel. A diode laser with a sculpted fiber can also be used. When using the chisel probe, the beveled surface is oriented parallel to the medial mucosal surface of the arytenoid. Beginning at the perimeter of the mass, a dissection plane is established between the granulation tissue and the underlying cartilage. The mass is completely freed up except for small remaining tags of attachment, and it is retrieved with 600-mm-long bronchoesophagoscopic grasping forceps. Any remaining small tags of loose tissue are subsequently débrided with the laser and removed with the forceps. Usually, a crater defect has been created with smooth mucosal margins that are firmly attached to underlying cartilage.

Exercise is restricted until the defect heals. Systemic nonsteroidal anti-inflammatory medication and a pharyngeal spray containing anti-inflammatory and antimicrobial medications may be useful in reducing inflammation.

EPIGLOTTIS

The epiglottis is an isosceles triangle–shaped structure with the tip projecting rostrally. It forms the floor of the entrance to the larynx. During normal breathing, the soft palate is positioned ventral to the epiglottis, with the free edge of the palate interfacing with the epiglottic base. The epiglottis is covered dorsally by a tightly adherent mucous membrane and ventrally by a loosely attached, somewhat redundant mucosa. The loosely folded ventral mucosa allows unrestricted dorsal and caudal movement of the epiglottis during swallowing. Endoscopically, the normal epiglottis is broad at the base, it narrows at the tip, and it has a dorsally convex surface that projects slightly above and parallel to the soft palate. The margins have distinct round serrations. The normal vascular pattern seen on the dorsal surface consists of a main vessel on either side that courses from the base toward the tip, parallel to and in from the margin approximately 8 to 10 mm (see Fig. 44-1). From these two major vessels, small perpendicular branches are seen coursing toward the epiglottic margin.

Epiglottic Entrapment

The aryepiglottic folds are thickened bands of mucous membrane that attach along the entire free edge of the epiglottis, blending in with the tightly adherent dorsal epiglottic mucosa and the mucosa covering the corniculate process of the arytenoid cartilage.[66] Ventral to the epiglottis, the mucosa is more loosely attached and compresses in accordion fashion when the horse is breathing normally with the epiglottis in a resting horizontal position. Epiglottic entrapment occurs when this loose mucous membrane located on the lingual epiglottic surface becomes abnormally positioned above the dorsal epiglottic surface. Epiglottic entrapment is a common cause of abnormal respiratory noise and exercise intolerance, particularly in Thoroughbred and Standardbred racehorses.[67-73] Other, much less frequent complaints are coughing and nasal exudate. Occasionally, epiglottic entrapment is an incidental endoscopic finding.

Diagnosis

On endoscopic examination, the general shape of the epiglottis is still visible, positioned above the soft palate (Fig. 44-18). However, because the epiglottis is covered with a fold of mucosa, the distinct serrated margins of the epiglottis and the dorsal epiglottic vascular pattern are obscured. The entrapping membranes may occasionally be intermittently relieved by swallowing, but in most cases they are persistent (Fig. 44-19). On the basis of subjective endoscopic observations, the entrapping membranes may be classified as being thin or thick, narrow (less than half the length of the epiglottis) or wide (greater than half the length of the epiglottis), and ulcerated or nonulcerated (Fig. 44-20). Mucosal ulceration can vary from minimal to extensive, with variable amounts of exposed granulation tissue and pale fibrous connective tissue proliferation around the

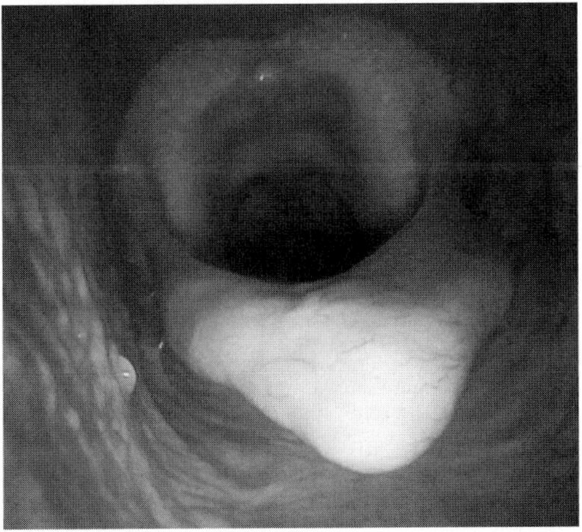

Figure 44-18. Endoscopic appearance of epiglottic entrapment showing a thin entrapping membrane where the outline of the epiglottis is still visible. (Courtesy M. Weishaupt, Zurich.)

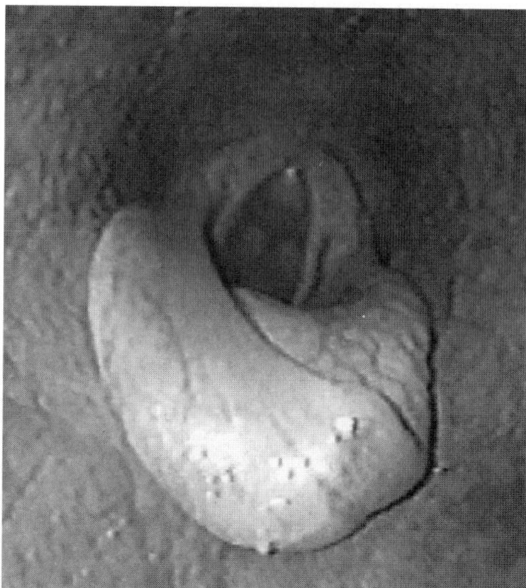

Figure 44-19. Endoscopic appearance of epiglottic entrapment where the fold partially entraps the epiglottis and is intermittently relieved by swallowing. (Courtesy J. Robertson, Ohio.)

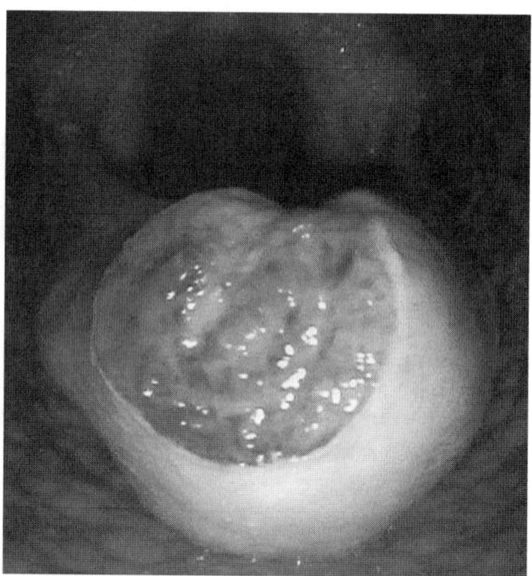

Figure 44-20 Ulcerated epiglottic entrapment in a Thoroughbred racehorse. (Courtesy M. Weishaupt, Zurich.)

perimeter of the ulcer (Fig. 44-21). Most epiglottic entrapments (97%) are persistent, most (98%) are thick, most (97%) are wide, and 45% are ulcerated.[67]

Horses with epiglottic entrapment may also suffer from varying degrees of epiglottic hypoplasia/flaccidity. On endoscopic examination, approximately 31% to 36% of horses with entrapment appear to have epiglottic hypoplasia.[67,71,74] Lateral laryngeal radiography is used to obtain accurate thyroepiglottic length and information about epiglottic thickness and contour. In one study of 9 Thoroughbreds with epiglottic entrapment, the thyroepiglottic length was 6.59 ± 0.33 cm,[75] and in another study of 35 Thoroughbreds it was 7.28 ± 0.67 cm.[74] Both measurements were significantly smaller than the thyroepiglottic length found in normal Thoroughbreds without entrapment,

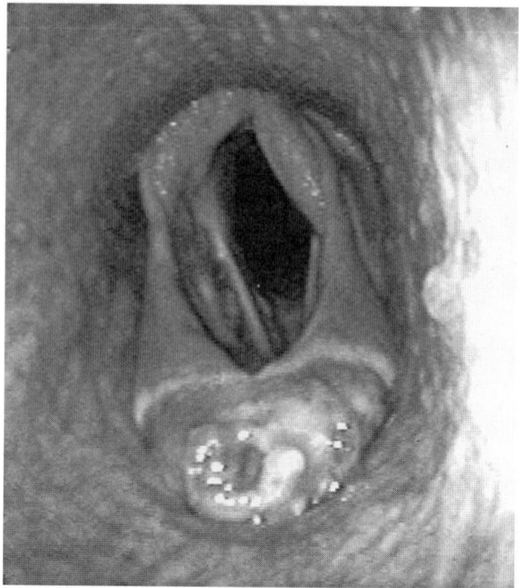

Figure 44-21. Endoscopic appearance of epiglottic entrapment with severe mucosal ulceration, showing exposed granulation tissue and pale fibrinous connective tissue proliferation around the perimeter of the ulcer.

which in two studies was 8.76 ± 0.38 cm and 8.56 ± 0.29 cm.[1,74] The thyroepiglottic length in 44 Standardbreds with entrapment was 7.21 ± 0.62 cm, which was also significantly smaller than the thyroepiglottic length of 8.74 ± 0.38 cm found in normal Standardbreds.[74] Among all Standardbred and Thoroughbred horses with epiglottic entrapment, those that also had endoscopically apparent epiglottic hypoplasia had significantly smaller thyroepiglottic lengths than horses with entrapment that appeared endoscopically normal.[74]

Treatment

Surgical correction of epiglottic entrapment has been described using transendoscopic contact Nd:YAG or diode laser axial division,[67,73] transnasal or transoral axial division using a curved bistoury,[68-71] transendoscopic electrosurgical axial division,[72] or surgical excision through a laryngotomy or a pharyngotomy.[66,69,71]

At one time, conventional side-to-side excision of the aryepiglottic folds performed through a laryngotomy was recommended[66]; however, dorsal displacement of the soft palate was a common sequela to this technique.[72] Currently, tissue-sparing techniques that preserve aryepiglottic fold mucosa and minimize scarring are preferred, in part because of the variable extent of underlying epiglottic hypoplasia found in many horses with epiglottic entrapment. Therefore, axial midline division of the aryepiglottic fold that allows the entrapping membranes to retract and heal in a normal ventral epiglottic position without removing any tissue is currently the technique of choice in most horses. The membranes can be divided with an Nd:YAG, a holmium:YAG, or a diode laser; a curved bistoury; or electrocautery, producing essentially the same effect.

With the laser, surgery can be safely performed transendoscopically on an outpatient basis with the horse standing sedated and the entrapping membranes topically anesthetized. Using the Nd:YAG laser as an example, a 600-μm sculpted fiber can be used to incise the membranes from caudal to rostral in contact fashion using approximately 12 W of power. Alternatively, a contact chisel probe attached to a 2.2-mm-outer-diameter fiber can be used to divide the membranes from rostral to caudal with 15 W of power. Using these two techniques, the re-entrapment rate in a series of over 500 cases was approximately 4%, and approximately 10% to 15% of horses experienced dorsal displacement of the soft palate.

Using a curved bistoury introduced either transnasally in the standing horse or transorally in the anesthetized horse (Fig. 44-22), the entrapping membranes can be incised on the midline from caudal to rostral. The reported re-entrapment rate ranges from 5% to 15%.[68-71] However, serious complications after *transnasal* axial division using a curved bistoury on conscious horses includes division of the soft palate and lacerations of the epiglottis or pharynx. Therefore, this technique is not recommended. Inadvertent incision of the soft palate can be avoided by performing the hook technique *through the mouth* with the horse anesthetized. The re-entrapment rate after transoral hook correction is approximately 10%, and approximately 10% of horses experienced dorsal displacement of the soft palate.[69-71] Transendoscopic electrosurgical division has the highest complication rate of the axial division techniques (in a series of five horses, it resulted in a 40% re-entrapment rate), and it has fallen into disuse.

Special Considerations

Excessively thickened, ulcerated, or fibrotic-appearing entrapping membranes are seen in approximately 5% of horses with epiglottic entrapment, and usually this condition is combined with severe epiglottic hypoplasia (Fig. 44-23). Horses with this endoscopic appearance are generally poor candidates for correction by axial division. Surgical excision of the central one third of these bulky membranes is recommended and can be performed through a laryngotomy, with the horse anesthetized and positioned in dorsal recumbency. Through the laryngotomy, the epiglottis is retroverted into view by placing traction on the aryepiglottic fold tissue with sponge or Allis tissue forceps. Applying traction directly to the epiglottic cartilage with forceps should be avoided. The aryepiglottic folds are placed under tension and stabilized in a fan shape with three evenly placed Allis tissue forceps, and the triangular shape of the epiglottis is identified by visual inspection and palpation. The outstretched aryepiglottic fold is incised on the midline with Metzenbaum scissors to within 2 to 3 mm of the epiglottic cartilage tip. The aryepiglottic fold is then cut for a length of about 1 to 1.5 cm parallel to each margin of the epiglottis. This cut angles out from each epiglottic edge, beginning adjacent to the cartilage and tapering to the free edge of the outstretched aryepiglottic fold. Two pieces of mucous membrane are thus excised out of the central portion of the aryepiglottic fold, debulking the membrane and, in most horses, preventing re-entrapment. The laryngotomy is left to heal by second intention, with routine cleaning provided twice daily. Exercise can be resumed after 4 weeks if healing progresses normally. Re-entrapment can occur and is treated by a second excision.

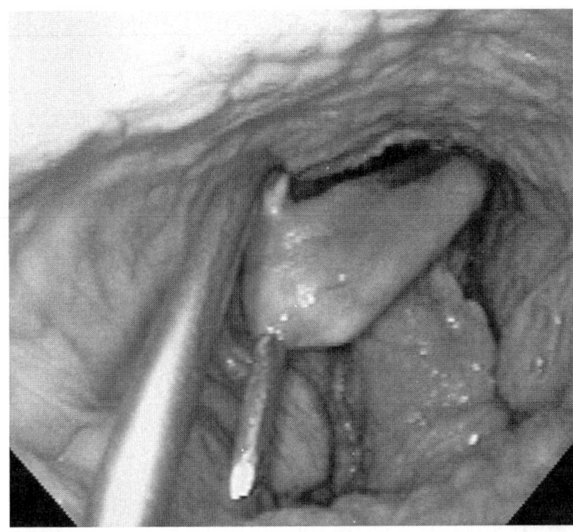

Figure 44-22. Endoscopic appearance of a curved bistoury axially dividing an entrapping membrane via an oral approach. Note the glossoepiglottic fold ventral to the epiglottis.

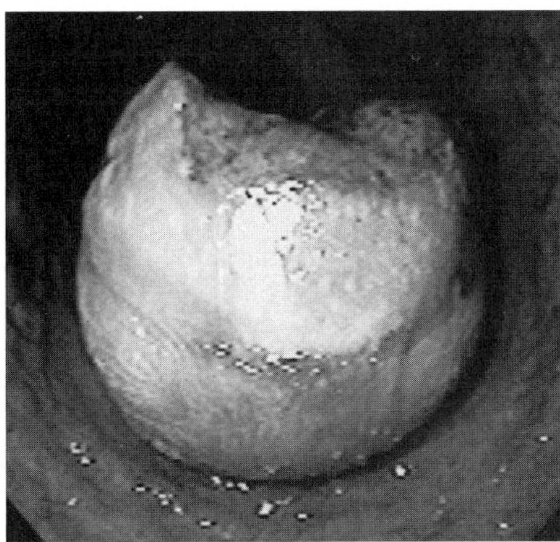

Figure 44-23. Endoscopic appearance of a thick, ulcerated epiglottic entrapment in a Thoroughbred racehorse. Surgical correction was achieved by excising the central third of the aryepiglottic fold through a laryngotomy.

Alternatively, the membrane can be debulked with the horse standing using transendoscopically guided laser excision via the nares. However, care must be taken to avoid thermal damage to the epiglottic cartilage because adhesions and indurated cicatrix often form between the entrapping membrane and the epiglottis, making their delineation difficult and often inducing complications. Owners should be warned that dorsal displacement of the soft palate may be a sequela to correction of epiglottic entrapment regardless of the technique performed, particularly in horses with severe epiglottic hypoplasia.

Acute Epiglottitis

Acute epiglottitis is manifested endoscopically by edema, reddening, and thickening of the epiglottis (Fig. 44-24). Occasionally, the cartilage tip of the epiglottis is exposed. There may be extensive reddening or purple swelling of the

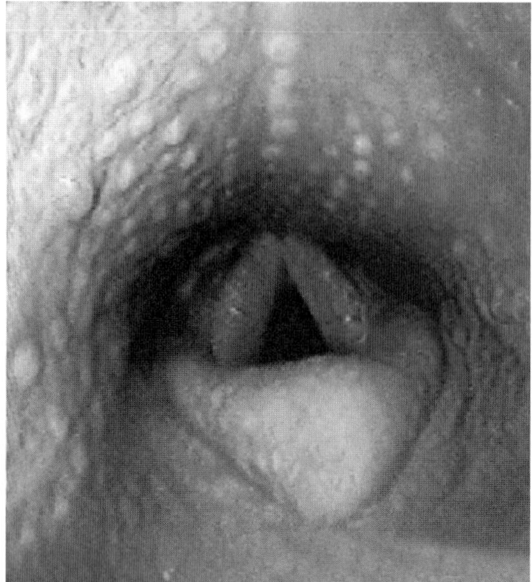

Figure 44-24. Endoscopic appearance of acute epiglottitis shows the typical edema, reddening, and thickening of the epiglottis with this condition. (Courtesy M. Weishaupt, Zurich.)

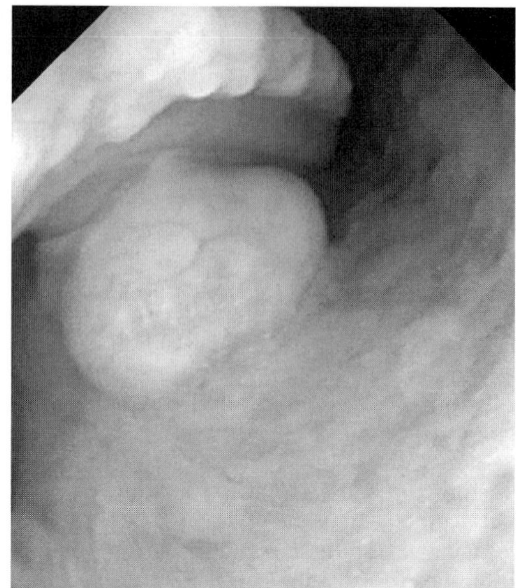

Figure 44-25. Endoscopic appearance of a large subepiglottic cyst in a foal; the cyst was resected via laryngotomy.

mucous membrane ventral to the epiglottis, elevating the epiglottis dorsally into an abnormal axis. The cause is unknown but the problem is seen most commonly in racehorses. The chief complaint is usually respiratory noise and exercise intolerance or coughing.

Exercise should be discontinued. Most horses respond well to systemic nonsteroidal anti-inflammatory and antimicrobial medications and pharyngeal sprays containing anti-inflammatory medication. Initially, systemic corticosteroids may be useful in reducing severe inflammation. Substantial improvement in endoscopic appearance is usually seen in 7 to 14 days. Most affected horses recover completely and successfully return to work. However, long-term complications occur about 50% of the time and include epiglottic deformity, epiglottic entrapment, or intermittent or persistent dorsal displacement of the soft palate.[76]

Subepiglottic Cysts

Subepiglottic cysts are particularly prevalent in young Thoroughbred and Standardbred racehorses, suggesting a possible congenital condition.[77,78] In young foals, subepiglottic cysts may cause coughing, dysphagia, and aspiration pneumonia.[79] Subepiglottic cysts may apparently be acquired, because they are occasionally diagnosed in older horses with no previous history of respiratory tract problems. Older horses are usually presented with a complaint of respiratory noise, coughing and even dysphagia if the cyst is large.[78]

Diagnosis

A diagnosis of a subepiglottic cyst is made on endoscopic examination. A round or oval, smooth, pink, fluctuant, mucosa-covered mass (15 to 40 mm) can be seen beneath the epiglottis (Fig. 44-25). The epiglottis may be asymmetrically elevated slightly above the soft palate by the cyst. Some larger, more fluctuant subepiglottic cysts may occasionally at rest or during swallowing slip beneath the soft palate into the oral pharynx, temporarily obscuring the cyst from view and causing the epiglottis to have a normal interface with the soft palate. Concurrent intermittent or persistent epiglottic entrapment by the aryepiglottic folds can occur. Lateral laryngeal radiography or contrast pharyngography may be useful in helping to define the location and size of the cyst.

An oral endoscopic and digital examination can reveal the exact size and position of the cyst. The horse is anesthetized, positioned in lateral recumbency, and nasotracheally intubated to allow unrestricted access to the oral pharynx. With a mouth speculum in position, the tongue is extended and the soft palate is digitally displaced above the epiglottis. The cyst can be felt beneath the epiglottis as a variably sized, smooth, fluctuant mass projecting from the area of the epiglottic base superficial to the hyoepiglotticus muscle. The cyst is submucosal in origin, hence the cyst base may be poorly defined (sessile) rather than reduced to a distinct narrow (pedunculated) stalk. Once the examination is complete, the horse may be placed in dorsal recumbency for approach via laryngotomy or left in lateral recumbency for an oral approach (see "Treatment," next). On histopathologic examination, subepiglottic cysts are usually lined with a combination of stratified squamous and pseudostratified columnar epithelium. Mucous glands, dilated ducts, and a homogeneous eosinophilic mucus are usually present.

Treatment

Removal of the secretory lining is important. If the cyst is merely punctured and drained, the cyst usually seals over and refills within days. Removal of an excessive amount of oral pharyngeal mucosa overlying the cyst may result in cicatrization beneath the epiglottis, possibly altering the normal range of motion or disrupting the normal synchrony between the epiglottis and the soft palate. Cicatrization after subepiglottic cyst removal may result in clinically significant problems with either intermittent or persistent dorsal displacement of the soft palate.[78]

Subepiglottic cysts may be removed through a laryngotomy with the horse positioned in dorsal recumbency under general anesthesia.[70,79] The epiglottis is gently retroverted into view by grasping the aryepiglottic folds with a sponge or Allis tissue forceps. By elevating the epiglottic tip, the cyst can be palpated on the ventral epiglottic surface. The mucosa is sharply incised over the cyst and the cyst is excised submucosally with Metzenbaum scissors. The mucosal incision is usually left to heal by second intention or it may be sutured with 3-0 to 5-0 synthetic absorbable suture. The laryngotomy is left open to heal by second intention with routine twice daily cleansing. Exercise is resumed in 3 to 4 weeks if the laryngotomy has healed routinely and follow-up endoscopy is normal.

Two techniques are available for excision of subepiglottic cysts via an oral approach.[78] The horse is anesthetized, positioned in lateral recumbency and nasotracheally intubated. After the cyst is evaluated by palpation, it is visualized on a television monitor with a videoendoscope. Traction is placed on the mucosa and the underlying cyst with 600-mm bronchoesophagoscopic grasping forceps (Universal bronchoesophagoscopic grasping forceps, 600-mm length, 8280.62, Richard Wolfe Medical Instrument Corporation, Rosemont, Ill). Using an Nd:YAG laser or a diode laser with a 600-μm sculpted fiber, a fusiform incision into the mucosa over the cyst is made transendoscopically with 15 to 18 W of power. Laser energy is then used to excise the cyst membrane submucosally. Occasionally, a small amount of digital dissection is necessary to free the cyst's final attachments. Alternatively, an electrocautery snare may be applied or a cyst snare can be fashioned from a mare urinary catheter and obstetrical wire and used to excise the cyst at its base, taking extreme caution to remove as little overlying mucosa as possible. In either technique, hemorrhage is minimal and the defect created is left to heal by second intention.

Transendoscopic laser or electrocautery excision can be performed with the horse sedated and cross-tied in stocks. This technique is usually reserved for small cysts that can be easily manipulated to a position above the palate. The cyst is anesthetized topically through polyethylene tubing introduced through the biopsy channel of the videoendoscope. Five to 10 mL of local anesthetic solution dripped over the cyst will induce local anesthesia in about 5 minutes. The 600-mm bronchoesophagoscopic forceps are introduced up the opposite nasal passage as the endoscope and the mucosa overlying the cyst is grasped. A fusiform mucosal incision and submucosal dissection of the cyst lining is then performed (as previously described under oral approach) using either an Nd:YAG or a diode laser and a 600-μm sculpted fiber.[73]

Aftercare

Postoperative inflammation and pain are controlled with a combination of corticosteroids, nonsteroidal anti-inflammatory medication, and pharyngeal sprays as needed (see "Postoperative Management," p. 574). Exercise is restricted until the pharynx appears endoscopically normal, which is usually within approximately 21 days. In horses with concurrent epiglottic entrapment, removal of the subepiglottic cyst usually corrects the epiglottic entrapment because of removal of a small portion of mucosa. Foals with concomitant aspiration pneumonia should be treated with broad-spectrum antimicrobial agents based on culture and sensitivity of tracheal aspirates before excision of the cyst.

Dorsal Epiglottic Abscess

Dorsal epiglottic abscess is a rare disease that causes coughing, respiratory noise, and exercise intolerance.[80] Palpation of the laryngeal cartilages may elicit pain. On endoscopic examination, there is a smooth, well-circumscribed, round or oval swelling on the dorsal epiglottic surface. Intermittent dorsal displacement of the soft palate may be observed. The abscess can be incised and drained transendoscopically on an outpatient basis with a contact Nd:YAG or diode laser using a sculpted fiber or chisel probe. After decompressing the abscess, débridement can be achieved with 600-mm-long bronchoesophagoscopic grasping forceps. The abscess cavity can be lavaged transendoscopically, if desired, with 240 polyethylene tubing and a dilute 1:10 chlorhexidine solution in physiologic saline.

Aftercare includes stall confinement and exercise restricted to hand-walking. Nonsteroidal anti-inflammatory medication and systemic antibiotics (procaine penicillin G given intramuscularly twice daily) are given at recommended dosages for 3 days. The abscess usually appears to be healed on endoscopic reexamination approximately 10 days postoperatively. In a small number of cases, clinical signs resolved and the horses resumed normal exercise without recurrence of the abscess.[80]

Subepiglottic Granulomas

Subepiglottic granulomas originate as an acute ulceration of the aryepiglottic fold in the ventral aspect of the epiglottis. In response to infection or chronic irritation, excessive granulation tissue forms. This tissue may be confused with subepiglottic cysts. Clinical signs usually include exercise intolerance and occasionally coughing and dysphagia. Large lesions may disrupt the normal interaction between the epiglottis and the soft palate.

Treatment

Small granulomas and ulcers respond to antimicrobial and anti-inflammatory medical therapy as long as the horse has received forced rest for approximately 4 to 6 weeks. In nonhealing ulcers, enlargement of the granulation tissue frequently occurs when the horses are returned to exercise. In these cases, excision either orally or through a ventral laryngotomy is indicated. Sharp surgical excision alone (performed through a ventral laryngotomy) may not result in complete resolution of the problem. Therefore, sterilization of this area with laser cautery of the surface after resection is indicated. Alternatively, laser photo ablation of the surface of the granulation tissue can be performed with the sculpted fiber using contact technique. It is imperative that extended periods of rest (up to 60 days) accompany any treatment of this condition.[81]

Epiglottic Hypoplasia/Flaccidity and Epiglottic Deformity

Diagnosis

Epiglottic hypoplasia/flaccidity and epiglottic deformity have been associated with dorsal displacement of the soft palate and epiglottic entrapment, both of which are causes for abnormal respiratory noise and exercise intolerance.[66-71,74,75,82-85] On endoscopic examination, the hypoplastic epiglottis in the adult horse appears short and narrow, particularly from midbody to the tip, or it may appear very thin (Fig. 44-26). The epiglottic contour may appear flaccid, conforming excessively to the shape of the underlying soft palate. In some horses, the epiglottic border is irregular or rounder and much flatter than normal. Occasionally, the epiglottis has a very shrunken, bumpy, or wrinkled and deformed appearance. Easily induced intermittent or persistent dorsal displacement of the soft palate may be observed during the endoscopic examination. Lateral laryngeal radiography and contrast pharyngography may provide additional information regarding thyroepiglottic length, epiglottic thickness and contour, and the relationship of the epiglottis to other adjacent pharyngeal structures. If the soft palate is persistently displaced dorsally, endoscopy and digital palpation of the epiglottis per os with the horse anesthetized, positioned in lateral recumbency, and nasotracheally intubated may provide useful information on the extent of the problem. Epiglottic hypoplasia severe enough to result in persistent dorsal displacement of the soft palate is associated with a guarded to poor prognosis for optimal exercise potential.[83,84] Other underlying problems causing dorsal displacement of the soft palate, such as epiglottic entrapment or subepiglottic cicatrix formation or granulation tissue, can also be fully assessed through a detailed endoscopic and digital oral examination. However, persistent dorsal displacement of the soft palate may occur secondary to severe epiglottic hypoplasia without any other underlying abnormalities or previous surgical intervention.[84]

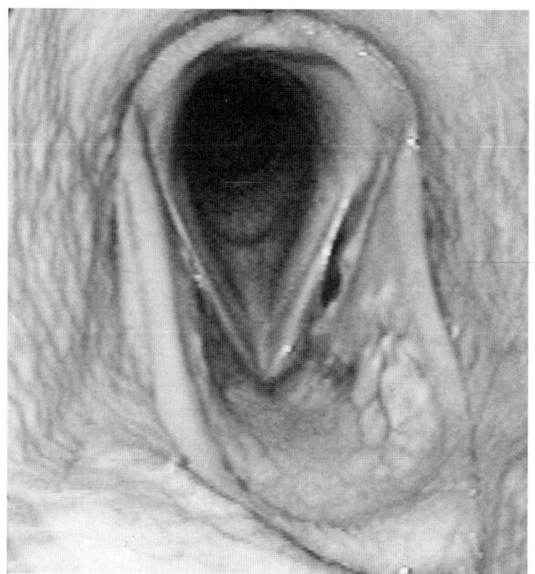

Figure 44-26. Endoscopic appearance of epiglottic hypoplasia/flaccidity, showing how the epiglottis appears very thin. (Courtesy J. Robertson, Ohio.)

Because epiglottic hypoplasia/flaccidity in adult horses is thought to contribute to epiglottic entrapment and intermittent dorsal displacement of the soft palate, the epiglottis is routinely scrutinized during pre-purchase endoscopic examinations in yearling Thoroughbreds. However, no correlation could be found between the appearance of a hypoplastic/flaccid epiglottis in the standing adult horse and dorsal displacement of the soft palate during exercise on a high-speed treadmill.[86] Additionally, these same visual epiglottic abnormalities in yearlings could not be significantly correlated with racing performance.[17] It is now recognized that the upper airway of yearling and adult horses differ. Compared with adult horses, yearlings have a shorter, narrower, and more flaccid-appearing epiglottis normally, and judgments about epiglottic appearance should be reserved until the horse reaches maturity, except in very severe cases.

Treatment

Epiglottic augmentation is performed only in the adult horse to increase the mechanical rigidity of the epiglottis and to make the hypoplastic/flaccid epiglottis more resistant to dorsal displacement of the soft palate. Several materials including collagen and autogenous and allogenous cartilage grafts have been evaluated, but epiglottic augmentation with polytetrafluoroethylene (Polytef Paste; Polytetrafluoroethylene Teflon paste, Mentor polytef paste for injection, Mentor O & O, Inc, Norwell, Mass) has proved to be the most useful.[87,88] Experimentally, in the normal epiglottis polytetrafluoroethylene paste injected submucosally on the ventral epiglottic surface through a laryngotomy (Fig. 44-27) using an Arnold-Bruning syringe (Arnold-Bruning intracordal injection syringe, catalog No. 7754, Stortz Instrument Company, St. Louis, Mo) (Fig. 44-28) resulted in an increased thickness of approximately 29% to 40% along the margins and midline[88] (Fig. 44-29). Epiglottic length was not increased. Polytetrafluoroethylene paste functions by inciting a sterile granulomatous reaction that is incorporated in fibrous connective tissue.

In two studies, an approach to management of intermittent dorsal displacement of the soft palate that most often combined surgical techniques and always included epiglottic augmentation improved racing performance in 66% of treated horses with poor racing performance attributable to epiglottic hypoplasia/flaccidity.[89,90]

Epiglottic Retroversion

Diagnosis

Epiglottic retroversion is a condition in which the epiglottis assumes a position dorsal to the soft palate and retroverts into the opening of the glottis during inspiration and returns to its normal position with each expiration.[91] Resting endoscopic examination of the pharynx and larynx can appear normal, or on occasion the epiglottis may project slightly above the soft palate. A high-speed treadmill exami-

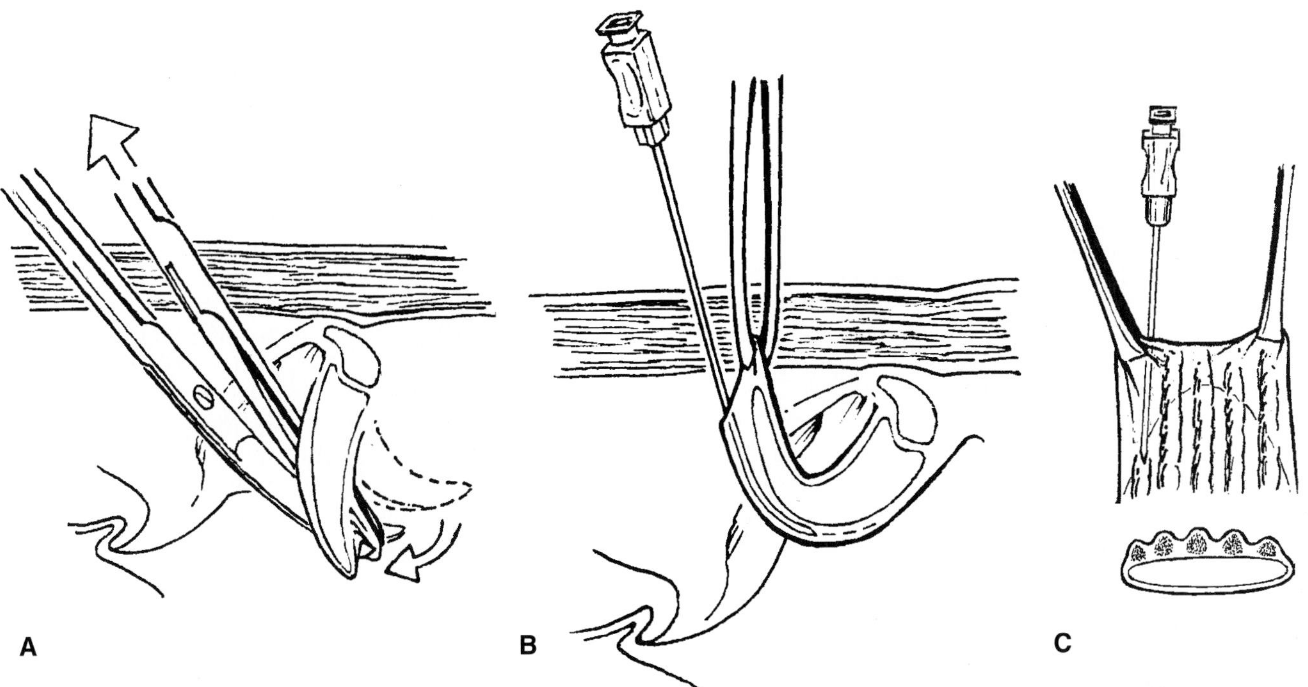

Figure 44-27. **A,** Technique used to evert the epiglottis through a laryngotomy incision. Curved scissors are used to evert the epiglottis until the epiglottic fold can be grasped with Allis tissue forceps. **B,** The endotracheal tube can be replaced and the ventral surface of the epiglottis is injected. **C,** Five linear injections are made equidistant from each other into the aryepligotic fold.

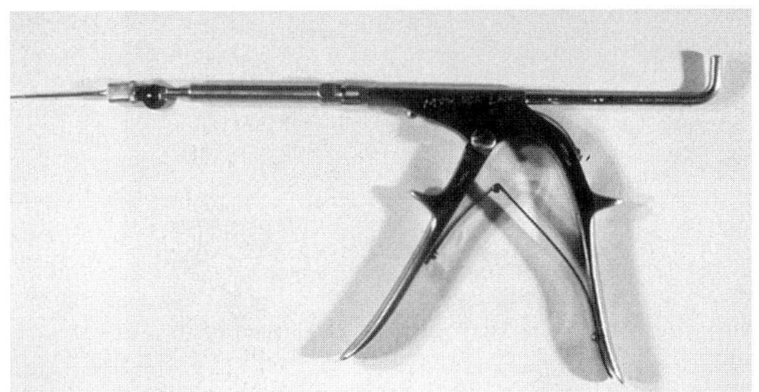

Figure 44-28. Photograph of Arnold-Bruning intracordal injection syringe, fully assembled.

nation is necessary to confirm the diagnosis (Fig. 44-30). Retroversion of the epiglottis enables visualization of the ventral (lingual) surface of the epiglottis, but at no time does the soft palate elevate or displace dorsal to the epiglottis. In one horse, the epiglottis rolled up in a tube-like fashion and pointed dorsally, but it did not retroflex into the glottis. During exercise, a respiratory noise may be heard.

Etiology

Experimentally, both local anesthesia of the geniohyoid muscle and local anesthesia of the hypoglossal nerves within the guttural pouch have produced epiglottic retroversion during exercise in normal horses.[92] Trauma or inflammation of the normal hyoid musculature or the hyoepiglotticus or geniohyoid muscles may precede epiglottic retroversion.

Treatment

Two horses with this rare problem were treated by epiglottic augmentation with polytetrafluoroethylene paste injected submucosally on the lingual epiglottic surface. One Standardbred was able to return to racing and competed successfully, including winning several races, and one Thoroughbred was retired when it continued to make noise during training after undergoing surgery. A prosthetic suture placed between the epiglottis and the thyroid cartilage was used to stabilize the epiglottis in a racing Standardbred, which allowed it to return to racing.[93]

Axial Deviation of the Aryepiglottic Folds

Diagnosis

Axial deviation of the aryepiglottic folds occurs during maximal exertion and causes dynamic upper respiratory tract obstruction. A diagnosis cannot be made during resting endoscopic evaluation but requires videoendoscopic examination during high-speed treadmill exercise (Fig. 44-31, *A*). It is a distinct entity from intermittent dorsal displacement. In a study of 15 affected horses, 80% were racing Thoroughbreds, 13% were racing Standardbreds, and 7% were racing Arabians. Abnormal respiratory tract noise and exercise intolerance were the most common clinical manifestations.[94] The condition is almost always bilateral, but unilateral involvement, if present, has been reported to be right-sided.[95]

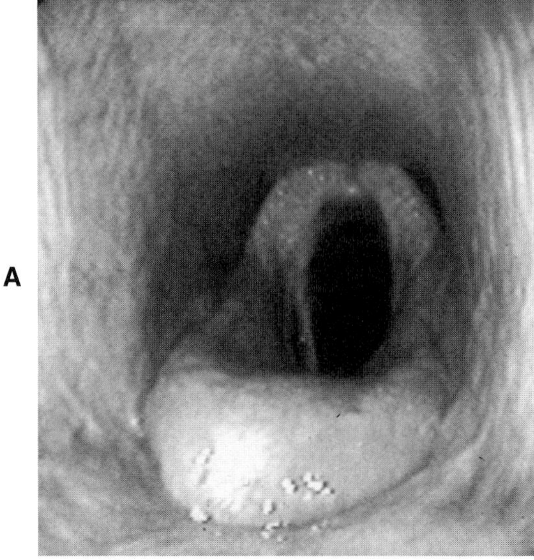

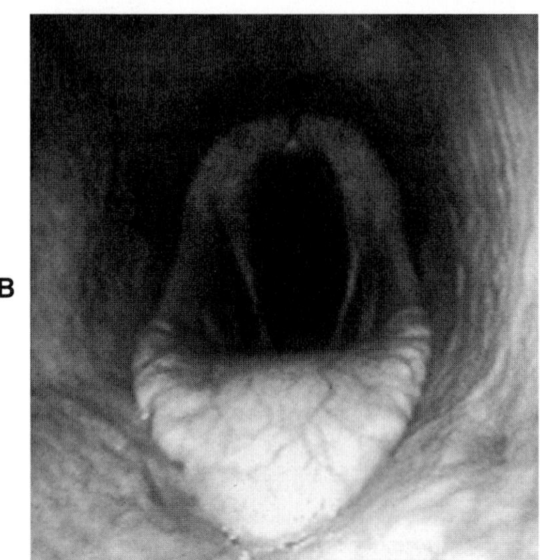

Figure 44-29. A, Twenty-four hours after Teflon injection in the epiglottic fold, the epiglottis becomes edematous. **B,** Thirty days after injection, the epiglottis is clearly thickened and more substantial when compared with its appearance before surgery (see Fig. 44-26). Video-endoscopic appearance of epiglottic retroversion during the high-speed treadmill examination.

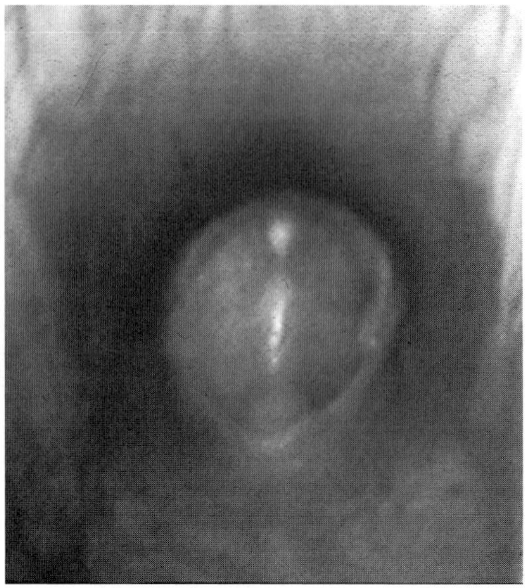

Figure 44-30. Epiglottic retroversion as seen during inspiration on a horse exercising on a high-speed treadmill.

Treatment

Transendoscopic laser surgery using an Nd:YAG or a diode laser with a 600-μm sculpted tip fiber in contact fashion can be performed on the conscious, standing horse or with the horse anesthetized. The tissue that is collapsing into the airway during exercise is grasped and placed under tension with 600-mm bronchoesophagoscopic grasping forceps, and an approximately 2-cm-wide triangle is excised transendoscopically.[73,94] Alternatively, this surgery can be performed through a laryngotomy in the anesthetized horse. Allis tissue forceps can be used to grasp the tissue, and Metzenbaum scissors are used to trim the redundant tissue (see Fig. 44-31, *B*). No suturing is necessary.

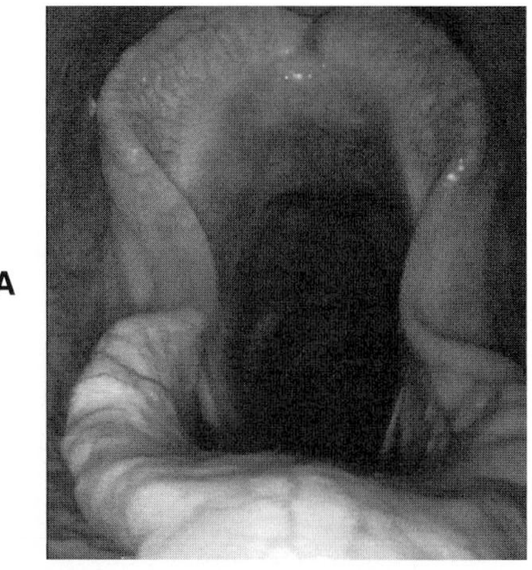

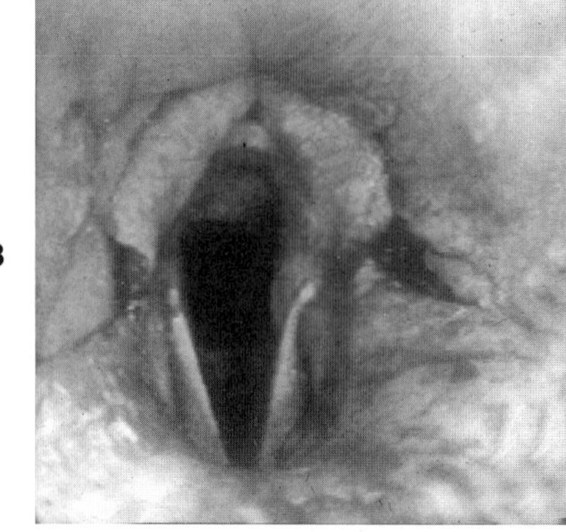

Figure 44-31. A, Videoendoscopic appearance of axial deviation of the membranous portions of the aryepiglottic folds during high-speed treadmill exercise. **B,** Immediate postoperative endoscopic appearance of the membranous portions of the aryepiglottic fold after excision through a laryngotomy. (**A** courtesy M. Weishaupt, Zurich.)

REFERENCES

1. Hare WCD: Equine respiratory system. In Getty R, editor: Sisson and Grossman's The Anatomy of Domestic Animal, ed 5, Philadelphia, 1975, WB Saunders.
2. Van Lunteren E, Strohl KP: Striated respiratory muscles of the upper airways. In Mathew OP, Sant'Ambrogia G, editors: Respiratory Function of the Upper Airway, vol 35, Lung Biology in Health and Disease, New York, 1988, Marcel Dekker.
3. Van Lunteren E: Upper airway effects on breathing. In Crystal RG, West JB, editors: The Lung: Scientific Foundations, ed 2, Philadelphia, 1996, Lippincott-Raven.
4. Sant'Ambrogio G, Mathew OP, Fisher JT, et al: Laryngeal receptors responding to transmural pressure, airflow, and local muscle activity, Respir Physiol 1983;54:317.
5. Woodall DL, Mathew OP: Effect of upper airway pressure pulses on breathing pattern, Respir Physiol 1986;66:71.
6. Duncan ID, Griffiths IR, McQueen A, et al: The pathology of equine laryngeal hemiplegia, Acta Neuropath 1974;27:337.
7. Duncan ID, Brook D: Bilateral laryngeal paralysis in the horse, Equine Vet J 1985;17:228.
8. Marks D, MacKay-Smith MP, Cushing LS, et al: Etiology and diagnosis of laryngeal hemiplegia in horses, J Am Vet Med Assoc 1970;157:429.
9. Baker GJ: Laryngeal hemiplegia in the horse, Comp Cont Educ Pract Vet 1983;5:S6.
10. Poncet PA, Montavon S, Gaillard C, et al: A preliminary report on the possible genetic basis of laryngeal hemiplegia, Equine Vet J 1989;21:137.
11. Cook WR: Diagnosis and grading of hereditary recurrent laryngeal neuropathy in the horse, J Equine Vet Sci 1988;8:432.
12. Goulden BE, Anderson LJ: Equine laryngeal hemiplegia: Part 1. Physical characteristics of affected animals, N Z Vet J 1981;29:150.
13. Beard WL, Hayes HM: Risk factors for laryngeal hemiplegia in the horse, Prev Vet Med 1993;17:57.
14. Hillidge CJ: Prevalence of laryngeal hemiplegia on a Thoroughbred horse farm, J Equine Vet Sci 1985;5:252.
15. Lane JG, Ellis DR, Greet TRC: Observations on the examinations of Thoroughbred yearlings for idiopathic laryngeal hemiplegia, Equine Vet J 1987;19:531.
16. Cook WR: Recent observations on recurrent laryngeal neuropathy in the horse: Applications to practice, Proc Am Assoc Equine Pract 1988;34:427.
17. Stick JA, Peloso JG, Morehead JP, et al: Endoscopic assessment of airway function as a predictor of racing performance in Thoroughbred yearlings: 427 cases (1997-2000), J Am Vet Med Assoc 2001;219:962.
18. Shappell KK, Derksen FJ, Stick JA, et al: Effects of ventriculectomy, prosthetic laryngoplasty, and exercise on upper airway function in horses with induced laryngeal hemiplegia, Am J Vet Res 1988;49:1760.
19. Tate LP, Corbett WT, Bishop BJ, et al: Blood gas tensions, acid base status, heart rates and venous profiles in exercising horses with laryngeal hemiplegia before and after corrective surgery, Vet Surg 1993;22:177.
20. Christley RM, Hodgson DR, Evans DL, et al: Cardio-respiratory responses to exercise in horses with different grades of idiopathic laryngeal hemiplegia, Equine Vet J 1997;29:6.
21. Robertson JT: Pharynx and larynx. In Beech J, editor: Equine Respiratory Disorders, Philadelphia, 1991, Lea & Febiger.
22. Attenburrow DP: Resonant frequency of the lateral ventricle and saccule and "whistling." In Snow DH, Persson SG, Rose RJ, editors: Equine Exercise Physiology, Cambridge, 1983, Granta Editions.
23. Dixon PM, McGorum BC, Railton DI, et al: Laryngeal paralysis: A study of 375 cases in a mixed-breed population of horses, Equine Vet J 2001;33:452.
24. Tulleners EP, Ross MW, Hawkins J: Management of right laryngeal hemiplegia in horses: 28 cases (1987-1996), Proc Am Coll Vet Surg Symp 1996;6:21.
25. Rakestraw PC, Hackett RP, Ducharme NG, et al: Arytenoid cartilage movement in resting and exercising horses, Vet Surg 1991;20:122-127.
26. Stick JA: Instrumentation and techniques in respiratory surgery, Vet Clin North Am Equine Pract 1996;12:351.
27. Strand E, Martin GS, Haynes PF, et al: Career racing performance in Thoroughbreds treated with prosthetic laryngoplasty for laryngeal neuropathy: 52 cases (1981-1989), J Am Vet Med Assoc 2000;217:1689.
28. Baker GJ: Laryngeal asynchrony in the horse: Definition and significance. In Snow DH, Persson SGB, Rose RJ, editors: Proceedings of the 1st International Conference on Equine Exercise Physiology, Cambridge, 1982, Granta.
29. Dixon PM, McGorum BC, Railton DI, et al: Clinical and endoscopic evidence of progression in 52 cases of equine recurrent laryngeal neuropathy (RLN), Equine Vet J 2002;34:29.
30. Derksen FJ, Stick JA, Scott EA, et al: Effect of laryngeal hemiplegia and laryngoplasty on airway flow mechanics in exercising horses, Am J Vet Res 1986;47:16.
31. Tetens J, Derken FJ, Stick JA, et al: Efficacy of prosthetic laryngoplasty with and without bilateral ventriculocordectomy as treatments for laryngeal hemiplegia in horses, Am J Vet Res 1996;57:1668.
32. Brown JA, Derksen FJ, Stick JA, et al: Ventriculocordectomy reduces respiratory noise in horses with laryngeal hemiplegia, Equine Vet J 2003;35:570.
33. Brown JA, Derksen FJ, Stick JA, et al: Laser vocal cordectomy fails to effectively reduce respiratory noise in horses with laryngeal hemiplegia, Vet Surg (in press).
34. Brown JA, Derksen FJ, Stick JA, et al: Effect of laryngoplasty on respiratory noise reduction in horses with laryngeal hemiplegia, Equine Vet J 2004;36:420.
35. Marks D, MacKay-Smith MP, Cushing LS, et al: Use of a prosthetic device for surgical correction of laryngeal hemiplegia in horses, J Am Vet Med Assoc 1970;157:157.
36. Speirs VC: Laryngeal surgery: 150 years on, Equine Vet J 1987;19:377.
37. Greet TRC, Maker GJ, Lee R: The effect of laryngoplasty on pharyngeal function in the horse, Equine Vet J 1979;11:153.
38. Russell AP, Slone DE: Performance analysis after prosthetic laryngoplasty and bilateral ventriculectomy for laryngeal hemiplegia in horses: 70 cases (1986-1991), J Am Vet Med Assoc 1994;204:1235.
39. Hawkins JF, Tulleners EP, Ross MW, et al: Laryngoplasty with or without ventriculectomy for treatment of left laryngeal hemiplegia in 230 race horses, Vet Surg 1997;26:484.
40. Dean PW, Nelson JK, Schumaker J: Effects of age and prosthesis material on in vitro cartilage retention of laryngoplasty prostheses in horses, Am J Vet Res 1990;51:114.
41. Dixon PM, McGorum BC, Railton DI, et al: Long-term survey of laryngoplasty and ventriculocordectomy in an older, mixed-breed population of 200 horses: Part 1. Maintenance of surgical arytenoid abduction and complications of surgery, Equine Vet J 2003;35:389.
42. Speirs VC, Boureke JM, Anderson GA: Assessment of the efficacy of an abductor muscle prosthesis for treatment of laryngeal hemiplegia in horses, Aust Vet J 1983;60:294.
43. Goulden BE, Anderson LG: Equine laryngeal hemiplegia: Part III. Treatment by laryngoplasty, N Z Vet J 1982;30:1.
44. Tulleners E: Management of failed laryngoplasty: 25 horses (1988-1993), Proc Ann Meet Am Coll Vet Surg 1994;29:24.
45. Wilson RG, Sutton RH, Groenendy KS: Rostral displacement of the palatopharyngeal arch in a Thoroughbred yearling, Aust Vet J 1986;63:99.
46. Goulden BE, Anderson LJ, Davies AS, et al: Rostral displacement of the palatopharyngeal arch: A case report, Equine Vet J 1976;8:95.
47. Klein H, Deegan E, Stockhofe N, et al: Rostral displacement of the palatopharyngeal arch in a seven-month-old Hanoverian colt, Equine Vet J 1989;21:382.

48. Dixon PM, McGorum BC, Else RW: Cricopharyngeal-laryngeal dysplasia in a horse with sudden clinical onset idiopathic laryngeal hemiparesis, N Z Vet J 1993;41:134.
49. Kraus BM, Parente EJ, Tulleners EP: Laryngoplasty with ventriculectomy or ventriculocordectomy in 104 draft horses (1992-2000), Vet Surg 2003;32:530.
50. Hawkins JF, Andrews-Jones L: Neodymium:yttrium aluminum garnet laser ventriculocordectomy in standing horses, Am J Vet Res 2001;62:531.
51. Tulleners E: Instrumentation and techniques in transendoscopic upper respiratory tract laser surgery, Vet Clin North Am Equine Pract 1996;21:373.
52. Fulton IC, Stick JA, Derksen FJ: Laryngeal reinnervation in the horse, Vet Clin North Am Equine Pract 2003;19:189.
53. Hengerer AS, Tucker HM: Restoration of abduction in the paralyzed canine vocal fold, Arch Otolaryngol 1973;97:247.
54. Tucker HM: Human laryngeal reinnervation, Laryngoscope 1976;86:769.
55. Fulton IC, Derksen FJ, Stick JA,, et al: Treatment of left laryngeal hemiplegia in Standardbreds, using a nerve muscle pedicle graft, Am J Vet Res 1991;52:1461.
56. Fulton IC: The nerve muscle pedicle graft for treatment of idiopathic equine laryngeal hemiplegia: current status, Proc Dubai Int Equine Symp 1997;2:407.
57. Fulton IC, Derksen FJ, Stick JA, et al: Histologic evaluation of nerve muscle pedicle graft used as a treatment for left laryngeal hemiplegia in Standardbreds, Am J Vet Res 1992;53:592.
58. Haynes PF, McClure JR, Watters JW: Subtotal arytenoidectomy in the horse: An update. Proc Am Assoc Equine Pract 1984;30:21.
59. White NA, Blackwell RB: Partial arytenoidectomy in the horse, Vet Surg 1980;9:5.
60. Tulleners EP, Harrison IW, Raker CW: Management of arytenoid chondropathy and failed laryngoplasty in horses: 75 cases (1979-1985), J Am Vet Med Assoc 1988;192:670.
61. Speirs VC: Partial arytenoidectomy in horses, Vet Surg 1986;15:316.
62. Belknap JK, Derksen FJ, Nickels FA, et al: Failure of subtotal arytenoidectomy to improve upper airway flow mechanics in exercising Standardbreds with induced laryngeal hemiplegia, Am J Vet Res 1990;51:1481.
63. Lumsden JM, Derksen, FJ, Stick JA, et al: Evaluation of partial arytenoidectomy as a treatment for equine laryngeal hemiplegia, Equine Vet J 1994;26:125.
64. Hay W, Tulleners EP: Excision of intralaryngeal granulation tissue in 25 horses using a neodymium:YAG laser (1986-1991), Vet Surg 1993;22:129.
65. Kelly G, Lumsden JM, Dunkerly G, et al: Idiopathic mucosal lesions of the arytenoid cartilages of 21 Thoroughbred yearlings: 1997-2001, Equine Vet J 2003;35:276.
66. Boles CL, Raker CW, Wheat JD: Epiglottic entrapment of arytenoepiglottic folds in the horse, J Am Vet Med Assoc 1978;172:338.
67. Tulleners EP: Transendoscopic contact neodymium:yttrium aluminum garnet laser correction of epiglottic entrapment in standing horses, J Am Vet Med Assoc 1990;196:1971.
68. Honnas CM, Wheat JD: Epiglottic entrapment: A transnasal surgical approach to divide the aryepiglottic fold axially in the standing horse, Vet Surg 1988;17:246.
69. Greet TRC: Experiences in treatment of epiglottal entrapment using a hook knife per nasum, Equine Vet J 1995;27:122.
70. Ross NW, Gentile DG, Evans LE: Transoral axial division, under endoscopic guidance, for correction of epiglottic entrapment in horses, J Am Vet Med Assoc 1993;203:416.
71. Lumsden JM, Stick JA, Caron JP, et al: Surgical treatment for epiglottic entrapment in horses: 51 cases (1981-1991), J Am Vet Med Assoc 1994;205:729.
72. Jann HW, Cook WR: Transendoscopic electrosurgery for epiglottal entrapment in the horse, J Am Vet Med Assoc 1985;187:484.
73. Tulleners EP: Transendoscopic laser surgery of the upper respiratory tract. In Traub-Dargatz JL, Brown CM, editors: Equine Endoscopy, ed 2, St Louis, 1997, CV Mosby.
74. Tulleners EP: Correlation of performance with endoscopic and radiographic assessment of epiglottic hypoplasia in racehorses with epiglottic entrapment corrected by use of contact neodymium:yttrium aluminum garnet laser correction, J Am Vet Med Assoc 1991;198:621.
75. Linford RL, O'Brien TR, Wheat JD, et al: Radiographic assessment of epiglottic length and pharyngeal and laryngeal diameters in the Thoroughbred, Am J Vet Res 1983;44:1660.
76. Hawkins JF, Tulleners EP: Epiglottis in horses: 20 cases (1988-1993), J Am Vet Med Assoc 1994;205:1577.
77. Koch DB, Tate LP: Pharyngeal cysts in horses, J Am Vet Med Assoc 1978;173:860.
78. Tulleners EP: Evaluation of per oral transendoscopic contact neodymium:yttrium aluminum garnet laser and snare excision of subepiglottic cysts in horses, J Am Vet Med Assoc 1991;198:1631.
79. Stick JA, Boles C: Subepiglottic cysts in three foals, J Am Vet Med Assoc 1980;177:62.
80. Tulleners EP: Use of transendoscopic contact neodymium:yttrium aluminum garnet laser to drain dorsal epiglottic abscess in two horses, J Am Vet Med Assoc 1991;198:1765.
81. Palmer SE: The use of lasers for treatment of upper respiratory tract disorders, Vet Clin Equine 2003;19:245.
82. Harrison IW, Raker CW: Sternothyrohyoideus myectomy in horses: 17 cases (1984-1984), J Am Vet Med Assoc 1988;193:1299.
83. Haynes PF: Dorsal displacement of the soft palate and epiglottic entrapment: Diagnosis, management and interrelationship, Comp Cont Educ Pract Vet 1983;5:S379.
84. Haynes PF: Persistent dorsal displacement of the soft palate associated with epiglottic shortening in two horses, J Am Vet Med Assoc 1981;179:677.
85. Anderson JD, Tulleners EP, Johnston JK, et al: Sternothyrohyoideus myectomy or staphylectomy for treatment of intermittent dorsal displacement of the soft palate in racehorses: 209 cases (1986-1991), J Am Vet Med Assoc 1995;206:1909.
86. Parente EJ, Martin BB, Tulleners EP, et al: Dorsal displacement of the soft palate in 92 horses during high-speed treadmill examination (1993-1998), Vet Surg 2002;31:507.
87. Tulleners EP, Mann P, Raker CW: Epiglottic augmentation in the horse, Vet Surg 1990;19:181.
88. Tulleners EP, Hamir A: Evaluation of epiglottic augmentation by use of polytetrafluoroethylene paste in horses, Am J Vet Res 1991;52:1908.
89. Tulleners EP, Stick JA, Leitch M, et al: Epiglottic augmentation for treatment of dorsal displacement of the soft palate in racehorses: 59 cases (1985-1994), J Am Vet Med Assoc 1997;211:1022.
90. Koch CM: Teflon augmentation of the epiglottis in the horse, Proc Am Assoc Equine Pract 1990;38:541.
91. Parente EJ, Martin BV, Tulleners EP: Epiglottic retroversion as a cause of poor performance in two horses, Equine Vet J 1997;30:270.
92. Holcombe SJ, Derksen FJ, Stick JA: Effects of bilateral hypoglossal and glossopharyngeal nerve blocks on epiglottic and soft palate position in exercising horses, Am J Vet Res 1997;58:1022.
93. Ducharme N: Personal communication.
94. King D, Tulleners EP, Martin B, et al: Transendoscopic Nd:YAG laser excision of the membranous portion of the aryepiglottic folds for treatment of axial deviation of the aryepiglottic folds in racehorses: 15 cases (1993-1996), Vet Surg 1997;26:418.
95. King DS, Tulleners E, Martin BB, et al: Clinical experiences with axial deviation of the aryepiglottic folds in 52 racehorses, Vet Surg 2001;30:151.

CHAPTER 45

Guttural Pouch

David E. Freeman
Joanne Hardy

ANATOMY

Guttural pouches are paired extensions of the eustachian tubes that connect the pharynx to the middle ear.[1] They are found in perissodactyls, such as equids, tapirs, some species of rhinoceros (except for the white rhinoceros), some bats, a South American forest mouse, and hyraxes.[2-4]

The pouches are separated from each other on the midline by the rectus capitis ventralis and the longus capitis muscles and the median septum.[1] Each is in close contact rostrally with the basisphenoid bone, ventrally with the retropharyngeal lymph nodes, pharynx, and the esophagus, caudally with the atlantooccipital joint, laterally with the digastricus muscle and the parotid and mandibular salivary glands, and dorsally with the petrous part of the temporal bone, tympanic bulla, and auditory meatus. Each guttural pouch is divided ventrally into a medial and a lateral compartment by the stylohyoid bone, and it communicates with the pharynx through the pharyngeal orifice of the eustachian tube. The pharyngeal orifice is a funnel-shaped opening in the dorsolateral aspect of the pharynx that forms an oblique slit, rostral and ventral to the dorsal pharyngeal recess. The small end of the funnel opens into the guttural pouch. The medial lamina of each opening is composed of fibrocartilage directed in a rostroventral-to-caudodorsal direction. The capacity of guttural pouches in adult horses is 472 +/− 12.4 mL and the lateral compartment is approximately one third of the capacity of the medial compartment.[5]

Clinical signs of important guttural pouch diseases are referable to injury of specific nerves and arteries in the guttural pouch and acoustic system. The internal carotid artery (ICA), cranial cervical ganglion, cervical sympathetic trunk, and vagus, glossopharyngeal, hypoglossal, and the spinal accessory nerves are all contained in a fold of mucous membrane along the caudal wall of the medial compartment[1] (Fig. 45-1). The cranial laryngeal nerve and the pharyngeal branch of the vagus nerve lie beneath the mucosa on the floor of the medial compartment[1] (see Fig. 45-1). The external carotid artery (ECA) lies along the wall of the lateral

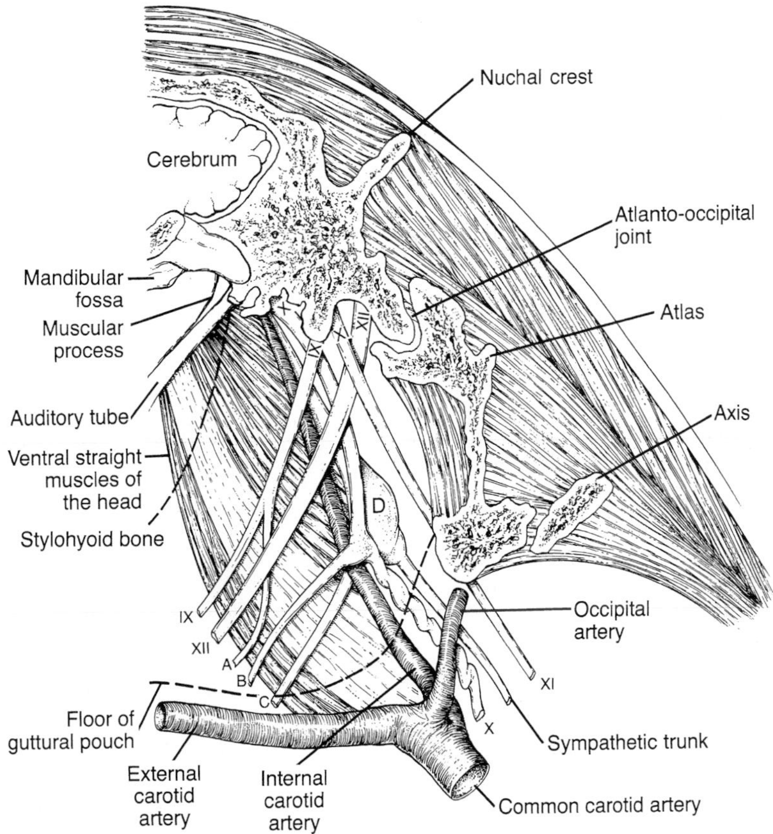

Figure 45-1. Interior of medial compartment of the left guttural pouch, viewed from the lateral aspect in a sagittal section of a horse's head. The section is cut through the styloid process of the petrous temporal bone on a line that divides the guttural pouch into medial and lateral compartments. (IX, glossopharyngeal nerve; X, vagus nerve; XI, accessory nerve; XII, hypoglossal nerve; A, pharyngeal branch of the glossopharyngeal nerve; B, pharyngeal branch of the vagus nerve; C, cranial laryngeal nerve; D, cranial cervical ganglion.) (Redrawn from Freeman DE, Donawick WJ: Occlusion of internal carotid artery in the horse by means of a balloon-tipped catheter: Clinical use of a method to prevent epistaxis caused by guttural pouch mycosis, J Am Vet Med Assoc 1980;176:236.)

compartment and gives off the caudal auricular artery and superficial temporal artery, and it continues as the maxillary artery (MA) along the roof of the guttural pouch. The facial nerve (CN VII) passes for a short distance over the caudal, dorsal aspect of the lateral compartment after it emerges from the stylomastoid foramen. The vestibulocochlear nerve (CN VIII) enters the internal acoustic meatus caudal to the facial nerve and divides into vestibular and cochlear branches that innervate components of the middle ear. This nerve does not enter the guttural pouch but can become involved in guttural pouch diseases that affect the middle ear (e.g., temporohyoid osteoarthropathy). The mandibular nerve, a branch of the trigeminal nerve (CN V), emerges from the foramen lacerum, passes close to the muscular process of the petrous part of the temporal bone, and continues rostrally along the roof of the lateral compartment of the guttural pouch.

The guttural pouch is lined with pseudostratified ciliated epithelium containing goblet cells[1] in both adults and foals.[6] The guttural pouch mucosa has the ability to clear foreign substances, but this ability varies among different regions of the epithelium.[6] In a study on the distribution of various immunoglobulin isotypes and sub-isotypes in the guttural pouch mucosa of healthy horses, IgGa was found in the guttural pouch mucosa, mucosal lymph nodules, and submucosal lymph nodules.[7] IgM was scattered in the mucosal lymph nodules and in the germinal centers of the submucosal lymph nodules. IgGc was recognized only in the submucosal lymph nodules, and IgA was detected in glandular epithelial cells and the surface layer of the mucosal epithelium.[7]

Possible functions of the guttural pouches include pressure equilibration across the tympanic membrane, contribution to air warming, a resonating chamber for vocalization, and a flotation device.[8] A role more recently proposed, on the basis of measurement of lower arterial temperatures in the cerebral side of the internal carotid artery compared with the cardiac side, is brain-cooling.[9,10] Based on cadaver studies, opening of the pharyngeal orifice of the guttural pouch involves the levator and tensor veli palatini muscles and the pterygopharyngeus and palatopharyngeus muscles. Passive opening of the auditory tube involves a reduced tone in the stylopharyngeus and pterygopharyngeus muscles, accompanied by increased inspiratory pressure.[11] Although guttural pouch filling was previously reported to occur on expiration, the latter study demonstrated that filling occurs on inspiration.[11]

EXAMINATION

The guttural pouches are examined by external palpation, endoscopy, and radiography. Enlargement caused by empyema (purulent material in the pouches), but particularly by tympany (air engorgement), can be palpated externally. Guttural pouch endoscopy provides the most information regarding guttural pouch disease. Nonspecific evidence of guttural pouch disease, such as collapse of the pharynx and blood or pus draining from the pharyngeal orifice, can be found on endoscopic examination of the pharynx. However, blood or pus from other respiratory sources may be aspirated into the guttural pouch opening and appear to drain from it, so that direct endoscopic examination of the pouches must be performed (Fig. 45-2). With the horse mildly sedated, the biopsy instrument is passed through the biopsy channel of the endoscope and used to guide the endoscope into the guttural pouch. The endoscope is placed so that the biopsy forceps is as close as possible to the lateral wall of the pharynx until successful insertion into the guttural pouch is achieved. Both pouches can be entered in this manner with the endoscope in the same nostril. Alternatively, the pharyngeal opening can be levered open with a Chamber's catheter to allow the endoscope to enter the pouches.

Lateral radiographic projections of the guttural pouches can demonstrate fluid lines, fractures and exostoses of the stylohyoid bone, radiopaque foreign bodies, and space-occupying masses.[12] Air distention, as in tympany, can increase dimensions of the affected guttural pouch, sometimes beyond the second cervical vertebra. A dorsoventral or ventrodorsal projection is best used to image the stylohyoid bones and temorohyoid articulation. Computed tomography can provide an alternate imaging modality,[13-16] especially for imaging of the stylohyoid bone, inner ear, and petrous temporal bone in cases of temporohyoid osteoarthropathy.[16] Ultrasonography can be used to demonstrate soft tissue lesions in the guttural pouches, such as tumors[17] or muscle damage and associated submucosal hemorrhage.[18]

A percutaneous centesis technique through Viborg's triangle has been described for guttural pouch lavage and collection of samples for cytologic and microbiologic examinations.[19] The normal cytologic pattern is less than 5% neutrophils, a large proportion of ciliated columnar epithelial cells, a few nonciliated cuboidal epithelial cells, and less than 1% monocytes, lymphocytes, and eosinophils.[20,21] The proportion of neutrophils is important, with less than 5% being considered normal and greater than 25% being considered abnormal. There is a high correlation between a high cytologic score and the presence of pathogenic bacteria such as *Streptococcus equi*.[20,21] The cytologic gradings and

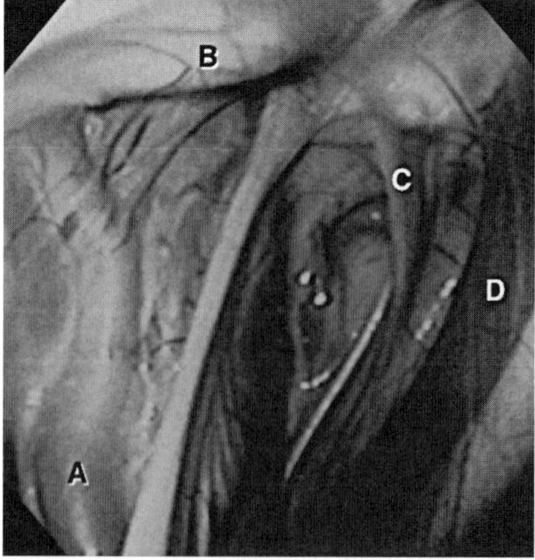

Figure 45-2. Normal endoscopic anatomy of right guttural pouch. The narrow pale structure that runs from dorsal to ventral is the stylohyoid bone that divides the caudoventral part into lateral (to left) and medial (to right) compartments. Sources of hemorrhage from the guttural pouch: A, external carotid artery; B, maxillary artery; C, internal carotid artery; D, ventral straight muscles.

neutrophil concentrations of guttural pouch washings are increased in horses whose heads are restrained for more than 12 hours, as would occur during long transportation.[22] Washings from these horses are more likely to contain bacteria and yield potentially pathogenic bacteria.[22]

DISEASES OF THE GUTTURAL POUCH

Tympany

Tympany, as the name implies, is the distention of the guttural pouches with air under pressure, sometimes accompanied with some fluid accumulation. This condition is usually unilateral but can be bilateral and is more common in fillies than in colts.[23] In 51 foals with guttural pouch tympany seen at a German clinic between 1994 and 2001, there were approximately three times as many fillies as colts,[24] regardless of breed.[25,26] There were significantly more Arabian and Paint horse foals compared with the breed distribution of hospitalized foals at the same clinic.[24] In the 27 Arabian purebred foals affected with guttural pouch tympany, many were from the same stud farm and some were full or half siblings. Complex segregation analysis showed that a polygenic and a mixed monogenic–polygenic model best explained the segregation of Arabian foals with this disease.[27]

Possible causes include a mucosal flap that acts as a one-way valve and traps air and fluid in the pouch, inflammation from an upper airway infection, persistent coughing, and muscle dysfunction.[28] In most cases, there is no gross anatomic abnormality at the guttural pouch opening.

Clinical Signs

Guttural pouch tympany develops in foals shortly after birth and up to 1 year of age. The affected guttural pouch is distended with air to form a nonpainful, elastic swelling in the parotid region. Although the swelling is most prominent on the affected side, it can extend across the neck and give the impression of bilateral involvement. Severe distention is usually well tolerated and does not interfere with growth and development, but it can cause dyspnea, dysphagia, and inhalation pneumonia. Secondary empyema is not uncommon.

Diagnosis

Diagnosis is based largely on clinical signs. On endoscopic examination, the pharyngeal openings usually appear normal, but the roof of the pharynx can be collapsed. Guttural pouch enlargement with air and fluid can be seen on radiographs. Distinguishing between unilateral and bilateral tympany can be difficult on radiographs, but usually they can be defined on direct endoscopy of each pouch.[29]

Treatment

Temporary alleviation can be achieved by needle decompression or by placing an indwelling catheter in the pharyngeal orifice; however, surgery is required for definitive treatment. The affected guttural pouch is usually entered through Viborg's triangle or through a modified Whitehouse approach (discussed later). The median septum can be fenestrated by removal of a 2-cm^2 segment to allow egress of trapped air from the tympanitic pouch through the normal side[28] (Fig. 45-3). A Chamber's mare catheter or, preferably, a lighted fiberoptic endoscope can be inserted into the healthy pouch to elevate the septum toward the incision and to demonstrate it (see Fig. 45-3). When bilateral involvement is suspected, the fenestration procedure can be

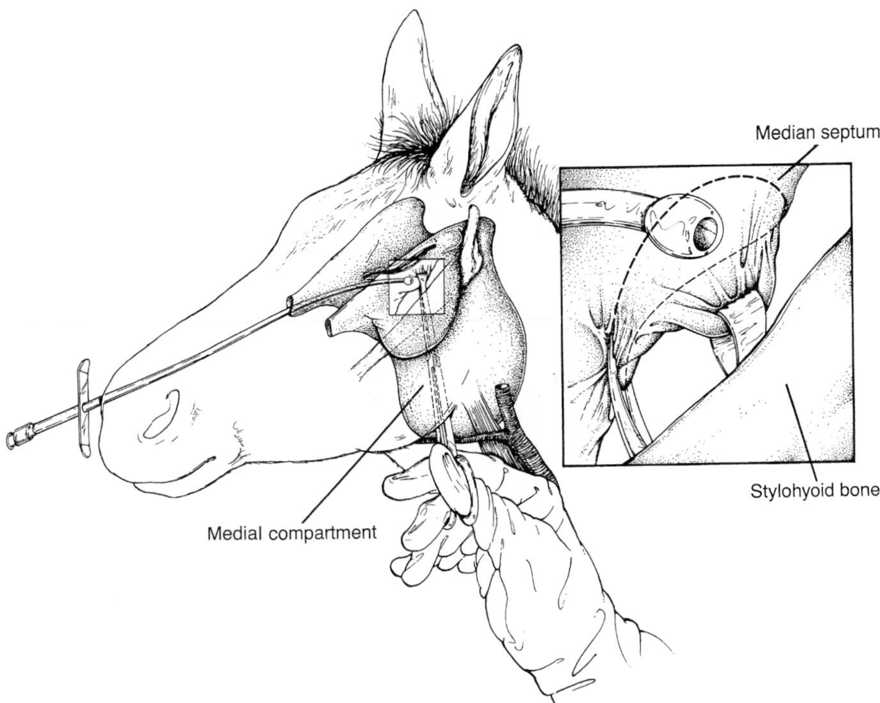

Figure 45-3. Method for creating a fenestration between the abnormal and normal guttural pouches in a foal with unilateral tympany. The affected guttural pouch (on the left side) is approached through an incision in Viborg's triangle, and a Chamber mare catheter in the right guttural pouch is used to elevate and expose the median septum. In the *expanded view,* a pair of scissors has been placed to start fenestration (*broken line*). (Redrawn from Milne DW, Fessler JF: Tympanitis of the guttural pouch in a foal, J Am Vet Med Assoc 1972;161:61; and Deen T: Surgically correcting guttural pouch tympany, Vet Med 1988;83:592.)

combined with removal of a small segment (1.5 × 2.5 cm) of the medial lamina of the eustachian tube and associated mucosal fold within the guttural pouch orifice[23,29]; this forms a larger opening into the pharynx. The approach incision can be closed or left open to heal by second intention. Systemic antibiotics are given if needed.

Transendoscopic electrocautery can be used to create a fenestration in the septum and to make a fistula into the guttural pouch through the pharyngeal recess.[28,30] A high-powered diode or a neodymium:yttrium-aluminum-garnet (Nd:YAG) laser can also be used through a transendoscopic approach to create the fenestration. This can be carried out as a standing procedure[31] or with the horse under general anesthesia.[29] An alternative and easier method is to create a salpingopharyngeal fistula using the laser under video-endoscopic control in the wall of the pharynx, caudal to the guttural pouch opening.[31] A Foley catheter is placed through the fistula for 7 to 10 days to act as a stent and to allow lavage of the guttural pouch.[31]

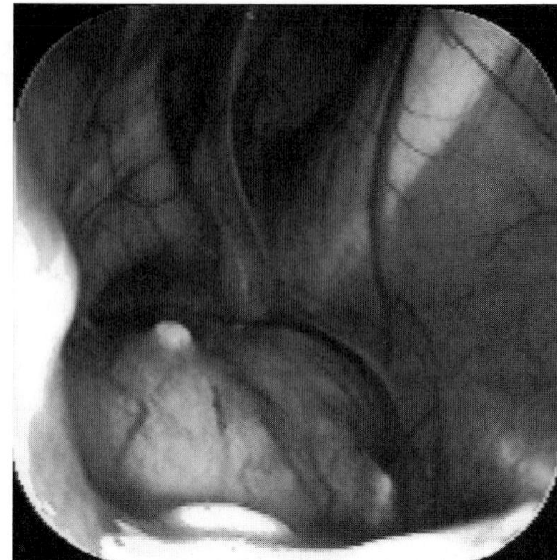

Figure 45-4. Endoscopic view of the interior of the right guttural pouch of a horse with enlargement and drainage from a retropharyngeal lymph node. Note purulent material on floor of the medial compartment.

Prognosis

The prognosis for complete recovery and a successful racing career is favorable after median septum fenestration by any method.[23,29] A surgical laser technique was used on 50 foals in one clinic and was successful in 35 foals after one treatment and in 15 foals after two treatments.[24] Long-term follow-up information, available for 44 of the 50 treated horses, revealed no deaths related to the disease or treatment and that all horses up to 2 years of age were healthy.[24]

Secondary empyema and pneumonia usually resolve spontaneously after successful treatment of the tympany; however, the prognosis is guarded for foals that have aspiration pneumonia and dysphagia secondary to nerve damage induced during surgical correction.[23] The fenestration procedure can fail if the newly created opening seals or the condition is bilateral.[23,29] Resection of the mucosal fold can fail if swelling and inflammation along the cut edges close the pharyngeal orifice.[32] The salpingopharyngeal fistula may seal if the catheter does not stay in place for the period required for the fistula to mature.[31] Horses treated with this method have responded favorably.[31]

Empyema

Empyema of the guttural pouches is defined as the presence of purulent material (Fig. 45-4), and chondroids within the one or both guttural pouches. Chondroids consist of inspissated purulent material (usually numerous individual round balls) that forms in some cases (Fig. 45-5). Empyema can affect horses of any age but usually occurs in young animals. Upper respiratory tract infections (especially those caused by *Streptococcus*), abscessation and rupture of retropharyngeal lymph nodes into the guttural pouch (see Fig. 45-4), infusion of irritant drugs, fracture of the stylohyoid bone, congenital or acquired stenosis of the pharyngeal orifice, and pharyngeal perforation by a nasogastric tube may cause empyema.[28,33] Persistence of guttural pouch infection in asymptomatic long-term carriers could be responsible for recurrent outbreaks of strangles.[34] In one study of 91 horses with guttural pouch empyema, 21% had chondroids, and the horses with chondroids were more likely to have retropharyngeal and pharyngeal swelling than those without this complication.[35] The number of chondroids present is variable, ranging from one to many (see Fig. 45-5), and both guttural pouches can be affected.[35] Duration of infection does not appear to correlate with development of chondroids.[35]

Clinical Signs

Clinical signs include intermittent nasal discharge in most cases, swelling of adjacent lymph nodes, parotid swelling and pain, extended head carriage, excessive respiratory noise, and difficulties in swallowing and breathing. In rare cases, guttural pouch empyema can cause pharyngeal and laryngeal paresis.[36]

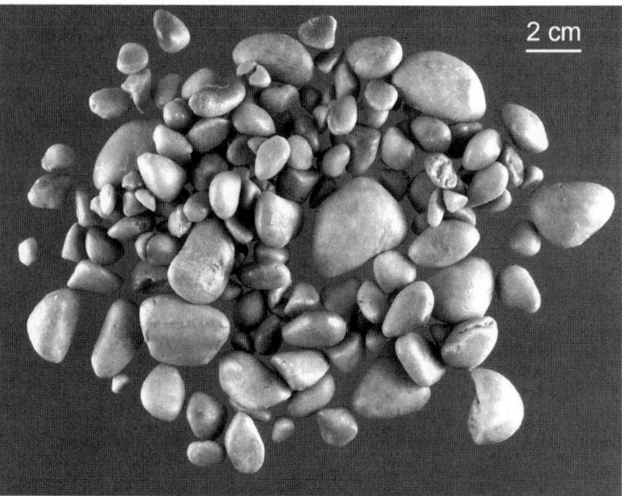

Figure 45-5. Guttural pouch chondroids removed through a modified Whitehouse approach.

Diagnosis

On endoscopic examination, a purulent discharge can be seen at the pharyngeal orifice of the affected side, with pharyngeal collapse in some horses. Fluid accompanied by masses seen within the guttural pouch on standing lateral radiographs is suggestive of chondroids.[37] Fluid aspirates or saline washings can be taken from the guttural pouch for culture and sensitivity testing; however, results should be interpreted with caution because microorganisms can be retrieved from the normal guttural pouch and upper respiratory tract. Horses that are carriers of, or are infected with, *S. equi* in the guttural pouches can be identified by culture and polymerase chain reaction tests with repeated swabs.[38]

Treatment

In acute cases, daily irrigation with physiologic saline solution is usually effective. An indwelling catheter, devised from polyethylene 240 tubing with heat-formed coils at one end, can be used for this purpose. Alternatively, a commercially available guttural pouch catheter (Cook Veterinary Projects, Bloomington, Ind; Mila International, Florence, Ky) or one fashioned from a polypropylene dog urinary catheter can be used. Coiled catheters can be straightened to facilitate insertion by inserting a coaxial wire or by passage through a larger curved catheter. The coiled end of the catheter is placed under endoscopic guidance within the pouch, and the free end is secured by a suture to the alar fold. A Foley catheter can also be used, but it should be advanced until the end is completely in the pouch because distention of the balloon within the pharyngeal opening could cause pressure necrosis. In larger horses, standard Foley catheters are not long enough to reach the guttural pouch. Alternatively, the pouch can be flushed through the biopsy channel of the endoscope, which has the advantage of delivery of the flush solution to areas coated with purulent material. After 7 to 10 days, irrigation should be interrupted briefly to assess the response, with the awareness that this treatment can cause some inflammation.

Hydrogen peroxide or concentrated antiseptic solutions should not be infused because they are irritating and can induce neuritis of the cranial nerves. Topical antibiotics are rarely effective because the contact period is too brief and many are inactivated by the products of inflammation present in the purulent material. Dilute povidone-iodine (1%) is more effective than concentrated solutions because free iodine dissociates more readily from the organic carrier at low concentrations; however, iodine can be neutralized by exudates.[39] In one horse with empyema that did not respond to saline lavage, infusion of acetylcysteine on four occasions appeared to hasten resolution.[40] However, despite its ability to disrupt disulfide bonds of mucoproteins, acetylcysteine did not alter the viscosity of purulent material in clot tubes compared with the use of saline alone.[40] Systemic antibiotics are rarely indicated unless the response to topical treatment is poor or the infection is severe. Drugs of choice are a potentiated sulphonamide, penicillin, or ceftiofur for at least 21 days.[38] Nonsteroidal anti-inflammatory drugs may be used as needed.

In severely dyspneic horses caused by guttural pouch distention, a tracheotomy should be performed. If the response to medical treatment is poor or if the purulent material becomes inspissated or forms chondroids, surgical drainage of the guttural pouch should be considered (discussed later). Chondroids can also be removed by maceration, followed by saline lavage or extraction by endoscopically guided grabbing forceps, a basket snare, or a memory-helical polyp retrieval basket (Cook Ltd, Bloomington, Ind).[38] Another technique involves repeated section of each mass by a diathermic snare (Olympus Optical Co, Irving, Tex) or a wire loop, with removal by suction, lavage, or extraction by basket-type endoscopic forceps (Gomco Equipment, Chemetron Medical Products, Buffalo, NY).[41] In one study, 44% of horses with chondroids were treated successfully by these noninvasive methods,[35] although removal by these methods can take a long time. If empyema is the result of occlusion of guttural pouch openings by adhesions, this occlusion may be relieved by blunt division through a surgical approach to the guttural pouch interior.[38] Chronic empyema of the guttural pouches, possibly unresponsive to medical therapy because of poor drainage through the pharyngeal ostia, can be successfully treated by using a laser to establish a permanent pharyngeal fistula into the guttural pouch.[42]

Prognosis

Response to medical treatment is usually satisfactory, and surgery is rarely indicated. Neurologic signs usually resolve once the infection is brought under control by medical or surgical treatment.

Guttural Pouch Mycosis

Guttural pouch mycosis affects the roof of one guttural pouch, rarely both. There is no apparent age, sex, breed, or geographic predisposition to this disease. The cause of guttural pouch mycosis is unknown, although *Aspergillus* can be identified in the lesion. The typical lesion of guttural pouch mycosis is a diphtheritic membrane of variable size, composed of necrotic tissue, cell debris, a variety of bacteria, and fungal mycelia.[28] Aneurysm formation does not appear to precede or follow arterial invasion consistently and, therefore, is not essential to the pathogenesis of arterial rupture.

Clinical Signs

The most common clinical sign is moderate-to-severe epistaxis, which is caused by fungal erosion of the internal carotid artery in most cases[43-46] (Fig. 45-6) and of the external carotid and maxillary arteries in approximately one third of cases[47,48] (Fig. 45-7, and see Fig. 45-2). However, any branch of the external carotid artery, such as the caudal auricular artery, can be affected. Several bouts of hemorrhage usually precede a fatal episode. Mucus and dark blood continue to drain from the nostril on the affected side for days after acute hemorrhage ceases.

The second most common clinical sign is dysphagia caused by damage to the pharyngeal branches of the vagus and glossopharyngeal nerves[44] (see Fig. 45-6). Aspiration pneumonia may develop in severe or protracted cases. Abnormal respiratory noise can arise from pharyngeal paresis or laryngeal hemiplegia, the latter as a result of recurrent laryngeal nerve damage.[44] Horner's syndrome may develop from damage to the cranial cervical ganglion and postganglionic sympathetic fibers. The classic signs associated with this denervation are ptosis, miosis, and enophthalmos; patchy sweating; and congestion of the nasal mucosa. The reason for equine sweat glands to increase their activity when denervated is unclear.[49] Equine sweat gland myoepithelium is predominantly under α_2-adrenergic control, with additional α-adrenergic input from receptors.[49] However, sweating after neurectomy may be caused by increased peripheral vasodilation, which increases blood flow and skin temperature.[49] Ptosis is caused by a decreased tone of the superior tarsus muscle, and it is assessed by observing eyelash angles from a frontal view.[49] Pupillary response to decreased sympathetic tone in horses is variable, and the maximal difference in pupil size is usually slight.[49] Enophthalmos, which is the result of decreased smooth muscle retrobulbar tone and unopposed activity of the striated retractor bulbi muscle, is rarely obvious and usually evident as a slight protrusion of the nictitating membrane.[49]

Less common signs of guttural pouch mycosis are parotid pain, nasal discharge, abnormal head posture, head shyness, sweating and shivering, corneal ulcers, colic, blindness, locomotion disturbances, facial nerve paralysis, paralysis of the tongue, and septic arthritis of the atlantooccipital joint.[43,44,50-53]

Diagnosis

Endoscopy is critical for diagnosis, and it should be combined with history and clinical signs. On endoscopic examination of a horse with epistaxis, blood can be seen draining from the pharyngeal orifice. In horses with dysphagia, the roof of the pharynx can be collapsed, the soft palate can be displaced, and the nasopharynx may contain food material. The lesion appears as a white, tan, and black diphtheritic membrane on the roof of the affected guttural pouch, and its size can vary but bears no relationship to the severity of clinical signs (see Fig. 45-6). Part of the diphtheritic membrane can coat the stylohyoid bone and the bone can be thickened, but clinical signs usually do not develop from this change. Fistulas may form into the opposite guttural pouch and pharynx.[46] The presence of serum antibodies to *Aspergillus fumigatus* detected by enzyme-linked immunosorbent assay (ELISA) cannot distinguish between horses with guttural pouch mycosis and healthy horses.[54]

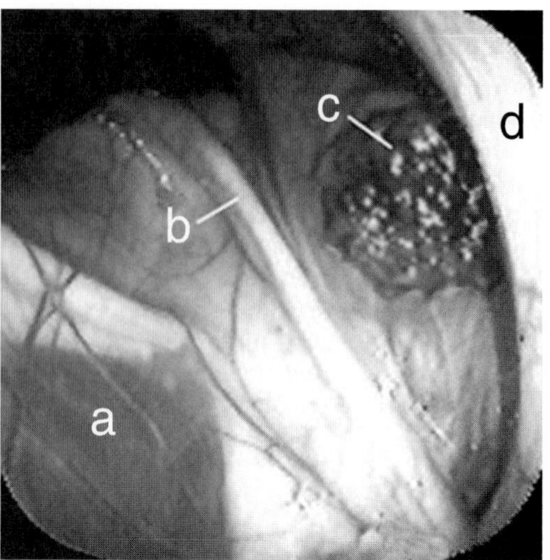

Figure 45-7. Roof of the left guttural pouch as viewed through retroflexion of the endoscope. a, insertion of ventral straight muscles of the head; b, cartilaginous flap of the eustachian tube; c, mycotic lesion on the left maxillary artery; d, dorsal edge of the stylohyoid bone. This approach provides an excellent view of these structures when the rostral end of the guttural pouch is obscured with hemorrhage.

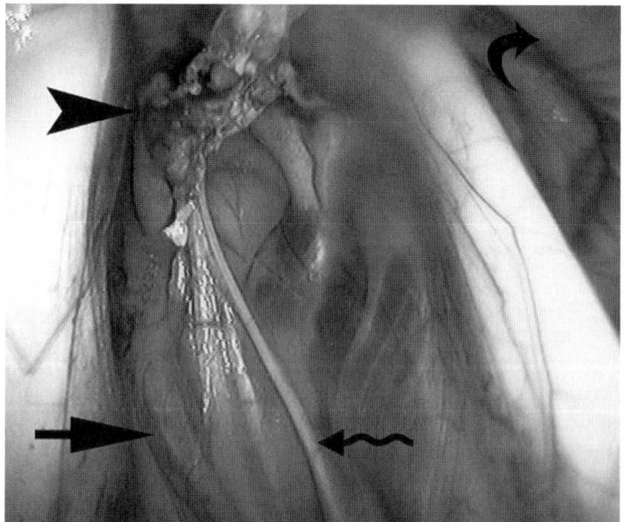

Figure 45-6. Guttural pouch mycosis in the typical location on the roof of the medial compartment (left guttural pouch), overlying the internal carotid artery. The *arrowhead* indicates the lesion, the *straight arrow* the internal carotid artery, the *wavy arrow* the mucosal reflection that contains the glossopharyngeal and hypoglossal nerves, and the *curved arrow* the maxillary artery lateral to the stylohyoid bone. This small lesion did not cause epistaxis but did cause dysphagia that necessitated euthanasia.

Treatment

NONSURGICAL TREATMENT

The response to topical treatment is generally slow and inconsistent. Daily direct lavage through the endoscope can macerate the diphtheritic membrane, and the biopsy forceps or cytology brush of the endoscope can be used to detach it, provided any eroded artery was occluded beforehand. Topical povidone-iodine or thiabendazole, with or without dimethyl sulfoxide, has been used with mixed results.[46,47,50,55] Nystatin, natamycin, and miconazole have little activity against *Aspergillus*,[56] but amphotericin B is effective against this organism, although its use in the horse is limited by its toxicity.[57]

Successful treatment of dysphagia from guttural pouch mycosis has been reported with a combination of itraconazole (5 mg/kg body weight PO) and topical enilconazole (60 mL of 33.3 mg/mL solution per daily flush) in one horse[55] and with topical enilconazole alone in another.[58] Itraconazole at 3 mg/kg twice a day in the feed can be effective against *Aspergillus* and other fungi in the nasal passage of horses, but treatment may be required for up to 4 or 5 months.[59] Bioavailability of another triazole antifungal agent, fluconazole, can be sufficiently high after oral and intravenous administration in horses to suggest a potential value in treatment of fungal infections.[60] The response to any treatment method that is measured solely by disappearance of the mycotic lesion should be interpreted with caution because spontaneous regression of the lesion over a variable time course is typical. Horses with blood loss should be treated with polyionic fluids and, if necessary, with blood transfusions, and horses with dysphagia should be fed by nasogastric tube or by esophagostomy and should receive nonsteroidal anti-inflammatory drugs to reduce neuritis.

SURGICAL TREATMENT

The diphtheritic membrane can be detached by gentle swabbing and lavage through a modified Whitehouse approach. This treatment does not eliminate the risk of hemorrhage completely, and it does not retard or reverse progression of neurologic signs, but it does carry the risk of iatrogenic nerve damage and hemorrhage. In horses with epistaxis, the affected artery should be identified by endoscopy and surgically occluded (discussed later). There is some anecdotal but widely accepted evidence that occlusion of the affected artery hastens spontaneous resolution of the mycotic lesion and thereby renders medical therapy unnecessary.[61]

Prognosis

Approximately 50% of horses with hemorrhage die from this complication,[44] but this risk can be abolished or considerably reduced by the occlusion procedures described later. These procedures must be performed as soon as possible after the first bout of hemorrhage to prevent subsequent bouts that could render the horse a poor candidate for anesthesia and surgery.

Although the mycotic lesion disappears with time, neurologic signs can persist. Laryngeal hemiplegia is usually permanent, but recovery has been reported.[43] Some horses with dysphagia do eventually recover, but 6 to 18 months may be required and recovery may be incomplete.[43,44] Horses can recover from Horner's syndrome and facial nerve paralysis.

Rupture of the Ventral Straight Muscles

Rupture of ventral straight muscles of the head (the longus capitis muscle and rectus capitis ventralis muscle) is usually caused by trauma, such as falling over backward, and it can cause severe epistaxis.[18] A nondisplaced impaction fracture at the basisphenoid–basioccipital junction associated with this injury can cause neurologic signs from subdural hemorrhage over the cerebral cortex and brain stem.[62] The same injury may occur without causing epistaxis.[62]

Clinical Signs and Diagnosis

Rupture of the ventral straight muscles causes severe epistaxis, as does guttural pouch mycosis.[18] Some horses may show ataxia and other neurologic signs, and hemorrhage from torn muscle into the retropharyngeal tissues can compress the pharynx and even the trachea and cause respiratory obstruction.[18]

Rupture of the ventral straight muscles is distinguished from guttural pouch mycosis by a history of trauma with the former, if such history is available, and by endoscopy.[18] In horses with rupture of the ventral straight muscles, the roof of the pharynx is collapsed and both guttural pouches are affected, usually more so on one side than on the other. Unlike in guttural pouch mycosis, the major arteries and the more caudal aspects of the guttural pouches are not involved, and there is no evidence of a diphtheritic membrane (Fig. 45-8). Although some dark blood can be seen in the most rostral aspect of the pouch, it usually obscures the view of this area. A more complete view of the source of hemorrhage and swollen muscle bellies can be seen by retroversion of the endoscope[18] (see Fig. 45-7). After swelling and inflammation from the original injury have subsided, any displaced bone fragment from a basisphenoid–basioccipital avulsion fracture can be seen on endoscopic examination of the medial compartment of the guttural pouch.[63]

On radiographs, partial obliteration of the guttural pouch by increased soft tissue density, soft tissue impingement on the roof of the pharynx, gas in soft tissues of the head and neck, and even avulsions of the basisphenoid bone may be evident[63] (Fig. 45-9). The size and extent of the hematoma and gas in soft tissues can be determined by an ultrasonographic examination.

Treatment and Prognosis

Treatment is stall rest for 4 to 6 weeks, and limiting head and neck movement that could disturb the damaged muscles and precipitate hemorrhage. Antibiotics are given to prevent secondary infections through the disrupted mucosa. The prognosis is good provided there are no neurologic signs, because these can be permanent and life threat-

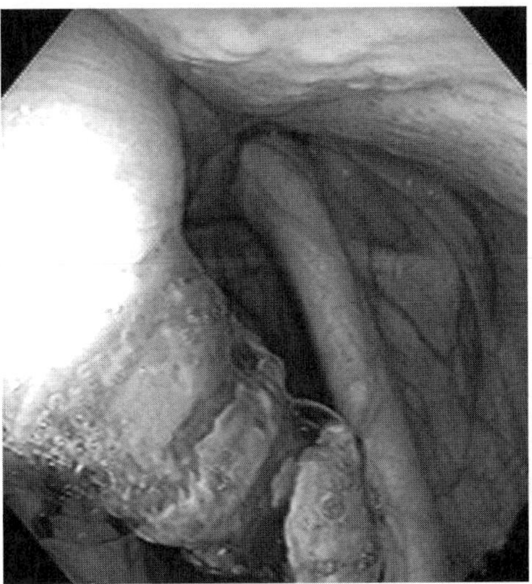

Figure 45-8. Endoscopic view of torn ventral straight muscles of the head in the left guttural pouch. The injury is rostral to the arteries in the caudal part of the guttural pouch. (Courtesy A. Walesby, Louisiana State University.)

ening.[18] Severe neurologic signs, such as inability to rise, depression, and sluggish menace response, may be caused by an associated subdural hemorrhage overlying the cerebral cortex and brain stem,[62] and warrant euthanasia.

Temporohyoid Osteoarthropathy (Middle Ear Disease)

Temporohyoid osteoarthropathy is a progressive disease of the middle ear and components of the temporohyoid joint, such as the stylohyoid bone, the cartilaginous tympanohyoid, and squamous portion of the temporal bone.[64] Horses of a wide age range and of any breed or either sex can be affected.[64] The cause is thought to be an inner or a middle ear infection of hematogenous origin that spreads to the aforementioned bones, causing them to thicken and the temporohyoid joint to fuse.[64] Other possible causes range from extension of otitis media/externa or guttural pouch infection to a nonseptic osteoarthritis.[64-68] Although guttural pouch mycosis can involve the same bony structures and temporohyoid articulation,[44] clinical signs of temporohyoid osteoarthropathy are rare with this disease.

Once the temporohyoid joint fuses and the associated bones thicken, forces generated by movement of the tongue and larynx during swallowing, vocalizing, combined head and neck movements, oral or dental examinations, and teeth floating may induce fractures of the petrous part of the temporal bone, resulting in facial nerve (CN VII) and vestibulocochlear nerve (CN VIII) dysfunction.[64-69] Severe new bone production and inflammation can damage the glossopharyngeal and vagus nerves where they leave the medulla caudal to the vestibulocochlear nerve.[1,70] After fracture of the petrous temporal bone, middle or inner ear infection could extend around the brain stem and involve additional cranial nerves and hindbrain structures.

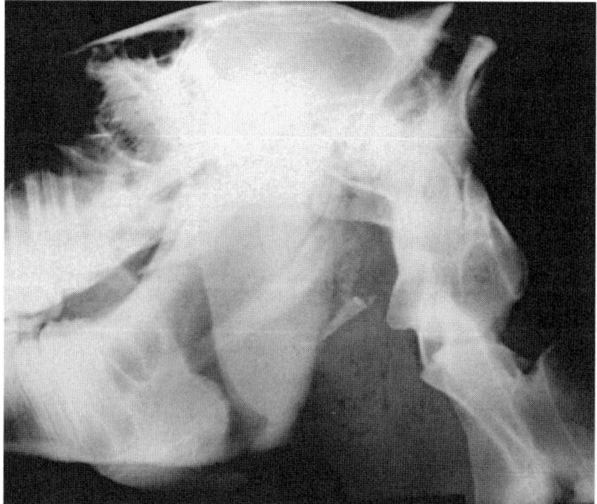

Figure 45-9. Radiograph demonstrating avulsion fracture of the basisphenoid bone, soft-tissue obliteration of the guttural pouch cavity, soft-tissue impingement on the pharynx, and gas in soft tissues in a horse with ruptured ventral straight muscles of the head. (Courtesy J. Foreman, Louisiana State University.)

Clinical Signs and Diagnosis

Early signs include head tossing, ear rubbing, refusing to take the bit, refusing to position the head properly when under saddle, resistance to digital pressure around the base of the ears or on the basihyoid bone, and other nonspecific behavioral changes.[64] The disease can cause an acute onset of signs consistently referable to the vestibulotrochlear nerve, including asymmetrical ataxia, head tilt with the poll to the affected side, and spontaneous nystagmus with the slow component to the affected side.[64] These signs can be revealed or exacerbated by blindfolding. Signs of facial nerve damage, including paresis or paralysis of the ear on the affected side, deviation of the upper lip away from the affected side, decreased tear production, and inability to close the eyes, are evident in most cases.[69,70] Decreased tear production and inability to close the eyes may cause corneal ulcers, keratoconjunctivitis sicca, and exposure keratitis.[69,70] Dysphagia is rare but can result from damage to the glossopharyngeal and vagus nerves.[64]

Radiographs of the skull may depict proliferation and osteitis of the affected bones; however, endoscopy of the guttural pouch is in most cases a more sensitive method for detection of stylohyoid bone and temporohyoid joint involvement and hence for making the diagnosis[71] (Fig. 45-10). Computed tomography can precisely demonstrate bony and soft tissue changes in the middle and inner ear.[16]

Treatment and Prognosis

Medical treatment includes broad-spectrum antibiotics for infection, nonsteroidal anti-inflammatory drugs to relieve pain and inflammation, and dimethyl sulfoxide to relieve inflammation.[64,72] Unilateral partial ostectomy of the stylohyoid bone has been used to create a pseudoarthrosis between the cut ends of the bone (Fig. 45-11), which decreases the forces on the ankylosed temporohyoid and thereby prevents skull fractures.[72] In this procedure, approximately 2 to 3 cm of the midbody of the stylohyoid bone is removed (see Fig. 45-11). Although this procedure appears to have merit as a prophylactic measure against more severe bone damage and associated neurologic consequences, it may cause transient dysphagia or injury to the hypoglossal nerve.[72] When performed as a bilateral procedure, it causes permanent problems with prehension.[72]

An additional complication of the partial ostectomy is regrowth of the stylohyoid bone approximately 6 months after surgical resection, and recurrence of clinical signs.[70] Because of this complication, a *ceratohyoidectomy* can be performed as a safer, easier, and more permanent surgical alternative[70] (see Fig. 45-11). For this, the horse is placed in dorsal recumbency and the ventral laryngeal region prepared aseptically. A 10- to 15-cm incision is made in the skin medial to the linguofacial vein on the affected side and centered on the basihyoid bone,[70] approximately 2 cm from the midline as it crosses the basihyoid bone. The fibers of the sternohyoideus muscle are separated bluntly until the basihyoid bone is exposed. Rostral to the basihyoid bone, the geniohyoid muscle is separated to expose the ceratohyoid bone and, lateral to it, the hypoglossal nerve. The ceratohyoid–basihyoid synovial joint is identified and disarticulated with cartilage scissors. The transected end of

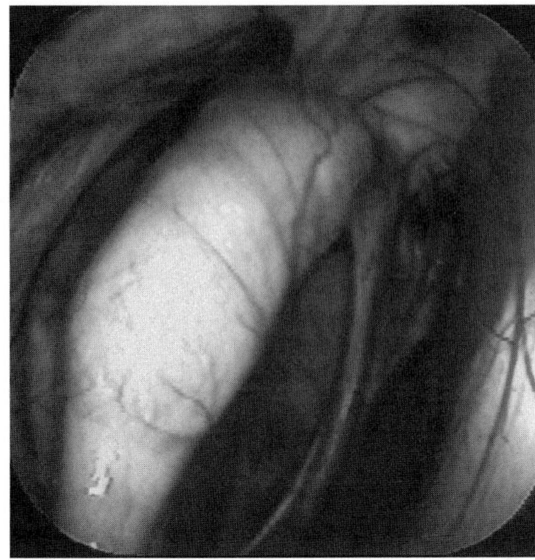

Figure 45-10. Thickened stylohyoid bone with involvement of the temporohyoid articulation in a horse with clinical signs of damage to the vestibulocochlear and facial nerves.

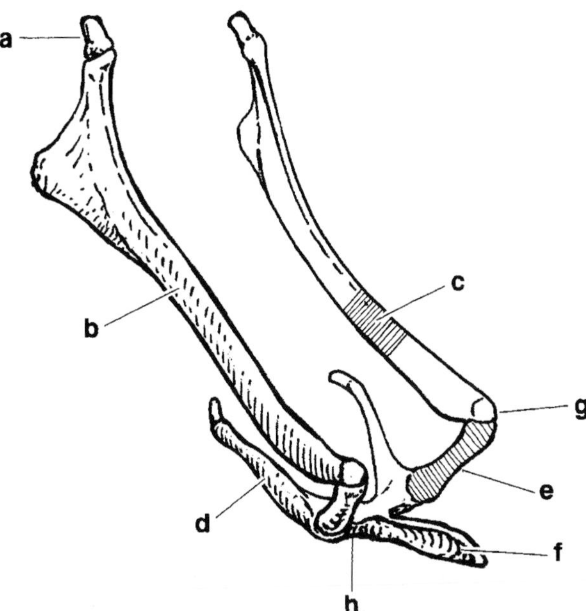

Figure 45-11. The hyoid apparatus, showing sites for ostectomy procedures *(shaded)* for horses with temporohyoid osteoarthropathy. a, tympanohyoid; b, stylohyoid bone; c, site for partial ostectomy of the stylohyoid bone; d, thyrohyoid bone; e, ceratohyoid bone; f, lingual process; g, articulation of ceratohyoid bone with stylohyoid bone and epihyoid; h, basihyoid bone.

the ceratohyoid bone is grasped and the ceratohyoid bone freed from its attachments to the ceratohyoideus, the hyoideus transversus, and the genioglossus muscles. The hypoglossal nerve and lingual branches of the mandibular and glossopharyngeal nerves are identified and gently retracted to protect them during these steps. The cartilaginous articulation between the ceratohyoid bone and the stylohyoid bone is cut by cartilage scissors, taking care to avoid tension on the bone and temporohyoid joint. The separated muscle fibers and subcutaneous tissues are then apposed using absorbable suture in a simple continuous fashion, and skin closure is routine.

Although the prognosis is good according to one report,[73] neurologic signs may persist,[71] especially if treatment is delayed. In general, the prognosis for stylohyoid arthropathy is based on the severity of the clinical signs. Some degree of facial nerve paresis can persist.[8] The corneal ulcers are difficult to treat, because there is an underlying problem with lid closure and tear production. A temporary tarsorrhaphy may help to manage the ocular complications until facial nerve function returns.

Miscellaneous

Although guttural pouch neoplasia is rare, squamous cell carcinoma,[74,75] round cell sarcoma,[12] fibroma,[76] hemangioma,[77] hemangiosarcoma,[78] and parotid melanoma have been described.[79,80] In one case, bilateral squamous cell carcinoma of the guttural pouches and the left middle ear was initially evident as protrusion of a mass in one external acoustic meatus, without other obvious clinical signs.[81]

Parotid melanomatosis can appear as multilobular or multiple individual firm lumps in the parotid region of Gray Horses with extension into the guttural pouches (Fig. 45-12) and may cause dyspnea and dysphagia from compression of the nasopharynx and larynx, and facial nerve paralysis from compression of the facial nerve.[79,80] In one case, a malignant amelanotic melanoma caused halitosis, nasal discharge and cough by undergoing central necrosis that extended from the guttural pouch into the pharynx.[17] The rate of growth of melanomas is variable and can be rapid after a prolonged initial growth,[80] but even clinically evident lesions can be well tolerated in sedentary horses and allow years of continued health.[79] Smaller lesions may not be evident externally, and it is not unusual to find small discrete and scattered submucosal black areas and even lumps in the guttural pouch of Gray Horses (see Fig. 45-12). These are unlikely to cause problems. Extensive tumors may infiltrate the parotid gland without apparent lymph node involvement. Surgical resection is rarely indicated and is usually impossible in most cases because of the extent of infiltration and the close association with vital structures.[80]

Fracture of the stylohyoid bone can be secondary to guttural pouch mycosis or trauma.[12,28] Bone necrosis can follow, and clinical signs include dysphagia, pharyngeal swelling, empyema, keratoconjunctivitis sicca, and abscessation.[12,44,69] Reported foreign bodies include segments of catheters and wire.[12,82] Cystic structures have been described as causes of guttural pouch swelling and dyspnea in young horses (Fig. 45-13) and respond favorably to surgical resection and fenestration in the median septum between the two guttural pouches.[83] The cause is unknown, but this lesion could be congenital or acquired.[83]

SURGICAL DRAINAGE OF THE GUTTURAL POUCH

The following approaches can be used to open the guttural pouch for removal of pus, mycotic plaques, and foreign bodies and to establish drainage.

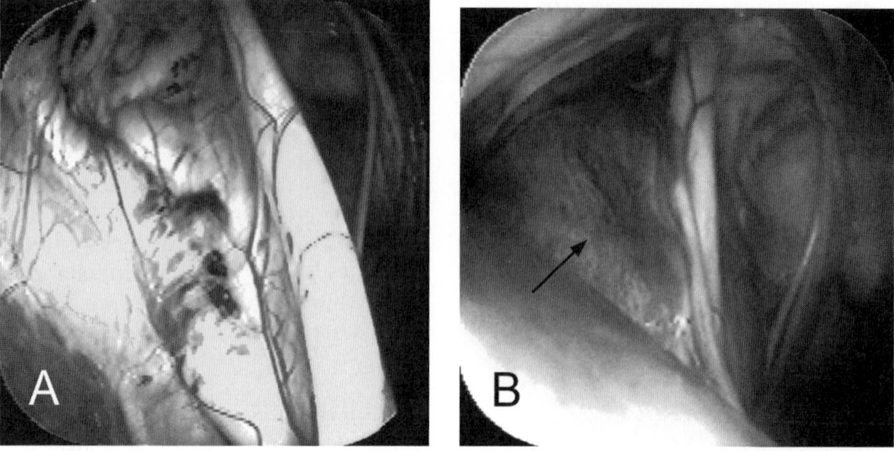

Figure 45-12. Endoscopic views of two horses with melanomas in the lateral compartments of their left guttural pouches that were not causing clinical problems. **A,** Typical melanin staining is scattered along the course of the external carotid artery and branches in an old gray horse without any external evidence of parotid involvement. **B,** A larger lesion *(arrow)* fills the lateral compartment and is evident externally as a firm mass over the parotid gland.

Hyovertebrotomy

A 10-cm-long incision is made 2 cm craniad to and parallel with the wing of the atlas (see Fig. 45-14). The dense parotid fascia is incised, and the parotid gland and overlying parotidoauricularis muscle are reflected cranially. The guttural pouch lining is exposed beneath a covering of areolar tissue and grasped with rat-toothed or Allis tissue forceps. It is punctured with the closed tips of scissors or a hemostat, and this opening is enlarged by spreading its edges with a hemostat or the fingers. To establish ventral drainage, the pouch is opened ventrally through an incision in Viborg's triangle, guided by a finger within the pouch. The hyovertebrotomy can be closed or left partly open for infusion of irrigating solutions.

Viborg's Triangle Approach

Viborg's triangle is bordered by the tendon of the sternocephalicus muscle, the linguofacial vein, and the vertical ramus of the mandible (see Fig. 45-14). A vertical or horizontal incision is made in this area, taking care to avoid the parotid duct and branches of the vagus nerve along the floor of the guttural pouch. The incision is usually kept open with a soft rubber drain to establish ventral drainage.

Whitehouse Approach

With the horse in dorsal recumbency, a skin incision is made on the ventral midline over the larynx (Fig. 45-14). Dissection is continued between the paired sternohyoideus

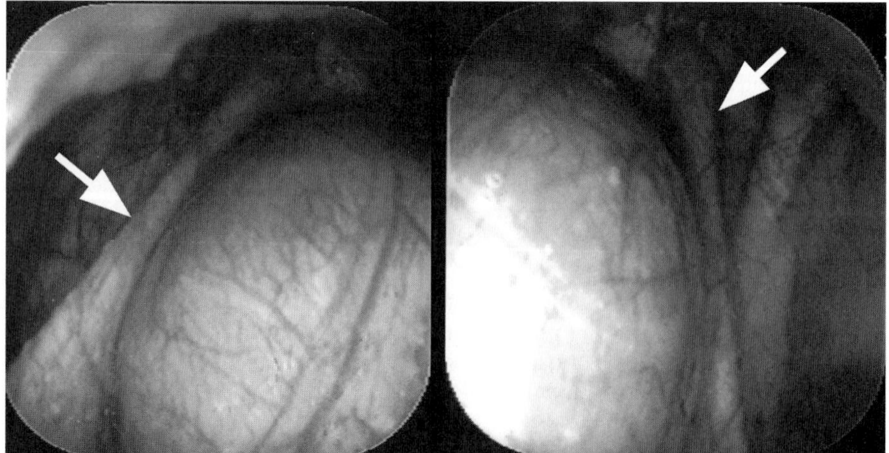

Figure 45-13. Bilateral guttural pouch cysts, each in the medial compartment of a Haflinger foal. *Arrows* point to the stylohyoid bones. This foal had nasal discharge, but the role of the cysts could not be established, there were no other clinical signs referable to them, and they were not treated.

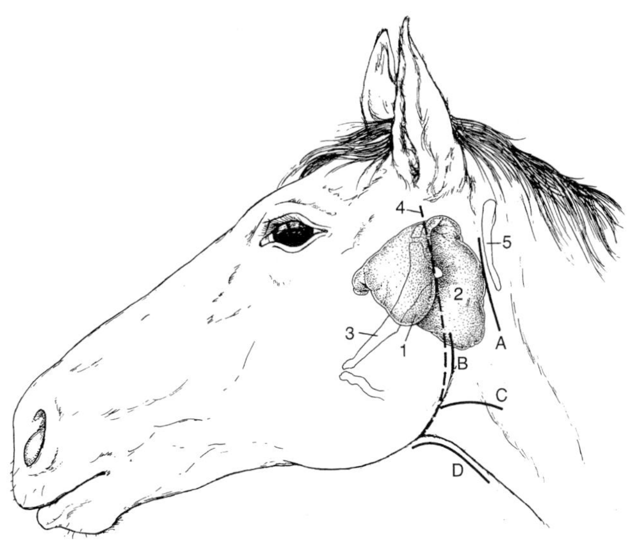

Figure 45-14. Surgical approaches to the guttural pouch. A, Hyovertebrotomy. B, Viborg's triangle. C, Modified Whitehouse. D, Whitehouse. 1, lateral compartment of the guttural pouch, which is partly separated from the medial compartment (2) by the stylohyoid bone (3); 4, vertical ramus of the mandible; 5, wing of the atlas. (Redrawn from Freeman DE: Diagnosis and treatment of diseases of the guttural pouch: Part II, Comp Cont Educ Pract Vet 1980;2:S25.)

and omohyoideus muscles and along the larynx to the affected guttural pouch. The guttural pouch is opened medial to the stylohyoid bone, and care is taken to avoid the pharyngeal branch of the vagus nerve and the cranial laryngeal nerve, which are close to the incision.

Modified Whitehouse Approach

In the modified Whitehouse approach, the skin incision is made along the ventral edge of the linguofacial vein and extends rostrally for about 12 cm from the jugular vein (see Fig. 45-14). The underlying fascia is incised to expose the lateral aspect of the larynx, and blunt dissection is continued until the guttural pouch cavity has been entered. The major advantage of this modification is that dissection is through a natural fascial plane and does not involve an incision between the sternohyoideus and omohyoideus muscles.

Advantages of both Whitehouse approaches are direct access to the roof of the guttural pouch, digital access to the lateral compartment, excellent ventral drainage, and simultaneous access through the septum to both pouches. Although both approaches involve deep dissection, they do not appear to have a higher rate of complications than other approaches.

General Comments

Surgery of the guttural pouch through any approach should be a last resort because of risks of iatrogenic nerve damage. Identification of the guttural pouch lining and underlying nerves is difficult, especially in cases in which there is no distention, and can be facilitated by a lighted endoscope inserted into the medial compartment. A fixed structure, such as the stylohyoid bone, should be used as a guide for deep dissection. The mucosa should not be incised with sharp instruments, and retractors should be applied with care to avoid nerve damage. Because all approaches enter the pouch cavity in the same approximate area, none provide less risk of nerve damage than others.

Open incisions in the guttural pouch are cleaned daily, and the guttural pouch cavity should be flushed daily with a nonirritating solution. Open incisions close spontaneously within 14 days, and the infection should also resolve within this time. Postoperative antibiotics can be given.

PROCEDURES FOR ARTERIAL OCCLUSION

In a horse with hemorrhage caused by guttural pouch mycosis, the involved artery or arteries should be occluded by one of the following procedures, or a combination of them, as soon as the diagnosis is made. The vessel to be occluded is determined by endoscopy. If accurate identification is impossible because landmarks are obscured by blood and diphtheritic membrane, all arteries in the pouch should be occluded, and this can be done safely.[48] Arteriography[84] may also be used to identify the affected vessel and to identify unusual anatomy, but it is not required in all methods or in all cases; however, it does allow more precise and selective occlusion.

Ligation of the Common Carotid Artery and Branches

In horses with guttural pouch mycosis, fatal or severe hemorrhage has followed ligation of the affected internal carotid artery (ICA) and could be attributed to occlusion of the wrong vessel or to retrograde flow from the cerebral arterial circle (circle of Willis).[43,45,85,86] A study was performed on six anesthetized adult horses to determine the effects of selective arterial occlusion on blood flow through the common carotid artery (CCA) and its branches, and to thereby establish the most effective ligation for horses with life-threatening hemorrhage from these vessels.[87] Compared with control values, flow through the left ICA was reduced to 38% by simultaneous occlusion of the left and right CCA and to 19% by occlusion of the left ICA.[87] Occlusion of the left mid-cervical CCA induced retrograde flow through the left ICA that was 40% greater than control flow.[87] In the same study, flow through the left ECA was reduced to 30% to 31% of control values by occlusion of the left mid-cervical CCA or by simultaneous occlusion of the left and right CCA.[87] Occlusion of the ECA or combined occlusion of the ECA and the major palatine artery reduced flow through the ECA to 1% of control values.[87] However, these data provide no information on blood pressure, which could remain sufficient after some of these ligations to cause substantial hemorrhage. Blood pressure in the segment of internal carotid artery in the guttural pouch is not reduced by ligation and is maintained for at least 3 days afterward at the same level as in the contralateral patent artery.[88]

Based on the preceding findings, ligation of the ipsilateral common carotid artery in a horse bleeding from the internal carotid artery would increase flow in the affected artery and would be contraindicated[87]; however, the same procedure may provide some immediate benefit in horses bleeding from the external carotid artery and its branches, although any such benefit could be temporary. Ligation of the affected ICA would decrease flow but not pressure, so bleeding could persist or recur; however, if access to definitive occlusion procedures is not immediate during a severe bleeding crisis, induction of general anesthesia to quiet the horse and ligation of the affected internal carotid artery could be attempted.

Success with *ligation of the internal carotid artery* can be attributed to thrombosis distal to the ligature at some time after surgery.[43,45] To prevent backflow, an additional ligature has been placed distal to the mycotic infection[86]; however, this is difficult because the artery must be ligated deep within the guttural pouch, where it is likely to be obscured by the diphtheritic membrane. The site for ligation of the ICA is immediately distal to its origin, outside the guttural pouch, using a similar but more ventral approach to a hyovertebrotomy (see Fig. 45-14). The ICA is identified on the cardiac side of the occipital artery and deep to that vessel. In some horses, both arteries arise as a single trunk. If necessary, both ICAs can be ligated simultaneously without any apparent risk.[45,85]

The *external carotid artery* can be ligated distal to the origin of the linguofacial trunk through an incision similar to that used for the internal carotid ligation but after extensive rostral dissection.[47] However, this procedure is generally unsuccessful because the external carotid and maxillary arteries have numerous collateral channels that allow retrograde flow to the affected segment.[1,48] Although ligation of the major palatine artery could prevent retrograde flow, a combination of this procedure with ligation of the external carotid and internal carotid arteries can cause ischemic optic neuropathy and permanent blindness.[89]

Balloon Catheter Occlusion of the Internal Carotid Artery

The balloon catheter technique allows immediate intravascular occlusion of the artery and prevents retrograde flow from the cerebral arterial circle.[46,90] Risk of retrograde flow is not diminished immediately by ligation alone, because this does not drop blood pressure in the distal segment of artery.[88]

The internal carotid artery is ligated close to its origin, and an arteriotomy is made distal to the ligature (Fig. 45-15). A size 6 French venous thrombectomy catheter (Fogarty-Edwards Laboratories, distributed by American V. Mueller, Chicago, Ill) is inserted through the arteriotomy for a distance of approximately 13 cm.[90] At this distance, the balloon tip of the catheter is arrested at the sigmoid flexure of the internal carotid artery, within the venous sinuses and distal to the site of infection (see Fig. 45-15). Fluoroscopy is not required to confirm placement, but intraoperative endoscopy can be helpful, although this can be difficult if landmarks are obscured by blood or the lesion. The catheter tip should be visible as it passes up the artery, and the balloon can be inflated at intervals to demonstrate its position. However, it does not distend the artery as dramatically as one would like, and this can make it difficult to locate. The balloon is inflated with sterile saline and secured in position by a ligature distal to the arteriotomy, and the redundant portion is buried as the incision is closed.

The horse may resume its usual activity when wound healing is complete and its packed cell volume has returned to normal. Perioperative antibiotics and nonsteroidal anti-inflammatory drugs can be used. It is not necessary to treat the fungal lesion or to remove the catheter after surgery, unless infection tracks along it and invades the surgical incision. For removal of the catheter, the horse is sedated and local anesthetic is infiltrated along and rostral to the original incision. A cut-down procedure is used to locate the coils of the catheter, which are then freed up and elevated. The balloon is deflated and the catheter is removed, usually

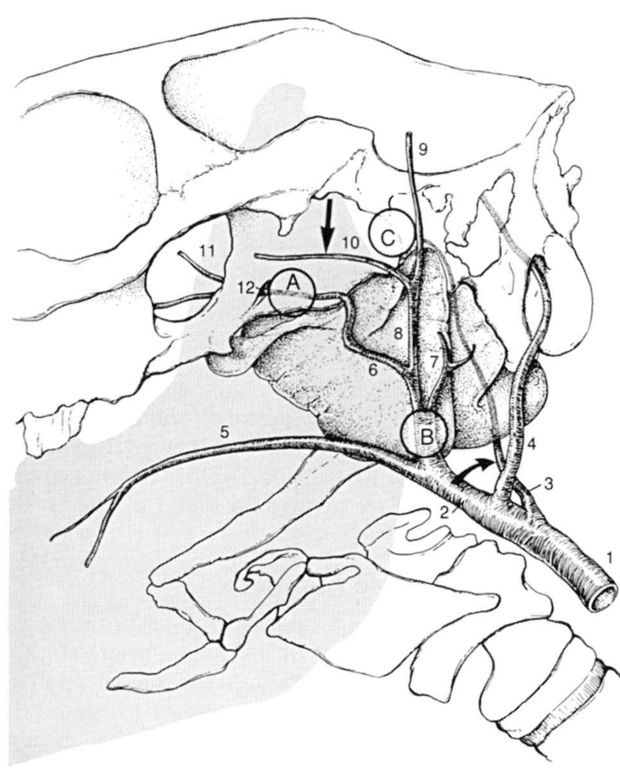

Figure 45-15. Diagram of major arteries close to and underlying the mucosa of the guttural pouch *(numbers)* and sites of balloon-catheter occlusion (*letters*). 1, common carotid artery; 2, external carotid artery; 3, internal carotid artery; 4, occipital artery; 5, linguofacial trunk; 6, maxillary artery; 7, caudal auricular artery; 8, 9 superficial temporal artery; 10, transverse facial artery; 11, external ophthalmic artery; 12, caudal alar foramen. A, Balloon inserted in the major palatine artery and guided in retrograde fashion to be inflated immediately caudal to the caudal alar foramen; B, balloon of catheter inserted into transverse facial artery (10) at arrow and directed into the external carotid artery, where it is inflated close to the floor of the guttural pouch; C, balloon in internal carotid artery at the sigmoid flexure, dorsal to the roof of the guttural pouch. This catheter is inserted into the internal carotid artery (3) at the *arrow*. A, B, C, and *arrow* on internal carotid artery are also the sites for obstruction with microcoils delivered through a catheter in the common carotid artery (1) in the upper third of the neck. (Redrawn from Caron JP, Fretz PB, Bailey JV, et al: Balloon-tipped catheter arterial occlusion for prevention of hemorrhage caused by guttural pouch mycosis: 13 cases [1982-1985], J Am Vet Assoc 1987;191:345; and Smith KM, Barber SM: Guttural pouch hemorrhage associated with lesions of the maxillary artery in horses, Can Vet J 1984;25:239.)

with considerable traction to get it through the ligature distal to the site of insertion.

Complications

Complications associated with this procedure are rare.[46,90] The catheter rarely penetrates the defect in the artery, and if it does, it can be withdrawn and redirected. Alternatively, the catheter can be left in place to obstruct the hole while another catheter is directed alongside it. This mishap can be detected by intraoperative endoscopy. Infection of the surgical site should be treated by removing the catheter and establishing drainage,[46,50] and it can be prevented by inflating the balloon to a sufficient diameter (at least 8 mm) to prevent displacement into the infected segment. Delayed prolapse of the catheter through the hole in the artery into the guttural pouch is favored by the normal pressure distal to the balloon and the loss of pressure proximal to it (heart side). The use of the more rigid commercially available catheters can also prevent this complication. Failure to prevent fatal hemorrhage in one case was caused by inadvertent catheterization and occlusion of an aberrant branch from the internal carotid artery, which left the affected segment of artery open to retrograde blood flow.[91] To prevent this mishap, approximately 6 cm of the ICA should be exposed to locate any aberrant branch. Such a branch should be ligated so that the catheter can be maintained in the internal carotid artery.[91]

It may be difficult to distinguish between the occipital and internal carotid arteries in some horses, especially those with a thick throatlatch and those in which both arteries arise as a single trunk and bifurcate at a variable distance from the common carotid artery. If both arteries arise in the normal fashion, the recommended method for identification is to dissect them both free for a couple of centimeters and then elevate each one gently with umbilical tape or a Penrose drain. It should be possible to demonstrate that the internal carotid artery lies deep to the occipital artery and that it courses more rostrally. The most troublesome anatomic aberration is an ICA that leads to the caudal cerebellar artery without following its usual pathway, and that places the inflated balloon in a position that causes neuronal necrosis of the brain stem. If a catheter cannot be inserted to the required distance or passes well beyond the 13-cm mark before it becomes arrested, then it is probably in an aberrant branch.

Balloon Catheter Occlusion of the External Carotid Artery and Its Branches

The most likely source of retrograde flow to the external carotid artery and its branches is the major palatine artery, which is a large continuation of the maxillary artery.[1,48] This joins the contralateral major palatine artery behind the upper row of incisor teeth to form a large arterial loop around the upper jaw.[1] Attempts to occlude the maxillary artery by a single balloon-tipped catheter in the external carotid artery have failed because the catheter tip can readily enter the superficial temporal artery rather than the maxillary artery[46,48] (see Fig. 45-15). The following procedure was developed to overcome these difficulties.

To prevent normograde flow, the external carotid artery is ligated after the linguofacial trunk and, to reduce retrograde flow, a size 6 French Fogarty venous thrombectomy catheter is inserted into the major palatine artery, 3 cm caudal to the corner incisor tooth.[48] This catheter is inserted retrograde for approximately 40 to 42 cm in a 450-kg horse, or the shortest distance from the arteriotomy to the articular tubercle of the temporal bone.[48] The balloon is partly inflated and the catheter is gently retracted until some resistance is encountered, at which point it is assumed that the balloon is at the caudal alar foramen[48] (see Fig. 45-15). It is subsequently fully inflated with sterile saline. At this site, the balloon can obstruct retrograde flow to the maxillary artery (see Fig. 45-15).

As an alternative to ligation, the external carotid artery can be occluded distal to the origin of the linguofacial trunk by a balloon catheter inserted through the transverse facial artery.[48] This obviates the difficulty of exposing the artery through a hyovertebrotomy and therefore is most useful in a horse that does not require ligation of the internal carotid artery. The catheter is inserted 3 cm rostral to the articular tubercle of the temporal bone and advanced in retrograde fashion until its tip enters the external carotid artery (approximately 12 cm from the arteriotomy site in a 450-kg horse)[48] (see Fig. 45-15). The balloon is inflated with saline. The redundant ends of catheters in the transverse facial and major palatine arteries are taped to the head or incorporated into a stockinette hood. These catheters are removed after 7 to 10 days without sedation or local anesthesia.

Although the maxillary artery has many collateral branches in the segment between the balloons,[1] this procedure has been effective to date and does not cause blindness, even when combined with occlusion of the internal carotid artery.[48] This difference from ligation of the major palatine artery[89] can be attributed to prevention of the "steal phenomenon" that occurs with ligation.[92] However, the owner should be warned of the risk of blindness.

Occlusion of the Internal Carotid Artery with Detachable Balloon Catheter Systems

A detachable, self-sealing, latex balloon can be used to successfully occlude the internal carotid artery,[93] without the need for catheter removal, as required in some cases treated with the nondetachable balloons. Combined with angiography, the detachable system can also be used to occlude aberrant vessels that originate at a distance from the origin of the ICA.[94]

The internal carotid artery is approached as described earlier (see Fig. 45-15), and a 3-cm segment, 1 to 2 cm distal to the origin of the internal carotid artery, is isolated between two Rummel tourniquets of umbilical tape and polyethylene tubing.[93] The balloon delivery system consists of a Tuohy-Borst adapter (Rotating Y Adapter, Medi-Tech, Natick, Mass) that is attached to an 8-F, 95-cm, nontapered, thin-walled guiding catheter (GC 8/95, Laboratoires Nycomed S.A., Paris, France; Yocan Medical Systems, Ontario, Canada). A 2-F, 135-cm, balloon-carrier microcatheter (Mini-Tourquer, CTFN 135, Laboratoires Nycomed; Yocan Medical) is placed through the adapter and guiding catheter, and an 8.5-mm-diameter, detachable, self-sealing, latex balloon (GoldValve Balloon, GVB 17, Laboratoiries Nycomed; Yocan Medical) inflated with 0.5 mL of a 1:1 solution of physiologic saline solution and 66.8% iothalamate sodium (Conray 400, Mallinckrodt Medical, Inc, St. Louis, Mo) is mounted onto the carrier microcatheter.[93] The balloon is then deflated, the carrier microcatheter is withdrawn so that the balloon is recessed 2 mm inside the guiding catheter, and the microcatheter is held in place by tightening the O-ring of the Tuohy-Borst adapter.[93]

A 19-gauge arterial access needle is inserted into the artery between the ligatures, and a 0.9-mm (0.035-inch) guide wire is placed through the needle into the artery.[93] The needle is withdrawn over the wire and an 8-F introducer sheath (Pinnacle Introducer Sheath, Medi-Tech, Natick, Mass) is advanced over the wire for 4 cm. The dilator and wire are removed, and retrograde blood flow from the cerebral arterial circle is confirmed by bleed-back through the ancillary fluid port of the introducer sheath. Continuous infusion of heparinized saline solution (4 U/mL, approximately 3 mL/min) is then maintained through the introducer sheath. The balloon delivery system is inserted through the flexible diaphragm of the introducer sheath and advanced approximately 13 cm into the internal carotid artery or until resistance is met. The carrier microcatheter is advanced 5 to 10 mm within the guiding catheter while the guiding catheter is retracted 1 cm over the microcatheter. The balloon is subsequently inflated with 0.5 mL of the radiopaque solution, and its appropriate positioning and degree of inflation are confirmed by a single lateral intraoperative radiograph. The balloon is detached by gentle traction on the carrier microcatheter, and all proximal ligatures are secured. All catheters are withdrawn from the introducer sheath and immediate occlusion of the distal internal carotid artery is confirmed by lack of retrograde blood flow through the ancillary fluid port of the introducer sheath. The introducer sheath is subsequently removed and the proximal Rummel tourniquet is replaced with two ligatures of no. 0 polypropylene. The subcutaneous tissues and skin are closed in layers.

Transarterial Coil Embolization

A transarterial coil embolization technique can selectively occlude the arterial segments involved in a mycotic lesion in horses with guttural pouch mycosis.[95-98] The coil embolization technique combines angiographic studies to image the affected vessels and identify any unusual vessels and sites of bleeding, followed by a selective embolization or occlusion of the affected vessels. Compared with the balloon catheter technique, transarterial coil embolization allows visualization of affected vessels throughout the procedure as it is performed under fluoroscopic guidance.[95] This is critical, because aberrant vasculature has been described in horses with guttural pouch mycosis, and failure to identify and occlude such aberrant branches may result in fatal hemorrhage.[91,99] Also, this procedure eliminates the need to protect redundant ends of catheters, which is necessary when nondetachable balloons are used. It is less invasive than the original balloon catheter procedures and requires shorter anesthesia and shorter hospitalization. Transarterial embolization can be performed during active bleeding. The surgical approach for all arteries in the guttural pouch is the common carotid artery exposed through a single incision.

Under general anesthesia, the horse is placed in lateral recumbency with the affected side uppermost, and the head and neck are placed on a radiolucent surface, such as a 30 × 30-cm sheet of Plexiglas, to allow intraoperative fluoroscopy to be performed[95] (Fig. 45-16). The fluoroscopy unit must be mobile and covered with a sterile cover if it is to be manipulated intraoperatively by the surgeon. All surgical and anesthesia personnel must wear protective lead aprons during fluoroscopy (see Fig. 45-16). The proximal aspect of the jugular groove is clipped and prepared and draped for aseptic surgery. Drapes must cover the front half of the horse, as catheters and guide wires used for the procedure are long and could get contaminated. All catheters, guide wires, and introducers are flushed with heparinized saline (10 IU/mL) and left soaking in a bowl containing heparinized saline until use. A single surgical approach is sufficient to allow access to all affected branches of the common carotid artery, such as the ICA, the ECA, the MA, and aberrant branches (see Fig. 45-16). In general, all four sites are occluded when lesions are extensive (see Fig. 45-15), or when preoperative hemorrhage precludes identification of the affected vessel. When the lesion is focal, only the affected vessel is occluded.

An 8-cm skin incision is made at the junction of the proximal and middle thirds of the neck, just above the jugular vein.[95] This distal location is important to avoid exposure of the surgeon's hands during fluoroscopy (see Fig. 45-16). The brachiocephalicus and omohyoid muscles are bluntly separated, and the carotid sheath is elevated by blunt finger dissection. The vagosympathetic trunk is

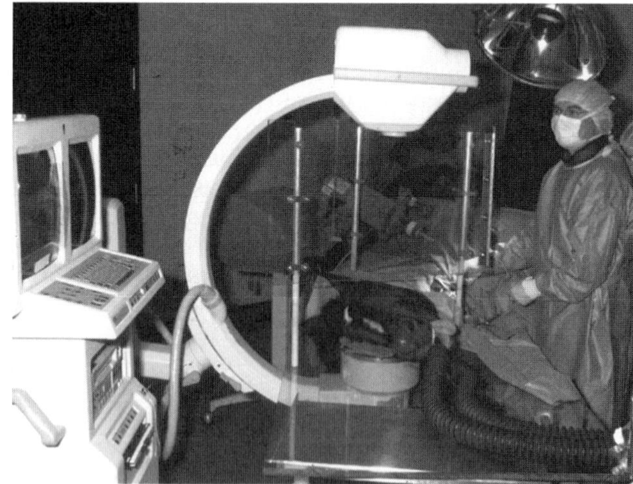

Figure 45-16. Room organization for coil embolization techniques. The horse's head rests on a thick Plexiglas sheet supported by the surgery table and a surgery cart so that the fluoroscopy unit can be positioned more accurately. The fluoroscopy head can be covered with a sterile drape if the surgeon is to manipulate it into position. The surgeon is directed by the image on the monitor to guide catheter advancement. Note the position of the radiation-shielding panels, and that the surgeon is wearing radiation protection beneath the gown. The horse's head is exposed for demonstration purposes but can be covered with a sterile drape to prevent contamination of the long catheters.

carefully separated from the carotid artery and replaced within the incision. Care must be taken to prevent tension on the nerves, which could result in postoperative complications such as Horner's syndrome or laryngeal hemiplegia. The carotid artery is elevated with umbilical tape and is punctured with an angiographic needle. A 6-F introducer system (Cook Inc, Bloomington, Ind) is inserted in the artery and guided toward the head (Fig. 45-17). The correct position of the introducer is verified by injection of contrast material before proceeding. Misdirection into the cranial thyroid artery precludes advancement of the angiography catheter and requires that the introducer be slightly withdrawn and repositioned into the CCA under fluoroscopic guidance. A 6-F single-end-hole nylon angiographic catheter (Cook Inc) is advanced rostrally into the common carotid artery to the level of the ICA under fluoroscopic guidance. Coils pass less readily through polyvinylchloride or vinyl catheters, so these should not be used. Angiography is performed during catheter advancement by hand-injection of 3 to 5 mL of a 1:2 solution of iohexol in heparinized saline, or iodinated contrast material, to identify the path of each vessel. All injections are made using a double-flush technique through a three-way stopcock. To avoid embolization of thrombi that may have formed within the catheter, heparinized saline is flushed and aspirated before injection of contrast material. Injection of air must be avoided by carefully expelling air from all syringes, and by performing injections with the piston of the syringes directed upward.

Preembolization angiography is mandatory for anatomic identification and location of the vessels, exclusion of vascular anomalies, abnormal vascular connections between the ICA and the occipital artery, and correct positioning of the embolization coils.[95] Small or aberrant arterial branches are present in up to one third of horses and require selective embolization. If a connection is present between two embolization sites, continued bleeding could still occur, and therefore such small branches must be occluded separately. The distal (cerebral) side of the lesion in the ICA is embolized first, to protect the cerebral circulation from any intraoperative errors such as air or clot embolization. The distal ICA is embolized at the level of its superimposition on the basisphenoid bone and caudal to the sigmoid flexure. To select a coil diameter, an estimate of the width of the artery at the embolization site is made by using the known diameter (3 mm) of the angiography catheter as a guide. For the distal ICA coil, diameters of 5 to 8 mm are usually necessary, although 3 mm may be needed in smaller horses or ponies. A Dacron fiber–covered, stainless steel, occluding spring embolization coil (Embolization Coils, Cook Inc) of proper diameter is introduced through the catheter, while its tip is in the desired location, and pushed into the ICA by the stiff end of a guide wire (Fig. 45-18). A coil slightly larger than the artery is placed first, and additional smaller imbricating embolization coils follow until complete occlusion is obtained. To imbricate the coils, the tip of the catheter is placed within the previous coil.

After occlusion is verified by injection of contrast material, the proximal (cardiac) side of the ICA is embolized next, midway between the first embolization site and its origin from the common carotid artery (Fig. 45-19). After occlusion of the ICA, the catheter is withdrawn into the common carotid artery and advanced to repeat the same procedure in the caudal MA and rostral ECA. The MA is embolized distal to the superficial temporal and proximal to the infraorbital, buccal, and mandibular alveolar arteries. Verification of correct identification of the maxillary artery is made by inserting the catheter further and imaging the ophthalmic artery. The catheter is subsequently withdrawn until it is within the alar foramen, just distal to the curvature of the maxillary artery, and cranial to the most cranial aspect of the guttural pouch outline. Coils of 8 to 12 mm in diameter are necessary at this location. The ECA is embolized next, on the caudal (cardiac) side of the origin of the caudal auricular artery. The ECA requires the largest size and greatest number of coils to achieve immediate and complete occlusion, usually 10 to 15 mm diameter.

After coil placement, the catheter and introducer system are removed.[95] The common carotid artery puncture site is closed using 5-0 silk in a cruciate pattern, and the muscle layers and skin are closed in three layers. Phenylbutazone is administered for 3 to 5 days after surgery to minimize

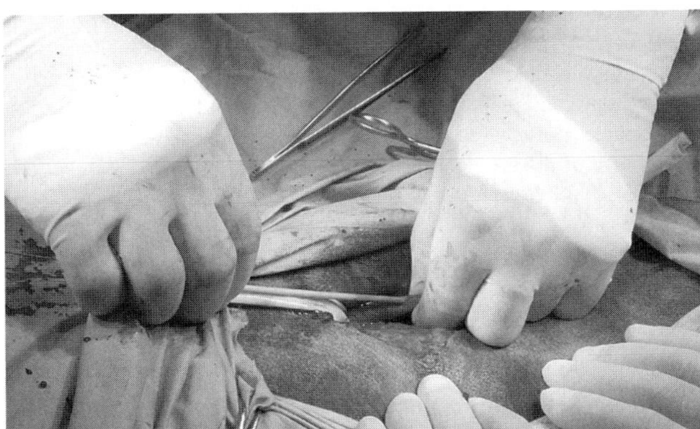

Figure 45-17. The carotid artery is elevated with umbilical tape and is punctured with an angiographic needle. A 6-F introducer system (Cook Inc, Bloomington, Ind) is inserted into the artery and guided toward the head.

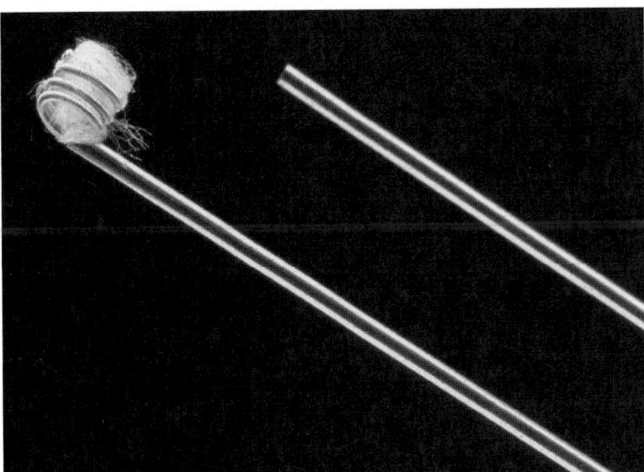

Figure 45-18. Microcoil used for coil embolization. The coils are made of stainless steel coated with Dacron fibers and presented in a stainless steel sheath. Coil formation is achieved by pushing the guide wire into the sheath *(right)* to deliver the coil *(left)* at the desired location.

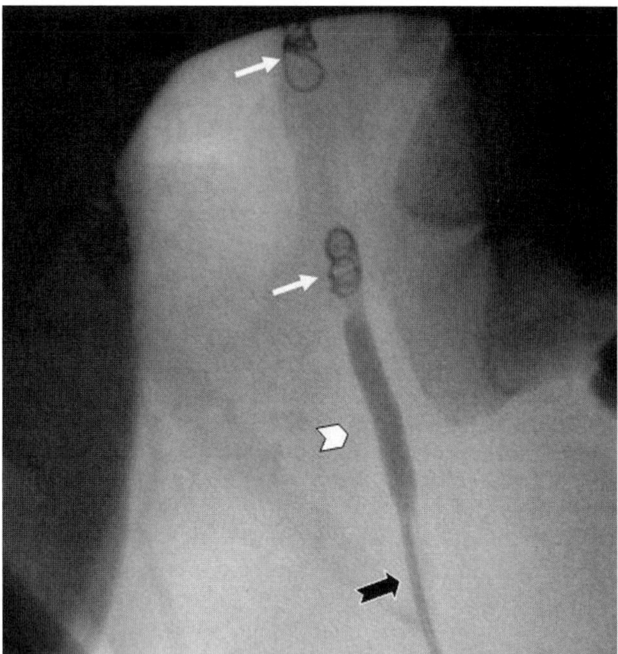

Figure 45-19. Fluoroscopic image obtained during coil embolization showing location of the distal and proximal coils within the internal carotid artery *(white arrows)*, the contrast material with complete occlusion of the artery *(arrowhead)*, and the angiography catheter within the internal carotid artery *(black arrow)*.

inflammation at the incision site. Horses are rested for 30 days and then gradually returned to use. This technique has been successful in 27 of 28 horses affected with guttural pouch mycosis, and the single failure was caused by unidentified abnormal anatomy and aberrant branching that resulted in continued hemorrhage. Such atypical anatomy may be more common than reported with this disease, so preocclusion angiography is critical. The ability to selectively occlude affected vessels with a minimally invasive approach makes transarterial coil embolization the preferred treatment.

The disadvantages of this technique are the need for fluoroscopy (and the specialized equipment and expertise involved), positioning of the horse's head for fluoroscopy, and radiation-shielding apparel and equipment. Although these disadvantages would limit this technique to a small number of well equipped hospitals, coils have been implanted in the internal carotid artery using *a cut-down procedure* similar to that for the balloon catheters.[96,97] Placement can be determined as for balloon catheters and confirmed by lack of back-flow through the arteriotomy and assessment of coil placement by radiography.[96] The same approach has been described with an allowance of 10 minutes after coil placement for a clot to form, followed by an injection of contrast material at 200 mm Hg for 3 seconds to determine occlusion.[97] This direct approach to the ICA also obviates the need for a proximal coil occlusion, because a ligature at the site of catheter insertion will prevent normograde flow. The major disadvantages of the cut-down procedure are failure to identify unusual anatomy and aberrant connections and to precisely position the microcoils.

REFERENCES

1. Sisson S: The ear. In Getty R, editor: Sisson and Grossman's The Anatomy of the Domestic Animal, ed 5, Philadelphia, 1975, WB Saunders.
2. Brandt JF: Bericht über eine Abhandlung, Untersuchung der Gattung Hyrax in anatomischer und verwandtschaftlicher Beziehung, Bull Acad Imp Sci 1863;5:508.
3. Endo H, Manglai D, Fujisawa M: The guttural pouch is not present in the white rhinoceros *(Ceratotherium simum)*: Morphology of the eustachian tube and nasopharynx, Anat Histol Embryol 1998;27:327.
4. Hinchcliffe R, Pye A: Variations in the middle ear of the Mammalia, J Zool 1969;157:277.
5. Manglai D, Wada R, Endo H, et al: Macroscopic anatomy of the auditory tube diverticulum (guttural pouch) in the Thoroughbred equine—a silicon mold approach, Okajimas Folia Anat Jpn 2000;76:335.
6. Manglai D, Wada R, Kurohmaru M, et al: Histological and morphometrical studies on the mucosa of the equine guttural pouch (auditory tube diverticulum), Okajimas Folia Anat Jpn 2000;77:69.
7. Manglai D, Wada R, Kurohmaru M, et al: Distribution of immunoglobulin isotypes and subisotypes in equine guttural pouch (auditory tube diverticulum), J Vet Med Sci 2000;62:1001.
8. Hardy J, Leveille R: Diseases of the guttural pouches, Vet Clin North Am Equine Pract 2003;19:123.
9. Baptiste KE: A function for guttural pouches in the horse, Nature 2000;403:382-383.
10. Baptiste KE: A preliminary study on the role of the equine guttural pouches in selective brain cooling, Vet J 1998;155:139-148.
11. Baptiste K: Functional anatomy observations of the pharyngeal orifice of the equine guttural pouch (auditory tube diverticulum), Vet J 1997;153:311-319.
12. Cook WR: The auditory tube diverticulum (guttural pouch) in the horse: Its radiographic examination, J Am Vet Radiol Soc 1973;14:51.
13. Sasaki M, Hayashi Y, Koie H, et al: CT examination of the guttural pouch (auditory tube diverticulum) in Przewalski's horse *(Equus przewalskii)*, J Vet Med Sci 1999;61:1019.
14. Tietje S, Becker M, Bockenhoff G: Computed tomographic evaluation of head diseases in the horse: 15 cases, Equine Vet J 1996;28:98.
15. Tucker RL, Farrell E: Computed tomography and magnetic resonance imaging of the equine head, Vet Clin North Am Equine Pract 2001;7:131.
16. Petzoldt S, Huskamp B: Computertomagraphische Untersuchungen bei der Otitis media und interna beim Pferd, Tierärztl Prax 2001;29:315.
17. Tyler RJ, Fox RI: Nasopharyngeal malignant amelanotic melanoma in a gelding age 9 years, Equine Vet Educ 2003:25.
18. Sweeney CR, Freeman DE, Sweeney RW, et al: Hemorrhage into the guttural pouch (auditory tube diverticulum) associated with rupture of the longus capitis muscle in three horses, J Am Vet Med Assoc 1993;202:1129.
19. Chiesa A, Lopez C, Domingo M, et al: A percutaneous technique for guttural pouch lavage, Equine Pract 2000;22:8.
20. Chiesa OA, Garcia F, Domingo M, et al: Cytological and microbiological results from equine guttural pouch lavages obtained percutaneously: Correlation with histopathological findings, Vet Rec 1999;144:618.
21. Chiesa OA, Vidal D, Domingo M, et al: Cytological and bacteriological findings in guttural pouch lavages of clinically normal horses, Vet Rec 1999;144:346.
22. Chiesa OA, Cuenca R, Mayayo E, et al: Cytological and microbiological findings in guttural pouch lavages of clinically normal horses with head restraint, Aust Vet J 2002;80:234.

23. McCue PM, Freeman DE, Donawick WJ: Guttural pouch tympany: 15 cases (1977-1986), J Am Vet Med Assoc 1989;194:1761.
24. Blazyczek I, Hamann H, Deegen E, et al: Retrospective analysis of 50 cases of guttural pouch tympany in foals, Vet Rec 2004;154:261.
25. Blazyczek I, Hamann H, Ohnesorge B, et al: Population genetic analysis of the heritability of guttural pouch tympany in Arabian purebred foals, Dtsch Tierarztl Wochenschr 2003;110:417.
26. Blazyczek I, Hamann H, Ohnesorge B, et al: Guttural pouch tympany in German Warmblood foals: Influence of sex, inbreeding and blood proportions of founding breeds as well as estimation of heritability, Berl Munch Tierarztl Wochenschr 2003;116:346.
27. Blazyczek I, Hamann H, Ohnesorge B, et al: Inheritance of guttural pouch tympany in the Arabian horse, J Hered 2004;95:195.
28. Cook WR: Diseases of the ear, nose, and throat in the horse: Part 1. The ear. In Grunsell CSG, editor: The Veterinary Annual, Bristol, UK, 1971, John Wright and Sons.
29. Tetens J, Tulleners EP, Ross MW, et al: Transendoscopic contact neodymium:yttrium aluminum garnet laser treatment of tympany of the auditory tube diverticulum in two foals, J Am Vet Med Assoc 1994;204:1927.
30. Sullins KE: Endoscopic application of cutting current for upper respiratory surgery in the standing horse, Proc Am Assoc Equine Pract 1990;36:439.
31. Tate LP, Blikslager AT, Little EDE: Transendoscopic laser treatment of guttural pouch tympanites in eight foals, Vet Surg 1995;24:367.
32. Milne DW, Fessler JR: Tympanitis of the guttural pouch in a foal, J Am Vet Med Assoc 1972;161:61.
33. Rashmir-Raven AM, DeBowes RM, Gift LJ, et al: What is your diagnosis? J Am Vet Med Assoc 1991;198:1991.
34. Newton JR, Wood JLN, Chanter N: Strangles: Long term carriage of *Streptococcus equi* in horses, J Equine Vet Educ 1997;9:98.
35. Judy CE, Chaffin MK, Cohen ND: Empyema of the guttural pouch (auditory tube diverticulum) in horses: 91 cases (1977-1997), J Am Vet Med Assoc 1999;215:1666.
36. Modransky PD, Reed SM, Barbee DD: Dysphagia associated with guttural pouch empyema and dorsal displacement of the soft palate, Equine Pract 1982;4:34.
37. Trostle SS, Rantanen NW, Nilsson SL, et al: What is your diagnosis? J Am Vet Med Assoc 2004;224:837.
38. Verheyen K, Newton JR, Talbot NC, et al: Elimination of guttural pouch infection and inflammation in asymptomatic carriers of *Streptococcus equi,* Equine Vet J 2000;32:527.
39. Harvey SC: Antiseptics and disinfectants; fungicides; ectoparasiticides. In Gilman A, Goodman LS, Rall TW, et al, editors: Goodman and Gilman's The Pharmacological Basis of Therapeutics, New York, 1985, Macmillan.
40. Bentz BG, Dowd AL, Freeman DE: Treatment of guttural pouch empyema with acetylcysteine irrigation, Equine Pract 1996;18:33.
41. Seahorn TL, Schumacher J: Nonsurgical removal of chondroid masses from the guttural pouches of two horses, J Am Vet Med Assoc 1991;199:368.
42. Hawkins JF, Frank N, Sojka JE, et al: Fistulation of the auditory tube diverticulum (guttural pouch) with a neodymium:yttrium-aluminum-garnet laser for treatment of chronic empyema in two horses, J Am Vet Med Assoc 2001;218:405.
43. Greet TRC: Outcome of treatment in 35 cases of guttural pouch mycosis, Equine Vet J 1987;19:483.
44. Cook WR: The clinical features of guttural pouch mycosis in the horse, Vet Rec 1968;83:336.
45. Church S, Wyn-Jones G, Park AH, et al: Treatment of guttural pouch mycosis, Equine Vet J 1986;18:362.
46. Caron JP, Fretz PD, Bailey JV, et al: Balloon-tipped catheter arterial occlusion for prevention of hemorrhage caused by guttural pouch mycosis: 13 cases (1982-1985), J Am Vet Med Assoc 1987;191:345.
47. Smith DM, Barber SM: Guttural pouch hemorrhage associated with lesions of the maxillary artery in two horses, Can Vet J 1984;25:239.
48. Freeman DE, Ross MW, Donawick WJ, et al: Occlusion of the external carotid and maxillary arteries in the horse to prevent hemorrhage from guttural pouch mycosis, Vet Surg 1989;18:39.
49. Hahn CN: Horner's syndrome in horses, Equine Vet Educ 2003:111.
50. Walmsley JP: A case of atlantooccipital arthropathy following guttural pouch mycosis in a horse: The use of radioisotope bone scanning as an aid to diagnosis, Equine Vet J 1988;20:219.
51. Hatziolos BC, Sass B, Albert TF, et al: Ocular changes in a horse with gutturomycosis, J Am Vet Med Assoc 1975;167:51.
52. McLaughlin BG, O'Brien JL: Guttural pouch mycosis and mycotic encephalitis in a horse, Can Vet J 1986;27:109.
53. Dixon PM, Rowlands AC: Atlanto-occipital joint infection associated with guttural pouch mycosis in a horse, Equine Vet J 1981;13:260.
54. Guillot J, Sarfati J, Ribot X, et al: Detection of antibodies to *Aspergillus fumigatus* in serum of horses with mycosis of the auditory tube diverticulum (guttural pouch), Am J Vet Res 1997;58:1364.
55. Davis EW, Legendre AM: Successful treatment of guttural pouch mycosis with itraconazole and topical enilconazole in a horse, J Vet Int Med 1994;8:304.
56. Utz JP: Chemotherapy of the systemic mycoses, Med Clin North Am 1982;66:221.
57. McMullan WC, Joyce RJ, Hanselka DV, et al: Amphotericin B for the treatment of localized subcutaneous phycomycosis in the horse, J Am Vet Med Assoc 1977;170:1293.
58. van Nieuwstadt RA, Kaalsbeek HC: Guttural pouch mycosis: Local treatment with an indwelling through-the-nose catheter with enilconazole, Tijd voor Diergeneeskunde 1994;119:3.
59. Korenek NL, Legendre AM, Andrews FM, et al: Treatment of mycotic rhinitis with itraconazole in three horses, J Vet Int Med 1994;8:224.
60. Latimer FG, Colitz CMH, Campbell NB, et al: Pharmacokinetics of fluconazole following intravenous and oral administration and body fluid concentrations of fluconazole following repeated oral administration in horses, Am J Vet Res 2001;62:1606.
61. Speirs VC, Harrison IW, van Veenendaal JC, et al: Is specific antifungal therapy necessary for the treatment of guttural pouch mycosis? Equine Vet J 1995;27:151.
62. Darien BJ, Watrous BJ, Huber MJ, et al: What is your diagnosis? J Am Vet Med Assoc 1991;198:1799.
63. Alexander K, Baird JD, Dobson H, et al: What is your diagnosis? J Am Vet Med Assoc 2002;220:297.
64. Blythe LL, Watrous BJ: Temporohyoid osteoarthropathy (middle ear disease). In Robinson NE, editor: Current Therapy in Equine Medicine, ed 4, Philadelphia, 1997, WB Saunders.
65. Blythe LL: Otitis media and interna and temporohyoid osteoarthropathy, Vet Clin North Am Equine Pract 1997;13:21.
66. Blythe LL, Watrous BJ, Schmitz JA, et al: Vestibular syndrome associated with temporohyoid joint fusion and temporal bone fracture in three horses, J Am Vet Med Assoc 1984;185:775.
67. Walker AM, Sellon DC, Cornelisse CJ, et al: Temporohyoid osteoarthropathy in 33 horses (1993-2000), J Vet Intern Med 2002;16:697.
68. Newton SA, Knottenbelt DC: Vestibular disease in two horses: A case of mycotic otitis media and a case of temporohyoid osteoarthropathy, Vet Rec 1999;145:142.
69. Spurlock SL, Spurlock GH, Wise M: Keratoconjunctivitis sicca associated with fracture of the stylohyoid bone in a horse, J Am Vet Med Assoc 1989;194:258.
70. Pease, AP, Van Biervliet J, Dykes NL, et al: Complication of partial stylohyoidectomy for treatment of temporohyoid osteoarthropathy and an alternative surgical technique in three cases, Equine Vet J 2004;36:546.
71. Hassel DM, Schott HC, Tucker RL, et al: Endoscopy of the auditory tube diverticula in four horses with otitis media/interna, J Am Vet Med Assoc 1995;207:1081.

72. Blythe LL, Watrous BJ, Shires GMH, et al: Prophylactic partial stylohyoidostectomy for horses with osteoarthropathy of the temporohyoid joint, J Equine Vet Sci 1994;14:32.
73. Blythe LL, Watrous BJ, Pearson EG, et al: Otitis media/interna in the horse: A cause of head shaking and skull fractures, Proc Am Assoc Equine Pract 1990;36:517.
74. Moulton JE, editor: Tumors in Domestic Animals, Los Angeles, 1978, University of California Press.
75. Trigo RJ, Nickels FA: Squamous cell carcinoma of a horse's guttural pouch, Mod Vet Pract 1981;62:456.
76. Merriam JG: Guttural pouch fibroma in a mare, J Am Vet Med Assoc 1972;161:487.
77. Greene HJ, O'Connor JP: Hemangioma of the guttural pouch of a 16-year-old Thoroughbred mare: Clinical and pathological findings, Vet Rec 1986;118:445.
78. Raker CW: The nasopharynx. In Mannsmann RA, McAllister ES, editors: Equine Medicine and Surgery, ed 3, Santa Barbara, Calif, 1982, American Veterinary Publications.
79. May KA, Howard RD: Exercise intolerance secondary to parotid melanomas in a mare, Equine Vet Educ 2001:246.
80. Fintl C, Dixon PM: A review of five cases of parotid melanoma in the horse, Equine Vet Educ 2001:43.
81. McConnico RS, Blas-Machado U, Cooper VL, et al: Bilateral squamous cell carcinoma of the guttural pouches and the left middle ear in a horse, Equine Vet Educ 2001:225.
82. Bayly WM, Robertson JT: Epistaxis caused by foreign body penetration of a guttural pouch, J Am Vet Med Assoc 1982; 180:1232.
83. Hance SR, Robertson JT, Bukowiecki CF: Cystic structures in the guttural pouch (auditory tube diverticulum) of two horses, J Am Vet Med Assoc 1992;200:1981.
84. Colles CM, Cook WR: Carotid and cerebral angiography in the horse, Vet Rec 1983;113:483.
85. McIlwraith CW, Turner AS: Equine Surgery: Advanced Techniques, Philadelphia, 1987, Lea & Febiger.
86. Owen R: Epistaxis prevented by ligation of the internal carotid artery in the guttural pouch, Equine Vet J 1974;6:143.
87. Woodie JB, Ducharme NG, Gleed RD, et al: In horses with guttural pouch mycosis or after stylohyoid bone resection, what arterial ligation(s) could be effective in emergency treatment of a hemorrhagic crisis? Vet Surg 2002;31:498.
88. Freeman DE, Donawick WJ, Klein L: Effect of ligation on internal carotid artery pressure in horses, Vet Surg 1994;23:250.
89. Hardy J, Robertson JT, Wilkie DA: Ischemic optic neuropathy and blindness after arterial occlusion for treatment of guttural pouch mycosis in two horses, J Am Vet Med Assoc 1990;196:1631.
90. Freeman DE, Donawick WJ: Occlusion of internal carotid artery in the horse by means of a balloon-tipped catheter: Clinical use of a method to prevent epistaxis caused by guttural pouch mycosis, J Am Vet Med Assoc 1980;176:236.
91. Freeman DE, Staller GS, Maxson AD, et al: Unusual internal carotid artery branching that prevented arterial occlusion with a balloon-tipped catheter in a horse, Vet Surg 1993;22:531.
92. Freeman DE, Ross MW, Donawick WJ: "Steal phenomenon" proposed as the cause of blindness after arterial occlusion for treatment of guttural pouch mycosis in horses, Am Vet Med Assoc 1990;197:811.
93. Cheramie HS, Pleasant RS, Robertson JL, et al: Evaluation of a technique to occlude the internal carotid artery of horses, Vet Surg 1999;28:83.
94. Cheramie HS, Pleasant RS, Dabareiner RM, et al: Detachable latex balloon occlusion of an internal carotid artery with an aberrant branch in a horse with guttural pouch (auditory tube diverticulum) mycosis: Evaluation of a technique to occlude the internal carotid artery of horses, Am Vet Med Assoc 2000;216:888.
95. Léveillé R, Hardy J, Robertson JT, et al: Transarterial coil embolization of the internal and external carotid and maxillary arteries for prevention of hemorrhage from guttural pouch mycosis in horses, Vet Surg 2000;29:389-397.
96. Matsuda Y, Nakanishi Y, Mizuno Y: Occlusion of the internal carotid artery by means of microcoils for preventing epistaxis caused by guttural pouch mycosis in horses, J Vet Med Sci 1998;61:221-225.
97. Ragle CA, Wooten TL, Tucker RL, et al: Microcoil embolization of the rostral portion of the internal carotid artery in the horse, Vet Surg 1997;26:425.
98. Lepage OM, Junot S, Desmiazieres LM, et al: Trans-arterial occlusion using embolization coils fro treatment of guttural pouch mycosis: A report of 7 cases, Vet Surg 2000;29:282.
99. Bacon Miller C, Wilson DA, Martin DD, et al: Complications of balloon catheterization associated with aberrant cerebral arterial anatomy in a horse with guttural pouch mycosis, Vet Surg 1998;27:450.

CHAPTER 46

Trachea

John A. Stick

Conditions that may require surgical intervention of the equine trachea include obstruction of the airway rostral to the trachea, perforation or rupture of the trachea, tracheal collapse, tracheal stenosis, bronchial foreign body, and mucosal granulomas within the trachea lumen. Surgical treatments include tracheotomy, tracheostomy (both temporary and permanent), tracheal resection and anastomosis, and tracheal reconstruction. Although conditions of the trachea requiring surgery are rare, successful surgical management requires knowledge of normal anatomy and physiology.

ANATOMY AND PHYSIOLOGY

The equine trachea is a membranous and cartilaginous tube extending from the larynx at the level of the 1st or 2nd cervical vertebra to the level of the 5th or 6th intercostal space, where it bifurcates into the principal bronchi dorsal to the base of the heart.[1] The trachea is median in position except for its very terminal thoracic part, where it is pushed to the right by the aortic arch. From just caudal to the larynx to its bifurcation, the equine trachea is about 70 to 80 cm long.

When operating on the trachea, its relationship to other structures is important. The arrangement of the muscles around the trachea should be noted, as well as nerve trunks, vessels, and the esophagus. The sternothyrohyoid muscles are located immediately ventral to the trachea, except at the most cranial extremity of the trachea, where it is related only to the sternohyoid muscle. The sternocephalic, omohyoid, and sternothyroid muscles are found lateral to the trachea near the larynx. An easy spot to perform a tracheotomy is where the sternocephalic muscle bellies diverge and the omohyoid muscle converges. From this area cranial to the larynx, the trachea can be easily palpated. The esophagus is located dorsolaterally to the trachea in the middle of the neck but comes to lie lateral to it in the caudal part of the neck and assumes a position ventral to the trachea at the thoracic inlet. This is another reason the tracheotomy should be performed in the proximal half of the trachea. The common carotid artery, vagosympathetic nerve trunk, and recurrent laryngeal nerve all are enclosed in the carotid sheath and lie alongside the dorsolateral aspects of the trachea. These structures come to lie more laterally near the thoracic inlet. Therefore, when surgery is performed in this area, caution needs to be taken. A tracheotomy cannot be performed blindly. In a young animal, the thymus may extend for a distance into the neck from the thoracic cavity and lie on the ventral and lateral aspects of the trachea. Additionally, in the proximal-most aspect of the trachea, the thyroid gland may have an isthmus that could be encountered if the trachea is surgically approached just caudal to the larynx.

The wall of the trachea can be divided into four layers: mucosa, submucosa, the musculocartilaginous layer, and the adventitia. The adventitia is a connective tissue layer that blends with the musculocutaneous layer and with the connective tissue surrounding the trachea. It is composed of loose areolar tissue that allows a considerable amount of movement of the trachea along its length. The musculocartilaginous layer consists of the cartilaginous plates, fibroelastic tissue (annular ligaments), and the tracheal muscle. The cartilaginous plates number between 48 and 60 and are composed of hyaline cartilage surrounded by perichondrium.[1] Vascular canals are consistently found within the cartilaginous plates and become obvious when they are traumatized or when incisions are made into the cartilaginous plates. These cartilaginous plates are curved and form incomplete hoops that are open dorsally. Tracheal muscle consisting of smooth muscle fibers extends transversely across the dorsal part of the wall and is attached to the inner surface of the tracheal plates. The tracheal lumen can vary considerably in size as the result of the action of the tracheal muscle, which is facilitated in the cervical region by overlapping of the cartilaginous rings when the muscle contracts. The submucosa contains many elastic fibers and fat cells and many small seromucous tubular glands,[2] which open into the lumen of the trachea.

The mucosa has numerous low longitudinal folds and is lined with pseudostratified columnar ciliated epithelium, which contains numerous goblet cells and rests on a basement membrane. The secretory cells and the mucous glands under the epithelium provide the mucous layer that covers the tracheal epithelium. As the cilia move in a coordinated fashion, they create a wave that carries the mucus and inhaled foreign particles orally, and this is referred to as the mucosal ciliary escalator. The rate at which tracheal mucus is transported orally has been determined to be 1.6 ± 0.24 cm/min.[3] This mucosal ciliary escalator is important as a pulmonary defense mechanism. Surgical interventions, as well as foreign bodies and endotracheal tubes, can disrupt this mechanism and may predispose the animal to pulmonary disease.

There is a wide variation in the extrathoracic tracheal cross-sectional shape in horses. In the adult horse, tracheal diameter varies from 5.5 cm cranially, where it is almost round, to up to 7 cm more distally, where it is flattened dorsoventrally.[1] It is recognized that as horses (particularly ponies) age, the trachea may undergo some torsion and additional flattening in the cervical area. This is important when performing permanent tracheostomies, as this surgery needs to be centered in the middle of the tracheal ring, which may become twisted with age.

In a recent cadaveric study of 33 freshly slaughtered horses, neither age nor weight of the horse had any influence on the mechanical properties of the trachea.[4] However, extension decreases the compressibility of the tracheal segments, and the shape of the cross-sectional area has a major influence on mechanical properties. Hyperextension of the neck partly facilitates respiration at high levels of ventilation by elongating the trachea and decreasing its collapsibility. Therefore, muscles that cranially retract the larynx (and hence the trachea) may provide some stability of the tracheal luminal diameter during inhalation. In addition, the tracheal cartilages themselves prevent tracheal collapse during inhalation when intraluminal pressures are lower than atmospheric pressure. The incomplete dorsal structure of the tracheal rings allows tracheal expansion when large volumes of air are exhaled, especially during periods of exercise. Although the fibroelastic annular ligaments positioned between consecutive tracheal rings allow considerable tracheal flexibility during neck movement, they become more stabilized whenever the trachea is elongated, and this probably occurs during exercise.

EXAMINATION

Preventing and managing complications of tracheal surgery in horses requires a thorough examination of the trachea. Preoperative evaluation should include manual palpation of the trachea. Its ventral aspect can easily be palpated in the cranial one half of the cervical trachea. The lateral aspects of the trachea and their rings can be palpated further distally in the neck, but it becomes increasingly more difficult as the musculature thickens in the neck near the thoracic inlet. Cartilaginous rings should be compressible except in older horses; if they are not, they may have become mineralized. However, any change in the amount of compressibility of the tracheal rings may indicate a diseased state.

The evaluation should also include direct flexible tracheoscopy, the goal being to identify other airway abnormalities such as laryngeal hemiplegia and to determine the extent of the tracheal disorder, thus allowing the surgeon to plan surgical management and achieve the best possible outcome for each patient. A technique for clinical bronchography has been developed in the horse using a barium sulfate powder and an ether vaporizer into which compressed air is blown.[5] Although the value of bronchoscopy as a diagnostic procedure has yet to be proven, the method of powder insufflation provides a safe and accurate means of evaluating bronchial conditions in the horse. This could have some application toward tracheal disease.

CONDITIONS REQUIRING TRACHEAL SURGERY

Rostral Upper Airway Obstruction

Surgery of the trachea is often an emergency procedure to bypass a life-threatening obstruction of the upper respiratory tract. It may also be conducted as a route for endotracheal intubation for general anesthesia when routine nasotracheal or orotracheal intubation limits access to the surgical field. Additionally, surgical interventions are performed to physically rest the upper respiratory tract on a temporary basis, or to simply bypass an inoperable upper respiratory tract obstruction (such as bilateral arytenoid chondritis).

Tracheotomy

Temporary tracheotomy and tracheotomy with an indwelling tracheal cannula (tracheostomy) may be performed with the horse standing or under general anesthesia. In the standing horse, the ventral midline of the neck is easier to locate (with regard to all tissue layers) and the dissection of the trachea is easier than in the anesthetized horse in dorsal or lateral recumbency, because the trachea shifts within the neck if the neck is not held in a perfectly vertical position. Tracheotomy is performed at the junction of the upper and middle thirds of the neck. The trachea is located superficially at this level. The horse is sedated in the stocks and the surgical site is prepared for aseptic intervention. Local anesthetic is injected on the ventral midline under the skin and into the paired sternothyrohyoid muscles prior to incision.

If the surgery is to be performed in the recumbent animal, a pad is placed under the head to place the neck in a slightly flexed position after the neck and the trachea have been placed in vertical position and as straight as possible. The objective is to align the skin so that it is in the position it will be after the horse recovers and is standing normally.

With the horse standing or in recumbency, a 10-cm incision is made through the skin, subcutaneous tissue, and cutaneus colli muscle. The paired sternothyrohyoid muscle bellies are bluntly divided along the ventral midline for a distance of about 8 cm and held in a retracted position with a self-retaining retractor (Fig. 46-1). The cartilage of the trachea can then be easily palpated. Although vertical and flap procedures are used in dogs, only the transverse tracheotomy technique is used in the horse to prevent problems with tracheal collapse and granulation tissue formation. Therefore, the annular ligament between two adjacent cartilage rings is incised parallel to the orientation of the rings. The incision between the rings is lengthened to allow placement of a tracheal cannula. The incision should not exceed one half the circumference of the trachea. A large hemostatic forceps or an index finger may be inserted between the rings to guide the tracheal tube in the lumen.

A variety of tracheal tubes are manufactured. Self-retaining tubes are popular because they do not require skin sutures for security. Short-cuff silicone tubes are a good choice (Fig. 46-2), because their compliance makes them more comfortable than rigid metal tubes. However, the cuff should not be inflated if the tubes are used long term, as they will produce mucosal erosions. Therefore, they are usually tied in place using the flanges on either side of the tubes.

In emergency situations, a segment of stomach tube, garden hose, or large plastic syringe casing with the tip

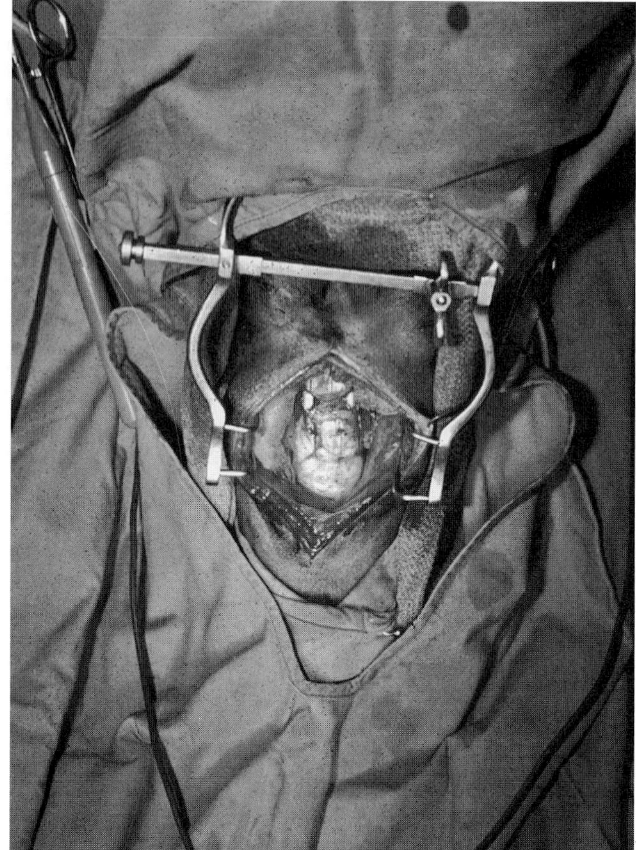

Figure 46-1. After the paired sternothyrohyoid muscles are bluntly divided along the ventral midline, they can be held in place with Weitlaner or baby Balfour retractors as shown. This provides good exposure to multiple tracheal rings.

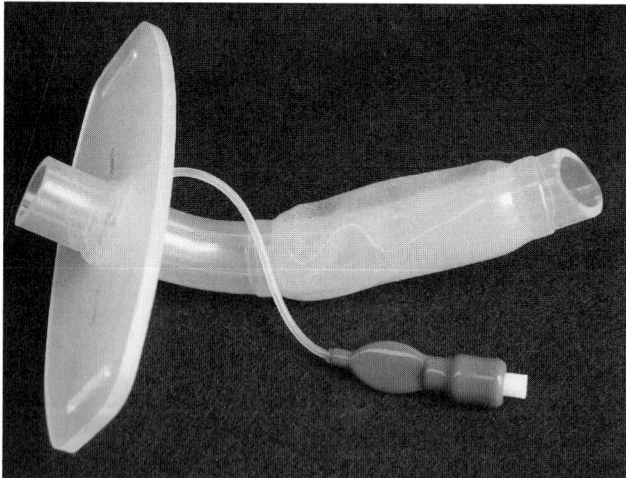

Figure 46-2. A short-cuff tracheal tube made out of silicone. The flanges are used to tie the tube in place.

removed may provide an airway until a better option is available. In an emergency situation, tracheotomy is difficult when performed on a horse that is struggling because of airway obstruction. It may be necessary to allow the horse to collapse; however, from that point forward, speed is imperative because the horse can die shortly after this stage is reached. The tracheotomy site should be cleaned and the indwelling cannula should be removed twice daily to remove accumulated tracheal secretions that could cause airway obstruction.

When direct tracheal intubation through a tracheotomy is carried out to avoid orotracheal or nasotracheal intubation, the procedure can be accomplished in the standing sedated or recumbent anesthetized horse. Precautions are taken to ensure that the skin incision is made on the ventral midline in the recumbent horse, because inappropriate positioning may create excessive skin tension or stoma obstruction at the tracheotomy site on recovery. The endotracheal tube should not extend past the carina, since endobronchial intubation will impair ventilation.

COMPLICATIONS

Early complications can be reduced by using aseptic technique and by performing minimal soft tissue dissection to limit the amount of dead space. Complications after aseptic tube placement are uncommon. Occasionally, the wound becomes infected or the horse develops subcutaneous emphysema. More commonly, obstruction of the tracheal cannula with mucous secretions occurs and needs clearing. This problem should be closely monitored and the tube replaced at least every 24 hours. Occasionally, the tracheal cannula is inadvertently placed peritracheally because of the loose areolar tissue around the trachea. This can be recognized immediately by the lack of air movement through the tube while the horse is breathing.

Long-term complications, including damage to tracheal cartilage or intraluminal granulation tissue and mucosal stricture, are extremely rare. Attention to the soft tissue dissection and aseptic technique whenever possible reduces these complications. Removal of the endotracheal cannula as soon as possible also reduces long-term complications. After the cannula is removed, the wound is left to heal by second intention with daily cleansing.

Tracheostomy

Permanent tracheostomy is used for correction of permanent impairment of the laryngotracheal apparatus such as bilateral laryngeal hemiplegia or chondritis. Permanent tracheostomy has been used to provide a large, stable, permanent tracheal stoma with minimal complications.[6] A retrospective study that followed 42 horses for an average of 4.8 years found that stomas remained functional and 91% of owners would have it done again.[7] The author has had good success with long-term function of tracheal stomas created in a number of adult horses.

Permanent tracheostomy can be performed with the horse sedated and standing or anesthetized and positioned in dorsal recumbency. The procedure should be performed under general anesthesia until the surgeon is comfortable with it before it is attempted in the standing horse.

SURGICAL TECHNIQUE WITH GENERAL ANESTHESIA

The horse is anesthetized and positioned in dorsal recumbency with the ventral cervical area prepared for surgery. A 10-cm ventral midline incision is made through the skin, subcutaneous tissues, and cutaneus colli muscle in the cranial third of the cervical region just caudal to the larynx (Fig. 46-3). The paired sternothyrohyoideus muscles are

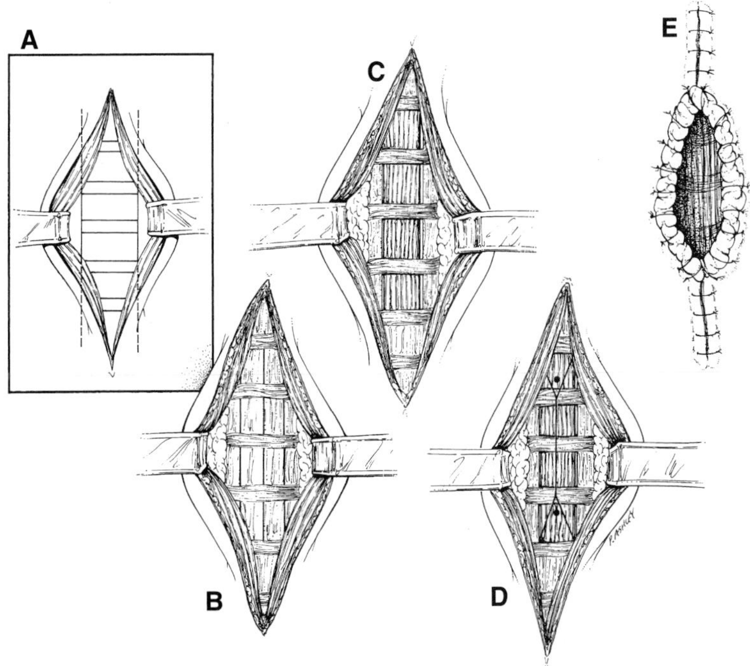

Figure 46-3. Surgical technique for permanent tracheotomy. **A,** Exposure of tracheal cartilage rings after separation of the sternothyrohyoideus muscles. **B,** Incision of tracheal cartilages. **C,** Removal of eight tracheal cartilage rectangles. **D,** Line of incision of tracheal mucosa and placement points for stay sutures *(circles)*. **E,** Mucosal epidermal apposition.

separated and retracted laterally to expose four tracheal rings. (The most cosmetic appearance is achieved if tracheal rings two to five are removed.) A 3-cm-wide band of each of these muscles is bluntly separated and transected on either side of the midline so that the skin will lie easily on the trachea without tension. The area is packed with gauze sponges to stem the bleeding as the rest of the surgery progresses. A ventral midline incision and two paramedian incisions 15 mm on either side of the midline are made through the tracheal cartilages without disrupting the tracheal mucosa underneath. The rectangular cartilage pieces are carefully dissected from the tracheal submucosa and removed. The tracheal mucosa and annular tracheal ligaments are incised in a double-Y pattern and stay sutures used to maintain mucosal traction. The intersection of the legs of each Y in the mucosa are elevated and sutured to the skin with 2-0 polypropylene in a simple-interrupted pattern. The main tracheal mucosa is apposed to the skin lateral to the stoma in a similar manner.

The stoma is cleaned twice daily until the sutures are removed and then once daily afterward. The sutures can be removed 10 to 14 days after surgery; however, by that time many of the sutures have sloughed and with time all of them will be extruded if they cannot be easily removed. This technique provides a cosmetically acceptable, structurally sound stoma, needing minimal aftercare (Fig. 46-4). The stoma is unlikely to be obstructed by accumulated secretions, even if daily cleaning is not done.

The stoma can be located at any site in the proximal third of the neck. However, for best cosmetic results, this stoma can be located beginning at the second tracheal ring. This often provides a permanent stoma that is not easily recognizable to the untrained observer. It is not recommended that the first tracheal ring be removed.

SURGICAL TECHNIQUE IN THE STANDING HORSE

If permanent tracheostomy is performed with the horse sedated and standing, the horse is restrained in stocks and cross-tied with the head extended. The horse is sedated and a local anesthetic infiltrated subcutaneously in an inverted-U pattern dorsal and lateral to the second through the fifth tracheal rings. The 6-cm-long incision is made through the skin centered over the ventral midline beginning 3 cm distal to the cricoid cartilage. The paired sternothyrohyoid muscles are isolated and removed as previously described. The tracheal mucosa is then desensitized by injecting 30 mL of 2% lidocaine with a 1-inch, 23-gauge needle into the lumen of the trachea proximal to the surgery site. The ventral third of the second through the fifth tracheal rings is resected as previously described, leaving the tracheal mucosa intact. The longitudinal double-Y incision is subsequently made through the tracheal mucosa and annular tracheal ligaments, and the stoma is completed by suturing the tracheal mucosa and the submucosa to the skin with simple-interrupted sutures of no. 0 polypropylene in the simple-interrupted pattern.

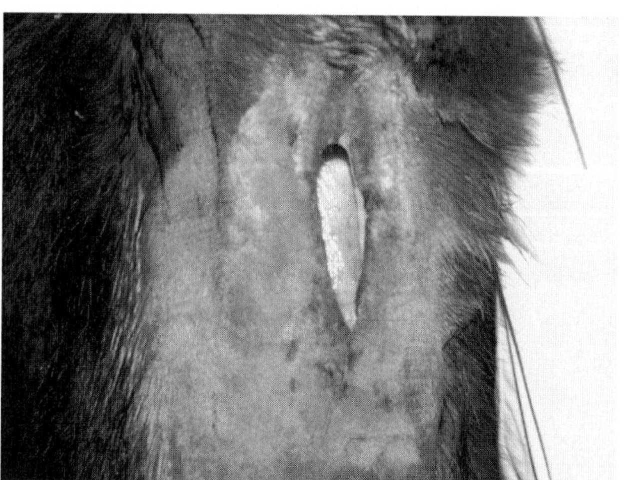

Figure 46-4. Permanent tracheostomy provides a cosmetically acceptable, structurally sound stoma requiring minimal aftercare.

COMPLICATIONS

Although the permanent stoma affects pulmonary defense mechanisms by reduced airway temperature control and altered humidification of inspired gases, the mucosal ciliary escalator continues to work, and mucus is continuously extruded through the stoma. Horses with existing pulmonary disease may have exacerbation of chronic pulmonary disease, or signs of respiratory disease may be induced, but this has not been the author's clinical experience.

Tracheal collapse will occur postoperatively if care is not taken to ensure that segments of the cartilage are removed from the ventral third of the cartilage rings only, and not close to the trachealis muscle. In older animals, the tracheal ring may become twisted, and if that is the case removing the center third of the cartilage ring is important even if it is off center. The amount of tension that is experienced from the skin can be adjusted by removing more of the sternothyrohyoid muscle if necessary. Also, to avoid tracheal collapse, no more than one third of the entire circumference of the ring should be removed.

Tracheal Perforation or Rupture

Disruption of the integrity of the tracheal lumen is usually caused by trauma. Clinical signs of tracheal trauma depend on the site of the tracheal injury, but trauma can cause tracheal perforation without concurrent cartilage damage or obvious skin damage or even rupture of the annular ligament (Fig. 46-5). Clinical signs include subcutaneous emphysema and harsh tracheal sounds. Often, the perforation or disruption is not recognized until regional subcutaneous emphysema develops. When these signs occur in mares separated from their foals by wire fences at weaning, tracheal trauma should be suspected. The subcutaneous swelling is usually nonpainful, soft, easily indented, mobile, and crepitant. When tracheal trauma is suspected, thoracic radiographs should be taken to check for pneumomediastinum. Continued leakage into the mediastinum may lead to pneumothorax. Small tissue perforations in the absence of cartilage damage may not be apparent on radiographs, but both large and small lesions are usually apparent with tracheoscopy (Fig. 46-6). Although the small tears rapidly form a fibrin seal, large ruptures should be treated promptly to avoid infection, obstruction from peritracheal tissue, progression of subcutaneous emphysema to the mediastinum, and development of pneumothorax. Small defects may respond to a pressure bandage over the affected region, which reduces the subcutaneous emphysema.

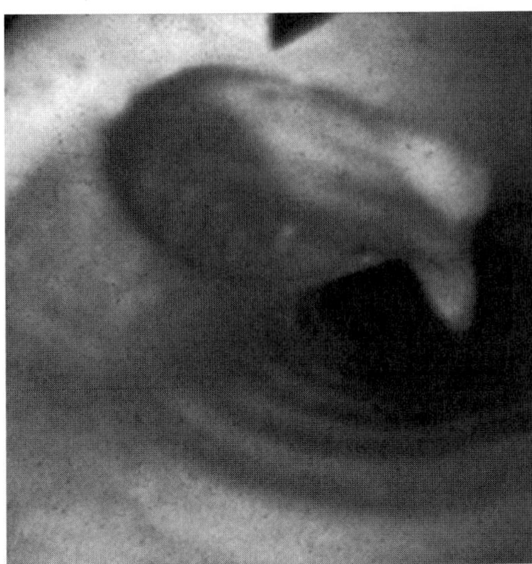

Figure 46-5. Endoscopic view of a tracheal rupture through the annular ligament. This horse had subcutaneous emphysema extending over the thorax.

Although small tears can be managed conservatively and generally resolve within 24 to 48 hours, the large tears should be managed surgically as soon as the horse's condition allows such an intervention. If there is a wound, the tears in the cervical trachea can be approached and directly sutured after débridement of devitalized tissue.[8] Wound margins are apposed in a simple-interrupted pattern of no. 0 absorbable suture material. Injuries that involve the trachealis muscle or the adventitia of the trachea, or that are rotational in nature, can be repaired by rotating the trachea to expose the dorsal surface. Closed suction drains are recommended in the postoperative period and should be removed every 48 to 72 hours, depending on the appearance of the wound and the amount of drainage. Once the tracheal defect is closed, the subcutaneous emphysema usually resolves in 7 to 10 days.

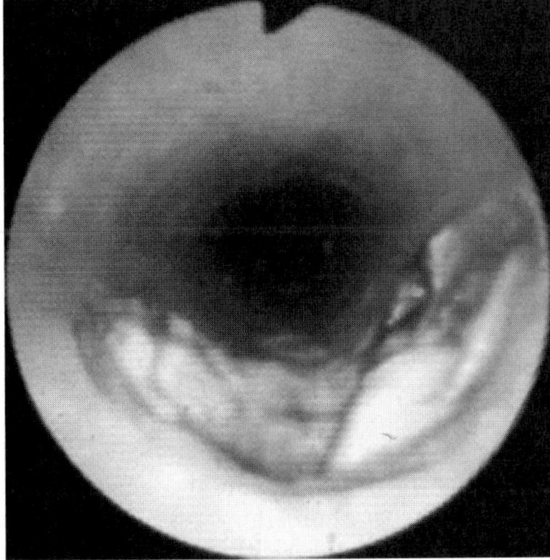

Figure 46-6. Endoscopic view of a tracheal perforation. Although this tear formed a fibrin seal, the presenting signs were subcutaneous emphysema.

Resection and Anastomosis

When tracheal trauma is extensive or when complete rupture occurs between tracheal rings, tracheal resection and anastomosis is indicated.[9-11] Before attempting a tracheal resection and anastomosis, the horse must be trained to wear a Martingale-type harness, which restricts dorsal movement of the head and reduces tension at the anastomotic site. This is particularly important if sections or rings need to be removed. If sections or rings do not need to be removed and the harness is quickly tolerated, the surgical preparation can occur immediately. Broad-spectrum antibiotics are administered prophylactically and the horse is anesthetized and positioned in dorsal recumbency.

The ventral cervical midline is prepared for aseptic surgery. A ventral midline cervical incision is made through the skin, subcutaneous tissue, and subcutaneous colli muscles over a distance of about 40 cm centered over the affected area. The sternothyrohyoid muscles are divided to expose the trachea. The trachea is separated from adjacent tissues along the entire cervical region within the incision site. If cartilage rings are to be removed, stay sutures are placed in tracheal cartilages adjacent to the segment to be removed. Up to five cartilages can be removed; however, tension on the anastomotic site will be excessive, and as few cartilages as possible should be removed (Fig. 46-7). Tracheal mucosa and annular ligament are incised to divide the trachea into proximal and distal segments. The endotracheal tube is removed and replaced in the distal segment. The tracheal mucosa is turned back over the open ends of the proximal tracheal segment and sutured to the adventitia. The same procedure is repeated on the distal segment, working around the endotracheal tube. The head is subsequently flexed at a right angle with the neck. The endotracheal tube is replaced through the mouth and advanced into the distal segment of the trachea. If this is not possible because of the distal location of the injury, the endotracheal tube needs to be placed through another tracheotomy incision proximal to the anastomotic site. Tracheal ends are apposed with towel clamps and anastomosed with 25-gauge stainless steel wire in a simple-interrupted pattern without mucosal penetration. After the anastomosis is complete, it is checked for air leaks prior to completely withdrawing the endotracheal tube. A continuous suction drain is placed in the soft tissue, and the remaining tissue layers are closed. The harness is applied before recovery and left in place for 3 weeks. Antibiotics are usually continued for 5 days. Complications include breakdown of the anastomosis and infection. Fistulation around the steel sutures persists if infection is present and development of intraluminal abscesses in the anastomotic site is possible. Therefore, these sutures may need to be removed if abscesses develop after the trachea is healed.

Tracheal Collapse

Tracheal collapse can be a sequela to peritracheal abscesses, tumors, any injury causing cartilage trauma, malformation of the cartilages, or chronic pneumonia.[12-15] An idiopathic primary collapse syndrome has also been reported in the horse.[16] Primary tracheal collapse is recognized by widespread or segmental dorsoventral flattening of tracheal cartilage rings. Neurologic, congenital, or nutritional

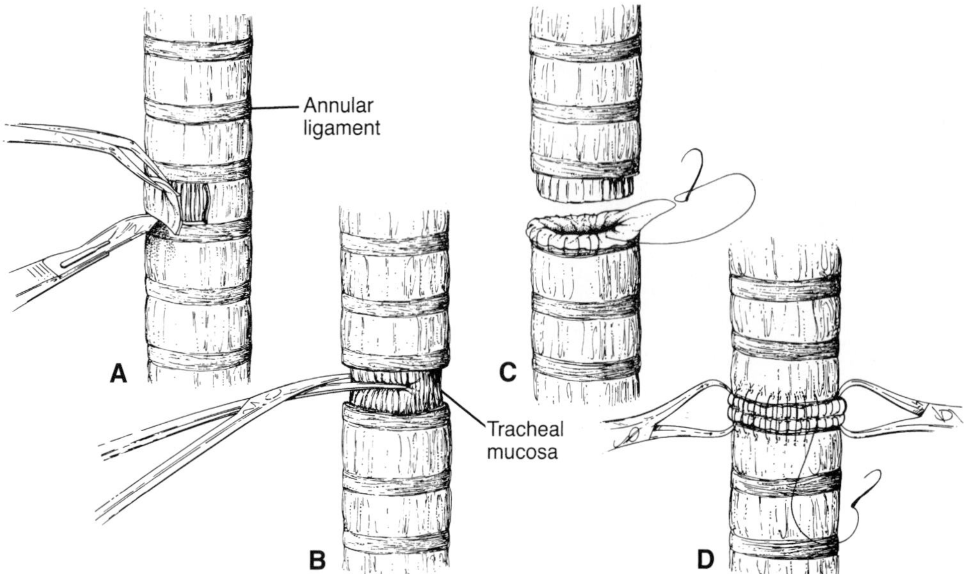

Figure 46-7. Surgical technique for tracheal anastomosis. **A,** Removal of a tracheal cartilage without penetration of mucosa. **B,** A 360-degree incision of mucosa between remaining cartilage rings. **C,** Eversion of mucosa, followed by suturing of mucosa to adventitia. **D,** Anastomosis of tracheal segments with stainless steel sutures.

abnormalities may cause collapse in other species. Tracheal collapse uncomplicated by trauma is reported only in mature horses. It also occurs after emergency tracheotomy when vertical incisions were made through the rings. When tracheal collapse occurs from dorsoventral flattening of the trachea in aged horses and particularly ponies, the tracheal rings form shallow arcs and the dorsal tracheal membrane is stretched, creating an elliptical rather than a circular cross-section.

Clinical signs vary with the degree of tracheal obstruction. Most animals experience varying degrees of respiratory distress and exercise intolerance and usually exhibit some stridor, although some animals may be asymptomatic until they become stressed. Diagnosis can be confirmed by auscultation, palpation, endoscopy, and radiography. Turbulent airflow may be auscultated within the cervical trachea and may thus allow localization of the site. Palpation may reveal the lateral edges of flattened tracheal rings in the jugular groove. Endoscopy will show the abnormal shape of the tracheal lumen, and lateral radiographs will depict the narrowed tracheal outline.

Treatment of tracheal collapse depends on the etiologic factors, length of the trachea involved, and accessibility of the affected area. Tracheal reconstruction has included complete replacement of tracheal segments with prostheses, external prostheses, imbrication of collapsed tracheal rings, plication of the trachealis muscle to reduce laxity of that structure, and resection of damaged cartilages with anastomosis of unaffected tracheal regions. The primary goal of the surgery is to restore the tracheal diameter without affecting the mucosal ciliary apparatus. This is best accomplished with an extraluminal prosthetic device that restores tracheal diameter by limiting redundant dorsal tracheal membrane and providing rigid support for the tracheal wall. Polyethylene syringe cases have commonly been used in ponies, but any nonreactive material of similar shape could be used. Partial chondrotomy is usually required on the ventral aspect of each collapsed tracheal ring to correct some deformities, which occur when this dorsoventral flattening has occurred over time. Failure of the prosthesis to work will result in resection and anastomosis as a second choice; however, no more than five rings can be removed, and frequently dorsoventral collapse of a chronic nature involves more rings than this.

Tracheal Stenosis

Tracheal stenosis refers to a narrowing or stricture of the tracheal lumen that can occur during healing of a tracheotomy made by transverse incision through more than 50% of the circumference of the annular tracheal ligament (Fig. 46-8). This produces instability and abnormal scarring. Other causes, particularly in foals, include *Streptococcus equi* abscesses in the peritracheal mediastinal lymph nodes and trauma. Tumors occur in this region, but tracheal collapse and stenosis secondary to tumors are unusual. Prolonged endotracheal intubation is associated with mucosal hemorrhage, necrosis, and stricture in people, and these lesions are frequently treated with surgery for removal of the circumferential fibrous tracheal stenosis.[17] Additionally, penetrating wounds that disrupt the tracheal mucosa, with or without infection, may lead to the development of tracheal stenosis.

Surgical procedures used in the treatment of tracheal stenosis include tracheal resection and anastomosis, extraluminal polypropylene prostheses, surgical drainage of peritracheal abscesses. and multiple tracheal ring chondrotomies with placement of retention sutures anchored to the skin.

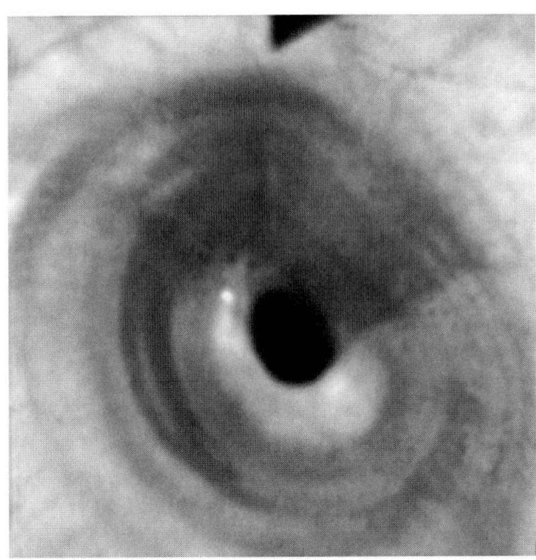

Figure 46-8. Endoscopic appearance of tracheal stenosis after transection of more than 50% of the annular ligament during temporary tracheostomy.

Foreign Body

Tracheal foreign bodies are uncommon in mature horses because of the size of the lumen of the trachea; however, endobronchial foreign bodies, although rare as well, are reported in equine patients.[18-21] They usually contain plant material, which may be inhaled accidentally, particularly during food prehension. The removal of foreign bodies from the respiratory tract is usually accomplished under general anesthesia and by way of tracheotomy. Frequently, removal involves endoscopic retrieval or endoscopically assisted surgical techniques. Foreign bodies in the tracheobronchial tree usually have thorns, which cause them to lodge in the bronchi. The clinical signs usually include coughing and epistaxis, and a bloody nasal discharge is not uncommon. Usually, despite the severity of bronchial lesions, improvement in the bronchial mucosa is observed very soon after removal of the plant material, and few long-term effects are reported.

Granulomas

Granulomatous nodules are occasionally observed in the trachea during endoscopic examination. Often these are in the proximal trachea near the larynx, but occasionally they are associated with healing tracheotomy incisions, foreign body irritation, or inappropriate passage of a stomach tube that damages the tracheal mucosa. Although they are usually an incidental finding and not associated with clinical signs, if they are of sufficient size to create airflow obstruction they can be removed using an endoscopically guided laser technique.

REFERENCES

1. Hare WCD: Equine respiratory system. In Getty R, editor, Sisson and Grossman's The Anatomy of the Domestic Animals, ed 5, Philadelphia, 1975, WB Saunders.
2. Widdicombe JH, Pecson IS: Distribution and numbers of mucous glands in the horse trachea, Equine Vet J 2002;34:630.
3. Nelson R, Hampe DW: Measurement of tracheal mucous transport rate in the horse, Am J Vet Res 1983;44:1165.
4. Art T, Lekeux P: The effect of shape, age and extension on the compliance of equine tracheal segments, Vet Res Commun 1991;15:135-146.
5. O'Callaghan MW, Sanderson GN: Clinical bronchography in the horse: Development of a method using barium sulphate powder, Equine Vet J 1982;14:282-289.
6. Shappell KK, Stick JA, Derksen FJ: Permanent tracheostomy in Equidae: 47 cases (1981-1986), J Am Vet Med Assoc 1988;192:939.
7. Rakestraw PC, Taylor TS, Schumacher J: Long-term outcome of horses undergoing permanent tracheostomy: 42 cases, Proc Am Assoc Equine Pract 2000;46.
8. Fubini SL, Todhunter RJ, Vivrette SL, et al: Tracheal rupture in two horses, J Am Vet Med Assoc 1985;187:69-70.
9. Tate LP Jr, Koch DB, Sembrat RF, et al: Tracheal reconstruction by resection and end-to-end anastomosis in the horse, J Am Vet Med Assoc 1981;178:253-258.
10. Scott EA: Ruptured trachea in the horse: A method of surgical reconstruction, Vet Med Small Anim Clin 1978;73:485-489.
11. Kirker-Head CA, Jakob TP: Surgical repair of ruptured trachea in a horse, J Am Vet Med Assoc 1990;196:1635-1638.
12. Shappell KK: Trachea. In Auer JA, Stick JA, editors: Equine Surgery, ed 2, Philadelphia, 1999, WB Saunders.
13. Rigg DL, Ramey DW, Reinertson EL: Tracheal compression secondary to abscessation of cranial mediastinal lymph nodes in a horse, J Am Vet Med Assoc 1985;186:283-284.
14. Robertson JT, Spurlock GH: Tracheal reconstruction in a foal, J Am Vet Med Assoc 1986;189:313-314.
15. Fenger CK, Kohn CW: Tracheal obstruction from tracheal collapse associated with pneumonia in a horse, J Am Vet Med Assoc 1992;200:1698-1700.
16. Tetens J, Hubert JD, Eddy AL, et al: Dynamic tracheal collapse as a cause of exercise intolerance in a Thoroughbred, J Am Vet Med Assoc 2000;216:722-724, 685.
17. Lesmo A, Ripamonti D: An unusual aspect of tracheal stenosis: Case report, Minerva Anestesiol 2003;69:861-867.
18. Brown CM, Collier MA: Tracheobronchial foreign body in a horse, J Am Vet Med Assoc 1983;182:280.
19. Duckett WM, Baum JL, Cook WR: Bronchial foreign body in a horse, Equine Pract 1983;5:8.
20. Ferrucci F, Croci C, Zucca E, et al: Case report: Use of a transendoscopic technique to remove a bronchial foreign body in a Standardbred colt, Equine Vet Educ AE 2003;15:228.
21. Greet TRC: Clinical commentary: Endoscopic retrieval of foreign bodies, Equine Vet Educ AE 2003;15:232.

CHAPTER 47

Thoracic Disorders

Joel Lugo

Thoracic disorders in horses amenable to surgical intervention include pleuropneumonia and pleural effusion (see Chapter 48), infectious or neoplastic masses, and thoracic trauma. This chapter's emphasis is on thoracic trauma and associated disorders, with some discussion on thoracic masses. Thoracic injuries in horses occur as a result of blunt or penetrating trauma. Blunt trauma is commonly seen in neonatal foals and believed to result from excessive compression of the pelvic canal of the dam during parturition.[1] In adult horses, penetrating trauma caused by collision with an object is most common.[2] Conditions associated with thoracic injuries include pneumothorax, hemothorax, rib fractures, flail chest, pulmonary contusion or laceration, and diaphragmatic hernias, and these can occur alone or in combination.

The pathophysiology of respiratory distress in horses with thoracic injury is complex. Pain associated with thoracic trauma restricts full expansion of the thorax during inspiration. This can induce rapid, shallow breathing, hypoventilation, and decreased clearance of pulmonary secretions that can eventually result in hypoxia and hypercarbia.[3] Pneumothorax, hemothorax, and contusion of pulmonary parenchyma can develop secondary to injury and can also contribute to respiratory insufficiency. Evaluation of a horse presented for thoracic trauma must be thorough but rapid, and, if necessary, potentially life-threatening conditions must be identified and immediately addressed. Emergency management of thoracic trauma patients (see Chapter 8) is directed at providing respiratory support to restore adequate ventilation and oxygenation, analgesia, and treatment of hypovolemic shock.

CLINICAL PRESENTATION

Horses with thoracic injuries may be presented with a range of signs, from stiffness at the walk or anxiety resulting from thoracic pain, to severe respiratory distress.[4] Clinical signs of respiratory distress include excessive respiratory effort, nostril flaring, tachypnea, dyspnea, accentuated thoracic excursion, and cyanotic mucous membranes.[5,6] Clinical signs may be subtle or dramatic, specific or nonspecific, and immediate or delayed in onset. This is especially true in horses with axillary wounds.[7] Initial evaluation of the respiratory system should include observation of the thoracic excursions, auscultation and palpation of the trachea and thorax, thoracic radiographs, thoracic ultrasonography, and arterial blood gas analysis.

DIAGNOSIS

Physical Examination and Triage

The physical examination of a horse with thoracic trauma should be both thorough and systematic. Observation of the rate, depth, and effort of respiration may help the clinician identify specific conditions. Rapidly developing respiratory distress is generally the result of pneumothorax or severe pulmonary contusion. Horses with hemothorax and pneumothorax develop a rapid and shallow respiratory pattern because of the restriction of lung expansion caused by the presence of fluid or air in the pleural cavity. A similar pattern of respiration can occur in horses with thoracic wounds or rib fractures, and this is most likely the result of restriction of thoracic wall movements because of pain. Paradoxical movement of the thoracic wall can be observed and is caused by collapse of a portion of the rib cage on inspiration when multiple rib fractures create an unstable flail chest wall.

Palpation of the thoracic wall should be performed to evaluate the potential presence of subcutaneous emphysema (crepitus), fractured ribs, hematomas, and unstable (flail) segments. Localized crepitus with or without a hematoma suggests the presence of fractured ribs, whereas more diffuse subcutaneous emphysema may indicate the presence of pneumothorax, pneumomediastinum, or axillary wounds.[7,8] Thoracic auscultation and percussion help determine the presence of pneumothorax and hemothorax. The absence of respiratory sounds and increased resonance on percussion strongly suggest pneumothorax. However, auscultation of the thorax should not be relied on as the sole means of diagnosing pneumothorax in horses. In a retrospective study, only 55% of the horses diagnosed with pneumothorax had decreased lung sounds dorsally.[7] When fluid accumulates in the pleural cavity, as with hemothorax, lung sounds are diminished ventrally, heart sounds resonate over a larger area, and a fluid line can be detected on percussion of the ventral thorax.[5] If crackling lung sounds are heard, pulmonary contusions should be suspected.

Several additional parameters should be monitored during the initial examination. The hematocrit and plasma total solids should be assessed at presentation and periodically afterward to determine if there is ongoing hemorrhage. Moreover, arterial blood gas analysis can help determine ventilatory function and the ability to oxygenate the tissues. If arterial blood cannot be obtained, a venous sample can allow assessment of ventilation. Hypoventilation is present if the P_{CO_2} is greater than 50 mm Hg, and hypoxemia is identified by an arterial P_{O_2} of less than 80 mm Hg. Frequent blood gas analyses can help assess if a horse's respiratory system is deteriorating or responding favorably to treatment.

Horses with thoracic trauma may suffer concurrent abdominal injury because of the close proximity of the abdomen to the thorax. Evaluation of the abdominal cavity is especially indicated when lacerations are present caudal to the 6th rib or when a deep penetration is suspected.[7] Abdominocentesis, ultrasonography, laparoscopy, or exploratory celiotomy can be used to rule out visceral involvement or rupture. Musculoskeletal injuries can also accompany thoracic trauma, but they are typically of secondary importance to systemic stabilization.

Radiography and Ultrasonography

Radiography and ultrasonography are valuable diagnostic tools for evaluation of the equine thorax. Pneumothorax is evident radiographically by the separation of the lung margins from the diaphragm caudally and the vertebral bodies dorsally, thus allowing the pleural surface of the collapsed lung to be observed (Fig. 47-1). Pneumomediastinum is diagnosed by the presence of air that outlines the mediastinal contents, and it can coexist with pneumothorax, usually secondary to trauma. Radiographs can also reveal other lesions, such as rib fractures, foreign objects, and diaphragmatic hernias. Intrathoracic and pulmonary masses may be seen as areas of increased soft tissue opacity that summate with or displace structures in the mediastinum, lung tissue, or thorax. Primary lung tumors tend to be well circumscribed and solitary. On the other hand, metastatic neoplasia is typically noted as multiple circular opacities of varying size and shape.

Thoracic ultrasonography is more valuable than radiography for confirming the presence of pleural fluid and for determining the best site for thoracentesis or placement of indwelling chest tubes. Ultrasonographic examination may permit the identification of foreign material, masses in the pulmonary parenchyma and cranial mediastinum, rib fractures, and diaphragmatic hernias.[9-13] Pneumothorax may be difficult to diagnose because free air in the dorsal thorax and aerated ventral lung lobes appear ultrasonographically similar. Thoracocentesis can be performed to obtain a sample of pleural fluid for analysis or to drain air or fluid from the pleural space. Aspirated fluid should be submitted for cytology studies, aerobic and anaerobic cultures, and antibiotic sensitivity testing. Sensitivity testing is important when hemothorax is caused by penetrating wounds, as the risk of contamination and subsequent infection is great.

Thoracoscopy

Equine thoracoscopy can be used to provide a more accurate diagnosis and prognosis of thoracic diseases when less invasive diagnostic tools fail to yield an accurate assessment. Common uses of thoracoscopy include the following[14-16]:

1. Exploration of the thorax of horses with suspected neoplasia or pleural effusion of unknown origin
2. Drain placement for relief of pleural effusion and abscesses
3. Transection of pleural adhesions
4. Pulmonary biopsy
5. Window pericardectomy

In addition, thoracoscopic surgery has been used to diagnose and assist in the repair of diaphragmatic hernias, and for exploration of the thorax in horses with open penetrating wounds.[17,18] Additional information on thoracoscopy can be found in Chapter 14.

Thoracoscopy can be performed with the horse standing or under general anesthesia. Thoracoscopy in the standing horse has proven to be safe, well tolerated, and associated with minimal detrimental effects to the cardiovascular and pulmonary function of healthy horses and horses with chronic lung disease.[19,20] The presence of a pneumothorax during thoracoscopy can cause a transient hypoxemia attributed to ventilation/perfusion mismatch and a slight decrease in cardiac output secondary to decreased venous return.[20,21] Analysis of arterial blood gases is considered essential to evaluate ventilation and oxygen exchange, especially in horses with compromised lung function.

For thoracoscopy in standing horses, the animal is restrained in stocks and sedated with xylazine (Rompum, Bayer Corporation, Shawnee, Mich) at 0.5 to 1.1 mg/kg IV, with detomidine (Dormosedan, Pfizer Animal Health, West Chester, Pa) at 8 to 10 µg/kg, or by use of a continuous IV drip infusion of detomidine (an 8-µg/kg loading dose followed by an administration rate of 0.3 to 0.5 µg/kg per minute until the desired effect is observed). During surgery, analgesia is provided by a single bolus of butorphanol tartrate (Torbugesic, Fort Dodge Laboratories, Fort Dodge, Iowa) (0.04 mg/kg IV) and local anesthesia of the skin, subcutaneous tissue, intercostal musculature, and costal pleura at each incision site. The thoracic chest wall is clipped and prepared for aseptic surgery. The sites for the telescope and instrument portals depend on the surgical intervention. The thoracic cavity can be better evaluated when the telescope is introduced into the thorax just cranial to the 10th to 12th intercostal spaces, avoiding the vessels and nerves located caudal to the ribs.[22] The mobility of the ribs at this location allows manipulation of the telescope for extensive exploration of the thorax. Selection of a thoracoscopic portal caudal to the 15th intercostal space can result in inadvertent injury of the diaphragm during insertion of the trocar–cannula system.[20] On the other hand, placing portals too far cranial at the eighth intercostal space causes some pain and discomfort during manipulation of the instruments or telescope as a result of distraction of the ribs.[22] A 1-cm stab incision should be made through skin and intercostal muscles just ventral to the epaxial muscles. To prevent damage to the lung by the trocar–cannula system through which the thoracoscope is inserted, a pneumothorax is induced by inserting a teat cannula into the thoracic cavity through the incision and the intercostal muscles into the pleural cavity.

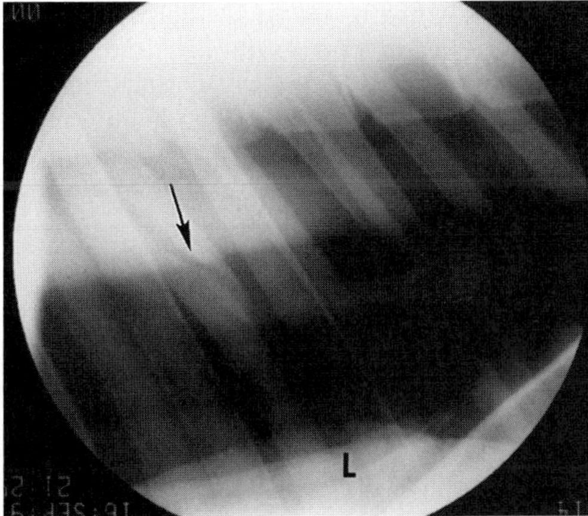

Figure 47-1. Thoracic radiograph of a horse with a rib fracture (*arrow*) that resulted in pneumothorax, as evidenced by air within the chest (appears black). The collapsed lung (L) lies ventral to the accumulated air.

After the pneumothorax is induced, the teat cannula is replaced by the trochar/cannula system. The trocar is then removed and replaced by the telescope. Once the telescope is inserted, a systemic exploration is performed and the desired surgical intervention is performed using triangulation technique. Multiple instrument portals are placed at least 10 to 15 cm apart (two to three intercostal spaces) to avoid obstruction of vision or restriction of instrument manipulations. Thoracoscopic viewing of the surgical field prevents injuries to thoracic structures during insertion of instrument and trocars. At the conclusion of the procedure, the thoracic cavity is inspected one final time and thoracic negative pressure is reestablished by removing all the air from the pleural cavity through a suction system connected to the thoracoscope cannula. Lung reinflation is observed through the telescope, which is retracted to the distal end of the endoscopic cannula, as inflation occurrs.[18] The telescope is removed and skin over the portals is closed with nonabsorbable suture material.

Thoracoscopy under general anesthesia is performed with the horse in either lateral or dorsal recumbency.[16,18] To perform the procedure under general anesthesia, positive-pressure ventilation is an absolute necessity, because bilateral pneumothorax is more common in the anesthetized than in the standing horse during thoracoscopy. After surgical preparation of the ventral aspect of the thorax, a pneumothorax is induced as previously described, and the telescope and instrument portals are made as dictated by the surgical intervention. On some occasions, CO_2 insufflation of the pleural cavity is utilized to facilitate surgical exposure. However, intrapleural pressure greater than 3 to 4 mm Hg can result in cardiovascular and pulmonary deterioration.[23] Thoracoscopy under general anesthesia improves the viewing of the ventral lung surfaces, ventral thoracic cavities, diaphragmatic surfaces, and lateral surface of the heart.[18]

Thoracoscopically guided lung biopsy has been described as safe and successful in the harvest of tissue samples for histologic and microbiologic examination.[20] Pulmonary tissue samples are collected from the caudodorsal aspect of the lung, because, when lung disease is diffuse, this site appears to be representative of the remainder of the horse's lung.[24] Direct observation of the surgical biopsy and excellent hemostasis enable surgeons to avoid complications reported by others when performing percutaneous lung biopsies.[25] Furthermore, multiple resections can be performed or larger wedge resections can be obtained when necessary. The main disadvantage of this technique is that the tissue access is limited to the periphery of the lung and therefore samples are useful only for peripheral lesions or diffuse interstitial diseases. If pulmonary lesions are seen during thoracoscopy on the broad surface of the lung, a biopsy can be performed with fine-needle aspirates, endoscopic biopsy forceps, or other biopsy instruments.

Thoracoscopically guided lung biopsy is performed with the horse standing under chemical restraint. The telescope portal is placed at the 12th or 13th intercostal space. One instrument portal is placed one or two intercostal spaces cranial and 15 cm ventral to the telescope, and the other instrument portal is located at the 15th intercostal space and approximately 10 cm ventral to the telescope portal. The caudal aspect of the caudal lung lobe can be grasped with atraumatic forceps (Babcock), and the wedge resection sample is obtained by the use of endoscopic staples (Fig. 47-2). When necessary, the atraumatic forceps and staple device are interchanged between portals to facilitate the approach to the tissue specimen. Because the tissue sample is usually too large to be withdrawn through the trocar–cannula system, it is withdrawn through the instrument portal with the cannula. The thoracic cavity and biopsy site are inspected for evidence of hemorrhage. Negative pressure of the thoracic cavity is reestablished by removing all the air from the chest, and the skin is closed routinely.

PNEUMOTHORAX AND HEMOTHORAX

Clinical Signs

Pneumothorax refers to the accumulation of air in the pleural cavity, which occurs as a result of pulmonary or chest wall injury.[26] When a communication between the atmosphere and the pleural space is created, a pressure gradient between the negative pressure in the pleural space and the alveolar or atmospheric pressure develops. Air enters the pleural cavity until the pressure gradient is eliminated or the communication is sealed. Consequently, the lung collapses to its minimal volume and this compromises pulmonary function. Meanwhile, the increase in pleural pressure causes a shift of the mediastinum to the contralateral side, enlarges the ipsilateral hemithorax, and depresses the diaphragm.[27] Pneumothorax in horses has been reported secondary to thoracic trauma, secondary to pleuropneumonia, and as a complication of upper airway surgery.[7] Traumatic pneumothorax can be classified by its physiologic nature as open or closed, or as a tension pneumothorax. Injury to the chest wall (e.g., from penetrating objects, wounds, gunshots) that creates a communication between the pleural cavity and the external environment produces an *open pneumothorax*. A

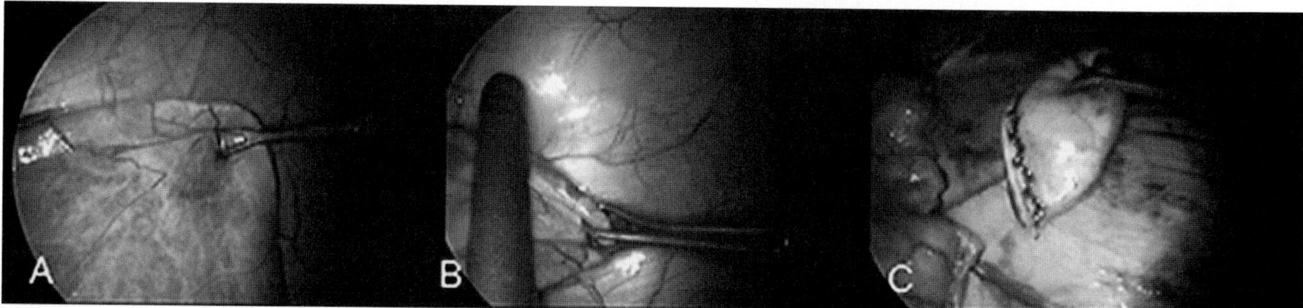

Figure 47-2. Thoracoscopically guided lung biopsy in a horse. The caudodorsal aspect of the lung lobe is grasped with Babcock forceps (**A**), and using endoscopic staples (**B**), the pulmonary wedge resection is performed (**C**).

closed pneumothorax results from leakage of air from the pulmonary parenchyma or an airway tear and commonly takes place after blunt trauma that is accompanied by fractured ribs that injure the lung parenchyma. *Tension pneumothorax* results when an air leakage, whether from the thoracic wall or lung parenchyma, acts like a one-way valve, allowing entry of air into the pleural cavity but not permitting its escape. Air continues to accumulate inside the pleural cavity during subsequent respiratory cycles, thus progressively increasing intrathoracic pressure to a point that it exceeds atmospheric pressure (positive pressure). Increasing intrathoracic pressure causes severe cardiovascular and pulmonary deterioration, and if not treated promptly and aggressively, this condition can be fatal.[27] Severe pleuropneumonia is another cause of pneumothorax in horses[7]. Slow leaks of air from necrotic pulmonary tissue or the formation of bronchopleural fistulas may be the source of pleural air in these horses.

The main physiologic consequences of pneumothorax are a decrease in the vital capacity of the lung and a decrease in the partial pressure of arterial O_2 (PaO_2).[27] Patients with pneumothorax have a reduced PaO_2 and an increased alveolar–arterial oxygen difference (A-a gradient). These physiologic changes appear to be caused by ventilation/perfusion mismatching (low V/Q ratio), intrapulmonary shunts, and alveolar hypoventilation.[27,28] Unless the mediastinum is sealed by another underlying inflammatory condition (e.g., pleuropneumonia, hemothorax), pneumothorax is frequently bilateral because an incomplete mediastinum exists in the horse.[29]

Clinical signs associated with pneumothorax include restlessness, cyanosis, tachypnea, dyspnea, unilateral expansion of the thorax, and accentuated respiratory excursions. In the absence of lower airway disease, the most probable cause of pneumothorax is trauma, and further examination may reveal evidence of a penetrating wound. Acute clinical signs are usually observed in horses with acute onset of pneumothorax or tension pneumothorax, whereas a more insidious onset of clinical signs is typical in horses with pleuropneumonia.[7] Decreased lung compliance and increased intrathoracic pressure increase the work of breathing.[26] To minimize the work of breathing, respiratory frequency increases, and the tidal volume decreases, producing the characteristic shallow, rapid breathing pattern observed in horses with pneumothorax.[5]

Hemothorax can develop secondary to any trauma that causes laceration of the intercostal blood vessels, myocardium, pulmonary parenchyma, or thoracic wall musculature. A horse with massive hemorrhage from laceration of the heart or one of the great vessels usually does not survive. Horses with hemothorax commonly present with signs of hypovolemic shock, anemia, and pain. Signs of respiratory distress develop once a large accumulation of blood in the pleural cavity restricts full expansion of the lungs, or when hemothorax is combined with pneumothorax.

Management

The emergency management of patients affected by pneumothorax is aimed at providing adequate ventilation, oxygenation, and systemic perfusion. Immediate therapy includes establishing a patent airway, reestablishing adequate alveolar ventilation by removal of the free air, and preventing recurrence. Supplemental oxygen therapy must be initiated for the treatment of hypoxemia (PaO_2 less than 80 mm Hg). Nasal insufflation of oxygenation at a flow rate of 15 L/min is recommended in adult horses to increase the inspired oxygen concentration.[5] In addition, patients with evidence of shock, such as tachycardia, weak peripheral pulses, peripheral vasoconstriction, and prolonged capillary refill time, require aggressive fluid volume replacement therapy.

Treatment of uncomplicated closed pneumothorax can be as simple as restriction of exercise and close monitoring. An open penetrating wound should be sealed immediately with a sterile, airtight bandage to convert the condition to a closed pneumothorax. Once sealed, thoracocentesis and reestablishment of negative pleural pressure can proceed. A large-gauge needle, teat cannula, or thoracostomy tube is inserted between the 12th and 15th intercostal spaces just below the epaxial muscles.[6] Air should be removed slowly from the pleural cavity, using a 60-mL syringe and a three-way stopcock or a suction device. Air leaks that recur after two to three needle aspirations require tube thoracostomy for intermittent or continuous evacuation. Thoracostomy tubes can be attached to a Heimlich valve for one-way flow (see Chapter 18), or to a pressure-regulated suction system such as the commercially available Pleuro-Evac (Genzyme Biosurgery, Fall River, Mass). Resolution of pneumothorax results in dramatic improvement in hemodynamic parameters, although abnormalities in gas exchange persist for 60 to 90 minutes after recovery and are associated with a decrease in pulmonary compliance.[28] After reinflation of the lung, some areas of V/Q mismatch and intrapulmonary shunts persist for several hours.

Unilateral pulmonary edema, also known as reexpansion pulmonary edema, can occur after rapid expansion of the lung following a period of collapse as the result of pneumothorax or pleural effusion.[30] Pulmonary edema acutely develops after reinflation and causes hypoxemia, decreased cardiac output, and transient hypotension, and may lead to death.[31,32] The pathophysiology is poorly understood; it appears that multiple factors contribute to increased vascular permeability in the alveolar capillary bed. The inflammatory response occurring after reexpansion of the lung is a strong predisposing factor for the development of pulmonary edema. The increase in capillary permeability is believed to be secondary to (1) mechanical vascular injuries to the alveolar capillary membrane and (2) reperfusion injury as blood flow returns to the now fully expanded lung.[33,34] Typically, the chance for development of reexpansion pulmonary edema is increased if the pneumothorax has been present for several days or when extremely negative pressure is used to evacuate the pleural cavity. A pressure of −20 mm Hg or less should be applied to the pleural cavity, and slow evacuation is recommended to minimize the chances of developing this complication.[35]

The rate of pleural air absorption can be accelerated by tracheal administration of 100% supplemental O_2.[36] When 100% O_2 is administered, the partial pressure of nitrogen in the pulmonary vessels is decreased to near zero, whereas the partial pressure of oxygen, carbon dioxide, and water remain unchanged. The absence of nitrogen in the dissolved gases in the pulmonary vessels establishes a diffusion gradient for nitrogen between the air in the pleural cavity and the gases in the pulmonary vessels. Once the nitrogen is absorbed, oxygen is 100% of the gas in the pleural cavity, which results in a gradient for uptake of oxygen. This gradient can increase the speed of absorption of free air to approximately 10 times the absorption achieved while breathing room air.[37] This therapy has been proven to be clinically effective in humans, but more investigations are necessary in horses.

Treatment of hemothorax involves restoration of the blood volume by use of intravenous fluids, blood transfusion, and pleural drainage. Removing the free blood from the thorax and reexpansion of the lung improves ventilation. In horses with open thoracic wounds, free blood should be removed to avoid the risk of developing septic pleuritis and pleural adhesions. Treatment of the simple hemothorax that is a complication of lung biopsy, thoracoscopy, or blunt trauma may be conservative unless the horse displays signs of respiratory distress, but careful monitoring is mandatory.[38] In these horses, absorption of blood occurs within days and pleural adhesions are unlikely.

Thoracocentesis is commonly used to reestablish adequate alveolar ventilation in patients with pneumothorax and pleural effusion. Evacuation of air or fluid from the chest improves ventilation/perfusion matching and reduces intrapulmonary shunting.[39] The site for thoracocentesis should be based on auscultation, or ideally on radiography and/or ultrasonography. In the case of both hemothorax and pneumothorax, both fluid and air can be evacuated from the same site. A large area over the selected site, usually the seventh and eighth intercostal space, should be clipped and prepared for an aseptic intervention. Local anesthetic is infiltrated into the skin, subcutaneous tissue, intercostal musculature, and costal pleura. A large-gauge needle, teat cannula, Chamber's catheter, or chest tube can be used for the procedure. The site for thoracocentesis is selected cranial to the rib to avoid the intercostal vessels located caudal to the rib. A small stab incision is made through the skin, and the selected instrument is advanced through the intercostal muscles until resistance is decreased as the pleural space is penetrated. At this moment, fluid or air can be drained and the catheter can be redirected if neither fluid nor air is aspirated. Thoracostomy tubes can be left in place after securing the tubes to the body wall with pursestring sutures. A Heimlich valve may be attached to the tube to provide one-way flow.

THORACIC WOUNDS

Etiology

Injury to the thorax in horses is uncommon but not rare, possibly because automobile accidents involving horses are infrequent. Most referral hospitals have one or two cases a year presented to them. Penetrating wounds to the thorax generally occur after an impact with sharp objects (e.g., trailers, gates, trees). Penetrating wounds are usually located in the lateral aspect of the thoracic wall or in the region of the thoracic inlet. The defect may look like a simple perforation requiring no specific treatment, or it may be extremely large. Open pneumothorax and subcutaneous emphysema are the most common clinical findings that develop subsequent to penetrating thoracic wounds.[2] The prognosis for horses with penetrating thoracic wounds is favorable if no other abdominal or musculoskeletal injury is present.[2] However, septic pleuritis can alter the prognosis in these horses.[2,40,41] Although a low incidence of septic pleuritis has been reported following thoracic trauma, approximately 50% of horses that developed pleuritis die or are euthanatized.[41]

Axillary wounds create interesting clinical signs for affected horses. The injury might not involve the thorax initially; however, marked subcutaneous emphysema may develop because the wounded tissue becomes a one-way valve for air as the horse moves. When extensive, this subcutaneous emphysema can migrate to the mediastinum (pneumomediastinum) and extend into the thorax, leading to life-threatening pneumothorax.[8] Therefore, horses with axillary wounds should be kept in strict confinement and monitored closely for signs of respiratory distress.

Management

Initial management of horses with thoracic wounds includes (1) the immediate covering of the wound with a sterile dressing to prevent any further ingress of air to the thoracic cavity and (2) assessment of the patient for intrathoracic injuries. Pneumothorax and hemothorax are likely to require treatment. If the wound is properly sealed, a one-time thoracocentesis or needle aspirate can alleviate the pneumothorax and associated ventilatory consequences. Any residual air in the pleural cavity will be reabsorbed within a few days. In horses with tension pneumothorax, emergency thoracocentesis is necessary to equilibrate pleural pressure with atmospheric pressure and relieve the respiratory insufficiency.

An important goal in the management of thoracic trauma is pain relief. All horses with thoracic wounds can have severe pain that limits chest wall excursions, and this often results in ventilatory impairment. Appropriate analgesia allows patients to maintain effective ventilation and oxygenation and to preserve the cough mechanism necessary to eliminate pulmonary secretions. Pain can be reduced by use of systemic analgesics and intercostal perineural anesthesia. Analgesics must be used carefully because of the potential for respiratory depression. Intercostal nerve blocks are performed with long-acting local anesthetic agents such as 5% bupivacaine. The block is performed dorsal and one to two intercostal spaces cranial and caudal to the injury to provide optimal local analgesia. Deeper infusion of local anesthetics is necessary to desensitize nonmyelinated C fibers located within the parietal pleura, which are a source of pain when stimulated by the penetrating object, fractured ribs, or wounds.[20]

Once life-threatening conditions are controlled, thoracic wound care consists of exploration, débridement, and closure. These manipulations can be accomplished with the horse standing under adequate analgesia or recumbent under general anesthesia. Treatment with the horse standing is preferred to avoid potential respiratory and cardiovascular complications that may develop under general anesthesia. General anesthesia is indicated for extensive wounds, for wounds that may involve underlying structures (e.g., the diaphragm), or for fractious animals. The horse must be stabilized by treating shock and respiratory impairments before the induction of anesthesia and, if necessary, the surgery should be delayed for 2 to 3 days. The wound must be thoroughly explored for the presence of foreign material and bone fragments, which can become the source of septic pleuritis or of recurrent purulent discharge. Thoracoscopy can be utilized to remove foreign objects while allowing a thorough inspection of thoracic structures.[42] The telescope is initially inserted into the thoracic cavity via a portal away from the wound, and a detailed thoracic exploration is performed. Meanwhile, pleural lavage with sterile saline solution can be performed. The wound can also be explored with the use of the telescope, but, to avoid further contamination of the pleural cavity, this is not recommended.

Immediate or delayed closure techniques may be used depending on the hemodynamic status of the patient, and the degree of contamination and tissue damage. The wound is irrigated with sterile saline solution and subjected to débridement. To facilitate assessment of damaged ribs, diaphragm, and lung lobes, the wound may need to be enlarged. Any foreign body is removed and ideally, primary closure of the wound is attempted. However, large thoracic defects may require reconstruction with primary muscle flaps, diaphragmatic advancement flaps, and/or prosthetic mesh. Creation of muscle pedicles from the longissimus dorsi and external abdominal oblique muscles to close a thoracic wall defect in a horse has been described.[43] If the wound defect cannot be closed, the wound is packed and sealed with moist, sterile laparotomy sponges to prevent the entry of air. A stent and thoracic bandage around the thorax holds the packing in place. Horses are also given broad-spectrum systemic antibiotics, nonsteroidal anti-inflammatory drugs, analgesic medications, and tetanus prophylaxis. The wound is allowed to heal by secondary closure with fresh bandage changes daily until the thoracic cavity seals.

FRACTURED RIBS

Rib fractures are common after thoracic trauma. Complications of rib fractures include underlying pulmonary contusion and thoracic wall pain. The most substantial physiologic impairment after rib fracture is a decrease in dynamic compliance, resulting in ventilatory impairment.[44] In addition, underlying pulmonary contusion renders a portion of the pulmonary parenchyma unavailable for adequate ventilation and oxygenation, resulting in hypercarbia and hypoxemia.[45]

Most isolated fractures heal spontaneously and surgical fixation is not necessary. The main goal for management of rib fractures is pain relief. Analgesia can be provided by administration of nonsteroidal anti-inflammatory drugs and by use of local intercostal nerve blocks. In the case of penetrating wounds, bone fragments are removed and rib edges are smoothed with rongeurs to prevent trauma to the pulmonary parenchyma.[4] The horse should be strictly confined and monitored for signs of respiratory distress.

Rib Fractures in the Neonate

A recent study revealed that approximately 21% of the foals up to 3 days of age have thoracic trauma, which can include rib fractures and costochondral dislocation.[1] In most foals, no clinical problems develop and the outcome is favorable. However, thoracic trauma and fractured ribs can have harmful effects and are a substantial contributor to morbidity and mortality in affected neonates.[11,46] Hemothorax, pneumothorax, diaphragmatic hernia, and even sudden death can result after laceration of intrathoracic vessels, lung parenchyma, and cardiac tissue by displaced fracture ribs. Underlying pulmonary contusion can also result in pulmonary insufficiency and predispose the foal to the development of pneumonia. Thoracic trauma in neonates usually involves three or more ribs, frequently occurs in one hemithorax, and is consistently located in the cranioventral aspect of the thorax.[47] The most common site for injury is the costochondral junction and the area immediately proximal to it. Dystocia and foaling in primiparous mares are two factors associated with thoracic trauma in foals.[11,47] These clinical findings and the occurrence of this condition during the first week of life suggest that injury occurs during parturition. The cause is believed to be pressure on the thorax during passage of the foal through the pelvic canal, but the thoracic circumference or the foal's weight does not appear to a factor in the development of thoracic trauma.

Clinical signs that may create suspicion of fractured ribs in foals include asymmetry of the thoracic cavity, groaning or grunting with respiration, plaques of subcutaneous emphysema overlying the ribs or ventral thorax, and crepitation or pain on palpation of the affected ribs. In a field study, 90% of affected foals were detected by palpation with the foal standing, but the thoracic cage asymmetry was better appreciated with the foal in dorsal recumbency.[1] Ultrasonography permits characterization of associated thoracic abnormalities. The presence of unilateral or bilateral pleural fluid, pulmonary contusion, or pericardial effusion, the number of fractured ribs, and the degree of fragment displacement are better evaluated with ultrasonography than with radiography.[46] Because more than three ribs are usually involved, affected foals can present with flail chest. Flail chest occurs when multiple ribs are fractured in two places (dorsal and ventral), resulting in loss of stability in a segment of the thoracic wall, known as the flail segment. The flail segment can also develop when ribs fracture in a single dorsal plane and the flexible costochondral junction becomes the second movement plane.[48] Respiratory efforts are hindered by the failure of the affected flail segment to expand and participate in the normal process of respiration. However, the underlying pulmonary contusion, not the mechanical disruption of the thoracic wall, causes the respiratory insufficiency.[49]

Management of foals with simple rib fractures consists of strict confinement for 1 to 4 weeks and supportive care with analgesics, anti-inflammatory drugs, antibiotics, and antiulcer medications. Foals with flail chest and concomitant pulmonary trauma are kept recumbent with the affected side down, and intranasal oxygenation is administered. Lateral recumbency with the affected lung down minimizes ventilatory impairment of the better-ventilated lung (on top).[11] Foals are kept in recumbency and sedated as necessary until the respiratory difficulties improve. However, lateral recumbency may lead to intrathoracic damage if axial displacement of the fracture is present. In these cases, foals can be placed in sternal recumbency. Surgical intervention is usually not necessary, but it has been pursued in foals when there is a potential for intrathoracic injury, as can occur with axial displacement of fracture fragments. There are reports of

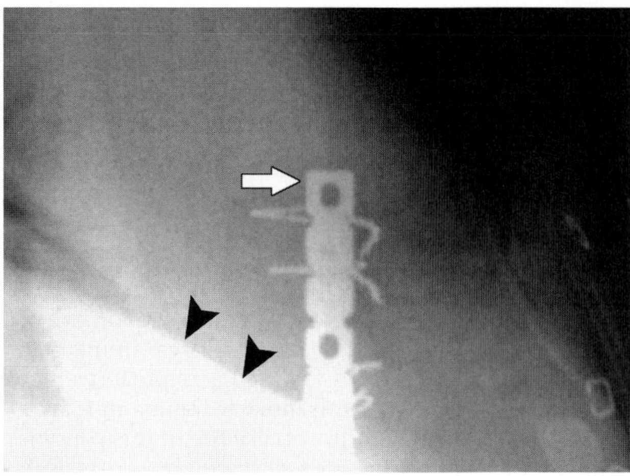

Figure 47-3. Postoperative radiograph of a fractured rib in a foal, repaired with a reconstructive plate *(white arrow)*, cortical screws, and cerclage wires. Note the caudal aspect of the distal humerus *(black arrows)*. (Courtesy Dr. F. Bellezzo.)

the use of both external coaptation and internal fixation of the affected ribs.[46,50] External coaptation was achieved by placing stainless steel suture material around the ribs and fixing the wires to cast material molded to the rib cage.

Internal fixation seems to be a better option to successfully manage foals with complicated rib fractures, or when the risk of intrathoracic injury is high. A recent report evaluated the repair of rib fractures using internal fixation techniques in 14 foals.[50] Surgical management was performed because the foals were considered at great risk for developing life-threatening injuries. A surgical procedure was performed on an average of two ribs (one to three ribs). After fracture reduction was achieved, a 2.7-mm reconstruction plate (Synthes, West Chester, Pa) was contoured to the rib and applied with 2.7-mm-diameter cortex screws engaging both cortices (Fig. 47-3). Four to six cortices of fixation on each fracture fragment were recommended. In addition, cerclage wire (18 to 22 gauge) was placed encircling the rib and plate at two sites above and two sites below the fracture. Application of the cerclage wire prevented implant failure from pullout of the cortex screws. Stall confinement was recommended from 4 to 6 weeks or until healing, which was evaluated with the use of ultrasonography. Of 14 foals treated using internal fixation, 12 were discharged from the hospital. Follow-up information on seven foals revealed that all were in good health and performing as expected, with the plates left in situ. Complications occurred in six foals and included implant failure, seroma formation, and subcutaneous hematoma.[50] Broad-spectrum systemic antibiotics, nonsteroidal anti-inflammatory drugs, and analgesic medications are also recommended.

REFERENCES

1. Jean D, Laverty S, Halley J, et al: Thoracic trauma in newborn foals, Equine Vet J 1999;31:149.
2. Laverty S, Lavoie JP, Pascoe JR, Ducharme N: Penetrating wounds of the thorax in 15 horses, Equine Vet J 1996;28:220.
3. Pate JW: Chest wall injuries, Surg Clin North Am 1989:69:59.
4. Laverty SH: Thoracic trauma. In Auer JA, Stick J, editors: Equine Surgery, ed 2, Philadelphia, 1999, WB Saunders.
5. Mason DE, Ainsworth DM, Robertson JT: Respiratory emergencies in the adult horse, Vet Clin North Am Equine Pract 1994;10:685.
6. Freeman DE: Standing surgery of the neck and thorax, Vet Clin North Am Equine Pract 1991;7:603.
7. Boy MG, Sweeney CR: Pneumothorax in horses: 40 cases (1980-1997), J Am Vet Med Assoc 2000;216:1955.
8. Hance SR, Robertson JT: Subcutaneous emphysema from an axillary wound that resulted in pneumomediastinum and bilateral pneumothorax in a horse, J Am Vet Med Assoc 1992;200:1107.
9. Lavoie JP, Fiset L, Laverty S: Review of 40 cases of lung abscesses in foals and adult horses, Equine Vet J 1994;26:348.
10. Reef VB, Boy MG, Reid CF, et al: Comparison between diagnostic ultrasonography and radiography in the evaluation of horses and cattle with thoracic disease: 56 cases (1984-1985), J Am Vet Med Assoc 1991;198:2112.
11. Byars T: Fractured ribs in neonatal foals. In American Association of Equine Practitioners Report, News, and Notes, 1997,
12. Dabareiner RM, White NA: Surgical repair of a diaphragmatic hernia in a racehorse, J Am Vet Med Assoc 1999;214:1517.
13. Byars TD, Dainis CM, Seltzer KL, et al: Cranial thoracic masses in the horse: A sequel to pleuropneumonia, Equine Vet J 1991;23:22.
14. Mackey VS, Wheat JD: Endoscopic examination of the equine thorax, Equine Vet J 1985;17:140.
15. Ford TS, Vaala WE, Sweeney CR, et al: Pleuroscopic diagnosis of gastroesophageal squamous cell carcinoma in a horse, J Am Vet Med Assoc 1987;190:1556.
16. Vachon AM, Fischer AT: Thoracoscopy in the horse: Diagnostic and therapeutic indications in 28 cases, Equine Vet J 1998;30:467.
17. Malone ED, Farnsworth K, Lennox T, et al: Thoracoscopic-assisted diaphragmatic hernia repair using a thoracic rib resection, Vet Surg 2001;30:175.
18. Klohnen A, Peroni JF: Thoracoscopy in horses, Vet Clin North Am Equine Pract 2000;16:351.
19. Peroni JF, Robinson NE, Stick JA, et al: Pleuropulmonary and cardiovascular consequences of thoracoscopy performed in healthy standing horses, Equine Vet J 2000;32:280.
20. Lugo J, Stick JA, Peroni J, et al: Safety and efficacy of a technique for thoracoscopically guided pulmonary wedge resection in horses, Am J Vet Res 2002;63:1232.
21. Peroni JF, Robinson NE, Stick JA, et al: Pleuropulmonary and cardiovascular consequences of thoracoscopy performed in healthy standing horses, Equine Vet J 2000;32:280.
22. Peroni JF, Horner NT, Robinson NE, et al: Equine thoracoscopy: normal anatomy and surgical technique, Equine Vet J 2001;33:231.
23. Daly CM, Swalec-Tobias K, Tobias AH, et al: Cardiopulmonary effects of intrathoracic insufflation in dogs, J Am Anim Hosp Assoc 2002;38:515.
24. Lugo J, Harkema J, deFeitjer-Rupp H, et al: Airway inflammation, mucous cell metaplasia, and mucus secretion in horses with heaves, Proc Am Assoc of Equine Pract 2004;50;348.
25. Savage CJ, Traub-Dargatz JL, Mumford EL: Survey of the large animal diplomates of the American College of Veterinary Internal Medicine regarding percutaneous lung biopsy in the horse, J Vet Intern Med 1998;12:456.
26. Leff AR, Schumacker PT: Respiratory Physiology: Basics and Applications, ed 1, Philadelphia, 1993, WB Saunders.
27. Gilmartin JJ, Wright AJ, Gibson GJ: Effects of pneumothorax or pleural effusion on pulmonary function, Thorax 1985;40:60.
28. Norris RM, Jones JG, Bishop JM: Respiratory gas exchange in patients with spontaneous pneumothorax, Thorax 1968;23:427.
29. Dyce KM, Sack WO, Wensing CJG: Textbook of Veterinary Anatomy, ed 1, Philadelphia, 1987, WB Saunders.
30. Pavlin J, Cheney FW Jr: Unilateral pulmonary edema in rabbits after reexpansion of collapsed lung, J Appl Physiol 1979;46:31.
31. Pavlin DJ, Raghu G, Rogers TR, et al: Reexpansion hypotension: A complication of rapid evacuation of prolonged pneumothorax, Chest 1986;89:70.

32. Pavlin DJ, Nessly ML, Cheney FW: Hemodynamic effects of rapidly evacuating prolonged pneumothorax in rabbits, J Appl Physiol 1987;62:477.
33. Pavlin DJ, Nessly ML, Cheney FW: Increased pulmonary vascular permeability as a cause of re-expansion edema in rabbits, Am Rev Respir Dis 1981;124:422.
34. Trachiotis GD, Vricella LA, Aaron BL, et al: As originally published in 1988: Reexpansion pulmonary edema. Updated in 1997. Ann Thorac Surg 1997;63:1206.
35. Light RW, Jenkinson SG, Minh VD, George RB: Observations on pleural fluid pressures as fluid is withdrawn during thoracocentesis, Am Rev Respir Dis 1980;121:799.
36. Zierold D, Lee SL, Subramanian S, et al: Supplemental oxygen improves resolution of injury-induced pneumothorax, J Pediatr Surg 2000;35:998.
37. Northfield TC: Oxygen therapy for spontaneous pneumothorax, Br Med J 1971;4:86.
38. Perkins G, Ainsworth DM, Yeager A: Hemothorax in 2 horses, J Vet Intern Med 1999;13:375.
39. Agusti AG, Cardus J, Roca J, et al: Ventilation-perfusion mismatch in patients with pleural effusion: Effects of thoracentesis, Am J Respir Crit Care Med 1997;156:1205.
40. Collins MB, Hodgson DR, Hutchins DR: Pleural effusion associated with acute and chronic pleuropneumonia and pleuritis secondary to thoracic wounds in horses: 43 cases (1982-1992), J Am Vet Med Assoc 1994;205:1753.
41. Mair TS, Lane JG: Pneumonia, lung abscesses and pleuritis in adult horses: A review of 51 cases, Equine Vet J 1989;21:175.
42. Lugo J: Personal communication, 2004.
43. Stone WC, Trostle SS, Gerros TC: Use of a primary muscle pedicle flap to repair a caudal thoracic wound in a horse, J Am Vet Med Assoc 1994;205:828.
44. McSwain N: Pulmonary chest trauma. In Moylan J, editor: Trauma Surgery, Philadelphia, 1988, JB Lippincott.
45. Craven KD, Oppenheimer L, Wood LD: Effects of contusion and flail chest on pulmonary perfusion and oxygen exchange, J Appl Physiol 47:729, 1979.
46. Sprayberry KA, Bain FT, Seahorn TL, et al: 56 Cases of rib fractures in neonatal foals hospitalized in a referral center intensive care unit from 1997-2001, Proc Am Assoc Equine Pract 2001;47;395.
47. Schambourg MA, Laverty S, Mullim S, et al: Thoracic trauma in foals: post mortem findings, Equine Vet J 2003;35:78.
48. Spackman CJ, Caywood DD: Management of thoracic trauma and chest wall reconstruction, Vet Clin North Am Small Anim Pract 1987;17:431.
49. Jackimczyk J: Blunt chest trauma, Emerg Med Clin North Am 1993;11:81.
50. Bellezzo F, Hunt RJ, Bain FT, Provost P: Surgical repair of rib fractures in 14 neonatal foals: case selection, surgical technique, and results, Equine Vet J 2004;36:557.

CHAPTER 48

Pleuropneumonia

Elizabeth A. Carr
Joel Lugo

Pleuropneumonia is a serious disease in the horse, and it has a significant economic impact on the equine industry. Treatment of horses with bacterial pleuropneumonia is frequently expensive, and it is time consuming. Resolution of the infection and response to therapy can be prolonged, even with early detection and aggressive treatment. Survival rates vary from 43% to 75% depending on the microbial pathogens involved, the rapidity of diagnosis and institution of appropriate treatment, and the development of secondary complications.[1-3] Many survivors are unable to return to their previous level of performance.[1]

RISK FACTORS

Bacterial pleuropneumonia most commonly occurs in horses subjected to physiologic stress, including long-distance transport, high-speed exercise, general anesthesia, and recent viral infection.[1,2,4,5] Horses subjected to long-distance transport have higher numbers of circulating neutrophils, an increased neutrophil-to-leukocyte ratio, elevated plasma cortisol levels, and decreased phagocytic function of peripheral blood neutrophils.[6,7] In addition, the practice of shipping horses with their heads secured in an elevated position results in increased bacterial and pollutant contamination of the lower airway compared with individuals allowed to lower their heads during transport.[8,9] Many horses refuse to drink appropriately during transport, and subsequent dehydration further compromises mucociliary clearance mechanisms.[10] During extended travel, periodic rest stops allowing the horse to lower its head and drink are necessary to resolve this contamination problem and to facilitate the correction of dehydration. However, rest stops may be infrequent with commercial hauling operations; consequently, the shipped horse is at increased risk of infection of the lower airway.

High-intensity exercise results in transient decreased peripheral blood neutrophil function and oxidative burst activity of pulmonary alveolar macrophages.[11,12] In the United States, Thoroughbred horses in race training are 4.3 times more likely to develop pleuropneumonia than nonracing Thoroughbreds, suggesting that career, not breed, is the risk factor.[5] In contrast, in Great Britain, show jumpers have the highest risk of developing pleuropneumonia.[13] The reason for this difference may be partly because most races are run on turf in the United Kingdom but on dirt in the United States. Additionally, European show jumpers frequently travel long distances for competitions, which may explain the increased risk in horses in this discipline.[13]

Endotracheal intubation, dorsal recumbency, and anesthetic-induced depression of the respiratory defense mechanisms may all increase the risk of lower airway contamination with general anesthesia. Respiratory viral infections result in damage to airway epithelium and breakdown of clearance mechanisms, further increasing the risk of bacterial colonization of the lower airway.[5] Penetrating thoracic injuries and pulmonary aspiration secondary to esophageal obstruction or upper airway dysfunction have also been associated with an increased risk of pleuropneumonia.[2,5,13]

CLINICAL SIGNS

Clinical signs vary depending on the chronicity and severity of disease and on the volume of pleural effusion. In the *peracute* stage, fever, inappetence, lethargy, depression, and exercise intolerance are common. Pleurodynia (pleural pain) secondary to pleural inflammation may be manifested by anxiety, pawing, reluctance to move, abduction of the elbows, and grunting when the thorax is percussed. A soft cough, dyspnea, tachypnea, and tachycardia may or may not be present during the peracute phase. Lung sounds vary depending on the severity of pulmonary and pleural changes, and a rebreathing examination is recommended to increase the depth of respiration and accentuate audible lung sounds. Although lung sounds may be relatively normal during the peracute stages, the patient often becomes distressed by the rebreathing examination (because of increased pleural pain) and may begin to cough violently.

With progression of the disease and accumulation of pleural effusion (*acute to chronic stages* of the disease), auscultation reveals ventral dullness with pleural friction rubs and adventitial sounds (crackles and wheezes) in the dorsal lung fields. Areas of dullness can also correlate with pulmonary or pleural abscessation. Cardiac sounds frequently radiate over a larger than normal area as a result of the pleural effusion and improved sound conduction. Nasal discharge can vary between absent and copious, and can range in consistency from serous to purulent. A chronic, brown, bloody nasal discharge may be indicative of pulmonary hemorrhage and infarction.[14] A foul, fetid odor to the breath is frequently associated with anaerobic infections.[15,16]

Accumulation of pleural effusion results in an increased respiratory effort with a slow prolonged pattern of inspiration and expiration. This pattern is the result of pleural fluid accumulation and its effects on lung volume and expansion of the chest wall.[17] Edema can frequently be palpated between the pectoral muscles and along the ventral midline, and it is a nonspecific finding with pleural effusion. Dramatic weight loss over a relatively short time results from the catabolic nature of the disease coupled with a decreased (or absent) appetite.

DIAGNOSIS

The diagnosis of bacterial pleuropneumonia is based on clinical findings (fever, pleural pain, abnormal lung sounds), complete blood count abnormalities, ultrasonographic and radiographic findings, coupled with positive bacterial culture of a tracheal wash and pleural fluid sample. Thoracic percussion can be used to detect and outline the extent of pleural effusion or pulmonary consolidation. The line of demarcation between resonant percussive sounds and dull sounds is usually the dorsal margin of pleural fluid accumulation. Fluid results in a horizontal line of percussion abnormality, whereas pulmonary consolidation without effusion generally results in a more irregular outline of dullness.

Thoracic ultrasound has largely replaced the need for percussion and is a simple and accurate way to assess the volume and type of effusion, if one is present (Fig. 48-1). Pleurocentesis is indicated if fluid is detected, and ultrasonography is used to determine the ideal site for the centesis. An ultrasonographic examination of the thorax in the peracute stage may reveal pleural irregularities (Fig. 48-2) without significant effusion or evidence of pulmonary consolidation. As the disease process progresses, pleural effusion generally increases and pulmonary consolidation becomes increasingly evident (Fig. 48-3). Because of the large reflection of ultrasound waves at an air–tissue interface, ultrasound is less useful in determining deep lung abscessation or consolidation if the superficial lung is aerated.[17] In this situation, thoracic radiography is a more effective tool for evaluating deeper pulmonary parenchymal

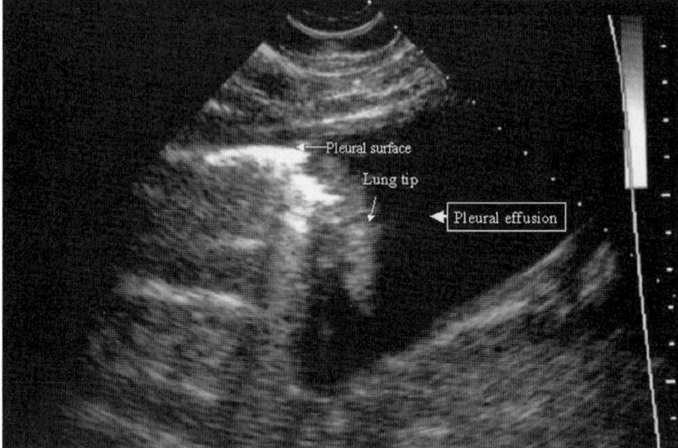

Figure 48-1. Ultrasonographic image of the left thoracic cavity of a horse with pleural effusion. A moderate volume of pleural effusion has resulted in collapse (atelectasis) of the ventral tip of the lung.

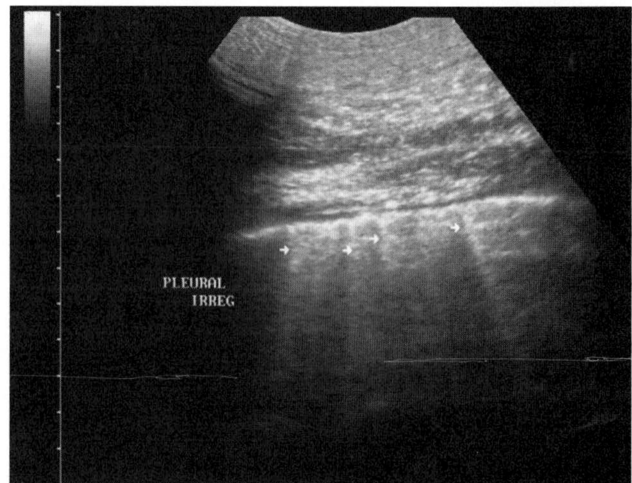

Figure 48-2. Ultrasonographic image of the left visceral pleura of a horse with peracute pleuropneumonia. The pleural surface casts irregular acoustic shadows or "comet tails" *(arrows)*. These irregular acoustic shadows are the result of pleural surface roughening. Subsequent reevaluation revealed progressive accumulation of pleural fluid and pulmonary consolidation.

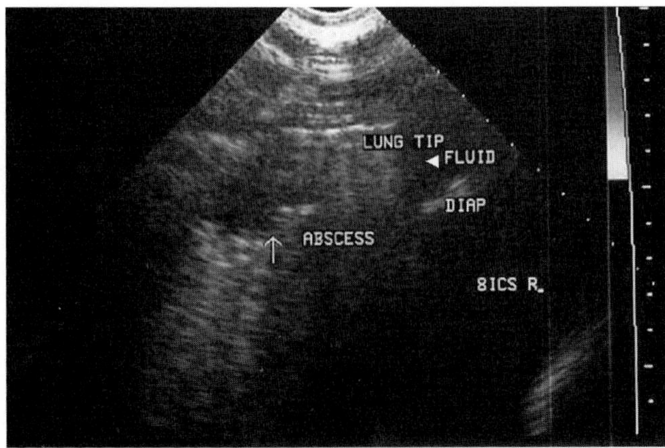

Figure 48-3. Ultrasonographic image of the right thorax of a horse with chronic pleuropneumonia. Minimal pleural effusion is evident *(arrowhead).* Consolidated or abscessed lung is evident by the break in the pleural surface and the ability to image the deeper parenchyma *(arrow).*

lesions (Fig. 48-4). Drainage of pleural effusion prior to thoracic radiography facilitates accurate evaluation since pleural fluid obscures the lung parenchyma, making it difficult to evaluate the extent or presence of consolidation or abscessation. Radiographs are useful, both to determine the extent of pulmonary consolidation and to evaluate progression over time; however, radiographic resolution of disease lags behind clinical resolution and, in the authors' experience, radiographic reevaluation is more useful in evaluating long-term progression than short-term changes.

Complete blood count and serum chemistry abnormalities are relatively nonspecific and reflect the chronicity and severity of the inflammatory processes. Hyperfibrinogenemia and a neutropenia with a toxic left shift are frequently seen in the acute stage of pleuropneumonia. Other common abnormalities may include hyperbilirubinemia (or anorexia) and azotemia (prerenal or renal). Neutrophilia is more commonly seen in the chronic stage of pleuropneumonia; an elevated serum globulin and anemia of chronic disease are also common. Although the abnormalities seen are nonspecific, they are useful in evaluating the response to treatment. A gradual decrease in serum fibrinogen and globulin levels, an improvement in the anemia, and a decrease in unconjugated bilirubin concentration (improved appetite) would be considered positive responses to therapy.

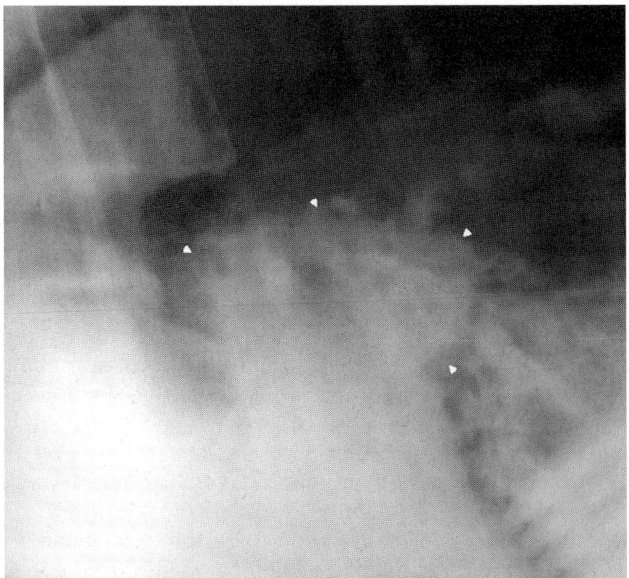

Figure 48-4. Thoracic radiographs of a horse with chronic pleuropneumonia and a large pulmonary abscess *(arrows).* Pleural effusion was removed via pleurocentesis prior to radiographic evaluation.

Both aerobic and anaerobic microbial culture of tracheal wash and pleural fluid samples should be performed prior to instituting antimicrobial therapy. Alternatively, antimicrobials can be withdrawn for 24 hours prior to sample collection. Tracheal wash samples can be collected percutaneously using a nested trocar or via endoscopic techniques. Both methods are effective in experienced hands. Complications of the percutaneous method include localized cellulitis and chondritis; therefore, the site should be monitored carefully for 48 hours after sample collection. If multiple samples cannot be obtained from the chest or if financial constraints exist, the tracheal wash is the preferred sampling technique, yielding positive results with a greater frequency than pleural fluid samples.[3] However, in some cases, only the pleural fluid yields bacterial growth. Consequently, when possible, it is best to submit both sample types for culture. The most common organisms isolated include *Streptococcus, Escherichia coli, Actinobacillus, Klebsiella, Pseudomonas,* and *Staphylococcus.*[1,3,13-15,19] Common anaerobes include *Bacteroides* and *Clostridium.* Anaerobic bacteria were isolated in 25% to 68% of cases.[2,3,16,19]

In addition to culture, cytologic analysis of a sample of transtracheal aspirate can be useful to assess the type of infectious process present, and to aid in determining the appropriate treatment protocol while awaiting culture results. For example, the presence of large, gram-positive coccobacilli from the transtracheal wash of a weanling foal may be indicative of a *Rhodococcus equi* infection. Alternatively, the presence of fungal elements, particularly if a horse has been on long-term antimicrobial treatment, may indicate infection with fungal agents.[20]

Pleural fluid cytology alone is of limited value in determining sepsis and should be coupled with the determination of pleural fluid glucose, pH, and lactate.[21] In general, septic effusions are expected to have a low pH and high lactate and low glucose levels when compared with plasma. The finding of sepsis is a clear indication for drainage. Serial pleural fluid protein measurements and cell counts are useful to determine progress and resolution of infection. A trend toward normalization of pleural fluid values is expected with appropriate treatment and control of the infectious agents.

MEDICAL MANAGEMENT

The cornerstone of medical treatment of bacterial pleuropneumonia is *early institution of appropriate antimicrobial therapy.* Treatment should be initiated with a broad-spectrum antimicrobial combination targeted against the most common bacterial pathogens isolated from equine pleuropneumonia cases, until specific culture results are available. A combination of a penicillin (or cephalosporin) and an aminoglycoside is a typical selection. Although many anaerobes found in equine pleuropneumonia are sensitive to penicillins, the addition of metronidazole is recommended if there is a lack of response to initial treatment or a resistant anaerobe (such as *Bacteroides fragilis*) is cultured. Depending on the chronicity of the disease, the type of sample cultured, and prior treatment, a culture may not always identify the pathogens involved; consequently, it is critical to monitor the patient's response to treatment. Repeat cultures or alternative antimicrobial therapy is indicated if the response to therapy is inadequate. In the authors' experience, a poor response to treatment typically occurs for one of three reasons: inappropriate antimicrobial treatment, inadequate pleural drainage, or the presence of abscessation or necrotic lung tissue. Therefore, daily assessment including by ultrasonography is critically important in the successful treatment of pleuropneumonia. When subcutaneous air prevents an accurate ultrasonographic evaluation, thoracoscopy is a useful and relatively safe tool to assess the development of pleural abscesses or necrotic lung tissue.

The second important part of medical management is *drainage of the pleural effusion*. In mild cases, with minimal effusion, antimicrobial therapy alone may be effective in resolution of the infection and the effusion. The need for drainage should be determined on an individual basis. Indications include large volumes of effusion with or without evidence of respiratory distress, purulent or septic effusions, the presence of gas echoes consistent with an anaerobic infection, and pleural abscessation or loculation. In the acute stages of pleuropneumonia, drainage of one hemithorax frequently results in bilateral resolution of the effusion. Over time, the accumulation of fibrin and debris results in closure of the mediastinal fenestrations, requiring bilateral thoracocentesis to remove bilateral effusion.

Drainage can be facilitated by ultrasound-guided placement of small cannulas or catheters that are temporarily placed into the pleural space and removed after completion of drainage, or via placement of a semipermanent indwelling tube. Indwelling tubes have the advantage of allowing frequently repeated drainage; however, in the authors' experience, over time these tubes become obstructed with fibrin or debris, necessitating removal and replacement. Attachment of a one-way valve allows continuous drainage, but this can be risky if the horse rolls or otherwise breaks the valve. Alternatively, the drain can be sealed and opened multiple times during the day to allow more control of the drainage. Localized cellulitis is a frequent complication of indwelling cannulas. Although this is generally not a life-threatening complication, it results in increased thoracic pain and is frequently associated with a poorer appetite and general demeanor. Depending on the severity of the underlying pulmonary parenchymal disease and the type of bacteria involved, drainage can become increasingly more difficult as fibrin is produced, and abscessation and loculation develop. Prior to the development of thoracoscopic techniques, one of us (EAC) successfully treated cases with multiple, mature, pleural abscesses by repeated ultrasound-guided pleurocenteses and drainage. Although this was time consuming, it can be a useful technique to manage cases with multiple abscesses or loculations.

The judicious use of anti-inflammatory and analgesic drugs is recommended to control pleural pain and fever, minimize malaise, and improve attitude and appetite. Nonsteroidal anti-inflammatories (NSAIDs) are potent analgesics and block production of inflammatory mediators that produce many of the systemic signs seen with pleuropneumonia. The value of NSAIDs in the treatment of pleuropneumonia needs to be weighed against the risks (nephrotoxicity and gastrointestinal ulceration), particularly in patients that are not eating or drinking adequately. The short-term use of small intramuscular doses or continuous-rate infusions (CRI) of the α_2 agonist detomidine, a potent analgesic, has been effective in controlling severe, non-responsive pleural pain in the experience of one of us (EAC).[22] Alpha-2 agonists should be avoided in febrile or hypovolemic patients until these conditions are corrected. Butorphanol, a potent opiate analgesic, can be administered intramuscularly or via CRI as well, and it may have the added benefit of suppression of the cough response.[23] Lidocaine infusions have also been reported to have an analgesic effect and may be an additional choice for pain control.[24] The use of combination therapies offers several advantages over single drug treatment protocols, including more effective pain control and the ability to minimize potential toxic side effects.

SUPPORTIVE CARE

Intravenous fluid therapy may be necessary in the initial treatment of the hypovolemic or dehydrated patient, but it is seldom required for chronic cases of pleuropneumonia. In addition to fluid therapy, nutritional support should be addressed. Many of these patients have a decreased (or absent) appetite, which, coupled with the catabolic nature of the disease, results in significant, often dramatic, weight loss if not addressed quickly. Feeding of palatable feeds, access to grass, and gradually increasing concentrates in the diet are important methods to increase caloric intake. The addition of corn oil or rice bran to the diet may also be of benefit. In some individuals, enteral supplementation via nasogastric intubation or parenteral nutrition may be required to adequately supply the patient's metabolic needs (see Chapter 6). Continued anorexia may be indicative of inadequate pain control, uncontrolled infection, or severe underlying lung pathology (pulmonary necrotic debris, abscessation, or neoplasia). Patients that continue to be anorexic despite aggressive therapy have a poor long-term prognosis.

SURGICAL TREATMENT

Surgical intervention is typically utilized to assist in the medical treatment of equine pleuropneumonia. Long-term antimicrobial therapy is rarely effective in penetrating and resolving large abscesses or loculations when substantial fibrosis or septic fluid is present.[25] Open and closed thoracotomy, with or without rib resection, has been successfully used for drainage of thoracic abscesses and resection of adhesions.[26-29] Surgical manipulations can be used to reduce excessive fibrin, which can result in loculations and adhesions, drain pulmonary or extrapulmonary abscesses, resect necrotic lung tissue, or perform pericardectomy in cases of septic pericarditis.[26,30-32]

Vachon and Fischer reported the use of *thoracoscopy* as a useful therapeutic tool in 16 cases of pleuropneumonia.[32]

Thoracoscopy facilitated the placement of thoracic drains in abscesses and loculated pleural effusion, and the transection of pleural adhesions to disrupt loculations, and it allowed direct evaluation of the lungs and pleural cavity (Fig. 48-5). Thoracoscopy provides a superior exploration of the pleural cavity compared with incisional thoracotomy.[33] Furthermore, the minimally invasive nature of thoracoscopy results in less morbidity and aftercare. This procedure can be performed in the standing, sedated horse with local anesthesia. (For surgical approaches to thoracoscopy, see Chapter 47.)

After establishing adequate pleural drainage, pleural lavage can be performed with isotonic balanced fluid solutions through the cannula system. Adhesions are more readily disrupted the first week after formation when the tissue is fibrinous rather than fibrous. Transection of mature, fibrous adhesions can be difficult and tedious, and it can cause profound hemorrhage. Therefore, conservative transection of mature adhesions is recommended. Careful insertion of instruments or portals into the thorax is mandatory in horses with severe pleuropneumonia and with extensive pleural adhesions or anaerobic infections. Adhesions between the lungs and the thoracic wall may not allow complete collapse of the lung, making the manipulation of the instruments more difficult and limiting the view of the pleural cavity. This can increase the risk of injury to vital organs (e.g., lungs, diaphragm).[32] Before introducing the trocar–cannula system in horses with possible adhesions, digital palpation of the lungs and pleura through the endoscope portal is recommended to avoid iatrogenic injury to these structures. In addition, the use of CO_2 insufflation (at less than 5 mm Hg) can facilitate and maintain collapse of the lung, improving surgical exposure.

Open drainage via *thoracotomy* should be considered for a chronic pleural effusion that has responded poorly to medical therapy, for localized or unilateral disease processes, for walled-off abscesses, or when tube drainage is inadequate.[25,34] Before performing open thoracic drainage, a horse's tolerance for pneumothorax must be assessed. This can be done with thoracoscopy or by inserting a large chest tube into the targeted cavity and leaving it open prior to thoracotomy.[32,34] If no respiratory distress is observed, the diseased pleural hemithorax is likely to be isolated from the rest of the thoracic cavity and is amenable to open drainage. Because these horses have compromised pulmonary function and are poor candidates for general anesthesia, the procedure is typically performed with the horse standing. However, general anesthesia with the horse in lateral recumbency is recommended to drain abscesses in the cranial mediastinum or when an abscess is not isolated from the rest of the pleural cavity.[35] Positive-pressure ventilation with a mechanical ventilator is mandatory. The use of isoflurane or sevoflurane is also recommended for gas anesthesia, because these drugs do not depress the equine myocardium as profoundly as halothane. Therefore, the combination of assisted ventilation, oxygen, and isoflurane or sevoflurane should be used to support horses undergoing a thoracotomy procedure when general anesthesia is required.

The preferred surgical approach to drain intrathoracic abscesses is determined by careful localization of the abscess by radiography and ultrasonography.[36] For the standing approach, local anesthesia is infiltrated into the skin, subcutaneous tissue, intercostal musculature, and costal pleura at the proposed incision site, and a local nerve block of the intercostals nerves is performed two intercostal spaces cranial and caudal to the site (see Chapter 47 for details). A 15- to 25-cm incision is made through the skin, intercostal musculature, and pleura over the selected intercostal space into the thorax. Manual exploration and débridement of the purulent material is followed by lavage with isotonic balanced saline solution. The incision is left open and the diseased cavity is irrigated twice daily until the surgical wound heals by second intention.

If thoracotomy with rib resection is elected, a 30-cm incision is made over the selected rib, through the skin to rib periosteum. In the cranial aspect of the thoracic wall, the cutaneus trunci muscle is incised at a right angle to its fibers. The latissimus dorsi and serratus muscles are then incised separately. The external thoracic vein is identified near the dorsal edge of the pectoral musculature, isolated, and retracted. Careful dissection of thoracic wall musculature avoids damage to the intercostal vessels and nerves, which are located at the caudal aspect of each rib. To expose the entire length of the rib, the fascia from the attachment of the external intercostal muscle is bluntly dissected. The periosteum is incised along the superficial surface of the rib for a distance of 25 cm and reflected circumferentially with

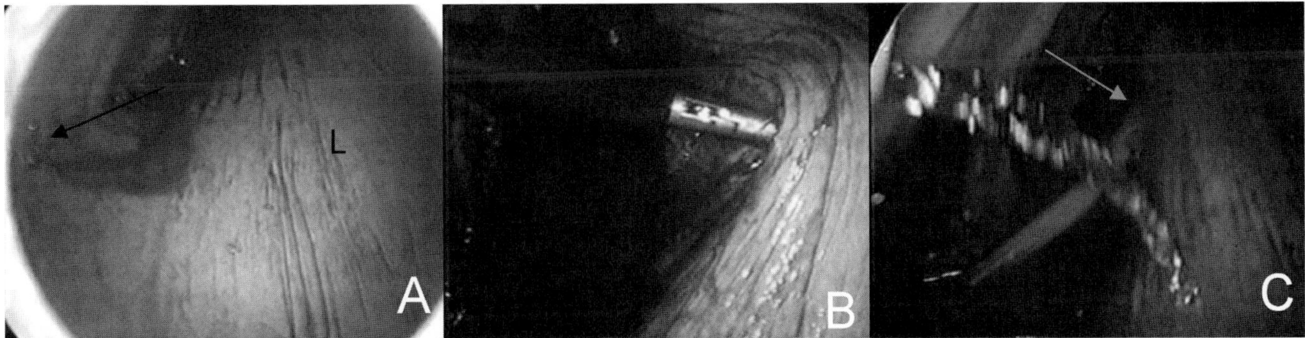

Figure 48-5. Thoracoscopic view of the left pleural cavity in a horse with pleuropneumonia. **A,** The collapsed lung (L) is adhered to the parietal pleura by fibrinous adhesions (*black arrow*). **B,** With the use of endoscopic instruments, the lung is separated from the adhered parietal pleura. **C,** After adequate drainage was established, a large chest tube (*arrow*) was introduced into the thorax and the pleural cavity was lavaged with isotonic saline.

a periosteal elevator (Fig. 48-6). The periosteum is separated from the rib, and an obstetric wire is passed around the most proximal aspect of the rib and transected. The rib is then disarticulated at the costochondral junction and removed. A small stab incision should be made through the periosteum and pleura, and the opening is enlarged with scissors. A Finochietto rib retractor can be used to separate the ribs for better surgical exposure, but this can cause discomfort in the standing horse. Thoracic exploration and débridement is then performed. Fluid and necrotic tissue are manually removed, taking care not to disrupt any mature adhesions.[36] If a localized abscess is encountered, a Foley catheter can be introduced from a separate stab incision through the thoracic wall into the abscess. The abscess can then be drained and lavaged, and the catheter can be removed or left in situ and secured to the chest wall for future irrigation. The thoracic incision is usually left open to heal by second intention.

If closure of the thoracotomy is performed, three layers of sutures are recommended. A rib contraction device (Bailey-Gibbon rib contractor, Standard model, Miltex, Inc, York, Pa) may facilitate the apposition of the thoracic wall. First, the periosteum is carefully apposed with size 0 or 1 absorbable suture material with a simple-interrupted pattern. The final suture in the first layer of the thoracic wall closure should be tightened while the lungs are fully inflated to reestablish the normal negative pressure of the pleural cavity. The intercostal musculature is subsequently closed in routine fashion with size 1 or 2 absorbable sutures. Finally, routine apposition of the skin edges with nonabsorbable suture material is recommended. Thoracic tubes are placed as necessary to alleviate pneumothorax or to drain pleural fluid.

Complications after thoracotomy include cardiac arrhythmias, thoracic wall abscesses, chronic draining tracts, and severe bilateral pneumothorax.[28,29] In contrast to thoracotomy, only mild discomfort during manipulation of instruments was reported during thoracoscopy in horses affected by pleuropneumonia.[32] However, thoracoscopy is not without risk; complications including injury to vital organs such as the lung and diaphragm have been reported.[37,38] In conclusion, surgical treatment does not replace medical management of equine pleuropneumonia but can, in selected cases, improve the prognosis of these horses.

PROGNOSIS

In retrospective reports, the survival rate for horses with bacterial pleuropneumonia varied from 43% to 75%.[1-3] The presence of anaerobic bacteria has been associated with a poorer survival rate in some studies but not others. Delay between the onset of clinical signs and the diagnosis and start of treatment is also associated with a poorer outcome.[19] The majority of horses that do not survive bacterial pleuropneumonia are euthanized for reasons including poor response to treatment, development of complications, expense involved in treatment, or a poor prognosis for return to performance. In a study of racehorses that survived pleuropneumonia, 61% returned to racing, with 56% of those winning at least one race. However, racing class was not examined in this report.[4] Complications associated with pleuropneumonia include bronchopleural fistulas, spontaneous pneumothorax, cranial thoracic abscessation, jugular vein thrombosis, pulmonary infarction, laminitis, and, rarely, pericarditis and peritonitis.[1-5,13-15,19,35]

A positive response to treatment is indicated by resolution of fever, return of appetite, and gradual reduction in the volume of effusion. Negative responses to treatment include recurrent fevers, continued inappetence and weight loss, continued effusion (particularly with progression of the effusion to an exudate), and development of the complications mentioned previously. These findings, coupled

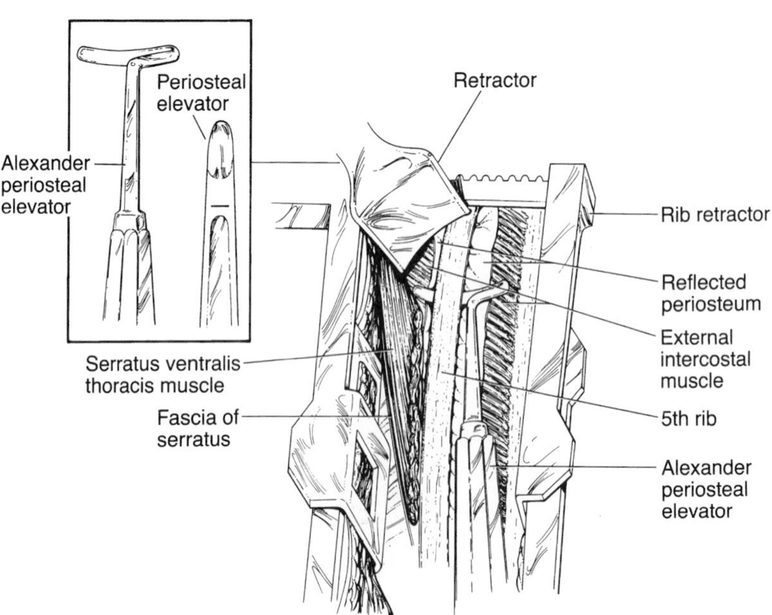

Figure 48-6. Surgical removal of the 5th rib with appropriate rib retractors and periosteal elevators. (Redrawn from the original by Gheorge M. Contantinescu, DVM, PhD, Drhc.)

with a continued elevation in serum fibrinogen and globulins and an abnormal white blood cell count, should stimulate careful reevaluation of the individual. Even with appropriate and early treatment, the response is often slow, with treatment durations ranging from 3 weeks to several months. After resolution of the underlying infection at least 3 to 6 months of recovery time should be allowed prior to return to training and performance.

REFERENCES

1. Raphel CF, Beech J: Pleuritis secondary to pneumonia or lung abscessation in 90 horses, J Am Vet Med Assoc 1982;181:808.
2. Collins MB, Hodgson DR, Hutchins DR: Pleural effusion associated with acute and chronic pleuropneumonia and pleuritis secondary to thoracic wounds in horses: 43 cases, J Am Vet Med Assoc 1994;205:1753.
3. Sweeney CR, Holcombe SJ, Barningham SC, et al: Aerobic and anaerobic bacterial isolates from horses with pneumonia or pleuropneumonia and antimicrobial susceptibility patterns of the aerobes, J Am Vet Med Assoc 1991;198:839.
4. Seltzer KL, Byars TD: Prognosis for return to racing after recovery from infectious pleuropneumonia in Thoroughbred racehorses: 70 cases (1984-1989), J Am Vet Med Assoc 1996;208:1300.
5. Austin SM, Foreman JH, Hungerford LL: Case-control study of risk factors for development of pleuropneumonia in horses, J Am Vet Med Assoc 1995;207:325.
6. Raidal SL, Bailey GD, Love DN: Effect of transportation on lower respiratory tract contamination and peripheral blood neutrophil function, Aust Vet J 1997;75:433.
7. Stull CL, Rodiek AV: Physiological responses of horses to 24 hours of transportation using a commercial van during summer conditions, J Anim Sci 2000;78:1458.
8. Raidal SL, Love DN, Bailey GD: Inflammation and increased numbers of bacteria in the lower respiratory tract of horses within 6 to 12 hours of confinement with the head elevated, Aust Vet J 1995;72:45.
9. Racklyeft DJ, Love DN: Influence of head posture on the respiratory tract of healthy horses, Aust Vet J 1990;67:402.
10. Friend TH, Martin MT, Householder DD, et al: Stress responses of horses during a long period of transport in a commercial truck, J Am Vet Med Assoc 1998;15:838.
11. Raidel SL, Love DN, Bailey GD, et al: The effect of high intensity exercise on the functional capacity of equine pulmonary alveolar macrophages and BAL-derived lymphocytes, Res Vet Sci 2000;68:249.
12. Raidel SL, Love DN, Bailey GD, et al: Effect of single bouts of moderate and high intensity exercise and training on equine peripheral blood neutrophil function, Res Vet Sci 2000;68:141.
13. Mair TS, Lane JG: Pneumonia, lung abscess and pleuritis in adult horses: A review of 51 cases, Equine Vet J 1989;21:175.
14. Carr EA, Carlson GP, Wilson DW, et al: Acute hemorrhagic pulmonary infarction and necrotizing pneumonia in horses: 21 cases (1967-1003), J Am Vet Med Assoc 1997;210:1774.
15. Sweeney CR, Divers TJ, Benson CE: Anaerobic bacteria in 21 horses with pleuropneumonia, J Am Vet Med Assoc 1985;187:721.
16. Reimer JM, Reef VB, Spencer PA: Ultrasonography as a diagnostic aid in horses with anaerobic bacterial pleuropneumonia and/or pulmonary abscessation: 27 cases, J Am Vet Med Assoc 1989; 194:278.
17. Black LF: Pleural effusion. In Staub NC, Taylor AE, editors: Edema, New York, 1984, Raven Press.
18. Reef VB, Boy MG, Reid CF, et al: Comparison between diagnostic ultrasonography and radiography in the evaluation of horses and cattle with thoracic disease: 56 cases, J Am Vet Med Assoc 1991;198:2112.
19. Racklyeft DJ, Love DN: Bacterial infection of the lower respiratory tract in 34 horses, Aust Vet J 2000;78:549.
20. Sweeney CR, Habecker PL: Pulmonary aspergillosis in horses: 29 cases (1974-1997), J Am Vet Med Assoc 1999;214:808.
21. Brumbaugh GW, Benson PA: Partial pressure of oxygen and carbon dioxide, pH, and concentration of bicarbonate, lactate and glucose in pleural fluid from horses, Am J Vet Res 1990;51:1032.
22. Daunt DA, Dunlop CI, Chapman PL, et al: Cardiopulmonary and behavioral responses to computer-driven infusion of detomidine in standing horses, Am J Vet Res 1993;54:2075.
23. Sellon DC, Monroe VL, Roberts MC: Pharmacokinetics and adverse effects of butorphanol administered by single intravenous injection or continuous intravenous infusion in horses, Am J Vet Res 2001;62:183.
24. Doherty TJ, Frazier DL: Effect of intravenous lidocaine on halothane minimum alveolar concentration in ponies, Equine Vet J 1998;30:300.
25. Raidal SL: Equine pleuropneumonia, Br Vet J 1995;151:233.
26. Boulton CH, Modranzki PD, Grant BD, et al: Partial equine lung resection using a stapling instrument, Vet Surg 1986;15:93.
27. Bernard-Strother S, Mansmann RA: Diagnosis and treatment of anaerobic bacterial pleuropneumonia in six horses, Comp Cont Educ Pract Vet 1985;7:S341.
28. Shearer DC, Slone DE, Moll HD: Rib resection and thoracotomy as a treatment of chronic pleuropneumonia, Proc Am Assoc Equine Pract 1985;31:393.
29. Carter GK, Ward DS, Taylor TS: Thoracotomy in the treatment of chronic equine pleuropneumonia, Vet Surg 1986;15:115.
30. Dechant JE: Combination of medical and surgical therapy for pleuropneumonia in a horse, Can Vet J 1997;38:499.
31. Colahan PT, Knight HD: Drainage of an intrathoracic abscess in a horse via thoracotomy, J Am Vet Med Assoc 1979;174:1231.
32. Vachon AM, Fischer AT: Thoracoscopy in the horse: Diagnostic and therapeutic indications in 28 cases, Equine Vet J 1998;30:467.
33. Peroni JF, Horner NT, Robinson NE, et al: Equine thoracoscopy: Normal anatomy and surgical technique, Equine Vet J 2001;33:231.
34. Schott HC, Mansmann RA: Thoracic drainage in horses, Comp Cont Educ Pract Vet 1990;12:251.
35. Byars TD, Dainis CM, Seltzer KL, et al: Cranial thoracic masses in the horse: A sequel to pleuropneumonia, Equine Vet J 1991;23:22.
36. Freeman DE: Standing surgery of the neck and thorax, Vet Clin North Am Equine Pract 1991;7:603.
37. Lugo J, Stick JA, Peroni J, et al: Safety and efficacy of a technique for thoracoscopically guided pulmonary wedge resection in horses, Am J Vet Res 2002;63:1232.
38. Peroni JF, Robinson NE, Stick JA, et al: Pleuropulmonary and cardiovascular consequences of thoracoscopy performed in healthy standing horses, Equine Vet J 2000;32:280.

SECTION **VII** NERVOUS SYSTEM

John A. Stick

CHAPTER 49

Anatomy and Physiology of the Nervous System

Robert J. MacKay

DEVELOPMENT AND ORGANIZATION OF THE NERVOUS SYSTEM

The nomenclature relating to embryologic, medical, and common description of the parts of the brain is inconsistently applied and can be confusing. Table 49-1 shows the principal naming systems used for the parts of the brain, Table 49-2 gives numeric and medical names for the cranial nerves, and Figure 49-1 depicts the locations of the cranial nerves on the ventral aspect of the brain.

The nervous system derives from a specialized strip of ectoderm, the neural plate, which runs along the dorsal midline of the developing embryo.[1] Ventral to the neural crest is the primordial vertebral organ, the notochord, which develops in concert with the central nervous system (CNS). The sides of the neural crest fold upward and medially to meet in the midline and form the neural tube.

Beginning at the brain–spinal cord junction, the neural tube closes progressively both rostrally and caudally to encircle the developing brain and spinal cord.[2] The rostral part of the neural tube buds large vesicles laterally on either side, which develop caudally and ventrally to form the hemispheres of the cerebrum (telencephalon), leaving the rest of the rostral tube to form the thalamus and hypothalamus (diencephalon) (see Table 49-1). The lumen of the neural tube (the neural canal) forms the interconnected ventricular system of the diencephalon (third ventricle) and cerebrum (lateral ventricles). Together, these structures become the *forebrain* (prosencephalon). Cranial nerves I and II arise from the forebrain (see Table 49-2). Successively more caudal dilations of the neural tube develop into the *midbrain* (mesencephalon) and *hindbrain* (rhombencephalon). The brain structures directly derived from the neural tube proper (namely, the diencephalon, midbrain, and hindbrain) make up the *brain stem*. As it develops, the neuropil, the dense feltwork of interwoven cytoplasmic processes of dendrites, neurons, and glial cells of the midbrain, encroaches on the neural canal until it is a narrow tube, the mesencephalic aqueduct. The rostral part of the hindbrain (metencephalon) develops into the pons and cerebellum, whereas the caudal part, which is contiguous with the spinal cord, forms the medulla oblongata (myelencephalon). Within the pons and medulla, the neural canal forms the fourth ventricle, connecting the mesencephalic aqueduct rostrally with the spinal (central) canal caudally. Cranial nerves III and IV (midbrain), V (pons), and VI to XII (medulla) develop in the ventrolateral brain stem.

Within the neural tube of the developing spinal cord, primitive neurons become organized into mantle and marginal layers that become white and gray matter, respectively.[2] Ventral mantle neurons grow through the surrounding marginal layer and course outside the neural tube to form ventral spinal nerve roots. Dorsal ganglia and roots form from the growth of neural crest cells centrally into the neural tube and distally to sensory structures. The developing gray matter becomes divided morphologically and functionally into dorsal, intermediate, and ventral columns. Ventral and dorsal roots and gray matter divide spinal cord white matter into three regions called funiculi. These are dorsal, lateral, and ventral on each side of the spinal cord (Fig. 49-2).

TABLE 49-1. Naming Systems for Principal Parts of the Brain

Primary Segments	Secondary Segments	Principal Divisions	Common Usage	Cavities
Prosencephalon (forebrain)	Telencephalon	Cerebrum	Brain	Lateral ventricle
	Diencephalon	Thalamus Hypothalamus	Brain stem	3rd ventricle
Mesencephalon (midbrain)	Mesencephalon	Midbrain	Brain stem	Mesencephalic aqueduct
	Metencephalon	Cerebellum	Brain stem*	
Rhombencephalon (hindbrain)		Pons	Brain stem	4th ventricle
	Myelencephalon	Medulla oblongata	Brain stem	

*Some authors exclude the cerebellum from definitions of the brain stem.

TABLE 49-2. Names of Cranial Nerves

Number	Name
I	Olfactory
II	Optic
III	Oculomotor
IV	Trochlear
V	Trigeminal
VI	Abducens
VII	Facial
VIII	Vestibulocochlear
IX	Glossopharyngeal
X	Vagus
XI	Accessory
XII	Hypoglossal

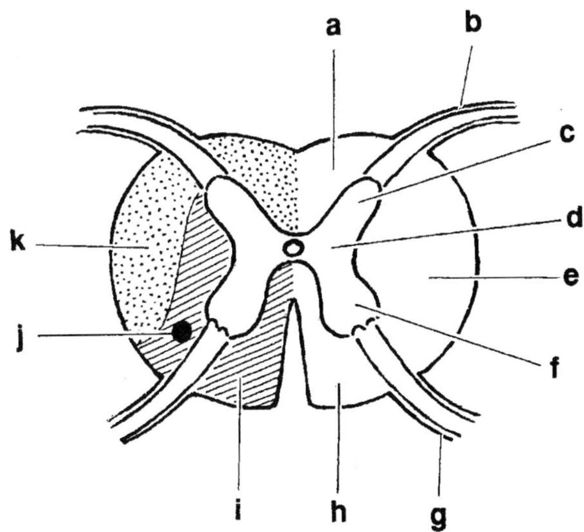

Figure 49-2. Simplified diagram of the functional *(left)* and anatomic *(right)* organization of the spinal cord at the level of the 7th cervical segment. a, Dorsal funiculus of the white matter; b, dorsal root; c, dorsal column of the gray matter; d, intermediate column of the gray matter; e, lateral funiculus of the white matter; f, ventral column of the gray matter; g, ventral root; h, ventral funiculus of the white matter; i, upper motor neuron (descending) tracts; j, sensory/pain (ascending) tracts; k, proprioceptive (ascending) tracts.

The Cranium

The cranium is made up of the occipital, sphenoid, ethmoid, interparietal, parietal, frontal, and temporal bones.[3,4] These bones enclose a cranial cavity with a volume of approximately 650 mL in an adult horse. The roof of the cranium features large rostral and caudal concavities, which accommodate the hemispheres of the cerebrum and cerebellum, respectively (Fig. 49-3). The internal occipital protuberance separates these cavities dorsally and provides attachment for the tentorium cerebelli, the tent-shaped extension of the dura mater that forms a partition between the cerebrum and cerebellum. The occipital and petrous temporal bones encase the cerebellum dorsally and laterally. The cerebrum is covered dorsally largely by the parietal bones, with smaller contributions from the interparietal bone caudally and the frontal bones rostrally. The rostral or nasal wall of the cranial cavity is formed by the cribriform plate of the ethmoid, which separates the cranium from the

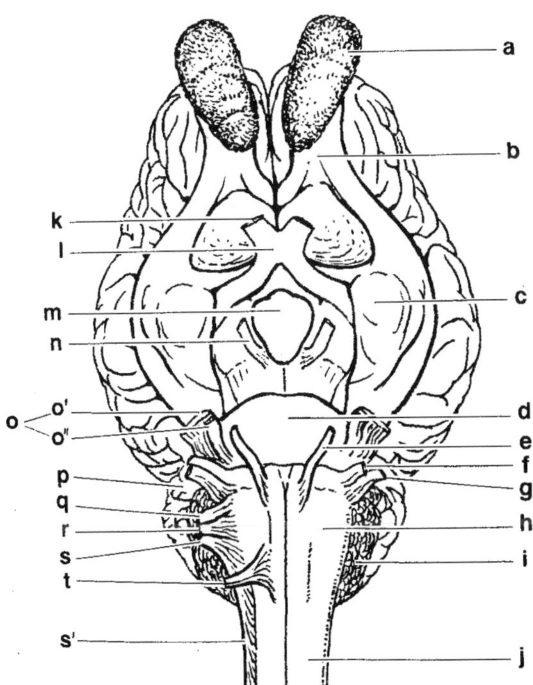

Figure 49-1. Base of the brain showing cranial nerve roots. a, Olfactory bulb; b, olfactory tract; c, optic tract; d, pons; e, abducens nerve; f, facial nerve; g, vestibulocochlear nerve; h, medulla oblongata; i, choroid plexus of the 4th ventricle; j, spinal cord; k, optic nerve; l, optic chiasm; m, pituitary; n, oculomotor nerve; o, trigeminal nerve (o′, motor root, o″, sensory root); p, cerebellum; q, glossopharyngeal nerve; r, vagus nerve; s, spinal accessory (medullary root); s′, spinal accessory (spinal root); t, hypoglossal nerve.

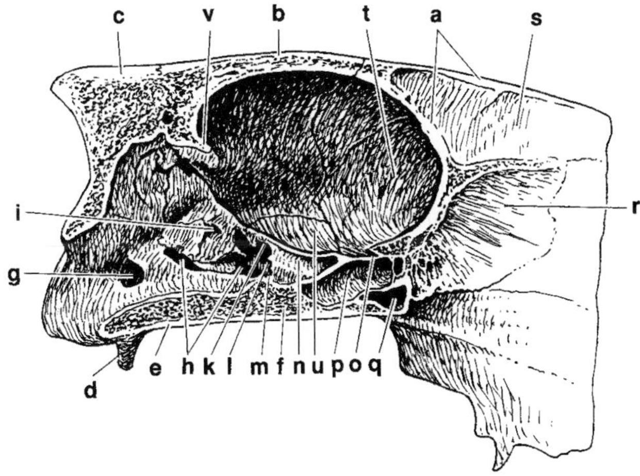

Figure 49-3. Sagittal section of cranium. a, Hypoglossal foramen; b, foramen lacerum; c, internal acoustic meatus; d, spinous notch; e, oval notch; f, carotid notch; g, groove for maxillary nerve; h, optic foramen; i, sphenoidal sinus; j, perpendicular plate of ethmoid bone; k, septum between frontal sinuses; l, orbital wing of sphenoid; m, temporal wing of sphenoid; n, internal occipital protuberance.

nasal cavity. It is perforated by numerous foramina through which olfactory nerve bundles pass. On the dorsal midline is the internal parietal crest, which furnishes attachment to the falx cerebri, the sickle-shaped fold of dura that separates the cerebral hemispheres. The forebrain may be injured by impact to the frontal/parietal area of the skull.[5] As a consequence of swelling, cerebral lobes may herniate under the falx or tentorium and compress other parts of the brain.

The floor of the cranial cavity is organized into three fossae.[4] The rostral fossa supports the frontal and olfactory parts of the cerebrum. It is formed chiefly by the sphenoid bone. Caudally in this fossa is a bony shelf that covers the entrance to the optic canals and supports the optic chiasm. The optic nerves are firmly attached within the optic canals and may be injured within the canals by the to-and-fro motion of the brain after skull impact.[6] From this point caudally to the junction between the basilar portions of the occipital and sphenoid bones is the middle fossa. This is the largest and widest part of the cranial cavity. In its middle is the hypophyseal fossa, and the caudal aspect supports the midbrain. On either side are two grooves. The medial one provides passage for cranial nerves III, IV, V (ophthalmic branch), and VI to the optic, trochlear, and orbital foramina; the lateral one leads to the foramen rotundum and contains the maxillary nerve (V). The posterior fossa is formed by the basilar part of the occipital bone. It supports the pons and medulla oblongata and continues dorsally to enclose the cerebellum. On either side of the basilar part of the occipital bone is the foramen lacerum, through which course cranial nerves V (mandibular branch), IX, X, and XI. Caudolaterally, on either side of the occipital condyles, is the hypoglossal foramen, through which passes cranial nerve XII. On the ventral aspect of the basilar bones, there are tubercles at the points of attachment of the large paired rectus capitis, ventralis major (longus capitis), and minor muscles. After poll impact, which typically results from a horse flipping over backwards, the wrenching action of these muscles may fracture or separate the basilar parts of the occipital or sphenoid bones and damage nerves in the adjacent foramen lacerum.[7]

The temporal bone forms most of the lateral wall of the cranium.[4] It is related to the occipital caudally, the parietal dorsally, the frontal rostrally, and the sphenoid bone ventrally. There are two distinct parts, the squamous and petrous bones. The squamous bone is platelike in shape and overlaps laterally much of the petrous bone. The petrous bone is a dense pyramid-shaped bone that forms the lateral margin of the foramen lacerum. The external acoustic meatus opens on the lateral side. Housed within the petrous temporal bone are the cavities and specialized bones of the auditory and vestibular systems, including the large ventrally projecting osseous bulla. Medially, the petrous temporal bone is related to the cerebellar hemisphere and transmits cranial nerves VII and VIII through the internal acoustic meatus. The temporal bone is vulnerable to fracture after poll impact.[5] A short rodlike projection, the hyoid process, projects from the base of the petrous slightly in front of the stylomastoid foramen, through which passes cranial nerve VII. The temporohyoid joint is formed by attachment of the hyoid process to the tympanohyoid cartilage and thus to the stylohyoid proper. A condition involving remodeling and fusion of this joint (temporohyoid osteoarthropathy) subjects the petrous bone to unusual stresses, which may result in fracture and signs of VII and VIII injury.[8]

The caudal fossa is continuous with the vertebral canal via the foramen magnum. As a result of increased pressure in the caudal fossa, the caudal part of the cerebellum may be squeezed through the foramen magnum (tonsillar herniation).[9]

Joints between the plates of the cranium are immobile synarthroses[4]; some, such as the joint between the basilar parts of the occipital and sphenoid bones, are bound together by cartilage (synchondroses), and others, such as the temporal–parietal joint, are united by fibrous tissue (sutures). These joints usually ossify and become completely fused. The sphenooccipital synchondrosis fuses at about 5 years of age. The suture between the parietal bones ossifies at 4 years, the parietooccipital suture at 5 years, and the parietotemporal suture at 12 to 15 years.

The Vertebral Column

The vertebral column extends from the skull to the end of the tail. There are five regions: cervical, thoracic, lumbar, sacral, and coccygeal (caudal). The typical formula for the horse is $C_7T_{18}L_6S_5Cy_{15\text{-}21}$.[3] Although regions of the spine vary as to details, the vertebral structure conforms to a common plan. Each vertebra comprises a body, an arch, and various processes. The body is a cylindrical mass oriented along the median plane and connected to other vertebrae by fibrocartilaginous discs. Together with the dorsal surface of the body, the arch completes the vertebral foramen, or ring. The arch consists of two lateral pedicles and a dorsal lamina. The intervertebral foramina, formed by the spaces between the arches of adjacent vertebrae, provide passage for spinal nerves and vessels. Successive vertebral rings are strung together by dorsal and ventral longitudinal ligaments to form the vertebral canal, a protective cylinder for the spinal cord, nerve roots, and cauda equina. The arch gives rise to articular processes at each end, a dorsal spinous process, and laterally projecting transverse processes. In some vertebrae, there are additionally mammillary or accessory processes, or costal facets. There are at least five centers of ossification in each vertebra: one body, two arches, and epiphyseal plates at either end of the body.

The spine can be modeled biomechanically as three "columns." The ventral column is composed of the ventral longitudinal ligament and the ventral half of the vertebral bodies and discs. The middle column is formed by the dorsal longitudinal ligament and the dorsal half of the bodies and discs, and the dorsal column consists of the arches, intervertebral joints, and associated ligaments.[10] The degree of instability after spinal injury increases as more columns are impacted, and the prognosis for recovery decreases correspondingly.

In its neutral position, the spine presents a series of curves in the median plane. The cranial part of the cervical spine is concave ventrally, the cervicothoracic junction is markedly concave dorsally, the thoracolumbar spine exhibits gentle ventral concavity, and the lumbosacral junction has more marked ventral concavity.[4] The vertebral canal varies in diameter as it progresses along the spine: within the atlas it is wide so as to house the dens and spinal cord, and there are cervicothoracic and lumbosacral dilations to accommodate the corresponding intumescences of the spinal cord. The sagittal diameters of the cervical vertebral foramina in horses of various sizes have been determined radiographically.[11] Mean sagittal diameters for horses heavier than 350 kg varied from 21.3 mm for C4 to 27.4 mm for C7.

The cervical vertebrae are relatively large and long. The arch is thick and strong and forms large articular processes. The cranial articular processes are directed dorsomedially; the posterior, ventrolaterally. Disordered vertebral development, possibly related to osteochondrosis, commonly causes malformation and arthropathy of the cervical vertebrae in young adult horses (see Chapter 51). These changes may cause cervical stenotic myelopathy with ataxia of the limbs and trunk. Horses with these clinical signs are commonly referred to as wobblers.

The first two cervical vertebrae are modified to accommodate the movements and weight of the head.[4] The atlas is composed of dorsal and ventral arches, lateral masses, and wings. The ventral arch has on its upper surface the fovea dentis, on which the dens rests. The dens projects forward from the body of the axis and is attached by strong transverse, alar, and apical ligaments to the atlas and occiput. The upper cervical area of performance and racing horses is prone to severe hyperflexion, hyperextension, and/or axial compressive forces caused by collisions at speed.[12] Such stresses may fracture any of the bony components of the upper (cranial) part of the neck or may separate the dens from the atlas.

Thoracic vertebrae are relatively constrained in their ranges of intervertebral movement. Added stability is provided to this region by the bracing action of the ribs and sternum. Perhaps because of the comparatively unconstrained movement of the cranial lumbar spine, fractures or dislocations of the vertebrae around the thoracolumbar joint occur quite commonly.

The sacrum is formed by the fusion of five sacral vertebrae.[4] It is wedged between and attached to the ilia. Branches of the first four sacral nerves course through the dorsal and ventral sacral foramina. Fusion proceeds from the front of the sacrum caudally and may not be complete even in adult horses. The sacrum houses the roots of the cauda equina and a small terminal part of the spinal cord that supplies the tail. These nerve roots are vulnerable to damage as a result of sacral fractures. Such injury may manifest as cauda equina syndrome (S2 to S5 roots)[9] or as gait abnormalities in the pelvic limbs (S1 to S2).

Cerebrospinal Fluid

Cerebrospinal fluid (CSF) envelops, bathes, and protects the CNS.[2,9] It is produced at a high rate by the choroid plexuses of the lateral, third, and fourth ventricles, and more generally by the meninges and ependyma. CSF passes from sites of production in the ventricles, out through the lateral apertures of the fourth ventricles, and it subsequently flows forward over the cerebrum and caudally over the spinal cord (Fig. 49-4). The rate of production is independent of CSF pressure. Absorption takes place in convoluted arachnoid structures, which project, mushroom-like, into cerebral veins or venous sinuses. Flow at these arachnoid villi is pressure dependent and unidirectional from CSF to blood.

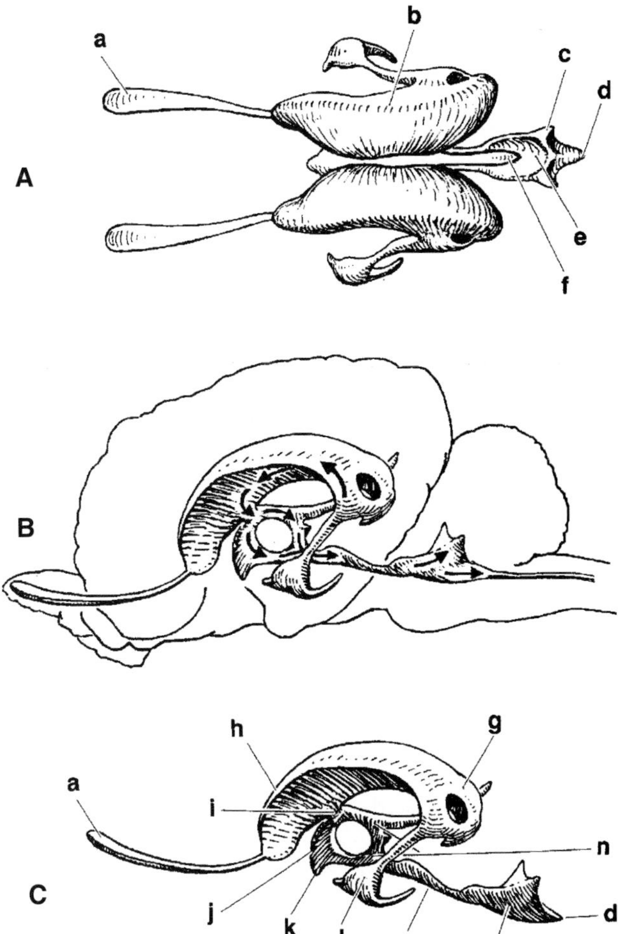

Figure 49-4. Ventricular system of the horse. **A,** Dorsal view. **B,** Lateral view showing direction of flow of cerebrospinal fluid. **C,** Lateral view. a, Cavity of olfactory bulb; b, lateral ventricle; c, lateral recess of the 4th ventricle; d, central canal; e, 4th ventricle; f, suprapineal recess, 3rd ventricle; g, body of the lateral ventricle; h, rostral horn of the lateral ventricle; i, interventricular foramen; j, optic recess; k, infundibular recess; l, caudal horn of the 4th ventricle; m, mesencephalic aqueduct.

The CSF plays an extremely important role in CNS homeostasis. Changes in CSF composition, as occur in subarachnoid hemorrhage[13] or bacterial meningitis, cause clinical changes out of proportion to the minor structural changes found in the underlying neuropil.

Cerebrospinal fluid is a modified transudate with lower potassium and calcium, and higher chloride, sodium, and magnesium concentrations than are found in plasma. Protein concentrations (60 mg/dL or greater) and cell counts (6 cells/μL or greater) are lower than in most other body cavities. In disease, changes in CSF composition are a useful diagnostic tool. CSF collection and analysis and myelography are described in Chapter 50.

The CNS is physically separated from circulating blood by an extensive blood–brain barrier and a relatively minor blood–CSF barrier.[14] The blood–brain barrier is formed by endothelial cells, support cells (such as astrocytes of the neuroglia and pericytes of the vascular system), and basal lamina. Endothelial cells of CNS capillaries are cemented together by continuous tight junctions. Foot processes of astrocytes (end feet) and long cytoplasmic processes of pericytes are closely adhered to the abluminal surfaces of CNS endothelial cells. These cells affect and support the barrier function of the endothelium. The basal lamina surrounds the endothelial cells and pericytes. A biochemical barrier against potentially injurious endogenous substances is provided by various endothelial enzymes including monoamine oxidases (e.g., epinephrine degradation) and aminopeptidases (e.g., enkephalins). Carrier and transport systems control traffic of some molecules across the blood–brain barrier. There is a Na/K-ATPase pump to regulate Na^+ and K^+, glucose transporters (including GLUT-1), amino acid transporters, and transcellular endocytosis systems for receptor-mediated transfer of insulin, immunoglobulin G, and transferrin into the CNS. Generally, diffusion of molecules across the blood–brain barrier depends on physicochemical properties such as lipid solubility, polarity, and molecular weight. There is a close association between lipid solubility of compounds and their ability to cross the blood–brain barrier. The free, non-protein-bound, nonionized form of most drugs can passively diffuse into the CNS.

In healthy animals, the blood–CNS barrier limits the passage of immunoglobulins, complement, and potentially injurious unconjugated bilirubin. Penicillin and aminoglycosides are excluded from the normal CNS; however, the blood–brain barrier reportedly allows passage of therapeutic amounts of sulfonamide-trimethoprim, chloramphenicol, enrofloxacin, and ceftriaxone into the CNS of horses.

PHYSIOLOGY OF NEUROTRANSMISSION

The transmission and processing of information in the nervous system depends on the presence and distribution of different ion channels in neurons, the localization of synaptic circuits, and the synaptic effects of neurotransmitters.[14]

The nervous system functions through propagation of electrical signals via changes in cell membrane potential. The resting membrane potential is determined by flow of K^+ through channels open at rest and by the activity of the Na/K-ATPase pump. In response to stimuli, neurons generate local potentials that can summate. When these potentials reach the threshold for opening voltage-gated Na^+ channels, an action potential is triggered. The opening of Na^+ or Ca^{2+} channels produces neuronal depolarization, whereas opening of K^+ and Cl^- channels decreases neuronal excitability.

Neurochemical pathways in the CNS can be divided into two main groups: relay systems and diffuse projection systems.[2] *Relay systems* include the long sensory and motor pathways that connect neurons of peripheral nerves to centers in the brain. Spinothalamic, visual, vestibulospinal, and reticulospinal pathways are examples of relay systems. *Diffuse projection systems* modulate brain function by distributing signals from individual nuclei to multiple other (usually higher) areas of the brain. They consist of cholinergic and monoaminergic neurons in nuclei of the brain stem and subcortical areas.

The excitatory neurotransmitter for relay systems is L-glutamate and, in some areas, aspartate. Local inhibitory circuits along these relay systems use gamma amino benzoic acid (GABA) or glycine. Numerous studies in experimental animals have implicated glutamatergic neurotransmission in toxicity associated with trauma, ischemia/reperfusion, and epilepsy. Experimental inhibitors of the glutamatergic system are being investigated as therapy for brain injury.[15] GABA is synthesized from glutamate by the action of glutamic acid decarboxylase (GAD). Impaired GABAergic transmission is involved in some forms of epilepsy, and autoantibodies against GAD are thought to be the cause of the spastic gait seen in horses with stiff-horse syndrome.[16]

Diffuse projection systems include cholinergic, dopaminergic, noradrenergic, serotonergic, and histaminergic neurons. These systems are targets for numerous drugs used for psychiatric and movement disorders in humans. Dysfunction of cholinergic neurotransmission is responsible for the signs of fluphenazine and metoclopramide reactions in horses.[17]

CLINICAL NEUROANATOMY

The remainder of this chapter is designed to group neurologic functions according to major areas of the CNS. It complements the information provided in Chapter 50.

Whole Brain

Level of Consciousness

One of the critical functions of the reticular formation of the brain stem is activation of the cerebral cortex for the awake state. This component of the formation, known as the ascending reticular activating system (ARAS), is an ill-defined meshwork of cells extending throughout the brain stem that receives afferent input from all parts of the CNS and projects excitatory stimuli cortically.

Lesions anywhere in the brain stem, whether they are focal or extensive, may reduce the level of consciousness, whereas cortical injury must be diffuse to cause noticeable obtundation. The ARAS is also involved in the initiation and maintenance of sleep. Abnormalities of production or action of hypothalamic arousal peptides (hypocretins/orexins)[18] or imbalances of brain stem neurotransmitters may result in narcolepsy/cataplexy sleep disorders.

Upper Motor Neuron System (Voluntary Movement)

The upper motor neuron (UMN) system is responsible for the initiation of voluntary movement and regulation of posture through support against gravity.[2] The latter is effected in part by modulation of the antigravity myotactic reflexes of the limbs. The component of the UMN system originating in the hypothalamus is responsible for the control of muscular activity associated with visceral functions (respiratory, cardiovascular, urinary).

Direct cortical influence over motor activity in the horse via the *pyramidal* system is largely limited to fine control of the muzzle and lips.[9] The much more important *extrapyramidal* system is a multisynaptic pathway from the brain to the lower motor neurons of the spinal cord and brain stem. The frontal and parietal lobes of the cerebrum, basal nuclei, diencephalon, midbrain, and hindbrain all contribute to the UMN system. Upper motor neurons, particularly those originating in the midbrain, are generally inhibitory to myotactic reflexes. Damage to the neurons or axons of these tracts, in the caudal midbrain, hindbrain, or spinal cord, increases extensor tonus and may result in limb spasticity ("stiffness"). With UMN injury there are also limb weakness, hyperactive extensor reflexes, and crossed extensor reflexes, all in the ipsilateral limbs.

Movement disorders are characteristic of UMN disease in the rostral brain stem. Abnormal involuntary movements include dystonia (writhing movements of the muscles of the head and spine), ballism (violent flailing of a limb), chorea (repetitive jerky movements of different muscle groups), and myoclonus (repetitive movements of a single muscle group).[14] Nigropallidal encephalomalacia is a disease of this type in horses that is caused by the chronic consumption of yellowstar thistle or Russian knapweed plants.[19] There is dystonia and rigidity of the muscles of the head resulting in lip retraction, tongue protrusion, and inability to prehend food. More generalized extrapyramidal syndromes in horses are reportedly associated with reactions to fluphenazine (an antipsychotic sedative drug) and metoclopramide (a prokinetic agent).

Forebrain

Behavior (Limbic System, Temporal Lobes)

Normal behavior requires integration of signals from the entire CNS, but it principally involves the forebrain. Most important in controlling intrinsic behavior is the limbic system, a connected series of structures in the cerebrum and diencephalon. A minor component is also found in the midbrain. Included are the amygdala, hippocampus, fornix, cingulate gyrus, and septal area. A closely associated region that is important in primate behavior is the temporal lobe of the cerebrum.[2] It is thought that behavior based on conditioning and experience (i.e., learning) is controlled by the temporal lobes. Structural, metabolic, or psychological disturbances affecting these areas may result in behavioral abnormalities (i.e., dementia). Dementia can be defined as changes in normal habits, personality, attitude, or reaction to the environment, or loss of learned skills. Some of the signs that may be seen include disorientation in a familiar environment, failure to recognize a handler or object, loss of the ability to be led, frequent yawning, head-pressing, irritability, unprovoked kicking or biting, compulsive walking or circling, and dramatic changes in eating or drinking habits.

Almost any disturbance of the forebrain can potentially cause dementia. Encephalitis, head trauma, space-occupying lesion, malformation, infarct, and metabolic disorders all are likely to cause changes in behavior. Important examples in horses include rabies, eastern equine encephalomyelitis (EEE), leukoencephalomalacia, neonatal encephalopathy (neonatal maladjustment syndrome), cerebral abscess, cholesterol granuloma, frontal/parietal trauma, postseizure encephalopathy, hepatic encephalopathy, hyperammonemia, and hydrocephalus. It is likely that structural or metabolic forebrain disease is the cause of dementia if other neurologic abnormalities are found by neurologic examination or imaging studies. In the absence of such supportive findings, abnormal behavior such as self-mutilation[20] may have a psychological basis.

Seizures

Seizures are sudden, transient attacks of abnormal motor or behavioral activity attributable to paroxysmal depolarization of part or all of the brain.[9] Depolarization occurs either simultaneously throughout the brain or originates from a hyperirritable focus somewhere in the forebrain. Seizures originating from a focus are likely to initially have asymmetric clinical signs, and there may be additional signs of forebrain disease between seizures that are revealed by neurologic examination.

Seizures frequently originate in the frontal (motor) cortex and involve muscle fasciculations and tremors around the head or abnormal movements of the jaws and tongue ("chewing gum fits"). Convulsions characteristic of neonatal encephalopathy often are of this type. In their severest (grand mal) form, seizures manifest as sudden recumbency, with a brief phase of extensor tonus, followed by clonic ("galloping") movements of the legs, loss of consciousness, and a variety of signs of autonomic discharge (e.g., sweating, urination, defecation, pupillary dilation). Mild motor seizures are often accompanied by behavioral signs such as obtundation, compulsive walking, hyperresponsiveness to stimuli, or other signs of dementia. Seizure foci in the forebrain may occur at sites of previous or current trauma or inflammation. Examples include skull trauma, equine protozoal myeloencephalitis (EPM), EEE, intracranial neoplasia, and aberrant parasite migration (see Table 49-3 for a more complete list). Causes external to the brain include hyperammonemia, hyponatremia, hyperthermia, and hepatic or renal failure. Juvenile epilepsy of Arabian foals occurs because of transiently increased susceptibility to seizures and manifests as repeated generalized seizures without other evidence of brain disease in foals 1 to 9 months old.[9]

Perception of Pain (Parietal Cortex, Cranial Nerve V)

Pain sensation is transmitted from the body to the brain in multisynaptic spinothalamic tracts.[2] Signals initiated by stimulation of pain receptors on one side of the body pass through spinothalamic tracts on both sides of the spinal cord. Axons in these tracts course rostrally to terminate in the thalamus. From there, cell bodies project axons to the sensory (somesthetic) cortex for conscious perception of pain or other sensory modalities. It is thought that the somesthetic cortex is located principally in the parietal lobe of the cerebrum.

The pathways for pain perception in the head pass through the maxillary, ophthalmic, and mandibular branches of the trigeminal nerve. The central component of this pathway is predominantly contralateral. Unilateral lesions of the sensory parts of the forebrain (thalamus, internal capsule, sensory cortex) thus cause contralateral facial hypalgesia. Because the central components of vision and facial pain perception are close anatomically, it is common to find unilateral facial hypalgesia and blindness (on the same side) in the same horse.

TABLE 49-3. Causes of Seizures in Horses

Classification	Possible Causes
Developmental/genetic	Hydrocephalus Hydranencephaly Portosystemic shunt Juvenile epilepsy of Arabians
Idiopathic	Unknown
Hypoxic/ischemic	Neonatal encephalopathy Intracarotid injection Air embolism Cribbing strap Thromboembolism Hypoxemia of any cause Arrhythmia
Inflammatory	Viral: EEE, WEE, VEE, West Nile, rabies, EHV-1, EIA Bacterial: meningitis, cerebral abscess Protozoal: *Sarcocystis neurona,** *Neospora hughesi** Parasitic: any, especially *Halicephalobus gingivalis*
Metabolic	Electrolytes: low Na, Ca; high Na; high/low pH Kernicterus Hypoglycemia Liver failure Renal failure
Neoplastic	Metastatic Primary
Toxic	Heavy metal: As, Pb, Hg Organophosphate Isopropyl alcohol Hyperammonemia (not liver) Fungal: fumonisins,† tremorgens‡ Bacterial: tunicamycin-like§
Traumatic	Acute brain injury Previous brain injury
Other	Cholesterol granuloma

* Cause of EPM.
† Cause of leukoencephalomalacia.
‡ Cause of perennial ryegrass, dallis grass, and Bermuda grass staggers.
§ Cause of annual ryegrass and blown grass staggers.
EEE, eastern equine encephalomyelitis; EHV-1, equine herpesvirus-1; EIA, equine infectious anemia; VEE, Venezuelan equine encephalomyelitis; WEE, western equine encephalomyelitis.

Diseases associated with abnormalities of facial pain perception are the same as those described later for disorders of vision perception.

Smell (Olfactory Bulbs, Cranial Nerve I)

Olfactory nerves pass through the cribriform plate and into the olfactory bulbs of the cerebrum. Information on smell is relayed through the thalamus to centers in the unconscious (limbic system) and conscious cerebrum.

Vision (Thalamus, Occipital Cortex, Cranial Nerve II)

In horses, 80% to 90% of optic nerve fibers from one eye cross at the optic chiasm, and 80% of fibers in the optic tracts synapse at the lateral geniculate nucleus in the thalamus.[2] The remainder course to the midbrain to function in the pupillary light reflex (see later). Neurons in the lateral geniculate nucleus project via the internal capsule to the visual cortex in the occipital lobe of the cerebrum. This area is caudal in the cerebrum, immediately rostral to the tentorium cerebelli, and caudal to the parietal cortex. The pathway from the eye to the contralateral visual cortex via the optic nerve, lateral geniculate nucleus, and internal capsule must be intact for normal vision. Lesions in the pathway caudal to the optic chiasm result in blindness in the opposite eye, and lesions in the optic nerve rostral to the chiasm affect vision in the ipsilateral eye. Damage to the cortex should not affect the pupillary reflex pathway.

Visual perception is evaluated by obstacle tests (with and without blindfolding of one eye) and by the menace response. The menace response requires the central visual pathway just described plus normal facial nerve function. Integrity of the cerebellar cortex is also needed, although it is not known if the pathway that mediates this response actually passes through the cerebellum. *It is important to note that the menace response does not develop in foals until they are 1 to 2 weeks old.*

Any disease that causes diffuse, severe cerebral dysfunction is likely to cause blindness. Examples include EEE, postseizure encephalopathy, hyperammonemia, leukoencephalomalacia, and frontal/parietal trauma. Asymmetric frontal/parietal skull trauma, EPM, cerebral abscess, and cholesterol granuloma are diseases that may cause unilateral visual deficits by affecting the forebrain on the opposite side. Arabian foals with cerebellar abiotrophy have normal vision, but menace responses are absent.[21]

Midbrain

Pupillary Light Response, Pupil Size (Midbrain, Cranial Nerves II, III)

In the normal horse, pupil size reflects the balance of sympathetic (dilator) and parasympathetic (constrictor) influences on the smooth muscle of the iris. Preganglionic neurons for sympathetic supply to the head arise in the gray matter of the first four thoracic segments of the spinal cord, and they then course rostrally in the cervical sympathetic trunk. After synapse in the cranial cervical ganglion adjacent to the guttural pouch, the postganglionic sympathetic neurons continue to the smooth muscle of the orbit and act to cause pupillary dilation. Emotional and other influences on sympathetic pupillary tone are governed by hypothalamic centers that act through UMN tracts descending from the midbrain.

Interruption of preganglionic or postganglionic sympathetic nerves to the eye causes Horner's syndrome, with miosis of the pupil, enophthalmos, ptosis, and spontaneous sweating and vasodilatation over the side of the face. Injury to the sympathetic UMN tracts in the brain or spinal cord not only may cause Horner's syndrome but also may result in increased sweating over the entire side of the body. Preganglionic neurons may be injured in the proximal thorax or along the neck in the vagosympathetic trunk. The cranial cervical ganglion and postganglionic neurons may be destroyed by fungal invasion in horses with guttural pouch mycosis.[22] Rarely, signs referable to interruption of sympathetic UMN tracts are found in horses with brain stem or spinal cord lesions (e.g., EPM, spinal cord trauma).

Parasympathetic preganglionic neurons arise in the midbrain and exit the skull in the oculomotor nerve (III). These neurons synapse behind the eye in the ciliary ganglion. Postganglionic neurons pass along the optic nerve to innervate the ciliary muscle and constrictor of the pupil. This system is responsive to the amount of light received by each eye. The afferent part of the pupillary light reflex passes via the optic nerves and optic tracts, past the thalamus, to terminate in the midbrain. There is extensive decussation of these tracts in both the chiasm and the midbrain, so light directed into one eye causes reflex pupillary constriction in both eyes.

Injury to an optic nerve renders the ipsilateral pupil unresponsive to direct light, but it remains responsive to light directed into the contralateral eye. In contrast, injury to the midbrain or oculomotor nerve causes mydriasis in the ipsilateral eye that is unresponsive to light directed into either eye. Focal diseases such as EPM, aberrant parasite migration, or midbrain hemorrhage could potentially involve the oculomotor nuclei, although this is rare. More commonly, the oculomotor nerves are compressed by swelling and subtentorial herniation of the cerebral hemispheres. Early in the process of cerebral injury, pupils are often miotic; progression to bilateral mydriasis is a grave prognostic sign.[2]

Midbrain/Hindbrain

Eye Position (Midbrain, Pons, Cranial Nerves III, IV, VI)

From nuclei in the midbrain and pons, the oculomotor, trochlear, and abducens nerves exit the cranial cavity through the orbital fissure and ramify in the periorbital tissues to innervate the rectus and oblique muscles of the eye. The oculomotor nerve also supplies the levator palpebrae and pupillary constrictor muscles, and the abducens nerve innervates the retractor bulbi muscle. Lesions in these nerves (or nuclei) cause abnormal eye position (strabismus). The direction of eye deviations resulting from specific nerve lesions is not known for the horse and cannot necessarily be inferred from data for other species.[9] Unlike vestibular strabismus, which can be corrected by rotating the head (usually in the direction of the lesion), strabismus caused by lesions in extraocular nerves persist in any head position. The finding of mydriasis (III) or defective eyeball retraction (VI) may provide additional information on lesion location in horses with strabismus.

Hindbrain

Mastication (Pons, Cranial Nerve V)

The lower motor neurons of the trigeminal nerve arise in the pons and pass through the petrous temporal bone and the foramen ovale adjacent to sensory trigeminal neurons and are distributed to the muscles of mastication: masseters, pterygoids, temporals, and rostral digastricus.

With unilateral damage to the trigeminal nucleus (or nerve), there is deviation of the lower jaw toward the normal side. By 2 weeks after injury, there is obvious muscular atrophy. Bilateral severe involvement of the trigeminal nuclei (or nerves) causes a dropped jaw, weak jaw tone, slight tongue protrusion, and inability to prehend or chew feed. Damage to the nucleus of V, either unilaterally or bilaterally, is found in some horses with EPM.[23]

Facial Expression and Movement (Medulla, Cranial Nerve VII)

Normal facial tone, expression, and movements are dependent on the integrity of the facial nerves. These nerves arise from nuclei in the rostral medulla (hindbrain) and exit the calvarium with cranial nerve VIII via the internal acoustic meatus. The nerve courses through the facial canal in the petrous temporal bone adjacent to the middle ear and emerges through the stylomastoid foramen. The facial nerve is distributed to the muscles of facial expression, including those of the ear, eyelid, nose, and lips, and the caudal belly of the digastric muscle.

The effects of interruption of this motor pathway depend on the site of damage. With involvement of the nucleus or proximal nerve, there is drooping of the ear and lip, ptosis, and collapse of the nostril, and the muzzle is pulled toward the normal side. Saliva often drools from the affected side of the mouth, and the horse has difficulty prehending food, especially grain. There may be exposure keratitis secondary to eyelid paralysis.

The facial nerve also contributes parasympathetic neurons to lacrimal glands (and some salivary glands). Damage to the facial nerve proximal to the middle ear is likely to affect tear production by this mechanism. Tear production can be measured and compared between sides using the Schirmer tear test. The sensory component of the facial nerve contains fibers from the tongue (taste) and middle ear.

Facial nerve motor function is evaluated by testing "flick" reflexes of the lip, eyelid and ear. These reflexes involve afferent sensory input via trigeminal neurons that terminate in the medulla on the lower motor neurons (LMNs) of the facial nerves. Note that these reflexes do not involve the forebrain and can thus occur without conscious perception. Because they are close together in the hindbrain and skull, the facial and vestibulocochlear nerves are often damaged together. Diseases that often affect both nerves include those that are central (West Nile virus encephalomyelitis, EEE, EPM, and migrating parasite) and those that are peripheral (polyneuritis equi, lightning strike, petrous temporal bone fracture, temporohyoid osteoarthropathy, and extramedullary neoplasm). To distinguish clinically between central and peripheral causes, it is important to look for other signs of brain disease. For example, a horse with a lesion in the medulla affecting the nuclei of cranial nerves VII and VIII may also be obtunded with weakness and ataxia of the ipsilateral limbs.

Balance and Equilibrium, Hearing (Medulla, Cranial Nerve VIII)

The vestibular system is responsible for orientation of the horse relative to gravity (Fig. 49-5). The receptor is in the bony labyrinth of the inner ear. The membranous labyrinth includes three semicircular ducts containing endolymph

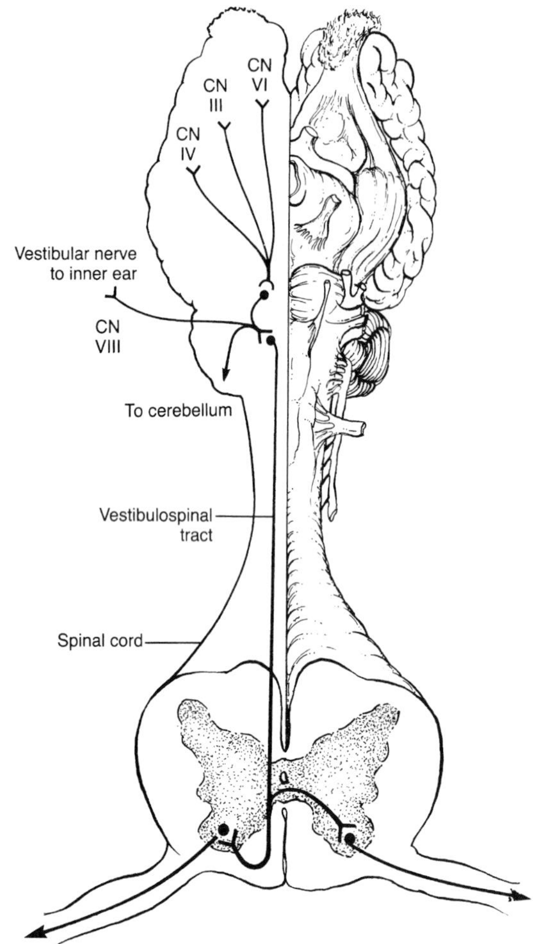

Figure 49-5. The vestibular system showing afferent input from the inner ear via cranial nerve VIII to the vestibular nuclei in the hindbrain. There is complex integrated output to the cranial nerves controlling extraocular muscles (III, IV, and VI), the cerebellum, and the trunk and limbs (vestibulospinal tracts).

that connect to vestibular nerve endings at the cristae ampullares. Vestibular neurons pass centrally through the internal acoustic meatus to penetrate the rostral medulla and terminate in four vestibular nuclei. These nuclei have numerous projections to the nuclei controlling extraocular muscles, the cerebellum, and the spinal cord.

The vestibular system controls the conjugate movements of the eyes during movement of the head through extensive connections with the nuclei of cranial nerves III, IV, and VI. Vestibular-cerebellar pathways pass through the caudal cerebellar peduncle. These pathways function to smoothly coordinate the movements of the eyeballs, trunk, and limbs with those of the head. Vestibulospinal tracts descend ipsilaterally to synapse on the LMNs and facilitate extensor muscles of the limbs while inhibiting flexor muscles. Some vestibulospinal tracts cross and reduce extensor tonus in contralateral limbs.

Unilateral disease involving the peripheral part of the vestibular system causes asymmetric ataxia *with preservation of strength*. The poll rotates toward the side of the lesion, and the head and neck may be turned toward the lesion. The body leans, falls, or rolls toward the side of the lesion, and the horse may stagger in tight circles. This type of circling should be distinguished from the compulsive walking in circles (without head tilt) that is characteristic of horses with asymmetric frontal cerebral lobe lesions. Because there is some visual compensation for vestibular ataxia, blindfolding exacerbates the signs and is a useful clinical test in mild cases of suspected vestibular disease.

In horses with central vestibular disease, there are usually additional signs of hindbrain disease (e.g., depression and *limb weakness*), and head tilt may be either toward or away from the side of the lesion. The latter presentation is known as paradoxical central vestibular disease and usually follows involvement of vestibular connections within the cerebellum. Unilateral vestibular disease often causes spontaneous or positional nystagmus, and physiologic (vestibular) nystagmus may be absent or abnormal. In peripheral disease, the nystagmus is always horizontal, rotatory, or arc shaped, with the fast phase away from the lesion. With central involvement of the vestibular system, nystagmus also may be vertical. Typically, the eye on the affected side rotates ventrally in the orbit while the eye on the normal side rotates dorsally (especially when the head is extended). This abnormal eye position is termed vestibular strabismus. Bilateral vestibular disease is characterized by severe symmetric ataxia and wide, sweeping movements of the head from side to side. In addition to the diseases described earlier that also affect the facial nerve, an idiopathic vestibular syndrome is reported to occur in the horse, possibly as a result of viral neuritis or labyrinthitis.[9]

Neurons of the cochlear division of cranial nerve VIII pass from receptors in the middle or inner ear to auditory centers in the midbrain and thalamus. A variety of local reflexes are initiated by stimulation of the cochlear nerve. In addition, there is projection of conscious pathways for hearing from the thalamus to the cortex (temporal lobe?). Deafness is rarely detected in the horse.

Taste (Cranial Nerves VII, IX, X)

Taste buds are found on the surface of the tongue and also in the soft palate, pharynx, lips, and cheeks. Sensory gustatory innervation is provided by the facial nerve (rostral two thirds of the tongue), glossopharyngeal nerve (caudal one third of the tongue), and vagus (pharynx and palate). General sensory innervation provided by the trigeminal nerve probably also contributes gustatory information. Perception of taste involves the forebrain, including the limbic system. Deficiencies in the sense of taste are very difficult to detect by clinical testing.

Movement of Pharynx and Larynx (Cranial Nerves IX, X, XI)

Motor innervation of the larynx and pharynx originates in neurons in the nucleus ambiguus, a fusiform structure extending the length of the medulla. This nucleus provides axons for the glossopharyngeal, vagus, and spinal accessory (internal branch) nerve roots. These roots form nerves that innervate the soft palate, pharynx, larynx, and cranial esophagus via the pharyngeal plexus and cranial and recurrent laryngeal nerves. The nucleus ambiguus is continued in the spinal cord as the nucleus of the external branch of the spinal accessory nerve (innervation of trapezius and parts of brachiocephalicus and sternocephalicus). The facial and hypoglossal nerves innervate several of the muscles that control movements of the hyoid apparatus; therefore, impaired movement of the hyoid apparatus caused by paralysis of these nerves could affect movements of the larynx and pharynx. Clinically, such effects are minor in horses at rest but can be revealed by intense exercise.

Unilateral (hemiplegia) or bilateral pharyngeal paralysis interferes with swallowing and manifests as signs of dysphagia: coughing and gagging during eating with return of saliva, feed, and water through the nostrils and mouth. With complete unilateral laryngeal hemiplegia (i.e., paralysis of adductors and abductors), there is exercise-induced respiratory stridor and aspiration of feed into the trachea. In horses with bilateral laryngeal paralysis, inspiratory stridor occurs at rest and there is aspiration pneumonia. Some to all of these pathways can be affected peripherally in horses with botulism, guttural pouch mycosis, extramedullary neoplasia, or basilar skull fracture. Examples of diseases affecting the hindbrain that may cause laryngeal or pharyngeal dysfunction are EEE, EPM, leukoencephalomalacia, bacterial meningitis, and West Nile viral encephalomyelitis.

Tongue Movement (Cranial Nerve XII)

The muscles affecting movement of the tongue are supplied by the hypoglossal nerve. Neurons of the hypoglossal nerve originate in the hypoglossal nucleus in the caudal aspect of the medulla and emerge from the medulla as a horizontal row of rootlets, which combine to form the nerve as it enters the hypoglossal foramen. After emerging from this foramen, the hypoglossal nerve runs forward and ventrally in association with the guttural pouch and the stylohyoid bone to innervate the geniohyoideus and muscles of the tongue.

Interruption of the hypoglossal pathways causes hemiparesis of the tongue, evident as deviation of the apex of the tongue toward the affected side. Within 2 to 4 weeks, atrophy of the tongue becomes noticeable. The peripheral nerve may be damaged by extramedullary neoplasia, upper cervical or caudal skull trauma, or guttural pouch mycosis. Tongue hemiplegia and atrophy has been seen in horses with EPM, although any cause of caudal hindbrain disease can damage the hypoglossal nuclei.

Cerebellum

The cerebellum sits in the caudal fossa of the skull and is separated from the cerebral hemispheres by the tentorium cerebelli. It is divided into the flocculonodular lobe, also known as the vestibular cerebellum, and the much larger body of the cerebellum. The cerebellar body consists of a median region, the vermis, and two lateral cerebellar hemispheres. Connections with the rest of the CNS are via three peduncles: efferent connections pass through the rostral peduncle and afferent pathways enter the cerebellum via the middle and caudal peduncles.

The cerebellum regulates and smoothes motor activity initiated by the UMN system. It also acts to maintain equilibrium and appropriate body posture during rest and motion. Proprioceptive information is gathered via afferent connections from the spinal cord (spinocerebellar tracts) and vestibular system and senses UMN activity via extensive connections with brain stem UMN nuclei (including the olivary nucleus). Efferent cerebellar neurons project to vestibular nuclei and other parts of the brain stem including the thalamus. There is virtually no projection of cerebellar efferents into the spinal cord.

Cerebellar disease is usually diffuse and manifests as symmetric ataxia without weakness. There is defective regulation of the rate, range, and force of movement. Limbs may appear spastic with excessive (hypermetric) or inadequate (hypometric) flexion during protraction. Signs are most obvious when there is a change in the force or direction of voluntary movement. At rest, the body may sway, laterally or backward and forward, and there may be coarse head bobbing or tremor that is exacerbated by voluntary movement, such as reaching the head out for food. Extensor muscle tone is increased and limb reflexes may be hyperactive. With diffuse cerebellar cortical disease, the menace response is absent, although vision is normal (see p. 636).

Signs of diffuse cerebellar disease are seen in Arabian horses[24] or Götland pony foals with cerebellar abiotrophy. This inherited disease manifests at any time from birth to 3 months of age and may be stable or progressive for weeks to months. Rarely, horses with poll trauma have a head bob indicating cerebellar injury. The rhabditid nematode *Halicephalobus gingivalis* has a propensity to invade the caudal fossa and cause cerebellar destruction.[25] Tremorgenic mycotoxins produced by parasitized perennial ryegrass or *Paspalum* species cause signs suggestive of cerebellar dysfunction, although other parts of the CNS are also affected.

Spinal Cord

Upper Motor Neuron (Muscle Tone and Voluntary Movement)

Axons of the UMN extrapyramidal and vestibular systems travel from cell bodies throughout the brain and pass predominantly in reticulospinal and vestibulospinal tracts to LMN in the ventral and intermediate columns of the gray matter of the spinal cord. As described previously (see "Upper Motor Neuron System" under "Whole Brain"), this system provides tonic support for the body against gravity and recruits spinal reflexes for the initiation of voluntary movement. UMNs act by influencing α and γ motor neurons in the spinal cord. These LMNs, in combination with afferent nerves and stretch receptors in the neuromuscular spindles and tendons, control muscle tone and movement by myotactic and antimyotactic reflexes. Most descending UMN tracts are inhibitory to extensor motor neurons. Removal of these influences by transection through the midbrain causes extension of head, neck, trunk, and limbs, signs that are characteristic of decerebrate rigidity.[2] Basic locomotor activity involves recruitment and control of these reflexes by distinct postural and voluntary UMN systems.

Interruption of UMN tracts in the spinal cord causes signs of ipsilateral weakness of the trunk and limbs. Signs of paresis range in severity from slight toe-dragging and delayed protraction, to recumbency and inability to rise. Because myotactic reflexes are released from inhibitory UMN influences, there may also be spasticity (stiffness) of limb movement. This is most obvious in the thoracic limbs, which may appear to float during walking. The stiff appearance reflects decreased flexion of the limb during the protraction phase of the stride. Interference with UMN may also manifest as delayed initiation of voluntary movement or alterations in gait cadence. For example, some horses with spinal cord disease may have a lateral "pacing" gait at walking speed. If LMNs are not affected, spinal reflexes (e.g., patellar) are either normal or exaggerated on the side of the spinal cord lesion, and crossed extensor reflexes may be seen. *It should be noted that crossed extensor reflexes are normal in newborn foals.*[9]

Spastic paresis is especially common with focal compression of the cervical spinal cord in horses with cervical stenotic myelopathy (CSM) or spinal cord trauma. Other significant causes of UMN disease (in the spinal cord) include EPM, equine degenerative myeloencephalopathy, spinal cord abscess or tumor, and aberrant parasite migration. In keeping with the basic principles of neuroanatomic localization, UMN lesions from C1 to T2 (inclusive) may cause neurologic signs in all four limbs, lesions from T3 to S2 can only affect the pelvic limbs, and lesions caudal to S2 do not directly affect gait. With external compression of the cervical spinal cord (as in CSM), signs are typically worse in the pelvic limbs than in the thoracic limbs. The principles of neuroanatomic localization of spinal cord lesions are discussed more fully in Chapter 50.

Lower Motor Neuron and Spinal Cord Reflexes

The function of the CNS is exerted entirely through the actions of LMN on striated (skeletal) and smooth muscle. Lower motor neurons to skeletal muscles are found in the ventral columns of the gray matter, whereas those of the autonomic nervous system are located in the intermediate columns. In the horse, there are 8 cervical, 18 thoracic, 6 lumbar, 5 sacral, and a variable number of coccygeal (caudal) spinal cord segments. LMNs originating in the gray matter of a segment form a ventral root, which then exits the vertebral canal through the intervertebral foramen of the vertebra of the same name. The ventral root joins with the dorsal sensory root to form the segmental spinal nerve. In the cervical vertebrae, this foramen is at the cranial end of each vertebra. For the remaining roots, the foramina are at the caudal end. The more caudal spinal cord segments have long nerve roots because the spinal cord segments are shifted cranially with respect to the vertebrae. The first three sacral segments are in the 6th lumbar vertebra, and the spinal cord ends within S2.[2]

The LMNs form the efferent part of spinal reflexes, which are central to the neurologic examination and the process of neuroanatomic localization. The neurons of the afferent (sensory) component of reflexes course from receptors in the skin, muscle, or tendon, through the spinal nerve and dorsal root, into the dorsal horn of the gray matter, where they terminate on interneurons. The interneurons then complete the pathway by passing to the LMN. An exception to this is the patellar reflex, wherein the sensory neuron terminates directly on the LMN in the ventral horn. Long (i.e., multisegment) spinal cord reflexes, including "slap" tests, cervicofacial and cutaneous trunci reflexes, and caudal reflexes, including anal and tail-clamp, are routinely evaluated during neurologic examination. Limb reflexes, including withdrawal, patella, and triceps, are always evaluated in neonatal foals and in older horses that are recumbent. The specifics of individual spinal cord reflexes are covered in Chapter 50.

Abnormalities of LMN (in gray matter, ventral root, peripheral nerve, or neuromuscular junction) manifest as flaccid muscle weakness (paresis, paralysis) with hypotonia and hyporeflexia. Within 1 to 2 weeks, muscle atrophy is noticeable, and this neurogenic muscle atrophy progresses rapidly.[9] Note that neurogenic atrophy is a consequence only of LMN disease; UMN involvement results in weakness without atrophy. Ventral nerve roots contribute to multiple peripheral nerves, and peripheral nerves are derived from multiple roots, so injury to gray matter of an individual segment or to a ventral nerve root produces less severe neurologic signs than does loss of function in a peripheral nerve.[2] Examples of conditions that affect the LMN in horses are botulism (neuromuscular junction), trauma, ischemia associated with recumbency, neuritis of the cauda equina/polyneuritis equi, EPM, postanesthetic myelomalacia, and equine motor neuron disease.

Proprioception

Through a system of receptors in muscles, tendons, and joints, the general proprioceptive system is able to monitor the position of the body or limbs in space. Proprioceptive information is passed centrally in sensory nerves that terminate in the dorsal gray column on cell bodies of neurons in the spinocerebellar tracts. These tracts pass cranially and provide information for the cerebellum to use in its role of regulating posture, muscle tone, locomotion, and equilibrium. Other proprioceptive pathways pass from the spinal cord to the somesthetic sensory cortex via relay nuclei in the midbrain and thalamus.

Interruption of spinal cord proprioceptive pathways interferes with recognition by the brain of the positions in space of the body and limbs. This is manifest as ataxia (incoordination). Signs of proprioceptive deficit in the horse include base-wide or base-narrow limb placement, swaying of the trunk and torso during walking (but not usually at rest), and overstriding, especially in the pelvic limbs. During circling, limb ataxia is evident as circumduction in the pelvic limbs and interference in the thoracic limbs.

Urination

Parasympathetic LMNs to the bladder's smooth muscle (detrusor) originate in the intermediate column of the gray matter of sacral segments 2 to 4. These neurons exit in ventral roots and contribute to the pelvic plexus, a network that supplies autonomic innervation to the smooth muscle of the bladder and rectum. Sympathetic LMNs to the bladder begin in the gray matter of L1-4, exit the vertebral canal, and course to the pelvic plexus. Postganglionic sympathetic neurons terminate on smooth muscle in the body and neck of the bladder and proximal urethra. These autonomic LMNs function in local reflexes. Afferent neurons pass from stretch receptors in the bladder wall and enter the spinal cord in dorsal sacral nerve roots to exert inhibitory influences on parasympathetic and sympathetic LMNs. Striated muscle of the urethra is innervated by somatic LMNs in the pudendal nerve. Urination occurs when there is stimulation of parasympathetic nerves to the detrusor muscle, inhibition of sympathetic nerves to the detrusor muscle, and inhibition of sympathetic and somatic nerves to the urethra. The net effect of this activity is contraction of the smooth muscle of the body of the bladder and relaxation of the proximal urethra. Centers in the midbrain and hindbrain receive sensory information from the bladder and modulate reflex activity via UMNs passing caudally in the spinal cord. Forebrain influence on these centers is responsible for initiation of voluntary voiding.

In horses with severe spinal cord disease cranial to S2, there may be loss of voluntary control of urination. Within 2 weeks, "spinal reflex bladder" function develops, which results in intermittent voiding with retention of small amounts of urine. Horses with severe CSM, EPM, vertebral trauma, or epidural abscess may be presented in this way. When there is a spinal cord lesion between L4 and S2, reflex pathways for inhibition of sympathetic activity may be interrupted, resulting in increased urethral tone and functional obstruction of urinary outflow. This is the case in some horses with equine herpesvirus-1 (EHV-1) myeloencephalopathy, although others have signs of LMN bladder (see later).[26]

With injury to the sacral spinal cord segments or nerves, the bladder and urethra are atonic and distended and there is overflow incontinence. Although a small amount of intrinsic reflex bladder contraction ("automatic bladder") may occur, it is ineffectual, and large volumes of urine and sediment remain. Trauma, epidural abscess or tumor, EHV-1 myeloencephalopathy, sorghum–Sudan grass toxicity, and neuritis of the cauda equina are diseases that can cause these signs. Idiopathic atonic bladder (also known as sabulous cystitis) is found in middle-aged geldings and some stallions and resembles the presentation of horses with cauda equina syndrome; however, the idiopathic syndrome does not appear to be caused by denervation of bladder muscle, and there are no other signs of cauda equina syndrome. In cases of LMN urinary incontinence, additional nonurinary signs of sacral nerve injury are expected. These are the signs of cauda equina syndrome and include fecal incontinence, paralysis of the anus, tail, and penis, and perineal analgesia.

Defecation

The smooth muscle of the rectum and anus is innervated by postganglionic parasympathetic neurons in a way that parallels that described for the bladder. Innervation of striated muscle of the anus is provided by the pudendal nerve. Spinal cord lesions cranial to S2 are unlikely to affect defecation; however, involvement of the sacral segments results in rectal obstipation and may cause colic. Diseases causing rectal paralysis are the same as those described under "Urination," earlier.

Sensation

Sensory information from pain, thermal, and touch receptors is conveyed to the spinal cord by peripheral nerves, spinal nerves, and dorsal roots. Branches pass several segments both cranially and caudally from the site of spinal cord penetration and terminate on spinothalamic neurons or interneurons involved in spinal reflexes. Spinothalamic pathways servicing a single dorsal nerve root course cranially on both sides of the spinal cord. Pain perception requires interpretation of afferent information by the forebrain and has already been described. The flexor (withdrawal) reflexes require only sensory nerves, contiguous spinal cord segments, and LMNs. In the thoracic limbs, spinal cord segments C6 to T2 are required, and L6 to S2 are involved in the pelvic limb reflex. Evaluation of sensation over the trunk and limbs requires knowledge of the common autonomous zones for sensory nerves. This will be described in more detail in Chapter 54.

REFERENCES

1. Sisken BF, Zwick M, Hyde JF, et al: Maturation of the central nervous system: Comparison of equine and other species, Equine Vet J Suppl 1993;14:31.
2. De Lahunta A: Veterinary Neuroanatomy and Clinical Neurology, ed 2, Philadelphia, 1983, WB Saunders.
3. Dyce KM, Sack WO, Wensing CJG: Textbook of Veterinary Anatomy, London, 2002, Elsevier.
4. Sisson S, Grossman JD, Getty R: Sisson and Grossman's The Anatomy of the Domestic Animals, Philadelphia, 1975, WB Saunders.
5. MacKay RJ: Brain injury after head trauma: Pathophysiology, diagnosis, and treatment, Vet Clin North Am Equine Pract 2004;20:199.
6. Martin L, Kaswan R, Chapman W: Four cases of traumatic optic nerve blindness in the horse, Equine Vet J 1986;18:133.
7. Stick JA, Wilson T, Kunze D: Basilar skull fractures in three horses, J Am Vet Med Assoc 1980;176:228.
8. Blythe LL, Watrous BJ, Schmitz JA, et al: Vestibular syndrome associated with temporohyoid joint fusion and temporal bone fracture in three horses, J Am Vet Med Assoc 1984;185:775.
9. Mayhew IG: Large Animal Neurology: A Handbook for Veterinary Clinicians, Philadelphia, 1989, WB Saunders.
10. Proctor MR: Spinal cord injury, Crit Care Med 2002;30(Suppl):S489.
11. Mayhew IG, De Lahunta A, Whitlock RH, et al: Spinal cord disease in the horse, Cornell Vet 1978;68(Suppl 6):1.
12. Reed SM: Medical and surgical emergencies of the nervous system of horses: Diagnosis, treatment, and sequelae, Vet Clin North Am Equine Pract 1994;10:703.
13. Qureshi AI, Tuhrim S, Broderick JP, et al: Medical progress: Spontaneous intracerebral hemorrhage, N Engl J Med 2001;344:1450.
14. Goetz CG: Textbook of Clinical Neurology, ed 2, London, 2003, Elsevier.
15. Royo NC, Shimizu S, Schouten JW, et al: Pharmacology of traumatic brain injury, Curr Opin Pharmacol 2003;3:27.
16. Nollet H, Vanderstraeten G, Sustronck B, et al: Suspected case of stiff-horse syndrome, Vet Rec 2000;146:282.
17. Brewer BD, Hines MT, Stewart JT, et al: Fluphenazine-induced Parkinson-like syndrome in a horse, Equine Vet J 1990;22:136.
18. Scammell TE: The neurobiology, diagnosis, and treatment of narcolepsy, Ann Neurol 2003;53:154.
19. Young S, Brown WW, Klinger B: Nigropallidal encephalomalacia in horses caused by ingestion of weeds of the genus *Centaurea,* J Am Vet Med Assoc 1970;157:1602.
20. Dodman NH, Normile JA, Shuster L, et al: Equine self-mutilation syndrome (57 cases), J Am Vet Med Assoc 1994;204:1219.

21. DeBowes RM, Leipold HW, Turner-Beatty M: Cerebellar abiotrophy, Vet Clin North Am Equine Pract 1987;3:345.
22. Firth EC: Horner's syndrome in the horse: Experimental induction and a case report, Equine Vet J 1978;10:9.
23. MacKay RJ, Granstrom DE, Saville WJ, Reed SM: Equine protozoal myeloencephalitis, Vet Clin North Am Equine Pract 2000;16:405.
24. Sponseller ML: Equine cerebellar hypoplasia and degeneration, Proc Am Assoc Equine Pract 1967;13:123.
25. Pletcher JM, Howerth E: *Micronema deletrix* infection in horses, J Am Vet Med Assoc 1980;177:1090.
26. Wilson WD: Equine herpesvirus 1 myeloencephalopathy, Vet Clin North Am Equine Pract 1997;13:53.

CHAPTER 50

Diagnostic Procedures

Robert J. MacKay

NEUROLOGIC EXAMINATION

A competent neurologic examination is not unlike an evaluation for lameness, where the initial evaluation is by systematic, "passive" examination and this is followed by an assessment of the gait. This chapter contains a description of an ordered approach to neurologic examination (Box 50-1 is a summary). There is considerable emphasis on evaluation of symmetry during each element of the examination. To accurately assess symmetry, it is essential that a mirror-image technique be used when comparing sides—that is, if the right hand of the examiner is used to test one side, the left hand should be used for testing the opposite side. The only equipment needed is a transilluminator, a hemostat, and a patella hammer (for neonatal examinations). The findings are used to localize a lesion or lesions. This is the basis for formulation of an initial rule-out list and for planning additional diagnostic tests.

BOX 50-1. Items for Neurologic Examination

Mentation
Orientation and coordination of the head
Muscles of mastication
Facial tone
Facial sensation
Menace response
Size of pupils and pupillary light reflex
Position and movement of the eyeballs
Swallowing
Tongue
General examination of the neck, trunk, and limbs
Slap test
Cervicofacial reflex
Cutaneus trunci reflex (panniculus)
Back reflexes
Tests for limb strength
Gait
Testing of recumbent horses
Tail and anus

In this discussion, all abnormal findings are interpreted in the context of a neurologic explanation. It is clear that many of these signs could be caused by lesions outside the nervous system. Full general physical and lameness examinations should also be performed to assess possible involvement of other body systems.

Mentation

Alertness and behavior are not evaluated by specific testing but are assessed from the history and general observation throughout the examination.

Alertness

Assess level of consciousness or alertness on a continuous scale from normal (i.e., bright and alert) to comatose. Progressive levels of obtundation are termed lethargy, stupor, semicoma, and coma. With *lethargy*, there is a somewhat blank facial expression with slight drooping of the ears and eyelids, sluggish responsiveness to stimuli, and reduced voluntary activity. It should be noted that some conditions cause horses to lose facial expression while maintaining normal alertness. Botulism is a disease of this type. A *stuporous* horse stands in one place with the head held low and responds only to strong stimuli. Stuporous horses that are recumbent are defined as *semicomatose*, and recumbent horses that do not respond to any stimulus are *comatose*. Some horses with reduced alertness appear irritable and anxious, walk compulsively, or otherwise interact abnormally with handlers. An obtunded horse showing such behavior may be termed *delirious*.

It is very unlikely that a horse with narcolepsy will have a sleep attack while being examined; thus, assessment of possible narcolepsy usually rests on description by the owner or video recordings of an attack. Occasionally, neonatal foals collapse during examination and briefly appear comatose. These are typically benign episodes of cataplexy and are probably an exaggerated version of the collapse response by which a normal foal can be cast into recumbency.

Behavior

Abnormalities of behavior are termed *dementia*. Behavior is assessed from history and general observation in the course of the examination. Typical abnormal behaviors resulting from central nervous system (CNS) disease include self-mutilation, head-pressing, compulsive walking (often in a circle), yawning, aggression (including unprovoked biting or kicking), timidity, loss of affinity of a foal for its dam, and loss of learned behaviors and skills. Inability or refusal of a trained horse to follow when being led is a form of dementia that may be obvious during neurologic examination.

Lesion Location

Obtundation reflects damage anywhere in the brain stem or diffusely in the cerebrum. Dementia is a sign of forebrain damage.

Associated Clinical Signs

Limb ataxia or weakness and signs of cranial nerve dysfunction are common in horses with obtundation secondary to brain stem disease. Compulsive turning of the head and neck in one direction, blindness, and seizures are other signs of forebrain dysfunction that may be seen in demented horses.

Orientation and Coordination of the Head

Examination

Evaluate the orientation of the head from directly in front. Any head tilt is described from the patient's perspective; thus, if the poll is rotated to the horse's left (i.e., clockwise from the examiner's point of view), the abnormality is described as a left head tilt. Repeatedly straighten and release the horse's neck and head and observe whether or not the head returns to one side. Asymmetric disease of the vestibular system causes the head to tilt *and* turn, whereas asymmetric cerebral disease may cause the head and neck to turn *without* tilting. Carefully blindfold the horse and observe the effect on head position (Fig. 50-1). Blindfolding removes visual input to head position and exacerbates abnormalities caused by either vestibular or cerebral disease. Observe the head and neck from the side. Persistent horizontal or low position of the head may indicate neurologic or muscular weakness of the neck, whereas extended head position may be found in horses with upper cervical vertebral problems or guttural pouch disease. Offer feed or a treat to the horse and observe the way in which the horse moves its head in response. Horses with cerebellar disease often make jerky or bobbing movements of the head as they move toward the offered feed.

Lesion Location

Head tilt suggests involvement of the vestibular labyrinth, nerve, or root peripherally, or the vestibular nuclei and connections in the medulla oblongata or cerebellum centrally. It has also been suggested that lesions in the proximal cervical nerves may cause signs suggestive of vestibular disease.[1] If the head is turned without tilting, involvement of the cerebrum is likely. Coarse or fine head bobbing, especially intentional, indicates diffuse cerebellar dysfunction.

Associated Clinical Signs

Because of the close association of cranial nerves VII and VIII, facial paralysis is often seen in horses with vestibular disease. With peripheral vestibular disease, there often is

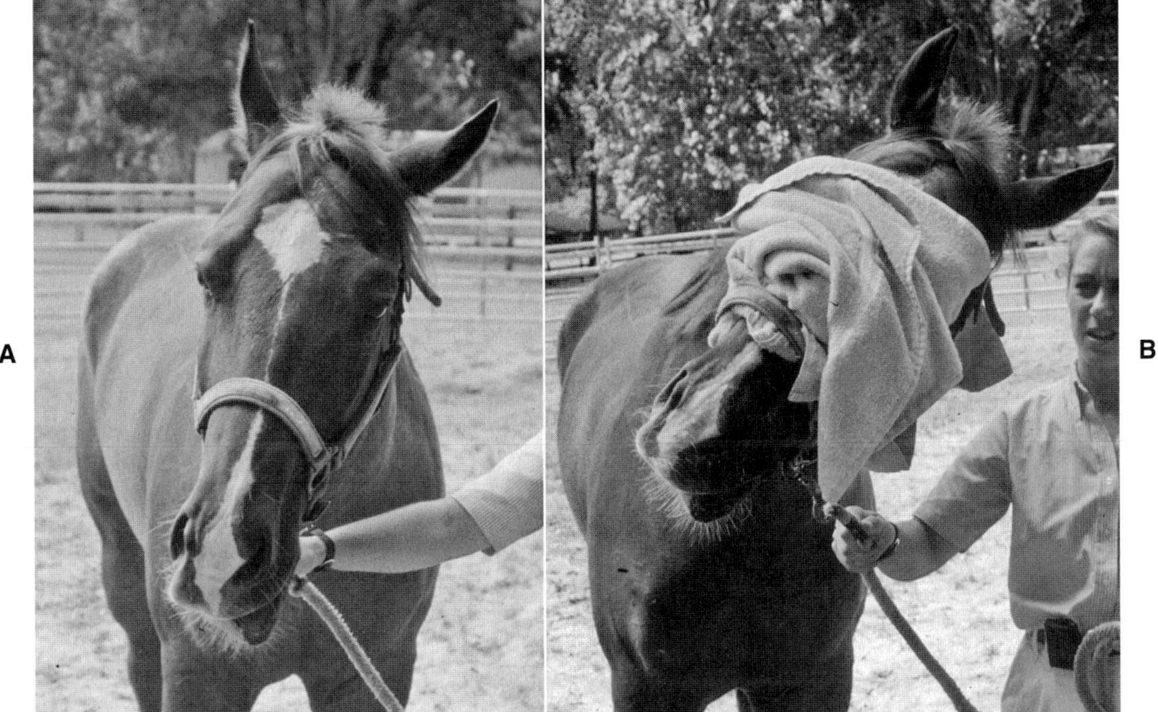

Figure 50-1. Head tilt associated with temporohyoid osteoarthropathy (THO). Six days earlier, this 7-year-old Quarter Horse gelding was presented with signs of acute-onset left-sided vestibular disease and facial paralysis. **A,** With anti-inflammatory therapy, the head tilt improved gradually to the time of presentation. **B,** Blindfolding removed visual input and exacerbated the head tilt.

spontaneous horizontal or arc-shaped nystagmus with the fast phase directed away from the side of the lesion. In horses with involvement of the central components of the vestibular system, there may be horizontal *or* vertical nystagmus. Damage to adjacent structures in the hindbrain may additionally cause obtundation, other signs of cranial nerve dysfunction such as dysphagia and masseter atrophy, and weakness or ataxia of the limbs on the side of the lesion. Horses with cerebellar cortical disease may lack menace responses despite having normal vision.

Muscles of Mastication

Examination

If the mouth hangs open and the tongue protrudes, there is probably bilateral paresis of the muscles that close the jaw (temporalis, masseter, and pterygoid). Grasp the upper and lower jaws at the level of the interdental space and attempt to pull the lower jaw downward. The jaws pull apart easily in horses with bilateral paresis of the masticatory muscles. Tuck the forelock behind one of the ears and compare the temporalis muscles from in front of the horse. Asymmetry may indicate neurogenic atrophy of the smaller side (Fig. 50-2). Turn the head from side to side and observe and palpate the masseter muscles. The pterygoid muscles and cranial belly of the digastricus muscle (the only muscle innervated by cranial nerve V that is devoted to opening the jaws) are located on the medial side of the mandible, so they are not readily palpable; however, atrophy of the pterygoids on one side is often evident as relative deepness of the supraorbital fossa on the same side. Peel back the upper and lower lips and examine the alignment of the symphyses of the upper and lower jaws. With acute unilateral paresis of the masticatory muscles, even before atrophy is apparent, the lower jaw may be deviated toward the normal side (see Fig. 50-2).

Lesion Location

Weakness or atrophy of the muscles of mastication indicates involvement of the motor division of the trigeminal nerve, its roots, or the trigeminal motor nucleus in the pons.

Associated Clinical Signs

Injury to the proximal part of the trigeminal nerve may also affect the sensory component, resulting in reduced facial sensation (hypalgesia) over one side of the face. With trigeminal damage at the level of the pons, there may be additional signs of hindbrain disease, such as obtundation, other signs of cranial nerve involvement (e.g., dysphagia, head tilt, or facial paralysis), and weakness and ataxia of the limbs on the same side.

Facial Tone

Examination

Examine the head carefully for symmetry of facial expression, particularly with respect to the ears, eyes, and muzzle. With complete unilateral facial paralysis, there is drooping of the ear, upper eyelid (ptosis), and lower lip, and immobility, narrowing, and lengthening of the affected external naris (Fig. 50-3). The muzzle is deviated away from the affected side, and saliva may drool from the mouth. Any or all of these components can be affected separately. Next, evaluate facial nerve function by testing "flick" reflexes on each side of the face. Each of these reflexes requires intact trigeminal sensory branches, central connections in the hindbrain, and functioning facial nerves. To test these reflexes, touch in turn the commissure of the lips, the medial and lateral canthi of the eye and the supraorbital fossa, and the ear. Appropriate responses are retraction of the commissure of the lip, blinking of the eye, and flick of the ear, respec-

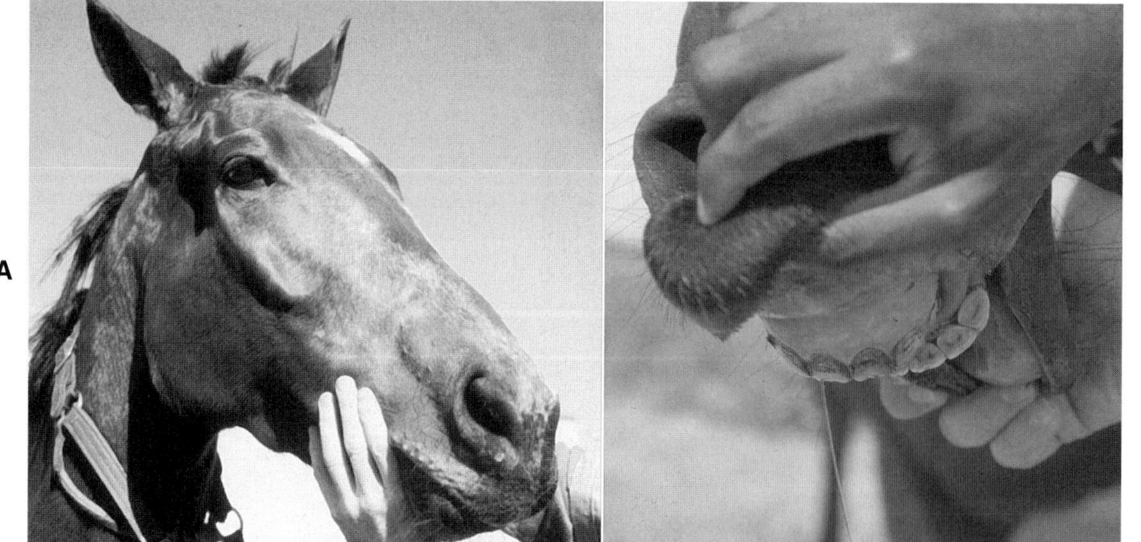

Figure 50-2. Atrophy of the muscles of mastication in a horse with equine protozoal myeloencephalitis. Beginning about a month after foaling, this 11-year-old Thoroughbred mare had an insidious onset of ataxia and limb weakness. **A,** Six weeks later, ataxia and weakness were worse, especially in the left limbs, and there was obvious atrophy of the masseter and temporalis muscles on the right side. **B,** The lower jaw was deviated away from the affected side.

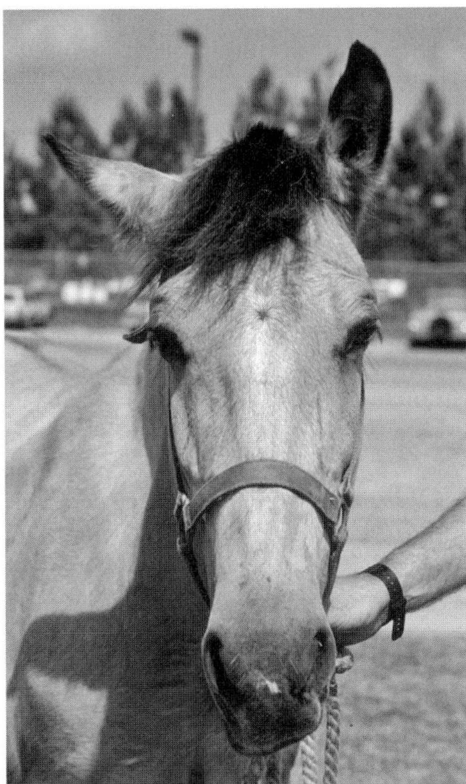

Figure 50-3. Facial paralysis in a horse with polyneuritis equi (neuritis of the cauda equina). Over the previous 2 weeks, this 13-year-old Quarter Horse mare had several exacerbations and remissions of right-sided facial paralysis. Beginning 3 days ago, there were also signs of cauda equina syndrome, including a weak tail and paralysis of the anus.

tively. It is helpful to have the handler cover the ipsilateral eye during testing of the lip and ear.

Test facial innervation of lacrimal glands by performing Schirmer tear tests. If tear production is reduced to less than 50% of normal on the side of the face that is paralyzed, there is likely to be a lesion affecting secretomotor fibers proximal (central) to the middle ear. Further test the symmetry of facial tone by using the thumbs or fingers to assess resistance simultaneously on both sides to retraction of lip commissures, elevation of upper eyelids, and forward extension of the ears. Examine the throat latch area. If there has been facial paralysis for more than 2 weeks, there usually is an obvious subcutaneous depression running ventrally from the base of the ear along the back of the mandible. This reflects atrophy of the parotidoauricularis muscle. Finally, test the cervicofacial reflex (see later) as part of the examination of long spinal reflexes. This reflex is not used as a primary test of facial nerve function but, clearly, its interpretation is affected by facial nerve paralysis.

Lesion Location

Abnormalities of facial tone reflect damage to the facial nucleus in the medulla oblongata, facial nerve root, or facial nerve or its motor branches, including dorsal and ventral buccal nerves, posterior and internal auricular and auriculopalpebral nerves, and the digastric nerve. If the Schirmer tear test gives a normal result on the affected side, the lesion is most likely at or peripheral to the middle ear; if tear production is reduced more than 50%, the lesion is central to the middle ear.

Associated Clinical Signs

Commonly there is also head tilt and spontaneous nystagmus because of involvement of the vestibular system. In horses with facial paralysis caused by brain disease, there may be other signs of hindbrain disorder such as obtundation, signs of abnormal cranial nerve function, such as dysphagia or masseter atrophy, or limb ataxia and weakness on the same side as the lesion. Nonneurologic signs include keratitis sicca (worse if tear production is reduced) and inspiratory stridor during exercise.

Facial Sensation

Examination

The sensory branches of the trigeminal nerve have already been tested as flick reflexes of the lip, eye, and ear. While standing in front of the horse, place the palm of the right hand on the muzzle, work the thumb into the right nostril, and touch the nasal septum on that side. In mirror-image fashion, use the left thumb to stimulate the left side of the septum. The normal response to this noxious stimulus is vigorous movement of the head away from the side of the stimulus. Compare the intensities of the response on each side. If there is obvious asymmetry of response, test cutaneous sensation at multiple locations over the face by pinching the skin with hemostats.

Lesion Location

The pathway for recognition of this noxious stimulus is input through the sensory division of the trigeminal nerve to the pons and thence to the somesthetic area of the contralateral cortex. If flick reflexes are normal, a reduced or absent response to a noxious stimulus suggests involvement of the contralateral forebrain, probably at the level of the parietal cortex. In contrast, hypalgesia and hyporeflexia of flick reflexes of part to all of one side of the head indicates involvement of the trigeminal nerve or branches.

Associated Clinical Signs

Cortical blindness, obtundation, and abnormal behaviors may be seen when hemifacial hypalgesia is a result of forebrain disease. Peripheral lesions of the trigeminal nerve may involve motor fibers and result in weakness and atrophy of masticatory muscles.

Menace Response

Examination

Test menace responses while standing in front of the horse. Use the palm of the hand to make a threatening gesture toward the eye. Test from both temporal and nasal directions on each side. Stimulate the horse just before each menace gesture by tapping the skin below the eye. For safety reasons, always hold the noseband of the halter with one hand while using the other for testing. A normal menace response is blinking of the eye, sometimes accompanied by evasive movement of the head and neck. Compare carefully the intensity of the menace responses elicited from each side. In this regard, menace should be considered a quantitative response. Unlike simple reflexes, which are assessed as present or absent, a menace response can be considered abnormal if it is less vigorous than that elicited from the opposite (normal) side.

Lesion Location

The menace response can be interrupted anywhere in its pathway from the eye via the optic nerve to the contralateral optic tract, diencephalon, internal capsule, and visual cortex. From the visual cortex, the menace response pathway continues to the facial nucleus and nerve on the side being tested and receives essential input from the cerebellum. If there is no other sign of cerebellar involvement, and if facial nerve function and pupillary light reflexes are intact, the lesion is contralateral, central to the optic chiasm, and most likely in the forebrain. In normal neonates and in older horses with diffuse cerebellar cortical disease, there is no menace response, but the horse can see. In these settings, vigorous threatening gestures toward the eye may cause evasive movements of the head without blinking of the eye.

Associated Clinical Signs

There may be other signs of asymmetric cerebral disease such as compulsive walking in circles, dementia, head and neck turn, obtundation, seizures, and facial hypalgesia on the side opposite the lesion (i.e., the same side as the defective menace). If the site of the lesion causing a menace deficit is the optic nerve or fundus of the eye, the pupillary light reflex on the same side should be abnormal. Head-bobbing, dysmetria, and ataxia are expected in horses with defective menace responses resulting from cerebellar dysfunction. If eyelid paralysis is preventing the menace response, the palpebral (eyelid flick) reflex should also be abnormal and there may be additional signs of facial paralysis.

Size of Pupils and Pupillary Light Reflex

Examination

If possible, examine the eyes in subdued or dim light so that the pupils are large enough to easily allow appreciation of reflex constriction. Stand in front of the horse while holding the noseband of the halter and swing the light back and forth from one side to the other so as to obliquely and briefly illuminate each eye without causing constriction of the pupils. Unequal pupillary size is termed *anisocoria,* a constricted pupil is *miotic,* and a dilated pupil is *mydriatic.* From this examination, determine whether or not the pupils are of equal size and if the diameter of each pupil is appropriate for the conditions. In this way, refine the diagnosis of anisocoria to miosis or mydriasis affecting a single eye.

Next, move closer to the horse and aim the light at the skin below one eye. Redirect the beam directly into the eye. This strong light should elicit both a *dazzle* reflex in the ipsilateral eye and pupillary light reflexes (PLRs) in both eyes. The dazzle response is an avoidance reaction to bright light. There is blinking, retraction of the eyeball, and movement of the head away from the light. A normal PLR is immediate constriction of the pupils of both eyes in response to light directed into one eye. If the direct (i.e., ipsilateral) pupillary light reflexes are normal on both sides, no further testing is necessary. If one is abnormal, then consensual (indirect) reflexes should be tested. To perform the consensual reflex, watch the pupil in one eye while an assistant shines the light into the opposite eye.

Lesion Location

The dazzle response is a subcortical reflex that is mediated via afferent input through the optic nerve to regions of the midbrain distinct from those required for the PLR and by efferent output along the facial nerve. It is possible for a horse to be cortically blind but still have dazzle reflexes, or to have PLRs but not dazzle reflexes. For a PLR, the stimulus pathway is via the optic nerves and optic tracts to the midbrain and thence to the efferent parasympathetic fibers of the oculomotor nerve. Fibers in the afferent limb of the reflex (i.e., optic nerve, optic tracts) pass on the same side *and* cross over at the optic chiasm and in the midbrain. Results of testing of menace responses along with direct and consensual PLRs usually allow anatomic localization of a lesion in the PLR pathways. In brief, without consideration of effects on consensual PLR, a lesion in an optic nerve affects the direct PLR and the menace on the same side; a lesion in an optic tract (rostral to the thalamus) affects the contralateral menace but does not affect direct PLR from either side, and a lesion in the midbrain or oculomotor nerve affects the ipsilateral PLR but not the menace responses.

Mydriasis is caused either by increased sympathetic dilator tone, by interference with the afferent arm of the PLR in the optic nerve, or by damage to the oculomotor nucleus or nerve. Mydriasis caused by sympathetic overstimulation is usually bilateral, and PLRs are normal. With a complete optic nerve lesion on one side, slight ipsilateral mydriasis is seen. Light directed into the opposite eye constricts the mydriatic pupil. With complete oculomotor nerve lesions, the ipsilateral pupil is fixed and dilated and unresponsive to light directed into either pupil; however, light directed into the fixed pupil causes reflex constriction of the pupil on the opposite side.

Miosis occurs because of removal of sympathetic dilator influence to the pupil or possibly because of excessive stimulation of pupillary constrictors. The sympathetic pathway can be affected anywhere along the three-neuron pathway from the midbrain to the eye. With damage anywhere along the preganglionic (2nd) or postganglionic (3rd) neurons of the sympathetic supply to the head, there are signs of Horner's syndrome in addition to ipsilateral miosis. If the lesion affects the 1st (upper motor) neuron, there most likely will be widespread areas of spontaneous sweating over one half of the head, neck, and torso, with additional signs of brain stem or spinal cord disease such as obtundation and ataxia and weakness of limbs. Early in the course of cerebral swelling, there often is miosis bilaterally. This is thought to be the result of either removal of sympathetic influences to the eyes or facilitation by upper motor neurons of the constrictor effects of oculomotor nerves.

Associated Clinical Signs

Horses with abnormal PLR because of cerebral swelling have other signs of forebrain disease such as obtundation, dementia, and cortical blindness. Within 4 weeks of optic nerve injury, abnormal pigmentation of the fundus develops and there is atrophy of the vasculature of the optic disc. In addition to miosis and ptosis, interruption of the sympathetic supply to the head causes other signs of Horner's syndrome, including spontaneous facial sweating and hyperemia of mucous membranes.

Position and Movement of the Eyeballs

Examination

While continuing to stand in front of the horse, observe the position and size of the pupils while the head is held level (i.e., a line through the center of each eyeball is parallel to the ground). While keeping the head level, lift the chin slowly. The eyeballs should remain stationary while the chin moves upward; thus, the eyes rotate ventrally *relative* to the long axis of the head. In horses with vestibular disease, abnormal eye positions are exaggerated by this maneuver.

If the pupils are in abnormal positions, try to position the head in such a way (usually by rotation) that the pupils are normally oriented *relative to the transverse axis of the head*. For example, a horse with vestibular disease often has ventral deviation of the eyeball on the side of the lesion and dorsal deviation on the opposite side (Fig. 50-4). Eye position can be normalized relative to the axis of the head simply by rotating the head in the direction of the ventrally deviated eye. The abnormal position of the eyes in horses with vestibular disease is termed *vestibular* strabismus. *True* strabismus is eye deviation that cannot be corrected by repositioning the head and usually reflects dysfunction of nerves to the extraocular muscles (i.e., oculomotor, trochlear, or abducens nerves). In horses with strabismus, the eyeball may be rotated medially or laterally, clockwise or counterclockwise. Newborn foals normally have slight dorsomedial rotation of the pupils compared with older horses.

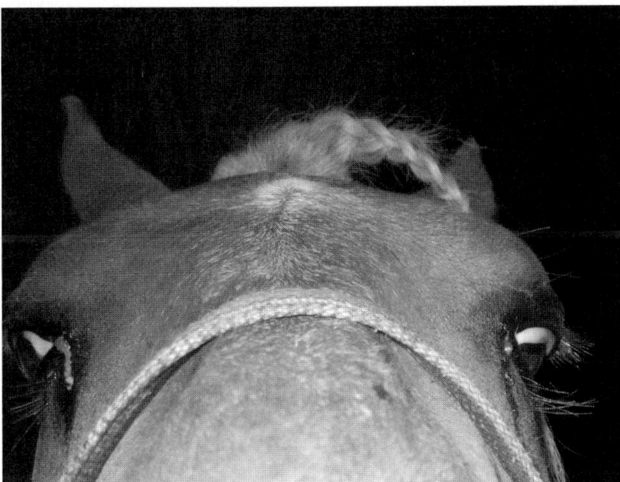

Figure 50-4. Vestibular strabismus in a horse with eastern equine encephalomyelitis (EEE). This yearling Quarter Horse presented initially with high fever and a left head tilt. When the head was straightened out and the chin lifted, the left eye deviated downward and the right eye upward.

Further assess abducens nerve function by performing a *modified corneal* reflex. Hold the eyelids closed and, through the eyelid, push the eyeball medially. The normal response to this maneuver is retraction (adduction) of the eyeball. This reflex requires intact sensory branches of the trigeminal nerve, central connections in the hindbrain, and motor fibers of the abducens nerve.

Move the horse's head in a horizontal arc from side to side and observe the movements of the eyeballs. Signs of *physiologic* nystagmus should normally be elicited—namely, a series of horizontal movements of the eyeball consisting of a rapid phase in the direction of head movement followed by a slow phase in the opposite direction. Each fast phase is accompanied by an eye blink. Physiologic nystagmus is normal and should be distinguished from eye movements characteristic of vestibular disease: *spontaneous* nystagmus, which occurs when the head is stationary and in a neutral position, and *positional* nystagmus, which occurs only when the head is moved to certain positions. In horses with asymmetric vestibular disease, physiologic nystagmus is often abnormal or absent when the head is moved toward the side of the lesion.

Lesion Location

For horses with vestibular strabismus, the causative lesion could be anywhere in the peripheral or central vestibular system (including connections with the cerebellum and nerves to the extraocular muscles), usually on the same side as the ventrally deviated eye (described more fully under "Orientation and Coordination of the Head," earlier). A horse exhibiting true strabismus most likely has a lesion in cranial nerve III, IV, or VI (or its roots or nuclei). These nerves exit the midbrain or hindbrain and pass a short distance to the oblique and rectus muscles of the eye.

Associated Clinical Signs

The roots of the nerves to the extraocular muscles are subject to dorsal pressure exerted by the cerebrum as it swells and herniates under the tentorium cerebelli. Other signs associated with cerebral swelling are obtundation, blindness, seizures, and fluctuant to dilated fixed pupils. There may also be jerky head movements as a result of pressure on the cerebellum. As compression of the midbrain and rostral hindbrain becomes more severe, obtundation progresses to coma with decerebrate posturing. With more focal lesions of the nerves or their nuclei, mydriasis (III) or defective modified corneal reflex (VI) is likely.

Swallowing

Examination

It is difficult to assess competence for swallowing during a physical examination. On the basis of history and observation, note whether feed, water, or saliva return through the nose, especially when the horse eats or drinks. Pass a nasogastric tube into the pharynx and assess effectiveness of swallowing movements as the horse attempts to move the tube into the esophagus.

Lesion Location

Involvement of the nucleus ambiguus in the hindbrain, or the roots or peripheral parts of one or both glossopharyngeal, vagus, or spinal accessory nerves, can cause dysphagia. These nerves are particularly vulnerable to damage as they pass over the guttural pouches.

Associated Clinical Signs

There is frequently coughing, especially during eating, and signs of pneumonia secondary to aspiration of feed. With bilateral laryngeal paresis because of involvement of the vagus nerves or branches, there may be inspiratory stridor at rest. At exercise, minor or unilateral laryngeal paresis (involvement of cranial nerve X or branches) may be evident as a "roaring" sound during inspiration; involvement of cranial nerve IX, X, or XI may lead to displacement of the soft palate and expiratory stridor. The slap test, which is described later, is negative on the paralyzed side.

Tongue

Examination

Pull the jaws slightly apart and observe the movements of the unrestrained tongue. With unilateral weakness, the tongue curls toward the weak side. Grasp the tongue from one side after inserting the hand through the interdental space. Note resistance of the tongue to being stretched and look for atrophy (Fig. 50-5) and muscular fasciculations. Gently pinch the side of the tongue with a hemostat and look for reflex retraction. Pull the tongue out one side of the mouth, release it, and look for retraction of the tongue back into the mouth. In normal horses, one or two chewing movements occur as the tongue is quickly retracted.

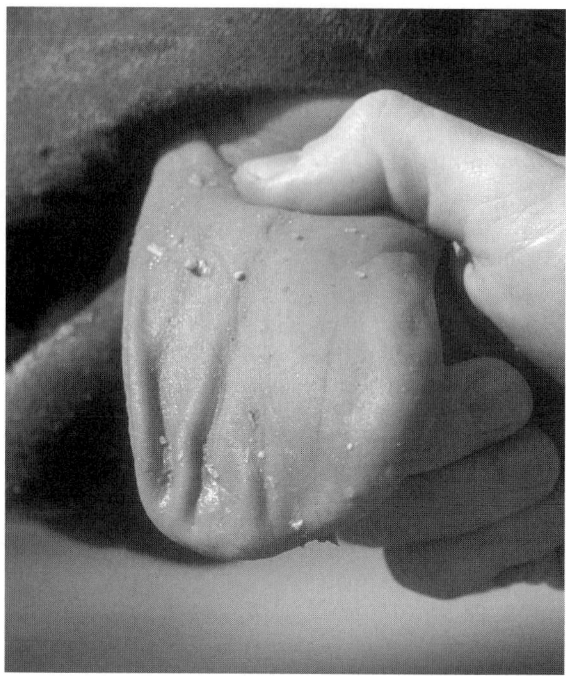

Figure 50-5. Unilateral tongue atrophy in a horse with possible equine protozoal myeloencephalitis. Note the characteristic longitudinal folds on the atrophied (right) side. The tongue intermittently deviated toward the right side when the mouth was held open.

Lesion Location

Tongue deviation, muscle atrophy, and/or fasciculations reflect involvement of a hypoglossal nerve or root. Delayed or absent retraction of the tongue back into the mouth can occur with any brain disease, probably because of involvement of upper motor neurons that regulate the actions of hypoglossal nerves.

Associated Clinical Signs

With delayed retraction caused by extensive brain disease, there is usually profound obtundation, often with ataxia and weakness of the trunk and limbs. Because the hypoglossal nerve is close to cranial nerves IX, X, and XI as they pass over the guttural pouch, signs of dysphagia and respiratory paralysis may accompany tongue atrophy in horses with guttural pouch disease.

General Examination of the Neck, Trunk, and Limbs

Examination

With the horse standing squarely, assess muscle mass, paying particular attention to asymmetries. Note any circumscribed or asymmetric areas of sweating. Firmly press the cranial edge of each of the cervical transverse processes from C3 to C6 on each side to test for a pain response. Put pressure on the C6-C7 intervertebral joints by pushing medial to the deep pectoral muscle in front of the shoulder on each side. Test lateral neck flexion by enticing the horse to move its head toward feed held at the point of the elbow.

Lesion Location

Neck pain revealed by palpation or reluctance to turn laterally may follow any neck trauma but usually reflects arthritis of intervertebral joints.

Severe or rapidly developing muscle atrophy indicates denervation and is a localizing sign. Neurogenic muscle atrophy is caused by damage to the lower motor neuron in the ventral column of the gray matter, nerve roots, or peripheral nerves supplying that muscle. Neurogenic atrophy of thoracic limb musculature results from lesions of the C6 to T2 spinal cord segments, brachial plexus, or peripheral nerves, whereas atrophy of pelvic limb muscles reflects involvement of L3 to S2. Anesthesia of a strip of skin is caused by loss of the segmental sensory nerve, dorsal nerve root, or connections in the spinal cord. Because sympathetic fibers are distributed with spinal nerves, spontaneous sweating may occur over denervated skin.

Associated Clinical Signs

Arthritic neck pain may be detected in wobblers, especially those older than 2 years. Neurogenic atrophy usually causes limb weakness and gait abnormality and may be associated with other signs of spinal cord disease. For example, there may be ataxia and weakness in a pelvic limb because of upper motor neuron damage at C6, and atrophy of the triceps and weakness of the thoracic limb on the same side because of a gray matter lesion in the same segment.

Slap Test

Examination

While standing on the left side, reach under the horse's neck and hook the index and middle fingers of the left hand over the highest palpable point of the larynx—the muscular process of the arytenoid. Have the handler move the head slightly to the left of midline. Gently strike the horse behind the withers several times with the palm of the right hand. The expected response is slight palpable movement (adduction) of the arytenoid in response to each slap. Repeat the procedure from the right side. More information on this test is found in Chapter 44.

Lesion Location

Sensory input to this reflex is the sensory nerves and roots under the area that is slapped (approximately T7 to T11). Central pathways are thought to cross to the other side at this level, and then they pass rostrally to the nucleus ambiguus. Next, efferent fibers pass out in the vagus nerve via the recurrent laryngeal nerve to innervate the contralateral laryngeal adductor muscles. Severe cervical spinal cord disease often affects this test bilaterally, and the vagus and recurrent laryngeal nerves may be affected at the guttural pouch or within the jugular groove. Variations in neck anatomy make this reflex easy to palpate in some horses but difficult or impossible in others.

Associated Clinical Signs

Other signs of cervical spinal cord disease include ataxia and weakness of the trunk and limbs. Dysphagia and aspiration pneumonia are further signs of guttural pouch disease, and Horner's syndrome may also be seen when there is involvement of the vagosympathetic trunk deep to the jugular groove.

Cervicofacial Reflex

Examination

Place the left index and middle fingers at the commissure of the left lip, then strike the skin over the brachiocephalicus muscle with the closed tip of the hemostat. Begin at the cranial end of the neck and continue back to the shoulder. The expected responses are facial contraction (detected as retraction of the commissure of the lip) and contraction of the brachiocephalicus and cutaneus colli (observed as shrugging of the shoulder, lateral jerking of the head, and twitching of the skin of the neck).

Lesion Location

Interruption of reflex components in the facial nerve (including the cervical sensory branch), cervical nerves or roots (sensory or motor), or local cervical spinal cord segments can affect the cervicofacial reflex. This reflex is typically reduced at the level of a cervical spinal cord lesion but is normal cranial and caudal to the lesion.

Associated Clinical Signs

There may be other signs of facial paralysis or cervical spinal cord disease (e.g., limb ataxia and weakness). With involvement of cervical sensory nerves or roots, there may be a strip of cutaneous anesthesia that corresponds to the area of diminished cervicofacial reflex. Asymmetric damage to the most cranial cervical nerves may lead to signs suggestive of peripheral vestibular disease.

Cutaneus Trunci Reflex (Panniculus)

Examination

When examining the reflex on the left side of the horse, use the extended right thumb to firmly prod the skin of the sensory field, beginning cranially just behind the shoulder and extending caudally to the last intercostal space. Check every intercostal space both ventrally and dorsally. For safety, firmly grasp the back of the mane with the left hand and face backward when testing the reflex, because horses that resent this test will try to kick the examiner. A normal response is twitching of the skin, with or without indication of conscious perception of the stimulus. Regardless of the site of stimulus, the twitch response is the same.

Lesion Location

The reflex pathway is input from sensory thoracic nerves to the ipsilateral spinal cord, where it courses rostrally via interneurons to end in the C8 and L1 segments, and thence via the brachial plexus to the lateral thoracic nerve and the cutaneus trunci muscle. Interruption of this pathway in the spinal cord white matter results in loss of the reflex from approximately the point of the lesion caudally. A lesion of the sensory nerve will affect only the reflex within the same dermatome (skin strip), whereas loss of lateral thoracic nerve function ablates the entire ipsilateral reflex.

Associated Clinical Signs

A strip of cutaneous anesthesia may overlay the cranial edge of the hyporeflexic zone when the spinal cord lesion affects interneurons coursing cranially *and* sensory connections from the segmental spinal nerve. Ataxia and weakness of the ipsilateral pelvic limb is usually found in such cases.

Back Reflexes

Examination

After making sure that the pelvic limbs are positioned equally and squarely, stroke the closed tip of the hemostat caudally along the skin over the longissimus muscle, from mid thorax caudally to the level of the tuber coxae. For safety, hold the back part of the mane with the other hand. The expected response is brisk extension of the back and pelvis followed quickly by return to normal posture. Next, stroke the hemostat caudally along the skin over the gluteal muscles. This should elicit flexion, followed by relaxation of the lumbar spine and pelvis. Common abnormal reactions to these tests include (1) partial collapse in the pelvic limbs, (2) wobbling of the pelvis from side to side, and (3) no response.

Lesion Location

Abnormal results of the back tests correlate with truncal and pelvic limb weakness and ataxia caused by spinal cord disease.

Associated Clinical Signs

Expect other signs of pelvic limb weakness and ataxia such as toe-dragging and circumduction.

Tests for Limb Strength

Examination

During the passive part of the examination, it is difficult to detect mild thoracic limb weakness. Only very weak horses buckle a thoracic limb in response to downward pressure exerted over the withers. The *hopping test* is more sensitive. From the left side, hold the halter with the left hand. Pick up the left leg then push the head toward the right side while leaning against the left shoulder (Fig. 50-6). Normal horses use the right limb to hop briskly around a circle centered on the pelvic limbs. With limb weakness, the response may be delayed so that the horse leans markedly before hopping, or the limb may buckle after landing.

Strength of the pelvic limbs is evaluated by resistance to pressure over the pelvis and to a sideways pull on the tail. Additional insight is provided by the back reflexes described earlier. To test resistance to dorsal pressure, stand on one side of the horse and hook the fingers over the opposite tuber sacrale. Use maximal effort to try to collapse the near limb. Only weak horses buckle in response to such pressure. The *tail-pull test* is done both at rest and while the horse is walking in a straight line. With the horse standing squarely, take the tail and pull sideways with gradually increasing force. After initial slight movement in the direction of pull, normal horses usually cannot be moved sideways, even with strong pressure. Next, pull sideways on the tail while the horse is walking in a straight line. Always work on the same side as the handler. Exert moderate lateral pressure during all phases of the stride, and then rhythmically increase pressure as the horse supports weight on the near leg. Normal horses of 450-kg bodyweight can be moved only slightly to the side. Response to this test varies according to the size and strength of the examiner and the bodyweight and temperament of the horse. Perform the test in mirror-image fashion from the right side (i.e., with the horse being led from the right side). Interpretation of this test requires practice and experience on the part of the examiner.

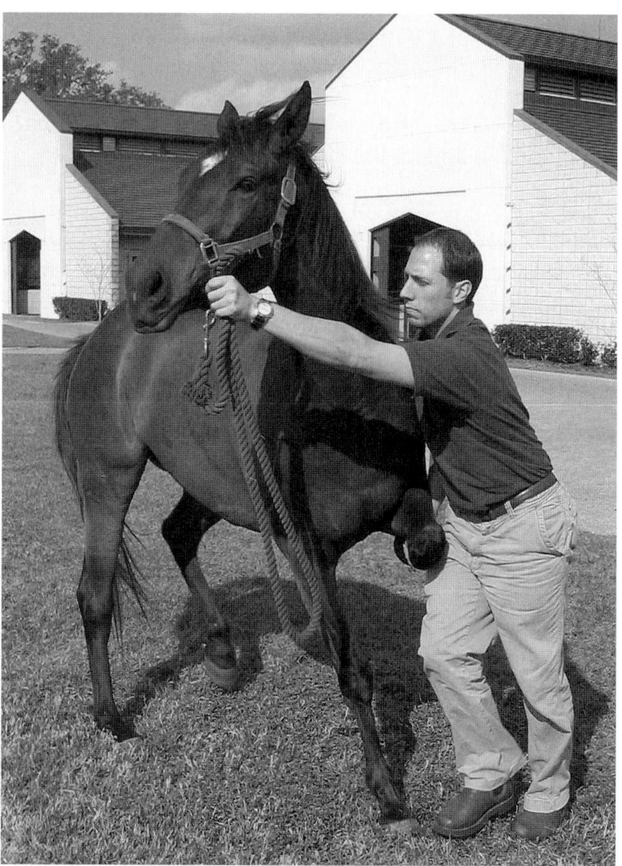

Figure 50-6. Force the horse to hop on each front limb to evaluate limb strength.

Lesion Location

If a full-size adult horse can easily be pulled sideways at rest, there is probably interruption of the antigravity myotactic reflex pathway. Practically, such a lesion most likely is located either in the ventral gray matter, or in the roots (L3 to L5) that form the femoral nerve, or in the femoral nerve itself. If cutaneous sensation over the saphenous vein is absent or reduced, the lesion is central to the ventral aspect of the shaft of the ilium (the site at which the sensory saphenous vein joints the femoral nerve). The much more common finding—namely, lack of resistance to tail-pull only during walking—is consistent with an ipsilateral spinal cord lesion affecting descending upper motor neurons anywhere from C1 to S2, inclusive.

Associated Clinical Signs

Depending on the location of the lesion, there may be interference with long spinal reflexes, hypalgesia of skin strips, spontaneous sweating of skin strips, or atrophy of musculature, in addition to alterations in gait.

Gait

Examination

Have the handler walk the horse in straight lines, leading alternately from the left and the right side. The handler should be instructed to keep the horse's head and neck as straight as possible during walking. When the horse turns its head to one side, there is reciprocal and potentially confusing movement of the pelvis toward the same side. Follow directly behind the horse. From this vantage point, evaluate leg position and stride symmetry. Also, watch for excessive (1) side-to-side (wobbling) movement of the pelvis, (2) up-and-down movement of the tuber coxae (pelvic roll), and (3) side-to-side rotation of an imaginary line from the tail-head to the tuber sacrale (pelvic yaw). Next, watch the gait from the side while walking in stride with the pelvic and then thoracic limbs. Note any toe-dragging, knuckling, stride-length asymmetries, and abnormal protractive movements such as hyperflexion, stiffness (hypometria), or excessive range of movement (hypermetria). Often, these signs are most obvious as the horse transitions from standing still to walking. Repeat this part of the examination with the horse's chin lifted and with the horse walking up and down a modest slope. These maneuvers exacerbate most gait abnormalities, especially stiffness of the thoracic limbs.

Take the horse in hand for the next part of the examination. Hold the lead rope with the left hand and, by walking backward, lead the horse in counterclockwise circles (Fig. 50-7). It is very important that the horse be always walking *forward* in these circles. Vary the diameter, making the circles alternately small and large. Observe carefully the motion of the right (outside) pelvic limb by looking under the horse's torso. This limb will often arc out widely on the outside of the circle (i.e., circumduct) in horses with spinal cord disease. In mirror-image fashion, lead the horse from the right side in clockwise circles.

Next, pull the horse sideways in *tight* circles in either direction. This is done from a position slightly behind the shoulder by pulling the lead rope at an angle sideways and caudally (Fig. 50-8). If done correctly in normal horses, the opposite thoracic limb should cross in front of the supporting limb and the pelvic limbs should move reciprocally, causing the horse to pivot around a point midway between the thoracic and pelvic limbs. Horses that are weak and ataxic tend to sag backward in the hindquarters before they start to move, and then pivot the front part of the body around one or both pelvic limbs. There is often also interference between or otherwise inappropriate placement of thoracic limbs.

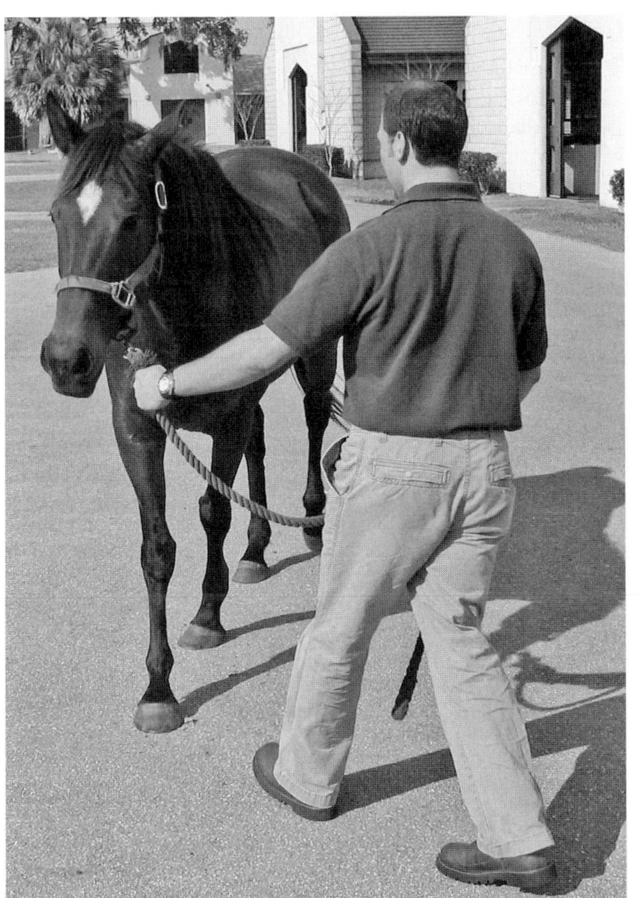

Figure 50-7. Testing for strength: walk backward and pull the horse in anticlockwise circles, then repeat in mirror-image fashion in clockwise circles.

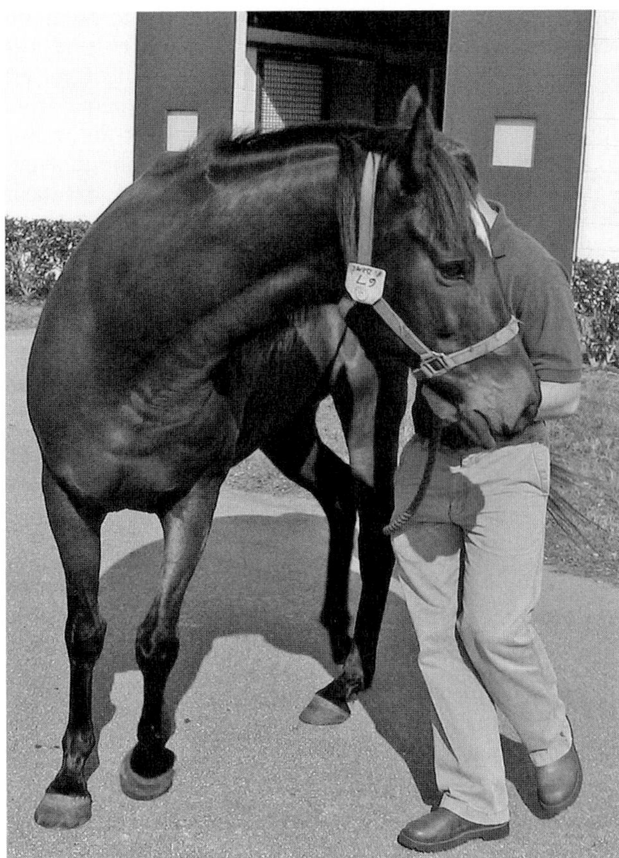

Figure 50-8. Gait analysis: pull the horse sideways and backward in tight circles so that it pivots around a point midway between the thoracic and pelvic limbs. Repeat on the right side.

Use the lead rope to push the horse straight backward. A normal horse should move backward in two-beat fashion, with simultaneous movement of diagonally opposite pairs of limbs (e.g., left thoracic and right pelvic limbs). A horse with spinal cord disease may sag backward before moving and slide its hooves along the ground rather than picking them up and placing them.

Lesion Location

Signs of limb weakness and ataxia suggest spinal cord (or, rarely, peripheral nerve) damage at or cranial to the affected limb. If there is obvious ataxia and weakness in thoracic *and* pelvic limbs, there is likely to be at least one lesion in the spinal cord somewhere between the front of the C1 and back of the T2 spinal cord segments. When the signs are caused by external compression of the cervical spinal cord (e.g., in cervical stenotic myelopathy), signs in the pelvic limbs are usually worse than those in the thoracic limbs. When, in such cases, the pelvic limb signs are mild, thoracic limbs may appear normal. In contrast, when thoracic limbs are normal but there is moderate or severe ataxia and weakness in the pelvic limbs, there is likely to be at least one lesion caudal to T2 and cranial to S3. If one or both thoracic limbs are abnormal in a horse that has normal pelvic-limb gait, the gray matter of the C6 to T2 spinal cord segments (without white matter involvement), the roots or nerves of the brachial plexus, or the peripheral nerves to the limbs are probably affected. Asymmetric lesions in the spinal cord cause signs that are more severe on the side of the lesion. Occasionally, there are signs of weakness without ataxia (e.g., botulism, equine motor neuron disease) or ataxia without weakness (e.g., cerebellar abiotrophy, peripheral vestibular disease). Additional signs, such as defective reflexes (cervicofacial, slap, or cutaneus trunci), neurogenic muscle atrophy, or cutaneus anesthesia, often help to localize the spinal cord lesion.

Associated Clinical Signs

Abnormal responses to tests for limb strength, reduced or absent long spinal reflexes, and strips of cutaneous anesthesia or spontaneous sweating may accompany lesions of the spinal cord or peripheral nerves.

Testing of Recumbent Horses

Examination

Note whether or not the horse moves its limbs voluntarily without stimulation. If possible, assist and stimulate the horse in such a way as to assess which of the following best describes the horse's maximal voluntary motor function: (1) lifts head off the ground; (2) rolls shoulders and chest into a sternal position, or (3) straightens thoracic limbs and assumes a "dog-sitting" position.

Check long spinal reflexes (cervicofacial, cutaneus trunci, slap) and test cutaneous sensation systematically over the limbs and torso. Test sensation at each site by grasping a fold of skin between the jaws of the hemostat and firmly squeezing the skin and watching for evidence of a conscious response by the horse. This is a behavioral reaction and must be distinguished from a reflex response. Sensory fields for some peripheral nerves of horses have been described.[2]

Test pelvic limb reflexes and function. First, assess extensor tone in the limb by testing resistance to passive flexion. Next, perform the flexion test by pinching skin on the distal limb with a hemostat. If there is no response, try pinching skin elsewhere on the leg. A normal response is flexion of the limb, usually with some evidence that the horse can feel the skin pinch. When abnormal, the flexor response may be reduced or absent, and it may be accompanied by reflex extension of the contralateral digit (*crossed extensor* reflex). To test the patellar reflex, hold the pelvic limb in a moderately flexed position, and strike the skin over the middle patellar ligament (Fig. 50-9). A twitch handle works well for this purpose in full-size horses; a patellar hammer or reversed hemostat can be used in foals. The expected response is brisk extension of the stifle. If the reflex is absent, move the leg into different positions and retest. Classify the response as absent, normal, or increased. Other extension reflexes in the pelvic limb cannot be elicited reliably but should be tested for comparison with the opposite leg. These include (1) the tibial reflex—tap just behind the greater trochanter; (2) the gastrocnemius reflex—strike the Achilles tendon close to its insertion; and (3) the anterior tibial reflex—strike the middle of the anterior tibial muscle.

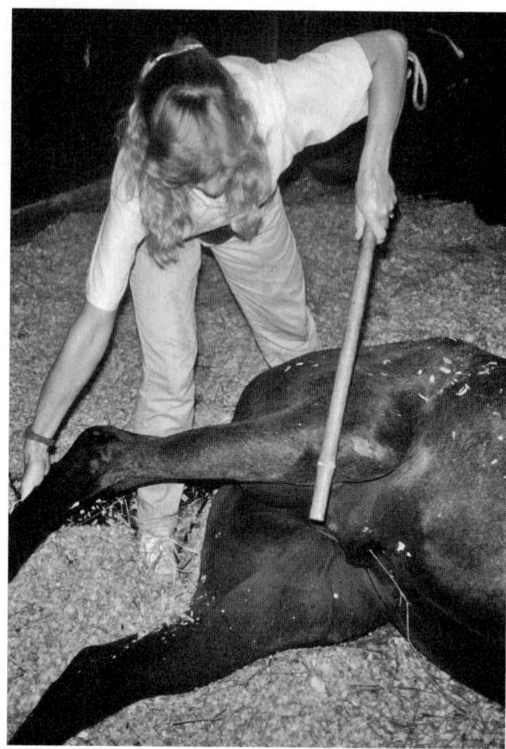

Figure 50-9. Testing the patellar reflex in a recumbent horse. The limb is held in a flexed and slightly abducted position, and the skin over the middle patellar ligament is struck with a twitch handle.

Test thoracic limb reflexes and function. Assess extensor tone and evaluate the flexor reflex as described for the pelvic limb. No other reflex can be obtained consistently in the thoracic limbs, but, for comparison with the opposite limb, test the following: (1) triceps reflex—with the limb in flexed position, strike the triceps muscle and watch for elbow extension; (2) biceps reflex—strike the front of the elbow and watch for extension of the shoulder and flexion of the elbow joint; and (3) strike the middle of the extensor carpi radialis muscle and look for extension of the carpus.

Lesion Location

If a horse can dog-sit, the principal spinal cord lesion is probably behind T2. Inability of a horse to roll from lateral into sternal recumbency is associated with severe lesions (usually involving gray matter) of the caudal cervical segments, whereas serious injury to the spinal cord in the rostral part of the neck may also prevent a horse from raising its head off the ground.

With involvement of lower motor neurons to limb muscles, there is reduced or absent extensor tone. Limb reflexes are reduced or abolished if the sensory nerves, motor nerves, or central components of the reflexes are affected. The afferent, central, and efferent parts of important reflexes are listed in Table 50-1. In contrast, extensor tone and limb reflexes may be exaggerated beginning several days after injury to descending upper motor neurons. For example, after trauma to the spinal cord at the T13 segment, patellar reflexes and pelvic extensor muscle tone may be exaggerated.

TABLE 50-1. Limb and Tail Reflexes

Reflex	Spinal Cord Segments	Peripheral Nerves
Flexor (thoracic)	C6-T2	Median, ulnar, axillary, musculocutaneous
Triceps	C7-T1	Radial
Biceps	C7-C8	Musculocutaneous
Patellar	L3-L5	Femoral
Flexor (pelvic)	L5-S2	Sciatic
Anal	S3-S4	Pudendal
Tail clamp	S3-S4	S1 to coccygeal segments

If there is no response to strong pinching of the skin over caudal regions of the body, there is probably catastrophic damage to the spinal cord cranial to the anesthetic area. If there is no response to deep pain for more than 24 hours, there is at least functional transection of the spinal cord.

Associated Clinical Signs

Large horses that remain recumbent for more than a few hours often have reduced skin sensation in the distal limbs secondary to pressure-induced injury of superficial sensory nerves. This complicates interpretation of tests for flexor reflexes and for presence of deep pain.

Tail and Anus

Examination

Assess tail strength by lifting (extending) the tail. Prod or pinch the skin adjacent to the anus and observe the anal contraction and tail-clamp reflexes. If these reflexes are abnormal or if the history suggests possible cauda equina syndrome, perform a rectal examination to assess rectal tone and bladder size and tone. Assess muscular symmetry of the tail and test cutaneous sensation over the tail and caudal structures.

Lesion Location

Anesthesia and areflexia of the tail, penis, and perineum and paralysis of the anus, rectum, bladder, and penis are signs of *cauda equina syndrome*. Lesions of the spinal cord or nerve roots caudal to the S2 spinal cord segment cause some or all of the signs of cauda equina syndrome. The bundled roots forming the cauda equina are vulnerable as they pass through the sacrum and proximal coccygeal vertebrae.

Associated Clinical Signs

With involvement of S2 and more cranial nerve roots, expect to see signs of pelvic limb weakness in addition to cauda equina syndrome. Colic caused by obstipation may be the presenting sign of rectal paralysis, and urinary overflow incontinence is a sign of bladder paralysis.

CEREBROSPINAL FLUID COLLECTION

Atlantooccipital (AO) cerebrospinal fluid (CSF) collection under general anesthesia is simple, and iatrogenic blood contamination is seldom a problem. Lumbosacral (LS) collection has the advantage of not requiring anesthesia, but the procedure is technically more challenging than AO collection and significant blood contamination may occur. Because CSF flows caudally over the spinal cord from sites of production in the brain, LS samples can theoretically reflect changes anywhere in the CNS, whereas AO samples may not reflect caudal spinal cord disease. In general, in cases where the horse's physical condition does not dictate the procedure used, select the collection site that is closest to the likely site of the lesion.

Atlantooccipital Cerebrospinal Fluid Collection

Anesthetize the horse (e.g., 1 mg/kg of xylazine and 2 mg/kg of ketamine, both given IV) and position it in lateral recumbency. *This procedure should not be performed in standing horses*. Clip and surgically prepare a rectangle of skin approximately 10 cm (4 inches) wide and 15 cm (6 inches) long centered on the dorsal midline and beginning just behind the forelock. Extend the prepared area on the side facing up so that a 2.5-cm (1-inch) strip is clipped over the cranial border of the wing of the atlas. In horses heavier than 150 kg bodyweight, use an 8.23-cm (3.5-inch) 18- or 20-gauge stiletted spinal needle.[3] In foals, use a regular 3.75-cm (1.5-inch) 20-gauge needle. Flex the atlantooccipital joint in the median sagittal plane to an angle of 90 degrees or less. This is conveniently done if the collector kneels in such a way as to flex the head with the inside of the knee while leaning over the neck to place the needle. The needle is inserted at the intersection of lines running along the front of the atlas and along the dorsal midline (Fig. 50-10). Insert the needle through the skin and then pass it in the median plane by aiming at the middle of the lower jaw. The needle is passed through the funicular part of the ligamentum nuchae and advanced until there is a popping sensation as the needle penetrates the atlantooccipital membrane, the cervical dura, and arachnoid mater. In practice, the stilette is withdrawn from the needle each time there is a popping

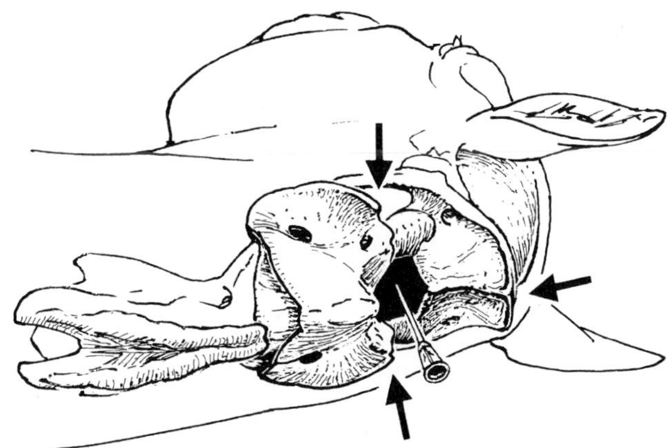

Figure 50-10. Atlantooccipital cerebrospinal fluid collection. The needle is inserted through the midline using the cranial border of the wings of the atlas and the nuchal crest of the skull *(arrows)* as landmarks.

sensation. CSF should flow freely from the hub when the subarachnoid space is entered. This can happen anywhere from 2.5 to 8.3 cm (1.0 to 3.5 inches) beneath the skin surface, depending on the size, sex, breed, and condition of the horse. Collect two or three aliquots of 1 to 5 mL of CSF, depending on need, either by aspirating drops as they fall from the hub of the needle or by attaching a syringe to the hub and aspirating directly. The last aliquot is least likely to be contaminated with blood and should be retained for analysis. Replace the stilette and withdraw the needle.

There is very little morbidity associated with this procedure; however, occasionally a horse will hold its head stiffly in an extended position for a few days afterward. This is not associated with fever (in which case infection would be likely) and may be analogous to the headache that occurs in some humans after CSF aspiration. The condition responds well to the use of a nonsteroidal anti-inflammatory drug (NSAID).

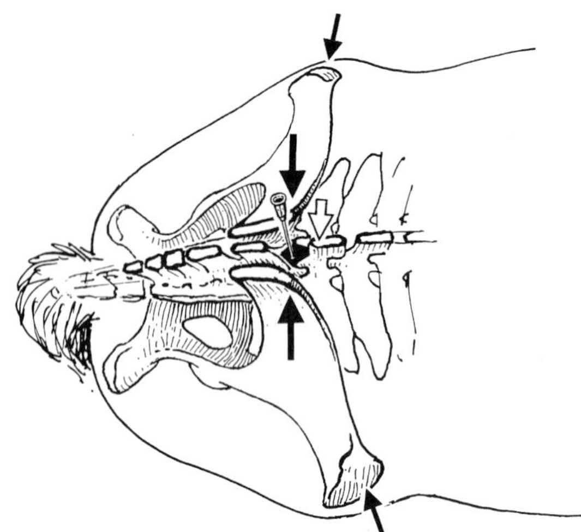

Figure 50-11. Lumbosacral cerebrospinal fluid collection. The caudal border of the tuber coxae *(small dark arrows)*, the cranial edge of the tuber sacrale *(large dark arrows)*, and the spine of L6 *(open arrow)* are used as landmarks.

Lumbosacral CSF Collection

This procedure is conveniently performed in stocks so that the collector can stand on a raised platform alongside the horse; however, it also can be done in a stall with the horse pushed against a wall. In either case, it is preferable that only a nose twitch be used. If a sedative must be given, use the lowest dose that controls the horse without causing the hindquarters to sway and wobble unduly.

The key landmarks for this procedure are the tuber sacrale and the dorsal spinous process of the 2nd sacral vertebra. The paired tubera sacrale are located near the midline and can be found between the caudal margins of the tuber coxae at approximately the highest point of the rump. The dorsal (superficial) edge of each sacral tuberosity can be palpated through the skin as a slender ridge beginning adjacent to the sacral spine and progressing cranially and slightly laterally for several centimeters. When viewed from above, the paired tubera sacrale thus form a V with the vertex caudal. The correct tap site is located on the midline within or slightly in front of the V. To find the site, palpate the dorsal spinous processes of the caudal sacrum with the thumb, then slide the thumb forward until a 2- to 3-cm-long depression is located on the midline (between the spinous processes of the 2nd sacral and 6th lumbar vertebrae). Clip and surgically prepare a rectangular section of skin centered on this site (Fig. 50-11).

Infiltrate 0.5 to 1.0 mL of local anesthetic into the skin of the tap site, and make a sagittally oriented stab through the skin with a no. 15 scalpel blade. Rest both forearms on the horse's back while holding the hub of the needle with both hands. The needle is inserted along the intersection of median and transverse planes. It is helpful to have an assistant watch from behind the horse to guide side-to-side orientation of the needle. Advance the needle until (1) a slight "pop" is felt as the needle traverses the ligamentum flavum, (2) there is an involuntary response from the horse (usually brisk extension of the tail and pelvis), or (3) the point of the needle strikes the bottom of the vertebral canal. Remove the stilette, attach a syringe, and apply gentle aspiration pressure. To obtain flow of CSF, it may be necessary to rotate the needle or slightly retract it (or both) during attempted aspiration. Advance the needle only if the stilette is in place. CSF may flow more easily if both jugular veins are occluded (thus increasing intracranial pressure). Collect an initial sample of 2 to 5 mL (or more if the sample is visibly contaminated with blood) to "clear" iatrogenic blood contamination; then collect another sample for analysis. Reinsert the stilette and remove the needle.

Rarely, horses are sensitive to touch near the tap site for several days after the procedure. Occasional cases of cauda equina syndrome have occurred because of development of epidural abscessation at the tap site.

CSF ANALYSIS

At least 1 mL of CSF anticoagulated with ethylenediaminetetra-acetic acid (EDTA) should be submitted for cytologic examination. A slide for this purpose should be prepared within 2 hours of collection by low-speed centrifugation of the sample. Alternatively, cell morphology can be preserved by mixing the sample with an equal volume of 50% ethyl alcohol. Standard chemistry analyses and immunoassays can also be performed on these samples. Normal values are shown in Table 50-2.[4,5] It is important to minimize blood contamination of the sample so that results do not reflect admixture of plasma and CSF. For most purposes, a red blood cell count of less than 50/μL is acceptable.

DIAGNOSTIC IMAGING EXAMINATION

Survey Radiographs

The primary reference for "Survey Radiographs" is reference 6.

Head

Lateral, oblique, and dorsoventral (in the standing animal) or ventrodorsal (in the anesthetized animal) views of the cranium and associated soft tissues can be obtained with portable film-screen or digital systems. On lateral radiographs, the ovoid shell of the cranial vault is seen. In foals

TABLE 50-2. Reference Values for Equine Cerebrospinal Fluid

Parameter	Adult (AO)*	Adult (LS)*	Neonate (AO)[†]
Specific gravity	1.004-1.008	1.004-1.008	—
WBC count (cells/μL)	0-7	0-7	—
RBC count (cells/μL)	<600	<600	—
Total protein (mg/dL)	10-120	10-120	109 ± 9.7
Albumin (mg/dL)	24-51	24-56	—
IgG (mg/dL)	3.0-8.0	3.0-10.5	—
Glucose (mg/dL)	30-80	40-75	98.8 ± 12.0
Creatine kinase (U/L)	0-8	0-8	—
LDH (U/L)	0-8	0-8	—
AST (U/L)	15-50	15-50	—
Lactic acid (mg/dL)	1.92 ± 0.12	2.3 ± 0.21	—
(mmol/L)	0.21 ± 0.01	0.26 ± 0.01	—
Sodium (mEq/L)	140-150	140-150	148.0 ± 7.2
Potassium (mEq/L)	2.5-3.5	2.5-3.5	3.01 ± 0.17
Chloride (mEq/L)	95-123	95-123	—
Calcium (mg/dL)	2.5-6.0	2.5-6.0	—
Phosphorus (mg/dL)	0.5-1.5	0.5-1.5	—
Urea nitrogen (mg/dL)	5-20	5-20	—

*From Green EM, Kroll RA, Constantinescu GM: Equine cerebrospinal fluid: Analysis, Comp Cont Educ Pract Vet 1993;15:288.
†From Furr MO, Bender H: Cerebrospinal fluid variables in clinically normal foals from birth to 42 days of age, Am J Vet Res 1994;55:781.
AO, from atlantooccipital cerebrospinal fluid; AST, aspartate transaminase; LDH, lactate dehydrogenase; LS, from lumbosacral cerebrospinal fluid, RBC, red blood cell; WBC, white blood cell.

less than 3 months of age, the dorsal profile of the cranial cavity is interrupted by the fontanel. Other relevant structures on lateral radiographs are the petrous temporal bone, basilar bones, occipital condyles, ethmoid turbinates and ethmoid plate, frontal sinus, hyoid apparatus, guttural pouches, soft palate, and epiglottis. Oblique radiographs are useful to separate the paired stylohyoid bones and petrous temporal bones. Ventrodorsal/dorsoventral views compare these structures more directly and also show the tympanic bullae.

The parietal-occipital suture and the synchondrosis between the basisphenoid and basioccipital bones disappear by 5 years of age.

Radiographs of the head are used to diagnose frontal/parietal fractures, fractures or separation of the basilar bones, fractures of the petrous temporal bone, hemorrhage into and around the guttural pouches, soft palate displacement, stylohyoid fractures, and orbital fractures.

Cervical Spine

Radiographic examination of the cervical spine is indicated when there is deformity or palpable abnormality of the neck, ataxia or weakness of the limbs, or neck trauma, stiffness, or pain.

Acceptable views of C1 to C6 are readily obtained in standing horses with the use of portable equipment, especially with fast rare-earth screens, grids, and appropriate film, newer imaging plates used for computed radiography, or direct digital systems. For normal 450-kg horses, more powerful equipment (75 to 100 kV, 75 to 100 mAs) is required for views of C7 to T1. Complete radiographic assessment of the cervical spine of a full-size horse requires four to five overlapping views: occiput and C1, C1 to C3, C3 to C5, C5 to C7, and C7 to T1 (Fig. 50-12). It is very important to obtain true lateral projections, since a slight obliquity complicates interpretation of the image. In anesthetized horses, additional views including lateral-flexed, lateral-extended, and ventrodorsal (C1 to C5 or C6), can be obtained.

The horse has seven cervical vertebrae. The cervical spine of the standing horse adopts a reverse-S shape when viewed from the left, with gradual flexion at the cranial end and extension caudally. Within each vertebra is a rectangular-appearing vertebral *foramen;* the continuous cylinder formed by these foramina is the vertebral *canal.* Absolute values for minimal sagittal diameter, sagittal ratio, and corrected minimal sagittal diameter of the cervical vertebral canal at various levels have been reported. Measurement of sagittal diameter is used to detect stenosis of the vertebral canal[7-9] and is described in detail in Chapter 51.

The atlas (C1) has no body or articular processes. The axis (C2) has a large dorsal spinous process and a cranially projecting dens (odontoid process). There are separate ossification centers for the dens, head, body, and caudal epiphysis of C2. The body of each of the C3 to C7 vertebrae has cranial and caudal epiphyses, and there is an extra center of ossification in the ventral processes of C6. The transverse processes of C6 differ from those of C3 to C5 by presenting an additional ventral process. This ventral process contributes to the ventral profile of C6 in lateral projections. The

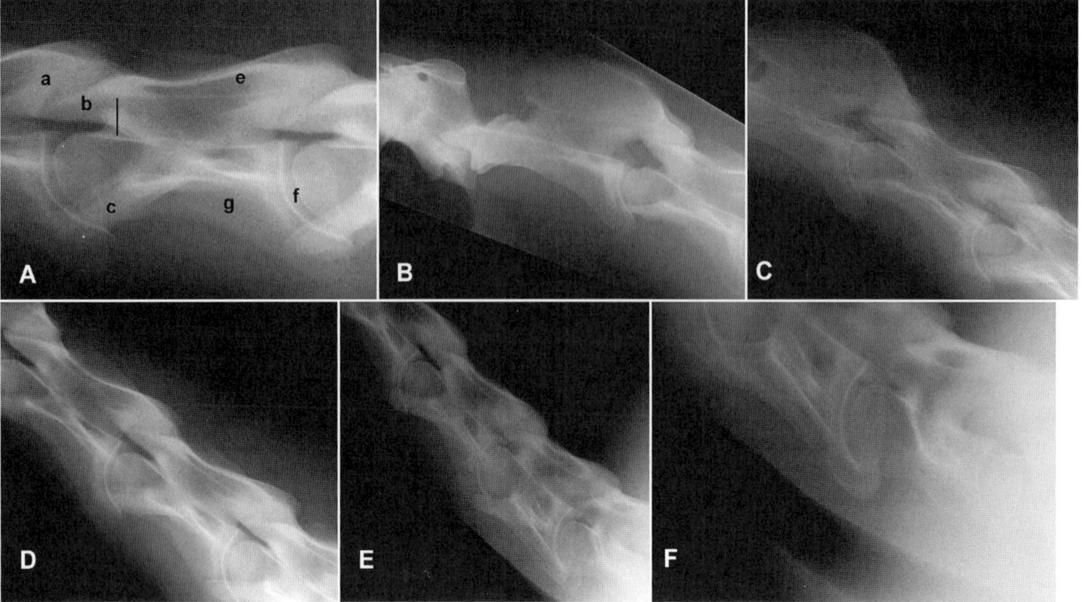

Figure 50-12. Survey radiographs of the neck of a standing normal horse. **A,** Fifth cervical vertebra. a, caudal articular process; b, cranial articular process; c, transverse process (cranial branch); d, vertebral body; e, dorsal lamina; f, intervertebral disc space; g, vertebral body. The *line* shows the sagittal diameter of the vertebral foramen. **B** to **F,** Five overlapping views of a complete cervical series. (Courtesy Dr. Greg Roberts, University of Florida.)

caudal aspect of each of the bodies of C3 to C7 is smoothly concave and accommodates the convex cranial aspect of the next vertebra caudally. Intervertebral discs are radiolucent and of uniform width dorsal to ventral. The cranial and caudal articular processes of C3 to C7 form pairs of true articulations (facet joints) that are visible as smooth ovoid radiodense structures at the dorsal aspect of each intervertebral foramen. C7 is a relatively short vertebra with a small dorsal spinous process. In most horses, the dens fuses with the head of C2 at about 7 months of age, and the cranial and caudal physes of C3 to C7 close by 2 and 5 years, respectively.

Vertebral abnormalities including occipitoatlantoaxial malformation, cervical stenotic myelopathy, degenerative arthritis of the facet joints, osteomyelitis, fracture, discospondylitis, and multiple myeloma are examples of cervical spinal diseases that can be diagnosed in plain radiographs (see Chapter 51).

Thoracolumbar Spine

Thoracolumbar radiography may be performed on horses that have a history of trauma to the back, deformity of the back, acute or chronic back pain, or signs of limb weakness and ataxia that localize to this area.

Radiography of this area of the spine is difficult and requires specialized and powerful (75 to 120 kV, 100 to 250 mAs) equipment, and fast rare-earth screens and grids or computed radiograph cassettes. With this equipment, it is technically possible to obtain lateral views from T1 to L3. Caudal to L3, superimposition of the ilial wings over the lumbar vertebrae precludes useful views. Ventrodorsal images from about T9 to L6 are possible in anesthetized horses. For all areas of the thoracolumbar spine, two lateral exposures are needed for film-screen systems: one optimized for the vertebral bodies and one for the dorsal spinous process. In some cases, separate processing algorithms can be used to obtain optimized images of bodies and spinous processes from a single exposure when a computed radiography system is used.

There are 18 thoracic vertebrae and usually six lumbar vertebrae. Some horses and all donkeys have only five lumbar vertebrae. Vertebral bodies are rectangular and the vertebral canal is of uniform sagittal diameter throughout. Disc spaces are curved and of uniform thickness, whereas facet joints vary over the length of the thoracolumbar spine. Thoracic and lumbar facet joints are difficult to image on lateral radiographs. In thoracic vertebrae, ribs articulate dorsal to the disc spaces. The dorsal spinous processes of the thoracic vertebrae increase in length to T6 or T7 and become shorter in the more caudally located vertebrae. Separate ossification centers are present in the dorsal spinous processes of T2 to T8. Thoracic dorsal spinous processes slope caudally, T15 is vertical (anticlinal), and the dorsal spinous processes of lumbar vertebrae slope cranially. The transverse processes of lumbar vertebrae are larger than those of the thoracic vertebrae and can be identified on lateral projections.

The cranial physes close by 12 months and the caudal physes by 4 years of age.

Degenerative joint disease, ossifying spondylosis, osteomyelitis, discospondylitis, and fractures and dislocations can be seen on plain films of the thoracolumbar vertebrae (see Chapter 52).

Sacrococcygeal Spine

Reasons for sacrococcygeal radiography include signs of cauda equina syndrome, and pain or deformity over the sacrum or tail. Lateral views of the sacrum may be obtained with techniques similar to those used for the lumbar

spine. The sacrum is usually poorly resolved because of overlying soft tissues, but the ventral profile can usually be seen as a straight horizontal line. The last segment of the sacrum (usually S5) is variably separated from the main body of the sacrum and may be confused with the first coccygeal vertebra. Ventrodorsal images can be obtained under anesthesia by using the pelvic technique described in Chapter 53. The sacroiliac joints can be seen on this projection.

Scout films of this area are most often useful in horses with signs of cauda equina syndrome caused by sacral or coccygeal fractures or dislocations.

Myelography

Myelography is the technique of introducing contrast material into the subarachnoid space to outline the spinal cord and adjacent structures. In the horse, cervical myelography is commonly used and is indicated when cervical survey films or clinical examinations have suggested the presence of a cervical spinal cord lesion.

Myelography should be performed under general inhalation anesthesia. An NSAID (preferably flunixin meglumine or ketoprofen) should be given prior to the procedure. All of the following views should be completed within 90 minutes, and preferably within 60 minutes. Begin in lateral recumbency and take plain lateral survey films. For these views, the head and neck need to be supported in horizontal position by radiolucent cushions. Perform atlantooccipital cisternal puncture with an 18-gauge 8.3-cm (3.5-inch) needle as described earlier. Connect a short extension tube to the needle and slowly withdraw 10 mL CSF per 100 kg bodyweight (i.e., 50 mL in a 500-kg horse). Retain a sample of CSF for analysis. Next, inject the same volume of contrast material (iopamidol or iohexol) into the subarachnoid space at constant rate over 5 minutes. Withdraw the needle, then elevate the head and neck at approximately 30 degrees from the horizontal and allow another 5 minutes for caudal flow of contrast material to occur. Bring the head and neck back to the horizontal position and repeat the radiographs of the cervical spine. Next, tie the horse's head in position to exert flexion pressure focused on the middle of the neck. Radiograph C1 to C5. Retie the head so that the caudal part of the neck is hyperextended, and radiograph C5 to C7 (Fig. 50-13). If indicated, position the horse in dorsal recumbency and take ventrodorsal views. Such views are possible from C1 to the cranial half of C6.

Neutral, flexed, and extended views are examined for evidence of dynamic or static vertebral canal stenosis or extradural compression by soft tissue. Typically, flexion reveals dynamic compression in the middle and cranial part of the neck, whereas extension views are best for dynamic compression in the caudal part of the neck. Criteria for interpretation of myelograms in cases of suspected cervical stenotic myelopathy have been reported and are described in Chapter 51.

NSAID therapy should be continued for 3 to 5 days after the procedure, and the horse should be closely observed and monitored during the first week. Fever and inappetence are common during this period if NSAIDs are not given, and they occasionally occur after NSAIDs are stopped. Seizures occur occasionally, usually within 24 hours of myelography. These are usually controlled with diazepam (0.05 to 0.1 mg/kg IV) and the horse is put on preventative antiseizure medication (e.g., phenobarbital, 5 mg/kg PO twice a day) for at least 7 days.

Computed Tomography

Computed tomography (CT) is a cross-sectional imaging method that provides additional diagnostic information in situations where survey radiography is unsatisfactory.[10] This is particularly true of the skull, where multiple soft-tissue and bony structures are superimposed on each other in two-dimensional radiographic images. Even in the cranial neck, where radiography is very useful, contrast-enhanced CT had

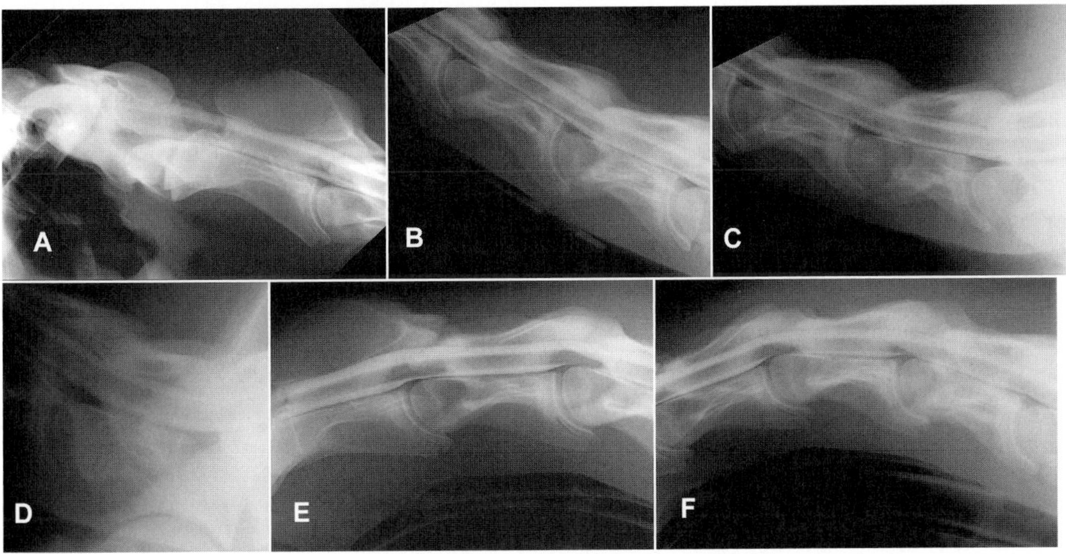

Figure 50-13. Cervical myelographic series in a normal horse. **A** to **C,** The neck is in a neutral position. Note that the transverse processes of C6 in this horse do not have the typical ventral extension. **D,** Now centered caudally, the neck is in extended position. **E** to **F,** Cranial and middle views of the neck in flexed position. (Courtesy Dr. Greg Roberts, University of Florida.)

better specificity for detection of spinal cord compression that did cervical myelography.[11] Compared to radiography, CT can discriminate much smaller differences in density (0.5% versus 10%). The gray matter of the brain can be distinguished from white matter, and acellular fluids can be distinguished from blood and pus.

The principles of CT have been reviewed[10] (see Chapter 75). In brief, CT images are produced in slices by an x-ray beam that rotates in a circular gantry around the object. The gantry and table carrying the patient move in precise relation to each other in a series of increments or slices. Slice thickness is typically 0.4 to 1.0 cm. As in radiographs, images are rendered in gray scale. Iodinated contrast media can be administered to enhance vascular mass lesions and to better detect diseases that disrupt the blood–brain barrier. Intravenous doses for equine CT contrast enhancement have been reported.[12] Data can be reconfigured to produce images in alternative planes or in three dimensions.

CT-based studies of the anatomy of the head in adult horses and foals have been reported.[13,14] The skull and first four or five cervical vertebrae can be imaged in adult horses, whereas the entire body of the neonatal foal can be passed through the gantry (50 to 60 cm in diameter). The technique has been used to detect or evaluate temporohyoid osteoarthropathy, brain abscess, cholesterinic granuloma of the choroid plexus, fracture of the basisphenoid and calvaria, and guttural pouch disease.[15]

Magnetic Resonance Imaging

Magnetic resonance imaging (MRI) of the skull and spine is a cross-sectional imaging technique that is less widely available than CT[10,15] (see Chapter 76). The strong magnets (0.5 to 1.5 tesla) required for this type of imaging preclude the use of "standing" units designed for imaging of distal limbs. Horses must be anesthetized and all metallic objects removed.

MRI provides a gray-scale map of the behavior of tissue protons in a strong magnetic field, and it yields cross-sectional slices in any plane. Data can be used to reconstruct images in three dimensions. T1-weighted images reveal fine anatomic detail but lack tissue contrast. T2-weighted images are grainier than T1-weighted images, but they are more useful for detection of fluid and pathologic change. Additional contrast during T1 pulse sequence can be provided by injection of gadolinium.

Reference studies for the head have been published, and cases of intracranial neoplasia, abscesses, temporohyoid osteoarthropathy, hydrocephalus, and cholesterinic granuloma have been diagnosed.[15] MRI is generally regarded as superior to CT for soft tissue images, whereas CT is better for bone images.

ELECTRODIAGNOSTIC TECHNIQUES

Electromyography

Needle electromyography (EMG) is the diagnostic recording of the electrical activity of muscle.[16] The EMG records spontaneous activity and response to needle insertion, voluntary or reflex muscle activity, and nerve stimulation. Abnormal results are consistent with muscle damage or motor denervation of at least 2 weeks' duration.[1] Use of the EMG allows objective mapping of the size and margins of involved muscle. This is discussed more fully in Chapter 87.

Electromyography requires needle electrodes, amplifier, cathode-ray oscilloscope, and speaker. Concentric and monopolar electrodes combine reference, ground, and exploring electrodes in different combinations. The examination can be performed standing, with or without sedation, or under general anesthesia. After the needle is pushed into muscle, insertional activity, motor unit action potentials (MUAPs) during muscle contraction, and abnormal spontaneous activity are measured. Normal and abnormal responses have been described for horses. Abnormal responses include fibrillations, fasciculation potentials, positive sharp waves, complex repetitive discharges, and myotonic discharges. Each of these has characteristic electrical profiles and sounds. Reference values for amplitude and duration of normal MUAPs in conscious horses have been published.[17,18] Values for horses with myopathies differed markedly from these normal values, and it is expected that values in denervated muscle would also be abnormal.

Nerve conduction studies combine nerve stimulation with EMG recording to evaluate conduction speeds in large motor nerves. These studies are performed under general anesthesia. Techniques have been described for the radial and median nerves in horses, and tibial nerve testing has been performed in horses with stringhalt.

Electroencephalography

Electrical activity arising from the cerebral cortex is recorded by subcutaneous electrodes inserted over the frontal/parietal area and displayed graphically on paper or captured for computerized analysis. Electroencephalography (EEG) is a useful tool for determining the presence, location, and extent of cerebral disease. Because of the expanded use of CT and MRI for evaluation of brain disease, the EEG is now used less frequently than it was 20 years ago.

Evoked Response Testing

The integrity of various parts of the central and peripheral nervous systems can be tested by providing a stimulus at one site and recording the electrical activity at another site. Techniques that have been used in horses include magnetic motor-evoked potentials, brain-stem auditory-evoked responses, and cortical somatosensory-evoked potentials.[19-21]

REFERENCES

1. Mayhew IG: The equine spinal cord in health and disease, Proc Am Assoc Equine Pract 1999;45:56.
2. Blythe LL, Kitchell RL: Electrophysiologic studies of the thoracic limb of the horse, Am J Vet Res 1982;43:1511.
3. Mayhew IG: Large Animal Neurology: A Handbook for Veterinary Clinicians, Philadelphia, 1989, WB Saunders.
4. Green EM, Kroll RA, Constantinescu GM: Equine cerebrospinal fluid: Analysis. Comp Cont Educ Pract Vet 1993;15:288.
5. Furr MO, Bender H: Cerebrospinal fluid variables in clinically normal foals from birth to 42 days of age, Am J Vet Res 1994;55:781.
6. Butler JA, Colles CM, Dyson SJ, et al: Clinical radiology of the horse, ed 2, Oxford, 2000, Blackwell Science.
7. Moore BR, Reed SM, Biller DS, et al: Assessment of vertebral canal

diameter and bony malformations of the cervical part of the spine in horses with cervical stenotic myelopathy, Am J Vet Res 1994;55:5.

8. van Biervliet J, Scrivani PV, Divers TJ, et al: Evaluation of decision criteria for detection of spinal cord compression based on cervical myelography in horses: 38 cases (1981-2001), Equine Vet J 2004;36:14.
9. Mayhew IG, Donawick WJ, Green SL, et al: Diagnosis and prediction of cervical vertebral malformation in Thoroughbred foals based on semi-quantitative radiographic indicators, Equine Vet J 1993;25:435.
10. Kraft SL, Gavin P: Physical principles and technical considerations for equine computed tomography and magnetic resonance imaging, Vet Clin North Am Equine Pract 2001;17:115.
11. Moore BR, Holbrook TC, Stefanacci JD, et al: Contrast-enhanced computed tomography and myelography in six horses with cervical stenotic myelopathy, Equine Vet J 1992;24:197.
12. Allen JR, Barbee DD, Boulton CR, et al: Brain abscess in a horse: Diagnosis by computed tomography and successful surgical treatment, Equine Vet J 1987;19:552.
13. Smallwood JE, Wood BC, Taylor WE, et al: Anatomic reference for computed tomography of the head of the foal, Vet Radiol Ultrasound 2002;43:99.
14. Morrow KL, Park RD, Spurgeon TL, et al: Computed tomographic imaging of the equine head, Vet Radiol Ultrasound 2000;41:491.
15. Tucker RL, Farrell E: Computed tomography and magnetic resonance imaging of the equine head, Vet Clin North Am Equine Pract 2001;17:131.
16. Andrews FM, Fenner WR: Indication and use of electrodiagnostic aids in neurologic disease, Vet Clin North Am Equine Pract 1987;3:293.
17. Wijnberg ID, Franssen H, Jansen GH, et al: Quantitative electromyographic examination in myogenic disorders of 6 horses, J Vet Intern Med 2003;17:185.
18. Wijnberg ID, Franssent H, van der Kolk JH, et al: Quantitative motor unit action potential analysis of skeletal muscles in the Warmblood horse, Equine Vet J 2002;34:556.
19. Nollet H, Deprez P, van Ham L, et al: Transcranial magnetic stimulation: Normal values of magnetic motor evoked potentials in 84 normal horses and influence of height, weight, age and sex, Equine Vet J 2004;36:51.
20. Mayhew IG, Washbourne JR: A method of assessing auditory and brainstem function in horses, Br Vet J 1990;146:509.
21. Strain GM, Taylor DS, Graham MC, et al: Cortical somatosensory-evoked potentials in the horse, Am J Vet Res 1988;49:1869.

CHAPTER 51

Developmental Vertebral Anomalies

Bonnie R. Rush

Cervical stenotic myelopathy (CSM) and occipitoatlantoaxial malformation (OAAM) are the most notable abnormalities of the vertebral column of the horse. Other congenital vertebral anomalies, such as hemivertebrae, block vertebrae, and spina bifida, occur rarely in horses, with individual reports involving a small number of foals. The pathogenesis of vertebral malformations is largely unknown, but it is suspected to be multifactorial, including heredity, dietary imbalance, and in utero insult (trauma and toxin). After a brief description of normal vertebral development, the clinical presentation and pathogenesis of vertebral malformations and anomalies are described.

NORMAL VERTEBRAL DEVELOPMENT

The critical phase of vertebral development is during gastrulation (the formation of the three primary germ layers: ectoderm, mesoderm, and endoderm) and neurulation (the formation of the notochord, neural crest, and the precursors of the nervous system).[1] The spine has its embryologic origins in the cell that is induced to migrate out of the somite, toward the notochord and the neural tube. A mass of sclerotomal cells collect segmentally at the embryonic midline, surrounding the neural tube and the notochord, and these cells begin to separate into a cranial portion and a caudal portion. Failure of segmentation produces a *block vertebra*. The cranial portion of each sclerotome recombines with the caudal portion of the directly superior sclerotome in a resegmentation process known as metameric shift. Failure of recombination produces *hemivertebrae*.[1] After the metameric shift, spinal nerves, which originally left the neural tube to go to the center of the sclerotome, are able to pass between the precartilaginous vertebral bodies to innervate the segmentation myotomes.

The atlas and axis form by a mechanism that is different from that of the other vertebral bodies. Part of the first cervical sclerotome plus the cranial portion of the second cervical sclerotome contribute cells to form the odontoid process and the arch of the atlas.[2] In the cervical region, eight cervical somites generate seven cervical vertebrae because the cranial portion of the first cervical sclerotome contributes to the formation of the occiput, and the caudal portion of the eighth cervical sclerotome contributes to T1. This is the process by which eight cervical spinal nerves become associated with seven cervical vertebrae.[1] Because the occiput, atlas, and axis are formed from shared sclerotomes, developmental abnormalities of these structures occur concomitantly, as in *occipitoatlantoaxial malformation* of Arabian foals. The first cervical spinal nerve passes between the base of the skull and the first cervical vertebra. The eighth cervical nerve exits below the seventh cervical vertebra and above the first thoracic vertebra. The reminder of the nerve roots exit below their corresponding vertebral bodies.

As the sclerotomes undergo shift to form the vertebral bodies, the adjacent visceral organs are differentiating, so that a noxious influence affecting development of a particular vertebral segment may affect adjacent organs at the same time. Hence, cardiac anomalies may occur with congenital malformation of the thoracic spine, and renal anomalies may be associated with congenital malformation of the lumbar spine. During axial embryogenesis, interdependence exists between the spinal cord and the axial skeleton. If this balance is distorted by genetic, traumatic, toxic, or nutritional factors, a malformation may occur. The type of malformation depends on the stage of development of the nervous system at the time of insult.[3] Vertebral anomalies can be divided into three categories from the standpoint of basic developmental pathogenesis: malformation, disruption, and deformation.[4]

Malformation results from a failure of embryologic differentiation of a specific anatomic structure, causing it to be absent or improperly formed during the embryonic stage of gestation. Hemivertebrae, butterfly vertebrae, and block vertebrae are examples of malformation abnormalities. Once the malformed vertebra is anatomically established, the defect may continue to adversely affect spinal development throughout the subsequent fetal and postnatal periods. The eventual type of malformation and its severity depend on the stage of the developmental or maturation cycle that is specifically affected.

Disruption is a structural defect resulting from destruction of an anatomic part during the fetal stage of gestation that formed normally during the embryonic period. This mechanism involves distal structures (e.g., flexural limb deformity or wry nose) more frequently than the axial skeleton.

Deformation is defined as alteration in the shape or structure of an individual vertebra or vertebral segment that had initially differentiated normally, during the fetal and/or postnatal periods (e.g., cervical stenotic myelopathy). Deformation abnormalities are not considered true congenital abnormalities.

CERVICAL STENOTIC MYELOPATHY

Etiology

Cervical stenotic myelopathy (CSM) (cervical vertebral malformation, wobbler syndrome) is a common cause of spinal ataxia in young horses. This developmental disorder is characterized by postnatal deformation of the cervical vertebrae, resulting in vertebral deformation, stenosis of the vertebral canal, and spinal cord compression.[5-7] The etiology of CSM appears to be multifactorial, and genetic predisposition and nutrition appear to play the most significant roles in the development of the disease.[7-9] Cervical stenotic myelopathy has been reported in most light and draft horse breeds, however, Thoroughbreds appear particularly predisposed. Male horses are more frequently affected than females by a ratio of 3:1. The age of onset is typically 6 months to 3 years, although mature horses (4 to 20 years) are identified with acute-onset of spinal cord compression because of cervical stenosis and arthropathy.[10] Affected horses often demonstrate rapid growth and are more likely to have developmental orthopedic disease of the appendicular skeleton than peers.[8]

Vertebral deformation associated with spinal cord compression includes flaring of the caudal epiphyses of the vertebral bodies, abnormal ossification of the articular facets, malalignment between adjacent vertebrae, osteoarthritis of the articular facets, and extension of the dorsal laminae.[11] In addition to these bony deformations, the vertebral canal is narrowed from C3 through C6, regardless of the specific site of spinal cord compression.[12] Spinal cord compression nearly always occurs in a dorsoventral plane, although lateral compression of the spinal cord has been demonstrated via computed tomography. Caudal epiphyseal flare occurs secondary to abnormal biomechanical forces on the vertebral growth plate because of subluxation and malalignment between adjacent vertebrae. Vertebral subluxation produces dynamic compression of the spinal cord during ventroflexion and is most commonly observed at C3-4, C4-5, and C5-6. Extension of the dorsal laminae contributes to spinal cord compression, because it ventrally displaces the roof of the vertebrae to produce a funnel shape, or "coning," of the vertebral canal.[11] Abnormal ossification of the articular facets often results from osteochondrosis of the joint surface, which quickly progresses to osteoarthritis.[11] Degenerative arthropathy of the articular processes occurs most frequently from C5 through C7 and is associated with spinal cord compression with the neck in the neutral (static) or hyperextended position.

Histopathologic evaluation of the spinal cord reveals necrosis of the white matter, with focal loss of neurons. Neuronal fiber (Wallerian) degeneration is observed in ascending tracts cranial to the site of compression and descending tracts caudal to the site of compression.[6]

Clinical Signs

The clinical signs of CSM result from focal compression of the cervical spinal cord between C1 and C7. Compression may occur at a single vertebral site or at more than one site in the same horse. Horses with CSM demonstrate upper motor neuron deficits to all four limbs, characterized by symmetric weakness, ataxia, and spasticity.[3] At rest, affected horses may have a base-wide stance and demonstrate delayed responses to proprioceptive positioning. At a walk, weakness is manifested by stumbling and toe dragging; horses with prolonged clinical signs of CSM may have hooves or shoes that are chipped, worn, or squared at the toe. Ataxia (proprioceptive loss) appears as truncal sway at a walk and is manifested by circumduction and posting (pivoting on the inside limb) of the hind limbs during circling. Moderate to severely affected horses have lacerations on the heel bulbs ("wobbler heels") and medial aspect of their forelimbs from overreaching and interference. Spasticity, characterized by a stiff-legged gait and decreased joint flexion, is often observed in moderately affected horses. Clinical signs can be exaggerated during the neurologic examination by manipulation such as tight circling, walking on a slope, or walking with the animal's head elevated. When prompted to back, horses may stand base-wide, lean backward, and drag their forelimbs. In most instances, the rear limbs are more severely affected than the forelimbs; neuronal tracts to the rear limbs are more superficial and thus susceptible to external compression. Occasionally, forelimb ataxia may be more severe in horses with stenosis of the caudal cervical vertebrae (C6 through C7) because of compression of the cervical intumescence.

Asymmetric ataxia may be observed in horses with dorsolateral compression of the spinal cord by proliferative, degenerative articular processes; periarticular soft tissue proliferation; or a synovial cyst.[13] Rarely, clinical signs of nerve root compression are seen, such as cervical pain, atrophy of the cervical musculature, cutaneous hypalgesia, and hyporeflexia of cervical reflexes adjacent to the site of spinal cord compression.[14] These signs are more commonly observed in horses over 4 years of age with moderate to severe arthropathy of the caudal cervical vertebrae (C5 through C7), and result from peripheral nerve compression by proliferative articular processes as the nerve root exits the vertebral canal through the intervertebral foramen.[5] In some instances, arthropathy of the caudal cervical vertebrae may produce cervical pain and forelimb lameness as a result of peripheral nerve compression, without producing clinical signs of spinal cord compression.[15] Affected horses typically travel with a short cranial phase of the stride and a low foot arc of one or both forelimbs, and they may stand or travel with their head and neck extended.

Diagnosis

The diagnosis of CSM requires collection of an accurate history, thorough physical and neurologic examinations, and radiographic evaluation of the cervical vertebrae.[7] The clinical signs of spinal cord compression often progress for a brief period and then stabilize.[5-7] Owners often report a traumatic incident with the onset of clinical signs of CSM. The traumatic incident may be the result of mild neurologic deficits, with the injury exacerbating the clinical signs of spinal cord compression. The following neurologic disorders should be considered differential diagnoses for cervical stenotic myelopathy: equine protozoal myeloencephalitis (EPM), equine degenerative myeloencephalopathy (EDM), equine herpesvirus myelitis, occipitoatlantoaxial malformation, spinal cord trauma, vertebral fracture, and vertebral abscess. Cerebrospinal fluid analysis may be performed during the diagnostic process, and it is usually unremarkable in horses with CSM. In CSM-affected horses with acute compression, mild xanthochromia or increases in protein concentration may be observed.

Assessment of plain film radiographs of the cervical vertebrae can determine the likelihood of CSM in horses with spinal ataxia.[12] Cervical radiographs should be evaluated for subjective assessment of vertebral deformation and objective determination of vertebral canal diameter. The five characteristic deformations of the cervical vertebrae in horses with CSM include flare of the caudal epiphysis of the vertebral body, abnormal ossification of the articular processes, subluxation between adjacent vertebrae, extension of the dorsal laminae, and osteoarthritis of the articular processes[16] (Figs. 51-1 and 51-2). Osteoarthritis of the caudal cervical vertebrae is the most frequent and severe deformation observed in CSM-affected horses. Nonetheless, degenerative arthropathy occurs in 10% to 50% of non-ataxic horses, and it is the most frequent and severe vertebral deformation in horses without CSM.[17] Therefore, subjective evaluation of osteoarthritis of the articular processes leads to a false-positive diagnosis of CSM. Although the presence of characteristic deformations supports the diagnosis of cervical stenotic myelopathy, subjective evaluation of cervical radiographs does not reliably discriminate between CSM-affected and unaffected horses.[18] Objective assessment of the vertebral canal diameter is more accurate than subjective

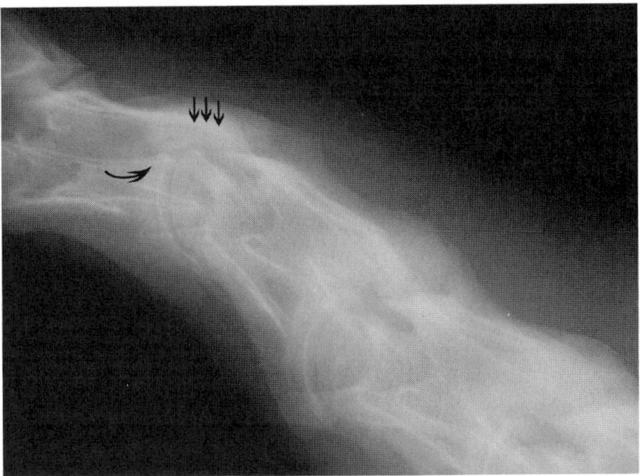

Figure 51-1. Lateromedial cervical radiograph of a 2-year-old Quarter Horse filly with spinal ataxia as a result of cervical stenotic myelopathy (CSM). Bony deformations consistent with CSM include flare of the caudal epiphysis *(curved arrow)*, caudal extension of the C3 dorsal lamina *(arrows)*, and malalignment of the C3-to-C4 articulation.

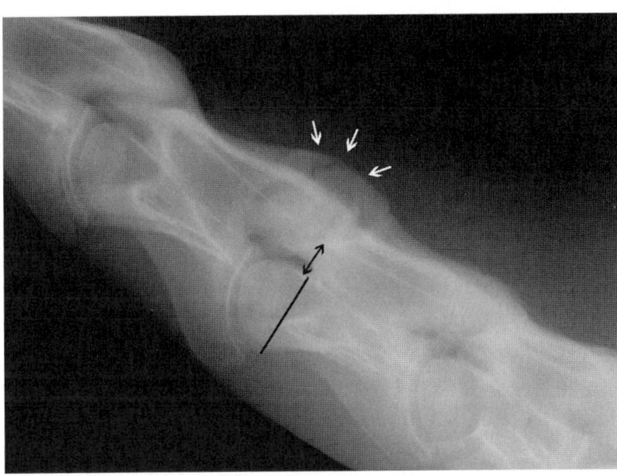

Figure 51-2. Lateromedial cervical radiograph of a 13-month-old Thoroughbred filly with spinal ataxia as a result of static spinal cord compression at C4-5. Severe osteoarthritis of the articular processes *(arrows)* is present at C4-5, and moderate osteoarthritis of the articular processes is seen at C5-6. The sagittal ratio is determined by dividing the intravertebral minimal sagittal diameter *(double arrow)* by the width of the vertebral body *(line)*, as demonstrated using C5 in this radiograph.

evaluation of vertebral deformation for identification of CSM-affected horses.

The sagittal ratio technique has been developed to objectively determine the vertebral canal diameter in horses.[12] The sensitivity and specificity of the sagittal ratio for identification of CSM-affected horses is approximately 89% for vertebral sites C4 through C7.[7] The accuracy of the sagittal ratio technique for identification of CSM-affected horses, without consideration of other bony malformations of the cervical vertebrae, suggests that generalized stenosis of the vertebral canal may be the most important factor in the development of CSM. The sagittal ratio is calculated by dividing the minimal sagittal diameter of the vertebral canal by the width of the vertebral body. The minimal sagittal diameter of the vertebral canal is obtained by determining the narrowest diameter measured from the dorsal aspect of the vertebral body to the ventral border of the dorsal laminae (see Fig. 51-2). The vertebral body width is measured perpendicular to the vertebral canal at the widest point of the cranial aspect of the vertebral body. Because the vertebral body is located within the same anatomic plane as the vertebral canal, determination of this proportion negates the effects of magnification that result from variability in object-to-film distance. The sagittal ratio should exceed 52% from C4 through C6, and 56% at C7 in horses greater than 320 kg. The clinician should interpret radiographic examination of the cervical vertebrae to classify the patient into one of the following categories:

1. Low sagittal ratio (less than 48% at C4 through C6), moderate to severe bony deformation. Perform myelographic examination to identify sites of spinal cord compression and classify lesions as static or dynamic.
2. Marginal sagittal ratio (48% through 56%), mild to moderate bony deformation. Perform myelographic examination to confirm or exclude CSM.
3. High sagittal ratio (greater than 56%), minimal bony deformation. Pursue alternative differential diagnoses.

The semiquantitative scoring system developed by Mayhew should be used in foals less than 1 year of age to assess cervical radiographs for diagnosis of CSM.[16] The scoring system combines the objective measurement of vertebral canal diameter and subjective evaluation of vertebral deformation. Stenosis of the vertebral canal is assessed by determination of the intervertebral and intravertebral minimal sagittal diameter (MSD). These values are corrected for radiographic magnification by dividing them by the length of the vertebral body. The maximal score for cervical vertebral stenosis is 10 points. Cervical vertebral deformation is determined by subjective assessment of five categories: encroachment of the caudal epiphysis of the vertebral body dorsally into the vertebral canal, caudal extension of the dorsal lamina to the cranial physis of the adjacent vertebra, angulation between adjacent vertebral bodies, abnormal ossification of the physis, and osteoarthritis of the articular processes. The maximal score allotted for each category of bony deformation is 5 points. A total score of 12 or higher (maximal total score, 35) confirms the radiographic diagnosis of CSM. Stenosis of the vertebral canal and malalignment between adjacent vertebrae are the most discriminating parameters in this scoring system to differentiate CSM-affected from normal foals.

Accurate assessment of cervical radiographs requires a precise lateral radiograph of the cervical vertebrae. Obliquity of the cervical vertebrae results in indistinct margins of the ventral aspect of the vertebral canal, producing erroneous values for MSD and vertebral body width. It is difficult to obtain precise lateral radiographs of the cervical vertebrae in recumbent horses. Plain film radiographs should be obtained in the standing sedated horse whenever possible.

Although plain film radiography can determine the likelihood of CSM, it cannot replace myelographic examination for definitive diagnosis, identification of the location, number of affected sites, and classification of spinal cord compressive lesions in horses with CSM. Spinal cord compression has been defined myelographically in three ways: (1) as a 50% or greater decrease in the sagittal diameter of the dorsal and ventral contrast columns,[19] (2) as a 20% reduction in the dural diameter,[20] or (3) as a dorsal contrast column of less than 2 mm.[19] Methods that use a relative decrease in contrast column as diagnostic criteria (i.e., 1 and 2) compare the suspected site to the mid-vertebral site, cranial or caudal to the compressed site. The ventral column, however, is often obliterated at the intervertebral space in normal studies, particularly in the flexed position. The author prefers to use a 20% reduction in the dural diameter as the diagnostic criterion for CSM. Most clinicians agree that the criterion of a less-than-2-mm dorsal contrast column is too rigid, resulting in a high number of false-negative diagnoses.

In addition to providing the definitive diagnosis of CSM, myelographic examination can differentiate between dynamic (type I) and static (type II) spinal cord compression.[19] Horses with dynamic spinal cord compression (type I) demonstrate narrowing of the dorsal and ventral contrast columns during ventroflexion of the neck, whereas spinal cord compression is not apparent with the neck in the neutral position (Fig. 51-3). Dynamic spinal cord compression usually occurs in younger horses (less than 2 years old) and is associated with instability of the cervical vertebrae, particularly from C3 through C6. Dorsal laminar extension, caudal epiphyseal flare, and abnormal ossification patterns often occur in horses with dynamic spinal cord compression. Static vertebral canal stenosis (type II) is characterized by constant spinal cord compression, regardless of cervical position (Fig. 51-4). Static compression usually occurs in slightly older horses (2 to 4 years) and results from osteoarthritis of the articular processes and proliferation of periarticular soft tissue structures. In some cases of caudal cervical arthropathy, flexion of the neck stretches the ligamentum flavum and relieves spinal cord compression, whereas extension exacerbates compression.

A complete myelographic study should include neutral and stressed (flexed and extended) views of the cervical

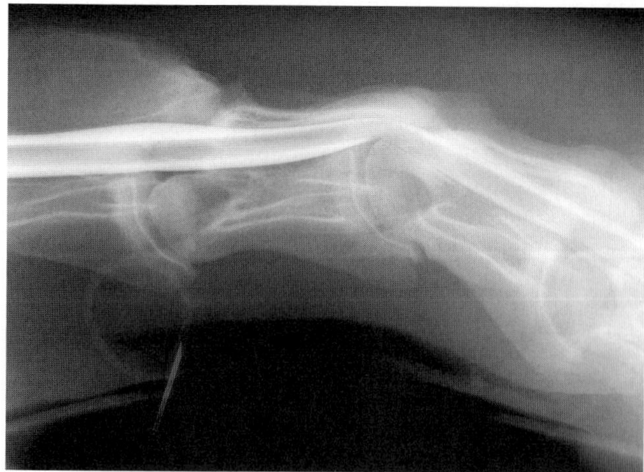

Figure 51-3. Myelographic examination of C2 through C4 of a 2-year-old Quarter Horse filly with dynamic spinal cord compression between the C3 and C5 articulations. The dorsal and ventral contrast columns are obliterated with the neck in the ventroflexed position. Spinal cord compression was not apparent with the neck in the neutral position (not shown).

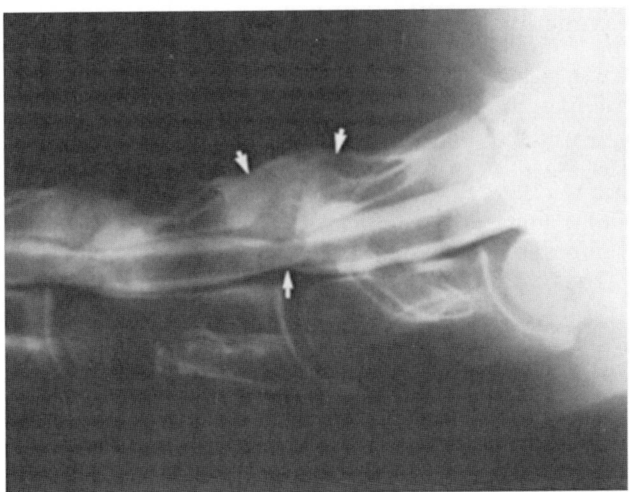

Figure 51-4. Osteoarthritis of the articular processes of C6-7 *(paired arrows)* producing static spinal cord compression *(lower arrow)*.

vertebrae.[19] In horses with obvious sites of spinal cord compression on neutral myelographic views, excessive flexion and extension of the neck should be avoided while obtaining dynamic views to prevent exacerbation of spinal cord injury. Horses should be monitored for 24 hours after the myelographic procedure for depression, fever, seizure, and worsening in neurologic status. Worsening of the neurologic status after myelography may result from spinal cord trauma during hyperflexion, iatrogenic puncture of the spinal cord, or chemical meningitis. Administration of phenylbutazone (4.4 mg/kg PO every 24 hours) 1 day prior to and through 1 day after the myelographic examination will attenuate fever and depression associated with chemical meningitis.

Treatment

Nutritional Adjustments

Successful conservative management of CSM has been achieved using the "paced diet" program in foals less than 1 year of age.[21] The goal of this dietary program is to retard bone growth, enhance bone metabolism, and allow the vertebral canal diameter to enlarge to relieve spinal cord compression. Serial radiographic examinations demonstrate improvement in the sagittal ratio; however, osteopenia may be observed. This dietary program is restricted in energy and protein (65% to 75% of National Research Council [NRC] recommendations) but maintains balanced vitamin and mineral intake (minimum, 100% of NRC recommendations). Vitamins A and E are provided at three times NRC recommendations and selenium is supplemented to 0.3 ppm. Roughage is provided by pasture or low-quality (6% to 9% crude protein) Timothy hay. Dietary regimens are individually formulated according to the age and weight of the foal. Solitary stall confinement is recommended to minimize repetitive spinal cord compression because of dynamic instability. This program of dietary management and restricted exercise has been successful for prevention of neurologic signs in foals with radiographic evidence of CSM and treatment of foals demonstrating clinical signs of CSM.[16]

Medical Management

Administration of glucocorticoids, dimethyl sulfoxide, and nonsteroidal anti-inflammatory drugs may reduce edema and provide transient improvement in neurologic signs. Spontaneous recovery from CSM without dietary management or surgical intervention is not reported.[22]

Horses with cervical pain and forelimb lameness as the result of cervical vertebral arthropathy may benefit from intra-articular administration of corticosteroids or chondroprotective agents, or both.[23] Arthrocentesis of the cervical vertebral articulations (facets) is performed with ultrasonographic guidance using a 15-cm (6-inch), 18-gauge spinal needle in the standing sedated or recumbent horse. The cranial facet of the caudal vertebrae appears superficial to the caudal facet of the cranial vertebrae. The articular space is accessed at the cranioventral opening of the articular facet, which is angled approximately 60 degrees from the ultrasound beam. The needle should be introduced 5 cm cranial to the facet and inserted at a 30-degree angle relative to the skin surface. Joint penetration should be confirmed by aspiration of synovial fluid. If the neck is extended, the transverse process of the cranial vertebrae may obscure the path to the articulation. Intra-articular triamcinolone (6 mg per joint) or methylprednisolone (100 mg per joint) has produced a positive clinical response in more than 50% of horses with arthrosis of the articular processes. The goal of intra-articular anti-inflammatory therapy should be to decrease cervical pain or eliminate forelimb lameness. It is unlikely that intra-articular therapy will significantly improve clinical signs of spinal ataxia.

Surgical Management

Surgical treatment of CSM is discussed in detail in Chapter 52.

OCCIPITOATLANTOAXIAL MALFORMATION

Occipitoatlantoaxial malformation occurs most frequently in Arabian foals, although it has been reported in Morgans, Appaloosas, and Thoroughbreds.[24-26] In Arabians, it is inherited in an autosomal recessive manner with no sex predilection.[24,25] In other breeds, a nongenetic congenital defect occurs at random during development of the vertebral column.[26]

In OAAM, the developmental error occurs during embryogenesis, before the end of the 6th week of gestation.[24-26] The atlas of affected foals is characterized by a small vertebral body, vertebral arches, and peglike transverse processes. The atlas is often fused to the occipital bone, resulting in synchondrosis or a barely detectable atlantooccipital joint (occipitalization of the atlas). The odontoid process of the axis (dens) is malformed and hypoplastic. In some cases, the axis may be luxated ventral to the atlas, leading to fracture of the dens. The fusion between the atlas and the occipital bones may be asymmetric, leading to the development of scoliosis (Fig. 51-5).

Clinical Signs and Diagnosis

OAAM may be obvious at birth or detected within the first few weeks of life. Affected animals demonstrate marked

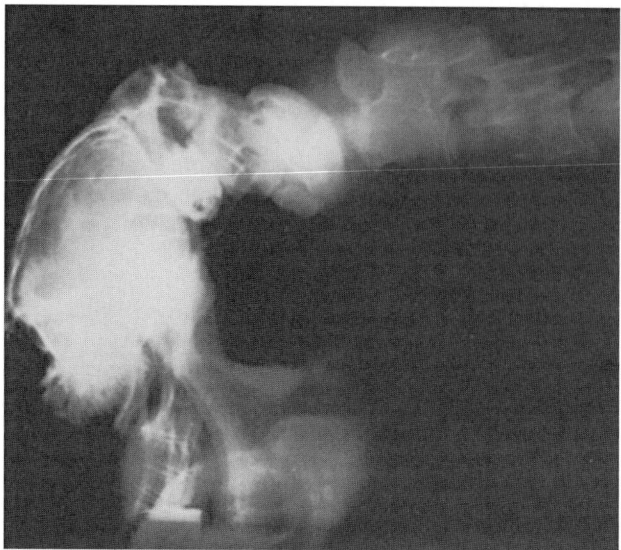

Figure 51-5. Atlantooccipital malformation in an Arabian foal. Note the atlantooccipital fusion, occipitalization of the atlas, and a hypoplastic dens.

weakness and ataxia when walking and may have an extended head and neck. A clicking sound may be elicited by manipulation of the head, resulting from the dens slipping under the body of the atlas.[24-26] Clinical signs worsen over time as a result of repetitive or persistent compression of the spinal cord. The malformed vertebrae lead to the formation of excess fibrous tissue within the atlantoaxial joint and adjacent ligaments, which in turn creates additional compression of the spinal cord.

Pathologic changes of the nervous system associated with OAAM include a dorsoventral flattening of the medulla oblongata and cranial cervical spinal cord. Histolopathologic evaluation of affected neuronal tissue reveals gliosis, astrofibrosis, neuronal fiber degeneration, and perivascular fibrosis.[24]

Treatment

In Arabian foals, euthanasia is recommended because of the heritable nature of the condition. In other breeds, surgical intervention may be used to correct atlantoaxial subluxation and scoliosis. Young horses and foals with malformation of the occiput, atlas, and axis should be managed conservatively if they do not demonstrate neurologic gait deficits.

ATLANTOAXIAL SUBLUXATION

Atlantoaxial subluxation (AAS) results from a developmental abnormality of the odontoid process of the axis (dens), such as malformation, absence, or separation from the axis. The excessive mobility of the atlantoaxial joint results in repetitive or constant spinal cord compression.[27] Congenital absence of the dens, the most extreme from of AAS, produces significant loss of stability between the atlas and the axis.

Clinical Signs and Diagnosis

The clinical signs of AAS include weakness, spasticity, and ataxia in all four limbs, consistent with focal compressive lesions of the cervical spinal cord.[27,28] Progression of signs is quite variable and depends on the degree of laxity between the axis and atlas. Clinical signs may be slowly progressive over weeks to months or may begin acutely, making spinal cord trauma an important differential diagnosis. Severe compression may produce tetraplegia.

The diagnosis may be confirmed by evaluating clinical signs, manipulating and palpating the head and neck, and taking lateral radiographs of the skull and proximal cervical region. A lateral radiograph should be obtained with the horse standing, with little manipulation of the head and neck. Widening of the space between the dorsal portion of the atlas and the axis, and a rounded cranial end of the axis are indicative of an abnormally shaped or absent dens. A myelogram is normally not required.

The prognosis for AAS is poor. Surgical stabilization of the atlantoaxial joint may be attempted as a salvage procedure. Subtotal dorsal laminectomy of the impinging dorsal arch of the atlas has been described in foals with a developmentally malformed dens.[29,30] In addition, a ventral approach for stabilization of AAS resulting from a Salter-Harris type II fracture of the odontoid process has been described[31,32] (see Chapter 53). Medical therapy (glucocorticoids and hyperosmotic agents) should be administered prior to surgical correction to reduce spinal cord swelling and edema. Affected foals should be maintained in a quiet environment with minimal handling to avoid additional trauma to the spinal cord.

ATLANTOAXIAL INSTABILITY

Atlantoaxial instability produces clinical signs in older foals and young horses.[29] Subluxation of the atlas relative to the axis occurs during extension of the head and neck because of malalignment of the atlas, resulting in caudal ventral tilting of the atlas relative to the vertebral canal. The subluxation results from ligamentous laxity and malarticulation. A congenital anomaly has been suggested, although trauma may be an important pathophysiologic factor. This syndrome emphasizes the importance of evaluating this area when examining a young horse with clinical signs of spinal ataxia localized to the cervical region. Treatment is not recommended.

Differential diagnoses for OAAM, AAS, and atlantoaxial instability include cervical trauma, vertebral osteomyelitis after neonatal septicemia, cervical vertebral stenotic myelopathy, and syringomyelia,[33] a congenital malformation of the spinal cord.[2,3]

HEMIVERTEBRAE

Hemivertebrae are wedge-shaped vertebral bodies in which the vertebral body apex may point dorsally, ventrally, or medially, resulting in kyphosis, lordosis, or scoliosis.[2,3,34-39] Moderate to severe angulation of the spine may result in animals with hemivertebrae, and the severity of the malalignment typically worsens during growth as a result of compression by adjacent vertebrae. Hemivertebrae can result from a hemimetameric shift of somites during recombi-

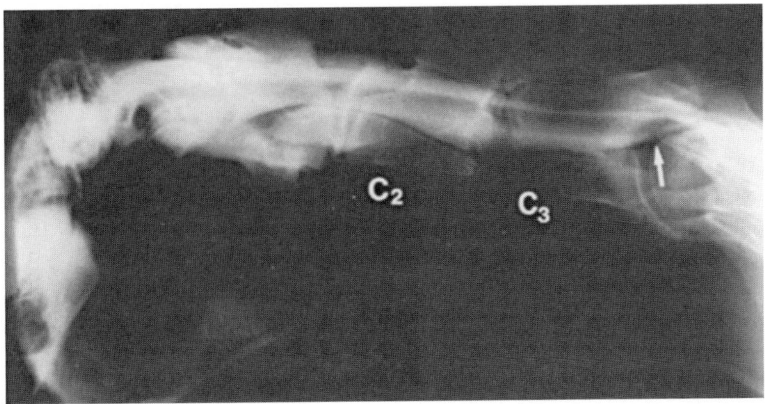

Figure 51-6. Block vertebrae involving C2-3. The block vertebrae are not associated with spinal cord compression, which is present at C3-4.

nation of sclerotomes to form primordial vertebrae,[1] or from a defect of the vascular supply at this developmental stage that results in a failure of half of the vertebral body to ossify.[3] If metameric shift is abnormal, one right and one left hemivertebra will be adjacent to each other. The vertebrae resulting from an alteration in vascular supply may appear as unilateral, dorsal, or ventral hemivertebrae.

In horses, hemivertebrae have been observed at C5, although in most species T7 and T9 are most commonly affected.[35] Clinical signs of hemivertebrae in foals are observed before 1 year of age. Foals demonstrate progressive vertebral malalignment, leading to kyphosis or scoliosis, with or without neurologic gait deficits. Hemivertebrae are often weaker than normal vertebrae; a sudden jump or fall may result in acute worsening of clinical signs.

THORACIC VERTEBRAL MALFORMATION

Malformation and compression of the thoracic vertebrae has been described in two unrelated horses.[40] Both horses appeared normal for the first year of life, with ages of onset being 13 and 28 months. Clinical signs included acute-onset pelvic limb weakness and ataxia in one horse, and severe spinal cord dysfunction and paralysis of the pelvic limbs in the other. Both horses demonstrated Schiff-Sherrington phenomena, characterized by hypertonicity of the thoracic limbs associated with focal thoracic spinal cord compression. This clinical sign has been described in humans and other animals with fracture of the thoracic vertebrae, although it is a rare finding in horses.[41] The malformation of the thoracic vertebrae was similar to malalignment and subluxation observed in horses with cervical stenotic myelopathy.

BLOCK VERTEBRAE

Block vertebrae are examples of improper somite segmentation and appear to be a result of incomplete separation of the vertebral bodies or arches, or both.[1] The length of a block vertebra is equivalent to the number of vertebral segments involved. Block vertebrae are generally stable and do not often result in clinical signs, although the rigid fixation may result in abnormal biomechanical forces on adjacent vertebrae. The sacrum is an example of a normal block vertebra. The most commonly reported location of block vertebrae in humans and animals is C2-3 (Fig. 51-6).

BUTTERFLY VERTEBRAE

Butterfly vertebra is a rare anomaly of the equine vertebral column. The embryonic notochord is normally obliterated with the development of the vertebral bodies and remains only as the vestige of the intervertebral disc. If the notochord persists, a dorsal-to-ventral cleft results, which results in a vertebra that resembles a butterfly on a dorsoventral radiograph. Butterfly vertebrae typically do not cause spinal cord compression and do not require treatment.[1,3]

VERTEBRAL DEFECTS

Spina bifida results from incomplete fusion of the dorsal components of the vertebrae during the neurulation process. It is often associated with a protrusion of the meninges (meningomyelocele) through the vertebral defect. Spina bifida (C5 through C6) with an accompanying meningomyelocele has been identified in a miniature horse foal that was unable to stand at birth.[42] The meningomyelocele appeared as a 5-cm, fluctuant mass of the dorsal aspect of the caudal cervical region. The colt also had hydrocephalus, which is present in the vast majority of children with meningomyelocele as part of the Arnold-Chiari malformation (protrusion of caudal cerebellar tissue through the foramen magnum with concomitant caudal displacement and elongation of the medulla oblongata, pons, and fourth ventricle).

Severe posterior ataxia as the result of a congenital cleft in the ventral aspect of a vertebral body (T5) has been described in an Arabian foal.[43] The foal had malformation and fusion of several thoracic vertebrae, with an intraspinal and extraspinal (intrathoracic) cyst. Therefore, a history of posterior paresis and ataxia present at birth should signal a need to perform a careful examination to search for malformation of the vertebral column in the thoracic region.

REFERENCES

1. Bailey CS: An embryological approach to the clinical significance of congenital vertebral and spinal cord abnormalities, J Am Anim Hosp Assoc 1975;11:426.
2. Vandeplassche M, Simoens P, Bouters R, et al: Aetiology and pathogenesis of congenital torticollis and head scoliosis in the equine fetus, Equine Vet J 1984;16:419.
3. Vandeplassche MM: The pathogenesis of dystocia and fetal malformation in the horse, J Reprod Fertil Suppl 1987;35:547.
4. Icenogle DA, Kaplan AM: A review of congenital neurologic malformations, Clin Pediatr 1981;20:565,
5. Wagner PC, Grant BD, Reed SM: Cervical vertebral malformations, Vet Clin North Am Equine Pract 1987;3:385.
6. Mayhew IG, deLahunta A, Whitlock RH, et al: Spinal cord disease in the horse, Cornell Vet 1978;68(Suppl 6):1.
7. Reed S, Bayly W, Traub J: Ataxia and paresis in horses: Part I. Differential diagnosis, Comp Cont Educ Pract Vet 1981;3:88.
8. Stewart RH, Reed SM, Weisbrode SE: The frequency and severity of osteochondrosis in cervical stenotic myelopathy in horses, Am J Vet Res 1991;52:873.
9. Falco MS, Whitwell K, Palmer AC: An investigation into the genetics of "wobblers disease" in Thoroughbred horses in Britain, Equine Vet J 1976;8:165.
10. Serena A, Murray RC, Blunden A, et al: An unusual cervical vertebral pathology causing ataxia in an aged horse, Ippologia 2002;13:41.
11. Powers BE, Stashak TS, Nixon AJ, et al: Pathology of the vertebral column of horses with cervical static stenosis, Vet Pathol 1986;23:392.
12. Rush Moore B, Reed SM, Biller DS, et al: Assessment of vertebral canal diameter and bony malformations of the cervical part of the spine in horses with cervical stenotic myelopathy, Am J Vet Res 1994;55:5.
13. Fisher LF, Bowman KF, MacHarg MA: Spinal ataxia in a horse caused by a synovial cyst, Vet Pathol 1981;18:407.
14. Rush Moore B, Holbrook, T, Reed, S, et al: Contrast-enhanced computed tomography in six horses with cervical stenotic myelopathy, Equine Vet J 1992;24:197.
15. Ricardi G, Dyson SJ: Forelimb lameness associated with radiographic abnormalities of the cervical vertebrae, Equine Vet J 1993;25:422.
16. Mayhew I, Donawick W, Green S, et al: Diagnosis and prediction of cervical vertebral malformation in Thoroughbred foals based on semi-quantitative radiographic indicators, Equine Vet J 1993;25:435.
17. Whitwell KE, Dyson S: Interpreting radiographs: 8. Equine cervical vertebrae, Equine Vet J 1987;19:8.
18. Papageorges M, Gavin PR, Sande RT, et al: Radiographic and myelographic examination of the cervical vertebral column in 306 ataxic horses, Vet Radiol 1989;28:53.
19. Neuwirth L: Equine myelography, Comp Cont Educ Pract Vet 1992;14:72.
20. Van Biervliet J, Scrivani P, Divers TJ, et al: Evaluation of diagnostic criterion for spinal cord compression during cervical myelography in horses, Proc Am Coll Vet Intern Med Forum 2002;20:769.
21. Donawick WJ, Mayhew IG, Galligan DT, et al: Recognition and non-surgical management of cervical vertebral malformation in foals, Proc Ann Surg Forum 1992;20:103.
22. Moore B, Reed S, Robertson J: Surgical treatment of cervical stenotic myelopathy in horses: 73 cases (1983-1992), J Am Vet Med Assoc 1993;203:108.
23. Grisel RG, Grant BD, Rantanen NW: Arthrocentesis of the equine cervical facets, Proc Am Assoc Equine Pract 1996;42;197.
24. Mayhew IG, Watson AG, Heissan JA: Congenital occipito-atlantoaxial malformations in the horse, Equine Vet J 1978;10:103.
25. Watson AG, Mayhew IG: Familial congenital occipitoatlantoaxial malformation (OAAM) in the Arabian horse, Spine 1986;11:334.
26. Wilson WD, Hughes SJ, Ghoshal NG, et al: Occipitoatlantoaxial malformation in two non-Arabian horses, J Am Vet Med Assoc 1985;187:36.
27. Guffy MM, Coffman JR, Strafuss AC: Atlantoaxial luxation in a foal, J Am Vet Med Assoc 1969;155:754.
28. Funk KA, Erikson EL: A case of atlantoaxial subluxation in a horse, Can Vet J 1968;9:120.
29. Nixon AJ, Stashak TS: Laminectomy for relief of atlantoaxial subluxation in four horses, J Am Vet Med Assoc 1988;193:677.
30. Slone DE, Bergfeld WA, Walker TL: Surgical decompression for traumatic atlantoaxial subluxation in a weanling filly, J Am Vet Med Assoc 1983;183:1266.
31. McCoy DJ, Shires PK, Beadle R: Ventral approach for stabilization of atlantoaxial subluxation secondary to odontoid fracture in a foal, J Am Vet Med Assoc 1984;185:545.
32. Sorzonen DC, Shires PK: Atlantoaxial instability: A ventral surgical technique for decompression, fixation and fusion, Vet Surg 1981;19:22.
33. Cho DY, Leipold HW: Syringomyelia in a Thoroughbred foal, Equine Vet J 1977;9:195.
34. Boyd JS: Congenital deformities in two Clydesdale foals, Equine Vet J 1976;8:161.
35. Klaassen JK, Wagner PC: Congenital vertebral abnormalities in a foal, Equine Pract 1981;3:11.
36. Leathers CW, Wagner PC, Milleson B: Cervical spina bifida with meningocele in an Appaloosa foal, J Vet Orthop 1979;1:55.
37. Rooney JR, Prickett ME: Congenital lordosis of the horse, Cornell Vet 1967;57:417.
38. Rooney JR: Congenital equine scoliosis and lordosis, Clin Orthop Rel Res 1969;62:25.
39. Stecher RM, Goss LJ: Ankylosing lesions of the spine of the horse, J Am Vet Med Assoc 1961;138:248.
40. Johnson P, Johnson G, Pace L: Thoracic vertebral malformation in two horses, Equine Vet J 1997;29:493.
41. Chiapetta JR, Baker JC, Feeney DA: Vertebral fracture, extensor hypertonia of thoracic limbs (Schiff-Sherrington) in an Arabian foal, J Am Vet Med Assoc 1985;186:387.
42. Rivas D, Hinchcliff K, Robertson J: Cervical meningomyelocele associated with spina bifida in a hydrocephalic miniature colt, J Am Vet Med Assoc 1996;209:950.
43. Doige CE: Congenital cleft vertebral centrum and intra- and extraspinal cyst in a foal, Vet Pathol 1996;33:87.

CHAPTER 52

Surgical Treatment of Developmental Diseases of the Spinal Column

Barrie D. Grant
Anja C. Schütte
George W. Bagby

Successful surgical treatments of developmental diseases of the spinal column depend on the most fundamental axiom of medicine: an early, complete, and accurate diagnosis. The etiology and diagnostic techniques have been discussed in Chapters 50 and 51. It is important to emphasize that successful treatment of localized cervical spinal cord compression depends on obtaining myelographic confirmation at the earliest possible time. There are many examples of horses that had had cord compression for 6 months to 1 year and improved dramatically with surgery.[1-4] However, the most gratifying experiences have been when patients were treated surgically within the first 2 to 3 weeks after the recognition of clinical signs. It would be incomplete not to perform cervical myelograms on an animal with neurologic signs attributable to pathology in the cervical cord, even with an obvious subluxation of C2-3 or C3-4 on scout films. It has been the author's (BDG) experience that the routine use of myelography may disclose multiple levels of compression, which play an important role in determining the feasibility of a surgical intervention, prognosis, and eventual outcome. Additionally, horses with clinical signs attributable to spinal cord compression with osteochondritic articular facets at C6-7 on survey radiographs may not suffer from cord compression, but rather may show signs of CNS disease caused by some other condition (e.g., protozoal myelitis).

After a thorough neurologic examination, survey radiographs and measurement of the vertebral-body-to-canal ratio, as well as location of any kyphosis, help to determine further procedures (Fig. 52-1). The authors found that in a majority of cases, when the ratio of the vertebral body width to vertebral canal width was found to be less than 0.5, the likelihood of cervical cord compression at this site is increased (Fig. 52-2). Although this is just a rough estimate, myelographic examinations can show the cervical cord compression at all sites reliably (Fig. 52-3).

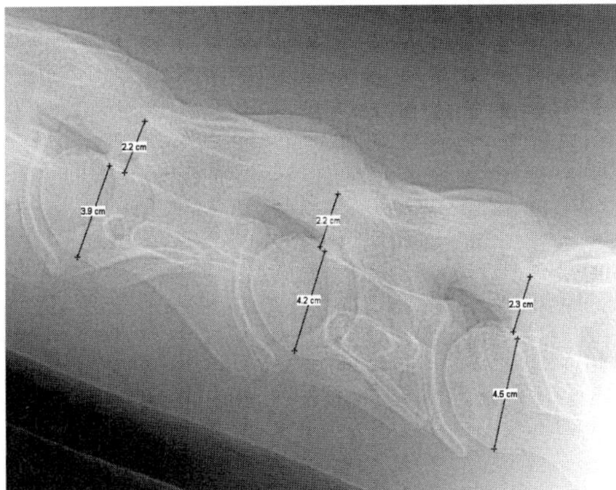

Figure 52-1. Survey radiographs of the cervical spine, showing normal measurements of vertebral-body-to-canal ratios.

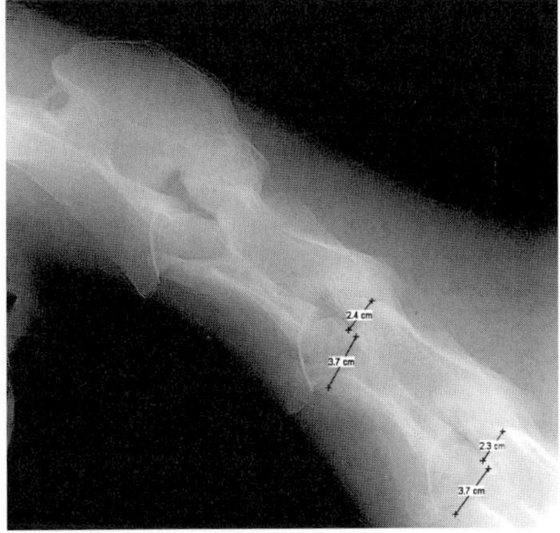

Figure 52-2. Survey radiographs of the cervical spine, showing abnormal vertebral-body-to-canal ratios (see Chapter 51).

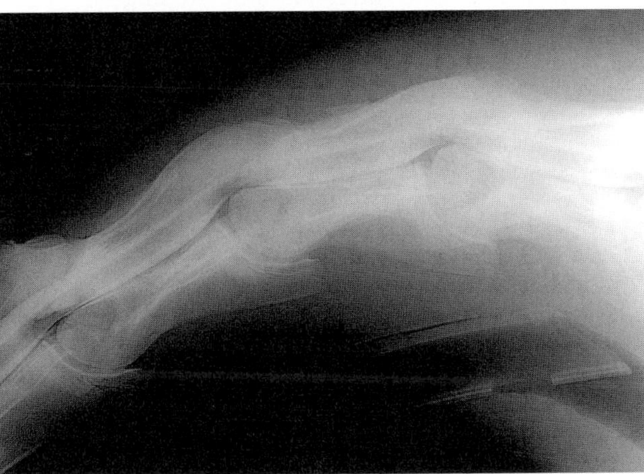

Figure 52-3. Myelogram showing severe cord compression. The prognosis for postsurgical outcome is less favorable than if there had been less cord compression.

CASE SELECTION FOR SURGERY

Once cervical cord compression is confirmed, other factors important to the successful outcome of the case are (1) number of sites of cord compression, (2) whether the cord compression is seen only in a flexed or extended position (i.e., is dynamic or static), (3) severity of the clinical signs, and (4) duration of clinical signs. The duration of the clinical signs may be shorter than the duration of compression, because the onset of clinical signs is not likely to be immediate. The temperament, age, and intended use of the animal also are important factors to consider when discussing surgical alternatives with the owner.

According to recent investigations, only severe myelographic cord compression also causes histopathologically recognizable lesions to the spinal cord.[5] Horses with mild to moderate compression have a more favorable prognosis for future use than horses with severe compression sites. Only 50% of severely affected horses could be ridden after surgery, whereas 68% with initially moderate compression and as many as 100% with mild myelographic compression were used in various riding disciplines after their surgery.[6]

In the ideal situation, an adolescent animal with a grade 1 to 2 ataxia (see Chapter 50) of less than 2 weeks' duration is presented with a single compressive lesion at C3-4, and the cord compression is seen only in a flexed position. The next most desirable case would be a horse with less than grade 2 ataxia, with only a moderate amount of cord compression at C5-6 or C6-7. On the other hand, some affected patients, despite having clinical signs of grade 3 or higher, multiple lesions, and duration of clinical signs extending from 3 weeks to 1 year, have raced and been successful sires or even performance horses after being surgically treated.[7] These, however, are the exception to the rule.

The temperament of the patient is important, because there are personality changes associated with cord compression (probably related to the anxiety of being ataxic): animals may become intractable and sometimes self-destructive. Young animals that have had little handling (e.g., have never had their feet picked up and trimmed) before the onset of clinical signs are at great risk for traumatic complications resulting from the restraint needed during diagnostic testing, anesthetic induction, recovery, and postoperative treatment. It is worth serious consideration to delay surgery for 4 or 5 days to work with an unbroken, adolescent horse to allow it to become confident with human assistance and restraint before surgery.

Surgery should not be performed on a patient heavily infested with parasites or suffering from pneumonia. Such conditions are aggravated by the stress of transportation and anesthesia, the latter being necessary for myelography and surgery. Therefore, a very thorough accurate physical examination, including necessary blood work, is essential prior to any diagnostic testing (e.g., myelography). Any economic or time benefits realized from performing surgery close to the time of myelography are hardly justified when the result is postoperative pleuropneumonia. Additionally, the location of the surgical incision makes it difficult to obtain a transtracheal wash sample for proper antimicrobial therapy and can sometimes compromise the healing of the initial incision.

Because of the association of osteochondrosis with the pathogenesis of developmental cervical cord compression, it is important to ensure that the other commonly involved articulations (e.g., the stifle, tarsus, fetlock, shoulder) are free from significant pathology.[8] If such concurrent pathology exists, the owner should be aware of its significance and possible effects on the outcome. Depending on its severity, osteochondrosis of the neck and stifle (see Chapter 51) can be treated concurrently or during separate surgical sessions with little significant change in the prognosis.

EXPECTATIONS OF SURGERY

It is important to understand the owner's expectations and desires in regard to the surgical intervention, and to put them into the context of what is possible. Owner compliance and commitment prior to surgery is essential. Some surgeons refuse to operate on a horse if the owner is not a willing participant. Owners must be completely informed of the risks, liability, and responsibilities of their decision. Their goals must be tempered with realism. Trainers and owners need to be patient, because full recovery may take up to 1 year or more, and a conscientious effort should be made to condition the patient, using a slow, gradually increasing training program. The majority of owners want to have horses that are capable of competing at high levels, even though they were initially emphatic about being satisfied with a pleasure horse or breeding animal. Interestingly, a long-term evaluation done 1 to 4 years after surgery revealed that as many as 90% of clients and referring veterinarians were satisfied with the outcome.[6]

Although some horses with grade 3 or 4 ataxia have gone on to race at a moderate level postoperatively, the percentage is low. It is possible for a horse with a grade 3 (out of 5) ataxia that has had clinical signs for only 2 to 3 weeks and only a single lesion present in severe flexion to return postoperatively to a barely detectable ataxic state and, therefore, to be able to compete. However, all other factors such as soundness, mental suitability, and overall health must be considered also. It is disappointing when horses that have undergone surgical correction do not recover enough to be handled safely or cannot be placed in a large pasture without extra observation. A mare should be able to stand for service; a stallion should be able to cover a mare naturally with only moderate assistance.

Based on an analysis of long-term results of 126 horses that had undergone ventral interbody fusion using the Seattle Slew implant (see later) between 2000 and 2003, 88% of the animals recovered at least 1 grade, and 60% are ridden successfully; 10% are used for breeding or were retired.[6]

SURGICAL APPROACHES AND TECHNIQUES

Ventral Interbody Fusion

The most frequently used technique today is a modification of the one developed by Cloward for use in humans.[2,6,9,10] This modification uses a threaded or partially threaded titanium implant that has multiple holes and an open end that leaves an isthmus of bone in the center to encourage faster fusion and reduce postoperative fractures and implant migration (Fig. 52-4).

Preoperative Medications

Preoperative antibiotics consisting of procaine penicillin and gentamicin are administered to the animal before induction of anesthesia, after surgery, and for the following 72 hours. Nonsteroidal anti-inflammatory drugs (NSAIDs), such as phenylbutazone or flunixin meglumine, are administered at therapeutic levels before induction and are continued as long as needed. Tetanus toxoid is routinely administered.

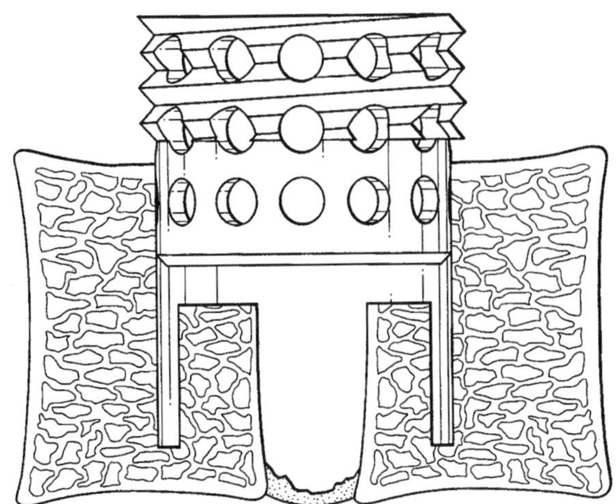

Figure 52-4. Drawing showing the Kerf Cut cylinder advancing into a prepared bone bed. Note the preserved peninsulas of bone, which remain inside the implant.

Prior to induction, an endoscopic examination of the upper airways is performed for detection of laryngeal hemiplegia. If this condition is identified, modifications should be made to the surgical approach, or the risk for bilateral laryngeal paralysis may be increased.

Anesthesia is begun with administration of xylazine, diazepam, or ketamine. Ataxic horses often show the desired effects with minimal doses of xylazine. Induction and recovery may be improved by slightly increasing the dose of diazepam.

Anesthesia

Positive-pressure-assisted inhalation of halothane, isoflurane, or sevoflurane is the preferred method of maintaining anesthesia, because it allows the surgeon to be minimally concerned for the horse's life while drilling close to the spinal cord. Some surgeons have performed this procedure with a thiopental drip regimen with apparently good success.[11] This technique requires an extremely efficient surgical method and practiced support personnel.

Common anesthesia problems are hypoxia, hypotension, and, because of the location of the surgical site, variable blood pressure readings if a facial artery is used (the authors recommend using the left facial artery, because the right carotid artery can be compressed with retractors during the procedure). Awareness of these possible complications allows early use of inotropic drugs; frequent arterial blood gas analyses and high oxygen flow rates should enable the anesthesiologist to react accordingly.

Patient Positioning

The animal is placed in dorsal recumbency, with the forelimbs tied in a moderately flexed position to allow adequate lateral stability without the excessive tension that could produce radial nerve dysfunction. A curved, heavy, 30-cm block of wood or metal is placed under the affected area (Fig. 52-5). The block helps with the extension of the cervical articulations and, at the same time, provides a stable surface to reduce excessive movement during drilling.

Identification of Surgical Site

The surgical site is identified after the ventral cervical area has been clipped, shaved, and disinfected. One or more 14-gauge needles are placed over the affected site and the articulation just cranial to it, and lateromedial radiographic projections are taken. The usual method of determining placement of the needles is to measure one hand width for each vertebra retrograde from the easily palpable wings

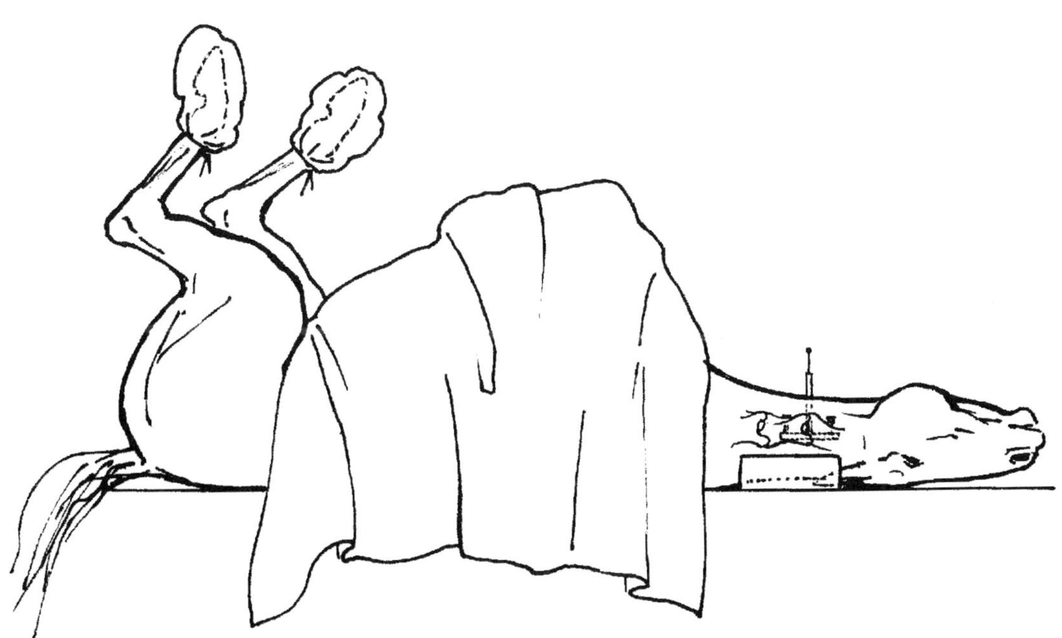

Figure 52-5. Schematic representation of a horse correctly positioned for surgery using a block of wood to extend the cervical articulations.

of the atlas (Fig. 52-6). The needles should be placed on the side of the neck closest to the x-ray cassette to avoid any undue distortion resulting from parallax, especially with smaller animals. Once it has been determined that the needles are at the correct level, preparation of the surgical site is completed and the entire horse is draped. The use of suction or electrocautery is not necessary, but both reduce intraoperative time. For intraoperative imaging and evaluation, the use of a C-arm is recommended, because it avoids delays for film development.

Surgical Technique

A 20-cm skin incision is used for a single-level fusion centered over the pre-placed needles. A towel clamp placed at this level serves as a landmark and obviates the need to constantly palpate through two or three levels of draping and towels to ensure the correct anatomic location. After the initial skin incision is made, the cutaneous musculature is incised with a scalpel blade. Skin and subcutaneous hemorrhaging is controlled with hemostats, ligatures, and hemoclips. The sternothyroideus muscles are separated longitudinally at their junction down to the trachea, and additional hemorrhage is controlled as needed. Once the trachea has been identified, blunt dissection is continued down the right side of the trachea, using scissors or sterile-gloved fingers, and exposure of the longus colli muscles, lying directly beneath the trachea and the carotid sheath, is rapidly achieved. Application of hand-held Deaver retractors by an assistant allows palpation of the ventral spines through the longus colli muscles. The recurrent laryngeal nerve must be identified and protected from excessive retraction or trauma.

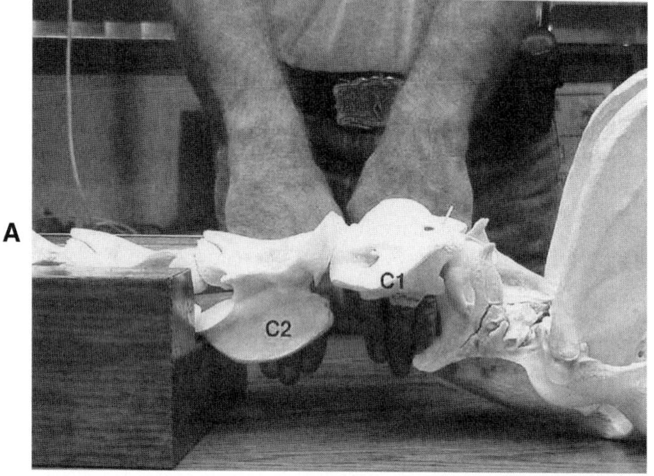

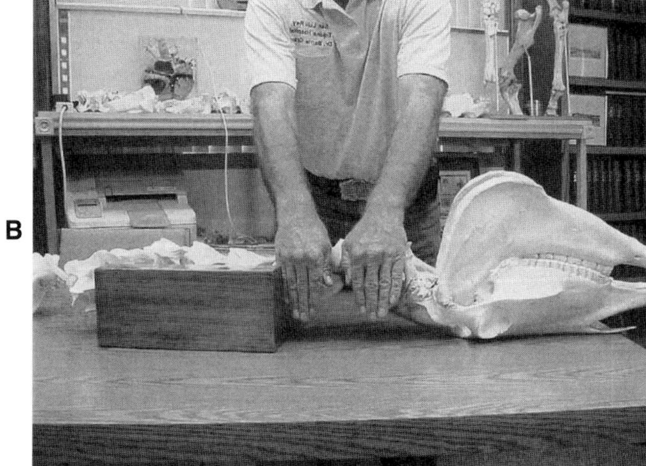

Figure 52-6. A horse skeleton is used to demonstrate disc location for surgery. Using the wing of the atlas (C1) as a palpable landmark, each vertebral body length is determined to be about one hand-width. **A,** Hands placed behind the vertebrae. **B,** Hands placed in front.

Usually, the ventral spinous processes (not present at C6-7) are readily identified. After making a 4-cm longitudinal midline incision over the ventral spine of the vertebra just cranial to the instability, the longus colli muscles are reflected from both sides with an osteotome or heavy dissection scissors. Self-retaining Inge retractors provide the best exposure of the ventral spine and reduce the effort needed from the assistant. The ventral spinous process is removed with a curved hand-osteotome and mallet down to the level of the body of the cervical vertebra. Bone hemorrhage is controlled with suction and with compression with sponges. The epiphyseal lines of the caudal aspect of the cranial vertebra can subsequently be identified.

A 16-mm drill guide is placed on the spine with its caudal surface on the old epiphyseal scar. Using a 16-mm drill, a test hole is drilled to a depth of 10 mm. A Hudson brace can be used, but a power reamer produces a more uniform hole. After the drill guide and drill are removed, it is usually easy to see the characteristic drab-white appearance of the intervertebral disc material. K-wires are then placed into the cranial and caudal aspects of the test hole, and an intraoperative radiograph is taken to assist in the placement of the 25-mm drill guide. Ideally, the drill guide should be perpendicular to the spinal canal and placed so that the joint space at the spinal canal is in the center of (or slightly caudal to) the guide (Fig. 52-7). Once this placement has been determined, the drill guide is hammered securely into place.

Using power equipment, the implant site is prepared by drilling with a series of drills starting with a narrow core saw, followed by a thicker core saw (Fig. 52-8) and a solid 25-mm drill to a depth of 15 mm. The implant site is initially widened with a no. 1 Kerf Cutter and followed by removal of the drill guide to allow the slightly larger no. 2 Kerf Cutter to finish the implant site to the desired depth (Fig. 52-9). This depth is usually 8 to 10 mm distant from the spinal canal. It has been the authors' experience that this shelf of bone should be left between the bottom of the hole and the spinal canal to provide overall strength to the articulation during the recovery process. It is important to use intraoperative imaging and repeated depth gauge measurements to confirm the proper depth. The approximate depth of the vertebral body can be determined on the preoperative radiographs, remembering that 1 or 2 mm of the enlargement has resulted from parallax. The depth of the drill hole may vary with the age of the patient. The drilling should be done by only one person, whose responsibility is to focus on the depth.

After the depth has been reached, the implant site is tapped with a large tap that matches the partially threaded

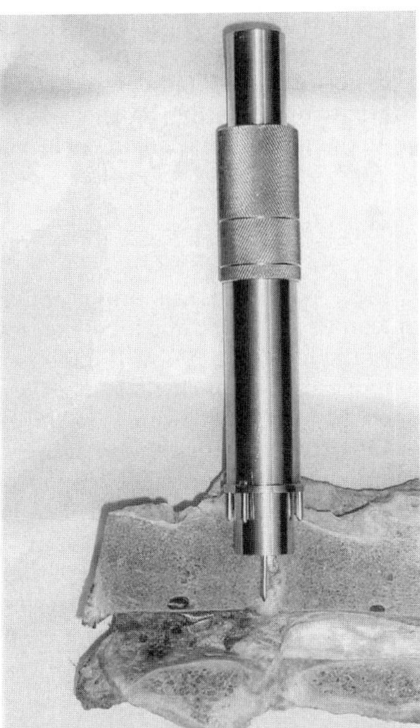

Figure 52-7. A cadaveric specimen showing correct placement of a solid cylinder placed over the guide pin, and a four-prong cylinder guide placed over it. The guide pin can be removed after the cylinder is tapped into place to act as a guide for the Kerf cutting process.

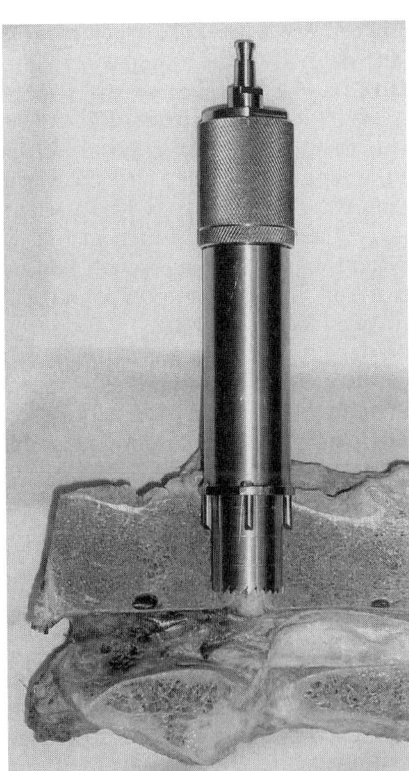

Figure 52-8. A cadaveric specimen showing the thin Kerf Cut saw advanced to the proper depth.

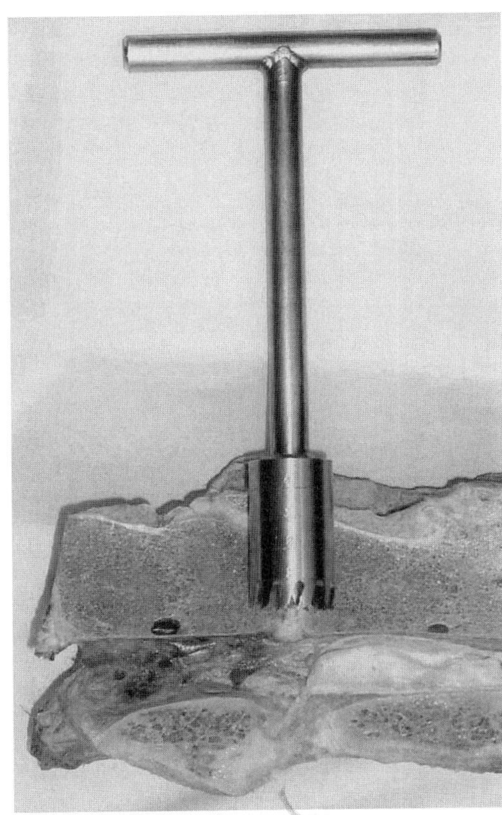

Figure 52-9. A cadaveric specimen showing the manual Kerf Cut widener and cleaner, which is used after the thin- and thick-cut saws.

Kerf implant. The implant is inserted until firm resistance is encountered (Fig. 52-10). A Hall drill is used to remove as much disc as possible to provide a bleeding surface of bone to encourage rapid acceptance of the bone graft. Bone graft material is prepared from the bone that is removed from the ventral spine and by the drilling process; the preparation involves dividing the dark red cancellous bone into small pieces. Small pieces of disc material, any periosteum, and excessive amounts of cortical bone should be excluded. The graft material should be covered with a blood-soaked sponge for optimal survival of the osteoblasts (see Chapter 82); it is not desirable to use saline, because its osmotic pressure may cause disruption of the osteoblasts.[12] The graft is secured in place with gentle pressure from the handle end of a curette or osteotome. For a multilevel fusion, this procedure is repeated at the desired locations (Fig. 52-11).

After liberal flushing of the entire surgical area and a careful count of all foreign materials (e.g., surgical sponges), the self-retaining retractors are removed. Closure of the longus colli muscle is carried out with no. 0 polydioxanone (PDS) in a two-layer mattress pattern to reduce dead space. The remaining ventral cervical muscles are closed with no. 0 PDS in a simple-continuous or Ford interlocking pattern (the surgeon's choice). No. 2-0 PDS is used on the subcutaneous tissue and staples on the skin. Application of drains is not essential. Even though seroma formation occurred in 4 of 126 cases, excessive seroma formation is a rare event.[6] In over 600 cases, the cosmetic appearance of the surgical area has been very satisfying 4 to 6 weeks after surgery,

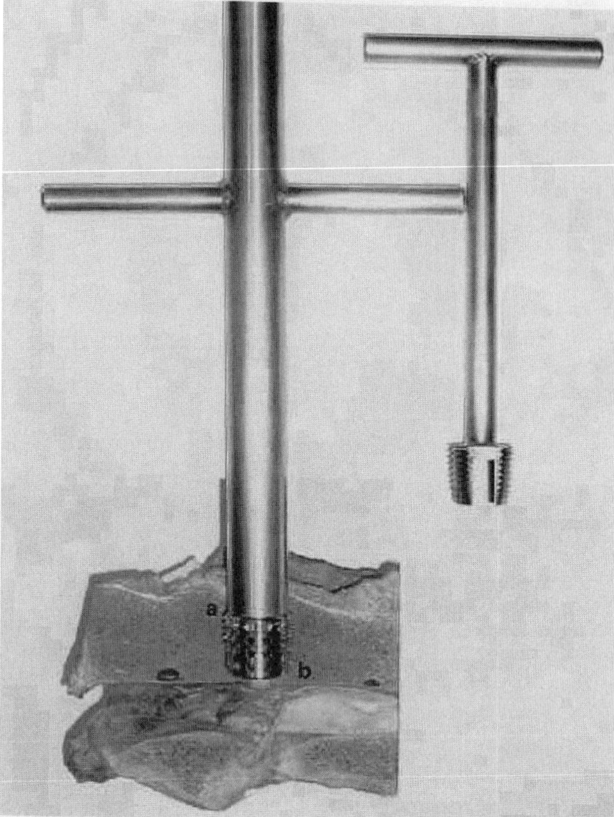

Figure 52-10. A cadaveric specimen showing the Kerf Cut cylinder (Seattle Slew implant) seated correctly and making complete contact with both the cranial (a) and caudal (b) vertebrae. The driver is still in place (left). The tap is shown (right).

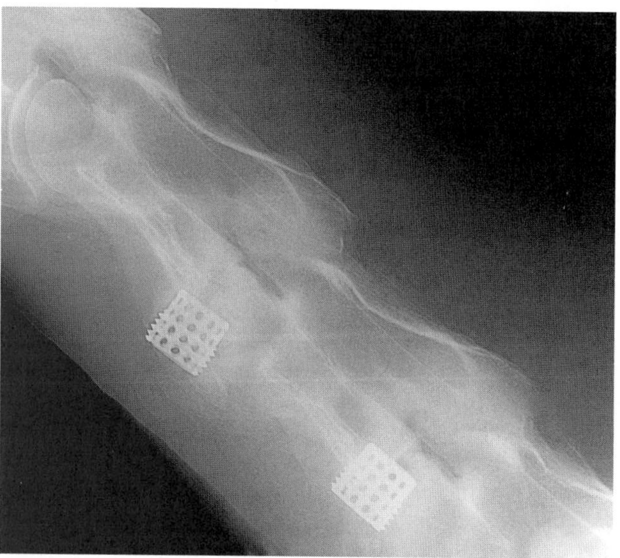

Figure 52-11. Cervical radiograph showing that the cranial implant is tilted slightly caudally and the caudal implant is well centered. This 6-month postsurgical radiograph shows good ossification and stabilization of both sites.

without the need for aspiration or drainage of any seroma. The incision is covered with a sterile towel or adhesive drape, and a postoperative radiograph is taken before removing the patient from the table so that there is a reference for any migration that might occur with a violent recovery.

Recovery

Recovery of these patients is an important aspect for a successful outcome. These ataxic patients are often unbroken, have had little handling, and will have some difficulty standing up under the best of circumstances. Violent recoveries are associated with migration of the implants and, as with most equine surgeries, anything that anesthetists and surgical personal can do to promote quiet, prolonged recoveries is beneficial. Hand recovery of all cases with a tail and head rope is important. The head rope must not be overused because of the likelihood that cervical traction will cause cervical fracture at the implant site. The head rope should be held by an experienced person who has respect for the dynamics of the surgery.

An extended period of recovery in lateral recumbency (40 to 90 minutes) is recommended. A combination of butorphanol and acepromazine in the early portions of the recovery to keep the horses comfortable and sensible has proved to be a good protocol. The onset of acepromazine is delayed compared with that of xylazine, so early administration is important, and excessive early movements can be directly controlled by the administration of very small xylazine dosages. Acepromazine has the advantage of inducing less severe ataxia than is produced by xylazine. Steroids are used only if the patient's ataxia is greater than grade 3-plus. Sling recoveries are sometimes necessary, especially for the patient with severe ataxia (grade greater than 3.5). Placing these candidates in the sling for 15 to 20 minutes a day for 1 to 2 days prior to surgery greatly enhances the usefulness of a sling postoperatively. Also, it is likely that if a sling was required after the myelogram, it will also be required after surgery. Older patients sometimes lie quietly for 75 minutes and then just stand up. A pool recovery system may not be indicated, because a compressive lesion at C6-7 may be disrupted as the head needs to be extended to keep from drowning.

After the patient is standing, a sterile dressing is applied to the incision site and is maintained with adhesive elastic tape applied in a circular fashion around the mane and neck. If there is a problem with stability and ataxia, a second dose of NSAIDs can be administered at this time. The patient should not return to the stall until the surgeon deems it stable enough to do so, and until the hallways leading to the stall are dry.

Postoperative Management

Postoperative antibiotic recommendations include penicillin or gentamicin intravenously for 3 days. NSAIDs (flunixin meglumine) are usually given intravenously for 3 days to reduce swelling and postoperative discomfort. Long-term oral use of NSAIDs (phenylbutazone), to reduce the cascading effect that compression causes in the spinal cord, is also recommended. Information[13] concerning the long-term effect of phenylbutazone on joint cartilage has resulted in modifying this recommendation, depending on the age and desired use of the patient.

Most patients are willing and eager to eat and move around. If possible, hay should be presented in a hanging net. Stretching the neck toward the floor is not ideal during the first week after surgery. The animal should be treated in the stall in a quiet, gentle manner to avoid sudden movements or falls. If the animal objects to intramuscular injections, switching to oral antibiotics and NSAIDs is indicated, or intravenous medications can be delivered by indwelling intravenous catheter. The bandage is left in place for the first 5 to 6 days postoperatively. It can be completely removed or replaced by a similar bandage if a good cosmetic appearance is desired in a short amount of time. The first 7 to 10 days after surgery are the most critical, so the animals are not walked out of the stall during this time.

A postoperative radiograph should be taken 4 to 5 days after surgery to evaluate any change in position of the implant. If there is any increase in swelling, discomfort, or ataxia, radiographs should be taken.

At least 45 days of stall confinement with a reduced caloric input is recommended to decrease the chance of some event occurring, such as a sudden fall, that would displace the implant. Hand-walking can start after 45 days. At 60 days, another radiograph and neurologic examination should be performed to help decide about increasing the amount of exercise and freedom. The fusion process is well underway at 60 days, and postoperative myelograms performed even on patients with static compression at C6-7 have normal dye columns at this time. The owner and trainer should be aware that the clinical signs will improve slowly for at least a year. Exercise will assist in retraining the spinal tracts. For the patients with greater than grade 2 ataxia, 4 to 6 month's paddock exercise is indicated. For patients with less than grade 2 ataxia, being ridden in an area with safe footing by an experienced rider with a helmet can be done.

The use of a treadmill on an incline can quickly increase the amount of strength in the pelvic appendages.

Complications

SEROMA FORMATION

The development of seromas after this procedure is usually associated with multiple-level fusions in older patients with heavier ventral cervical muscles that require more extensive dissection and retraction. Although drains can be used, the majority of cases resolve with time and without constant aspiration or lancing. If the seroma develops into an abscess, open drainage is encouraged to avoid seeding the implant with bacteria. Effective control of hemorrhage during surgery will keep the number of postoperative seromas low.

INFECTION

The incidence of postoperative infection of the soft tissues or the implant is very low (less than 1%). Soft tissue infection usually produces a febrile response with a firm, painful enlargement at the surgical site, leukocytosis, and increased fibrinogen concentration. Treatment consists of drainage (best done under ultrasonographic monitoring), administration of appropriate antibiotics, and hot packing. Infection of the implant produces the same clinical response, but, in addition, the patient is unwilling to move the cervical area and may show increased neurologic signs compatible with meningitis. In one case of suppurative meningitis (from infection with *Klebsiella*), a postoperative myelogram taken when the patient was tetraparetic demonstrated a uniform narrowing of both dye columns of the entire cervical area. The signs resolved after retrieval of the implant and the application of methylmethacrylate bone cement impregnated with cephalosporin antibiotic powder.

FRACTURES

The occurrence of fractures of the adjacent vertebrae at the time of surgical implantation or during the immediate recovery period is less than 1% and is generally related to overdrilling the implant hole, leaving only a thin plate of bone between the end of the implant and the spinal canal. The resulting structure cannot withstand the force of a violent recovery or a severe fall during the early postoperative period. In most instances, the only clinical signs associated with nondisplaced fractures are an increase in the rigidity of the neck. Severe fractures can result in clinical signs that range from paralysis (when displaced fragments cause severe cord compression) to obvious seroma formation and ventral displacement of the trachea as the implant migrates ventrally.

Fractures are confirmed by radiographic examination, although subtle fracture lines may be difficult to detect immediately, requiring repeat radiographs after 10 days. It may be necessary to perform a myelogram to determine whether the spinal canal diameter has been compromised.

Conservative treatment is indicated in most cases because revision with unstable vertebral bodies is very difficult, and the majority of cases resolve with the passage of time (Fig. 52-12).

Complication Rates

Minor complications associated with this procedure include ventral migration of the implant, laryngeal hemiplegia (LH), and Horner's syndrome. Ventral migration was found on postoperative radiographs of 3.5% of patients and tended to occur within the first 7 days after surgery.[10] The risk of LH was less than 1%, and transient Horner's syndrome was observed in 1.5%. Fatal complications include esophageal rupture (1.5%), laryngospasm (0.8%), and fractures (0.8%).[6]

Preliminary results show that the partially threaded Kerf cylinder implant procedure, if correctly performed, allows a faster fusion and reduces the chances of vertebral fractures and ventral migration, which has been associated with the Bagby Basket (Fig. 52-13).

Subtotal Dorsal Decompression Laminectomy

Indications

Subtotal dorsal decompression laminectomy, in which the dorsal caudal aspect of the cranial vertebra and the dorsal cranial aspect of the caudal vertebra are removed, is indicated

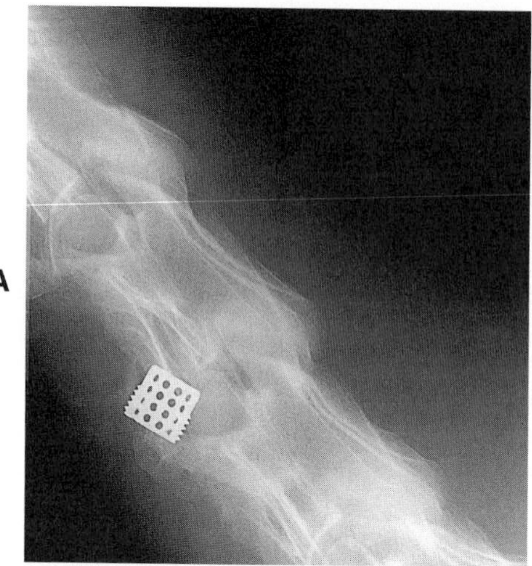

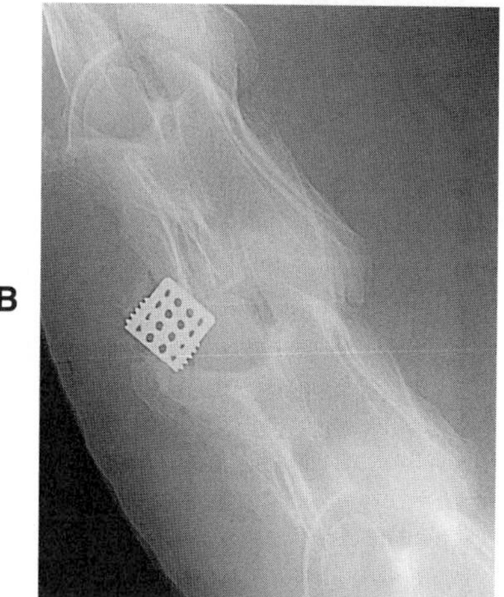

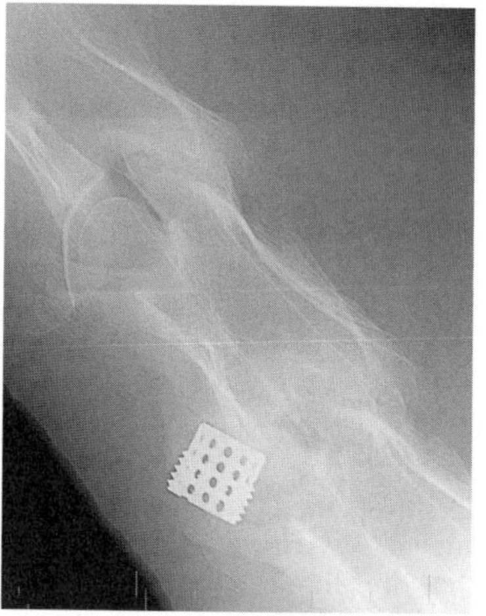

Figure 52-12. A, Cervical radiograph taken 1 day after surgery. This horse experienced a fracture cranial to the implant. **B,** The same fracture 1 week after surgery. **C,** The fracture healed after 8 weeks of stall rest.

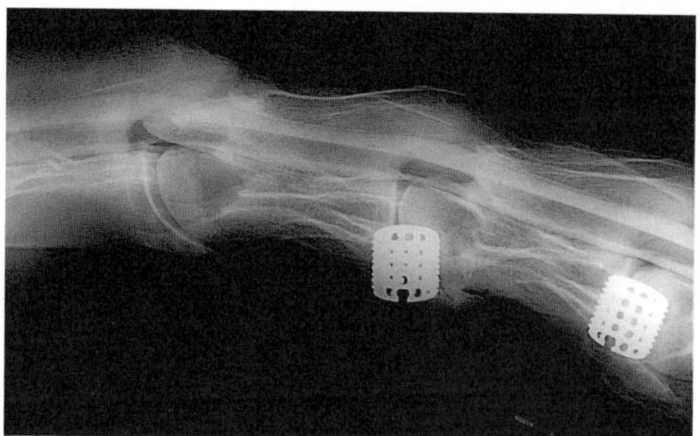

Figure 52-13. Cervical radiograph showing extrusion of the cranial implant, which occurred with a Bagby Basket implant. (This is the same patient shown in Fig. 52-2.)

in cases of intramedullar or extramedullar enlargements with resulting cord compression, meningeal infiltration of metastatic malignant melanomas, presence of excessive synovial villi from the osteoarthritic facets, and hypertrophic dorsal lamina, resulting in extramedullar cord compression. Abscesses, parasitic granulomas, and intramedullar neoplasms may also be approached with this method if the diagnosis is reliable (Fig. 52-14).

Subtotal dorsal decompression laminectomy is not indicated for the removal of dorsal arches that result from fractures, or for the removal of dorsal arches that may play a part in cord compression resulting from the ankylosed hyperflexed joints seen in C2-3. There is even some question as to whether it is indicated for the presence of a hypertrophic dorsal longitudinal ligament or when disc material protrudes into the ventral aspect of the spinal canal.

Surgical Positioning

Once the decision has been made to perform a subtotal dorsal decompression, positioning of the patient is the most important factor contributing to the success or failure of the procedure. A number of surgical positions have been tried, including (1) placing the animal in ventral recumbency with all limbs flexed on a table and extending the head, (2) "hanging" the horse from the vertical surgical table under general anesthesia, and (3) placing the patient in a sling, inducing general anesthesia, and supplementing the suspension of the animal by locating the table under the sternum. Currently, the third method and a lateral recumbency

A

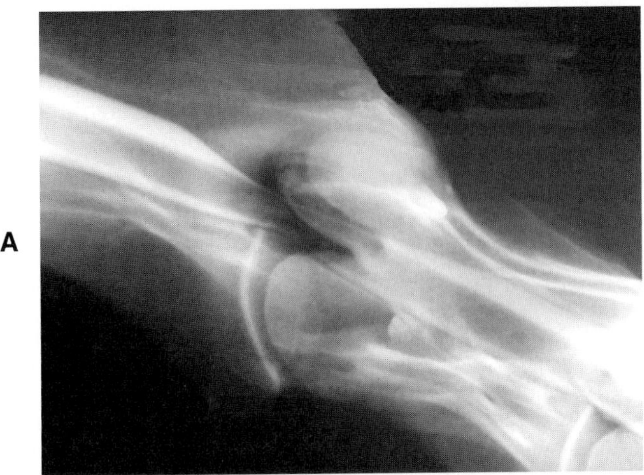

B

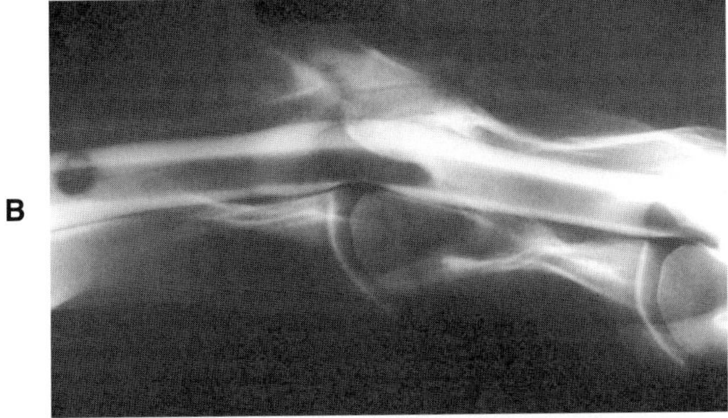

Figure 52-14. A, Myelogram of a 6-year-old Thoroughbred hunter that was falling during competition and was grade 2 (out of 5) ataxic. **B,** A 6-month follow-up myelogram performed after a subtotal dorsal decompression was performed to remove a space-occupying mass later identified as a lymphoma.

approach with the neck in full flexion[14,15] are the most widely used. The choice of position usually rests with the surgeon, who should have practiced it (at least on several cadavers) prior to applying it to a clinical case.

Preoperative Preparation

Uneventful induction and recovery can be facilitated, especially in younger animals, if 2 or 3 days prior to surgery the animal can be accustomed to the use of a sling. The usual standard operative procedures of preventive medicine, including administration of anthelmintic medication and vaccination against upper respiratory infections, are strongly recommended to reduce the incidence of postoperative complications. The day before surgery, the mane is clipped and the animal is given a bath with a medicated shampoo. In addition, scrubbing of the dorsal neck surface with a bacteriostatic detergent is indicated. The perioperative use of NSAIDs and antibiotics is strongly recommended. The use of a depilatory agent 1 or 2 hours before surgery further aids in the removal of small hairs in the many creases of the dorsal aspect of the cervical arch. Some animals tend to show an inflammatory response to the depilatory agents, so these should be selected with caution.

Surgical Technique

After the animal is placed in the position most familiar to the surgeon, a large area extending from the summit to the intra-thoracic vertebrae (T4-5 to C2-3) is disinfected, draped, and toweled. A long incision (30 to 40 cm) is made through the usually thickened skin on the dorsal midline. After the initial profuse hemorrhage is controlled, the skin edges are toweled. Although it is not always necessary, application of the towels and towel clamps helps reduce any further capillary hemorrhage. Using a fresh scalpel blade, the subcutaneous tissue and fat overlying the funicular part of the ligamentum nuchae is sharply incised, exposing the dense white fibrous tissue of the ligamentum. Sometimes three or four small linear incisions are required to find the separation between the lamellar halves of the ligamentum nuchae, but as soon as this division is found, the two halves can be separated by blunt manual dissection. The incision needs to be of considerable length because of the depth of the field and the inelastic quality of the ligamentum nuchae. One or two sets of large, self-retaining retractors of the Finochietto or Balfour type will facilitate retraction in this area.

At this point, it should be possible to palpate the small spinal processes on the dorsal aspect of the vertebra. The location of the dorsal decompression at C6-7 is facilitated by palpating the 3- to 4-cm dorsal spinous process that often exists at the first thoracic vertebra. Radiographic markers (needles), applied before draping in the manner previously described, help confirm the proper location. The overlying epaxial muscles and soft tissues are removed from the dorsal arch with the combined use of periosteal elevators, large curettes, and rongeurs. The use of scalpel blades in this area should be avoided, if possible, because incising the many small blood vessels produces hemorrhage that is often difficult to control, greatly obscures vision, and increases the surgical time. After the soft tissue is removed from the vertebral arches, the white cortical bone is removed using a combination of a Hall drill, cranial drills, and rongeurs.

The original description advocated the use of Gigli wire inserted between one dorsal foramen and the next foramen. In the authors' experience, horses with stenotic hypertrophic vertebrae often have no discernible dorsal foramina because they have been encroached on by the hypertrophic bone, and attempts to pass a Gigli wire as described is not recommended. It is important to remember that that the majority of these compressive lesions are the result of proliferation of dorsal bone, which is often much thicker than on normal specimens. This proliferative bone increases the surgical time, and it is important to be patient during the careful, tedious removal of this bone. A rapid, forceful puncture through the dorsal arch with an instrument can result in cord trauma that will exacerbate the already existing neurologic signs. A recommended technique is to identify the remains of any dorsal foramen and work cranially and caudally from this aspect with a Hall or cranial drill. After the inner cortical layer of bone appears, reverse-cutting rongeurs help remove the dorsal arch while protecting the cord. Proliferative or hypertrophic soft tissue arising from osteoarthritic articular facets can be removed with rongeurs and long scissors.

The appearance of epidural fat over the top of the bright, shiny dura indicates that decompression of the spinal cord has been completed. Removal of the bone over the affected site must be adequate, especially on the caudal aspect. If cord compression was caused by a metastatic melanoma, all the discolored tissue should be removed. After the bone has been removed and the edges have been smoothed with a Hall drill, bone wax is applied to the bleeding edges of bone to reduce the amount of hemorrhage and the risk of clot formation around the spinal cord.

After careful inspection of the surgical site, all sponges and instruments are removed and a drain is secured into the tissues directly overlying the decompression site. The drain should exit through the lateral aspects of the cervical muscles. The drain is secured to the soft tissue surrounding the laminectomy with a 2-0 absorbable suture, which facilitates removal with gentle traction after 4 to 5 days.

With removal of the self-retaining retractors, the laminar portions of the ligamentum nuchae fall together and need to be apposed only on the most superficial aspect with a continuous Ford interlocking pattern using absorbable monofilament suture material. The funicular portion of the ligamentum nuchae, the subcutaneous tissue, and skin are all apposed using absorbable sutures in a continuous Ford interlocking pattern. Finally, stent bandages are applied to provide protection for the incision from excessive trauma that could occur during a violent recovery. Firmly applying bandages around the entire neck is discouraged, because this produces pressure that is directly transmitted to the exposed cord and can result in noticeable discomfort to the patient and increased ataxia.

Postoperative Management and Aftercare

Immediate postoperative management consists of antibiotics for 36 hours or longer, depending on surgical time and the possibility of breaks of aseptic technique during the procedure. The continued use of NSAIDs is indicated, especially in the severely ataxic patient, to reduce any sudden falls, because one of the more frequent complications of this procedure is fracture of the articular facets because of the destabilizing effect that the procedure has on the dorsal arches. The drain site should be continually bandaged or protected with antiseptic swabs and the drain left in place until there is a noticeable reduction in the amount of fluid obtained, usually 24 to 36 hours postoperatively. Hand-walking and resumption of physical therapy can begin within 10 days; the judgment of the surgeon or neurologist is the most important factor in determining this time.

Subtotal dorsal decompression laminectomy is not widely used because of its degree of difficulty, the amount of surgical time involved and surgical expertise required to perform it efficiently, and the development of a number of postoperative complications (e.g., articular facet fractures, compressive hematomas, and suppurative meningitis), which often result in the death of the patient.[12,16]

REFERENCES

1. Wagner PC, Bagby GW, Grant BD, et al: Surgical stabilization of the equine cervical spine, Vet Surg 1979;8:7.
2. Wagner PC, Grant BD, Bagby GW, et al: Evaluation of cervical spinal fusion as a treatment in equine wobbler syndrome, Vet Surg 1979;8:84.
3. DeBowes RM, Grant BD, Bagby GW, et al: Cervical interbody fusion in the horse: A comparative study of bovine xenografts supported by stainless steel baskets, Am J Vet Res 1984;45:191.
4. Grant BD, Barbee DD, Wagner PC, et al: Long term results of surgery for equine cervical vertebral malformation, Proc Am Assoc Equine Pract 1985;31:91.
5. van Biervliet J, Scrivani PV, Divers TJ, et al: Evaluation of decision criteria for detection of spinal cord compression based on cervical myelography in horses: 38 cases (1981-2001), Equine Vet J 2004;36:14-20.
6. Grant BD, Trostle S, Rantanen N, et al: Preliminary results using an improved implant for cervical interbody arthrodesis in the horse, Proc Eur Coll Vet Surg 2003;12:138.
7. Grant BD, Hoskinson JJ, Barbee DD, et al: Ventral stabilization for decompression of caudal cervical spinal cord compression in the horse, Proc Am Assoc Equine Pract 1985;31:75.
8. Rush Moore B, Reed SM, Robertson JT: Surgical management of cervical stenotic myelopathy in horses: 73 cases (1983-1992), J Am Vet Med Assoc 1993;203:108.
9. McAfee PC: Interbody fusion cages in reconstructive operations on the spine, J Bone Joint Surg Am 1999;81:859.
10. Trostle SS, Grant BD, Bagby G, Rantanen N: Clinical results of Kerf Cylinder (Seattle Slew Implant) to reduce implant migration and fracture in horses undergoing cervical interbody fusion, Vet Surg 2003;32:5.
11. Lewis R: Personal communication, 2004.
12. Grant BD: Surgical treatment of developmental disorders of the spinal column. In Auer JA, Stick JA, editors: Equine Surgery, ed 2, Philadelphia, 1999, WB Saunders.
13. Stevenson S: Bone grafting. In Slatter DH, editor: Textbook of Small Animal Surgery, Philadelphia, 1985, WB Saunders.
14. Nixon AJ, Stashak TS: Surgical therapy for spinal cord disease in the horse, Proc Am Assoc Equine Pract 1985;31:61.
15. Nixon AJ, Stashak TS: Dorsal laminectomy in the horse. I. Review of the literature and description of a new procedure, Vet Surg 1983;12:172.
16. Nixon AJ, Stashak TS: Dorsal laminectomy in the horse: III. Results in horses with cervical vertebral malformation, Vet Surg 1983;12:184.

CHAPTER 53

Traumatic Disorders of the Spinal Column

James T. Robertson
Valerie Samii

Trauma to the spinal column in horses occurs most frequently in the cervical and thoracolumbar vertebrae, and the reported incidence varies.[1-3] Vertebral fractures may be present with or without neurologic signs, depending on the area of the spine and the portion of the vertebra that sustains the trauma. Confirming a diagnosis of spinal trauma is complicated by the variation in clinical signs. Foals are more susceptible to vertebral fractures than adults, and the cervical vertebrae are more likely to be affected. The most common injuries in foals involve luxations, subluxations, and physeal separations of the cervical vertebrae.[2,3] In adult horses, the injuries tend to involve both the cervical and the thoracolumbar regions.[3-5]

Causes of spinal trauma include rearing and falling over backward, collisions with immoveable objects, kicks from other horses, hyperflexion or hyperextension of the neck when falling, slipping on wet or muddy footing, and violently sitting backward on the ground or against solid objects.[1-3] Injury to the spinal cord can occur without radiographic evidence of osseous damage, making the history of possible trauma important for arriving at a diagnosis.

This chapter describes the traumatic spinal injuries that are amenable to surgical correction, although in the horse the number is limited, for many reasons. The size of the horse presents unique technical challenges from a diagnostic and surgical standpoint, and it is difficult to maintain fracture fixation during the anesthetic recovery and rehabilitation period. Innovation is required during the surgical repair to achieve success, and there certainly are not many case reports in the literature from which to draw information when formulating a surgical plan.

TRAUMATIC INJURIES TO THE CERVICAL SPINE

Fracture of the Axial Dens with Atlantoaxial Subluxation

This injury is most commonly seen in foals younger than 6 months.[3,6-8] The dens or odontoid process originates embryologically from the body of the first cervical vertebra and is attached to the axis by a physis. This physis closes by 8 to 12 months of age. Fracture occurs when a foal falls with the neck in hyperflexion (somersaulting) or when the fall is violent, as in halter breaking incidents. The fracture most often occurs through the cranial physis of the axis, separating the dens from the body of the vertebrae (Fig. 53-1). The dens remains attached by its ligaments to the atlas, and the axis moves ventrally. This results in cord compression at the atlantoaxial joint.

The degree of neurologic deficit depends on the degree and force of the spinal impact at the time of the injury. Neurologic deficits range from a stiff gait and splinted neck to total tetraparesis or even sudden death.[3,6-8] In most cases, the foal becomes ambulatory almost immediately, with signs of neck splinting, ataxia, and tetraparesis developing gradually. Manipulation of the neck produces pain as well as palpable and audible crepitation. There may be an obvious axial malalignment in the atlantoaxial area.[3] Lateral radiographs with the horse under sedation confirm the separation (widening) of the cranial physis of the axis and cranioventral luxation of that vertebra.[3,6-8] If ventrodorsal radiographs can be obtained, asymmetry in the atlantoaxial articulation may be noted.

The prognosis for recovery from this type of injury can be roughly correlated with the severity of the spinal cord

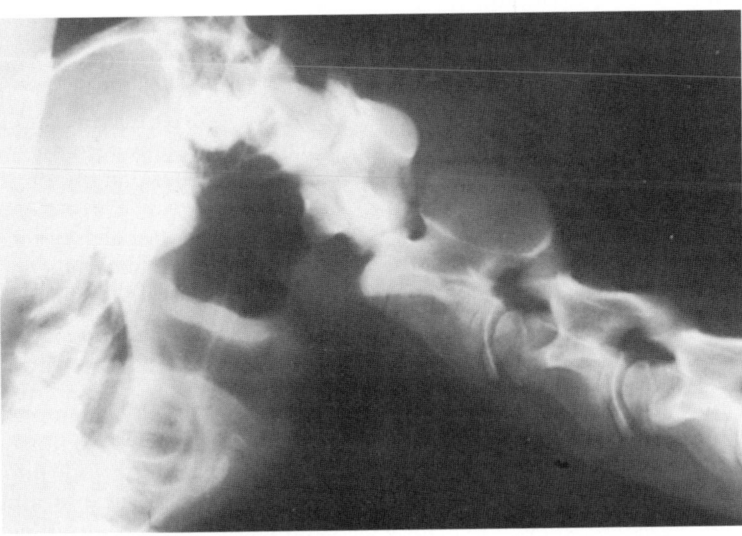

Figure 53-1. Fracture of the dens, which occurs through the cranial physis of C2.

damage. If there is motor function of all four limbs, with only paresis rather than paralysis, the prognosis for survival is favorable. If there is paralysis but the foal still shows conscious pain responses in all four limbs, the prognosis is guarded. If there is no conscious pain response, the prognosis is grave.

The method of treatment varies depending on the stability of the fracture and, to some extent, on the intended use of the horse. Nonsurgical management includes stall rest and the judicious use of anti-inflammatory drugs when foals exhibit splinting of the neck and relative instability at the atlantoaxial junction. Worsening of signs may become apparent if a fall occurs and further displacement of the axis relative to the atlas results. With time, a fibrous union of the dens to the axis may develop and the neurologic deficits will decrease. However, late-developing neurologic deterioration, in a patient that showed initial improvement, indicates that a proliferative bony callus or soft tissue hypertrophy is causing cord compression.[3]

Surgical repair is warranted if deterioration in the foal's clinical signs is noted, preferably before the foal becomes recumbent. Although the prognosis is guarded to poor if the foal is presented in recumbency, it may be improved with surgery. The goal of surgery is to provide decompression at the fracture site by realigning the vertebrae and providing stability with some form of fixation. Surgical techniques for repair of fracture-luxations include external fixation using Steinmann pins, compression plating, ventral atlantoaxial fusion, and dorsal laminectomy of the caudal atlas.[3,6-8]

One report described the placement of two, six-hole, broad dynamic compression plates on the ventral surface of the atlas and axis.[6] The approach and exposure for this technique are the same as those described for ventral interbody fusion (Chapter 52). After exposing the ventral surfaces of the atlas and axis, the alignment of the vertebrae is corrected and maintained with bone-holding forceps. The ventral spinous processes are removed using rongeurs to create a smooth bed for the two plates. One plate is placed to each side of the midline and anchored using short, 4.5-mm cortex screws.

Another report described a ventral stabilization of the atlantoaxial junction by inserting two, 6.5-mm cancellous screws across the articulation after removal of cartilage from the articular surfaces. Removal of the fractured dens prior to stabilization is optional. Care must be taken during drilling of the screw holes in the vertebral arches of the atlas to avoid the spinal canal axially, and the vertebral arteries and first cervical nerves abaxially. A bone graft is placed in the articulation to promote fusion and a polyvinylidine plate is applied to the ventral surface of the atlas and axis to provide additional stability.[3]

In the first of these two reports, at 12 months after the surgery, ataxia was no longer apparent and radiography showed fusion of C1 to C2. One complication of surgery was right-sided laryngeal hemiplegia that did not resolve.[6] The author of the second report warns of reduced lateral motion of the cranial portion of the neck after atlantoaxial fusion.[3] Implants need be removed only if there is loosening or lysis of bone.

Various arrangements of Steinmann pins and variations in the application of Kirschner apparatuses in a through-and-through pattern have been reported. Four pins placed through the vertebral bodies of the atlas and axis, anchoring the dens with one pin and securing the pins with plates at the skin surface have been used. Care was taken to avoid the vertebral arteries. The animal recovered completely.[8]

Atlantoaxial Subluxation and Luxation

Subluxation of the atlantoaxial articulation, without fracture of the dens, is a rare condition seen in young horses up to 3½ years of age.[3,9-11] The condition can be congenital in origin or the result of a traumatic incident. A combination of stretching or tearing of the ligamentous attachments of the dens and the fibrous atlantoaxial joint capsule leads to instability and spinal cord compression that is exacerbated with neck extension and relieved with flexion. The neurologic signs can be acute or chronic, and they vary in severity from mild ataxia to recumbency.[11] The horse may have abnormal head and neck carriage and local swelling if the injury is acute, and it may resent neck manipulation. On plain radiographs, there may be a malalignment of the atlas and axis and, possibly, bony changes of the atlas secondary to trauma. On the extended views, further evidence of subluxation is a lengthening of the space between the articular surfaces of the atlas and the axis ventrally, whereas the space between the dorsal arch of the atlas and the spinous process of the axis is shortened.[3,7] The spinal cord compression is documented with myelography. Computed tomography (CT) scanning of the atlas and axis may help in further defining the nature of the luxation.

Complete luxation of the atlantoaxial articulation resulting in displacement of the dens so that it lies ventral to the atlas is very rare (Figs. 53-2 through 53-5). For a complete luxation to develop, there needs to be complete disruption of the ligamentous attachments of the dens. Reportedly, horses with atlantoaxial luxation may have some stiffness of the neck but relatively few neurologic deficits.[3] The diagnosis is confirmed by radiography. With the horse under general anesthesia, efforts can be made to reduce the luxation with head and neck manipulation, but this is likely to be successful only if the injury is acute.[3] In foals, there is also a significant risk of traumatizing the spinal cord during the reduction attempts.

Horses with atlantoaxial subluxation can be successfully treated with subtotal dorsal laminectomy[3,11] (see "Subtotal Dorsal Decompression Laminectomy," in Chapter 52). Surgery is certainly recommended if the horse is showing neurologic deterioration or if neurologic deficits persist despite conservative treatment. Removing the caudal two thirds of the dorsal arch of the atlas relieves the spinal cord compression and allows the range of motion of the atlantoaxial articulation to be maintained. A portion of the dorsal atlantoaxial ligament is left intact. Although the compression may be relieved, persistent instability represents a potential threat for several weeks after surgery. In a report of four horses with atlantoaxial subluxation treated with dorsal laminectomy, two horses recovered completely and a third showed satisfactory improvement. One was lost to follow-up. No surgical treatment has been reported for complete atlantoaxial luxation.

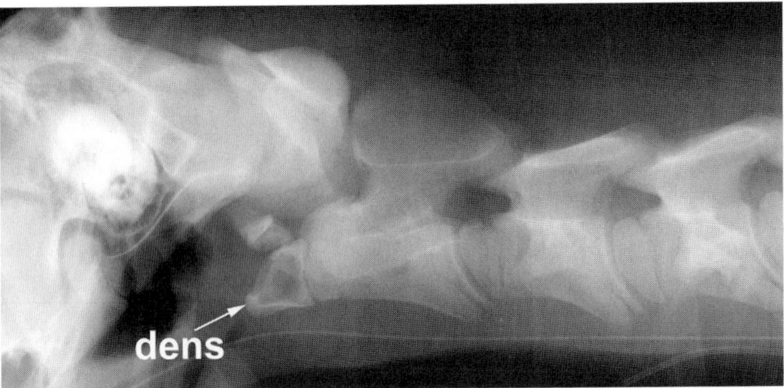

Figure 53-2. Lateral radiograph of the cranial cervical spine in a 1-week-old foal. There is luxation of C2 ventrally, relative to C1. The odontoid process (dens) is abnormally angled in a ventral direction. The body of C1 is rotated relative to the caudal cervical spine.

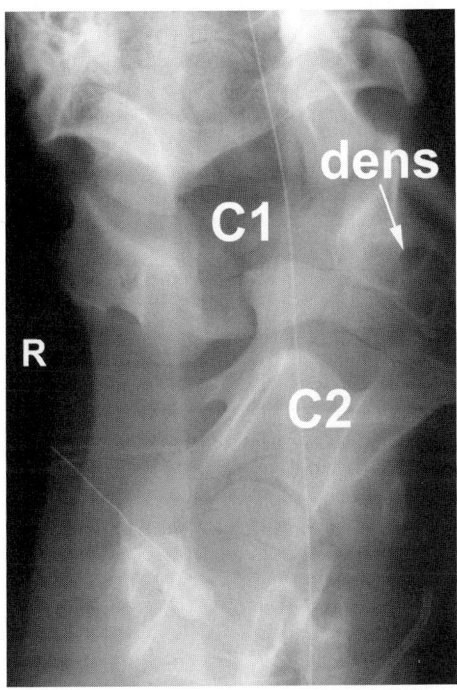

Figure 53-3. Ventrodorsal radiograph of the C1-2 articulation in a 1-week-old foal. There is leftward luxation of C2 relative to C1. The odontoid process (dens) is abnormally conformed and contains cystlike cavities.

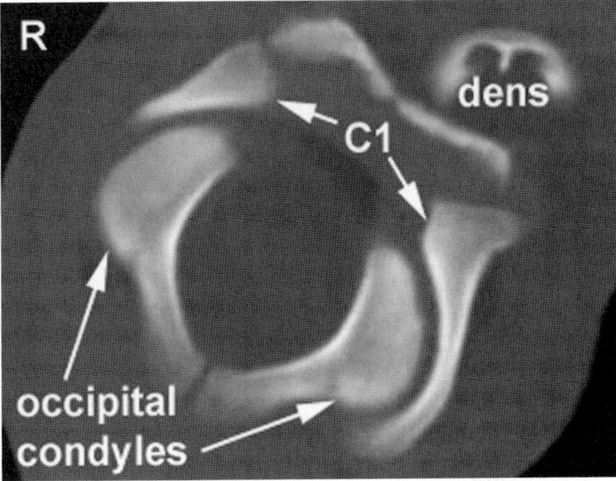

Figure 53-4. Transverse computed tomographic image at the level of the atlantooccipital articulation. The dens is displaced ventral to C1 and to the left, and it is of abnormal shape, containing cystlike cavities.

Fractures of the Atlas and the Axis

Fractures involving the atlas and the axis (other than fractures of the dens) occur occasionally. Fractures of the atlas produce neck pain and stiffness, but the degree of ataxia depends on the nature of the fracture and the degree of spinal cord impingement. In some patients, there are no neurologic deficits associated with a fracture of the atlas. Standing radiographs, including a dorsoventral view, are used to make a definitive diagnosis. In the foal, the growth plates and their closure times must be taken into consideration when interpreting the films.[12]

Fracture of the ventral arch of the atlas and disruption of the ligaments that secure the dens can lead to the formation of a bony callus that impinges on the vertebral canal and produces a later onset of ataxia.[3] Myelography and, if available, CT scanning should subsequently be performed to further document and evaluate the nature of the compression. A dorsal laminectomy of the caudal half to two thirds of the dorsal arch of the atlas can relieve the spinal cord compression created by the fracture callus and may result in a long-term improvement in the neurologic status of the horse.[3] Fractures of the axis (other than those involving the dens) occur but reports of surgical repair are rare.[2,3] There is a case report of a successful lag screw fixation of an oblique fracture of the body of C2 in a yearling warmblood stallion that was accomplished with the aid of computed tomography.[13]

Cervical Vertebral Fractures (C3 to C7)

Cervical spinal fractures in the adult horse are rare, but of the spinal fractures reported in the horse approximately 50% involved the cervical vertebrae.[2,4,5,13] Compression

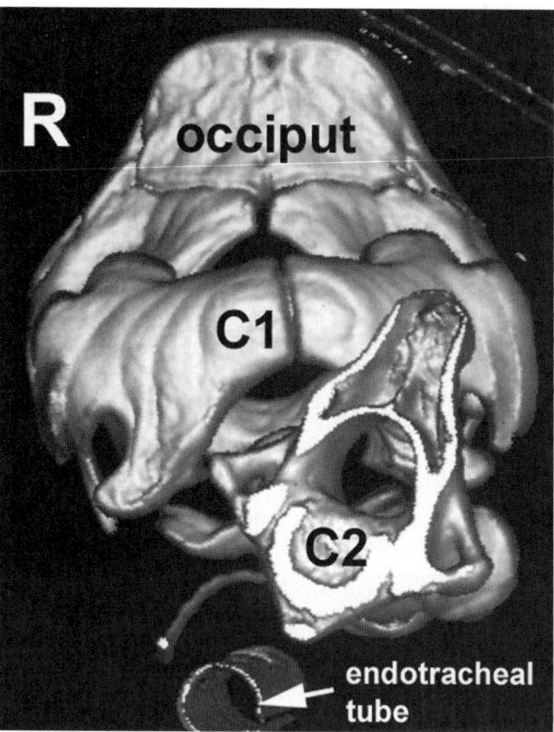

Figure 53-5. Caudodorsal, three-dimensional computed tomographic reconstruction demonstrating the relationship of C2 to C1.

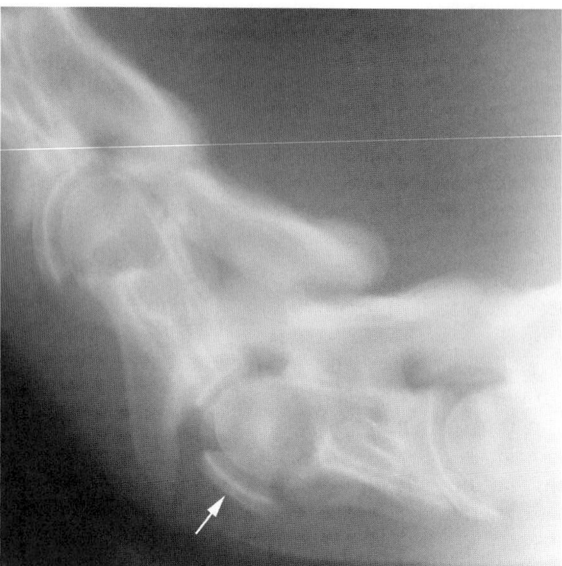

Figure 53-6. Standing lateral radiograph after an acute de-roofing injury at C4-5. The caudal endplate of C5 is fractured and there is fracture/subluxation of the C4-5 articular processes and C4 dorsal lamina, resulting in acute cervical hyperextension at this level. Note that the ventral portion of the caudal epiphysis of C4 remains attached to the C5 vertebra *(arrow)*. Motion artifact, secondary to the horse's acute neurologic deficits, is evident on the image. The horse remained standing and subsequently healed with minimal neurologic deficits.

fractures of the vertebral body are most frequently diagnosed, followed by articular facet fractures.[2] These injuries result from head-on collisions or falling over jumps or obstacles. Falls in which the neck is severely hyperextended can result in fracture through the ventral half of the caudal end plate of the vertebral body. The ventral portion of the epiphysis remains attached to the caudal vertebra by the strong fibrocartilaginous disc (Fig. 53-6). The caudal cervical vertebral body physes in horses are not closed until 4 to 5 years of age, although, practically, the cranial and caudal physes do not separate from the vertebral body in fractures or luxations after the horse is 2 years old.[2,3] If trauma is severe, pedicles of the caudal facets fracture and elevate, effectively de-roofing the spinal canal (Fig. 53-7, and see Fig. 53-6). Although the fractures can produce severe angulation of the spine, the neurologic effects are diminished as a result of the de-roofing.

Cervical vertebral body fractures can also occur after intervertebral stabilization, particularly at C5-6 and C6-7 (regardless of the fusion technique).

Clinical signs depend on the degree of bony disruption and instability at the fracture site, and on the severity of the trauma to the cord. If the fracture is displaced and the spinal cord is compressed, neurologic signs vary from mild ataxia to quadriplegia and, in some cases, sudden death.[2] Because of damage to the central portion of the spinal cord with trauma, the innervation to the forelimbs is severely affected. When compression involves dorsal nerve roots, pain and torticollis are the principal signs. Sympathetic dysfunction, exhibited by Horner's syndrome and skin hyperthermia, may be present.

The diagnosis of cervical vertebral fracture is confirmed by radiography. However, it can be very difficult in thick-necked

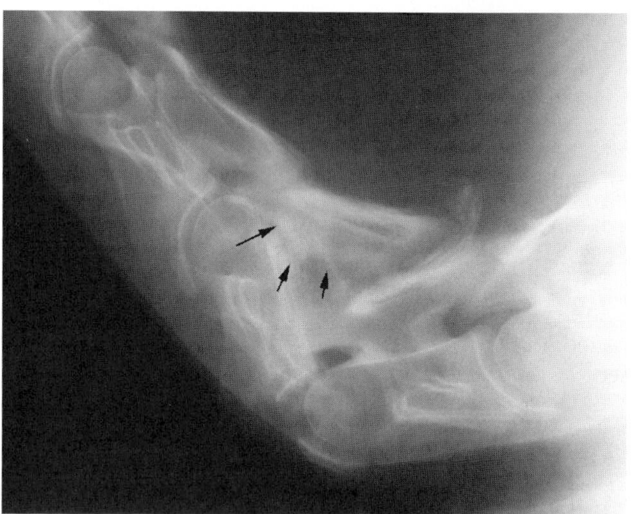

Figure 53-7. Standing lateral radiograph 40 days after injury. There is periarticular proliferative remodeling at the C4-5 articular processes representing an advanced stage of intervertebral fusion. Proliferative osseous remodeling is also present at the C4 dorsal lamina fracture *(arrows)* summating, and possibly extending into, the vertebral canal. The intervertebral disc space at C4-5 is wedged, and there is static hyperextension of the C4-5 articulation. The fractured ventral portion of the caudal epiphysis of C4 remains attached to the C5 vertebra.

horses, even if the horse is in lateral recumbency, to get diagnostic radiographs if there is minimal disruption of the fracture fragments or there is a great deal of swelling in the neck. Fracture lines may be poorly visualized. If the horse is standing, every effort should be made to get diagnostic standing radiographs. This allows a diagnosis without subjecting the horse to anesthesia and recovery, which may displace the fracture fragments, causing more damage to the spinal cord. If the horse is already recumbent, or there is progressive neurologic deterioration despite aggressive medical therapy, the horse can be anesthetized to obtain the radiographs. High-quality radiographs, including oblique and ventrodorsal views, or CT scans are necessary to gain an appreciation for the fracture configuration, particularly of vertebral body fractures where there can be multiple fracture lines and minimal displacement. The more distal portion of the neck (C5 to C7) in a large horse may be too large to be accommodated by the portal of the CT scanner. If more than one vertebra is fractured, a myelogram may be useful to determine the site or sites of spinal cord compression. When the fracture is amenable to some form of fixation, the surgeon must be prepared to immediately follow the radiographic studies with the surgical repair. The risk of further spinal cord damage if the horse is allowed to recover and be repaired at a later date is too great.

If the horse remains standing and is not showing progressive deterioration, conservative treatment is usually the treatment of choice. Some horses with pedicle fracture(s) experience further neurologic deterioration, with the formation of a healing callus that impinges on the dorsolateral aspect of the spinal canal causing cord compression[3] (Figs. 53-8 and 53-9). Horses with an articular facet fracture can also develop torticollis that becomes permanent as a result of vertebral malalignment. There is a report of coaptation cast application used successfully to immobilize noncomminuted proximal cervical vertebral fractures in foals.[14] These types of casts can be difficult to apply properly and safely.

If enough intact bone exists in the vertebral body to allow secure implant fixation, some types of recent fractures can be realigned and stabilized with screws or with plate and screw fixation, possibly in combination with ventral intervertebral stabilization.[3] Each case needs to be considered on its own merit with regard to the type of fixation required for a successful repair. Intraoperative radiographic control of the drilling depth and screw positioning is critical to avoid penetration of the vertebral canal. It is difficult to get a secure screw purchase in vertebral bone, particularly in foals. There is a report of a successful repair of a cranial articular process and lateral neural arch fracture of C4 using a combination of an intervertebral fusion procedure followed by the ventral application of a broad DC plate that spanned the bodies of C3 and C4.[3] The prognosis for recovery from any form of surgical repair is related directly to the severity of the initial neurologic deficits and the long-term stability of the repair.[3]

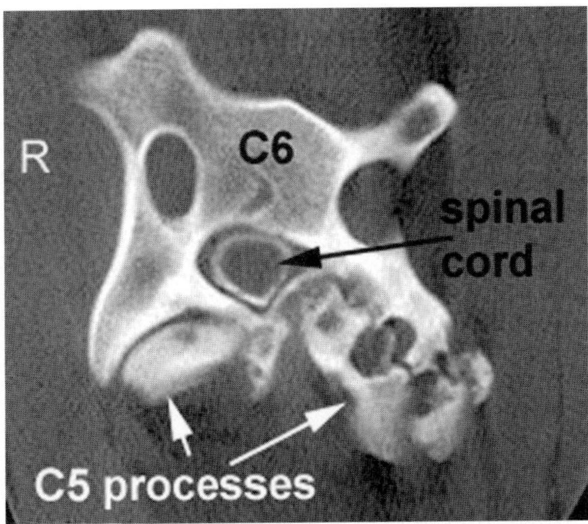

Figure 53-9. Transverse computed tomographic image through the cranial aspect of C6 after myelography. Severe degenerative remodeling and subchondral cystic change of the articular processes of C5-6 is seen on the left. Mild remodeling and subchondral cystic change is also seen at the axial aspect of the C5-6 articulation on the right. The spinal cord is outlined by a contrast-filled subarachnoid space. Note the left-sided, dorsal compression of the spinal cord secondary to the articular process remodeling.

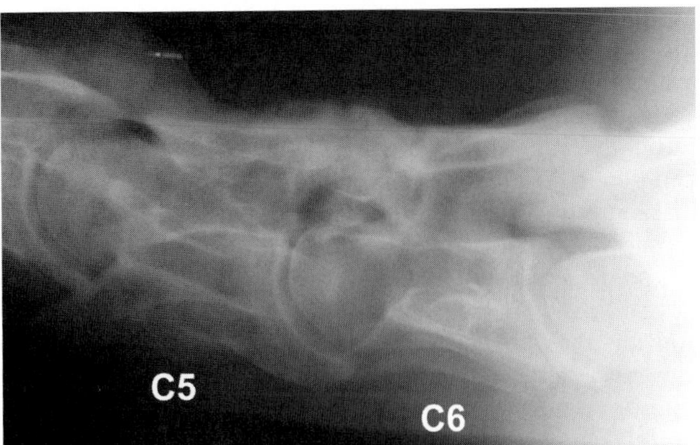

Figure 53-8. Standing oblique lateral radiograph of the C5-6 articulation in a yearling. There is severe proliferative remodeling of the articular processes at C5-6. Lateralization of the observed remodeling could not be determined radiographically.

In horses that have pedicle fractures that develop exuberant bony callus impinging on the spinal canal or the lateral foramen, signs of spinal cord compression or nerve root impingement may develop. One author suggests that surgical intervention is indicated, in the form of either a dorsal laminectomy or a ventral stabilization.[3] Removal of the dorsal lamina and reduction of the bony callus at the compressed site produces immediate decompression, but the procedure is difficult and tedious, and there is a risk of refracture of the affected pedicle and worsening of the neurologic signs as a result of surgical trauma. Ventral intervertebral fusion leads to reduction in the size of the articular facets and the bony callus over a 3-month period after the surgery. Although there is not an immediate decompression, as produced with dorsal laminectomy, there is much less risk associated with the surgery.

TRAUMATIC INJURIES TO THE THORACOLUMBAR SPINE

Thoracolumbar vertebral injuries are more common in adult horses than in foals.[4] Horses that engage in jumping activities are most often affected with life-threatening vertebral fractures.[4,15] The incidence of these types of lesions cannot be accurately assessed because some fractures are never identified. For instance, in many racing jurisdictions, it is not mandatory to perform postmortem examinations on those horses that are euthanized at the racetrack. Fracture of the thoracic dorsal spinal processes is often associated with the horse rearing, falling backward, and striking the withers. In a report of 22 cases of thoracolumbar vertebral fractures, 15 involved the vertebral body or neural arch and produced severe neurologic signs that necessitated euthanasia. The remaining seven horses had fractures of the dorsal spinous processes and exhibited no neurologic signs.[15] The more common sites of fracture of vertebral bodies include the first three thoracic vertebrae, around T12 (the area of greatest lateral bending and axial rotation), and the lumbar vertebrae.[16] Dorsal spinous process fractures tend to occur at or near T6. In a foal, a thoracic vertebral body fracture occurred at T11 after an electric shock.[17] Abscess formation in the vertebral body as a result of septicemia in foals can predispose to fracture.

The clinical signs associated with a thoracolumbar vertebral fracture depend on the portion of the vertebra that is fractured and the degree of bony disruption. Severe compressive fracture of the vertebral body may result in paraplegia if the fragments displace, in delayed onset of paraplegia if the fragments do not displace until after continued movement, and, finally, in no paraplegia if displacement remains minimal. Only the group with little or no displacement of fragments has a chance of total recovery with conservative management.

The diagnosis of a thoracolumbar vertebral body fracture in an adult horse is complicated by the fact that radiography of this area is generally unrewarding because of the massive musculature around the vertebrae. The clinician must often rely on the physical examination and neuroanatomic localization of the lesion to make a presumptive diagnosis. In the horse with a healing fracture, scintigraphy may be useful for localizing the affected vertebra. In foals, CT scanning can be used to assess the thoracolumbar spine, and myelography is used to document the extent of the spinal cord compression—information that is necessary for determining the length of decompression required if a dorsal laminectomy is being considered.[3]

Thoracolumbar laminectomy and fracture stabilization has been described in the foal and should be attempted only if the foal has evidence of deep pain recognition or some voluntary movement of the hindlimbs.[3] A dorsal laminectomy of the affected area is performed with the foal in sternal recumbency. Steinmann pins are placed into the adjacent vertebral bodies, the vertebrae are manipulated into alignment, and polyvinylidine plates are applied to the dorsal spinous processes. Polymethylmethacrylate is used to connect the pins and produce rigid fixation. The plates and pin fixation are removed in 3 to 6 months. The author stated that the prognosis for foals with thoracolumbar fractures is generally grave, although surgical treatment may improve the outcome in selected cases.[3] Adult horses that are recumbent and have severe neurologic signs as a result of thoracolumbar spinal fracture are euthanized. In those horses where the signs are limited to back pain and rear limb incoordination, conservative management can be successful.[15]

The diagnosis of fracture of the dorsal spinous processes is not difficult. The height of the spine is decreased, because the most proximal aspect of the spine fractures and moves laterally. The area becomes swollen and painful to the touch. Radiographs are helpful in confirming fractures of the dorsal spines and the extent of the damage (Fig. 53-10).

Figure 53-10. A radiograph of fractured dorsal spinous processes of the thoracic vertebrae.

Fractures of the dorsal spines usually do not require surgery unless the bone fragments become sequestered or their position, after fracture, precludes the use of a saddle. A defect in the withers area may necessitate a special saddle pad. If surgery is required or elected, the same procedure used for treatment of overriding dorsal spinous processes is employed.[18]

With the horse in lateral recumbency and the displaced processes uppermost, a long, slightly curved incision is centered over the fragments. The incision extends through the skin, the subcutis, and the supraspinous ligament. Bone fragments are identified and removed by freeing them from underlying muscle and ligamentous attachments. If the bone has sequestered or if infection is present, appropriate drainage exits are created to facilitate gravitational drainage. The area will heal enough to resume riding after 8 to 12 weeks; however, special saddle pads may need to be used to prevent abrasion by the saddle. Internal fixation of spinous process fractures with plates and screws has been performed, but the procedure carries the risk of prolonged anesthetic time and a difficult recovery from anesthesia.

TRAUMATIC INJURIES TO THE SACRAL SPINE

Trauma to the sacral area occurs when the horse suddenly dog-sits or falls over backward, landing on the croup area.[20] Subluxation where the sacrum articulates with the iliac crests causes chronic pain that may originate with one traumatic event or may be caused by repetitive jarring of the spine in this area during work. Compressive lesions of the sacrum involve the cauda equina with loss of function to the sacral and caudal nerve roots and the pudendal, caudal, and parasympathetic pelvic nerves that originate from these nerve roots.[21] The resultant clinical signs include pain and swelling over the croup and tail head, tail weakness or paralysis, decreased anal tone, retention of feces, bladder distention, and urine dribbling. There may be analgesia of the tail, anus, and perineal region, and the surface of the penis in males. The diagnosis of a sacral compressive lesion is based on the clinical signs, palpation of the sacral area per rectum, radiography, and, if the horse is small enough, CT scanning.[3,22] Scintigraphy may be useful for initially localizing an injury to the sacrum. More extensive injuries that involve the caudal lumbar and sacral regions can produce marked hind limb weakness, ataxia, and neurogenic muscle atrophy of the hindquarters. This may be documented by electromyography and muscle biopsy.

Acute injury should be treated with anti-inflammatory drugs, and up to 10 days should be allowed for signs of recovery. During this time, evacuation of the rectum several times daily and topical treatment of the tail and perineal region to prevent scalding is part of the management required. If there is no improvement within 10 days, the prognosis is unfavorable for recovery, and either surgical intervention or euthanasia should be considered. Surgical decompression of the sacrum can be achieved by removing the spinous processes and dorsal laminae of the sacral vertebrae. Even with surgery, the prognosis is guarded. In acute cases, stabilization after decompression is necessary and can be accomplished by using plates and screws.[3] In foals where stabilization was accomplished using long plates attached to dorsal spinous processes, the plates must be removed within months of the repair to prevent development of lordosis in the lumbosacral region.[3]

One of the authors examined a 6-week-old foal that had a compressive spinal lesion at L6 and S1 as a result of trauma at birth. The foal underwent a dorsal decompression of L6 and S1 and there was some improvement in clinical signs after surgery. A follow-up CT scan 4 months after surgery showed good decompression at the dorsal laminectomy site, but stenosis of several of the nerve root canals probably contributed to the ongoing muscle weakness. To date, some 5 years after surgery, the horse has residual ataxia and muscle weakness but has learned to adapt remarkably well as a nonathletic companion animal. In horses with persistent tail paralysis, the tail may need to be amputated.[22]

TRAUMATIC INJURIES TO THE COCCYGEAL VERTEBRAE

Horses have an average of 18 coccygeal vertebrae. Trauma to the more distal vertebrae may well go unnoticed. Coccygeal fractures generally occur as a result of the horse falling back onto the tail or backing into an immoveable object. Other causes of tail injury include entrapment in a door, bite wounds by other animals, and improperly placed tail wraps. If the tail distal to the site of trauma loses its blood supply, necrosis occurs, requiring amputation.

Trauma to the base of the tail (Ccy 1 to 3) may cause fracture to the vertebrae as well as soft tissue injury, and neuropraxia of the motor nerves in this area. In most horses, the fractures are closed, but the fracture may be comminuted with displacement of the fracture fragments.[23] The nerve injury can result in an inability to move the tail and defecate properly. Urine (in females) and fecal scalds can develop. Muscle atrophy over the tail head is consistent with neurogenic atrophy. Manipulation of the tail produces pain, and there is palpable crepitus at the tail base. Distal to the lesion there is loss of motor function. Lateral or oblique lateral radiographs confirm the presence of a vertebral fracture. Nuclear scintigraphy may be useful for identifying concurrent bony trauma, such as a sacral fracture.

Most horses with fractures of the coccygeal vertebrae are managed conservatively with stall rest and the use of anti-inflammatory drugs. The fractures can be relatively slow to heal, and there may be permanent neurologic damage as well as conformational changes as a result of the muscle atrophy and callus formation.[23] Some form of stabilization or fixation, such as the placement of Steinmann pins across the fracture or the use of the pinless external fixator (see Chapters 81 and 103), might hasten healing and reduce the irritation to nerves in the area, thereby allowing a quicker return of tail function.

REFERENCES

1. Jeffcott LB: Disorders of the thoracolumbar spine of the horse: A survey of 443 cases, Equine Vet J 1980;12:197.
2. Pinchbeck G, Murphy D: Cervical vertebral fracture in three foals, Equine Vet Educ 2001;13:8.
3. Nixon AJ: Equine Fracture Repair, Philadelphia, 1996, WB Saunders.
4. Mayhew IG, MacKay RJ: The nervous system. In Equine Medicine and Surgery, ed 3, Santa Barbara, Calif, 1982, American Veterinary Publications.
5. Tyler CM, Davis RE, Begg AP, et al: A survey of neurological diseases in horses, Aust Vet J 1993;70:445.
6. McCoy DJ, Shires PK, Beadle R: A ventral approach for stabilization of atlantoaxial subluxation secondary to an odontoid fracture in a foal, J Am Vet Med Assoc 1984;185:545.
7. Slone DE, Bergfeld WA, Walker TL: Surgical decompression for traumatic atlantoaxial subluxation in a weanling filly, J Am Vet Med Assoc 1979;174:1234.
8. Owen RR, Smith-Maxie LL: Repair of a fractured dens of the axis in a foal, J Am Vet Med Assoc 1978;173:854.
9. Funk KA, Erikson ED: A case of atlantoaxial subluxation in a horse, Can Vet J 1968;9:120.
10. Guffy MM, Coffman JR, Strafuss AC: Atlantoaxial luxation in a foal, J Am Vet Med Assoc 1969;155:754.
11. Nixon AJ, Stashak TS: Laminectomy for relief of atlantoaxial subluxation in four horses, J Am Vet Med Assoc 1988;193:677.
12. Maierl J, Zechmeister R, Schill W, et al: Radiologic description of the growth plates of the atlas and axis in foals, Tierarztl Prax Ausg G Grosstiere Nutztiere 1998;26:341.
13. Barnes HG, Tucker RL, Grant BD, et al: Lag screw stabilization of a cervical vertebral fracture by use of computed tomography in a horse, J Am Vet Med Assoc 1995;206:221.
14. Schneider JE: Immobilization of cervical vertebral fractures, Proc Am Assoc Equine Pract 1981;27:253.
15. Jeffcott LB, Whitwell KE: Fractures of the thoracolumbar spine of the horse, Proc Am Assoc Equine Pract 1976;22:91.
16. Townsend HG, Leach DH, Doige CE, et al: Relationship between spinal biomechanics and pathological changes in the equine thoracolumbar spine, Equine Vet J 1986;18:107.
17. DeBowes RM, Wagner PC, Gavin PR, et al: Vertebral compression fracture in a foal following electrical shock, J Vet Orthop 1981;2:14.
18. Walmsley JP, Pettersson H, Winberg F, et al: Impingement of the dorsal spinous processes in two hundred and fifteen horses: Case selection, surgical technique and results, Equine Vet J 2002;34:23.
19. Vlahos T: Personal communication, 2004.
20. Wagner PC, Long GG, Chatburn CC, et al: Traumatic injury of the cauda equina in the horse. A case report, J Equine Med Surg 1977;1:282.
21. Chaffin MK, Honnas CM, Crabill MR, et al: Cauda equina syndrome, diskospondylitis, and a paravertebral abscess caused by *Rhodococcus equi* in a foal, J Am Vet Med Assoc 1995;206:215.
22. Collatos C, Allen D, Chambers J, et al: Surgical treatment of sacral fracture in a horse, J Am Vet Med Assoc 1991;198:877.
23. Tutko JM, Sellon DC, Burns GA, et al: Cranial coccygeal vertebral fractures in horses: 12 cases, Equine Vet Educ 2002;14:197.

CHAPTER 54

Peripheral Nerve Injury

Robert J. MacKay

ETIOLOGY AND PATHOGENESIS

Mechanical injuries to peripheral nerves occur because of compression, entrapment, transection, laceration, ischemia, crushing, stretching, and chemical or burn damage.[1,2] These injuries are usually categorized according to the degree of damage to a single axon. However, compound nerves contain numerous fascicles, and each fascicle is made up of many axons within a connective tissue sheath. The functional effect of damage is seldom as straightforward as single-fiber classifications would suggest, and usually reflects differing degrees of damage across a nerve.

Damage to individual axons fall into two major functional categories. Type 1 injury refers to loss of function without loss of axonal continuity. Type 2 injury represents damage to axonal structures such that Wallerian degeneration of the axon ensues distal to the site of injury; the proximal axonal segment and the cell body remain intact. Retrograde degeneration of the proximal nerve occurs if connectivity is not reestablished. A well-accepted classification system that divides the spectrum of injury into five categories[3] is shown in Figure 54-1.

Type 1 or *neurapractic lesions* are characterized by a failure of conduction of the action potential across the injured axonal segment.[4] Normal muscle action potentials are evoked by stimulation of the nerve anywhere distal to the lesion, but they are absent when the nerve is stimulated proximal to the injury. The pathologic basis for these reversible injuries could be nerve compression, damage to the myelin sheath, or alteration of the functions of the axonal cell membrane or its channel proteins.

Type 2 injuries are characterized by axonal interruption, or *axonotmesis*. This is equivalent to the Sunderland type II injury. If there is disruption of components of the connective tissue sheath and axon, the process is termed *neurotmesis*. According to the Sunderland classification system, there are three grades of neurotmesis (III, IV, and V), reflecting disruption of endoneurium, perineurium, and epineurium. Recovery by axonal regrowth is unlikely after neurotmesis.[5] Immediately after axonotmetic injury, the distal axonal segment is competent to conduct action potentials; however, within 3 to 8 days after injury, the distal segment degenerates and no longer responds to electrical stimulation. In this way, neurapractic (type 1) and axonotmetic (type 2) injuries of greater than 8 days' duration can theoretically be distinguished. Longstanding axonotmetic injuries result in retrograde degeneration of the neuronal cell body and secondary demyelination of the proximal axonal segment. After axonotmesis of motor nerves, muscle reinnervation occurs by two separate mechanisms: collateral sprouting and axonal regrowth.[1] If there is incomplete loss of axons to a muscle, surviving motor axons generate sprouts from their nerve terminals, which can establish competent junctions with adjacent denervated muscle units. Reinnervation of muscle units by this process occurs within days to weeks. However, if the motor axons to a muscle are severed, reinnervation occurs by growth of collateral sprouts from the proximal stump. Axonal sprouts grow at a rate of 1 mm per day (approximately 1 inch per month). Regeneration occurs under the influence of growth factors including neurotrophic growth factor, brain-derived neurotrophic factor, and ciliary neurotrophic factor.[6] Successful reinnervation thus may take many months. Because of progressive fibrous replacement of denervated muscle and retrograde degeneration of the proximal parts of affected motor neurons, it has been suggested that reinnervation may not be possible if more than 12 months have elapsed since the original injury. However, reinnervation surgery has been successful when performed on human patients 20 years or more after denervation.[7]

Large-diameter myelinated fibers are most sensitive to compression forces. The largest sensory axons, including afferent fibers conveying touch-pressure, vibration, and proprioception, are larger than motor axons and are usually damaged first.

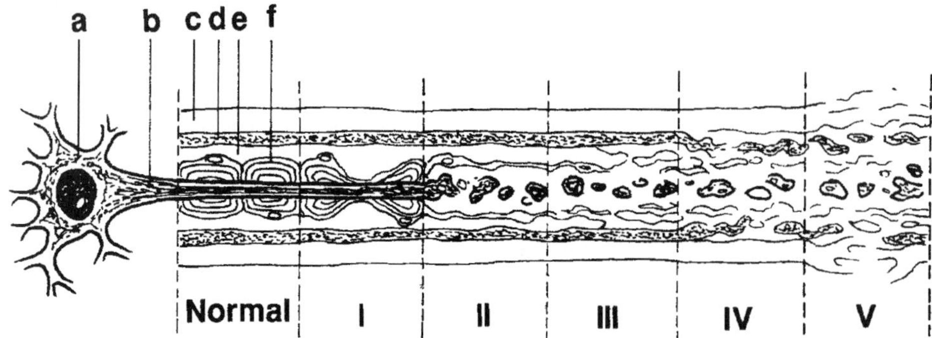

Figure 54-1. Sunderland classification of nerve injury. a, cell body; b, axon; c, epineurium; d, perineurium; e, endoneurium; f, myelin sheath; I, first degree (neurapraxia); II, second degree (axonotmesis); III, third degree; IV, fourth degree; V, fifth degree.

CLINICAL SIGNS

Peripheral nerve injuries are characterized by weakness of the innervated muscle, accompanied within 2 to 4 weeks by appreciable atrophy. When the injured nerve supplies important extensor muscles of the limbs (e.g., radial, femoral, sciatic, peroneal), there is obvious alteration of gait. Areas of cutaneous anesthesia occasionally accompany peripheral nerve injuries. Over the neck and trunk, cutaneous sensory innervation occurs in defined bands associated with segmental dermatomes. Damage to a peripheral spinal nerve or dorsal nerve root results in cutaneous anesthesia/hypalgesia over the supplied dermatome. With damage to the pudendal nerve or its sacral nerve roots, there is anesthesia/hypalgesia of the perineal area. In contrast, relatively small autonomous zones have been defined for sensory components of the ulnar, musculocutaneous, median, femoral, tibial, and peroneal nerves[8,9] (Fig. 54-2). Sympathetic fibers are distributed with peripheral nerves, so denervated skin also may be evident as circumscribed spontaneous sweating. The most common and important syndromes of mechanical injury to peripheral nerves of the limbs are described later.[9-11]

Suprascapular Nerve

The suprascapular nerve arises from the 6th and 7th cervical spinal cord segments and courses laterally and ventrally between the supraspinatus and subscapularis muscles before coursing around the front of the scapula about 7 cm proximal to the scapular tuberosity and ramifying in the supraspinous and infraspinous fossae.

Suprascapular nerve injury occurs most commonly when a horse collides at speed with another horse or with inanimate objects, such as fences, trees, or doorways. It may also occur when a galloping horse stumbles over uneven ground. In each of these situations, there is likely to be stretching or direct compression (or both) of the suprascapular nerve as it curls around the front of the neck of the scapula under cover of the supraspinatus muscle. The muscles innervated by the suprascapular nerve, the supraspinatus and infraspinatus, normally provide lateral support for the shoulder joint. Consequently, when the nerve is injured, there immediately is laxity and lateral instability of the shoulder joint, which bows out or "pops" as the affected limb bears weight. Although subluxation of the shoulder joint does occur after the suprascapular nerve is blocked at the scapular neck, it has been suggested that other nerves (e.g., axillary, pectoral, subscapular, brachial plexus roots) and muscles (e.g., pectoral, subclavius, subscapularis) are usually damaged with this type of injury, thus contributing to shoulder instability and subluxation.[10] Within 2 to 4 weeks of injury, there is obvious atrophy of the supraspinatus and infraspinatus muscles. Wasting of these muscles becomes complete over the ensuing several months. The condition is known as *sweeney*.

Neurapractic damage to the suprascapular nerve should heal within several days to several weeks. After partial nerve damage, sprouts from the neuromuscular terminals of surviving fibers should find denervated muscle and restore function within several weeks. In either of these settings (neurapraxia or partial nerve damage), severe muscle atrophy should not occur before recovery begins. More complete axonal injury results in sweeney, and any recovery depends on regrowth of axonal sprouts from the proximal stump of the suprascapular nerve. Successful reinnervation is evident as recovery of muscle bulk in the ventral part of the

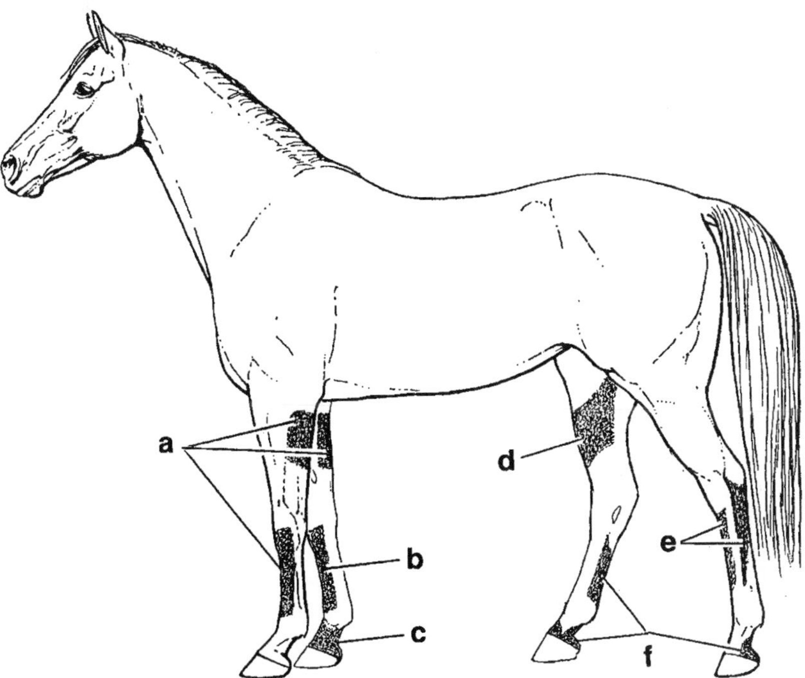

Figure 54-2. Areas of anesthesia/hypalgesia (autonomous zones) associated with injury to the major peripheral nerves of the limbs of the horse. a, Ulnar n. dermatomes; musculocutaneous n. dermatome; c, median n. dermatome; d, femoral n. dermatome; e, peroneal n. dermatomes; f, tibial n. dermatomes.

supraspinatus muscle beginning within 3 months of injury. Maximal recovery takes an additional 3 to 12 months. Regrowth of the suprascapular nerve can be facilitated by surgery to resect scar tissue (external neurolysis) and reduce tension on the nerve as it crosses the front of the scapula (see Chapter 98).[12,13] The surgery can either be performed preemptively when soft tissue swelling has subsided, or 3 to 6 months after injury when it is clear that spontaneous re-innervation is not occurring.

Radial Nerve

The radial nerve innervates a flexor of the shoulder and the extensors of the elbow, carpal, and digital joints. It arises chiefly from the 1st thoracic root of the brachial plexus. The nerve travels for a short distance with the ulnar nerve as it passes between the long and medial heads of the triceps. From there, it winds downward and outward around the humerus in the musculospiral groove, crosses the lateral aspect of the elbow joint, and ramifies in the extensor muscles of the digit.

The nerve is well protected by surrounding muscles and therefore not normally damaged unless there is severe injury to adjacent tissues. The T1 nerve root may be lacerated by fracture of the C7 or T1 vertebra or the first rib. Likewise, the proximal part of the nerve is commonly damaged as a result of humeral fracture.[14] The radial nerve (or the roots that form it) may be injured with other components of the brachial plexus by trauma to the shoulder region. Rarely, the nerve is injured when the upper leg gets wedged (e.g., in a tub or between the rails of a fence) and the horse struggles to release it. The radial nerve and triceps muscles are vulnerable to damage when horses are positioned in lateral recumbency, usually under general anesthesia. The risk is particularly high in large, muscular horses on poorly padded surfaces, and it increases with the duration of the procedure. Experimental studies have shown that ½ to 1 hour of ischemia produces neurapractic conduction failure, and greater than 3 hours of ischemia causes permanent changes.[15] The lower part of the nerve is in close proximity to the lateral aspect of the elbow, under cover of the lateral head of the triceps, and it may be damaged by direct trauma to this site or by dislocation or fractures that involve the elbow.

Horses with complete radial paralysis stand with the shoulder extended and the rest of the joints flexed. The elbow is "dropped" (i.e., lower than normal) and the dorsum of the hoof rests on the ground. When forced to walk, the horse may partially protract the limb by exaggerated extension of the shoulder; however, the toe drags and the horse collapses on the limb during the weight-bearing phase of the stride. If the site of damage is distal to the branches to the heads of the triceps (middle third of the humerus), the shoulder is held in normal position and the elbow is not usually dropped. Such horses can bear weight if the hoof is placed flat on the ground. If reflexes can be tested while the horse is recumbent, it is expected that the triceps reflex will be absent but the flexor (withdrawal) reflex will be normal. Although the radial nerve has numerous cutaneous sensory branches, injury to this nerve does not result in any consistent area of cutaneous anesthesia.

Beginning at 2 to 4 weeks, there is progressive atrophy of the extensor muscles of the limb distal to the site of injury. The principles just described for neurapractic and axonotmetic injuries apply. With regrowth of axonal sprouts from the proximal stump of the radial nerve, the triceps muscle is expected to recover function before the digital extensors.

Musculocutaneous Nerve

The musculocutaneous nerve arises near the suprascapular nerve from the part of the brachial plexus supplied by the 7th and 8th cervical roots. It descends on the medial surface of the coracobrachialis muscle and forms a loop with the median nerve directly beneath the brachial artery before terminating in branches to the biceps brachii, pectoral, and brachialis muscles. The musculocutaneous nerve supplies flexors of the elbow.

Injury to the nerve is rare and causes only transient toe-dragging. The shoulder may be held in a flexed position and the elbow in an extended position. The diagnosis can be made by finding hypalgesia/anesthesia over the dorsomedial aspect of the carpal region and proximal metacarpus (see Fig. 54-2), beginning immediately after the injury, and by appreciating obvious atrophy of the biceps and brachialis muscles, beginning 2 to 4 weeks after injury. Injury to the musculocutaneous nerve eliminates the biceps reflex, although this reflex is difficult to obtain even in normal horses. The flexor reflex should be intact, although elbow flexion may be weak.

Median and Ulnar Nerves

The median nerve is the largest branch of the brachial plexus and receives input from the 8th cervical and 1st thoracic nerves. After exchanging fibers with the musculocutaneous nerve, it descends along the medial aspect of the leg in association with major arteries and terminates in palmar and cutaneous branches. The ulnar nerve arises from the thoracic part of the brachial plexus, passes downward and backward over the medial epicondyle of the humerus (deep to the medial head of the triceps), and passes along the palmar aspect of the metacarpus under cover of the digital flexors to terminate in branches that contribute to the lateral palmar nerve and cutaneous sensation. These nerves supply muscles that extend the elbow, and flex the carpus and digits.

Injury to either or both nerves can be caused by injury at the brachial plexus or along the medial aspect of the upper limb. Experimental section of the nerves causes a "tin soldier" gait, with decreased flexion and dragging of the toe during the protraction phase of the stride. There is hypalgesia/analgesia of the skin of the caudal forearm, lateral metacarpus, and medial phalangeal areas. When flexor reflexes are tested by pinching the skin of an area with unimpaired sensation (e.g., over the lateral metacarpophalangeal [MCP] joint), there is an intact flexor response, but it is weak compared with the normal side. Even without recovery of nerve function, interference with gait at the walk decreases over time and is minimal by 3 months after the injury. The reason for this adaptation is unclear, although it has been suggested that fibers contributed by the musculocutaneous nerve may take over some of the functions from the median nerve. Atrophy of the carpal and digital flexor muscles is apparent after 2 to 4 weeks.

Femoral Nerve

The femoral nerve arises principally from the 4th and 5th lumbar nerve roots, courses backward and ventrally between the psoas major and minor muscles, and then runs between the sartorius and iliopsoas muscles lateral to the external iliac artery. It terminates as branches to the heads of the quadriceps. The saphenous nerve, a branch with both motor and sensory function, joins the femoral nerve at the point of emergence from the psoas muscles. The femoral nerve innervates muscles that flex the hip and extend the stifle.

The nerve courses too deeply to be directly affected by an external blow to the pelvic limb; however, it can be damaged by ilial, femoral, or vertebral fractures. Ischemic injury caused by prolonged stretch or increased tissue pressure during anesthesia in dorsal recumbency may cause bilateral femoral neurapraxia.[16] A similar presentation, presumably caused by compression of nerve roots by the foal in the birth canal, is seen in mares after severe prolonged dystocia.

With unilateral paralysis of the femoral nerve, the pelvic limb adopts a flexed posture, usually with the foot flat on the ground. When the horse tries to bear weight, the limb buckles. During walking, there is obvious lameness, with a relatively brief and ineffectual weight-bearing phase over the affected limb. This can be quite subtle in horses with partial femoral nerve paralysis. In the case of bilateral involvement, the horse is either unable to rise or gets to its feet with difficulty, and then stands briefly and uncomfortably in a crouched position.

If the nerve injury occurs proximal to the saphenous branch, there is anesthesia/hypalgesia of the skin over the medial surface of the thigh (see Fig. 54-2). Atrophy of the quadriceps muscle is evident within 2 to 4 weeks. The flexor reflex should be normal, but the patellar reflex is weak or absent.

Sciatic Nerve

The sciatic nerve is the largest nerve in the body. It is derived principally from the 6th lumbar and 1st sacral nerves but also receives a branch from the 5th lumbar nerve. The nerve passes caudally and ventrally on the sacrosciatic ligament before turning between the greater trochanter and tuber ischii. It courses ventrally in the thigh between the biceps femoris laterally and the adductor, semimembranosus, and semitendinosus medially. It continues as the tibial and peroneal nerves. The sciatic nerve supplies important extensors of the hip and flexors of the stifle.

Sciatic nerve damage is usually a result of deep injections into the caudal thigh ventral to the greater trochanter. Such injections may injure the nerve by direct laceration, injection of material into the nerve, or through secondary inflammation or compression from scarring induced by previous deposition of the drug close to the nerve.[1] In most cases, the neurologic deficits are apparent within a few minutes. A delayed onset suggests the development of perineurial or endoneurial inflammation or fibrosis. The nerve may also be injured by fractures of the ilium or ischium, or by sacroiliac and coxofemoral dislocations.

The posture of the affected limb is characteristic: it is held slightly caudal with the dorsum of the hoof resting on the ground. The stifle and tarsus are more extended than normal, whereas the distal joints are flexed. During walking, the leg is dragged forward by the actions of the quadriceps and biceps femoris muscles. These muscles, in concert with the reciprocal apparatus, allow the horse to bear some weight on the limb if the foot is first placed in normal position.

There is cutaneous hypalgesia/anesthesia over most of the limb except for the medial thigh. If the flexor reflex is tested by pinching the skin over the medial thigh, the response is intact, but weak compared with the normal side.

Peroneal Nerve

The peroneal nerve arises from the sciatic trunk deep to the biceps femoris and descends on the lateral head of the gastrocnemius. It crosses the lateral aspect of the femorotibial joint and terminates in superficial and deep branches, which course ventrally between the long and lateral digital extensors. The nerve provides motor innervation to the flexors of the tarsus and the extensors of the digit.

Paralysis results in extension of the tarsus and flexion of the distal joints of the pelvic limb. At rest, the limb is held slightly caudally with the distal joints in flexed position and the dorsum of the hoof contacting the ground. During walking, the limb is moved erratically. The toe is dragged along the ground during the weak protraction phase, and then pulled caudally as the horse attempts to bear weight. As is the case with sciatic involvement, the limb can support weight if the foot is placed in normal position.

There is progressive atrophy of the cranial tibial and long and lateral digital extensors and immediate cutaneous hypalgesia/anesthesia over the lateral metatarsus. The flexor reflex is intact and usually appears normal.

Tibial Nerve

The tibial nerve represents the direct continuation of the sciatic nerve. It runs between the bellies of the gastrocnemius muscle and passes distally on the medial aspect of the leg immediately dorsal to the superficial flexor tendon before terminating in the medial and lateral plantar nerves. The tibial nerve innervates the gastrocnemius (extensor of the tarsus) and digital flexors.

With tibial neuropathy, the resting limb is held more flexed than is normal and, although the foot contacts the ground in normal position, the MCP joint often partially collapses into a flexed position (i.e., "knuckles"). The foot is moved in stringhalt-like fashion, with exaggerated flexion of the tarsus and stifle during protraction, followed by sudden extension to the weight-bearing phase of the stride.

There is atrophy of the gastrocnemius and cutaneous hypalgesia/anesthesia of the caudal metatarsal region and bulbs of the heels. The flexor reflex is tested by pinching the skin over the dorsal aspect of the MCP joint. The reflex is present but weaker than on the normal side.

DIAGNOSIS

The diagnosis of peripheral nerve injuries is normally made by careful observation of clinical signs, including testing of reflexes and cutaneous sensation. It may not be possible to discern the effects of nerve damage until fractures are stabilized and soft tissue swelling subsides. The examination must carefully document the location and severity of weakness, atrophy, and sensory and reflex alterations. The findings should be documented thoroughly and recorded at each examination so that progression can be determined.

Beginning 2 to 4 weeks after injury, progressive atrophy becomes apparent in large muscles supplied by the damaged nerve. Beginning about 2 weeks after injury, the distribution of muscular denervation can be determined objectively by needle electromyography in the sedated or anesthetized patient. This is particularly helpful in cases of apparent suprascapular or radial neuropathy to determine whether there is singular involvement of a particular peripheral nerve or injury at the level of the brachial plexus.

Nerve stimulation can be used to assess location, severity, and recovery from nerve injury. With both neurapraxia and axonotmesis, nerve conduction across the lesion is affected. Thus, when the proximal segment of the motor nerve is stimulated electrically, the amplitude of the evoked muscle action potential is reduced in proportion to the severity of the injury. It is technically possible to distinguish signs of neurapraxia from those that are the result of physical interruption of the axons of the nerve. Because axonal injury leads to degeneration of the distal nerve segment, electrical stimulation of the nerve distal to the injury site fails to evoke motor action potentials, or they are of reduced amplitude, when tested at least 9 days after the injury.[1] In contrast, nerves blocked by neurapraxia evoke normal muscle responses after stimulation. It must be remembered that an injured nerve frequently has a mixture of neurapractic and axonotmetic lesions, and the findings may not clearly distinguish between the two types of injury. Sensory nerve conduction studies are performed in humans by electrically stimulating peripheral sensory axons at one point and recording sensory nerve action potentials at a more proximal point. This technique is useful for distinguishing lesions of the dorsal root from those involving peripheral parts of the nerve.

Nerve conduction procedures are not well established in the horse but "proof-of-principle" studies have been published for selected nerves in normal horses.[8,17-19] High-resolution ultrasonography[20] or magnetic resonance imaging may be used to help pinpoint the location of peripheral nerves and aid in precise stimulation and recording.

MANAGEMENT

Nonsurgical Management

The objectives of medical treatment of peripheral nerve injury are (1) reduction of swelling and inflammation at the site of injury, (2) support and stabilization of the denervated area, and (3) maintenance of the general health of the animal.

In the case of lacerating trauma, the general principles of wound management apply. The wound should be cleaned, irrigated, débrided, and dressed and ventral drainage established. If severed nerve ends are visible, they can be tagged for later identification. Medical therapy for inflammation and swelling should be initiated, especially if there is obvious tissue swelling. This may include any combination of a cyclooxygenase inhibitor (e.g., flunixin meglumine, 1.1 mg/kg IV, IM, or PO once or twice daily), dimethyl sulfoxide (DMSO) (1 g/kg as a 10% solution IV or by nasogastric tube once or twice daily), and a glucocorticoid (e.g., dexamethasone, 0.05 mg/kg IV or IM once daily, or 0.1 mg/kg PO once daily). Additional anti-inflammatory effect can be provided by cold water hydrotherapy or local application of skin-permeant drugs such as DMSO or diclofenac. If there is an open wound or other risk for bacterial infection, broad-spectrum antimicrobial therapy should be initiated. This can be directed by culture results, if available.

Fractured or dislocated bones that have the potential to further injure nerves must be reduced and stabilized. Stall rest is essential to prevent further injury. In the case of paralyzed limbs, a protective wrap may be necessary to prevent damage caused by dragging or improperly placing the limb. A support wrap or light cast should be maintained on a leg affected with radial paralysis so as to prevent limb contracture. A support wrap should also be placed on the opposite limb to protect against breakdown caused by increased weightbearing. If the horse has difficulty alternating between recumbency and standing, it should be supported as necessary in an abdominal sling until it is able to rise unassisted. Because of the buoyancy provided by water, horses may be able to exercise affected limbs in swimming pools. Skin over bony prominences should be padded to prevent decubital injury; such injuries must be treated aggressively if they occur.

In foals, passive range-of-motion exercises should be performed on paralyzed limbs in an attempt to preserve joint flexibility and prevent contracture. Faradic or galvanic electrical muscle stimulation has been advocated for denervated muscle to help preserve muscle mass, and units designed for use in horses are available. This practice is controversial, however, and may possibly delay nerve regrowth into muscle.[21] Hyperbaric oxygen is an approved adjunctive treatment for acute traumatic ischemic reperfusion injury of humans and theoretically could help horses with post-recumbency neuropathies.

Surgical Management

Because neurosurgery in horses is at a rudimentary stage, it is difficult to provide precise rules for assessment and intervention after mechanical nerve injury. The following guidelines are based on comparable situations in human medicine.[1,2]

- In clean lacerating injuries in which the nerve ends are visible or when clinical examination reveals obvious motor and sensory deficits resulting from the injury at the laceration, primary repair may be indicated. In general, results of primary repair (within 3 to 4 days) are better than results of secondary repair (after 2 to 3 weeks).
- In nerve transections resulting from blunt lacerating trauma, secondary repair has a better surgical result. This allows time for control of infection and resolution of soft tissue swelling.
- Injuries that do not demonstrate evidence of early spontaneous recovery should be explored surgically. This applies especially to traumatic injury of the suprascapular nerve or injection injury of the sciatic nerve. Empirically, the outer time limit for exploration can be estimated from the observations that muscle must be reinnervated within 12 months and that nerve regrows at the rate of 1 inch per month. According to these precepts, the length in inches

from the injury site to the muscle supplied plus the time in months since the injury should not exceed 12. For example, if the peroneal nerve were injured 6 inches from its entry into the anterior tibial muscle, no more than 6 months should be allowed for spontaneous recovery of innervation.

Anastomosis

If the nerve is ruptured or severed, the retracted ends should be identified.[22] With the help of an operating microscope, the damaged portions of the nerve should be trimmed and the proximal and distal stumps aligned as accurately as possible by *epineurial repair*. Coaptation is achieved by simple-interrupted epineurial sutures (8-0 to 10-0 monofilament nylon or silk) around the circumference of the anastomosis. A perfect superficial alignment can be achieved using epineurial vessels as landmarks, but the internal orientation of fascicular bundles and individual fascicles may not be correct (Fig. 54-3). The more technically difficult *fascicular repair* technique involves alignment and attachment of individual fascicular groups. Epineurial tissue is resected from around the circumference of the nerve, and fascicular groups are subsequently coapted with single sutures in the perineurium or connective tissue surrounding groups of fascicles. Nonsuture methods have been described and include wrapping the nerve, gluing the ends together with plasma clot or fibrin glue, or using a carbon dioxide laser to weld the nerve ends together.[23]

Tension at the anastomosis site must be minimized by mobilization of the nerve ends and postoperative immobilization and rest. If the gap between the ends is too large to permit anastomosis without tension, a *conduit technique* may be considered, wherein the defect is bridged in such a way as to support axonal growth toward the distal nerve segment. For this purpose, either a tube or a graft is used. Silicone tubes, freeze-thawed muscle tubes, and collagen-based nerve gap conduits have been used. Nerve autografts

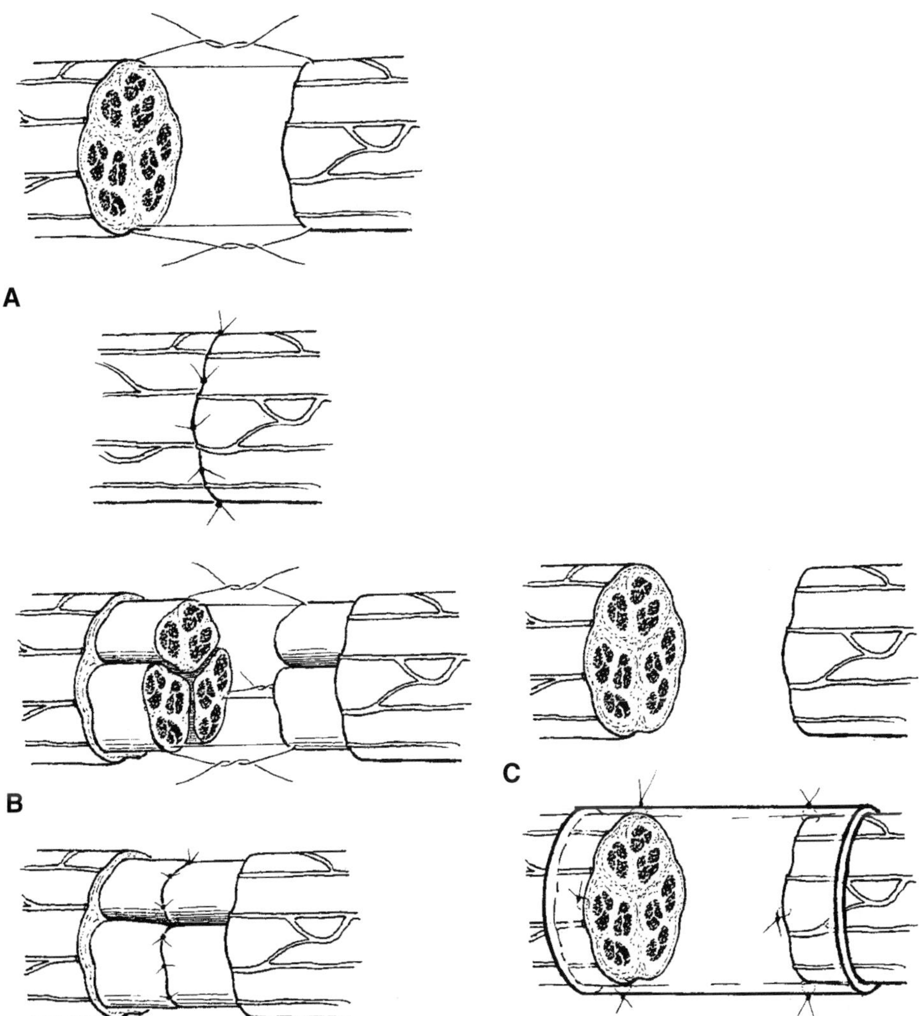

Figure 54-3. End-to-end repair of peripheral nerves. **A,** Epineural suture. Coaptation is achieved by single sutures in the epineurium around the circumference of the nerve. **B,** Group fascicular suture. Epineural tissue has been resected, and fascicular groups are coapted with single sutures in the perineurium or connective tissue surrounding groups of fascicles. **C,** Tubular repair. (Modified from Lundborg GA: 25-year perspective of peripheral nerve surgery: Evolving neuroscientific concepts and clinical significance, J Hand Surg Am 2000;25:391.)

from a remote donor site (e.g., sural nerve) also could be used for bridging a long nerve gap. In nerve injuries in which the proximal segment cannot be used for grafting, the distal segment theoretically can be implanted in end-to-side fashion into an epineurial window on an adjacent uninjured nerve. Similarly, the technique of direct neurotization of muscle has been validated experimentally in settings where nerve has been traumatically avulsed from muscle. A similar technique has been used in horses with left laryngeal hemiplegia. In this technique, a narrow strip of muscle with an intact nerve supply (the neuromuscular pedicle graft) is removed from the omohyoid muscle and inserted into the paralyzed dorsal cricoarytenoid muscle.[24] Over the subsequent months, the dorsal cricoarytenoid muscle becomes reinnervated and is stimulated to contract during exercise.

After surgical exploration of a nonregenerating nerve, the damaged section can be removed and the ends anastomosed using one of the techniques described earlier.

Neurolysis

External neurolysis refers to the dissection of the nerve from a bed of scar tissue.[1] This is indicated if there is obvious compression from fibrous tissue, and it is performed routinely in horses with suprascapular neuropathy.[12] This procedure is described in Chapter 98. *Internal neurolysis* involves an incision of the epineurium and resection of scar tissue from between nerve fascicles.

COMPLICATIONS

In response to trophic factors produced at the site of nerve injury, misdirected axonal sprouting and Schwann cell proliferation may produce bulblike *neuromas,* either at the proximal stump of a transected nerve (end-neuroma) or within a partially disrupted nerve (neuroma-in-continuity).[25] End-neuromas are a common complication of palmar digital neurectomy in horses suffering from navicular syndrome.[26,27] Neuroma-in-continuity or fibrous entrapment at the site of injury or surgical repair is associated with a variety of pain syndromes in humans. The local sensitivity and reaction to touch that occur are described as dysesthesia (unpleasant abnormal sensation, whether spontaneous or evoked), allodynia (pain as a result of a stimulus that does not normally provoke pain), or hyperpathia (excessive reaction to painful stimuli). Disruption of sensory, motor, and autonomic fibers together can result in causalgia syndromes with sustained burning pain, vasomotor and sudomotor dysfunction, and later trophic changes of the skin. On the basis of the documented painful local effect of neuromas after palmar digital neurectomy, it is likely that similar syndromes occur in horses.

In attempts to reduce neuroma formation in nerved horses, the proximal stump has been exposed to CO_2 laser energy or injected with doxorubicin.[26,27] Neuroma treatment in humans generally involves excision of the neuroma and proximal translocation of the nerve stump into adjacent fat or into a burr hole created in bone.[25]

In addition to permanent degenerative changes in muscle, fibrous replacement and contracture may result in reduced range of motion and permanent flexion of involved joints. Such an outcome is particularly likely after radial paralysis in the horse. Proper management by prolonged stall rest, orthotic support, and passive range-of-motion exercises may help prevent such an outcome. The use of electrical stimulation of muscle is controversial. Recent studies have indicated that the function of denervated muscle can be preserved only if use-specific stimulation paradigms are developed.[21] Previous evidence suggested that electrical stimulation may reduce nerve regrowth into denervated muscle.

PROGNOSIS

With suprascapular neuropathy secondary to confirmed or suspected shoulder trauma, restoration of shoulder stability occurred within 3 to 12 months in seven out of eight horses treated only with stall rest.[28] Atrophy of the infraspinatus and supraspinatus muscles resolved in only two of these horses. Although there is no comparative study to show any additional effect of procedures to relieve entrapment of the suprascapular nerve,[12,13] it is expected that these procedures should improve recovery of muscle mass. Data for outcome of radial nerve neuropathy are not published; however, it is reasonable to assume that the prognosis for complete recovery from signs of radial paralysis induced by positioning in lateral recumbency, soft tissue trauma, and humeral fracture is good (greater than 80%), fair, and poor, respectively. Injection-associated neuropathy (usually sciatic) usually resolves in days.

It is reported that approximately 70% of end-to-end nerve repairs and 50% of graft repairs performed in humans achieve good functional results.[2]

REFERENCES

1. Hermann RC Jr: Mechanical nerve injuries. In Noseworthy JH, editor: Neurological Therapeutics: Principles and Practice, London, 2003, Martin Dunitz.
2. Spinner RJ, Kline DG: Surgery for peripheral nerve and brachial plexus injuries or other nerve lesions, Muscle Nerve 2000;23:680-695.
3. Sunderland S: Nerves and Nerve Injuries, Edinburgh, 1978, Churchill Livingstone.
4. Grant GA, Goodkin R, Kliot M: Evaluation and surgical management of peripheral nerve problems, Neurosurgery 1999;44:825-839.
5. Schwartz SI: Principles of Surgery, New York, 1999, McGraw-Hill.
6. Frostick SP, Yin Q, Kemp GJ: Schwann cells, neurotrophic factors, and peripheral nerve regeneration, Microsurgery 1998;18:397-405.
7. Tucker HM: Human laryngeal reinnervation, Laryngoscope 1976;86:769-779.
8. Blythe LL, Kitchell RL: Electrophysiologic studies of the thoracic limb of the horse, Am J Vet Res 1982;43:1511-1524.
9. Mayhew IG: Large Animal Neurology: A Handbook for Veterinary Clinicians, Philadelphia, 1989, WB Saunders.
10. Hahn CN, Mayhew IG, MacKay RJ: Diseases of the peripheral (spinal) nerves. In Colahan PC, Mayhew IG, Merritt AM, Moore JN, editors: Equine Medicine and Surgery, ed 5, St Louis, 1999, Mosby.
11. George LW: Peripheral nerve disorders. In Smith BP, editor: Large animal internal medicine, ed 3, St Louis, 2002, Mosby.
12. Adams OR, Schneider RK, Bramlage LR, et al: A surgical approach to treatment of suprascapular nerve injury in the horse, J Am Vet Med Assoc 1985;187:1016-1018.
13. Schneider JE, Adams OR, Easley KJ, et al: Scapular notch resection for suprascapular nerve decompression in 12 horses, J Am Vet Med Assoc 1985;187:1019-1020.

14. Rooney JR: Radial paralysis in the horse, Cornell Vet 1963;53:328-337.
15. Schmelzer JD, Zochodne DW, Low PA: Ischemic and reperfusion injury of rat peripheral nerve, Proc Natl Acad Sci U S A 1989;86:1639-1642.
16. Dyson S, Taylor P, Whitwell K: Femoral nerve paralysis after general anaesthesia, Equine Vet J 1988;20:376-380.
17. Blythe LL, Engel HN Jr, Rowe KE: Comparison of sensory nerve conduction velocities in horses versus ponies, Am J Vet Res 1988;49:2138-2142.
18. Henry RW, Diesem CD: Proximal equine radial and median motor nerve conduction velocity, Am J Vet Res 1981;42:1819-1822.
19. Whalen LR, Wheeler DW, LeCouteur RA, et al: Sensory nerve conduction velocity of the caudal cutaneous sural and medial cutaneous antebrachial nerves of adult horses, Am J Vet Res 1994;55:892-897.
20. Alexander K, Dobson H: Ultrasonography of peripheral nerves in the normal adult horse, Vet Radiol Ultrasound 2003;44:456-464.
21. Kern H, Hofer C, Modlin M, et al: Denervated muscles in humans: Limitations and problems of currently used functional electrical stimulation training protocols, Artif Organs 2002;26:216-218.
22. Lundborg G: A 25-year perspective of peripheral nerve surgery: evolving neuroscientific concepts and clinical significance, J Hand Surg Am 2000;25:391-414.
23. Neblett CR, Morris JR, Thomsen S: Laser-assisted microsurgical anastomosis, Neurosurgery 1986;19:914-934.
24. Fulton IC, Derksen FJ, Stick JA, et al: Treatment of left laryngeal hemiplegia in Standardbreds, using a nerve muscle pedicle graft, Am J Vet Res 1991;52:1461-1467.
25. Hazari A, Elliot D: Treatment of end-neuromas, neuromas-in-continuity and scarred nerves of the digits by proximal relocation, J Hand Surg Br 2004;29:338-350.
26. Haugland LM, Collier MA, Panciera RJ, Bellamy J: The effect of CO_2 laser neurectomy on neuroma formation and axonal regeneration, Vet Surg 1992;21:351-354.
27. Fubini SL, Cummings JF, Todhunter RJ: The use of intraneural doxorubicin in association with palmar digital neurectomy in 28 horses, Vet Surg 1988;17:346-349.
28. Dutton DM, Honnas CM, Watkins JP: Nonsurgical treatment of suprascapular nerve injury in horses: 8 cases (1988-1998), J Am Vet Med Assoc 1999;214:1657-1659.

SECTION **VIII** EYE AND ADNEXA

Jörg A. Auer

CHAPTER 55

Principles of Ophthalmic Surgery

Nicholas J. Millichamp

Ocular surgery, unlike general surgery, often requires microsurgical instrumentation and techniques. Anesthesia must provide immobility of the eye. Additionally, the potential loss of vision because of ocular inflammation that occurs after most ocular procedures makes it essential that preoperative and postoperative pharmacologic control of inflammation be used.

PHARMACOLOGIC PREPARATION

Various drugs are used routinely before surgery on the eye, although corneal and intraocular procedures require more vigorous therapy.

Antibiotics

Antibiotics are used topically for 24 to 48 hours prior to intraocular procedures to sterilize the cornea and conjunctiva, which cannot be scrubbed. In view of the normal bacterial flora of the horse,[1-5] a suitable antibiotic combination for preoperative topical use is neomycin sulfate, polymyxin B sulfate, and gramicidin (Neomycin, Burroughs Wellcome Company, Raleigh, NC) applied three or four times a day.

When corneal infection is suspected, a culture and sensitivity of the corneal lesion should be performed before or at the time of surgery. Because there is a shift from gram-positive to gram-negative organisms in many cases of conjunctivitis or keratitis,[6,7] antibiotics such as gentamicin, tobramycin, and amikacin may be more appropriate.[8] Fortified antibiotic solutions are indicated perioperatively in cases of severe or chronic nonresolving deep ulcerative keratitis (Box 55-1). Ciprofloxacin (Ciloxan, Alcon Laboratories Inc, Fort Worth, Tex) and ofloxacin (Ocuflox, Allergan Pharmaceuticals Inc, Irvine, Calif), although not licensed for use in horses, have occasionally been used for severe and resistant bacterial infections. These drugs have a fairly broad antibacterial spectrum and may penetrate well into the eye. Postoperative endophthalmitis has been reported as a complication of intraocular surgery in the horse and warrants perioperative antibiotic therapy. Despite this precaution, postoperative bacterial infections may still occur.[9] Interestingly, despite the prevalence of fungal organisms in the conjunctival sac of the horse,[7,10] fungal endophthalmitis associated with surgery appears to be rare.

Systemic antibiotics are rarely needed for nonperforating corneal procedures. For intraocular surgery, systemic antibiotics are indicated. Procaine penicillin G and trimethoprim/sulfamethoxazole are reasonable choices when ocular inflammation exists or is caused surgically, because these drugs cross the blood–aqueous barrier in reasonable concentrations. The author often uses systemic doxycycline prior to intraocular surgery in horses.

Anti-inflammatory Drugs

Topical corticosteroids are indicated prior to intraocular surgery to control uveitis, unless corneal ulceration is a complicating factor (e.g., corneal or conjunctival surgery for therapy of corneal ulceration). Recommended preparations are dexamethasone 0.1% suspension (Maxidex, Alcon Laboratories) or prednisolone acetate 1.0% (EconoPred Plus, Alcon Laboratories) TIL or QID.

Drugs that inhibit the cyclo-oxygenase (COX) pathway of arachidonic acid metabolism are beneficial in limiting inflammation during and after ocular surgery. Experiences in other species suggest that prostaglandins are involved in the breakdown of the blood–aqueous barrier and cause miosis in the surgically traumatized eye.[11] Flunixin meglumine (Banamine, Schering Corporation, Kenilworth, NJ) administered intravenously (IV) or per os (PO) (1.0 mg/kg) is particularly effective in limiting ocular inflammation. Phenylbutazone, 2 g/kg PO once a day, may be used for a longer term than flunixin meglumine, but clinically it does not have as potent an anti-inflammatory effect on ocular tissues. Flunixin meglumine is ideal for an acute, perioperative anti-inflammatory effect in equine ocular surgery. Flurbiprofen (0.03%) (Ocufen, Allergan Pharmaceuticals; not licensed for use in the horse) is very effective in maintaining mydriasis during intraocular surgery, and in limiting ocular inflammation after surgery. Other COX-inhibiting NSAIDs—diclofenac Na (Voltaren, Novartis, New York, NY) and ketorolac (Acular, Allergan Pharmaceuticals)—are available in the United States or Europe. One to two drops are applied to the cornea four times a day or administered via subpalpebral lavage. These drugs may slow corneal epithelialization and limit corneal neovascularization, and they should be used with caution in cases of deep corneal ulceration, in which vascularization of the cornea is required for healing.

Mydriatics

Mydriatics are required to limit miosis and development of posterior synechia in inflamed eyes. Atropine sulfate

BOX 55-1. Preparation of Fortified Antibiotic Eyedrops

PENICILLIN G

1. Remove 5 mL "tears" from a 15-mL tear-substitute squeeze bottle.
2. Add 5 mL "tears" to 1 vial penicillin G (5 million U).
3. Replace 5 mL reconstituted penicillin into tear squeeze bottle (10 mL + 5 mL = 15 mL).
4. Final concentration of penicillin = 333,000 U/mL.

OXACILLIN

1. Remove 7 mL "tears" from a 15-mL tear-substitute squeeze bottle.
2. Add 7 mL tears to 1 ampule oxacillin (1 g).
3. Replace 7.2 mL reconstituted oxacillin into tear squeeze bottle (8 mL + 7.2 mL = 15.2 mL).
4. Final concentration of oxacillin, 66 mg/mL.

CARBENICILLIN

1. Reconstitute 1 vial carbenicillin (1 g) with 9.5 mL sterile water.
2. Add 1 mL reconstituted carbenicillin into 15-mL tear-substitute squeeze bottle (15 mL + 1 mL = 16 mL).
3. Final concentration of carbenicillin, 6.2 mg/mL.

TICARCILLIN

1. Reconstitute 1 vial ticarcillin (1 g) with 10 mL sterile water.
2. Add 1 mL reconstituted ticarcillin into 15-mL tear-substitute squeeze bottle.
3. Final concentration of ticarcillin, 6.3 mg/mL.

CEPHALORIDINE

1. Remove 2 mL "tears" from a 15-mL tear-substitute squeeze bottle and discard.
2. Add 2 mL sterile saline to 1 ampule cephaloridine (500 mg).
3. Replace 2.4 mL reconstituted cephaloridine into tear squeeze bottle (13 mL + 2.4 mL = 15.4 mL).
4. Final concentration of cephaloridine, 32 mg/mL.

CEFAZOLIN

1. Remove 2 mL "tears" from a 15-mL tear-substitute squeeze bottle and discard.
2. Add 2 mL sterile saline to ampule cefazolin (500 mg).
3. Replace 2.2 mL reconstituted cefazolin into tear squeeze bottle (13 mL + 2.2 mL = 15.2 mL).
4. Final concentration of cefazolin, 33 mg/mL.

VANCOMYCIN

1. Remove 9 mL "tears" from a 15-mL tear-substitute squeeze bottle and discard.
2. Add 10 mL sterile water to 1 vial vancomycin (500 mg).
3. Replace 10.2 mL of reconstituted vancomycin into tear-substitute squeeze bottle.
4. Final concentration of vancomycin, 31 mg/mL.

GENTAMICIN

1. Add 2 mL parenteral gentamicin to the 5-mL dropper bottle of commercial ophthalmic gentamicin.
2. Final concentration of gentamicin, 15 mg/mL.

TOBRAMYCIN

1. Remove 2 mL "tears" from a 15-mL tear-substitute squeeze bottle and discard.
2. Add 2 mL parenteral tobramycin (80 mg) to tear-substitute squeeze bottle (13 mL + 2 mL = 15 mL).
3. Final concentration of tobramycin, 5 mg/mL.

AMIKACIN

1. Remove 2 mL "tears" from a 15-mL tear-substitute squeeze bottle and discard.
2. Add 2 mL parenteral amikacin (100 mg) to tear-substitute squeeze bottle (13 mL + 2 mL = 15 mL).
3. Final concentration of amikacin, 6.7 mg/mL.

BACITRACIN

1. Remove 9 mL "tears" from a 15-mL tear-substitute squeeze bottle.
2. Add 3 mL tears to each of 3 commercial vials of bacitracin (50,000 U each).
3. Replace 9.6 mL reconstituted bacitracin into tear squeeze bottle (9.6 mL + 6 mL = 15.6 mL).
4. Final concentration of bacitracin, 9600 IU/mL.

NEOMYCIN

1. Remove 2 mL "tears" from a 15-mL tear-substitute squeeze bottle.
2. Add 2 mL tears to 1 vial neomycin (500 mg).
3. Replace 2 mL reconstituted neomycin into tear squeeze bottle (13 mL + 2 mL = 15 mL).
4. Final concentration of neomycin, 33 mg/mL.

PIPERACILLIN

1. Reconstitute 1 vial piperacillin (2 g) with 10 mL sterile water.
2. Add 1 mL reconstituted piperacillin into a 15-mL tear-substitute squeeze bottle.
3. Final concentration of piperacillin, 12.5 mg/mL.

From Baum JL: Antibiotic use in ophthalmology. In Tanan W, Duane AE, editors: Clinical Ophthalmology, Philadelphia, 1996, Lippincott-Raven.

(Isopto Atropine, Alcon Laboratories) 1% is adequate when applied topically four times a day. In adult horses, when ocular inflammation is severe, 3% can be used, although care should be taken not to administer an overdose of this drug to avoid systemic absorption, which may lead to development of gastrointestinal stasis. In general, 1% atropine is most commonly used in horses and should be used *to effect*—that is, use as little as needed to achieve mydriasis. Sympathomimetics including Neo-Synephrine and cocaine have been used in horses. Neo-Synephrine has limited mydriatic activity. Cocaine and atropine injected subconjunctivally may aid in mydriasis in cases where posterior synechiae are beginning to form. Once posterior synechiae are established (as in many cases of equine recurrent uveitis), pharmacologic mydriasis is never effective.

Cycloplegia (paralysis of the ciliary muscle) is necessary when performing corneal or intraocular surgery to reduce painful spasms of the ciliary muscle. Atropine used for mydriasis achieves cycloplegia.

GENERAL ANESTHESIA

Routine and specific anesthetic procedures should be reviewed (see Chapters 19 to 22).

Of particular importance is maintaining anesthesia at a depth that adequately provides both ocular surface analgesia and ocular immobility. These objectives can be achieved in various ways without taking the animal to a potentially unsafe plane of general anesthesia. Topical anesthesia using proparacaine hydrochloride (Ophthaine, ER Squibb & Sons, Princeton, NJ) applied to the corneal and conjunctival surface reduces the requirement for deep general anesthesia when performing superficial corneal and conjunctival surgery.

For surgery involving deep corneal ulcers, in which traction on the globe could cause globe rupture, or for intraocular procedures, the use of muscle relaxants is recommended in any setting in which adequate intermittent positive-pressure ventilation and anesthetic monitoring are available. Muscle relaxants reduce ocular movement, including nystagmus, and by abolishing contraction of the extraocular muscles, they reduce pressure on the globe. This is especially important when performing cataract surgery in the horse to avoid collapse of the opened eye or vitreous prolapse.

Retrobulbar nerve blocks are occasionally used to avoid the need for systemic paralysis during intraocular surgery. Lidocaine 1% is injected into the retrobulbar space. Care must be taken to avoid the globe and the optic nerve. Inaccurate needle placement can have severe and even fatal consequences.

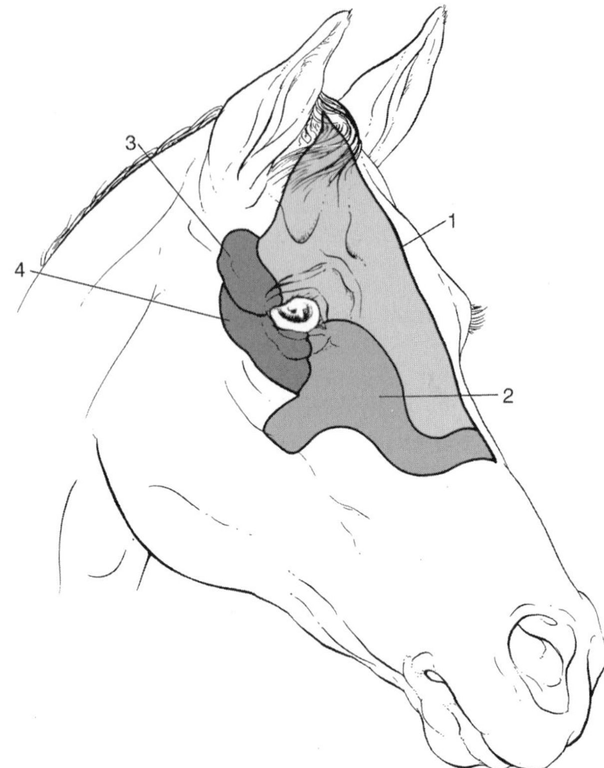

Figure 55-1. Distribution of sensory innervation of the periocular skin of the horse. (1) Frontal nerve, (2) infratrochlear nerve, (3) lacrimal nerve, and (4) zygomatic nerve.

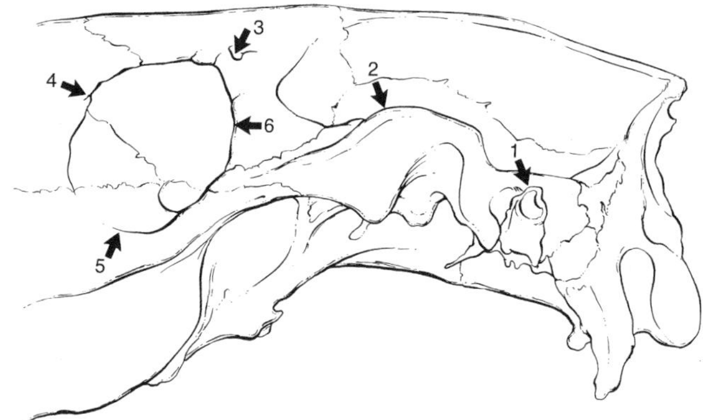

Figure 55-2. Sites for regional sensory and motor nerve blocks around the eye of the horse. (1) Auriculopalpebral nerve, (2) palpebral nerve, (3) frontal nerve emerging from supraorbital foramen, (4) infratrochlear nerve, (5) zygomatic nerve, and (6) lacrimal nerve.

REGIONAL ANESTHESIA

Regional anesthesia may be required to perform an adequate ocular examination or to enable minor surgical procedures to be performed on the eye or eyelids. In particular, regional anesthesia is suitable for biopsy and for removal or cryotherapy of small eyelid or ocular neoplasms. Sedation is necessary prior to examining the eye. Xylazine (Rompun, 100 mg/mL, Mobay Corporation, Shawnee, Kan) administered at 0.4 mg/kg IV is suitable in most cases. If painful procedures are anticipated, butorphanol, 0.02 mg/kg IV (Torbugesic, Fort Dodge Laboratories, Inc, Fort Dodge, Iowa) can be used in conjunction with local nerve blocks. Detomidine hydrochloride (10 µg/mL), at a routine dose of 20 µg/ kg IV (dependent on the patient the dosage may be selected from 10 to 40 µg/kg) (Dormosedan, Norden Laboratories, Lincoln, Neb) provides good sedation and analgesia for many minor ocular and periocular procedures in the horse. Anesthesia of the corneal and conjunctival surfaces must be achieved independently with topical proparacaine.

Sensory Nerves

The sensory innervation of the head in the periocular region is shown in Figure 55-1. The most frequently used sensory regional nerve block in the horse is the frontal nerve block, to anesthetize the central two thirds of the upper lid (Fig. 55-2). This block is needed when placing a subpalpebral lavage. The nerve is anesthetized either within or as it emerges from the supraorbital foramen, which can easily be palpated as a small depression approximately 2.5 cm (1 inch) above the free margin of the supraorbital process in an adult horse. A 25-gauge, 15-mm needle can often be inserted into the foramen (Fig. 55-3) and 1 to 2 mL Xylocaine can be injected.[12] Care should be taken not to inject local anesthetic into the frontal artery or vein, which runs alongside the nerve.

The other nerves innervating the skin around the eye are the infratrochlear, lacrimal, and zygomatic nerves, which

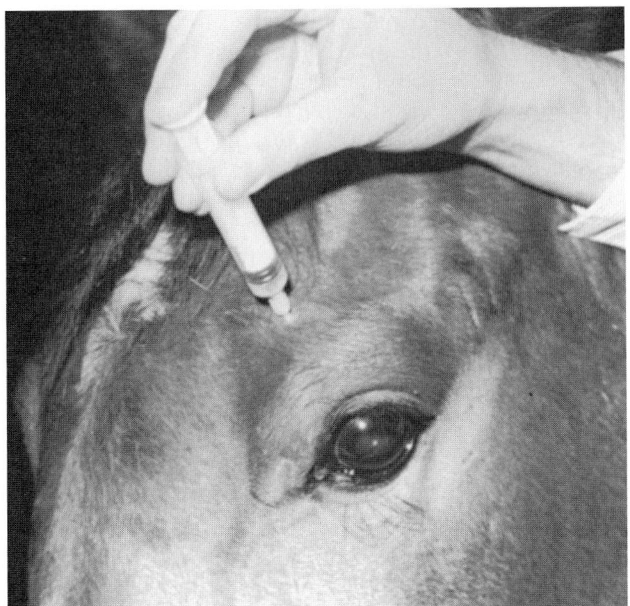

Figure 55-3. Site at which the frontal nerve is blocked as it emerges from the supraorbital foramen.

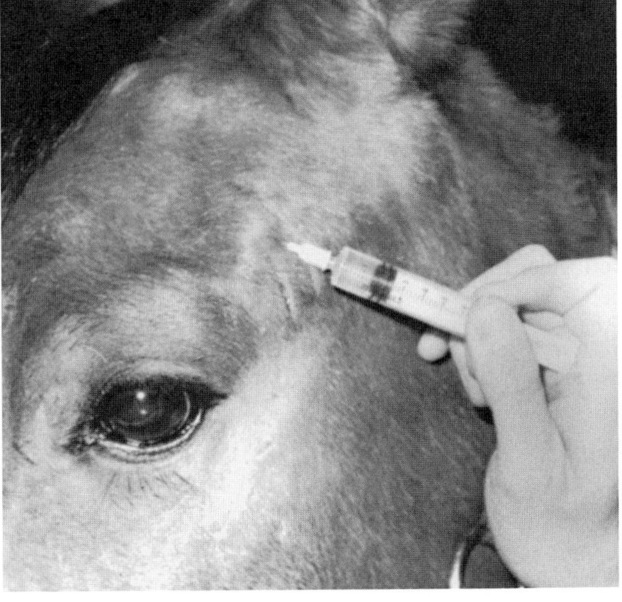

Figure 55-4. Site at which the palpebral nerve is blocked as it runs along the zygomatic arch halfway between the eye and the ear.

can be blocked as they cross the rim of the orbit (see Fig. 55-2).[12] Anesthesia at these sites may be necessary for local excision of small tumors. In addition, local infiltration of 2% lidocaine may be used to augment these specific nerve blocks.

Motor Nerves

The most frequently anesthetized motor nerve is the auriculopalpebral nerve (see Fig. 55-2). The auriculopalpebral nerve innervates several of the periocular cutaneous muscles, particularly the orbicularis oculi muscle, which encircles the eyelids and is responsible for closure of the lids. To facilitate examination of a painful eye, especially one in danger of rupture because of a penetrating corneal laceration or a deep corneal ulcer, it is essential that the auriculopalpebral nerve be blocked.[12] This nerve can be blocked at one of two sites (see Fig. 55-2): (1) in the depression where a line along the dorsal border of the zygomatic arch intersects with a vertical line drawn along the posterior border of the ramus of the mandible, or (2) at the palpebral nerve where it crosses the superior margin of the zygomatic arch, halfway between the eye and the ear (Fig. 55-4). At the latter site, the nerve can readily be palpated. Three to 6 mL of lidocaine hydrochloride 2% (Xylocaine, Astra Pharmaceutical Products, Westborough, Mass) is injected at either site. Anesthesia at the more posterior site occasionally results in temporary facial paralysis, with drooping of the lip on the injected side.

Local and general anesthesia may be combined to limit eye movement during surgery and to abolish the oculocardiac reflex. Retrobulbar anesthesia of the extraocular muscles can be used. A 7.5-cm (3-inch), 20-gauge needle is used to deposit 5 to 10 mL of lidocaine into the four quadrants of the orbit.[13] The needle passes superiorly through the center of the upper lid and is directed parallel to the globe. Temporally, the needle passes through the lateral canthus skin and follows the globe posteriorly. Distally, the needle passes through the skin or bulbar conjunctiva posteriorly and nasally to avoid the optic nerve. Nasally, the needle passes through the base of the elevated third eyelid and posteriorly into the orbit. However, this technique should not be used when performing intraocular surgery or when repairing a defect in the cornea (laceration or ulcer), in which anesthetic injected into the orbit may put pressure on the globe. Use of a modified Peterson's block has been reported in the horse, but it rarely has an application in ocular surgery.[14]

SURGICAL PROCEDURE

Positioning

For most ophthalmic procedures, the horse should be positioned in lateral recumbency, with the nose tilted upward so that the palpebral fissure is as near to horizontal as possible. This can usually be achieved with the help of sandbags. Space should be available adjacent to the animal for the surgeon to sit comfortably and position the operating microscope, if it is used. The surgeon's arms should be supported either by an arm rest attached to an adjustable stool or by the patient's head.

Surgical Site Preparation

The periocular area should be clipped and cleaned with three applications of povidone-iodine solution (Betadine solution, Purdue Frederick Company, Norwalk, Conn) diluted to 50% with sterile saline. This diluted povidone-iodine solution is also applied to the clipped eyelid margins and conjunctival cul-de-sac. Before intraocular surgery, the author uses three applications to the conjunctival sac and around the eyelids of sterile 5% povidone-iodine solution (Alcon Laboratories) The area is rinsed with sterile physiologic saline or a sterile ophthalmic irrigating solution (Dacriose, IOLAB, Claremont, Calif).

Draping

Cotton or paper quarter drapes are applied around the eye, and a fenestrated, disposable, plastic-coated paper drape (Convertors Eye Sheet, no. 8441, Baxter Healthcare Corporation, Deerfield, Ill) of a size large enough to cover at least the head and neck is applied over the quarter drapes. Finally, a disposable plastic barrier drape (Steri-Drape Surgical Drape, 3M Corporation, St. Paul, Minn), with an ellipse cut out the size of the eye, is applied over the other drapes and periocular exposed skin.

Illumination

For adnexal surgery, regular operating room lights are suitable. For corneal, conjunctival, and intraocular surgery, either a head-mounted focal light source or coaxial lighting built into the operating microscope is essential to reduce reflections from the eye.

Magnification

For all microsurgical procedures, an operating microscope is recommended. For eyelid and conjunctival surgery, a powerful magnifying loupe with 2 to 4 times magnification and a focal length of 20 to 30 cm is needed.

Instrumentation

Particular attention should be paid to the quality of the instruments purchased for ophthalmic microsurgery. In this specialty, it is false economy to use cheap instrumentation. Ophthalmic instruments are designed to be held with the fingers, with movements accomplished by the fingers and wrist and with the lower arm supported at the elbow.

Two forceps are recommended for routine use. A straight tissue forceps with teeth (e.g., Bishop-Harmon forceps) is suitable for handling the lids and episcleral fascia. A fine forceps with teeth (e.g., Castroviejo or Troutman-Barraquer corneal utility forceps) is needed for handling the conjunctiva or cornea. Iris forceps may occasionally be required for intraocular surgery (Fig. 55-5).

Scissors used for ocular procedures include the Stevens tenotomy scissor, the wide flat blades and rounded tips of which are ideal for conjunctival dissection. The Castroviejo corneal section scissors (left and right) are required for cutting corneal tissue; in the horse, as in other species, the corneal thickness requires initial outlining of the corneal incision with a scalpel. Bard-Parker scalpels and handles are suitable for many ophthalmic surgeries, especially for the adnexa, in the horse (see Chapter 12). Additionally, for corneal and intraocular surgery, the more delicate Beaver scalpel handle and blades (R. Beaver, Inc., Waltham, Mass) are recommended. In particular, Beaver blades nos. 75, 64, and 6900 may be useful (see Fig. 55-5).

Two sizes of needle holders are required for ocular surgery. The Alabama-Green needle holder or its equivalent is suitable for needle sizes used in the eyelids. For suturing conjunctival and corneal areas, a fine straight or curved holder, such as the Barraquer or Castroviejo needle holder, is recommended (see Fig. 55-5).

Ophthalmic instruments should be stored in a tray that keeps instruments separated on felt or rubber mats or in

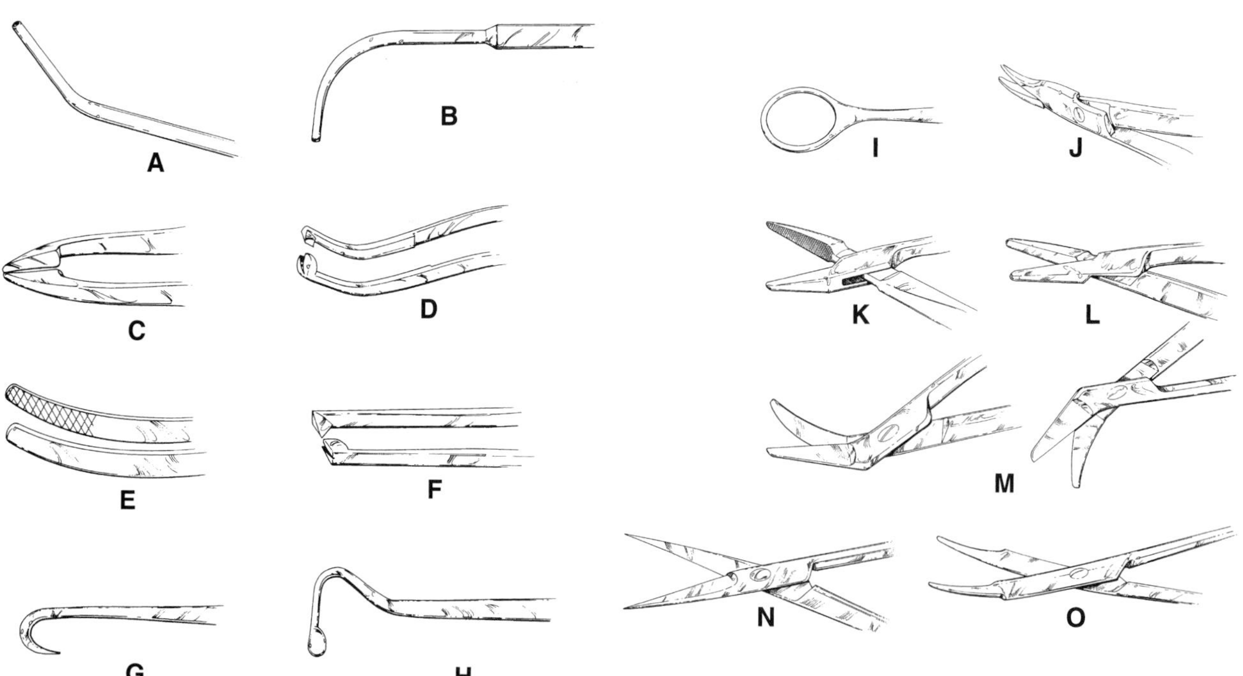

Figure 55-5. Instruments for ophthalmic surgery. **A,** 27-gauge injection cannula; **B,** lacrimal cannula; **C,** Barraquer cilia forceps; **D,** Troutman-Barraquer corneal utility forceps; **E,** Gill curved iris forceps; **F,** Bishop-Harmon straight tissue forceps; **G,** Maumenee iris hook; **H,** Jameson muscle hook; **I,** Lewis lens loop; **J,** Barraquer curved needle holder; **K,** Alabama-Green needle holder; **L,** Castroviejo straight needle holder; **M,** Castroviejo corneal section scissors (left and right); **N,** straight iris scissors; **O,** curved Stevens tenotomy scissors.

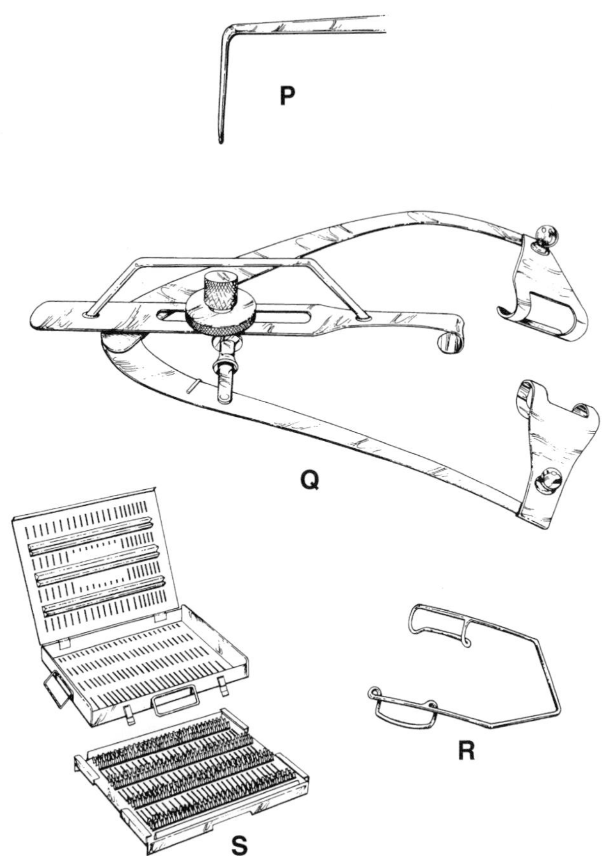

Figure 55-5, cont'd. P, Castroviejo cyclodialysis spatula; **Q,** Guyton-Park eyelid speculum; **R,** Barraquer eyelid speculum; **S,** microsurgical instrument tray.

polyester foam compartments. Tips of forceps, scissors, and needle holders should be protected when not in use.

Instruments should be cleaned very carefully with fine brushes. To avoid corrosion, never autoclave ophthalmic microsurgical instruments, particularly scissors. Air-dry instruments and, if possible, use ethylene oxide gas for all instrument sterilization. Hot-air, dry-heat sterilization at 160° C (320° F) for 4 hours, or 180° C (356° F) for 2 hours is adequate.[15]

Suture Materials

Both nonabsorbable and absorbable suture materials are used in ophthalmic surgery. Nonabsorbable materials that may be used are silk 4-0 to 6-0 for eyelid procedures, 8-0 for scleral incisions, nylon 7-0 to 8-0 for corneal sutures, and nylon or polypropylene monofilament 4-0 to 6-0 for eyelid procedures.

Absorbable suture materials are most often used for conjunctival or corneal surgery. In particular, polyglycolic acid (Dexon, Davis and Geck, Manati, Puerto Rico), polyglactin 910 (Vicryl, Ethicon, Somerville, NJ), and polydioxanone (PDS, Ethicon) provide excellent material handling in these tissues. For conjunctival or corneal sutures, 6-0 to 9-0 is recommended. The author has found that 9-0 monofilament polyglycolic acid (Vicryl) appears to result in less suture reaction than the larger-gauge multifilament sutures. For corneal suturation, 9-0 monofilament material is suitable.

Needles

A reasonable selection of suture needles for ocular surgery are reverse-cutting needles for most eyelid procedures (CE-2, Davis and Geck; GE-3, Ethicon), micropoint reverse-cutting needles for sclera and conjunctiva (G-1, Ethicon), and micropoint spatula needles (TG-140-8, Ethicon) for corneal sutures. (Additional information on suture materials and needles can be found in Chapter 17.)

Supplemental Equipment

Additional equipment that may be required are cellulose sponges (Weck Cel Surgical Spears, Edward Weck and Company, Inc, Raleigh, NC), ocular and intraocular irrigating solution (B.S.S., Alcon Laboratories, Surgical Products Division), and cautery. Regular cautery units may be needed for eyelid procedures. Fine-tip disposable cautery units are ideal for microsurgical application (Disposable cautery no. 6821 Fine Tip, Edward Weck and Company).

Cryotherapy units used in general surgery are appropriate for ophthalmic work. Liquid nitrogen, nitrous oxide, or carbon dioxide cryotherapy units are used for tumor therapy in the horse.

Butylcyanoacrylate tissue adhesive (Ophthalmic Nexaband, CRX Medical, Raleigh, NC) may be used in the treatment of various types of corneal ulcer.

Various substances have been used in horses for the support of deeper corneal ulcers—usually some form of collagen matrix. These include porcine small intestinal submucosa (Vet Biosist, Global Veterinary Products Inc. New Buffalo, Mich),[16] porcine urinary bladder (Corneal Discs and Lyophilized Sheets, ACell Vet Inc, Jessup, Md) bovine endocardium and dura mater (Dura Guard, Synovis Surgical Innovations, St. Paul, Minn). These vary in their thickness and the degree of support that they provide.

Contact lenses may be used to promote healing of indolent corneal ulcers in the horse. Various sizes are available (OcularVision, Buellton, Calif).[17,18]

Viscoelastic substances including sodium hyaluronate (Healon, Pharmacia Ophthalmics, Pasadena, Calif; AmVisc, IOLAB Corporation), sodium chondroitin sulfate–sodium hyaluronate (Viscoat, Cooper Vision, Bellevue, Wash), and hydroxypropyl methylcellulose (Occucoat, Storz Pharmaceuticals, St. Louis, Mo) may be used to protect the corneal endothelium during intraocular surgery and may help maintain the anterior chamber if a sufficient volume is used.[19]

Surgical equipment that is finding applications in equine ophthalmic surgery includes the carbon dioxide laser, the Nd:YAG laser (Surgical Laser Technologies, Malvern, Pa) and the diode laser (DioVet, Iris Medical, Mountain View, Calif). Laser therapy has been used in horses for treatment of iris cysts[20] and glaucoma and may be a better therapeutic approach to glaucoma in this species in view of the poor response to medical therapy.[21] The approach to cyclophotocoagulation with the Nd:YAG or diode laser has been recently reviewed.[22] Laser sites for diode laser cyclophotocoagulation have been described for the horse.[23]

Exposure

Adequate exposure is achieved by using an eyelid speculum. In many cases, a simple large wire speculum of the Barraquer type is adequate. A Guyton-Park eyelid speculum may provide better exposure in adult horses.

Fixation of the globe for conjunctival, corneal, and intraocular surgery may require the use of stay sutures (4-0 silk, reverse-cutting needle) inserted into the perilimbal episcleral fascia. Sutures may be tagged and attached to the adjacent drape for fixation.

APPLICATION OF MEDICATIONS

Medications can be applied in liquid or ointment formulations. Application of solutions and suspensions to the equine eye from a dropper bottle is extremely difficult, especially if this is to be carried out by the owner. Use of ointment tubes carries the risk of inadvertent corneal injury. These problems are compounded in a horse with a painful eye either before or after surgery.

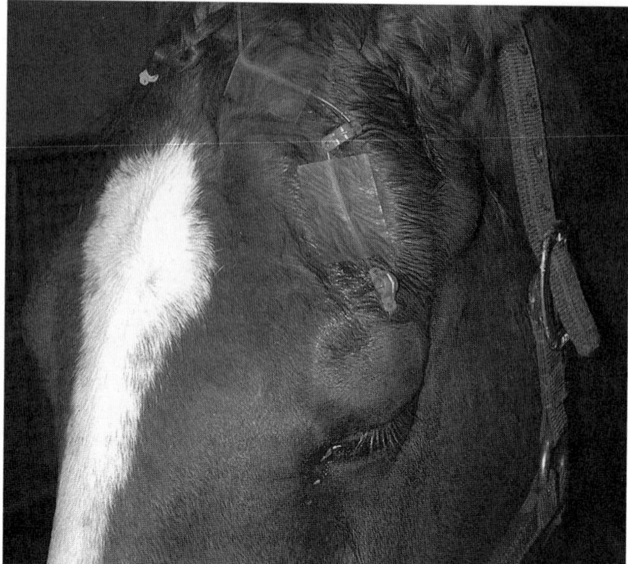

Figure 55-6. Silastic tubing with attached Silastic footplate for single-hole lavage placement.

Subpalpebral Lavage

Use of a subpalpebral lavage is the most satisfactory solution to the problem of ocular medicine application in the horse, enabling delivery of adequate medication over an extended period of time with minimal risk to horse or owner. The technique described here has been found to be most reliable.

To place a subpalpebral lavage tube, the horse must be sedated with xylazine or detomidine hydrochloride. Xylazine may be supplemented with butorphanol tartrate for analgesia. Despite these measures, a twitch may be needed. The auriculopalpebral and frontal nerves should be anesthetized. Additionally, a small bleb of 1 mL of 2% Xylocaine should be applied at two sites in the upper lid at which the lavage placement needles will penetrate the skin. Proparacaine hydrochloride is squirted under the upper lid into the conjunctival fornix using a 1-mL syringe and the hub (the needle broken off) of a 25-gauge needle.

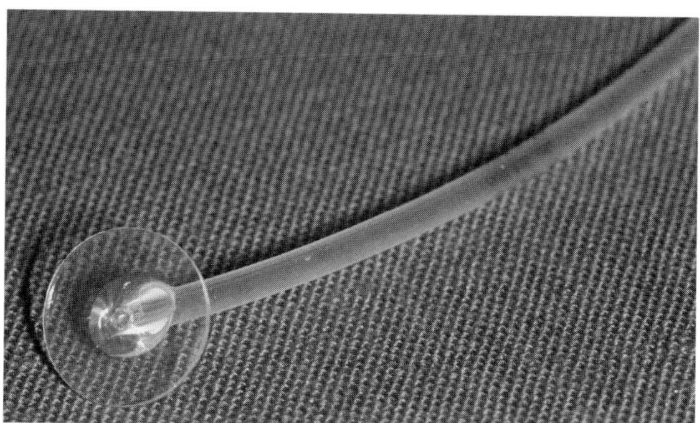

Figure 55-7. Single-hole subpalpebral lavage with footplate-style Silastic tubing in a horse.

The lavage can be performed in various ways: The simplest approach is to place a lavage tube with a soft footplate into the upper lateral or medial conjunctival fornix, well away from the corneal surface (Fig. 55-6). The author has used a commercially available subpalpebral eye lavage kit, supplied complete with 12-gauge needle, Silastic tubing, and silicone footplate (Mila International, Inc, Erlanger, Ky) (Fig. 55-7).

Others have used an inferomedial placement of the lavage tubing with a homemade footplate that resides in the space between the lower palpebral conjunctiva and the anterior surface of the third eyelid. This placement may reduce the incidence of corneal damage from the lavage tubing.[24]

For upper lid placement, the upper lid is grasped centrally and elevated away from the globe. A 7- to 8-mm, 12-gauge needle, detached from the hub, is directed laterally or medially up into the recess of the upper conjunctival fornix as far as possible. The needle is advanced through the full thickness of the lid, emerging laterally above the upper eyelid, near the rim of the orbit (which can be felt with the needle) (Fig. 55-8). A piece of folded gauze sponge helps grasp the needle as it is pushed through the tough lid skin. An assistant can apply counterpressure with the opened ends of a needle holder, over the tented area of the lid where the needle will emerge. Keeping the needle away from the cornea, Silastic tubing (Dow Corning Silastic Medical-Grade Tubing, cat. no. 602-175; 0.030-inch ID by 0.065-inch OD) is passed through the needle from the blunt to the pointed end (see Fig. 55-8). When the tubing emerges from the point of the needle, the needle and tubing are pulled through the lid using needle holders to grasp the needle. Silastic tubing is preferable to polyethylene tubing because the latter is less pliable and more likely to irritate the cornea. The footplate is seated as far dorsally in the conjunctival fornix as possible.

If only Silastic tubing is available and no footplate is attached, a loop of tubing can be seated in the conjunctival fornix. The procedure is essentially identical to that just described for the lateral penetration of the tube into the conjunctival fornix. Once the tubing is placed in the upper lateral part of the lid, the procedure is repeated medially. The entry (lateral) and exit (medial) holes should be placed

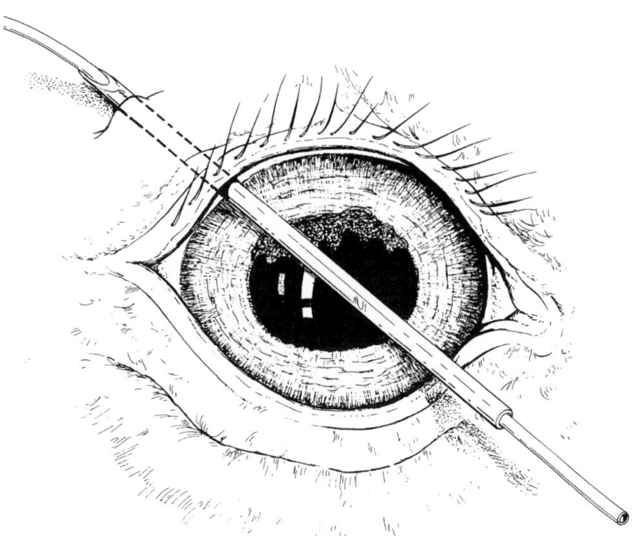

Figure 55-8. Silastic tubing is threaded through the needle.

4 to 5 cm apart, and the tubing should enter and emerge from the respective holes at an angle to prevent the tubing inside the lid from hanging down and rubbing the cornea (Fig. 55-9). The end of the Silastic tubing that emerges medially is tied on itself several times to prevent the tube from slipping out (Fig. 55-10). The end with the knot is pulled out from the eyelid, and the tube is laid back over the eyelid skin with the knot adjacent to the lateral insertion hole (Fig. 55-11). The middle point of the tube in the conjunctival sac can then be judged, and three to five holes are placed in the Silastic tube close together at the center of the conjunctival portion of the tubing using a 23-gauge needle (Figs. 55-12 and 55-13). Wide spacing of these holes along the tube may result in subcutaneous leakage of medications,

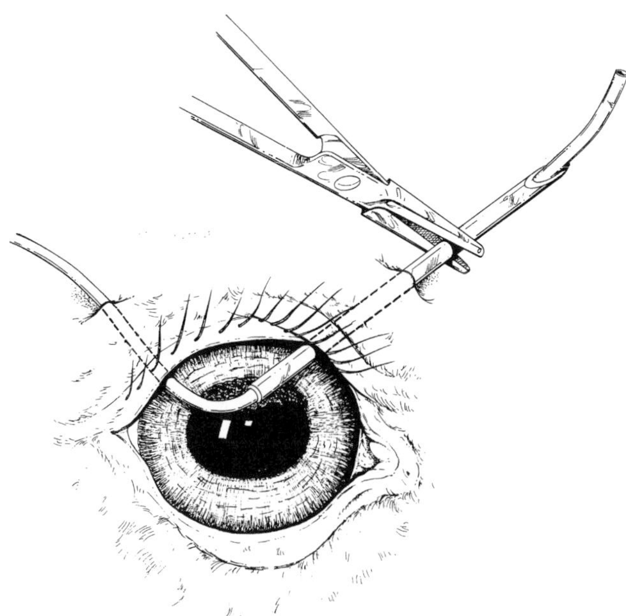

Figure 55-9. The needle is placed high enough in the fornix to avoid corneal irritation from the Silastic tubing.

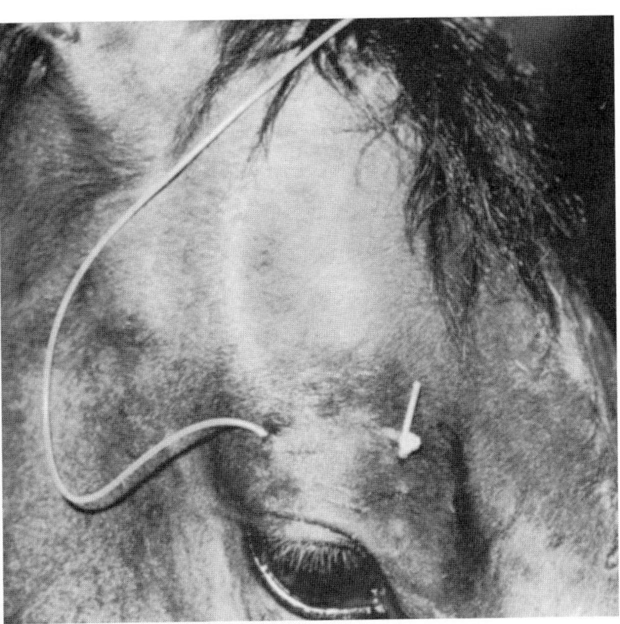

Figure 55-10. A knot is tied consisting of two half-hitches adjacent to its medial exit from the eyelid.

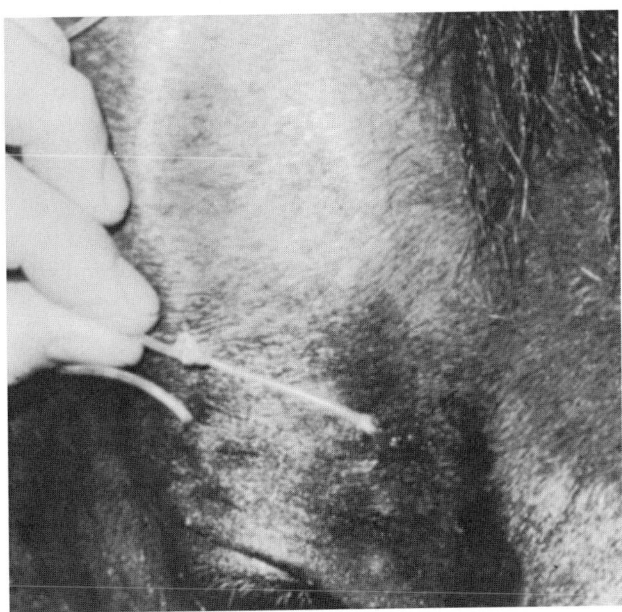

Figure 55-11. The medial end is pulled from the fornix and laid back over the lid to the lateral needle hole to assess the central point of the tube.

which may cause tissue reactions. The tubing is subsequently repositioned. A piece of waterproof white tape is attached to the tubing adjacent to the lateral exit hole and halfway between the eye and the poll. The tape may be sutured to the head skin with nonabsorbable monofilament sutures using a regular cutting needle, although this is not essential (Fig. 55-14). The Silastic tubing runs through the braided forelock and along the base of braids in the mane to the withers, or from the mane behind the ears onto a halter (see Fig. 55-14). A feline indwelling catheter (20-gauge, with 22-gauge needle, Sherwood Medical, Ireland) is inserted

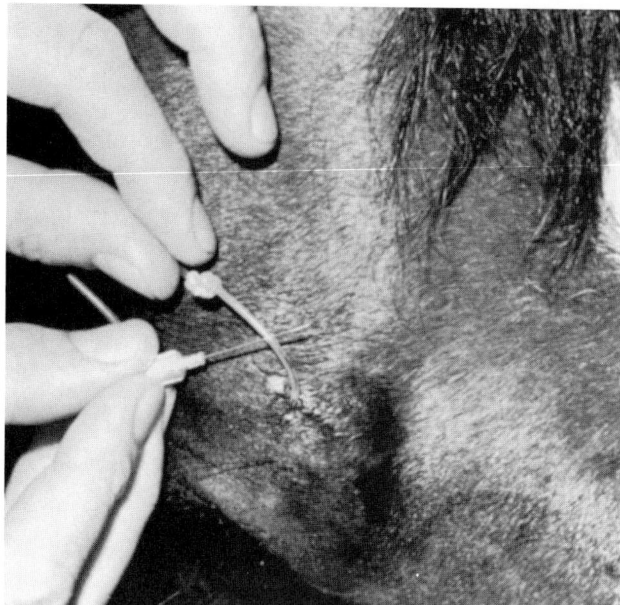

Figure 55-12. Several holes are made in the central area of the tube with a 23-gauge needle.

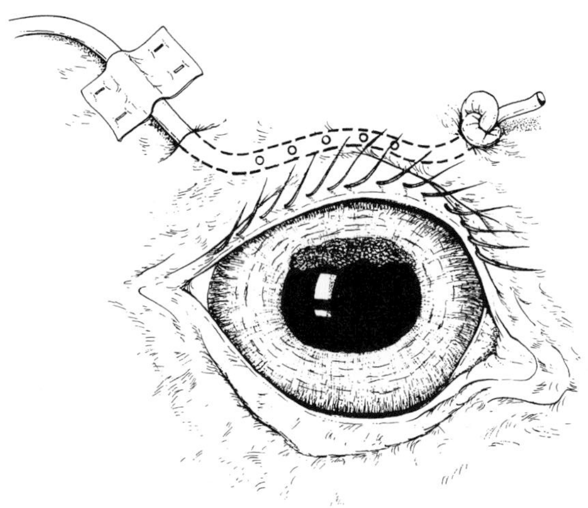

Figure 55-13. The needle holes should be closely clustered together in the conjunctival fornix to avoid subcutaneous leakage.

1 cm into the free end of the Silastic tubing, and the catheter is attached to a tongue depressor with tape. An injection cap is applied to the catheter. The tongue depressor and catheter can be taped either to the halter or to the mane at the withers (see Fig. 55-14).

Medications can be injected through the remote catheter and flushed to the eye with 1 to 2 mL of air. Alternatively, if several medications are to be used and there are no incompatibilities between them, they can be used sequentially in the tubing and the tubing always kept primed with medication, or all of the medications can be mixed in one bottle in the appropriate concentrations. Subconjunctivally implanted micro-osmotic pumps have been successfully evaluated for continuous release of medications into the conjunctival sac in the horse and may provide a reasonable alternative to a subpalpebral lavage in some cases.[25]

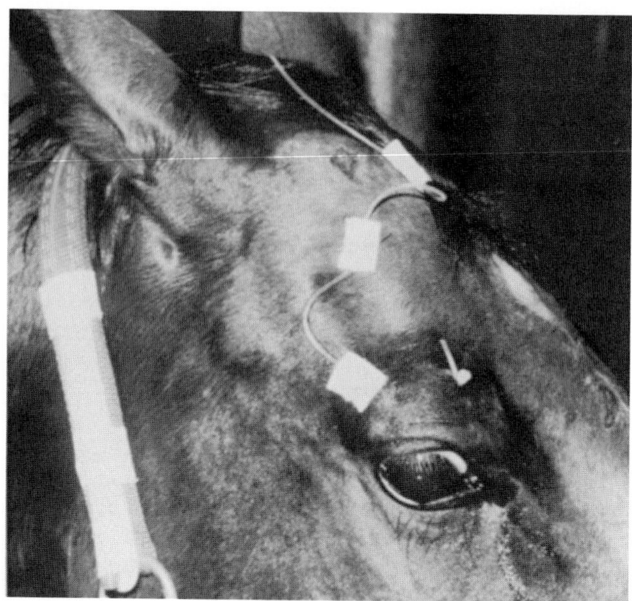

Figure 55-14. The lavage tubing is sutured to the head and attached to the halter or threaded through braids in the mane to the withers.

All horses in which a lavage system is installed should be given a tetanus toxoid booster. The tubing should be placed high enough in the cul-de-sac of the upper eyelid to avoid rubbing the cornea. Loosening of the lateral pieces of tape should be noted immediately and the tape replaced if needed. If the openings of the tubing move from the conjunctival sac into the subcutaneous tissue, medications may be deposited at this site, resulting in considerable reaction and swelling. If this occurs, medications should be discontinued by lavage and systemic antibiotics and nonsteroidal anti-inflammatory drugs administered for 24 to 48 hours until the swelling subsides. The tubing should be adjusted to ensure that the medications discharge only into the conjunctival sac.

Occasionally, a horse breaks the tubing somewhere on the head. If this happens, a new tube can be joined to the old piece remaining in the upper lid with 2 to 3 cm of a Tomcat catheter and the new tube pulled through the lid, laterally to medially, and reattached. Neck cradles may help prevent this problem. When placement of a lavage system in the upper lid is for any reason impractical, the same technique can be used in the lower eyelid after the appropriate sensory and motor nerves are blocked.

Other techniques have been described to apply medications to the equine eye. A size 8 French 105-cm infant feeding tube may be passed up the nasolacrimal duct and used to deliver medications to the eye.[26]

Subconjunctival Injections

Subconjunctival injections are useful when the horse can be medicated only infrequently. With adequate sedation, an auriculopalpebral block, and topical proparacaine anesthesia, a 25-gauge needle is advanced beneath the bulbar conjunctiva a few millimeters behind the limbus, where the drug is injected. The drug should not be injected beneath the palpebral conjunctiva because it will be rapidly absorbed systemically with minimal benefit to the eye itself.

The antibiotics most commonly applied in this manner are amikacin (25 mg), gentamicin (25 to 50 mg), ampicillin (250 mg), cephaloridine (100 mg), and penicillin G (500,000 IU). In eyes where difficulty is encountered maintaining mydriasis or cycloplegia, 15 mg (1 mL) of atropine (L.A. Injectable) can be used. Topical atropine solutions should not be injected subconjunctivally. For uveitis therapy, subconjunctival betamethasone acetate and betamethasone sodium phosphate (Betavet, Upjohn, Kalamazoo, Mich) application has proved successful. Methylprednisolone acetate, which is a long-acting drug, leaves subconjunctival plaques, potentially causing conjunctival irritation. Additionally, these drugs are contraindicated in eyes that postoperatively develop corneal ulcers or endophthalmitis. Most of these subconjunctival therapies should be repeated daily. Dosages of other drugs for subconjunctival injection have been listed elsewhere.[27]

AFTERCARE

Postoperative medication is usually similar to that initiated prior to surgery. During recovery from anesthesia, tear production and blinking may be reduced and topical petrolatum and mineral oil ointment (LacriLube, Allergan Pharmaceuticals) should be applied to the corneal and conjunctival surfaces.

Dimethyl sulfoxide (Domoso 90%, Syntex Animal Health Inc, West Des Moines, Iowa) may be applied to the outside of the eyelids to reduce swelling after eyelid surgery, surgical placement of a silicone intraocular prosthesis, or enucleation.

If a horse attempts to rub the eye after surgery, the application of a neck cradle or cross-tying is an option. Often, these methods are not needed if adequate attention is paid to analgesia. Flunixin meglumine administered intravenously or in the feed may keep the horse comfortable after ocular surgery. Protective hoods are available in various sizes that cover the periocular area and prevent direct trauma to the eye (Veterinary Protective Hood, Equestrian Care Products, Leesburg, Fla).

REFERENCES

1. Lundvall RL: The bacterial and mycotic flora of the normal equine conjunctival sac in the horse, Proc Am Assoc Equine Pract 1967;13:101.
2. Whitley RD, Moore CP: Microbiology of the equine eye in health and disease, Vet Clin North Am Large Anim Pract 1984;6:451-466.
3. Whitley RD, Burgess EC, Moore CP: Microbial isolates of the normal equine eye, Equine Vet J Suppl 1983;2:138.
4. Andrew SE, Nguyen A, Jones GL, Brooks DE: Seasonal effects on the aerobic bacterial and fungal conjunctival flora of normal Thoroughbred brood mares in Florida, Vet Ophthalmol 2003;6:45-50.
5. Moore CP, Heller N, Majors LJ, et al: Prevalence of ocular microorganisms in hospitalized and stabled horses, Am J Vet Res 1988;49:773-777.
6. Moore CP, Collins BK, Fales WH: Antibacterial susceptibility patterns for microbial isolates associated with infectious keratitis in horses: 63 cases (1986-1994), J Am Vet Med Assoc 1995;207:928-933.
7. McLaughlin SA, Brightman AH, Helper LC, et al: Pathogenic bacteria and fungi associated with extraocular disease in the horse, J Am Vet Med Assoc 1983;182:241-242.
8. Moore CP, Collins BK, Fales WH, Halenda RM: Antimicrobial agents for treatment of infectious keratitis in horses, J Am Vet Med Assoc 1995;207:855-862.
9. Millichamp NJ, Dziezyc J: Cataract phacofragmentation in horses, Vet Ophthalmol 2000;3:157-164.
10. Rosa M, Cardozo LM, da Silva PJ, et al: Fungal flora of normal eyes of healthy horses from the State of Rio de Janeiro, Brazil, Vet Ophthalmol 2003;6:51-55.
11. Miranda OC, Bito LZ: The putative and demonstrated miotic effects of prostaglandins in mammals, Prog Clin Biol Res 1989;312:171-195.
12. Manning JP, St Clair LE: Palpebral, frontal, and zygomatic nerve blocks for examination of the equine eye, Vet Med Small Anim Clin 1976;71:187-189.
13. Lavach JD: Handbook of Equine Ophthalmology, Fort Collins, Colo, 1987, Giddings Studio.
14. Raffe MR, Bistner SI, Crimi AJ, Ruff J: Retrobulbar block in combination with general anesthesia for equine ophthalmic surgery, Vet Surg 1986;15:139.
15. Bistner SI, Aguirre GD, Batik G: Atlas of Veterinary Ophthalmic Surgery, Philadelphia, 1977, WB Saunders.
16. Bussieres M, Krohne SG, Stiles J, Townsend WM: The use of porcine small intestinal submucosa for the repair of full-thickness corneal defects in dogs, cats and horses, Vet Ophthalmol 2004;7:352-359.
17. Wada S, Yoshinari M, Mizuno Y: Practical usefulness of a therapeutic soft contact lens for a corneal ulcer in a racehorse, Vet Ophthalmol 2000;3:217-219.
18. Tammeus J, Krall CJ, Rengstorff RH: Therapeutic extended wear contact lens for corneal injury in a horse, J Am Vet Med Assoc 1983;182:286.
19. Wilkie DA, Willis AM: Viscoelastic materials in veterinary ophthalmology, Vet Ophthalmol 1999;2:147-153.
20. Gemensky-Metzler AJ, Wilkie DA, Cook CS: The use of semiconductor diode laser for deflation and coagulation of anterior uveal cysts in dogs, cats and horses: A report of 20 cases, Vet Ophthalmol 2004;7:360-368.
21. Whigham HM, Brooks DE, Andrew SE, et al: Treatment of equine glaucoma by transscleral neodymium:yttrium aluminum garnet laser cyclophotocoagulation: A retrospective study of 23 eyes of 16 horses, Vet Ophthalmol 1999;2:243-250.
22. Wilkie DA, Gilger BC: Equine glaucoma, Vet Clin North Am Equine Pract 2004;20:381-391, vii.
23. Miller TL, Willis AM, Wilkie DA, et al: Description of ciliary body anatomy and identification of sites for transscleral cyclophotocoagulation in the equine eye, Vet Ophthalmol 2001;4:183-190.
24. Giuliano EA, Maggs DJ, Moore CP, et al: Inferomedial placement of a single-entry subpalpebral lavage tube for treatment of equine eye disease, Vet Ophthalmol 2000;3:153-156.
25. Blair MJ, Gionfriddo JR, Polazzi LM, et al: Subconjunctivally implanted micro-osmotic pumps for continuous ocular treatment in horses, Am J Vet Res 1999;60:1102-1105.
26. Lavach JD, Roberts SM, Severin GA: Current concepts in equine ocular therapeutics, Vet Clin North Am Large Anim Pract 1984;6:435-449.
27. Baum JL: Antibiotic use in ophthalmology. In Duane TD, editor: Clinical Ophthalmology, Philadelphia, 1986, Harper & Row.

CHAPTER 56

Eyelids

Thomas R. Miller

ANATOMY

The eyelids should fit closely to the globe, with the exception of a recess medially that forms the lacrimal lake. A fleshy prominence, the lacrimal caruncle, is found at the medial canthus. The caruncle is frequently pigmented. The lacrimal puncta are small (2 mm), slit-like openings on the conjunctival surface adjacent to the eyelid margin, approximately 8 mm from the medial canthus on the upper and lower eyelids.

Distinct cilia (eyelashes) are present on the upper eyelid only, and they extend over the lateral two thirds of the eyelid. Vibrissae (tactile hairs) are present at the base of the upper eyelid medially, and along the base of the lower eyelid.

The eyelids consist of four major layers. From the external surface, they are skin, muscle, tarsal plate, and conjunctiva (Fig. 56-1). The skin, covered by fine hair, with small sebaceous and sweat glands, is thin and freely moveable, except adjacent to the eyelid margin, where it is firmly attached to the underlying tissue.[1] The subcutaneous tissue consists of irregular connective tissue and is devoid of fat.[2]

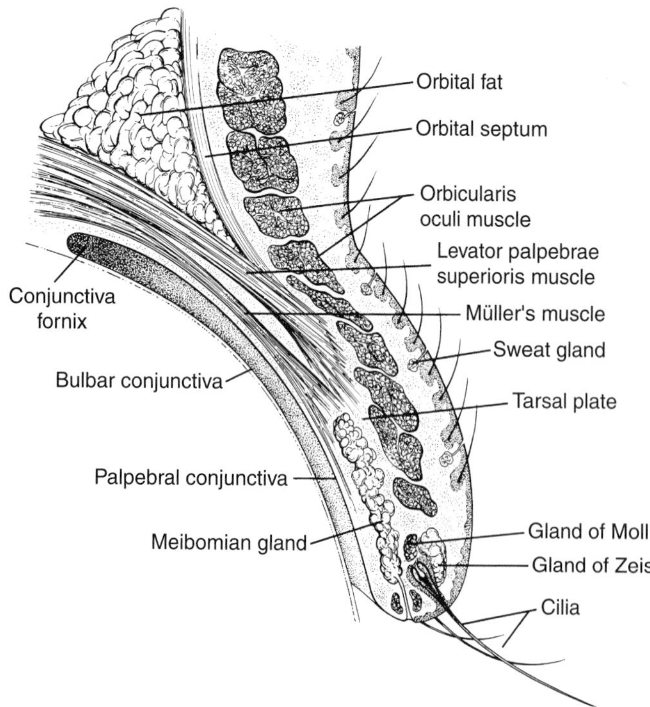

Figure 56-1. Cross-sectional anatomy of the normal upper eyelid.

The subcutaneous connective tissue blends with the orbicularis oculi muscle, which is composed of striated muscle fibers interspersed with dense connective tissue. This tissue is continuous with the deep and intermediate orbital fascial sheaths.

Deep to the orbicularis oculi muscle are the tarsal or meibomian glands, surrounded by a plate of connective tissue. The tarsal plate is not as well developed in the horse as in humans. Tarsal glands resemble modified sebaceous glands and may be seen from the conjunctival surface as a palisade of yellow glands measuring 5 mm by 1 mm, oriented perpendicular to the eyelid margin.[3] The ducts of the glands open on the eyelid margin. The tarsal glands produce the oily secretion that forms the superficial layer of the tear film, which provides tear stability.

There are additional glandular structures at the eyelid margins that are associated with the cilia. The apocrine glands (glands of Moll) and sebaceous glands (glands of Zeis) resemble the glands associated with all hair follicles.[4] The inner surface of the eyelid is lined by conjunctiva, a two-layered tissue consisting of nonkeratinized stratified columnar epithelium interspersed with goblet cells, and the deeper substantia propria, a loose connective tissue layer.

Musculature and Motor Control

The orbicularis oculi muscle is a flat, elliptical muscle that surrounds the orbit and functions as a sphincter, acting to close the eyelids (Fig. 56-2). Attachments by the palpebral ligaments prevent a circular closure. The medial palpebral ligament is a defined fibrous band connecting the orbicularis oculi muscle with the lacrimal tubercle. The lateral palpebral ligament is less distinct, formed by decussating muscle fibers.[2] The orbicularis oculi muscle is innervated by the palpebral branch of the facial nerve (cranial nerve [CN] VII).

Opening of the eyelid fissure is a function of several muscles, exerting a force perpendicular to that of the orbicularis oculi muscle. One is the levator palpebrae superioris muscle, which arises from the pterygoid crest and passes

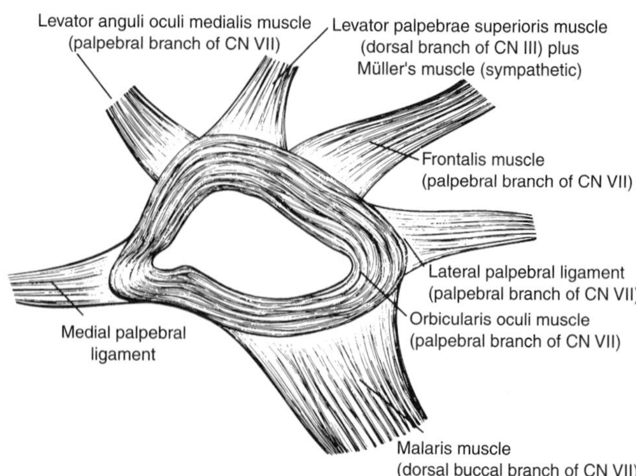

Figure 56-2. Muscles and motor innervation of the equine eyelids.

posterior to the orbicularis oculi muscle, ending before it reaches the eyelid margin. Innervation is provided through the dorsal branch of the oculomotor nerve (CN III).[5] Another is Müller's muscle, which is a smooth muscle closely associated with the levator palpebrae superioris muscle and is thought to be under sympathetic innervation.

The small levator anguli oculi medialis muscle also serves to raise the upper eyelid. Originating at the base of the zygomatic process, it spreads over the medial upper eyelid, blending with the orbicularis oculi muscle.[6] The action of this muscle is responsible for the angle at the junction of the medial and middle third of the upper eyelid. It is innervated by the palpebral branch of the facial nerve (CN VII).

The frontalis muscle inserts laterally on the upper eyelid. It, too, is innervated by the palpebral nerve.

The malaris muscle originates from the rostral fascia of the lower eyelid, spreads as a thin muscle to insert on the ventral orbicularis oculi muscle, and functions to depress the lower eyelid. Innervation is provided by the dorsal buccal branch of the facial nerve.

The upper eyelid is the larger and more mobile section, and it therefore provides much of the blinking function.

Sensory Innervation of the Eyelids

The sensory innervation of both the upper and lower eyelids is provided by the ophthalmic and maxillary branches of the trigeminal nerve. The ophthalmic branch enters the orbit through the orbital fissure and divides into several branches—the frontal, lacrimal, and nasociliary nerves. The frontal branch passes rostrally through the periorbital fascia and exits the orbit through the supraorbital foramen. As the supraorbital nerve, it ramifies over the forehead and innervates much of the upper eyelid. The lacrimal nerve passes in association with the dorsal rectus and levator palpebrae superioris muscle to ramify in the lacrimal gland and the upper eyelid in the area of the lateral canthus. The nasociliary nerve gives rise to the infratrochlear nerve, which passes under the dorsal rectus muscle to ramify medially, providing sensory innervation to the eyelids at the medial canthus, as well as to the lacrimal caruncle, third eyelid, nasolacrimal puncta and ducts, and areas of the conjunctiva.[7]

The lower eyelid derives most of its innervation from the zygomatic nerve, a branch of the maxillary nerve, which ramifies temporally in conjunction with the lacrimal nerve to supply the lateral region of the lower eyelid.[5,7] Anatomic landmarks and injection techniques for regional analgesia were discussed in Chapter 55.

Vascular Supply

Eyelids are extremely vascular, deriving blood supply from the facial, transverse facial, and supraorbital arteries and the malar branch of the infraorbital artery. These vessels anastomose fully, creating tarsal arterial arcs, which are located in the orbital septum superficial to the tarsus.[8,9] Vessels arising from these arcs penetrate the tarsus to supply the palpebral conjunctiva.[8] Blood vessels are located in both the deep and the superficial layers of the conjunctiva. As a result of this abundant vascularity, eyelids tend to bleed profusely during surgery.[9]

DIAGNOSTIC PROCEDURES

Clinical Examination

As in making any diagnosis, an accurate history, including information on the duration of the problem, changes in appearance, previous therapy, and response to therapy, is essential. It is important to perform a preliminary evaluation of the eyelids before the administration of sedatives, regional nerve blocks, or topical anesthesia. This evaluation permits an accurate assessment of conformation, eyelid function, and neurologic reflexes.

The size of the palpebral fissure should be evaluated. It may appear small in cases of microphthalmos, ankyloblepharon, symblepharon, or ptosis, or enlarged in cases of glaucoma or exophthalmos. The shape and position of the eyelid margin should be assessed for the presence of entropion or ectropion. The angulation of the upper eyelid should be assessed. Exaggerated notching may suggest decreased intraocular pressure, phthisis bulbi, or enophthalmos.[10,11] The position of the eyelid may be evaluated by examining the angle of the cilia in relation to the globe.

Eyelids should move freely while fitting tightly to the globe. Movement may be restricted by the presence of blepharospasm, adhesions, neoplasia, blepharoedema, or neurologic deficits.[11]

Neurologic function of the eyelids may be assessed in three ways—by the palpebral, the menace, and the corneal reflexes. The palpebral reflex is elicited by touching the eyelid or tactile hairs. The trigeminal nerve forms the afferent pathway. The facial nerve is the efferent pathway, causing a blink reflex. The corneal reflex is similar, except that the reflex is tested by touching the cornea with a wisp of cotton to elicit the blink response, thereby allowing assessment of corneal innervation rather than eyelid sensitivity. The menace response uses a visual stimulus to elicit a blink response. The retina and optic nerve start the afferent pathway, which continues through the lateral geniculate nucleus to the visual cortex. The efferent pathway starts in the visual cortex and travels to the cerebellum through the internal capsule and pontine nucleus and continues to the facial nucleus to activate the orbicularis oculi muscles.

After evaluation of neurologic and motor function of the eyelid, it may be necessary to sedate the horse or perform a palpebral nerve block to allow further examination. Eyelids should be palpated in a closed position to detect and define any swelling or presence of masses. Eyelid edema associated with circulatory stasis can be differentiated from inflammation, because edema is usually cool to the touch, whereas inflammatory swelling is warmer than normal and often painful. A more detailed inspection of lesions using magnification and focal illumination may be beneficial in some cases, such as in suspected ectopic cilia or conjunctival masses. This may be provided by a magnifying head-loupe and a transilluminator, or a hand-held slit-lamp biomicroscope.

Laboratory and Histopathologic Examination

Definitive diagnosis of eyelid lesions may be provided by cultures, exfoliative cytology, fine-needle aspiration, or biopsy and histopathology. The collection of samples may be facilitated by the use of sedation, a palpebral nerve block to immobilize the eyelids, or both. Any draining tract or penetrating wound should be cultured. In granulomatous or deep blepharitis, culture of excised tissue within the lesion may be preferable to simple swabbing.

Cytology samples may be collected using a platinum Kimura spatula, cytology collection brushes, or, more simply, the butt-end of a Bard-Parker scalpel blade. Specimens should be spread on glass slides and air-dried. It is preferable to collect several slides to allow the preparation of a variety of staining techniques, such as the Gram stain, fungal stains, and appropriate cytology stains.

Excisional biopsy for histopathology requires analgesia provided by infiltration with a local anesthetic or by the appropriate regional nerve blocks (see Chapter 55). Excision of large lesions requiring extensive reconstruction is frequently performed with the horse under general anesthesia. This is also true for deep lesions or penetrating injuries that require surgical exploration. In such cases, survey radiographs or ultrasonography may be useful to localize the lesion and assist in identifying a foreign body. The injection of contrast material into fistulous tracts may also be useful in delineating the lesion.

SURGICAL DISORDERS

Congenital eyelid anomalies are relatively uncommon in horses. Disorders such as eyelid agenesis and dermoids (see Chapters 57 and 60) are rare but may require surgical correction when they are present.[12] Ankyloblepharon (fusion of the eyelids) is abnormal in foals and may be corrected readily by applying digital traction on the eyelids.[13] In difficult cases, a scissor blade can be inserted medially in the fissure, and advanced laterally by sliding, *not* cutting, to aid in eyelid separation.[5]

Acquired eyelid disorders in the horse are frequent and arise as a result of neoplasia, trauma, or inflammatory disorders.

Entropion

Entropion is defined as an inward rolling of the eyelid, allowing facial hair to rub on the cornea. Irritation causes blepharospasm and excessive tearing. Keratitis and corneal ulcers are common sequelae. Entropion is more often seen in young foals and may be hereditary,[14] or secondary to a variety of factors, such as blepharospasm, loss of eyelid turgor, and enophthalmia.[15-17] Because many cases of entropion in foals are seen in dehydrated or septicemic patients, acquired entropion seems more likely.[17] Therefore, surgical correction may not be indicated or desirable as primary therapy.

Nonsurgical Management

In acute cases, manual repositioning of the eyelids, repeated as required, combined with an ophthalmic ointment to lubricate and protect the cornea may be all that is required.[5] Temporary eversion of the eyelid may be achieved by injection of procaine penicillin G into the eyelid.[18] A 20-gauge, 2.5-cm (1-inch) needle is inserted into the lower eyelid above the ventral orbit. A 0.5 to 1 mL bleb is injected at the base of the affected area, and massaged up to the eyelid margin. The resultant swelling persists for up to 48 hours and may alleviate the entropion. Injection of liquid paraffin has also been reported[19] but is not recommended because of the risk of recurring inflammation.[5]

Surgical Management

EVERTING SUTURE

An entropion that fails to respond to manual correction may be managed by the use of everting sutures (Fig. 56-3). Sutures should be placed in a vertical mattress pattern. Two or more sutures may be required, depending on the severity of the entropion. Correct placement of these sutures is essential for success. To ensure adequate eversion of the eyelid, the suture should be placed as close as practical to the eyelid margin (approximately 3 mm). Secondly, the span of the suture should not be so great as to produce overcorrection. The ectropion caused by this error may interfere with proper eyelid closure. Also, the increased tension may cause the suture to cut through the skin, leading to failure of the procedure and increased scar formation. Nonabsorbable suture material, such as monofilament nylon or silk (3-0 or 4-0) is preferred. Sutures are left in place for 7 to 10 days. This method is frequently adequate to correct the entropion permanently if predisposing factors are corrected.

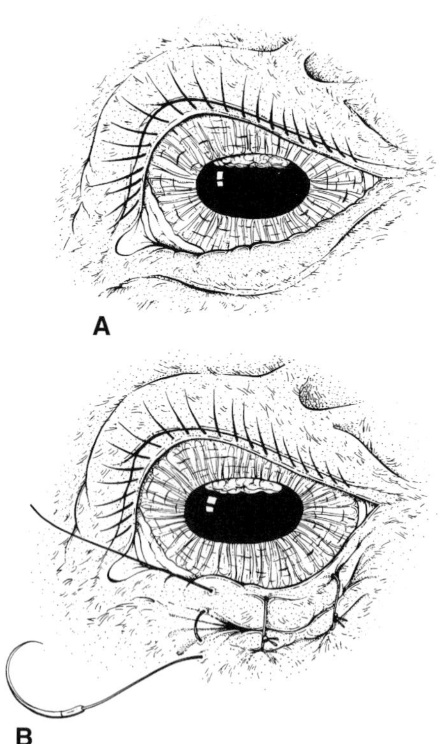

Figure 56-3. A, Entropion of the lower eyelid. **B,** Temporary stay sutures for correction of entropion. Vertical mattress sutures are placed perpendicular to the eyelid margin. The initial bite is taken close (2 to 3 mm) to the eyelid margin. Sutures should be pre-placed to distribute tension equally. Knots should be placed away from eyelid margin to avoid contact with the cornea.

RECONSTRUCTIVE TECHNIQUES

An acquired entropion in older horses is usually associated with cicatrix formation and requires permanent surgical correction. Horses with large areas of eyelid involvement are best treated using a modified Hotz-Celsus technique (Fig. 56-4). In this procedure, a crescent-shaped area of skin and orbicularis oculi muscle is removed. The initial incision is made close to the eyelid margin (3 mm). The width and length of the excised skin should be determined prior to induction of anesthesia. Incisions are made with a no. 15 scalpel blade. A Jaeger eyelid plate or sterile tongue depressor inserted into the conjunctival fornix stabilizes the skin and facilitates the excision.[20] After the skin is incised, the skin and orbicularis oculi muscle are undermined and dissected free using scissors.

Closure is achieved with a single layer of simple-interrupted sutures using a fine (4-0) nonabsorbable suture material, such as silk or monofilament nylon. Sutures may be removed after 10 days.

When an entropion is associated with a localized eyelid lesion, such as a cicatrix, a Y-to-V repair may be the best surgical option (Fig. 56-5). The arms of the Y should extend slightly beyond the extent of the lesion. The height of the Y is determined by the degree of eversion required. The adjoining skin should be undermined. The underlying scar tissue should be dissected from the skin and orbicularis oculi and excised.

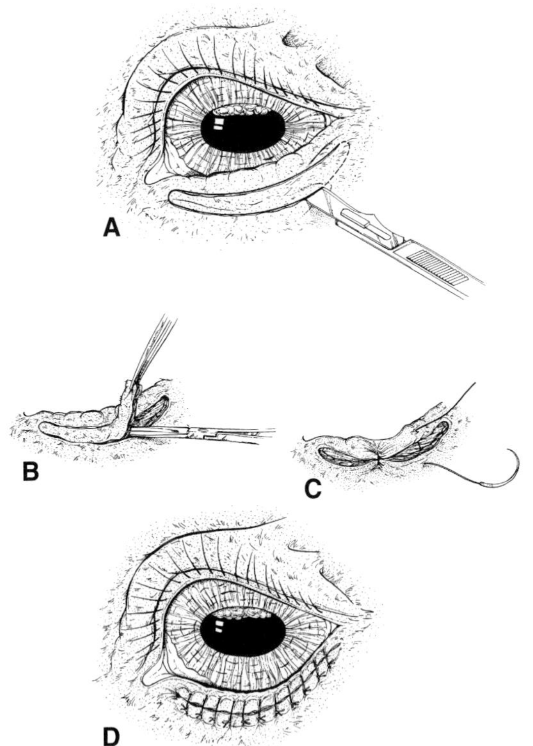

Figure 56-4. Modified Hotz-Celsus procedure for entropion repair. **A,** The initial incisions of the skin and orbicularis oculi muscle are made with a scalpel. **B,** The skin and superficial orbicularis oculi muscle are excised with scissors. **C,** A single-layer closure, starting at the center, incorporates both skin and orbicularis oculi muscle. **D,** Postoperative appearance.

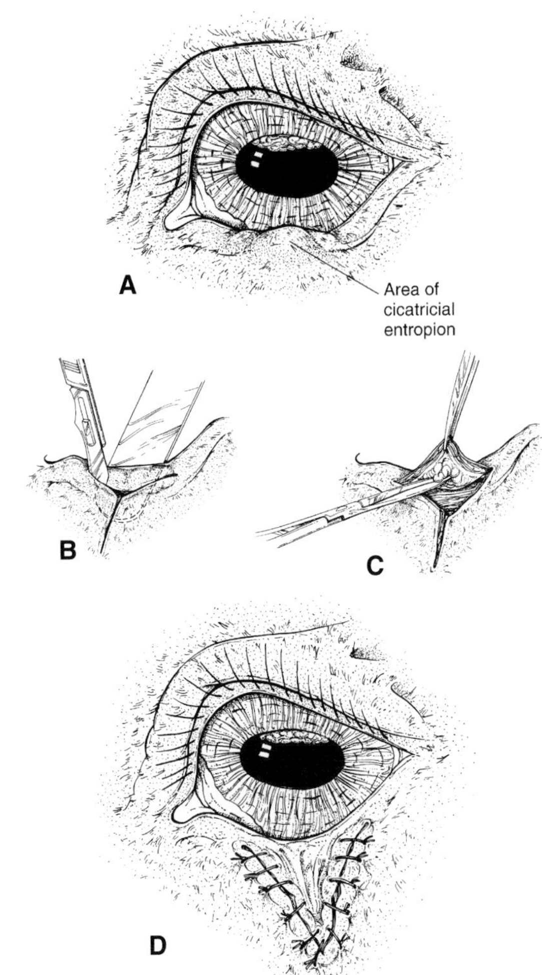

Figure 56-5. Y-to-V correction for entropion repair. **A,** The affected portion of eyelid is identified. **B,** The Y-incision is made with a scalpel. The arms of the Y should extend slightly beyond the extent of the lesion. Support of the eyelid may facilitate skin incision. **C,** Cicatricial tissue should be dissected free using scissors. **D,** The incision is sutured in a V-closure, creating eversion of the eyelid margin.

Ectropion

Ectropion represents an outward rolling of the eyelid, resulting in increased exposure of the globe or conjunctiva. In horses, it is frequently associated with cicatrix formation. Although a variety of surgical techniques have been described for correction of ectropion in dogs, the most useful technique in horses is the V-to-Y procedure (Fig. 56-6). As in entropion repair, the V should span the extent of the affected eyelid area, with enough height to release the tension creating the ectropion. The underlying cicatricial scar tissue should be excised.

Trichiasis

Abnormal cilia are rare in horses. Trichiasis, an eyelash or hair growing from a normal follicle directed onto the cornea, is the most common and is usually associated with cicatrix formation. The ideal treatment is appropriate

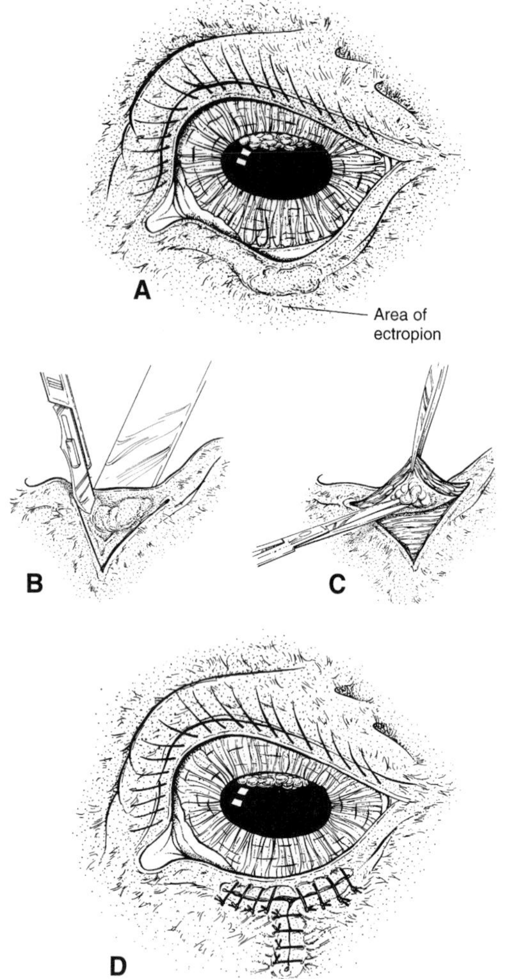

Figure 56-6. V-to-Y correction for ectropion. **A,** The area of ectropion is identified. **B,** The V-incision is made with a scalpel. **C,** The skin flap is elevated, and underlying cicatricial tissue is excised using scissors. **D,** The skin flap is advanced to relieve skin tension. Closure is performed in a Y pattern.

blepharoplasty to reconstruct the eyelid defect. An alternative procedure, such as electroepilation or cryoepilation, may be used to remove offending hairs.[5] For cryoepilation, the cryoprobe should be centered at the base of the meibomian glands. Freezing should continue until the iceball extends beyond the gland openings on the eyelid margin. Permanent depigmentation may result.

Distichiasis

Distichiasis, a cilium arising from tarsal glands, and districhiasis, multiple cilia arising from a single follicle, are rare and may be removed by electroepilation or cryosurgery.

Eyelid Trauma

Because of the propensity of horses for tossing their head when frightened, eyelid trauma is common. Blepharoedema and hematomas occur readily because of the lack of dermal fatty tissue in the eyelid.[5] Ice packs, dimethyl sulfoxide applied to the eyelid, and flunixin meglumine (Banamine, Schering, Kenilworth, NJ) (1 mg/kg IV) may reduce the severity of the lesion. If eyelid function is impaired, a third eyelid flap or temporary tarsorrhaphy may be necessary to protect the globe. If eyelid abrasions are present, topical antibiotic ointments are indicated. The globe should be examined carefully to rule out traumatic injury.

Eyelid lacerations should be thoroughly flushed with saline and explored to remove any foreign material. To improve the surgical results, longstanding infected wounds are packed with an antibiotic dressing such as nitrofurazone ointment for 24 to 48 hours before attempting closure.

Surgery may be performed with the horse under general anesthesia or with sedation and nerve blocks, depending on the extent of the injury. Surgical preparation is performed with diluted povidone-iodine solution (see Chapter 55). Necrotic tissue should be excised, but débridement should not be excessive. In particular, an attempt should be made to preserve as much of the eyelid margin as possible. Defects involving up to one third of the eyelid margin may be closed by direct suturing without creating excessive tension. Larger defects require other blepharoplastic techniques. Closure is performed in two layers. The palpebral conjunctiva is closed using 4-0 to 6-0 absorbable suture material such as polyglactin 910 (Vicryl, Ethicon, Somerville, NJ) in a simple-interrupted or continuous pattern, starting near the eyelid margin. Knots should be buried to avoid corneal irritation (Fig. 56-7).

Closure of the skin should always start at the eyelid margin to ensure optimal apposition and proper eyelid function. A simple-interrupted suture pattern using 4-0 or 5-0 nonabsorbable material provides maximal apposition of the wound edges. A figure-eight suture placed at the eyelid margin (see Fig. 56-7) allows the placement of the suture directly at the eyelid margin but avoids a knot being placed at the margin, which could cause corneal irritation. Alternatively, a simple-interrupted suture can be placed at the margin, with long suture ends left on the knot. These ends can be incorporated into the knot of the second suture to direct the first knot away from the cornea.

Habronema

Adult *Habronema*—before the introduction of ivermectin, a frequent problem in horses—live in the equine stomach, where they are generally asymptomatic. Larvae are passed in the feces, where they are ingested by house fly or stable fly larvae, which act as intermediate hosts. The *Habronema* larvae develop to an infective third-stage larva (L_3) in the pupating fly. As the adult fly feeds on the horse, L_3 may be deposited in wounds or periocular structures, which may lead to clinical habronemiasis (summer sores).

Adnexal habronemiasis may be unilateral or bilateral and is most common during the summer months. Clinical signs include nodular or ulcerative blepharitis and conjunctivitis. The presence of multiple yellow "sulfur granules" within the conjunctiva is considered pathognomonic.[21-23] The medial canthal area is frequently involved, and nasolacrimal duct involvement caused by migration of larvae may result in a circular lesion 1 to 5 cm below the canthus. Corneal ulceration caused by abrasion of conjunctival masses is common.

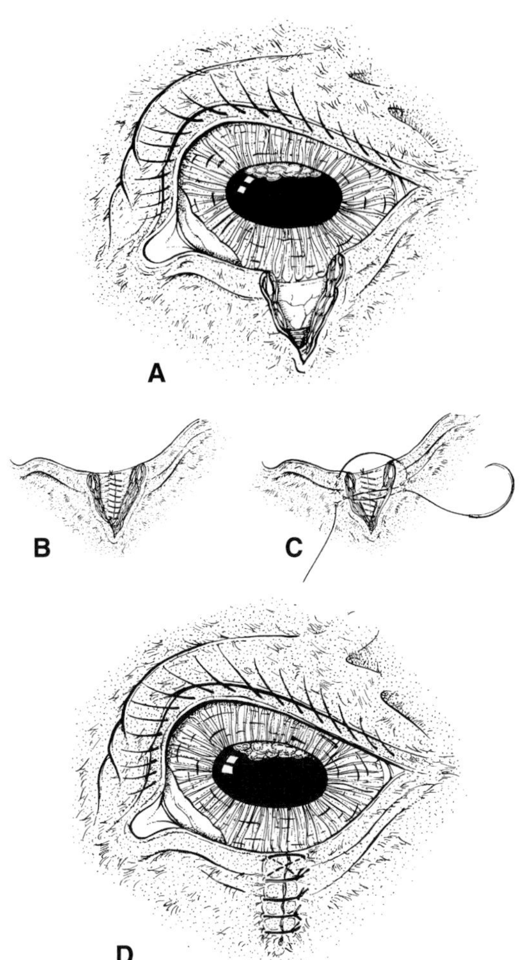

Figure 56-7. Repair of eyelid laceration. **A,** Minimal débridement is performed. **B,** Closure is performed in two layers, starting at the eyelid margin to ensure optimal alignment. **C** and **D,** Skin closure is accomplished with simple-interrupted sutures (4-0 or 5-0). A figure-eight suture pattern is useful for closure of the eyelid margin, since it allows suture placement on the eyelid margin, with placement of the knot away from the globe.

Although the granulomatous nature of these lesions is frequently characteristic, histopathology or fine-needle aspiration is recommended to distinguish these lesions from squamous cell carcinoma, sarcoids, or other palpebral neoplasias. Mast cells and eosinophils are frequently present in high numbers.

Medical management is directed toward removing the aberrant larvae and controlling secondary infection and inflammation. Topical ophthalmic antibiotics and corticosteroids (in the absence of corneal ulcers) are often helpful. Echothiophate iodide 0.03%, applied topically twice daily, is larvicidal for conjunctival infections. A variety of concoctions have been suggested for external eyelid lesions[5]: a mixture of 135 g of nitrofurazone ointment, 30 mL of 12.3% oral trichlorphon solution, 30 mL of 0.2% dexamethasone, and 30 mL of 90% dimethyl sulfoxide is a representative sample.[22] Ivermectin (Eqvalan, MSD-AGVET, Rahway, NJ) at 0.02 mg/kg IM, has a larvicidal effect. Oral diethylcarbamazine at 6 mg/kg daily for 21 days may also be effective and may be used prophylactically during fly season.

Probably the most practical medical therapy is the systemic use of ivermectin as a larvicide, with an antibiotic plus corticosteroid preparation applied topically. The use of ointments provides longer contact time than ophthalmic solutions. Systemic or intralesional corticosteroids may be indicated to help control the hypersensitivity reaction to the larvae.[5,21-23] Fly control to prevent reinfection is recommended.

Recovery may be hastened by surgical intervention. Removal of granulomatous lesions from conjunctival surfaces may prevent the development of secondary corneal ulcers. Débridement of palpebral lesions removes necrotic debris as well as *Habronema* larvae, which act as an antigenic source, and speeds their resolution.

Eyelid Neoplasia

A number of eyelid tumors have been reported in the horse, including squamous cell carcinomas, equine sarcoids, fibromas, schwannomas, melanomas, basal cell carcinomas, papillomas, hemangiosarcomas, lymphosarcomas, mastocytomas, and adenocarcinomas.[24-28] Of these, squamous cell carcinoma is by far the most common tumor in the horse associated with the eye, followed by sarcoids. All other tumor types are rare. Histopathology or fine-needle aspiration for cytology is recommended to differentiate tumor types and to distinguish them from inflammatory lesions. Papilloma, the third most common eyelid tumor, is usually seen in young horses. It is usually self-limiting and does not require treatment.

Squamous Cell Carcinoma

Squamous cell carcinoma may involve the eyelid, the third eyelid, and the globe. Lesions are not uncommonly bilateral but are not necessarily symmetric. Draft breeds may be predisposed to this tumor.[29,30] Horses with nonpigmented eyelids may possibly be at increased risk as well. The average age of affected horses is 8 to 11 years.[29,30]

The clinical appearance of squamous cell carcinoma is variable. Early tumors resemble a mild inflammatory reaction. As the tumor progresses, it may appear proliferative or ulcerative. Tumors are locally invasive with a high rate of recurrence and a significant rate of systemic metastasis (6% to 15%).[28,31]

Modes of therapy include excision, alone or in combination with other procedures; hyperthermia; cryotherapy; radiation therapy; immunotherapy; chemotherapy; and laser therapy. Excision of masses involving removal of up to one third of the eyelid margin may be repaired by simple closure. More extensive excisions require reconstructive efforts (see "Blepharoplasty," p. 709). All surgical margins should be examined histopathologically.

HYPERTHERMIA

Hyperthermia is easily performed and well tolerated by ocular tissue.[32] Large tumors should be debulked prior to hyperthermia.[33] Surface probes should be pressed against the tumor to ensure contact adequate to provide uniform heating (RF-22 Thermoprobe, Hach Chemical Company, Loveland, Colo). Treatment is maintained for 30 seconds after 50° C (122° F) is reached. Many units have an audible signal when the therapeutic temperature is reached, which may startle the horse during standing procedures. Deep palpebral lesions require the use of piercing probes, which should be applied at 2- to 3-mm intervals.[33] Most eyelid tumors slough within 7 to 10 days, leaving a granulating wound. Cosmetic results are usually good, although depigmentation may occur. A high rate of regression has been reported.[33] The usefulness of this procedure is limited by tumor size.

CRYOTHERAPY

Cryotherapy has the advantages of sparing normal tissues and of possibly stimulating the immune system against the neoplastic cells. Liquid nitrogen is the preferred cryogen because of its ability to produce a fast, deep freeze (see Chapter 15). The use of nitrous oxide is limited to smaller, more superficial masses (See "Sarcoids," later). Success rates are approximately 80% with a single treatment.[34-37]

RADIATION THERAPY

Radiation therapy may be divided into teletherapy, interstitial therapy, and β-radiation. Teletherapy is capable of delivering high doses of radiation but has the disadvantage of requiring fractionation of the dose, necessitating repeated weekly general anesthesia. Strontium-90 may be applied topically as a source of β-radiation. Although β-radiation is useful for tumors involving the globe, it may be limited in palpebral tumors because of its poor penetration. For this reason, tumors should be debulked to a thickness of less than 2 mm.[38,39] Recurrence rates may be as low as 11%.[38] Although β-radiation is well tolerated, chronic keratopathy has been reported.[40]

Interstitial therapy, which has been reported with iridium-192, gold-198, and cobalt-60,[41-45] has the advantage of direct placement of the radiation source into the tumor, providing a high radiation dose to the mass. The continuous irradiation may increase the efficacy of radiation therapy.[41] The use of interstitial implantation is restricted to licensed facilities and operators. The horse must be considered a radiation hazard during the period of implantation, which is usually 7 to 10 days, necessitating quarantine. Success rates of 73% to 90% have been reported.[41-45] Cosmetic results are generally good, with alopecia and depigmentation representing common side effects. Eyelid fibrosis, cataract, and keratitis with corneal ulcers are also possible complications, the incidence of which is radiation dose dependent.[42]

IMMUNOTHERAPY

Immunotherapy of equine squamous cell carcinoma using local infiltration of bacille Calmette-Guérin (BCG) cell wall emulsion has been described.[46] In a single case report, there was regression of both the primary periocular tumor and an untreated metastatic lymph node lesion.

CHEMOTHERAPY

Cisplatin has been used to treat squamous cell carcinoma and equine sarcoid by intratumoral injection.[47] Emulsions in sesame oil, containing 3.3 mg of cisplatin per milliliter of emulsion, were injected into the tumor at a dosage of 1 mg cisplatin per cubic centimeter of tumor mass. Injections were repeated four times at 2-week intervals, perfusing a treatment field that encompassed a 1-cm margin around the gross lesion. Tumor regression was seen in all cases, and complete regression was seen in 5 of 7 squamous cell carcinomas and in 4 of 4 squamous cell papillomas, with a mean relapse-free interval of 14 months (see Chapter 29).

LASER EXCISION

Ablation by a carbon dioxide laser has been reported for the treatment of limbal squamous cell carcinoma.[48] General anesthesia is preferred to local anesthesia because inadvertent tissue burns associated with patient movement may be avoided. A defocused laser beam is applied to provide ablation rather than cutting. Laser ablation may provide advantages of improved control of hemorrhage and decreased discomfort postoperatively, and it may serve to enhance the antitumor immune response. Disadvantages include prolonged wound healing time and high cost of equipment.

Sarcoids

Sarcoids are locally invasive fibroblastic tumors with a variable epithelial component. The sarcoid is the most common skin tumor in the horse, second only to squamous cell carcinoma in frequency of eyelid involvement.[24-26,49-51] The histopathologic classification of sarcoids is controversial. Some authors consider a sarcoid to represent a distinct pathologic entity,[26,27] and others make no distinction between sarcoids and other fibrous tumors. Biopsy is recommended for diagnosis. Clinically, the sarcoid may be classified as verrucous, fibroblastic, or mixed types, occurring in two growth patterns—sessile or pedunculated[50] (see Chapter 29). Electron microscopic studies and viral cultures support a viral cause for the tumor.[52] The retrovirus suggested by initial studies[53] was later characterized as an endogenous virus.[54] More recent studies suggest a bovine papilloma virus as a causative agent.[55-57] Sarcoids may be transferred experimentally.[58] Younger horses are more commonly affected, with a mean age of 3 to 5 years.[26,51,57] There may also be an association between increased incidence and recurrence rates and equine leucocyte antigens.[59,60]

Sarcoids may be treated by a variety of methods, including surgical excision, hyperthermia, cryotherapy, irradiation, immunotherapy, and chemotherapy.

SURGICAL EXCISION

Surgical excision by itself has a high recurrence rate (up to 50%).[5,50] However, surgical debulking is frequently performed when using other treatment modalities. Combination therapy may be particularly helpful when the involvement of the eyelid precludes total excision.

Laser ablation or excision can also be performed. Tissue handling can be reduced, and cosmetic results are usually good. However, wound healing may be prolonged. The recurrence rate has been reported to be comparable to that of conventional excision when used as the sole modality of treatment,[59] but other reviews suggest there may be a definite advantage to using laser.[57]

HYPERTHERMIA

Hyperthermia can be used after debulking, alone in small masses or with the use of piercing probes. Horses with deep sarcoids, larger than 5 mm diameter, are poor candidates. Tissue temperature of 50° C (122° F) should be maintained for 30 seconds per site. Treatment should be repeated at 1- to 2-week intervals until the sarcoid is in remission. The tumor will slough, leaving a granulating wound.[5,34,60]

CRYOTHERAPY

The goal of cryotherapy is to destroy the sarcoid in situ, causing the tumor to slough and healing to occur by granulation. Scar formation is usually minimal.[60] When using the spray technique, it is necessary to shield the globe and surrounding normal tissue with insulators, such as polystyrene, to prevent inadvertent freezing. Caution is recommended to avoid run-off of liquid nitrogen under shields.[61] Overfreezing may lead to cicatrix formation. Additional information on cryosurgery can be found in Chapter 15.

Other complications include temporary facial paralysis caused by freezing masses adjacent to the facial nerve,[62] as well as poliosis (depigmentation of hair), similar to freeze-branding. Poliosis is common and may be permanent. Healing may take several weeks, and general nursing care of the wound is required. Repeated freezing may be required in 8 to 12 weeks. Success rates of up to 75% have been reported.[34,37,62-65]

RADIATION THERAPY

Radiation therapy is a successful mode of therapy for sarcoids. Brachytherapy involves the application of radioactive isotopes, such as ^{192}Ir, ^{198}Au, cesium-137, radon-222, or ^{90}Sr, on or into affected tissues. This method allows the delivery of a high dose of radiation to a localized area, with a low dose delivered to surrounding normal tissue.

The use of radioimplants is restricted to approved facilities and certified operators. The hazards and expense limit this method of therapy to referral institutions. However, it can be an effective therapy, with reported success rates of over 90% after 1 year.[5,38,61]

IMMUNOTHERAPY

Immunotherapy involves the stimulation of the patient's immune response to tumor cell membrane antigen, leading to rejection of the tumor. Various preparations, including autogenous bacterins, sarcoid vaccine, live BCG administration, BCG cell wall in oil, and *Corynebacterium parvum* intralesional vaccine, have been recommended.[63,66-75] BCG cell wall in oil may be the most efficacious of all and, because it is available commercially as a licensed product (Ribigen E, RIBI Immunochem Research, Inc, Hamilton, Mo), it may be the most practical.

Injection of sarcoids requires sedation of the horse or general anesthesia. Pedunculated or large necrotic masses should be debulked before injecting the BCG vaccine. The tumor is injected using a 25-gauge needle at a dose of 1 mL/cm^2 tumor surface, attempting to saturate the tumor base. Injections should be repeated at 3- to 4-week intervals until the sarcoid is resolved.

The immune response produces swelling and exudation, with eventual sloughing at the tumor site. The severity of the inflammatory response often correlates positively with the response to therapy. Tissue reaction is more severe after the second or third injection. Inflammation should be allowed to subside before the injection is repeated.

Proper use of BCG should resolve all periocular sarcoids.[57,67] (Lesions on other sites, especially on the limbs, may be more refractory to treatment.[67]) Usually, complications or disfigurements are minimal.[69] Previous cryotherapy may reduce the efficacy of BCG injections.[75] However, because the average horse requires four injections, treatment time may be prolonged. Additionally, there is a risk of inducing anaphylaxis with BCG, usually after the second injection. Therefore, it is prudent to monitor all cases following injection. Premedicating with flunixin meglumine (1 mg/kg IV) and corticosteroids such as prednisolone (2 mg/kg IM) 30 minutes prior to the second or subsequent BCG injections has been recommended.[76] The rate of anaphylaxis with a purified cell wall fraction may be less than with whole cell preparations.[74]

In horses with multiple sarcoids, treatment of each lesion may not be required. Treatment of the larger masses by BCG injection or cryotherapy may enhance the remission of the untreated lesions. Spontaneous remission may occur in any untreated horse. This may be associated with increased cell-mediated immunity against sarcoid cells.[77]

CHEMOTHERAPY

Intratumoral injection of cisplatin can be used for the treatment of equine sarcoids, as described for periocular squamous cell carcinoma. Regression was seen in all cases and was complete in 18 of 19 cases. The mean relapse-free interval was 21.6 months. The 1-year relapse-free rate was 87%.[47]

OTHER METHODS

Other methods of removing sarcoids have appeared in the literature, such as topical 5-fluorouracil,[73] topical idoxuridine,[73] and topical podophyllum application.[78] These therapies have not gained general acceptance.[78]

Special Surgical Techniques

Blepharoplasty

Reconstructive blepharoplasty is indicated in any horse in which trauma or surgical excision has removed more than one third of the eyelid margin. This type of surgery is best performed under general anesthesia. It should be remembered that although the eyelid skin is pliable, the surrounding facial skin is relatively inelastic and may not stretch readily to provide donor skin.

SLIDING SKIN FLAP

The simplest form of blepharoplasty is the sliding skin flap (Fig. 56-8). After excision of affected tissue, the incisions are extended vertically for twice the height of the excised portion. Slightly diverging incisions allow for wound contracture. Triangular pieces of skin should be excised at the end of each incision. These triangles facilitate closure without skin folds (dog-ears) and help to distribute tension. The sides of the triangle should approximate the height of the excised portion. Surrounding skin should be undermined with scissors to provide skin mobility. Adjacent conjunctiva should also be mobilized to cover the defect, if possible. Skin closure should begin at the eyelid margin using a 4-0 nonabsorbable suture material. A slight overcorrection—that is, bringing the flap slightly beyond the desired level of the eyelid margin—may result in a better cosmetic result after wound contracture occurs. The flap should be sutured to the underlying conjunctiva along the eyelid margin with 6-0 absorbable suture (e.g., polyglactin 910) in a simple continuous pattern. If tension exists on the skin flap, additional support may be provided by performing a temporary tarsorrhaphy.

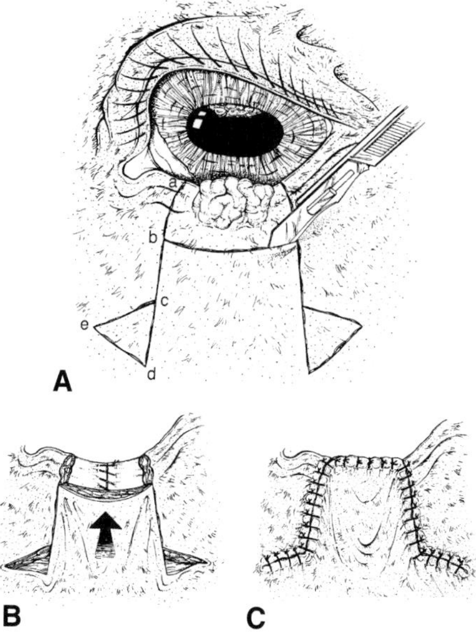

Figure 56-8. Sliding skin flap to repair eyelid defects. **A,** Proportions of incisions should be ab = bc = cd = de. **B,** Equilateral triangles of skin are excised, as is the affected portion of eyelid. The skin flap and adjacent skin are undermined with scissors. Adjacent conjunctiva is mobilized and closed with absorbable suture (polyglactin 910 [6-0 Vicryl]). **C,** The skin flap is advanced, and the leading edge of the flap is sutured to the conjunctiva and skin.

CONJUNCTIVAL ADVANCEMENT FLAP

In cases with extensive conjunctival involvement, a conjunctival advancement flap from the opposing eyelid may be required (Fig. 56-9). The conjunctiva should be incised 3 to 4 mm from the eyelid margin, and it is undermined to create a flap, which is sutured to the opposing conjunctiva. The skin flap is performed as already described. A temporary tarsorrhaphy is required to relieve tension on the conjunctival flap. A second surgical procedure is required to cut the conjunctival flap to restore the eyelid margin. This procedure should not be performed for at least 1 month after the primary surgery.

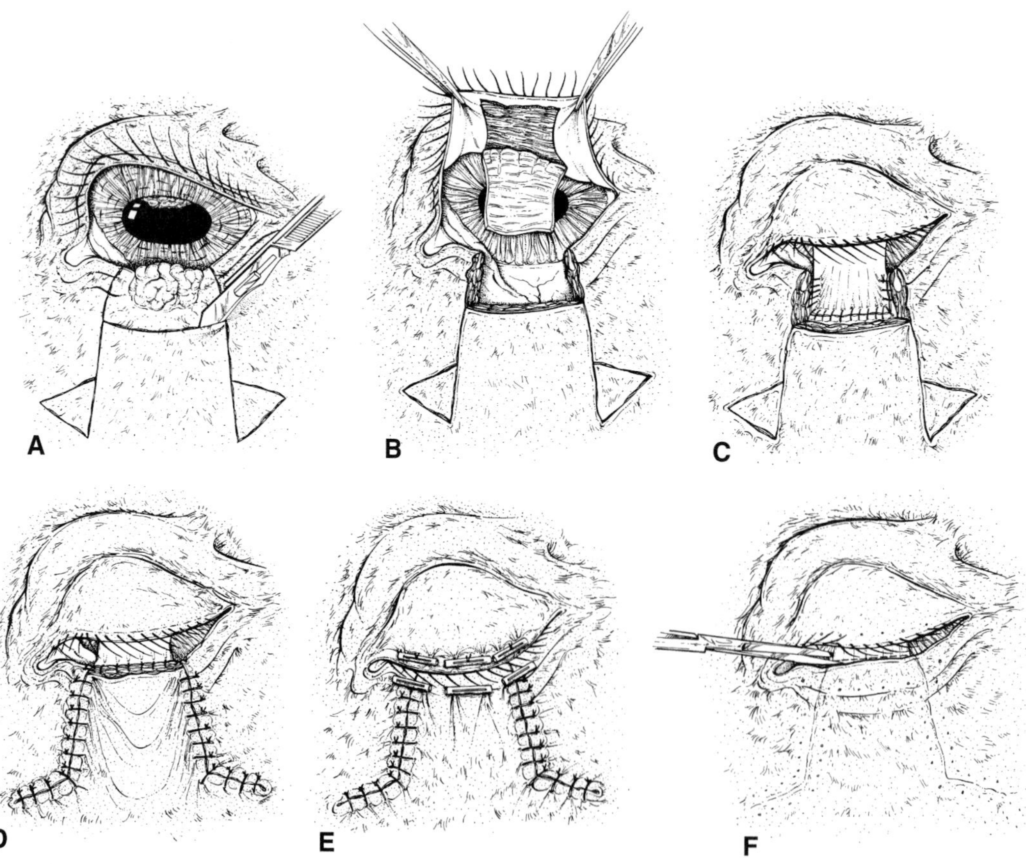

Figure 56-9. Tarsoconjunctival advancement flap. **A,** A skin advancement flap is prepared as in Figure 56-8. **B,** Conjunctiva of the upper eyelid opposite the defect is incised 3 to 4 mm from the eyelid margin and is undermined to create a flap. **C,** The conjunctival flap is advanced and sutured into the defect. **D,** The skin flap is advanced and sutured in place. **E,** A temporary tarsorrhaphy relieves tension on the flaps. The use of stents helps to distribute tension. **F,** After 4 weeks, the tarsorrhaphy is removed and the conjunctival flap is severed at the level of the eyelid margin. The conjunctiva and skin are apposed with a continuous pattern of 6-0 or 7-0 absorbable suture.

FULL-THICKNESS EYELID GRAFT

A full-thickness eyelid graft may be required because of the poor mobility of facial skin (Fig. 56-10). This technique is best suited for a graft for a lower eyelid defect, because the upper eyelid is larger and more mobile, providing a better donor flap. The width of the graft should approximate the width of the defect. In extensive defects, a lateral canthotomy to release tension may be helpful. The opposing eyelid is incised approximately 5 mm above the eyelid margin to avoid the tarsal glands. Splitting the graft into skin-muscle and tarsoconjunctival layers improves mobility, reducing the size of the graft required.[79] A sliding skin flap is prepared on the lower eyelid. The tarsoconjunctival layers are closed with 6-0 absorbable sutures, with knots buried to prevent corneal contact. The skin is closed with 4-0 nonabsorbable sutures, such as silk or nylon. The bridge is sutured to the graft to prevent retraction. The flap is left in place until tension has dissipated, which may take several weeks. In a second procedure, the flap is transected along the new eyelid margin and sutured to the bridge. The new eyelid margin is sutured with 6-0 absorbable sutures to appose conjunctiva and skin.

RHOMBOID GRAFT FLAP

A rhomboid graft flap for repairing defects involving more than 50% of the eyelid has been described[80] (Fig. 56-11). The rhomboid is an equal-sided parallelogram and can be constructed with sides at 90 degrees (square) or at 60 and 120 degrees. One side of the rhomboid assumes the position of the eyelid margin. The replacement flap is constructed by two incisions, the first being an extension of the diagonal of the rhomboid and equal in length to the sides of the rhombus. The second incision is made parallel to the rhombus for an equal distance. Conjunctiva from the eyelid or globe should be identified for use in closure. The skin is undermined and rotated to fill the defect. The skin is closed with simple-interrupted 4-0 nonabsorbable sutures. The conjunctiva is sutured to the skin flap to form an eyelid

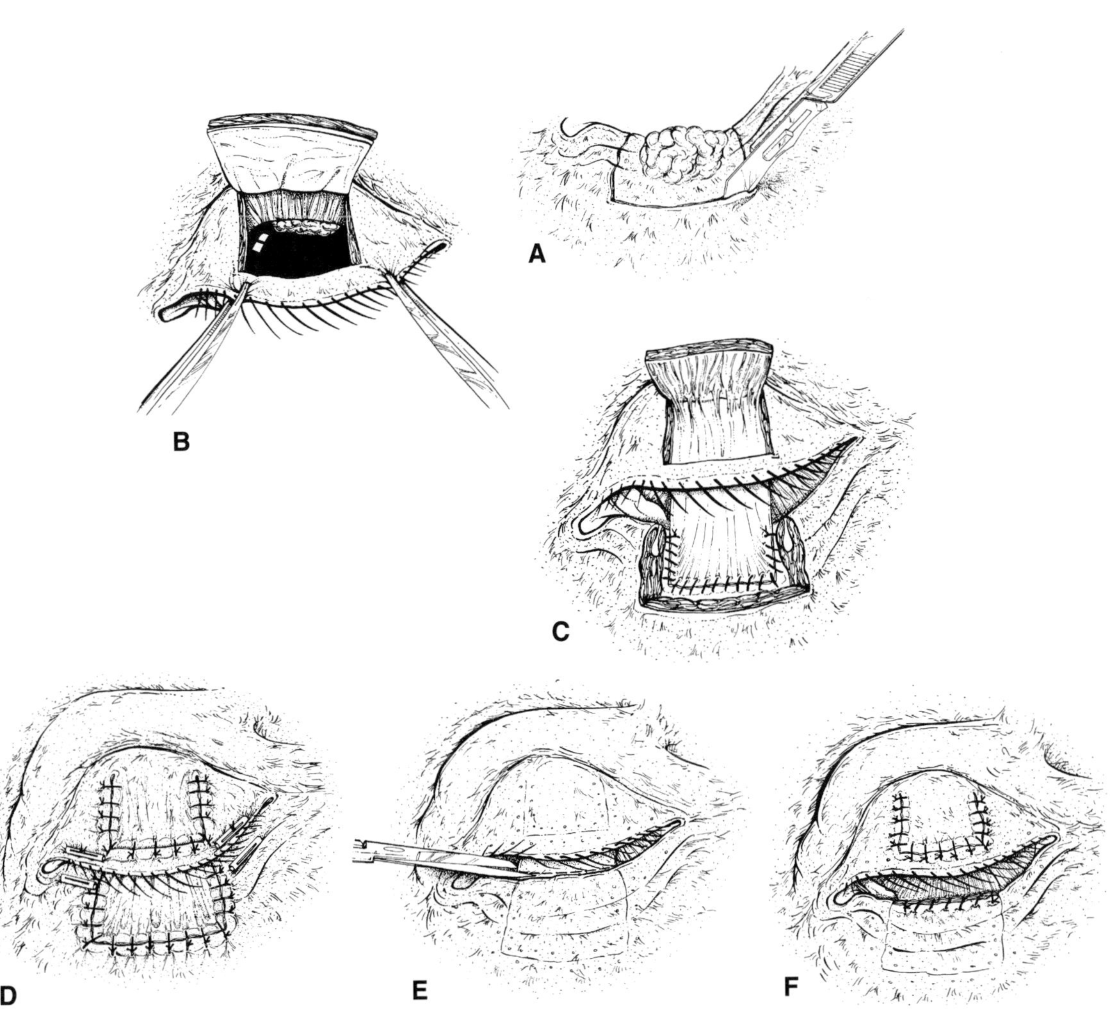

Figure 56-10. Full-thickness eyelid graft. **A,** The area of affected lower eyelid is excised. **B,** The upper eyelid is excised 5 mm above the eyelid margin opposite the defect. **C,** The graft is split into skin and tarsoconjunctival layers. The graft is advanced under the eyelid margin and sutured in place. **D,** The bridging eyelid margin is sutured to the graft. A temporary tarsorrhaphy alleviates tension on the graft. **E,** After adequate healing has occurred, the graft is severed along the intended eyelid margin. **F,** The conjunctiva and skin are apposed along the eyelid margin with a continuous suture pattern. The skin flap is sutured to the bridge to complete the closure.

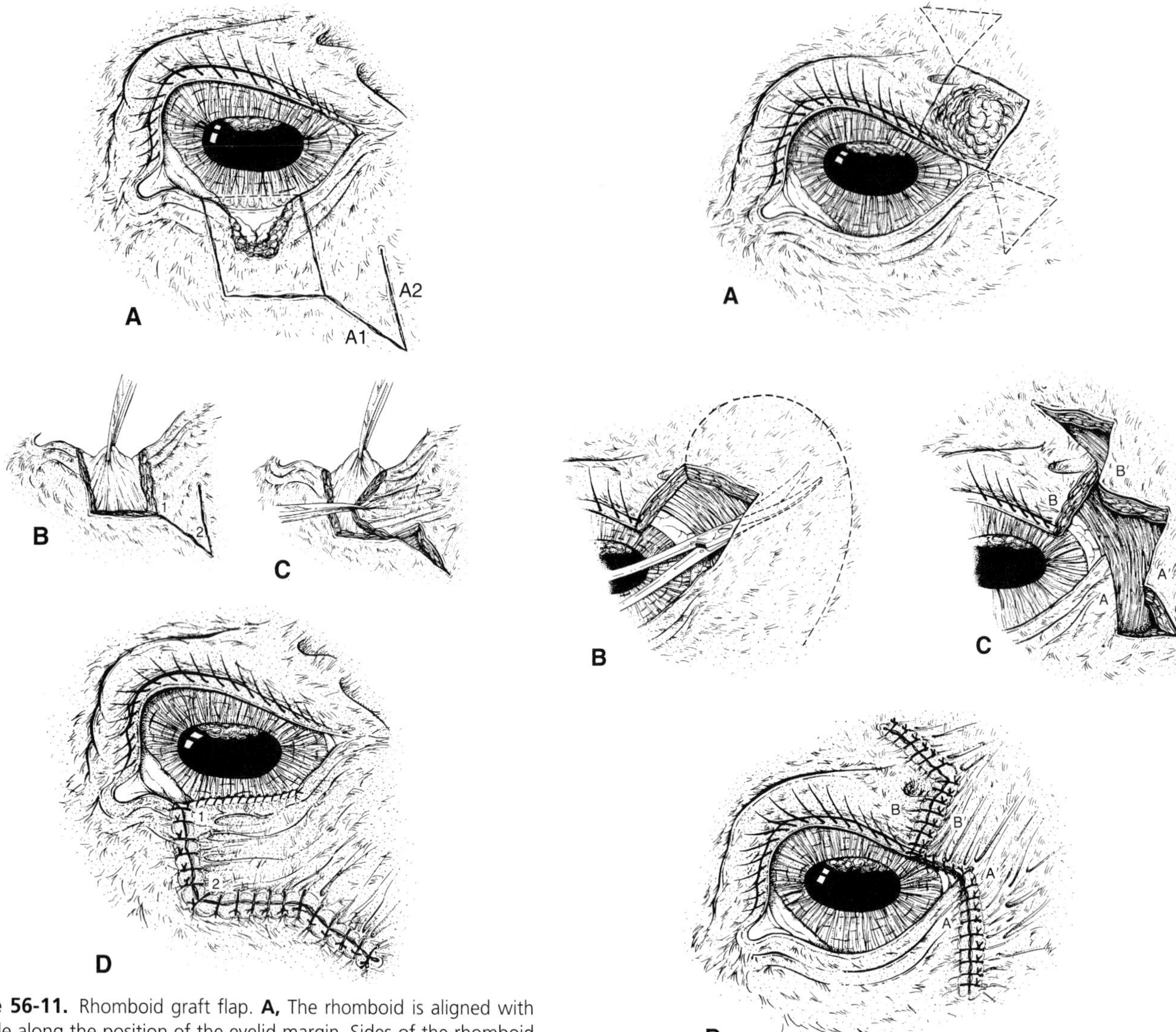

Figure 56-11. Rhomboid graft flap. **A,** The rhomboid is aligned with one side along the position of the eyelid margin. Sides of the rhomboid are equal. The replacement flap is incised on a line (A1) continuous with the diagonal of the rhomboid, for a distance equal to the sides of the rhomboid. The second incision (A2) is also equal in length, and is placed parallel to the side of the rhomboid. **B,** The lesion is excised and conjunctiva is mobilized to cover the replacement flap. **C,** The flap is dissected free from underlying tissue and rotated into position. **D,** The flap is sutured in position with the leading edge forming the new eyelid margin. (Angles 1 and 2 are indicated on **B** and **D** to aid in orientation.)

Figure 56-12. Sliding Z flap. **A,** Growths of the lateral eyelid can be removed en bloc. The triangular areas of skin to be removed adjacent to the defect are marked. Excision of these flaps facilitates skin mobilization. (The bases of the triangles align with the diagonal of the defect.) **B,** Adjacent skin is undermined. **C,** Equivalent triangles of skin are excised. (Cut edges A, A′, B, and B′ are shown to aid in orientation for advancement of the flap.) **D,** The flap is advanced and sutured in place.

margin using 6-0 absorbable suture material in a simple-continuous pattern. It is advisable to draw the proposed incisions on the skin with a surgical marker prior to surgery for optimal results.

SLIDING Z FLAP

Defects in the lateral upper eyelid can be closed with a sliding Z flap (Fig. 56-12). After excision of the lesion, adjacent conjunctiva is undermined and apposed with 6-0 absorbable sutures. The surrounding skin is undermined. Triangles of skin are excised above and below the defect. The bases of these triangles are aligned on the diagonal of the defect, and the sides are equal to the width of the defect. Again, it may be helpful to draw the proposed incision lines on the skin with a surgical marker prior to beginning surgery to ensure proper orientation of incisions.

Other types of skin flaps and reconstructive techniques applicable to the horse may be found in human and small animal ophthalmology texts, or in equine surgical case reports.[81,82]

PARTIAL ORBITAL RIM RESECTION

In cases requiring radical resection of the periocular tissue combined with enucleation or exenteration, there may be inadequate tissue to close the skin using conventional reconstructive techniques. In this technique, the caudal portion of the dorsal orbital rim is resected after enucleation to reduce the wound size and reduce tension on the closure. Extensive undermining of adjacent skin and mesh skin expansion are required to permit advancement and closure of the wound.[83]

Tarsorrhaphy

Tarsorrhaphies may be temporary or permanent, depending on whether the eyelid margins are excised prior to suturing. A tarsorrhaphy is indicated for protection of the cornea in cases of facial paralysis or when eyelid swelling causes the loss of the ability to close the eye; after corneal surgery, to provide additional support to the globe; and after eyelid surgery, to allow the normal eyelid to "splint" the affected eyelid to reduce the risk of wound dehiscence or eyelid distortion.

TEMPORARY TARSORRHAPHY

A temporary tarsorrhaphy is adequate for most cases and can be performed in the standing animal with the use of sedation, regional nerve blocks, and topical anesthesia. Preparation of the eye region for aseptic surgery should be performed. Three or four horizontal mattress sutures are spaced along the palpebral fissure to distribute the tension. It is usually helpful to leave the medial canthus slightly open to facilitate drainage. A relatively heavy nonabsorbable suture material (e.g., 2-0 or 3-0 monofilament nylon or silk) should be placed in partial thickness to avoid contact with the cornea (Fig. 56-13). The use of rubber tubing or button stents helps to prevent sutures cutting into the eyelid.

PERMANENT TARSORRHAPHY

If extended closure is anticipated, such as in facial paralysis, a permanent tarsorrhaphy is recommended (Fig. 56-14). This is similar to the temporary tarsorrhaphy, except that the eyelid margin is excised at the site of each suture placement. This method facilitates eyelid adhesion along these sites after the sutures are removed. It can be left for prolonged periods while waiting for neurologic improvement. When the tarsorrhaphy is no longer required, the adhered regions of eyelid margin can be incised with scissors to restore the palpebral fissure.

AFTERCARE

The principles of aftercare for eyelid surgery are the same as for surgical procedures elsewhere on the skin. Perioperative topical and systemic broad-spectrum antibiotics are frequently indicated. The placement of a subpalpebral lavage system or a nasolacrimal medication catheter may greatly facilitate topical therapy.

Postoperative swelling may be minimized by the use of ice packs in the immediate postoperative period. If swelling is present for more than 24 to 48 hours after surgery, warm compresses may reduce swelling and discomfort. The use of flunixin meglumine at 1 mg/kg IV immediately prior to surgery greatly reduces postoperative swelling. Dimethyl sulfoxide applied to the periorbital skin also reduces post-

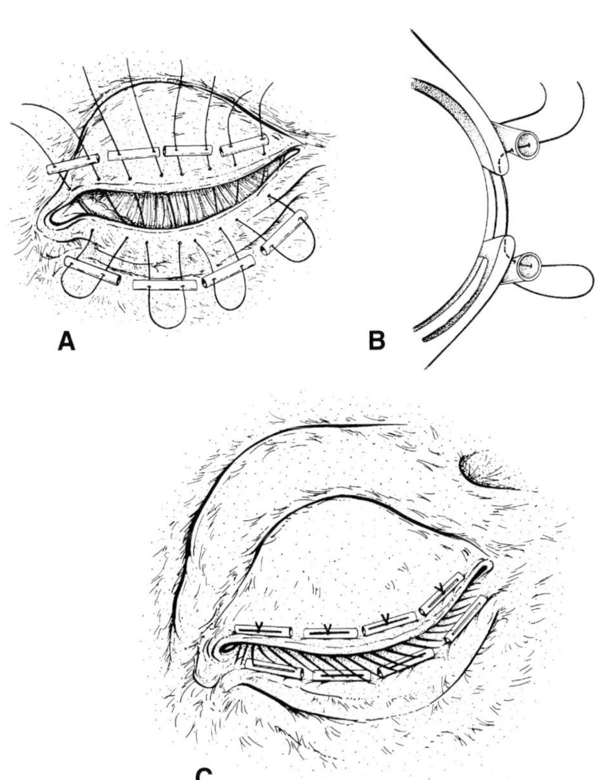

Figure 56-13. Temporary tarsorrhaphy. **A,** Sutures should be preplaced to distribute tension. **B,** Sutures should be placed at partial thickness, crossing the eyelid margin at the level of the meibomian gland openings. **C,** Sutures are tied. The use of stents reduces the risk of sutures cutting into the eyelids.

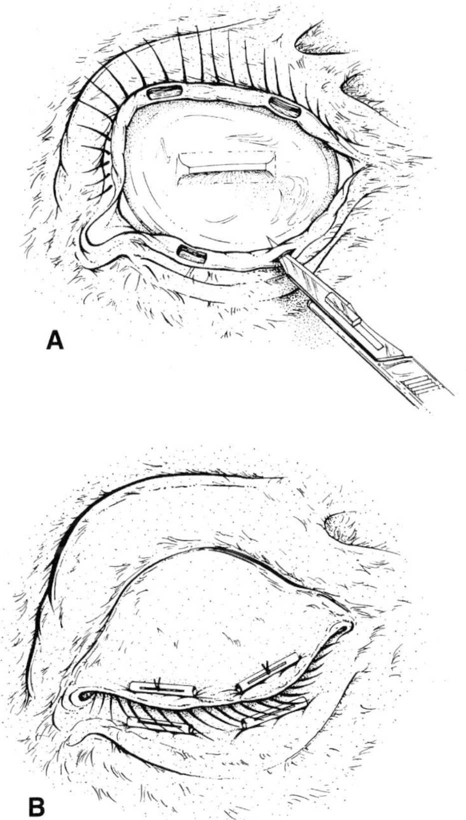

Figure 56-14. Permanent tarsorrhaphy. **A,** Opposing areas of eyelid margin (approximately 3 mm long) are excised with a #11 Bard-Parker scalpel blade. **B,** Sutures are placed in the areas of excised margin. Sutures should be left in place for 3 weeks to allow eyelid adhesion.

operative inflammation. Care should be taken to avoid inadvertent application to the eye.

In procedures such as cryotherapy and immunotherapy, which create granulating wounds, removal of exudate by frequent cleaning and fly control are important for patient comfort. Fly control may be achieved by wiping fly repellent around the surgical site, by allowing the horse to wear a fly screen face cover, or by using fly-repellent halter strips.

If discomfort occurs, the surgical site must be protected against rubbing and self-mutilation. Neck cradles or cross-tying may restrict activity adequately. A hood with an eyecup is also helpful (Eyesaver, Pasadena, Calif).

In many cases, skin sutures may be removed as early as 7 to 10 days postoperatively. Sutures in horses with tension on skin flaps, for example, must remain longer.

REFERENCES

1. Dellman HD: Veterinary Histology: An Outline Text-Atlas, Philadelphia, 1971, Lea & Febiger.
2. Diesem C: The organ of vision. In Getty R, editor: Sisson and Grossman's Anatomy of the Domestic Animals, ed 5, Philadelphia, 1975, WB Saunders.
3. Habel RE: Applied Veterinary Anatomy, ed 2, Ithaca, NY, 1978, RE Habel.
4. Martin CL, Anderson BG: Ocular anatomy. In Gelatt KN, editor: Veterinary Ophthalmology, Philadelphia, 1981, Lea & Febiger.
5. Lavach JD: The Handbook of Equine Ophthalmology, Fort Collins, Colo, 1987, Gidding Studio.
6. Sisson S: Equine myology. In Getty R, editor: Sisson and Grossman's Anatomy of the Domestic Animals, ed 5, Philadelphia, 1975, WB Saunders.
7. Godinks HP, Getty R: Cranial nerves. In Getty R, editor: Sisson and Grossman's Anatomy of the Domestic Animals, ed 5, Philadelphia, 1975, WB Saunders.
8. Rooney JR, Sack WO, Habel RE: Guide to the Dissection of the Horse, Ithaca, NY, 1967, WO Sack.
9. Schmidt GM, Coulter DB: Physiology of the eye. In Gelatt KN, editor: Veterinary Ophthalmology, Philadelphia, 1981, Lea & Febiger.
10. Gelatt KN: The eye. In Mannsman RA, McAllister ES, Pratt PW, editors: Equine Medicine and Surgery, ed 3, Santa Barbara, Calif, 1982, American Veterinary Publications.
11. Schmidt V: Diseases of the eye. In Dietz O, Weisner E, editors: Diseases of the Horse, Basel, 1984, S Karger.
12. Priester WA: Congenital ocular defects in cattle, horses, cats and dogs, J Am Vet Med Assoc 1972;160:1504.
13. Fox LM, Thurmon JC: Bilateral ankyloblepharon congenita in a newborn foal, Vet Med Small Anim Clin 1969;64:237.
14. Barnett KC: The eye of the newborn foal, J Reprod Fert Supp 1969;23:701.
15. Peiffer RL, Williams R, Schenk M: Correction of congenital entropion in a foal, Vet Med Small Anim Clin 1977;72:1219.
16. Latimer CA: Diseases of the adnexa and conjunctiva. In Robinson NE, editor: Current Therapy in Equine Medicine, ed 2, Philadelphia, 1987, WB Saunders.
17. Severin GA: Veterinary Ophthalmic Notes, ed 2, Ft. Collins, Colo, 1976, Colorado State University.
18. Senk GW: Ocular discharge in young horses. In Robinson NE, editor: Current Therapy in Equine Medicine, ed 2, Philadelphia, 1987, WB Saunders.
19. Craven JR: Significance of lesions of the cornea and lens in the examination of horses for soundness, Equine Vet J 1971;3:141.
20. Vestre WA, Brightman AH: Correction of cicatricial entropion and trichiasis in the horse, Equine Pract 1980;2:13.
21. Glaze MB: Equine adnexal habronemiasis, Equine Vet J Suppl 1983;2:71.
22. Moore CP, Sarazan RD, Whitley RD, Jackson WF: Equine ocular parasites: A review, Equine Vet J Suppl 1983;2:76.
23. Rebhun WC, Mirro EJ, George ME, Kern TJ: Habronemic blepharoconjunctivitis in horses, J Am Vet Med Assoc 1981;179:469.
24. Sundberg JP, Burnstein T, Page EH, et al: Neoplasms of Equidae, J Am Vet Med Assoc 1977;170:150.
25. Cotchin E: A general survey of tumors in the horse, Equine Vet J 1977;9:16.
26. Lavach JD, Severin GA: Neoplasia of the equine eye, adnexa, and orbit: A review of 68 cases, J Am Vet Med Assoc 1977;170:202.
27. Baker JR, Leyland A: Histological survey of tumors of the horse, with particular reference to those of the skin, Vet Rec 1975;96:419.
28. Blodi FC, Ramsey FK: Ocular tumors in domestic animals, Am J Ophthalmol 1967;64:627.
29. Schwink K: Factors influencing morbidity and outcome of equine ocular squamous cell carcinoma, Equine Vet J 1987;19:198.
30. Dugan SJ, Curtis CR, Roberts SM, Severin GA: Epidemiologic study of ocular/adnexal squamous cell carcinoma in horses, J Am Vet Med Assoc 1991;198:251.
31. Gelatt KN, Myers VS, Perman V, Jessen C: Conjunctival squamous cell carcinoma in the horse, J Am Vet Med Assoc 1974;165:617.
32. Neumann SM, Kainer RA, Severin GA: Reaction of normal equine eyes to radiofrequency current-induced hyperthermia, Am J Vet Res 1982;43:1938.
33. Grier RL, Brewer WG, Paul SR, Theilen GH: Treatment of bovine and equine ocular squamous cell carcinoma by radiofrequency hyperthermia, J Am Vet Med Assoc 1980;177:55.
34. Joyce JR: Cryosurgical treatment of horses and cattle, J Am Vet Med Assoc 1976;168:226.
35. Harling DE, Peiffer RL, Cook CS: Excision and cryosurgical treatment of five cases of squamous cell carcinoma in the horse, Equine Vet J Suppl 1983;2:105.
36. Hilbert BJ, Farrell RK, Grant BD: Cryotherapy of periocular squamous cell carcinoma in the horse, J Am Vet Med Assoc 1977;170:1305.
37. Farris HE, Fraunfelder FT, Mason CT: Cryotherapy of the equine sarcoid and other lesions, Vet Med Small Anim Clin 1976;71:325.
38. Fraunfelder HC, Blevins WE, Page EH: ^{222}Rn for treatment of periocular fibrous connective tissue sarcomas in the horse, J Am Vet Med Assoc 1982;180:310.
39. Owen LN, Barnett KC: Treatment of equine squamous cell carcinoma of the conjunctiva using a strontium 90 applicator, Equine Vet J Suppl 1983;2:125.
40. Moore CP, Couvin LA, Collier LL: Keratopathy induced by beta radiation therapy in a horse, Equine Vet J Suppl 1983;2:112.
41. Gavin PR, Gillette EL: Interstitial radiation therapy of equine squamous cell carcinomas, J Am Vet Rad Soc 1978;19:138.
42. Theon AP, Pascoe JR: Iridium-192 interstitial brachytherapy for equine periocular tumors: Treatment results and prognostic factors in 115 horses, Equine Vet J 1994;27:117.
43. Turrel JM, Stover SM, Gyorgyfalrey J: Iridium-192 interstitial brachytherapy for equine sarcoid, Vet Radiol 1985;5:20,
44. Wyn-Jones G: Treatment of equine cutaneous neoplasia by radiotherapy using iridium-192 linear sources, Equine Vet J 1983;5:361.
45. Wyn-Jones G: Treatment of periocular tumors of horses using radioactive gold 198 grains, Equine Vet J 1979;11:3.
46. McCalla TL, Moore CP, Collier LL: Immunotherapy of periocular squamous cell carcinoma with metastasis in a pony, J Am Vet Med Assoc 1992;200:1678,
47. Theon AP, Pascoe JR, Carlson GP, Krag DN: Intratumoral chemotherapy with cisplatin in oily emulsion in horses, J Am Vet Med Assoc 1993;202:261.
48. English RV, Nasisse MP, Davidson MG: Carbon dioxide laser ablation for treatment of limbal squamous cell carcinoma in horses, J Am Vet Med Assoc 1990;196:439.

49. Slatter DH: Fundamentals of Veterinary Ophthalmology, Philadelphia, 1981, WB Saunders.
50. Ragland WL, Keown GH, Spencer GR: Equine sarcoid, Equine Vet J 1970;2:2.
51. Strafuss AC, Smith JE, Dennis SM, Anthony HD: Sarcoid in horses, Vet Med Small Anim Clin 1973;68:1246.
52. England JJ, Watson RE, Larson KA: Virus-like particles in an equine sarcoid cell line, Am J Vet Res 1973;34:1601.
53. Cheevers WP, Roberson SM, Brassfield AL, et al: Isolation of a retrovirus from cultured equine sarcoid tumor cells, Am J Vet Res 1982;43:804.
54. Fatemi-Nainie S, Anderson LW, Cheevers WP: Culture characteristics and tumorigenicity of the equine sarcoid-derived MC-1 cell line, Am J Vet Res 1984;45:1105.
55. Angelos JA, Marti E, Lazary S, Carmichael LE: Characterization of BPV-like DNA in equine sarcoids, Arch Virol 1991;119:95.
56. Nasir L, Reid SW: Bovine papilloma virus gene expression in equine sarcoid tumors, Virus Res 1999;61:171.
57. Marti E, Lazary S, Antczak DF, et al: Report of the first international workshop on equine sarcoid, Equine Vet J 1993;25:397.
58. Voss JL: Transmission of equine sarcoid, Am J Vet Res 1969;30:183.
59. Lazary S, Marti E, Szalai G, et al: Studies on the frequency and association of equine leucocyte antigens and summer dermatitis, Anim Genet 1994;25:75.
60. Bostrom H: Equine sarcoids: A clinical and epidemiological study in relation to equine leucocyte antigens (ELA), Acta Vet Scand 1995;36:223.
61. Carstanjen B, Jordan P, Lepage OM: Carbon dioxide laser as a surgical instrument for sarcoid therapy: A retrospective study on 60 cases, Can Vet J 1997;38:773.
62. Hoffman KD, Kainer RA, Shideler RK: Radiofrequency current-induced hyperthermia for the treatment of equine sarcoid, Equine Pract 1983;5:24.
63. Houlton JEF: Treatment of periocular equine sarcoids, Equine Vet J Suppl 1983;2:117.
64. Lane JG: The treatment of equine sarcoids by cryosurgery, Equine Vet J 1977;9:127.
65. Fretz PB, Barber SM: Prospective analysis of cryosurgery as the sole treatment for equine sarcoids, Vet Clin North Am Large Anim Pract 1980;10:847.
66. Lewis RE: Radon implant therapy of squamous cell carcinoma and equine sarcoid, Proc Am Assoc Equine Pract 1964;10:217.
67. Lavach JD, Sullins KE, Roberts SM, et al: BCG treatment of periocular sarcoid, Equine Vet J 1985;17:445.
68. Klein WR, Rutten VP, Steerenberg PA, Ruitenberg EJ: The present status of BCG treatment in the veterinary practice, In Vivo 1991;5:605.
69. Murphy JM, Severin GA, Lavach JD, et al: Immunotherapy in ocular equine sarcoid, J Am Vet Med Assoc 1979;174:269.
70. Wyman M, Rings MD, Tarr MJ, et al: Immunotherapy in equine sarcoid: A report of two cases, J Am Vet Med Assoc 1977;171:449.
71. Page EH, Tiffany LW, Russell HT: Use of an autogenous equine fibrosarcoma vaccine, J Am Vet Med Assoc 1967;150:177.
72. Schwartzman SM, Cantrell JL, Ribi E, et al: Immunotherapy of equine sarcoid with cell wall skeleton (CWS): Trehalose dimycolate (TDM) biologic, Equine Pract 1984;6:13.
73. Roberts WD: Experimental treatment of equine sarcoid, Vet Med Small Anim Clin 1970;65:67.
74. Owen RR, Jagger DW: Clinical observations on the use of BCG cell wall fraction for treatment of periocular and other equine sarcoids, Vet Rec 1987;120:548.
75. Webster CJ, Webster JM: Treatment of equine sarcoids with BCG, Vet Rec 1987;120:131.
76. Winston T, Rings M, Wyman M: Treatment of equine sarcoids (Letter), J Am Vet Med Assoc 1979;175:775.
77. Brostrom H, Bredberg-Raden U, England J, et al: Cell-mediated immunity in horses with sarcoid tumors against sarcoid cells in vitro, Am J Vet Res 1979;40:1701.
78. Metcalf JW: Improved technique in sarcoid removal, Proc Am Assoc Equine Pract 1971;17:45.
79. Riis RC: Equine ophthalmology. In Gelatt KN, editor: Veterinary Ophthalmology, Philadelphia, 1981, Lea & Febiger.
80. Blanchard GL, Keller WF: The rhomboid graft-flap for the repair of extensive ocular adnexal defects, J Am Anim Hosp Assoc 1976;12:576.
81. Gelatt KN: Blepharoplastic procedures in horses, J Am Vet Med Assoc 1967;151:27.
82. Peyton LC: Reconstructive surgical techniques in the horse, J Am Vet Med Assoc 1981;179:460.
83. Beard WL, Wilkie DA: Partial orbital rim resection, mesh skin expansion, and second intention healing combined with enucleation or exenteration for extensive periocular tumors in horses, Vet Ophthalmol 2002;5:23.

CHAPTER 57

Conjunctiva

Nicholas J. Millichamp

ANATOMY

The conjunctiva is a thin mucous membrane that extends from the limbus of the eye to the margin of the eyelids. The part of the conjunctiva covering the anterior portion of the sclera is the bulbar conjunctiva. It is reflected at the conjunctival fornix to line the inner surface of the eyelids as the palpebral conjunctiva and to cover the third eyelid. The space bordered by the conjunctival and corneal surfaces is the conjunctival sac (Fig. 57-1).

The palpebral conjunctiva is firmly attached to the underlying tarsal collagenous connective tissue. At the medial canthus, horses, unlike small animals, have a small fleshy protrusion, the lacrimal caruncle, which consists of modified skin surrounded by palpebral conjunctiva. The bulbar conjunctiva is loosely attached to the globe except near the limbus, where its deeper layer blends with the attachments of the underlying Tenon's capsule (a thin fascial coat that envelops the globe). Dissection of the conjunctiva from the globe is therefore more difficult immediately behind the limbus. The conjunctiva of the upper lid near the fornix is penetrated by 12 to 16 ducts of the lacrimal gland.

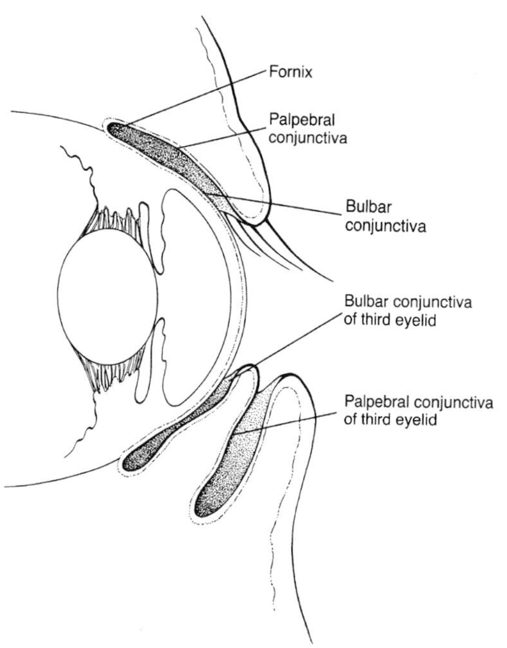

Figure 57-1. Areas of the conjunctiva. (Redrawn from Slatter DH: Fundamentals of Veterinary Ophthalmology, ed 2, Philadelphia, 1990, WB Saunders.)

The conjunctiva is divided histologically into two layers: a superficial layer of stratified columnar epithelium, which is continuous with the stratified squamous epithelium of the cornea, and a deeper substantia propria. The substantia propria at the fornices is complemented by fascial attachments of the eyelid and extraocular muscles that hold the fornices in place. The palpebral conjunctival epithelium contains goblet cells that are particularly numerous at the fornices and over the base of the anterior surface of the third eyelid. The conjunctival epithelium may be variably pigmented and is particularly so in the horse near the limbus and at the margin of the third eyelid.

The substantia propria has a superficial glandular layer and a deeper layer of loose fibrous tissue. Two layers of lymphatics are present, one at the depth of the superficial blood vessels and the other in the deep fibrous layer. Lymph follicles are especially numerous in the bulbar conjunctiva of the third eyelid and fornices.[1]

Surgically, the conjunctiva can be divided into the superficial epithelial layer and the subepithelial fibrous layer, to which the epithelial layer is anchored by subepithelial fibers. A potential space, the episcleral space, lies between the fibrous layer and the globe, ending a few millimeters behind the limbus where the conjunctiva and Tenon's capsule fuse.

The blood supply to the conjunctiva is derived from the anterior ciliary arteries and the vascular arcades of the eyelids. The deep anterior ciliary vessels, which are straight and deep red, can be seen beneath the bulbar conjunctiva near the limbus, where they communicate with the finer, pinker, and more tortuous superficial conjunctival blood vessels. These conjunctival vessels radiate from the limbus toward the fornix.

The conjunctiva receives sensory innervation from the trigeminal nerve.

PATHOPHYSIOLOGY

The conjunctiva responds to injury with vascular dilatation and edema. Lacerations heal quickly. The edges of the defect adhere to the underlying palpebral tarsus or episclera and Tenon's capsule. Epithelial cells slide into the area of the defect, and the conjunctival surface is subsequently reformed by mitosis of adjacent basal cells.

The dense vascular arcades and lymphatics in the conjunctiva predispose it to become inflamed in response to many irritants and infectious organisms. In acute conjunctivitis, the conjunctiva is injected or hyperemic and edematous, and inflammatory cell infiltration may be seen histologically. In chronic conjunctivitis, the conjunctiva becomes hypertrophic and lymphoid follicles become enlarged and prominent. Pseudodiphtheritic and diphtheritic membranes may develop. Hyperemia of deep ciliary vessels can be differentiated from superficial vessels in the bulbar conjunctiva by their deeper red color, straight course, and immobility when the bulbar conjunctiva is moved. Application of topical 2.5% phenylephrine (Mydfrin, Alcon Laboratories, Inc, Fort Worth, Tex) frequently blanches superficial but not deeper blood vessels. Conjunctival swelling may be caused by edema (chemosis) and inflammatory or neoplastic cell infiltrates.

DIAGNOSTIC PROCEDURES

The conjunctiva should be examined with a good light source for color change, irregularities of the surface, and swellings. The conjunctiva is best examined after performing an auriculopalpebral nerve block (see Chapter 55). The lids should be retracted from the globe to allow examination of the conjunctival fornices for foreign bodies and irregularities. After applying topical proparacaine hydrochloride, the conjunctival surface can be palpated gently with the index finger. This is especially important when assessing the extent of spread of conjunctival neoplasms, which may be better felt than seen.

Conjunctival cytology and subconjunctival aspiration can be valuable in cases where conjunctivitis or conjunctival masses are present. After applying topical anesthetic, the conjunctival surfaces are scraped using either a platinum Kimura spatula, the hub end of a scalpel blade, or a cotton-tipped applicator. Smears are made and stained using the Giemsa and Gram technique.

Conjunctival biopsies are essential in making a diagnosis in cases of potential neoplasia and may be of value diagnostically in some cases of conjunctivitis (for instance, habronemiasis). After applying topical proparacaine, a small area of a lesion can be excised with tenotomy scissors.

CONJUNCTIVAL SURGERY

The layers of conjunctiva sectioned during surgery depend on the procedure being performed. In preparing a conjunctival flap, the dissection should involve only the epithelial layer, with as little subepithelial fibrous tissue as possible. The epithelial layer has an extensive surface area and considerable elasticity. Incorporation of the underlying fibrous layer reduces the elasticity and consequently promotes tearing of the flap after surgery. The epithelial layer, however, is thin and can easily be torn or perforated during dissection by rough tissue handling. For removal of conjunctival neoplasms, resection of the conjunctiva to the episcleral space is recommended.

Dissection

Dissection of the conjunctiva requires fine-toothed forceps (Colibri forceps) and semiblunt-tipped scissors (Stevens tenotomy scissors). Incisions into the conjunctiva can be made either with short strokes of a rounded blade or with the scissors. Incisions with scissors should, whenever possible, be carried out with the scissor tip to avoid pulling excess tissue into the scissor blades as they are closed because of the elastic nature of the epithelial layer. At sites where the conjunctiva is anchored, and particularly adjacent to the limbus, there is a greater tendency to perforate the tissue during dissection. Small instrument excursions when cutting the subepithelial fibers reduce the risk of perforations. Additionally, elevation of the conjunctiva tenses the subepithelial fibers and increases the ease with which fibers are cut, reducing the risk of drawing the epithelial layer into the path of the scissor blade.[2]

Suturing

Suturing the conjunctiva requires fine-tipped forceps and absorbable 6-0 to 7-0 suture material (polyglycolic acid or polyglactin 910). Nonabsorbable sutures are rarely used in the horse for conjunctival suturing because of the inconvenience of later removal. Swaged-on taper-point or spatula needles are used.

Conjunctival Flaps

To prepare a conjunctival flap, a portion of the conjunctiva is incised from the limbus or fornix, dissected from underlying tissues, and advanced over the corneal surface. When covering a corneal defect, a conjunctival flap provides blood supply and nutrition and potentiates the immune response against infectious agents attacking the cornea. Rarely is a conjunctival flap thick enough to provide any significant physical support for a thinned cornea. General anesthesia is essential to place a conjunctival flap.

Conjunctival flaps are indicated for ulcerative keratitis when the corneal ulcer extends into the corneal stroma. Although conjunctival flaps can be used for superficial corneal ulcers that are refractory to medical therapy, this is usually not necessary. The value of conjunctival flaps for deep corneal ulcers is debatable, particularly if the ulcer extends to Descemet's membrane (descemetoceles). Because conjunctival flaps provide little support for the cornea, techniques that move corneal tissue to provide support are more appropriate for descemetoceles of more than a few millimeters in diameter. If the descemetocele is less than 5 mm in diameter, a conjunctival flap is often sufficient if surgical rather than medical therapy is elected. When a deep corneal ulcer cannot be intensively medicated (frequently around the clock), surgical therapy should be considered. The decision to proceed with surgical therapy has to be weighed against the risk of corneal perforation that might occur during anesthetic induction or recovery. Corneal ulcers that undergo rapid stromal enzymatic breakdown (melting ulcers) would benefit from a conjunctival flap, but rarely do they have healthy-enough corneal tissue to hold sutures of a pedicle or 180-degree conjunctival flap. A 360-degree flap that does not involve suture placement in the cornea is more appropriate in this situation.

Various types of conjunctival flaps can be used in horses, including pedicle flaps (dissected from either bulbar or tarsal conjunctiva), bridge flaps of bulbar conjunctiva, and 180-degree hood flaps. Complete (360-degree) flaps of bulbar conjunctiva can be used, although because of the friable nature of the equine conjunctiva, they are more difficult to dissect than in small animals and are more prone to retract soon after surgery.

Pedicle Flap

A pedicle flap of bulbar conjunctiva is indicated for a corneal ulcer involving the peripheral cornea in any quadrant. The bulbar conjunctiva is grasped 1 to 2 mm behind the limbus with Colibri corneal fixation forceps and is slightly elevated, and a small conjunctival incision is made with tenotomy scissors. The tips of the scissors are used to open the incision and bluntly dissect the conjunctival epithelium from the underlying fascia. The incision is continued parallel to the limbus for about one third of the corneal circumference, centered adjacent to the corneal ulcer (Fig. 57-2). The bulbar conjunctiva is subsequently dissected bluntly with tenotomy scissors from the underlying fascia back toward the fornix. At one end of the limbal incision, the conjunctiva is incised in a radial direction at 90 degrees to the limbus for a distance equal to the width of the flap required.

Dissection of the flap is completed by continuing the incision parallel to the initial limbal incision to create a pedicle of conjunctiva with a wide base. The width of the pedicle is largely determined by the width of the corneal ulcer and should be large enough to cover the defect and a few millimeters of healthy cornea on either side, without undue stretching of the tissues involved. The extra width allows for contraction after surgery without applying excessive tension on the sutures. The incision farthest from the limbus should be shorter than the first incision to ensure that the base of the flap has an adequate blood supply from radially oriented conjunctival vessels. If dissected well, the conjunctival flap will be a thin, semitransparent layer that will cover the ulcer when reflected onto the cornea without stretching or retraction. The area of corneal epithelium 1 to 2 mm around the corneal ulcer is débrided with a Beaver blade to expose stroma to which the conjunctival flap can adhere. The flap is sutured to the cornea using absorbable sutures, 6-0 or 7-0 polyglycolic acid or polyglactin 910, with a swaged-on micropoint spatula needle penetrating from half to two thirds of the corneal depth. The needle should pass through the conjunctiva, enter the edge of the ulcer, and emerge from the cornea 2 to 3 mm from the ulcer edge. Usually, four to eight sutures are adequate. The exposed area of bulbar conjunctiva from where the flap was dissected can be closed with the same suture material in a simple-continuous pattern. Small defects in the bulbar conjunctiva can be left to heal by second intention.

Tarsoconjunctival pedicle grafts can also be used to provide blood supply and support to a deeply ulcerated or perforated cornea.[3] A pedicle of tarsoconjunctiva is excised from the middle third of the inside of the upper eyelid, leaving an attachment at the eyelid margin. The flap is rotated so that the deep tarsoconjunctival tissue faces the cornea, and the graft is sutured over the area of the corneal lesion with absorbable sutures. After 2 to 3 weeks, the flap is transected from the upper eyelid, and loose excess tissue is excised from the corneal attachments.

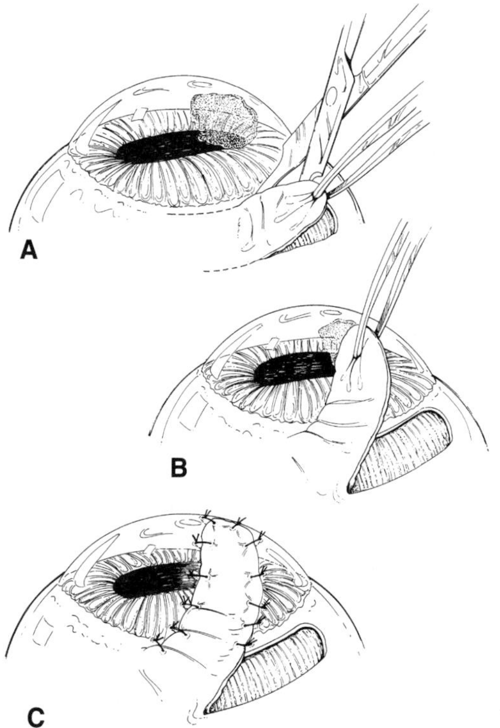

Figure 57-2. Pedicle conjunctival flap. **A,** The pedicle is bluntly dissected from underlying fibrous tissue. **B,** The pedicle should lie over the corneal defect without undue tension. **C,** The pedicle is sutured around the edge of the corneal lesion.

Bridge Flap

A bridge flap is indicated for central corneal ulcers. Ideally, the flap is dissected from the lateral bulbar conjunctiva so that it is oriented vertically across the corneal surface. This way, tension on the flap and sutures is reduced during movement of the eyelids over the flap surface. The conjunctiva is dissected free from the limbus from 160 to 180 degrees and bluntly dissected back toward the fornix with tenotomy scissors. Care must be taken to keep the dissection of the conjunctiva as superficial as possible. A second incision is made with tenotomy scissors, parallel to the first one and abaxially, except at the ends, where it diverges away from the first incision toward the fornix (Fig. 57-3). The distance between the two parallel incisions (i.e., the width of the flap) is determined by the width of the corneal lesion to be covered. As with a pedicle flap, the second incision should be no longer than the perilimbal incision to allow blood vessels to enter the flap. The flap, attached at two

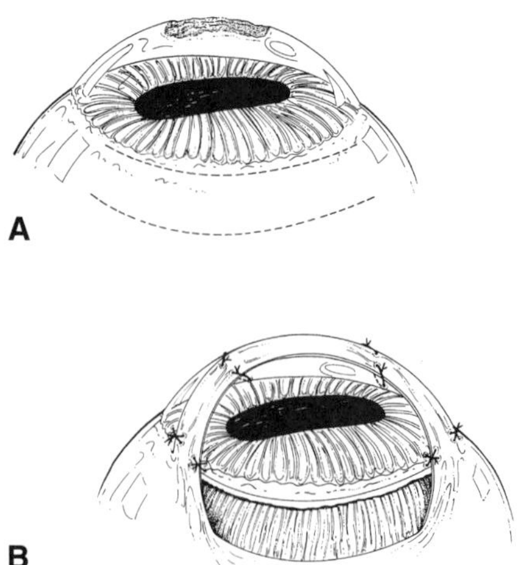

Figure 57-3. Bridge conjunctival flap. **A,** A strip of conjunctiva is incised and bluntly dissected from the bulbar conjunctiva. **B,** The bridge of conjunctiva is sutured to the cornea around the edge of the corneal ulcer.

ends, is subsequently transferred to the cornea and sutured around the edges of the corneal ulcer with simple-interrupted sutures of 6-0 or 7-0 polyglycolic acid or polyglactin 910. Additional sutures are placed in the episclera adjacent to the limbus at either end of the flap. The exposed area of sclera behind the limbus from which the flap was dissected is covered with bulbar conjunctiva pulled from the fornix and sutured to the perilimbal episclera with the same suture material in a simple-continuous pattern. Bridge and pedicle flaps can be dissected medially to cover medial corneal lesions if necessary, although the manner in which the bulbar conjunctiva is reflected onto the inner surface of the third eyelid may hinder dissection.

Both pedicle and bridge flaps are left in place for 14 to 21 days, or longer, until the area of the corneal ulcer is vascularized and granulation tissue can be seen around the edge of the flap. The flap often adheres to the edges of the ulcer. Some flaps may retract from the cornea on their own, and others may become cornea-like in appearance. Conjunctival flaps, however, can easily be removed from the cornea once their presence is no longer needed. Using sedation, an auriculopalpebral nerve block, and topical proparacaine anesthesia of the cornea and conjunctiva, the flap is trimmed away around the area of the ulcer and redundant conjunctival tissue excised.

The 180-Degree Flap

The 180-degree conjunctival flap is indicated for the treatment of a large area of corneal ulceration involving the peripheral cornea. A 180-degree incision is made into the conjunctiva 1 to 2 mm behind the limbus. Using tenotomy scissors, the conjunctiva is gently undermined toward the fornix (Fig. 57-4). It is especially important to keep the flap as thin as possible and not to incorporate subepithelial fascia when dissecting a 180-degree flap. If the flap is dissected satisfactorily, it can be advanced onto the cornea. Minimal flap retraction will occur. If the flap is too thick and has subepithelial fascia incorporated, undue tension will be needed to move the flap over the corneal surface, resulting in retraction of the flap within a few days of surgery. A flap containing too much subepithelial fibrous tissue should have the fibrous tissue gently dissected from the epithelial layer before attempting to suture it to the cornea. The flap is sutured to the episclera at the ends of the incision and to the cornea with several sutures of 6-0 or 7-0 polyglycolic acid or polyglactin 910 using a swaged-on micropoint spatula needle penetrating one half to two thirds of the corneal depth. The flap will retract as the sutures are absorbed, or it can be released after 14 to 21 days by removing the sutures.

The 360-Degree Flap

Conjunctival flaps of 360 degrees are dissected in the same way as 180-degree flaps, but the incision is extended around the entire limbus (Fig. 57-5). The conjunctival flaps from the superior and inferior hemispheres are advanced onto the cornea and sutured together using interrupted horizontal mattress sutures of 6-0 silk. Using a 360-degree flap avoids the need to place sutures into the cornea itself. The silk sutures are removed after 10 to 14 days and the conjunctiva is allowed to retract.

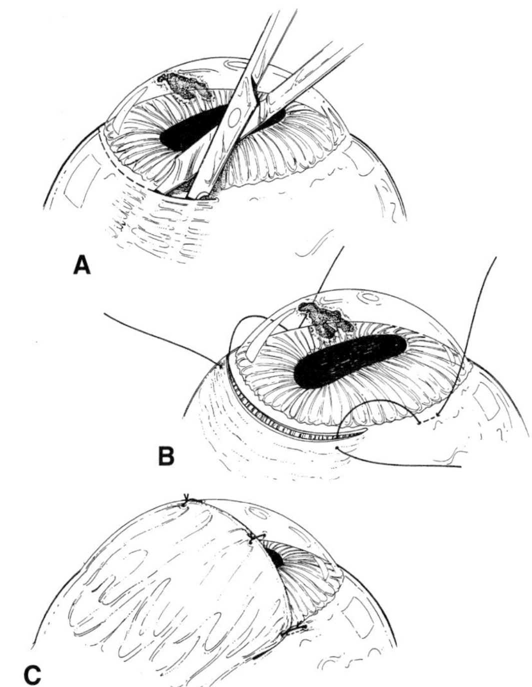

Figure 57-4. A 180-degree conjunctival flap. An incision is made adjacent to the limbus. **A,** The bulbar conjunctiva is undermined toward the fornix. **B,** The flap is sutured to the episclera at the edges of the incision. **C,** The flap is sutured to the cornea.

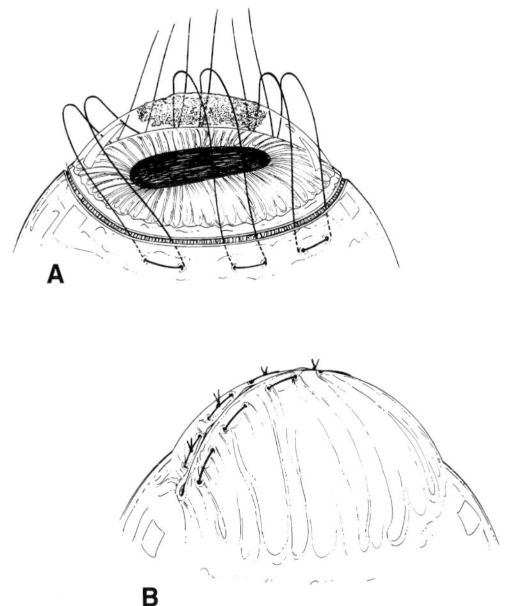

Figure 57-5. A 360-degree conjunctival flap. **A,** The bulbar conjunctiva is incised circumferentially around the limbus and is undermined toward the fornix. **B,** The apposing sides of the flap are sutured together with mattress sutures.

Limbal-Based Flap

Limbal-based flaps involve making incisions into the conjunctiva at some distance between the limbus and the fornix and inverting the conjunctiva (hinged at the limbus) over the cornea so that its exterior surface contacts the corneal surface. These flaps are used less in veterinary than in human ophthalmology, although there is no reason why they cannot be applied in horses.

SURGICAL DISORDERS

Dermoids

Dermoids are occasionally seen in horses (Fig. 57-6). Although these need not cause significant impairment of vision, some involving the conjunctiva may encroach onto the cornea and pigment it, causing some visual handicap. Dermoids are excised from the cornea with a superficial keratectomy, and areas of involved conjunctiva are excised using tenotomy scissors. The exposed episclera can be repaired by apposing the edges of bulbar conjunctiva with absorbable suture (polyglactin 910 or polyglycolic acid) in a simple-continuous suture pattern.

Lacerations

Small lacerations of the conjunctiva require no surgical treatment and heal rapidly by second intention. Large defects can be repaired by suturing the cut edges with absorbable suture. Lacerations involving the palpebral (tarsal) conjunctiva should be sutured using a simple-continuous pattern with buried knots to avoid having the suture material abrade the cornea. This can be performed quite simply in lacerations involving the entire lid thickness by suturing the tarsoconjunctival layer before closing the skin-orbicularis muscle layer of the lid (see Chapter 56).

Neoplasia

Squamous Cell Carcinoma

The most common tumor to involve the conjunctiva is squamous cell carcinoma. The incidence of the tumor affecting the globe and periocular structures has varied from 0.2% to 0.6% of equine cases seen at two veterinary schools.[4,5] The mean age of occurrence is 8 to 10 years.[6-12] Breed predisposition most likely reflects the indigenous population sampled, although draft breeds and horses with light-colored eyes and eyelids may be predisposed to the disease.[9,13] Squamous cell carcinoma may be the most common tumor in geographic areas receiving high levels of ultraviolet radiation.[9] The disease may be bilateral and asymmetric.

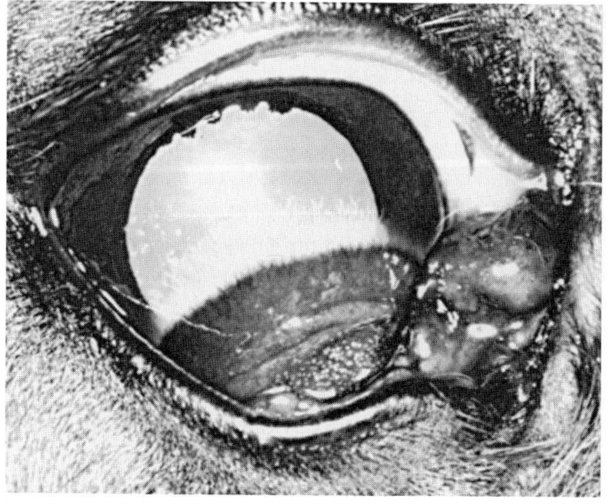

Figure 57-6. Conjunctival and corneal dermoid with associated malformation of the medial canthus.

The tumor often involves other ocular structures in the horse (particularly the nictitating membrane, corneosclera, and eyelids), and the site of the tumor influences the means of therapy. The reader is referred to the chapters on these other sites for discussion of the appropriate therapy.

Squamous cell carcinoma of the conjunctiva is initially seen as an area of conjunctival hyperemia that may ulcerate or progress to become a pink, slightly raised, and roughened area of the conjunctiva. These tumors may also appear as pigmented masses.[14] The tumor may have a cobblestone and papillomatous appearance or, if untreated, may become an unsightly granulomatous-appearing mass. Affected eyes usually have associated conjunctivitis and ocular discharge. Squamous cell carcinoma may involve both palpebral conjunctiva and the eyelids, or bulbar conjunctiva and cornea. Local invasion of ocular and periocular tissues occurs and may involve the globe and adnexa, the bony orbit, paranasal sinuses, and brain.[15] It is often impossible from the clinical appearance to determine whether the tumor has started to invade adjacent structures. Digital palpation of the conjunctival sac after auriculopalpebral and topical anesthesia is a useful means of determining the extent of the conjunctival involvement. Skull radiography or computed tomography (where available) aids in determining whether the tumor has invaded adjacent orbital bone. Metastasis occurs to regional lymph nodes, parotid salivary glands, and lymph nodes of the cervical chain and mediastinum in up to 15% of cases.[15] The primary differential diagnoses for conjunctival squamous cell carcinoma are habronemiasis, conjunctivitis, and other neoplasms.[7,16,17]

All lesions suspected as being squamous cell carcinomas should undergo biopsy for histopathology. The tumor is often quite friable, and impression smears may be used for an early diagnosis. The clinical appearance of squamous cell carcinoma is not diagnostic per se, and confirmation must rely on histopathologic examination.

TREATMENT

Treatment of conjunctival squamous cell carcinoma depends on the size of the tumor and involvement of other ocular structures. It includes surgical excision, radiation therapy, orbital exenteration, cryotherapy, and hyperthermia.

Surgical excision

Small areas of conjunctival tumor can be removed by excision.[10] Care should be taken to excise as wide a margin as possible (at least 3 mm). The margins of the conjunctiva can be sutured prior to irradiation to reduce the conjunctival reaction.

Radiation therapy

Radiation therapy is a valuable additional means of treating conjunctival squamous cell carcinoma. For debulked conjunctival squamous cell tumors, γ-irradiation with a strontium-90 probe is suitable when the tumor bed is no more than 1 to 2 mm thick.[5,18] Doses have ranged from 2000 to 45,000 cGy per site. A reasonable dose in most cases is probably 100 cGy.[5] Nonrecurrence rates using ^{90}Sr probes for ocular squamous cell carcinoma have ranged from 87.5% to 89% over 1 to 6 years of follow-up.[4,5] Radiation-induced keratopathy has been reported in one horse after ^{90}Sr irradiation of a limbal squamous cell carcinoma.[19]

More extensive conjunctival squamous cell carcinomas can be irradiated with interstitial implant radiotherapy. This is particularly true for squamous cell carcinomas that cannot reliably be debulked to a thickness of less than 2 mm. Various modalities of interstitial therapy have been used for ocular and periocular squamous cell carcinoma, including radon-222, gold-198, iridium-192, cobalt-60, cesium-137, and iodine-125.[5,20-23] Minimal total doses of 3600 to 10,000 cGy have been used, with reported nonrecurrence rates of 60% to 87% with follow-up periods between 3 months and 2 years in different studies.[5,20-23] Implants are placed in periocular eyelid skin after debulking the tumor and performing a complete, temporary tarsorrhaphy (Fig. 57-7). The author uses a dose of 5000 to 7000 cGy over 5 to 7 days.

Orbital exenteration and radiation therapy

Invasive conjunctival squamous cell carcinoma should be treated by orbital exenteration and radiation with interstitial implant radiotherapy. Implants are inserted into the eyelid skin after it is closed over the exenterated orbit.

Cryotherapy

Cryotherapy can be used for conjunctival squamous cell carcinoma. Cure rates of 66% to 97% have been reported in cattle and horses, although the period of follow-up has not always been well defined. Care must be taken to limit the extent of freezing if only the conjunctiva is involved. A polystyrene cup can be used to shield the cornea during freezing, and petrolatum ointment can be applied to the cornea and ocular adnexa. Use of a probe rather than a spray limits the effects on surrounding tissues (see Chapter 15). A thermocouple should be used to monitor tissue temperatures during freezing to ensure adequate therapy.[24] The cryogens most frequently used are liquid nitrogen and CO_2. The lesion is frozen rapidly to −20° to −30° C and allowed to thaw slowly. The tissue is then frozen again rapidly.[24-27]

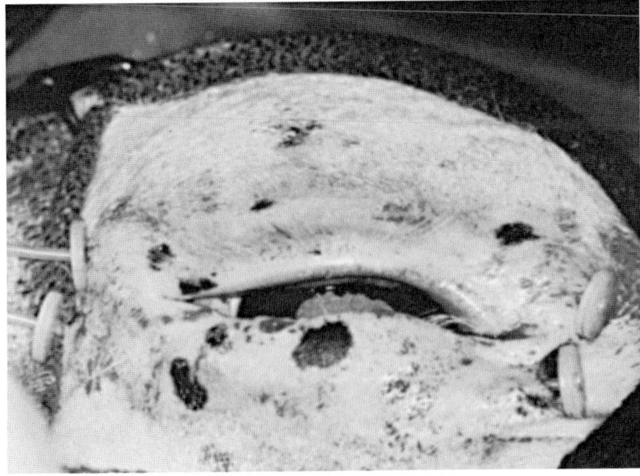

Figure 57-7. Interstitial radiation therapy. Tubes containing radioactive substances are placed subcutaneously in the eyelid skin.

Hyperthermia

Radiofrequency hyperthermia has been used for conjunctival squamous cell carcinomas in horses and cattle.[5,28-30] Tumors should be debulked if thicker than 3 mm or wider than 25 mm.[28,29] Electric current of 2 MHz is passed between two electrodes applied to the tissue. The tissue temperature is raised to 50° C for 30 seconds.[29]

Other Tumors

Other reported neoplasms that involve the conjunctiva in the horse are angiosarcomas,[9,31-32] hemangiosarcomas,[15,32,33] lymphosarcomas,[32,34] and melanomas.[32,35-37] Angiosarcomas arise in the conjunctiva of aging horses, are locally invasive, and eventually metastasize to regional lymph nodes. The prognosis for angiosarcomas is unfavorable.[31] Surgical excision or reduction of tumor size is the most appropriate means of both diagnosis and therapy. When the neoplasia has extensively involved the conjunctiva and globe, enucleation is the most appropriate therapy. The orbit should be exenterated if there is any doubt as to the extent of local invasion. Depending on the type of tumor, interstitial implant radiotherapy may be indicated.

Conjunctival melanomas are less common than intraocular melanomas in the horse. In two case reports, they responded to either local excision or excision with combined cryotherapy.[35,36] In another case, repeated local excision and cryotherapy was unsuccessful in preventing local invasion of the melanoma into the cornea and sclera. Exenteration of the orbit was effective in treating the disease.[37]

Conjunctival Pseudotumors

Unilateral raised pink smooth masses involving the bulbar conjunctiva or the third-eyelid conjunctiva have been reported in horses 5 to 8 years of age. These may be flat and diffuse or focal and nodular in appearance. Histologically, these contain large numbers of lymphocytes and may represent an immune-mediated disease (similar to fibrous histiocytoma or nodular fasciitis in dogs). These masses can usually be treated effectively by surgical excision or debulking and/or topical or intralesional use of anti-inflammatory drugs (corticosteroids).[38]

Conjunctival Papillary Endothelial Hyperplasia

A single report exists of conjunctival papillary endothelial hyperplasia (IPEH) affecting the perilimbal conjunctiva of a horse. By its appearance, the lobulated, raised, red mass could be mistaken for a malignant vascular tumor. Surgical excision of the mass and adjacent bulbar conjunctiva was curative.[39]

Aftercare

Postoperative care of corneal ulceration treated with a conjunctival flap is discussed in Chapter 60. In all cases when conjunctival flaps are deemed necessary for therapy of corneal ulceration, the author recommends a subpalpebral lavage as the most effective method of applying medications (see Chapter 55).

Postoperative therapy for conjunctival neoplasia should include antibacterial agents and a mydriatic/cycloplegic drug if uveitis is present.

Complications

Failure to close the conjunctiva over an area of sclera from which a flap has been dissected may result in postoperative infection, although clinical experience indicates that this is a rare occurrence. Exposed sclera in the horse appears to heal with more vascularization and granulation tissue formation than in small animals. If topical antibacterial drugs are used after surgery, this should not be a problem.

Radiation therapy may result in injury to other ocular structures in isolated cases, and it definitely occurs if careful attention is not given to the dose of radiation being delivered. Complications of interstitial radiation therapy have included temporary corneal opacification and edema, epithelial desquamation, and necrosis. The complications are rarely severe enough to warrant enucleation.[20,22,23]

REFERENCES

1. Prince JH, Diesem CD, Eglitis I, Ruskell GL: Anatomy and Histology of the Eye and Orbit in Domestic Animals, Springfield, Mass, 1960, CC Thomas.
2. Eisner GG: Eye Surgery, Berlin, 1980, Springer Verlag.
3. Holmberg DL: Conjunctival pedicle grafts used to repair corneal perforations in the horse, Can Vet J 1981;22:86-89.
4. Frauenfelder HC, Blevins WE, Page EH: 90Sr for treatment of periocular squamous cell carcinoma in the horse, J Am Vet Med Assoc 1982;180:307-309.
5. Walker MA, Goble D, Geiser D: Two year nonrecurrence rates for equine ocular and periorbital squamous cell carcinoma following radiotherapy, Vet Radiol 1986;27:146.
6. Runnells RA, Benbrook EA: Epithelial tumors of horses, Am J Vet Res 1942;3:176.
7. Junge RE, Sundberg JP, Lancaster WD: Papillomas and squamous cell carcinomas of horses, J Am Vet Med Assoc 1984;185:656-659.
8. Strafuss AC: Squamous cell carcinoma in horses, J Am Vet Med Assoc 1976;168:61-62.
9. Lavach JD, Severin GA: Neoplasia of the equine eye, adnexa, and orbit: A review of 68 cases, J Am Vet Med Assoc 1977;170:202-203.
10. Gelatt KN, Myers VS Jr, Perman V, Jessen C: Conjunctival squamous cell carcinoma in the horse, J Am Vet Med Assoc 1974;165:617-620.
11. Dugan SJ, Roberts SM, Curtis CR, Severin GA: Prognostic factors and survival of horses with ocular/adnexal squamous cell carcinoma: 147 cases (1978-1988), J Am Vet Med Assoc 1991;198:298-303.
12. Dugan SJ, Curtis CR, Roberts SM, Severin GA: Epidemiologic study of ocular/adnexal squamous cell carcinoma in horses, J Am Vet Med Assoc 1991;198:251-256.
13. Schwink K: Factors influencing morbidity and outcome of equine ocular squamous cell carcinoma, Equine Vet J 1987;19:198-200.
14. McCowan C, Stanley RG: Pigmented squamous cell carcinoma of the conjunctiva of a horse, Vet Ophthalmol 2004;7:421-423.
15. Lavach JD: Handbook of Equine Ophthalmology, Fort Collins, Colo, 1987, Giddings Studio.
16. Blodi FC, Ramsey FK: Ocular tumors in domestic animals, Am J Ophthalmol 1967;64(Suppl):33.
17. Brooks DE: Equine ophthalmology. In Gelatt KN, editor: Veterinary Ophthalmology, Philadelphia, 1999, Lippincott, Williams & Wilkins.
18. Owen LN, Barnett KC: Treatment of equine squamous cell carcinoma of the conjunctiva using a strontium 90 applicator, Equine Vet J Suppl 1984;2:125.
19. Moore CP: Keratopathy induced by beta radiation therapy in a horse, Equine Vet J Suppl 1984;2:112.
20. Lewis RE: Radon implant therapy of squamous cell carcinoma and equine sarcoid, Proc Am Assoc Equine Pract 1964;10:217.
21. WynJones G: Treatment of periocular tumors of horses using radioactive gold 198 grains, Equine Vet J 1979;11:3.
22. Turrell JM: Techniques of afterloading iridium192 interstitial brachytherapy in veterinary medicine, Vet Radiol 1983;24:278.
23. Gavin PR, Gillette EL: Interstitial radiation therapy of equine squamous cell carcinomas, J Am Vet Radiol Soc 19:138, 1978.
24. Joyce JR: Cryosurgical treatment of tumors of horses and cattle, J Am Vet Med Assoc 1976;168:226.
25. Hilbert BJ, Farrell RK, Grant BD: Cryotherapy of periocular squamous cell carcinoma in the horse, J Am Vet Med Assoc 1977;170:1305.
26. Farris HE, Fraunfelder FT: Cryosurgical treatment of ocular squamous cell carcinoma of cattle, J Am Vet Med Assoc 1976;168:213.
27. Harling DE: Excision and cryosurgical treatment of five cases of squamous cell carcinoma in the horse, Equine Vet J 1983;2:105.
28. Grier RL, Brewer WG Jr, Paul SR, Theilen GH: Treatment of bovine and equine ocular squamous cell carcinoma by radiofrequency hyperthermia, J Am Vet Med Assoc 1980;177:55-61.
29. Kainer RA, Stringer JM, Lueker DC: Hyperthermia for treatment of ocular squamous cell tumors in cattle, J Am Vet Med Assoc 1980;176:356.
30. Neumann SM, Kainer RA, Severin GA: Reaction of normal equine eyes to radio-frequency current-induced hyperthermia, Am J Vet Res 1982;43:1938-1944.
31. Moore PF, Hacker DV, Buyukmihci NC: Ocular angiosarcoma in the horse: Morphological and immunohistochemical studies, Vet Pathol 1986;23:240-244.
32. Barnett KC, Crispin SM, Lavach JD, Matthews AG: Color Atlas and Text of Equine Ophthalmology, London, 1995, CV Mosby.
33. Vestre WA, Turner TA, Carlton WW: Conjunctival hemangioma in a horse, J Am Vet Med Assoc 1982;180:1481.
34. Rebhun WC, Bertone A: Equine lymphosarcoma, J Am Vet Med Assoc 1984;184:720.
35. Hirst LW, Jabs DA, Stoskopf M, Strandberg JD, Kempski S: Benign epibulbar melanocytoma in a horse, J Am Vet Med Assoc 183:333-334, 1983.
36. Hamor RE, Ramsey DT, Wiedmeyer CE, et al: Melanoma of the conjunctiva and cornea in a horse, Vet Comp Ophthalmol 1997;7:52.
37. Moore CP, Collins BK, Linton LL, Collier LL: Conjunctival malignant melanoma in a horse, Vet Ophthalmol 2000;3:201-206.
38. Moore CP, Grevan VL, Champagne ES, et al: Equine conjunctival pseudotumors, Vet Ophthalmol 2000;3:57-63.
39. Herrera HD, Duchene AG, Croxatto JO, et al: Intravascular papillary endothelial hyperplasia of the conjunctiva in a horse, Vet Ophthalmol 2003;6:269-272.

CHAPTER 58

Third Eyelid

Nicholas J. Millichamp

ANATOMY

The third eyelid (membrana nictitans, nictitating membrane, or plica semilunaris conjunctivae) is situated inferomedially in the anterior part of the orbit between the eyelids and the globe. The structure is a T-shaped to irregularly-shaped piece of elastic cartilage that is covered by a fold of conjunctiva reflected from both the palpebral and bulbar conjunctiva. The cartilage is curved to conform to the anterior curvature of the globe. The top of the T ends a few millimeters behind and supports the free, often pigmented, margin of the third eyelid. The gland of the third eyelid, serous in nature in horses, surrounds the base of the cartilage. In dogs, the gland secretes into the conjunctival sac via ductules on the bulbar surface of the third eyelid, and the same is presumably true in the horse. Some horses may also have glandular tissue on the convex (palpebral) side of the third eyelid[1,2] (Fig. 58-1).

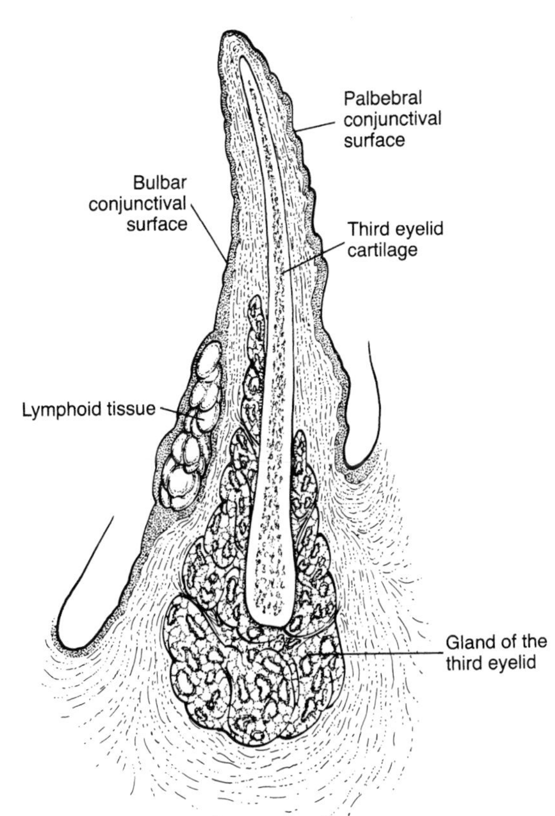

Figure 58-1. Histologic section of the third eyelid.

The surfaces and apex of the third eyelid are covered by stratified squamous epithelium, which becomes columnar epithelium containing mucus-secreting goblet cells and intraepithelial glands at the third-eyelid base.[3] A substantia propria of loose connective tissue, which is associated with blood vessels, is located beneath the epithelium. Lymphatic nodules are clustered in the substantia propria of the bulbar surface of the third eyelid. The third eyelid receives blood vessels from the malar artery, a branch of the internal maxillary artery. Large blood vessels pass through the lymphoid follicles on the bulbar surface of the third eyelid. Sensory innervation is derived from the trigeminal nerve.[1] Anesthesia of the conjunctival surface can be achieved with topical application of proparacaine hydrochloride. For anesthesia of the deeper structures, local infiltration of the base of the third eyelid is required.

In horses, movement of the third eyelid occurs passively, depending on retraction of the globe into the orbit by the retractor bulbi muscles, which pushes orbital fat and the third eyelid forward. The third eyelid is capable of covering most of the cornea when protracted.[1,2]

PATHOPHYSIOLOGY

The third eyelid may protrude unilaterally from its normal position whenever there is an orbital space-occupying lesion present. A mass located inferomedially outside the cone of extraocular muscles is especially likely to cause third eyelid protrusion. The third eyelid also protrudes when the eye is retracted because of ocular pain (e.g., in uveitis or corneal ulceration) or if the globe is smaller than normal (either a congenital microphthalmia or an acquired phthisis bulbi secondary to uveitis or glaucoma). Occasionally, the third eyelid may protrude in horses with Horner's syndrome.[4] Bilateral protrusion may occur in some systemic diseases with infiltration of the orbit (lymphosarcoma) or in debilitated animals with loss of orbital fat and recession of the globe in the orbit. In horses with tetanus, the third eyelid may be visible and rapidly move across the eye in response to stimuli to the head.[5,6]

In cases of conjunctivitis, the third-eyelid conjunctiva is involved with the palpebral and bulbar conjunctiva. Hyperplasia of the lymphoid follicles on the bulbar surface of the third eyelids is often obvious, although lymphoid tissue on other conjunctival surfaces also may be enlarged.

DIAGNOSTIC PROCEDURES

The third eyelid should be examined carefully in any horse with conjunctivitis or keratitis. The anterior surface can be examined by pressing the globe posteriorly into the orbit with digital pressure applied through the upper eyelid. The third eyelid will passively protrude, enabling examination of its anterior surface. To examine the folds of conjunctiva at the base of the anterior surface or to examine the bulbar surface of the third eyelid, proparacaine hydrochloride is applied to the eye and the cross-bar of the T cartilage is grasped with serrated forceps. The third eyelid can then be drawn from the conjunctival sac and reflected anteriorly to expose the bulbar surface. Examination behind the third eyelid is important in locating foreign bodies and conjunctival parasites, including *Thelazia*. The margin of the eyelid should not be held with forceps because it will tear easily if the horse pulls away during examination. The eyelid can also be palpated for masses after application of topical anesthetic.

Conjunctival lesions can be cultured and scrapings taken for cytology the same way as for other conjunctival lesions. Masses on the conjunctiva should undergo biopsy for histopathologic examination. This can usually be achieved with an auriculopalpebral nerve block and topical anesthesia alone. For potentially deep masses, local infiltration of anesthetic should supplement topical anesthesia.

For surgery on the third eyelid in a sedated standing animal, topical proparacaine hydrochloride is applied to the eye. Local analgesia is achieved by lacrimal and zygomatic nerve blocks. The third eyelid is elevated and 5 to 10 mL of 2% Xylocaine hydrochloride is injected along the base.

SURGICAL TECHNIQUES

Third Eyelid Flap

The third eyelid is often used as a flap to cover lesions of the cornea and, in particular, corneal ulcers. The rationale for using a third-eyelid flap is as follows: the flap, when placed correctly, provides physical protection for the cornea and may bring blood supply (from the conjunctiva covering the third eyelid) into close apposition with the corneal lesion and promote healing. No controlled study has been performed in any species to determine whether third-eyelid flaps promote healing of corneal lesions. It is possible that corneal ulcers that heal with a third-eyelid flap in place would have healed as well with medical therapy alone. Potential disadvantages of the third-eyelid flap include the following:

1. A third-eyelid flap applied over the cornea obscures any view of the cornea, making it difficult to evaluate improvement or deterioration of the corneal lesion (unless sutures are tied in such a way as to allow the flap to be lowered periodically).
2. If poorly applied, the third-eyelid flap may apply pressure to the cornea and, in cases of deep corneal ulceration, may actually promote perforation of the cornea.
3. The third-eyelid flap may prevent topically applied medications from reaching the corneal lesion in adequate concentrations to combat infection.

When deep stromal corneal ulcers, melting ulcers, or descemetoceles are present, conjunctival flaps or corneal grafts (including the corneoscleral transposition) are better means of treating the problem. These techniques allow the eye to be easily examined and effectively medicated, they provide a good blood supply to the cornea, and they may offer some support for a thin area of the cornea.

Third-eyelid flaps may be used in horses for superficial corneal ulcers that cannot be medicated by the owner. The flap is placed under general or local anesthesia with sedation. Three or four horizontal mattress sutures of nonabsorbable 2-0 to 3-0 material are used. The sutures are inserted from the skin into the upper conjunctival fornix. The sutures pass through the palpebral surface of the third eyelid 4 to 5 mm behind its free margin. The cartilage of the third eyelid may be encircled by the suture but probably should not be penetrated by the needle or the suture. The suture is again passed through the upper eyelid via the fornix. Stents of polyethylene tubing may be used over the upper eyelid to distribute pressure. Tension on the third-eyelid flap is relieved by performing a temporary tarsorrhaphy at the same time. It is recommended that, whenever possible, the third-eyelid flap be placed along with a subpalpebral lavage system (see Chapter 55) to medicate the eye effectively. The sutures of the flap may be tied with a bow to allow lowering of the flap and evaluation of the progress of corneal healing or deterioration.

Excision

Excision of the third eyelid can be performed either under general anesthesia or in the standing animal with adequate local anesthesia and analgesia. The latter requires sedation with xylazine or detomidine; auriculopalpebral, infratrochlear, and zygomatic nerve blocks; and infiltration of local anesthetic at the base of the third eyelid (Fig. 58-2). Topical proparacaine hydrochloride should be applied to the conjunctiva.

The third eyelid is grasped at either end of the T of the cartilage with Allis tissue forceps or towel clamps and elevated from the fornix. Two hemostats are clamped across the base of the third eyelid as far from the visible margins of the tumor as possible. The hemostats form a V with the tip at the base of the eyelid and should be clamped below the cartilage. The distal part of the third eyelid is excised with either a scalpel or scissors, taking care to include the cartilage and third-eyelid gland. The hemostats are left in place for a few minutes. Usually there is no need to suture the cut conjunctival edges, although this can be done with 6-0 absorbable suture if prolapse of orbital fat is a problem. The excised tissue should be submitted for histopathologic examination, with the request that the borders of the excised tissue be examined.

SURGICAL DISORDERS

Lacerations

Lacerations of the third eyelid may involve only the conjunctiva or the cartilage. Even if the cartilage is torn, the goal of repair is to restore apposition of the edges of the conjunctiva and, in particular, to repair the third-eyelid margin.

Sutures should start at the third-eyelid margin and progress toward the base for accurate apposition of the margin. Absorbable 6-0 to 8-0 sutures are used with an atraumatic needle. Sutures should emerge on the palpebral surface of the third eyelid, and knots should be buried. Care must be taken not to allow suture material to emerge through the bulbar surface and abrade the cornea. The cartilage should be completely covered by conjunctiva to avoid corneal damage by exposed cartilage.

Neoplasia

Squamous Cell Carcinoma

The third eyelid is the most common site of ocular squamous cell carcinoma in the horse.[7-13] Details of the disease affecting the equine eye are found in Chapter 57.

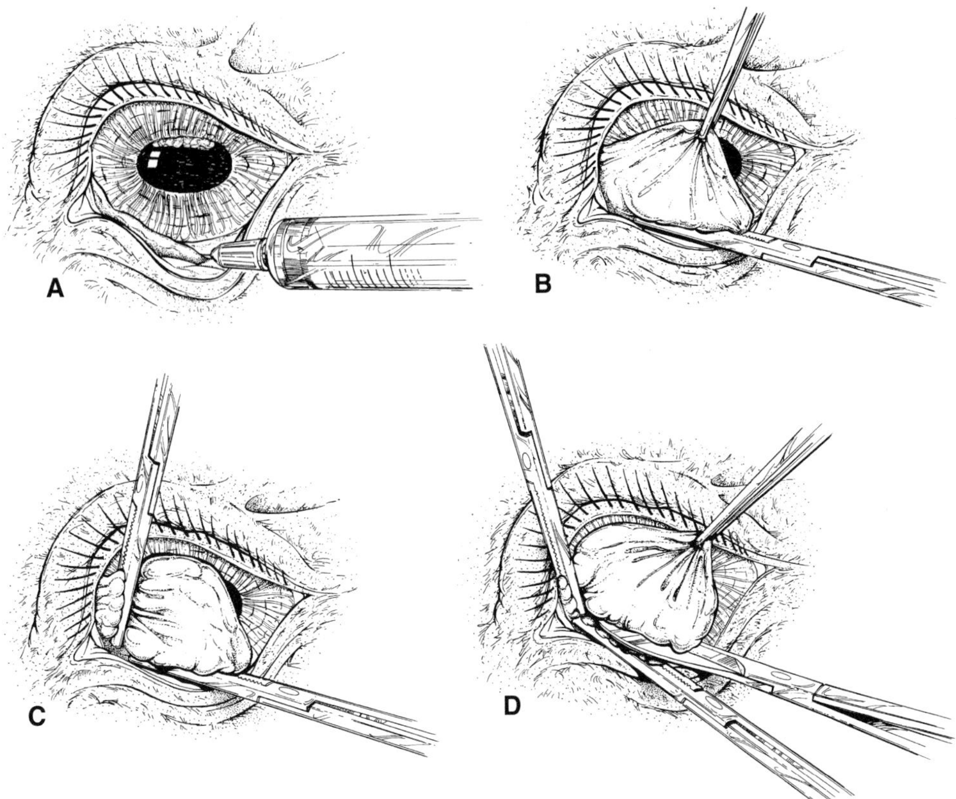

Figure 58-2. Surgical removal of the third eyelid. **A,** Local anesthetic is injected at the base of the third eyelid. **B,** The nictitating membrane is lifted from the fornix with forceps. **C,** Two hemostats are placed across the base of the third eyelid. **D,** The third eyelid is excised along the two hemostatic forceps.

The tumor affecting the third eyelid initially appears as an area of hyperemia. The lesion becomes raised and occasionally has a papillomatous appearance (Fig. 58-3). The diagnosis is confirmed by impression smears or biopsy.

Treatment of squamous cell carcinoma of the third eyelid usually requires removal of the entire structure. Small lesions may be excised from the conjunctival surface while sparing the third eyelid as a whole; however, histopathology should be used to ensure that margins of the excised tissues are free of tumor tissue. If the margins are not clear of tumor, the third eyelid should be completely removed. If the tumor appears extensive or there is any doubt as to how much of the conjunctival surface is involved, complete excision of the eyelid is recommended. Horses rarely appear to have any significant problems after nictitans removal, and this is definitely a better option than tumor extension into tissues around the third eyelid.

Alternatively, excision of the visible tumor from the conjunctiva can be followed by γ-irradiation[14,15] or cryotherapy[16,17] over and adjacent to the biopsy site to provide an added safeguard against tumor recurrence. Radiofrequency hyperthermia has also been used with some success to treat squamous cell carcinoma of the third eyelid in horses.[13,18]

In extensive cases of squamous cell carcinoma involving the third eyelid, the nictitating membrane should be excised and other therapies used in the surrounding tissues. In view of the potential local spread of tumor tissue in the distomedial fornix, cryosurgery may be difficult to achieve practically. Radiotherapy is a valuable technique for treatment of squamous cell carcinoma in this relatively inaccessible site.[13,19] The author has used γ-irradiation at this site by inserting radiation sources in the eyelids at the medial canthus. Options for irradiation of the conjunctiva are discussed in Chapter 57.

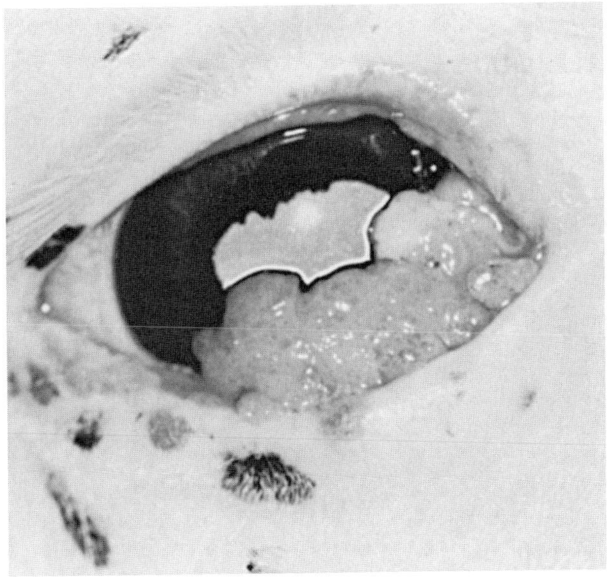

Figure 58-3. Squamous cell carcinoma of the third eyelid.

Other Tumors

Other reported third-eyelid tumors in horses include sebaceous adenocarcinomas,[20] squamous papillomas,[9,10] basal cell tumor,[21] and lymphosarcomas.[22] Localized lesions are best treated by excision for histopathology coupled with either cryosurgery or radiotherapy.[23]

Aftercare

Horses that have undergone third-eyelid surgery should receive topical antibacterial agents BID or TID. Parenteral antibiotics are recommended after excision of the third eyelid. If sutures have been used in or around the third eyelid, the cornea should be observed closely for any evidence of suture irritation.

Complications

Protrusion of the cartilage of the third eyelid after local excision of neoplasms could result in corneal irritation. The cartilage should be removed completely when the third eyelid is excised. Although no cases of chondrosarcoma affecting the third-eyelid cartilage have been reported, the propensity of the horse to develop tumors of damaged cartilage at other sites should promote caution when performing surgery on the third eyelid.

Herniation of orbital fat after excision of the third eyelid may be prevented by suturing the inferomedial conjunctival defect, although in this author's experience this is rarely necessary. Hemorrhage from conjunctival or orbital vessels is rarely a problem when removing the third eyelid and rarely justifies attempts at hemostasis. If this is a concern, cautery can be applied to the stump of conjunctiva when hemostats are removed.

REFERENCES

1. Prince JH, Diesem CD, Eglitis I, Ruskell GL: Anatomy and Histology of the Eye and Orbit in Domestic Animals, Springfield, Mass, 1960, CC Thomas.
2. Samuelson D: Ophthalmic anatomy. In Gelatt K, editor: Veterinary Ophthalmology, Philadelphia, 1999, Lippincott, Williams & Wilkins.
3. Dhingra LD: Histological and certain histochemical studies on the nictitating membrane of the donkey, Haryana Agr Univ J Res 1971;1:93.
4. Bacon CL, Davidson HJ, Yvorchuk K, Basaraba RJ: Bilateral Horner's syndrome secondary to metastatic squamous cell carcinoma in a horse, Equine Vet J 1996;28:500-503.
5. Green SL, Little CB, Baird JD, et al: Tetanus in the horse: A review of 20 cases (1970 to 1990), J Vet Intern Med 1994;8:128-132.
6. Stiles J: Ocular manifestations of systemic disease: Part 3. Horse. In Gelatt K, editor: Veterinary Ophthalmology, Philadelphia, 1999, Lippincott, Williams & Wilkins.
7. Gelatt KN, Myers VS Jr, Perman V, Jessen C: Conjunctival squamous cell carcinoma in the horse, J Am Vet Med Assoc 1974;165:617-620.
8. Strafuss AC: Squamous cell carcinoma in horses, J Am Vet Med Assoc 1976;168:61-62.
9. Lavach JD, Severin GA: Neoplasia of the equine eye, adnexa, and orbit: A review of 68 cases, J Am Vet Med Assoc 1977;170:202-203.
10. Junge RE, Sundberg JP, Lancaster WD: Papillomas and squamous cell carcinomas of horses, J Am Vet Med Assoc 1984;185:656-659.
11. Dugan SJ, Roberts SM, Curtis CR, Severin GA: Prognostic factors and survival of horses with ocular/adnexal squamous cell carcinoma: 147 cases (1978-1988), J Am Vet Med Assoc 1991;198:298-303.
12. Dugan SJ, Curtis CR, Roberts SM, Severin GA: Epidemiologic study of ocular/adnexal squamous cell carcinoma in horses, J Am Vet Med Assoc 1991;198:251-256.
13. King TC, Priehs DR, Gum GG, Miller TR: Therapeutic management of ocular squamous cell carcinoma in the horse: 43 cases (1979-1989), Equine Vet J 1991;23:449-452.
14. Frauenfelder HC, Blevins WE, Page EH: 90Sr for treatment of periocular squamous cell carcinoma in the horse, J Am Vet Med Assoc 1982;180:307-309.
15. Owen LN, Barnett KC: Treatment of equine squamous cell carcinoma of the conjunctiva using a strontium 90 applicator, Equine Vet J Suppl 1984;2:125.
16. Hilbert BJ, Farrell RK, Grant BD: Cryotherapy of periocular squamous cell carcinoma in the horse, J Am Vet Med Assoc 1977;170:1305.
17. Harling DE: Excision and cryosurgical treatment of five cases of squamous cell carcinoma in the horse, Equine Vet J 2:105, 1983.
18. Grier RL, Brewer WG Jr, Paul SR, Theilen GH: Treatment of bovine and equine ocular squamous cell carcinoma by radiofrequency hyperthermia, J Am Vet Med Assoc 1980;177:55-61.
19. Walker MA, Goble D, Geiser D: Two year nonrecurrence rates for equine ocular and periorbital squamous cell carcinoma following radiotherapy, Vet Radiol 1986;27:146.
20. Kunze D, Schmidt G, Tvedten H: Sebaceous adenocarcinoma of the third eyelid of a horse, J Am Anim Hosp Assoc 1979;3:452.
21. Baril C: Basal cell tumour of third eyelid in a horse, Can Vet J 1973;14:66-67.
22. Rebhun WC, Bertone A: Equine lymphosarcoma, J Am Vet Med Assoc 1984;184:720.
23. Lavach JD: Handbook of Equine Ophthalmology, Fort Collins, Colo, 1987, Giddings Studio.

CHAPTER 59

Nasolacrimal System

Joan Dziezyc

ANATOMY

Tears are produced by the lacrimal gland, located in the orbit between the supraorbital process and the superotemporal aspect of the globe, separated from the globe by the periorbita. There are 12 to 16 excretory ducts opening into the temporal conjunctival sac near the fornix.[1] Tears are also produced by the nictitating gland found at the base of the nictitans membrane.

The lacrimal puncta drain tears from the conjunctival sac. The two puncta are located on the conjunctival surface of the upper and lower eyelid, near the free edge, about 8 mm from the medial canthus (Fig. 59-1). Each is a small (2-mm) slit-like opening that empties into a canaliculus, and the canaliculi converge to form the lacrimal sac. The lacrimal sac sits in the funnel-like opening of the bony lacrimal canal and leads into the (common) nasolacrimal duct, which passes along the outer wall of the frontal sinus and nasal cavity.[1] Proximally, the duct is enclosed in bone for 7 to 8 cm; distally, it lies in the lacrimal groove of the maxilla, covered by cartilage. Further distally, it is covered only by the mucous membrane of the middle meatus.[1,2] The external opening of the nasolacrimal duct, the distal punctum, is situated on the floor of the nasal cavity , about 5 cm into the nostril. The opening is seen at the junction of the skin and the mucous membrane (Fig. 59-2). Accessory openings may be present farther back.[1] In mules, the distal punctum opens on the lateral part of the floor or the lateral wall of the nostril.[1]

The precorneal tear film, which is essential for the maintenance of a transparent cornea and healthy conjunctiva, is composed of three layers. The *outer layer* consists of an oily secretion produced by the meibomian or tarsal glands. This layer decreases evaporation of the aqueous layer and prevents tear overflow. The *middle layer* is the aqueous layer derived from the lacrimal and nictitating glands. This layer provides lubrication for the lids, flushes foreign material from the conjunctival sac, and allows atmospheric oxygen to be transferred to the cornea. Antibodies and leukocytes can be found in this layer. The *deep layer* consists of mucin secreted by conjunctival goblet cells. Mucous threads allow lubrication and coat foreign bodies to protect the cornea. Mucin contributes stability to the preocular tear film, as does the outer layer, and furnishes an attachment of tear film to cornea and conjunctiva. Mucin on the surface of corneal epithelial cells acts to reduce surface tension. In the aqueous phase, mucin acts to smooth and spread the tear film.[3]

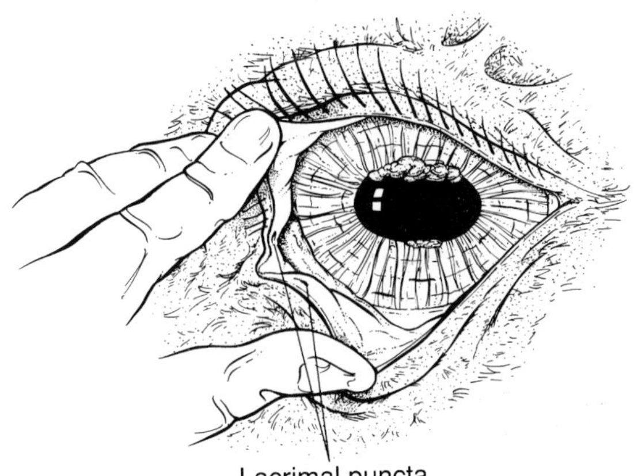

Figure 59-1. Upper and lower puncta of the equine eyelid.

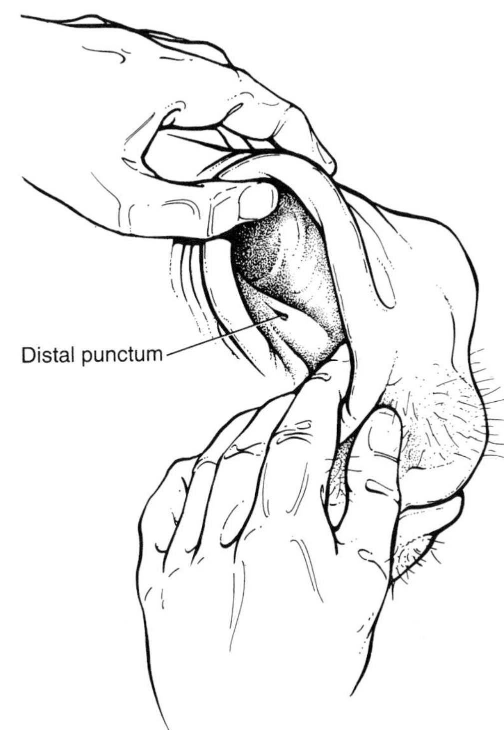

Figure 59-2. The distal punctum of the nasolacrimal duct located inside the horse's nostril.

PATHOPHYSIOLOGY

Abnormalities of the lacrimal and nasolacrimal systems include insufficient production of the preocular tear film, which can include both quantitative and qualitative abnormalities, and insufficient drainage of tears. Insufficient production of the preocular tear film is uncommon in horses.

Abnormalities of drainage are seen as an overflow of tears known as epiphora. This must be distinguished from an increased production of tears that overwhelms the capacity of the normal nasolacrimal duct.

DIAGNOSTIC PROCEDURES

Tear Production

Abnormalities of the oily or mucous layers of the precorneal tear film have not been described in horses, whereas abnormalities of the aqueous layer have been described[4,5] but are uncommon. This is in contrast to dogs, where low tear production causing keratoconjunctivitis sicca is common.

Aqueous tear production is measured using Schirmer Tear Test strips (Cooper Vision, San German, Puerto Rico). Commercially available Schirmer Tear Test strips measuring 5×35 mm have been used to measure tear values in horses. In 50 normal horses, the mean wetting was 24.8 mm in 60 seconds.[6] Schirmer Tear Test strips can also be made by cutting Whatman no. 41 filter paper into 5×40 mm strips and placing a notch 5 mm from one end.

Culture

The nasolacrimal system is cultured, when necessary, by retrograde flushing of the nasolacrimal duct. When purulent material is seen at a punctum, a Culturette (Becton Dickinson and Co., Cockeysville, Md) is used to harvest this material. Aerobic and anaerobic cultures should be performed.

Dye Passage

Patency of the nasolacrimal duct is most easily assessed by instilling fluorescein into the conjunctival cul-de-sac and examining for its appearance at the distal punctum. Either a moistened fluorescein strip is touched to the bulbar conjunctiva or a freshly made fluorescein solution is instilled into the conjunctival sac. Fluorescein should be seen at the distal punctum within a few minutes.

Nasolacrimal Duct Irrigation

If fluorescein dye does not traverse the nasolacrimal duct, flushing of the duct should be performed. The horse is restrained, the distal punctum identified, and a catheter passed up the nasolacrimal duct (see Fig. 59-2). Occasionally, the tip of the catheter hits a blind end several centimeters from the punctum, corresponding to an area of the duct compressed by the medial accessory cartilage.[2] If the catheter is directed laterally, this can be avoided. Six to 10 mL of saline or irrigating solution (Dacriose, Iolab, Claremont, Calif) are flushed into the catheter while holding a finger over the punctum to prevent backflow. An open-ended tomcat catheter or a no. 8 polyethylene catheter is ideal for this procedure. If the punctum cannot be located, the nasolacrimal duct can be flushed from one of the proximal puncta. The auriculopalpebral nerve should be blocked and the conjunctiva anesthetized with a topical ophthalmic anesthetic such as proparacaine hydrochloride. A 20-gauge nasolacrimal cannula can be used to cannulate either the upper or the lower punctum, and saline or an irrigating solution may be used to flush the duct.

Dacryocystorhinography

If the nasolacrimal duct cannot be flushed, dacryocystorhinography[2] is the best way to determine the site of the obstruction. Dacryocystorhinography refers to the radiographic study of the nasolacrimal duct using a positive contrast medium. The horse must be under general anesthesia to perform this study. The nasolacrimal duct is cannulated at the eyelid, and 2 to 5 mL of a radio-opaque contrast material (ethiodized poppy seed oil, Ethiodol, or propyliodone oil, Dionosil Oily) is injected. Care is taken to avoid getting the oil into the conjunctival cul-de-sac. Lateral and dorsoventral or oblique radiographic views are taken. A normal dacryocystorhinogram is shown in Figure 59-3. Computed tomography and magnetic resonance imaging are potentially useful in diagnosing nasolacrimal duct problems.

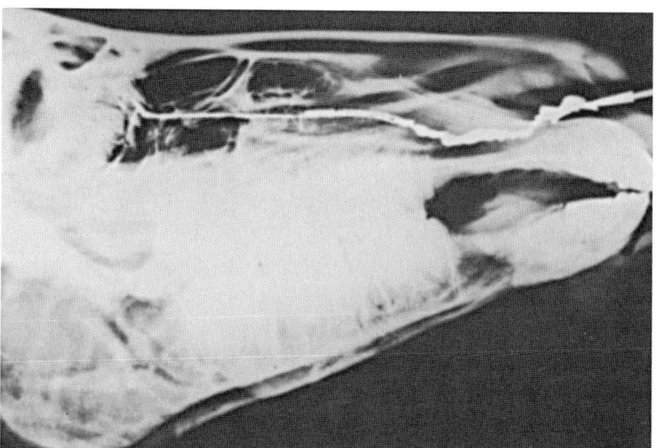

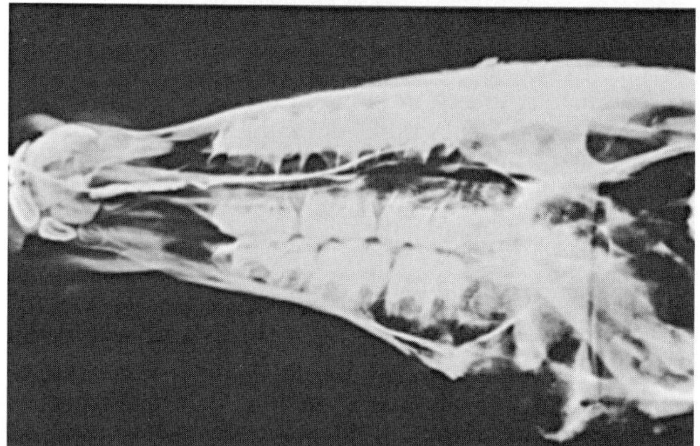

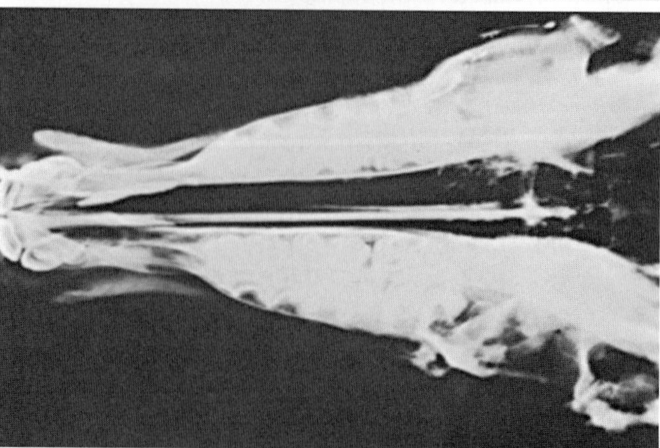

Figure 59-3. Normal dacryocystorhinograms of a foal. **A,** Lateral view. **B,** Oblique view. **C,** Dorsoventral view.

SURGICAL DISORDERS

Punctal Atresia

The most common congenital nasolacrimal disorder is atresia of the distal punctum. Clinical signs include persistent epiphora or mucopurulent discharge, usually noticed from birth on,[7,8] although occasional horses do not show severe clinical signs until they are 1 to 2 years old.[9] In most cases, the duct opening is covered by only a thin layer of mucosa.

The duct can be filled with saline after cannulating a proximal punctum and the mucosa incised over the saline bleb with a scalpel blade. This can usually be performed in a standing sedated foal. Alternatively, it may be easier to identify the end of the duct by passing a catheter through a proximal punctum and incising over the tip of the catheter. A no. 6 cardiac catheter with a guide wire is often effective for this purpose. After the nasolacrimal duct is opened, the guide wire is removed and the catheter sutured to the face near the eyelids and to the floor of the nostril (Fig. 59-4). Alternatively, an incision can be made in the lateral wall of the nostril, and the catheter can be pulled through the incision and sutured to the chin or the face. The catheter should be left in place for 2 weeks.

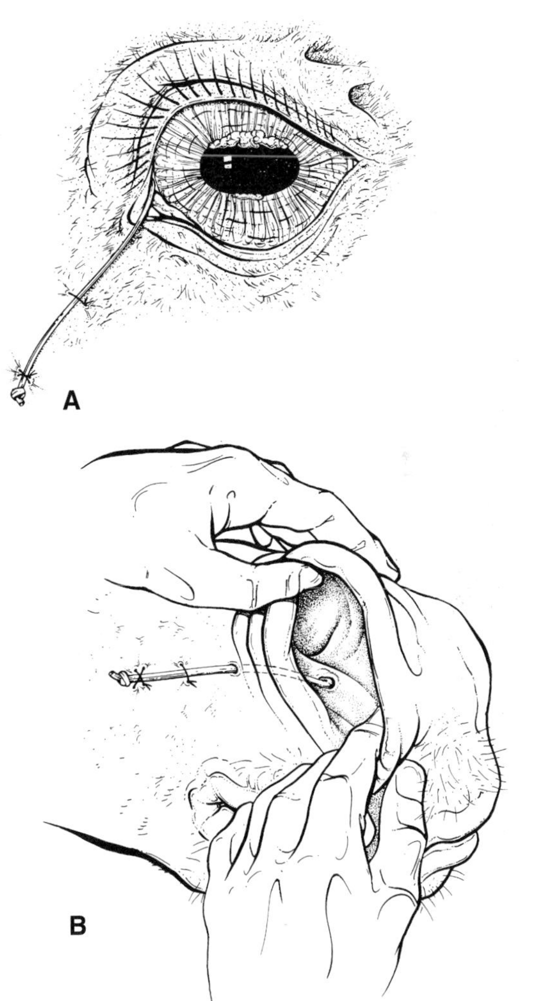

Figure 59-4. A catheter is sutured to the face (**A**) and floor (**B**) of the nostril after cannulating and opening an imperforate nasolacrimal duct.

Horses may also suffer from atresia of the upper or lower eyelid punctum.[9] The absence of the punctum can be seen with magnification, or a bleb can be raised when the duct is cannulated from the nose and saline is instilled. In this case, the duct is easily opened with a scalpel blade. Fastening a stent is ideal, but ducts sometimes heal open without a stent.

If the imperforate punctum cannot be identified, dacryocystorhinography should be performed to delineate the existing nasolacrimal duct. The surgical approach can then be determined.

Lacerations

Lacerations of the nasolacrimal system, usually seen at or near the eyelids and possibly involving the nasolacrimal puncta, require expert repair. The lacerated canaliculus must be cannulated to identify the severed ends and to allow primary closure to maintain patency (Fig. 59-5). This can be achieved by passing a Worst pigtail probe through the unaffected punctum and rotating the probe out of the severed canaliculus. A fine suture material (e.g., 6-0 silk) is threaded into the probe, and the probe is withdrawn, placing the suture from the laceration through the normal punctum. The probe is then passed through the punctum of the lacerated canaliculus. The suture is threaded into the probe, and the probe is withdrawn, drawing the suture through the second punctum. A tapered silicone tubing is tied to the suture and drawn into one punctum, through the canaliculi, and out through the second punctum. The canaliculus and the laceration are sutured with 6-0 silk or nylon. The tube is sutured to itself and left in place for several weeks to maintain patency as the canaliculus heals.[10]

Alternatively, a nasolacrimal duct cannulation can be performed if a Worst probe cannot be passed successfully. Monofilament nylon (2-0) can be passed from the distal nasal punctum retrograde through the nasolacrimal duct to exit the lacerated canaliculus. The Worst probe is used to draw the suture through the proximal portion of the severed canaliculus. The suture is tied to fine silicone tubing, and the tubing is drawn normograde through the canaliculus and the nasolacrimal duct. The tubing is sutured to the skin at the puncta and at the nasolacrimal orifice.

Dacryocystitis

Dacryocystitis refers to inflammation of the nasolacrimal duct and is seen infrequently in horses. Clinical signs include chronic conjunctivitis, with mucopurulent to purulent discharge from the eye. Purulent material can be expressed at the proximal punctum with manipulation or flushing. Occasionally, foreign bodies can be irrigated from the duct and are the likely cause of the inflammation, but most cases do not have a determinable etiology.

Treatment of dacryocystitis in horses is similar to that in other species. A culture is taken of the purulent material expressed or flushed from the nasolacrimal punctum. Topical antibiotics may be applied, but appropriate systemic

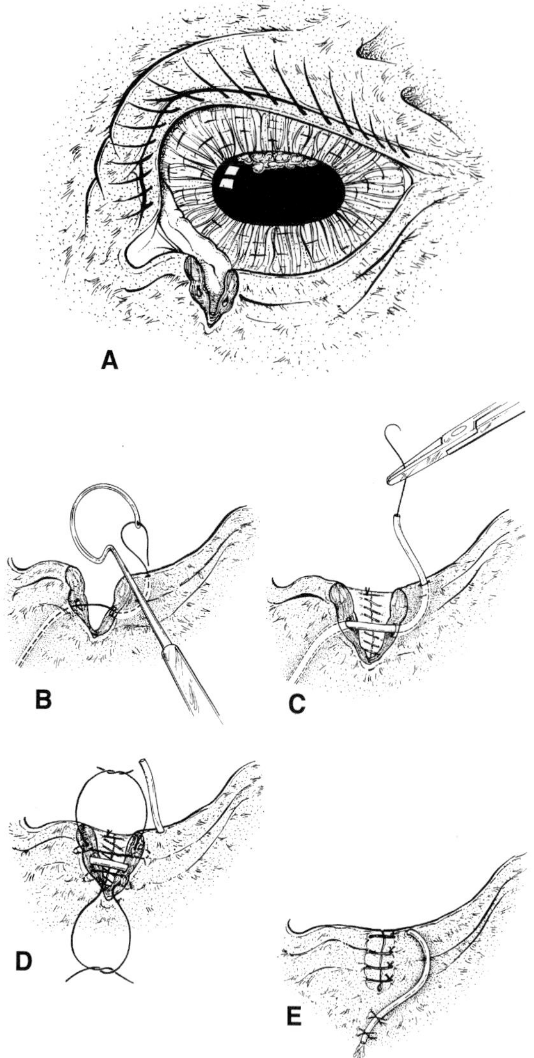

Figure 59-5. Repair of the severed lacrimal canaliculus. **A,** Laceration of the lower eyelid, severing the lacrimal canaliculus. **B,** A 2-0 nylon suture is passed through the nasolacrimal duct and exits through the wound. A Worst probe is passed through the ventral punctum and draws the suture through the distal portion of the severed canaliculus. **C,** A fine silicone tube is cut to a taper, tied to the suture, and pulled through the canaliculi. **D,** The canaliculus and wound are sutured with 6-0 nylon silk. **E,** The tubing is sutured to the skin of the eyelid and at the nasal end. It is left in place for 3 weeks.

antibiotics often must be used to effect a cure. Additionally, the distal portion of the nasolacrimal duct can be cannulated, the cannula sutured into place (see earlier discussion), and an appropriate antibiotic solution flushed through the duct daily.

Blockage of the Nasolacrimal Duct

Acquired blockage of the nasolacrimal duct is seen commonly in the horse. Frequently, epiphora is the only clinical sign, although with chronicity a mucopurulent discharge may be seen.

Patency can be checked with fluorescein dye, and if the duct is not patent, it is flushed from the distal punctum. If flushing is unsuccessful, dacryocystorhinography should be performed.

Causes of acquired nasolacrimal duct blockage include trauma,[11] foreign bodies, and swelling of the duct wall because of inflammation. Diseases of adjoining structures may cause blockage or stenosis of the duct. These include chronic rhinitis or sinusitis, neoplasms of the nasal passages or sinuses, and osteomyelitis from actinomycosis or periodontitis.[12]

Canaliculorhinostomy has been described in the horse for treating an acquired blockage of the nasolacrimal duct. This surgery created a fistula running from the lower lid canaliculus to the rostral maxillary sinus.[11] Conjunctivorhinostomy has been described in dogs and cats as another treatment for blocked nasolacrimal ducts.[13] A permanent mucous membrane–lined fistula is created between the inferonasal conjunctival sac and the nasal cavity. This procedure may have applicability in horses but has not been described in this species.

Keratoconjunctivitis Sicca

Keratoconjunctivitis sicca refers to the abnormal drying of the cornea and conjunctiva caused by a decrease in the aqueous phase of the precorneal tear film. Clinical signs in horses include a chronic tenacious mucopurulent discharge and chronic corneal ulceration.[4,14,15] Schirmer Tear Test values in affected horses have ranged from 0 to 8 mm wetting.[4,5,14,16] Causes of keratoconjunctivitis sicca described in horses include eosinophilic dacryoadenitis,[14,16] locoweed poisoning,[17] and trauma to the nerves that innervate the gland.[5,18] The lacrimal gland is innervated by parasympathetic fibers of the facial nerve (cranial nerve VII). Damage to cranial nerve VII may cause additional clinical signs of ipsilateral ear droop, ptosis, and deviation of the muzzle to the contralateral side. Sulfonamide toxicity has been described in dogs to induce keratoconjunctivitis sicca, and it is theoretically possible that chronic sulfonamide therapy in horses could do the same.

Parotid duct transposition has been described as a treatment for keratoconjunctivitis sicca in horses.[4] This procedure involves moving the parotid salivary duct to the conjunctival sac of the affected eye. Saliva is subsequently continuously secreted onto the eye. Although it is not a perfect tear substitute, saliva is a reasonable alternative to tears and is usually effective in moistening the ocular surface. Topical cyclosporine has also been used successfully to treat keratoconjunctivitis sicca in a horse.[5,16]

REFERENCES

1. Sisson S, Grossman JD: The Anatomy of the Domestic Animals, ed 4, Philadelphia, 1959, WB Saunders.
2. Latimer CA, Wyman M: Radiographic and gross anatomy of the nasolacrimal duct of the horse, Am J Vet Res 1984;45:451.
3. Records RE: The tear film. In Duane TD, Jaeger EA, editors: Biomedical Foundations of Ophthalmology, vol 2, Philadelphia, 1986, Harper & Row.
4. Wolf ED, Meredith R: Parotid duct transposition in the horse, J Equine Vet Sci 1981;1:143.

5. Reilly L, Beech J: Bilateral keratoconjunctivitis sicca in a horse, Equine Vet J 1994;26:171.
6. Marts BS, Bryan GM, Prieur DJ: Schirmer Tear Test measurements and lysozyme concentration of equine tears, J Equine Med Surg 1977;1:427.
7. Munroe GA, Barnett KC: Congenital ocular disease in the foal, Vet Clin North Am Large Anim Pract 1984;6:516.
8. Latimer CA, Wyman M: Atresia of the nasolacrimal duct in three horses, J Am Vet Med Assoc 1984;184:989.
9. Brooks DE: Equine ophthalmology. In Gelatt KN, editor: Veterinary Ophthalmology, Philadelphia, 1999, Lippincott, Williams & Wilkins.
10. Slatter DH: Fundamentals of Veterinary Ophthalmology, St Louis, 2001, Elsevier Science.
11. McIlnay TR, Miller SM, Dugan SJ: Use of canaliculorhinostomy for repair of nasolacrimal duct obstruction in a horse, J Am Vet Med Assoc 2001;218:1323.
12. Riis RC: Equine ophthalmology. In Gelatt KN, editor: Textbook of Veterinary Ophthalmology, Philadelphia, 1981, Lea & Febiger.
13. Covitz D, Hunziker J, Kick SA: Conjunctivorhinostomy: A surgical method for the control of epiphora in the dog and cat, J Am Vet Med Assoc 1977;171:251.
14. Spiess BM, Wilcock BP, Physick-Sheard PW: Eosinophilic granulomatous dacryoadenitis causing bilateral keratoconjunctivitis sicca in a horse, Equine Vet J 1989;21:226.
15. Spurlock SL, Spurlock GH, Wise M: Keratoconjunctivitis sicca associated with fracture of the stylohyoid bone in a horse, J Am Vet Med Assoc 1989;194:258.
16. Collins BK, Johnson PJ, Moore CP, et al: Immune-mediated keratoconjunctivitis sicca in a horse, Vet Comp Ophthalmol 1994;4:61.
17. Van Kampen KR, James LF: Ophthalmic lesions in locoweed poisoning of cattle, sheep, and horses, Am J Vet Res 1971;32:1293.
18. Joyce JR, Bratton GR: Keratoconjunctivitis sicca secondary to fracture of the mandible, Vet Med Small Anim Clin 1973;68:619.

CHAPTER 60

Cornea and Sclera

Mark P. Nasisse
Vivian E. Jamieson
Dennis E. Brooks

Of the domestic large-animal species, the horse demonstrates the greatest predisposition toward ocular diseases requiring surgical therapy. Because of the relatively large globe size, the normal protrusion of the corneal surface, and the environment in which horses exist, ocular trauma is common.[1-3] The direct effects of ocular trauma or the secondary complications mediated by infectious agents often mandate surgical intervention. The tendency of aged horses to develop limbal neoplasms provides further indication for surgery of the corneal and scleral tissues. Successful preservation of vision in such cases depends on the ability of the equine surgeon to apply the principles of corneal and scleral surgery.

ANATOMY

The cornea forms the anterior one fourth of the outer fibrous tunic of the globe and is continuous with the sclera.[4,5] It is horizontally elliptical, being slightly more narrow laterally. The diameter is greater horizontally than vertically (32 to 38 and 26 to 28 mm, respectively), and the radius of curvature is approximately 17 mm. As in other animal species, the cornea is the major refractive surface of the globe (refractive index = 1.37). The thickness of the equine cornea varies from 0.56 mm centrally to 1 mm peripherally.

Histologically, the cornea consists of four layers (Fig. 60-1). The anterior layer is nonkeratinized, stratified squamous epithelium, approximately 10 to 15 cell layers thick, with a thin basement membrane. The substantia propria (stroma) makes up 90% of the corneal thickness and is composed of regularly arranged collagen lamellae, which are separated by a ground substance of mucopolysaccharides that vary according to corneal region, and

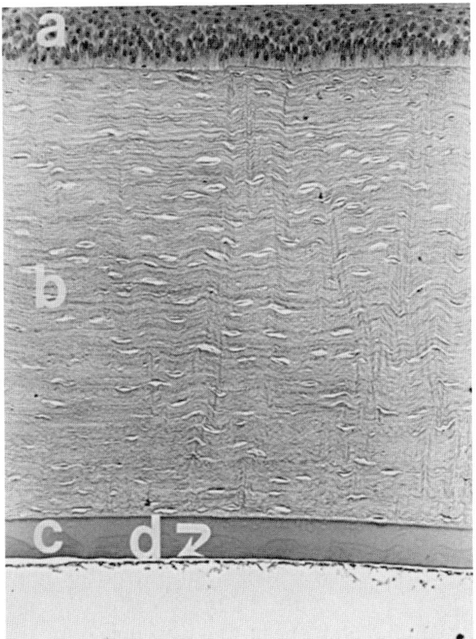

Figure 60-1. Photomicrograph of normal equine cornea. The four layers include the epithelium (a), the stroma (b), Descemet's membrane (c), and the endothelium *(arrow)* (d). (H & E, ×170.)

specialized fibrocytes (keratocytes). A rich supply of sensory nerves, originating from the ophthalmic branch of the trigeminal nerve, extends radially into the midstroma. Nerves branch extensively to terminate as a plexus of free nerve endings in the superficial stroma and epithelial layer. Descemet's membrane is a tough, elastic basement membrane secreted by the deepest layer of the cornea, the posterior epithelium (endothelium). It is 21 microns thick in the adult horse. The endothelium is a monolayer of hexagonally shaped epithelial cells.

A pigmented limbus marks the transition between the cornea and the sclera. A scleral "shelf," which is wider dorsally and ventrally, projects into the superficial corneal stroma at the limbus and obscures the view of the insertion of the pectinate ligaments onto Descemet's membrane. The sclera is thickest anterior to the equator (1.3 to 3 mm) and thinnest at the insertion of the extraocular muscles. Histologically, the sclera is composed of a superficial vascular layer called the episclera, a thicker central layer called the stroma, and an innermost pigmented layer called the lamina fusca. The random arrangement of the sclera's collagen bundles and the relative lack of corneal hydration account for its lack of transparency.

PATHOPHYSIOLOGY

Uncomplicated Corneal Wounds

The process by which corneal wounds heal varies considerably with the size, location, and depth of the injury. After an acute *epithelial* wound that is uncomplicated by secondary infection, the healing process begins with migration of adjacent epithelial cells. Cells of the epithelium's basal layer send out cytoplasmic processes within 1 hour of the injury as they prepare to slide over the defect.[6-8] Within several days of the injury, the same cells increase their mitotic activity as they begin regenerating new epithelium. Complete re-epithelialization of a 12-mm defect may occur in as little as 7 days (0.6 mm/day). Rapid healing of a noninfected superficial ulcer is often followed by a lag phase of slow epithelial movement. Healing of defects involving the epithelial basement membrane takes longer, because hemidesmosomes, which attach the basal epithelial cells to the basement membrane, require several weeks to re-form.

Healing of *stromal* wounds is considerably more complex and time consuming. In a corneal laceration, the process begins with fibrin filling the stromal defect. Leukocytes, whose principal source is the tear film, are quick to migrate to the lesion (usually within several hours) to serve phagocytic and nutritional functions in the damaged tissue. At the same time, epithelial cells bridge the defect as previously described. Keratocytes adjacent to the wound are eventually stimulated to differentiate into fibroblasts and begin secreting collagen. Once the stromal defect is filled, the slow process of wound remodeling, often requiring weeks to months, ensues as stromal cellularity decreases, fibroblasts cease metabolic activity, and collagen fibrils reorient in a parallel direction. Because the perfect lamellar arrangement of the original collagen fibrils can never be duplicated, healing of stromal wounds invariably results in scar formation, the extent of which is commensurate with the degree of stromal damage.

Complicated Corneal and Scleral Wounds

When factors obstruct restoration of corneal or scleral structural integrity or prevent restoration of functional vision after healing of the fibrous tunic is complete, wounds are referred to as "complicated." The most common complicating factor in corneal wounds is the establishment of secondary microbial infection. In the normal equine conjunctival sac, gram-positive bacteria predominate. In several studies, *Corynebacterium* species have been reported to be most frequently encountered; however, β-hemolytic streptococci, staphylococci, and bacilli are also commonly isolated.[9-11] Even *Pseudomonas,* well known for corneal pathogenicity, is occasionally isolated from normal conjunctiva. Fungal hyphae have been isolated from the conjunctiva of 95% of normal horses.[12] Those recovered most commonly were *Aspergillus* and *Penicillium*. Studies reporting microbial isolates from diseased eyes indicate that gram-negative organisms, particularly *Pseudomonas, Enterobacter,* and *Acinetobacter,* are most pathogenic.[13] Other reported pathogenic species include streptococci, especially the devastating β-hemolytic streptococcal species, *Corynebacterium*, staphylococci, and *Salmonella*.[14-18] *Aspergillus* is the most commonly reported fungal pathogen, followed by *Fusarium*.[19-22] Other fungi, such as *Penicillium, Phycomycetes, Pseudallescheria boydii,* and *Cylindrocarpon destructans,* have also been described.[21-23]

The ubiquitous exposure of the equine cornea to microorganisms demonstrates the importance of some predisposing event in the establishment of infection. That event, in most instances, is traumatic disruption of corneal epithelium; bacteria and fungi that are not normally pathogenic become so when access to the corneal stroma is provided.[24,25] The chronic use of topical antibiotics, which may shift the resident flora from being predominantly gram positive to gram negative, may also play a role. Replication of microorganisms that have established a foothold in the damaged corneal tissue has several significant adverse effects. First, the production of collagenolytic enzymes (proteases) from microorganisms and degenerating corneal cells precipitates the clinical phenomenon of corneal melting[26-29] (Fig. 60-2). Melting may be associated with no infection in foals, but it tends to be more severe with bacterial than fungal infection. In cases of rapidly melting corneal ulceration, perforation can occur in as little as 48 hours. Fungi, in contrast to bacteria (which remain confined to the corneal surface), are capable of migrating through the corneal stroma. Tear film instability may precede fungal invasion of the equine corneal epithelium. Endophthalmitis, therefore, is a potential and significant complication of keratomycosis. Even if organisms have not gained access to the anterior chamber, corneal sepsis provides a strong stimulus for secondary intraocular changes. Release of chemotactic factors and toxins may cause the formation of sterile hypopyon (accumulation of inflammatory cells in the anterior chamber). Breakdown of the blood ocular barrier, evidenced by aqueous flare (increased protein) and miosis, is mediated by stimulation of the sensory corneal nerves (branches of the ophthalmic division of cranial nerve V) that results in antidromic release of substance P and other polypeptides to the iris.

In the event that a globe becomes perforated, whether by sharp injury or perforation of an infected corneal ulcer,

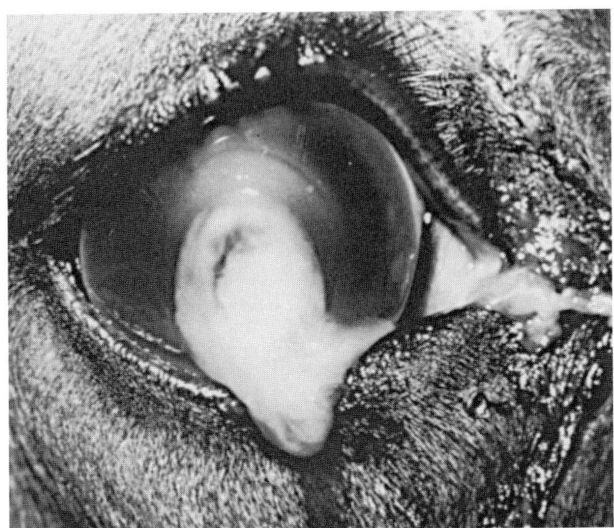

Figure 60-2. Melting corneal ulcer in a horse. Corneal infection by *Pseudomonas aeruginosa* has resulted in extensive liquefaction of the corneal collagen.

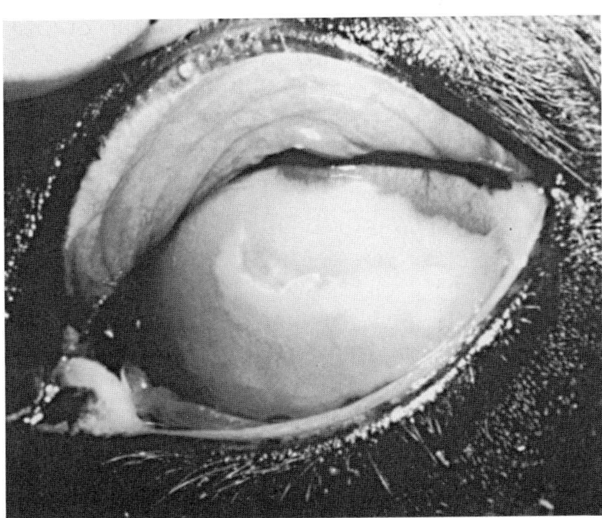

Figure 60-3. Typical appearance of keratomycosis in a horse. The cornea is extensively edematous. There is deep vascularization; and fungus-infected tissue is visible on the corneal surface.

copious amounts of fibrin spill into the aqueous humor. Fibrin normally has a protective effect by plugging the corneal wound, often with the help of entrapped uveal tissue. In the event this corneal plug is ineffective and aqueous humor continues to leak from the wound, a persistent state of hypotony follows that may result in uveal atrophy and, eventually, phthisis bulbi. Ciliary atrophy and phthisis bulbi also may occur as the direct effects of ocular trauma.

DIAGNOSTIC PROCEDURES

Ophthalmic Examination

The ophthalmic examination should proceed in a systematic anterior-to-posterior fashion. The eyelids are first scrutinized with magnification for foreign bodies, neoplasms, or traumatic lesions. The most important abnormalities to be considered when examining the cornea are edema, vascularization, cellular infiltrates, neoplastic growths, foreign bodies, and alterations in structural integrity (Fig. 60-3, and see Fig. 60-2). Structural integrity is assessed first with the application of fluorescein (Fluorets ophthalmic strips) to detect disruptions in the epithelial barrier. Fluorescein should be applied at full strength and not diluted. It is important that excess stain be thoroughly rinsed from the eye to avoid misinterpreting stain pooled in an epithelialized stromal defect as an active ulcer. Rose bengal stain should be applied to detect tear film instability in all horses with painful eyes. The hydrophilic rose bengal dye stains epithelial cells or stains the stroma in the absence of the tear mucin layer or epithelial cells, respectively. Perforation of the cornea can be difficult to detect, but it is usually indicated by one of several clinical signs. Because uveal prolapse consistently accompanies the leakage of aqueous humor, the presence of pigmented tissue in or adjacent to the corneal wound is indicative of perforation (Fig. 60-4). Organized fibrin is usually present, often in large quantities, and frequently obscures the corneal defect (Fig. 60-5). In such cases, it becomes necessary to rely on other clinical signs. By viewing the anterior chamber obliquely from the limbus, it is possible to determine if the iris is displaced forward. Applanation tonometry is useful for documenting extremely low intraocular pressure (less than 10 mm Hg), which is suggestive of aqueous humor leakage. Finally, Seidel's test may be used to confirm leakage of aqueous humor: after the tear film is heavily saturated with fluorescein stain, the area of the suspected perforation is examined under magnification with a cobalt blue light for a change in color, indicating a mixture of aqueous humor with the tear film.

Examination of the anterior chamber should include a deliberate effort to detect increased protein (flare), inflammatory cells (hypopyon), and blood (hyphema). As men-

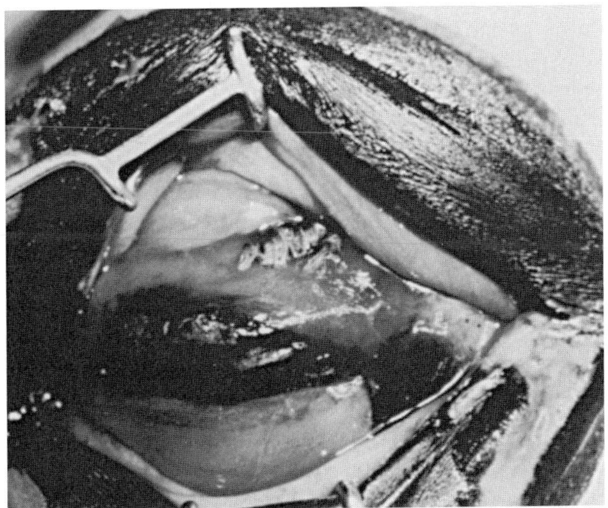

Figure 60-4. A globe rupture by blunt trauma. The cornea has been ruptured from the medial to the lateral limbus, and massive uveal tissue protrudes from the wound.

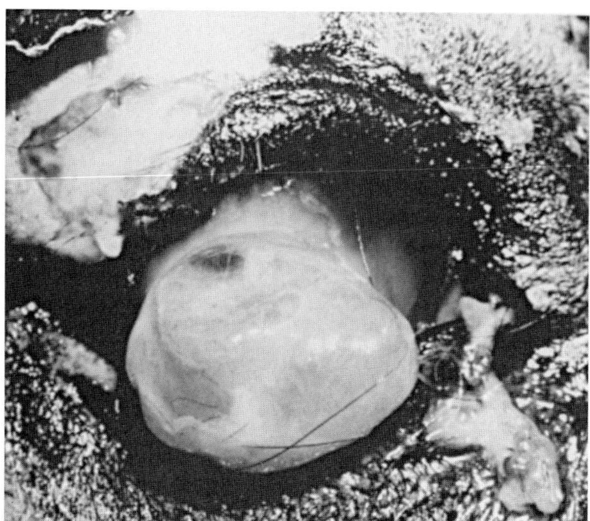

Figure 60-5. Corneal perforation in a horse secondary to bacterial ulceration. A large fibrin clot protrudes from the wound. The intraocular tissues, however, were minimally damaged.

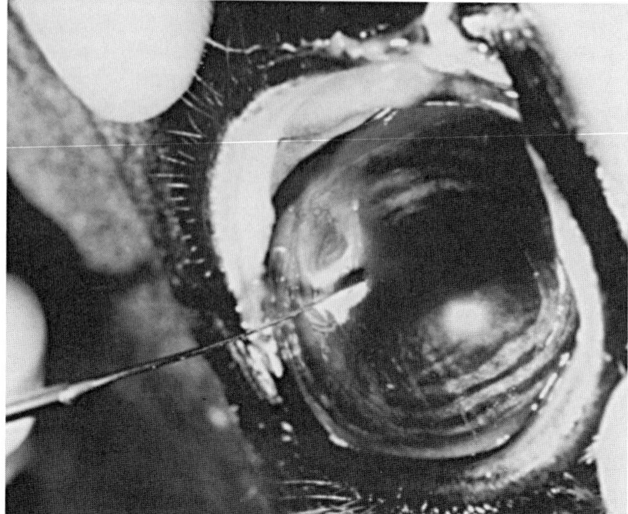

Figure 60-6. Technique for acquiring corneal samples for cytology and culture. The corneal surface is aggressively scraped with a Kimura platinum spatula.

tioned previously, the presence of hypopyon in the absence of corneal perforation may not suggest a poor prognosis. If its presence is secondary to bacterial keratitis, the hypopyon is sterile and will readily resolve with proper antimicrobial therapy. In fungal infections, because the organisms can migrate through Descemet's membrane, the presence of hypopyon has potentially graver significance, but the hypopyon is still generally aseptic.

Laboratory Procedures

If corneal infection is suspected, supportive laboratory tests are indicated. The preferred method for obtaining specimens in such instances is to collect tissue directly from the corneal surface with a Kimura platinum spatula (Fig. 60-6). If this instrument is unavailable, a dulled scalpel blade or the blunt end of a scalpel handle may be used. Ideally, corneal specimens are collected before the instillation of topical anesthetics that may inhibit microbial growth.[30] Unless there is a descemetocele or the eye is perforated, aggressive scraping can be performed with little chance of damaging the globe. It is imperative to collect samples both from the center of the lesion and its periphery, since fungi and bacteria, respectively, are most likely to be found at these sites. Particularly in cases of fungal keratitis, scraping from the deeper corneal tissues must be aggressive to obtain diagnostic samples. Material obtained from the first sampling should be inoculated directly onto blood and Sabouraud agar plates. If culture media are unavailable, a commercial Culturette (Becton Dickinson and Co, Cockeysville, Md) offers a more practical, although less desirable, alternative. Subsequent samples are smeared onto glass slides for cytologic evaluation (Figs. 60-7 and 60-8). Separate specimens should be stained with the Gram and the modified Wright-Giemsa (Leukostat; Fisher Diagnostics, Norcross, Ga) techniques. Identification of fungal hyphae is facilitated by using specific stains such as the Gomori methenamine silver, periodic acid–Schiff, and new methylene blues. When fungal infection is strongly suspected but corneal cytology and culture fail to identify organisms, corneal biopsy by lamellar keratectomy is recommended.

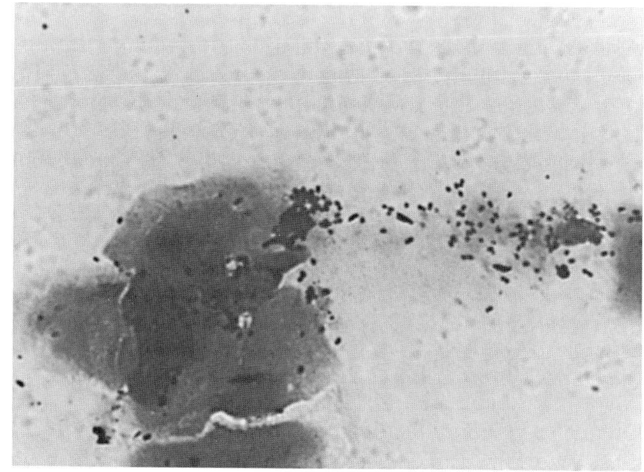

Figure 60-7. Cytologic appearance of corneal scraping from an eye with a bacterial ulcer. Numerous gram-positive organisms are visible. (Gram stain, ×1100.)

PRINCIPLES OF CORNEAL AND SCLERAL SURGERY

Patient Preparation

Horses with corneas that are perforated or have deep stromal ulcers require special care during preparation for surgery. Anesthetic induction must be performed carefully, preferably with the eye to be operated on protected from injury by padded headgear. Cleansing of the eye must likewise be gentle to avoid perforating deep corneal ulcers and to prevent the dislodging of fibrin plugs that may be sealing an already perforated cornea. Care must be taken to avoid putting pressure on the globe when swabbing the adnexa and conjunctival sac with surgical scrub solutions (see Chapter 55).

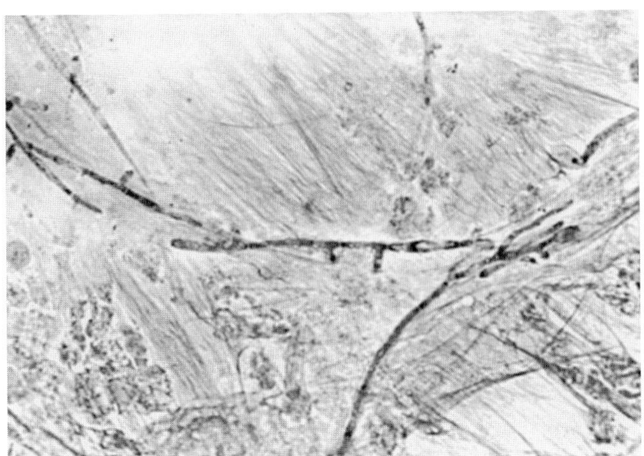

Figure 60-8. Cytologic appearance of corneal scrapings from an eye with a fungal ulcer. Branching hyphae are visible. (Modified Wright-Giemsa stain, ×700.)

Because the large extraocular muscle mass of horses exerts considerable tension on the globe, intraoperative corneal perforation invariably results in anterior displacement of vitreous humor and anterior chamber collapse. Excessive intraocular tension can be prevented either by administering an orbital injection of anesthetic or by augmenting the therapeutic regimen with a neuromuscular blocking agent[31] (see Chapter 55). The placement of scleral stay sutures is a common and accepted method of stabilizing the globe during surgery. Stay sutures must be used with caution in cases involving corneal perforation, however, since the tension created by the suture, particularly during forced ductions of the globe, can have potentially adverse intraocular effects. Therefore, either neuromuscular blockage or orbital anesthesia is superior to scleral stay sutures.

Surgeon Preparation

Accurate and atraumatic manipulation of corneal tissue requires the surgeon to be in a sitting position, with arms supported by the arm rests of a chair designed for microsurgery, by the patient's head, or by both. Magnification is essential and may be provided by inexpensive (approximately $25) head loupes with plastic lenses (Optivisor; Donegan Optical, Lenexa, Kan), or high-quality loupes with glass lenses (Jena Company, East Germany; approximate cost, $500). A threefold magnification is comfortable for most corneal procedures; increased magnification is helpful only if the optical quality of the instrument is equally high. Without question, the optimal source of magnification for corneal surgery is an operating microscope.

Selection of Suture Material

Proper suture selection is perhaps the single most important variable in successful corneal and scleral surgery.[32,33] The suture and, more important, the needle must be sufficiently small that damage created during placement of the suture does not outweigh the intended benefits. An appropriate suture size for equine corneal and scleral work is 7-0 to 8-0. When excessive tension is encountered, 6-0 suture may be more appropriate. There is rarely an indication for placing sutures larger than 6-0 in the fibrous tunic of the eye; the exception is the scleral stay suture, in which case 5-0 is often used.

It is imperative that the suture be armed with a needle designed for corneal surgery. The micropoint spatula needle is ideal because, after having been passed to the appropriate tissue depth, the spatula shape allows it to slip between the cornea's collagen lamellae and prevent further penetration. The shape of the needle is strictly a matter of preference; one type is the Ethicon TG140-8 type (Ethicon Inc, Somerville, NJ). The choice of suture is also a matter of surgeon preference, as nylon, silk, and polyglactin 910 all have inherent advantages and limitations (see Chapter 55). Polyglactin 910 has the practical advantage of not requiring removal.

Instrumentation

The reader is referred to Chapter 55 for a detailed discussion of ophthalmic instrumentation. For corneal surgery, there are several specific and important considerations. Because the cornea may be severely damaged by handling with improper instruments, there is no effective substitute for properly designed corneal forceps. Many different styles are available, but they all have a 1-to-2 interdigitating tooth design of sufficiently small size to minimize corneal damage. Tooth sizes used for corneal work range from 0.12 to 1.5 mm, with the 0.12- and 0.3-mm teeth being most appropriate for the equine cornea. The Colibri and Castroviejo-Colibri forceps are popular choices that are available with 0.12-mm teeth.

The second most important choice of instrument for corneal surgery is that of the needle holder. Because it is impossible to place micropoint needles accurately with a conventional needle holder, a microsurgical needle holder is essential. As its rounded handle facilitates digital manipulation, the Troutman-Barraquer needle holder with nonlocking handle is a very good choice. Other less critical but necessary instruments are multipurpose forceps and scissors. For manipulation of the sclera, a forceps with larger teeth is sometimes desired, and for this purpose the Bishop-Harmon forceps is ideal. Corneal section scissors are occasionally necessary for corneal débridement and graft preparation. Other cutting needs in corneal surgery are adequately met with tenotomy scissors (Stevens or Westcott). At least one suture-tying forceps is necessary, and the Harm tying forceps is adequate. Miscellaneous instruments used in the subsequently described procedures include an iris spatula, a corneal intralamellar dissector, an irrigation bulb, and an eyelid speculum.

Suturing Techniques and Suture Patterns

Because wound dehiscence and leakage of aqueous humor have potentially devastating consequences, correct technique is imperative when suturing corneal and scleral tissues. Corneal sutures are placed by grasping the tissue adjacent to the area intended to receive the suture with corneal forceps (Fig. 60-9). The upper teeth of the forceps are imbedded through the epithelium, and the ventral teeth enter the cross-section of corneal stroma at the junction of the middle and deep one third of the cornea. The needle is inserted into the distal cornea at a distance of 1 to 2 mm from the cut

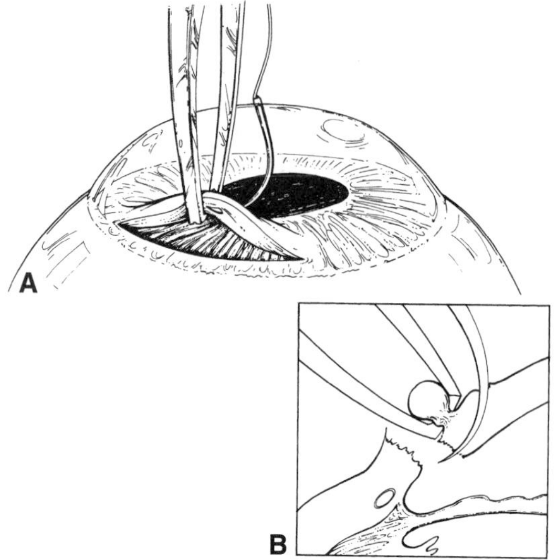

Figure 60-9. Correct technique for placing corneal sutures. **A,** The cornea is grasped at its margin with the forceps' opposing teeth entering the epithelial surface and the exposed stroma. **B,** The needle extends to, but not past, Descemet's membrane.

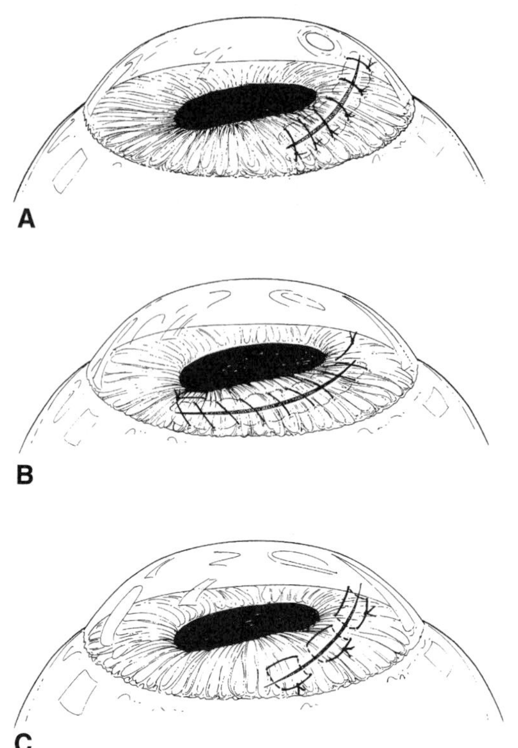

Figure 60-10. Basic suture patterns used to close corneal defects: **A,** Interrupted pattern. **B,** Continuous pattern. **C,** Horizontal mattress sutures.

edge, depending on the type and intention of the suture pattern being used, in a perpendicular direction. This is important because vector forces limit accurate and controlled needle movement to planes that are perpendicular or parallel with the collagen lamellae.[34] After reaching the desired stromal depth, which ideally is close to but not through Descemet's membrane, the needle is redirected parallel with the collagen lamellae to exit the deep corneal stroma. Placement of the proximal suture is generally easier because less resistance is offered by the exposed stromal cross-section than by the corneal surface. The tissue on the near side of the wound may be immobilized with the same forceps technique used to make the first bite or by resting the closed forceps against the cornea adjacent to the intended site of needle exit.

Tying forceps, rather than needle holders, are used to tie corneal sutures to prevent suture damage and loss of tensile strength. The Castroviejo corneal forceps are designed with tying platforms for this purpose. In general, a double or triple suture loop is used in the first throw, with two single-loop throws completing the knot. In continuous suture patterns, a fourth throw is indicated to increase knot security. Suture tags are cut to a length of approximately 0.5 mm. For polyglactin 910 (Vicryl, Ethicon, Johnson & Johnson, Somerville, NJ), suture texture limits the tension that can be placed on the knot. For nylon suture, however, it is possible to over-tighten knots, thus decreasing suture strength. The proper knot tension is achieved by tightening the second throw to the point of the maximal tension that does not cause the linear arrangement of the first double throw to deviate.

The choice of suture pattern used to close corneal and scleral wounds is dictated primarily by the size of the defect and the health of the surrounding tissue (Fig. 60-10). In simplest terms, acute lacerations with relatively healthy surrounding cornea are usually best closed with a continuous pattern, whereas for large corneal defects in which tension is anticipated or when the ability of the cornea to hold sutures is in question, simple-interrupted patterns, mattress patterns, or both, are necessary. The prime advantage of a continuous suture pattern is that equal tension is applied to all areas of the suture line. Interrupted sutures, in contrast, concentrate the tension in a plane directly between the needle tracks, thus creating uneven tension along the suture line. A continuous pattern, therefore, more effectively seals a corneal incision or wound. The interrupted pattern offers the clear advantage of not relying on only a single knot to provide security. Mattress sutures are usually reserved for occasions when excessive tension on the wound is anticipated. The most common example is the deep stromal ulcer, the closure of which is accomplished with alternating horizontal mattress and simple-interrupted sutures. The choice of suture pattern is also influenced by the suture material being used. Nylon, by virtue of its elastic properties, is less prone to breaking in the event of trauma and is, therefore, better suited for continuous use than polyglactin 910 or silk.

Keratectomy

Lamellar keratectomy is commonly carried out in horses for the removal of dermoids and limbal squamous cell neoplasms, to obtain diagnostic corneal biopsies, and in the formation of autogenous corneal grafts. Regardless of the indication, keratectomy is initiated with a corneal incision. The depth and shape of the incision are dictated by the shape of the tissue to be excised. For removal of surface lesions and biopsies, a depth of one third of the corneal thickness is adequate. When fashioning lamellar grafts, incision depth ranges from one third to two thirds of the corneal thickness. Although most experienced surgeons judge incisional depth by tactile impression, corneal trephines and blades are available with adjustable depth gauges. The shape of a corneal incision to remove limbal lesions is generally triangular, with the apex in the central cornea. Lamellar keratectomy for graft retrieval is performed in either a rectangular or circular configuration.

Despite the thinness of the cornea, the lamellar arrangement of the collagen lamellae makes accurate separation a relatively simple task. After the proper depth has been achieved, collagen lamellae are separated by moving a flat instrument, held parallel with the lamellar plane, in a back-and-forth motion. If the instrument is kept parallel with the cornea, the interlamellar position is maintained and depth is not changed. Corneal dissectors (Martinez, Troutman) designed specifically for this purpose have a flat head, a semi-sharp tip, and a curvature that matches that of the cornea. A commercial blade that is sharpened on both sides and at the tip (Beaver 6900 Mini-Blade; R. Beaver, Inc, Waltham, Mass) can be used, but this is not ideal.

Lamellar and Penetrating Keratoplasty

Although the term *keratoplasty* refers to any procedure designed to reshape the cornea, only lamellar and perforating keratoplasties are routinely performed on horses, most often to treat large corneal defects. The autogenous lamellar keratoplasty is performed by excising a section of cornea that is one half to two thirds of its thickness, either from a normal portion of the recipient eye or from the patient's opposite eye.[35-37] The graft is trimmed and sutured into the recipient bed. Penetrating keratoplasty, in contrast, uses a full-thickness corneal button as the donor tissue.[38,39] Because penetrating keratoplasty requires considerable surgical skill and the ready availability of healthy donor tissue, the procedure is not used routinely to treat equine corneal diseases. However, penetrating and split-thickness keratoplasty have been shown to be useful for treating chronic stromal abscesses in horses.[40] The application of each procedure is described in the following section.

SURGICALLY MANAGED DISORDERS

Dermoids

Congenital dermoids are effectively removed by one-third-depth lamellar keratectomy. The corneal incisions are usually made in clear cornea, extending from the limbus adjacent to the lesion to an apex point in clear cornea. Lamellar dissection is started at the apex of the keratectomy site, ending at the limbus. For dermoids that involve the sclera, the keratectomy is continued across the limbus into superficial sclera and Tenon's capsule. Once beyond the margins of the dermoid, corneal section scissors are used to transect the base of the tissue to be removed.

Lacerations

Lacerations of the equine cornea and sclera are among the most common corneal problems requiring surgical management. For penetrating lacerations with little adjacent corneal damage, correction is easily effected by closure in a simple-continuous pattern. Because the cornea is not perforated, 8-0 suture material is adequate. Perforating lacerations with little secondary corneal or uveal damage may be closed in an identical fashion, particularly if the wound is small.

Perforating corneal lacerations with uveal prolapse are managed by first gently removing adhered fibrin from the incarcerated uveal tissue with thumb forceps. Care must be taken to avoid traumatizing the iris and inducing hemorrhage. The integrity of the corneal seal, however, should not be broken until the wound margins are fully visualized, the problem is assessed, and a decision is made as to the appropriate surgical procedure. The decision of whether to amputate prolapsed uveal tissue is then made. The increased potential for uveal hemorrhage, hyphema, and postoperative uveitis mandates that iridectomy be performed only if the prolapsed tissue is excessive or necrotic. Uveal tissue that has been prolapsed for as long as 3 to 4 days, if protected by a fibrin cover, can be safely returned to the anterior chamber. If uveal amputation is necessary, cautery is the preferred method because hemorrhage is minimized. If scissors must be used, and hemorrhage does occur, gentle intraocular irrigation with a dilute (1:10,000) epinephrine borate solution is beneficial.

Before the placement of corneal sutures, it is critical that uveal adhesions be broken sufficiently to allow visualization of the corneal stroma and to prevent incarceration of uvea in the sutured wound. An iris spatula is useful for this procedure: it is gently passed between the iris and the corneal margins. It is imperative that uveal manipulation be minimized to prevent significant postoperative uveitis. If the prolapse is small, it is gently tucked into the anterior chamber prior to wound closure. Ideally, an effort should be made to minimize anterior synechiae. All too often, however, iris swelling precludes wound closure without contact between iris and endothelium. It is important to appreciate that focal anterior synechiae are far less significant complications than the uveitis induced by aggressive uveal manipulation. The corneal wound is closed with 7-0 polyglactin 910 in a simple-interrupted or simple-continuous suture pattern, depending on the size of the wound (Fig. 60-11). If uveal tissue attempts to escape from the wound during closure, it is necessary to pre-place interrupted sutures while an assistant depresses the uveal tissue with an iris spatula.

When the corneal wound is securely closed, the anterior chamber depth is assessed. This is important because iridocorneal adhesions, if extensive, may result in postoperative angle closure, leading potentially to glaucoma development.

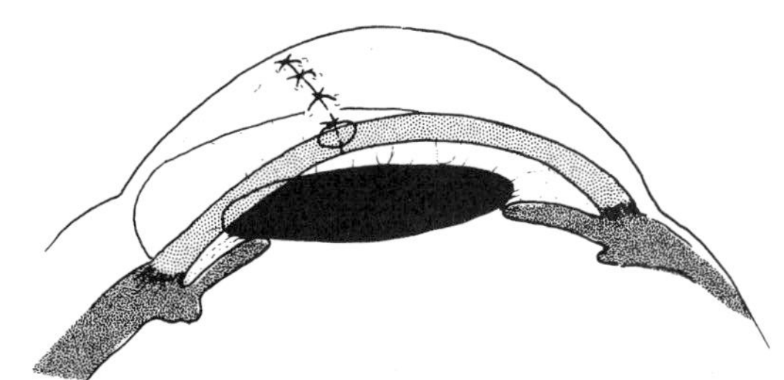

Figure 60-11. Appearance of a corneal laceration immediately after surgical correction.

In many cases, particularly if the wound is small and the injury acute, the anterior chamber will have filled with aqueous humor by the time surgery is complete. If it has not, it should be filled by injection of irrigation solution (saline, balanced salt solution, or lactated Ringer's solution) or with the more viscous hyaluronic acid (Hylartin V, Pfizer Animal Health, New York, NY). If the anterior chamber is extremely shallow, a small air bubble is injected to keep the iris from contacting the cornea; air is superior to fluid under these circumstances because it will not be forced through the iridocorneal angle by increased intraocular pressure. The chamber is filled, by injecting either through the wound with a 30-gauge injection cannula or through the limbus with a 27-gauge needle. Hyaluronic acid can be injected with a 20-gauge needle at the limbus. The latter technique will maintain the anterior chamber depth for a longer time.

Large corneal lacerations are handled in an identical fashion, except that uveal presentation is more difficult to manage, and corneal closure may require the use of mattress sutures to improve wound security. If the cornea is weakened by the effects of inflammation, the sutured defect should be covered with a conjunctival graft or filled with a corneal graft. Wounds involving the sclera are handled similarly. It is important to distinguish, however, between corneal and scleral lacerations and globe ruptures. The fibrous tunic of horses is prone to rupture on impact with blunt objects. The injury may appear grossly similar to a sharp laceration, except that these "blow-out" injuries tend to be larger, often extending from limbus to limbus, and are invariably associated with considerable hyphema.[41] In such cases, enucleation or evisceration and intraocular prosthesis implantation are more appropriate choices of therapy.

Corneal Foreign Bodies

Small cylindric objects of plant origin are the most common corneal foreign bodies seen in horses. They may penetrate the stroma to varying degrees or actually perforate the eye. When foreign bodies are suspected, slit-lamp biomicroscopic examination is essential to determine the depth and location of the object.

Superficial foreign bodies are often easily extracted with only topical anesthetic. For this purpose, a jeweler's forceps is ideal. For removal of deeper penetrating foreign bodies, general anesthesia is necessary. To reach the foreign body, it is often necessary to enlarge the corneal wound. This is accomplished by making a linear incision of 2 to 4 mm that extends on either side of the object. After removal of the object, the incision is closed with 8-0 polyglactin 910 sutures in a continuous pattern. Foreign bodies that penetrate the anterior chamber are removed in the same way, except that the postoperative considerations differ, taking into account management of postoperative uveitis as discussed later in this chapter.

Ulcerative Keratitis

The need for surgical therapy of corneal ulcers varies, depending on the depth of the lesion and the rate of corneal melting. For most ulcers that are up to, but no deeper than, three fourths of the corneal thickness, conjunctival flaps are generally preferred (see Chapter 57).

Corneal Suturing

Corneal sutures may be used to close deep ulcers and descemetoceles that are less than 2 mm in diameter. The choice of suture pattern depends on the degree of anticipated tension and suture-holding ability of the cornea; however, in general only interrupted sutures are used for this purpose. The closure is initiated by pre-placing two horizontal mattress sutures across the corneal defect. Because considerable suture tension is anticipated, 6-0 suture material may be necessary. The normal intraocular pressure exerts considerable tension on the cornea, which makes it difficult to appose the ulcer margins without creating excessive suture tension. In addition to suture breakage, the pressure may cause the suture to cut through the tissue. This problem is handled in one of two ways. First, the mattress sutures may be tied in a gradually alternating fashion over a several-minute period. This allows aqueous humor to be forced through the iridocorneal angle and the anterior chamber to decrease in size. Alternatively, a 25-gauge needle is inserted into the anterior chamber, and 0.25 mL of aqueous humor is withdrawn to relieve the tension. The mattress sutures are subsequently alternated with simple-interrupted sutures. The anterior chamber is re-inflated, if necessary, as described for corneal lacerations.

Corneal Grafting

Perhaps the most difficult corneal injury to manage is the deep corneal ulcer that exceeds 5 mm in diameter. Because the defect is too large for direct suturing, a grafting technique is necessary. If corneal transparency is not a surgical objective, conjunctival grafts may be used[42,43]; however, corneal grafts are preferable because they provide greater structural support.

SLIDING LAMELLAR CORNEAL GRAFTS

A sliding lamellar graft (Figs. 60-12 and 60-13) is started by preparing the recipient bed. Because most ulcers are circular, this usually involves little more than débriding loose and necrotic corneal tissue from the ulcer margins with a no. 64 Beaver blade. If the ulcer has irregular margins, corneal scissors should be used to trim the edges to make them as smooth as possible. The decision of whether to harvest the graft from tissue directly adjacent to the defect, leaving bulbar conjunctiva attached, or from a distant corneal site, is left to the surgeon. The primary advantage of harvesting the graft from tissue adjacent to the ulcer is that the graft depth can be accurately judged against the depth of the ulcer. In this case, the graft is prepared by extending parallel corneal incisions from the ulcer's widest margin to the nearest limbus. The graft thickness should be one half to two thirds the thickness of the cornea. Using scissors, the incisions are extended into the conjunctiva along a line slightly diverging from the corneal incisions. The graft is then lifted free of the underlying cornea by lamellar dissection, as described for keratectomy. When the limbus is reached, the dissection is beveled in a superficial direction to connect with the subconjunctival space, thus creating a corneal–conjunctival transposition flap. Dissection may be directed deeper into the sclera to create a corneal and scleral transposition flap[35]; however, postoperative corneal opacification tends to be greater. After the conjunctiva is undermined by blunt dis-

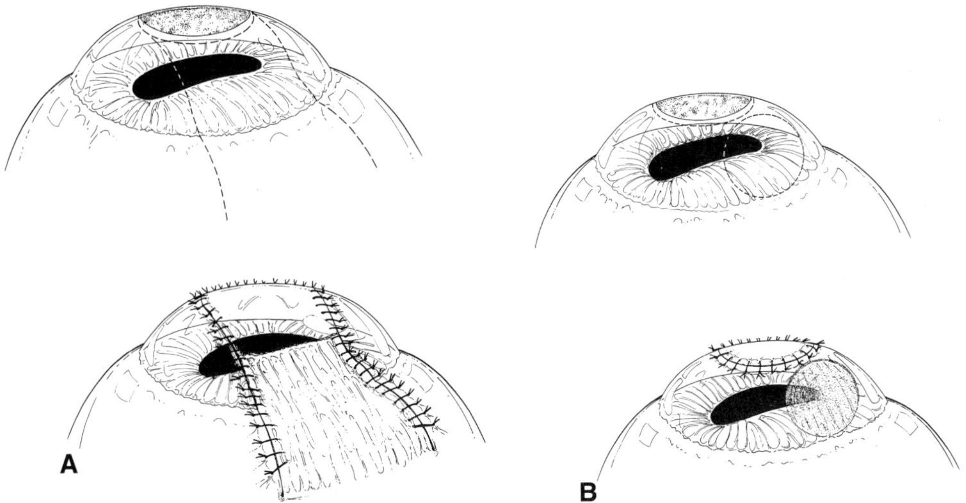

Figure 60-12. Lamellar keratoplasty. **A,** In the corneal-conjunctival transposition technique, the cornea is left attached to the conjunctiva. **B,** Alternatively, the donor corneal tissue may be harvested from a site distant to the defect to be closed.

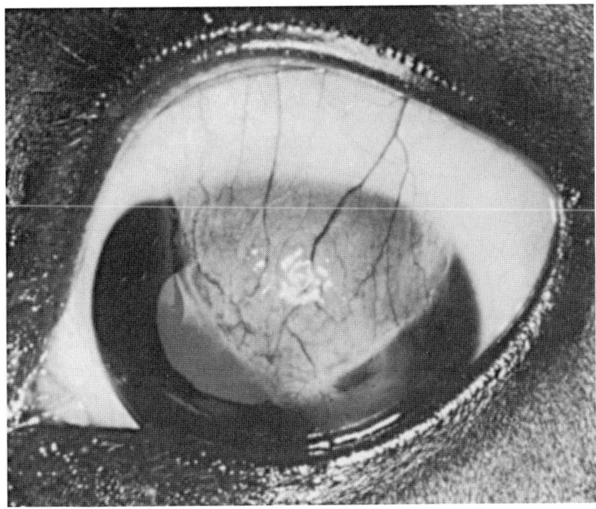

Figure 60-13. Appearance of a lamellar corneal graft after surgical correction. (Courtesy Dr. Nicholas J. Millichamp.)

section, the graft's leading margins are sculpted to conform to the contour of the recipient bed. The graft is subsequently sutured into place with 7-0 or 8-0 polyglactin 910 sutures in a simple-interrupted pattern.

The sliding lamellar graft may also be used to reconstruct perforated ulcers. A uveal prolapse is managed as a laceration (described earlier). Creating an effective corneal seal, however, is difficult in these cases, because leaking aqueous humor from the perforation site readily undermines the graft and gains access into the subconjunctival space. This is prevented by suturing the conjunctiva, at the graft margin, to the underlying cornea. Sutures should not be so numerous, however, to obstruct the blood supply to the graft.

FREE LAMELLAR CORNEAL GRAFTS

When performing a free lamellar graft, tissue should be harvested from the inferior medial cornea so that the donor bed is protected postoperatively by the nictitating membrane. The donor button may either be excised with a corneal trephine or by scalpel incision. If a trephine is used, the donor button should have a diameter that is 1 mm larger than the area to be grafted. When using a blade to collect the graft, a rectangular button is excised and then trimmed to fit the defect.

CORNEAL TRANSPLANTATION

Corneal transplantation is a viable and successful surgical technique in the horse. Full-thickness penetrating keratoplasty (PK) may be performed for melting ulcers, iris prolapse or descemetoceles, and full-thickness stromal abscesses.[44] Deep lamellar endothelial keratoplasty (DLEK) and posterior lamellar keratoplasty (PLK) are split-thickness penetrating keratoplasties used for deep stromal abscesses with clear overlying anterior stroma. Frozen donor grafts can be used successfully for transplants in the horse eye. Corneal transplants in horses are associated with high success rates, good visual outcomes (greater than 80%), and shorter treatment times than medical treatment alone for these eye problems, but the corneal transplants in horses do vascularize, have some degree of opacity, and thus exhibit some degree of graft rejection.

PENETRATING KERATOPLASTY

Penetrating keratoplasty involves full-thickness removal and replacement of a portion of the cornea. Corneal sutures are necessarily utilized to heal a vertical stromal incision with an associated disruption of the corneal surface and topography. Topical serum and cyclosporine A are added postoperatively. The surgical approach for PK in horses is as follows.

Donor corneal material is harvested preferentially from fresh or frozen equine cadaver eyes (i.e., within 24 hours of death). The size of the lesion is determined with calipers. A full-thickness button of cornea that is 1 mm larger than the recipient bed is trephined from the endothelial to the epithelial side of the donor cornea. The ideal graft size in horses is 6 to 8 mm in diameter, but larger grafts are possible. The donor button is grasped with fine-toothed forceps (while paying particular attention to the orientation of the epithelium and endothelium), placed on a gauze sponge, and kept moistened with lactated Ringer's solution. The epithelium is not removed from the corneal donor button.

The recipient globe is stabilized with scleral fixation sutures of 5-0 nylon (Ethicon, Johnson & Johnson). A corneal trephine of appropriate size (i.e., 6 to 8 mm or greater) is centered over the diseased area and then rotated with minimal downward pressure to obtain a clear-cut, round incision with vertical sides. The incision with the trephine approaches to just near Descemet's membrane.

The remaining intact deep stromal tissue is vertically incised with a no. 65 Beaver blade to enter the anterior chamber, being careful to avoid the iris, corpora nigra, and lens. The button of diseased host tissue is then removed with corneal section scissors. The keratectomy button is processed for culture and sensitivity, cytology, and histopathology.

Bulging of the iris and the corpora nigra into the incision site may occur. Adhesions or synechia between the abscess and iris may be present. The anterior chamber is re-formed by injecting hyaluronic acid solution into the anterior chamber. The viscoelastic solution also moves the iris posteriorly and breaks down any adhesions between the abscess and the iris. Direct contact with the lens capsule is also avoided by re-forming the anterior chamber with the viscoelastic solution.

The donor cornea is removed from the moistened gauze swab and placed in the recipient bed, and four cardinal sutures of 8-0 polyglactin 910 or 9-0 nylon are placed at the 12-, 6-, 9-, and 3-o'clock positions. Simple-interrupted sutures are placed to fill in the remaining sectors in each quadrant, or alternatively, a simple-continuous suture pattern can be placed to hold the graft. Once the donor cornea is sutured into place (Fig. 60-14), viscoelastic solution may again be injected via a limbal incision to re-form the anterior chamber.

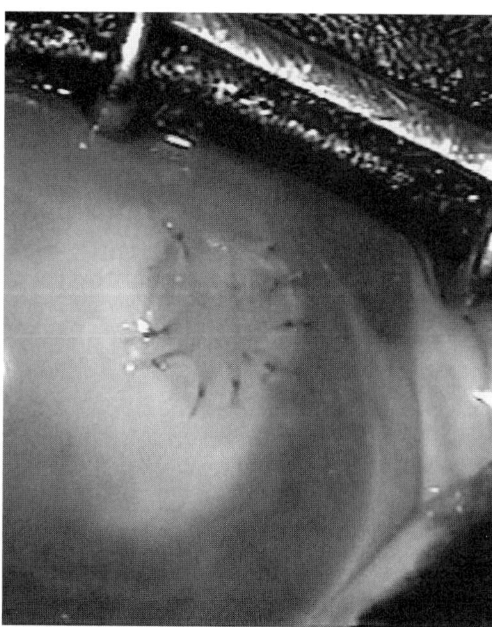

Figure 60-14. A penetrating keratectomy (PK) graft sutured into place.

SPLIT-THICKNESS PENETRATING KERATOPLASTY

In some deep stromal abscesses, the superficial cornea is vascularized but otherwise normal. For horses with deep stromal abscesses and anterior chamber fungal invasions that persist, or even progress, with severe pain and vision-threatening uveitis in the face of aggressive medical therapy, surgical removal of the posterior stroma and endothelium containing the abscess by corneal transplantation is warranted.

The inherent philosophy of split-thickness or lamellar surgery is to replace only the diseased portion of the cornea, leaving the normal tissue intact—in other words, to do the least amount of resection for the greatest amount of benefit.[44,45] Both the PLK and DLEK surgical methods are forms of split-thickness PK, because they avoid removal of superficial normal tissue but do surgically enter the anterior chamber.[44,45] These surgical methods are important for resolving deep stromal abscesses with anterior chamber invasion in horses.

POSTERIOR LAMELLAR KERATOPLASTY

Posterior lamellar keratoplasty is recommended for deep stromal abscesses in the central cornea that are 8 mm or less and that have a clear overlying anterior stroma. Topical serum and cyclosporine A are added postoperatively. The surgical approach for PLK in horses is as follows.

A rectangular, anterior lamellar corneal flap, hinged on one side, is constructed by hand dissection to two thirds of the stromal thickness over the stromal abscess. A Martinez corneal dissector is used to undermine and elevate the superficial corneal layers to expose the abscess. The flap is gently raised, and a trephine, a no. 65 Beaver blade, and corneal scissors are used to remove the posterior stromal abscess, Descemet's membrane, and endothelium. The anterior chamber is re-formed with viscoelastic solution. A circular graft (of posterior stroma, Descemet's membrane, and endothelium) 1 mm larger than the defect is cut from donor tissue using a trephine. The graft is placed in the corneal defect and sutured every 2 mm using 8-0 absorbable suture material in a simple-interrupted pattern (Fig. 60-15). The three-sided superficial flap is then sutured in place using 8-0 absorbable suture material. A partial temporary

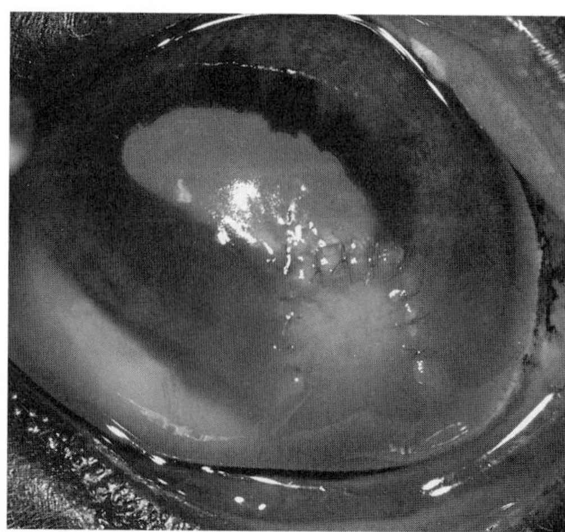

Figure 60-15. Three-sided posterior lamellar keratoplasty (PLK) immediately after surgery.

tarsorrhaphy is always placed to protect the graft during recovery.

The PLK is associated with a shorter surgery and treatment time than the PK.[46] Complications of PLK include superficial suture abscesses, suture incision leaks, flap ulcers, and flap edema. The donor graft remains transparent for up to 7 days and then opacifies. Partial graft rejection and scar formation have been unavoidable for both the PK and PLK procedures. PLK and PK result in similar scars, which are typically vascularized and eventually opaque. The visual outcome is greater than 90% for the eyes that have the PLK procedure.[44]

DEEP LAMELLAR ENDOTHELIAL KERATOPLASTY

The deep lamellar endothelial keratoplasty is recommended for deep stromal abscesses in the peripheral cornea that are 6 mm or less and have a clear overlying anterior stroma. It avoids the superficial incisions and suturing of the central cornea. The DLEK transfers healthy endothelium while preserving the corneal surface integrity. A fully intact epithelium with no corneal sutures is present postoperatively. The surgical approach for DLEK in horses is as follows.

A two-thirds depth, limbal incision up to 23 mm in length is made with a no. 64 Beaver blade. A stromal pocket is formed over the deep stromal abscesses with a Martinez corneal dissector. Bleeding from the vascularized cornea is controlled with electrocautery. The superficial corneal flap is gently retracted, and the abscess is removed with a trephine, a no. 65 Beaver blade, and corneal scissors. The anterior chamber is re-formed with viscoelastic solution. The anterior two thirds of the donor cornea is removed by hand dissection, and a trephine 1 mm larger in diameter than the recipient site used to obtain the circular donor graft from the remaining split-thickness cornea. The superficial corneal flap is partially sutured with 8-0 polyglactin 910. The donor graft is inserted into place with Utrata forceps, and the limbal incision is closed (Fig. 60-16). The graft adheres to the recipient stroma by action of the endothelial pump, but it may need to be positioned in place by a needle inserted between the flap sutures, or at the limbus. The graft is supported by the viscoelastic solution in the anterior chamber, which can be safely left in situ. A partial temporary tarsorrhaphy is always placed to protect the surgical site during recovery. Medical therapy postoperatively includes topical atropine, cyclosporine A, autogenous serum, topical antifungals and antibiotics, systemic antibiotics, and nonsteroidal anti-inflammatory drugs.

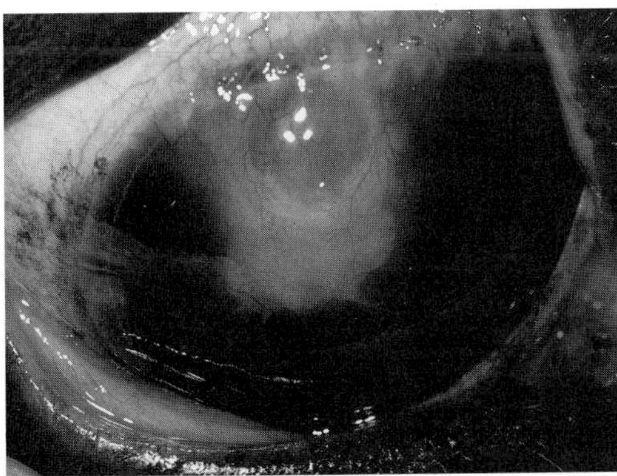

Figure 60-16. Deep lamellar endothelial keratoplasty (DLEK) with clear oval graft and opaque superficial stroma.

Neoplasia (Squamous Cell Carcinoma)

The most common tumor requiring corneal surgery is squamous cell carcinoma[47-50] (Fig. 60-17). Because these tumors generally occur at the limbus, both cornea and sclera are generally involved. Numerous surgical options are available.

Lamellar Keratectomy

Lamellar keratectomy is predictably successful because intraocular tumor extension is inhibited by the dense collagen arrangement of the corneal stroma. One-third-depth keratectomy is therefore usually adequate.[51]

Cryotherapy

Cryosurgery is also effective for destroying limbal tumors.[52-54] Liquid nitrogen, the preferred cryogen, may be applied either as a fine spray or via a copper contact probe. The objective is to reduce the tissue temperature to −20° C (−4° F). Because thermocouples are unsuitable for corneal implantation, the extent of freezing must be judged subjectively. The ice-ball should be allowed to extend 1 to 2 mm beyond the visible margins of the tumor. A double freeze–thaw cycle is recommended. The primary disadvantage of cryosurgery is the potential for nonselective destruction of normal tissue; corneal stromal and endothelial damage are potential complications.

Laser Ablation

The effective use of carbon dioxide laser ablation in treating limbal squamous cell carcinomas has been described.[55] The carbon dioxide laser emits a beam in the infrared spectrum (10,600 nm) that exerts a thermal tissue effect whose physical characteristics are determined by the power density of the beam. If the beam is focused, the tissue is incised,

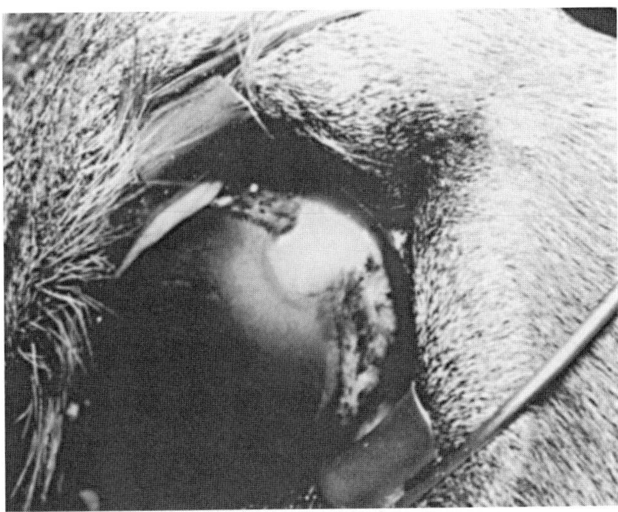

Figure 60-17. Typical appearance of a limbal squamous cell carcinoma in a horse. The tumor is slightly raised and extends into the cornea from the limbus.

whereas a defocused beam of lower energy density diffusely vaporizes the exposed tissue. The latter application is ideally suited for excision of superficial neoplasms. Treatment may be performed with local anesthesia; however, general anesthesia is recommended. The laser is operated in the continuous mode with power settings of 3 to 8 W. Either continuous energy release or timed bursts may be applied, depending on the surgeon's preference. The tumor tissue is ablated until charred superficial stroma remains, and healing occurs in 30 days (Fig. 60-18). For very large tumors, the mass may be debulked by conventional excision prior to laser applications. Advantages of laser vaporization of neoplasms include (1) simultaneous coagulation of small vessels, (2) coagulation of nerve endings, resulting in minimal postoperative discomfort, (3) predictable excision depth without damage to adjacent normal tissue, and (4) the stimulation of a beneficial immune response.

Other Techniques

Small (less than 5 cm) limbal squamous cell carcinomas also may be treated successfully with radiofrequency hyperthermia.[56,57] In this procedure, contact probes are placed on either side of the tumor, and tissue is destroyed by raising its temperature to 50° C (122° F). Limbal squamous cell carcinomas are amenable to brachytherapy with strontium-90 probes; a radiation dose of 25,000 rad has been recommended.[58-61] However, ^{90}Sr therapy is effective only for tumors less than 2 mm in thickness. Immunotherapy with bacillus cell wall extract, used successfully to treat squamous cell neoplasms at other sites, is not applicable for limbal tumors.

AFTERCARE

Medical Therapy

For surgical procedures involving the cornea and sclera specifically, topical antibiotics are always indicated. The choice of drug, vehicle, and administration route, however, varies with the surgical procedure and needs of the patient.

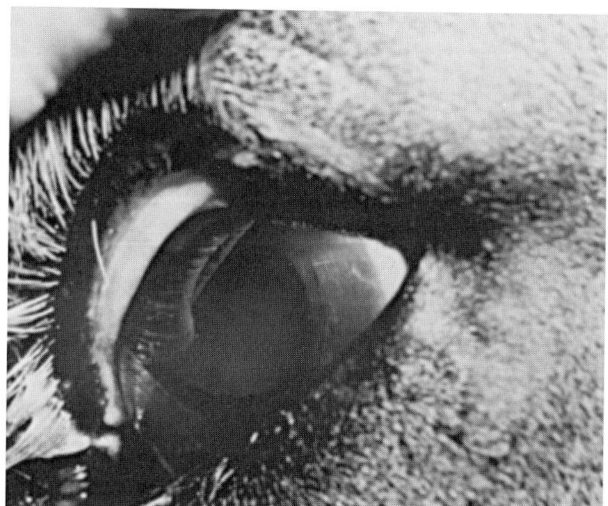

Figure 60-18. Appearance of the eye in Figure 60-17, 1 month after carbon dioxide laser therapy. No tumor is visible, and the cornea is clear.

For elective procedures performed on intact globes (e.g., keratectomy, cryosurgery, and CO_2 laser ablation), broad-spectrum antibiotics are applied four times a day. Because of its wide antimicrobial spectrum and predictable efficacy against gram-positive organisms, triple antibiotic (neomycin, bacitracin, and polymyxin) is preferred.[62] Solutions are difficult to administer to horses without the benefit of some type of lavage catheter,[63-66] so ointment is preferred for topical therapy of low frequency. Acute lacerations are also adequately treated with topical therapy with triple antibiotic ointment four times a day. For subacute lacerations and ulcers requiring surgery, however, topical therapy may be indicated from every 4 hours to every 1 hour, depending on the severity of corneal infection. In these cases, an antibiotic solution is applied through a subpalpebral lavage catheter (see Chapter 55). The choice of antibiotic is based on cytologic and culture results. For gram-positive organisms, triple antibiotic is indicated, and for gram-negative organisms, an aminoglycoside (gentamicin [Gentocin ophthalmic solution or ointment] or tobramycin [Tobrex]) is preferred.[67,68] The current drug of choice for *Pseudomonas* infections that are resistant to aminoglycosides is ciprofloxacin (Ciloxan; ciprofloxacin 0.3%, Alcon Labs, Ft. Worth, Tex).

Subconjunctival antibiotics are usually administered only if significant corneal sepsis is present, such as melting corneal ulcer, or if intraocular infection is suspected. Systemic antibiotics are not indicated unless corneal perforation has occurred. The mucolytic agent acetylcysteine, advocated as an addition to antibiotic solutions to inhibit stromal melting, is insufficiently beneficial to warrant its use. Antiproteases such as topical serum, 0.17% ethylenediaminetetra-acetic acid (EDTA), and 0.1% doxycycline are critical to the healing of horses after corneal injury and surgery. They inhibit tear film protease digestion of the absorbable sutures used in equine corneal surgery.[45]

Concurrent parasympatholytic therapy is generally indicated to relieve the pain associated with ciliary spasm and to prevent synechia formation, particularly in cases of corneal perforation. The use of 1% to 2% atropine, as either an ointment or a solution, is the preferred agent, and 0.1 mL (approximately 1 drop) is applied at the lowest frequency necessary to maintain mydriasis. Although intensive therapy (every 2 to 4 hours) is often necessary in the acute postoperative period, rarely is treatment required more frequently than QID thereafter. Colic, traditionally described as a complication of ophthalmic atropine therapy in the horse, is an insignificant problem when parasympatholytic therapy is prescribed responsibly.[69]

For cases accompanied by severe pain, particularly when associated with perforation and uveal injury, systemic anti-inflammatory therapy is beneficial (flunixin meglumine at 1 mg/kg orally QID [Banamine]).[70,71]

Adjunctive Therapy

Contact Lenses

Hydrophilic corneal contact lenses (Equus, The Cutting Edge, Santa Clara, Calif) in diameter sizes of 26 to 34 mm (base curve, 15 to 18 mm) are available for horses at an approximate cost of $60. Contact lenses can be used to protect ulcerated or lacerated corneas and may be used postoperatively to protect sutured corneas.[72] Contact lenses are contraindicated, however, for use in infected ulcers and are poorly effective for managing ulcers with impending perforation. A major limitation of contact lenses in animals is the tendency for them to become dislodged by movement of the nictitating membrane.

COMPLICATIONS

The most important complications of corneal and scleral surgery are related to concurrent intraocular tissue damage or to dehiscence of sutured wounds. As mentioned previously, phthisis bulbi is a common sequela to traumatic globe injuries and particularly to traumatic globe rupture. If the globe is going to undergo significant phthisis, it will generally be apparent within 30 days of the injury. Enucleation should not be elected hastily, as horses possess a unique ability to undergo partial phthisis and still retain vision. Wound dehiscence most commonly occurs after closure of corneal and scleral perforations, particularly if the wound was infected at the time of the surgery. If, in the surgeon's opinion, vision is potentially salvageable, the wound should be closed again and supported with a conjunctival flap, or a corneal graft should be applied. If wound dehiscence is chronic or associated with large uveal perforation, enucleation is often the most practical alternative. Intraocular infection appears to be the least common complication of corneal or scleral surgery. This is because of the efficacy of prophylactically applied antibiotics, as well as the tendency of fibrin and uveal tissue to seal corneal and scleral defects effectively at the time of perforation. When intraocular infection does occur, however, it almost always necessitates enucleation, because of the difficulty in achieving effective intraocular antibiotic concentrations.

REFERENCES

1. Brooks DE, Wolf ED: Ocular trauma in the horse, Equine Vet J Suppl 1983;2:141.
2. Bistner SI: Traumatic panophthalmitis in a horse, Cornell Vet 1971;61:415.
3. Gertsen K, Wales L, Dawson H: Care of traumatic corneal lesions in Thoroughbred racehorses, Vet Med Small Anim Clin 1973;68:156.
4. Prince JH, Diesem I, Eglitis I, Ruskell GL: Anatomy and histology of the eye and orbit in domestic animals, Springfield, Ill, 1960, Charles C. Thomas.
5. Peiffer RL: Foundations of equine ophthalmology: Clinical anatomy and physiology, Equine Pract 1979;1:39.
6. Kuwabara T, Perkins DG, Cogan DG: Sliding of the epithelium in experimental corneal wounds, Invest Ophthalmol Vis Sci 1976;15:4.
7. Matsuda H, Smelser GK: Electron microscopy of normal wound healing, Exp Eye Res 1973;16:427.
8. Neaderland MH, Riis RC, Rebhun WC, et al: Healing of experimentally induced corneal ulcers in horses, Am J Vet Res 1987;48:427.
9. Whitley RD, Moore CP: Microbiology of the equine eye in health and disease, Vet Clin North Am Large Anim Pract 1984;6:451.
10. Whitley RD, Bugers EC, Moore CP: Microbial isolates of the normal equine eye, Equine Vet J Suppl 1983;2:138.
11. Moore CP, Heller N, Majors LJ, et al: Prevalence of ocular microorganisms in hospitalized and stabled horses, Am J Vet Res 1988;49:773.
12. Samuelson DA, Andresen TL, Gwin RM: Conjunctival fungal flora in horses, cattle, dogs, and cats, J Am Vet Med Assoc 1984;184:1240.
13. Moore CP, Fales WH, Whittington P, et al: Bacterial and fungal isolates from Equidae with ulcerative keratitis, J Am Vet Med Assoc 1983;182:600.
14. McLaughlin SA, Brightman AH, Helper LC, et al: Pathogenic bacteria and fungi associated with extraocular disease in the horse, J Am Vet Med Assoc 1983;182:241.
15. Gelatt KN: *Pseudomonas* ulcerative keratitis and abscess in a horse, Vet Med Small Anim Clin 1974;69:1309.
16. Divers TJ, George LW: Hypopyon and descemetocele associated with *Pseudomonas* ulcerative keratitis in a horse: A case report and review, J Equine Vet Sci 1982;2:104.
17. Rebhun WC: Bacterial ulcers of the equine cornea, Equine Pract 1981;3:40.
18. Adamson PJW, Jang SS: Ulcerative keratitis associated with *Salmonella arizonae* infection in a horse, J Am Vet Med Assoc 1985;186:1219.
19. Mitchell JS, Attleberger MH: *Fusarium* keratomycosis in the horse, Vet Med Small Anim Clin 1973;68:1257.
20. Kern TJ, Brooks DE, White MM: Equine keratomycosis: Current concepts of diagnosis and therapy, Equine Vet J Suppl 1983;2:33.
21. Friedman DS, Schoster JV, Pickett JP, et al: *Pseudallescheria boydii* keratomycosis in a horse, J Am Vet Med Assoc 1989;195:616.
22. Gwin RM: Equine fungal keratitis: Diagnosis and treatment, J Equine Vet Sci 1981;1:66.
23. Hendrix DVH, Chmielewski NT, Smith PJ, et al: Keratomycosis in four horses caused by *Cylindrocarpon destructans*, Vet Comp Ophthalmol 1996;6:253.
24. Ramphal R, McNiece MT, Polack FM: Adherence of *Pseudomonas aeruginosa* to the injured cornea: A step in the pathogenesis of corneal infections, Ann Ophthalmol 1981;13:421.
25. Reed WP, Williams RC: Bacterial adherence: First step in pathogenesis of certain infections, J Chronic Dis 1978;31:67.
26. Brown SI: Cell origin of collagenase in normal and wounded corneas, Arch Ophthalmol 1970;83:74.
27. Slansky HH, Gnadinger MC, Itoi M, et al: Collagenase in corneal ulcers, Arch Ophthalmol 1969;82:108.
28. Brown SI, Hook CW: Isolation of stromal collagenase in corneal inflammation, Am J Ophthalmol 1971;72:1139.
29. Brown SI, Bloomfield SE, Tam WI: The cornea-destroying enzyme of *Pseudomonas aeruginosa*, Invest Ophthalmol Vis Sci 1974;13:174.
30. Kleinfeld J, Ellis PP: Effects of topical anesthetics on growth of microorganisms, Arch Virol 1966;76:712.
31. Hildebrand SV, Holland M, Copland VS, et al: Clinical use of the neuro-muscular blocking agents atracurium and pancuronium for equine anesthesia, J Am Vet Med Assoc 1989;195:212.
32. Troutman RC: Microsurgery of the Anterior Segment of the Eye: Vol I. Introduction and Basic Techniques, St Louis, 1974, CV Mosby.
33. Troutman RC: Microsurgery of the Anterior Segment of the Eye: Vol II. The Cornea: Optics and Surgery, St Louis, 1974, CV Mosby.
34. Eisner G: Eye Surgery: An Introduction to Operative Technique, Berlin, 1980, Springer-Verlag.
35. Parshall CJ: Lamellar corneal-scleral transposition, J Am Anim Hosp Assoc 1973;9:270.
36. McLaughlin SA, Brightman AH, Brogdon JD: Autogenous, partial-thickness corneal graft for repair of a perforated corneal ulcer in a horse, Equine Pract 1985;7:34.
37. Hekmati P, Schels H: Lamellar corneal transplantation in the horse, Vet Rec 1976;99:46.
38. Jakobiec FA, Sigelman J: Advanced Techniques in Ocular Surgery, Philadelphia, 1984, WB Saunders.
39. Brightbill FS: Corneal Surgery: Theory, Technique, and Tissue. St Louis, 1986, CV Mosby.
40. Whittaker CJG, Smith PJ, Brooks DE, et al: Therapeutic penetrating keratoplasty for deep corneal stromal abscesses in eight horses, Vet Comp Ophthalmol 1997;7:19.
41. Lavach JD, Severin GA, Roberts SM: Lacerations of the equine eye: A review of 48 cases, J Am Vet Med Assoc 1984;184:1243.
42. Holmberg DL: Conjunctival pedicle grafts used to repair corneal perforations in the horse, Can Vet J 1981;22:86.

43. Schoster JV: Using conjunctival flaps to prevent rupture of deep corneal ulcers, Vet Med Small Anim Clin 1989;84:307.
44. Brooks DE, Kallberg ME, Ollivier FJ, et al: Penetrating keratoplasty, deep lamellar endothelial keratoplasty, and posterior lamellar keratoplasty in the horse: Visual outcome in 105 cases (1993-2004), Vet Ophthalmol 2004;7:425.
45. Ollivier FJ, Brooks DE, Kallberg ME, et al: Evaluation of various compounds to inhibit activity of matrix metalloproteinases in the tear film of horses with ulcerative keratitis, Am J Vet Res 2003;64:1081.
46. Brooks DE: Equine Ophthalmology, Jackson Hole, Wyo, 2002, Teton NewMedia.
47. Strafuss AC: Squamous cell carcinoma in horses, J Am Vet Med Assoc 1976;168:61.
48. Lavach JD, Severin GA: Neoplasia of the equine eye, adnexa, and orbit: A review of 68 cases, J Am Vet Med Assoc 1977;170:202.
49. Gelatt KN, Myers VS, Periman V, et al: Conjunctival squamous cell carcinoma in the horse, J Am Vet Med Assoc 1974;165:617.
50. Gelatt KN: Corneolimbal squamous cell carcinoma in a horse, Vet Med Small Anim Clin 1975;70:53.
51. Koch SA, Cowles RR: Surgical removal of a squamous cell carcinoma of the equine eye, Vet Med Small Anim Clin 1971;66:327.
52. Harling DE, Peiffer RL, Cook CS: Excision and cryosurgical treatment of five cases of squamous cell carcinoma in the horse, Equine Vet J Suppl 1983;2:105.
53. Hilbert BJ, Farrell RK, Grant BD: Cryotherapy of periocular squamous cell carcinoma in the horse, J Am Vet Med Assoc 1977;170:1305.
54. Joyce JR: Cryosurgical treatment of tumors in horses and cattle, J Am Vet Med Assoc 1976;168:226.
55. English RV, Nasisse MP, Davidson MG: Carbon dioxide laser ablation of limbal squamous cell carcinoma in horses, J Am Vet Med Assoc 1990;196:439.
56. Grier RL, Brewer WG, Paul SR, et al: Treatment of bovine and equine ocular squamous cell carcinoma by radiofrequency hyperthermia, J Am Vet Med Assoc 1980;177:55.
57. Neumann SM, Kainer RA, Severin GA: Reaction of normal equine eyes to radio-frequency current-induced hyperthermia, Am J Vet Res 1982;43:1938.
58. Frauenfelder HC, Blevins WE, Page EH: 90^{Sr} for treatment of periocular squamous cell carcinoma in the horse, J Am Vet Med Assoc 1982;180:307.
59. Owen LN, Barnett KC: Treatment of equine squamous cell carcinoma of the conjunctiva using a strontium 90 applicator, Equine Vet J Suppl 1983;2:125.
60. Walker MN, Goble G, Geiser D: Two year non-recurrence rates for equine ocular and periocular squamous cell carcinoma following radiotherapy, Vet Radiol 1986;27:146.
61. Moore CP, Corwin LA, Collier LL: Keratopathy induced by beta radiation therapy in a horse, Equine Vet J Suppl 1983;2:112.
62. Havener WH: Ocular Pharmacology, ed 5, St Louis, 1983, CV Mosby.
63. Brooks D: Further development of an indwelling nasolacrimal cannula for the administration of medication to the equine eye, Equine Pract 1987;9:12.
64. Gelatt KN: A modified subpalpebral system for the horse, J Am Anim Hosp Assoc 1979;3:141.
65. Gelatt KN: Postoperative subpalpebral medications in horses and dogs, Vet Med Small Anim Clin 1967;62:1165.
66. Raphel Sweeney C, Hammel EP, Martin BB: A new method for placement of the subpalpebral lavage apparatus, Equine Pract 1984;6:23.
67. Smolin G, Okumoto M, Wilson FM: The effect of tobramycin on gentamicin resistant strains in pseudomonas keratitis, Am J Ophthalmol 1974;77:583.
68. Omerod LK, Heseltine PNR, Alfonso E, et al: Gentamicin-resistant pseudomonal infection: Rationale for redefinition of ophthalmic antimicrobial sensitivities, Cornea 1989;8:195.
69. Williams M, Spiess B: Systemic effects of topically applied ophthalmic atropine in equine. Presented at the 17th Annual Meeting of American College of Veterinary Ophthalmologists and Scientific Program of the International Society of Veterinary Ophthalmology, 1986.
70. Krohne SDG, Vestre WA: Effects of flunixin meglumine and dexamethasone on aqueous protein values after intraocular surgery in the dog, Am J Vet Res 1987;48:420.
71. Cooley PL, Milvae R, Riis RC, et al: Effects of flunixin meglumine on prostacyclin accumulation in the equine eye, Am J Vet Res 1984;45:1383.
72. Tammeus J, Krall J, Rengstorff RH: Therapeutic extended wear contact lens for corneal injury in a horse, J Am Vet Med Assoc 1983;182:286.

CHAPTER 61

Intraocular Surgery

Joan Dziezyc

ANATOMY

Iris

The iris comprises the most anterior part of the uveal (vascular) tract. The colors of the equine iris vary from blue to dark brown. The pupil is horizontally oriented with large corpora nigra (granula iridica) superiorly and much smaller corpora nigra inferiorly (Fig. 61-1).

The iris is composed of an anterior border layer with fibroblasts and melanocytes (in pigmented irides), the stroma (making up the bulk of the iris), and a double layer of posterior pigmented epithelium.[1] The stroma contains the smooth muscle of the pupillary sphincter as well as melanocytes (in pigmented irides), collagen fibrils, fibroblasts, nerves, and blood vessels. At the level of the last ciliary process runs the incomplete major arterial circle of the iris (incomplete at 12 and 6 o'clock), which is a continuation of the long posterior ciliary arteries.[2] Radial vessels from this incomplete circle pass to the pupil and also to the ciliary body. There is another incomplete arterial circle at the level of the sphincter muscle, with small arterioles continuing into the corpora nigra. The capillary endothelium is not fenestrated and probably represents the anatomic blood–aqueous barrier in the iris.[3] A double layer of pigmented epithelium lines the posterior surface of the iris. The anterior layer of cells forms the iris dilator muscle, which is poorly developed in the horizontal axis. Proliferations of the two layers of epithelium form the corpora nigra.

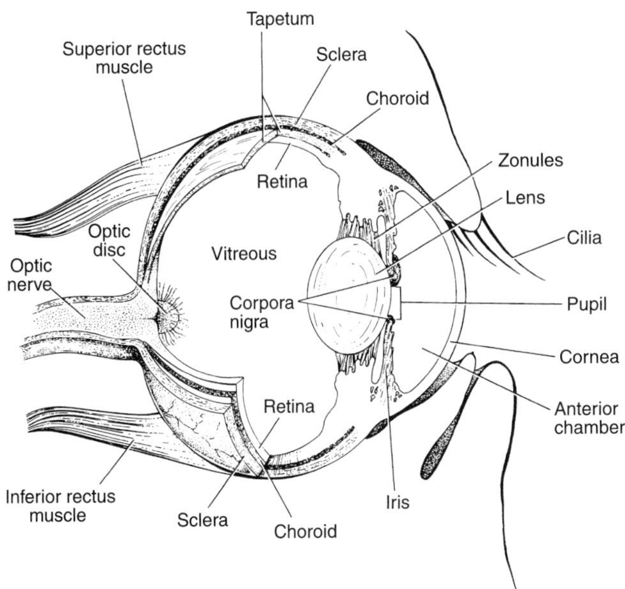

Figure 61-1. A cross-section of an equine eye.

Ciliary Body

The ciliary body is the midportion of the uveal tract found between the iris and the choroid plexus. It is made up of the ciliary processes anteriorly (pars plicata) and a flattened area posteriorly (pars plana). Zonular fibers insert on the pars plicata and pass to the pars plana.

The ciliary body is lined with a double layer of epithelium: the inner layer is nonpigmented, and the outer layer pigmented. Junctions between the apical ends of the nonpigmented epithelium probably represent the anatomic blood–aqueous barrier in the ciliary body.[3]

The ciliary body stroma is made up of connective tissue, numerous blood vessels, nerves, and melanocytes. Capillaries contain fenestrated endothelium. The radial ciliary muscle, which opens the drainage angle and alters the shape of the lens, is poorly developed in the horse.

Lens

The lens is positioned behind the iris and held in place by numerous zonules, which run from the ciliary body and insert at the lens circumference. The lens consists of the lens capsule, anterior and equatorial epithelium, and lens fibers. The horse's lens measures about 20 mm in diameter and 13 mm in depth anteroposteriorly.

The lens in young animals is very elastic and changes shape with differing zonular tension. This in turn is controlled by the action of the ciliary muscles. The focusing ability of horses is much less than that of humans.

The lens capsule completely surrounds the lens and is the basement membrane of the lens epithelium. Only the anterior surface of the capsule is lined by epithelium in the mature lens. Lens epithelial cells at the lens equator continue to divide during life, creating new cells that elongate to form lens fibers. The most recently formed lens fibers are found under the lens capsule (in the lens cortex), and the oldest fibers are found in the center of the lens (in the lens nucleus). Lens suture lines are most easily seen in young animals and represent the junctions between the ends of the lens fibers that have become apposed as the fibers grow toward opposite sides of the lens.

The posterior segment of the eye is filled with vitreous. The vitreous is mostly made up of water with a collagen–hyaluronic acid network and a few cells called *hyalocytes*. The vitreous is attached to the eye at the optic disc, by the vitreous base at the ora ciliaris retinae, and by the hyaloideocapsular ligament at the posterior lens capsule.

The posterior area of the globe is made up of retina, choroid, and sclera. The sclera is the outer fibrous layer of the globe, continuous with the cornea at the limbus. The choroid is the posterior uveal (vascular) layer, continuous with the ciliary body anteriorly. The choroid consists mainly of blood vessels, which provide nutrition to the retina and optic nerve. Arteries are branches of the short posterior ciliary arteries that enter the globe near the optic nerve. Capillaries are fenestrated. The choroid also contains melanocytes and fibroblasts, collagen and elastic fibers, and the tapetum. In horses, the tapetum is mainly acellular, composed of lamellae of collagen fibrils. The tapetum is found in the superior half of the fundus.

The retina represents the inner layer of the posterior globe and is divided into two layers: (1) the neurosensory, inner retina, which contains photoreceptors and neurons, including ganglion cells whose axons form the optic nerve; and (2) the retinal pigment epithelium, the outer layer, which is important in the maintenance of the photoreceptors. Retinal detachments occur between the neurosensory layers and the retinal pigment epithelium. The intraocular optic nerve in horses is nonmyelinated and is seen as a large oval in the nontapetal region, just below the tapetal–nontapetal junction. The retina of a horse is paurangiotic, with retinal vessels extending only a short distance from the optic disc.

IMMUNOLOGY

The major problem associated with intraocular surgery in horses is postoperative inflammation (uveitis). The act of incising the eye, or performing a paracentesis, causes a cascade of events that, if not modified, may end in a phthisic eye. Inflammatory mediators that are released include prostaglandins, leukotrienes, and prostacyclin.[4] These mediators cause miosis, dilation and increased permeability of uveal blood vessels, and production of a plasmoid aqueous (a breakdown of the blood–aqueous barrier). Opening the lens capsule during cataract surgery causes inflammation by exposing the eye to large amounts of lens proteins. Normally, lens protein is semisequestered from the body by the lens capsule. Low levels of circulating lens antigens normally maintain a tolerance to these proteins.[5] When large amounts of lens protein are liberated or normal tolerance is altered, autologous lens protein can initiate immune-mediated uveitis.[6]

Unless the inflammatory response is altered by drugs, sequelae can be expected, including posterior synechiae, cataract formation, corneal edema, chorioretinitis, retinal detachment, and phthisis bulbi.

Additional information on other causes of uveitis and its control can be found in Chapters 62 and 64.

DIAGNOSTIC PROCEDURE: PARACENTESIS

Paracentesis pertains to the removal of either aqueous from the anterior chamber (anterior chamber paracentesis) or removal of liquefied vitreous from the posterior segment of the eye (vitreal paracentesis). Paracentesis is a procedure used in the diagnosis of uveitis when conventional diagnostic aids have failed and therapy is unrewarding. It is valuable when endophthalmitis is suspected. Paracentesis is not without risks; the potential for damage to the eye exists. Also, paracentesis is often unrewarding in terms of making a diagnosis. However, if a diagnosis cannot be made any other way and the eye is not improving with treatment, paracentesis should be performed. A paracentesis should be followed up with an injection of an antibiotic, an antifungal agent, and a tissue plasminogen activator (to dissolve fibrin deposits) if any of these treatments are indicated.

Anterior chamber paracentesis can be performed under general anesthesia, or with eyelid blocks in a heavily sedated horse. General anesthesia carries less risk to the eye but more risk to the horse. A lid speculum is used to open the eyelids. Topical anesthetic is applied to the cornea and conjunctiva. Subconjunctival lidocaine should be injected over the paracentesis site in a sedated horse. The conjunctiva is grasped near the limbus with small-toothed forceps, and a 25-gauge (or smaller) needle attached to a 1-mL syringe is inserted under the conjunctiva, through the limbus, and into the anterior chamber (Fig. 61-2). The needle should be directed parallel to the plane of the iris. No more than 0.5 mL should be removed. For a vitreal aspirate, a 22- to 23-gauge needle is used. The author has performed these aspirates only under general anesthesia. The needle is inserted 10 mm behind the limbus at the 12-o'clock position, through conjunctiva, sclera, and the pars plana of the ciliary body, and directed toward the posterior pole of the eye to avoid traumatizing the lens. Because the needle often cannot be observed, vitreous paracentesis carries a greater risk of injury to the eye.

Aspirates should be cultured for aerobic as well as anaerobic bacteria, and fungal cultures should be performed if appropriate. Cytology of the aspirate may be most informative. In cases of suspected endophthalmitis, antibiotics should be injected into the vitreous. Antibiotics may sterilize the eye, but enucleation may still be necessary because of intractable uveitis.

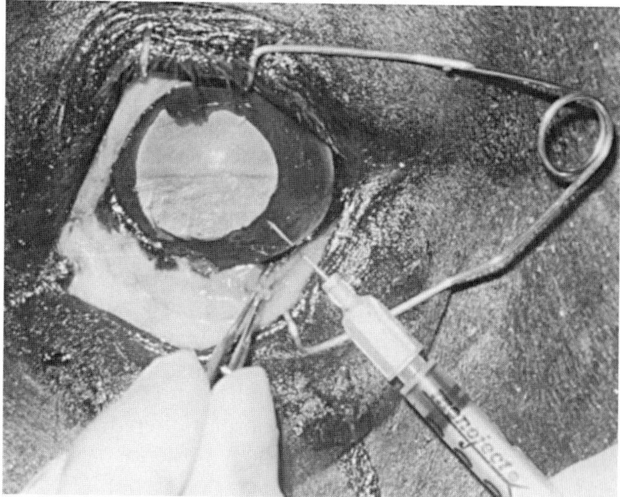

Figure 61-2. Paracentesis of the anterior chamber. A 25-gauge needle attached to a 1-mL syringe is inserted into the anterior chamber at the limbus, and fluid is withdrawn.

SURGICALLY MANAGED DISORDERS

For intraocular surgery to be successful in any species, several requirements have to be satisfied. First, the surgeon must be trained in microsurgery and must perform enough intraocular procedures to stay competent. Second, a means of magnification, usually an operating microscope, and microsurgical instruments must be available. Third, close work with anesthesiologists is necessary because a motionless eye is very important in intraocular procedures, which may require concomitant use of inhalation anesthesia, muscle relaxants, and narcotics. Finally, patient selection and follow-up therapy are especially important. Horses' eyes are more reactive than eyes of other domestic species, and close follow-up with changes in therapy, when appropriate, is extremely important. For example, equine cataract patients often remain hospitalized for 3 to 4 weeks to ensure adequate postoperative therapy.

Iris and Ciliary Body

Surgery of the equine iris and ciliary body is performed rarely. Iridectomy has been described for treatment of an iris melanoma.[7] The use of lasers allows manipulation of the anterior uvea without entering the eye. Both the Nd:YAG and diode lasers have been used to shrink or destroy anterior uveal tumors in horses. The diode laser also has an endoprobe that can be used in the anterior chamber through a small incision.

Epithelial Iris Cysts

Occasionally, horses are presented with visual deficits secondary to iris cysts associated with the corpora nigra. These can be opened in several ways. Under general anesthesia, a 20-gauge needle can be inserted into the anterior chamber through the limbus and used to lacerate the cysts. Alternately, the use of lasers allows opening of the cysts without entering the eye and therefore carries a better prognosis. Lasers can also be used on a standing, sedated horse, eliminating the need for general anesthesia. Nd:YAG, argon, or diode lasers have been used. One report[8] describes treating eight horses with large corpora nigra cysts with the Nd:YAG laser. Clinical signs, including vision problems, resolved after laser therapy

Lens

Cataract

Cataracts are optical opacities in the lens. They range in size from minute opacities that can be seen only with magnification, to opacities that involve the entire lens. Vision may (or may not) be impaired, depending on the size and location of the cataract.

Cataracts can be seen in animals of any age and have a number of different causes. In horses, cataracts most commonly develop secondary to periodic ophthalmia (equine recurrent uveitis, moon blindness). Another common cause is trauma, usually either a perforating or a concussive injury. Congenital cataracts are seen less frequently. Most congenital cataracts are assumed to occur spontaneously, although inherited congenital cataracts have been described in the Belgian Draft horses, associated with aniridia[9]; in Morgan horses, where cataracts were nuclear and affected animals had no visual deficits[10]; and in the Rocky Mountain horse with nuclear cataracts associated with multiple anterior segment anomalies.[11] Often, congenital cataracts are associated with varying degrees of microphthalmia.

Patient selection is an important part of cataract removal in horses. The best candidate is a horse with a cataract uncomplicated by any other ocular problems. Uncomplicated cataracts are seen more frequently in young animals with congenital cataracts than acquired cataracts in adult horses. Ocular problems that worsen the prognosis but are not a contraindication for surgery include (1) microphthalmia; (2) evidence of perforating trauma, such as a full-thickness corneal scar, or small synechiae; and (3) evidence of mild uveitis, such as a darkened iris or a pupil that does not dilate as well as the normal eye. Evidence of periodic ophthalmia (equine recurrent uveitis, moon blindness) is a contraindication for cataract surgery in the author's clinic. Signs of periodic ophthalmia include corneal edema, multiple posterior synechiae, aqueous flare, retinal detachment, chorioretinal scars (especially around the optic disc), and phthisis bulbi.

If the retina cannot be seen through clear areas of the lens (i.e., when the cataract is mature), ultrasonography is used to image the posterior aspect of the eye. Ultrasonography can detect retinal detachments, posterior capsular ruptures, lenticonus, vitreal abnormalities,[12] and optic nerve colobomas.[13]

Preoperative and postoperative treatments include topical mydriatics or cycloplegics, such as atropine; topical anti-inflammatory drugs such as corticosteroids (prednisolone acetate 1.0%, dexamethasone 0.1%); a nonsteroidal anti-inflammatory drug (flurbiprofen); and topical antibiotics. In addition, systemic antibiotics are used perioperatively, and systemic nonsteroidal anti-inflammatory drugs (flunixin meglumine) are used. These drugs are used to dilate the pupil, to decrease the inflammation induced by the surgery, to decrease pain, and to attempt to sterilize the surgical site. Drugs are used for 1 to 2 days before surgery in quiet eyes, and for as long as necessary in eyes with low-grade uveitis. Drugs are used postoperatively for at least 3 weeks and often longer.

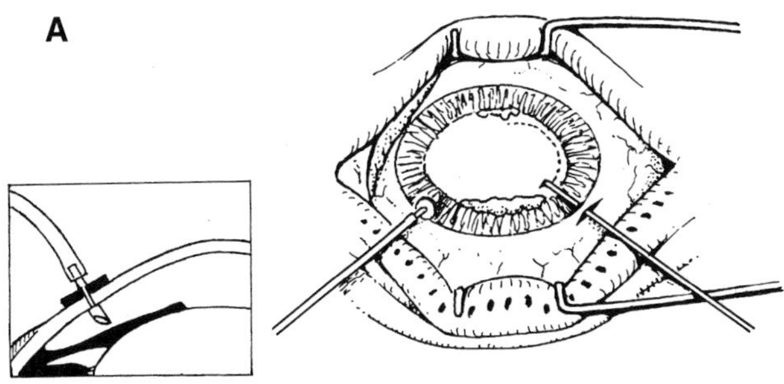

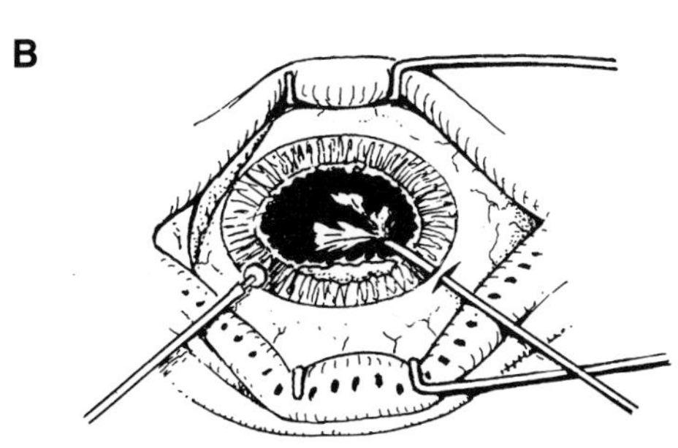

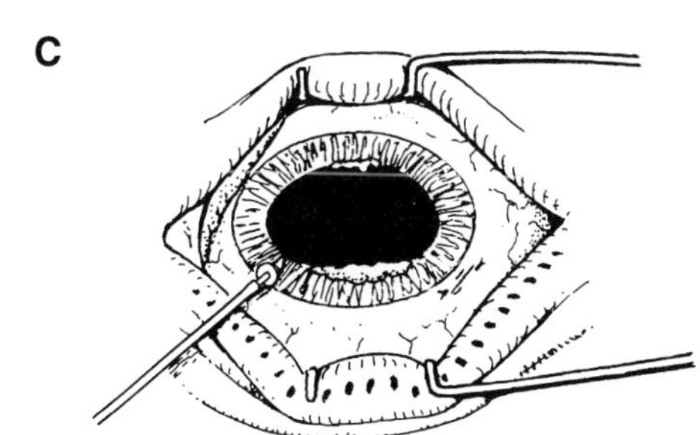

Figure 61-3. Phacofragmentation in the horse. **A,** The cystotome on the right tears the anterior capsule while lactated Ringer's solution is infused through the irrigation cannula (see *insert*) on the left. **B,** Phacofragmentation of the lens cortex is carried out through the phacofragmentor needle *(right)*. **C,** The incision on the right is sutured while continuing the infusion through the irrigation cannula *(left)*.

PHACOFRAGMENTATION

Surgery is performed using phacofragmentation[14] (Fig. 61-3). Phacofragmentation refers to the use of ultrasonic waves to break up the lens. The lens particles are subsequently aspirated from the eye. Various techniques for phacofragmentation are used in different clinics. The technique used by the author is described.

The horse is positioned in lateral recumbency. A 19-gauge irrigating cannula is inserted through a clear corneal incision. Lactated Ringer's solution is continuously infused through this cannula. A limbal-based conjunctival flap is dissected, a partial-thickness limbal incision is created, and the anterior chamber is entered with a stab incision. A cystotome, made by bending the tip of a 23-gauge needle, is inserted through the incision and used to tear and remove the majority of the anterior lens capsule (see Fig. 61-3). A 17-gauge, 4-cm, blunt-tipped needle with a 30-degree bevel attached to the handpiece of a modified lithotriptor (Fibrasonics Lithotriptor, Fibrasonics, Chicago, Ill) is inserted into the eye and held by the surgeon's dominant hand. Aspiration is performed by a phacoemulsifier aspiration unit (Model 8000[V] Cavitron/Kellman Phaco-Emulsifier Aspirator, Cooper Vision, Irvine, Calif) attached to the handpiece. Ultrasonic waves break up the lens into particles, which are aspirated from the eye. When the entire lens cortex and nucleus are removed, the lithotriptor needle is removed from the eye. The corneal incisions are closed with two or three simple-interrupted sutures of 7-0 polyglactin (Vicryl, Ethicon, Somerville, NJ) to provide a watertight seal. The conjunctival incision is closed with a simple-continuous pattern using the same suture material. A subpalpebral lavage system (see Chapter 55) is placed.

When a modified lithotriptor is not available, veterinary ophthalmologists using standard human phacofragmentors, whose tips are too short to cross the entire lens capsule of a horse, may have to make more than one corneal incision to remove all the lens material.[15]

Phacofragmentation works well in horses because only a small incision is used, perfusion is constant, and the eye does not collapse. Additionally, all lens fibers can be removed from the eye, eliminating this potentially antigenic material. The use of muscle relaxants such as pancuronium or atracurium establishes a motionless eye with minimal vitreal and posterior capsular movement. This results in a considerable shortening of the operative time and a decrease in the amount of irrigating solution used.

PROGNOSIS

Several recent publications have looked at the success (in horses) of lens removal by phacofragmentation. Fifty-one eyes in 36 horses were operated on at the institution of this author.[14] Useful vision was restored in 30 horses in the immediate postoperative period. At 1 year or longer, 16 out of 19 horses were visual. Three of these horses were followed for 5 years or longer. Postoperative complications included corneal ulcers, excessive anterior chamber fibrin deposition, diffuse corneal edema, elevated intraocular pressure, and most devastatingly, endophthalmitis in four eyes of three horses. *Streptococcus zooepidemicus* was cultured from three of these eyes. Tissue plasminogen activator (25 μg) was injected into the aqueous of eight eyes and successfully caused dissolution of fibrin in these eyes.

In a report from The Ohio State University, 47 eyes in 39 horses were operated on with phacofragmentation. Similar postoperative complications were reported, including one eye with panophthalmitis. At last follow-up (ranging from 1 day to longer than 1 year), 88% of the horses were visual.[16] One horse was operated on for a morgagnian cataract and had useful vision at 7 months postoperatively.[17]

Despite the lack of postoperative visual correction, horses have useful vision after successful surgery. Working horses such as roping horses or polo ponies are able to work as well as they had before the development of cataracts. In foals, vision is more difficult to evaluate, but foals with congenital cataracts should probably be operated on as soon as possible to allow visual pathway development. Equine research in this area has not been conducted, but work in cats shows that visual deprivation in kittens between the ages of 4 to 12 weeks leads to abnormalities in the development of the visual pathway and behavioral blindness.[18] In visually deprived humans, the same signs are seen. The critical period in humans begins soon after birth and ends in the 3rd year.[19]

Pseudophakia

Pseudophakia is the replacement of the cataractous lens with a synthetic intraocular lens (IOL). The normal lens in a human supplies about a third of the total refractive power of the eye; lenses in animals also supply a good deal of the refractive power of the eye. Removing this lens, without implanting an IOL, would leave the patient with greatly reduced visual acuity. Therefore, IOLs are commonly implanted in people and dogs after cataract removal, with the goal providing emmetropia (the rays of light entering the eye are all brought in focus on the retina; 0D or 20/20 in the United States). Streak retinoscopy is a method of determining the focusing ability of the eye without having subjective responses from the patient (i.e., without the patient reading an eye chart). Streak retinoscopy of three aphakic equine eyes gave a mean value of +9.94D (hyperopia [far-sightedness]), whereas normal horse refraction was +0.25D (close to emmetropia).[14]

A pilot study using donated horses with cataracts investigated a prototype IOL of +25D. In that study, two eyes with clear media were refracted at −4.75D and −9.5D (myopia [near-sightedness]). Clearly, this +25D IOL did not allow the horses to be emmetropic, but the assumption is that decreasing the power of this IOL would lead to an emmetropic eye. However, because of intraoperative and postoperative complications associated with the large limbal incision, IOLs are presently not implanted in horses. Further work is needed to optimize lens power, and perhaps an injectable lens will be devised for the horse in the future.

Traumatic Lens Rupture

Perforating injuries occasionally involve the lens. If the capsular laceration of the lens is small, it can seal with only a small opacity developing in the injured area. If the laceration is large, aqueous humor can enter the lens, causing a very rapidly developing cataract. The uveitis seen with a large laceration is unresponsive to medication, probably because of the large amount of foreign protein that continues to be presented to the immune system. As in other species, the treatment of choice is lens removal. The lens should be removed as soon after the injury as possible. All injuries of this type carry a guarded prognosis.

In a series of seven horses with penetrating corneal and lenticular trauma, most eyes were enucleated.[20] In one eye with an acute history, removal of the lens using phacofragmentation was performed, but the eye remained blind after surgery as a result of retinal detachment.[20]

Spontaneous lens rupture is also seen. In one case seen at the authors' clinic, a ruptured lens of several months' duration was discovered ultrasonographically in a quiet eye with a cataract, during a cataract workup. Unfortunately, the horse was lost to follow-up.

Vitreous and Retina

Most retinal detachments in horses develop secondary to equine recurrent uveitis, and these are not amenable to surgical therapy. Treatment of rhegmatogenous detachments (detachments with a retinal tear) has not been described in the horse. Chapter 62 has more information on vitreal surgery and vitreal and suprachoroidal cyclosporine implants for treating recurrent uveitis.

Glaucoma

Although glaucoma in horses is uncommon, this condition is as difficult to treat in this species as in any other. Normal intraocular pressure in horses is similar to that in other species and should be less than 30 mm Hg. Applanation tonometers are easiest to use in this species. Both the Nd:YAG[15,21] and diode lasers[22] have been used successfully in horses to reduce intraocular pressure. Fifty-five applications of the Nd:YAG laser 5 to 6 mm from the limbus with 10 W for a duration of 0.4 second per site have been recommended.[15] For the diode laser, 1500 mW and 1500 msec per site has been described, varying from 30 to 80 sites at 4 to 6 mm from the limbus.[15]

Filtration gonioimplants have been used successfully by the author as well as by others[15] to improve aqueous drainage. In blind eyes with uncontrolled intraocular pressure or buphthalmia, either an enucleation should be performed or an intraocular prosthesis should be implanted to eliminate the chronic discomfort associated with these eyes.

Intraocular Prostheses

An intraocular prostheses can be useful for horses with blind, painful eyes, such as eyes affected with equine recurrent uveitis or glaucoma (see Chapter 63).

REFERENCES

1. Samuelson DA: Ophthalmic embryology and anatomy. In Gelatt KN, editor: Textbook of Veterinary Ophthalmology, ed 2, Philadelphia, 1991, Lea & Febiger.
2. Anderson BG, Anderson WD: Vasculature of the equine and canine iris, Am J Vet Res 1977;38:1791.
3. Butler JM, Unger WG, Grierson I: Recent experimental studies on the blood-aqueous barrier: The anatomical basis of the response to injury, Eye 1988;2(Suppl):S213.
4. Cooley PL, Milvae R, Riis RC, Laratta LJ: Effect of flunixin meglumine on prostacyclin accumulation in the equine eye, Am J Vet Res 1984;45:1383.
5. Marak GE, Font RL, Alepa FP: Immunopathogenicity of lens crystallins in the production of experimental lens-induced granulomatous endophthalmitis, Ophthalmol Res 1978;10:30.
6. Spencer WH: Lens. In Spencer WH, editor: Ophthalmic Pathology, ed 3, Philadelphia, 1985, WB Saunders.
7. Latimer CA, Wyman M: Sector iridectomy in the management of iris melanoma in a horse, Equine Vet J 1983;2(suppl):101.
8. Gilger BC, Davidson MG, Nadelstein B, Nasisse M: Neodymium:yttrium-aluminum-garnet laser treatment of cystic granula iridica in horses: Eight cases (1988-1996), J Am Vet Med Assoc 1997;211:341.
9. Eriksson K: Hereditary aniridia with secondary cataract in horses, Nord Vet Med 1955;7:773.
10. Beech J, Aguirre G, Cross S: Congenital nuclear cataracts in the Morgan horse, J Am Vet Med Assoc 1984;184:1363.
11. Ewart SL. Ramsey DT, Xu J, Meyers D: The horse homolog of congenital Aniridia conforms to codominant inheritance, J Hered 2000;91:93.
12. Scotty NC, Cutler TJ, Brooks, DE, Ferrell E: Diagnostic ultrasonography of equine lens and posterior segment abnormalities, Vet Ophthalmol 2004;7:127.
13. Bildfell R, Watrous B, Maxwell S, et al: Bilateral optic disc colobomas in a Quarter Horse filly, Equine Vet J 2003;35:325.
14. Millichamp NJ, Dziezyc J: Cataract phacofragmentation in horses, Vet Ophthalmol 2000;3:157.
15. Brooks DE: Equine ophthalmology. In Gelatt KN, editor: Textbook of Veterinary Ophthalmology, ed 3, Philadelphia, 1999, Lippincott Williams & Wilkins.
16. Fife TM, Gemensky-Metzler AJ, Colitz CMH, et al: Clinical features and outcomes of phacoemulsification in 39 horses: A retrospective study (1993-2003). Abstract of 35th annual conference of the American College of Veterinary Ophthalmologists, Washington, DC, 2004.
17. Hardman C, McIlany TR, Dugan SJ: Phacofragmentation for morgagnian cataract in a horse, Vet Ophthalmol 2001;4:221.
18. Hubel DH, Weisel TN: The period of susceptibility to the physiological effects of unilateral eye closure in kittens, J Physiol 1970;206:419.
19. Tyler CW, Scott AB: Binocular vision. In Duane TD, Jaeger EA, editors: Biomedical Foundations of Ophthalmology, Philadelphia, vol 2, 1986, Harper & Row.
20. Grahn BH, Cullen CL: Equine phacoclastic uveitis: The clinical manifestations, light microscopic findings, and therapy of 7 cases, Can Vet J 2000;41:376.
21. Miller TR, Brooks DE, Gelatt KN, et al: Equine glaucoma: Clinical findings and response to treatment in 14 horses, Vet Comp Ophthalmol 1995;5:170.
22. Cullen CL, Grahn BH: Equine glaucoma: A retrospective study of 13 cases presented at the Western College of Veterinary Medicine from 1992 to 1999, Can Vet J 2000;41:470.

CHAPTER 62

Surgical Management of Equine Recurrent Uveitis

Brian C. Gilger
Bernhard M. Spiess

Equine recurrent uveitis (ERU), also known as moon blindness, iridocyclitis, and periodic ophthalmia, is one of most common causes of blindness in horses. This immune-mediated pan-uveitis has an approximately 2% prevalence in horses in the United States. ERU is characterized by episodes of intraocular inflammation that develop weeks to months after an initial uveitis episode. Not every case of uveitis is ERU, but instead, ERU is a syndrome of chronic recurrent uveitis that differs from primary uveitis. ERU is diagnosed only when typical clinical signs of uveitis are coupled with a documented history of recurrence of inflammation. Therefore, ERU cannot be diagnosed after a single episode of inflammation.

Typical clinical signs of active uveitis include blepharospasm, epiphora, and photophobia. There is corneal edema and aqueous humor flare and fibrin accumulation. The pupil is usually miotic. After recurrent episodes, posterior synechiae and dyscoria may be noted. Ocular hypotony may be palpated or assessed by applanation tonometry. If the pupil can be pharmacologically dilated, capsular and subcapsular cataracts may be seen. Vitreal opacities and peripapillary chorioretinal scars are additional clinical signs. The diagnosis of uveitis is based on clinical signs and ocular hypotony.

Medications typically used to treat ERU (i.e., corticosteroids, mydriatics, and nonsteroidal anti-inflammatory drugs [NSAIDs]) are used to reduce inflammation and minimize permanent ocular damage at each episode of active uveitis, but they are not effective in preventing recurrence of disease. Corticosteroids are used topically or subconjunctivally, together with topical 1% atropine sulfate. NSAIDs are usually administered systemically. Intracameral injection of tissue plasminogen activator may be used to dissolve organized fibrinous exudates in the anterior chamber. Other medications, such as aspirin, phenylbutazone, and various herbal treatments, used by some clinicians to possibly prevent or decrease the severity of recurrent episodes of uveitis, have limited efficacy and potentially detrimental side effects when used chronically in the horse.

Cyclosporine sustained-release devices and pars plana vitrectomy offer new and promising avenues for long-term control of equine recurrent uveitis. In this chapter, treatment of recurrent ophthalmia with the help of these novel techniques is described.

SUSTAINED-RELEASE MEDICATION DEVICES FOR ERU

Ocular devices that provide sustained release of medications have many advantages over more traditional methods of drug administration to the eye.[1] These include the delivery of a constant therapeutic level of medication directly to the site of inflammation, bypassing some of the blood–ocular barriers, and eliminating the need to rely on the owners to treat their horses. Release rates are typically well below toxic levels of the drug, and higher concentrations of the drug are achieved in the eye while systemic side effects are avoided. Devices also have the benefit of being more convenient for the patient and reducing the risk involved with frequent intravitreal or periocular injections.[1]

Cyclosporine A (CsA) is a 1.2-kD cyclic peptide that blocks the transcription of interleukin (IL)-2 and the responsiveness of the T-cell.[2,3] It may be the ideal drug to prevent the activation of T-lymphocytes and the recurrence of uveitis. Because CsA is hydrophobic and does not penetrate into the eye when applied topically, currently available methods of delivery to the eye are inadequate.[4-6] The pharmacokinetics of oral cyclosporine have not been determined in horses, but systemic treatment with cyclosporine may promote serious side effects such as renal, hepatic, and neurologic toxicity.[7] Also, it is very costly to administer to a horse.

Intravitreal Cyclosporine Devices

A polyvinyl alcohol and silicone–coated intravitreal CsA sustained-delivery device was shown to produce a sustained level of CsA in ocular tissues of rabbits.[8,9] Similar intravitreal CsA devices (Fig. 62-1) were implanted into normal horse eyes for up to 1 year and were not associated with ocular inflammation or complications.[10] In equine eyes with experimentally induced uveitis, eyes with CsA-releasing devices decreased the duration and severity of inflammation, cellular infiltration, tissue destruction, and level of transcription of proinflammatory cytokines.[11] In a study using CsA devices in horses with naturally occurring ERU,[12] horses with frequent recurrence of uveitis without vision-threatening ocular changes (e.g., cataracts, retinal degeneration) or systemic illnesses were selected to receive the device. Although the device prevented the development of recurrent episodes in 81% of horses, complications were noted after surgery that included intraocular hemorrhage, progression of cataract formation, and retinal detachment.[12] The surgical intervention in fragile ERU eyes was thought to be the source of the observed complications, so less invasive methods were evaluated for the constant release of cyclosporine.

Suprachoroidal Cyclosporine Devices

A new device that allowed constant release of cyclosporine (or other selected immunosuppressive medications) was developed to be placed in the suprachoroidal space directly adjacent to the ciliary body (Fig. 62-2). Horses with chronic, documented ERU as determined after complete ophthalmic examination, and that have little or no active inflammation but are experiencing frequent recurrences or early relapse of active ERU after stopping medications were considered appropriate candidates for surgical placement of a suprachoroidal CsA device. Horses whose actively inflamed eyes could not be controlled with anti-inflammatory medications were not considered good candidates for CsA implantation because CsA has poor anti-inflammatory properties (its immunosuppressive properties help prevent new recurrent episodes), and inflamed eyes were considered to

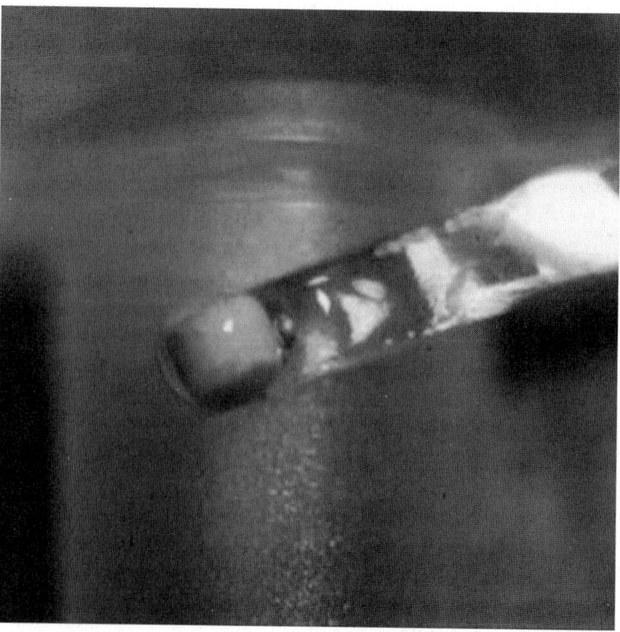

Figure 62-1. Silicone-coated pellet of cyclosporine A used for intravitreal placement for the control of equine recurrent uveitis.

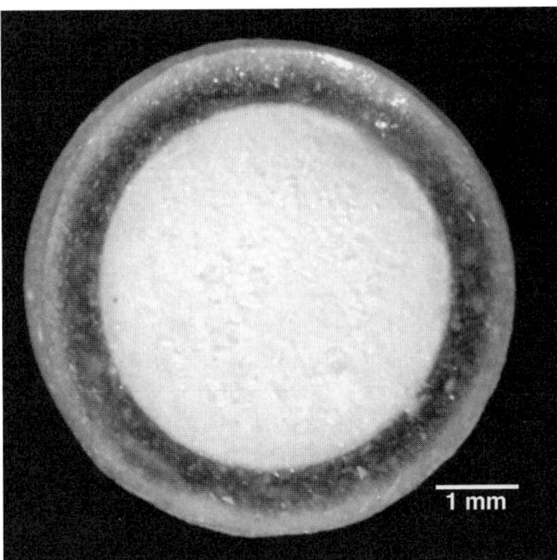

Figure 62-2. Cyclosporine A–containing device for placement in the suprachoroidal space for long-term treatment of equine recurrent uveitis. (Photograph courtesy of Dr. Mike Robinson.)

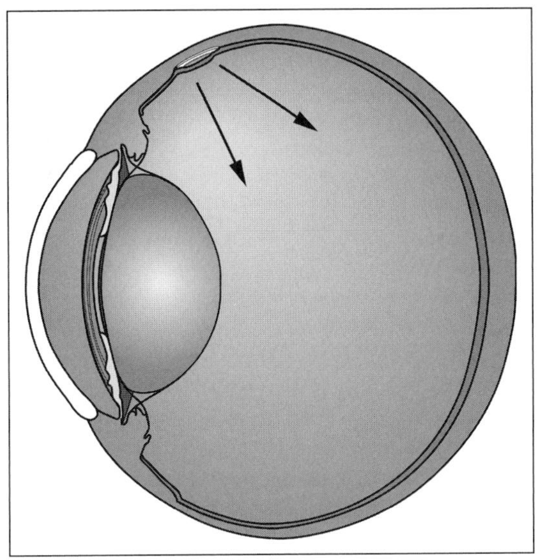

Figure 62-3. Location of the placement of a suprachoroidal drug delivery device. Drug delivery is in the direction of the *arrows*.

be more prone to surgical and postsurgical complications. Equine patients with evidence of significant cataract formation or other ocular conditions (e.g., glaucoma) were also considered poor candidates for surgery. *Leptospira* titers should be performed in endemic areas, and systemic antibiotic therapy (e.g., doxycycline, 10 to 20 mg/kg PO BID for 30 days) should be administered prior to considering surgical therapy for ERU.

The surgical technique for suprachoroidal device implantation requires that the horse be placed under general anesthesia. A 1-cm conjunctival incision is made in the dorsolateral bulbar conjunctiva. A 7-mm-wide scleral flap is prepared, exposing the uveal tract (i.e., the black uvea is visible) approximately 8 mm posterior to the limbus and just lateral to the insertion of the dorsal rectus muscle (Fig. 62-3). The CsA-containing device is placed into the incision, in contact with the uveal tract (Fig. 62-4). The incision is closed with the scleral flap over the implant using 5-0 to 6-0 polyglactin 910 or similar absorbable suture material in a simple-interrupted pattern (Fig. 62-5). Recommended postoperative medications include flunixin meglumine (500 mg PO once a day) for 5 days, topical triple antibiotic ophthalmic ointment BID for 10 days, and topical atropine ointment SID for 7 days. A few horses were noted to have a mild flare-up following discontinuation of the flunixin meglumine, so additional systemic anti-inflammatory medication may be needed after 5 days.

Preliminary results from a clinical trial of over 100 horses with documented ERU suggest that it takes 30 to 45 days after implantation of the device to get adequate ocular levels of CsA. Approximately 75% of horses have had complete control of the uveitis 30 days after implantation. If recurrent episodes occur after implantation, traditional treatment with systemic NSAIDs, topical steroids, and atropine is recommended. Those horses that had recurrences of the uveitis, subjectively, required less medication to control the active inflammation, and the duration of their inflammatory episodes was shorter. More important, the suprachoroidal implant is not associated with any vision-threatening complications such as retinal detachment. The duration of delivery of medication from the current devices is approximately 24 to 30 months. Evaluation of the results from a multicenter clinical trial is currently underway; if the results are favorable, approval by the U.S. Food and Drug Administration and commercial manufacture of the device will follow. A similar device is being tested for effectiveness for chronic control of canine keratoconjunctivitis sicca. Other immunosuppressive medications may also be evaluated in similar devices, such as tacrolimus (FK506), sirolimus, and rapamycin.[13,14]

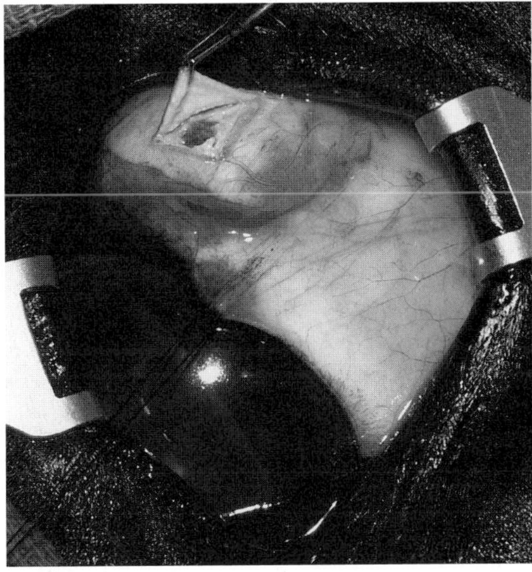

Figure 62-4. A 7-mm-wide scleral flap is made exposing the uveal tract (the black uvea is just visible through the sclera) approximately 8 mm posterior to the limbus and just lateral to the insertion of the dorsal rectus muscle.

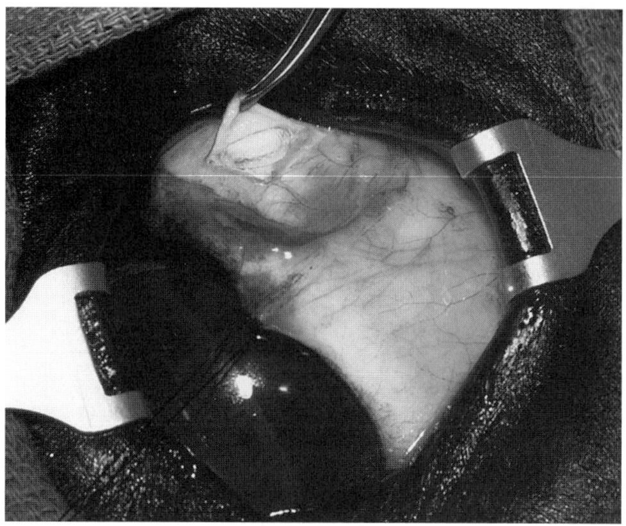

Figure 62-5. The cyclosporine A–containing device is placed into the incision, in contact with the uveal tract. The scleral flap and conjunctival incision is closed with 6-0 polyglactin 910 suture material in a simple-interrupted pattern followed by closure of the conjunctiva over the scleral incision.

PARS PLANA VITRECTOMY

For more than 25 years, pars plana vitrectomy (PPV)[15] has been used in the management of chronic endogenous uveitis (CEU) in humans.[16-20] The main goal was to improve vision by clearing the media or removing membranes. However, it turned out that PPV in eyes with CEU also altered or diminished the severity as well as the frequency of attacks.[18] There is evidence that PPV has a beneficial effect on the clinical course of chronic endogenous posterior uveitis, possibly by physically removing any resident inflammatory cells with the vitreous.[21] Despite the reported complications (i.e., vitreal hemorrhage, cataract formation, retinal detachment) after PPV, an overwhelming majority of the patients were able to be switched from rigorous systemic preoperative medication to simple eye drops or no treatment at all.[20]

Vitrectomy has been studied in experimental, protein-induced uveitis in rabbits,[22,23] but it was not until 1991 that PPV has been described in the management of equine recurrent uveitis.[24] PPV has since been increasingly employed in the treatment of ERU in Europe.[25,26] Similar to in humans, the most common complications reported in horses are transient hypopyon, vitreal or retinal hemorrhage, retinal detachment, and cataract formation.

In the majority of reported cases in Europe, *Leptospira* species have been identified in serum and diluted vitreous samples. This indicates that ERU is probably often a sequel of systemic *Leptospira* infection. The presence of intact *Leptospira* and specific antibodies in eyes affected with ERU indicates a local antibody production to *Leptospira* organisms and/or their antigens.[27-30]

Patient Selection

Because of the possible serious complications of PPV, patient selection is of great importance. All patients are examined by slit-lamp biomicroscopy, indirect and direct ophthalmoscopy, and applanation tonometry. Ultrasonography is performed in cases with opaque media. The diagnosis of ERU is based on the typical signs of acute or chronic uveitis and a documented history of recurrent episodes of acute uveitis. Horses ideally are operated in the quiescent stage of the disease. Because of the transpupillary visualization of the vitrectomy probe during the procedure, the optical media (i.e., cornea, anterior chamber, lens) should be as transparent as possible. The pupil should dilate maximally with no or few posterior synechiae. Preexisting focal cataracts are likely to progress after PPV. This should be taken into consideration. In patients with secondary glaucoma, phthisis bulbi, or preexisting retinal detachment, PPV should not be recommended. Owners should be carefully informed about the surgery, and in particular about the possible intraoperative and postoperative complications.

Preoperative and Postoperative Medication

Topical 0.1% dexamethasone drops in combination with neomycin and polymyxin B are administered QID beginning 1 week prior to surgery. Systemic NSAIDs (e.g., vedaprofen, flunixin meglumine) are administered beginning 3 days preoperatively.

The pupil is dilated with 1% atropine drops on the day of surgery.

Postoperatively, topical dexamethasone/neomycin/polymyxin B eye drops are continued 3 days a week for 2 weeks and then tapered over another 4 weeks.

Systemic NSAIDs are continued for 1 week.

Surgical Technique

A standard two-port PPV is performed in lateral recumbency under general inhalation anesthesia. The eye is prepared for intraocular surgery. After draping, an eyelid speculum is inserted. A lateral canthotomy may improve exposure of the globe. With a special manipulator, the globe is rotated to expose the dorsal bulbar conjunctiva. Alternatively, a limbal stay-suture may help globe manipulation. A limbal-based conjunctival flap is prepared and the sclera exposed medially and laterally to the dorsal rectus muscle. Using a CO_2 laser, a sclerotomy is performed 10 mm posterior to the limbus. A right-handed surgeon places this first entry to the left of the rectus muscle. The irrigation port is inserted and secured to the sclera with a 4-0 polyglactin 910 suture (Fig. 62-6). With the vitrectomy unit in continuous irrigation mode and the fluid-containing bottle positioned 85 cm higher than the surgical site, the intraocular pressure will be around 40 mm Hg. Physiologic saline solution with 40 mg of gentamicin added per 500 mL is used as irrigation fluid. A second laser sclerotomy is performed, again 10 mm posterior to the limbus and to the right of the rectus muscle (Fig. 62-7). The vitrectomy probe is carefully inserted and advanced in the direction of the center of the vitreous. The sclerotomy may be enlarged with a lacrimal dilator if necessary. Care is taken to avoid touching the lens when inserting the probe (Fig. 62-8). The probe tip should be held with the aspiration port facing the surgeon. In this position, the port can be visualized through the pupil using the light of an indirect binocular ophthalmoscope (Fig. 62-9).

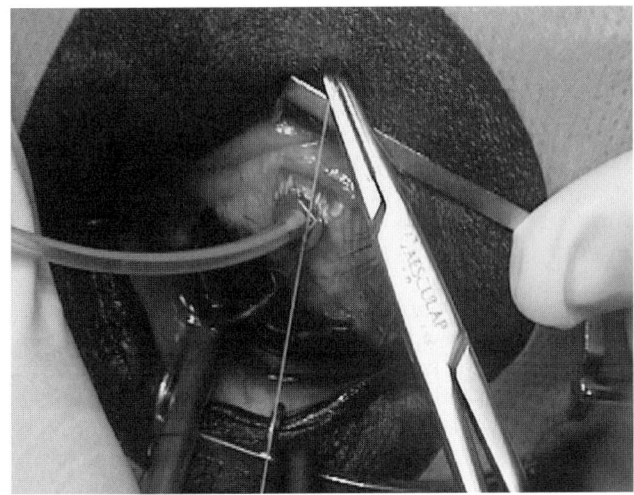

Figure 62-6. The irrigation port of the two-port vitrectomy unit is anchored to the sclera using 4-0 Vicryl.

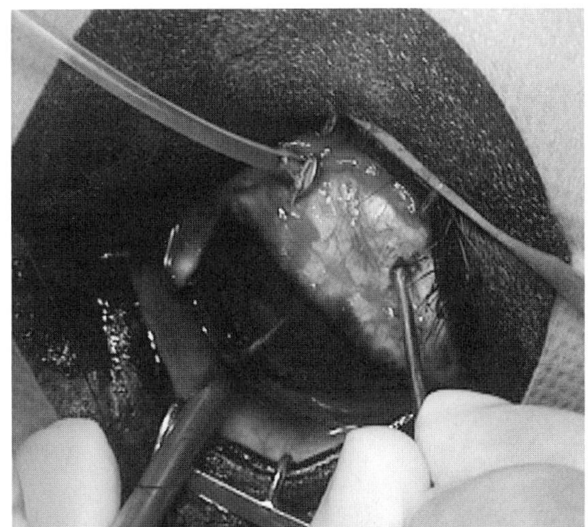

Figure 62-8. The custom-made vitrectomy hand piece is advanced into the center of the vitreous cavity.

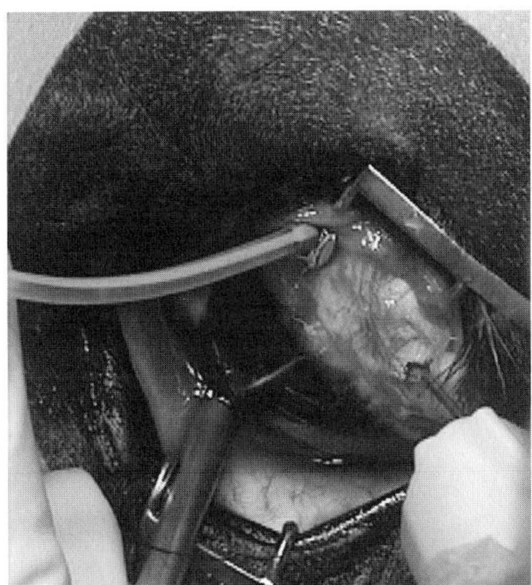

Figure 62-7. CO_2 laser sclerotomy for the vitrectomy hand piece.

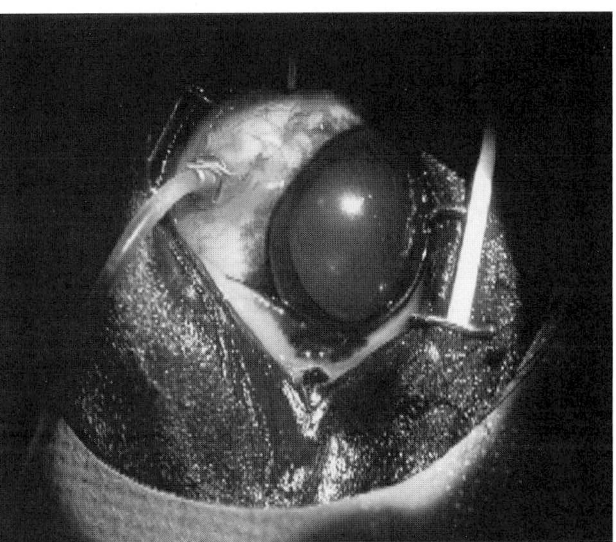

Figure 62-9. Vitrectomy is performed in a darkened operating theater using a binocular indirect ophthalmoscope and a 20D lens. The vitrectomy probe can be visualized through the dilated pupil. (Courtesy Dr. B. Wollanke.)

With a 20D lens in the left hand and the vitrectomy probe in the right, vitrectomy is started. Aspiration of vitreous can easily be seen. Again, care is taken to avoid the lens. Estimating the distance between the probe and its shadow cast onto the retina helps the surgeon avoid touching the retina. Throughout the entire procedure, the intraocular pressure (IOP) should be maintained at approximately 40 mm Hg. Slight wrinkling of the retina, seen with the aid of the ophthalmoscope, indicates that the IOP may be too low. Vitrectomy should be interrupted until a normal IOP is restored. The procedure is continued until all turbid vitreal material has been removed. Under continuous irrigation, the vitrectomy probe is removed and the sclerotomy closed with one or two pre-placed simple interrupted sutures using 4-0 polyglactin 910. Subsequently, the irrigation port is removed. Remaining vitreous will usually prevent fluid from escaping through this sclerotomy, which is closed with 4-0 polyglactin 910. The conjunctiva is closed with polyglactin 910 in a continuous pattern. The canthotomy is closed with a figure-of-eight suture using 4-0 nonabsorbable suture materials.

At the end of surgery, 20 mg of methylprednisolone is injected subconjunctivally into the inferior bulbar conjunctiva.

Technical Aspects

To avoid uveal hemorrhage both sclerotomies are performed using a CO_2 laser in continuous mode at 50 W. Commercially available vitrectomy probes are too short for use in horses. A custom-made 55-mm oscillating vitrectomy probe is used at 6.5 Hz, at an aspiration vacuum of 240 mm Hg, and at a flow rate of 20 mL/min (Fig. 62-10). A custom-made globe manipulator is used to position the globe (Fig. 62-11).

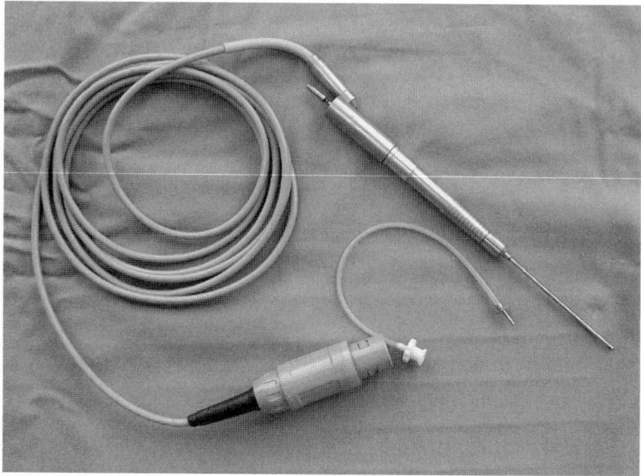

Figure 62-10. Custom-made vitrectomy hand piece with a 55-mm shaft and independent irrigation port.

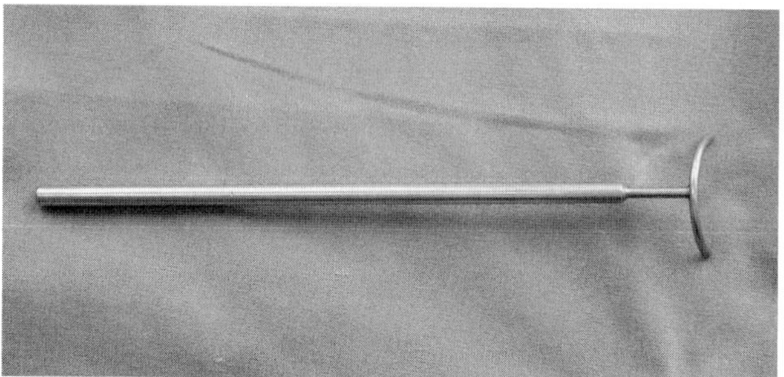

Figure 62-11. Custom-made globe manipulator to facilitate globe rotation during laser sclerotomy.

Complications

Intraoperative complications include vitreal/retinal hemorrhage and retinal detachment. Maintaining IOP at around 40 mm Hg and using a CO_2 laser for the sclerotomies instead of surgical blades can avoid hemorrhage. Touching the retina should also be avoided as it results in immediate hemorrhage and subsequent detachment.[24-26]

Early postoperative complications (less than 3 months) include cataract formation and retinal detachment. Late complications occurring after 3 months include cataract formation as well as recurrence of active uveitis.[21,26]

Long-term Results

In one study of 38 cases, five eyes showed recurrence of uveitis between 10 days and 3 years postoperatively.[26] Thirty-three eyes showed no recurrence during a follow-up period of up to 5 years. Vision remained stable in 28 eyes and improved in one eye. The remaining eyes showed marked vision loss as a result of cataracts (3), phthisis bulbi (1), or unknown causes (1). Of the five eyes with recurrent uveitis two demonstrated marked loss of vision, and three maintained preoperative vision.

In an earlier study of 43 eyes after PPV, 42 remained free of recurrent uveitis during the follow-up period of 67 months, and of these eyes, 70% retained some vision.[31] The most common complication was cataract formation in 19 of 43 eyes, followed by phthisis bulbi in six eyes, and retinal detachment in four eyes.

The authors' results are similar to those of other groups. Episodes of recurrent uveitis were reported to us in only 3% and vision was retained in 50% of the patients. Complications causing visual impairment or blindness include phthisis bulbi in 15%, cataract formation in 15%, retinal detachment in 10%, and corneal calcific degeneration in 10%.

Most veterinary ophthalmologists agree that long-term prognosis for ERU with medical therapy alone is poor. Even aggressive therapy is often insufficient to prevent recurrent painful inflammatory episodes. Cumulative intraocular damage often leads to phthisis bulbi, glaucoma, or loss of vision as a result of cataract formation or retinal detachment.

In selected patients with consenting owners, PPV offers a promising alternative to conventional therapy. With few exceptions, eyes show no recurrence of uveitis after PPV. However, a significant number of postoperative complications cause visual impairment or blindness. The most common long-term postoperative complication appears to be cataract formation. It is unclear whether preexisting lenticular opacities progress despite PPV or whether the progression is caused by the procedure. Touching the posterior lens capsule during PPV invariably leads to focal cataracts, which very often progress.

Retinal and vitreal hemorrhage is the most common intraoperative complication. Maintaining a high normal IOP, careful manipulation of the vitrectomy probe, and avoidance of touching the retina usually prevents such complications. Choroidal hemorrhage can be avoided with the use of a CO_2 laser instead of a surgical blade.

REFERENCES

1. Davis J, Gilger BC, Robinson M: Novel approaches to ocular drug delivery, Curr Opin Mol Ther 2004;6:44.
2. Kay JE: Inhibitory effects of cyclosporin A on lymphocyte activation. In Thomson AW, editor: Cyclosporine: Mode of Action and Clinical Application, Dordrecht, 1989, Kluuver Academic.
3. Granelli-Piperno A: Cellular mode of action of cyclosporin A. In Bach JF, editor: T-Cell Directed Immunointervention, Oxford, 1993, Blackwell Scientific.
4. BenEzra D, Maftzir G: Ocular penetration of cyclosporine A in the rat eye, Arch Ophthalmol 1990;108:584,.
5. BenEzra D, Maftzir G: Ocular penetration of cyclosporin A: The rabbit eye, Invest Ophthalmol Vis Sci 1990;31:1362.
6. BenEzra D, Maftizir G, de Courten C, et al: Ocular penetration of cyclosporin A: III. The human eye, Br J Ophthalmol 1990;74:350.
7. Svenson K, Bohman SO, Hallgren R: Renal interstitial fibrosis and vascular changes. Occurrence in patients with autoimmune diseases treated with cyclosporine, Arch Intern Med 1986;146:2007,.
8. Jaffe GJ, Yang CS, Wang XC, et al: Intravitreal sustained-release cyclosporine in the treatment of experimental uveitis, Ophthalmology 1998;105:46.
9. Enyedi LB, Pearson PA, Ashton P, et al: An intravitreal device providing sustained release of cyclosporine and dexamethasone, Curr Eye Res 1996;15:549.
10. Gilger BC, Malok E, Stewart T, et al: Long-term effect on the equine eye of an intravitreal device used for sustained release of cyclosporine A, Vet Ophthalmol 2000;3:105.
11. Gilger BC, Malok E, Stewart T, et al: Effect of an intravitreal

cyclosporine implant on experimental uveitis in horses, Vet Immunol Immunopathol 2000;76:239.
12. Gilger BC, Wilkie DA, Davidson MG, et al: Use of an intravitreal sustained-release cyclosporine delivery device for treatment of equine recurrent uveitis, Am J Vet Res 2001;62:1892.
13. Kulkarni P: Review: uveitis and immunosuppressive drugs, J Ocul Pharmacol Ther 2001;17:181.
14. Sakurai E, Nozaki M, Okabe K, et al: Scleral plug of biodegradable polymers containing tacrolimus (FK506) for experimental uveitis, Invest Ophthalmol Vis Sci 2003;44:4845.
15. Becker MD, Harsch N, Ziehut M, et al: Therapeutische Vitrektomie bei Uveitis Aktueller Stand und Empfehlungen, Ophthalmologe 2003;100:787.
16. Diamond JG, Kaplan HJ: Lensectomy and vitrectomy for complicated cataract secondary to uveitis, Arch Ophthalmol 1978;96:1798.
17. Diamond JG Kaplan HJ: Uveitis: Effect of vitrectomy combined with lensectomy, Ophthalmology 1979;86:1320,.
18. Binder S, Freyler H: Vitrektomie bei entzundlichen Erkrankungen des hinteren Augenabschnittes, Klin Monatsbl Augenheilk 1983;183:86.
19. Werry H. Honegger H: Pars-plana Vitrektomie bei chronischer Uveitis, Klin Monatsbl Augenheilk 1987;191:9,.
20. Kloti R: Pars-plana Vitrektomie bei chronischer Uveitis, Klin Monatsbl Augenheilk 1988;192:425.
21. Scott RA, Haynes RJ, Orr GM, et al: Vitreous surgery in the management of chronic endogenous posterior uveitis, Eye 2003;17:221.
22. Kaplan HJ, Diamond JG, Brown SA: Vitrectomy in experimental uveitis. II. Method in eyes with protein-induced uveitis, Arch Ophthalmol 1979;97:336.
23. Kaplan HJ, Diamond JG, Brown SA: Vitrectomy in experimental uveitis: I. Operative technique in rabbits, Arch Ophthalmol 1979;97:331.
24. Werry H, Gerhards H: Möglichkeiten und Indikationen zur chirurgischen Behandlung der equinen rezidivierenden Uveitis (ERU), Pferdeheilkunde 1991;7:321.
25. Werry H, Gerhards H: [The surgical therapy of equine recurrent uveitis], Tieraerztl Prax 1992;20:178.
26. Frühauf B, Ohnesorge B, Deegen E, et al: Surgical management of equine recurrent uveitis with single port pars plana vitrectomy, Vet Ophthalmol 1998;1:137.
27. Brem S, Gerhards H, Wollanke B, et al: Intraokularer Leptospirennachweis bei 4 Pferden mit rezidivierender Uveitis (ERU). Berl Munch Tierarztl Wochenschr 1998;111:415.
28. Brem S, Gerhards H, Wollanke B, et al: 35 Leptospirenisolationen aus Glaskorpern von 32 Pferden mit rezidivierender Uveitis (ERU). Berl Munch Tierarztl Wochenschr 1999;112:390.
29. Wollanke B, Rohrbach BW, Gerhards H: Serum and vitreous humor antibody titers in and isolation of *Leptospira* interrogans from horses with recurrent uveitis, J AmVet Med Assoc 2001;219:795.
30. Wollanke B, Gerhards H, Brem S, et al: Etiology of equine recurrent uveitis (ERU): Autoimmune disease or intraocular leptospiral infection? Pferdeheilkunde 2004;20:327.
31. Winterberg A, Gerhards H: Longterm results of pars plana vitrectomy in equine recurrent uveitis, Pferdeheilkunde 1997; 13:377.

CHAPTER 63

Orbit

Dennis E. Brooks

ANATOMY AND PHYSIOLOGY

The diagnosis and treatment of soft tissue and osseous orbital disease in the horse requires a clear understanding of the normal equine globe and orbital anatomy. The adult equine orbit is 62.1 mm in width, 59.4 mm in height, and 98.3 mm in depth.[1] The globe of the equine eye is larger in the horizontal (48.4 mm) than in the vertical (47.6 mm) diameter.[1,2] The mean anterior-to-posterior diameter is 43.7 mm.[1] The volume of the equine globe ranges between 45.0 and 50.9 mL.[3] The orbits and globes of the horse skull are directed anteriorly, slightly dorsally, and are positioned 80 degrees lateral to the midline to allow wide panoramic vision.[1,2] The orbits are bony cavities formed by the frontal, lacrimal, zygomatic, temporal, sphenoid, and palatine bones, and they function to protect the globe[1-5] (Fig. 63-1). The orbits of the horse are open anteriorly and closed posteriorly, they possess a soft tissue–covered ventral floor, and they contain osseous canals, fissures, and foramina.[1-5] Sinuses surround the orbit.

The anterior rim of the bony orbit is complete in the horse[1-5] (see Fig. 63-1). The nasal wall is extensive and formed by the frontal, lacrimal, and presphenoid bones. The roof or dorsal wall is formed by the frontal and, to a small degree, the lacrimal bone. The orbital floor or ventral wall consists anteriorly of the zygomatic bone and the zygomatic

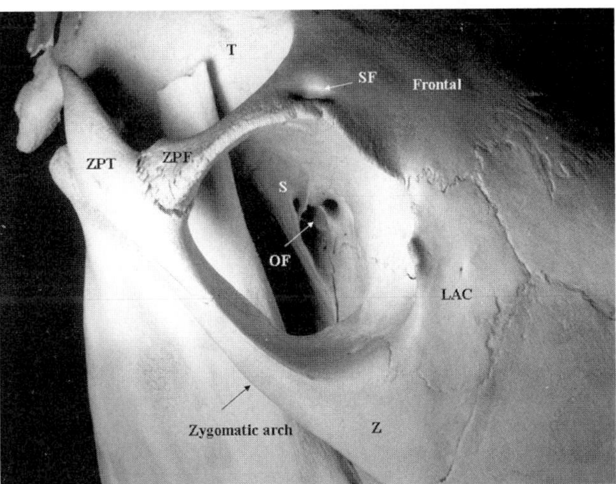

Figure 63-1. A normal skull, demonstrating the complete anterior bony orbital rim of the horse. The pertinent bones that form the orbit of the horse are labeled. LAC, lacrimal bone; OF, orbital foramina including ethmoid, optic, orbital fissure, and rostral alar; S, sphenoid bone; SF, supraorbital foramen; T, temporal bone; Z, zygomatic bone; ZPF, zygomatic process of the frontal bone; ZPT, zygomatic process of the temporal bone.

process of the temporal bone, with the larger posterior orbital floor consisting of soft tissue formed by periorbital fascia.[2,4,6] The zygomatic arch, formed by the zygomatic process of the frontal bone, the frontal process of the zygomatic bone, and the zygomatic process of the temporal bone, closes the temporal orbital wall.[1,4] Trauma to the prominent zygomatic arch of the horse skull may result in severe skin lacerations because the anterior edge of the zygomatic arch facial crest is quite sharp.

The zygomatic process of the frontal bone contains the supraorbital foramen, which carries sensory nerve fibers to the upper eyelid.[1,2,4,5] The lacrimal bone forms the nasal part of the anterior orbital rim. The anterior ventral surface contains the entrance to the lacrimal canal, and it is the site of origin for the ventral oblique muscle.[1,2,4] The sphenoid bones form the nasal, posterior, and ventral orbital boundaries.[1,2,4] The optic nerve and internal ophthalmic artery pass in the optic canal of the presphenoid bone and enter the orbit at the optic foramen. The basisphenoid bone is associated with the orbital and round foramina, the alar canal, the maxillary artery and nerve, and the cavernous sinus.[2,4]

The extreme posterior orbit contains the ethmoidal foramen with the ethmoidal vessels and nerve, the optic foramen with the optic nerve and internal ophthalmic artery, the orbital foramen with cranial nerves III through VI, the round foramen and the maxillary nerve, and the rostral alar foramen with the external ophthalmic and maxillary arteries.[1,2,4] The maxillary, sphenopalatine, and major palatine foramina and their associated blood vessels and nerves are found ventral to the anterior portion of the orbital cavity in the pterygopalatine fossa.[1,2,4]

The orbital system functions as a precise and complex unit.[7] An extensive system of orbital connective tissues forms a framework for the compartmentalization and support of all orbital structures to maintain appropriate anatomic relationships and to allow the precise and coordinated globe movements.[5,7] The essential components of the orbital connective tissues are the periorbita, the orbital septum, and the episcleral fascia or Tenon's capsule.[1,4,5]

Periosteum lines the orbital bones and the optic and orbital foramina.[2,4,5,7] Attached to the surface of the periosteum are multiple layers of orbital connective tissue called the periorbita. The inner layers of the periorbita continue anteriorly as the orbital septum, which separates from the periosteum at the lid margin to continue into the lid as the tarsal plate. The optic nerve is contained within a dural sheath that is continuous at the orbital apex with the periosteum of the optic canal. Well-developed fascial slings of the orbital septum form suspensory complexes with orbital fat to maintain precise extraocular muscle alignment as the globe moves.[7] Tenon's capsule, also termed episcleral fascia, is located between the conjunctiva and sclera. Tenon's capsule begins anteriorly at the perilimbal sclera and extends around the globe to the optic nerve, where it blends with fibers of the dural sheath and sclera.[2,4,5,7] It is firmly adherent to the episcleral tissue anterior to the scleral insertions of the rectus muscles.[1,4,5]

The frontal sinus is located dorsal and ventral to the medial orbit.[4] The maxillary sinus is located ventral and nasal to the orbit. The bony plate between the orbit and maxillary sinus is very thin.[4] The anterior maxillary sinus can be located just ventral to the intersection of (1) a line between the medial canthus and infraorbital foramen and (2) a perpendicular line from the fourth cheek tooth.[3] Trephination dorsal to a line drawn between the infraorbital foramen and the medial canthus may result in nasolacrimal duct damage (see Chapter 42). The center of a line drawn between the medial canthus and the facial crest indicates the location of the caudal maxillary sinus.[3] The sphenopalatine sinus is located medial and ventral to the orbit. All sinuses in the horse communicate with the nasal cavity either directly or via the maxillary sinus.[3,4] In horses, sinus disease involving the frontal, maxillary, or sphenopalatine sinuses may intrude on the orbit.[3,8]

The lacrimal gland, orbital fat, and connective tissue fascia completely fill the orbital spaces between the globe, extraocular muscles, optic and other cranial nerves, and orbital vascular elements of horses to provide a cushion that protects these delicate structures from injury during ocular movements. The lacrimal gland is situated dorsolaterally between the zygomatic process and the globe.[4,5] It is separated from the globe by periorbital fascia, and it opens via 12 to 16 small ducts along the lateral part of the conjunctival sac in a line anterior to the dorsal conjunctival fornix.[5] Care should be taken when preparing conjunctival flaps or when placing subpalpebral lavage systems in this area, since damage to these ducts could result in a tear insufficiency problem. There is no orbital salivary gland in the horse.[4] A cushion of fat lies in the ventral equine orbit.[4]

The horse has seven extraocular muscles.[1-5] The dorsal rectus muscle rotates the globe dorsally, and the ventral rectus muscle rotates the globe ventrally. The medial and lateral rectus muscles rotate the eye medially and laterally, respectively. The dorsal oblique muscle rotates the dorsal part of the eye medially and ventrally along an anterior–posterior axis, and the ventral oblique muscle rotates the ventral part of the eye medially and dorsally. The retractor bulbi muscle pulls the globe into the orbit to allow passive movement of the nictitating membrane to protect the globe. All extraocular muscles except the ventral oblique arise near the optic foramen. The sites of scleral insertion of the equine extraocular muscles are listed in Table 63-1.[2,3] The oculomotor nerve innervates the ventral oblique muscle and the dorsal, ventral, and medial rectus muscles. The abducens nerve innervates the lateral rectus and retractor bulbi muscles. The trochlear nerve innervates the dorsal oblique muscle.

PATHOPHYSIOLOGY

Orbital disease processes may occur within the extraocular muscle cone (intraconal), between the muscle cone and the periorbital sheath, or external to the periorbital sheath (subperiosteal).[9] Orbital diseases can result in exophthalmos caused by space-occupying orbital lesions, or in enophthalmos if the volume of the orbital contents becomes reduced as a result of malnutrition or disease.[3,9,10] The degree and direction of exophthalmos depends on the size and location of the lesion. Intraconal lesions cause anterior displacement of the globe.[9] Lesions of the medial orbit displace the globe laterally. Exposure keratitis may result because of the inability of the lids to cover the cornea in a severe case of exophthalmos. Large space-occupying masses such as tumors or bone fragments can limit ocular motility

TABLE 63-1. Extraocular Muscle Scleral Insertion Sites in the Horse

Extraocular Muscle	Scleral Insertion Sites*
Dorsal rectus	9-13 (11.2) mm from limbus
Ventral rectus	8 (8.0) mm from limbus
Medial rectus	10 (14.2) mm from limbus
Lateral rectus	12 (4.0) mm from limbus dorsally, 5 mm ventrally
Dorsal oblique	14 (14.2) mm from limbus dorsally, 23 mm ventrally
Ventral oblique	21 (4.8) mm from limbus dorsally, 3 mm ventrally
Retractor bulbi	37 mm from limbus dorsally 18 mm from limbus ventrally 18 mm from limbus medially 22 mm from limbus laterally

Values for the distances from the limbus for the muscle insertions are from references 2 (in parentheses) and 3.

and impair ocular circulation. The globe size of the exophthalmic eye is normal and should not be confused with the globe enlargement (buphthalmos) noted in advanced equine glaucoma. The nictitating membrane may protrude with exophthalmos or enophthalmos.

Infectious, traumatic, inflammatory, or neoplastic disease processes involving the eyelids, paranasal sinuses, tooth roots, guttural pouch, or nasal cavity may extend into the orbit to cause exophthalmos.[3,6,8-21] Fractures of the walls of the paranasal sinuses and orbit can result in enophthalmos, facial deformity, and orbital emphysema. Tooth root abscesses may cause sinus and orbital disease.

DIAGNOSTIC PROCEDURES

The diagnosis of orbital disease may require special diagnostic procedures in addition to a complete ophthalmic examination.

Retrobulbar Needle Aspiration

Aspiration of fluid or biopsy of a mass behind the globe should be performed for culture, cytology and/or histopathology for differentiation of space occupying masses in cases of exophthalmos (Fig. 63-2). An 18-gauge, 10-cm, slightly curved needle is inserted 1 cm lateral to the lateral canthus and directed posteriorly in a line parallel to the medial canthus. Care is taken to prevent damage to the globe or optic nerve. This technique may be varied in selected cases by making a small skin incision and obtaining a large-needle core biopsy from the supraorbital fossa behind the globe.

Retrobulbar Nerve Blocks

Orbital or retrobulbar anesthesia can reduce eye and third eyelid movement, and it can decrease corneal sensation for short ophthalmic procedures such as eyelid laceration repair, nictitans removal, corneal foreign body removal, intraocular injections or aqueocentesis, or iris cyst laser ablation in standing horses and horses under general anesthesia. Retrobulbar nerve blocks can reduce the depth of general anesthesia required for enucleation surgery. A 22-gauge, 6.25-cm spinal needle is inserted through the skin prepared for aseptic surgery of the orbital fossa, just caudal to the posterior aspect of the bony dorsal orbital rim. The needle is advanced until it reaches the retrobulbar muscle cone. This can be detected by slight dorsal movement of the eye. Once positioned, 10 to 12 mL of 2% lidocaine is injected into the orbit. Slight exophthalmos occurs. The lidocaine takes effect in 5 minutes and lasts 1 to 2 hours.[22]

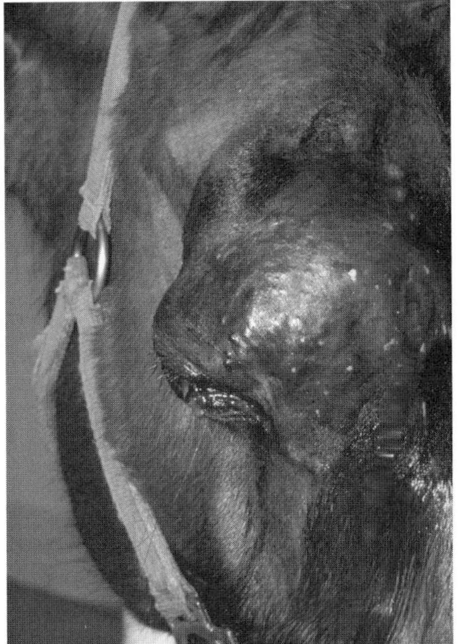

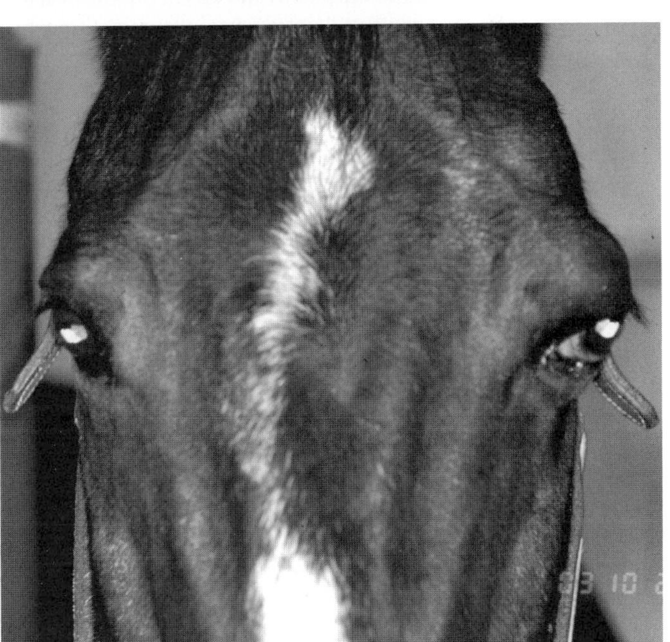

Figure 63-2. A, Progressive exophthalmos as a result of an osteoma of the frontal bone in this 12-year-old mare. The horse still had vision in this eye. **B,** Exophthalmos in aged gelding. Computed tomography (see Fig. 63-4, *B*) revealed a sinus tumor to be the cause of the orbital disease.

Radiography

Radiography is especially useful in fracture localization and diseases associated with bony destruction. Meticulous attention to detail in film handling and patient positioning, and a thorough knowledge of normal equine orbital anatomy are required for radiographic examination of the horse with signs of orbital disease.[9] Good-quality films can be obtained with portable radiographic equipment and rare earth screens.

Radiographs should be taken using lateral, ventrodorsal, oblique, and dorsoventral views to attempt to identify ocular and orbital foreign bodies, tumors, fractures, or the extent of soft tissue or bony lesions (Fig. 63-3). Oblique views should be oriented to silhouette the area of greatest soft tissue swelling, with a contralateral (normal) oblique view used for comparison. Special attention should be directed to examination of the nasal cavity, paranasal sinuses, tooth roots and calvarium. Dorsoventral views reveal nasal cavity or bony nasolacrimal duct problems. In the evaluation of unilateral lesions, the involved portion should be placed against the film cassette. Most lateral, dorsoventral, and oblique views of the equine orbit can be obtained with the use of xylazine sedation. Ventrodorsal views of the orbit require general anesthesia. A Flieringa ring placed at the limbus can help localize the globe and orbit. Orbital aspirates and biopsies may be performed after the radiographic study of the orbital region so as not to introduce artifactual changes into the radiographic image. The reader might want to review the normal radiographic orbital anatomy of the horse.[23]

The multiple superimposed bones, teeth, soft tissue, and air shadows in a skull radiograph of a horse may initially appear to be nothing more than a confusing mass of shadows. Increased soft tissue densities and lytic bone changes are associated with neoplasia and chronic inflammatory diseases. Calcification of soft tissues may develop as a result of orbital cellulitis and tumors.

The advent of high-resolution computed tomography (CT) and magnetic resonance imaging (MRI) has dramatically enhanced orbital evaluation in humans and small animals, and it is the procedure of choice in these species.[24,25] In the horse, CT and MRI are more limited because of the ratio of the size of the animal to size of the imaging units.[18,24] Foals can be easily evaluated by these methods. Utilization of these techniques in equine ophthalmology continues to increase (Fig. 63-4).

Ultrasonography

Ocular ultrasonography is a noninvasive diagnostic procedure that can qualitatively and quantitatively evaluate various globe and orbital abnormalities. It is indicated for evaluation of an exophthalmic globe or a globe obscured by opacities of the cornea, lens, or vitreous.[25,26] Differentiation

A

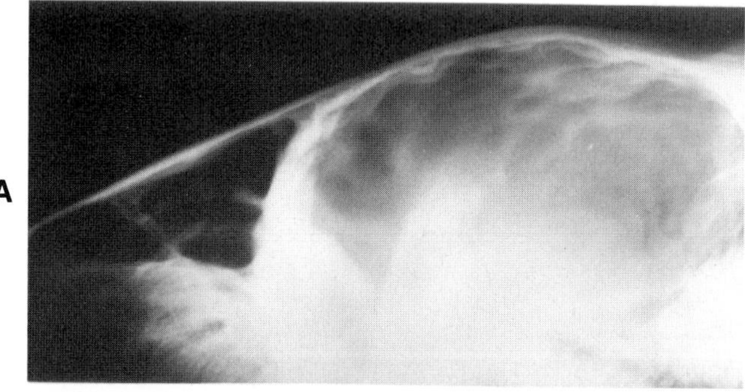

B

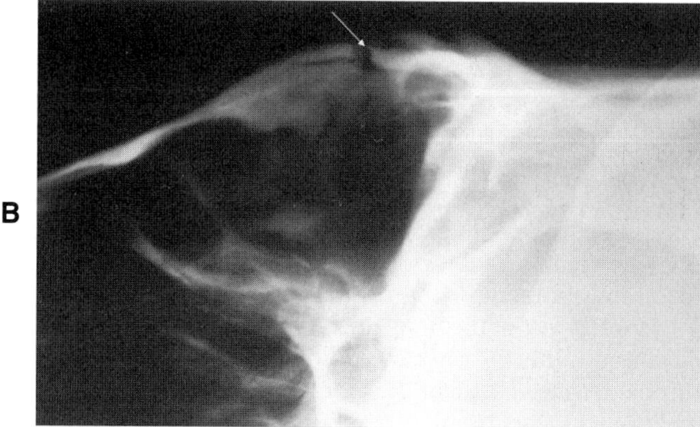

Figure 63-3. An orbital fracture is difficult to visualize on a lateral skull radiograph (**A**), but it is easily seen *(arrow)* on an oblique view (**B**).

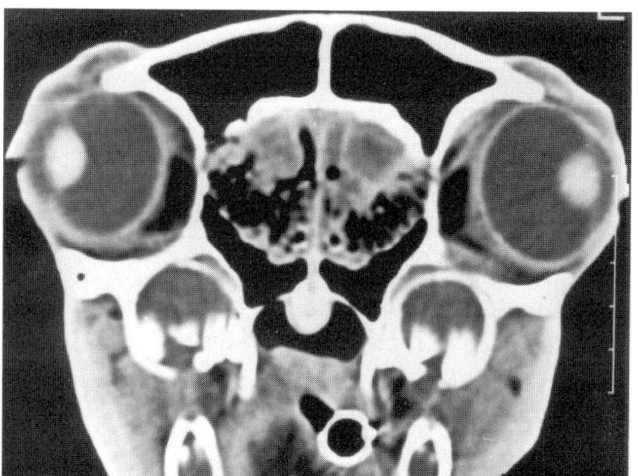

A

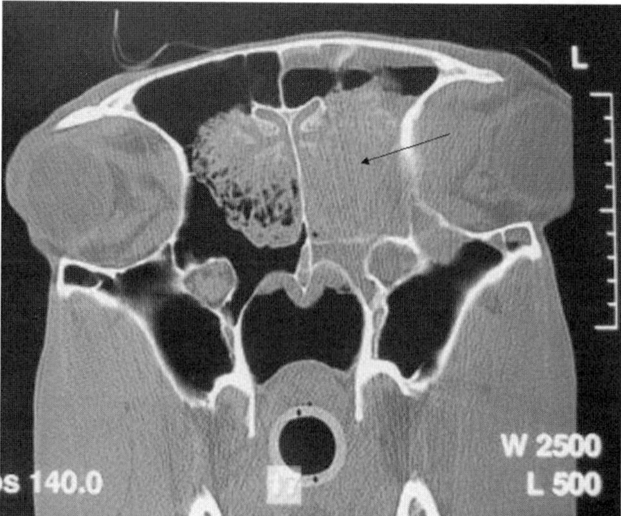

B

Figure 63-4. A, The globes, intraocular contents and extraocular muscles are shown at the level of the orbit in a transverse computed tomography (CT) of a normal horse. **B,** A CT image demonstrates a sinus tumor that has invaded the orbit *(arrow)* in an old horse (see Fig. 63-2).

of solid soft orbital tissue masses versus cystic orbital masses (Fig. 63-5), determination of the size of various globe or orbital components, and localization of orbital foreign bodies are possible. Real time B-scan ultrasound units emit focused sound waves to produce a two-dimensional cross-section of orbital tissues, with ultrasound probes of 7.5 or 10 MHz providing the best resolution. The ultrasonic transducer can be placed in contact with the eyelids via a methylcellulose coupling agent to evaluate the globe and anterior orbit, or it can be placed in gentle contact with the cornea after instillation of a topical anesthetic to evaluate the posterior orbit. For the evaluation of the orbital structures, the ultrasonic beam is angled so that it enters the orbit between the globe and the bony orbital wall. This bypasses the lens, which tends to attenuate the sound beam and maximizes the echo intensity. Most orbital lesions exhibit lower reflectivity and less sound attenuation than the normal orbital contents. Foreign bodies are hyperechoic in many cases. The opposite globe and orbit provide a normal "control" for comparison purposes (see Fig. 63-5, *C*).

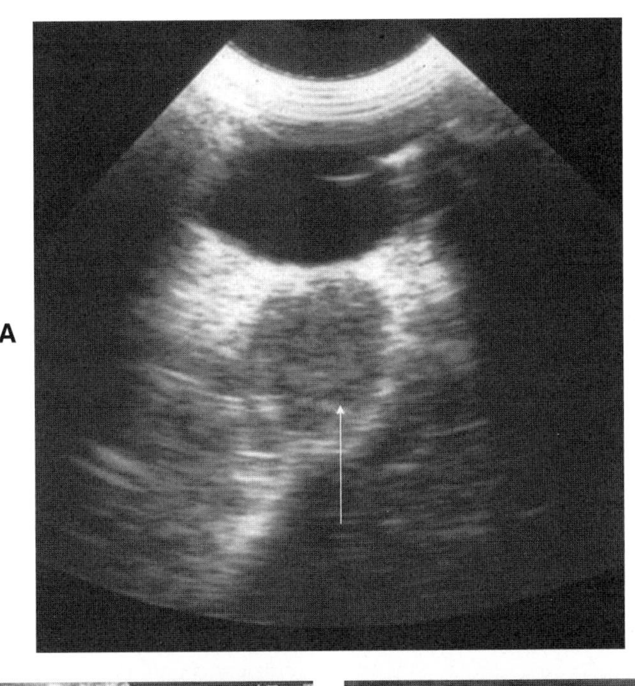

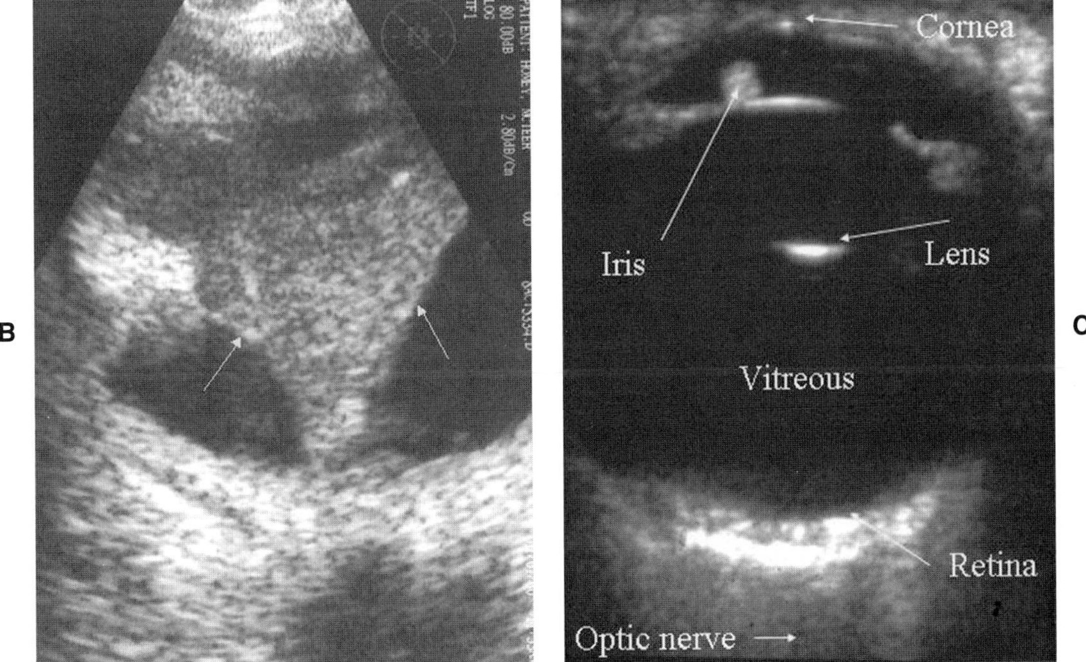

Figure 63-5. A, B-scan ultrasonographic view reveals an orbital optic nerve tumor *(arrow)*. **B,** This ultrasonographic scan reveals a retinal detachment that resulted from severe eye trauma *(arrows)*. The vitreous is opaque from hemorrhage. **C,** A normal B-scan ultrasonographic image is shown for comparison.

SURGICAL TECHNIQUES

The instruments needed for orbital surgeries such as enucleation, exenteration, and evisceration (Fig. 63-6) are the standard instruments utilized for soft tissue surgeries. Some magnification via head loupe is helpful. If the zygomatic arch or other orbital bones need to be removed, osteotomes, an oscillating bone saw, and pneumatic drill are required.

Exenteration

Indication and Surgical Technique

Orbital exenteration is a surgical technique used to remove large malignant tumors of the orbit that are unresponsive to chemotherapy or radiotherapy[9,27] (see Fig. 63-6, *B*). In this procedure, the entire orbital contents, including periorbita and globe, are surgically removed. The eyeball or globe is enucleated first (see Fig. 63-6, *A*). Periosteal elevators may be needed to remove the periorbital fascia. The remaining tissue is excised using scalpel or scissors. Bleeding is controlled with ligation and cautery. A skin graft can be used to cover the open socket if excessive eyelid skin must be removed, or the socket can be left to granulate and epithelialize in rare cases. A permanent tarsorrhaphy is performed to cover the orbital cavity if the lids were not involved in the disease process.

Aftercare

Postoperative care should include pressure dressings on the head to reduce swelling and the use of a tamponade if hemorrhage was severe. Systemic antibiotics and nonsteroidal anti-inflammatories are indicated. Inadvertent entry into a paranasal sinus may require trephination of the sinus, lavage, and drainage.

Evisceration

Evisceration refers to the surgical removal of the iris, lens, ciliary body, choroids, vitreous and retina. The cornea, the sclera, and their extraocular muscle attachments are left intact[9,27-30] (see Fig. 63-6, *C*). This is performed prior to placement of an intrascleral silicone implant or a prosthesis. Evisceration is not generally recommended for an eye suspected of having an intraocular tumor or infection, or for eyes with severe corneal disease. Horses beginning to undergo globe atrophy or phthisis bulbi are good candidates. This surgery is performed mainly for cosmetic purposes.

Surgical Procedure

A 180-degree limbal peritomy is performed with tenotomy scissors. The conjunctiva is then undermined so that the sclera near the limbus is free of conjunctiva and fascia. A no. 15 blade is used to make a 180-degree full-thickness incision in the sclera 4 to 5 mm from the limbus. Suction and cautery are used to control extensive hemorrhage and visualize the incision. A lens loop or evisceration spoon is used to remove all the intraocular contents while the globe is fixed with toothed forceps. Care is taken to avoid scraping the corneal endothelium. A silicone implant of suitable size (usually 34 to 44 mm) is inserted into the sclera so that suturing the sclera can be accomplished without undue tension. Preoperative ultrasonic measurement of the normal eye aids in the selection of the proper-size implant. The anterior face of the implant can be trimmed to create a flatter surface in the part of the implant that is apposed to the cornea.[28,29] Simple-interrupted sutures of 6-0 absorbable suture are placed in the sclera, and a simple-continuous pattern of 6-0 absorbable suture is placed in the conjunctiva.

Aftercare

Topically applied antibiotics and systemically administered antibiotics and nonsteroidal anti-inflammatories should be used postoperatively. A temporary tarsorrhaphy protects the cornea while postoperative eyelid swelling subsides.

Complications

The main complications are extrusion of the implant as a result of rubbing of the head, and postoperative infection.[28] Enucleation is the only recourse if these occur. Protective headgear helps prevent irritation from head rubbing. Placement of too small an implant results in a cosmetically unacceptable eye. Owners should be warned that corneal opacification and vascularization also may occur in some animals and cause problems with ocular cosmesis. Corneal opacification in show horses can be masked for short times with tinted contact lenses. Healing time of intrascleral implants is typically 6 to 8 weeks.

Enucleation

Indication and Types

Enucleation refers to surgical removal of the globe, conjunctiva, and nictitating membrane (see Fig. 63-6, *A*) because of severe corneal infection and endophthalmitis, corneal or adnexal neoplasia, orbital neoplasia, or severe ocular trauma causing a painful, blind eye. This procedure does not necessarily indicate a failure of ophthalmic care; it may be a necessary and planned treatment for specific conditions. The two basic approaches to enucleation in the horse are the transpalpebral and subconjunctival techniques.[27] Orbital silicone implants may be placed with either method to reduce "pitting" of the eyelid skin after enucleation.[28]

Transpalpebral Enucleation Technique

The transpalpebral technique (see Fig. 63-6, *D* through *G*) is most useful for cases of severe corneal infection, endophthalmitis, and widespread neoplasia of the conjunctiva, nictitating membrane, cornea, or orbit. It does leave a large orbital soft tissue defect.[9,27] In this approach, dissection into the orbit is made external to the extraocular muscles. The conjunctiva, globe, and nictitating membrane are completely removed en masse.

The eyelids are sutured together with a simple-continuous suture and the ends held with hemostatic forceps (see Fig. 63-6, *D* through *G*). An incision 5 mm from the eyelid margin (where the skin hair begins) is made with a no. 15

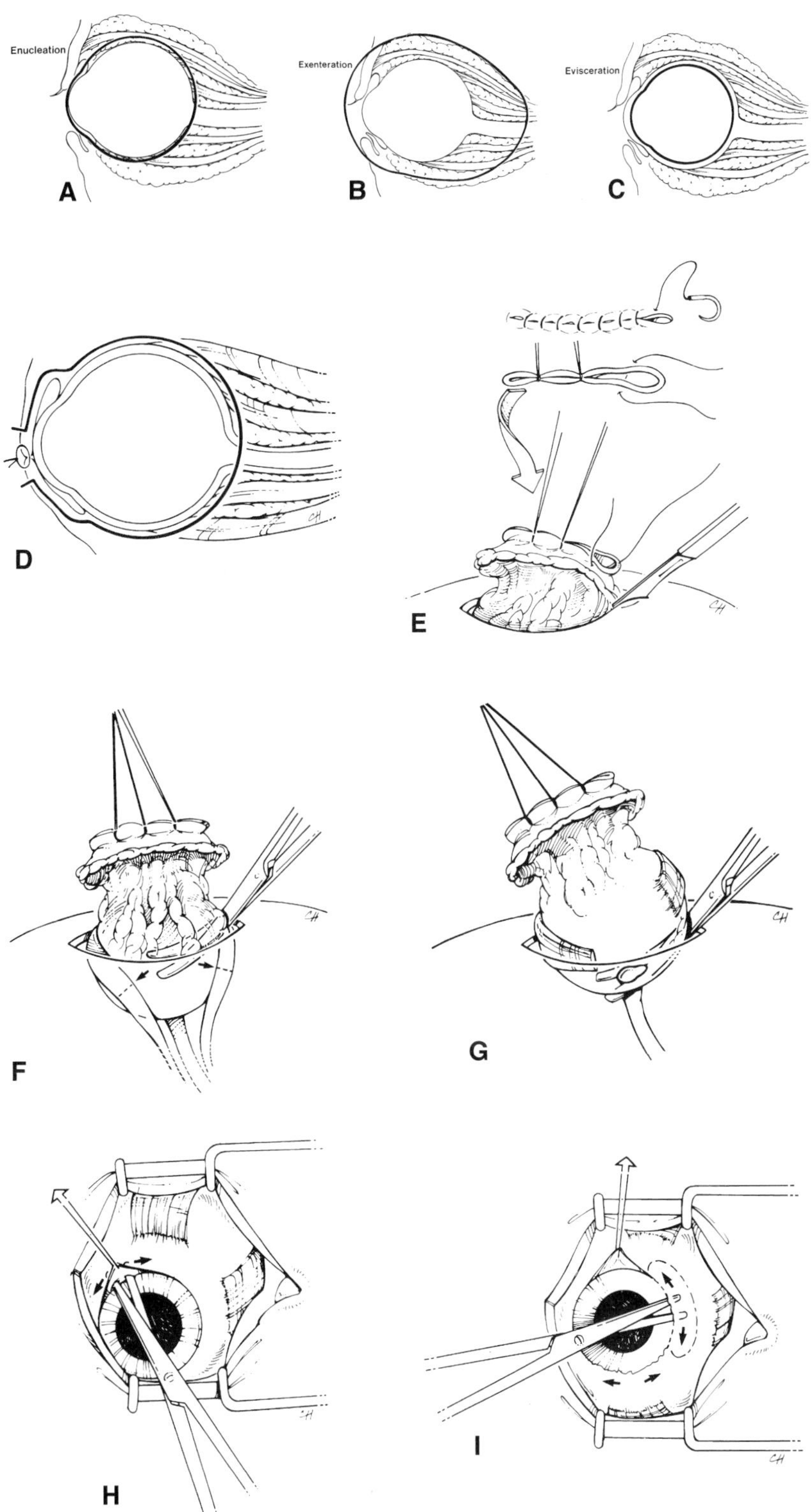

Figure 63-6. The surgical techniques for enucleation (**A**), exenteration (**B**), and evisceration (**C**)., Enucleation by the transpalpebral method involves closure of the lids, an incision around the eyelid margin, and blunt dissection posteriorly without breaking into the conjunctival sac (**D** through **G**). The subconjunctival enucleation technique (**H** and **I**) involves subconjunctival dissection posteriorly. *Continued*

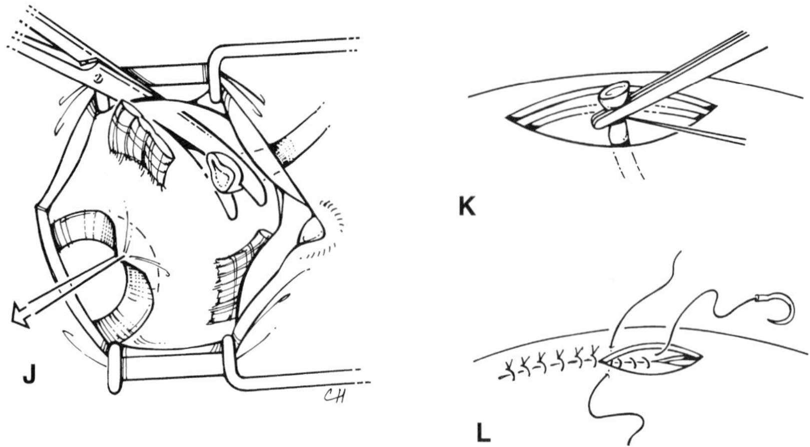

Figure 63-6, cont'd. In both methods, the extraocular muscles are transected and the optic nerve is subsequently clamped (**J** and **K**). A two-layer skin closure is performed (**L**).

scalpel blade. The angularis oculi vein located near the medial canthus should be avoided. Blunt subcutaneous dissection with Metzenbaum scissors is performed posteriorly, taking care to avoid breaking into the conjunctival sac. The medial and lateral canthal ligaments are transected with the blade. A large curved Rochester-Carmalt hemostat (20 to 25 cm) or Satinsky vascular clamp (27.3 mm) is used to crush the optic nerve, and curved scissors are used to transect the optic nerve between the globe and the clamp (see Fig. 63-6, *J* and *K*). The optic nerve is best approached from the nasal side of the orbit. Care should be taken not to pull on the optic nerve, as tension at the optic chiasm may result in damage to the contralateral eye. A ligature may be placed on the transected optic nerve stump, and the nerve tissue is cauterized (see Fig. 63-6, *J* and *K*). Soft tissues of the orbit are closed in a simple-continuous pattern with 3-0 absorbable suture to minimize postoperative "pitting" of the eyelids. A silicone prosthesis can be inserted prior to closure of the muscle, fascial, and eyelid skin layers to reduce the postenucleation orbital tissue defect. Simple-interrupted sutures of 4-0 nylon or silk are used to permanently close the skin incision (see Fig. 63-6, *L*).

AFTERCARE

All enucleated globes should be submitted in fixative for histologic evaluation. Some postoperative swelling is to be expected. Slight epistaxis may occur postoperatively. Systemically administered antibiotics and nonsteroidal anti-inflammatory drugs are beneficial.

COMPLICATIONS

Complications of enucleation include intraoperative rupture of the globe (causing orbital contamination with microbes or tumor cells into the orbit and circulation), severe intraoperative and postoperative hemorrhage, orbital cyst formation resulting from failure to remove all secreting orbital and ocular tissues, and blindness from stretching of the contralateral optic nerve as a result of pulling on the affected optic nerve intraoperatively. Rupture of an infected eye may result in orbital infection and cellulitis. In such cases, the orbit should be irrigated with povidone-iodine solution, and intraoperative cultures should be obtained. Broad-spectrum systemic antibiotics should also be administered and the regimen modified according to the sensitivities of the organism isolated. A drain should be placed if contamination is severe. Surgical transection of the optic nerve may result in severe intraoperative hemorrhaging. Wet-field cautery or careful ligation should result in hemostasis. Metal hemoclips can also be used to control bleeding. Eyelid tamponade and head bandaging suppresses slight postoperative hemorrhaging. An orbital silicone implant should not be placed if infection or a tumor is found in the orbit at enucleation.

Subconjunctival Enucleation Technique

The subconjunctival approach (see Fig. 63-6, *H* and *I*) is quicker and associated with less hemorrhage. It should be used when a cosmetic shell is to be placed to maintain the integrity of the lid margin. A lateral canthotomy may be necessary to increase exposure. A 360-degree limbal peritomy is performed using sharp scissors. All four quadrants are undermined posteriorly with tenotomy or Metzenbaum scissors (see Fig. 63-6, *H* and *I*). The extraocular muscles are isolated and transected. The medial and lateral canthal ligaments are transected with a blade. Cautery is used to control bleeding.

A large, curved Rochester-Carmalt hemostat (20 to 25 cm) or Satinsky vascular clamp (27.3 mm) is used to crush the optic nerve, and curved scissors are used to transect the optic nerve between the globe and the clamp (see Fig. 63-6, *J* and *K*). The optic nerve is best approached from the nasal side of the orbit. Care should be taken not to pull on the optic nerve, as tension at the optic chiasm may result in damage to the contralateral eye. A ligature may be placed on the transected optic nerve stump, and the nerve tissue cauterized. The nictitating membrane and its gland are carefully removed with scissors. Three to 5 mm of the lid margin is excised with scissors. The conjunctiva is stripped from the remaining lid, and the subcutaneous fascia and orbital septum are closed with a simple-continuous suture pattern of 3-0 absorbable suture material to produce a tissue bridge across the front of the orbit. This minimizes postoperative eyelid "pitting." The lid incision is permanently closed with simple-interrupted sutures of 4-0 nylon or silk. A silicone prosthesis can be inserted prior to closure of the muscle, fascia, and skin layers to reduce the orbital defect.

Prosthetic Implants

Intrascleral Prosthetic Implants

The intrascleral prosthesis (ISP) or intraocular silicone prosthesis has been used in horses as a cosmetic alternative to enucleation.[3,9,10,27-29] The ISP replaces the intraocular contents, which are removed by evisceration. Implants of 34 to 44 mm in diameter are recommended for adult horses but, as mentioned before, should not be placed in eyes with severe corneal disease, intraocular neoplasia, or infectious panophthalmitis. The ISP provides a cosmetically acceptable, nonpainful eye that has normal lid movements, normal tear function and normal globe motility.[28,29]

Intraorbital Prostheses

Intraorbital prostheses are used to prevent severe pitting of the skin over the orbital cavity after exenteration or enucleation.[3,27-29] The use of intraorbital implants in the presence of orbital neoplasia and/or infection is controversial. Implants for horses are available from Jardon Eye Prosthetics (Southfield, Mich). A silicone orbital implant specifically designed to reduce postenucleation eyelid skin "pitting" is now available from Veterinary Ophthalmic Specialties (Moscow, Idaho).

Extrascleral Shell Prostheses

Extrascleral shell implants or conformers consist of hydroxyapatite, porcelain, or methylmethacrylate shells made by ocularists to cover a disfigured or phthisical globe.[30] The surface of the shell is painted and the prosthesis is placed into the conjunctival sac. The lids and nictitating membrane hold the conformer in place. Daily cleaning and high costs are the main limitations to their use, but the results are quite extraordinary[30] (Fig. 63-7). Ocular conformers are available from Jardon Eye Prosthetics or can be custom made for horses by Dallas Eye Prosthetics (Dallas, Tex).

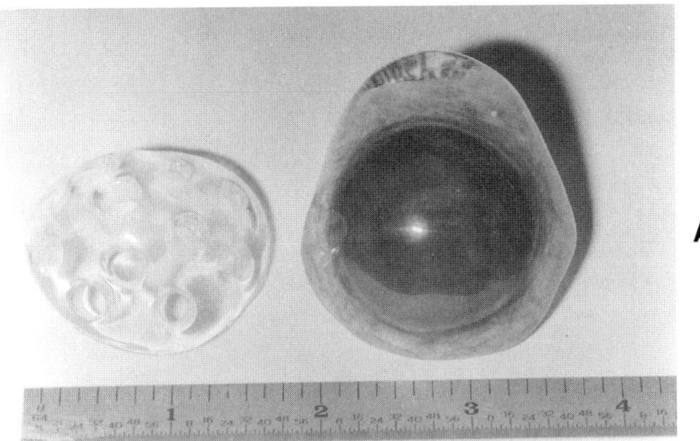

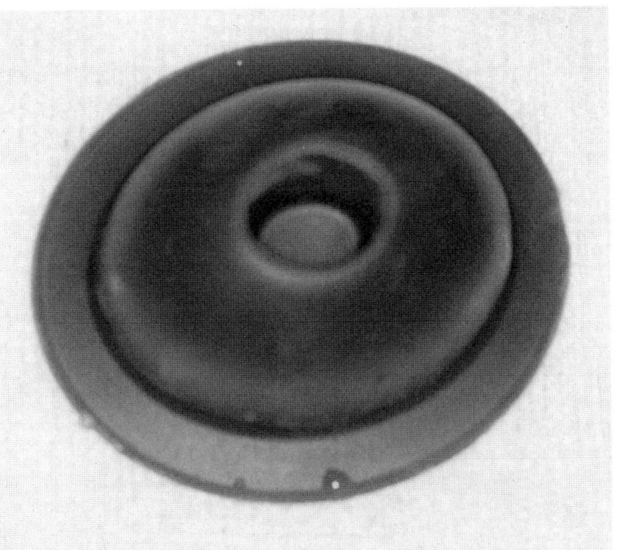

Figure 63-7. A, This methylmethacrylate cosmetic shell *(right)* was custom made to fit anterior to an orbital silicone implant in a horse. The impression tray *(left)* was used to make the initial mold for the shell. **B,** This orbital implant is designed to reduce "pitting" after enucleation.

Orbitotomy

Indication

Orbitotomy is indicated for biopsy or excision of orbital masses, drainage of infectious processes that are nonresponsive to medical therapy, or retrieval of foreign bodies. Orbital surgery may also be necessary in the horse to repair periorbital fractures.[6,20]

Surgical Procedures

Surgical procedures used for orbital exploration in the horse include a dorsal orbitotomy approach[15,20] and approaches that require an osteotomy of the zygomatic, temporal, and frontal components of the zygomatic arch.[6,16,17] The dorsal orbitotomy approach involves a slightly curved skin incision over the dorsal orbital region just lateral to the external sagittal crest of the frontal and parietal bones, extending laterally caudal to the zygomatic process of the frontal bone. Lateral retraction of the attachments of the frontoscutularis, interscutularis, and temporal muscles to the temporal and frontal bones allows exposure of the extraocular muscle cone.[4]

An alternative orbitotomy procedure in horses involves resection of the zygomatic, temporal, and frontal components of the zygomatic arch[6,16,17] (Fig. 63-8). A lateral canthotomy is performed for exposure. A slightly curved skin incision is made over the length of the zygomatic process of the frontal bone, being careful to preserve the sensory nerve fibers to the upper eyelid from the supraorbital foramen and the laterally located motor fibers to the orbicularis oculi muscle from the palpebral branch of the facial nerve. The periosteum of the cranial rim of the zygomatic process is incised along its length and the aponeurosis of the frontoscutularis, interscutularis, temporal, and masseter muscles reflected. A wedge of the zygomatic process of the frontal bone is removed with an oscillating bone saw or osteotome to expose the dorsolateral orbit. The lesion is drained, or biopsied and debulked.

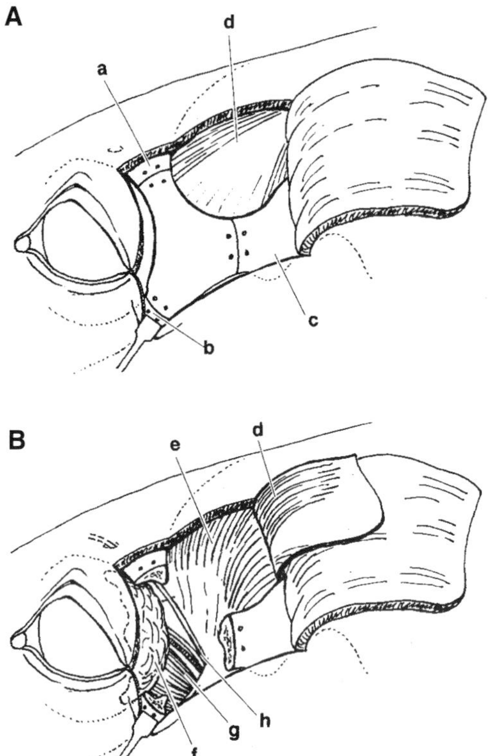

Figure 63-8. Diagrammatic orbitotomy technique* involving zygomatic arch transection to remove orbital masses. A, The positions where the zygomatic arch and zygomatic process of the frontal bone are drilled prior to transection of the arch are illustrated. B, The extraocular muscle cone is exposed after removal of the zygomatic arch and temporal muscle. a, zygomatic process of frontal bone; b, zygomatic arch; c, zygomatic process of temporal bone; d, scutular muscles; e, temporal muscle; f, retrobulbar muscle cone; g, lacrimal gland; h, supraorbital nerve). (*Technique modified from Goodhead AD, Vener IJ, Nesbit JW: Vet Comp Ophthalmol 1997;7:96.)

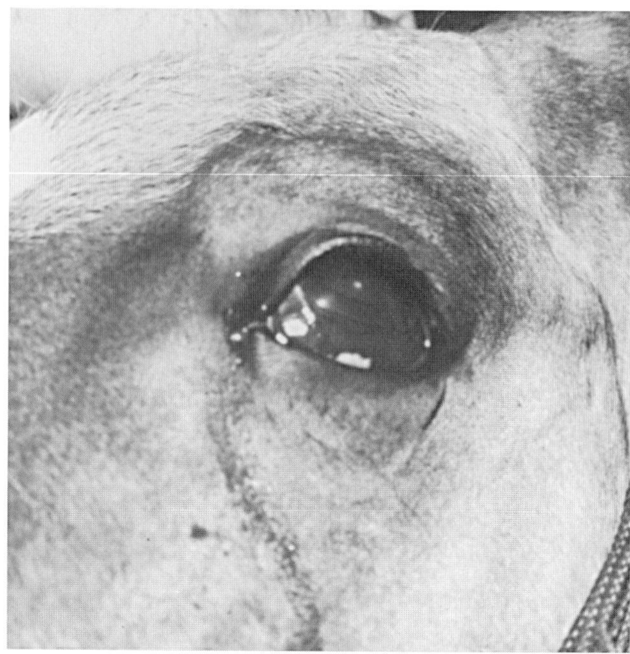

Figure 63-9. Dorsal strabismus caused by an orbital traumatic proptosis in this horse.

Iridium seeds can be implanted or cisplatin injected into the tumor mass.

The bone wedge is then replaced and fixed into position with 20-gauge stainless steel wire through predrilled 2-mm holes. The periosteum and subcutaneous tissues are closed with simple-interrupted absorbable sutures. The skin incision and canthotomy are closed with simple-interrupted nonabsorbable sutures.

SURGICAL DISORDERS OF THE ORBIT

Congenital Orbital Disease

Strabismus

Strabismus refers to a deviation of the globe from its normal position. In the neonatal foal, the horizontal axis of the pupil and globe is deviated slightly medially and ventrally, and the eye reaches the normal adult position by 1 month of age.[31] Strabismus in adult horses may be associated with visual difficulties and abnormal head posture[3,10] (Fig. 63-9). Surgical correction of strabismus by rectus muscle transposition is infrequently performed in veterinary ophthalmology. Muscles can be weakened by moving the muscle insertion posteriorly, or they can be strengthened by shortening the muscle or advancing the insertion site anteriorly, or muscle insertions can be transposed to different locations to alter the functional pull of the muscles. The reader is advised to consult the literature and a veterinary or physician ophthalmologist prior to attempting correction of strabismus in the horse.

Microphthalmos

Microphthalmos refers to a congenitally small globe. This differs from phthisis bulbi, in which a normal-size globe degenerates because of severe injury. If microphthalmos is associated with other ocular defects, it is termed a complicated microphthalmos. If the globe is simply small and functional, it is termed a pure microphthalmos.[32] The microphthalmic globe may be so small that a secondary entropion occurs, causing ulcerative keratitis and pain. Enucleation and orbital implant surgery is indicated in some cases to prevent skull deformities associated with abnormal skull growth caused by severe microphthalmos.[10]

Acquired Orbital Disease

Orbital Cellulitis or Sinusitis

Inflammatory, infectious, and neoplastic diseases of the sinuses and guttural pouch, teeth problems, foreign bodies, and trauma may result in orbital cellulitis or abscess formation.[3,10] Orbital cellulitis is manifested by blepharoedema, swelling of the supraorbital fossa, exophthalmos, orbital pain, epiphora, and nictitating membrane protrusion.

Orbital cellulitis can damage the globe and optic nerve of the horse within a short time. Treatment should be timely and aggressive. Topically applied and broad-spectrum systemically administered antibiotics are always indicated. Ultrasonography and radiography may help localize the site of inflammation. Trephination into a paranasal sinus for culture of exudate, irrigation, and drainage is indicated if sinusitis is involved. Fluid-filled swellings should be aspirated and specimens submitted for microbiologic culture and cytology. Orbital cellulitis caused by traumatic orbital contusions may be associated with fractures of the orbital rim. Retrobulbar hemorrhage from trauma can result in exophthalmos.[24]

Orbital Neoplasia

Tumors reported from the equine orbit include lipoma, fibroma, paraganglioma, osteoma, adenocarcinoma, lymphosarcoma, melanoma, sarcoid, squamous cell carcinoma, meningioma, hemangiosarcoma, sarcoid, multilobular osteoma, neurofibroma, medulloepithelioma, schwannoma, and neuroendocrine tumors.[3,10-19] Progressive exophthalmos, orbital swelling, blindness, strabismus, anisocoria, and behavioral abnormalities are reported symptoms of horses with orbital tumors.[3,10-19] If the tumor is extensive and the eye incapable of vision, it should be enucleated and the orbit exenterated. Intralesional iridium implantation or cisplatin chemotherapy into the orbital tumor may be beneficial in some types of neoplasia. The presence of a sighted eye and a retrobulbar mass in the horse requires that an orbitotomy be considered for diagnosis and possible therapy.*

Other Orbital Conditions

Hydatid cysts in the orbit have been reported to cause exophthalmos and optic nerve atrophy in horses in Europe.[33] Fungal infections can affect the horse orbit.[8]

Orbital fat may herniate through weakened episcleral fascia or from trauma to cause lobular subconjunctival masses that mimic tumors.[3,34] Aspiration, biopsy, and cytologic evaluation of these masses reveals the presence of adipose cells. The lesion can be simply observed, or the affected tissue can be excised and the wound sutured to prevent recurrent herniation.[3,34]

Traumatic Proptosis

The complete bony orbital rim of the horse protects against traumatic globe proptosis, but this problem does occasionally occur after orbital injuries.[10] Miosis with severe hypotony and hyphema indicates severe trauma and has a poor prognosis for a viable globe. Corneal ulcers, corneal desiccation, and keratomalacia can be minor or severe. The horse eye tolerates little disruption of its intraocular blood supply, and severe intraocular hemorrhage usually results in phthisis bulbi. The globe with proptosis should be replaced into the orbit with the horse under general anesthesia. A temporary tarsorrhaphy will protect the cornea. Topically applied antibiotics and atropine, and systemically administered nonsteroidal anti-inflammatories and antibiotics will decrease swelling and minimize infection. The globe should be reexamined when lid swelling has subsided, and the cornea and globe integrity reevaluated.

Orbital Fractures

Fractures of the bones of the orbit (Fig. 63-10) may be manifested by asymmetry of the globes or face, epistaxis, exophthalmos, proptosis, eyelid and conjunctival swelling, depression or concavity of the periorbital region, crepitus, and sometimes pain on periorbital palpation. Damage to the intraosseous nasolacrimal duct, globe, optic nerve, or paranasal sinuses can also occur.[6,20,21] All cases of suspected orbital fractures should be examined and evaluated by radiography. Ophthalmic complications include corneal ulcers, iridocyclitis, entrapment of the globe by bone fragments, and blindness.[20,21]

Periorbital fractures should be repaired quickly, because fibrous union of the fractured pieces begins within 1 week after the injury to make elevation and realignment very difficult.[6,20] Minor orbital rim fractures seldom require surgical correction unless they are contributing to continued proptosis. Small bone fragments should be removed to prevent sequestrum formation. Bony fragments near fractures of the medial canthus can impinge and entrap the globe. Fragments may be palpated at the conjunctival fornix.[20,21] Open fractures should be lavaged and débrided to remove necrotic tissues. Necrotic bone should be curetted to a bleeding surface. Surgical exploration may reveal fractures to be more extensive than were detected radiographically.[20,21] Incomplete fractures may not be visible without subperiosteal dissection. Failure to repair large fractures may result in permanent facial deformity.[20,21] Fracture sites should be approached by slightly curved skin incisions adjacent to the fracture site.[20] Monofilament stainless steel wire suture (20- to 22-gauge), cerclage wire, small pins and orthopedic bone plates (Fig. 63-11), and cancellous bone

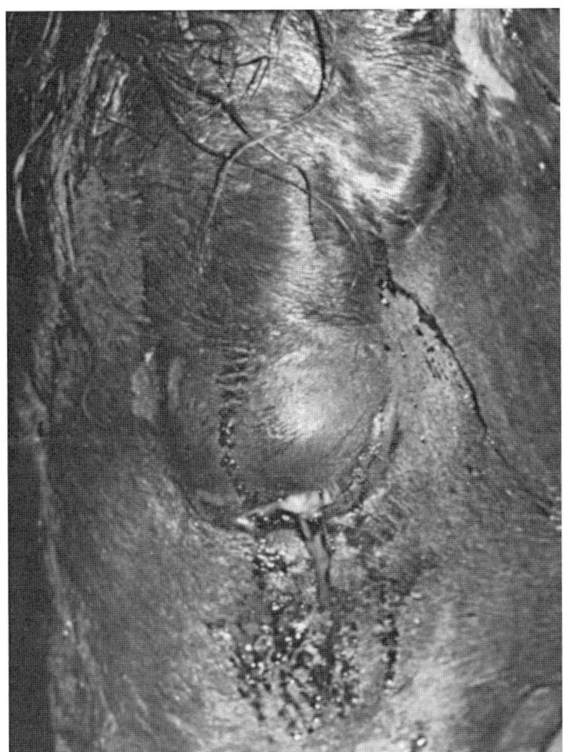

Figure 63-10. Severe eyelid swelling in a horse with a periorbital fracture.

*References 3, 6, 7, 13, 15, 16.

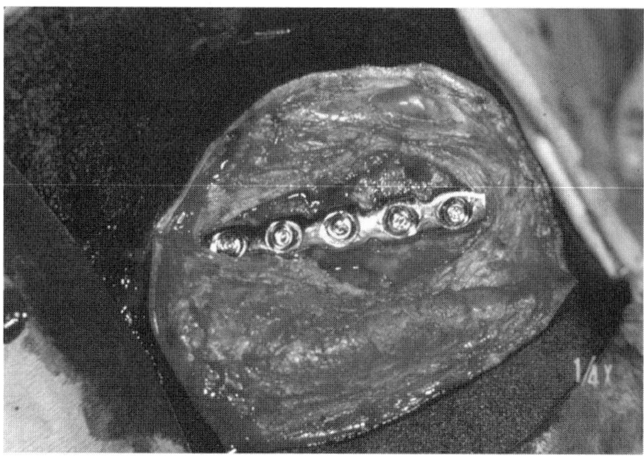

Figure 63-11. A 2.7-mm-diameter five-hole bone plate was used to repair this supraorbital process fracture.

grafts are utilized to stabilize bone fragments, and to immobilize and repair extensive orbital fractures.[6,20,21] Fractures that are difficult to elevate may be reduced by drilling trephine holes at the fracture periphery and using angled probes to elevate the fragment (see Chapter 103). Postoperative antibiotics and nonsteroidal anti-inflammatory drugs are indicated to reduce infection, inflammation, and discomfort. Concurrent corneal ulcers, uveitis, lid lacerations, and other associated eye problems should also be treated appropriately.

REFERENCES

1. Samuelson DA: Ophthalmic anatomy. In Gelatt KN, editor: Veterinary Ophthalmology, ed 3, Philadelphia, 1991, Lippincott Williams and Wilkins.
2. Prince JH, Diesem C, Eglitis I, Ruskell G: Anatomy and Histology of the Eye and Orbit in Domestic Animals, Springfield, Ill, 1960, Charles C Thomas.
3. Lavach JD: Handbook of Equine Ophthalmology, Ft Collins, Colo, 1987, Giddings.
4. Diesem C: Organs of vision. In Getty R, editor: Sisson and Grossman's The Anatomy of the Domestic Animals, ed 5, Philadelphia, 1975, WB Saunders.
5. Diesem C: Gross anatomic structures of equine and bovine orbit and its contents, Am J Vet Res 1968;29:1769.
6. Koch DB, Leitch M, Beech J: Orbital surgery in two horses, Vet Surg 1980;9:61.
7. Dutton JJ: Clinical and surgical orbital anatomy, Ophthalmol Clin North Am 1996;9:527.
8. Scott EA, Duncan JR, McCormack JE: Cryptococcosis involving the postorbital area and frontal sinus in a horse, J Am Vet Med Assoc 1974;165:626.
9. Slatter DH: Fundamentals of Veterinary Ophthalmology, Philadelphia, 1981, WB Saunders.
10. Brooks DE: Equine Ophthalmology Made Easy. Jackson Hole, Wyo, 2002, Teton NewMedia.
11. Lavach J, Severin G: Neoplasia of the equine eye, adnexa and orbit, J Am Vet Med Assoc 1977;170:202.
12. Rebhun WC: Equine lymphosarcoma, J Am Vet Med Assoc 1984;184:720.
13. Richardson DW, Acland HM: Multilobular osteoma (chondroma rodens) in a horse, J Am Vet Med Assoc 1983;182:289.
14. Sweeney CR, Beech J: Retrobulbar melanoma in a horse, Equine Vet J Suppl 1983;2:123.
15. Basher AW, Severin GA, Chavkin MJ, Frank AA: Orbital neuroendocrine tumors in three horses, J Am Vet Med Assoc 1997;210:668.
16. Goodhead AD, Vener IJ, Nesbit JW: Retrobulbar extra-adrenal paraganglioma in horse and its surgical removal by orbitotomy, Vet Comp Ophthalmol 1997;7:96.
17. Colitz C, Gilger BC, Davidson MG: Orbital fibroma in a horse, Vet Ophthalmol 2000;3:213.
18. Davis JL, Gilger BC, Spaulding K, et al: Nasal adenocarcinoma with diffuse metastases involving the orbit, cerebrum, and multiple cranial nerves in a horse, J Am Vet Med Assoc 2002;221:1460.
19. Scotty NC, Ford M, Williams F, et al: Exophthalmia associated with paranasal sinus osteoma in a Quarterhorse mare, J Vet Diagn Invest 2004;16:155.
20. Caron JP, Barber SM, Bailey JV, et al: Periorbital skull fractures in five horses, J Am Vet Med Assoc 1986;188:280.
21. Blogg JR, Stanley RG, Philip CJ: Skull and orbital blow out fractures in a horse, Equine Vet J Suppl 1990;10:5.
22. Gilger BC, Davidson MG: How to prepare for ocular surgery in the standing horse, Proc Am Assoc Eq Pract 2002;48:266.
23. Schebitz H, Wilkens H: Atlas of Radiographic Anatomy of the Horse, ed 3, Philadelphia, 1978, WB Saunders.
24. Morgan RV, Daniel GB, Donnell RL: Magnetic resonance imaging of the normal eye and orbit of the horse, Prog Vet Comp Ophthalmol 1993;3:127.
25. Boroffka S, van den Belt A: CT/ultrasound diagnosis-retrobulbar hematoma in a horse, Vet Radiol Ultrasound 1996;37:441.
26. Rogers M, Cartee RE, Miller W, et al: Evaluation of the extirpated equine eye using B-mode ultrasonography, Vet Radiol 1986;27:24.
27. Gelatt KN, Gelatt JP: Small Animal Ophthalmic Surgery, Oxford, 2001, Butterworth-Heinemann.
28. Hamor RE, Roberts SM, Severin GA: Use of orbital implants after enucleation in dogs, horses, and cats: 161 cases (1980-1990), J Am Vet Med Assoc 1993;203:701.
29. Provost PJ, Ortenburger AI, Caron JP: Silicone ocular prosthesis in horses: 11 cases (1983-1987), J Am Vet Med Assoc 1989;194:1764.
30. Gilger BC, Pizzirani S, Johnston LC, et al: Use of a hydroxyapatite orbital implant in a cosmetic corneoscleral prosthesis after enucleation in a horse, J Am Vet Med Assoc 2003;3:343.
31. Adams R, Mayhew I: Neurologic examination of newborn foals, Equine Vet J 1984;16:306.
32. Dziezyc J, Kern TJ, Wolf ED: Microphthalmia in a foal, Equine Vet J Suppl 1983;2:15.
33. Barnett KC, Cotrell BD, Rest JR: Retrobulbar hydatid cyst in the horse, Equine Vet J 1988;20:136.
34. Munroe GA, Belgrave JOS: Surgical repair of an episcleral prolapse of orbital fat in a foal, Equine Vet J 1988;20:131.

CHAPTER 64

Ocular Emergencies and Trauma

Dennis E. Brooks

Many ophthalmic emergencies in the horse are related to trauma.[1-5] The active physical nature of the horse in a stable, trailer, race track, or pasture environment leaves the large prominent orbit, eye, and adnexal structures vulnerable to traumatic injury. Ocular emergencies in the horse can provide some of the most challenging experiences for the veterinarian, in preserving sight, relieving pain, and restoring cosmesis. In general, any acute change in appearance, comfort, or vision of the eye should be considered an emergency. Consultation with a veterinary ophthalmologist is advisable in horses with extensive corneal disease, severe globe damage, marked orbital fractures, and periorbital soft tissue damage.[2,3,5]

Failure to look beyond the obvious when assessing the equine patient presented for ocular trauma can prevent recognition of associated subtle and concurrent eye problems.[1,3] Vision is to be cherished, and it is important to initiate aggressive medical and surgical therapy of trauma-damaged horse eyes.

EVALUATION OF THE TRAUMATIZED EYE

Adequate restraint is very important in evaluating the traumatized eye of the horse. The pain may be so intense that examination or manipulation of the orbital area is difficult. The eyelids may be so swollen that the globe cannot be examined. The eyelids should never be forcibly opened, because rupture of the eye and expulsion of intraocular contents may occur through a full-thickness corneal or scleral laceration. Topically applied anesthetics, supraorbital sensory and auriculopalpebral motor nerve blocks, a nose or ear twitch, and intravenous sedation facilitate examination of the horse with a damaged eye. The fluorescein and rose bengal dye tests should be an integral part of every ocular examination of horses with traumatized eyes. General anesthesia may be necessary in some horses for thorough ophthalmic examination, and it is definitely required for the meticulous repair of many injuries of the eye and periocular region.

ORBITAL CONTUSION AND PERI-ORBITAL FRACTURES

Etiology and Diagnosis

The anterior rim of the bony orbit is complete in the horse. Orbital contents are cushioned by orbital fascia, fat, and the extraocular muscles.[1,3] Periorbital fractures of the orbital rim, zygomatic arch, and supraorbital process can occur from collisions with inanimate objects, or from kicks or blows to the head.[2,5] Orbital fractures can be identified by palpation, facial deformity, ultrasonography, radiography, and computed tomography. Fractures may be accompanied by blepharoedema, epistaxis, orbital emphysema, corneal ulcers, uveitis, and limitations of global motility caused by entrapment of bone fragments.[1,2,5] Retrobulbar hemorrhage and cellulitis associated with orbital trauma may cause exophthalmos. Proptosis of the globe is rare but can occur after penetrating orbital injury.[3]

Treatment

Treatment of orbital soft tissue trauma depends on the specific ocular area damaged, the degree of dysfunction or displacement, and the involvement of adjacent orbital tissues. Systemically administered antibiotics and nonsteroidal anti-inflammatory drugs are indicated to minimize infection and to reduce pain and eyelid swelling. Topically applied corticosteroids should be used only in the presence of an intact corneal epithelium. Cold compresses in acute cases and hot compresses in more chronic cases of orbital trauma may speed a reduction in eyelid swelling. Dimethyl sulfoxide can be applied topically to reduce swelling in edematous eyelids. Minor orbital rim fractures may not require surgical correction unless fracture fragments are impinging on the globe. Interosseous wiring with stainless steel suture, bone plating, and cancellous bone grafts may be necessary to immobilize and repair extensive orbital fractures.[2,5]

EYELID AND NICTITANS INJURIES

Etiology and Diagnosis

Eyelid lacerations are common in the horse.[3] Damage to the upper eyelid is more significant, because most lid movement occurs in the upper eyelid. Medial canthal lacerations may result in damage to the nasolacrimal canaliculi. Lid lacerations may be accompanied by orbital cellulitis, periorbital fractures and bony sequestration, and severe to minor corneal ulceration. Careful examination of the globe for corneal integrity, anterior chamber clarity and depth, and scleral continuity is essential.

Treatment

Small eyelid punctures can cause an infectious retrobulbar cellulitis or abscess with fever and exophthalmos. These eyelid wounds should be cultured for bacteria and fungi, bony or other foreign bodies removed, necrotic tissue surgically débrided, and the area covered with warm compresses. Systemically administered antibiotics and nonsteroidal anti-inflammatory drugs will aid in resolving the condition. In some cases, surgical drains may need to be placed (Fig. 64-1).

Eyelid lacerations need to be repaired quickly to avoid eyelid infection, reduce eyelid edema, minimize scarring of the lid, and prevent corneal desiccation and ulceration. Small lid lacerations can be repaired under local anesthesia and mild sedation. Débridement is rarely necessary because of the abundant eyelid circulation, but when it must be

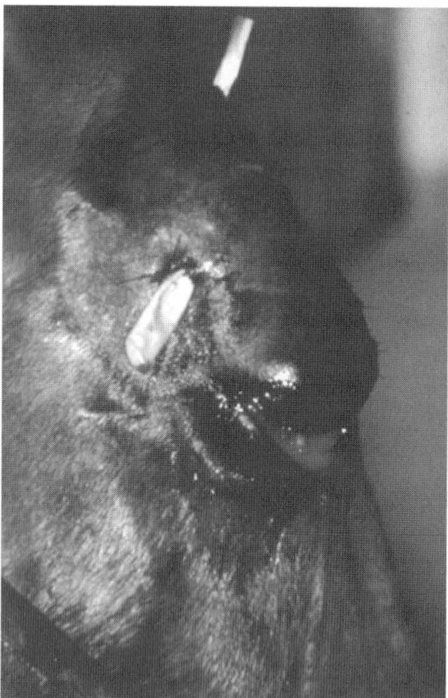

Figure 64-1. Orbital drainage is necessary after orbital penetration through the upper lid.

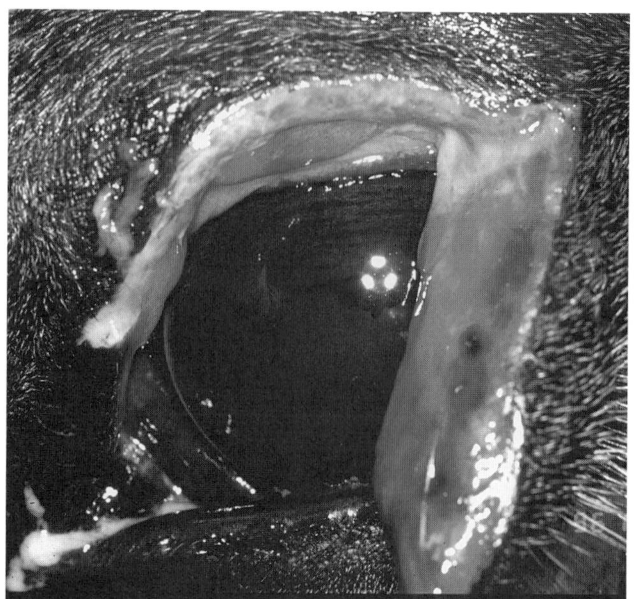

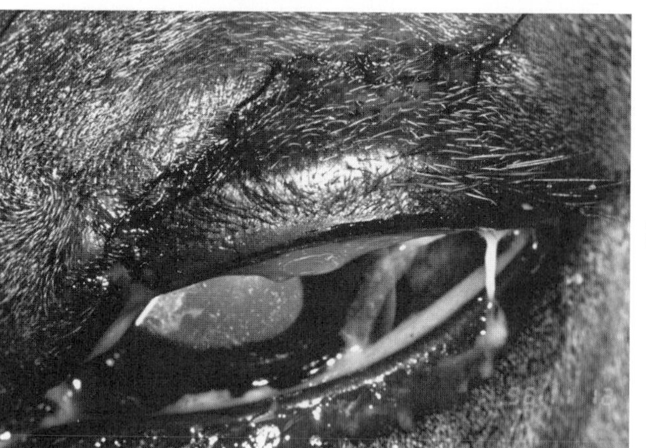

Figure 64-2. Severe lid laceration. **A,** The entire upper eyelid margin of this horse was traumatically lacerated so that it is attached by only a small pedicle at the lateral canthus. **B,** The laceration was successfully repaired with a two-layer closure.

done, it should be performed carefully to avoid functional abnormalities of the eyelids.[3] Lacerations that involve a significant amount of eyelid tissue but still retain a vascular supply should be repaired (Fig. 64-2). Failure to repair a laceration, or amputating a torn eyelid pedicle rather than a surgically repairing it, can cause moderate to severe exposure-induced corneal ulceration. Accurate two-layer closure of the deep tarsal-to-conjunctival and superficial skin-to-orbicularis muscle layers speeds healing and rapid return to function because it minimizes lid cicatrization and deformity. The eyelid margin should be carefully apposed—a very important step in eyelid repair. Large eyelid lacerations with loss of tissue require general anesthesia and sophisticated blepharoplastic grafting procedures for successful repair.

Lacerations of the margin or body of the nictitating membrane should be carefully repaired to avoid corneal irritation. Removal of the entire nictitating membrane should be performed only if it is severely damaged. The area adjacent to the cornea posterior to the nictitating membrane should always be examined for foreign bodies.

CORNEAL INJURIES

Indication

Corneal trauma can range from simple ulcers to full-thickness perforations with iris prolapse. Posttraumatic corneal infection and iridocyclitis are always major concerns for even the slightest corneal ulcerations. The type of medical or surgical treatment, or both, is determined by the type and extent of corneal disease and the ocular complications that have occurred. *All* corneal injuries should be fluorescein stained to detect corneal ulcers.

Abrasions and Ulcers

Diagnosis

Small corneal abrasions are detected through the use of illumination with a light source and fluorescein dye retention. The cornea may be cloudy, the conjunctiva red, and the eye painful. The upper eyelashes may droop. Topically applied antibiotics may help retard bacterial infectious processes but should be used carefully. *Staphylococcus, Streptococcus,* and *Pseudomonas* are frequent pathogens of the horse cornea.[6] The use of topically applied corticosteroids in treating corneal ulcers in the horse is *contraindicated* because the environment of the horse contains many saprophytic fungi, such as *Fusarium* and *Aspergillus,* that are capable of causing devastating fungal keratitis. *This fact cannot be overemphasized.*[4]

Tear film neutrophils and some bacteria and fungi are associated with highly destructive protease and collagenase enzymes that can result in rapid corneal stromal melting and perforation in the horse[3] (Fig. 64-3, *A*). Cytologic examination and microbiologic culturing of deep or rapidly progressing ulcers are imperative.

Treatment

Appropriate topically applied antibiotics, such as the triple-antibiotic ophthalmic solutions, and mydriatics or cycloplegics, such as 1% atropine ophthalmic solution, are recommended for equine corneal ulcers. Autologous serum has anticollagenase activity to aid corneal healing, and it should be used topically on ulcers in the horse to minimize stromal melting and speed healing.[3] Systemically administered nonsteroidal anti-inflammatory agents, such as phenylbutazone (2 to 4 mg/kg twice a day, PO) and flunixin meglumine (1 mg/kg twice a day, IM or PO), are also beneficial. Conjunctival grafts provide nutrition, fibroblasts, physical support, and endogenous plasma or serum to the melting ulcer, and they are strongly recommended (see Fig. 64-3, *B* and *C*).

A descemetocele can be recognized as a dark clearing at the bottom of a deep ulcer (Fig. 64-4, and see Fig. 64-3, *D* and *E*). It does not retain fluorescein dye, whereas the stroma of deep ulcers does retain the dye. Conjunctival or corneal grafts are preferred over nictitans flaps for surgical therapy for a descemetocele. Topically applied antibiotics, serum, and atropine are indicated, as well as systemically administered anti-inflammatory drugs.

Corneal Lacerations and Perforations

Treatment

Corneal lacerations may perforate a partial thickness or the full thickness of the horse cornea, but they are always accompanied by degrees of iridocyclitis.[3] Medical therapy should be sufficient for superficial, nonperforating lacerations. Topically applied broad-spectrum antibiotics, mydriatics or cycloplegics, and serum are recommended. Topically applied serum reduces enzymatic collagen breakdown of the cornea and prevents rapid dissolution of absorbable corneal sutures. Systemic nonsteroidal anti-inflammatories are strongly indicated.

Small full-thickness corneal perforations may be detected using Seidel's test. Clear aqueous humor leaking from the anterior chamber through a corneal fistula will dilute fluorescein dye placed on the cornea, causing it to be clear or green in Seidel's test (see Fig. 64-3, *F*). All such full-thickness lesions must be surgically repaired, or infection and/or phthisis bulbi will occur. Deep or irregular corneal partial-thickness lacerations or melting ulcers require surgical support of the cornea and more aggressive therapy for corneal disease and iridocyclitis (Fig. 64-5). Direct corneal suturing, and corneal and conjunctival grafts are indicated to more

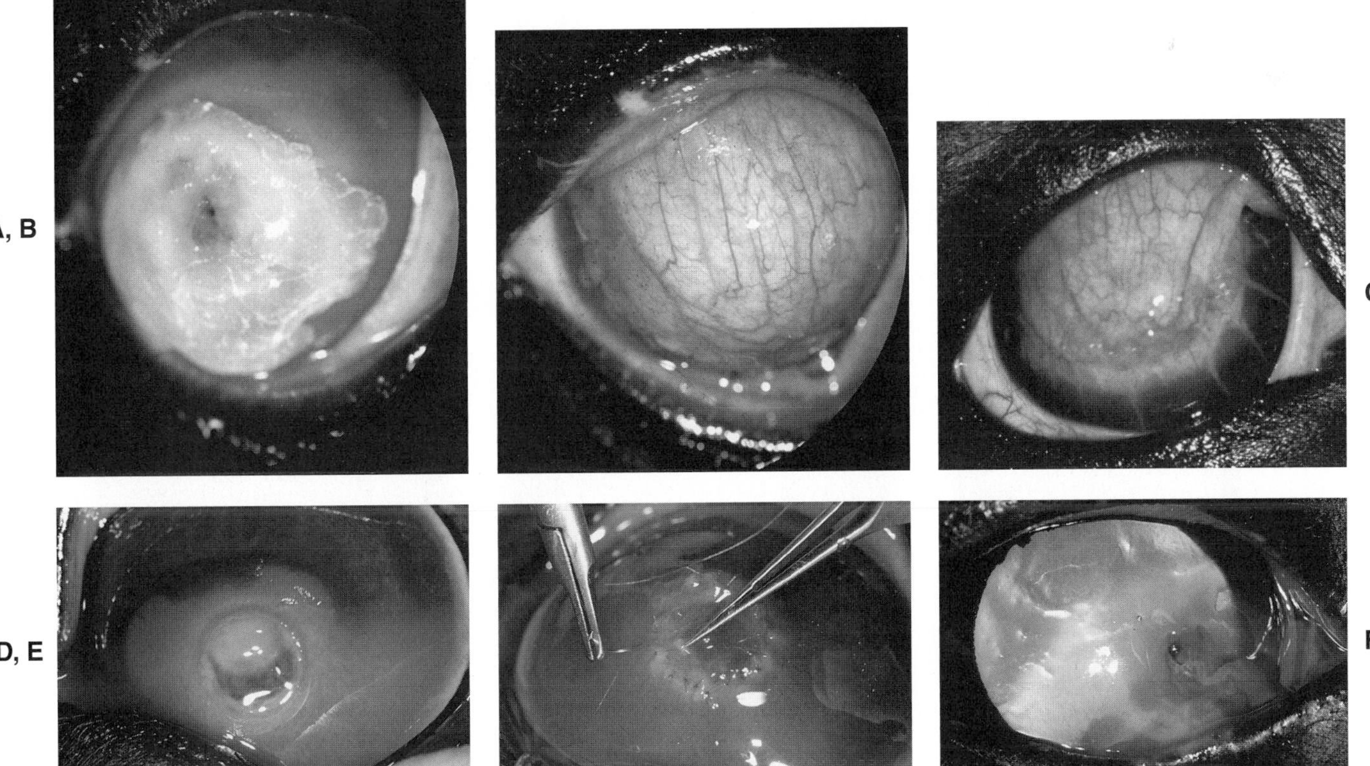

Figure 64-3. A, A melting ulcer caused by a *Staphylococcus*. A small descemetocele is seen in the center. **B,** A conjunctival flap was placed and removed after 2 weeks. **C,** The horse retained vision in the eye at 3 months, despite the large corneal scar. A tinted contact lens masks the scar when the horse is at a horse show. **D,** A melting ulcer with a crescent-shaped descemetocele. **E,** The ulcer in **D** was treated successfully with a corneal transplant. **F,** A corneal fistula is revealed by positive Seidel's test in this horse with a fungal ulcer.

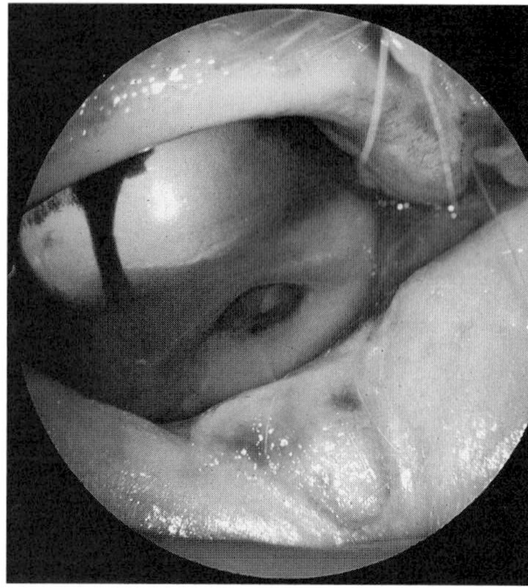

Figure 64-4. Thermal keratitis and blepharitis after neodymium:yttrium-aluminum-garnet laser removal of a tumor of the nictitating membrane. The very deep corneal ulcer became a descemetocele associated with a *Pseudomonas* infection. A conjunctival flap protected the cornea, and topically applied amikacin (1%) was used to stop the infection. The horse recovered completely.

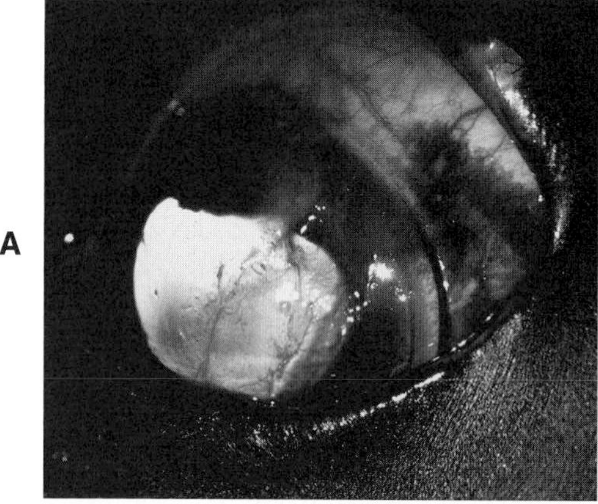

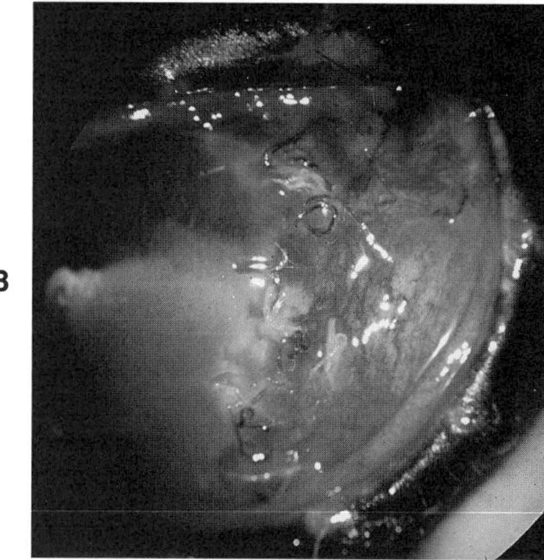

Figure 64-5. A, Jagged corneal laceration. The large denudation of the corneal epithelium was caused by a rock accidentally thrown into the eye. **B,** The conjunctival flap is shown 10 days later. The knots anchoring the flap to the cornea are loose, but the flap adhered to the cornea and was cut off with scissors. The horse recovered with a corneal scar.

rapidly restore corneal integrity (see Chapters 57 and 60). Topically applied antibiotics, mydriatics or cycloplegics, and serum, as well as systemically administered anti-inflammatory drugs, are used until healing is complete.

Full-thickness corneal perforations are usually associated with shallow anterior chambers and iris prolapse (Fig. 64-6). Hyphema and fibrin may be present in some eyes (Fig. 64-7). If the corneal lesion extends to the limbus, the sclera should also be carefully checked for perforation, because a scleral tear can be obscured by conjunctival chemosis and hemorrhage. Failure to detect such a scleral rupture results in chronic hypotony and globe atrophy (phthisis bulbi).[1,3]

Both small and large corneal perforations should be surgically repaired. Complications include infection, iris prolapse, anterior and posterior synechiae, cataract formation, and persistent iridocyclitis. Both small and large corneal or scleral defects can result in phthisis bulbi if left untreated.[1,3] Successful surgical repair of the iris prolapse and corneal perforation requires good illumination, good magnification, and proper microsurgical instrumentation. Eyes with an iris prolapse present for over 2 weeks, secondary to infected or sterile melting ulcers, and associated with corneal lacerations greater than 15 mm in length generally have a poor outcome in reference to sight and may result in enucleation as a result of endophthalmitis or phthisis bulbi.[7]

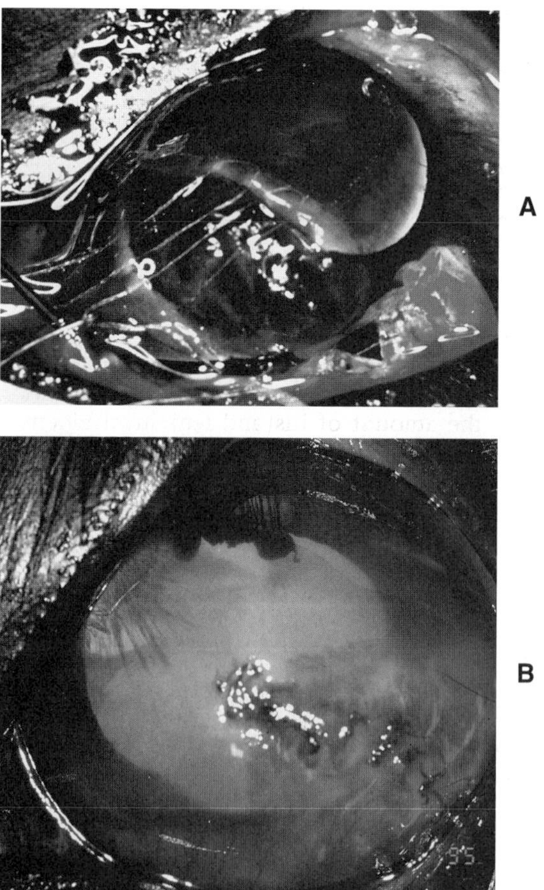

Figure 64-6. Corneal laceration and iris prolapse. **A,** A large corneal laceration and iris prolapse are surgically repaired. **B,** Successful repair is evident 3 weeks postoperatively.

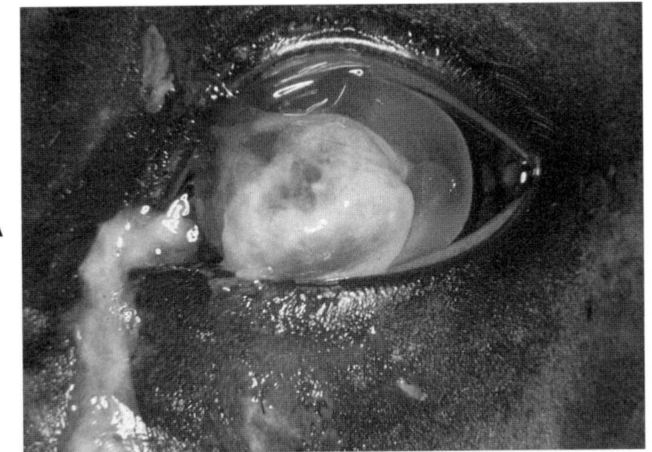

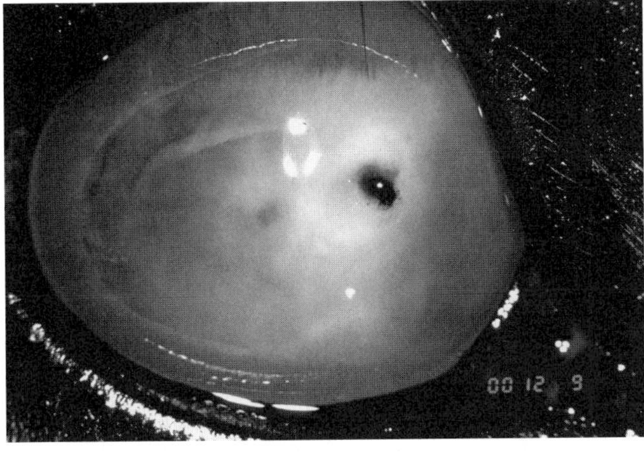

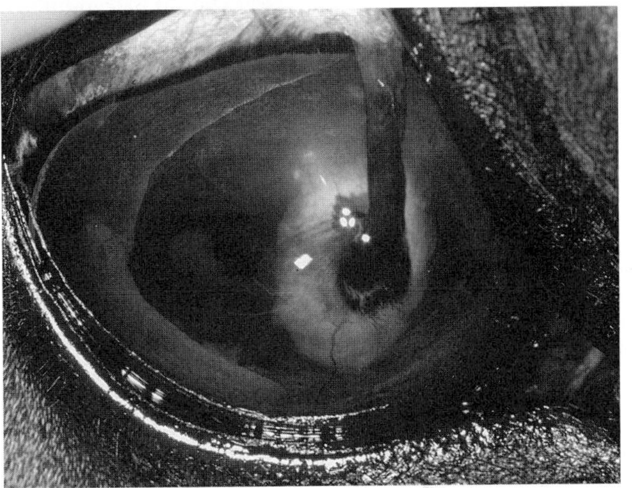

Figure 64-7. A, A large iris prolapse. The iris is encapsulated in fibrin. The globe was enucleated because of the large amount of protruding iris. **B,** A small iris prolapse as a result of a corneal ulcer. The anterior chamber is filled with fibrin. **C,** A corneal transplant and conjunctival flap were placed over the lesion (see Fig. 64-7, *B*), and the horse's vision is restored 1 year postoperatively.

Prognosis

The prognosis of a full-thickness corneal perforation depends on the duration and size of the wound (see Fig. 64-6), the amount of iris and lens involvement, and the presence of infection and hemorrhage.[1,3,7] A horse with a traumatic corneal perforation that defies repair and that has extensive extrusion of intraocular contents, severe intraocular hemorrhage, or evidence of bacterial infection should have the affected globe enucleated (see Fig. 64-7). Severe intraocular hemorrhage usually results in phthisis bulbi, because the eye of the horse does not tolerate much damage to its vasculature. Septic intrusion into the globe results in painful endophthalmitis. Such infection can spread to surrounding soft tissues and necessitates enucleation.

CHEMICAL BURNS

Etiology

Chemical burns are among the most urgent of ocular emergencies and may involve the eyelids, conjunctiva, and cornea.[8] Insecticide sprays or ointments, antiseptic solutions containing detergents, dermatologic creams containing alcohol, grooming soaps, and other caustic substances can cause blepharospasm, epiphora, and corneal ulceration. The extent of damage and prognosis for recovery after chemical injury of the eye depend on a multiplicity of factors, including the type and amount of the agent involved, its pH, and the duration of contact.[8] Alkali injuries are more damaging to the globe than injuries caused by acids. Alkalis are water-soluble substances that release hydroxyl ions and have a basic pH. The higher the pH, the greater the damage to the eye, with the most significant injuries occurring at a pH of 11 or higher.[8] Alkalis saponify corneal and conjunctival epithelial cell membranes and intercellular bridges, which facilitates rapid penetration into the deeper corneal stroma. In the corneal stroma, alkalis cause damage and necrosis by binding to mucopolysaccharides and collagen.[8] Leukocytes are attracted and release high levels of proteinases.[5] Alkali-induced ulcers resemble the collagenase ulcers caused by *Pseudomonas* bacteria.[3,8] Corneal perforation is highly likely in alkali injuries.

Acids dissociate in water to form hydrogen ions. Free hydrogen ions cause cellular necrosis. The intact corneal and conjunctival epithelia offer moderate protection against penetration of dilute or weak acids, allowing little damage unless the pH is 2.5 or lower.[8] Acids quickly denature proteins in the corneal stroma, forming precipitates that retard additional penetration. Acidic chemicals thus generally yield more superficial, sharply demarcated, and self-limiting corneal lesions.[8]

Treatment

Chemical burns should be quickly lavaged to bring the pH to normal levels with copious quantities of saline or water until the offending substance is removed. This may be the most important determinant for the ultimate prognosis of the insult to the eye. Topically applied antibiotics, atropine, and large amounts of antiproteinases, such as endogenous serum or ethylenediaminetetra-acetic acid (EDTA; 0.2%), are used until healing is complete.[3,8] Severe cases may warrant continuous perfusion of medication through a subpalpebral lavage system. The conjunctival fornices should be carefully flushed to remove any sequestered chemical. Systemically administered antibiotics, nonsteroidal anti-inflammatory agents, and analgesics are also beneficial. Topically applied corticosteroids interfere with the corneal healing process and are contraindicated. Therapeutic soft contact lenses may help heal ulcerated corneas (Keragenix, available at sales@keragenix.com). Conjunctival transplants from the contralateral eye are indicated for severely damaged conjunctival and corneal tissue.[8] The eye of a chemically burned horse should be watched closely for development of tear insufficiency caused by conjunctival scarring. Cicatricial eyelid disease may also occur.

UVEITIS

Etiology and Diagnosis

Blunt trauma to the globe can result in hyphema and iridocyclitis.[1,3] If severe, both hyphema and iridocyclitis can quickly lead to hypotony and phthisis bulbi in the horse.[1,3] Hyphema indicates uveal vascular trauma and is a sign of anterior uveitis. Miosis, aqueous flare, hypopyon, fibrin formation in the anterior chamber, and the presence of synechiae are also signs of anterior uveitis. Posterior uveitis (choroiditis) may lead to retinal detachment. Chronic uveitis after trauma may be associated with infectious agents, retained intraocular foreign bodies, lens capsule disruption and exposure of lens proteins, or autosensitization against uveal proteins or pigment.[1,3]

Trauma-induced hyphema has a reasonable prognosis for recovery if hemorrhage fills less than one-half the anterior chamber. The existence of hyphema itself is not an ocular emergency, but its presence generally implies severe ocular disease.

Treatment

Topically administered atropine (1%) should be used two to four times a day to attempt to dilate the pupil and minimize formation of synechiae in horses with anterior uveitis. Topically applied atropine is absorbed systemically and can cause enough intestinal hypomotility to result in colic in the horse, and it should always be used carefully. Most horses can tolerate the use of topically applied atropine three to four times per day with no problem, although a minority may develop colic with as little as one dose per day. Topically applied corticosteroids (dexamethasone or prednisolone acetate, four times a day) and systemically administered anti-inflammatory drugs (phenylbutazone, 1 g twice a day, PO) are also needed to suppress inflammation. This author has successfully used tissue plasminogen activator (TPA; Activase, Genentech, South San Francisco, Calif) for a horse suffering from traumatic uveitis when a severe amount of fibrin was present in the anterior chamber. TPA can digest blood clots and should not be used in the presence of hyphema. A dose of 50 to 100 µg of TPA is injected into the affected eye.

THERMAL BURNS

Fire can cause damage to the adnexa, cornea, and conjunctiva in horses. After copious irrigation and débridement, superficial cutaneous injuries are allowed to granulate during the healing process.[9] Antibiotic ointments and non-adherent dressings are used for wound coverage and as a prophylaxis for infection. Artificial tear ointments may be needed to lubricate the cornea if lagophthalmos is present. When deep dermal injuries occur in association with severe third-degree burns, the wound should be gently cleaned and carefully débrided. The early application of a meshed or split-thickness skin graft reduces subsequent scarring and ectropion. A tarsorrhaphy should be performed to provide corneal protection and to keep the eyelids tightly against the globe until swelling subsides. The vigorous use of antibiotic ointments is essential in the early phase of wound healing to prevent infection. Cicatricial entropion and ectropion (Fig. 64-8) may occur and may require skin grafting, skin advancement flaps, or other extensive blepharoplastic procedures.

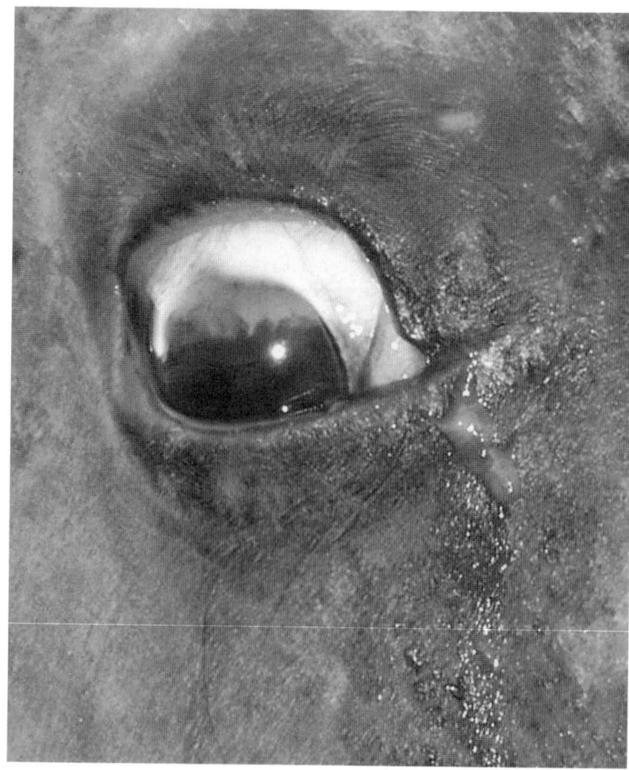

Figure 64-8. Cicatricial ectropion in a horse that escaped a barn fire.

FOREIGN BODIES

Etiology and Diagnosis

The effect of a foreign body on the eye depends on its size, its location, the type of material, and the length of time in the eye.[1] Iron, copper, and vegetative material are poorly tolerated intraocularly. Infectious agents can cause severe damage when associated with foreign material in the eye.[3] Foreign bodies may be found in the eyelids, in conjunctival fornices, behind the nictitating membrane, in the cornea, and intraocularly. Corneal, conjunctival, and eyelid foreign bodies can cause nonhealing superficial corneal ulcers (Fig. 64-9, *A* and *B*). Vitreal or retinal foreign bodies are difficult to identify and nearly impossible to remove at the present level of sophistication in equine ophthalmology. Metallic foreign bodies can be confirmed by skull radiography and ocular ultrasonography (see Fig. 64-9, *C* and *D*). It is rarely feasible or beneficial to remove a gunshot pellet from within the eye or orbit.

Treatment

Superficial corneal foreign bodies can be quickly removed with topical anesthesia, sensory and motor nerve blocks, and sedation (see Fig. 64-9, *A* and *B*). Penetrating or deep foreign bodies may need to be removed under general anesthesia. The corneal puncture wound caused by a foreign body should be treated with topically applied antibiotics. Systemically administered antibiotics, anti-inflammatory agents, and topical mydriatics or cycloplegics are also beneficial. Topically applied corticosteroids are contraindicated in corneal lesions associated with vegetative matter.[3] A foreign body in the anterior chamber or lens may be removed through a limbal incision. If a foreign body is of nonreactive material and if the ocular tissues penetrated do not react to the insult, surgical removal may be contraindicated when the surgical procedure would create more inflammation than the foreign body itself.

ENDOPHTHALMITIS

Etiology and Diagnosis

Severe endophthalmitis can result from septicemia, orbital surgery, intraocular surgery, corneal perforations, ruptured descemetoceles or ulcers, lens capsule rupture, or entrapped vitreal foreign bodies. It may be of a septic or sterile nature. Intraocular infections causing endophthalmitis, whether bacterial or fungal, are devastating in the horse. Culture of aqueous and vitreous aspirates is imperative for the correct diagnosis and should be carried out immediately.

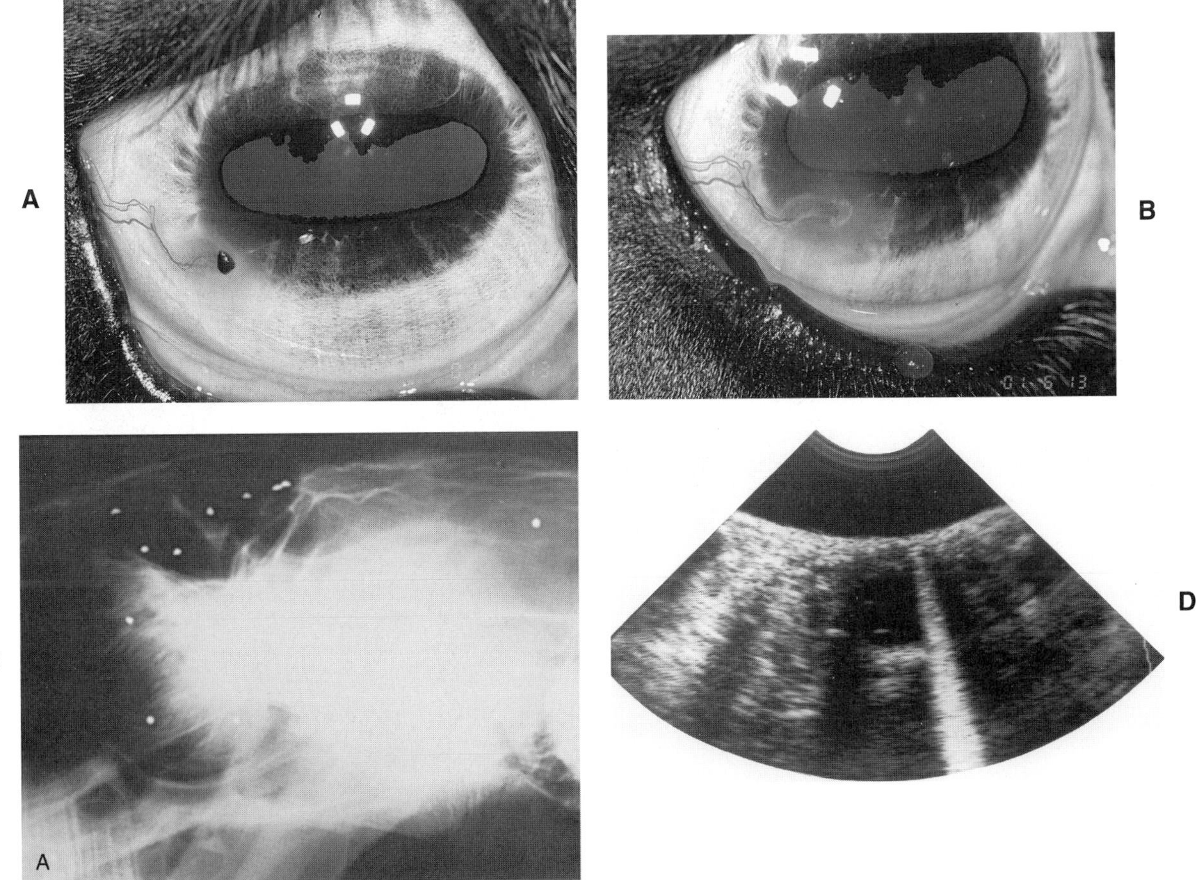

Figure 64-9. A, Small dark corneal foreign body has induced corneal vascularization. **B,** When the foreign body is removed, a small fluorescein-positive ulcer is present that requires therapy. **C,** Radiograph showing an orbital foreign body. Gunshot pellets are present near the orbit. **D,** Ultrasonography was used to locate the intraorbital and intraocular pellets.

Treatment

A dosage of 2 to 5 mg of gentamicin in 0.1 mL of solution is injected intravitreally if gram-negative organisms are isolated; in gram-positive infections, 2.2 μg of intravitreally applied cefazolin is recommended.[10] In fungal endophthalmitis, fluconazole (10 mg/kg of body weight) is administered intravenously or orally. Medical therapy must be aggressive and may require systemic antibiotics and repeated intravitreal antibiotic injections. Vitrectomy should also be considered. Painful blind globes with endophthalmitis should be enucleated.

BLINDNESS

Etiology and Diagnosis

It is critical for the veterinarian to assess whether the horse truly became acutely blind. An ocular examination and a carefully assembled history helps determine this factor. Acute blindness associated with head or ocular trauma may result from glaucoma, cataracts, intraocular hemorrhage, retinal or optic nerve disease, or brain injury.[3,11]

The optic nerve is contained within a dural sheath that is continuous at the orbital apex with the periosteum of the optic canal. Traumatic optic neuropathy occurs in the optic canal where the dural sheaths and the periosteum are fused. Concussive shock waves focused on the optic canal may result in optic nerve damage because the nerve is fixed and experiences the same force as the surrounding bone. Stretching, shearing, or avulsion of the equine optic nerve or chiasm can result in optic nerve atrophy and blindness from concussive cranial injuries.[4] Fractures of orbital bones, cerebral edema, and vascular infarction in the horse may also play a role in blindness as a result of head trauma.[10]

Chorioretinal degeneration and optic nerve atrophy are also reported secondary to acute blood loss caused by trauma or surgery in the horse.[3] Surgery to eliminate epistaxis induced by guttural pouch mycosis using the ligation technique for the internal and external carotid and the greater palatine arteries can be associated with ischemic optic neuropathy and sudden irreversible blindness in horses.[11]

Treatment

Systemically administered nonsteroidal anti-inflammatory agents and dimethyl sulfoxide may be beneficial in treating or preventing blindness in cases of acute head injury. A thorough ophthalmic and physical examination is necessary to identify the cause of the blindness for specific therapy.

REFERENCES

1. Brooks DE, Wolf ED: Ocular trauma in the horse, Equine Vet J Suppl 1983;2:141.
2. Caron JP, Barber SM, Bailey JV, et al: Periorbital skull fractures in five horses, J Am Vet Med Assoc 1986;188:280..
3. Brooks DE: Ophthalmology for the Equine Practitioner, Jackson, Wyo, 2002, Teton NewMedia.
4. Martin L, Kaswan R, Chapman W: Four cases of traumatic optic nerve blindness in the horse, Equine Vet J 1986;18:133.
5. Blogg JR, Stanley RG, Philip CJ: Skull and orbital blow out fractures in a horse, Equine Vet J Suppl 1990;10:5.
6. Moore CP, Fales WH, Whittington P, et al: Bacterial and fungal isolates from Equidae with ulcerative keratitis, J Am Vet Med Assoc 1983;182:600.
7. Chmielewski NT, Brooks DE, Smith PJ, et al: Visual outcome and ocular survival following iris prolapse in the horse: A review of 32 cases, Equine Vet J 1997;29:31.
8. Ralph RA: Chemical injuries of the eye. In Tasman W, Jaeger EA, editors: Duane's Clinical Ophthalmology on CD-ROM, Philadelphia, 2003, Lippincott Williams and Wilkins.
9. Karesh JW: The evaluation and management of ocular trauma. In Tasman W, Jaeger EA, editors, Duane's Clinical Ophthalmology on CD-ROM, Philadelphia, 2003, Lippincott Williams and Wilkins.
10. Stern GA, Engel HM, Driebe WT: The treatment of postoperative endophthalmitis: Results of differing approaches to treatment, Ophthalmology 1989;96:62.
11. Hardy J, Robertson JT, Wilkie DA: Ischemic optic neuropathy and blindness after arterial occlusion for treatment of guttural pouch mycosis in two horses, J Am Vet Med Assoc 1990;196:1631.

SECTION IX REPRODUCTIVE SYSTEM

Jörg A. Auer

CHAPTER 65

Testis

James Schumacher

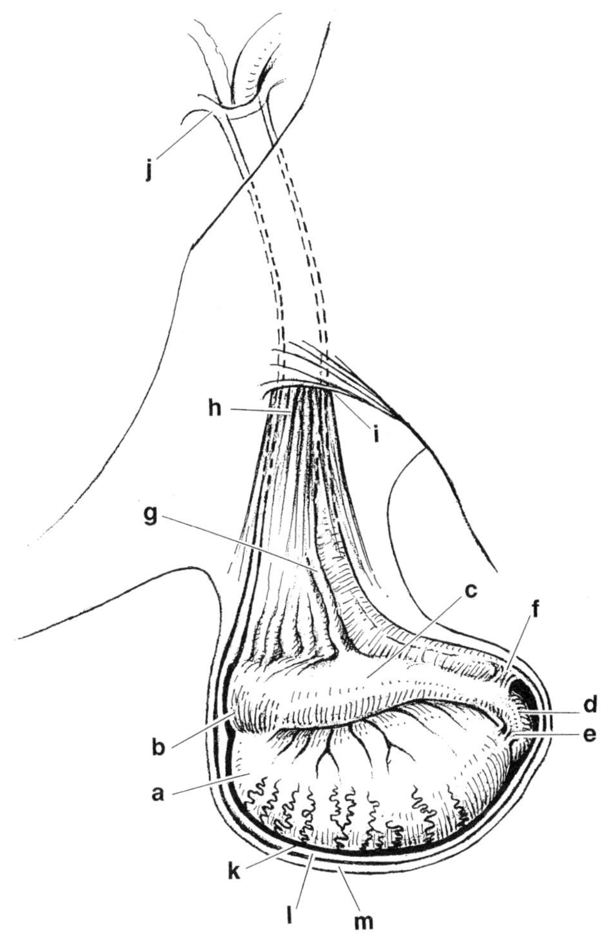

Figure 65-1. Right testis and epididymis of a stallion, lateral aspect. a, testis; b, head of epididymis; c, body of epididymis; d, tail of epididymis; e, proper ligamentum testis; f, ligament of the tail of the epididymis; g, spermatic cord; h, cremaster muscle; i, external inguinal ring; j, vaginal ring; k, visceral tunic; l, vaginal cavity; m, parietal tunic.

ANATOMY AND PHYSIOLOGY

Scrotum

The scrotum is a prepubic diverticulum of skin that contains the testes, their associated ducts, and the distal portion of the spermatic cords.[1] It is divided on the midline by the scrotal raphe, which is continuous with the raphae of the prepuce, penis, and perineum.[1,2] The skin of the scrotum is thin, sparsely covered with fine hair, and contains an unusually high number of sweat glands.

Intimately adherent to the scrotal skin is a layer of connective tissue and involuntary muscle, the tunica dartos.[1,3,4] This muscle relaxes with heat and contracts with cold to regulate testicular temperature, thus varying the size of the scrotum.[1] At the median plane, the tunica dartos sends a sagittal septum into the scrotal sac, dividing the scrotum into right and left pouches, each of which contains a testis.[1,4]

The vascular supply to the scrotum originates from the external pudendal vessels.[1,3,4] The nervous supply descends into the scrotum on the outer surface of the tunica vaginalis via the genitofemoral nerve.[1,4] Lymphatic vessels from the scrotum drain to the superficial inguinal lymph nodes.[3]

Epididymis and Testis

The testes produce spermatozoa and hormones.[5] The hormones govern spermatogenesis, sexual differentiation, secondary sexual characteristics, and libido.[6] The testes are oval and, depending on the age and breed of the horse, weigh between 150 and 300 g each.[1,2] The left testis is usually larger, suspended more ventrally, and situated further caudally than the right testis.[1] The long axis of the testis is nearly horizontal but raised slightly cranially.[1-4] The epididymis attaches to the dorsolateral border of the testis (i.e., the attached or epididymal border) and overlaps the lateral surface slightly, forming a testicular bursa between the testis and epididymis (Fig. 65-1). Opposite the attached border is the free border, and opposite the lateral surface is the medial surface. The epididymis is an elaborately coiled tube consisting of three parts: the head (caput), body (corpus), and tail (cauda).[1] The head lies at the cranial pole of the testis, and the body is positioned on the lateral surface of the testis. The tail projects beyond the caudal border of the testis, wraps around to the medial side, and continues proximally as the ductus deferens.[1,3,4,7]

The testis is covered by the tunica albuginea, a tough, inelastic capsule of dense fibrous tissue.[1,3] Trabeculae and septa of connective tissue from the tunica albuginea penetrate the testis to subdivide the parenchyma into lobules. Each lobule consists of convoluted seminiferous tubules lined by spermatogonia, from which spermatozoa arise, and Sertoli cells (also called sustentacular cells), which supply mechanical and nutritive support for the developing spermatozoa.[1,5] The primary spermatogonia are attached to the basement membrane of the tubule, and the more mature spermatozoa are pushed toward the lumen. Follicle-stimulating hormone produced by the hypophysis stimulates spermatogenesis. The seminiferous tubules make up over 70% of the parenchyma of the testis.[8]

Located between the seminiferous tubules are interstitial cells, known as the cells of Leydig, which produce androgens in response to interstitial cell–stimulating hormone (which is similar or identical to luteinizing hormone), produced by the hypophysis.[5] The testis of the stallion produces an unusually high concentration of estrogen in comparison to other domestic species, and the source of this estrogen is the cells of Leydig.[9]

The seminiferous tubules converge to form the tubules of the rete testis, which pierce the tunica albuginea at the dorsocranial border of the testis to become the efferent ductules.[4] The dozen or more efferent ductules unite in the head of the epididymis to form a single coiled tube, over 70 m long, that continues to become the body and tail of the epididymis and ascends with the testicular vessels as the ductus deferens.[1,2] Spermatozoa mature in the epididymal duct, and the duct's tortuous course allows the storage of a large number of spermatozoa.[5]

Inguinal Canal

The inguinal canal is an oblique passage in the abdominal wall through which traverse the *ductus deferens,* nerves, and vessels that enter or exit the scrotum and testis.[10] The internal opening of the inguinal canal, the deep inguinal ring, is a dilatable slit, about 16 cm long in the average-size horse, bordered cranially by the caudal edge of the internal abdominal oblique muscle, ventromedially by the rectus abdominis muscle and prepubic tendon, and caudally by the inguinal ligament.[1,4] The external opening of the inguinal canal, the superficial inguinal ring, is a 10- to 12-cm-long slit in the external abdominal oblique muscle.[1,10]

The medial border of the superficial inguinal ring lies directly below the medial border of the deep inguinal ring, making the medial wall of the inguinal canal very short.[4] The superficial inguinal ring is directed craniolaterally, and the deep inguinal ring is directed dorsolaterally, making the lateral angles of the rings widely divergent. The length of the canal in a medium-size horse is about 15 cm when measured along the spermatic cord.[7] The wall of the inguinal canal is lined by peritoneum, which forms the tunica vaginalis.[10]

Tunics

The tunica vaginalis, derived from the abdominal peritoneum, continues through the inguinal canal to line the interior of the scrotum and envelope the testis and its associated ducts and spermatic cord[1,11] (Fig. 65-2). The tunica vaginalis consists of a visceral tunic (tunica vaginalis propria) and a parietal tunic (tunica vaginalis communis). The visceral tunic adheres firmly to the tunica albuginea and covers the testis and associated ducts, except at the dorsal border of the testis, where vessels and the epididymis enter or leave the testis.[1,3,4,11] The parietal tunic is continuous with the parietal peritoneum of the abdomen at the deep inguinal ring and forms a sac that lines the scrotal cavity.[1,3,11] This sac is referred to as the vaginal process or vaginal sac, and its opening at the deep inguinal ring is the vaginal ring. The vaginal ring is found, during examination per rectum in the average-size horse, 10 or 12 cm abaxial to the linea alba and 6 or 8 cm cranial to the iliopectineal eminence.[1] The

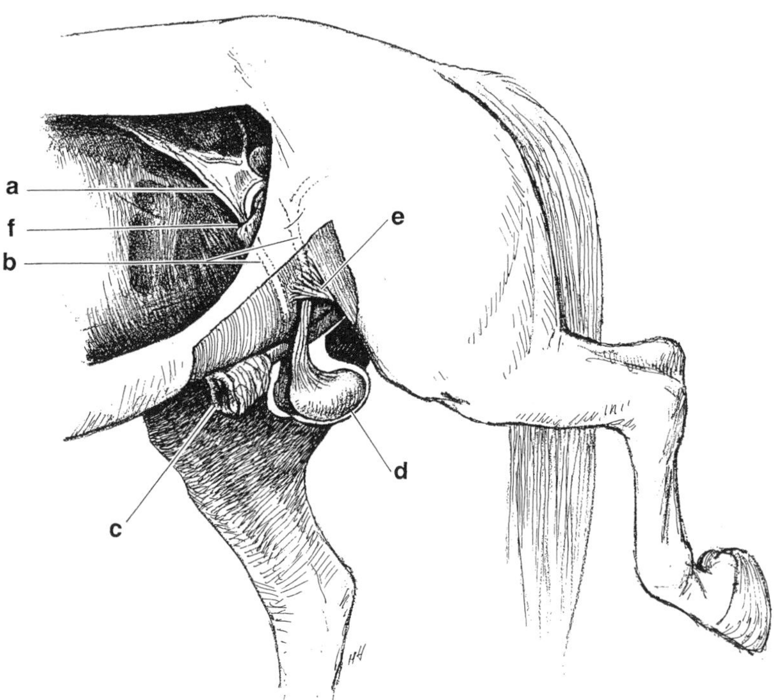

Figure 65-2. Graphic representation of the reproductive tract of the stallion, left-sided view. a, testicular artery and vein; b, spermatic cords with their inguinal canal; c, external lamina of the prepuce; d, testis within scrotum; e, external inguinal ring; f, internal inguinal (vaginal) ring.

diverticulum of the peritoneal cavity between the parietal and visceral tunics is the vaginal cavity.[1,11] This cavity communicates with the peritoneal cavity and normally contains only a small quantity of serous fluid, which serves as a lubricant to facilitate movement of the testis. The right and left vaginal cavities do not communicate.

Gubernaculum

The gubernaculum testis is a fetal, retroperitoneal, mesenchymal cord that extends between the caudal pole of the fetal testis and the scrotum and guides the fetal testis in its descent from the ventral surface of the kidney to its final position in the scrotum[10] (Fig. 65-3). The gubernaculum testis can be divided into three parts: the cranial part, which lies between the testis and the epididymis; the middle part, which lies between the epididymis and the point at which the gubernaculum penetrates the abdominal wall at the inguinal rings; and the caudal or scrotal part, which extends from the abdominal wall at the site of the future inguinal canal to the scrotum. The cranial part becomes the *proper ligament of the testis* and connects the tail of the epididymis to the testis.[3,4,10] The middle part becomes the *ligament of the tail of the epididymis* (also known as the caudal ligament of the epididymis) and connects the tail of the epididymis to the parietal tunic. The caudal part becomes the *scrotal ligament* and connects the parietal tunic to the bottom the scrotum. The scrotal ligament of an abdominally retained testis is sometimes referred to as the inguinal extension of the gubernaculum testis.[12] These ligaments may be abnormally long if the testis fails to descend.[13] Improper function of the gubernaculum may result in abdominal or inguinal retention of a testis.[14,15]

Descent of the Testis

The gonads arise retroperitoneally from the gonadal ridges caudal to the kidney and differentiate into testes at 40 days of gestation.[16,17] By gestational day 55, the testis is suspended cranially by the cephalic (suspensory) ligament and dorsally by the mesorchium. The interstitial cells begin multiplying at 6 weeks of gestation, causing the testis to hypertrophy until, at 5 months of gestation, the testis is nearly as large as that of a mature stallion and contacts both the kidney and the deep inguinal ring. This phase of testicular hypertrophy corresponds with a period of a high serum concentration of estrogen in the mare.[18]

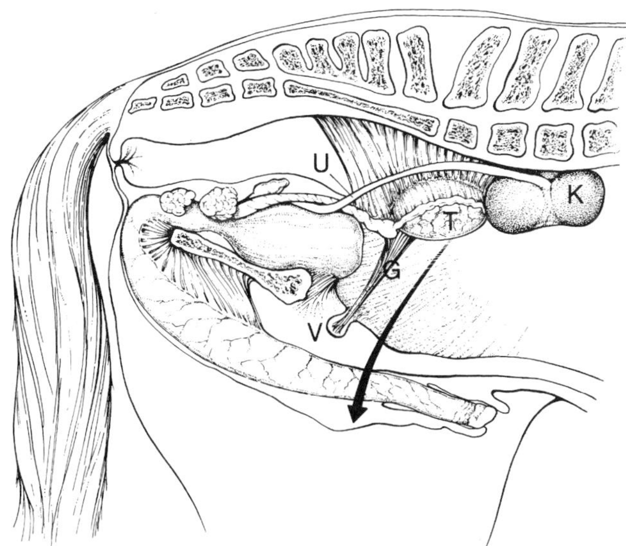

Figure 65-3. Descent of the testis. G, gubernaculum; K, kidney; T, testis; U, ureter; V, vaginal ring.

The gubernaculum extends from the caudal end of the testis to the inguinal canal and ends in a knoblike expansion between the differentiating internal and external oblique abdominal muscles.[14,16] On gestational day 45, the peritoneum invades the subperitoneal tissue around this extra-abdominal expansion of the gubernaculum to form the vaginal process. At about 5 months of gestation, the cephalic ligament atrophies, and the epididymis descends into the vaginal process while the testis remains in the abdomen.[16,17]

At 8½ months of gestation, the gubernaculum begins to shorten. Simultaneously, the testis regresses in size, mainly because of loss of interstitial cells, until during the last month of gestation, when it becomes one-tenth its former size.[16] The epididymis and subperitoneal gubernaculum expand in diameter, thus dilating the vaginal ring and inguinal canal. This, along with an increase in intra-abdominal pressure, allows the testis to pass into the inguinal canal at between 270 and 300 days of gestation.[7,14,16,17] The mass of extra-abdominal gubernaculum prevents the testis from moving directly into the scrotum so that, at birth, most testes lie in the inguinal canal. *This extra-abdominal portion of gubernaculum can be quite large at birth and easily mistaken for a testis.* The vaginal rings contract to approximately 1 cm in diameter during the first few weeks of neonatal life and become so fibrous that the testis cannot be forced through from either direction.[16]

Spermatic Cord

The spermatic cord consists of structures carried ventrally by the testis in its migration through the inguinal canal from the abdomen to the scrotum.[1,10] The spermatic cord begins at the deep inguinal ring, where its constituent parts converge. It extends obliquely and ventrally through the inguinal canal, passes beside the penis, and terminates at the dorsal border of the testis.[1] The structures that make up the cord are the tunica vaginalis; the vessels, nerves, and lymphatics of the testis; and the ductus deferens.[1,10,11] Technically, the cremaster muscle is not included as a component of the cord because it lies external to the parietal tunic.[3,15] The neurovascular components of the cord are enclosed in the mesorchium, a fold of serous membrane formed by invagination of the parietal tunic along its caudal wall (Fig. 65-4). The mesorchium extends from the origin of the testicular vessels to the testis. The mesoductus deferens is a caudomedially located fold of the parietal tunic containing the ductus deferens and the deferential vessels.[1,3,4] The mesoductus deferens is continuous with the mesorchium. The mesofuniculum is the thin part of the mesorchium between the mesoductus deferens and the parietal tunic.

The ductus deferens is a direct continuation of the epididymal duct.[1] It stores spermatozoa, and during ejaculation, it propels spermatozoa from the epididymis to the pelvic urethra.[5] The ductus deferens is somewhat convoluted

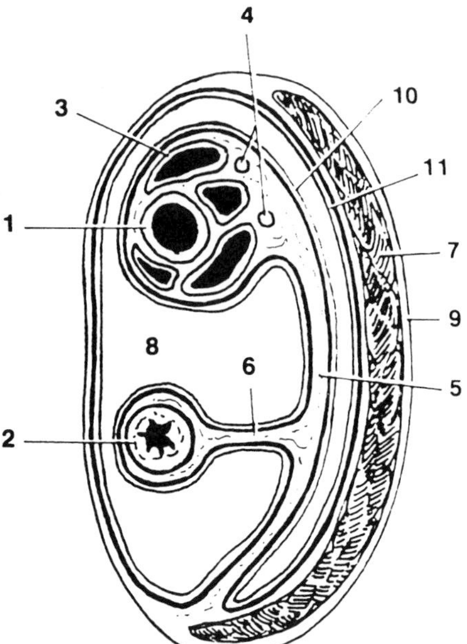

Figure 65-4. Transverse section of the spermatic cord. 1, testicular artery; 2, ductus deferens; 3, pampiniform plexus; 4, testicular nerves and lymphatic vessels; 5, mesorchium; 6, mesoductus; 7, cremaster muscle; 8, vaginal cavity; 9, spermatic fascia; 10, visceral layer of vaginal tunic; 11, parietal layer of vaginal tunic.

near the epididymis but straightens as it continues dorsally.[1,2] At the vaginal ring, it separates from other constituents of the spermatic cord and turns caudomedially into the pelvic cavity, where it lies in the genital fold. Dorsal to the bladder, it increases in diameter and forms the ampulla, which in the stallion is 15 to 20 cm long and about 1 to 2 cm in diameter. The ampulla is not nearly as pronounced in geldings. Beyond the ampulla, the ductus deferens narrows and opens with the ducts of the seminal vesicles at the ejaculatory orifices on the colliculus seminalis, a protuberance on the dorsal wall of the urethra, located about 5 cm caudal to the internal urethral orifice. The ductus deferens is supplied by the deferential artery, a branch of the umbilical artery.[3]

The testicular artery, a branch of the abdominal aorta, descends in the cranial part of the cord.[1] As the artery descends in the inguinal canal, it becomes greatly convoluted. At the testis, it continues caudally with the epididymis, turns ventrally around the caudal pole of the testis, and travels cranially on the free border, sending off branches to the medial and lateral surfaces.[1,19] Testicular veins ascend from the dorsal border of the testis. Small veins coalesce into larger veins about 10 cm proximal to the testis.[20] These larger veins contain valves that prevent retrograde flow of blood. The veins divide and convolute to form the pampiniform plexus, which lies around the coiled testicular artery and forms the bulk of the spermatic cord.[1,3,4,7] The veins unite within the abdomen to become the testicular vein. The right testicular vein usually joins the caudal vena cava, and the left testicular vein usually joins the left renal vein.[1] The lymphatic vessels of the testis and epididymis ascend directly to the medial iliac and lumbar lymph nodes.[1,3,4] A plexus of autonomic and visceral sensory nerves accompany the blood vessels to supply the testis and epididymis.

The cremaster muscle, a slip of the internal abdominal oblique muscle, lies on the caudolateral surface of the parietal tunic and attaches to this tunic at the caudal pole of the testis.[1,10] Its blood supply is the cremaster artery.[3,4] Contraction of the cremaster muscle retracts the testis.[1]

PATHOPHYSIOLOGY

Congenital Monorchidism

Horses possessing one descended testis and one that has failed to descend are sometimes described incorrectly as being monorchids.[20] The term *monorchidism* should be reserved to describe the more uncommon situation of complete absence of one testis. Horses in possession of only one testis usually reach this state from failure of a surgeon to remove both testes at the time of castration, but the condition can also occur from unilateral testicular agenesis or when a vascular insult, presumably caused by torsion of the spermatic cord, causes an abdominally located testis to degenerate.[21-26]

Monorchidism of an apparently congenital nature is usually caused by testicular degeneration rather than by atresia,[22] and the vascular insult responsible for the degeneration may occur before or after birth.[21,22,27] Torsion of the spermatic cord of the abdominal testis may cause the horse to show moderate to severe signs of abdominal pain,[28] but some similarly affected horses do not demonstrate any signs of pain (author's observation).[27]

Congenital absence of testicular tissue or absence of testicular tissue caused by testicular degeneration is discovered when, during inguinal or abdominal exploration to locate a cryptorchid testis, the tail of the epididymis is found attached to both the ligament of the tail of the epididymis and the ductus deferens, but the testis is absent.[21,22] More rarely, the epididymis or even the ductus deferens may also be missing. Monorchidism can be confirmed with a human chorionic gonadotropin (hCG)-stimulation test, after the contralateral testis is removed and the horse has recovered from surgery, but determining whether monorchidism was caused by degeneration, atresia, or surgical excision of the testis may be difficult.[22] The presence of a vaginal process suggests that monorchidism was acquired, and identifying remnants of the cremaster muscle, ductus deferens, and testicular vessels within the inguinal canal suggests that the testis was excised.

Cryptorchidism

Cryptorchidism is an anomaly of testicular position and is the most prevalent, nonlethal developmental defect of the horse.[16,29,30] Abnormal testicular location occurs when one testis or both testes fail to descend completely from the fetal position in the sublumbar area through the inguinal canal into the scrotum.[16] The term *cryptorchid* refers to the nondescended testis (by extension, a horse with this condition is also termed a cryptorchid), and removal of a cryptorchid testis is sometimes referred to as cryptorchidectomy. Colloquial terms for the cryptorchid include *rig, ridgling,* or *original.*[31-33] If a testis and its epididymis are both abdominally retained, the horse is termed a complete abdominal cryptorchid. If the epididymis, but not the testis, has descended through the vaginal ring, the horse is termed a partial or incomplete abdominal cryptorchid.[31,33,34] An inguinal cryptorchid or "high flanker" is a horse with a testis retained within the inguinal canal.[31-34]

Cryptorchidism of stallions is of considerable economic significance, because the seminiferous tubules of the cryptorchid testis are rudimentarily developed and incapable of producing sperm.[16] Unilateral cryptorchids are usually fertile but have reduced production of sperm,[35] and horses affected with bilateral testicular retention are sterile.[16] The androgen-producing cells of Leydig of a cryptorchid testis are functional and produce testosterone, although at reduced concentrations, so that the cryptorchid horse exhibits sexual behavior. Exposure of the testis to the high temperature of the abdomen or inguinal canal appears to be responsible for hypoplasia of the seminiferous tubules and results in a small, soft testis. Location of the testis at sites other than the scrotum complicates removal of the testis. Because malfunction of descent may be inherited, cryptorchid horses are generally considered genetically unsound.[29] For this reason, registration of cryptorchid stallions is disallowed by some breed associations.

An epidemiologic survey investigating the prevalence of equine cryptorchidism found that approximately one of six (i.e., about 17%) 2- to 3-year-old colts presented to a veterinary medical teaching hospital was cryptorchid.[29] Groups most commonly represented were Percherons, American Saddlebreds, American Quarter Horses, ponies, and crossbred horses. Thoroughbreds had the lowest prevalence of cryptorchidism.

Etiology

Improper function of the gubernaculum has been postulated to cause failure of testicular descent.[14,16] Failure of the subperitoneal portion of the gubernaculum to enlarge may result in failure of the vaginal ring to expand sufficiently to allow the testis to pass. Excessive enlargement of the subperitoneal portion of the gubernaculum, followed by its failure to regress adequately, may also inhibit passage of the testis into the inguinal canal.[15] Fetal endocrinologic events that control proper growth of the gubernaculum and regression are obscure, but studies of testicular descent in the pig indicate that the fetal Sertoli cells or primitive germ cells may be responsible for enlargement of the gubernaculum, and that fetal estradiol may be responsible for regression of the gubernaculum. The source of fetal estradiol is unknown. Fetal testosterone and fetal gonadotropins do not appear to be essential for normal testicular descent.

The testis may fail to descend if it does not regress to a sufficiently small size to traverse the vaginal ring.[16,18] A testicular cyst or teratoma or persistence of the suspensory ligament of the testis during gestation may account for failure of testicular descent.[33,36]

Although genetic studies of cryptorchid horses indicate that in many instances the condition is hereditary, no definitive studies have supported a plausible genetic mechanism. The effects of maternal environment and mechanical factors (e.g., dystocia) in the etiology of cryptorchidism have not been examined.[29] The conflicting observations of numerous studies of genetic transmission of equine cryptorchidism suggest that the mechanism of inheritance is complex and most likely involves several genes.[37] One of the most frequently cited investigations is a thesis published in 1943 on the genetic nature of cryptorchidism of several species of domestic animals. The Technical Development Committee of Great Britain (1954), citing this thesis, concluded that equine cryptorchidism is transmitted by a dominant factor.[38] Other researchers, citing the same thesis, reported that the investigation had determined that equine cryptorchidism is caused by a simple autosomal recessive gene.[39] A German study of 21 cryptorchid stallions postulated that at least two genetic factors are involved, one of which is located on the sex chromosomes.[39] Another German study, however, concluded that equine cryptorchidism is transmitted as an autosomal dominant gene.[39]

Researchers at Texas A&M University found that 56 of 58 colts sired by a cryptorchid American Quarter Horse stallion had both scrotal testes.[40] The other two colts were unavailable for assessment of testicular location. This stallion was unlikely to have carried a dominant autosomal gene for cryptorchidism, unless the gene had low penetrance. If equine cryptorchidism is caused by an autosomal recessive gene, the frequency of the recessive gene in the dams of these 56 colts would have had to have been nearly zero.

Cryptorchidism is often a feature of intersexuality.[41,42] For example, the testes of the male pseudohermaphrodite are often located within the inguinal canals or the abdomen.[6,43] Cryptorchidism may also be a manifestation of an abnormal karyotype.[41,42] Horses that are cryptorchid because of an aberration of genetic sex, however, are usually easily identified by their intersexual phenotypes.[6,42] The prevalence of horses that are cryptorchid because of intersexuality appears to be quite low; in a study of 5018 cryptorchid horses, only nine were intersexes.[29]

Incidence

Retrospective studies of large numbers of cryptorchid horses indicate that failure of right and left testicular descent occurs with nearly equal frequency.[44-46] Right-sided testicular retention predominates in young cryptorchid ponies, but the incidence of right-to-left retention decreases as the ponies age.[45] The decrease in incidence of right testicular retention is probably the result of descent of the right testis from an inguinal location.

A study of 350 cryptorchid horses and another of 205 cryptorchid horses found abdominal testicular retention to be more common than inguinal testicular retention.[44,46] Another study of 500 cryptorchid horses, however, found inguinal cryptorchidism to be more common than abdominal cryptorchidism.[45]

The study of 350 cryptorchid horses found that 75% of left, undescended testes were located within the abdomen, whereas only 42% of right, undescended testes were retained abdominally.[46] The reason for this difference may be that the right testis is smaller than the left during the stage of testicular regression.[17] Consequently, if the gubernaculum fails to expand sufficiently to dilate the vaginal ring, or if the testes incompletely regress in size, the larger left testis is more likely to be incapable of traversing the vaginal ring. Because this difference in testicular size remains after birth, the smaller right testis is more apt to be inguinally retained. Increase in testicular size with the onset of puberty may cause an inguinally retained testis to descend into the scrotum.[44,45]

In one study, 14% of cryptorchid horses were bilaterally affected, and most of these (60%) had abdominal testicular retention.[46] Another study found a 9% incidence of bilateral testicular retention among cryptorchid horses, but in that study, most bilaterally retained testes (67%) were inguinally located.[44] The incidence of cryptorchid horses with one inguinally located testis and one abdominally located testis was quite low in both studies (i.e., when both testes of a horse had failed to descend into the scrotum, the testes were usually either both inguinal or both abdominal).

Inguinal Herniation and Rupture

Inguinal herniation occurs when intestine, usually a portion of the ileum or a loop of the distal portion of jejunum, protrudes through the vaginal ring into the inguinal canal. If the contents extend into the scrotum, the condition is sometimes referred to as scrotal herniation (Fig. 65-5), but the terms are used interchangeably.[47,48] Inguinal hernias are sometimes called *indirect hernias,* a term borrowed from descriptions of the comparable condition in humans.[47]

A ruptured inguinal hernia occurs when intestine protrudes through the vaginal ring and then passes through a rent in the parietal tunic and scrotal fascia so that it lies subcutaneously in the inguinal or scrotal region[49] (Fig. 65-6). The term *inguinal rupture* describes a similar condition, which occurs when intestine protrudes through a rent in the peritoneum and transverse fascia adjacent to the vaginal ring, causing intestine to reside subcutaneously beside the vaginal process[47] (Fig. 65-7). Inguinal ruptures have been referred to as *direct hernias,*[50] but this term is derived from descriptions of hernias in humans and inaccurately describes the condition in horses.[47] In humans, the transverse fascia adjacent to the vaginal ring becomes weakened and protrudes, forming a peritoneum-lined sac. In horses, the integrity of the tissue adjacent to the vaginal ring is disturbed, and the intestine passing through the rent is not surrounded by peritoneum. The purported direct hernias of horses are actually ruptures, not hernias.[47,51]

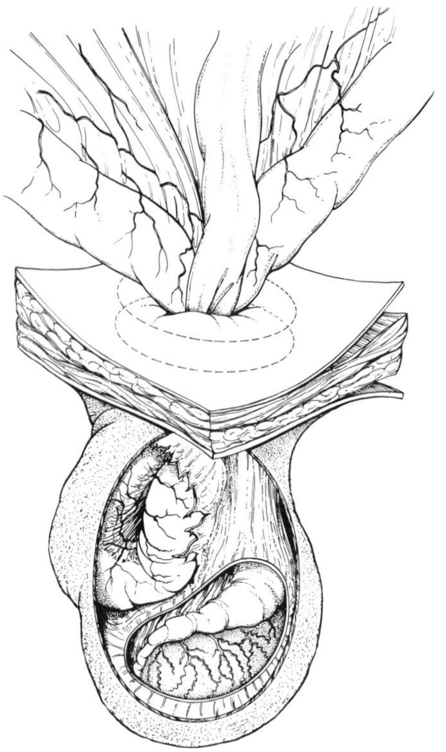

Figure 65-6. Ruptured inguinal hernia. Intestine protrudes through the vaginal ring and passes through a rent in the parietal tunic and scrotal fascia so that it lies subcutaneously in the inguinal or scrotal region.

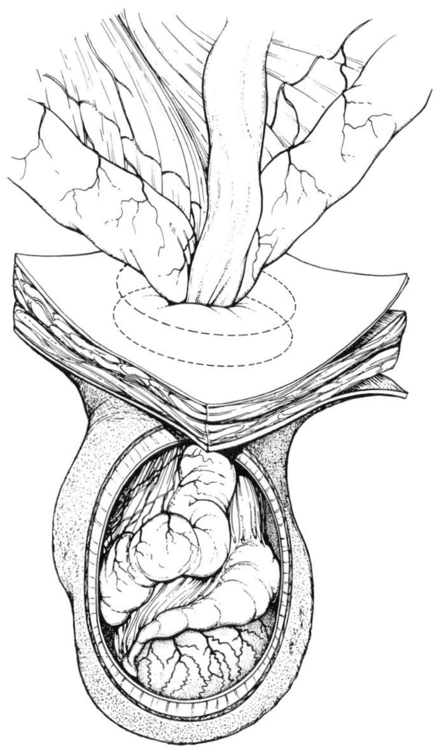

Figure 65-5. Inguinal hernia. Intestine protrudes through the vaginal ring into the inguinal canal or scrotum. The intestine lies within the vaginal cavity.

Etiology

Inguinal herniation and rupture occur almost exclusively in stallions,[48,49,52] but inguinal herniation has been reported in a few geldings[48,53,54] and a mare.[55] Geldings seldom develop inguinal herniation, because the vaginal rings decrease in size soon after castration.

Inguinal hernias of foals are congenital, and most are hereditary.[6] The left inguinal canal is most often involved.[56] Congenital inguinal herniation may be caused by excessive outgrowth of the extra-abdominal part of the gubernaculum, which results in a vaginal process with an unusually wide neck.[7,14] Congenital inguinal hernias may occur unilaterally or bilaterally, are usually reducible, cause no strangulation, and spontaneously resolve by the time the foal is 3 to 6 months old.[47,54] Longstanding, congenital, inguinal hernias may lead to testicular atrophy.[54]

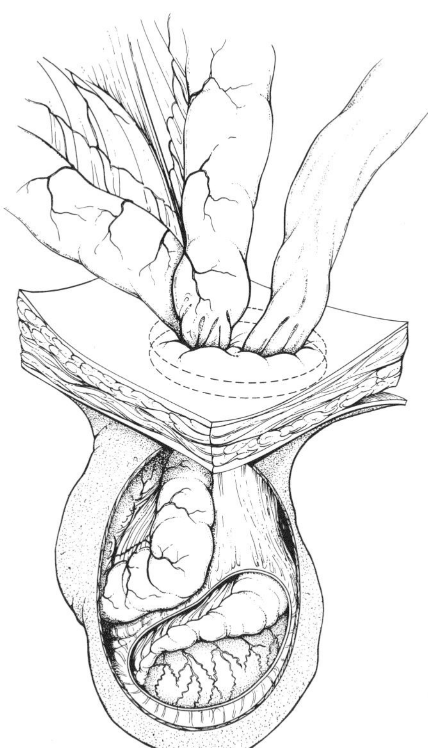

Figure 65-7. Inguinal rupture. Intestine protrudes through a rent in the peritoneum and transverse fascia outside the vaginal sac but adjacent to the vaginal ring.

Inguinal hernias occurring in adult horses are usually acquired and can occur during exercise or copulation, either of which may contribute to herniation by altering the anatomy of the inguinal canal and increasing abdominal pressure.[48] The incidence of acquired inguinal herniation in Standardbreds is reported to be higher than that of the general equine population.[57] Other breeds with anecdotal evidence of increased incidence of inguinal herniation are Tennessee Walking Horses and American Saddlebreds.

An acquired inguinal hernia of an adult horse commonly results in strangulation of small intestine and represents a surgical emergency.[48] Clinical signs are usually referable to obstruction of the small intestine and include recovery of nasogastric reflux after nasogastric intubation and rectally palpable, distended small intestine.[48,52] Strangulation of herniated intestine is caused by constriction of the intestine by the vaginal ring.[52] An acquired inguinal hernia usually causes obstruction of the vasculature of the spermatic cord, which leads to edema of the external genitalia and testicular degeneration or necrosis.

Abdominal compression during parturition may be responsible for ruptured inguinal herniation in foals.[49,58] Ruptured inguinal herniation appears to occur much less commonly in adults than in foals. In adults, inguinal rupture is primarily traumatic in origin, but in foals, it occurs much less commonly than does ruptured inguinal herniation.[47] With an inguinal rupture or a ruptured inguinal hernia, the intestine that protrudes through the rent may become strangulated or may adhere to subcutaneous tissue, and the separation of the skin from its blood supply may reduce the viability of the skin.

Torsion of the Spermatic Cord

Torsion of the spermatic cord occurs when the attached testis rotates on its vertical axis.[59] The condition is sometimes improperly referred to as testicular torsion. Torsion of the spermatic cord causes the testicular vessels to twist, producing venous and often arterial obstruction, which leads to testicular congestion and edema in mild cases and complete testicular infarction in severe cases[27,59,60] (Fig. 65-8). Clinically significant torsion of the spermatic cord in the horse occurs rarely, and few reports of the condition can be found.[27,61-64] This condition is reported to occur most commonly in trotting Standardbreds.[6]

Torsion of the spermatic cord of 360 degrees or more is accompanied by signs of acute pain, which may resemble signs of colic pain, and enlargement of the affected testis and cord.[61] The condition is a surgical emergency that usually requires removal of the affected testis, because the testis is rarely salvageable. Torsion of the spermatic cord of an abdominally located testis may cause the affected horse to show mild signs of colic pain,[28] but acute torsion of the spermatic cord has been recognized during cryptorchidectomy of several apparently normal horses that apparently displayed no signs of colic (author's observation).[27] Evidently, torsions less than 180 degrees cause no clinical abnormalities and are considered an incidental finding. Evaluation of testicular blood flow of stallions using color Doppler ultrasonography, however, shows that 180-degree torsion of a spermatic cord may cause retrograde blood flow and suggests that torsion of this degree may have a detrimental effect on testicular function, even in the absence of clinical signs of substantial vascular compromise.[65]

Torsion of the spermatic cord of 180 degrees is relatively easy to diagnose because it causes the tail of the epididymis to reside in the cranial portion of the scrotum, rather than in its normal caudolateral position in the scrotum. Torsion of the spermatic cord may be difficult to determine when the spermatic cord is twisted 360 or 720 degrees, because the tail of the epididymis resides in its normal caudolateral position in the scrotum. Torsion of the spermatic cord of 360 degrees or more may be accompanied by so much scrotal, testicular, and epididymal swelling that palpation of the epididymis is not possible.

Torsion of the spermatic cord of the descended testis of horses apparently occurs intravaginally (i.e., within the vaginal process).[61,64] Torsion may occur because the ligament of

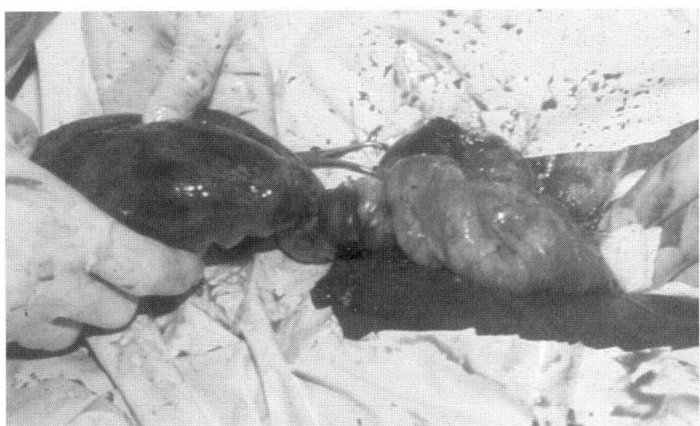

Figure 65-8. Torsion of the spermatic cord has caused necrosis of the testis and the portion of the cord distal to the torsion.

the tail of the epididymis (caudal ligament of the epididymis) or the proper ligament of the testis is abnormally long. The ligaments of the contralateral testis may also be abnormally long, making that spermatic cord also prone to torsion.[64] To prevent torsion of the contralateral spermatic cord, the contralateral testis can be fixed permanently in position (orchiopexy) by placing a nonabsorbable suture through the tunica albuginea and the dartos tissue at the cranial and caudal poles of the testis.

The spermatic cord of an abdominal testis may be more apt to develop torsion than the spermatic cord of a descended testis, because the proper ligament of the testis and sometimes the ligament of the tail of the epididymis of an abdominal testis are abnormally long.[25,27,35] None of 350 cryptorchid horses in one study, however, developed torsion of the spermatic cord.[46]

Hydrocele (Vaginocele) and Hematocele

A *hydrocele,* or vaginocele, is an abnormal collection of serous fluid between the visceral and parietal layers of the tunica vaginalis.[66,67] Hydroceles form when fluid normally secreted by the vaginal tunic is produced at a rate greater than that at which it can be absorbed by the lymphatic vessels and veins of the spermatic cord.[68] The cause of the discrepancy between the rate of production and the rate of resorption of the fluid is usually idiopathic.[67] Hydroceles may accompany testicular neoplasia or orchitis, and because the vaginal and peritoneal cavities communicate, some hydroceles could be caused when fluid present in excess in the abdominal cavity enters the vaginal cavity.[69] Migration of parasites through the vaginal cavity, 180-degree torsion of the spermatic cord, trauma, and a hot climate in conjunction with lack of exercise have been implicated as causes of hydroceles.[67,70] Hydroceles may develop acutely or insidiously. They are generally considered to cause temperature-induced dysfunction of spermatogenesis by insulating the testis and epididymis, but one investigation found they caused no important effect on semen quality.[67] A hydrocele can occasionally be a complication of castration, but only when the parietal tunic is retained (i.e., after an open castration).

Palpation of a hydrocele usually causes no apparent discomfort to the horse, and the involved testis is freely moveable and feels as though it resides within a compressible, fluid-filled bag.[69] Anechoic to semi-echoic fluid surrounding the involved testis and epididymis is seen during ultrasonographic examination of the scrotum, and a yellowish, clear fluid is obtained during aspiration of the vaginal cavity. The involved testis of a chronically affected horse may be abnormally small.

The size of a hydrocele may reduce temporarily with exercise, and some hydroceles may spontaneously resolve when the affected horses are moved to a cooler environment.[67,69] Fluid usually re-forms quickly after aspiration. Treatment of a horse for hydrocele should be aimed at removing the inciting cause, but because the cause can rarely be identified, the usual treatment of horses affected with persistent, unilateral hydrocele is removal of the affected testis and parietal tunic. The testis and tunic should be removed before spermatogenesis of the contralateral testis becomes affected by increased scrotal temperature. Prognosis for fertility is guarded if bilateral hydroceles persist, but some stallions affected with hydrocele retain normal spermatogenesis.[67]

Sclerotherapy, using either a 2.5%, a 5%, or a 10% solution of tetracycline injected into the vaginal cavity, has been used successfully to treat men affected with a hydrocele,[71] but sclerotherapy has not been evaluated as a treatment for stallions with a hydrocele.

A *hematocele* may resemble a hydrocele, but it is characterized by a collection of blood within the vaginal cavity.[72,73] Hematoceles are usually caused by testicular or scrotal trauma, but they may occur as an extension of hemoperitoneum.[35] Ultrasonographic examination of the scrotum and its contents and aseptic aspiration of the vaginal cavity may help differentiate other causes of scrotal enlargement, such as hydrocele, from hematocele.

A horse with a hematocele may be treated successfully by aspiration of blood from the vaginal cavity followed by lavage of the cavity with a balanced electrolyte solution, provided that the tunica albuginea is not ruptured.[73] This treatment may minimize the insulating effect of blood and reduce the formation of adhesions between the visceral and parietal layers of the tunica vaginalis. If torn, the tunica albuginea should be sutured, or the testis should be removed.

Varicocele

A varicocele is an abnormally distended and tortuous pampiniform plexus.[66,74] Valvular incompetence of the testicular vein, where it empties into the vena cava or renal vein, may increase hydrostatic pressure in the pampiniform plexus by causing reflux of caval or renal blood into the testicular vein.[74] Varicoceles disturb countercurrent exchange of heat from the arterial to the venous blood, causing temperature-induced dysfunction of spermatogenesis.[66,74] Although varicoceles are known to cause infertility in men and rams, their effect on fertility of horses has not been evaluated, perhaps because varicoceles of stallions are so infrequently encountered. Unilateral varicoceles have been noted in some stallions with normal ejaculates.[75] Varicoceles of stallions usually occur unilaterally and, when palpated, do not cause the horse to display signs of pain. The affected spermatic cord has the texture of a "bag of worms," and the neck of the scrotum on the affected side may be wider than usual.

Treatment of stallions with varicoceles is removal of the affected cord and testis, but treatment is not necessary if the varicocele does not affect seminal quality. Humans affected with varicocele have been treated by ligation of the venous loops of the pampiniform plexus.[76]

Testicular Neoplasia

The classification of testicular neoplasms of horses is far less extensive than that of humans. Primary testicular tumors are usually divided into germinal and nongerminal types. Germinal neoplasms arise from germ cells of the spermatic epithelium, and nongerminal neoplasms arise from testicular stromal cells. Reported germinal testicular tumors of the horse include the seminoma, teratoma, teratocarcinoma, and embryonic carcinoma. Nongerminal testicular tumors of the horse are the Sertoli cell and Leydig cell tumors. Secondary tumors (i.e., tumors that are the result of metastases) of the equine testis are extremely rare.[59,77,78]

The prevalence of primary testicular neoplasia in horses is unknown but is probably low, perhaps because most stallions are castrated while young, before neoplasia has had an opportunity to develop,[77,79] and perhaps because testes removed from apparently normal stallions are seldom examined closely for the presence of neoplasia.[80] Consequently, the few acknowledged characteristics of testicular neoplasms of horses have been established by collecting information gathered from a small number of case reports. Characteristics of equine testicular neoplasms, such as hormonal effects, tendency toward malignancy, and relationship to cryptorchidism, have been inferred from characteristics of testicular neoplasms of other species more commonly affected, such as humans and dogs. Characteristics of testicular neoplasms differ among species, so extrapolating characteristics of testicular neoplasms of other species to horses may result in mistaken assumptions.

Testicular enlargement is the primary presenting sign of testicular neoplasia when the neoplastic testis is located scrotally.[81] Usually, the enlargement is of an insidious nature. Signs of tenderness during palpation are uncommon but may be a feature of the neoplastic testis.[77,82] The surface of the neoplastic testis may be characterized by multiple, irregular bumps, and the consistency of the testis may be firmer than normal.[82,83] Horses with neoplastic abdominal testes may be presented for examination because of intermittent signs of colic.[81,84] Metastases may cause weight loss or dyspnea. Identifying a tumor is difficult without histologic examination of either the entire testis or tissue obtained by biopsy.[82] Metastatic spread of testicular tumors is uncommon, but when it occurs, metastases can sometimes be palpated as an enlargement of the sublumbar lymph nodes.[35]

Seminoma

Seminomas arise from the germinal cells of the seminiferous tubules and are the most common testicular tumors of horses.[77,81] These tumors probably do not produce hormones.[35] As in other species, seminomas of the horse seem to appear with greater frequency in cryptorchid testes and are most commonly found in old horses[81-83,85-87]

Although most equine seminomas behave benignly, they have a higher incidence of malignancy than do some of the other types of testicular neoplasms, and they metastasize more frequently.[77,78,81] The relative risk of a seminoma in a human becoming malignant is highest if the testis is abdominal,[88] but no such correlation has been made between the location of a seminoma in the horse and malignancy. All seminomas of horses should be considered potentially malignant, because clear histologic differentiation between benign and malignant seminomas is almost impossible.[79] Abdominal invasion should be suspected if an enlarged spermatic cord can be palpated externally.[77] Thoracic metastasis has been reported.[78,86] The sectional surface of a seminoma is lobulated, homogeneous, and white or grayish

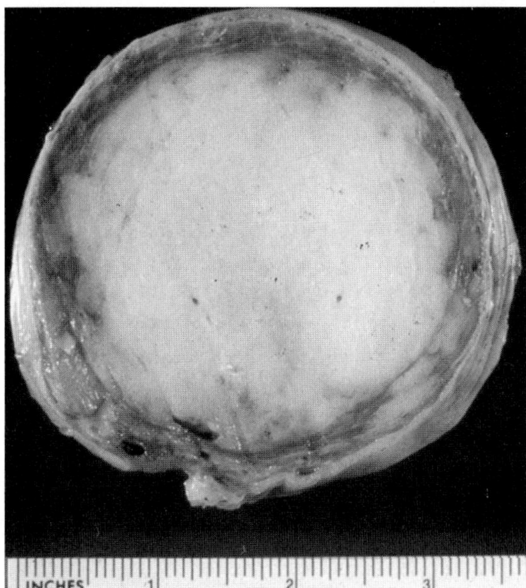

Figure 65-9. Cross-section of a testis containing a seminoma. The seminoma has replaced the parenchyma of the testis.

white (Fig. 65-9). The tumor is soft to moderately firm, and when squeezed, the surface may exude a milky fluid.[35,86]

Sertoli Cell Tumor

The Sertoli cell or sustentacular cell tumor of the horse arises from the nonspermatogenic cells of the seminiferous tubules.[35] Sertoli cell tumors of horses are less frequently encountered than are other types of testicular tumors.[79,89,90] Their biologic behavior in horses is unknown because of the small number of reports, but in dogs and people, these tumors often cause hyperestrogenism and feminization.[59]

Malignant Sertoli cell tumors of dogs are rare,[59] but of the few Sertoli cell tumors of horses that have been reported, several were malignant.[91,92] A malignant Sertoli cell tumor that had metastasized to many organs was found in a descended testis of a horse,[91] and a malignant Sertoli cell tumor that also had metastasized to many organs was found in an abdominal testis of another horse believed previously to be a gelding.[92] Whether cryptorchidism is a predisposing factor to development of the Sertoli cell tumor cannot be determined from the few reports.[77] The sectional surface of a Sertoli cell tumor is firm, white or tan, and homogeneous.[90,91]

Leydig Cell Tumor

The interstitial or Leydig cell tumor is an infrequently reported equine testicular tumor.[77,79,93,94] Although these tumors arise from the androgen-producing cells of the testis, evidence of production of androgenic hormones by these tumors is lacking in horses and other animals.[35,79,80] Because the Leydig cells of the testes of horses secrete a large amount of estrogen, in addition to androgenic hormones, the hormonal effect of Leydig cell tumors in the horse could vary.[9,95] Cryptorchidism may be associated with this neoplasm on the basis of the observation that, in a study of nine stallions affected unilaterally or bilaterally with Leydig cell tumor, the tumors in all but one horse were found in one or both undescended testes.[80]

Most Leydig cell tumors of horses are benign, and metastasis is rare.[35] The sectional surface of the tumor is yellow to brown, which may help grossly to differentiate this tumor from other types of testicular tumors.[77,80] The demarcation between the tumor and adjacent normal parenchyma is poor.[80]

Teratoma

Teratomas are tumors of multiple tissues whose embryologic origin is different from that of the tissue in which they arise,[79] and evidence indicates that they develop from pluripotential tumor cells capable of giving rise to any type of tissue found in the body.[96] Most teratomas occur in the gonads.[59] Histologic examination of equine testicular teratomas shows that they are benign, slow growing, and composed of mixed, well-differentiated tissues.[97] Derivatives from all three germinal layers, such as bone, cartilage, brain, and respiratory and glandular epithelium, may be present within the testis.[79,98] Occasionally, teeth can be found.[26,79] Teratomas that consist primarily of cysts lined by squamous epithelium and contain hair have incorrectly been referred to as dermoids or dermoid cysts. The term *dermoid*, however, should not be used when referring to a teratoma, because unlike dermoids, teratomas display progressive growth.[26]

The teratoma is the second most common form of equine testicular neoplasia.[77,79] It is found in both descended and cryptorchid testes, but some investigators believe it occurs more frequently in the latter.[89,99-101] Others dispute this claim, stating the opposite.[79,102] Failure of descent of a testis, rather than being a predisposing factor in the formation of a teratoma, may more probably be a result of the teratoma itself.[89,100]

Teratocarcinoma and Embryonal Carcinoma

Teratocarcinomas are similar to teratomas but contain undifferentiated embryonic tissue interspersed among the disarranged mix of differentiated tissues.[103,104] Embryonal carcinomas resemble teratocarcinomas but are composed entirely of undifferentiated embryonic tissue.[104] The undifferentiated embryonic tissue is responsible for the malignant properties of teratocarcinomas and embryonal carcinomas. Teratocarcinomas and embryonic carcinomas of the horse are evidently quite rare but appear to be rapidly fatal.

Intersex

Because male and female reproductive organs arise from the same embryonic structures, errors of development may result in a horse that possesses sexual structures common to both sexes.[59] An individual whose sexual identity is confused because of congenital anatomic abnormalities of the genital organs is called an intersex.[6,41,59] An animal's sexual identity can be defined according to its genetic makeup, the type of its gonads, or the morphology of its accessory genitals. A normal animal is the same sex in all three categories, but the intersex differs in one of the categories.

Intersexes are divided into three main classes: "true" hermaphrodites, female pseudohermaphrodites, and male pseudohermaphrodites. Hermaphrodites are usually defined on the basis of gonadal sex, with true hermaphrodites having both testicular and ovarian tissue.[6,41,105] Pseudohermaphrodites have gonads of only one sex and are classified as male or female, depending on whether the gonads are testes or ovaries.

The true hermaphrodite is much rarer than the pseudohermaphrodite.[6,41,105,106] One gonad of a hermaphrodite may be a testis and the other an ovary, or one or both gonads may consist of both ovarian and testicular tissue (i.e., ovotestes). The hermaphrodite's external as well as internal genitalia usually represent both sexes, but its external genitalia may tend toward either the male or female. Some cases of equine hermaphrodism have been attributed to chimerism resulting from double fertilization or fusion of blastocysts, but other equine hermaphrodites are one genetic sex.[42,106]

Gonads of the pseudohermaphrodite are of one sex, but the external genitalia resemble those of the opposite sex.[6,41,105] The male pseudohermaphrodite is by far the most common intersex of horses and typically has hypoplastic testes within the abdomen or inguinal canal and a penis-like structure, which often resembles a clitoris, emerging from a rudimentary prepuce (Fig. 65-10). The rudimentary "penis" and prepuce are positioned anywhere on the midline from the perineum to a scrotal or abdominal location.[6,43] Although the phenotypic appearance of a male pseudohermaphrodite is often that of a female, sexual behavior is

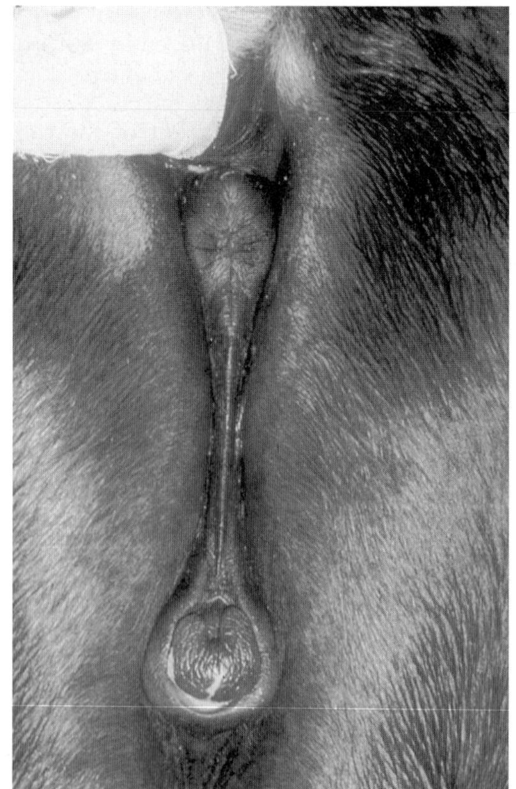

Figure 65-10. Male pseudohermaphrodite. A rudimentary penis and prepuce are positioned in the perineal region. (Courtesy of E. Behrens, MV.)

that of a male.[105] Most equine male pseudohermaphrodites appear to be masculinized, genetic females (64, XX).[6,41,59,105,107] The contradiction between gonadal and genetic sex has not been fully explained.

DIAGNOSTIC PROCEDURES

History and Physical Examination

History pertaining to problems of the testes and related structures may include such information as infertility, history of unilateral or bilateral testicular retention, enlargement in the inguinal or scrotal areas, testicular pain, and changes in testicular size. Knowledge of events surrounding the onset of testicular pain or increase in testicular size, such as occurrence after exercise or copulation, is sometimes helpful in making a diagnosis. Other considerations include previous urogenital surgery, illnesses, and drug therapy.

Physical examination of the testes and associated structures should include inspection and palpation. Notice should be given to the size, shape, texture, and temperature of the testes, and the horse should be observed for evidence of pain when the testes are palpated. Right and left testes should be compared. The scrotum of a normal stallion usually appears asymmetric, because the left testis has a longer spermatic cord and is, therefore, often more pendulous than the right. With cryptorchidism, the scrotum on the involved side is poorly developed. Scrotal scars should be noted, bearing in mind that a scrotal scar may mean only that an orchidectomy was attempted, not that it was accomplished. Occasionally, scrotal edema may be noted. This does not usually imply disease related to the genitalia but is more likely a consequence of general retention of fluid associated with disease of other systems.

The testes should feel smooth and elastic. Irregularities in size and texture may indicate orchitis, torsion of the spermatic cord, thrombosis of the testicular artery, inguinal herniation, or neoplasia. Often, a neoplastic testis is insensitive to digital compression that would cause a normal horse to show signs of pain. Insidious increase in testicular size is suggestive of neoplasia, whereas acute increase in size may suggest torsion of the spermatic cord, inguinal herniation or rupture, or orchitis. As a testicular neoplasm grows, it may seem to replace the entire organ. The neoplastic testis characteristically feels heavier than the normal testis. Because neoplasia may be associated with inguinal or pelvic lymphadenopathy, palpation per rectum of internal lymph nodes should, if possible, accompany examination for testicular enlargement.

The testes of the prepubescent stallion are often quite small, retractile, and therefore often difficult to palpate. Before declaring the stallion a cryptorchid, a tranquilizer or sedative should be administered to relax the cremaster muscles and thus facilitate palpation. The medial crus of the superficial inguinal ring is easily palpated if the palm of the hand is turned toward the abdomen.[4] If the palm is turned toward the thigh, the fingers may pass into the inguinal canal without encountering the ring, because the lateral border of the ring is not as readily palpated. Because the average-size stallion's canal is about 15 cm in depth,[32] only the most ventral part of the inguinal canal can be palpated. An inguinal testis lies with its long axis oriented vertically and is preceded in its descent by the tail of the epididymis. A partial abdominal cryptorchid can be easily mistaken for an inguinal cryptorchid if the epididymis within an everted vaginal process is, by chance, palpated and mistakenly identified as a small testis. The vaginal rings can be palpated only by examination per rectum.

The epididymis, located on the dorsolateral surface of the descended testis, should be easily identifiable. The tail of the epididymis should be easily palpated on the caudal pole of the testis. If the tail of the epididymis is located cranially in the scrotum, the spermatic cord has rotated 180 degrees. Torsions of 180 degrees or less probably cause no clinical problems. When palpating the scrotum of a foal to ascertain if testicular descent is complete, the epididymis should be identified so that the remnant of the gubernaculum is not mistaken for a descended testis.

A bulge in the spermatic cord or scrotum may suggest the presence of an inguinal hernia, hydrocele, or hematocele. Because the intestinal contents of most acquired inguinal hernias are strangulated, palpation of the scrotum and examination of the vaginal rings per rectum should be part of the physical examination of every adult stallion with signs of intestinal obstruction. Unapparent, congenital inguinal hernias may become apparent after castration. Examining the inguinal area of foals before castration for the presence of a congenital inguinal hernia is especially important to avoid evisceration. If a scrotal hernia is present, palpation may elicit a sensation of crepitus. Occasionally, peristalsis may be noted by movement of the skin overlying the bulge.[52] A ruptured inguinal hernia or an inguinal rupture should be suspected if the skin over the inguinal or scrotal swelling is cold, edematous, or macerated. A strangulated inguinal hernia or rupture should be suspected when a stallion develops signs of colic after copulation or exercise, especially if a testis and its spermatic cord are swollen and tender. A varicocele should be suspected if the spermatic cord appears larger than normal and has the texture of a "bag of worms." A hydrocele should be suspected if the scrotum appears to be smooth, nontender, and fluid filled, and the testis is smaller than normal. The presence of a fluid-filled, nontender scrotum after castration is also indicative of a hydrocele.

Examination per Rectum

Examination per rectum of the vaginal rings and structures that traverse them may be helpful in the diagnosis and evaluation of some genital abnormalities, such as cryptorchidism, inguinal or scrotal herniation, scirrhous cord, and testicular neoplasia. The vaginal rings and associated structures are located about 6 or 8 cm cranial to the iliopectineal eminence and 10 to 12 cm abaxial to the linea alba in the average-size horse.[1] The vaginal ring is palpable in geldings as a slight depression, but in stallions it is large enough to insert a finger.[108]

The risk of rectal injury should be weighed against the value of the diagnostic information to be gained before performing an examination per rectum. For example, examination per rectum is probably not necessary before removing a cryptorchid testis by an inguinal approach, provided that the owner is confident that orchidectomy has not been attempted previously. If, during surgery, the testis is not encountered in the inguinal canal, it can usually be extracted from the abdomen through the vaginal ring or through a parainguinal incision. Even though mares are more commonly subjected to examination per rectum, the incidence of rectal injury in geldings and stallions is higher, perhaps because males are less accustomed to the procedure and resist it more forcibly.[109] Most cryptorchid stallions presented for examination are young, and the small size and fractious nature of young horses predispose them to rectal injury during examination per rectum.

To palpate the vaginal rings, the examiner introduces a hand into the rectum until the lateral aspect of the wrist rests on the pubic brim at the pelvic symphysis.[110] The examiner may find it advantageous to palpate the right vaginal ring with the left hand and the left vaginal ring with the right hand. The fingertips are flexed and pressed against the lateral aspect of the abdominal wall, and fingers are extended in a downward and forward direction against the abdominal wall until a finger enters the vaginal ring. If the search is made with a backward flexing motion of the finger, the medial border of the deep inguinal ring tends to close, causing the finger to slide over the vaginal ring. When the vaginal ring is located, the components of the spermatic cord can be felt as a cordlike structure entering the canal. The ductus deferens is more readily palpated at the ring than are the testicular vessels,[4] and it can be palpated on the caudomedial aspect of the ring, if the testis or epididymis has descended.[26]

The vaginal rings should always be examined for evidence of intestinal incarceration when examining a colicky stallion. Palpating distended loops of intestine and a loop descending through the vaginal ring indicates that intestine has become inguinally incarcerated. Traction on the loop usually causes a painful reaction from the horse. For horses with septic funiculitis, thickening of the spermatic cord at the vaginal ring is evidence of ascension of infection into the abdominal cavity. For horses with testicular neoplasia, thickening of the spermatic cord at the vaginal ring suggests that the neoplasm has metastasized. The lymph nodes surrounding the terminal portion of the aorta and its branches should also be palpated for evidence of metastasis.

For a horse with an unknown history of castration that displays masculine behavior, or for a stallion known to be cryptorchid, examination per rectum may be useful in determining whether a testis has traversed the vaginal ring.[110] Determining the location of a retained testis prior to orchidectomy is especially important if a flank or paramedian approach is to be used, because an inguinally retained testis is difficult to remove using any approach other than the inguinal one. Palpating an abdominal testis per rectum is difficult, because the testis is small and flaccid, and because the proper ligament of the testis is usually elongated, allowing the testis a wide range of movement. Palpation of an abdominal testis per rectum by an inexperienced examiner should be regarded as a fortuitous occurrence, and failure to palpate an abdominal testis should not be relied on diagnostically. The vaginal ring cannot be palpated in horses with complete abdominal testicular retention, but palpation of the vaginal ring is evidence that the testis or at least its epididymis has descended through the ring into the inguinal canal. Unfortunately, a partial abdominal cryptorchid cannot be distinguished from a horse whose testes have descended through the vaginal ring by examining the vaginal rings per rectum.

Testicular Biopsy

Testicular biopsy is indicated when less invasive diagnostic methods have failed to provide an etiologic or pathologic diagnosis of testicular disease, and when a diagnosis is essential to determine treatment and prognosis.[111] An obviously neoplastic testis should be removed rather than biopsied, because biopsy may disseminate neoplastic cells. Testicular biopsy has been used to a limited extent in the horse, perhaps because of fear of the complications reported after incisional (especially) or needle biopsy of the testes in other species.[112,113] Because horses are usually able to maintain breeding soundness after removal of one testis, obviously diseased testes have often been removed rather than biopsied, even though the testicular disease has not been definitively identified.

Biopsy provides the only method for directly assessing stages of spermatogenesis and rates of sperm production and for determining the identity of space-occupying lesions.[113] Biopsy may be helpful in differentiating among causes of testicular enlargement, such as septic orchitis, neoplasia, or trauma. Despite complications reported to occur in other species, aspiration and needle biopsies have been performed successfully in a small number of horses.[112,114,115]

Aspiration Biopsy

Aspiration biopsy presents little risk to the horse because decreased spermatogenesis is not a likely complication.[111] Although an aspiration biopsy is less damaging to the testis than a needle biopsy, an aspiration biopsy usually does not offer useful information about spermatogenesis.[113] Its main use is to help determine the cause of testicular enlargement. Aspiration biopsy can be performed by inserting a 23- or 25-gauge needle into the testicular parenchyma.[111] Local anesthesia of scrotal skin is unnecessary. A 12-mL syringe is attached to the needle, and the plunger is withdrawn. The needle is retracted without exiting the parenchyma and is reinserted into several areas. The plunger is released, and the needle is removed from the testis. Although hemorrhage after biopsy is uncommon, digital pressure maintained over the puncture site for several minutes ensures hemostasis. Aspirated material is expelled onto a glass slide, smeared, dried, and stained. Aspirated material should be smeared gently, because cells collected from the testis by aspiration are extremely fragile. The slides should be examined by an experienced cytologist, because normally developing spermatocytes have cytologic characteristics that could lead to a mistaken diagnosis of malignancy.

Needle Biopsy

The needle biopsy provides the most useful information about spermatogenesis, and the technique is unlikely to have deleterious effects on the testis.[111,112,114] Needle biopsy of a testis can be performed using a 12- or 14-gauge Vim-Silverman needle[112] or a 12- or 14-gauge automated biopsy needle (Biopty Biopsy Instrument, CR Bard, Inc, Covington, Ga)[114] (Fig. 65-11). Biopsy can be performed with the horse standing and sedated. The scrotum is prepared as if for aseptic surgery, and a small volume of local anesthetic solution is injected subcutaneously at the proposed site of biopsy using a 25-gauge needle. The site of biopsy should be the craniolateral quarter of the testis, away from the head of the epididymis, where the vasculature is the least prominent, unless there is a particular area of interest. The biopsy needle can be guided ultrasonographically to sample a discrete lesion. The testis is held tightly against the scrotal skin, and a small stab incision is created on the lateral surface of the scrotum, down to and through the parietal tunic. The Vim-Silverman needle or automated biopsy needle is inserted through the visceral tunic and tunica albuginea into the testicular parenchyma. Two or three samples are collected through the same skin incision but at slightly different angles. Pressure is maintained over the incision for several minutes, and the cutaneous incision is closed with a single suture. Samples are fixed in Bouin's solution for 6 to 12 hours, washed, and stored for about 12 hours in 70% ethanol. They are then shipped to a laboratory in 50% ethanol.

Complications associated with needle biopsy of the testis in other species include transient scrotal edema; intratesticular hemorrhage resulting in pressure necrosis; immune reaction to spermatozoa caused by disruption of the blood–testis barrier; dissemination of neoplastic cells if a tumor is biopsied; formation a hematoma between the testis and the parietal tunic or between the parietal tunic and scrotum, which can result in insulation-induced damage to the seminiferous epithelium; and transient decrease in semen quality.[111] Formation of antisperm antibodies and decrease in semen quality reported to occur in other species after testicular needle biopsy have not been reported to occur in the horse.[111,114]

Hormonal Assays

Occasionally, physical examination is inadequate to determine whether a horse possesses a retained testis, in which case a hormonal assay may be necessary to distinguish between psychic and hormonal causes of persistent masculine behavior. Concentration of testosterone in the plasma or serum can be used to distinguish between geldings and horses with extrascrotal testicular tissue.[116-121] Stallions with descended testes (sometimes referred to as "entire stallions") and cryptorchid stallions have significantly higher concentrations of androgens and estrogens in the serum or plasma than do geldings.

In several studies, basal concentration of testosterone in castrated horses was generally less than 40 pg/mL of serum, and that of entire stallions was greater than 100 pg/mL.[116,117] The concentration of testosterone of entire stallions was often 1000 to 2000 pg/mL, although the concentration during winter was often as low as 200 pg/mL.[117] In one study, geldings were found to have a testosterone concentration in serum of less than 240 pg/mL, and horses with testicular tissue had a concentration of greater than 440 pg/mL.[118] Another investigation found the concentration of testosterone in the serum of ponies with testicular tissue to be 440 to 1550 pg/mL; 6 weeks after castration, the concentration had decreased to an average of 40 pg/mL.[120] These studies found the concentration of testosterone in the serum of stallions to be dependent on the age of the horse and the season, with the concentration being lowest in horses younger than 3 years and during the winter.[116-118]

Some investigators noted that cryptorchid stallions generally had a slightly lower concentration of testosterone than did entire stallions.[117,120,121] In contrast, other investigators observed that mature, bilateral, cryptorchid stallions and hemi-castrated stallions (i.e., unilateral cryptorchid horses whose scrotal testis had been removed) had a similar or higher concentration of testosterone in the serum than did entire stallions.[118] These authors suggested that retained abdominal testes may produce as much or more testosterone than do scrotal testes.

Wide variations in basal concentration of testosterone occasionally lead to confusion.[116,117,119-121] Because the concentration of testosterone in some entire stallions is exceptionally low and that in some geldings is exceptionally high, values may overlap, causing erroneous conclusions to be drawn as to whether a horse possesses testicular tissue. One investigator reported 14% error using basal

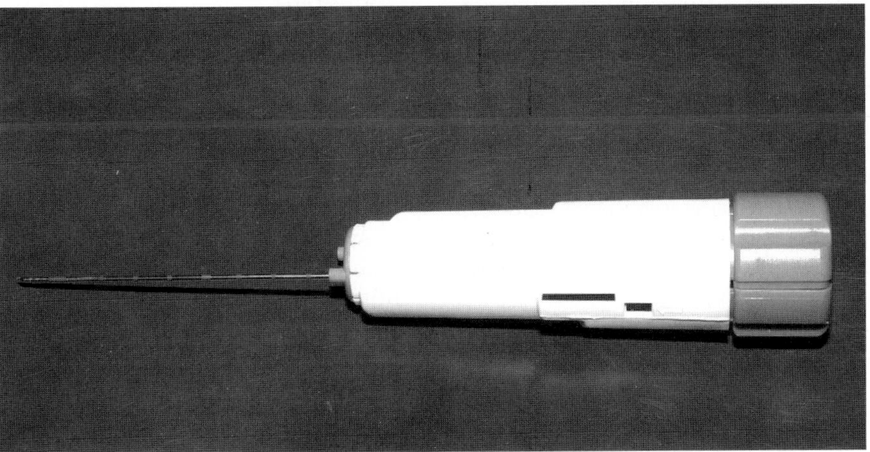

Figure 65-11. An automated biopsy needle (Monopty Biopsy Instrument, C.R. Bard, Inc, Covington, Ga) for performing needle biopsy of the testis. (Courtesy John Schumacher.)

concentration of testosterone to differentiate geldings from horses with testicular tissue.[117] These wide variations in concentration of testosterone were not observed in another study, which found basal concentrations of testosterone to be accurate in predicting the presence of testicular tissue.[118] That study found an error of only 5%.

A rise in the concentration of testosterone in response to stimulation by administration of hCG increases the accuracy of detecting cryptorchidism.[116,117,120,121] Investigators reported increased concentration of testosterone in cryptorchid stallions at any time between 30 and 120 minutes after intravenous administration of 6000 or 12,000 units of hCG.[116,117] Horses were classified as cryptorchid if the concentration of testosterone both before and after administration of hCG was greater than 100 pg/mL, or as geldings if the concentration in both samples was less than 40 pg/mL. The hCG-stimulation test was 94.6% accurate in predicting the presence of testicular tissue. Response to hCG was poor in horses less than 18 months old and during the winter.[116] Other investigators found that response of bilateral cryptorchid stallions and hemi-castrates to hCG was minimal, but that best results were achieved if poststimulation samples were obtained at 24 hours rather than at 1 hour.[118] Other investigators found that administration of hCG to entire stallions induced an increase in concentration of testosterone that lasted about 10 days, and they suggested that for detection of a retained testis a poststimulation sample should be taken at 2 to 3 days.[119]

In one study, quantification of total, free (i.e., unconjugated) estrogen alone was superior to quantification of total androgens, with or without hCG stimulation, for detecting retained testicular tissue.[121] Although other investigators were unable to confirm superiority of free estrogens for detecting testicular tissue, they found a high correlation between the presence of testicular tissue and the concentration of conjugated estrogen (e.g., estrone sulfate) if cryptorchid horses younger than 3 years and cryptorchid donkeys of any age were excluded from the study.[116,117] The investigators found that young cryptorchid horses and cryptorchid donkeys did not consistently produce enough conjugated estrogens to yield reliable results. Quantification of conjugated estrogen was 96% accurate when these animals were excluded from the study. Although cryptorchid horses produced less estrogen than did entire stallions, the lower threshold of conjugated estrogen for a cryptorchid horse was higher than that of testosterone. Horses with a concentration of estrone sulfate less than 50 pg/mL in plasma or serum were determined to be geldings. A concentration in excess of 400 pg/mL indicated cryptorchidism. Another investigation also revealed a high correlation between the concentration of conjugated estrogens and the presence of testicular tissue in horses older than 3 years.[118] In that investigation, geldings had a concentration of estrone sulfate less than 120 pg/mL, and cryptorchid stallions had a concentration greater than 1000 pg/mL.

Knowing the laboratory's standards for normal hormonal concentrations of geldings and horses with testicular tissue is important when evaluating results of hormonal assays. Comparing test results with values from a known gelding may be necessary, if the laboratory cannot furnish standards. False-positive results from hormonal assays to determine the presence of testicular tissue have not been reported.[122] The clinician can be confident that a horse has testicular tissue if the result of a hormonal assay indicates that testicular tissue is present.

Other Diagnostic Tests

Ultrasonographic examination may delineate abnormalities within the testis and associated structures or assist in determining the location of a cryptorchid testis. To ultrasonographically image an inguinal testis, a 5-MHz, transrectal transducer is placed longitudinally over the superficial inguinal ring.[123] To image an abdominal testis, the transducer is inserted rectally, cranial to the pelvic brim, and the abdomen is scanned in a to-and-fro pattern as the transducer is advanced cranially. Inguinal ultrasonography is ineffective in locating an abdominal testis, and furthermore, abdominal ultrasonography is ineffective in locating an inguinal testis. The echotexture of the cryptorchid testis is less dense than that of a normal descended testis.

Serum concentrations of biochemical markers, such as α-fetoprotein and hCG, are measurable in minute quantities using radioimmunoassay and have been used to monitor the response of humans to treatment for testicular neoplasia.[88] Apparently, no such markers have been used to detect testicular neoplasia of horses or to monitor for the presence of metastatic neoplasms after a neoplastic testis has been removed.

Cytologic examination of peritoneal fluid may be valuable in diagnosing certain diseases of the testes and associated structures, because changes in the fluid within the vaginal cavity may be reflected in the peritoneal fluid. Semen evaluation may be valuable in diagnosing orchitis, epididymitis, or seminal vesiculitis. Thermographic examination of the scrotum may detect a variation in temperature between the testes. A horse with morphologic abnormalities suggestive of intersexuality, such as cryptorchidism accompanied by ambiguous genitalia, can be karyotyped to determine its genetic sexual identity.

SURGICAL PROCEDURES

Castration

Indications

Synonyms for castration include orchidectomy, emasculation, gelding, and cutting. Castration is one of the most common equine surgical procedures and is usually performed to sterilize horses unsuitable for the genetic pool and to eliminate masculine behavior. By removing the primary source of androgens, castration renders the horse more docile and manageable.

Although stallions can be safely castrated at any age, managerial convenience usually governs the age at which a horse is castrated. Typically, a horse is castrated simply because facilities are insufficient to safely contain a stallion. Most horses are castrated when they are 1 to 2 years old, when masculine behavior becomes intolerable to the owner. Sometimes castration is delayed until a masculine feature, such as a crest on the neck, has developed or until it becomes apparent that the horse is unsuitable for breeding.

Castration may be performed to alter conformation. Bulls castrated prior to puberty grow to a greater height because castration delays closure of the growth plates of their long bones,[124] and the same may be true of stallions castrated before puberty. Orchitis, epididymitis, testicular neoplasia, hydrocele, varicocele, testicular damage caused by trauma, torsion of the spermatic cord, or inguinal herniation may necessitate unilateral or sometimes bilateral orchidectomy. Impotent or infertile breeding stallions may be salvaged for other uses by castration.

Preoperative Considerations

A general physical examination of the horse should precede castration, and the scrotum, especially that of very young horses, should be inspected for inguinal herniation and for the presence of both testes. Discovery of inguinal herniation or cryptorchidism may affect the choice of anesthesia and the surgical approach. Preoperative sedation of a fractious horse usually permits safe palpation of the scrotal and inguinal areas and occasionally facilitates palpation of an inguinal testis by causing the cremaster muscles to relax.

Standing Castration

CASE SELECTION

Castration performed with the horse standing can be difficult and dangerous to the surgeon if candidates for the procedure are not selected prudently. Standing castration of horses with poorly developed testes and of ponies is mechanically difficult. Donkeys and mules can be dangerous to castrate while they are standing because of their athletic agility. Stallions that elicit a hostile or evasive response to genital palpation may best be castrated while they are anesthetized. Docile stallions with well-developed testes whose genitalia can be palpated without being sedated are usually the safest candidates for standing castration.

PREPARATION OF THE HORSE

Sedating the horse to be castrated while standing is optional but advisable. Drugs commonly used, either alone or in combination, are xylazine HCl, detomidine, pentazocine, and butorphanol tartrate. Acetylpromazine, although commonly administered to tranquilize stallions before castration, can result, on rare occasion, in priapism or penile paralysis, and so its use in stallions should be avoided.

The scrotum must be anesthetized on each side of the scrotal raphe from the cranial to the caudal pole of the testis along the proposed lines of incision. The spermatic cords can be anesthetized by injecting local anesthetic solution, usually 15 to 30 mL, through a 22- to 20-gauge needle directly into each cord. This anesthetic technique ensures good anesthesia of the cord but occasionally causes a hematoma that interferes with application of the emasculator. Alternatively, about 25 mL of local anesthetic solution (without epinephrine) can be injected directly into the parenchyma of each testis through an 18-gauge, 1½-inch needle. The anesthetic solution diffuses proximally into each spermatic cord. The horse's tail should be wrapped to prevent it from contaminating the surgical field, and the scrotum should be scrubbed before and after administering the local anesthetic solution.

RESTRAINT

The horse should be restrained by a competent handler, and to ensure adequate immobilization, application of a lip twitch may be necessary. The standing castration should be performed with both the surgeon and the handler positioned on the same side of the horse, usually the left side for the right-handed surgeon. The surgeon should be positioned at the horse's shoulder well out of kicking range with his or her head and shoulder pressed firmly into the horse's flank.

Standing castration can be performed safely and efficiently if candidates are selected prudently, if the horse is adequately sedated, if the spermatic cord and scrotum are properly desensitized with a local anesthetic agent, and if the surgeon is technically proficient. A standing castration requires less expense and assistance, and it is often less time consuming because the surgeon need not wait for the horse to recover from general anesthesia. Risks to the horse that attend general anesthesia are avoided. Because the spermatic cords and scrotum are locally desensitized, measures to rectify immediate postoperative complications, such as hemorrhage, can be accomplished without reanesthetizing the horse.

Recumbent Castration

ANESTHESIA

To castrate a horse in the recumbent position, a clean, safe area in which to anesthetize and recover the horse is a prerequisite. A variety of intravenous anesthetics, alone or in combination, can be administered to provide safe and predictable anesthesia of sufficient duration. A thiobarbiturate administered as a bolus produces rapid anesthesia characterized by moderate analgesia and muscular relaxation, particularly if the horse has been sedated with xylazine.[125] Recovery is usually satisfactory if repeated administration of the thiobarbiturate is not necessary. Ketamine, administered after sedating the horse with xylazine, provides 10 to 15 minutes of surgical anesthesia. Muscular relaxation and analgesia are only moderate but can be enhanced if butorphanol tartrate or diazepam is added to the preanesthetic regimen.[125-127] If necessary, anesthesia can be extended by administering half the dosage of xylazine and ketamine combined in one syringe. Guaifenesin (5% to10%), in combination with ketamine or a thiobarbiturate, provides smooth induction and recovery and good analgesia with excellent muscular relaxation, but guaifenesin must be administered in large volumes.[128] Succinylcholine, a muscle relaxant, has been widely employed as a chemical restraint for recumbent castration, but because it provides no analgesia, its use alone for castration is inhumane. Additional information on anesthesia can be found in Chapters 19 and 20.

POSITIONING

The horse is anesthetized and positioned in lateral recumbency with its upper rear limb pulled forward and secured with rope. The right-handed surgeon generally finds the recumbent castration most easily performed with the horse positioned in left lateral recumbency, and vice versa.

Approach

SCROTAL INCISION

For the standing castration and one technique of recumbent castration, the testes are removed through a scrotal incision. If the horse is anesthetized, and if the testes are small and difficult to grasp, as is often the case with prepubescent stallions, the scrotum can be safely incised by pulling the cranial end of the prepuce craniad and upward to tense the scrotal raphe (Fig. 65-12). Another method of incising the scrotum is to compress the testes against the bottom of the scrotum. Two parallel 8- to 10-cm-long incisions are made 2 cm on either side of the raphe. The incision should be sufficiently long to provide adequate postoperative drainage. To ensure adequate drainage, many surgeons prefer to partially ablate the scrotum, which can be accomplished by connecting the two parallel incisions cranially and caudally and removing the portion of scrotum between the incisions.

Another method of removing the bottom of the scrotum is to grasp the scrotal raphe between the thumb and forefinger, and while applying traction to the bottom of the scrotum, to excise a portion of the tented tissue with a scalpel (Fig. 65-13). When surgery is performed with the horse standing, stab wounds to the horse or surgeon that could result from sudden movement by the horse are avoided by incising with a scalpel blade held between the fingers rather than attached to a handle. A large portion of

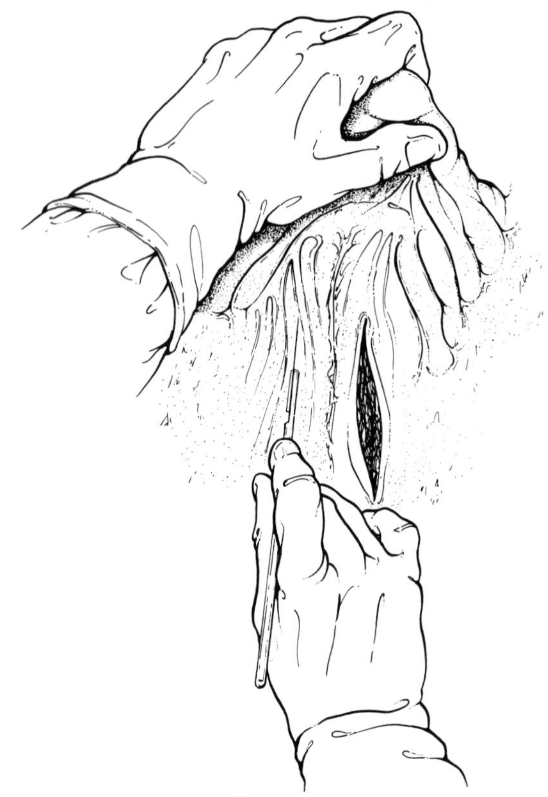

Figure 65-12. Incising the scrotum for castration. If the testes are difficult to grasp, the cranial end of the prepuce can be pulled craniad and upward to tense the scrotal raphe.

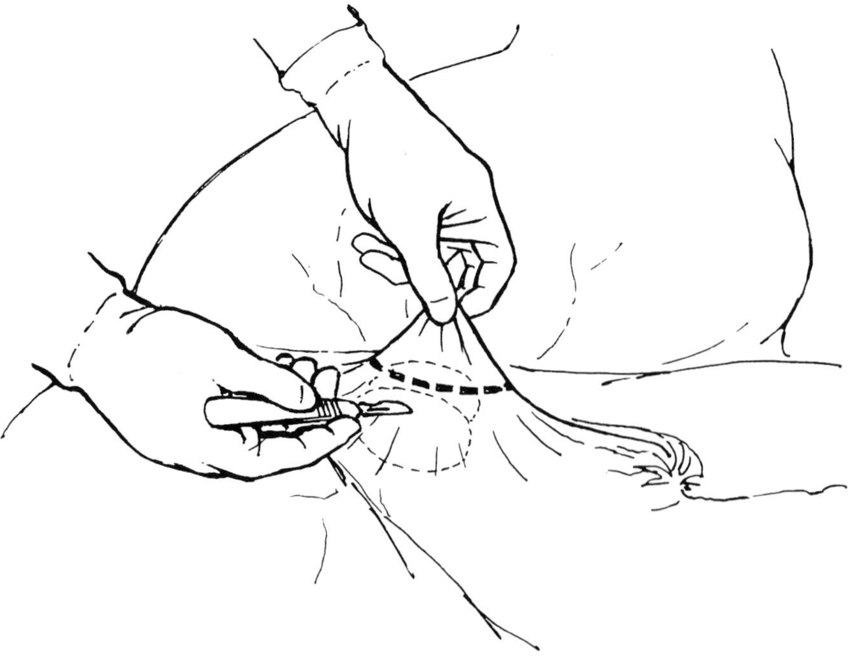

Figure 65-13. The bottom of the scrotum is removed by placing traction on the scrotal raphe with a thumb and forefinger and excising a portion of the tented tissue with a scalpel.

the scrotum should be excised to ensure adequate drainage. To avoid cutting large vessels, the dissection should remain close to the scrotal skin. The testes are then isolated using digital dissection.

INGUINAL INCISION

For the inguinal approach, the horse is anesthetized and positioned in dorsal recumbency. The superficial inguinal ring is exposed through an 8- to 15-cm skin incision (depending on the horse's size) made directly over the superficial inguinal ring.

EMASCULATORS

The emasculator models most commonly used are the improved White's, the Reimer, and the Serra emasculators[129] (Fig. 65-14). The Reimer emasculator crushes the cord, and a separate handle and blade sever the cord distally. Because the cord is severed with a separate handle, there is no danger of cutting the cord before it is satisfactorily crushed. The extra handle on the Reimer emasculator makes the instrument somewhat unwieldy for standing castration. The jaws of the Serra emasculator are curved, so that the cord is evenly crushed, and the grooves on the crushing blades are oriented parallel to the cord, decreasing the chance of accidentally transecting the cord with the crushing portion of the jaws[20] (Fig. 65-15). A type of emasculator used more commonly in Europe than in North American has no cutting component and only crushes the cord (Fig. 65-16). The cord must be severed distal to the crushed segment with a scissors or scalpel blade.

Surgical Techniques

Techniques of orchidectomy are the open, closed, and half-closed techniques, regardless of whether the horse is castrated while standing or recumbent, or whether the approach is inguinal or scrotal. With the open technique of castration, the parietal (or common vaginal) tunic is retained. With the closed and the half-closed techniques, the portion of the parietal tunic that surrounds the testis and distal portion of the spermatic cord is removed.

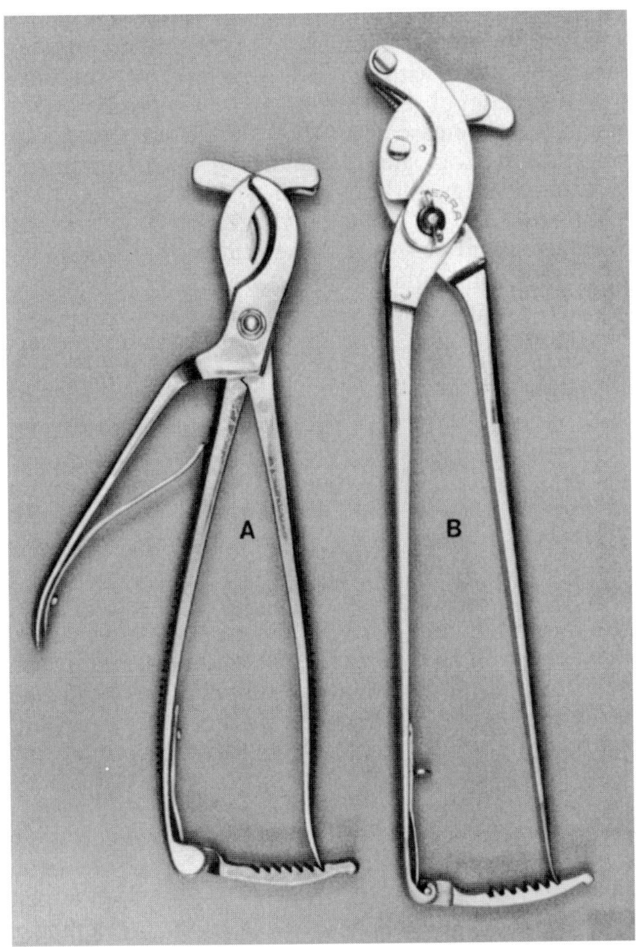

Figure 65-14. Reimer (**A**) and Serra (**B**) emasculators. The Reimer emasculator severs the cord with a blade on a separate handle so that the cord is not accidentally cut before it is satisfactorily crushed.

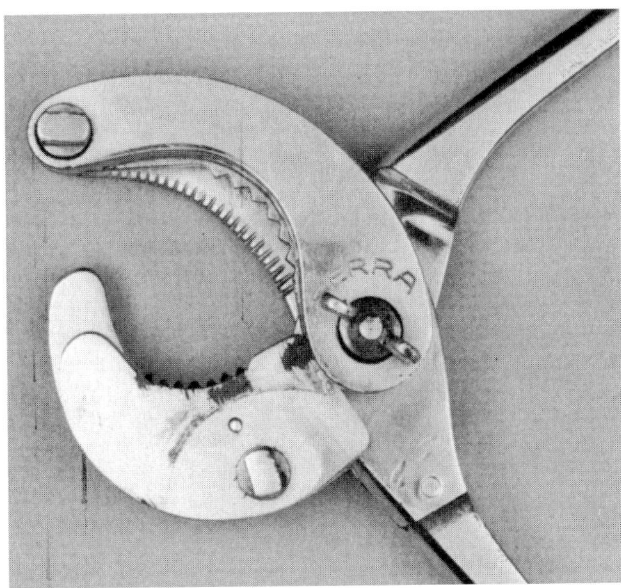

Figure 65-15. Serra emasculator. The grooves of the crushing blade are oriented vertically to prevent the blade from accidentally cutting the cord.

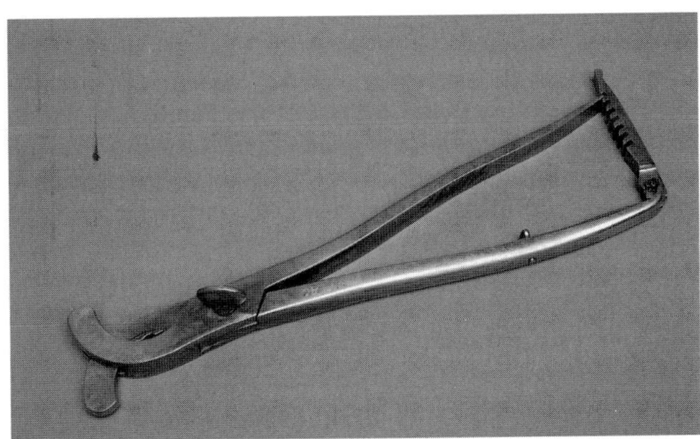

Figure 65-16. An emasculator without a cutting blade. The spermatic cord must be severed distal to the emasculator with a scissors or scalpel blade.

OPEN TECHNIQUE

When performing the open technique of castration, the parietal tunic of testis is incised. The ligament of the tail of the epididymis (caudal ligament of the epididymis), which attaches the parietal tunic to the epididymis, is severed or bluntly transected. By transecting the fold of the mesorchium and mesofuniculum, the testis, epididymis, and distal portion of the spermatic cord are completely freed from the parietal tunic and removed using an emasculator. The open technique of castration is probably the most commonly used technique.[129]

CLOSED TECHNIQUE THROUGH A SCROTAL APPROACH

With the closed technique, the parietal tunic is not incised, so it also is removed along with the testis and a portion of the cord. Using digital dissection, the parietal tunic surrounding the testis is freed from the scrotal ligament and scrotal fascia, and by placing mild traction on the testis with one hand, the parietal tunic surrounding the cord is separated from fascia surrounding the spermatic cord with the other hand. After the parietal tunic is separated from the surrounding fascia, it and its contents are removed using an emasculator. Care should be taken, when separating the fascia from the spermatic cord, to include the large pudendal vessels that lie within the fascia, so that these vessels are not included in the jaws of the emasculator.

HALF-CLOSED TECHNIQUE

The closed technique just described can be converted to a half-closed technique by making a 2- to 3-cm vertical incision through the exposed parietal tunic at the cranial end of the testis or the distal end of the spermatic cord. A thumb (the left thumb if the operator is right-handed) is inserted through the incision into the vaginal cavity. The testis and a portion of the spermatic vasculature are prolapsed through the incision by applying downward traction on the tunic with the thumb while simultaneously using the fingers of the same hand to push the testis through the incision. The fundus of the parietal tunic inverts and follows the testis through the incision because of its attachment to the testis by the ligament of the tail of the epididymis. Traction is applied to the parietal tunic with the index and middle fingers, which are placed into the sac formed by the inverted fundus. Traction can also be applied to the parietal tunic and the testis by applying a large Carmalt or Allis forceps to the parietal tunic before prolapsing the testis from the vaginal cavity. The half-closed technique should be considered a closed technique because the parietal tunic is removed along with the testis and the distal portion of the spermatic cord.

For each technique, the emasculator is applied at a right angle to the spermatic cord, loosely closed to avoid incorporation of scrotal skin, and slid further proximally. The emasculator is applied so that the crushing component is proximal to the cutting blade. When correctly applied, the wing-nut of the emasculator is oriented distally toward the testis, and the emasculator is said to be positioned "nut to nut." This positioning is not critical when using an emasculator that does not have a cutting blade. The scrotal skin is pushed toward the abdomen with one hand (with the spermatic cord positioned between the index and middle fingers) toward the horse's abdomen, and the jaws of the emasculator are inspected to ensure that they do not contain scrotal skin. The tension on the cord is relieved, and the handles of the emasculator are compressed completely to crush and sever the cord. The time that should elapse before the emasculator is removed from the spermatic cord depends on the size of the cord being severed and the dependability of the emasculator used, but applying the emasculator for about 1 minute is usually sufficient to achieve hemostasis. If the cord is exceptionally large, the emasculator can be applied for a longer time, or the parietal tunic and cremaster muscle can be crushed and severed separately from the testicular vessels and the ductus deferens. The cutting blade of the emasculator should not be so sharp that the cord is completely severed but rather should be slightly dull so that the cord must be torn, although with only slight effort, from the blade. If a noncutting emasculator is used, the cord is severed with a scalpel blade 2 to 3 cm distal to the emasculator. The emasculator should be elevated toward the horse's inguinal area before the cord is released, so that the testicular vessels do not recoil. It is customary, and perhaps prudent, when performing a standing castration to leave the scrotal wound unsutured. Loose scrotal fascia protruding from the scrotal opening is trimmed with scissors.

A technique (i.e., the Zurich technique) frequently used in Europe to ensure adequate scrotal drainage involves suturing a 30-cm-long gauze drain to the stump of one of the cords with heavy catgut suture.[130] The drain that exits the scrotal wound is removed 2 days after castration by rupturing the catgut suture with a sharp tug on the drain.

SELECTION OF TECHNIQUE

An advantage of the closed and half-closed techniques of castration is that removal of the parietal tunic decreases the incidence of postoperative complications, such as septic funiculitis and hydrocele[32,34] (see "Postoperative Complications of Testicular Surgery," p. 802). The half-closed technique permits inspection of the components of the cord and allows a greater portion of the ductus deferens and testicular vasculature to be exteriorized. For horses at risk of having an unapparent inguinal hernia, such as Standardbreds, evisceration can be avoided by using a closed technique and placing a ligature proximal to the proposed site of transection.

The closed technique of castration has no advantage over the open technique in preventing evisceration if a ligature is not applied to the cord proximal to the site of transection. The closed and half-closed techniques are indicated for disease conditions that may involve the parietal tunic, such as neoplasia and orchitis. The closed and half-closed techniques require more dissection than does the open method of castration, and this may be a disadvantage when performing a standing castration on a fractious stallion.

Primary Closure of the Incision

By convention, scrotal incisions are usually left unsutured to heal by secondary intention. Primary closure, however, speeds healing and recovery, eliminates infection, and decreases edema, pain, and muscular stiffness.[131-134] Primary closure may be particularly useful if vigorous exercise cannot be enforced postoperatively. Primary closure decreases convalescence but is time consuming and requires meticulous hemostasis and strict adherence to aseptic technique. In one study, no complications were encountered when the spermatic cords were simply transected with an emasculator.[133] Hemorrhage from a cord into the sutured scrotum, however, even if only a small amount, risks formation of a hematoma, and therefore, ligation of the cord proximal to the point of division with the emasculator ensures good hemostasis and should be considered an important part of the procedure.

One investigator, pointing out the importance of eliminating dead space, closed the subcutaneous tissue with multiple rows of absorbable suture.[133] Another investigator, however, found multiple-layer closure unnecessary and reported minimal postoperative complications when only the scrotal skin was sutured.[131] The cutaneous incision is best closed with an absorbable 2-0 monofilament suture using a simple-continuous intradermal suture pattern. Because the cutaneous incision is sutured intradermally, removal of cutaneous sutures is not necessary.

The testes can be removed *per primam* through an inguinal incision created over each spermatic cord.[135] This technique is frequently used in Europe when castrating horses 2 years old or older to avoid evisceration, because the vaginal rings of these horses are thought by some surgeons to be wider than those of younger horses. Using this technique, the inguinal fascia is separated digitally to expose the superficial inguinal ring. The fascia must be separated bluntly to avoid lacerating large branches of the external pudendal vessels. Blunt dissection is continued until the spermatic cord is encountered. The parietal tunic surrounding the cord is freed from surrounding fascia and incised longitudinally for 5 cm.

Using an index finger, the testicular vessels and ductus deferens are exteriorized through the incision, and using gentle traction on these structures, the testis is pulled from the vaginal cavity. The ligament of the tail of the epididymis, which attaches the testis to the parietal tunic, is identified and transected. Bleeding vessels are cauterized to prevent hemorrhage into the vaginal cavity. Two transfixing ligatures are applied 1 cm apart, as far proximally as possible, to the testicular vasculature and ductus deferens, using an absorbable, heavy monofilament suture. The vasculature and ductus deferens are severed 2 cm distal to the distal ligature, and the stump is replaced into the vaginal cavity. If this technique of *per primam* castration is performed with the expectation of preventing incarceration of intestine in the inguinal canal, a ligature should be applied to each spermatic cord proximal to the site of transection.[136]

The incision in the parietal tunic and the subcutaneous tissue are each sutured with an absorbable 2-0 monofilament suture using a simple-continuous pattern. The cutaneous incision is closed with the same suture using a simple-continuous intradermal suture pattern.

Aftercare

All horses not previously immunized with tetanus toxoid should receive both tetanus antitoxin and toxoid. The previously immunized horse should receive a booster vaccination if more than a year has passed since its last vaccination.[137] The horse's activity should be restricted for the first 24 hours after castration to avoid hemorrhage from the severed testicular and scrotal vessels. After this period, the horse should be exercised to the degree necessary to prevent excessive preputial and scrotal edema. A large, grass-covered field is an ideal environment for postoperative recuperation, but the owner should be cautioned that turning a horse into a field does not ensure that it will receive adequate exercise.

Antimicrobial treatment is probably unnecessary if clean surroundings are provided, but a survey of practitioners, undertaken to determine the type and frequency of complications that occur after castration, found that horses may be less likely to develop infection at the castration site if they receive perioperative antimicrobial treatment.[129] The operative site can be hosed vigorously, if the horse permits it, to keep the scrotal wound clean, open, and draining, but this same survey found that horses that receive hydrotherapy after castration may be more prone to develop excessive swelling and infection of the scrotum.

Protecting the wound against flies is usually unnecessary, even during fly season, if the horse's tail-hairs are long enough to reach the scrotal area. The horse should be isolated from mares for at least 2 days after castration. Ejaculates are highly unlikely to contain sufficient spermatozoa to cause impregnation after 2 days.[138] The castration wound should be nearly healed by 3 weeks.

Laparoscopic Castration

Ligating and transecting the blood supply and ductus deferens of scrotal testes laparoscopically with the horse standing or anesthetized results in avascular necrosis of the testicular parenchyma with the testes in situ.[139,140]

The standing approach is preferred by most surgeons, when the horse is castrated laparoscopically. To safely insert a laparoscopic sleeve and cannula into the abdomen, the abdomen can be insufflated through a Veress needle, IV catheter, teat cannula, chest drain, or metal uterine catheter introduced into the abdomen through a stab incision created slightly dorsal to the crus of the internal abdominal oblique muscle, midway between the last rib and the tuber coxae. The abdomen can also be insufflated, using the same devices, through a stab incision created on the linea alba. The abdomen is insufflated using a gas, such as carbon dioxide, nitrous oxide, or helium, until the intra-abdominal pressure rises to 8 to10 mm Hg. Care should be taken to avoid insufflating the retroperitoneal space. After the abdomen is inflated, the insufflation device is removed, and a laparoscopic sleeve with a guarded trocar is inserted through an incision in the flank. The laparoscopic sleeve and guarded trocar can also be inserted safely, without insufflating the abdomen, by allowing air to enter the abdomen through a blunt cannula, such as a chest drain, inserted into the abdomen through the flank. Air entering the abdomen causes the viscera to fall away from the body wall, allowing safe introduction of the laparoscopic sleeve and trocar. The trocar is removed, and the laparoscope, which is attached to a fiberoptic light source and a video camera and viewing monitor, is introduced into the abdomen. The laparoscope is directed caudally to view the inguinal areas. A 10-mm-diameter instrument portal is created 8 to 10 cm cranioventral to the laparoscopic portal, and another is created 8 to

10 cm caudoventral to the laparoscopic portal. A third, 5-mm-diameter instrument portal is created 8 to 10 cm caudodorsal to the laparoscopic portal.

The testicular vessels and ductus deferens are identified in the mesorchium as they course toward the vaginal ring. A ligating loop is placed through the 5-mm instrument portal, and a right-angle dissecting forceps is inserted through the cranioventral portal and the ligating loop. The ductus deferens and testicular vessels are grasped with the forceps. Using a bipolar cautery forceps placed through the caudoventral instrument portal, the ductus deferens and testicular vessels are coagulated distal to the forceps. The cautery instrument is removed and replaced with a laparoscopic scissors, which is used to transect the ductus deferens and spermatic vessel immediately distad to the site of coagulation. The ligating loop is now slid over the right-angle forceps onto the coagulated stump of the ductus deferens and testicular vessels, tightened, and tied, and the ends of the ligature are cut. After releasing the forceps, the stump is inspected for hemorrhage.

By elevating the small colon manually per rectum, the contralateral testis can be removed using the same portals and technique. Removing the contralateral testis using portals created on the contralateral side, however, may be faster and easier.

The testes, deprived of their blood supply, swell during the first week and then begin to decrease in size. The atrophied testes can be palpated in the scrotum for at least several months,[140] but by 5 months the remnants are no longer palpable.[139] Within 7 days after the testicular vessels are ligated, the concentration of testosterone falls to that expected of a horse with no functional testicular tissue. The epididymis remains viable, but because it has no contribution to masculine behavior, the horse behaves as a gelding. Swelling and discomfort observed after laparoscopic castration seem to be less severe than is seen after routine castration.[140] A testis whose blood supply has been interrupted can revascularize, however, apparently by peritesticular angiogenesis, before the testis becomes completely necrotic, resulting in preservation of stallion-like behavior.[141] The owner should be warned of this uncommon complication.

Vasectomy

A stallion used for detecting estrous (i.e., a teaser stallion) can be vasectomized to render it incapable of ejaculating spermatozoa and thus from accidentally impregnating mares. A stallion can be vasectomized through an incision created over each spermatic cord or through a single incision created over one testis.[142] To transect a portion of the ductus deferens through a single incision in the scrotal area, the horse is anesthetized, positioned in dorsal or lateral recumbency, and the scrotum is prepared for surgery. A 2-cm, longitudinal, cutaneous incision is made on the medial aspect of one testis, and the incision is extended through the dartos and parietal tunic. The ductus deferens, which is identified as a white, 2- to 3-mm-diameter, cordlike structure, is exteriorized and separated for a length of several centimeters from its mesorchium, using a curved hemostat. Two ligatures of 2-0 absorbable or nonabsorbable suture are placed around the most proximal aspect of the exposed portion of the ductus deferens, and a third ligature is placed around the most distal aspect of the exposed portion of the ductus deferens. The segment of ductus deferens between the two proximal ligatures and the distal ligature is removed. Double-ligating the proximal end minimizes the likelihood of spontaneous reanastomosis and formation of a sperm granuloma.

The incision in the parietal tunic is sutured with an absorbable 2-0 suture using a simple-continuous pattern. The ductus deferens on the medial aspect of the other testis is then palpated through the cutaneous incision and exposed by incising the scrotal septum and overlying parietal tunic. A segment of the ductus deferens is exteriorized, ligated, and transected as described. The incision in the parietal tunic and the subcutaneous tissue are each sutured with an absorbable 2-0 suture using a simple-continuous pattern. The cutaneous incision is closed with the same suture using a simple-continuous intradermal suture pattern.

Immunologic Castration

Immunization against luteinizing hormone–releasing hormone (LHRH), a neuropeptide produced by the hypothalamus, was used in a cryptorchid stallion to decrease serum concentration of testosterone,[143] and immunization against gonadotropin-releasing hormone (GnRH) was used experimentally to suppress testicular function of entire stallions.[144,145] Repeated immunization was necessary to maintain a sufficient binding titer for complete neutralization of LHRH or GnRH and inhibition of the reproductive endocrine axis. Immunization against GnRH caused decreased concentrations of testosterone and estrogen in the serum, diminished sexual behavior, and decreased testicular size, and it had a negative effect on semen quality. Stallions varied in response to immunization, and in one study, libido was not totally suppressed.[144]

If a vaccine against LHRH or GnRH becomes commercially available, unwanted male sexual behavior by cryptorchid or entire stallions can be prevented temporarily. A vaccine against GnRH may enable a stallion to perform at its peak ability at athletic competitions, by decreasing undesirable sexual behavior, until the stallion's genetic potential can be determined, while allowing the stallion to retain its ability to produce progeny. The time required for recovery of libido and semen quality needs to be determined before a vaccine against LHRH or GnRH is used clinically for temporary diminution of male sexual behavior.

Cryptorchid Castration

A retained testis can be removed through an inguinal, parainguinal, suprapubic paramedian, or flank approach. For each of these approaches, except the flank approach, the horse must be anesthetized. The approach is termed noninvasive if the testis can be removed by introducing only one or two fingers into the abdominal cavity, and an approach that requires insertion of a hand into the abdomen is considered invasive. Only the inguinal and parainguinal approaches allow noninvasive removal of a cryptorchid testis.

Inguinal Approach

For the inguinal approach, the horse is anesthetized and positioned in dorsal recumbency. The superficial inguinal ring is exposed through an elliptical, scrotal incision or through an 8- to 15-cm skin incision (depending on the horse's size) made directly over the superficial inguinal ring. A cryptorchid testis and the contralateral scrotal testis (or two cryptorchid testes) can be removed from one incision if the incision is created over the scrotum rather than over the superficial inguinal ring.

The inguinal fascia is separated digitally to expose the superficial inguinal ring. An inguinal testis is readily encountered when the superficial inguinal ring is exposed. The vaginal sac should always be opened and its contents examined to avoid mistaking the descended tail of the epididymis of a partial abdominal cryptorchid for a small, inguinal testis. If the testis has already been removed, the stump of the spermatic cord is encountered as it exits the canal. Finding a stump of a severed ductus deferens, the remnant of spermatic vessels, and a well-developed cremaster muscle indicates that the horse has been castrated.[22,116]

After the superficial inguinal ring has been exposed, an abdominal testis can be retrieved using one of several noninvasive techniques. One noninvasive technique requires locating the rudimentary common vaginal tunic, or vaginal process. This structure contains a portion the epididymis or sometimes a portion of the gubernaculum testis. The body of the epididymis can be exposed through a small incision in the vaginal process and traced to the tail of the epididymis, which is connected to the testis by the proper ligament of the testis. By placing traction on this ligament, the abdominal testis can be exteriorized through the vaginal ring. The key to this technique is locating the vaginal process. The vaginal process of the partial abdominal cryptorchid lies everted within the inguinal canal and is readily encountered during inguinal exploration. The vaginal process of the complete abdominal cryptorchid lies inverted within the abdominal cavity, along with the epididymis and testis, and difficulty may be encountered in locating and everting it into the canal.

An inverted vaginal process can be everted into the inguinal canal by exerting traction on the scrotal ligament, which is also known as the inguinal extension of the gubernaculum testis (IEGT)[12] (Fig. 65-17). This ligament is a remnant of the gubernaculum testis and attaches the vaginal process to the scrotum. The IEGT is located by

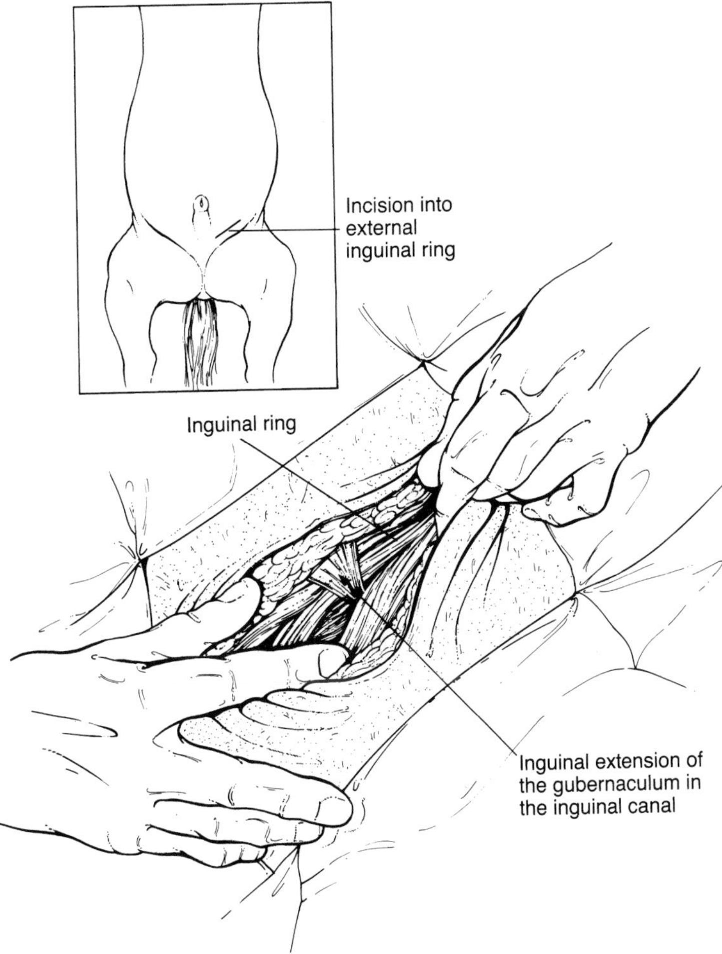

Figure 65-17. An inverted vaginal process can be everted into the inguinal canal by exerting traction on the inguinal extension of the gubernaculum testis. This ligament is a remnant of the gubernaculum and attaches the vaginal process to the scrotum.

carefully examining the margin of the superficial inguinal ring for a fibrous band that descends into the canal. The IEGT can be found on either the medial or lateral aspect of the ring, usually at the junction of the middle and cranial third of the ring. The genitofemoral nerve courses through the canal and can be mistaken for the IEGT. This nerve usually lies further caudally, in the middle or caudal third of the superficial inguinal ring. The IEGT is most easily located by grasping and retracting loose fascia at the junction of the middle and cranial thirds of the ring with the thumb and index finger of one hand and tracing it into the canal with the index finger and thumb of the other hand. The fascia tears if the IEGT is not contained within the fascia, but if the IEGT lies within this fascia, traction causes the inverted vaginal process to evert into the canal, where it and the epididymis or gubernaculum contained within can be seen and palpated. The everted process is a glistening, white structure, usually about the size of a fingertip. A hypoplastic cremaster muscle can be seen attached to the lateral aspect of the vaginal process.

An inverted vaginal process can also be everted using a sponge forceps.[26] A finger is inserted through the vaginal ring into the inverted vaginal process, and a 25-cm, curved sponge forceps is introduced beside the finger. The jaws of the forceps are opened and closed to grasp the apex of the vaginal process. Traction applied on the forceps everts the inverted vaginal process. The difficulty of this technique is locating the vaginal ring. The ring can usually be found beneath the third finger when four fingers are inserted into the inguinal canal.

After the vaginal process is everted and stripped of inguinal fascia, it is incised longitudinally (a no. 12 scalpel blade works best for this) to expose a portion of the epididymis contained within (Fig. 65-18, *A*). The epididymis is grasped with a hemostat and exteriorized until the tail of the epididymis is located (see Fig. 65-18, *B*). The proper ligament of the testis connects the tail of the epididymis to the caudal pole of the testis (Fig. 65-19), and by applying traction to this structure, the testis can be pulled through the vaginal ring and exteriorized for removal (Fig. 65-20). Stretching the vaginal ring to accommodate passage of the testis may not be necessary if the stallion is immature. Usually though, the vaginal ring must be stretched to allow passage of the testis, and this is accomplished by inserting a finger through the incision in the vaginal process and through the vaginal ring. The finger is inserted through the vaginal ring to the level of the second joint, and by flexing the finger, the ring is dilated. The vaginal ring of a mature stallion is usually much more difficult to dilate than that of an immature stallion.

Rarely, the vascular pedicle of the testis is so short that placing an emasculator proximal to the testis and epididymis is impossible. The cord must then be crushed and transected using an écraseur or severed with scissors after occluding the testicular vasculature with one or two ligatures. The contralateral testis is then removed, and the skin incision is sutured or left to heal by secondary intention.

PREVENTING EVISCERATION

The vaginal ring should be re-palpated after the abdominal testis is removed. If the ring accommodates no more than the tips of the index and middle fingers, the horse can be recovered, and unrestricted activity can be safely allowed after several days. If the ring has been dilated beyond this diameter, one of two measures must be taken to prevent evisceration. To avoid evisceration, the inguinal canal can be packed to the level of the vaginal ring with sterile gauze for 24 to 36 hours. The pack is maintained in the canal by partially suturing the skin incision. Evisceration may follow removal of the pack, especially if gauze has been inadvertently inserted through the vaginal ring into the abdomen. Not only does gauze in the abdomen prevent the vaginal ring from contracting but it also becomes adhered to viscera. Evisceration can be avoided by palpating the vaginal ring per rectum after the pack is inserted and before it is removed to ensure that gauze has not entered the abdomen. After the pack is removed, the horse's activity should be restricted to hand-walking for several days before forced exercise is imposed. Jumping, cantering, and galloping should not be allowed for 3 weeks.

Although the deep inguinal ring is inaccessible for suturing, the superficial inguinal ring can be closed with an interrupted or continuous pattern of heavy, absorbable suture to prevent evisceration. A hernia or kidney needle is the needle of choice for suturing the inguinal ring. Not only does suturing the superficial inguinal ring provide better security against evisceration than does packing the canal with gauze but it also allows primary closure of the inguinal fascia and skin. Although viscera can enter the inguinal canal, incarceration of intestine by the vaginal ring has not been reported. Inguinal fascia and skin can be sutured after closure of the superficial inguinal ring or allowed to heal by secondary intention. Activity should be restricted to hand-walking for several days before forced exercise is imposed. Heavy exercise should not be allowed for 3 weeks after surgery.

Parainguinal Approach

If the vaginal process cannot be located using the previously described techniques, the testis can be removed noninvasively by converting the inguinal approach to a parainguinal approach.[146] A 4-cm incision is made in the aponeurosis of the external abdominal oblique muscle, 1 to 2 cm medial and parallel to the superficial inguinal ring (Fig. 65-21). The incision is centered over the cranial aspect of the ring. The internal abdominal oblique muscle underlying the aponeurosis is spread in the direction of its fibers, and the peritoneum is penetrated with a sharp thrust of the index and middle fingers. The vaginal ring is palpated caudolateral to the point of entry into the abdomen (Fig. 65-22). The epididymis, ductus deferens, and gubernaculum are situated near the ring, and by sweeping the region with a finger, one of these structures can be grasped between the index and middle fingers and exteriorized. The body of the epididymis is followed to the tail. Traction on the proper ligament of testis pulls the testis through the incision.

If difficulty is encountered in locating the epididymis or associated structures, or if exteriorizing the testis is difficult, the incision can be enlarged to accommodate a hand. After excising the testis, the incision in the aponeurosis of the external abdominal oblique muscle is apposed using heavy absorbable sutures in an interrupted or continuous pattern. The subcutaneous tissue and skin can be sutured or left unapposed to heal by secondary intention. The horse can

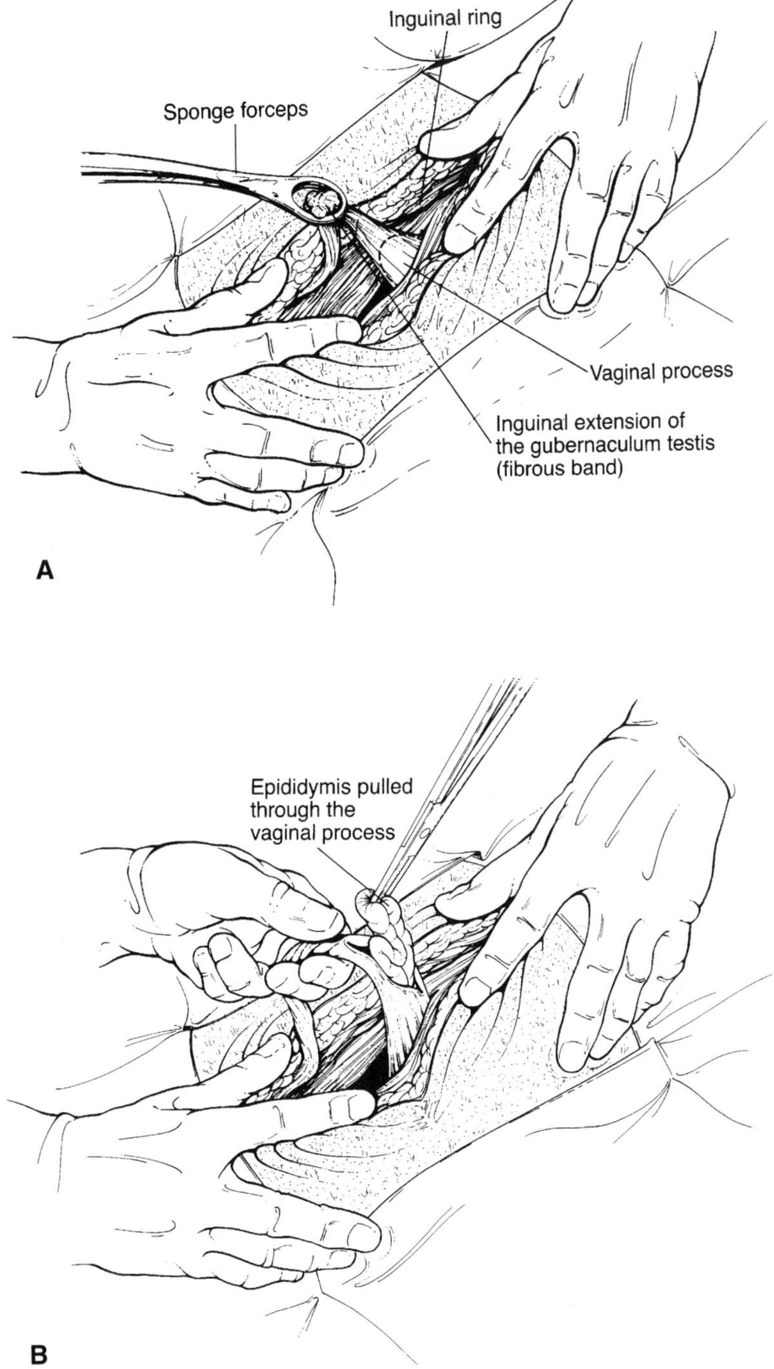

Figure 65-18. A, The everted vaginal process is stripped of inguinal fascia and longitudinally incised. **B,** The epididymis contained within is grasped with a hemostat and exteriorized.

receive exercise after surgery, excluding cantering and galloping, provided that the parainguinal incision was short enough that it could accommodate only several fingers. Unrestricted activity is allowed 3 weeks after surgery.[146]

The parainguinal approach is preferred over the inguinal approach by some surgeons because the vaginal ring is not disrupted.[146] The aponeurosis of the external abdominal oblique muscle is more easily sutured than the superficial inguinal ring.

Suprapubic Paramedian Approach

For the suprapubic paramedian approach, an 8- to 15-cm, longitudinal skin incision is made 5 to 10 cm lateral to the ventral midline.[147-149] The incision begins at the level of the preputial orifice and extends caudally. The large subcutaneous vessels encountered caudally in the incision are ligated. The abdominal tunic and the closely adherent ventral sheath of the rectus abdominis muscle are incised longitudinally, and the underlying fibers of the rectus

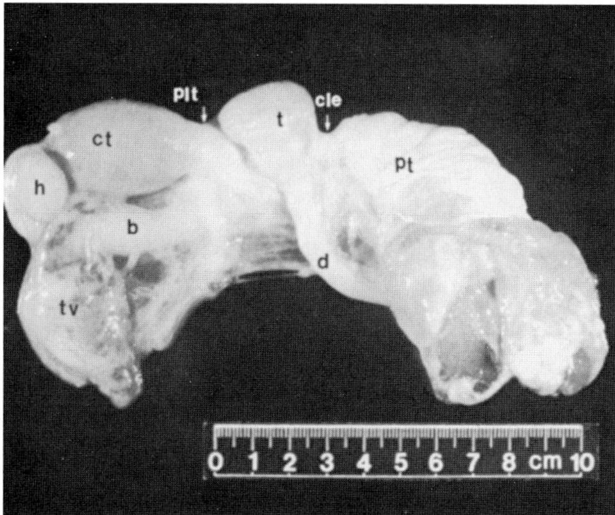

Figure 65-19. Cryptorchid testis. b, body of epididymis; cle, caudal ligament of the epididymis; ct, cryptorchid testis; d, ductus deferens; h, head of epididymis; plt, proper ligament of the testis; pt, parietal tunic; t, tail of epididymis; tv, testicular vessels.

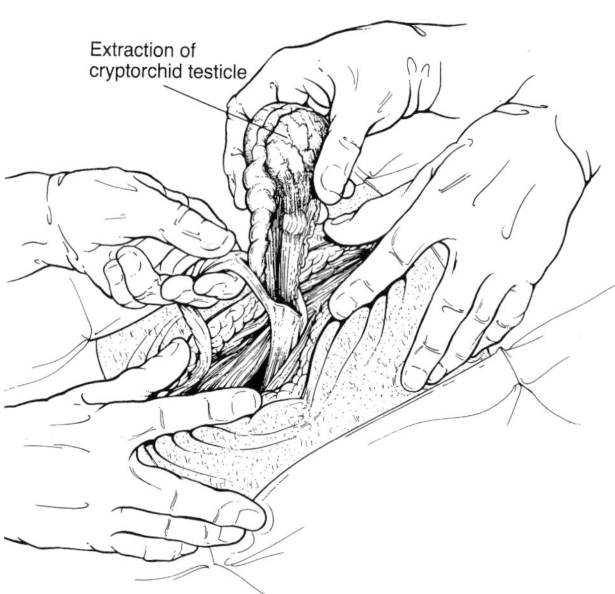

Figure 65-20. With traction on the proper ligament of the testis, the testis is pulled through the vaginal ring.

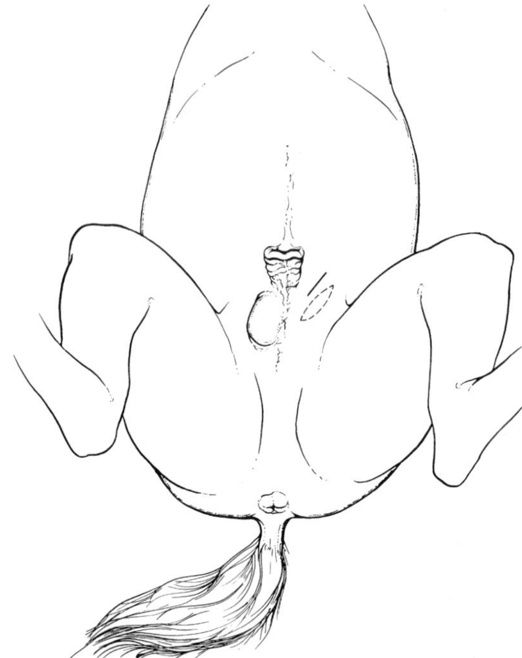

Figure 65-21. Parainguinal approach to cryptorchidectomy. A 4-cm incision is made in the aponeurosis of the external abdominal oblique muscle 1 to 2 cm medial and parallel to the superficial inguinal ring. The incision is centered over the cranial aspect of the ring.

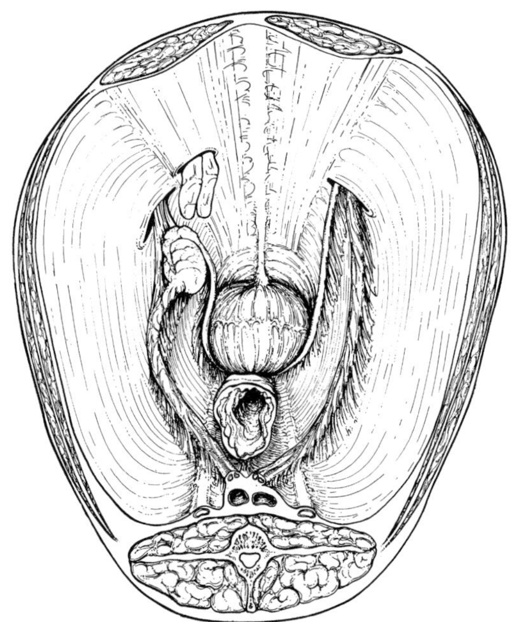

Figure 65-22. Parainguinal approach to cryptorchidectomy. The vaginal ring is palpated caudolateral to the point of entry into the abdomen. Either the epididymis, gubernaculum, or ductus deferens is located at the vaginal ring and exteriorized.

abdominis muscle are bluntly separated in the same direction. The dorsal rectus sheath, retroperitoneal fat, and peritoneum are penetrated with a finger. The perforation is bluntly enlarged, and a hand is introduced into the abdomen.

The testis is usually encountered near the vaginal ring. If the testis cannot be palpated, accessory structures at the vaginal ring can be located and followed to the testis, or the ductus deferens can be found in the genital fold of the bladder and traced to the testis. Both testes of a bilateral cryptorchid can be removed through one incision, but the contralateral testis is difficult to exteriorize, and its cord usually must be transected with an écraseur. After removing the testis, the abdominal tunic, the subcutis, and skin are each closed separately with interrupted or continuous sutures.

Flank Approach

For the flank approach, a 10- to 15-cm incision is made through the skin and subcutis in the paralumbar fossa of the affected side with the horse standing or recumbent.[150] In a standing horse, the incision site must be anesthetized before the surgery. The external abdominal oblique muscle is transected in the direction of the skin incision, and the peritoneum is exposed by splitting the internal abdominal oblique and transversus abdominis muscles in the direction of their fibers. The peritoneum and retroperitoneal fat are perforated with a finger to enter the abdomen. The testis is located and exteriorized as described for the paramedian approach. If the testis cannot be exteriorized, an écraseur is used to transect the testicular vasculature. After the abdominal testis is removed, the internal and external abdominal oblique muscles, subcutis, and skin are each closed separately with interrupted or continuous sutures. Closing the peritoneum and transversus abdominis muscle is difficult and not necessary.

Selection of Approach

The paramedian and flank approaches allow removal of only an abdominal testis, because retraction of an inguinal testis into the abdomen can usually be accomplished only with difficulty. Abdominal testicular retention should be confirmed before either of these approaches is used, but often testicular location cannot be determined reliably. The inguinal approach allows removal of either an abdominal or an inguinal testis. Because an inguinal testis is quickly encountered using an inguinal approach, prior determination of testicular location is not necessary. If the testis is not encountered in the inguinal canal using an inguinal approach, the testis can be removed from the abdomen noninvasively through the vaginal ring or through a small parainguinal incision in the abdominal musculature.

Because the inguinal and parainguinal approaches allow removal of an abdominal testis through a finger-size abdominal perforation, surgery is rapid, and convalescence is short. The lengthy incision required for the suprapubic paramedian and flank approaches prolongs surgery and convalescence. The paramedian approach also increases the risk of postoperative evisceration or herniation. Rarely, an invasive approach is necessary to remove a large, neoplastic, abdominal testis. An abdominal testis can be removed with the horse standing using a flank approach, when general anesthesia is not practical.

Laparoscopic Technique of Cryptorchidectomy

An abdominal testis can be removed laparoscopically with the horse standing or recumbent, but fractious stallions should be anesthetized. Food should be withheld for at least 12 hours before surgery to allow the colon to empty, to decrease the risk of penetrating a viscus when instruments are introduced, and to optimize visualization of intra-abdominal structures.[151-153]

To perform laparoscopic removal of an abdominal testis with the horse standing, the horse is restrained in stocks and sedated.[151-154] The flank region is prepared for surgery, and proposed sites for inserting the laparoscope and grasping forceps are infiltrated subcutaneously and intramuscularly with a local anesthetic agent. The surgical approach is identical to the one described for laparoscopic castration.

The testis is located by inspecting the region surrounding the vaginal ring. The vaginal ring and associated structures are easier to see when the horse is standing than when it is anesthetized and recumbent, because the abdominal contents fall away from the inguinal area. The contralateral vaginal ring can be observed by manipulating the laparoscope under the descending colon, or by passing the laparoscope through a small perforation created in the mesocolon of the descending colon, or by elevating the descending colon, either with an instrument placed through an abdominal portal or with a hand per rectum.[155] The mesorchium, which contains the testicular vasculature, can be seen coursing caudally from the area of the kidney to the area of the deep inguinal ring. An abdominal testis can be observed to lie anywhere between the kidney and the vaginal ring,[140] but most commonly it is located cranioventral to the ring. The testis is attached to the tail of the epididymis by the proper ligament of the testis, and the epididymis is attached to the vaginal ring and sac by the caudal ligament of the epididymis (ligament of the tail of the epididymis).

The testis and mesorchium are desensitized by injecting a local anesthetic agent into the mesorchium or the testis, using a 30-cm-long, 18-gauge needle introduced through the flank.[153,154] Desensitizing the testis and mesorchium may not be necessary, especially if caudal epidural anesthesia, using either a combination of 2% mepivacaine (5 mL) and xylazine (0.18 mg/kg), or xylazine (0.18 mg/kg) diluted to 10 to 15 mL with physiologic saline solution, is administered before surgery.[155]

An instrument portal close to the vaginal ring is created caudal and ventral to the laparoscopic portal.[151-154] The testis is grasped and exteriorized using grasping forceps inserted through this portal. If triangulation is inadequate, a new portal for the laparoscope can be created between the last two ribs using laparoscopic control.[156] The testicular vessels and ductus deferens are ligated and cut, or crushed and transected using an emasculator, and the stump is returned to the abdomen and inspected through the laparoscope for hemorrhage. If the contralateral testis is also located abdominally, the laparoscopic procedure is repeated on the contralateral side. The abdomen is decompressed by opening the cannula. The abdominal fascia and skin are sutured.

The testicular vessels and ductus deferens of an abdominal testis can also be transected intra-abdominally, with the horse standing, before removing the testis.[155] This technique requires the use of a third portal, created close to the other portals, to introduce instruments used to occlude and transect the testicular vasculature and ductus deferens.

The scrotal testis of a unilateral cryptorchid or an inguinal testis is removed through a scrotal incision, or its ductus deferens and vasculature can be ligated and severed intra-abdominally, which causes the testis to atrophy in the scrotum or inguinal canal.[140] Palpable but nonfunctional remnants of the testis may be detectable in the scrotum several months after the testis is destroyed by ligation of the testicular artery and vein. A scrotal testis of a juvenile stallion or an inguinal testis can be retracted into the abdomen for intra-abdominal transection of the ductus deferens and testicular vessels. The testis is retracted into the abdomen by placing traction on the mesorchium, after enlarging the vaginal ring with scissors. Retracting the testis into the abdomen inverts the vaginal tunic into the abdomen and the exposed ligament of the tail of the epididymis, which attaches the vaginal tunic to the tail of the epididymis, is severed. The incision in the vaginal ring can be closed with staples or left open.[140,157]

To perform laparoscopic removal of an abdominal testis with the horse anesthetized, the horse is positioned in dorsal recumbency.[151-153,157] After preparing the ventral aspect of the abdomen for aseptic surgery, a stab incision is made through the umbilicus, and through this incision the abdomen is insufflated to 10 to 15 mm Hg as described earlier. A laparoscopic sleeve with a guarded trocar is inserted through the incision into the abdominal cavity. The trocar is removed and replaced with a laparoscope. The horse is tipped into Trendelenburg position (i.e., head down approximately 30 degrees) to displace the viscera cranially,[151-153,157] and the laparoscope is directed caudally to view the inguinal areas. Because the hindquarters are elevated, positive-pressure ventilation is necessary. If the testis is not readily visible, it can be located by following the ductus deferens cranially over the lateral ligament of the bladder to the inguinal ring. Traction on the ductus deferens elevates the testis into view.

The testis can be removed prior to occluding and transecting the testicular vessels and ductus deferens,[151-153] or the testicular vessels and ductus deferens can be occluded and transected intra-abdominally before the testis is removed.[151-153,157] If the testis is to be exteriorized prior to transecting the testicular vessels and ductus deferens, the instrument portal is created 4 cm cranial and axial to the superficial inguinal ring, on the side of testicular retention. The testis is exteriorized using a grasping forceps introduced into the abdomen through this incision.[151-153] The exteriorized testicular vessels and ductus deferens are ligated and cut, or crushed and transected using an emasculator, and the stump is returned to the abdomen. Both testes of a horse with bilateral, abdominal, testicular retention can be viewed from one portal, but a portal must be created cranial and axial to each inguinal ring to remove each testis. The abdomen is deflated through the laparoscopic cannula, and the portals are closed by suturing the external lamina of the rectus abdominis muscle, the subcutaneous tissue, and skin.

To occlude and transect the testicular vessels and ductus deferens intra-abdominally with the horse anesthetized and positioned in dorsal recumbency, a grasping forceps for manipulating the testis is introduced through a cannula inserted 8 to 10 cm axial and cranial to the superficial inguinal ring.[157] A third instrument portal is created at the cranial, abaxial edge of the sheath to introduce instruments used to occlude and transect the testicular vasculature and ductus deferens. The testicular vessels and ductus deferens can be occluded using an endoscopic clip or an endoscopic ligating loop and transected using an endoscopic scissor or monopolar or bipolar electrocoagulation or a harmonic scalpel, or they can be occluded and transected using an endo-GIA stapler (Endo-GIA 30, United States Surgical Co., Norwalk, Ct).[157] Severing the mesorchium and ductus deferens with monopolar or bipolar electrocoagulation alone provides adequate control of hemostasis.[158] The risk of accidental thermal injury to adjacent viscera is far greater when using monopolar electrocoagulation than when using bipolar electrocoagulation. The testis is removed from the abdomen by expanding the skin incision over the portal through which the grasping forceps was introduced. Placing the testis in a retrieval bag facilitates exteriorization of the testis and eliminates the risk of dropping it into the abdomen.[158]

An advantage of intra-abdominal transection over extra-abdominal transection is that with intra-abdominal transection, the severed stump of the vasculature can be inspected before the testis is removed from the abdomen. Exteriorizing a testis causes loss of insufflation, which impairs visibility. A hemorrhaging stump is more easily noted and ligated when the abdomen is still inflated. Insufflation of the abdomen can be preserved during bilateral cryptorchidectomy by occluding and transecting the ductus deferens and vessels of each testis before either testis is removed from the abdomen.

Laparoscopic cryptorchidectomy simplifies locating the cryptorchid testis, avoids disruption of the vaginal ring, which minimizes the likelihood of evisceration, and permits early return to exercise because the incisions are small.[151-153,159] Laparoscopy may be particularly useful in evaluating a horse that displays stallion-like behavior but has the appearance of a gelding, especially when the presence or absence of testicular tissue cannot be determined conclusively by hormonal assay.[152] Laparoscopy is also useful for removing an abdominal testis when the side of the testicular retention is not known.

A disadvantage of laparoscopic cryptorchidectomy is the expense of the equipment.[151-153] A viscus, a large vessel, or the spleen can be penetrated inadvertently if the instruments are not inserted carefully into the abdomen.[160,161] Improper use of electrosurgical coagulation during the procedure may also result in perforation of a viscus.[157] If the procedure is performed with the horse anesthetized, the hindquarters must be elevated to displace the viscera cranially, making positive-pressure ventilation necessary. Familiarity with laparoscopic equipment and experience in laparoscopic techniques are required.

Repair of Inguinal Hernias and Ruptures

Nonsurgical Management

The majority of inguinal hernias are congenital, cause no distress, and spontaneously reduce by the time the foal is 3 to 6 months old.[52,162] Repeated manual reduction may encourage spontaneous reduction, and applying a truss after manually reducing the hernia may speed resolution.[75] To apply a truss, the foal is sedated and positioned in dorsal recumbency. The hernia is reduced, and the superficial inguinal ring is packed with rolled cotton. The cotton is maintained within the ring with elastic gauze and tape wrapped over the back and over both inguinal rings in a figure-eight (Fig. 65-23). The bandage can be left in place for up to a week. Surgical reduction of a congenital inguinal hernia is not necessary unless contents of the hernia become incarcerated or unless the hernia fails to regress.

Horses with an acquired inguinal hernia or an inguinal rupture usually require immediate treatment, because the intestine that has escaped through the vaginal ring or hole in the peritoneum is likely to become strangulated. Nonsurgical reduction of inguinal hernias by external

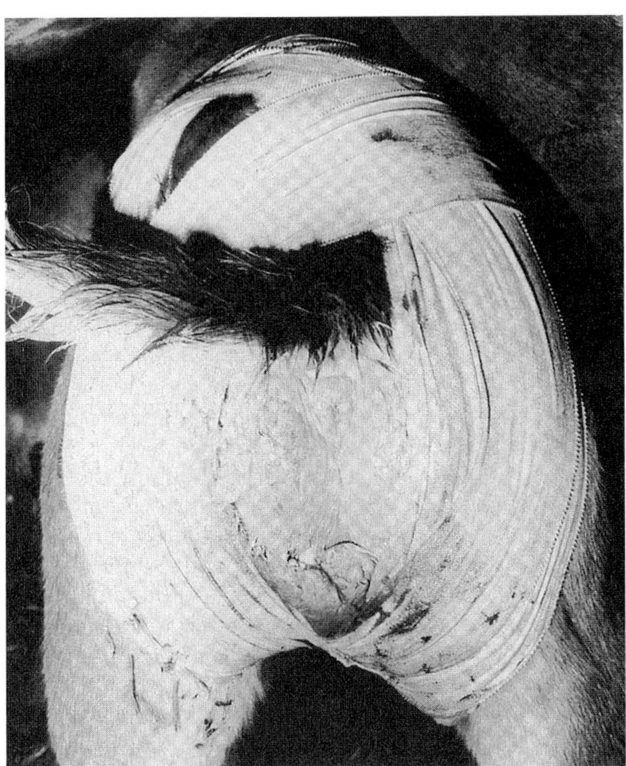

Figure 65-23. Application of a truss after manual reduction of a congenital hernia.

manipulation or rectal traction can be attempted if herniation is diagnosed soon after the onset of signs.[162] Nonsurgical reduction should not be attempted if the viability of the incarcerated intestine is in doubt, or if ruptured inguinal herniation or inguinal rupture is suspected.

To replace hernial contents into the abdomen by external manipulation, the horse is sedated, and the testis of the affected side is grasped and pulled downward so that the vaginal sac is tensed into a rigid, tube-like configuration.[160] With the second hand, the cord is grasped above the testis and slid proximally until herniated intestine is encountered. The second hand maintains traction on the cord and prevents herniated intestine from slipping downward. The first hand releases the testis and grasps and squeezes the cord above the second hand to force the contents of the hernia proximally. The hands are alternated in this manner until the intestine has been returned through the vaginal ring into the abdomen.

If reduction by external manipulation fails, it may be possible to retract the incarcerated loop of intestine into the abdomen by grasping the incarcerated loop per rectum as it enters the vaginal ring and applying traction.[162,163] The horse should be sedated, and an epidural anesthetic administered to minimize the risk of rectal injury or damage to incarcerated intestine. Administering propantheline bromide or hyoscine to relax the rectum may be helpful. The horse should be observed closely after nonsurgical reduction of an inguinal hernia, because the health of the reduced intestine cannot be assessed directly. Intestinal viability should be monitored by periodically evaluating the horse's peritoneal fluid.

Surgical Management

A congenital inguinal hernia of a foal should be reduced surgically if the hernia cannot be reduced, has escaped into subcutaneous tissue through a rent in the vaginal sac, fails to resolve or enlarges, or is so large that spontaneous resolution is unlikely.[164] To surgically correct inguinal herniation, the foal is anesthetized and positioned in dorsal recumbency. An incision is made directly over the superficial inguinal ring of the affected side, and the vaginal sac is isolated from surrounding fascia using blunt dissection. The scrotal ligament, which attaches the vaginal sac to the scrotum, is transected. While applying traction to the testis, the intestinal contents of the vaginal sac are milked back into the abdomen. Twisting the spermatic cord may facilitate replacement of intestine into the abdomen. The cord is ligated and resected proximal to the superficial inguinal ring. Ligating the cord prevents re-herniation, but for added security, the superficial inguinal ring can be closed with absorbable suture placed in a continuous or interrupted pattern. The skin and subcutaneous tissue can be left open to heal by secondary intention or closed primarily.

Nonstrangulating congenital inguinal hernias of foals can be corrected using laparoscopic technique.[164,165] The contents of the hernia are reduced into the abdominal cavity laparoscopically, with the foal anesthetized, and the testis of the affected side is retracted from the vaginal cavity into the abdominal cavity and removed, after ligating and transecting the testicular vessels and ductus deferens. The vaginal ring is closed using a laparoscopic stapling device. The testis of the nonaffected side can also be removed in this manner. Nonstrangulating congenital inguinal hernias can be corrected using a similar laparoscopic technique without removing the testes.[164] Advantages of laparoscopic herniorrhaphy are the quickness of the procedure and the rapid return of the foal to normal activity.

Emergency surgery is usually indicated for horses with an inguinal rupture or a ruptured inguinal hernia and for horses with an acute inguinal hernia that cannot be reduced by nonsurgical manipulation. Surgical correction of inguinal hernias is always indicated if viability of the testis or incarcerated intestine is questionable, because surgery allows these structures to be assessed visually.

Fluids should be administered intravenously in volumes sufficient to combat shock. The horse should be positioned in dorsal recumbency, and the ventral aspect of the abdomen and inguinal area should be prepared for aseptic surgery. The vaginal sac and its contents are exposed and isolated by blunt dissection through an incision created over the superficial inguinal ring. The vaginal sac is opened to expose its hernial contents and the testis. Devitalized intestine may be resected at the inguinal wound, but resection and anastomosis are usually more easily accomplished through a celiotomy. Dilating the vaginal ring and applying traction to the intestine through a ventral midline, paramedian, or parainguinal celiotomy may assist reduction of the herniated intestine. The affected testis should be removed if it appears nonviable or even if its viability is questionable.

If the testis is removed, re-herniation through the inguinal canal can be prevented by ligating the spermatic cord and the vaginal tunic as proximally as possible with absorbable suture. For additional security, the inguinal canal can be packed with gauze for 24 to 48 hours, or the superficial inguinal ring can be closed with heavy absorbable suture. Suturing the superficial inguinal ring gives greater security against re-herniation than does packing the inguinal canal. The inguinal fascia and skin can be closed primarily or left unsutured to heal by secondary intention. The celiotomy is closed in routine fashion.

Reherniation through the inguinal canal can be prevented, while at the same time trying to preserve a viable testis, by partially suturing the superficial inguinal ring around the spermatic cord.[166] Suturing starts at the cranial aspect of the ring and ends near the middle of the ring to give a snug, but not tight, closure around the spermatic cord. Difficulty arises in closing the ring adequately to prevent reherniation while still maintaining blood supply to the testis. A more certain method of salvaging the testis is laparoscopic inguinal herniorrhaphy. One method of laparoscopic inguinal herniorrhaphy entails implanting a polypropylene mesh beneath the peritoneum over the deep inguinal ring and the ductus deferens and testicular vessels that enter it, with the horse anesthetized and in the Trendelenburg position.[163] A less sophisticated but apparently effective technique of laparoscopic inguinal herniorrhaphy involves inserting a coiled polypropylene mesh through the enlarged vaginal ring into the inguinal canal.[167] The coiled mesh is pushed into the inguinal canal until the proximal edge of the mesh is distal to the vaginal ring and allowed to uncoil. The mesh is fixed to the inguinal canal with endoscopic staples. Fibrous reaction to the mesh obliterates the canal, preventing intestine from entering it. The procedure can be performed with the horse standing.

SPECIAL CONSIDERATIONS

Hemicastration

Fertility is maintained after hemicastration of normal horses. Testes undergo compensatory hypertrophy after hemicastration in response to increased secretion of interstitial cell–stimulating hormone from the hypophysis.[168] A hydrocele, neoplasia, or orchitis of one testis can cause temperature-induced dysfunction of spermatogenesis of the other testis, but removing the diseased testis may allow the remaining testis to regain normal spermatogenesis.[72] Postponing removal of the diseased testis can result in permanent dysfunction of the nondiseased testis.

The descended testis of a cryptorchid should never be removed without first removing the nondescended testis. Failure to find and remove the nondescended testis after the descended testis has been removed enables an unscrupulous owner to fraudulently represent the horse as a gelding and may complicate subsequent surgery, especially if there is no written record of which testis was removed. Compensatory hypertrophy of the nondescended testis occurs after hemicastration and may complicate removal of an abdominal testis.[18] Removing the descended testis has been advocated to promote descent of the cryptorchid testis,[169] but descent of an abdominal testis becomes impossible within several weeks after birth.[16,170] There is no proof that hemicastration actually results in descent of an inguinal testis. An inguinally retained testis is located easily during inguinal exploration and should be removed along with the descended testis.

Hormonally Induced Testicular Descent

Because testicular descent is hormonally controlled, treatment of a horse for cryptorchidism with hormones would seem to be an attractive mode of therapy. Hormonal factors responsible for testicular descent are still obscure, however, and no specific therapy has been developed to correct the hormonal defect responsible for testicular retention. GnRH and hCG have been administered separately and in combination to bring about testicular descent, but evidence of efficacy is lacking.[171] If a cryptorchid testis of a human descends into the scrotum or is surgically placed in the scrotum, degenerative changes within the testis can reverse so that the testis becomes capable of producing sperm, but for degenerative changes to reverse, the cryptorchid testis must enter the scrotum while the child is very young.[172] The age of the horse at which a cryptorchid testis must descend into the scrotum to contribute to fertility has not been determined.

After the first few weeks of neonatal life, the vaginal rings contract, reducing the likelihood of descent of an abdominal testis.[16] Hormonal therapy, therefore, is likely to have no effect on descent of an abdominal testis. Testicular growth, brought about by onset of puberty, may bring about descent of an inguinal testis,[18] and this supports the rationale for administration of GnRH or hCG. The effect of exogenous hormones on descent of inguinal testes, however, is unclear. Because genetic studies of equine cryptorchidism indicate that testicular retention is probably hereditary, hormonal therapy to bring about testicular descent is no more ethical than surgically placing the testis in the scrotum.

POSTOPERATIVE COMPLICATIONS OF TESTICULAR SURGERY

Hemorrhage

Excessive hemorrhage is usually the result of an emasculator that is improperly applied or is in imperfect working order. Reversing the emasculator (i.e., placing the cutting edge toward the abdomen) usually results in severe hemorrhage, because the cord is crushed distal to the site of transection. The emasculator should be applied perpendicular to the cord, because transection of the cord other than at a right angle increases the diameter of the severed ends of the testicular vessels. The blade of the emasculator should not be so sharp that the testicular vessels are severed before they are crushed properly. A blade that is too sharp can be dulled by using it several times to cut rope.[166]

The testicular vessels may be insufficiently crushed if scrotal skin is inadvertently included in the emasculator's jaws. The thick cords of a mature stallion may require double emasculation to sufficiently crush the vessels. Using this technique, the parietal tunic and cremaster muscle are crushed and transected separately from the testicular vessels and ductus deferens.

A ligature placed around the entire spermatic cord or around the testicular vessels alone can be used alone, or in conjunction with an emasculator, to prevent hemorrhage. Although a ligature, with or without an emasculator, may be more effective than the emasculator alone in preventing hemorrhage, the use of a ligature may increase the incidence of infection at the surgery site.[129] The increase in risk of infection associated with the use of a ligature is likely to be the result of reduced resistance of tissue contaminated with bacteria to infection in the presence of foreign material, especially if a nonabsorbable suture is used.

Dripping of blood from the wound for several minutes after emasculation is expected and should cause no concern. Unabated streaming of blood for 15 to 30 minutes is a signal for alarm. The testicular artery is the usual source of severe hemorrhage.[20] Because testicular veins are valved, hemorrhage from these vessels is usually mild. Hemorrhage from scrotal vessels is usually not serious and soon ceases spontaneously. If, after allowing the horse to stand quietly for 15 to 30 minutes, hemorrhage does not diminish, the end of the cord can be grasped using fingers and stretched to allow application of a crushing forceps or an emasculator. A crushing forceps with curved jaws, such as a kidney clamp, is easier to apply and maintain in position than a straight forceps. If the horse was castrated while standing, the end of the cord is likely to still be desensitized, and the forceps or emasculator can usually be applied without causing serious discomfort to the horse. The forceps is removed the next day. If the horse was castrated while recumbent, the cord is not desensitized, so to safely grasp and crush the end of the cord, the horse may need to be reanesthetized.

If the end of the cord is inaccessible through the scrotal incision, hemorrhage can be stopped by ligating the testicular vessels intra-abdominally using the procedure described for laparoscopic removal of an abdominal testis.[173,174] Laparoscopic surgery to stop hemorrhage after castration can be performed with the horse standing or anesthetized and positioned in dorsal recumbency. The testicular artery can be coagulated using electrocoagulation, or occluded with a laparoscopic suture loop or a vascular clip.

If the end of the cord is inaccessible, and if intra-abdominal ligation of the testicular vessels using laparoscopy is not an option, sterile gauze can be packed tightly into the inguinal canal and scrotum, and the scrotum closed with sutures or towel clamps. The pack is removed the next day.

Ten percent formalin (i.e., a 4% aqueous solution of formaldehyde gas created by diluting a 37% to 40% solution of formaldehyde gas with 9 parts of water) has been used with questionable success to stop hemorrhage. In one study, 8 to 16 mL of 4% to 12% formaldehyde solution administered intravenously to average-size horses decreased time of coagulation by 67% for 24 hours.[175] However, another study demonstrated no variation in time of coagulation after intravenous administration of formaldehyde solution.[176]

Formaldehyde solution is pyretogenetic and accelerates pulse and respiration.[175] Other side effects include restlessness, lacrimation, salivation, elevation of the tail, nasal discharge, increased peristalsis with frequent defecation, sweating, quivering of muscles, signs of severe abdominal pain, and tenesmus. Physical reaction is minimal when 10 mL of 4% formaldehyde solution (i.e., 10% formalin), diluted in a liter or more of physiologic saline solution, is administered intravenously. This author has observed dramatic reduction of hemorrhage, with no clinically apparent side effects, within minutes after intravenously administering this amount, but convincing scientific evidence of the safety and efficacy of a formaldehyde solution in reducing hemorrhage is lacking.

Evisceration

An uncommon but potentially fatal complication of castration is evisceration through the vaginal ring and open scrotal incision. Horses that eviscerate after castration may have a pre-existing, unapparent, congenital, inguinal hernia.[56] Most unapparent inguinal hernias resolve by the time the horse is 3 to 6 months old,[164] so horses castrated before they are 6 months old may be at greater risk of eviscerating after castration than are horses castrated after they are 6 months old. Standardbreds and Draft Horses may be more frequently affected by postoperative evisceration, because they have a higher incidence of congenital inguinal herniation.[129,136] Based on anecdotal evidence and unpublished data, Tennessee Walking Horses and American Saddlebreds may also have a higher incidence of congenital inguinal herniation and so may be predisposed to evisceration after castration.[177]

To decrease the likelihood of evisceration after castration, the horse's inguinal area should be palpated for the presence of an inguinal hernia before the horse is castrated, and the owner should be questioned as to whether the horse suffered from a congenital inguinal hernia as a foal. If the horse has or has had an inguinal hernia, is less than 6 months old, or is a member of a breed that has an increased incidence of inguinal herniation, the surgeon should consider taking measures to prevent evisceration. Some clinicians examine the vaginal rings per rectum before castrating a horse deemed to be at risk for evisceration because of its breed.[178] The vaginal ring of stallions is normally large enough to accommodate the tip of one finger. According to some clinicians, precautions to prevent evisceration should be taken if a vaginal ring is larger than two fingers. The risk of rectal injury should be weighed against the value of the diagnostic information to be gained before performing examination of the vaginal rings per rectum.

For horses that have a higher than normal risk for evisceration, castration should be performed with the horse anesthetized. The testes should be removed using a closed technique, and the spermatic cord should be ligated. The cremaster muscle should be isolated from the cord before the cord is ligated, so that it is not included in the ligature. Including the cremaster muscle in the ligature could cause the ligature to loosen when the cremaster muscle contracts. The closed technique of castration does not diminish the incidence of evisceration unless a ligature is applied to the cord proximal to the site of transection.[136]

Evisceration usually occurs within 4 hours after castration and may be precipitated by attempts to rise from anesthesia.[56,179] Evisceration has occurred up to 6 days after castration,[56] and one horse was reported to have herniated into its sutured scrotum and vaginal cavity 12 days after castration.[180] After intestine enters the canal, peristalsis encourages further protrusion, and intestinal strangulation accompanied by severe signs of colic rapidly ensues. Treatment of a horse that has eviscerated through the inguinal canal is similar to emergency treatment of horses with acquired inguinal herniation. The horse should be anesthetized immediately to prevent contamination of and damage to the herniated intestine. Torn mesentery should be repaired, and the intestine should be meticulously cleaned, copiously irrigated, and replaced into the abdomen as rapidly as possible to avoid ischemic damage. Dilating the vaginal ring and applying traction to the intestine through a celiotomy may assist reduction of the intestine. Parenteral antimicrobial therapy should be initiated, and peritoneal fluid should be examined postoperatively if the horse displays signs of septic peritonitis.

Protrusion of greater omentum through the scrotal incision after castration causes no immediate distress to the horse and need not be considered a dire emergency (Fig. 65-24). The horse should be examined per rectum to determine the size of the vaginal ring and to confirm that intestine has not entered the inguinal canal. Exposed omentum is transected as proximally as possible using an emasculator. This can usually be accomplished with the horse standing. To prevent further protrusion of omentum, the horse should be forced to stand in a stall for 48 hours. Suturing the superficial inguinal ring or packing the inguinal canal and scrotum gives additional security against evisceration but may not always be necessary, because omentum occupying the vaginal ring prevents intestine from entering the canal. If omentum continues to exit the scrotal incision, the superficial inguinal ring should be sutured.

Edema

Preputial and scrotal edema develops after nearly every castration and is generally greatest around the fourth postoperative day.[20] Excessive edema, reported to be the most common complication of castration,[129] can usually be avoided by removing a generous portion of the scrotum during castration and by vigorously exercising the horse for several weeks to promote drainage from the open wound. Without vigorous exercise, the scrotal skin may seal and trap fluid containing bacteria or inflammatory products within the scrotal cavity. Excessive edema can usually be relieved by opening the sealed wound with scrotal massage or by inserting a gloved finger into the scrotal cavity and enforcing vigorous exercise. High-pressure lavage of the scrotal wound with tap water administered using a garden hose may assist in keeping the wound open and clean, but a survey of practitioners (performed to determine the type and frequency of complications that occur after castration) indicated that horses that receive hydrotherapy after castration may be more prone to develop excessive swelling and infection of the scrotum.[129]

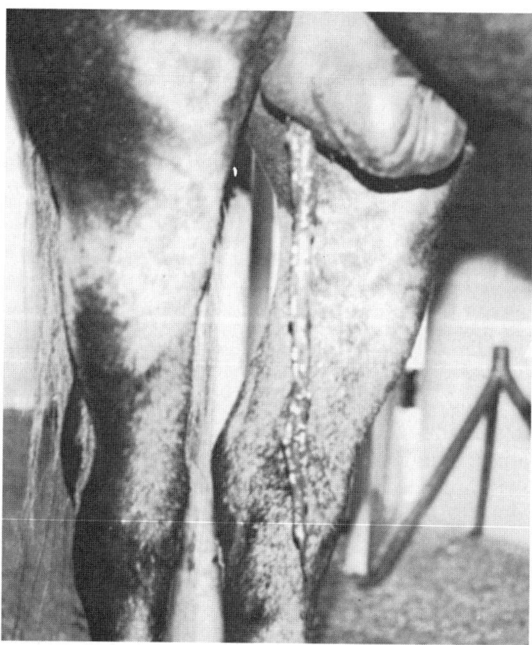

Figure 65-24. Protrusion of greater omentum through the scrotal incision after castration.

Septic Funiculitis

A scrotal wound, like any other wound left unsutured to heal by secondary intention, becomes contaminated and may subsequently become infected. The infection remains confined to the scrotal cavity as long as the scrotal incision remains open and draining, and it resolves as the scrotum heals. Septic funiculitis, or infection of the spermatic cord, can occur from extension of the scrotal infection, especially if the scrotal cavity does not properly drain. Septic funiculitis can also be caused by a contaminated emasculator or ligature. The open method of castration, in which the vaginal tunic and cremaster muscle are not removed, may predispose the horse to septic funiculitis.[34] The condition is characterized by preputial and scrotal edema, pain, pyrexia, and sometimes lameness.[66] Septic funiculitis may resolve with antimicrobial therapy and re-establishment of drainage, but occasionally, removal of the infected stump is required, especially if the cord has been ligated.

Champignon (French for "mushroom") is a term used to describe a type of septic funiculitis of the stump of the cord caused by infection with *Streptococcus*.[20] Champignon is characterized by purulent discharge and a mushroom-shaped mound of granulation tissue that protrudes from the scrotal incision.[181] This was a common complication of castration before the invention of the emasculator, when hemorrhage was controlled by ligatures or "clams," but now its importance is mostly historical.[20]

A stump chronically infected with pyogenic bacteria is commonly referred to as a scirrhous cord.[32,59] Scirrhous cord, caused by *Staphylococcus*, is sometimes referred to as botryomycosis.[20,59] The scrotal incision of a horse affected with septic funiculitis may eventually heal, but if the septic funiculitis does not resolve, the cord enlarges with granulation tissue and abscesses, which may eventually discharge through sinus tracts. The cord is hard, often painless, and adhered to scrotal skin. The stump may become so large that it mechanically interferes with locomotion of the rear limb. In extreme cases, infection may ascend the cord into the abdomen, where a hard mass can be palpated per rectum at the deep inguinal ring.[33] Occasionally, the lesion does not become apparent for several years after castration.[20,182] Treatment is removal of the infected mass. The horse is anesthetized and positioned in dorsal recumbency. An incision is made over the superficial inguinal ring, and the infected cord is isolated from normal tissue (Fig. 65-25). The cord is transected proximal to the mass, using an

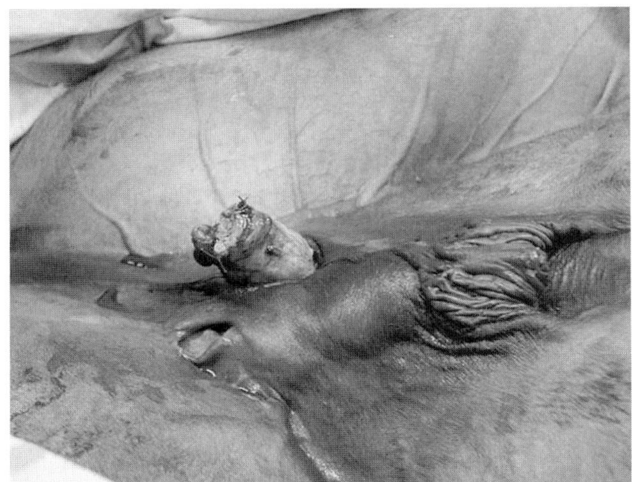

Figure 65-25. The exteriorized portion of the spermatic cord is thickened and hardened from infection. The demarcation between normal and abnormal portions of the cord is obvious. A thick, hard, infected cord after castration is commonly referred to as a scirrhous cord.

emasculator or écraseur, and the wound is left unsutured to heal by secondary intention.

Clostridial Infection

Clostridial infection of the castration wound is particularly severe, because tissue necrosis and toxemia produced by clostridial organisms may lead to death within several days. Specific systemic signs of clostridial infection vary according to the clostridial species involved. *Clostridium tetani* causes general spasms and paralysis of the voluntary muscles. Horses develop a characteristic "saw-horse" stance and protrusion of the third eyelid.[183] *Clostridium botulinum* causes flaccid paralysis, and early signs include decreased tone of the eyelids and tail, weakened gait, muscular tremors, and dysphagia.[184] *Clostridium septicum, Clostridium perfringens, Clostridium chauvoei,* and *Clostridium fallax* have been identified as etiologic agents of malignant edema, a highly fatal disease characterized by fever, depression, toxemia, subcutaneous accumulation of gas, and fulminating cellulitis.[185] Treatment of horses for clostridial infection at the castration site includes administration of high doses of penicillin and nonsteroidal anti-inflammatory and analgesic drugs, supportive therapy, radical débridement of all necrotic scrotal tissue, and establishment of scrotal drainage. Horses infected with *C. botulinum* and *C. tetani* can also be treated with antitoxin.[184,186]

Septic Peritonitis

Subclinical, nonseptic peritonitis occurs in many horses after castration because the peritoneal and vaginal cavities communicate.[187] Postoperative, intra-abdominal hemorrhage may be responsible, at least in part, for nonseptic peritonitis, because free blood in contact with the peritoneum causes inflammation.[188] A concentration of nucleated cells greater than 10,000/μL in the peritoneal fluid indicates peritoneal inflammation. A concentration greater than 10,000/μL can be found routinely in peritoneal fluid for at least 5 days after uncomplicated castration, and a concentration greater than 100,000/μL is not uncommon.[187]

Septic peritonitis occurs when peritoneal inflammation is accompanied by bacterial infection. Signs of septic peritonitis include colic, pyrexia, tachycardia, diarrhea, weight loss, and reluctance to move.[189] Septic peritonitis should not be diagnosed on the basis of the concentration of nucleated cells in the peritoneal fluid alone, because a concentration greater than 10,000/μL merely indicates that the peritoneum is inflamed.[187] The presence of degenerated neutrophils or intracellular bacteria in the peritoneal fluid is more indicative of bacterial peritonitis, especially when accompanied by clinical signs.[190] Treatment of horses for septic peritonitis includes administration of antimicrobial and nonsteroidal anti-inflammatory and analgesic drugs, supportive therapy, and peritoneal lavage. Proper drainage of the scrotum must be established. The occurrence of septic peritonitis after castration is rare, perhaps because the funicular portion of the vaginal process is collapsed as it courses obliquely through the abdominal wall,[191] and because mesothelial cells of the vaginal process are phagocytic.[68]

Penile Damage

The surgeon may encounter the shaft of the penis while separating scrotal fascia in search of an inguinal testis and, if inexperienced in orchidectomy, may mistake it for the testis. A portion of the shaft of the penis may be stripped of fascia, partially exteriorized, and amputated before its true identity is recognized (Fig. 65-26). Even if the penile shaft is recog-

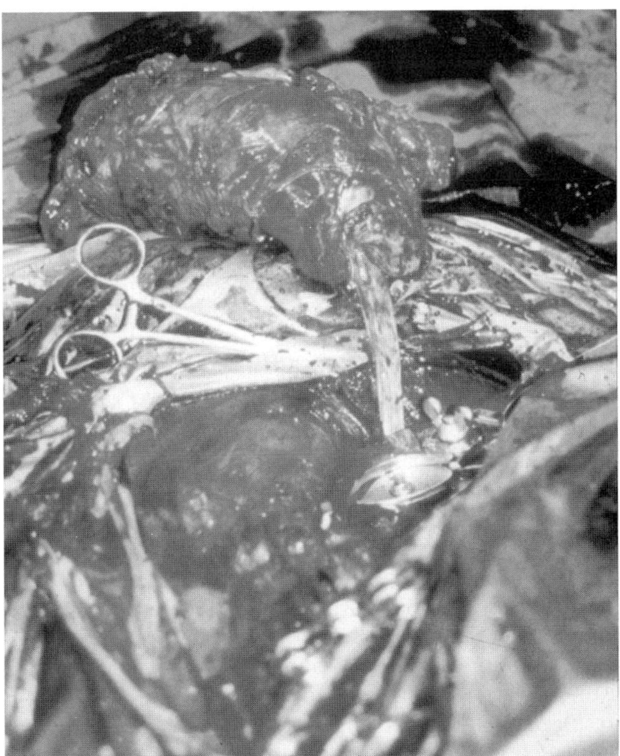

Figure 65-26. Stump of penis emerging from a scrotal incision. Much of the shaft of the penis was inadvertently removed during a standing castration.

nized before the penis is damaged, damage to the penile fascia created by dissection can result in excessive edema and even paraphimosis. Damage to the urethra during sharp dissection results in severe necrosis of tissue from extravasation of urine into surrounding tissue.[192,193] Penile damage is easily avoided if the surgeon possesses some familiarity of genital anatomy and proper techniques of castration.

Excessive edema after castration can result in protrusion of the penis from the preputial cavity, and if the protruded penis is improperly cared for, its integument can be irreparably damaged. Prolonged penile protrusion can result in permanent penile paralysis.[166] Administering a phenothiazine-derivative tranquilizer as a preanesthetic agent can result in priapism or penile paralysis. Penile paralysis and priapism are described in detail in Chapter 66.

Hydrocele (Vaginocele)

A hydrocele, or vaginocele, is a fluid-filled, painless swelling in the scrotum that may appear months or years after castration and is the result of the accumulation of sterile, amber-colored fluid in the vaginal sac.[20] The fluid can often be reduced into the abdomen. The condition is uncommon and idiopathic, but open castration predisposes to the condition because the vaginal tunic is not removed. Hydroceles may occur more frequently in mules than in horses after castration.[194] Enlargement of the scrotum with fluid may give the horse the appearance of an entire stallion, or the horse may appear to have an inguinal hernia.

If the hydrocele does not increase in size, is not aesthetically displeasing to the owner, and does not inconvenience the horse, no treatment is necessary; otherwise, the hydrocele should be surgically removed. Drainage only temporarily alleviates the condition. To remove the hydrocele, the horse is anesthetized, placed in dorsal recumbency, and prepared for aseptic surgery. Skin is incised directly over the fluid-filled vaginal sac, the sac is bluntly separated from adherent fascia, and the scrotal ligament, which attaches the vaginal sac to the scrotum, is severed. The sac is transected, using a scissors or an emasculator, as proximally as possible. The wound can be sutured or left open to heal by secondary intention.

Continued Masculine Behavior

Castration is not always successful in completely eliminating objectionable masculine behavior, and some geldings may display sexual behavior, such as genital investigation, erection, mounting, and even copulation. Objectionable masculine behavior of geldings is especially common in spring and early summer. Geldings with objectionable sexual libido and aggressive temperament characteristic of stallions are sometimes referred to as *false rigs*.[195]

Persistent masculine behavior of false rigs has been attributed to failure to remove all epididymal tissue during castration, and geldings that display masculine behavior as a result of retention of epididymal tissue are said to be *proud cut*.[195] Epididymal tissue is unlikely to be inadvertently left with the horse, because the epididymis is intimately attached to the normal, descended testis. Regardless, androgens are neither produced nor released by the epididymis, and therefore, the presence or absence of epididymal tissue should not influence masculine behavior.[120] Because masculine behavior of a false rig cannot be justly attributed to retention of epididymal tissue, there is no such thing as a proud cut horse.[195]

Masculine behavior of a false rig has also been attributed to production of testosterone by the adrenal cortex.[120] The circulating concentration of luteinizing hormone is increased after castration in response to the falling concentration of testosterone, and the rise in luteinizing hormone concentration may produce some adrenal hypertrophy. False rigs, however, have no higher concentration of testosterone or dihydrotestosterone in serum than do normal, quiet geldings, and the presence of significant concentration of any other androgen is unlikely.[195] Moreover, administering hCG to false rigs produces no discernable rise in concentration of testosterone in serum.

Heterotopic testicular tissue has been incriminated as a cause of continued masculine behavior after castration.[196] Failure of embryonic primordial germ cells to migrate caudally and dispersion of the cells of the embryonic germinal epithelium from trauma have been theorized as causes of transplantation of testicular tissue throughout the peritoneal cavity of pigs.[196] The occurrence of heterotopic testicular tissue in horses, however, has not been reported. Administering hCG to a horse with heterotopic testicular tissue would probably produce a rise in concentration of testosterone in the serum.

Objectionable masculine behavior after castration is most likely innate and not caused by extragonadal production of testosterone.[195,197] Masculine behavior of false rigs is probably part of the normal social interaction between horses.[195] About 20% to 30% of castrated horses can be expected to display stallion-like sexual interest in mares and aggression toward other horses, and about 5% can be expected to display stallion-like aggression toward people.[197] Because the prevalence of masculine behavior of horses castrated as juveniles is similar to that of horses castrated as adults, castration before puberty is no more effective in preventing objectionable behavior than castration after puberty. These percentages should be considered the normal prevalence of masculine behavior in geldings.

Amputating the stumps of the spermatic cords was reported to abolish objectionable masculine behavior in 75% of 18 false rigs,[198] but no satisfactory rationale was offered to account for the success of this procedure. Because spermatic cords contain no Leydig cells and are incapable of producing androgens, the efficacy of shortening cords to eliminate libido seems doubtful. Limiting social interaction with other horses or imposing stricter discipline may be more successful in eliminating or diminishing undesirable masculine behavior.[195]

Incomplete Cryptorchid Castration

The tail of the epididymis of the partial abdominal cryptorchid lies within the inguinal canal, enclosed in a well-developed vaginal process. Excessive length of the proper ligament of the testis and body of the epididymis may allow the tail of the epididymis to descend through the inguinal canal. A surgeon unfamiliar with testicular anatomy and the mechanism of testicular descent may amputate the tail of

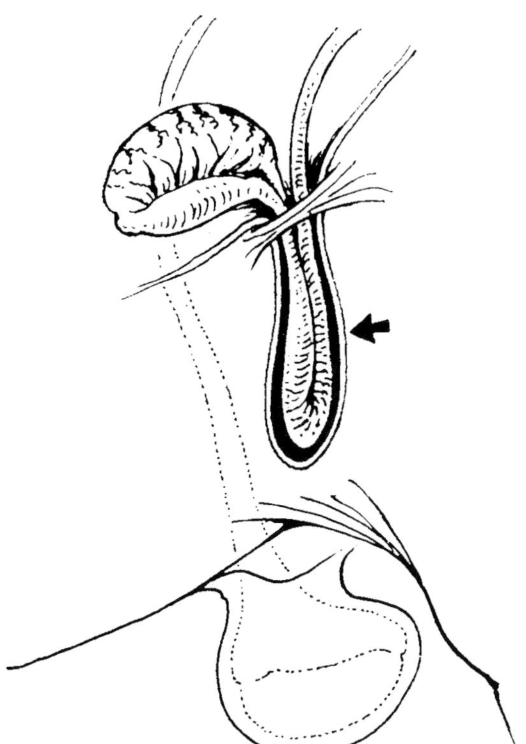

Figure 65-27. *Arrow* points to the epididymis of a partial abdominal cryptorchid. A portion of the epididymis lies within the inguinal canal, enclosed within the vaginal process. This portion of the epididymis could be mistaken for an inguinal testis by an inexperienced surgeon, and amputated.

the epididymis after mistaking it for a hypoplastic inguinal testis (Fig. 65-27). The horse naturally continues to display objectionable, stallion-like behavior.

The vaginal tunic should be opened before removing a structure presumed to be an inguinal testis to ensure that a testis, and not just the epididymis, is contained within. An hCG-stimulation test differentiates a horse with testicular tissue from a false rig. Locating both the end of the epididymis and the stump of the ductus deferens in the inguinal canal at surgery identifies a horse as a partial abdominal cryptorchid whose epididymis has been partially resected.[13]

REFERENCES

1. Sisson S, Grossman JD: The Anatomy of the Domestic Animals, ed 4, Philadelphia, 1953, WB Saunders.
2. Schummer A, Nickel R, Sack WO: The Viscera of the Domestic Mammals, ed 2, Berlin, 1979, Paul Parey.
3. Habel RE: Applied Veterinary Anatomy, ed 2, Ithaca, NY, 1981, self-published.
4. de Lahunta A, Habel RE: Applied Veterinary Anatomy, Philadelphia, 1986, WB Saunders.
5. Breazile JE: The male reproductive system. In Breazile JE, editor: Textbook of Veterinary Physiology, Philadelphia, 1971, Lea & Febiger.
6. Roberts SJ: Veterinary Obstetrics and Genital Diseases, ed 2, Ithaca, NY, 1971, self-published.
7. Budras KD, Sack WO: Anatomy of the Horse, ed 2, London, 1994, Mosby-Wolfe.
8. Johnson L, Neaves W: Age related changes in the Leydig cell population, seminiferous tubules, and sperm production in the stallion, Biol Reprod 1981;24:703.
9. Amann RP: A review of anatomy and physiology of the stallion, J Equine Vet Sci 1981;1:83.
10. Ashdown RR: The anatomy of the inguinal canal in the domesticated mammals, Vet Rec 1963;75:1345.
11. Rooney JR, Sack WO, Habel RE: Guide to the Dissection of the Horse, Ithaca, NY, 1967, WO Sack.
12. Valdez H, Taylor TS, McLaughlin SA, et al: Abdominal cryptorchidectomy in the horse using inguinal extension of the gubernaculum testis, J Am Vet Med Assoc 1979;174:1110.
13. Trotter GW, Aanes WA: A complication of cryptorchid castration in three horses, J Am Vet Med Assoc 1981;178:246.
14. Wensing CJG, Colenbrander B, van Straaten HWM: Normal and abnormal testicular descent in some mammals. In Hafez ESE, editor: Descended and Cryptorchid Testis, Boston, 1980, Martinus Nijhoff.
15. Ellenport CR: General urogenital system. In Getty R, editor: Sisson and Grossman's The Anatomy of the Domestic Animals, Philadelphia, 1975, WB Saunders.
16. Bergin WC, Gier HT, Marion GB, et al: A developmental concept of equine cryptorchidism, Biol Reprod 1970;3:82.
17. Smith JA: The development and descent of the testes in the horse, Vet Ann 1975;15:156.
18. Arthur GH: The surgery of the equine cryptorchid, Vet Rec 1961;73:385.
19. Smith JA: Biopsy and the testicular artery of the horse, Equine Vet J 1974;6:81.
20. Cox JE: Surgery of the Reproductive Tract in Large Animals, Liverpool, 1987, Liverpool University Press.
21. Santschi EM, Juzwiak JS, Stone DE: Monorchidism in three colts, J Am Vet Med Assoc 1989;194:265.
22. Parks AH, Scott EA, Cox JE, Stick JA: Monorchidism in the horse, Equine Vet J 1989;21:215.
23. Rebar A, Fessler JF, Erb R, et al: Testicular teratoma in a horse: A case report and endocrinologic study, J Equine Med Surg 1979;3:361.
24. Martin GS, Archer RM, Cho DY: Identification of a severely atrophic testicle during castration of a horse: A case report, Vet Surg 1985;14:194.
25. Arthur GH, Tavernor WD: Spontaneous emasculation of an equine cryptorchid, Vet Rec 1960;72:445.
26. Adams OR: An improved method of diagnosis and castration of cryptorchid horses, J Am Vet Med Assoc 1964;145:439.
27. Parker JE, Rakestraw PC: Intra-abdominal testicular torsion in a horse without signs of colic, J Am Vet Med Assoc 1997;210:375.
28. Hunt RJ, Hay W, Collatos C, et al: Testicular seminoma associated with torsion of the spermatic cord in two cryptorchid stallions, J Am Vet Med Assoc 1990;197:1484.
29. Hayes HM: Epidemiological features of 5009 cases of equine cryptorchidism, Equine Vet J 1986;18:467.
30. Priester WA, Glass AG, Waggoner NS: Congenital defects in domesticated animals: General considerations, Am J Vet Res 1970;31:1871.
31. Genetsky RM, Shire MJ, Schneider EJ, et al: Equine cryptorchidism: Pathogenesis, diagnosis and treatment, Comp Cont Educ Pract Vet 1984;6:S577.
32. Frank ER: Veterinary Surgery, ed 7, Minneapolis, 1964, Burgess.
33. O'Connor JJ: Dollar's Veterinary Surgery, ed 3, Chicago, 1938, Alexander Eger.
34. Bishop MWH, David JSE, Messervy A: Some observations on cryptorchidism in the horse, Vet Rec 1964;76:1041.
35. Jubb KVF, Kennedy PC: Pathology of Domestic Animals, vol 1, ed 2, New York, 1970, Academic Press.
36. Wilson DG, Nixon AJ: Case of equine cryptorchidism resulting from persistence of the suspensory ligament of the gonad, Equine Vet J 1986;18:412.
37. Kieffer N: Personal communication, Texas A&M University, 1989.

38. Couvreux R: Cryptorchidie et Heredite. Thesis, Paris, 1943. Cited by the Technical Development Committee of Great Britain. Cryptorchidism with special reference to the condition in the dog, Vet Rec 1954;66:482.
39. Leipold HW, De Bowes RM, Bennett S, et al: Cryptorchidism in the horse: Genetic implications, Proc Am Assoc Equine Pract 1986;31:579.
40. Kieffer NM, Webb G: Observation on the testicular descent of the progeny of a cryptorchid Quarter Horse stallion, Department of Animal Science, Texas A&M University, unpublished data.
41. McIlwraith CW, Owen R, Ap R, et al: An equine cryptorchid with testicular and ovarian tissues, Equine Vet J 1976;8:156.
42. McFeely RA, Kanagawa H: Intersexuality. In Hafez ESE, editor: Reproduction in Farm Animals, ed 3, Philadelphia, 1974, Lea & Febiger.
43. Bracken FK, Wagner PC: Cosmetic surgery for equine pseudohermaphroditism, Vet Med Small Anim Clin 1983;78:879.
44. Cornellyn M, De Moor A, Bouters R, et al: Clinical, morphological and endocrinological aspects of cryptorchidism in the horse, Theriogenology 1981;16:489.
45. Cox JE, Edwards GB, Neal PA: An analysis of 500 cases of equine cryptorchidism, Equine Vet J 1979;11:113.
46. Stickle RL, Fessler JF: Retrospective study of 350 cases of equine cryptorchidism, J Am Vet Med Assoc 1978;172:343.
47. Cox JE: Hernias and ruptures: Words to the heat of deeds, Equine Vet J 1988;20:155.
48. Schneider RK, Milne DW, Kohn CW: Acquired inguinal hernia in the horse: A review of 27 cases, J Am Vet Med Assoc 1982;180:317.
49. van der Velden MA: Ruptured inguinal hernia in new-born colt foals: A review of 14 cases, Equine Vet J 1988;20:178.
50. Vasey JR: Simultaneous presence of a direct and indirect hernia in a stallion, Aust Vet J 1981;57:418.
51. Kersjes AW, Nemeth F, Rutgers LJE: Atlas of Large Animal Surgery, Baltimore, 1985, Williams and Wilkins.
52. van der Velden MA: Surgical treatment of acquired inguinal hernia in the horse: A review of 51 cases, Equine Vet J 1988;20:173.
53. Bickers RJ, Lewis RD, Hays T, et al: Acquired inguinal hernia in a gelding, Equine Pract 1998;20:28.
54. Wright JG: The surgery of the inguinal canal in animals, Vet Rec 1963;75:1352.
55. Umstead JA, Nyack B, Padmore CL: Inguinal ring herniation in a female Shetland pony, Comp Cont Educ Pract Vet 1986;8:S164.
56. Hutchins DR, Rawlinson RJ: Eventration as a sequel to castration of the horse, Aust Vet J 1972;48:288.
57. Sembrat RF: The acute abdomen in the horse: Epidemiologic considerations, Arch Am Coll Vet Surg 1975;4:34.
58. Spurlock GH, Robertson JT: Congenital inguinal hernias associated with a rent in the common vaginal tunic in five foals, J Am Vet Med Assoc 1987;193:1087.
59. Smith HA, Jones TC, Hunt RD: Pathology, ed 4, Philadelphia, 1972, Lea & Febiger.
60. Muschat M: The pathological anatomy of testicular torsion, Surg Gynecol Obstet 1932;54:758.
61. Pascoe JR, Ellenburg TV, Culbertson MR, et al: Torsion of the spermatic cord in a horse, J Am Vet Med Assoc 1981;178:242.
62. Horney FD, Barker CAV: Torsion of the testicle in a Standardbred, Can Vet J 1975;16:272.
63. Behrens E, Reyes C: Un testiculo enfermo produce perdidas, Protinal 1988;41:36.
64. Threlfall WR, Carleton CL, Robertson J, et al: Recurrent torsion of the spermatic cord and scrotal testis in a stallion, J Am Vet Med Assoc 1990;196:1641.
65. Pozor MA, McDonnell SM: Color Doppler ultrasound evaluation of testicular blood flow in stallions, Theriogenology 2004;61:799.
66. Keller H: Diseases of male reproductive organs in non-breeding horses. In Wintzer HJ, editor: Equine Diseases, New York, 1986, Springer-Verlag.
67. Henry M, Amaral D, Tavares FF, et al: Hydrocele of the vaginal cavity of stallions, J Reprod Fertil Suppl 2000;56:13.
68. Leeson TS, Adamson L: The mammalian tunica vaginalis testis: Its fine structure and function, Acta Anat 1962;51:226.
69. Varner DD, Schumacher J, Blanchard TL, et al: Diseases and Management of Breeding Stallions, Goleta, Calif, 1991, American Veterinary Publications.
70. Teuscher H: Diseases of the male genital organs and hermaphroditism. In Dietz O, Wiesner E, editors: Diseases of the Horse, New York, 1982, Karger.
71. Hu KN, Khan AS, Gonder M: Sclerotherapy with tetracycline solution for hydrocele, Urology 1984;24:572.
72. Gygax AP, Donawick WJ, Gledhill BL: Haematocoele in a stallion and recovery of fertility following unilateral castration, Equine Vet J 1973;5:128.
73. Blanchard TL, Varner DD, Brinsko SP: Theriogenology question of the month: Scrotal hematocele, J Am Vet Med Assoc 1996;209:2013.
74. Compaire FH: Evaluation and treatment of varicocele. In Santen RJ, Swerdloff RS, editors: Male Reproductive Dysfunction: Diagnosis and Management of Hypogonadism, Infertility and Impotence, New York, 1986, Marcel Dekker.
75. Varner DD: Personal communication, Texas A&M University, 1997.
76. Szabo R, Kressler R: Hydrocele following internal spermatic vein ligation: A retrospective study and review of the literature, J Urol 1984;132:924.
77. Caron JP, Barber SM, Bailey JV: Equine testicular neoplasia, Comp Cont Educ Pract Vet 1985;7:S53.
78. Pandolfi F, Roperto F: Seminoma with multiple metastases in a zebra *(Equus zebra)* X mare *(Equus caballus)*, Equine Vet J 1983;15:70.
79. Moulton JE: Tumors of the genital system. In Moulton JE, editor: Tumors in Domestic Animals, Berkeley, 1978, University of California Press.
80. Gelberg HB, McEntee K: Equine testicular interstitial cell tumors, Vet Pathol 1987;24:231.
81. Vaillancourt D, Fretz P, Orr JP: Seminoma in the horse: Report of two cases, J Equine Med Surg 1979;3:213.
82. Knudsen O, Schantz B: Seminoma in the stallion: A clinical, cytological, and pathologicoanatomical investigation, Cornell Vet 1963;53:395.
83. Peterson DE: Equine testicular tumors, J Equine Vet Sci 1984;4:25.
84. Parks AH, Wyn-Jones G, Cox JE, et al: Partial obstruction of the small colon associated with an abdominal testicular teratoma in a foal, Equine Vet J 1986;18:342.
85. Becht JL, Thacker HL, Page EH: Malignant seminoma in a stallion, J Am Vet Med Assoc 1979;175:292.
86. Gibson GW: Malignant seminoma in a Welsh Pony stallion, Comp Cont Educ Pract Vet 1984;6:S296.
87. Trigo FJ, Miller RA, Torbeck RL: Metastatic equine seminoma: Report of two cases, Vet Path 1984;21:259.
88. Presti JC, Stoller ML, Carroll PR: Primary tumors of the testis. In Tierney LMJ, McPhee SJ, Papadakis MA, editors: Current Medical Diagnosis and Treatment, ed 37, Stamford, Conn, 1998, Appleton and Lange.
89. Cotchin E: A general survey of tumors in the horse, Equine Vet J 1977;9:16.
90. Rahaley RS, Gordon BJ, Leipold HW, et al: Sertoli cell tumor in a horse, Equine Vet J 1983;15:68.
91. Duncan RB: Malignant Sertoli cell tumour in a horse, Equine Vet J 1998;30:355.
92. Pratt SM, Stacy BA, Whitcomb MB, et al: Malignant Sertoli cell tumor in the retained abdominal testis of a unilaterally cryptorchid horse, J Am Vet Med Assoc 2003;222:486.
93. Smith HA: Interstitial cell tumor of the equine testis, J Am Vet Med Assoc 1954;124:356.

94. Hay WP, Baskett A, Gregory CR: Testicular interstitial cell tumour and aplasia of the head of the epididymis in a cryptorchid stallion, Equine Vet Educ 1997;9:240.
95. May KA, Moll HD, Duncan RB, et al: Unilateral Leydig cell tumour resulting in acute colic and scrotal swelling in a stallion with descended testes, Equine Vet J 1999;31:343.
96. Martin GR: Teratocarcinomas and mammalian embryogenesis, Science 1980;209:768.
97. Smyth GB: Testicular teratoma in an equine cryptorchid, Equine Vet J 1979;11:21.
98. Innes JRM: Tumors of the testis. North Am Vet 1952;33:623.
99. Williams WL: The Diseases of the Genital Organs of Domestic Animals, ed 3, Worcester, Mass, 1943, Ethel Williams Plimpton.
100. Stick JA: Teratoma and cyst formation of the equine cryptorchid testicle, J Am Vet Med Assoc 1980;176:211.
101. Innes JRM: Neoplastic diseases of the testis of animals, J Pathol Bacteriol 1943;54:485.
102. Willis RA, Rudduck HB: Testicular teratomas in horses, J Pathol Bacteriol 1943;55:165.
103. Shaw DP, Roth JE: Testicular teratocarcinoma in a horse, Vet Pathol 1986;23:327.
104. Valentine BA, Weinstock D: Metastatic testicular embryonal carcinoma in a young horse, Vet Path 1986;23:92.
105. Stabenfeldt GH, Hughes JP: Reproduction in horses. In Cole HH, Cupps PT, editors: Reproduction in Domestic Animals, ed 3, New York, 1977, Academic Press.
106. Dunn HO, Smiley D, Duncan JR, et al: Two equine true hermaphrodites with 64, XX/64, XY and 63, XO/64, XY chimerism, Cornell Vet 1981;71:123.
107. Fretz PB, Hare WC: A male pseudohermaphrodite horse with 63X0?/64XX/65XXY mixoploidy, Equine Vet J 1976;8:130.
108. Greatorex JC: Rectal exploration as an aid to the diagnosis of some medical conditions in the horse, Equine Vet J 1968;1:26.
109. Stauffer VD: Equine rectal tears: A malpractice problem, J Am Vet Med Assoc 1981;178:798.
110. O'Connor JP: Rectal examination of the cryptorchid horse. Ir Vet J 1971;25:129.
111. Schumacher J, Moll HD: A Manual of Equine Diagnostic Procedures, Jackson, Wyo, 2004, Teton NewMedia.
112. Galina CS: An evaluation of testicular biopsy in farm animals, Vet Rec 1971;88:628.
113. Blanchard TL, Varner DD, Schumacher J, et al: Manual of Equine Reproduction, ed 2, St Louis, 2003, Mosby.
114. Faber NF, Roser JF: Testicular biopsy in stallions: Diagnostic potential and effects on prospective fertility, J Reprod Fertil Suppl 2000;56:31.
115. Threlfall WR, Lopate C: Testicular biopsy, Presented at Annual Meeting of The Society of Theriogenology, 1987:65.
116. Cox JE: Experiences with a diagnostic test for equine cryptorchidism, Equine Vet J 1975;7:179.
117. Cox JE, Redhead PH, Dawson FE: Comparison of the measurement of plasma testosterone and plasma oestrogens for the diagnosis of cryptorchidism in the horse, Equine Vet J 1986;18:179.
118. Arighi M, Bosu WTK: Comparison of hormonal methods for diagnosis in horses, J Equine Vet Sci 1989;9:20.
119. Silberzahn P, Zwain I, Guerin P, et al: Testosterone response to human chorionic gonadotrophin injection in the stallion, Equine Vet J 1988;20:61.
120. Crowe CW, Gardner RE, Humburg JM, et al: Plasma testosterone and behavioral characteristics in geldings with intact epididymides, J Equine Med Surg 1977;1:387.
121. Ganjam VK: An inexpensive, yet precise, laboratory diagnostic method to confirm cryptorchidism in the horse, Proc Am Assoc Equine Pract 1977;23:245.
122. Burba DJ, Sedrish SA, Paccamonti DL: Theriogenology question of the month, J Am Vet Med Assoc 1996;209:1705.
123. Jann HW, Rains JR: Diagnostic ultrasonography for evaluation of cryptorchidism in horses, J Am Vet Med Assoc 1990;196:297-300.
124. Purchas RW, Burnham DL, Morris ST: Effects of growth potential and growth path on tenderness of beef longissimus muscle from bulls and steers, J Anim Sci 2002;80:3211.
125. Geiser DR: Practical equine injectable anesthesia, J Am Vet Med Assoc 1983;182:574.
126. Butera TS, Moore JN, Garner HE, et al: Diazepam/xylazine/ketamine combination for short-term anesthesia in the horse, Vet Med Small Anim Clin 1978;32:490.
127. Tranquilli W, Thurmon JC, Turner TA: Butorphanol tartrate as an adjunct to xylazine-ketamine anesthesia in the horse, Equine Pract 1983;5:26.
128. Hubbell JAE, Robertson JT, Muir WW, et al: Perianesthetic considerations in the horse, Comp Cont Educ Pract Vet 1984;6:S401.
129. Moll HD, Pelzer KD, Pleasant RS, et al: A survey of equine castration complications, J Equine Vet Sci 1995;15:522.
130. Zindel W: Die Kastration des Hengstes unter besonderer Berücksichtigung der an der Veterinär-Chrirurgischen Klinik der Universität Zürich seit mehr als dreissig Jahren geübten Methode, Zürich, Veterinär-chirurigsche Klinik der Universität Zürich, Universität Zürich, 1945.
131. Cox JE: Castration of horses and donkeys with first intention healing, Vet Rec 1984;115:372.
132. Lowe JE, Dougherty R: Castration of horses and ponies by a primary closure method, J Am Vet Med Assoc 1972;160:183.
133. Barber SM: Castration of horses with primary closure and scrotal ablation, Vet Surg 1985;14:2.
134. Palmer SE, Passmore JL: Midline scrotal ablation technique for unilateral cryptorchid castration in horses, J Am Vet Med Assoc 1989;190:283.
135. Kaegi B, Furst A, Struchen CH, et al: Experience with primary closure of the incisions following castration in horses, Proc Eur Coll Vet Surg 1994;3:119-120.
136. Shoemaker R, Bailey J, Janzen E, et al: Routine castration in 568 draught colts: Incidence of evisceration and omental herniation, Equine Vet J 2004;36:336.
137. Liefman CE: Active immunization of horses against tetanus including the booster dose and its application, Aust Vet J 1981;57:57.
138. Shideler RK, Squires EL, Voss JL: Equine castration—disappearance of spermatozoa, Equine Pract 1981;3:31.
139. Rijkenhuizen ABM: Castration of the stallion: Preferable in the standing horse using laparoscopy? Proc Eur Coll Vet Surg 1998;7:199.
140. Wilson DG, Hendrickson DA, Cooley AJ, et al: Laparoscopic methods for castration in equids, J Am Vet Med Assoc 1996;209:112.
141. Bergeron JA, Hendrickson DA: Viability of an inguinal testis after laparoscopic cauterization and transection of its blood supply, J Am Vet Med Assoc 1998;213:1303.
142. Selway SJ, Kenney RM, Bergman RV, et al: Field technique for vasectomy, Proc Am Assoc Equine Pract 1977;27:355.
143. Schanbacher BD, Pratt BR: Response of a cryptorchid stallion to vaccination against luteinising hormone releasing hormone, Vet Rec 1985;116:74.
144. Dowsett KF, Knott LM, Tshewang U, et al: Suppression of testicular function using two dose rates of a reversible water soluble gonadotrophin releasing hormone (GnRH) vaccine in colts, Aust Vet J 1996;74:228.
145. Malmgren L, Andresen O, Dalin A-M: Effect of GnRH immunisation on hormonal levels, sexual behavior, semen quality, and testicular morphology in mature stallions, Equine Vet J 2001;33:75.
146. Wilson DG, Reinertson EL: A modified parainguinal approach for cryptorchidectomy in horses: An evaluation in 107 horses, Vet Surg 1987;16:1.

147. Cox JE, Edwards GB, Neal PA: Suprapubic paramedian laparotomy for equine abdominal cryptorchidism, Vet Rec 1975;97:428.
148. Lowe JE, Higginbotham R: Castration of abdominal cryptorchid horses by a paramedian laparotomy approach, Cornell Vet 1969;59:121.
149. DeMoore A, Verschooten F: Paramedian incision for removal of abdominal testicles in the horse, Vet Med Small Anim Clin 1967;62:1083.
150. Swift PN: Castration of a stallion with bilateral abdominal cryptorchidism by flank laparotomy, Aust Vet J 1972;48:472.
151. Ragle CA, Schneider RK, Southwood LL: Abdominal laparoscopy in horses, Comp Cont Educ Pract Vet 1996;18:1231.
152. Wilson DG: Laparoscopy as an aid in the surgical management of the equine hemicastrate, Proc Am Assoc Equine Pract 1989;35:347.
153. Fischer AT Jr, Vachon AM: Laparoscopic cryptorchidectomy in horses, J Am Vet Med Assoc 1992;201:1705.
154. Davis EW: Laparoscopic cryptorchidectomy in standing horses, Vet Surg 1997;26:326.
155. Hendrickson DA, Wilson DG: Laparoscopic cryptorchid castration in standing horses, Vet Surg 1997;26:335.
156. Walmsley JP: Personal communication, Liphook Equine Hospital, Liphook, Hampshire, UK, 2004.
157. Fischer AT, Vachon AM: Laparoscopic intra-abdominal ligation and removal of cryptorchid testes in horses, Equine Vet J 1998;30:105.
158. Hanrath M, Rodgerson DH: Laparoscopic cryptorchidectomy using electrosurgical instrumentation in standing horses, Vet Surg 2002;31:117.
159. Walmsley JP: Review of equine laparoscopy and an analysis of 158 laparoscopies in the horse, Equine Vet J 1999;31:456.
160. Ragle CA, Southwood LL, Schneider RK: Injury to abdominal wall vessels during laparoscopy in three horses, J Am Vet Med Assoc 1998;212:87.
161. Desmaizieres L-M, Martinot S, Lepage OM, et al: Complications associated with cannula insertion techniques used for laparoscopy in standing horses, Vet Surg 2003;32:501.
162. Goetz TE, Boulton CH, Coffman JR: Inguinal and scrotal hernias in colts and stallions, Comp Cont Educ Pract Vet 1981;3:S272.
163. Fischer AT Jr, Vachon AM, Klein SR: Laparoscopic inguinal herniorrhaphy in two stallions, J Am Vet Med Assoc 1995;207:1599.
164. Marien T, Hoeck FV, Adriaenssen A, et al: Laparoscopic testis-sparing herniorrhaphy: a new approach for congenital inguinal hernia repair in the foal, Equine Vet Educ 2001;13:32.
165. Klohnen A, Wilson DG: Laparoscopic repair of scrotal hernia in two foals, Vet Surg 1996;25:414.
166. Vaughan JT: Surgery of the testes. In Walker DF, Vaughan JT, editors: Bovine and Equine Urogenital Surgery, Philadelphia, 1980, Lea & Febiger.
167. Marien T: Standing laparoscopic herniorrhaphy in stallions using cylindrical polypropylene mesh prosthesis, Equine Vet J 2001;33:91.
168. Hoagland TA, Ott KM, Dinger JE, et al: Effects of unilateral castration on morphological characteristics of the testis in one-, two-, and three-year-old stallions, Theriogenology 1986;26:397.
169. Chambers F: Castration of horses, Vet Rec 1973;93:497.
170. Cox JE: The castration of horses: Castration of half a horse? Vet Rec 1973;93:425.
171. O'Grady JF: Treatment of cryptorchidism in the horse with Pregnyl. Ir Vet J 1952;6:505.
172. Allen TD: Impact of cryptorchidism on fertility. In Negro-Vilar A, editor, Male Reproduction and Fertility, New York, 1983, Raven Press.
173. Trumble TN, Ingle-Fehr J, Hendrickson DA: Laparoscopic intra-abdominal ligation of the testicular artery following castration in a horse, J Am Vet Med Assoc 2000;216:1596.
174. Waguespack R, Belknap J, Williams A: Laparoscopic management of postcastration hemorrhage in a horse, Equine Vet J 2001;33:510.
175. Roberts SJ: The effects of various intravenous injections on the horse, Am J Vet Res 1943;4:226.
176. Morris DL: Unpublished data, Texas A&M University, 1982.
177. Adair HS: Personal communication, University of Tennessee, 2004.
178. Schramme M: Personal communication, Cornell University, 2004.
179. Hunt RJ, Boles C: Postcastration eventration in eight horses (1982-1986), Can Vet J 1989;30:961.
180. Boussauw B, Wilderjans H: Inguinal herniation 12 days after a unilateral castration with primary wound closure, Equine Vet Educ 1996;8:248.
181. Wright JG: Champignon and scirrhous cord (Abstract), J Am Vet Med Assoc 1964;144:402.
182. Fitch G, Schumacher J: Infection of the spermatic cord of a pony gelding, Equine Vet Educ 1996;8:251.
183. Ansari MM, Matros LE: Tetanus, Comp Cont Educ Pract Vet 1982;4:S473.
184. Bernard W, Divers TJ, Whitlock RH, et al: Botulism as a sequel to open castration in a horse, J Am Vet Med Assoc 1987;191:73.
185. Perdrizet JA, Callihan DR, Rebhun WC, et al: Successful management of malignant edema caused by *Clostridium septicum* in a horse, Cornell Vet 1987;77:328.
186. Muylle E, Oyaert W, Ooms L, et al: Treatment of tetanus in the horse by injections of tetanus antitoxin into the subarachnoid space, J Am Vet Med Assoc 1975;167:47.
187. Schumacher J, Schumacher J, Spano JS, et al: Effects of castration on peritoneal fluid constituents in the horse, J Vet Intern Med 1988;2:22.
188. Shearman DJC, Finlayson NDC: Diseases of the Gastrointestinal Tract and Liver, New York, 1982, Churchill Livingston.
189. Dyson S: Review of 30 cases of peritonitis in the horse, Equine Vet J 1983;15:25.
190. Adams SB, Fessler JF, Rebar AH: Cytologic interpretation of peritoneal fluid in the evaluation of equine abdominal crises, Cornell Vet 1980;70:232.
191. Shively MJ: Veterinary Anatomy, College Station, Tex, 1984, Texas A&M University Press.
192. Todhunter RJ, Parker JE: Surgical repair of urethral transection in a horse, J Am Vet Med Assoc 1988;193:1085.
193. Yovich JV, Turner AS: Treatment of postcastration urethral stricture by phallectomy in a gelding, Comp Cont Educ Pract Vet 1986;8:393.
194. White GR: Animal Castration, Nashville, 1947, self-published.
195. Cox JE: Behaviour of the false rig: Causes and treatments, Vet Rec 1986;118:353.
196. Todd C, Nelson LW, Migaki G: Multiple heterotopic testicular tissue in the pig: A report of seven cases, Cornell Vet 1968;58:614.
197. Line SW, Hart BL, Sanders L: Effect of prepubertal versus post-pubertal castration on sexual and aggressive behavior in male horses, J Am Vet Med Assoc 1985;186:249.
198. Smith JA: Masculine behavior in geldings, Vet Rec 1974;94:160.

CHAPTER 66

Penis and Prepuce

James Schumacher

ANATOMY AND PHYSIOLOGY

Penis

The penis is the male organ of copulation and is composed of erectile tissue that encases the extrapelvic portion of the urethra[1-4] (Fig. 66-1). The penis of the horse is musculocavernous and can be divided into three parts: the root, the body or shaft, and the glans penis. The penis originates caudally at the root, which is fixed to the lateral aspects of the ischial arch by two crura (leg-like parts) that converge to form the shaft of the penis. The shaft constitutes the major portion of the penis and begins at the junction of the crura. It is attached caudally to the symphysis ischii of the pelvis by two short suspensory ligaments that merge with the origin of the gracilis muscles (Fig. 66-2). The glans penis is the conical enlargement that caps the shaft. The urethra passes over the ischial arch between the crura and curves cranioventrally to become incorporated within erectile tissue of the penis.

The mobile shaft and glans penis extend cranioventrally to the umbilical region of the abdominal wall.[3] The body is cylindrical but compressed laterally. When quiescent, the penis is soft, compressible, and about 50 cm long.[4] Fifteen to 20 cm lie free in the prepuce. When maximally erect, the penis is up to three times longer than when it is in a quiescent state.[5]

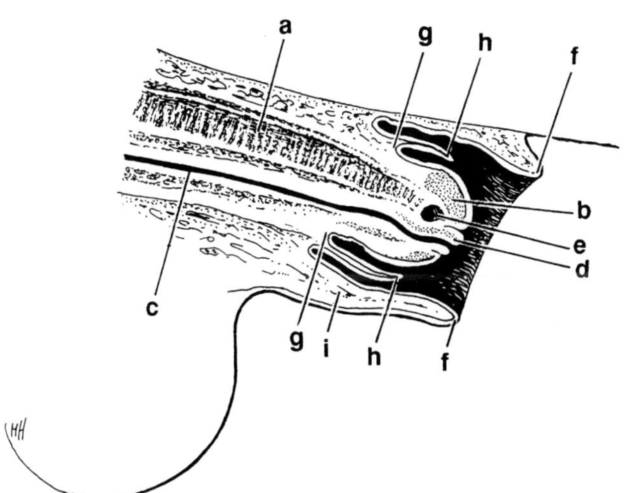

Figure 66-1. The cranial end of the penis in median section in situ in the horse, medial aspect. a, corpus cavernosum penis; b, corpus spongiosum glandis; c, urethra; d, urethral process; e, fossa glandis; f, external preputial orifice; g, preputial cavity (internal); h, plica preputialis; i, prepuce.

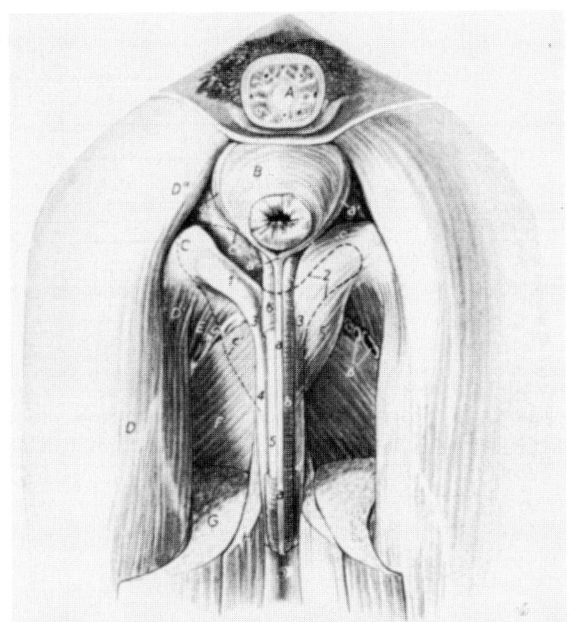

Figure 66-2. Perineum of stallion, deep dissection, caudal aspect. A, cross-section through root of tail; B, external anal sphincter; C, tuber ischiadicum; D, semitendinosus; D′, short head from tuber ischiadicum; D″, vertebral head; E, obturator externus; F, adductor; G, ventral stump of semimembranosus (the dorsal part of the muscle has been removed); H, gracilis; J, caudal wall of scrotum; a, penile part of retractor penis; a′, a″, rectal part of retractor penis; b, bulbospongiosus, partly removed on the left side to expose the urethra; c, right ischiocavernosus, covering right crus penis *(broken line);* c′, outline of left ischiocavernosus, which has been removed to expose left crus penis; 1, left crus penis; 2, outline of right crus penis under cover of ischiocavernosus; 3, union of crura penis; 4, corpus cavernosum penis; 5, urethra, surrounded by corpus spongiosum; 6, muscular branches of obturator vessels. (From Nickel R, Schummer A, Seiferle E, Sack WO: The Viscera of the Domestic Mammals, Oxford, UK, 1973, Blackwell.)

Erectile Bodies

Two cavernous spaces make up the majority of the penile shaft: the dorsally located corpus cavernosum penis (CCP), which is responsible for erection, and the ventrally located corpus spongiosum penis (CSP), formerly termed the corpus cavernosum urethrae[3,4] (Fig. 66-3). The CCP originates below the ischial arch at the union of the crura, which attach to the ischial arch, and makes up the bulk of the shaft.[2,3] It ends distally in one long central and two blunt ventrolateral projections[3] (Fig. 66-4). Along the ventral surface of the CCP runs the urethral groove or urethral sulcus.

The CSP lies in the urethral groove of the CCP and surrounds the urethra[2-4] (see Fig. 66-3). The bulb of the penis is the proximal enlargement of the CSP. At its distal termination, the CSP expands into the glans penis, which caps the central projection of the CCP (see Fig. 66-4). The tunica albuginea of the glans is thinner than that of the rest of the penis, making it softer in the erect state than the CCP.[5] A long dorsal process of the glans penis extends 10 cm proximally on the dorsum of the CCP. The circular edge of the glans penis is termed the corona glandis, and the collum glandis represents the constriction behind it. The convex, cranial surface of the glans contains a deep

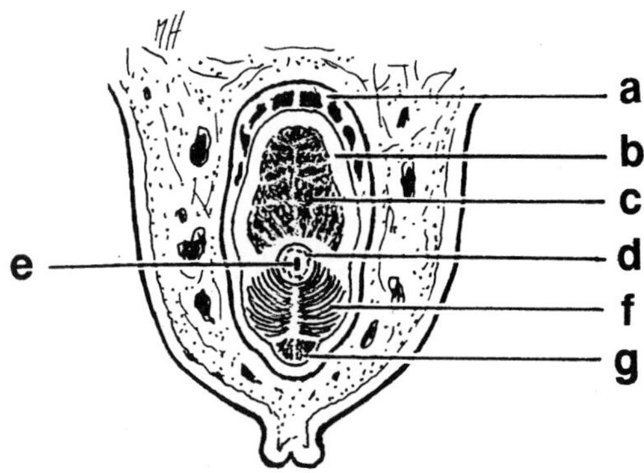

Figure 66-3. Cross-section of the penis. a, dorsal veins of penis; b, tunica albuginea; c, corpus cavernosum penis with dividing trabeculae; d, corpus spongiosum; e, urethra; f, bulbospongiosus; g, retractor penis muscle.

depression, the fossa glandis, into which the urethra protrudes 1.5 to 3.0 cm as a free tube surrounded only by thin integument[1,3,4,6] (Fig. 66-5). This tubular protrusion of the urethra is termed the urethral process. A dorsal diverticulum of the fossa glandis, the urethral sinus, is often filled with smegma, a caseous mass of sebaceous matter and epithelial debris. A collection of hardened smegma in the urethral sinus is termed a bean. Large beans have been purported to interfere with urination. Two ventrolateral recesses also project from the fossa glandis.[4] The fossa glandis and its recesses can harbor bacteria capable of producing venereal disease.[7]

The erectile bodies are surrounded by the thick, fibroelastic tunica albuginea, which sends fibrous trabeculae inward to form the supporting framework of the cavernous spaces.[1,2,6] The CSP has thinner trabeculae with larger,

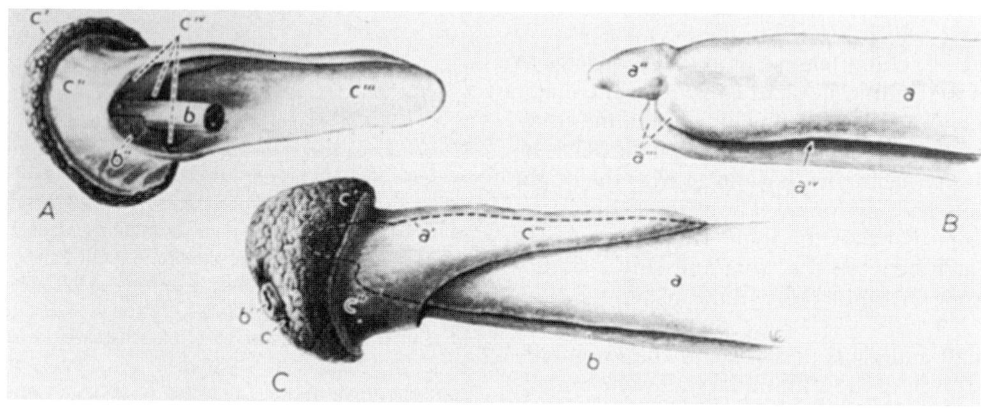

Figure 66-4. Distal end of the penis of the horse. A, caudoventral aspect of the glans, and of the terminal part of the urethra with corpus spongiosum; B, ventrolateral aspect of corpus cavernosum; C, lateral aspect of tip of the penis (the skin of the penis has been removed proximal to the corona glandis); a, a′, corpus cavernosum; a″, dorsomedian process of corpus cavernosum; a‴, ventrolateral processes of corpus cavernosum; a^{iv}, urethral groove; b, urethra, surrounded by corpus spongiosum; b′, urethral process and external urethral orifice; b″, stump of bulbospongiosus; c, fossa glandis; c′, corona glandis; c″, collum glandis; c‴, dorsal process of glans; c^{iv}, recesses on the interior of the glans for the three processes (a″, a‴) of the corpus cavernosum. (From Nickel R, Schummer A, Seiferle E, Sack WO: The Viscera of the Domestic Mammals, Oxford, UK, 1973, Blackwell.)

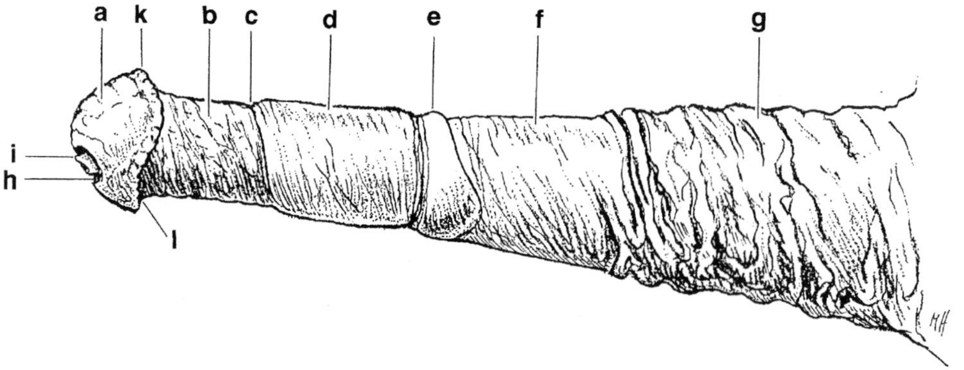

Figure 66-5. Extended penis of a stallion (protruded from the prepuce), left lateral aspect. a, glans penis; b, free part of the penis; c, attachment of the inner lamina of the preputial fold to penis; d, inner lamina of the preputial fold; e, preputial ring; f, outer lamina of the preputial fold; g, internal lamina of the external fold of the prepuce; h, fossa glandis; i, urethral process; k, corona glandis; l, collum glandis.

veinlike cavernous spaces than seen in the CCP. The tunica albuginea of the CSP is thin and elastic and merges distally with the integument of the glans.[4] The cavernous spaces are lined with endothelial cells and longitudinally oriented bundles of smooth muscle. Tonus of these muscular trabeculae and the retractor penis muscles maintains the nonerect penis within the prepuce. Decrease in tonus, as during micturition, causes the nonerect penis to protrude from the prepuce.

Mechanism of Erection

Penile erection is a neurovascular phenomenon, and the primary hemodynamic event leading to erection is increased arterial flow to the cavernous spaces.[4] Sexual excitement stimulates parasympathetic outflow from the sacral portion of the spinal cord and results in dilation and straightening of the helicine arteries (coiled branches of the deep artery of the penis) and relaxation of the sinusoidal smooth muscles, enabling blood to pass into the sinusoidal spaces.[4,8] Engorgement of the cavernous spaces, which is controlled and finally stopped by the unyielding tunica albuginea and trabeculae, lengthens and stiffens the penis.

Obstruction of venous return from the CCP appears to be important during erection in the stallion.[9,10] Circulation to and from the CCP passes between the ischium and the ischiocavernosus muscles. Contraction of the ischiocavernosus muscles from stimulation of the pudendal nerves occludes arterial and venous flow against the ischium, making the CCP a closed system during peak erection. Compression of the crura by the ischiocavernosus muscles forces blood into the CCP to produce high pressures. In one study, the mean pressure within the quiescent CCP measured 13 mm Hg, but it rose to 107 mm Hg during sexual arousal, and finally to 6530 mm Hg during coitus.[10] Anesthesia of the ischiocavernosus muscles caused diminution of erection by reducing the peak pressure in the CCP to a value close to that of the systemic blood pressure.

During coitus, increased arterial blood flow into the CSP and contraction of the bulbospongiosus muscles lead to increased pressure within the CSP and considerable distention of the glans penis.[11] The glans penis is greatly distensible and may become so large before coitus that the stallion is unable to accomplish intromission. In one study, mean pressure within the CSP was 17 mm Hg during the quiescent state, 76 mm Hg on arousal, and finally, 994 mm Hg during coitus.[11] Contractions of the bulbospongiosus muscles were likely responsible for the high pressure, because anesthesia of these muscles greatly reduced pressure in the CSP during coitus. The CSP remains an open system during erection because vessels entering the bulb of the penis do not pass between an osseous structure and the bulbospongiosus muscles.[11] Blood passes down the CSP to the glans penis and out through the dorsal veins.

Detumescence occurs after ejaculation because parasympathetic impulses diminish, and because sympathetic impulses that facilitate emission of semen also cause the helicine arteries to return to their coiled state, thus restricting inflow of arterial blood. Sympathetic impulses also decrease venous compression and allow emissary veins to open, thereby increasing venous outflow.[4,8,12,13]

Muscles

The short, paired, ischiocavernosus muscles that arise from the tuber ischii and the adjacent part of the sacrotuberous ligament attach to the crura and adjacent parts of the body of the penis[3,4] (see Fig. 66-2). Contraction of these muscles elevates the erect penis, bringing it into position for intromission. By compressing the penis against the ischium, the ischiocavernosus muscles assist in producing and maintaining erection by impeding venous return from the CCP.

The urethralis muscle surrounds the pelvic urethra and the bulbourethral glands and, by its contractions, forces release of seminal fluid during ejaculation as well as emptying of the last of the urine during urination.[3] The bulbospongiosus muscle, formerly termed the bulbocavernosus muscle, covers the CSP ventrally and extends nearly the entire length of the penis[4] (see Fig. 66-2). It originates near the bulbourethral glands, where it is continuous with the urethralis muscle, and ends at the free part of the penis near the glans penis. It sends transversely directed fibers from the edges of the urethral groove to meet at a median septum. Rhythmic contractions of the bulbospongiosus muscle during ejaculation force blood from the bulb, causing a pressure wave to be sent down the CSP to forcefully expel semen from the urethra.[3,11]

The ischiourethral muscles extend from the ventral surface of the ischium and crura, pass around the ischial arch into the pelvic cavity, and end at the ventral layer of the urethralis muscle.[3,4] They may assist erection by compressing the dorsal veins of the penis. The paired, longitudinal retractor penis muscles arise on the ventral surface of the first few coccygeal vertebrae and pass ventrally on each side of the rectum to form a loop beneath the terminal end of the rectum and anus[3,4] (see Fig. 66-2). From the loop, the muscles pass distally along the bulbospongiosus muscle and end at the glans penis. They retract the penis into the prepuce after erection or protrusion.

Blood Vessels, Nerves, and Lymphatics

Arteries supplying the penis include the terminal branches of the internal pudendal, obturator, and external pudendal arteries.[1-3] The external pudendal artery supplies the cranial artery of the penis, a major source of blood for erectile tissue.[2] It supplies a branch to the scrotum and continues as the caudal superficial epigastric artery, which provides branches to the prepuce.[2,4] The deep arteries of the penis originate from the obturator arteries and supply the CCP.[9] The internal pudendal artery supplies the pelvic portion of the urethra and terminates in the CSP as the artery of the bulb of the penis, which supplies the CSP.[2,4] Blood flows from the penis through a venous plexus on the dorsum and sides of the penis.[2,3] The venous plexus is emptied by the external pudendal and obturator veins; blood is carried from the root by the internal pudendal veins.[3]

Nervous supply to the penis is primarily via the pudendal nerves and the pelvic plexus of the sympathetic nervous system.[3] The pudendal nerves branch into the dorsal nerves of the penis, and the sympathetic fibers supply the smooth muscle of the vessels and the erectile tissue. The deep perineal and caudal rectal nerves supply the bulbospongiosus, ischiocavernosus, and retractor penis muscles.[4] Efferent lymphatics of the penis carry lymph to the superficial and deep inguinal lymph nodes.

Accessory Genital Glands

The accessory genital glands of the horse are the paired seminal vesicles, the prostate, the paired bulbourethral glands, and the paired ampullae of the ductus deferens[3,4,14] (Fig. 66-6). The accessory genital glands are fully developed in the sexually mature stallion but resume their juvenile size in the gelding.[5] The ducts of these glands empty into the pelvic urethra and provide the major portion of the ejaculate and serve to transport, nourish, and buffer spermatozoa.[8]

The distal 10 to 15 cm of each deferent duct widens to form an ampulla, the wall of which is thickened with secretory glands.[5,15] Each ampulla is evident as an enlargement near the midline of the pelvic floor. The seminal vesicles are two hollow, pear-shaped glands that lie on the dorsal surface of the neck of the bladder lateral to the ampullae.[3,4] They are often difficult to palpate per rectum, but identification can be enhanced if the stallion is sexually aroused prior to palpation.[14] Each vesicle of the stallion is 10 to 15 cm long and 3 to 6 cm wide, but those of geldings are much smaller. The seminal vesicles narrow as they converge toward the midline, and each forms a single excretory duct, which travels beneath the prostate and opens together with or beside the ipsilateral ampulla on the colliculus seminalis. The combined terminal portion of the ampulla and excretory duct of the seminal vesicle is termed the ejaculatory duct. The seminal vesicles are true glandular structures and not just reservoirs for the storage of spermatozoa, as was once thought.[8] The secretions of the seminal vesicles are viscous and contribute the major portion of the volume of ejaculate.[3,4,8] Secretions from the seminal vesicles are the last to enter the urethra.[5] Seminal vesiculitis, a rare but important problem in stallions, may be associated with infertility. Surgical removal of chronically infected vesicles has been described.[16]

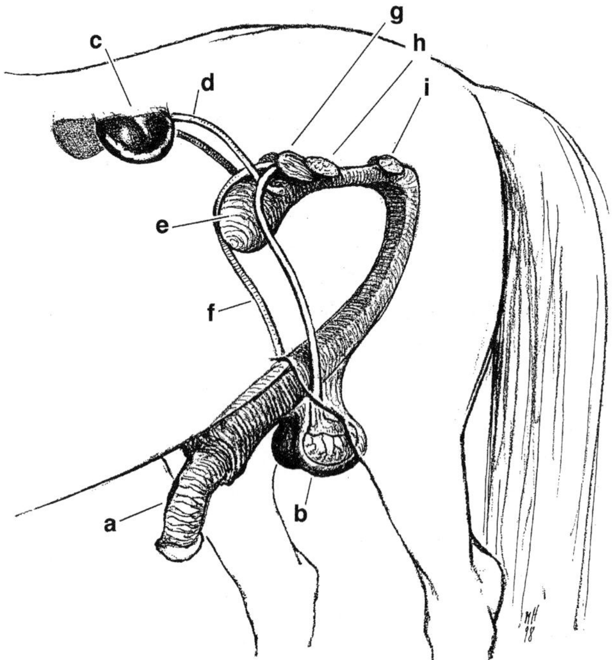

Figure 66-6. Graphic representation of the urogenital tract of the stallion. a, penis; b, testes; c, kidneys; d, ureters; e, urinary bladder; f, ductus deferens; g, seminal vesicles; h, prostate gland; i, bulbourethral glands.

The prostate is a nodular, bilobed gland that lies dorsal to the neck of the bladder.[3,4] The prostate of a stallion can, with some difficulty, be palpated per rectum, especially if the horse is sexually aroused. Each lobe is 5 to 9 cm long, 3 to 6 cm wide, and about 1 cm thick; the lobes are connected across the midline by a 3-cm-long isthmus. Prostatic secretion from each lobe is carried through 15 to 20 prostatic ducts, which open into the urethra through small, slit-like openings located lateral to the colliculus seminalis. The prostate produces a watery, alkaline secretion that neutralizes the acidity of fluid entering the urethra from the ductus deferens.[8]

The two bulbourethral (or Cowper's) glands are situated on the dorsolateral surface of the urethra at the ischial arch, 2 to 3 cm caudal to the prostate.[1-5] Each is covered by a bulboglandularis muscle. The bulbourethral glands of the stallion are 4 to 5 cm long and 2.5 cm wide and are difficult to palpate per rectum. Six to eight excretory ducts from each gland open in two longitudinal rows of small papillae on the dorsal surface of the pelvic urethra caudal to the openings of the prostatic ducts. The bulbourethral glands produce an alkaline, mucinous secretion that clears the urethra of urine prior to ejaculation and lubricates the urethra for the passage of seminal fluid.[8]

Prepuce

The prepuce, or sheath, is a voluminous, folded "sleeve" of integument covering the mobile portion of the quiescent penis.[3] The prepuce consists of the haired external lamina, which is continuous with the skin of the abdominal wall, and an internal lamina, which is in contact with the penis[3,4,6] (see Fig. 66-5). The external lamina extends cranially from the scrotum to within 5 to 8 cm of the umbilicus and is continuous with the internal lamina at the opening of the prepuce, the preputial orifice[3] (see Fig. 66-1). Close to the cranial extent of the external lamina are two rudimentary teats. The preputial raphe, a cranial continuation of the scrotal raphe, divides the external lamina sagittally on its ventral midline. The prepuce is supported by an elastic suspensory ligament that lies within the external lamina and is derived from the abdominal tunic.[17] When the horse trots or canters, movement of the penis within the prepuce often creates a sucking noise.

The prepuce of the horse differs from that of other species in that it is formed by a double fold of preputial skin, one inside the other.[2-4,6] When the penis is retracted, the internal lamina doubles on itself to form a cylindrical internal fold, the plica preputialis or preputial fold. The preputial cavity is thus divided into external and internal cavities, of which the external is the more spacious.[4] The opening of the plica preputialis is termed the preputial ring. When the plica preputialis unfolds during erection, the preputial ring can be recognized as a thickened band on the extended penis.[1,2]

The penis is not free in the preputial cavity at birth, because epithelium of the internal lamina of the prepuce and epithelium of the free part of the penis are fused into a single lamina. The lamina is split into external and internal laminae by a cytolytic process that forms vesicles that coalesce to form the preputial cavity.[18,19] Separation of the internal and external laminae occurs in the first month after birth and is controlled by androgens.

DIAGNOSTIC PROCEDURES

History

Most preputial and penile abnormalities are easily diagnosed from the horse's history and during physical examination, and further studies are not required. History pertaining to problems of the penis and prepuce may include such information as copulatory performance, drug therapy, behavioral changes, conception rates, duration of disability, and previous injuries, illnesses, or urogenital surgery.

Clinical Examination

Urination

Physical examination of a horse with a penile or preputial disorder should include observation of urination. The horse can sometimes be stimulated to urinate by placing it in a freshly bedded stall; shaking the bedding while whistling may increase the horse's urge to urinate. If this technique fails, intravenously administered furosemide generally results in urination within 15 minutes. If the horse makes painful and unsuccessful attempts to urinate, urethral obstruction should be suspected, and the bladder should be palpated per rectum. If the bladder is distended, it should be catheterized to relieve its distention and to determine the location of urethral obstruction. A large accumulation of hardened smegma within the fossa glandis can produce stranguria by distorting the urethral process, but this accumulation is readily identified and easily removed.

Erection and Ejaculation

A breeding stallion that is experiencing difficulty with erection or ejaculation should be observed servicing a mare. Inability of a sexually excited stallion to achieve erection could be caused by a vascular shunt from the CCP to a vessel outside the tunica albuginea, or by fibrosis of cavernous tissue from an unresolved episode of priapism. Shunts between the CCP and one or more dorsal veins of the penis could result from a congenital anomaly or from laceration or rupture of the tunica albuginea. Damage to the CCP caused by priapism (persistent erection without sexual excitement) can be assessed by palpating the cavernous tissue. Fibrous, noncompliant cavernous tissue indicates that the CCP has been permanently damaged. A stallion that is reluctant to ejaculate or displays pain during ejaculation may suffer from urethritis or seminal vesiculitis. If so, semen should be examined for the presence of blood, and the urethra should be endoscopically inspected for evidence of seminal vesiculitis or a urethral abnormality.

Palpation

The penis can be palpated as it lies retracted in the prepuce by inserting a gloved and lubricated hand through the preputial orifice and preputial ring. This may be the only method of physically evaluating the penis and internal preputial lamina of a horse with phimosis (an inability to protrude the penis from the prepuce because of a stricture of the preputial orifice or preputial ring). The external and internal preputial cavities, preputial ring, and free part of the penis, including the urethral sinus and process, can be evaluated by palpation. Beans within the urethral sinus can usually be palpated by compressing the tip of the penis. Dense, brown-black, greasy smegma is normally encountered at the preputial fornix.

Visual Inspection

To ascertain the exact nature and extent of penile or preputial abnormalities, visual inspection of the horse's penis and internal preputial lamina is usually necessary. The stallion's penis can be protruded by administering xylazine HCl or preferably by stimulating sexual arousal. Administration of phenothiazine-derivative tranquilizers to stallions should be avoided because of association of these tranquilizers with penile paralysis and priapism. The gelding's penis can be protruded by administering a tranquilizer or sedative or by placing a loop of gauze behind the corona glandis and with steady traction overcoming the pull of the retractor penis muscles. Producing penile protrusion by chemical means is preferable to pulling the penis from the prepuce, because traction on the penis is resented by the horse and could damage the penis.

The penis can be desensitized and extruded by anesthetizing the pudendal nerves at the level of the ischial arch.[2,20] The point of injection is 2 cm dorsal to the ischial arch and an equal distance lateral to the anus. The needle is inserted at an angle until its point contacts the ischial arch on the midline where the pudendal nerves course around the ischium. The penis usually protrudes within 5 minutes after deposition of 3 to 5 mL of a local anesthetic agent adjacent to each nerve. Unless prolonged penile desensitization is required, a short-acting local anesthetic, such as lidocaine HCl, should be used to avoid prolonged penile protrusion. Desensitization and extrusion of the penis and internal lamina of the prepuce by anesthetizing the right and left pudendal nerves where they are embedded in the sacrotuberous ligament is described, but this pudendal nerve block is difficult.[21]

The urethral process and fossa glandis should be inspected for lesions of cutaneous habronemiasis. With the penis extended, the entire internal preputial lamina is visible and can be evaluated for wounds, scars, hematomas, neoplasia, and granulomas. Penile and preputial wounds should be closely examined to determine if they penetrate the tunica albuginea or invade the urethra. Leakage of urine from a traumatized area may be noted, especially when the horse urinates. A hematoma should be differentiated from an abscess. Physical findings of hematoma include penile swelling and ecchymosis, particularly noticeable in nonpigmented areas. Aspiration of a hematoma confirms the diagnosis. Examination of a horse with paraphimosis (an inability to retract the protruded penis into the prepuce) should include an evaluation of penile sensory innervation, because protrusion accompanied by penile paralysis may be permanent.

If preputial or penile neoplasia is suspected, the entire external genitalia should be examined meticulously for other primary lesions, and the inguinal regions should be palpated to detect enlarged lymph nodes. Superficial inguinal lymph nodes may enlarge initially from inflammation but later from malignant infiltration. Lymph nodes adhered to overlying skin or with fistulous tracts have most likely been infiltrated by malignant emboli. Metastases to internal lymph nodes may be detected by palpation per rectum. Recognition of carcinoma of the external genitalia should lead to examination of other structures commonly affected by carcinoma, such as the third eyelids and the perineum.

Other Diagnostic Procedures

Endoscopy

Endoscopy may be useful for identifying the source of hemorrhage noted to occur during urination or ejaculation. Endoscopy of the urethra and bladder is performed with the horse standing and sedated using a sterile, 100-cm (or longer), flexible endoscope with a diameter no larger than 12 mm. The vasculature and cavernosal spaces surrounding the urethra are prominent, especially in the proximal portion of the urethra, and should not be mistakenly interpreted as inflammation. The lumen of the seminal vesicles can be examined for evidence of infection by passing the insertion tube of a small-diameter endoscope into the ducts at the colliculus seminalis.[22]

Ultrasonography

Ultrasonography can be used to assess the physical status of cavernous tissue and to identify urethral lesions, such as calculi or stenosing scars. Ultrasonographic examination of a penile hematoma may identify a rupture of the tunica albuginea. Abnormality of an accessory sex gland can sometimes be detected using transrectal ultrasonography.[14] The glands can be more readily identified if the stallion has been sexually aroused before ultrasonographic examination.

Cavernosography

Cavernosography may be useful for determining the cause of persistent impotence. Contrast medium (100 to 200 mL of iohexol, a 24% water-soluble, organic iodine radiographic contrast medium) is injected into the CCP, and serial radiographs of the penis are obtained. If shunts are present, contrast medium appears in the nutrient vessels of the penis and prepuce. If trabeculae are damaged, the sinusoidal spaces fill incompletely with contrast medium. Cavernosography also may be useful in identifying a rupture or laceration of the tunica albuginea of the CCP.

Miscellaneous Diagnostic Procedures

Urethral and ureteral catheterization may be useful for determining the source of hemorrhage observed to occur during urination or ejaculation or to obtain fluid expressed from the seminal vesicles for cytologic examination and culture.[22] Cytologic or histologic evaluation of penile and preputial lesions may be necessary to distinguish between various diseases, such as cutaneous habronemiasis and squamous cell carcinoma.

PENILE AND PREPUTIAL DISORDERS

Penile and Preputial Injuries

Etiology

Horses can lacerate their penis while jumping barriers or attempting to breed a mare over a fence, by falling on sharp objects, or during coitus from the mare's tail hairs or a loosely tied "breeding stitch." Stallion rings that are too small or improperly cleaned may cause erosions of the shaft.[23] Penile hematomas are usually caused by trauma to the erect penis and can occur when stallions are pastured with other horses or permitted to breed improperly restrained mares. Severe bending of the penile shaft during coitus or semen collection may cause tearing of a corporeal body or subfascial vessels on the surface of the penis.

Penile lacerations or erosions are usually superficial, but lacerations into the cavernous tissue and urethra have been reported.[24-28] A tear in the urethral sinus leading directly into the CSP caused severe penile hemorrhage in a stallion during coitus,[25] and improper castration of two horses caused urethral damage and necrosis of tissue at the scrotum from escape of urine.[26,27]

Hematomas usually arise from rupture of the extensive vascular plexus located subfascially on the surface of the penis,[29] but occasionally, a hematoma may originate from a torn corporeal body.[30] Rupture of the CCP is sometimes referred to as fracture of the penis. Rupture of the bulb of the penis, presumably from a blow, eventually led to the death of a stallion by causing urethral stenosis and subsequent rupture of the bladder.[31] A hematoma confined within the intact tunica albuginea of the CCP, apparently caused by a breeding accident, resulted in deviation of a stallion's penis during erection, presumably from disruption of blood flow through the cavernous structure.[32] Aspiration of the hematoma, using ultrasonographic guidance, resulted in straightening of the penis.

Pathophysiology

Unsutured preputial lacerations inevitably become infected, and migration of infection through the loose preputial connective tissue results in cellulitis and generalized swelling. If cellulitis and swelling become severe, the penis and internal lamina of the prepuce protrude through the preputial orifice. Superficial wounds, if properly treated, heal without complication, but large unattended wounds that heal by cicatrization may restrict action of the prepuce. An unsutured wound into cavernous tissue may lead to impotence caused by creation of a shunt between the cavernous tissue and the superficial penile vasculature. Although longitudinal urethral lacerations generally heal without stricture when left to heal by secondary intention, unsutured, transecting urethral lacerations usually heal with obstructing stenosis. An improperly attended urethral injury could result in a cutaneous-urethral or cavernosourethral fistula.

Rupture of superficial penile vessels or corporeal bodies causes extravasation of blood into the loose preputial fascia. Extreme preputial swelling may occur within minutes of injury and may prevent the horse from retracting its penis into the preputial cavity. The penis may rapidly enlarge to several times its normal size. The hematoma may interfere with venous and lymphatic drainage by impinging on undamaged veins and lymphatic vessels, thus exacerbating the swelling,[23] or the hematoma may interfere with urination by impinging on the urethra.[31]

Treatment

OPEN WOUNDS

To avoid infection, fresh penile and preputial wounds should be débrided and sutured. Sutures can be either absorbable or nonabsorbable but should be soft and nonirritating. Infected wounds should be frequently cleansed with a mild antiseptic solution several times daily and covered with an antimicrobial ointment. If the urethra is completely disrupted, it should be reapposed with absorbable suture; stenting the urethral lumen with a male urinary catheter during surgery simplifies the anastomosis. Stenosis of the urethra caused by cicatrix formation after injury can sometimes be relieved by transendoscopic laser ablation.[33] Often, penile amputation is the most expedient means of treating complete urethral disruption accompanied by severe trauma of surrounding tissue, especially if the injured horse is a gelding.[28]

HEMATOMAS

Treatment of a horse with a penile hematoma should be instituted immediately after injury and aimed at decreasing hemorrhage. Compressing the penis and internal lamina of the prepuce with a pneumatic bandage or tight wrap may relieve edema and minimize hemorrhage. To compress the penis and prepuce, the horse is anesthetized, and starting at the distal end of the penis, the penis and internal lamina of the prepuce are wrapped snugly from the glans to the preputial orifice with an elastic bandage.[34] The wrapped penis and prepuce and the preputial orifice are massaged until the wrap loosens from the decrease in size of the penis and prepuce. The process is repeated until maximal decrease in size is achieved. The penis and internal lamina of the prepuce should then be supported against the abdomen or within the external prepuce to diminish hemorrhage and edema. Hydrotherapy with cold water may hasten vasoconstriction. If the hematoma continues to expand despite treatment, the area of the hematoma should be examined ultrasonographically for evidence of a rent in the tunica albuginea, or surgically explored. Failure to repair a rupture of the tunica albuginea could result in formation of a shunt between the damaged erectile body and the dorsal veins of the penis.

Aftercare

To avoid erection and more hemorrhage, a horse with a penile or preputial injury should not be subjected to sexual stimuli. Because exercise may exacerbate hemorrhage, the horse should initially be closely confined. After 5 or 6 days, when hemostasis is ensured, the horse should be lightly exercised to decrease the edema. Hot packs applied to the penis at this time stimulate vasodilatation and thus resorption of the hematoma.

Paraphimosis

Etiology

Paraphimosis, or the inability of the horse to retract its protruded penis into the prepuce, occurs most frequently from preputial edema caused by genital trauma, such as preputial laceration, penile hematoma, or castration. Paraphimosis may be a manifestation of disease characterized by extensive edema, such as dourine and purpura hemorrhagica,[23,35] or it may be caused by damage to penile innervation. Penile denervation has been associated with spinal disease, trauma, and infectious diseases, such as equine herpes virus I and rabies.[23,36] Paralysis associated with priapism and debilitation has been reported[37,38] (Fig. 66-7). Penile paralysis has followed administration of

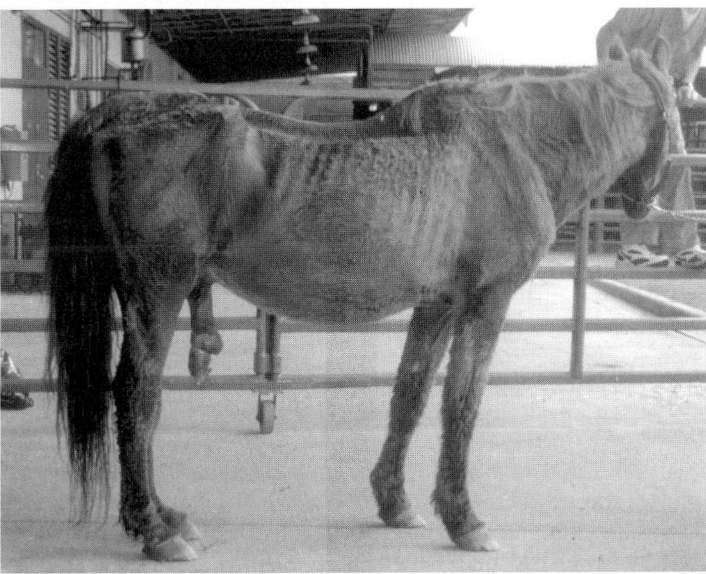

Figure 66-7. Paraphimosis caused by severe debilitation. The preputial ring has become a constricting cuff.

phenothiazine-derivative tranquilizers, most notably propiomazine (formerly termed propiopromazine).[39,40]

Pathophysiology

Tonus of the retractor penis muscles and the smooth muscle of the cavernous spaces normally maintains the penis within the prepuce.[37] With penile or preputial injury, edema develops in loose connective tissue between the penis and the internal lamina of the prepuce, and the weight of edema causes muscular fatigue, followed by protrusion of the penis and internal preputial lamina from the preputial cavity. The relationship between debilitation and penile paralysis is obscure, but general debilitation may cause loss of muscular tonus, allowing the penis to protrude and the pudendal nerves to become contused or stretched at the ischial arch.[37,41,42] Penile paralysis occurring after administration of a phenothiazine-derivative tranquilizer may likewise be caused by mechanical damage to the pudendal nerves from prolonged penile protrusion and not from direct damage to penile innervation by the tranquilizer, as suggested by one investigator.[39] Motor innervation of the retractor penis muscles is probably supplied solely by α-adrenergic fibers, and phenothiazine-derivative tranquilizers block these α-adrenergic fibers.[1] The retractor penis muscles can, however, be transected without causing the penis to protrude. Tranquilization may also block sympathetic impulses to the smooth muscle of the cavernous tissue, allowing the sinusoidal spaces to fill with blood and the penis to drop from the preputial cavity.[36]

Prolonged protrusion itself produces edema of the penis and prepuce by impairing venous and lymphatic drainage. As the penis and internal preputial lamina swell from edema, the preputial ring becomes a constricting cuff that compounds swelling distally. After several days, fluid begins to seep diffusely through the penile and preputial epithelium. Edema increases fragility of tissues, and because the exposed penis is subjected to trauma and effects of temperature, the penile and preputial epithelia soon become extensively excoriated.

Bacterial invasion of excoriated epithelium causes inflammation of the penis and prepuce, or balanoposthitis, and bacterial migration through the loose preputial connective tissue causes cellulitis. Eventual invasion of edematous and inflamed tissue by fibroblasts results in fibrosis of the penile integument and fascia, causing permanent impairment of the normal telescoping action of the prepuce.[37] The pendulous weight of the penis may eventually damage the pudendal nerves.[40,41]

The protruded penis becomes curved with the glans penis pointing caudoventrally. Urination is usually unimpeded.[40] Paralysis is usually accompanied by loss of erectile function, but ejaculatory capability is often still preserved.[23]

Treatment

Treatment of a horse affected with paraphimosis should be directed toward controlling edema and preventing further trauma. To preserve normal venous and lymphatic drainage and to protect against injury, the penis should be retained within the external preputial lamina. The penis can be temporarily retained with sutures or towel clamps placed across either the preputial orifice or preputial ring, but these devices should not be relied on for more than several days, because they damage the prepuce. Prolonged, atraumatic support can be provided by a nylon net or hosiery suspended at the preputial orifice by a crupper and surcingle made of rubber tubing (Fig. 66-8).

If the protruded penis is too edematous to be replaced within the external preputial lamina, it should be compressed against the abdomen with a bandage until edema subsides. A pneumatic bandage or a tight bandage applied directly to the penis may also be effective in reducing edema. Applying a nonirritating, hydrophilic agent, such as glycerin, or sulfa-urea to the penis may increase the effectiveness of the compressive bandage. Massaging the penis between bandage changes is helpful for dissipating edema. Applying an antimicrobial ointment to the penis prevents epithelial maceration and infection, and a systemically administered nonsteroidal anti-inflammatory drug reduces inflammation. The horse should be lightly exercised to reduce edema.

If the relatively inelastic preputial ring prevents penile retraction or impedes venous and lymphatic drainage, a

A

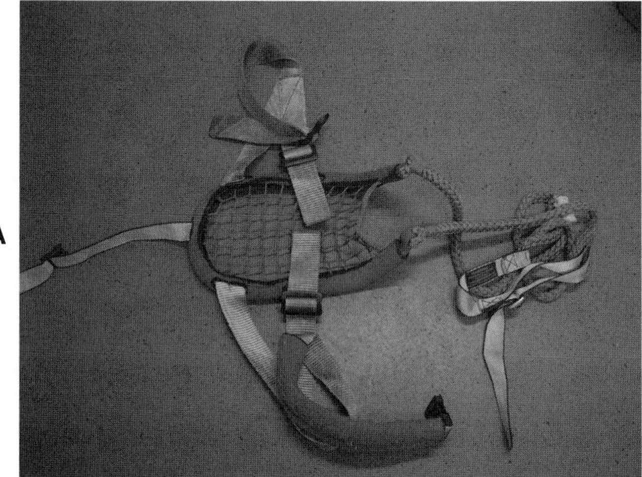

B

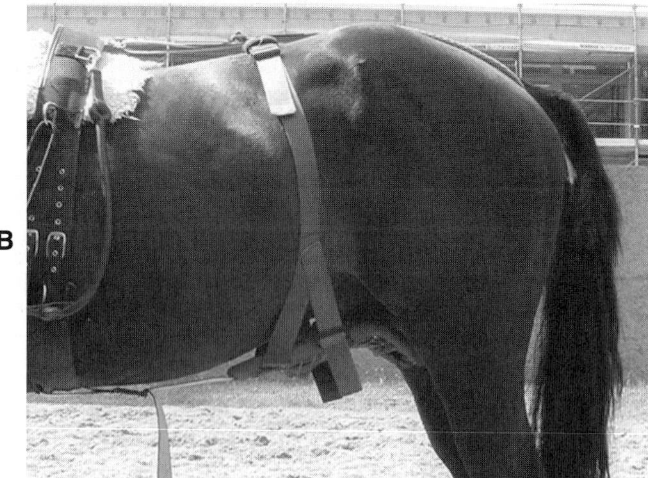

Figure 66-8. A, Suspensory device manufactured from a lightweight aluminum tube and nylon net. **B,** The device mounted on a horse. (Courtesy A. Fürst and R. Keller, University of Zurich.)

preputiotomy can be performed. The preputial ring is severed with a longitudinal incision after administration of local or general anesthesia, and the incision is allowed to heal by secondary intention.[36]

With prompt treatment, paraphimosis resulting from acute trauma usually resolves within several days. Even after initial swelling and inflammation subside, preputial cicatrization may restrict normal telescoping action of the prepuce. Excision of restrictive cicatricial tissue by segmental posthetomy (reefing) may be necessary to restore normal preputial function (see "General Surgical Procedures," p. 827). Horses with chronic paraphimosis accompanied by penile paralysis or generalized preputial fibrosis are unlikely to regain the ability to retract the penis. Stallions with penile paralysis generally retain their libido but are unable to achieve erection.[23,39] For some stallions, however, ejaculation may still be possible. Penile paralysis need not necessarily end a stallion's breeding career, if the stallion can be trained to ejaculate into an artificial vagina (provided that the horse's breed registry permits artificial insemination). The horse can be salvaged for purposes other than breeding by permanently retracting its penis into the preputial cavity or by amputating its penis (see "General Surgical Procedures," p. 827).

Phimosis

Etiology

Phimosis refers to the inability of the horse to protrude its penis from the prepuce because of a congenital or acquired stricture of the preputial orifice or preputial ring. Discounting the normal fusion of the internal lamina of the prepuce to the free part of the penis present during the first month after birth, congenital phimosis rarely, if ever, occurs in horses.

Acquired phimosis can result from tumors or cicatrizing lesions at the preputial orifice or preputial ring (Fig. 66-9) or from impairment of the normal telescoping action of the prepuce. When the horse cannot protrude its penis, urine enters the preputial cavity and produces mucosal inflammation that may eventually lead to more cicatrization and occlusion of the preputial orifice or preputial ring. An unusual cause of phimosis occurred when a gelding's penis became entrapped in a rent in the suspensory ligament of the prepuce. The ligament had apparently been torn when the horse was castrated.[17]

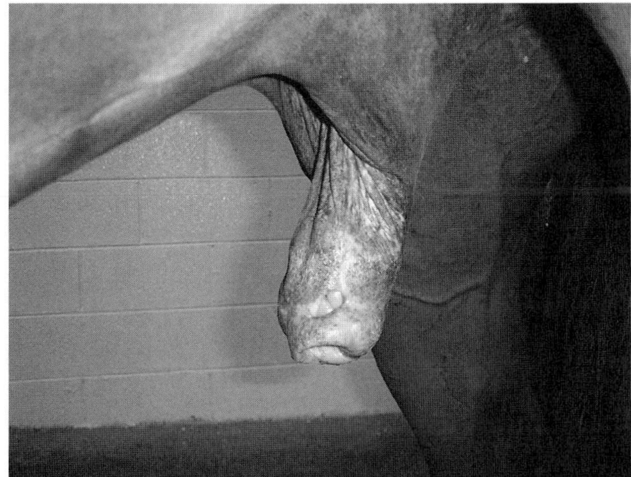

Figure 66-9. Phimosis in a horse caused by a cicatrix at the preputial ring.

Treatment

If phimosis is caused by constriction of the preputial orifice, a wedge of external preputial lamina based toward the preputial orifice is removed.[43] The internal and external preputial laminae are joined with a row of closely spaced, interrupted sutures. If phimosis is caused by constriction of the preputial ring, a similar wedge can be removed from the internal preputial fold, and after the penis is exposed, the constricting cicatrix can be removed by segmental posthetomy (reefing) (see "General Surgical Procedures," later). Phimosis caused by rupture of the suspensory ligament of the prepuce is corrected by suturing the torn ligament.[17]

Priapism

Priapism, or persistent erection without sexual excitement, occurs when the erect penis fails to detumesce.[44] The condition derives its name from the Greek god Priapus, symbol of fertility, but a frequent outcome of the condition in all species in which it occurs is infertility resulting from impotency.

Etiologic Factors

Etiologic factors in the development of priapism in men include hematologic diseases that cause vascular sludging, such as sickle cell anemia and leukemia; administration of antihypertensive or antidepressant drugs, especially when combined with alcohol; perineal trauma; spinal cord injury; and inflammatory disorders of the urogenital tract.[44] The cause of priapism in about half of all affected men is idiopathic.[45] Priapism of horses usually occurs after administration of a phenothiazine-derivative tranquilizer, usually acetylpromazine.[46] Phenothiazine-derivative tranquilizers may cause failure of detumescence by blocking α-adrenergic impulses that mediate detumescence.[47] Other, less commonly reported causes of priapism of horses include general anesthesia,[48] nematodiasis of the spinal cord,[49] and neoplasia of the pelvic canal.[50] Priapism occurs in both stallions and geldings, but stallions are more commonly affected, perhaps because of a direct influence of androgens on development of the condition, or perhaps because stallions develop erections more frequently.[50,51]

Pathophysiology

During normal erection, the rate of flow of blood into the CCP equals the rate of flow of blood from the structure. The precise mechanisms by which priapism occurs are unknown, but basically, priapism is a result of a disturbance of either the arterial inflow or the venous outflow to the CCP, causing the erect penis to fail to detumesce.[44] Priapism in men is classified as being either high flow or low flow. High-flow priapism occurs when arterial blood flow to the cavernosal tissue is increased, usually as a result of a traumatically induced arteriocavernosal shunt, and venous drainage cannot compensate for this increase.[52] Low-flow priapism occurs when the neural impulses that mediate detumescence are altered or when vascular or hematologic alterations mechanically interfere with venous drainage. High-flow priapism of men almost always results from trauma to the perineum or penis.[52] Low-flow priapism occurs in men much more commonly than does high-flow priapism, and it is the only type of priapism reported to occur in horses.

Low-flow priapism, regardless of its etiology, is characterized by stasis of blood within the CCP (Fig. 66-10). Blood aspirated from the CCP of men affected with low-flow priapism has a low pH (typically, less than 7.25), a low partial pressure of O_2 (typically, less than 30 mm Hg), and a high partial pressure of CO_2 (typically, greater than 60 mm Hg).[53] High partial pressure of CO_2, caused by vascular stasis, causes erythrocytes to sickle and causes endothelial damage to the vessels and trabeculae in the CCP. The sickled erythrocytes occlude the venous outflow from the CCP, eventually irreversibly.[54] Endothelial damage and occlusion cause trabecular edema, which eventually progresses to fibrosis, thereby decreasing the size of the sinusoidal spaces in the CCP and the capacity of the CCP to expand during erection. Arterial flow to the CCP remains patent during early stages of priapism, but ultimately, it too becomes occluded permanently by clots, edema, or fibrosis.[54] Protracted erection in the horse may also damage the pudendal nerves, presumably from tension on the nerves or from compression of the nerves against the ischium, causing paralysis of the penis.[50] The end result of unresolved priapism in the horse is impotence caused by loss of both erectile function and sensitivity of the glans and shaft of the penis.

Clinical Signs

A horse suffering from priapism may not have a full erection, causing the penis to appear to be paralyzed or merely protruded rather than erect. Turgidity of the CCP can be detected when the penis is palpated, however, and the engorged penis cannot be reduced manually into the prepuce. Unless properly cared for, the penis and the internal lamina of the prepuce become edematous soon after the onset of priapism.[51] Although uncommon, dysuria may be a feature of the condition. The CCP of a horse chronically affected by priapism feels fibrous, and during ultrasonographic examination, it appears to be densely echogenic. A chronically affected horse may not respond when a noxious stimulus is applied to the distal portion of the penis or internal lamina of the prepuce.[50]

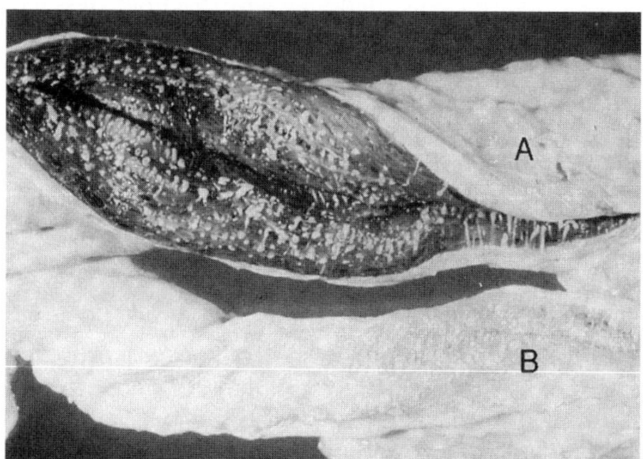

Figure 66-10. A, Longitudinal section of corpus cavernosum penis (CCP) of a stallion with longstanding priapism. The CCP is hemorrhagic and edematous. B, Longitudinal section of the CCP of a normal gelding.

Treatment

MEDICAL

Horses with priapism have been treated by massaging the penis, by applying an emollient dressing to the penis, and by compressing the penis against the body wall with a sling.[51] These treatments, although important in preventing preputial edema and damage to the penile and preputial integument, have no effect on re-establishing normal circulation in the erectile tissue of the CCP. To re-establish normal venous drainage impaired by drugs that cause α-adrenergic blockade, such as acetylpromazine, affected horses have been treated by administration of benztropine mesylate.[44,48,55-57] Benztropine mesylate is a synthetic drug created by combining the active portions of atropine and diphenhydramine.[48] This drug is most successful in resolving priapism if treatment is initiated soon after the onset of priapism.[48,55] The effects of the drug on horses affected with priapism are attributed to its anticholinergic effects.[48] The usual dose for a horse of average size is 8 mg, administered by slow intravenous injection. Side effects seen at higher dosages could include paralytic ileus, impaction, dysuria, and muscular weakness.

Alpha-adrenergic agents, such as adrenalin and phenylephrine, are often injected into the CCP of men in the early stages of priapism to achieve detumescence by promoting contractility of cavernous and arterial smooth muscle.[12,44,53,56] Instillation of 10 mg of phenylephrine diluted in 10 mL physiologic saline solution directly into the erect CCP is sometimes effective in resolving priapism of horses, provided that treatment is initiated soon after onset of priapism.[58] Phenylephrine can be injected safely into the cavernous tissue of men every 15 minutes until detumescence occurs,[12] and the same is probably true for horses. Horses chronically affected by priapism experience only temporary detumescence after this treatment.

IRRIGATION OF THE CORPUS CAVERNOSUM PENIS

A horse that does not respond within a few hours to cholinergic blockage or to three or more intracavernosal injections of an α-adrenergic agent, such as phenylephrine, should be treated by irrigation of its CCP with heparinized, physiologic saline solution (PSS).[38] Irrigation of the CCP not only removes sickled erythrocytes, it also improves the acidotic environment within the CCP. The CCP can be irrigated with the horse standing, but the procedure is most easily accomplished with the horse anesthetized and in dorsal recumbency. After preparing the penis and perineal area for aseptic surgery, PSS containing 10 IU heparin/mL is introduced into the CCP under pressure through a large-bore needle (e.g., a

12-gauge needle) inserted into the turgid CCP just proximal to the glans penis. The PSS, along with the stagnant blood, is exited 10 to 15 cm caudal to the scrotum, either through one or two large-bore needles inserted into the CCP or through a stab incision into the CCP. The CCP is irrigated until fresh blood appears in the efflux. Failure of arterial blood to appear in the efflux after stagnant blood has been evacuated indicates that the arteriolar supply to the CCP is permanently damaged and that the horse is likely to be impotent. The stab incision in the tunica albuginea of the CCP is sutured after irrigation is complete.

CREATION OF A SHUNT

Erection recurs after irrigation if venous outflow remains occluded, provided that arteriolar inflow vessels remain patent. If erection fails to resolve after several irrigations of the CCP, blood trapped in the CCP should be removed by creating a shunt between the CCP and the corpus spongiosum penis (CSP). The CSP offers a convenient exit for blood trapped in the CCP, because in contrast to the CCP, the CSP does not act as a closed system during erection.[44,45] Shunting should be performed before the cavernous tissue or the pudendal nerves become irreversibly damaged, but the time at which damage to the cavernosal tissue becomes irreversible after the onset of priapism has not been determined for horses.

The shunt is probably best performed in the perineal region of the horse. It could be created further distally, but creating it in the perineal region allows a more thorough evacuation of the stagnant blood by irrigation and provides drainage of blood from a greater length of the CCP. Because the CSP is thickest in the perineal region, the urethra is less likely to be perforated during the procedure. To create the shunt, the horse is anesthetized and positioned in dorsal recumbency. The penis and inguinal and perineal regions are prepared for aseptic surgery, and a stallion catheter is inserted into the urethra. A 15-cm incision is created along the perineal raphe, about 4 to 8 cm caudal to the base of the scrotum to expose the penis, and the retractor penis muscle is retracted to expose the bulbospongiosus muscle, which covers the ventral aspect of the CSP. The right or left edge of the bulbospongiosus muscle is elevated from the edge of the urethral groove to expose 4 to 5 cm of the underlying tunica albuginea of the CSP. A 3-cm longitudinal incision is made through the tunica albuginea of the CCP adjacent to the CSP to expose the sinusoidal spaces of the CCP, and stagnant blood is evacuated from the cavernous spaces of the CCP through this incision using irrigation as described earlier (Fig. 66-11).

A matching 3-cm longitudinal incision through the tunica albuginea of the CSP is created adjacent to the 3-cm incision into the CCP. The urethral catheter compresses the sinusoidal spaces of the encircling CSP, so the CSP must be incised carefully to avoid extending this incision into the lumen of the urethra. Bright red blood hemorrhages from the incised CSP, and at this point in the procedure, suction is usually required to maintain visibility. The medial edge of the incision in the tunica albuginea of the CCP is sutured to the lateral edge of the incision in the tunica albuginea of the CSP with 3-0 or 2-0 absorbable suture using a simple-continuous suture pattern. To complete the shunt, the lateral edge of the incision into the CCP is sutured to the medial edge of the incision into the CSP using a simple-continuous suture pattern. The bulbospongiosus muscle is sutured to its origin on the tunica albuginea of the CCP at the edge of the urethral groove, and the subcutaneous tissue and skin are apposed. Horses appear to suffer no discomfort after the surgery, and swelling is minimal.[57] The stallion should receive no sexual stimulation for at least a month after surgery.

Complications of the cavernosal shunt in men include urethrocavernous or urethrocutaneous fistula, penile gangrene, infection, and a painful CSP during erection.[45] Men receiving a shunt for treatment for priapism may become impotent from failure to achieve or maintain pressure in the CCP required for intromission,[44,45] and this failure can be the result of damaged cavernous tissue or from the shunt itself.[45] The shunt may close as normal blood outflow in the CCP resumes, but whether closure is essential for return of potency is not known. Bulls may become impotent after developing a trauma-induced shunt between the CCP and CSP,[36,59] but a shunt created surgically between the CCP and

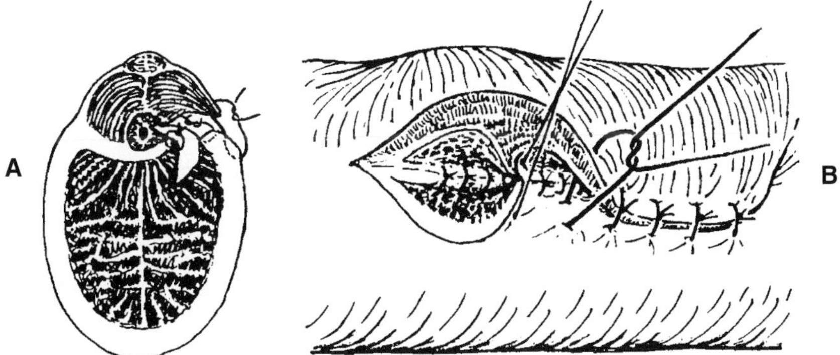

Figure 66-11. Cross-sectional view (**A**) and three-dimensional view (**B**) showing creation of a vascular shunt between the corpus cavernosum penis (CCP) and corpus spongiosum penis (CSP). 1, retractor penis muscle (not shown in B); 2, bulbospongiosus muscle; 3, CSP surrounding the urethra; CCP; 5, tunica albuginea of CSP; 6, tunica albuginea of CCP. The medial portion of the incision through the tunica albuginea of the CCP is sutured to the lateral portion of the incision through the tunica albuginea of the CSP. The medial portion of the incision through the tunica albuginea of the CSP is sutured to the lateral portion of the incision through the tunica albuginea of the CCP. The bulbospongiosus muscle is sutured to the tunica albuginea of the CCP.

the CSP of normal stallions does not seem to interfere with subsequent erection and ejaculation, even if the shunt does not close.[57] In one report, a stallion that developed penile paralysis after suffering from priapism for several days regained normal erectile and ejaculatory function within 1 year after resolution of priapism, even though the horse had received two shunts between the CCP and the CSP.[60] Failure of a stallion affected by priapism to develop a normal erection after creation of a shunt between the CCP and the CSP is most likely the result of damage to erectile tissue caused by protracted priapism, rather than by the shunt.

Erectile function in men with cavernosal tissue damaged by protracted priapism has been enhanced by injecting a vasoactive drug, such as papaverine, phenoxybenzamine, or phentolamine, into the cavernosal tissue.[44,61] Administering a vasoactive drug into the cavernous tissue may likewise be useful for enhancing erectile function of horses with damaged erectile tissue. Some stallions with damaged erectile tissue may regain the ability to achieve intromission if they are assisted in placing their penis into the vagina of the mare, and some may be trained to ejaculate into an artificial vagina. If a stallion has decreased penile sensitivity resulting from damage to the pudendal nerves caused by priapism, an antidepressive drug, imipramine, can be administered before breeding to lower the stallion's ejaculatory threshold.[62]

PHALLECTOMY

Phallectomy may be necessary if all other treatments to relieve priapism fail[51,63] (see "General Surgical Procedures," p. 829). Hemorrhage during or after phallectomy may be no worse than that expected during and after amputation of the penis of a horse not affected by priapism.

Intersex

Clinical Features

Anomalous development of the external genitalia of intersexes confuses their sexual identification. The most common intersex, the male pseudohermaphrodite, usually has a rudimentary penis, which resembles an enlarged clitoris, and prepuce, which resembles a vulva, situated on the midline somewhere between the ischial arch and the normal, ventral abdominal location of the preputial orifice (see Fig. 65-10).[43,64-66] Its testes are usually located within the abdomen or inguinal canals or hidden subcutaneously beneath a moderately developed udder (see Chapter 65). Despite its deceptive feminine appearance, the intact male pseudohermaphrodite displays masculine behavior and is even capable of achieving an erection of the rudimentary penis.

Treatment

If the genitalia are located close to the ischium, the pseudohermaphrodite's appearance can be altered to more closely resemble that of a female by amputating the rudimentary penis and constructing a vulva using the prepuce.[43] Alternatively, if the genitalia are less than 15 cm caudal to the inguinal area, the male pseudohermaphrodite's appearance can be altered to more closely resemble that of a male by cranially rotating the genitalia to a more normal position caudal to the umbilicus.[64] The horse should be castrated 4 to 6 weeks before surgery.

Neoplasia

Incidence and Etiology

The incidence of neoplasia of the external genitalia is second only to that of the skin.[67] Neoplasms of the penis and prepuce include squamous papillomas, squamous cell carcinomas, sarcoids, melanomas, mastocytomas, and hemangiomas.[68-71] Melanomas are occasionally found on the prepuce of old gray horses,[23] and squamous papillomas, the benign counterparts of squamous cell carcinoma, are often found on the external genitalia of young horses[72] or adjacent to penile or preputial carcinomas of old horses.[73] Squamous cell carcinoma is by far the most common penile and preputial neoplasm.[68,73] Genital squamous cell carcinoma may arise de novo or from malignant transformation of a squamous papilloma.[72,73] Any papillomatous lesion present on the penis or prepuce of a horse should be considered to be premalignant.

Squamous cell carcinoma is usually found on old horses, especially those of breeds with nonpigmented genitalia, such as Appaloosas and American Paint horses.[36,69,74] Lack of preputial or penile pigmentation seems to predispose to carcinoma, even though the external genitalia are not exposed to direct sunlight.[75] One study performed on mice showed that squamous cell carcinoma may be caused by unidentified carcinogenic agents in smegma,[76] but another study, also performed on mice, which used human smegma, was not able to substantiate this finding.[77] Regardless of whether smegma contains a carcinogenic agent, it may stimulate neoplastic changes in penile and preputial integument by causing chronic irritation. Geldings and old horses, therefore, may be predisposed to development of genital squamous cell carcinoma, because they produce a greater amount of smegma than do young horses and stallions.[75,76]

Squamous cell carcinoma occurs most commonly on the glans and internal lamina of the prepuce.[73,74] Penile and preputial squamous cell carcinomas are locally invasive but have a low grade of malignancy and grow surprisingly slowly for carcinomas.[69,73,74] Metastasis to the superficial and deep inguinal lymph nodes occurs late in the disease. In one study, 12% of 48 horses affected with penile or preputial squamous cell carcinoma had metastatic involvement of the inguinal lymph nodes.[73]

Diagnosis

Most affected horses are presented for examination when the owner observes the lesion, but some may be presented because of a malodorous, purulent, blood-stained, preputial discharge.[73,74] The duration of disease is usually unknown but lengthy, because most owners inspect their horse's penis infrequently.[74] Precancerous lesions may appear as a small, heavily keratinized plaque, and cancerous lesions may first appear as a shallow, flat ulceration with an indurated base.[69,74,78] Longstanding carcinomas may attain a cauliflower-like excrescence, containing areas of necrosis, ulceration, and hemorrhage, that can interfere with coitus or normal protrusion and retraction of the penis[79] (Fig. 66-12). The

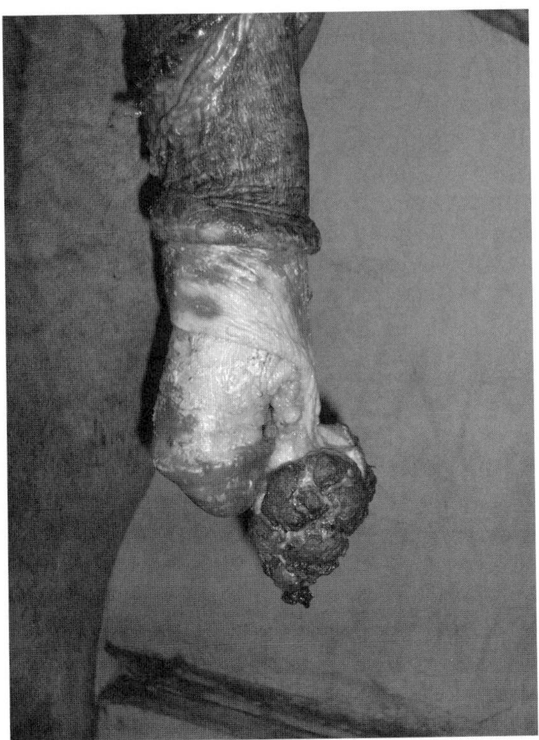

Figure 66-12. Squamous cell carcinoma of the inner lamina of the preputial fold.

tumor can cause dysuria by impinging on the urethra. Most affected horses are also affected by balanoposthitis.[71,74]

Metastatic spread of penile and preputial squamous cell carcinoma can sometimes be palpated as an enlargement of the inguinal lymph nodes, but mild, metastatic enlargement of the inguinal lymph nodes may be difficult to differentiate from lymphadenopathy secondary to balanoposthitis.[73] Penile or preputial squamous cell carcinoma can metastasize to internal organs without causing gross enlargement of the inguinal lymph nodes.[80]

Treatment

A variety of treatments for horses affected with squamous cell carcinoma of the penis or prepuce have been described, including surgical excision, cryosurgery, chemotherapy, and hypothermia.

SURGICAL EXCISION

A small lesion on the prepuce can be excised and the wound sutured. Using a carbon dioxide laser to locally excise squamous cell carcinoma from the external genitalia may decrease the incidence of recurrence of the neoplasm.[81] Using a laser to excise a neoplasm not only decreases postoperative swelling by sealing lymphatic vessels but also has a thermal, killing effect on marginal tumor cells.[82] Horses with extensive neoplastic lesions of the external genitalia require preputial reefing or phallectomy (see "General Surgical Procedures," p. 827). Occasionally, neoplasms become so extensive that prescrotal urethrostomy combined with en bloc resection of the penis, prepuce, and inguinal lymph nodes becomes necessary.[83]

CRYOTHERAPY

Cryotherapy is a useful treatment of horses with early lesions of squamous cell carcinoma. Cryotherapy can be performed using liquid nitrogen administered as a spray or through a cryoprobe, or using CO_2 administered through a cryoprobe. Thermocouple needles and a pyrometer (i.e., tissue temperature indicator) are used to monitor the depth and degree of freezing. A double, fast-freeze–slow-thaw cycle gives the best results.[84] More information on cryosurgery is found in Chapter 15.

CHEMOTHERAPY

Horses with small genital lesions of squamous cell carcinoma have been treated successfully by applying 5% 5-fluorouracil to the lesions at 14-day intervals.[85] Lesions need not be debulked, provided that the lesion is raised no more than to 2 to 3 mm above the surrounding integument. Up to seven treatments may be required to effect resolution of lesions. The drug is also effective in causing regression of preneoplastic lesions to which it is applied.

Horses with squamous carcinoma of the external genitalia have been treated by intratumoral injection of cisplatin in sesame oil.[86,87] The drug is administered at a dosage of 1 mg/cm^3 tissue every 2 weeks, usually until the tumor has been injected four times. Intratumoral chemotherapy with cisplatin can be used alone for treatment of horses with small tumors or in combination with surgery for treatment of horses with large tumors. Tumor cells still present after the tumor has been excised or debulked are stimulated into active proliferation and hence are more susceptible to cisplatin. Administration of cisplatin treatments intra-operatively and at 2-week intervals appears to result in a better outcome, at least for horses with tumors that have a high proliferation index, than does delaying chemotherapy until the wound has healed.[87] Injecting the tumor bed and a margin of normal tissue with cisplatin at the time of surgery and during all phases of wound healing does not have clinically apparent detrimental effects on healing of wounds closed primarily or wounds left open to heal by secondary intention.[86,87] (For more information on skin tumor treatments, and chemotherapy in general, see Chapter 29.) Topical or intratumoral chemotherapy is impractical for treatment of horses affected with squamous cell carcinoma that has metastasized to internal organs. Horses affected with metastatic squamous cell carcinoma can be treated with a systemically administered chemotherapeutic agent, such as doxorubicin or piroxicam,[88] but little information is available on the efficacy of systemically administered chemotherapy to treat horses for neoplasia.

HYPOTHERMIA

Radiofrequency-induced hyperthermia has been used to treat horses with sarcoids and cattle and horses suffering from ocular neoplasia.[89,90] Although its use to treat horses with genital neoplasia has not been reported, radiofrequency-induced hyperthermia could be useful for treatment of horses with genital neoplasia. Intratumoral hyperthermia is induced by a radiofrequency current of 2 MHz. Using this treatment, the tumor is heated to approximately 50° C for 30 seconds. Large tumors are heated in sections. Multiple treatments are required, but the length of the interval between treatments is determined subjectively.

Prognosis

In one study of 48 male horses with genital carcinoma, 64.5% of horses were alive 18 months after surgical therapy.[73] In another study, about 81% of 45 affected horses survived at least 1 year after surgical therapy with no evidence of recurrence of the disease.[74] Both studies found that prognosis for survival was poor if squamous cell carcinoma had metastasized to the inguinal lymph nodes.[73]

Invasion of the cavernous tissue by squamous cell carcinoma is a pejorative prognostic factor for survival in men[91] and is likely to be so in horses as well, because neoplastic invasion into a corporeal body may be more likely to result in hematogenous spread of the neoplasm. In one study, three of four horses that had metastases of penile carcinoma to the abdomen had gross or histologic evidence that the neoplasm had invaded the cavernous tissue.[74] Horses that have corporeal invasion by a carcinoma seem to have a high likelihood of abdominal metastases, and therefore, laparoscopic examination of the abdomen of a horse that has neoplastic invasion of a corporeal body may be prudent. Because lesions of squamous cell carcinoma sometimes recur, horses should be monitored periodically for recurrence of disease after apparently successful treatment.

Habronemiasis

Etiology

Cutaneous habronemiasis, also known as "summer sore" or granular dermatitis, is a granulomatous, mildly pruritic disease caused by cutaneous migration and encystment of the larvae of the equine stomach worm *Habronema*.[78,92] Larvae passed in the feces are ingested by fly maggots, and after the maggot pupates, the larvae are deposited on wounds from the feeding fly. The disease appears in spring and summer, when flies are prevalent, and usually disappears with onset of cold weather. The penis and prepuce are common sites of infestation by these larvae because moisture on these structures attracts flies. Horses that tend to extend their penis while resting and horses that receive anthelmintic drugs infrequently may be more prone to developing genital habronemiasis.[92]

Pathophysiology

Infestation stimulates an acute granulomatous reaction characterized by exuberant granulation tissue that contains numerous small, yellow, hard, caseous granules composed of eosinophils, nuclear remnants, and larvae. The larvae may excrete a substance lytic to the host's tissue,[78] but a local hypersensitivity reaction to the larvae resulting from repeated reinfestation is probably responsible for the extreme granulomatous response.[92] The presence of mature *Habronema* in the stomach may induce a state of general hypersensitivity, because horses affected by cutaneous habronemiasis are almost always heavily parasitized by adult worms. Some horses appear to be more susceptible and are plagued by yearly recurrence of lesions.

Clinical Signs

The preputial ring and urethral process are the genital sites of predilection. Preputial lesions may appear as ulcerated, red areas demarcated by edges of depigmentation.[78] Lesions may be granulomatous and extensive (Fig. 66-13). The infested urethral process may be enlarged from periurethral fibrosis, and hyperemic prolapsed mucous membrane may protrude from the urethral orifice.[93] Preputial lesions may mechanically impede the telescoping action of the preputial laminae, and lesions of the urethral process may cause partial obstruction to the flow of urine.[93] A horse with a distorted urethral process may spray itself or show signs of discomfort during urination. Erosions into the CSP may result in hemorrhage at the end of urination or ejaculation.[94] Horses with a genital lesion of cutaneous habronemiasis may have lesions of cutaneous habronemiasis elsewhere on the body.

Diagnosis

Cutaneous habronemiasis of the external genitalia is usually diagnosed by its typical appearance, but lesions can be confused with squamous cell carcinoma, exuberant granulation tissue, or phycomycosis.[92] A nonhealing, granulating wound accompanied by marked circulating eosinophilia is suggestive of the disease. Squeezing the lesion may cause granules to extrude, and occasionally a larva may be found if exudate is squeezed onto a slide and examined microscopically. Eosinophils, multinucleated giant cells, granules, and, sometimes, cross-sections of larvae can be seen by examining affected tissue histologically.[93,95]

Treatment

NONSURGICAL TREATMENT

Lesions are resolved by eliminating the larvae or by reducing the horse's hypersensitivity to them.[92] Ivermectin, administered orally at 200 µg/kg, or organophosphates administered topically, orally, or intravenously have been effective in destroying the larvae.[96] Prednisolone, administered orally at 1.5 mg/kg once a day for 10 to 14 days, or diethylcarbamazine, administered orally at 1.5 mg/kg twice a day for

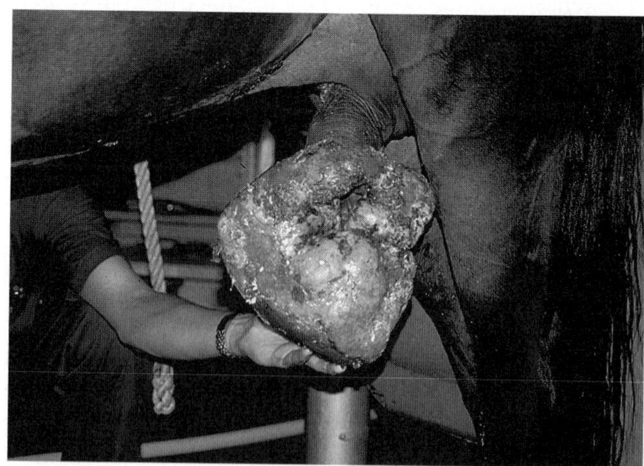

Figure 66-13. Massive granuloma on the internal preputial lamina caused by cutaneous habronemiasis. This mass was removed by segmental posthetomy.

7 to 14 days, has brought about resolution of lesions by diminishing the body's response to the larvae. Daily topical application of a cream containing an organophosphate, such as trichlorfon, and a corticosteroid, such as dexamethasone, may bring about resolution of small granulomatous lesions caused by cutaneous habronemiasis.

SURGICAL TREATMENT

Elliptical or circumferential resection of fibrotic areas of the internal lamina of the prepuce caused by chronic infestation may be required to restore normal preputial function, and amputation of an affected urethral process may be required to restore normal urination or to prevent hemospermia.[93]

Hemospermia

Etiology

Hemospermia, or blood in the ejaculate, is an important cause of infertility of stallions and has been attributed to bacterial urethritis occurring usually at the area of the ejaculatory ducts; habronemiasis or neoplasia of the urethral process; improperly fitted stallion rings; seminal vesiculitis; and trauma to the urethral process or glans penis.[25,97,98] Viral urethritis has been suspected, but not proven, to cause hemospermia.[99] Hemospermia has been reported to occur from urethral rents, the etiology of which is unknown.[100] The source of voluminous hemorrhage in the ejaculate is usually the CSP. Hemorrhage from the CSP typically occurs at the end of ejaculation when contraction of the bulbospongiosus muscle causes pressure within the CSP to increase from 17 to nearly 1000 mm Hg.[11]

Red blood cells in the ejaculate are associated with reduced fertility, even though seminal quality appears otherwise unaffected, because red blood cells are spermicidal.[98] The condition may be more common in Quarter Horses,[101] and frequently bred stallions are more often affected.[98]

Diagnosis

Stallions affected by hemospermia may require several mounts to ejaculate and sometimes exhibit pain during erection or ejaculation.[101] Blood in the semen is most easily identified by collecting the stallion's ejaculate with an artificial vagina. Semen of affected horses is usually pink to red, but because blood in amounts too minute to be detected grossly can cause infertility, microscopic examination of the semen may be necessary to detect the condition.[22] Microscopic examination of semen may also reveal a large number of white blood cells if septic seminal vesiculitis is the cause of hemospermia.

Septic seminal vesiculitis, an occasional cause of hemospermia, may be detected by identifying numerous clumps of purulent material in the semen and by finding blood in the gel fraction of the ejaculate.[102] A thickened vesicle filled with echogenic fluid may be seen during transrectal ultrasonographic examination of a septic seminal vesicle. The causative organism of septic, seminal vesiculitis can be cultured from fluid obtained directly from the infected seminal vesicle.

Rents in the urethra, a common cause of hemospermia, can be detected by examining the urethra with a sterilized, flexible endoscope that is at least 100 cm long. A urethral tear into the CSP appears endoscopically as a 5- to 10-mm-long, linear defect on the convex surface of the urethra, distal to the openings of the bulbourethral glands, near the level of the ischial arch.[100] The shaft of a hypodermic needle can be introduced percutaneously into the lumen of the urethra at the level of the ischial arch during endoscopic examination to confirm the location of the defect (Fig. 66-14). By endoscopically examining the urethra of a horse affected with hemospermia immediately after ejaculation, the examiner may be able to observe blood emanating from an otherwise undetectable rent.[22]

Urethrography to diagnose urethral lesions has been described.[98,99] The penis is radiographed after injecting 180 mL of barium suspension into the urethra. The barium is allowed to drain, 180 mL of air is injected to provide double contrast, and the penis is again radiographed. Bacterial and viral cultures and biopsy and histologic examination of urethral lesions may establish the cause of urethritis.

Treatment

NONSURGICAL TREATMENT

Sexual abstinence seems to be important in the treatment of stallions affected with hemospermia, regardless of the origin, because erection and contractions of the bulbospongiosus muscle during ejaculation dilate and further traumatize the urethra.[98,101] Medical treatment of affected horses has included intravenous administration of formaldehyde solution, oral administration of methenamine, and systemic administration of antimicrobial drugs.[99]

Horses affected with hemospermia caused by septic seminal vesiculitis should receive antimicrobial therapy that is effective against the causative organism. Systemic

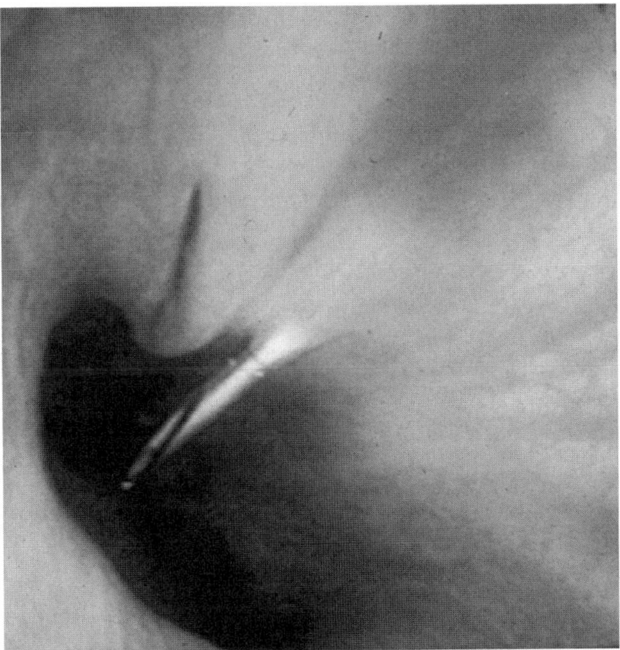

Figure 66-14. Endoscopic view of a urethral rent. The shaft of a hypodermic needle has been inserted percutaneously into the lumen of the urethra at the level of the ischium to pinpoint the location of the defect.

administration of antimicrobial drugs to stallions affected with septic seminal vesiculitis is often ineffective because antimicrobial drugs diffuse poorly into the gland. Infusing the appropriate antimicrobial drug directly into the seminal vesicles after the vesicles have been lavaged may be a more effective treatment.[102] Horses with low-grade hemospermia can sometimes be managed by adding an extender to the semen to dilute the effect of the red blood cells on the spermatozoa.[97,103]

SURGICAL TREATMENT

Temporary perineal urethrostomy combined with sexual rest has been effective in eliminating hemospermia caused by a urethral lesion.[99-101] Eleven of 15 affected horses were successfully treated by temporary subischial urethrostomy and daily installation of suppositories of nitrofurazone and hydrocortisone into the urethra, although two stallions developed a urethral fistula.[101] These investigators offered no sound rationale for the relatively high incidence of success of temporary urethrostomy, but other investigators implied that topical application of antimicrobial drugs to lesions of bacterial urethritis is responsible for resolution of hemospermia.[98] More likely, success of temporary subischial urethrostomy in eliminating hemospermia should be attributed to decreased pressure in the CSP and diversion of blood flow from the urethral lesion. When the bladder has been emptied, the bulbospongiosus muscle contracts to expel urine that remains in the urethra. Incising the CSP at the ischium decreases cavernosal pressure at the end of urination and diverts blood flow from the urethral lesion to the temporary urethrostomy, thus permitting healing of the urethral mucosa and underlying tunica albuginea of the CSP. Simply incising the convex surface of the tunica albuginea of the CSP at the ischium, without exposing the lumen of the urethra, may be as effective as temporary urethrostomy for eliminating hemospermia, and the risk of the stallion's developing a urethral fistula is eliminated. This theory, however, has not been clinically evaluated.

Hematuria

Etiology

Hematuria can originate from the kidney, ureter, bladder, urethra, or reproductive organs.[94,97] Causes of hematuria include renal, ureteral, vesicular, or urethral calculi; renal, and vesicular neoplasia; and pyelonephritis. Terminal hematuria (i.e., hematuria that occurs at the end of urination) is associated with a lesion located at the proximal portion of the urethra and the trigone of the bladder. Hematuria associated with a rent of unknown cause at the proximal portion of the urethra has been observed in geldings.[100] The urethral rent appears to be identical to that often seen in stallions with hemospermia (see "Hemospermia," earlier).

The cause of urethral rents is idiopathic, but the reason why the rent occurs invariably at the level of the ischial arch may be explained by the anatomy of the urethra. The diameter of the urethral lumen is approximately 1 to 1.5 cm at the origin of the urethra.[3] The lumen dilates to 3.5 to 5 cm in the pelvic portion of the urethra (i.e., at the pars pelvina) and decreases dramatically in diameter to 1 to 1.5 cm where the urethra bends sharply as it crosses the ischial arch. The sharp turn and the narrowing of the urethral lumen in the area of the ischial arch may expose the convex surface of the urethra at the level of the ischial arch to hydrodynamic forces not encountered by other portions of the urethra.

Pathophysiology

Because urethral rents communicate with the CSP, hemorrhage through the rent into the urethral lumen was thought to occur when pressure within this cavernosal space increases at the end of urination when the bulbospongiosus muscle contracts to expel the last vestige of urine.[100] Recent research, however, showed that the rise in pressure within the CSP associated with contraction of the bulbospongiosus muscle is slight. Investigators theorized that the most likely explanation for hemorrhage at the end of micturition in horses with a urethral rent is that the intraluminal urethral pressure suddenly decreases at the end of urination while the pressure in the CSP remains high.[104]

Even though the lesion in stallions is identical in appearance to that responsible for hematuria of geldings, the lesion in stallions rarely causes macroscopic hematuria.[94,100] The reason for the difference in clinical signs between stallions and geldings is probably that during urination, pressure within the CSP of geldings is nearly double that of stallions.[104] The CSP of geldings is not as well developed as that of stallions, and the difference in volume of the cavernosal space between geldings and stallions results in different pressures in the CSP at the end of urination.

Diagnosis

Blood in urine that results from a urethral rent is characteristically discharged at the end of urination (i.e., terminal hematuria).[100] Occasionally, a horse with a urethral rent may show signs of dysuria, such as tenesmus at the end of urination. Endoscopic examination of the urethra reveals a 5- to 10-mm linear urethral defect on the convex surface of the urethra, distal to the openings of the bulbourethral glands, near the level of the ischial arch. Gross evidence of inflammation around the defect is not observed.

Treatment

Some urethral rents heal spontaneously,[105] but horses with hematuria caused by a urethral rent can be treated successfully by temporary perineal urethrostomy (see "Temporary Perineal Urethrostomy," p. 833, for a description of the surgical technique).[94,100,101] Surgery eliminates hematuria, presumably by reducing vascular pressure in the CSP, which prevents escape of blood through a rent at the end of urination, thereby allowing the rent to heal. A perineal incision that extends into the CSP but does not penetrate the urethra seems to be as effective as temporary urethrostomy in eliminating hematuria and may reduce the risk of complications associated with temporary urethrostomy, such as development of a urethral fistula[101] or stricture.[106] Although horses may bleed substantially from the perineal wound, especially at the end of urination, macroscopic hemorrhage from the urethral orifice and evidence of pain during urination are not observed after surgery.

GENERAL SURGICAL PROCEDURES

Segmental Posthetomy

Indications

Segmental posthetomy, or resection of a circumferential segment of the internal preputial lamina, is indicated for removal of preputial neoplasms, granulomas, or scars so extensive that simple excision of the lesion is impossible. Other terms for the procedure include posthioplasty, circumcision, and reefing.[107] Provided that the preputial lesions do not involve the underlying tunica albuginea, penile amputation can be avoided by segmental posthetomy. With removal of most of the internal lamina of the prepuce, a paralyzed penis can be maintained permanently within the preputial cavity.

Surgical Technique

Segmental posthetomy can be performed with the horse standing after anesthetizing the pudendal nerves (see "Diagnostic Procedures," earlier), but the procedure is most easily and safely accomplished with the horse anesthetized and positioned in dorsal or lateral recumbency. The urethra is catheterized, and the penis is extended by traction on gauze looped around the collum glandis. A tourniquet placed proximal to the surgical site may facilitate surgery. Parallel circumferential incisions through the preputial epithelium are created distal and proximal to the lesion, and these incisions are connected by a longitudinal incision (Fig. 66-15). Care must be taken to avoid severing the large, longitudinal, subcutaneous branches of the external pudendal arteries and veins that lie superficial to the tunica albuginea.

In cases where segmental posthetomy is performed to maintain a paralyzed penis within the external lamina of the prepuce, the distal circumferential incision should be made through the penile epithelium at the level where the internal preputial lamina inserts on the free body of the penis. The proximal circumferential incision should be made close to the preputial orifice.[108]

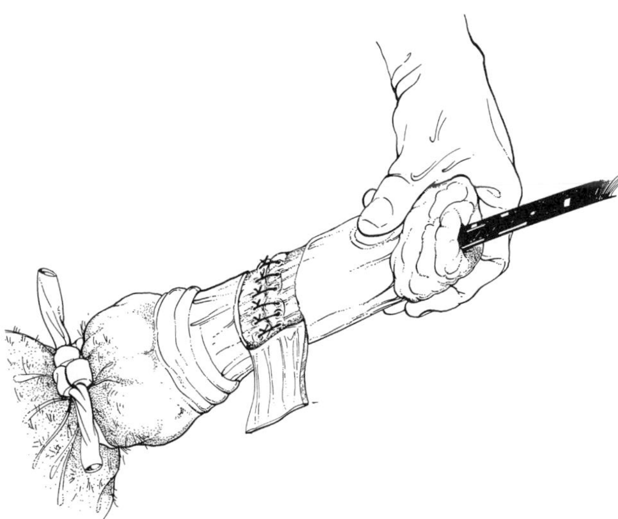

Figure 66-15. Segmental posthetomy. A cuff of epithelium is removed from the shaft of the penis.

The cuff of integument between the incisions is dissected from the penis with scissors, taking care to avoid the large vessels. Normal alignment of tissue is maintained by placing four sutures at equidistant points around the circumference of the penis before the cuff of tissue is removed. The tourniquet is released, and all bleeding vessels are identified and ligated with absorbable sutures or cauterized. Loose adventitia is apposed with interrupted 2-0 absorbable sutures. The epithelium is apposed with interrupted no. 0 or 2-0 absorbable or nonabsorbable sutures.

Aftercare

Stallions should wear a stallion ring for at least 2 weeks and must be isolated from mares for 2 to 4 weeks.[109] Regular exercise reduces postoperative edema. Nonabsorbable sutures should be removed 10 to 12 days postoperatively.

Bolz Technique of Phallopexy

Indication

The Bolz procedure is a technique used to permanently retract a paralyzed penis into the preputial cavity and is performed to avoid phallectomy.[40] This method of permanent retraction cannot be used if the penis or internal lamina of the prepuce is badly damaged or if the horse is still capable of attaining an erection. Damaged sections of prepuce, however, can be removed by segmental posthetomy during the same procedure.

Surgical Technique

The horse is anesthetized and positioned in dorsal recumbency. The urethra should be catheterized for easy identification. A 10-cm longitudinal incision is made on the perineal raphe just caudal to the scrotum (Fig. 66-16, *A*), and the penis is bluntly separated from surrounding fascia, taking care to avoid damaging the surrounding large pudendal vessels (see Fig. 66-16, *B*). The penis is retracted until the annular ring of the reflection of the internal preputial lamina onto the free body of the penis is visible at the cranial extent of the incision (see Fig. 64-16, *C*). The penis is anchored in this position with two heavy, nonabsorbable percutaneous sutures through the annular ring on each side of the penis.

The anchoring sutures should penetrate the skin 2 to 4 cm from the incision at about the level of the middle of the incision. The sutures are inserted through the annular ring on the lateral surface of the penis, taking care to avoid entering the preputial cavity, the urethra, or cavernous tissue. An assistant should palpate the fornix of the preputial cavity during placement of the sutures through the annular ring to ensure that the sutures do not penetrate the preputial epithelium. The sutures exit the skin 2 to 3 cm from their entry points. They are tightened until the glans penis is flush with the preputial orifice and tied over rolls of gauze or large buttons to prevent the suture from cutting through the skin (see Fig. 66-16, *D*). The subcutaneous tissue and skin are each closed separately.

The percutaneous anchoring sutures are removed after 10 to 12 days; at this time, adhesions of sufficient strength to maintain the penis in its retracted position have formed.

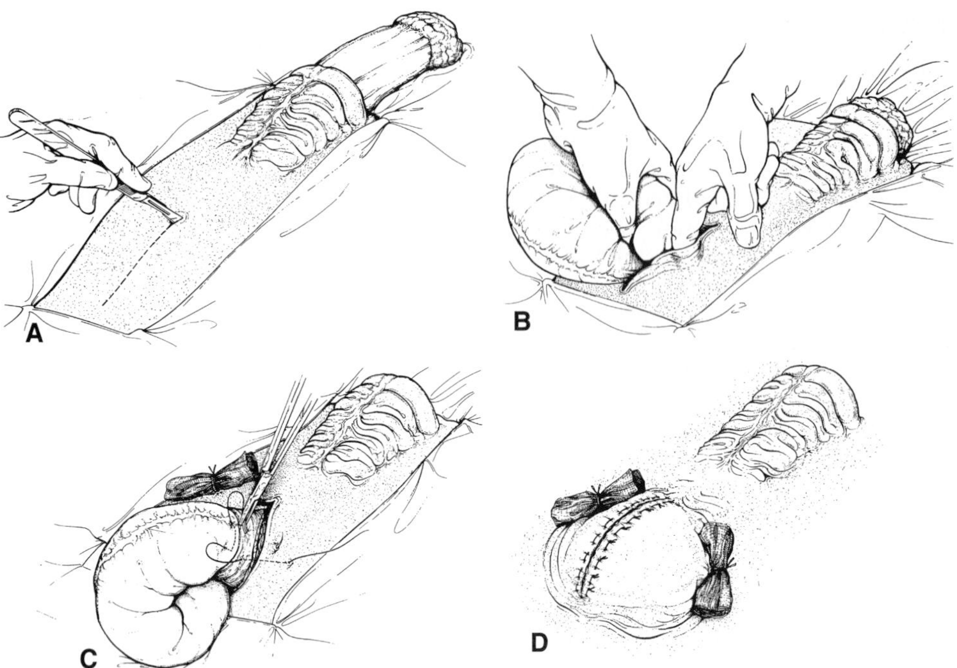

Figure 66-16. **A,** Bolz technique of phallopexy. A 10-cm incision is made on the perineal raphe just caudal to the scrotum. **B,** The penis is bluntly separated from surrounding fascia, taking care to avoid damaging the surrounding large pudendal vessels. **C,** The penis is retracted until the annular ring of the reflection of the internal preputial lamina onto the free body of the penis is visible at the cranial extent of the incision. The penis is fixed in this position with two heavy nonabsorbable percutaneous sutures through the annular ring on each side of the penis. **D,** The sutures are tightened until the glans penis is flush with the preputial orifice and tied over rolls of gauze or large buttons to prevent the suture from cutting through the skin. The subcutaneous tissue and skin are closed separately.

Necrosis of skin beneath the rolls of gauze is inevitable, but the technique allows adjustment of tension on the percutaneous sutures and repositioning of the penis. Precise positioning of the penis in the prepuce is important because, if the penis is inadequately retracted, the glans penis may protrude excessively through the preputial orifice, or if the penis is excessively retracted, the horse may develop urine scald from urinating in the preputial cavity. Two heavy absorbable sutures, substituted for the nonabsorbable percutaneous sutures, can be used to anchor the annular ring to the subcutaneous fascia.[110] Necrosis of skin is avoided, but the sutures cannot be adjusted after surgery.

Aftercare

The horse should be walked daily to minimize swelling, and heavy exercise can be resumed 2 to 3 weeks after skin sutures have been removed. Retraction distorts the penis into a sigmoid curvature with acute bends, but penile blood supply and urination remain unaffected. The horse can be castrated during the same procedure, using either an inguinal or a scrotal approach. The incision should be sutured because an open inguinal or scrotal wound may interfere with healing around the anchoring sutures. If the horse is castrated before the procedure and the scrotal wound is left unsutured to heal by secondary intention, the surgeon is confronted with the tedious task of caring for the protruded penis for several weeks while the scrotal incision heals.

Amputation of the Urethral Process

Indications

The urethral process is most commonly excised to remove a granuloma caused by cutaneous habronemiasis, when the affected horse fails to respond to medical therapy.[93] The urethral process is sometimes excised to remove a neoplastic lesion.[97]

Patient Preparation

The urethral process can be amputated with the horse standing and sedated after infiltrating the base of the urethral process with a local anesthetic agent, but the procedure is most easily and safely accomplished with the horse anesthetized and in dorsal recumbency.[93] The penis is prepared for aseptic surgery, and a urinary catheter is passed into the urethra. After placing traction on the urethral process with one or two Allis tissue forceps, two small-gauge needles (e.g., 23 or 25 gauge) are placed through the urethral process and the catheter at right angles to each other, proximal to the diseased portion of the urethral process (Fig. 66-17). These needles anchor the urethral process to

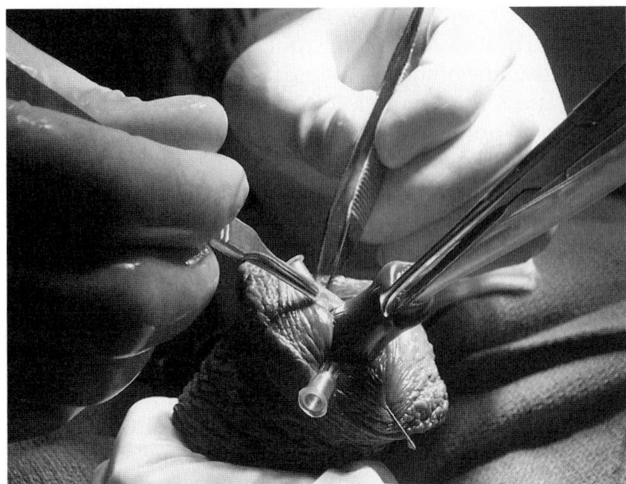

Figure 66-17. This urethral process was amputated to eliminate hemospermia caused by carcinoma of the urethral mucosa. The urethral process was stretched with tissue forceps, and two small-gauge needles were placed through the urethral process and the catheter at right angles to each other, proximal to the diseased portion of the urethral process, to anchor the urethral process to the catheter.

the catheter, making the incised margin of the process more stable and accessible for suturing.

Surgical Technique

A circumferential incision extending through the skin, CSP, and urethral mucosa is made around the base of the urethral process proximal to the affected tissue and distal to the anchoring hypodermic needles. The urethral mucosa is apposed to the epithelium of the remaining stump of the process with simple-interrupted or simple-continuous sutures of 4-0 or 5-0 absorbable suture.[97] The sutures should be closely spaced to compress the erectile tissue of the CSP. A simple-continuous suture pattern is probably more effective than a simple-interrupted suture pattern in compressing the erectile tissue of the CSP. The entire length of the process can be removed.

Aftercare

Stallions and recently castrated geldings should be isolated from mares for at least 3 weeks. Hemorrhage from the stump of the process, especially at the end of urination, should be expected for at least several days after amputation of the urethral process.

Phallectomy

Indications

Phallectomy is indicated when permanent penile paralysis is accompanied by irreparable penile damage, and more commonly, when neoplasia has invaded the tunica albuginea or is so extensive that more conservative treatment by cryosurgery, hyperthermia, local excision, or segmental posthetomy is impossible. For geldings, phallectomy may be the most expedient means of treating urethral stenosis distal to the preputial orifice. Phallectomy of stallions is generally performed to salvage the horse for purposes other than breeding, but amputation of just the glans penis may not interfere with copulation.[111]

Patient Preparation

A stallion should be castrated 3 to 4 weeks prior to phallectomy, if possible, to avoid postoperative erection, which leads to hemorrhage and dehiscence. The procedure can sometimes be performed with the horse standing and sedated after anesthetizing the pudendal nerves (see "Diagnostic Procedures," earlier),[28] but the procedure is most easily performed with the horse anesthetized and positioned in lateral or, preferably, dorsal recumbency. The urethra is catheterized with an equine male urinary catheter, and the penis is extended with gauze looped around the collum glandis. A tourniquet placed proximal to the proposed site of transection facilitates surgery.

Surgical Techniques

VINSOT'S TECHNIQUE OF PHALLECTOMY

One of the simplest techniques of phallectomy is Vinsot's procedure.[43,112] A triangular section of tissue that includes epithelium, fascia, bulbospongiosus muscle, and CSP is removed from the ventrum of the penis proximal to the proposed site of transection, taking care not to enter the urethral lumen (Fig. 66-18). The triangle has a 2.5-cm base and 4-cm sides. Its apex points distally and is located about 4 or 5 cm proximal to the proposed site of transection. The exposed urethra is incised on its midline from the base to the apex of the triangle, and the incised edges of the urethra and the triangle's epithelial border are apposed with simple-interrupted or simple-continuous absorbable sutures. The sutures should include the tunica albuginea of the CSP, and they should be closely spaced to compress the erectile tissue

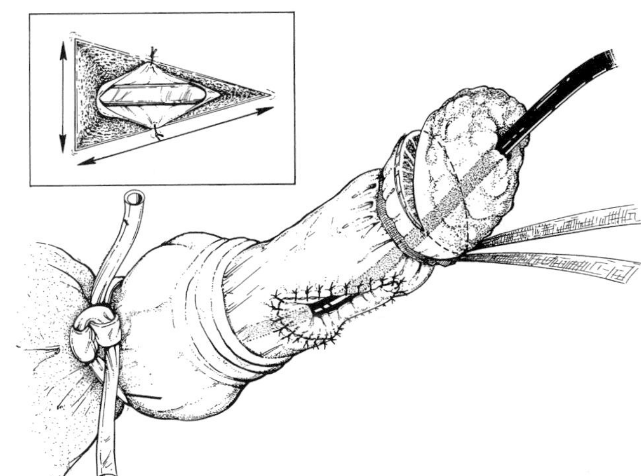

Figure 66-18. Vinsot's technique of phallectomy. A triangular section of tissue is removed from the ventrum of the penis proximal to the proposed site of transection, taking care not to enter the urethral lumen. The exposed urethra is incised on its midline from the base to the apex of the triangle, and the incised edges of the urethra and the triangle's epithelial border are apposed with simple-interrupted, absorbable sutures. A nonabsorbable ligature is placed around the penis distal to the apex of the triangle, and the penis is severed distal to the ligature.

of the CSP. A simple-continuous suture pattern is probably more effective than a simple-interrupted suture pattern in compressing the erectile tissue of the CSP. The diseased portion of the penis is removed 4 to 5 cm distal to the urethrostomy using a wedge-shaped incision. Large vessels on the dorsal and lateral aspects of the tunica albuginea are ligated with absorbable suture, and the corporeal bodies are compressed with absorbable sutures placed through the tunica albuginea in an everting or appositional pattern. The penile or preputial integument is sutured with absorbable or nonabsorbable sutures placed in an everting or appositional pattern.

Instead of suturing the end of the stump, the surgeon can leave it unsutured to heal by secondary intention. To prevent hemorrhage from the corporeal bodies, a tightly fixed, nonabsorbable ligature is placed around the penis 2 to 3 cm distal to the apex of the triangle, before the penis is transversely severed 1 to 2 cm distal to the ligature.

Rather than removing a triangle of tissue overlying the urethra, the technique can be simplified by making a 4- to 5-cm longitudinal incision into the urethral lumen.[113] The incised edges of the urethra and the integument are apposed with simple-interrupted or simple-continuous absorbable sutures. These sutures incorporate and compress the cavernous tissue of the CSP. Vinsot's technique, especially its modification,[113] can often be performed with the horse standing. A primary disadvantage of the technique, or its modification, is the tendency of the urethra to stricture.[43]

WILLIAMS' TECHNIQUE OF PHALLECTOMY

The likelihood of urethral stricture is decreased when the Williams' technique of phallectomy is employed.[111] With this technique, a triangle of tissue with similar dimensions to those described in Vinsot's technique is removed from the ventrum of the penis (Fig. 66-19, *A*). The triangle's apex is directed proximally, rather than distally, and the base of the triangle is the site of penile transection. The urethra is split on its midline from the base to the apex of the triangle, and the incised edge of the urethra and the triangle's epithelial edge are apposed with simple-interrupted or simple-continuous absorbable sutures. These sutures incorporate and compress the cavernous tissue of the CSP: A simple-continuous suture pattern is probably more effective than a simple-interrupted suture pattern in providing compression.

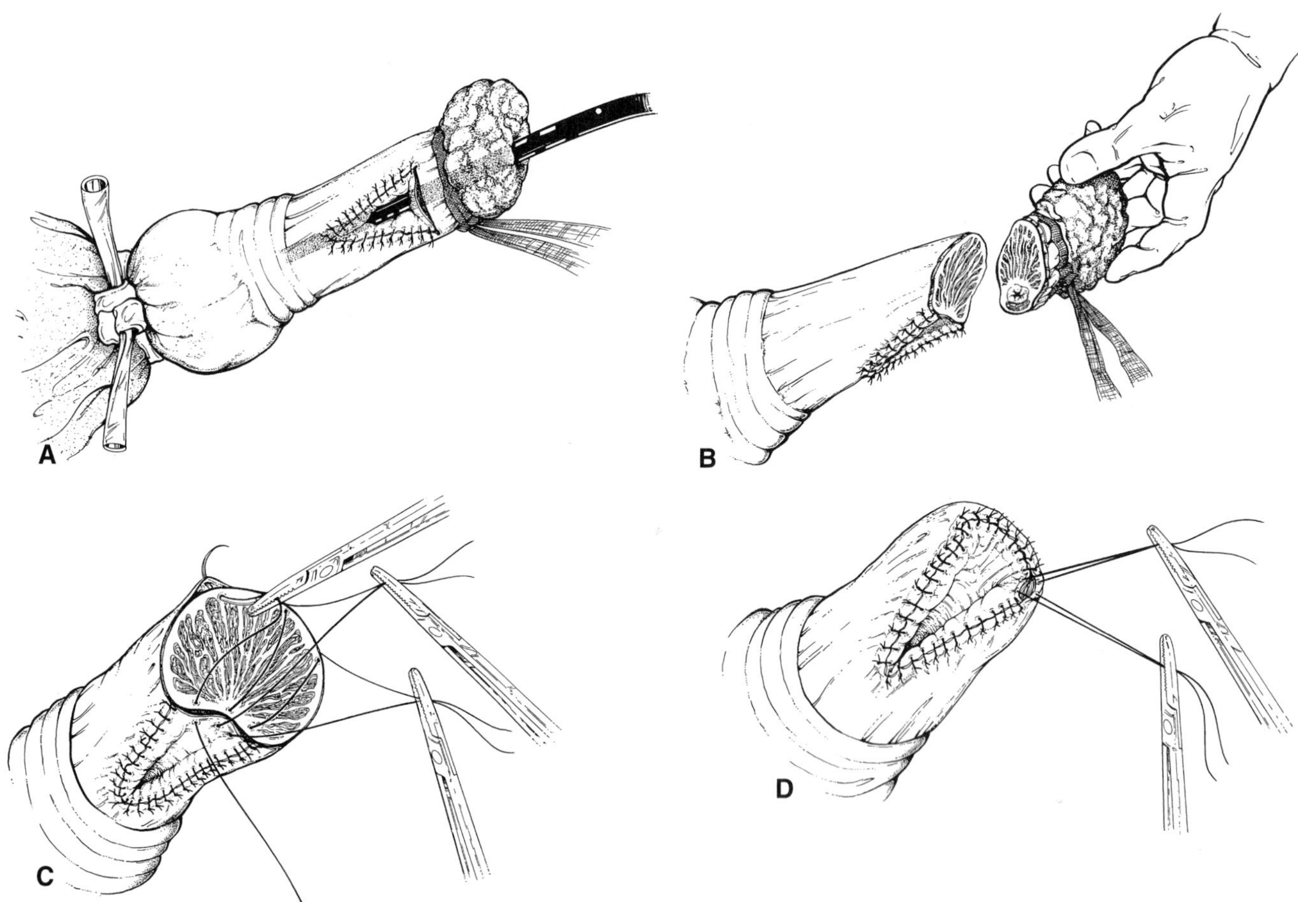

Figure 66-19. A, Williams technique of phallectomy. A triangle is removed from the ventrum of the penis. The triangle's apex is directed proximally. The urethra is split on its midline from the base to the apex of the triangle, and the edges of the urethra and the triangle's epithelial edges are apposed with simple-interrupted absorbable sutures. **B,** The base of the triangle is left unsutured. The urethral catheter is removed, and the penis is obliquely transected at the base of the triangular urethrostomy in a craniodorsal direction. **C,** The stump is closed with interrupted sutures that pass through the urethra, the tunica albuginea of the urethral groove, and the tunica albuginea of the dorsum of the corpus cavernosum penis (CCP) and the penile or preputial epithelium. The sutures should be pre-placed at equidistant intervals for an even closure. **D,** The sutures are tightened and tied, compressing the cavernous spaces, and the epithelium is apposed to the urethral mucosa.

The base of the triangle is left unsutured. The urethral catheter is removed, and the penis is obliquely transected at the base of the triangular urethrostomy in a craniodorsal direction, so that the dorsum of the penile stump is longer than the ventrum (see Fig. 66-19, *B*). Large branches of the external pudendal vessels that reside in loose fascia on the dorsal and lateral aspects of the tunica albuginea are ligated with absorbable suture.

The stump is closed with interrupted absorbable or nonabsorbable sutures that pass through the urethra, the tunica albuginea of the urethral groove, and the tunica albuginea of the dorsum of the CCP and the penile or preputial epithelium (see Fig. 66-19, *C*). The sutures should be pre-placed at equidistant intervals for an even closure. When these sutures are tightened and tied, the erectile bodies are compressed, and the epithelium is apposed to the urethral mucosa (see Fig. 66-19, *D*). Alternatively, the stump can be closed in two layers by first suturing the tunica albuginea of the dorsum of the CCP to the tunica albuginea of the urethral groove with interrupted absorbable sutures placed at bisecting intervals and by suturing the penile or preputial integument to the urethral mucosa with interrupted absorbable or nonabsorbable sutures.

SCOTT'S TECHNIQUE OF PHALLECTOMY

With this technique, a circumferential transverse incision through the epithelium of the body of the penis or prepuce is made at the intended site of transection, and branches of the external pudendal vessels are ligated.[79] Dissection is continued through the CCP to the urethral groove. The CSP is circumferentially incised to the urethra, which is easily identified by the urinary catheter in its lumen, and a 4- to 5-cm segment of urethra is dissected free from the amputated section of penis (Fig. 66-20, *A*).

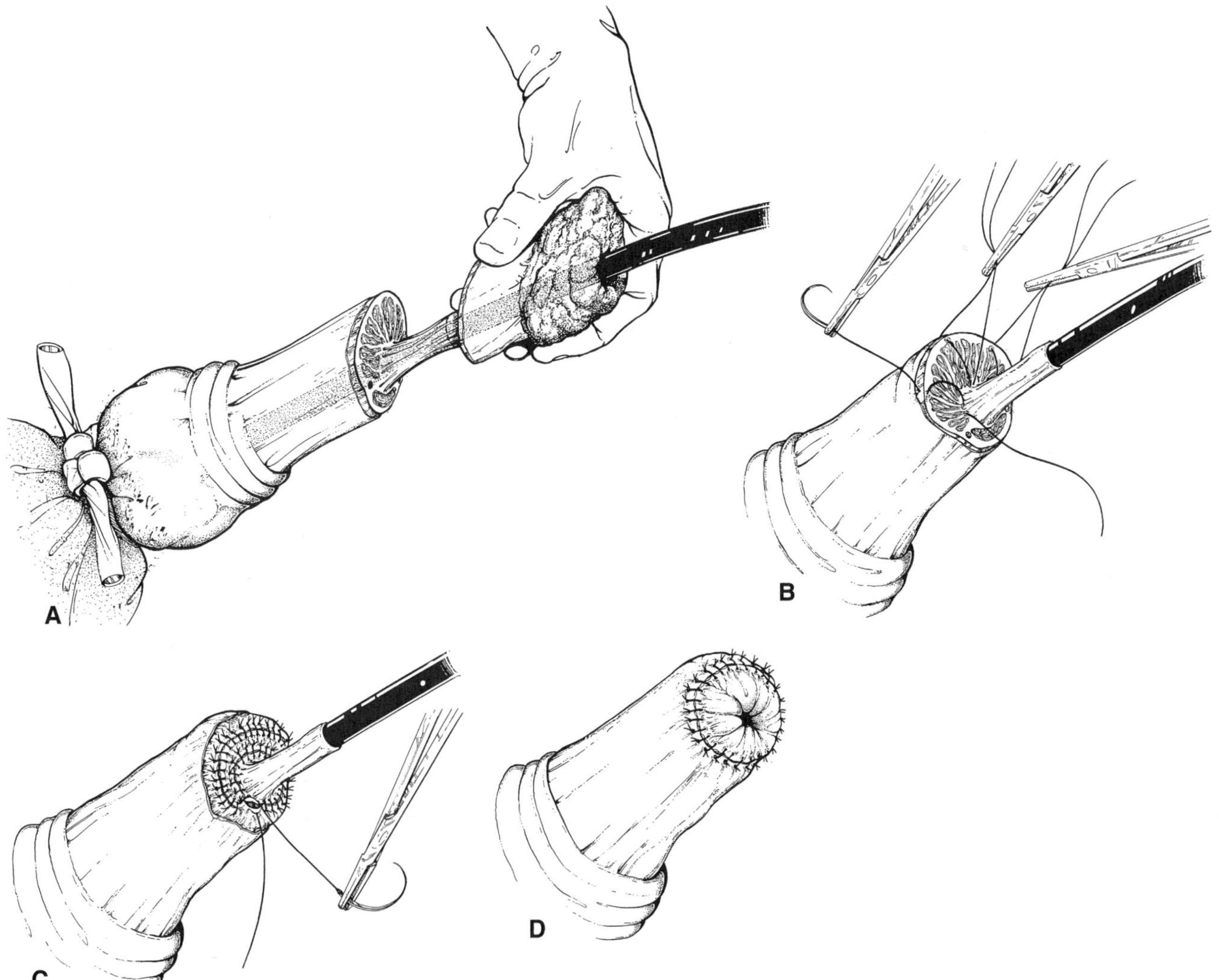

Figure 66-20. Scott's technique of phallectomy. **A,** A circumferential transverse incision through the epithelium of the body of the penis or prepuce is made at the intended site of transection. Dissection is continued through the corpus cavernosum penis (CCP) to the urethral groove. The corpus spongiosum penis (CSP) is circumferentially incised to the urethra, and a 4- to 5-cm segment of urethra is dissected free from the amputated section of penis. **B,** The stump of the CCP is closed by apposing the outer perimeter of its tunica albuginea to the tunica albuginea of the urethral groove with interrupted absorbable sutures pre-placed at equidistant intervals. **C,** The sinusoidal spaces of the CSP are closed by suturing the tunica albuginea surrounding the CSP to the submucosa of the urethra with interrupted absorbable sutures. **D,** The urethral stump is stretched and folded back over the end of the penis, where it is sutured to the penile or preputial epithelium and underlying tunica albuginea.

The stump of the CCP is closed by apposing the outer perimeter of its tunica albuginea to the tunica albuginea of the urethral groove with interrupted absorbable sutures pre-placed at equidistant intervals (see Fig. 66-20, *B*). The sinusoidal spaces of the CSP are closed by suturing the tunica albuginea surrounding the CSP to the submucosa of the urethra with interrupted absorbable sutures (see Fig. 66-20, *C*). The urethral stump is divided into three equal triangular segments, with the apex of each triangle pointing distally. These segments are intermeshed with similarly prepared segments of penile or preputial integument and are apposed with simple-interrupted absorbable or non-absorbable sutures. Sutures should include underlying tunica albuginea. Instead of dividing the urethral stump into three triangles, the urethral stump can be stretched and folded back over the end of the penis, where it is sutured to the penile or preputial epithelium and underlying tunica albuginea (see Fig. 66-20, *D*).

PHALLECTOMY BY EN BLOC RESECTION WITH PENILE RETROVERSION

Removal of the free portion of the penis, the internal lamina and external lamina of the prepuce, and regional lymph nodes may be indicated when these structures are extensively affected with neoplasia.[83] With this technique of phallectomy, a fusiform incision is created around the preputial orifice. The incision begins 6 cm cranial to the orifice and ends 10 cm caudal to it. The incision is carried to the deep fascia of the abdominal tunic, and if neoplasia has metastasized to the superficial lymph nodes, dissection is extended through this plane to both superficial inguinal rings, and the superficial inguinal lymph nodes are removed. The penis is amputated approximately 6 to 8 cm caudal to the fornix of the prepuce, and the amputated portion of the penis and the prepuce are removed en bloc. The penile shaft is amputated using a method similar to that described by Scott, so that 4 cm of urethra is left protruding from the penile stump[79] (Fig. 66-21, *A*). The technique can be modified by amputating the penis using Williams' or Vinsot's technique of phallectomy.[114]

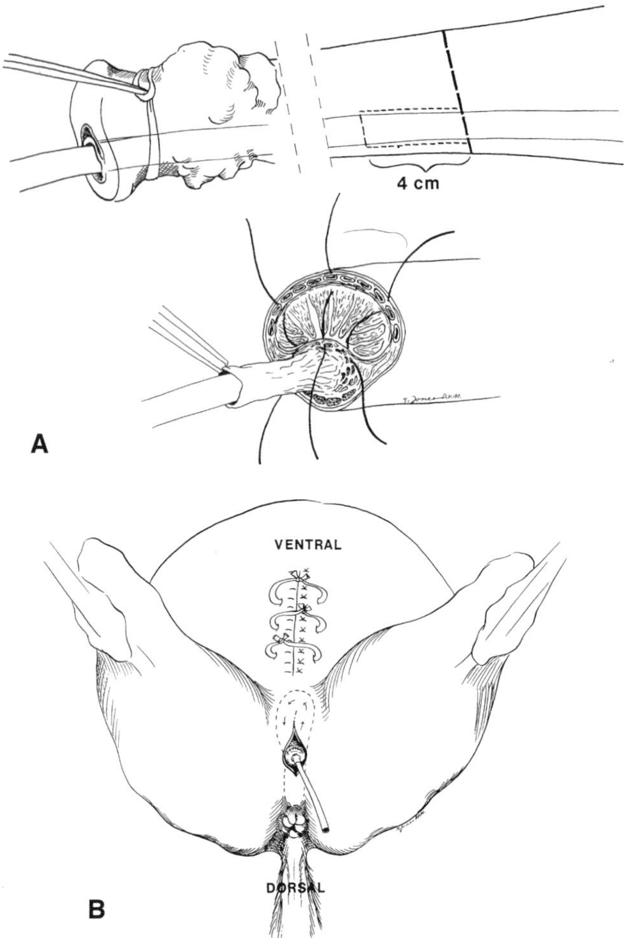

Figure 66-21. En bloc resection of the penis. **A,** Four centimeters of urethra is left beyond the penile stump. **B,** The position of the penile stump when retroverted is demonstrated. (From Markel MD, Wheat JD, Jones K: Genital neoplasms treated by en bloc resection and penile retroversion in horses: 10 cases 1977-1986. J Am Vet Med Assoc 1988;192:396.)

By bluntly separating penile fascia, the stump of the penis is retroverted through a 6-cm subischial incision created approximately 20 cm ventral to the anus, so that its distal end points caudally and extends just beyond the subischial incision (see Fig. 66-21, *B*). The tunica albuginea of the CCP and the fascia of the penis are sutured to the subcutaneous tissue of the subischial incision. The ventral aspect of the urethra is incised longitudinally over its 4-cm length, and the edges of the urethra are sutured to the surrounding edges of the incised subischial skin. Penrose drains are placed deeply at the cranial incision, and the subcutaneous tissue and skin are each closed separately.

PHALLECTOMY BY EN BLOC RESECTION WITHOUT PENILE RETROVERSION

This technique of phallectomy is similar in many respects to phallectomy by en bloc resection with penile retroversion, but with this technique, the stump of the penis is not retroverted but is maintained in its normal ventral position.[115] With this technique, a fusiform incision is created on the midline beginning at the umbilicus. The incision extends caudally on each side of the preputial orifice and continues on the midline to a point 10 cm caudal to the preputial orifice. The caudal portion of the incision is extended and deepened to expose and remove the inguinal lymph nodes, if neoplasia has metastasized to these structures.

Blunt dissection is continued into the loose areolar tissue of the prepuce, ligating large vessels as they are encountered. After the shaft of the penis is exposed, dissection is redirected along the shaft of the penis in a plane superficial to the loose subcutaneous tissue overlying the vasculature of the penis. At least 10 cm of the shaft should be exposed. A tourniquet is applied around the shaft of the penis proximal to the site of amputation. The dorsal arteries and veins of the penis are ligated and transfixed to the tunica albuginea. The penis is transected caudal to the fornix of the prepuce, using the method described by Williams.[111] After the tourniquet is removed, the stump is fixed to the body wall on the midline with heavy absorbable interrupted sutures. The subcutaneous tissue cranial to the penile stump surrounding the exposed penile shaft is apposed. Skin is sutured to the tunica albuginea and the urethral mucosa of the new urethral orifice. The skin cranial and caudal to the urethral orifice is sutured.

This technique of en bloc resection requires a smaller incision and results in less alteration to the appearance of the horse than does the retroversion technique, while still allowing the surgeon to remove extensive portions of the penis and extirpate the regional lymph nodes.[115]

Aftercare

Because the procedure is generally performed to salvage the horse for purposes other than breeding, stallions should be castrated several weeks in advance of phallectomy. Stallions and recently castrated geldings should be isolated from mares for 2 to 3 weeks and should wear a stallion ring on the penile stump during this time.

Complications

Hemorrhage from the penile stump, especially at the end of urination, should be expected for at least several days after phallectomy. Hemorrhage usually emanates from the CSP. Phallectomy of geldings is attended by less hemorrhage than phallectomy of stallions. Excessive hemorrhage may be accompanied by minor dehiscence, which is usually of no consequence. Dehiscence of sutured erectile tissue may lead to the formation of a large hematoma. Other complications of phallectomy in the immediate postoperative period include pain, infection of the surgical wound, edema of the prepuce, and acute urinary obstruction caused by edema of the urethra.[73,74,83,115] Long-term complications include cystitis, urine scalding, dysuria caused by urethral stricture, recurrence of neoplasia at the site of amputation, and neoplastic metastases to inguinal lymph nodes and internal organs.

Temporary Perineal Urethrostomy

Indications

Temporary urethrostomy at the ischial arch is performed to provide access to small cystic calculi, for treatment of horses affected with hemospermia or hematuria, and to divert the flow of urine from the penile urethra for such conditions as urethral laceration or urethral urolithiasis.

Surgical Technique

Temporary perineal urethrostomy is best performed with the horse standing and sedated after administering epidural anesthesia or infiltrating the tissue at the proposed site of incision with a local anesthetic agent. A 6- to 8-cm vertical incision is created on the perineal raphe about 2 to 3 cm below the anus. The incision is extended through the skin, the retractor penis and bulbospongiosus muscles, the CSP, and the urethral mucosa (see Fig. 66-2).

Preoperative insertion of a large-bore urethral catheter facilitates identification of the urethra. The perineal incision should "funnel" to a short urethral incision as it deepens to avoid postoperative pocketing of urine in the tissues. If the incision strays from the midline, profuse hemorrhage can result from laceration of branches of the external pudendal artery.[36] The urethrostomy is generally allowed to heal by secondary intention; development of clinically apparent urethral stenosis after this procedure is rare. The urethrostomy normally heals within 2 weeks.[104]

REFERENCES

1. de Lahunta A, Habel RE: Applied Veterinary Anatomy, Philadelphia, 1986, WB Saunders.
2. Habel RE: Applied Veterinary Anatomy, ed 2, Ithaca, NY, 1981, self-published.
3. Sisson S, Grossman JD: The Anatomy of the Domestic Animals, ed 4, Philadelphia, 1953, WB Saunders.
4. Schummer A, Nickel R, Sack WO: The Viscera of the Domestic Mammals, ed 2, Berlin, 1979, Paul Parey Verlag.
5. Budras K-D, Sack WO, Rock S: Anatomy of the Horse, An Illustrated Text, ed 2, Philadelphia, 1994, Mosby-Wolfe.
6. Rooney JR, Sack WO, Habel RE: Guide to the Dissection of the Horse, Ithaca, NY, 1967 WO Sack.
7. Rossdale PD, Ricketts SW: Equine Stud Farm Medicine, ed 2, Philadelphia, 1980, Lea & Febiger.
8. Breazile JE: The male reproductive system. In Breazile JE, editor: Textbook of Veterinary Physiology, Philadelphia, 1971, Lea & Febiger.
9. Bartels JE, Beckett DS, Brown BG: Angiography of the corpus cavernosum penis in the pony stallion during erection and quiescence, Am J Vet Res 1984;45:1464.
10. Beckett SD, Hudson RS, Walker DF, et al: Blood pressures and penile muscle activity in the stallion during coitus, Am J Physiol 1973;225:1072.
11. Beckett SD, Walker DF, Hudson RS, et al: Corpus spongiosum penis pressure and penile muscle activity in the stallion during coitus, Am J Vet Res 1975;36:431.
12. Muruve N, Hosking DH: Intracorporeal phenylephrine in the treatment of priapism, J Urol 1996;155:141.
13. Weiss HD: The physiology of human penile erection, Ann Intern Med 1972;76:793.
14. Weber JA, Woods GL: Transrectal ultrasonography for the evaluation of stallion accessory sex glands, Vet Clin North Am Equine Pract 1992;8:183.
15. Dyce KM, Sack WO, Wensing CJG: Textbook of Veterinary Anatomy, Philadelphia, 1987, WB Saunders.
16. Taylor TS, Varner DD: Diseases of the accessory sex glands of the stallion. In Auer JA, editor: Equine Surgery, ed 1, Philadelphia, 1992, WB Saunders.
17. Swanstrom OG, Krahwinkel DJ: Preputial hernia in a horse, Vet Med Small Anim Clin 1974;69:870.
18. Ashdown RR, Done SH: Color Atlas of Veterinary Anatomy. The Horse, Philadelphia, 1987, JB Lippincott.
19. Faulkner LC, Pineda MH: Male reproduction. In McDonald LE, editor: Veterinary Endocrinology and Reproduction, ed 2, Philadelphia, 1975, Lea & Febiger.
20. Magda II: Local anesthesia in operations on the male perineum in horses (Abstract), J Am Vet Med Assoc 1948;113:559.
21. Schumacher J, Bratton GR, Williams JW: Pudendal and caudal rectal nerve blocks in the horse: An anesthetic procedure for reproductive surgery, Theriogenology 1985;24:457.
22. Varner DD, Blanchard TL, Brinsko SP, et al: Techniques for evaluating selected reproductive disorders of stallions, Anim Reprod Sci 2000;60:493.
23. Neely DP: Physical examination and genital diseases of the stallion. In Morrow DA, editor: Current Therapy in Theriogenology, Philadelphia, 1980, WB Saunders.
24. Munger RJ, Meagher DM: Surgical repair of a fistula of the urethral diverticulum in a horse, Vet Med Small Anim Clin 1976;71:96.
25. Pascoe RR: Rupture of the corpus cavernosum penis of a stallion, Aust Vet J 1971;47:610.
26. Yovich JV, Turner AS: Treatment of postcastration urethral stricture by phallectomy in a gelding, Comp Cont Educ Pract Vet 1986;8:S393.
27. Todhunter RJ, Parker JE: Surgical repair of urethral transection in a horse, J Am Vet Med Assoc 1988;193:1085.
28. Perkins JD, Schumacher J, Waguespack RW, et al: Penile

retroversion and partial phallectomy performed in a standing horse, Vet Rec 2003;153:184.

29. Cox JE: Surgery of the Reproductive Tract in Large Animals, Liverpool, 1987, Liverpool University Press.
30. Boyer K, Jann HW, Dawson LJ, et al: Penile hematoma in a stallion resulting in proximal penile amputation, Equine Pract 1995;17:8.
31. Firth EC: Dissecting hematoma of corpus spongiosum and urinary bladder rupture in a stallion, J Am Vet Med Assoc 1976;169:800.
32. Hyland J, Church S: The use of ultrasonography in the diagnosis and treatment of a haematoma in the corpus cavernosum penis of a stallion, Aust Vet J 1995;72:468.
33. Blikslager AT, Tate LP Jr, Jones SL: Neodymium:yttrium-aluminum-garnet laser ablation of a urethral web to relieve urinary outflow obstruction in a horse, J Am Vet Med Assoc 2001;218:1970.
34. Boero MJ: A simple technique for conservative therapy of acute traumatic paraphimosis in the horse, Proc Am Assoc Equine Pract 1990;36:625.
35. Henning MW: Animal Diseases in South Africa, ed 3, Pretoria, South Africa, 1956, Central News Agency Ltd.
36. Walker DF: Surgery of the penis. In Walker DF, Vaughan JT, editors: Bovine and Equine Urogenital Surgery, Philadelphia, 1980, Lea & Febiger.
37. Simmons HA, Cox JE, Edwards PA, et al: Paraphimosis in seven debilitated horses, Vet Rec 1985;116:126.
38. Schumacher J, Hardin DK: Surgical treatment of priapism in a stallion, Vet Surg 1987;16:193.
38. Wheat JD: Penile paralysis in stallions given propriopromazine, J Am Vet Med Assoc 1966;148:405.
40. Bolz W: The prophylaxis and therapy of prolapse and paralysis of the penis occurring in the horse after the administration of neuroleptics, Vet Med Rev Leverkusen 1970;4:255.
41. Teuscher H: Diseases of the male genital organs and hermaphroditism. In Dietz O, Wiesner E, editors: Diseases of the Horse, New York, 1982, Karger.
42. Nie GJ, Pope KC: Persistent penile prolapse associated with acute blood loss and acepromazine maleate administration in a horse, J Am Vet Med Assoc 1997;211:587.
43. Frank ER: Veterinary Surgery, ed 7, Minneapolis, 1964, Burgess.
44. Pohl J, Polt B, Kleinhans G: Priapism: A three phase concept of management according to aetiology and progress, Br J Urol 1986;58:113.
45. Cosgrove MD, La Rocque MA: Shunt surgery for priapism, Urol 1974;4:1.
46. Gerring EL: Priapism and ACP in the horse, Vet Rec 1981;109:64.
47. Dorman WB, Schmidt JD: Association of priapism in phenothiazine therapy, J Urol 1976;116:51.
48. Wilson DV, Nickels FA, Williams MA: Pharmacologic treatment of priapism in two horses, J Am Vet Med Assoc 1991;119:1183.
49. Oyamada T, Miyajima K, Kimura Y, et al: Priapism possibly caused by spinal nematodiasis in a stallion, J Equine Sci 1997;8:101.
50. Blanchard TL, Schumacher J, Edwards JF, et al: Priapism in a stallion with generalized malignant melanoma, J Am Vet Med Assoc 1991;198:1043.
51. Pearson H, Weaver BMQ: Priapism after sedation, neuroleptanalgesia and anaesthesia in the horse, Equine Vet J 1978;10:85.
52. Stock KW, Jacob AL, Kummer M, et al: High-flow priapism in a child: Treatment with superselective embolization, Am J Roentgenol 1996;166:290.
53. Lue TF, Hellstrom WJG, McAninch JW, et al: Priapism: a refined approach to diagnosis and treatment, J Urol 1986;136:104.
54. Hinman F: Priapism: Reason for failure of therapy, J Urol 1960;83:420.
55. Sharrock AG: Reversal of drug-induced priapism in a gelding by medication, Aust Vet J 1982;58:39.
56. van Driel MF, Hesselink JW: [Priapism in the stallion and in man], Tijdschr Diergeneeskd 2003;128:255.
57. Schumacher J, Varner DD, Crabill MR, et al: The effect of a surgically created shunt between the corpus cavernosum penis and corpus spongiosum penis of stallions on erectile and ejaculatory function, Vet Surg 1999;28:21.
58. Varner DD: Personal communication, Texas A&M University, 2004.
59. Wolfe DF, Hudson RS, Walker DG, et al: Failure of penile erection due to vascular shunt from corpus cavernosum penis to the corpus spongiosum penis in a bull, J Am Vet Med Assoc 1984;184:1511.
60. Boller M, Fürst A, Ringer S, et al: Complete recovery from long standing priapism in a stallion after propionylpromazine/xylazine sedation, Equine Vet Educ 2004 (in press).
61. Virag R: Intracavernous injection of papaverine for erectile failure, Lancet 1982;2:938.
62. McDonnell SM: Oral imipramine and intravenous xylazine for pharmacologically-induced ex copula ejaculation in stallions, Anim Reprod Sci 2001;68:153.
63. Van Harreveld PD, Gaughan EM: Partial phallectomy to treat priapism in a horse, Aust Vet J 1999;77:167.
64. Bracken FK, Wagner PC: Cosmetic surgery for equine pseudohermaphroditism, Vet Med Small Anim Clin 1983;78:879.
65. Roberts SJ: Veterinary Obstetrics and Genital Diseases, Ithaca, NY, 1971, self-published.
66. McFeely RA, Kanagawa H: Intersexuality. In Hafez ESE, editor: Reproduction in Farm Animals, ed 3, Philadelphia, 1974, Lea & Febiger.
67. Baker JR: Histological survey of tumours of the horse, with particular reference to those of the skin, Vet Rec 1975;96:419.
68. Cotchin E: Neoplasms of the Domesticated Mammals, England, 1956, Commonwealth Agricultural Bureaux.
69. Jubb KVF, Kennedy PC: Pathology of Domestic Animals, vol 1, ed 2, New York, 1970, Academic Press.
70. Keller H: Diseases of male reproductive organs in non-breeding horses. In Wintzer HJ, editor: Equine Diseases, New York, 1986, Springer-Verlag.
71. Moulton JE: Tumors in Domestic Animals, Berkeley, 1978, University of California Press.
72. Junge RE, Sundberg JP, Lancaster WD: Papillomas and squamous cell carcinomas of horses, J Am Vet Med Assoc 1984;185:656.
73. Howarth S, Lucke VM, Pearson H: Squamous cell carcinoma of the equine external genitalia: A review and assessment of penile amputation and urethrostomy as a surgical treatment, Equine Vet J 1991;23:53.
74. Mair TS, Walmsley JP, Phillips TJ: Surgical treatment of 45 horses affected by squamous cell carcinoma of the penis and prepuce, Equine Vet J 2000;32:406.
75. Akerejola OO, Ayivor MD, Adams EW: Equine squamous-cell carcinoma in Northern Nigeria, Vet Rec 1978;103:336.
76. Plaut A, Kohn-Speyer AC: The carcinogenic action of smegma, Science 1947;105:91.
77. Reddy DG, Baruah IK: Carcinogenic action of human smegma, Arch Pathol 1963;75:414.
78. Montes LF, Vaughan JT: Atlas of Skin Diseases of the Horse, Philadelphia, 1983, WB Saunders.
79. Scott EA: A technique for amputation of the equine penis, J Am Vet Med Assoc 1976;168:1047.
80. Patterson LJ, May SA, Baker JR: Skeletal metastasis of a penile squamous cell carcinoma, Vet Rec 1990;126:579.
81. McCauley CT, Hawkins JK, Adams SB, et al: Use of a carbon dioxide laser for surgical management of cutaneous masses in horses: 32 cases (1993-2000), J Am Vet Med Assoc 2002;220:1192.
82. Palmer SE: Instrumentation and techniques for carbon dioxide laser in equine surgery, Vet Clin North Am Equine Pract 1996;12:397.
83. Markel MD, Wheat JD, Jones K: Genital neoplasms treated by en bloc resection and penile retroversion in horses: 10 cases (1977-1986), J Am Vet Med Assoc 1988;192:396.
84. Joyce JR. Cryosurgery for removal of equine sarcoids, Vet Med Small Anim Clin 1975;70:200.

85. Fortier LA, MacHarg MA: Topical use of 5-fluorouracil for treatment of squamous cell carcinoma of the external genitalia of horses: 11 cases (1988-1992), J Am Vet Med Assoc 1994;205:1183.
86. Theon AP, Pascoe JR, Carlson GP, et al: Intratumoral chemotherapy with cisplatin in oily emulsion in horses, J Am Vet Med Assoc 1993;202:261.
87. Theon AP, Pascoe JR, Galuppo LD, et al: Comparison of perioperative versus postoperative intratumoral administration of cisplatin for treatment of cutaneous sarcoids and squamous cell carcinomas in horses, J Am Vet Med Assoc 1999;215:1655.
88. Moore AS, Beam SL, Rassnick KM, et al: Long-term control of mucocutaneous squamous cell carcinoma and metastases in a horse using piroxicam, Equine Vet J 2003;35:715.
89. Grier R, Brewer W, Paul S, et al: Treatment of bovine and equine ocular squamous cell carcinoma by radiofrequency hyperthermia, J Am Vet Med Assoc 1980;177:55.
90. Hoffman KD, Dainer RA, Shideler RK, et al: Radio-frequency current-induced hyperthermia for the treatment of equine sarcoid, Equine Pract 1983;5:24.
91. Soria JC, Theodore C, Gerbaulet A: Carcinome epidermoide de la verge, Bull Cancer 1998 ;85:773.
92. McMullan W: Habronemiasis, Proc Am Assoc Equine Pract 1976;22:295.
93. Stick JA: Amputation of the equine urethral process affected with habronemiasis, Vet Med Small Anim Clin 1979;74:1453.
94. Schumacher J, Schumacher J, Schmitz D: Macroscopic haematuria of horses, Equine Vet Educ 2002;14:201.
95. Stick JA: Surgical management of genital habronemiasis, Vet Med Small Anim Clin 1981;76:410.
96. Herd RP, Donaham JC: Efficacy of ivermectin against cutaneous *Drashia* and *Habronema* infection (summer sores) in horses, Am J Vet Res 1981;42:1952.
97. Bedford SJ, McDonnell SM, Tulleners E, et al: Squamous cell carcinoma of the urethral process in a horse with hemospermia and self-mutilation behavior, J Am Vet Med Assoc 2000;216:551.
98. Pickett BW, Voss JL, Squires EL, et al: Management of the Stallion for Maximum Reproductive Efficiency, General Series 1005, Fort Collins, Colo, Colorado State University Experiment Station & Animal Reproduction Laboratory, 1981.
99. Voss JL, Pickett BW: Diagnosis and treatment of hemospermia in the stallion, J Reprod Fertil Suppl 1975;23:151.
100. Schumacher J, Varner DD, Schmitz DG, et al: Urethral defects in geldings with hematuria and stallions with hemospermia, Vet Surg 1995;24:250.
101. Sullins KE, Bertone JJ, Voss JL, et al: Treatment of hemospermia in stallions: A discussion of 18 cases, Comp Cont Educ Pract Vet 1988;10:S1396.
102. Macpherson ML: Hemospermia. In Brown CM, Bertone J, editors: The 5-Minute Veterinary Consult, Equine, Philadelphia, 2002, Lippincott Williams & Wilkins.
103. Blanchard TL: Use of a semen extender containing antibiotics to improve the fertility of a stallion with seminal vesiculitis due to *Pseudomonas aeruginosa*, Theriogenology 1987;28:541.
104. Taintor J, Schumacher J, Schumacher J: Comparison of pressures in the corpus spongiosum penis during urination between geldings and stallions, Equine Vet J 2004;36:362.
105. Schott HC: Hematuria. In Reed SM, Bayly WM, editors: Equine Internal Medicine, Philadelphia, 1988, WB Saunders.
106. Laverty S, Pascoe JR, Ling GV, et al: Urolithiasis in 68 horses, Vet Surg 1992;21:56.
107. Peyton LC: The reefing operation in large animals (a pictorial essay), Vet Med Small Anim Clin 1980;75:112-114.
108. Wheat JD: Personal communication, University of California, 1988.
109. Vaughan JT: Surgery of the prepuce and penis, Proc Am Assoc Equine Pract 1972;18:19.
110. Kersjes AW, Nemeth F, Rutgers LJE: Atlas of Large Animal Surgery, Baltimore, 1985, Williams & Wilkins.
111. Williams WL: The Diseases of the Genital Organs of Domestic Animals, ed 3, Worcester, Mass, 1943, Ethel Williams Plimpton.
112. Riggs E: Diagnosis and treatment of penile conditions in horses, In Pract 1996;18:488.
113. Joyce JR: Personal communication, Texas A&M University, 1996.
114. Archer DC, Edwards GB: En bloc resection of the penis in five geldings, Equine Vet Educ 2004;16:12.
115. Doles J, Williams JW, Yarbrough TB: Penile amputation and sheath ablation in the horse, Vet Surg 2001;30:327.

CHAPTER 67

Vulva, Vestibule, Vagina, and Cervix

Brett Woodie

The caudal aspect of the reproductive tract is composed of the vulva, vestibule, vagina, and cervix. These structures are susceptible to a variety of injuries during breeding and foaling. Conformational abnormalities of the caudal reproductive tract may predispose the mare to pneumovagina, urovagina, and other problems. Ultimately, problems associated with the caudal reproductive tract can lead to infertility.

ANATOMY

The external genitalia of the mare are composed of the perineum and the vulva. The *perineum* is the region bound dorsally by the base of the tail, laterally by the semimembranosus muscles and sacrosciatic ligaments, and ventrally by the ventral commissure of the vulva[1] (Fig. 67-1). The fibromuscular perineal body lies between the anus and the vulva. Fibers of the external anal sphincter and the constrictor vulvae muscles form the perineal body (Fig. 67-2).

The *vulva* includes the two labia and the clitoris. The external orifice of the vulva is typically 12 to 15 cm long.[2] When the architecture of the external genitalia of the mare is normal, the labia of the vulva are vertical and meet dorsally to form the dorsal commissure, which is located just ventral to the anus. The labia meet ventrally to form the ventral commissure, which is located caudal and ventral to the ischial arch. Approximately two thirds of the vulvar cleft is ventral to the ischial arch.[3] Normally, the labia of the vulva are muscular and resist manual separation, as a result of the paired constrictor vulvae muscles, which lie deep to the skin of the labia. The internal pudendal vessels provide

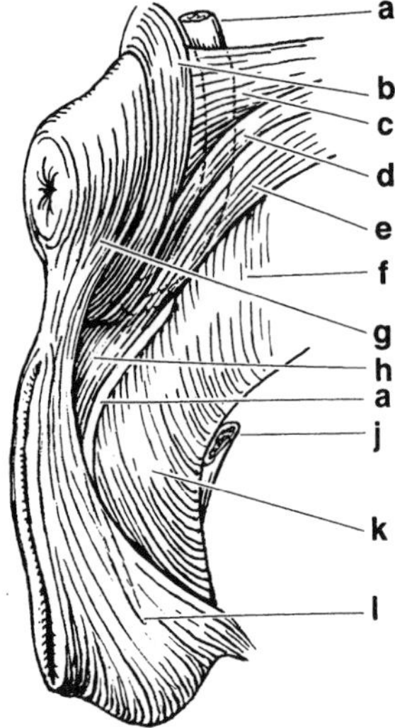

Figure 67-1. Muscles of the perineal region. a, M. retractor clitoridis; b, M. external anal sphincter (cranial superficial part); c, M. levator ani; d, subanal loop of M. levator ani; e, ventral part of M. levator ani; f, M. urethralis; g, external anal sphincter (caudal superficial part); h, perineal septum; j, crus clitoridis (cut); k, M. constrictor vestibuli; l, constrictor vulvae.

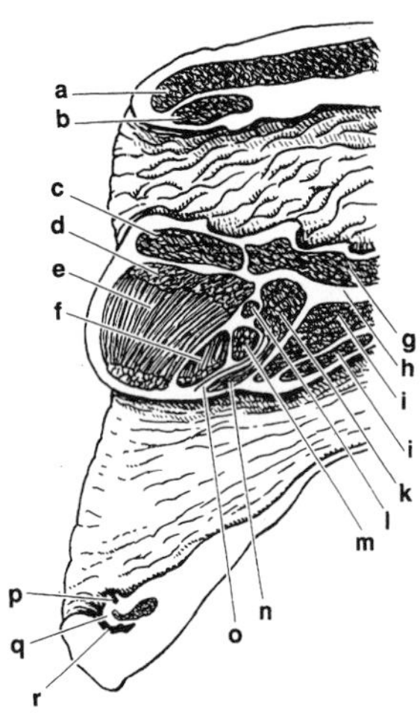

Figure 67-2. Muscles that are part of the vulvar and vestibular sphincters, and the perineal body. a, external anal sphincter; b, internal anal sphincter; c, internal anal sphincter; d, external anal sphincter; e, muscular fibers from external anal sphincter to constrictor vulvae; f, cranial superficial part and deep part of external anal sphincter; g, rectal musculature; h, rectovaginal septum; i and j, vaginal musculature; k, rectal part of retractor clitoridis; l, clitorial part of retractor clitoridis; m, subanal loop of levator ani; n, decussation of retractor clitoridis; o, perineal septum; p, clitoral sinus; q, glans clitoris; r, clitoral fossa.

the vascular supply to the vulva, its labia, and the clitoris. The pudendal and caudal rectal nerves provide motor innervation to the muscles of the vestibule and vulva.[4] These nerves also supply sensory fibers to the mucous membrane of the vulva and the skin of the labia.[4]

The clitoris in the mare is the homolog of the penis in the male. It is located at the ventral commissure of the vulvar labia. The clitoral glans is approximately 2.5 cm in diameter and contains erectile tissue similar to that of the corpus cavernosum penis. The clitoral fossa that surrounds the glans is located laterally and ventrally. The body of the clitoris is approximately 5 cm in length and is attached to the ischial arch by two crura.[2]

The *vestibule* is the terminal part of the internal genital tract. It is a tubular structure approximately 12 to 15 cm long that connects the vulva to the vagina.[2] The normal configuration of the vestibule is a ventrodorsal slope in the rostrad direction.[5] The cranial extent of the vestibule ends at the level of the transverse fold, which is located dorsal to the external urethral orifice. The lateral and ventral surface of the vestibule is covered by the constrictor vestibuli muscles, which dorsally are incomplete.[1] The paired constrictor vestibuli muscles blend caudally with the constrictor vulvae muscles. The constrictor vestibuli muscles, the pillars of the hymen, and the floor of the pelvis meet to form the vestibular sphincter.[6]

The *vagina* is a tubular structure extending cranially from the transverse fold of the external urethral orifice to the vaginal fornix around the cervix. The vagina is related to the rectum dorsally, to the bladder and urethra ventrally, and laterally to the pelvic wall. The majority of the vagina is located retroperitoneally, but a small cranial portion of the ventral aspect and larger portions of the dorsal aspect are always covered with peritoneum.[2] The extent to which the cranial part of the vagina is covered with peritoneum is related inversely to the fullness of the rectum and bladder.[4] The vascular supply of the vagina is derived from the internal pudendal vessels. Since there is no skeletal muscle present in the vagina, there is no motor innervation. Multiple sympathetic ganglia are present in the vaginal wall.[7]

The cervix is an extension of the uterine body, with the caudal portion positioned in the cranial aspect (fornix) of the vagina. The caudal portion of the cervix is referred to as the external cervical os, and it is covered by vaginal mucosa. The cervix is a tubular muscular structure lined with mucosa that forms many longitudinal folds. It functions as a sphincter, separating the caudal reproductive tract from the uterus.

There are essentially three protective barriers in the caudal reproductive tract. The constrictor vulvae muscles of the labia form the first barrier, the second is the vestibular sphincter, and the cervix is the third. When any of these barriers becomes incompetent, contamination of the reproductive tract may occur and result in infertility.

PATHOPHYSIOLOGY

Failure of the protective barriers in the caudal reproductive tract can be caused by numerous factors. Mares with conformational abnormalities, such as a flat croup, a sunken anus, or underdeveloped vulvar labia, are predisposed to pneumovagina[8] (Fig. 67-3). Poor perineal conformation is often found in older multiparous mares that are thin in body condition.

A large percentage of the injuries to the caudal reproductive tract occur secondary to trauma from breeding or foaling. Some of the injuries are readily apparent in the immediate postpartum period, but others can go unnoticed until it is time to rebreed the mare. Injuries that occur during foaling include cervical lacerations, cervical contusions, perineal lacerations, rectovestibular fistulas, urinary bladder eversion or prolapse, urinary bladder rupture, vaginal contusions, vaginal lacerations, vestibular lacerations, and uterine

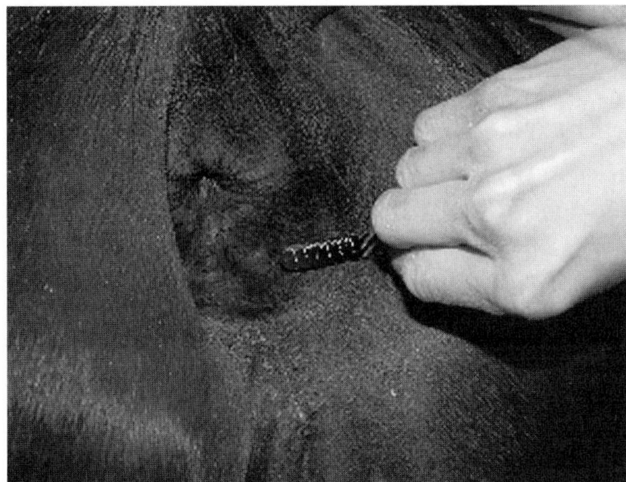

Figure 67-3. A mare with poor perineal conformation. The anus has a sunken appearance and is accompanied by cranial sloping of the vulva. There is evidence of a previously performed Caslick procedure.

prolapse or rupture.[9-11] The severity of these injuries ranges from minor to severe, and not all require intervention. However, extensive surgical repair may be necessary to restore normal anatomic function. Without repair of the injured tissue, infertility is often the result. When an injury has been identified, a thorough examination is necessary to ensure that more than one anatomic structure does not need surgical repair.

Injuries during breeding do not occur frequently, but they may require medical or surgical treatment.[12] When perforation of the vagina occurs (usually during intromission), the lesion is typically located at the cranial aspect of the vagina adjacent to the cervix. Predisposing factors for this type of injury include an overly vigorous stallion or a large stallion breeding a small mare.[12] Depending on the location and depth of penetration, the peritoneal cavity may be entered. Semen is not sterile and peritonitis may develop secondary to ejaculation into the peritoneal cavity.[13,14] Eventration can occur through a tear in the vaginal wall.[15] The development of an abscess in the pelvic cavity may result from an injury that does not involve the peritoneal cavity.[16] Inadvertent entry of the stallion's penis into the mare's rectum during breeding can result in rectal injury or perforation. This type of accident, which does not occur commonly, has been associated with poor vulvar conformation, a small vulvar opening after a Caslick procedure, and a relaxed anal sphincter after palpation per rectum.[12]

DIAGNOSTIC PROCEDURES

Examination of the reproductive tract of the mare should progress from an external to an internal evaluation. Visual evaluation of the conformation of the perineum and vulva as well as looking for evidence of vulvar discharge is a logical starting point. Examination of the external genitalia for diseases such as neoplasia and intersex conditions should be performed. The conformation of the vulva is very important because this anatomic structure is the first line of defense in protecting the reproductive tract from contamination (see Fig. 67-3). The labia should be evaluated for symmetry, position, angle, and tone. Pascoe's Caslick index is an objective scoring system that can be used to determine the risk for ascending infection to the reproductive tract.[5] The length of the vulva (in centimeters) is multiplied by the angle of declination of the vulvar lips. Higher pregnancy rates have been reported in mares that had a Caslick index of less than 150.[3]

The vestibule, vagina, and cervix should be examined digitally as well as visually, using a speculum. Samples for endometrial biopsy, culture, and cytology should be taken. The reproductive tract should be assessed by palpation and ultrasonography per rectum.

Chemical Restraint

The majority of diagnostic and surgical procedures that are performed on the caudal reproductive tract of the mare are accomplished in the standing mare using chemical restraint, usually supplemented with local and/or regional anesthesia for surgical procedures. The drugs used for chemical restraint provide variable degrees of sedation and analgesia. A number of sedative-hypnotic, tranquilizing, and opioid agents are available for use in the horse (see Chapter 20). Selection is based on personal preference and the type of surgical procedure that is being performed. The use of combinations of drugs often optimizes restraint and analgesia as compared with the use of an individual drug.

The use of acetylpromazine, a phenothiazine tranquilizer, produces sedation without analgesia. The peak effect of sedation after intravenous administration (0.04 mg/kg) is approximately 30 minutes, and sedation may last for 1 to 3 hours depending on dosage and route of administration.[17] The phenothiazine tranquilizers do not produce analgesia and should be used in combination with an analgesic agent if a surgical procedure is to be performed.

Xylazine and detomidine are the most commonly used sedative-hypnotic drugs for standing chemical restraint. These drugs produce varying degrees of sedation, muscle relaxation, analgesia, and ataxia, depending on the dosage administered. Both drugs induce diuresis, which may warrant placement of a urinary catheter.[18] Detomidine has a longer duration of action and greater potency than xylazine.[19] Each of these drugs can be used in combination with an opiate such as butorphanol. This typically produces more profound sedation and analgesia. Reduced dosages for chemical restraint should be considered when working on Draft breeds, because they appear to respond more intensely than light breeds.[20]

Epidural Anesthesia

Epidural anesthesia is achieved when the local anesthetic solution is deposited between the dura mater and the periosteum of the spinal canal, which blocks conduction in the caudal nerve roots. The goal of caudal epidural anesthesia is to induce temporary neutralization of sensory innervation while maintaining motor control of the hind limbs. However, the tail should be tied overhead to support the horse in case ataxia develops. The sacrocaudal (first intercoccygeal) vertebral space is selected as the site for injection for epidural anesthesia.[21] This location is found by grasping the tail and moving it up and down and palpating the first articulation caudal to the sacrum; this is the first intercoccygeal space. The site should be clipped and aseptically prepared. The epidural should be administered using aseptic technique.

Various injection techniques and drug combinations can be used to achieve epidural anesthesia. The mare should be sedated and restrained in stocks during administration of the epidural. A small skin bleb of local anesthetic can be deposited at the proposed injection site to facilitate placement of the spinal needle. A 20-gauge, 7.5-cm spinal needle should be positioned just cranial to the dorsal spinous process of the second coccygeal vertebra. The needle is inserted through the skin at an angle of 30 degrees relative to the tail and advanced cranially. If bone is encountered, the needle should be redirected. Once the needle is placed, the stylet should be withdrawn and the hub of the needle filled with the local anesthetic to be injected. If the needle is positioned in the epidural space, the fluid will be aspirated into the needle (hanging drop technique). Minimal resistance is encountered during epidural injection. Mares that have had previous epidural injections may develop fibrous scar tissue over the intercoccygeal space, making needle placement difficult.[21] After the injection, the needle should be removed. Caution should be exercised during placement of the spinal needle, since some mares kick during the procedure. An epidural catheter can be placed to facilitate re-administration of anesthetic agents if needed during the surgery.[20] Loss of anal sphincter tone is common when epidural anesthesia is achieved.

The type of blockade (motor and/or sensory) and the duration of effect depends on the drug type and the volume that is administered. Local anesthetics produce motor and sensory blockade, whereas only sensory innervation is lost with other drug treatments. The use of 5 to 7 mL of 2% lidocaine hydrochloride per 500 kg of body weight should produce analgesia within 5 to 15 minutes, and the duration of analgesia should be 60 to 90 minutes.[21] Two percent mepivacaine hydrochloride given at the same dosage produces analgesia in 10 to 30 minutes and provides analgesia for 90 to 120 minutes.[21] Ataxia is a complication when using local anesthetics.

Epidural administration of α_2-adrenergic agonists such as xylazine provides profound analgesia without the complication of ataxia.[22,23] The recommended dosage of xylazine is 0.17 mg/kg. The onset of action is 10 to 30 minutes, and the duration of analgesia is 2½ to 4 hours.[21] The xylazine should be diluted in saline to a total volume of 6 to 10 mL. Epidural administration of detomidine (30 to 60 μg/kg) provides analgesia lasting for 2 to 3 hours but produces sedation and ataxia.[21,22] The combination of lidocaine (0.22 mg/kg) and xylazine (0.17 mg/kg) produces significantly longer analgesia (approximately 5 hours) with only mild ataxia when compared with lidocaine used alone.[23]

Preparation of the Surgical Site and the Mare

The rectum should be evacuated prior to starting any surgical procedure on the caudal reproductive tract. The tail should be wrapped and secured so that it does not interfere during surgery. The perineum and buttocks should be scrubbed with a nonirritating soap. A dilute antibacterial solution of 1% Betadine can be used to cleanse the vestibule and vagina. All fluid should be removed from the vestibule and vagina before beginning surgery.

Tetanus prophylaxis should be administered if necessary. The use of perioperative antibiotics and anti-inflammatory drugs is at the discretion of the surgeon.

Instrumentation

Special instruments are needed to perform certain surgical procedures on the caudal reproductive tract. Illumination of the surgical field is crucial. Options include a light source that can be attached to the self-retaining retractor, a head-lamp, or overhead surgical lights that can be adjusted. Retractors are needed to provide exposure to the surgical site. A modified Finochietto retractor with long blades (Sontec Instruments, Englewood, Colo) (Fig. 67-4) is very helpful in repairing cervical lacerations. Balfour retractors are useful for surgical procedures caudal to the vestibulovaginal junction. Positioning the retractor with the retaining mechanism so that it is dorsal to the anus, and securing it to the tail head using umbilical tape keeps the retractor in place and out of the surgical field. Hand-held instruments need to be longer than conventional instruments (Fig. 67-5). Scalpel handles, scissors, thumb forceps, Allis tissue forceps, and needle holders should be 25 to 30 cm in length.[24]

DISORDERS REQUIRING SURGERY

Pneumovagina

Pneumovagina leads to chronic inflammation and infection of the vagina and uterus and is one cause of infertility in the mare. The most common cause of aspiration of air into the vagina is poor perineal conformation (see Fig. 67-3). Pneumovagina may develop secondary to foaling trauma with scar tissue formation, excessive stretching of the vulvar tissues from foaling, or poor body condition.[8] Sinking of the anus into the pelvic canal causes the dorsal commissure of

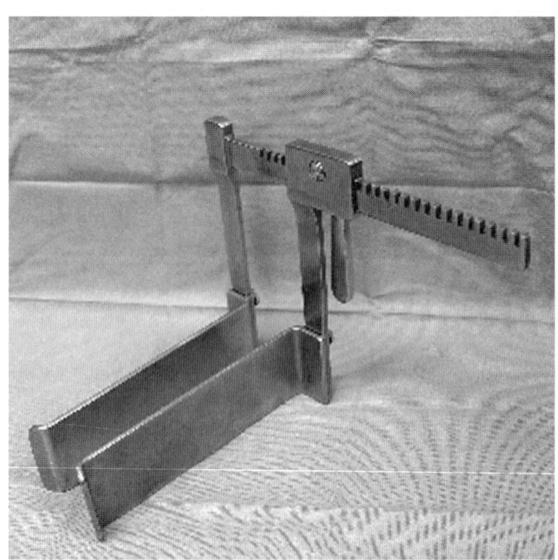

Figure 67-4. Modified Finochietto retractor with long blades. This retractor is very useful for certain surgical procedures of the caudal reproductive tract, such as repair of a cervical laceration.

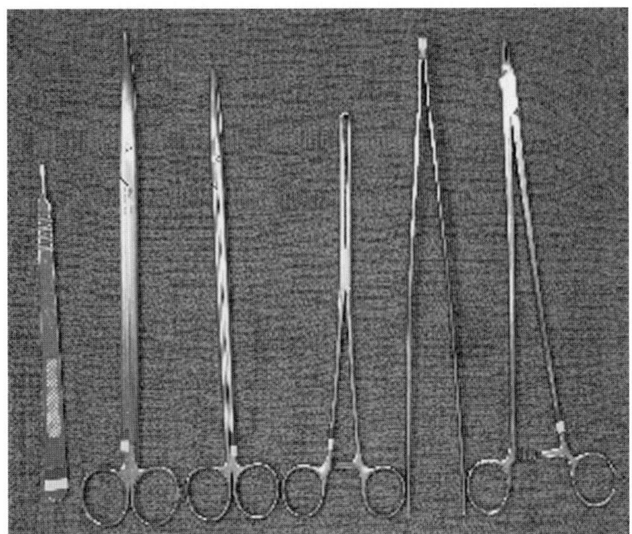

Figure 67-5. Long-handled instruments are necessary for adequate handling of tissues in many of the surgical procedures on the female caudal reproductive tract.

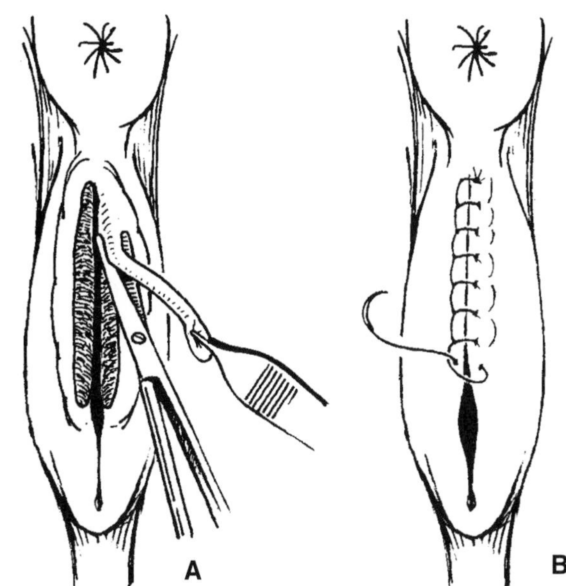

Figure 67-6. The Caslick procedure. **A,** Removal of a narrow strip of tissue from the mucocutaneous junction. **B,** Closure, using Ford interlocking suture pattern.

the vulva to tip forward and have a horizontal orientation as opposed to vertical. This can disrupt the vulvar seal and lead to pneumovagina as well as fecal contamination of the caudal reproductive tract. If manually separating the labia results in an inrushing of air, the mare is predisposed to pneumovagina. In some mares, pneumovagina occurs only during estrus when perineal tissues are more relaxed.[25] Urovagina can result from the same causes as pneumovagina, and the mare should be evaluated to determine if more than one surgical procedure is necessary.

Episioplasty

CASLICK PROCEDURE

The most common surgical method for correction of pneumovagina is the Caslick procedure, first described in 1937.[6,16] The intent of this surgery is to form a seal to prevent aspiration of air or fecal material into the vestibule. This is accomplished by incising the labia or excising a thin strip of tissue from the labial borders and then suturing the labia together. Pneumovagina can be prevented in most cases by suturing the labia together to the level of the ventral border of the ischial arch. The ventral limit is determined by palpating the ischial arch just lateral to the opening of the vulva.[25] The mare should be sedated and restrained so that the clinician is protected from a kick injury. The perineum is prepared, and local anesthesia is infiltrated into the labial margins extending from the ischial arch to the dorsal commissure. A 4- to 8-mm-wide strip of mucosa is excised with a pair of scissors along the mucocutaneous junction on each labium (Fig. 67-6). It is important to include the dorsal commissure of the vulva in the excision, so that a seal at the dorsal aspect is achieved. Alternatively, a scalpel can be used to incise the labia at the mucocutaneous junction rather than to excise any tissue. The incision must be of sufficient depth so that a tissue gap of 4 to 8 mm is achieved.

Closure is achieved using 2-0 absorbable or nonabsorbable suture material in a continuous pattern.[26] Stainless steel skin staples can be used for the closure instead of suture material.[27] The sutures or staples should be removed 10 to 12 days later, and the surgery site should be evaluated for fistula formation. Because fistula formation can lead to aspiration of air and fecal material and negate the effects of the procedure, it should be repaired.[28]

A mare requiring a Caslick procedure will very likely continue to need the procedure done for the rest of her broodmare life, so care should be taken to remove only as much tissue as necessary to achieve a complete seal between the labia.[25] Excessive removal of tissue will make subsequent Caslick procedures more difficult because of fibrosis and loss of tissue. Older mares that have had numerous Caslick procedures occasionally develop enough fibrous tissue or lose enough skin to make closure difficult as a result of tension. This may lead to dehiscence of a routine Caslick procedure. In such cases, a three-layer closure can be used. The inner layer consists of the mucosa of the two labia, which is apposed using 2-0 absorbable suture material in a continuous horizontal mattress pattern. Then, the constrictor vulvae muscles are apposed using 2-0 absorbable suture material in a similar pattern. Finally, the cutaneous layer is apposed using 2-0 or 0 absorbable or nonabsorbable suture material in a continuous pattern.

A breeding stitch is often placed at the ventral limits of the suture line to protect the Caslick procedure at subsequent breeding.[28] This consists of an interrupted suture of small-width umbilical tape or large-diameter suture material that is placed 2 to 3 cm lateral to both sides of the mucocutaneous border of the labia[26] (Fig. 67-7). The suture must be positioned so that it does not interfere with the stallion's penis during intromission. Natural cover of the mare can be achieved with the suture in place by manually elevating the vulvar opening and guiding the stallion's penis. The breeding stitch is removed once the mare is confirmed to be pregnant.

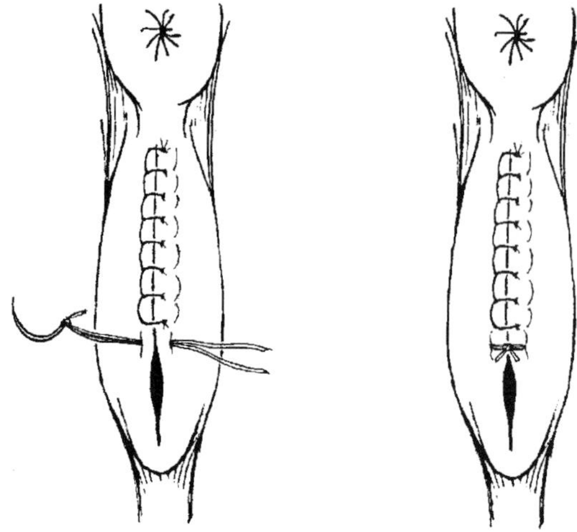

Figure 67-7. A breeding stitch placed ventral to a Caslick suture.

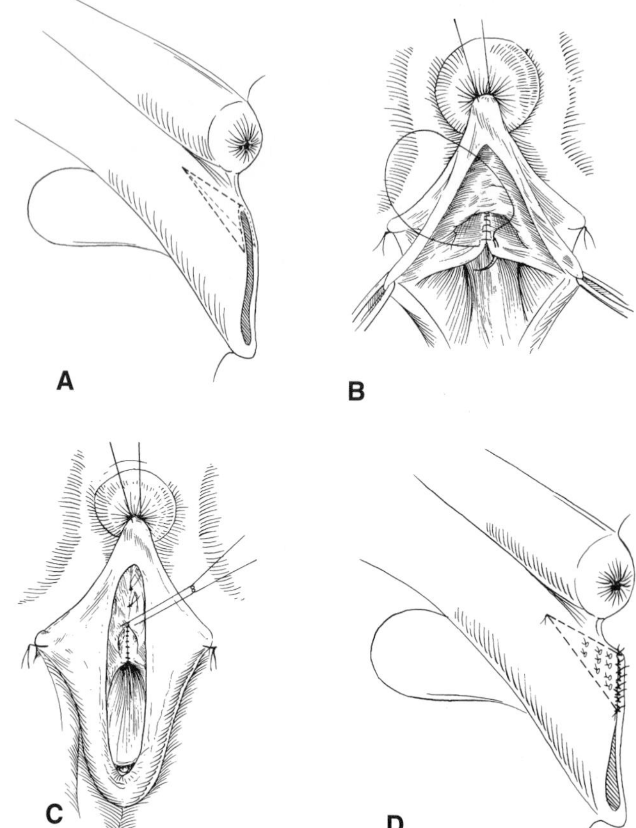

Figure 67-8. Perineal body repair. **A,** The triangular piece of mucosa to be excised from the dorsal vestibule is outlined. **B,** The dorsal portion of the vulva and vestibule are retracted caudally, and the vestibular mucosa is closed. **C,** Submucosal tissues are apposed with a series of interrupted absorbable sutures. **D,** The vulva should be in a more vertical position.

Urovagina may result from excessive closure of the vulvar cleft.[29] Closure is considered excessive if a tube speculum cannot be readily passed.[28] Some mares have such poor perineal conformation that performing a Caslick procedure predisposes them to urovagina. In such cases, an alternative surgical procedure to correct the pneumovagina or a procedure to correct urovagina is necessary (see later).

In mares that have had a Caslick procedure, an episiotomy should be performed 2 weeks prior to foaling to prevent damage to the vulva and perineum during the foaling process.

PERINEAL BODY RECONSTRUCTION

Reconstruction of the perineal body is useful when the vulvar and vestibular constrictor muscles have become ineffective.[25] Damage to the perineal body occurs from repeated stretching of these muscles in older multiparous mares, or from foaling trauma (second-degree rectovestibular injury). The goal of this surgery is restoration of the integrity of the dorsal aspect of the vestibule and return of vestibular sphincter function. The surgical procedure is termed an episioplasty, the Gadd technique, or perineal body reconstruction.[30]

The surgery is performed with the mare sedated and restrained in stocks. Epidural anesthesia or local infiltration is used to desensitize the surgery site. The labia are retracted to the side using towel clamps or stay sutures. An incision is made along the mucocutaneous junction of the labia in a dorsoventral direction and extending craniad along the dorsal commissure of the vestibule to the level of the vestibulovaginal sphincter. Dissection is continued submucosally from the dorsal and dorsolateral aspects of the vestibule. The triangular tissue flaps of mucosa are excised, and this approximates the shape of the perineal body. Using caudal dorsal retraction on the stay sutures, a position for closure of the tissues is chosen so that the vulva will have a more vertical orientation after the procedure is completed (Fig. 67-8).

Closure of the tissue layers begins with closure of the vestibular mucosa using 2-0 or 0 absorbable suture material in a horizontal mattress pattern, inverting the mucosa into the vestibule. The submucosal tissue is closed beginning at the cranial aspect of the vestibule using No. 0 or 1 absorbable suture material in an interrupted pattern. The labial skin is apposed as for the Caslick procedure. Four weeks of sexual rest is recommended after surgery. Since the diameter of the vestibule has been decreased by this procedure, some mares require an episiotomy at the time of foaling.[31]

PERINEAL BODY TRANSECTION

This technique is used to treat both pneumovagina and urovagina by the separation of muscular and ligamentous attachments between the rectum and the caudal reproductive tract.[32] The objective of this surgery is to return the vulva to a more natural conformation. The mare is sedated and restrained in stocks and epidural anesthesia or local infiltration of the perineal body is performed. A 4- to 6-cm horizontal skin incision is made midway between the ventral aspect of the anus and the dorsal commissure of the vulva. This incision is continued ventrad for 3 to 4 cm on both sides of the vulva. A combination of blunt and sharp dissection is utilized to extend the dissection in a cranial direction through the muscles of the perineal body. The dissection is continued cranially for 8 to 14 cm until the connections between the rectum and caudal reproductive tract have been severed.[30] Placing a hand in the vestibule to help guide the dissection helps prevent inadvertent entry into the rectum or peritoneal cavity. The dissection should be continued until the vulva has attained a normal vertical position without applying traction (Fig. 67-9). No attempt is made to close the resulting dead space between the rectum and reproductive tract. Closure of the skin, either transversely or in a T-shaped configuration, has been suggested.[32,33] An alternative involves allowing the wound to heal by secondary intention, which should occur within 3 weeks.[25] Natural cover should be delayed until the surgery site has healed (3 weeks). Mares may be bred by artificial insemination immediately.

Urovagina

Vesicovaginal reflux is the accumulation or pooling of urine in the vaginal fornix of the mare.[29] *Urovagina* and *urine pooling* are terms that have also been used to describe this condition. This abnormality is most often seen in thin, multiparous mares in which the cranial vagina slopes ventrally. Stretching and relaxation of the supporting ligaments of the urogenital tract lead to the excessive cranioventral sloping of the vagina. Mares often have a sunken appearance to their anus and dorsal vulva and frequently have had a Caslick procedure performed.[34] Excessive closure of the dorsal vulva during a Caslick procedure may contribute to urine reflux by causing back-splash of urine into the vagina.[35] In young fillies that are experiencing urovagina, an ectopic ureter must be ruled out.[29]

The chronic presence of urine in the cranial vagina leads to vaginitis, cervicitis, and endometritis. These inflammatory conditions can interfere with the ability of the mare to conceive and carry a foal to term.[36]

Urovagina is diagnosed by finding an accumulation of urine in the fornix of the vagina during vaginoscopy. It is best to perform a speculum examination of the vagina during estrus, because some mares pool urine only when the reproductive tract is under the influence of increased circulating levels of estrogen.[29] Examination of the mare on several occasions and finding urine in the cranial aspect of the vagina confirms the diagnosis. The differential diagnosis of urine poling should include uterine infection with accumulation of exudate in the cranial vagina. Evaluation of the accumulated fluid using laboratory tests and cytology is often necessary. A cytologic evaluation of the fluid involves checking for bacteria, white blood cells, and calcium carbonate crystals. Creatinine and urea nitrogen testing can be performed on the fluid. Creatinine levels in accumulated urine can be expected to be at least two to three times serum creatinine levels.[29]

Surgical intervention is usually required for treatment of urine pooling.[35,37-39] Mares with poor body condition and the resulting abnormal perineal conformation can benefit from weight gain. Manual evacuation of urine from the cranial aspect of the vagina prior to breeding may improve conception rates, but this does not address the long-term negative side effects of urovagina. Definitive surgical treatment for vesicovaginal reflux involves modification of the external urethral orifice.

Caudal Relocation of the Transverse Fold

Caudal relocation of the transverse urethral fold was first described in 1972 by Monin. The Monin technique is beneficial only when the reflux and abnormal perineal conformation are minimal.[29,39] This procedure does not resolve severe vesicovaginal reflux and can make subsequent surgical procedures such as a urethral extension more difficult.

A Balfour retractor or stay sutures are utilized to provide access to the transverse fold of the external urethral orifice. The center of the fold is grasped with an Allis tissue forceps and retracted caudally toward the surgeon (Fig. 67-10). The transverse fold is incised in a horizontal plane, splitting it into dorsal and ventral shelves. Thumb forceps are used to

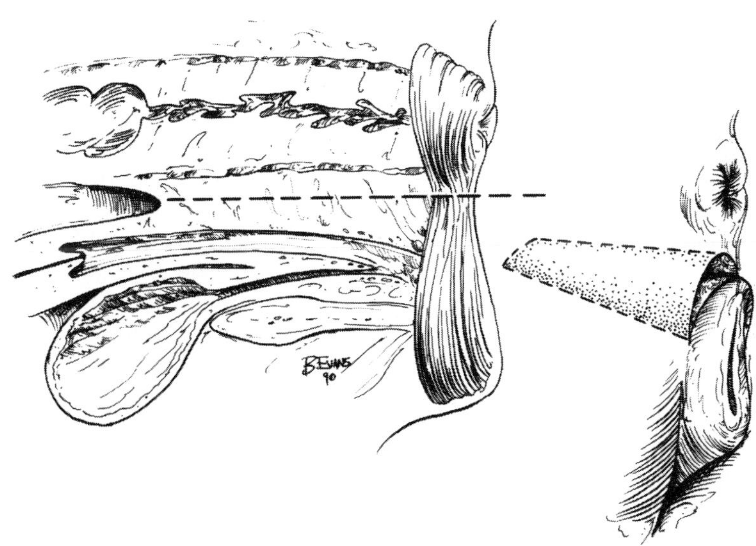

Figure 67-9. Perineal body transaction. Dissection between the rectum and caudal reproductive tract is performed until the vulva assumes a more vertical orientation.

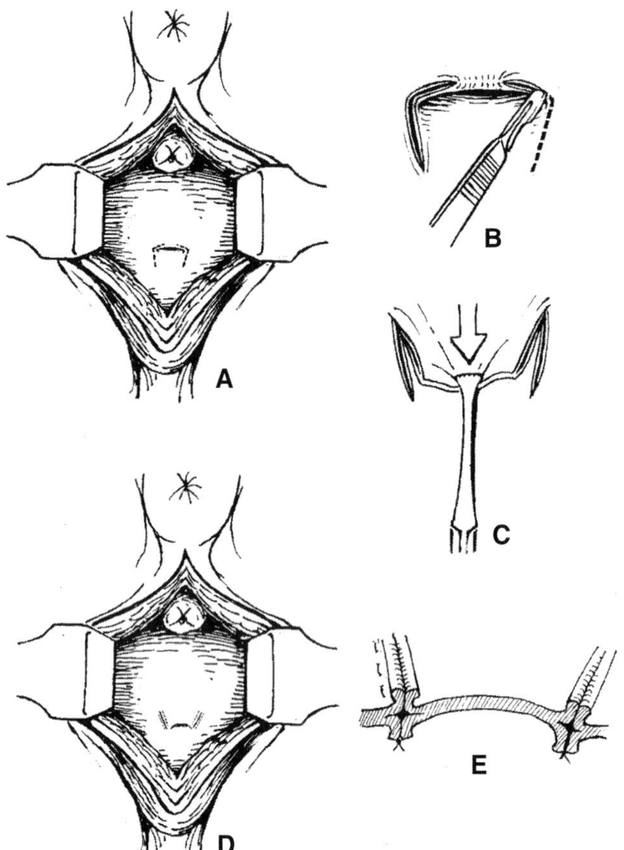

Figure 67-10. Monin urethroplasty. **A,** Incision of transverse fold of the urethra. **B,** Mucosal incisions are extended into the walls of the vestibule. **C,** Caudal retraction of the transverse fold in preparation for suturing. **D,** Completed Monin urethroplasty. **E,** Close-up cross-sectional view of the two-layer closure using a horizontal mattress pattern.

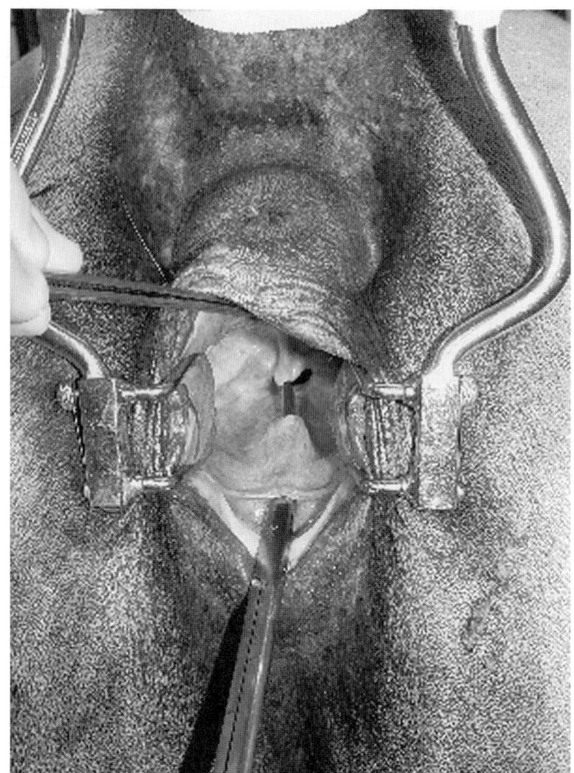

Figure 67-11. A failed urethral extension with fistula formation. The tips of scissors are sticking through the fistula.

position the transverse fold along the ventrolateral walls of the vestibule. Mucosal incisions are then made in the walls of the vestibule at the proposed site of attachment. The transverse urethral fold is sutured to the vestibular floor in the retracted position, creating the extension. A one- or two-layer closure may be performed using 2-0 absorbable suture material.[39] This technique creates a urethral orifice that opens 2.5 to 5 cm more caudally after completion of the procedure. It is important to position the transverse fold so that it is not placed under excessive tension. This technique is simple to perform but it has the disadvantage of not being able to extend the urethral opening as far caudally as other urethral extension procedures.[40]

Urethral Extension

Several urethral extension procedures have been described, and all have the advantage of being able to extend the urethral opening as far caudally as necessary.[35,37] A common pitfall of urethral extension procedures is fistula formation along the suture line.[40] In most instances, fistula formation must be repaired. However, the surgeon should wait until tissue inflammation has subsided before attempting another repair (Fig. 67-11).

The mare should be sedated and restrained in stocks, and epidural anesthesia should be administered to desensitize the perineum. Balfour retractors or stay sutures can be used to provide access to the surgical site. When self-retaining retractors are used, excessive lateral retraction should be avoided because this makes apposition of the vestibular mucosa more difficult. Insertion of a no. 30 French Foley catheter into the bladder ensures an adequate lumen diameter of the urethral extension and helps prevent urine contamination of the surgery site.

BROWN TECHNIQUE

The first urethral extension procedure, described in 1978, involves creating tissue flaps beginning at the level of the transverse urethral fold and continuing to just inside the labia.[35] The free edge of the transverse urethral fold is incised with a scalpel in a horizontal plane, creating dorsal and ventral tissue flaps of equal thickness (Fig. 67-12). It is important not to create holes in the flaps during the dissection. The transverse incision is continued caudally along the vestibular wall to create a dorsal and ventral shelf of vestibular mucosa and submucosa. Dissection dorsally and ventrally allows the flaps to be apposed on the midline without any tension. It is critical that the dissection generate tissue flaps large enough to result in a urethral tunnel of adequate diameter. The ventral shelves of tissue from opposing sites are sutured using 2-0 absorbable material in a continuous horizontal mattress pattern that inverts the mucosa of the ventral shelf into the new urethral lumen. The submucosa is closed using 2-0 absorbable suture material in a continuous

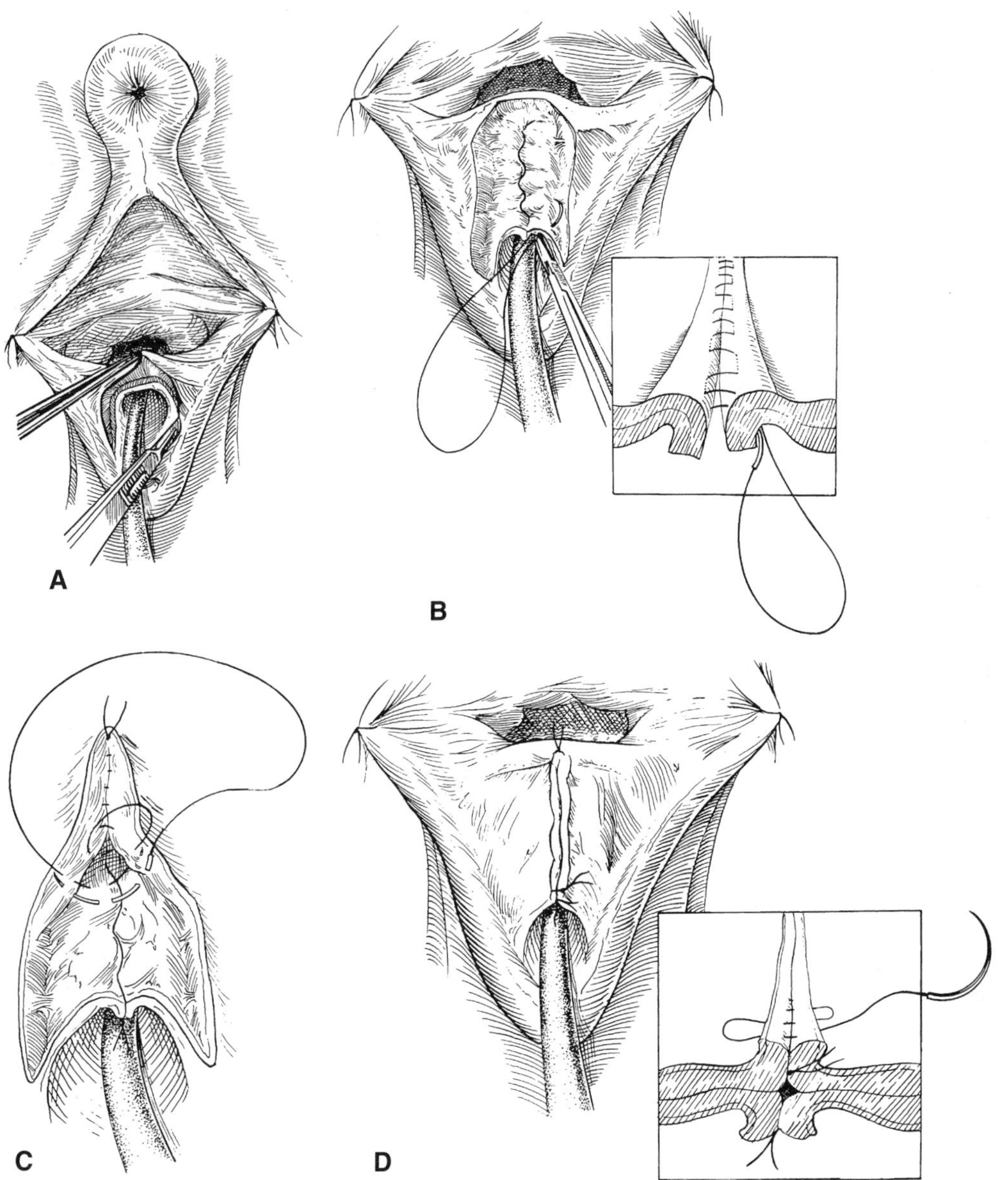

Figure 67-12. Brown technique for urethral extension. **A,** The transverse fold is split into dorsal and ventral shelves, and the incisions are continued caudally along the ventrolateral walls of the vestibule. **B,** The first suture line inverts the vestibular mucosa into the new urethral lumen. **C,** The second suture line apposes the submucosal tissues. **D,** The third suture line everts the vestibular mucosa into the vestibule.

pattern. The dorsal shelves are sutured using 2-0 absorbable suture material in a continuous horizontal mattress pattern that everts the mucosa into the vestibule. In the original description, urine pooling was resolved in 16 of 18 mares.[35] After surgery, 11 mares were bred and 7 of them conceived.[35]

SHIRES TECHNIQUE

The Shires technique also creates a urethral tunnel using mucosa from the floor of the vestibule around a Foley catheter placed in the bladder.[38] A No. 30 French Foley catheter is inserted through the urethral orifice into the bladder, and the balloon is inflated to secure the catheter (Fig. 67-13). Interrupted horizontal mattress sutures using 2-0 or 0 absorbable suture material are placed in the ventral vestibular mucosa and tied so that a tunnel is formed over the catheter. The sutures must be positioned so that there is minimal tension on the mucosa over the catheter. The tunnel must begin cranial to the urethral orifice and extend caudally to a point approximately 2 to 3 cm cranial to the vulva. The everted ridges of mucosa dorsal to the horizontal mattress sutures are excised using a scissors after the completion of the tunnel. The cut edges of the mucosa are apposed using 2-0 absorbable suture material in a continuous pattern. This procedure is relatively easy to perform and has been reported to be successful after a single surgery in 12 of 15 mares.[38]

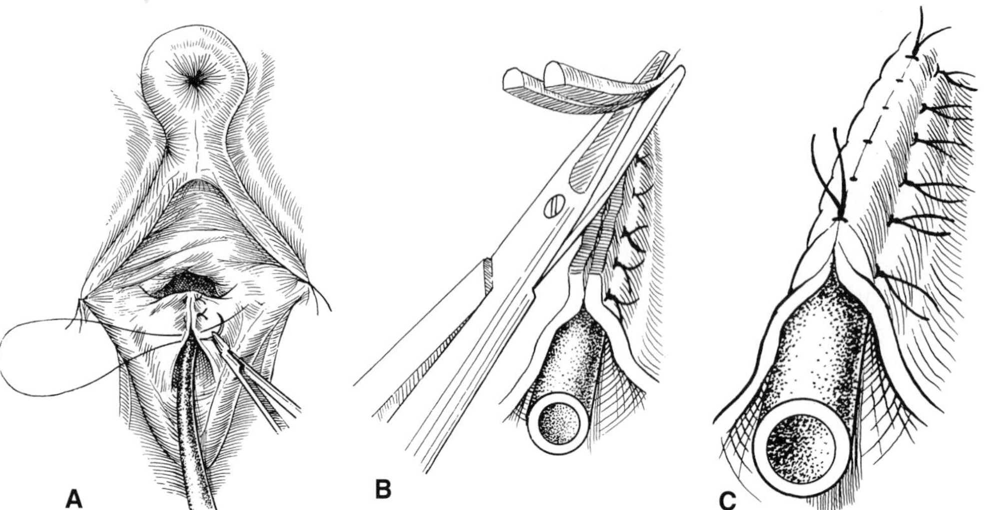

Figure 67-13. Shires technique for urethral extension. **A,** Vestibular mucosa is apposed over a Foley catheter using horizontal mattress sutures. **B,** The everted mucosal ridge is excised. **C,** The exposed submucosa is apposed using a continuous suture pattern.

MCKINNON TECHNIQUE

The McKinnon technique, described in 1988, results in a larger and stronger urethral tunnel than obtained by the Brown and Shires techniques.[37] A horizontal incision is made in the mucosa of the transverse fold of the urethra 2 cm cranial to the caudal free edge (Fig. 67-14). Incisions are made in the lateral walls of the vestibule approximately one-half the distance from the floor of the vestibule. Dissection of the tissue flaps continues in a ventral direction until the flaps can be apposed on midline without tension. The tissue flaps are sutured using a one-layer technique of 2-0 absorbable suture material in a continuous horizontal mattress pattern, inverting the mucosa into the lumen of the urethral tunnel. The initial dissection over the transverse urethral fold results in the cranial aspect of the closure assuming a Y-shaped pattern before the two suture lines meet on midline. Correction of urovagina using this technique was achieved in 32 of 34 mares, with fistula formation occurring in 5 of 34 mares.[37] Fistula formation is most common at the junction of the Y-suture pattern. The exposed submucosal tissue heals by secondary intention. Mares may be bred 1 month postoperatively.

COMBINED MCKINNON AND BROWN TECHNIQUE

Combining the McKinnon and Brown techniques for urethral extension has been reported.[36] The initial dissection is similar to that in the Brown technique. The caudal free edge of the transverse fold of the urethral orifice is incised into dorsal and ventral shelves of equal thickness (Fig. 67-15, *A* and *B*). It is important that no holes be created in these tissue layers during dissection. The incisions are continued caudally along the ventrolateral walls of the vestibule to a point approximately 2 cm cranial to the labia. Submucosal dissection is performed to create dorsal and ventral vestibular tissue flaps that can be apposed on midline and create a urethral lumen of adequate diameter. A no. 30 French Foley catheter can be inserted into the bladder to help determine the location of the incisions and prevent urine contamination of the surgical field (see Fig. 67-15, *C*). The dissection of the vestibular walls is not as dorsal as described for the McKinnon technique.

Closure of the tissue flaps is performed as follows. The midpoint of the caudal free edge of the transverse urethral fold is grasped with an Allis tissue forceps and retracted caudally (see Fig. 67-15, *D*). Suturing begins at the junction of the right ventral flap of the transverse fold and the right ventral flap of the vestibular wall. A continuous horizontal mattress pattern using 2-0 absorbable suture material is used (see Fig. 67-15, *D*). The mucosa of the ventral flaps should be inverted into the lumen of the urethral extension. During closure, it is important to retract the transverse fold caudally. This suture pattern is continued caudally to the midpoint of the transverse fold, and the suture is tied. The right dorsal flap of the transverse fold and the right dorsal flap of the vestibular wall are sutured next, using a continuous horizontal mattress pattern of 2-0 absorbable suture material that everts the mucosa into the vestibule (see Fig. 67-15, *E* [a]). The procedure is repeated for the left side. The remainder of the roof of the urethral tunnel is created by first suturing the right and left ventral vestibular tissue flaps and then the dorsal flaps. The ventral flaps are apposed using 2-0 absorbable suture material in a continuous horizontal mattress pattern, inverting the mucosa into the urethral lumen (see Fig. 67-15, *E*). The dorsal flaps are apposed using 2-0 absorbable suture material in a continuous horizontal mattress pattern, everting the mucosa into the vestibular lumen (see Fig. 67-15, *E* [c]). The most difficult part of the repair is at the junction of the Y of the three tissue layers—transverse urethral fold and right and left vestibular tissue flaps. This location is most prone to dehiscence and fistula formation. Therefore, a third layer of sutures using 2-0 absorbable suture material placed in a simple-continuous everting pattern around the circumference of the Y is used as shown in Figure 67-15, *E* (b). Maintaining a urinary catheter postoperatively for some time is based on surgeon preference (see Fig. 67-15, *F* and *G*).

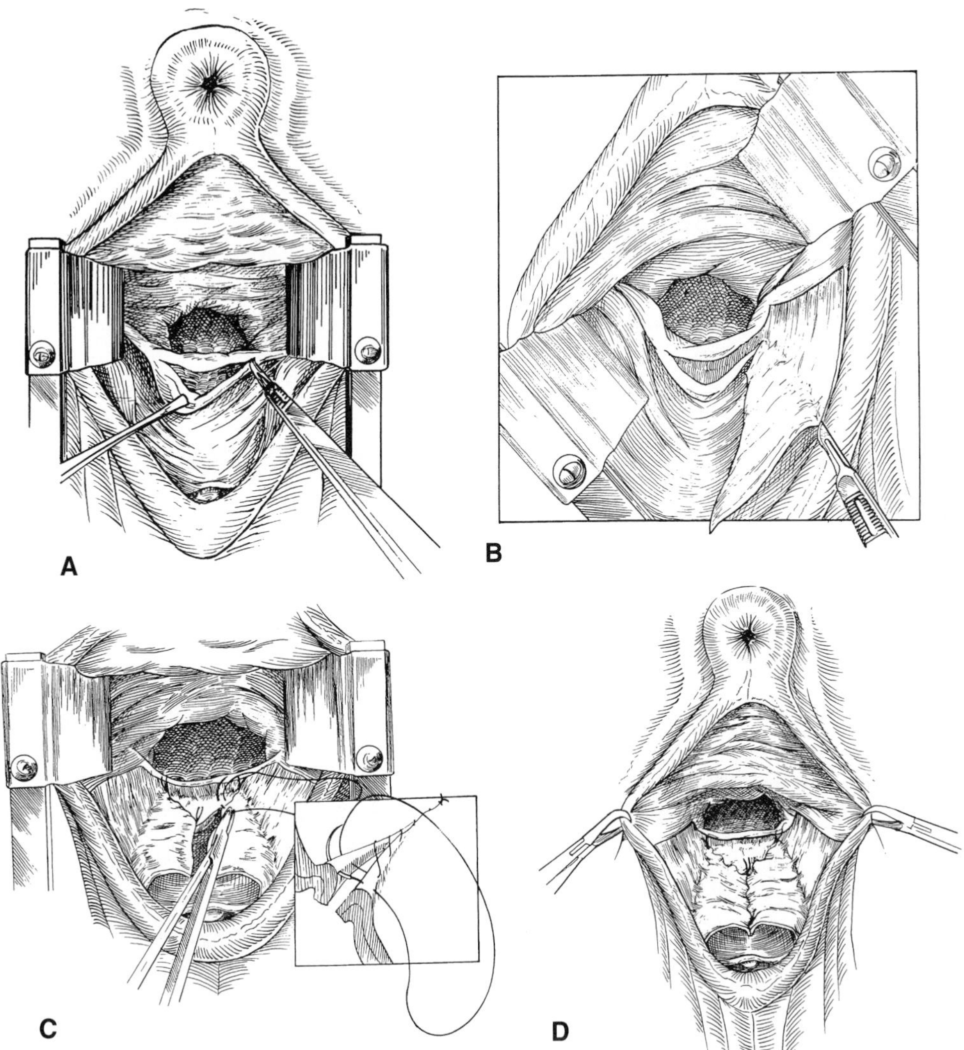

Figure 67-14. McKinnon technique for urethral extension. **A,** Horizontal incision in the mucosa of the transverse fold. **B,** Dissection is continued caudally high along the vestibular wall to create large tissue flaps. **C,** Apposition of the tissue flaps using a continuous horizontal mattress pattern. **D,** Completed urethral extension.

Foaling Injuries

Numerous types of injuries may be associated with parturition in the mare. Injuries caused by foaling and the resulting complications make up a large percentage of injuries to the perineum and cervix. Most injuries are obvious after foaling, but some are not apparent until it is time to rebreed the mare.

Perineal Lacerations

Perineal lacerations typically occur during unassisted foaling, most commonly in primiparous mares. These injuries are most likely caused by the prominence of the vestibulovaginal sphincter and remnants of the hymen in mares foaling for the first time.[41] It is hypothesized that the forefoot of the foal catches on the dorsal transverse fold of the vestibulovaginal junction, and the mare's abdominal press forces the foal's foot into the roof of the vestibule. Perineal lacerations have been classified into first-, second-, and third-degree lacerations, based on the extent and severity of the injury.[11,42] First-degree perineal lacerations involve the mucosa of the vestibule and the skin of the dorsal commissure of the vulva. Second-degree perineal lacerations involve vestibular mucosa and submucosa and continue into the muscles of the perineal body, including the constrictor vulvae muscle. These injuries do not involve the anal sphincter or rectum. This injury compromises the closure of the labia, predisposing the mare to pneumovagina.

Third degree perineal lacerations are complete disruptions of the rectovestibular shelf, penetrating the rectum, perineal body, and anal sphincter. These injuries result in a common opening between the rectum and the vestibule (Fig. 67-16) and often occur in primiparous mares that have an excitable temperament. Fetal malposition, large fetal size, or aggressive assistance during delivery may play a role in the development of a third-degree perineal laceration. However, when the foal's foot perforates the vestibule and enters the mare's rectum, a rectovestibular fistula results if a

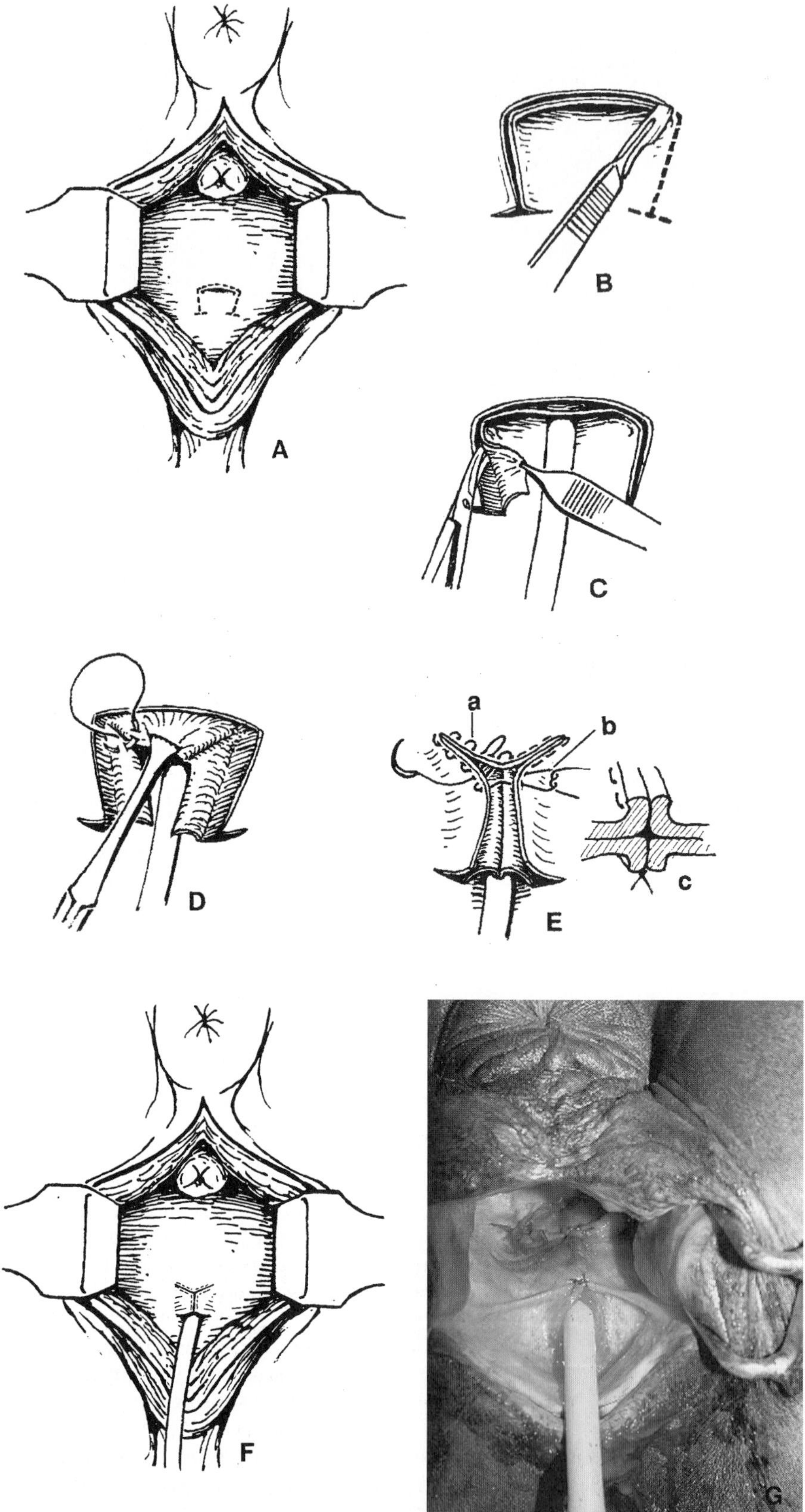

Figure 67-15. A, The scalpel is used to split the free edge of the transverse fold into dorsal and ventral shelves. **B** and **C,** Dorsal and ventral mucosal shelves are created by undermining the vestibular mucosa. The dissection should allow the shelves to meet on the midline without tension. **D,** The midpoint of the horizontal shelf is retracted caudally, and the ventral shelf is closed using a continuous horizontal mattress pattern to invert the tissue into the newly created urethral tunnel in a Y pattern. **E,** (a) The dorsal shelves are sutured using a continuous horizontal mattress pattern to evert the tissue into the vestibule. (b) An additional continuous everting suture is placed around the three portions of the Y and tied at the end to provide further support to this very vulnerable location. (c) Close-up view of the new urethral shelf with the two everting patterns. **F,** The completed urethral extension. **G,** A clinical case showing the urinary catheter in place.

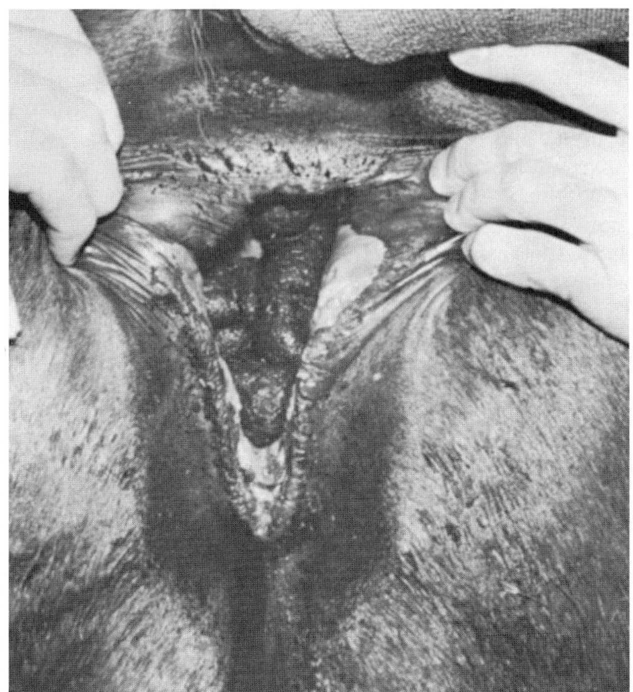

Figure 67-16. Third-degree perineal laceration with fecal contamination of the vestibule. Contamination of the vagina and uterus will occur if the vestibulovaginal sphincter is dysfunctional.

foaling attendant is present to replace the foal's foot back into the vestibule or if the foal retracts its foot; otherwise, a third-degree perineal laceration ensues as foaling continues with the foot in the rectum.

First-degree injuries typically do not require surgical intervention. If needed, a Caslick procedure can be performed. Repair of second-degree injuries requires a Caslick procedure and reconstruction of the perineal body. The mare will develop a sunken perineum and be predisposed to pneumovagina and urovagina if the perineal body is not reconstructed.[43] All third-degree perineal lacerations require surgical repair. The management is divided into two parts: immediate treatment and delayed surgical repair. Repair of a third-degree perineal laceration in the acute stage should not be attempted. The tissue is very edematous and contaminated with feces, and some tissues may not be viable (Fig. 67-17). Repair should be delayed at least 3 to 4 weeks, or longer if possible, to allow healing of the injured tissues (Fig. 67-18). Initial therapy should include daily wound care and cleaning of the contaminated tissues. Third-degree perineal lacerations result in continuous bacterial contamination of the vagina and uterus. However, the inflammatory uterine changes are reversible after surgical repair. A uterine biopsy is not needed because preoperative uterine biopsy grades do not correlate with conception data after surgery.

Initially, dietary changes may be necessary so that the mare has soft feces without an excessive amount of water content, to limit uterine contamination. Many methods can be used to soften the feces. Pasturing the mare on lush green grass, administering laxatives such as mineral oil or magnesium sulfate via a nasogastric tube, and feeding wet bran mashes are a few examples. Additional dietary changes should be instituted well before surgery so the fecal consistency is soft by the date of surgery. If the mare has firm formed feces, the surgery should be postponed because dehiscence of the surgical repair is likely. Often, the surgery is delayed until the foal is weaned, so that the foal does not have to enter the hospital environment. However, the timing of the surgery may be dictated by the urgency to get the injury repaired and the mare rebred.

Surgery is performed with the mare sedated and restrained in stocks. The use of epidural anesthesia is necessary. After surgery, soft fecal consistency should be maintained for at least 2 to 3 weeks.

TWO-STAGE REPAIR

The Aanes technique or a two-stage repair is designed to minimize obstipation, which can lead to failure of the repair.[42] In the first stage of the repair, the rectovestibular shelf is reconstructed without repair of the perineal body. Three to 4 weeks later, the second stage, or perineal body repair, is performed.

Balfour retractors or stay sutures can be used to provide access to the surgical site. Initial dissection begins cranially in a frontal plane at the level of the rectovestibular shelf.

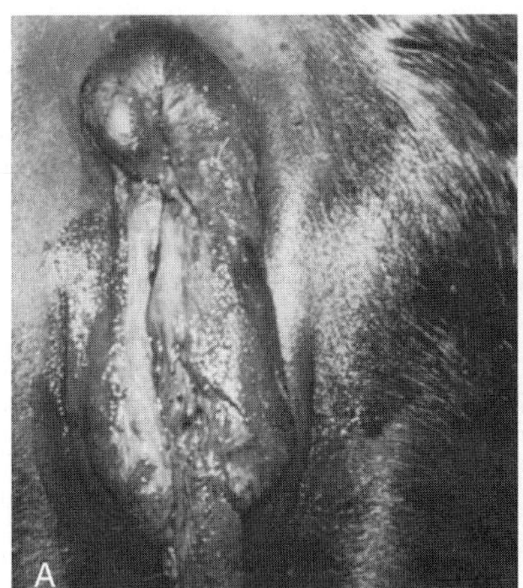

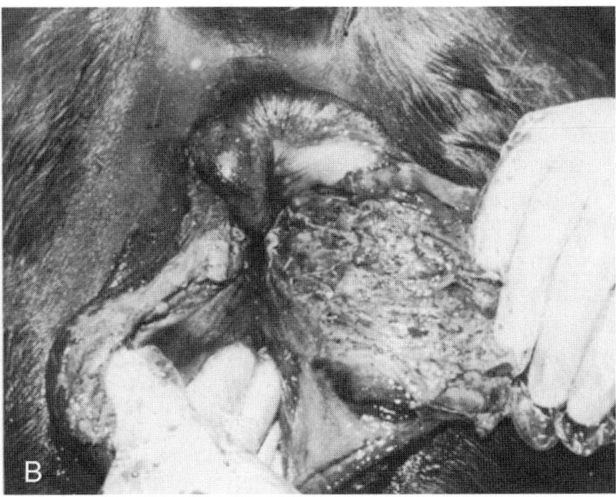

Figure 67-17. A, The vulva and perivulvar tissues are very edematous. **B,** Third-degree perineal laceration with edematous and necrotic tissue.

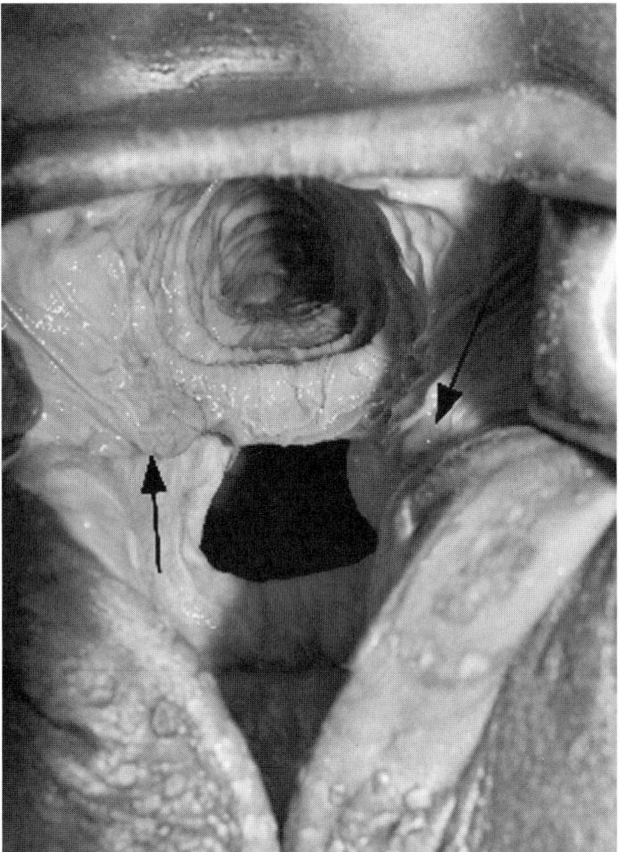

Figure 67-18. Third-degree perineal laceration ready for repair. The rectal mucosa overhangs the intact shelf at the cranial extent of the laceration. *Arrows* point to the junction of the rectal mucosa and the vestibular mucosa.

Thumb forceps can be used to place tension on the rectovestibular shelf to facilitate dissection. A combination of sharp and blunt dissection is used to divide the tissue into rectal and vestibular shelves (Fig. 67-19). The rectal shelf should make up two thirds of the thickness, and the vestibular shelf one third. The plane of dissection is continued cranially for a distance of 3 to 5 cm. The cranial dissection is important to relieve tension at the tissue edges. The incisions are continued laterally and caudally through the scar tissue that has formed at the junction of the rectal mucosa and the vestibular mucosa. The dissection is continued laterally until the tissue shelves can be apposed on the midline without tension. Hemostasis using ligatures can be performed if necessary. Once sufficient dissection has been achieved, reconstruction of the tissue shelves can commence.

The first stage of the repair is composed of two suture lines. The first suture line apposes the vestibular shelves. A continuous horizontal mattress pattern of no. 1 or 2 absorbable suture material is used to invert the vestibular mucosa into the vestibule. This pattern should be interrupted when approximately one quarter to one half of the vestibular defect is closed. This allows easier access for placement of the second line of sutures, which is placed dorsal to the first in an interrupted fashion in the perirectal and perivestibular tissues. Absorbable suture material (no. 1 or 2) is placed in a four-bite pursestring fashion.[41] It is crucial that the rectal mucosa not be penetrated. The four-bite pursestring is placed by taking the first bite in the subrectal mucosal layer on the right; the second, in the subvestibular mucosal tissue on the right; the third, in the subvestibular tissue on the left; and the fourth, in the subrectal mucosal tissue on the left, followed by tying of the knot. These two suture lines are continued caudally in an alternating fashion until the level of the dorsal commissure of the vulva is reached. Neither the anal sphincter nor the perineal body is repaired.

The second stage of the repair is performed 3 to 4 weeks later. It consists of removing the epithelium from the triangular surface of the perineal body and apposing these tissues on midline (Fig. 67-20) as was described in the section on perineal body reconstruction. The function of the anal sphincter is gained by suturing the tissues of the perineal body. No attempt is made to isolate and suture the muscle fibers of the anal sphincter. A Caslick procedure is performed, if necessary.

SINGLE-STAGE REPAIR

The initial dissection is the same in the single-stage repair as in the two-stage repair. The Goetze modification of the single-stage repair utilizes a six-bite suture pattern (Fig. 67-21). The suture is typically no. 2 absorbable material, and it is placed in an interrupted pattern. The first suture is placed at the cranial edge of the dissected shelf and follows this sequence:

The first bite is deep in the left vestibular flap in a ventral-to-dorsal direction.

The second bite is in the left rectal submucosa, taking care not to penetrate the rectal mucosa.

The third bite is in the right rectal submucosa.

The fourth bite is through the right vestibular flap in a dorsal-to-ventral direction.

The fifth bite re-enters the right vestibular shelf axial to the fourth bite in a ventral-to-dorsal direction.

The sixth bite is in the left vestibular flap from dorsal to ventral and is positioned axial to the first bite.

When the suture is tied, the rectal edges should be apposed and the vestibular edges should be everted into the lumen of the vestibule. The sutures should be placed approximately 1.5 cm apart. Any sutures that are loose or placed too far apart should be replaced; failure to do so will compromise the repair. Closure of the rectal mucosa has been proposed but is not necessary.[43] This repair is continued to a point approximately 4 to 6 cm cranial to the cutaneous perineum. At this point, the perineal body is repaired as previously described. A Caslick operation is performed if necessary.

The single-stage repair can be performed using the Aanes reconstruction technique as described for the two-stage repair. Another modification of the single-stage repair uses a three-layer closure that includes a continuous horizontal mattress suture in the vestibular submucosa and rectal submucosa, inverting each mucosa into its respective lumen.[44] Simple-interrupted sutures are placed in the connective tissue shelf between the rectum and vestibule. All three sutures are started cranially and continue in an alternating fashion toward the vulva.

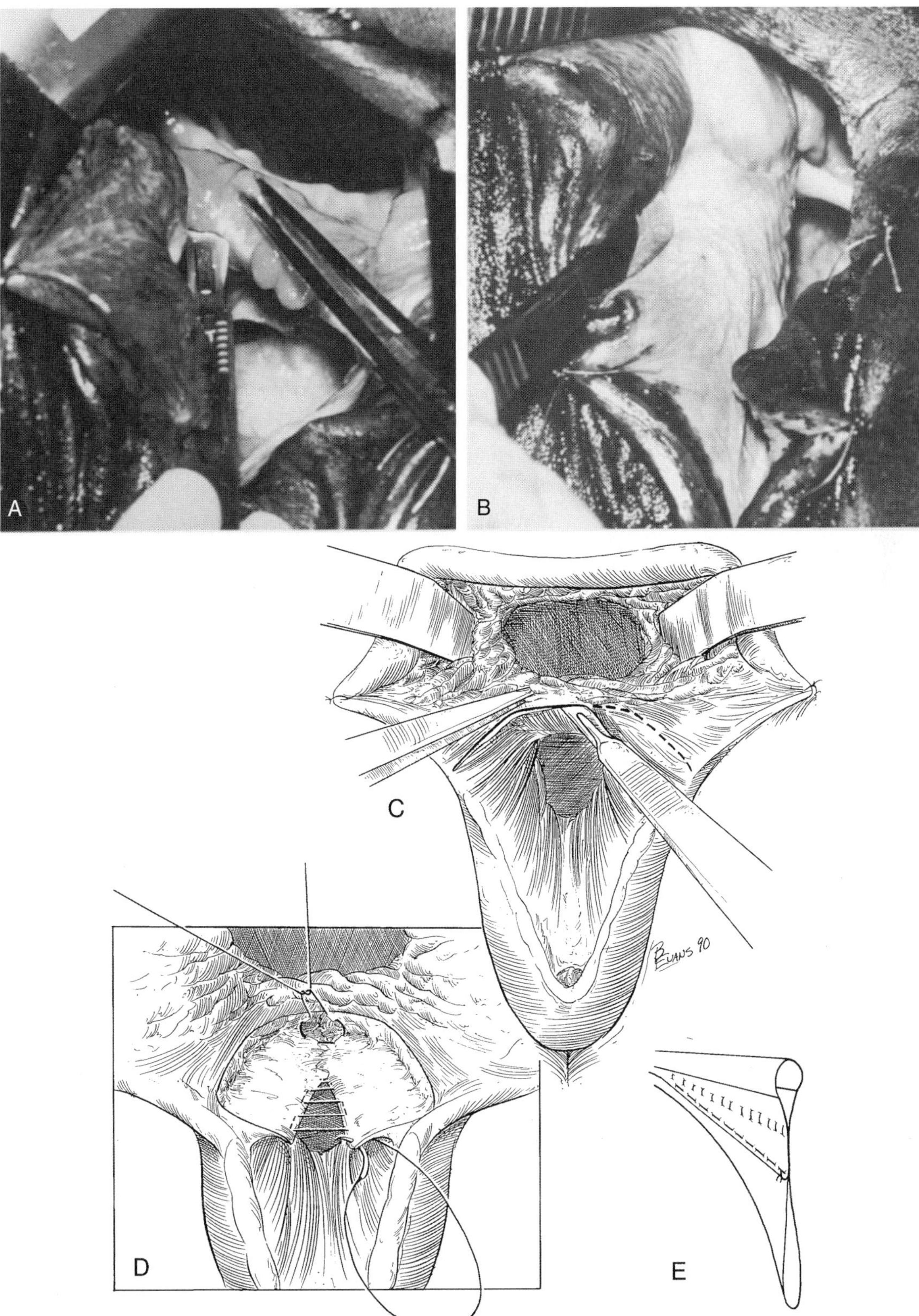

Figure 67-19. First stage of two-stage repair of a third-degree perineal laceration. **A,** The cranial-most extent of the rectovestibular shelf is incised in a horizontal plane. **B,** The junction between the rectal mucosa and the vestibular mucosa is delineated by a thin line of scar tissue. **C,** Vestibular and rectal tissue flaps are created by dissecting along the line of scar tissue. **D,** The vestibular mucosa is inverted into the vestibule using a continuous horizontal mattress pattern. The submucosal tissues are apposed using an interrupted pattern. **E,** Completed first-stage repair.

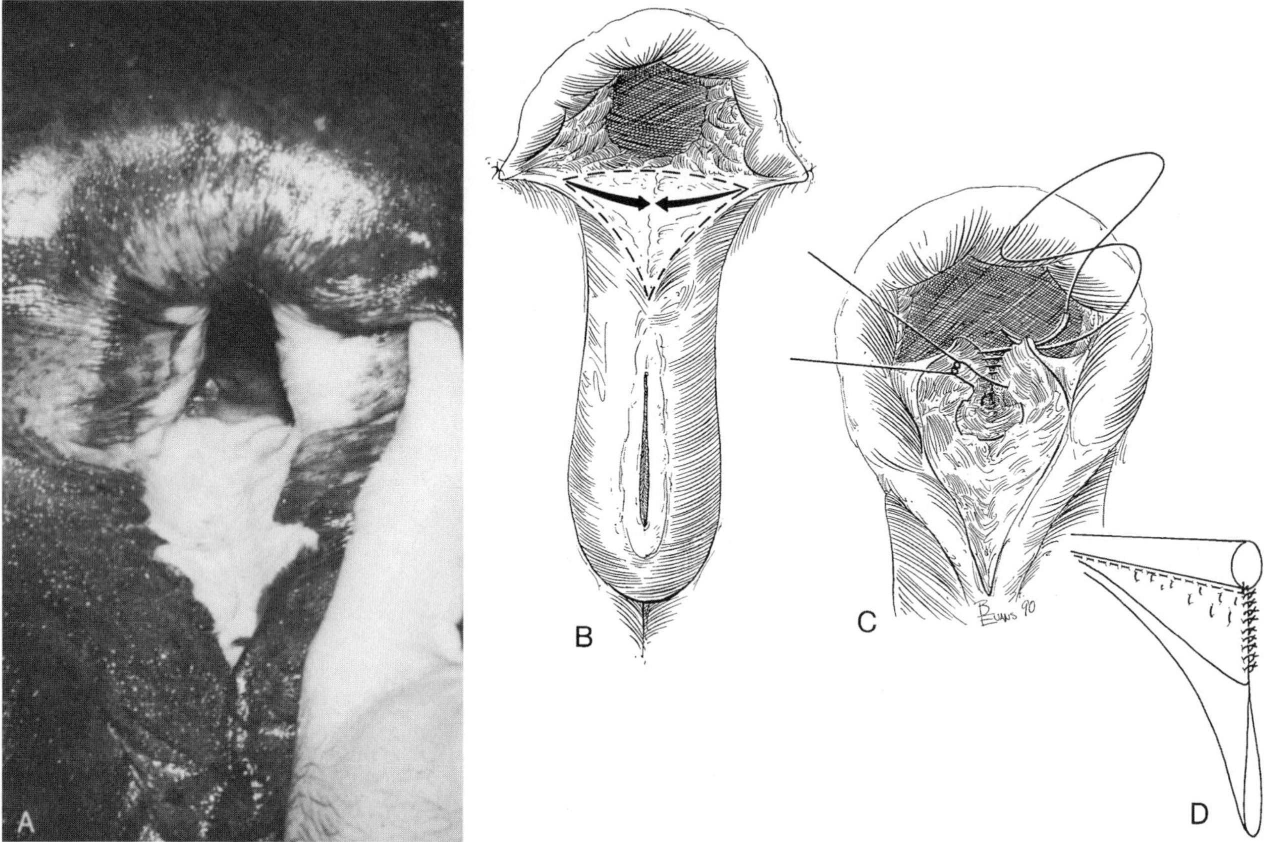

Figure 67-20. Second stage of a two-stage repair of a third-degree perineal laceration: **A,** The first stage of the repair has healed and the mare is ready for the second stage of the repair. **B,** The area of epithelialized tissue that is to be excised is outlined. **C,** The submucosal tissues are apposed using interrupted pursestring sutures. This reconstructs the perineal body. **D,** Completed second stage of repair.

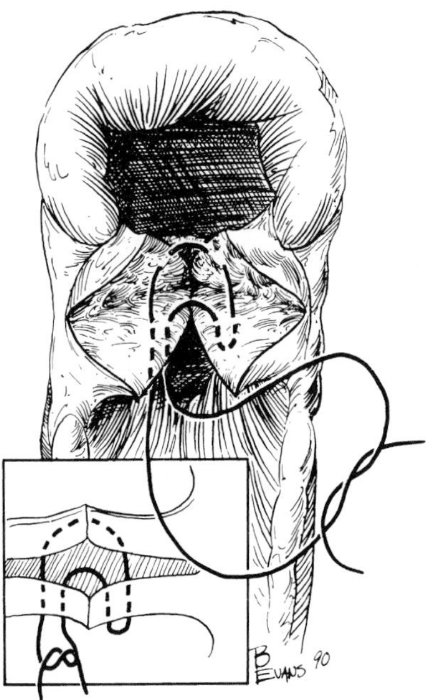

Figure 67-21. Drawing of the six-bite suture pattern used to appose tissues in a single-stage repair.

Rectovestibular Fistula

Rectovestibular fistula formation is the result of a perineal laceration from the dorsum of the vestibule into the rectum, without disruption of the anal sphincter (Fig. 67-22). These fistulas can form secondary to an unsuccessful repair of a third-degree rectovestibular laceration. Small fistulas sometimes close with conservative therapy, but larger ones require surgical repair.[40] Fistulas are most commonly 3 to 5 cm in diameter and located cranial to the perineal body.[43] Surgical approaches include conversion of the fistula into a third-degree perineal laceration, a horizontal approach through the perineal body, and a direct suturing technique.

A horizontal skin incision is made midway between the ventral aspect of the anus and the dorsal commissure of the vulva (Figs. 67-23 and 67-24, *A*). A combination of blunt and sharp dissection is used to separate the perineal body. This plane of dissection is continued through the fistula for a distance of 3 cm. Stay sutures or Allis tissue forceps can be used to help retract the tissue during dissection. It is important not to penetrate into the rectum or vestibule before reaching the fistula. The dissection should be such that the rectal shelf of tissue is thicker (two thirds of the thickness) than the vestibular shelf (one third of the thick-

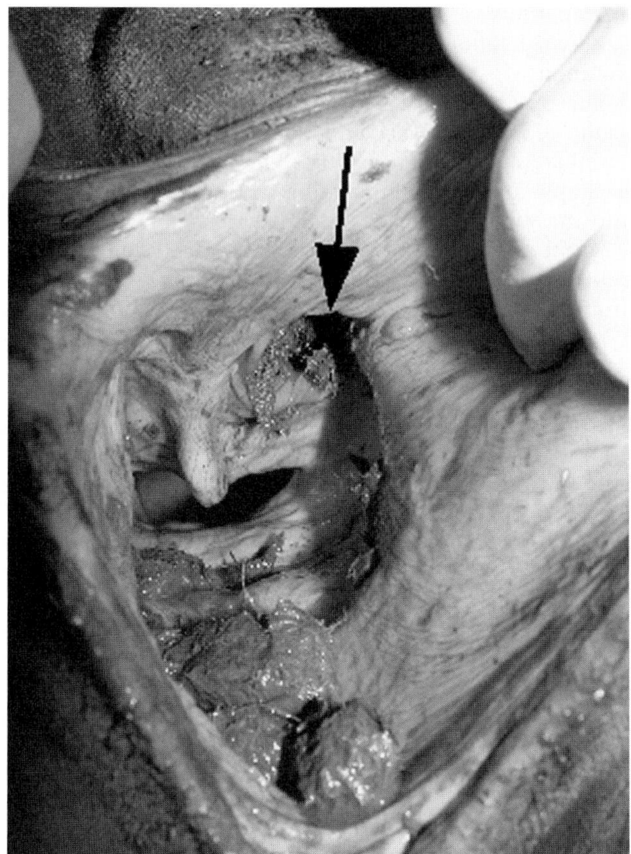

Figure 67-22. Rectovestibular fistula with manure contaminating the vestibule. *Arrow* points to the fistula.

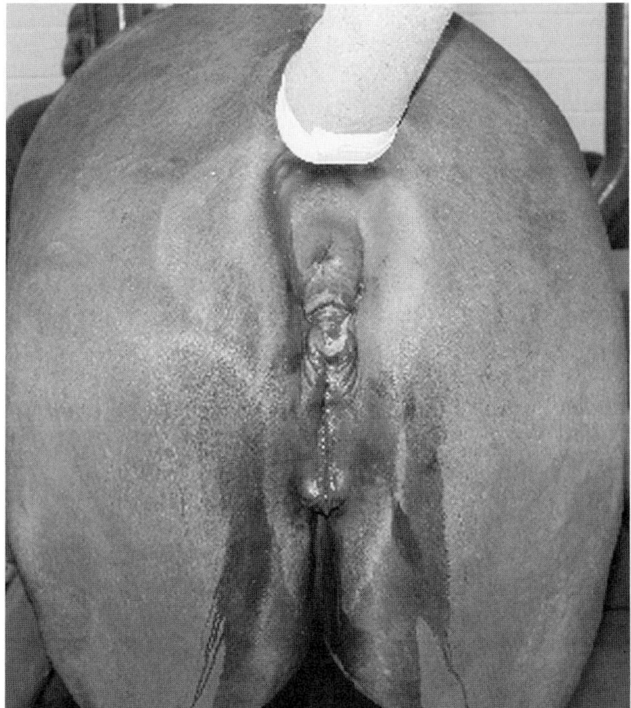

Figure 67-23. The perineal body approach for rectovestibular fistula repair.

ness). The fistula in the rectal tissue is closed transversely using an interrupted Lembert pattern of no. 0 absorbable suture material. The fistula in the vestibular shelf is closed longitudinally in a continuous horizontal mattress pattern. This results in the suture lines being oriented at right angles to one another (see Fig. 67-24, *C*). The dead space created by the approach is closed using interrupted pursestring sutures. The skin is closed with a continuous or an interrupted pattern. An alternative is to allow the dead space and skin to heal by secondary intention.[11]

Direct suturing techniques have been described for successful repair of rectovestibular fistulas.[45,46] Recently, a mucosal pedicle flap technique for repair of rectovestibular fistulas was described.[47] This technique is performed as a standing procedure. The edges of the fistula are débrided by full-thickness excision of 2 mm of the margin of the fistula. The fistula dimensions are assessed and a dorsally based U-shaped mucosal and submucosal pedicle flap is dissected from the vestibular wall. The flap is rotated 90 degrees so

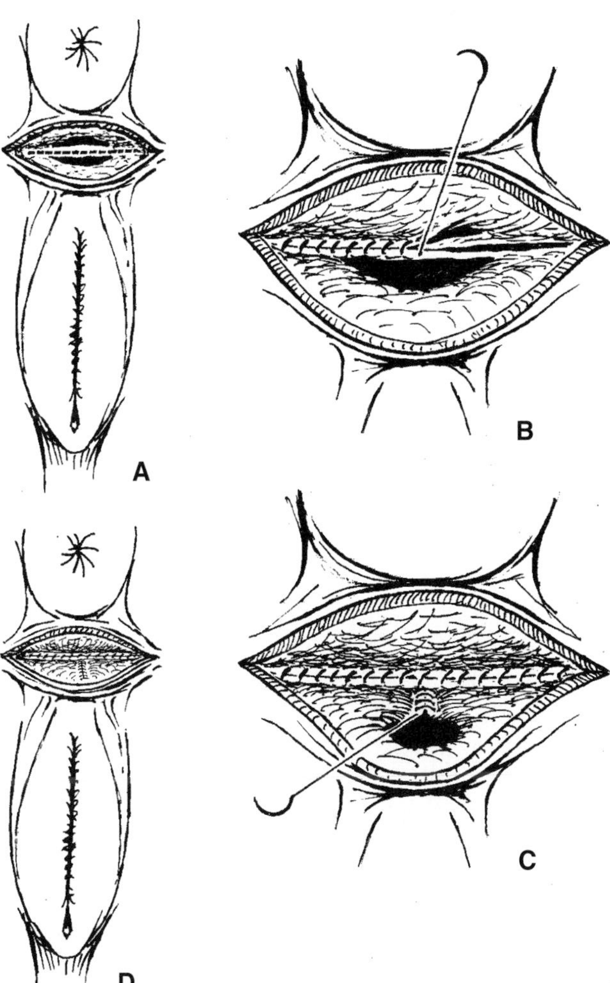

Figure 67-24. Repair of a rectovestibular fistula. **A,** Completed dissection showing the fistula divided into rectal and vestibular shelves. **B,** The rectal shelf is sutured transversely. **C,** The vestibular shelf is sutured longitudinally. **D,** The rectovestibular fistula is repaired. The dead space created by the approach can now be closed.

that the vestibular mucosa is continuous with the rectal mucosa covering the fistula. The flap is sutured in place using absorbable suture material placed in an interrupted pattern. Two of the three horses treated with this technique healed by primary intention. The third horse required additional sutures to repair a partial dehiscence.[47]

Cervical Injuries

Injuries to the cervix usually occur during foaling. They result from stretching, tears, and lacerations and have significant adverse effects on fertility. Cervical injuries can be placed into three categories related to their repair: lacerations, adhesions, and incompetence.

Lacerations

Lacerations of the cervix occur during foaling, as a result of excessive stretching until the musculature tears, often along with the mucosa. Cervical injury is more likely to develop during dystocia or in association with a fetotomy.[48] Cervical lacerations have been reported to occur during normal parturition and during the abortion of a relatively small fetus.[24] Laceration of the cervix has also been reported following breeding.[24] The incidence of cervical lacerations is reported to be higher when parturition is induced.[42] This may be the result of the cervix not relaxing adequately prior to foaling.

The most common clinical signs associated with cervical lacerations are failure to conceive, endometritis, early fetal abortion, and persistent infertility. All mares that have undergone dystocia should have their cervix examined approximately 21 days postpartum[49] (Fig. 67-25). Palpation of the cervix is crucial to making a diagnosis of a cervical laceration. Lacerations can be easily missed on visual examination alone, because the mucosa will have healed over the lacerated or separated musculature of the cervix. Lacerations can even be missed on palpation, especially if the mare is near estrus and has a relaxed cervix. Therefore, diestrus is the optimal time to evaluate the cervix. During this stage of the reproductive cycle, the cervix should be constricted in size, which allows an accurate determination of cervical continuity.

The cervix is evaluated in the follow manner. The perineum should be washed and prepared for examination. The examiner should wear a sterile glove or sleeve and apply an ample amount of lubricating jelly. The hand is inserted into the vagina of the mare and the cervix is identified at the most cranial aspect of the vaginal fornix. When using the right hand to examine the cervix, the examiner places the thumb in the lumen of the cervix and uses the index finger to palpate the cervix from the most dorsal aspect to the most ventral aspect of the right side of the cervix. To examine the left side of the cervix, the examiner inserts the index finger into the lumen and uses the thumb to palpate the cervix from the most dorsal to the most ventral aspect of the left side of the cervix. If a cervical laceration is present, the severity and extent should be determined. Not all cervical lacerations require surgical repair. It has been reported that surgery is unnecessary if 50% or less of the vaginal cervix is involved.[50] However, the economic impact of fetal loss must be considered, and if it is possible to improve the chances that a mare will conceive and carry the foal to term, surgical intervention is warranted.

Surgery should be performed during diestrus and at least 3 weeks postpartum. Alternatively, the repair can be performed immediately after the mare is bred (just after ovulation). The mare is sedated and restrained in stocks, and epidural anesthesia is used. A modified Finochietto retractor with long blades (Sontec Instruments) is very helpful in repairing cervical lacerations. Surgical interventions on the cervix should be performed in a caudally retracted position to bring it closer to the surgeon. Methods for retracting the cervix include Knowles cervical forceps and stay sutures (Fig. 67-26). The Knowles cervical forceps are more traumatic than stay sutures and are not necessary. Three stay sutures using large-diameter (no. 2) suture material are placed in the external cervical os by hand or with the aid of long needle holders. The stay sutures must be positioned to accentuate the cervical defect and so as not to interfere with

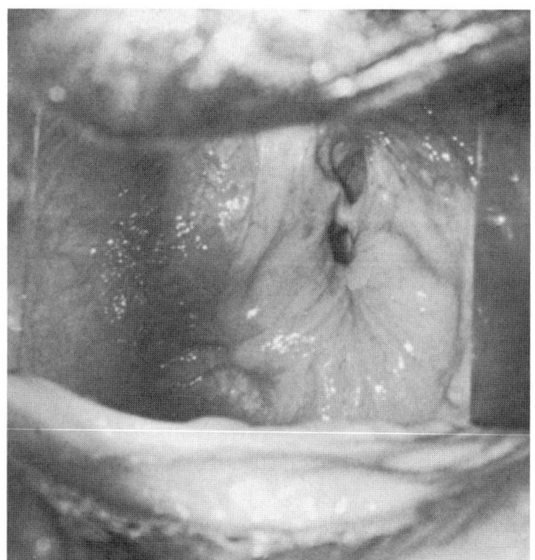

Figure 67-25. A dorsal cervical laceration as seen at speculum examination. Not all cervical lacerations are visible.

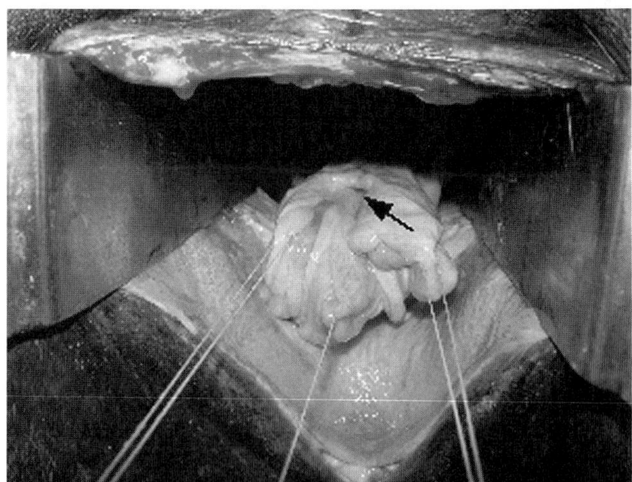

Figure 67-26. Stay sutures are used to retract the cervix into the vestibule to facilitate repair. The sutures are placed to accentuate the defect in the cervix. The *arrow* points to the defect.

the dissection and repair of the defect. The long ends of the stay sutures should be tagged with a hemostat and the needle removed. An assistant should apply gentle, steady caudal traction on the stay sutures so that the surgeon has access to the cervix. The cervix can usually be retracted to the level of the vestibulovaginal junction. Allis tissue forceps are used to grasp the caudal-most extent of the scar tissue on each side of the cervical laceration. The scar tissue is excised using a scalpel blade or a scissors. Following excision of the scar tissue, the three layers of cervical tissue should be evident.

Repair of the defect is accomplished by a three-layer closure. The first layer, the inner cervical mucosa, is the most difficult to close and probably the most important. This layer is closed using no. 0 or 1 absorbable suture material in a continuous horizontal mattress pattern to invert the mucosa into the cervical lumen, beginning at the most cranial aspect of the defect and working caudally. After each bite, the surgeon should check whether the cervical lumen was penetrated and to ensure the patency of the cervical lumen. The second layer in the cervical muscle is apposed using no. 1 absorbable suture material placed in a simple-continuous pattern. The third layer, the outer cervical mucosa, is closed using no. 1 absorbable suture material placed in a simple-continuous pattern. In a report of 53 mares, a 75% pregnancy rate was achieved after surgical repair of cervical lacerations.[51] The mare should not be bred for at least 30 to 45 days after surgery, unless breeding was completed just before repair.

Adhesions

Transluminal adhesions interfere with the normal opening and closing of the cervix.[49] Less severe adhesions may lead to infertility, whereas more severe adhesions can result in mucometra or pyometra.[16] Adhesions may form secondary to cervical trauma or cervical laceration repair. The more extensive the adhesions, the worse is the prognosis. Transluminal adhesions can be broken down manually or surgically. Daily topical application of steroid-based ointment to the cervical lumen has been recommended as a means of preventing the adhesions from re-forming.[16] Adhesions from the vaginal wall to the cervical os can be relieved by sharp and blunt dissection. The surgeon must be careful not to perforate the vaginal wall and enter the peritoneal cavity when working in the cranial aspect of the vagina.

Incompetence

Incompetence of the cervix can result from a tear that cannot be effectively repaired, it can result from muscle atony from repeated stretching, or it may be a congenital anomaly.[16,52,53] Mares with an incompetent cervix may fail to conceive or experience early fetal abortion. Correction of these cervical problems has met with varied success.[16] The use of a buried retention suture or a nonabsorbable suture used in purse-string fashion around the base of the external os has been described.[54] The authors recommended that the suture be placed during the first 48 hours after breeding and ovulation. The suture must be removed prior to foaling. The success of this type of procedure is not known.

Clitoral Disorders

Abnormal conditions of the clitoris are rare. Squamous cell carcinoma has been reported to affect the clitoris.[55] Smegma can become impacted in the clitoral sinuses.[56] The sinuses of the clitoris can harbor *Taylorella equigenitalis,* the causative agent of contagious equine metritis (CEM).[57]

Extirpation of the clitoral sinuses has been recommended as a treatment of mares affected by CEM. Sinusectomy is completed as a standing procedure using local anesthesia. The glans clitoridis is not excised. The frenulum clitoris, which is a fold of tissue overlying the clitoral sinuses, is retracted dorsally, and submucosal dissection is used to remove all clitoral sinus mucosa.[57] The resulting surgical wounds are left open to heal by secondary intention.

Congenital Anomalies

Congenital anomalies do not occur very often. Persistent hymen is the most frequently observed developmental anomaly of the mare's tubular genital system[58] (Fig. 67-27). The hymen may be imperforate or may be persistent in varying degrees because of failure of the caudal sections of the müllerian duct to fuse with the urogenital sinus. Failure of proper fusion of the müllerian ducts may result in a dorsoventral band in the cranial aspect of the vagina coursing across the external os of the cervix.[59] Surgical removal easily resolves both of these problems.

Developmental anomalies of the cranial vagina, cervix, and uterus are the result of partial or complete inhibition of müllerian ducts. These anomalies are rare but occur more frequently in the cervix than in the vagina or uterus. Reports of congenital cervical anomalies include cervical aplasia,

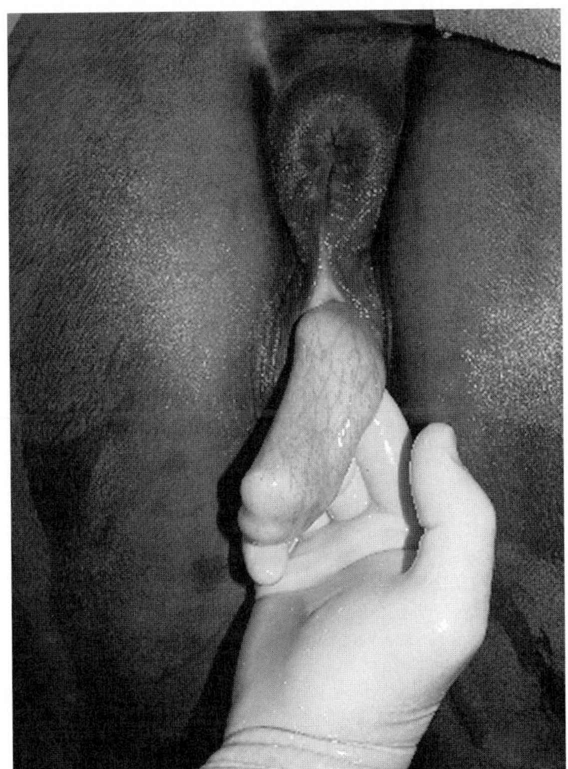

Figure 67-27. A young mare with an exteriorized persistent hymen.

double cervix, and congenitally incompetent cervix.[52,53] Segmental aplasia of portions of the reproductive tract are rarely seen and may be associated with mucometra.[16] Ovariohysterectomy is recommended as a salvage procedure.

Incomplete separation of the urorectal septum leads to the formation of a rectovestibular fistula.[60] This is often seen in conjunction with atresia ani. In addition to urogenital abnormalities, other anomalies may be present. Atresia ani may be a heritable condition in the horse; therefore, salvage of affected foals for breeding purposes is not advised.

REFERENCES

1. Habel RE: The perineum of the mare, Cornell Vet 1953;43:249.
2. Sisson S: The Anatomy of the Domestic Animals, ed 5, Philadelphia, 1975, WB Saunders.
3. Pascoe RR: Observations on the length and angle of declination of the vulva and its relation to fertility in the mare, J Reprod Fertil Suppl 1979;27:299.
4. Kainer RA: Reproductive organs of the mare. In McKinnon AO, Voss JL, editors: Equine Reproduction, Philadelphia, 1993, Lea & Febiger.
5. Ley WB: Examination of the vulva, vestibule, vagina, and cervix. In Wolfe DF, Moll HD, editors: Large Animal Urogenital Surgery, Baltimore, 1999, Williams & Wilkins.
6. Caslick EA: The vulva and the vulvo-vaginal orifice and its relation to genital health of the Thoroughbred mare, Cornell Vet 1937;27:178.
7. Ley WB: Anatomy and physiology of the female reproductive system. In Wolfe DF, Moll HD, editors: Large Animal Urogenital Surgery, Baltimore, 1999, Williams & Wilkins.
8. Vaughan JT: The female genital system. In Oehme FW, editor: Textbook of Large Animal Surgery, ed 2, Baltimore, 1988, Williams & Wilkins.
9. Jones PA, Sertich PS, Johnston JK: Uroperitoneum associated with ruptured urinary bladder in a postpartum mare, Aust Vet J 1996;74:354.
10. Rodgerson DH, Spirito MA, Thorpe PE: Standing surgical repair of cystorrhexis in two mares, Vet Surg 1999;28:113.
11. Embertson RE, Robertson JT: Parturient perineal and rectovestibular injuries. In Robinson NE, editor: Current Therapy in Equine Medicine, ed 2, Philadelphia, 1987, WB Saunders.
12. Pascoe JR, Pascoe RR: Displacements, malpositions, and miscellaneous injuries of the mare's urogenital tract, Vet Clin North Am Equine Pract 1988;4:439.
13. Hinchcliff KW, MacWilliams PS, Wilson DG: Seminoperitoneum and peritonitis in a mare, Equine Vet J 1988;20:71.
14. Simpson RB, Burns SJ, Snell JR: Microflora in stallion semen and their control with a semen extender, Proc Am Assoc Equine Pract 1975;21:257.
15. Blue MG: Genital injuries from mating in the mare, Equine Vet J 1985;17:297.
16. Vaughan JT: Equine urogenital system. In Jennings PB, editor: The Practice of Large Animal Surgery, Philadelphia, 1984, WB Saunders.
17. LeBlanc PH: Chemical restraint for surgery in the standing horse, Vet Clin North Am Equine Pract 1991;7:521.
18. Thurmon JC, Steffey EP, Ainkl JG, et al: Xylazine causes transient dose-related hyperglycemia and increased urine volume in mares, Am J Vet Res 1984;45:224.
19. Lowe JE, Hilfiger J: Analgesic and sedative effects of detomidine compared to xylazine in a colic model using IV and IM routes of administration, Acta Vet Scand 1986;82(Suppl):85.
20. Pleasant RS, McGrath CJ: Anesthetic techniques. In Wolfe DF, Moll HD, editors: Large Animal Urogenital Surgery, Baltimore, 1999, Williams & Wilkins.
21. Robinson EP, Natalini DD: Epidural anesthesia and analgesia in horses, Vet Clin North Am Equine Pract 2002;18:61.
22. LeBlanc PH, Caron JP, Patterson J, et al: Epidural injection of xylazine for perineal analgesia in horses, J Am Vet Med Assoc 1988;193:1405.
23. Grubb TL, Riebold TW, Huber MJ: Comparison of lidocaine, xylazine, and xylazine/lidocaine for caudal epidural analgesia in horses, J Am Vet Med Assoc 1992;201:1187.
24. Aanes WA: Surgical management of foaling injuries, Vet Clin North Am Equine Pract 1988;4:417.
25. Trotter GW, McKinnon AO: Surgery for abnormal vulvar and perineal conformation, Vet Clin North Am Equine Pract 1988;4:395.
26. Purswell BJ, Moll HD: Surgery of the vulva and perineum. In Wolfe DF, Moll HD, editors: Large Animal Urogenital Surgery, Baltimore, 1999, Williams & Wilkins.
27. Caudle AB, Purswell B, Williams DJ, et al: Skin staples for nonscarified Caslick procedures, Vet Med Small Anim Clin 1983;78:782.
28. Witherspoon DM: Some reflections concerning Caslick's surgery, ultrasonography and the treatment of uterine cysts, Equine Pract 1989;11:12.
29. Easley KJ: Diagnosis and treatment of vesicovaginal reflux in the mare, Vet Clin North Am Equine Pract 1988;4:407.
30. Trotter GW: The vulva, vestibule, vagina, and cervix. In Auer JA, Stick JA, editors: Equine Surgery, ed 2, Philadelphia, 1999, WB Saunders.
31. Trotter GW: Surgery of the perineum in the mare. In McKinnon AO, Voss JL, editors: Equine Reproduction, Philadelphia, 1993, Lea & Febiger.
32. Pouret EJM: Surgical technique for the correction of pneumo- and urovagina, Equine Vet J 1982;14:249.
33. Ricketts SW: Perineal conformation abnormalities. In Robinson NE, editor: Current Therapy in Equine Medicine, ed 2, Philadelphia, 1987, WB Saunders.
34. Madison JB: Surgery of the urinary tract. In Wolfe DF, Moll HD, editors: Large Animal Urogenital Surgery, Baltimore, 1999, Williams & Wilkins.
35. Brown MP, Colahan PT, Hawkins DL: Urethral extension for treatment of urine pooling in mares, J Am Vet Med Assoc 1978;17:1005.
36. Emberston RM: Urovagina. In White NW, Moore JN, editors: Current Practice of Equine Surgery, Philadelphia, 1990, JB Lippincott.
37. McKinnon AO, Belden J: A urethral extension technique to correct urine pooling (vesicovaginal reflux) in mares, J Am Vet Med Assoc 1988;192:647.
38. Shires GM, Kaneps AJ: A practical and simple surgical technique for repair of urine pooling in the mare, Proc Am Assoc Equine Pract 1986;32:51.
39. Monin T: Vaginoplasty: A surgical treatment for urine pooling in the mare, Proc Am Assoc Equine Pract 1972;18:99.
40. Beard WL: Standing urogenital surgery, Vet Clin North Am Equine Pract 1991;7:669.
41. LeBlanc MM: Third-degree rectovestibular lacerations and fistulas. In White NW, Moore JN, editors: Current Techniques in Equine Surgery and Lameness, ed 2, Philadelphia, 1998, WB Saunders.
42. Aanes WA: Surgical management of foaling injuries, Vet Clin North Am Equine Pract 1988;4:417.
43. Moll HD, Slone DE: Perineal lacerations and rectovestibular fistulas. In Wolfe DF, Moll HD, editors: Large Animal Urogenital Surgery, Baltimore, 1999, Williams & Wilkins.
44. Stickle RL, Fessler JF, Adams SB: A single-stage technique for repair of rectovestibular lacerations in the mare, Vet Surg 1980;9:66.
45. Huber MJ: Modified technique for single stage rectovestibular fistula closure in three mares, Equine Vet J 1998;30:82.
46. Adams S, Benker F, Brandenburg T: Direct rectovestibular fistula repair in five mares, Proc Am Assoc Equine Pract 1996;42:156.
47. Schonfelder AM, Sobiraj A: A vaginal mucosal pedicle flap technique for repair of rectovaginal fistula in mares, Vet Surg 2004;33:517.
48. Moll HD, May KA: Surgery of the vestibule, vagina, and cervix. In Wolfe DF, Moll HD, editors: Large Animal Urogenital Surgery, Baltimore, 1999, Williams & Wilkins.

49. Easley KJ, Osborne J, Thorpe PE: Surgery for conditions causing decreased fertility in mares: Case selection, Vet Clin North Am Equine Pract 1988;4:381.
50. Brown JS, Varner DD, Hinrichs K, et al: Surgical repair of the lacerated cervix in the mare, Theriogenology 1984;22:351.
51. Miller C, Embertson R, Smith S: Surgical repair of cervical lacerations in Thoroughbred mares: 53 cases (1986-1995), Proc Am Assoc Equine Pract 1996;42:154.
52. Blanchard TL, Evan LH, Kenney RM, et al: Congenitally incompetent cervix in a mare, J Am Vet Med Assoc 1982;181:266.
53. Allen WE: A cervical anomaly in an Arabian filly, Equine Vet J 1981;13:268.
54. Evans LH, Tate LP, Cooper WL, Robertson JT: Surgical repair of cervical lacerations and the incompetent cervix, Proc Am Assoc Equine Pract 1979;25:483.
55. Cox JE: Surgery of the Reproductive Tract in Large Animals, ed 3, Liverpool, 1987, Liverpool University Press.
56. Bigby NJ, Ricketts SW: A method for clitoral sinusectomy in mares. In Practice 1982;4:145.
57. Zent WW: Surgical removal of the clitoral sinus(es) for elimination of the contagious equine metritis carrier state in mares. In Proc Int Symp Equine Venereal Diseases, 1979:43.
58. McEntee K: Reproductive Pathology of Domestic Animals, San Diego, 1990, Academic Press.
59. Hughes JP: Developmental anomalies of the female reproductive tract. In McKinnon AO, Voss JL, editors: Equine Reproduction, Philadelphia, 1993, Lea & Febiger.
60. Robertson JT, Embertson RM: Surgical management of congenital and perinatal abnormalities of the urogenital tract, Vet Clin North Am Equine Pract 1988;4:359.

CHAPTER 68

Ovaries and Uterus

Rolf M. Embertson

ANATOMY

The ovaries in the mare are about 70 to 80 mm long and 40 to 60 mm wide, but the size varies depending on the season and stage of the estrous cycle.[1] The ovaries are generally kidney shaped, with a palpable indentation representing the ovulation fossa. The cranial aspect of the broad ligament, which contains the ovarian blood supply, the ovarian branch of the ovarian artery, suspends the ovaries.[1]

The funnel-shaped infundibulum of the oviduct is positioned adjacent to the ovulation fossa of the ovary. The oviduct (uterine tube) becomes very tortuous as it courses to the tip of the uterine horn, where it enters the uterus at the tubal papilla.[1]

The uterine horns, which lie entirely within the abdominal cavity, extend caudally to the uterine body. Part of the uterine body is positioned in the peritoneal cavity and part is retroperitoneal. The uterine body ends caudally as the thick-walled muscular cervix, which projects into the cranial vagina. The uterus is suspended in the caudal abdomen by the broad ligament, which contains vessels, nerves, lymphatics, fat, connective tissue, and some smooth muscle. It receives its blood supply via the uterine branch of the vaginal artery, the vaginal artery, and the uterine branch of the ovarian artery.[1]

DIAGNOSTIC PROCEDURES

Advanced diagnostic procedures used to evaluate the cranial reproductive tract of the mare have improved the general understanding of the potential disease processes involved. Competence with these procedures, particularly ultrasonography and endoscopy, has permitted more rapid and accurate diagnoses, yielding more successful treatment regimens. Despite the benefit gained from these technologies, a complete history and a thorough physical examination are still the foundation of the diagnostic workup. Palpation often provides as much, if not more, information than visualization of some disorders. This includes rectal, vaginal, and external palpation. The results of blood work, culture, cytology, and histology are commonly used diagnostic aids. Ultrasonography has been used extensively in evaluating the reproductive tract and the abdomen for abnormalities. Hysteroscopy is now a routine technique, and the uses of the laparoscope are well recognized.

PREPARATION FOR SURGERY

Decreasing the volume of ingesta within the intestinal tract generally facilitates elective procedures involving the abdomen, so withholding food for about 24 hours is recommended. However, disruption of a horse's routine may increase the risk of developing intestinal abnormalities. Many of the disorders involving the uterus are of an emergency nature, requiring well-trained personnel to assist in the management of these conditions.

Anesthesia and Analgesia

Standing surgery of the cranial reproductive tract requires profound sedation, visceral analgesia, and local anesthesia. Xylazine, detomidine, and butorphanol are often used in combination for sedation and analgesia. Epidural anesthesia may help facilitate some procedures. Many of the procedures used for the cranial reproductive tract require general anesthesia. However, there is concern about the effects of inhalation anesthetic agents on the fetus in mares with dystocia and those undergoing a cesarean section (C-section). Therefore, total IV anesthesia (guaifenesin, ketamine, and detomidine) has been recommended for these mares, at least until the foal is delivered.[2]

For mares that have dystocia, the author has had consistently good results using xylazine, diazepam, and ketamine for induction, and halothane or isoflurane in oxygen for maintenance of anesthesia. Isoflurane has become the inhalant agent of choice for the horse because of its availability, cost, and anesthetic properties (see Chapter 19). Rapid delivery of the live foal combined with immediate neonatal care provides the best opportunity for the foal's survival when the mare has dystocia. Anesthesia should be induced rapidly and maintained at a light surgical plane, allowing the procedure to proceed as quickly as possible.

Laparotomy

The standing flank approach to the abdomen is primarily used to perform an ovariectomy or to correct a uterine torsion. The mare is preferably placed in stocks with moveable sidebars. Routine skin preparation for aseptic surgery and draping are used. A modified grid approach is made through the body wall in the appropriate flank of the horse (see Chapter 33). Complications encountered with this technique include an uncooperative mare, the inability to resolve the disorder (e.g., uterine torsion), and incisional infection.

General anesthesia is required to perform a ventral laparotomy. This procedure can be performed safely, on an elective or an emergency basis, in most surgical facilities by properly trained equine surgeons because of the number of colic surgeries treated at most facilities. The ventral approach to the abdomen, midline or paramedian, provides better access than other approaches and allows faster and safer resolution of most cranial reproductive tract abnormalities. Complications include anesthetic, recovery, and incisional problems.

Laparoscopy

The most common use of the laparoscope for the mare's reproductive tract has been for ovariectomy.[3] It has also become useful as a diagnostic tool, and with time, more applications will be developed. Laparoscopy requires special equipment and instruments, an in-depth knowledge of the abdominal and reproductive anatomy, and just as important, extensive surgical training.[3]

Generally, procedures are performed in the standing horse, with the laparoscope placed through the flank. A ventral approach to the abdomen is occasionally used. Complications generally relate to abdominal organ trauma as a result of placement of the cannula for the telescope and the instruments.

THE OVARIES

The most common surgical procedure involving the ovary is resection. This is performed for various conditions and by applying various methods. The procedure used for ovariectomy depends on the reason for their resection, the temperament of the mare, the experience of the surgeon, and the cost to the client.

Neoplastic Conditions

Granulosa cell tumors (GCTs) are the most common ovarian neoplasm.[4-6] Affected mares may show anestrus, intermittent or continuous estrus, nymphomania, or stallion-like behavior. Generally, the ovary is enlarged, sometimes quite massively, and the contralateral ovary is usually small and inactive. The ultrasonographic appearance is usually that of a multiple cystic structure, although this can vary. Testosterone levels are generally elevated. Inhibin levels are more consistently elevated but not always. Repeated palpation of the ovary may be useful to help rule out other causes of the enlargement.

A GCT most commonly develops unilaterally, but it can occur bilaterally; it is usually benign, but it may exhibit metastases.[4,5,7,8] The tumor can develop in mares of all ages, and a juvenile form has been reported in the neonate.[4,9] Unusual abnormalities associated with GTCs have been noted, including hemoperitoneum, adhesions to adjacent organs, and small colon strangulation obstruction.[9-13] Ovariectomy is usually needed to resolve these conditions.

Other neoplastic conditions of the ovary are rare. They include teratoma, cystadenoma, adenocarcinoma, lymphosarcoma, melanoma, dysgerminoma, and arrhenoblastoma.[5,6,14-20]

Nonneoplastic Conditions

An enlarged ovary may have nonneoplastic causes.[6,21,22] Occasionally, hematomas and cysts become quite large and adversely affect ovarian architecture. Abscessation can cause an enlarged, painful ovary. Ovariectomy is usually needed to resolve these conditions.

Abnormal behavior is occasionally encountered in show mares during estrus. If hormone therapy is unsuccessful, bilateral ovariectomy can be used to correct this behavior.

Ovariectomy

Colpotomy

Ovariectomy via a colpotomy has been used primarily for bilateral ovariectomy, either to effect an improvement in a mare's behavior or for research applications. The procedure has been used for years and has changed little, except for improvements such as surgical gloves and anesthetics and analgesics.[6,23-25]

The mare is sedated and placed in stocks, and the tail is wrapped. Epidural anesthesia is generally recommended. The rectum is evacuated, and the bladder is emptied if it is distended. The tail is tied upward and the perineal region is prepared for surgery. A pointed bistoury or guarded scalpel is used to make a small incision through the cranial vaginal wall, 4 to 5 cm caudal to the cervix. The incision is made at the 2- or 4-o'clock position if the surgeon is right handed, or at the 8- or 10-o'clock position if the surgeon is left handed. These sites avoid inadvertent penetration of the bladder, rectum, and uterine branch of the urogenital artery laterally. The peritoneum is penetrated with a thrust from closed blunt-pointed scissors. This small incision is enlarged digitally until the entire hand can pass into the peritoneal cavity (Fig. 68-1). Lidocaine-soaked gauze sponges, tethered with a long strand of umbilical tape, are held around the ovarian pedicle for 1 minute. The chain loop of the écraseur is placed around an ovary, with care taken to exclude other tissues and slowly (over 3 to 4 minutes) tightened until the ovary falls into the surgeon's hand (see Fig. 68-1, *B*). The

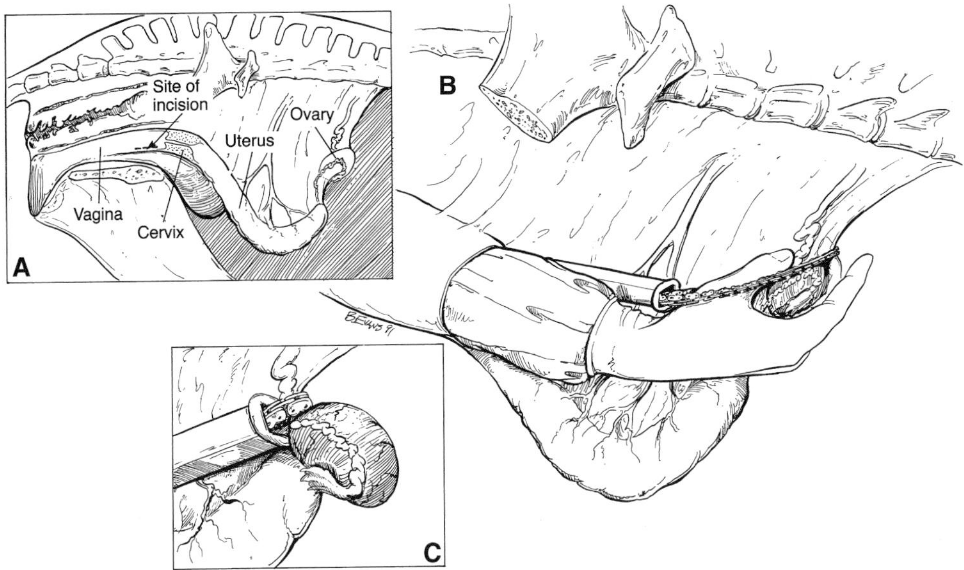

Figure 68-1. Colpotomy approach to ovariectomy. **A,** The site for the vaginal incision is along the ventrolateral wall of the vagina and 4 to 5 cm caudal to the cervix. **B,** The chain loop of the écraseur is positioned over the hand so that the ovary can be grasped and drawn inside the loop. **C,** After ensuring that the ovarian pedicle is within the chain loop, écrasement proceeds over 3 to 4 minutes

ovary is removed from the abdomen and the procedure is repeated on the other ovary.

The vaginal incision is allowed to heal as an open wound and the mare is kept standing for 2 to 3 days to prevent the rare case of eventration. Loose apposition of the wound edges with large absorbable sutures may lessen the anxiety level of the surgeon postoperatively. Broad-spectrum antibiotics and anti-inflammatory drugs are administered for 5 days postoperatively, and the mare is walked daily for 2 weeks before resuming previous activities.

Possible complications include excessive (possibly fatal) bleeding from the ovarian pedicle and eventration through the vaginal surgery site.

Laparotomy

Ovariectomy via a laparotomy allows the ovary to be exteriorized under visual control, which facilitates direct hemostasis. A flank approach can be used in the standing mare if the ovary is less then 10 cm in diameter and there is concern about general anesthesia. A flank approach may also be used with the mare under general anesthesia. A grid approach through the abdominal muscles is used to access the abdomen. Occasionally, a seroma forms postoperatively at the surgery site.

As mentioned, a ventral approach to the abdomen can be via a midline, paramedian, or diagonal paramedian incision.[4,6,24-26] The ventral midline incision is best for very large ovarian tumors with an ovarian pedicle of adequate length. The diagonal paramedian laparotomy approach is, however, the most useful. The incision is positioned directly over the ovary, so less tension is applied to the ovarian pedicle during vessel ligation than with other procedures.

The mare is anesthetized and placed in dorsal recumbency, and the surgery site is prepared for aseptic surgery. A 12- to 15-cm incision is made starting about 5 cm cranial to the mammary gland and nearly bisecting the angle formed by the ventral midline and the inguinal depression. An attempt is made to avoid any large subcutaneous vessels. The incision is continued through the external rectus sheath. The rectus abdominis muscle fibers are bluntly separated, and the internal rectus sheath is opened carefully with scissors. A hand is introduced into the peritoneal cavity, and the ovary is found and carefully exteriorized. Stay sutures are placed in the ovary. Distended follicles may need to be aspirated to allow passage of the enlarged ovary through the incision. Smaller ovaries can be pushed up to the incision per rectum by an assistant.[27] Ligatures are placed around the cranial and caudal margins of the ovarian pedicle and used as stay sutures. A 90-mm thoracoabdominal stapling device (TA 90; United States Surgical Corp, Norwalk, Conn) is placed across the ovarian pedicle and discharged.[28] The ovarian pedicle is transected between the rows of staples and the ovary, which is removed from the surgery site (Fig. 68-2).

After removal of the stapling device, tension is relieved on the end of the ovarian pedicle while still holding the stay sutures, and the transection site is checked for bleeding. Extra ligatures are used as needed. In very large GCTs that are difficult to exteriorize out of the abdomen, some surgeons prefer to separate the tumor from the pedicle in the abdomen with the help of an écraseur. Care must be taken to leave approximately a 2-cm stump of the pedicle with the tumor. Separation through the écraseur should be accomplished over a 3- to 4-minute period. After the tumor is removed from the abdomen, the large vessels in the pedicle are ligated or closed with staples to prevent postoperative hemorrhage. The ovarian pedicle is placed back into the abdomen and the abdomen is closed. The rectus abdominis muscle fibers are reapposed with no. 2 absorbable suture in an interrupted cruciate pattern. The external rectus fascia is closed with no. 2 absorbable suture in a continuous pattern, the subcutaneous tissue with no. 1 absorbable suture in a continuous pattern, and the skin with no. 0 absorbable suture in a continuous pattern. An

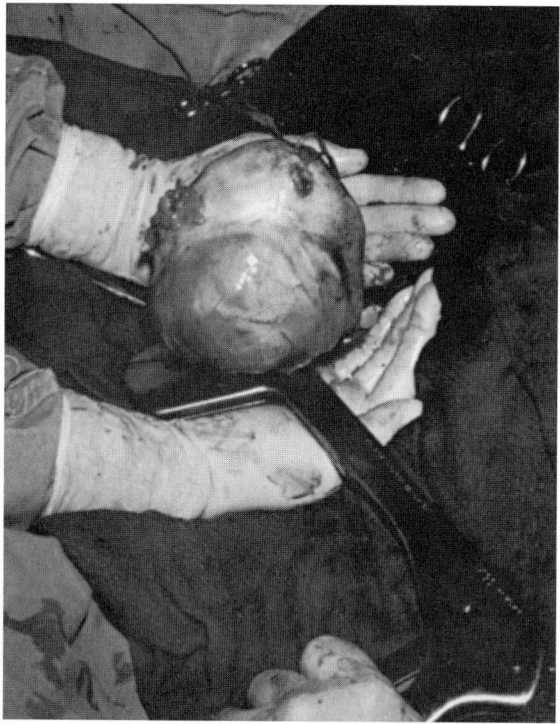

Figure 68-2. After placement of two stay sutures in the ovarian pedicle, a commercial stapling unit can be used successfully for hemostasis of the ovarian pedicle.

experienced surgeon is able to perform this procedure bilaterally, if needed, in a relatively short time.[29]

Postoperative instructions include 1 week of hand-walking, followed by 2 weeks of small-paddock turn-out and subsequent routine care. The rare postoperative complications include postoperative abdominal pain and incisional infection.

Laparoscopy

Ovariectomy using the laparoscope is the treatment of choice in some hospitals.[3,29-38] The laparoscope allows visualization and manipulation of the ovary in situ. Various methods of hemostasis can be applied with minimal tension on the ovarian pedicle. There are reports of performing an ovariectomy under general anesthesia using a ventral approach.[38] However, a distinct advantage of using the laparoscope is to perform the procedure in the standing mare.

The mare is sedated, usually with detomidine and butorphanol, and placed in stocks, and the surgery sites are prepared for aseptic surgery. Local anesthesia is used at the laparoscopic portal sites in the flank. For a bilateral ovariectomy, three small incisions are made in the left flank, which is safer for the initial approach because it minimizes the risk of cecal trauma. The dorsal incision is initially used to pass a cannula with a blunt trocar through the peritoneal lining. The abdomen is subsequently insufflated with CO_2. The laparoscope is placed through this cannula, and the other portals are used for instruments. Lidocaine is administered through a laparoscopic injection needle (Karl Storz Veterinary Endoscopy, Goleta, Calif) to desensitize the ovarian pedicle.

Various methods have been used for hemostasis and resection of the ovary, including the neodymium:yttrium-aluminum-garnet (Nd:YAG) laser, laparoscopic scissors and stapling instruments, ligatures tied in a modified Roeder knot or Tayside slipping knot, electrocoagulation, and ultrasonic instruments that cut and coagulate. One of the ventral portals is enlarged to remove the ovary. If the ovary is much larger than 10 cm in diameter, a hand-assisted laparoscopic technique can be used in the standing mare. In a recent report, ovaries up to 40 cm in diameter were removed using this technique.[35] The procedure is repeated on the contralateral side if a bilateral ovariectomy is to be performed. The incisions are closed after deflating the abdomen and removing the cannulas.

Postoperative care includes antibiotics and anti-inflammatories for 2 to 3 days, and 2 weeks of hand-walking before returning to routine care. As after a laparotomy, complications are uncommon but include postoperative abdominal discomfort and incisional infection.

THE UTERUS

Uterine Cysts

Uterine or endometrial cysts are most commonly found in older mares and are usually diagnosed by ultrasonography. If many are present, they may have an adverse affect on fertility. If the cysts are suspected to be the cause of infertility, they should be removed. Methods of cyst removal have included mechanical curettage, cyst rupture with endometrial biopsy forceps, uterine lavage with a hypertonic saline or magnesium sulfate solution, electrocoagulation of the cyst, and laser ablation.[39,40] In the author's opinion, laser ablation has been the most successful and most accepted technique.

The mare is sedated and placed in stocks, and the perineal region is prepared for hysteroscopy. A 1-m videoendoscope that has been cold-sterilized and rinsed with sterile water is passed through the cervix into the uterus. The uterus is distended with air to allow visualization of the body and both horns. The uterine cysts are first opened and drained. A diode laser, set at 14 W, is used to ablate the cysts. Lasing is continued until the remaining cystic tissue is shriveled and burned. Smoke and fluid often need to be evacuated from the uterus a few times during the procedure. Immediately after the procedure, the uterus is lavaged or infused with antibiotics. An ultrasonographic examination of the uterus should be performed prior to breeding. A recent report of the use of the Nd:YAG laser to ablate endometrial cysts in 55 barren mares demonstrated improved fertility.[40]

Uterine Neoplasia and Pyometra

Uterine neoplasia and chronic pyometra are rare conditions that are treated by ovariohysterectomy.[25,39,41-49] The most commonly encountered uterine tumors are leiomyoma and leiomyosarcoma, and botryoid rhabdomyosarcoma has also been reported. Chronic pyometra is generally the result of an obstruction of complete drainage. Drainage of the uterine contents prior to surgery is advisable.

Partial ovariohysterectomy has been used to remove a focal uterine tumor and ovarian masses with adhesions to the uterine horn.[22,46,47,49] The approaches have included a caudal ventral midline and paramedian laparotomy and a standing flank laparoscopy. Live foals have been produced by mares after partial ovariohysterectomy.[42,46,49]

Total ovariohysterectomy is best approached through a caudal ventral midline incision. The ovarian pedicles are ligated, and dissection continues through the broad ligament, ligating large vessels in the process. The body of the uterus is transected as far caudal as possible, with care taken to avoid contamination of the peritoneal cavity. The uterine stump is closed with a double-inverting suture pattern. The abdomen is closed in routine fashion.

Uterine Torsion

Mares with uterine torsion are initially examined for signs of colic. Affected mares usually exhibit mild to moderate, intermittent abdominal pain. The diagnosis is usually made by rectal examination. In most cases, a taut broad ligament is palpable, coursing dorsal to the caudal aspect of the uterus in the direction of the torsion. An ultrasonographic examination may provide useful information about fetal viability, status of the uterus, and other abdominal abnormalities.

Uterine torsion can affect mares of all ages, usually during the last 2 months of gestation, although this varies.[50-58] The direction of the torsion may be clockwise or counterclockwise, and the majority are turned 180 degrees. Uterine torsion is usually diagnosed in its acute stage, although chronic uterine torsion has been reported.[59] Nonsurgical management usually requires general anesthesia and rolling of the mare. The few mares that are at term may be successfully corrected by passing a hand into the uterus, grasping the fetus, and gradually rocking it, together with the uterus, in larger and larger arcs until it untwists.[50,54]

The procedure for rolling involves anesthetizing the mare and rolling her 360 degrees in the direction of the torsion. A long wooden plank, firmly placed across the mare's flank, is helpful in keeping the gravid uterus in the same position while the mare is rolled around it. This method of management has been quite successful.[52-54] However, uterine rupture in a mare at term has been reported.[53]

Surgical management of uterine torsion is frequently used. The standing flank approach has been more popular than the ventral midline approach.* The mare is sedated and placed in stocks. Local anesthesia is administered and routine surgical preparations are made. The flank incision is made on the side toward which the uterus is twisted. A modified grid approach is made through the body wall. An arm is introduced and a hand is placed under the gravid uterine horn. The uterus is gradually rocked back and forth, eventually allowing the uterus to flip back into its normal position. The status of the fetus and of the uterus should be evaluated. Closure is routine.

A ventral midline approach should be used if uterine rupture, tearing, or devitalization is suspected, if the foal is known to be dead and the mare is preterm, and if attempts at standing correction are unsuccessful.[25,51] If the mare is in a surgical facility where many abdominal surgeries are performed, the ventral midline approach should be considered instead of the flank approach, since it is more versatile.

The most frequently referenced review of uterine torsions (1981) revealed 19 of 26 (73%) of the mares survived, and of 20 foals determined viable at surgery, 12 (70%) were foaled normally.[51] The success rates for mare and foal survival are likely to have improved since that review.

Uterine Prolapse

Uterine prolapse in the mare rarely occurs.[25,39,58] It tends to occur more frequently after dystocia and when fetal membranes are retained. Tension placed on the placenta and the use of excessive oxytocin have also been implicated.[39] Although rare, the condition may be complicated by bladder prolapse, uterine tear, intestinal herniation, or uterine vessel rupture.

In the initial stages, this is quite painful for the mare. Sedation is indicated. Tocolytic agents, if available, may help decrease straining and discomfort. Prompt treatment is important. The uterus should be cleaned with saline and any placenta not directly attached to the uterus resected. Keeping the uterus elevated and protected in a plastic bag until definitive treatment is started reduces swelling, contamination, trauma, and straining.

Occasionally, the uterus can be replaced in the standing mare if it is heavily sedated. Copious amounts of lubricant are used, and the uterus is gradually pushed back into its normal position. The use of fingertips should be avoided. The author does not use epidural anesthesia, since it does not tend to eliminate all straining, and its use is contraindicated if general anesthesia is needed. If standing uterine replacement is unsuccessful, the mare is anesthetized and her hind limbs hoisted. Then, the uterus can be replaced relatively easily into its normal position. Care is taken to ensure that the uterine horns are fully extended. The vulva is sutured, except for a small ventral opening, and the mare is recovered. The mare is treated with antibiotics, anti-inflammatories, and IV fluids if needed. Uterine lavages commence the next day. Although oxytocin is recommended by some,[58] the author avoids its use for 2 to 3 days.

Uterine Rupture

Uterine rupture or tear usually occurs during a dystocia or normal foaling, but rarely it can also occur with uterine torsion or hydramnios.[51,60] Most tears are not appreciated for 24 to 72 hours postpartum.[25,39] Uterine or vaginal tears are infrequently associated with evisceration of bowel during foaling. In this situation, the bowel should be cleansed and replaced in the abdomen prior to delivering the foal. The tear should then be identified and a plan formulated for repair. Very rarely, a fetus may gain access to the abdomen through a uterine tear, necessitating abdominal surgery to deliver the foal and repair the uterus.

Tears in the uterine body are sometimes found relatively early postpartum by palpation of the cervix and caudal vagina during uterine lavage. However, palpation of a tear at

*References 25, 39, 50, 51, 54, 55.

that site can be difficult postpartum because of the swelling and folding of the uterine lining.

Most uterine ruptures are diagnosed 1 to 3 days postpartum, when the mare presents with depression, fever, and mild abdominal discomfort. In the presence of an elevated peritoneal fluid white blood cell count and protein level, uterine rupture becomes the most likely diagnosis.

Uterine rupture can be fatal, but with prompt diagnosis and treatment the prognosis for survival is good. In a study of postpartum mare death over a 2-year period, 6 of 98 mares died from a perforated uterus.[61] Earlier reports of mares with uterine rupture yielded survival rates of 39% and 60%.[62,63] A more recent study of 33 mares revealed an 80% survival rate.[64] Although medical management may occasionally be successful, surgical repair yields a more consistently successful result.

Information obtained from the more recent study just mentioned revealed that 73% of the perforations occurred in the uterine horn and 27% in the uterine body[64] (Fig. 68-3). Interestingly, only 10 of the 33 mares had encountered dystocia. All of the uterine tears in this study were repaired surgically. All of the uterine horn and some of the uterine body tears were accessed through a caudal ventral midline celiotomy. These defects were closed using a simple-continuous pattern and oversewn with a continuous inverting pattern, both using no. 1 multifilament absorbable suture. The abdomens were lavaged during surgery and for 2 to 3 days postoperatively. Uterine lavage started 1 day postoperatively and continued for 3 to 4 days. Some perforations in the caudal body of the uterus were repaired in the standing mare per vagina. Closure consisted of a single layer of simple-interrupted or continuous sutures.

Uterine Artery Hemorrhage

Hemorrhage from the uterine arteries (i.e., the uterine branch of the vaginal artery), the uterine artery, and the uterine branch of the ovarian artery is the most common cause of death of the postpartum mare. A study of 98 mares that died postpartum revealed that 40 died from a ruptured uterine artery.[61] It is uncommon for these arteries to rupture at times other than in the first several days postpartum.

The condition is usually seen in older mares. Affected mares are often initially in quite an amount of pain, especially if the blood is contained within the broad ligament. The rectal examination in these mares generally reveals a fluctuant mass in the broad ligament. If the broad ligament ruptures and the blood gains access to the abdominal cavity, the mare may not exhibit as much pain. On rectal examination, the broad ligament has a more edematous feel. These mares generally have very pale mucous membranes, a weak pulse, and an elevated heart rate, and they are anxious and often sweating.

Treatment varies depending on the clinician, but it essentially follows the approach taken for hemorrhagic shock (see Chapters 1 and 4).[58] Attempts to ligate the ruptured artery have met with limited success.

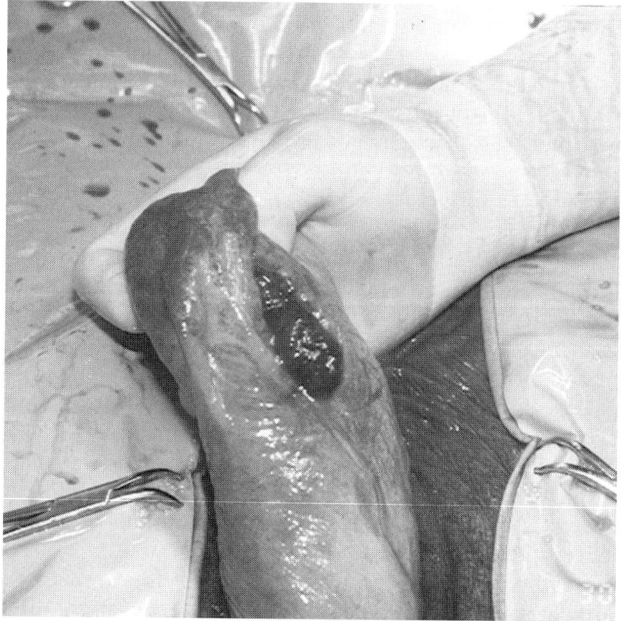

Figure 68-3. Typical appearance of a uterine tear at the tip of the uterine horn.

Cesarean Section

Elective C-Section

Candidates for an elective C-section include mares that have a compromised birth canal as a result of a previous pelvic fracture or a soft tissue injury within the reproductive tract, and mares that have previously had a difficult dystocia or a severe uterine artery hemorrhage. This surgery has also been used to produce gnotobiotic foals for research purposes.[65] The surgery must be well timed to yield a viable foal and have minimal adverse effects on the mare, so it is important to perform it as close as possible to the natural foaling time. The mare should be hospitalized 7 to 10 days prior to her due date. Her physical status is checked frequently to determine udder development, softening of her perineal tissues, and behavior. Concentrations of electrolytes in the mammary secretions are very helpful for timing the surgery.[66] Decreasing sodium and increasing potassium and calcium levels are good indicators of impending parturition. The surgery, when performed, should proceed rapidly, with knowledgeable staff waiting to resuscitate the anesthetized foal on delivery. The fetal survival rate following elective C-section is about 90%.[67-69]

Emergency C-Section

The most common reason to perform a C-section in the mare is to resolve a dystocia.[25,66,67,69-72] This is truly an emergency situation and once the decision is made, the C-section should proceed rapidly. The team of people involved should be well organized and prepared for this situation. Other circumstances potentially needing an emergency C-section include a near-term mare undergoing colic surgery or correction for uterine torsion. Ideally, if the mare has a good prognosis to survive, the fetus should remain in the mare until normal parturition. A C-section should be performed if the mare has a guarded prognosis. A recent study showed only 3 of 8 (38%) term foals delivered during colic surgery survived to discharge.[69] It would be rare to encounter significant incisional complications during parturition after a recent abdominal surgery.

Surgical Technique

As the obstetrical manipulations for controlled vaginal delivery are being performed, the ventral midline of the mare is being prepared for a possible C-section.[25] Once the decision is made, the surgery room is set up and the mare is positioned on the surgery table and readied for surgery. The time from the decision to perform a C-section to the delivery of the foal should be no more than 20 minutes.[25] This is the same for elective and emergency C-section. If the foal is known to be dead, this time is not as critical.

The two most commonly used approaches for C-section in the mare are the modified low flank (Marcenac) and the ventral midline. The modified low flank approach, which positions the horse in lateral recumbency, used to be popular in Europe.[70] The most rapid approach to the abdomen, and the approach most commonly used in North America, is the caudal ventral midline approach.[25,66-69,72]

The mare is positioned in dorsal lateral recumbency with the ventral midline tilted toward the surgeon. A 35- to 40-cm incision is made into the abdomen beginning 10 cm caudal to the umbilicus and extending craniad. The gravid uterine horn, which usually contains the hind limbs of the fetus, is located and exteriorized. One stay suture is placed in a cruciate pattern near the tip of the uterine horn, close to the position of the fetal feet, and another toward the body of the uterus, close to the position of the fetal hocks. An assistant surgeon handles the stay sutures during the procedure to minimize contamination of the abdomen with uterine fluids and to help facilitate closure. An extra impermeable drape is placed over the other drapes on the surgeon's side of the abdomen.

An incision is made through the uterine wall and chorioallantois from the level of the fetal hocks to the feet, creating a straight incision between the stay sutures (Fig. 68-4). During extraction of the fetus, it is not uncommon to have the uterine wall tear slightly at the end of the uterotomy incision. The amniotic membrane, which has collapsed around the foal, is elevated and incised. The surgeon grasps the hind limbs and lifts the fetus up and out of the uterus. The hind limbs are handed to a third assistant, and the surgeon pulls the body up and out of the uterus. In this manner, the fetus is pulled from the mare rapidly. The umbilical cord is clamped and transected and the neonate is quickly transferred to a table set up just outside the surgery room for resuscitation and evaluation. The chorioallantois is separated from the endometrium for 3 to 4 cm along the incised edge of the uterine wall. If the placenta separates easily from the uterus, it may be entirely removed at that time. However, it is usually still well attached.

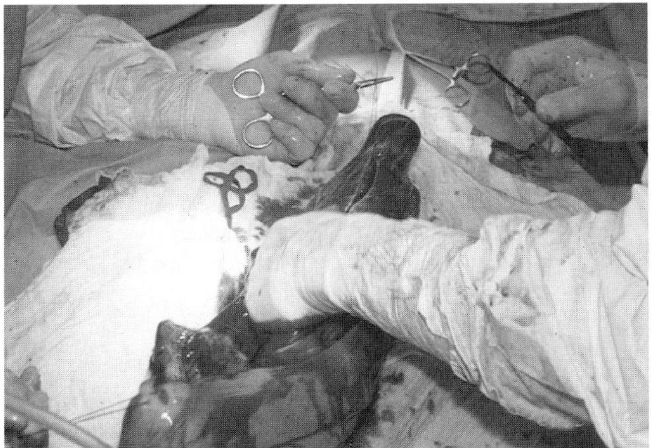

Figure 68-4. Uterotomy with stay sutures in place. The amnion is partially incised near the point of the hock.

Infrequently, the hind limbs are not present in a uterine horn, making it extremely difficult to exteriorize any part of the uterus. The uterine incision is then made at the base of a horn and body of the uterus with the uterus in the abdomen. This causes significant concern about the amount of contamination occurring during surgery. (After closure of the uterus, the abdomen will be lavaged with copious amounts of saline.)

The incised edge of the uterine wall bleeds profusely. A continuous suture line is placed along this edge to provide some hemostasis. Large vessels are individually ligated. The need for the hemostatic suture line has recently been questioned.[73] This author feels that it lessens the risk of bleeding enough to warrant the 10 minutes needed for its placement. The assistant elevates and tenses the stay sutures to facilitate closure of the uterus, which is performed in 2 layers with no. 1 or 2 absorbable suture material. A continuous Connell pattern is used for the first layer, and a continuous Lembert for the second layer. After uterine closure, the uterus is lavaged and 40 units of oxytocin is administered IV. This quickly stimulates contraction of the uterus and aids expulsion of the placenta. The stay sutures are removed and the uterus is replaced into its normal position in the abdomen.

The extra impermeable drape is removed, the drape surface around the incision is lavaged, and the surgeon's gown and gloves are changed if needed. The abdomen is lavaged with 10 to 15 L of warm saline, which is removed by suction. An abdominal drain for subsequent lavage may be placed if deemed necessary. A crystalline penicillin solution is instilled into the abdomen, which is closed in routine fashion for a ventral midline celiotomy.

Terminal C-Section

Significant concern for a foal in a mare with a terminal illness may require a C-section. Examples include mares recumbent as a result of neurologic abnormalities, severe laminitis, or other potentially fatal or debilitating conditions. If euthanasia is planned for the mare after the surgery, sterility is not a high priority but speed of delivery is. Most of these surgeries can be performed quickly through a low flank approach after induction of anesthesia.

Aftercare

Postoperative care for a C-section mare is very similar to that for any mare after abdominal surgery, with special attention paid to the reproductive tract.[25] Some mares pass their placenta in the recovery stall. If the placenta has not passed, oxytocin is again administered 2 to 3 hours postpartum.[25] The initial dose is 40 U in 1 L of lactated Ringer's solution given IV over 30 to 60 minutes. Since this often causes abdominal pain, the rate of administration is dictated by the response of the mare. In refractory cases, 80 U is used every 4 to 6 hours. Usually, the placenta passes within 8 hours postpartum. Manual rupture of the chorioallantoic membrane and exteriorization of the amniotic membrane per vagina may be needed to initiate placental expulsion after an elective C-section. Uterine lavage is started soon after the placenta is passed, or simultaneously if it is retained. The uterus is generally lavaged once daily for 3 to 4 days.

Systemic antibiotics and flunixin meglumine are administered for 3 to 5 days after the delivery, depending on the degree of contamination and tissue trauma encountered. Intravenous fluids are administered as needed to maintain adequate hydration and vascular volume and to correct electrolyte imbalances. Abdominal surgery, even without manipulation of the intestines, combined with possible bruising of the small colon or cecum from the dystocia, can result in transient postoperative ileus. Swollen and painful pelvic tissues may lead to retention of feces. The postpartum diet should reflect concern for these potential problems. Water is offered freely. The mare is walked and allowed to graze on green grass the first postoperative day. A bran mash with mineral oil may be beneficial. Discharge instructions include hand walking 2 to 3 times each day, with or without small-paddock turn-out for 3 to 4 weeks.

DYSTOCIA

Dystocia in the mare is one of the few true emergencies an equine practitioner may encounter.[74] Prompt action increases the probability of survival of the foal and decreases the degree of reproductive trauma to the mare.[74] There are four procedures to resolve dystocia: assisted vaginal delivery, in which the mare is awake and is assisted in the vaginal delivery of an intact foal; controlled vaginal delivery (CVD), in which the mare is anesthetized and the clinician is in complete control of the delivery of an intact foal vaginally; fetotomy, in which the dead fetus is divided into more than one part for removal from the uterus per vagina in an awake or an anesthetized mare; and C-section, in which the fetus is removed through an incision in the uterus.

The goal of dystocia resolution is to deliver a live foal in a manner resulting in a reproductively sound mare.[74] This is usually accomplished at the farm. However, referral hospitals need to be prepared for difficult cases, and the clinician must be able to perform whatever procedure is necessary to resolve any dystocia. Currently, emergency clinicians, who are usually trained as surgeons or internists, tend to perform C-sections at these hospitals. Thus, these clinicians should also be familiar with CVD and fetotomy techniques. No single procedure is right for every situation.

Once the mare is in the hospital, dystocia requires prompt action. The mare is anesthetized shortly after arrival to attempt CVD. The hind limbs are hoisted upward until the pelvis is about 3 feet above the ground (Fig. 68-5). Decreased straining, gravity, and lubrication usually enable resolution of the dystocia. If the foal cannot be delivered within 15 minutes, a C-section or fetotomy should be considered. C-section techniques were described earlier. Fetotomy techniques are described elsewhere.[75]

Results of dystocia resolved in a referral hospital in an area with a high concentration of broodmares were recently examined.[72] Of 247 cases of dystocia, 71% were resolved by CVD, 25% by C-section, and 4% by fetotomy. A live foal was delivered in 42% of cases, and 30% were discharged from the hospital, with 91% of the mares surviving to discharge.

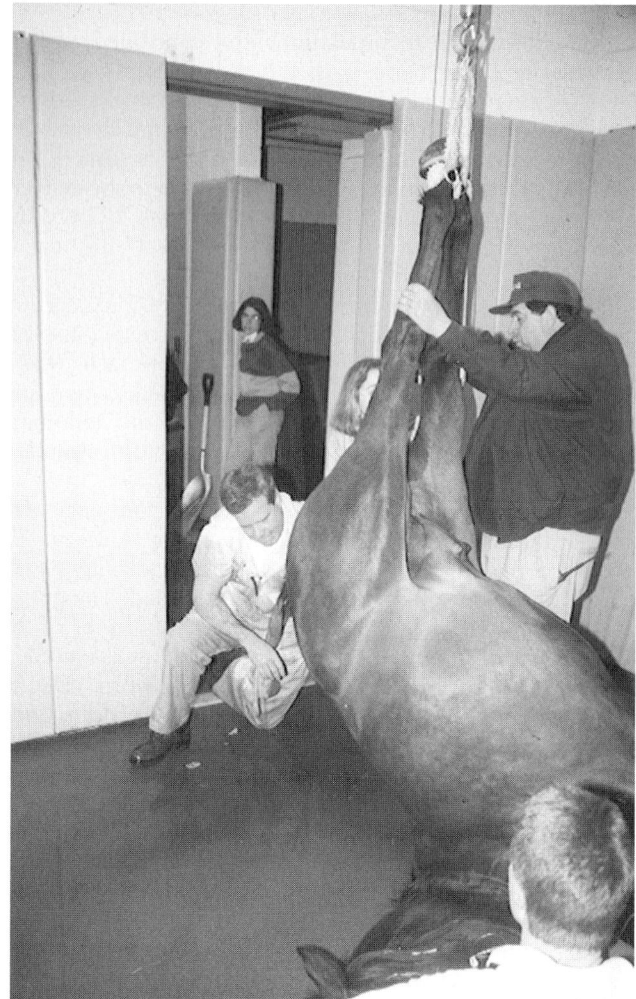

Figure 68-5. The hind limbs of the mare are hoisted to facilitate controlled vaginal delivery.

The elapsed time from chorioallantoic membrane rupture to delivery for foals alive at discharge (mean of 72 minutes) was significantly less than for foals not surviving (mean of 85 minutes). The effect on fertility after dystocia was examined in Thoroughbreds in this study. It was shown to be decreased, although still respectable: the pre-dystocia live foaling rate was 84%, whereas the rate after dystocia was 67%.

REFERENCES

1. Ley WB: Anatomy and physiology of the female reproductive system. In Wolfe DF, Moll HD, editors: Large Animal Urogenital Surgery, Baltimore, 1999, Williams and Wilkins.
2. Cornick-Seahorn J: Anesthesia of the critically ill equine patient, Vet Clin North Am Equine Pract 2004;20:127.
3. Fischer AT: Diagnostic and surgical laparoscopy. In Traub-Dargatz JL, Brown CM, editors: Equine Endoscopy, ed 2, St Louis, 1997, Mosby.
4. Meagher DM, Wheat JD, Hughes JP, et al: Granulosa cell tumors in mares: A review of 78 cases, Proc Am Assoc Equine Pract 1977;23:133.
5. Pugh DG, Bowen JM, Gaughan EM: Equine overview tumors, Comp Cont Educ Pract Vet 1985;7:710.

6. Moll HD, Slone DE: Surgery of the ovaries. In Wolfe DF, Moll HD, editors: Large Animal Urogenital Surgery, Baltimore, 1999, Williams and Wilkins.
7. Turner TA, Manno M: Bilateral granulosa cell tumor in a mare, J Am Vet Med Assoc 1983;182:713.
8. Gift LJ, Gaughan EM, Schoning P: Metastatic granulosa cell tumor in a mare, J Am Vet Med Assoc 1992;200:1525.
9. Green SL, Specht TE, Dowling SC, et al: Hemoperitoneum caused by rupture of a juvenile granulosa tumor in an equine neonate, J Am Vet Med Assoc 1988;193:1417.
10. Gatewood DM, Douglass JP, Cox JH, et al: Intraabdominal hemorrhage associated with a granulosa-thecal cell neoplasm in a mare, J Am Vet Med Assoc 1990;196:1827.
11. Rembags BPS, Stout TAC, Rijkenhuizen ABM: Ovarian granulosa cell tumors adherent to other abdominal organs; surgical removal from two Warmblood mares, Equine Vet J 2003;35:627.
12. Wilson DA, Foreman JH, Boero MJ, et al: Small-colon rupture attributable to granulosa cell tumor in a mare, J Am Vet Med Assoc 1989;194:681.
13. Evard JH, Fischer AT, Greenwood LD: Ovarian strangulation as a cause of small colon obstruction in a foal, Equine Vet J 1988;20:217.
14. Frazer GS, Robertson JT, Boyce BW: Teratocarcinoma of the ovary in a mare, J Am Vet Med Assoc 1988;193:953.
15. Hinrichs K, Frazer GS, de Gannes RUG, et al: Serous cystadenoma in a normally cyclic mare with high plasma testosterone values, J Am Vet Med Assoc 1989;194:381.
16. Held JP, Buergelt C, Colahan D: Serous cystadenoma in a mare, J Am Vet Med Assoc 1982;181:496.
17. Morris DD, Acland HM, Hodge TG, et al: Pleural effusion secondary to metastasis of an ovarian adenocarcinoma in a horse, J Am Vet Med Assoc 1985;187:272.
18. Van Camp SC, Mahler J, Roberts MC, et al: Primary ovarian adenocarcinoma associated with teratomatous elements in a mare, J Am Vet Med Assoc 1989;194:172.
19. Lock TF, Macy DW: Equine ovarian lymphosarcoma, J Am Vet Med Assoc 1979;175:72.
20. Mills JHL, Fretz PB, Clark EG, et al: Arrhenoblastoma in a mare, J Am Vet Med Assoc 1977;171:754.
21. Nie GJ, Momont H: Ovarian mass in three mares with regular estrous cycles, J Am Vet Med Assoc 1992;201:1043.
22. Adams SB: Oophoritis in a horse, Vet Surg 1981;10:67.
23. White GR: Animal Castration, Chicago, 1920, American Veterinary Publishing.
24. Walker DF, Vaughan JT: Bovine and Equine Urogenital Surgery, Philadelphia, 1980, Lea & Febiger.
25. Trotter GW, Embertson RM: The uterus and ovaries. In Auer JA, Stick JA, editors: Equine Surgery, ed 2, Philadelphia, 1999, WB Saunders.
26. Moll HD, Slone DE, Juzwick JS, et al: Diagonal paramedian approach for removal of ovarian tumors in the mare, Vet Surg 1987;16:456.
27. Santschi EM, Troedsson MHT: How to perform bilateral ovariectomy in the mare through two paramedian incisions, Proc Am Assoc Equine Pract 2001;47:420.
28. Doran R, Allen D, Gordon B: Use of stapling instruments to aid in the removal of ovarian tumors in mares, Equine Vet J 1988;20:37.
29. Palmer SE: Standing laparoscopic laser technique for ovariectomy in five mares, J Am Vet Med Assoc 1993;203:279.
30. Ragle CA, Southwood LL, Hopper SA, et al: Laparoscopic ovariectomy in two horses with granulosa cell tumors, J Am Vet Med Assoc 1996;209:1121.
31. Hanson CA, Gallupo LD: Bilateral laparoscopic ovariectomy in standing mares: 22 cases, Vet Surg 1999;28:106.
32. Marien T, De Clercq T, Adriaenssen F, et al: Standing laparoscopic ovariectomy in mares using monopolar electrocoagulation and extracorporeal Tayside slipping knot technique, Equine Vet Educ 2000;12:202.
33. Rodgerson DH, Belknap JK, Wilson DA: Laparoscopic ovariectomy using sequential electrocoagulation and sharp transection of the equine mesovarium, Vet Surg 2001;30:572.
34. Hand R, Rakestraw P, Taylor T: Evaluation of a vessel-sealing device for use in laparoscopic ovariectomy in mares, Vet Surg 2002;31:240.
35. Rodgerson DH, Brown MP, Watt BC, et al: Hand-assisted laparoscopic technique for removal of ovarian tumors in standing mares, J Am Vet Med Assoc 2002;220:1503.
36. Dusterdieck KA, Pleasant RS, Lanz OI, et al: Evaluation of the harmonic scalpel for laparoscopic ovariectomy in mares, J Am Vet Med Assoc 2004;225:1598.
37. Alldredge JG, Hendrickson DA: Use of high-power ultrasonic sheers for laparoscopic ovariectomy in mares, J Am Vet Med Assoc 2004;225:1598.
38. Ragle CA, Schneider RK: Ventral abdominal approach for laparoscopic ovariectomy in horses, Vet Surg 1995;24:492.
39. Ley WB, Santschi EM: Examination and surgery of the uterus. In Wolfe DF, Moll HD, editors: Large Animal Urogenital Surgery, Baltimore, 1999, Williams and Wilkins.
40. Griffin RL, Bennett SD: Nd:YAG laser photoablation of endometrial cysts: A review of 55 cases (2000-2001), Proc Am Assoc Equine Pract 2002;48:58.
41. Torbeck RL, Kittleson SL, Leathers CW: Botryoid rhabdomyosarcoma of the uterus in a filly, J Am Vet Med Assoc 1980;176:914.
42. Lofstedt RM, Spurlock G, Willimas R, et al: Leiomyosarcoma in the uterus of a mare, Comp Cont Educ Pract Vet 1987;9:93.
43. Romagnoli SE, Momont HW, Hilbert BJ, et al: Multiple recurring uterocervical leiomyomas in two half-sibling Appaloosa fillies, J Am Vet Med Assoc 1987;191:1449.
44. Hooper RN, Taylor TS, Behrens EA, et al: Use of an écraseur for ovariohysterectomy in mares, Vet Surg 1992;21:374.
45. Broome TA, Allen D, Baxter GM, et al: Septic metritis secondary to torsion of a pedunculated uterine fibroleiomyoma in a filly, J Am Vet Med Assoc 1992;200:1685.
46. Santschi EM, Slone DE: Successful pregnancy after partial hysterectomy in two mares, J Am Vet Med Assoc 1994;205:1180.
47. Rotting AK, Freeman DE, Doyle AJ, et al: Total and partial ovariohysterectomy in seven mares, Equine Vet J 2003;35:29.
48. Delling U, Howard RD, Pleasant RS, et al: Hand-assisted laparoscopic ovariohysterectomy in the mare, Vet Surg 2004;33:487.
49. Janicek JC, Rodgerson DH, Boone BL: Use of a hand-assisted laparoscopic technique for removal of a uterine leiomyoma in a standing mare, J Am Vet Med Assoc 2004;225:911.
50. Vandeplassche M, Spincemaille J, Bowters R, et al: Some aspects of equine reproduction, Equine Vet J 1972;4:105.
51. Pascoe JR, Meagher DM, Wheat JD: Surgical management of uterine torsion in the mare: A review of 26 cases, J Am Vet Med Assoc 1981;179:351.
52. Guthrie RG: Rolling for correction of uterine torsion in a mare, J Am Vet Assoc 1982;181:66.
53. Wichtel JJ, Reinertson EL, Clark TL: Nonsurgical treatment of uterine torsion in seven mares, J Am Vet Med Assoc 1988;193:337.
54. Taylor TS, Blanchard TL, Varner DD, et al: Management of dystocia in mares: Uterine torsion and cesarean section, Comp Cont Educ Pract Vet 1989;11:1265.
55. Perkins NR, Robertson JT, Colon LA: Uterine torsion and uterine tear in a mare, J Am Vet Med Assoc 1992;201:92.
56. Ruffin DC, Schumacher J, Comer JS: Uterine torsion associated with small intestinal incarceration in a mare at 126 days of gestation, J Am Vet Med Assoc 1995;209:329.
57. Doyle AJ, Freeman DE, Sanberli DS, et al: Clinical signs and treatment of chronic uterine torsion in two mares, J Am Vet Med Assoc 2002;220:349.
58. Frazer GS: Postpartum complications in the mare: Part 1. Conditions affecting the uterus, Equine Vet Educ 2003;15:45.
59. Vivrette SL: Parturition and postpartum complications. In Robinson NE, editor: Current Therapy in Equine Medicine, ed 4, Philadelphia, 1997, WB Saunders.

60. Honnas CM, Spensley MS, Laverty S, et al: Hydramnios causing uterine rupture in a mare, J Am Vet Med Assoc 1988;193:334.
61. Dwyer R: Post partum deaths of mares, Equine Dis Q 1993;2:5.
62. Hooper RN, Schumacher J, Taylor TS, et al: Diagnosing and treating uterine rupture in mares, Vet Med 1993;88:263.
63. Fischer AT, Phillips TN: Surgical repair of a ruptured uterus in five mares, Equine Vet J 1986;18:153.
64. Sutter WW, Hopper S, Embertson RM, et al: Diagnosis and surgical treatment of uterine lacerations in mares (33 cases), Proc Am Assoc Equine Pract 2003;49:357.
65. Edwards GB, Newcombe JR: Elective caesarean section in the mare for the production of gnotobiotic foals, Equine Vet J 1974;6:122.
66. Santschi EM: Surgery of the uterus. In Wolfe DF, Moll HD, editors: Large Animal Urogenital Surgery, Baltimore, 1999, Williams and Wilkins.
67. Juswiak JS, Slone DE, Santschi EM, et al: Cesarean section in 19 mares: Results and postoperative fertility, Vet Surg 1990;19:50.
68. Watkins JP, Taylor TS, Day WC, et al: Elective cesarean section in mares: Eight cases (1980-1989), J Am Vet Med Assoc 1990;197:1639.
69. Freeman DE, Hungerford LL, Schaeffer D, et al: Caesarean section and other methods for assisted delivery: Comparison of effects on mare mortality and complications, Equine Vet J 1999;31:203.
70. Vandeplassche M, Bouters R, Spincemaille J, et al: Caesarean section in the mare, Proc Am Assoc Equine Pract 1977;23:75.
71. Embertson RM: The indications and surgical techniques for caesarean section in the mare, Equine Vet Educ 1992;4:31.
72. Byron CR, Embertson RM, Bernard WV, et al: Dystocia in a referral hospital setting: Approach and results, Equine Vet J 2002;35:82.
73. Freeman DE, Johnston JK, Baker GJ, et al: An evaluation of the haemostatic suture in hysterotomy closure in the mare, Equine Vet J 1999;31:208.
74. Embertson RM: Dystocia management, Proc Am Assoc Equine Pract 2003;49:6.
75. Frazer GS: Fetotomy technique in the mare, Equine Vet Educ 2001;13:195.

SECTION **X** URINARY SYSTEM

John A. Stick

CHAPTER 69

Principles of Urinary Tract Surgery

James D. Lillich
Richard M. DeBowes

PATIENT EVALUATION

History

A complete patient history should be obtained as part of any evaluation of a horse with suspected urinary tract disease. Contrary to popular opinion, horses with clinically significant disease of the kidneys or proximal urinary tract typically do not exhibit back pain as a principal clinical sign.[1] Veterinarians should be alert for signs of low-grade abdominal pain, weight loss, stranguria, dysuria, hematuria, oliguria, or incontinence.[1-3] Of all the primary signs reported by owners of horses with suspected urinary tract disease, abdominal discomfort accompanied by oliguria, anuria, or hemorrhage from the urethra is the most urgent and demands prompt investigation.

Physical Examination

All horses with urologic signs should undergo a complete physical examination. Horses with suspected urinary tract disease should be evaluated for general health status and fitness not only for the diagnosis of the urologic pathology, but also before surgical intervention. Systemic consequences of the urinary tract condition as well as the presence of concurrent systemic disease may have profound effects on the anesthetic course and postoperative care. Patients that are toxemic or suffering from severe electrolyte or acid–base derangements are particularly susceptible to anesthetic crises.

The perineum, tail, and medial surface of the hindlimbs should be inspected for the presence of dried urine, urine scald dermatitis, or blood. If possible, micturition should be observed to establish the presence of abnormal urine flow, incontinence, hematuria, or dysuria. Stranguria is usually accompanied by tail switching or flagging during urination. The volume and quality of the urine should be determined. Finally, all external portions of the urogenital tract should be palpated.

Rectal Examination

A rectal examination is indicated to evaluate the pelvic urethra, bladder, and left kidney. Size, consistency, and position of organs, as well as pain on manipulation, should be noted during palpation. The bladder can be palpated dorsal and slightly cranial to the pubic bone. When the bladder is greatly distended, the cranial edge is usually far forward and off to one side of the abdominal midline. Palpation of the bladder is of greatest value when it is relatively empty. Special attention should be given to evidence of thickening or swellings, as well as intraluminal concretions or calculi. Usually, the ureters and right kidney are not palpable[4] unless significant pathology alters their size or position within the abdomen. Distal ureteral calculi are palpable in the trigone region. Ureteral calculi cause dilation and distention proximal to the obstruction. Right renal hydronephrosis or neoplasia can result in renal enlargement or caudal displacement sufficient to permit palpation per rectum. The left kidney is generally palpated medial to the spleen and ventral to the lumbar spine.[4] Typically, it is a smooth-surfaced, bean-shaped structure that can be moved to the left body wall to permit percutaneous biopsy[5,6] (see Chapter 70).

Clinical Pathology

Preoperative laboratory examinations of surgical patients should include a complete blood count; determination of serum urea nitrogen, creatinine, and electrolyte values; and urinalysis. When reduced renal function is suspected, urine glutamyl transpeptidase levels and sodium sulfanilate clearance may be determined.[3,7-10] Fractional excretion of electrolytes is also important in determining renal function. Evaluation of blood pH and base excess may be helpful, particularly in surgical cases involving uroperitoneum. Preoperative identification and correction of metabolic acidemia and electrolyte anomalies are often important to patient survival; foals suffering from cystorrhexis (ruptured bladder) and uroperitoneum frequently develop severe metabolic acidemia and hyperkalemia,[11] which may result in anesthetic or postanesthetic death of cardiac origin.[12]

Imaging Techniques

Radiography and Nuclear Scintigraphy

A variety of modalities are available for imaging the distal urinary tract. Radiography is effective for evaluation of the proximal urinary tract of foals and young horses. In adult horses, large patient size and technical problems—associated with radiation scatter and definitive radiographic interpretation—generally preclude effective imaging of proximal urinary tract diseases. Positive-, negative-, or double-contrast cystography enhances the value of a radiographic examination of pediatric or young adult patients suspected of suffering from distal urinary obstruction or hemorrhage. When a diagnosis of ectopic ureter is suspected, intravenous pyelography is potentially useful for identification of the abnormal course and insertion of the involved ureters.[13]

Intravenous contrast agents should be used with caution because of reports of acute renal failure in humans.[14,15] Presumably, many of these problems are the result of organ ischemia subsequent to vascular occlusion of the arteries by injection catheters, a situation not likely to occur during the performance of an excretory urogram. Kidneys affected in this way demonstrate intense and prolonged staining characteristics.

Recently, nuclear scintigraphy has been used to determine renal function in horses. The use of technetium-99m–labeled diethylenetriamine penta-acetic acid or iodine-131-ortho-iodohippuric acid has permitted measurement of glomerular filtration rate, renal plasma, and blood flow in horses.[16,17] Nuclear scintigraphy can be used to confirm the lack of blood flow or loss of function to the pathologic kidney while simultaneously documenting the health of the contralateral kidney prior to nephrectomy (Fig. 69-1).

Ultrasonography

Ultrasonographic examination of the equine urinary tract has value in the diagnosis of a variety of clinical conditions.[18,19] This imaging modality permits evaluation of the kidneys for changes in size, shape, and consistency or echogenicity. It aids in the diagnosis of renal calculi, ureteral obstruction, hydroureter, hydronephrosis, renal cysts, abscesses, tumors, and developmental anomalies. Typically, a 3-MHz transducer with a 15- to 20-cm field of view is required for transmural ultrasonography of adult horse kidneys.[16] The right kidney can be imaged at the 15th, 16th, or 17th intercostal space below the level of the transverse processes. The left kidney is imaged through the 17th intercostal space or immediately caudal to the 18th rib, where it lies deep to the spleen (Fig. 69-2). Transrectal scanning techniques can be used with 5- to 10-MHz transducers for detailed evaluation of the renal pelvis or ureters.[19]

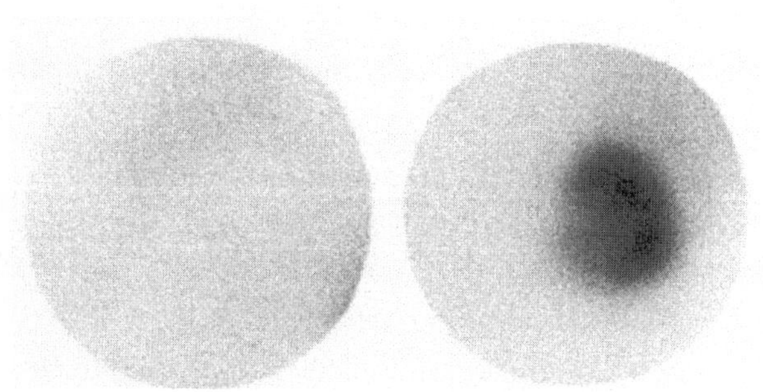

Figure 69-1. Nuclear scintigraphic image of the kidney region of a 7-year-old Quarter Horse mare with a history of granulosa cell tumor removal and chronic abdominal discomfort. Results indicate a lack of blood flow and urine production of the left kidney, which was confirmed at necropsy to contain metastatic disease.

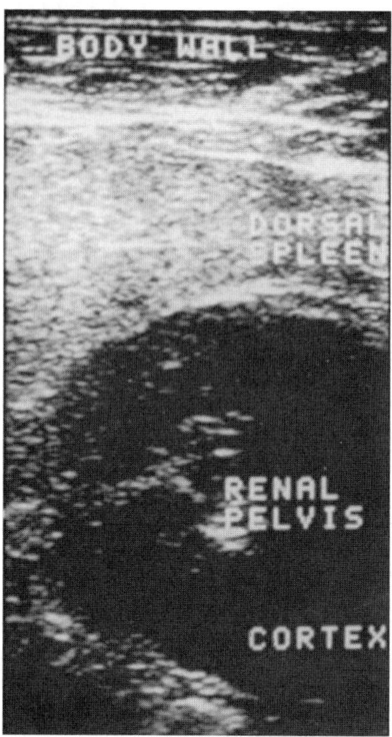

Figure 69-2. Left lateral abdominal transcutaneous ultrasonogram. The dorsal lateral body wall is located at the top of the figure. The fluid-dense renal cortex is immediately evident deep to the spleen.

Ultrasonography is especially useful for guided needle biopsy of the kidney, where the needle can be directed toward areas of altered renal echogenicity or tissue of questionable integrity.[18,19] This ability to identify and avoid renal vasculature reduces the likelihood of perirenal hematoma formation.[18] Whenever unilateral renal or ureteral disease has been identified and resection of the affected kidney alone or together with the proximal ureter is contemplated, the contralateral kidney should be ultrasonically imaged and biopsied. Additionally, analysis of urine from the individual kidneys facilitated by catheterization of ureters may also be required to determine that the contralateral kidney is normal and free of degenerative processes.[5,18]

Evaluation of the foal bladder and umbilical remnants with ultrasonographic examination has generally replaced standard and contrast radiography as the imaging modality of choice. Normal limits for size of umbilical structures and fetal remnants have been established[20-22] (see Chapter 71). Pathologic increases in the cross-sectional area and echogenic appearance of these fetal structures is commonly seen with bacterial infections. In addition, rents through the bladder can be identified by urinary catheter placement and ultrasonographic "bubblegram" (Fig. 69-3).

Endoscopy

The distal urinary tracts of male and female horses of nearly all ages can be examined with fiberoptic or videoendoscopic instruments. The short, wide urethra of the female permits indirect inspection with either rigid scopes or flexible

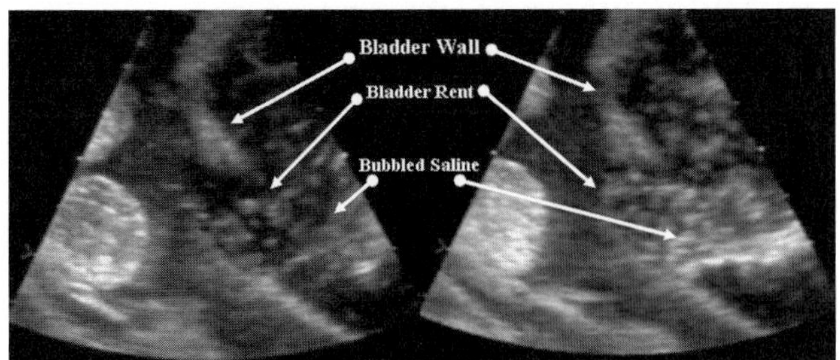

Figure 69-3. Ultrasonographic "bubblegram" of a 3-day-old Quarter Horse colt with uroperitoneum. Bubbled saline is seen moving through the rent. The rent in the urinary bladder was detected and repaired in surgery.

fiberoptic endoscopes. Endoscopes with a diameter of less than 1 cm and a working length of 120 to 140 cm are generally adequate for examination of adult male horses. The narrow diameter of the young male patient's urethra prohibits the introduction of most of these diagnostic instruments except via perineal percutaneous urethroscopy. The ureters in the female horse (or in the male horse via perineal urethrostomy) can be examined with a smaller bronchoscope with a diameter of less than 4 mm and working length of 40 to 60 cm.

Endoscopy has been used to identify lesions in the bladder and urethra, including ruptures, cystic and urethral calculi, and urethral erosions.[17] Endoscopy should be used for examination of the trigone to confirm the periodic efflux of urine from both ureteral openings at regular intervals.[2,23] Clinically, normal horses sedated with xylazine (Rompun; Haver, Shawnee, Kan) demonstrate a 20- to 45-second interval between peristaltic discharges of urine. In horses with nonfunctional kidneys or obstructive disease of the proximal urinary tract, the ureteral passage of urine can be irregular or nonexistent. Direct observation of ureteral discharge facilitates identification of unilateral proximal urinary tract disease and may complement or augment previous ultrasonographic findings. Catheterization of each ureter with polyethylene tubing and collection of urine for laboratory analyses (e.g., fraction excretion, culture) assist in the determination of renal function or disease.

SURGERY

Instruments

It is useful to have a broad selection of long, slender surgical instruments suitable for operating in the narrow confines of a deep midline or dorsal flank incision.[24] Broad-bladed self-retaining retractors are essential for effective surgical access to the renal pelvis. For electrosurgery, the use of fine-needle electrodes and scalpels is appropriate. Anastomotic procedures and intra-operative stenting of the urethra or ureters can be facilitated by using sterile flexible rubber urethral catheters or silicon or polyethylene cannulae. (However, the use of catheter stents is controversial,[25] and chronic placement appears to promote stricture formation of anastomosed ureters.[25] If stent catheters are used, they should probably be removed as soon as possible, preferably within 5 to 7 days after surgery.[26]) A magnifying loupe or an operating microscope and adequate lighting are useful for repair of ureteral defects.

Suture Material

Suture materials in a variety of sizes and strengths are required when performing urinary tract surgery. Tissues, such as the neonatal bladder, may be weak or friable, whereas bladders containing cystic calculi may be chronically thickened. Sutures should be selected with some appreciation of specific tissue strength and regenerative capacity. The bladder is considered to be one of the weakest tissues in the human body.[27] Nevertheless, bladders and ureters have a high regenerative capacity and heal readily.[25,28] For these reasons, sustained strength typically associated with the use of nonabsorbable suture materials is not required.[29]

In fact, nonabsorbable sutures should not be used for closure of any structure of the urinary tract. Nonabsorbable sutures serve as a nidus for formation of urinary concretions.[24] As a technical point of urinary tract surgery, no suture material of any type should be placed in such a fashion that it penetrates the urinary epithelium and is exposed to urine.[26,27] When synthetic absorbable sutures are exposed to alkaline urine (commonly found in herbivores or carnivores with urinary tract infections),[30] suture hydrolysis may be accelerated.

A comparative study of bursting strength of rat bladders sutured with 5-0 polyglycolic acid, 6-0 surgical gut, and 7-0 chromic gut suggested that infusion pressures of up to 550 mm Hg are required to induce failure.[31] Voiding pressures of most mammals are considerably lower.[32] The voiding pressures of adult ponies and mares have been determined to be approximately 90 mm Hg.[33] The use of 2-0 or 1-0 suture material is adequate to maintain primary closure of incisions in the pressurized portions of the equine distal urinary tract.

Absorbable staples may provide an alternative method of closure of hollow organs, including the bladder. Bladders closed with absorbable staples must be oversewn with a continuous inverting pattern to reduce the formation of adhesions.[34] The use of nonabsorbable staples in the bladder is not recommended based on the formation of a urolith in one case report.[35]

Laparoscopy

The use of the laparoscope as a minimally invasive procedure in equine surgery has greatly expanded over recent years. The horse is well suited to laparoscopic techniques because of its size and the anatomic limitations in dealing with several urologic surgical procedures. Standard laparoscopic equipment and instrumentation (described in Chapter 14) can be used for several surgical procedures of the urinary tract, including, but not limited to, exploratory laparotomy, nephrectomy, renal biopsy, umbilical remnant resection, cystic calculi removal, and urinary bladder repair. Hand-assisted techniques combine the benefits of laparoscopic and open surgical approaches. Advantages over laparoscopic techniques alone are seen in the ability to perform manual dissection and retraction, as well as an increase in the safety factor when controlling hemorrhage. As experience is gained and applications are contemplated, additional surgical techniques utilizing the laparoscope for urological disorders are likely to be developed.

Pharmacologic Considerations

The kidney is a major excretory pathway for many drugs that are administered systemically. As a consequence of its normal filtration and concentrating activities, the kidney is exposed to high levels of drugs and drug metabolites. Therefore, the renal effects of all drugs administered to surgical patients must be considered.[36]

ANESTHESIA

When planning anesthesia for a patient with renal impairment, it is important to minimize the period of surgical anesthesia and any related hypotension. All the fluorinated gas anesthetics are nephrotoxic to some degree; methoxyflurane is the most toxic, followed in decreasing order by enflurane, isoflurane, and halothane.[24] A newer inhalant anesthetic, sevoflurane, has cardiopulmonary effects similar to those of isoflurane, and it has the theoretical possibility of creating both hepatic and renal toxicity through the formation of compound A via the interaction between metabolites and CO_2 absorbents.[37,38] Despite the potential for the formation of toxic metabolites, sevoflurane has been used on over 120 million human patients without one report of renal-induced toxicity.[38] Halothane undergoes more hepatic metabolism than other inhalants, but formation of toxic waste products appears to be minimal.[39] Halothane is a widely used anesthetic agent for horses.[40] Its reduced degree of metabolism renders it relatively less toxic for use in renally impaired horses. Alternatively, isoflurane is useful in critically ill horses and has few renal effects,[41] which are limited to an increase in urine flow and an increase in serum glucose.[43]

The kidney is sensitive to hypoperfusion resulting from hypotension. Anesthesia often produces variable degrees of depression of myocardial contractility, heart rate, and cardiac output. Several commonly used anesthetic agents also produce some degree of peripheral vasodilation, which may result in reflex renal vasoconstriction, and associated renal perfusion.[43] Renal damage may be avoided by maintaining renal blood flow and minimizing the duration and magnitude of hypotension associated with general anesthesia. Intraoperative administration of balanced fluids enhances perfusion of the functional kidney by improving cardiac output.

Selective vasopressors such as dobutamine or dopamine increase cardiac output and enhance renal perfusion.[44,45] The use of an α-blocker as a premedication reduces the degree of catecholamine-induced vasoconstriction and improves renal perfusion in some anesthetized patients.[46]

Xylazine is a sedative hypnotic agent commonly administered to horses to facilitate examination or as a preanesthetic medication. Xylazine has a dose-dependent diuretic effect.[47] Horses with uncomplicated obstructive disease of the lower urinary tract that are at risk for acute cystorrhexis could be further compromised by the use of sedatives or tranquilizers with diuretic properties.

ANTIMICROBIAL AGENTS

Antibiotics are frequently administered to horses undergoing urinary tract surgery. Aminoglycoside antibiotics require special consideration when administered to dehydrated or renally impaired patients. Excretion of aminoglycosides occurs essentially via glomerular filtration without biotransformation.[48] As a result, these compounds are retained and concentrated within the renal cortex to levels 20 times that found in plasma.[49] Aminoglycosides bind to the brush border of renal tubular cells and produce proximal tubular disease.[46,50] Although all aminoglycosides demonstrate some degree of nephrotoxicity, neomycin is the most toxic.[51] Kanamycin, gentamicin, tobramycin, amikacin, and streptomycin follow in order of decreasing toxicity.[51,52] Other antimicrobials, notably polymyxin B, selected cephalosporins, and tetracycline degradation products, are variably nephrotoxic and should be avoided unless specifically indicated.[48,53]

Horses requiring the administration of drugs should be well hydrated and carefully monitored for exacerbation of renal impairment.[48] Periodic evaluation of patient hydration, serum urea nitrogen, and creatinine is appropriate. Evaluation of the urine for protein, blood, tubular casts, and γ-glutamyl transpeptidase is also reasonable. Serum drug levels can be monitored for peak and trough concentrations. Trough serum levels of gentamicin greater than 2 μg/mL in humans have been associated with increased nephrotoxicity.[54] This has led to the alteration of dosage and time for administration of gentamicin and other aminoglycosides. Currently, the recommendation of 6.6 mg/kg of gentamicin IV every 24 hours is considered to be safe and efficacious in the horse. It has also been documented in clinical cases that gentamicin at 4 mg/kg IV every 24 hours is safe and will result in peak plasma levels of greater than 2 μg/mL, which is required for antimicrobial effectiveness.[55]

ANTI-INFLAMMATORY DRUGS

Nonsteroidal anti-inflammatory drugs (NSAIDs) are routinely administered to equine patients undergoing general anesthesia for major surgery and present a risk to renally impaired patients. For many years, NSAID nephropathy has been recognized as a cause of renal papillary necrosis in rats,[56] humans receiving aspirin,[57] and horses administered phenylbutazone.[58] Nonselective NSAID administration reduces the levels of all prostaglandins, including those responsible for maintenance of renal vasculature and perfusion. Therefore, renally impaired horses requiring NSAID medications should receive reduced dosages, ranging from one-fifth to one-third the normal dosage, in an effort to reduce thromboxane concentration without altering renal prostaglandins.[59]

REFERENCES

1. Brown CM: Examination of the urinary system. In Robinson NE, editor: Current Therapy in Equine Medicine, ed 2, Philadelphia, 1983, WB Saunders.
2. DeBowes RM, Nyrop KA, Boulton CH: Cystic calculi in the horse, Comp Cont Educ Pract Vet 1984;6:S268.
3. Adams R: Acute renal failure. In Robinson NE, editor: Current Therapy in Equine Medicine, ed 2, Philadelphia, 1983, WB Saunders.

4. Nickel R, Schummer A, Seiferle E: Viscera of Domestic Mammals, New York, 1979, Springer-Verlag.
5. Bayly WM, Paradis MR, Reed SM: Equine renal biopsy: Indications, technic, interpretation and complications, Mod Vet Pract 1980;9:763.
6. Osborne CA, Fahning ML, Schultz RH, Perman V: Percutaneous renal biopsy in the cow and horse, J Am Vet Med Assoc 1968;153:563.
7. Bertone JJ, Traub-Dargatz JL, Fettman MJ, et al: Monitoring the progression of renal failure in a horse with polycystic kidney disease: Use of the reciprocal of serum creatinine concentration and sodium sulfanilate clearance half-time, J Am Vet Med Assoc 1987;191:565.
8. Brobst DF, Carrol RJ, Bayly WM: Urinary enzyme concentrations in normal horses, Cornell Vet 1986;76:299.
9. Brobst DF, Bramwell K, Kramer JW: Sodium sulfanilate clearance as a method of determining renal function in the horse, J Equine Med Surg 1978;2:500.
10. Adams R, McClure JJ, Gossett KA, et al: Evaluation of a technique for measurement of γ-glutamyl transpeptidase in equine urine, Am J Vet Res 1985;46:147.
11. Richardson DW: Urogenital problems in the neonatal foal, Vet Clin North Am Equine Pract 1985;1:179.
12. Manning M, Dubiolizeg R, McGuirk S: Postoperative myositis in a neonatal foal: A case report, Vet Surg 1995;24:69.
13. Modransky PD, Wagner PC, Robinette JD, et al: Surgical correction of bilateral ectopic ureters in two foals, J Vet Surg 1983;12:141.
14. Brady TM, Singer D, Weiss CA, et al: Angiographic nephrectomy using iodinated contrast agent, Invest Radiol 1982;17:479.
15. Wagoner RD: Acute renal failure associated with contrast agents, Arch Intern Med 1978;138:353.
16. Walsh DM, Royal HD: Evaluation of a single injection of ^{99m}Tc-labeled diethylenetriaminepentaacetic acid for measuring glomerular filtration rate in horses, Am J Vet Res 1992;53:776.
17. Held JP, Daniel GB: Use of nonimaging nuclear medicine techniques to assess the effect of flunixin meglumine on effective renal plasma flow and effective renal blood flow in healthy horses, Am J Vet Res 1991;52:1619.
18. Modransky PD: Ultrasound guided renal and hepatic biopsy techniques, Vet Clin North Am Equine Pract 1986;2:115.
19. Rantanen NW: Diseases of the kidneys, Vet Clin North Am Equine Pract 1986;2:89.
20. Reef, VB, Collatos CA: Ultrasonography of umbilical structures in clinically normal foals, Am J Vet Res 1988;49:2143.
21. Reef, VB, Collatos CA: Clinical, ultrasonography and surgical findings in foals with umbilical remnant infections, J Am Vet Med Assoc 1988;195:69.
22. Reef VB. Sonographic diagnosis of uroperitoneum in foals and horses, Proc Vet Med Forum 1995:13.
23. Sullins KE, Traub-Dargatz JL: Endoscopic anatomy of the equine urinary tract, Comp Cont Educ Pract Vet 1984;6:S663.
24. Christie BA: Principles of urinary tract surgery. In Slatter DH, editor: Textbook of Small Animal Surgery, Philadelphia, 1985, WB Saunders.
25. Peacock EE: Healing and repair of viscera. In Peacock EE, editor: Wound Repair, ed 3, Philadelphia, 1984, WB Saunders.
26. Robertson JT, Spurlock GH, Bramlage LR, et al: Repair of ureteral defect in a foal, J Am Vet Med Assoc 1983;183:779.
27. Van Winkle W, Hastings JC: Considerations in the choice of suture material for various tissues, Surg Gynecol Obstet 1972;135:113.
28. Rasmussen F: Biochemical analysis of wound healing in the urinary bladder, Surg Gynecol Obstet 1967;124:553.
29. Brannan W, Ochsner MG, Pond HS III, et al: Laboratory and clinical experience with polyglycolic acid suture in urogenital surgery, J Urol 1973;110:551.
30. Kaminski JM, Katz AR, Woodward SC: Urinary bladder calculus formation on sutures in rabbits, cats, and dogs, Surg Gynecol Obstet 1978;146:353.
31. Adams H, Narmes R, Small C, Hadley H: Suture and bladder wound healing in the experimental animal, Invest Urol 1975;12:267.
32. Christie BA: Incidence and etiology of vesico-ureteral reflux and pyelonephritis in apparently normal dogs, Invest Urol 1973;10:459.
33. Clark ES, Semrad SD, Bischel P, Oliver JE: Cystometrography and urethral pressure profiles in healthy horses and pony mares, Am J Vet Res 1987;48:552.
34. Rashmir-Raver AM, DeBowes RM: Unpublished data, 1990.
35. Edwards RB, Ducharme NG, Hackett RP: Laparoscopic repair of a bladder rupture in a foal, Vet Surg 1995;24:60.
36. Bennett WM, Singer I, Golper T, et al: Guidelines for drug therapy in renal failure, Ann Intern Med 1977;86:754.
37. Clarke KW. Desflurane and sevoflurane: New volatile anesthetic agents, Vet Clin North Am Small Anim Pract 1999;29:793.
38. Anders MW. Formation and toxicity of anesthetic degradation products, Ann Rev Pharmacol Toxicol 2005;45:147.
39. Lowe G, Motulsky H, Trudell J, et al: Quantum chemical studies of the metabolism of the inhalation anesthetics methoxyflurane, enflurane, and isoflurane, Mol Pharmacol 1979;10:406.
40. Steffey EP: Enflurane and isoflurane anesthesia: A summary of laboratory and clinical investigations in horses, J Am Vet Med Assoc 1978;121:367.
41. Steffey EG, Howland D: Comparison of circulatory and respiratory effects of isoflurane and halothane anesthesia in horses, Am J Vet Res 1980;41:821.
42. Watson ZE, Steffey EP, VanHoogmoed LM, et al: Effect of general anesthesia and minor surgical trauma on urine and serum measurements in horses, Am J Vet Res 1999;63:1061.
43. Deutsch S, Pierce EC, Vandam LD: Effects of anesthesia with thiopental, nitrous oxide and neuromuscular blockers on renal function in normal man, Anesthesiology 1968;20:184.
44. Linder A: Synergism of dopamine and furosemide in oliguric acute renal failure, Nephron 1983;33:121.
45. Swanson CR, Muir WW, Bednarski RM, et al: Hemodynamic responses in halothane-anesthetized horses given infusions of dopamine or dobutamine, Am J Vet Res 1985;46:365.
46. Cousins MJ, Mazze RI: Anaesthesia surgery and renal function, Anaesth Intens Care 1973;1:355.
47. Thurmon JC, Benson GJ: Injectable anesthetics and anesthetic adjuncts, Vet Clin North Am Equine Pract 1987;3:15.
48. Davis LE: Adverse drug reactions in the horse, Vet Clin North Am Equine Pract 1987;3:153.
49. Luft FC, Patel V, Yum MN, et al: Experimental aminoglycoside nephrotoxicity, J Lab Clin Med 1975;86:213.
50. Just M, Erdmann G, Habermann E: The renal handling of polybasic drugs: 1. Gentamicin and aprotinin in intact animals, Naunyn Schmiedebergs Arch Pharmacol 1977;300:57.
51. Edwards DJ, Love DN, Raus J, et al: The nephrotoxic potential of neomycin in the horse, Equine Vet J 1989;21:206.
52. Appel GB, Neu HC: The nephrotoxicity of antimicrobial agents, N Engl J Med 1977;296:722.
53. Riviere JE, Traver DS, Coppoc GL: Gentamicin toxic nephropathy in horses with disseminated bacterial infection, J Am Vet Med Assoc 1982;180:648.
54. Sojka JE, Brown SA: Pharmacokinetic adjustment of gentamicin dosing in horses with sepsis, J Am Vet Med Assoc 1986;189:784.
55. Tudor RA, Papich MG, Reddine WR: Drug disposition and dosage determination of once daily administration of gentamicin sulfate in horses after abdominal surgery, J Am Vet Assoc 1999;215:503.
56. Nanra RS, Kincaid-Smith P: Papillary necrosis in rats caused by aspirin and aspirin-containing mixtures, Br Med J 1970;3:559.
57. Kincaid-Smith P: Pathogenesis of the renal lesion associated with the abuse of analgesics, Lancet 1967;1:859.
58. Gunson DE: Renal papillary necrosis in horses, J Am Vet Med Assoc 1983;182:263.
59. Patrignani P, Filabozzi P, Patrono C: Selective cumulative inhibition of platelet thromboxane production by low dose aspirin therapy in healthy subjects, J Clin Invest 1982;69:1366.

CHAPTER 70

Kidneys and Ureters

James D. Lillich
Andrew T. Fischer, Jr.
Richard M. DeBowes

ANATOMY

The kidneys of the horse are located retroperitoneally in the left and right lumbar regions.[1] The left kidney lies deep to the lumbar fascia of the psoas musculature in a paramedian position between the 17th rib and the 3rd lumbar vertebra. Laterally, the left kidney is related to the spleen and the renosplenic ligament; ventrally, to the jejunum and descending colon; and medially, to the adrenal glands and left lobe of the pancreas. The right kidney is located in a right paramedian position, more cranial than the left kidney, and between the 16th rib and the 1st lumbar vertebra. Dorsally, the right kidney is related to the right crus of the diaphragm; medially, to the adrenal gland and pancreas; and ventrally, to the cecum. Only the lateral aspect of the right kidney is covered by peritoneum. The renal arteries, which arise from the aorta, frequently branch before penetrating the renal parenchyma. Accessory branches of the renal arteries that penetrate the cranial or caudal poles of the kidney are found occasionally.

The ureters arise from the renal pelvis of each kidney and course laterally and retroperitoneally from their dorsal paramedian origin to the trigone of the bladder, where they insert in a dorsolateral position cranial to the renal crest. In the mare, the caudal ureters can be found in the attached border of the lateral ligaments of the bladder.[2] The ureters of the adult horse are typically 70 cm long and have a diameter of 0.5 to 1 cm.[1]

DISORDERS REQUIRING SURGERY

Surgery of the proximal urinary tract of the horse is both tedious and difficult. Postmortem findings in 364 horses suggest that the frequency of renal disease is 3.84%.[3] The frequency of renal or ureteral disease treatable by surgical methods is presumably lower. Furthermore, candidates for renal surgery (other than elective biopsy) must have renal pathology confined to one kidney. Horses with unilateral renal pathology treatable with surgery are a select minority.[4,5] Patients with bilateral renal disease such as polycystic kidneys or chronic renal failure secondary to obstructive disease are generally not candidates for renal surgery.[6] Possible indications for renal surgery include the presence of renal calculi,[7-10] neoplasia,[11-13] hydronephrosis, unilateral pyelonephritis,[14] ectopic ureter,[15,16] and renal dysplasia.[17]

Surgical disease of the equine ureter is also uncommon.[10,15,16,18-21] Reports of ureteral surgery are infrequent, because ureteral disease rarely exists as an isolated entity. Potential surgical indications include ureteral calculi,[10,21,22] ureterorrhexis,[23,24] ectopic ureter,[15,16,18-20,25] or rare conditions such as ureteropelvic polyps.[17]

Renal and Ureteral Calculi

Urinary calculi are formed from hydrated crystals of calcium carbonate. Although uncommon, these calculi can become large and produce extensive damage to the kidney, either by causing an obstructive hydronephrosis[4,9,10] or by direct encroachment on the renal parenchyma.[4,7] Select cases, diagnosed early in the course of the disease, can be treated by nephrotomy or nephrostomy.[22] Chronic cases can involve calculi of exceptional size and require treatment by nephrectomy.[7,8] It is possible for smaller calculi to move distally and lodge in the distal ureter, resulting in obstructive hydroureter and hydronephrosis.[5,10]

Clinical signs of obstructive renal or ureteral disease are often nonspecific and subtle. Horses are usually asymptomatic until advanced renal disease is present. Weight loss, anorexia, lethargy, and colic are more commonly associated with upper urinary tract obstructive disease rather than with altered urination and hematuria.[4,5]

Rectal identification of a nephrolith is difficult and unlikely unless the calculus is large and located within the left kidney. The diagnosis of nephrolithiasis (or ureterolithiasis) is made most commonly from clinical signs supported by ultrasonographic and endoscopic findings.[15,22,26] Percutaneous ultrasonographic examination of an affected kidney is characterized by an echogenic interface with acoustic shadowing deep to the urolith (Fig. 70-1). Kidneys may be enlarged or smaller than expected on ultrasonographic examination.[4] Ureteral calculi can be identified with rectal palpation. Endoscopic examination of the trigone of

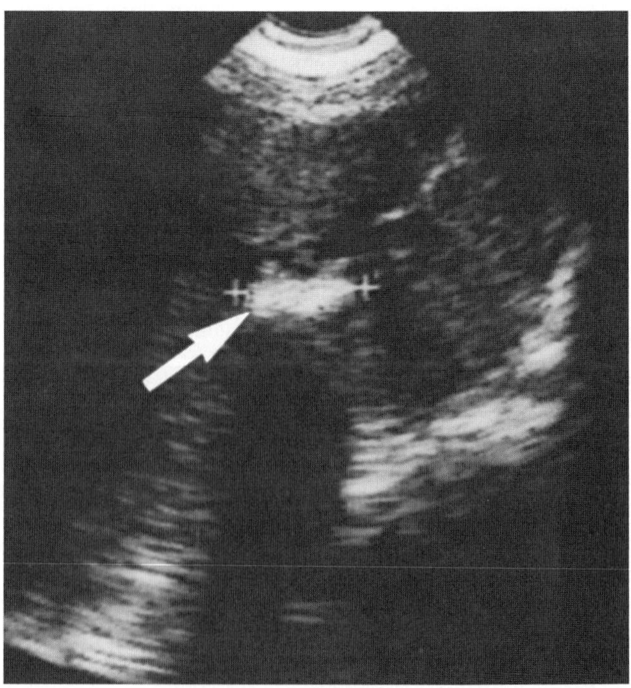

Figure 70-1. A solitary hyperechoic nephrolith is evident *(arrow)* on this transcutaneous ultrasonographic study of the right kidney.

affected horses evaluates the ureters for periodic elimination of urine.[21] Hemorrhage or cloudy discharge at the ureteral openings and failure to observe periodic elimination of urine from ureteral openings are suggestive of a proximal obstruction. Select cases of ureteroliths are usually treated surgically, but there is one case report of successful resolution using electrohydraulic lithotripsy.[27]

Renal Neoplasia and Dysplasia

Renal neoplasia, either primary or metastatic, is rare in horses. However, renal adenomas, primary renal cell carcinomas, undifferentiated renal sarcomas, and metastatic hemangiosarcomas have been documented[11-13,28] A metastatic granulosa cell tumor has been observed by one author. These tumors are typically large and not detected until late in the course of the disease. Renal dysplasia has been reported in the horse and may be secondary to obstruction from benign ureteropelvic polyps. Unilateral disease may be successfully treated with ipsilateral nephrectomy and ureterectomy.[17]

Renal neoplasia is usually diagnosed in older horses and associated with weight loss, anorexia, or hematuria. Primary tumors may metastasize via the renal vein to the lungs, via the renal lymphatics to the regional lymph nodes, or by transperitoneal exfoliation to other abdominal organs. Primary neoplasia of the ureters has not been described.

Pyelonephritis

Pyelonephritis is an uncommon disease of horses. Horses with unilateral involvement that is refractory to medical therapy, or with discrete, singular renal abscesses are treated by nephrectomy.[14,29] Horses with disseminated bilateral septic nephritis are not candidates for nephrectomy.

Ureterorrhexis

Ureterorrhexis is a relatively rare condition in which the ureter develops a mural defect and leaks urine.[23,30,31] Presumably, this condition results from a congenital defect,[23] and fillies are predisposed.[30,31] In small domestic animals, trauma or obstruction is the most common cause. Acquired defects can result from trauma or obstructive disease in horses, as described in one case report.[26] There is also one case report of urine leakage from the renal pelvis secondary to renal calculi.[4]

Diagnosis of uroperitoneum is made from the clinical history, physical examination findings, and abdominocentesis. The specific site is identified by excretory urography, ultrasonography, or surgical exploration. Although retroperitoneal extravasation of sterile urine is not considered problematic in humans, extravasation of septic urine or the concurrent presence of urine and bacteria in the tissue results in fulminant septic cellulitis.

Ectopic Ureter

Ectopic ureter is an uncommon developmental condition of horses and results from faulty differentiation of the metanephric duct.[23] There is neither sex nor breed predisposition in horses,[16,18,19] which is not the case in dogs.

Typically, the anomalous ureters insert distal to the trigone, resulting in urinary incontinence. A history of urinary incontinence since birth leads to the diagnosis, which is confirmed by endoscopy, contrast radiography (Fig. 70-2), or surgical exploration.[17,19,20,23] Affected individuals should be evaluated for the concurrent problems of hydronephrosis and hydroureter (Fig. 70-3). Timely diagnosis appears to be important for successful treatment. Older patients are more difficult to operate on because of their larger size and an increased incidence of acquired hydronephrosis or ascending urinary tract infection. The surgical approaches for the management of ureteral ectopia include ureteral transplantation and neoureterostomy.[19,20] Success is obtained in large

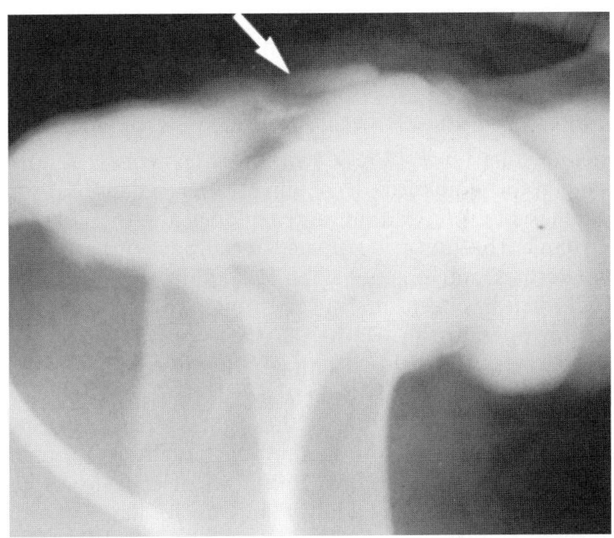

Figure 70-2. A lateral radiographic projection of the lower urinary tract was made during an excretory urogram of a foal with urinary incontinence. An ectopic ureter can be seen *(arrow)* emptying into the pelvic urethra, distal to the trigone.

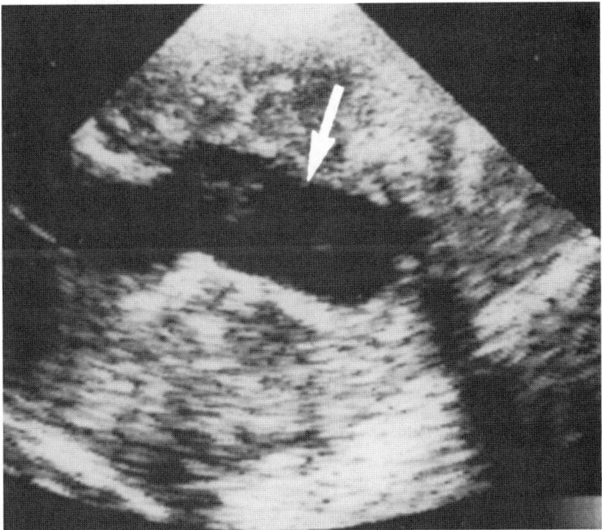

Figure 70-3. A dilated hypoechoic renal pelvis *(arrow)* and ureter are evident on this transrectal ultrasonographic examination of a horse with hydronephrosis and hydroureter. (Courtesy Norman Rantanen, DVM, MS.)

horses with proper patient positioning and visceral retraction.[32] Horses with a unilateral ectopic ureter have been managed successfully by ipsilateral nephrectomy.[16,17]

SURGICAL PROCEDURES

Renal Biopsy

Biopsy of the kidney is used to complete the diagnostic evaluation of suspected renal disease and to evaluate the contralateral kidney before unilateral nephrectomy. It may provide diagnostic information not afforded by ultrasonographic examination or excretory urography. Surgical techniques for biopsy of the kidney are based on anatomic landmarks[33,34] or directed ultrasonic guidance.[35] Ultrasonic guidance provides the added benefit of biopsy of selected areas of sonographically abnormal renal tissue while avoiding major vascular structures.

Simple Percutaneous Technique

Percutaneous renal biopsy (without the benefit of ultrasonographic guidance) is obtained after sedation of the horse, aseptic preparation, and regional anesthesia of the left flank. The horse is palpated rectally by one operator, who locates and positions the left kidney over a biopsy needle that has been introduced through the left flank by a second operator.[33,34] Either a Vim Tru-Cut (Travenol Laboratories, Deerfield, Ill) or a Vim-Silverman (Mueller Company, Chicago, Ill) biopsy needle is used. It is considerably less safe to biopsy the right kidney using this technique, because it is located more cranially and difficult to palpate. The operator's ability to selectively biopsy discrete regions of the kidney and avoid large vascular structures is minimal.

Ultrasonographically and Laparoscopically Guided Percutaneous Techniques

Ultrasonographically guided needle biopsy of the kidney is obtained with the horse restrained in stocks and prepared as described earlier. The left kidney is imaged at the 17th intercostal space or immediately caudal to the 18th rib and identified deep to the spleen. The right kidney is imaged at the 15th or 16th intercostal space immediately ventral to the transverse processes of the lumbar vertebrae. A 3-MHz transducer produces images of both the kidney and the biopsy instrument. Imaging of the left kidney is particularly enhanced by the presence of the spleen interposed between the body wall and the renal parenchyma. Typically, renal parenchyma has a homogeneous low-amplitude image surrounding a more echogenic collecting system.

When the kidney has been located and identified by ultrasonographic scanning, a biopsy needle is introduced through the desensitized skin of the flank and into the deeper tissues. Typically, the scanning plane is oriented in a longitudinal direction, and the biopsy needle is identified (Fig. 70-4). Passage of the biopsy needle through the tissues and into the kidney is monitored, and large vascular structures and loops of bowel are avoided. Because the operator is able to visualize and direct the biopsy needle to specific regions of the kidney under ultrasonic guidance, selected areas of the kidney can be biopsied where altered echogenicity is consistent with renal pathology.

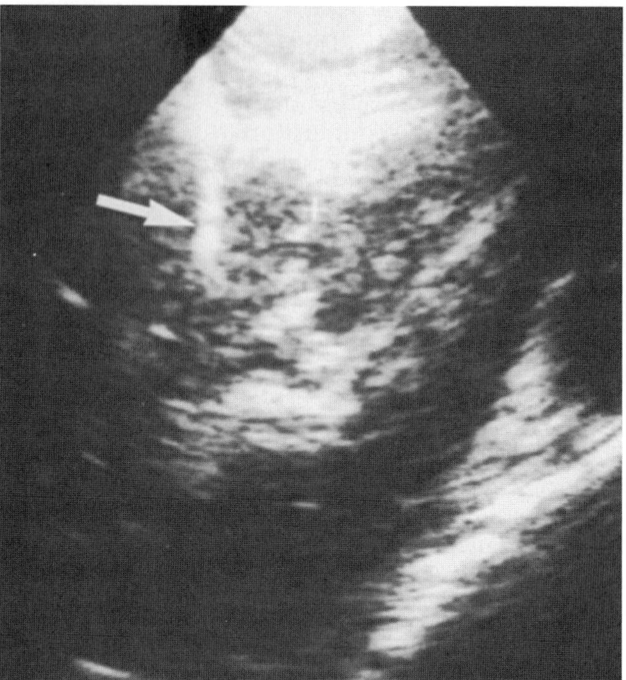

Figure 70-4. A renal biopsy can be obtained readily under ultrasonic control. The hyperechoic biopsy needle *(arrow)* can be observed in the renal cortex. (Courtesy Norman Rantanen, DVM, MS.)

If the ultrasonographic examination identifies gross abnormalities to the architecture of the kidneys or the kidneys cannot be accurately identified, laparoscopic exploration should be considered. Standard equipment and approaches to the abdomen have been described in Chapter 14. In general, an ipsilateral approach is used for laparoscopic assisted biopsies. Biopsy forceps are visually introduced in to the abdomen through a separate stab incision made 5 to 10 cm ventral or dorsal to the laparoscope. Perirenal fat may inhibit access to the parenchyma. The biopsy site is checked for hemorrhage and the abdomen is deflated and skin incisions are closed routinely.

Complications

Complications of renal biopsy include hemorrhage (predominantly) and infection.[34] Biopsies collected without the benefit of ultrasonographic guidance are periodically associated with perirenal hemorrhage and hematoma formation (Fig. 70-5), the severity of which can vary significantly. Patients that suffer a laceration of a larger vessel may develop a perirenal hematoma. No treatment is required unless active hemorrhage fails to stop. Transfusions or procoagulant therapy is rarely necessary. Some patients develop transient hematuria after renal biopsy, but usually this problem resolves spontaneously within 24 to 36 hours after the biopsy procedure.[33,34] Infection is rare if aseptic principles are strictly followed. The use of antibiotics after renal biopsy should be considered if a break in surgical technique occurs or a perirenal hematoma develops.

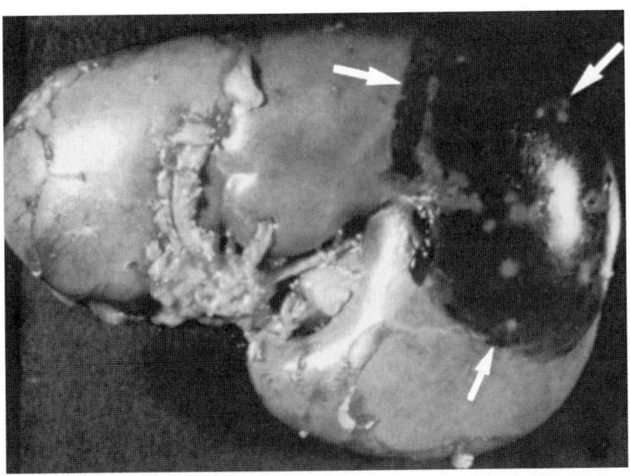

Figure 70-5. Subcapsular hematoma *(arrows)* is a possible complication of renal biopsy performed without the benefit of ultrasonic guidance.

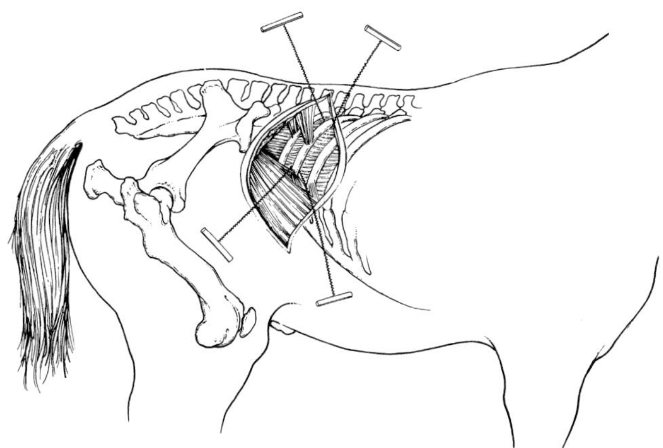

Figure 70-6. Right 17th rib resection permits surgical access for right nephrectomy or nephrotomy procedure.

Nephrectomy

Nephrectomy is the surgical treatment of choice for unilateral hydronephrosis, abscessation, neoplasia, ureteropelvic polyp, and ectopic ureter. Severe cases of unilateral obstructive ureterolithiasis or nephrolithiasis may also require nephrectomy.

Unilateral right nephrectomy is performed through a right 16th or 17th rib resection or, alternatively, at the 16th and 15th intercostal spaces.[36] Depending on the degree of anatomic variation, the most cranial approach can create a plane of dissection across the dorsal aspect of the costophrenic angle and through the diaphragm to the kidney. Although transthoracic approaches have been used successfully, they are more complicated than the right 17th rib resection and are not recommended.

In the *transcostal* approach, the animal is anesthetized, placed in lateral recumbency, clipped, and prepared for aseptic abdominal surgery. A 30- to 40-cm skin incision is made over the 16th or 17th rib. Dissection is continued deep to divide the musculature and expose the rib. The periosteum is incised and elevated around the rib, taking care to avoid injury to the intercostal vasculature. The rib is transected 2 to 5 cm distal to the costovertebral articulation using a bone saw, Gigli wire, or an osteotome (Fig. 70-6). Ventrally, the rib is disarticulated at the costochondral junction. Proximally, the ends of the parent bone are smoothed with a bone rasp. The medial costal periosteum is longitudinally incised, and the kidney is exposed by blunt dissection through the retroperitoneal fat. If additional exposure is required, the incision can be extended ventrally.

The kidney is mobilized by digital circumferential dissection through perinephric fat to expose the ureterovascular pedicle and penetrating capsular vessels (Fig. 70-7). Small capsular vessels and accessory renal arteries are electrocauterized and ligated, respectively. The ureterovascular pedicle is isolated, and the artery, vein, and ureter are individually double-ligated (Fig. 70-8). The use of hemostatic vascular clips or staples facilitates removal of the kidney and provides adequate access for suture ligation of major vascular elements.

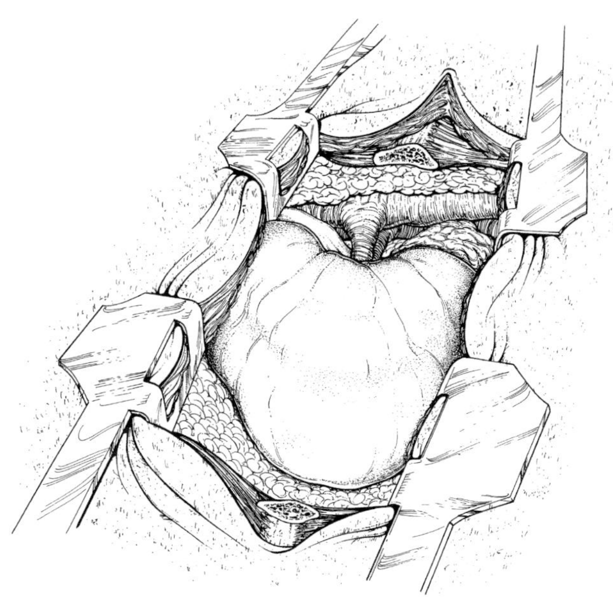

Figure 70-7. Perirenal fat is removed by blunt dissection to permit access to the ureterovascular pedicle.

After removal of the affected kidney, the renal fossa is lavaged and again evaluated for evidence of hemorrhage. The ureter is mobilized, ligated as far distally as possible, and transected. (Resection of the pelvic ureter is not possible when using a flank approach for nephrectomy.) Either Penrose or closed suction drains are placed after resection of the kidney to evacuate blood accumulating in the dead space or to manage urine-contaminated tissues.

The periosteum of the rib and deep fascia are closed with a synthetic absorbable suture material placed in simple-interrupted fashion. The subcutaneous tissues and skin are closed routinely. Unilateral left nephrectomy of the horse is performed in similar fashion using either a 17th or 18th rib resection or a dorsal flank incision.[16,37,38]

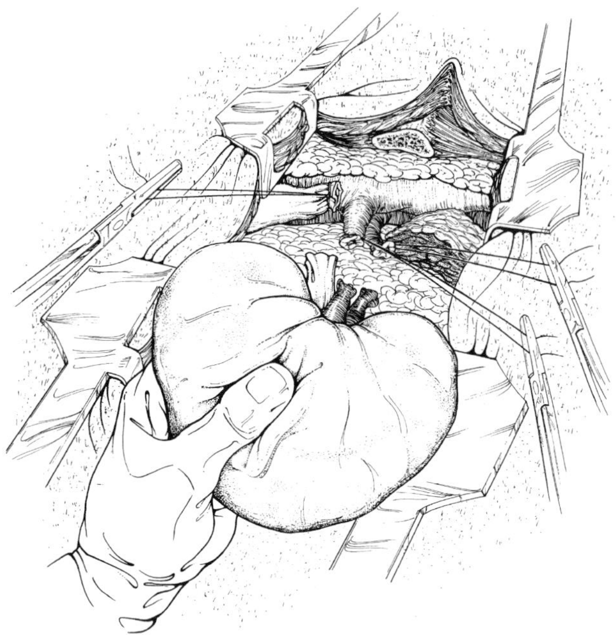

Figure 70-8. The renal artery, vein, and ureter are ligated with transfixing ligatures before resection of the kidney.

Laparoscopic Nephrectomy by Hand-Assisted Techniques

Laparoscopic nephrectomy in the horse has been described.[39] An ipsilateral flank approach is used for removal of the respective kidney. At least three portals are required: the first between the 17th and 18th ribs ventral to the tuber coxae, and the second and third in the paralumbar fossa caudal to the 18th rib. A 0-degree laparoscope is utilized. The procedure for removal of the left kidney starts with injection of epinephrine (1 mg in 10 mL of saline) in three or four sites at the dorsal border of the spleen to create splenic contraction. The perirenal fascia is injected dorsally with 20 mL of 2% mepivacaine. An electrocautery hook blade is used to create a plane of dissection dorsal to the kidney. Perirenal fat is dissected and removed with curved laparoscopic scissors. The hilus of the kidney is carefully dissected to identify the vessels. Specialized (clockwise and counterclockwise) laparoscopic ligation instruments (Richard Wolf Company, Germany) are used to ligate the renal artery, vein, and ureter, in that order. The area is checked for hemorrhage prior to making a small flank incision to retrieve the kidney. Complications include pneumothorax and bleeding from accessory renal arteries. It should be noted that while the procedure holds promise, it is technically demanding and requires practice before attempting it on clinical patients.

The first hand-assisted nephrectomy in human medicine was described in 1997.[40] The hand-assisted laparoscopic surgical technique has been described for the left kidney in the standing horse.[41] Preparation of the horse for this surgery includes withholding feed for at least 12 hours, and administration of perioperative antibiotics and analgesics. The left paralumbar fossa is clipped and surgically prepared for aseptic surgery. Administration of a systemic α_2-agonist provides sedation, and local infiltration with mepivacaine provides anesthesia. Because of the open approach, insufflation of the abdominal cavity is not necessary. A 10- to 12-cm skin incision is made in the paralumbar fossa beginning 5 to 8 cm below the dorsal border of the internal abdominal oblique muscle. The external abdominal oblique muscle is sharply incised and a modified grid approach is used to gain access to the peritoneal cavity. The peritoneum is sharply incised. A laparoscopic viewing portal is made dorsal to the proximal border of the flank incision, and an instrument portal is created dorsal and cranial to the viewing portal.

A 0-degree laparoscope is utilized for viewing the surgical site, and a hand within the abdomen is used for retraction and blunt dissection. The retroperitoneal space caudoventral to the kidney is infiltrated with 15 to 20 mL of mepivacaine followed by digital massage to facilitate distribution. The peritoneum is sharply incised via an instrument portal and then bluntly, manually dissected to expose the left kidney. Careful manual dissection is used to completely identify all of the vascular structures entering and leaving the kidney. The renal artery and vein are double-ligated, separately using no. 2 polyglactin 910 with one-handed ties. The vessels are transected and the kidney is delivered out of the flank incision. The ureter is double-ligated and the incisions are closed routinely.

The most immediate and severe complication is uncontrollable hemorrhage, which generally originates from a torn accessory branch of the renal artery. Benefits from hand-assisted procedures include: smaller surgical incision, decreased surgical time, and less surgical morbidity, in addition to eliminating the need for general anesthesia. Although this procedure has not been applied clinically on a large scale, the procedure holds significant promise.

Nephrotomy

Nephrotomy is not considered a benign or potentially less complicated surgical procedure than nephrectomy. In dogs, it results in a 20% to 40% reduction in renal function.[42] In equine patients, nephrotomy is performed less commonly than nephrectomy because indications are fewer, and the degree of technical difficulty is substantially greater.

The surgical approach for nephrotomy is similar to that used for nephrectomy. The procedure is technically difficult, given the depth and dimensions of the surgical field and the reduced intraoperative visualization of the tissues, complicated by hemorrhage from the penetrating capsular vessels. In canine patients, the approach is through a longitudinal sagittal incision in the convex lateral surface of the kidney.[42] To make such an incision, the kidney must be dissected free from the perirenal fat. This disrupts multiple small penetrating capsular vessels that require hemostasis.

Once the kidney is mobilized, it may be pivoted about the ureterovascular pedicle to expose the convex surface. Before incising the cortex, major renal vessels are temporarily occluded with noncrushing vascular forceps or Rummel's tourniquets. The renal incision is extended to expose the collecting system and the renal pelvis. Obstructive lesions of the renal pelvis (e.g., renal calculi) are removed, and the collecting system is lavaged. The associated ureter should be cannulated with a no. 10 to 15 French polyethylene catheter to ensure patency.

Canine nephrotomy incisions are closed by gently pressing the renal halves together with sustained pressure.[42]

However, capsular sutures or parenchymal mattress sutures should be considered for closure of the equine kidney. Although pyelotomy has been suggested as a reasonable approach to the canine renal pelvis, its small size increases the risk of accidental transection of an interlobar artery. Likewise, the close proximity of the renal artery and veins would make pyelotomy a difficult and risky procedure to perform in equine patients.

Ureterotomy

Indications for ureterotomy in the horse are limited principally to obstructive urolithiasis. Presentation of uncomplicated cases of ureteral calculi for surgical treatment is rare. Horses are often chronically affected and have developed some degree of renal pathology. Some horses with sufficient renal mass remain asymptomatic, and the condition is diagnosed at necropsy as an incidental finding.

Horses with identifiable ureteral pathology may be explored through a flank laparotomy, or through caudal ventral midline laparotomy in the mare. Exposure is difficult and extremely limited over the posterior course of the ureter. Typically, lesions are located in the proximal third of the ureter. When lesions can be identified and exposed, the ureter is incised proximal to the obstruction, and the contents are evacuated with surgical suction. The urolith is removed and the ureter closed in a simple-continuous pattern with synthetic absorbable sutures. Silastic tubing may be introduced into the ureter as a stent over which the ureteral repair may be performed. When direct surgical intervention is not possible, the use of a grasping basket (Dormia Stone Dislodger, V. Mueller Company, McGow Park, Ill) can facilitate closed dislodgment of a ureterolith.[43] The instrument is introduced into the ureteral orifice by direct insertion (mares) or under videoendoscopic control using a perineal urethrotomy (males) (see Chapter 72). Guidance by rectal palpation is desirable to manipulate the dislodger into a position proximal to the urolith. The dislodger is subsequently opened and retracted to ensnare the urolith and displace it distally using slow, gentle traction.

Repair of ureterorrhexis is approached in similar fashion.[23,24] In a case report, successful repair of a traumatic ureteral tear in a postpartum mare was accomplished with an indwelling polyethylene stent tubing (outside diameter, 1.90 mm).[24] The salient presurgical features of the case included profound uroperitoneum and associated electrolyte abnormalities (hyponatremia, hyperkalemia). A ventral midline celiotomy was utilized; however, because of the accumulation of urine around the ureter and broad ligament, the rent within the ureter could not be identified for primary repair. The surgery was assisted with the use of videoendoscopy of the urinary bladder. This allowed the surgeon to accurately place the stent within the ureter past the presumptive location of the rent. The stent was checked for urine production and then anchored to the vaginal mucosa and perineal skin and kept in place for 21 days. Although a few prosthetic constructs are available for use as ureteral stents in human medicine, the optimal size (no. 7 to 9 French in humans) and material have yet to be determined for the horse and will likely not be determined scientifically because of the rarity of the condition.

Neoureterostomy

Neoureterostomy techniques are used in the horse to manage ectopic ureters. In human and canine patients, vesicoureteral anastomosis has traditionally been the method of choice for treatment of ectopic ureters and selected cases of ureteral avulsion. Complications with these techniques in equine patients[20] prompted treatment of foals by unilateral nephrectomy, assuming that the contralateral kidney was normal.[16,17] Surgical success can be obtained, however, in large horses.

The surgical approach is made through a caudoventral midline incision, extended to the pubis for exposure of the bladder. The viscera are packed off cranially in the abdomen, and the ureter is identified as it traverses the dorsolateral bladder. The ectopic ureter can be identified by retrograde catheterization. If the ectopic ureter is in close proximity to the dorsal bladder, a side-to-side or end-to-side extravesicoureteral anastomosis may be performed to create a new ureteral opening along the dorsolateral cranial base of the bladder. The distal ureter is ligated and dissected free unless it is in an intramural location and surgically inaccessible.

Alternatively, if the ectopic ureter is not in close proximity to the bladder, the ureter may be ligated distally and neoureterostomy achieved by intravesicular anastomosis (Fig. 70-9). Tunneling the ureter creates a functional equivalent of a distal ureteral valve, which reduces the likelihood of vesicoureteral reflux.[44] Apposition of the ureteral and vesicular mucosa with small (3-0, 4-0) synthetic absorbable suture material is ideal (Fig. 70-10).

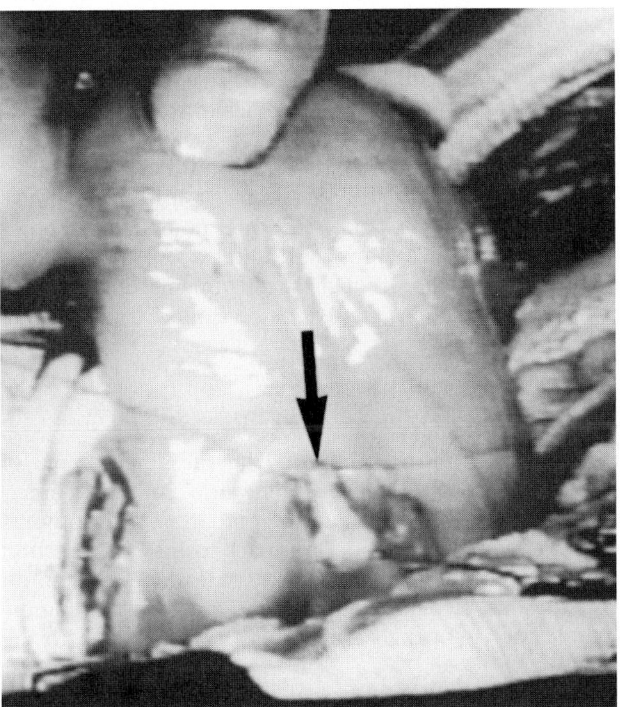

Figure 70-9. Ligatures are placed to secure a ureter *(arrow)* after translocation to the bladder from an ectopic site. The ureter has been tunneled through the seromuscular layer of the bladder to prevent vesicoureteral reflux. (Courtesy Candace Lundin, DVM.)

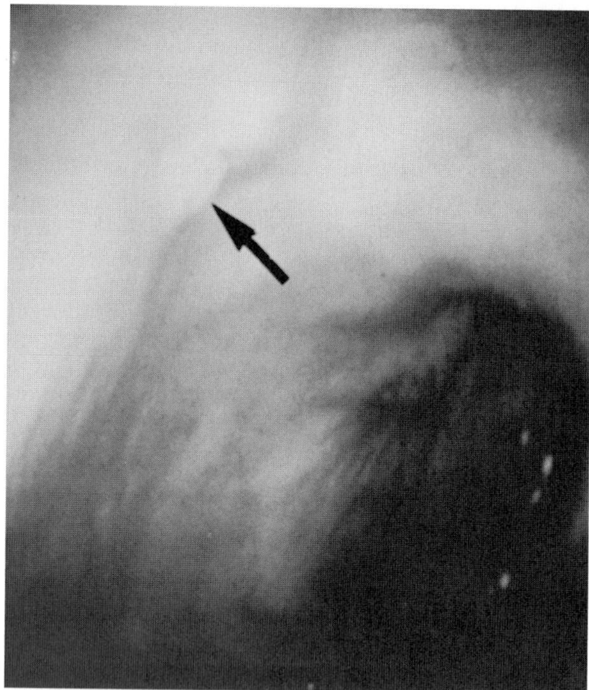

Figure 70-10. Endoscopic appearance of the ureterovesicular anastomosis demonstrated in Figure 70-9. The ureteral stoma can be observed on the dorsolateral wall of the bladder *(arrow)*. (Courtesy Candace Lundin, DVM.)

Aftercare

After all renal surgery, horses should be evaluated for water consumption and urine production and supported with intravenous fluids. Serum electrolytes and clearance ratios may reveal transient imbalance in electrolyte clearance after nephrectomy, particularly with regard to potassium. Fluid therapy should be adjusted accordingly.

Prophylactic antibiotics are indicated during the perioperative period because this is a clean-contaminated surgery. When septic conditions are encountered, antibiotic therapy should be directed by the results of intraoperative culture and sensitivity analysis. When potentially nephrotoxic antibiotics must be used, dosages should be adjusted for the reduction in renal mass. Depending on the drug, serum levels can be monitored for peak and trough levels to minimize the possibility of renal damage.[45]

Complications

The patient should be monitored for the development of pneumothorax during surgical dissection. Although inherently a part of the transthoracic approach, pneumothorax can develop when a flank approach using rib resection disrupts the crura of the diaphragm. Access to a mechanical ventilator may be required immediately in the event that the pleural space is opened during the flank approach to the kidney.[34]

Other complications of renal surgery include postoperative hemorrhage and infection. Management of postoperative hemorrhage is based on prevention through application of good surgical technique for isolation and cautery or ligation of contributing and emerging vessels. Assessment of packed cell volume and coagulation defects is appropriate before undertaking renal biopsy or excisional techniques. Surgical drainage is appropriate whenever diffuse hemorrhage, seroma, or bacterial contamination is anticipated.

REFERENCES

1. Nickel R, Schummer A, Seiferle E: Viscera of Domestic Mammals, New York, 1979, Springer-Verlag.
2. Rooney JR, Sack WO, Habel RE: Guide to the Dissection of the Horse, Ithaca, NY, 1967, Veterinary Textbooks.
3. Zhirik MG: Frequency of kidney disease among slaughtered animals (horses, cattle, sheep, pigs), Veterinariya Moscow 1974;7:94.
4. Ehnen SJ, Divers TJ, Gillette D, et al: Obstructive nephrolithiasis and ureterolithiasis associated with chronic renal failure in horses: Eight cases (1981-1987), J Am Vet Med Assoc 1990;197:249.
5. Laverty S, Pascoe JR, Ling GV, et al: Urolithiasis in 68 horses, Vet Surg 1992;21:56.
6. Ramsay G, Rothwell TLW, Gibson KT, et al: Polycystic kidneys in an adult horse, Equine Vet J 1987;19:243.
7. Jackson OF: Renal calculi in a horse, Vet Rec 1972;91:7.
8. Juzwiak JS, Bain FT, Slone DE, et al: Unilateral nephrectomy for treatment of chronic hematuria due to nephrolithiasis in a colt, Can Vet J 1988;29:931.
9. Johnson BP, Klingborg DJ, Heitman JM, et al: A horse with one kidney, partially obstructed ureter, and contralateral urogenital anomalies, J Am Vet Med Assoc 1976;169:217.
10. Hope WD, Wilson JH, Hager DA, et al: Chronic renal failure associated with bilateral nephroliths and ureteroliths in a two-year-old Thoroughbred colt, Equine Vet J 1989;21:228.
11. Sundberg JP, Burnstein T, Page EH, et al: Neoplasms of Equidae, J Am Vet Med Assoc 1977;170:150.
12. Berggren PC: Renal adenocarcinoma in a horse, J Am Vet Med Assoc 1980;176:1252.
13. Haschek WM, King JM, Tennant BC: Primary renal cell carcinoma in two horses, J Am Vet Med Assoc 1981;179:992.
14. Irwin DHG, Howell DW: Equine pyelonephritis and unilateral nephrectomy, J S Afr Vet Assoc 1980;51:235.
15. Sullins KE, McIlwraith CW, Yovich JV, et al: Ectopic ureter managed by unilateral nephrectomy in two female horses, Equine Vet J 1988;20:463.
16. Houlton JEF, Wright IM, Matic S, et al: Urinary incontinence in a Shire foal due to ureteral ectopia, Equine Vet J 1987;19:244.
17. Jones SL, Langer DL, Sterner-Kock A, et al: Renal dysplasia and benign ureteropelvic polyps associated with hydronephrosis in a foal, J Am Vet Med Assoc 1994;204:1230.
18. Ordridge RM: Urinary incontinence due to unilateral ureteral ectopia in a foal, Vet Rec 1976;98:384.
19. Christie B, Haywood N, Hilbert B, et al: Surgical correction of bilateral ureteral ectopia in a male Appaloosa foal, Aust Vet J 1981;57:336.
20. Modransky PD, Wagner PC, Robinette JD, et al: Surgical correction of bilateral ectopic ureters in two foals, Vet Surg 1983;12:141.
21. DeBowes RM, Nyrop KA, Boulton CH: Cystic calculi in the horse, Comp Cont Educ Pract Vet 1984;6:S268.
22. Byars TD, Simpson JS, Divers TJ, et al: Percutaneous nephrostomy in short term management of ureterolithiasis and renal dysfunction in a filly, J Am Vet Med Assoc 1989;195:499.
23. Robertson JT, Embertson RS: Surgical management of congenital and perinatal abnormalities of the urogenital tract, Vet Clin North Am Equine Pract 1988;4:359.
24. Voss ED, Taylor DS, Slovis NM: Use of a temporary indwelling ureteral stent catheter in a mare with a traumatic ureteral tear, J Am Vet Med Assoc 1999;214:10.
25. Bilkslager AT, Green EM, MacFadden KE: Excretory urogram and ultrasonography in the diagnosis of bilateral ectopic ureters in a foal, Vet Radiol Ultrasound 1992;33:41.

26. Rantanen NW: Diseases of the kidney, Vet Clin North Am Equine Pract 1986;2:89.
27. Rodger LD, Carlson GP, Moran ME, et al: Resolution of a left ureteral stone using electrohydraulic lithotripsy in a Thoroughbred colt, J Vet Intern Med 1995;9:280.
28. Geelen SW, Sloet van Oldruitenborgh MM: A pony with a metastasized hemangiosarcoma, Tijdschr Diergeneeskd 1996;121:544.
29. Trotter GW, Brown CM, Ainsworth DM: Unilateral nephrectomy for treatment of a renal abscess in a foal, J Am Vet Med Assoc 1984;184:1392.
30. Robertson JT, Spurlock GH, Bramlage LR, et al: Repair of ureteral defect in a foal, J Am Vet Med Assoc 1983;183:799.
31. Divers TJ, Byars TD, Spirito M: Correction of bilateral ureteral defects in a foal, J Am Vet Med Assoc 1988;192:384.
32. Squire KR, Adams SB: Bilateral ureterocystostomy in a 450-kg horse with ectopic ureters, J Am Vet Med Assoc 1992;201:1213.
33. Osborne CA, Fahning ML, Schultz RH, et al: Percutaneous renal biopsy in the cow and horse, J Am Vet Med Assoc 1968;153:563.
34. Bayly WM, Paradis MR, Reed SM: Equine renal biopsy: Indications, technic, interpretation, and complications, Mod Vet Pract 1980;61:763.
35. Modransky PD: Ultrasound-guided renal and hepatic biopsy techniques, Vet Clin North Am Equine Pract 1986;2:115.
36. DeBowes RM: Surgical management of urolithiasis, Vet Clin North Am Equine Pract 1988;4:461.
37. Walker DF, Vaughan JT: Bovine and Equine Urogenital Surgery, Philadelphia, 1980, Lea & Febiger.
38. Slone DE, Vaughan JT, Garrett PD, et al: Vascular anatomy and surgical technique for bilateral adrenalectomy in the equid, Am J Vet Res 1980;41:829.
39. Mariën T: Laparoscopic nephrectomy in the standing horse. In Fischer AT Jr, editor: Equine Diagnostic and Surgical Laparoscopy, Philadelphia, 2002, WB Saunders.
40. Nakada SY, Moon TD, Gist M: Use of a pneumosleeve as an adjunct in laparoscopic nephrectomy, Urology 1997;49:612.
41. Keoughan CG, Rodgerson DH, Brown MP: Hand-assisted laparoscopic left nephrectomy in standing horses, Vet Surg 2003;32:206.
42. Gahring DW, Crowe DT, Powers TE, et al: Comparative renal function studies of nephrotomy closure with and without sutures in dogs, J Am Vet Med Assoc 1977;171:537.
43. MacHarg MA, Foerner JJ, Phillips TN, et al: Two methods for the treatment of ureterolithiasis in a mare, J Vet Surg 1984;13:95.
44. Christie BA: Kidneys. In Slatter DH, editor: Textbook of Small Animal Surgery, vol 2, Philadelphia, 1985, WB Saunders.
45. Sojka JE, Brown SA: Pharmacokinetic adjustment of gentamicin dosing in horses with sepsis, J Am Vet Med Assoc 1986;189:784.

CHAPTER 71

Bladder

James D. Lillich
Andrew T. Fischer, Jr.
Richard M. DeBowes

ANATOMY AND PHYSIOLOGY

The equine bladder is a pear-shaped organ free at its apex and supported at its base by paired lateral ligaments and a ventral median ligament.[1] Within the free margins of the lateral ligaments of the bladder, fibrous remnants of the umbilical arteries remain as the round ligaments of the bladder. Distention of the bladder results in cranial displacement of the apex to a position cranial and ventral to the pubic bone,[1] and this displacement may be found on either side of the ventral midline.

The urinary bladder is the storage organ of the urinary tract and has a large capacity. It is composed of two interwoven layers of smooth muscle and lined with transitional epithelium supported by a thick, compliant submucosa.[1,2] The inner layer of muscle is oriented in a circular fashion and the outer muscular layer is oriented longitudinally, except over the dorsal cranial bladder, where the circular layer is external.[2] The importance of this anatomic difference is considerable, because when perinatal cystorrhexis occurs, the bladder commonly ruptures in this dorsal cranial region.[3,4] A small amount of disorganized scar tissue is located at the ventral cranial bladder, a remnant of the fetal urachus.

The urachus is a tube-shaped organ responsible for the conduction of urine from the primitive embryonic bladder through the umbilical cord to the allantoic sac. On separation of the umbilical cord shortly after parturition, the urachus degenerates along its intra-abdominal course and is replaced by fibrous tissue.

DISORDERS REQUIRING SURGERY

Pathologic conditions affecting the equine bladder that are amenable to surgical intervention include cystorrhexis,[2-25] persistent urachus,[5,6,15-17,26-28] cystic calculus,[6,16,29-47] eversion,[48] and transitional cell carcinoma.[6] Cystorrhexis and persistent urachus are the most common indications for surgery of the bladder and typically affect young or newborn foals. Cystic calculi and neoplastic diseases are less commonly observed and usually affect only adult horses. Eversion of the bladder occurs exclusively in females.

Uroperitoneum

Uroperitoneum is a serious condition that results in the development of uremia and severe electrolyte and acid–base imbalances.[3-5,11] Although uroperitoneum is the result of urinary bladder rupture, a variety of congenital or traumatic defects of the proximal urinary tract are reported.[49,50] Rupture of the foal's bladder occurs because of congenital defects[2-5] or compressive forces associated with parturition.[3-5] The rupture occurs along the dorsal or dorsocranial margin of the foal's bladder (Fig. 71-1) because of the inherently thin wall in that area.[2] With less frequency, cystorrhexis has also been diagnosed in adult horses with uroperitoneum,[7-9,51] and it may be secondary to obstructive disease of the urethra.

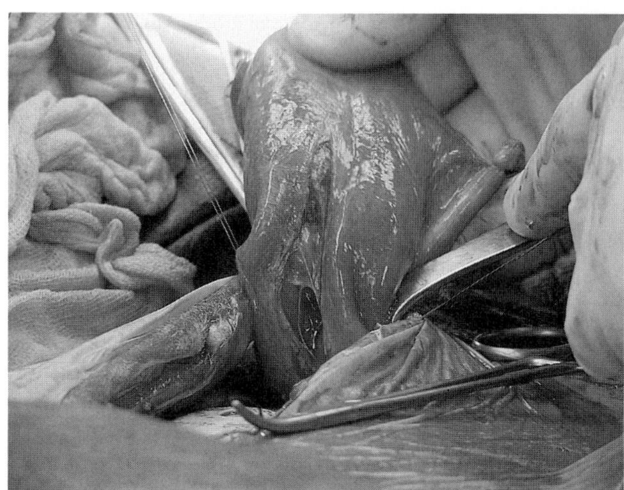

Figure 71-1. Rupture of the pediatric equine bladder usually occurs longitudinally along the dorsal or dorsocranial aspect.

Foals 1 to 5 days old are affected.[3-5,10] Although the majority are male, the problem may also occur in females.* Foals are initially normal in clinical appearance and usually become symptomatic by 1 to 3 days of age. Clinical signs include depression, progressive anorexia, and abdominal distention with mild to moderate colic.[3-5,17] Some foals that experience severe abdominal distention become dyspneic. Affected foals are capable of voiding a stream of urine, although increased frequency and reduced volume of urine flow can be expected.[5]

The diagnosis of uroperitoneum is suspected from the history and findings on physical examination.[3-6,8-12,17,18,51] Confirmation of the diagnosis of uroperitoneum in foals of all ages can usually be achieved through abdominocentesis, as well as through dye studies, contrast radiography, ultrasonography, and cystoscopy.[9]

Clinicopathologic evaluation commonly reveals evidence of marked hyperkalemia, hyponatremia, and hypochloremia.[3,4,11,12] Dehydration and metabolic acidemia are commonly observed, particularly in older foals. Although serum and peritoneal creatinine and urea nitrogen values are often elevated, creatinine is the most meaningful parameter to evaluate.[3,5,11,52] *Serum-to-peritoneal creatinine ratios* should be determined in all patients suspected of having uroperitoneum and are considered diagnostic when they are greater than 1:2.[3]

Peritoneal fluid from affected individuals has a variable volume of a clear, yellow, odorless fluid with a low specific gravity (less than 1.008). Urinary calcium carbonate crystals have been identified on microscopic evaluation of fluid harvested by abdominocentesis,[9] but this finding would not be typical in foals with uroperitoneum.

Sterile solutions of methylene blue, fluorescein, or neoprontosil may be instilled into the bladder of foals suspected of having uroperitoneum secondary to cystorrhexis. Identification of instilled dye in abdominal fluid recovered from drains or abdominocentesis confirms the diagnosis. Alternatively, a lateral abdominal radiographic examination after retrograde contrast medium instillation (Renografin-76, Squibb Diagnostics, New Brunswick, NJ) into the bladder identifies the presence of a rupture (Fig. 71-2). Cystoscopic examination of the bladder is valuable for identification of bladder ruptures in adult horses.[9] Its value in foals is limited by the sex of the foal and the size of the endoscope. Ultrasonographic examination may also be used to identify a rent in the urinary bladder. In addition, a "bubblegram" (sterile saline shaken and instilled in to the bladder during the ultrasonic examination) can confirm the existence of a rent (see Fig. 69-3).

Foals with uroperitoneum must be medically stabilized before anesthetic induction and should be examined for the presence of concurrent disease.[17,18,53] Dehydration should be managed by the administration of 0.9% or 1.8% to 2.5% sterile saline for dehydrated or rehydrated foals, respectively. Foals with moderate to severe abdominal distention may require peritoneal drainage to improve their cardiovascular and ventilation status. Correction of pre-existing electrolyte abnormalities is important, particularly of hyperkalemia, which is arrhythmogenic.[54] Drainage of the peritoneal urine or peritoneal dialysis with concurrent volume expansion and supplementation of sodium chloride and bicarbonate should be sufficient.[13] Supplementation of serum sodium levels is important because hyponatremia potentiates the cardiotoxicity of hyperkalemia.[3,54] Once stabilized, affected individuals are managed by midline celiotomy for abdominal exploration and cystorrhaphy (see "Cystorrhaphy," p. 881). Severely debilitated patients are suboptimal candidates for general anesthesia. Foals with uroperitoneum because of small tears in the bladder wall can be managed conservatively by medical support and closed continuous suction drainage of the bladder.[14] Likewise, adults with uroperitoneum from bladder leakage secondary to obstructive urolithiasis have been managed with perineal urethrostomy and temporary urine diversion with a Foley catheter. This management should be considered a viable option when no definitive tear is appreciated on cystoscopic examination.[51]

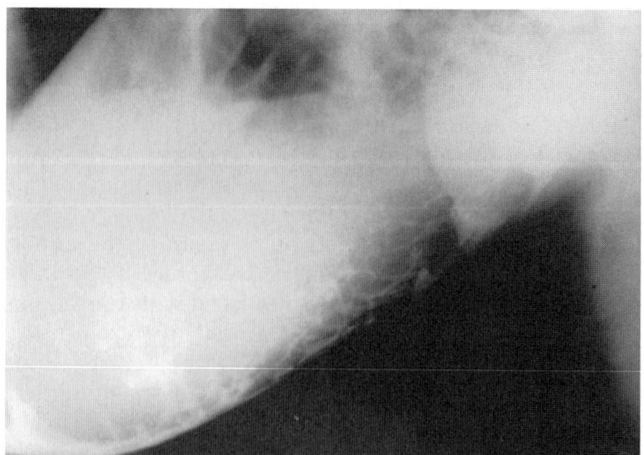

Figure 71-2. Lateral radiographic view of the abdomen of a foal with cystorrhexis. Positive-contrast medium is apparent along the ventral aspect of the abdomen after positive-contrast cystography.

*References 3, 4, 12, 17, 18, 22.

Persistent or Patent Urachus

Persistent or patent urachus is a condition of young foals in which the urachus fails to close spontaneously at or shortly after parturition.[5,6,15-17,27,28] The pathogenesis could be either excessive traction on the umbilicus as a congenital problem or the development of omphalophlebitis as a contributing postnatal problem.[5,17,26] Patent urachus has been associated with development of septic arthritis, septic physitis, and septicemia complex.[17,27,52,55] *Streptococcus* species, *Actinobacillus* species, and *Escherichia coli* have been implicated in septicemic extensions of umbilical infections.[26]

Affected foals show moisture around the navel region[5,15,17] (Fig. 71-3). Some foals drip or stream urine from the umbilicus when posturing to urinate. In chronic cases, urine scald may be present around the navel. Foals should be evaluated for the presence of a complete and patent urethra. Foals with septic omphalophlebitis may have grossly enlarged navels (Fig. 71-4) and purulent drainage associated with the urachal fistula.[17,27] When deep urachal infection is present, as determined by bacterial culture and sensitivity tests, systemic antibiotic therapy should be initiated.[17,27] If the foal develops symptoms consistent with septicemia, further evaluation and application of additional therapies, including surgery, are warranted.[17,18,27]

The diagnosis of persistent or patent urachus is frequently assumed from the history and findings on physical examination. Positive-contrast radiographic examination confirms the presence of a patent urachus by documenting the clearance of contrast agent through the urachus after retrograde cystography. Foals suspected of having urachal disease or omphalophlebitis should be evaluated by ultrasonographic examination[17,28] (Fig. 71-5). Identification of vesicourachal patency is confirmatory, and identification of an umbilical or urachal abscess necessitates prompt surgical intervention.[17,28]

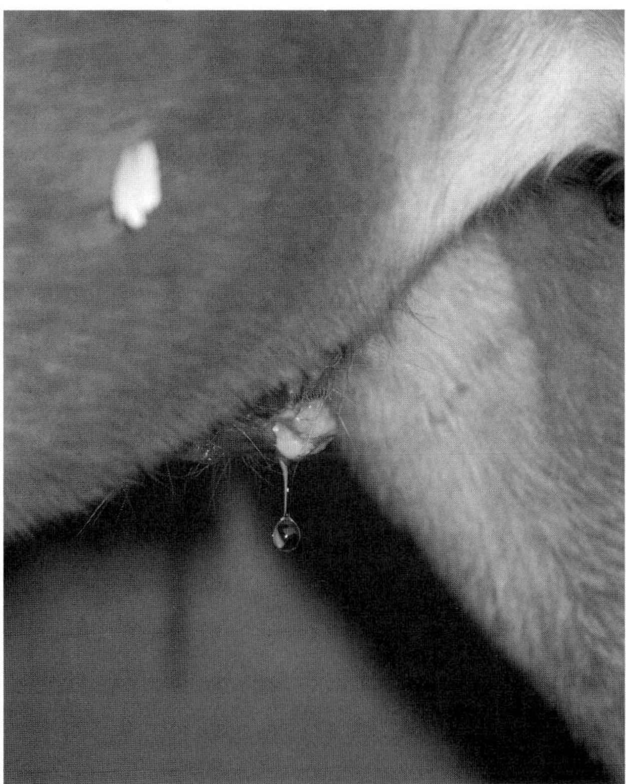

Figure 71-3. A patent or persistent urachus is usually recognized by its moist and fistulous appearance.

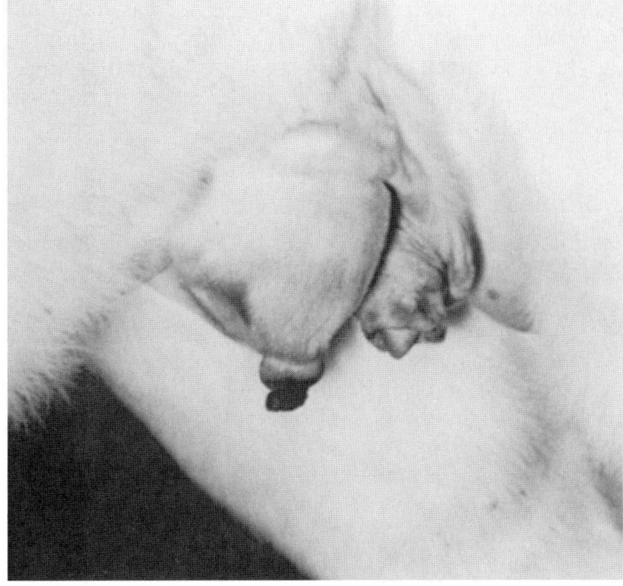

Figure 71-4. Marked enlargement of the umbilicus is evident in this male foal with septic omphalophlebitis and patent urachus.

Most uncomplicated cases of congenital patent urachus are treated medically by systemic antimicrobial therapy and topical application of cauterizing or astringent compounds such as phenol, Lugol's iodine, or silver nitrate.[3,6,15-17] Foals with uncomplicated congenital patent urachus typically respond after a few days of therapy. If resolution has not occurred after 5 to 7 days of treatment, surgical therapy is recommended.[5,17]

Individuals requiring surgical management are operated on through a modified midline celiotomy for exploration, evaluation, and resection of the urachus with its associated

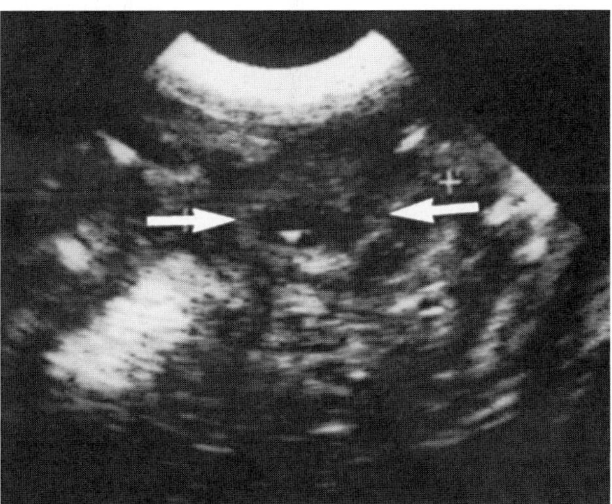

Figure 71-5. A transcutaneous ultrasonographic examination of a foal with patent urachus and suspected umbilical abscess reveals urachal enlargement *(arrows)*. (Courtesy Norman Rantanen, DVM, MS.)

umbilical vascular elements[5,16,17] (see "Cystoplasty," p. 883). Foals with patent urachus and septic omphalophlebitis (see Fig. 38-2) or urachal abscess that are treated with surgery and antibiotics appear to survive more frequently and with lower morbidity than foals treated with antibiotics alone.[17,27]

Urolithiasis

Urolithiasis is a potentially serious but relatively uncommon disease of horses.[6,16,29-47,56-59] Renal,[56,57,60] ureteral,[15,33,47,56] urethral,[56,61] and cystic calculi[33,45,47,56] all can occur, but cystic calculi are the most common. The etiopathogenesis of urolithiasis has not been thoroughly defined. A dietary etiology has not been demonstrated. Mineral content of drinking water, infection, and nonsteroidal anti-inflammatory drug use have been suspected of playing a major role in the development of uroliths. Hyperhydrated forms of calcium carbonate crystals may precipitate and coalesce into a nidus within the urinary tract.[29,30] Desquamated epithelial cells, mucoproteins, or aggregations of white blood cells may also serve as a nidus that promotes calculus formation.[16] Calculi develop in horses of both sexes but are more commonly diagnosed in males.[33,45,47] This sex predilection occurs because the anatomy of female urethra permits the mare to void small calculi and remain asymptomatic (with few exceptions). Horses with cystic calculi are adults, usually older than 10 years, with only occasional cases reported in animals younger than 2 years.[47] In contrast, five of eight horses with renal calculi in one report were between 2 and 3 years of age.[62]

Two types of calculi occur in equine patients. The more common calculus (type I) is a soft, yellow-green urolith composed of a variety of hydrated salts of calcium carbonate (Fig. 71-6). The spiculated surface of the type I urolith is responsible for producing traumatic cystitis.[47] The second form of urolith (type II) is composed of hydrated calcium carbonate salts admixed with phosphate and magnesium. The type II calculi tend to be smooth, firm, and white.[47]

Clinical signs of cystic calculi include hematuria, tenesmus, incontinence, dysuria, stranguria, and oliguria.* Affected horses spend prolonged periods posturing as if to urinate, with minimal results. Urine scald dermatitis of the adductor surfaces of the hindlimbs is common in chronically affected patients. Affected horses may vocalize while urinating; however, intermittent abdominal discomfort is more commonly associated with calculi of the upper urinary system.[56,62]

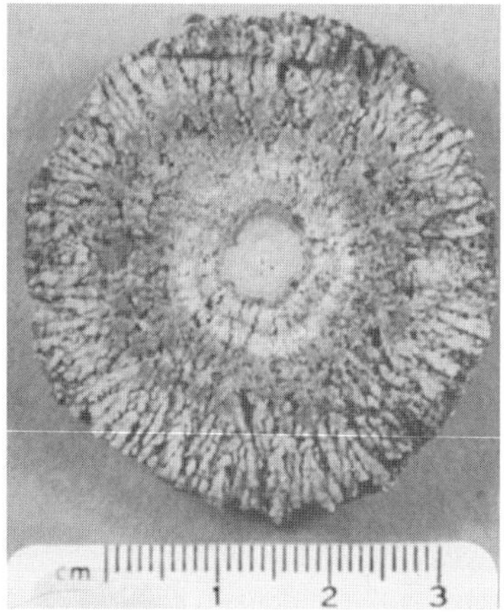

Figure 71-6. The type I urolith is readily recognized by its spiculated appearance and yellow-green color.

Diagnosis is made from the history and findings on physical examination, supported by a rectal examination. Palpation of the bladder is definitive for diagnosing cystic urolithiasis. A cystoscopic examination provides additional information on the number and type of stones, the patency of the ureters, and the presence and severity of traumatic cystitis.[47,63] A variety of surgical approaches have been suggested for removal of cystic calculi.† Laparocystotomy is the treatment of choice for removal of the calculus after effective cleansing and evacuation of the bladder[15,16,37-44,47] (see "Cystotomy," p. 881).

Electrohydraulic lithotripsy or mechanical crushing offers an alternative therapeutic approach.[58,59] Male patients may be sedated, blocked (epidural), and prepared for a standing perineal urethrostomy (see Chapter 72). The bladder is emptied and the calculus identified by cystoscopy. A lithotripsy probe (Electrohydraulic Lithotripter, Richard Wolf Medical Instruments Corp, Rosemont, Ill) or lithotrite is passed through the urethrostomy into the bladder. Electrical current is applied to the calculus to produce fragmentation. Pieces of the calculus may be removed by grasping forceps or by warm sterile saline lavage. Perioperative complications of removal of cystic calculi via perineal urethrostomy include rectal tear, perforation of the pelvic urethra, orchitis, peritonitis, and tenesmus, all of which may be the result of excessive surgical trauma.[56] Long-term complications include stricture with fibrosis and urethral diverticulum formation.[61] In female patients, calculi can be removed manually through the urethral sphincter or with the aid of sphincterotomy. Large calculi may require mechanical crushing before removal.

Shockwave, dye-pulsed, and holmium:yttrium-aluminum-garnet (holmium-YAG) laser lithotripsy have also been reported.[64-66] Detailed descriptions are available, and the techniques have merit for providing surgical resolution of the clinical signs with mild surgical morbidity. Although these applications minimize surgical trauma over conventional surgical approaches, the availability and expense of the equipment limit large-scale use. Additionally, failure of the holmium-YAG laser to completely pulverize the cystic calculi has been reported.[66]

Bladder Eversion

Bladder eversion may occur in the female horse.[48] It is associated with parturition and third-degree perineal lacerations. Diagnosis is made on the basis of the history and physical examination findings. Typically, the bladder is everted through the urethral sphincter, so that exposed mucosa extends beyond the ventral commissure of the vulva (Fig. 71-7). Visceral contents can be contained within an everted bladder. Manual reduction followed by pursestring suture placement around a Foley catheter is the treatment of choice. In chronic cases, however, the exposed bladder

*References 6, 15, 16, 33, 45, 47, 56.
†References 6, 15, 16, 31, 32, 47.

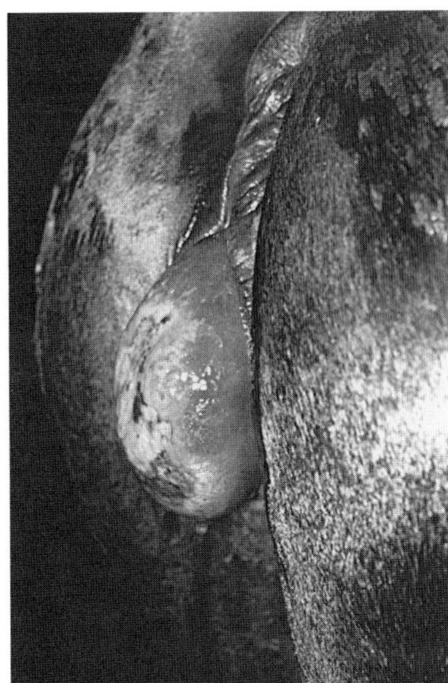

Figure 71-7. Everted bladder in a postpartum 4-year-old Standardbred mare. (Courtesy Warren L. Beard, DVM, MS.)

mucosa can become edematous and necrotic, requiring partial cystectomy. Partial cystectomy can be accomplished in a standing patient with sedation, epidural anesthesia, and incremental resection of the diseased bladder.[48] Care should be taken to identify and exclude the ureteral openings from surgical manipulation.

Neoplasia

Neoplasia of the equine bladder is rare but includes squamous cell carcinomas, transitional cell carcinomas, leiomyomas, and leiomyosarcomas,[6] with squamous cell carcinomas being the most common.[67] Clinical signs include hematuria and stranguria. Solitary lesions of the apex of the bladder may be amenable to resection cystoplasty. Disseminated lesions have probably developed beyond the point where surgical management would be effective.

SURGICAL PROCEDURES

Cystorrhaphy

Cystorrhaphy is indicated for disruption of the bladder.[5,6,15-18] The anesthetized patient is positioned in dorsal recumbency. An appropriate-size rubber catheter (Sherwood Medical Industries, St. Louis, Mo) is passed through the urethra and secured in the bladder to ensure outflow of urine and to permit intraoperative lavage of the base of the bladder. The prepuce in males is cleansed and closed with suture or towel clamps to reduce the possibility of incisional contamination. The abdomen is aseptically prepared for a ventral midline incision.

In the adult female patient, the surgeon should make a 15- to 18-cm caudal midline incision that extends caudally from a point 2 to 5 cm cranial to the umbilicus. In foals, the incision should be directed abaxially to create an elliptical incision around the umbilicus for removal. In the male patient, the cranial aspect of the incision is identical; however, the skin and subcutaneous layers of the caudal incision should be directed 2 to 4 cm paramedian to the prepuce (Fig. 71-8). The prepuce can be mobilized and retracted to expose the posterior midline for deep incision.

After the peritoneal cavity has been opened, peritoneal fluid should be cultured and suctioned. The bladder is exposed by maintaining traction on the urachus if present (Fig. 71-9). Large, self-retaining retractors (Balfour, Finochietto) may be used to facilitate the abdominal exploration. The bladder and urachus should be inspected to identify the site of rupture. The site of rupture in the foal may be the urachus as well as the dorsal or ventral bladder[18] (Fig. 71-10). Urachal rupture is a sequela of urachal infection, especially in septicemic foals[17,18] (Fig. 71-11). Ventral tears run longitudinally along the ventral bladder to the neck, making surgical access difficult.[17]

If the origin of the uroperitoneum is not evident,[18] the bladder may be distended by retrograde introduction of a sterile solution of fluorescein or methylene blue through the urethral catheter. This method identifies thin or attenuated areas in the bladder wall that may be leaking, typically on the dorsocranial surface of the bladder.

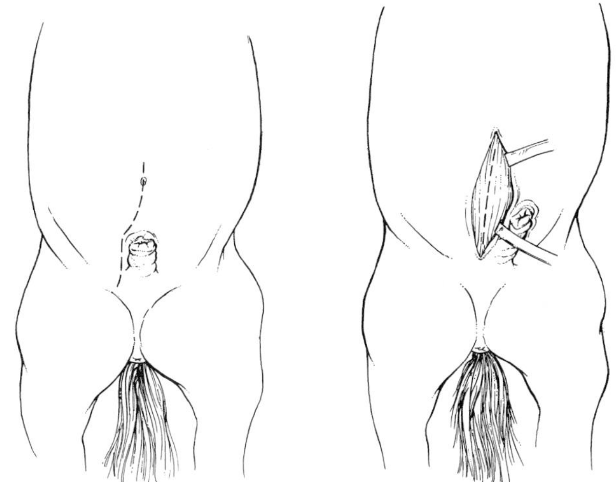

Figure 71-8. In male horses or foals, the posterior aspect of the cutaneous caudal midline incision and subcutaneous dissection is directed abaxially to avoid the prepuce and penis.

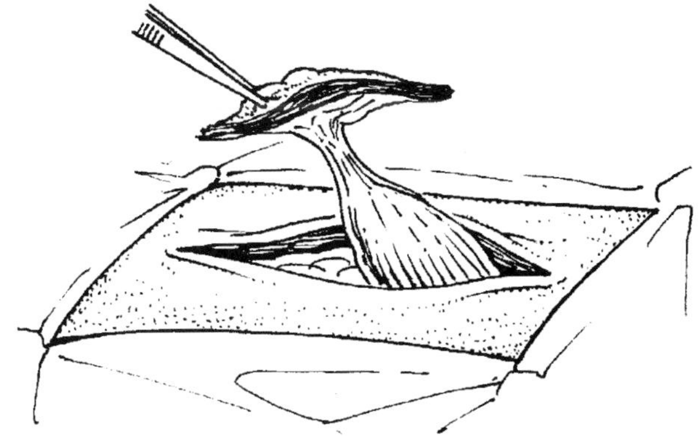

Figure 71-9. After completing the midline incision and mobilizing the umbilicus and urachal remnant from the abdominal wall, the bladder is exposed by careful traction on the umbilicus. When the bladder is exposed, the tissues are retracted caudally.

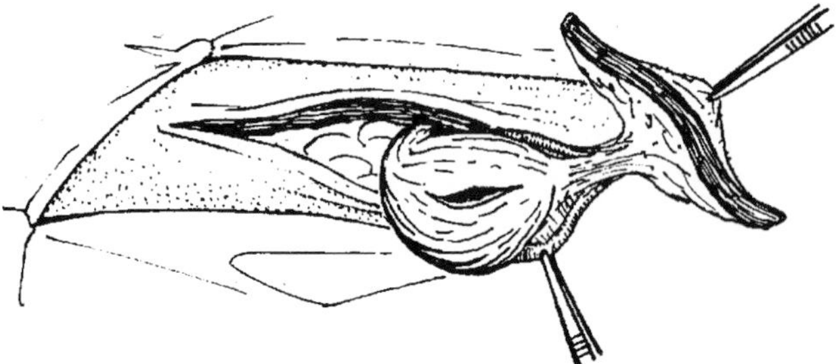

Figure 71-10. The bladder is retroflexed to permit visualization of the tear on the dorsocranial border.

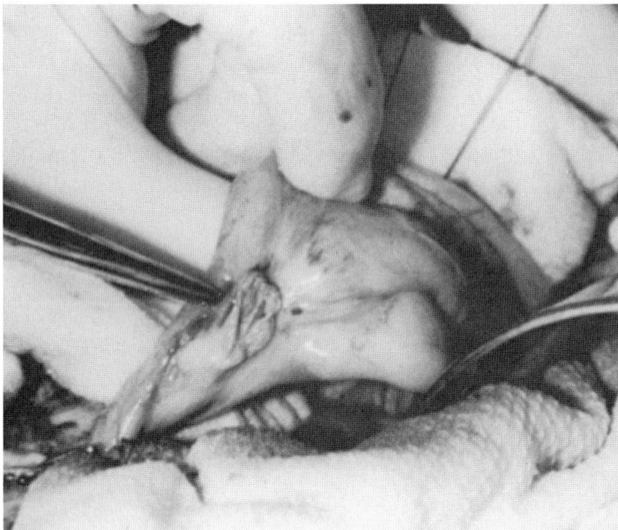

Figure 71-11. A rupture of the urachus (located at the tip of the hemostatic forceps) is readily apparent on inspection of the cranial bladder.

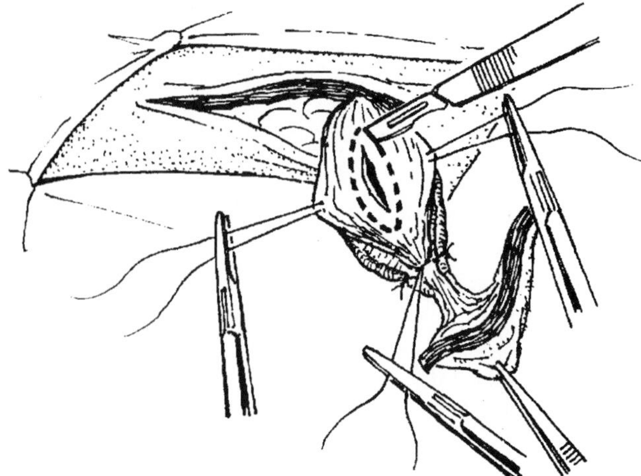

Figure 71-12. Tissues surrounding a tear in the bladder should be débrided before primary repair.

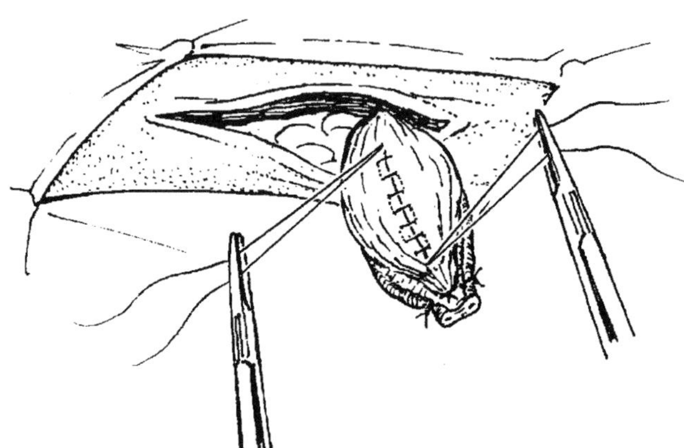

Figure 71-13. A two-layer inverting continuous closure is appropriate for repair of a bladder rupture.

Once the tear is identified, the wound margins are débrided (Fig. 71-12). Culture and histopathologic evaluation of the débrided margins of the tear in septic foals should be considered.[18] The use of monofilament stay sutures to support the bladder during primary repair is recommended. Surgical closure of the tear should be accomplished in two layers: an interrupted pattern in the first layer, followed by a continuous inverting pattern[16] (Fig. 71-13). Small-size (2-0, 3-0) synthetic absorbable suture (chromic catgut, polyglycolic acid, polyglactin 910, or polydioxanone) on a taper-point atraumatic needle is used. Care should be taken to avoid suture penetration of the vesicular mucosa, because when sutures penetrate the bladder mucosa (of rabbits) in the presence of alkaline urine, the result is the formation of cystic calculi.[53]

After repair, the bladder should be distended with sterile saline to evaluate for leakage along the suture line. In a young foal in which the urachus is present, the urachus should be resected, cultured, and removed with the umbilicus after primary repair of the tear (see "Cystoplasty," p. 883). Before abdominal closure, the peritoneal cavity is lavaged with warm sterile saline solution. Indwelling drains (Argyle Trochar Catheter, Sherwood Medical Industries, St. Louis, Mo) may be placed if septic processes are present or anticipated. Despite the irritative nature of urine, clinically significant peritonitis is rare unless concurrent septic disease processes such as omphalophlebitis or neonatal septicemia are present.[16-18] The midline incision is closed with no. 1 or no. 2 synthetic absorbable suture placed in simple-continuous fashion. The subcutaneous tissues and skin are closed with 3-0 synthetic absorbable sutures and skin staples, respectively.

Urinary bladder repair in the standing postparturient mare can also be accomplished by prolapsing the bladder either through a vaginal incision or urethrotomy and sphincterotomy.[68,69] Clinical signs are consistent with uroperitoneum and diagnostic tests confirm the presence of a rent. Horses should be stabilized and the uroperitoneum, which is usually profound, sterilely drained. Caudal epidural anesthesia is utilized. For the *vaginal approach,* a rigid urinary catheter is placed to identify the location of the urethra and bladder under the vaginal mucosa. A 2-cm incision is made 5 to 10 cm caudal to the cervix. Blunt dissection increases the size of the incision, which facilitates the delivery of the bladder into the vaginal vault. Alternatively, a linear *urethrotomy* and *sphincterotomy* can be preformed. A 5-cm incision is made in the urethral sphincter on the dorsal midline. The surgeon places a hand in the bladder and everts the bladder out of the vulva. Care is taken to identify the ureter openings. Rents are closed with a single- or double-layer closure. The bladder is replaced and the vaginal incision or sphincterotomy closed in a simple-continuous pattern with absorbable 2-0 or 0 suture material.

Cystoplasty

Cystoplasty is the technique of choice for patent or persistent urachus.[5,6,15-18] Before anesthesia induction, the bladder is catheterized and emptied. The foal is anesthetized, prepared, positioned, and draped as described earlier (see "Cystorrhaphy"). If the urachus is open and draining, the margins may be oversewn with a continuous inverting suture pattern before aseptic preparation.

A 15-cm caudoventral midline incision is made. The incision extends caudally from a point 8 cm cranial to the umbilicus. An elliptical incision is created at the umbilicus for its removal. In male patients, the posterior aspect of the skin and subcutaneous incisions are directed 2 to 4 cm lateral to the prepuce (see Fig. 71-8). The prepuce can be mobilized and retracted to expose the posterior midline for deep incision.

The umbilicus and urachus are dissected free from the body wall. The falciform ligament and umbilical vein are ligated and resected as far craniad as possible. Occasionally, the midline incision must be extended cranially to permit adequate resection of the umbilical vein. The affected urachus may be thickened and distorted (Fig. 71-14). Adhesions may exist between the urachus or its associated vascular structures and the surrounding viscera.[17,18] Care should be taken to identify and transect adhesions that involve the urachus before manipulation of the bladder.

Exposure of the bladder is achieved by sustained traction on the urachus. Traction should be applied with caution because of the friable nature of the tissue and the possibility of rupture. Sterile moistened laparotomy pads are used to pack off intestines and assist in positioning the bladder. Stay sutures are placed at the ventrolateral margins of the bladder

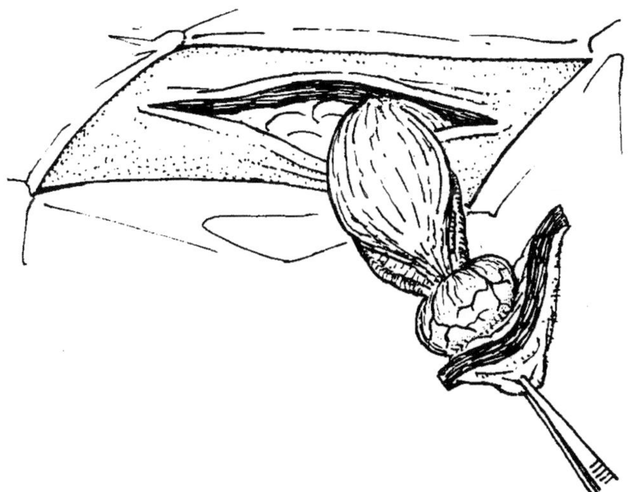

Figure 71-14. After mobilization and retraction of an umbilical or urachal abscess, the abdomen should be explored for adhesions or additional foci of abscessation.

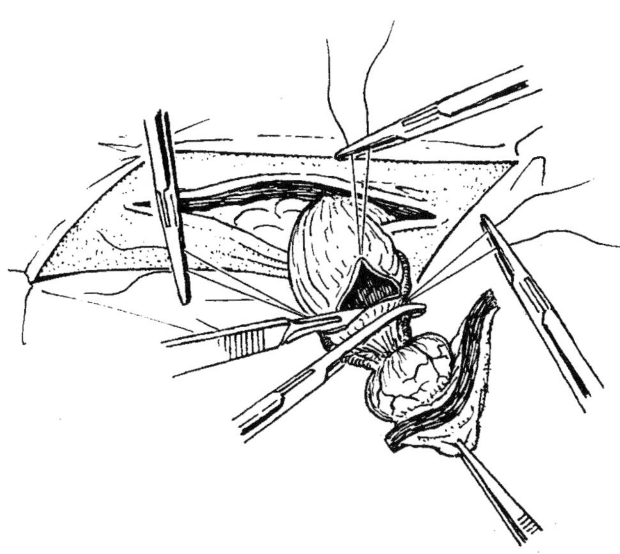

Figure 71-15. Before urachal-umbilical resection, a clamp is applied to prevent spillage of urachal contents into the peritoneal cavity. Here, the bladder has been stabilized by stay sutures transfixed as ligatures around the round ligaments of the bladder (umbilical arteries).The urachus and umbilical tissues are removed by sharp dissection. The cranial edge of the bladder is closed by the two-layer inverting continuous techniques demonstrated in Figure 71-13.

for additional support and control of the bladder after resection of the urachus. The umbilical arteries (around the ligaments of the bladder) are ligated with a transfixing suture at the level of urachal resection.

An occluding forceps is used to isolate the urachus and apex of the bladder (Fig. 71-15). A transverse incision is made across the apex of the bladder to remove the urachus and vesicular apex (see Fig. 71-15). The urachus is removed and submitted for culture and sensitivity tests. Traction is applied to the previously positioned stay sutures to elevate the apex of the bladder and to prevent spillage of urine. Suction is used to remove the residual urine or pus from the bladder. Closure is accomplished using a two-layer inverting suture pattern with 2-0 or 3-0 synthetic absorbable suture material, taking care not to penetrate the lumen. Alternatively, a simple-continuous closure of the first layer may be followed by an inverting suture pattern.[17] The abdomen is lavaged with warm sterile saline before closure. Unless significant spillage of urine or exudate has occurred, abdominal drains are not necessary. Broad-spectrum antibiotics are administered routinely for 3 to 5 days because of the potential for abdominal contamination from urachal bacterial contaminants.

Cystotomy

Cystotomy is the treatment of choice for cystic calculi.* After anesthesia induction, the horse is positioned in dorsal recumbency. A urinary catheter is passed into the bladder and sutured in place. The prepuce is cleaned and sutured or closed with towel clamps. The abdomen is aseptically prepared for a ventral midline approach.

*References 6, 15, 16, 33, 38, 47.

A 20- to 25-cm skin incision is made along the caudal ventral midline of the abdomen. In male horses, the skin incision is directed lateral to the prepuce (see Fig. 71-8). With continued dissection of the subcutaneous tissues, the prepuce is mobilized and retracted to expose the posterior midline. The surgeon should identify and avoid the large superficial caudal epigastric and external pudendal vessels when dissecting deep to the prepuce to expose the posterior midline. In mares, the incision is made on the midline from the umbilicus caudally to the prepubic tendon.

The bladder is identified by palpation in the pelvic canal. Sustained gentle traction is required to exteriorize the bladder[33,45,47] (Fig. 71-16). Once it is exposed, moistened laparotomy pads are used to pack off the bowel and elevate the bladder in the surgical field. Large-diameter stay sutures should be positioned at the ventrolateral aspects of the bladder to facilitate control of the cystotomy incision and to reduce urine spillage. A transverse incision is made across the ventral bladder to expose the urolith. Frequently, the urolith is closely adherent to the bladder mucosa, particularly in the case of a type I urolith. The mucosal layer of the bladder must be peeled back from the urolith to permit removal of the calculus (Fig. 71-17). After its removal, a full-thickness biopsy should be taken from the margin of the cystotomy incision for culture and histopathology. The bladder is lavaged extensively in an effort to remove small fragments of calcular material and blood clots. Irrigation of the bladder by retrograde introduction of sterile saline through the urinary catheter flushes small fragments of the urolith from the neck of the bladder toward the incision, where they can be evacuated through suction.

The cystotomy is sutured with a two-layer closure of synthetic absorbable suture material. Continuous inverting suture patterns such as the Cushing and Lembert patterns are preferred. The suture should not penetrate the urinary mucosa to the lumen. The bladder may be distended with sterile saline to evaluate the closure for leakage. The abdomen is lavaged with sterile balanced saline solution and suctioned. The midline incision is closed with no. 2 synthetic absorbable suture material in continuous or interrupted fashion. If the caudal limit of the incision was made in a paramedian location, the fascial closure is completed in two layers by suturing the deep and superficial layers of the rectus sheath separately. Of the two layers, the superficial sheath is the more critical to the security of the abdominal closure.[15,16,34,70] The subcutaneous tissues and skin are closed in routine fashion.

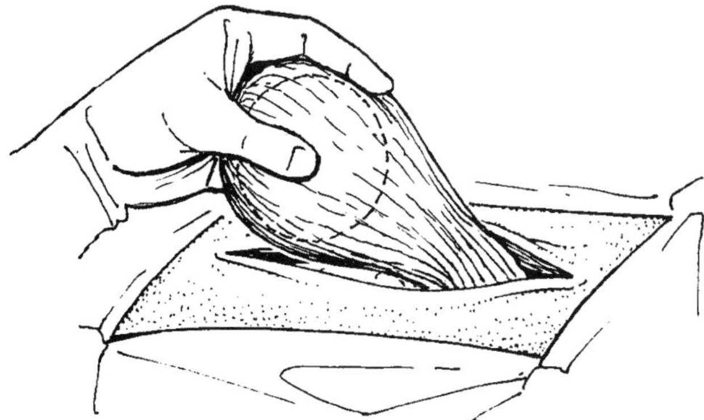

Figure 71-16. The bladder and urolith are delivered into the surgical field by gentle, sustained traction.

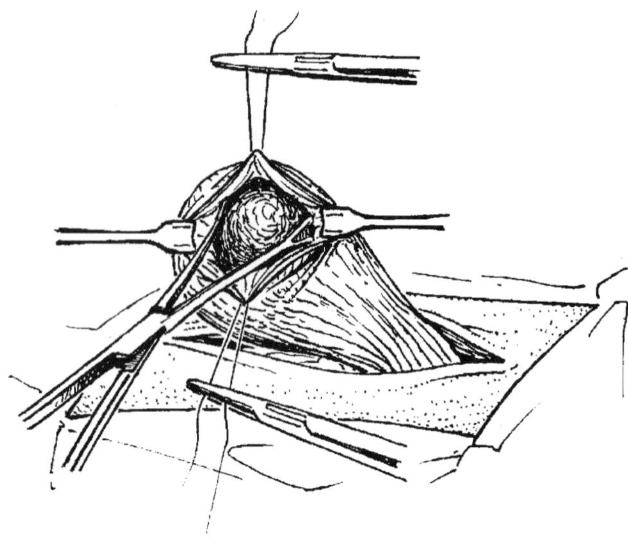

Figure 71-17. The urolith can be grasped with sponge forceps for expedient removal.

Parainguinal Approach

Another surgical approach to the urinary bladder in the adult male horse has been described—the parainguinal approach.[71] This approach eliminates the need to reflect the prepuce and reduces the chances of encountering large vessels prior to gaining access to the urinary bladder. With the horse in dorsal recumbency and the penis sterilely catheterized, the inguinal region is clipped and prepared for aseptic surgery. A 12- to 14-cm skin incision is made starting 2 cm cranial to the left external inguinal ring and continuing in a caudomedial direction toward the midline (Fig. 71-18). Subcutaneous tissues and fat are bluntly and sharply dissected to reveal the aponeurosis of the external abdominal oblique muscle. The aponeurosis is sharply incised, starting

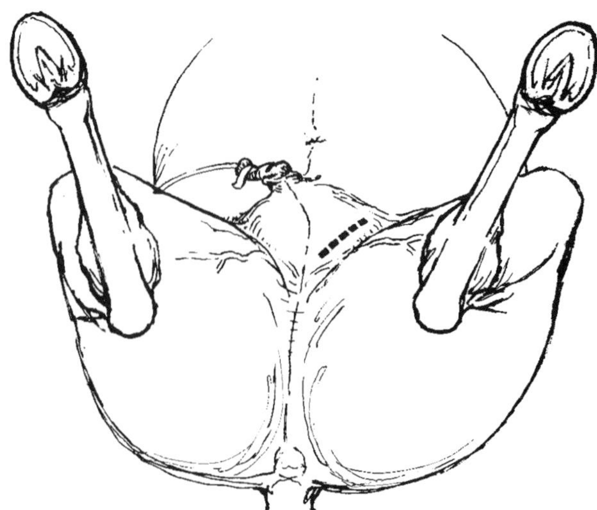

Figure 71-18. Patient preparation and location of the incision for the parainguinal laparocystotomy approach.

at the midline and continuing laterally roughly parallel to the skin incision for 12 to 14 cm. Retraction is used to gain access to the internal abdominal oblique muscle, which is separated along its fibers. The peritoneum is bluntly entered with the surgeon's finger. The bladder is identified and exteriorized with steady traction. The surgical field can be isolated and the bladder twisted to maintain exteriorization to complete the cystotomy. Double-layer closure of the bladder is recommended. Closure of the abdomen is routine, with attention paid to the aponeurosis of the external abdominal oblique muscle. An interrupted cruciate, near-far-far-near, or a simple-interrupted pattern is recommended. None of the nine geldings that underwent this approach developed incisional complications, including herniation.

Laparoscopic Techniques

Laparoscopic techniques have been described for repair of cystorrhexis, persistent urachus, and umbilical infections in the foal.[72,73] Patient preparation including appropriate diagnostic examinations and perioperative therapeutics do not differ from those used for foals undergoing conventional surgical approaches. Foals are placed in dorsal recumbency with the pelvic limbs elevated. This position usually demands that intermittent positive-pressure ventilation be available. The ventral midline is prepared routinely for aseptic surgery.

Because the foal's body wall is thin, it is recommended that insufflation be done with a teat cannula and that lower (1 to 2 L/minute) insufflation rates be used. A 1.5-cm incision is made 5 cm lateral to ventral midline and 10 to 15 cm cranial to the umbilicus for placement of the laparoscopic cannula. A 30-degree laparoscope telescope is used to explore the abdomen. Additional portals are made 8 to 10 cm lateral and 5 cm cranial to the umbilicus.

For *cystorrhexis,* urine accumulation needs to be evacuated prior to insufflation. Once the telescope is placed, the entire bladder should be inspected. Two working portals are required to freshen the edges of the rent and repair the bladder with absorbable sutures using intracorporeal suturing techniques. It is prudent to test the bladder for leaks before deflating the abdomen.

For *resection of umbilical remnants,* or umbilical remnant infection, the umbilical vein and arteries are isolated with endoscopic scissors and dissected free to facilitate ligation. A large ligation clip or loop can be utilized. Several clips may be necessary to ensure proper ligation, especially when structures appear large or pathologic. Once the umbilical vein and arteries have been transected, an elliptic incision is made around the umbilicus through the body wall under laparoscopic guidance. The end of the bladder is exteriorized and resected. A two-layer closure in the bladder is recommended.

Closure of the body wall is routine. Closure of the portal is performed with no. 1 absorbable material in an inverted cruciate pattern in the external fascia. Intradermal sutures can complete the procedure. Overall, good visualization with minimal intervention is obtained with laparoscopic techniques. The use of nonabsorbable linear staples for repair of a tear in the bladder is discouraged, because the staples may serve as nidus for urolith formation.[72]

Laparoscopic techniques for *removal of cystic calculi* in the adult male horse have also been described.[74] The horse is placed in dorsal recumbency with the pelvic limbs elevated. Additional preparation steps include placement of a urinary catheter and caudal retraction of the penis, the latter being secured between the patient's legs. The bladder is lavaged and drained until clear saline irrigation solution is obtained.

A standard umbilical portal is made after insufflation. Five instrument portals are made to complete the procedure. The instrument portals are in a radiant line centered on the sheath. A laparoscopic electrocautery tip is inserted into the cranial right portal and is used for suction when the cystotomy incision is made. A retrieval bag is also placed in the abdomen, which is positioned below the bladder. The cystotomy incision is made just long enough to remove the calculus. A retractable metal loop forceps aids in the removal of the urolith and placement into the retrieval bag. Suction is used to remove residual debris. Closure of the bladder is accomplished with an auto-suture device. A double-layer closure is recommended. The bladder is tested for leaks prior to deflation of the abdomen. The umbilical portal is enlarged to retrieve the calculus within the retrieval bag. The linea and portal incisions are closed routinely.

Complications of this technique include intraoperative hemorrhage from the instrument portals, and obstructed visualization from falciform fat. It should be noted that practice is required to become proficient in using the auto-suturing devices. With proper preparation, cystic calculi can be removed safety and cleanly in the adult male horse.

Aftercare

Antibiotics are commonly administered after surgery of the bladder. In cases of cystorrhexis or persistent urachus, sepsis represents a risk,[18] so antibiotics are routinely administered to reduce the risk of septic peritonitis and may be continued for several days or weeks postoperatively.[17,18,27] In adult patients with urolithiasis, the risk of urine spillage during removal of cystic calculi is considerable.[34,47] However, antibiotics are continued for only 48 to 72 hours unless clinical signs of infection develop.

Postoperative abdominal drainage is indicated if surgical findings suggest the presence of peritonitis or if gross soilage of the peritoneum from an urachal abscess has occurred. Generally, abdominal drainage is not required after cystorrhaphy or cystoplasty. Unless significant spillage with fragments of uroliths has occurred, the need for peritoneal drainage in urolithiasis patients is not necessary. Patients with abdominal drains should remain on prophylactic antibiotic therapy.

Typically, patients are administered low doses of nonsteroidal anti-inflammatory drugs to control postoperative and incisional discomfort. Patients recovering from cystorrhaphy and cystoplasty often require intravenous fluids to correct dehydration and acid–base and electrolyte imbalances. All patients should be routinely monitored for urine output after surgery. Foals that are at risk for sepsis or that are subjected to intensive medical care after surgery are candidates for development of gastric ulceration. Use of a type II histamine blocker (Zantac, Glaxo Inc, Research Triangle Park, NC) and a mucosal protectant (Carafate, Marion Labs Inc, Kansas City, Mo) is indicated in these cases.

Complications

Clinically significant complications of bladder surgery are rare. The most acute and striking complication is the development of severe ventricular arrhythmias in the anesthetized foal with uroperitoneum.[3,5] Postoperative myositis resulting in death has also been documented.[75] Correction of electrolyte and acid–base status before surgery minimizes the risk of developing these problems.

In foals, contamination of the peritoneal cavity with urine is common and may result in the development of chemical peritonitis.[18] Although most foals with cystorrhexis have a chronic history of uroperitoneum and presumably some degree of chemical peritonitis, the incidence of septic peritonitis is low[16] unless concurrent septic omphalophlebitis or other septic processes are present simultaneously.[17,18] In one retrospective study of celiotomy for the treatment of uroperitoneum, several foals had positive culture results for *Mucor* and *Candida* species.[18] All foals with uroperitoneum and concurrent septic disease should be monitored closely for clinical evidence of septicemia or septic arthritis and physitis after surgery.

Adhesions have also been reported as a consequence of abdominal surgery in foals for correction of uroperitoneum.[18] The development of septic peritonitis can result in an increased incidence of adhesion formation, particularly in the posterior abdomen near the bladder.[17]

Contamination of the midline incision with urine or bacteria may lead to the formation of incisional edema and drainage. In adult male horses operated on for cystic calculi, preputial edema occurs occasionally.[47] Although generally responsive to anti-inflammatory agents and local wound therapy, it may require temporary placement of peri-incisional drains. Surgical failures of the cystotomy incision after cystoplasty and exploratory cystotomy have been reported.[8,19] Typically, these are not a problem.[19]

REFERENCES

1. Nickel R, Schummer A, Seiferle E: The Viscera of the Domestic Mammals, New York, 1979, Springer-Verlag.
2. Rooney JR: Rupture of the urinary bladder in the foal, Vet Pathol 1971;8:445.
3. Richardson DW, Kohn CW: Uroperitoneum in the foal, J Am Vet Med Assoc 1983;182:267.
4. Hackett RP: Rupture of the urinary bladder in neonatal foals, Comp Cont Educ Pract Vet 1984;6:S488.
5. Richardson DW: Urogenital problems in the neonatal foal, Vet Clin North Am Equine Pract 1985;1:179.
6. Hackett RP, Vaughan JT, Tennant BC: The urinary system. In Mannsman RA, editor: Equine Medicine and Surgery, ed 3, Santa Barbara, Calif, 1982, American Veterinary Publications.
7. Firth EC: Dissecting hematoma of corpus spongiosum and urinary bladder rupture in a stallion, J Am Vet Med Assoc 1976;169:801.
8. Pankowski RL, Fubini SL: Urinary bladder rupture in a two-year-old horse: Sequel to a surgically repaired neonatal injury, J Am Vet Med Assoc 1987;191:560.
9. Nyrop KA, DeBowes RM, Cox JH, et al: Rupture of the urinary bladder in two postparturient mares, Comp Cont Educ Pract Vet 1984;6:S510.
10. Madigan JE: Diagnosing and treating the foal with bladder rupture, Equine Pract 1987;9:1048.
11. Behr MJ, Hackett RP, Bentinck-Smith J, et al: Metabolic abnormalities associated with rupture of the urinary bladder in neonatal foals, J Am Vet Med Assoc 1981;178:263.
12. Colahan PT, Mayhew IG, MacKay RJ: Hyperkalemia due to uremic acidosis in a foal with a ruptured bladder. Florida Vet J 1980;9:22.
13. Kritchevsky JE, Stevens DL, Christopher J, et al: Peritoneal dialysis for presurgical management of ruptured bladder in a foal, J Am Vet Med Assoc 1984;185:81.
14. Lavoie JP, Harnagel SH: Nonsurgical management of ruptured urinary bladder in a critically ill foal, J Am Vet Med Assoc 1988;192:1577.
15. Walker DF, Vaughan JT: Bovine and Equine Urogenital Surgery, Philadelphia, 1980, Lea & Febiger.
16. McIlwraith CW, Turner AS: Surgery of the urogenital system. In McIlwraith CW, Turner AS, editors: Equine Surgery: Advanced Techniques, Philadelphia, 1987, Lea & Febiger.
17. Robertson JT, Embertson RS: Congenital and perinatal abnormalities of the urogenital tract, Vet Clin North Am Equine Pract 1988;4:359.
18. Adams R, Koterba AM, Cudd TC, et al: Exploratory celiotomy for suspected urinary tract disruption in neonatal foals: A review of 18 cases, Equine Vet J 1988;20:13.
19. Pascoe RR: Complications following a ruptured bladder in a 60-day old foal, Aust Vet J 1976;52:473.
20. Crowhurst RC: Abdominal surgery in the foal, Equine Vet J 1974;6:22.
21. Darbishire HB: Operation to repair rupture of the bladder in the young foal, Vet Rec 1961;73:693.
22. duPleisse JL: Rupture of the bladder in the newborn foal and its surgical correction, J S Afr Vet Assoc 1958;29:261.
23. Genetzky RM, Hagemoser WA: Physical and clinical pathological findings associated with experimentally induced rupture of the equine urinary bladder, Can Vet J 1985;26:391.
24. Hodgson DR: Rupture of the urinary bladder. In Robinson NE, editor: Current Therapy in Equine Medicine, Philadelphia, 1986, WB Saunders.
25. Koterba AM, Adams R, McClure JR, et al: Renal and urinary tract function and dysfunction in the neonatal foal, Proc Am Assoc Equine Pract 1985;31:659.
26. Modransky PD: Neoplastic and anomalous conditions of the urinary tract. In Robinson NE, editor: Current Therapy in Equine Medicine, ed 2, Philadelphia, WB Saunders, 1987.
27. Adams SB, Fessler JF: Umbilical cord remnant infections in foals: 16 cases (1975-1985), J Am Vet Med Assoc 1987;190:316.
28. Reef VB: Ultrasonographic diagnosis of umbilical infections in the foal, Proc Am Vet Med Forum 1988;5:462.
29. Sutor DJ, Wooley SE: Animal calculi: An x-ray diffraction study of their crystalline composition, Res Vet Sci 1970;11:299.
30. Greuberg W: Karbonat-Harnsteine herbivorer Säugetiere, Zentralbl Vet Med A 1971;18:767.
31. Lowe JE: Long-term results of cystotomy for removal of uroliths from horses, J Am Vet Med Assoc 1965;147:147.
32. Firth EC: Urethral sphincterotomy for delivery of vesical calculus in the mare: A case report, Equine Vet J 1976;8:99.
33. Holt PE, Pearson H: Urolithiasis in the horse: A review of 13 cases, Equine Vet J 1984;16:31.
34. DeBowes RM: Surgical management of urolithiasis, Vet Clin North Am Equine Pract 1988;4:461.
35. Larsen LH: Laparotomy and cystectomy in a Thoroughbred mare, Aust Vet J 1954;30:307.
36. Usenik EA, Larson LL, Sauer F: Cystotomy and removal of urolith in a Shetland mare, J Am Vet Med Assoc 1956;128:453.
37. Menon MN, Lingam UM: Laparo-cystotomy in a horse, Indian Vet J 1958;35:482.
38. Lowe JE: Suprapubic cystotomy in a gelding, Cornell Vet 1960;50:510.
39. Wright JC, Neal PA: Laparo-cystotomy for urinary calculus in a gelding, Vet Rec 1960;72:301.
40. Williams KR: Laparo-cystotomy in a gelding, Vet Rec 1964;76:83.
41. Reed DG: Suprapubic cystotomy in a stallion, Can J Comp Med Vet Sci 1964;28:95.

42. Wharrier J: Cystic calculus in the horse, Vet Rec 1964;76:187.
43. Williams PFB: Removal of an urinary calculus from a gelding, N Z Vet J 1979;27:223.
44. Belling TH: Equine laparocystotomy, Equine Pract 1983;5:16.
45. DeBowes RM: Obstructive urinary tract disease. In Robinson NE, editor: Current Therapy in Equine Medicine, ed 2, Philadelphia, WB Saunders, 1987.
46. Snyder JR, Pascoe JR, Williams JW: Rectal prolapse and cystic calculus in a burro, J Am Vet Med Assoc 1985;187:421.
47. DeBowes RM, Nyrop KA, Boulton CH: Cystic calculi in the horse, Comp Cont Educ Pract Vet 1984;6:S268.
48. Squire KR, Adams SB, Conley R: Postpartum partial cystectomy through the vagina in a mare with everted partially necrotic bladder, J Am Vet Med Assoc 1992;200:1111.
49. Stickle RL, Wilcock BP, Huseman JL: Multiple ureteral defects in a Belgian foal, Vet Med Small Anim Clin 1975;70:819.
50. Robertson JT, Spurlock GH, Bramlage LL, Landry SL: Repair of ureteral defect in a foal, J Am Vet Med Assoc 1983;183:799.
51. Gibson KT, Trotter GW, Gustafson SB: Conservative management of uroperitoneum in a gelding, J Am Vet Med Assoc 1992;200:1692.
52. Evans LH: Surgical treatment of the polyarthritis-septicemia complex in young foals, Arch Am Coll Vet Surg 1977;6:44.
53. Kaminski JM, Katz AR, Woodward SC: Urinary bladder calculus formation on sutures in rabbits, cats and dogs, Surg Gynecol Obstet 1978;146:353.
54. Christy JH, Clements SD: Electrolytes and the heart. In Hurst HW, editor: The Heart, New York, 1979, McGraw-Hill.
55. Roberts MC: Ascending urinary tract infection in ponies, Aust Vet J 1979;55:191.
56. Laverty S, Pascoe JR, Ling GV, et al: Urolithiasis in 68 horses, Vet Surg 1992;21:56.
57. Hutchins DR: Abdominal surgery in horses, Aust Vet J 1956;32:149.
58. MacHarg MA, Foerner JJ, Phillips TN, et al: Electrohydraulic lithotripsy for treatment of a cystic calculus in a mare, J Vet Surg 1985;14:325.
59. Eustace RA, Hunt JM, Brearley MJ: Electrohydraulic lithotripsy for the treatment of cystic calculus in two geldings, Equine Vet J 1988;20:221.
60. Jackson OF: Renal calculus in a horse, Vet Rec 1972;91:7.
61. Trotter GW, Bennett DG, Behm RJ: Urethral calculi in five horses, J Vet Surg 1981;10:159.
62. Ehnen SJ, Divers TJ, Gillette D, et al: Obstructive nephrolithiasis and ureterolithiasis associated with chronic renal failure in horses: Eight cases (1981-1987), J Am Vet Med Assoc 1990;197:249.
63. Sullins KE, Traub-Dargats JL: Endoscopic anatomy of the equine urinary tract, Comp Cont Educ Pract Vet 1984;6:S663.
64. Howard R, Pleasant R, May K: Pulsed dye laser lithotripsy for treatment of urolithiasis in two geldings, J Am Vet Med Assoc 1998;212:1600.
65. Judy C, Galuppo L: Endoscopic-assisted disruption of urinary calculi using a holmium YAG laser in the standing horse, Vet Surg 2002;31:245.
66. May KA, Pleasant RS, Howard RD, et al. Failure of holmium:yttrium-aluminum-garnet laser lithotripsy in two horses with calculi in the urinary bladder, J Am Vet Med Assoc 2001;219:957.
67. Pringle JK, Schott HC: Miscellaneous disorders of the urinary tract. In Robinson NE, editor: Current Therapy in Equine Medicine, ed 4, Philadelphia, 1997, WB Saunders.
68. Rodgerson DH, Spirito MA, Thrope PE, Hanson RR: Standing surgical repair of cystorrhexis in two mares, Vet Surg 1999;28:113.
69. Higuchi T, Nanao Y, Senba H: Repair of urinary bladder rupture through a urethrotomy and urethral sphincterotomy in four postpartum mares, Vet Surg 2002;31:344.
70. Adams SB: Surgical approaches to and exploration of the equine abdomen, Vet Clin North Am Large Anim Pract 1982;4:89.
71. Beard WL: Parainguinal laparocystotomy for urolith removal in geldings, Vet Surg 2004;33:386.
72. Edwards RB, Ducharme NG, Hackett RP: Laparoscopic repair of a bladder rupture in a foal, Vet Surg 1995;24:60.
73. Fischer AT: Laparoscopically assisted resection of umbilical structures in foals, J Am Vet Med Assoc 1998;214:1813.
74. Ragle C: Laparoscopic removal of cystic calculi. In Fischer AT Jr, editor: Equine Diagnostic and Surgical Laparoscopy, Philadelphia, 2002, WB Saunders.
75. Manning M, Dubielzig R, McGuirk S: Postoperative myositis in a neonatal foal: A case report, Vet Surg 1995;24:69.

CHAPTER 72

Urethra

James D. Lillich
Richard M. DeBowes

ANATOMY

The urethra, a muscular tube lined by mucosa, serves as the normal conduit for urine flow to the exterior of the body after birth.[1,2] In the mare, the urethra is 5 to 8 cm long and 2 to 3 cm wide, and it connects the caudal bladder to the cranial limits of the vestibule.[1]

The male urethra connects the bladder to the glans of the male penis and consists of pelvic and extrapelvic segments. The pelvic urethra is 10 to 12 cm long and expands to a width of 3 cm caudal to the prostate.[1] Dorsally, the pelvic urethra receives the ducts of the seminal vesicles and the vas deferens in the paramedian diverticula lateral to the colliculus seminalis. Lateral and slightly caudal to the colliculus, numerous small ducts of the prostate enter the urethra. Distally, the ducts of the bulbourethral glands enter the pelvic urethra, arranged in two parallel rows of six to eight openings. The pelvic urethra and bulbourethral glands are enveloped in the urethralis muscle, which contracts to evacuate the urethra at the end of micturition or ejaculation. The pelvic urethra narrows caudally as it courses ventrally and cranially at the caudal margin of the ischial arch.

The extrapelvic male urethra is 1.5 cm wide and of variable length, depending on the presence or absence of an erection. The extrapelvic urethra courses distally through the male penis supported by the bulbospongiosus muscle and the corpus spongiosum penis to its distal limits, where it terminates at the glans as the urethral process.[1]

PHYSIOLOGY

The urethra functions as a conduit for the propulsion of urine distally during contraction of the detrusor muscle of the bladder.[3] The urethra is enveloped in smooth muscle and is protected by muscular sphincters under voluntary and involuntary control. Since the urethra represents the only pathway for urinary outflow in the adult patient, its prolonged obstruction results in serious consequences, including cystorrhexis, uroperitoneum, and associated metabolic derangements.[4,5]

Either a loss of neuromuscular control of the urethral sphincters or the presence of selected developmental anomalies can result in clinical urinary incontinence of urethral origin. Although it is not acutely life threatening, urinary incontinence can be a difficult problem to resolve, and it often is associated with ascending urinary tract infection.[6]

DISORDERS REQUIRING SURGERY

Disorders of the equine urethra that require surgery are urolithiasis (primary urethral or secondary to cystic calculi), soft tissue obstructions (mucosal webbing), contusions, and lacerations.[4,5,7-12] Traumatic injuries to the distal penis and urethra are the most common conditions. In stallions, kicks and self-trauma associated with fencing or housing commonly result in injury. Hematuria and hemospermia can also be considered disorders requiring surgery, because affected individuals may respond to temporary urinary diversion via perineal urethrostomy.[9,13]

Urethral Obstruction

Acute urethral obstruction in the male horse results from occlusion with urinary calculi[5,8,9] or, less commonly, from extraurethral compression associated with soft tissue problems of contusion,[10,11] hematoma,[4,14,15] stricture,[16] parasitic granuloma,[17,18] or neoplasia[8,9] (see Chapter 66). Affected individuals may require temporary or permanent urinary diversion as part of their definitive therapy.

Urolithiasis

The etiology of equine urolithiasis is discussed in Chapter 71. Although large calculi can be accommodated by the bladder with few clinical signs, small (0.5 to 1.0 cm) calculi are capable of passing through the trigone and into the proximal urethra, occluding the equine male urethra and thus blocking urine outflow.[5,8,9] The most common area of obstruction is at the junction of the wide pelvic urethra with the more narrow extrapelvic urethra. In contrast, mares rarely develop this condition because of the short length and wide diameter of the female urethra.

Horses demonstrate signs of moderate to severe colic related to distention of the urinary bladder, which must be differentiated from discomfort of intestinal origin. Horses with an obstruction assume the posture to urinate but pass little or no urine.[5,8,9] Spontaneous urethral hemorrhage is commonly observed in these patients.[5,8-10] Occasionally, affected individuals are refractory to analgesic therapy.

Close examination of the patient reveals a complete lack of clinical signs referable to endotoxemia. Tachycardia, tachypnea, and ileus may be observed but are probably the result of visceral discomfort associated with distention of the urinary bladder. Rectal examination reveals moderate to severe distention of the bladder. Passage of a rubber urinary catheter, a flexible urethral probe, or a fiberoptic endoscope identifies a urethral obstruction distal to the trigone[5,8,9,19,20] (Fig. 72-1). Horses with the aforementioned history that become acutely asymptomatic should be suspected of having cystorrhexis and should be evaluated for uroperitoneum.

Medical treatment for urethrolithiasis includes sedatives, muscle relaxants, and analgesics, followed by attempted manipulation of the offending calculus.[5,8,9] Caution should be used when selecting xylazine as a sedative because of its diuretic effect, which substantially increases the formation of urine.[21] Phenothiazine-derivative tranquilizers have minimal diuretic effect, but their use in intact male horses may result in penile paralysis. Therefore, the use of sedation should always accompany the establishment of urine outflow and bladder decompression. Distention of the urethra with a solution of sterile saline, sterile lubricant, and mepivacaine hydrochloride can facilitate ballottement of the calculus with a sterile urinary catheter. Temporary relief may be achieved with dislodgment and retrograde displacement of the obstructing urolith into the bladder, which permits the temporary evacuation of urine. Calculi managed in this fashion must ultimately be removed through either laparocystotomy or perineal urethrotomy.[5,8,9] Calculi that cannot be dislodged retrograde in this fashion must be removed through perineal urethrotomy. Distally lodged uroliths may be removed by using laparoscopic or arthroscopic grasping forceps with the aid of endoscopic examination. Care should be taken not to further damage already irritated mucosa (Fig. 72-2).

Obstructive Soft Tissue Lesions

Obstructive soft-tissue lesions of the urethra are diagnosed infrequently. They include neoplasia,[8,10] scar tissue,[16] hematoma,[4,14,15] and parasitic granuloma,[17,18] with the latter two conditions being most commonly observed.

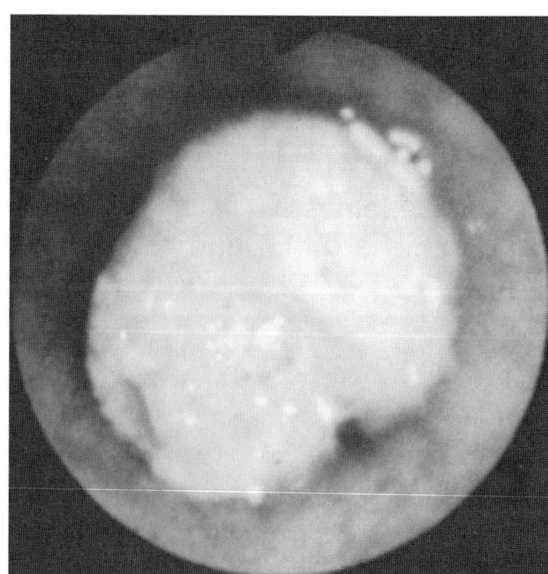

Figure 72-1. Endoscopic examination of the urethra reveals a type I urolith.

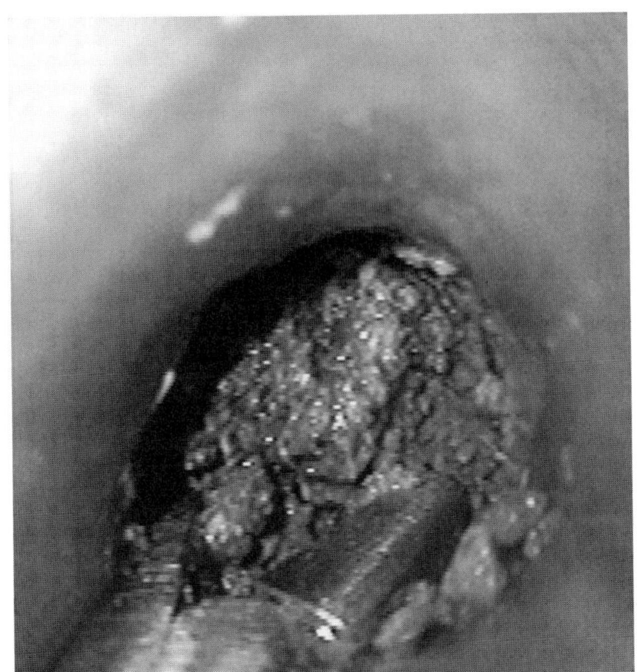

Figure 72-2. An endoscopic image of an obstructive type I urolith being removed from the distal urethra with a Ferris-Smith rongeur. (Courtesy Carolyn Arnold, DVM.)

Squamous cell carcinoma is the most frequently diagnosed neoplasm associated with the penis or prepuce of the horse.[10] Melanoma and sarcoids are found also, but with a lower frequency.[8,10,19] Although most of these problems are nearly unique to the male patient, squamous cell carcinoma of the mare's perineum and vulva may extend to involve the distal urethral tissues.

The offending mass is usually located along the distal penis, glans, or urethral process. Either distal proliferative lesions or deep invasive lesions of the penile shaft can encroach on, distort, and occlude the extrapelvic urethra.[8,18] In contrast to patients with obstructive urethrolithiasis, horses with soft tissue obstructions are not acutely obstructed and colicky. More commonly, these animals have a chronic history of unthriftiness and dysuria. Some individuals may have dirty or malodorous sheaths. Often, affected animals soil the medial surfaces of their hindlimbs (males) or perineum (females) with urine. During micturition, the urine stream may be severely distorted.

Mass lesions are readily recognized on physical examination, but identification is often difficult to make on gross appearance alone. Typically, cytologic impressions and excisional or fine-needle biopsy is required to arrive at a definitive diagnosis. The diagnosis of hematoma is made without difficulty on the basis of the history and physical examination, and ultrasonographic evaluation confirms its presence, size, and potential importance.

Damage to the urethral mucosa can lead to *scar formation* within the lumen of the urethra, which may result in an outflow obstruction. For lesions that involve the mucosa alone, the webbing can be ablated with the neodymium:yttrium-aluminum-garnet laser through the endoscope. In one case report, a noncontact technique was utilized with 2- to 3-second bursts at 40 W.[22]

Periurethral *hematomas* result from direct blunt trauma to the extrapelvic urethra, typically in the region of the perineum.[4,14,15] Large hematomas are capable of occluding the urethra until cystorrhexis occurs.[4] Hematomas are treated with rest and hydrotherapy. An alternative treatment regimen consists of draining the hematoma using an appropriate method for the specific case, or as dictated by the horse's ability to urinate. Large hematomas that occlude or nearly occlude the urethra should be either drained or bypassed by temporary urinary diversion via perineal urethrotomy. Parasitic granulomas are readily managed by the administration of ivermectin or organophosphate pharmaceutical agents.[8,10] Parasitic lesions respond to routine systemic therapy and rarely require surgical débridement. Affirmatively diagnosed neoplastic lesions are treated by local resection.[8,19,23] When distal urethral amputation or phallectomy is required, a spatulated urethroplasty can be performed (see Chapter 66).[18,19,23,24]

Cutaneous habronemiasis (larval *Habronema* species) is the most common parasitic infestation affecting the mucocutaneous junction of the distal urethral orifice, It results in a pyogranulomatous reaction and the formation of proliferative granulation tissue.[9,10,21]

Urethrorrhexis

Urethrorrhexis, or urethral laceration, is observed periodically in horses after kicks or wire trauma involving the perineum or inguinal region.[8,9,25] The extrapelvic urethra is particularly susceptible at the level of the ischial arch because of its superficial and relatively unprotected position. Urethral injury can occur as a result of inadvertent iatrogenic urethral injury associated with routine scrotal orchidectomy.[19,25]

A pronounced soft tissue inflammatory reaction develops in the perineal and inguinal regions in response to the presence of extravasated urine. Edema of the prepuce, inguinal region, and hindlimbs may result.[25] When a full-thickness urethral laceration is present, urine is observed leaking from the wound,[25] and the skin surrounding the wound is soiled and inflamed.

The diagnosis can be made from a careful physical examination. When open wounds over the urethra are believed to communicate with the urethral lumen, retrograde infusion of sterile saline and methylene blue confirms urethral luminal compromise. Confirmation of a diagnosis of closed urethrorrhexis is more difficult and requires either direct visualization by urethroscopic examination[20] or imaging by positive-contrast radiographic or ultrasonographic examination. Retrograde distention of the urethra with sterile saline enhances its visualization and identification of its defect on ultrasonic examination. The literature suggests that in cases of suspected urethral trauma, radiographic confirmation is superior to urethral instrumentation (catheterization or urethroscopy).[26,27]

Therapy is directed at controlling regional inflammation and diverting the flow of urine through a urinary catheter.[8,19] The urethral epithelium has a relatively high potential for regeneration,[28] and closed crushing injuries of the urethra

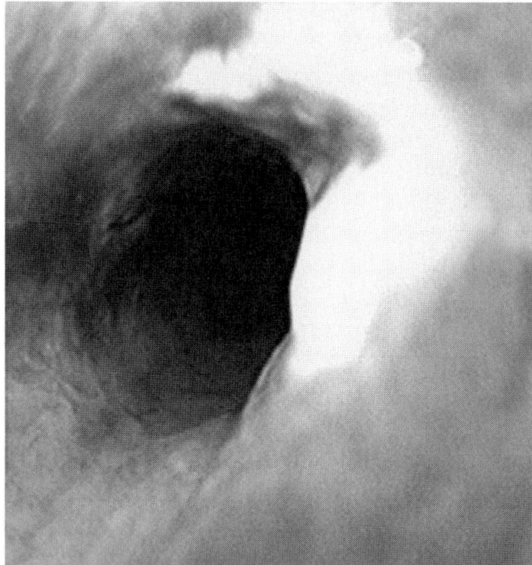

Figure 72-3. An endoscopic image of a 2-year-old Quarter Horse gelding, 6 weeks after the urethra was repaired. The horse was referred for repair of iatrogenic inadvertent complete transection of the penile urethra during castration. (Courtesy James Bryant, DVM.)

may be treated by placement of a sterile urinary catheter for 5 to 7 days.[8,9,25,28] Primary repair of a urethral laceration may not be necessary unless the urethra is completely transected.[9,25] Inadvertent iatrogenic urethral transaction may not be appreciated for a few days. Urine accumulation within the scrotal tissues is usually evident. Repair of the urethra can be assisted with endoscopy and/or normograde passage of a urinary catheter through a perineal urethrotomy. Periurethral tissues should be débrided and the urethral mucosa apposed to reduce secondary-intention healing and stricture formation. With proper apposition of the mucosa, primary healing can be obtained with preservation of lumen diameter (Fig. 72-3).

Hematuria and Hemospermia

Hematuria in geldings and hemospermia in stallions have been related to urethral defects that communicate with the corpus spongiosum penis. Linear urethral defects are identified with endoscopic examination, typically located at the level of the ischial arch. The origin of urethral defects is unknown. Treatment with temporary urethrostomy that does not enter the urethral lumen has been successful.[29] This procedure is thought to lower vascular pressure of the corpus spongiosum penis during micturition. The technique, alone in the gelding and with sexual rest in the stallion, allows healing of the mucosal defect.

SURGICAL PROCEDURES

Perineal Urethrotomy

Perineal urethrotomy is typically performed for temporary urine diversion in male patients with obstructive urinary outflow disease.* In patients requiring chronic urinary diversion, a permanent urethrostomy may be created.[29] For perineal urethrotomy or urethrostomy, the patient is sedated and confined in stocks for a standing surgical procedure.[5,8,19] The administration of detomidine hydrochloride (Dormosedan, SmithKline Beecham, Lincoln, Neb) or a combination of xylazine (Rompun, Haver-Lockhart, Shawnee, Kan) and butorphanol tartrate (Torbugesic, Fort Dodge Laboratories, Fort Dodge, Iowa) is usually adequate. An epidural injection of mepivacaine hydrochloride (Carbocaine, Winthrop Laboratories, New York, NY) is administered to desensitize the perineal region. When epidural anesthesia is ineffective, the application of an inverted-V block is usually sufficient to desensitize the skin and superficial tissues of the perineal region. A rubber urinary catheter is advanced proximally through the urethra to aid in intraoperative identification of the urethra. The operative field is clipped and aseptically prepared for surgery.

A 6- to 8-cm longitudinal midline skin incision is made in the perineum extending from a point 10 to 15 cm ventral to the anus ventrally to the ischial arch[5,8,19] (Fig. 72-4). The distal limit of the incision should not be located ventral to the ischial arch. The subcutaneous tissues are divided, and the longitudinal incision is continued deep to divide the bulbospongiosus muscle and corpus spongiosum.[12,19] The urethra is exposed by retraction of these muscles. The urethra is identified and stabilized by palpation of the urinary catheter (Fig. 72-4, *B*). A longitudinal incision is made along the caudal surface of the urethra, and the mucosa is reflected abaxially. Intraluminal obstructions such as uroliths may be manipulated and removed by urinary catheters or forceps inserted through the perineal urethrotomy incision.[12]

For temporary diversion of urine, the wound is managed with local care during the process of secondary-intention wound healing (Fig. 72-5). A urinary catheter may be placed through the temporary urethrotomy incision and secured with stay sutures for 2 to 4 days after surgery. Typically, a urethrotomy wound heals in 14 to 21 days with minimal complications.[19] If a permanent urethrostomy is desired, the muscles of the ventral penis are sutured along their cut edges with a continuous suture of 3-0 synthetic absorbable suture to control hemorrhage. The urethral mucosa and skin are approximated using interrupted sutures of 2-0 or 3-0 synthetic monofilament nonabsorbable suture (Fig. 72-6). Care must be taken to ensure accurate, tensionless apposition of the perineal skin and urethral mucosa.

Distal Urethrotomy

Distal urethral calcular obstruction can be approached with grasping forceps with the aid of endoscopy. For uroliths that cannot be removed in this manner, a scrotal or prescrotal urethrotomy may be required. Horses must be anesthetized and positioned in dorsal recumbency. Technically, the surgical procedure is similar to that for perineal urethrotomy. If the lesion is sufficiently distal, a tourniquet may be applied to assist with hemostasis and improve intraoperative visualization. Incisions are made over or slightly proximal to the urethral calculus to permit the insertion of grasping forceps. After removal of the calculus, the incision is closed in anatomic fashion using 3-0 synthetic absorbable suture. It is important to accurately reconstruct the corpus spongio-

*References 5, 8, 9, 11, 12, 19.

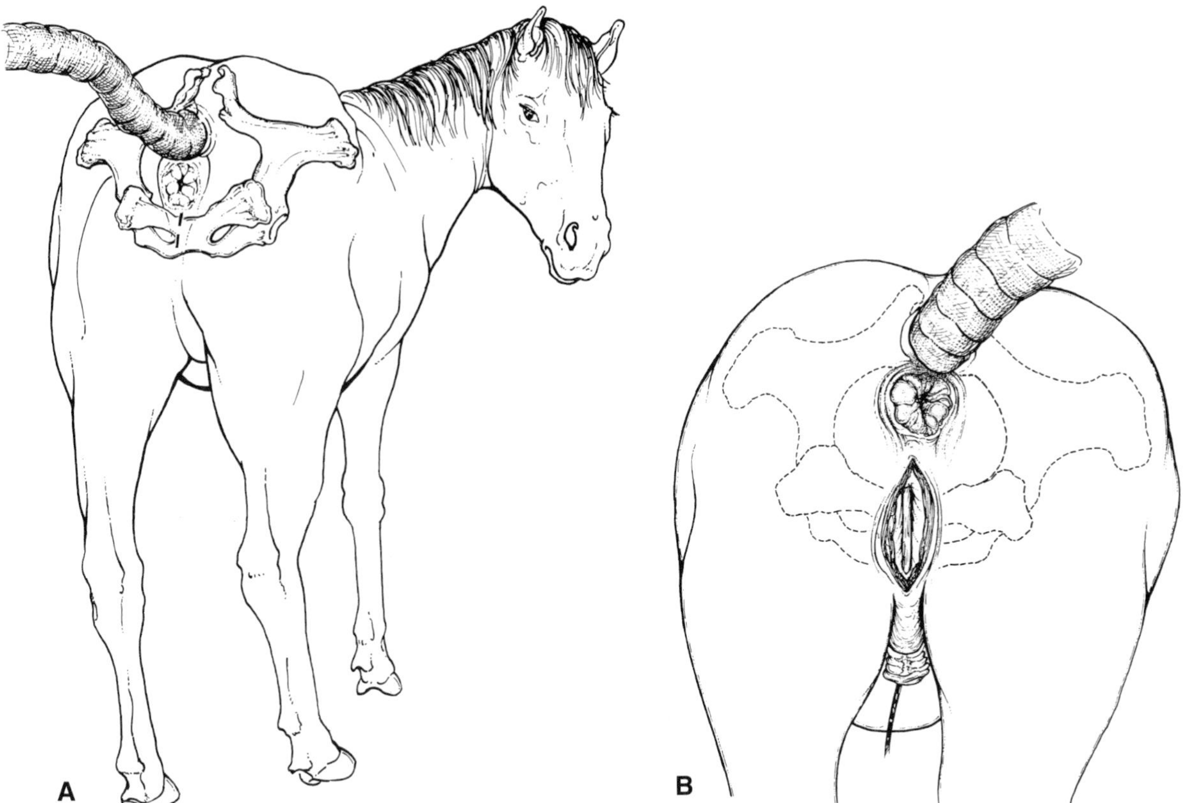

Figure 72-4. A, The incision for a perineal urethrotomy or urethrostomy must be located immediately dorsal to the ischium to reduce the likelihood of postoperative urine scalding. **B,** Preoperative placement of a urinary catheter facilitates intraoperative identification and exposure of the urethra.

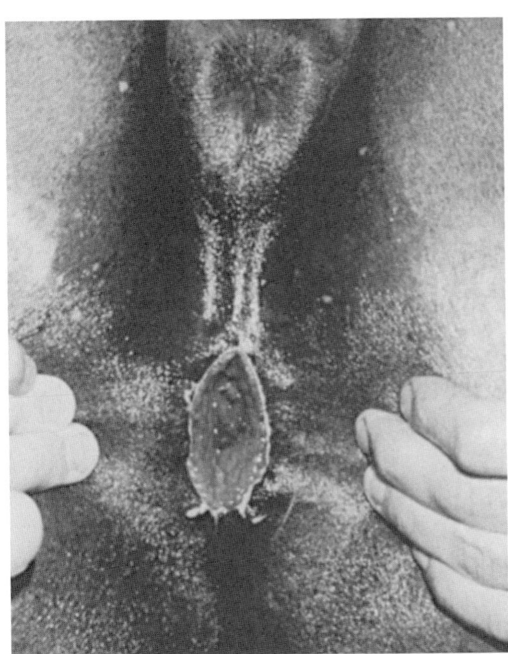

Figure 72-5. Perineal urethrotomy for temporary urinary diversion will heal by secondary intention with minimal complications.

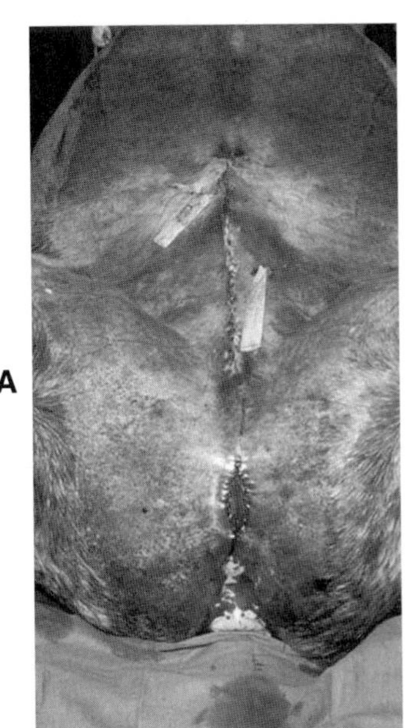

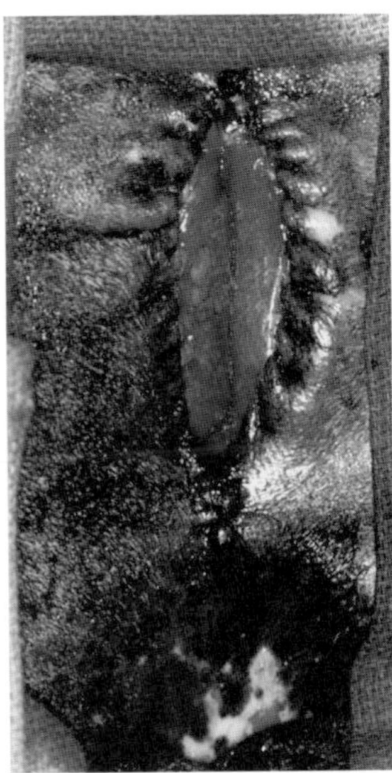

Figure 72-6. A, Permanent perineal urethrostomy for chronic urinary diversion to bypass extensive preputial and penile squamous cell carcinoma. **B,** Accurate apposition of mucosal and cutaneous layers is essential to minimize postoperative complications.

sum and bulbospongiosus muscle to reduce the risk for urine leakage and development of cellulitis. Approximation of the retractor penis muscle provides additional security for the closure.

Urethroplasty

The patient is sedated, restrained, and prepared for standing surgery as described. Repair of a urethral laceration is consistent with the repair of any other hollow viscus. Careful attention to wound débridement, lavage, and preservation of intrinsic vascular and neural supply is important. Fully circumferential lacerations may be repaired by end-to-end anastomosis. Fine (3-0) absorbable suture material such as polyglactin 910 (Vicryl, Ethicon, Somerville, NJ) should be used. The use of an intraluminal stent (urinary catheter) for the repair of a lacerated urethra is considered acceptable.[31]

Aftercare

After surgery of the urethra, the patient should be observed to ensure that urination occurs without difficulty. Antibiotics and nonsteroidal anti-inflammatory drugs may be administered as required. There is little need for prolonged postoperative analgesia. In cases in which urine was extravasated, the use of surgical drains is appropriate.[9,25]

The literature is unclear on the value of chronic catheter placement after urethral repair. Traditionally, catheters were left in place after primary repair of a traumatized urethra.[28] More recently, chronic placement of urinary catheters has been discouraged because of locally increased inflammatory response and subsequent stricture formation.[28] Postoperative stricture is minimized by limiting the duration of catheterization, by accurate tissue repair, by effective hemostasis, and by adequate drainage of the periurethral tissues.[9,25] Because the chronic use of indwelling urinary catheters is controversial, they should be removed as soon as possible.[6,19,28,30,31] Foley catheters may be secured in place with stay sutures during the first 48 to 96 hours. Foley catheters distended with saline or another salt solution are better tolerated than those distended with air.

The potential for urine soilage of the ventral perineum and subsequent urine scalding is great. Care of the healing urethrotomy incision should include local cleansing for removal of accumulated urinary salts or exudate. The skin of the ventral perineum, inguinal region, and adductor surfaces of the hindlimbs should be cleansed daily and protective emollients applied.

Complications

Mild tenesmus and discomfort are expected after surgery. The effect of urine contamination of tissues is usually minimal unless tissue trauma is advanced or sepsis is present. Antibiotic and anti-inflammatory therapy is appropriate in such cases. Partial dehiscence of urethrostomy incisions occurs infrequently and may be managed with local tissue therapy, débridement, and delayed closure.[9,25-27] Stricture of the urethra is a common postoperative finding[31]; stricture is most commonly observed in distal urogenital surgeries such as posthioplasty or subtotal phallectomy.[23] Surgical procedures involving the distal urethra may require spatulation to reduce the likelihood of stricture formation (see Chapter 66).[19,23,24] Less commonly, thin veils of urethral mucosa may form in such a fashion as to partially occlude the urethral lumen, requiring further surgical revision.[12]

REFERENCES

1. Sisson S, Grossman JD: Equine urogenital system. In Getty R, editor: The Anatomy of the Domestic Animals, ed 5, Philadelphia, 1975, WB Saunders.
2. Rooney JR, Sack WO, Habel RE: Guide to the Dissection of the Horse, Ithaca, NY, 1969, WO Sack.
3. Guyton AC: Renal disease, diuresis and micturition. In Guyton AC, editor: Textbook of Medical Physiology, ed 6, Philadelphia, 1981, WB Saunders.
4. Firth EC: Dissecting hematoma of the corpus spongiosum and urinary bladder rupture in a stallion, J Am Vet Med Assoc 1976;169:800.
5. Trotter GW, Bennett DG, Behm RJ: Urethral calculi in five horses, J Vet Surg 1981;10:159.
6. Robertson JT, Embertson RS: Surgical management of congenital and perinatal abnormalities of the urogenital tract, Vet Clin North Am Equine Pract 1988;4:359.
7. Laverty S, Pascoe JR, Ling GV, et al: Urolithiasis in 68 horses, J Vet Surg 1992;21:56.
8. Hackett RP, Vaughan JT, Tennant BC: The urinary system. In Mannsman RA, McAllister ES, editors: Equine Medicine and Surgery, vol 2, ed 3, Santa Barbara, 1982, American Veterinary Publications.
9. Robertson JT: Conditions of the urethra. In Robinson NE, editor: Current Therapy in Equine Medicine, ed 2, Philadelphia, 1984, WB Saunders.
10. Gatewood DM, Cox JH, DeBowes RM: Diagnosis and treatment of acquired pathologic conditions of the equine penis and prepuce, Comp Cont Educ Pract Vet 1989;11:1498.
11. Clem MF, DeBowes RM: Paraphimosis in horses: Part II. Comp Cont Educ Pract Vet 1989;11:S184.
12. Dyke TM, Maclean AA: Urethral obstruction in a stallion with possible synchronous diaphragmatic flutter, Vet Rec 1987;121:425.
13. Voss JL, Wotowey JL: Hemospermia, Proc Am Assoc Equine Pract 1972;18:103.
14. Gibbons WJ: Hematoma of the penis, Mod Vet Pract 1974;45:76.
15. Pascoe RR: Rupture of the corpus cavernosum penis of a stallion, Aust Vet 1971;47:610.
16. Yovich JV, Turner AS: Treatment of a postcastration urethral stricture by phallectomy in a gelding, Comp Cont Educ Pract Vet 1986;8:S393.
17. Finocchio EJ, Merriam JC: Surgical correction of myiasitic urethritis granulosa, Vet Med Small Anim Clin 1976;71:1629.
18. Stick JA: Amputation of the equine urethral process affected with habronemiasis, Vet Med Small Anim Clin 1979;74:1453.
19. Sullins KE, Traub-Dargatz JL: Endoscopic anatomy of the equine urinary tract, Comp Cont Educ Pract Vet 1984;6:S663.
20. Thurmon JC, Benson GJ: Injectable anesthetics and anesthetic adjuncts, Vet Clin North Am Equine Pract 1987;3:15.
21. Walker DF, Vaughan JT: Bovine and Equine Urogenital Surgery, Philadelphia, 1989, Lea & Febiger.
22. Blikslager AT, Tate Jr LP, Jones SL: Neodymium:yttrium-aluminium-garnet laser ablation of urethral web to relieve urinary outflow obstruction in an adult horse, J Am Vet Med Assoc 2001;218:2.
23. Welch RD, DeBowes RM: Surgical techniques for treatment of pathologic conditions of the equine penis, Comp Cont Educt Pract Vet 1989;11:1505.

24. Turner AS, McIlwraith CW: Techniques in Large Animal Surgery, ed 2,Philadelphia, 1989, Lea & Febiger.
25. Todhunter RJ, Parker JE: Surgical repair of urethral transection in a horse, J Am Vet Med Assoc 1988;193:1085.
26. Weems W: Urology. In Hardy JC, editor: Hardy's Textbook of Surgery, Philadelphia, 1983, JB Lippincott.
27. Glenn JF, Weinerth JL: The male genital system. In Sabiston DC, editor: Textbook of Surgery: The Biological Basis of Modern Surgical Practice, ed 12, Philadelphia, 1981, WB Saunders.
28. Peacock EE: Healing and repair of viscera. In Peacock EE, editor: Wound Healing, ed 3, Philadelphia, 1984, WB Saunders.
29. Schumacher J, Varner DD, Schmitz DG, et al: Urethral defects in geldings with hematuria and stallions with hemospermia, J Vet Surg 1995;24:250.
30. Smith CW: Surgical disease of the urethra. In Slatter DE, editor: Small Animal Surgery, Philadelphia, 1988, WB Saunders.
31. Layton CE, Ferguson HR, Cook JE, et al: Intrapelvic urethral anastomosis: A comparison of three techniques, J Vet Surg 1984;16:175.

SECTION XI Selected Topics of the Lameness Examination

Jörg. A. Auer

CHAPTER 73

Gait Analysis

Michael A. Weishaupt
H. H. Florian Buchner

Lameness is a symptom and can be defined as an alteration of the normal gait pattern caused by a functional or structural disorder in the locomotor system. Clinicians assess lameness by mentally comparing the gait of the lame horse with movements of normal subjects, by matching the symmetry of movements of the left with the right body side, and by comparing the gait before and after an intervention such as a stress test or a diagnostic nerve block. Visual assessment carries all risks that are inherent in subjectivity, and therefore, interpretation of clinical signs depends directly on the expertise of the observer.[1] Because gait compensations made by lame horses may occur very rapidly or subtly, the temporal resolution of the human eye can easily be overtaxed.

Quantitative gait analysis offers a higher spatial and temporal resolution and allows objective characterization of intermittent and mild lamenesses or of gait alterations involving more than one limb. The benefit of clinically applied gait analysis is the reliable documentation of individual locomotion patterns, the degree of lameness, and the result of diagnostic anesthesia, as well as being a quantitative assessment of drug efficacy and specific interventions such as shoeing or surgical procedures.

METHODOLOGY

Biomechanics involves the application of mechanical laws to living structures. Two complementary methods are used to study the body in motion: kinematics and kinetics.[2]

Kinematic Analysis

Kinematic analysis measures the geometry of movement without considering the forces that cause the movement.

The movements are quantified by linear and angular variables in relation to a timeline. The current techniques of choice are digital videography combined with commercial marker tracking software or opto-electronic systems (Table 73-1). Light-reflective markers are placed over specific bony landmarks or joint centers and filmed at 50 to 2000 frames per second (Fig. 73-1, *A*). In contrast to videographic systems where whole-image information is processed, opto-electronic cameras selectively record the marker points by emitting and capturing selected wavelengths of the light (e.g., in the infrared spectrum). Body-marker tracking is performed either manually or automatically and results in the two-dimensional coordinates of the marker's center. A multi-camera setup (see Fig. 73-1, *B*) allows the reconstruction of the three-dimensional trajectory coordinates of the various body markers by merging numerous two-dimensional views using direct linear transformation (see Fig. 73-1, *C*).

By combining kinematic data with a segmental body model of a standard horse,[3,4] the three-dimensional movement of the body center of mass (BCM) can be reconstructed.[5] The BCM is a key factor in the analysis of equine locomotion, since its position and trajectory determine the distribution of loads within the limbs.

Kinetic Analysis

Kinetic analysis studies the forces that are responsible for a movement. Kinetics distinguishes between internal and external forces and torques. Human sensory perception is not able to derive kinetic information from visual gait assessment.

External forces—that is, the forces acting between the hoof and the ground (ground reaction force [GRF])—can be measured directly by using a force plate[6-8] or a force shoe,[9-14] or on a force-measuring runway such as the Equine Gait Analysis system.[15-17] The most established technique is the force plate embedded in a runway. Standard force plates (see Table 73-1) are able to split the force vector into its three orthogonal components, the transverse-horizontal (F_x), the longitudinal-horizontal (F_y), and the vertical force (F_z) component. However, repeated recording sessions are necessary to obtain a sufficient number of representative strides of the different limbs. A treadmill equipped with a dynamometric platform combines the benefits of kinetic analysis with the advantages of the treadmill, such as control of movement velocity and data acquisition over multiple consecutive motion cycles of all four limbs simultaneously[18] (Fig. 73-2). Controlling velocity of movement is a prerequisite for accurate gait analysis, since kinematic and kinetic parameters are known to be velocity dependent.[19-22] The instrumented treadmill is fully operational in a clinical setup. Typically, up to 50 strides per limb, at both walk and trot, are recorded within less than 5 minutes. The calculation of the vertical force traces starts during data acquisition, and force curves are presented in real time on a computer screen. Fourteen force, and 11 temporal and 6 spatial parameters are

TABLE 73-1. Manufacturers

Equipment	Product Name	Address
Videographic systems and analysis software	SIMI Motion	SIMI Reality Motion Systems GmbH, Unterschleissheim, Germany (www.simi.com)
	MaxTRAQ, MaxMATE	Innovision Systems Inc, Columbiaville, Mich (www.innovision-systems.com)
	Peak Motus	Peak Performance Technologies Inc, Centennial, Colo (www.peakperform.com)
	APAS	Ariel Dynamics (www.arielnet.com)
Optoelectronic systems	ProReflex	Qualisys Medical AB, Gothenburg, Sweden (www.qualisys.se)
	Vicon	Vicon Motion Systems Ltd., Oxford, UK (www.vicon.com)
	Motion Analysis	Motion Analysis Corporation, Santa Rosa, Calif (www.motionanalysis.com)
	CODA Motion	Carnwood Dynamics Ltd, Leicestershire, UK (www.charndyn.com)
	Optotrak	Northern Digital Inc, Waterloo, Canada (www.ndigital.com)
Ultrasound-based kinematic system	CMS-HS	Zebris, Isny im Allgäu, Germany (www.zebris.de)
Force plates		AMTI, Watertown, Mass (www.amtiweb.com)
		Bertec Corporation, Columbus, Ohio (www.bertec.com)
		Kistler Instrumente AG, Winterthur, Switzerland (www.kistler.com)

derived from the raw data and presented graphically a few seconds after completion of the measurement. This allows instantaneous assessment of diagnostic blocks (Fig. 73-3).

Modeling of Movement

Mathematical concepts that involve applying the dynamic laws of Newton and defining the body as a linked multi-segment model provide a noninvasive way to study the forces within the body based on kinematic and kinetic data (inverse dynamics) or to simulate movement of a horse based on known forces (forward dynamics).[23]

Inverse dynamic analysis is used to calculate the internal forces acting on the joints (joint moments) as well as tendon forces and bone strains. Tendon force and joint moment profiles of the distal limb have been established during stance and swing phase, during various gaits, and while jumping.[24-27] In the stance phase dynamics of one limb, a static equilibrium is assumed between the external forces (represented by the ground reaction force vector) and the tendon forces acting on the limb joints. Radiography of the specific anatomic region supplies the geometric information (e.g., moment arm of the tendons at the coffin and fetlock joint). Kinematic measurements provide the joint angles and the position of the joint rotation centers in relation to the GRF vector. During the swing phase, in the absence of external forces, inertial parameters (mass, center of mass, moments of inertia) combined with the kinematic data permit the calculation of the power flow along the limb joints.[28]

CLINICAL APPLICATION OF GAIT ANALYSIS

The principal clinical application of gait analysis is the quantification of locomotor performance and lameness. The unloading of a painful limb will lead to a redistribution of load and to visible compensatory movements of specific body parts. Load redistributions are closely related to changes in stride timing and coordination between limbs.

Kinematics of the Lame Horse

In weight-bearing lamenesses, the most consistent changes are observed in the vertical displacement and maximal vertical acceleration of the head and sacrum, as well as in the maximal metacarpophalangeal (MCP) hyperextension and the maximal distal interphalangeal flexion angle. At the trot, asymmetric vertical head nodding is probably the most obvious sign of weight-bearing asymmetry between forelimbs.[29-32] Correspondingly, the vertical movement of the sacrum shows less lowering and lifting during the stance phase of the lame hindlimb.[31] The tuber coxae shows a biphasic movement during an entire stride cycle, with a slightly smaller amplitude of motion during the stance, than during the swing phase of the limb.[33] Lameness amplifies the difference between these two amplitudes in the affected hindlimb: the vertical amplitude is diminished or even absent during the stance phase and enlarged during the swing phase.[31,34] Maximal MCP hyperextension was shown to be an indirect measure for the vertical ground reaction force[35,36] and is reduced in the lame limb at midstance proportionally to the degree of lameness. In a group of horses with moderate to severe lameness, MCP hyperextension decreased on average by 10 degrees, which corresponded to a reduction in peak vertical force of 27%.[37,38] In the contralateral, sound limb, a minimal compensatory increase of MCP hyperextension could be observed.[39] This may be attributed to increased longitudinal braking forces, which extend beyond midstance.[37,40] In proximal joints, such as the shoulder and tarsal joints, flexion increases in the lame limb, indicating smooth limb loading controlled by extensor muscles.[41,42]

A

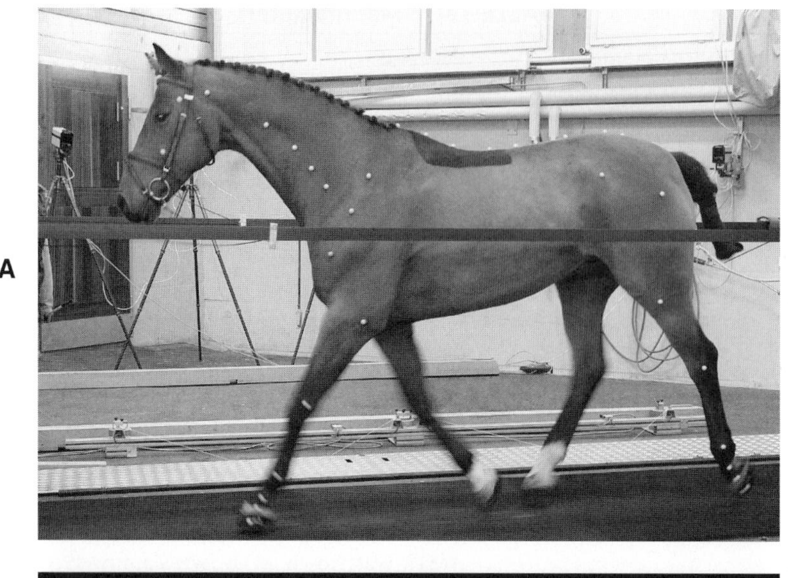

B

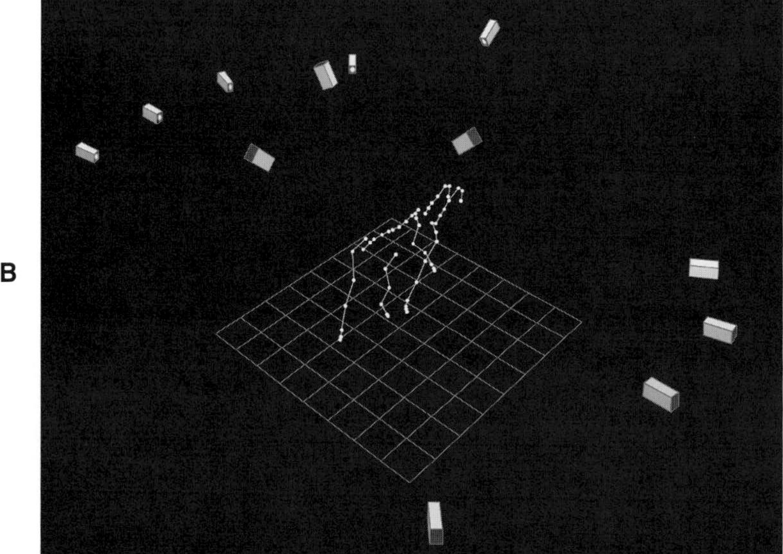

C

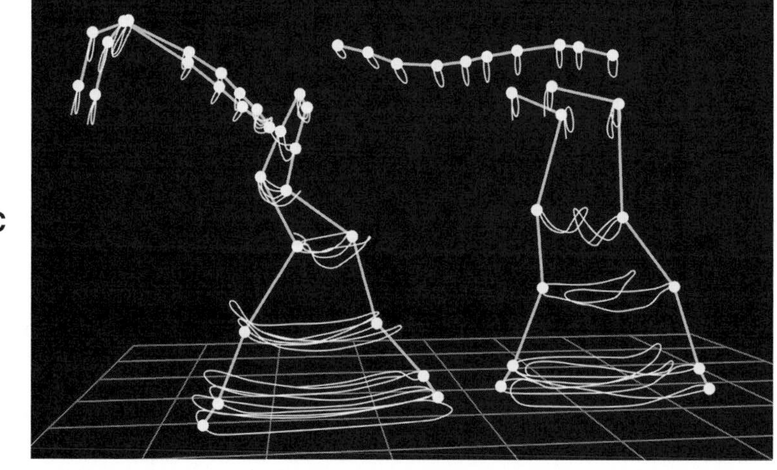

Figure 73-1. Kinematic gait analysis. **A,** The different joints of the forelimbs and hindlimbs, as well as of the neck and selected dorsal spinous processes, are marked with light-reflective spheres. **B,** Multi-camera setup of the Qualisys ProReflex system (Qualisys Medical AB, Gothenburg, Sweden). Cameras are connected in series to a personal computer. **C,** The three-dimensional reconstruction of the marker trajectories during a trot phase. (Courtesy SDS Equine Motion Research Cooperation, Uppsala-Utrecht-Zurich.)

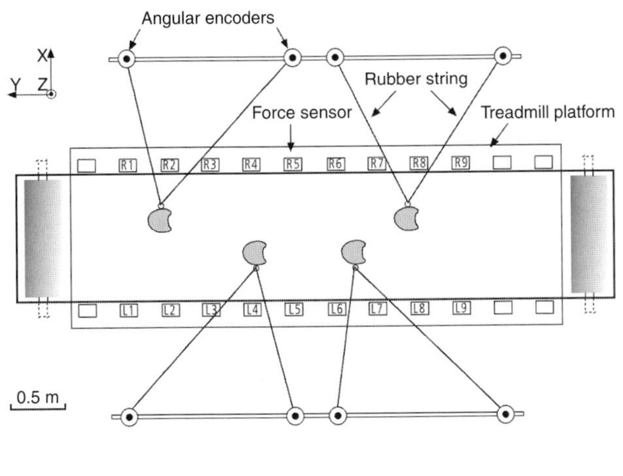

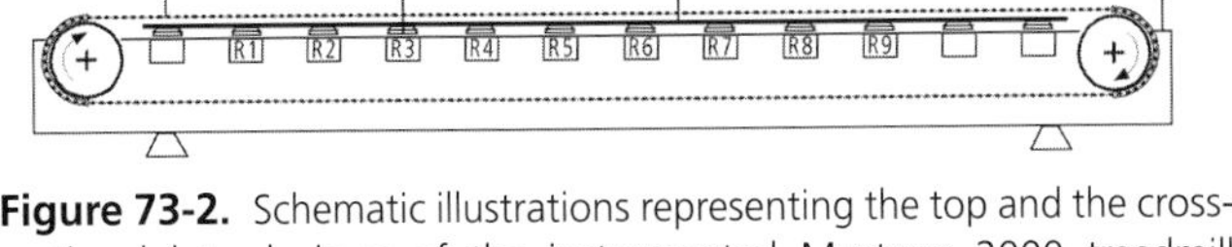

Figure 73-2. Schematic illustrations representing the top and the cross-sectional lateral views of the instrumented Mustang 2000 treadmill (Kagra AG, Fahrwangen, Switzerland) for use in determination of vertical ground reaction forces of all four limbs simultaneously. Notice the 18 force sensors and the four triangulation units used to determine the hoof coordinates. (From Weishaupt MA, Hogg HP, Wiestner T, et al: Am J Vet Res 2002;63:520.)

The mixed lameness is defined as a lameness where pain or pain reactions are obvious during the stance and swing phases. During the stance phase, the previously mentioned typical changes of a weight-bearing lameness can be observed. During the swing phase, flexion of the affected and linked joints is decreased. Both the maximal flexion and the total range of motion are restricted, which may give the impression of a stiff leg.

Compensatory movements of supporting forelimb lameness can be observed at the sacrum or croup, and those of supporting hindlimb lameness, at the head. These movements may mislead the observer during visual gait assessment and suggest a false lameness in a sound limb without structural or functional lesions. In moderate and more accentuated hindlimb lamenesses, a distinct head nod can be observed during the diagonal stance that includes the lame hindlimb, suggesting a lameness in the ipsilateral forelimb.[34,43,44] This compensatory head movement is reported to be more distinguishable than the compensations made by the hind quarter as a consequence of forelimb lameness.[31,45,46] This transmission may occur ipsilaterally as well as along the diagonal.[31,45]

Kinetics of the Lame Horse

At the walk, in unilateral forelimb as well as hindlimb lamenesses, reduced loading of the lame limb is compensated primarily by the contralateral limb and to a lesser extent by concurrently loaded limbs.[47]

At the trot, four compensatory mechanisms serve to reduce structural stress—that is, peak vertical force on the affected limb[48,49]:

1. With increasing lameness, horses reduce the total vertical impulse per stride by increasing stride frequency.
2. The diagonal vertical impulse decreases selectively in the lame diagonal, which causes a shortened suspension phase and a faster transition from the lame to the sound diagonal stance.
3. In forelimb lameness, the impulse is shifted within the lame diagonal limbs to the hindlimb and in the sound diagonal to the contralateral forelimb.[17,40] In hindlimb lameness, the impulse shift occurs predominantly from the affected to the contralateral hindlimb.

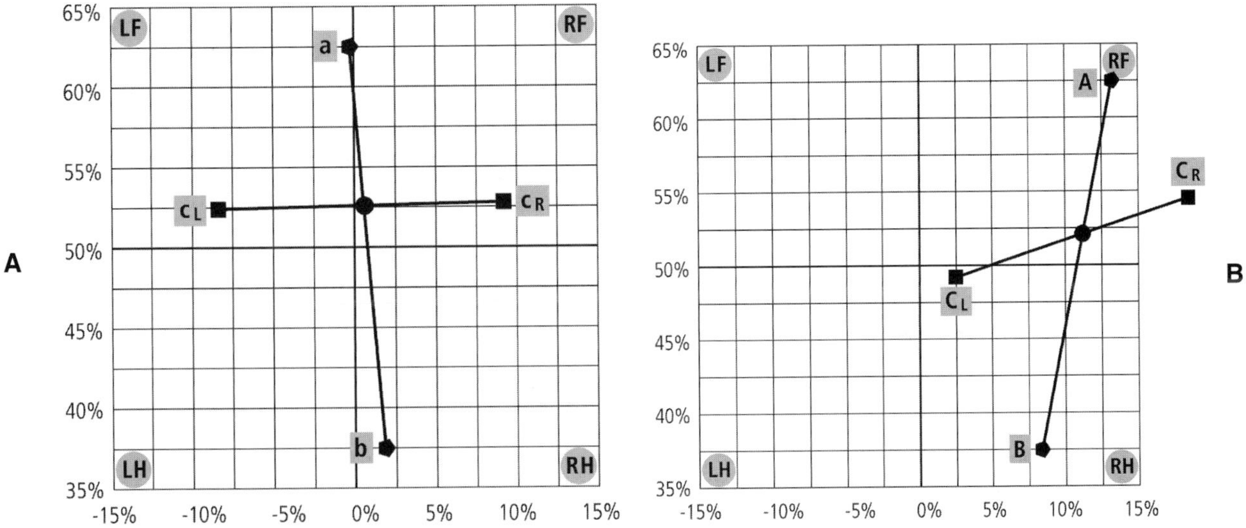

Figure 73-3. Force symmetry plots. **A,** Distribution of peak vertical ground reaction forces (Fz_{peak}) in a sound horse. **B,** The same in a horse with moderate left forelimb lameness. In the lame horse (**B**), the absolute differences in Fz_{peak} are 764 N between forelimbs and 440 N between hindlimbs. This accounts for a 13.5% Fz_{peak} asymmetry in the forelimbs and a 8.3% compensatory asymmetry in the hindlimbs. Comparing both diagonal stances, load is shifted forward during the right diagonal stance (c_R) and backward during the left diagonal stance (c_L). a, forelimb asymmetry index; (LF – RF)/0.5(LF + RF). b, hindlimb asymmetry index; (LH – RH)/0.5(LH + RH). c, distribution of Fz_{peak} within the diagonal limb pair at midstance (percentage carried by the forelimb); c_L, during the left diagonal stance, (LF)/(LF + RH); c_R, during the right diagonal stance, (RF)/(RF + LH).

The weight-shifting mechanism along the longitudinal axis of the horse corresponds to the changes in body center of mass movement[50] and is compatible with the conclusions drawn from the modeling of compensatory head movements in lame horses.[51] The reduction or even suppression of the downward head acceleration during the lame diagonal stance phase decreases the momentum in the trunk, thus unloading the lame forelimb but increasing the loading of the diagonal hindlimb. During the sound diagonal stance, the distinct vertical head nod, together with the higher horizontal braking forces in the contralateral forelimb,[37,40] produces a momentum in the trunk, that increases the loading of the contralateral forelimb and decreases that of the ipsilateral hindlimb.

4. The rate of loading and the peak forces are reduced by prolonging the stance duration in the affected as well as in the contralateral limb.

Except in moderate forelimb lameness, where peak vertical forces increase slightly in the diagonal hindlimb, no compensatory increase in peak vertical force can be observed in other limbs[49] (Fig. 73-4). Likewise, in mild and moderate hindlimb lameness, no compensatory increase in peak vertical force can be observed in other limbs.[48]

Applied Inverse Dynamic Analysis

In clinical studies on horses suffering from superficial digital flexor tendinitis, the specific pattern of the limb joint moments, the load distribution between all flexor tendons, and the effects of therapeutic shoeing were evaluated.[52] Heel wedges were not beneficial for the treatment of superficial digital flexor tendinitis, because the effects of the wedges were limited to the distal interphalangeal joint. In another study, tendon load distribution and limb movement adaptations before and after desmotomy of the accessory ligament of the deep digital flexor tendon were evaluated.[53] Analysis of the gait pattern after surgery showed intra-limb compensation for the lost accessory ligament function through the superficial digital flexor tendon and the suspensory ligament. In a study on sound horses and horses suffering from navicular disease, the forces acting on the deep digital flexor tendon and the navicular bone were measured using inverse dynamic analysis. An unexpected increase in load on the distal sesamoid bone during the initial phase of stance was found in lame horses.[54] This load was reduced by about 24% through orthopedic shoeing using 6-degree heel wedges, whereas eggbar shoes did not reduce the maximal load on the distal sesamoid bone.[55] Similarly, various horseshoe types, which are believed to ease breakover, such as natural balance shoes or quarter-clip shoes, do not reduce distal interphalangeal joint moment or the force on the distal sesamoid bone.[56] However, the ratio of heel to toe height, and the angles of the distal phalanx are well correlated to the forces applied to the foot.[57]

Applied Forward Dynamic Analysis

Forward dynamic analysis is opposite to the approach of inverse dynamics and uses given internal forces combined with segmental data to predict external forces and move-

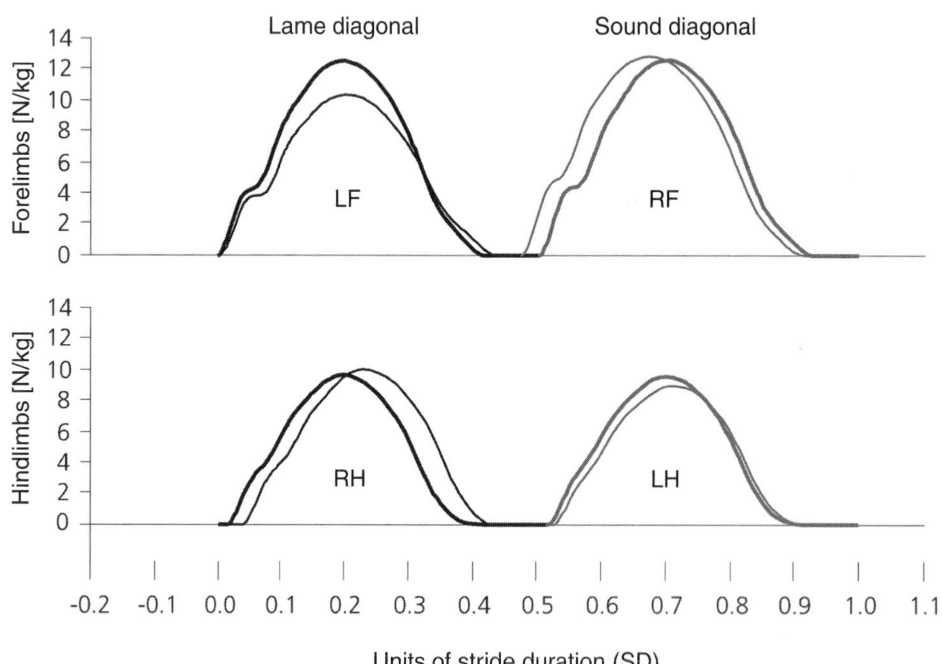

Figure 73-4. Representative vertical force curves of a horse trotting on an instrumented treadmill before and after inducing lameness by applying pressure to the sole. Timeline normalized to units of stride duration. *Bold line,* sound condition; *thin line,* moderate left forelimb lameness. *Black,* lame diagonal (left front [LF] – right hind [RH]); *grey,* sound diagonal (right front [RF] – left hind [LH]). In the affected limb (LF) the reduced impact force and rate of loading in the first half of stance, the lower peak vertical force, and the prolongation of stance duration are obvious. In the contralateral limb (RF), only the prolonged stance duration and therefore an enlarged impulse could be observed. In the diagonal limb (RH), peak vertical force increased slightly, whereas it decreased in the ipsilateral limb (LH). (From Weishaupt MA, Weistner T, Hogg HP, et al: Vet J [in press].)

ments. Both total body movement and specific joint loading during various interventions or loading scenarios can be simulated.[58,59] The accuracy of the model output depends on the complexity of the model and the accuracy of the input data.

Finite element modeling (FEM) is a method adopted from engineering. Modeling a complex object as a composition of numerous single elements with known material properties and interactions allows the calculation of the effect of external forces on internal stress. FEM has been used to simulate bone or hoof loading patterns.[60-62] Depending on the degree of conformity between the introduced properties and the real diversity of microscopic structure, the effects of interventions such as various shoeing can be estimated. For example, several variations of nail or clip placement were tested and their influences on strain and displacement of different hoof wall segments were assessed.[61]

To answer practical relevant questions, future clinically applied locomotor research will have to combine kinematic and kinetic analysis techniques with complementary methods such as saddle pressure measurements (Fig. 73-5) (see Chapter 77). Further efforts should focus on localizing the precise site of lameness and on evaluation of interventions, not only in terms of changes in locomotion pattern but also on the mechanical effects on internal structures such as tendons and joints, using inverse dynamic analysis. Additionally, basic statements used generally among riders, such as "collecting the horse" can be objectively evaluated and statements can be made in regard to their abilities as riders.

Predictive models of mechanical function will aid surgical decision making and drive rehabilitation of gait by providing normative indications and feedback on efficacy of treatment.

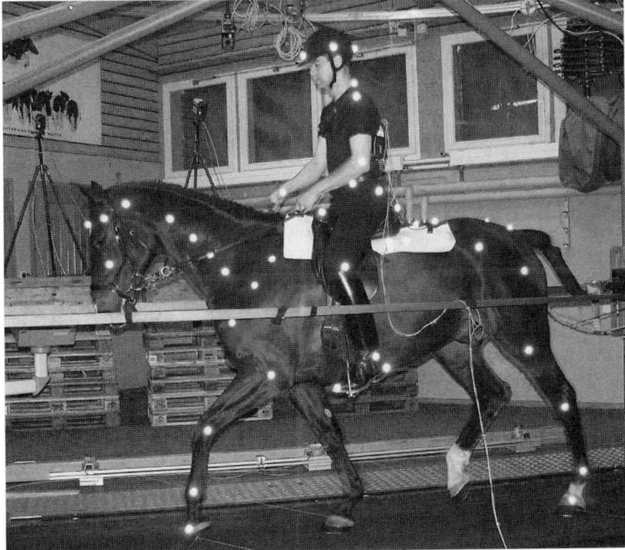

Figure 73-5. Combined kinematic, kinetic, and saddle pressure analysis in a study assessing the rider's influence on the biomechanics of the horse. (Courtesy SDS Equine Motion Research Cooperation, Uppsala-Utrecht-Zurich.)

REFERENCES

1. Keegan KG, Wilson DA, Wilson DJ, et al: Evaluation of mild lameness in horses trotting on a treadmill by clinicians and interns or residents and correlation of their assessments with kinematic gait analysis, Am J Vet Res 1998;59:1370.
2. Clayton HM, Schamhardt HC: Measurement techniques for gait analysis. In Back W, Clayton HM, editors: Equine Locomotion, London, 2001, WB Saunders.
3. Kubo K, Sakai T, Sakuraoka H, et al: Segmental body weight, volume and mass center in Thoroughbred horses, Jpn J Equine Sci 1992;3:149.
4. Buchner HHF, Savelberg HH, Schamhardt HC, et al: Inertial properties of Dutch Warmblood horses, J Biomech 1997;30:653.
5. Buchner HHF, Obermüller S, Scheidl M: Body centre of mass movement in the sound horse, Vet J 2000;160:225.
6. Koch A: Zeit und Belastungsmessungen an den Vorderhufen des Pferdes mittels der Mehrkomponenten-Kraftmessplatte "Kistler," Veterinary Medicine Thesis, University of Zurich, 1973.
7. Pratt GW, O'Connor JT: Force plate studies of equine biomechanics, Am J Vet Res 1976;37:1251.
8. Steiss JE, Yuill GT, White NA, et al: Modifications of a force plate system for equine gait analysis, Am J Vet Res 1982;43:538.
9. Hugelshofer J: Vergleichende Kraft- und Belastungszeit-Messungen an den Vorderhufen von gesunden und an Podotrochlose erkrankten Pferden, Veterinary Medicine Thesis, University of Zurich, 1982.
10. Barrey E: Investigation of the vertical hoof force distribution in the equine forelimb with an instrumented horseboot, Equine Vet J Suppl 1990;9:35.
11. Dohne W, Werner KH, Hertsch B, et al: Vorstellung eines neuartigen Messsystems zur dynamographischen Untersuchung der Bewegung des Pferdes, Pferdeheilkunde 1990;6:265.
12. Ratzlaff MH, Hyde ML, Grant BD, et al: Measurement of vertical forces and temporal components of the strides of horses using instrumented shoes, J Equine Vet Sci 1990;10:23.
13. Roepstorff L, Drevemo S: Concept of a force-measuring horseshoe, Acta Anat (Basel) 1993;146:114.
14. Kai M, Aoki O, Hiraga A, et al: Use of an instrument sandwiched between the hoof and shoe to measure vertical ground reaction forces and three-dimensional acceleration at the walk, trot, and canter in horses, Am J Vet Res 2000;61:979.
15. Auer JA, Butler KD: An introduction to the Kaegi equine gait analysis system in the horse, Proc Am Assoc Equine Pract 1985;31:209.
16. Huskamp B, Tietje S, Nowak M, et al: Fussungs- und Bewegungsmuster gesunder und strahlbeinkranker Pferde: Gemessen mit dem Equine-Gait-Analysis-System (EGA-System), Pferdeheilkunde 1990;6:231.
17. Tietje S: Das EGA-System (Equine Gait Analysis): Eine Möglichkeit zur Bewegungsanalyse und Lahmheitsuntersuchung beim Pferd, Veterinary Medicine Thesis, University of Munich, 1992.
18. Weishaupt MA, Hogg HP, Wiestner T, et al: Instrumented treadmill for measuring vertical ground reaction forces in horses, Am J Vet Res 2002;63:520.
19. McLaughlin RM, Gaughan EM, Roush JK, et al: Effects of subject velocity on ground reaction force measurements and stance times in clinically normal horses at the walk and trot, Am J Vet Res 1996;57:7.
20. Khumsap S, Clayton HM, Lanovaz JL: Effect of walking velocity on ground reaction force variables in the hind limb of clinically normal horses, Am J Vet Res 2001;62:901.
21. Khumsap S, Clayton HM, Lanovaz JL: Effect of walking velocity on hindlimb kinetics during stance in normal horses, Equine Vet J Suppl 2001;33:21.
22. Khumsap S, Clayton HM, Lanovaz JL, et al: Effect of walking velocity on forelimb kinematics and kinetics, Equine Vet J Suppl 2002;34:325.

23. Meershoek LS, van den Bogert A: Mechanical analysis of locomotion. In Back W, Clayton HM, editors: Equine Locomotion, London, 2001, WB Saunders.
24. Bartel DL, Schryver HF, Lowe JE, et al: Locomotion in the horse: A procedure for computing the internal forces in the digit, Am J Vet Res 1978;39:1721.
25. Clayton HM, Lanovaz JL, Schamhardt HC, et al: Net joint moments and powers in the equine forelimb during the stance phase of the trot, Equine Vet J 30:384, 1998.
26. Colborne GR, Lanovaz JL, Sprigings EJ, et al: Forelimb joint moments and power during the walking stance phase of horses, Am J Vet Res 1998;59:609.
27. Meershoek LS, Schamhardt HC, Roepstorff L, et al: Forelimb tendon loading during jump landings and the influence of fence height, Equine Vet J Suppl 2001;33:6.
28. Lanovaz JL, Clayton HM, Colborne GR, et al: Forelimb kinematics and net joint moments during the swing phase of the trot, Equine Vet J Suppl 1999;30:235,:
29. Peloso JG, Stick JA, Soutas-Little RW, et al: Computer-assisted three-dimensional gait analysis of amphotericin-induced carpal lameness in horses, Am J Vet Res 1993;54:1535.
30. Weishaupt MA, Schatzmann U, Straub R: Quantifizierung der Stützbeinlahmheit mit Hilfe akzelerometrischer Messungen am Kopf des Pferdes, Pferdeheilkunde 1993;9:375.
31. Buchner HHF, Savelberg HH, Schamhardt HC, et al: Head and trunk movement adaptations in horses with experimentally induced fore- or hindlimb lameness, Equine Vet J 1996;28:71.
32. Keegan KG, Wilson DJ, Wilson DA, et al: Effects of anesthesia of the palmar digital nerves on kinematic gait analysis in horses with and without navicular disease, Am J Vet Res 1997;58:218.
33. Buchner F, Kastner J, Girtler D, et al: Quantification of hind limb lameness in the horse, Acta Anat (Basel) 1993;146:196.
34. May SA, Wyn-Jones G: Identification of hindleg lameness, Equine Vet J 1987;19:185.
35. Riemersma DJ, Schamhardt HC, Hartman W, et al: Kinetics and kinematics of the equine hind limb: In vivo tendon loads and force plate measurements in ponies, Am J Vet Res 1988;49:1344.
36. Ratzlaff MH, Wilson PD, Hyde ML, et al: Relationship between locomotor forces, hoof position and joint motion during the support phase of the stride of galloping horses, Acta Anat (Basel) 1993;146:200.
37. Clayton HM, Schamhardt HC, Willemen MA, et al: Kinematics and ground reaction forces in horses with superficial digital flexor tendinitis, Am J Vet Res 2000;61:191.
38. McGuigan MP, Wilson AM: The effect of gait and digital flexor muscle activation on limb compliance in the forelimb of the horse *Equus caballus*, J Exp Biol 2003;206:1325.
39. Buchner HHF, Savelberg HH, Schamhardt HC, et al: Limb movement adaptations in horses with experimentally induced fore- or hindlimb lameness, Equine Vet J 1996;28:63.
40. Morris EA, Seeherman HJ: Redistribution of ground reaction forces in experimentally induced equine carpal lameness. In Gillespie JR, Robinson NE, editors: Equine Exercise Physiology, Davis, Calif, 1987, ICEEP Publications.
41. Hjerten G, Drevemo S, Eriksson L-E: Shortening of the hind limb in the horse during the stance phase, Equine Vet J Suppl 1994;17:48.
42. Back W, Schamhardt HC, Savelberg HH, et al: How the horse moves: 2. Significance of the graphical representations of equine hind limb kinematics, Equine Vet J 1995;27:39.
43. Clayton HM: Cinematographic analysis of the gait of lame horses IV: Degenerative joint disease of the distal intertarsal joint, J Equine Vet Sci 1987;7:274.
44. Stashak TS: Examination for lameness. In Stashak TS, editor: Adams' Lameness in Horses, Philadelphia, 2002, Lippincott Williams & Wilkins.
45. Uhlir C, Licka T, Kubber P, et al: Compensatory movements of horses with a stance phase lameness, Equine Vet J Suppl 1997;23:102.
46. Audigie F, Pourcelot P, Degueurce C, et al: Kinematic analysis of the symmetry of limb movements in lame trotting horses, Equine Vet J Suppl 2001;33:128.
47. Merkens HW: Quantitative evaluation of equine locomotion using force plate data, PhD Thesis, Utrecht University, 1987.
48. Weishaupt MA, Wiestner T, Hogg HP, et al: Compensatory load redistribution of horses with induced weightbearing hindlimb lameness trotting on a treadmill, Equine Vet J 2004;36:727.
49. Weishaupt MA, Wiestner T, Hogg HP, et al: Compensatory load redistribution of horses with induced weight-bearing forelimb lameness trotting on a treadmill, Vet J (in press).
50. Buchner HHF, Obermüller S, Scheidl M: Body centre of mass movement in the lame horse, Equine Vet J Suppl 2001;33:122.
51. Vorstenbosch MA, Buchner HHF, Savelberg HH, et al: Modeling study of compensatory head movements in lame horses, Am J Vet Res 1997;58:713.
52. Clayton H, Willemen MA, Lanovaz JL, et al: Effects of a heel wedge in horses with superficial digital flexor tendonitis, Vet Comp Orthop Traumatol 2000;13:1.
53. Buchner HHF, Savelberg HH, Becker CK: Load redistribution after desmotomy of the accessory ligament of the deep digital flexor tendon in adult horses, Vet Q 1996;18(Suppl)2:70.
54. Wilson AM, McGuigan MP, Fouracre L, et al: The force and contact stress on the navicular bone during trot locomotion in sound horses and horses with navicular disease, Equine Vet J 2001;33:159.
55. Willemen MA, Savelberg HH, Barneveld A: The effect of orthopaedic shoeing on the force exerted by the deep digital flexor tendon on the navicular bone in horses, Equine Vet J 1999;31:25.
56. Eliashar E, McGuigan MP, Rogers KA, et al: A comparison of three horseshoeing styles on the kinetics of breakover in sound horses, Equine Vet J 2002;34:184.
57. Eliashar E, McGuigan MP, Wilson AM: Relationship of foot conformation and force applied to the navicular bone of sound horses at the trot, Equine Vet J 2004;36:431.
58. van den Bogert AJ: Computer simulation of locomotion in the horse, PhD Thesis, Utrecht University, 1989.
59. Peham C, Schobesberger H: Influence of the load of a rider or of a region with increased stiffness on the equine back: A modelling study, Equine Vet J 2004;36:703.
60. Les CM, Keyak JH, Stover SM, et al: Development and validation of a series of three-dimensional finite element models of the equine metacarpus, J Biomech 1997;30:737.
61. Hinterhofer C, Stanek C, Haider H: Finite element analysis (FEA) as a model to predict effects of farriery on the equine hoof, Equine Vet J Suppl 2001;33:58.
62. Thomason JJ, McClinchey HL, Jofriet JC: Analysis of strain and stress in the equine hoof capsule using finite element methods: Comparison with principal strains recorded in vivo, Equine Vet J 2002;34:719.

CHAPTER 74

Diagnostic Anesthesia

Anton E. Fürst

In a lameness examination, diagnostic analgesia is carried out to assist in the determination of the anatomic site of lameness. It is generally used in horses that are obviously lame or that show a positive response to a flexion or other provocation tests. A detailed discussion of diagnostic analgesia can be found in the textbooks dealing mainly with lameness.[1,2] Perineural anesthesia is preferred over intra-articular anesthesia because it generates less morbidity.

TECHNICAL ASPECTS

General Considerations

Injectable solutions, needles, and syringes must be sterile. It is advantageous to use new needles for each injection, and the gauge of needle should be as small as practicable. Diagnostic anesthesia of the distal limb up to the tarsus or carpus is carried out with the affected limb held in a nonweightbearing position by the clinician, if possible, whereas the limb is usually bearing weight for proximal analgesia. For temperamental horses, the limb may be held up for analgesia of the proximal regions as well.

Mechanism of Action

Injury is transmitted to the central nervous system by peripheral nerves. There are specific roles for thinly myelinated A-delta and nonmyelinated C-fibers in signaling pain sensation. Local anesthetics block nerve conduction by preventing the increase in membrane permeability to sodium ions. Local anesthetics exert their effect by inhibiting the rapid inward flow of sodium ions, thereby inhibiting depolarization of the membrane. This can be done by the dissociation of local anesthetic, which alters the electrical forces across the membrane. The order and degree of neural blockade correlate with the diameter and type of nerve fiber and the degree of myelinization. The first nerve fibers blocked are the B-fibers; the A-delta and C-fibers are next, and the last nerves blocked are A-gamma, A-beta, and A-alpha.[3] For more details on pain management see Chapter 23.

Choice of Local Anesthetic Agent

Mepivacaine is the local anesthetic agent of choice for perineural and intrasynovial analgesia.[3] Its duration of action is 2 to 3 hours, and it causes less tissue irritation than other local anesthetics. Once a bottle of local anesthetic is opened, the efficacy of the drug diminishes rapidly, so it should be used within a few days. Generally, 2% solutions (20 mg/mL) of local anesthetic are used. Sensory nerves are the first to be desensitized, followed by sympathetic and eventually motor nerves.[3] As a rule, because of the irritant properties of anesthetic agents, as little should be injected as is necessary to obtain anesthesia. In severely inflamed or abnormal tissues, a higher concentration or amount of local anesthetic is frequently needed to achieve the desired effect. Local anesthetics penetrate membranes less effectively in an acidotic area, such as an infected wound.[3] Diffusion of the anesthetic to its intended site of action is diminished in edematous or scarred tissues, and the anesthetic effect is therefore less reliable.

Adrenalin at a low concentration is often added to a local anesthetic when it is used for perineural anesthesia to induce some vasoconstriction.[4] Although it provides a longer duration of analgesia, adrenalin also imparts a more selective analgesia. Thus, adjacent structures including other nerves and ligaments are affected to a lesser degree.[3] However, the disadvantage of adrenalin is that severe swelling may occur 1 day later. Adrenalin may be responsible for the occurrence of skin necrosis and white hair, which are sometimes observed after diagnostic analgesia.

Perineural Anesthesia

Long or dirty hair should be trimmed with a no. 40 clipper blade, and all injection sites should be thoroughly cleaned with antiseptic soap and gauze sponges. A combination of 70% alcohol and chlorhexidine is often used for this purpose. Aseptic preparation of the skin is required before injection of synovial spaces. The clinician's hands must also be clean because they are used to palpate and locate the nerves under the skin immediately prior to injection.

Synovial Anesthesia

Anesthesia of synovial spaces is performed only after thorough cleaning of the relevant area. Hair should be clipped and the skin cleaned first with a surgical scrub, such as chlorhexidine, followed by a disinfectant as described previously. The skin should be cleaned for 5 to 10 minutes. Clipping the hair has two advantages: it aids in cleaning the skin and in identifying the injection site. However, in two studies, infection rates after perineural anesthesia were not decreased by clipping or shaving the hair.[5,6]

Anesthesia of synovial spaces requires sterile gloves, needles, and syringes. Generally, the synovial space is injected using an 18-gauge (1.2-mm-diameter) or 20-gauge (0.9-mm-diameter) needle. Large-gauge needles are better for the collection of synovial fluid, but horses tolerate their placement less well than smaller-gauge needles. The needle is inserted alone without the syringe attached. Depending on the temperament of the horse, a twitch may be used for restraint. This is particularly useful when needles are inserted through large muscles masses—for example, over the shoulder, elbow, and hip joints. A twitch also should be used when injecting complex joints such as the stifle. The operator should always use a competent assistant to restrain the horse, so that sudden movements, which may result in damage to the joint cartilage or needle breakage, are prevented. When the needle is to be inserted over a large distance (shoulder or hip joint), the skin over the injection site should be anesthetized using a small amount of anesthetic and a small-gauge needle. For certain procedures, a spinal needle is used because it is flexible and less likely to break. After injection of the synovial space, the horse is walked to promote distribution of the anesthetic agent.

Needle Positioning for Intrasynovial Anesthesia

For most synovial spaces, the needle is correctly positioned when synovial fluid flows spontaneously out of the back of the needle. Sometimes, the needle must be turned several times until synovial fluid flows out. When this fails, aspiration of synovial fluid may be attempted, although this rarely works because the synovial villi become lodged in the tip of the needle, thereby blocking flow. Injection of air often produces a characteristic bubbling of synovial fluid in the joint, and a larger amount of injected air sometimes results in backflow of foamy synovial fluid. Another indication of correct needle placement is minimal resistance to the injection of local anesthetic. In special cases, the joint can be radiographed after intrasynovial injection of contrast medium (see Chapter 75).

Animal Restraint

Whenever possible, horses should not be sedated for diagnostic anesthesia because the risk of injury while working on the hindlimbs is high. A twitch applied to the nose is an excellent restraining method and makes diagnostic anesthesia easier and safer. However, sedation may be necessary in intractable horses. Detomidine (1 mg/kg intravenously) is ideal and can be reversed.[7] Alternatively, acepromazine (5 mg per horse intravenously) may be used. The use of α_2-agonists for sedation is not recommended because the horse may react violently when the needle is inserted. Additionally, these drugs have two other effects that may be confusing during a lameness evaluation: they induce some analgesia and they produce ataxia.

EVALUATION OF ANESTHESIA

Testing

The clinician must determine whether the diagnostic anesthesia has achieved the desired effect and the nerve in question has been desensitized before re-evaluation of lameness. A pointed instrument, such as a ballpoint pen, can be used to assess the sensitivity of the skin and deeper structures including tendons and ligaments. A convenient device consists of a stick approximately 1 m long, with a blunt nail positioned at one end. The nail can be conveniently placed on the region of temporarily neutralized sensory innervation of the horse to test the efficacy of analgesia without bending down. Lameness can be evaluated only when the nerve has been correctly desensitized.

Onset and Duration of Effect

Depending on the site, lameness should be re-evaluated 5 to 50 minutes after the injection of local anesthetic. Not waiting long enough leads to false-negative results. Local anesthetic effects begin within a few minutes after injection, but it takes variable periods of time for the horse to become sound. The first re-evaluation of lameness should always be done 5 to 10 minutes after injection. Before performing the next nerve block in the distal limb, the clinician should wait a minimum of 20 minutes, and for the proximal limb, a minimum of 45 minutes. Generally, the horse is re-evaluated 5 to 60 minutes after analgesia of a synovial space, although this time depends greatly on the joint—for example, as little as 5 minutes for desensitization of small synovial spaces such as the distal interphalangeal joint, and up to 60 minutes for the desensitization of large synovial spaces such as the stifle joint. The goal of intrasynovial analgesia is desensitization of the nerve fibers of synovial structures. Studies show that additional structures outside the synovial space are also desensitized.[8] This occurs because of the close proximity of large nerves to the synovial space and the rapid diffusion of the anesthetic agent into the surrounding tissue. Therefore, the selectivity of joint analgesia comes into question; in a cadaveric study, it was shown that 15 minutes after injection of mepivacaine with an added radiodense dye into one synovial space, mepivacaine was present in adjacent synovial spaces.[9]

Interpretation

Lameness is re-evaluated after each injection of anesthetic. The horse should be walked and trotted "in hand" on a hard flat surface. Tests (flexion, moving the horse in a tight circle, hyperflexion, extension) that were positive in the initial examination should be repeated. If required, the horse can also be lunged on soft ground (see later). The response to diagnostic anesthesia can be negative, positive with residual lameness, positive, or positive with lameness in the contralateral limb. A positive response with residual lameness may be difficult to interpret. The most difficult interpretation is that of a lameness that gradually improves after each injection. The results of diagnostic anesthesia may be incorrectly assessed, yielding false-positive or false-negative results.[10] Negative results, in particular, must be carefully interpreted; failure to desensitize a nerve may be caused by an individual variation in the course of a nerve in some horses, or by loss of efficacy of the local anesthetic agent. Furthermore, excessive diffusion of the anesthetic agent may lead to erroneous results. Certain types of lameness may become less pronounced during the evaluation, as a result of a warming-out effect (some arthritic conditions are less painful as exercise progresses and the horse is said to "warm out" of the lameness), or the lameness may be overshadowed by agitation of the patient. Sometimes, the horse must be re-evaluated the next day.

PRECAUTIONS

Interpretation of the results of perineural anesthesia in horses treated with analgesics can be difficult. Therefore, diagnostic analgesia should not be performed until the effects of the systemic analgesics have worn off.

Horses Suspected of Having Incomplete Fractures

In severely lame horses (e.g., with tendon rupture, bone fracture), the cause can usually be diagnosed without diagnostic anesthesia, and in these cases, the area is merely radiographed or examined ultrasonographically. In selected cases, diagnostic analgesia may be carried out before or after radiography to confirm a diagnosis. However, incomplete fractures can progress into complete fractures with displacement after diagnostic anesthesia. Therefore, the horse with a suspected fracture should be walked or trotted in a straight line, in hand, for only a few strides to determine the effects of the anesthetic.

With mild to moderate lameness, the question always arises as to whether horses should be lunged after diagnostic anesthesia. In the author's experience, several displaced fractures have developed in horses that were lunged after perineural anesthesia. Interestingly, the hindlimbs were more often affected than the forelimbs. The bones most commonly affected are the proximal first phalanx and the distal MCIII/MTIII. Fractures of other bones after lunging are rare. The following general rules should be observed:

- Horses with acute lameness (up to 6 weeks) should not be lunged.
- The horse must be quiet and under the control of the examiner during lunging; otherwise, lunging should be discontinued.
- Trotting the horse in hand in a straight line is always safer than lunging in a circle.

Every diagnostic anesthetic injection proximal to the palmar digital nerve block increases the risk of fracture; therefore, if an incomplete fracture of the proximal phalanx is suspected, blocks should not be continued above this point.

Bandaging and Stall Rest

At the end of the diagnostic analgesia procedure, a bandage moistened with disinfectant solution should be applied to the leg for 12 to 24 hours. This is to prevent swelling associated with the injections in the distal limb. The horse should remain in a box stall for 24 hours. Under no circumstances should a horse be turned out after diagnostic analgesia. Horses should be rested for 3 days after intrasynovial analgesia.

COMPLICATIONS

Swelling often occurs for a few days in limbs that have had multiple perineural anesthetic injections. In these cases, the limb must be kept under bandages for several days.

In fractious horses, the needle may break and remain under the skin. Whenever possible, an attempt should be made to remove the part of the needle buried in the tissues.

Adjacent structures may be damaged; however, the risk of this is low if a correct approach and proper injection technique are applied.

Infection of synovial structures or cellulitis after perineural or intrasynovial anesthesia is very rare, particularly when aseptic technique has been followed. The risk of cartilage damage and joint infection or inflammation is also very low provided that intrasynovial analgesia is performed correctly. Thus, it usually is unnecessary to advise the owner explicitly of these risks (in the author's opinion). Joint hemorrhage, which occurs frequently, does not appear to have any adverse effects.[11]

APPLICATION

Perineural analgesia must be carried out in a systematic and logical manner. The aim is to be specific and exact, while avoiding an excessive number of nerve blocks. Generally, the procedure is begun distally, and it progresses proximally. The more distal the nerve block, the more specific is the diagnostic anesthesia. Perineural anesthesia is usually applied medially and laterally at the specific location at the same time. In addition to perineural anesthesia, which usually desensitizes a single nerve (medially and laterally), ring blocks are frequently used to block the entire region distal to the anesthetized area.

Nomenclature

The names of the various diagnostic nerve blocks vary depending on the literature consulted. Because of this confusion, a simple classification system was chosen for the tables and figures in this chapter. "F" corresponds to forelimb and "H" to hindlimb. Numbers indicate perineural injection of a nerve or nerve pair. When a ring block is used, it is referred to by the number of the nerve anesthetized.

Perineural Anesthesia in the Forelimb

In the forelimb, a palmar digital block is carried out, followed by a low palmar block and a high palmar block.[8,12-16] These are followed by an ulnar nerve block and by desensitization of the medial and cutaneous nerves of the antebrachium. Each positive perineural anesthesia can be followed by a more specific anesthesia, such as intrasynovial anesthesia or anesthesia of a specific nerve after the effect of the previous anesthetic has worn off. In some instances, it may be helpful to block only the medial or lateral palmar digital nerve. The detailed information for these nerve blocks is summarized in Table 74-1 and illustrated in Figures 74-1 to 74-3.

Perineural Anesthesia in the Hindlimb

Perineural anesthesia in the distal hindlimb is similar to that described for the forelimb.[17] However, there are important differences in innervation, such as the dorsal metatarsal nerves, which must be taken into consideration. Safety of the examiner and horse handler is crucial, so in most cases diagnostic anesthesia is started further proximally, provided that a lower limb problem is not suspected. In some instances, where a problem is expected distal to the metatarsophalangeal joint, a nerve block is first performed in the pastern region, and this is followed by a nerve block proximal to the metatarsophalangeal joint. These blocks are followed by a high plantar nerve block, and by fibular and tibial nerve blocks. The detailed information for these nerve blocks is summarized in Table 74-2 and illustrated in Figures 74-4 and 74-5.

Text continued on p. 909.

TABLE 74-1. Perineural Analgesic Blocks of the Forelimb

Number	Nomenclature	Desensitized nerves resp. Region	Injection site	Gauge (G) of needle and amount of 2% local anesthetic agent	Testing the analgesia	Desensitized nerves or region	Differential diagnosis, remarks
F1 (Fig.74-1)	Distal palmar digital nerve block, palmar digital block	Lateral and medial palmar digital nerves	The needle is inserted subcutanously directly over the nerve, just proximal to the cartilages of the foot	24 G, 2 ml per site	Deep pain is assesed with hoof testers; loss of skin sensation proximal to the heels	80% of the hoof and a large part of the digit	Navicular disease, disorders of the distal interphalangeal and proximal interphalangeal joint, fissure fractures and fractures of distal, middle, or proximal phalanx, pedal osteitis, abscess in the hoof capsule, pododermatitis, laminitis, hoof cracks, tendinitis and insertional desmitis of the deep digital flexor tendon, cysts in the distal, middle, or proximal phalanx
F2 (Fig.74-1)	Proximal palmar digital nerve block, basis sesamoid block, mid pastern ring block, pastern nerve block	Lateral and medial palmar digital nerves and dorsal branches	The needle is inserted in the mid pastern region directly over the nerve and subsequently advanced further dorsally; the nerve is easily palpated	24 G, 3-5 ml per site	Hoof testers are used to assess entire hoof; loss of skin sensation proximal to the bulbs of the heel	100% of the hoof and also the dorsal pastern region	The same as F1 (see above) and distal sesamoidean desmitis
F3 (Fig.74-1)	Abaxial sesamoid block, mid sesamoid block	Lateral and medial palmar digital nerves and dorsal branches	The needle is inserted subcutanously directly over the nerve on the abaxial side of the proximal sesamoid bones	24 G, 3 ml per site	Loss of skin sensation over the pastern region	The same as F2 and parts of the metacarpophalangeal joint: foot, digit, metacarpophalangeal joint, proximal sesamoid bones	Often performed in combination with other nerve blocks; other than that, rarely performed because interpretation is difficult

F4 (Fig.74- 1)	Low metacarpal nerve block	Medial and lateral palmar metacarpal nerves	With the limb held up, the needle is inserted between MCIII and the distal free end of MCII and MCIV, respectively, and advanced subcutaneously, axially, and subfascially, or the needle is inserted just at the distal aspect of the MCII/MCIV, and directed axially, where the metacarpal nerves course more superficially.	22 G, 5 ml per site	Loss of skin sensation in the metacarpopha-langeal area	The entire phalangeal region including parts of the metacarpophalangeal joint and the proximal sesamoid bones	This nerve block is predominantly performed in conjunction with other more distal nerve blocks
F3, F4 (Fig. 74-1)	Low four point, abaxial sesamoid block and low palmar metacarpal nerve block, low palmar anaglesia or block, low palmar ring block, distal metacarpal nerve block	F3 and F4	F3 and F4	22 G, 5 ml per site	Forceful flexion of the interphalangeal joints; loss of skin sensation distal to the injection site	The same as with F3 and F4	The same as with F3 and F4

Continued

TABLE 74-1. Perineural Analgesic Blocks of the Forelimb—cont'd

Number	Nomenclature	Desensitized nerves resp. Region	Injection site	Gauge (G) of needle and amount of 2% local anesthetic agent	Testing the analgesia	Desensitized nerves or region	Differential diagnosis, remarks
F5 (Fig. 74-1)	High palmar nerve block	Lateral and medial palmar nerves	Local anesthetic is first deposited subfascially on the lateral aspect, immediately proximal to the flexor tendon sheath bewteen the deep digital flexor and the suspensory ligament. The needle is then advanced and the injection is repeated on the medial aspect of the limb.	20 G, 5 ml per site	Loss of skin and tendon sensation distal to the injection site	As for F3 plus parts of the flexor tendon sheath, parts of the superficial and deep flexor tendons, and the suspensory ligament	
F4, F5 (Fig. 74-1)	High palmar metacarpal nerve block, mid four point, mid palmar ring block, middle metacarpal nerve block	F4 and F5	F4 and F5	20 G, 5 ml per site	Loss of skin sensation distal to the injections	The same as with F4 and F5	The same as with F4 and F5
F6 (Figs.74-1 and 74-2)	High palmar nerve block	Lateral and medial palmar nerves	The needle is inserted between the suspensory ligament and the deep digital flexor tendon 2 cm distal to the carpometacarpal joint	20 G, 5 ml per site	Pressure applied to the flexor tendons	Parts of the flexor tendons	

F7 (Fig.74-2)	Lateral and medial palmar metacarpal nerve analgesia or infiltration of the origin of the suspensory ligament	Lateral and medial palmar metacarpal nerves	The needle is inserted axial to the splint bones just abaxial to the suspensory ligament, 2 cm distal to the carpometacarpal joint and advanced to the palmar cortex of the MCIII	20 G, 3-5 ml per site; aseptic procedure is required because synovial structures like the carpometacarpal joint and the carpal calanal may be penetrated	Pressure applied to the origin of the suspensory ligament	Suspensory ligament, parts of the carpal joints, carpal canal, intermetacarpal ligament	
F6, F7 (Fig. 74-2)	High four point, high palmar ring block, subcarpal block, proximal metacarpal nerve block	F6 and F7	F6 and F7	20 G, 5-10 ml per site; aseptic procedure is required because synovial structures are penetrated	Loss of sensation in the area distal to the injection site	The entire limb distal to the injection site and parts of the carpal joints and the carpal flexor tendon sheath	Disorders of the distal sesamoidean and suspensory ligaments, metacarapal ligament, MCIII, carpal joint, carpal flexor tendon sheath, metacarpal fascia
F8 (Fig. 74-2)	Lateral palmar nerve block	Parts of the median and ulnar nerves	With the carpus flexed 90 degrees, the needle is inserted just distal to the accessory carpal bone at the distal border of the ligament between MCIV and the accessory carpal bone	22 G, 3 ml	Pressure applied to the distal sesamoidean and suspensory ligaments should elicit no response	Suspensory ligament, carpal canal	Insertion desmopathy of the suspensory ligament

Continued

TABLE 74-1. Perineural Analgesic Blocks of the Forelimb—cont'd

Number	Nomenclature	Desensitized nerves resp. Region	Injection site	Gauge (G) of needle and amount of 2% local anesthetic agent	Testing the analgesia	Desensitized nerves or region	Differential diagnosis, remarks
F9 (Figs. 74-2 and 74-3)	Ulnar nerve block, ulnar block	Ulnar nerve	With the limb held up or weight bearing, the needle is inserted between the flexor carpi ulnaris and the ulnaris lateralis muscles, 5-10 cm proximal to the accessory carpal bone on the caudal aspect of the antebrachium and advanced to a depth of approximately 2 cm	20 G, 10 ml	Loss of skin sensation along the lateral aspect of the carpus to the metacarpophalangeal joint	Parts of the suspensory ligament, carpal canal, carpal joints, deep and superficial flexor tendons	
F10 (Fig. 74-3)	Median nerve block	Median nerve	Caudal to the radius, just distal to the superficial pectoral muscle, approximately 4 cm deep	20 G, 10-20 ml	Loss of skin sensation distal to the injection site	Parts of the suspensory ligament, carpal canal, carpal joints, deep and superficial flexor tendons, distal radius	
F11 (Fig. 74-3)	Cutaneous nerve block; cutaneous antebrachial block	Medial cutaneous antebrachial nerve	On the cranial and caudal aspects of the accessory cephalic and cephalic veins, between the carpus and elbow	20 G, 10 ml		Only skin innervation	
F9, F10, F11 (Fig. 74-3)	Triple block	Ulnar nerve, median nerve, and medial cutaneous antebrachial nerve	F9, F10, F11; see above	F9, F10, F11; see above	F9, F10, F11; see above	Loss of sensation to all parts of limb distal to the mid radius	

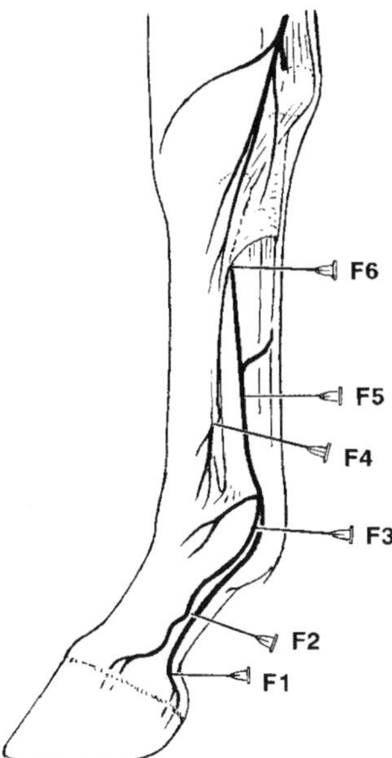

Figure 74-1. The lateral aspect of the left distal forelimb, with location of needle placement for perineural anesthesia. For an explanation of each needle position, see Table 74-1. F1, distal palmar digital nerve block; F2, proximal palmar digital nerve block; F3, abaxial sesamoid block; F4, low metacarpal nerve block; F5 and F6, high palmar nerve block.

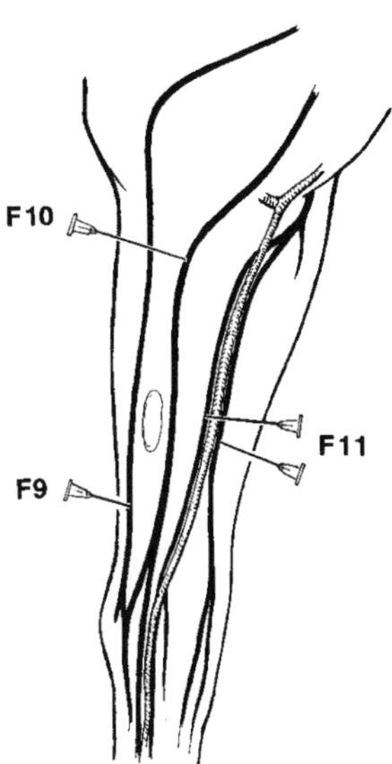

Figure 74-3. The medial aspect of the left antebrachium, with location of needle placement for perineural anesthesia. For an explanation of each needle position, see Table 74-1. F9, ulnar nerve block; F10, median nerve block; F11, cutaneus nerve block.

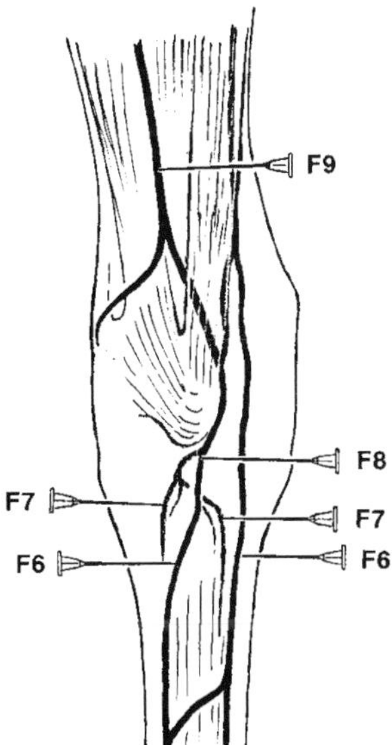

Figure 74-2. The left palmar aspect of the carpus, with location of needle placement for perineural anesthesia. For an explanation of each needle position, see Table 74-1. F6, high palmar nerve block; F7, high metacarpal nerve block; F8, lateral palmar nerve block; F9, ulnar nerve block.

Local Infiltrations

The detailed information for the different local infiltration sites is summarized in Table 74-3.

INTRASYNOVIAL ANESTHESIA

Intrasynovial Anesthesia in the Forelimb

The detailed information for the different intrasynovial injection sites in the forelimb is summarized in Table 74-4 and illustrated in Figures 74-6 to 74-9.

Intrasynovial Anesthesia in the Hindlimb

The detailed information for the different intrasynovial injection sites in the hindlimb is summarized in Table 74-5 and illustrated in Figures 74-10 to 74-14.

TABLE 74-2. Perineural Analgesic Blocks of the Hindlimb

Number	Nomenclature	Desensitized nerves resp. Region	Injection site	Gauge (G) of needle and amount of 2% local anesthetic agent	Testing the analgesia	Desensitized nerves or region	Differential diagnosis, remarks
H1 (Fig. 74-4)	Low plantar nerve block, plantar digital block	Digital plantar nerve	The same as F1	24 G, 6 ml	The same as F1	The same as F1	
H2 (Fig. 74-4)	Mid pastern ring block, pastern nerve block	Digital plantar nerve and its dorsal branch; deep branch of the fibular nerve	As for F1 plus lateral and medial to the long digital extensor tendon	22 G, 16 ml	The same as F2	The same as F2	
H3 (Fig. 74-4)	Abaxial sesamoid block, basis sesamoid block	Digital plantar nerve and its dorsal branch; deep branch of the fibular nerve	As for F1 plus lateral and medial to the long digital extensor tendon	22 G, 12 ml	Loss of skin sensation below the injection site	The same as F3	
H4 (Fig. 74-4)	Low metatarsal nerve block	Medial and lateral plantar metatarsal nerves	The same as F4	22 G, 6 ml	See F4	See F4	
H5 (Fig. 74-4)		Superficial and deep fibular nerves	Lateral and medial to the long digital extensor tendon	22 G, 6 ml	Loss of skin sensation below the injection site	Skin below the injection site	This anaesthesia is never carried out on its own

H3, H4, H5 (Fig. 74-4)	Low plantar ring block, distal metatarsal nerve block	Medial and lateral plantar nerves, medial and lateral plantar metatarsal nerves, dorsal metatarsal nerves	H3, H4, H5; see above	22 G, 15-20 ml	Forceful flexion of the interphalangeal joints	All structures distal to the injection sites: hoof, interphalangeal joints, metatarsophalangeal joint
H6 (Fig. 74-4)	High plantar nerve block	Medial and lateral plantar metatarsal nerves	The same as F5	22 G, 12 ml	The same as F5	The same as F5
H4, H5, H6 (Fig. 74-4)	Middle plantar ring block, middle metatarsal nerve block	H4, H5, H6	H4, H5, H6; see above	22 G, 15-20 ml	Forceful flexion of the interphalangeal joints	All structures distal to the injection sites: hoof, interphalangeal joints, metatarsophalangeal joint, and parts of the tendons
H7 (Fig. 74-4)		Medial and lateral plantar nerves	The needle is inserted 3 cm into the subcutaneous tissue, distal to the tarsometatarsal joint axial to MTII and MTIV, respectively	20 G, 2 × 5 ml		
H8 (Fig. 74-4)		Medial and lateral plantar metatarsal nerves	The needle is inserted 3 cm distal to the tarsometatarsal joint axial to MTII and MTIV until contact is made with MTIII	20 G, 2 × 5 ml		

Continued

TABLE 74-2. Perineural Analgesic Blocks of the Hindlimb—cont'd

Number	Nomenclature	Desensitized nerves resp. Region	Injection site	Gauge (G) of needle and amount of 2% local anesthetic agent	Testing the analgesia	Desensitized nerves or region	Differential diagnosis, remarks
H5, H7, H8 (Fig. 74-4)	High plantar ring block, proximal metatarsal nerve block	The same as H7 and H8	The needle is inserted 3 cm distal to the tarsometatarsal joint axial to MTII and MTIV until contact is made with MTIII; the needle is withdrawn and a second depot is injected subfascially; the needle is subsequently advanced subcutaneously farther dorsally to the long digital extensor tendon	20 G, 6 x 5 ml	Forceful flexion of the interphalangeal joints; deep palpation of the tendons	All structures distal to the injection sites, hoof, interphalangeal joints, metatarsophalangeal joint, most of the tendons, part of the tarsometatarsal joint, part of the tarsal sheath	
H9 (Fig. 74-5)	Analgesia of the tibial nerve, tibial nerve block	Tibial nerve; the nerve lies in a groove between the calcaneal tendon and the deep digital flexor tendon	The needle is inserted 8 cm proximal to the calcaneus, from medial (or lateral); the anesthetic should be injected into a larger region subfascially. Caution is advised because horses can react violently to the injection. It is preferable to pick up the ipsilateral forelimb. The nerve can be palpated as a firm cord-like structure with the tarsus flexed.	20 G, 20 ml	Loss of skin sensation on the plantar surface of the tarsus	Plantar structures of the tarsus	

H10 (Fig. 74-5)	Analgesia of the fibular nerve, fibular nerve block	Superficial and deep fibular nerves; fibular nerve	The needle is inserted approximately 10 cm proximal to the tarsal joint, between the long digital extensor muscle and the lateral digital extensor muscle. First, 10 ml is injected subcutanously, and then the needle is inserted slightly caudal to the tibia. Analgesia of the deep fibular nerve is not always satisfactory; the superficial nerve can be easily palpated.	20 G, 2 × 10 ml	Loss of skin sensation on the dorsal tarsus and dorsolaterally on the tarsus and metatarsus		
H11 (Fig. 74-5)	Analgesia of the saphenous nerve	Saphenous nerve	Cranial and caudal to the saphenous vein, approximately 15 cm proximal to the tarsus	20 G, 2 × 10 ml	Loss of skin sensation dorsomedially on the tarsus and metatarsus		
H9, H10, H11 (Fig. 74-5)	Triple block	H9, H10, H11; see above	H 9, H10, H11; see above	H9, H10, H11; see above		Entire distal hindlimb, tarsus, and distal tibial region	Useful analgesia to differentiate disorders located distal and proximal to the tarsus

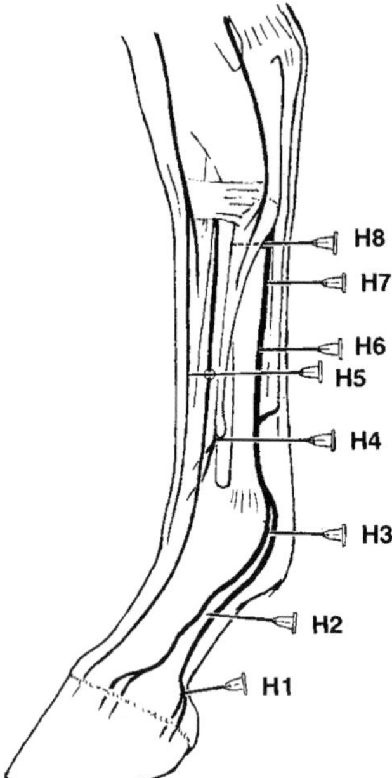

Figure 74-4. The lateral aspect of the left distal hindlimb, with location of needle placement for perineural anesthesia. For an explanation of each needle position, see Table 74-2. H1, low plantar digital nerve block; H2, high plantar digital nerve block; H3, abaxial sesamoid block; H4, low metatarsal nerve block; H5, mid third metatarsal fibularis nerve block; H6 and H7, high plantar nerve block; H8, high metatarsal nerve block.

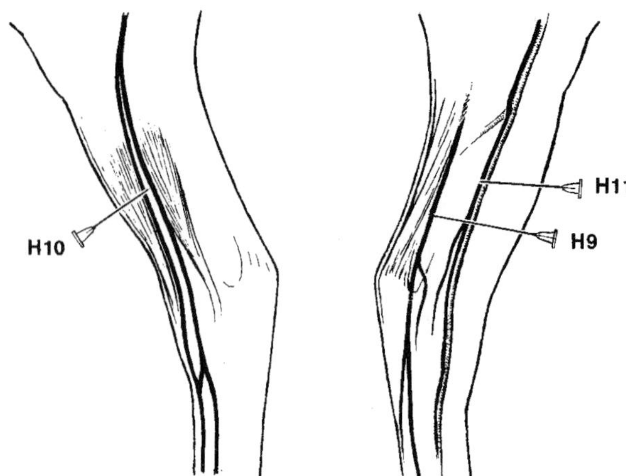

Figure 74-5. The lateral and medial aspects of the left hindlimb, with location of the needle end point for perineural anesthesia. For an explanation of the needle position, see Table 74-2. H9, tibial nerve block; H10, fibularis nerve block; H11, saphenous nerve block.

TABLE 74-3. Local Infiltrations

Nomenclature	Desensitized nerves resp. Region	Injection site	Type of needle and amount of 2% local anesthetic agent	Testing the analgesia	Desensitized nerves or region	Differential diagnosis, remarks
Analgesia of the interspinal ligament	Dorsal spinous process	The needle is inserted along the dorsal midline and directed ventrally into the interspinous space; the interspinous space can be palpated as a depression	20 G, 9 cm, 5-10 ml for interspinal space		Dorsal spinous processes, interspinal ligament	The horse must be lunged or ridden to allow judgment
Analgesia of the splint bones	Splints	The needle is inserted along the proliferative lesion between the skin and bone	20 G, 5-10 ml	Local palpation	Region around the bony proliferation	Splints, tissues distal to the infiltration

TABLE 74-4. Intrasynovial Analgesia in the Forelimb

Name of the joint, bursa, or tendon sheath	Location for injection	Alternative approach	Technique	Type of needle and amount of local anesthetic agent	Onset of effect	Important anatomic structures that are often partly or completely anesthetized
Distal interphalangeal joint	1 cm dorsal to the coronary band, abaxial from, or through, the common digial extensor tendon, horizontally or slightly distally (Fig. 74-6, *A*)	Lateral or palmar approach to the distal interphalangeal joint	The limb is held up and flexed or the limb may be weight bearing	20 G, 5-10 ml	5-10 minutes	Proximal interphalangeal joint, navicular bone, hoof capsule, insertion of the deep digital flexor tendon
Navicular bursa	Palmar midline approach (Figs. 74-6, B, and 74-7)	Proximal palmar injection technique, lateral or medial approach	The hoof is positioned in the Hickman block and thus slightly flexed. The needle is inserted through the palmar midline, just proximal to the coronary band, and directed toward the distal sesamoid bone, which is located 1-2 cm distal to and halfway between the dorsal and palmar aspects of the coronary band	20 G, spinal needle, 9 cm long, 3-5 ml	5-15 minutes	Distal sesamoid bone, parts of the hoof caspule, insertion of the deep digital flexor tendon
Proximal interphalangeal joint	The needle is inserted 1 cm proximal to the joint space in the midline, or slightly paramedian, and directed horizontally or slightly distally into the joint space (Fig. 74-6, C)	Proximal palmar pouch	The limb is held up and flexed, or the limb may be weight bearing	20 G, 5-10 ml	5-15 minutes	

Continued

TABLE 74-4. Intrasynovial Analgesia in the Forelimb—cont'd

Name of the joint, bursa, or tendon sheath	Location for injection	Alternative approach	Technique	Type of needle and amount of local anesthetic agent	Onset of effect	Important anatomic structures that are often partly or completely anesthetized
Metacarpophalangeal joint	Proximopalmar or proximoplantar pouch (Fig. 74-6, D)	Dorsal pouch, distopalmar pouch	With the limb held up and flexed, the needle is inserted immediately proximal to the condyle of MCIII between MCIII and the lateral branch of the suspensory ligamant and directed distally	20 G, 10-15 ml	10-20 minutes	Proximal sesamoid bones, branch of the suspensory ligament
Digital flexor tendon sheath	Outpouching of the sheath proximal to the palmar annular ligament (Fig. 74-6, E)	Between the proximal and distal digital annular ligaments; distal to the proximal sesamoid bones, between the palmar annular ligament and the proximal digital annular ligament	With the limb held up and flexed, the needle is inserted directly into the outpouching	20 G, 10-20 ml	10-20 minutes	Distal and proximal interphalangeal joints, metacarpophalangeal joint, navicular bursa
Middle carpal joint	Lateral or medial to the extensor carpi radialis tendon, Fig. 74-8, F	Palmar pouch of the middle carpal joint	With the limb held up and flexed, the needle is inserted in a palmar direction into the joint	20 G, 10-15 ml	10-20 minutes	Middle carpal joint, origin of suspensory ligament, palmar metacarpal nerves
Antebrachiocarpal joint	Lateral or medial to the extensor carpi radialis tendon (Fig. 74-8, G)	Palmarolateral pouch of the antebrachiocarpal joint	With the limb held up and flexed, the needle is inserted in a palmar direction approximately 2 cm into the joint	20 G, 10-15 ml	10-20 minutes	Antebrachiocarpal joint
Carpal flexor tendon sheath	Proximal aspect of the carpal sheath (Fig. 74-8, H)	Distal aspect of the carpal sheath	The needle is inserted proximal to the accessory carpal bone between the lateral digital extensor and ulnaris lateralis tendons	20 G, 10-20 ml	10-20 minutes	Origin of the suspensory ligament

Elbow joint	Proximolateral aspect of the caudal pouch (Fig. 74-9, I)	Cranial pouch	With the limb weight bearing, the needle is inserted 3-4 cm caudal to the lateral epicondyle and advanced 4-8 cm in a distal, slightly cranial and medial direction	20 G, 10-20 ml	20-40 minutes	
Shoulder joint	Lateral pouch of the joint (Fig. 74-7, J)	No alternatives	The needle is inserted cranial to the infraspinatus tendon in the notch between the cranial and caudal eminences of the greater tubercle of the humerus, in a caudomedial direction (about 45 degrees) and slightly distally	20 G, spinal needle, 9 cm long, 10-20 ml	20-40 minutes	Bicipital bursa
Bicipital bursa	Lateral pouch of the bursa (Fig. 74-9, K)	Proximal approach	The needle is inserted 3-4 cm proximal to the tibial tuberosity, cranial to the humerus, and is directed proximally, medially, and slightly cranially	20 G, spinal needle, 9 cm long, 10-20 ml	20-40 minutes	Bicipital bursa

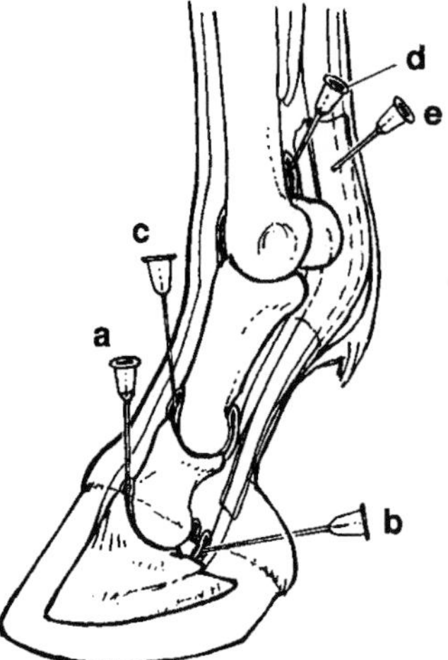

Figure 74-6. Intrasynovial injection sites. a, distal interphalangeal joint; b, navicular bursa; c, proximal interphalangeal joint; d, metacarpophalangeal joint; e, digital flexor tendon sheath.

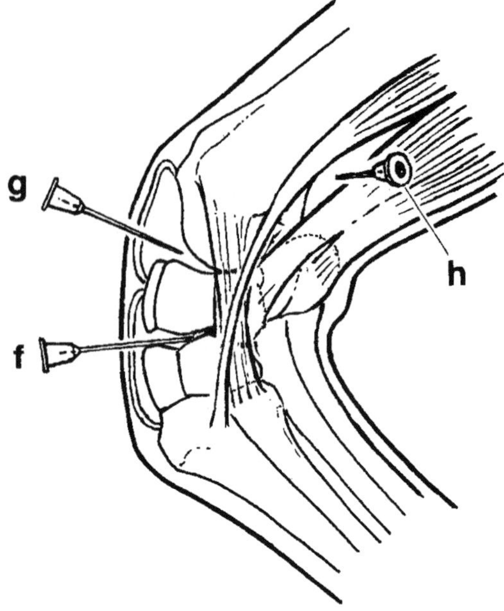

Figure 74-8. Intrasynovial injection sites. f, middle carpal joint; g, antebrachiocarpal joint; h, carpal flexor tendon sheath.

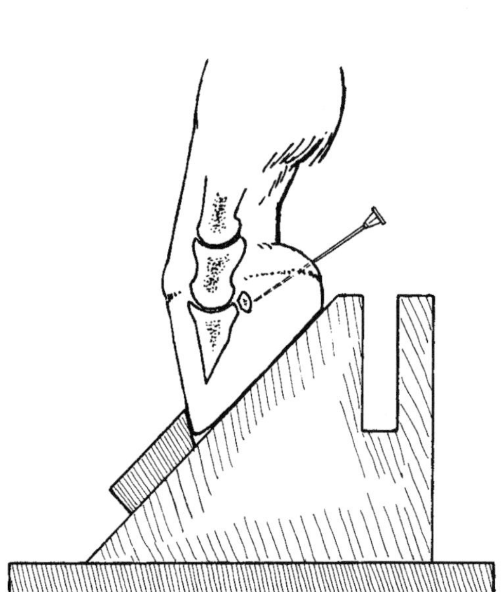

Figure 74-7. Injection of the navicular bursa.

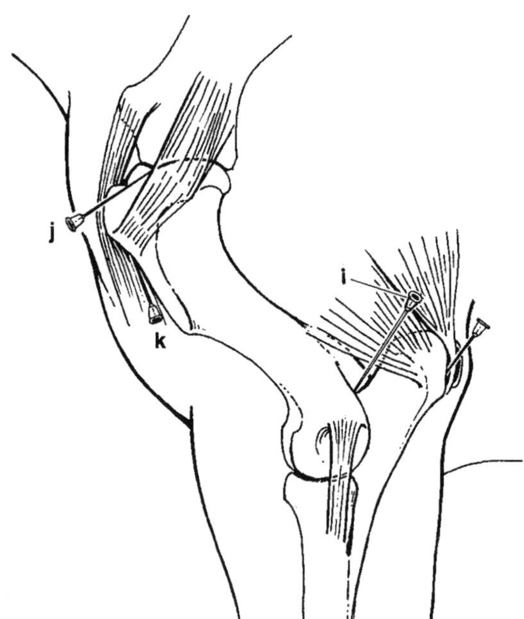

Figure 74-9. Intrasynovial injection sites. i, elbow joint; j, shoulder joint; k, bicipital bursa.

TABLE 74-5. Intrasynovial Analgesia in the Hindlimb

Name of the joint, bursa, or tendon sheath	Location for injection	Alternative approach	Technique	Type of needle and amount of local anesthetic agent	Onset of effect	Important anatomic structures that are often partly or completely anesthetized
Tarsometatarsal joint	Lateral approach (Fig. 74-11, L)		The needle is inserted just proximal to MTIVe, at the level of the palpable depression, in a craniomedial and distal direction	20 G, 3-6 ml	10-20 minutes	Origin of suspensory ligament, proximal aspect of MTIII
Distal intertarsal joint	Medial approach (Fig. 74-10, M)		The needle is inserted horizontally between the fused first and second tarsal bones and the third and central tarsal bones in a small depression just distal to the cunean tendon; this is halfway between the talus and the head of MTIV.	22 G, 3-6 ml	10-20 minutes	Distal intertarsal joint
Tarsocrural joint	Dorsomedial outpouching (Fig. 74-10, N)	Dorsolateral and plantar pouches	Medial (or lateral) to the saphenous vein	20 G, 20-30 ml	20 minutes	Proximal intertarsal joint
Cuneal bursa	Medial approach (Fig. 74-10, O)		The needle is inserted between the distal tarsal bones and the medial branch of the cranial tibial tendon at the distal edge of the tendon	22 G, 3-6 ml	20 minutes	
Calcaneal subtendinous bursa	Medial or lateral approach (Fig. 74-11, P)		The needle is inserted proximal or distal to the tuber calcanei in the lateral or medial outpouching	20 G, 10 ml	20-40 minutes	
Tarsal sheath	Medial or lateral approach (Fig. 74-11, Q)		The needle is inserted in the proximal or distal outpouching of the tarsal sheath	20 G, 20 ml	20-40 minutes	

Continued

TABLE 74-5. Intrasynovial Analgesia in the Hindlimb—cont'd

Name of the joint, bursa, or tendon sheath	Location for injection	Alternative approach	Technique	Type of needle and amount of local anesthetic agent	Onset of effect	Important anatomic structures that are often partly or completely anesthetized
Femoropatellar joint	Craniomedial or craniolateral approach (Fig. 74-12, R)	Lateral approach, subpatellar site in a flexed position	The needle is inserted either lateral or medial to the middle patellar ligament until the needle tip contacts the articular cartilage of the distal femur; the needle is then withdrawn slightly.	20 G, 20 ml	20-60 minutes	Lateral and medial femorotibial joint
Medial compartment of the femorotibial joint	Medial approach (Fig. 74-12, S)	Cranial approach	The needle is inserted just caudal to the medial patellar ligament, 1-2 cm proximal to the medial tibial plateau, perpendicular to the skin	20 G, 20 ml	20-40 minutes	Lateral femorotibial joint, femoropateral joint
Lateral compartment of the femorotibial joint	Lateral approach (Fig. 74-12, T)	Cranial approach	The needle is inserted caudal to the long digital extensor tendon, 1-2 cm proximal to the lateral tibial plateau, horizontally and slightly cranially	20 G, 20 ml	20-40 minutes	Medial femorotibial joint, femoropateral joint
Coxofemoral joint	Lateral approach (Fig. 74-13, U)		The spinal needle is inserted between the caudal and short cranial processes of the greater trochanter of the femur in a slightly craniomedial direction and slightly distally until the joint capsule is penetrated.	Spinal needle, 20-30 ml	20-40 minutes	
Sacroiliac joint	Medial approach; middle or caudal third of the sacroiliac joint (Fig. 74-14, V)	Cranial third of the sacroiliac joint	The needle is inserted 2 cm cranial to the opposite sacral tuberosity and directed to the midpoint of the distance between the cranial aspect of the tuber coxae and the greater trochanter	Spinal needle, 15-18 G, 20-25 cm, 20-30 ml	20-40 minutes	

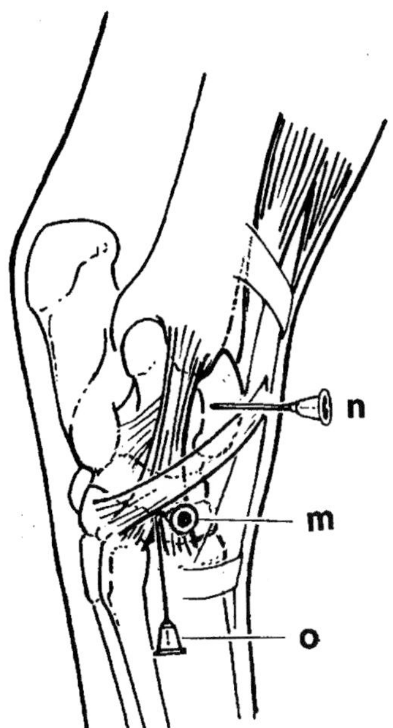

Figure 74-10. Intrasynovial injection sites. m, distal intertarsal joint; n, tarsocrural joint; o, cuneal bursa.

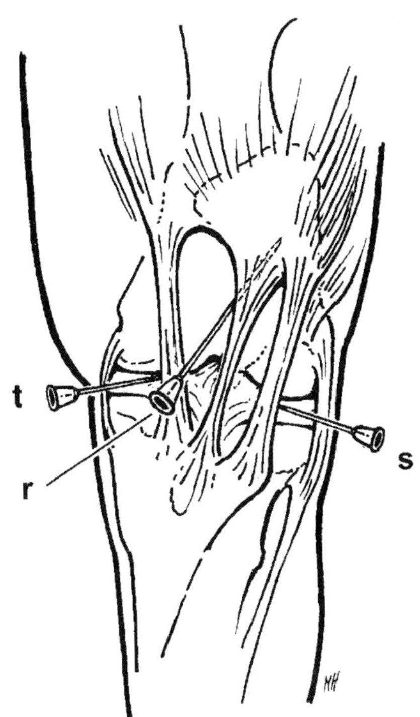

Figure 74-12. Intrasynovial injection sites. r, lateral femorotibial joint; s, femoropatellar joint; t, medial femorotibial joint.

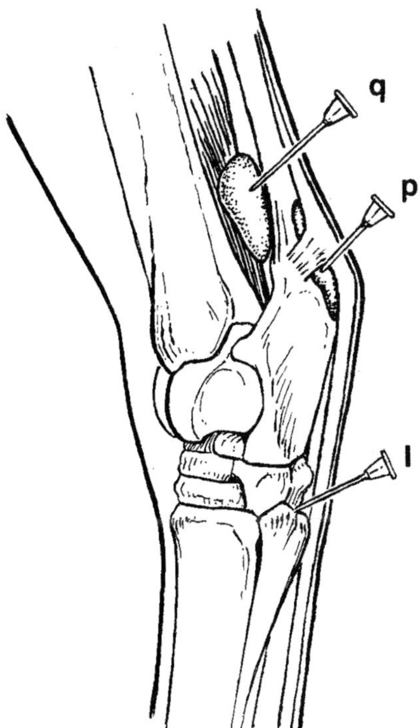

Figure 74-11. Intrasynovial injection sites. l, tarsometatarsal joint; p, calcaneal bursa; q, tendon sheath of long digital extensor (muscle).

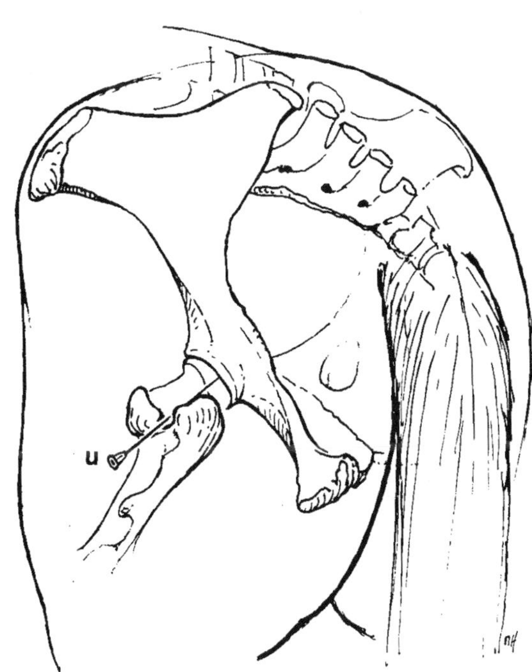

Figure 74-13. Intrasynovial injection sites. u, coxofemoral joint.

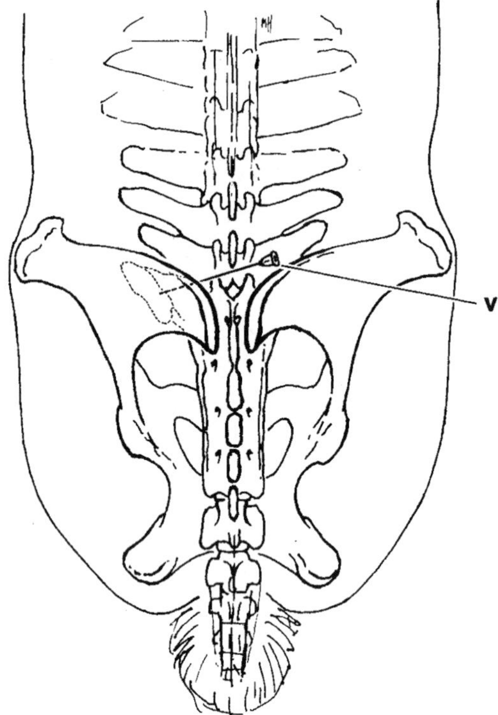

Figure 74-14. Intrasynovial injection sites. v, sacroiliac joint.

REFERENCES

1. Bassage LH, Ross MW: Diagnostic analgesia. In Ross MW, Dyson SJ, editors: Diagnosis and Management of Lameness in the Horse, Philadelphia, 2003, WB Saunders.
2. Stashak TS: Examination for lameness. In Stashak TS, editor: Adams' Lameness in Horses, ed 5, Philadelphia, 2002, Lippincott Williams & Wilkins.
3. Day TK, Skarda RT: The pharmacology of local anesthetics, Vet Clin North Am Equine Pract 1991;7:489.
4. Spoormakers TJ, Donker SH, Ensink JM: Diagnostic anaesthesia of the equine lower limb: A comparison of lidocaine and lidocaine with epinephrine, Tijdschr Diergeneeskd 2004;129:548.
5. Hague BA, Honnas CM, Simpson RB, et al: Evaluation of skin bacterial flora before and after aseptic preparation of clipped and nonclipped arthrocentesis sites in horses, Vet Surg 1997;26:121.
6. Zubrod CJ, Farnsworth KD, Oaks JL: Evaluation of arthrocentesis site bacterial flora before and after 4 methods of preparation in horses with and without evidence of skin contamination, Vet Surg 2004;33:525.
7. Buchner HHF, Kubber P, Zohmann E, et al: Sedation and antisedation as tools in equine lameness examination, Equine Vet J Suppl 1999;30:227.
8. Schumacher J, Steiger R, de Graves F, et al: Effects of analgesia of the distal interphalangeal joint or palmar digital nerves on lameness caused by solar pain in horses, Vet Surg 2000;29:54.
9. Gough MR, Mayhew G, Munroe GA: Diffusion of mepivacaine between adjacent synovial structures in the horse: Part 1. Forelimb foot and carpus, Equine Vet J 2002;34:80.
10. Dyson S: Problems associated with the interpretation of the results of regional and intra-articular anaesthesia in the horse, Vet Rec 1986;118:419.
11. Zeman DH, Roberts ED, Shoji H, et al: Experimental haemarthrosis in rhesus monkeys: Morphometric, biochemical and metabolic analyses, J Comp Pathol 1991;104:129.
12. Schumacher J, Wilson AM, Pardoe C, et al: In vitro evaluation of a novel prosthesis for laryngoplasty of horses with recurrent laryngeal neuropathy, Equine Vet J 2000;32:43.
13. Schumacher J, Schumacher J, de Graves F, et al: A comparison of the effects of local analgesic solution in the navicular bursa of horses with lameness caused by solar toe or solar heel pain, Equine Vet J 2001;33:386.
14. Schumacher J, Livesey L, DeGraves FJ, et al: Effect of anaesthesia of the palmar digital nerves on proximal interphalangeal joint pain in the horse, Equine Vet J 2004;36:409.
15. Schumacher J, de Graves F, Steiger R, et al: A comparison of the effects of two volumes of local analgesic solution in the distal interphalangeal joint of horses with lameness caused by solar toe or solar heel pain, Equine Vet J 2001;33:265.
16. Schumacher J, Gillette R, DeGraves F, et al: The effects of local anaesthetic solution in the navicular bursa of horses with lameness caused by distal interphalangeal joint pain, Equine Vet J 2003;35:502.
17. Engeli E, Haussler KK, Erb HN: Development and validation of a periarticular injection technique of the sacroiliac joint in horses, Equine Vet J 2004;36:324.

CHAPTER 75

Diagnostic Medical Imaging

Barbara Kaser-Hotz
Gottlieb Ueltschi

Equine surgery depends heavily on various imaging procedures. Imaging plays important roles—first, in diagnosing and localizing a disease process; second, in assessing the surgical intervention; and third, in the follow-up evaluation of a patient. Many imaging techniques are available. In this chapter, the basic principles of image production and interpretation are discussed.

RADIOGRAPHY

Production of X-Rays

Every radiographic examination is based on the fact that x-rays are attenuated when passing through matter. The chemical and physical properties of matter are the decisive factors in the attenuation process. The attenuated x-ray beam can be registered by appropriate imaging systems. X-ray tubes are used for the production of high-velocity electrons. This highly evacuated glass tube contains the positive (anode) and the negative pole (cathode). The cathode produces the electrons by heating a tungsten filament. The electron cloud is accelerated toward the positive pole of the x-ray tube when a very high voltage is applied.

The applied high voltage dictates the velocity of the electrons. The impact of the electrons on the anode generates the desired x-rays (deceleration x-ray beam emittance), but also it produces undesirable interactions that cause high thermal loading of the anode material (Fig. 75-1).

Several techniques are used to remove the heat from the anode. In the stationary x-ray tube, the anode consists of a small plate of tungsten, embedded in a large block of copper. The copper removes the heat from the tungsten target by conduction. In the rotating-anode x-ray tube, the anode consists of a tungsten alloy disk that is rotated by an electric motor during the exposure. The anode disk has a very high heat capacity, and the area exposed to the impinging electrons changes continuously during the exposure, so heat is distributed. Because heat is dissipated only by convection, it is radiated to the adjacent glass envelope and the surrounding cooling oil. In the rotating anode, the focal spot becomes a focal ring, which, depending on exposure time, is irradiated in part or totally. The metallic tube housing containing the cooling oil surrounds the x-ray tube and shields against the x-ray radiation. The cooling oil also is used as an electrical insulator against the high voltage. A small aperture allows passage of the x-ray beam through the glass envelope in which the x-ray beam is attenuated. The x-ray beam contains a variety of different x-ray intensities. The lower intensities are removed from the beam by appropriate filters, because they increase the radiation burden on the patient but do not have enough energy to penetrate the patient.[1-3] Today, every x-ray tube has at least a 2-mm-thick aluminium filter. At the tube housing, a light beam diaphragm with special lead diaphragms is attached. The light beam diaphragm limits the x-ray beam and serves as an aiming device, showing with cross-hairs the position of the central beam (center) (Fig. 75-2).

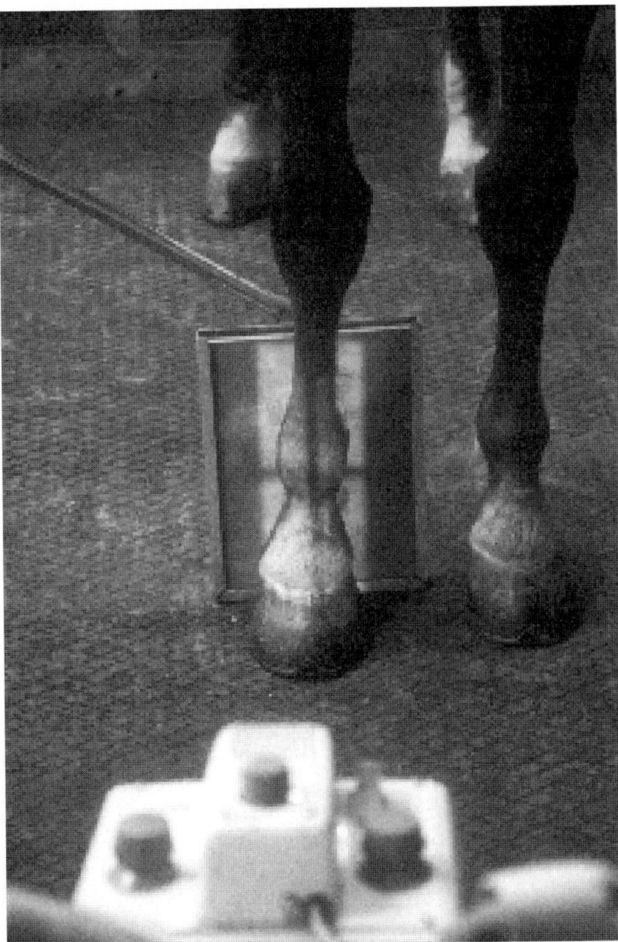

Figure 75-2. The light beam indicates with cross-hairs the center of the beam. The light diaphragm limits the x-ray beam to the region of interest. A lead letter is placed on the lateral aspect of the radiograph to identify the limb of interest.

Image Formation and Storage

Film and Screen Combinations

After passage through the patient, the attenuated x-ray beam is registered by a combination of intensifying screens and specially adapted x-ray film. The most popular imaging system is photographic film that is exposed by the x-rays directly or indirectly through the light emission of the intensifying screens. A so-called latent image of the intensity distribution of the x-ray beam is generated in the film. The image becomes visible after development, fixation, and drying of the film. The intensifying screens contain substances (phosphors) that belong chemically to the rare earth group of elements. They convert the x-ray photons much more efficiently than the formerly used calcium tungstate. The intensification of the screens is divided into three groups. The groups are calibrated so that, from one class to the next, the exposure must be either doubled or divided by two. High-intensifying or high-speed screens have the highest emission of fluorescent light and therefore the highest possible amplification, but resolution is limited (greater than 0.3 mm). Resolution is best described as the ability to discern two neighboring structures. Regular screens are the compromise between high intensification and resolution. High-resolution screens have good resolution (0.1 mm), but their sensitivity is quite low.[4] In equine radiography, high-resolution screens should be used to demonstrate bony structures. The evaluation of the navicular

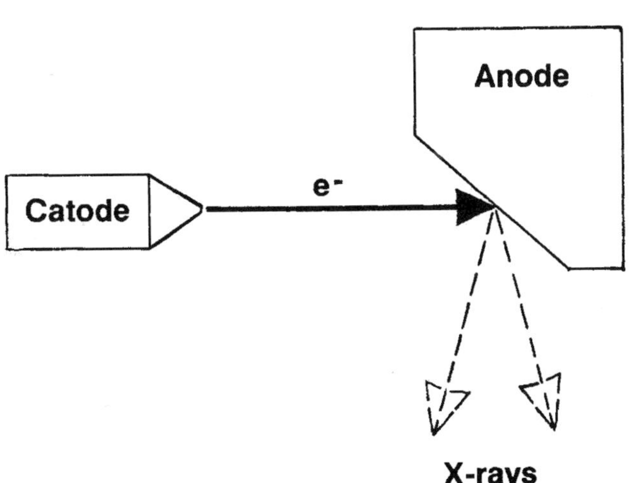

Figure 75-1. Production of x-rays. Electrons are emitted from the cathode and impinge on the anode where x-rays are produced.

bone requires particularly high resolution imaging systems similar to those used in mammography.

Digital Radiography

The altered x-ray beam after passage through the patient can be captured with specially designed systems. The most commonly used method is the imaging plate, where the storage phosphor consists of europium-activated fluorohalides. Not only does irradiating the imaging plate cause blue fluorescence but also the larger part of the x-ray energy is absorbed by the phosphor, whereby the electrons are lifted to a higher energy level. The exposed imaging plate can store the latent image without loss of details for several hours. In the "reader," the stored energy of the phosphors is emitted upon irradiation with red laser light. The emitted fluorescence is blue and is seen by a photomultiplier tube, which converts the light intensities into electric signals. An analog-to-digital converter digitizes the signals and stores them in a computer in form of a matrix. (Because the matrix is stored in a computer, this technology is sometimes referred to as computerized radiography.) The final x-ray image is produced when the data of the image matrix are converted to analog brightness signals by the use of a look-up table.

The x-ray picture can be obtained as a hardcopy on special film or displayed on a monitor screen. The stored image data can be displayed in many ways using different look-up tables. Mostly, images are displayed as conventional radiographs, but image frequencies can be altered to better visualize certain structures such as subchondral cystic lesions or fissure lines. Also edge enhancement can be used to delineate linear structures more clearly. The image data can be stored and later reused. The memory necessary to store a common 24×30-cm radiographic picture lies between 6 and 8 MB. This considerable memory requirement often leads to compression of the image data, but compression always means loss of information. The compression ratio dictates the information loss.

Apart from the storage phosphor technique, other systems exist that are able to store and convert the information of the x-ray beam as modified by the patient. Nearly all systems are based on the same principle: A luminescence screen converts the energies of the x-ray photons into visible light. Using one or several charged-coupled devices, the fluorescent image is converted to electrical signals and thereafter digitized and stored in a matrix. Another method functions like a thin film transistor display. Here, the sensitive photo elements are directly coupled to the luminescent screen. These systems are usually called direct digital radiography (DDRx). The display of the final image also takes place on a monitor screen or as a hardcopy on special film. DDRx is too expensive to be used in equine orthopedics. Storage phosphor systems are available in several versions and are used in several equine clinics.[5]

A third method is used to convert the x-ray beam into a visible image. The signal of the image intensifier tube may be digitized, stored, and converted by a computer in a way similar to that used by the other digital methods. The only shortcoming of this method is the limited resolution capacity of the image intensifier. The use of the image intensifier in equine practice is quite restricted because of the size and construction of the equipment.

Image Quality

Apart from the resolution, as discussed earlier, image contrast plays an important role. Contrast is defined as the difference of neighboring intensities. High contrast means clear-cut and intense changes of brightness, whereas in low-contrast images the transition from one light intensity into the next is less pronounced and more blurred.

The contrast is mainly influenced by the scattered radiation. Scatter radiation is produced in the examined volume of the patient by the Compton process. The amount of scatter radiation can be drastically diminished by reducing the volume irradiated (the exposure field). This is accomplished by collimation of the beam (Fig. 75-3). In addition, scatter grids can be used to remove, in part, the effect of the generated scattered radiation. The grid consists of a large number of lead foil strips separated by x-ray–transparent spaces. The grid allows passage of the primary beam only. The lead foil strips of the grid absorb radiation that is not perpendicular to the screen. For areas producing a large amount of scatter radiation, grids have to be used to obtain optimal contrasts. Remember the following rule of thumb: if the object to be examined is thicker than 10 cm, the use of a grid is indicated. The use of a grid requires higher exposure values, so collimation of the beam should be done at the same time to reduce scatter radiation of the assisting personnel. The grid ratio is defined as the quotient of the height of the lead strips divided by the length of the interspace through which the primary radiation passes. The grid ratios useable in equine radiography range from 8:1 to 10:1, and the suitable number of lines per centimeter should be not less than 30. Parallel grids are easier to use than parallel focused ones. Crisscrossed grids are best for extremely thick body portions such as the pelvis and femoropatellar joint region (Fig. 75-4).

Inconsistency of image quality also may stem from film development. An automatic processor does all development, fixation, and drying steps. This does not mean that manual processing of the radiographic film is inferior, but it is more susceptible to underexposure, overexposure, and other mistakes.

Basic Image Interpretation

Every radiograph contains the information of a three-dimensional object, and this is compressed into a two-dimensional image. Therefore, every x-ray examination should consist of at least two planes that are oriented at right angles to each other. In many situations, these two standard imaging planes are not sufficient to allow correct interpretation, and additional (e.g., oblique) projections of the x-ray beam have to be used. Image interpretation is easiest when the same standard projections are routinely performed for a given region or joint. On the radiograph, the name of the owner; the age, breed, and sex of the horse; the examination date; and name of the hospital, practice, or institution must be clearly identified. Lead marks for right or left limb are placed in the proximal, dorsal or cranial, upper

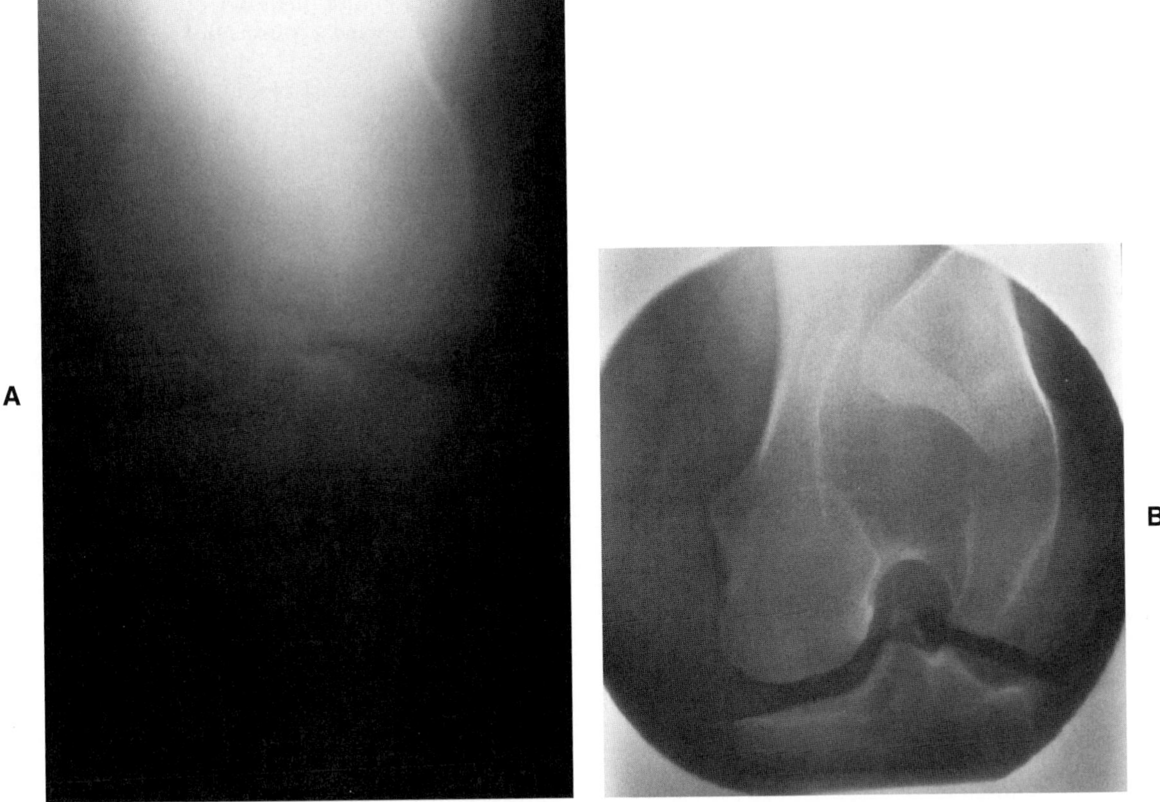

Figure 75-3. A, Caudocranial view of the femorotibial joint without collimation. **B,** The identical radiographic view with tight collimation. The amount of scatter radiation produced within the large muscle mass is dramatically reduced, improving image quality.

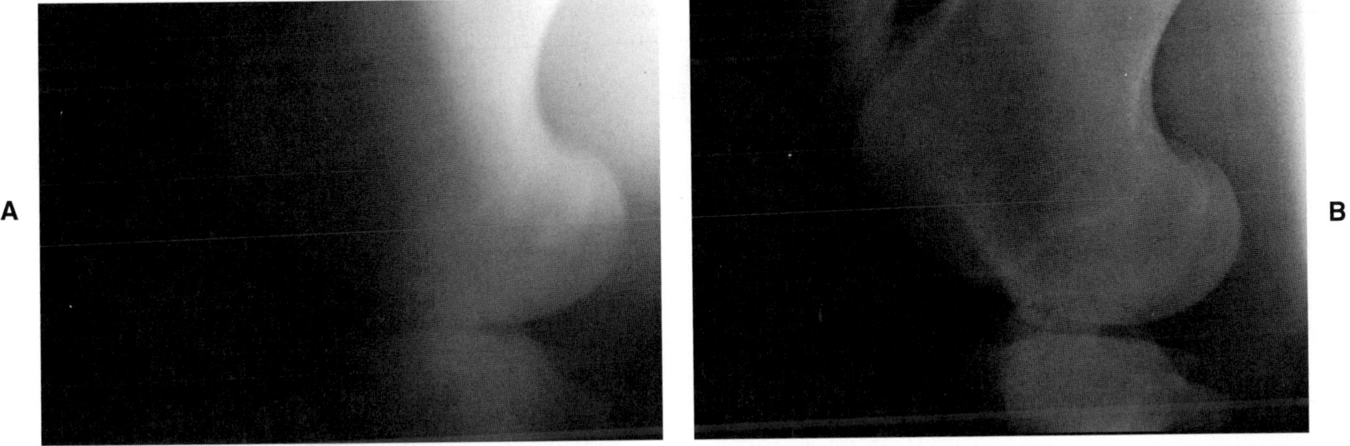

Figure 75-4. A, Lateral radiographic projection of the femorotibial joint without a grid. **B,** The identical projection with a parallel grid. The image contrast is improved by reduction of scatter radiation.

corner on a lateral radiograph, and in the proximal, lateral corner in a dorsopalmar, dorsoplantar, or any oblique radiograph. The first step to radiographic interpretation is to assess whether image quality is appropriate and whether the anatomic region of interest is fully depicted on the imaging study. Once this has been done, the actual reading of the radiograph can start.[6]

A radiograph is a reflection of the different absorptions and attenuations of the x-ray beam in matter. Only five different radiologic densities can be demonstrated on a radiograph—those of gas, fat, water or soft tissue, bone, and metal. Radiographic density or opacity depends on these physical and chemical properties, as well as on the thickness of a given object. Fat is helpful in separating muscle bellies and tendinous structures from one another. Reading a radiograph means identifying abnormalities in texture, contour, and structure of the five different densities visible on a radiograph. Radiographs are read in a standard way, and whether this is done from left to right or from top to bottom, or in a more anatomic method from joint to joint, is not important. However, using the same routine all the time helps prevent the oversight of some lesions, particularly when the reader finds an obvious abnormality and stops reading the entire film. Then the various abnormalities are summarized to form a radiographic impression or diagnosis.

Radiography is often the first imaging study used to arrive at a diagnosis, and if the reading is equivocal, further imaging studies may be suggested. These may include additional views in different projections and the application of negative or positive contrast agents. With the introduction of ultrasonography, computed tomography (CT), and magnetic resonance imaging (MRI), the use of contrast procedures to assess joint cartilage and synovial membrane has gradually diminished. Abnormal communication of a synovial space and the surrounding soft tissue can be analyzed with an arthrogram, fistulogram, tendonogram, or bursogram (Fig. 75-5). Aseptic centesis of a synovial space should be done and the contrast agent instilled slowly. It is important to bring the contrast agent to body temperature, because viscosity is heavily dependent on temperature of the contrast agents. Nonionic contrast media are less irritating than ionic contrast agents, but they are also more expensive. For larger joints, ionic contrast agents are sufficient. Depending on the joint space, 5 to 20 mL of contrast medium is injected. There is a tendency to use too small an amount of contrast medium, but image interpretation is more difficult when a joint is not fully distended. The joint should be flexed and then the same radiographs are repeated. The contrast medium will be absorbed through lymph and venous drainage quite rapidly.

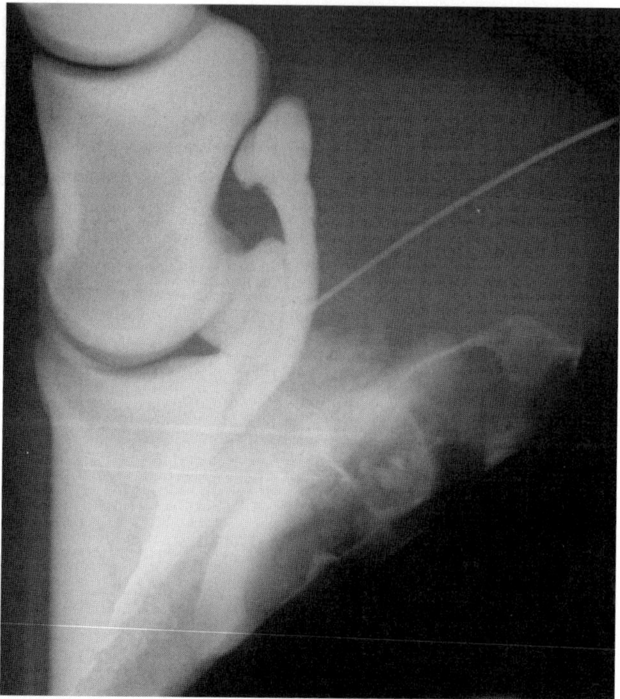

Figure 75-5. Lateral radiograph of the distal phalanx. Contrast medium has been instilled into the navicular bursa. Contrast leaks out through a tract that penetrated the solar hoof wall.

ULTRASONOGRAPHY

Ultrasonography is an established technique in the diagnostic workup of the flexor tendons, the suspensory ligament, and the check ligament (Fig. 75-6). Ultrasonography of other ligaments, joints, bursae, tendon sheaths, and muscles is becoming more routine. The biggest drawback of ultrasonography is operator dependence. Although it represents a cross-sectional imaging technique, the planes are individually set, and multiple artifacts can make interpretation difficult for the inexperienced operator. Nevertheless, ultrasonography has become an integral part of equine surgery because it is noninvasive.

Image Formation

Diagnostic ultrasonography uses high-frequency sound waves between 2 and 12 MHz. The sound waves are produced in a transducer, and a series of ultrasound pulses are transmitted into the patient. The ultrasound waves are propagated but also reflected to form an image by transforming the returning ultrasound energy into electrical energy. The reflected signal, which corresponds to the anatomy of the structure producing the reflecting signal, is converted into an image and projected onto a monitor. The brightness of a dot on the monitor screen correlates to the amplitude of the returning echo. Different shades of gray are assigned to different echo strengths. The propagation speed of an ultrasound wave is determined by the density and stiffness of a given tissue. The propagation speed is highest in solid tissues such as bone, it is lower in fluid-filled structures, and it is lowest in air. It is the interface between tissues that allows the differentiation of one structure from another. Large differences exist between soft tissue and bone,

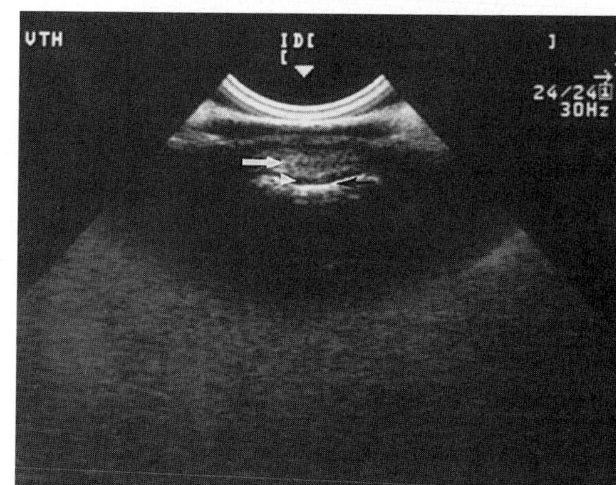

Figure 75-6. From the dorsolateral aspect of the metacarpophalangeal joint, the lateral digital extensor tendon *(white arrow)*, articular cartilage *(arrowhead)*, and cortex of the MCIII *(black arrow)* are shown on this sonogram.

or soft tissue and air. The various soft tissue densities differ only minimally and, therefore, tendon structures are easier to distinguish from one another when a fluid-filled tendon sheath surrounds the tendon. Ultrasound waves are also attenuated, scattered, reflected, and refracted. The combination of these interactions of ultrasound waves with tissue creates an image.

The resolution of an ultrasonographic image depends on, among other things, the axial and lateral resolution. *Axial resolution* is the ability to distinguish the dots along the ultrasound path. This is determined by the pulse length, which depends on the frequency of the transducer. The higher the frequency is, the better the axial resolution. However, the price for the higher resolution is a loss of depth in tissue penetration. Therefore, superficial lesions can be scanned with high frequencies, whereas deep-seated structures have to be examined with low frequencies. *Lateral resolution* is the minimum distance two dots can be from one another and still be distinguished from one another in a plane perpendicular to the sound wave. This is determined by the diameter of the ultrasound beam. The lateral resolution typically decreases with distance from the transducer, since the beam diverges with distance. Lateral resolution is best in the focal zone. Usually, axial resolution is superior to lateral resolution.

For most structures to be scanned in equine surgery, a high-frequency transducer with good resolution can be used. Various types of transducers exist. Linear probes provide good-quality images and the best overview, but they need a large footprint (surface area on the probe). This may be a problem when curvy, irregular surfaces have to be scanned. Fluid-filled stand-off pads may improve tissue contact. Sector scanners have a smaller footprint.

Ultrasound waves are produced by mechanically oscillating or rotating one or more crystals. Phased-array transducers do not excite the crystals mechanically but use an electrical signal to excite them. One crystal after the other is excited in a timely (or phased) fashion. These transducers have the smallest footprint, but they have less penetration than sector scanners. Color and power Doppler sonography are newer techniques that rely on the Doppler shift as the ultrasound wave is reflected off a moving target, typically red blood cells. Power Doppler ultrasonography is promising for the evaluation of vascularity—or example, in the tendon healing process.

Image Interpretation

Before interpreting an ultrasonographic image, the operator should know the various control buttons on the machine. The amplitude of the returning signal is steered by the power control, which delivers a specific amount of energy to the emitted ultrasound waves. Only the returning signals can be amplified by using the gain setting. Preferentially, the echoes returning from the far field are amplified the most, and the returning signals in the near field are not augmented. When all settings are set correctly, image interpretation is made easier and structures (e.g., the flexor tendons) are assessed for their contour, echo texture, and relative echogenicity. The terms to describe a lesion are relative terms, such as *hypoechoic, hyperechoic,* and *isoechoic*.

NUCLEAR MEDICINE

Equipment

Scintigraphic examinations of equine patients became possible about 30 years ago. Scintigraphy is an imaging method used to detect inflammation in tissues, which usually represents the source of lameness in the musculoskeletal tissues. This special imaging method detects gamma rays emanating from the patient who has been injected with a radiolabeled compound, and converts them into visible light. This light is recognized by photomultiplier tubes (PMTs) in a gamma camera and converted into electrical signals, which are thereafter amplified. The detector of the gamma camera consists of a large but thin NaJ(Tl) crystal and a large number of PMTs. The PMTs are interconnected with each other in a resistance matrix, so the scintillation event can be localized in the crystal. In front of the NaJ crystal, a collimator is placed to select the incident gamma radiation according to the direction of the holes. Depending on the construction of the collimator, only radiation with right-angle incidence or obliquely angled gamma rays can pass through. The size and the number of the holes and the thickness of the septa or "walls of the holes" are the determining factors. The collimators have to be adapted to the energy of the gamma isotopes and the desired resolution. Increasing the resolution always causes a lengthening of the acquisition time. Therefore, collimators with larger holes are often used because their better counting rate makes the duration of the examination shorter. The detector head shields the delicate crystal and the electronic circuitry from external radiation and mechanical shocks.

The gamma camera was developed for the human patient, and using the camera to examine the horse poses some problems. Most cameras consist of two separate elements: the detector head and the acquisition unit that consists of the computer storing the acquired data and a display unit. For the equine patient, scintigraphic application requires special positions for the gamma camera, and many mounting solutions have been developed and used. The best ones seem to be gimbals mounted on an electrically driven cart, or a hydraulic crane mounted to the ceiling of the examination room. Many clinics use only the gamma camera in the standing animal, which reduces the potential of the nuclear examination method quite drastically. The size of the camera also plays an important role. A large-field gamma scintillation camera may cover a large anatomic region but may be very cumbersome to position correctly. Usually, large-field cameras have rectangular or circular fields of view. The very large circular detector head is difficult to position over extremities. A large part of the examination field is not used. The age of the camera is important, too. Many improvements have been made in the design and construction of the collimators. Modern equipment offers better resolution and higher sensitivity.

Image Production and Quality

Examinations are always influenced by the duration of the acquisition, which is limited by the animal's motion. Image quality is in turn affected by the number of counts available: a higher number of counts produces a better image (Fig. 75-7).

In the standing animal, the examination should be as short as possible, so that motion, which interferes with image quality, can be minimized. On the other hand, it is evident that larger count numbers improves the scintigraphic image. A compromise has to be made between short examination duration and the total count number. The easiest way to reduce movement of the patient is adequate sedation or tranquilizing of the horse. Correct handling of the animal is also very important for avoiding motion. Mathematical motion correction programs do exist, but they can be applied only with dynamic studies, and only minor movement errors can be resolved. Examination of the anesthetized patient in lateral recumbency allows longer examination times, and together with the use of high-resolution collimators, this permits delineation of deep structures with more detail.

The source of the gamma radiation is the metabolized radioactive label, and technetium-99m is used as a source of the gamma radiation. ^{99m}Tc has a short half-life of only 6 hours and a suitable gamma ray energy of 140 keV. The radioisotope can be eluted with physiologic saline from a generator system. The mother isotope of ^{99m}Tc is molybdenum-99. The eluate contains pertechnetate-99m, which is the oxide of technetium and has the chemical formula TcO_4. ^{99m}Tc can be coupled to specific organic or inorganic compounds. For example, ^{99m}Tc coupled to phosphates will be concentrated in the skeleton, and bone imaging will become possible. Denaturized albumin tagged with ^{99m}Tc will stay in the vascular bed. The complex of ^{99m}Tc and sulfur colloid will mark the liver, the bone marrow, and the spleen. The quantity of the marker in a vial used in human nuclear medicine is usually sufficient to allow visualization of the desired organs in the horse. However, the activity of ^{99m}Tc for a horse has to be increased at least five times. Approximately 4.5 to 7.5 GBq of ^{99m}Tc is commonly used for an adult horse. Labeling agents are usually applied by intravenous injection in the jugular vein. In the first phase, the labeling agent circulates in the blood system and can be monitored with a fast dynamic study.

After a few minutes, the label leaves the large vessels and is found mostly in the extracellular fluid and soft tissue. This intermediate stage is called pool phase. After about 2 hours, the target organ (e.g., bone) becomes clearly visible via the uptake of the radioactively tagged imaging agent. The soft tissue activity interferes with the bone activity and decreases image detail. However, soft tissue activity decreases more rapidly than the bone activity, which is primarily the result of decay of the radio-isotope. A large proportion of the imaging label is excreted by the kidneys. This activity will accumulate in the bladder. Therefore, it is useful to empty

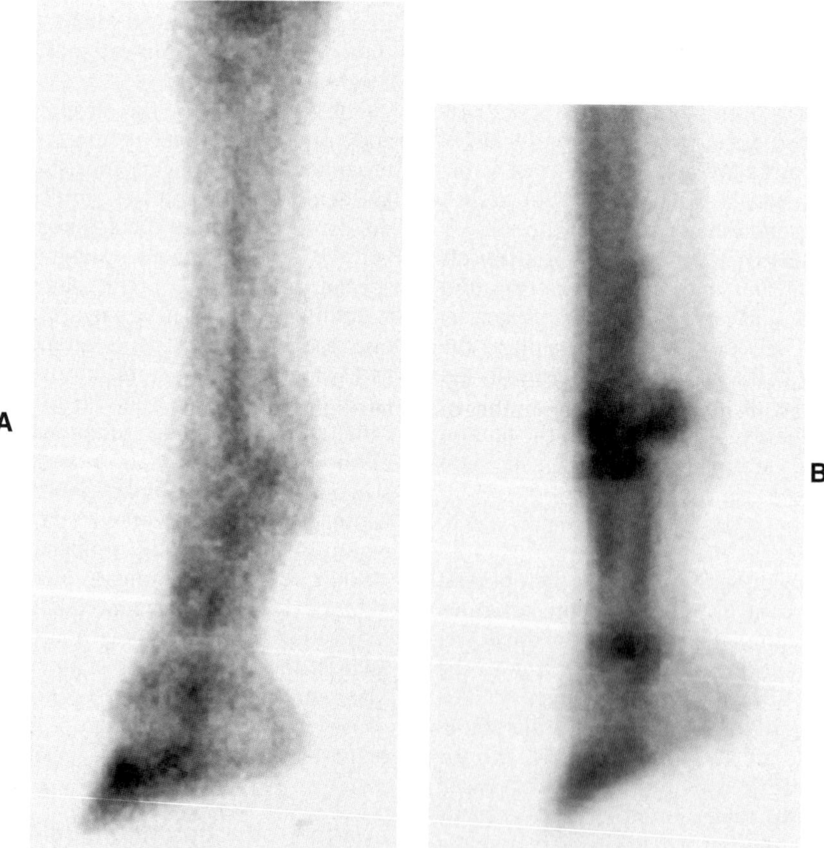

Figure 75-7. Bone scan of the left phalangeal region with 200,000 counts. **A,** Anatomic detail is poor because of the low count rate. **B,** Bone scan of the same region with 600,000 accumulated counts, which improved the image quality. A normal uptake pattern is present.

the bladder by catheterization if the pelvic region has to be examined.

Examination Procedure

The horse receives the radioactive substance by intravenous injection. A catheter is recommended because depots of the marker behind or around the jugular vein lead to low-count images of the regions of interest. Also, examination of the cervical region becomes difficult or impossible when paravenous deposits of radioactivity are present.

In moderate and cold climates, bandaging of the legs to be investigated at least 12 hours prior to the examination improves uptake of the radioactive agent. The mechanism involved is not clearly understood. At the authors' institution, felt pads are wrapped around the legs. If the hoof region has to be examined, bandages are also applied there. The shoes are removed to access the solar region, too.

For the pool phase, hoof images are acquired after 2 minutes. The contralateral side should be investigated for comparison. After 2 hours, the late or metabolic phase images can be registered. Usually, in the standing, tranquilized animal, only the lateral views of the phalanges and the proximal extremities can be attained without difficulty. In the anesthetized horse, dorsopalmar and palmarodorsal views of the limbs are possible. With a low-energy ultrahigh-sensitivity or high-sensitivity collimator, 300,000 (300 k) to 400,000 (400 k) counts can be registered in the lower phalanges. Over large joints, 500 k and greater are easily collectable in most cases. In the pelvic and back region, the limit lies around 1,000 k. For the visualization of the spine, a general-purpose collimator should be used to visualize the spinous processes. In the cervical region, less than 500 k can be gathered without movement of the standing patient even with the high-sensitivity collimator. The amount of collected counts is more important for a correct evaluation than a preset collection time with variable count numbers.

Image Analysis

The distribution of the radioactive label in the patient's body can be observed in different ways. The count sampling technique is based on the acquisition of a certain number of counts (preset counts—the preferred method) or limiting the observation period by time (preset time). This procedure is referred to as a static planar study.

It is also possible to register a number of static images with predefined time intervals (e.g., one frame per second, one frame every third second, and so on). The single images are usually called frames. The set of static images is designed as a dynamic study. The data are stored in a dedicated computer that is capable of displaying the results in a dynamic fashion and that allows image manipulation.

With any of these methods, the radioactive data are stored on the hard disk of a computer with dedicated nuclear medicine software. The data are gathered in a matrix representing the field of view of the detector. The matrix sizes for nuclear medicine purposes lie between 64×64 and 256×256. Finer matrices are of no practical value, because the intrinsic resolution of nearly all gamma cameras is larger than 3 or 4 mm. Under practical conditions, the resolution of deeper structures is about 10 mm. So the 128×128 matrix is optimal in most cases. Earlier gamma cameras had only limited memory and hard disk space, so the number of counts storable in a matrix element was also limited. This restriction does not exist in more modern equipment.

The image manipulation programs of modern nuclear medicine software allow filtering of image data, definition of thresholds with upper and lower limits, demonstration of activity profiles whereby the width of the slice can be chosen, and definition of regions of interest (ROI). In the ROI, the number of pixels, the average counts, and the lowest and highest count numbers are displayed. The ROI technique is very useful, allowing calculation of uptake ratios that allow a reference area of interest to be compared with other ROIs. The quotient of the ROI in question and the reference ROI is known as the uptake ratio. The display of the activity distribution on the monitor can be freely chosen to be black and white, white and black, or different color scales. In the authors' experience, the best recognition of anatomic details and structures is achieved with a black and white or the inversed black and white display.

COMPUTED TOMOGRAPHY

CT is a radiologic examination method that delivers information in the form of cross-sectional or transverse images. Unlike in conventional radiography, where the image is the sum of all structures penetrated by the primary x-ray beam, CT demonstrates the object free of superimposition by neighboring structures. First, a topogram is made, which produces an overview of the body portion to be scanned, and the position of the patient can be checked and changed if necessary. Then tomograms, which are transverse sections through the topogram, are recorded. After the acquisition of the first transverse section, the patient is moved a small distance and the scanning begins again. This procedure is repeated until the previously defined anatomic field in the topogram is completely examined. CT for horses requires a table that can hold much more weight than commercially available tables. Also, moving the horse and the special table at a constant speed into the gantry is not an easy task. Therefore, a topogram is not usually obtained for horses, and only tomograms are acquired. Instead of moving the table, the gantry can be moved over a fixed table (Fig. 75-8).

The introduction of CT in the early 1970s was a revolutionary step. In the first CT models, the x-ray tube rotated around the patient, emitting a pencil-thin x-ray beam at predefined positions. The tube was coupled to a detector system that registered the altered primary beam. Based on the attenuated primary beam, the attenuation coefficient was calculated according to a simple object model. So, for every direction of the primary beam, a special relationship could be derived, and for the whole series, a set of linear equations for calculating the attenuation coefficients was generated. Further development of CT resulted in larger, fanlike x-ray beams and larger detector elements. The calculation of the attenuation coefficients was no longer done by iterative methods but by convolution and back-projection techniques. In the first 10 years, new generations of CT models were developed in quick succession. An important step forward was the introduction of the spiral CT at the end of the 1980s. With this procedure, the patient is continually scanned, and the x-ray tube and the axial translation are

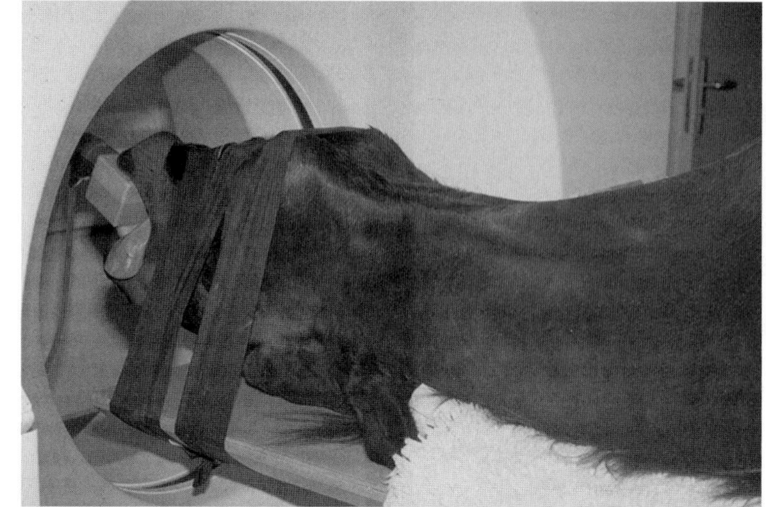

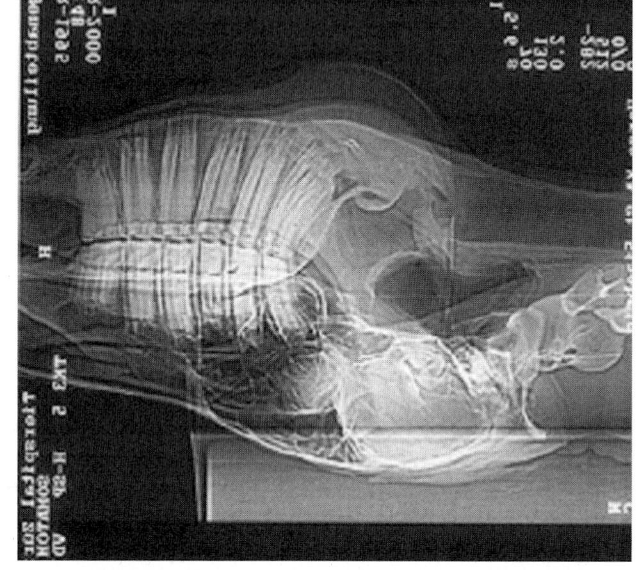

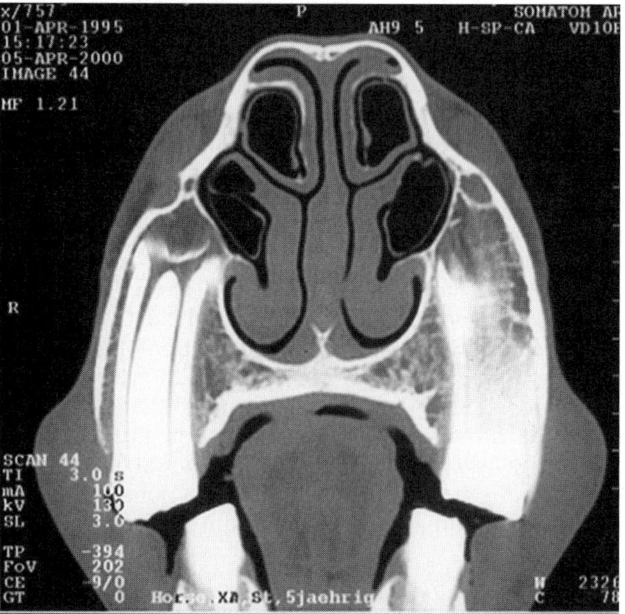

Figure 75-8. A, The head of a patient is fixed to the table for a computed tomography study. **B,** The initial topogram of the area to be studied allows the area of interest to be centered. **C,** Normal cross-sectional image.

coupled. In multislice CTs (MSCT), up to 64 different cross-sections can be acquired during one rotation of the x-ray tube. The rotation time of the x-ray tube is only 0.5 second. With this technique and breath holding by the patient, even dynamic processes, such as the beating heart, can be observed. In veterinary medicine, such sophisticated CTs are rare exceptions. However, single-slice CT (SSCT) is used in many clinics and private practices. In SSCT, a single slice is scanned, followed by translation of the patient, and this step is repeated until the object is completely examined as just described. SSCT is less expensive, but examination times are much longer than with a MSCT. Resolution is also less than with MSCT, but by using overlapping slices, 1-mm-thick sections are possible.

The major advantages of CT over routine radiography are the acquisition of transverse or cross-sectional images and superior low-contrast differences. This latter advantage allows the delineation of different soft tissue structures. The acquired density datasets permit reconstruction of the object in a longitudinal or an oblique direction. Three-dimensional reconstruction is also possible (Fig. 75-9). The registered datasets can be stored on a variety of different storage media (MO, DVD, CD, hard disk).

The CT examination can be enhanced with special contrast agents that allow increased soft tissue differentiation and demonstration of tissue perfusion.

CT examinations of animals differ from human examinations in one aspect: animals are examined under general anesthesia. In horses, the examinations are limited to the extremities, neck, and head by the dimensions of the gantry. CT is particularly useful in the evaluation of the equine head, where the cross-sectional images provide much more information than multiple radiographic projections. Occult tooth abnormalities, skull fractures, and ethmoidal hematomas are common indications for CT of the equine head. Because of the anesthesia required, CT is not routinely

A

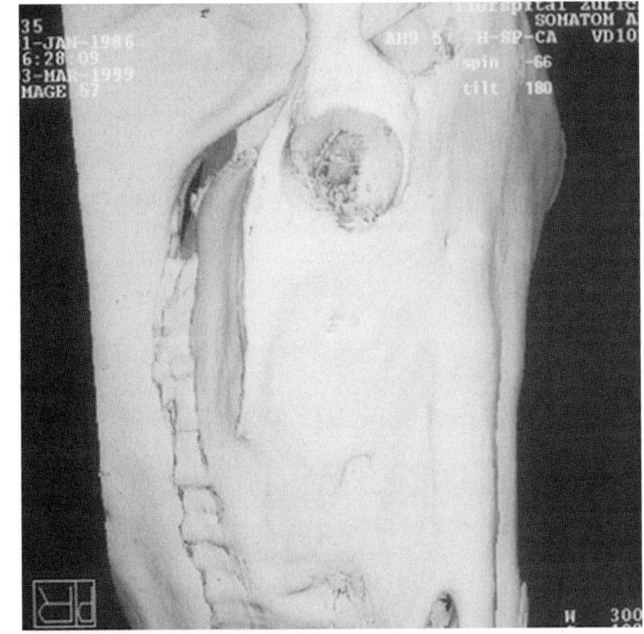

B

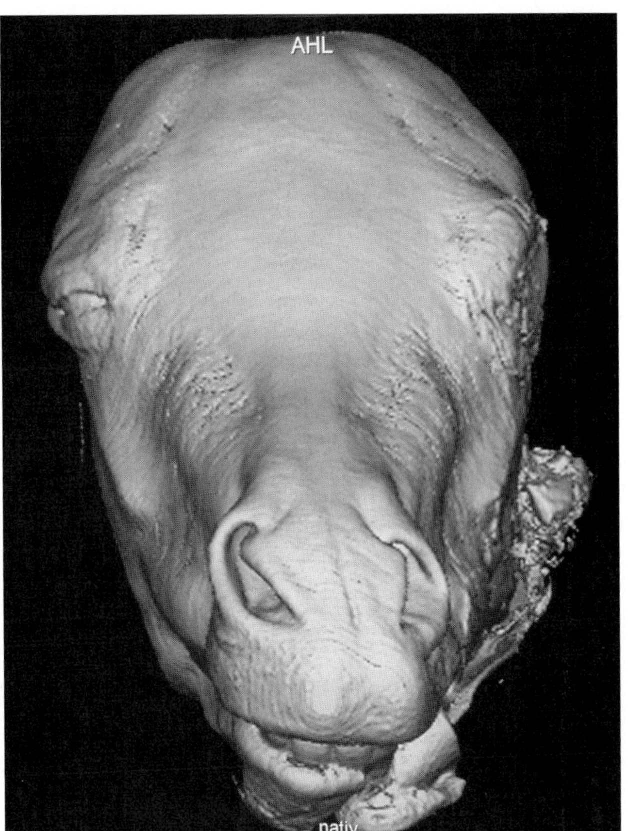

Figure 75-9. A, Three-dimensional reconstruction of the skull using computed tomography. **B,** Three-dimensional reconstruction of the soft tissue–covered surfaces of an equine head.

used to evaluate complex problems of the limb. However, it gives very good information about bony abnormalities and about soft tissue structures of the phalanges, carpus, and tarsus. Once multislice CT scanners become more common, shorter anesthesia time may allow CT of the lower limb to become more routine.

MAGNETIC RESONANCE IMAGING

MRI generates cross-sectional images of the patient using the nuclear spins of certain atoms. This modality does not use ionizing radiation. Any moving electrical charge is an electrical current and generates a magnetic field. Atomic nuclei with uneven proton and neutron numbers have a rotational motion (nuclear spin) like that of a spinning top. The nuclear spin consists of the single-spin elements of the nuclear components such as the neutrons and protons. The spin of the nucleus produces a magnetic moment. The simplest nucleus is the hydrogen nucleus with one proton. Hydrogen is very abundant in biologic material.

Under normal conditions, the spins of the hydrogen nuclei are randomly distributed and the mean magnetic moment is zero. In a strong magnetic field, the orientation of the spins becomes either parallel or antiparallel to the magnetic field lines. The orientation of the spins in the parallel field direction is slightly larger than in the antiparallel one. Therefore, a measurable magnetic moment exists. This surplus causes an observable magnetic moment. It can easily be influenced by an additional magnetic field such as the one generated by radiofrequency (RF) coils. The MRI machine generates a radiofrequency pulse that is specific to hydrogen. The protons absorb the energy of the pulse, and this causes them to spin or precess in a direction different from that of the original magnetic field. The specific frequency, called the Larmour frequency, depends on the strength of the main magnetic field and the tissue under examination. When the RF pulse is turned off, the protons of the hydrogen slowly return to the original alignment within the magnetic field. When this happens, they release the stored energy. The released energy is picked up by the RF coil as an electric signal and transmitted to the computer system. The coils are designed in such a way that they closely fit the body contours of the patient. Many different RF coils are available for the different body parts. At approximately the same time that the RF coil is activated, the three gradient magnets jump into action. They are arranged in such a way inside the main magnet that when they are switched on and off very rapidly, they change the main magnetic field locally in a specific manner. This means that a desired area in the patient can be selected and imaged. The slices in MRI are very precise and a few millimeters thick. The orientation of the slices in the patient can be chosen freely. This is a huge advantage over all other imaging modalities.

The relaxation times describe the return of proton spin into the equilibrium situation in the main magnetic field. The relaxation is influenced by spin-lattice interactions and the neighboring atomic structures. Spin-lattice relaxation produces thermal equilibrium, reflecting the parallel or antiparallel orientation of the protons. The spin-lattice relaxation time is also called T1. The influence of the precessing protons on each other depends on the fluctuating intermolecular magnetic fields. The parallel orientation among the protons subsides with a time constant T2. T2 is usually much shorter than T1. With T1 and T2 image modalities, tissue properties can be characterized, so they are used to differentiate between tissue and tumor. As with all other imaging modalities, the signal-to-noise ratio limits the resolution. Therefore, the volumes of voxel chosen have to be large enough to get a reasonable signal-to-noise ratio using acceptable imaging times. As in classical radiology, contrast agents can be used to improve the contrast behavior of certain tissues. Usually paramagnetic substances containing metallo complexes are used. MRI contrast works by altering the local magnetic field in the tissue under examination. Normal and abnormal tissues respond differently to this slight alteration, giving different magnetic signals. These altered signals are transferred to the images, which allows visualization of various types of tissue abnormalities and disease processes.

MRI is the ideal imaging modality for soft tissues. Tumors in the brain and infections of the brain, spine, and joints are much better demonstrated by MRI than by any other method. Ligaments and tendons can be investigated in detail. Torn ligaments and damaged tendon tissue can be localized exactly and the extent of the lesion visualized.

The major shortcoming of MRI for the equine patient is the necessity of general anesthesia to use its full potential. Small stationary MRI units have been developed for the examination of the lower equine limb, but the limiting factor is patient movement. Additional information of MRI physics and clinical examples of MR images are found in Chapter 76.

CLINICAL APPLICATION OF DIAGNOSTIC MEDICAL IMAGING

Distal Interphalangeal Joint

The distal interphalangeal joint is radiographed with the horse's hoof placed on a wooden block. Routinely, a horizontal lateral view and an angled dorsopalmar or dorsoplantar view is obtained first. Oblique projections at 45-degree angles from dorsomedial and dorsolateral, respectively, may be added. Rarely, a horizontal dorsopalmar or dorsoplantar view is obtained. This projection allows visualization of the joint space but is also the only projection in which the thickness of the medial and lateral hoof wall can be measured. This is sometimes helpful for the farrier when hoof balance is in question. A dorsopalmar or dorsoplantar view at a 60-degree angle to the floor with the horse's hoof placed forward is routinely taken to assess the distal phalanx. Additional, oblique 45-degree views are taken when a fracture of the distal phalanx is suspected.

It is advisable to obtain four views, a dorsopalmar or dorsoplantar, a lateral, and two oblique views, when a nondisplaced fracture is suspected. The distal interphalangeal joint may be altered by osteoarthritis, typically seen as new bone formation at the extensor process, the medial and lateral aspects of the articular surfaces, and the articular margins of the distal sesamoid (navicular) bone. The joint space may become incongruent. Rarely, subchondral bone sclerosis can be visualized. Cystlike lesions may be present in the subchondral bone of the distal or the middle phalanx. A variety of different types of fractures of the distal phalanx can be diagnosed (Fig. 75-10). The solar border of the distal phalanx may become very irregular and lucent with pedal osteitis. On scintigrams, an increased uptake is seen in the pool phase, most accentuated in the dorsal aspect of the normal distal phalanx. This occurs because of the naturally occurring hyperthermia of this region. The dorsal hoof wall is evaluated in laminitis. The dorsal contour of the hoof wall and the distal phalanx in the lateral projection is no longer parallel when a rotation of the distal phalanx has occurred. Pododermatitis causes focal increased accumulation of the bone label in the toe region. Most often, the pool phase shows localized hyperperfusion. Extremely high concentrations in the toe region are seen in laminitis. The highest accumulation of the bone tracer is seen with fractures of the distal phalanx.

Distal Sesamoid Bone

The distal sesamoid bone requires the best possible image quality to identify subtle lesions. High-resolution screens, collimation, and good positioning techniques help achieve this goal. For the evaluation of navicular disease, both distal sesamoid bones are routinely radiographed. A lateral radiograph is obtained with the horse's hoof placed on a wooden block. The central beam is directed in an imaginary line representing the continuation of the deep digital flexor, approximately 2 cm below the coronary band. It is very important that the central beam hit the cassette parallel to the bulbs of the heels. Otherwise, the distal sesamoid bone is projected obliquely, and this makes interpretation more difficult. The second view is taken with the hoof placed on a specially constructed wooden block. The angle of the block to the floor is 55 degrees. The central beam is directed horizontally or 5 degrees downward in the midline, approximately 1 cm above the coronary band. To avoid artifacts,

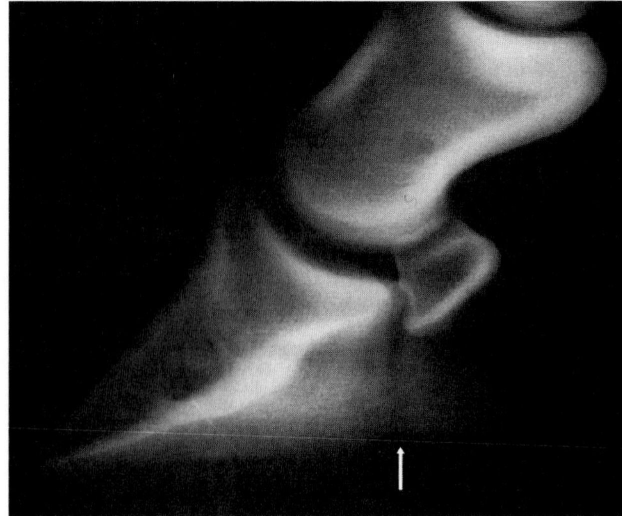

Figure 75-10. A fracture line in the distal phalanx *(arrow)* is visible in this poor-quality lateral radiographic view only because the x-ray beam is oriented perpendicular the fracture line.

the collateral sulci of the frog are filled with a tissue-equivalent material (playdough). The third projection, the tangential view, is performed with the horse's hoof placed under its belly. This limb is not bearing weight, and the x-ray tube is positioned under the horse's belly. The tube-to-cassette distance therefore is usually less than 1 m, but this depends on the size of the horse. Approximately the same distance should be used for both forelimbs. This palmaroproximal–dorsodistal view is performed with an angle of 45 degrees to the floor (Fig. 75-11). With a very steep pastern, this angle is increased to 55 degrees; horses with a sloping metacarpophalangeal or metatarsophalangeal angle require a flattening of the angle to 35 degrees to avoid superimposition of the palmar or plantar aspect of the metacarpophalangeal or metatarsophalangeal joint. The beam is centered over the deepest point between the bulbs of the heel. There is a tendency to center the beam too far palmar or plantar. To avoid backscatter from the hoof and the floor, tight collimation is used.[7]

The lateral view gives information not only about the navicular beam itself but also about the limb axis and particularly about the distal interphalangeal joint and the distal phalanx. The articular surface of the distal sesamoid bone should be smooth; the spongiosa should be regular and fine and clearly delineated from the subchondral bone of the flexor surface. The flexor surface itself is smooth. On a perpendicular view, the sagittal ridge of the distal sesamoid bone is visible. Sometimes, there is a small indentation in the sagittal ridge slightly distal to the middle portion. This is a normal variation and should not be misinterpreted as an abnormality. The dorsopalmar or dorsoplantar view depicts the distal sesamoid bone superimposed on the middle phalanx. This should be noted because (1) lesions in the middle phalanx may be falsely attributed to changes in the distal sesamoid bone, and (2) smaller lesions in the distal sesamoid bone may not become apparent. The distal sesamoid bone normally has a regular bony pattern. The proximal and distal borders should be smooth. Typically, two contours are recognizable, one for the articular surface and the other for the flexor surface. The tangential or skyline view is the best to depict subtle or early changes. The distal sesamoid bone is superimposed only over the palmar processes, and the center region, where most pathology is seen, is free of superimposition. Again, artifacts may occur because of the frog. The distal sesamoid bone normally has a smooth flexor surface, with a more or less pointed sagittal ridge. The subchondral bone of this flexor surface should have the same thickness from medial to lateral. There may be a crescent-shaped small lucency in the area of the sagittal ridge, which represents the indentation described earlier.

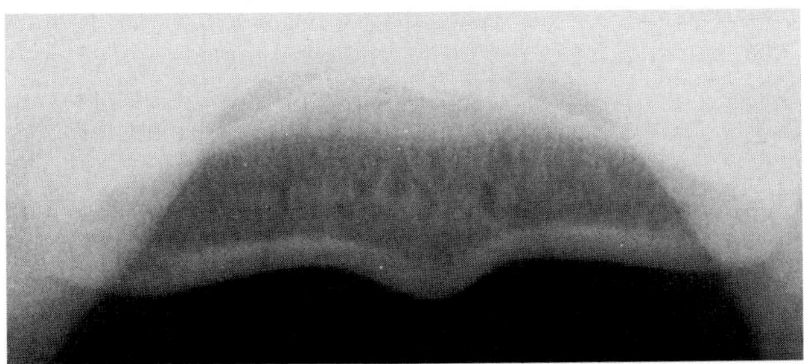

Figure 75-11. Normal radiographic appearance of the distal sesamoid bone in the tangential projection taken at a 45-degree angle relative to the floor.

The most common reason to radiograph the distal sesamoid bones is suspected navicular disease (Figs. 75-12 and 75-13). This term includes a variety of radiographic findings. The most typical radiographic pattern found in navicular disease is a defect or lucency in the subchondral bone in the sagittal ridge region (Fig. 75-14). In these cases, the spongiosa in this region is sclerotic, and the junction between the spongiosa and the subchondral bone plate becomes indistinct. This may or may not be accompanied by distention of the channels at the distal (and less frequently at the proximal) border of the distal sesamoid bone. The so-called channels represent synovial invaginations of the distal interphalangeal joint. Spurring at the lateral (and less frequently at the medial) proximal distal sesamoid bone border may be present. Sometimes, small fragments at the distal aspect of the distal sesamoid bone, usually medially

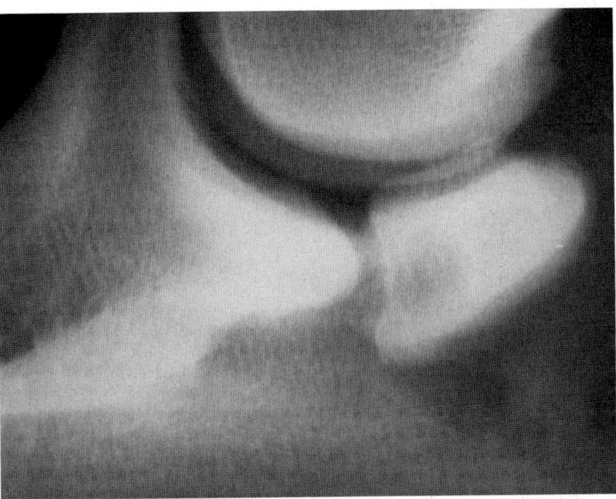

Figure 75-12. Lateral radiographic view of a distal sesamoid bone with marked sclerosis of the spongiosa in the proximal region of the bone. No delineation between the flexor cortex and the spongiosa is visible.

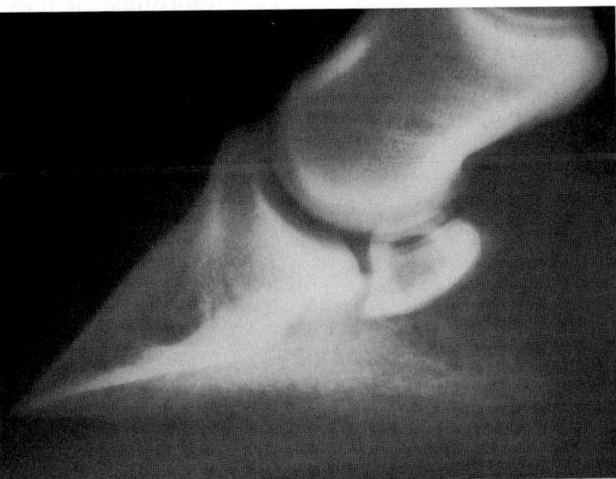

Figure 75-13. Lateral radiograph of a distal sesamoid bone with a cyst within the spongiosa. This is a very rare finding and is attributed to the osteochondrosis complex.

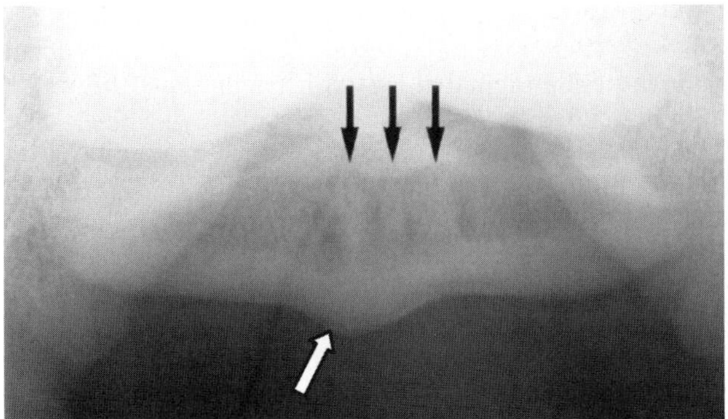

Figure 75-14. Tangential view of a distal sesamoid bone with focal sclerosis of the spongiosa *(black arrows)* and indistinct differentiation near the flexor surface. Note a very thin, flat lucency in the flexor cortex in the region of the sagittal ridge *(white arrow)*. This may develop into a larger lytic lesion.

and laterally to the sagittal ridge, may be present. They most likely stem from separate centers of ossification. True avulsion fractures of the distal or proximal edge of the distal sesamoid bone are rare and typically cause lameness.[8-13] Sagittal or parasagittal fractures of the distal sesamoid bone are rare. Rarely, bipartite distal sesamoid bones may pose a problem in the diagnosis of a fracture. Small spikes on the flexor surface can be seen with high-quality radiographs. Such spikes most likely represent calcifications and are probably secondary to navicular bursitis. With septic navicular bursitis, the flexor cortex appears lucent approximately 7 days after the insult (e.g., a penetrating wound). The navicular bursa can be imaged ultrasonographically, but the procedure is demanding and requires softening of the solar region of the hoof.

MRI and CT are very good tools for the evaluation of the distal sesamoid bone. MRI in the standing sedated horse produces adequate images, but it is susceptible to artifacts, mostly because of motion. Scintigraphic scanning of the distal sesamoid bone is carried out with the horse's hoof placed on the scanning head and from the lateral aspect with the horse positioned on a block of wood (Fig. 75-15). Very intense uptake in the distal sesamoid bone is usually associated with radiographic changes compatible with navicular disease.[14] However, in some cases, this imaging pattern is the only obvious finding. When the image is not well demarcated, inflammation of the distal sesamoid bone is usually the cause. This is quite often observed together with accumulation of the bone label in the deep digital flexor tendon. Prognosis appears to be more favorable with this finding than when the uptake is more intense.

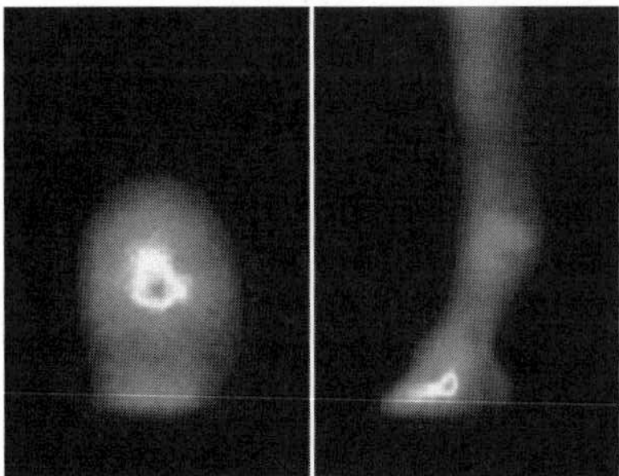

Figure 75-15. Scintigraphic views of the distal sesamoid bone. Clinically, navicular bursitis was suspected. Radiographs were normal. There is intense increased uptake in the center of the distal sesamoid bone. This is also visible on the lateral view. A lesion of the flexor surface is suspected.

The insertion of the deep digital flexor tendon can be the site of high uptake, suggesting tearing. By combining the pool and late phase images, the lesion can be further evaluated. Increased perfusion is seen with soft tissue involvement and hyperemia. Lack of hyperemia in the early imaging phase can be interpreted as only bony involvement. The enhanced accumulation at the insertion site seems to have a fair prognosis. Radiographically, often no abnormalities are found with this condition.

The lateral scintigraphic view quite often allows better localization of the exact site of increased uptake. Uptake at the insertion of the deep digital flexor tendon (DDFT) can easily be distinguished from other pedal bone disorders. Uptake in the distal sesamoid bone region is not always easily distinguished from active ossification of the cartilage of the pedal bones. The solar view or the dorsal view helps in such situations.

Sometimes the ossified cartilages of the pedal bones are fractured. In the bone scan, a line of intense uptake is seen.

Proximal Interphalangeal Joint

The radiographic technique for the proximal interphalangeal joint is less demanding than for the metacarpophalangeal or metatarsophalangeal joint. Again, lateral and dorsopalmar, dorsoplantar radiographs are obtained, as well as two oblique views at 45 degrees. The angle of the dorsopalmar view is less than that for the distal interphalangeal joint, approximately 10 degrees, because the angulation of the joint is less. The most common finding of this joint is osteoarthritis. Large osteophytes, enthesiophytes, and periosteal proliferations (ringbone) at the dorsal aspect of the proximal and middle phalanx, and various degrees of joint incongruity are common. Subchondral bone cysts may be found, both in the distal epiphysis of the proximal phalanx and in the proximal aspect of the middle phalanx. Fractures do occur in the middle phalanx but seem to be less frequent than in the proximal phalanx.[15]

Scintigraphy is less rewarding in the middle phalanx. Cystlike lesions can cause increased uptake, but quite often only normal or reduced bone metabolism can be detected. Periarticular new bone formation around the proximal interphalangeal joint shows little bone activity. Sometimes the insertion of the superficial digital flexor tendon is associated with increased uptake as a result of tearing. Osteoarthritis of the proximal interphalangeal joint is easily recognized by a clearly delineated enhanced uptake. The tendon sheath, the flexor tendons, and the distal sesamoidean ligaments are best imaged with ultrasonography. CT and MRI have been described but are not routinely performed.

Metacarpophalangeal and Metatarsophalangeal Joints

The metacarpophalangeal and metatarsophalangeal joints are two of the most commonly radiographed regions of the horse. The radiographic technique appears to be simple;

however, it is quite difficult to obtain properly positioned radiographs. This can be explained by the lack of clear anatomic landmarks that can be used for positioning the limb and centering the x-ray beam. The minimal standard investigation consists of two imaging planes at right angles to each other. A good lateral view should show the articulation without any distortion, and the articular radius of the metacarpal condyle with the proximal phalanx is smaller than the radius for the condylar articular surface near the sesamoid bones. The dorsopalmar projection should be taken in the direction of the sagittal plane of the forelimb. The central beam is directed approximately 20 degrees from proximal to distal to avoid superimposition of the distal border of the joint with the sesamoid bones. A dorsopalmar radiograph is orthogonal to the joint when an imaginary line between the sesamoid bones falls into the sagittal groove of the proximal phalanx (Fig. 75-16). If this is not the case, the medial and lateral aspects of the articular surfaces become more pointed, and this is often misread as osteophytosis.

Two additional oblique views should be obtained to assess not only the sesamoid bones but also the articular margins of the joint. The dorsal aspect of the sagittal ridge of MCIII/MTIII can best be demonstrated by a lateral

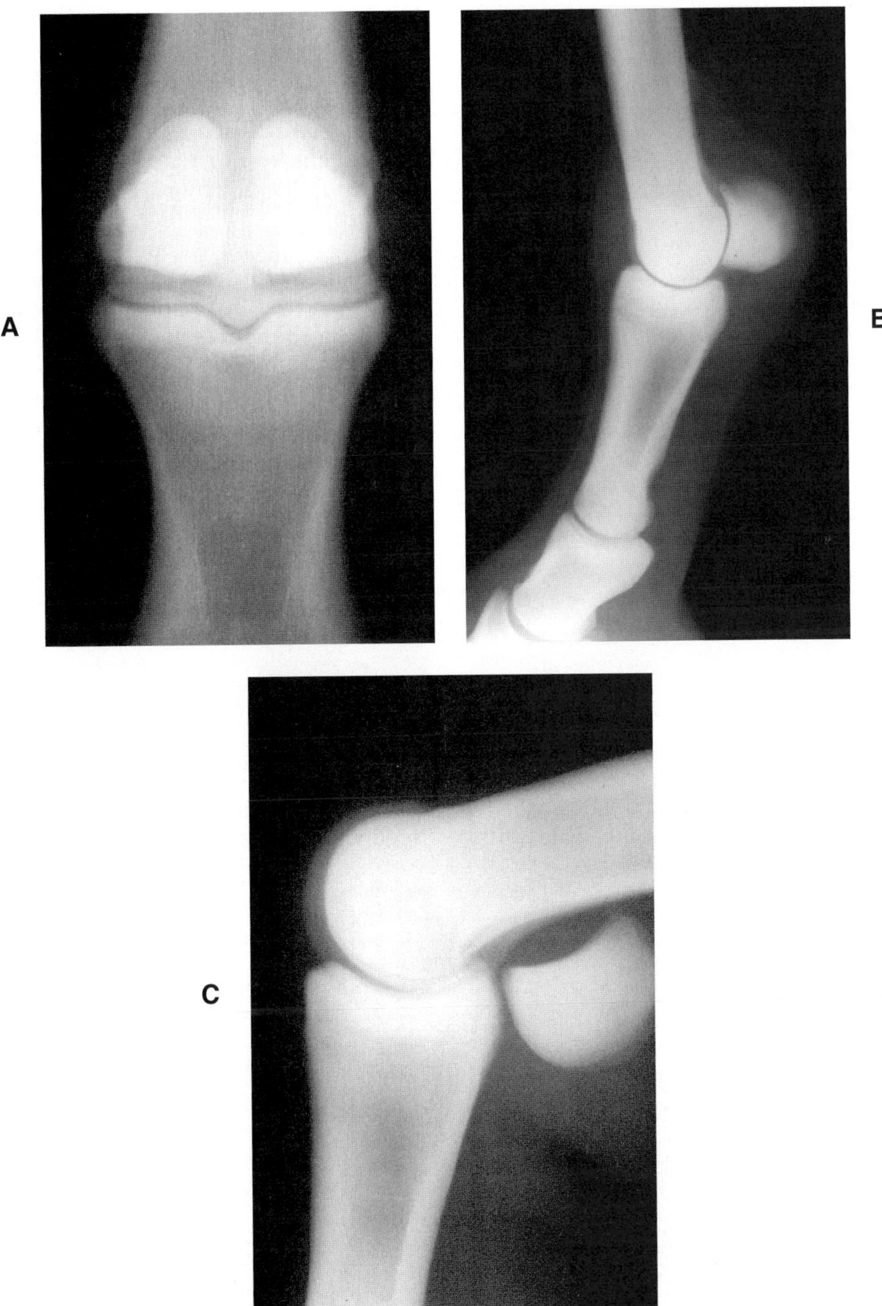

Figure 75-16. Dorsopalmar (**A**), lateromedial (**B**), and flexed lateral (**C**) radiographs of a normal metacarpophalangeal joint. Note the correct positioning enabling easier image interpretation.

projection with the joint flexed. A number of additional oblique projections with proximodistally tilted x-ray beams allows identification of unusual disorders of the proximal sesamoids and plantar fractures of the proximal phalanx (Fig. 75-17). A special dorsopalmar projection with the limb positioned on a farrier's stand enables inspection of the caudal joint space, mostly to detect condylar fractures. Sometimes, multiple oblique views are necessary to completely characterize fractures of the proximal phalanx before surgical intervention.

For the evaluation of the metacarpophalangeal or metatarsophalangeal joint, the following radiographic criteria should be checked: soft tissue shadows, articular space, joint margins, subchondral bone density, articular surface continuity, marginal osteophytes, intracapsular and intra-articular new bone formation (enthesiophytes), and the presence of osteochondral fragments.

Subchondral sclerosis, osteophytes, and enthesiophytes (usually at the dorsal articular surface) are quite common findings. The high frequency of these signs makes the evaluation of their clinical significance quite difficult. If clinical signs are localized to this joint, these radiographic signs are more likely the result of osteoarthritis.[16]

Intra-articular fragments are found quite frequently, especially in the younger horse. The frequency of bony fragments in the dorsal part of the joint is higher. In a recent study, the authors found that the presence of bone fragments in the dorsal joint space was twice as likely than in the palmar or plantar space.[17] Some fragments represent avulsion fractures, and their origin may show a fracture bed.

Free fragments in the dorsal joint space are more likely to represent osteochondritis dissecans, and quite often the dorsal sagittal ridge of the third metacarpus or third metatarsus has an irregular bony contour representing the fragment bed. For most of the other osteochondral fragments, no fracture bed can be demonstrated with radiographs.

Circumscribed radiolucent areas in the subchondral bone may represent cystlike lesions (Fig. 75-18). They can be observed in the bone plate of the mid-sagittal groove of the proximal phalanx or in the condyles of the third metacarpus or third metatarsus. Fine radiolucent discontinuities originating from the dorsal part of the sagittal groove of the proximal phalanx in horses with moderate or severe lameness represent fissure fractures.[18] For the evaluation of the proximal sesamoid bones, the borders and the bone structure are assessed. Irregular bone margins and radiolucent areas are signs of recent bone trauma. Avulsions of bony fragments occur at the apex as well as at the base of the proximal sesamoid bones. The fracture bed is usually easily located. Enthesiophytes of the distal and proximal articular surface of the sesamoid bones is associated with osteoarthritis.

Ultrasonography is commonly performed in the metacarpophalangeal or metatarsophalangeal region. Certainly, the flexor tendons, the short and long distal sesamoidean ligaments, the annular ligament, and the dorsal aspect of the joint, including the bony surfaces of the metacarpal or metatarsal condyle and the proximal phalanx, can be visualized. A detailed description of ultrasonographic changes of the flexor tendons is presented in Chapter 86.

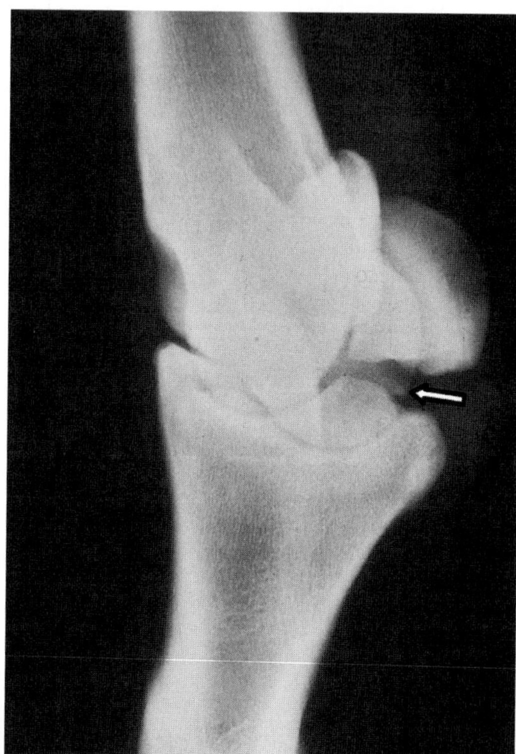

Figure 75-17. An oblique projection angled 45 degrees from proximal to distal to visualize the plantar aspect of the metatarsophalangeal joint. Note the small fragment located at the plantar articular rim.

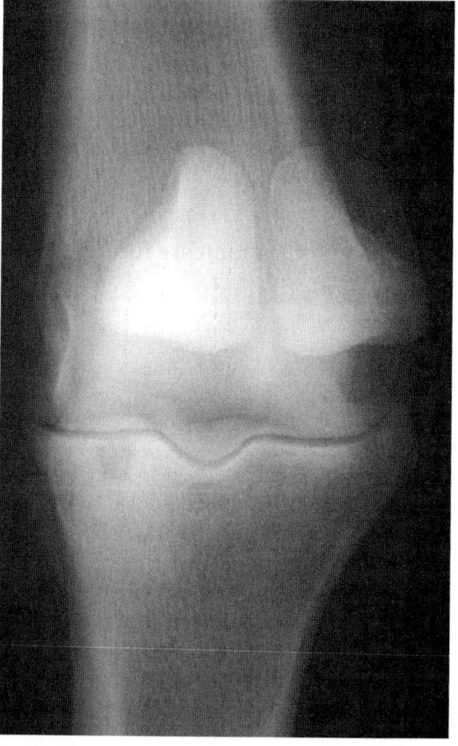

Figure 75-18. Oblique dorsopalmar view of a metacarpophalangeal joint. There is a focal lucency, surrounded by sclerosis at the medial proximal aspect of the proximal phalanx. Diagnosis: cystlike lesion.

On scintigraphy, the metacarpophalangeal or metatarsophalangeal joint very often shows quite intriguing findings, e.g., increased uptake in the dorsal aspect of the joint, linear or multifocal uptake along the joint surface, and uptake in the proximal sesamoid bones. The proximal phalanx can also show abnormal uptake at the insertions of the ligaments. Not all of these signs have clinical significance or show radiologic alterations, and only a thorough lameness examination may prove their clinical relevance. Typically, the metacarpophalangeal or metatarsophalangeal region is examined scintigraphically with a lateral approach. Dorsal views can be easily achieved by holding the front hoof on a farrier's stand and positioning the camera dorsally onto the limb. This view allows the detection of abnormal uptake in the subchondral bone plate and in the sagittal groove of the proximal phalanx. The evaluation of the distribution of the bone label in the proximal sesamoid bones is not so simple with this view, because of superimposed articular structures. The true distribution of the bone label of the proximal sesamoid bones is therefore best performed with palmar views, which are rarely possible in the standing animal. Findings detected in the proximal sesamoid bones include increased or reduced uptake in the apex, at the base, or near the articular surface.

Metacarpus and Metatarsus

A special location to evaluate in the metacarpal or metatarsal region is the origin of the suspensory ligament (the interosseus muscle) at the palmar or plantar aspect of the MCIII or MTIII, respectively. Radiographically, an avulsion fragment may be present in the acute phase; more chronically, the bone pattern in the plantar or palmar aspect of the MTIII/MCIII is irregular and sclerosed. Ultrasonography may (or may not) depict any lesion on the proximal suspensory ligament. Acute lesions have hypoechoic regions of various sizes; more chronic injuries are recognized by an altered fiber pattern, increased diameter of the ligament, and calcification.[19] CT depicts these changes even more clearly; however, the need for general anesthesia often precludes the use of CT.

Scintigraphy is used to detect metabolic bone changes in this region. Trauma produces intense focal accumulation of the bone label. Uptake ratios can be calculated to compare ROI of the origin with an adjacent ROI of the cannon bone or with soft tissue. High ratios (bone, 4:1; soft tissue, 12:1) signify a fresh lesion.[20] The metacarpus is assessed with a lateral and a dorsal view. The most frequent abnormalities are linear, focal, or multifocal concentrations of the labeling agent in or along the splint bones. The clinical significance of such signs is usually quite low. MCIII/MTIII show one or two linear regions of higher uptake representing the dorsal and caudal cortices. Stress fractures show intense linear uptake in an oblique direction. It is not uncommon to see intense focal spots in the medullary cavity of MCIII/MTIII. This behavior is known as enostosis. Their significance is controversial.

Carpus

The carpus is a very complex anatomic structure, so it is necessary to use multiple beam angles for radiographic evaluation. The simplest views are the dorsopalmar and the lateromedial projections. However, these views may not demonstrate lesions of the small cuboidal bones in the proximal and distal row. Two oblique views, one at an angle of approximately 30 degrees from dorsomedial and the other 45 degrees from dorsolateral, are used to depict the dorsal contour and to visualize the accessory carpal bone and the vestigial metacarpal bones. Special skyline views are added when the third carpal bone or the radial and intermediate carpal bones have to be assessed. The flexed lateromedial projection allows the best visualization of the deeper aspects of the middle carpal and the antebrachiocarpal joints. This view is also very helpful in separating lesions of the small cuboidal bones, which are superimposed on the straight lateral view. Therefore, if a practitioner has only two radiographic cassettes, the dorsopalmar, lateromedial oblique and flexed lateromedial views should be taken to get the most information on carpal pathology.

Several anatomic variations should not be read as pathologic findings. For example, the remnant of the styloid is the first carpal bone, which is present in approximately 40% of all horses. An irregular, almost cystlike pattern in the accessory carpal bone is also normal. The radiographic changes seen in the carpus depend heavily on the use of the horse. Racehorses commonly suffer from various forms and degrees of carpal disorders, including slab fractures and sclerosis of the third carpal bone, as well as osteochondral fractures of the distal aspect of the radial and intermediate carpal bone. The other small cuboidal bones are less frequently affected. Hyperextension injuries and repeated trauma to the carpus result in periosteal and articular reactions, mostly at the dorsal surface of the carpal bones. This is accompanied by dorsal soft tissue swelling, which often includes joint effusion. Fractures of the accessory carpal bone may occur both in racehorses and in jumping or event horses. The fracture may be articular or nonarticular. Horses not used for racing are far less commonly affected with carpal injuries. Osteoarthritis is sometimes seen in the antebrachiocarpal joint and will be recognized by enthesiophytosis of the lateral and mostly medial aspects of the distal radius and radial and ulnar carpal bones, respectively. The subchondral bone density increases, and the joint space becomes irregular. Osteochondrosis lesions are rare in the carpal region, but when present, they usually appear as subchondral cystic lesions in the distal radial epiphysis.

Ultrasonography is a good technique for evaluating the tendons at the dorsal carpal area and the carpal sheath. Typically, radiography is performed first, followed by ultrasonography to distinguish articular distention from tendon sheath abnormalities. In addition, the integrity of the individual tendons and collateral ligaments can be analyzed.[21]

Although ultrasonography is usually the modality of choice because it can be performed in the standing horse, it lacks the topographic overview, and CT and MRI are superior and easier to interpret.[22] Both bony and soft tissue structures can be assessed at the same time. Limitations are cost and the need for anesthesia.

Scintigraphy seems to play a less important role in the carpal region. It is mostly used to detect occult fractures. In the medullary cavity of the distal radius, an increased uptake can be found, which is called enostoses and is similar to panosteitis in dogs. Fissure and stress fractures in the distal radius are easily diagnosed with bone scanning.

Tarsus and Tibia

The radiographic examination of the equine tarsus is based on at least two projections at a right angle to each other. Additional oblique views facilitate the radiographic interpretation. The x-ray beam should always be centered over the distal intertarsal joint, because this is the joint most frequently affected. The direction of the x-ray beam of the lateral view is not really at 90 degrees to the median plane but rather at an angle of 105 to 110 degrees. It is important that the limb under examination be weightbearing. For the oblique and dorsoplantar views, this can be achieved by holding up the front leg on the examination side. For the lateral view, two possible positions are used. In the first one, the contralateral side is held up by an assistant and the x-ray beam is oriented parallel to the floor. In the second method, the horse is standing squarely on its rear legs but the projection of the x-ray beam is slightly angled downward (7 degrees). The centered beam is still aimed at the distal intertarsal joint. High-resolution rare-earth intensifying screens are recommended. If images with more detail are desired, a scatter grid is a necessity.

The equine tarsus exhibits some anatomic variations that make interpretation difficult.[23,24] In-depth knowledge of the anatomy is an important prerequisite. For instance, the sometimes very impressive osteophytes on the proximal dorsal metatarsus or at the distal end of the medial trochlear ridge of the talus are often considered pathologic. However, if the borders of these proliferations are smooth and well mineralized, they have no clinical significance.

The tarsal regions most likely to have radiographic changes are the distal intermediate ridge of the tibia, the lateral trochlear ridge of the talus (both frequent locations of osteochondrosis [OC] lesions), and the intertarsal articulations. The OC fragments of the distal intermediate ridge of the tibia may appear radiographically separated, but they are frequently held in place by the articular cartilage or soft tissue. Loose fragments are usually situated in the lowest part of the joint cavity, which extends all the way down to the level of the proximal row of tarsal bones. The use of a high-intensity examination light may be helpful to detect poorly mineralized bony fragments. In the talocrural joint, OC may cause degenerative changes. The dorsomedial to plantarolateral view is best for depicting the lateral trochlear ridge and its osteochondritis dissecans fragments. At the distal end of the medial trochlear ridge, one may occasionally find a small, calcified shadow, which does not seem to cause any clinical signs. Cystlike lesions are rare but have been observed at the base of the talus. Compression of the third or central tarsal bone can be found in foals. Slab fractures of the third and central tarsal bones may be diagnosed in racing breeds. Avulsion fractures of the articular borders of the medial or lateral malleolus quite often occur in the jumping and the cutting horse. The exact position of the fragment should be identified with oblique radiographs before surgical removal.[25]

The most common disorder of the tarsus is osteoarthritis of the distal and proximal intertarsal and tarsometatarsal joints. Changes of the distal intertarsal joint are most frequently observed, followed in frequency by changes of the tarsometatarsal and proximal intertarsal joints. The typical radiographic alterations are subchondral sclerosis, marginal osteophyte or enthesiophyte formation, alterations in the width of the articular space, and deformations, especially of the dorsal contours of the third and central tarsal bones. One of the most valuable signs for the evaluation of the diseased tarsal joints is narrowing and disappearance of the synovial groove. This sign is very reliable, but is easily seen and inspected only in radiographs of excellent quality and positioning. In general, only the synovial grooves of the distal intertarsal and the tarsometatarsal articulations are clearly demonstrated. The groove of the proximal intertarsal joint is usually not sufficiently depicted. In osteoarthritis, the synovial groove becomes unapparent because of newly formed bone.

In the assessment of tarsal radiographs, the talocalcaneal articulation and the sustentaculum tali should not be overlooked. The talocalcaneal joint is normally seen as a discrete, straight, radiolucent line. The articular space becomes irregular, and subchondral sclerosis and osteolysis are present in the case of osteoarthritis. This finding is clinically relevant. The sustentaculum tali is usually affected in conjunction with inflammation of the tarsal sheath. A special skyline view can be taken to evaluate the surface of the sustentaculum tali. The surface becomes irregular and roughened when the sheath is chronically affected. The radiographs of the tarsus are an important part of the prepurchase examination, because the clinical examination sometimes seems to be inconspicuous even when marked joint alterations are present.

Whereas radiography is commonly used to find bony changes, ultrasonography adds information on the soft tissues. The plantar ligament, the tarsal sheath, and the calcaneal bursa are the most commonly affected structures. Ultrasonography may be very useful to assess joint fluid and synovial hypertrophy of the tarsocrural joint. Again, CT gives even better anatomic detail.[26]

Scintigraphy is used to detect early osteoarthritis, and trauma and tears at the insertion of collateral ligaments. Focally increased concentrations of the imaging agent may be observed in the joint spaces (distal intertarsal, tarsometatarsal, and occasionally the proximal intertarsal joint), representing well-developed chronic osteoarthritis with no apparent radiographic alterations.

Fatigue or stress fractures of the tibia are very difficult to visualize in the early stage on radiographs. Stress fractures of the tibia produce a distinct uptake pattern.

Focal uptake in the medullary cavity may represent enostosis. In the proximal part of the tibia, very intense and well-delineated regions of high uptake can be caused by avascular areas or bone infarcts. Smaller uptake regions of similar intensity can also be observed in fissures of the tibial plateau.

Proximal Limb

The large joints, such as the femoropatellar, femorotibial, coxofemoral, and scapulohumeral joints, are best radiographed under general anesthesia. Although it is possible to examine the most proximal joints in the limbs in a standing sedated horse and accept lower image quality, it is not advised to radiograph the coxofemoral joint without general anesthesia. The scatter radiation to which assisting personnel will be exposed must be taken very seriously. Protective lead aprons and gloves reduce the radiation only partially. Because large soft tissue masses have to be penetrated by the x-rays, a large amount of scatter radiation is produced, which in turn decreases image contrast. To improve image quality, grids have to be used and tight collimation is mandatory. Cones and other x-ray beam limiters are useful, particularly in the stifle region.

Cubital Joint and Humerus

The radiographic examination of the cubital joint is easier than that of the scapulohumeral joint. General anesthesia is not necessary. The mediolateral view is obtained with the leg pulled forward and downward. The craniocaudal view is taken with the leg positioned slightly cranially to allow room for the cassette to be placed caudal to the olecranon. The central beam is angled slightly downward. The most frequent findings in the elbow region are various types of fractures of the olecranon. Subchondral bone cysts may be found in the proximal radius. Primary degenerative disease is rare.

The collateral ligaments are accessible for ultrasonographic scanning and may show alterations in fiber alignment, size, and echogenicity.

Scintigraphy may be helpful in the detection of smaller subchondral bone cysts (Fig. 75-19). The anconeal process can be traumatized, producing a very high tracer uptake. Finally, stress fractures may occur. Their usual site is the distal part of the humerus. In the acute phase, the uptake region is very clearly delineated.

Scapulohumeral Joint

Most examiners image the shoulder in the standing tranquilized horse with the affected leg extended cranially. The beam is centered from medial to lateral, with a slight angle from cranial to avoid superimposition of the contralateral shoulder region. Oblique and skyline views can be taken to outline the tubercles. The resulting images may be of

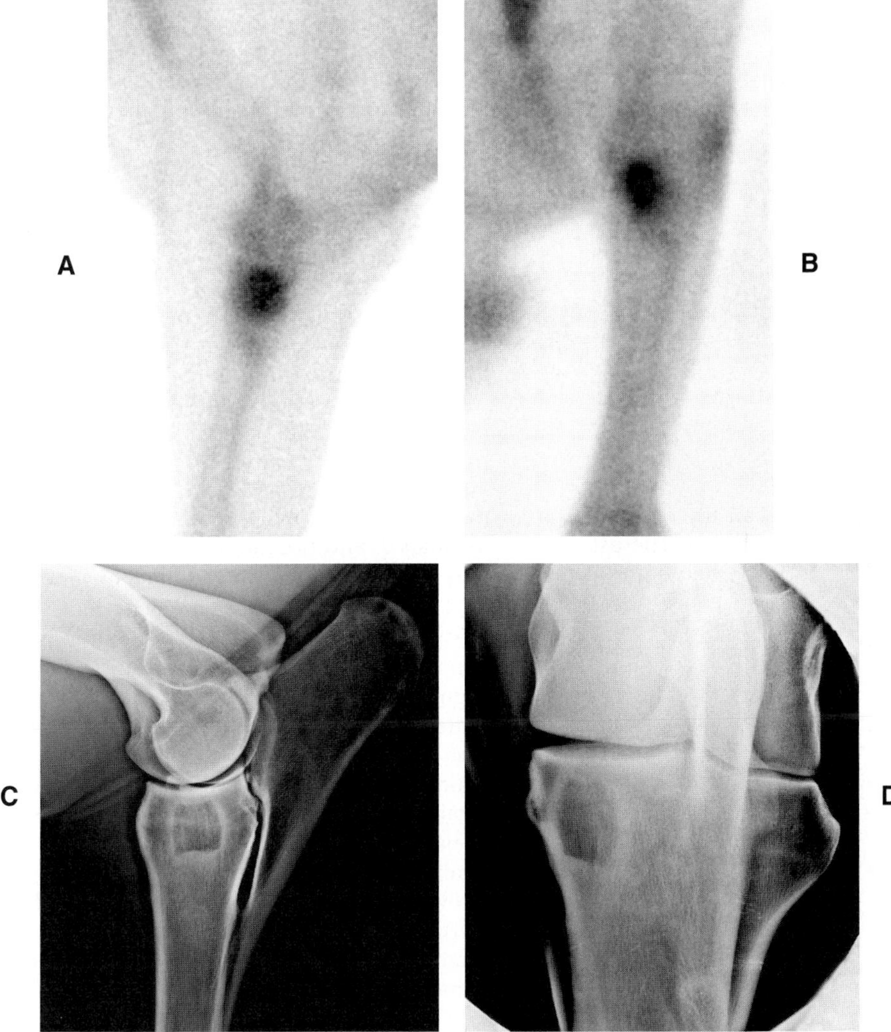

Figure 75-19. Lateral (**A**) and craniocaudal (**B**) scintigraphic view of the cubital joint. There is marked focal uptake of the bone tracer in the proximal radius. Mediolateral (**C**) and craniocaudal (**D**) radiographs document a large subchondral bone cyst in the proximal radius.

satisfactory quality and allow a radiographic diagnosis. If this is not possible, the horse should be anesthetized lying with the side under examination on the imaging system. This allows the use of the scatter grids, small examination fields, and screens with higher resolution. The positions of the standing and of the anesthetized horse are identical; the limb has to be pulled cranially and upward. The central x-ray beam is aimed at a point just below the cervical spine at the base of the thoracic inlet. If everything has been done correctly, the resulting image shows the shoulder joint lying in the shadow of the trachea, free from the rib cage and below the cervical spine. The articular space with the proximal humerus and the distal part of the scapula will be visible. The most common findings include fractures of the supraglenoid tubercle, and of the greater, intermediate, or lesser tubercle. Very rarely, luxations of the scapulohumeral joints are seen. Osteochondrosis may be present in the form of cartilage flaps of the humeral head or cystlike lesions of the glenoid of the scapula. Osteoarthritis is usually secondary to trauma or OC and typically shows a flattening and elongation of the humeral head with subchondral sclerosis of the glenoid of the scapula.

Ultrasonography can be successfully used to diagnose alterations in the biceps tendon and bursa. The sheath may contain an abnormal amount of fluid, and there may be calcification in or around the tendon.

Scintigraphy may provide additional information on the scapulohumeral joint (Fig. 75-20). The chronically affected joint usually develops intense uptake adjacent to the actual joint space. But in some cases, negative contrast is found. Subchondral cystic lesions usually produce increased focal accumulation of the bone label. The attachment of the joint capsule may show increased uptake. Focal uptake can also be observed in the caudal region of the greater tubercle, representing insertion problems of the infraspinatus muscle or bursitis (bursa infraspinati). The proximal cranial aspect of the humerus may be the site of enhanced, mostly clearly delineated uptake, representing inflammatory disorders of the bicipital bursa or the biceps tendon.

Fractures of the deltoid tuberosity are not always localized clinically, but on scintigrams will show up as a region of intense uptake.

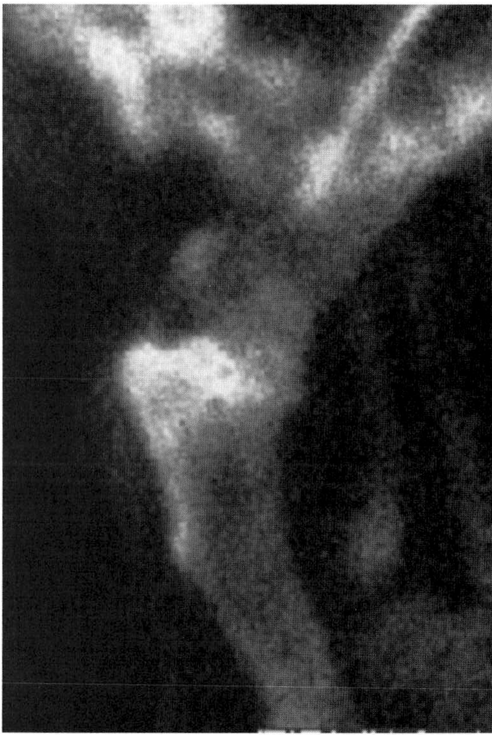

Figure 75-20. Scintigraphic image of the shoulder region of a horse with sudden unwillingness to jump obstacles. Radiographs were normal. There is a focal increased accumulation of the bone tracer in the region of insertion of the supraspinatus muscle and the lateral ligaments. Acute tearing of these insertions was suspected.

Femoropatellar and Femorotibial Joints

A caudocranial and a mediolateral (or lateromedial in the standing horse) view are the standard imaging projections. When using a cone of 8 cm in diameter, two sets of caudocranial images are necessary to image both the joint and the patella. Additional oblique views to image the femoral condyles and the tibial plateau can be added.

The most common radiographic findings include fractures of the patella, tibial plateau, or intercondylar eminence; osteochondrosis; and osteoarthritis. Osteoarthritis is often secondary to meniscal injuries and cruciate ligament ruptures. The radiographs of the stifle are viewed to identify an abnormal amount of soft tissue, changes in the bony contours, and bone density. An increase of the soft tissue shadow may be caused by periarticular swelling or distended joint capsules. Increased articular filling of the femoropatellar joint can sometimes be observed. The outlines of the bones may be disrupted by an avulsion fracture at the attachment of ligaments or by fractures of the patella or the tibial crest. The contour of the trochlear ridges can be impaired by OC. Irregular contours of the lateral trochlear ridge are commonly found accompanied by flaplike fragments and irregular bone density in the affected region. Subchondral cystic lesions are commonly found in the medial femoral condyle as circular or ellipsoid radiolucent areas. The borders may be more radiodense. Cystlike lesions in the lateral condyle or the tibial plateau are rare. Most cystlike lesions have a connection to the articular space. The articular surface may be flattened or indented.

The attachment of the cruciate ligaments can be easily observed on the lateral views. Alterations of the bone margin and its structure of the medial eminence are convincing signs of tearing of the cranial cruciate ligament (Fig. 75-21). Often, avulsion fragments are also observed. Damage to the ligaments results in joint instability and produces fibrillation of the articular cartilage.[27] The consequence is formation of articular marginal osteophytes, which can best be viewed on caudocranial projections. The outlines of the eminence may be quite heavily modified by bony outgrowth. At the margins of the tibial and femoral articular surfaces, rounded bone proliferations can be seen. Loose bony fragments may be seen in the femoropatellar or the femorotibial joint. They result either from avulsion fractures or OC.

Infections of the femoropatellar or femorotibial joint occur most commonly in foals. The result is increased synovial filling of the femoropatellar joint, causing a larger joint

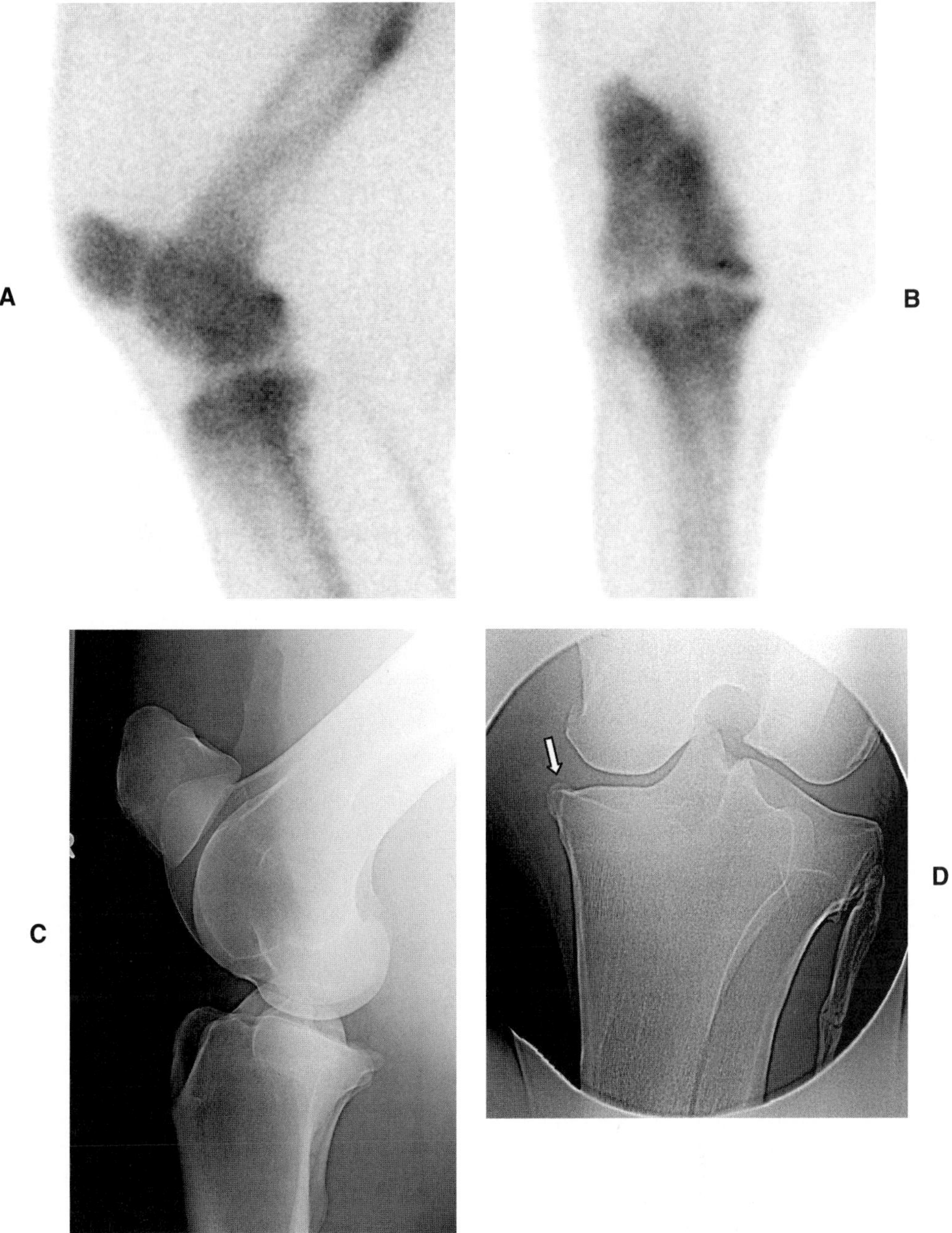

Figure 75-21. Lateral (**A**) and caudocranial (**B**) scintigraphic images of a femorotibial joint of a horse with chronic intermittent lameness. There is increased uptake in the femoral condyles in the lateral projection, which can be localized to the medial side when the caudocranial view is added. There is also increased tracer uptake on the medial aspect of the tibial plateau and the intercondylar eminence. On the lateromedial radiograph (**C**), a caudal displacement of the tibia is noted, which is characteristic for anterior cruciate ligament rupture. On the caudocranial radiograph (**D**), osteophytes at the medial aspect of the femorotibial joint *(white arrow)* indicate osteoarthritis.

space between the patella and the trochlear ridges. The enlarged joint capsule may become visible. In later stages of the infection, circular lytic regions may develop in the subchondral bone.

Ultrasonography is useful in evaluating the medial and lateral collateral ligaments, the patellar ligament, the cruciate ligaments, and the menisci. The bony contours, especially the cartilage of the trochlear ridges, can also be assessed quite easily.

Bone imaging of the femoropatellar or the femorotibial joint is very rewarding, since many discrete alterations can be visualized. It is best performed in the anesthetized animal, which allows acquisition of high count numbers and the use of collimators for better resolution.

Occult subchondral bone cysts usually produce focal areas of intense uptake. The attachment of the cruciate and meniscal ligaments can be visualized. Osteoarthritis produces increased uptake at the joint margins. It is very important in the evaluation of femoropatellar and femorotibial joint problems to obtain two scintigraphic views: a lateral and a craniocaudal. The patellar ligaments also may provoke accumulation of the bone label at their attachment sites.

Coxofemoral and Sacroiliac Joints

Several techniques have been described in the literature for the demonstration of the coxofemoral articulation in the standing horse. All result in a high radiation burden for the assisting personnel. Image quality is usually impaired by the choice of the fast intensifying screens, which have to be used to avoid patient movement. The use of a scatter grid is not possible. Therefore, it is strongly suggested that this examination be performed only in the anesthetized horse, where the patient can be positioned onto the imaging system allowing a true ventrodorsal projection. This view can be completed by additional oblique views of the coxofemoral joint. The side under examination is lowered onto the image plate. Use of x-ray beam limiting devices such as a cone greatly increases the details in the image, but positioning becomes critical. When the horse is lying on its back, the cleft in the gracilis muscle can be palpated. A point of this cleft about 10 to 12 cm from the midline serves as a landmark for centering the x-ray beam onto the coxofemoral joint.

In the normal horse, the acetabular structures and the femoral head can be seen. In the acetabulum, a shallow groove can always be discerned. In the normal articulation of the femoral head, a radiolucent area is visible where the round ligament is attached.

Arthritic changes are sometimes observed in the form of enthesiophytes. These may deform the articular head and the articular margins (Fig. 75-22). The bone density and the articular contour may become irregular. Very often, the attachment site of the round ligament becomes more pronounced. Cystlike lesions also have been observed at the site of the capital femoral physis.

Epiphyseal detachment (traumatic epiphysiolysis) is usually diagnosed before epiphyseal closure, but sometimes it is observed even after closure in well-developed colts and fillies.

The radiographic examination of the coxofemoral region should always be preceded by a pelvic overview image, allowing interpretation of the adjacent bony structures. Fractures of the ischium, ilium, tuber sacrale, and other pelvic structures may be diagnosed. Fractures of the ischial process and the third trochanter may mimic hip joint disorders. Luxations of the femur are rare events and usually easily diagnosed by the displaced femoral head.

Scintigraphic evaluation of the pelvis is particularly useful because of the limitations of radiography (Fig. 75-23).

The local activity and the shape of the anatomic landmarks are compared. The sacroiliac joints, the tuber ischii, the lumbosacral joints, and the tuber coxae are most frequently affected. High focal uptake of the bone label in the sacral region is not infrequent. Fissures do occur in the

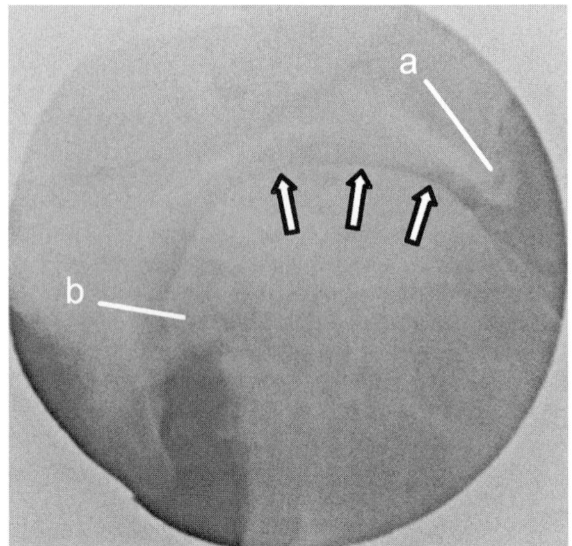

Figure 75-22. Coned-down radiographic view of the coxofemoral joint of a Friesian stallion. Severe osteoarthritis is indicated by flattening of the femoral head *(arrows)*, and by marked osteophyte production on the acetabular rims (a and b). Interestingly, the horse was only moderately lame.

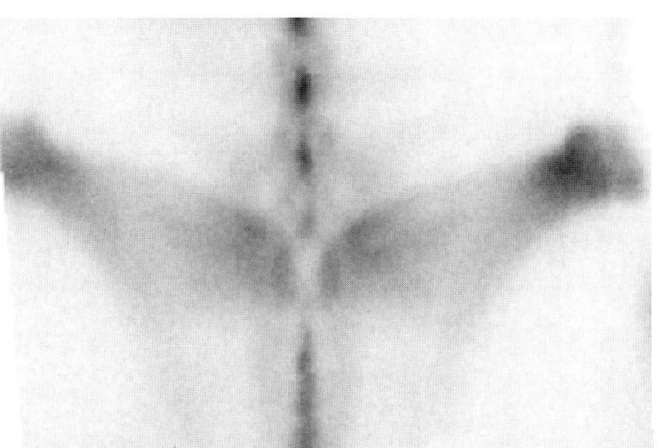

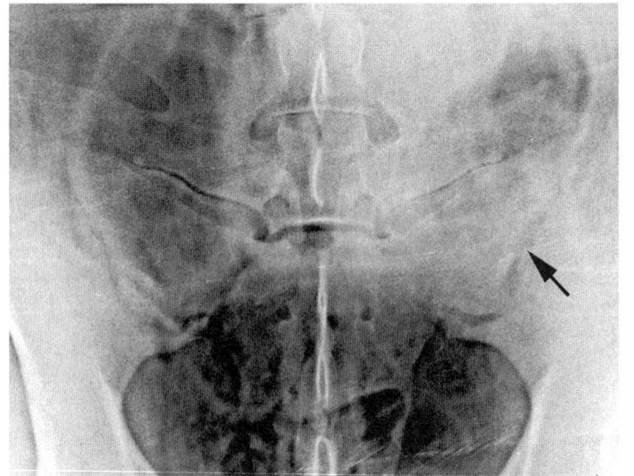

Figure 75-23. A, Bone scan of the sacroiliac region. The increased uptake in the medial aspects of the sacroiliac joints is more pronounced on the left side. **B,** Ventrodorsal radiograph of the same area documents osteophyte formation, joint irregularity, and enlargement of the sacral wings *(arrowhead)*, more evident on the left side.

proximal half of the femur, producing linear increased uptake patterns. Fracture of the third trochanter provokes high focalized activity. Enostosis in the femur is visualized by intense focal uptake.

Spine

The techniques used for the radiographic visualization of the equine spine vary for different regions. For the cervical spine, the examination is best performed in the standing animal. The quite large and broad cervical vertebrae have a more normal position in the standing horse. Distortion as a result of oblique positioning of the vertebrae may occur under anesthesia but can be avoided. With the horse standing, it also is possible to obtain oblique views of the cervical column, which make interpretation of the cervical facet joints much easier.

Usually, the horse is slightly tranquilized. A cassette stand is used for holding the cassettes in place. For the lateral views, a scatter grid and screens of medium speed are advisable. When using a cassette size of 30×40 cm, three views are necessary to cover the entire cervical column. The first view is centered on the articulation of the first and second vertebrae, the second view on the fourth vertebra, and the third on the intervertebral joint of C5-6. The oblique views are made at an angle of 45 to 55 degrees to the x-ray tube, either from below or from above. It is advisable to take the oblique views of the cervical spine from both sides.

In foals, malformation of the occiput and the first and second vertebrae have been observed and reported in the literature (see Chapter 51). The involvement of the different vertebrae and the degree of the malformation vary. Malformations are reported to occur in some Arabian families. The authors have seen some cases in Warmblood horses. Fracture of the dens of the second vertebra occurs in the young animals, usually along the unfused physis as a sequela of trauma. Subluxation may be observed between the first and second and between the third and fourth cervical vertebra. The extent of the abnormal angulation is the decisive diagnostic criterion. Small angular deviations seem to have no significance, whereas larger ones usually cause cervical stenosis and impairment of the spinal cord (wobbling).

Common radiographic findings in adult horses are enlargement of the joint facets, especially in the lower cervical region, subluxations, OC-related arthritic changes, and osteoarthritis.

In young animals, malformations are mostly seen in the proximal cervical spine. Fractures of the vertebral bodies or the articular processes are observed occasionally. In horses with ataxia and forelimb lameness, the enlargement of the facet joints in the last three vertebrae plays an important role (Fig. 75-24). The incidence of such lesions and the correlation with the clinical signs are very high.[28,29] Suspected space-occupying lesions (e.g., enlarged joint capsules of the facet joints) can be further evaluated by myelography.

Only the spinous processes of the thoracic spine can be radiographed in the standing animal. Many clinicians are satisfied with these images, but the thoracic spine is not well investigated by this method. If more details are desired, the examination has to be performed in the anesthetized horse in lateral recumbency. Because large masses of soft tissue have to be penetrated by the x-ray beam, scatter radiation is a big problem. Therefore, a two-step examination using smaller exposure fields and scatter grids is strongly recommended.[30,31] Fine-to-medium screens can be used to demonstrate the spinous processes in the saddle region. In the more posterior parts of the spine, the highest screen speeds are important. Only small fields are exposed (10×30 cm); the cassette is shielded with lead plates to eliminate scatter radiation from reaching the film. The x-ray beam is partially attenuated by a specially formed filter (SAAB Dodger, Trollhättan, Sweden). To demonstrate the intervertebral articulations, only a narrow strip of the 30×40-cm cassette is exposed. Together with the scatter grid and high-speed screens, it is possible to visualize the articular structures. To cover the most affected regions of the thoracic spine, usually three views of 30×40-cm film are necessary. Positioning of the animal is important to reduce distortion of the spine and superimposition of the rib cage. Only the three cranially situated vertebrae of the lumbar spine are demonstrable. The caudal part is overlaid by the pelvis.

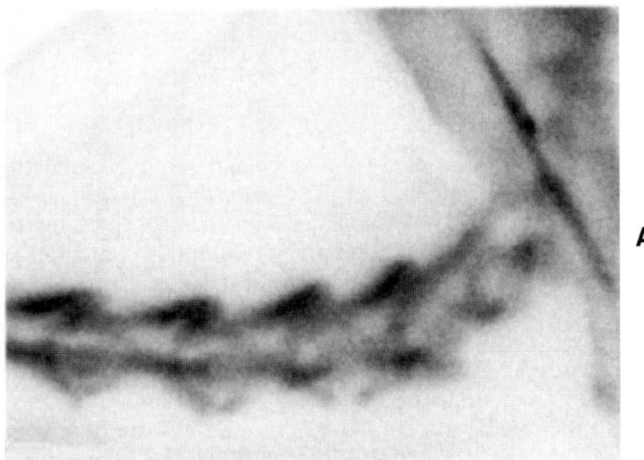

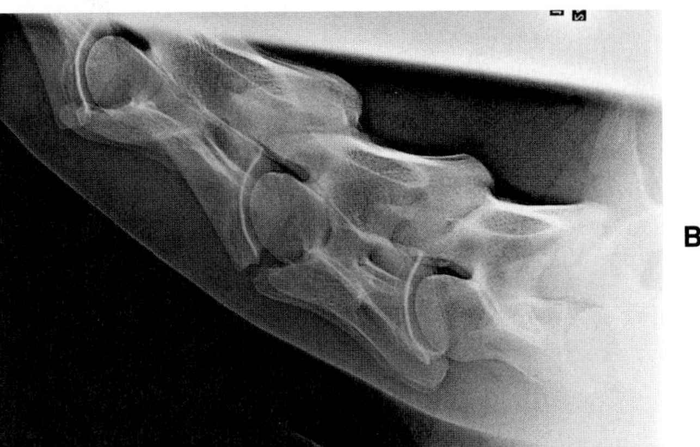

Figure 75-24. A, Bone scan of the lower cervical spine. The dorsal intervertebral articulation of C5-6 and C6-7 accumulates the tracer. Normally, these articulations are less visible because of the absorption of the gamma rays by the large muscle mass in this region. **B,** Radiographically, the dorsal intervertebral articulations of C6-7 are enlarged and sclerosed, and the joint space is irregular and narrowed. The intervertebral foramen is also narrowed.

The principal radiographic signs of changes of the spinous processes consist of deformations, narrowing of the interspinous spaces, sclerotic borders, facet formation, and spinal arthritis. In advanced cases, debris cysts and vacuum phenomena may also be observed.

The alterations of the intervertebral joints include the usual radiographic findings of subchondral sclerosis, irregular joint spaces and margins, enlargement of the articular surfaces, subchondral radiolucent areas, and in some horses, even ankylosis. The most affected vertebrae are the last three thoracic ones.

The sacroiliac region can be radiographed only in the ventrodorsal projection under general anesthesia. The imaging system with a scatter grid is placed under the horse and the horse turned onto it. The intestines can be moved by forced ventilation during the exposure. More powerful x-ray generators allow prolonged exposure times of up to 5 seconds. This allows at least two forced expirations. With this procedure, the margins of the intestines with their contents become blurred. The sacral wings of the pelvis and the lumbosacral joints can be observed. Enlargement and gross alterations of the contours of the sacral wings are very common. Changes of the lumbosacral joints consist of irregular articulations and subchondral sclerosis. Sometimes, even the dorsal intervertebral joints of the last lumbar vertebrae are visible and can be inspected.

Indications for bone imaging of the spine include clinical signs such as painful back, loss of performance in jumping and dressage horses, and lameness in the hindlimbs.[32] General anesthesia is necessary, as is the use of high-resolution collimators and high total count numbers.

The lumbar and thoracic spine is demonstrated by dorsal oblique views. It is recommended that the camera be placed on the right side to avoid superimposition of the right kidney over thoracic vertebral structures. Very small anatomic details can be demonstrated with the HRLE collimator at 2,000 k for the lumbar spine and 3,000 k for the posterior thoracic spine. It is not necessary to examine the spine from both sides.

In the lumbar spine, the uptake pattern (focal increased uptake) and the shape of the dorsal and lateral processes are investigated. Very frequently the fourth and fifth dorsal spinous processes show high focal uptake when they are contacting each other. Very often, the uptake of the kidneys disturbs the interpretation of the lumbar and thoracic spine. Modern nuclear medicine computers permit drawing an ROI around the kidneys, which can then be subtracted from the image, allowing better visualization of bone structure.

The most frequent pathologic finding is increased uptake in the sacroiliac and lumbosacral joints.[33,34] Ankylosis of the dorsal intervertebral joints occurs first in the lumbar spine. Trauma to the lumbar spine (e.g., fracture) may produce very intense circumscribed accumulation within the affected region.

The thoracic spine is the most affected part of the equine back. Two different structures seem to play an important role in the equine back pain syndrome: the spinous processes and the dorsal intervertebral joints (Fig. 75-25). The alterations of the spinous processes consist of deformation, enlargement of the proximal part, and increased focal or bifocal uptake at the sites where new joints are formed or overriding of the spinous processes occurs. Increased joint activity can be observed affecting the whole joint by producing one single area of activity. As a second pattern, sometimes increased activity in either one or both joint facets producing one or two smaller focal uptake areas is seen. Ankylosis of joints occurs mostly in the posterior section of the thoracic spine. In the bone scan, this can be perceived by enlargement of the joint or formation of an extra-articular bridge. The highest frequency of joint alterations is observed between the 15th and the 17th thoracic vertebrae. Alterations of the spinous processes are most frequently seen in the region of 13th to 16th thoracic vertebrae.

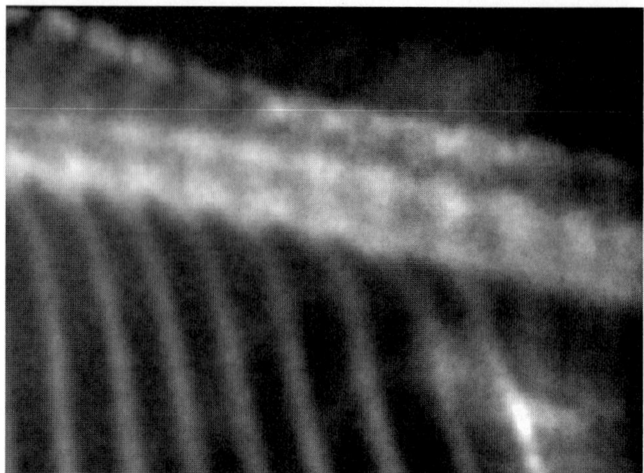

Figure 75-25. Lateral scintigraphic image of the caudal thoracic spine. There is markedly increased uptake in the dorsal spinous processes, particularly of the last thoracic vertebra. The dorsal intervertebral joints also have increased uptake, indicating osteoarthritis.

Interpretation of the true bone activity is sometimes very difficult, especially when the whole spine shows increased tracer accumulation. For a more objective evaluation, a special ROI technique has been developed. A reference ROI is placed on the middle part of the 16th or 17th rib. Subsequently, ROIs of similar size are defined over the intervertebral joints and the spinous processes. The actual size of the ROIs is not very important, because only the average values (total counts of a specific ROI per number of pixels in the ROI) are used. The uptake ratio of a particular joint is obtained by dividing it by the reference ROI. In normal horses, the uptake ratios for the dorsal intervertebral joints are less than 2.0, and the spinous processes have values less than 1.5.

In the recumbent animal, the cervical spine can be examined with the high-resolution or a GP collimator. The resolution of the GP collimator is not as good as that of the HRLE. The dorsal intervertebral joints can be evaluated by bone scans. The activity of the joints of C5 through C7 should be less than of the joints in the more cranial region because of the attenuation by the overlaying muscle mass. High activity in the lower cervical spine represents active arthropathy. Quite often, the joint surfaces are so enlarged that this can be recognized in the bone scan.

REFERENCES

1. Curry TS, Dowdey JE, Murry RC: Christensen's Physics of Diagnostic Radiology, ed 4, Philadelphia, 1990, Lea & Febiger.
2. Farr RF, Allisy-Roberts PJ: Physics for Medical Imaging, Philadelphia, 1997, WB Saunders.
3. Johns HE, Cunningham JR: The Physics of Radiology, ed 4, Springfield, Ill, 1983, Charles C. Thomas.
4. Pizzutiello RJ, Cullinan JE: Introduction to Medical Radiographic Imaging, Rochester, NY, 1993, Eastman Kodak.
5. Bushberg JDT, Seibert JA, Leidholdt EM, Boone JM: The Essential Physics of Medical Imaging, ed 2, Philadelphia, 2002, Lippincott Williams & Wilkins.
6. Thrall DE: Textbook of Veterinary Diagnostic Radiology, ed 3, Philadelphia, 1998, WB Saunders.
7. Kaser-Hotz B, Ueltschi G: Radiographic appearance of the navicular bone in sound horses, Vet Radiol 1992;33:9.
8. Kaser-Hotz B, Ueltschi G, Hess N: Navicular bone fracture in the pelvic limb in two horses,Vet Radiol 1991;32:283.
9. Thompson KN, Rooney JR, Petrites-Murphy MB: Considerations on the pathogenesis of navicular disease, J Equine Vet Sci 1991;11:4.
10. Viitanen M, Bird J, Smith R, et al: Biochemical characterisation of navicular hyaline cartilage, navicular fibrocartilage and the deep digital flexor tendon in horses with navicular disease, Res Vet Sci 2003;75:113.
11. Svalastoga E, Reimann I, Nielsen K: Changes of the fibrocartilage in navicular disease in horses. A histological and histochemical investigation of navicular bones, Nord Vet Med. 1983;35:372.
12. Wright IM: A study of 118 cases of navicular disease: Clinical features, Equine Vet J 1993;25:488.
13. Williams GE: Locomotor characteristics of horses with navicular disease, Am J Vet Res 2001;62:206.
14. Ruohoniemi M, Makela O, Eskonen T: Clinical significance of ossification of the cartilages of the front feet based on nuclear bone scintigraphy, radiography and lameness examinations in 21 Finnhorses, Equine Vet J 2004;36:143.
15. Nilsson G, Persson L: Changes in the synovial fluid of equine fetlock joints with lesions in the cartilage and joint capsule: A study in the Standardbred horse, Acta Vet Scand Suppl 1973;44:99.
16. Chateau H, Degueurce C, Denoix JM: Three-dimensional kinematics of the equine distal forelimb: Effects of a sharp turn at the walk, Equine Vet J 2005;37:12.
17. Von Saldern C: Retrospektive Studie an arthroskopierten Fessel- und Sprunggelenken beim Pferd: Vergleich der klinischen, radiologischen und arthroskopischen Befunde. Thesis, 2005, University of Berne.
18. Chateau H, Degueurce C, Denoix JM: Evaluation of three-dimensional kinematics of the distal portion of the forelimb in horses walking in a straight line, Am J Vet Res 2004;65:447.
19. Tnibar M, Kaser-Hotz B, Auer JA: Ultrasonography of the dorsal and lateral aspects of the equine carpus: Technique and normal appearance, Vet Radiol Ultrasound 1993;34:413.
20. Kaser-Hotz B, Sartoretti-Schefer S, Weiss R: Computed tomography and magnetic resonance imaging of the normal equine carpus, Vet Radiol Ultrasound 1994;35:457.
21. Kaser-Hotz B: Sonographische Diagnostik orthopädischer Erkrankungen beim Grosstier. In Knesevic P, editor: Orthopädie bei Huf-und Klauentieren, Stuttgart, 1995, PF Schattauer.
22. Ueltschi G: Zur Diagnose von Interosseusläsionen an der Ursprungsstelle, Pferdeheilkunde 1988;5:65.
23. Harasen G: Arthrodesis: Part II. The tarsus, Can Vet J 2002;43:806.
24. Lanovaz JL, Khumsap S, Clayton HM, et al: Three-dimensional kinematics of the tarsal joint at the trot, Equine Vet J Suppl 2002;34:308.
25. Vinayak A, Weigel JP, Henry GA, et al: What is your diagnosis? Avulsion fracture of the plantar aspect of the distal end of the calcaneus and plantar proximal intertarsal subluxation, J Am Vet Med Assoc 2004;224:39.
26. Tomlinson JE, Redding WR, Berry C, et al: Computed tomographic anatomy of the equine tarsus, Vet Radiol Ultrasound 2003;44:174.
27. Bukowiecki CF, Sanders-Shamis M, Bramlage LR: Treatment of a ruptured medial collateral ligament of the stifle in a horse, J Am Vet Med Assoc 1988;193:687.
28. Hett A: Untersuchungen zur Objektivierung der Röntgendiagnostik an der arthrotisch veränderten Halswirbelsäule des Pferdes, Thesis, 1999, University of Berne.
29. Ricardi G, Dyson SJ: Forelimb lameness associated with radiographic abnormalities of the cervical vertebrae, Equine Vet J 1993;12:422.
30. Gundel M, Schatzmann U, Ueltschi G: Back-problems in the horse: A comparison of diagnostic imaging with clinical examination, Pferdeheilkunde 1997;13:659.
31. Ueltschi G: Radiographie und Szintigraphie der Wirbelsäule. In Knezevic P, editor: Orthopädie bei Huf- und Klauentieren, Stuttgart, 1995, PF Schattauer.
32. Weaver MP, Jeffcott LB, Nowak M: Back problems: Radiology and scintigraphy, Clin North Am Equine Pract 1999;15:113.
33. Dyson SJ, Murray R, Branch M, et al: The sacroiliac joints: Evaluation using nuclear scintigraphy: Part I. The normal horse. Equine Vet J 2003;35:226.
34. Erichsen CH: Diagnostic imaging of the equine thoracolumbar spine and sacroiliac joint region, Thesis, 2003, Oslo.

CHAPTER 76

Magnetic Resonance Imaging of the Equine Distal Limb

Sarah N. Sampson
Robert K. Schneider
Russell L. Tucker

Magnetic resonance imaging (MRI) uses the hydrogen protons in the body to produce detailed images of bone and soft tissue structures.[1] The images (slices) that are obtained can provide a variety of different information from the same anatomy by varying the imaging sequences. Depending on the type of lesion suspected, different imaging sequences are chosen to highlight a specific tissue type. A typical protocol used to look at anatomy and pathology in the distal limb of a horse is composed of a variety of sequences. In this way, visualization of inflammation, edema, or irregularity of signal in soft tissue structures and bone is possible. Because the MRI unit generates a radiofrequency pulse that is specific to hydrogen atoms, it is capable of detecting subtle abnormalities in tissues when the field strength of the magnet is greater than 1.0 tesla.

Magnetic resonance imaging is a continuously evolving technology because the imaging techniques and slice planes are constantly being refined. Initially, MRI sectional anatomy was described for the equine foot and metacarpophalangeal regions using cadaveric limbs.[2,3] However, as more detailed information regarding sectional anatomy and observations of pathology in the distal limb has been related to lameness in live horses, this technology has achieved practical clinical application. MRI is extremely complex, and the goal of this chapter is to provide an introductory basis for understanding it in a clinical environment as it applies to equine lameness diagnoses.

PHYSICS OF MRI

Magnetic resonance results from the effect of magnetic properties of atoms found in biologic tissues. These atoms consist of a central nucleus containing both protons and neutrons, surrounded by orbiting electrons. The spinning motion of specific nuclei in tissue, called MR active nuclei, form the basis of MRI. These spinning nuclei acquire a magnetic moment, enabling them to interact with an external magnetic field. The positive charge of protons and the spinning motion generate a magnetic field of their own.[1]

The most common MR active nucleus found in all tissues is that of the hydrogen atom, which contains one positively charged proton.[1] The abundance of hydrogen in tissue and its relatively large magnetic moment make it the optimal choice for clinical MRI. Because of the high concentration of available hydrogen in fat and water, these substances contribute the majority of the signal in MRI. When an animal or its extremity is placed into the bore of a magnet, all the available hydrogen atoms that are normally randomly oriented align with the external magnetic field. At this time, a short-duration radiofrequency pulse that can be programmed to disrupt the aligned protons is applied to the area. This disruption will be best when the pulse has the same frequency as the aligned protons, causing generation of a signal through an exchange of energy. From the collected signals, images are obtained. Signal intensity is shown on the images in grayscale, where high-signal areas are white and low-signal areas are black.

A multitude of pulse sequences can be created to highlight specific tissues by modifying the signal intensity, but sampling time and image quality must be taken into consideration when determining the optimal sequences to use. The collected signal is called an echo, and it is detected by a radiofrequency receiver coil placed around the tissue of interest. Multiple echoes are necessary to provide all the information necessary to create an MR image. Fast spin echo sequences are typically used in horses to shorten scan time and reduce the length of time under general anesthesia. Magnetic field gradients within the magnet allow tissue sampling in a chosen orientation. This creates the ability to look at one slice at a time. With MRI, the generation of an image of a specific, thin cross section of the body is possible. These slices can be obtained in standard anatomic planes (e.g., transverse, sagittal, dorsal), or the slice plane can be oriented in any direction through the horse's limb. The number of slices and the thickness of the slices can also be varied. Additional information on MRI physics is found in Chapter 75.

APPLICATION TO THE HORSE

Magnetic resonance imaging has been routinely used to evaluate horses with lameness problems in the distal limb at Washington State University Veterinary Teaching Hospital since 1997.[4-6] In the last 8 years, MRI has proven to be a valuable diagnostic tool for making specific diagnoses in horses with performance-limiting lameness problems in the distal limb.[7-10] It is especially valuable in the equine foot because it allows evaluation of soft tissue structures within the hoof capsule that are difficult to visualize with other imaging modalities.[11-13] It also allows multiplane images through the foot, enabling soft tissue and bone structures to be seen in ways not previously possible.

Radiography has for a long time served as the gold standard for evaluating horses with lameness localized to the foot, providing excellent evaluation of osseous structures but minimal information on soft tissue structures.[14] Ultrasonography of the foot is limited because of the hoof capsule and the difficulty in achieving good scan-head contact through the sole or frog.[15] Nuclear scintigraphy (see Chapter 75) can be used to evaluate the foot, but it is of limited value in detecting abnormalities in soft tissue structures and in detecting small areas of abnormalities in the bone; it is best for finding fractures and acute bone injuries that involve enough bone that increased metabolic bone activity can be detected.[16] When compared with scintigraphy, MRI is more sensitive and specific for both bone and soft tissue injury.[17] High-field magnets (1 to 1.5 tesla) are able to image forelimbs of horses from the foot to the distal radius, hindlimbs from the foot to the distal tibia, and the head to the first few cervical vertebrae. It is also possible to image most other areas in small foals or miniature horses.

Image quality and resolution increase with increasing magnetic field strength, so high-field magnets have more detailed images than low-field magnets. "Open" magnets have an opening along one side of the magnet. However, magnetic field strength is most uniform in "closed" magnets, which are cylindrical, with openings at both ends. Therefore, image quality is superior with closed, high-field magnets when compared with low-field open or closed magnets. High-field magnets of 1.0 tesla or higher are necessary to obtain quality images in live horses.

LOGISTICS OF MRI FOR HORSES

Magnetic resonance imaging of horses requires general anesthesia if a high-field magnet is used. Image quality deteriorates when the area being imaged is not within the isocenter of the magnet. High-field magnets designed for humans have a long, narrow bore that makes it difficult for the limbs of a horse to be placed in the isocenter. However, high-field, short-bore magnets with flared ends are available that allow the horse's limbs to be better positioned. Therefore, imaging of the proximal limb is limited only by how far the horse can be pulled into the magnet. For horses with shorter limbs and thicker bodies, it may be possible to provide more room by removing the table from within the bore of the magnet.

Horses undergoing MR scanning must have all shoes and nails removed to avoid artifacts from ferrous material. If feet are being scanned, a 60-degree dorsopalmar radiograph must be taken prior to scanning to avoid artifacts from small pieces of horseshoe nails that might be left in the hoof wall after the shoes are removed. All limbs are placed in obstetrical sleeves to decrease debris in the magnet. Thorough cleaning of the frog sulci and sole of the foot is needed to prevent foreign material from causing magnetic susceptibility artifacts.

High-field magnets are constructed in a room shielded from radiofrequency waves, and ferromagnetic material cannot be used. Horse transport tables are currently custom built without ferromagnetic materials, but with the capability of supporting horses weighing up to 2000 pounds. Anesthesia equipment should contain as little ferromagnetic material as possible and have a position in the shielded room that is far enough from the magnet so as not to interfere with the magnetic field. Induction and transport of horses to and from the magnet requires a team of experienced people. The horse can be maintained on injectable anesthetics during transport and then connected to a vaporizer once in the shielded room.

CASE SELECTION

Magnetic resonance imaging is indicated when other diagnostic modalities fail to yield a diagnosis of the horse's lameness problem. Although MRI provides useful information in many clinical conditions, the authors have restricted its use to horses with lameness problems that are localized to an anatomic area but that do not have radiographically or ultrasonographically detectable abnormalities. This has been implemented because of the length and expense of the procedure and the need for general anesthesia. It is important to localize the source of the lameness prior to performing MRI, because the length of time required to image one area of the distal limb and the contralateral limb is approximately 45 to 60 minutes. Additional time is required for anesthetic induction, transport, and positioning of the horse in the magnet. Scanning more of the horse's limb than is necessary not only increases the time to perform the sequences but also requires repositioning of both the coil on the limb and the horse within the magnet. Therefore, prolonged anesthesia can be avoided if a lameness examination with diagnostic blocks is used to localize the source of the problem in the distal limb of the horse.

IMAGING PROTOCOLS

Until more experience with MRI of horses improves the present knowledge of variations of normal, MRI should always be performed on both limbs, even in horses with a unilateral lameness. This allows the evaluator to compare the affected limb to the contralateral limb.

The standard protocols include proton density (PD), T2-weighted (T2), short tau inversion recovery (STIR), and three-dimensional gradient echo (3D) sequences (Table 76-1). *Proton density* sequences provide images that clearly show anatomic structure, and therefore they are the easiest images to evaluate for ligament and tendon symmetry. These images display any change in the density of protons as a change in signal intensity, causing each tissue to produce different signal intensities. *T2-weighted* sequences produce images with high fluid contrast but minimal shades of gray, resulting in an image that is more difficult to evaluate for definition of soft tissue structures. T2-weighted images are useful when looking for fluid within soft tissues and for determining whether areas of high signal within soft tissue are fibrous tissue or inflammatory fluid. *Short tau inversion recovery* sequences produce images that are of high contrast and low clarity, but they provide the best sequence for finding fluid within bone and soft tissue structures. This sequence is useful for diagnosing inflammatory bone lesions. *Gradient echo* sequences produce images with good definition of bone structure but poor definition of some soft tissue structures. These can be set up with or without fat suppression and are the most time-efficient scans to run. Areas of fluid within the bone may be seen with these scans, but they are not as sensitive as the STIR sequences.

The majority of MRI series performed in the horse have been done on the foot, phalangeal, metacarpophalangeal (MCP) and metatarsophalangeal (MTP), and metacarpal and metatarsal regions. This chapter describes pathologic abnormalities observed in horses limbs distal to the carpus and tarsus.

MRI OF THE FOOT

Magnetic resonance imaging has allowed veterinarians to understand the interrelationships of the internal soft tissue structures in the horse's foot for the first time. In addition to

TABLE 76-1. Imaging Protocols for Horses Using 1.0 Tesla Gyroscan Magnet

Slice Plane	Sequence	TR (msec)	TE (msec)	FA	FOV/rFOV	Matrix Size	Slice #/Width	Gap (mm)	Time (min)
FOOT									
Transverse	TSE T2	2116	100	90	15/10	256×512	30/4 mm	0.5	2:34
Transverse	TSE PD	2116	10.5	90	15/10	256×512	30/4 mm	0.5	2:34
Transverse	STIR	1725	35	90	15/10	192×256	30/3.5 mm	1.0	4:42
Transverse	3D GE	47	9	25	10/10	192×256	30/1.5 mm	−0.5	3:13
Sagittal	TSE T2	3395	110	90	14/10	256×512	22/4 mm	0.5	2:21
Sagittal	TSE PD	3395	13.8	90	14/10	256×512	22/4 mm	0.5	2:21
Sagittal	STIR	1500	35	90	14/10	256×256	22/3.5 mm	0.5	5:48
Dorsal	3D GE	47	6	25	10/10	192×256	30/1.5 mm	−0.5	3:13
PASTERN/FETLOCK									
Transverse	TSE T2	2143	100	90	15/12	256×512	30/4.5 mm	0.5	1:57
Transverse	TSE PD	2143	10.5	90	15/12	256×512	30/4.5 mm	0.5	1:57
Transverse	STIR	1725	35	90	15/12	192×256	30/4 mm	1.0	5:17
Sagittal	TSE T2	1899	110	90	14/12	256×512	24/3.2 mm	0.4	2:22
Sagittal	TSE PD	1899	13.8	90	14/12	256×512	24/3.2m	0.4	2:22
Sagittal	STIR	1500	35	90	14/12	192×256	24/3.0 mm	0.6	5:12
Dorsal	3D GE	47	8.3	25	11/10	192×256	40/1.5 mm	−0.5	4:41
METACARPUS/METATARSUS									
Transverse	TSE T2	2143	100	90	15/10	256×512	30/4.5 mm	0.5	1:57
Transverse	TSE PD	2143	10.5	90	15/10	256×512	30/4.5 mm	0.5	1:57
Transverse	STIR	1725	35	90	15/10	192×256	30/4 mm	1.0	5:17
Sagittal	TSE T2	1899	110	90	14/10	256×512	24/3.2 mm	0.4	2:22
Sagittal	TSE PD	1899	13.8	90	14/10	256×512	24/3.2m	0.4	2:22
Sagittal	STIR	1500	35	90	14/10	192×256	24/3.0 mm	0.6	5:12
Dorsal	3D GE	47	8.3	25	11/10	192×256	40/1.5 mm	−0.5	4:41

TI for STIR sequences is 140 msec; the T2 and PD sequences are collected together during the TSE scan.
FA, flip angle; FOV, field of view; Gap, space between slices; PD, proton density; rFOV, relative field of view; STIR, short tau inversion recovery; TE, echo time; time, actual scanning time for each sequence; TR, repetition time; TSE, turbo spin echo; T2, T2-weighted; width, thickness of slice; 3D GE, three-dimensional gradient echo.

soft tissue structures, the ability to section the limb in any plane has also allowed better visualization of the osseous and synovial structures in the equine foot. All of this has improved the ability to derive specific diagnoses in horses with lameness problems originating in the foot and has led to better treatment decisions and case management.[18]

Deep Digital Flexor Tendinitis

The deep digital flexor tendon (DDFT) is a low-signal (black), well-defined structure with two symmetrical lobes that become fan shaped at their insertion onto the distal phalanx. Lesions in the DDFT are typically found at three locations in the foot of the horse: the insertion to the distal phalanx (Fig. 76-1), at the level of the distal sesamoid bone (Fig. 76-2), and proximal to the distal sesamoid bone (DSB)[14] (Fig. 76-3). Horses may suffer from lesions at one, two, or all three locations at one time, and some have lesions extending from the insertion on the distal phalanx proximally to the MCP joint.

Deep digital flexor tendon lesions are commonly seen as high-signal (white) areas within the tendon (core lesion), as roughened, irregular surfaces along the dorsal edge of the tendon, or as small vertical splits that are often located at the insertion of the DDFT or at the level of or proximal to the DSB. Lesions can also be seen as an enlargement of the tendon in which the signal remains low but tendon thickening or an irregular shape is observed. The high-signal lesions are usually well defined and run longitudinally within the tendon, in one or both lobes, and there is typically enlargement of the tendon (Fig. 76-4).

Tendinitis of the DDFT is a common finding in horses that present with heel pain. Affected horses may show a unilateral or bilateral lameness with clinical signs that mimic navicular disease. In many cases, this is the primary abnormality observed with MRI. Horses that suffer from tendinitis without DSB abnormalities have treatment options that differ from those of horses with chronic DSB degeneration.

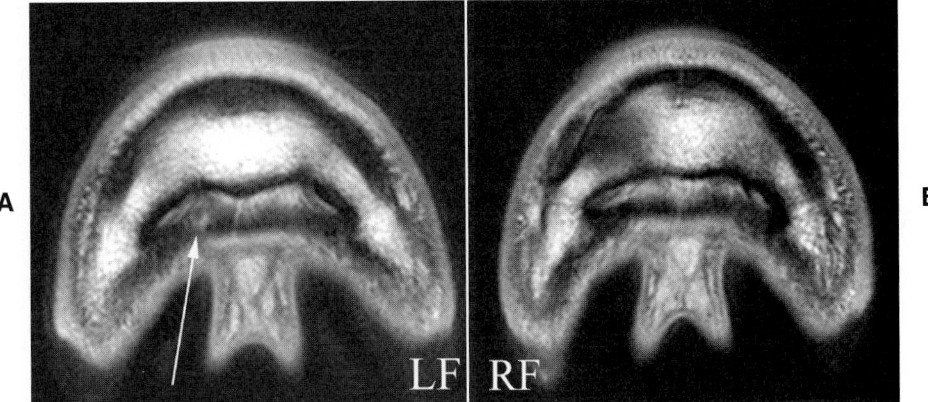

Figure 76-1. Axial proton density images through the distal phalanx and the deep digital flexor tendon (DDFT) proximal to its insertion on the distal phalanx. **A,** The lame left front foot has abnormal high-signal intensity *(arrow)* as a result of a tear in the medial aspect of the DDFT. **B,** The normal right front foot for comparison.

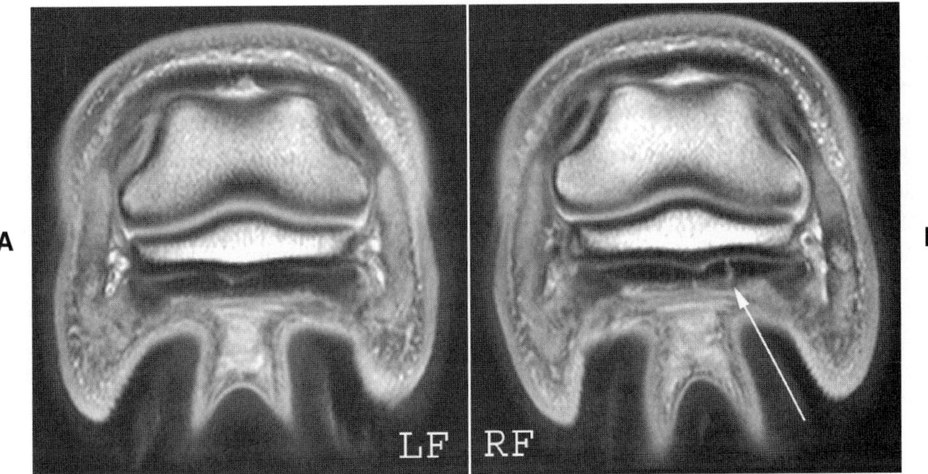

Figure 76-2. Axial proton density sequences from a horse with a right front limb lameness that blocks to a palmar digital nerve block. **A,** The normal left front foot for comparison. **B,** A full-thickness, high-signal-intensity vertical tear is seen in the enlarged bundle of the deep digital flexor tendon of the right front foot *(arrow)*. The sections are through the distal aspect of the middle phalanx and the distal sesamoid bone of both feet.

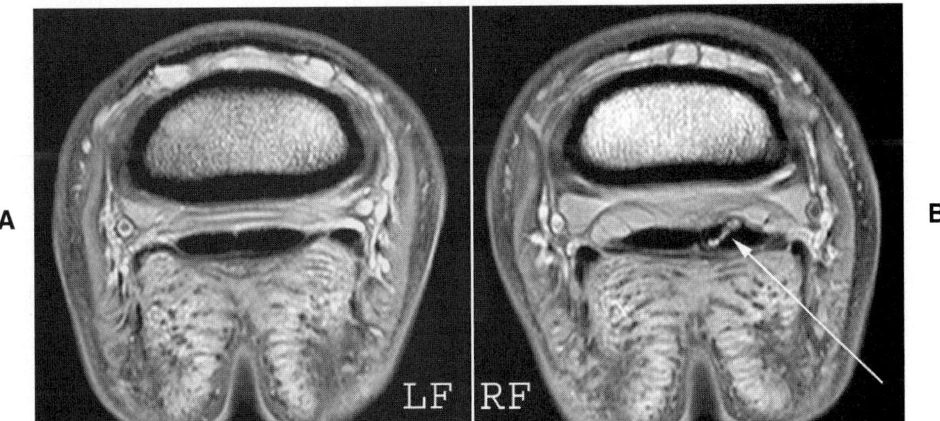

Figure 76-3. Axial proton density images through the proximal aspect of the middle phalanx from a horse with right front limb lameness. **A,** The normal left front foot for comparison. **B,** There is abnormal high-signal intensity in the deep digital flexor tendon *(arrow)* of the right foot and increased fluid in the digital flexor tendon sheath.

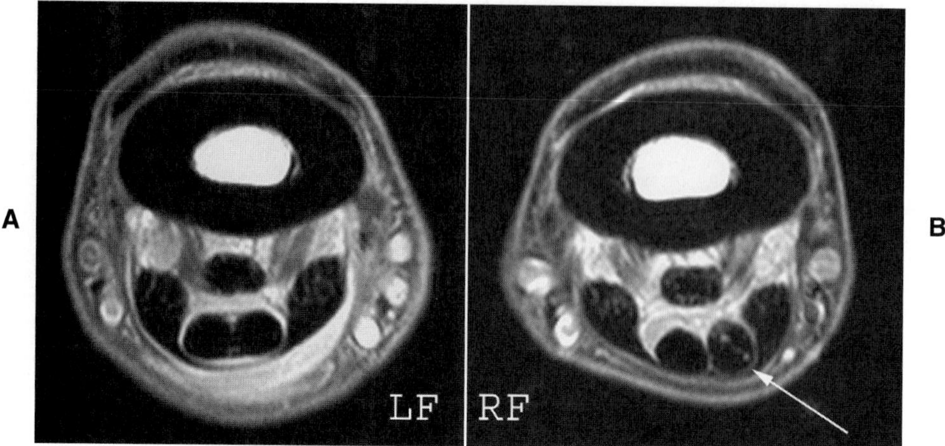

Figure 76-4. Axial proton density images from a horse with lameness of the right front limb. **A,** The normal left front foot for comparison. **B,** There is enlargement and two areas of abnormal high signal in the deep digital flexor tendon *(arrow)* of the right front limb. The sections are through the distal aspect of the proximal phalanx.

Observations in Horses with Clinical Signs of Navicular Disease

Distal Sesamoid Bone, Fluid, and Sclerosis

In many horses with navicular disease, abnormal fluid is observed in the DSB. The fluid can be classified as mild to severe based on the amount observed. *Bone edema* is a term that is used to describe abnormal fluid within the DSB. It is most visible when the high signal of fat is suppressed, as in the STIR imaging sequences (Fig. 76-5). Fluid accumulates in areas of inflammation, and the high signal from fluid in the bone is likely to be the result of inflammation. In horses with acute lameness, the fluid may be caused by bone injury—for example, hemorrhage secondary to a contusion.

In the DSB, fluid is most often seen at its distal aspect proximal to the insertion of the impar ligament (IL) (Fig. 76-6). The accumulation of fluid commonly extends proximally along the palmar half of the bone to the insertion of the navicular suspensory ligament (NSL). More severe involvement of the DSB results in diffuse fluid throughout the medullary cavity.

Low-signal intensity (black areas) is indicative of bone sclerosis and is observed in the medullary cavity of the DSB on palmarodorsal images. Sclerosis or increased bone density observed in the DSB results from the bone's response to increased load (Wolff's Law) or to injury. Horses that suffer from bone injury in other locations, including

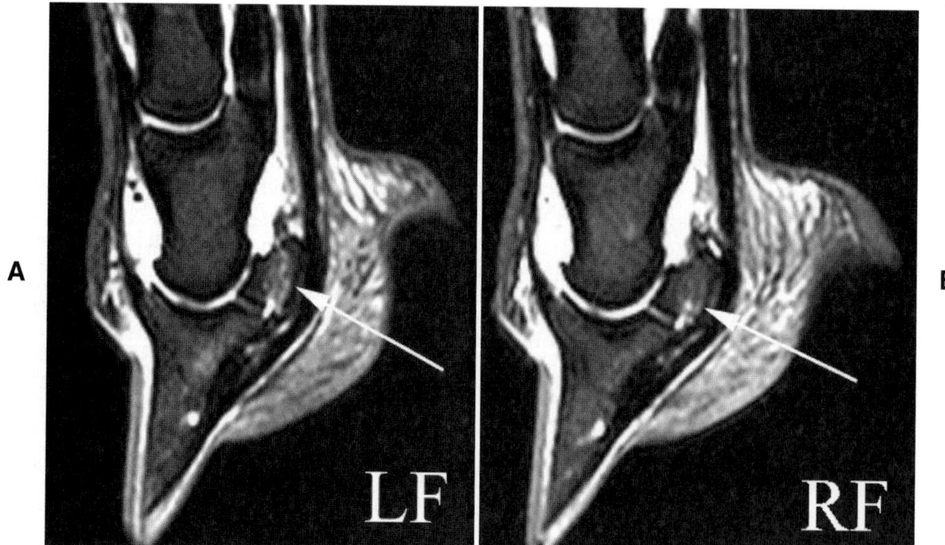

Figure 76-5. Sagittal short tau inversion recovery (STIR) images of the front feet of a horse with diffuse high signal *(arrows)* in the palmar half of the distal sesamoid bone (DSB) extending from the insertion of the impar ligament to the proximal DSB, more severe on the left front foot (**A**) and less severe on the right front foot (**B**). This is a frequent finding in horses with signs of navicular disease.

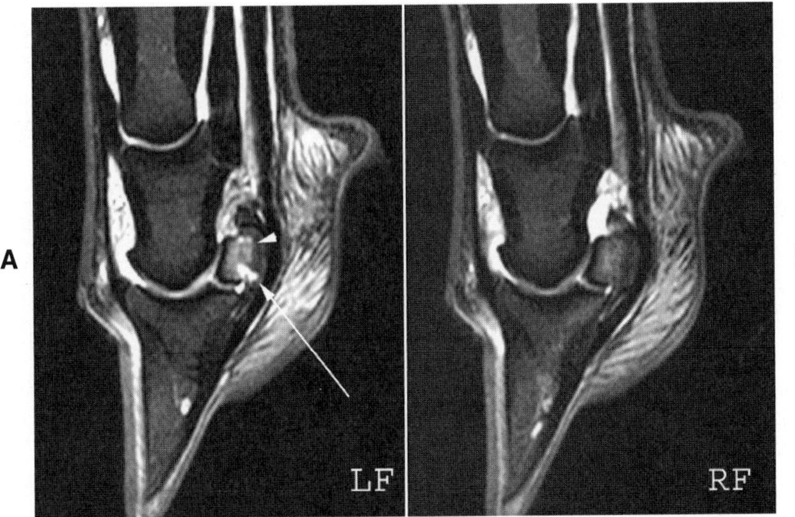

Figure 76-6. A, Sagittal short tau inversion recovery (STIR) image of a horse with abnormal fluid in the left front foot distal sesamoid bone. There is an area of high-signal-intensity fluid in the distal third of the bone *(arrow)* on the left front foot. **B,** The normal right front foot for comparison.

horses with fractures, develop sclerosis or increased bone density around the injury, and abnormal areas of low-signal intensity are observed on palmarodorsal images. Although the cause for sclerosis of the DSB remains speculative, it seems logical that it is a response to repetitive injury. Sclerosis can be observed along with areas of fluid, but it is also seen in bones where no inflammatory fluid is present. In a DSB that has undergone severe trauma, large portions of the entire bone of one foot are sclerotic. Sclerosis can occur diffusely throughout the DSB (Fig. 76-7), or it can be localized to one area, most commonly in the central region (Fig. 76-8). Some horses have either fluid or sclerosis of the DSB as the only abnormal finding. Sound horses do not have edema or sclerosis in their navicular bones.

Erosion of the flexor cortex (Fig. 76-9) is well visualized with MRI; subchondral defects most commonly occur along the palmar distal half of the bone and are most often seen centrally, or on one (Fig. 76-10) or both sides of the sagittal ridge. Adhesion of the DDFT to the DSB can be clearly observed in some horses, but injection of fluid into the navicular bursa may be necessary to clearly define adhesions in other horses.

Navicular Suspensory Ligament Desmitis

One of the abnormalities observed in horses with navicular disease is desmitis of the NSL of the DSB. This is seen as thickening that can be localized either to the body or to

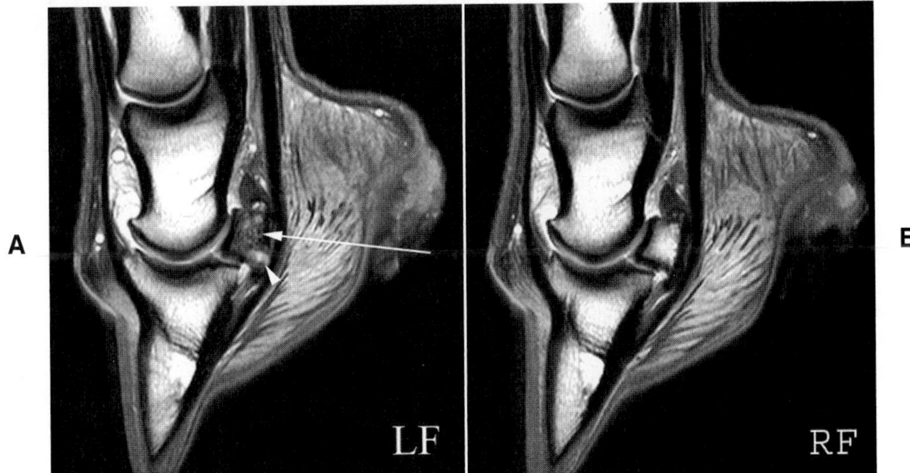

Figure 76-7. A, Sagittal proton density (PD) image of the front feet of a horse with diffuse sclerosis (low signal intensity shows as black) of the medullary cavity of the distal sesamoid bone (DSB) in the left front foot. The darkness of the medullary cavity is caused by increased bone density when observed on PD sequences. A small area of high signal intensity in the DSB at the insertion of the impar ligament indicates inflammatory fluid *(arrowhead)*. **B,** The normal right front foot for comparison.

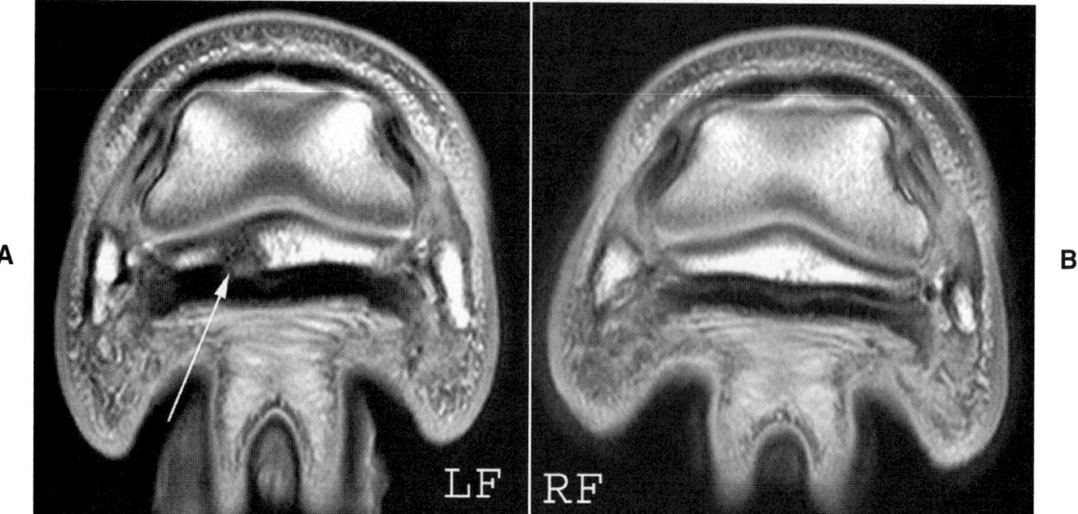

Figure 76-8. A, Axial proton density images of a horse with focal sclerosis in the medial aspect of the distal sesamoid bone *(arrow)* of the left front foot. **B,** The normal right front foot for comparison.

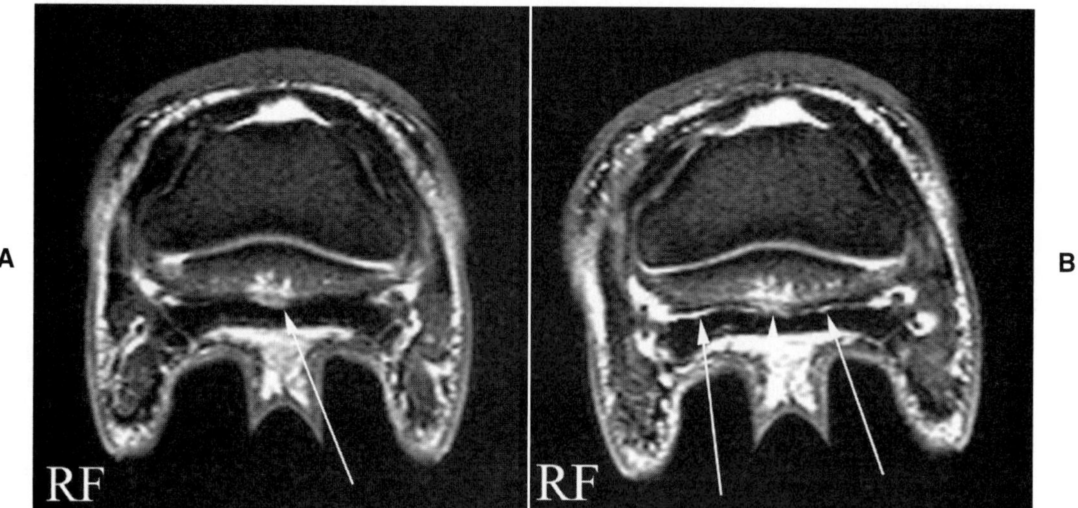

Figure 76-9. Axial short tau inversion recovery (STIR) images of the same foot of a horse before (**A**) and after (**B**) injection of the navicular bursa with hyaluronic acid and cortisone. The fluid space between the deep digital flexor tendon and the distal sesamoid bone *(arrows)* makes the tissue-dense adhesion *(middle arrowhead)* easier to observe in the image on the right.

the collateral branches, or it shows up as a diffuse signal throughout the entire ligament. Enlargement of this ligament is a finding consistent with chronic desmitis. High-signal intensity in the body of the ligament has been seen in some horses, most commonly on transverse slices, and it is indicative of acute inflammation and/or tearing of the ligament (Fig. 76-11). The acute history in these patients is consistent with a ligament injury.

Thickening of the NSL is also a common finding in horses that have multiple abnormalities associated with navicular disease. Desmitis of the NSL is currently evaluated as mild, moderate, or severe on the basis of the amount of thickening observed in the ligament. Avulsion fracture of the proximal aspect of the DSB has also been visualized with MRI.

Impar Ligament (IL) Desmitis

Impar ligament desmitis is another abnormality observed in horses that present with clinical signs of navicular syndrome. Lesions in this ligament are seen as discrete or diffuse high-signal lesions. Thickening of the ligament, with or without changes in signal, also occurs (Fig. 76-12). Abnormal fluid signal is observed at its origin on the distal aspect of the DSB or at its insertion on the palmar or plantar

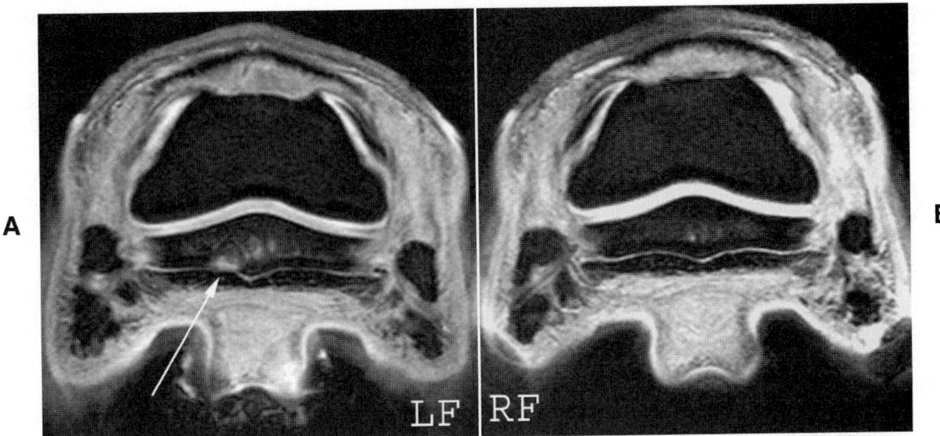

Figure 76-10. Axial gradient echo image from the left front foot (**A**) clearly shows a defect in the flexor cortex *(arrow)* of the distal sesamoid bone (high signal) when compared with the normal right front foot (**B**).

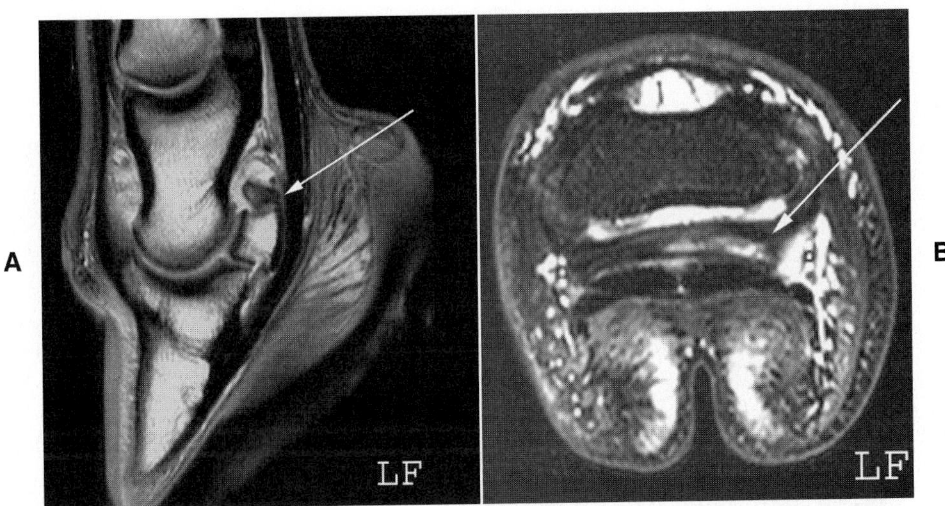

Figure 76-11. Sagittal proton density (**A**) and axial short tau inversion recovery (STIR) (**B**) images of the left front foot of a horse with enlargement of the proximal suspensory ligament of the distal sesamoid bone. There is high signal intensity in the ligament *(arrow)* on the axial section that is consistent with active inflammation and thickening of the ligament seen on both images.

distal phalanx. Avulsion fractures at the distal aspect of the DSB have been observed. Irregularity in the IL can also be seen as a part of multiple abnormalities found in horses with navicular disease.

Navicular Bursitis and Distal Interphalangeal Joint Synovitis

The amount of fluid in the synovial structures can be evaluated most easily with STIR and T2 sequences. Joint injury, osteoarthritis, and inflammation usually cause synovial effusion. Magnetic resonance images are evaluated for increased fluid in the distal interphalangeal joint (Fig. 76-13) and the navicular bursa (Fig. 76-14). Fibrous scar tissue (adhesions) is observed between the DSB and the DDFT in horses with chronic DSB degeneration and erosion of the flexor cortex. Fibrous scar tissue is also observed in the proximal aspect of the navicular bursa and may be the result of chronic inflammation in this area. Adhesions within the navicular bursa, between the NSL and DDFT or between the IL and DDFT, can be visualized. Navicular bursal fluid distention can also outline adhesions of the DDFT to the flexor cortex of the DSB, as well as defects within the flexor cortex. Fluid distention of the navicular bursa is observed in some horses and is an MRI finding consistent with inflammation and bursitis.[18]

Distal Navicular Bone Fractures

A slice plane oriented from proximal to distal through the DSB allows avulsion fractures to be clearly seen in the insertion of the IL to the DSB (Fig. 76-15). When seen in lame horses, there is fluid at the fracture site indicating active inflammation.

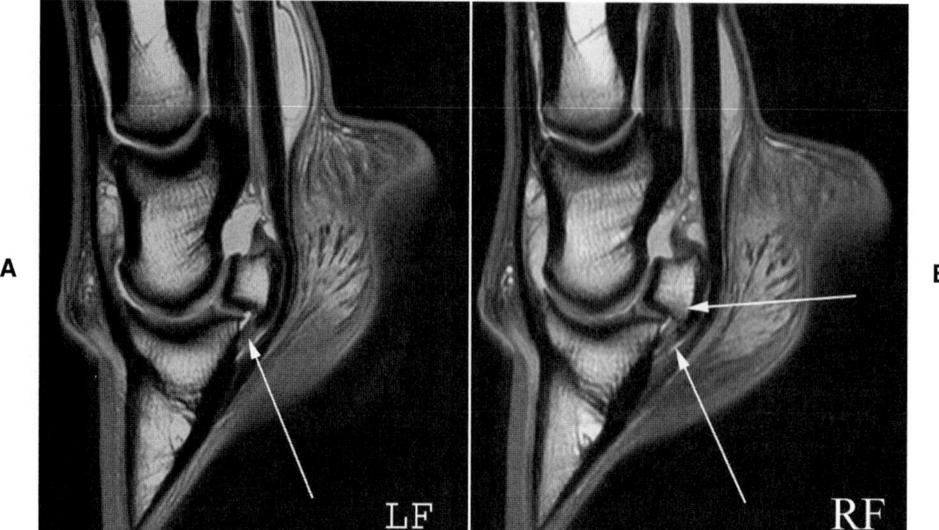

Figure 76-12. Sagittal proton density images from a horse with clinical signs of navicular disease. There is enlargement and irregular diffuse high signal intensity located in the impar ligament (IL) of the left front foot (**A**) and right front foot (**B**) *(arrows)*. There is also an area of mild sclerosis in the distal sesamoid bone at the IL attachment in the right front foot *(upper arrow in* **B***)*.

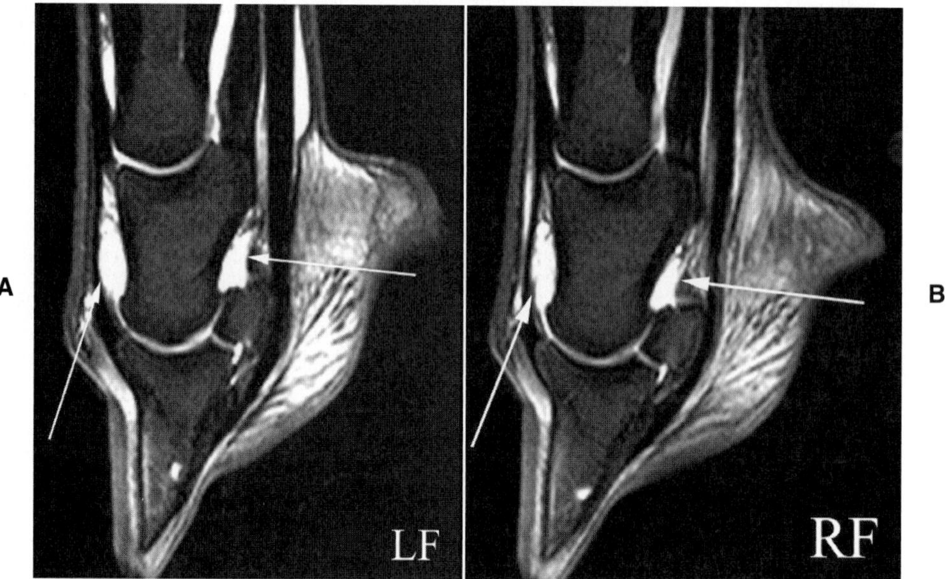

Figure 76-13. Sagittal short tau inversion recovery (STIR) images from a horse that has effusion in the distal interphalangeal joint in the left front foot (**A**) and right front foot (**B**). The high signal intensities *(arrows)* on the image represent synovial fluid in the dorsal and palmar pouches.

Other Abnormalities Observed in Horses with Lameness Localized to the Foot

Collateral Ligament Desmitis

Damage to the collateral ligaments has been observed in a number of horses with lameness localized to the foot. On the basis of the authors' experience and that of others,[19] it appears that this is an important cause of lameness in some horses. Inflammation and fiber disruption cause higher signal intensity within or around the affected ligament (Fig. 76-16), and there may be concomitant bone disruption at the origin or insertion sites. Bilateral desmitis of the collateral ligaments of this joint has been observed in some horses. The medial collateral ligament is affected more commonly than the lateral collateral ligament.[19]

Osteochondral Abnormalities

Lesions within the subchondral bone show areas of fluid accumulation or sclerosis, indicating injury and inflammation in the bone. At joint surfaces, MRI can define cartilage defects with or without underlying subchondral bone damage that are not visible with radiography.[8] Synovial fluid

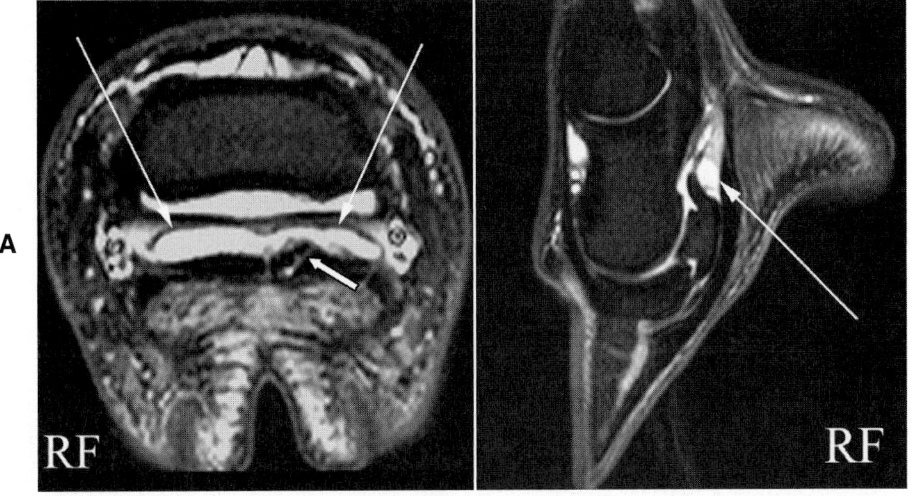

Figure 76-14. Axial (**A**) and sagittal (**B**) short tau inversion recovery (STIR) images, both of the right front foot, in a horse that has increased fluid in the navicular bursa *(arrows)*. The horse also has deep digital flexor tendinitis, seen on the axial section *(short arrow)*.

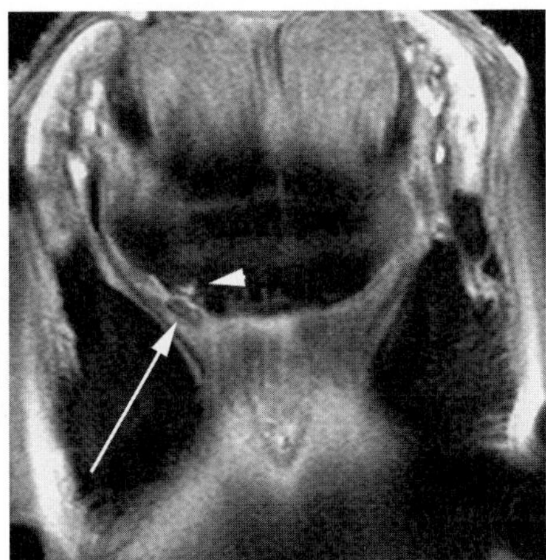

Figure 76-15. A gradient echo coronal section through the distal sesamoid bone (DSB) in a horse with a small avulsion fracture *(arrow)* at the distal border of the right front foot DSB. Fluid in the DSB *(arrowhead)* indicates inflammation and fluid in the defect.

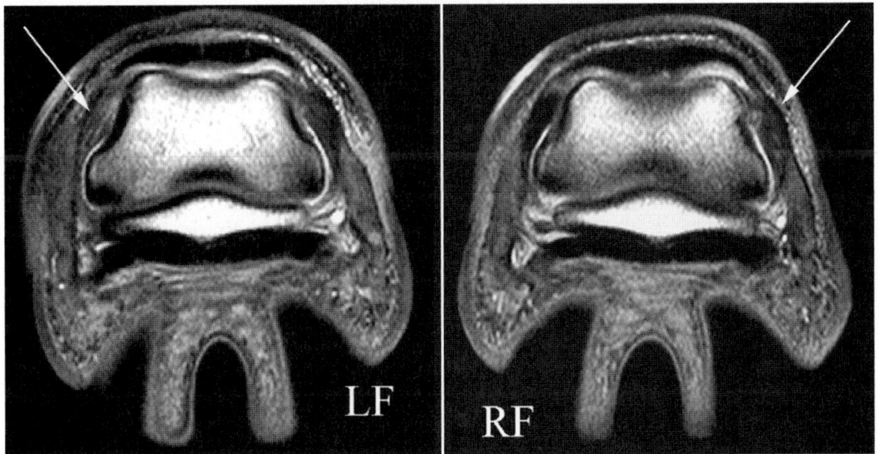

Figure 76-16. Axial proton density sections through the condyles of the middle phalanx of the left front foot (**A**) and right front foot (**B**) show diffuse high signal intensity in the medial collateral ligaments *(arrows)* of the distal interphalangeal joint.

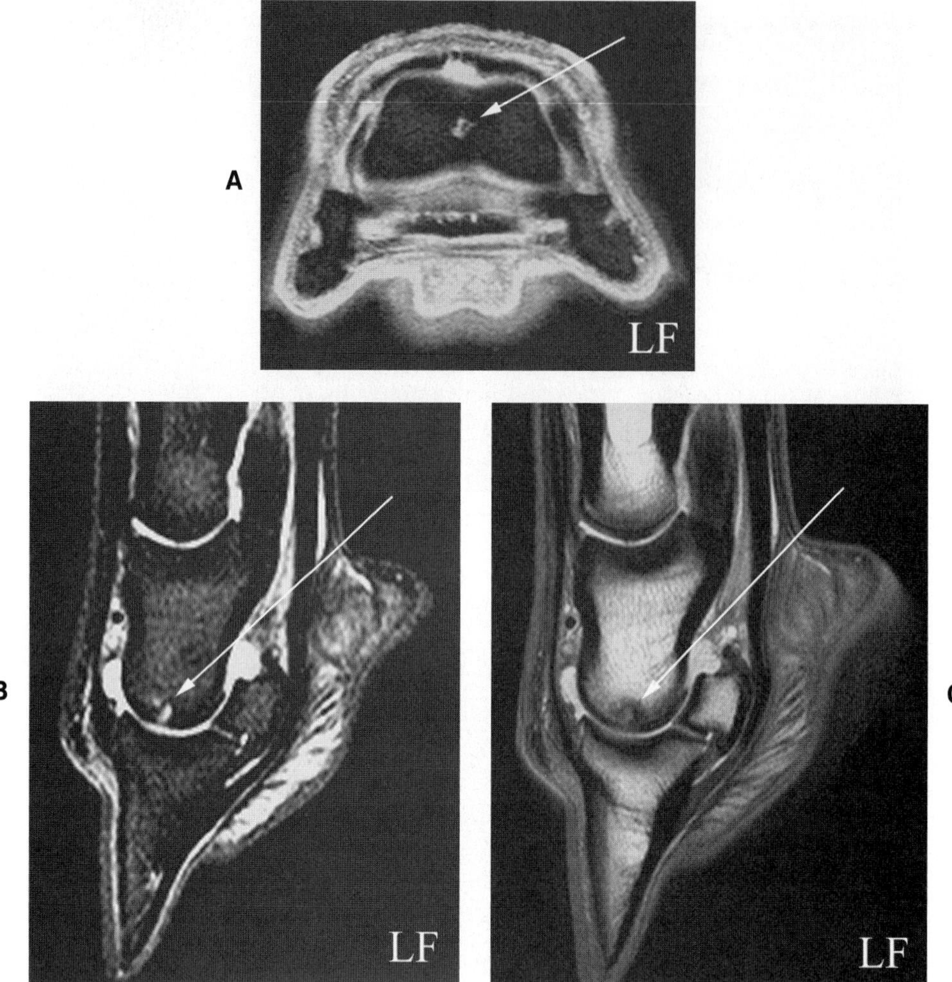

Figure 76-17. Axial gradient echo (**A**) and sagittal short tau inversion recovery (STIR) (**B**) sections from a horse that has a fluid signal in the subchondral bone of the distal middle phalanx with a chondral defect in the joint surface *(arrow)*. The sagittal proton density image (**C**) shows the abnormality in the subchondral bone with surrounding sclerosis *(arrow)* in the same location.

will enter defects in cartilage, resulting in a high signal within the articular cartilage and in the corresponding subchondral bone when full-thickness articular cartilage damage or defects occur (Fig. 76-17). Trauma to the subchondral bone may occur without overlying cartilage damage, as is seen with bone bruising and trabecular bone microfractures. The high signal in these cases may be caused by hemorrhage in the subchondral bone and medullary cavity.

Osteoarthritis of the Distal and Proximal Interphalangeal Joints

Inflammation of synovial structures results in joint effusion, which can be easily visualized with MRI. Periarticular bone proliferation is evident on MR images in sagittal, dorsal, and transverse imaging sequences.

Penetrating Injuries and Wounds

Magnetic resonance imaging of horses with puncture wounds in the sole or frog has been beneficial, because it provides an evaluation of affected structures (Fig. 76-18). This is important in making treatment decisions as well as for prognosis. The depth and penetration of the injury can be accurately determined, and the synovial and osseous structures that may have been entered can be seen (Fig. 76-19). MRI has the ability to determine if a laceration has damaged the collateral ligaments of the distal interphalangeal joint or other soft tissue structures in this area.

MRI OF THE METACARPOPHALANGEAL AND METATARSOPHALANGEAL REGIONS

Subchondral Bone and Cartilage Damage

Subchondral bone damage in the MCP and MTP joints has been identified as areas of fluid accumulation in the bone or as sclerosis.[8] Multiple areas of subchondral bone and cartilage damage have been observed in the MCP and MTP joints (Figs. 76-20 and 76-21), although a common location is the palmar or plantar condyle.

Bone bruises show an area of fluid or an area of sclerosis in the bone, but the overlying cartilage can be intact. Fluid accumulation in the bone appears more commonly in acute injuries, whereas chronic bone damage is more frequently

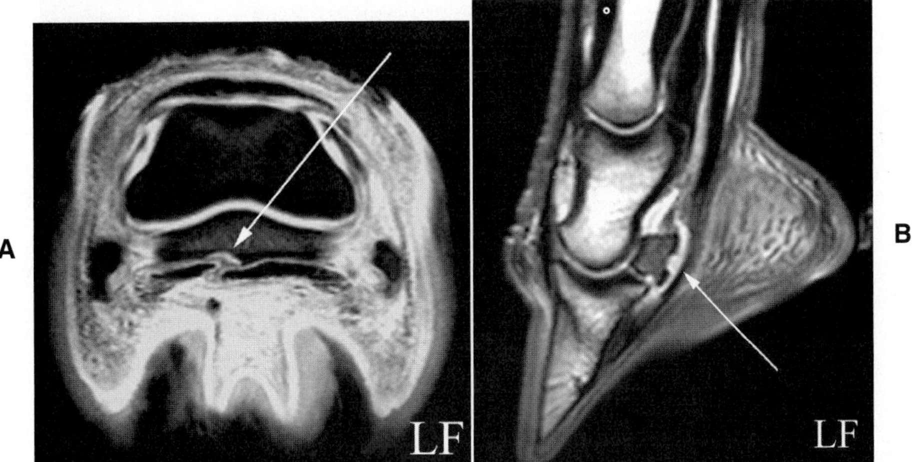

Figure 76-18. Axial gradient echo (**A**) and sagittal proton density (PD) (**B**) images of the left front foot of a horse that suffered a nail puncture of the frog. The nail penetrated the deep digital flexor tendon and damaged the flexor cortex of the distal sesamoid bone (DSB) *(arrows)*. The sagittal PD image also shows diffuse sclerosis of the medullary cavity of the DSB.

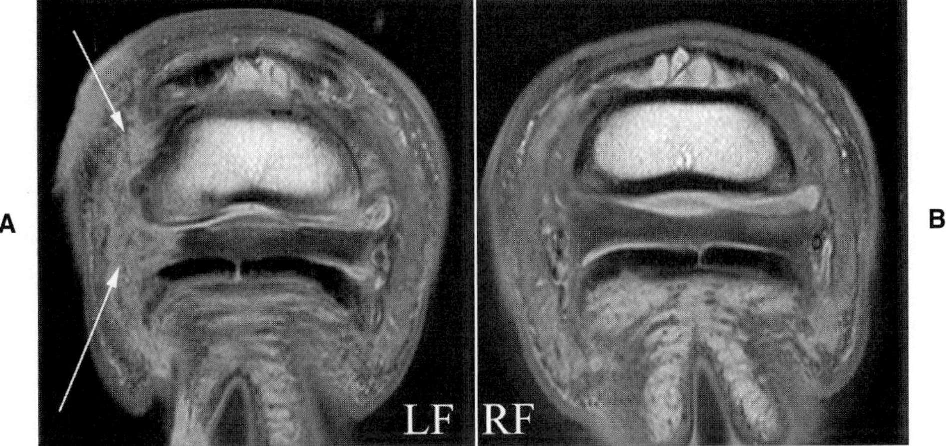

Figure 76-19. A, Axial proton density section through the condyles of the distal aspect of the middle phalanx of the left front foot shows the marked thickening and abnormal signal observed in the damaged medial collateral ligament and navicular suspensory ligament in a horse with a laceration proximal to the coronary band. **B,** The more normal right front foot for comparison.

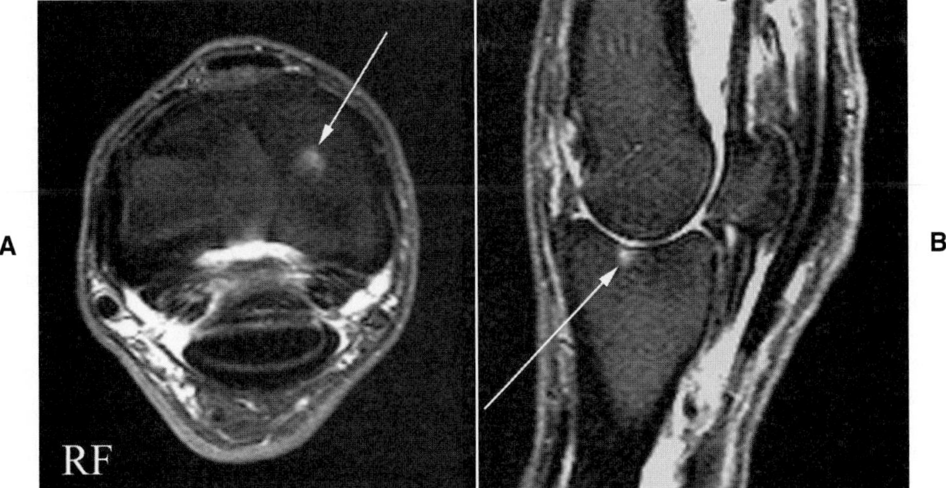

Figure 76-20. Axial (**A**) and sagittal (**B**) short tau inversion recovery (STIR) images of the right front limb from a horse with a high-signal-intensity area of fluid in the subchondral bone of the proximal aspect of the proximal phalanx *(arrows)*. An area of osteochondral damage was found on arthroscopic evaluation of the joint.

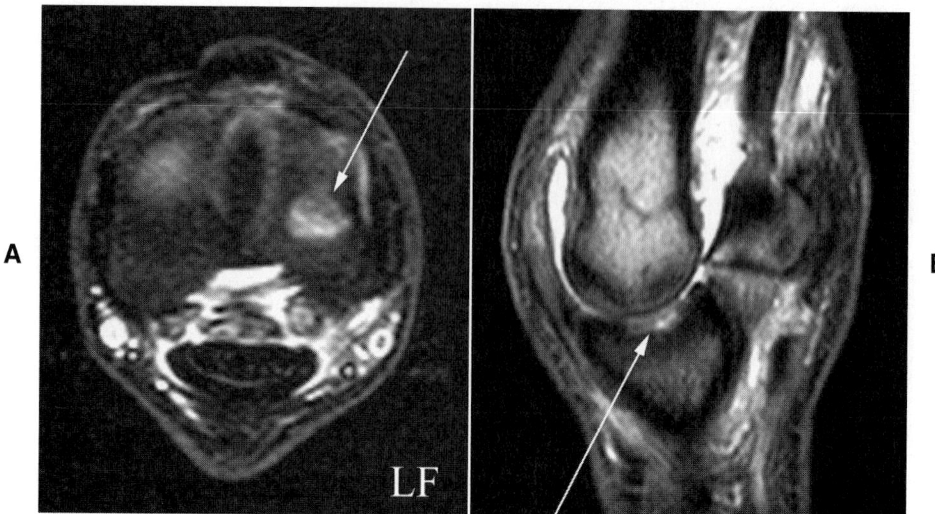

Figure 76-21. An axial short tau inversion recovery (STIR) (**A**) and sagittal proton density (**B**) image showing high signal intensity in the subchondral bone of both the proximal phalanx *(arrows)* and the opposing condyle of the distal third metacarpal bone. Because of the acute history of lameness, subchondral bone injury (bruising) was diagnosed.

observed as sclerosis as the bone responds to the injury. These observations with MRI have resulted in an expansion of the concept of bone injury beyond macroscopic fractures.

Subchondral bone damage may occur prior to, at the same time as, or after cartilage damage. Bone injuries may likely cause a larger number of lameness problems than was previously thought because most of the subchondral bone lesions observed with MRI are not visible on radiographs. Before MRI was available, these horses were diagnosed as suffering from a soft tissue injury of unknown origin.

Oblique and Straight Distal Sesamoidean Ligament Desmitis

The oblique distal sesamoidean ligaments (ODSL) have a homogeneous appearance on MR images, except where they originate from the base of the proximal sesamoid bones. In this area, the ligaments often appear striated with areas of low- and high-signal intensity. Both branches are low-signal, ovoid to triangular structures that form a single structure as they insert on the distopalmar aspect of the proximal phalanx. The straight distal sesamoidean ligaments (SDSL) have a heterogeneous appearance, with multiple low- and high-signal areas spread throughout most of its length. Lesions within the ODSL and SDSL can result in discrete or diffuse high-signal areas within or along the edge of the ligament. Enlargement of the ligament also can occur, usually with a moderate increase in signal density (Fig. 76-22). Desmitis of the ODSL can affect one or both branches (Fig. 76-23).

Distal sesamoidean ligament desmitis is not a new cause of lameness in horses, but it was previously difficult to definitively diagnose. Desmitis of the ODSL and SDSL involves injuries that can cause forelimb and hindlimb lameness in many types of performance horses. The lameness varies from mild to severe depending on the amount of damage to the ligament and the duration of the injury prior to diagnosis. Most of these horses do not have a palpable enlargement or swelling over the mid-phalangeal region, so MRI has proven valuable for diagnosing injury to the distal sesamoidean ligaments.[10]

Superficial Digital Flexor Tendinitis

Superficial digital flexor tendon lesions can be diagnosed with MRI in the phalangeal region. These lesions are most commonly seen distal to the bifurcation in the proximal phalangeal region (Fig. 76-24). The tendon gradually separates into two lobes, and lesions in one or both lobes can be observed as high-signal enlargements of the branches of the tendon proximal to its insertion on the middle phalanx.

Suspensory Ligament Desmitis

Clinical examination and ultrasonography have been used to diagnose horses with suspensory ligament injuries, a common problem in many types of performance horses. However, MRI has enabled diagnoses that were not possible before, including abnormalities in suspensory ligament branches (Figs. 76-25 and 76-26), insertion of the ligament on the proximal sesamoid bones, and insertion of the proximal suspensory ligament on the third metacarpals and third metatarsal bones (MCIII/MTIII). In the experience of the authors, MRI has proven superior to ultrasound for detecting desmitis in the equine suspensory ligament.

MRI OF THE METACARPUS AND METATARSUS

Proximal Suspensory Ligament Desmitis

The normal suspensory ligament (SL) does not contact the MCIII/MTIII at any point other than at its origin, and thickening caused by desmitis often results in a decrease or loss of the space between the SL and the MCIII/MTIII. Inflammation of the origin and body of the SL results in

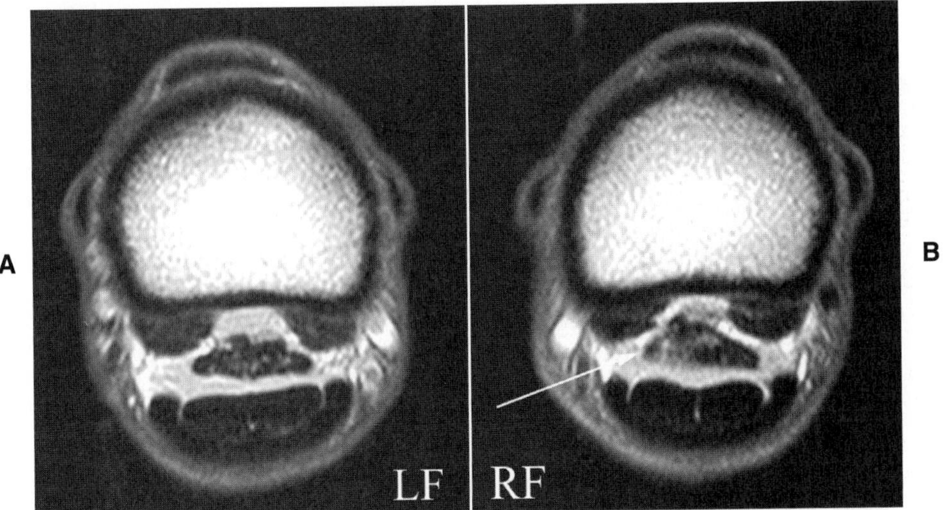

Figure 76-22. **A,** The normal left front limb for comparison. **B,** Axial proton density image of a horse with enlargement and an area of high signal intensity *(arrow)* in the straight distal sesamoidean ligament of the right front limb.

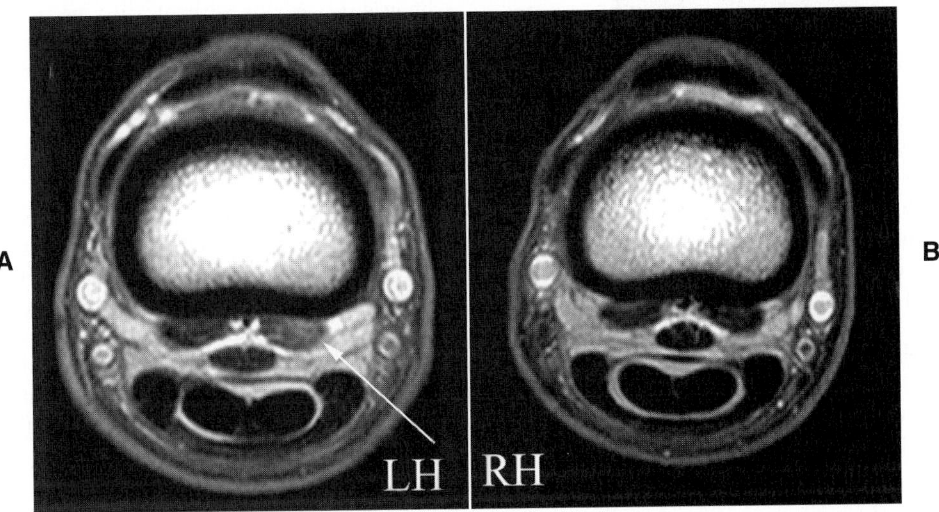

Figure 76-23. **A,** Axial proton density image of a horse with high signal intensity *(arrow)* in the lateral branch of the oblique distal sesamoidean ligament in the left pastern region. The abnormal ligament should be compared with the low signal intensity (dark) in the medial branch of the left hindlimb (**A**) and both branches of the right hindlimb (**B**), which serves as a normal control. These sections are through the middle aspect of the proximal phalanx.

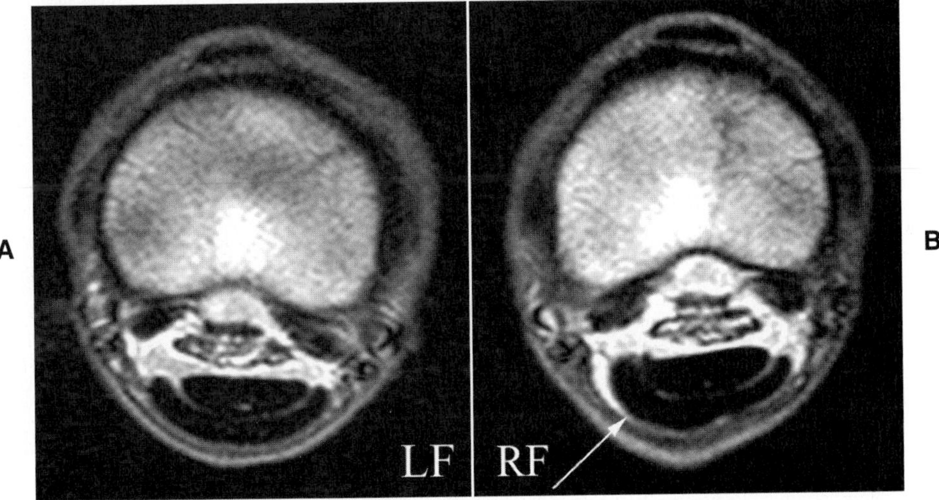

Figure 76-24. **A,** The normal left front image for control. **B,** Axial proton density image of a horse with enlargement of the lateral branch of the superficial digital flexor tendon *(arrow)* of the right front pastern.

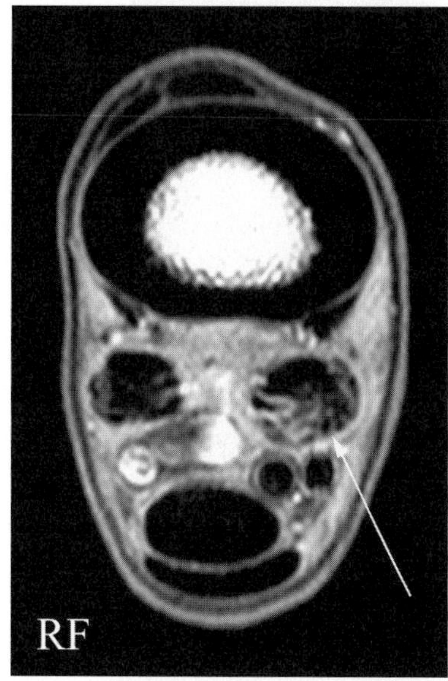

Figure 76-25. An axial proton density image from a horse with diffuse high signal intensity *(arrow)* in the axial aspect of the medial suspensory ligament branch proximal to its insertion on the proximal sesamoid bone. Clinical palpation of the horse's suspensory ligament did not detect this abnormality.

disruption of the fiber pattern with or without thickening of the ligament. Diffuse or discrete thickening can occur, and in severe cases of proximal SL desmitis, bone fluid has been seen at its origin (Fig. 76-27). Desmitis of the SL is an important cause of lameness in all types of performance horses. MRI has detected desmitis that was difficult to identify with other imaging modalities[9] (Fig. 76-28).

The ability to visualize margins of the entire suspensory ligament with MRI has enabled definitive diagnosis of adhesions between it and exostoses of MCII/IV and MTII/IV.[9] Adhesions are visible as low-signal fibers connecting the suspensory ligament to the axial aspect of the vestigial metacarpal or metatarsal bones. In many cases, ultrasonography cannot definitively determine whether adhesions in this area exist.[9] MRI can provide information on the suspensory ligament, location of adhesions, and size of exostoses on the axial surface of the vestigial metacarpal or metatarsal bones. Thickening and linear tears in the suspensory branches and adhesion between the suspensory body and MCII/IV and MTII/IV can be documented (Fig. 76-29).

Desmitis of the Accessory Ligament of the Deep Digital Flexor Tendon

Inflammation of the accessory ligament of the deep digital flexor tendon (ALDDFT) is most often seen as diffuse enlargement of the middle to proximal aspect of the ligament, with or without discrete or diffuse areas of high signal. A comparison can be made between the unaffected and the affected limb (Fig. 76-30). Mild desmitis of the ALDDFT is difficult to palpate and the diagnosis is made after MR scanning.

Magnetic resonance imaging enables the definitive diagnosis of a variety of equine distal limb lameness problems. It can be of great value when localization of lameness is not specific enough, or when more information is necessary for the selection of the best treatment modality or an accurate prognosis. MRI can identify lesions not apparent on radiographs or with ultrasonography and can define causes of lameness that can be localized only to an area on the limb. It is an invaluable diagnostic aid for the accurate diagnosis and treatment of equine lameness problems.

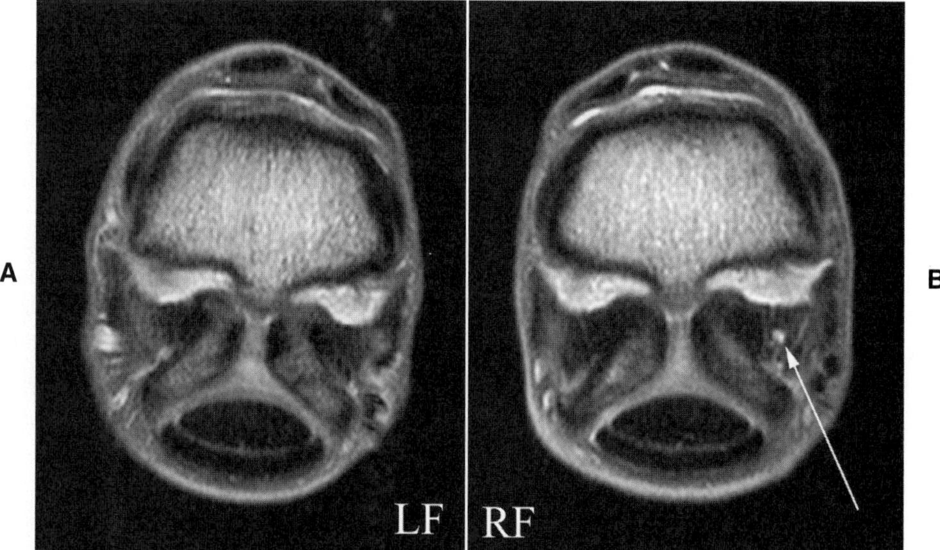

Figure 76-26. **A,** The normal left front limb for comparison. **B,** Axial proton density image of a Thoroughbred race horse with high signal intensity *(arrow)* at the insertion of the medial suspensory ligament branch to the proximal sesamoid bone of the right front metacarpophalangeal region.

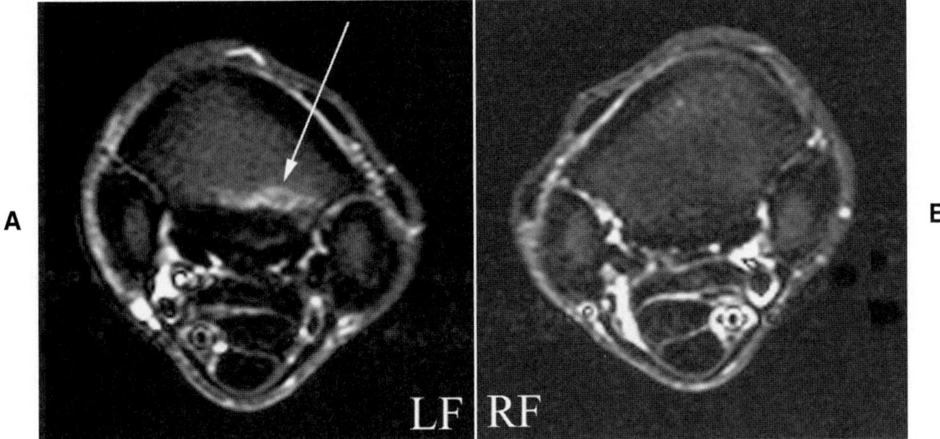

Figure 76-27. A, Axial short tau inversion recovery (STIR) image of a horse with high signal intensity *(arrow)* indicating fluid in the left front third metacarpus at the insertion of the proximal suspensory ligament. **B,** The normal right front limb shown for comparison. Note the vascular flow artifact running across the palmar aspect of the image.

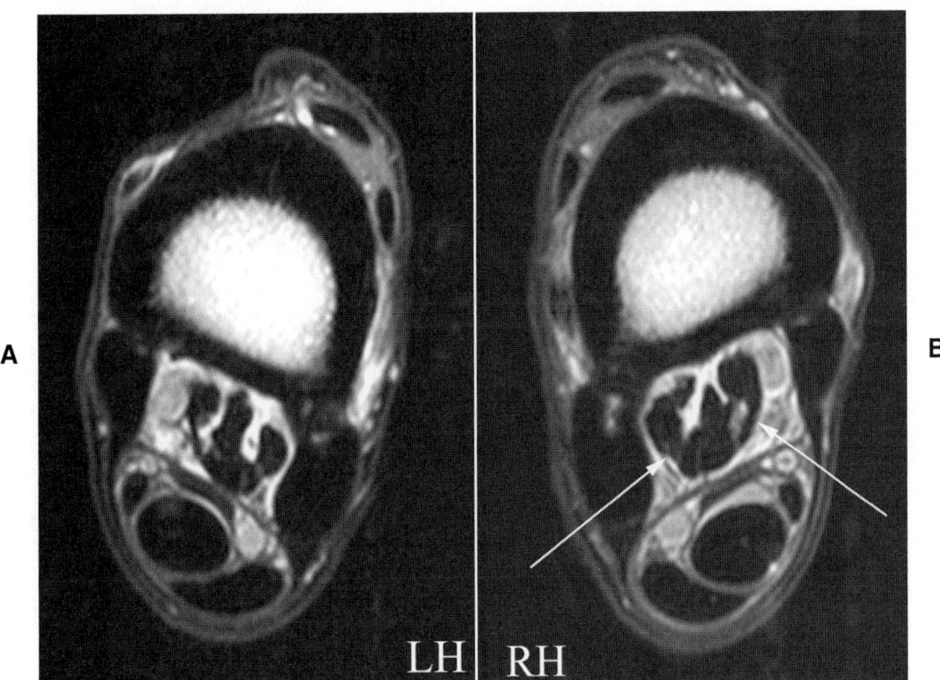

Figure 76-28. A, The normal left hindlimb is depicted for comparison. **B,** Axial proton density image from a horse with mild enlargement of the proximal suspensory ligament *(arrows)* of the right hindlimb.

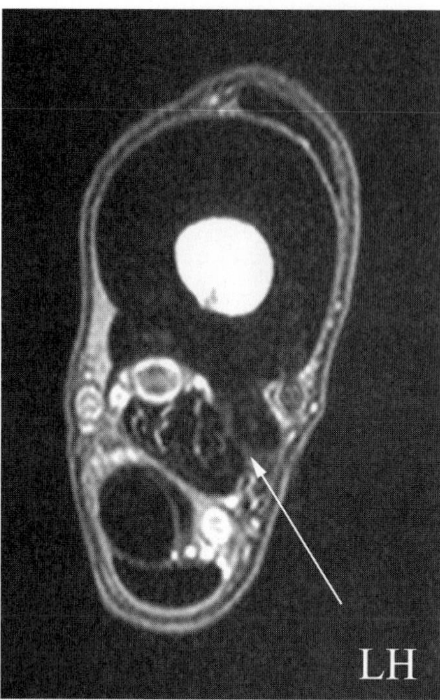

Figure 76-29. An axial proton density image of a horse with enlargement of the suspensory ligament and adhesion to the fourth metatarsal bone. (MTIV). Tissue is observed between MTIV and the suspensory ligament *(arrow)*.

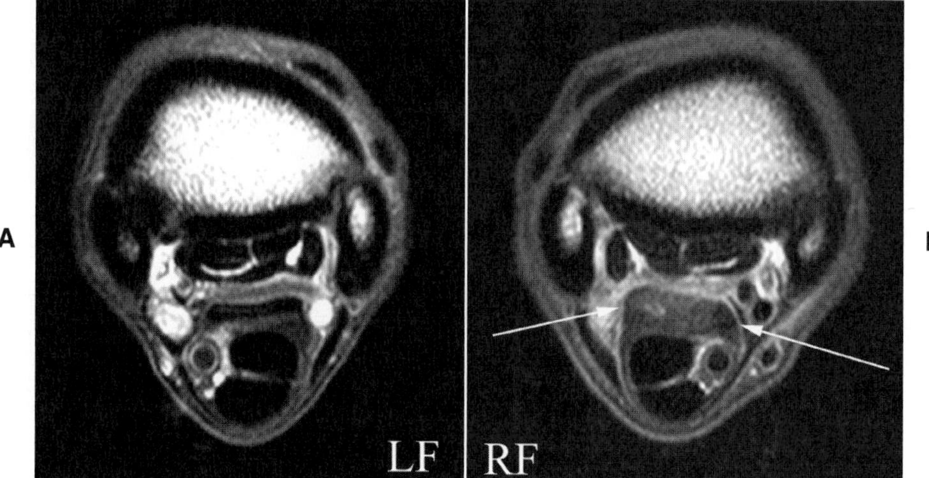

Figure 76-30. A, The normal left front limb for comparison. **B,** Axial proton density image of a horse with enlargement and high signal intensity in the accessory ligament of the deep digital flexor tendon (ALDDFT) of the right front metacarpus *(arrows)*. The abnormal ligament (**B**) should be compared with the dark, compact structure of the ALDDFT of the contralateral limb (**A**).

REFERENCES

1. Westbrook C, Kaut C: MRI in Practice, ed 2, Malden, Mass, 1998, Blackwell Science.
2. Snow VE, Rantanen NW: Sectional Anatomy of the Equine Digit with MRI, Buellton, Calif, 1996, Santa Ynez Valley Printing and Lithography.
3. Denoix JM: The Equine Distal Limb: An Atlas of Clinical Anatomy and Comparative Imaging, London, 2000, Manson.
4. Kraft SL, Gavin PR: Physical principles and technical considerations for equine computed tomography and magnetic resonance imaging, Vet Clin North Am Equine Pract 2001;17:115-130.
5. Tucker RL, Sande RD: Computed tomography and magnetic resonance imaging in equine musculoskeletal conditions, Vet Clin North Am Equine Pract 2001;17:145-157.
6. Schneider RK, Gavin PR, Tucker RL: What MRI is teaching us about navicular disease, Proc Am Assoc Equine Pract 2003;49:210-218.
7. Mehl ML, Tucker RL, Ragle CA, et al: The use of MRI in the diagnosis of equine limb disorders, Equine Pract 1998;20:14-17.
8. Zubrod CJ, Schneider RK, Tucker RL, et al: Use of magnetic

resonance imaging for identifying subchondral bone damage in horses: 11 cases (1999-2003), J Am Vet Med Assoc 2004;224:411-418.
9. Zubrod CJ, Schneider RK, Tucker RL: Use of magnetic resonance imaging to identify suspensory desmitis and adhesions between exostoses of the second metacarpal bone and the suspensory ligament in four horses, J Am Vet Med Assoc 2004;224:1815-1820.
10. Sampson SN, Schneider RK, Tucker RL, et al: Oblique and straight distal sesamoidean ligament desmitis diagnosed with MRI in horses with lameness: 27 cases (1998-2004) (in preparation).
11. Murray RC, Dyson SJ, Schramme MC, et al: Magnetic resonance imaging of the equine digit with chronic laminitis, Vet Rad Ultrasound 2003;44:609-617.
12. Dyson S, Murray R, Schramme M, et al: Magnetic resonance imaging of the equine foot: 15 horses, Equine Vet J 2003;35:18-26.
13. Busoni V, Snaps F, Trenteseaux, RT, et al: Magnetic resonance imaging of the palmar aspect of the equine podotrochlear apparatus: Normal appearance, Vet Rad Ultrasound 2004;45:198-204.
14. Turner TA, Kneller SK, Badertscher RR, et al: Radiographic changes in the navicular bones of normal horses, Am Assoc Equine Pract 1986;32:309-313.
15. Busoni V, Denoix JM: Ultrasonography of the podotrochlear apparatus in the horse using a transcuneal approach: technique and reference images, Vet Radiol Ultrasound 2001;46:534-540.
16. Dyson SJ: Subjective and quantitative scintigraphic assessment of the equine foot and its relationship with foot pain, Equine Vet J 2002;34:164-170.
17. Dyson SJ, Murray RC, Schramme MC, Branch MW: Magnetic resonance imaging in 18 horses with palmar foot pain, Proc Am Assoc Equine Pract 2002;48:145-154.
18. Schneider RK, Tucker RL, Gavin PR, et al: Magnetic resonance imaging of the front feet of horses with clinical signs of navicular disease without radiographic abnormalities (in preparation).
19. Dyson SJ, Murray RC, Schramme MC, et al: Collateral desmitis of the distal interphalangeal joint in 18 horses (2001-2002), Equine Vet J 2004;36:160-166.

CHAPTER 77

Saddle Evaluation: Poor Fit Contributing to Back Problems in Horses

Brigitte von Rechenberg

Back problems from thoracolumbar soreness in horses have become a frequent complaint in equine practice and represent a challenge for the practitioner.[1-8] If there are clear radiographic signs of changes at the spine, such as impingement of the dorsal spinous processes ("kissing spines"), spondylopathies of the vertebral bodies, or narrowing of the spinal canal in the cervical area, the diagnosis is relatively straightforward, although the situation is not always easily resolved for the patient. However, in most cases, the cause is more obscure, and pain cannot be easily attributed to changes in the bony skeleton. Complaints of the owners are unspecific and usually consist of problems related to riding rather than lameness. Owners often complain about "unexplainable" resistance of the horses to perform, mental problems of the horses, such as subtle changes of character, and in more severe cases, slight lameness of the hindlimbs or even the forelimbs. In these cases of slight lameness, frequent staggering can become a problem, apart from on-and-off lameness. Very often, owners have sought veterinary help to no avail, especially when radiographs of joints or the spine are normal. Frequently, horses have gone through osteopathic, chiropractic, and acupuncture therapy with a short period of improvement, but the problems are usually not solved in the long term.[9,10]

Although horses today are kept mainly for horseback riding in leisure or sports activities, veterinarians are reluctant to look into problems related to their use connected to the riding style or equestrian equipment. This may be partly because many equine veterinarians are not horseback riders themselves and simply cannot make educated recommendations. It may also be related to a lack of the courage needed to tell their prospective horse clients that their riding style or equipment needs improvement. Fortunately, antique beliefs that horses do not have back problems have vanished altogether. It is impossible to evaluate today whether horses in older times really did not suffer from back problems or whether symptoms were simply ignored. Nevertheless, the increasing frequency of the complaint of back problems in horses may be related to an increased awareness of horse owners and veterinarians, but also to the attempts of many horse owners to take shortcuts in basic horse education. Therefore, careful training, especially of young sport horses, is neglected. This means that they are not given enough time to learn how to move with a rider on their back, and they are forced into positions of the head and back that the osseous and soft tissue structures of their backs are not quite ready to accept. For example, dressage horses are frequently forced into collection by their owners using all kind of support reins, whips, spurs, and other questionable riding gear.

In addition, the increasing frequency of back problems in horses may be the result of the modern breeding of horses, which (at least in Warmblood horses) has changed considerably. Not only has the size of horses become enormous (e.g., Hanoverian horses), but also the percentage of Thoroughbred and Arabian blood in their breeding has increased. The huge size of the Warmblood horses renders riding them in collection more problematic, and the character and mentality of Thoroughbreds and Arabian horses do not permit the forceful riding style that the older type of Warmblood horses seems to have accepted.

Hence, to make an accurate assessment of back pain caused by poor saddle fit, a careful clinical examination should be carried out, and an in-depth anamnesis of the problems encountered by the rider during riding gathered. Ideally, the horse should also be presented under saddle and tack.

SIGNS OF BACK PAIN ATTRIBUTABLE TO POOR SADDLE FIT

Signs of horses with back pain attributable to poor saddle fit may be obvious, such as saddle pressure soreness mainly in the area of the withers. However, most signs are much more subtle and need careful evaluation.[3-7,11-14] Therefore, the first evaluation should be an assessment of riding style.

Regardless of the type of horseback riding used (e.g., English, Western, Spanish), a rider usually tries to ride the horse "in collection." This means that the horse, in response to the aids given by the rider, bends its head at an angle of 95 degrees to the vertical line of the ground and places the hindlimbs under the rump, resulting in a lifting of the back toward the saddle. In rider jargon, this is referred to as the horse "giving" its back. If a horse is collected properly under the rider, guidance of the horse through fine weight-shifting of the rider in the saddle and subtle signals through the reins becomes very easy and smooth. A well-ridden horse responds to these aids swiftly and to a pull at the reins of only 100 to 200 g. Also, the horse moves forward easily and, in most instances, keeps chewing on the bit, producing visible saliva on its lips.

Unfortunately, often horses are ridden very differently. Riders without patience force the horses to collect, so that they pull their heads down into collection with the reins, using a force up to kilogram levels. Quite often, this false collection is aided by all kinds of support reins. Although these horses may look collected to the observer, in reality the situation is the opposite of being ridden under collection. These horses work against the reins and hands of the rider, and they do not place their hindlimbs under their rump. The gaits of these horses seem choppy, their strides are shortened, and very often their hindlimbs seem to move independently and out of rhythm with the forelimbs. These forceful riding styles can be diagnosed by "counting" the rhythm and looking at the placement of the limbs of the horse, first while being lunged without a rider, and comparing this with the rhythm of the horse moving under the rider. In addition, horses that go against the hand of the rider (or are pulled back forcefully) have pain in the parotid salivary gland regions when they are palpated. Often, these glands are swollen as well. Especially in dressage horses, pain at the proximal insertion of the nuchal ligament on the head supports this diagnosis.

Forceful riding styles alone can be responsible for horses being unresponsive to given aids, especially after they develop back soreness. However, these signs are presented very often in combination with ill-fitting saddles. Most likely, the ill-fitting saddle is disturbing the muscle action of the back by eliciting undue pressure under the saddle. The horses try to evade the pain through pulling the head up and not bending the back upward toward the saddle. These actions cause shortening of the strides and wrong placement of the limbs during the movements mentioned. An impatient and ignorant rider worsens the problem for the horse considerably. If these horses are ridden with a well-fitting saddle, improvement in movement and riding actions is instantaneous. If a horse is unresponsive to the aids, the rider often refers to a horse as being "hard mouthed" and not "bending" easily into curves or volts (tight circles) required in basic dressage exercises. Therefore, dressage riders, especially, include these symptoms in their anamnesis, together with other behavioral problems of their mounts.

Changes in temperament include frequent and unexplainable attempts of the horse to run off while being ridden. Dressage horses are reported to "hollow the back" from underneath the saddle, which makes it impossible to collect the horse at the reins and bend them smoothly into volts or to perform on a higher level (e.g., the piaffe). It becomes difficult for the rider to elicit smooth transitions between gaits without the horse pulling its head up and losing collection. Often, affected horses become "hard" in the mouth, stop salivating while being ridden, and are difficult to be guided or ridden smoothly. When observed during riding, and especially in collection, horses frequently do not overreach with their hindlimbs (as viewed from the side), and they deviate to one side (mostly to the right side if the rider is right handed) with their hindlimbs (as viewed from the back). If the latter gait abnormality disappears when the horse is ridden with loose reins, it indicates that these problems may be connected to the riding style (e.g., forceful collection) alone. However, if related to poor saddle fit, especially in the lumbar area, the signs usually persist during more relaxed movements. Holding the tail to one side during (or with repeated attempts at) urination may also indicate saddle problems as well as pain. When transitions are made from a collected to a relaxed riding style, horses may pull their heads up instead of stretching their necks and heads forward and downward (in rider jargon, "finding their way to the ground"). However, this may also be related to riding style, with or without a relationship to poor saddle fit. When horses are observed during saddling, they often pull back their ears, move away from underneath the saddle, or, in severe cases, even try to bite the owners.

Close inspection of the hair coat shows broken hair and sometimes swollen hair follicles in particular areas—normally, either the withers or the lumbar area. Both indicate too much pressure, or movement of the saddle, during riding. Muscle atrophy, mainly in the area of the withers or just behind, is often associated with narrow saddles. Soft palpation of the muscles using just the fingertips reveals tension and muscle soreness, especially in the lumbar area. Normal horses do not contract their muscles in response to this type of palpation. Sore spots on the neck, mainly at the interface between the cleidomastoid part of the sternocephalic muscle and the brachiocephalic muscle, may be attributed to ill-fitting saddles, but they are more often the result of the rider technique ("hard hand") or the use of support reins (e.g., sliding reins). Finally, dorsiflexion, lateroflexion, and ventral flexion are severely impaired in horses with back soreness.[10,15,16]

Back problems caused by the saddle can be associated with the type of riding because they are linked with certain reins, additional aids, and type of saddles. As an example, Western saddles are usually longer than English saddles and, depending on the size of the horse, may cause problems in the lumbar area (Arabian horses frequently have shorter backs—one less lumbar vertebra—and are therefore ill suited to most Western saddles). The baroque or Iberian style of riding is connected to a specific construction of a saddle (the Spanish type of bar saddle) that distributes the main pressure of the saddle on two main areas (the withers and lumbar areas), which not all horses are strong enough and suited to tolerate without developing back soreness. Additionally, when saddles are bought according to the rider's preference, and not adapted to the needs of the horse, the saddle may be the center of a back problem. One saddle is often used for several horses, despite the fact that the sizes and the conformations of their backs may be very different (e.g., V-shaped or U-shaped). With racehorses, the saddle comes with the jockey but is never adapted to the young horse.

Ideally, the comfort of both rider and horse should be taken into consideration. A saddle should *never* be purchased without fitting it to the horse's back. Ideally, a good saddle maker is present to consider the needs of the rider *and* the horse. The horse's back has a certain conformation and cannot adapt to a saddle; rather, the saddle should be adapted to the back of the horse. It is the configuration of the back (where the saddle is positioned), the distribution of the pressure the saddle exerts on the underlying muscles, and the conditioning (or lack thereof) of the back muscles that interact to cause of back problems.

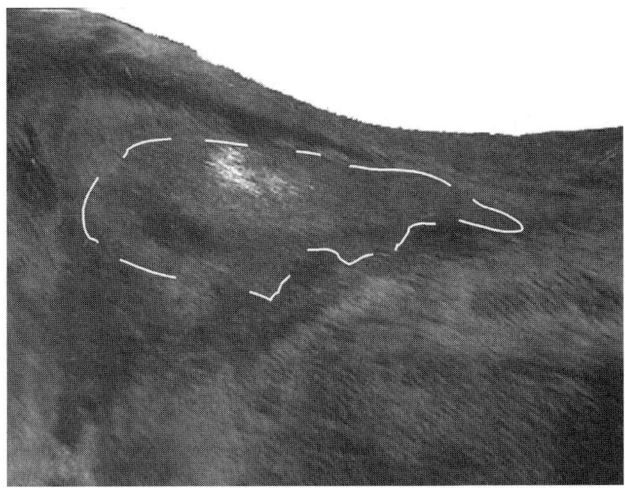

Figure 77-1. The saddle was removed from this horse immediately after exercise. Apart from a former saddle pressure sore (indicated by white hair), it can be seen that the horse did not sweat under the saddle at the slope of the shoulder *(encircled area)*. This indicates that the saddle was too tight and was not adapted properly to the slope of the shoulder.

SADDLE EVALUATION

Saddle evaluations should start with a good physical examination. The radius of the horse's back and the curve of the saddle have to correlate well (Fig. 77-1). Freedom for shoulder movement and dorsal spinal processes of the thoracic vertebrae must be allowed with all types of saddles (Fig. 77-2, *A*). The outward rotation of the saddle tree (or twist) at the front end of the saddle allows room for the shoulder musculature (Fig. 77-2, *B*). The angle of the saddle cushions should correspond to the shape of the back.

A variety of equipment is available to assist in determining the shape of the back for saddle fitting. The aids range from more complicated computer-driven topographic devices (Saddletech gauges) to simple flexible rods and calipers. This equipment is useful for purchasing a saddle, but generally it cannot be used to evaluate back problems related to poor saddle fit. The most reliable equipment is an electronic saddle mat that allows dynamic pressure

A

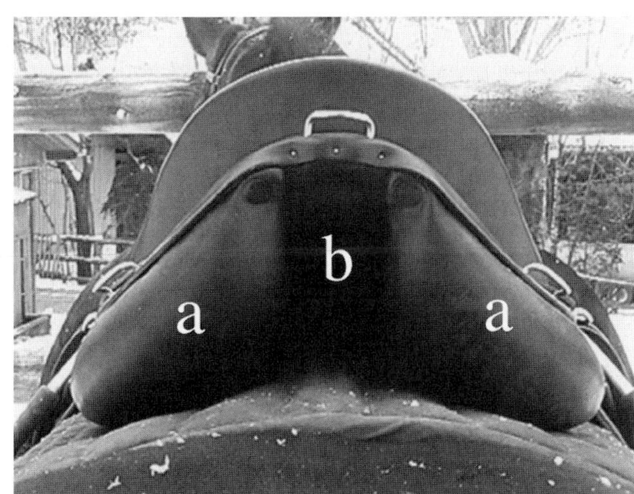

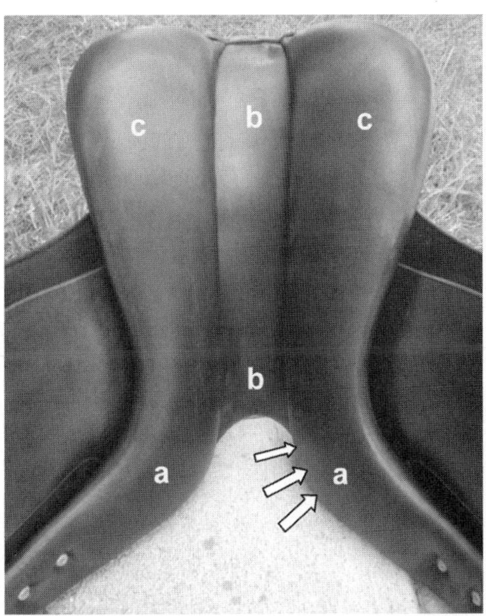

B

Figure 77-2. A well-fitting saddle seen from behind (**A**) and from underneath (**B**). The saddle has cushions (a) with even, soft upholstery; a large gulch (b) with an appropriate height in the withers area to prevent pressure on the dorsal spinal processes; and wide extensions (c) in the lumbar area. Furthermore, there is an outward rotation (twist) at the shoulder area *(arrows)* to accept the slope of the shoulder of the horse. Note that the cushions are fixed only at the cranial and caudal ends, leaving them more flexible to adapt to the angle of the horse's back.

measurements to be taken while the horse is in motion.[17-20] (Pressure measurements under the saddle taken during the stance phase is of limited value.) The Pliance saddle system (Novel GmbH, Munich, Germany) is one of the most sophisticated and useful systems to record pressure measurements during motion.[15,16]

The Pliance mobile 16HE system consists of two thin 2.6-mm saddle mats (dimensions, 169×105×45 mm), weighing 800 g. These mats are equipped with 112 (English saddle) or 128 (Western saddle) sensors on each side of the saddle that allow measurements between 10 and 60 kPa. The analyzer (Pliance-16 analyzer) is connected to the saddle mats by wires, and it is carried on the rider's back with a special belt (Fig. 77-3). The data are transferred to the computer either by a computer memory card or via Bluetooth wireless. Several software programs (Novel-Win, Novel GmbH, Munich, Germany) are available for data analysis, each with characteristics that demonstrate one particular feature of the measurements. Either they use two- (Axis, Isobar) or three-dimensional (Mountain Magic) color pictures indicating the individual sensors, or they use curves (Value Master, Emed-*sf*) over the entire measurement period, where maximal, minimal, or mean values are exhibited (Fig. 77-4). The Novel player allows synchronization with videos taken at the time of measurements. Each program has the ability to show the measured area either as a single, virtually calculated picture or in the time sequence as it was measured in real time. The scanning rate of the sensors is 10,000 frames per second (44 frames per second).

Colors (black, blue, green, yellow, pink, red) can be assigned to the pressure values, facilitating interpretation of the data. The maximal pressure picture (MPP) is a virtual picture that gives this value for each sensor during the entire measurement period. The mean value picture (MVP) is the calculated mean value over time and includes all sensors that were loaded at one time. The maximal area picture (MAP) is the frame where the measured area was highest. The maximal force picture (MFP) is the frame where the sum of all forces is the highest.

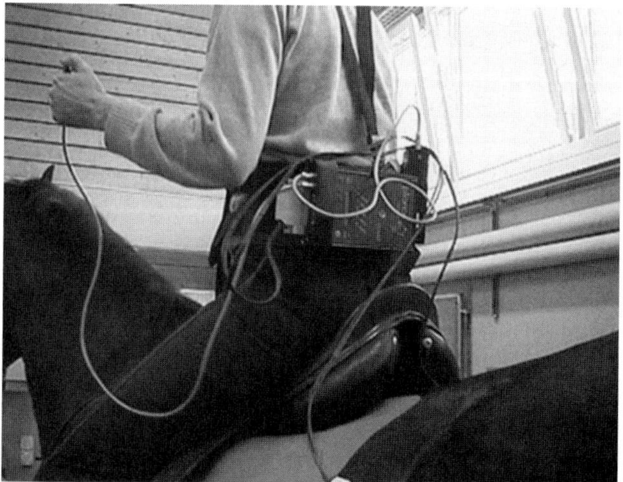

Figure 77-3. The Pliance mobile HE16 system mounted on rider and horse. The analyzer is carried on the back of the rider using a special harness, and it is connected to the electronic saddle mat by wires. The measurement is sent to a laptop computer via Bluetooth wireless.

The development of a new database allows direct capturing of the data measured, and the editing and printing of the results according to an individually customized computer macro.

Apart from the different software programs, a generalized feature is available that allows the entire mat to be divided into smaller areas called masks. This allows predefined local areas to be calculated separately (Fig. 77-5). Additional features are included to statistically evaluate individual measurements.

INTERPRETATION OF THE DATA

The Pliance system measures not only the pressure under the saddle and its distribution over the saddle area but also the direction of forces, which provides a better understanding of the interaction between the rider, the saddle, and the horse. The system is easy to use and delivers reliable and repeatable data in normal horses, horses with back pain, and horses before and after osteopathic or chiropractic treatment.[10,15,16]

For a more detailed evaluation, the pressure recording is divided into six masks. On each side a cranial, middle, and caudal mask are defined (see Fig. 77-5). Evaluation of saddles on 500 different horses using the six masks proved to be a reliable method to assess saddle fit.[10,16] It was shown that horses tolerate higher pressures in the cranial part of the saddle corresponding to the withers area than in the caudal part representing the lumbar area. Saddles exceeding MPP values of 34.5 kPa in the cranial, 30.3 kPa in the middle, and 31.0 kPa in the caudal third of the saddle were always connected to back problems diagnosed according to a clinical scoring system for back pain.[15] The same was found for the MVP, for which values greater than 13.2 kPa for the cranial, 11.4 kPa for the middle, and 10.0 kPa for the caudal part were related to back problems.[15,16]

Absolute pressure values played a significant role. However, the distribution of peak pressures was equally important. Independent of saddle type, if high peak pressure values occurred in a small area close to the spine or in the lumbar area, back problems were generally more severe than when the same pressures were distributed equally over a larger area (Fig. 77-6). Saddles resulting in relatively uniform pressure recordings during the entire trotting cycle (or, more precisely, where at least two thirds of the entire saddle area continuously registered pressure data during the entire evaluation period) showed lower pressure values and the horses experienced fewer back problems.[15] The presence of a high variability in the cranial and caudal aspects of the saddle indicated wiggling of the saddle, usually caused by the radius of the saddle being smaller than the radius of the horse's back (Fig. 77-7). This was often combined with a very irregular center of gravity for the rider as recorded in the axis program (Fig. 77-8).

Bridging of the saddles (i.e., the front and back of the saddle make contact with the horse's back, but not the middle) was observed if the radius of the saddle was larger than the radius of the horse's back, and this resulted in very high pressure values in the cranial and caudal parts of the saddle and relatively low values in the middle part (Fig. 77-9). In severe cases, pressure values up to 60 kPa were seen, which inevitably correlated to severe muscle pain and sensitivity of the dorsal spinal processes of the spine in the

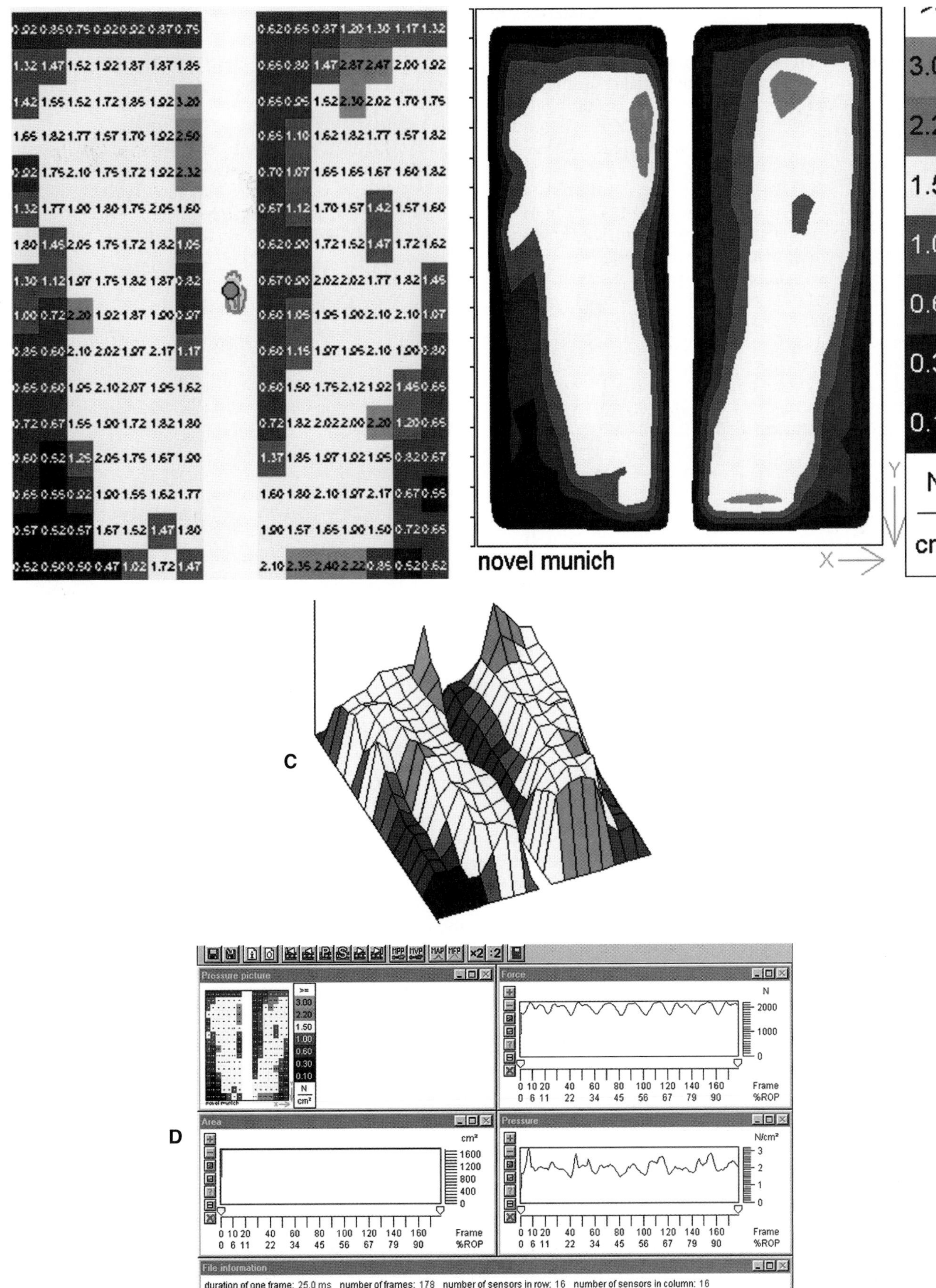

Figure 77-4. Different graphics produced by software programs used with the Pliance mobile system. **A,** Axis. **B,** Isobar. **C,** Magic Mountain. **D,** Value Master, and Emed-*sf*. Although Axis, Isobar, and Magic Mountain have good visual effects and are well suited to explain pressure values to owners, the Value Master and Emed-*sf* programs are better suited for scientific analysis.

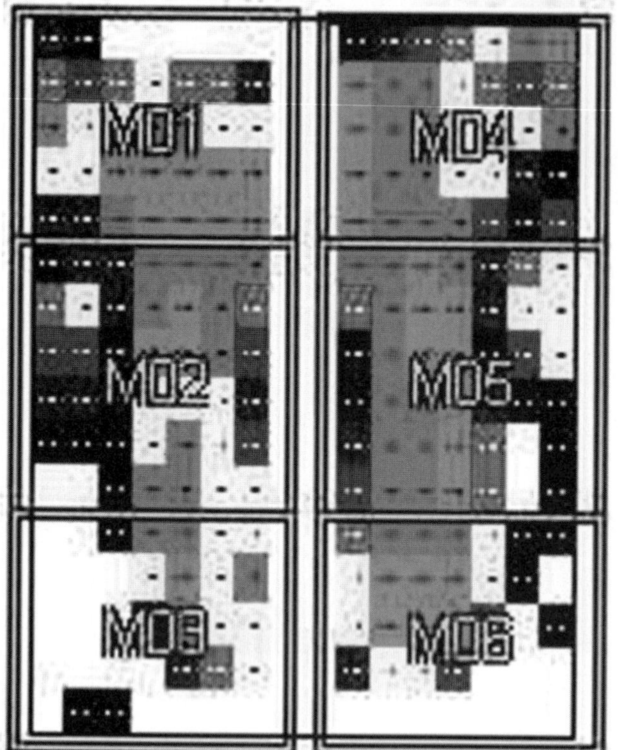

Figure 77-5. The pressure recordings of a saddle can be divided into left (MO1 to MO3) and right (MO4 to MO6) sides, as well as into cranial (MO1 and MO4), middle (MO2 and MO5) and caudal (MO3 and MO7) masks. This facilitates the correlation of the values measured to back pain in localized areas.

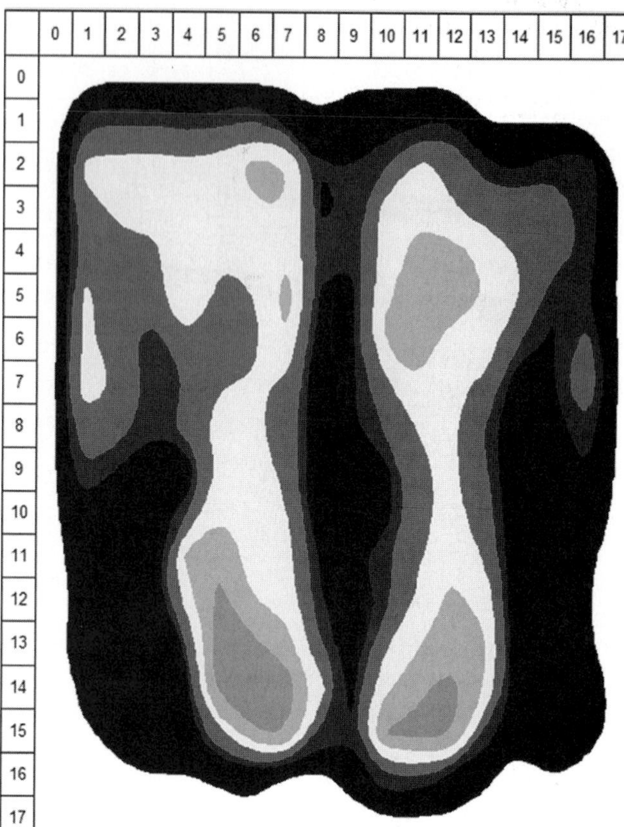

Figure 77-6. Maximal pressure picture (MPP) of saddle measurements with peak pressures in a small and very localized area. Horses are more sensitive to peak pressures in a small area, as indicated in this MPP graph using the Isobar representation.

lumbar area, as identified during the physical examination.[16] The bridging effect was considered one of the most severe faults in saddle fit. In Western saddles, high pressures were more obvious in the shoulder area, often restricting free movement of the forelimbs.[21] In race saddles, the peak pressures were often seen over the dorsal spinal processes and directly caudal from the withers. However, even in racehorses, high pressure values were seen in the lumbar area, especially with the training saddles. The occurrence of back pain and other signs in race horses could be correlated to their age of training and also to pressure values found with the saddles.[16]

Significantly different pressure patterns and high pressure values were always found in saddles with narrow widths of the gullet and missing freedom of the shoulder, not only in the withers but also in the lumbar area[16] (Fig. 77-10). Significantly lower pressure values were observed with custom-fit saddles than with off-the-shelf saddles. High pressure values were found in horses with neck problems, and with painful cervical and lumbar muscles in association with abnormalities of all flexion tests of the back and the neck. Significant correlations were demonstrated between back muscle atrophy and MPP values, saddle repairs, freedom of the shoulder, and length of the saddle tree. This was also true for saddle pressure and symmetry as well as padding of the saddle cushions. The harder the cushions, the higher were the pressure values. Significant correlations were also found between the caudal positioning of the center of the saddle seat (moved toward the lumbar area) and cervical and lumbar muscle sores. Pain on palpation of the dorsal processes was always correlated with the width of the gulch and caudal positioning of the center of the saddle seat. Problems of the iliosacral joint were associated with the width of the gulch as well as the length of the saddle tree. If supporting aids such as sliding reins were used, forcing the horse into false collection, the pressure values (MPP and MVP) were increased up to 8 kPa (MPP) and 3 kPa (MVP) in the cranial part of the saddle. This pressure increase amounts to approximately 30% of the allowed pressure values for both the MPP and the MVP.[22]

OPTIMAL SADDLE FIT

As a result of the studies with the Pliance system, pressure values for an optimal saddle fit were calculated.[15,16] If MPP values were lower than 34.5 kPa in the cranial, 30.3 kPa in the middle, and 31.0 kPa in the caudal part, and MVP values were below 13.2 kPa for the cranial, 11.4 kPa for the middle, and 10.0 kPa for the caudal part of the saddles, horses were normally free of saddle-induced back pain. A good saddle shows symmetric distribution of the saddle area, and MAP values greater than 900 cm^2 during the unloaded phase and 1200 to 1400 cm^2 during the loaded phase (with the rider). In the loaded phase, the weight of the rider is fully in the saddle, whereas during the unloaded phase, the rider's weight is not in the center of the saddle (e.g., in posting, in

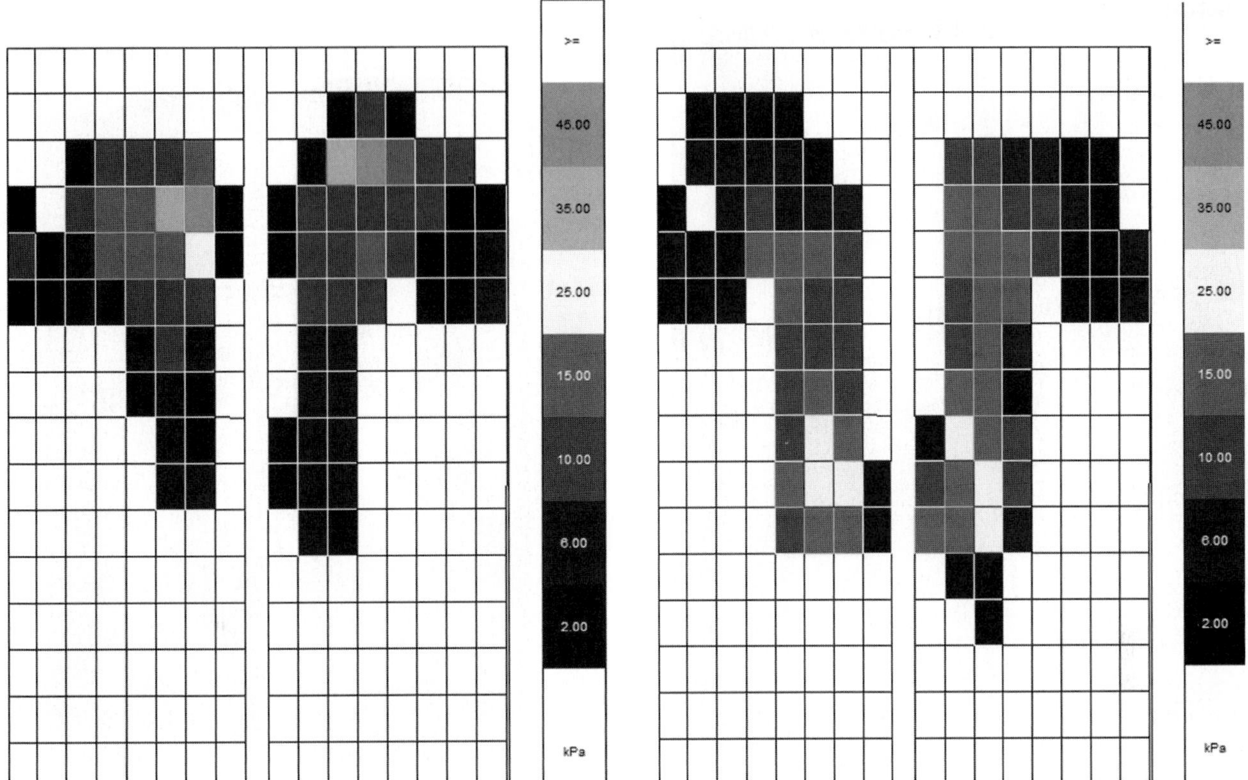

Figure 77-7. Consecutive frames of a saddle measurement. In this case, the saddle had a smaller radius than the radius of the horse's back. During movement (English trot), the saddle wiggles and loses contact with the shoulder and the lumbar areas. **A,** Mean value picture (MVP) values are shown while the rider is standing in the stirrups (standing phase). **B,** The weight is distributed over a larger area while the rider is seated in the saddle (sitting phase). Note the shift of the area and weight of the rider to the lumbar area and compare with the standing phase, where high peak pressures are shown in the shoulder area.

the swinging phase of the movement). Good saddle panels for the horse's back are large, they have a soft and even padding, they have no stitches facing the horse's back, they are wide in the lumbar area, and they optimally are fixed to the saddle body only in the front and the back (see Fig. 77-2). They leave a wide, symmetric gulch of even width from the cranial to the caudal aspect of the saddle. A well-fitting saddle is placed with its front end at the caudal edge of the scapula; the center of the seat should be positioned over the 12th thoracic rib, and the length of the saddle should not reach farther than the last thoracic vertebrae. In smaller horses, such as Arabians, ponies, and Haflinger horses, this may be a problem depending on the size of the saddle seat (which depends on the size of the rider) and the overall construction of the saddle (e.g., a Western saddle).

An optimal saddle fit is difficult or impossible to achieve if the radius of the saddle and the horse's back do not match. The same is true if the center of the saddle seat is not in the middle part of the saddle but is shifted toward the caudal aspect. This may be related, at least in the English saddle, to the saddle model and the construction of the saddletree (including the head-iron, which determines the fit at the shoulder and over the withers), as well as to the width and height of the saddle gullet in the front of the saddle. In some cases, it may be possible to correct the twist of the saddle, but generally this is not successful. With the shift of the center of the saddle seat toward its caudal aspect, the distance between the suspension of the stirrups and the center of the seat becomes too long (Fig. 77-11). Ideally, this distance does not exceed 1.5 times the width of the hand of the rider. If it is longer, the rider is placed in a so-called chair-seat, which induces unduly high pressures on the horse's lumbar area and "moves the rider behind the horse."

This feature is very difficult to correct in a saddle. When the width of the saddle in the shoulder area is too narrow, correction can be made by replacing the head-iron with a new and larger one, as long as the height of the saddle gulch permits it. If it does not, the saddle may touch the dorsal spinal processes of the withers and cause new and severe problems. Sometimes, a saddle correction can be easily made by renewing the saddle panels with new, soft padding. Restuffing the old saddle panels is not recommended, because they end up being harder than the original ones, the symmetry of the saddle cushions often cannot be achieved, and the padding itself is not of even consistency. In an earlier research study using the Pliance system, it was shown that upholstering the cushions was correlated with higher pressure values and mild muscle sores.

A total of 25 horses presented with back pain were followed after saddle corrections were performed by a skilled saddle maker, or after purchase of a new saddle, and an evaluation was performed with the Pliance system. The absolute pressure values given earlier could be confirmed in this study.[23] If corrections resulted in lower values, the back pain of the horses resolved in all cases, normally within 4 to 6 months after changing the saddles and without any further

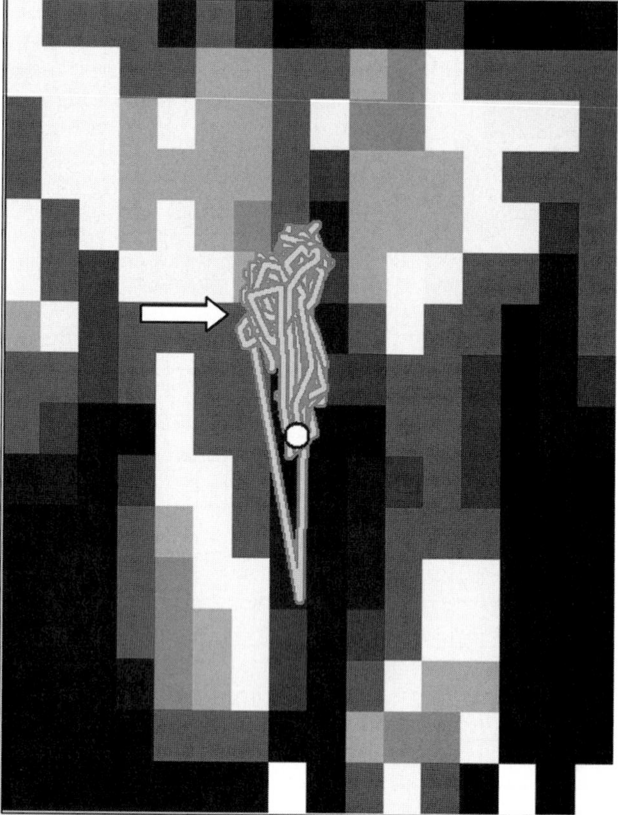

Figure 77-8. Maximal pressure picture (MPP) presented in the Axis program, showing the excursions made by the rider's center of gravity *(arrow)* during a trot. The *white circle* represents the center of gravity when the rider is standing in the saddle. A good saddle automatically places even an inexperienced rider in its center. The better the saddle and the rider, the smaller is the excursion of the center of gravity.

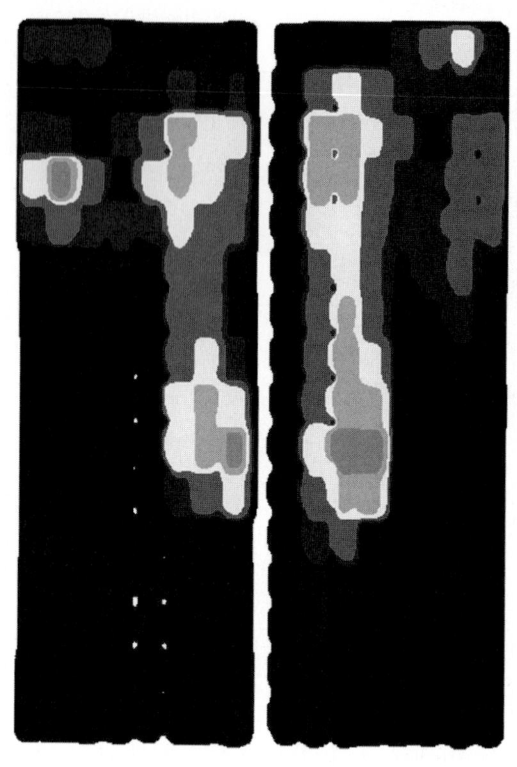

Figure 77-9. The bridging effect of a saddle. High pressure values are recorded at the withers and the lumbar regions but not in the middle of the saddle area. The bridging effect occurs because the radius of the saddle is larger than the radius of the horse's back. The bridging effect shown is severe.

treatment modalities. If horses showed severe pain mainly in the lumbar area, the owners were directed to rest them on pasture for at least 4 weeks before riding with the new or corrected saddle was resumed. In most cases, the corrections were most critical for the lumbar area, since corrections normally included a cranial shift of the center of saddle seat away from the lumbar region and toward the middle or wither area of the horse's back. Although both the corrected and the newly purchased saddles fulfilled these criteria of optimal saddle pressures, the values obtained with corrections of the saddles were better than those of the new saddles. This may just highlight the fact that saddle makers generally have a better knowledge of optimal saddle fit than the salesperson in the average equestrian equipment shop. In all cases, owners were highly satisfied with the results and commented on the improved motivation, willingness, and ease of their horses to perform according to their wishes.

SADDLE EVALUATIONS IN EQUINE VETERINARY PRACTICE

Evaluation of saddle fit in relation to back problems in horses has a definite place in equine veterinary practice. Without a well-fitting saddle, good riding and performance cannot be expected. Since horseback riding is the main reason that horses are kept and brought to the veterinarian, saddle evaluations should be routinely offered in specialized equine veterinary practices. Surgeons, who diagnose obscure lameness in horses, especially when no correlation between radiographic findings and clinical examinations can be found, should also be aware of this. Before horses are subjected to alternative therapies, such as manipulations of the spine using osteopathy, chiropractic manipulations, and acupuncture, a thorough saddle evaluation should be performed by an experienced clinician. The saddle should be inspected from all sides and then placed on the horse to see if it fits properly. The horse should be observed with the saddle and with the rider at a walk and trot. If a computer system that allows evaluation during movement of the horses at the walk, posting and sitting trot, and gallop on both hands is available, electronic pressure measurements can provide objective data and help to identify the reason for the back problems or uncooperative handling during riding.

Once the saddle in combination with riding problems (e.g., false collection) is resolved, the alternative treatment modalities may support the rehabilitation of the horse's back.[9,10] However, they can never counteract an ill-fitting saddle or the corrupt riding style of an impatient rider. Although the many corrective saddle pads and wedges available to correct ill-fitting saddles may help to overcome an immediate problem, none of them can replace a genuinely well fitting saddle. Saddles of good quality are normally expensive, especially custom-made ones. However,

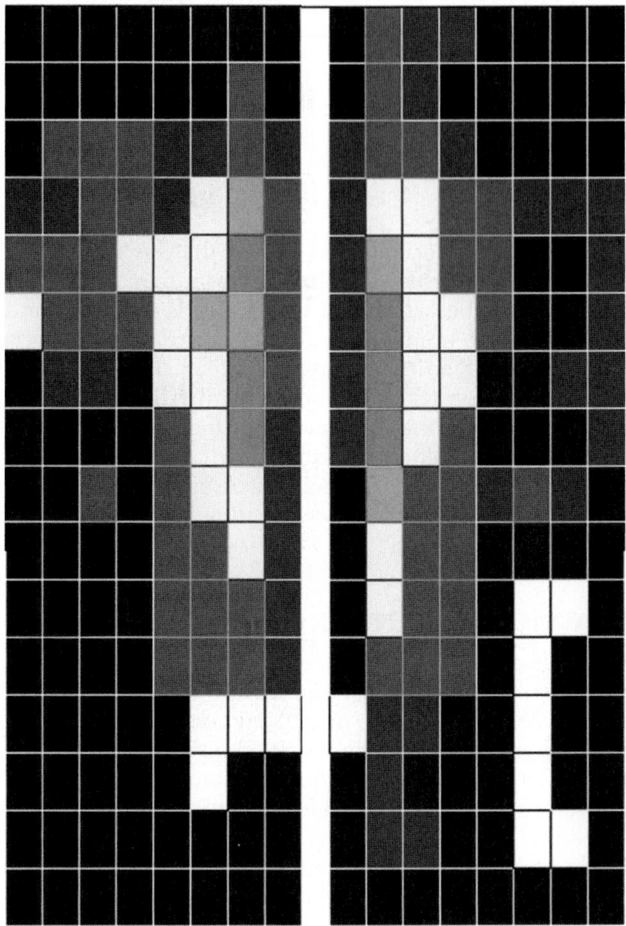

Figure 77-10. Maximal pressure picture (MPP) of a saddle with a narrow gulch of low height in the withers area. The high pressure values are distributed immediately adjacent to the spine in the region of the withers, indicating a narrow gulch. This saddle causes problems of the dorsal spinal processes.

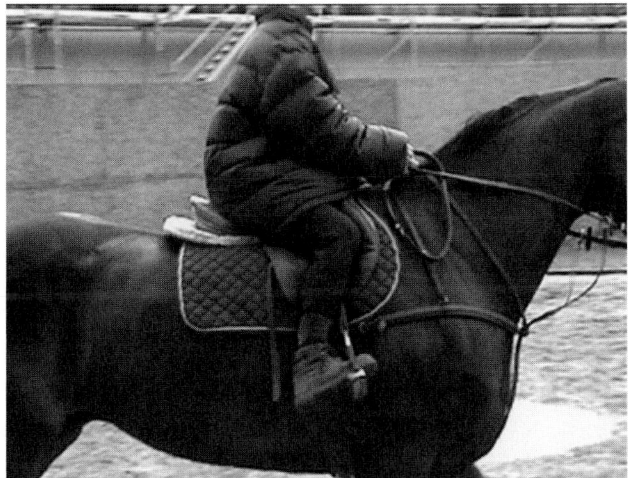

Figure 77-11. A rider with "chair-seat" caused by the construction of the saddle. The distance between the suspension of the stirrups and the center of the saddle seat should not exceed 1.5 times the width of the rider's hand. If it exceeds this, the rider has "chair-seat," which impairs the rider's balance as the horse moves. This leads to increased pressure in the lumbar area, which is poorly tolerated by most horses and results in contractions and muscle pain in this area.

owners save money on veterinary care and alternative treatment modalities in the long run. In addition, clients are very grateful to their veterinarians when their horses no longer object to the daily riding routine. In the long run, saddle mats are a sound investment for equine hospitals, especially if the veterinarians have built up a good collaboration with knowledgeable saddle makers, riding instructors, and salespersons of new saddle and riding equipment.

REFERENCES

1. Jeffcott LB: Klinische und röntgenologische Diagnostik der Wirbelsäulenerkrankungen des Pferdes, Prakt Tierarzt 1978;4:272.
2. Jeffcott LB: Back problems in the horse: A look at past, present and future progress, Equine Vet J 1979;11:129.
3. Jeffcott LB: Back problems in the horse: A method of clinical examination, Vet Rec 1979;5:4.
4. Jeffcott LB: The examination of a horse with a potential back problem. From The Proceedings of the Thirty-first Annual Convention of the American Association of Equine Practitioners, 1986.
5. Jeffcott LB: Rückenprobleme des Athleten "Pferd": 1. Ein Bericht über das Erkennen und die Möglichkeiten der Diagnose, Pferdeheilkunde 1993;9:143.
6. Jeffcott LB: Rückenprobleme des Athleten "Pferd": 2. Mögliche Differentialdiagnosen und Therapiemethoden, Pferdeheilkunde 1993;9:223.
7. Jeffcott LB: The approach to the back of the horse. In Knezevic PF, editor: Orthopädie bei Huf- und Klauentieren, Stuttgart, 1995, FK Schattauer Verlagsgesellschaft GmbH.
8. Gundel M, Schatzmann U: Rückenprobleme beim Pferd: 1. Eine Literaturzusammenfassung zur klinischen Untersuchung, Pferdeheilkunde 1997;13:199.
9. Harman J: Backs, performance, and acupuncture, Proc Am Assoc Equine Pract vol 337, 1992.
10. Buess C: Auswirkung einer manuellen Osteotherapie auf die "Losgelassenheit" des Pferdes während der Arbeit im Dressurviereck, ermittelt mit einer elektronischen Druckmessung unter dem Sattel, Thesis, 2003, University of Zurich.
11. Harman J: Practical saddle fitting: Part 3. Equine Athlete 1995:8:17.
12. Harman J: Practical saddle fitting: Part 2. Equine Athlete 1995;8:14.
13. Harman J: Practical saddle fitting: Part 1. Equine Athlete 1995;8:10.
14. Harman J: Tack and saddle fit, Vet Clin North Am 1999;15:247.
15. Werner D, Nykos S, Kalpen A, et al: Druckmessungen unter dem Sattel: Eine Studie mit einem Messsystem (Novel GmbH), Pferdeheilkunde 2002;18:125.
16. Nykos S, Werner D, Müller JA, et al: Elektronische Satteldruckmessungen im Zusammenhang mit Rückenproblemen bei Pferden, Pferdeheilkunde 2005;21:187.
17. Jeffcott LB, Holmes MA, Townsend HG: Validity of saddle pressure measurements using force-sensing array technology: Preliminary studies, Vet J 1999;158:113.
18. Pullin JG, Collier MA, Durham CM, et al: Use of force sensing array technology in the development of a new equine saddle pad: Static and dynamic evaluations and technical considerations, J Equine Vet Sci 1996;16:207.
19. Harman JC: Practical use of a computerized saddle pressure measuring device to determine the effects of saddle pads on the horse's back, J Equine Vet Sci 1994;14:606.
20. Harman, JC: Measurement of the pressures exerted by saddles on the horse's back using a computerized pressure measuring device, Pferdeheilkunde 1997;13:129.
21. Müller J: Personal observations, 2003.
22. Rechenberg BV: Personal observations, 2004.
23. Mönkemöller S, Keel R, Hambsch D, et al: Eine Folgestudie über elektronische Anpassung der Sattelsituation, Pferdeheilkunde 2005;21:102.

SECTION XII MUSCULOSKELETAL SYSTEM

Jörg. A. Auer

CHAPTER 78

Emergency Treatment and Transportation of Equine Fracture Patients

Anton E. Fürst

In horses, the initial treatment of injuries to skin, muscles, joints, tendons, tendon sheaths, and bones greatly affects the chances for perfect healing. Particularly for long bone fractures, a successful surgical outcome is forfeited with improper initial care. Unfortunately, most fractures are exposed to substantial additional trauma during the transportation of the injured horse. In certain situations, it is necessary to use a rescue net and crane or even a helicopter to rescue a horse from a dangerous location. A large-animal rescue unit operating in Switzerland and Liechtenstein specializes in the rescue of large animals involved in automobile accidents or trapped in wells, ditches, gullies, lakes, or rivers.

Rescue efforts can be conducted with the animal standing or in lateral or dorsal recumbency. Rescuing horses is a very complex procedure that must be well planned and calmly executed. A veterinarian experienced with horses should be on hand to prepare and accompany the horse during the rescue operation. Additionally, sedation or short-term anesthesia may be required. Although every rescue operation must be carried out as quickly as possible, time is of secondary importance. In emergency situations, it is imperative to remember that the horse may be in pain, and hastily improvised rescue methods will probably be inadequate and result in additional trauma. For example, narrow, flat, belly bands are painful for the horse and usually fail because the animal slips out of the bands and cannot be rescued or falls out while being lifted, resulting in severe additional injury or even death.

EXAMINATION OF THE PATIENT

A thorough clinical examination is mandatory for horses with fractures.[1] Lacerations or lesions that are overlooked can affect the diagnosis and prognosis considerably. A fracture is often suspected because of the severity of the lameness and the acute onset. When there is doubt, the horse should be treated and handled as a fracture patient. All too often, the assessment of injuries is incorrect, and incomplete and nondisplaced fractures are initially overlooked. This is particularly true in horses that have been kicked in a region where the bone lies directly beneath the skin—for example, the scapular spine, the major tubercle of the humerus, the deltoid tuberosity, the cutaneous plane of the radius, the metacarpus, the metatarsus, the tuber coxae, the third trochanter, the sustentaculum of the talus, the calcaneus, and the tibia[2] (Fig. 78-1).

TREATMENT OR EUTHANASIA

Despite great advances in veterinary orthopedic surgery and anesthesia, there are several injuries and fractures in horses that can only rarely be treated successfully. When the prognosis is hopeless, the horse should be euthanized immediately. A smooth and quiet euthanasia is of utmost importance for the owner and for potential spectators of the procedure.[3] In all cases, a veterinarian should examine the horse before carrying out the euthanasia.

However, the number of injuries and fractures that have a good prognosis with state-of-the-art treatment is increasing. Radiography is necessary to establish an exact diagnosis as well as to arrive at a prognosis for many fractures. Therefore, adequate emergency treatment is the initial step in the treatment, and the horse is then referred to a clinic that specializes in managing such problems.[4] Once it has been determined that the prognosis is probably favorable and euthanasia is not an option, it is imperative that the patient

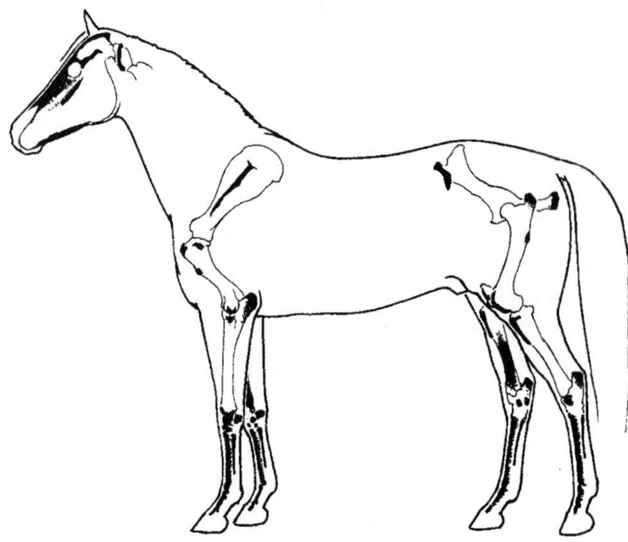

Figure 78-1. Sites on the horse *(dark spots)* where bones are covered only by skin with no muscle protection, making them susceptible to open fractures.

be given the opportunity to receive optimal care and treatment. However, time and time again, horses with fractures are transported without adequate emergency treatment, which not only compromises or eliminates the chance of a successful surgical repair but also is extremely painful for the horse.

Optimal emergency treatment includes the following:

- Initial wound management
- Prophylaxis of infection
- Proper analgesia
- Intravenous fluid therapy
- Sedation and possibly anesthesia
- Stabilization of the fracture
- Careful and safe rescue with proper transportation

Wound Management

Skin wounds must be treated with care. The hair around the wound is removed after covering the wound with water-soluble ointment. Then, a general cleaning of the area is completed with mild soap and water. The wound is cleaned thoroughly, disinfected, and covered with a bandage. A water-soluble antibiotic ointment and sterile dressing should be applied under the bandage. With open fractures, the bone must be cleaned also and covered with a sterile dressing.

Antibiotic Therapy

Immediate administration of systemic antibiotics is indicated in horses with open fractures or large wounds. Otherwise, antibiotic therapy can be delayed until the time of surgery. Antibiotics administered intravenously immediately prior to a surgical intervention achieve effective blood and tissue concentrations within approximately 20 minutes. The regimen of choice is a combination of 30,000 IU/kg of crystalline penicillin and 7 mg/kg of gentamicin sulfate, both administered intravenously. (For details on surgical site infection and antimicrobial use, see Chapter 7.)

Analgesia

Systemic analgesics should be given to the horse as soon as the fracture is stabilized. Nonsteroidal anti-inflammatory drugs such as flunixin meglumine (1.1 mg/kg IV) and phenylbutazone (4 mg/kg IV) may be used. However, when fracture stabilization is inadequate, the use of a potent analgesic is absolutely contraindicated, because this leads to an overload of the injured limb with associated complications. On the other hand, in many cases, good stabilization of the fracture relieves the pain, and analgesics are not necessary.

Intravenous Fluid Therapy

Fractures are rarely associated with severe hemorrhage. However, pain and shock lead to a substantial loss of fluid, which should be replaced using intravenous fluid therapy. After an indwelling intravenous catheter is placed and secured to the skin, a solution of electrolytes and glucose (up to 10% of body weight) should be administered with the drip rate set at maximum. (See Chapter 3 for details on fluid administration.) Horses out in the open should be kept warm with a horse blanket or an aluminum emergency blanket. (See Chapter 8 for details on triage of the trauma patient.)

Sedation

General rules for the use of sedatives cannot be given. What is indicated for one horse may be hazardous to another. The use of sedatives depends on the fracture and, in particular, the type and character of the horse. In most cases, judicious use of a sedative makes the examination and emergency treatment of an acutely traumatized horse much easier, especially when the horse is already stressed from competing in an event or is in pain. Furthermore, horses do not tolerate external coaptation well, especially when the fixation extends above the carpus or tarsus. The use of a sedative may be necessary to induce acceptance of the external coaptation device. Alpha-2 agonists are the drugs of choice, because they have few side effects and provide some analgesia and reliable sedation. Xylazine HCl is suitable for short procedures and detomidine HCl is used for longer sedation. For additional sedation and analgesia, a morphine derivative can be administered as well. Butorphanol tartrate has a wide variety of applications in horses and is an ideal drug for this scenario.

The dosage of these drugs varies according to the type of emergency. Agitated horses usually respond poorly to sedatives and require a higher dosage. In contrast, a lower dosage is needed when the horse's condition is compromised by shock or severe blood loss. After intravenous injection of the sedative, a minimum of 5 minutes is required for sedation to occur. This time period may seem quite long in an emergency situation, but it is prudent to wait without interfering with the horse to avoid overdosage and an unstable patient. It should be remembered that cold-blooded horses require less sedative on a per weight basis, and the dosage should not exceed that used for a 550-kg horse. Foals usually require heavy sedation to enable good stabilization of a fracture, and it is advantageous to have them restrained in lateral recumbency when a splint is applied.

A combination of detomidine HCl (Dormosedan) and butorphanol tartrate (Torbugesic or Morphasol) is favored by the author. The two drugs can be combined in one syringe and given intravenously or intramuscularly. A 400- to 1000-kg horse should receive 0.5 mL of Dormosedan together with 2.5 mL of Morphasol or 1 mL of Torbugesic (butorphanol tartrate, 0.02 mg/kg), intravenously. Xylazine can be used instead of detomidine; the onset of effects is more rapid but less reliable. The addition of a neuroleptic agent such as acepromazine (0.02 mg/kg) can substantially increase the duration of sedation. However, acepromazine should not be used in stallions or physiologically compromised patients.

Anesthesia

For certain rescue procedures or for the application of a cast, short-term anesthesia may be necessary. Various drug combinations, such as xylazine-diazepam-ketamine or xylazine-myolaxin-ketamine, provide reliable anesthesia even in an emergency situation. (See Chapter 20 for more on anesthesia.)

FRACTURE STABILIZATION

Stabilization of the fractured limb in an anatomically normal position is the most important aspect of the initial treatment. This allows the patient to bear some weight without undue damage to the fracture ends and the soft tissues. A very important additional effect of fracture stabilization is the diminution of anxiety and pain for the patient, thereby preventing complications.

Goals of Stabilization

To Reduce Stress and Anxiety and Provide Weightbearing

Pain from instability is extremely stressful for the fracture patient. Effective stabilization of the fracture alone substantially improves the general well-being of the animal. The fractured limb should be stabilized so that the horse is able to bear some weight on it.[1]

When the pain is reduced, the patient is in better physiological condition for referral and can undergo surgical repair more rapidly. Horses attempt to move the fractured limb constantly in an effort to find a stable position. Therefore, the horse is much quieter once stabilization has been provided (Fig. 78-2).

To Prevent Complications

Horses cannot balance well on three limbs and will repeatedly attempt to use the fractured limb. Continued movement of the fractured bones not only traumatizes the fragment ends, thus preventing anatomic reconstruction of the bone, but also injures the soft tissues, whose integrity is critical for fracture healing. The skin of horses is quite thin, and the worst complication is perforation of the skin by sharp bone fragments, resulting in contamination of the bone ends. Horses with open fractures of long bones have a very poor prognosis, and the use of modern and expensive antibiotics do not change this situation significantly. Thus, all efforts must be made to prevent such a complication. Perforation of the skin occurs quite readily in the distal region of the limb and the medial aspects of the radius and tibia because there is little additional tissue between the bone and the skin.

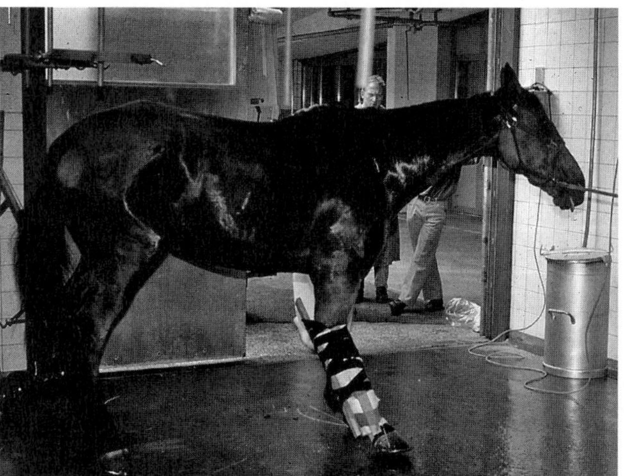

Figure 78-2. Inadequate and counterproductive attempt at stabilization of a radial fracture. The fracture remains unstable and weighted now by the inadequate splint bandage, and there is additional bone and soft tissue trauma. The patient is profusely sweating—a clear sign of pain and anxiety.

To Immobilize Adjacent Joints

The joints above and below the fracture must be immobilized, and the stabilization must extend well beyond the fracture line. In no case should the splint end near the fracture line, because it then acts like a lever. A cast should not end at the mid diaphysis, and, when possible, it should include the hoof. For example, splints should not be applied for fractures of the humerus and femur. These requirements sharply limit the number of fractures that can be stabilized with external coaptation techniques.

Types of Stabilization

For emergency stabilization of fractures, robust materials must be used.

Robert Jones Bandage

A Robert Jones bandage consists of many layers of cotton, each held in place and tightened by elastic gauze. Each layer is applied more tightly than the previous one. The finished Robert Jones bandage for a normal-size horse requires 10 to 15 rolls of cotton, and its diameter is about three times the diameter of the limb. This type of bandage can be used for a short period of immobilization. However, it cannot be used to stabilize the limb for long without the addition of splints. When splints are added, the bandage does not have to be as thick.

Splints

A variety of splints are suitable for stabilization of fractures in horses. Splints must be applied to the cranial, caudal, lateral, or medial aspects of the limb and held in place with nonelastic tape. For optimal stabilization, the splints are applied in two planes at right angles (90 degrees) to each other. Sufficient padding and good fixation are necessary to prevent slippage of the splint. The splints can be applied in one or two layers.

Polyvinyl chloride (PVC) splints are very stable and inexpensive but difficult to mold. The commercially available Fraktomedsplint (Fraktomedschiene, Verbandstoff-Fabrik Zürich AG, Fällanden/Zürich), made of a polyvinyl alcohol polymer, is also suitable for immobilization of a fracture but is rarely available in an emergency situation. This type of splint is very rigid when cold and must be heated in steam to facilitate molding it to fit the limb. Within a few minutes, the splint hardens and becomes stable. The Fraktomedsplint is expensive but can be reused many times. Splints can also be improvised using metal rods, broom handles, wooden boards, and other sturdy materials. The Thomas splint is generally unsuitable for horses and should not be used to splint a fractured limb, especially in an emergency.

Cast

The equine cast, also referred to as a synthetic splint, is formed from fiberglass tape impregnated with a polyurethane resin. These materials are very well suited for immobilizing equine limbs. Although it is expensive, it is very strong, cures quickly, is easy to apply, and is very light. While the cast is being applied, the horse should stand quietly to prevent the occurrence of microfractures and folds in the cast, which can reduce its strength and cause pressure sores. This can be helped somewhat if the horse can be supported in a special harness inside an emergency trailer, because there it is usually much quieter. In some situations, this may be difficult, so splints are usually the first choice of stabilization.

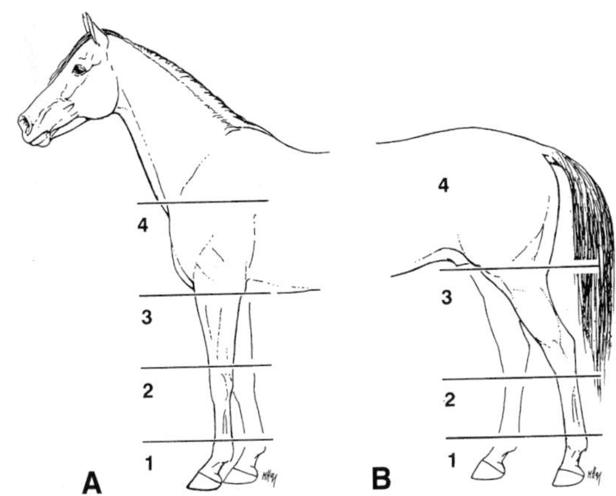

Figure 78-3. A, Biomechanically important divisions of the forelimb from distal to proximal: (1) distal to the distal quarter of MCIII, (2) from the distal MCIII to the distal radius, (3) from the distal radius to the elbow joint, and (4) from the elbow joint to distal scapula. **B,** Biomechanically important divisions of the hindlimb from distal to proximal: (1) distal to the distal quarter of MTIII, (2) from the distal MTIII to the tarsus, (3) from the tarsus to the stifle joint, and (4) proximal to the stifle joint. (From Bramlage LR: Com Cont Educ Pract Vet 1983;5:S564.)

Principles of Stabilization

Prevention of Soft Tissue Damage

Good stabilization does not inflict additional damage to the limb. Swelling of the surrounding tissues is common after an injury and may result in pressure and friction sores as well as tissue strangulation if the splint or cast is not sufficiently padded. The padding should be layered, with each layer being tightened with nonadhesive gauze. Layers that are too thick (2 to 4 cm) allow movement of the bone fragments or slippage of the splint. Ideally, the thickness of each layer of the padding should be about 1 cm.

Regional Immobilization

Techniques for immobilization of equine long bone fractures have been established.[5] The limbs can be divided into four distinct regions for stabilization techniques[5] (Fig. 78-3). The regions for the forelimb are (1) the hoof to the distal metacarpus, (2) the distal metacarpus to the distal radius, (3) the distal radius to the elbow joint, and (4) the elbow joint to the distal scapula. The regions for the hindlimb are (1) the hoof to the distal metatarsus, (2) the distal metatarsus to the tarsus, (3) the tarsus to the stifle, and (4) the region proximal to the stifle.

Specific Applications

Fractures of the Proximal, Middle, and Distal Phalanges, and the Distal Sesamoid Bone

Incomplete and complete fractures of the proximal, middle, and distal phalanx and the distal sesamoid bone are easily stabilized with either a cast or a splint.[4] With fractures of the proximal or middle phalanx, the third metacarpus and third metatarsus (MCIII/MTIII) and the proximal and middle phalanx must be stabilized in an almost straight line to prevent movement in the frontal plane at the fracture line. To achieve this, the heels are raised with a wedge, which also serves to facilitate the attachment of the cast distally. With the limb in this position, a cast is applied from the heels to the proximal end of the MCIII/MTIII. To obtain optimal stabilization, the entire hoof, or at least the heels, should be included in the cast. If nonmoldable splints are used instead of a cast, they are preferably fixed dorsally (see Fig. 18-17).

Holding the forelimb off the ground makes application of the synthetic splint easier because the horse is less likely to move. However, this is not possible with the hindlimb because of the reciprocal apparatus, which causes flexion of all the joints when the limb is held off the ground. However, with proper sedation, most horses will stand quietly for a few minutes with the injured limb lightly touching the ground and in a fairly normal position. Various other splints such as the Kimzey (Fig. 78-4) or monkey splint (Fig. 78-5) can be used instead of a cast.

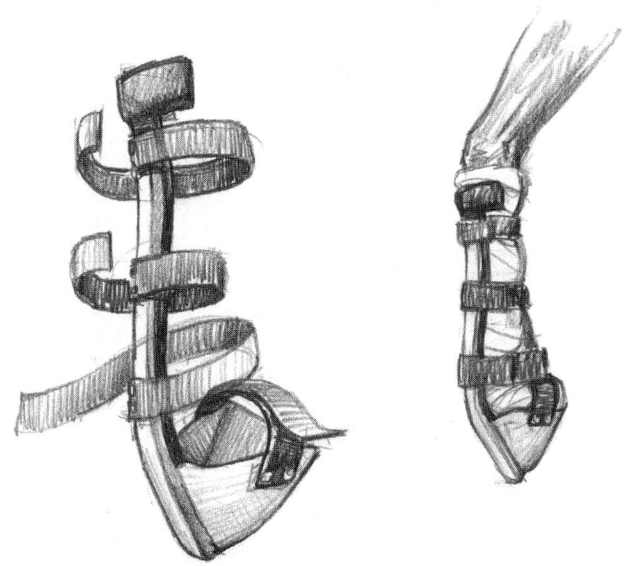

Figure 78-4. A Kimzey splint applied to the distal limb of a horse. These splints are well suited for first aid for disruptions of the suspensory apparatus.

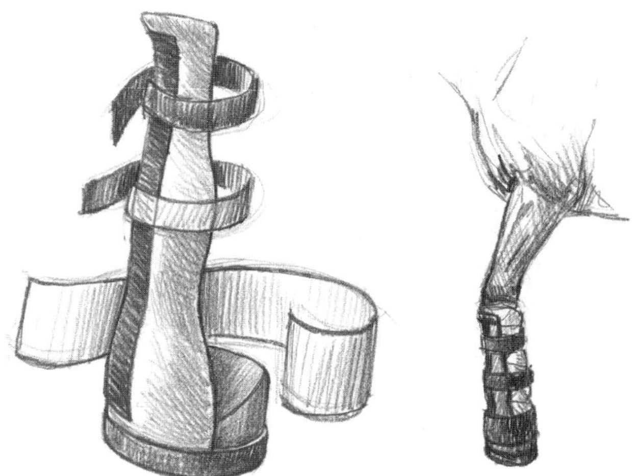

Figure 78-5. A monkey splint applied to the distal limb of a horse. These splints align the phalanges and MCIII into one plane.

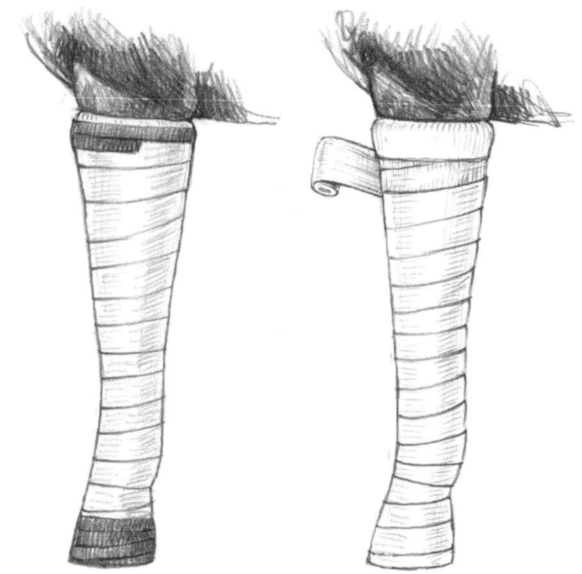

Figure 78-7. Application of a full forelimb cast using the technique described in Figure 18-17 but extending over the entire forelimb up to the elbow joint. Care is taken to apply the cast material evenly along the entire limb and to fold back the stockinette over the top of the cast, incorporating it into the last layer to provide a smooth top edge.

Fractures of the Third Metacarpal, Third Metatarsal, Carpal, and Tarsal Bones

With fractures of the MCIII/MTIII, a cast or splint is applied from the hoof to the elbow or stifle joint, respectively (Figs. 78-6 through 78-8). Depending on the temperament of the horse and the location of the fracture, the splint or cast may reach only the top of the calcaneus for fractures of the metatarsus. However, this does not produce optimal stabilization and should be looked at as an exception rather than the rule. Extending the external coaptation above the tarsus should always be the goal and should in most cases be possible with the use of adequate sedation.

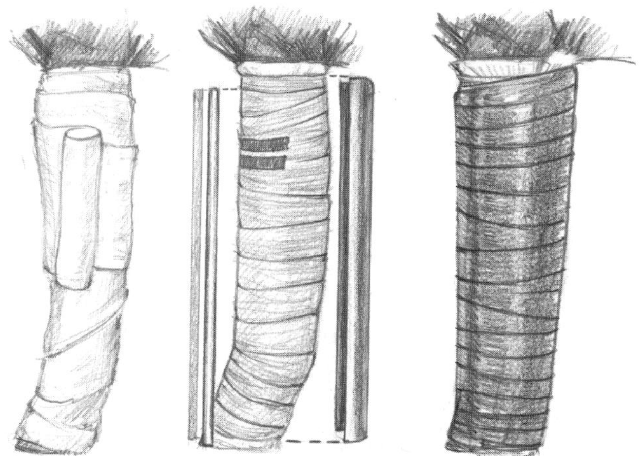

Figure 78-6. Application of a full forelimb splint. The padding is applied evenly in several layers over the entire limb, and each layer is tightened separately. A PVC-pipe splint is applied to the caudal aspect of the bandage and augmented with one pole medially and laterally. The splints are incorporated into the bandage with tape.

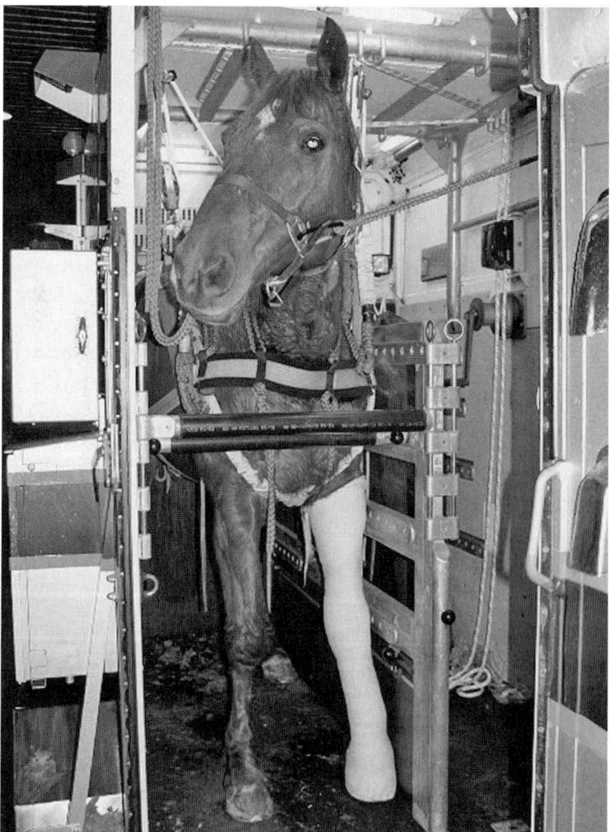

Figure 78-8. A horse with a fracture of the metacarpus, which has been stabilized with a full limb cast. The horse is loaded in an emergency trailer and is ready for the transport. The harness supports the patient during the transport.

Fractures of the Radius and Tibia

Fractures of the radius and tibia present special difficulties because the large muscle masses prevent fixation of the elbow and stifle joints. Furthermore, contraction of the extensor tendons, located craniolaterally on the limb, causes abduction of the limb below the fracture line, which can produce skin perforation on the medial aspect of the radius or tibia (Fig. 78-9, *A* and *B*). Therefore, stabilization up to the elbow or stifle is not sufficient and will not prevent abduction. In these fractures, a stable splint or cast should first be applied up to the elbow or stifle joint (see Fig. 78-9, *C*). This should then be augmented with an additional splint applied laterally and reaching from the hoof to the point of the shoulder or hip, respectively. Additional padding is added to the splint so that it conforms to the contour of the limb. Immobilization is difficult in the hindlimb because of the reciprocal apparatus (see Fig. 18-15). Flexion of the stifle, which cannot be prevented, results in flexion of the hock via the superficial digital flexor muscle and the peroneus tertius muscle. This results in large forces acting on the tibia so that dislocation of the fragments is unavoidable. Regardless, these fractures are stabilized as well as possible using this technique.

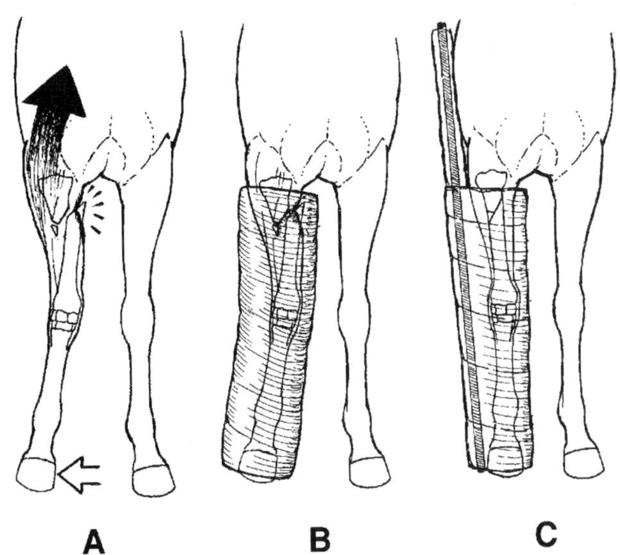

Figure 78-9. Splinting of a proximal radial fracture. **A,** All the muscles are arranged cranially, laterally, and caudally, which results in a lateral deviation of the limb when the muscles contract to provide support to the fractured limb. This may result in perforation of the skin at the medial aspect of the limb by sharp bone edges. **B,** A Robert Jones dressing or cast has been applied to the limb. It ends near the fracture site and provides only limited support. Also, it increases the leverage arm, causing more tissue damage. **C,** The incorporation of long splint or wooden plank to the lateral aspect of the bandage effectively counteracts the valgus-inducing forces and adds significant stability to the splint bandage. With such a splint, the patient may load the fractured limb.

Fractures of the Ulna

Fractures of the ulna result in failure of the passive stay apparatus of the forelimb (triceps apparatus), which allows the horse to stand with little muscular effort for prolonged periods of time. Therefore, the limb should be stabilized with a splint that extends the carpus so that the horse can bear weight on the limb. The splint should be applied caudally and should extend from the metacarpophalangeal region to the level of the elbow joint (Fig. 78-10).

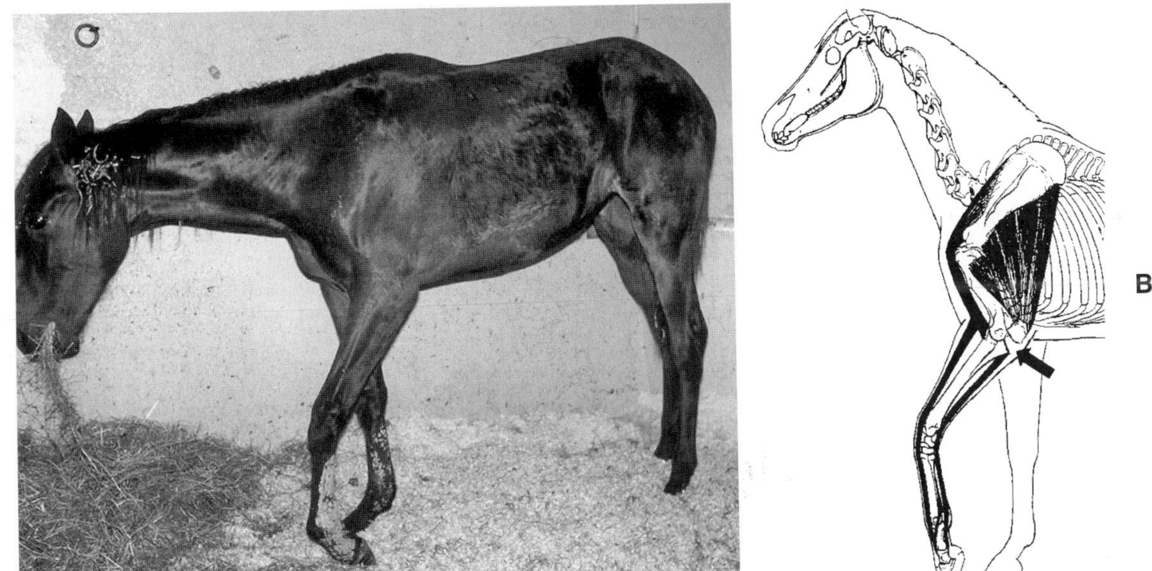

Figure 78-10. A, Typical posture of a horse with a fracture of the olecranon process of the ulna. **B,** The carpus cannot be maintained in a straight position because the triceps muscle pulls on only the proximal fragment, which results in the formation of a fracture gap *(arrow)*.

Fractures of the Humerus and Femur

Fractures of the humerus and femur do not require a bandage or a splint because they cannot be adequately immobilized and there is enough muscle mass to protect the bone. These fractures are rarely open and a bandage would be counterproductive, because it would only add weight without providing stabilization. In some cases, fractures of the humerus or neck of the scapula can be helped with a splint that extends the carpus, similar to the situation with fractures of the ulna.

TRANSPORTATION OF THE HORSE

The injured horse must be transported carefully and humanely, according to animal welfare legislation.[6,7] It is advantageous to have a specialized large-animal trailer or van and the support of an experienced veterinarian or assistant.[6] However, some controversy exists: there are those who think that this kind of transportation can be accomplished with normal horse trailers that are slightly adapted.[8] In the experience of the authors, horses with a fracture should be transported by a specialized large-animal trailer built for the transportation of injured horses.

Equipment

The emergency trailer or van should have enough room for two standing horses (Fig. 78-11, *A*) or one recumbent horse.[3] Ideally, there should be enough space to handle the horse from all sides. The trailer should be approximately 30 cm higher than standard horse vans, and it should be equipped with a nonslip floor (see Fig. 78-11, *B*). It should be well ventilated and spacious with a good lighting system for night transport. Additionally, the vehicle should be solidly built, preferably of aluminum. The loading and unloading ramps should be long enough that the slope is minimal, which is especially important for horses wearing a splint. The ramp must have an even nonslip surface, and the end must be flush with the ground. The vehicle must be equipped with a winch and a strong frame to support a harness. Different sizes of suspensory harnesses are required with a minimum carrying weight of 1200 kg. Other requirements are a gurney or a mat on which a recumbent animal can be pulled into the trailer. Curtains or movable, lightweight walls are helpful when the working area needs to be blocked off from the view of spectators. For safety reasons, the driver must be able to observe what is going on via a video camera and able to have audio contact with the support assistants caring for the horse during the transport. The vehicle should be equipped with a heater and the floor should be well padded (e.g., with an air mattress) to minimize vibrations during the transport of a recumbent animal. The interior installations should be adjustable to accommodate horses of different breeds and sizes. The emergency trailer or van should be stocked with all the necessary medical supplies for various emergency treatments including shock therapy.

Loading Injured Horses

It is best to maneuver the vehicle as close to the injured horse as possible to spare it unnecessary walking.[3] As the steepness of the loading ramp increases, so must the interior height of the trailer (minimum height, 2.35 to 2.50 m), particularly when a forelimb is injured. Increasing the height of the trailer jack will lower the height of the ramp

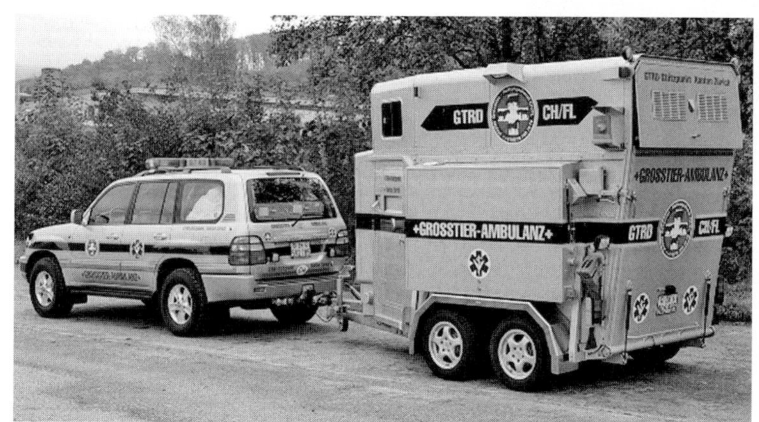

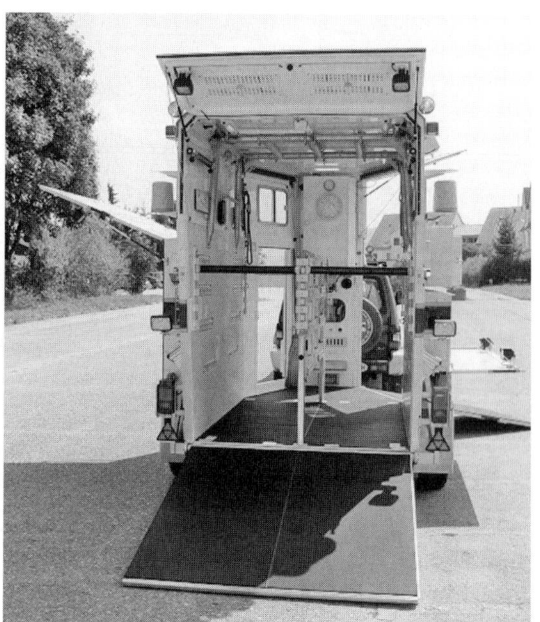

Figure 78-11. Ideal emergency vehicle. **A,** The SUV is equipped with blinking lights and all the necessary emergency equipment for rescuing horses. Additional equipment is stored on the side of the trailer. **B,** The trailer has an axle constructed close to the ground, which results in a ramp with a gentle slope. This ramp angle makes loading a patient wearing a splint easy. The roof is reinforced to allow the installation of a support harness. A winch is built into the front wall to allow a recumbent patient to be pulled into the trailer.

somewhat. Horses also load better when the trailer is positioned so that the horse can walk in the same direction as the barn. The horse should be acclimated to the cast or splint by walking a few steps before being loaded.

Application of a bridle over a halter is recommend for better control during loading. In this way, fractious horses can be better controlled by a handler walking on the side. Two readily available lunge lines are tied to either side of the trailer and are used to direct the horse into the vehicle. For injured horses, the stall partition should be moved to one side to provide the maximal amount of space for loading. Before loading, the service door and the front-unloading door should be opened and the interior lights turned on at night to illuminate the interior as much as possible. Two assistants hold the lunge lines and move slowly toward each other, progressively narrowing the space between them. Touching the horse with the lines may help loading and is not necessarily discouraged. As soon as the horse is in the trailer, the rump bar is replaced, the ramp is closed, and the service door and the front-unloading door are closed. The stall partition and chest bar are the last barriers to be put in place.

It has been recommended that horses with forelimb fractures be transported facing backward[9] in an attempt to relieve the stress on the forelimbs during braking. However, almost all standard European two-horse transporters do not provide enough space for the horse to comfortably stand backward; when the chest and rump bars are in place, the horse would have to keep its head either very high or turned to the side because of the ramp (the back door) in front of it. This would be very uncomfortable for the horse. Furthermore, the head and neck are important for balance but they have to be free to perform this function properly. Finally, it is very difficult if not impossible to load an injured horse backward or to turn it around once it is inside the trailer. Loading the horse via the front unloading ramp is not practical because the space is limited and the slope of the front ramp is usually steeper than that of the rear ramp. For a horse standing backward in the trailer, the injured forelimb would then be positioned at the back of the transporter between the rear axle and the ramp, where the ride is the roughest.

The horse has to balance not only during braking but also during acceleration and in curves. Therefore, the driver must take the time to ensure a comfortable ride for the horse. A video camera in the trailer is very helpful. An assistant in the trailer with the horse helps to calm it and relay any developing problems directly to the driver. For horses with hindlimb injuries, the driving speed must be as slow as possible, because the ride is the roughest behind the rear axle.

Transport in a Supporting Harness

A harness should be used to transport horses with severe injuries.[10] Many horses allow the harness to support their entire weight during transport. Most horses alternately rest one limb and then the other. After some time, horses with a properly splinted limb frequently bear some weight on the fractured limb while being supported by a harness, thereby resting the healthy contralateral limb. Transportation in a harness can provide tremendous relief for an injured horse. For this type of transport, a person experienced in large animal rescue operations should always be present in the trailer to provide optimal care for the patient. In extreme cases, a veterinarian may be required to travel with the horse as well. The harness must be fitted so that it does not interfere with the horse's respiration and balance. It allows the horse to rest its limbs during transport, which reduces anxiety and pain and improves the general attitude of the patient. Horses that are transported with a harness arrive at the hospital in much better general condition than those that are not. Most horses can be easily positioned in a harness provided that it is applied snugly and gives support to the patient from the front as well as from the back. During transportation, the bellyband is tightened several times, and the front and hind belts are adjusted until the horse is comfortable. It is imperative that everything be checked repeatedly throughout the transport, so that problems can immediately be identified and corrected (Fig. 78-12).

Unloading Fracture Patients

In general, the horse should get off the trailer using the sound limbs first. With a forelimb injury, the horse should be backed off the transporter. With hindlimb injuries, the horse should be unloaded via the front ramp. As for loading,

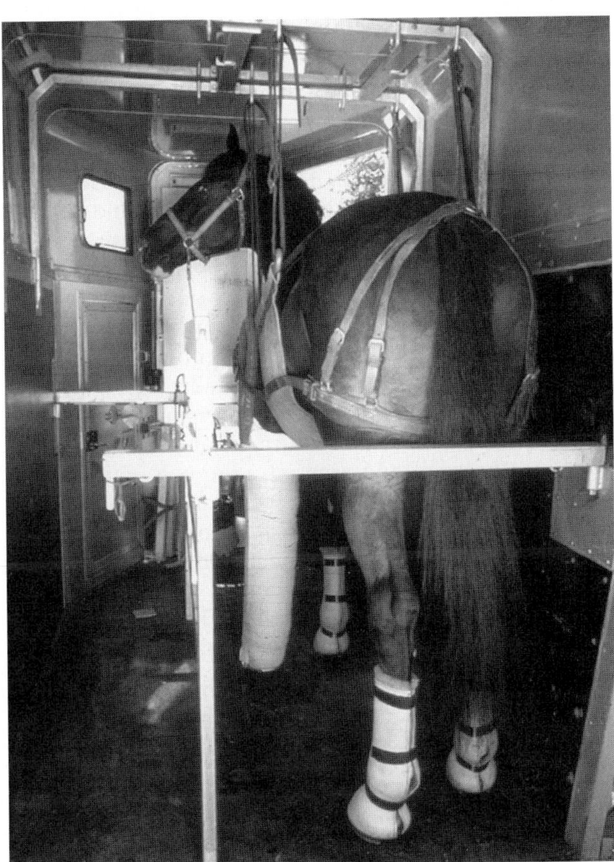

Figure 78-12. A fracture patient supported by a harness is ready to be transported to a specialty clinic.

the trailer jack can be adjusted to provide the optimal ramp angle for unloading.

Injured horses, particularly those with fractures, should be lightly sedated for unloading. Most horses feel insecure when they are presented with new surroundings and when forced to use the injured limb after having been supported in a harness. This stress may result in hectic or hesitant and uncontrolled movements during unloading. Sedation dampens these reactions, and unloading is safer for both the horse and the handlers.

Transport of Recumbent Horses

It is a general rule that horses should be transported standing whenever possible. Horses that are unable to stand are transported in lateral recumbency, and anesthesia may be induced for the ride to the clinic.[7] Transportation of horses under general anesthesia is rare; the anesthesia must be carried out and maintained by a veterinarian, who must travel with the horse. The duration of transportation in such cases must be as rapid as possible, perhaps assisted by a police escort, and it should not exceed 90 minutes.

A mechanical or electric winch, transport mat, insulated air mattress, head protection for the horse, and hobbles are some of the equipment needed for transportation of recumbent horses.

Once the decision has been made that the horse is to be transported in recumbency, an indwelling intravenous catheter is placed and intravenous fluids are started. This is the only way of ensuring rapid treatment at any time. Horses that cannot rise are sedated and those that can rise are anesthetized so they can be transported in recumbency. After induction, anesthesia must be maintained during the entire transport period. General anesthesia is usually induced and maintained using injectable drugs, some of which can be administered via a drip (see Chapter 20). The van is positioned as close to the horse as possible, and the stall partition is placed to one side so that the entire interior space can be used. The winch wire is pulled out to the desired length and the horse is placed on the rubber transport mat or another device so that it can be pulled into the van. Either a hand or electric winch can be used, but there should be a backup if the electric one fails.

For recumbent horses, leather boots are placed on the hooves to reduce the risk of injury, and hobbles are put on all limbs. The head and especially the eyes must be well protected. This is best achieved with padded leather headgear, after the halter has been removed to prevent damage to the facial nerves. The horse can be pulled into the van using a slide mat.

Recently, special air mattresses have been developed for the transport of recumbent horses; these mattresses are used by the large-animal rescue unit operating in Switzerland and Liechtenstein (Herr Ruedi Keller, Embrach).[6] Before inflation, the air mattress is placed between the horse and the transport mat, which are then pulled into the van together. The mattress is then inflated using compressed air. This procedure takes about 2 minutes and ensures a comfortable ride for the patient. Horses can be transported great distances without the risk of pressure necrosis or nerve damage (Fig. 78-13). Often, the amount of drugs used to sedate the horse can be reduced as well.

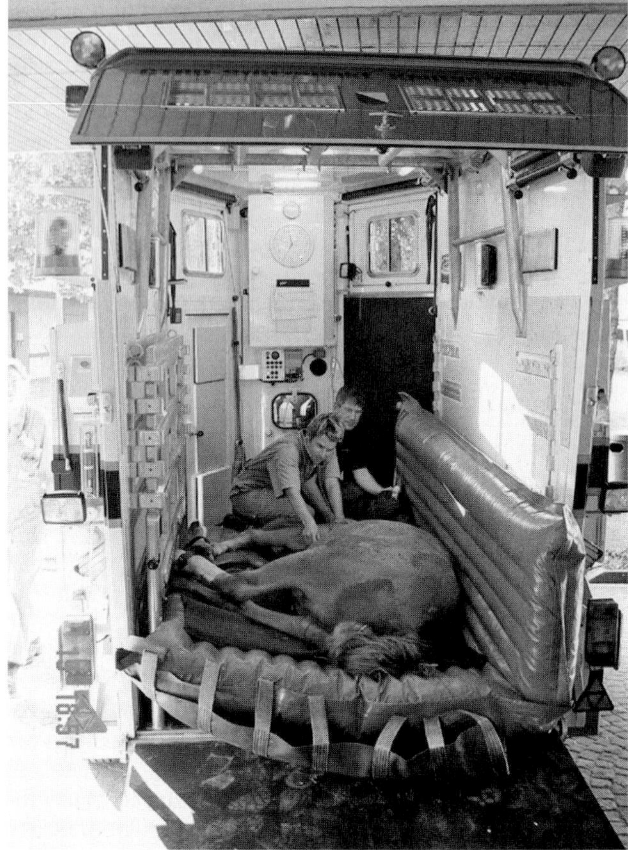

Figure 78-13. A recumbent patient was pulled into the trailer and rests comfortably on an air mattress. Two assistants help with anesthesia.

The journey should begin as soon as the horse is in the van, because transportation time is critical. In special circumstances, a police escort should be arranged. A veterinarian or veterinary assistant should accompany the horse so that sedation or anesthesia can be maintained. An audio-video system helps to ensure the safety of the personnel accompanying the horse. For long distances, a mobile anesthetic machine operated by experienced assistants may be necessary. This enables the administration of intravenous fluids and air supplemented with oxygen (approximately 2 to 12 L of oxygen per minute). Unloading the recumbent horse is straightforward and is achieved by pulling the transport mat out of the van with a winch or crane or by hand.

REFERENCES

1. Walmsley J: Management of a suspected fracture. In Dyson S, editor: A Guide to the Management of Emergencies at Equine Competitions, Newmarket, Suffolk, 1996, British Equine Veterinary Association.
2. Derungs S, Fürst AE, Haas C, et al: Fissure fractures of the radius and tibia in 23 horses: A retrospective study, Equine Vet Educ 2002;16:313.
3. von Salis B: Olyckfalls-och amulansberedskap (rid-och körsport), Svensk Veterinärtidining 1989;41:104.
4. Fürst AE, Kaegi B, Auer JA: Die Erstversorgung von Pferden mit Frakturen, Tierärztl Praxis 1993;24:21.
5. Bramlage L: Emergency first aid treatment and transportation of

equine fracture patients. In Auer JA, Stick JA, editors: Equine Surgery, Philadelphia, 1999, WB Saunders.
6. Keller R, Fürst AE: Erste Hilfe und Transport von Unfallpferden. Submitted Schweiz Arch Tierheilk, 2005.
7. Keller R: Personal communication, 2004.
8. Ellis D: Transporting an injured horse. In Dyson S, editor: A Guide to the Management of Emergencies at Equine Competitions, Newmarket, Suffolk, 1996, British Equine Veterinary Association.
9. Bramlage L: Grundlagen für Erste-Hilfe-Massnahmen und Transport von Frakturpferden, Pferdeheilkunde 1989;5:3.
10. von Salis B: An injured horse: What now? In 11th FEI General meeting, Bern, 1980.

CHAPTER 79

Molecular Biology Techniques in Musculoskeletal Research

Brigitte von Rechenberg
Michael O. Hottiger

BACKGROUND

Molecular biology is the branch of science devoted to studies of the structure, function, and reactions of DNA, RNA, proteins, and other molecules in connection with life processes. In 1953, Watson and Crick were the first to determine the true crystalline structure of deoxyribonucleic acid. DNA is the elementary template carrying the essential genetic code for every living organism. In the eukaryotic cells that make up plants, animals, and other multicellular organisms, most of the DNA is found in the chromosomes, which are located in the cell nucleus. Once the structure of DNA was identified, the mechanisms behind inheritance, information flow, and gene function fell into place. In 1958, Crick described the paradigm of molecular biology in which the flow of information is depicted as DNA → RNA → protein. DNA is replicated (i.e., DNA is synthesized from DNA), whereas RNA is transcribed from DNA. It is called transcription because the same type of "language" is used in DNA as in RNA—that is, nucleic acids. In some cases, RNA may be used to make complementary DNA (cDNA) (i.e., reverse transcription) using a particular enzyme called reverse transcriptase. Protein is synthesized from messenger RNA (mRNA) by translation. This is called translation because a different language is used—that is, amino acids instead of nucleic acids. Once protein has been synthesized from RNA, the information is trapped. In other words, there is no known mechanism that allows information to flow back into RNA from protein.

Thousands of genes are being discovered for the first time by sequencing the genomes of model organisms, a reminder that much of the natural world remains to be explored at the molecular level. With the recent completion of the sequencing of the different genomes, it appears that now a map of a defined being exists. In a genetic map, the location of the genes is assigned to the different chromosomes. A gene is the functional and physical unit of heredity passed from parent to offspring. Most genes contain the information to synthesize a specific protein. However, it is the proteins of those genes that interact with each other in the context of a cell (or more appropriately, in the context of a whole organism, unicellular or multicellular). In eukaryotes, certain proteins are targeted to particular compartments within the cell (e.g., organelles (such as mitochondria), endoplasmic reticulum). Where a particular protein will go can be predicted by the signal sequence that is encoded by the gene. However, a genetic map by itself cannot describe how proteins will interact with one another.

Genomics refers to the study of genes and genomes, whereas proteomics is the study of proteins (i.e., protein structure and function, and their interactions in an organism). Now that several genomes have been sequenced, research focuses on protein structures and interactions (primarily for the purpose of medically relevant information).

Molecular techniques alone, however, are not sufficient to explain complex cell mechanisms, which always warrant a combination of biochemistry, chemistry, and other life science fields such as cell biology. Molecular techniques used for applications in cartilage resurfacing or bone augmentation and enhancement usually involve scientists who provide basic scaffolds or carriers for tissue engineering[1-3] and engineers who construct the necessary bioreactors where tissues are grown in vitro.[4-8] Molecular techniques have led to explanations of how biomechanical forces (e.g., compression, strain, tension) induce signaling pathways on a cellular level in fibrous tissue, cartilage, bone, and tendons. Almost 110 years after Wolff wrought "the law of transformation of bone according to mechanical load,"[9-11] molecular biology provided the foundation to understand what causes this transformation on a molecular level.

The introduction of molecular biology into the field of musculoskeletal research has opened new avenues for understanding the pathophysiology of musculoskeletal structures, including bone, cartilage, tendons, periosteum, paratenon, and perimysium. Through molecular techniques, signal pathways and signal molecules involved in synthesis and degradation of matrix macromolecules can be identified and manipulated for diagnostic and therapeutic purposes.[12,13-20] For example, once the pathway of pathologic articular cartilage degradation is better understood, the use of molecular techniques aimed at downregulating DNA/RNA expression of degradative protein concentrations,[21,22] and the use of knockout or transgenic mice to upregulate protective mechanisms, will be possible.[23,24] Furthermore, molecular technology has provided novel therapy through the use of genetic vectors,[15,25-28] application of growth factors,[29-32] and the implantation of tissues grown in vitro (e.g., for cartilage resurfacing).[1] Growth factors are used to influence multipotent stem cells in vitro and in vivo to facilitate differentiation of cells in a desired direction, or to discourage de-differentiation of cell lines or tissue-engineered products.[33]

INTERACTION OF DIAGNOSTICS AND RESEARCH

The introduction of molecular biology has made it possible to study cellular mechanisms in tissues harvested from patients, either from biopsies or during surgery. Recently, the search for biomarkers that allow early detection of, for example, cartilage destruction, fracture healing, and bone resorption has become very popular, not only in research[34] but also in clinical settings.[35-37] For example, antibodies against epitopes in degraded collagen type II or cleaved procollagen fibrils can be measured in synovial fluids of patients[35,36] as well as in dissolved cartilage tissue, cell, or explant cultures. Antibodies against epitopes (BC-3, epitope 846) of proteoglycans[38,39] allow the measurement of glycosaminoglycan (GAG) concentrations. Similarly, the enzymatic activity of matrix metalloproteinases, nitric oxide, prostaglandin (PG) E_2, and GAG concentrations are being studied for their suitability as biomarkers to predict early cartilage degeneration in equine patients.[40-43] Some of the most useful methods for diagnosis of and research into musculoskeletal disorders are described here.

Methods of Detecting Gene Regulation

Analysis of the DNA/Genome: Whole Genome Application

Advancements in technology have made it possible to sequence the bases in a section of the DNA of any organism in a short time. The purpose of such sequencing is to *determine* the sequences of the chemical base pairs that make up DNA, to *store* this information in databases, and to *identify* all genes in a desired species. The DNA Isolation Kit for Cells and Tissues permits the rapid, large-scale isolation of DNA from cells and tissues. Even small amounts of tissue such as those found in thin sections can be used. Several procedures provide a quick, easy, and safe method for removing contaminating RNA and proteins, resulting in purified genomic DNA ranging in size from 50 to 150 kilobases (kB). The procedure includes sample homogenization followed by cellular lysis, in the presence of a strong anionic detergent and proteinase K. RNA is eliminated with an RNase treatment, and proteins are removed by selective precipitation and centrifugation. The purified DNA is subsequently recovered by isopropanol precipitation.

To understand the role and function of genes, complete information on their RNA transcripts and proteins is needed. Unfortunately, exploring protein functions is difficult because of their complicated and unique three-dimensional structures and the lack of efficient technology. To overcome this difficulty, a technique is used that focuses on the mRNA molecules produced by the genes of interest (gene expression), and this information is used to investigate the functional roles of the genes. This idea stimulated the development of the micro-array technique—a method to study the interactions between thousands of genes based on their mRNA transcript level.

DNA micro-arrays provide a natural vehicle for the exploration of genome-wide surveys of gene expression patterns or functions. The results should be viewed as maps that reflect the order and logic of the genetic program rather than as the physical order of genes on chromosomes (genetic map). Exploration of the genome using DNA micro-arrays and other genome-scale technologies should improve our knowledge of gene function and molecular biology.

Applications of micro-arrays range from the study of gene expression in different tissues under different environmental stress conditions to the comparison of gene expression profiles for tissues with pathophysiologic changes. This approach involves the use of fluorescently labeled reverse transcribed mRNAs (also called complementary DNA [cDNA]), which contains only the coding part of the sequence, complementary to its corresponding mRNA transcript. Micro-arrays are a form of microscopic chip containing hundreds to thousands of immobilized DNA samples. The main function of a micro-array chip is to detect and quantify the concentration of a specific mRNA transcript or its cDNA respectively. The chips are overlayed in a solution containing the fluorescently labeled cDNAs to allow them to hybridize with their complementary DNA sequences, previously placed on the micro-array chip. Because the cDNA on the chip is fluorescently labeled, every spot emits light in the ultraviolet spectrum corresponding to the amount of hybridized cDNA. The variable intensity of the ultraviolet dye at different spots allows the comparison of the gene expression patterns under different experimental conditions (case-control studies). The hybridized array is typically scanned with a system that uses lasers as a source of excitation light and photomultiplier tubes as detectors. This system is capable of differentiating the fluorescently labeled probes. Initial data obtained from DNA micro-arrays are in the form of scanned images. Coding the gene expression by means of colors can be helpful for building genetic maps and graphic data processing. An expression gene map is presented in the form of a table, the rows of which correspond to the consecutive genes and columns representing different samples, such as under multiple experimental conditions or for different patients.

This approach provides a way to directly use the growing body of sequence information for parallel experimental investigations. Because of the combinatorial nature of the chemistry and the ability to synthesize small arrays containing hundreds of thousands of specifically chosen oligonucleotides, the method is readily scalable to monitor tens of thousands of genes simultaneously. After the scanning of the micro-array chips for fluorescence, a grid must be placed on the image and the spots representing the arrayed genes must be identified. The data must be normalized to allow a comparison of the separate arrays. With multiple experimental conditions (e.g., time-points or drug doses), the genes are often grouped into clusters that behave similarly under the different conditions. Gene clusters are visualized with trees or color-coded matrices by placing genes with similar patterns of expression into a clustered group.

Several providers manufacture arrays to monitor the global activities of genes. In addition, custom expression arrays can be designed for other model organisms, proprietary sequences, or specific subsets of known genes. For human arrays, expressed sequences from databases are collected and clustered into groups of similar sequences. Using clusters as a starting point, sequences are further subdivided into subclusters representing distinct transcripts. This categorization process involves alignment to the human genome, which reveals splicing variants.

Presently, apart from the human and mice genome, an equine-specific gene chip is being developed for research purposes offering up to 3000 equine genes normally involved in musculoskeletal diseases (Affymetrix, Santa Clara, Calif, is presently developing a Genechip System).

Analysis of the DNA Genome: Gene-Specific Applications

Micro-array analysis of gene expression does have limitations. They include the impact of mRNAs that are spliced alternatively or the limited ability to detect unstable mRNAs. Therefore, differential gene expression results must be confirmed through direct examination of selected genes. These analyses typically occur at the level of RNA blot or quantitative real-time polymerase chain reactions (qRT-PCR) to examine transcripts of a specific gene. The technique of qRT-PCR is a powerful method for studying gene expression in various species and tissues. Competitive PCR for quantitative measurement of absolute levels of mRNA molecules has been applied to different genes and species. Moreover, total RNA isolated from individual microbiopsy samples may be successfully used for micro-array–based gene expression analysis of any discretely localized cellular group, which can be identified functionally or morphologically.

In many laboratories, these technologies are being used to detect gene regulation of disease after treatment with stimulating or inhibiting substances. Northern blots,[44] followed by densitometry measurements or the more advanced TaqMan system,[45,46] are used. For both techniques, mRNA probes (of about 100 to 120 base pairs) have to be developed out of cDNA using reverse transcription methods based on the isolation of total mRNA from the specific tissues in question.

Obtaining high-quality, intact RNA is the first and often the most critical step in performing many fundamental molecular biology experiments. The isolation and use of purified RNA in the laboratory is complicated by the fact that, chemically and biologically, RNA is significantly more labile than DNA. The choice and optimization of RNA purification methods are important for successful isolation of quality RNA and consistent performance of downstream applications. To avoid damage or loss of RNA, nuclease contamination of the RNA samples during preparation and handling should be avoided. The process of isolating intact total RNA from certain tissues is even more difficult. Fibrous tissues and tissues rich in protein are challenges for total RNA isolation because of the DNA and nucleases present. These tissues require more manipulation during the RNA isolation procedure. Finding the most appropriate method of cell or tissue disruption for the specific starting material is important for maximizing the yield and quality of RNA preparation.

Research into optimizing RNA analyses has identified two points in the RNA isolation process that can be improved: treatment and handling of tissue or cells prior to RNA isolation, and storage of the isolated RNA. During tissue disruption for RNA isolation, it is crucial that the denaturant be in contact with the cellular contents at the moment the cells are disrupted. This is difficult to achieve when the tissue and cells are hard (e.g., bone) and when samples are numerous, making rapid processing difficult. A common solution to these problems is to freeze the tissue/cells in liquid nitrogen or on dry ice. The samples are then ground with a mortar and pestle into a fine powder, which is added to the denaturant. This freezing and grinding process allows the postponement of RNA isolation, but it is time consuming and laborious. The last step in every RNA isolation protocol, whether for total or mRNA preparation, is to resuspend the purified RNA pellet. After carefully preparing an RNA sample, the RNA is suspended and stored in a safe, RNase-free solution.

Therefore, on a practical level, whenever tissues from patients or experimental animals are harvested with the aim of isolating mRNA levels, collection has to occur without delay at surgery, after euthanasia, or after slaughter, and tissues need to be preserved immediately. Apart from the freezing of the tissues as just described, storage of the tissues for PCR in RNAlater (Qiagen, Valencia, Calif), has worked well in the authors' laboratory for cartilage and soft tissue. The tissue should be no thicker than 0.5 cm and should be kept in no less than 10 µL RNAlater per milligram of tissue. The tissues should be stored at +4° C for 24 to 48 hours for fixation, and afterward stored at −20° C, where they are stable indefinitely. If this method is chosen, it is not necessary to use liquid nitrogen or to store at −80° C. To extract the RNA from fibrous tissue, cartilage, and bone, Trizol combined with the RNeasy kit (Qiagen) in a Polytron mixer works well in the authors' experience. When preparing samples for testing using PCR, tissue should be handled with sterile instruments and surgical gloves (without glove powder).

In Situ Hybridization on Microscopic Sections

The qRT-PCR, cDNA, and RNA micro-arrays make it possible to follow the presence of, and the gene expression patterns in, tissues from clinical patients, explant cultures, or specific cell lines in cell cultures.[47,48] With the exception of the cell culture systems, however, they do not allocate certain gene patterns to one specific cell type at a particular location. For example, if cartilage tissue harvested en bloc from a joint is minced, and total RNA is extracted for qRT-PCR to assess the expression of matrix metalloproteinases (MMPs), it is not possible to track down the upregulation of MMPs to the superficial, middle, or deep zone of the entire cartilage. The data will show only that mRNAs of particular genes are upregulated in the cartilage.

In some instances, however, it is important to know which cell type regulates these gene patterns and, above all, where it is regulated, to understand the whole cascade of events. For this, the technique of in situ hybridization can be used.[49-52] Although this technique can be used for localizing DNA, it usually is applied for detection of mRNA. Specific

RNA probes are hybridized to mRNA directly in tissue sections and visualized with special detection systems. The mRNA probes are ideally longer (about 400 to 600 base pairs) compared with the qRT-PCR or micro-array techniques and are coupled to the detection systems. These can consist of fluorescent substances, digoxenin, or radioisotopes (^{35}S, ^{32}P, ^{3}H). In the case of digoxenin, a secondary antibody is normally used for detection of the probes (e.g., alkaline phosphatase), whereas for visualization of radioisotopes, techniques similar to autoradiography are applied. The technique of in situ hybridization is quite demanding and its successful use depends on the individual tissue and probes. Whereas in cartilage, muscle, or other soft tissue related to the musculoskeletal system, it can be relatively easily performed, application in bone structures is very difficult. In situ hybridization for cartilage and soft tissue can be performed using either frozen (cryosections) or paraffin-embedded tissue sections. In the latter, only small tissue samples should be prepared, which are fixed in buffered, freshly made 4% paraformaldehyde for only a short time (30 minutes to 12 hours). The ideal time has to be determined for each particular probe and tissue section. If tissue is fixed too long in paraformaldehyde, the collagen linkage may be too strong for the probe to penetrate the tissue and hybridize the mRNA in question. This may lead to false interpretations. Therefore, it is wise to run qRT-PCR parallel to or even in advance of in situ hybridizations.

Alternative studies often include alteration of gene function with targeted gene deletion by the application of RNA interference (RNAi) on the cellular level. Posttranscriptional gene silencing or RNAi is the technique in which introduction of a double-stranded RNA (dsRNA) suppresses the expression of the homologous gene. Longer dsRNA molecules are reduced in vivo to 21- to 23-nucleotide small interfering RNAs (siRNAs), which are the mediators of the RNAi effect. Introduction of 21 nucleotides siRNAs with two nucleotide 3′ overhangs does not stimulate the antiviral response in mammalian cells and can effectively target specific mRNAs for gene silencing. Such molecules can be prepared by chemical synthesis or in vitro transcription. Being a highly specific and efficient knockdown technique, RNAi not only is a powerful tool but also holds promise for gene therapy. The interesting biology as well as the remarkable technical value has been drawing widespread attention to this exciting new field.

Methods of Detecting Proteins

In gene expression, the correlation between induced mRNA and induced levels of protein is not always clear. Translational and posttranslational regulatory mechanisms that impact the activity of various cellular proteins are not examined by DNA micro-arrays, although the emerging field of proteomics is beginning to address this issue.

Analysis of Proteins: Global Analysis

Proteomics is the study of the overall protein content of a subcellular compartment, cell, tissue, or organism at a particular moment in time and under certain environmental conditions. There are more proteins than genes in an organism by orders of magnitude. On the basis of alternative splicing (several per gene) and posttranslational modifications (over 100 known), there are estimated to be a million or more different proteins. Proteonomics is a powerful field of study to compare different states of a biologic system—for example, normal versus diseased. The success of proteome analysis is largely built on three techniques: two-dimensional (2D) polyacrylamide gel electrophoresis, mass spectrometry (MS), and genomic sequences.

A broad range of technologies are used in proteomics, but the central paradigm has been the use of 2D gel electrophoresis (2D-GE) followed by mass spectrometry (MS). 2D-GE is used to first separate the proteins by isoelectric point and then by size. Individual proteins are subsequently removed from the gel, prepared, and finally analyzed by MS to determine their identity and characteristics. Various types of mass analyzers are used in proteomics MS. The recent development of soft-ionization techniques, namely matrix-assisted laser desorption ionization and electro-spray ionization, have allowed large biomolecules to be introduced into the mass analyzer without completely decomposing their structures, or even without breaking them at all, depending on the design of the experiment.

Analysis of Specific Proteins

Protein function refers to the variety of mechanisms by which proteins are activated or inactivated in vivo. The study of protein function includes assays to detect and quantitate the activity of specific proteins in vitro and in vivo. With the emergence of functional proteomics in the postgenomic era, an expanded view of protein function exists, with each protein operating as a component of an intricate web of interacting molecules.

To study protein function, purified proteins may be delivered into cells to determine the conditions under which they are active. Signal transduction, the communication of extracellular signal to intracellular activation of proteins, may be examined by specific detection of activation states of key regulatory proteins.

Detection of Protein Expression Levels

Antibodies (monoclonal and polyclonal) have been successfully applied in musculoskeletal research. Antibodies allow following signaling molecules on a protein level—that is, assessing whether translation into proteins has occurred. Depending on the antibody and available commercial tests, the identification and determination of concentrations of certain proteins can be conducted by Western blot or ELISA.[53] Unfortunately, commercially available antibodies and ELISA are normally designed for antibodies in humans, mice, rats, or rabbits and may not be valid for use in equine tissues. However, in molecules where high homology is conserved between species, antibodies may cross-react with antibodies from humans, rats, or mice.[54] Furthermore, if money is available and collaborations are sought with molecular biology departments, antibodies and ELISA can be custom designed for equine patients.

Antibodies also make it possible to label cells, since many cells expose specific CD receptors at their surface (e.g.,

CD44).[55,56] For example, to find out which cell types are involved in certain tissue reactions, tissues are digested, and the cells are carefully isolated, labeled with specific antibodies, and subjected to fluorescence-activated cell sorter (FACS) analysis (see later). The FACS machine sorts cells according to their label and displays their distribution in the cell suspensions.

Immunohistochemical techniques are used to demonstrate antibodies bound to antigen in tissue sections. A secondary antibody directed against the antigen-specific antibody coupled with a fluorescent dye, digoxenin, biotin, or avidine generates a strong signal and thus allows visualization of the distribution of the antigen in the tissue section using a light microscope. Immunohistochemistry is used to type collagen (collagen types I, II, III, IX, or X), to detect the epitopes of collagen degradation or cleavage products of procollagen,[35,36] and to demonstrate the presence of MMPs 1, 2, 3, 8, 9, and 13[57] and their tissue inhibitors (TIMP) in different cartilage zones.

Depending on the homology of proteins between species, antibodies can be used across species (e.g., antibodies to inducible nitric oxide synthase [iNOS], prostaglandin [PG] E_2, factor VIII, tumor necrosis factor [TNF]-α).[58,59] The pitfalls are unexpected cross-reactions and misinterpretation of data. If antibodies have not been validated for horses beforehand, the surgeon should collaborate with immunologists. It should be determined in advance whether the antibodies can be used in paraffin sections or cryosections (further detail follows).

Detection of Enzymatic Activities

Sometimes it is not possible to visualize or measure proteins from tissue or body fluids using antibodies because the proteins are either inactive or irreversibly bound through other proteins. It may also be that the protein is ubiquitously present in a latent form but is only of interest in an activated form. For example, some MMPs are irreversibly bound by either α-microglobulins or TIMP-1, 2, or 3).[60,61] In these cases, it is possible to use fluorescein quenchers bound to a peptide, which release the fluorescein upon degradation and thus give an indirect measure of the enzyme's activity.[41,42]

Several methods are available to study the multiplication or expression of a certain gene or protein, such as bromodeoxyuridine labeling of proliferating tissue[62] or bioluminescence imaging using luciferase with either cell cultures or living animals.[63,64] (The latter, however, is applicable only in laboratory mice.) Another possibility involves the insertion of a reporter plasmid carrying the green fluorescent protein (GFP) reporter gene under the control of a constitutive activated promoter that is randomly incorporated in the genome and later can be visualized by confocal imaging and fluorescence microscopy.[65,66] To study the incorporation of a plasmid and the later expression on a transcriptional level, plasmids encoding enhanced GFP can also be introduced into cells and followed by visualizing the expression of GFP with fluorescent microscopy.[66-68] Apart from studying proliferation of cells or expression of proteins, these methods may also be used to track migration of cells within specific tissues.

Cellular Analysis

Cell sorting based on labeling of specific cell structures has become routine in cell biology. Sophisticated machines allow identification of cells according to previously applied labels. In addition to the FACS cell sorter (Becton-Dickinson), there is a flow cytometer by Coulter Electronics and the MoFlow by Cytomation. They all use the technique of flow cytometry to quantify components or structural features of cells, primarily by optical means. Although the measurements are made on one cell at a time, the machines process thousands of cells in a few seconds. The cells may be alive or fixed at the time of measurement, but they must be in a *monodispersed* (single-cell) suspension. The sample is passed through a laser beam in a continuous flow of a fine stream of the suspension. Each cell scatters some of the laser light, and it also emits fluorescent light excited by the laser. Light scatter alone is often quite useful. This technique is commonly used to exclude dead cells, cell aggregates, and cell debris from the fluorescence data. Light scatter has been used in the authors' facility to quantitate aggregation of living cells.

Fluorescent probes are used to study the quantities of specific components of cells, whereas fluorescent antibodies are used to study the densities of specific surface receptors and thus to distinguish subpopulations of differentiated cell types, including cells expressing a transgene. By antibodies fluorescent, the binding of hormones to surface receptors can be measured. Intracellular components can also be determined by fluorescent probes, including total DNA per cell (allowing cell cycle analysis), newly synthesized DNA, specific nucleotide sequences in DNA or mRNA, filamentous actin, and any structure for which an antibody is available. Flow cytometry can also monitor rapid changes in intracellular free calcium, membrane potential, pH, or free fatty acids.

Methods Involving Whole Animals

Molecular biology can be used to investigate gene function in living animals. Through genetic and appropriate breeding manipulations, either knockout[23,24,69] or transgenic mice with overexpression of a certain gene[70] are produced. Depending on the importance of the gene in body function or morphology, these mice may not grossly differ phenotypically from their normal siblings (the wild type *[wt]* mice).[71] These knockout or overexpression mice are usually recognized by an addition to their homozygous or heterozygous state (−/−, −/+, +/+). If these animals are compared with their *wt* groups, the effect of a gene can be studied, especially after stimulation with critical substances. For instance, it was demonstrated that the development of collagen-induced osteoarthritis was delayed in iNOS knockout mice, or in *wt* mice treated with a potent iNOS inhibitor, compared with the untreated *wt* mice.[72]

Animal experiments with genetically modified mice have clarified cell mechanisms in the musculoskeletal system. However, the bone structure of rodents is different from that of other animals and, therefore, results have to be interpreted with some caution. Rodents seem to be more sensitive than other animals in their response to fracture healing, the application of growth factors, and heterotopic bone formation or cartilage healing of defects. Some reported results obtained in rodents were not repeatable in higher animals and thus may have created some confusion in the field of bone enhancement.

Difficulties Related to Hard Tissue Structures

Although these molecular biologic and immunohistochemical methods are routinely used in soft tissue without difficulty, their use in cartilage and bone is more complex. The isolation of RNA from cartilage and bone tissue can prove tricky because of the low number of cells per sample weight and the heavy interference of the extracellular matrix. This is especially true for bone, for which double or triple the amount of tissue must be used and extra purification steps are needed if routine RNA isolation kits are used. Automated isolation procedures for obtaining total RNA can be used for cell cultures of osteoblasts and chondrocytes only, not for bone or cartilage tissue. Bone and cartilage tissues must be manually ground using a plotter, which is time consuming.

Problems also arise when using immunohistochemical and in situ hybridization methods for cartilage and bone of animals other than laboratory mice and rats. As long as cartilage samples can be embedded in paraffin, routine immunohistochemistry and even in situ hybridization procedures can be conducted. However, if cryosections are required, problems may be encountered related to the attachment of the sample to the glass slide. In these cases, there should be extra cartilage sections in reserve. Immunohistochemical and in situ hybridization methods in undecalcified bone samples of horses embedded in plastic sections have proved to be impossible in the authors' laboratory, even if special acrylic resins as embedding medium are used (LR-White, Polyscience, UK; HistoDur, Leica, Switzerland). Although these materials may be sufficient for rodents and small dogs and cats, they are not hard enough for horse (or sheep) bone to be cut in thin sections. In addition, epitopes may be distorted or hidden in the plastic embedding media, so that no reactions can occur despite prior deplastification of the sections. As for in situ hybridization, the probes may be too long to penetrate the tissue in the plastic, and they are hindered by the hydroxyapatite crystals. Recommended decalcification methods using 4% to 14% ethylenediaminetetra-acetic acid (EDTA) for horse (or sheep) bone samples render the process a lengthy procedure (7 to 12 months), especially if the material does not allow cutting thin slices (2 to 3 mm) in a fresh-harvested state. The use of formic acid for decalcification accelerates the process significantly, although epitopes may be destroyed, rendering the decalcified bone samples unsuitable for most antibodies used in immunohistochemistry. A mixture of formic and citric acids for decalcification (ratio of 40% to 20%), however, is more gentle for the tissue and is suitable for at least some antibodies used in immunohistochemistry. Cryosections with equine bone are not possible even if special cryostat knives are used. The hydroxyapatite crystals make it almost impossible to cut the bone in a frozen state, because they break the tissue. Not only is bone histomorphology impossible to perform but also the background noise makes it impossible to interpret immunohistologic sections correctly.

Besides the myriad technological problems of bone tissues, problems concerning the availability of gene sequences and antibodies specific for the horse are prominent. Equine libraries of DNA primers are being established, and even equine gene chips are under construction. However, depending on the molecule, the sequence (i.e., primer) or the antibody (in the case of proteins) has to be established first on an individual basis before it can be used in a research project.

MOLECULAR BIOLOGY IN CLINICAL THERAPY OF THE MUSCULOSKELETAL SYSTEM

Molecular biology has gained wide acceptance for therapeutic interventions in the musculoskeletal system. The delivery of recombinant growth factors (e.g., bone morphogenetic protein [BMP]-2) to enhance defect healing[73-77] in cartilage or bone[73-77] has finally become a clinical reality, at least in humans[78] where cost issues are not as prohibitive as in veterinary medicine. The possibility of using recombinant technologies to produce these factors has further stimulated this type of research for clinical applications. For many years, a single growth factor was sought as a solution for delayed fracture healing or nonunion. More recently, however, researchers have fine tuned this type of biological enhancement so that combinations of growth factors and timely sequences as well as release patterns are sought after.[20,32,76]

Biotechnology,[79,80] an emerging field in musculoskeletal research and in clinics, generally involves a combination of molecular technology (mostly growth factors and DNA plasmids), natural or synthetic scaffolds or carrier substances, appropriate release systems, and engineering in the form of bioreactors with or without mechanical stimulation and final implantation in the body system.[81] Molecular techniques are used to produce the appropriate growth factors applied in these systems, and to investigate the cellular synthesis of macromolecules under these conditions. It was shown for cartilage and vertebral discs created in bioreactors that functional loading during in vitro incubation increased the production of extracellular matrix significantly.[82] In fact, transplantation of cartilage discs created in vitro has already become a clinical reality, used in focal cartilage lesions, such as in osteochondritis dissecans lesions in humans.[83,84]

Importance of Biomaterials

Biomaterials play a major role in the field of biotechnology apart from cell culture methods with the appropriate cell culture media and incubation conditions for different cell types (e.g., bioreactors, mechanical stimulation).[3,85,86] Bioresorbable materials, such as tricalcium phosphate (TCP)[87,88] or similar ceramics,[89] scaffolds based on polyglycolic or lactic acids,[32,90] polyester urethane foam (DegraPol),[91] and other materials,[3,92,93] are often used for cell seeding or incorporation of substances that enhance tissue healing. The biocompatibility of the biomaterials—not only the finished product but also the intermediate degradation products—must be tested for toxicity and tissue-specific immunologic reactions while the scaffolds are being resorbed.[89] Immediate, short-term, and long-term results of biomaterials in the tissues must be investigated to avoid unpleasant surprises.

Purified silk is a new alternative to one of the oldest surgical materials.[94] Silk used as suture material is accompanied by modest inflammatory reactions, but new molecular techniques allow purification of the fibroin fibers, leading to a highly biocompatible biomatrix for synthetic replacement of bone, ligaments, tendon, and possibly (in the future) cartilage.[8,95-97] Using purified silk is an innovative approach that means that the same scaffold material can be adapted to the local requirements in strength, structure, pore size, and composition. Furthermore, it can be modified by adding release systems and additional structural components such as crystals (for example, in bone).

Recently, hydrogels have been successfully introduced as carrier matrices for bone- and cartilage-enhancing substances, without or in combination with calcium phosphate granules.[75,98-101] Calcium phosphate is needed for structural purposes, because defect healing in bone may not be achieved with bone-enhancing substances alone. However, linking bone-enhancing substances to the hydrogels allows retracted release of the molecules, and it thus avoids premature clearing of the substances from the field of action.

Additional information about biomaterials is presented in Chapter 9.

Growth Factors

Several techniques have been used successfully to enhance bone and cartilage healing with growth factors, mostly in mice, rats, and rabbits,[102-104] and considerably less in higher animal species.[30,105,106] The synthesis of growth factors has been greatly facilitated by recombinant technology in molecular biology, which made it possible to seek commercial applications in tissue healing, mainly in bone and cartilage. Platelet-derived growth factor (PDGF), acid and basic fibroblast growth factor (FGF), insulin-like growth factor (IGF)-II, transforming growth factor (TGF)-β, and BMPs are the most widely used. Among these, the BMP family is probably the most established and meanwhile also is clinically applied grouping humans and animals (Genzyme, Cambridge, Mass). Some of these factors (TGF, IGF, BMP) are abundantly present in bone matrix, and others occur naturally during fracture healing (PDGF, FGF).[20] These growth factors appear in concert and in a timely sequence, which may be one of the reasons that surgical application of just one factor in a relatively high concentration may not be as beneficial for bone healing in higher animals as originally hoped. Therefore, modern approaches concentrate on combinations of growth factors, careful selections of dosages, and respect for the natural sequences of these factors.

In recent years, it was demonstrated that low doses of parathyroid hormone (PTH) applied systemically could counteract the negative effects of osteoporosis in postmenopausal women.[107] As a consequence, the local application of PTH_{1-34} incorporated in a fibrin-based hydrogel structure with granules consisting of a mixture of tricalcium phosphate/hydroxyapatite (HA/TCP)-β at a 60%-to-40% ratio was investigated in a critical mid-shaft tibia defect in experimental sheep (Kuros Biosurgery, Switzerland). A dose-dependent increase of callus formation and bridging of the original defects could be demonstrated, with the best results being close to the gold standard, the autogenic bone grafts[108] (see Chapter 92).

Release Systems and Drug Delivery

As when only a single growth factor was applied, results were discouraging if growth factors were injected locally in the form of proteins via a single dose at the time of the initial surgery or during fracture healing. This was attributed to the fast clearance of the growth factor through the local vasculature, and a short incubation time with the local cells. Therefore, release systems were studied that allowed protracted or burst releases of these growth factors at later times.[32,75,90,109,110] Microspheres consisting of polyglycolic acid are capable of directing the local release of BMP-2[110] and IGF-II[32] and improve results considerably. Along the same line, nonviral vectors, such as liposomes or magnetofection are reported in the literature for enhancing bone healing, although only in experimental animals.[111-113] Drug delivery is possible using polymer nanoparticles or superparamagnetic iron oxide nanoparticles (SPIONs) coated with a suitable polymer (dextran, silicon, PVA, PEI) that are functionalized with either pharmaceutical substances, proteins, or peptides, and also DNA plasmids.[114,115] If plasmids are delivered with SPIONs, the process is called magnetofection.[113]

Gene Transfections

Gene transfections using viral and nonviral vectors have been attempted in synovial membranes of horses, and also in equine chondrocytes in culture.[116-119] For therapeutic purposes, an attempt has been made to introduce plasmids into the genomic information of these cells to affect their biologic behavior. These gene transfections can be performed in vivo or ex vivo.[120] In the latter method, autogeneic cells are harvested from the animal, kept in culture under appropriate conditions, transfected using a viral or nonviral vector, and finally reintroduced into the site of harvest. For example, the gene transfection of equine synovial membranes with interleukin-1 receptor antagonist (IL-1ra) by means of an adenoviral vector inhibited the development of osteoarthritis in an established equine model of osteoarthritis.[118]

Pitfalls of Molecular Biology Techniques in Therapeutic Interventions

Molecular biology techniques have a place in musculoskeletal research but not yet in equine therapy. The cost is prohibitive for veterinary medicine, Also, clinical reports in which healing of cartilage or bone after application of growth factor could not be seriously demonstrated or could not be repeated, raised criticism of their use. Finally, the long-term effects and safety issues of the application of growth factors (proteins, peptides, or plasmids) are controversial. Research must focus on these issues before safe and routine clinical use can be advocated.

Potential of Applying Molecular Biology in Musculoskeletal Research

Although molecular biology is still an emerging field in musculoskeletal research, the tools are established in diagnostics and increasingly becoming so in basic clinical research. Recombinant technology allows the development of equine-specific gene chips and antibodies that will open avenues in musculoskeletal research. Some techniques have to be adapted and modified in hard tissues such as calcified cartilage and bone, but the potential benefit for important research in the field of cartilage and bone development is unlimited. In fact, this technology makes it possible to answer research questions that could not be solved with other methods, and to use tissues harvested from patients to explain pathophysiologic mechanisms leading to disease. In addition, this technology can save lives of experimental animals, since diseased tissues of patients can be compared with controls without having to conduct animal experiments. Studies of tissues harvested from subchondral cystic lesions in horses during surgery are an example. Incubating tissues as explant cultures, the determination of pro-inflammatory and local mediators, and measuring the regulation of cytokines IL-1 and IL-6 using qRT-PCR and in situ hybridization demonstrated the inflammatory nature of the lesions without sacrificing horses as experimental animals[121,122] (see Chapter 92).

The future of molecular biology techniques in equine therapy, possibly in combination with surgery or chemotherapy, is promising. Already, treatment of equine melanomas with cytokines,[123] or filling surgically débrided cystic lesions with hydrogels enriched with bone-enhancing molecules,[124] points to a successful clinical application.

Research of the musculoskeletal system depends on collaborations with scientists from other fields. Surgeons interested in clinical research in this field need a solid background in molecular biology, biochemistry, and cell biology. Graduate courses and postgraduate training are mandatory. This field of research has a great potential to change the future of musculoskeletal diagnostics and therapy in horses and humans.

REFERENCES

1. Boyan BD, Lohmann CH, Romero J, et al: Bone and cartilage tissue engineering, Clin Plast Surg 1999;26:629.
2. Caplan AI, Goldberg VM: Principles of tissue engineered regeneration of skeletal tissues, Clin Orthop 1999;S12.
3. Wintermantel E, Mayer J, Blum J, et al: Tissue engineering scaffolds using superstructures, Biomaterials 1996;17:83.
4. Darling EM, Athanasiou KA: Articular cartilage bioreactors and bioprocesses, Tissue Eng 2003;9:9.
5. Edgington SM: New horizons for stem-cell bioreactors, Biotechnology (N Y) 1992;10:1099.
6. Freed LE, Martin I, Vunjak-Novakovic G: Frontiers in tissue engineering: In vitro modulation of chondrogenesis, Clin Orthop 1999;S46.
7. Lee DA, Martin I: Bioreactor culture techniques for cartilage-tissue engineering, Methods Mol Biol 2004;238:159.
8. Meinel L, Karageorgiou V, Fajardo R, et al: Bone tissue engineering using human mesenchymal stem cells: Effects of scaffold material and medium flow, Ann Biomed Eng 2004;32:112.
9. Wolff J: Das Gesetz der Transformation der Knochen, Berlin, 1882, A. Hirschwald.
10. Burger EH, Klein-Nulen J: Responses of bone cells to biomechanical forces in vitro, Adv Dent Res 1999;13:93.
11. Cullinane DM, Salisbury KT, Alkhiary Y, et al: Effects of the local mechanical environment on vertebrate tissue differentiation during repair: Does repair recapitulate development? J Exp Biol 2003;206:2459.
12. Bateman JF: The molecular genetics of inherited cartilage disease, Osteoarthritis Cartilage 2001;9(Suppl A):S141.
13. Belknap J: Molecular biology in equine medicine: Current and future applications, Comp Cont Ed 1997;19:224.
14. Hegemann N, Kohn B, Brunnberg L, et al: Biomarkers of joint tissue metabolism in canine osteoarthritic and arthritic joint disorders, Osteoarthritis Cartilage 2002;10:714.
15. Uusitalo H, Hiltunen A, Ahonen M, et al: Induction of periosteal callus formation by bone morphogenetic protein-2 employing adenovirus-mediated gene delivery, Matrix Biol 2001;20:123.
16. Poole AR, Paul D: Biological markers in rheumatoid arthritis, Sem Arthritis Rheum 1994;17.
17. Poole AR, Nelson F, Dahlberg L, et al: Proteolysis of the collagen fibril in osteoarthritis, Biochem Soc Symp 2003;(70):115.
18. Poole AR: Can serum biomarker assays measure the progression of cartilage degeneration in osteoarthritis? Arthritis Rheum 2002;46:2549.
19. Poole AR, Nelson F, Hollander A, et al: Collagen II turnover in joint diseases, Acta Orthop Scand Suppl 1995;266:88.
20. Bourque WT, Gross M, Hall BK: Expression of four growth factors during fracture repair, Int J Dev Biol 1993;37:573.
21. Hollander AP, Heathfield TF, Liu JJ, et al: Enhanced denaturation of the alpha (II) chains of type-II collagen in normal adult human intervertebral discs compared with femoral articular cartilage, J Orthop Res 1996;14:61.
22. Billinghurst RC, Dahlberg L, Ionescu M, et al: Enhanced cleavage of type II collagen by collagenases in osteoarthritic articular cartilage, J Clin Invest 1997;99:1534.
23. Suda N, Shibata S, Yamazaki K, et al: Parathyroid hormone-related protein regulates proliferation of condylar hypertrophic chondrocytes, J Bone Miner Res 1999;14:1838.
24. Lapvetelainen T, Hyttinen M, Lindblom J, et al: More knee joint osteoarthritis (OA) in mice after inactivation of one allele of type II procollagen gene but less OA after lifelong voluntary wheel running exercise, Osteoarthritis Cartilage 2001;9:152.
25. van Lent PL, Holthuysen AE, Sloetjes A, et al: Local overexpression of adeno-viral IL-4 protects cartilage from metallo proteinase-induced destruction during immune complex-mediated arthritis by preventing activation of pro-MMPs, Osteoarthritis Cartilage 2002;10:234.
26. Goomer RS, Maris TM, Gelberman R, et al: Nonviral in vivo gene therapy for tissue engineering of articular cartilage and tendon repair, Clin Orthop 2000;S189.
27. Stove J, Fiedler J, Huch K, et al: Lipofection of rabbit chondrocytes and long lasting expression of a lacZ reporter system in alginate beads, Osteoarthritis Cartilage 2002;10:212.
28. Bonadio J, Smiley E, Patil P, et al: Localized, direct plasmid gene delivery in vivo: Prolonged therapy results in reproducible tissue regeneration, Nat Med 1999;5:753.
29. Mastrogiacomo M, Cancedda R, Quarto R: Effect of different growth factors on the chondrogenic potential of human bone marrow stromal cells, Osteoarthritis Cartilage 2001;9(Suppl A):S36.
30. Marx RE, Carlson ER, Eichstaedt RM, et al: Platelet-rich plasma: Growth factor enhancement for bone grafts, Oral Surg Oral Med Oral Pathol Oral Radiol Endod 1998;85:638.
31. Henson FMD, Davenport C, Butler L, et al: Effects of insulin and insulin-like growth factors I and II on the growth of equine fetal and neonatal chondrocytes, Equine Vet J 1997;29:441.

32. Meinel L: Delivery of insulin like growth factor I for bone repair, Thesis, 2001, Swiss Federal Institute of Technology.
33. Boden SD: Bioactive factors for bone tissue engineering, Clin Orthop 1999;S84.
34. Billinghurst RC, Brama PA, van Weeren PR, et al: Significant exercise-related changes in the serum levels of two biomarkers of collagen metabolism in young horses, Osteoarthritis Cartilage 2003;11:760.
35. Hollander AP, Heathfield TF, Webber C, et al: Increased damage to type II collagen in osteoarthritic articular cartilage detected by a new immunoassay, J Clin Invest 1994;93:1722.
36. Hollander AP, Pidoux I, Reiner A, et al: Damage to type II collagen in aging and osteoarthritis starts at the articular surface, originates around chondrocytes, and extends into the cartilage with progressive degeneration, J Clin Invest 1995;96:2859.
37. Laverty S, Ionescu M, Marcoux M, et al: Syovial fluid markers of cartilage metabolism in horses with osteochondrosis, Vet Surg 1995;24:429.
38. Hughes CE, Caterson B, Fosang AJ, et al: Monoclonal antibodies that specifically recognize neoepitope sequences generated by "aggrecanase" and matrix metalloproteinase cleavage of aggrecan: Application to catabolism in situ and in vitro, Biochem J 1995;305:799.
39. Chu Q, Lopez M, Hayashi K, et al: Elevation of a collagenase generated type II collagen neoepitope and proteoglycan epitopes in synovial fluid following induction of joint instability in the dog, Osteoarthritis Cartilage 2002;10:662.
40. Rechenberg BV, McIlwraith CW, Akens M, et al: Spontaneous production of nitric oxide (NO), prostaglandin E2 (PGE2) and neutral metalloproteinases (NMPs) in media of explant cultures of equine synovial membrane and articular cartilage, Equine Vet J 2000;32:140.
41. Brama PA, van den Boom R, DeGroott J, et al: Collagenase-1 (MMP-1) activity in equine synovial fluid: Influence of age, joint pathology, exercise and repeated arthrocentesis, Equine Vet J 2004;36:34.
42. van den Boom R, Brama PA, Kiers GH, et al: The influence of repeated arthrocentesis and exercise on matrix metalloproteinase and tumour necrosis factor alpha activities in normal equine joints, Equine Vet J 2004;36:155.
43. van den Boom R, Brama PA, Kiers GH, et al: Assessment of the effects of age and joint disease on hydroxyproline and glycosaminoglycan concentrations in synovial fluid from the metacarpophalangeal joint of horses, Am J Vet Res 2004;65:296.
44. Darbre PD: Introduction to Practical Molecular Biology, New York, 1988, John Wiley & Sons.
45. Leutenegger CM, Mislin CN, Sigrist B, et al: Quantitative real-time PCR for the measurement of feline cytokine mRNA, Vet Immunol Immunopathol 1999;71:291.
46. Livak K, Marmaro J, Flood S: Guidelines for designing TaqMan fluorogenic probes for 5¢ nuclease assays, PE Appl Biosyst Res News 1995.
47. Zhang H, Liew CC, Marshall KW: Microarray analysis reveals the involvement of beta-2 microglobulin (B2M) in human osteoarthritis, Osteoarthritis Cartilage 2002;10:950.
48. Connor JR, Kumar S, Sathe G, et al: Clusterin expression in adult human normal and osteoarthritic articular cartilage, Osteoarthritis Cartilage 2001;9:727.
49. Alberts B, Bray D, Lewis J, et al: Recombinant DNA Technology: Molecular Biology of the Cell, New York, 1994, Garland.
50. Höfler H: Principles of in situ hybridization. In Polak JM, McGee JOD, editors: In Situ Hybridization: Principles and Practice, Oxford, 1990, Oxford University Press.
51. Angerer LM, Angerer RC: Localization of mRNAs by in situ hybridization, Methods Cell Biol 1991;35:37.
52. Leitch AR, Schwarzacher T, Jackson D, et al: In situ Hybridization: A Practical Guide, London, 1994, Bios Scientific.
53. Darbre PD: Introduction to Practical Molecular Biology, New York, 1988, John Wiley & Sons.
54. Semevolos SA, Brower-Toland BD, Bent SJ, et al: Parathyroid hormone-related peptide and Indian hedgehog expression patterns in naturally acquired equine osteochondrosis, J Orthop Res 2002;20:1290.
55. Seemayer CA, Kuchen S, Kuenzler P, et al: Cartilage destruction mediated by synovial fibroblasts does not depend on proliferation in rheumatoid arthritis, Am J Pathol 2003;162:1549.
56. Knudson CB, Knudson W: Hyaluronan and CD44: Modulators of chondrocyte metabolism, Clin Orthop 2004;S152.
57. Lark M, Williams H, Hoerrner L, et al: Development of an antibody against a metalloproteinase generated neo-epitope in human aggrecan, Proc Orthop Res Soc 1994;19, section 2:313.
58. Riitano MC, Pfister H, Engelhardt P, et al: Effects of stimulus with proinflammatory mediators on nitric oxide production and matrix metalloproteinase activity in explants of cranial cruciate ligaments obtained from dogs, Am J Vet Res 2002;63:1423.
59. Bertone AL, Palmer JL, Jones J: Synovial fluid cytokines and eicosanoids as markers of joint disease in horses, Vet Surg 2001;30:528.
60. Evans CH: The role of proteinases in cartilage destruction. In Parnham MJ, Bray MA, Berg WB, editors: Drugs in Inflammation, Berlin, 1991, Birkhaeuser Verlag.
61. Birkedal-Hansen H: Role of matrix metalloproteinases in human periodontal diseases, J Periodont 1993;64:474.
62. Breitbart AS, Grande DA, Kessler R, et al: Tissue engineered bone repair of calvarial defects using cultured periosteal cells, Plast Reconstr Surg 1998;101:567.
63. Luker GD, Bardill JP, Prior JL, et al: Noninvasive bioluminescence imaging of herpes simplex virus type 1 infection and therapy in living mice, J Virol 2002;76:12149.
64. Luker GD, Sharma V, Pica CM, et al: Noninvasive imaging of protein-protein interactions in living animals, Proc Natl Acad Sci U S A 2002;99:6961.
65. Hirschmann F, Verhoeyen E, Wirth D, et al: Vital marking of articular chondrocytes by retroviral infection using green fluorescence protein, Osteoarthritis Cartilage 2002;10:109.
66. Yakhnin AV, Vinokurov LM, Surin AK, et al: Green fluorescent protein purification by organic extraction, Protein Expr Purif 1998;14:382.
67. Chalfie M, Tu Y, Euskirchen G, et al: Green fluorescent protein as a marker for gene expression, Science 1994;263:802.
68. Tsien RY: The green fluorescent protein, Annu Rev Biochem 1998;67:509.
69. Iotsova V, Caamano J, Loy J, et al: Osteopetrosis in mice lacking NF-kappaB1 and NF-kappaB2, Nat Med 1997;3:1285.
70. Chambers MG, Kuffner T, Cowan SK, et al: Expression of collagen and aggrecan genes in normal and osteoarthritic murine knee joints, Osteoarthritis Cartilage 2002;10:51.
71. Poli V, Balena R, Fattori E, et al: Interleukin-6 deficient mice are protected from bone loss caused by estrogen depletion, EMBO J 1994;13:1189.
72. Cuzzocrea S, Chatterjee PK, Mazzon E, et al: Beneficial effects of GW274150, a novel, potent and selective inhibitor of iNOS activity, in a rodent model of collagen-induced arthritis, Eur J Pharmacol 2002;453:119.
73. Gordh M, Alberius P, Johnell O, et al: Effects of rhBMP-2 and osteopromotive membranes on experimental bone grafting, Plast Reconstr Surg 1999;103:1909.
74. Kirker-Head CA: Recombinant bone morphogenetic proteins: Novel substances for enhancing bone healing, Vet Surg 1995;24:408.
75. Schmoekel H, Schense JC, Weber FE, et al: Bone healing in the rat and dog with nonglycosylated BMP-2 demonstrating low solubility in fibrin matrices, J Orthop Res 2004;22:376.
76. Schmokel HG, Weber FE, Seiler G, et al: Treatment of nonunions with nonglycosylated recombinant human bone morphogenetic protein-2 delivered from a fibrin matrix, Vet Surg 2004;33:112.
77. Wozney JM: Overview of bone morphogenetic proteins, Spine 2002;27:S2.

78. Geesink RG, Hoefnagels NH, Bulstra SK: Osteogenic activity of OP-1 bone morphogenetic protein (BMP-7) in a human fibular defect, J Bone Joint Surg Br 1999;81:710.
79. Reddi AH: Symbiosis of biotechnology and biomaterials: Applications in tissue engineering of bone and cartilage, J Cell Biochem 1994;56:192.
80. Reddi AH: Morphogenetic messages are in the extracellular matrix: Biotechnology from bench to bedside, Biochem Soc Trans 2000;28:345.
81. Vunjak-Novakovic G: The fundamentals of tissue engineering: Scaffolds and bioreactors, Novartis Found Symp 2003;249:34.
82. Sucosky P, Osorio DF, Brown JB, et al: Fluid mechanics of a spinner-flask bioreactor, Biotechnol Bioeng 2004;85:34.
83. Schreiber RE, Ilten-Kirby BM, Dunkelman NS, et al: Repair of osteochondral defects with allogeneic tissue engineered cartilage implants, Clin Orthop 1999;S382.
84. Yaylaoglu MB, Yildiz C, Korkusuz F, et al: A novel osteochondral implant, Biomaterials 1999;20:1513.
85. Warren SM, Sylvester K, Chen CM, et al: New directions in bioabsorbable technology, Orthopedics 2002;25:S1201.
86. Wang M: Developing bioactive composite materials for tissue replacement, Biomaterials 2003;24:2133.
87. Rose PL, Auer JA, Hulse D, et al: Effect of B-tricalcium phosphate in surgically created subchondral bone defects in male horses. Am J Vet Res 1988;49:417.
88. Deiss E, Fuerst A, Haas C, et al: Symptomatik, Diagnostik und Therapie von 5 Pferden mit traumatischen subchondralen Knochenzysten, Wien Tierarztl Mschr 2001;88:1.
89. Apelt D, Theiss F, El-Warrak AO, et al: In vivo behavior of three different injectable hydraulic calcium phosphate cements, Biomaterials 2004;25:1439.
90. Gander B, Meinel L, Walter E, et al: Polymers as a platform for drug delivery: Reviewing our current portfolio on poly(lactide-co-glycolide) (PLGA) microspheres, Chimia 2001;55:212.
91. Saad B, Kuboki Y, Welti M, et al: DegraPol-foam: A degradable and highly porous polyesterurethane foam as a new substrate for bone formation, Artif Organs 2000;24:939.
92. Kokubo T, Kim HM, Kawashita M: Novel bioactive materials with different mechanical properties, Biomaterials 2003;24:2161.
93. Riminucci M, Bianco P: Building bone tissue: Matrices and scaffolds in physiology and biotechnology, Braz J Med Biol Res 2003;36:1027.
94. Kaplan DL: Spiderless spider webs, Nat Biotechnol 2002;20:239.
95. Meinel L, Hofmann S, Karageorgiou V, et al: The inflammatory responses to silk films in vitro and in vivo, Biomaterials 2004;26:147.
96. Gosline J, Lillie M, Carrington E, et al: Elastic proteins: biological roles and mechanical properties, Philos Trans R Soc Lond B Biol Sci 2002;357:121.
97. Bini E, Knight DP, Kaplan DL: Mapping domain structures in silks from insects and spiders related to protein assembly, J Mol Biol 2004;335:27.
98. Mauro S, Orlando L, Panzoni R, et al: Platelet gel biotechnology applied to regenerative surgery of intrabony defects in patients with refractory generalized aggressive peridontitis: Case report, Minerva Stomatol 2003;52:401.
99. Hendrickson DA, Nixon AJ, Grande DA, et al: Chondrocyte-fibrin matrix transplants for resurfacing extensive articular cartilage defects, J Orthop Res 1994;12:485.
100. Bhanot S, Alex JC: Current applications of platelet gels in facial plastic surgery, Facial Plast Surg 2002;18:27.
101. Bonucci E, Marini E, Valdinucci F, et al: Osteogenic response to hydroxyapatite-fibrin implants in maxillofacial bone defects, Eur J Oral Sci 1997;105:557.
102. Forell EB, Straw RC: Bone morphogenetic proteins and bone derived growth factors, Vet Comp Orthop Traumatol 1993;6:166.
103. Bland YS, Critchlow MA, Ashhurst DE: Exogenous fibroblast growth factors-1 and -2 do not accelerate fracture healing in the rabbit, Acta Orthop Scand 1995;66:543.
104. Critchlow MA, Bland YS, Ashhurst DE: The effect of exogenous transforming growth factor-beta2 on healing fractures in the rabbit, Bone 1995;16:521.
105. Gerhart TN, Kirker-Head CA, Kriz MJ, et al: Healing segmental femoral defects in sheep using recombinant human bone morphogenetic protein, Clin Orthop 1993;317.
106. Ripamonti U, Duneas N, Heever B, et al: recombinant transforming growth factor-beta 1 induces endochondral bone in the baboon and synergizes with recombinant osteogenic protein-1 (bone morphogenetic protein-7) to initiate rapid bone formation, J Bone Min Res 1997;12:1584.
107. Miyakoshi N: Effects of parathyroid hormone on cancellous bone mass and structure in osteoporosis, Curr Pharm Des 2004;10:2615.
108. Schense J: Personal communication, 2005.
109. Zimmermann H, Hillgartner M, Manz B, et al: Fabrication of homogeneously cross-linked, functional alginate microcapsules validated by NMR-, CLSM- and AFM-imaging, Biomaterials 2003;24:2083.
110. Weber FE, Eyrich G, Gratz KW, et al: Slow and continuous application of human recombinant bone morphogenetic protein via biodegradable poly(lactide-co-glycolide) foamspheres, Int J Oral Maxillofac Surg 2002;31:60.
111. Dokka S, Toledo D, Shi, X, et al: High-efficiency gene transfection of macrophages by lipoplexes, Int J Pharm 2000;206:97.
112. Goomer RS, Deftos LJ, Terkeltaub R, et al: High-efficiency non-viral transfection of primary chondrocytes and perichondrial cells for ex-vivo gene therapy to repair articular cartilage defects, Osteoarthritis Cartilage 2001;9:248.
113. Scherer F, Anton M, Schillinger U, et al: Magnetofection: Enhancing and targeting gene delivery by magnetic force in vitro and in vivo, Gene Ther 2002;9:102.
114. Chastellain M, Petri A, Gupta A, et al: Superparamagnetic silica-iron oxide nanocomposites for application in hyperthermia, Adv Eng Mat 2004;6:235.
115. Chastellain M, Petri A, Hofmann H: Particle size investigations of a multistep synthesis of PVA coated superparamagnetic nanoparticles, J Colloid Interface Sci 2004;278:353.
116. Hidaka C, Goodrich LR, Chen CT, et al: Acceleration of cartilage repair by genetically modified chondrocytes over expressing bone morphogenetic protein-7, J Orthop Res 2003;21:573.
117. Nixon AJ, Brower-Toland BD, Bent SJ, et al: Insulinlike growth factor-I gene therapy applications for cartilage repair, Clin Orthop 2000;S201.
118. Frisbie DD, Ghivizzani SC, Robbins PD, et al: Treatment of experimental equine osteoarthritis by in vivo delivery of the equine interleukin-1 receptor antagonist gene. Gene Ther 2002;9:12.
119. Frisbie DD, McIlwraith CW: Evaluation of gene therapy as a treatment for equine traumatic arthritis and osteoarthritis, Clin Orthop 2000;S273.
120. Evans CH, Robbins PD: Introduction: Why gene therapy for arthritis? In Wolff JA, editor: Gene Therapy for Arthritis, Boston, 1994, Birkhauser.
121. Rechenberg B, Leutenegger CM, Zlinszky K, et al: Upregulation of mRNA of interleukin-1 and 6 in subchondral cystic lesions of four horses, Equine Vet J 2000;33:143.
122. Rechenberg B, McIlwraith CW, Guenther H, et al: Fibrous tissue of subchondral cystic lesions (scl) in horses produce inflammatory mediators and matrix metalloproteinases and cause bone resorption in vitro, Vet Surg 1998;27:520.
123. Feige K, Müller J: Personal communication, 2005.
124. Fürst A, Watson J, Schense J, et al: Personal communication, 2005.

CHAPTER 80

Bone Biology and Fracture Healing

Mark D. Markel
Mandi J. Lopez

As in all vertebrate species, the skeleton is a major component of the horse's body, since it provides structural protection to the internal organs and rigid links for muscular attachment to allow for muscle action and body movement. It also acts as a reservoir for calcium and phosphorus—a dynamic mineral reserve.[1-3] Bone is the principal component of the skeleton, and it is composed of an orderly deposition of mineral on an organic matrix substrate giving it the viscoelastic properties required to serve its function.[4] Bone has many unique features that allow it to fulfill these functions. It is the third hardest substance in the body, after dentin and enamel. Bone has orderly micro- and macrostructural properties that are constantly turned over in response to physical and biochemical demands. Bone is a highly vascular tissue with an excellent capacity for self-repair. In this chapter, the structure and function of bone including its biomechanical characteristics and the specific forces that lead to particular fracture types is discussed. The necessity for establishing stability after fracture and the biologic reaction and healing of bone, including how to clinically evaluate a fracture's healing to determine when to remove external coaptation or to return a horse to exercise, is described.

STRUCTURE AND FUNCTION OF BONE

Macroscopically, bone can be divided into two broad types, compact or cortical bone and cancellous or trabecular bone. Compact bone is present in the shafts of the long bones, whereas cancellous or trabecular bone occupies the cavities within bone that contain either hematopoietic or fatty marrow. Cancellous bone is composed of a fine network of interlacing partitions called trabeculae, and it is found in most of the axial skeleton and in the ends of the long bones.

The appendicular skeleton generally consists of long cylindrical structures with narrow, predominately cortical midsections. The relatively long length of equine bones increases the moment arm of each limb, enhancing a horse's power and speed. The expanded ends of the bones distribute stresses across the joint surface, thereby diminishing the loads to the articular surface.

All long bones, except regions covered by articular cartilage or where ligaments, tendons, or joint capsules are attached, are covered by periosteum[4,5] (Fig. 80-1). Periosteum is made up of two layers: an outer fibrous layer that acts in a supportive capacity, and an inner osteogenic layer that provides the cells necessary for fracture healing, or that during growth is responsible for appositional bone formation before skeletal maturity. In immature animals, the osteogenic layer of the periosteum is thick and highly vascular. As the animal matures, this layer thins and becomes only loosely adhered to the bone.

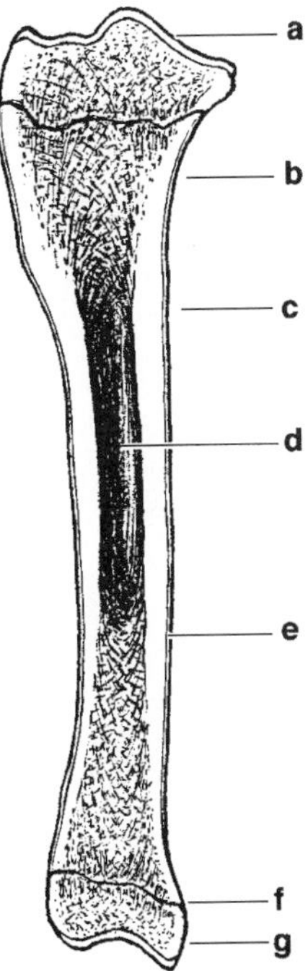

Figure 80-1. A growing equine tibia showing the different regions of the long bone. a, articular cartilage; b, metaphysis; c, diaphysis; d, medullary cavity; e, periosteum; f, growth plate; g, epiphysis.

On a microstructural level, bone can be divided into three principal components that are intimately associated with each other to allow rapid responses to both the mechanical and the homeostatic requirements of the body. These components are the cells, the organic extracellular matrix, and the inorganic portion of bone.

Of the cellular component, osteoblasts, osteocytes, and osteoclasts are the predominant cell types in bone. *Osteoblasts* develop from fibroblastic osteoprogenitor or mesenchymal cells and cover the majority of bone surfaces.[5-8] They are responsible for the formation of the organic matrix of bone called osteoid. Osteoblasts deposit osteoid on bone surfaces, incorporating themselves in osteoid seams. Approximately 10% of the osteoblasts become enclosed in matrix and are then referred to as *osteocytes*. Compared with osteoblasts, osteocytes have less endoplasmic reticulum and fewer cytoplasmic organelles.[6] Osteocytes have numerous cytoplasmic processes that extend into the matrix and fill the canaliculi of bone (Fig. 80-2). These processes contact adjacent osteocyte processes and osteoblasts to form an intricate transport and communication system within bone. This interconnecting framework regulates the flow of mineral ions from the extracellular space surrounding the osteoblasts to the osteocytes and then from the osteocytes to the extracellular fluid surrounding them. This arrangement allows the large surface area of the osteocyte population to regulate mineral ion exchange between the extracellular fluid and the bone by the canalicular system.

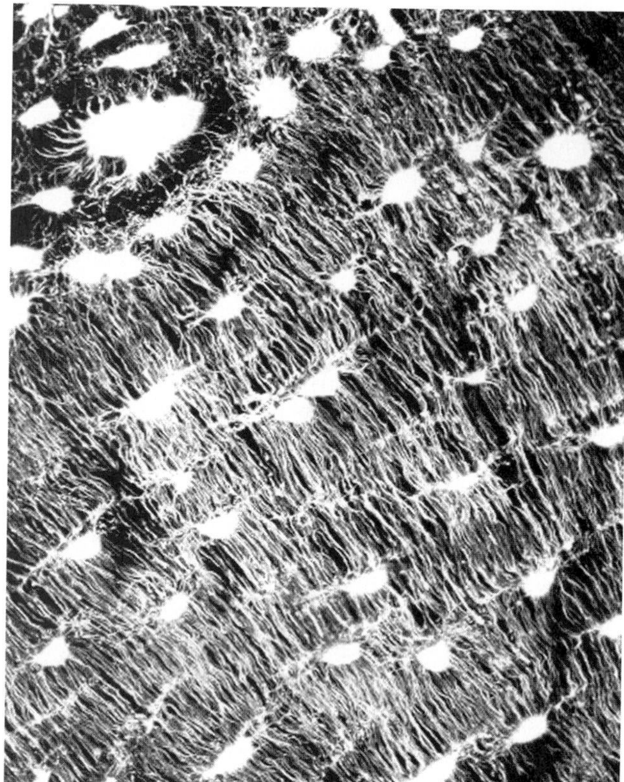

Figure 80-2. Grayscale composite Z-stacked confocal photomicrograph of cortical bone demonstrating a dense syncytial network of vital osteocytes and their canaliculi, bulk-stained with basic fuchsin. (Courtesy Peter Muir, University of Wisconsin, Madison.)

Osteoclasts are the cell type responsible for the majority of bone resorption.[6] These cells are large, multinucleated, and are found on or near bone surfaces that occupy concavities on their surface called Howship's lacunae. Osteoclasts originate from blood monocytes, which arrive at their destination in bone through the vascular system. Osteoclasts produce acid phosphatase and collagenase to first dissolve mineral and then to remove the organic matrix underneath the cells. In the extracellular space between the osteoclasts and the surface of the bone, both hydroxyapatite crystals and collagen fibers can be observed; they are degraded and taken up via endocytosis, transported across the cell, and finally extruded into the extracellular space.

The organic extracellular matrix is composed principally of collagen, proteoglycans, and glycosaminoglycans. Overall, the organic matrix makes up approximately 21% of bone by wet weight, with the remainder of the bone composed of inorganic material (71%) and water (8%).[5] Of the organic matrix, 95% is collagen, with type I collagen being the predominant type. Collagen is the most abundant protein in mammals, accounting for 20% to 50% of the dry weight of adult long bones. Type I collagen is exceedingly strong in tension and is composed of three tightly folded polypeptide chains called α-chains (Fig. 80-3). The basic unit of collagen is tropocollagen, which is composed of three procollagen polypeptides coiled into a left-handed helix, and they are further coiled around each other into a right-handed triple helix. Triple helical collagen molecules polymerize into larger collagen fibrils with covalent bonds and cross-links

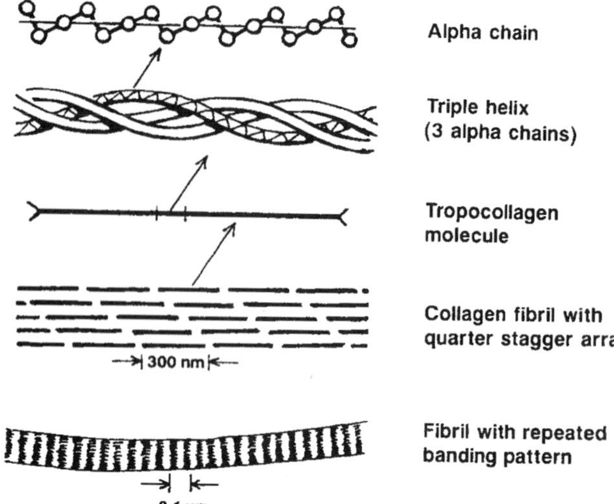

Figure 80-3. The molecular features of type I collagen from the alpha chain to the collagen fibril. (Adapted with permission from Markel MD: In Nixon AJ, editor: Equine Fracture Repair, Philadelphia, 1996, WB Saunders.)

forming between these molecules, adding to the fibrils' high tensile strength. Individual α-chains of type I collagen consist of repeating tripeptides of glycine, proline, hydroxyproline, and hydroxylysine. Glycine accounts for approximately one third of all constituent amino acids in type I collagen because it is the only amino acid small enough to fit into the center of the triple helix of collagen.

The remaining 5% of the organic matrix in bone is ground substance, consisting of proteoglycans and glycosaminoglycans. Proteoglycans are high-molecular-weight substances or molecules that provide flexibility and resilience to the connective tissue matrix.[5] Proteoglycans are made up of a central core protein, with glycosaminoglycan side chains that are attached covalently. These side chains are composed of repeating basic and acidic disaccharides. In addition to serving as the major constituent of the side chains of proteoglycans, glycosaminoglycans also serve as the cementing substance between layers of mineralized collagen fibers in lamellar bone.

The inorganic portion of bone consists primarily of calcium and phosphate, mainly in the form of hydroxyapatite crystals. The combination of the triple helical structure of type I collagen in intimate apposition with the small crystals of hydroxyapatite is responsible for the bone's mechanical strength.

BIOMECHANICAL DEFINITIONS

The strength and stiffness of bone are its most important mechanical properties, and they can be assessed best by evaluating the response of bone to externally applied forces called loads.[3] When these forces act on a structure like bone, deformation occurs, which is defined as a change in dimension such as decreased or increased length. When a load is applied to a structure, the deformation of the structure can be measured and plotted on a load-deformation curve. A typical load-deformation curve is illustrated in Figure 80-4.[3] The initial linear portion of the curve, called the *elastic*

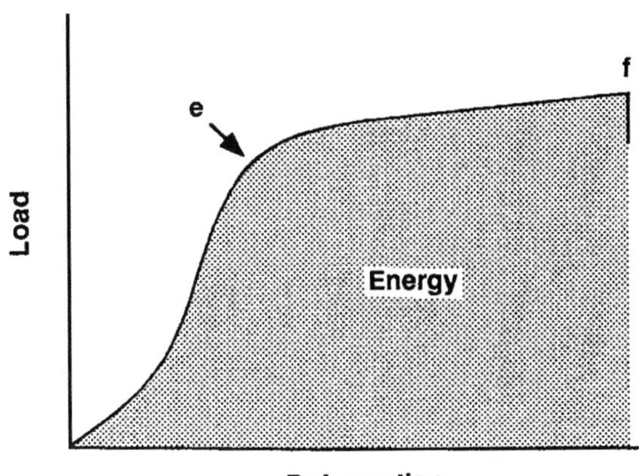

Figure 80-4. Typical load-deformation curve of a viscoelastic substance such as bone. The ultimate failure point (f) is the load at which fracture occurs. The stiffness of the structure is the slope of the elastic region of the curve (before the yield point, e, which is the change from elastic to plastic deformation). The area underneath the curve defines the energy absorption of the bone as it is loaded.

region, is a measure of the stiffness or elasticity of the structure. If the bone is loaded only through this elastic region, it will return to its original shape when the load is removed. As loading continues beyond the elastic region, yield begins to occur, which is defined as permanent deformation. When the load exceeds this yield point, the structure exhibits plastic behavior, known as the *plastic region* on the load-deformation curve. In this region, the bone deforms to a much greater extent per given load—that is, the structure is *less stiff* than in the elastic region of the curve.

With progressively increasing loads, the bone eventually fails at what is defined as the ultimate failure point. The *toughness* of a structure is defined as the energy stored by the structure during loading and is equivalent to the area under the curve. Toughness is important to the bone's mechanical properties, because the more energy that is stored in a bone prior to failure, the greater the comminution or soft tissue damage that will be caused when a fracture occurs.

The load-deformation curve is extremely useful for determining the mechanical properties of whole structures such as an entire bone or when determining the biomechanical properties of fixation devices. This type of gross structural testing does not allow determination of local material properties of bone. To conduct such testing, a stress-strain curve must be generated typically utilizing machined, standardized bone specimens.

Stress is defined as the amount of force per unit area that develops on a plane surface within a structure in response to an externally applied load. Normal stress is the magnitude of the internal force perpendicular to a plane that passes through a point in the body. Tensile stress is defined as positive and compressive stress as negative. Commonly used units are pounds per square inch (psi), or pascals [Pa] (1 Pa = 1 newton per meter squared [N/m^2]), and 1 megapascal [MPa] = 10^6 Pa = 1 N/mm^2 = 145 psi.

Strain is the magnitude of the internal forces parallel to a plane that passes through a point in the body, and it is also expressed as force per unit area. Strain is defined as the localized change in dimension that occurs within a structure as it responds to externally applied loads. The two basic types of strain that are described are linear strain, which causes a change in the length of the structure, and shear strain, which causes a change in the angular relationships within the structure. Linear strain is a measure of localized deformation divided by the original length of the structure, and therefore it is dimensionless and expressed as a percentage. Shear strain is measured as the amount of angular deformation (γ) of a right angle lying in the plane of interest in the sample. Shear strain is expressed in radians and therefore also is dimensionless.

The stress-strain curve typically looks very similar to the previously described load deformation curve. Typically, standardized specimens are machined into a cylinder or cube and then loaded until failure. Stress is typically plotted along the ordinate and strain along the abscissa (Fig. 80-5). The elastic region of the stress-strain curve in compression or tension is defined as Young's modulus, whereas when the test is carried out under pure shear forces, the slope of the elastic region is called the shear modulus. As for the load-deformation curve, stress or strain beyond the yield point results in plastic deformation of the structure. Deformation within the elastic region of the curve is defined as elastic, and that which occurs in the plastic region of the curve is defined as plastic deformation. A ductile material has the ability to deform plastically to a great extent before fracturing. In contrast, a brittle material can sustain very limited strain prior to fracture.

The mechanical properties of bone differ significantly between the two macroscopic bone types. Cortical bone is *stiffer* than cancellous bone and fails at approximately 2% strain, whereas cancellous bone fails at 75% strain.[9] Cancellous bone has the ability to store significantly more energy prior to failure than cortical bone, because of its ductility. Cortical bone tends to be a fairly brittle material and by definition can sustain only limited strain before fracture. Bone as a structure performs differently depending on the orientation of loading. For example, bone is significantly stronger in compression than in tension, a property known as *anisotropy.* In contrast, a material that exhibits neither structural orientation nor dependency on loading orientation is said to be *isotropic.*

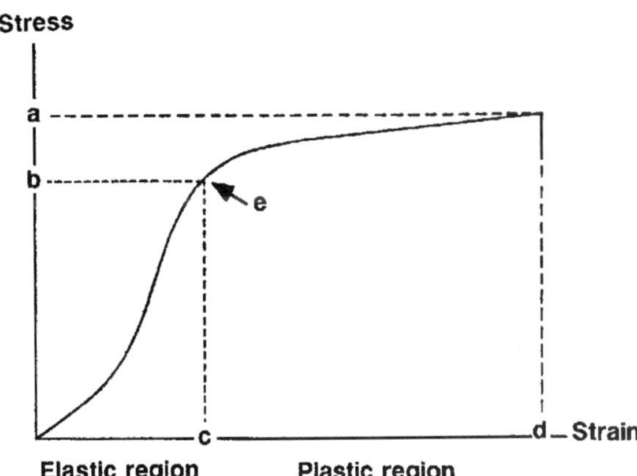

Figure 80-5. Typical stress–strain curve of a bone sample. The slope of the linear elastic region of the curve defines Young's modulus in tension and compression and the shear modulus in pure shear. As for the load–deformation curve, stress or strain beyond the yield point results in permanent deformation of the specimen.

The biomechanical response of bone to load depends on many factors including the geometry of the bone, the loading mode applied (for example, tension, compression), the material properties of the bone, and the frequency of loading. During normal daily activities, bone is subjected to various loading conditions including tension, compression, bending, shear, torsion, and, in many instances, a combination of these loads (Fig. 80-6).

During *tensile loading,* equal and opposite loads are applied to the ends of the structure, resulting in tensile stresses and strains within the structure. Maximal tensile stresses occur on a plane perpendicular to the applied load and tension. Tensile loading both lengthens and narrows the bone. Failure results from osteons debonding along cement lines; causing osteon pullout. Typically, tensile loading results in transverse fractures as occur in the proximal ulna, the proximal sesamoid bones, the patella, and the calcaneus (Fig. 80-7). Tensile fractures occur along the plane of maximal tensile stress, which is usually transverse to the tensile load.

When a bone is loaded in *compression,* equal and opposite loads are applied at the end of the structure, resulting in compressive stresses and strains (see Fig. 80-7). Maximal compressive stress occurs on a plane perpendicular to the applied load. In contrast to a bone's response to tensile loading, the bone shortens and widens under compression, with failure occurring obliquely through the osteons, corresponding to the plane of maximal shear stress (at a 45-degree angle to the orientation of the compressive load). The bone fails along the maximal shear-stress plane because bone as a material is strongest in compression and weakest in tension, with shear strength being intermediate between compressive and tensile strengths. Pure compressive fractures are rare in horses but include Y-shaped fractures of the distal humerus and femur.

Bending, a very common loading mode in the appendicular skeleton, results in a combination of tension and compression (see Fig. 80-7). Typically, tensile stresses act on one side of the bone and compressive stresses act on the

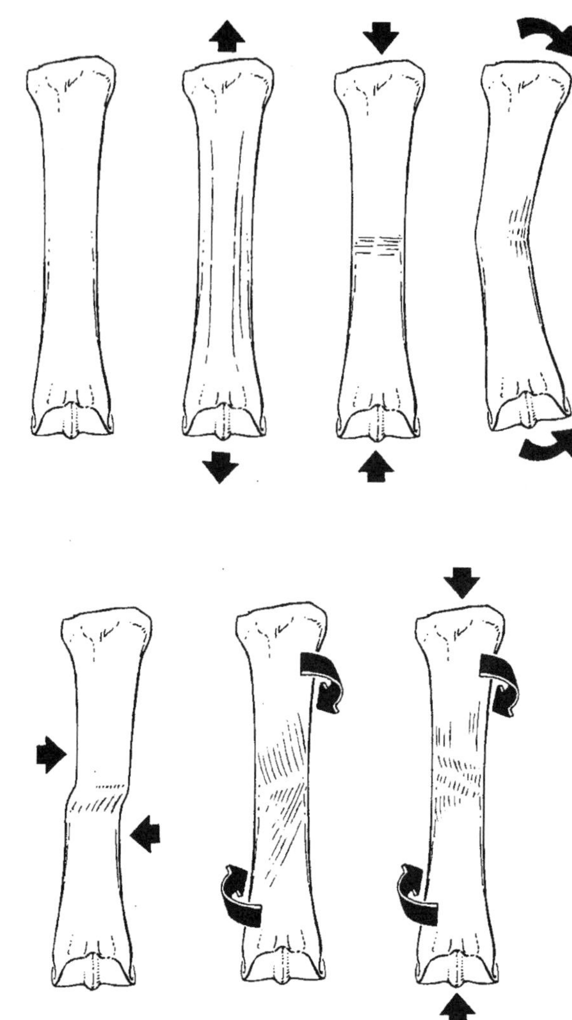

Figure 80-6. The various loading conditions that bone is subjected to during normal daily activities. From top to bottom and left to right: no load, tension, compression, bending, shear, torsion, and compression and torsion.

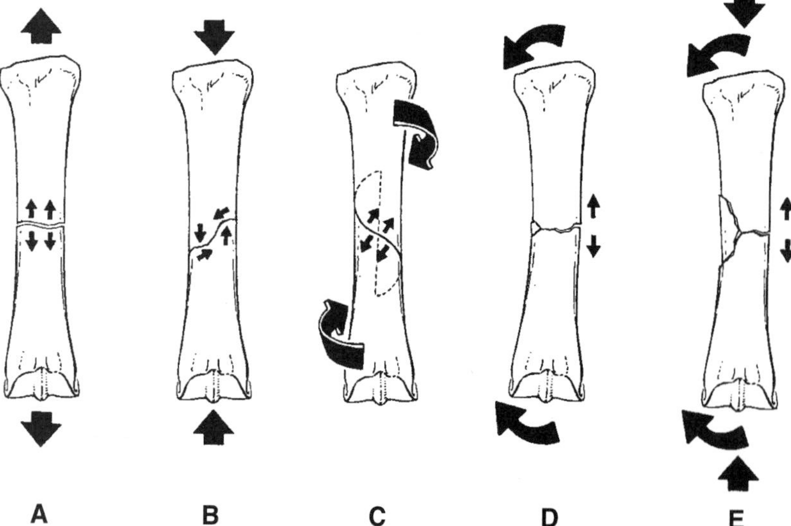

Figure 80-7. Long bone fracture configurations associated with the typical forces that result in fracture. **A,** In pure tension, the bone fails transversely. **B,** In compression, the bone fails obliquely along the maximal shear plane. **C,** In torsion, the fracture initiates in shear along the surface of the bone and then propagates in tension in a spiral manner. **D,** In pure bending, the bone initially fails in tension *(small arrows),* and the fracture propagates toward the compressive surface, resulting in a small butterfly fragment. **E,** In combined compression and bending, the bone initially fails in tension *(small arrows),* and the fracture propagates toward the compression surface, resulting in a large butterfly fragment along the maximal shear plane.

opposite cortex. The neutral axis is defined as the plane within the bone that is not subjected to tension or compression. The farther from the neutral axis, the greater the magnitude of the tensile and compressive stresses. Both clinically and experimentally, bending can be three-point or four-point bending (Fig. 80-8). Three-point bending occurs when three forces act on a bone to produce two equal maximal bending moments. The bending stress is concentrated at the point of load application, and fractures typically occur at this point. A typical three-point bending fracture in a horse occurs at the top of a cast or when the horse steps in a hole. Since adult bone is weakest in tension, failure begins on the tensile surface of the bone and subsequently progresses to the surface along the maximal tension plane until shear forces acting on 45-degree planes become sufficiently high to cause a butterfly fracture at the compressive surface of the bone.

Four-point bending is caused by two force couples or four forces (two central and two peripheral) acting on a structure to produce two equal moments (see Fig. 80-8). The region between the two central application points is subjected to a uniform bending moment, and the bone fractures through the weakest portion of the bone in this central region. Four-point bending rarely results in a fracture clinically, but it is often used when experimentally determining the biomechanical properties of bone.

Torsion occurs when a load is applied to a structure and results in twisting around an axis, causing torque to be produced within the structure (see Fig. 80-7, *C*). When a bone is subjected to torsion, shear stresses are distributed over the entire structure. As with bending loads, the magnitude of these stresses is proportional to their distance from the neutral axis (usually the central axis of rotation). Therefore, the periosteal surface of bone is typically subjected to the highest shear stresses when a bone is loaded in torsion. Maximal tensile and compressive stresses always act on a plane at 45 degrees relative to the maximal shear-stress plane as a result of the large shear stresses that occur on the surface of the bone. A bone loaded in torsion first fails in shear along its outer surface with the formation of cracks parallel to the long axis of the cortex. Subsequent cracks then form along the plane of maximal tensile stress, causing a spiral fracture to occur.

The most common loading pattern that occurs during normal daily activities is combined loading. Bones are regularly subjected to complex loads in multiple directions that occur simultaneously. This results in varying strains in different orientations depending on the surface of the bone evaluated, the geometry of the bone, and the portion of the bone being examined.

An extremely important property of bone is its *rate dependency*. Since bone is viscoelastic, the faster the bone is loaded, the greater are its stiffness, strength, and energy absorption during loading. Therefore, if a bone is rapidly loaded and then fails, this greater energy absorption is released during fracture, causing greater comminution as well as greater soft tissue injury. At lower loading rates, bone is less stiff, fails at a lower load, and stores less energy prior to failure, typically resulting in simple fractures with little comminution and less displacement of the bone fragments.

Fractures can occur as a result of a single incident or secondary to repeated loading cycles. Bones that fail secondary to *repeated cyclic loading* are typically viewed as failing secondary to a fatigue fracture (Fig. 80-9). Under cyclic loads, the susceptibility of bone to fracture is related to its crystal structure and collagen orientation reflected by its viscoelastic properties. Cortical bone is particularly

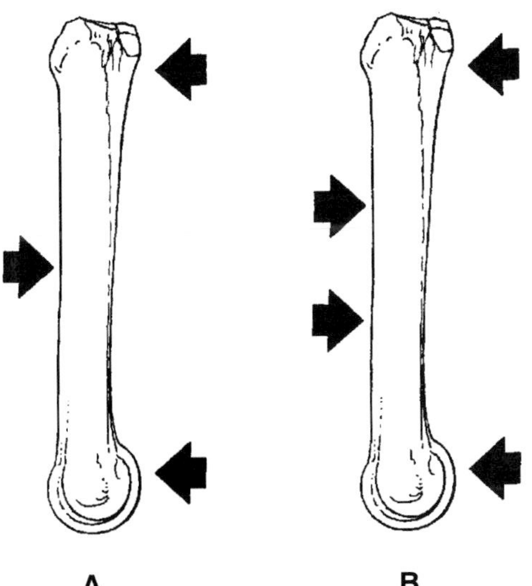

Figure 80-8. Two types of bending to which the equine bone might be subjected. **A,** Three-point bending. **B,** Four-point bending.

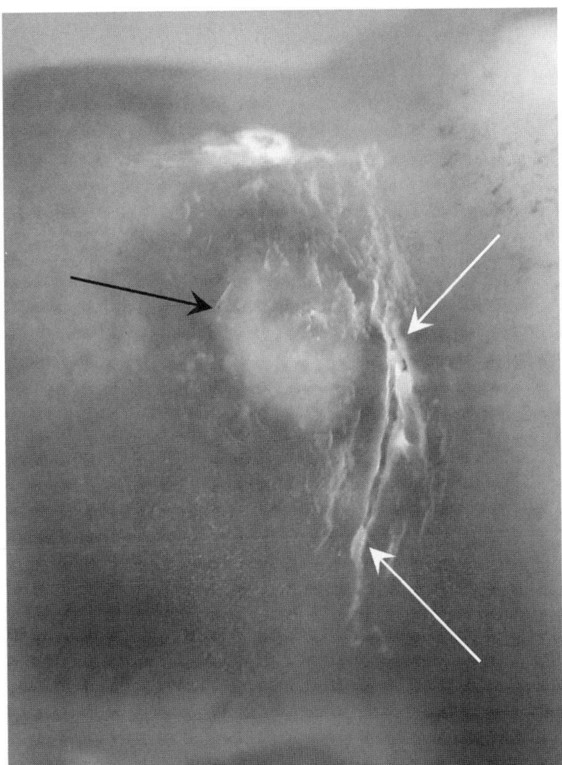

Figure 80-9. The parasagittal region of the distal end of the third metacarpal bone from a racing Thoroughbred. The predominant parasagittal linear subchondral crack *(white arrows)* is a result of fatigue loading of the articular surface and is also located on the axial margin of a subchondral erosion in the palmar region of the lateral condyle *(black arrow)*. (Courtesy Peter Muir, University of Wisconsin, Madison.)

vulnerable to both tensile and compressive cyclic stresses. Fatigue load under certain strain rates can cause progressive microdamage accumulation in cortical bone (Fig. 80-10). If this process continues, the bone may eventually fail through coalescences and propagation of these cracks. Although cortical bone is relatively brittle and has poor fatigue resistance in vitro, it is a living tissue that can remodel and repair during and after loading, as occurs in shin splints in horses. Periosteal new bone formation near microcrack formation can arrest crack propagation by reducing the stresses encountered at the tip of the crack. In a fatigue test, the endurance limit of a bone is the stress level under which no fractures can develop regardless of the number of loading cycles applied. For this repair process to be effective following fatigue-induced microcracks, relatively low loads must be present and be maintained to allow sufficient time for the repair process to occur.

BIOLOGIC REACTION AND HEALING OF BONE

To successfully treat fractures, knowledge of bone biology and of the causes, management strategies, and healing of fractures is essential.[2] Fracture healing typically results in the return of the injured bone to its original form and function and involves a number of significant processes that can be regarded as temporary reversion to the embryonic state.[10,11] Skin, muscle, and tendon tissue, unlike bone, are unable to fully regenerate after injury, but rather heal with a permanent scar.

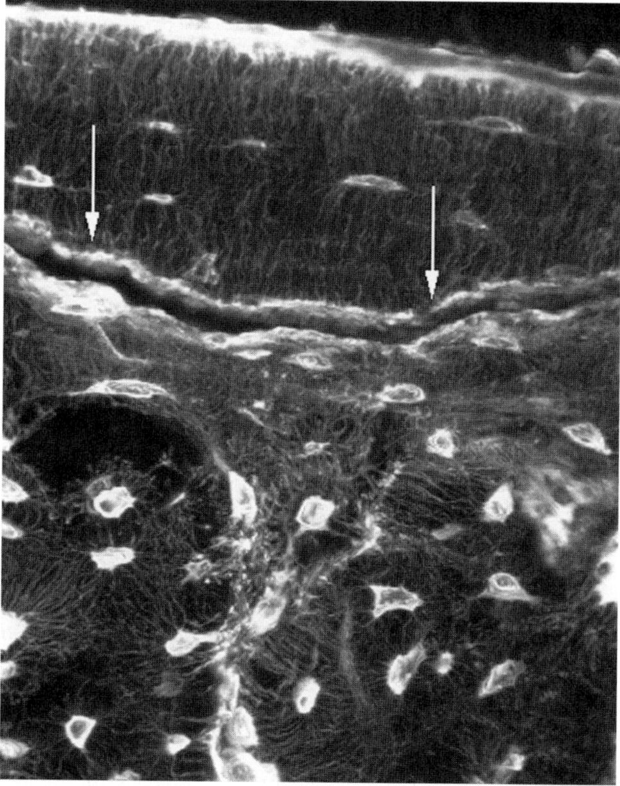

Figure 80-10. Grayscale composite Z-stacked confocal photomicrograph of a bone 7 days after fatigue loading bulk-stained with basic fuchsin. The osteocyte syncytium in this region has lost its normal canalicular network and has become devitalized (see Fig. 80-2). A prominent microcrack is clearly visible in the cortical bone.

Fracture healing involves a series of overlapping processes that occur in the majority of fractures. These stages are typically referred to as the inflammatory phase, the reparative phase, and the remodeling phase.[12] The *inflammatory phase* is a critical prerequisite for the reparative phase of fracture healing and usually occurs during the first 2 to 3 weeks after injury.[13] If impairment of the inflammatory phase occurs, fracture healing is compromised.[13] During the inflammatory phase, several cellular mechanisms responsible for repair of the fracture and protection of the healing tissue from infection are activated. Various chemical mediators cause vasodilation, migration of leukocytes, and chemotaxis. Platelets contribute cytokines that assist in mesenchymal cell proliferation and angiogenesis. After migration to the injured site, granulocytes ingest and destroy bacteria but do not contribute to repair. Macrophages and to a smaller extent lymphocytes also aide in the destruction of bacteria and stimulate repair by releasing both cell growth factors and angiogenic factors.[13]

The *reparative phase* follows and overlaps with the inflammatory phase. During the reparative phase of fracture healing, the bone is highly susceptible to mechanical factors such as interfragmentary motion between fracture fragments. The reparative phase can take between 2 and 12 months to be completed. Without immobilization, the natural course of fracture healing begins with interfragmentary stabilization by both periosteal and endosteal callus formation.[14] This process restores continuity of the bone and union occurs by endochondral and intramembranous ossification (Fig. 80-11).

The *remodeling phase* occurs during and after the reparative phase. The vascular and necrotic regions of bone are replaced through *osteonal remodeling* (Fig. 80-12). Alignment of the fragments can be corrected to a certain extent by remodeling of the healed bone. During loading, convex surfaces carry a positive charge and attract osteoclasts, whereas concave surfaces carry a negative charge and attract osteoblasts. Therefore, bone is laid down on concave surfaces and removed from convex surfaces, helping to straighten a malaligned bone. Over 40 years ago, it was discovered that rigid compression plating of a fracture inhibited callus formation, allowing bone ends to unite via *haversian remodeling*

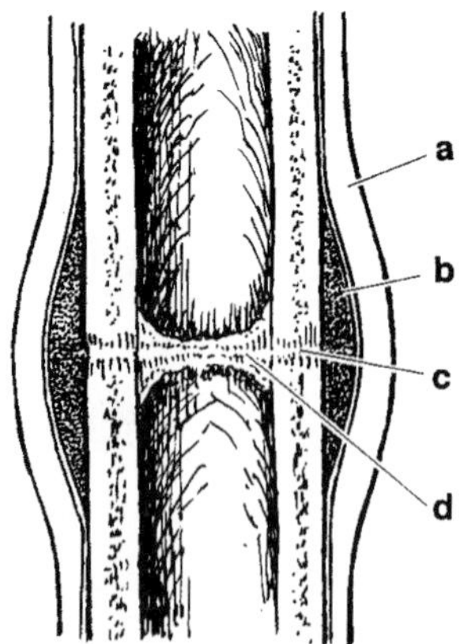

Figure 80-11. The typical soft tissue response associated with normal fracture healing. a, external soft tissue reaction; b, periosteal reaction; c, cortical reaction; d, bone marrow reaction. (Adapted with permission from Markel MD: Fracture healing and its noninvasive assessment. In Nixon AJ, editor: Equine Fracture Repair, Philadelphia, 1995, WB Saunders.)

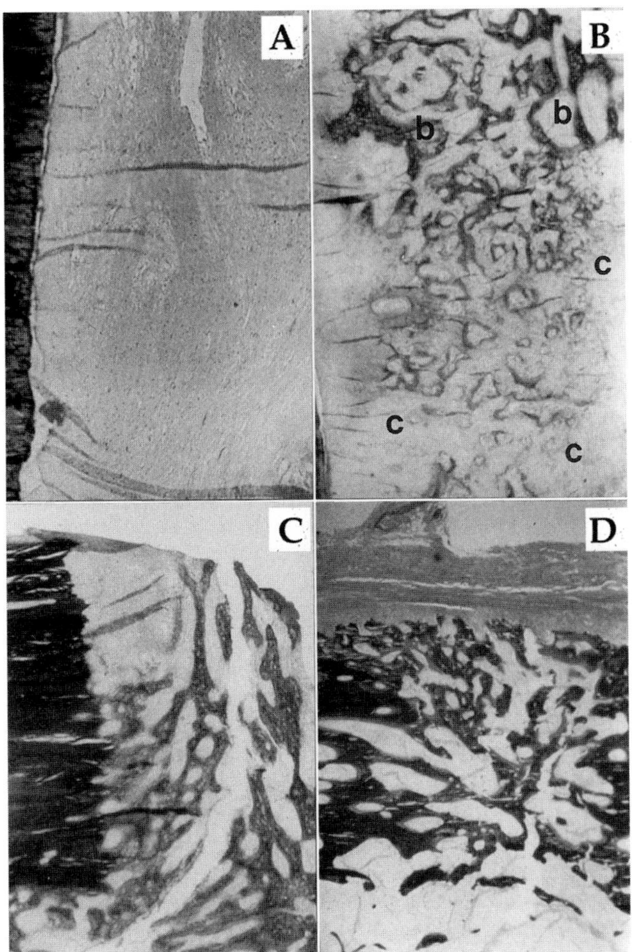

Figure 80-12. Light microscopic images of a 5-µm undecalcified specimen of a fracture gap (Goldner stain, ×20). **A,** Two weeks after fracture healing, the gap has filled with undifferentiated mesenchymal tissue. **B,** Four weeks after fracture healing, with islands of cartilage (c) and bone (b). **C,** Eight weeks after fracture, with porous woven bone filling the gap. **D,** Twelve weeks after fracture healing, with the cortex united (but with porous bone that is in the process of being remodeled).

in contact areas (contact healing) and noncontact areas (gap healing).[15] Fracture healing was subsequently divided into two distinct patterns, including primary (or direct) bone healing and secondary (or indirect) fracture healing. Indirect fracture healing, which requires healing by periosteal and endosteal callus formation, is considered secondary because either fibrous tissue or fibrocartilage is formed initially between the fracture fragments, which is subsequently replaced by new bone.[10]

The ultimate goal of fracture healing is to reconstruct the original cortical bone (see Fig. 80-12). The cortical ends of the fracture site become avascular and necrotic immediately after the fracture. Fortunately, this vascular compromise does not prevent the avascular ends from serving important biomechanical roles as supportive elements for a fracture fixation device. Haversian remodeling of the uniting fracture serves two principal functions—the revascularization of necrotic bone at the fracture site and the reconstitution of the interfragmentary gaps. There are three specific requirements for haversian remodeling to occur across a fracture site. These include adequate reduction, rigid fixation, and sufficient blood supply. Haversian remodeling of the fracture typically begins in the second to third month after fracture healing. It is unknown exactly what factors initiate the dramatic increase in secondary osteon formation, which occurs during fracture healing, but it has been postulated that the activation of haversian remodeling is related to tissue damage at the fracture site.[10]

Progression of secondary osteons from one fracture fragment to another does not require intimate contact of fracture fragments. Even with perfect reduction and rigid internal fixation, there are incongruencies at the fracture site that result in small gaps between areas of contact. These gaps are typically filled within weeks after the fracture occurs by direct lamellar or woven new bone. Secondary osteons use this gap tissue as a scaffold to grow from one fragment to another. Although growth and progression of these secondary osteons are critical for final union, the growth typically results in a transitory reduction of cortical bone density because of increased porosity.[16]

As highlighted, fracture healing can follow any number of pathways to the final stage of union. The choice of which path to follow depends on many factors, including the surgeon's expertise and experience. There is certainly not one fixation technique that is superior to all others for all fractures. Many clinical factors, such as the animal's age, prospective use, value, and attitude, and fracture configuration play important roles in the selection of a fixation method. Fortunately, fracture healing appears to have a high level of tolerance and adaptability to even the most adverse conditions.

EVALUATION OF HEALING FOR CLINICAL JUDGMENTS

Determination of effective osseous fracture union can be a diagnostic challenge. Clinical assessment requires comprehensive consideration of numerous factors including initial trauma, healing period length, fracture site pain, palpable callus, lameness, and stability on manual examination. For bones underlying deep tissue, clinical assessment is often qualitative.

Radiographic evaluation is the standard modality by which fracture healing is assessed. Secondary bone healing is the most common mechanism of equine fracture healing, and radiographic changes coincide with the three phases of fracture repair described earlier. Up to a week after the initial trauma, sharp fracture margins are typically visible.[17] Once the locally mediated inflammation of the inflammatory phase is established, necrotic bone is removed by osteoclasts and phagocytes. During this period, approximately 2 to 3 weeks after fracture, the fracture gap appears to widen and its margins become indistinct.

During the ensuing reparative phase, periosteal, endosteal, and intercortical calluses become evident, although they vary in radiographic visibility depending on the degree of mineralization, which in turn depends on local blood supply and tissue oxygenation. Initial callus formation occurs within 5 days after trauma, but bony callus requires adequate mineralization to be radiographically evident. As healing progresses, fracture lines disappear and the external callus increases in opacity relative to adjacent bone. The size and shape of an external callus is significantly influenced by motion at the fracture site, with greater motion resulting in a larger callus. In the remodeling phase, the woven and cancellous bone of the callus transition to lamellar bone. As remodeling progresses, the callus is revised to the original conformation of the bone. Traditionally, bony unions are characterized radiographically by a bony callus, obliteration of the fracture line by bony trabeculae, and cortical bone bridging the fracture gap.[18]

Development of methods to improve evaluation of equine bone healing is an area of ongoing research. Nuclear scintigraphy is one modality that has been used to evaluate equine fracture healing.[19-21] It is advantageous in that it provides a clear assessment of fracture vascularity for prognostic purposes. Both computed tomography and nuclear scintigraphy have been used to detect and assess equine fractures, although computed tomography has not been applied extensively to assess fracture healing.[19,22-25] Dual x-ray absorptiometry (DEXA), magnetic resonance imaging (MRI), and ultrasonography are gaining in popularity for evaluating fracture healing in human and small animal patients, but they are not routinely applied to the horse.[26-28] Methods for enhancement of traditional radiography to assess the degree of equine fracture healing will most likely become more common with development of equine-specific equipment and methodology.

COMPLICATIONS

Complications of equine fracture healing include infection, fixation failure, delay or failure of bony union, and stress-induced laminitis. These are broad generalizations that represent some common problems associated with fracture repair. Each fracture and patient is unique and subject to individual variation and associated complications. Complications should be specifically addressed as they arise.

Perioperative antibiotic administration and improved surgical techniques and equipment have significantly reduced the incidence of nosocomial equine orthopedic infections, but severe soft tissue damage often associated with the initial injury can result in exposed bone and severe contamination. In spite of appropriate surgical débridement and antibiotic administration, compromised blood supply, swelling, edema, and necrotic tissues provide an ideal environment for bacterial proliferation. Local infection can easily proceed through the cortex, marrow, and articulations of bones involved. Treatment of osteomyelitis after fracture stabilization requires individualized assessment and therapy. Additional information on bone infections can be found in Chapter 88.

Many factors are associated with delay or failure of fracture union, including, but not limited to, infection, inadequate reduction, inadequate immobilization, and soft tissue disruption. *Delayed union* refers to the situation in which healing is not complete within an adequate time interval for fracture union. Healing progresses, but at a slower rate than normal. Typically, long bone fractures are expected to heal within approximately 4 months in adult horses and 3 months in foals. *Nonunion* occurs when fracture repair ceases prior to restoration of the bony structure. Three types of nonunion have been identified—vascular, avascular, and infected nonunions. Treatment depends on the specific condition present.

Stress-induced laminitis is a compounding factor in many fracture repairs. The basic cause of the condition is related to continued severe lameness after fracture fixation. The primary goal of any form of fracture stabilization is return to comfortable weightbearing on the affected limb as quickly as possible. In spite of appropriate, stable reduction and analgesic administration, continued pain in some fractured limbs results in increased weightbearing on the contralateral limb. Stress-induced laminitis generally does not have a metabolic component. It can result in rotation and even sinking of the distal phalanx as the germinal layers separate from the horny tissues in the hoof.

Fixation failure, either of external coaptation or of the surgical implant, can occur in the horse for any number of reasons, not the least of which are the forces inherent to the equine limb. External coaptation is not used routinely for fracture stabilization but usually for protection of surgical reduction and stabilization in the postoperative period. Transfixation casts are used on occasion. Cast complications, pin breakage, fracture through pin holes, and pin-track infections are problems associated with such stabilization. Surgical implant complications are often associated with the strength of the fixation construct relative to the mechanical demands placed on it. Catastrophic fracture construct failure may occur when it is exposed to forces that exceed the implant strength, such as during recovery, or when the rate of bone healing is slower than the implant fatigue life. Implant loosening as a result of localized implant or bony failure can result in an unstable fracture and delayed healing. Although no amount of caution can prevent all fixation-associated problems, appropriate preoperative planning, fracture stabilization, and postoperative care improve chances of success considerably.

DISTRACTION OSTEOGENESIS

Distraction osteogenesis is the formation of new bone by controlled separation of stabilized bone ends on each side of a corticotomy or osteotomy.[29,30] To achieve bone formation, there must be adequate fixator stability, adequate periosteal and medullary blood supply, minimal soft tissue disruption, and physiologic use of the bone.[31,32] Bone formation also depends on the appropriate distraction rate and rhythm, the length of distraction, and the number of distraction increments every 24 hours. New bone, referred to as regenerate bone, forms according to a general principle called the tension-stress effect.[33] Specifically, early callus tissue subjected to slow steady traction is metabolically stimulated to differentiate and proliferate in the distraction gap.

The process of distraction osteogenesis is divided into three periods—latency, activation, and consolidation.[29,30] The *latency period* is the time between bone transection and the initiation of distraction, which is postulated to enhance cellular and vascular responses and improve osteogenesis. The *activation period* is characterized by bony in-growth as distraction is applied. Within 3 to 7 days after bone transection, osteoblast or osteoclast progenitor cells on the bone surface differentiate according to the mechanical and biologic environment and begin to proliferate. Osteoid is laid down in parallel columns extending centrally from each bone surface.[33] Lamellar bone typically develops within the columns, but fibrous tissue formation may occur if the fracture site is sufficiently unstable. The distraction device remains in place to serve as rigid skeletal fixation until maturation of new bone is achieved during the *consolidation period*. Metaphyseal cancellous bone does not heal the same way cortical bone does, because trabecular bone is inherently more stable.[34] Periosteal callus formation does not occur unless there is significant instability. Instead, osteoblasts deposit new bone on trabeculae, and the fracture gap fills with woven bone, bridging the trabeculae prior to cortical union. As with any fracture, individualized distraction osteogenesis must be based on patient age and health, the bone involved, the osteotomy type and location, and the degree of soft tissue trauma.

Distraction osteogenesis has limited potential for equine application. Circular external fixator strength is usually inadequate for stabilization of equine long bones, with the possible exception of small foals. Successful correction of a deviated nasal septum and premaxilla in a yearling filly bas been accomplished with distraction osteogenesis, and distraction osteogenesis may be useful for mandibular elongation to treat equine brachygnathism in both juvenile and adult patients.[35,36] With careful case selection and appropriate external or internal fixator construction, it is possible that distraction osteogenesis may be a useful treatment in certain equine patients.

STIMULATION OF BONE HEALING

Enhancement of fracture healing for rapid restoration of skeletal function could greatly benefit the equine patient. Both biologic and mechanical methods to accelerate the process of bone repair have been evaluated in the horse. Local biologic methods for enhancement of fracture healing most frequently include the use of autogenous cancellous and cortical bone grafts, though both autogenous and allogeneic demineralized bone matrix and allogeneic bone have also been used to facilitate bone repair.[21,37,38] Grafts have varying capacities to provide cells for active bone formation (osteogenesis), to induce bone formation by host cells (osteoinduction), and to provide a substrate for bone formation (osteoconduction). Successful graft incorporation requires an appropriate match between the biologic graft activity, the surrounding host tissues, and the mechanical environment (see Chapter 82).

A number of growth-promoting substances involved in regulation of fracture repair have been identified. They are generally categorized into two groups: growth factors and immunomodulatory cytokines. These substances have been investigated for promotion of equine articular cartilage repair, but to date, augmentation of equine fracture repair by exogenous administration of growth-promoting substances is not well investigated (see Chapter 79).[39,40]

One of the most highly investigated mechanical techniques to stimulate fracture healing in the horse is the application of electric and electromagnetic fields.[41-45] The premise for such treatment is based on Wolff's law: living bone adapts its structure in response to mechanical stress by producing electric potentials that optimize bone growth. There is a large body of evidence that metabolic activity and mechanical deformation in living bone generate steady direct current and time-varying electric fields, respectively.[46] Numerous basic research and clinical investigations surrounding stimulation of bone repair with energy application have been conducted across species. There are anecdotal reports of treatment success in the horse, but clinical efficacy has yet to be clearly established.[41,47]

REFERENCES

1. Hayes WC, Carter DR: Biomechanics of bone. In Simmons DJ, Kunin AS, editors: Skeletal Research: An Experimental Approach, New York, 1979, Academic Press.
2. Markel MD: Fracture biology and mechanics. In Auer JA, editor: Textbook of Equine Surgery, Philadelphia, 1992, WB Saunders.
3. Nordin M, Frankel VH: Biomechanics of bone. In Nordin M, Frankel VH, editors: Basic Biomechanics of the Musculoskeletal System, Philadelphia, 1989, Lea & Febiger.
4. Arnoczky SP, Wilson JW: The connective tissues. In Whittick WG, editor: Canine Orthopedics, Philadelphia, 1990, Lea & Febiger.
5. Boskey AL: Connective tissues of the musculoskeletal system. In Slatter DH, editor: Textbook of Small Animal Surgery, Philadelphia, 1985, WB Saunders.
6. Fetter AW: Structure and function of bone. In Newton CD, Nunamaker DM, editors: Textbook of Small Animal Orthopaedics, Philadelphia, 1985, JB Lippincott.
7. Marks SC: The origin of osteoclasts: Evidence, clinical implications and investigative challenges of an extra-skeletal source, J Oral Pathol 1983;12:226-256.
8. Simmons DJ, Kent GN, Jilka RL, et al: Formation of bone by isolated, cultured osteoblasts in Millipore diffusion chambers, Calcif Tissue Int 1982;34:291-294.
9. Behrens F, Johnson WD, Koch TW, Kovacevic N: Bending stiffness of unilateral and bilateral fixator frames, Clin Orthop 1983;178:103-110.
10. Schenk RK: Histophysiology of bone remodeling and bone repair. In Lin OCC, Chao EYS, editors: Perspectives on Biomaterials, Amsterdam, 1986, Elsevier Science.
11. Sevitt S: Healing of fractures in man. In Owen R, Goodfellow J, Bullough P, editors: Scientific Foundation of Orthopedics and Traumatology, Philadelphia, 1980, WB Saunders.
12. Cruess RL, Dumont J: Fracture healing, Can J Surg 1975;18:403-413.
13. Hunt TK: Can repair process be stimulated by modulators (cell growth factors, antigenetic factors, etc.) without adversely affecting normal processes? J Trauma 1984;24:S39-S49.
14. Ham AW: A histological study of the early phases of bone repair, J Bone Joint Surg 1930;12:827-844.
15. Schenk R, Willenegger H: Zum histologischen Bild der Sogenannten Primarheilung der Knochenkompakta nach experimentellen Osteotomien am Hund, Experientia 1963;19:593.
16. Aro H, Kelly PJ, Lewallen DG, Chao EYS: Comparison of the effects of dynamization and constant rigid fixation on rate and quality of bone osteotomy union in external fixation, Transactions 34th Annual Meeting of Orthopaedic Research Society, Atlanta, 1988:303.
17. Sande R: Radiography of orthopedic trauma and fracture repair, Vet Clin North Am Small Anim Pract 1999;29:1247-1260.
18. Panjabi MM, Walter SD, Karuda M, et al: Correlations of radiographic analysis of healing fractures with strength: A statistical analysis of experimental osteotomies, J Orthop Res 1985;3:212-218.
19. Markel MD, Snyder JR, Hornof WJ, et al: Nuclear scintigraphic evaluation of third metacarpal and metatarsal bone fractures in three horses, J Am Vet Med Assoc 1987;191:75-77.
20. Devous MD Sr, Twardock AR: Techniques and applications of nuclear medicine in the diagnosis of equine lameness, J Am Vet Med Assoc 1984;184:318-325.
21. Kawcak CE, Trotter GW, Powers BE, et al: Comparison of bone

healing by demineralized bone matrix and autogenous cancellous bone in horses, Vet Surg 2000;29:218-226.
22. Barnes HG, Tucker RL, Grant BD, et al: Lag screw stabilization of a cervical vertebral fracture by use of computed tomography in a horse, J Am Vet Med Assoc 1995;206:221-223.
23. Martens P, Ihler CF, Rennesund J: Detection of a radiographically occult fracture of the lateral palmar process of the distal phalanx in a horse using computed tomography, Vet Radiol Ultrasound 1999;40:346-349.
24. Rose PL, Seeherman H, O'Callaghan M: Computed tomographic evaluation of comminuted middle phalangeal fractures in the horse, Vet Radiol Ultrasound 1997;38:424-429.
25. Ruggles AJ, Moore RM, Bertone AL, et al: Tibial stress fractures in racing Standardbreds: 13 cases (1989-1993), J Am Vet Med Assoc 1996;209:634-637.
26. Moed BR, Kim EC, van Holsbeeck M, et al: Ultrasound for the early diagnosis of tibial fracture healing after static interlocked nailing without reaming: Histologic correlation using a canine model, J Orthop Trauma 1998;12:200-205.
27. Njeh CF, Kearton JR, Hans D, et al: The use of quantitative ultrasound to monitor fracture healing: A feasibility study using phantoms, Med Eng Phys 1998;20:781-786.
28. Markel MD, Chao EY: Noninvasive monitoring techniques for quantitative description of callus mineral content and mechanical properties, Clin Orthop 1993;293:37-45.
29. Shaw WC, Mandall NA, Mattick CR: Ethical and scientific decision making in distraction osteogenesis, Cleft Palate Craniofac J 2002;39:641-645.
30. Stallings JT, Lewis DD, Welch RD, et al: An introduction to distraction osteogenesis and the principles of the Ilizarov method, Vet Comp Orthop Traumatol 1998;11:59-67.
31. Ilizarov GA: The tension-stress effect on the genesis and growth of tissues: Part II. The influence of the rate and frequency of distraction, Clin Orthop 1989;239:263-285.
32. Ilizarov GA: The tension-stress effect on the genesis and growth of tissues: Part I. The influence of stability of fixation and soft-tissue preservation, Clin Orthop 1989;238:249-281.
33. Delloye C, Delefortrie G, Coutelier L, et al: Bone regenerate formation in cortical bone during distraction lengthening: An experimental study, Clin Orthop 1990;250:34-42.
34. Aronson J, Shen X: Experimental healing of distraction osteogenesis comparing metaphyseal with diaphyseal sites, Clin Orthop 1994;301:25-30.
35. Puchol JL, Herran R, Durall I, et al: Use of distraction osteogenesis for the correction of deviated nasal septum and premaxilla in a horse, J Am Vet Med Assoc 2004;224:1147-1150.
36. Gaughan EM, DeBowes RM: Congenital diseases of the equine head, Vet Clin North Am Equine Pract 1993;9:93-110.
37. Fackelman GE, von Rechenberg B, Fetter AW: Decalcified bone grafts in the horse, Am J Vet Res 1981;42:943-948.
38. Jones RD, Milne DW, Fetter AW: Cortical bone allografting in the horse, Vet Surg 1981;10:1-11.
39. Nixon AJ, Brower-Toland BD, Bent SJ, et al: Insulinlike growth factor-I gene therapy applications for cartilage repair, Clin Orthop 2000;379(Suppl):S201-S213.
40. Hidaka C, Goodrich LR, Chen CT, et al: Acceleration of cartilage repair by genetically modified chondrocytes over expressing bone morphogenetic protein-7, J Orthop Res 2003;21:573-583.
41. Auer JA, Burch GE, Hall P: Review of pulsing electromagnetic field therapy and its possible application to horses, Equine Vet J 1983;15:354-360.
42. Collier MA, Rendano VT, Kallfelz FA: Repair of a delayed-union stress fracture of the dorsal cortex of a metacarpal bone in a horse, J Am Vet Med Assoc 1985;187:1040-1043.
43. Collier MA, Brighton CT, Norrdin R, et al: Direct current stimulation of bone production in the horse: Preliminary study with a "gap healing" model. Am J Vet Res 1985;46:610-621.
44. Collier MA, Brighton CT, Rendano VT, et al: Direct current stimulation of bone production in the pony: Observations with a diaphyseal osteotomy model, Am J Vet Res 1985;46:600-609.
45. Sanders-Shamis M, Gabel AA: Surgical reconstruction of a ruptured medial collateral ligament in a foal, J Am Vet Med Assoc 1988;193:80-82.
46. Otter MW, McLeod KJ, Rubin CT: Effects of electromagnetic fields in experimental fracture repair, Clin Orthop 1998;355(Suppl):S90-104.
47. Sanders-Shamis M, Bramlage LR, Weisbrode SE, et al: A preliminary investigation of the effect of selected electromagnetic field devices on healing of cannon bone osteotomies in horses, Equine Vet J 1989;21:201-205.

CHAPTER 81

Principles of Fracture Treatment

Jörg A. Auer

Fractures are diagnosed in practically every bone of the horse and encountered at all ages. Fractures vary in clinical presentation and significance, ranging from exercise-induced fractures causing only relatively minor lameness, such as chip fractures of the carpus, to fractures causing a nonweightbearing lameness, such as a transverse failure of the third metacarpal bone (MCIII). The management of intra-articular chip fractures and osteochondrosis lesions will be discussed in Chapters 84 and 91, respectively. In this chapter, the principles of fracture treatment, nonsurgical and surgical, are presented.

Fracture treatment in the horse follows the same basic guidelines developed for humans[1] and small animals.[2] Many techniques can be derived from them, but some principles in the treatment of equine long bone fractures are unique.[3,4] These differences are discussed in detail, with emphasis given to surgical fracture treatment, including internal fixation and external coaptation.

NONSURGICAL MANAGEMENT

Some fractures heal sufficiently with nonsurgical management to allow the animal to return to an athletic career. Nonsurgical management techniques include stall rest and external coaptation.

Stall Rest

Frequently, horses are admitted in a "fracture-lame" state without a visible or palpable fracture. According to the anamnesis, these patients were found on pasture with the non-weightbearing lameness, or they did not return to the stable in the evening with the other horses. The physical examination may reveal a small wound over a vestigial metacarpal or metatarsal bone, the radius, or the tibia. In the case of splint bone fracture, radiography may reveal a fracture or even multiple fractures. In selected cases, these fractures are amenable to nonsurgical management with a bandage alone. Additional information on the treatment of these fractures is found in Chapter 95.

Other fractures amenable to management by stall rest include fractures of the deltoid tubercle, nonarticular patellar fractures, and fractures of the scapular spine. However, for the vast majority of fractures, nonsurgical management is not the treatment of choice and should not be advocated.

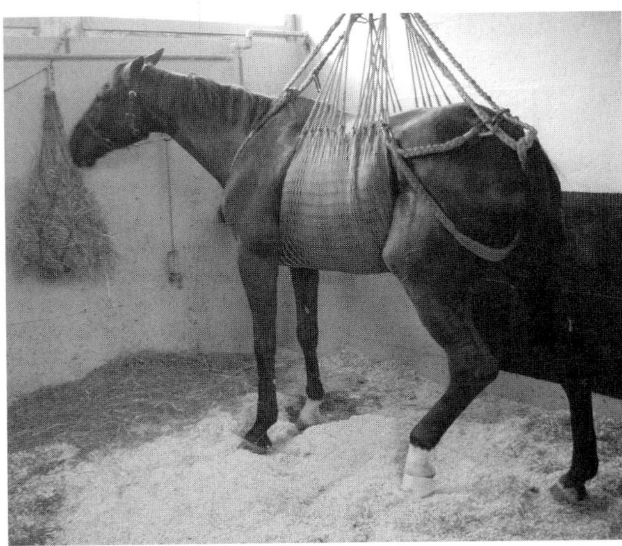

Figure 81-1. An adult horse suffering from a fissure fracture of the tibia, supported by a rescue net. The net, which is applied relatively snugly to allow the horse to apply some weight to it, is tolerated very well.

External Coaptation

For a detailed description of the indications and applications of external coaptation devices, such as fiberglass casts and splints, please review Chapter 18. In this chapter, external coaptation is discussed as it pertains to fracture treatment.

Splints

The indications for limb splints as a sole means of fracture treatment are limited. More commonly, they are used as a form of emergency fixation (see Chapter 78). This type of external coaptation may be employed in fissure fractures of the diaphysis of the radius and tibia, or as adjunct treatment to internal fixation of a fracture, either during the immediate postoperative period or as an intermediary step after removal of a cast.

In acute fissure fractures of the radius and tibia, radiography may not show a fracture. Affected animals are usually reluctant to bear any weight on the limb. Initial management should include not only the application of a splint bandage but prevention of the animal from lying down. It is frequently during the process of lying down or getting up that these fissure fractures evolve into complete fractures. Tying the horse with a short rope and providing a filled hay net to allow them to eat is an effective management method. Nonsteroidal anti-inflammatory agents are indicated to provide some comfort. However, the dosages should not be so high that they abolish the lameness completely. A complementary or independent management option involves the application of sling or rescue net (Fig. 81-1). Usually, the animals tolerate these slings very well. They allow the patient to rest their intact limbs for some time by lowering their abdomen into the sling. It is important that the sling be installed such that the body has to be lowered only a few centimeters to allow it to rest in the sling. If the body has to be lowered too much, complete fractures of the bone may still occur.

If initially no fracture can be found on radiography, additional images should be taken a few days later. Usually, at this point, fractures may be seen radiographically (Fig. 81-2). Depending on the configuration of the fissure fracture and the width of the fracture gap, the management may be modified. When the fissure lines are small with a barely visible gap, no bandages are needed, but the animal is maintained in the sling for 2 to 3 weeks. If the fracture line is long and associated with a significant gap, the splint bandage should be maintained.

Splint bandages should be changed every 3 to 4 days, and in hot and humid climates they should be changed more frequently. Caution should be used during the process because weightbearing on the limb without the splint or bandage could have deleterious effects on fracture healing.

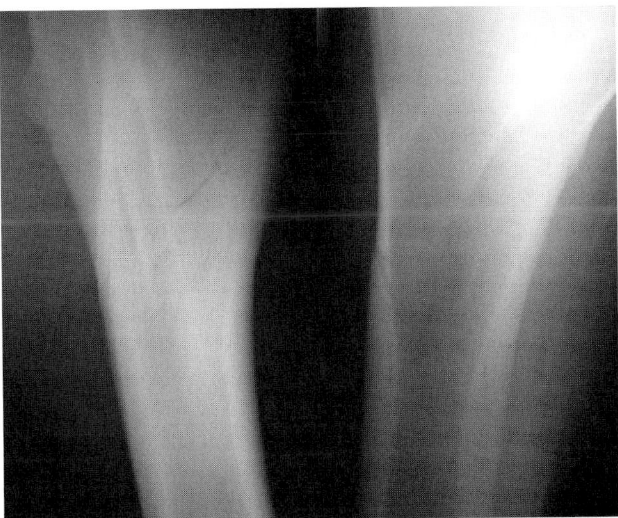

Figure 81-2. Craniocaudal and lateromedial radiographic views of a fissure fracture in the proximal metaphysis of the tibia of an adult horse.

Casts

External coaptation using fiberglass cast material as the primary treatment technique of a fracture may initially be considered as a conservative, less expensive type of treatment. However, the frequent cast changes usually necessitated by soft tissue problems must usually be carried out under general anesthesia. The costs of several anesthetic events, cast materials, and professional fees add up rapidly and may soon exceed the costs of a state-of-the-art internal fixation performed on admission. Additionally, the advantages of early return to function, achieved through internal fixation, are lost. Cast materials selected for fracture treatment should be of the fiberglass type, because this material allows the skin and the limb underneath the cast to breathe. Also, it is lighter in weight, so the animal is more comfortable.

Casts should be palpated daily and evaluated for hot areas. Any odor from the cast should be investigated, and weightbearing on the limb should be evaluated. Sudden changes in weightbearing patterns, edema above the proximal cast end, and a foul odor or wet spots on the cast are signals of skin damage and possible necrosis underneath the cast. The same is true when hot areas develop in the fetlock region or at the dorsal aspect of the cast in the region of the proximal MCIII or third metatarsus (MTIII). All of these signs signal the need for cast removal.

The first cast should be changed after a few days, because during this the time initial swelling has subsided, resulting in a loose cast that is ineffective in stabilizing the initial fracture and may even cause some additional damage to the soft tissues. Casts applied to foals should be changed at 10- to 14-day intervals and eliminated as soon as possible. In adult animals, longer intervals are tolerated. If the condition of the skin beneath the cast and the weightbearing patterns permit, up to 5 or 6 weeks may be allowed before the cast is changed. Longer intervals reduce costs and, in most cases, are followed by better results. Some horses have thinner and more sensitive skin, therefore are more subject to skin trauma, and hence require shorter intervals between cast changes.

Complications

Nonsurgical management of fractures is associated with various complications (see Chapter 18). When internal fixation is not applied, the fracture fragments are not stable. The resulting callus formation often impinges on soft tissue structures or tendons and may prevent future athletic use. However, bone remodeling after fracture healing may reduce such a callus, eliminating impingement on the soft tissue structures.

Skin trauma from casts and splints can be severe enough to endanger the outcome of fracture healing. It is important that the skin remain dry and healthy. Development of cast sores should be monitored. If they do develop, casts must be changed frequently and padded so that the pressure on the skin is redistributed.

If infection develops underneath the cast, swelling causes increased pressure within the tissues. Because the skin cannot expand beyond the inner limitations of the cast, a compartment syndrome develops, resulting in tissue necrosis. Additionally, drainage from the limb accumulates within the cast, and the skin will be damaged by enzymes. Hosing down the cast with copious amounts of water on a daily basis prolongs its usefulness and postpones a change, but an infected limb should be maintained under a cast only if no alternative exists.

During the time that the limb is maintained in the cast, the joints are unable to move and the articular cartilage is poorly nourished. This results in loss of proteoglycans and subsequent degeneration of the cartilage. Additionally, the soft tissue structures surrounding the joint are not flexed and stretched, which causes them to become weak and inelastic. When prolonged external coaptation is used, these pathologic changes are exacerbated and are referred to as "cast disease."

If a foot is maintained under a cast while a fracture in the limb is allowed to heal, it is prevented from expanding during weightbearing and the structures underneath the hoof wall constrict. After the cast is removed and the limb is loaded once again, the foot expands, which causes pain for several days.

Flexing of the joints after a prolonged fixation in one position causes pain and an initial unwillingness to bear weight. This, however, is overcome after a few days in most cases and can be facilitated with anti-inflammatory drugs.

SURGICAL MANAGEMENT

Equine bone reacts to trauma and fracture with active new bone formation and subsequent remodeling. Many osteons are mobilized to facilitate remodeling of the cortex. However, fracture healing in the horse occurs at a slower pace than in most other animals, especially ruminants, small animals, and humans.[5] Therefore, any adjunct treatment that benefits bone healing is advantageous.

External Fixation

External fixation using intraosseous or transosseous pins and clamps is common in humans[6] and small animals[7] but less so in the horse. This type of fixation is employed frequently as emergency treatment in open or in severely comminuted fractures when anatomic reduction, reconstruction, and internal fixation of the fracture are not possible. External fixation techniques can be applied using three types of constructs: transfixation-pin casts, an external fixator, or an external skeletal fixation device.

Transfixation-Pin Casting

Nemeth and Back popularized transfixation-pin casting among equine specialists.[8] This efficient and relatively easily applied treatment method is indicated for comminuted fractures of the phalanges, the distal MCIII/MTIII, and breakdown injuries of the metacarpophalangeal joint.[9] A retrospective study involving more than 50 horses and ponies treated by means of transfixation-pin casting showed that comminuted fractures had better results (86% healed) than simple fractures (23% healed).[8] It is assumed that the micromotion between the fragments after fixation was distributed between more fragments in the comminuted fracture and therefore was decreased compared with simple transverse fracture, where distribution was not possible.

Under aseptic conditions two to three cross-pins of 4 to 6 mm in diameter are introduced in the metaphyseal region of the bone. The use of positive-profile pins (IMEX Veterinary Inc, Longview, Tex) is preferred.[9] A 30-degree divergence of the pins in the frontal plane results in a stronger fixation and lower risk for postoperative fracture.[10,11] The pins should be separated by 2 to 4 cm. A stab incision is made down to the bone and, using tissue protection, the predetermined-size hole is prepared. An effective method of heat control is to initially drill a smaller hole, followed by stepwise enlargement through larger drill bits. Production of heat is associated with bone necrosis around the pin and its subsequent loosening.

A pin with a diameter that is 0.1 mm larger than the prepared hole (radial preload of 0.1 mm) provides the best pin holding strength with the least weakening of the bone surrounding the implant.[1] If positive-threaded pins are used, appropriate threads have to be cut in the pre-drilled hole prior to pin insertion. Newer pin generations are equipped with a self-tapping device at the beginning of the threaded part. Care has to be taken to engage the threaded pin portion with both cortices. Protruding portions of the pins are cut off at a length of 3 to 5 cm from the limb, which allows their incorporation into the cast.

After applying a double layer of stockinet, followed by a double layer of resin-impregnated foam padding (3M Corporation, St. Paul, Minn), a 5-mm layer of fiberglass cast is applied as described in Chapter 18. The ends of the pins can be covered by hoof acrylic and incorporated in an additional layer of fiberglass cast tape (Fig. 81-3). An alternative approach involves the application of dowels over the pin ends, fastened with fixation screws on the pins, just adjacent to the layer of casting tape. These dowels are subsequently covered by an additional solid layer of cast material. These two methods prevent migration of the pins after loosening, because they are fixed within the cast. A recent in vitro study revealed that the fixation of the pin within the cast plays a minor role.[12] The fiberglass cast material appears to be the major determinant of axial stability. However, because it was an in vitro study, the long-term effect of such a fixation could not be evaluated. Therefore, an additional fixation device, as described earlier, may still have some merit.

The incorporation of horizontal pins in a U-bar fastened around the distal limb has been advocated.[8] This technique was thought to allow some weightbearing, but this has been disproven.[13] A combination of transfixation-pin casting and strategic lag screw placement across major fracture lines to ensure anatomic reduction of intra-articular fractures may speed up fracture healing.

Centrally threaded, positive-profile transfixation pins have greater resistance to axial extraction in the diaphysis than in the metaphysis of equine MCIII bone in vitro.[14] Again, this observation resulted from an in vitro study and may lead to the conclusion that it is advantageous to introduce the pins into the diaphyseal region of the long bone. However, the author's experience is that diaphyseal pins lead to more complications, which include ring sequestrum formation and subsequent pathologic fractures.

Advantages of transfixation-pin casting include no load on the fracture site and minimal distraction and movement between the fragments. Also, the tissues are spared additional trauma and further disruption of the blood supply. All the disadvantages of external coaptation, such as the development of cast disease, osteoporosis, contracted feet, and tendon laxity, apply to this type of treatment. Pin tract infection with ring sequestrum formation can occur and is preceded by a sudden onset of lameness. This usually occurs in heavy horses (greater than 500 kg of bodyweight) and warrants immediate removal of the proximal transfixation pin. Another pin can be inserted at a different location to prolong unloading of the fracture, or, alternatively, the limb can be placed in a new cast without the proximal-most pin. A new pin can be expected to form a similar sequestrum within the next 2 weeks, and the procedure can be repeated. If three pins are inserted initially, transfixation may be maintained for 6 to 8 weeks, before simple casting is applied. At that time, a full-limb cast is applied to prevent rotation of the MCIII/MTIII. (Rotation can occur in a half-limb cast and may lead to a fracture across a pin tract.)

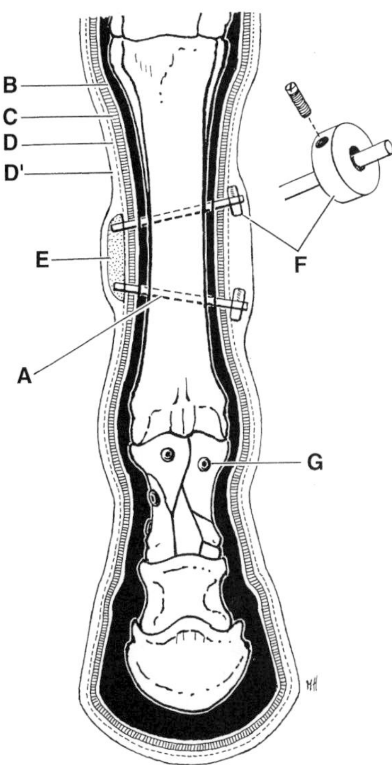

Figure 81-3. Transfixation cast for the treatment of a comminuted fracture of the proximal phalanx, partially managed by strategically placed lag screws. A, obliquely inserted Steinmann pins; B, stockinet; C, custom foam; D, initial, and D', second layer of fiberglass cast; E, hoof acrylic covering the Steinmann pin ends on the left side; F, custom-made dowels with set screw stabilizing the ends of the Steinmann pins on the right side. G, Cortex screws placed in lag fashion to reduce fracture fragments.

External Fixator

Application of an external fixator allows immediate, although subnormal, weightbearing on the limb. The Steinmann pins and Schanz screws used with this fixation device create minimal additional trauma to the injured soft tissue. Because in most cases no external coaptation is used, there is easy access to an open wound, which facilitates débridement and management. Application of an external fixator also allows additional correction and fracture alignment after the initial operation, whereas a fracture treated with internal fixation can be adjusted only through an additional surgery. However, this technique has not been very successful in equine patients.

An external fixator utilizes transversely inserted (cross) Steinmann pins or Schanz screws (Steinmann pins with a threaded end) proximal and distal to the fracture site. These pins are firmly connected to external rods through special clamps, which may be applied in many configurations.[9] An in vitro study showed that the best results are achieved with an elaborate three-dimensional design, including three Steinmann pins proximal and distal to the osteotomy, inserted at different angles in the frontal plane and obliquely from proximal to distal, and connected to four external rods.[15] Such a configuration is expensive and very heavy and therefore not practical.

To improve the bone-holding properties of Schanz screws, a new design has been developed by the AO/ASIF group. It has the features of the ideal pin with a 0.1-mm greater diameter than the hole drilled for it (larger radial preloads result in microfractures and deformation of the bone surrounding the pin, with subsequent loosening[1]). The Seldrill Schanz screw is manufactured of pure titanium and stainless steel and has a self-drilling, self-tapping tip.[16] This implant is inserted through a stab incision without predrilling the bone or pretapping the hole, even in hard equine bone. The Seldrill Schanz screw contains a relatively thick core and thin threads and includes a portion with a built-in radial preload of 0.1 mm, immediately adjacent to the self-drilling, self-tapping tip. Because the sharp tip should not exit the opposite cortex, this implant is to be used in half splints (type I), where the external tube or rod is located only on one side of the bone. Additionally, this device can be used in three-dimensional (type III) configurations, where a half splint is connected to a full, bilateral splint (type II), which uses nonthreaded pins.

A modification of an external fixator, the Pinless external fixator, is available for selected fractures in large animals.[17] This device is manufactured in three sizes and configurations of clamps, which are applied over a bone without completely penetrating the cortex (Fig. 81-4). The clamps are fastened through a connection rod and clamps to an external fixator tube or carbon rod. This device is not rigid enough to support weightbearing of a large animal with a fractured limb, but it is effective in stabilizing mandible fractures in cattle and horses (see Chapter 103) and fractures of the tail in the horse (see Chapter 53). In vivo studies show that the clamping force is maintained over several weeks while inducing only minor bony changes where the clamps contact the bone.[18] Animals tolerate the device well. The advantage of this type of external fixator is the minimal damage to bone and tooth roots.

External Skeletal Fixation Device

The external skeletal fixation device (ESFD) was developed for horses with severely comminuted fractures of the phalanges, fractures of the distal MCIII/MTIII, and "breakdown injuries" of the metacarpophalangeal joint: The ESFD uses two to three transfixation pins in the intact bone proximal to the fracture, and sidebars and a base plate. Weightbearing forces are transmitted via the pins and sidebars around the fracture to the ground, allowing the animal to immediately bear full weight without loading the fracture.[19-21] The original report described the device and 15 cases, only four of which survived long term.[19] Through a meticulous study of the design, an effective ESFD transfixation system has been developed and is commercially available.[18] Early complications included fractures through the pin tract while the device was worn, or during recovery after implant removal. These complications were almost completely abolished with the latest generation ESFD.[21] Removal of the device on the sedated, standing animal eliminates some problems

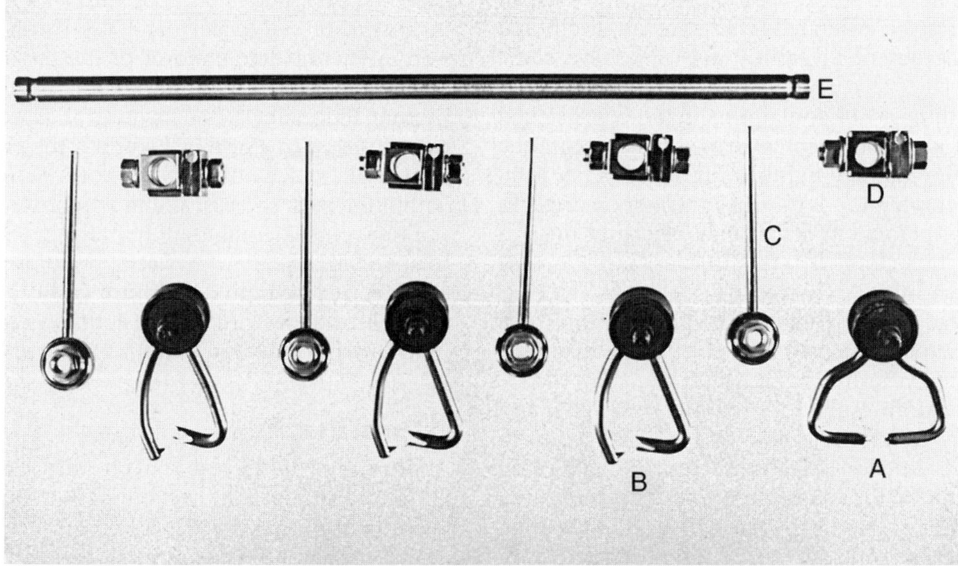

Figure 81-4. One symmetric (A) and three asymmetric (B) titanium Pinless fixator clamps are shown with connecting rods (C), clamps (D), and longitudinal rod (E). This configuration is used for treatment of mandibular fractures.

encountered after device removal, but the risk of fracture while wearing the device continues.[21]

Up to 90% of the stresses generated at the bone–pin interface contribute directly to pin bending, resulting in uneven stress distribution, with peak stresses concentrated at the outer bone cortex.[22] The new design has been modified to minimize transcortical pin bending with weightbearing. It enhances overall fixation stiffness and minimizes complications at the bone–pin interface. Large-diameter, tapered sleeves are applied over the transfixation pins (biaxially loaded in tension and shear) and are incorporated in a stronger, lighter frame[23] (Fig. 81-5). In vitro tests applying cyclic loading show that significant increases in stiffness, reduced bending, and increases in load-to-failure-of-bone could been achieved with the new sleeved-pin design.[23] Since bone failure occurs at a finite strain level, it appeared that the larger loads to failure were indicative of lower strains in the bone at the working stress level.

Aftercare

Application of an external fixator or ESFD allows easy wound management of open fractures. Débridement should be performed under aseptic conditions, and every measure must be taken to prevent additional contamination. Broad-spectrum antibiotic coverage is indicated in any horse treated with external fixation during the entire time the device is in place. The skin around the cross pins should be cleaned daily with alcohol-soaked swabs and dried before reapplication of the bandage. Internal fixation of the fracture may be considered once the infection has subsided and healthy granulation tissue has formed. At that time, the external fixation device is removed.

Any sudden changes in weightbearing patterns are indications for close scrutiny of the fracture and the fixation device. Radiographs should be taken at the onset of any complication and repeated in routine fashion at 2- to 4-week intervals without complications. Once fracture healing has occurred, the device is removed. The abrupt change in stability caused by removal of the external fixator can be minimized through partial destabilization of the device. This is best achieved by moving the vertical connecting bars farther away from the limb. An alternative approach involves the strategic removal of one or two pins at 2- to 3-week intervals. After a few weeks in this configuration, the device is removed.

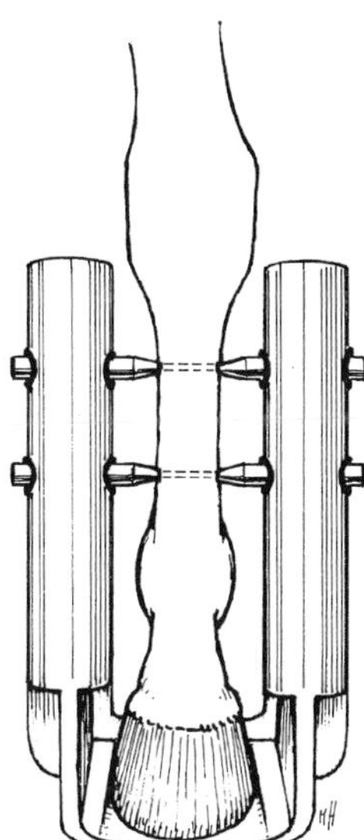

Figure 81-5. Graphic representation of the state-of-the-art design of the external skeletal fixation device developed by Nunamaker and coworkers.[19] Two tapered transosseous pins are incorporated into the U-shaped apparatus, providing additional stability.

Complications

Loosening of the pins, infected pin tracts, and fracture through a pin hole are the main complications of external fixation in horses.[13] Loosening of cross pins is the most frequent complication of external fixation.[7,24] Weightbearing on the affected limb causes osteolysis around the pins, followed by infection of the pin tract and subsequent loosening.[24] Once a pin loosens, pain develops. A loose pin should be removed immediately, because it no longer serves a useful function, and infection around it will not subside as long as the pin remains in situ. Curetting and flushing of the tract facilitates cessation of draining within a few days. If drainage persists, the skin should be reopened, followed by an additional curettage of the pin tract. Removal of a loose pin destabilizes the fixation. Depending on the degree of fracture healing, it is important that pins be removed one at a time. Premature removal of the implants results in total instability.

Removal of a loose transfixation pin is performed on the standing, sedated horse. If external coaptation was used, cast material immediately adjacent to the pin is removed and the pin pulled out. The tract is flushed and the hole filled with a surgical sponge soaked in an antiseptic solution and fixed in place with tape. If the pin is fixed within the cast through a dowel or a hoof acrylic pad (see Fig. 81-3), a complete cast change under general anesthesia is necessary.

Osteomyelitis may develop as an extension of pin tract infection or at the open ends of the fracture. Treatment of orthopedic infections is discussed in Chapter 88. When osteomyelitis is rampant and uncontrollable, euthanasia may be the only alternative.

Soft tissue swelling occurs frequently in animals wearing an external fixator. This is a normal reaction to the implants, local insult, trauma, and controlled infection. Therefore, adequate distance between the skin and the vertical bars and clamps has to be allowed to accommodate the swelling. This will prevent skin necrosis near contact areas of the clamps.

Pathologic fracture is a common problem encountered in horses treated with the external skeletal fixation device[19] or external fixator.[25,26] Frequently, a doughnut-shaped cylinder of bone is walled off around the pin (Fig. 81-6). This creates a relatively large defect in the bone and significantly reduces its strength. The bone within the fixator becomes weakened by osteoporosis (disuse atrophy depending on the duration of fixation), and weightbearing on the limb can result in failure through one of the pin tracts (see Fig. 81-6). If the animal is not euthanized at once after failure, the fracture must be treated immediately by either internal fixation or a full-limb cast. Changing the design of the Steinmann pins as well as the threads may limit the recurrence of this complication.[23]

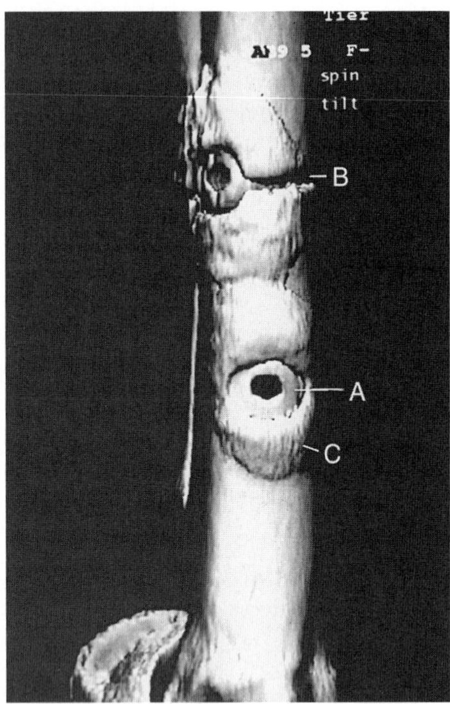

Figure 81-6. Three-dimensional reconstruction of a computed tomographic study of MCIII showing ring sequestra (A) as a result of transfixation pinning and a pathologic fracture (B) through the proximal pin tract or ring sequestrum. Periosteal new bone formation (C) surrounds the ring sequestra.

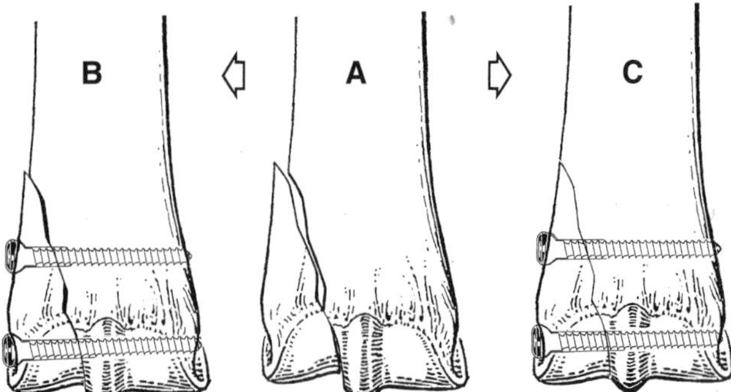

Figure 81-7. A, A displaced articular fracture of the lateral condyle of distal MCIII. **B,** Inadequate reduction was achieved after interfragmentary compression via two cortex screws applied in lag technique. The articular surface is not congruent, which would lead to osteoarthritis. **C,** Adequate anatomic reduction was achieved prior to screw fixation reestablishing the articular surface and normal bone-to-bone contact.

Internal Fixation

At the turn of the 20th century, compression in rigid fixation was recognized as an important component of rapid fracture healing. Rigid internal fixation became an important step in reaching the goal of early return to full function for the fractured limb and the patient.[27,28] The devastating effects of prolonged external coaptation—"cast disease"—were avoided when this goal was attained. Early return to function allows movement of the joints, associated nourishment of the articular cartilage, and prevention of proteoglycan loss. Additionally, disuse osteoporosis is avoided, and the soft tissues surrounding the fractured bone are maintained in physiologic condition. Early return to function is achieved through anatomic reduction of the fracture and stable internal fixation.[1]

Internal fixation is achieved through opening of the skin. This may occur through a stab incision, as with intramedullary pinning, transcutaneous interlocking, and minimally invasive plating techniques, or through opening the skin over a greater distance, followed by separation of the soft tissues surrounding the fractured bones when bone plates are applied.

Principles

Fracture fragments fixed to each other under compression heal without callus formation.[5] Precise anatomic reduction of the fracture is of paramount importance for this type of bone healing (primary union). It is also critical when the articular surface is involved, because if the reconstruction is not nearly perfect, osteoarthritis will develop (Fig. 81-7).

In the last 50 years, tremendous progress has been made in the art of equine fracture treatment. The greatest influence on this achievement can be ascribed to the AO/ASIF group. Founded in 1958 by four Swiss surgeons, the AO (Arbeitsgesellschaft für Osteosynthesefragen) quickly developed into a worldwide organization.[1] In 1984, the AO Foundation was established, to which all the rights for royalty income were bestowed. Recently, the three manufacturers that supplied surgeons with a large variety of sophisticated, high quality implants (Mathys AG, Bettlach, Switzerland; Stratec Medical, Oberdorf, Switzerland [formerly Institut Strauman, Waldenburg]; and Synthes USA, Paoli, Pa) have merged to form a worldwide single company, Synthes Inc., with its headquarters in Solothurn, Switzerland. For every implant sold, Synthes Inc. pays a certain amount to the AO Foundation to support teaching and the development of new instruments—a genuine approach to the improvement of fracture fixation. Techniques developed for human patients were quickly adopted by veterinarians, and many are applied in daily practice with good success.[1-3]

The implants, their function, and their application as discussed in this chapter are mainly those developed by the AO group. Included are screws, plates, pins, wires, and specially designed plates and nails. Only the instruments and implants used in equine fracture treatment will be discussed.

Approach to and Manipulation of Bone

Before surgically approaching the bone, a careful radiographic study should be conducted that includes multiple views from a variety of angles. Along with standard radiography, computed tomographic scans may aid in the selection of the locations where implants are applied and the direction of their insertion. Potential interference of interfragmentary screws and plates with soft tissue structures must be considered. In articular fractures, reconstruction of the joint should be the deciding factor in the decision of how to approach the fracture and apply the implants. For some fractures, surgery should not be attempted—for example, a comminuted fracture of the radius with substantial defects in the caudal cortex has no chance to heal because continuous cycling of the implants eventually leads to implant failure. It is prudent to conduct a detailed discussion with the owners of equine patients about the chances for a successful surgical outcome, the potential complications, and the costs of the particular fracture repair prior to surgery. Availability of all implants and instruments needed at the time of surgery is an absolute prerequisite for a successful result. The approach to the bone should be carried out rapidly carefully and with respect for Halsted's principles of good surgical technique. Special attention should be paid to the blood supply, with severance of major blood vessels avoided. The periosteum should be maintained with the underlying bone whenever possible. Periosteum is stripped off the bone only immediately under implants such as plates. Recently developed plates such as the limited contact dynamic compression plate (LC-DCP), the PC-Fix, and the locking compression plate (LCP) are applied over the periosteum (see later). Massive dissection should be avoided, because it facilitates the accumulation of blood and serum. Planning the approach relative to the application of selected implants is of great importance for a successful outcome of the surgery. For example, the approach to the MCIII is made through longitudinal splitting of the common or lateral digital extensor tendon, which facilitates secure closure of the soft tissues and skin over the implants after the fracture is repaired.[29,30]

In human and small animal osteosynthesis, biological fracture fixation has become very popular.[31] This technique abandons the dogma of anatomic reconstruction and accepts that proper axial and rotational alignment of the bone, despite incomplete reconstruction, followed by fixation of the fracture with strategically placed implants is preferred. Longer plates are used, providing better leverage conditions. Screws are inserted through the holes that are most important biomechanically, but not all holes in a plate are filled with screws. If possible, the plate is pre-bent (to conform to the shape of the contralateral intact bone), slid along the fractured bone through a small incision, and fixed with screws implanted through stab incisions. Such minimal fixation cannot be used successfully in horses. However, the principle of applying the implant by a minimally invasive technique is applicable to the horse, even if the implant has to be modified to meet the demands placed by the horse's size.

Instruments

Basic instruments used for fracture treatment include a variable-speed air or electric drill with forward and reverse gears. To facilitate mechanical preparation of the threads in the bone, switching between forward and reverse should be easy. Drill bits and guides of different types and sizes are needed (Table 81-1). Drill guides allow application of concentric pressure, they stabilize the drill bit, and, in doing so, they prevent breakage. They protect tissues around the hole from frictional trauma generated by the drill bit and the tap. It has been shown that drilling at maximal speed (about 90 psi of air pressure) results in less heat production than drilling at low speeds.[3] The drill bits should be sharp and should be exchanged frequently, because dull drill bits create heat in the hard and dense equine bone. This is especially true in adult animals. Continuous application of saline solution throughout the drilling procedure is important to reduce heat production.[3] The drill bits are designed to allow penetration of the fluid along their outside perimeter, which facilitates lubrication and reduction of friction. However, not enough water can be flushed into the drill hole to effectively cool the drill bit. Frequent cleansing of the drill bit to remove the swath material is the single most important factor in reducing heat production. During drilling, axial pressure is applied to the drill bit without bending it. Bending causes the drill bit to become dull too rapidly because of interference with the drill guide. More importantly, the hole will be of a larger diameter than intended. Adequate but not excessive pressure should be applied. The instruments used for screw insertion are discussed in the paragraphs about the lag technique, later. Other instruments such as various drill guides, special reduction forceps, bone clamps, rongeurs, curets, osteotomes, and a mallet (for more information, see Chapter 12) aid in bone handling as well as in maintaining compression during fracture reduction and the insertion of the desired implants.[27]

Implants

SCREWS

Various types of screws were developed by the AO together with Synthes Inc. (see Table 81-1) and have different functions. The parts of a screw include the head, shaft, core, and thread. Its attributes include pitch, shaft length, thread length, and total screw length.

Screw types

Cortex screws have a 0.7-mm thread width, and a thread length that depends on the screw length (see Table 81-1). A cortex screw does not contain a shaft portion and is referred to as a fully threaded screw. The shaft screw (see Table 81-1) is an exception and therefore a special cortex screw. The shaft screw contains a shaft portion of the same diameter as the outside diameter of the threads.[32] The threads have the same geometry as the cortex screws. Shaft screws are available in various shaft and thread lengths. Because of the smooth shaft portion, these screws are ideally suited for lag screw fixation, especially through plates.

Cancellous screws have a wider thread diameter than the cortex screws and they have a different pitch (see Table 81-1). This screw is designed to improve holding power in soft cancellous bone, but it is only rarely used in equine internal fixation.

Cannulated screws contain a central canal for a guide wire[33] (see Table 81-1). The design resembles the cancellous screw, because it has a thinner shaft and a wider thread portion. The 7.3-mm cannulated screw contains a self-drilling and self-tapping tip, as well as a reverse cutting device at the back end of the threads[34] (Fig. 81-8). A recent in vitro study using equine cadaveric femora revealed that the 6.5-mm cancellous and the 7.3-mm cannulated screws vary in insertion properties (the 7.3-cannulated screw requires significantly greater insertion torques), but they have similar pullout properties in the mid, proximal, and distal metaphyses of foal femora.[35] Both screw types have greater holding power at the mid-diaphyseal location than at metaphyseal locations. Because of the overall similar

TABLE 81-1. Veterinary Large Animal Screw, Drill Bit, and Tap Chart

Screw Name	3.5 mm Cortex	4.5 mm Cortex	4.5 mm Shaft	4.5 mm Cannulated	5.0 mm Locking	5.5 mm Cortex	6.5 mm Cancellous	7.3 mm Cannulated
Screw ø	3.5	4.5	4.5	4.5	5	5.5	6.5	7.3
Gliding hole ø	3.5	4.5	4.5	4.5 None	None	5.5	4.5	7.3
Thread hole ø	2.5	3.2	3.2	3.2	4.3	4	3.2	5
Tap ø	3.5	4.5	4.5	4.5	None	5.5	6.5	7.3 Optional
Screw shape								
Cannulation guide pin	—	—	—	150 mm long/ 1.6 mm O	—	—	—	300 mm long / 2.8 mm O
Type thread	Cortical	Cortical	Cortical	Cancellous	Cortical narrow	Cortical	Cancellous	Cancellous
Pitch	1.25	1.75	1.75	1.75	1	2	1.75	2.75
Screw head ø	6	8	8	6.5	6.6	8	8	8.2
Special head design	—	—	—	—	Conical threaded	—	—	—
Thread length	Fully threaded	Fully threaded	Variable	⅓ of Length/ Fully threaded	Fully threaded	Fully threaded	16 mm/32 mm/ Fully threaded	16 mm/32 mm/ Fully threaded
Shaft O	—	—	4.5	3.1	—	—	4.5	4.8
Core ø	2.4	3.1	3.1	2.7	4.4	4	3	4.5
Self-tapping	Yes	Yes	Yes	Yes	Yes	Yes	No	Yes
Self-drilling	No	No	No	Yes	Available	No	No	Yes

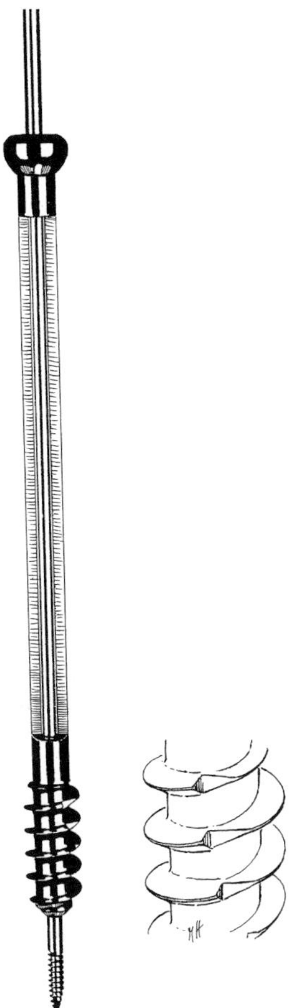

Figure 81-8. Schematic drawing of 7.3-mm cannulated screw with the guide pin inserted and half of the shaft removed. *Insert:* The reverse-cutting design of threads, which facilitates screw removal after healing of the fracture. (From Nixon AJ: Equine Fracture Repair, Philadelphia, 1996, WB Saunders.)

holding powers of 6.5-mm cancellous and 7.3-mm cannulated screws, it is unlikely that increasing the screw diameter beyond 6.5 mm will provide increased holding power in foal femoral bone. The use of the 7.3-mm cannulated screw should be considered for foal femoral fracture repair when greater accuracy is needed, or when bone threads for the 6.5-mm cancellous screw have been stripped.[35]

Self-tapping cortex screws contain the same thread-cutting device at the tip as the tap, obviating one step of the standard screw insertion technique[36] (see Table 81-1). These screws are popular in human surgery and are gaining more acceptance in equine surgery.[37] A recent in vitro study revealed that the mechanical properties of regular and self-tapping 4.5-mm cortex screws are similar with regard to pullout from the adult equine MCIII, and that the self-tapping cortex screws require less than half the total insertion time required by standard screws.[38] Interestingly, bone failure and bone comminution during the pullout tests were more commonly associated with self-tapping screws.[38]

Locking head screws were introduced with the less invasive stabilization system (LISS) and subsequently also applied in the locking compression plates by Synthes Inc. (Fig. 81-9). The conical shape of the PC-Fix screw (which is no longer

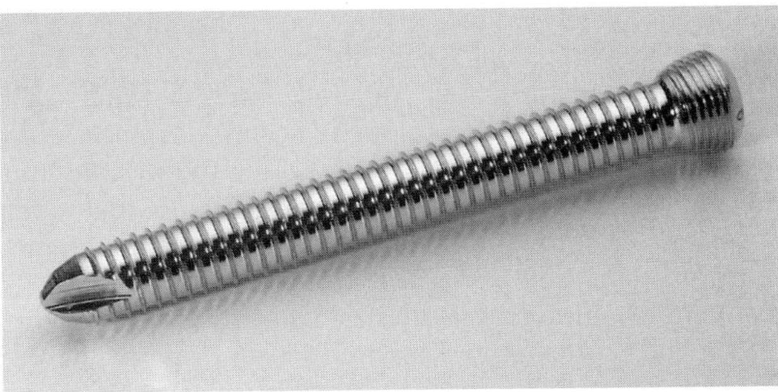

Figure 81-9. A self-tapping locking-head screw. Note the threads manufactured into the conically shaped screw head. These interlock with complementary threads in the plate. The self-tapping ends are visible at the tip of the screw.

manufactured) served as a basis for the new design.[39] The screw head was modified with a threaded profile, which complemented the one in the LISS plate hole. This design provided a stable angular fixation of the screw–plate (fixator) junction: the screw head is self-centering in the hole, and it keeps the screw from backing out of the LISS and LCP fixator (see later). The pitch of the threads at the screw head is identical to that of the threads on the shaft. Because of the larger diameter of the screw head, the pitch seems larger than on the shaft. However, the threads on the screw head catch after turning only 180 degrees instead of 360 degrees in the shaft. This facilitates faster fixation of the screw head in the plate and reduces the development of plate deformation through tightening of the screw.

The screw was also adapted to the unique mechanical demands of an internal fixator. The core diameter of the screw was enlarged to resist the increased bending moments and higher shear forces induced by a fixator.[37] This, plus the threaded screw–plate interface, allows the use of unicortical screw fixation in the diaphysis. The stability of unicortical fixation with locking head screws was established in a cadaveric biomechanical study.[40]

Unicortical screw fixation, in turn, allows the application of self-drilling or self-tapping screws, which was made possible by reducing the thread pitch and adding drill and tap sections to the screw tip[39] (see Table 81-1). These design changes have additional benefits: screw length determination is no longer needed because all diaphyseal screws can be the same length; therefore, screw lengths are not needed in increments of 2 mm, which results in a smaller inventory; pre-drilling and tapping are no longer needed, and the thread profile cut into the bone is more precise (because each screw is used once and therefore the drill and tap parts are sharp), which results in a better anchorage of the screw in the bone.[39]

In the horse, self-drilling and self-tapping screws are rarely used because of their high price, and screws are usually inserted bicortically. Therefore, most of the advantages just listed do not apply to this species. However, self-tapping screws are used in the horse in bicortical applications.

Other screws include the Herbert screw (Zimmer Orthopedics, Warsaw, Ind), an example of a self-contained compression screw.[41] This screw is fully threaded and contains threads not only over its entire length but also on the head. The head is wider than the rest of the screw and can be completely buried in the bone. It has been used in condylar fractures of MCIII/MTIII.

Recently, a cannulated, tapered, variable-pitch, self-compressing screw was developed (Acutrack Equine Screw, Acumed Veterinary, Hillsboro, Ore). This screw is 45 mm long, and it has a diameter of 6.5 mm at its base that tapers to a diameter of 5.0 mm at its apex. Because of the tapered shape, no glide hole is needed. The screw is manufactured of titanium. Biomedical studies comparing Acutrack to 4.5-mm AO cortex screws inserted in lag fashion revealed that the screws had similar biomedical shear properties.[42] The self-compressing action of the Acutrack screw provided only 70% of the compression force achieved with the 4.5-mm AO cortex screw.[43] The pushout strength was higher in the Acutrack screw.[43] Simulated mid-body fractures of the medial proximal sesamoid bone repaired with Acutrack compared with 4.5-mm AO cortex screws showed mechanically comparable strengths.[44] Both constructs were mechanically inferior to intact limbs.[44]

Sizes

The size of a screw is determined by the outside diameter of the threads. The standard screws for the horse are the 4.5- and 5.5-mm cortex screws. Pertinent data on each screw type as well as drill sizes needed are summarized in Table 81-1. For compact equine bone, the 5.5-mm screw was developed. This screw has advantages in adult horses over the 4.5-mm screw.[45-47] The 6.5-mm cancellous screw is available in three different configurations: with a thread length of 16 mm, with a thread length of 32 mm, and as a fully threaded screw. Since the introduction of the 5.5-mm cortex screw, the 6.5-mm cancellous screw has diminished in importance, because the 5.5-mm screw can also be inserted when a 4.5-mm hole has been stripped. A stripped 5.5-mm hole can still be engaged by a 6.5-mm cancellous screw. Cannulated screws are manufactured in 3.5-, 4.5-, 7.0-, and 7.3-mm diameters, but only the latter two sizes are interesting for the equine surgeon, and they can be used if a 6.5-mm cancellous screw is stripped.

The 3.5-mm cortex screw is used to achieve interfragmentary compression of certain fractures, such as third carpal bone slab fractures. It is also applicable for anatomic reduction of long bone fractures and interfragmentary compression of the fragments. The screw has such a small head that it can be completely buried in bone, which allows plating over the screw.[30] This is a great advantage, especially if two plates have to be applied.

The recently developed locking-head screws are the strongest screws available for equine fracture treatment, because of their large core diameter (4.3 mm). These screws can be applied only through the LISS and the LC-plates. They are available as nontapping; self-tapping; and self-drilling, self-tapping screws. Only the first two types are of interest for equine surgeons. The self-drilling, self-tapping screw is very expensive, and because of its design it is impossible to predetermine the depth of the screw hole. Also, in equine fracture treatment it is important to achieve screw purchase in both cortices. If a self-drilling, self-tapping screw were inserted, the sharp self-drilling part of the screw would protrude out of the *trans*-cortex, which could produce soft tissue damage.

Functions

Screws can be used as *lag screws, position screws,* and *plate screws.*[48] There is a difference between a partially threaded cancellous or cannulated screw, which automatically produces a lag effect, and a cortex or shaft screw used in lag fashion.[3] The cancellous and cannulated screws are inserted in such a manner that all of the threads pass the fracture line. Thus, tightening of the screw provides interfragmentary compression[1-3] (Fig. 81-10, *A*). If the threads of a cancellous screw bridge the fracture gap, however, no compression can be achieved (see Fig. 81-10, *B*). The same holds true for a cortex screw placed as a position screw (i.e., with no lag effect): its threads engage bone on both sides of a fracture, and because no glide hole was prepared in the near cortex, no interfragmentary compression is achieved. A plate screw lags the plate to the bone.[2] The lag technique may, however, also be applied through a plate hole. In this case, the screws are inserted through the plate *and* they cross the fracture line.[1-3]

The preparation of the screw surface plays an important role in the holding power of the implant.[46] Special surface preparation of stainless steel and titanium screws showed superior holding characteristics over the plain stainless steel and titanium screws.[49]

The *lag technique* is used to place cortex screws so that they act in lag fashion. This technique is not necessary when using partially threaded screws (such as cancellous or cannulated screws) as lag screws when applied as discussed in later paragraphs. The *cis-cortex* or *near cortex* is drilled with a drill bit having the same diameter as the outside thread diameter of the screw (Fig. 81-11, *A*). This is referred to as overdrilling. Therefore, at insertion of the screw, the threads do not engage bone in that cortex but glide through, so this portion of the hole is called the *glide hole.* The *insert drill*

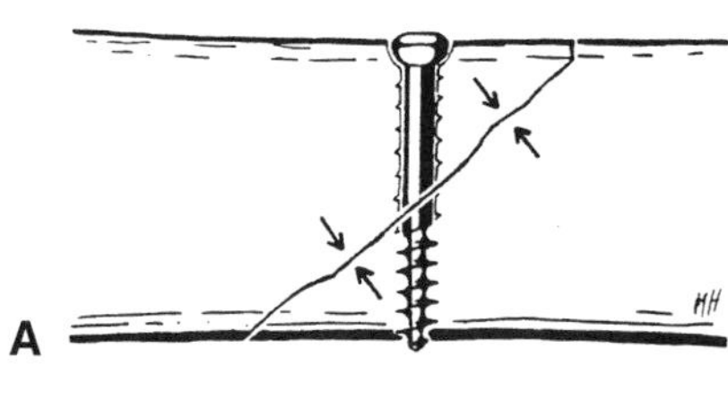

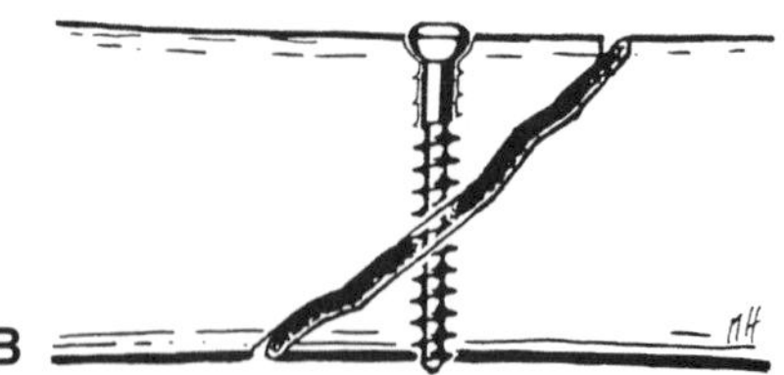

Figure 81-10. Lag screw technique. **A,** A cancellous screw of the correct thread length. All threads are located past the fracture plane, allowing interfragmentary compression. **B,** Selection of a cancellous screw with too long a thread length. Threads are located on both sides of the fracture plane, preventing interfragmentary compression. (From Nixon AJ: Equine Fracture Repair, Philadelphia, 1996, WB Saunders).

sleeve is designed to have an outside diameter that is the same as that of the glide hole, and an inside diameter that is the same as that of the smaller drill bit, which has a diameter identical to that of the core of the screw. Insertion of this drill sleeve into the glide hole ensures concentric drilling and accurate reduction of the fracture (see Fig. 81-11, *B*). The hole drilled through this sleeve across the *trans-cortex* or *far cortex* is referred to as the *thread hole*.

To allow a greater contact area between the screw head and the bone, a depression is created at the near cortex using the *countersink* (see Fig. 81-11, *C*). This decreases stress concentration at the screw head–bone interface. It is important to use the countersink in a 360-degree motion rather than in a to-and-fro motion; otherwise, an imperfect indentation is cut, preventing proper seating of the head. Countersinking is especially important in screws inserted at nonorthogonal angles relative to the surface of the bone. Care is taken to insert the nozzle at the tip of the countersink axially into the glide hole, and to remove the bone making contact with the instrument. If this is not done, tightening of the screw results in stress accumulation at the screw–thread junction, and bending of the screw head is possible.

The *depth gauge* is then used to determine the total length of the screw, including the head (see Fig. 81-11, *D*). Therefore, the length of the screw is measured to include the head. The depth gauge has a small hook at the end of its thin shaft that is inserted through the thread hole. By slightly tilting the instrument to one side, the hook catches the opposite cortex, and by sliding the movable portion toward the countersink depression, the exact length of screw is determined. Using the *tap sleeve* to protect the soft tissues as well as to help guide the *tap*, the tap is inserted into the glide hole and the threads are cut into the thread hole (see Fig. 81-11, *E*). The threads are cut by advancing the tap three half-turns clockwise, followed by one half-turn counterclockwise. The counterclockwise action allows transport of the swath material into the flutes of the tap and ensures precise cutting of the threads without interference of the swath material cut from previous threads. An experienced surgeon may tap the thread hole with the air drill (power tapping) to speed up the procedure. This is especially advantageous when many screws are to be inserted. It requires experience, however, or serious complications may arise, such as stripping of the thread holes, cross threading of

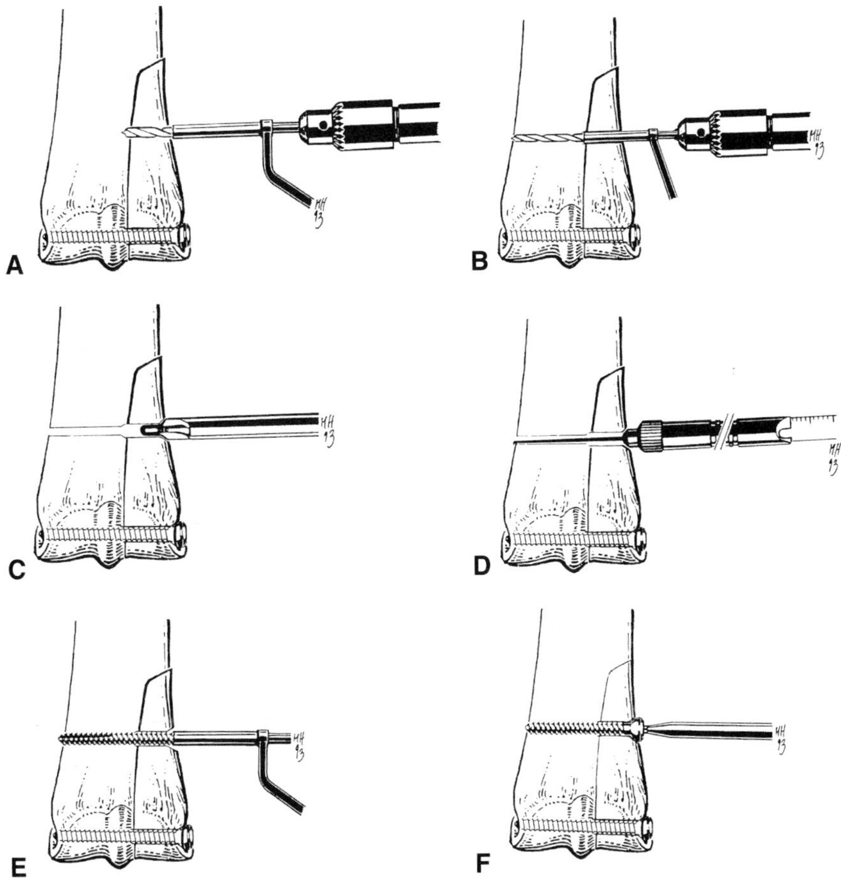

Figure 81-11. Lag technique, shown on a lateral condylar fracture of the distal MCIII. **A,** The *cis*-cortex is overdrilled. **B,** The insert drill bit is placed into the glide hole and advanced past the fracture plane, and the concentric thread hole is drilled across the *trans*-cortex. **C,** A depression for the screw head is prepared with the countersink. **D,** The required length of the screw is determined with the depth gauge. **E,** The threads are cut into the thread hole with the tap. **F,** The screw of predetermined length is inserted and solidly tightened with the hexagonal-tipped screwdriver. (From Nixon AJ: Equine Fracture Repair, Philadelphia, 1996, WB Saunders.)

the tap, and instrument breakage. If a self-tapping screw is used, this step is not necessary. The small AO air drill is not powerful enough to insert a self-tapping screw without applying a to-and-fro "power-tapping" technique. The AO compact air drill, however, has one third more strength and easily inserts self-tapping screws without to-and-fro activity.

Once the hole has been tapped, it is flushed to clean the hole and to provide lubrication. A screw of the predetermined length is inserted, using the hexagonal tipped *screwdriver* (see Fig. 81-11, *F*) either by hand or with an air drill. Final tightening is always carried out by hand. Care is taken to avoid excessive force, which may result in failure of the screw head, or in stripping of the threads cut into the thread hole.[48] This is not a common problem in dense equine bone. The shaft screw is inserted by applying the identical lag technique. However, care has to be taken that the glide hole is made slightly longer than the screw shaft. If the shaft is longer than the glide hole, no interfragmentary compression is achieved.

In the *lag screw technique,* a lag screw (either a partially threaded cancellous screw or a cannulated screw) is inserted after using a drill bit of only one size across the entire bone. Threads are cut along the total length of the hole with the cancellous tap, and the lag screw is inserted. The threads in the *cis*-cortex should not be engaged by the screw threads but only those of the *trans*-cortex, allowing achievement of interfragmentary compression.[1-3] Because the hardness of equine bone makes screw insertion difficult, it may be advisable to enlarge the *cis*-cortex with a 4.5-mm-diameter drill bit after first drilling the entire hole with the 3.6-mm drill bit.

Insertion of cannulated screws employs the same technique. However, the initial step involves placement of a guide wire in the desired location.[34] A special drill sleeve allows insertion of parallel screws close together. It is advisable to pre-drill equine cortical bone with a small drill bit before insertion of the guide wire to avoid bending it. All instruments are cannulated to accept the guide wire. The size of the drill bit depends on the size of the screw to be implanted and the size of the guide wire. Once the guide wire is in place, the measuring device is placed over the portion protruding out of the bone. The length of guide wire located in the bone is determined, and this is the length of screw required. It is advisable to select a screw 5 mm shorter than the length of the guide wire, to ensure secure seating of the wire throughout the implantation procedure. Subsequently, the cannulated drill bit is placed over the guide wire and the hole of predetermined length is prepared. The hole is tapped and finally the selected screw is inserted and firmly tightened (Fig. 81-12). At the end, the guide wire is removed.

The 7.3-mm cannulated screw has a self-drilling and self-tapping tip. Therefore, a screw of predetermined length is inserted without drilling a thread hole. Because of the initial insertion of the guide pin and the ability to select a screw of correct length, the danger of implanting a screw that is too long and protrudes out of the opposite side of the bone is negligible. In equine bone, insertion occurs in the same manner as tapping, meaning that the screw is advanced three half-turns, followed by a half-turn in the opposite direction. Care has to be taken with power insertion.[30]

The *position screw* is used to maintain two pieces of bone at a certain distance apart and to prevent interfragmentary

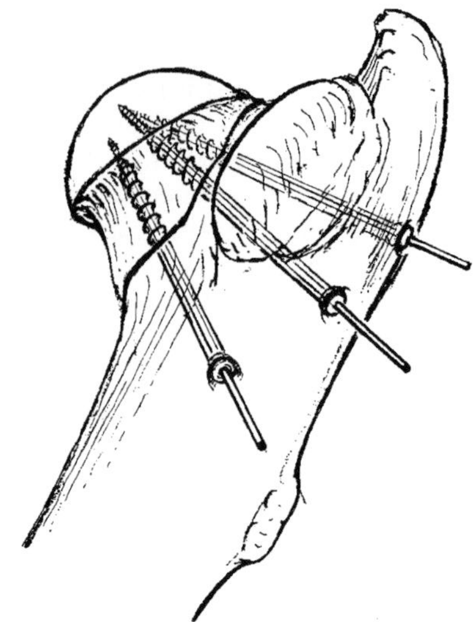

Figure 81-12. A capital femoral fracture is repaired with three cannulated screws. After the screws are inserted over a guide pin and tightened, the guide pins (which penetrated further than the screws) are removed.

compression. This is achieved by drilling a hole of only one size (thread hole) across both cortices, followed by tapping. Only fully threaded cortex screws may be inserted as position screws. Because the threads catch in the *cis*- and *trans*-cortex, interfragmentary compression is prevented. No lag effect is achieved.

The *plate screw* is inserted by the technique described for the position screw. Any type screw may be used in this manner. With the plate screw, the plate hole serves as a glide hole and allows compression of the plate onto the underlying bone, providing friction and stability.

Screw removal

Cortex and locking-head screws are easily removed because of their fully threaded design. Similarly, shaft screws are easy to remove, because the shaft completely fills the glide hole. However, after a fracture has healed, a cancellous screw may be impossible to remove from hard equine bone, because during fracture healing, the pre-cut threads in the *cis*-cortex fill in with solid bone. Removal of the screw necessitates that the threads cut their own way through the bone, a task for which they are not designed. This frequently results in the screw breaking, usually at the head–shaft or the shaft–thread junction. Therefore, cancellous screws should not be used when implant removal may be necessary at a later stage. Smaller cannulated screws have the same problem as cancellous screws. The 7.3-mm cannulated screw, however, contains a reverse-cutting edge at the caudal end of the threads, which facilitates re-cutting of the bone threads during screw removal[33] (see Fig. 81-8).

Occasionally, the hexagonal indentation in the screw head may be stripped during screw removal. This occurs if the screwdriver is improperly inserted in the hexagonal hole. Alternatively, if the hole is partially filled with tissue, the screwdriver cannot be inserted completely. Subsequent application of extraction force (counterclockwise motion on the screwdriver) may strip the hole. This problem is mainly encountered with the 3.5-mm screw because of its smaller screw head. A special screw retrieval instrument has been designed for such situations (Fig. 81-13). A shaft with a conical, threaded tip is inserted into the hexagonal indentation of the screw head. The threads of the tip have a reversed orientation compared with the screw threads. Therefore, when the cone is tightened in the screw head with a counterclockwise motion, an extraction force is applied to the screw, allowing it to be easily removed. These screw-retrieval devices are available for all sizes of screws.

When a screw head is broken off, a special hollow drill bit is available to remove the bone surrounding the screw. Because it rotates counterclockwise, the threads on the inside of the hollow drill bit interlock with the screw, and advancing the drill bit removes the broken screw.

PLATES

The first plates to contain an axial compression device were developed by Danis in 1947.[50] They consisted of a plate with an oblong hole on one end. At the head of the plate, a compression screw could be introduced, which pushed the screw placed through the oblong plate hole toward the fracture line and in doing so provided axial compression to the fractured bone ends (Fig. 81-14). Ten years later, Bagby introduced an impacting bone plate.[51] The heads of the screws he designed had a conical underside. If the screw was inserted eccentrically into the plate hole, the conical underside made contact with the edge of the plate hole. By tightening the screw, the bone into which the screw was implanted was displaced toward the fracture site and thus induced axial compression (Fig. 81-15). The first plates developed by the AO in 1958 contained round holes[52] (Fig. 81-16). Axial compression was applied with the help of a tension device (see later). Plate hole designs are shown in Figure 81-16 and described in the following paragraphs.

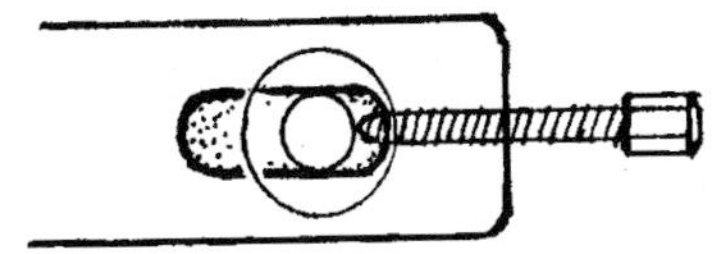

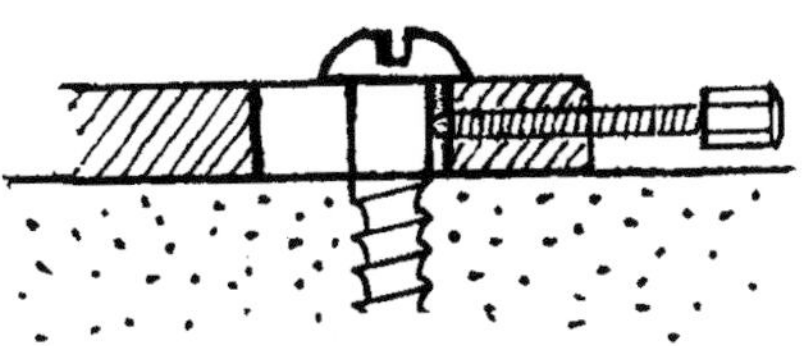

Figure 81-14. Redrawing of the Danis plate, developed in 1947. The plate screw is inserted into an oblong hole, and by tightening a smaller screw placed parallel to the long axis of the plate, the initial screw is displaced, providing axial compression of the fracture.

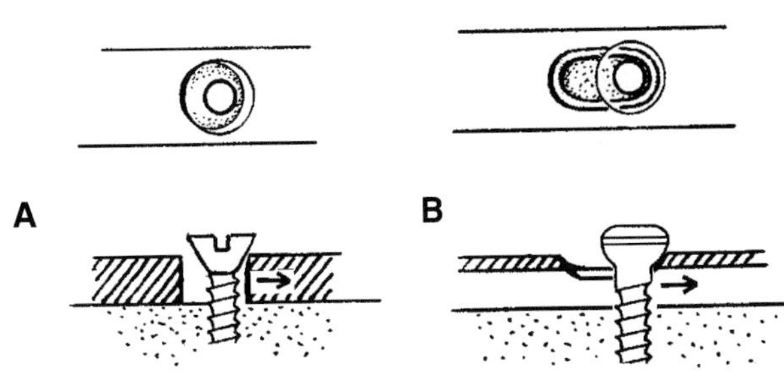

Figure 81-15. Redrawing of the Bagby plate, developed in 1958. **A,** A screw with slanted screw head is inserted under load conditions into a larger plate hole, and through tightening of the screw, the axial compression is achieved across the fracture, similar to the DCP principle shown in **B.**

Standard plates: LC-DCP

The dynamic compression plate (DCP), up to now the workhorse for equine fracture treatment, is being replaced by the limited contact dynamic compression plate (LC-DCP), especially in the United States. Studies in human medicine showed the DCP to cause osteoporosis development under the plate, although this is not encountered in equine surgery[1] (see later). This led to the development of biologically improved plates.

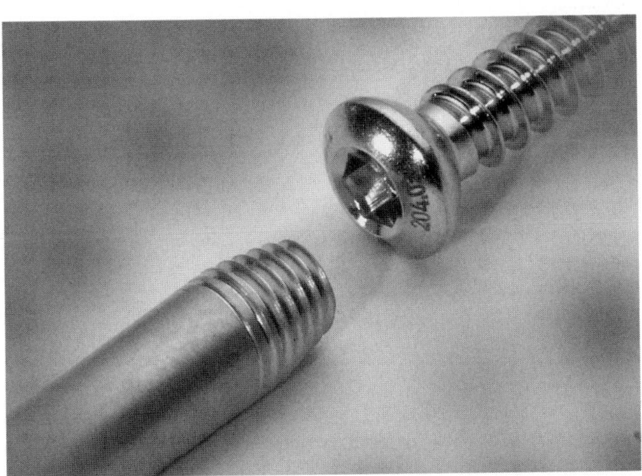

Figure 81-13. Removal device for stripped 3.5-mm screw heads. An intact hexagonal hole in the screw head is shown. It is smaller than the tip of the screw. However, once the hole in the screw head is stripped, the tip of the device (whose threads are oriented in the direction opposite to those in the screw) will fit.

In the conventional DCP, the plate holes provided the least resistance to failure. This problem was somewhat offset in equine fracture treatment by inserting screws through all plate holes. By designing a plate that contained at each cross-section along its entire length the same amount of metal, an implant of uniform bending stiffness was developed.[49] To achieve this, half-moon–shaped pieces of metal were removed from the underside of the plate. This resulted in limited contact between bone and the plate, which led to the name of the plate: LC-DCP (Fig. 81-17). The limited contact surface was welcomed in human surgery to fight the problem of osteoporosis developing under the plate.[49] Extensive tests comparing the LC-DCP with the conventional DCP revealed that the LC-DCP had an equal bending stiffness and a 50% increase in the continuity of the bending stiffness.[49] This reduces local stress concentration near fracture gaps. Additionally, the blood supply of the bone under the plate was significantly improved.[53] Mechanical tests revealed that the design of the LC-DCP provided increased resistance to cycling failure compared with the DCP.[52] The undercuts of the plate allow the development of some callus bridges over the fracture gap, which lead to a

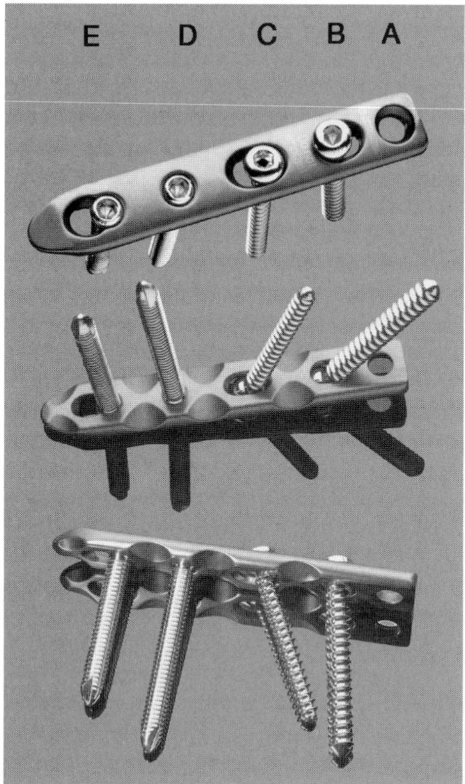

Figure 81-16. The plate holes designed for Synthes plates. A, The initially developed round hole. B, The dynamic compression plate hole, which allows compression from one side. The screws can be angulated axially up to 25 degrees. C, The dynamic compression unit hole, which allows compression from either side and is used in the LC-DCP. The screws can be angulated axially up to 40 degrees. The plates have undercuts. D, Locking head plate holes used in the LISS plate, allowing only orthogonal insertion of the screws. The plates have undercuts. E, The Combi-Hole used in the locking compression plate allows the insertion of locking head screws—as shown here—and standard screws. The plates have undercuts and a pointed end that allows minimally invasive insertion through a small incision.

significant increase in stability, despite the fact the these bridges are small. The trapezoidal cross-section allows the formation of shorter but stronger bone lamellae on either side. Also, it prevents the bone from growing over the plate. The dynamic compression unit (DCU) hole design in the LC-DCP, which allows axial compression to be applied from either side of the hole, replaced the conventional DCP hole design (see Fig. 81-16). This allows the distribution of the plate holes evenly along the entire plate and obviated the need for a center in the plate. The DCU hole is also undercut at each end to allow the insertion of screws up to a 40-degree angle relative to the orthogonal direction. In the DCP hole, only a 25-degree angulation can be achieved.[52]

There are two plate widths: the narrow, with the holes arranged in a straight line, and the broad, with alternating offset holes. Pertinent data on width, length, and hole distribution in these plates are summarized in Table 81-2. Recently, a special equine LC-DCP (see Table 81-2) made from thicker plate stock was developed for application during arthrodesis of the metacarpophalangeal joint (see Chapter 85). This plate is available in all sizes and will undoubtedly be very popular among equine orthopedic surgeons.

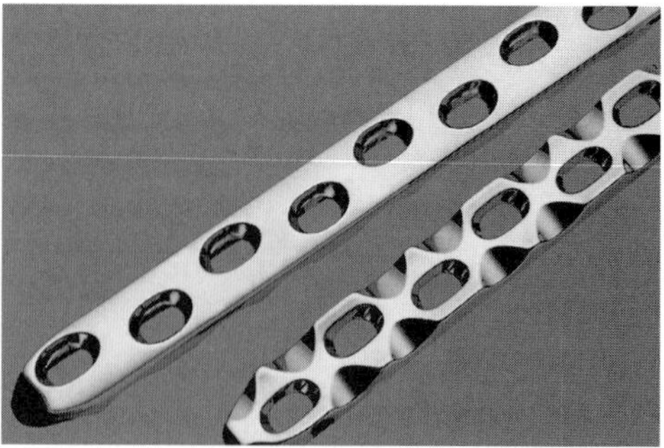

Figure 81-17. 5.5 LC-DCP. The ends are pointed, the screw holes are arranged in two slightly offset rows (top side of plate shown above), evenly distributed along the plate, and the underside of the plate (shown below) contains undercuts.

The DCU holes are specially designed to allow dynamic compression as the screw is tightened. The holes are arranged according to the spherical gliding principle, with an incline, or slope, toward the center portion of the plate[52,54] (Fig. 81-18). When a screw is inserted in a far (load) position (offset 1 mm from the center of the hole), the screw head contacts the plate at the top of this incline. With tightening, the screw head "slides down the slope" until it comes to rest at the bottom of the incline, in the center of the oblong screw hole. Because the screw is introduced into the bone, screw movement toward the fracture line results in compression of the fractured bone ends. This offset drilling can be carried out on either side of each hole and therefore on either side of the fracture line[52] (see Fig. 81-15). The application of the LC-DCP requires the use of the special LC-DCP double drill guide identified by its undercuts on the handle, identical to the ones under the plate itself (Figs. 81-19 to 81-21). (Note: the DCP drill guide should not be used with the LC-DCP.) An alternative to the LC-DCP drill guide is the universal drill guide, which contains a spring-loaded tip (see Fig. 81-19). Pressing down on the drill guide places it near the center of the hole (Fig. 81-22). Placing the spring-loaded tip on the far end of the DCU hole relative to the fracture line allows a 1-mm compression of the fracture line.

The *technique of application* is as follows. The fracture is reduced (Fig. 81-23, *A*), and it is maintained in that config-

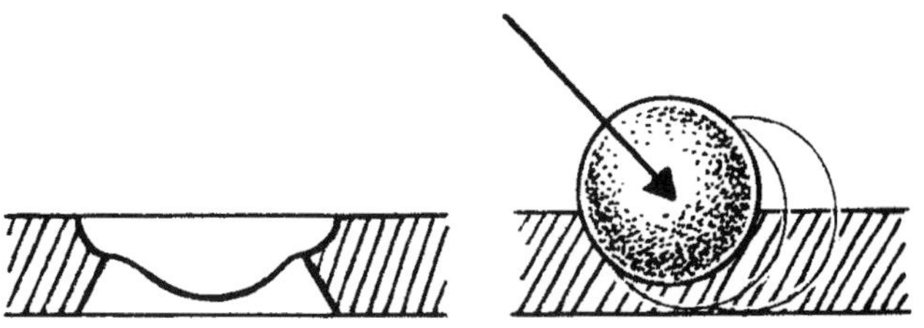

Figure 81-18. Design of the dynamic compression unit (DCU). Both sides of the hole are shaped like an inclined cylinder. Like a ball, the screw head slides down the incline. Because the screw head is fixed to the bone via the shaft, it can move only vertically relative to the bone. The horizontal movement of the head, as it impacts against the angled side of the hole, results in movement of the bone fragment relative to the plate and leads to compression of the fracture. With the DCU, compression can be achieved on either side, obviating the need for the plate to have a center, as in the dynamic compression plate.

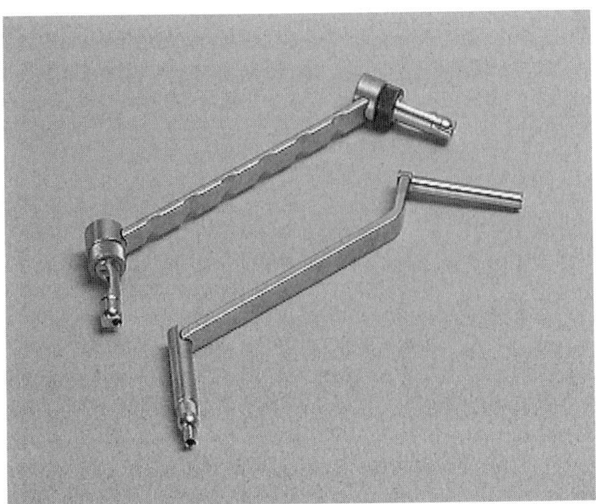

Figure 81-19. The LC-DCP double drill guide *(top)* contains undercuts like those of the corresponding plate to distinguish it from the DCP double drill guide. The dark ring represents the neutral (green) guide, the light ring the load (yellow) guide. The universal drill guide (bottom) contains a spring-loaded guide for the thread hole and a larger guide of the glide hole. The universal drill guide is available for the different screw sizes.

uration initially with pointed reduction forceps until one or two interfragmentary cortex screws 3.5 or 4.5 mm in diameter can be applied in lag fashion (see Fig. 81-23, *B*). The plate is then contoured, overbent at the fracture site, and applied to the bone (see Fig. 81-23, *C*). The first screw hole is drilled toward one end of the plate in neutral position (green LC-DCP drill guide or pressed-down universal drill guide). The screw is inserted but not completely tightened. This allows the plate to be pulled into a loaded position. The same can be achieved by drilling the initial hole through the load (yellow) LC-DCP guide or the universal drill guide placed at the far end of the hole, and maintaining the plate in the same position (see Fig. 81-23, *D*). The hole for the second screw is drilled on the other side of the fracture line through a plate hole near the other end, using the load drill guide (see Fig. 81-23, *E*), if additional compression is needed. Care is taken to ensure correct plate position prior to drilling the second hole. The hole is prepared for the screw, which is subsequently inserted. Interfragmentary compression is achieved through alternate tightening of the two screws (see Fig. 81-23, *F*). More screws may be applied in the loaded position on either side of the fracture. A maximum of two screws can be placed under load conditions on either side of the fracture line. Therefore, a maximal compression of 4 mm can be achieved. Before the second loaded screw is completely tightened, the first one on the same side has to be slightly loosened. This allows the additional compression to be applied. Without this loosening, no additional compression is achieved and the two screws that are "compressed" toward each other are stressed.

The remaining screws are implanted in neutral position. Any screw placed through a plate across a fracture line is introduced using the lag technique (see Fig. 81-23, *G*). All the screws are finally tightened (see Fig. 81-23, *H*). A cortex screw inserted through a plate in lag fashion perpendicularly across a fracture may not achieve the desired effect, because the threads in the glide hole cut into the cortex and prevent any gliding.[52] To correct this undesirable effect, the shaft screw was developed. The shaft, which fills out the glide hole completely, does not cut into the cortex.

Any cortex or shaft screw can be inserted under load (at the far end of the oblong plate hole) or in neutral position (at the center) of each plate hole. Under load, 1-mm centripetal displacement or compression of the fracture gap is implemented. In neutral position, 0.1-mm compression is achieved. If double plating is applied, only two screws are placed under load in the second plate, which in most cases is arranged at 90 degrees relative to the first plate.

Plates are contoured with the help of a plate-bending press to fit the surface of the bone. A perfectly contoured plate, however, compresses only the cortex immediately under the plate, whereas the opposite cortex remains decompressed (Fig. 81-24, *A*). By slightly overbending the plates at the fracture site (see Fig. 81-24, *B*), compression is achieved along the entire circumference of the bone[1-3] (see Fig. 81-24, *C*).

Axial interfragmentary compression under a plate may also be implemented with the help of a tension device (Fig. 81-25). The plate is applied to the bone with several screws in neutral position on one end of the fracture. The tension device is hooked into last hole on the other end of the plate and attached to the underlying bone through a unicortically applied 4.5-mm cortex screw. With the help of a wrench, the tension device is tightened, which pulls the plate toward the tension device and thus applies compression to the fracture site. Once adequate compression is applied, screws are inserted on the other side of the fracture through the plate in neutral position and tightened. The tension device is subsequently removed and the remaining screws are inserted in empty plate holes.

The stability of the fixation is derived from friction between the implants and the bone. A technique called plate luting has been developed to obtain 100% plate–bone contact by applying bone cement (methylmethacrylate) between the plate and the bone.[55] This is achieved after all the screws of the plate are inserted. All the screws are then loosened, the plate is lifted off the bone, the soft bone cement is placed underneath it, and the screws of the plate are retightened, preferably with the power drill. Entrance of bone cement into the fracture line must be prevented because it retards or prevents bony union in that area. Once the screws are tightened, the soft cement fills the oblong plate holes around the screw heads and provides additional support, making the fixation extremely rigid.[55-57] When only the oblong plate holes are filled with bone cement, a similar but lesser increase in strain protection occurs.[57] Excess bone cement is rapidly and carefully removed. Plate luting is especially useful on bones with anatomically complex surfaces that make contouring of the plate difficult.[57] The addition of gentamicin into the bone cement facilitates long-term release of this antibiotic and provides effective protection against postoperative infections (see Chapter 88). Plate luting is not used in humans and small animals because vascular necrosis of the bone develops under the plate, resulting in pathologic fractures after implant removal. This complication has not been reported in horses.

Screws should be inserted perpendicular to the surface of the bone. If a second plate is used, it should be positioned to allow the screw holes to be located between the screws of the other plate.[29,58,59] This reduces the likelihood of

TABLE 81-2. Standard and Special Plates Used in the Horse

Name	LC-DCP 3.5	LC-DCP 3.5 Broad	LC-DCP 4.5	LC-DCP 4.5 Broad	LC-DCP 5.5 Broad	LC-DCP 3.5 Veterinary
Plate type	Standard	Standard	Standard	Standard	Standard	Special
Plate cross-section						
Width (mm)	11	13.5	13.5	17	16	12
Thickness (mm)	3.3	4.2	4.2	5.2	5.7	3.6
Length (mm)	25 (2 holes) to 259 (20 holes)	90 (7 holes) to 285 (22 holes)	34 (2 holes) to 394 (22 holes)	106 (6 holes) to 394 (22 holes)	188 (10 holes) to 332 (18 holes)	86 (7 holes) to 266 (22 holes)
Plate angle	Straight	Straight	Straight	Straight	Straight	Straight
Angled portion	—	—	—	—	—	Barrel 25 mm long
Screw size (mm)	3.5, 4.0	3.5, 4.0	4.5, 5.5, (6.5)	4.5, 5.5, (6.5)	4.5, 5.5, (6.5)	3.5, 4.0
Hole arrangement	Straight	Staggered	Straight	Staggered	Staggered	Straight
Hole spacing	13	13	18	18	18	12
Hole design	DCU	DCU	DCU	DCU	DCU	DCP
Plate mid-section	No	No	No	No	No	Yes
Hole spacing in plate mid-section	—	—	—	—	—	13

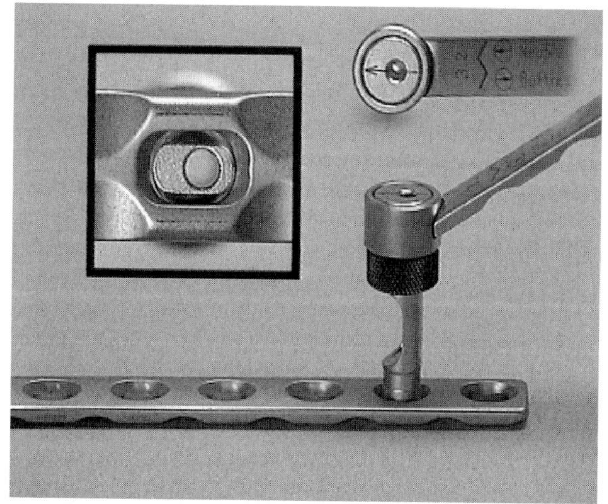

Figure 81-20. The neutral LC-DCP drill guide inserted into a dynamic compression unit (DCU) hole *(bottom)*. From below the plate, it can be seen that there is a gap between the right end of the DCU hole and the drill guide hole *(top left)*. From the top, the *arrow* pointing toward the fracture line is visible *(top right)*. In the DCP neutral guide, there is *no* arrow.

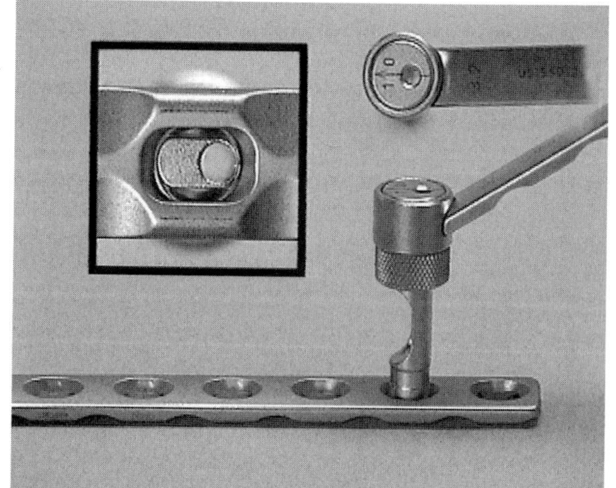

Figure 81-21. The load LC-DCP drill guide inserted into a dynamic compression unit (DCU) hole *(bottom)*. From below the plate, it can be seen that there is no gap between the right end of the DCU hole and the drill guide hole *(top left)*. From the top, the *arrow* pointing toward the fracture line is visible *(top right)*.

TABLE 81-2. Standard and Special Plates Used in the Horse—cont'd

DCP 4.5 Broad	DCS Plate	DHS Pate	LCP 3.5	LCP 4.5	LCP 4.5 Broad	One Third Tubular Plate
Special	Special	Special	Special	Special	Special	Special
16	16	19	11	13.5	17.5	9
4.8	5.4	5.8	3.4	4.5	5.4	1
103 (6 holes) to 359 (22 holes)	114 (6 holes) to 370 (22 holes)	46 (2 holes) to 270 (16 holes)	33 (2 holes) to 293 (22 holes)	44 (2 holes) to 440 (24 holes)	116 (6 holes) to 440 (24 holes)	28 (2 holes) to 148 (12 holes)
Straight	95°	135° (140°, 145°, 150°)	Straight	Straight	Straight	Straight
—	Barrel 25 mm long	Barrel 25 and 38 mm long	—	—	—	—
4.5, 5.5, (6.5)	4.5, 5.5, (6.5)	4.5, 5.5, (6.5)	3.5, 4.0 3.5 LS	4.5, 5.5, (6.5) 5.0 LS	4.5, 5.5, (6.5) 5.0 LS	3.5, 3.5 LS
Staggered	Staggered	Staggered	Straight	Straight	Staggered	Straight
16	16	16	13	18	18	12
DCP	2 Round, rest DCP	DCP	Combi-Hole	Combi-Hole	Combi-Hole	Oval, round w/collar
Yes	No	No	Yes	Yes	Yes	Yes
25	—	—	LO-LO 9 DCU-DCU 15	LO-LO 13 DCU-DCU 20	LO-LO 13 DCU-DCU 20	16

A
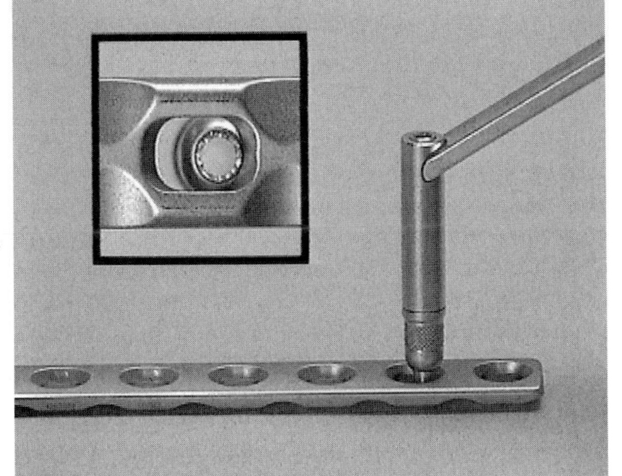

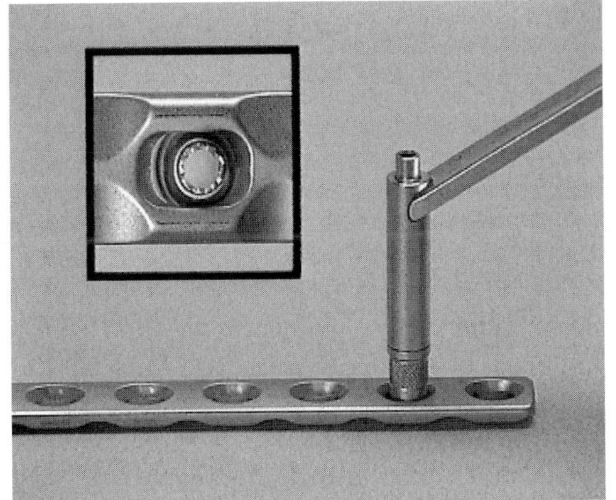
B

Figure 81-22. A, The universal drill guide placed into a dynamic compression unit (DCU) hole without applying pressure onto the guide. Viewed from below, the hole in the guide can be seen very close to the right end of the DCU hole. **B,** The universal drill guide placed into a DCU hole under pressure. The spring-loaded part of the guide is sticking out on top. From below, a gap can be seen between the hole in the guide and the right end of the DCU hole.

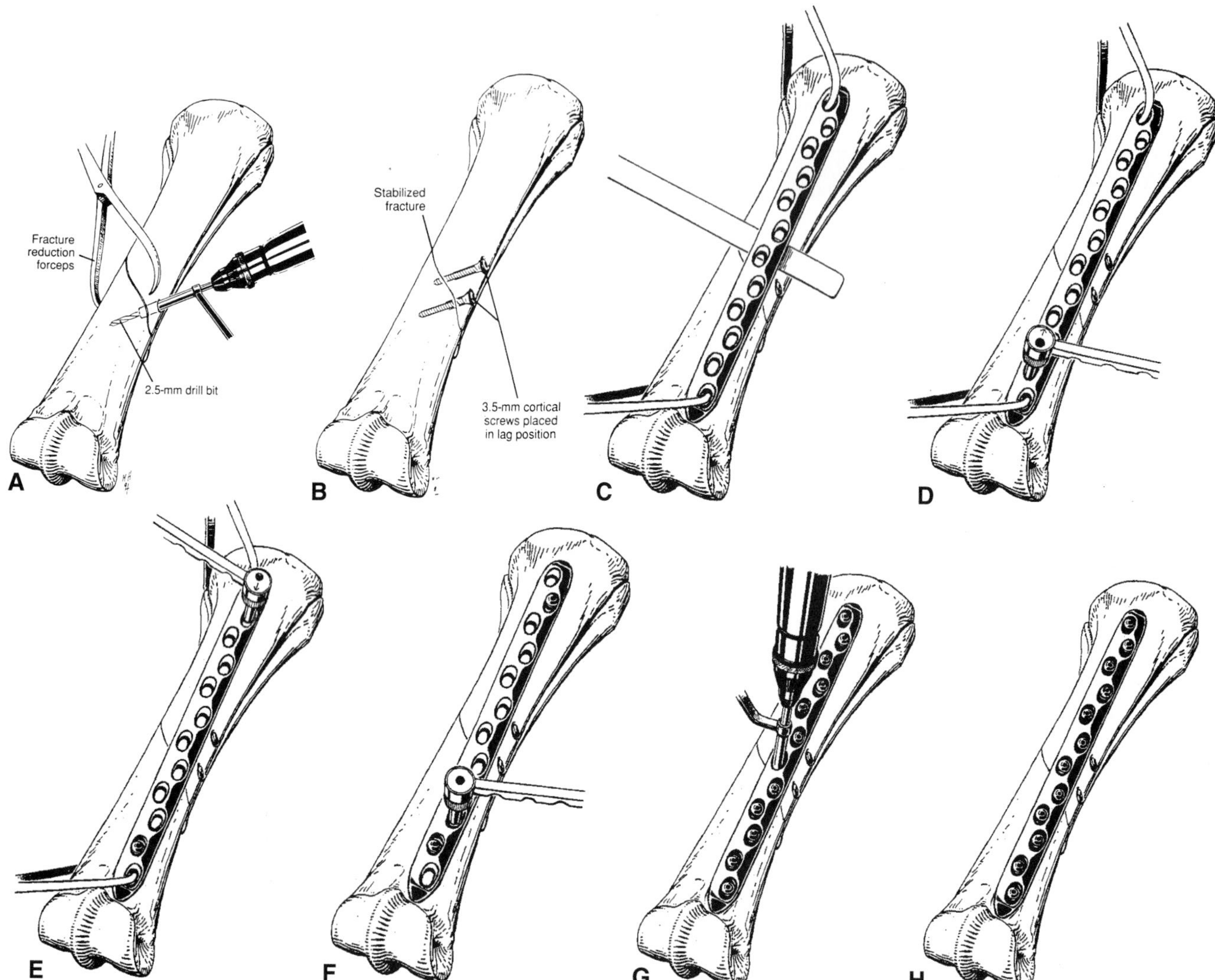

Figure 81-23. Repair of a simple oblique MCIII fracture with two cortex screws applied in lag technique combined with a broad LC-DCP as neutralization plate. **A,** The large pointed reduction forceps maintains alignment of the fractured bone during implantation of the two 3.5-mm cortex screws. **B,** The two screws are implanted and the reduction forceps removed. **C,** A 10-hole broad DCP is applied to the dorsolateral aspect of the bone, distal from the two interfragmentary 3.5-mm cortex screws. The plate was overbent at the fracture site, allowing introduction of an aluminum template between the bone and the plate. **D,** A thread hole is drilled across the bone through the second most distal plate hole with the help of the yellow, load drill sleeve. **E,** The screw is inserted but not completely tightened, followed by preparation of an identical hole at the opposite end of the plate. **F,** The second screw is inserted and both are alternately tightened, placing the fracture under axial compression. The remaining screw holes are prepared through the green, neutral drill guide. **G,** A lag screw is implanted across the fracture plane. **H,** All the screws are tightened. (From Nixon AJ: Equine Fracture Repair, Philadelphia, 1996, WB Saunders.)

inadvertent contact between the screws of the two plates. Every hole in a plate should be filled with a screw.[29] Should a hole traverse a fracture line, the lag technique should be applied by overdrilling of the *cis*-cortex, and the screw should be directed in such a way that it engages the opposite cortex next to the fracture line. Where no support can be achieved in a cortex, bone cement may be placed and the screw implanted. After the cement hardens, the screw will be solidly fixed.

Application of 4.5-mm screws through a 4.5-mm plate allows angulation in the longitudinal direction of about 40 degrees, and 7 degrees laterally.[52] Application of a 5.5-mm screw through the same hole allows an angulation of only about 25 degrees in the longitudinal direction. The plates applied for fixation of a long bone fracture ideally extend over the entire length of the bone.[4] Shorter plates must be staggered to ensure plate coverage of the total length of the bone. The most distal end of the proximal fragment in an oblique long bone fracture should be wedged between a plate and the opposing distal fragment. Therefore, the configuration of a fracture dictates to a certain extent the location of the plate to be applied (not just the tension side of the bone; see later).[29] Implants should be applied at a distance from severely bruised skin or areas of frank skin defects.

Plate *functions* include compression, neutralization, tension-band, and buttressing. The design of a plate does not dictate its function, because the same plate may be used for different functions and a plate may serve more than one

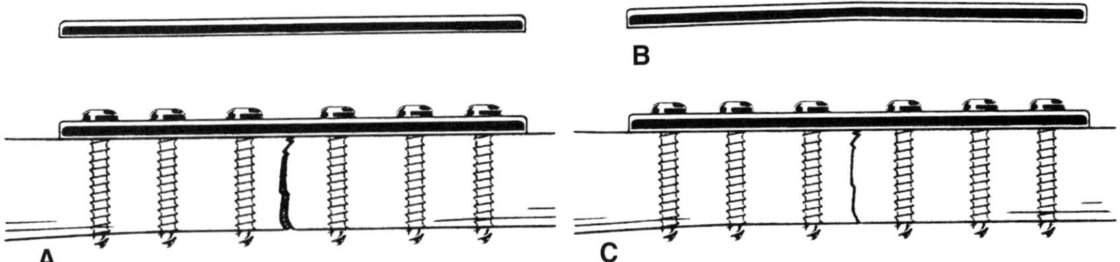

Figure 81-24. Application of a plate onto a bone. **A,** If a plate is perfectly contoured to the surface of the bone, a narrow gap develops at the fracture site opposite the plate after insertion and tightening of the screws. **B,** To overcome this problem, the plate is overbent (prestressed) about 1 mm, right at the fracture site. **C,** When the screws are reinserted the entire circumference of the fracture is under compression.

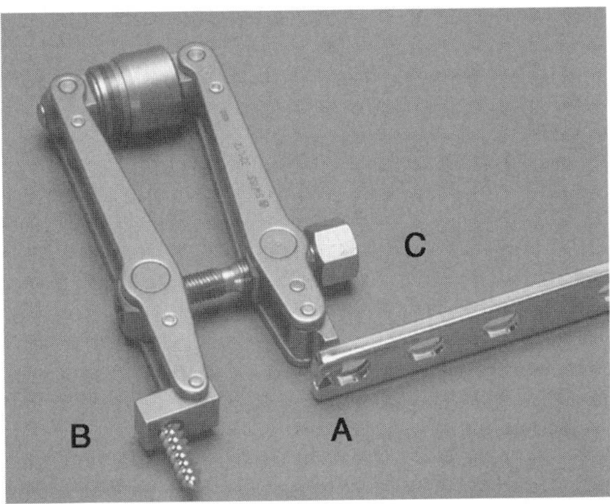

Figure 81-25. A, The tension device is hooked in the last plate hole. **B,** The device is attached to the bone with a short screw. **C,** Twisting of the hexagonal screw head pulls the plate toward the left side and applies axial compression to the underlying fracture.

function at a time. The compression and neutralization functions are the most frequently applied. When a plate serves in *compression* function, two screws on either side of the fracture line are placed under a load.[3] A plate serves a *neutralization* function after anatomic reconstruction and interfragmentary compression of a simple or comminuted fracture is accomplished by several screws placed in lag fashion.[1-3,29] The various diverging shear, bending, and rotational torque forces converging on these screws are neutralized by one or two plates. Such plates effectively bridge the proximal and distal aspects of the bone and protect the fixed fracture. The screws are inserted in the neutral position. Application of neutralization plates has to be planned ahead of time to avoid interfering with the reduction screws or eliminating options for their placement. Most plates applied satisfy both compression and neutralization functions.

A plate applied in the tension-band function transforms the tensile forces applied to the fractured bone underneath into compressive forces. The classic example of such a plate is one that is applied to fix an olecranon fracture. Because these plates are subjected mainly to tensile forces, smaller plates may be applied in these situations than for plates used in compression or neutralization functions.

Cortical bone defects that persist after anatomic reconstruction of the fracture cause instability of the repair because of stress concentration. Such areas need to be protected and bridged by an implant, maintaining length by preventing collapse of the fixation (Fig. 81-26). A plate applied in such a fashion is called a *buttress plate*. It is advisable to fill the defect in the bone with a cancellous bone graft or bone replacement material. Any screw placed through the plate in the region of the defect should engage the *trans*-cortex. All the other principles for plate fixation are applied.

Special plates

The *DCP*, as mentioned, has played a key role in establishing the guideline for plate fixations of fractures in humans, small animals, and horses.[1-3,29,30] After being replaced by the LC-DCP as the standard plate, its use will diminish. Table 81-2 summarizes the pertinent data of the most frequently used DCPs. These plates may be applied in all situations described for the LC-DCP. The DCP holes contain an incline on one side, which allows 1 mm of compression to be applied by drilling an eccentric hole (see Fig. 81-16).

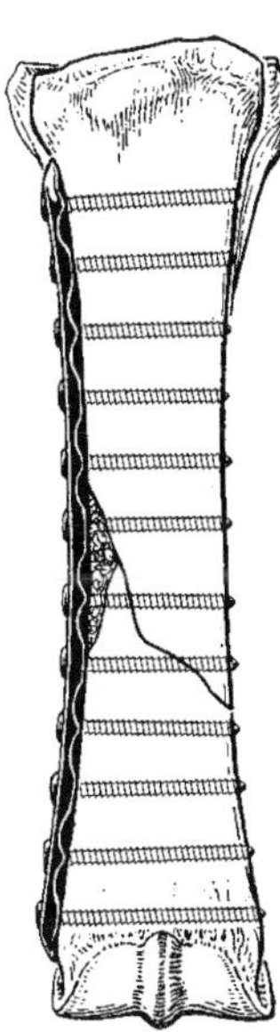

Figure 81-26. Comminuted mid-shaft fracture of MCIII showing a bone defect. The defect is filled with cancellous bone graft and a broad 12-hole LC-DCP is applied over the defect in buttress function. For better visualization, the dorsally applied LC-DCP, routinely used in a clinical case, is not shown.

Therefore, the plates have a center, on either side of which the DCP holes are arranged such that the incline is located at the far end of the holes. The plates have to be applied so that the center of the plate is positioned over the fracture site whenever possible.

One-third tubular plates are very thin and, depending on the size of the hole, may be applied with a 3.5- or a 4.5-mm screw (see Table 81-2). The 3.5-mm plate is applied, using standard technique, in fracture treatment of proximal MCII, MCIV, MTII, and MTIV fractures in adult horses, and of nondisplaced ulnar fractures in very young foals.

T-plates are available for 4.5- and 5.5-mm screws as well as in a smaller version for the 3.5-mm screws. These plates are suited to areas where tension is applied without bending and sufficient space is not available for the application of a straight, regular plate. T-plates have been used for arthrodeses of the tarsometatarsal and distal intertarsal joints.

Dynamic condylar screw (DCS) and *dynamic hip screw (DHS) plates* are used in implant systems that were developed on the principles of the angled blade plate (ABP).[60] These plates consist of a long lag screw with a 12.5-mm thread width, a 25-mm thread length, and an 8-mm shaft diameter. The shaft is flattened on two opposing sides to prevent rotation of the screw after it is introduced into the barrel of the plate. The DCS/DHS screw is inserted at a predetermined angle (95 degrees for the DCS plate and 135 degrees [standard] for the DHS plate) (see Table 81-2). The most important step in the application of the DCS and DHS plate systems is the correct insertion of the 2.5-mm guide pin. Drill guides aid in the placement of the guide pin, which is best verified intraoperatively with an image intensifier. (Intraoperative radiographs, despite being more time consuming, are satisfactory as well.) Pre-drilling of the cortex with a 2.5-mm drill bit facilitates insertion of the guide pin. Care has to be taken that all of the four points on the base of the drill guide under the handle are in contact with the bone during drilling, even if the drill guide tip does not make contact with the underlying bone (Fig. 81-27, *A*). Tilting of the drill guide with its tip down to bone results in false orientation of the DCS screw, which prevents the plate from making contact with the bone. This will require complicated adjustments of the plate angulations to make the plate contact the bone and will prolong the surgical procedure. If the plate barrel junction is not in direct contact with the bone, the gap may be bridged with polymethylmethacrylate (PMMA). Once the guide pin is correctly placed, the subsequent steps are easily accomplished because all instruments are hollow and accept the guide pin.

The measuring device is placed over the guide pin, and its depth in the bone is determined (see Fig. 81-27, *A*). The triple reamer placed over the guide pin allows simultaneous drilling of the core hole, the portion for the plate barrel, and the beveled plate-barrel interface (see Fig. 81-27, *B*). The reamer is assembled and adjusted to a length measuring 5 mm less than the pin portion located within the bone. This ensures persistence of the pin in its position throughout the screw insertion procedure. After preparing the screw hole, the threads are cut using routine technique (see Fig. 81-27, *C*), and the screw of appropriate length is introduced, followed by application of the plate (see Fig. 81-27, *D*). Once the shaft of the screw and the barrel are aligned, the barrel slides easily over the shaft and the plate position can be adjusted before impacting it onto the bone (see Fig. 81-27, *E*). The barrel has the same inside diameter as the screw shaft cross-section (8 mm and flattened at two opposite sides). The DCS plate has a barrel length of 25 mm, whereas the standard DHS has a barrel length of 38 mm. A special version of the DHS plate has a 25-mm barrel length as well. After their implantation, the lag screw and the plate are joined with a connecting screw, making the two components work as one unit (see Fig. 81-27, *F*). Tightening of the connecting screw creates interfragmentary compression, provided the lag screw has passed the fracture line.

Currently, the DHS plate is the strongest plate available in the AO-System.[60] The DCS and DHS plates are versatile, rapidly implanted, and a real asset to large animal surgery, especially when treating long bone fractures in adult horses.[61,62] The DCS system is useful in metaphyseal fractures of the MCIII or MTIII (Fig. 81-28), the proximal radius, and even the femur. The DHS may be applied for arthrodesis of the metacarpophalangeal joint (see Fig. 85-8) and in selected femoral fractures.[61] Combined with 5.5-mm screws, these plates produce extremely strong fixations.

The *PC-Fix* plate, which is presently not manufactured, is mentioned here for historical purposes, because it represented the first type of *internal fixator* developed by Synthes Inc.[63,64] It was manufactured from pure titanium, and it had round, conical screw holes, evenly distributed along the plate, and a specially designed underside that represents a further development of the LC-DCP. One row of points is arranged along either side of the plate, with the points being located between two plate holes. Between two points, the plate is undercut in an arcuate pattern, similar to the LC-DCP but to a greater extent. The short unicortical screws contained a conical head that locked in the plate hole while being tightened, forming a solid unit between plate and screws, without applying any load onto the screw threads (Fig. 81-29). The first clinical tests conducted with the PC-Fix were done on large animals, mainly cattle[65] (Fig. 81-30). The subsequently developed PC-Fix II was manufactured only as a 3.5-mm implant system. It had a slightly altered plate design and was applied with self-tapping screws.[66] A special plate-bending device was developed to prevent altering of the plate holes during bending. Development of this system led to the next generation of titanium implants: the LISS.

The *less invasive stabilization system (LISS)* consists of a forged titanium plate, which cannot be bent, and self-cutting, self-tapping titanium screws of predetermined length. The shape of the plate is predetermined and forged accordingly.[39,67] A guide system for transcutaneous insertion of the screw is mounted on the plate head (Fig. 81-31, *A*). This bar also facilitates insertion of the plate through a small surgical approach at one end of the bone and subsequent advancement of the plate along the periosteum, therefore bridging the approximately reduced fracture. Once in place, the last plate hole is approached through a stab incision and connected through the last hole in the aiming device with a drill sleeve, which is threaded into the plate. This establishes a solid frame, which maintains its angles during screw application and ensures that the screws are inserted orthogonally relative to the long axis of the plate and may be threaded into the plate holes. The remaining screws are inserted transcutaneously through stab incisions. An

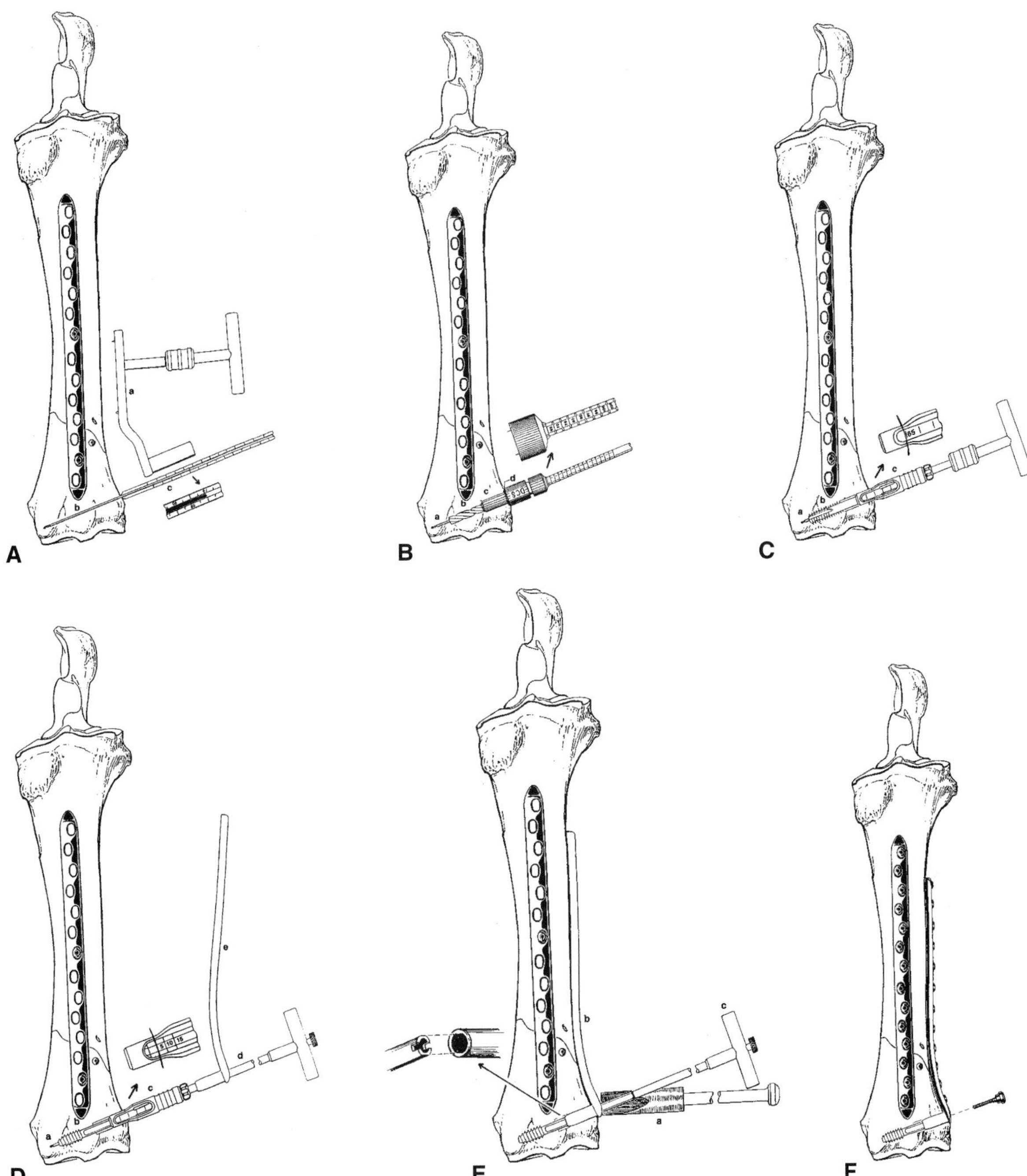

Figure 81-27. Application of an LC-DCP and a dynamic condylar screw (DCS) plate to a radius fracture. **A,** The fracture is initially repaired with two interfragmentary 3.5-mm cortex screws, applied in lag fashion. Subsequently, a 14-hole LC-DCP is applied to the cranial bone surface (tension side) under compression. The guide pin (b) is applied through the special drill guide (a). The measuring device (c) applied over the guide pin allows determination of the length of the pin inserted in the bone (70 mm). **B,** The DCS-triple reamer is assembled and set for the 65-mm drilling depth, which is 5 mm less than the pin length in the bone and ensures maintenance of the pin during DCS screw insertion. The triple reamer is placed over the guide pin (a) and the shaft hole for the DCS screw (b), the barrel hole for the plate (c), and the barrel–plate junction (d) are prepared. **C,** The DCS centering sleeve (c) is placed over the tap (b), which is subsequently placed over the guide pin (a). After inserting the centering sleeve into the barrel hole, the tap is advanced to the desired depth (65 mm). **D,** The DCS coupling screw (d) is placed through the T-handle and the DCS plate (e) is selected (12-hole), and connected to the DCS screw (b) of the desired length (60 mm). The centering sleeve (c) is applied over the coupling screw. After placing the assembly over the guide pin, the screw is inserted to a depth of 65 mm, which is marked on the centering sleeve as 5 mm. **E,** After tightening the screw and adjusting the horizontal bar of the T-handle parallel to the long axis of the bone, the DCS plate is seated over the shaft of the DCS screw with the help of the DCS impactor (a) and a mallet (not shown). Orientation of the instruments and implants is important, because the DCS screw *(left insert)* and the plate barrel *(right insert)* contain complementary parallel contours, which have to be aligned to allow sliding of the barrel over the screw shaft. **F,** The DCS compression screw is inserted through the plate barrel, inserted into the back end of the DCS screw, and tightened. This unites the three components (DCS screw, DCS plate, and connecting screw) into one unit. Insertion of all remaining screws and tightening of them completes the procedure.

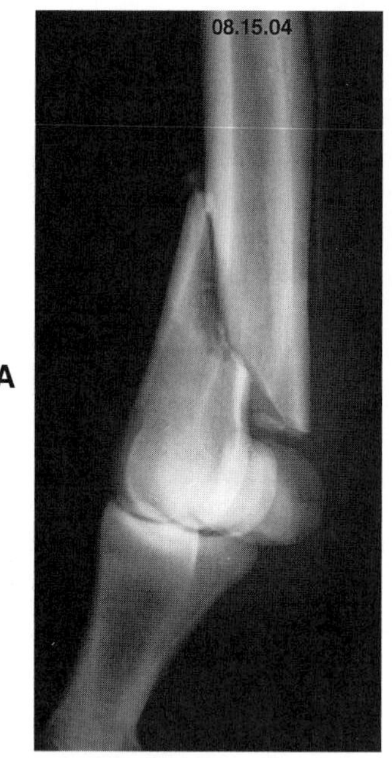

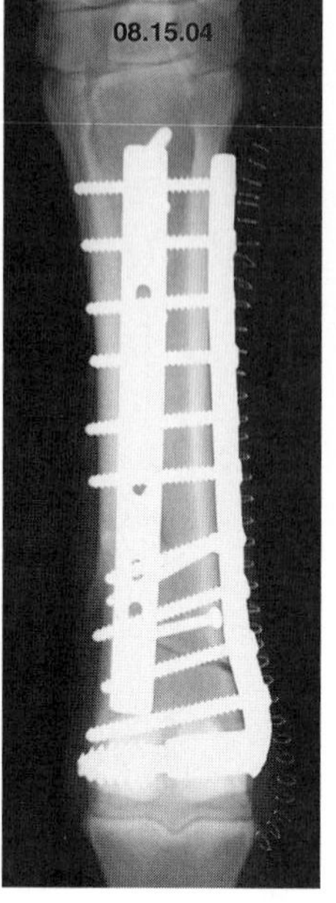

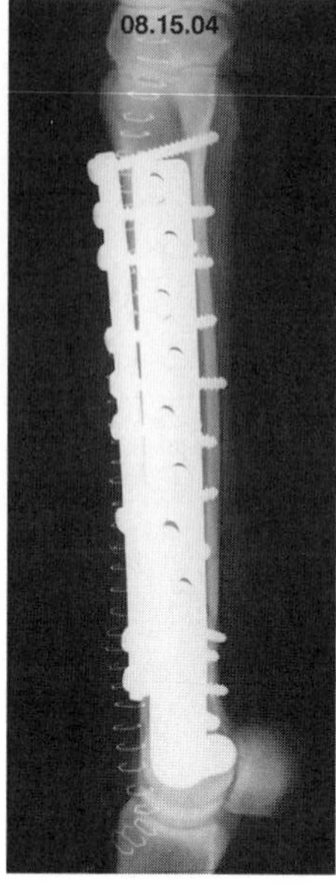

Figure 81-28. Preoperative (**A**) and postoperative (**B** and **C**) radiographs of a metaphyseal MCIII fracture in an adult Icelandic pony. The fracture was repaired with a laterally applied DCS plate and a shorter dorsal DCP.

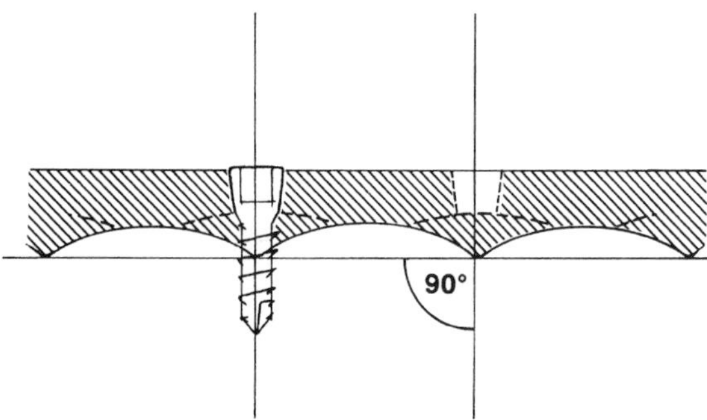

Figure 81-29. Side view of PC-Fix. The arcs under the plate are easily recognized and lead to the points in contact with the bone. The unicortical screws are implanted perpendicularly to the long axis of the plate, where the conical screw heads lock within the plate holes. This is an internal fixator. The plate is applied over the periosteum.

anatomic plate–bone interface is not important, because the screw heads interlock through a thread system with the plate, establishing a solid internal fixator. If the correct implant is selected, implantation of the system is efficient. This system is especially well suited to foals. A successful fixation has been accomplished in a tibial fracture in a calf[68] (see Fig. 81-31).

The *locking compression plate (LCP)* is an implant system that combines the two treatment methods in one implant: compression plating and internal fixators.[69] The individual construction elements in this new implant system have individually proved extremely valuable in clinical practice in human and veterinary applications alike. The combination of these elements into one implant system has been made compatible with the majority of existing instruments and conventional screws. The surgeon is free to select the function best suited for the fracture to be treated.

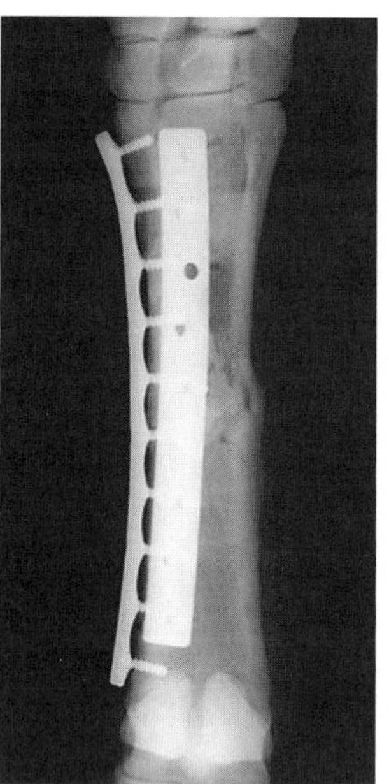

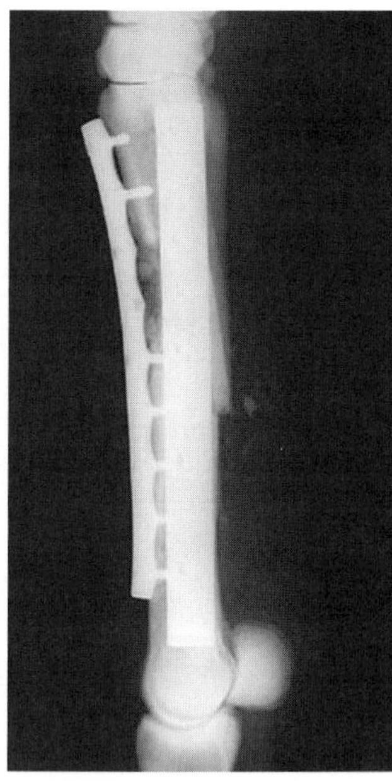

Figure 81-30. Two PC-Fix plates are applied at a right angle relative to each other in a comminuted and open MCIII fracture in a horse. Note the different configurations of the plates and the unicortical screws. With time, the empty spaces under the plate were filled with bone.

The LCP uses a Combi-Hole, which is a combination between a DCU and a LISS hole (see Fig. 81-16). The surgeon may select the type of screw to be inserted at any given place—either a 4.5-mm or a 5.5-mm cortex screw (or even a cancellous screw) at an axial angle up to 40 degrees, or a locking head screw with a thick core and thin threads and additional threads at the screw head. The locking head screw, however, has to be inserted orthogonally relative to

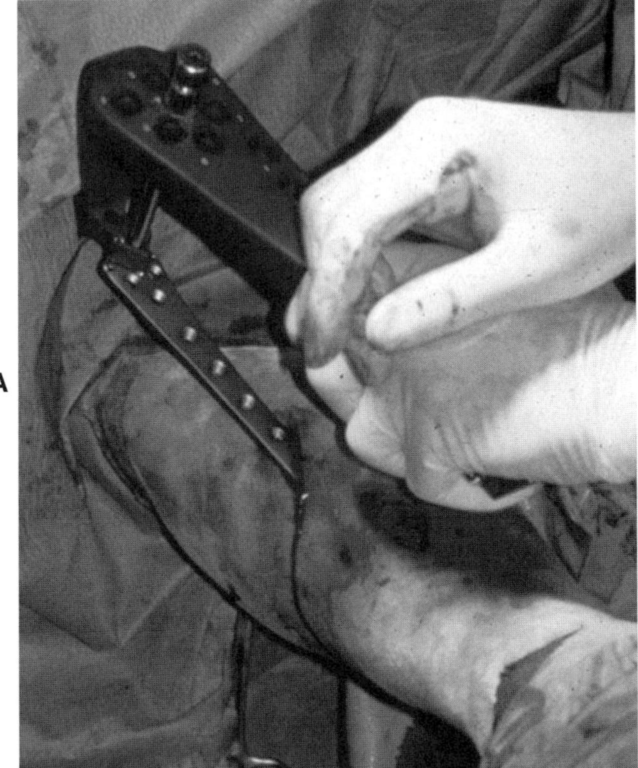

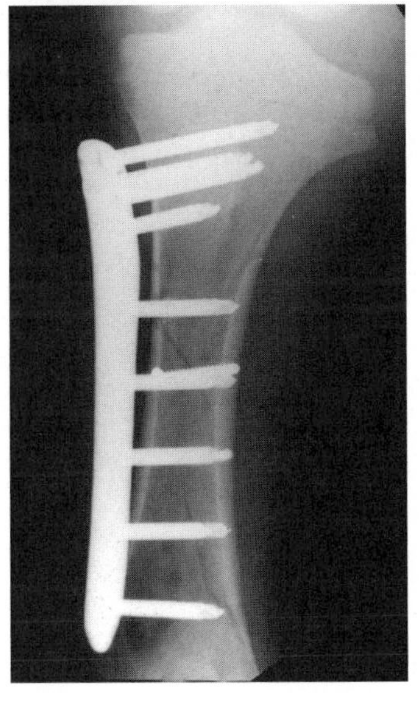

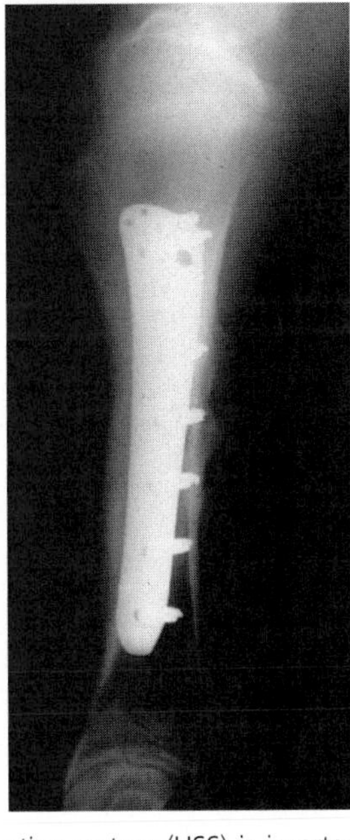

Figure 81-31. A, A less invasive stabilization system (LISS) is inserted through a small proximal incision to repair a tibial fracture. **B** and **C,** Postoperative radiographs show the plate attached to the bone, but only the screws make contact with the bone. The fracture healed without problems.

the long side of the plate. The plate contains also a beveled end at either side to allow insertion through a small incision and sliding of the plate along the periosteum of the fractured bone. A special tissue spreader has been developed to prepare the future plate bed. The thin beveled end separates the soft tissues from the periosteum. The screws may subsequently be implanted through minimally invasive stab incisions.

The clinically available LCP represents a breakthrough in internal fixation (Fig. 81-32). The implants are available in stainless steel in all sizes (see Table 81-2). The fracture fixation has to be planned ahead, because the locking screws cannot be angled in an ideal direction and therefore require solid cortical bone for purchase. Because the strength of a screw is dependent mainly on the core diameter and not thread width,[64] the thicker core of the locking screws and the thin threads make the screw several times stronger than the conventional cortex screws. A recent study revealed that the LCP is significantly stiffer than the DCP, the equine LC-DCP, and the clamp-rod internal fixator (not discussed here), making it the implant of choice for most long bone fractures if cost is not a factor.[70] Alternatively, attempts are presently underway to develop the PC-Fix as a veterinary-implant-only, with costs compatible with equine surgery.[68]

Addendum

Thorough knowledge of the basic principles of internal fixation, as well as familiarity with the instruments and numerous implants, is a prerequisite for successful surgery. Everyone interested in treating long bone fractures should register for a basic and advanced AO/ASIF course on internal fixation.

CERCLAGE WIRE

Cerclage wire is used frequently in humans and small animals.[71,72] Tension-band fixations with pins and wire are often carried out in dogs and cats. Cerclage wires are also applied around oblique long bone fractures in small animals. This type of fixation has not been successful in horses because of a lack of stability and breakdown of the fixation. However, cerclage wires may be applied in a few situations. Proximal sesamoid fractures can be successfully treated with cerclage wires.[73] Also, this type of fixation has been used in connection with small Steinmann pins to provide temporary stabilization of comminuted long bone fractures prior to plate and lag screw application.[3]

One frequent application of cerclage wire is growth retardation surgery, even though the wire is not applied in cerclage fashion (see Chapter 89). Cerclage wires have been used to treat nondisplaced ulnar fractures in foals.[74,75] The wires are passed through holes placed in the frontal plane across the proximal and distal fragments of the ulna. A small loop created before entering the hole in the distal fragment allows even tightening on both sides of the bone after the wire is applied in figure-eight fashion, and the ends are twisted together. This type of fixation results in reduced trauma to the ulna and radius, and it avoids inadvertent fixation of the ulna to the radius, which can occur when using a plate in a young foal. (This may induce subluxation of the cubital joint.) A total of three to four figure-eight wires are applied.

Cerclage wire is used in arthrodeses of the fetlock joint.[76] In comminuted fractures of the proximal sesamoid bones associated with complete breakdown of the suspensory apparatus, a tension band is inserted in figure-eight fashion through the palmar/plantar aspect of the metacarpophalangeal joint, prior to applying the dorsal plate[76] (see Chapter 85).

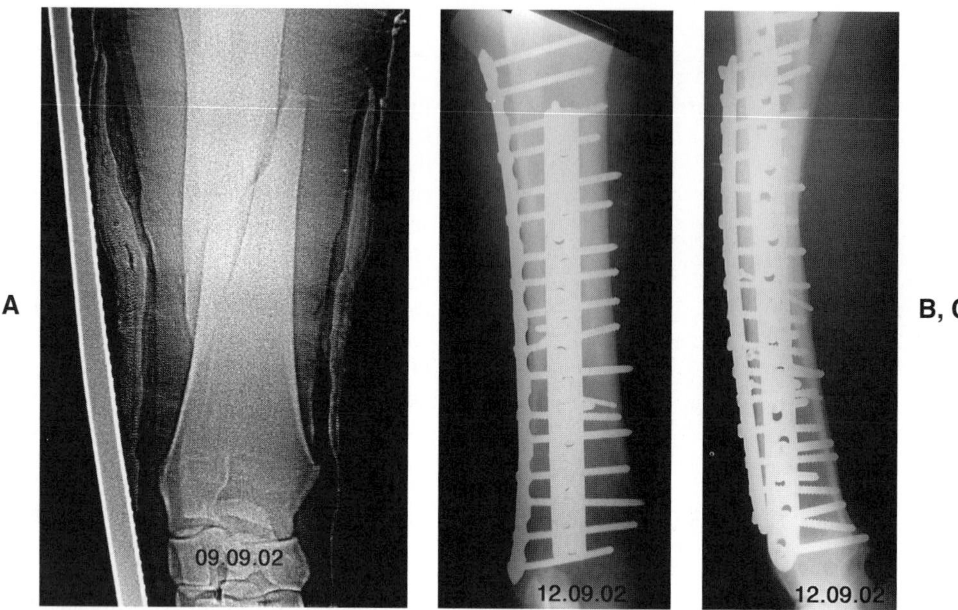

Figure 81-32. Preoperative (**A**) and postoperative (**B** and **C**) radiographs of an oblique, spiral radial fracture. The fracture was repaired with a 17-hole LC-LCP laterally and a 14-hole 5.5 DCP preliminary arthrodesis plate cranially. The undercuts of the LCP are easily recognized under the lateral plate.

Wire tightening is carried out with utmost prudence. Initially, the wires are loosely twisted by hand. Then, with a pair of flat pliers, the two ends are grabbed, pulled at a right angle away from the bone and, while decreasing the pulling force, evenly twisted around each other. Care must be taken not to twist one wire end around the straight end of the other wire (this type of fixation slips off under tension). Overtightening may result in wire breakage and breakdown of the fixation.

CABLES

Two types of cables have been introduced into orthopedic surgery as treatment modality for specific fractures. Ultra-high-molecular weight polyethylene (UHMWPE) cable (Securos, Charlton, Mass) has been tested in an in vitro model for the repair of proximal sesamoid bone fractures and compared against the commonly used stainless steel cerclage wire (SSCW). The ultimate tensile strength of UHMWPE cable constructs was 34% greater than that of SSCW constructs. Fatigue strength was 2 to 20 times greater for UHMWPE cable constructs than for SSCW constructs. Separation of fragments was 153% less for limbs repaired by the cable construct compared with those repaired by the transfixed cerclage technique.[77] These cables may also be beneficial in the use of fetlock breakdown injuries, as a palmar figure-eight tension band.

Another type of cable consists of multiple weaved stainless steel, titanium alloy, or cobalt chromium alloy strands (Synthes, Paoli, Pa). It is available as 1.0- and 1.7-mm-diameter cables, consisting of a central bundle of 19 strands surrounded by eight outer bundles of seven strands each (Fig. 81-33). It is designed to be used with all Synthes stainless steel and titanium plates. Specially designed positioning pins are used in empty plate holes and the cable is threaded through an oblong hole in the pin. Once the cable is tightened, the pin cannot move because it is pressed into the plate hole and therefore confined. A special tensioning device is used to tighten the cable before it is crimped with the help of a cable crimper. Care should be taken to not exceed 50 kg of tension. Applying tension at levels higher than 50 kg may cause the cable to cut through soft or osteopenic bone (which is not a problem in horses). This product is used mainly in human orthopedic surgery in the management of periprosthetic fractures in elderly adults, where other internal fixation devices are not successful.[78] Additionally, it is used in the tension-band function in the management of patellar fractures and olecranon osteotomies. Indications for these cables are similar to those for the UHMWPE cables in horses.

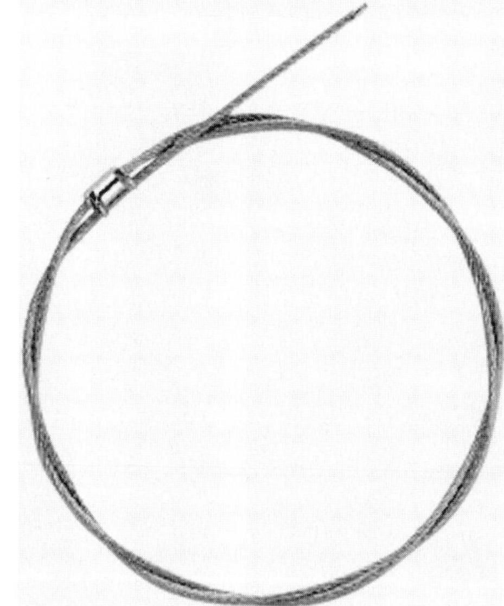

Figure 81-33. The Synthes 1.7-mm stainless steel cable with the crimp device placed over it.

PINS

Steinmann pins

Steinmann pins are not frequently used in fracture treatment in horses, mainly because they do not provide stability.[79] They are used as transfixation pins in conjunction with external coaptation (see earlier discussion).

Intramedullar application of Steinmann pins is used only in humeral fractures in foals.[79] Multiple pins are introduced parallel to each other to fill the entire medullary space at its isthmus at the distal third of the bone. This "stacked pin" method is presently the treatment of choice in these fractures. For additional stability, these pins may be encircled by cerclage wires and placed into the medullary cavity, possibly through a cortical defect or a drill hole. The wires are subsequently tightened. In cases with a cortical defect, the cerclage may also be applied intramedullarly. The advantage of the stacked pin method is an increase in rotational and bending stability. A single pin provides no rotational stability. Collapse of the fracture along the single pin is a frequent complication.

Application of multiple pins across a capital femoral physeal fracture has been advocated and has met with some success. Steinmann pins have also been used in the treatment of olecranon fractures in the very young foal in combination with a tension band made of multiple cerclage wires.[79]

Rush pins

The Rush pin method of fracture treatment was popular before bone plating was introduced. Fracture fixation using these devices is an art.[80] The slightly pre-bent pins are introduced obliquely into the distal fragment and advanced toward the opposite cortex. The tip, which is flattened on one side, slides off the opposite cortex and is redirected toward the *cis*-cortex. The pin length has to allow the tips to engage in the *cis*-cortex both proximally and distally to the fracture, providing four-point contact. Usually, two pins are introduced, one from each side of the bone. When performed correctly, rotational stability is achieved with a minimum of implants and surgical trauma. The Rush pin fixation technique is not applicable to comminuted or open fractures.

NAILS

Intramedullary nails have a place in equine long bone fracture repair, but the ideal implant has not been developed despite recent efforts.[9,33] Initially, intramedullary nails manufactured for human application were tried in equine fractures with mixed success.[81] For example, in two reports, a solid titanium nail was inserted through the middle carpal joint after removing the articular cartilage of the middle carpal and carpometacarpal joints.[82,83] The joints were fused to facilitate solid fixation. Transfixation was achieved with 4.5-mm screws inserted through the proximal aspect of the nail. Although good results were achieved, the fact that the joints had to be fused to facilitate healing of MCIII was undesirable. Healing of these fractures can be achieved with plating techniques without fusing a joint.

A system of intramedullary interlocking nails (IIN) has been developed for equine humeral and femoral fractures[84-87] (Fig. 81-34). Comparison of this method of fracture repair to fracture plating have been met with mixed results in experimental studies. A cadaveric in vitro biomechanical study on immature equine femurs revealed that a diaphyseal osteotomy fixed with two DCPs at 90 degrees relative to each other provided superior strength and stiffness compared with an IIN and a construct of an IIN and cranially applied DCP.[85] In another in vitro study on osteotomized tibias, a construct composed of a 16-mm stainless steel nail with a

A

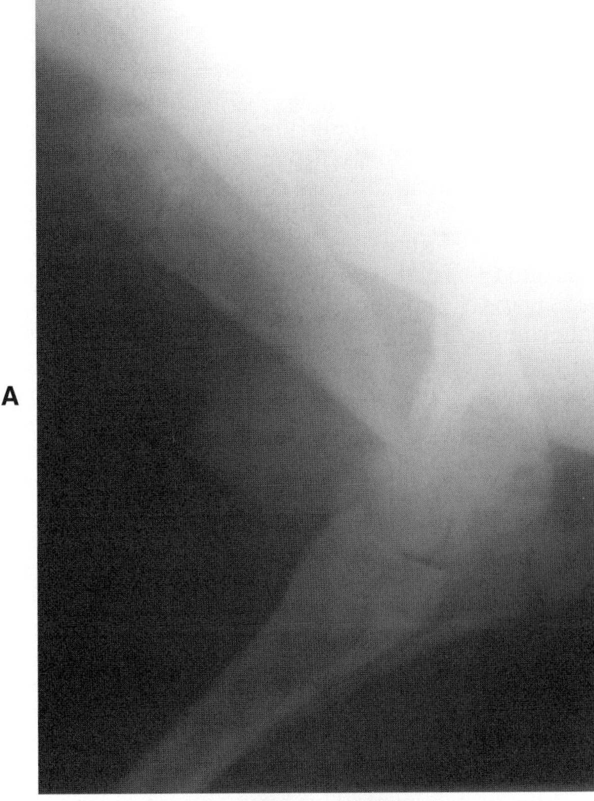

B

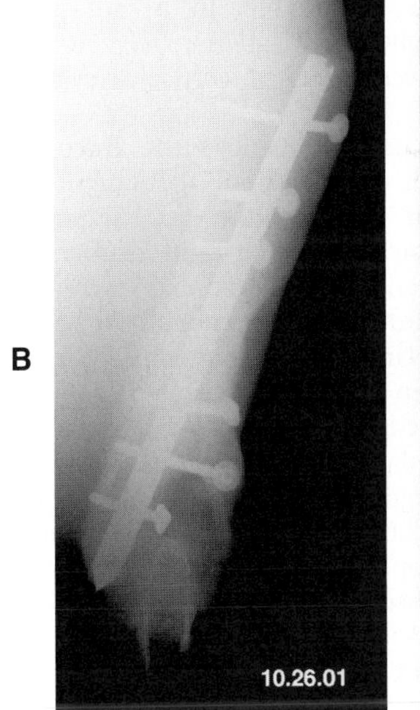

C

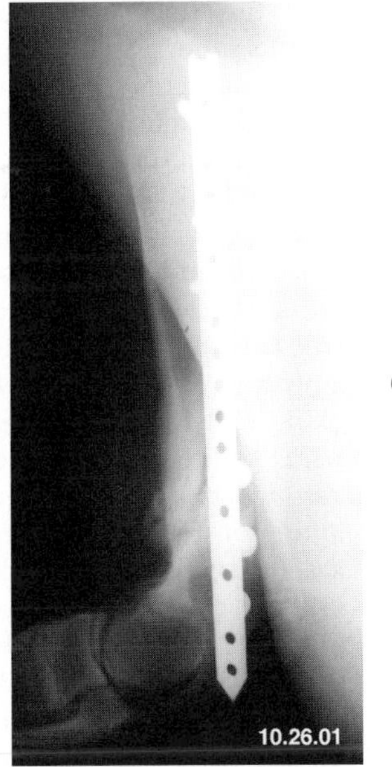

Figure 81-34. This long oblique humeral fracture (**A**) was treated with an intramedullary interlocking nail. To provide a greater screw-bone contact area, washers were used. The craniocaudal (**B**) and lateromedial (**C**) 2-month follow-up radiographs show progressive bone healing in the fracture gap. Bone length is maintained. (Courtesy J. P. Watkins, Texas A&M University.)

wall thickness of 4 mm and four 8-mm interlocking screws was compared with a human interlocking nail (UFN, Synthes Inc., Solothurn, Switzerland) and to tibias treated by means of double plating.[88] The interlocking nails achieved similar loads until failure, but the plates demonstrated higher yield loads. Recent in vitro cadaveric studies tested several interlocking nail configurations in MCIII and femora in foals,[89,90] and in MCIII with and without a gap in adult horses.[91,92] All constructs were weaker than the intact bone, and the parallel alignment of the holes for the interlocking screws were stronger than the offset screws.[91] One study compared IIN with a combination of an IIN and a DCP, and with two DCPs in a 1-cm gap model in foals, showing the double-plating construct to be closest to the intact bone in most aspects, followed by the combination and the IIN alone.[90]

Several application principles have been advocated in foals for the presently used equine IIN.[93] The location and configuration of the fracture significantly affects the ultimate outcome of the repair. If possible, three interlocking screws should be inserted on either side of the fracture. Fractures near the epiphysis are less readily stabilized with an IIN, and the epiphyseal segment is at an increased risk for secondary fracture through the interlocking screw holes. In these instances, some type of supplemental fixation is desirable to decrease the potential of catastrophic failure of the fixation. In long oblique fractures, the IIN should be positioned to allow one or two interlocking screws placed in lag fashion across the fracture plane, if possible. In a nail–plate construct, the plate is applied 90 degrees relative to the interlocking screws. Whenever possible, bicortical screws are inserted through the plate.

A lateral approach is used to expose the fractured humerus and femur. Prior to reduction, the fracture is débrided and the medullary cavity of the distal fragment reamed. Reaming is accomplished with rigid reamers of increasing size to arrive at an ultimate hole diameter of 13 mm. This procedure destroys the intramedullary blood supply and slows healing. Unreamed intramedullary interlocking nails have not been successfully applied in living horses. Additional exposure is usually necessary to provide access to the proximal end of the bone for normograde reaming of the proximal segment. After both fragments are reamed, the fracture is reduced and held in that position with bone clamps. An appropriate-length nail is chosen, and with the targeting jig attached, the nail is inserted into the reamed medullary canal. Washers are used to prevent the conical heads of the cortex screws from penetrating the cortical bone. A successful result was achieved with an IIN in 5 of 10 foals with humerus fractures; the foals ranged in weight from 136 to 204 kg. They attained athletic soundness and performed their intended purpose without complications. Three out of three neonates with femoral fractures healed after IIN fixation. Four out of six older foals with short oblique femur fractures also were successfully treated in this manner. In these foals, a DCP was applied to the cranial aspect of the bone in addition to an IIN.

AFTERCARE

After fracture fixation with any of the internal fixation devices and techniques described here, overlying soft tissues and skin are closed in routine fashion. Application of continuous suture patterns is advocated to reduce surgery time. Depending on the type of fixation and the technique of recovery from anesthesia, application of some type of external coaptation may be considered, because the animal has to be able to get up and place weight on the limb immediately after surgery. If a pool recovery is implemented, the limb and skin incision is in most cases protected only by a plastic adhesive sheet (Ioban 2, 3M Health Care, St. Paul, Minn) after applying cyanoacrylate Superglue to the skin incision. This sheet is covered with elastic adhesive tape (Elasticon, 3M Health Care), which is exchanged for a regular bandage or splint bandage after successful recovery from anesthesia (see Chapters 18 and 22).

External coaptation may consist of a fiberglass cast or a heavy splint bandage (see Chapter 18). Depending on the type of fixation, external coaptation is maintained for a few days to weeks. A fiberglass cast can be applied over a bandaged limb, and after the cast has cured, it can be split in half along the frontal plane. These "half shells" are reapplied using nonelastic adhesive tape. Such coaptation allows evaluation and, if necessary, wound management of the limb underneath. The unaffected contralateral limb should be protected and supported by a pressure bandage. In young foals, too much support is to be avoided to prevent temporary weakness of the flexor tendons. It is important to keep the patient comfortable with the help of moderate amounts of anti-inflammatory and analgesic drugs. These drugs should be used judiciously to prevent toxic reactions and to allow some residual amount of pain, so the patient will protect the injured limb. If a nonweightbearing lameness lasts for a prolonged period, other problems develop in the healthy limbs.

Application of a frog pad in adult horses may prevent the development of laminitis in the contralateral foot. Laminitis is the major complication that occurs after fracture repair. Again, administration of anti-inflammatory drugs in moderate amounts may prevent this problem. As early as possible, the animals should be allowed to walk. Although controlled exercise is advocated, free pasture exercise is discouraged. This is especially important if a weightbearing fixation was performed and the animal is not placed in an external coaptation device. Patients with casts should not be exercised at all.

Implant Removal

Implants are foreign bodies and may have to be removed, particularly in young athletes. Therefore, implant removal depends on the use of the horse, the type of fracture treated, the type of implants employed, and the potential development of complications, including postoperative infection. Lag screws are not removed in horses unless they produce pain or bone reactions. Recently, the practice of removing lag screws in young racehorses has gained popularity. Frequently, the reason for implant removal is a request by the owner. Cerclage wire used for fracture fixation does not need to be removed unless the wire breaks, as it does frequently in the treatment of transverse fractures of the proximal sesamoid bones.[71] Plates applied to long bones of horses should be removed in most cases. This is especially important if the animal enters or resumes an athletic career. Implants applied to the femur or olecranon and for arthrodesis purposes are left in place. This presupposes that no problems are encountered with the implants.

When to remove implants after the fracture has healed depends on the age of the animal, the type of fracture treated, and the implants used. In a condylar or stress fracture of MCIII/MTIII, screws may be removed about 2 months postoperatively. Plate removal in foals may be carried out at an average of 4 to 6 months after fracture treatment. Staggered removal of the implants is advocated if two plates were applied, because it reduces the risk of refracturing the bone through one of the screw holes. (Filling the empty screw holes in the bone with a bone graft has been recommended in humans.[64])

An important reason for implant removal is infection surrounding the implants. An infection, once established around implants, persists and does not resolve until after the implants have been removed, even in the presence of broad-spectrum antimicrobials.[29] Fractures can heal in the presence of infection if rigid internal fixation is maintained. However, it is frequently a race between loosening of the implants caused by the infection, and healing of the fracture. Once an infected fracture is healed, the implants are removed to allow resolution of the infection. If the implants are removed too early, before adequate healing of the fracture has occurred, refracture of the bone is likely. In one case, however, where titanium implants were applied to a comminuted open fracture of the proximal MTIII in a Thoroughbred foal, a postoperative infection resolved completely prior to implant removal (Fig. 81-35).

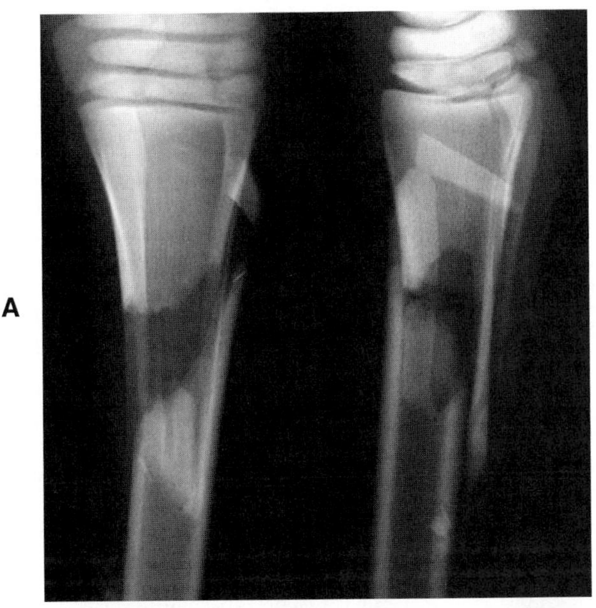

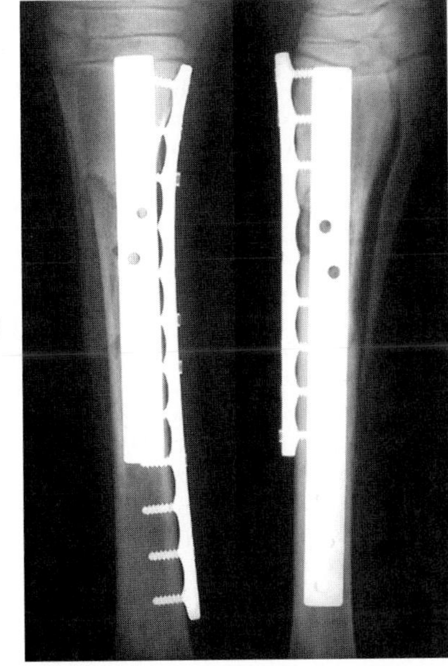

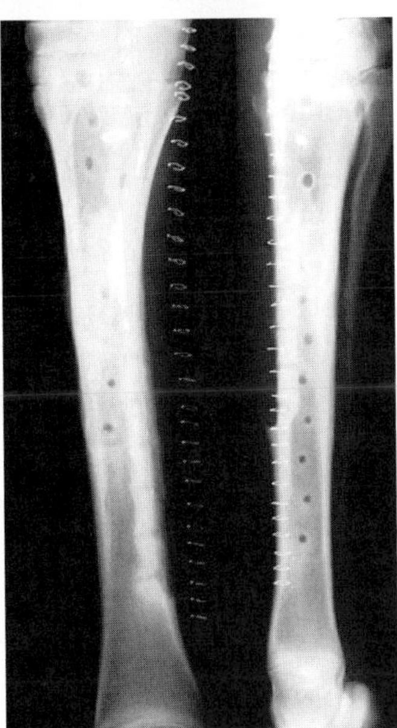

Figure 81-35. A 2-month-old Thoroughbred colt was admitted with a comminuted fracture of MTIII. **A,** The fracture was treated with two PC-Fix plates applied over the periosteum. **B,** This prevented adequate visualization and resulted in suboptimal fracture reduction. An infection developed, which was managed with parenteral broad-spectrum antibiotics, daily flushing of the surgical site, and local antibiotic application. Within a month, the infection had resolved. **C,** Bacterial cultures taken at the time of implant removal revealed no growth. The foal developed into a successful racehorse.

REFERENCES

1. Müller ME, Allgöwer M, Schneider R, Willenegger H: Manual of Internal Fixation, ed 3, Berlin, 1990, Springer Verlag.
2. Johnson AL, Houlton JEF, Vannini R: AO Principles of Fracture Management in the Dog and Cat, Stuttgart, 2005, Thieme.
3. Fackelman GE, Auer JA, Nunamaker DM: AO Principles of Equine Osteosynthesis, Stuttgart, 2000, Thieme.
4. Auer JA: Internal fixation. In Mayhew IG, Merritt AL, Colahan P, Moore JN, editors: Equine Medicine and Surgery, ed 5, St Louis, 1999, Mosby.
5. Schenk RK, Wilenegger H: Zum histologischen Bild der sogenannten Primärheilung der Knochenkompakta nach experimentellen Osteotomien am Hund, Experientia 1963;19:593.
6. Hierzolzer G, Allgöwer M, Rüedi TH: Fixateur Externe-Osteosynthese, Berlin, 1985, Springer-Verlag.
7. Egger EL: Static strength evaluation of six external skeletal fixation configurations, Vet Surg 12:130, 1983.
8. Nemeth F, Back W: The use of the walking cast to repair fractures in horses and ponies, Equine Vet J 1991;23:32.
9. Nixon AJ, Watkins JP, Auer JA: Principles of fracture treatment. In Nixon AJ, editor: Equine Fracture Repair, Philadelphia, 1996, WB Saunders.
10. Taylor DS, Stover SM, Willits N: The effect of differing pin size on the mechanical performance of transfixation in the equine third metacarpal bone, Proc Vet Orthop Soc Lake Louise, Canada, 1993;20:2.
11. McClure SR, Watkins JP, Bronson DG, Ashman RP: In vitro comparison of the effect of parallel and divergent transfixation pins on breaking strength of equine third metatarsal bones, J Am Vet Res 1994;55:1327.
12. McClure SR, Watkins JP, Hogan HA: In vitro evaluation of four methods of attaching transfixation pins into a fiberglass cast for use in horses, Am J Vet Res 1996;57:1098.
13. McClure SR, Watkins JP, Bronson DG, Ashman RP: In vitro comparison of the standard sort limb cast and three configurations of short limb transfixation casts in equine fore limbs, J Am Vet Res 1994;55:1331.
14. McClure SR, Hillberry BM, Fisher KE: In vitro comparison of metaphyseal and diaphyseal placement of centrally threaded, positive-profile transfixation pins in the equine third metacarpal bone, Am J Vet Res 2000;61:1304.
15. Matter G: Mechanische Untersuchung verschiedener Fixateur externe Konfigurationen am Röhrenbein des Pferdes: Eine in vitro Studie, Thesis, Zurich, Switzerland, 1993, University of Zurich.
16. Frigg R: Development of new products at the AO ASIF Development Institute, Proc Am Coll Vet Surg, Large Animal Vet Symp, Chicago, 1995;5:229.
17. Lischer CJ, Fluri E, Kaser-Hotz B, et al: Pinless external fixation of mandible fractures in cattle, Vet Surg 1997;26:14.
18. Frigg R: The development of the pinless external fixator: From the idea to the implant—Introduction, Injury 1992;23:S3.
19. Nunamaker DM, Richardson DW, Butterweck DM, et al: A new external skeletal fixation device that allows immediate weight bearing: Application in the horse, Vet Surg 1986;15:345.
20. Richardson DW, Nunamaker DM, Sigafoos RD: Use of an external skeletal fixation device and bone graft for arthrodesis of the metacarpophalangeal joint in horses, J Am Vet Med Assoc 1987;191:316.
21. Nunamaker DM, Richardson DW: External skeletal fixation in the horse, Proc Am Assoc Equine Pract 1992;37:549.
22. Huiskes R, Chao EYS, Crippen TE: Parametric analysis of pin-bone stresses in external fracture fixation devices, J Orthop Res 1985;3:341.
23. Nash RA, Nunamaker DM, Boston R: Evaluation of a tapered-sleeve transcortical pin to reduce stress at the bone-pin interface in metacarpal bones obtained from horses, Am J Vet Res 2001;62:955.
24. Bignozzi L, Gnudi M, Masetti L, et al: Half pin fixation in 2 cases of equine long bone fractures, Equine Vet J 1981;13:64.
25. Sullins KE, McIlwraith CW: Evaluation of 2 types of external skeletal fixation for repair of experimental tibia fractures in foals, Vet Surg 1987;16:255.
26. Rahn B: Personal communication, 1989.
27. Lambotte A: Chirurgie opératoire des fractures, Paris, 1913, Masson.
28. Danis R: Théorie et pratique de l'ostéosynthèse, Paris, 1947, Masson.
29. Bramlage LR: Long bone fractures, Vet Clin North Am Large Anim Pract 1983;5:285.
30. Auer JA: Surgical equipment and implants for fracture repair. In Nixon AJ, editor: Equine Fracture Repair, Philadelphia, 1996, WB Saunders.
31. Farouk O, Krettek C, Miclau T, et al: Minimally invasive plate osteosynthesis and vascularity: Preliminary results of a cadaver injection study, Injury 1997;28(Suppl 1):S-A7.
32. Rahm C, Ito K, Auer J: Lagscrew fixation of equine cannon bone fractures: A biomechanical comparative study of shaft and shaftless cortical screws, Vet Surg 2000;29;564.
33. Auer JA, Watkins JP: Instrumentation and techniques in equine fracture fixation, Vet Clin North Am Equine Pract 1996;12:283.
34. Fackelman GE, Auer JA: The AO/ASIF 7.3 mm cannulated screw in a model of the equine distal limb, Equine Pract 1996;18:15.
35. Johnson NL, Galuppo LD, Stover SM, et al: An in vitro biomechanical comparison of the insertion variables and pullout mechanical properties of AO 6.5-mm standard cancellous and 7.3-mm self-tapping, cannulated bone screws in foal femoral bone, Vet Surg 2004;33:691.
36. Baumgart FW, Cordey J, Morikawa K, et al: AO/ASIF selftapping screws (STS), Injury 1995;24(Suppl 1):S1.
37. Schnewlin M, Auer JA: The AO/ASIF self-tapping 4.5 mm screws (STS), Proc Ann Symp Am Coll Vet Surg 1995;5:231.
38. Andrea CR, Stover SM, Galuppo LD, et al: Comparison of insertion time and pullout strength between self-tapping and nonself-tapping AO 4.5-mm cortical bone screws in adult equine third metacarpal bone, Vet Surg 2002;31:189.
39. Frigg R, Appenzeller A, Christensen R, et al: The development of the distal femur less invasive stabilization system (LISS), Injury 2001;32;SC24.
40. Fankhauser C, Frenk A, Marti A: A comparative biomechanical evaluation of three systems for internal fixation of distal femur fractures, Orthopaedic Research Society Poster Presentation, 1999, Anaheim.
41. Herthel DJ, Moody JL, Lauper I: The repair of condylar fractures of the third metacarpal bone and the third metatarsal bone using the Herbert compression screw in nine Thoroughbred racehorses, Equine Pract 1995;19:6.
42. Galuppo LD, Stover SM, Jensen DG, et al: A biomechanical comparison of headless tapered variable pitch and AO cortical bone screws for fixation of simulated lateral condylar fractures in equine third metacarpal bones, Vet Surg 2001;30:332.
43. Galuppo LD, Stover SM, Jensen DG: A biomechanical comparison of equine third metacarpal condylar bone fragment compression and screw pushout strength between headless tapered variable pitch and AO cortical bone screws, Vet Surg 2002;31:201.
44. Eddy AL, Galuppo LD, Stover SM, et al: A Biomechanical comparison of headless tapered variable pitch compression and AO cortical bone screws for fixation of a simulated midbody transverse fracture of the proximal sesamoid bone in horses, Vet Surg 2004;33:253.
45. Yovich JV, Turner AS, Smith FW: Holding power of orthopedic screws in equine third metacarpal and metatarsal bones: Part I. Foal bone, Vet Surg 1985;14:221.
46. Yovich JV, Turner AS, Smith FW: Holding power of orthopedic screws in equine third metacarpal and metatarsal bones: Part 2. Foal bone, Vet Surg 1985;14:230.

47. Yovich JV, Turner AS, Smith RX, Davis DM: Holding power of orthopedic screws: Comparison of self-tapped and pre-tapped screws in foal bone, Vet Surg 1986;15:55.
48. Nunamaker DM, Perren SM: Force measurements in screw fixation, J Biomech 1976;9:669.
49. Olmstead ML, Schenk R, Pohler O, et al: Bone screw holding power: The effect of surface character and metal type, Vet Surg 15:128, 1986.
50. Danis R: The operative treatment of bone fractures, J Int Chir 1947;7:318.
51. Bagby GW, Janes JM: An impacting bone plate, Mayo Clinic Proc 1957;32:55,
52. Perren SM, Allgöwer M, Brunner H, et al: Das Konzept der biologischen Osteosynthese unter Anwendung der Dynamischen Kopmressionsplatte mit limitiertem Kontakt (LC-DCP), Injury Suppl 1991;22:1.
53. Monney G, Cordey J, Rahn B: Untersuchungen über die Blutzufuhr nach der Plattenosteosynthese mit DCP und LC-DCP, Injury Suppl 1991;22:18.
54. Allgöwer M, Matter P, Perren SM, Rüedi T: The dynamic compression plate DCP, Berlin, 1973, Springer-Verlag.
55. Nunamaker DM, Bowmann KF, Richardson DW, Herring M: Plate luting: A preliminary report on its use in horses, Vet Surg 1986;15:289.
56. Turner AS, Cordey JR, Nunamaker DM, et al: In vivo strain patterns of the intact equine metacarpus and metatarsus following plate luting, Vet Comp Orthop Traumatol 1990;3:84.
57. Turner AS, Smith FW, Nunamaker DM, et al: Improved plate fixation of unstable fractures due to bone cement around the screw heads, Vet Surg 1991;20:349.
58. Auer JA, Watkins JP: Treatment of radial fractures in adult horses: An analysis of 15 cases, Equine Vet J 1987;19:103.
59. Sanders-Shamis M, Bramlage LR: Radius fractures in the horse: A retrospective study of 47 cases, Equine Vet J 1986;18:432.
60. Regazzoni P, Rüedi T, Allgöwer M: The dynamic hip screw implant system, Berlin, 1987, Springer-Verlag.
61. Auer JA: Application of the dynamic condylar screw (DCS)-dynamic hip screw (DHS) implant system in the horse, Vet Comp Orthop Traumatol 1988;1:18.
62. Hunt DA, Snyder JR, Morgan JP, Pascoe JR: Femoral capital physeal fractures in 25 foals, Vet Surg 1990;19:41.
63. Miclau T, Martin RE: The evolution of modern plate osteosynthesis, Injury 1997;28(Suppl 1):A3.
64. Tepic S, Perren SM: The biomechanics of the PC-Fix internal fixator, Injury 1995;26(Suppl 2):S-B5.
65. Auer JA, Lischer C, Kaegi B, et al: Application of the point contact fixator in large animals, Injury 1995;26(Suppl 2):B37.
66. Savoldelli D, Montavon P: Clinical handling: Small animals, Injury 1995;26(Suppl 2):B47.
67. Marti A, Fankhauser C, Frenk A, et al: Biomechanical evaluation of the less invasive stabilization system (LISS) for fixation of distal femur fractures, J Orthop Trauma 2001;14:133.
68. Auer JA: Internal fixators, Proc Eur Coll Vet Surg 2004;13:202.
69. Frigg R: Locking compression plate (LCP): An osteosynthesis plate based on the dynamic compression plate and the point contact fixator (PC-Fix), Injury 2001;32:B63-66.
70. Florin M, Arzdorf M, Linke B, et al: Assessment of stiffness and strength of four different implants available for equine fracture treatment: A study on a 20 degree oblique long bone fracture model using a bone substitute, Vet Surg 2005;34:231.
71. Blass CE, Caldarise SG, Torzin PA, et al: Mechanical properties of three orthopedic wire configurations, Am J Vet Res 1985;46:1725.
72. Hulse DA, Nelson J, Herron M: Cerclage, hemicerclage and tension band application, Texas Vet Med Assoc J 1988;50:23.
73. Martin BB, Nunamaker DM, Evans LH, et al: Tension band repair of mid body and large base sesamoid fractures in 15 horses, Vet Surg 1991;20:9.
74. Richardson DW: Ulnar fractures. In White NA, Moore JN, editors: Current Practice of Equine Surgery, Philadelphia, 1990, JB Lippincott.
75. Nixon AJ: Fractures of the ulna. In Nixon AJ, editor: Equine Fracture Repair, Philadelphia, 1996, WB Saunders.
76. Bramlage LT: Arthrodesis of the fetlock joint. In Mansman RA, McAlister GS, editors: Equine Medicine and Surgery, ed 2, Santa Barbara, Calif, 1982, American Veterinary Publications.
77. Rothaug PG, Boston RC, Richardson DW, et al: A comparison of ultra-high molecular weight polyethylene cable and stainless steel wire using two fixation techniques for repair of equine midbody sesamoid fractures: An in vitro biomechanical study, Vet Surg 2002;31:454.
78. Parvizi J, Venkat R, Rapuri JJ, et al: Treatment protocol for proximal femoral periprosthetic fractures, J Bone Joint Surg 2004;78A(Suppl 2):8.
79. Turner AS: Equine orthopedics. In Jennings PB, editor: The practice of large animal surgery, Philadelphia, 1984, WB Saunders.
80. Foerner JJ: The use of Rush pins in long bone fractures, Proc Am Assoc Equine Pract 1977;23:223.
81. Fröhlich D: Versuche zur intramedullären Osteosynthese des Metacarpus beim Pferd. Thesis, 1973, University of Zürich, Switzerland.
82. Herthel DJ, Lauper L, Rick MC, et al: Comminuted MCIII fracture treatment using titanium static interlocking intramedullary nails, Equine Pract 1996;18:26.
83. Herthel DJ: Application of the interlocking intramedullary nail. In: Nixon AJ, editor: Equine Fracture Repair, Philadelphia, 1996, WB Saunders.
84. Watkins JP: Intramedullary interlocking nail fixation in foals: Effects on normal growth and development of the humerus, Vet Surg 1990;19:80.
85. Watkins JP, Ashman RB: Intramedullary interlocking nail fixation in transverse humeral fractures: An in vitro comparison with stacked pin fixation. Proc Vet Orthop Soc 1991;18:54.
86. Radcliffe RM, Lopez MJ, Turner TA, et al: An in vitro biomechanical comparison of interlocking nail constructs and double plating for fixation of diaphyseal femur fractures in immature horses, Vet Surg 2001;30:179,
87. Nixon AJ, Watkins JP: Fractures of the humerus. In Nixon AJ, editor: Equine Fracture Repair, Philadelphia, 1996, WB Saunders.
88. McDuffee LA, Stover SM, Taylor KT, Les CM: In vitro biomechanical investigation of an interlocking nail for fixation of diaphyseal tibial fractures in adult horses, Vet Surg 1994;23:219.
89. Fitch GL, Galuppo LD, Stover SM, et al: An in vitro biomechanical investigation of an intramedullary nailing technique for repair of third metacarpal and metatarsal fractures in neonates and foals, Vet Surg 2001;30:422,
90. Radcliffe, Lopez, MJ, Turner TA, et al: An in vitro biomechanical comparison of interlocking nail constructs and double plating for fixation of diaphyseal femur fractures in immature horses, Vet Surg 2001;30:179.
91 Lopez MJ, Wilson DG, Trostle SS, et al: An in vitro biomechanical comparison of two interlocking-nail systems for fixation of ostectomized equine third metacarpal bones, Vet Surg 2001;30:246.
92. Galuppo LD, Stover SM, Aldridge A, et al: An in vitro biomechanical investigation of an mp35n intramedullary interlocking nail system for repair of third metacarpal fractures in adult horses, Vet Surg 2002;31:211.
93. Watknis JP: Personal communication, 2003.

CHAPTER 82

Bone Grafts and Bone Replacements

Brigitte von Rechenberg
Jörg A. Auer

Biologic bone grafts are distinguished from synthetic bone replacements because they come from different sources and require a variety of pretreatments.[1,2] However, the mechanism by which both are integrated into host bone is similar. All grafts are eventually replaced with host tissue by a process called creeping substitution.[1,3] Mesenchymal stem cells or osteoprogenitor cells and capillary sprouts from either adjacent bone marrow, periosteum, endosteum, or surrounding soft tissues grow into the porous structure of the grafts. There, stimulated by various local substances, they differentiate into osteoblasts, producing new mineralized osteoid that is deposited either on the old matrix or on the synthetic ceramic structure. Osteoclasts are recruited from the vascular system, and they differentiate for later physiologic remodeling to mature lamellar bone.[1,3,4] Pretreatment of allogeneic or xenogeneic bone grafts is necessary to reduce antigenicity that could lead to graft rejection.[1]

TYPES AND DEFINITIONS

A distinction is made between fresh biologic bone grafts and preserved ones. A bone graft may be transferred immediately from the donor to the implant site, in which case it is a *fresh graft*. *Preserved grafts* include specially prepared pieces of dead bone—for example, decalcified, freeze-dried, irradiated, or sterilized bone. In a third category are artificial bone replacements, which consist of ceramics such as tricalcium phosphate (TCP) or hydroxyapatite (HA)[5] (see Chapter 9).

Bone grafts can be classified according to their origin. A graft harvested from one site and applied to another in the same individual is an *autograft*. An *allograft* refers to tissue removed from one individual and given to a genetically different individual in the same species. Tissue transferred between two members of different species is a *xenograft*. If the transferred tissues are applied in an anatomically similar location, the graft is an *orthotopic* graft; if the implantation site is dissimilar, the graft is referred to as *heterotopic*. Bone grafts may be composed of purely *cancellous* or *cortical* bone, or they may be composed of a combination—for example, a *corticocancellous* graft or, in combination with articular cartilage, an *osteochondral* graft. In equine orthopedic surgery, fresh bone grafts are always autografts. The most frequently used fresh grafts are autogenous cancellous bone grafts, but cortical chips taken from the fracture site, free cortical grafts, and vascularized cortical bone grafts may be used. Free cortical grafts depend on the ingrowth of host vessels for their nutrition, whereas vascularized cortical bone grafts are harvested with their blood vessels to be anastomosed to the local blood supply.

Preserved grafts are pretreated with either freezing alone, freeze-drying, radiation, sterilization, or complete or surface decalcification.[1,6] The process of pretreatment kills viable bone cells, reducing antigenicity considerably, and allows safe and sterile storage of the bone grafts. These grafts are kept in bone banks, which makes them easily available on request.[6,7] Their ease of accessibility avoids a second surgery to harvest the autografts and thus decreases surgery time.

Bone grafts are used most often to facilitate healing after long bone fracture repair, arthrodeses, and comminuted phalangeal fractures in the horse, and autogenous cancellous bone grafts are the most frequently applied type.[8] Therefore, the major emphasis in this chapter is on this technique. Bone banking is discussed for the sake of completeness. In humans and small animals, a variety of bone grafts are used, most of which are not readily applicable to the horse.

BONE GRAFTS

Functions

Depending on the type of bone grafts, their main function is osteoinduction or osteoconduction.[1] Osteoinduction refers to the local triggering of osteogenesis (new bone formation), whereas in osteoconduction, the matrix of the graft acts as a scaffold into which mesenchymal cells grow.[6] In fresh, autogenous grafts, osteogenesis occurs partially as the result of the activity of viable osteoblasts aligned on the surface of the living bone graft. Therefore, the greater the surface is, the more living cells are available and the greater is the osteogenic activity that is observed. However, up to 90% of living cells die after bone graft transfer, with only the surface cells surviving. Therefore, the greater the number of surface cells transferred, the larger is the number of osteogenic cells that survive in the graft bed. Therefore, loosely arranged cancellous bone grafts are the most desirable in the horse. The number of surviving cells is also influenced by the handling of a graft during surgery, where dehydration and compacting of the graft are to be avoided.[6]

Some systemic influences and local factors, such as local and systemic cytokines, inflammatory mediators, and growth factors, are very important for the mechanism of osteoinduction.[9-11] Cytokines are polypeptide molecules capable of signal transduction in cells through specific surface cell receptors. Inflammatory mediators elicit changes in cell metabolism through activating either cyclic guanylate cyclase (cGMP) or cyclic adenosine monophosphate (cAMP).[10,12] Cytokines, such as interleukins and tumor necrosis factors, and inflammatory mediators, such as nitric oxide and prostaglandin E_2, may be produced either by local mesenchymal, fibrous, or vascular tissue cells. On one hand, these signals attract and recruit undifferentiated mesenchymal cells from the environment to the local area; on the other hand, they also induce bone resorption, facilitating bone graft replacement (creeping substitution). Through the locally invading cells and ongoing bone matrix resorption, a myriad of local growth factors are released that allow the mesenchymal cells to proliferate and differentiate. Through various cell generations, the graft undergoes enchondral ossification into woven bone. This bone is replaced later with mature lamellar bone. Growth factors (GFs) involved in fracture healing and graft incorporation are platelet-derived GF (PDGF), fibroblast GF (FGF), insulin GF (IGF), transforming GF (TGF), and the bone morphogenetic proteins (BMP), including osteogenic proteins (OPs).[9] The BMPs and OPs belong to the TGF-β super family.[11] Various BMPs are now produced synthetically by recombinant processes with molecular biology technologies.

Support, another important function of bone grafts, is mainly derived from corticocancellous or osteochondral bone grafts. These grafts may be transferred as fresh autogenous, vascularized grafts or as allogenous grafts. With allogenous cortical grafts, there are fewer surviving cells than with cancellous bone grafts, and nutrition depends on the formation of new haversian and Volkmann's canals and canaliculi, which means it is a slow remodeling process that may take longer than 1 year, depending on the size of the graft.[13] This type of bone grafting is not very important in fracture repair in horses.

The successful incorporation of a bone graft depends on the interplay of the following six parameters[6,7]: (1) the host bed, (2) the viability of the bone graft, (3) the volume of bone to be grafted, (4) the growth factor activity of the host bed, (5) the metabolic activity index (MAI), and (6) the homostructural function of the bone graft.

The condition and location of the *host bed* determines the response to osteoprogenitor cells and perivascular connective tissue. Different bones exhibit different fracture healing rates, depending on local blood flow and bone marrow activity. The more viable and uncompromised the host bed, the better the acceptance of the bone graft.

The better the *viability* of the bone graft is, the better the acceptance of the graft. Therefore, cancellous and vascularized corticocancellous or cortical bone grafts may have the greatest chance of acceptance.

The larger the *volume* of bone to be grafted, the longer it takes to become completely incorporated into and remodeled by the host tissue. The longer the time needed for complete incorporation, the greater is the likelihood for development of complications. In large defects, there is a greater need for incorporation of a bone graft with a large surface, such as a cancellous graft. Such a graft demands absolutely rigid internal fixation until structural rigidity is achieved.

Growth factor activity of the host bed and bone graft induces proliferation of perivascular connective tissue, facilitating osteogenesis. Augmentation of the bone graft can be achieved by GFs through recruitment of additional cell populations as well.

The MAI, which is composed of parameters such as heart rate, blood flow, basic metabolic rate, respiratory rate, and body temperature, is correlated with the capacity to incorporate bone grafts, repair fractures, and respond to local growth factors.[7] The MAI of humans is 1.0, which is close to the MAI of the dog (1.5). The MAI of the horse has not yet been determined. The closer the MAI of two species, the better is the correlation of the factors influencing bone healing and the more meaningful are comparative studies conducted between them.

The *homostructural function* of a bone graft, such as "spacer" function or support function, together with the fixation technique, influences the incorporation of the graft considerably. It may take years until it is completely incorporated or rejected.[7]

Surgical Techniques

Fresh Bone Grafts

GENERAL GUIDELINES

It is advisable to use a separate surgical team for harvesting the cancellous bone graft and to plan it in such a way as to allow its immediate embedding into the recipient site by the surgeons repairing the fracture.[14] If there is any time lag between harvesting and implantation, the graft should be stored in blood-soaked sponges. It has been shown that the exposure to air or to saline-soaked sponges is harmful to the survival of cells.[14] Additionally, exposure of the bone graft to antibiotics before and during harvesting is also detrimental to survival of the cells.[15]

The bone graft should be lightly packed into the host site (Fig. 82-1). Excessive packing should be avoided to allow the host tissues and fluids ingress to nourish the graft. The graft should be exposed as much as possible to bone marrow and endosteum of the parent portion of the bone.[1] It is of paramount importance to ensure rigid internal fixation of the fracture in the presence of a bone graft to allow adequate ingrowth of a healthy vasculature. Otherwise, the cells in the bone graft may not survive, as a result of the lack of oxygen, compounded by mechanical damage.[14] Absolute asepsis is a prerequisite for successful application of a bone graft.

LOCATIONS

The principal donor sites for cancellous bone grafts in the horse include the tuber coxae (Fig. 82-2, *A*), the sternum (see Fig. 82-2, *B*), and the medial aspect of the tibia (see Fig. 82-2, *C*). All these sites are easily accessible, and large amounts of (viable) cancellous bone may be harvested.[16] There is little danger of a fracture through a cortex portal in the proximal tibia, provided the holes are appropriately located.[17] Cancellous bone samples from these conventional donor sites were evaluated for the presence of osteoprogenitor cells to those taken from the fourth coccygeal vertebra and tibial periosteum.[18] Sternal and tibial bone yielded viable osteogenic cells from 25% and 50% of horses, respectively, whereas yields from tuber coxae, coccygeal

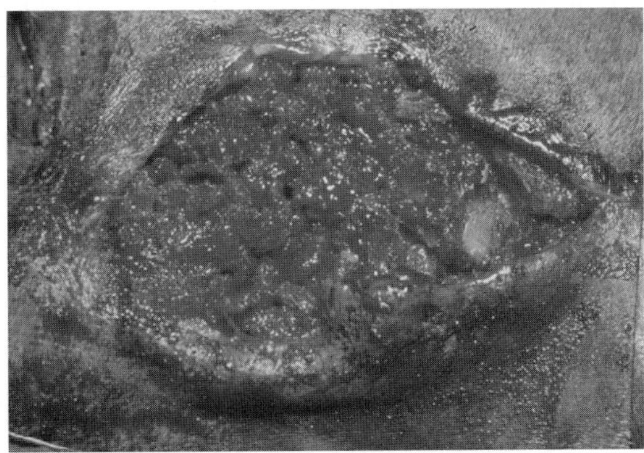

Figure 82-1. A cancellous bone graft placed in a bone defect of the skull.

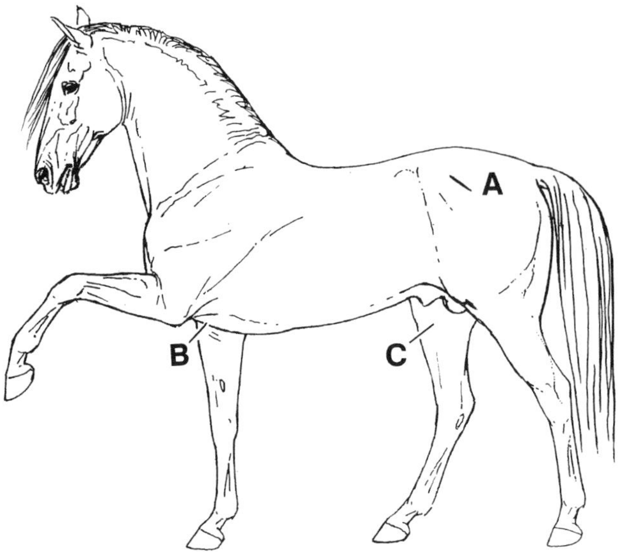

Figure 82-2. Skin incision sites used for harvesting cancellous bone for autologous bone grafting purposes. A, Tuber coxae, the most frequently used site. B, The sternum, ideal when the horse is positioned in dorsal recumbency. C, The proximal and medial aspect of the tibia.

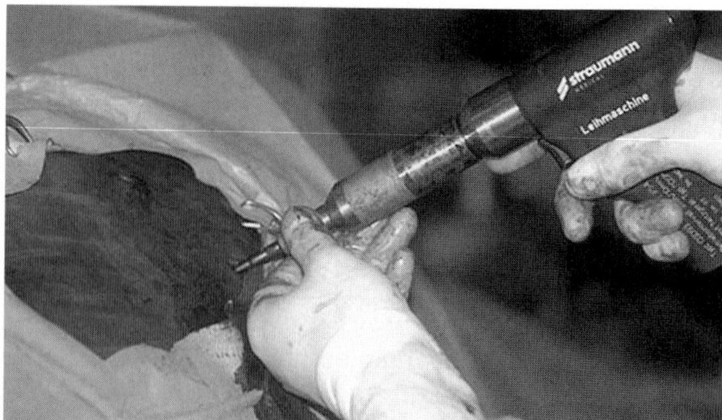

Figure 82-3. The bone graft harvesting drill with 4.0-mm-inside-diameter hollow drill bits is shown being applied to the tuber coxae of an anesthetized horse.

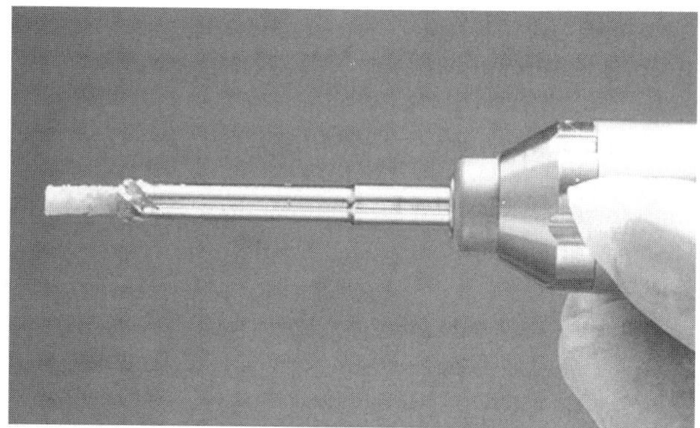

Figure 82-4. A 4.0-mm-diameter cancellous bone plug is shown protruding from the hollow drill bit.

vertebra, and periosteum were 75%, 100%, and 100%, respectively. Tuber coxae and tibial periosteum had significantly greater numbers of osteoprogenitors compared with the fourth coccygeal vertebra.[18] Although a recent study proposed the proximal humerus as an additional graft site, it is not recommended as a viable option.[19]

Tuber coxae

A straight 3-cm skin incision should be made over the tuber coxae, through the fat pad and subcutaneous tissues to the bone[20] (see Fig. 82-2, *A*). Using a 5.5-mm drill bit passed through the 5.5-mm drill guide, a hole is prepared across the thin cortex. With the help of a curet, the cancellous bone located within the ilium is harvested in the quantity needed. Care is taken to avoid breaking through the thin inner cortex of the ilium, which could cause complications. If needed, additional holes may be drilled adjacent to the first one at a different angle. The fat and subcutaneous tissues are closed over the bone in a simple-continuous pattern; an interrupted tension-relieving pattern is used in the skin. In selected cases, stapling of the skin may also be used. A stent bandage, consisting of a gauze sponge rolled up tightly and placed in a longitudinal direction, is sutured over the incision. This bandage protects the skin edges and reduces undue movement in this region, facilitating skin healing. It might be advisable to cover this area with additional padding, especially during the recovery phase and in horses with a tendency to rest in a recumbent position.

Recently, a bone graft–harvesting drill (Fig. 82-3) was introduced (Institute Straumann, Waldenburg, Switzerland). With this device, 4-mm-diameter cancellous bone plugs can be harvested through a stab incision (Fig. 82-4). These plugs are an ideal size when implanted into drill holes of the same diameter during arthrodesis of the distal intertarsal joint (see Chapter 99).

Sternum

The sternum is an especially advantageous donor site, because, when the animal is placed in dorsal recumbency, access is easy for the harvesting[21] (see Fig. 82-2, *B*). The sternum may also be approached with the animal in lateral recumbency; however, this is somewhat more cumbersome and the surgeon may have to perform the surgery in a less desirable position. Fracture treatment in a forelimb using internal fixation augmented by an autograft of cancellous bone from the sternum would be difficult to perform with two surgical teams working simultaneously, because of the proximity of the two surgical incisions. A straight incision is made on the midline until the sternum is encountered. The hyaline cartilage is split longitudinally with the scalpel, and with the help of a periosteal elevator, the sternebrae are identified. The cancellous bone graft is harvested from each sternebra that is isolated. Care is taken not to incorporate hyaline cartilage within the bone chips. If more cancellous bone is needed than is contained within one of the sternebrae, the next nucleus may also be excavated and used as a graft. There are six to seven usable nuclei within the sternum, allowing an adequate amount of high-quality cancellous bone graft to be harvested for any type of fracture. Closure consists of an initial simple-continuous layer along the border of the cartilage, through which the two cartilage flaps are united, followed by routine closure of the subcutaneous tissues and skin. It may be advisable to install a suction or Penrose drain for 24 hours. Additionally, the skin incision should be protected with a stent bandage, because otherwise this region is very difficult to protect.

Proximal tibia

A straight incision is made over the medial aspect of the proximal tibia through skin, subcutaneous tissues, and periosteum[17] (see Fig. 82-2, C). Using a 5.5-mm drill bit, the cortex is penetrated in one or two places, depending on the amount of cancellous bone graft needed. In a recently reported technique, two holes were drilled next to each other so that they became one hole 8 to 9 mm long.[18] This allowed access of a rather large curet, and a large amount of high quality cancellous bone graft could be harvested. Closure of the incision is routine. Again, a stent bandage is applied over the incision to stabilize the skin edges.

Proximal humerus

The quantity of cancellous bone collected from the proximal humerus with traditional harvesting instruments is comparable to that collected from other sites in horses. The procedure is associated with minimal postoperative incisional complications or lameness. However, because one horse suffered a catastrophic humerus fracture, further research is required to assess the effects of this procedure on humeral breaking strength. On the basis of the risk of catastrophic fracture, this technique cannot be recommended for use in clinical cases, especially if an unassisted recovery from general anesthesia is planned.[19]

Bone Banking

CORTICAL BONE

Cortical bone banks have never been very popular in equine surgery. Nevertheless, it is possible, and in selected instances even desirable, to develop a bank for certain horse bones. Donor horses should be free of any systemic disease, and the grafts should be harvested using aseptic technique.[22] Harvesting can be performed after the animal is euthanized, or from the anesthetized horse before it is euthanized. It may be possible to collect several bones from the same donor horse to allow greater flexibility at a later stage.[1] The bones should be radiographed after harvesting and identified as to the particular animal, bone and limb of origin, and age of the donor animal. It is advisable to add a small piece of bone to each of the separately packed donor bones. This piece of bone is cultured prior to implantation of the donor bone, and its sterility is checked. Once the bone is harvested, the desired banking technique is chosen: ethylene oxide sterilization, irradiation, freeze-drying, or decalcification. After irradiation and gas sterilization techniques, the double-wrapped donor bone can be stored at ambient temperature. The shelf life of a bone graft prepared using these methods is up to 2 years. After freeze-drying and freezing, the bone is double-wrapped and placed in a freezer, where it is maintained at −70° C. This is a very efficient way of storing a bone. Once the donor bone is needed, it is rapidly thawed in warm saline solution. This thawing process should take place while the surgical repair is being carried out, allowing the implant to be ready for implantation.[1]

ACID-DECALCIFIED GRAFTS

Acid-decalcified grafts or demineralized freeze-dried bone allografts are effective osteoinductive materials. Ribs (11th to 17th) or other corticocancellous bones may be chosen as the donor bone. Harvesting of the grafts is carried out under aseptic conditions as described for the other bone banking procedures.[22] All of the periosteum is removed from the donor bone, and the corticocancellous graft material is washed thoroughly. Decalcification is achieved using baths of 0.6N HCl at 2° C. The solution is changed daily until the bone pieces are completely decalcified, which takes between 14 and 21 days, depending on the size of the bone and the thickness of the cortex. Throughout the process, the bone is handled under aseptic conditions. The final product is stored in sterile, sealed plastic containers and subsequently frozen or freeze-dried. As with cancellous bone grafts, these grafts do not have any support function. Acid-decalcified, frozen grafts are easily applied and contoured because of their rubbery consistency after thawing.

Bone Replacements

FUNCTIONS

Bone replacement with synthetic materials has been advocated in human surgery to avoid the danger of transmitting infectious diseases (e.g., human immunodeficiency virus) through bone taken from bone banks and to avoid donor site morbidity. Therefore, new materials have been developed with a similar structure and composition to bone (i.e., they contain calcium and phosphorus)[23] (see Chapter 9). Despite the materials used, bone replacements are meant to function in a manner similar to cortical bone grafts—for example, serving as scaffolds for new bone formation and acting as a "spacer" surrounded by the host bone. Thus, synthetic bone replacements have a purely osteoconductive effect (Fig. 82-5). For large implants (greater than 1 cm in diameter), time is needed for the center portion of the graft to be invaded by blood vessels and osteogenic cells. This process may be enhanced by incubating the synthetic bone graft for a short period of time with a bone marrow aspirate mixed with blood.[4] During fracture repair, if the synthetic graft is placed into the medullary cavity, access to pluripotent mesenchymal cells has to be provided. The environment of the medullary cavity in the immediate vicinity of the fracture may be altered through trauma, and there may be no viable cells present. Therefore, bone marrow aspirates from more distant areas may be obtained with the help of a long needle inserted through one of the fracture ends and added to the synthetic bone scaffold. Moreover, the addition of fresh autogenous cancellous bone to the synthetic replacement may facilitate bone healing and provide living cells, especially when mixed with a granular product.[24] The graft and granules may be mixed prior to implantation, but with the advantage of not having to harvest a fresh, cancellous bone graft at surgery, some osteoinduction may be lost.

BONE REPLACEMENTS IN COMBINATION WITH ANTIBIOTICS

Chronic osteomyelitis is one of the most challenging conditions in orthopedic surgery. Because of the high degree of fibrosis and reduced vascularity, systemic antibiotics are of only limited value. Therefore, bone cement impregnated

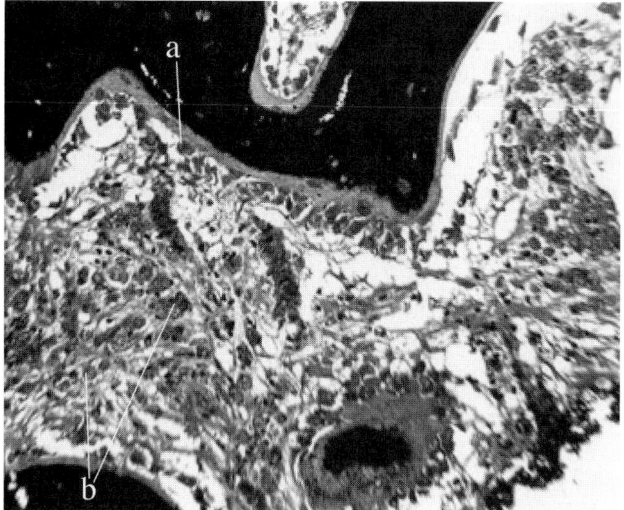

Figure 82-5. Histologic view of a synthetic injectable bone cement (chronOS Inject) 2 months after implantation. This biphasic brushite hydraulic cement has served as a scaffold on which osteoprogenitor cells have grown and formed new bone. Active seams of osteoblasts (*a*) are seen in the mineralized bone matrix. Nests of the cement are visible in the soft tissue of the cancellous bone, where macrophages (*b*) have ingested the particles. Like all bone replacements, the cement is replaced by "creeping substitution." (5-μm section of undecalcified bone sample embedded in acrylic resin, stained with von Kossa/McNeal, ×20.)

with antibiotics can be used to combat infection locally (see Chapter 88).

Traditionally, nonresorbable chains of polymethylmethacrylate (PMMA) beads are used in combination with antibiotics. When implanted, the antibiotic is gradually eluted over variable time periods. Gentamicin, amikacin, and cephalosporins have been proven to be effective in this manner.[25]

TCP impregnated with gentamicin is being evaluated as bone replacement for contaminated or infected areas. Use of this product in open fractures in the horse has had promising results. The gentamicin is released over a period of 90 days.[26] Gentamicin-impregnated TCP granules were inserted into the medullary cavity immediately prior to final reduction of the fracture. Newer compositions with liquid, resorbable bone cement mixed with gentamicin and TCP are still under investigation. The resorbable bone replacements or cements impregnated with antibiotics have an advantage in that they do not require a second procedure for removal but will be eventually replaced by normal bone tissue.[26,27]

BONE REPLACEMENTS USING THE BIOTECHNOLOGY APPROACH

In recent years, major advances have been made in the field of biotechnology.[28,29] In contrast to using synthetic bone replacements alone (Fig. 82-6), biotechnology has allowed the combination of a carrier or scaffold material either with

A

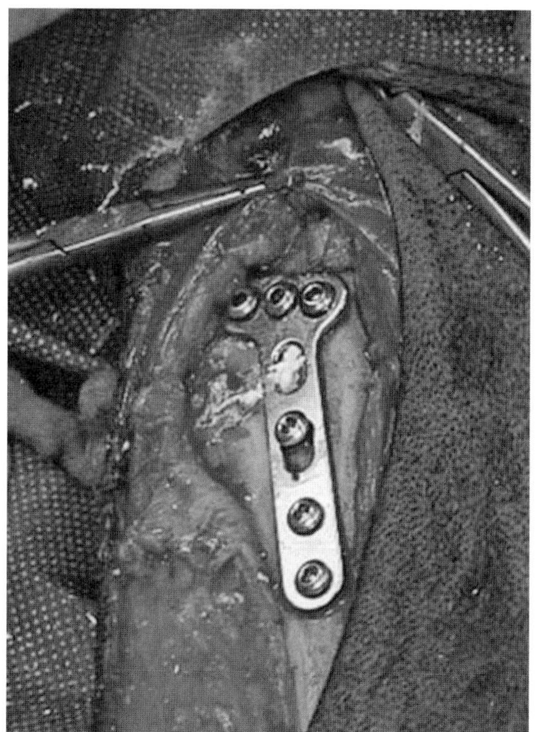

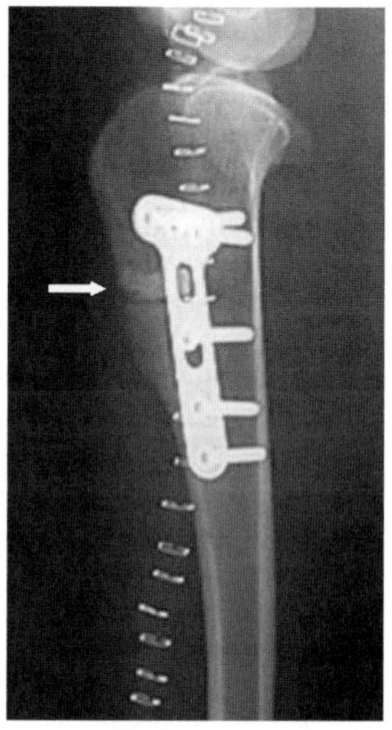

B

Figure 82-6. The proximal tibia of an experimental sheep with an injectable cement (chronOS Inject) in situ at the time of surgery (**A**) and at the time of sacrifice at 4 weeks after implantation (**B**). New bone has covered the original cement, and only remnants are visible underneath the plate.

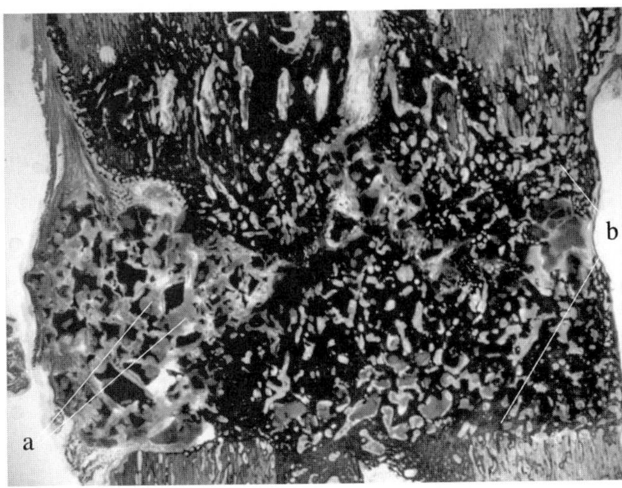

Figure 82-7. Histologic view of a 1-cm tibial defect filled with a composite consisting of calcium phosphate granules, fibrin-based hydrogel, and parathyroid hormone (PTH)-1-34 as a bone growth-enhancing factor. At 12 weeks, granules (a) are still present and serve as a nidus where new bone is deposited. The hydrogel is mostly resorbed, and the original fracture ends are well embedded in a hard callus. Extensive bone remodeling (b) is ongoing at the callus, as well as at the fracture ends (ground section, 30 to 40 μm) of undecalcified bone samples embedded in acrylic resin.

a gel-like matrix or with additional bone-enhancing substances[30-33] (Fig. 82-7). Polymers alone[34] or as composites with ceramic substances have had impressive results and are being used in clinical applications in human patients.[35-37] Additionally, the use of mesenchymal stem cells in addition to the material composites are being advocated and used in experimental and a few clinical applications.[38] Various kinds of bioreactors have been developed, where composites are incubated with mesenchymal stem[38,39] or periosteal cells.[40] Furthermore, modern diagnostic imaging procedures and the modern polymers allow rapid prototyping of materials prior to surgery with[41,42] or without[43] additional incubation of stem cells. Finally, modern purification processes have revived one of the oldest surgical materials—namely, silk[44]—so that it no longer causes inflammatory tissue reactions and can be customized in its structure to local requirements of bone architecture.[45,46]

Although some of these materials may be too expensive to be used in veterinary surgery at the moment, others are already being applied in clinical trials in horses and will be on the veterinary market in the near future. Composite materials that release bone-enhancing factors in small concentrations over a protracted period of time will be superior to simple bone replacements, enhancing bone healing, especially in large bony defects.

REFERENCES

1. Stevenson S: Bone grafting. In Slatter DH, editor: Textbook of Small Animal Surgery, Philadelphia, 1986, WB Saunders.
2. Heppenstall RB: Bone grafting. In McCollister-Evarts C, editor: Surgery of the Muscoskeletal System, New York, 1983, Churchill-Livingston.
3. Schenk RK: Mikroskopische Untersuchungen über die Gewebe- und Knochenreaktion, Proc Ceros Symp Bettlach, R. Mathys, 1987:2.
4. Nade S, Armstrong L, McCartney G, Baggaley B: Osteogenesis after bone and bone marrow transplantation, Clin Orthop Rel Res 1983;181:255.
5. Fackelman GE, Auer JA: Bone graft biology and autogenous grafting. In Fackelmann GE, Auer JA, Nunamaker DM, editors: AO Principles of Equine Osteosynthesis, Stuttgart, 1999, Thieme Verlag.
6. Burchardt H: Biology of cortical bone graft incorporation. In Aebi M, Regazzoni P, editors: Bone Transplantation, Berlin, 1989, Springer-Verlag.
7. Urist MR: Introduction to update on allograft surgery. In Aebi M, Regazzoni P, editors: Bone Transplantation, Berlin, 1989, Springer-Verlag.
8. Bramlage LR: Autologous cancellous bone grafting in the horse, Proc Am Assoc Equine Pract 1981;27:243.
9. Bourque WT, Gross M, Hall BK: Expression of four growth factors during fracture repair, Int J Dev Biol 1993;37:573.
10. Lorenzo JA: The role of cytokines in the regulation of local bone resorption, Crit Rev Immunol 1991;11;195.
11. Mundy GR: Cytokines and growth factors in the regulation of bone remodelling, J Bone Min Res 1993;8:S505.
12. Ralston SH, Grabowski PS: Mechanisms of cytokine induced bone resorption: Role of nitric oxide, cyclic guanosine monophosphate, and prostaglandins, Bone 1996;19:29.
13. Burchardt H: The biology of bone graft repair, Clin Orthop Rel Res 174 23, 1983.
14. Bassett CAL: Clinical implications of cell function in bone grafting, Clin Orthop Rel Res 1972;87:49.
15. Gray JC, Elves MW: Osteogenesis in bone grafts after short term storage and topical antibiotic treatment, J Bone Joint Surg 1981;63B:441.
16. Auer JA: Bone grafting. In Colahan P, Mayhew IG, Merritt AL, Moore JN, editors: Equine Medicine and Surgery, St Louis, 1999, Mosby.
17. Boero MJ, Schneider JE, Mosier JE, et al: Evaluation of the tibia as the source of autogenous cancellous bone in the horse, Vet Surg 1989;18:323.
18. McDuffee LA, Anderson GI: In vitro comparison of equine cancellous bone graft donor sites and tibial periosteum as sources of viable osteoprogenitors, Vet Surg 2003;32:455.
19. Harriss FK, Galuppo LD, Decock HEV, et al: Evaluation of a technique for collection of cancellous bone graft from the proximal humerus in horses, Vet Surg 2004;33:293.
20. Stashak TS, Adams OR: Collection of bone grafts from the tuber coxae of the horse, J Am Vet Med Assoc 1975;167:397.
21. Richardson GL, Pool RR, Pascoe JR, Wheat JD: Autogenous cancellous bone grafts from the sternum in horses: Comparison with other donor sites and results of use in orthopedic surgery, Vet Surg 1986;15:9.
22. Fackelman GE, von Rechenberg B, Fetter AW: Decalcified bone grafts in the horse, Am J Vet Res 1981;27:243.
23. Müller W: Ceros 80/82-eine Einführung, Proc Ceros Symp Bettlach, R Mathys, 1987:2.
24. Rose PL, Auer JA, Hulse D, et al: Effect of beta-tricalcium phosphate in surgically created subchondral bone defects in male horses, Am J Vet Res 1988;49:417.
25. Tobias KMS, Schneider RK, Besser TE: Antibiotic impregnated polymethyl methacrylate: A review of the literature. J Am Vet Med Assoc 1996;208:841.
26. Auer JA, Schenk RK, Gillis JP, Rose PL: The use of ceramic implants in articular and cortical bone defects in horses: A comparison of three different materials and their clinical application, Proc Vet Orthop Soc 1988;15:37.
27. Auer JA, Schenk R: The application of tricalcium phosphate cylinders in articular and cortical defects in the horse, Vet Surg 1989;18:73.

28. Vunjak-Novakovic G: The fundamentals of tissue engineering: Scaffolds and bioreactors, Novartis Found Symp 2003;249:34.
29. Kokubo T, Kim HM, Kawashita M: Novel bioactive materials with different mechanical properties, Biomaterials 2003;24:2161.
30. Meinel L, Zoidis E, Zapf J, et al: Localized insulin-like growth factor I delivery to enhance new bone formation, Bone 2003;33:660.
31. Kirker-Head CA, Gerhart TN, Armstrong R, et al: Healing bone using recombinant human bone morphogenetic protein 2 and copolymer, Clin Orthop Relat Res 1998;349:205.
32. Hallman M, Nordin T: Sinus floor augmentation with bovine hydroxyapatite mixed with fibrin glue and later placement of nonsubmerged implants: A retrospective study in 50 patients, Int J Oral Maxillofac Implants 2004;19:222.
33. Schmokel HG, Weber FE, Seiler G, et al: Treatment of nonunions with nonglycosylated recombinant human bone morphogenetic protein-2 delivered from a fibrin matrix, Vet Surg 2004;33:112.
34. Lutolf MP, Lauer-Fields JL, Schmoekel HG, et al: Synthetic matrix metalloproteinase-sensitive hydrogels for the conduction of tissue regeneration: Engineering cell-invasion characteristics, Proc Natl Acad Sci U S A 2003;100:5413.
35. Yuan X, Mak AF, He F: [Hydrolysis of poly(L-lactic acid) fibers and formation of low crystalline apatite on their surface by a biomimetic process], Sheng Wu Yi Xue Gong Cheng Xue Za Zhi 2003;20:404.
36. Kawashita M, Nakao M, Minoda M, et al: Apatite-forming ability of carboxyl group-containing polymer gels in a simulated body fluid, Biomaterials 2003;24:2477.
37. Chang MC, Ko CC, Douglas WH: Preparation of hydroxyapatite-gelatin nanocomposite, Biomaterials 2003;24:2853.
38. Bensaid W, Triffitt JT, Blanchat C, et al: A biodegradable fibrin scaffold for mesenchymal stem cell transplantation, Biomaterials 2003;24:2497.
39. Meinel L, Karageorgiou V, Fajardo R, et al: Bone tissue engineering using human mesenchymal stem cells: Effects of scaffold material and medium flow, Ann Biomed Eng 2004;32:112.
40. Breitbart AS, Grande DA, Kessler R, et al: Tissue engineered bone repair of calvarial defects using cultured periosteal cells, Plast Reconstr Surg 1998;101:567.
41. Schantz JT, Teoh SH, Lim TC, et al: Repair of calvarial defects with customized tissue-engineered bone grafts: I. Evaluation of osteogenesis in a three-dimensional culture system, Tissue Eng 2003;9(Suppl 1):S113.
43. Schantz JT, Hutmacher DW, Lam CX, et al: Repair of calvarial defects with customised tissue-engineered bone grafts: II. Evaluation of cellular efficiency and efficacy in vivo, Tissue Eng 2003;9(Suppl 1):S127.
44. Wang Z, Teng Y, Li D: [Fabrication of custom-made artificial semi-knee joint based on rapid prototyping technique: Computer-assisted design and manufacturing], Zhongguo Xiu Fu Chong Jian Wai Ke Za Zhi 2004;18:347.
45. Kaplan DL: Spiderless spider webs, Nat Biotechnol 2002;20:239.
46. Meinel L, Hofmann S, Karageorgiou V, et al: The inflammatory responses to silk films in vitro and in vivo, Biomaterials 2004;26:147.

CHAPTER 83

Synovial Joint Biology and Pathobiology

David D. Frisbie

The function of synovial joints depends on the integrity of normal anatomy and cellular function of each of its components. Bone, articular cartilage, synovial fluid, synovial membrane, fibrous joint capsule, and ligamentous structures make up these components (Fig. 83-1). On either side of a synovial joint, subchondral bone is covered by articular cartilage, providing the nearly frictionless contact surfaces of the joint. Synovial membrane and ligamentous joint capsule surround the cartilage and attach to bone on either side of the joint, providing stability and a reservoir for the synovial fluid. The synovial joint is further stabilized by ligamentous and muscular structures that surround the joint; these structures are extracapsular in most instances. Three different classifications of joints exist: synarthroses (immovable), amphiarthroses (slightly movable), and diarthrodial (movable). Diarthrodial joints account for the greatest

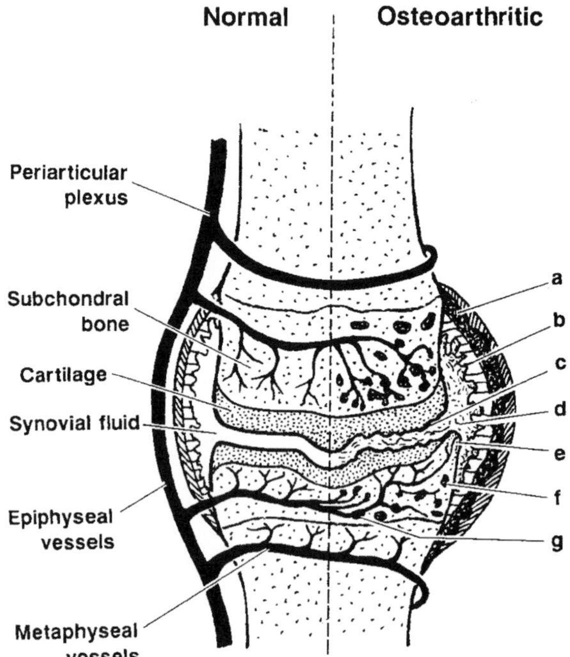

Figure 83-1. A normal synovial joint, including articular cartilage, synovial fluid, and synovial membranes, together with changes seen in a joint with osteoarthritis. In an osteoarthritic joint, the following can be identified: a, capsular fibrosis; b, synovitis; c, cartilage failure; d, depolymerized hyaluronic acid; e, osteophytes; f, subchondral cysts; g, vascular engorgement. (Modified from March L: In Sambrook P, editor: The Musculoskeletal System, New York, 2001, Churchill Livingstone.)

number in the body and will be the focus of this chapter. The articulations of diarthrodial joints provide for movement of the rigid skeleton. A healthy joint provides a frictionless system with efficiency that is an order of magnitude superior to the best bearing surfaces known to modern engineering.[1] When pathologic states arise, it is usually because of dysfunction of one or more components. Because the health of the synovial joint depends on the sum of its parts to be working in unison, it is often referred to as an organ system, as all components must be functional for the health of the "organ." This chapter will explore in more detail each component of the synovial joint both in health and disease.

ANATOMY OF SYNOVIAL JOINTS

Synovial Membrane and Synovial Fluid

The synovial membrane, or synovium, lines the joint cavity and is made up of two layers: intimal and subintimal. The intimal layer is largely responsible for the content of the synovial fluid, is typically one to four cell layers thick, and does not have a basement membrane. The lack of basement membrane is relevant with respect to the role the synovium plays in determining the content of the synovial fluid in the joint and will be covered in more detail later. The subintimal layer is made up of fibrous, areolar, and fatty tissues. A very good blood supply is present in the subintimal tissue, as well as innervation originating from both peripheral and muscular nerve branches[2,3] (Fig. 83-2). In fact, using an arthroscope close up and focused directly on normal synovial membrane, one can see individual red blood cells coursing through the capillary network of the villi. When viewed both grossly and arthroscopically, the synovium has areas that are flat intermixed with areas of loose collections of villi. These areas of villi are often described as "seaweed-like" when viewed arthroscopically in a fluid medium. The two appearances of the synovium are thought to be related to biomechanical characteristics of the joint area, since

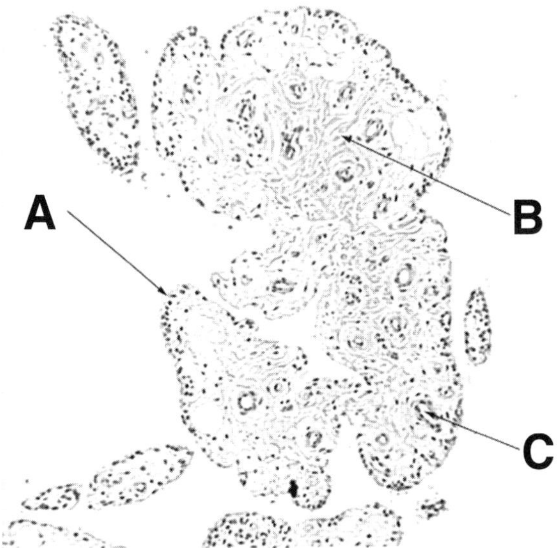

Figure 83-2. Photomicrograph of a 5-μm section of normal synovial membrane (H&E). A, the intimal layer; B, the subintimal layer; C, a vessel in the subintima.

they remain relatively unchanged throughout the life of healthy joints.

The cellular population of the intimal layer is based on two basic functions: phagocytosis and protein secretion. The cell types have historically been classified as type A or B synoviocytes on the basis of ultrastructure and immunohistologic characteristics. Cells engaged in phagocytosis or pinocytosis are termed type A synoviocytes, while those responsible for protein secretion have been referred to as type B.[4] More recently, the description of type C cells has been reported, and these cells are thought to represent a cell type between type A and B. Because type A and B cells have demonstrated functions assigned to the other cell type, and because synoviocytes have been shown to be dynamic, it is likely that type C cells represent synoviocytes in a transition from type A to B, or vice versa.[5,6]

When the focus is on the function of the intimal layer of synoviocytes, the importance of its role in both health and disease of the joint becomes apparent. One function is phagocytosis—the mechanism whereby unwanted particles can be cleared from the joint. However, a central role of the synoviocytes is the secretion of proteins that contribute to both the anabolic and the catabolic metabolism of the joint as a whole. Like many other metabolic processes, when checks and balances are in place, these metabolic processes are part of normal turnover, but when unregulated or aberrant regulation occurs, these same processes can lead to the development of disease. The synoviocytes are responsible for the secretion of a diverse array of proteins that contribute to the synovial membrane proper, as well as to the composition of the synovial fluid, and they include hyaluronan, collagen, lubricin, matrix pro-metalloproteinases (pro-MMPs), interleukins, and eicosanoids (e.g., prostaglandin E_2).[7,8] The breadth of these proteins in the pathophysiology of the joint underscores the importance of this tissue.

Another important role of the synovial membrane is to regulate the composition of synovial fluid. Synovial fluid is often referred to as an ultrafiltrate of the plasma. This term implies a more passive process, but is actually very dynamic and inter-related with many factors, including the molecules composing synovial fluid (e.g., hyaluronan size and concentration), degree of inflammation, and lymphatic drainage. Components of the plasma, such as glucose, oxygen, carbon dioxide, and proteins, typically less than 10 kDa in size, are allowed through the endothelium of the subintima and contribute to the composition of the synovial fluid, whereas large molecules are excluded. Routine cytologic examination techniques, as well as normal and disease state levels of the constituents, will be reported later. Most laboratories consider levels of less than 500 cells per deciliter of synovial fluid normal.

Molecules such as hyaluronan and lubricin are contributed to the synovial fluid directly by the synoviocytes. These molecules are thought to be important in the steric exclusion of larger molecules from the synovial cavity, thus regulating synovial fluid composition (Fig. 83-3), and as boundary lubrication of the joint surfaces. The regulation of size and concentration of hyaluronan within the synovial fluid is unknown, but these two factors do affect the functional properties assigned to the molecule. A variety of methods have been used to determine both the concentration and the molecular weight (or size) of hyaluronan.

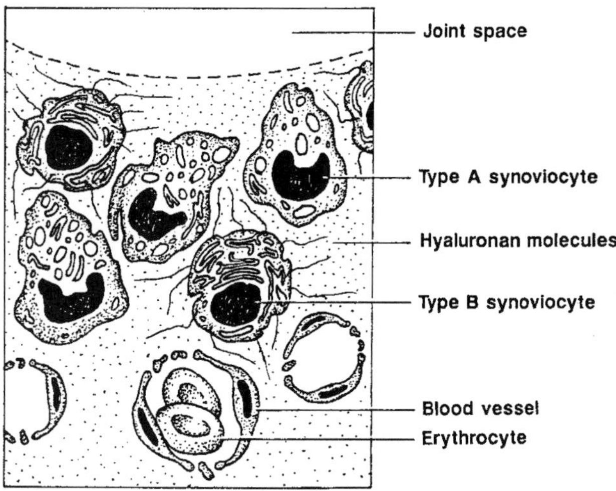

Figure 83-3. Hyaluronan secretion from type B synoviocytes, and its close association with the synovium, where it is thought to aid in excluding leukocytes and other solutes from the joint space through steric hindrance. (Adapted from Howard RD, McIlwraith CW: Hyaluronan and its use in the treatment of equine joint disease. In McIlwraith CW, Trotter GW, editors: Joint Disease in the Horse, Philadelphia, 1996, WB Saunders.)

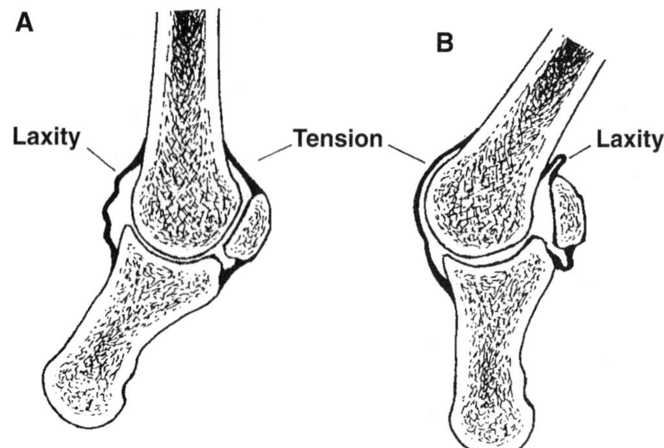

Figure 83-4. Synovial and joint capsule laxity or tension based on the anatomic position of the joint. The dorsal aspect of the joint capsule is lax in fetlock extension (**A**) and under tension in flexion (**B**). This figure also illustrates the change in joint congruity thought to occur during loading. In an unloaded position (**B**), it is thought that joints are not completely congruous, but as load is applied, a more congruous joint is formed. (**A,** adapted from McIlwraith CW: In Stashak TS, editor: Adams' Lameness in Horses, ed 5, Oxford, 2002, Blackwell; **B,** from Koopman WJ, editor: Arthritis and Allied Conditions: A Textbook of Rheumatology, vol 1, ed 13, Baltimore, 1997, Williams & Wilkins.)

The diversity of methods has provided a wide range of normal values, 0.33 to 1.5 mg/mL and several thousand kilodaltons, respectively.[7,9] The half-life of endogenous hyaluronan has been estimated by injecting radiolabeled hyaluronan into the joint and tracking both its degradation and its clearance. It appears that the majority of exogenous hyaluronan is cleared within 48 hours through the synovium and lymphatics, with degradation occurring in both the synovium and the liver.[7]

Periarticular Ligaments and Joint Capsule

Periarticular ligaments, the fibrous joint capsule, and surrounding muscles provide stability to synovial joints. The contribution to stability afforded by each of these structures differs according to its anatomic location. Joints higher in the limb obtain more stability from muscle than those lower in the limb, so the contour of the joint surface and stability from the joint capsule are more important in the lower limb, although muscular stabilization is a factor. The role of muscular stabilization cannot be overemphasized. For example, even with all periarticular ligaments and the joint capsule intact, desensitization of the suprascapular nerve results in subluxation of the shoulder joint.

The ligamentous and capsular configurations within a joint are different depending on the specific joint and the location within the joint, presumably based on range of motion and other biomechanical considerations. For example, in extension, the dorsal aspect of the metacarpophalangeal joint has capsular redundancy,[10] but in flexion, the same region of the capsule is under tension[11] (Fig. 83-4). It is easy to see how a decrease in compliance of the joint capsule because of increased fibrous tissue deposition could limit the range of motion within a particular joint.

The ligaments and fibrous joint capsule are composed mainly of type I collagen with some elastin fibers, accounting for 75% of the organic solids, with 23% being proteoglycan.[12] The organization is mainly in parallel fascicles with occasional fibrocytes and blood vessels. Most of the innervation of a joint is seen in association with perivascular structures.[10] The attachment of these structures to bone has been compared to Sharpey's fibers, because the collagen fibers course through both fibrocartilage and calcified cartilage prior to their insertion in bone. This type of transition is credited with the biomechanical pullout properties (the amount of force needed to pull a ligament from the bone attachment) of the ligaments and joint capsule.[13] It is important to note that these tissues are metabolically active and undergo hypertrophy with activity and atrophy with immobilization. Immobilization has been shown to affect the microscopic, enzymatic, and biomechanical properties of ligaments, suggesting that immobilization should be used temporarily to maintain joint stability during a controlled return to use after injury, as is used in human medicine in the form of function splints (knee braces).[14]

Subchondral Bone

The subchondral bone plate, along with epiphyseal bone, provides contour and stability to the articular cartilage. The subchondral bone plate consists of cortical bone with the haversian system running parallel to the joint surface, unlike the diaphyseal cortical bone, where the haversian system runs perpendicular to joint surface. The biochemical and histologic appearance of subchondral bone is similar to bone in other locations. In humans, the subchondral bone plate has been shown to be approximately 10 times more deformable than the cortical shaft.[10] Remodeling or stiffening of the subchondral bone plate has been noted to occur with osteoarthritis in humans and is considered deleterious to the joint function.[15] This has sparked similar exploration in horses, and, although remodeling and subchondral bone sclerosis is easily documented, especially in areas such as the third carpal bone, deleterious changes in proteoglycan content in this location have not been documented to date.[16] However, subchondral bone microcracks and other forms of bone remodeling have been demonstrated in this area in response to exercise, although their relationship to pathophysiology is not well defined.[17] The subchondral bone plate is integral to joint function as a whole; research in this area is quite active and may provide insights into its role in disease.

Articular Cartilage

Articular cartilage is the central structure that constitutes the joint surface and ultimately its function. In conjunction with the synovial fluid, articular cartilage is credited with providing the nearly frictionless movement of the synovial joint. Although other components of the joint, such as the subchondral bone, synovial membrane, joint capsule, and ligamentous structures, are integral for proper function and continued health of the joint, it is the state of the articular cartilage that is typically used to define joint health. Furthermore, although it is likely that disease may start in components of the joint other than the articular cartilage (e.g., subchondral bone or ligamentous structures), the degeneration and slow or poor healing response of the cartilage usually defines the level and progression of the joint disease.

On gross appearance, the articular cartilage appears smooth or glasslike (hence the term *hyaline*). In most areas, the articular cartilage has an opaque white color, with areas of thin articular cartilage appearing slightly pink because of the underlying subchondral bone color showing through. Although grossly the surface of articular cartilage appears flawless, a scanning electron microscope reveals it to be gently undulating with depressions that appear to correlate with surface chondrocytes. These depressions have been estimated to be 20 to 40 µm in diameter and have a density of about 430/mm^2.[10] The thickness of articular cartilage varies by joint, location (related to the degree of weight-bearing), and age, but it is in the 1- to 4-mm range.

The lack of vascular, lymphatic, and neural supply makes cartilage a unique tissue and dictates a dependency on diffusion for nutrient supply and waste removal. The nutritional supply is provided via the synovial fluid. The nutritional solutes diffuse from subintimal vessels through the intimal layer of the synovium to the synovial fluid, then through the articular cartilage matrix, until they finally reach the chondrocytes. The ultrastructure of the chondrocytes supports a diffusion gradient; for example, a decrease in the number of mitochondria in deeper chondrocytes suggests that they are less dependent on oxygen than chondrocytes located more superficially.

The chondrocyte content of articular cartilage typically accounts for 1% to 12% of the volume of the cartilage, with the remaining component being termed *extracellular matrix*.[7] The extracellular matrix is somewhat complex but can be broken down into three main components: collagens, proteoglycans, and water. Water is the most abundant molecule of the extracellular matrix, making up about 70% of the wet weight in adults and closer to 80% in young and immature animals. On a dry weight basis, the extracellular matrix is composed of approximately 50% collagen, 35% proteoglycan, 10% glycoprotein (e.g., growth factors, cartilage oligomeric protein [COMP], proteinases), 3% minerals, 1% lipids, and 1% miscellaneous substances.[7]

Microscopic Appearance

On the basis of the microscopic appearance of both the chondrocytes and collagen orientation, articular cartilage has been historically divided into four contiguous zones (Fig. 83-5):

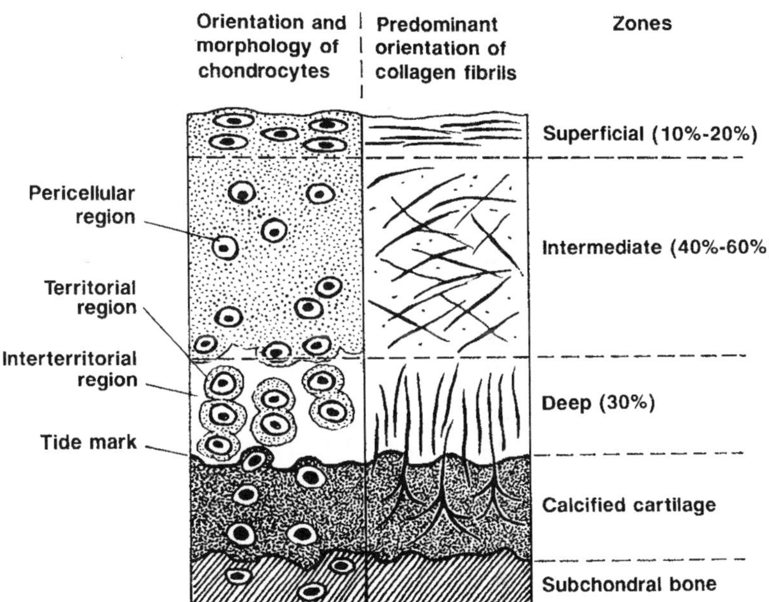

Figure 83-5. Normal articular cartilage with orientation and morphology of the chondrocytes, orientation of the collagen fibrils, and the relative contribution of the zone or layer. (Adapted from March L: In Sambrook P, editor: The Musculoskeletal System, New York, 2001, Churchill Livingstone.)

1. The superficial (tangential) zone has the highest density of chondrocytes. These chondrocytes appear flattened and are oriented with the long axis of the cell parallel with the joint surface. The collagen here is more densely packed than in deeper layers, and the orientation of the fibers is also parallel with the joint surface. Recently, there has been acceptance of a previously described but refuted acellular layer of collagen called the lamina splendens. This layer has fibril diameters that are distinctly different from those of the traditional cellular portion of the superficial zone and that can be consistently separated from the cellular portion of the superficial zone without damage to the collagen network. The lamina splendens is only loosely connected to the fibrous structure in the adjacent layer beneath. It is, however, firmly connected to the deeper cartilage matrix at the vicinity of the synovium, where it undergoes transition to synovial tissue.[18]
2. The intermediate (transitional) zone is characterized by larger, more ovoid to round chondrocytes.
3. The deep (radiate) zone has the largest chondrocytes, and the long axis of the cell is oriented perpendicular to the joint surface.
4. The calcified zone consists of mineralized cells and matrix. The *tidemark* refers to the junction of the noncalcified and calcified cartilage, which is a distinct transition seen on histologic sections. More recently, the tidemark has also been described arthroscopically.[19]

Cartilage Collagens

Collagen is considered the component of articular cartilage that provides the framework or lattice in which all other matrix molecules are constrained. It is also the component attributed to the counteraction of tensile stresses seen at the joint surface. As described previously, the architecture of the collagen differs depending on its zone or depth within the cartilage. In 1925, Benninghoff described an arcade configuration of articular cartilage collagen, which is helpful in understanding the function of the cartilage. Although the overall accuracy of his model has been challenged, it is useful for demonstration purposes[1] (Fig. 83-6). The superficial pattern of the collagen framework was described as "armor plating," referring to the tough, resilient, skinlike cartilage surface. The collagen content in this area is higher and the fibrils are of smaller diameter (about 31 nm) with an orientation parallel with the joint surface, which is different from collagen in deeper zones. Based on this configuration, minute openings exist in the superficial layer of cartilage, which have been calculated to be around 6 nm in diameter. This pore size would preclude large proteins such as hyaluronan from entering the cartilage from the synovial fluid in any significant quantities. However, small ions and molecules such as glucose could readily pass through an opening of this size.[20] As previously mentioned, the collagen fibrils of the intermediate zone are oriented in a more random pattern and are between 40 and 100 nm in diameter. The collagen fibrils of the deep zone have the largest diameter, are oriented perpendicular to the joint surface, and cross the calcified zone prior to attaching within the subchondral bone. This pattern of collagen orientation is supported by light and electron microscopy, with further confirmation by an interesting phenomenon called the Hultkrantz line, which appears when the articular surface is penetrated with a pin and stained with India ink.[21] The round hole made by the pin appears as an elongated slit, and the axis of the slit has been found to run perpendicular

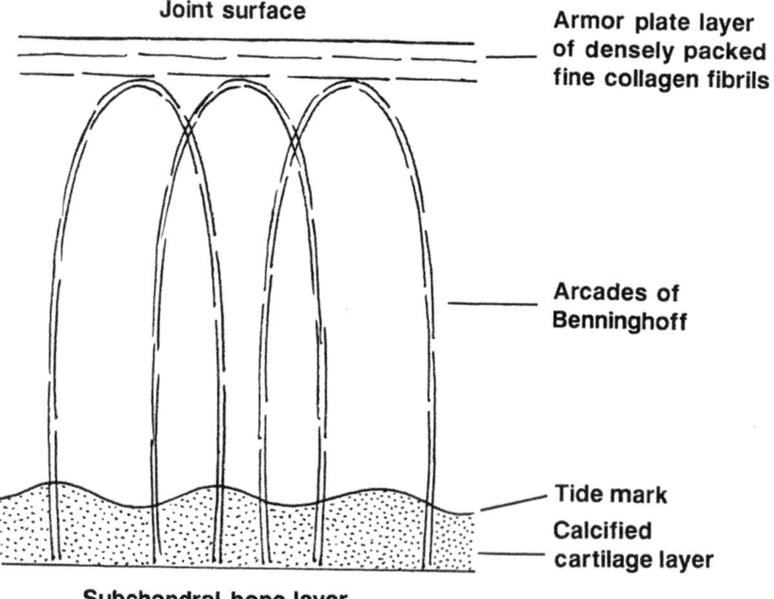

Figure 83-6. Simplistic illustration of the biomechanical function of the collagen fibrils in the different areas of articular cartilage. The tightly packed, smaller-diameter collagen fibrils are near the surface in the superficial layer, notably in the lamina splendens. The larger-diameter, more loosely spaced fibrils of the deep layer traverse the calcified layer and are anchored in the subchondral bone. (Adapted from Daniel DM, Pedowitz RA, O'Connor JJ, et al, editors: Daniel's Knee Injuries: Ligament and Cartilage Structure, Function, Injury, and Repair, ed 2, Philadelphia, 2003, Lippincott Williams & Wilkins.)

to the collagen fibril orientation and to the maximal surface tensile strains.[22] This method is currently the preferred test to determine the orientation of collagen in articular cartilage (Fig. 83-7).

At least 16 different collagens have been described in mammalian species, and they are divided into two main categories on the basis of their primary structure and supramolecular assembly: fibril-forming collagens (including types I, II, III, V, and XI) and non-fibril-forming collagens.[23] Collagen turnover is much like that of other fibrous connective tissues, but it tends to be slower than that of other matrix components of the articular cartilage. It has been shown that significant collagen synthesis occurs in adult cartilage, although not much is understood about the process by which orientation is controlled in response to remodeling.

TYPE II COLLAGEN

The primary collagen of articular cartilage is type II and is produced by the chondrocytes. It constitutes 90% to 95% of the total collagen content.[24] The principal differences between type II and type I collagen (the latter found in the majority of other musculoskeletal tissues) are the number of hydroxylysine molecules and an increase in glycosylation. Type II collagen is a homotrimer composed of three identical collagen molecules that are constructed in such a manner that the start of each molecule is offset from the next by 25%, or by a "quarter stagger" (see Fig. 80-3). Of the other types of collagen found in articular cartilage, types IX and XI are thought to be integral in the organization and mechanical stability of the type II collagen fibrillar network (Fig. 83-8) and are intimately associated with type II collagen.

MINOR COLLAGENS

The content of type IX collagen in articular cartilage decreases from being around 10% of the collagen protein in fetal tissue to being about 1% in the adult. This molecule is found on the outer surface of the type I triple helix and is thought to provide a covalent interface between the surface of the type II collagen fibril and other type II fibrils as well as the interfibrillar proteoglycan domain, thus providing mechanical stability of the fibrillar network.[1] Types VI, XII, and XIV collagen also are thought to have roles in the association between fibrillar collagen and other matrix components.[25,26] Type XI collagen, on the other hand, is found within the type II triple helix and acts as a core filament on which the type II molecules are deposited during formation.[27] Type XI collagen accounts for about 3% of mature collagen protein. Type VI collagen binds both hyaluronan and fibronectin and has been identified in the perilacunar area.[1]

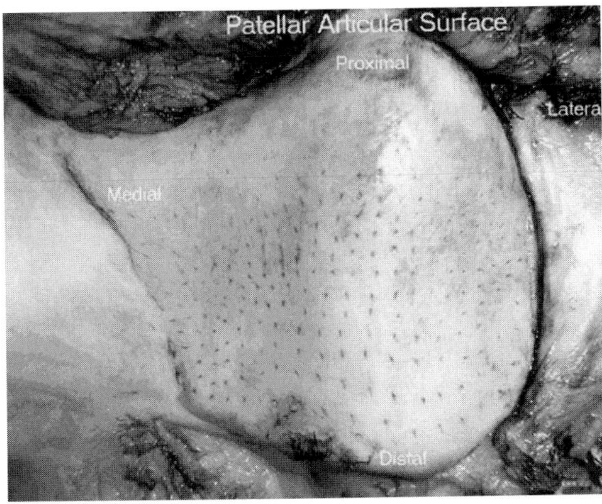

Figure 83-7. Gross photo demonstrating Hultkrantz lines in an equine patella following round perforations of the articular cartilage. (Courtesy Dr. Chris E. Kawcak and Dr. Chad Lewis.)

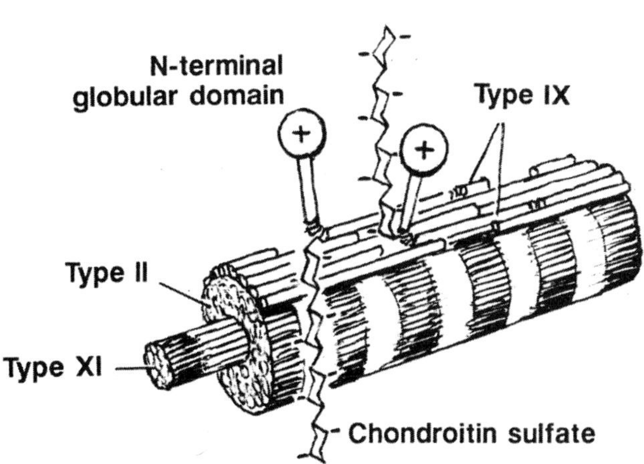

Figure 83-8. Arrangement of types II, XI, and IX collagen in articular cartilage. (Adapted from Eikenberry EF, Mendler M, Burgin R, et al: In Kuettner KE, Schleyerbach R, Peyron JG, et al, editors: Articular Cartilage and Osteoarthritis, New York, 1992, Raven Press.)

Proteoglycans

Proteoglycans make up the other major component of the articular cartilage extracellular matrix, about 35% on a dry weight basis. As the name implies, these molecules are a combination of protein (*proteo* for the core protein to which glycosaminoglycans are attached) and glycosaminoglycan (*glycan* for the repeating disaccharide or polysaccharide). At first glance, the nomenclature of proteoglycans appears somewhat complex, but when broken down into its components it is relatively straightforward, and it is important to understand its evolution. The proteoglycan molecule aggrecan makes up about 85% of the proteoglycans that in turn make up the extracellular matrix, and it is mainly responsible for providing the resistance to compressive forces within the articular cartilage. The other proteoglycans are less studied but function in interactions with collagens and in various metabolic roles in cartilage.

AGGRECAN

A single (monomer) aggrecan molecule is made up of two main components: the core protein, which acts as the backbone of aggrecan, and the glycosaminoglycans (GAGs) that attach radially to the core protein. The three main GAG molecules (Fig. 83-9) that make up aggrecan are chondroitin-4-sulfate, chondroitin-6-sulfate, and keratan sulfate. Their ratio differs with age. Of note is an increase in chondroitin-6-sulfate over chondroitin-4-sulfate as the cartilage becomes more mature. The GAGs covalently attach to the core

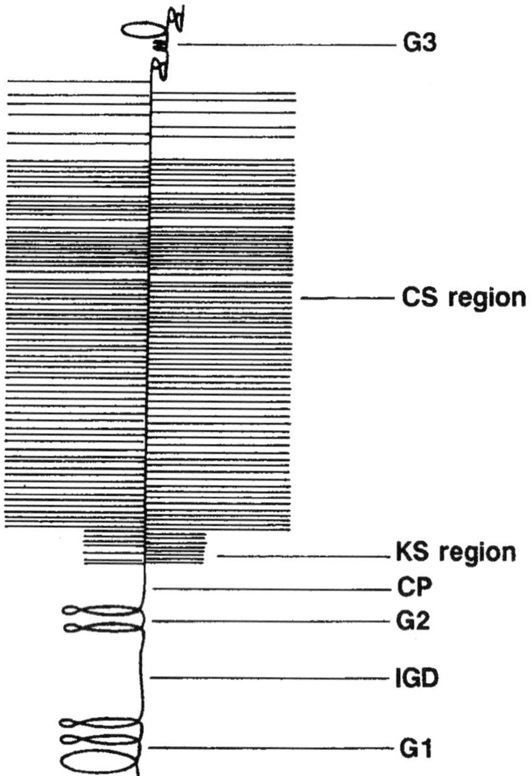

Figure 83-9. An aggrecan monomer consisting of a central core protein (CP) interrupted by three globular domains (G1, G2, and G3). Peripherally on the molecule are the keratan sulfate (KS) and chondroitin sulfate (CS) regions. Proteolytic cleavage of the molecule in vivo first occurs in the interglobular domain (IGD). (From Koopman WJ, editor: Arthritis and Allied Conditions: A Textbook of Rheumatology, vol 1, ed 13, Baltimore, 1997, Williams & Wilkins.)

protein, and about 100 chondroitin sulfate molecules preferentially attach at the carboxy end of the molecule. Likewise, approximately 100 keratan sulfate molecules are preferentially found closer to the *N*-terminal region of the aggrecan monomer.[11] These regions are sometimes described as chondroitin- or keratan-rich regions. Because of the high negative charge associated with the GAGs, they tend to repel each other (chemical expansive stresses) and attract water, creating positive pressure (Donnan osmotic pressure). The combination of these two forces has been termed *cartilage swelling pressure* and is roughly the equivalent of tire pressure.[28]

Current research has focused on delineating various functional and structural domains along the core protein. These regions or domains have been shown to help define the breakdown of various catabolic enzymes involved in normal and pathologic processes—for example, the cleavage site of aggrecanase is different from that of stromelysin, two molecules important in aggrecan turnover. Three main domains have been defined: G1, G2, and G3. The G1 region of the core protein interacts with hyaluronan, and this interaction is involved in arranging about 100 aggrecan monomers along a hyaluronan backbone. The G2 region is located on the *N*-terminal side of the keratan sulfate–rich region and is a key target of enzymes that break down aggrecan.[29] The G3 region is on the "end" or carboxy side of the aggrecan molecule and in fact is present in only some aggrecan molecules, suggesting a less important role.[30]

Aggrecan (proteoglycan) aggregates

Aggrecan monomers are further organized into large aggregates around a hyaluronan molecule. These aggregates can be in the range of 200 million daltons in size and comprise over 100 aggrecan monomers.[31] The noncovalent bond between the aggrecan monomers and hyaluronan is stabilized by a small group of link proteins[1] in conjunction with the G1 domain of the core protein (Fig. 83-10).

SMALL PROTEOGLYCANS

About 5% of the articular cartilage proteoglycans are termed small proteoglycans or nonaggregating proteoglycans. Like aggrecan, they consist of a protein core and attached glycosaminoglycan chains. As the name implies, these molecules are smaller than aggrecan—in fact, the core protein is about 25% of that found in an aggrecan molecule. Examples are biglycan, decorin, and fibromodulin. Decorin and fibromodulin are found associated with collagen molecules in the superficial zones of the articular cartilage. Decorin has been shown to inhibit type I and II collagen formation, and fibromodulin inhibits fibrillogenesis. Biglycan and decorin have been shown to bind transforming growth factor-beta (TGF-β), thus making it unavailable to perform its biologic function. This may play an important role in the healing process of articular cartilage and needs to be better understood to improve intervention in cartilage healing.[1] The overall condition of the extracellular matrix is presented graphically in Figure 83-11.

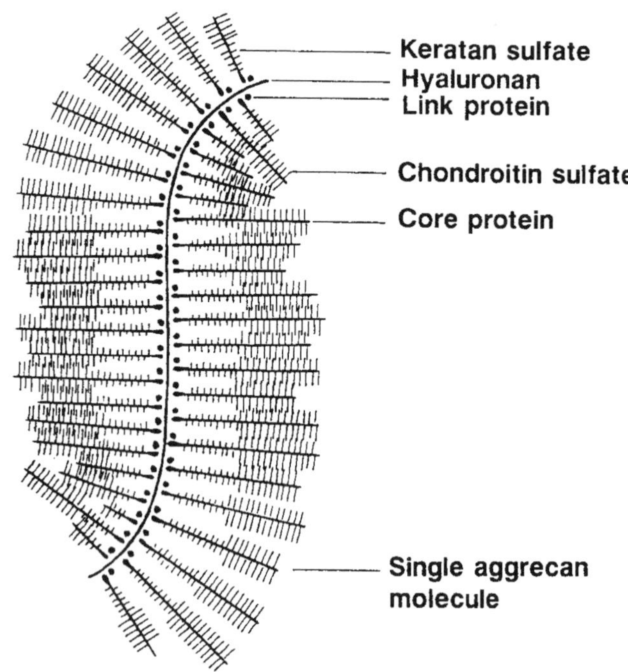

Figure 83-10. An aggregate containing many aggrecan molecules that are linked to hyaluronan via a noncovalent bond associated with the link protein. (Adapted from Daniel DM, Pedowitz RA, O'Connor JJ, et al, editors: Daniel's Knee Injuries: Ligament and Cartilage Structure, Function, Injury, and Repair, ed 2, Philadelphia, 2003, Lippincott Williams & Wilkins.)

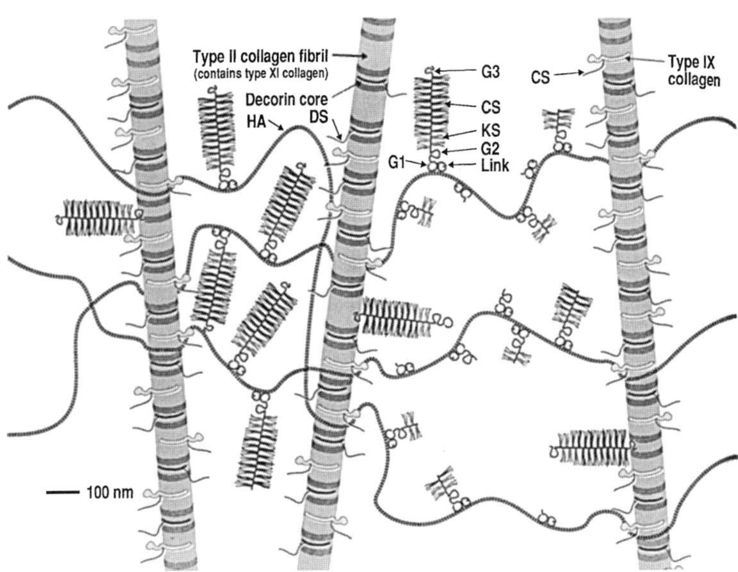

Figure 83-11. Organization of the major extracellular matrix components in articular cartilage. The principal collagen of cartilage is type II, and a network of these fibrils provides much of the tensile strength of the tissue. Aggrecan consists of a linear protein with three globular domains (G1 to G3), to which are attached numerous glycosaminoglycan chains of chondroitin sulfate (CS) and keratan sulfate (KS). Supramolecular aggregates are formed by the noncovalent interaction of aggrecan with hyaluronan (HA) and stabilized by a link protein (Link). The negatively charged glycosaminoglycans (CS and KS) attract several times their weight in water, and this proteoglycan–water composite is responsible for the compressive stiffness of cartilage. Cartilage also has a number of minor proteoglycans and collagens (e.g., decorin and dermatan sulfate [DS]) whose functions are not fully characterized. Fragments of aggrecan, remaining bound to HA, are shown to illustrate the effects of proteolytic activity in cartilage. (From Koopman WJ, editor: Arthritis and Allied Conditions: A Textbook of Rheumatology, vol 1, ed 13, Baltimore, 1997, Williams & Wilkins.)

Chondrocytes

The chondrocytes, as previously mentioned, represent a small proportion of the total volume of the articular cartilage. The morphology and metabolism of the chondrocytes vary according to their depth within the cartilage, and the presence of lacunae represents a microenvironment around the chondrocytes that is more prevalent in the deeper layers. Chondrocytes have cytoplasmic processes that extend into the interterritorial region and appear to sense the biochemical and biomechanical environment, but, unlike the cytoplasmic processes of osteocytes, they do not make contact with cellular processes of other chondrocytes. These cytoplasmic processes may represent one mechanism through which the chondrocytes respond to articular cartilage loading. It appears that at a low level of mechanical stress, chondrocyte metabolism favors the catabolic processes, whereas at normal physiologic levels, anabolic processes are favored, and a balance of metabolism is possible. In contrast, at super-physiologic levels, the metabolism favors catabolism, potentially as a result of an overwhelmed anabolic pathway.[32] Alterations in extracellular matrix pressure caused by biochemical changes may also direct chondrocyte metabolism.

Turnover of the proteoglycan portion of the extracellular matrix occurs faster than the collagen component. Specifically, proteoglycan turnover has been estimated at about 300 days in dogs and rabbits, versus an estimated 350 days for total turnover of the collagen in humans and 120 in dogs.[11] These rates can be upregulated in disease states—in fact, upregulation of anabolism of both aggrecan and collagen synthesis appears to be one of the earliest changes detected in osteoarthritic processes.[33] More detail on cytokines and regulation of articular cartilage metabolism will be covered in subsequent sections.

PHYSIOLOGY OF SYNOVIAL JOINTS

Intra-articular Volume and Pressure

The volume of the synovial space or joint cavity varies with its anatomic location, and, because of the elasticity of the joint capsule, it can change depending on various factors (e.g., disease, level of exercise). As an example, horses exercising at an increased level are often noted to have synovial effusion, notably in the fetlock and tarsocrural joints, without pathology being present. Some data on the "normal" synovial volume have been published, but, as previously noted, this can be somewhat subjective depending on the degree of joint capsule distention that is perceived as typical.[34] The mechanism by which intra-articular volume and pressure are regulated are poorly understood. Most synovial joints are reported as having negative pressure in a neutral position, whereas at the extremes of flexion and extension the intra-articular pressure increases up to 30 psi in the human knee. These pressures are also sensitive to synovial effusion; increased pressures can be translated to the innervation of the joint capsule and subsequently to joint pain during range-of-motion activities.

Joint Mechanics

Joint mechanics are unique and very complex, largely because of the articular cartilage and its response to loading. The study of the loading properties of synovial joints is a very active field whose scope is beyond the reach of this chapter, but it is summarized here. Joint mechanics are dependent on three aspects: kinematics, kinetics, and joint lubrication. Kinematics involves the study of the motion of the articulating surfaces in relation to each other. Kinetics relates to the forces that are created during the motion of the joint and the loads that are created across the articular surface. Joint lubrication provides a nearly frictionless movement of the soft tissues and articular cartilage.

Kinematics

The kinematics of a particular joint are a function of the geometry of the joint surface—specifically, of the articular cartilage and the underlying subchondral bone, as well as the periarticular supporting structures such as ligaments and muscles. The types of motion that occur in joints fall into three categories: translational, rolling, and sliding motions. *Translational* motion refers to movement without rotation, where two surfaces move past each other. This type of motion somewhat describes the movement in the spine and shoulder. Both rolling and sliding imply some degree of rotational component, which adds another dimension and makes the mathematical models and understanding of these motions complex. Pure *rolling* motion implies that the instant center of rotation is always at the point of contact between the two surfaces, and that the distance over which contact occurs is similar on both opposing surfaces. In *sliding* motion, the point of contact is not the instant center of rotation, and the areas of contact during the motion are not equal on both surfaces (Fig. 83-12). Most synovial joints have some component of sliding and translational motion, and pure rolling motion is just theoretical.

Another factor that affects the kinematics of synovial joints is the observation that joint surfaces that are relatively congruent possess thinner articular cartilage than those with incongruent surfaces. Furthermore, in some joints, overall joint congruity appears less when they are unloaded than when they are under load. This is thought to allow better distribution of forces over a larger surface with increasing loads[10] (see Fig. 83-4). It becomes quickly apparent that loss of any component of the synovial joint will alter the normal motion of a joint and its ultimate function.

Kinetics

The analysis of joint forces is even more complex, because it is dependent on the kinematics of the joint as well as on any change of normal position, which then alters the forces as they are applied to the joint. Kinetics takes into account the muscle forces pulling across a joint, the superimposed body weight, the force of the floor or surface pushing back against the joint in question, and the force felt by the cartilage in any given load-bearing situation (termed the J-force).[35] Joint modeling has been a focus in human research for some years and is currently being conducted in the equine carpus. This may provide valuable insight into the joint as a whole organ in the years to come.

Lubrication

Lubrication of the synovial joint can be broken down into two main components, that of the soft tissue and that of the articular cartilage. From a pure point of view, two types of lubrication function in the synovial joint: boundary and fluid-film lubrication. Boundary lubrication prevents adhesion and abrasions of two surfaces and is independent of the physical properties of the lubricant or contacting surfaces. Hyaluronan and lubricin (secreted by the synovial membrane) are believed to be the main boundary lubricants of the diarthrodial joint. Boundary lubrication is the main way of decreasing friction between soft tissue and bone, but it is believed to be relatively ineffective at providing a frictionless surface between articular cartilage surfaces at physiologic loads.[35]

Fluid-film mechanisms are believed to provide the low friction environment for the articular cartilage at physiologic loads, accomplished by creating a wedge of fluid between the two bearing surfaces. Several models have been proposed, including squeeze film, hydrodynamic, and elastohydrodynamic models (Fig. 83-13). The elastohydrodynamic model, which is accepted as best representing lubrication of the articular cartilage, is based on the attraction of water by aggrecan molecules at the porous articular surface. In this model, when load or pressure is applied to the surface, water is squeezed from the articular surface and interposed between the bearing surfaces. With joint movement, a wedge

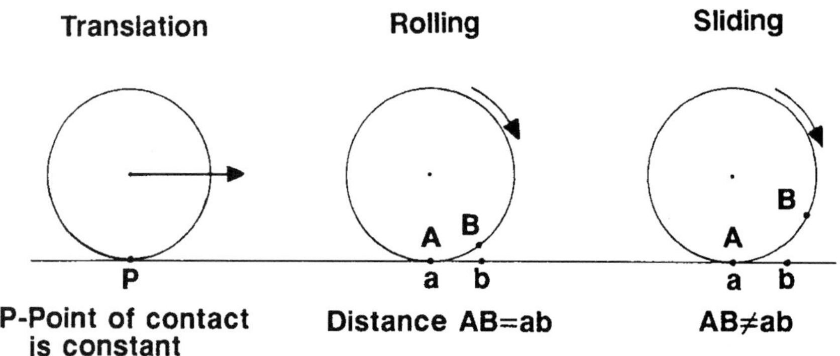

Figure 83-12. The three types of joint motion. (Adapted from Delahay JN: In Wiesel SW, Delahay JN, editors: Principles of Orthopaedic Medicine and Surgery, Philadelphia, 2001, WB Saunders.)

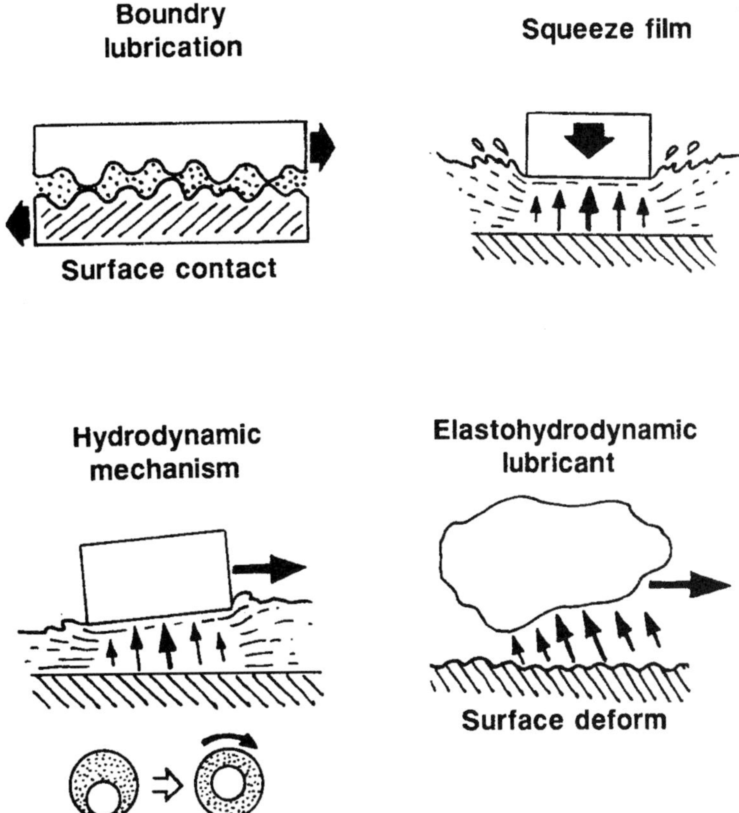

Figure 83-13. Models of lubrication: boundary, squeeze film, hydrodynamic, and elastohydrodynamic (a combination of squeeze film and hydrodynamic). (Adapted from Delahay JN: In Wiesel SW, Delahay JN, editors: Principles of Orthopaedic Medicine and Surgery, Philadelphia, 2001, WB Saunders.)

of fluid is created, the leading edge of which is wider and exudes fluid, and at the thinner trailing edge, fluid is thought to be resorbed. Stated another way, as load is applied to the bearing surface of the articular cartilage, fluid is squeezed from the cartilage, separating the surfaces, and is resorbed as the load decreases on the backside of the motion.[35] The material properties responsible for the fluid flow in the articular cartilage have been studied in detail.

Akeson used an analogy of an air tent (like those used to cover tennis courts) as a very effective way to understand the biomechanical function of the articular cartilage as it relates to the components of the cartilage matrix and fluid flow.[1] The components required for the proper function of the air tent are a pump (intake portal and fan), an inflation medium (air), and some form of fabric enabling containment of the inflation medium, thus creating a pressurized system. These tents are engineered to have small openings in the fabric, which require the pump to move more air inward than is escaping to keep the tent inflated. In articular cartilage, the pump corresponds to the proteoglycans; their ability to attract solutes based on their strong negative charge is the driving force of the pump. The inflation medium is solutes from the synovial fluid made up mainly of water, and the containment material, or fabric, is the network of collagen. Instead of entering through a single intake port of a mechanical pump, solutes gain access to the articular cartilage through the fine network of pores formed in the superficial layer of collagen, and likewise these molecules exit via these pores. Both systems (air tent and articular cartilage) depend on all components functioning appropriately and in unison. For example, if a tear in the containment material is too large, the pump cannot continue to pressurize the tent and the system collapses; likewise, if the pump fails, the normal egress of inflation media ultimately ends in a collapse of the tent.

In a state of equilibrium, the articular cartilage maintains a balance of pressure created by the interaction of aggrecan and water that is counteracted by the constraints of the collagen network. When an external load is applied to the articular surface, water flows out of the surface pores until a new equilibrium is reached. This process is relatively complex and not linear in nature. For example, as water egresses out of the articular cartilage as a result of increased surface load, the proteoglycans are forced closer together and generate greater repulsive pressures as they come closer to each other, much like similar poles of magnets repel each other with increasing proximity. Such fluid movement in and out of the articular cartilage is of great interest, because it is integral to the lubrication of the joint surface, load bearing functions of the articular surface, and nutrition of the chondrocytes.

The nutritional supply of the articular cartilage is thought to be provided through the exchange of solutes present in the synovial fluid during loading and unloading of the articular surface. Maroudas and colleagues calculated that based on this type of supply, the articular cartilage was limited to 6 mm of thickness for chondrocyte viability to be maintained, a calculation that appears to be accurate in terms of synovial joints.[35]

The term *viscoelastic* is used to describe the biomechanical properties of articular cartilage, and as the name implies, it is a combination of viscous, or fluid, and elastic biomechanical properties. When a static load is applied in a laboratory setting, there is an initial rapid movement of water out of the cartilage in the fluid phase, followed by a slower loss of water and compression of the collagen known as the creep phase. A time-deformation curve is used to graphically represent the response of the cartilage to loading after the static application of a load (Fig. 83-14). The loss of water and compression of the tissue, forcing the proteoglycans or aggrecans into closer proximity and repelling the forces of the proteoglycans from one another, also contributes to opposing the loading force in the creep phase. It has been estimated that 2- to 4-mm-thick cartilage can take 4 to 16 hours to reach creep equilibrium.[36]

PATHOPHYSIOLOGY OF OSTEOARTHROPATHY

Osteoarthropathy is a general term defined as any disease of the joints and bones. It is derived from the Greek words *osteo* ("bone or bones") and *arthron* ("joint"). A more specific term that relates to disease of the articular cartilage is *osteoarthritis,* defined as a disorder of movable joints characterized by degeneration and loss of articular cartilage. The suffix *itis* is somewhat misleading because it suggests a central inflammatory role, which is not present in many joint diseases of both horses and humans. Human rheumatoid arthritis is a notable exception and does have a central inflammatory role. Some definitions of osteoarthritis even state that it is a noninflammatory disease process, which is also somewhat misleading because inflammatory factors do play a part in most arthropathies (defined as any joint disease). Because of these discrepancies, several terms are used to describe similar disease processes. Other common terms are *degenerative joint disease* (DJD), which circumvents these issues but is often not favored as a scientific term. *Osteoarthrosis* is also sometimes used, correctly not emphasizing the inflammatory component, but this is defined as a chronic condition, which is not always accurate. *Osteoarthritis* is, in the author's experience, the currently accepted term describing degeneration of the equine articular cartilage. Therefore, this term will be used in this chapter.

Many texts define specific mechanisms as being responsible for the pathogenesis of osteoarthritis. For example, Caron describes three proposed mechanisms for osteoarthritis,[37] the first being fundamentally defective cartilage with abnormal biomechanical properties. Thus, the cartilage fails under normal loading conditions. An example of abnormal biomechanical properties is the genetic defect described in humans that results in a type II collagen that is unable to withstand normal joint loading.[38] The second mechanism involves abnormal change in the subchondral bone. It is accepted that subchondral bone typically undergoes remodeling in response to exercise or to changes in load. It is thought that in some cases, the bone increases its density to a pathologic level, which in turn results in a stiffer or less compliant bone–cartilage unit that is prone to failure. The third proposed mechanism revolves around normal cartilage that is exposed to abnormal forces—for example, those that may be seen with abnormal joint congruity

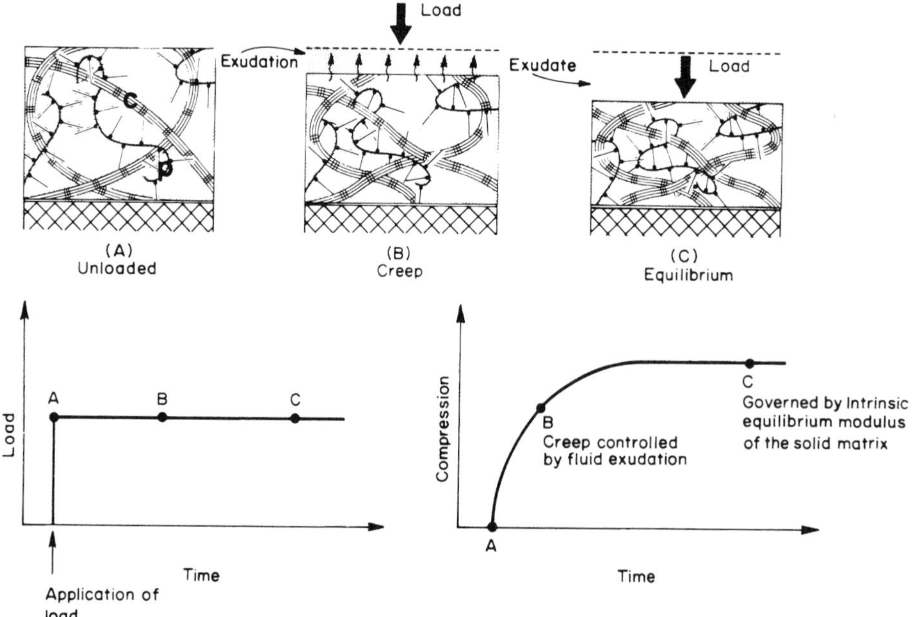

Figure 83-14. Schematic representation of time-dependent deformation of cartilage. The steep portion of the curve (A to B) represents initial loading. Subsequently, in the creep phase, there is further deformation of the matrix, which is a result of a slower flow of water through the matrix, until the equilibrium stage is reached. (From Myers ER, Mow VC: Biomechanics of cartilage and its response to biomechanical stimuli. In Hall BK, editor: Cartilage, vol 1, New York, 1983, Academic Press.)

resulting from a collateral ligament strain. In this mechanism, abnormal forces overwhelm the normal metabolic repair mechanisms in the articular cartilage and ultimately lead to its failure.

McIlwraith[8] has also outlined discrete mechanisms whereby osteoarthritis may ensue, and many similarities exist. More recently, he gave an example of a scenario that could lead to osteoarthritis and described how the different joint tissues may be involved, but he did not elaborate on previously defined mechanisms.[11] This trend for more general pathogenic descriptions is favored by the author. It is probable that most cases of equine joint disease have some involvement of most joint tissues: subchondral bone, articular cartilage, synovial fluid, synovium, ligamentous joint capsule, and external stabilizers of the joint such as ligaments, tendons, and muscles. This is not to say that specific components do not play a leading role, and initial failure of a single component or tissue is not often the case, but rather each component has some capacity for repair, and clinical disease usually is characterized by involvement of multiple joint tissues in some degree of pathology.

Metabolism of Arthritic Cartilage

It is widely accepted that all joint tissues have normal metabolic turnover, and the turnover is a balance of anabolic and catabolic pathways. Osteoarthritis at its origin may be defined by the predominance of the catabolic pathway, which leads to the ultimate failure of the tissue. Two interrelated factors should be considered in the pathogenesis of osteoarthritis: abnormal mechanical loads and metabolic tissue failure. Abnormal mechanical loads may be in the form of mechanical instability that can overwhelm the normal repair process of the tissues it is acting on. It may range from microdamage because of slight imperfections in conformation, to a single traumatic event leading to immediate catastrophic failure. Microdamage is believed to accumulate over time, leading to failure of the tissue after a failed reparative effort, and it may be likened to microcracks in an airplane wing that ultimately lead to failure if not repaired in time. On the other end of the spectrum, immediate damage to the cartilage could occur with a single impact without chance for repair, such as an articular fracture caused by a traumatic event. Metabolic tissue failure revolves around normal tissue metabolism and the fact that all the tissues of the joint have some capability for normal turnover and thus repair. However, some tissues, such as bone, are very adept at repair, whereas others, such as articular cartilage, are less adept. Thus, osteoarthritis could be defined as the point at which the anabolic repair process is overwhelmed by the catabolic processes. As described earlier, the imbalance and failure can be initiated by mechanical forces or by an inherent defect caused by a genetic imperfection, such as a type II collagen defect. A continuum of disease severity and involvement of multiple joint tissues is often the case in osteoarthritis; the etiology is most likely multifactorial, and at some stage, it includes some degree of both abnormal mechanical loads and metabolic tissue failure. The current understanding for normal metabolism and, in the case of osteoarthritis, response to injury for each joint tissue is described in the following paragraphs.

Mechanisms of Articular Cartilage Matrix Depletion

Synovial Membrane and Ligamentous Joint Capsule

The involvement of the synovial membrane and joint capsule in the pathogenesis of osteoarthritis is often not emphasized, with more focus being on the articular cartilage and bone. The synovium is a very dynamic tissue that has an integral role in influencing the joint environment, especially through the constituents of the synovial fluid, and thus it can have an especially significant effect on the articular cartilage. The highly vascular nature of the synovium allows it to act as the conduit and regulator for inflammatory cells and peripheral mediators that influence metabolic processes, especially in the release of catabolic substances affecting the joint. Likewise, the synoviocytes themselves, much like the chondrocytes, are capable of producing a wide variety of anabolic and catabolic enzymes, including prostaglandins, cytokines, and matrix MMPs.[8] In vitro experiments have shown the importance of mediators released specifically from the synovial membrane in regard to the degradation of articular cartilage. A limitation in determining the relative quantitative and temporal contributions of the synovial membrane to disease in vivo is our inability to identify the origin of the mediators in situ as being synovial or chondrocytic. To avoid redundancy, a more detailed description of the mediators and their role in osteoarthritis will be presented next, under "Chondrocytes."

Primary synovitis or capsulitis is thought to result from biomechanical damage, which may be on a continuum of repetitive trauma from discrete incidents. Severe trauma can lead to an effect on the joint capsule's role in joint stability and thus joint-wide abnormal biomechanical forces. The response of the joint capsule to injury is to form a fibrous repair tissue that is not biomechanically equivalent to the original tissue and can often result in a decreased range of motion for the particular joint. It is conceivable that this may have long-term ramifications of altered use of the joint and overall abnormal biomechanical forces to the joint tissues. Although the synovium is not thought to have any biomechanical stabilizing properties, it does respond to injury through cellular and enzymatic pathways. It is worth noting that synovitis and capsulitis can be secondary to other abnormalities in the joint. Synovitis may be secondary to other damage within the joint such as occurs with an osteochondral fragment in the carpus. In this example, physical damage to the tissues as well as liberation of debris and mediators from the damaged cartilage and bone will affect the synovial membrane and capsule. In concert with the lymphatic drainage of the joint, the synovial membrane is responsible for clearing debris from the synovial space. Neutrophils, macrophages, and mononuclear cells can also be routinely found in inflamed synovial membrane, contributing to both the phagocytic role of the membrane and the production of enzymatic mediators.

Histologic abnormalities seen in the synovial membrane can be characterized by edema, hyperplasia of the intimal cell lining, hypervascularity, cellular infiltration of inflammatory cells, and fibrosis of the subintima. The order in which these events appear loosely corresponds to the appearance of the abnormalities in a equine model of osteoarthritis and presumably in naturally occurring disease.[39] Changes documented histologically support alterations seen in other areas of the joint. For example, an increase in vascularity is typically associated with some degree of synovial effusion and an increased protein concentration in the synovial fluid. The increase in protein and fluid is thought to be associated with "gaps or leakiness" of the endothelial cell layer. Although ill defined, alterations in the lymphatic drainage of the synovial space is most likely a component of synovial effusion, with one proposed mechanism being an increased fluid pressure allowing less egress via the lymphatics. Intimal cell hyperplasia is also seen in cases of synovitis and is believed to be associated with a substantial metabolic response by the synoviocytes and most likely contributes to the central pathophysiologic events in osteoarthritis.

Chondrocytes

The joint chondrocytes are responsible for maintaining their surrounding environment through a complex interaction of anabolic and catabolic mediators as well as mechanical stimuli. In osteoarthritis, the net outcome favors the catabolic pathways, and degeneration of the articular cartilage ensues with loss of the key matrix components, including aggrecan and type II collagen. There has been a long-raging debate over the definition of the earliest sign of osteoarthritis as it relates to aggrecan or type II collagen loss (reminiscent of the chicken-or-egg argument). Both in vitro and in vivo studies have documented loss of aggrecan as an initial biochemical event.[33,40-42] Furthermore, it appears that upregulation of the synthetic pathways is one of the earliest metabolic manifestations, although the net loss of aggrecan and collagen prevail. The quality and quantity of both matrix components are affected, with an increase in water content and surface fibrillation also being early events in articular cartilage degeneration. This, in turn, will affect the mechanical properties of the cartilage, making it less able to withstand normal loads, perpetuating the disease process, and inciting changes in other tissues such as bone and synovial membrane as the cartilage loses its functionality.

The proteolytic enzymes synthesized by the chondrocytes and synoviocytes, and their role in cartilage breakdown, have been extensively studied. They are described by their catalytic mechanisms and include MMPs, aspartic proteinases, cysteine proteinases, and serine proteinases, with the MMPs thought to be most involved in the pathogenesis of osteoarthritis.[8,43]

Matrix Metalloproteinases

The MMPs are grouped together by a requirement for zinc in their active binding site and are typically described either by a descriptive name or by a numerical MMP assignment. To date, 25 different MMPs have been described.[44] The descriptive name is often based on the substrate the MMP was first observed to degrade—such as collagenases, stromelysins, and gelatinases. The MMPs are secreted in an inactive "pro" form and collectively possess the ability to degrade all of the major components in the articular cartilage; thus, they play a major role in both health and disease of the articular cartilage. The synoviocytes and chondrocytes as well as other cell types are capable of MMP production. Increasing concentrations of MMPs have been correlated to areas of histologic abnormalities, signifying their active role in cartilage degradation.[45,46] The major MMPs that have been incriminated in osteoarthritis include collagenase 1 (MMP-1), collagenase 2 (MMP-8), collagenase 3 (MMP-13), stromelysin 1 (MMP-3), and two gelatinases (MMP-2 and MMP-9). A family of enzymes called "a disintegrin and metalloproteinase" (ADAM) is structurally and functionally related to the MMPs and is also a major factor in aggrecan cleavage. A summary of the nomenclature and function of the MMPs and related proteinases can be found in Table 83-1.

TABLE 83-1. Matrix Metalloproteins (MMPs) Implicated in Cartilage Matrix Degradation

Enzyme	MMP Number	Function	TIMP Number
COLLAGENASES			
Interstitial collagenase (collagenase 1)[‡]	MMP-1[§]	Collagens II and X (not IX and XI), denatured type II, aggrecan, link protein	TIMP-1>TIMP-2
Neutrophil collagenase[‡]	MMP-8	Collagen II, aggrecan, link protein	TIMP-1, TIMP-2
Collagenase 3[‡‖]	MMP-13[§]	Collagens II, IV, IX, X; aggrecan; fibronectin	TIMP-3
STROMELYSINS			
Stromelysin 1[‡]	MMP-3[§]	Aggrecan, fibronectin; denatured collagen II	TIMP-1>TIMP-2
Stromelysin 2[‡]	MMP-10	Collagens IV, IX, X, XI; procollagens; link protein; decorin; elastin; laminin Same as for stromelysin 1	TIMP-3
GELATINASES			
Gelatinase A (72 kD)[‡]	MMP-2[§]	Denatured collagen II, collagens X and XI, elastin	TIMP-2>TIMP-1
Gelatinase B (92 kD)[‡]	MMP-9[§]	Aggrecan, fibroconectin, collagens IX and XI, procollagens, link protein, decorin, elastin	—

‡ Expressed by chondrocytes. All are expressed in synovium.

§ MMPs characterized in the horse.

‖ MMP-13 expression is relatively weak in equine system.

Interstitial or tissue collagenase (MMP-1) is able to break intact type II collagen molecules by cleaving all three collagen α-chains of the triple helix at a specific amino acid sequence (residues 775-776).[8] Collagenase 2 or human neutrophil collagenase (MMP-8) is released from polymorphonuclear leukocytes (PMNs) and was first shown to be active in human osteoarthritis[47] but has more recently been identified as having activity in equine cartilage.[48] Collagenase 3 (MMP-13) has been shown to be more aggressive in type II collagen degradation, cleaving it 10 times faster than MMP-1. Also found in higher concentrations in diseased cartilage of horses and humans, MMP-13 is upregulated by interleukin-1 (IL-1) and tumor necrosis factor (TNF), key enzymes at the top of the articular cartilage catabolic pathway.[46,49] Stromelysins have been studied most notably for their ability to break down proteoglycans, but partially degraded collagen and other minor cartilage proteins can be substrates. Much of the credit for breaking down aggrecan in osteoarthritic cartilage has recently been given to members in the ADAMs family of enzymes, specifically aggrecanases.[43] It is currently thought that aggrecanases play a pivotal role in proteoglycan depletion in disease cartilage. The gelatinases also have a diverse range of substrates, including partially degraded collagens and elastins.[8]

Cytokines

Historically, the term *cytokine* denoted small regulatory proteins that were associated with catabolic pathways. More recently, the term has been broadened and is now considered to define catabolic, modulatory, and anabolic proteins that are produced by one cell while acting on another. Cytokine pathways are relatively complex, and more in-depth knowledge of these pathways, as well as their interactions with other molecules, is being published. These mediators play a pivotal role in the metabolism of the synovial membrane and articular cartilage in health and disease.

Most notable of the *catabolic cytokines* are IL-1 and TNF-α, which can be secreted from chondrocytes and synoviocytes. Both have been demonstrated to be upregulated beyond a normal level in osteoarthritis, promoting production of MMP, nitric oxide, and prostaglandin E_2 (PGE_2), as well as inhibiting aggrecan and type II collagen synthesis.[8] Although both IL-1 and TNF have relatively similar actions, it is thought that IL-1 is the most important of the proinflammatory cytokines.[50] In vitro, the two molecules do appear to potentiate each other, and TNF has been shown to stimulate IL-1.[51] In addition to having these effects, IL-1 has also been shown to inhibit the production of natural antiarthritic molecules such as the MMP inhibitors (tissue inhibitor of matrix metalloproteinase, or TIMP) and interleukin-1 receptor antagonist (IL-1Ra), which potentates the catabolic cascade.

The *modulatory* or *regulatory cytokines*, such as IL-4, IL-10, and IL-13, have actions that balance or modulate the proinflammatory cytokines, namely IL-1 and TNF. They have been shown to inhibit the synthesis of IL-1 as well as to promote the synthesis of the natural inhibitors, specifically the TIMPs and IL-1Ra. IL-6 has a mixed mode of action that includes magnifying the effects of IL-1 while promoting synthesis of the TIMPs.[52]

Cytokines that promote the *anabolic* cascade of cartilage metabolism, such as insulin-like growth factor (IGF) and transforming growth factor (TGF), play a role in osteoarthritis. These molecules have been shown to promote chondrocyte production of matrix molecules such as proteoglycans and type II collagen. Thus, anabolic cytokines can be helpful in reparative attempts in diseased joints. The use of anabolic cytokines in treatment protocols of osteoarthritis is an area of current research.[53,54]

Although not classified as cytokines, nitric oxide (as well as other oxygen-derived free radicals) and prostaglandins are increased in joints with osteoarthritis. Free radicals play a role in the degradation of hyaluronan and collagen. Cells have been shown to produce nitric oxide in response to IL-1, and its production has been related to inhibition of chondrocyte anabolic activities. Association with activation of MMPs and the reduction in the natural inhibitors has also been observed with nitric oxide, although this molecule's specific role in osteoarthritis is still somewhat controversial.[55,56] Also associated with decrease in anabolic synthesis is the E series of prostaglandins. PGE_2 has been shown to be increased in the synovial fluid of horses with osteoarthritis and has been correlated with both synovitis and clinical lameness as well as being produced after stimulation with IL-1 and TNF in vitro.[8]

Natural Inhibitors of MMPs and Cytokines

The biologic response to IL-1 and TNF occurs after the molecules bind to a specific receptor. Both molecules have at least one mechanism by which their activity is blocked by a natural inhibitor. One example of a natural inhibitor of IL-1 is IL-1Ra, which has affinity for the IL-1 receptor, but when it binds to the receptor, it does not elicit a biologic response, and thus it acts as a natural inhibitor of IL-1. In the case of TNF, the membrane-bound receptors can be secreted or solubilized (in this form, there is no way to signal a biologic response once bound to TNF). They maintain the affinity for the TNF molecule and, in thus binding the molecule, prevent it from binding a membrane bound receptor. Numerous in vitro and in vivo studies have been carried out using natural inhibitors of the cytokines with very promising results[57,58] (see Chapter 84).

Like the cytokines, natural inhibitors of the MMPs also exist, termed TIMPs. Four different TIMPs have been described, three of which (TIMP-1, TIMP-2, and TIMP-3) are thought to be active in inhibition of joint-related functions. Synthesized by numerous cells that include chondrocytes and synoviocytes, these inhibitors bind one-to-one with MMPs to form an inactive complex.[59,60] Believed to play an important role in the normal regulatory mechanism of the joint environment, these inhibitors have been shown to be present in abnormal levels in human osteoarthritic cartilage.[61,62] Therapeutic intervention using TIMPs has not appeared to advance as rapidly as cytokine inhibitor therapy, which may suggest a less global role in osteoarthritis, although more research is needed.[63]

In summary, a vast number of mediators are involved in joint metabolism in both health and disease. This chapter has only outlined the major molecules and the current level of understanding. Given the discovery of new mediators and common pathways, substantial changes in our understanding of osteoarthritis should be expected in the next decade. Additional information on this subject can be found in Chapter 79.

Clinical Manifestations of Osteoarthritis

Sources of Pain

Joint-related problems account for the greatest single economic loss to the horse industry, much of which can be related to osteoarthritic pain. Although the articular cartilage is devoid of innervation, the surrounding tissues are rich in unmyelinated C fibers. The capsule, synovium, tendons, ligaments, periosteum, and bone have all been defined as sources of pain in osteoarthritic cases. Sensory nerves are known to respond both to mechanical stimuli, such as stretching, and to chemical mediators. Mediators such as kinins and the neuropeptides (e.g., substance P) have been shown to stimulate pain fibers directly. These mediators, along with others, such as PGE_2 and IL-1, sensitize fibers to be more reactive after mechanical stimulation. Upregulation of pain receptors and involvement of the central nervous system (i.e., the spinal nerves) has also been demonstrated in osteoarthritis.[64] Elevated levels of substance P have been observed in both equine and human patients with osteoarthritis, and they can stimulate monocytes to release other pro-inflammatory cytokines such as IL-1 and TNF.[65-67]

In both horses and humans, correlation between clinical signs and disease severity is poor. In humans, there is an increased chance of reporting pain with increasing radiographic changes consistent with osteoarthritis, but a significant number of people report pain despite normal radiographs, and many individuals with unequivocal knee osteoarthritis deny having pain. Similar parallels can be drawn from equine patients, although anatomic location in both horses and humans appears to play a part in the correlation between clinical pain and the objective parameters. One explanation for the lack of association between pain and structural damage is the lack of sensitivity of outcome parameters, such as radiographs. Many of the soft tissue structures responsible for the pain, such as joint capsule, ligaments, and menisci, are poorly imaged using radiographs. In fact, the importance of soft tissue in joint health is underscored by the fact that quadriceps weakness is a risk factor for human knee osteoarthritis. Multiple studies have shown that strengthening exercises are an effective method of reducing pain and improving function in people with osteoarthritis.[68-70]

It is also believed that the periosteum and bone can play a significant role in osteoarthritic pain. People report focal pain in the area of osteophyte growth, and it is believed that growth of the osteophyte may result in elevation and stretching of the richly innervated periosteum.[64] In some cases, the subchondral bone plate appears to be a source of pain, although not all horses with subchondral cystic lesions demonstrate clinical lameness.[71] Increases in intraosseous pressure have been demonstrated in osteoarthritis, and there is evidence to link this with pain in people, especially following reduction of symptoms after cortical fenestration.[64] Similar mechanisms have been proposed for horses, and decompression of cystic lesions has led to improved lameness scores.

Clinical Parameters

An increase in synovial fluid or synovial pressure is a common finding, especially in joints with excessive joint distention. Thought to be initiated by inflammatory events occurring in the joint, synovial effusion is in part a result of increased vascular permeability (ingress) and a decrease in lymphatic drainage (egress). This net increase in fluid results in an abnormal usage of the joint for both mechanical and pain-related reasons. If not controlled, the inflammatory process may lead to changes in the synovium and the joint capsule, which are often observed as a decreased range of motion. Although an increase in synovial fluid can be solely responsible for decreases in range of motion, edema and a decreased pain threshold most likely also contribute. More chronic changes, such as fibrosis in the synovial membrane and joint capsule, can also be observed histologically.

Changes in the content of the synovial fluid are also observed in most cases of osteoarthritis, and reduction in viscosity is one of the oldest measures of a diseased joint. A rough evaluation of viscosity is often made by handling a tenacious string of synovial fluid between the evaluator's fingers. The loss in viscosity is typically attributed to a decease in hyaluronan concentration as well as to depolymerization or shortening of the molecule.[72] The large variation in scientific methods and the time-consuming nature of measuring synovial fluid viscosity often make this measurement clinically impractical. The addition of acetic acid leading to precipitation of mucin or a "mucin clot" is a quick and easier but less specific or sensitive way to measure synovial fluid quality. This, in combination with gross observation of the synovial fluid, which is usually pale yellow to clear and free of flocculent material, has been used in the field to assess quality. In a laboratory setting, the determination of synovial fluid total protein is often useful in relation to the degree of synovitis and also has been correlated to articular cartilage damage arthroscopically.[73] Cytologic examination of the synovial fluid also is routinely performed in the laboratory. Although synovial fluid total protein and cytology is not diagnostically very specific or sensitive, it can be useful in some cases, especially those with extreme values (Table 83-2).

Recently, more sophisticated methods of measuring cartilage-specific (aggrecan and type II collagen) synthetic and degradation molecules have become available for use on synovial fluid and serum of horses with osteoarthritis. These biomarkers show promise in early detection and staging of equine joint disease, although more clinical research is needed.[33,73]

As previously mentioned, the usefulness of radiographs is somewhat limited in osteoarthritis, but, because of their ease, they have historically been a method for evaluating joint disease. Although often not correlated to the severity of clinical signs, periarticular osteophytes, joint-space narrowing, subchondral bone sclerosis or lysis, and the presence of osteochondral fragments are typical features that can be present radiographically in an osteoarthritic joint (Table 83-3).

Other imaging modalities such as ultrasonography and magnetic resonance imaging (MRI) have more recently gained acceptance in veterinary medicine. The ability of ultrasonography to image soft tissues, including articular cartilage, makes it an especially useful adjunctive diagnostic

TABLE 83-2. Synovial Fluid Cytology Corresponding to Various Clinical Conditions and Diagnostic or Therapeutic Manipulations

Parameter	Normal	Mild Synovitis (e.g., OCD)	Osteo-arthritis	Septic Arthritis*	Arthrocentesis	Balanced Electrolyte Solution	Local Anesthetics†‡	Gentamicin†	DMSO† (10% Solution)
Total leukocytes (/μL)	50-500	20-250	≤1 × 10?	20-200 × 10^3	1-4 × 10^3	6-45 × 10^3 (typically 20 × 10^3)	2-10 × 10^3	8-40 × 10^3	6-20 × 10^3
Neutrophils (%)	<10	<10	<15	>90 (variable toxic changes)	50	80	60	50	>50
Mononuclear cells (%)	>90	>90	>85	<10	50	20	40	50	<50
Total Proteins (g/dL)	0.8-2.5	0.8-3	0.8-3.5	4.0-8+	1.5-2.5	3-4	2.5-4	4.5-6	2.5-4

Listed ranges are approximate. Considerable variability exists in published reports.
*Significant elevations in leukocyte counts and total protein concentration occur within the first 12 hours in experimentally inoculated joints. Values shown represent those observed at 24 hours.
†Leukocyte counts and total protein concentrations correspond to the maximum values that typically occur within the first 24 hours.
‡Synovial response to lidocaine and mepivacaine are comparable

TABLE 83-3. Radiographic Features of Osteoarthritis

Radiographic Feature	Pathogenic mechanism*
Periarticular osteophytosis	Endochondral ossification occurring at bony margins of unknown cause. Possible repair attempt modulated by altered cytokine milieu.
(Asymmetrical) joint space thinning	Cartilage degeneration and loss.† Usually at areas of weight bearing or high stress. May be absent when focal cartilage loss occurs.
Subchondral sclerosis	Deposition of new bone as a response to changes in force transmission and from healing of trabecular microfractures. Corresponds to areas of maximum stress. Significant sclerosis often corresponds to full-thickness cartilage loss.
Subchondral lysis	Less common change of uncertain pathogenesis. Possibly pressure necrosis from synovial fluid gaining access to subchondral plate via fissures, or related to pressure necrosis from trauma to bone.
Osteochondral bodies	Disintegration of joint surfaces or fractured osteophytes. May represent inciting lesions (e.g., osteochondral fracture).
Advanced remodeling/ ankylosis	Articular response to advanced degeneration. Environment more consistent with fracture than synovial joint.

*Specific pathophysiologic mechanisms and reasons for disproportionate representation of changes among and between joints remain unclear.
†Seldom used as a marker of disease progression because of problems with technical aspects of radiographic positioning and focal-film distance.

tool in osteoarthritis. The level of sophistication and general knowledge in equine ultrasonographic joint anatomy has greatly increased in the last decade, making joint ultrasonography a standard tool.[74] Likewise, with increased knowledge of normal anatomy and increased availability of equine-dedicated MRI units, this modality will surely gain greater acceptance. The use of MRI in the human orthopedic field is commonplace, largely because of the ability to image all of the joint tissues in a three-dimensional space.

Cartilage Repair

An observation made in 1743 that "cartilage once destroyed never heals" is still accurate today.[75] Modern nomenclature defines healing as the restoration of structural and functional integrity, whereas regeneration suggests the tissue will be identical to that of the original. Repair, on the other hand, has a more limited meaning and suggests that cells and tissue structures replace the damaged tissue, but that the tissue does not necessarily return to its original structure or function. The degree of damage to normal articular cartilage is typically described by the dimensions of the lesion and its depth into the tissue; both of these factors, as well as anatomic location and weightbearing, play a significant role in the degree of healing and return to normal function.

It is important to note discrepancies in the cartilage repair literature regarding the definition of full-thickness defects. This term has been used by some to describe lesions including only the noncalcified cartilage (superficial, intermediate, and deep, but not the calcified cartilage layers) all the way to lesions that extend past the subchondral bone plate. Until recently the true depth was known only if histologic confirmation was performed. However, after studies using arthroscopic visualization of experimental cartilage defects were correlated directly to histologic sections, some degree of confidence about the depth of defects can be made. Today, most authors use full-thickness articular cartilage defects to describe a lesion through the calcified cartilage layer but not involving the subchondral bone plate.

It is believed that full-thickness defects greater than 3 to 5 mm^2 in surface area have a poor capacity for repair. In general, defects of this size range are difficult to identify grossly 1 year after they are created, whereas larger defects show good initial healing but degenerate within a year's time.[76,77] Partial-thickness defects are believed to have some minor capacity for healing, but typically they appear neither to be progressive nor to compromise joint function, and they are, therefore, not the focus of most cartilage repair procedures. Clinically, partial-thickness lesions are débrided of any surface fibrillation without débriding deeper. This is because currently used cartilage-repair processes do not provide a repair tissue that is clearly better than the tissue in a partial-thickness defect.

Historically, two different repair mechanisms are described for articular cartilage: intrinsic and extrinsic. Intrinsic, as the name implies, occurs from within the cartilage. Thus, intrinsic repair relies on the limited capacity of the chondrocytes to divide and repair the damage. A type of intrinsic repair termed *matrix flow* describes healing lesions that have chondrocytes and surrounding matrix that appear to flow from the peripheral cartilage edges into the defect in an attempt to fill the lesion. Small defects appear to repair via this process. Extrinsic repair derives cells and other factors contributing to the repair process from sources other than the chondrocytes. One example is repair following surgical perforation of the subchondral bone plate, which is believed to allow stem or progenitor cells as well as growth factors access to the defect, thus enhancing the repair of large defects, which would otherwise exhibit poor healing.[19] The currently accepted method of subchondral perforation is called subchondral bone microfracture. Contrary to historic beliefs, mounting evidence suggests that progenitor cells may exist in the surface layer of articular cartilage,[78] thereby challenging the distinction of intrinsic and extrinsic healing, although it is still accepted that large lesions most likely derive most of their reparative capacity from extrinsic sources. Another example of extrinsic repair is through the implantation of chondrocytes obtained from an external source, which are typically suspended in some form of scaffold and secured into the defect. Greater detail on specific cartilage repair procedures can be found in Chapter 84.

Repair of clinically significant lesions (i.e., greater than 5 mm in diameter), which requires extrinsic repair methods, appears to be hampered by a less-than-optimal aggrecan, type II collagen content, and re-formation of normal subchondral bone and calcified cartilage layers. As was previously described, all of these components are integral to the normal function of articular cartilage and hence the joint. Significant improvements in re-establishment of the type II collagen content and to some degree aggrecan have been made recently, but little has been done to improve, enhance, or even control the re-formation of the subchondral bone plate or calcified cartilage layer. Experimental defects have been shown to heal through an influx of granulation tissue, which is characterized by types I and III collagen, and by little proteoglycan or aggrecan in the first 6 weeks. The granulation tissue is then slowly replaced with increasing amounts of type II collagen and aggrecan by chondrocyte-like cells.[79] At best, a hyaline-like tissue is formed, and the biomechanical and biochemical properties of this tissue leave much to be desired. Although modern science has made great leaps in improving the in vitro character of tissue-engineered cartilage, the absence of normal physiologic mechanical stimuli appears to be a rate-limiting step in vivo, given the critical role it plays in tissue integration and long-term survival of these creations. Interestingly, it has been observed in humans that the quality of the repair tissue is not always directly correlated to the functional outcome of the patient. Thus, less emphasis is now being placed on the regeneration of the articular cartilage and more on long-term improvement in function. In some older human patients, 5 years of dramatic pain relief, thus delaying joint replacement, is considered a success.[80]

REFERENCES

1. Akeson WH: Articular cartilage and its exacting characteristics: The benchmark for all attempts to achieve articular cartilage regeneration or repair. In Daniel DM, Pedowitz RA, O'Connor JJ, et al, editors: Daniel's Knee Injuries: Ligament and Cartilage Structure, Function, Injury, and Repair, ed 2, Philadelphia, 2003, Lippincott Williams & Wilkins.
2. Dee R: The innervation of joints. In Sokoloff L, editor: The Joints and Synovial Fluid, New York, 1978, Academic Press.
3. Gronblad M, Korkala O, Liesi P, et al: Innervation of synovial membrane and meniscus, Acta Orthop Scand 1985;56:484-486.
4. Henderson B, Pettipher ER: The synovial lining cell: Biology and pathobiology, Semin Arthritis Rheum 1985;15:1-32.
5. Norton WL, Lewis DC, Ziff M: Electron-dense deposits following injection of gold sodium thiomalate and thiomalic acid, Arthritis Rheum 1968;11:436-443.
6. Roy S, Ghadially FN, Crane WA: Synovial membrane in traumatic effusion: Ultrastructure and autoradiography with tritiated leucine, Ann Rheum Dis 1966;25:259-271.
7. Todhunter RJ: Anatomy and physiology of synovial joints. In McIlwraith CW, Trotter GW, editors: Joint Disease in the Horse, Philadelphia, 1996, WB Saunders.
8. McIlwraith CW: General pathobiology of the joint and response to injury. In McIlwraith CW, Trotter GW, editors: Joint Disease in the Horse, ed 1, Philadelphia, 1996, WB Saunders.
9. Howard RD, McIlwraith CW: Hyaluronan and its use in the treatment of equine joint disease. In McIlwraith CW,Trotter GW, editors: Joint Disease in the Horse, Philadelphia, 1996, WB Saunders.
10. Mankin HJ, Radin EL: Structure and function of joints. In McCarty DJ, editor: Arthritis and Allied Conditions: A Textbook of Rheumatology, ed 2, Philadelphia, 1993, Lea & Febiger.
11. McIlwraith CW: Diseases of joints, tendons, ligaments, and related structures. In Stashak TS, editor: Adams' Lameness in Horses, ed 5, Philadelphia, 2002, Williams & Wilkins.
12. Gamble JG, Edwards CC, Max SR: Enzymatic adaptation in ligaments during immobilization, Am J Sports Med 1984;12:221-228.
13. Ralphs JR, Benjamin M: The joint capsule: Structure, composition, ageing and disease, J Anat 1994;184:503-509.
14. Thornton GM, Shrive NG, Frank CB: Healing ligaments have decreased cyclic modulus compared to normal ligaments and immobilization further compromises healing ligament response to cyclic loading, J Orthop Res 2003;21:716-722.
15. Radin EL, Paul IL, Tolkoff MJ: Subchondral bone changes in patients with early degenerative joint disease, Arthritis Rheum 1970;13:400-405.
16. Richardson DW, Yound DR, Clark CC: The relationship of subchondral bone stiffness to overlying cartilage morphology and biochemistry, Orthop Res Soc 1993:720.
17. Kawcak CE, McIlwraith CW, Norrdin RW, et al: Clinical effects of exercise on subchondral bone of carpal and metacarpophalangeal joints in horses, Am J Vet Res 2000;61:1252-1258.
18. Teshima R, Otsuka T, Takasu N, et al: Structure of the most superficial layer of articular cartilage, J Bone Joint Surg Br 1995;77:460-464.
19. Frisbie DD, Trotter GW, Powers BE, et al: Arthroscopic subchondral bone plate microfracture technique augments healing of large chondral defects in the radial carpal bone and medial femoral condyle of horses, Vet Surg 1999;28:242-255.
20. McCutchen C: The frictional properties of animal joints, Wear 1962;5:1.
21. Hultkrantz W: Uber die Spaltrichtungen der Gelenkknorpel, Verh Anat Ges 1898;12:248.
22. Pauwels F: Structure of the tangential fibrous layer of the articular cartilage in the scapular glenoid cavity as an example of an unsubstantiated strain field, Z Anat Entw Gesch 1959;121:188.
23. van der Rest M, Garrone R: Collagen family of proteins, FASEB J 1991;5:2814-2823.
24. Vachon AM, Keeley FW, McIlwraith CW, et al: Biochemical analysis of normal articular cartilage in horses, Am J Vet Res 1990;51:1905-1911.
25. Kielty CM, Whittaker SP, Grant ME, et al: Type VI collagen microfibrils: Evidence for a structural association with hyaluronan, J Cell Biol 1992;118:979-990.
26. Stallcup WB, Dahlin K, Healy P: Interaction of the NG2 chondroitin sulfate proteoglycan with type VI collagen, J Cell Biol 1990;111:3177-3188.
27. Eikenberry EF, Mendler M, Burgin R, et al: Fibrillar organization in cartilage. In Kuettner KE, Schleyerbach R, Peyron JG, et al, editors: Articular Cartilage and Osteoarthritis, New York, 1992, Raven Press.
28. Ogston A: The biological functions of the glycosaminoglycans. In Balazs EA, editor: Chemistry and Molecular Biology of the Intercellular Matrix, New York, 1970, Academic Press.
29. Mehmet H, Scudder P, Tang PW, et al: The antigenic determinants recognized by three monoclonal antibodies to keratan sulphate involve sulphated hepta- or larger oligosaccharides of the poly(*N*-acetyllactosamine) series, Eur J Biochem 1986;157:385-391.
30. Flannery C, Stanescu V, Morgelin M, et al: Variability in the G3 domain content of bovine aggrecan from cartilage extracts and chondrocyte cultures, Arch Biochem Biophys 1992;297:52-60.
31. Lohmander S: Proteoglycans of joint cartilage: Structure, function, turnover and role as markers of joint disease, Baillieres Clin Rheumatol 1988;2:37-62.
32. March L: Articular cartilage in health and disease. In Sambrook P, editor: The Musculoskeletal System, New York, 2001, Churchill Livingstone.

33. Frisbie DD, Al-Sobayil F, Billinghurst RC, et al: Serum biomarkers distinguish exercise from osteoarthritic pathology, Osteoarthritis Cartilage 2001;10(Suppl A):S53.
34. Ekman L, Nilsson G, Persson L, et al: Volume of the synovia in certain joint cavities in the horse, Acta Vet Scand 1981;22:23-31.
35. Delahay JN: Biomechanics and biomaterials. In Wiesel SW, Delahay JN, editors: Principles of Orthopaedic Medicine and Surgery, Philadelphia, 2001, WB Saunders.
36. Mow VC, Hung CT: Biomechanics of articular cartilage. In Nordin M, Frankel VH, editors: Basic Biomechanics of the Musculoskeletal System, ed 3, Philadelphia, 2001, Lippincott Williams & Wilkins.
37. Caron JP: Osteoarthritis. In Ross MW, Dyson SJ, editors: Diagnosis and Management of Lameness in the Horse, Philadelphia, 2003, WB Saunders.
38. Knowlton RG, Katsenstein PL, Moskowitz RW, et al: Genetic linkage of a polymorphism in the type II procollagen gene (COL2A1) to primary osteoarthritis associated with mild chondrodysplasia, N Engl J Med 1990;322:526-530.
39. Frisbie DD, Kawcak CE, Trotter GW, et al: The effects of 6-alpha methylprednisolone acetate on an in vivo equine osteochondral fragment exercise model, Am J Vet Res 1998;12:1619-1628.
40. Altman RD, Tenenbaum J, Latta L, et al: Biomechanical and biochemical properties of dog cartilage in experimentally induced osteoarthritis, Ann Rheum Dis 1984;43:83-90.
41. Curtin WA, Reville WJ: Ultrastructural observations on fibril profiles in normal and degenerative human articular cartilage, Clin Orthop 1995:224-230.
42. Maroudas A, Ziv I, Weisman N, et al: Studies of hydration and swelling pressure in normal and osteoarthritic cartilage. Biorheology 1985;22:159-169.
43. Little CB, Flannery CR, Hughes CE, et al: Aggrecanase versus matrix metalloproteinases in the catabolism of the interglobular domain of aggrecan in vitro, Biochem J 1999;344:61-68.
44. Woessner JF Jr: MMPs and TIMPs: An historical perspective, Mol Biotechnol 2002;22:33-49.
45. Okada Y, Shinmei M, Tanaka O, et al: Localization of matrix metalloproteinase 3 (stromelysin) in osteoarthritic cartilage and synovium, Lab Invest 1992;66:680-690.
46. Caron JP, Tardif G, Martel-Pelletier J, et al: Modulation of matrix metalloprotease 13 (collagenase 3) gene expression in equine chondrocytes by interleukin 1 and corticosteroids, Am J Vet Res 1996;57:1631-1634.
47. Billinghurst RC, Dahlberg L, Ionescu M, et al: Enhanced cleavage of type II collagen by collagenases in osteoarthritic articular cartilage, J Clin Invest 1997;99:1534-1545.
48. Billinghurst RC, O'Brien K, Poole AR, et al: Inhibition of articular cartilage degradation in culture by a novel nonpeptidic matrix metalloproteinase inhibitor, Ann N Y Acad Sci 1999;878:594-597.
49. Trumble TN, Trotter GW, Oxford JR, et al: Synovial fluid gelatinase concentrations and matrix metalloproteinase and cytokine expression in naturally occurring joint disease in horses, Am J Vet Res 2001;62:1467-1477.
50. Yaron I, Meyer FA, Dayer JM, et al: Some recombinant human cytokines stimulate glycosaminoglycan synthesis in human synovial fibroblast cultures and inhibit it in human articular cartilage cultures, Arthritis Rheum 1989;32:173-180.
51. Meyer FA, Yaron I, Yaron M: Synergistic, additive, and antagonistic effects of interleukin-1 beta, tumor necrosis factor alpha, and gamma-interferon on prostaglandin E, hyaluronic acid, and collagenase production by cultured synovial fibroblasts, Arthritis Rheum 1990;33:1518-1525.
52. Martel-Pelletier J, Alaaeddine N, Pelletier JP: Cytokines and their role in the pathophysiology of osteoarthritis. Front Biosci 1999;4:D694-703.
53. Malemud CJ, Islam N, Haqqi TM: Pathophysiological mechanisms in osteoarthritis lead to novel therapeutic strategies, Cells Tissues Organs 2003;174:34-48.
54. Steinmeyer J: Cytokines in osteoarthritis—current status on the pharmacological intervention, Front Biosci 2004;9:575-580.
55. Cao M, Westerhausen-Larson A, Niyibizi C, et al: Nitric oxide inhibits the synthesis of type-II collagen without altering Col2A1 mRNA abundance: Prolyl hydroxylase as a possible target, Biochem J 1997;324:305-310.
56. Oh M, Fukuda K, Asada S, et al: Concurrent generation of nitric oxide and superoxide inhibits proteoglycan synthesis in bovine articular chondrocytes: Involvement of peroxynitrite, J Rheumatol 1998;25:2169-2174.
57. Frisbie DD, McIlwraith CW: Evaluation of gene therapy as a treatment for equine traumatic arthritis and osteoarthritis, Clin Orthop 2000:S273-287.
58. Moreland LW: Inhibitors of tumor necrosis factor for rheumatoid arthritis, J Rheumatol Suppl 1999;57:7-15.
59. Su S, Grover J, Roughley PJ, et al: Expression of the tissue inhibitor of metalloproteinases (TIMP) gene family in normal and osteoarthritic joints, Rheumatol Int 1999;18:183-191.
60. Zafarullah M, Su S, Martel-Pelletier J, et al: Tissue inhibitor of metalloproteinase-2 (TIMP-2) mRNA is constitutively expressed in bovine, human normal, and osteoarthritic articular chondrocytes, J Cell Biochem 1996;60:211-217.
61. Dean DD, Azzo W, Martel-Pelletier J, et al: Levels of metalloproteases and tissue inhibitor of metalloproteases in human osteoarthritic cartilage, J Rheumatol 1987;14:43-44.
62. Dean DD, Martel-Pelletier J, Pelletier JP, et al: Evidence for metalloproteinase and metalloproteinase inhibitor imbalance in human osteoarthritic cartilage, J Clin Invest 1989;84:678-685.
63. Baker AH, Edwards DR, Murphy G: Metalloproteinase inhibitors: Biological actions and therapeutic opportunities, J Cell Sci 2002;115:3719-3727.
64. Creamer P: Osteoarthritis. In Wall PD, Melzack R, editors: Textbook of Pain, ed 4, New York, 1999, Churchill Livingstone.
65. Caron JP, Bowker RM, Abhold RH, et al: Substance P in the synovial membrane and fluid of the equine middle carpal joint, Equine Vet J 1992;24:364-366.
66. Lotz M, Carson DA, Vaughan JH: Substance P activation of rheumatoid synoviocytes: Neural pathway in pathogenesis of arthritis, Science 1987;235:893-895.
67. Marshall KW, Chiu B, Inman RD: Substance P and arthritis: Analysis of plasma and synovial fluid levels, Arthritis Rheum 1990;33:87-90.
68. Chamberlain MA, Care G, Harfield B: Physiotherapy in osteoarthrosis of the knees: A controlled trial of hospital versus home exercises. Int Rehabil Med 1982;4:101-106.
69. Dekker J, Tola P, Aufdemkampe G, et al: Negative affect, pain and disability in osteoarthritis patients: The mediating role of muscle weakness, Behav Res Ther 1993;31:203-206.
70. Fisher NM, Gresham GE, Abrams M, et al: Quantitative effects of physical therapy on muscular and functional performance in subjects with osteoarthritis of the knees, Arch Phys Med Rehabil 1993;74:840-847.
71. Baxter GM: Subchondral cystic lesions in horses. In McIlwraith CW, Trotter GW, editors: Joint Disease in the Horse, Philadelphia, 1996, WB Saunders.
72. Tulamo RM, Houttu J, Tupamaki A, et al: Hyaluronate and large molecular weight proteoglycans in synovial fluid from horses with various arthritides, Am J Vet Res 1996;57:932-937.
73. Frisbie DD, Ray CS, Ionescu M, et al: Measurement of synovial fluid and serum concentrations of the 846 epitope of chondroitin sulfate and of carboxy propeptides of type II procollagen for diagnosis of osteochondral fragmentation in horses. Am J Vet Res 1999;60:306-309.
74. Denoix J-M: The equine distal limb: Atlas of clinical anatomy and comparative imaging, Ames, 2000, Iowa State University Press.
75. Hunter W: Of the structure and diseases of articulating cartilages, Philosoph Trans 1743;470:514-521.

76. Convery FR, Akeson WH, Keown GH: The repair of large osteochondral defects, Clin Orthop 1972;82:253-262.
77. Hurtig MB, Fretz PB, Doige CE, et al: Effects of lesion size and location on equine articular cartilage repair, Can J Vet Res 1988;52:137-146.
78. Dowthwaite GP, Bishop JÇ, Redman SN, et al: The surface of articular cartilage contains a progenitor cell population, J Cell Sci 2004;117:889-897.
79. Frisbie DD, Oxford JT, Southwood L, et al: Early events in cartilage repair after subchondral bone microfracture, Clin Orthop 2003:215-227.
80. Kinner B, Spector M: Cartilage: Current applications. In Caplan AI, Goldberg VM, editors: Orthopedic Tissue Engineering: Basic Science and Practices, New York, 2004, Marcel Dekker.

CHAPTER 84

Principles of Treatment of Joint Disease

David D. Frisbie

Over the last decade, significant advancements have been made in the understanding of medical and surgical treatment of equine joint disease. Many of these advances originally were aimed at helping humans, but the principles have been adapted for use in the horse. Advances in understanding pathophysiology, novel surgical techniques, improved surgical equipment, and more-sophisticated imaging modalities have led to improved treatment of joint disease.

It is important to focus on the two main treatments for joint disease: the relief of pain to regain functional use of the diseased joint and the arrest of disease progression. In many cases, generalized osteoarthritis (OA) is treated using medical management and exercise protocols, whereas full-thickness articular cartilage damage usually involves some surgical intervention.

SURGICAL TREATMENT

Diagnostic and Surgical Arthroscopy

Equine arthroscopy was first described as a diagnostic tool to visualize lesions that were undetectable using x-ray or other routine imaging procedures, but it was soon employed for therapeutic purposes, such as surgical removal of osteochondral fragments. Arthroscopy is now considered part of routine equine surgery and has, for the most part, replaced arthrotomy. It allows better visualization of the joint anatomy and inflicts less damage to the joint capsule and surrounding tissues, leading to quicker return to use and a more favorable outcome for the horse.[1] Since the 1980s, various publications have described arthroscopy in the horse; many of the early publications only described various techniques and approaches to joints, with more-specific outcomes and prognosis for specific pathologies following in subsequent publications. Most of the published work has been compiled in equine-specific texts.[1,2] The equipment used for arthroscopy and the surgical technique is discussed in Chapter 14.

Arthroscopy has a diagnostic and a therapeutic function in joint disease. Even with modern imaging modalities, it is still considered the gold standard for diagnosing equine joint problems. The cost and availability of arthroscopic equipment, along with arthroscopy's specificity and sensitivity when compared to more complex imaging modalities such as computed tomography (CT) and magnetic resonance imaging (MRI) and the expertise needed to perform definitive joint ultrasound, will likely keep arthroscopy in the forefront of diagnostics for equine joint disease for many years. This is especially true in cases that show no demonstrable or questionable joint lesions using traditional imaging modalities, even though the horse has localized clinical pain based on diagnostic analgesia.

In recent years more joint pathology, such as meniscal and cruciate lesions, has been described. This may be because diagnostic arthroscopy, especially in the stifle joint, has become more accepted. Therefore, these types of lesions, which are not detectable using radiography, are being recognized more often. With an increased awareness of how often these types of lesions occur, further work is being focused on therapeutic treatments. This is especially true in the field of cartilage resurfacing and meniscal pathology, with many of the therapeutic avenues pursued in equine practice representing the current state of the art in human medicine.

Another advantage of the use of arthroscopy is the potential benefit of lavage. Arthroscopy is often performed using fluid to distend the joint for better visualization. The accompanying egress of joint fluid, which potentially contains cytokines and cartilage wear particles, may be therapeutically beneficial, even when lavage is performed as a sole treatment in cases of osteoarthritis. However, the benefit of lavage is controversial, and it does not work in cases with significant definable disease such as meniscal tears. Research also has shown that when lavage is performed with large-gauge needles (14 gauge), it is not as effective as using arthroscopic cannulas.[3-5] Distention of the joint can be accomplished using inert gas, which can be especially helpful if bleeding of intrasynovial tissues impairs visualization when a fluid medium is being used.

In general, arthroscopy is of more therapeutic benefit in acute than in chronic cases. For example, removing a fresh osteochondral fragment before osteoarthritis can develop typically produces a better outcome after surgery than removing a chronic osteochondral fragment after osteoarthritis has developed. However, there are some exceptions, such as osteonecrosis and cartilage fibrillation of the third carpal bone, which can be successfully managed using arthroscopy.

Another consideration regarding arthroscopic surgery is the documentation of the surgical procedure. Since the 1990s, reduction in cost and increases of availability of video and still-capture devices have allowed real-time documentation of arthroscopic surgery to be made and kept as part of the medical record. This real-time information is embraced by trainers and owners as a means of understanding the pathology and treatment procedures, as well as providing more specific information about the surgery. Detailed drawings of many intra-articular surfaces can also be helpful in documenting surgical findings (Fig. 84-1).

Removal of Osteochondral Fragments

In most instances, osteochondral fragments are removed when they are diagnosed in conjunction with clinical lameness. Some fragments are considered relatively benign, and removal is not indicated without clinical lameness.[1,6,7] The routine use of arthroscopy has improved the outcome of osteochondral fragment removal as compared to removal using arthrotomy. Outcomes related to osteochondral fragment removal are presented in Table 84-1, and specific arthroscopic approaches to anatomic joints can be found detailed in this text and in published references.[1]

In general, diagnostic visualization of the entire joint cavity is performed prior to fragment removal. When multiple fragments are present, typically the smaller fragments are removed first. This postpones the need to increase the size of the instrument portal and delays the potential for subsequent reduced visualization until the end of the surgery. Very large fragments can be broken into smaller pieces using a rongeur or osteotome to avoid excessive portal size. Hand curets are typically used to débride the parent bone down to the appropriate level as well as to smooth any edges to prevent trauma to opposing joint surfaces postoperatively. Prior to finishing arthroscopic surgery, typically the joints are lavaged with fluids while a final inspection of the joint is completed to ensure all debris has been removed. Debris often accumulates in certain locations within a specific joint, and knowledge of these locations often aids in finding debris that has inadvertently escaped removal by lavage alone.

Reconstruction of Intra-articular Fractures

Once damaged, bone can be repaired so that it is indistinguishable from the original tissue. However, articular cartilage does not have the same ability to heal. Therefore, correct anatomic alignment and reconstruction of the fracture gap, especially the articular component, is integral to the repair process and determines the long-term resolution of intra-articular fractures.

Arthroscopic visualization during the reconstruction of the articular component of the fracture is recommended to ensure the best possible outcome in a high-motion joint. In many cases, loose debris is débrided and flushed from around and in the fracture gap, allowing more anatomically correct reduction and better stabilization of the fracture. In some cases, such as with slab fractures of the third carpal bone, assessment of the articular component dictates the surgical procedure, namely repair or removal of the fracture fragment.

Common intra-articular fractures encountered in equine athletes are condylar fractures of the third metacarpal (MCIII) and third metatarsal (MTIII), third carpal bone slab fractures, and sagittal fractures involving the proximal phalanx. Most cases of intra-articular fractures are repaired using internal fixation and lag-screw principles. These are covered in other chapters of the text, but some treatments and outcomes are listed in Table 84-2.

Synovectomy

Equine synovium is occasionally removed locally (partial synovectomy) to help arthroscopic visualization, but synovectomy can also be performed as a therapeutic treatment, most often in cases of septic arthritis. With sepsis, the synovial membrane can be laden with fibrin. Fibrin is thought to harbor bacteria; thus removal of the involved synovium is thought to aid in treatment and potentially prevent recurrence of the septic process. Some septic equine joints appear to produce more fibrin than others (tarsocrural, distal phalangeal, and elbow joints are among the most prolific), which requires visualization of the joint space and synovectomy rather than ingress-egress flushing using large-gauge needles. In some cases of chronic osteoarthritis, marked hypertrophy of the synovium can be encountered, and current practice is to perform a subtotal or complete synovectomy of the affected membrane to reduce cytokine production as well as physical impingement. The carpal joints and the metacarpophalangeal and metatarsophalangeal joints appear to benefit clinically from this type of treatment.[54]

The role that the synovial membrane plays in equine joint disease is not as well characterized as it is in humans. In human osteoarthritis, the synovial membrane is thought to play a secondary role to the cartilage lesion in the pathogenesis. Conversely, in rheumatoid arthritis, the synovial membrane is thought to be the primary instigator and to propagate the ongoing degeneration of the cartilage. Thus, an effective method of controlling rheumatoid arthritis in people is through synovectomy, although it has a limited duration of clinical effectiveness.[55-58] A rheumatoid condition has not been identified in the horse.

Different methodologies have been used to accomplish synovectomy, including use of surgery, chemicals, and radioisotopes. Typically, surgical methods in horses use motorized synovial resection. Experimentally, synovectomy has been performed in normal horses and has shown no ill effects, but the regeneration of the synovial membrane was slower than expected when compared to other species.[54,59,60]

Joint Resurfacing

Partial-thickness lesions and full-thickness articular cartilage lesions greater than 5 mm in diameter do not heal spontaneously in the horse. In spite of the recent interest in assessing treatments for chondral defects, efforts have been under way for more than 250 years to heal articular cartilage with only moderate progress.[61] The reason is related to the highly specialized nature of articular cartilage and the need for an intact structure to perform its biochemical and physiologic functions.

Damage to articular cartilage is common in horses and typically is described in two forms, chronic degenerative

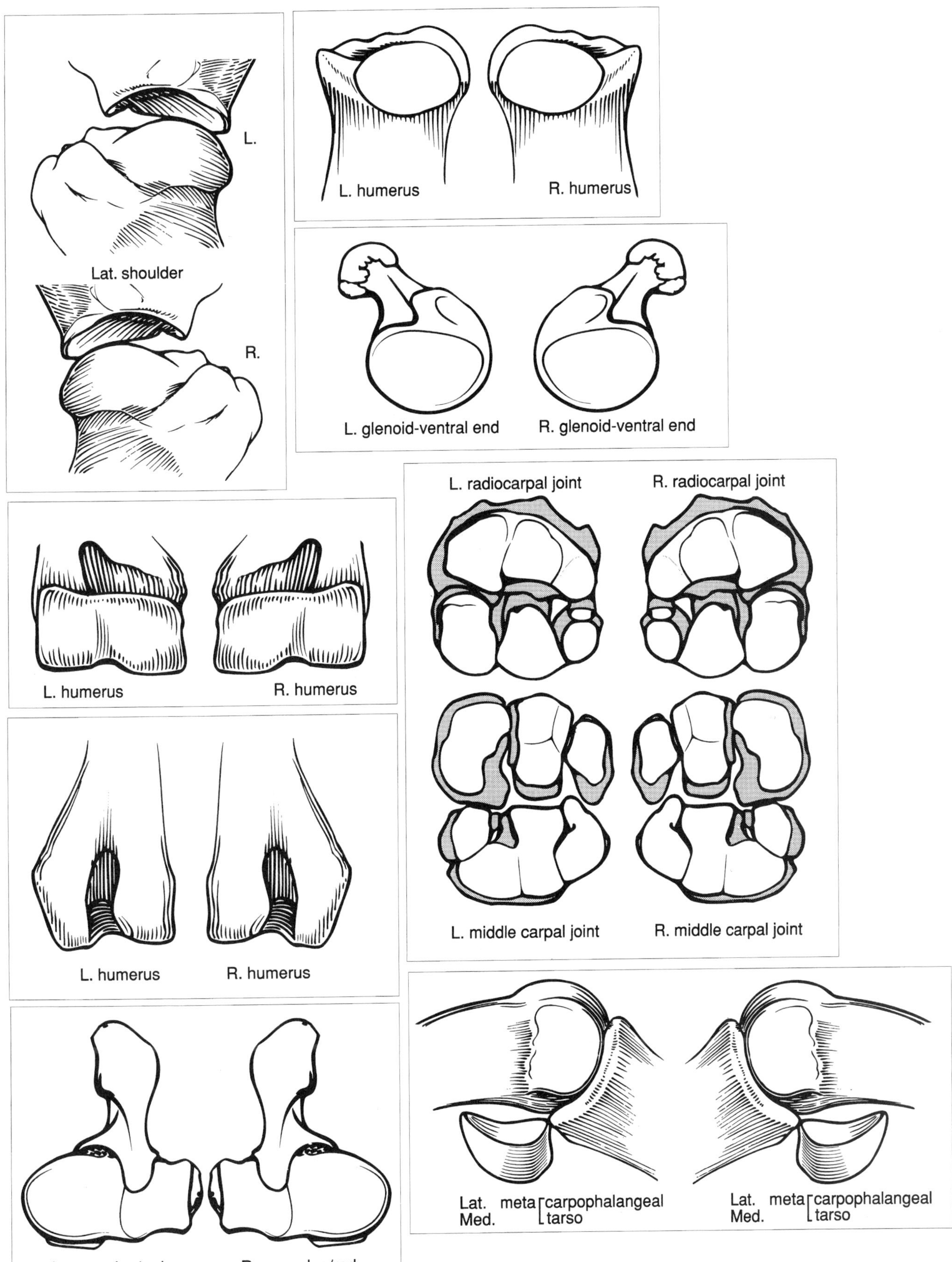

Figure 84-1. Diagrams of equine joints for marking the locations and sizes of cartilaginous lesions observed arthroscopically.

Continued

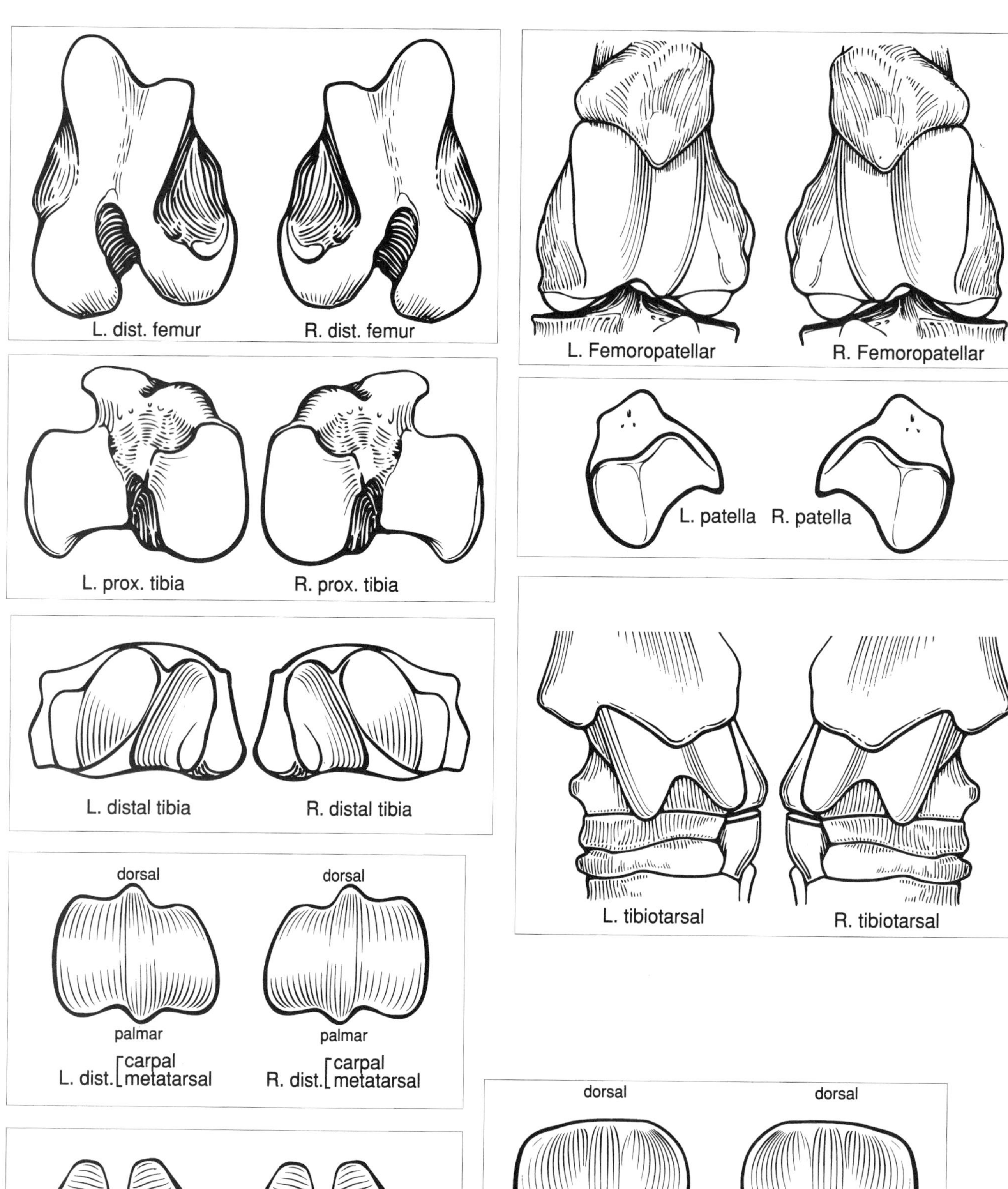

Figure 84-1, cont'd.

TABLE 84-1. Prognosis* for Racing or Athletic Soundness Given by Various Authors for Intra-articular Osteochondral (Chip) Fractures[†] in Various Locations and Joints

Fracture Location	Treatment	Prognosis	Reference
Extensor process of P3	M or S[A]	Guarded	8, 9, 10
	M or S[A]	Poor	11
	M or S[A]	Good	12
P2 (not involving DIP joint)	S[A]	Guarded to good[‡]	13, 14
	S[A]	Guarded	11, 15, 16
P2 (involving DIP joint)	M or S[A]	Poor	11
Dorsal frontal P1	S[A] (displaced)	Good	17
	M (nondisplaced)	Good	17
Proximodorsal P1	S[A]	Excellent	18
	—	Good	19
	S[B]	Excellent	16, 20, 21
Plantar P1	S[A]	Excellent	22
	S[A]	Good	23
	S[B]	Excellent	12
	S[B]	Good	24
Palmar P1	M	Guarded	22
	S[A]	Excellent	25
	S[B]	Excellent	12, 26
	S[B]	Good	27
Apical sesamoid	M	Poor	28
	S[A]	Good	28, 29
	M or S[A]	S better than M	30
	S[B]	Good	31, 32
Abaxial sesamoid	S[B]	Good	33
Basilar sesamoid	M or S[A]	Guarded	34, 35
	S[B]	Guarded	36
Distal radius	M	Guarded	12
	S[A]	HR=1[§]	34
	S[A]	Guarded to good[‡]	37
	S[B]	Good	20
Proximal RC	S[A]	Good	37
	S[A]	HR=2[§]	20, 38
	S[B]	Good	20
Proximal IC	S[B]	Good	20
Distal RC	S[A]	Guarded	37, 35
	S[A]	HR=1[§]	38
	S[B]	Guarded	35, 20
Distal IC	S[B]	Good	20
C3	S[A]	Guarded to good[‡]	36, 39
	S[B]	Guarded	36, 39
	S[A]	HR = [§]	20, 38

*The prognoses have been graded as excellent (80% to 90% chance of athletic soundness), good (60% to 80%), guarded (40% to 60%), and poor (<40%) and usually refer to the ability to race after injury. These are approximate percentages extrapolated from the literature because these categories are not always used by each author and a definition of these categories is not usually given. "Favorable" has been graded with "good." In general, the prognosis given is for horses with no radiographic signs of osteoarthritis (i.e., the horse is given its best chance of recovery).

[†]These fractures do not cause major joint instability.

[‡]Guarded to good used when the percentages spanned 2 ranges.

[§]Hazard ratio was used to compare the racing performance of the treated with that of a control group, taken from the race horse registry for the same period. A hazard ratio of approximately 1 means that the same number of treated horses dropped out of racing as the controls. A hazard ratio of 2 means that twice as many treated horses were lost as the controls.

A, Arthrotomy; B, arthroscopy

C3, 3rd carpal bone; DIP, distal interphalangeal; HR, hazard ratio; IC, intermediate carpal bone; M, medical; P, phalanx; RC, radial carpal bone; S, surgical.

Adapted from Caron JP: In Auer JA, Stick J, editors: Equine Surgery, Philadelphia, 1999, WB Saunders.

TABLE 84-2. Prognosis* for Racing or Athletic Soundness Given by Various Authors for Intra-articular Fractures

Fracture Location and Type	Treatment†	Prognosis	Reference
Distal phalanx (all except fractures of extensor process fractures)	M	Good (horses <3 y old)	8
Distal phalanx (intra-articular, except extensor process fractures)	S	Good (horses >3 y old)	8
P3 (type II)	M	Guarded	11, 40
Middle phalanx (comminuted)	M or S	Guarded	11
	S	Poor to guarded‡	15
	M	Poor	15
Proximal phalanx (simple, nondisplaced)	M or S	Good	11, 17, 41, 42, 43, 44
Proximal phalanx (noncomminuted, displaced)	S	Good	17, 45
Proximal phalanx (comminuted)	S	Poor	11, 43
Proximal sesamoid (midbody)	M or S	Poor	34, 43
MCIII/MTIII (noncomminuted)	S	Good	34, 46, 47
MCIII/MTIII (with comminution)	S	Guarded	34
	S	Good	48
MTIII (medial condyle)	S	Good	49
MCIII/MTIII (displaced)	M or S	Poor	41
MCIII/MTIII (complete, nondisplaced)	S	Good	41
MCIII/MTIII (incomplete, nondisplaced)	S	Excellent	41
	M	Excellent	41
C3 slab (frontal)	S (TB)	Guarded to good‡	50
	S	Guarded to good‡	12, 51
		Guarded	52
	M	Poor	53
	M or S (SB)	Good	50
C3 slab (sagittal)	M	Guarded	12, 45

*The prognoses have been graded as excellent (80% to 90% chance of athletic soundness), good (60% to 80%), guarded (40% to 60%), and poor (<40%) and usually refer to the ability to race after injury. These are approximate percentages extrapolated from the literature because these categories are not always used by each author and a definition of these categories is not usually given. Favorable has been graded with good. In general, the prognosis given is for horses with no radiographic signs of osteoarthritis (i.e., the horse is given its best chance of recovery).

†Articular fractures of long bones (except for the metacarpus and metatarsus) have not been included because of insufficient numbers from which to derive prognoses or other complicating factors, or both.

‡All fractures repaired surgically with stab incisions or arthrotomies, or both, except C3 slabs, in which repair was guided by arthroscopic visualization. Two grades given when percentages spanned two categories.

C3, third carpal bone; M, medical; MC, metacarpus; P, phalanx; S, surgical; SB, Standardbred; TB, Thoroughbred.

Adapted from Caron JP: In Auer JA, Stick J, editors: Equine Surgery, Philadelphia, 1999, WB Saunders.

lesions and acute damage. Chronic lesions are often considered osteoarthritis, and whereas these lesions would benefit from joint resurfacing, this type of lesion is the most challenging in which to achieve long-term repair because of generalized joint pathology that is not addressed with most current joint-resurfacing techniques. Conversely, acute lesions typically comprise a discrete or focal area of cartilage loss without other chronic manifestations of joint degeneration. Such lesions are currently best treated with equine joint-resurfacing techniques.

The outcome of cartilage repair is typically assessed on biochemical content (including type II collagen and aggrecan), histologic appearance (resemblance to hyaline cartilage), biomechanical properties, and functional outcome of the joint and patient. As a general rule, it appears that cartilage in younger patients has a better capacity for repair compared to that of older patients.

When intra-articular osteochondral fragmentation occurs in the horse, surgical treatment involves removal of the fragment and débridement of the damaged cartilage and subchondral bone. In general, because of a generalized poor regenerative response, articular cartilage is usually minimally débrided, doing no more than is necessary to remove damaged cartilage. Partial-thickness cartilage lesions are typically not converted into full-thickness lesions, but rather the fibrillated cartilage is removed, leaving the intact cartilage below the fibrillated cartilage in place. In the case of a full-thickness lesion, the edges of the damaged articular cartilage are débrided until cartilage that is firmly attached to the subchondral bone plate is reached. The edges of the cartilage are débrided so that they have a sharp vertical border. The bone is always débrided down to a level of the subchondral bone plate so as to fully remove the calcified cartilage, which has been shown to impede the repair process. When necrotic bone is encountered, it is débrided aggressively to ensure that healthy bleeding bone is being left in the lesion.

The previous chapter covered general concepts regarding treatment based on the lesion depth, size, and basic repair or treatment options. Two basic approaches are historically thought of in joint resurfacing: stimulated endogenous repair and transplantation or grafting of tissues. Although these techniques are covered as separate entities, many cutting-edge approaches are combining the techniques as well as augmenting either or both techniques with growth factor supplementation.

Stimulated Endogenous Repair

Because bone marrow has a good supply of both stem cells and growth factors thought to be integral to cartilage health and repair, direct communication of articular lesions to these elements beneath the subchondral bone plate has been a cornerstone of stimulated cartilage repair. Growth factors believed to be important in cartilage repair include insulin-like growth factor-1(IGF-1), transforming growth factor-β (TGF-β), and bone morphogenetic proteins (BMP) 2 and 7. Access to these marrow elements has been facilitated by various surgical techniques including abrasion arthroplasty, which involves débridement to the level of the subchondral plate; spongialization, which is débridement past the subchondral plate into cancellous bone; focal drilling to the depth of cancellous bone in discrete locations throughout the cartilage lesion (osteostixis); and subchondral bone microfracture, which also penetrates to the level of the subchondral bone in discrete locations. Current literature and clinical practice do not favor spongialization, in part because it is thought to destabilize the subchondral bone plate.

Based on the human and equine literature, the current recommendations for stimulated endogenous repair of an articular lesion are débridement of lesions to the level of the subchondral bone plate (abrasion arthroplasty) alone or in conjunction with subchondral bone microfracture. If the lesion crosses the subchondral bone plate into the cancellous bone, the addition of subchondral bone microfracture is probably not necessary. In the presence of sclerotic bone, the lesion is débrided to a depth that produces petechial bleeding (in the absence of fluid pressure) but does not enter the cancellous bone. In this case, subchondral bone microfracture is also used.

Currently, subchondral bone plate drilling is not widely used based on subsequent formation of subchondral bone cysts and poor histologic appearance of repair tissue, especially when compared to other, more recently developed techniques such as subchondral bone microfracture.[62,63] The greater depth of penetration, smooth penetration through the bone, and heat generated with the drilling process probably contribute to the less-than-optimal repair tissue. Bone cyst formation associated with the drilling technique is probably a result of synovial fluid movement into the bone through the drill holes (see Chapter 92).

Subchondral bone microfracture allows access to the cells and growth factors beneath the subchondral plate, without destabilization of the subchondral plate's biomechanical stability. In addition, the penetration of the stainless steel bone awl causes cracks in the bone as well as spicules of bone that protrude from the penetration site, both of which are believed to aid in the attachment of the repair tissue. Experimental studies have demonstrated that large articular cartilage defects (1 to 2 cm in diameter) débrided to the level of the subchondral bone have significantly greater volume of healing tissue following subchondral bone microfracture compared to defects that were débrided to the level of the subchondral bone plate but did not undergo microfracture. Biochemical analysis of the repair tissues also has shown a greater type II collagen content in repair tissue of microfractured defects in two experimental studies, although histologic appearance of the repair tissues was similar.[64,65]

Further improvement in the repair tissue obtained following subchondral bone microfracture has been achieved by supplementing IGF-1 and interleukin-1 (IL-1) receptor antagonist using gene transfer.[66] Experimental work assessing subchondral bone microfracture has also confirmed the poor attachment of repair tissue in areas where the calcified cartilage layer had been incompletely removed. Confirmation of the level of débridement can be achieved using a micro-arthroscope or focusing close to the defect margins with a standard arthroscope. A granular appearance of the defect should be evident, differentiating the subchondral bone plate from the glasslike appearance of the calcified cartilage layer. Following débridement of the lesion, microfracture holes are spaced 2 to 3 mm apart, avoiding communication between sites and penetrating approximately 2 mm into the bone (Fig. 84-2).

To date, no long-term follow-up on clinical results after resurfacing therapy have been published relating specifically to horses, although anecdotal reports have been promising. However, recent human data compared long-term follow-up

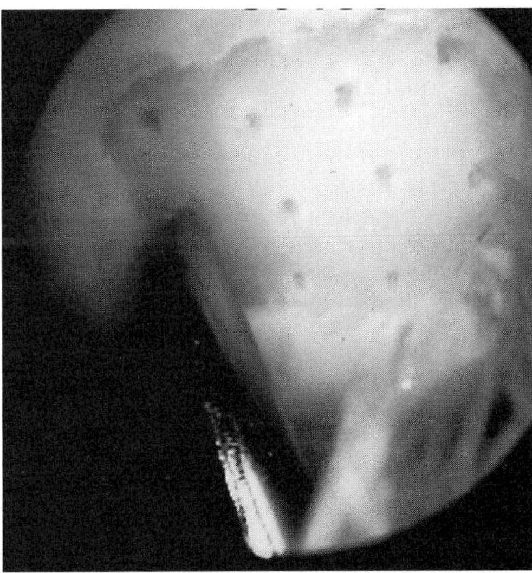

Figure 84-2. Arthroscopic image of microfracture spacing on the medial femoral condyle.

of the most commonly used cartilage resurfacing techniques,[67] autologous cartilage implantation (ACI) as described by Brittberg[68] and subchondral bone microfracture first described by Steadman.[69] The short-term and long-term results of this study show minor significant improvement with subchondral bone microfracture, with no significant differences in histologic appearance of repair tissue or patient outcome between the two techniques. Both of these techniques are considered better than débridement alone for most human and equine patients. Because subchondral bone microfracture does not require a second surgery and is less technically challenging compared to ACI, it is favored by most equine surgeons.

Articular Grafting

Many different tissues have been transplanted or grafted into cartilage defects; they include periosteal and perichondrial autografts, osteochondral, chondral, or isolated chondrocyte autografts or allografts, and stem cell transplants from bone marrow or fat. Periosteal and perichondrial grafts have been performed in laboratory animals with some success, but results in the horse have been very disappointing and are no longer a focus of ongoing research.[70,71]

Osteochondral grafting procedures have been well developed for use in people, but they have had limited success in the horse. Early work in the horse demonstrated short-term success but resulted in long-term failures.[72-74] Many of the failures with osteochondral grafting have been attributed to lack of congruity of the recipient and donor tissues as well as difficulties with surgical technique. Some concern also revolves around morbidity in the donor graft site. Typically, in people, a nonweightbearing region is used for donor harvest, reducing morbidity, but lack of suitable nonweightbearing donor tissue has been a limitation in horses. More recently, with the advent of specialized surgical tools designed for human osteochondral grafting, studies are under way using this technique in the horse. Surgical technique and donor site selection are the main hurdles yet to be overcome before this technique will reach mainstream practice.[75-78]

Chondrocyte transplantation has been a very active area of equine research since the 1990s. Techniques using both allografts and autografts have been reported, but most work, especially in humans, has focused on autografts. The technique described by Brittberg and marketed by Genzyme is the most well studied grafting technique.[68] This technique uses autologous chondrocytes harvested from a nonweightbearing region, usually the trochlea of the distal femur, followed by a four-week in vitro expansion of chondrocytes. The expanded cell population is then implanted during a second surgical procedure and held in the defect beneath autologous periosteum, which is sutured to the cartilage bordering the defect to create a watertight seal. Although this technique has been performed in horses with outcomes similar to those seen in people, the cost, laboratory facilities, need for multiple surgeries, and technical challenges of the procedure have limited its usefulness in clinical cases.

Techniques using frozen chondrocytes harvested from neonatal foals, which are implanted in a fibrin glue to help retain the cells in the chondral defect, have had some success in a limited number of chondral defects. The technique is being used more commonly in cystic defects to date.[79] Other materials used to fill cystic lesions are discussed in Chapter 92.

Techniques using autologous chondrocytes harvested from the nonweightbearing region of the lateral trochlea of the distal femur, implanted into 15-mm diameter defects, have been successful in experimental equine trials. One of the tested procedures uses fibrin glue holding minced cartilage to a bioresorbable scaffold, which is subsequently stapled to the subchondral bone of the defect in a one-step surgical procedure.[80,81] In comparable equine experimental trials this technique has been superior to the ACI technique. This technique is now undergoing human clinical trials, and because of the ease, cost, and promising results in equine experimental trials, it is likely to be used in equine clinical cases in the near future.

Considerable research is being directed toward the use of mesenchymal stem cells for implantation in cartilage defects. This cell population has been shown to improve healing in experimental animals, but gaining access to a sufficient number of stem cells without in vitro expansion is a hurdle yet to be resolved in horses.[79]

Arthrodesis

Assisted fusion of a joint is sometimes indicated when destruction to the joint is beyond any other treatment. Although most commonly achieved through surgical methods typically involving internal fixation, arthrodesis can be carried out using chemical or laser-based methods as well.[2,82-84]

In high-motion joints, such as the radiocarpal, midcarpal, metacarpophalangeal, and distal phalangeal joints, surgical fusion using internal fixation is required (see Chapter 85). The expectation of this procedure is to alleviate the pain associated with movement of the joint and to salvage the animal for nonathletic function. Conversely, arthrodesis of low-motion joints often carries a reasonable prognosis for athletic soundness and can be accomplished using surgical, chemical, or laser-based techniques. This is especially true for the proximal interphalangeal, tarsometatarsal, and distal intertarsal joints. Some risks have been identified with chemical fusion of joints because unexpected anatomic communications with other synovial and nonsynovial structures can be encountered. Thus, contrast studies outlining the structure and extent of the communication should be performed prior to chemical fusion, and caution should be used not to create further injury by overdistending the joint capsule.

In the distal tarsal joints, some initial studies have been performed comparing surgical drilling to ablation of the joint space using a laser in both clinical and experimental cases. Early results indicate that some decrease in time to resolution of clinical lameness may be seen for the laser-based procedure, but actual bony union of the joint space appears to occur more quickly with drilling. Further research comparing these techniques is needed, but the morbidity associated with the early reports using the laser favors the continued use of surgical arthrodesis in the distal tarsal joint, using the modified drilling technique. Further discussion of the principles of arthrodesis can be found in more detail in Chapter 85.

Joint Replacement

When reparative surgical procedures have failed, and the patient is unresponsive to medical management, many end-stage cases of osteoarthritis in people are treated using joint replacements, especially in the knee and hip. Joint replacement procedures are typically postponed until the patient is old enough that the implant will not fail during the expected remaining lifetime. Implant wear is improving, but it is still in the 10- to 20-year range, depending on the location and type of implant. Even in humans, where a large number of joint replacements are carried out annually, relatively high morbidity is associated with such procedures, especially related to implant loosening. With respect to equine joint replacement, cost of implant design and manufacturing, difficulties with prolonged nonweightbearing, and surgical morbidity continue to keep equine joint replacement out of mainstream clinical practice.

Aftercare

The aftercare for surgical joint treatment is often as important as the central treatment itself. Treatment goals and pathophysiology of healing tissue should be kept in mind when the aftercare protocol is being designed. Each aftercare protocol varies depending on the procedure, but a common focus is to minimize the duration to full return to function without compromising the athletic soundness of the patient. Following surgery, the goals are to provide support to the weakened areas, often through bandaging, casts, and controlled exercise, which can range from strict stall rest to specific graded exercise programs.

It is also well accepted that decreasing postoperative inflammation is beneficial in the healing process, as is controlling postoperative pain. Given that maximal inflammation in a surgical wound typically occurs 3 to 5 days postoperatively, systemic nonsteroidal anti-inflammatory medication is administered for at least this time period. The postoperative use of corticosteroids, although providing potent anti-inflammatory activities, is often contraindicated in the first 4 weeks because of their role in decreased cell metabolism, which affects healing time, as well as the decreased ability of the immune system to combat infection.

Other medications believed to have chondro-enhancing or chondroprotective qualities, such as hyaluronan or polysulfated glycosaminoglycans (Adequan), have also been studied in an attempt to demonstrate enhanced postoperative healing. However, they have not shown significant benefit in most studies, with the exception of decreasing adhesions in tendon sheaths.[85-87]

MEDICAL TREATMENT

There are two main goals for medical treatment of OA in the horse: reducing pain (lameness) and minimizing progression of joint deterioration. When formulating a treatment plan, the optimization of these goals will be influenced by an accurate and specific diagnosis, the stage of disease, severity, available treatment modalities, and rehabilitation time. Clinicians realize that treating joint disease is an art and does not follow any specific recipe.

Nonsteroidal Anti-Inflammatory Drugs

The use of NSAIDs for inhibiting the arachidonic acid cascade has been a mainstay for the treatment of joint disease for many decades. NSAIDs are typically used in cases of acute injury and are often accompanied by other treatment modalities. The renal and gastrointestinal side effects associated with NSAID administration limit their long-term use for treatment of joint disease. NSAIDs inhibit the production of prostaglandins and thromboxanes, especially the prostaglandin E (PGE) series, which is thought to be intimately involved in pain, altered cartilage metabolism, and ongoing inflammation in damaged joints (Fig. 84-3).

Traditionally, inhibition of PGEs and the resulting symptomatic pain relief has been viewed as a beneficial goal in treating OA (Fig. 84-4). Although relatively recent research has offered some suggestion that this inhibition may have

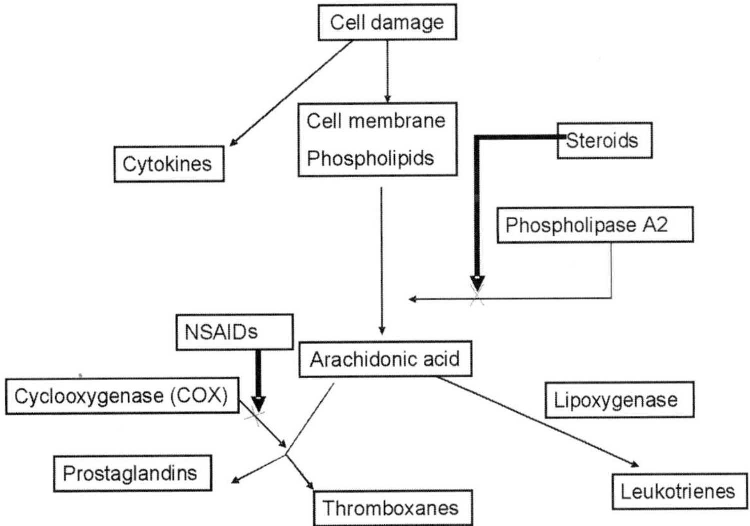

Figure 84-3. Schematic representation of inhibition of the inflammatory cascade by nonsteroidal anti-inflammatory drugs (NSAIDs) and corticosteroids.

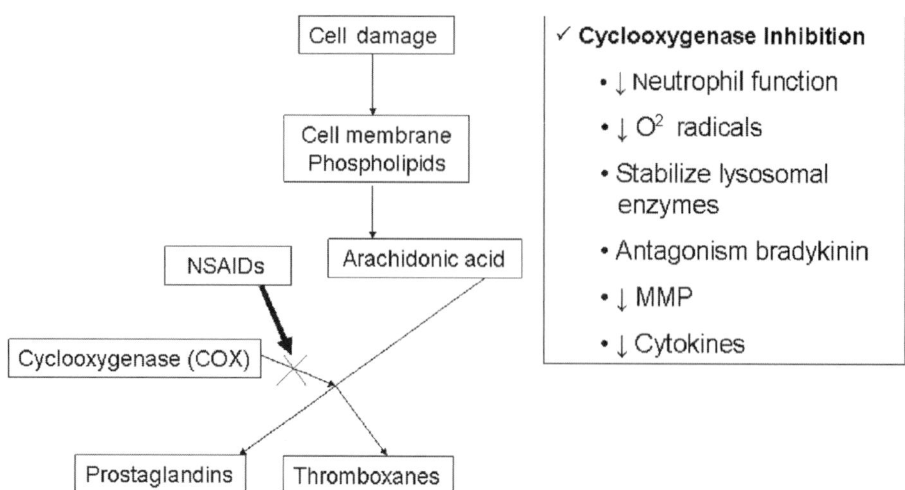

Figure 84-4. Schematic representation of effects associated with the administration of nonsteroidal anti-inflammatory drugs (NSAIDs).

long-term unfavorable effects on cartilage metabolism[88] and does warrant further investigation, the current level knowledge of these unfavorable effects most likely will not alter the use of NSAIDs in clinical practice. Research has also suggested that NSAIDs may have a role in mediating joint pain at the level of the spinal cord as well as locally,[89] although specific research in this area has not been performed in the horse to date. In the early 1990s, a major advancement in NSAIDs for treatment of OA occurred with the identification of isoenzymes for the cyclo-oxygenase (COX) pathway (COX-1 and COX-2), and this does have current equine implications.

COX-1 has been associated with the housekeeping functions of the cyclooxygenase pathway. It is known to be constitutively produced and important in the balance of normal physiologic function of the gastrointestinal and renal systems, although it has a lesser role in the inflammatory cascade. COX-2 has mainly been associated with inflammatory events, especially those driven by macrophages and synovial cells, and has only minor roles in normal physiology, thus its "bad" or inducible role (Fig. 84-5). These findings have led to a paradigm that the anti-inflammatory properties of NSAIDs are mediated through the inhibition of the COX-2 enzyme, whereas the untoward effects occur as a result of their action on COX-1.

The protective role of COX-1 for the gastroduodenal mucosa has been shown both experimentally in laboratory animals and in human clinical trials. Furthermore, studies have shown that the greatest degree of damage to the gastroduodenal mucosa is generally caused by NSAIDs that preferentially inhibit COX-1. In fact, the preferential COX-2 inhibitor rofecoxib (Vioxx) was shown in human patients to induce ulceration that was actually lower than that produced in a randomized placebo group.[90]

As with most biologic systems, complete inhibition of COX-2 may not be optimal; some value, albeit minimal, has been shown from expression of COX-2 as well as some demonstrable negative effects of COX-1 expression. More specifically, some low level of COX-1 expression is inducible during stress or inflammatory periods. Likewise, some constitutive expression of COX-2 has been demonstrated by the brain, kidney, and pancreatic islet cells, and it has a function in bone resorption. Furthermore, COX-2 suppression has been shown to delay gastric ulcer healing in rats. Thus, as Oscar Wilde said, "The pure and simple truth is rarely pure and never simple."

To summarize: COX-1 is mainly responsible for the protective prostaglandins, but COX-2 plays some accessory role that is more important than previously thought. However, these facts still might not outweigh the beneficial effects of selective COX-2 inhibition in joint disease.

Research in humans has indicated that topical NSAID application can be clinically beneficial and may reduce systemic side effects.[91] The effect of topical application of diclofenac liposomal suspension has been evaluated in an equine clinical trial with promising results.[92] This product is indicated for horses with a finite number of affected joints, especially if prolonged treatment is not necessary.

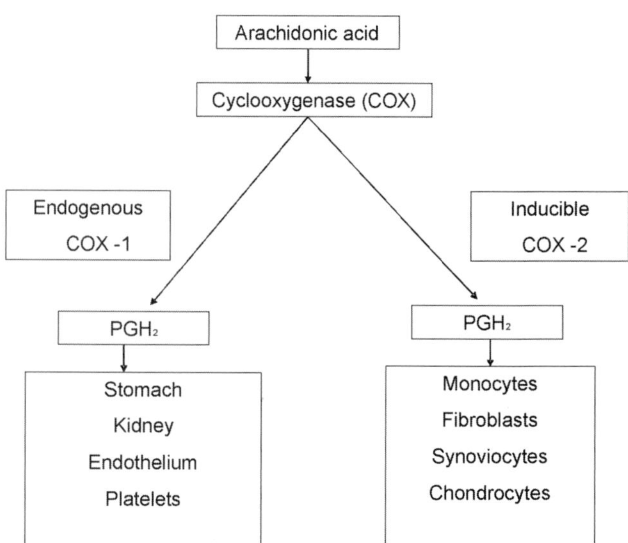

Figure 84-5. Schematic representation of the cyclooxygenase isoenzymes and target tissues.

Of products currently on the market, phenylbutazone remains one of the most popular NSAIDs for musculoskeletal pain in horses. Its cost, ease of administration, and relatively few side effects during short-term administration make it a good therapeutic choice. Flunixin meglumine and ketoprofen both have uses in treatment of equine OA, especially with some reports of fewer side effects; however the cost-to-benefit ratio often limits their use. The use of the first-generation COX-2 inhibitor carprofen is indicated in horses experiencing side effects or when extended treatment periods are predicted or side effects have been encountered with traditional NSAIDs.

Continued use of NSAIDs for treating acute inflammation associated with joint disease is likely for the foreseeable future. Selective COX-2 inhibitors will most likely be used more clinically as more information specific to the horse becomes available and the cost of these agents decreases. The currently applied NSAIDs in the horse are summarized in Table 84-3.

Corticosteroids

More equine-specific research has been published on intra-articular (IA) administration of corticosteroids than any other equine joint medication. Since the introduction of IA corticosteroid use in the mid 1950s, controversy has existed over the risk-to-benefit ratio of this class of medication. Much of this controversy has been fueled from unsubstantiated statements in both the scientific and lay press. Studies showing potentially detrimental effects of corticosteroids on articular cartilage have been conducted using normal cartilage. Current research[93] suggests that inflamed or abnormal joints do not exhibit the detrimental effects seen in normal joints when corticosteroid is administered, potentially explaining some discrepancies seen in experimental studies conducted on normal tissues compared to clinical impressions.

It is well documented that corticosteroids inhibit the arachidonic acid cascade by blocking phospholipase A2 and that they are selective COX-2 inhibitors.[94] The selective COX-2 inhibition, and low incidence of side effects, may be one of the reasons this class of medication is so useful in the horse. The use of corticosteroids for joint disease often brings up three main questions: which preparation to use, at what dose, and the appropriate rest period.

Currently, three main corticosteroid preparations are available to the equine clinician: methylprednisolone acetate (Depo-Medrol), triamcinolone acetonide (Vetalog), and compounded betamethasone sodium phosphate and betamethasone acetate (Celestone Soluspan, formerly Betavet) (Table 84-4). Compounded betamethasone has been difficult to obtain commercially in the United States, but it remains available in other countries. As a result, it has been compounded by various pharmacies; however, significant problems have resulted from the use of some of these formulations.

Experimental studies[95-97] have provided a relatively good comparison of these three products and found that they are not equivalent. The three preparations were tested using a relatively similar osteochondral fragment model. Results of this work indicated that the most beneficial effects were seen with triamcinolone, and some protective effects were associated with this preparation. Methylprednisolone did have beneficial effects, but detrimental effects on the articular cartilage were also demonstrated. Compounded betamethasone had no measured effects, which suggests that this

TABLE 84-3. Partial Listing of Currently Available NSAIDs*

Generic Name	Product Name	Formulations	Recommended Dose (mg/kg)	Standard Availability	Cost
Phenylbutazone	Equipharphenylbutazone	1 g tablet	4.4 bid for one day, 2.2 bid for 4 days, 2.2 sid	Bottle 100 tabs	$9.71
	Equipharphenylbutazone injection 20%	Injectable 20% (cs/12)	2.2-4.4 bid (5 days)	100 mL	$5.81
	Phenylzone paste	200 mg/g (20% paste), 12 g Rx	1-2.2 bid (4 days)	60 g	$7.08
	Phenylzone paste	200 mg/g (20% paste), 6 g Rx	1-2.2 bid (4 days)	30 g	$4.78
Carprofen	Rimadyl	Injectable or tablets	0.7 daily (IV, PO)	Bottle of 180 tablets	$1.26/tablet
Flunixin meglumine	FluNix Rx (Flunixamine)	Injectable	1.1 daily (5 days) (IV, IM)	100 mL 200 mL	$25.51 $54.55
	Banamine Paste	Paste	1.1 daily (5 days)	30-g tube	$88.20
Meclofenamic acid	Arquel	Granules	2.2 daily (5-7 days), then 2.2 daily or less (PO)	20 mg, bottle of 500	$92.25
Ketoprofen	Ketofen	Injectable	2.2 daily (5 days) (IV)	100 mL 50 mL	$103.38 $62.67

*Availability and costs are as of spring of 2004.
bid, twice daily; IM, intramuscular; IV, intravenous; PO, by mouth.

TABLE 84-4. Corticosteroids Commonly Used for Intra-articular Administration

Corticosteroid	Product Name	Manufacturer	Concentration (mg/mL)	Dose (mg)	Potency Relative to Hydrocortisone
Betamethasone sulfate	Celestone Soluspan	Schering-Plough	6	3-18	30
Triamcinolone acetonide	Vetalog	Solvay	6	6-18	5
Flumethasone	Flucort	Syntex	0.5	1.25-2.5	120
Isoflupredone acetate	Predef 2X	Pharmacia and Upjohn	2	5-20	50
Methylprednisolone acetate	Depo-Medrol	Pharmacia and Upjohn	40	40-120	5

preparation has a less potent effect on joint tissues compared to triamcinolone and methylprednisolone. Compounded betamethasone might not have caused significant improvement because the newly developed experimental model might not have elicited sufficient lameness to evaluate a difference. These in vivo studies coupled with in vitro work have fueled the recommendation to use triamcinolone, especially in *high-motion joints*.

Recent research has also focused on low-dose corticosteroid administration for the treatment of equine joint disease. It appears to take about a 10-fold change in concentration to alter in vitro effects of corticosteroids. As an example, joint concentrations between 1 mg and 10 mg of triamcinolone or between 20 mg and 200 mg of methylprednisolone would respond in a relatively similar manner. However, in vitro studies have indicated that lower concentrations of these corticosteroids might not inhibit the catabolic pathways driving joint disease.[98] The currently recommended doses (see Table 84-4) appear to be within an acceptable range given in published information.

Corticosteroids combined with hyaluronan are very commonly administered. This combination is based on limited scientific evidence but good clinical responses. Combination treatment was supported by 50% to 80% of recently polled equine practitioners, reinforcing the favorable clinical response.[99]

The exercise or rest period following treatment with IA corticosteroids is also somewhat controversial. The controversy is based on the ability of some corticosteroids to transiently decrease the anabolic metabolism of chondrocytes and potentially blunt the normal metabolic responses to exercise. Although this is a concern, it is most likely overstated. A decrease in chondrocyte anabolic rate has not been proved to be detrimental. Furthermore, studies have not identified gross or histologic lesions subsequent to IA corticosteroid administration and exercise; however, changes in biochemical and biomechanical parameters have been identified. Changes induced by methylprednisolone have been noted to last for more than 21 days, and this information has influenced exercise recommendations for all other corticosteroids. Anecdotal recommendations for rest periods after IA corticosteroid injection vary widely from immediate return to work to more than 30 days of rest. Even a relatively aggressive protocol, involving a high dose of corticosteroids repeated at 14 days along with concurrent strenuous exercise, has failed to demonstrate definitive detrimental effects.[95-97] Thus, a rest period might not be absolutely necessary. Anecdotal clinical impression does suggest that confinement to a box stall and run for 7 to 10 days, with a slow return to full work in the subsequent week, can prolong the duration of action following injection, but it does not appear to alter the effect of the treatment.

Some consideration should be given to the reported incidence of corticosteroid-induced laminitis; however, no direct association has been proved. It has been suggested that the total body dose of triamcinolone should not exceed 18 mg, methylprednisolone should not exceed 200 mg, and compounded betamethasone should not exceed 30 mg. These numbers are based on some fact and some fiction, but one of the main goals is to eliminate corticosteroid-induced laminitis. A recent study with long-term follow-up on 205 clinical cases of joint injections using either 40 mg or 80 mg of triamcinolone acetonide found that the incidence of laminitis was effectively 0.5%.[100] Because it is not possible to have a consistent model of laminitis following corticosteroid injection, we must rely on clinical reports and anecdotal suggestions for dosing regimens.

Hyaluronan

Hyaluronan (HA) is a normal and necessary component of synovial fluid and proteoglycan aggregates (aggrecan) (see Fig. 83-10). Based mainly on in vitro work, both the concentration and molecular weight (degree of polymerization) appear to be important in the normal function of HA. Although the exact mechanism through which endogenous or exogenous HA exhibits an effect is not known, additional effects of exogenous HA administration have been documented to include anti-inflammatory activity such as inhibition of chemotaxis, inhibition of phagocytosis of granulocytes and macrophages, and reduction in the stimulation, proliferation, and migration of lymphocytes. Hyaluronan has also been shown to decrease the formation and release of prostaglandins from macrophages and to scavenge oxygen-derived free radicals in a dose-dependent manner.[101] Researchers also hypothesize that exogenous administration of HA increases the synthesis of high molecular weight hyaluronate by the synoviocytes, a theory that is yet to be definitively proved. In addition, some questions exist about the molecular weight requirement for effectiveness of exogenous HA.

Previous research has suggested that molecular mass less than 500 kDa has little effect, whereas HA with a larger molecular mass demonstrates a dose-dependent response. Other studies have failed to correlate molecular mass to outcome parameters. Summarizing the current literature,[102] it appears that some basal molecular mass is needed for effectiveness. The author therefore uses products with molecular mass greater than 500 kDa and selects products with yet higher molecular mass based more on economic consideration of the client (Table 84-5).

Crossed-linked exogenous HA has been introduced in an attempt to improve viscosupplementation of joints. Briefly, viscosupplementation refers to the injection of HA or its derivative in an attempt to return the elasticity and viscosity of the synovial fluid to normal or higher levels. Cross-linked HA has been developed as an improvement to other synthetic HA. Because its rheologic properties are increased, it has a longer retention time in the synovial space and appears to be more resistant to free radicals. Hylan G-F20 (Synvisc), a cross-linked HA with a molecular mass on average greater than 6 MDa, has demonstrated favorable results in large multicenter human clinical studies, showing effectiveness as a nonsteroidal medication. An experimental study conducted in the horse failed to show beneficial effects of hylan, but it does cite the difference in acute experimental synovitis compared to the more chronic OA (in the human trial) as one possible explanation for the study outcome. The authors also mention that the severity of the model may have been too harsh to observe a significant treatment effect. Further work on case selection for viscosupplementation (cross-linked HAs) is needed.

The dosage of conventional HA (0, 1, 10, 20, and 40 mg per joint) has been tested using an equine OA model.[103] This study demonstrated that a dose of 20 mg per joint was needed to demonstrate improvement in degree of lameness measured using a force plate. Dose-frequency studies are based on work in human clinical patients, suggesting that at least 3 doses are required (administered one week apart) to see significant effects in clinical parameters of pain and effusion. The current recommended equine HA treatment protocol is 20 mg of HA once a week for 3 weeks. Clinical equine reports have generally supported the use of HA, but many of these published evaluations have been subjective,

TABLE 84-5. Partial Listing of Available Hyaluron Products*

Product Name	Manufacturer	Concentration	Molecular Weight (Daltons)	How Supplied	Recommended Dose* (for Small to Medium-Size Joints)	SA	Cost
Hylartin V	Pharmacia and Upjohn	10 mg/mL	3.5×10^6	2 mL syringe 20 mg	20 mg	Each	$51.70
MAP-5 (used intra-articularly at this dose)	Vetrepharm	10.3 mg/mL (2mL) 5 mg/mL (10 mL)	7.5×10^5	2 mL vial 10 mL vial	20 mg	10 cc 2 cc	$44.71 $19.12
Legend (Hyonate) Intravenous/ intra-articular use	Bayer Corporation	10 mg/mL	3×10^5	4 mL vial	40 mg (IV)	Box of 6	$55.59
Hyalovet (Hyalovet-20)	Fort Dodge/ Vetrepharm	10 mg/mL	$4\text{-}7 \times 10^5$	2 mL syringe	20 mg	2 cc	$30.17
Hycoat (used intra-articularly)	Neogen	5 mg/mL	$>1.0 \times 10^6$	6 mL vial	30 mg	10 cc	$41.64
Hyvisc	Vetmedica	11 mg/mL	2.1×10^6	2 mL syringe	20 mg	B100 B20 B50 each	$3,595 $819 $1897 $44.95
HY-50	Bexco Pharma	17 mg/mL	—	3 mL syringe	51 mg	—	—
Equron	Solvay Animal Health	5 mg/mL	$1.5 - 2.0 \times 10^6$	2 mL syringe	10 mg	—	—
Equiflex	Chesapeake Biological	5 mg/mL	1×10^6	5 mL vial	10 mg	—	—
Synacid	Schering-Plough	10 mg/mL	$0.15\text{-}0.20 \times 10^6$	5 mL vial	50 mg	—	—

*Availability and costs are as of spring 2004.

and the definitions of criteria for successful treatment are absent. It appears that HA may be more effective when used in cases of mild synovitis or capsulitis and not as effective in severe synovitis or capsulitis and chronic OA.[104]

The use of intravenous (IV) HA in the treatment of joint disease is very common. An experimental study documented improvement in clinical lameness and synovial membrane histology, as well as better synovial fluid parameters such as lower PGE_2 and total protein levels in a carpal chip model.[105] These improvements were seen 42 days following the last of three treatments (40 mg) that were given 1 week apart.

Research to elucidate the mechanism of action for IV HA has been conducted, although relatively few answers have been found. A recent survey of 20 equine practitioners did not reflect an overwhelming usefulness of IV HA; however, case selection or objective outcome parameters were not clearly defined.[99] From both scientific and anecdotal reports, it appears that the use of IV HA in cases of acute synovitis could yield a better chance for success than in cases of chronic OA, where significant cartilage loss is present.

The prophylactic use of IV HA has also been studied in both Quarter and Thoroughbred racehorses. The Quarter Horse study enrolled 140 horses; subjects received either IV saline or HA every 2 weeks for the duration of the 9-month study.[106] HA-treated horses tended to race longer before requiring the first joint injection and to have a better speed index, higher average number of starts, and more money earned compared to placebo-treated horses. A similar study has been conducted in Thoroughbred racehorses to alleviate confounding variables introduced with the multiple trainers used in the Quarter Horse study, but data on performance outcomes is not yet available. Anecdotal reports from trainers in various equine disciplines have been positive regarding the prophylactic use of IV HA.

Polysulfated Polysaccharides

Polysulfated polysaccharides include polysulfated glycosaminoglycan (PSGAG; Adequan), GAG peptide complex (Rumalon), and pentosan polysulfate Cartrophen Vet; Pentequin). These drugs have been referred to as exhibiting chondroprotective effects or, by more recent definitions, are slow-acting disease-modifying osteoarthritic drugs (SAMOADs). Such agents are meant to prevent, retard, or reverse the morphologic cartilaginous lesion of OA.

PSGAG is made from bovine lung and trachea extracts containing mainly chondroitin sulfate. Numerous equine studies have been carried out in vitro and in vivo using PSGAG and have had contradictory results. Some studies have shown PSGAG to inhibit many of the key enzymes or cytokines involved in OA including IL-1, matrix metalloproteinases (MMPs), and PGE_2, as well as affecting proteoglycan synthesis and degradation. Because the testing systems, duration of experiments, and dosages varied from study to study, direct comparisons are difficult. The precise mechanisms of action of PSGAG are uncertain and the interaction of PSGAG with cytokines involved in joint disease has not been well defined.[102]

Some of the earliest work involving IA PSGAG in the horse investigated the effects of administering 250 mg biweekly for 3 weeks in clinical cases. This study and others using models of acute synovitis have shown improvements in clinical disease parameters following PSGAG treatment. One study also looked at cartilage histology, observing improvement in chondrocyte morphology. The same authors, using a similar model, also tested PSGAG via an IM route with less-impressive results.[102] In a group of ponies with experimentally induced osteochondral lesions, IA PSGAG (250 mg once a week for 5 weeks) significantly improved clinical lameness, radiographic progression of OA, and joint capsule parameters compared with untreated ponies. However, PSGAG also reduced the endogenous repair of the cartilaginous lesions.[105] Therefore, care should be taken when using PSGAG in cases where significant cartilage lesions exist on weightbearing surfaces.

In an experimental study, IM PSGAG administered every 4th day for 28 days, starting 14 days following OA induction, demonstrated some improvement in clinical lameness 56 days after initiation of treatment.[107] Although PSGAG-treated horses did show biochemical improvements compared to placebo-treated horses, overall more impressive improvements were observed with shock wave treatment of the affected joint (see "Extracorporeal Shock Wave Therapy").

A survey[104] to assess the perceived efficacy of PSGAG by 1522 equine practitioners was published in 1996. Practitioners treating Thoroughbred racehorses gave the highest efficacy scores, and practitioners treating pleasure horses gave the lowest efficacy scores. PSGAG was considered more effective than sodium hyaluronate for the treatment of subacute OA and less effective for idiopathic joint effusion and acute synovitis. The authors of the survey concluded that the efficacy of PSGAG for incipient and chronic forms of OA is comparable to that of sodium hyaluronate.

Important information has been published indicating that a lower bacterial inoculation is needed to establish septic arthritis when PSGAG is administered IA. This result is abolished with the addition of 125 mg amikacin with the PSGAG treatment. Therefore, administration of amikacin with PSGAG administered IA is strongly recommended.

Like PSGAG, pentosan polysulfate (PPS) is a heparinoid compound, but it is unique in that it is derived from beechwood hemicellulose instead of animal or bacterial sources as with PSGAGs. These products have been administered mainly in horses in Australia, although efficacy reports have been anecdotal. To the author's knowledge, sodium pentosan polysulfate has been used only parenterally in horses. Although a form has been complexed with a calcium salt and tested in other species, the results indicate that pentosan appears to be bioavailable following oral administration. Clinical studies in dogs and people with OA have shown convincing evidence of clinical efficacy.[108] In the horse, an unpublished study using an experimental model of OA has shown favorable results.[109] In this model, parenteral PPS showed significant improvement in reducing articular cartilage fibrillation and a strong trend for overall improvement in the histologic appearance of cartilage. Furthermore, most parameters showed numerical improvements (lameness, joint flexion, synovial fluid total protein, synovial fluid collagen degradation products, and aggrecan synthesis), although statistical significance of greater than 95% was not obtained.

Clinically, PPS could be used to treat horses with mild or early-stage OA, particularly with multiple joint involvement, because it is a systemic therapy. At this time, a dose of

3 mg/kg IM once weekly for 4 weeks is recommended for treatment of equine OA.

Oral Joint Supplements

A vast number of different oral supplements are available for the horse. Many of these work on the premise of providing building blocks of molecules that are integral in the articular cartilage or joint fluid. Although the formulation, concentration, and source of the products differ widely, most contain chondroitin sulfate, glucosamine, or hyaluronan, or some combination of these. Chondroitin sulfate has been assessed using radioisotope tracking and shown to be absorbed through the gastrointestinal tract, but it is thought to be in a smaller monomeric form compared to the ingested molecule. Glucosamine is even more bioavailable when compared to chondroitin sulfate.[109-113]

A study was conducted to document absorption specifically in the horse, but how these levels relate to clinically therapeutic levels is yet to be determined.[110] Double-blinded controlled studies in humans have indicated that these substances are efficacious in the treatment of joint disease.[114-117] Unfortunately, only limited, poorly controlled equine clinical studies have been performed to date, but anecdotal reports and in vitro tests are favorable for the use of glucosamine and chondroitin sulfate.[118]

Oral hyaluronan products are relatively new on the market and have been tested less compared to chondroitin sulfate or glucosamine. However, a controlled experimental in vivo trial comparing IV Legend and Conquer, an oral hyalronan, is under way. An interesting report in the human literature compared the label ingredient with the independent testing of the products and found little correlation to label claim and content or price and content. This potentially emphasizes the use of trusted brands that have at least undergone some testing.

Extracorporeal Shock Wave Therapy

Recent experimental evidence and anecdotal clinical impressions of extracorporeal shock wave therapy (ESWT) for the treatment of OA have been reported.[119-121] Unpublished clinical studies in the dog have shown promising results, as have anecdotal reports of treating shoulder, pastern, and coffin joint OA in horses.[107] An equine-specific-controlled experimental OA study has been completed comparing ESWT to PSGAG and sham treatments. The study used an established short-term (70 days) OA model where an osteochondral fragment was created at time zero and treatments were initiated 14 days later.[97] IM PSGAG treatment was administered every 4 days for 28 days. ESWT was administered on days 14 and 28 using a VersaTron (High Medical Technologies, Lengwil, Switzerland) 12 mm probe, and a sham shockwave procedure was performed on the control horses on days 14 and 28. In the ESWT group, 2000 shock waves at the E4 energy level were administered on study day 14 and 1500 shock waves at the E6 level on study day 28. The energy was delivered mainly to the middle carpal joint capsule attachment, but some energy (approximately 20%) was delivered to the area of fragmentation. Significant improvement in clinical lameness, decreased synovial fluid total protein (as a marker of synovitis), and less GAG release into the bloodstream were observed with ESWT compared to both control and PSGAG-treated horses. These results appear to show promise for this type of therapy for use in localized joint disease in horses, although clinical studies are still needed.

Challenges of Medical Management in Equine Joint Disease

Some of the considerations in treating equine joint disease have been presented in this chapter. Challenges that equine clinicians face are numerous, but the rapid evolution of knowledge of joint disease pathophysiology, the relative lack of specific equine research, economic considerations of the owner, and rules imposed by governing bodies of sanctioned equine events pose a unique set of challenges. More specifically, the pathophysiology of joint disease is extremely complex, the multifactorial nature of the disease makes it challenging to study, and at best it is only partly understood in any species.[122,123] Even with the greatest understanding of the disease being in people, human physicians do not agree upon a course of treatment based on joint affected, stage of disease progression, or age of the patient. Further removed is the equine practitioner, who is often making therapeutic decisions based on extrapolated data from people, a comparison that is not always justifiable.

The lack of specific equine research often drives the need to extrapolate from other species on the class of substance to use, specific compound within a class (such as which specific corticosteroid), dose, frequency of administration, or whether a combination of medications should be employed. The equine clinician is often left to make a plan based on anecdotal information rather than substantial evidence showing safety or efficacy of a specific regimen. Advances in equine-specific studies are occurring, thus confirming or refuting many anecdotal or uncontrolled published studies although, as expected, much work is left to be completed.

Other factors do play a real role in defining a therapeutic plan, but some of them have little to do with the defined treatment goals. Economic consideration and medication rules governing many sanctioned equine events are just two such examples. The coordination of all of the presented factors and issues into a sound, effective therapeutic plan are what makes treatment of equine joint disease challenging. Through an understanding of the historic and current literature, anecdotal information, and up-to-date rules pertinent to equine events, advancements can be realized in the treatment of equine joint disease.

Future Therapies

Since the 1990s, research has led to a greater understanding of joint disease pathophysiology and identification of major mediators driving the disease process. Also, the identification of naturally occurring antagonists or synthetic analogs with the ability to block these degenerative mediators has been realized. Numerous novel medical treatments are being tested in vivo after successful in vitro trials.[124,125] Furthermore, in the long term, the field of tissue engineering is burgeoning with the promise of being able to recreate organ systems.[126] Realistically, in the short term, the subdiscipline of cartilage engineering is most likely to make the biggest impact on the treatment of equine joint disease and is an active area of research at several equine orthopedic research facilities.

Treatment of generalized OA using novel methods of administering antiarthritic therapeutic proteins will most likely be the first advance that changes the future of treating equine joint disease.[126-128] Given that the inhibition of IL-1 and tumor necrosis factors has been shown to be clinically beneficial, in vivo practical methods of administering these therapeutics are being explored. Specific examples that have shown clinical success in people with either rheumatoid arthritis or OA are the administration of IL-1 receptor antagonist (IL-1Ra, a natural antagonist of interleukin-1), soluble receptors to tumor necrosis factor (receptors that bind the parent molecule but have no further biological action), and antibodies directed at tumor necrosis factor.

In one study conducted in the horse, gene therapy was shown to be an effective treatment in an experimental model of osteoarthritis.[129] Briefly, the gene sequence for equine IL-1Ra was delivered to the affected joint by direct IA injection of a nonpathogenic virus. This virus was engineered to deliver the genetic information to overproduce equine Il-1Ra protein within joint tissues without causing adverse effects on the cell. In this study, the ability to decrease clinical lameness and slow the progression of induced joint disease was more profound than any other medication tested (including corticosteroids, PSGAG, PPS, HA, or ECSWT). Advancement in delivering genes or recombinant proteins to specific target cells and the ability to turn on and off the protein production is being realized. Furthermore, this technology is being used in combination with surgical techniques to improve cartilage healing and treatment of osteoarthritis.[130,131]

REFERENCES

1. McIlwraith CW: Diagnostic and Surgical Arthroscopy in the Horse, ed 2, Philadelphia, 1990, Lea & Febiger.
2. Nixon AJ: Equine Fracture Repair, ed 1, Philadelphia, 1996, WB Saunders.
3. Ike RW, Arnold WJ, Rothschild EW, et al: Tidal irrigation versus conservative medical management in patients with osteoarthritis of the knee: A prospective randomized study. Tidal Irrigation Cooperating Group, J Rheumatol 1992;19:772-779.
4. Bradley JD, Heilman DK, Katz BP, et al: Tidal irrigation as treatment for knee osteoarthritis: A sham-controlled, randomized, double-blinded evaluation, Arthritis Rheum 2002;46:100-108.
5. Kalunian KC, Moreland LW, Klashman DJ, et al: Visually-guided irrigation in patients with early knee osteoarthritis: A multicenter randomized, controlled trial, Osteoarthritis Cartilage 2000;8:412-418.
6. Kane AJ, McIlwraith CW, Park RD, et al: Radiographic changes in Thoroughbred yearlings. Part 2: Associations with racing performance, Equine Vet J 2003;35:366-374.
7. Kane AJ, Park RD, McIlwraith CW, et al: Radiographic changes in Thoroughbred yearlings. Part 1: Prevalence at the time of the yearling sales, Equine Vet J 2003;35:354-365.
8. Pettersson H: Fractures of the pedal bone in the horse, Equine Vet J 1976;8:104-109.
9. Haynes PF, Adams OR: Internal fixation of fractured extensor process of third phalanx in a horse, J Am Vet Med Assoc 1974;164:61-63.
10. Dechant JE, Trotter GW, Stashak TS, et al: Removal of large fragments of the extensor process of the distal phalanx via arthrotomy in horses: 14 cases (1992-1998), J Am Vet Med Assoc 2000;217:1351-1355.
11. Gabel AA, Bukowiecki CF: Fractures of the phalanges, Vet Clin North Am Large Anim Pract 1983;5:233-260.
12. Foerner JJ, McIlwraith CW: Orthopaedic surgery in the racehorse, Vet Clin North Am Large Anim Pract 1990;6:147.
13. Schneider JE, Carnine BL, Guffy MM: Arthrodesis of the proximal interphalangeal joint in the horse: A surgical treatment for high ringbone, J Am Vet Med Assoc 1978;173:1364-1369.
14. Doran RE, White NA 2nd, Allen D: Use of a bone plate for treatment of middle phalangeal fractures in horses: Seven cases (1979-1984), J Am Vet Med Assoc 1987;191:575-578.
15. Colahan PT, Wheat JD, Meagher DM: Treatment of middle phalangeal fractures in the horse, J Am Vet Med Assoc 1981;178:1182-1185.
16. Yovich JV, Stashak TS, Sullins KE: Bilateral hindlimb pastern arthrodesis in a horse, Equine Vet J 1986;18:79-81.
17. Markel MD, Richardson DW, Nunamaker DM: Comminuted first phalanx fractures in 30 horses: Surgical vs nonsurgical treatments, Vet Surg 1985;14:135-140.
18. Speirs VC: Assessment of the economic value of orthopaedic surgery in Thoroughbred racehorses, Vet Clin North Am Large Anim Pract 1983;5:391-401.
19. Bramlage LA: Complications of orthopedic surgery, Proc Am Assoc Equine Pract 1979; 25:219.
20. McIlwraith CW, Yovich JV, Martin GS: Arthroscopic surgery for the treatment of osteochondral chip fractures in the equine carpus, J Am Vet Med Assoc 1987;191:531-540.
21. Elce, YA, Richardson DW: Arthroscopic removal of dorsoproximal chip fractures of the proximal phalanx in standing horses, Vet Surg 2002;31:195-200.
22. Barclay WP, Foerner JJ, Phillips TN: Lameness attributable to osteochondral fragmentation of the plantar aspect of the proximal phalanx in horses: 19 cases (1981-1985), J Am Vet Med Assoc 1987;7:855-858.
23. Pettersson H, Ryden G: Avulsion fragments of the caudoproximal extremity of the first phalanx, Equine Vet J 1982;14:333-335.
24. Simon O, Laverty S, Boure L, et al: Arthroscopic removal of axial osteochondral fragments of the proximoplantar aspect of the proximal phalanx using electrocautery probes in 23 Standardbred racehorses, Vet Surg 2004;33:422-427.
25. Bukowiecki CF, Bramlage LR, Gabel AA: Palmar/plantar process fractures of the proximal phalanx in 15 horses, Vet Surg 1986;15:383-388.
26. Fortier LA, Foerner JJ, Nixon AJ: Arthroscopic removal of axial osteochondral fragments of the plantar/palmar proximal aspect of the proximal phalanx in horses: 119 cases (1988-1992), J Am Vet Med Assoc 1995;206:71-74.
27. Whitton RC, Kannegieter NJ: Osteochondral fragmentation of the plantar/palmar proximal aspect of the proximal phalanx in racing horses, Aust Vet J 1994,71:318-321.
28. Spurlock GH, Gabel AA: Apical fractures of the proximal sesamoid bones in 109 Standardbred horses, J Am Vet Med Assoc 1983;183:76-79.
29. Buckowiecki CF, Bramlage LA, Gabel AA: Proximal sesamoid bone fractures in horses: Current treatments and prognoses, Comp Cont Educ Pract Vet 1985;7:S684.
30. Fretz PB, Barber SM, Bailey JV, et al: Management of proximal sesamoid bone fractures in the horse, J Am Vet Med Assoc 1984;185:282-284.
31. Palmer SE: Arthroscopic removal of apical and abaxial sesamoid fracture fragments in five horses, Vet Surg 1989;18:347-352.
32. Boure L, Marcoux M, Laverty S, et al: Use of electrocautery probes in arthroscopic removal of apical sesamoid fracture fragments in 18 Standardbred horses, Vet Surg 1999;28:226-232.

33. Southwood LL, Trotter GW, McIlwraith CW: Arthroscopic removal of abaxial fracture fragments of the proximal sesamoid bones in horses: 47 cases (1989-1997), J Am Vet Med Assoc 1998;213:1016-1021.
34. Copelan RW, Bramlage LR: Surgery of the fetlock joint, Vet Clin North Am Large Anim Pract 1983;5:221-231.
35. Parente EJ, Richardson DW, Spencer P: Basal sesamoidean fractures in horses: 57 cases (1980-1991), J Am Vet Med Assoc 1993;202:1293-1297.
36. Southwood LL, McIlwraith CW: Arthroscopic removal of fracture fragments involving a portion of the base of the proximal sesamoid bone in horses: 26 cases (1984-1997), J Am Vet Med Assoc 2000;217:236-240.
37. Lindsay WA, Horney FD: Equine carpal surgery: A review of 89 cases and evaluation of return to function, J Am Vet Med Assoc 1981;179:682-685.
38. Speirs VC, Anderson GA, Bourke JM: Assessment of prognosis for racing after carpal surgery in 210 Thoroughbreds, Equine Vet J 1986;18:187-192.
39. Raidal SL, Wright JD: A retrospective evaluation of the surgical management of equine carpal injury, Aust Vet J 1996;74:198-202.
40. O'Sullivan CB, Dart AJ, Malikides N, et al: Nonsurgical management of type II fractures of the distal phalanx in 48 Standardbred horses, Aust Vet J 1999;77:501-503.
41. Rick MC, O'Brien TR, Pool RR, et al: Condylar fractures of the third metacarpal bone and third metatarsal bone in 75 horses: Radiographic features, treatments, and outcome, J Am Vet Med Assoc 1983;183:287-296.
42. Fackelman GE: Sagittal fractures of the first phalanx (P 1) in the horse: Fixation by the lag screw principle, Vet Med Small Anim Clin 1973;68:622-636.
43. Ellis DR, Simpson DJ, Greenwood RE, et al: Observations and management of fractures of the proximal phalanx in young Thoroughbreds, Equine Vet J 1987;19:43-49.
44. Holcombe SJ, Schneider RK, Bramlage LR, et al: Lag screw fixation of noncomminuted sagittal fractures of the proximal phalanx in racehorses: 59 cases (1973-1991), J Am Vet Med Assoc 1995;206:1195-1199.
45. Fischer AT Jr, Stover SM: Sagittal fractures of the third carpal bone in horses: 12 cases (1977-1985), J Am Vet Med Assoc 1987;191:106-108.
46. Meagher DM: Lateral condylar fractures of the metacarpus and metatarsus in horses, Proc Am Assoc Equine Pract 1976; 22:147.
47. Barclay WP, Foerner JJ, Phillips TN: Axial sesamoid injuries associated with lateral condylar fractures in horses, J Am Vet Med Assoc 1985;186:278-279.
48. Adams S, Turner T, Blevins W, et al: Surgical repair of metacarpal condylar fractures with palmar osteochondral communication in two Thoroughbred horses, Vet Surg 1985;14:32.
49. Richardson DW: Medial condylar fractures of the third metatarsal bone in horses, J Am Vet Med Assoc 1984;185:761-765.
50. Stephens PR, Richardson DW, Spencer PA: Slab fractures of the third carpal bone in Standardbreds and Thoroughbreds: 155 cases (1977-1984), J Am Vet Med Assoc 1988;193:353-358.
51. Richardson DW: Technique for arthroscopic repair of third carpal bone slab fractures in horses, J Am Vet Med Assoc 1986;188:288-291.
52. Martin GS, Haynes PF, McClure JR: Effect of third carpal slab fracture and repair on racing performance in Thoroughbred horses: 31 cases (1977-1984), J Am Vet Med Assoc 1988;193:107-110.
53. Bramlage LR: Surgical diseases of the carpus, Vet Clin North Am Large Anim Pract 1983;5:261-274.
54. Roneus B, Andersson AM, Ekman S: Racing performance in Standardbred trotters with chronic synovitis after partial arthroscopic synovectomy in the metacarpophalangeal, metatarsophalangeal and intercarpal (midcarpal) joints, Acta Vet Scand 1997;38:87-95.
55. Doets HC, Bierman BTM, Soesbergen RMV: Synovectomy of the rheumatoid knee does not prevent deterioration, Acta Orthop Scand 1989;60:523-525.
56. Goldenberg D, Cohen A: Synovial membrane histopathology in the differential diagnosis of rheumatoid arthritis, gout, pseudogout, systemic lupus erythematosus, infectious arthritis and degenerative joint disease, Medicine (Baltimore) 1978;57:239-252.
57. Haraoui B, Pelletier JP, Cloutier JM, et al: Synovial membrane histology and immunopathology in rheumatoid arthritis and osteoarthritis. In vivo effects of antirheumatic drugs, Arthritis Rheum 1991;34:153-163.
58. McEwen C: Early synovectomy in the treatment of rheumatoid arthritis, N Engl J Med 1968;279:420-421.
59. Doyle-Jones PS, Sullins KE, Saunders GK: Synovial regeneration in the equine carpus after arthroscopic mechanical or carbon dioxide laser synovectomy, Vet Surg 2002;31:331-343.
60. Yarbrough TB, Lee MR, Hornof WJ, et al: Evaluation of samarium-153 for synovectomy in an osteochondral fragment-induced model of synovitis in horses, Vet Surg 2000;29:252-263.
61. Caplan AI, Elyaderani M, Mochizuki Y, et al: Principles of cartilage repair and regeneration, Clin Orthop Relat Res 1997;(342):254-269.
62. Vachon A, Bramlage LR, Gabel AA, et al: Evaluation of the repair process of cartilage defects of the equine third carpal bone with and without subchondral bone perforation, Am J Vet Res 1986;47:2637-2645.
63. Shamis LD, Bramlage LR, Gabel AA, et al: Effect of subchondral drilling on repair of partial-thickness cartilage defects of third carpal bones in horses, Am J Vet Res 1989;50:290-295.
64. Frisbie DD, Oxford JT, Southwood L, et al: Early events in cartilage repair after subchondral bone microfracture, Clin Orthop Relat Res 2003;(407):215-227.
65. Frisbie DD, Trotter GW, Powers BE, et al: Arthroscopic subchondral bone plate microfracture technique augments healing of large chondral defects in the radial carpal bone and medial femoral condyle of horses, Vet Surg 1999;28:242-255.
66. Morisset S, Frisbie DD, Robbins PD, et al: Healing of full thickness chondral defects treated with arthroscopic subchondral bone plate microfracture and IL-1Ra/IGF-1 delivered through gene transfer, Proc Am Coll Vet Surg 2004:E16.
67. Knutsen G, Engebretsen L, Ludvigsen TC, et al: Autologous chondrocyte implantation compared with microfracture in the knee. A randomized trial, J Bone Joint Surg Am 2004;86-A:455-464.
68. Brittberg M, Lindahl A, Nilsson A, et al: Treatment of deep cartilage defects in the knee with autologous chondrocyte transplantation, N Engl J Med 1994;331:889-941.
69. Steadman JR, Rodkey WG, Singleton SB, et al: Microfracture technique for full-thickness chondral defects: Technique and clinical results, Oper Tech Orthop 1997;7:300-304.
70. Sullins KE, McIlwraith CW, Powers BE, et al: Evaluation of periosteal grafts in articular cartilage repair in horses, Vet Surg 1985;14:66-67.
71. Vachon A, McIlwraith CW, Trotter GW, et al: Neochondrogenesis in free intraarticular, periosteal, and perichondrial autografts in horses, Am J Vet Res 1989;50:1787-1794.
72. Vachon AM, McIlwraith CW, McFadden P, et al: Sternal cartilage autografts for repair of large osteochondral defects in the horse. Transactions of the Thirty-seventh Annual Meeting of the Orthopaedic Research Society, 1991;16:327.
73. Howard RD, McIlwraith CW, Trotter GW, et al: Sternebral cartilage autografts in the repair of osteochondral defects in horses: Long term fate and effects of exercise, Vet Surg 1992;21:393.
74. Howard RD, McIlwraith CW, Trotter GW, et al: Long-term fate and effects of exercise on sternal cartilage autografts used for repair of large osteochondral defects in horses, Am J Vet Res 1994;55:1158-1167.

75. Evans PJ, Miniaci A, Hurtig MB: Manual punch versus power harvesting of osteochondral grafts, Arthroscopy 2004;20:306-310.
76. Hurtig M, Pearce S, Warren S, et al: Arthroscopic mosaic arthroplasty in the equine third carpal bone, Vet Surg 2001;30:228-239.
77. Pearce SG, Hurtig MB, Boure LP, et al: Cylindrical press-fit osteochondral allografts for resurfacing the equine metatarsophalangeal joint, Vet Surg 2003;32:220-230.
78. von Rechenberg B, Akens MK, Nadler D, et al: The use of photooxidized, mushroom-structured osteochondral grafts for cartilage resurfacing: A comparison to photooxidized cylindrical grafts in an experimental study in sheep, Osteoarthritis Cartilage 2004;12:201-216.
79. Nixon AJ: Advances in cell-based grafting, Proc Am Coll Vet Surg 2001;11:128-131.
80. Frisbie DD, Colhoun HA, Bowman S, McIlwraith CW: PDS/PGA staples compared to suture fixation of autologous chondrocyte constructs. In 49th Annual Meeting of the Orthopaedic Research Society, New Orleans, 2003:712.
81. Frisbie DD, Colhoun HA, Bowman S, et al: In vivo evaluation of autologous chondrocytes seeded on a collagen scaffold. In 50th Annual meeting of the Orthopaedic Research Society, San Francisco, March 7-10, 2004:703.
82. Bohanon TC, Schneider RK, Weisbrode SE: Fusion of the distal intertarsal and tarsometatarsal joints in the horse using intra-articular sodium monoiodoacetate, Equine Vet J 1991;23:289-295.
83. Dechant JE, Baxter GM, Southwood LL, et al: Use of a three-drill-tract technique for arthrodesis of the distal tarsal joints in horses with distal tarsal osteoarthritis: 54 cases (1990-1999), J Am Vet Med Assoc 2003;223:1800-1805.
84. Hague BA, Guccione A: Laser-facilitated arthrodesis of the distal tarsal joints, Clin Tech Equine Pract 2002;1:32-35.
85. Todhunter RJ, Minor RR, Wootton JA, et al: Effects of exercise and polysulfated glycosaminoglycan on repair of articular cartilage defects in the equine carpus, J Orthop Res 1993;11:782-795.
86. Barr ARS, Duance VC, Wotton SF, et al: Influence of intra-articular sodium hyaluronate and polysulphated glycosaminoglycans on the biochemical composition of equine articular surface repair tissue, Equine Vet J 1994;26:40-42.
87. Gaughan EM, Nixon AJ, Krook LP, et al: Effects of sodium hyaluronate on tendon healing and adhesion formation in horses, Am J Vet Res 1991;52:764-773.
88. Dingle JT: Prostaglandins in human cartilage metabolism, J Lipid Mediat 6:303-312.
89. Malmberg AB, Yaksh TL: Hyperalgesia mediated by spinal glutamate or substance P receptor blocked by spinal cyclooxygenase inhibition, Science 1992;257:1276-1279.
90. Laine L, Harper S, Simon T, et al: A randomized trial comparing the effect of rofecoxib, a cyclooxygenase 2-specific inhibitor, with that of ibuprofen on the gastroduodenal mucosa of patients with osteoarthritis. Rofecoxib Osteoarthritis Endoscopy Study Group, Gastroenterology 1999;117:776-783.
91. Caldwell FJ, Mueller PO, Lynn RC, et al: Effect of topical application of diclofenac liposomal suspension on experimentally induced subcutaneous inflammation in horses, Am J Vet Res 2004;65:271-276.
92. Bertone JJ, Lynn RC, Vatistas NJ, et al: Clinical field trial to evaluate the efficacy of topically applied diclofenac liposomal cream for the relief of joint lameness in horse. Proc Am Assoc Equine Pract 2002;48:190-193.
93. Todhunter RJ, Fubini SL, Vernier-Singer V, et al: Acute synovitis and intra-articular methylprednisolone acetate in ponies, Osteoarthritis Cartilage 1998;6:94-105.
94. Masferrer JL, Seibert K: Regulation of prostaglandin synthesis by glucocorticoids, Receptor 1994;4:25-30.
95. Foland JW, McIlwraith CW, Trotter GW, et al: Effect of betamethasone and exercise on equine carpal joints with osteochondral fragments, Vet Surg 1994;23:369-376.
96. Frisbie DD, Kawcak CE, Trotter GW, et al: The effects of 6-alpha methylprednisolone acetate on an in vivo equine osteochondral fragment exercise model, Am J Vet Res 1998;12:1619-1628.
97. Frisbie DD, Kawcak CE, Trotter GW, et al: The effects of triamcinolone acetate on an in vivo equine osteochondral fragment exercise model, Equine Vet J 1997;29:349-359.
98. Dechant JE, Baxter GM, Frisbie DD, et al: Effects of dosage titration of methylprednisolone acetate and triamcinolone acetonide on interleukin-1–conditioned equine articular cartilage explants in vitro, Equine Vet J 2003;35:444-450.
99. Caron JP, Genovesse RL: Principles and practices of joint disease treatment. In Ross MW, Dyson SJ, editors: Diagnostics and Management of Lameness in the Horse, Philadelphia, 2003, Elsevier Science.
100. McCluskey MJ, Kavenagh PB: Clinical use of triamcinolone acetonide in the horse (205 cases) and the incidence of glucocorticoid induced laminitis associated with its use, Equine Vet Educ 2004;16:86-89.
101. Howard RD, McIlwraith CW: Sodium hyaluronate in the treatment of equine joint disease, Compend Contin Educ Practicing Vet 15:473-481, 1993.
102. McIlwraith CW, Trotter GW: Joint disease in the horse, ed 1, Philadelphia, 1996, WB Saunders.
103. Auer J, Fackelman G: Treatment of degenerative joint disease of the horse: a review and commentary, Vet Surg 1981;2:80-90.
104. Caron JP, JB Kaneene JB, Miller R: Results of a survey of equine practitioners on the use and perceived efficacy of polysulfated glycosaminoglycan, J Am Vet Med Assoc 1996;209:1564-1568.
105. Kawcak CE, Frisbie DD, McIlwraith CW, et al: Effects of intravenously administered sodium hyaluronate on equine carpal joints with osteochondral fragments under exercise, Am J Vet Res 1997;58:1132-1140.
106. McIlwraith CW, Goodman NL, Frisbie DD: Prospective study on the prophaylactic value of intravenous hyaluronan in 2-year-old racing Quarter Horses, Proc Am Assoc Equine Pract 1998;44:269-270.
107. Frisbie DD, Kawcak CE, McIlwraith CW: Evaluation of Extracorporeal Shock Wave Therapy for Osteoarthritis. In 50th Annual Convention Am Assoc Equine Practitioners, Denver, 2004:261-263.
108. Ghosh P: The pathobiology of osteoarthritis and the rationale for the use of pentosan polysulfate for its treatment, Semin Arthritis Rheum 1999;28:211-267.
109. Baici A, Diczhazi C, Neszmelyi A, et al: Inhibition of the human leukocyte endopeptidases elastase and cathepsin G and of porcine pancreatic elastase by *N*-oleoyl derivatives of heparin, Biochem Pharmacol 1993;46:1545-1549.
110. Du J, White N, Eddington ND: The bioavailability and pharmacokinetics of glucosamine hydrochloride and chondroitin sulfate after oral and intravenous single dose administration in the horse, Biopharm Drug Dispos 2004;25:109-116.
111. Palmieri L, Conte A, Giovannini L, et al: Metabolic fate of exogenous chondroitin sulfate in the experimental animal, Arzneimittelforschung 1990;40:319-323.
112. Reichelt A, Forster KK, Fischer M, et al: Efficacy and safety of intramuscular glucosamine sulfate in osteoarthritis of the knee: A randomised, placebo-controlled, double-blind study, Arzneimittelforschung 1994;44:75-80.
113. Setnikar I, Palumbo R, Canali S, et al: Pharmacokinetics of glucosamine in man, Arzneimittelforschung 1993;43:1109-1113.
114. Bourgeois P, Chales G, Dehais J, et al: Efficacy and tolerability of chondroitin sulfate 1200 mg/day vs chondroitin sulfate 3 × 400 mg/day vs placebo, Osteoarthritis Cartilage 1998;6(Suppl A):25-30.
115. Bucsi L, Poor G: Efficacy and tolerability of oral chondroitin sulfate as a symptomatic slow-acting drug for osteoarthritis (SYSADOA) in the treatment of knee osteoarthritis, Osteoarthritis Cartilage 1998;6(Suppl A):31-36.
116. Pavelka K, Gatterova J, Olejarova M, et al: Glucosamine sulfate use

and delay of progression of knee osteoarthritis: A 3-year, randomized, placebo-controlled, double-blind study, Arch Intern Med 2002;162:2113-2123.
117. Reginster JY, Deroisy R, Rovati LC, et al: Long-term effects of glucosamine sulphate on osteoarthritis progression: A randomised, placebo-controlled clinical trial, Lancet 2001;357(9252):251-256.
118. Hansen RR: Oral glycosaminoglycans in the treatment of degenerative joint disease in horses, Equine Pract 1996;18:18.
119. Coombs R, Schaden W, Zhou SSH: Musculoskeletal Shockwave Therapy, ed 1, London, 2000, Greenwich Medical Media.
120. Scheuch B, Whitcomb MB, Galuppo L, et al: Clinical evaluation of high-energy extracorporeal shock waves on equine orthopedic injuries, Proc Am Assoc Equine Sports Med 2000;19:18-20.
121. McCarroll GD, Hague B, Smitherman S, et al: The use of extracorporal shock wave lithotripsy for treatment of distal tarsal arthropathies of the horse, Proc Am Assoc Equine Sports Med 1999;18:40-41.
122. McIlwraith CW: General pathobiology of the joint and response to injury. In McIlwraith CW, Trotter GW, editors: Joint Disease in the Horse, Philadelphia, 1997, WB Saunders.
123. Poole AR: Cartilage in health and disease. In McCarty DJ, editor: Arthritis and Allied Conditions: A Textbook of Rheumatology, Philadelphia, 1993, Lea & Febiger.
124. Chikanza I, Fernandes L: Novel strategies for the treatment of osteoarthritis, Expert Opin Investig Drugs 2000;9:1499-1510.
125. Evans CH, Robbins PD: Gene therapy of arthritis, Intern Med 1999;38:233-239.
126. Hunziker B: Articular cartilage repair: Basic science and clinical progress. A review of the current status and prospects, Osteoarthritis Cartilage 2002;10:432-463.
127. Davis JC Jr, Van Der Heijde D, Braun J, et al: Recombinant human tumor necrosis factor receptor (etanercept) for treating ankylosing spondylitis: A randomized, controlled trial, Arthritis Rheum 2003:48:3230-3236.
128. Keystone EC, Kavanaugh AF, Sharp JT, et al: Radiographic, clinical, and functional outcomes of treatment with adalimumab (a human anti-tumor necrosis factor monoclonal antibody) in patients with active rheumatoid arthritis receiving concomitant methotrexate therapy: A randomized, placebo-controlled, 52-week trial, Arthritis Rheum 2004;50:1400-1411.
129. Frisbie DD, Ghivizzani SC, Robbins PD, et al: Treatment of experimental equine osteoarthritis by in vivo delivery of the equine interleukin-1 receptor antagonist gene, Gene Ther 2002;9:12-20.
130. Haupt JL, Frisbie DD, McIlwraith CW, et al: Dual transduction of insulin-like growth factor-I and interleukin-1 receptor antagonist protein controls cartilage degradation in an osteoarthritic culture model, J Orthop Res 2005;23:118-126.
131. Nixon AJ, Haupt JL, Frisbie DD, et al: Gene-mediated restoration of cartilage matrix by combination of insulin-like growth factor-I/interleukin-1 receptor antagonist therapy. Gene Ther 2005; 12:177-186.
132. Caron JP: Principles of treatment of joint disease. In Auer JA, Stick JA, editors: Equine Surgery, Philadelphia, 1999, WB Saunders.

CHAPTER 85

Arthrodesis Techniques

Jörg A. Auer

It is every surgeon's goal to maintain or reestablish joint integrity to allow optimal function after treatment and subsequent healing of an injury. Unfortunately, in many instances this is not attainable, and degenerative changes limit the horse's use as an athlete or a pleasure animal.

However, in selected joint disorders arthrodesis is an option to maintain a useful horse despite sacrificing a joint. By definition, arthrodesis involves surgical fixation of a joint by a procedure designed to promote fusion of the joint surfaces.[1] Ankylosis involves achievement of immobility and consolidation of a joint damaged by disease, injury, or a surgical procedure. Therefore, an arthrodesis may be thought of as a type of ankylosis.

In most cases, surgical arthrodesis is carried out to salvage valuable breeding stock. However, certain joints can be fused without unduly compromising the animal's performance.

GENERAL GUIDELINES

The articular cartilage of opposing bones should be removed for achievement of an effective arthrodesis within the shortest time.[2-5] Persistence of cartilage between the bone ends delays bone union. Immobility of a joint with persistent articular cartilage results in malnutrition of the cartilage and its eventual degeneration. This is a very slow process, and islands of articular cartilage can persist between bone bridges across a joint for several years. However, removing minimal cartilage, by drilling across a joint surface, for example, can result in a joint with minimal movement and produce a functional arthrodesis with relief of pain symptoms. This procedure can be performed in the small tarsal articulations.[6] As a general rule, as much cartilage as possible should be removed, allowing maximum bone-on-bone contact.

Fusion of the joint is facilitated by drilling several holes of 2.5 to 3 mm in diameter across the dense subchondral bone plate of each of the opposing bone ends.[5,6] This type of osteostixis promotes ingrowth of blood vessels across the bone plate and hastens fusion. Incorporation of a cancellous bone graft, tricalcium phosphate granules,[7,8] or injectable biodegradable bone cement or hydrogel[9-11] enhances fusion of the joint as well.

Arthrodesis requires joint immobility, and this is accomplished by means of multiple screws placed in lag fashion, application of a bone plate, or implantation of a transarticular Bagby basket. The principal techniques used for arthrodesis of the distal and proximal interphalangeal joints, metacarpophalangeal joint, and carpal and tarsal region are discussed in detail in this chapter. Additionally, the arthrodesis technique applied in the scapulohumeral joint is briefly discussed.

DISTAL INTERPHALANGEAL JOINT ARTHRODESIS

Indications

Disorders that are not responsive to massive anti-inflammatory therapy and neurectomy might be candidates for distal interphalangeal (DIP) joint arthrodesis. The indications include advanced osteoarthritis and luxation of the DIP joint after rupture of the deep digital flexor tendon at the level of the distal sesamoid bone. This surgical intervention is a salvage procedure and does not permit the patient to assume any form of athletic competition. However, the horse might be useful for breeding.

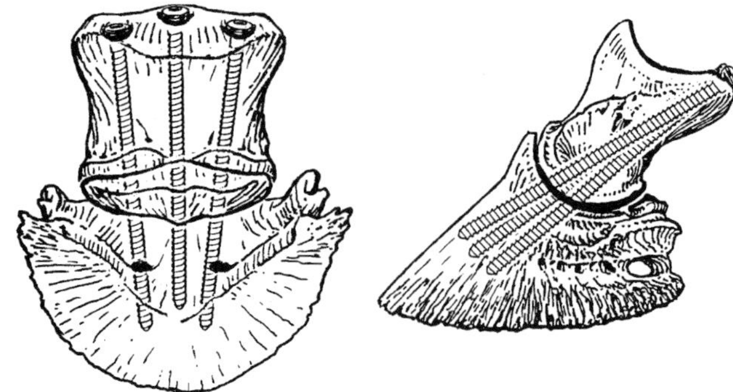

Figure 85-1. Graphic illustration of an arthrodesis of the DIP joint using three parallel 5.5-mm cortex screws placed between the proximal and palmar aspect of the middle phalanx and the distal phalanx.

Surgical Techniques

For this arthrodesis, two surgical approaches are necessary.[12] Through a *dorsal approach* to the DIP joint, as much articular cartilage as possible is removed and the implants are inserted through a palmar approach to the proximal and palmar aspect of the middle phalanx. An 8-cm semi-circumferential horizontal skin incision is made 1 cm proximal and parallel to the coronary band, centered over the midline of the foot. The incision is extended through the common digital extensor tendon into the dorsal pouch of the DIP joint. The incision is extended through the joint capsule and the collateral ligaments until the joint can be subluxated. Approximately 70% of the articular cartilage can be removed with a curet through this approach, but the distal sesamoid bone and the palmar aspect of the middle phalanx cannot be accessed for cartilage removal.

The *palmar approach* involves an 8-cm skin incision parallel to the long axis of the limb in the median plane centered over the proximal interphalangeal (PIP) joint. The incision is extended into the digital tendon sheath, where the deep digital flexor tendon is transected and reflected. Three stab incisions through the distal sesamoidean ligament provide access to the proximal palmar rim of the middle phalanx.

While maintaining the DIP joint in reduction, the first thread hole is prepared under fluoroscopic control across the middle phalanx in a distodorsal direction into the distal phalanx. The thread hole across the middle phalanx is enlarged to a glide hole, with the joint opened to prevent inadvertent enlargement of part of the thread hole in the distal phalanx. Then two more glide holes across the middle phalanx are made parallel to the first one. The center hole is finished using routine lag screw technique, and a 5.5-mm cortex screw of correct length is inserted and solidly tightened. Care should be taken to make sure that the screw does not impinge on the blind end of the thread hole, because this would prevent effective compression of the joint surface. The other two 5.5-mm cortex screws are implanted using routine technique (Fig. 85-1). If a cancellous bone graft or an alternate osteoinductive material (see Chapter 82) is used, the screws may be loosened temporarily so that the material can be placed through the dorsal aspect of the joint.

The dorsal incision is closed in three layers: extensor tendon and joint capsule, subcutaneous tissue, and skin. Although an attempt should be made to suture the ends of the deep digital flexor tendon with interrupted sutures of no. 0 polydioxanone, the tendon ends often retract, making accurate anatomic reconstruction impossible. The palmar incision is closed in two layers: tendon sheath and subcutaneous tissues in one layer followed by closure of the skin layer. The limb is placed into a half-limb cast for 3 months, ideally with only one cast change. Routine anti-inflammatory therapy and antibiotic prophylaxis are used.

In one horse that suffered from nonresponsive progressive arthritis of the DIP joint, this technique resulted in sold fusion. The horse was able to ambulate with a mechanical lameness but was pain free for more than a year.[12]

PROXIMAL INTERPHALANGEAL JOINT ARTHRODESIS

Indications

Indications for arthrodesis of the PIP joint include osteoarthritis (high ring-bone),[13,14] comminuted fractures of the proximal or middle phalanx,[5,15] and luxation or subluxation of the PIP joint.[5] Fractures entering the PIP joint through either the proximal or the middle phalanx often result in osteoarthritis or subluxation.

Because of the low-motion and high-load nature of this joint and the lack of interdigitation, attempts to manage the majority of common conditions of the PIP joint by methods other than arthrodesis usually fail to provide long-term success. Therefore, arthrodesis is often performed as part of the definitive treatment of the fracture. In comminuted fractures of the proximal phalanx, the middle phalanx serves as the distal fragment, achieving additional stability for the fixation. Conversely, the proximal phalanx can serve as the proximal fragment in comminuted middle phalanx fractures.

Recent Developments

Over the years, a variety of techniques have been advocated for PIP joint arthrodesis.[16-19] The technique most often applied since the 1980s used three transarticular cortex screws placed in lag fashion in a parallel or diverging pattern.[16-18]

This technique has several disadvantages.[20] The almost linear alignment of the screws in the frontal plane provide minimal stability, especially at the dorsal aspect of the joint. This has resulted in patient discomfort because of excessive new bone formation that has impinged on the extensor tendon or the coffin joint, or both. The screw tip can protrude at the middle aspect of the palmar or plantar cortex of the middle phalanx, which can interfere with the dynamics of the distal sesamoid bone. The bone can fail at the dorsal aspect of the proximal phalanx distal to the glide holes because of the acute angle at which the screws are inserted. The period of external coaptation is prolonged: 6 to 8 weeks postoperatively in cast, which is advocated by most surgeons. Therefore, new techniques were needed and have been developed.

A recent in vitro study compared interfragmentary cortex screws applied in lag fashion in fore- and hindlimbs[21]; three parallel 4.5-mm cortex screws were compared to two parallel 5.5-mm cortex screws in three-point bending to failure. The bending moments were greater in the forelimbs than in the hindlimbs. The difference between the two techniques was not statistically significant. However, more 4.5-mm cortex screws failed than 5.5-mm.

An arthrodesis technique using an axial plate in conjunction with two abaxial transarticular lag screws was also tested in vitro.[22,23] A substantial increase in stability across the dorsal aspect of the PIP joint was recorded in addition to a significantly longer fatigue life compared to the method using three transarticular screws. Clinical results gained on horses suffering from osteoarthritis, subluxations, and some stable middle phalanx fractures confirmed the in vitro results.[24] Postoperatively, the patients were more comfortable on the limb and the cast was removed earlier compared to patients treated with the three parallel 5.5-mm cortex screws. No difference was found in the number of horses returning to soundness. Based on these studies, the author recommends the plate technique.

Surgical Techniques

Preparation

The joint is approached through an inverted-T skin incision that begins just distal to the level of the metacarpophalangeal (MCP) or the metatarsophalangeal (MTP) joint and ends at a horizontal skin incision made 1.5 cm proximal to the coronary band. The horizontal incision extends 4 cm on either side of the midline. The subcutaneous tissue is separated sharply down to the common digital extensor tendon. The two triangular skin flaps are dissected free from the common digital extensor tendon with the help of scissors and sutured to the intact skin on either side of the incision.

The common digital extensor tendon is transected with an inverted V-shaped tenotomy at the level of the insertion of the extensor branches of the suspensory apparatus[17] (Fig. 85-2). The proximal tendon stump is reflected proximally using scissors, taking care to spare the attachments of the extensor branches of the suspensory ligament. The distal tendon stump is sharply incised along its lateral and medial sides and reflected distally, exposing the PIP joint.

The dorsal attachments of the PIP joint capsule are sharply incised parallel to the joint surface, the collateral ligaments are transected, and the joint is disarticulated. As much cartilage as possible is removed from both articular surfaces with a curet. By removing the articular cartilage layers, the radii of the two opposing bones are altered

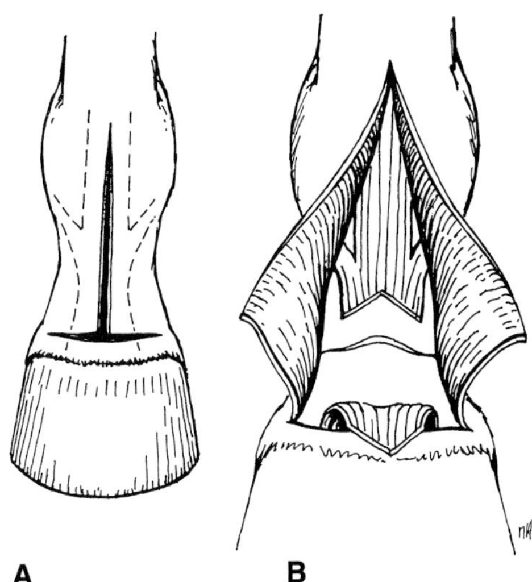

Figure 85-2. **A**, The surgical approach for arthrodesis of the proximal interphalangeal joint involves an inverted T skin incision with the horizontal portion located 1 cm proximal to the coronary band. A sagittal vertical incision is extended to the level of the metacarpophalangeal joint. **B**, An inverted V tenotomy of the common digital extensor tendon, just distal to the insertion of the extensor branches of the suspensory ligament, allows access to the joint.

Fig. 85-3, *A*); the radius of the proximal phalanx is reduced, whereas that of the middle phalanx is increased. This results in reduced contact between opposing bones (see Fig. 85-3, *B*). By rasping the subchondral bone of the distal articular surface of the proximal phalanx, the contact area can be increased (see Fig. 85-3, *C*).

The use of a 2.5-, 3.2-, or 4.5-mm drill bit between the two articular surfaces to remove part of the cartilage is discouraged because it results in partial bone loss, asymmetry, and decreased contact surface. As a direct result, stability of the arthrodesis is reduced and the implants are subjected to excessive cycling stress, eventually leading to implant failure.

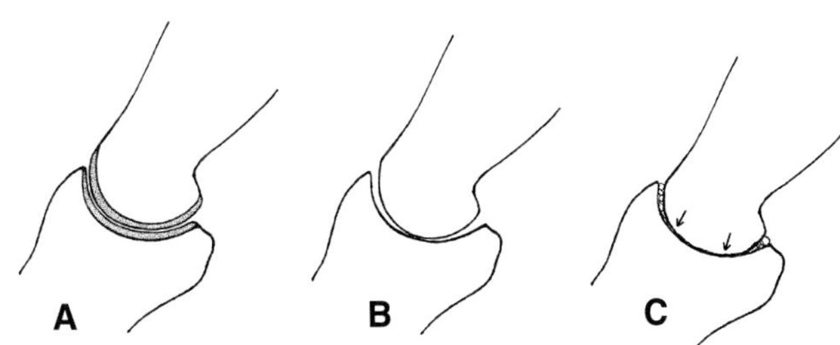

Figure 85-3. **A**, The articular cartilage covering the two opposing bones normally allows congruency of the surfaces during joint loading and maximum contact surface. **B**, Removal of the articular cartilage from the bone ends results in an incongruity between the two surfaces. Insertion of three lag screws after this type of preparation results in an inadequate fixation because of cyclic screw failure. **C**, Rasping of the distal subchondral surface of the proximal phalanx (between the two *arrows*) substantially enlarges the contact surface. Cancellous bone may be placed between the two bone ends.

Arthrodesis

The preferred technique for arthrodesis of the proximal interphalangeal joint involves the application of a three-hole narrow limited-contact dynamic compression plate (LC-DCP) in conjunction with two additional transarticular cortex screws[11] (Fig. 85-4). The plate is temporarily placed axially over the joint, with the single hole positioned at the proximal and dorsal aspect of the middle phalanx. This permits the size of the screw heads to be taken into account while the location of the two holes for the transarticular lag screws are marked on the distal aspect of the proximal phalanx.

With the joint opened, drilling of the 5.5-mm glide hole for the first lag screw is started perpendicular to the bone surface, followed by a gradual redirection of the drill to the desired oblique orientation. Because the middle phalanx is wider than the proximal phalanx, the drill holes are prepared in slightly diverging directions. Drilling is continued until the drill bit enters the joint to ensure lag effect without drilling into the palmar and proximal aspect of the middle phalanx. The hole should enter the joint midway between the dorsal and palmar or plantar cortices. The same procedure is repeated on the other side for the second lag screw. The 3.2-mm drill bit, protected by the corresponding drill guide, is used to prepare several osteostixis holes across the subchondral bone plate of the middle and proximal phalanx. By waiting with this procedure until the two glide holes have been prepared, the osteostixis holes can be placed so that they do not interfere with the glide holes.

With the joint remaining open and using the 4.0-mm drill bit placed through the neutral drill guide, a thread hole is prepared parallel to the joint surface in the proximal aspect of the middle phalanx for placement of the distal plate screw. By positioning the plate proximally, interference between the extensor process of the distal phalanx and the distal end of the plate is prevented. Additionally, the risk of inadvertent injury to the distal sesamoid bone at the palmar or plantar aspect of the middle phalanx is reduced. A 5.5-mm cortex screw of correct length is inserted through the distal single hole in the plate and into the middle phalanx, but it is only partially tightened. The joint is closed to its normal anatomic position.

The countersink is used to prepare depressions in the bone for the heads of the lag screws. Care is taken to work predominantly on the proximal rim. The plate is displaced proximally, and with the help of the load drill guide the thread hole is drilled through the middle plate hole perpendicular to the long axis of the proximal phalanx. The selected 5.5-mm cortex screw is inserted but not fully tightened. The thread hole for one of the lag screws is finished and the screw is inserted and tightened. The second screw is implanted in the same manner. The two plate screws are now tightened as well, bringing about transarticular compression. Finally, the most proximal screw is inserted in the neutral position parallel to the center screw. Only the dorsal cortex of the proximal phalanx is used for this screw (Fig. 85-5).

This technique has a biomechanical advantage over a single plate: it provides compression across the entire joint because the tensile forces, which develop at the palmar aspect of the joint and are caused by the plate, are neutralized by the two oblique transarticular lag screws. It has a similar advantage over the three-screw technique because the dorsal joint instability seen with that technique is obviated by the plate.

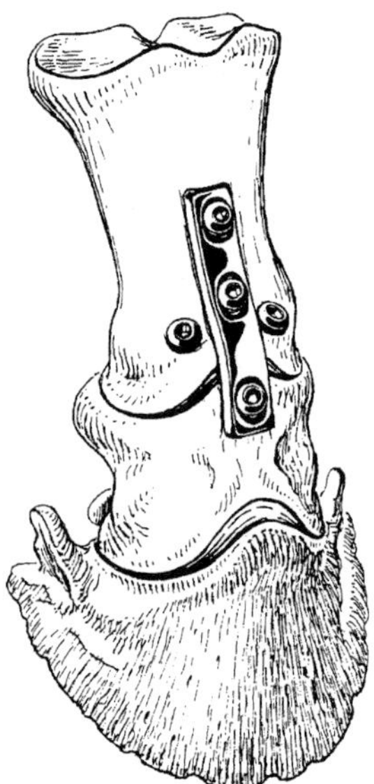

Figure 85-4. Graphic illustration of an arthrodesis of the proximal interphalangeal joint using a 3-hole narrow dynamic compression plate (DCP) and one 5.5-mm cortex screw applied in lag fashion across the joint on either side of the plate. The plate is applied axially over the dorsal aspect of the joint with the most distal screw inserted into the proximal aspect of the middle phalanx.

Closure and Aftercare

Closure of the V plasty of the tendon is accomplished with no. 1 polydioxanone suture using a simple continuous pattern, and the skin is apposed using a combination of no. 0 polypropylene (Prolene) and skin staples. A standard distal limb cast is applied for the immediate postoperative period to protect the fixation during recovery and, most importantly, to support healing of the soft tissues. The cast is removed at about 2 weeks, and every other skin suture is taken out at that time, with the patient standing. The limb is protected with a bandage, and the remaining sutures are removed at the next bandage change. The horse is discharged from the clinic about 3 weeks postoperatively. Owners are advised to limit exercise to hand-walking for the next 3 months.

Discussion

When treating fractures of the middle or proximal phalanx with an arthrodesis technique, it may be advisable to apply two plates, one dorsomedially and one dorsolaterally, once the bone has been reconstructed with strategically placed lag screws[16,19] (Fig. 85-6). Care is taken to prevent interference of the interfragmentary lag screw heads with the plates. Therefore, 3.5-mm cortex screws are often used because they permit the screw heads to be buried within the cortex

A biomechanical in vitro study compared two seven-hole, 3.5-mm broad DCPs with two five-hole 4.5-mm narrow DCPs. The DCPs were placed dorsomedially and dorsolaterally, respectively. No significant difference was detected

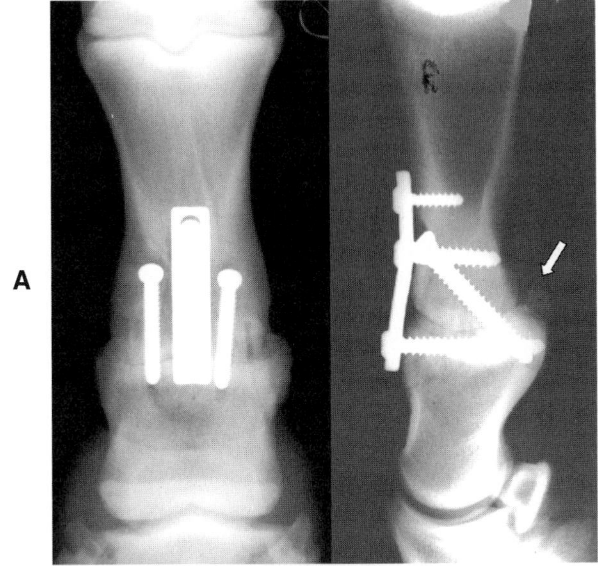

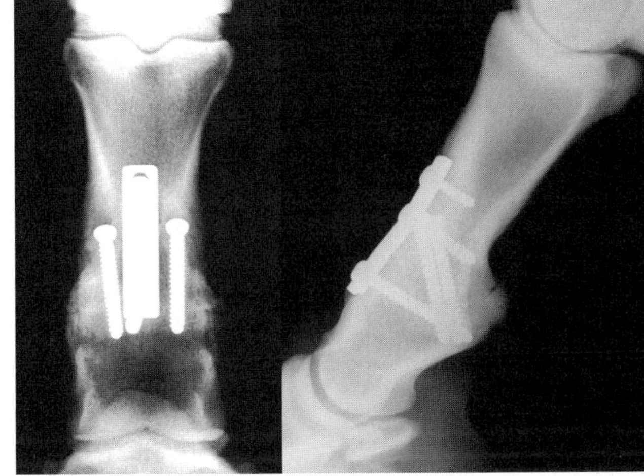

Figure 85-5. **A,** Immediate postoperative dorsopalmar and lateromedial radiographs of a PIP joint arthrodesis in a 2-year-old Thoroughbred filly with a proximal palmar fracture of the middle phalanx. The arthrodesis was accomplished with a three-hole narrow DCP and two 5.5-mm cortex screws. The plate used two loaded bicortical 5.5-mm screws and a single unicortical 4.5-mm screw in the proximal hole. The two transarticular 5.5-mm cortex screws were inserted in lag fashion to provide plantar compression. The *arrow* points to the palmar fragment of the middle phalanx. Note the slightly radiolucent osteostixis holes in the distal aspect of the proximal phalanx. **B,** The 11-month follow-up dorsopalmar and lateromedial radiographs show complete fusion of the joint, with negligible periarticular new bone formation. (Courtesy J. Watkins, Texas A&M University.)

either in composite stiffness or maximal bending moment between the two fixation techniques.[25] Therefore, either plate size could be used for arthrodesis of the PIP after fractures to the pastern.

The closure of soft tissues after this technique involves a simple continuous suture of the tenotomy incision along the reflected tendon stumps, and an additional simple continuous pattern of 2-0 or 3-0 absorbable monofilament suture material placed subcutaneously, intradermally, or both, followed by skin closure. A cast is applied after all

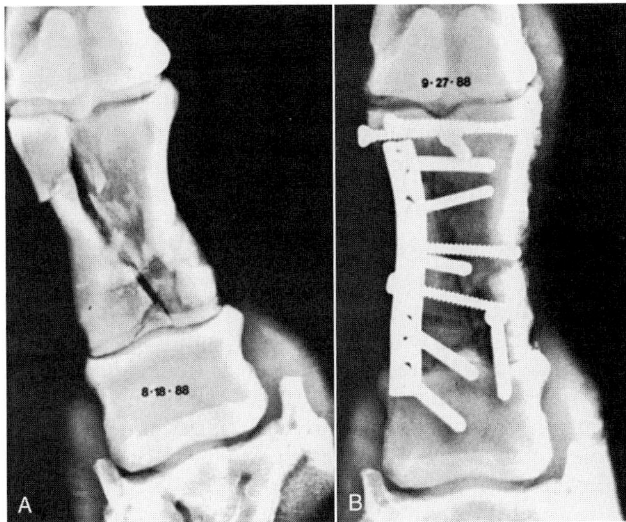

Figure 85-6. **A,** Dorsopalmar radiograph of a comminuted proximal phalanx fracture. **B,** The fracture has been repaired with several lag screws and a six-hole narrow DCP as a neutralization plate. To gain stability and to prevent osteoarthritis in the proximal interphalangeal joint, an arthrodesis was performed. Two cortex screws were placed transarticularly in lag fashion. A second plate could have been applied to the dorsomedial aspect of the proximal and middle phalanx for even greater stability. In this case, six 5.5-mm and five 4.5-mm screws were used.

arthrodeses for the initial postoperative period. When a cast is used after fracture reconstruction, the time period will vary depending on stability of the repair and healing.

Long-term follow-up results after arthrodeses of the proximal interphalangeal joint from one study reported success rates of 67% and 80% in the forelimbs and hindlimbs, respectively.[20,24] Another retrospective study on 39 proximal interphalangeal joint arthrodeses performed using two parallel 5.5-mm cortex screws applied in lag fashion on 34 horses revealed a success rate of 85% in the forelimbs and 89% in hindlimbs.[26] The increased bending moment recorded in the front limbs compared to the rear limbs by Watt and colleagues[21] could explain the clinical observation that hindlimb arthrodeses have a better prognosis for return to soundness.

METACARPOPHALANGEAL OR METATARSOPHALANGEAL JOINT ARTHRODESIS

Indications

MCP or MTP joint arthrodesis is performed for breakdown injuries of the suspensory apparatus. This injury occurs almost exclusively in the forelimbs of Thoroughbred racehorses, although it can be suffered by any horse running at high speed.[3,5,27] Fatigue of the digital check ligaments and flexor muscles supporting the fetlock and digit leads to higher stresses in all components of the suspensory apparatus and permits development of the injury. Comminuted proximal phalanx fractures,[9] advanced osteoarthritis, and severe flexural deformities of that region represent other indications for the arthrodesis.[5] In flexural deformities, an osteotomy might be needed to achieve an acceptable joint angle before arthrodesis.

The major physical finding is dorsiflexion or hyperextension (dropping) of the fetlock joint as the horse attempts to bear weight. Many horses become anxious or even frantic as they attempt to control the injured limb. The disruption can occur as a result of fracture of both proximal sesamoid bones in the injured limb or, less often, rupture of the distal sesamoidean ligaments of the two suspensory ligament branches.

Breakdown of the suspensory apparatus should always be considered a career-ending injury. Because of the massive trauma that occurs with this injury, a myriad of complications is expected. It is therefore important to explain the situation to the owner so that an informed decision can be made concerning treatment. Most horses can be saved as pasture-sound or breeding animals, but treatment is often prolonged and expensive, despite the therapeutic approach selected.

Surgical Techniques

Dorsal Plate Technique

The most frequently applied technique for MCP or MTP arthrodesis involves implanting a dorsal plate and creating a tension band on the palmar aspect[27] (Fig. 85-7). Dorsal plating without a tension band on the palmar aspect of the fetlock usually results in failure, because the plate cycles in bending on the joint's dorsal surface and eventually breaks. The different techniques used to create the tension band depend on the type of breakdown injury.

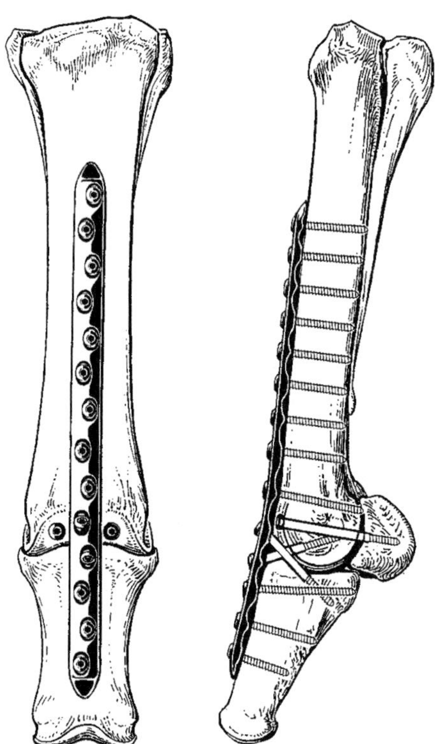

Figure 85-7. Graphic illustration of an arthrodesis of the metacarpophalangeal joint using a dorsally applied 14-hole 5.5 LC-DCP. Two cortex screws are implanted transarticularly, and an additional cortex screw is inserted from the dorsal aspect of the MCIII into each proximal sesamoid bone. An additional cortex screw on either side of the plate may be implanted transarticularly from the proximodorsal aspect of the proximal phalanx into the palmar or plantar aspect of the MCIII with disruption of the suspensory ligament proximal to the sesamoid bones. Both ends of the plate are tapered to reduce the risk of skin perforation under the cast, especially at the proximal end.

A straight skin incision is made between the common and lateral digital extensor tendon, extending from the proximal aspect of the third metacarpus or third metatarsus (MCIII or MTIII) to the proximal interphalangeal joint. The incision is carried through the periosteum.

A 5-cm sagittal strip of the proximal phalanx is denuded of periosteum. The joint capsule of the MCP or MTP joint is transected parallel to the articular surface. Transection of the lateral collateral ligament, as well as the lateral metacarposesamoidean or metatarsosesamoidean ligament, allows disarticulation of the joint and removal of all articular cartilage from the proximal phalanx, the distal MCIII or MTIII, and the proximal sesamoid bones.

The cartilage is removed with a curette, and multiple osteostixis holes are drilled across the subchondral bone plates of all of the bones. With an osteotome, the proximal dorsal end of the proximal phalanx and the intermediate ridge of the distal MCIII or MTIII are contoured to accept a 14-hole, 5.5 LC-DCP (see Fig. 81-17), which is slightly bent at an angle of about 8 to 10 degrees. Because compression can be applied on either side of all plate holes of the LC-DCP (dynamic compression unit [DCU] architecture), placement of the plate is not critical. The plate is applied with the three or four most distal screws inserted in neutral position into the proximal phalanx. The hole adjacent to the joint should at this point be left without a screw.

With an intact suspensory apparatus, one 5.5-mm cortex screw is placed in lag fashion from the dorsal aspect of the distal MCIII or MTIII into each proximal sesamoid bone. For that procedure, the joint is maintained in a slightly flexed position. Using the tension device, the plate is tightened across the joint, and two screws are inserted in a neutral position through proximal plate holes into the MCIII or MTIII. Forcing the MCP or MTP joint into a slightly extended position tightens the distal sesamoidean ligament, which accepts the tension band function and protects the dorsally applied plate.

The tension device is removed, and the remaining plate holes are filled with screws except the two screws immediately adjacent to the joint. These screws are implanted transarticularly in lag fashion. Care must be taken to direct the screws so that they do not interfere with each other. Additionally, one cortex screw may be inserted from the proximal phalanx in a proximal palmar or plantar direction into the MCIII or MTIII medial and lateral to the plate.

With comminuted proximal sesamoidean fractures, insertion of screws into the proximal sesamoid bones is not possible. Also, in cases where the distal sesamoidean ligaments are ruptured, inserting the lag screws into the proximal sesamoid bone does not produce a tension band across the palmar or plantar joint surface. In such cases, a double strand of 1.5-mm diameter cerclage wire is placed in figure-eight fashion across the palmar or plantar aspect of the joint. A 3.2-mm hole is drilled in a frontal plane parallel to the joint surface at about 4 to 6 cm proximal and distal to the joint surface across the MCIII or MTIII and the proximal phalanx, respectively.

The wire is guided through these holes and directed toward the palmar or plantar joint surface with the help of the large wire passer (Synthes Inc, Solothurn, Switzerland). The wires are passed around the suspensory apparatus in a figure-eight pattern such that the two wires can be twisted together into one unit. Wires are tightened with the joint maintained in slightly flexed position. One set of wire ends is tightened on the lateral side of the MCIII or MTIII and the other set on the medial side of the bone. Prior to final tightening, all the slack has to be taken out of the wire to ensure the development of an effective tension band function. The remainder of the procedure is identical to the one described earlier.

A 16-hole 5.5 LC-DCP may be used to treat a severely comminuted proximal phalangeal fracture when an arthrodesis of the MCP or MTP joint and the PIP joint is desired (Fig. 85-8).

Dynamic Hip Screw Plate Technique

An alternative technique involves application of a dynamic hip screw (DHS) plate[5,28] (Fig. 85-9). Plate application is identical to the dynamic condylar screw (DCS) plate application described in Chapter 81. The lateral aspect of the MCP or MTP joint is prepared for plate application. The palmarolateral or plantarolateral aspect of the distal condyle is removed with an osteotome or an oscillating saw. A 2.5-mm hole is drilled from the level of the MCP or MTP joint into the proximal phalanx after aligning the joint at the desired angle. A drill guide with the preset screw angle facilitates placement of the drill hole. Correctness of the drill hole is monitored by intraoperative radiographs or the use of a fluoroscope.

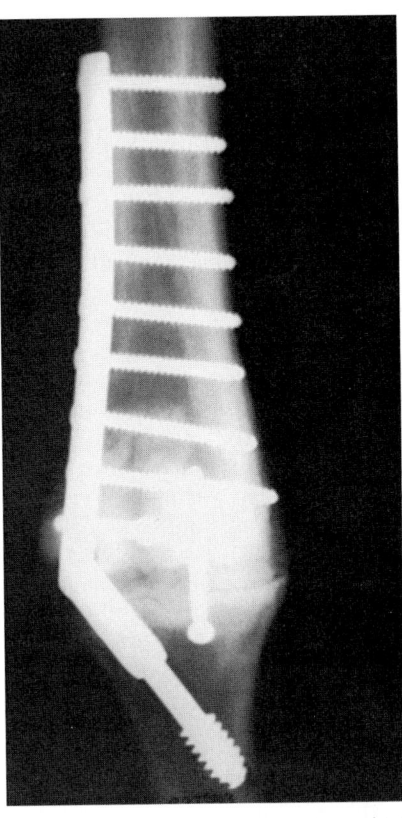

Figure 85-9. Arthrodesis of the metacarpophalangeal joint using the DHS implant system. The large distally oriented screw, which is fed through the barrel of the plate, provides the major amount of stability. An additional screw is placed transarticularly in lag fashion, and one additional screw is placed into each proximal sesamoid bone.

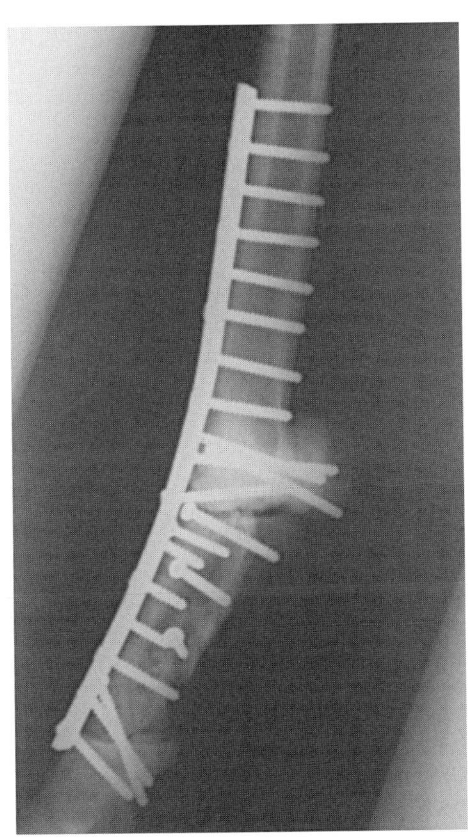

Figure 85-8. Radiograph of a comminuted proximal phalanx fracture repaired with an 18-hole DCP. The plate was applied to the dorsal aspect and spanned the proximal interphalangeal and metacarpophalangeal joint. This repair is used as a salvage procedure.

When the position is correct, the 2.5-mm guide pin is introduced into the predrilled hole and seated in the opposite cortex. The guide pin has an inadequate cutting edge and is incapable of self-cutting, so a 2.5-mm drill bit is used to create its hole through dense equine bone. The length of the screw to be inserted is determined using the measuring device, and with the triple reamer for the DHS plate set at the correct distance (5 mm shorter than the pin length as measured to be located in the bone), the shaft and the barrel hole are prepared.

Using the tap placed over the guide pin, the threads for the lag DHS screw are cut. Care is taken to engage the opposite cortex; otherwise adequate stability will not be achieved. The plate is placed over the screw shaft and aligned along the axis of the bone. The connecting screw is subsequently inserted and tightened, followed by the insertion of the 5.5-mm-diameter cortex bone screws into the MCIII or MTIII. Two additional transarticular cortex screws are placed from the proximal aspect of the proximal phalanx in a proximopalmar or proximoplantar direction into the MCIII or MTIII using lag technique. Additionally, cortex screws may be inserted in lag fashion into the proximal sesamoids if the injury allows application. Alternatively, a tension band wire as described earlier may be applied prior to plate application in cases where no natural tension band can be established along the palmar or plantar joint surface. The subcutaneous tissues and skin are closed using routine technique. Application of a cast for 3 to 4 weeks is indicated.

Other Techniques

An arthrodesis technique using a prototype of an intramedullary pin plate (IMPP) has been compared in vitro with a dorsal DCP technique.[29] The study revealed a significantly greater mean yield load, yield stiffness, and failure load (axial compression, torsional loading) of the IMPP compared with the DCP system. Mean cycles to failure for axial compression was significantly greater for the IMPP compared with the DCP system. The IMPP was superior to the DCP system in resisting the biomechanical forces most likely to cause failure of MCP joint arthrodesis. Therefore, the IMPP implant might represent an interesting alternative for MCP arthrodesis in horses with traumatic disruption of the suspensory apparatus in the future.

Description of the modified Cloward technique for MCP/MTP arthrodesis has been proposed, but it has not been pursued lately. This approach, however, does not represent an improvement over the techniques described here.

CARPAL ARTHRODESIS

Indications

In the carpal region, two types of arthrodeses are performed: the pancarpal arthrodesis, where all the joints in the carpus are fused,[30] and the subtotal or partial arthrodesis involving only one or two of the joints.[31] Carpal arthrodeses are indicated for treatment of comminuted carpal fractures as well as luxations and subluxations of this region. In most animals, these operations should be viewed as salvage procedures, with the exception of animals with carpometacarpal luxations. Partial carpal arthrodeses are recommended in cases in which the distal row of carpal bones has comminuted fractures and accurate anatomic reconstruction is impossible or in luxations of the carpometacarpal and the middle carpal joints.

Surgical Techniques

Partial Carpal Arthrodesis

Depending on the injury, partial carpal arthrodesis involves either fixing the proximal row of carpal bones to the distal row and MCIII or fixing the distal row of carpal bones to the MCIII (Fig. 85-10). Additionally, partial carpal arthrodesis can be used for antebrachiocarpal luxations, where the proximal row of carpal bones is fastened to the distal radial epiphysis or metaphysis. For these arthrodesis techniques, a variety of plates may be used. Selection depends on availability of the plates and preference of the surgeon. The surgical incision is made in the region in which the plate

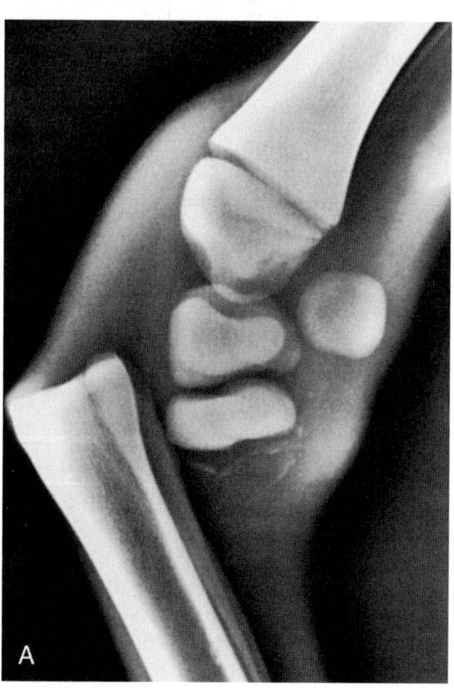

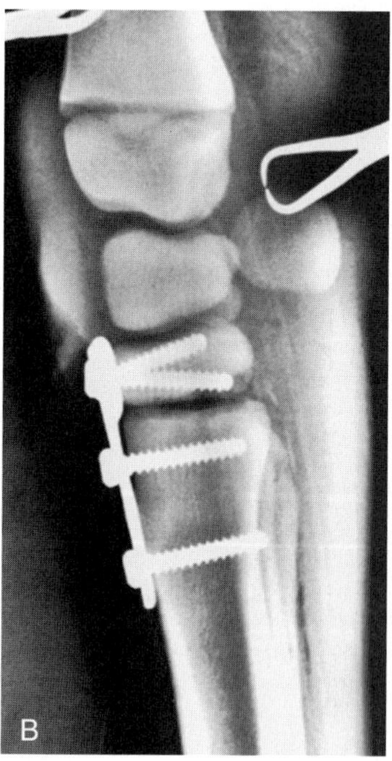

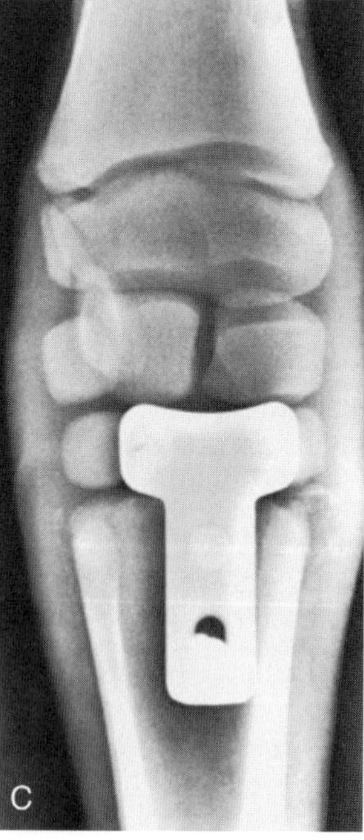

Figure 85-10. A, Lateromedial radiograph of a carpometacarpal luxation in a 2-week-old foal. Lateromedial (**B**) and dorsopalmar (**C**) radiographs of the repair depicting a 2-hole T-plate applied to the dorsal aspect of the distal row of carpal bones and the proximal aspect of MCIII. (From Auer JA, Taylor JR, Watkins JP, et al: Vet Comp Orthop Traumatol 1990;3:51.)

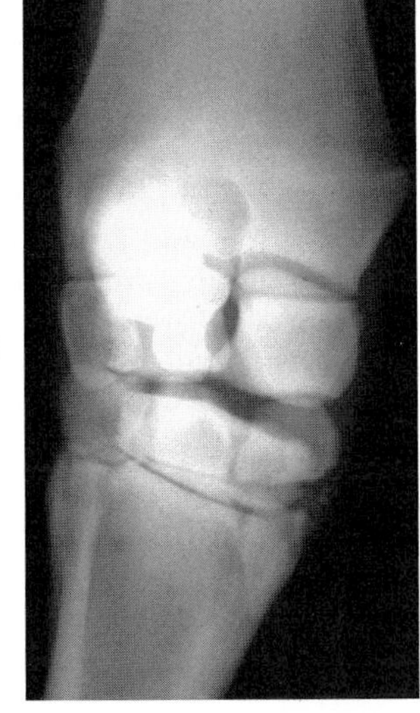

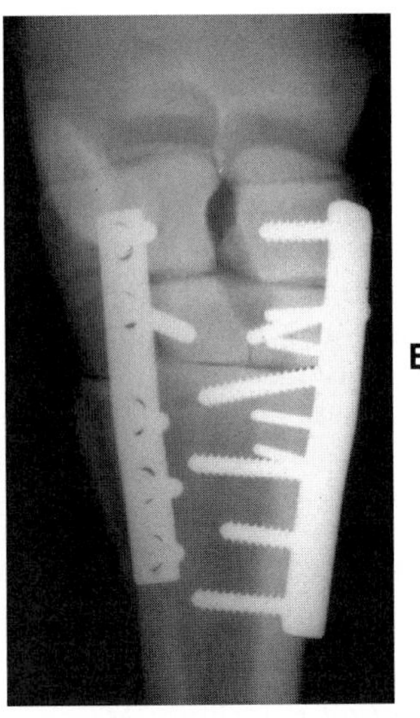

Figure 85-11. **A,** Dorsopalmar radiographic view of subluxation of the middle carpal joint in a 6-year-old brood mare. Note the avulsion fracture at the medial aspect of the carpometacarpal joint. The 2nd carpal bone is also partially luxated. **B,** Postoperative dorsopalmar radiographic view showing a broad six-hole 4.5 DCP applied to dorsomedial aspect and a narrow five-hole 4.5 DCP applied to the dorsal aspect of the carpal region to achieve a partial carpal arthrodesis.

will be applied. General surgical and specific anatomic considerations guide the surgeon in selecting the proper approach.[18]

Whenever possible, articular cartilage should be removed to allow fusion of the joint surfaces. Performance of osteostixis as well as a cancellous bone graft, tricalcium phosphate granules, or high molecular weight gel inserted into the joint are indicated to facilitate fusion. In comminuted carpal bone fractures, strategically placed interfragmentary screws inserted in lag fashion contribute considerably to stability of the joint. In most cases, it is prudent to maintain alignment by applying one or two bone plates across the joint involved. The same holds true for selected subluxations with signs of avulsion fractures and displacement of specific bones (Fig. 85-11).

In a mare with severely comminuted fractures, all the fragments of the distal row of carpal bones were removed, with subsequent fixation of the proximal row of carpal bones to the MCIII.[26] After 3 months in a tube cast, the mare developed fusion in the arthrodesis site and served for several years as a successful brood mare.[31]

Pancarpal Arthrodesis

Pancarpal arthrodesis using two long, broad DCPs or leg-lengthening plates is advocated for comminuted fractures involving both rows of carpal bones[29] (Fig. 85-12) and for severe degenerative carpal joint disease in older horses that develop carpus valgus. The 5.5 LC-DCP, DHS, or DCS plates are excellent alternatives to these implants, because they are stronger. Simple cast application is not effective in these cases.[29]

In severely comminuted fractures, the purpose of the plates is to buttress the unstable limb and maintain a straight axis. In these cases, the leg-lengthening plates may be superior to the routine LC-DCPs, because they do not contain holes in the middle portion. Occasionally a plate hole must be left open in severely comminuted fractures because the size of the underlying fragment may be inadequate to accept a screw. These plate holes are a site of decreased strength and can doom the repair to failure.

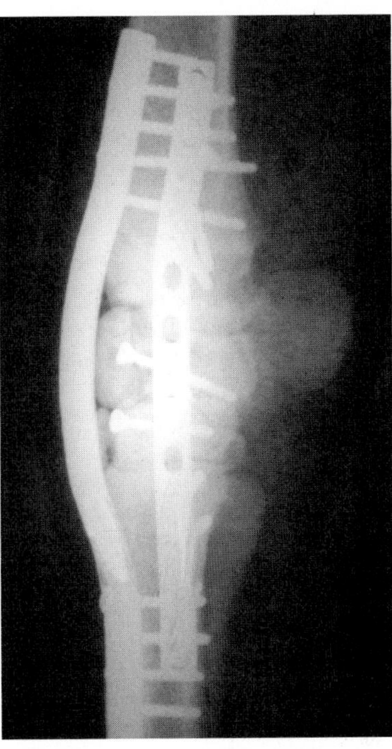

Figure 85-12. Lateromedial radiograph depicting pancarpal arthrodesis used to repair a comminuted carpal fracture. A 12-hole broad DCP bone-lengthening plate (Synthes, Inc, Paoli, Pa) was applied to the dorsal/cranial aspect of the limb, and a narrow 12-hole DCP was applied laterally. Cortex screws were used to provide interfragmentary compression across slab fractures.

Plate luting[32] is indicated in pancarpal arthrodeses (see Chapter 81). The plates might have to be inserted through two separate approaches, which, after application of the implants, are closed using routine techniques. Splints or casts may be necessary, depending on the injury that led to the partial or pancarpal arthrodeses.

SCAPULOHUMERAL JOINT ARTHRODESIS

Indications

Advanced osteoarthritis and persistent luxations and subluxations of the scapulohumeral (SH) joint in Shetland or Icelandic ponies may be treated by arthrodesis with the aim to render the animals free from painful lameness.[45] This technique is not well suited for horses, because the quality of bone in this region is inadequate to withstand the tremendous mechanical forces that would be exerted on the implants

Surgical Technique

A 10- or 11-hole, 4.5-mm narrow LC-DCP or DCP and 4.5-mm cortex screws are applied to the cranial surface of the scapula and cranial surface of the humerus after

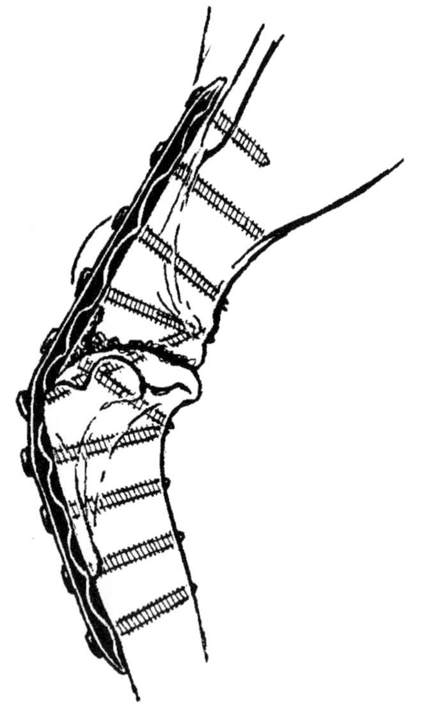

Figure 85-13. Graphic illustration of a scapulohumeral arthrodesis using a bone plate applied to the cranial aspect of the bones.

osteotomy of the intermediate tubercle (Fig. 85-13). A broad 3.5 LC-DCP or a reinforced 3.5 DCP are alternative implants. They have the same cross-sectional area as the narrow 4.5 DCP, but more screws can be inserted through these other plates, which provides a biomechanically superior fixation. In most horses, one or two plate holes over the joint should be filled with transarticular screws inserted in lag fashion.

A report of four miniature horses suffering from SH osteoarthritis, some with concurrent shoulder luxation or subluxation, described SH arthrodesis as a successful technique, despite some complications.[45] The animals developed a mechanical lameness but were able to ambulate well after surgery.

TARSAL ARTHRODESIS

Indications

The primary indication for tarsal arthrodesis is osteoarthritis (spavin) of the tarsometatarsal, distal, and possibly proximal intertarsal joints that is unresponsive to medical therapy.[2,33-36] Occasionally, luxations of the tarsus, especially involving the tarsometatarsal and distal intertarsal joints, necessitate arthrodesis. Talocalcaneal arthrodesis has been described as a promising treatment for talocalcaneal osteoarthritis.[37,38]

Distal Intertarsal Arthrodesis

Chemical Arthrodesis

Some time ago, chemical arthrodesis through intra-articular injection of 100 mg of monoiodoacetic acid (MIA) was introduced as a treatment for osteoarthritis of the tarsometatarsal and distal intertarsal joints.[39,40] Pronounced synovitis occurs for 12 to 24 hours after injection and is managed with sedation and analgesia with detomidine. Patients are pretreated with phenylbutazone before injection. MIA is injected three times at 10-day intervals. Joints fuse within 6 months; some residual lameness can persist.

The severe inflammation induced by MIA causes destruction of the articular cartilage, which is followed by bone union. Because of the reaction caused by the drug, it is essential that *only* the joints to be fused are injected. Occasionally, communication exists between the distal and proximal intertarsal joint, and the communication permits the drug to enter the tarsocrural joint with fatal consequences. Therefore, a positive contrast arthrogram of the joint or joints to be treated before MIA injection is strongly advised to assess ectopic communications. For additional information on this technique, see Chapter 99.

Surgical Techniques

The animal is positioned in lateral recumbency, providing access to the dorsomedial aspect of the tarsus involved. If the procedure is performed in both hindlimbs at the same time, the horse is positioned in dorsal recumbency. After routine preparation of the surgical site for aseptic surgery, a 10- to 15-cm straight skin incision is made, centered over the tarsometatarsal joint. The saphenous vein, which crosses the surgical field diagonally, is isolated and retracted. Placement of a Penrose drain around the vein facilitates its manipulation during the surgical procedure. The cunean tendon is dissected and approximately 5 cm of its length within the surgical field is removed. During preparation and resection, the cunean bursa is inevitably opened and partially destroyed. The tarsometatarsal and distal intertarsal joints are identified with hypodermic needles. Several techniques merit discussion.[36]

DRILLING TECHNIQUE

A 3.2- or 4.0-mm drill bit is passed into the joint space in three directions from a single entry point on the medial aspect of the hock, creating a fan-like pattern of holes extending dorsolaterally, laterally, and plantarolaterally for 2 to 3 cm[6] (Fig. 85-14). Frequent cleaning of the bit and use of a new bit for each horse is recommended to decrease the potential for bit breakage. The holes fill first with blood, then with fibrous tissue, and ultimately with bone, effectively bridging the joint in spot-weld fashion. This technique causes little pain and allows about 80% of the horses to return to soundness within 6 to 9 months.[34-36,39,40]

Drilling too deeply can penetrate the tarsal canal, resulting in unnecessary periosteal reaction or profuse hemorrhage from disruption of the perforating branch of the cranial tibial artery. Excessive drilling causes instability, severe pain, and prolonged recumbency and is associated with excessive periosteal new bone formation.[41] Most of the horses in which excessive drilling has been performed never regain complete soundness.[41]

Local cartilage destruction of these joints also has been achieved with the help of surgical lasers.[42] The results are similar to the drill hole technique. However, some experience is necessary because excessive cartilage destruction using the laser also leads to massive new bone formation and prolonged lameness.

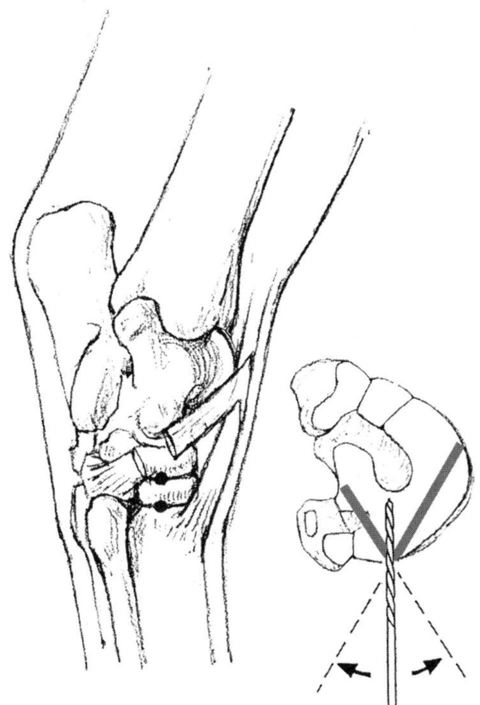

Figure 85-14. Graphic illustration of the drilling technique for tarsal arthrodesis. Three diverging drill holes are made along the articular surfaces of the distal tarsal joints after cunean tenectomy.

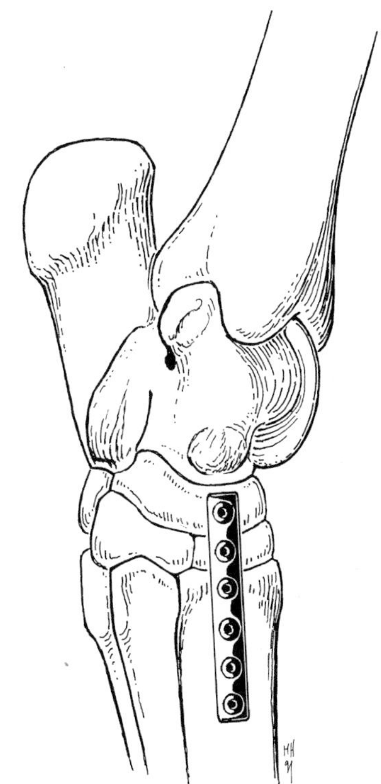

Figure 85-15. Graphic illustration of a tarsal arthrodesis with a six-hole narrow DCP applied medially. One screw penetrates both the central and third tarsal bones. The remaining screws are placed into proximal MTIII.

FIXATION TECHNIQUES

One technique consists of application of a narrow DCP over the medial aspect of the tarsal region (Fig. 85-15). Fibrous covering of the dorsomedial aspects of the joints together with any exuberant exostoses are partially removed with an osteotome and mallet. This facilitates identification of the joint spaces involved, provides a greater plate–bone contact area, and allows less contouring of the plate. The proximal intertarsal joint space is identified through placement of two hypodermic needles or two 2-mm drill bits. Either a radiographic examination is conducted at that stage or the image intensifier is applied to verify correct location.

As an optional procedure, two drill holes 4.0 mm in diameter are prepared along each of the joints as previously described.[41] These holes may be filled with a bone graft plug harvested from the proximal tibia or the tuber coxae. Placement of such a plug, hydroxyapatite granules, or biodegradable bone cement will enhance osseous union of the two articulations by means of spot welds.

The desired five-hole narrow 4.5-mm DCP is applied to the arthrodesis site. The thread hole for the most proximal plate screw is drilled with the 4.0-mm drill bit protected by the corresponding drill guide within the body of the central tarsal bone, parallel to the joint surfaces. In smaller horses, 4.5-mm screws may be used instead of 5.5-mm. In that case, a 3.2-mm thread hole will be prepared. (It is important to use 5.5-mm cortex screws whenever possible, because they resist cyclic loading better than 4.5-mm screws. Screws 4.5 mm in diameter often fail in an adult horse.)

After tapping the thread hole, a 30- to 40-mm long cortex screw is inserted through the most proximal plate hole and tightened. Care is taken to avoid impacting the selected screw upon the dead-end hole. The tension device is applied subsequently at the distal end of the plate, secured to MTIII, and tightened. One or two plate screws are subsequently inserted into the third metatarsal bone. After the tension device is removed, the remaining plate holes are filled with screws. If the distal intertarsal and tarsometatarsal joints are to be fused, one screw is inserted into the central tarsal bone and one into the third tarsal bone (Fig. 85-16).

After flushing the surgical site, the subcutaneous tissues and the skin are closed in routine fashion. The surgical site is covered by a bandage.

Postoperatively, the limb is kept under a bandage for 2 to 3 weeks. The skin sutures or staples are removed 10 days after the surgery. Lameness can persist for several months. Rehabilitation must be conducted gradually over several months.

An alternative technique involves implantation of perforated stainless steel cylinders filled with autogenous cancellous bone in the distal tarsal joints.[43] This technique was applied in four horses. Graft cell survival was poor 2 weeks after surgery in one horse. In two horses at 10 months, there was partial arthrodesis of the joints with incorporation of the implants into the osseous union. The implants were filled with vascularized woven bone. These two horses were sound 9 months after surgery, but one horse fractured its third tarsal bone and was still positive to a hock flexion test 12 months after surgery.

A more involved technique that is occasionally used in tarsal luxations involves the application of a 12- to 14-hole

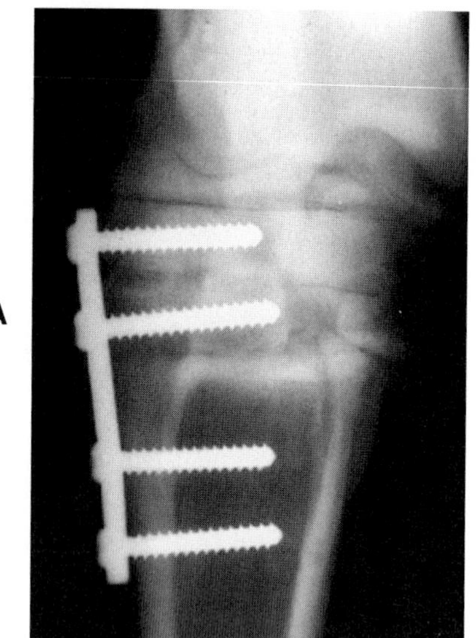

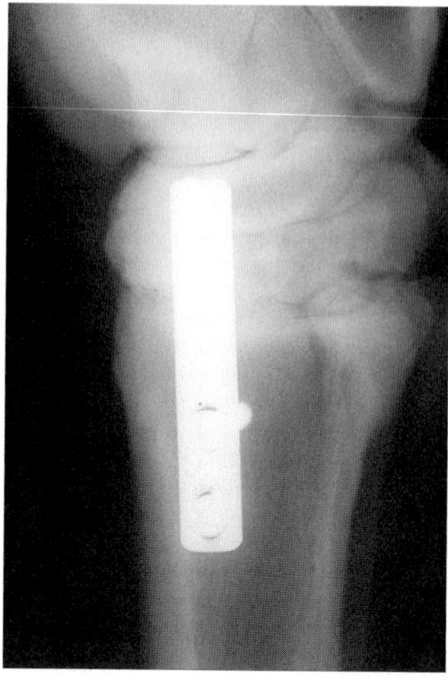

Figure 85-16. Dorsoplantar (**A**) and lateromedial (**B**) 4-week postoperative radiographic views of a tarsal arthrodesis using a four-hole narrow DCP in a 9-year-old Andalusian gelding. One 5.5-mm cortex screw is inserted into both the central and the third tarsal bones. Two identical screws are placed into the proximal MTIII. Note that the drill holes into the two distal joints are already filling in with new bone and becoming less obvious on these radiographs.

5.5 LC-DCP or broad DCP to the plantarolateral aspect of the calcaneus and proximal MT region (Fig. 85-17). This technique allows extension of the plate farther proximally, resulting in a stronger arthrodesis. In selected cases, MTIV is removed before plate application. However, care must be taken to avoid damage to the greater metatarsal artery coursing between MTIII and MTIV. The surgical approach is more extensive than that for the technique described earlier, and the surgery itself is more demanding. Care must be taken to avoid penetration of the tarsocrural joint with a screw. Selected screws can be placed in lag fashion across the more distally located joints, facilitating interfragmentary fixation.

Talocalcaneal Arthrodesis

For talocalcaneal arthrodesis,[37] the horse is placed under general anesthesia in lateral recumbency, with the affected limb positioned uppermost. Application of a tourniquet proximal to the tarsus is optional. A slightly curved incision is made over the distal half of the calcaneus, and the tissues are sharply divided down to the bone.

Needle markers are used to determine under fluoroscopic control the correct angulation of the future screws. Computer-assisted guidance greatly facilitates preparation of the drill holes (see Chapter 14). The drill bit is aimed toward the plantaromedial aspect of the medial trochlear ridge of the talus, avoiding penetration of the tarsocrural joint at the intertrochlear groove.

Two or three 5.5-mm cortex screws are inserted in lag fashion across the lateral facet, using routine technique

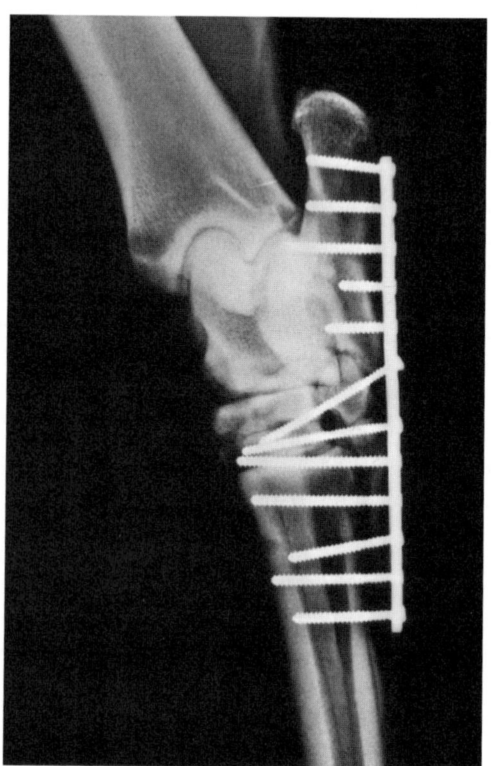

Figure 85-17. Oblique postoperative radiographic view of the tarsal region of a horse that suffered luxation of the proximal intertarsal joint. A 12-hole broad DCP was applied palmarolaterally to the calcaneus and proximal MT region. Some minor displacement is still present. (Courtesy J. P. Watkins, Texas A&M University.)

(Fig. 85-18). There is an adequate amount of solid bone present to achieve solid transarticular compression. By slightly altering the direction of the screws, an increased compressive effect can be achieved. To prevent weakening of the calcaneal bone, washers may be applied, which negate the need for countersinking.[37] Alternatively, the screws may be inserted through a plate contoured to the calcaneal surface. Once the screws are in place and solidly tightened, the incision is closed using routine technique.[37]

A slightly different technique was presented in another paper, where two clinical cases were also treated with 5.5-mm cortex screws applied in lag fashion. In a pony, three parallel screws were inserted through a dorsomedial arthrotomy to the talus across the medial facet into the calcaneus; in a horse, identical screws were augmented with two additional screws similarly inserted as described in the first technique.[38] Both techniques resulted in successful fusion.[6,44] Talocalacaneal arthrodesis could develop into an effective treatment for local talocalcaneal osteoarthritis. Early results are encouraging.

COMPLICATIONS

Complications include postoperative infection, implant failure, laminitis in the opposite limb, long-term lameness, and development of angular limb deformities. Accidental insertion of bone screws into a joint space can provide a continuous source of pain and should be avoided. This can be done by meticulous surgical technique and careful intraoperative radiographic control.

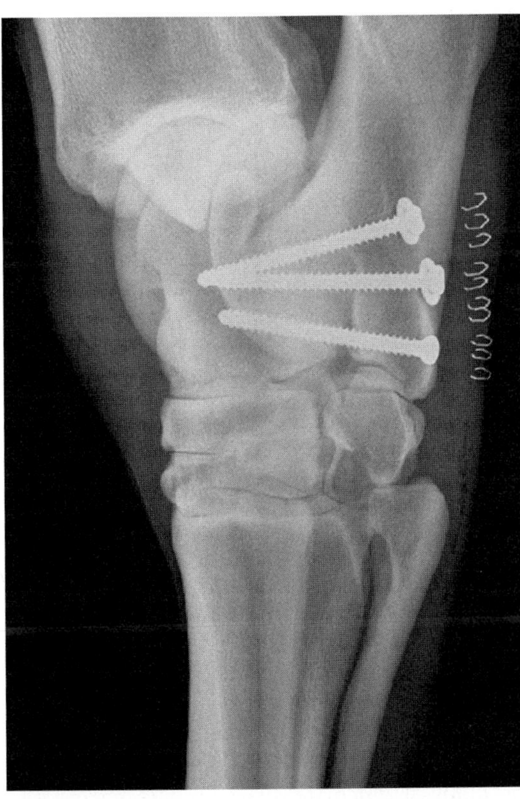

Figure 85-18. Oblique postoperative radiographic view of a talocalcaneal arthrodesis performed through three converging 5.5-mm cortex screws inserted in lag fashion across the lateral facet of the talocalcaneal joint. Washers were used in the two proximal screws to increase the contact area of the implants and reduce stress concentration at the bone–screw head junction. (Courtesy R. Smith, Royal Veterinary College, London.)

REFERENCES

1. Dorland's Illustrated Medical Dictionary, ed 30, Philadelphia, 2003, WB Saunders.
2. Adams OR: Surgical arthrodesis for treatment of bone spavin, J Am Vet Med Assoc 1970;157:1480.
3. Bramlage LR: Arthrodesis of the fetlock joint. In Mansmann RA, McAllister GS editors: Equine Medicine and Surgery, ed 3, Santa Barbara, CA, 1982, American Veterinary Publications.
4. Turner AS: Large animal orthopedic surgery. In Jennings P, editor: Textbook of Large Animal Surgery, Philadelphia, 1984, WB Saunders.
5. Auer JA: Arthrodesis techniques, In Auer JA, Stick JA, editors: Equine Surgery, ed 2, Philadelphia, 1999, WB Saunders.
6. McIlwraith CW, Turner AS: Equine Surgery: Advanced Techniques, Philadelphia, 1987, Lea & Febiger.
7. Deiss E, Fuerst A, Haas C, et al: Symptomatik, Diagnostik und Therapie von 5 Pferden mit traumatischen subchondralen Knochenzysten, Wien Tierärztl Mschr 2001;88:1.
8. Fuerst A, Kaegi B, Rechenberg BV, et al: Die Behandlung von 5 Pferden mit subchondralen zystoiden Defekten im Fesselbein, Pferdeheilkunde 1997;13:147.
9. Auer J: Personal observations, 2001.
10. Fuerst A, Derungs S, von Rechenberg B, et al: Use of a parathyroid hormone (PTH_{1-34})-enriched hydrogel for the treatment of a subchondral cystic lesion in the proximal interphalangeal joint of a warmblood filly. Submitted to Vet Surg 2005.
11. Schmökel HG: Treatment of nonunions with nonglycosylated recombinant human bone morphogenetic protein-2 delivered from a fibrin matrix, Vet Surg 2004;33:112.
12. Schneider RK, Bramlage LR, Hardy J: Arthrodesis of the distal interphalangeal joint in 2 horses using 3 parallel 5.5mm cortical screws, Vet Surg 1993;22:122-128.
13. Schneider EJ, Carnine BL, Guffy MM: Arthrodesis of the proximal interphalangeal joint in the horse: A surgical treatment for high ringbone, J Am Vet Med Assoc 1978;173:1364.
14. Trotter GW, McIlwraith CW, Norrdin RW, et al: Degenerative joint disease with osteochondrosis of the proximal interphalangeal joint in young horses, J Am Vet Med Assoc 1982;180:1312.
15. Gabel AA, Bukowiecki CF: Fractures of the phalanges, Vet Clin North Am Large Anim Pract 1983;5:233.
16. Watkins JP: Fractures of the middle phalanx. In Nixon AJ, editor: Equine Fracture Repair, Philadelphia, 1996, WB Saunders.
17. Genetzky RM, Schneider EJ, Butler HC, et al: Comparison of two surgical procedures for arthrodesis of the proximal interphalangeal joint in horses, J Am Vet Med Assoc 1981;179:464.
18. Schneider RK: Arthrodesis of the proximal interphalangeal joint—three screw method. AO/ASIF Basic Equine Course. Internal Fixation of Fractures, Columbus, Ohio, 1997.
19. Crabill MR, Watkins JP, Schneider RK, Auer JA: Double plate fixation of comminuted middle phalangeal fractures in horses (1985-1993), J Am Vet Med Assoc 1995;207:1458.
20. Martin GS, McIlwraith CW, Turner AS, et al: Long term results and complications of proximal interphalangeal arthrodesis in horses, J Am Vet Med Assoc 1984;184:1136.
21. Watt BC, Edwards RB III, Markel M, et al: Arthrodesis of the equine proximal interphalangeal joint: A biomechanical comparison of three 4.5-mm and two 5.5-mm cortical screws, Vet Surg 2001;30: 287.
22. Easter JL, Watkins JP: Unpublished data. College Station, 1997, Texas A&M University.

23. Eastman TG, Watkins JP: Unpublished data. College Station, 1999, Texas A&M University.
24. Schaer TP, Bramlage LR, Emertson RM, et al: Proximal interphalangeal arthrodesis in 22 horses, Equine Vet J 2001;33:360.
25. Watt BC, Edwards RB III, Markel MD, et al: Arthrodesis of the equine proximal interphalangeal joint: A biomechanical comparison of two 7-hole 3.5-mm broad and two 5-hole 4.5-mm narrow dynamic compression plates, Vet Surg 2002;31:85.
26. MacLellan KNM, Crawford WH, MacDonald DG: Proximal interphalangeal joint arthrodesis in 34 horses using two parallel 5.5-mm cortical bone screws, Vet Surg 2001;30:454.
27. Bramlage LR: Fetlock arthrodesis. In Nixon AJ, editor: Equine Fracture Repair, Philadelphia, 1996, WB Saunders.
28. Auer JA: Application of the dynamic condylar screw (DCS) and dynamic hip screw (DHS) implant system in the horse, Vet Comp Orthop Traumatol 1988;1:18.
29. Sod GA, Martin GS: An in vitro biomechanical comparison of a prototype intramedullary pin-plate with a dynamic compression plate for equine metacarpophalangeal arthrodesis, Vet Surg 2004;33:83.
30. Bertone AL, Schneiter HL, Turner AS, Shoemaker RS: Pancarpal arthrodesis for the treatment of carpal collapse in the adult horse: A report of two cases, Vet Surg 1989;18:353.
31. Auer JA, Taylor JR, Watkins JP, et al: Partial carpal arthrodesis in the horse, Vet Comp Orthop Traumatol 1990;3:51.
32. Nunamaker DM, Bowmann KF, Richardson DW, Herring M: Plate luting: A preliminary report on its use in horses, Vet Surg 1986;15:289.
33. Edwards GB: Surgical arthrodesis for the treatment of bone spavin in 20 horses, Equine Vet J 1982;14:117.
34. Wyn-Jones G, May GS: Surgical arthrodesis for the treatment of osteoarthrosis of the proximal intertarsal, distal intertarsal and tarsometatarsal joints in 30 horses: A comparison of four different techniques, Equine Vet J 1986;18:59.
35. Barneveld A: Die Arthrodese der distalen Tarsalgelenke, Pferdeheilkunde 1986;3:35.
36. Stashak TS: The tarsus. In Stashak TS, editor: Adams' Lameness in Horses, ed 4, Philadelphia, 1987, Lea & Febiger.
37. Smith RKW, Dyson SJ, Schramme MC, et al: Osteoarthritis of the talocalcaneal joint in 18 horses, Equine Vet J 2005;37:166.
38. Pauwels FE, Adams SB, Blevins WB: Arthrodesis of the talocalcaneal joint for the treatment of two horses with talocalcaneal osteoarthritis, Vet Comp Orthop Traumatol 2005;17:7.
39. Schneider RK: Arthrodesis of the tarsus by other means. AO/ASIF Basic Equine Course: Internal Fixation of Fractures, Columbus, Ohio, 1997.
40. Bohanon TC: The tarsus. In Auer JA, Stick JA, editors: Equine Surgery, ed 2, Philadelphia, 1999, WB Saunders.
41. Barber SM: Arthrodesis of the distal intertarsal and tarsometatarsal joints in the horse, Vet Surg 1984;13:227.
42. Hague B, Guccione A: Laser-facilitated arthrodesis of the distal intertarsal joints, Clin Tech Equine Pract 2002;1:32.
43. von Salis B, Auer JA, Fackelman GE: Small tarsal joint arthrodesis. In Fackelman GE, Nunamaker DM, Auer JA, editors: AO Principles of Equine Osteosynthesis: An Electronic Manual of the AO/ASIF Technique, Stuttgart, 1999, Thieme Verlag.
44. Archer RM, Schneider RK, Lindsay WA, et al: Arthrodesis of the equine distal tarsal joints by perforated stainless steel cylinders, Equine Vet J Suppl 1988;6:125.
45. Semevolos SA, Watkins JP, Auer JA: Scapulohumeral arthrodesis in miniature horses, Vet Surg 2003;32:416.

CHAPTER 86

Diagnosis and Management of Tendon and Ligament Disorders

Charlotte S. Davis
Roger K. W. Smith

TENDON BIOLOGY

Structure of Tendons and Ligaments: From Molecule to Organ

Tendons and ligaments are complex organs built up in a hierarchical arrangement of increasingly smaller subunits (Fig. 86-1). Tendon is highly hydrated, having a water content of around 70%, and the remaining 30% (the dry weight) is composed predominantly of type I collagen. Collagen is synthesized as procollagen molecules consisting of an α-helical chain and amino-terminal and carboxy-terminal extensions that are cleaved by procollagenases immediately before three α-chains are combined to give a single collagen fibril. This process appears to take place postnatally outside the cell, but recent evidence has suggested that the original structural template for tendon formation is laid down by cells in the embryo that secrete formed fibrils into the extracellular space.[1] Thereafter, growth of the tendon occurs via a "seed-and-feed" mechanism, whereby collagen fibrils form extracellularly and accrete onto the sides of the template fibrils.

The function of the tendon depends on the spatial organization of the collagen fibrils and their crosslinking. The determination of collagen fibril size, organization, and crosslinking is provided by an array of noncollagenous proteins, many of which are yet to be characterized fully. The next most abundant protein in young tendon is cartilage oligomeric matrix protein (COMP),[2] which is believed to be involved in the organization of the collagen fibril framework during formation and growth. In support of this proposed action, recent experimental data showed that COMP accelerated collagen fibril formation in vitro.[3] From these data, it was proposed that COMP molecules bring together

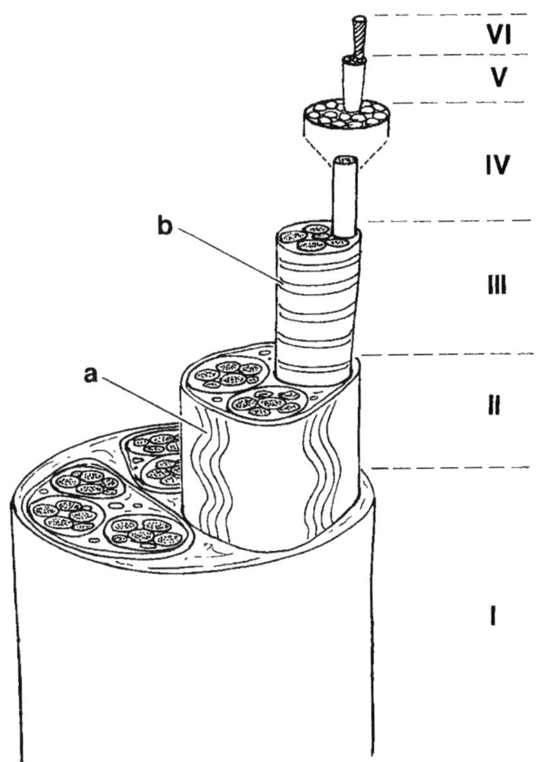

Figure 86-1. The structural hierarchy of tendon. The tendon is composed of increasingly smaller subunits, from fascicles visible to the naked eye (see Fig. 86-3), to fibers seen under light microscopy, to individual collagen fibrils seen by electron microscopy.

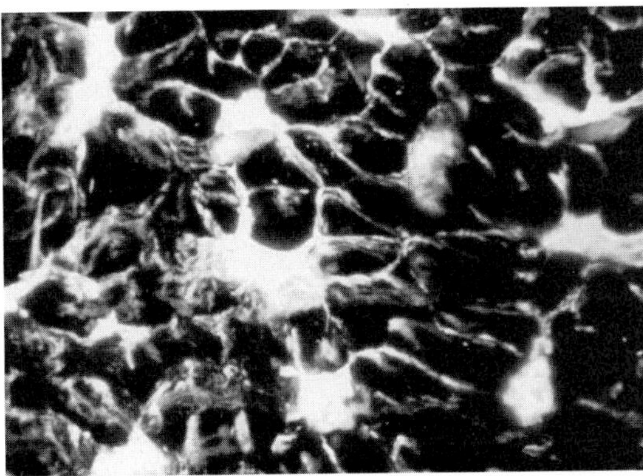

Figure 86-2. Transverse section of tendon stained to show the cytoplasmic membrane of the tenocytes. Note the large cell bodies and the extensive network of cytoplasmic extensions, which connect adjacent cells via gap junctions to produce a syncytium capable of orchestrating coordinated responses to loading. (Courtesy Dr. Jim Ralph, Cardiff University, UK.)

five separate collagen molecules in the "quarter-stagger" that is characteristic of collagen fibrils. Once these collagen molecules have formed a fibril, COMP no longer functions in binding and is displaced from the collagen fibril. In keeping with this role, levels of COMP in equine digital flexor tendons increase dramatically during growth, peak at around 2 years of age in the metacarpal region of the equine digital flexor tendons, and then decline once growth ceases and the animal ages.[2] The importance and relevance of this protein during growth is suggested by a correlation between tendon ultimate tensile strength and the level of COMP at skeletal maturity.[4]

Tendons also contain a wide variety of other noncollagenous proteins, many of which have yet to be characterized. The composition varies along the length of the tendon, reflecting the biomechanical environment. Hence, the small proteoglycans (decorin, fibromodulin, lumican, and mimecan) predominate in the tensional regions, whereas the large proteoglycans (aggrecan and versican) are mainly, but not exclusively, located in the regions of the tendon that are subjected to compression as the tendon changes direction over a bony prominence (e.g., the deep digital flexor tendon at the level of the metacarpophalangeal joint).[5,6]

Bundles of collagen fibrils are grouped together into fibers that are separated by cytoplasmic extensions of the cellular components of tendon, known as tenocytes[7] (Fig. 86-2). Little is known about these cells, although several different types are identified on light microscopy on the basis of their nuclear morphology.[8,9] These different nuclear shapes may represent stages of activation or differently differentiated cells. Type I cells, which have thin, spindle-shaped nuclei characteristic of adult tendon, are most likely to be relatively inactive forms of the type II cells, whose nuclei are more oval and that are abundant in young, growing tendon. In adult digital flexor tendon, where the tendon changes direction over the palmar/plantar aspect of the metacarpophalangeal/metatarsophalangeal (MCP/MTP) joint, external compression results in a matrix that is more like that of fibrocartilage. Reflecting this matrix, type III cells have round nuclei characteristic of chondrocytes. Other cell types are found within the endotenon (see later) and are associated with aging changes (e.g., chondroid metaplasia).

On a large scale, collagen fibers are grouped together in increasingly larger subunits divided by looser connective tissue known as the endotenon. It is these subunits, known as fascicles, that are visible to the naked eye on a cut section of tendon (Fig. 86-3). In relaxed tendon, the fascicles have a waveform known as crimp, which is best seen under polarized light. The endotenon carries blood vessels and nerves and is the location of a different type of cell, one that has a more rounded shape; these cells are believed to be the source of mesenchymal stem cells within the tendon. This compartment of the tendon contains higher levels of certain growth factors, such as transforming growth factor (TGF)-β, than within the fascicles.[10]

The endotenon is continuous with the layer of connective tissue surrounding the outside of the tendon, known as the epitenon. Outside this layer, around tendons that are not contained within a tendon sheath, is a thicker layer known as the paratenon, which is able to stretch considerably and is therefore rarely ruptured when a tendon suffers a strain injury. This layer is believed to play particularly important roles both in reducing frictional forces between the tendon and the surrounding soft tissues and as a supplier of new blood vessels and cellular elements for repair. It is hypothesized that the lack of this layer intrathecally and the synovial fluid environment results in slower healing of these regions.

Where tendon changes direction over a joint, the tendon usually is enclosed within a tendon sheath (Fig. 86-4). This structure provides a synovial environment for the smooth

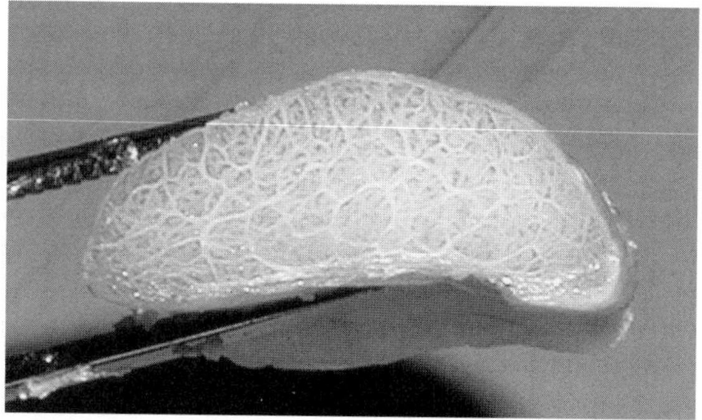

Figure 86-3. Cut surface of a frozen piece of superficial digital flexor tendon revealing the extensive interfascicular tissue, the endotenon, which contains the internal vascular and nervous supply to the tendon and is responsible for interfascicular gliding movements (where most of the tendon's stretch occurs). (From Smith RKW, Goodship AE: Tendon and ligament physiology. In Hinchcliff KW, Kaneps AJ, Geor RJ, editors: Equine Sports Medicine and Surgery, Philadelphia, 2004, WB Saunders.)

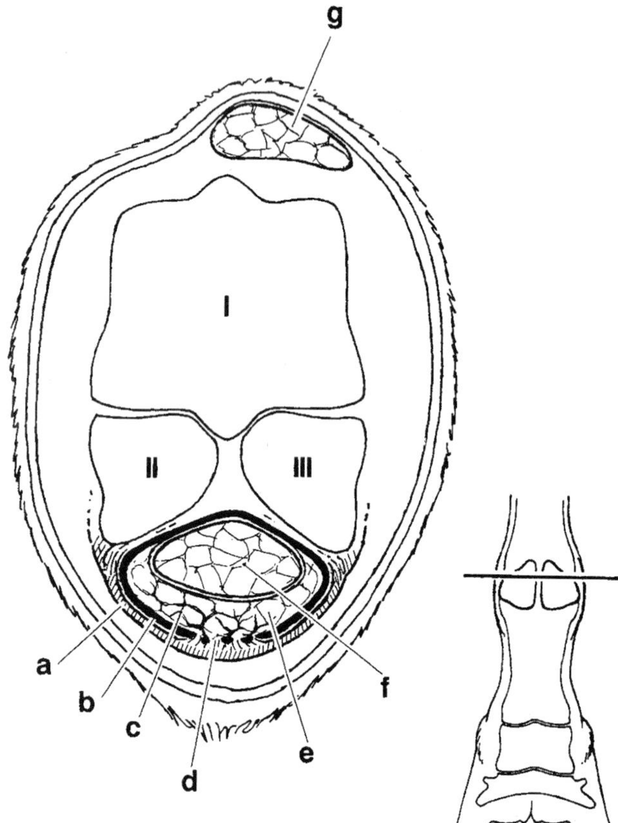

Figure 86-4. The anatomy of a tendon within a tendon sheath. Note the absence of a paratenon and the presence of mesotenon attachments, which are incomplete along the length of a sheath, through which blood supply gains access to the tendon. (From McIlwraith CW: Diseases of joints, tendons, ligaments, and related structures. In Stashak TS, editor: Adams' Lameness in Horses, ed 5, Oxford, 2002, Blackwell.)

gliding of tendon over a bony prominence. Associated with this sheath, there is usually a smooth fibrocartilaginous pad covering the bony prominences, best exemplified by the scuta of the distal limb—the proximal scutum or intersesamoidean ligament at the level of the MCP/MTP joint, the middle scutum attached to the middle phalanx, and the distal scutum attached to the distal sesamoid (navicular) bone. The tendon sheath, like a joint, consists of an outer fibrous wall and an inner synovial membrane, which also surrounds the tendons within the tendon sheath. Dividing the sheath into complete or incomplete compartments are a number of mesotenons that are composed of two layers of synovium and frequently, but not always, carry the blood supply to the tendon.

Blood Supply

The blood supply to the tendon comes from its muscular origin and osseous insertion and variably from accessory ligaments, the paratenon, and mesotenon attachments. However, work on equine digital flexor tendons showed that stripping the paratenon failed to cause any ischemic damage to the tendon,[11,12] indicating the importance of the intratendinous supply for this tendon. Based on the microvascular anatomy determined by microradiographs,[13] this intratendinous supply is most abundant around the periphery of the tendon, which has led to the hypothesis that the central region of the tendon is relatively hypoxic, and that this is one of the reasons for the common manifestation of tendon disease as a central core lesion. However, there is little supporting evidence for this hypothesis and, in fact, the superficial digital flexor tendon has a blood supply, as determined by xenon clearance, similar to that of resting skeletal muscle and is capable of increasing flow during exercise and after injury.[14]

Functional Characteristics of Tendon and Ligament

Tendon and ligaments have a variety of functions: they transmit forces to move the equine skeleton, or they provide support of the distal limb in the case of the digital flexor tendons, or, as ligaments, they maintain joint integrity. Their structure is optimized to play these mechanical roles.

Tendons and ligaments have viscoelastic properties, which means that their mechanical properties vary as they are stretched. A typical force–elongation curve for tendon is shown in Figure 86-5. Initially, the tendon stretches under relatively little load, which is associated with the elimination of crimp in the fascicles. Thereafter, the curve is almost linear. It is from this area of the curve that the structural property of stiffness is determined (load divided by deformation). As the load increases further, there is a change in the gradient such that the tendon becomes less stiff. This is known as the *yield point,* and it is thought to arise from covalent crosslink rupture and slippage of collagen fibrils. If the tendon is stretched past this point, irreversible damage occurs. If loading is continued past this point, the tendon ruptures, which for the equine superficial digital flexor tendons (SDFT) is approximately 12 kilo-newtons (kN) or 1.2 tons (ultimate tensile strength).[15,16]

If the cross-sectional area and length of the tendon is known, then the stress (force per unit area) can be plotted against strain (change in length over original length), from which the material properties of ultimate tensile stress (N/mm^2) and Young's modulus of elasticity (E [MPa]) can be calculated. The approximate ultimate tensile stress of 100 MPa for the equine SDFT is similar to previously documented figures in other species (20 to 144 MPa).[17,18]

In vitro, equine flexor tendons can extend 10% to 12% of their length before they rupture (ultimate tensile strain), and values of up to 20% have been reported.[8] However, the ultimate tensile strain reflects only the final strain before rupture and includes the yield portion of the stress–strain curve that represents irreversible damage to the tendon tissue. The normal strains in the digital flexor tendons, recorded in vivo, are in the region of 3% to 8% at the walk, 7% to 10% at the trot, and 12% to 16% at the gallop.[19] Such strains, far greater than usually expected in tendons from most other species, may reflect the importance of the digital flexor tendon as an elastic energy store, where maximal deformation stores the most energy but also makes them operate close to their functional limit.

In addition to these basic functional characteristics, tendon has other mechanical properties of potentially important biologic relevance. There is a difference between the stress–strain relationship when the tendon is loaded and the relationship when it is unloaded, which is known as hysteresis (see Fig. 86-5). The area between these two curves represents the energy lost during the loading cycle. This is usually about 5% in equine tendons. Much of this energy is lost as heat and is responsible for the rise in temperature in the tendon core when the horse exercises. These temperatures can rise to as high as 44° C, which is potentially damaging to both tendon matrix and tenocytes. However, tenocytes recovered from the center of equine SDFT remain viable when subjected to rises in temperature of this magnitude, whereas those recovered from the periphery of the tendon do not.[20] This property is also present in fetal tenocytes, which suggests that the tendon has an inherent genetic adaptation to this physical process.

The loading rate has only a minimal effect on tendon biomechanics: a rapid loading rate results in a stiffer tendon, whereas repeated loading, in contrast, results in a less stiff tendon, a process known as *conditioning* (see Fig. 86-5). This effect appears to occur in vivo[21] and the change is recoverable but significant resting time is necessary.[8]

The Relationship of Structure to Function

It would appear that all tendons are formed in utero in a similar fashion and with a similar composition, analogous to the "blank joint" concept for articular cartilage.[6,22,23] However, as soon as the animal is born and stands, tendons and ligaments receive very different mechanical loading. It is believed that different mechanical environments drive growth and differentiation of tendons so that at skeletal maturity, different tendons have different compositional and structural properties that relate to their function. Thus, mature tendons are not all composed of the same material and hence do not all have the same functional characteristics. Furthermore, different loading patterns induce anisotropy within certain tendons. Thus, where the digital flexor tendons change direction across the palmar aspect of the MCP/MTP joint and are subjected to external compression, they develop a cartilage-like matrix.[24]

The horse's distal limb is designed like a spring to store energy from weightbearing for the subsequent stride.[25] The horse essentially bounces up and down on its forelimbs, whereas its hindlimbs provide propulsive force. This system is optimized by having a hyperextended MCP joint and by the energy being stored in the palmar soft tissue structures, principally the SDFT and suspensory ligaments (Fig. 86-6). The superficial digital flexor muscle contains a high proportion of fibrous tissue, and recent data have indicated that its maximal contraction shortens the muscular unit by only 2 mm.[25] Hence, the muscle acts not to flex the MCP joint but rather to fix the origin of the SDFT and dampen high-frequency damaging oscillations. Although the muscle within the suspensory ligament is considered vestigial, it may also have a similar role in dampening the damaging oscillation during high-speed exercise.

Consequently, these two structures have very similar matrix compositions and configurations: both have high COMP levels and a combination of small and large collagen fibrils. In contrast, the common digital extensor tendon (CDET), a low-load tendon, and the deep digital flexor

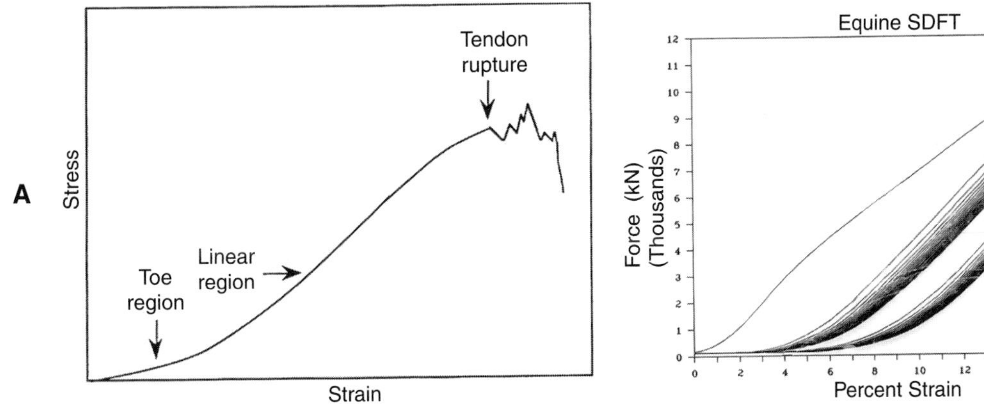

Figure 86-5. A, The stress–strain curve for tendon showing its viscoelastic properties. The toe region is associated with elimination of "crimp," and the linear region is where the tendon is operating in an elastic fashion. At the end of the linear region, the yield point is reached, where irreversible damage starts to occur before the tendon ruptures completely. **B,** Hysteresis and conditioning. The loading and unloading curves are not the same, resulting in an energy loss, which is represented by the area between the two curves (hysteresis loop). If the tendon continues to be loaded repeatedly, the curve moves to the right until it reaches a steady state, when the tendon is more elastic. (From Smith RKW, Goodship AE: Tendon and ligament physiology. In Hinchcliff KW, Kaneps AJ, Geor RJ, editors: Equine Sports Medicine and Surgery, Philadelphia, 2004, WB Saunders.)

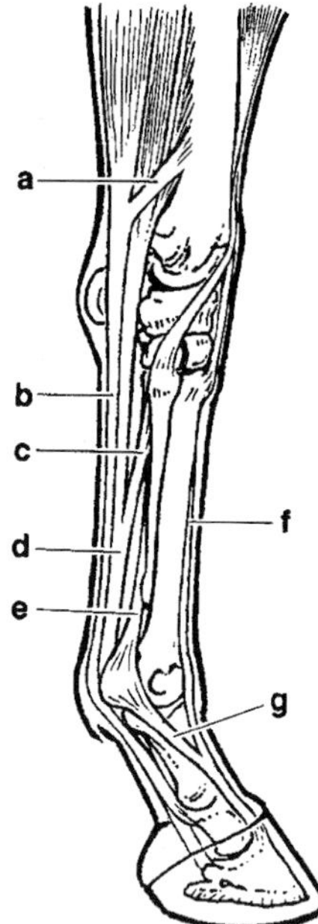

Figure 86-6. The anatomy of the equine distal limb showing the important weight-bearing tendons and ligament on the palmar aspect of the limb. It is these structures that most frequently suffer strain-induced injury.

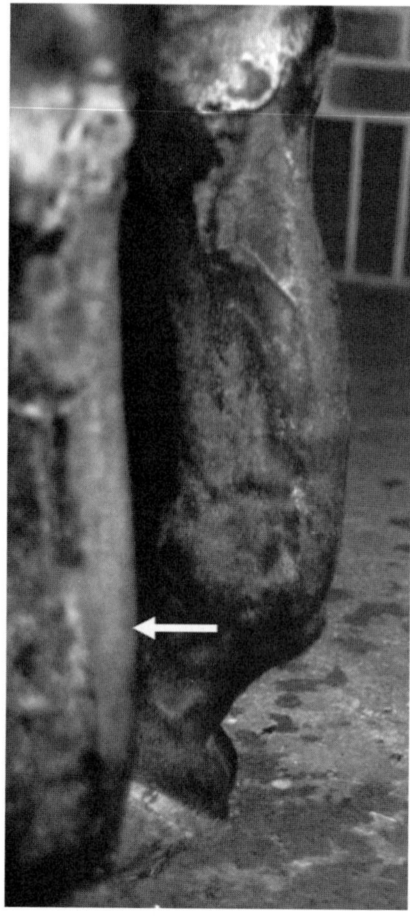

Figure 86-7. Superficial digital flexor tendinitis. Note the bowing, or swelling, of the palmar border of the right limb. Careful attention must also be given to the contralateral limb, which may exhibit a smaller swelling that can be easily missed *(arrow)*.

tendon (DDFT), which also has a different role, have lower levels of COMP and predominantly large collagen fibrils. These compositional differences are reflected in their mechanical properties. Tendons can be divided into weight-bearing tendons that function like springs (and are less stiff, or more elastic) and those that position the skeleton (which requires greater stiffness). Thus, the CDET is almost twice as stiff a material as the SDFT.

Etiopathogenesis of Tendon Injury

Tendons and ligaments can be injured in one of two ways: by overstrain or percutaneously. Overstrain injuries are believed to occur by one of two mechanisms. They can result from a sudden overloading of the structure, which overwhelms its resistive strength. This type of injury is probably the mechanism for most ligament and some DDFT injuries in the horse. However, for the most common strain-induced injuries in the horse, involving the palmar soft tissue structures of the metacarpal region, the clinical injury is believed to be preceded by a phase of molecular degeneration ("molecular inflammation"[26]), which induces neither a clinically evident inflammatory reaction nor any reparative response, but instead progressively weakens the tendon.[22,27] The evidence for this degeneration is based on four observations:

"Asymptomatic" lesions are present both grossly and microscopically in postmortem studies of normal horses.[28] However, analysis of these lesions suggests that they are the result of healing of low-grade clinical injuries rather than true degeneration.[29]

Most clinical strain-induced tendinopathies are bilateral, but one limb is more severely affected than the other (Fig. 86-7). Careful ultrasonographic examination often reveals changes in the contralateral limb. Furthermore, in seemingly unilateral cases, blood flow studies have demonstrated increases in the "normal" contralateral tendon, which would suggest that it is not totally unaffected.

Epidemiologic studies in both horses and humans have shown strong associations between injury rates and age.[30-32]

A number of experimental exercise studies and postmortem analyses of normal tendons have indicated that increasing age and amounts of exercise induce tendon matrix degeneration rather than adaptation in the adult horse.[27]

Response of Tendons to Aging and Exercise

When evaluating the gross mechanical properties of the SDFT in a large group of normal horses, there is a reduction in tendon strength with age, but this is statistically insignificant because of high variance. Thus, in a population of normal horses, there is more than a twofold variation in ultimate tensile strength of the SDFT. This high variance arises from inaccuracies in measuring ultimate tensile strength in vitro and the true variation in tendon strength, which is influenced by genetic components, but probably most importantly by environmental factors of aging and exercise.

The collagen crimp angle and length showed a regional reduction in the central core with exercise and age, both acting synergistically.[33,34] This results in the central fibers being straightened first under loading, and hence they are the most likely to rupture first, giving rise to a possible mechanism for the generation of the "core lesion" frequently seen clinically (Fig. 86-8).

Within the matrix, regional differences in collagen fibril diameter are seen in long-term exercised older horses but not in short-term exercised, or younger, horses.[35] The higher proportion of small fibrils in the central region of long-term exercised horses does not appear to be associated with increased collagen content, and the collagen-related fluorescence (a measure of collagen age) is unaltered, suggesting that this change results from disassembly of the larger-diameter fibrils.

Collagen content varies little with age and exercise, but the noncollagenous component of tendon is much more labile, with changes evident in longer-term exercised and older horses. Thus, in the center of the tendon where clinical injury is seen, there is an accelerated loss of glycosaminoglycans (GAG) and COMP. This is in contrast to the central discolored regions seen as an occasional coincidental finding at postmortem, which contain higher hydration and increased GAG levels more suggestive of reparative (scar) tissue formation.[29]

In contrast, exercise in immature horses appears to stimulate tendon formation and adaptation, and experimental long-term exercise studies have failed to induce any degenerative changes.

From the results of these studies, it is hypothesized that the mid-metacarpal region of the equine SDFT can adapt to exercise during skeletal development but has poor or no ability to do so after skeletal maturity.[22,27] After skeletal maturity, the synergistic effect of aging and exercise causes an inevitable accumulation of microdamage (degeneration). In support of this hypothesis, analysis of matrix gene expression in bovine digital flexor tendons has shown prominent matrix gene expression at birth and during growth, but a dramatic reduction in the tensile (but not compressed) regions after skeletal maturity.[36]

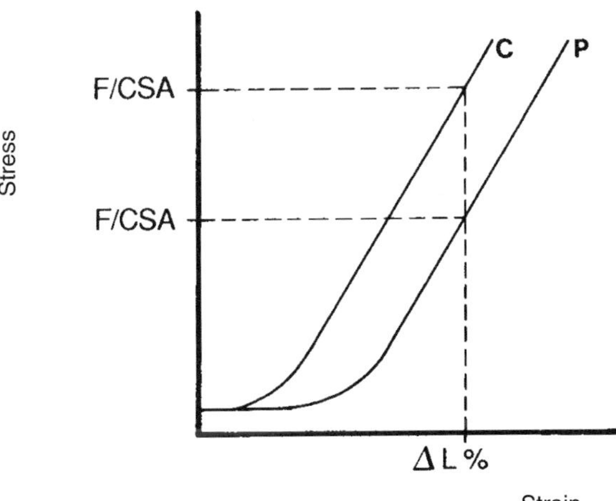

Figure 86-8. One possible explanation for the occurrence of a core lesion in the superficial digital flexor tendon. With aging and exercise, the central (C) crimp pattern, which is responsible for the toe region on a stress–strain curve (see Fig. 86-5), is reduced more than that in the periphery (P). Consequently, as the tendon is loaded, the central fibers are loaded first and take the most load for a given strain. Hence, it would be expected that they would rupture first, giving rise to a core lesion. (From Wilmink J, Wilson AM, Goodship AE. Functional significance of the morphology and micromechanics of collagen fibers in relation to partial rupture of the superficial digital flexor tendon in racehourses, Res Vet Sci 1992;53:355.)

Mechanisms for Tendon Degeneration

Cumulative tendon microdamage arises from the induction of tendon matrix damage and the failure of the resident cell population to repair this damage. The mechanism for the failure of tenocytes to repair or adapt to exercise-induced microdamage in the adult is unclear but possibly involves both an absence of appropriate growth factor stimulus and a degree of cellular senescence. Investigations into the synthetic response by equine tenocytes to mechanical load (biaxial stretch) and growth factors (e.g., TGF-β) in vitro have demonstrated that tenocytes recovered from aged flexor tendons do demonstrate a small, but significant, reduced response.[37] Interestingly, this age effect is not apparent in tenocytes recovered from digital extensor tendons, which appear to continue to remodel and adapt during maturity.

The mechanism of degeneration of the tendon is currently unknown, but there are several possibilities. The close association between age and exercise suggests that the number of loading cycles is important, and it is logical to presume that the highest loading rates are likely to be the most damaging, so the amount of time spent at the fastest gaits (canter and gallop) are likely to most contribute to degeneration. The actual mechanisms can be either physical or metabolic. The physical energy imparted to the tendon under weight-bearing load can produce direct damage to the matrix by disrupting crosslinks or actual matrix proteins. An indirect physical effect of weightbearing is via the energy lost through hysteresis.[38] This results in a temperature rise at the center of the tendon, which has been recorded to be as high as 44° C at the gallop (Fig. 86-9). Although tenocytes in the SDFT have been shown to be resistant to these temperature rises,[20] this temperature could still be damaging to matrix proteins. Cyclical loading of tendon explants in vitro

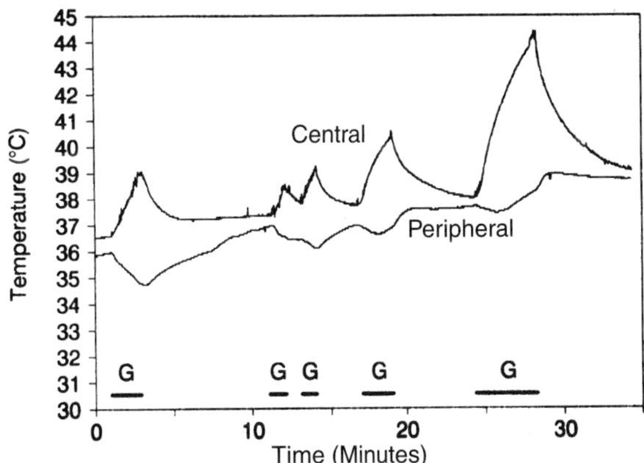

Figure 86-9. The hyperthermia theory of tendinitis. When the horse is galloped (G), the temperature in the superficial digital flexor tendon rises as high as 44° C, which could damage the tendon matrix and be responsible for tendon degeneration. (Courtesy Dr. Alan Wilson.)

induces the upregulation of both synthesis and activity of proteolytic enzymes, and this can induce a reduction in strength.[39] Furthermore, cleaved matrix proteins, generated either from direct physical forces or from enzymatic cleavage, can also provoke further matrix degradation, giving rise to an exercise-induced cycle of matrix degeneration.[40] Further work is necessary to elucidate the mechanisms of soft tissue degeneration so that preventative strategies can be developed.

Mechanisms of Clinical Injury

STRAIN-INDUCED INJURY

Degeneration is usually the first phase of tendinopathy. Any change in the structural properties of the tendon does not have to be great, as the tendon is already operating close to its tolerance limit. Clinical injury occurs when the highest stresses encountered by the tendon overwhelm its structural integrity, resulting in irreversible damage. At heel strike, the loads rise most quickly in the soft tissue structures that support primarily the metacarpophalangeal joint: the SDFT and the suspensory ligament (SL)[8] (Fig. 86-10). The load in the DDFT rises later during stance, which may help to explain why the SDFT and the SL are the most prone to injury.

Once the peak load on the tendon overcomes its structural strength, there is physical disruption to the tendon matrix. The clinical injury varies in degree from fibrillar slippage, with breakage of crosslinking elements, to fibrillar rupture and, in some cases, complete separation of tendon tissue. Once this occurs, the damage created induces a repair process not dissimilar to that found in other soft tissues, such as skin, characterized by inflammation followed by fibroplasia (scar tissue formation).

This process allows the incorporation of risk factors that have been identified for inducing tendinitis. These risk factors act to increase the peak loads on the SDFT, thereby increasing the risk of structural disruption. One of the most important factors is the speed of the horse. The faster the horse is going, the greater the risk of developing tendinitis.

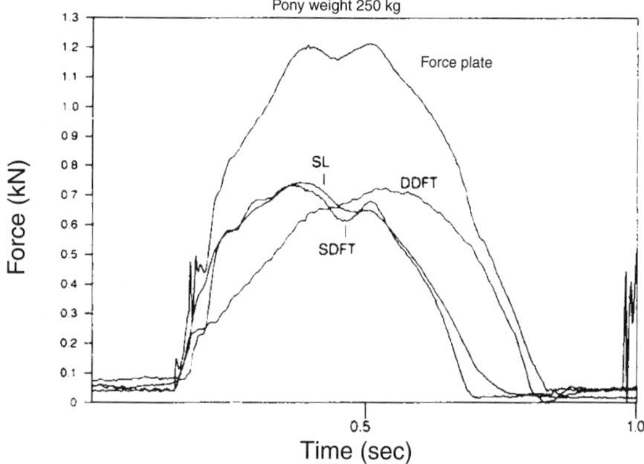

Figure 86-10. The force of individual tendons and ligaments of the equine distal limb during stance. Note the rapid rise in loading in the superficial digital flexor tendon and suspensory ligament (including what is thought to be damaging high-frequency "transients" at foot placement), whereas loading rises more slowly in the deep digital flexor tendon. This may help explain why injuries are much more common in the superficial digital flexor tendon and suspensory ligament than in the deep digital flexor tendon. (Courtesy Dr. Alan Wilson.)

Thus, a hard track surface is associated with tendinitis, since it increases the speed of the horse and also increases the peak impact loading.[31] Slower surfaces (including soft track surfaces) tend to be protective. Other factors, such as the weight the horse is carrying, fatigue, and the shoeing, can all influence peak tendon loads in this way. Heel elevation has been shown to decrease the load on the DDFT and increase the degree of extension in the MCP joint,[41,42] with toe elevation having the opposite effect. It may be thought, therefore, that low heels would be protective of tendinitis. However, epidemiologic studies have shown an association between low heel and long toe conformation and orthopedic injury, of which the most common were tendon and ligament injuries.

TENDON TEARS

The mechanism for the generation of tendon or ligament tears within synovial cavities is much less clear. The most common site is the DDFT (mainly in the forelimb) and the manica flexoria (predominantly in the hindlimb) in the proximal digital sheath (Fig. 86-11). For the former, higher pressures within the compressed portion of the DDFT as it passes over the palmar aspect of the MCP joint may cause "bursting" of the lateral (or, less commonly, of the medial) borders of the tendon. For manica tears, it is possible that the manica gets caught as it passes into the fetlock canal, and, as some of these tears have been seen after a prolonged period of tenosynovitis, this may be exacerbated by synovial hypertrophy within the sheath (making this passage even more restricted) or, less commonly, by the presence of adhesions.

PERCUTANEOUS TENDON INJURY

Percutaneous tendon injuries arise most frequently from trauma to the distal limb because of the minimal soft tissue cover. These injuries are usually associated with considerable contusion. Traumatic injuries involving over-reaches, wires, jumping injuries, and kicking injuries are the most frequent causes. Tendon laceration usually requires the tendon to be taut, so tendons are most frequently partially or fully severed when under weight-bearing load. The exception to this is the lacerations caused when limbs are caught (e.g., in wire), when repeated attempts to free the limb can saw through any associated tendon or ligament.

The most serious consequences follow trauma to the palmar aspect of the metacarpus or pastern. Up to 50% of the tendon can be lacerated and still provide full tendon function at the walk. In contrast, extensor tendon lacerations on the dorsal aspect of the distal limb, although common (especially in hindlimbs caught in wire), rarely have long-term functional consequences.

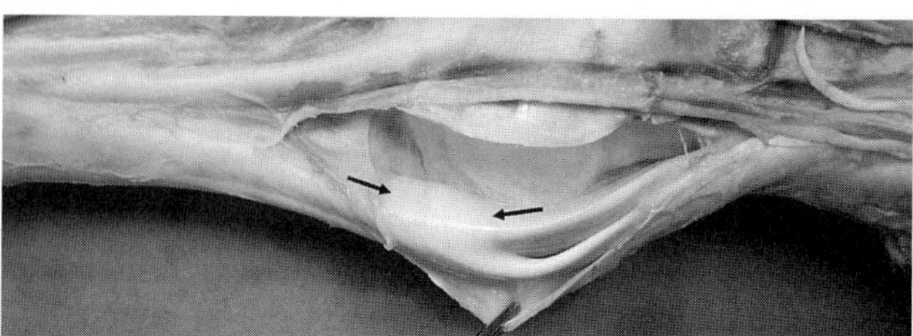

Figure 86-11. The manica flexoria (between *arrows*).

Pathophysiology of Tendon Repair

Once the tendon suffers clinical injury with disruption of the tendon matrix, there is intratendinous hemorrhage initially, usually followed rapidly by a pronounced inflammatory reaction (Fig. 86-12). This inflammatory reaction results in an increase in blood flow, the development of edema, the infiltration of neutrophils, macrophages, and monocytes, and the release of proteolytic enzymes. Although this is the earliest stage of repair, designed to remove damaged tendon tissue, the response is thought to be excessive, causing further damage to the tendon. The inflammatory phase is usually short-lived, and it overlaps the reparative phase, which begins within a few days and lasts several months. This phase is associated with a pronounced angiogenic response and fibroblastic cellular infiltration (extrinsic repair). It is believed that intrinsic repair mechanisms (i.e., from the tendon itself) are limited. The result is the synthesis of scar tissue that has a composition that is different from that of tendon, with a higher ratio of collagen types III: I (about 50% compared with 10% for normal tendon), a higher hydration, and higher levels of GAGs[29] (see Fig. 86-12).

The reparative phase of tendon healing merges with the remodeling phase, during which there is a gradual but incomplete transformation to a higher proportion of type I collagen as the scar tissue matures[44] (see Fig. 86-12). The new collagen fibrils become thicker and crosslinked. Although mature scar tissue tends to be less stiff as a material than tendon, because large amounts are formed, the scarred tendon often results in a stiffer tendon than the original. As a result, the healed tendon becomes strong but it is functionally inferior to normal tendon and is thus predisposed to reinjury, often at sites adjacent to the original injury, which potentially reduces performance.

This process is less efficient when injuries occur to an intrathecal tendon, which is thought to be the consequence of the absence of a paratenon and reduced extrinsic repair. In addition, any surface defect within a tendon sheath will be bathed in synovial fluid, which will slow or even halt repair.

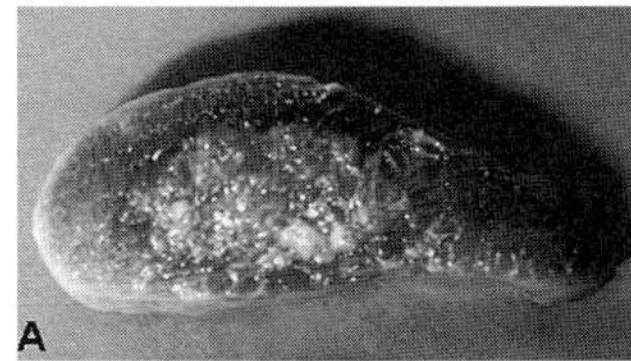

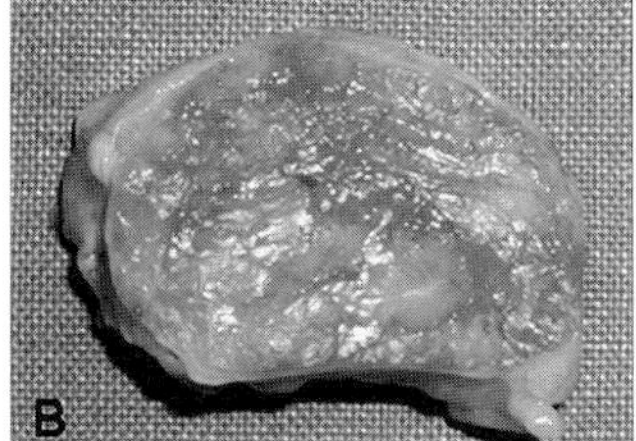

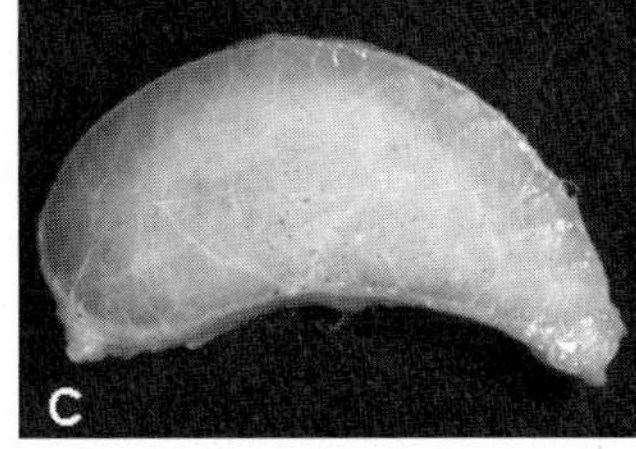

Figure 86-12. The different stages of superficial digital flexor tendinitis. **A,** acute. **B,** subacute. **C,** chronic. Note the replacement of tendon tissue with white fibrous tissue in **C**.

DIAGNOSIS

Clinical Evaluation

Diagnosis of strain-induced tendon injury is usually based on history (frequently a preceding period of exercise) and the development of the signs of inflammation (pain, heat, swelling, and lameness) over the affected structure. Lameness, which is often severe in the early stages, is not always evident when a patient is presented to a clinician, and it tends to be related to the degree of inflammation rather than to the degree of damage. Similarly, once the inflammatory phase has passed (within 1 or 2 weeks), lameness usually resolves rapidly.

The posture and function of the limb may be altered depending on the structure damaged and on the severity of the injury. In the case of severe superficial digital flexor tendinitis, resting MCP joint angle may be normal because of the action of the other supporters of this joint (SL and DDFT). However, when loading on the limb increases (e.g., when the contralateral limb is raised off the ground), the affected limb shows greater than normal overextension of the MCP joint (Fig. 86-13). Severe damage to the SL has a greater effect on MCP joint extension. Complete disruption of the peroneus tertius produces a characteristic mechanical lameness because of disruption of the reciprocal apparatus. This allows tarsal extension when the stifle is flexed. Similarly, complete rupture of the extensor carpi radialis tendon results in hyperflexion of the carpus during limb protraction.

For subtle cases, careful palpation of the tendons and ligaments in the limb should be made with the limb both weightbearing and raised. Careful attention should be given to pain response, subtle enlargement, and consistency of the structure (soft after recent injury; firm after healing). The horse must be relaxed so that muscle activity does not tense the tendons and make them appear artificially firm. Careful visual assessment of bowing of the palmar contour of the

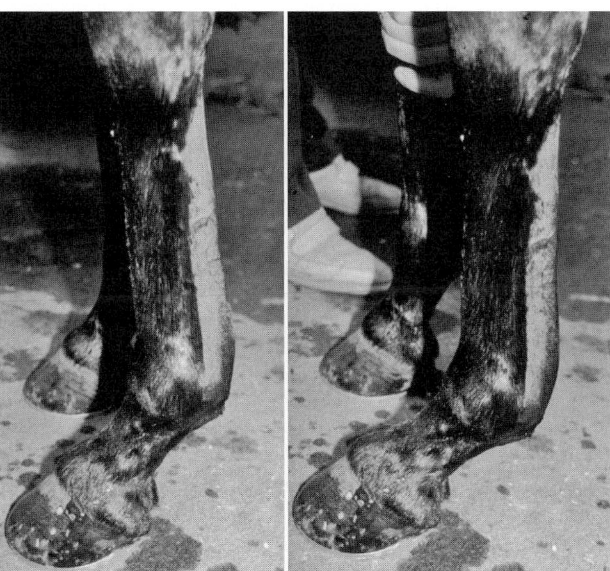

Figure 86-13. Demonstration of significant damage to the superficial digital flexor tendon (and/or suspensory ligament). Increasing the load on the affected limb by lifting the contralateral limb causes an abnormal increase in the metacarpophalangeal joint extension.

metacarpal region can help to identify subtle superficial digital flexor tendinitis. This assessment also should include the contralateral limb, since many strain-induced injuries are bilateral but with one limb more severely affected than the other.

Percutaneous tendon injuries are usually associated with moderate to severe lameness and may or may not have a concurrent wound. If a wound is present, it should be initially cleaned and then explored digitally with sterile gloves to ascertain which structures are damaged. Small wounds may hinder full evaluation, because the site of the tendon laceration, sustained under full weight-bearing load, is unlikely to be visible in the wound when the horse is severely lame. In such cases, concurrent ultrasonographic examination is very helpful. Penetration injuries or partial severance of a tendon does not alter the function of the tendon, so, other than lameness, there are few alterations of limb conformation. Complete transection, however, is associated with significant alterations in limb conformation under loading (see later). If the laceration is complete, the proximal part of a lacerated tendon often recoils as a result of the action of the associated muscle. It is necessary to assess whether any synovial structures have been penetrated, since this is a common complication of trauma to the distal limbs.

Ultrasonography

For strain-induced tendinopathies, clinical examination, however, may not detect the most subtle injuries, and it provides a poor objective assessment of severity. Since prognosis is most dependent on the severity of the initial injury,[45] it is prudent to evaluate the damaged area ultrasonographically, and this is best carried out approximately 1 week after the onset of the injury, since many lesions may expand during the initial few days. Modern ultrasound machines with a 7.5- to 10-MHz linear transducer produce excellent-quality images of the flexor tendons and SL. Although the metacarpal region can be evaluated ultrasonographically without clipping the hair, it is best to prepare the limb by clipping and washing (with a surgical scrub and alcohol) to obtain the best-quality images. The horse should stand square, and both transverse and longitudinal images should be obtained in a methodical fashion throughout the length of the region containing the injured tendon. For the metacarpal region, the area is divided up into seven zones, each with characteristic anatomy (Fig. 86-14). Alternatively, the distance between the transducer and the accessory carpal bone can be recorded. The palmar soft tissue structures of the metacarpus can be evaluated satisfactorily from the palmar aspect of the limb, except for the SL branches, which should be evaluated from the medial and lateral aspects of the limb, respectively. Both limbs should *always* be examined, since many cases of strain-induced tendon injury have bilateral components but with one limb more severely affected than the other.

Acute tendon pathology is manifest ultrasonographically by enlargement, hypoechogenicity (focal or generalized), reduced striated pattern in the longitudinal images, and changes in shape, margin, or position (Fig. 86-15). Chronic tendinopathy is associated with variable enlargement and

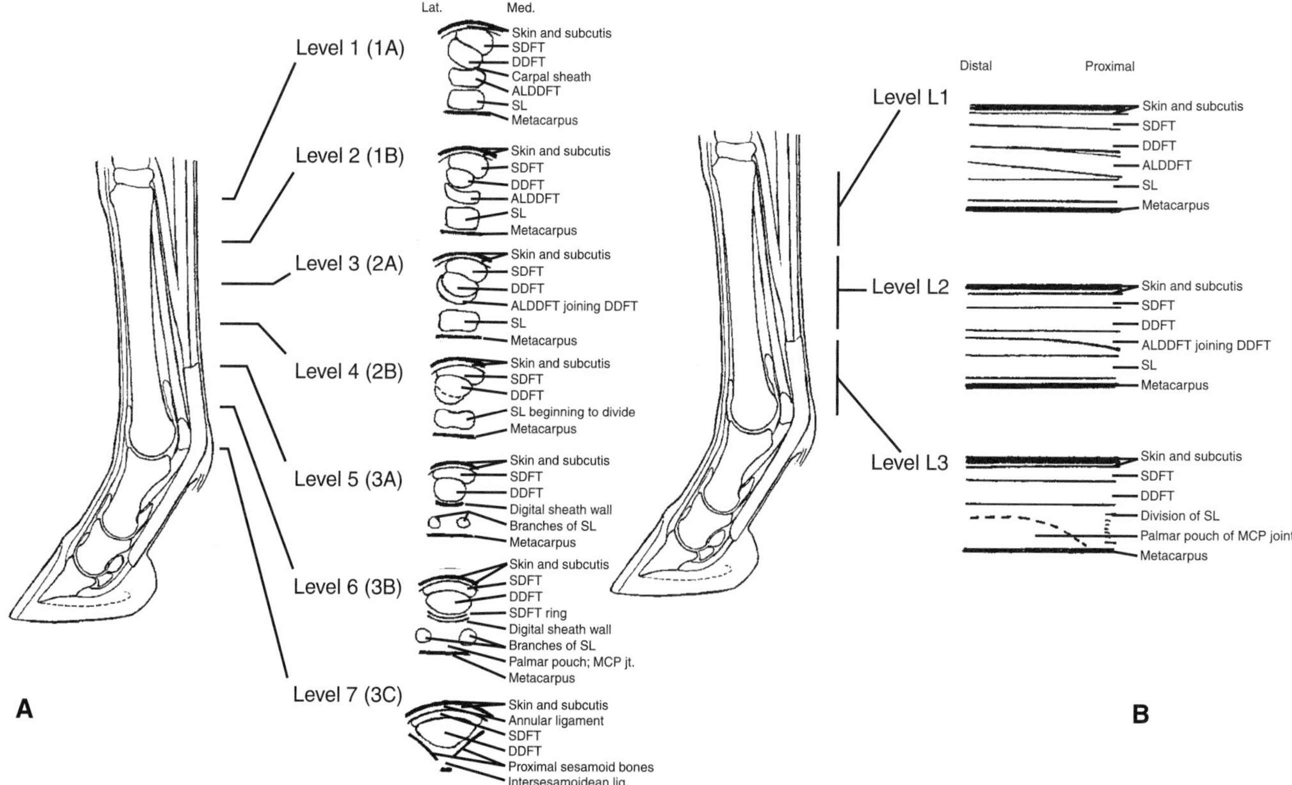

Figure 86-14. Line drawings of the cross-sectional (**A**) and longitudinal (**B**) ultrasonographic anatomy of the third metacarpal region. *SDFT,* Superficial digital flexor tendon; *DDFT,* deep digital flexor tendon; *ALDDFT,* accessory ligament of the deep digital flexor tendon; *SL,* suspensory ligament; *MCP,* metacarpophalangeal joint. (**A** from Smith RKW, Webbon PM: Diagnostic imaging in the athletic horse: musculoskeletal ultrasonography. In Hodgson DR, Rose RJ, editors: The Athletic Horse, Philadelphia, 1994, WB Saunders; **B** from Smith RKW, Webbon PM: Soft tissue injuries of the pastern. In Robinson NE, editor: Current Therapy in Equine Medicine, Philadelphia, 1997, WB Saunders.)

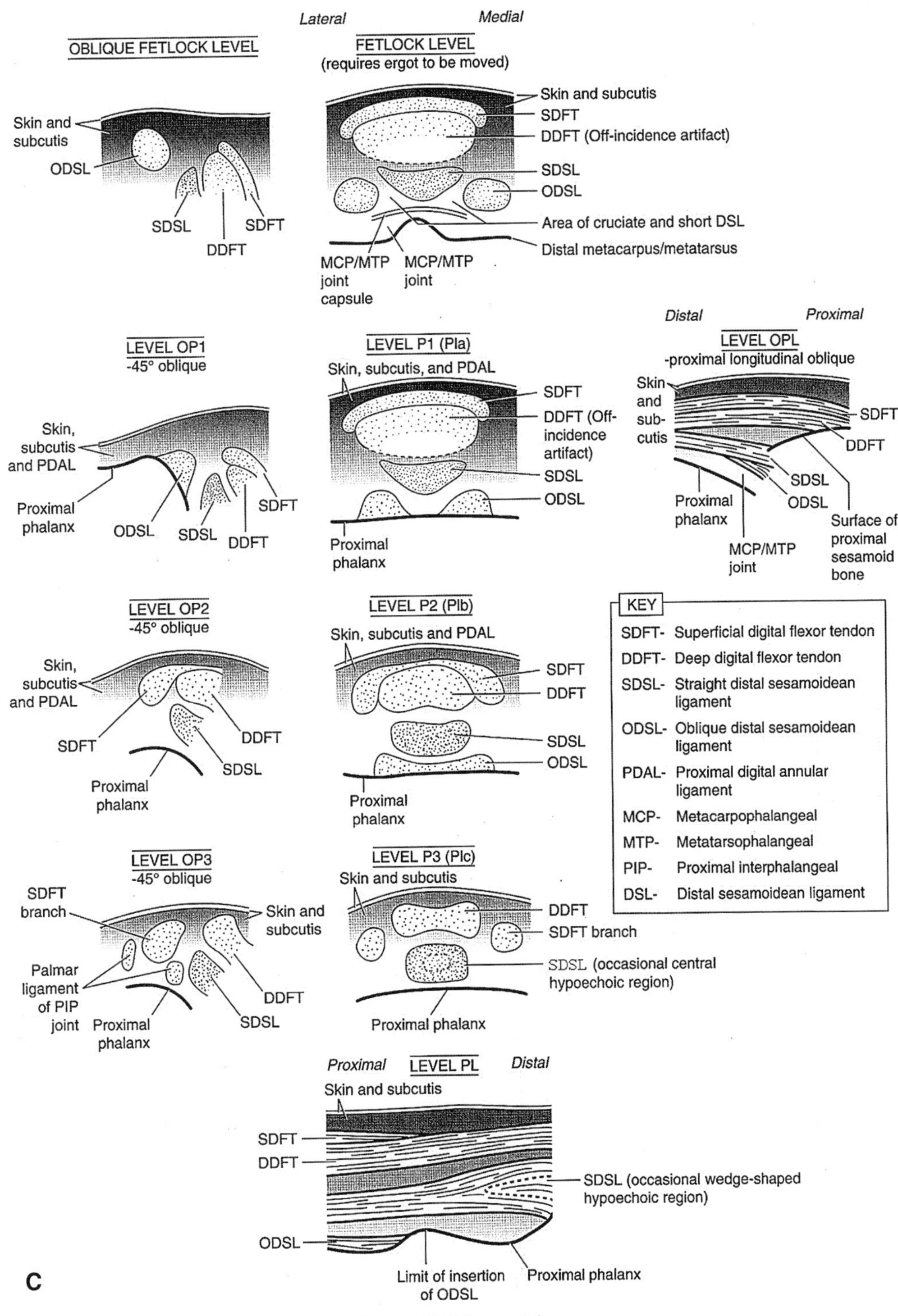

Figure 86-14, cont'd.

echogenicity (often heterogeneous), and an irregular striated pattern is indicative of fibrosis (see Fig. 86-15).

Ultrasonography is particularly useful for the assessment of tendon lacerations, which are associated with small wounds that limit digital exploration. However, ultrasonographic assessment may be impeded because of air artifacts and skin contusions.

Molecular Markers

Molecular markers have the potential to contribute four useful parameters to the evaluation of equine tendon disease. First, they may be used to provide a diagnosis when other diagnostic tests are negative (rarely needed for first-time injuries of the SDFT, but may be useful for detecting re-injury). In this respect, they also may be useful for screening

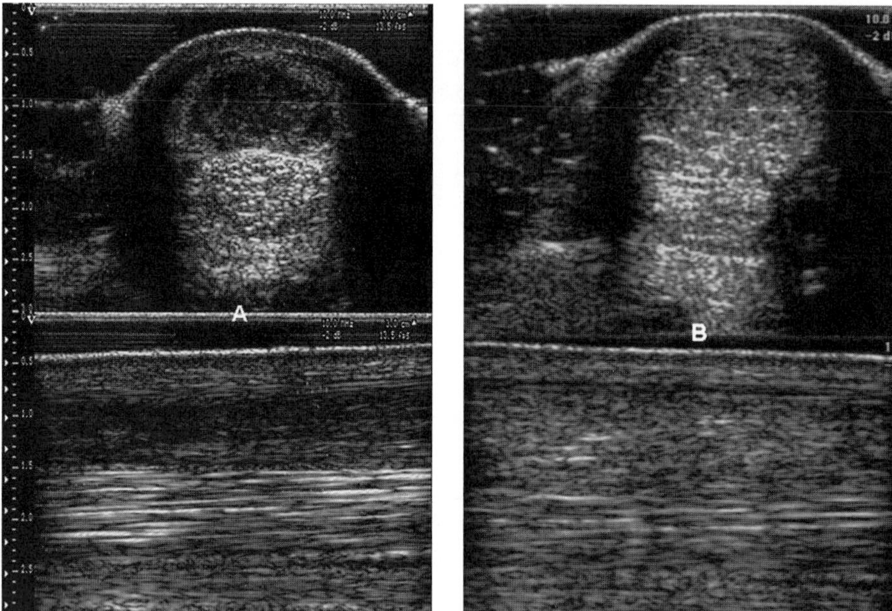

Figure 86-15. Ultrasonographic appearance of superficial digital flexor tendinitis. **A,** Acute injury is manifested by enlargement, a reduction in echogenicity (especially centrally), and a disrupted striated pattern on longitudinal views. **B,** Chronic injury. The tendon is variably echogenic (usually heterogenous), enlarged, and has a poorer striated pattern than normal tendon, which is thought to represent the quality of the healed tendon.

as part of a preventative strategy: early detection may enable preventative measures (e.g., altered training) to be introduced to minimize the risk of provoking a career-ending injury. Second, they may allow a more objective assessment of the severity of the pathology and therefore help to determine prognosis. Third, they may give information about the stage of the disease process, optimizing rehabilitation protocols. Finally, they may assist in the choice of treatment and provide an objective assessment of its efficacy.

To date, the diagnosis and assessment of stage, severity, and prognosis of equine tendinitis have been correlated to semiquantitative ultrasonographic changes,[45] but this procedure is time consuming and has a relatively low sensitivity. In contrast, molecular markers have the potential to reflect specific processes, anabolic or catabolic, within the tissue of interest. Initial investigations assessed markers of both collagen I synthesis (carboxy-terminal propeptide of type I collagen [PICP]) and degradation (crosslinked carboxy-terminal telopeptide of type I collagen [ICTP]) after tendon injury.[46] Tendinitis resulted in a significant rise in PICP concentrations, whereas ICTP concentrations were not different from those in the control group. These results indicated that serum concentrations of PICP are able to reflect changes in type I collagen formation in healing connective tissue in one area of the body. The results also suggest that PICP is not an entirely bone-specific marker if repair in tissues other than bone can contribute to concentrations in serum.

Another candidate, COMP, which is abundant in young tendon, also has been assessed.[47] Synovial fluid levels were more than 10-fold higher than serum levels, and they were significantly raised only when tendon damage or sepsis was present within the tendon sheath. However, serum COMP levels were not significantly elevated with tendon disease, which is related to high natural levels of COMP in blood. Longitudinal studies with this marker have shown variable results, but rather than reflecting specific tendon pathology, serum COMP levels might be more useful for detecting joint disease or for determining whether training levels are too excessive and are damaging multiple soft tissues.

Clinical Characteristics of Specific Strain-Induced Injuries

For the SDFT, the clinical injury may be focal or generalized, one of the more common manifestations being a centrally located region of injury (the so-called core lesion seen ultrasonographically). Usually, the most severe level is located just below the mid-metacarpal region, but it can extend throughout most of the length of the metacarpal extrasynovial tendon and give rise to swelling on the palmar aspect of the metacarpal region (the "bowed" limb). Regions of the SDFT enclosed within a tendon sheath (carpal sheath proximally, digital sheath distally) are much less often affected, although this can be more common when the metacarpal region was previously injured.

Desmitis of the accessory ligament of the DDFT may occur as an isolated injury or in conjunction with superficial digital flexor tendinitis. Although ponies rarely suffer strain-induced tendinopathies, they do have a relatively high incidence of desmitis of the accessory ligament of the DDFT. Lameness is often mild, or even absent, in this injury. Swelling is restricted to the proximal half of the palmar metacarpus, immediately dorsal to the SDFT and surrounding the DDFT.

The SL can fail at any site along its length. Injury to its proximal region at its attachment onto the palmar/plantar aspect of the third metacarpus/metatarsus is often restricted to this area, whereas injuries to the branches usually occur separate from proximal suspensory desmitis and may extend into the body of the ligament. Some branch injuries may also "tear" into the MCP/MTP joint and result in persistent joint effusion and lameness (Fig. 86-16). Furthermore, the synovial fluid environment dramatically slows down healing processes (see earlier).

In contrast to the SDFT and the SL, the DDFT is most frequently injured within the digital sheath. It is not known whether these injuries have a preceding phase of tendon degeneration, but many are potentially the result of single excessive loading cycles. Two manifestations are seen clinically. The first arises within the substance of the tendon (although it may extend to the borders of the tendon) and is similar to other clinical manifestations of tendinitis.[48] The second arises at the medial or lateral borders of the tendon, usually in the region of the MCP joint.[49] Both lesions are invariably associated with a distended digital sheath, but the latter can be difficult to identify ultrasonographically if the tear does not extend into the body of the tendon (Fig. 86-17).

Other tendons can suffer from strain-induced injury, although much less commonly than that affecting the palmar soft tissue structures of the metacarpus. Ligament injuries tend to occur when the joint they span is loaded inappropriately, resulting in a degree of subluxation or even complete luxation.

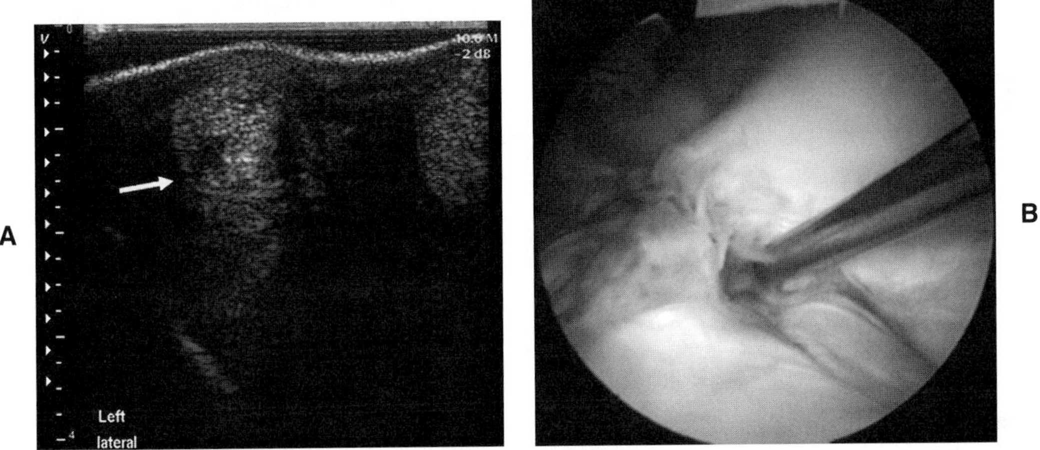

Figure 86-16. A, A hypoechoic defect *(arrow)* in the lateral suspensory ligament branch, which communicates with the metacarpophalangeal joint, causing joint distention, persistent lameness, and slow healing. **B,** This communication was confirmed by arthroscopy.

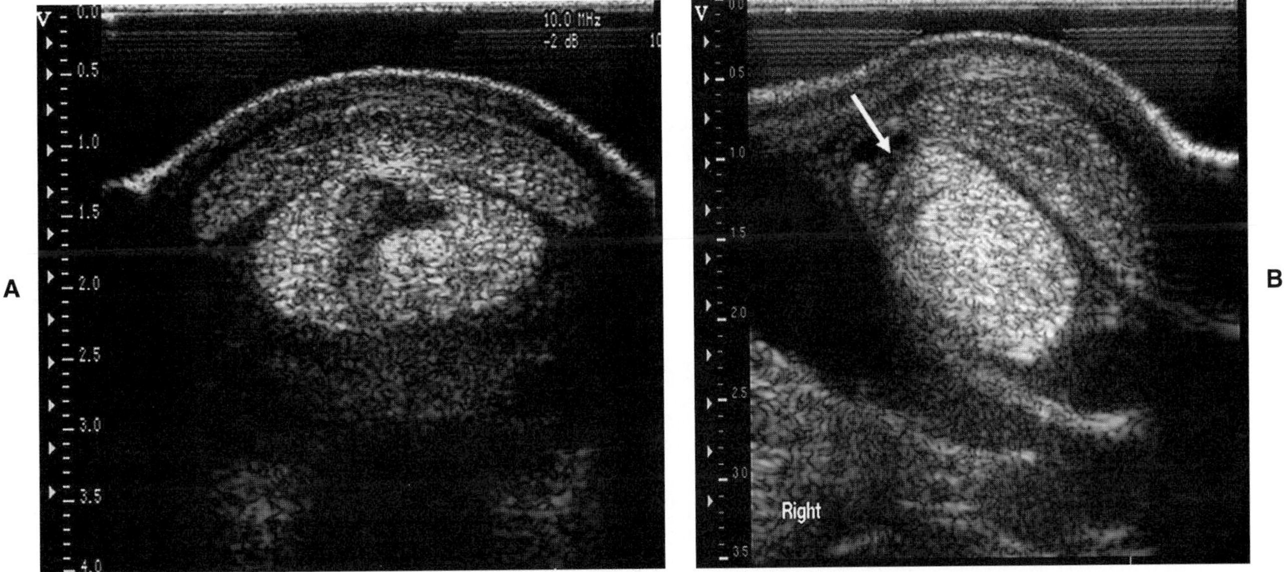

Figure 86-17. Deep digital flexor tendon injury. **A,** Mid-substance strain injury, **B,** Surface tear. The surface tear can be easily missed with ultrasonography and requires tenoscopy for confirmation and débridement.

Clinical Characteristics of Specific Tendon Lacerations

Complete transection of specific palmar metacarpal tendons and ligaments produces characteristic alterations in limb conformation, which may indicate the tendon or ligament that has been lacerated (Fig. 86-18). With SDFT laceration, the MCP/MTP joint is hyperextended (dropped) relative to the normal limb when the limb is loaded, but in the standing horse can appear symmetrical to the joint in the contralateral limb. If the SDFT and DDFT are lacerated concurrently, in addition to the signs described for SDFT laceration, the toe will be raised from the ground. If the SL is completely transected in addition to the SDFT and the DDFT, there is complete loss of support of the MCP/MTP joint, which is hyperextended to the extent that the MCP/MTP joint contacts the ground during the stance phase. Complete loss of MTP/MCP joint support often causes the horse to be severely distressed.

Extensor tendon lacerations frequently involve the metacarpal and metatarsal regions, although lacerations proximal to the dorsal aspect of the carpus involving the extensor carpi radialis or common digital extensor tendons are not uncommon. Lacerations proximal to the tarsus may involve the cranialis tibialis, the long digital extensor tendon, or the peroneus tertius tendon. Lacerations of the extensor tendons generally do not result in significant gait abnormalities or lameness, although they may cause the horse to stumble onto the dorsal aspect of the MTP/MCP joint region at a walk and to be unable to protract the limb completely.

TREATMENT OF TENDON AND LIGAMENT INJURIES

Strain-Induced Tendinopathy (Tendinitis)

In 1964, Asheim described the common treatment of tendon and ligament injuries as "phlebotomy, local cooling, plaster bandaging and rest."[50] Over the last 4 decades, many treatments have been proposed for the management of tendon injury, although few, if any, have convincing supporting evidence of efficacy, and some can even be considered deleterious or detrimental to healing. However, the basic principles described by Asheim of cooling, support, and rest remain integral parts of the management protocol. Acute tendon and ligament injuries are medical emergencies requiring prompt and appropriate treatment to reduce inflammation rapidly, since persistent inflammation may be responsible for further damage to the tendon.

Nonsurgical Therapies

PHYSICAL THERAPIES

Cold therapy

In the acute inflammatory phase of tendon injury, cold therapy is an important aspect of treatment because it is both anti-inflammatory and analgesic, largely through its ability to cause vasoconstriction, decrease enzymatic activity, reduce the formation of inflammatory mediators, and slow down nerve conduction.[51] The optimal frequency and duration of cold treatment for musculoskeletal disorders in horses has not been determined. The authors recommend

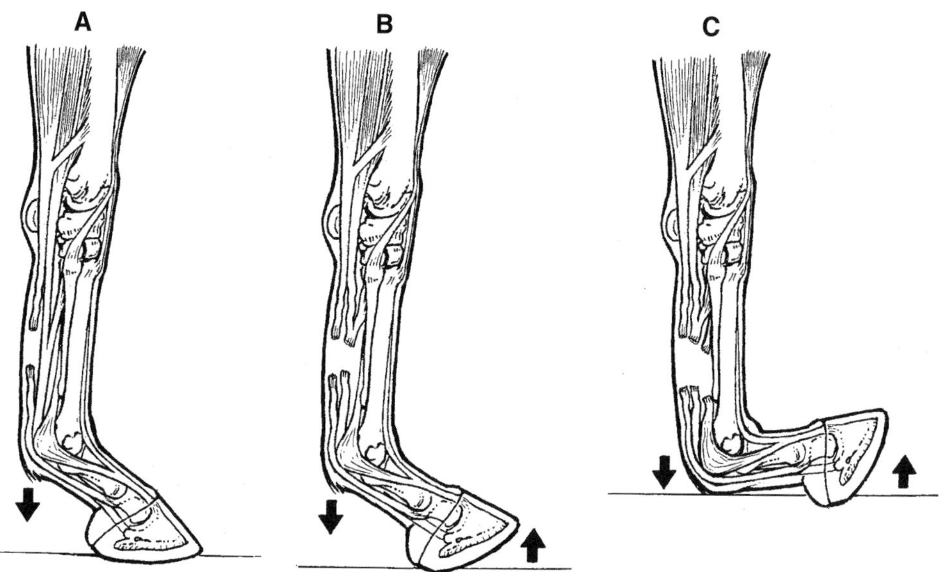

Figure 86-18. A, The relative degree of hyperflexion of the metacarpophalangeal joint when the superficial digital flexor tendon has been transected proximal to the joint. **B,** Relative hyperextension of the joint and elevation of the toe off the ground when both the superficial and the deep digital flexor tendons are transected. **C,** Complete loss of metacarpophalangeal joint support when both digital flexor tendons and the suspensory ligament have been disrupted.

20 minutes of cold hosing several times daily during the acute phase of tendon and ligament injuries.

Research data have indicated that cold hydrotherapy is superior to the use of ice packs because of the increased contact and evaporation.[52] It is also less likely to cause adverse effects such as superficial tissue damage and cold-induced nerve palsy. Prolonged exposure to cold temperatures can also cause a reflex vasodilation, which can accentuate tissue swelling and edema. For this reason, it is recommended not to apply cold therapy for periods longer than 30 minutes. One highly effective way of providing cold hydrotherapy is the use of equine spas, which are currently gaining popularity. They provide both cold and compression using hypertonic saline at 5° to 9° C.[53] In addition to equine spas, underwater treadmills, used as part of controlled exercise programs in tendon and ligament injury rehabilitation, allow conditioning of the musculoskeletal system with minimal concussive forces.

Compression and coaptation

In the acute phase of injury, pressure applied to the affected limb reduces inflammation and edema formation by increasing interstitial hydrostatic pressure. A modified Robert Jones bandage is suitable in most cases of acute tendon and ligament injury.

In severe injuries when there is hyperextension of the MCP joint, a palmar/plantar splint or cast may be applied to the bandaged limb to provide MCP joint support (Fig. 86-19). A palmar splint can be fashioned from two rolls of 7.5-cm (5-inch) casting tape. One roll is layered on top of itself over a length that matches the length of the limb from the carpus to the bulbs of the foot. This is placed on the palmar aspect of a 2.5-cm-thick support bandage on the contralateral limb. The contralateral limb can be used as a template for making the splint, since it has the optimal degree of extension at the MCP joint. A second roll is wrapped around the palmar splint and bandage and left to set. The palmar splint is then cut away from the bandage using a cast saw and applied to the palmar aspect of the bandaged affected limb. A similar effect can be achieved more easily with the specially designed boot, although this is not yet available commercially.[54] A full distal limb cast may be used as an alternative in the most severe cases, such as suspensory ligament rupture, when all MCP joint support has been lost.

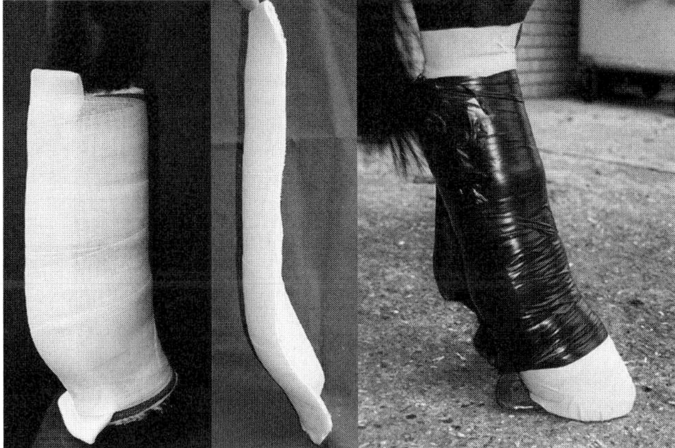

Figure 86-19. The use of a palmar splint to protect overloading of the superficial digital flexor tendon or suspensory ligament. The splint is fashioned out of casting tape on the back of a bandaged limb with normal conformation (either the contralateral limb or a "dummy," as shown here). It is then cut from the limb, the edges are smoothed off, and it is taped to the palmar aspect of the bandaged affected limb. This limb has also been fitted with a heel extension shoe to protect the deep digital flexor tendon, since this was damaged concurrently.

Immediate controlled mobilization

Immediate controlled mobilization of the limb has been advocated in the acute phase of tendon and ligament injury to reduce inflammation and improve healing.[55] This mobilization is obtained by early passive and active movement of the injured tissues. To be successful, the degree or frequency of mobilization must remain below the patient's pain threshold. The mobilization is administered by a 15 minute session of gentle physical therapy, involving series of 10 to 30 passive carpal and MCP joint flexions, interspersed with short breaks, for the first 72 hours.

Controlled exercise

Controlled exercise is an intrinsic part of the rehabilitation of tendon and ligament injuries, helping to resolve residual inflammation, maintain gliding function, and promote optimal collagen remodeling.[56] Most SDFT injuries require at least 8 to 9 months of rehabilitation before resumption of full athletic function, although some may require up to 18 months. It is rarely necessary to prolong rehabilitation longer than this, because healing appears to be complete by this stage.

A suitable exercise rehabilitation program should be created on the basis of the severity of the ultrasonographic appearance of the lesion. The aim of the program is to provide a controlled and ascending exercise regimen that optimizes scar tissue function without causing further injury. Since this is difficult to predict because of variability between animals, the program should be adapted on the basis of serial ultrasonographic monitoring and clinical signs such as lameness, heat, and swelling.

Ultrasonographic monitoring of the tendon or ligament injuries should include measurements of tendon cross-sectional area (CSA). An increase in CSA of greater than 10% between examinations would suggest a degree of reinjury, and in such cases the level of exercise should be reduced. Because there is a sudden increase in strain levels in the SDFT and SL with an upward transition in gait from walk to trot, trot to canter, and canter to gallop, ultrasonographic examinations before and after these transitions can help to determine if the injured tendon or ligament can withstand the increased strain levels.

The importance of a controlled exercise program was illustrated by Gillis, who demonstrated that of 28 Thoroughbred racehorses with SDFT tendinitis placed in a controlled exercise program, 71% returned to racing, compared with only 25% of 8 horses managed with uncontrolled turnout.[56] An example of rehabilitation programs for racehorses and sports horses is shown in Table 86-1.

TABLE 86-1. Typical Exercise Program* after Tendon Injury

Exercise Level	Weeks	Duration and Nature of Exercise
0	0-2	Box rest
1	3	10 minutes walking daily
1	4	15 minutes walking daily
1	5	20 minutes walking daily
1	6	25 minutes walking daily
1	7	30 minutes walking daily
1	8	35 minutes walking daily
1	9	40 minutes walking daily
1	10-12	45 minutes walking daily
WEEK 12: REPEAT ULTRASOUND EXAMINATION		
2	13-16	40 minutes walking and 5 minutes trotting daily
2	17-20	35 minutes walking and 10 minutes trotting daily
2	21-24	30 minutes walking and 15 minutes trotting daily
WEEK 24: REPEAT ULTRASOUND EXAMINATION		
2	25-28	25 minutes walking and 20 minutes trotting daily
2	29-32	20 minutes walking and 25 minutes trotting daily
WEEK 32: REPEAT ULTRASOUND EXAMINATION		
3	33-40	45 minutes exercise daily with slow canter, gradually increasing in amount
3	41-48	45 minutes exercise daily with fast work three times a week
WEEK 48: REPEAT ULTRASOUND EXAMINATION		
4	48+	Return to full competition/ race training

*This program is shortened or lengthened depending on the severity of the lesion and the progress of the patient.

Extracorporeal shock wave therapy

Extracorporeal shock wave therapy (ECSWT) has been established for a number of years for the treatment of human orthopedic conditions, especially insertional desmopathies. ECSWT involves the use of shock or pressure waves that are transmitted into the tissues to which the hand piece is applied. Both focused and nonfocused units have been used, although the data that compare these machines are too limited to indicate a significant difference. The mechanism of action of ECSWT on tissues is unclear, but it is most likely related to induction of analgesia through an effect on sensory nerves.[57] The most frequently reported use of ECSWT in horses has been for the treatment of proximal SL desmitis, and a significant improvement in prognosis over conservative treatment for chronic hindlimb proximal SL desmitis has been reported. Investigation into ECSWT as a treatment for chronic SL desmitis resulted in 41% of hindlimb cases returning to full work within 6 months of diagnosis,[58] compared with the previously reported 13% for conservatively managed cases.[59]

Therapeutic ultrasound, laser, and magnetic fields

The effect of ultrasound, laser, and magnetic fields on tissues is not completely understood. It is thought that the main effect of ultrasound is the conversion of sound energy into thermal energy. Although there is a paucity of scientifically convincing research into the effects of ultrasound for the treatment of equine musculoskeletal disorders, a study by Morcos and Aswad showed that in experimentally split equine tendons, the use of therapeutic ultrasound resulted in increased vascularization and fibroblastic proliferation compared with controls.[60]

Low-level laser (light amplification by stimulated emission of radiation) therapy has been shown to stimulate cellular metabolism and to enhance fibroblast proliferation and collagen synthesis in vitro.[61] However, there are no clinical trials demonstrating a significant difference between laser-treated and control cases of tendinitis or desmitis.

Magnetic therapy has not been demonstrated in any clinical trials to enhance tendon or ligament healing, despite its widespread use by horse owners and anecdotal reports of its efficacy.

Counter-irritation

Counter-irritation, in the form of chemical or thermal cauterization, has long been used in equine practice for the treatment of tendon and ligament injuries. Topical iodine and mercury-based compounds have been used for chemical cauterization or "blistering" of tendon injuries. Thermal cauterization (or "firing") is performed under general anesthesia or standing sedation with local analgesia, using heated bars or pins, which are applied to the skin over the injured tendon or ligament. In some cases, the tendon is penetrated with the heated pins. Studies have shown that there is no histologic difference between the collagen arrangement in the scar in cases of tendinitis treated with firing and that of the controls.[62] It has been postulated that any benefits from firing result from the enforced rest, the local release of inflammatory cytokines, or a protective "bandage" of fibrous tissue or skin that supports the tendon. However, it has been demonstrated that firing causes thinner and weaker skin in the region that was cauterized.[62] The limited controlled studies that have been performed on firing have concluded that it is not an effective treatment for tendon and ligament injuries.

PHARMACOLOGIC MANAGEMENT

Systemic medication

Both systemic corticosteroids and nonsteroidal anti-inflammatory drugs can be considered for the management of tendon or ligament inflammation in the acute stages. Phenylbutazone is commonly used at a dose of 2.2 mg/kg twice daily, but the clinical effects of this drug appear to be more analgesic than anti-inflammatory.[63] Systemic steroids can be administered within the first 24 to 48 hours after injury, but they should be avoided after this time because they also inhibit fibroplasia and hence repair of the tendon. The most commonly used systemic steroid is dexamethasone at 0.1 mg/kg as a single dose. The induction of laminitis with systemic steroids represents a small, but nevertheless real, risk. Topical or intravenous dimethyl sulfoxide (DMSO) may reduce the inflammation, but a study has shown that 40% to 90% topical medical grade DMSO may weaken normal tendon tissue.[64]

Intralesional medication

Various intralesional treatments have been advocated for the management of tendinitis. These treatments include polysulfated glycosaminoglycans (PSGAGs), hyaluronan (HA), and beta-aminopropionitrile fumarate, with recent interest being focused on novel growth factor and cell-based therapies. Intralesional tendon and ligament treatment can be performed under standing sedation and local analgesia, or under general anesthesia. Weightbearing potentially assists injection, since the tendons are then taut. Although the technique is frequently performed blindly, by injecting where the least resistance in the tendon is detected, accurate placement of the needle in the center of the lesion is best achieved using ultrasonographic guidance. The skin overlying the tendon or ligament to be injected should be clipped and aseptically prepared, and if ultrasonographic guidance is used, a sterile sleeve should be placed over the probe. A 2.5-cm, 23-gauge hypodermic needle can be used for most intratendinous treatments, but this depends on the viscosity of the agent. Intralesional treatment should not be administered until 3 days after the injury, because there is the potential to increase hemorrhage. The volume injected into the tendon or ligament will depend on the extent of the lesion. Large volumes can be damaging to the healing tendon.[65]

PSGAGs have been shown to inhibit collagenases and metalloproteinases and to inhibit macrophage activation,[5] but they were shown to have no effect on fibroblasts.[66] Hence, this drug can be viewed as a soft tissue anti-inflammatory agent. PSGAGs have been widely used for the treatment of tendinitis and desmitis, both intralesionally and intramuscularly. In one study of 73 horses, treatment with PSGAG either intramuscularly or intralesionally resulted in 76% of horses returning to work versus 46% of the control animals, although these results were not statistically significant.[67] Another study demonstrated improved echogenicity of collagenase-induced superficial digital flexor tendinitis treated with intralesional PSGAGs, with faster resolution of core lesions.[68] However, Dyson demonstrated no significant difference in reinjury rates between horses treated with PSGAGs and those treated with controlled exercise alone.[69]

HA consists of repeating units of D-glucuronic acid and repeating units of *N*-acetyl-D-glucosamine and is a component of the tendon matrix. HA has been administered peritendinously, intralesionally, and systemically to treat tendinitis. A study by Dyson showed no significant difference between the reinjury rates of horses with SDFT tendinitis treated with intralesional HA and those treated conservatively.[69] In a study of collagenase-induced digital flexor tendinitis, HA was found to minimize tendon enlargement compared with controls, although histopathologic examination of the tendons failed to demonstrate a significant difference in the degree of inflammation.[70] Peritendinous HA has been shown to have no effect on ultrasonographic or histologic appearance, biomechanical properties, or molecular composition of tendons in collagenase-induced tendinitis compared with controls, although it did appear to reduce lameness.[71]

HA has been shown to decrease the extent of adhesions when administered intrathecally to treat collagenase-induced deep digital flexor tendinitis within the digital sheath.[72] Horses treated with intrathecal HA showed decreased inflammatory cell infiltrate and less intratendinous hemorrhage than controls.[72]

Methylprednisolone injected into and around normal equine tendons has been shown to cause dystrophic tissue mineralization and tissue necrosis, most likely a consequence of the carrier.[73] Hence, the local use of this steroid should be avoided. Nondepot preparations may be used peritendinously with caution.

Intralesional *beta-aminopropionitrile fumarate* (BAPN) has been used to treat tendinitis 30 to 60 days after injury. BAPN (derived from *Lathyrus odoratus* [sweet pea]), inhibits the enzyme lysyl oxidase, which normally forms crosslinks between collagen fibers. The rationale for its use is to allow exercise to promote alignment of newly formed collagen fibrils while preventing them from being fixed in a haphazard fashion by crosslinking. BAPN does not hasten the resolution of the tendinitis but aims to improve the structure of the repaired tendon.

Initial studies by Genovese on the effect of BAPN for the treatment of tendinitis demonstrated that 80% of tendons treated with BAPN had normal ultrasonographic echogenicity 20 weeks after injury, compared with only 29% of control cases.[74] However, long-term follow-up results of horses with SDFT tendinitis treated with BAPN based on return to racing showed less favorable results: 67% (56/84) of horses returned to racing, with 50% (42/84) of horses racing five times or more.[75]

Although in collagenase-induced models of tendinitis, both the ultrasonographic appearance[76] and the histologic collagen alignment were superior in BAPN-treated horses compared with controls,[77] more recent concerns have been raised over its efficacy, based on observations that BAPN reduces collagen synthesis[78] and showed no improvement over controls in a rabbit model of tendinitis.[79] Nevertheless, Dyson compared the re-injury rate of horses with SDFT tendinitis treated with either BAPN or PSGAGs combined with controlled exercise, with the re-injury rate of controlled exercise alone, and the use of BAPN resulted in a decreased re-injury rate; however, the long-term injury rate of the untreated limb was high.[69] On the basis of this information, Dyson recommended treatment of both limbs even if there was no ultrasonographic evidence of tendon damage on the contralateral limb.[69] BAPN treatment is most appropriate in cases of severe tendinitis with an extensive core lesion, when there is potentially a greater volume of scar tissue that will be synthesized.

New advances: Tissue engineering approaches

The use of *growth factors* is a relatively recent approach. Insulin-like growth factor-1 (IGF-1) has been investigated to assess its effect on tendon healing both in vitro and in collagenase-induced models of tendinitis.[80] IGF-1 stimulates extracellular tendon matrix synthesis, and it is also a potent mitogen.[80] In collagenase-induced models of tendinitis, initial swelling was decreased after intralesional injections of IGF-1 compared with controls, although no differences were found at later time points and there was no difference between the quantities of type I and type III collagen synthesized.[80] There are no published long-term follow-up data regarding reinjury rates of tendinitis treated with IGF-1.

Recombinant equine growth hormone administered intramuscularly has demonstrated a negative effect on the biomechanical properties (decreased yield point and ultimate tensile strength) of the SDFT during the early phases of healing in collagenase induced tendinitis.[81] However, these properties were assessed at 6 weeks after treatment, which may have been too soon to detect any beneficial effects.

TGF-β has been considered as another appropriate growth factor treatment, but clinical experience has been limited. Treated horses showed significant enlargement of the tendon and, although reinjury rates were similar to those in conservatively managed horses, these reinjuries were all on contralateral, untreated, limbs.[82]

A Cell Vet is a novel intralesional treatment for tendinitis using acellular tissue components derived from porcine urinary bladder submucosa. This preparation has been suggested to deliver appropriate growth factors to the injured tissue and to attract mesenchymal stem cells. There is only anecdotal evidence that this treatment improves tendon and ligament healing, and controlled clinical trials are required to further assess efficacy.

Treatment with intralesional *bone marrow* has been investigated for SL desmitis.[83] The aim was to stimulate ligament regeneration rather than scar tissue formation by the delivery of stem cells to the damaged tendon or ligament. Bone marrow is a rich source of growth factors[84] but contains very few stem cells (1 in 10^4 nucleated cells). Hence, this treatment more closely resembles a growth factor treatment.

In a survey of clinical cases, 84% of horses treated with intralesional bone marrow were reported to return to the preinjury level of exercise, whereas only 15% of control cases achieved this.[83] However, no information was provided about the specific location of the SL injury, or whether lesions were located in the hindlimb or forelimb, which has a significant effect on prognosis. Furthermore, the large volumes of bone marrow used (30 to 50 mL) and the presence of other cells and material may have deleterious effects on the healing tendon or ligament tissue surrounding the lesion.

The use of autologous mesenchymal stem cells (MSCs) for intralesional treatment of SDFT and SL lesions is currently being investigated. MSCs have the potential to differentiate into tenocytes and to regenerate tendon matrix, thereby creating a repair that is functionally superior to fibrous scar tissue. Initial studies have included the isolation of MSCs from either bone marrow or fat, followed by either direct implantation or expansion of MSC numbers in vitro before implantation.[85] No controlled studies have been published to prove efficacy, although anecdotal clinical evidence has been encouraging.

Surgical Therapies

TENDON SPLITTING

Tendon splitting was first performed in the 1940s and the technique was published in 1967.[86] It was initially advocated as a treatment for chronic tendinitis to improve blood flow to damaged tendon tissue that is relatively avascular. The technique fell out of favor when subsequent research demonstrated extensive granulation tissue formation, and increased trauma to the tendon tissue and persistent lameness after treatment.[87] Tendon splitting is therefore no longer recommended for the treatment of chronic tendinitis but is now thought to be more relevant to the management of acute cases when there is an anechoic core lesion evident on ultrasonographic examination, indicating the presence of a seroma or hematoma. It has been hypothesized that the presence of a core lesion within a tendon produces a compartment syndrome, resulting in decreased perfusion and ischemia of the region.[88] The aim of tendon splitting in acute cases is therefore to decompress the core lesion by evacuating the serum or hemorrhage and to facilitate vascular ingrowth.[88] Removal of the fluid in the core lesion may also reduce proximodistal propagation of the lesion. In a collagenase-induced model of tendinitis in six horses, tendon splitting using the knife technique resulted in a faster resolution of the core lesion, quicker revascularization of the lesion, and increased collagen deposition than in controls.[89]

Tendon splitting may be performed under standing sedation or under general anesthesia. It can be done blindly or using ultrasonographic guidance, which minimizes damage to normal tendon tissue by enabling the needle or knife to be inserted at a point where the core lesion is closest to the periphery of the tendon. A no. 11 scalpel blade or double-edged blade is inserted into the tendon and "fanned" proximally and distally (Fig. 86-20). Alternatively, the procedure can be achieved with multiple insertions of a 23-gauge needle, possibly with less damage to the remaining, relatively intact, tendon tissue. Furthermore, needle splitting may be combined with various intralesional treatments.

After tendon splitting has been performed, a modified Robert Jones bandage should be applied and the horse rested in a stall for 10 to 14 days, after which a controlled exercise program should be initiated.

DESMOTOMY OF THE ACCESSORY LIGAMENT OF THE SDFT

Superior check ligament desmotomy was first described as a treatment for SDFT tendinitis by Bramlage in 1986.[90] The aim of the surgery is to produce a functionally longer musculotendinous unit to reduce strain on the SDFT. However, it has been shown in equine cadaver models that desmotomy of the accessory ligament of the SDFT (DALSDFT) actually increases the strain on the SDFT during loading because of increased extension of the MCP joint.[91] The biomechanical alterations of DALSDFT thus are complex, and studies using cadaver limbs may not represent the biomechanical events in a fatigued galloping racehorse. However, increased risk of injury of the suspensory ligament after the DALSDFT has been performed has also been demonstrated in vivo.[92]

Initial results from Bramlage demonstrated that 79% of horses suffering from superficial digital flexor tendinitis

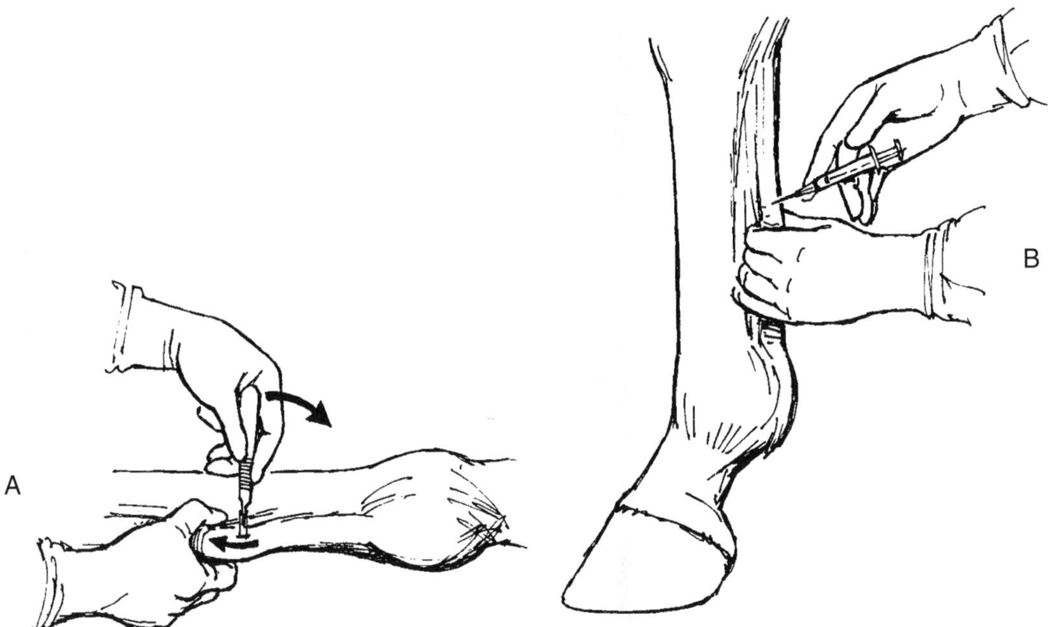

Figure 86-20. Tendon splitting can be performed with a blade (**A**) or with needles (**B**). With needles, the splitting procedure can be combined with an intratendinous treatment, if appropriate.

treated with DALSDFT competed in two races without recurrent tendinitis.[90]

DALSDFT can be performed with the horse in lateral or dorsal recumbency. A 10-cm skin incision is made between the cephalic vein and the caudal radius on the medial aspect of the limb. The incision should extend from the level of the medial malleolus of the radius, to mid-chestnut proximally (see Fig. 90-14). A transverse branch of the cephalic vein may require ligation to improve access. The cephalic vein is retracted caudally to expose the flexor carpi radialis (FCR) sheath, which is incised to reveal the FCR tendon. The FCR tendon is retracted caudally to expose the accessory ligament of the SDFT, which is located adherent to and deep to the lateral aspect of the FCR sheath. Both the transverse and the deeper oblique fibers of the accessory ligament of the SDFT are transected sharply with or without the assistance of forceps to elevate the latter. Ideally, the artery and vein of the proximal SDFT are identified on the proximal border of the accessory ligament and preserved.[93]

The FCR sheath and the fascia should be closed in two layers using a simple-interrupted pattern and with 2-0 or 0 synthetic absorbable suture material for each layer (e.g., polyglactin 910). The skin is then closed with a simple-interrupted or vertical mattress suture pattern using 2-0 or 0 nonabsorbable material (e.g., monofilament nylon).

A well-padded bandage capable of providing compression is applied over a sterile dressing for 10 to 14 days to reduce the risk of seroma formation at the surgical site, which is a common complication of this procedure. The initial rehabilitation period involves 2 weeks of stall rest, followed by a controlled exercise program as previously described.

More recently, this procedure has been carried out tenoscopically through the carpal sheath.[94] With the affected limb uppermost and partially flexed, an arthroscopic portal is created into the carpal sheath 2 cm proximal to the distal radial physis on the lateral side of the limb (Fig. 86-21). An instrument portal is made immediately proximal to the distal radial physis. With the limb in 90 degrees of flexion, the accessory ligament is visualized on the medial aspect of the sheath and cut using a no. 10 scalpel blade on a long handle, or meniscectomy knife. The very proximal portion of the ligament cannot be visualized directly but is transected by careful dissection using punch biopsy forceps, taking care to avoid the perforating blood vessel at the proximal limit of the accessory ligament.

TENOSCOPY

The increasingly widespread use of tenoscopy has demonstrated a high frequency of intrathecal tendon tears that are associated with tenosynovitis and lameness. Hence, horses presenting with tenosynovitis with pain on palpation of the proximal digital sheath and lameness should always be considered candidates for tenoscopic evaluation. Based on a recent survey of cases, tears in the DDFT are more commonly found in forelimb digital sheaths, whereas tears to the manica flexoria are more commonly found in hindlimbs (Fig. 86-22). Ultrasonographic evaluation usually reveals nonspecific changes of synovial hypertrophy, and it is frequently not possible to identify tears on ultrasonographic examination with confidence. However, when a tendon tear extends into the center of the tendon, it can be identified as an anechoic lesion (since it is filled with synovial fluid). Manica tears are particularly difficult to identify ultrasonographically, but occasionally disruption of the attachment of the manica to the SDFT can be demonstrated. In addition, tears can also be found and débrided tenoscopically in the SDFT and in the distal sesamoidean ligaments within the digital sheath. Tears of other tendons and ligaments communicating with a synovial cavity have been seen to be associated with synovial distention and lameness (e.g., in

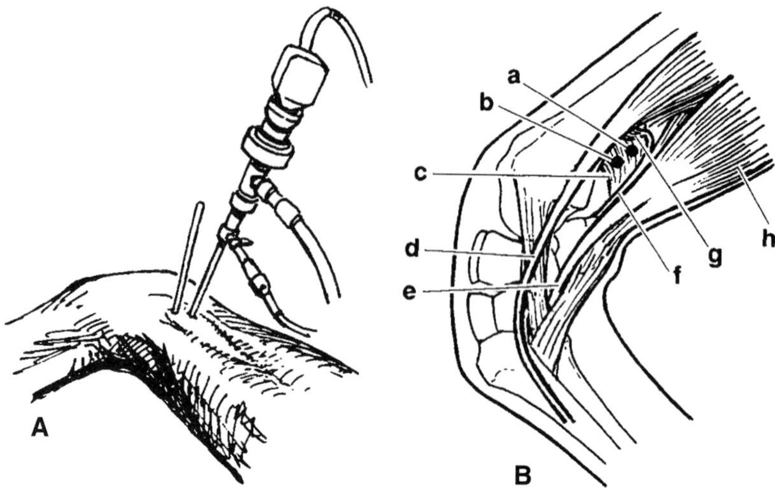

Figure 86-21. Site for tenoscopic transection of the accessory ligament of the superficial digital flexor tendon (superior check ligament desmotomy). a. arthroscopic portal; b, egress/instrument portal; c, accessory ligament of the tendon of the superficial digital flexor muscle; d, tendon of the laterall digital extensor muscle; e, tendon of the ulnaris lateralis muscle; f, tendon of the deep digital flexor muscle; g, radial head of deep digital flexor muscle; h, superficial digital flexor muscle. (From Southwood LL, Stashak TS, Kainer RA: Tenoscopic anatomy of the equine carpal flexor synovial sheath, Vet Surg 1998;27:152.)

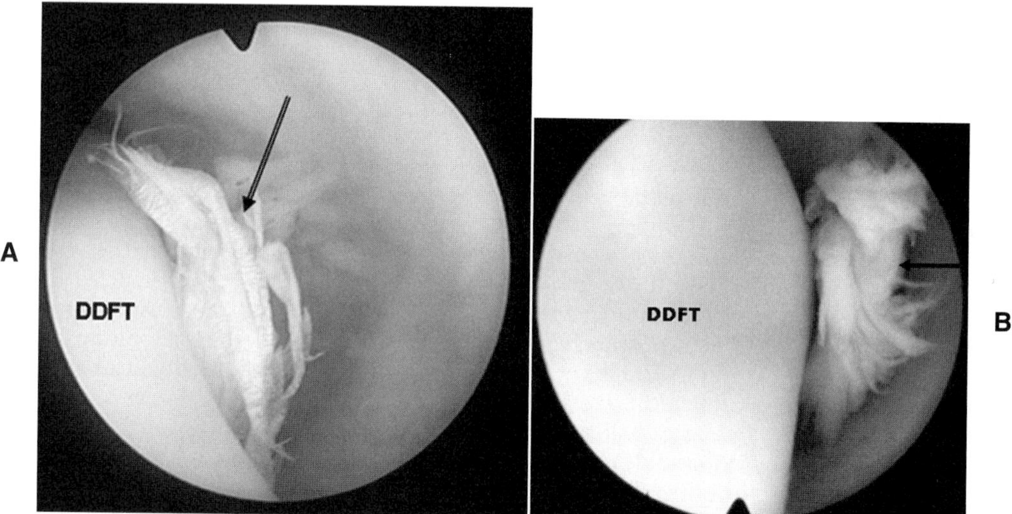

Figure 86-22. Common abnormalities detected as causing tenosynovitis of the digital sheath. **A,** Surface tear of the deep digital flexor tendon, most commonly found in forelimb tenosynovitis. **B,** Rupture of the attachments of the manica flexoria, most frequently seen in hindlimb tenosynovitis.

the suspensory ligament branches into the MCP/MTP joint) (see Fig. 86-16).

Tenoscopy of the digital sheath requires general anesthesia and can be performed in lateral or dorsal recumbency. However, dorsal recumbency allows easier access to both sides of the digital sheath and is recommended. Arthroscopic portals are created immediately distal to the proximal sesamoid and 1 to 2 cm palmar/plantar to the neurovascular bundle[95] (Fig. 86-23). This allows evaluation of the proximal and distal parts of the digital sheath, although distal visualization can sometimes be easier with the arthroscope inserted through a portal in the proximal digital sheath (e.g., as for a proximal instrument portal). Instrument portals are created where appropriate to allow débridement of any tendon tears with a mechanical resector. This may require the instrument portals to be extended through the synovial reflection that attaches to the proximal border of the manica flexoria to allow access to DDFT tears located within or proximal to the manica. Although manica tears can also be débrided as is done for DDFT tears, this has been associated with poorer outcome than complete removal. As no adverse effects have been observed with complete removal, this is recommended for all but the most minor manica tears. Removal requires transection of both medial and lateral attachments to the SDFT, as well as transection of the synovial attachment to the proximal border of the manica. This is facilitated by an assistant who maintains tension on the manica with rongeurs through the contra-axial proximal instrument portal. Transection can be achieved with arthroscopic scissors, bistoury, or a hook knife.

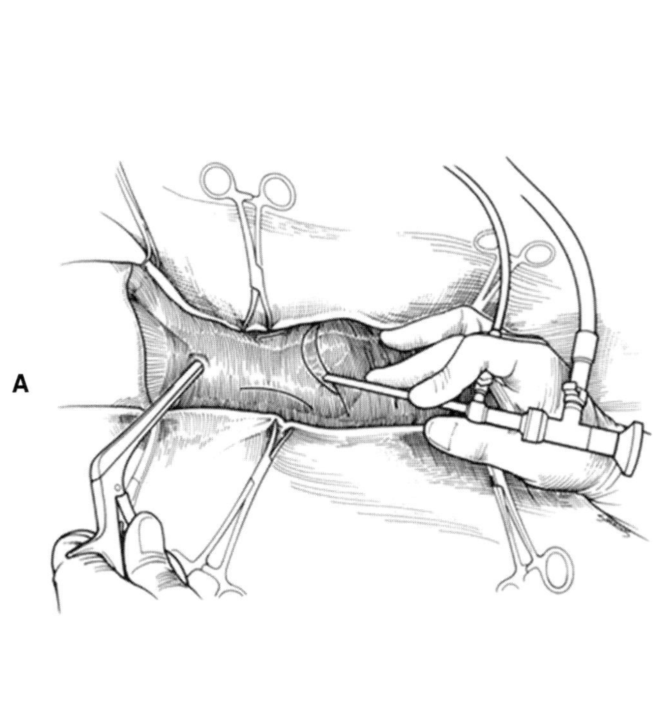

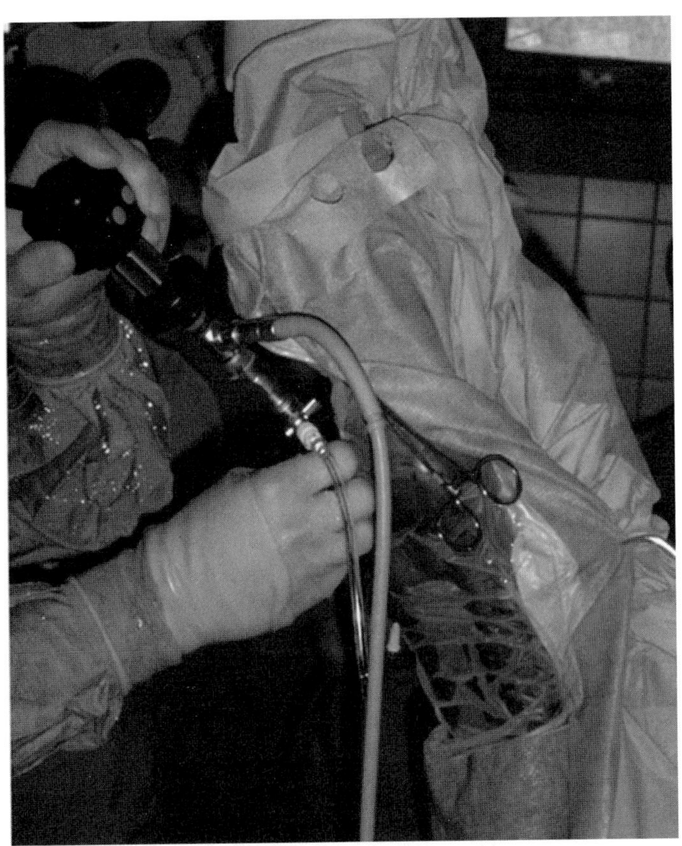

Figure 86-23. Tenoscopy of the digital sheath, now a routine procedure. **A,** The original description was in lateral recumbency, and the arthroscope was introduced into the digital sheath immediately distal to the palmar annular ligament, 1 to 2 cm palmar to the neurovascular bundle. **B,** However, dorsal recumbency allows more flexibility to evaluate both sides of the digital sheath and easier bilateral approach for surgical removal of the manica flexoria. (From Nixon AJ: Endoscopy of the digital flexor tendon sheath in horses, Vet Surg 1990;19:267.)

Chronic tenosynovitis can be associated with synovial masses attached to the synovial plicae in the proximal digital sheath. These, together with isolated adhesions, can also be resected during tenoscopic evaluation and the palmar or plantar annular ligament transected if it is believed to be involved in the pathology (Fig. 86-24). Postoperatively, the horse should be strictly rested for at least 2 weeks, after which hand-walking can be started and gradually increased over a period of at least 6 weeks. Thereafter, the duration of rehabilitation depends of the severity of the injury. The prognosis for simple DDFT tears (about 40%) is worse than for simple manica tears (about 80%).[96]

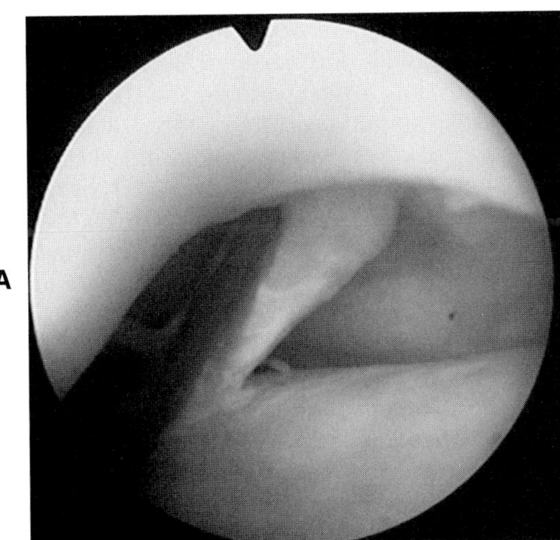

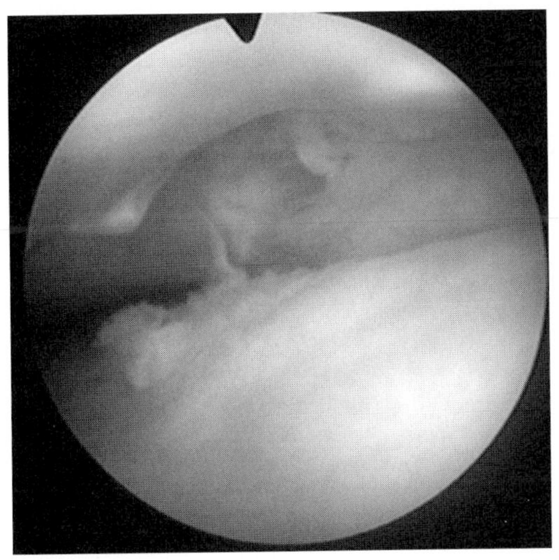

Figure 86-24. Tenoscopic resection of an adhesion. If adhesions are isolated findings (**A**), they can be removed using a mechanical resector (**B**). Care should be taken to avoid disrupting large areas of the synovium, or adhesion formation may be even more exaggerated after surgery.

ANNULAR LIGAMENT DESMOTOMY

Annular ligament desmotomy has been advocated for the management of DDFT and SDFT lesions in the region of the MCP and MTP joints. The procedure is indicated if the annular ligament is impeding the normal gliding function of the flexor tendons. Annular ligament desmotomy is performed under general anesthesia and is ideally performed tenoscopically using a hook knife with or without a slotted cannula (Fig. 86-25), rather than via closed or open techniques, because it is less traumatic, ensures accurate transection of only the palmar or plantar annular ligament, and allows evaluation of the tendons to identify any surface defects. For a more detailed discussion of annular ligament desmotomy and its indication, please review Chapter 94.

FASCIOTOMY AND NEURECTOMY OF THE DEEP BRANCH OF THE LATERAL PLANTAR NERVE FOR THE TREATMENT OF PSLD

Surgery has been advocated in cases of proximal suspensory ligament desmitis (PSLD) of the hindlimb that are unresponsive to conservative management. It has been reported that horses have returned to high-level competition after tibial neurectomy to treat PSLD.[97] However, a more specific neurectomy of the deep branch of the plantar nerve has recently been described.[98] This is performed under general anesthesia with the horse in dorsal recumbency. A 4- to 6-cm incision is made adjacent to the lateral border of the SDFT, originating proximally from the level of the chestnut (Fig. 86-26). The plantar metatarsal fascia is incised and the incision extended deep to the SDFT by blunt dissection, facilitated by retraction of the SDFT. The lateral plantar nerve is located in connective tissue, the deep branch is identified and transected using a scalpel, and a 3-cm section is removed. The connective tissue fascia covering the suspensory ligament is cut (fasciotomy) adjacent to the lateral splint bone to decompress the origin of the suspensory ligament, since hindlimb proximal suspensory desmitis is believed to be associated with a compressive compartment syndrome involving the plantar metatarsal nerves.

Postoperatively, only a short period of strict rest is needed (about 2 weeks) to allow the surgical incisions to heal. Thereafter, the horse can gradually begin a controlled ascending exercise program. Nonpublished reports have suggested that this technique is associated with a high level

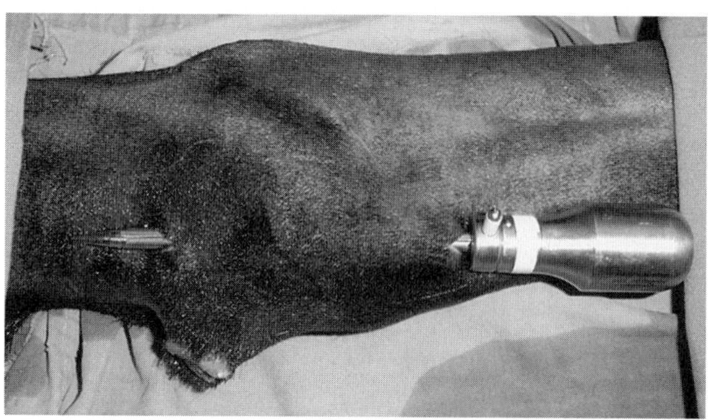

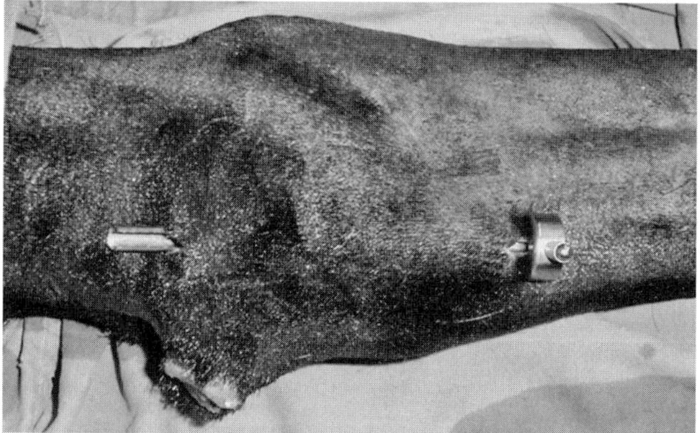

Figure 86-25. The use of the slotted cannula for transection of the palmar annular ligament. The cannula is guided through the sheath from proximal to distal under arthroscopic control to ensure that it does not lie inside the manica flexoria. The central obturator is removed and a hook knife is introduced to cut the palmar annular ligament via the slot in the cannula. This can be introduced from either a proximal or a distal direction, with the arthroscope (without its sleeve) in the opposite end to view the procedure. This technique allows closed and accurate transection of the ligament without damaging other structures.

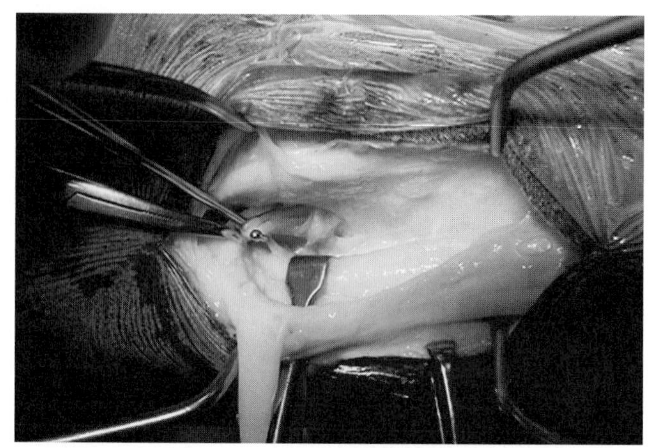

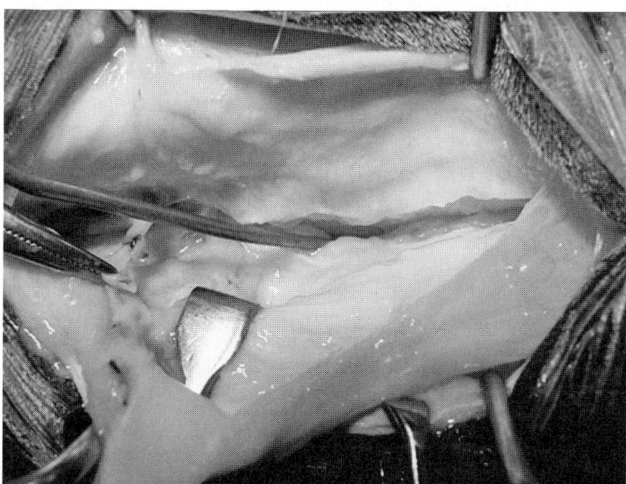

Figure 86-26. Neurectomy of the deep branch of the lateral plantar nerve (**A**) combined with fasciotomy (**B**) for treatment of proximal suspensory desmitis of the hindlimb. The hook has isolated the deep branch. A 3-cm section of nerve is removed using the guillotine method. Note that these figures were prepared in a cadaveric limb using a large incision to demonstrate the procedure; the normal incision length is usually 5 to 6 cm. (Courtesy M. Schramme, North Carolina State University.)

of success in returning affected animals to full work with minimal risk of exacerbating the desmitis.

ACCESSORY LIGAMENT OF THE DDFT DESMOTOMY/DESMECTOMY

Conservative treatment is usually successful for the treatment of accessory ligament of the DDFT (ALDDFT) desmitis. However, in some cases, desmitis may be recurrent or cause adhesions between the ALDDFT and the SDFT, or a flexural deformity. In such cases desmotomy, or preferably desmectomy, of the accessory ligament of the DDFT can be considered.[99]

ALDDFT desmotomy is performed under general anesthesia in lateral recumbency. The ALDDFT can be approached medially or laterally. A medial approach results in improved cosmesis but an increased risk of vascular damage to the medial palmar artery, and the lateral technique has the opposite effect. After aseptic preparation of the surgical site, a skin incision is made in the proximal half of the metacarpus adjacent to the palmar border of the DDFT (see Fig. 90-11). The incision is continued deeper by blunt dissection to expose the ALDDFT. The ALDDFT is elevated using forceps and is transected with a scalpel. Greater exposure can allow complete removal of the accessory ligament if necessary. The wound is closed in two layers—first, the fascia with a simple-continuous pattern using an absorbable suture material, and second, the skin. A modified Robert Jones bandage should be applied to the distal limb postoperatively for 3 to 4 days.

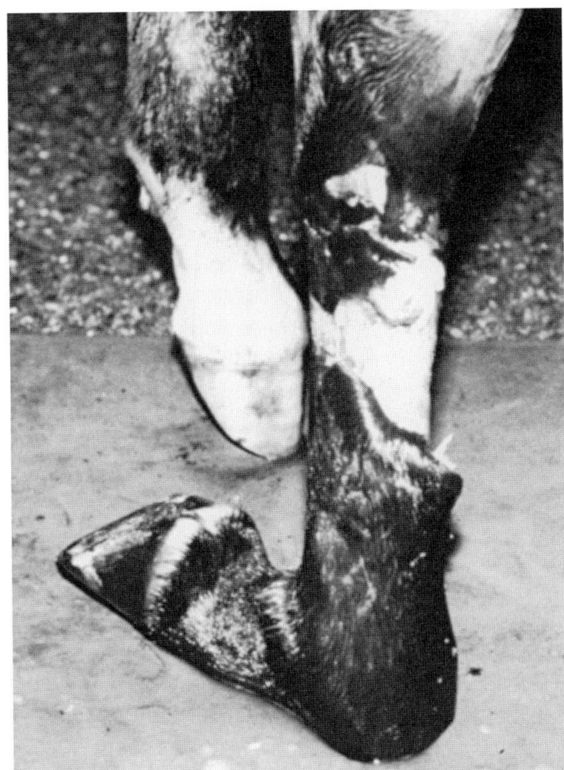

Figure 86-27. Loss of digital extensor function secondary to extensor tendon laceration, resulting in weightbearing on the dorsum of the hoof and phalangeal region.

Tendon Lacerations

Lacerations of the digital extensor tendons can result in the partial or complete loss of protraction of the distal limb, or the animal may place the limb in an abnormal position (Fig. 86-27). However, many cases show minimal signs. In contrast, horses suffering from flexor tendon lacerations are usually in severe pain and need immediate attention.

Emergency Treatment of Tendon Lacerations

The limb should be stabilized before the horse is moved to an appropriate place for treatment. It is important that the limb be supported to ensure the comfort of the horse by restoring some biomechanical function of the limb and to prevent further tissue damage. It is particularly important to avoid further trauma to the neurovascular structures of the distal limb. For flexor tendon lacerations, a palmar or dorsal splint or a commercial splint (e.g., a Kimsey splint [see Fig. 78-4]) should be applied. Any difficulty in limb protraction with an extensor tendon laceration can be managed with a simple splint bandage. For more information on the first aid of traumatized horses, review Chapter 78.

Surgical Repair

FLEXOR TENDONS

Surgical repair of flexor tendon lacerations involves débridement, suturing of the tendon, and closure of the wound and is usually performed under general anesthesia in lateral or dorsal recumbency. The aims of tenorrhaphy are to restore tendon gliding function, minimize gap formation between the tendon ends, minimize adhesion formation, and preserve functional vasculature. If the laceration is complete, the tendon may have recoiled, requiring proximal and distal extension of the skin wound in an elongated S shape to locate both tendon ends (Fig. 86-28). Flexing of the MCP/MTP joint may facilitate locating the distal tendon end. The wound and tendon ends should be débrided and lavaged. If the tendon ends can be apposed, tenorrhaphy can

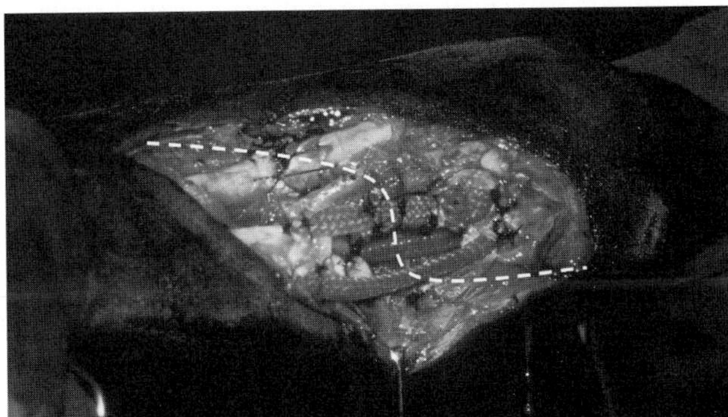

Figure 86-28. The use of poly-L-lactic acid (PLLA) to repair extensive defects in the digital flexor tendons. This horse suffered a transverse wound to the plantar aspect of the mid-metatarsal region, which transected both the superficial and deep digital flexor tendons and the lateral branch of the suspensory ligament. The wound was resected and the area exposed by using an S-shaped incision *(dotted line)*. After débridement of the tendons, a 5-cm defect was present in both tendons, which was bridged with two PLLA implants sutured to each end of the tendons. The lateral branch of the suspensory ligament was apposed using a three-loop pulley suture (see Fig. 86-29).

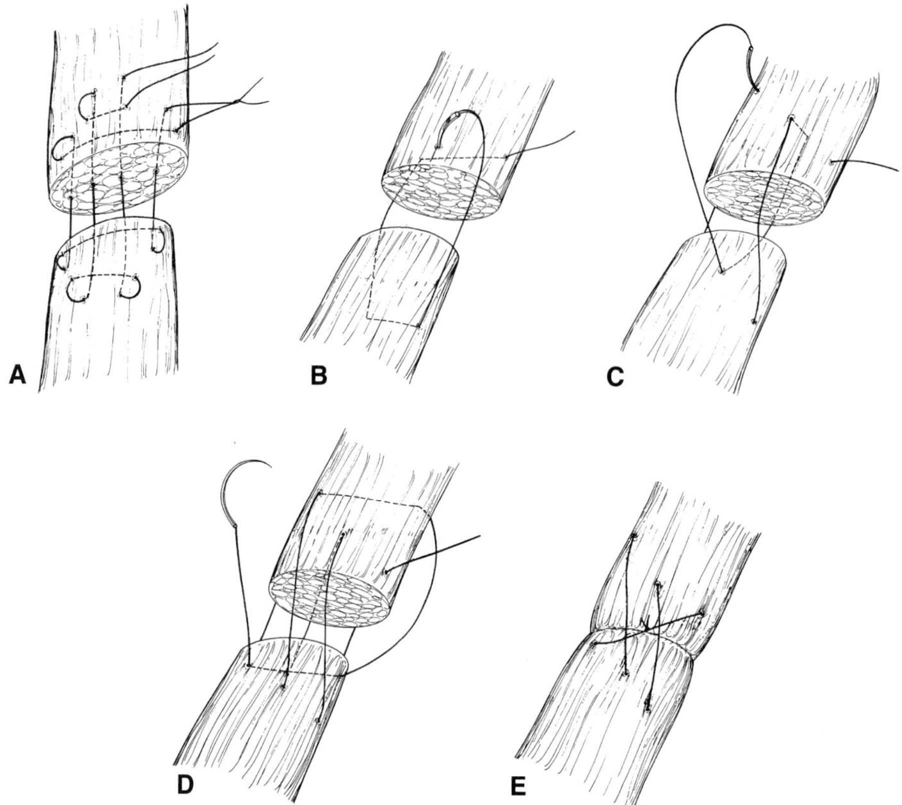

Figure 86-29. A, A modified compound locking-loop suture pattern. Bites perpendicular to the tendon fibers are superficial relative to bites that are aligned parallel to the fibers. **B** to **E,** The three-loop pulley suture pattern with each loop oriented 120 degrees relative to the others. The first loop is in a near-far pattern (**B**), the second loop is equidistant from the transected ends (**C**), and the third loop is placed in a far-near pattern (**D** and **E**). (From Watkins JP: Tendon and ligament disorders. In Auer JA, Stick JA, editors: Equine Surgery, ed 2, Philadelphia, 1999, WB Saunders.)

be performed using a monofilament absorbable suture (e.g., polydioxanone or polyglyconate). Nonabsorbable materials should be avoided, since they can result in shearing between the healed tissue and the suture material and may be responsible for persistent lameness. Two suture patterns are commonly used, the three-loop pulley and the interlocking loop (Fig. 86-29). The three-loop pulley prevents distraction of the ends of the tendon under loading (i.e., gapping), whereas the interlocking loop has little suture material outside the tendon and is therefore the recommended technique for repair of intrathecal lacerations. The interlocking-loop pattern can be supplemented with simple-continuous sutures to reduce gap formation between the tendon ends. A single locking-loop suture is not as strong as a double- or triple-locking loop or a three-loop pulley pattern.[100]

Frequently the injury is associated with significant blunt trauma to the tendon ends, which precludes direct apposition of the tendon ends. In this situation, the tendon ends can be left after débridement, the wound closed, and the limb cast, or an implant can be used to maintain the alignment of the tendon ends. The ideal tendon implant material would have biomechanical properties similar to those of normal tendon. Various implant materials have been used to repair lacerated flexor tendons including carbon fiber, terylene (polyester), autologous extensor tendon grafts, and poly-L-lactic acid (PLLA).[101] Carbon fiber implants were associated with persistent lameness postoperatively, which may have been caused by tenalgia resulting from shear forces between inelastic carbon fibers and the healed tendon tissue. The use of autologous grafts using extensor tendons to bridge the deficit between two ends of a lacerated tendon has never gained popularity. The advantage of PLLA is that it supports fibroblast growth on its surface and loses its strength over several months, thereby being able to match its mechanical properties with the tendon. Implants are anchored in each end of the lacerated tendon by fixing the ends in V-shaped incisions created in the tendon ends with sutures of monofilament absorbable sutures. Implants are not recommended as a treatment for strain-induced tendinitis.

Partial lacerations involving less than 50% of the tendon may need only local débridement. Lacerations involving greater than 50% are probably best sutured, since this can prevent the generation of longitudinal splits between loaded and unloaded parts of the tendon.

Flexor tendon lacerations require a protracted rehabilitation period. A distal limb cast should be placed with forelimb lacerations postoperatively. In the hindlimb, a full-limb cast is required after flexor tendon laceration to immobilize the forces of the reciprocal apparatus. However, distal limb casts can be used in the hindlimb to avoid the increased risk of complications of full-limb casts, unless an implant has been placed, in which case the result is usually that one end is pulled out of the tendon. Casting is required for a minimum of 6 to 8 weeks and no more than 12 weeks, thereby often necessitating one cast change under general anesthesia, as studies have shown that the breaking strength of the tendon repair at 6 weeks approximates the bodyweight of the horse.[102]

Support of the MCP/MTP joint using a palmar/plantar splint with a modified Robert Jones bandage and caudal shoe extensions (for DDFT lacerations) can help protect the repair after cast removal. Continued box stall rest is necessary for a further 2 to 3 months, after which walking exercise followed by an ascending exercise regimen can be initiated. Ultrasonographic monitoring of tendon healing is useful to assess the integrity of the tendon repair. A minimum of 8 to 12 months is usually required before full athletic function can be resumed.

The prognosis for flexor tendon injuries is guarded, with approximately 45% of horses returning to athletic function in one study[102]; in another study, the prognosis was 59% for flexor tendon lacerations.[103] In the second study, the prognosis for return to soundness was not increased if the DDFT and SDFT were simultaneously lacerated compared with involvement of only a single structure.[103] Complications of tendon lacerations include necrotic tendinitis (which occurs as a result of infection or damage to the vascular supply), concurrent synovial sepsis, cast complications, adhesions resulting in continued pain and lameness, exuberant granulation tissue formation, flexural deformity, and reinjury.

EXTENSOR TENDONS

Extensor tendon lacerations heal remarkably well without tenorrhaphy and respond well to conservative management. The wound should be débrided and the primary wound closed if appropriate. If the extensor tendon has been lacerated within the confines of a tendon sheath (e.g., for extensor lacerations over the dorsal aspect of the carpus), the area should be lavaged, and elimination of sepsis from the tendon sheath needs to be addressed. Fibrous scar tissue gradually forms an attachment between the two tendon ends. A period of 4 to 6 weeks of box stall rest until the wound has healed is usually all that is required. A cast can be used to assist soft tissue healing if contusion has been extensive. The prognosis for extensor tendon lacerations is good, with about 72% of horses returning to athletic function,[104] and other sources report an 80% good prognosis.[103] The prognosis for extensor tendon lacerations is better than for flexor tendon lacerations because the extensor tendon bears considerably less load and has a minimal effect on the gait, with most protraction of the limb and digit arising from the upper limb and momentum of the foot. Indeed, a recent publication reported the successful management of septic common digital extensor tenosynovitis by complete resection of the tendon.[105] Stumbling may be evident at the walk until the tendon has healed, but this can be reduced by shortening the toe of the hoof and rolling the toe of the shoe or by fitting a Natural Balance type of shoe. If extension cannot be maintained spontaneously, a toe extension can be fitted to the shoe to prevent secondary contracture, although this may make stumbling more severe.

The most common complications associated with extensor tendon lacerations include exuberant granulation tissue and sequestrum formation associated with underlying damage to the bone, although acquired flexural deformities can occur.

REFERENCES

1. Canty EG, Lu Y, Meadows RS, et al: Coalignment of plasma membrane channels and protrusions (fibripositors) specifies the parallelism of tendon, J Cell Biol 2004;24:553.
2. Smith RKW, Zunino L, Webbon PM, et al: The distribution of cartilage oligomeric matrix protein (COMP) in tendon and its variation with tendon site, age, and load, Matrix Biol 1997;16:255.
3. Rosenberg K: Cartilage oligomeric matrix protein (COMP): Functions in collagen binding and assembly, PhD thesis, Sweden, 2001, University of Lund.
4. Smith RKW, Gerard M, Dowling B, et al: Correlation of cartilage oligomeric matrix protein (COMP) levels in equine tendon with mechanical properties: A proposed role for COMP in determining function-specific mechanical characteristics of locomotor tendons, Equine Vet J Suppl 2002;34:241.
5. Dowling BA, Dart AJ, Hodgson DR, et al: Superficial digital flexor tendonitis in the horse, Equine Vet J 2000;32:369.
6. Smith RKW, Goodship AE: Tendon physiology. In Hinchcliff KW, Kaneps AJ, Geor RJ, editors: Equine Sports Medicine and Surgery, Philadelphia, 2004, WB Saunders.
7. McNeilly CM, Banes AJ, Benjamin M, et al: Tendon cells in vivo form a three dimensional network of cell processes linked by gap junctions, J Anat 1996;189:593.
8. Goodship AE, Birch HL, Wilson AM: The pathobiology and repair of tendon and ligament injury, Vet Clin North Am Equine Pract 1994;10:323.
9. Smith RKW, Webbon PM: The physiology of normal tendon and ligament. In Rantanen NW, Hauser ML, editors: Dubai Equine International Symposium Proceedings: The Equine Athlete—Tendon, Ligament, and Soft Tissue Injuries, Dubai, United Arab Emirates, 1996.
10. Cauvin ERJ: An investigation into the roles of transforming growth factor-beta (TGFβ) in the development, adaptation and repair of equine tendons, PhD thesis, 2001, University of London.
11. Kraus-Hansen AE, Fackelman GE, Becker C, et al: Preliminary studies on the vascular anatomy of the equine superficial digital flexor tendon, Equine Vet J 1992;24:46.
12. Kraus BLH, Kirker-Head CA, Kraus KH, et al: Vascular supply of the tendon of the equine deep digital flexor muscle within the digital sheath, Vet Surg 1995;24:102.
13. Strömberg B, Tufvesson G: Lesions of the superficial flexor tendons in racehorses: A microangiographic and histopathologic study, Clin Orthop 1969;62:113.
14. Jones AJ: Normal and diseased equine digital flexor tendon: Blood flow, biochemical and serological studies, PhD thesis, 1993, University of London.
15. Denoix J-M: Functional anatomy of tendons and ligaments in the distal limb (manus and pes), Vet Clin North Am Equine Pract 1994;10:273.
16. Crevier-Denoix N, Collobert C, Pourcelot P, et al: Mechanical properties of pathological equine superficial digital flexor tendons, Equine Vet J Suppl 1997;23:23.
17. Ker RF, Wang XT, Pike AV: Fatigue quality of mammalian tendons, J Exp Biol 2000;203:1317.
18. Ker RF: The implications of the adaptable fatigue quality of tendons for their construction, repair and function, Comp Biochem Physiol A Mol Integr Physiol 2002;133:987.
19. Stephens PR, Nunamaker DM, Butterweck DM: Application of a Hall-effect transducer for the measurement of tendon strain in horses, Am J Vet Res 1989;50:1089.
20. Birch HL, Wilson AM, Goodship AE: The effect of exercise-induced localised hyperthermia on tendon cell survival, J Exp Biol 1997;200:1703.
21. Maganaris CN. Tendon conditioning: An artefact or property, Proc R Soc Lond B Biol Sci 2003;270(Suppl 1):S39.
22. Smith RKW, Birch HL, Goodman S, et al: The influence of ageing and exercise on tendon growth and degeneration: Hypotheses for

the initiation and prevention of strain-induced tendinopathies, Comp Biochem Physiol A Mol Integr Physiol 2002;133:1039.
23. Batson EL, Paramour RJ, Smith TJ, et al: Are the material properties and matrix composition of equine flexor and extensor tendons determined by their functions? Equine Vet J 2003;35:314.
24. Vogel KG, Koob TJ: Structural specialisation in tendons under compression, Int Rev Cytol 1989;115:267.
25. Wilson AM, McGuigan MP, Su A, van Den Bogart AJ: Horses damp the spring in their step, Nature 2001;414:895.
26. Tsuzaki M, Guyton G, Garrett W, et al: IL-1 beta induces COX2, MMP-1, -3 and -13, ADAMTS-4, IL-1 beta and IL-6 in human tendon cells, J Orthop Res 2003;21:256.
27. Smith RKW, Birch HL, Patterson-Kane J, et al: Should equine athletes commence training during skeletal development? Changes in tendon matrix associated with development, ageing, function and exercise, Equine Vet J Suppl 1999;31:201.
28. Webbon PM: Post mortem study of equine digital flexor tendons, Equine Vet J 1977;9:61.
29. Birch HL, Bailey AJ, Goodship AE: Macroscopic "degeneration" of equine superficial digital flexor tendon is accompanied by a change in extracellular matrix composition, Equine Vet J 1998;30:534.
30. Pickersgill C: Epidemiological studies into orthopaedic conditions of the equine athlete, MVM thesis, 2000, University of Glasgow.
31. Williams RB, Harkins LS, Hammond CJ, et al: Racehorse injuries, clinical problems and fatalities recorded on British racecourses from flat racing and National Hunt racing during 1996, 1997, and 1998, Equine Vet J 2001;33:478.
32. Kasashima Y, Takahashi T, Smith RK, et al: Prevalence of superficial digital flexor tendonitis and suspensory desmitis in Japanese Thoroughbred flat racehorses in 1999, Equine Vet J 2004;36:346.
33. Patterson-Kane JC, Firth EC, Goodship AE, et al: Age-related differences in collagen crimp patterns in the superficial digital flexor tendon core region of untrained horses, Aust Vet J 1997;75:39.
34. Patterson-Kane JC, Wilson AM, Firth EC, et al: Exercise-related alterations in crimp morphology in the central regions of superficial digital flexor tendons from young Thoroughbreds: A controlled study, Equine Vet J 1998;30:61.
35. Patterson-Kane JC, Wilson AM, Firth EC, et al: Comparison of collagen fibril populations in the superficial digital flexor tendons of exercised and nonexercised Thoroughbreds, Equine Vet J 1997;29:121.
36. Perez-Castro AV, Vogel KG: In situ expression of collagen and proteoglycan genes during development of fibrocartilage in bovine deep flexor tendon, J Orthop Res 1999;17:139.
37. Goodman SA, May SA, Heinegard D, et al: Tenocyte response to cyclical strain and transforming growth factor beta is dependent upon age and site of origin, Biorheology 2004;41:613.
38. Wilson AM, Goodship AE: Exercise induced hyperthermia as a possible mechanism for tendon degeneration, J Biomech 1993;27:899.
39. Dudhia J, Scott C, Pitsillides AP, et al: Personal communication, 2004.
40. Johnson A, Smith R, Saxne T, et al: Fibronectin fragments cause the release and degradation of collagen-binding molecules from equine explant cultures, Osteoarthritis Cartilage 2004;12:149.
41. Crevier-Denoix N, Roosen C, Dardillat C, et al: Effects of heel and toe elevation upon the digital joint angles in the standing horse, Equine Vet J 2001;33(Suppl):74.
42. Eliashar E, McGuigan MP, Wilson AM: Relationship of foot conformation and force applied to the navicular bone of sound horses at the trot, Equine Vet J 2004;36:431.
43. Pinchbeck GL, Clegg PD, Proudman CJ, et al: Horse injuries and racing practices in National Hunt racehorses in the UK: The results of a prospective cohort study, Vet J 2004;167:45.
44. Watkins JP, Auer JA, Gay S, et al: Healing of surgically created defects in the equine superficial digital flexor tendon: Collagen type transformation and tissue morphologic reorganization, Am J Vet Res 1985;46:2091.
45. Genovese RL, Rantanen NW, Simpson BS, et al: Clinical experience with quantitative analysis of superficial digital flexor tendon injuries in Thoroughbred and Standardbred racehorses, Vet Clin North Am Equine Pract 1990;6:129.
46. Jackson BF, Smith RKW, Price JS: A molecular marker of type I collagen metabolism reflects changes in connective tissue remodelling associated with injury to the equine superficial digital flexor tendon, Equine Vet J 2003;35:211.
47. Smith RKW, Heinegård D: Cartilage oligomeric matrix protein levels in digital sheath synovial fluid and serum with tendon injury, Equine Vet J 2000;32:52.
48. Barr AR, Dyson SJ, Barr FJ, et al: Tendonitis of the deep digital flexor tendon in the distal metacarpal/metatarsal region associated with tenosynovitis of the digital sheath in the horse, Equine Vet J 1995;27:348.
49. Wright IM, McMahon PJ: Tenosynovitis associated with longitudinal tears of the digital flexor tendons in horses: A report of 20 cases, Equine Vet J 1999;31:12.
50. Asheim A: Surgical treatment of tendon injuries in the horse, J Am Vet Med Assoc 1964;145:447.
51. Petrov R, MacDonald H, Tesch AM, et al: Influence of topically applied cold treatment on core temperature and cell viability in equine superficial digital flexor tendons, Am J Vet Res 2003;64:835.
52. Kasashima Y, Eto D, Kusano K: Comparison of the method of cold therapy to equine limbs after training, with the aim of preventing tendonitis, Jpn J Equine Sci 2001;12:96.
53. Hunt ER: Response of twenty-seven horses with lower leg injuries to cold spa bath hydrotherapy, J Equine Vet Sci 2001;21:188.
54. Smith RKW, McGuigan MP, Hyde JT, et al: In vitro evaluation of nonrigid support systems for the equine metacarpophalangeal joint, Equine Vet J 2002;34:726.
55. Buckwalter JA: Effects of early motion on healing of musculoskeletal tissues, Hand Clin 1996;12:13.
56. Gillis CL: Rehabilitation of tendon and ligament injuries, Proc Am Assoc Equine Pract 1997;43:306.
57. Bolt, DM, Burba DJ, Hubert JD, et al: Evaluation of cutaneous analgesia after non-focused extracorporeal shock wave application over the 3rd metacarpal bone in horses, Can J Vet Res 2004;68:288.
58. Crowe OM, Dyson SJ, Wright IM, et al: Treatment of chronic or recurrent proximal suspensory desmitis using radial pressure wave therapy in the horse, Equine Vet J 2004;36:313.
59. Dyson SJ: Proximal suspensory desmitis in the hindlimb: 42 cases, Br Vet J 1994;150:279.
60. Morcos MB, Aswad A: Histological studies of the effects of ultrasonographic therapy on surgically split flexor tendons, Equine Vet J 1978;10:267.
61. Henninger R: Treatment of superficial digital flexor tendonitis, Vet Clin North Am Equine Pract 1994;10:409.
62. Silver IA, Brown PN, Goodship AE, et al: Biochemistry and pathology of tendon injury and healing. In Silver IA, Rossdale PD, editors: A Clinical and Experimental Study of Tendon Injury, Healing and Treatment in the Horse, Equine Vet J 1983;Suppl 1.
63. May SA, Lees P: Non-steroidal anti-inflammatory drugs. In Mcillwraith CW, Trotter GW, editors: Joint Disease in the Horse, Philadelphia, 1996, WB Saunders.
64. Albrechsen SJ, Harvey JS: Dimethyl sulfoxide biomechanical effects on tendons, Am J Sports Med 1982;10:177.
65. van den Belt AJM, Keg PR, Dik KJ: The correlation between the dose distribution of intratendinous fluid injections in the flexor tendons of the horse: A pilot study, Vet Radiol Ultrasound 1992;33:120.
66. Dahlgren LA, Rosenbusch RF, Booth LC: The effect of polysulphated glycosaminoglycan on the production of proteoglycan by equine tendon fibroblasts on monolayer culture, Vet Comp Orthop Traumatol 1998;11:136.
67. Marr CM, Love S, Boyd JS, et al: Factors affecting the clinical outcome of injuries to the superficial digital flexor tendon in

National Hunt and point-to-point racehorses, Vet Rec 1993;132:476.
68. Redding WR, Booth LC, Pool RR: ACVS Abstract: Effects of polysulphated glycosaminoglycans on the healing of collagenase induced tendonitis of the equine superficial digital flexor tendon, Vet Surg 1992;21:403.
69. Dyson SJ: Medical management of superficial digital flexor tendinitis: A comparative study in 219 horses (1992-2000), Equine Vet J 2004;36:415.
70. Gift LJ, Gaughan EM, DeBowes RM, et al: The influence of intratendinous sodium hyaluronate on tendon healing in horses, Vet Comp Orthop Traumatol 1992;5:151.
71. Foland JW, Trotter, GW, Powers BE, et al: Effect of sodium hyaluronate in collagenase-induced superficial digital flexor tendinitis in horses, Am J Vet Res 1992;53:2371.
72. Gaughan EM, Nixon AJ, Krook LP, et al: Effects of sodium hyaluronate on tendon healing and adhesion formation in horses, Am J Vet Res 1991;52:764.
73. Pool RR, Wheat JD, Ferraro GL: Corticosteroid therapy in common joint and tendon injuries of the horse: Parts I and II. The effects on tendons, Proc Am Assoc Equine Pract 1980;26:397.
74. Genovese RL: Sonographic response to intralesional therapy with beta-aminopropionitrile fumarate for clinical tendon injuries in horses, Proc Am Assoc Equine Pract 1992;38:65.
75. Reef VB, Genovese RL, Davis WM: Initial long-term results of horses with superficial digital flexor tendonitis treated with intralesional beta-aminoproprionitrile fumarate, Proc Am Assoc Equine Pract 1997;43:301.
76. Reef VB, Genovese RL, Byrd JW, et al: Treatment of superficial digital flexor tendon injuries with beta-aminoproprionitrile fumarate (BAPN-F): sonographic evaluation of early tendon healing and remodelling. In Rantanen NW, Hauser ML, editors, Dubai International Equine Symposium: The Equine Athlete—Tendon, ligament and soft tissue injuries, 1996, Matthew R. Rantanen Design, USA.
77. Alves ALG, Rodrigues MAM, Aguiar AJA, et al: Effects of beta-aminopropionitrile fumarate and exercise on equine tendon healing: Gross and histological aspects J Equine Vet Sci 2001;21:335.
78. Dahlgren LA, Nixon AJ, Brower-Toland BD: Effects of beta-aminopropionitrile on equine tendon metabolism in vitro and on effects of insulin-like growth factor-1 on matrix production by equine tenocytes, Am J Vet Res 2001;62:1557.
79. Yamamoto E, Hata D, Kobayashi A, et al: Effect of beta-aminopropionitrile and hyaluronic acid on repair of collagenase-induced injury of the rabbit Achilles tendon, J Comp Pathol 2002;126:161.
80. Dahlgren LA, van der Meulen MCH, Bertram JEA, et al: Insulin-like growth factor-I improves cellular and molecular aspects of healing in a collagenase-induced model of flexor tendinitis, J Orthop Res 2002;20:910.
81. Dowling BA, Dart AJ, Hodgeson DR, et al: The effect of recombinant equine growth hormone on the biomechanical properties of healing superficial digital flexor tendons in horses, Vet Surg 2002;31:320.
82. Bathe AP: Personal communication, 2003.
83. Herthel DJ: Enhanced suspensory ligament healing in 100 horses by stem cells and other bone marrow components, Proc Am Assoc Equine Pract 2001;47:319.
84. Smith JJ, Scott CM, Ross MW, Smith RKW: Anabolic effects of acellular bone marrow, platelet rich plasma, and serum on equine ligament fibroblasts in vitro, Vet Surg 2003;32:496.
85. Smith RKW, Korda M, Blunn GW, et al: Isolation and implantation of autologous equine mesenchymal stem cells from bone marrow into the superficial digital flexor tendon as a potential novel treatment, Equine Vet J 2003;35:99.
86. Asheim A, Knudsen O: Percutaneous tendon splitting, Proc Am Assoc Equine Pract 1967;13:255.
87. Stromberg B, Tufvesson G, Nilsson G: Effect of surgical splitting on vascular reactions in the superficial flexor tendon of the horse, J Am Vet Med Assoc 1974;164:57.
88. Dabareiner RM, Carter GK, Chaffin MK: How to perform ultrasound-guided tendon splitting and intralesional tendon injections in the standing horse, Proc Am Assoc Equine Pract 2000;46:176.
89. Henninger RW, Bramlage LR, Bailey M, et al: Effects of tendon splitting on experimentally-induced acute equine tendonitis, Vet Comp Orthop Traumatol 1992;5:1.
90. Bramlage LR: Superior check desmotomy as a treatment for superficial digital flexor tendinitis: Initial report, Proc Am Assoc Equine Pract 1986;32:365.
91. Shoemaker RS, Bertone AL, Mohammad LN, et al: Desmotomy of the accessory ligament of the superficial digital flexor muscle in equine cadaver limbs, Vet Surg 1991;20:245.
92. Gibson KT, Burbidge HM, Pfeiffer DU: Superficial digital flexor tendonitis in thoroughbred race horses: Outcome following non-surgical treatment and superior check desmotomy, Aust Vet J 1997;75:631.
93. McIlwraith CW, Robertson JT: Superior check ligament desmotomy (after Bramlage). In Equine Surgery Advanced Techniques, ed 2, Baltimore, 1998, Williams and Wilkins.
94. Southwood LL, Stashak TS, Kainer RA, et al: Desmotomy of the accessory ligament of the superficial digital flexor tendon in the horse with use of a tenoscopic approach to the carpal sheath, Vet Surg 1999;28:99.
95. Nixon AJ: Endoscopy of the digital flexor tendon sheath in horses, Vet Surg 1990;10:266.
96. Smith MRW, Wright IM: Personal communication, 2005.
97. Dyson SJ: Proximal suspensory desmitis in the forelimb and the hindlimb, Proc Am Assoc Equine Pract 2000;46:137.
98. Bathe AP: Plantar metatarsal neurectomy and fasciotomy for treatment of hindlimb proximal suspensory desmitis, Vet Surg 2003;32:480.
99. Boswell JC, Schramme MC: Desmitis of the accessory ligament of the deep digital flexor tendon in the hindlimb in a horse, Equine Vet Educ 2000;12:129.
100. Easley KJ, Stashak TS, Smith FW, et al: Mechanical properties of four suture patterns for transacted equine tendon repair, Vet Surg 1990;19:102.
101. Eliashar E, Schramme MC, Schumacher J, et al: Use of a bioabsorbable implant for the repair of severed digital flexor tendons in four horses, Vet Rec 2001;148:506.
102. Bertone AL: Tendon lacerations, Vet Clin North Am Equine Pract 1995;11:293.
103. Foland JW, Trotter GW, Stashak TS, et al: Traumatic injuries involving tendons of the distal limbs in horses: A retrospective study of 55 cases, Equine Vet J 1991;23:422.
104. Belknap JK, Baxter GM, Nickels FA: Extensor tendon lacerations in horses: 50 cases (1982-1988), J Am Vet Med Assoc 1993;203:428.
105. Booth TM, Abbot J, Clements A, et al: Treatment of septic common digital extensor tenosynovitis by complete resection in seven horses, Vet Surg 2004;33:107.

CHAPTER 87

Biology and Management of Muscle Disorders and Diseases

John G. Peloso

STRUCTURE AND FUNCTION OF MUSCLES

Of the three types of muscle in the body—skeletal, smooth, and cardiac—skeletal muscle makes up about 40% of the body weight.[1,2] All movement is the result of contraction of skeletal muscle, and most patients with neuromuscular disease exhibit abnormal movement. Skeletal muscle consists of a central fleshy muscle belly and a tendon at each end. The tendon at one end of the muscle originates on one bone, and the tendon at the other end inserts on a different bone, with a movable joint interposed. When activated by a motor neuron, a skeletal muscle can only contract (or shorten). Movement occurs when the central muscle belly shortens, causing the two tendons and their bones of attachment to move with respect to each other around a central joint. A muscle returns to its original longer length by the pull of its antagonistic pair, a muscle that traverses the joint on the opposite side. Some muscles increase joint angle (extensors), and some muscles decrease joint angles (flexors).

Anatomy

Skeletal muscle has several levels of organization (Fig. 87-1). Each muscle belly is made up of thousands of muscle cells (also called muscle fibers). Each muscle fiber contains thousands of myofibrils that are arraged in parallel along its length, and each myofibril is made up of a series of repeating sarcomeres. The sarcomere is the basic contractile unit of the muscle fiber.[1,2]

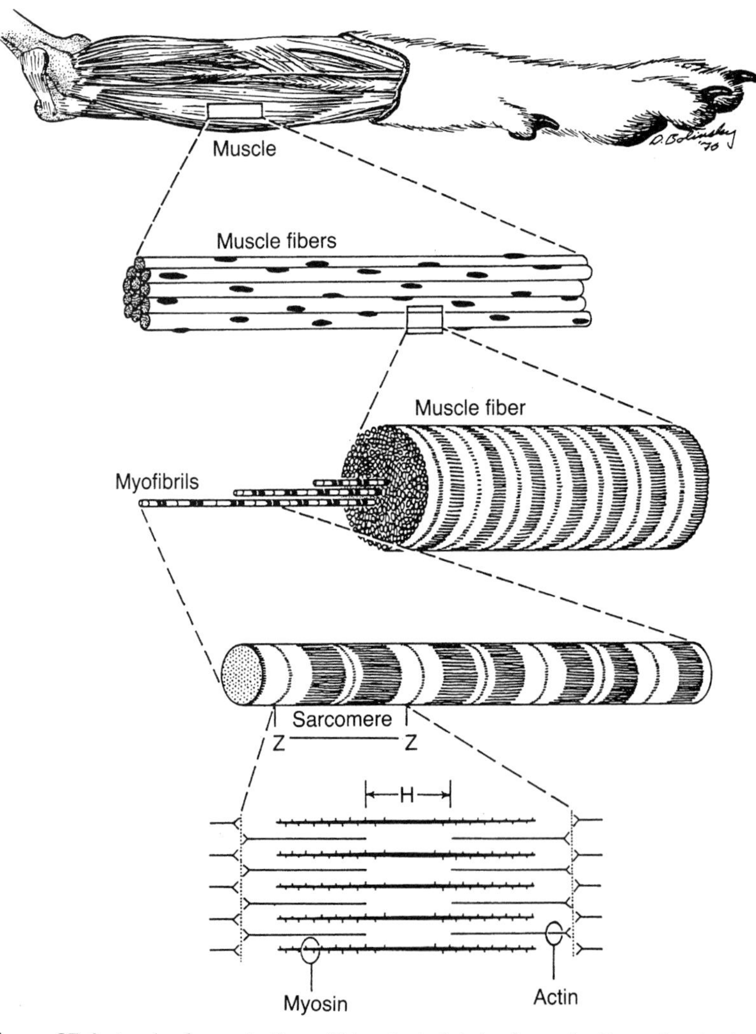

Figure 87-1. Levels of organization within a typical skeletal muscle. (From Cunningham JG: Textbook of Veterinary Physiology, ed 3, Philadelphia, 2002, WB Saunders.)

Myofibrils have an arrangement of alternating thick and thin filaments. The thick filaments are composed of the protein myosin, and the thin filaments are composed of the proteins actin, tropomyosin, and troponin.[1,2] Myofibrils are surrounded by membranes in the form of tubules. These tubules are composed of a transverse tubular system and the sarcoplasmic reticulum, and collectively they are called the sarcotubular system. Each muscle fiber is innervated by a terminal branch of a motor nerve fiber. The junction between the nerve and the muscle fiber is the neuromuscular junction. All muscle fibers that are innervated by a single nerve fiber are called a motor unit because all of the muscle fibers within a unit are excited simultaneously and contract in unison.

Physiology of Contraction

It is at the neuromuscular junction that action potentials are generated. The resting membrane potential of the sarcolemma is excited by a synaptic transmission at the neuromuscular junction. Via transverse tubules, the action potential reaches the sarcoplasmic reticulum throughout the muscle fiber.

Skeletal muscle cells (muscle fibers) convert chemical energy into mechanical energy. At rest, calcium ions are maintained within the sarcoplasmic reticulum of the muscle cell. The arrival of an action potential to the sarcoplasmic reticulum causes the release of calcium ions. These calcium ions perfuse the sarcomere and bind with troponin. This alters the actin filament, allowing it to react with the myosin filament. Although a detailed molecular explanation of the sliding filament mechanism is not known, the altered actin molecule is now able to slide along the myosin molecule, causing a physical shortening of the sarcomere (Fig. 87-2). As the action potential passes, calcium ions are returned to the sarcoplasmic reticulum, allowing the sarcomere to relax.

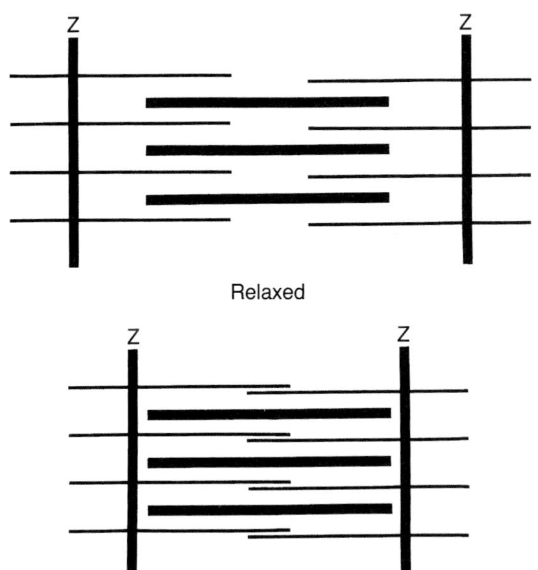

Figure 87-2. The sliding of actin along the myosin molecule results in the physical shortening (contraction) of the sarcomere. (From Cunningham JG: Textbook of Veterinary Physiology, ed 3, Philadelphia, 2002, WB Saunders.)

Therefore, in the presence of calcium ions and ATP, actin and myosin molecules slide over one another. This results in a physical shortening of the sarcomere and ultimately of the myofibril and the muscle belly. The cumulative effect of a shortened sarcomere is a reduction in the distance between the two tendon ends, and their bones of attachment move with respect to each other around a central joint.

Adenosine triphosphate is needed for this contraction, and creatinine phosphate can be used to replenish ATP stores from ADP. The enzyme creatine phosphokinase (CPK) catalyzes this conversion and is found in high concentrations within muscle cells. During muscle cell damage, the CPK that is normally contained within intact muscle cells can leak into the bloodstream. Therefore, identification of an abnormally high concentration of serum CPK is used routinely to assess skeletal muscle necrosis. Muscle contraction is only about 40% efficient in converting chemical energy to mechanical energy, and most of the energy is lost as heat. This phenomenon is exploited during shivering to raise core body temperatures. During shivering, antagonistic muscle groups are activated so that they produce no useful work. The chemical energy lost as heat is transferred to the body core to increase temperature.

Muscle Repair

Muscle has a very limited capacity for regeneration. In some muscles, stellate cells have been identified that can form new muscle fibers. For practical purposes, however, new muscle fibers are not formed after birth. Enlargement and growth of muscle occur via enlargement of fibers caused by formation of additional myofibrils. Repair of damaged muscle occurs by replacement with connective tissue. Muscle has a good blood supply and a ready source of fibroblasts. Healing of damaged muscle with scar tissue is usually rapid, but replacement of damaged muscle with large amounts of scar tissue can restrict muscle length and function.

SPECIFIC MUSCLE DISORDERS

Fibrotic Myopathy

The classic description of fibrotic myopathy is that of a unilateral hindlimb gait abnormality, in which the cranial phase of the stride is shortened and there is a rapid caudal movement of the limb during the caudal phase of the stride as the foot slaps the ground (Fig. 87-3). This condition is most evident when the horse is observed at the walk from a lateral perspective.[2-11] The overall prevalence of the disease is low: of the 167,132 horses examined by 22 university veterinary hospitals in North America over the 10 years from 1979 to 1988, 102 horses (0.06%) were diagnosed with fibrotic myopathy.[2]

Pathophysiology

In most horses, traumatic injuries that cause adhesions and fibrosis of the semitendinosus muscle are responsible for the condition. Less commonly, injury to the semimembranosus, biceps femoris, and gracilis muscles have been identified.[7] Trauma may result from lacerations, slipping while exercising, and entrapment of a foot in halters, lead shanks, or fences. In one study, 5 of 18 horses with fibrotic

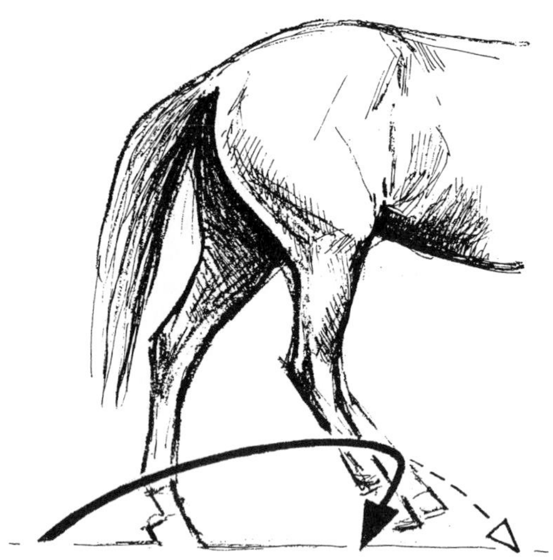

Figure 87-3. Motion of the rear limb of a horse affected with fibrotic or ossifying myopathy. The limb is jerked backward just before hitting the ground.

myopathy developed the condition secondary to intramuscular injections.[6] Tearing the insertion of the semitendinous muscle during activities that create extreme tension on the caudal aspect of the hindlimb (barrel racing, the slide of a reining horse) has also been incriminated. The characteristic gait of horses with fibrotic myopathy can occur temporarily after transportation in a trailer; in this case, it is caused by a localized myositis of the semitendinosus muscle because of prolonged pressure by the rear rope or bar on the muscle. Fibrotic myopathy in the neonate is speculated to be caused by trauma at or soon after birth, although the exact etiology is unknown in congenital cases.[8] Horses born with the gait characteristic of fibrotic myopathy have a taut semitendinosus muscle and tendon, but they do not have palpable fibrosis of the muscle. In a small series of horses, traumatic or degenerative neuropathy causing denervation of the distal semitendinous muscle resulted in fibrotic myopathy.[12] The underlying neuropathy is the most likely cause in horses when the condition progresses to involve both limbs. If bone forms in the affected tissue, the condition is termed ossifying myopathy.

Diagnosis

The diagnosis of fibrotic myopathy is made by observing the abnormal gait and by palpating the fibrotic or ossified muscle areas. Lameness is usually most apparent at the walk and is characterized by an abrupt cessation of the cranial phase of the stride of the affected limb, with the foot suddenly jerked caudally just before it hits the ground (see Fig. 87-3). This gait abnormality is not painful and is caused by mechanical restriction (either fibrous or osseous) of the affected thigh muscles. The gait abnormality is evident on every stride, is nonresponsive to analgesics, and is not altered by manipulative tests.

The fibrotic or ossified areas of the affected muscles may be palpated on the caudal aspect of the thigh at the level of the stifle joint or immediately above it. Ultrasonography may be helpful in defining areas of fibrosis, whereas radiography is more useful to demonstrate areas of ossification.

Treatment

Several surgical procedures for the correction of this disorder have been described. These techniques include semitendinosus myotomy, semitendinosus myotenectomy, or semitendinosus tenotomy at the tibial insertion of the muscle.* Earlier treatments described for these conditions include resection of the fibrous or ossified part of the semitendinosus muscle and removal of adhesions to surrounding muscles.[3,6] Myotomy and myotenectomy are no longer recommended because of the relative high rate of postoperative complications, including prolonged hemorrhage, wound dehiscence, high recurrence rate, and noncosmetic outcomes.

Semitendinosus tenotomy is presently the treatment of choice for fibrotic myopathy of the semitendinosus muscle.[8,10] This procedure is performed under general anesthesia in lateral recumbency with the affected limb down, providing access to the medial aspect of the tibia. Landmarks for surgery include the tibial insertion of the muscle on the caudomedial aspect of the tibia just distal to the medial femorotibial joint and caudal to the saphenous vein overlying the gastrocnemius muscle. An 8-cm vertical skin incision is made directly over the palpable tendon, and through the subcutaneous and crural fascia until the tendon is exposed. A large forceps, such as a curved Kelly or Crile, is passed under the tendon to isolate it from the muscle, and the tendon is transected (Fig. 87-4). Resection of a 3-cm segment of the tendon may delay recurrence of the gait abnormality. Facial layers are closed with interrupted or continuous synthetic absorbable sutures, and the skin is closed with interrupted or continuous nonabsorbable suture material.

When the affected limb is pulled forward during surgery, the tendon of insertion of the semitendinosus muscle onto the calcaneal tuber may become very taut in some horses.[2] An additional 3- to 4-cm-long incision has been recommended directly over the taut tendon, which is then isolated and transected. This incision is caudal and slightly distal to the first incision. Tenotomy is technically easier than the other procedures and eliminates an incision into diseased muscle.

Prognosis

With myectomy and myotomy, improvement is usually noticed immediately, but it may take up to 7 days for maximal improvement. Standing myotomy resulted in partial recurrence of the gait abnormality after surgery in approximately one third of 39 horses treated.[11] The tenotomy procedure alone results in fewer complications than the other techniques, including less predisposition for reformation of the fibrous band, but it may not result in complete resolution of the gait abnormality.[8] If a degenerative neuropathy is the cause of the condition, recurrence of clinical signs is likely, regardless of the surgical technique employed.

Stringhalt

Stringhalt is a hindlimb gait abnormality characterized by involuntary and exaggerated flexion of one or both

*References 3, 5, 6, 8, 10, 11.

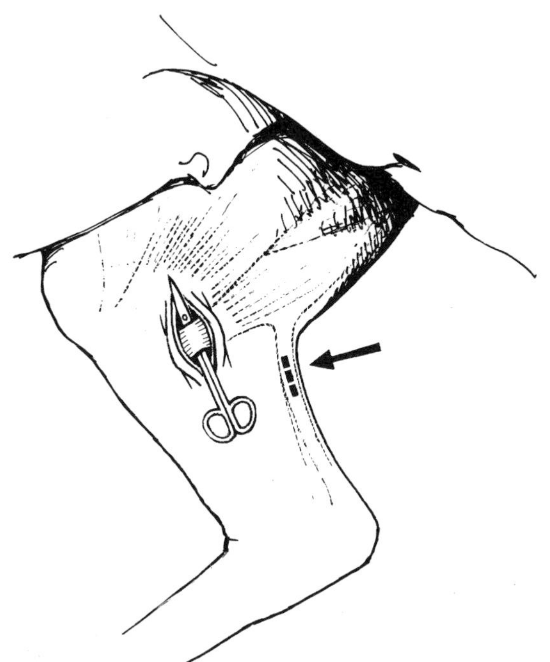

Figure 87-4. Semitendinosus tenotomy. The tendon of the tibia insertion has been isolated on the medial side of the proximal tibia and is ready to be severed. The *dashed line (arrow)* indicates the location for the second incision, which is performed if the insertion of the tendon on the tuber calcis is taut.

limbs.[13-19] During the cranial phase of the stride, the limb is jerked toward the abdomen (Fig. 87-5). There may be a wide variation in the severity of the signs that occur during every walk stride. The gait abnormality has a classic appearance, but it should be differentiated from mild forms of intermittent upward fixation of the patella. The patella catches on the medial trochlea of the distal femur in intermittent upward fixation of the patella, and when it releases it gives the appearance of a horse with stringhalt.

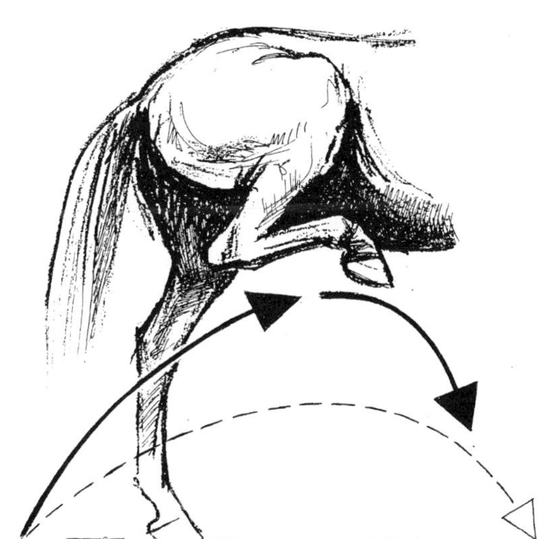

Figure 87-5. Exaggerated flexion of the rear limb is a characteristic sign in horses with stringhalt.

Pathophysiology

Two forms of stringhalt have been described: a conventional (sporadic) form and an Australian (outbreak) form. In North America, the disease is usually seen as the sporadic form; it involves a single hindlimb and occurs as isolated cases.[2,16-18] In Australian and New Zealand, the disease is usually observed in both hindlimbs and occurs epidemically.[13-15] The occurrence of conventional stringhalt is rarely seen as a bilateral condition. The cause has been attributed to an overextension injury of the tarsus and metatarsus[19]; metatarsal, tarsal, and stifle injuries; foot pain; spinal cord disease; and tendon adhesions.[14] Although the true etiology for the condition is unknown, sporadic stringhalt is suggested to be caused by an underlying neuropathy.[18] One author reports that all muscle or peripheral nerve isolates from horses with sporadic stringhalt had histologic evidence of neuropathy or degenerative myopathy.[18] This form of stringhalt usually has not been associated with the spontaneous recovery that is seen in the Australian form.

Australian stringhalt is recognized predominantly during the summer or fall in horses on pasture, and it often follows drier-than-normal summer months. Its etiology has been clearly shown to involve an underlying neuropathy.[16] Although the toxic principle is not known, it occurs in groups of horses on pastures containing dandelions known as flatweeds *(Hypochoeris radica)*. Evaluation of nerve samples from horses with Australian stringhalt has demonstrated widespread neuropathy. Lesions occur in the left recurrent laryngeal nerve in approximately 60% of these horses.[15] The lameness in Australian stringhalt is caused by a peripheral neuropathy and neurogenic muscle atrophy of the long digital extensor, lateral digital extensor, and gastrocnemius muscles. Many horses recover without treatment.

Diagnosis

The diagnosis is based on observation of the characteristic gait caused by exaggerated flexion of one or both hindlimbs. The abnormalities are usually bilateral in Australian stringhalt. The onset is often sudden. Some horses show a very mild flexion of the hock during walking, and others show a marked jerking of the foot toward the abdomen, with the foot actually hitting the abdomen in severe cases (see Fig. 87-5). The abnormal gait is usually evident with each step. Rest and cold weather tend to accentuate the gait, and in some horses, the gait may return to normal with exercise. All breeds can be affected.

Treatment

Horses with Australian stringhalt often recover spontaneously. Removal from the incriminated pasture may be curative, although recovery can take from months to years and may not be complete. In one study, 78% of the horses recovered over a period ranging from a few days to more than 18 months.[15] Although surgical treatment is not recommended for horses with Australian stringhalt, good results were recently reported in 11 horses.[16] Five horses were able to walk normally immediately after the surgery (described later) in both hindlimbs, whereas only partial improvement was noted immediately postoperatively in the remaining six horses. Five of them resumed a normal gait in 4 to 12 weeks postoperatively. The last horse suffered a relapse several weeks postoperatively and eventually recovered spontaneously 9 months after surgery.[16] Because conventional stringhalt is rarely associated with spontaneous recovery, lateral digital extensor tenectomy and partial myectomy is the treatment option for these horses.[20]

The objective of lateral digital extensor (LDE) tenectomy and partial myectomy is to remove the distal 2 to 10 cm of the LDE muscle, and the entire tendon, from the muscle to its attachment to the long digital extensor tendon. The procedure may be performed using local anesthesia when removing small portions of muscle belly, or under general anesthesia when removing large portions of the muscle belly. For the standing procedure, a 2-cm line of local anesthetic is injected over the LDE tendon just proximal to its junction with the long digital extensor tendon on the lateral aspect of the metatarsus. This site is easily palpable just below the tarsometatarsal joint. Local anesthetic also is infiltrated directly into the muscle belly of the LDE, about 2 cm above the lateral malleolus of the tibia.

The distal incision is made directly over the tendon just proximal to its junction with the long digital extensor tendon. The tendon is subsequently exposed by bluntly dissecting beneath the tendon with a curved Kelly or Ochsner forceps. The proximal incision is located on the lateral aspect of the limb approximately 6 cm above the lateral malleolus of the tibia. It extends through the skin, subcutaneous tissue, and fascia directly over the lateral digital muscle in a vertical direction, parallel with the muscle fibers. The muscle belly is exposed using blunt dissection, and a heavy curved instrument is placed underneath it (Fig. 87-6).

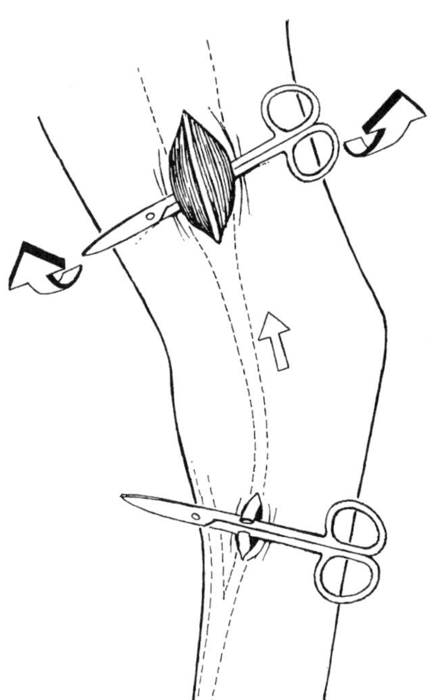

Figure 87-6. The muscle belly and tendon of the lateral digital extensor muscle have been isolated through two separate incisions. The distal part of the muscle and adjacent tendon are removed between these two incisions by transecting the tendon at the distal incision and pulling it out through the proximal incision *(arrows)*. The distal 2 cm of the muscle with the attached tendon are subsequently severed, and the incisions are closed.

Before severing the tendon, the surgeon should ensure that the tendon in the distal incision corresponds to the muscle belly in the proximal incision. The tendon is severed in the distal incision and is pulled through the tendon sheath by traction on the proximal portion with a curved Ochsner forceps or Mayo scissors. Removing the tendon from its sheath is a maneuver that requires substantial force, particularly if adhesions are present. After the entire length of the tendon has been exteriorized, the muscle is severed at the proximal aspect of the incision, thereby ensuring that at least 2 cm of the muscle is removed.

The heavy fascia of the proximal incision is closed with a simple-interrupted or continuous pattern of no. 0 synthetic absorbable suture material. The subcutaneous tissue is closed with 2-0 synthetic absorbable suture using a simple-continuous pattern, and the skin is closed with nonabsorbable suture material in a simple-continuous pattern. The distal incision is closed with skin sutures only. The wounds are covered with a sterile dressing, and the entire limb is bandaged for 10 to 14 days to control seroma formation. The horse is confined to a stall for this time, after which the sutures can be removed. The horse is then given 1 week of controlled hand-walking, and normal exercise can resume 3 to 4 weeks after surgery.

Complications of surgery include dehiscence; infection, which may enter the open tendon sheath of the LDE tendon; and failure of improvement of the lameness.

Prognosis

The prognosis for Australian stringhalt is fair. Many horses recover spontaneously, although a few have stringhalt of such severity that they are euthanized. The prognosis for conventional stringhalt is guarded to favorable, because surgery is unpredictable and can result in partial to complete recovery. Many horses show improvement after surgery, but the degree of improvement varies from slight to a complete remission.[6] Improvement may occur immediately or take several months.

Peroneus Tertius Disorders

The peroneus tertius is an entirely tendinous muscle. It originates in the extensor fossa on the cranial lateral aspect of the distal femur with the long digital flexor tendon. It courses distally over the cranial aspect of the tibia, and it divides distally into branches that surround the tendon of insertion of the tibialis cranialis muscle. At the dorsal aspect of the tarsus, it divides into a lateral branch that inserts on the calcaneal and fourth metatarsal bones, and a medial branch that inserts on third metatarsal and third tarsal bones. The tarsocrural joint is actively flexed by the contraction of the tibialis cranialis muscle and the passive pull of the tendinous peroneus tertius muscle. The peroneus tertius is an important part of the reciprocal apparatus of the hindlimb, which coordinates flexion of the hock and stifle (see Figs. 99-2 and 99-3).

Injury to the peroneus tertius is a relatively rare condition that has been reported in two locations: avulsion at the origin (most commonly seen in foals),[21-23] and in the distal third of the body (most commonly seen in adults).[24,25] It has been speculated that foals may be more likely to suffer avulsion injuries as a result of inherent weakness in their bones.[22]

Pathophysiology

By virtue of the anatomy described earlier, flexion and extension of the tarsus and stifle must occur simultaneously. Rupture of the peroneus tertius tendon is usually the result of overextension of the tarsus with normal stifle flexion. This may occur when the horse slips with a hindlimb extended backward, during the exertion of a rapid start, or when the limb is trapped and the horse struggles to free it.[24] A full limb cast extending to the proximal tibia may cause rupture if the horse slips with the leg extended behind, or struggles against the cast.[4]

Diagnosis

Although the peroneus tertius tendon may rupture anywhere along its length, it does so most commonly in the distal third of the tibia just proximal to the tarsus. The classic sign of a complete rupture is the ability to extend the hock while the stifle is flexed. A characteristic dimple forms in the common calcaneal tendon on the caudal lateral aspect of the crus, just proximal to the calcaneal tuber (Fig. 87-7). When standing, the horses may bear weight normally, but during the caudal phase of the stride during the walk or trot, the distal limb appears abnormally flaccid. With avulsion injuries, horses can be severely lame initially, and there may be accompanying distention of the femorotibial and femoropatellar joints.[22,23] In the acute phases of a rupture, digital palpation may reveal some swelling and pain in the craniolateral aspect of the crus, but typically there is little or no evidence of pain.

When the horse is walked, the tarsus may be noted to extend more than usual, and at the trot the horse is seen to be severely lame. A delay in the cranial phase of the stride can be easily identified because of an inappropriate degree of extension in the tarsus. Although there are usually no radiographically apparent signs of rupture, the peroneus tertius tendon is the most echogenic structure on the craniolateral aspect of the crus, and it is readily identified by ultrasonography. Radiography is necessary for diagnosing avulsion fractures.

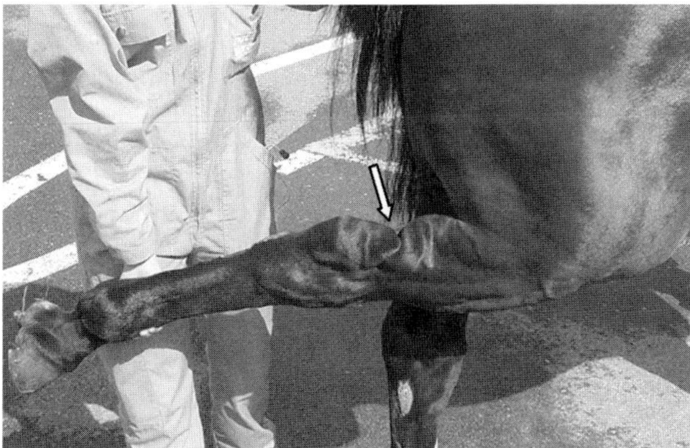

Figure 87-7. A horse with rupture of the peroneus tertius. The hock is extended while the stifle is flexed. Note the characteristic dimple in the contour of the caudal distal aspect of the crus.

Treatment

Horses with avulsion injuries of the origin of the peroneus tertius muscle are best evaluated arthroscopically.[22,23] Small bone fragments can be removed, but large bone fragments that are encapsulated by the joint capsule are better left in place. Six weeks of stall rest followed by controlled exercise for 3 months is recommended.

Peroneus tertius rupture is best treated with 3 months of restricted exercise in a box stall. Resumption of exercise starting with hand-walking usually results in a total resolution of clinical signs, and surgical intervention is unnecessary.

Prognosis

Horses with avulsion injuries have a guarded prognosis for full soundness, but successful outcomes have been reported.[22-24] Minor disruptions may heal, but outcomes are contingent on concurrent injuries. Most horses with ruptures of the body are able to return to full athletic function.[24,25]

Rupture of the Extensor Carpi Radialis Tendon

Rupture of the extensor carpi radialis tendon is usually the result of a traumatic insult, such as a kick or laceration at the distal cranial aspect of the radius, stumbling and falling on a road (coronation), or contact between a forelimb and a sharp object.

Diagnosis

Horses suffering from a rupture of the extensor carpi radialis tendon have a peculiar gait. Protraction of the involved forelimb results in hypermetric elevation, because the flexor muscles are not opposed by their main antagonist, the extensor carpi radialis muscle (Fig. 87-8). Palpation of the cranial aspect of the carpal and distal radial region reveals a defect in the area of the missing tendon. In cases with a laceration, the distal tendon stump is often seen in the injury site.

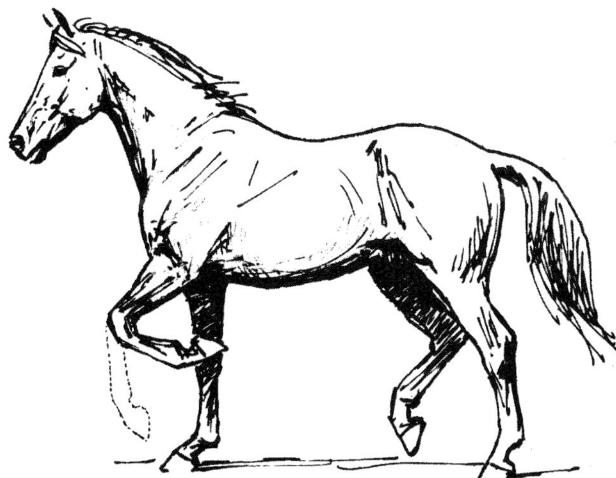

Figure 87-8. Drawing of a horse demonstrating the exaggerated flexion and forward movement of the left forelimb as a result of a traumatic rupture of the extensor carpi radialis tendon. The *dotted outline* of normal forelimb flexion is shown for comparison.

Treatment

Lacerations should be carefully débrided and closed, and a drain should be placed for the initial few days. If possible, the tendon should be repaired with three-loop pulley or a locking loop technique (see Fig. 86-29). The laceration should be sutured using routine wound repair techniques and the limb placed in a splint bandage that prohibits carpal flexion for 6 weeks. The bandage should be changed after 3 days and the drain removed. The horse is restricted to a box stall and the splint bandage is changed at regular intervals. If no open wound is present or the wound does not involve the sheath of the extensor carpi radialis tendon, the tendon is not sutured, but the limb is kept in a splint bandage for 6 weeks, followed by bandaging the limb for an additional 3 weeks. Hand-walking is initially the only exercise, and it is gradually increased. Local wound management should be applied to superficial wounds.

Prognosis

Generally, a good prognosis for return to a successful athletic career is given for rupture of the extensor carpi radialis tendon. Complications include infection of the tendon sheath and dehiscence of the sutured tendon or sutured laceration. In such cases, conservative management involving daily wound care and bandage changes is required. The prognosis in complicated cases is guarded for return to an athletic career.

Cribbing and Aerophagia

Etiology

Cribbing or crib biting in the horse is a vice characterized by the placement of the upper incisors on a solid object, arching the neck, depressing the tongue, elevating the larynx, and pulling backward.[26-35] If the horse swallows air, the process is called aerophagia, or "wind sucking," and an audible grunt can be heard. The sequelae to this habit are poor performance, weight loss, erosion of the incisors, and chronic colic. The principal reason that horses with this vice are presented to a veterinarian is because the behavior is objectionable and irritating to owners, and it results in an unacceptable level of property destruction. The habit is learned or acquired and is usually associated with stabled horses, although once learned it can continue in the pasture. Another reason patients are presented is that pressure is exerted on the owner by owners of horses stabled in the same barn, who are afraid their horses will acquire the vice as well. It is not known what causes horses to initiate this activity, but the most common explanation is boredom or frustration. Aerophagia may also be a pleasurable sensation to horses experiencing gastrointestinal discomfort.[27] Cribbing and windsucking may be acquired vices or may be learned from other horses, although learning the vice has not been proven.[27] It has also been associated with genetic factors.[28]

Treatment

NONSURGICAL MANAGEMENT

Horses that are stalled continuously may limit or discontinue the behavior when they are moved to pasture.[26,27] Removing fixed objects that are grasped while cribbing may deter horses that have just learned the vice. Management changes rarely deter horses with established habits, some of which are capable of aerophagia without grasping a fixed object. Cribbing straps are perhaps the most common nonsurgical means used to control cribbing or windsucking. Leather straps with or without a ventrally located piece of articulating metal are placed snugly around the throatlatch of the horse to discourage contraction of the ventral neck muscles and arching of the neck. More severe straps have metal prongs that pierce the skin when the neck is flexed. Cribbing straps are adjusted to allow the horse to eat and breathe normally and are worn at all times except during exercise. Acupuncture may be useful for eliminating or decreasing cribbing and aerophagia.[30] Aversion (shock) therapy has also been used to treat horses that crib.[22]

SURGICAL MANAGEMENT

Three surgical procedures are described for the control of cribbing and aerophagia: the Forssell procedure, a modified Forssell procedure, and bilateral neurectomy of the ventral branch of the spinal accessory nerve.[26,28,32-35] The original procedure was developed by Dr. Forssell in 1920 and involves the surgical removal of portions of the sternomandibularis, sternothyrohyoideus, and omohyoideus muscles.[26,32,33] A modification of Dr. Forssell's original surgery, developed to produce a better cosmetic appearance, is the treatment of choice for wind sucking when used in combination with neurectomy.[28] The technique of bilateral neurectomy of the ventral branches of the spinal accessory nerves (11th cranial nerves) is modified from the technique described by Hamm.[34] The ventral branches provide motor innervation to the sternomandibularis muscles, which are the major muscles used by the horse to flex its neck. Because of the poor results achieved with this procedure alone, it is now described as a part of the modified Forssell procedure.[28]

Modified Forssell procedure

The horse under general anesthesia is placed in dorsal recumbency with the head tilted at a 30-degree angle to the horizon.[20] After surgical preparation, a 30-cm incision is made on the ventral midline of the neck through the skin, the edges of which are retracted laterally, exposing the ventral surface of the paired bellies of the omohyoideus and the sternothyrohyoideus, and the cranial aspect of the sternomandibularis muscle. Careful attention to hemostasis minimizes staining of the areolar tissue and thus simplifies identification of the nerve. A plane of dissection is created on the medial aspect of the sternomandibularis muscle about 5 cm caudal to the musculotendinous junction. The ventral branch of the spinal accessory nerve is located on the dorsomedial aspect of this muscle by carefully rolling the muscle belly laterally. Curved hemostatic forceps are placed under the nerve, which is elevated until a sizable portion of it can be exteriorized. Contraction of the muscle after the nerve is pinched with hemostat forceps confirms isolation of the correct nerve. A large portion (6 to 12 cm) of nerve is removed. This same procedure is then repeated on the opposite side of the neck.

After the bilateral neurectomy, the myectomy is performed. A 30-cm section of the combined bellies of the omohy-

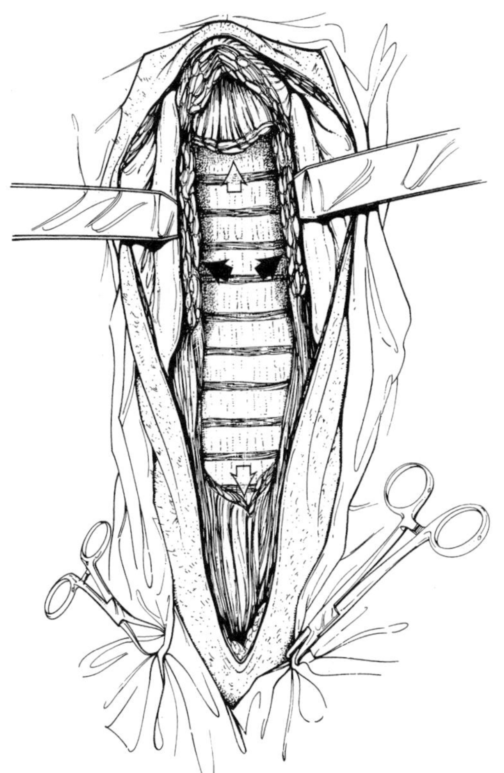

Figure 87-9. The modified Forssell procedure for cribbing is performed by a myectomy of the omohyoideus and sternothyrohyoideus muscles and by a neurectomy of the ventral branch of the spinal accessory nerve. *Closed arrows,* omohyoideus muscle stumps; *open arrows,* stumps of the sternothyrohyoideus muscles.

oideus and sternothyrohyoid muscles is removed (Fig. 87-9). These muscles are identified in the cranial aspect of the incision, just ventral to the larynx, and they are freed from the larynx and fascial attachments to the linguofacial vein and thyroid gland. Curved scissors or other curved instruments are passed under the muscles to ensure inclusion of all parts of the muscle bellies, which are then transected. These muscles bellies are then grasped and "peeled" caudally. The areolar connective tissue connecting them to the trachea is sharply dissected. The omohyoideus muscles are sectioned obliquely and the sternohyoid bands transversely at the caudal aspect of the incision. The sternothyroid bands of the sternothyrohyoideus muscles are elevated from the trachea and removed. Special attention is given to hemostasis of the muscle stumps to prevent hematoma formation.

A Penrose drain is inserted in the wound and brought out through separate stab incisions on both ends of the incision. The subcutaneous tissues are closed with a simple-continuous suture pattern using no. 0 synthetic absorbable suture material, and the skin is closed with any suitable pattern and material. To help eliminate dead space, a stent bandage is sutured over the incision to provide constant pressure to the wound and to protect it during the initial phase of healing.

After surgery, the horse is confined to a stall or small paddock for 2 weeks. Unless it is soiled earlier, the stent bandage is removed 2 or 3 days postoperatively. The Penrose drain is removed 4 to 6 days later, followed by the skin sutures 10 to 14 days postoperatively. Exercise can be resumed after 21 days. Hematomas or seromas, although rarely encountered, can be managed conservatively or by drainage. Antibiotic therapy initiated preoperatively can be applied until the drain is removed.

Prognosis

The modified Forssell procedure produces a good cosmetic appearance after surgery, and rapid healing of the wound.[29] A review of 35 horses that underwent the modified Forssell procedure revealed that 57% had complete remission, 31% had improvement, and 12% had no improvement.[29]

Calcinosis Circumscripta

Pathophysiology

Calcinosis circumscripta (tumoral calcinosis) is an uncommon condition that is identified more commonly in the young horse.[36-40] Although the etiology of these lesions is unknown, it has been suggested that prolonged repeated trauma may be the cause.[38] These horses have normal serum calcium and phosphorus concentrations.[41] Histologically, these masses are calcified granular amorphous material that induces a fibrous reaction.[36] They are surrounded by a thick fibrous capsule that contains deposits of gritty material. They are typically located in the subcutaneous tissue close to joints or tendon sheaths. The lateral aspect of the stifle adjacent to the fibula is an area of predilection,[36-38] although they also can be found on the dorsal lateral aspect of the tarsus, and around the neck and shoulder.[36] In 14 affected horses, the characteristic feature was a 3- to 12-cm dense subcutaneous mass located at the lateral aspect of the gaskin, adjacent to the stifle.[36,40]

Diagnosis

Rarely is lameness or pain associated with the condition. Typically, these horses present for cosmetic reasons and do not have any lameness.[41] Owners notice an unsightly lesion that may be increasing in size. Lesions are usually hard, are occasionally bilateral, are well circumscribed, do not involve the overlying skin, and are tightly adherent to the underlying tissue. Radiographs demonstrate a circumscribed mineralized tissue lying close to the lateral aspect of the femorotibial joint with a density that is similar to that of cortical bone.

Treatment

Treatment is indicated only if the cosmetic appearance is unacceptable to the owner, or if there is lameness caused by the mass. When required, surgical excision is the recommended treatment option. Attention to aseptic technique is imperative, since some masses attach to the femorotibial joint capsule, which may be accidentally entered during surgery. Closing dead space during surgery, and snug limb bandages or stent bandages will prevent postoperative seroma formation, since wound dehiscence and septic arthritis are potential complications.

Prognosis

For horses that are not treated, the mass remains and may not cause complications. A good result can be expected after surgical excision, and regrowth has not been reported. Wound healing is important if the joint capsule is entered during surgery.

REFERENCES

1. Cunningham JG: The physiology of muscle. In Cunningham JG, editor: Textbook of Veterinary Physiology, ed 2, Philadelphia, 1997, WB Saunders.
2. Adams SB: Biology and treatment of specific muscle disorders. In Auer JA, Stick JA, editors: Equine Surgery, ed 2, Philadelphia, 1999, WB Saunders.
3. Adams OR: Fibrotic myopathy in the hindlegs of horses, J Am Vet Med Assoc 1961;139:1089.
4. Stashak TS: Lameness. In Stashak TS, editor: Adams' Lameness in Horses, ed 4, Philadelphia, 1987, Lea & Febiger.
5. Pickersgill CH, Kriz N, Malikides N: Surgical treatment of semitendinosus fibrotic myopathy in an endurance horse: Management, complications and outcome, Equine Vet Educ 2000;12:320.
6. Turner AS, Trotter GW: Fibrotic myopathy in the horse, J Am Vet Med Assoc 1984;184:335.
7. Bishop R: Fibrotic myopathy of the gracilis muscle of a horse, Vet Med Small Anim Clin 1972;7:270.
8. Bramlage LR, Reed SM, Embertson RM: Semitendinosus tenotomy for treatment of fibrotic myopathy in the horse, J Am Vet Med Assoc 1985;186:565.
9. Irwin DHG, Howell DW: Fibrotic myopathy, haematomas, and scar tissue in the gaskin area of the Thoroughbred, J South Afr Vet Assoc 1981;52:65.
10. Bramlage LR: Fibrotic myopathy, diagnosis and treatment, Proc Am Coll Vet Surg Vet Symp Large Anim 1996;6:90.
11. Magee AA, Vatistas NJ: Standing semitendinous myotomy for the treatment of fibrotic myopathy in 39 horses (1989-1997), Proc Am Assoc Equine Pract 1998;44:263.
12. Valentine BA, Rousselle SD, Sams AE, et al. Degenerative atrophy in three horses with fibrotic myopathy, J Am Vet Med Assoc 1994;205:332.
13. Slocombe RF, Huntington PJ, Friend SCE, et al: Pathological aspects of Australian stringhalt, Equine Vet J 1992;24:174.
14. Cahill JI, Goulden BE, Pearce HG: A review and some observations on stringhalt, N Z Vet J 1985;33:101.
15. Huntington PJ, Jeffcott LB, Friend SCE, et al: Australian stringhalt: Epidemiological, clinical and neurological investigations, Equine Vet J 1989;21:266.
16. Torre F: Clinical diagnosis and results of surgical treatment of 11 cases of Australian stringhalt (1991-2002), Proc. Eur Coll Vet Surg 2003;12:208.
17. Cahill JI, Goulden BE, Jolly RD: Stringhalt in horses: A distal axonopathy, Neuropathol Appl Neurobiol 1986;12:459.
18. Crabill MR, Honnas CM, Taylor DS, et al: Stringhalt secondary to trauma to the dorsoproximal region of the metatarsus in horses: 10 cases (1986-1991), J Am Vet Med Assoc 1994;205:867.
19. Valentine BA. Mechanical lameness in the hindlimb. In Ross MW, Dyson SJ, editors: Diagnosis and Management of Lameness in the Horse, Philadelphia, 2003, WB Saunders.
20. Bramlage LB: Personal communication.
21. Turner AS, McIlwraith CW: Techniques in Large Animal Surgery, Philadelphia, 1989, Lea & Febiger.
22. Blikslager AT, Bristol DG: Avulsion of the origin of the peroneus tertius tendon in a foal, J Am Vet Med Assoc 1994;204:1483.
23. Holcombe S, Bertone AL: Avulsion fracture of the origin of the extensor digitorum longus in a foal, J Am Vet Med Assoc 1994;204:1652.
24. Hogan PM, Watkins JP, Schneider RK: Avulsion fractures of the extensor fossa of the distal femur in 6 foals, Proc Annu Conf Vet Orthop Soc 1996;23:38.
25. Szabuniewicz M, Titus RS: Rupture of the peroneus tertius in the horse, Vet Med Small Anim Clin 1967;62:993.
26. Dyson SJ: Other soft tissue injuries. In Ross MW, Dyson SJ, editors: Diagnosis and Management of Lameness in the Horse, Philadelphia, 2003, WB Saunders.
27. Monin T: Surgical management of crib biting in the horse, Comp Cont Educ Pract Vet 1982;4:S69.
28. Houpt KA: Stable vices and trailering problems, Vet Clin North Am: Equine Pract 1986;2:623.
29. Turner AS, White N, Ismay J: Modified Forssell operation for crib biting in the horse, J Am Vet Med Assoc 1984;184:309.
30. Vechiotti GG, Galanti R: Evidence of heredity in cribbing, weaving, and stall walking in Thoroughbred horses, Lifest Prod Sci 1986;14:91.
31. Kuusaari J: Acupuncture treatment of aerophagia in horses, Am J Acupunct 1983;11:363.
32. Baker GJ, Kear Colwell J: Aerophagia (windsucking) and aversion therapy in the horse, Proc Am Assoc Equine Pract 1974;20:127.
33. Forssell G: The new surgical treatment against crib biting, Vet J 1926;82:538.
34. Hamm D: A new surgical procedure to control crib biting, Proc Am Assoc Equine Pract 1977;23:301.
35. Firth EC: Bilateral ventral accessory neurectomy in windsucking horses, Vet Rec 1980;106:30.
36. Owen RR, McKeating FJ, Jagger DW: Neurectomy in windsucking horses, Vet Rec 1980;106:134.
37. Dodd DC, Raker CW: Tumoral calcinosis (calcinosis circumscripta) in the horse, J Am Vet Med Assoc 1979;57:968.
38. Goulden BE, O'Callaghan MW: Tumoral calcinosis in the horse, N Z Vet J 1980;28:217.
39. O'Connor JP, Lucey MP: Tumoral calcinosis (calcinosis circumscripta) in the horse, Irish Vet J 1977,31:173.
40. Thompson SW, Sullivan DJ, Pedersen RA: Calcinosis circumscripta: A histo-chemical study of the lesion in man, dogs, and monkeys, Cornell Vet 1959;49:265-285.
41. Hutchins DR: Tumoral calcinosis in the horse, Aust Vet J 1972;48:200-202.

CHAPTER 88

Synovial and Osseous Infections

Robert K. Schneider

Orthopedic infection is a more serious clinical problem in horses than in many other species, because its consequences can induce permanent lameness and result in loss of use of the horse or in death. Infection in a joint causes severe inflammation that can lead to irreversible cartilage damage and continued degeneration of the joint even after the infection is resolved.[1,2] Pain from osteoarthritis causes lameness that prohibits the return of the horse to active use. Lower joint forces and adjustment to a less active lifestyle make this same result of less consequence in human and canine patients. Infection of a fracture site, especially after surgical repair, greatly complicates treatment and frequently results in failure of the fracture to heal.[3] It is difficult to rigidly immobilize fractured bones with available implants in an animal the size of a horse. The combination of infection and minor movement at the fracture usually results in failure of the fracture to heal and ultimately to humane destruction of the horse. The treatment of orthopedic infection in horses is also more difficult because of the high incidence of laminitis in the opposite limb from increased weightbearing while the infection is being treated. Chronic increased weightbearing on the normal limb eventually results in failure of the laminae in the foot, laminitis, and separation of the distal phalanx from the hoof wall. Laminitis may occur at any time during treatment and can result in treatment failure even when the infected fracture heals or the joint infection resolves.

The treatment of orthopedic infection in horses has greatly improved over the last 20 years. Early recognition, improved methods of delivering high concentrations of antibiotics to the site of infection,[4-9] and techniques used to achieve effective drainage[10] have improved the clinician's ability to successfully eliminate the infecting bacteria. The prognosis for a horse with a septic joint to return to athletic function is no longer hopeless.[2,10] Despite the advances in treatment, limitations persist. Not every infection can be eliminated, and complications such as opposite-limb laminitis because of delayed fracture healing still result in death of the animal. In addition, the cost of treating horses with orthopedic infection is high. In a review of 38 horses with fractures that developed infection after surgical repair, the average duration of hospitalization was 142 days.[11] The costs of hospitalization and treatment make humane destruction the treatment of choice for some horse owners. However, the treatment of orthopedic infection has been successful even in complicated cases, and euthanasia should be considered only after treatment options have been explored, many of which were not considerations 20 years ago.

SEPTIC ARTHRITIS

Etiology

The etiology, diagnosis, and treatment principles are the same for other synovial structures, such as tendon sheaths and bursas, as they are for joint infections. Infection of a joint occurs when microorganisms colonize the joint after a penetrating wound, joint injection, surgery, or hematogenous localization. Hematogenous infection is common in foals, but it can also occur in adult horses. In a review of 192 horses with synovial sepsis, 12 adult horses developed an infected joint or a tendon sheath without a history of previous injury or treatment.[2] Two of these horses had a primary infection in another anatomic location in the body, but in 10 horses infection occurred without signs of infection in any other location. Joint infection should be considered in the differential diagnosis of any horse with an acute onset of joint swelling and lameness. Intra-articular injection or a penetrating wound is the most common cause of infectious arthritis or synovitis in adult horses. Therefore, horses with a wound over a synovial structure should be carefully evaluated to determine whether the synovial space has been penetrated.

Clinical Signs

Bacterial invasion of a joint induces rapid pathologic changes[12,13] that result in joint effusion and severe lameness. The degree of lameness varies depending on the size of the horse (foals typically bear some weight on the limb), the duration of the infection, and the pathogenicity of the infecting organism. Some horses may walk almost normally, whereas others support little or no weight on the affected limb. Distention of the involved joint is a consistent sign that can be detected visually, by palpation of the joint pouches, or both. In some horses, increased joint fluid may not be detectable because of overlying soft tissues (i.e., at the shoulder) or the small size of the joint capsule (i.e., at the distal two tarsal joints). Periarticular edema, cellulitis, or both may make palpation of joint effusion difficult. Horses with a joint infection have pain on palpation and usually respond to digital pressure applied over the joint capsule. Horses with open joint lacerations through which synovial fluid is draining are frequently not as lame as horses with closed joint infections.

Horses with septic arthritis usually have a fever at some point after the initial infection. However, fever may not be present, especially if the animal has been treated or placed on nonsteroidal anti-inflammatory medication. On the other hand, fever is one of the earliest and most consistent observations in horses that develop an infection after joint surgery. In a retrospective study of 25 horses with postoperative joint infection, a body temperature above 39° C (101° F) was the most consistent clinical observation and appeared at an average of 9 days after surgery.[2]

Diagnosis

A diagnosis of septic arthritis or synovitis is confirmed by obtaining fluid for cytology and analysis. Synovial fluid is obtained through arthrocentesis using aseptic technique. Synovial fluid from infected joints averages a total white blood cell (WBC) count of more than 75,000 cells/dL, predominantly neutrophils, and contains more than 5 g/dL total protein.[2] Normal synovial fluid has fewer than 300 cells, fewer than 10% neutrophils, and less than 2.5 g/dL protein.[14] When the gross appearance of the synovial fluid is cloudy or turbid, infection is likely. A total WBC count of less than 10,000 cells/dL does not rule out an infected joint; some joints have relatively low WBC counts because of sequestration of the WBCs within fibrin deposits in the joint. One of the most consistent findings in the synovial fluid is a shift to more than 80% to 90% neutrophils.[2,13]

Bacteria may be seen during cytologic evaluation, but only 24% of fluid samples have bacteria observed on a direct smear. Although chemical irritants injected into a joint may cause similar abnormalities in the synovial fluid, there are few, if any, other causes of these synovial fluid abnormalities in horses. Immune-mediated inflammatory arthropathies are rare in horses but should be considered in adult animals with multiple affected joints. Horses exhibiting the described abnormalities in their synovial fluid analysis and cytology should be treated as if they have a septic joint or tendon sheath until proven otherwise.

Before treating a horse with an infected joint or tendon sheath, it is important to obtain a sample of synovial fluid for culture. Synovial fluid is aspirated and placed in blood culture medium.[15,16] Ideally, 5 mL is obtained for culture, but any volume that is aspirated is used. The use of blood culture techniques maximizes the chance of incubating the infecting organism or organisms and obtaining antimicrobial sensitivity results, which help in the selection of effective antimicrobial drugs.[15] There is no advantage to obtaining a synovial membrane biopsy for culture because bacterial isolation rates in clinical cases[16] and experimental trials[15] have been as high or higher with synovial fluid. If the horse has been previously treated with antibiotics, obtaining synovial fluid for culture is still recommended, although the presence of antibiotics decreases the chances for a positive culture. It is important to list the type of antibiotic used on the laboratory request form. In joints with a small volume of fluid, such as the tarsometatarsal joint, it may be necessary to first inject the joint with sterile saline before a sample can be aspirated for culture.

Radiography

Radiographic examination is recommended for every horse with an infected joint or tendon sheath to evaluate the bones for signs of osteitis or osteomyelitis and to rule out fractures and associated joint pathology. This is essential in foals and horses with chronic joint infections. The presence of osteomyelitis in subchondral epiphyseal bone or in the physis in foals complicates treatment and may decrease the prognosis for soundness based on the anatomic location (e.g., beneath a weight-bearing articular surface). The subchondral bone and, in young horses, the surrounding physes should be evaluated for local bone lysis (Fig. 88-1).

Treatment

Aggressive and early treatment is recommended to eliminate an infection in synovial structures as soon as possible. Treatment is always initiated before culture results are known. Because in 25% of synovial fluid samples, an organism may not be isolated,[2] it is important to aim antimicrobial therapy at the most likely infecting organism using broad-spectrum antimicrobial agents. The source of the joint infection should be considered. Horses that develop sepsis after surgery or intra-articular injection are likely to be infected with staphylococcus, especially *Staphylococcus aureus.*[2] Horses that develop infection after a wound are more likely to have an *Enterobacter* species isolated from the synovial fluid; cultures from these joints frequently have multiple organisms identified, including *Staphylococcus, Streptococcus, Pseudomonas,* and anaerobes.[2] The most common bacteria isolated from a group of equine orthopedic patients in one hospital were Enterobacteriaceae, *Streptococcus, Staphylococcus,* and *Pseudomonas,* in decreasing order of incidence.[4] Broad-spectrum bactericidal drugs should be administered by the intravenous route to maximize penetration into the synovial fluid.

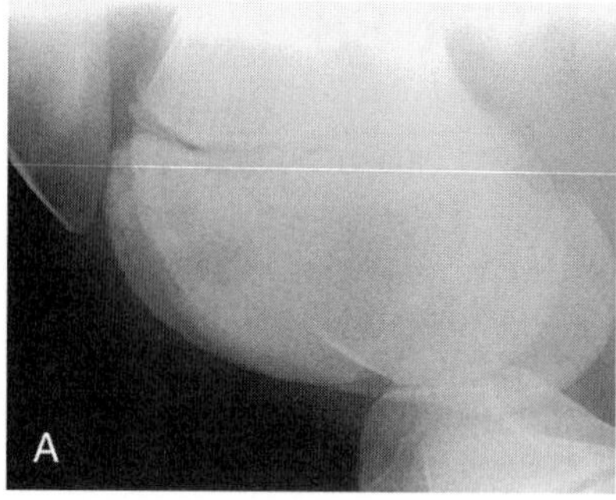

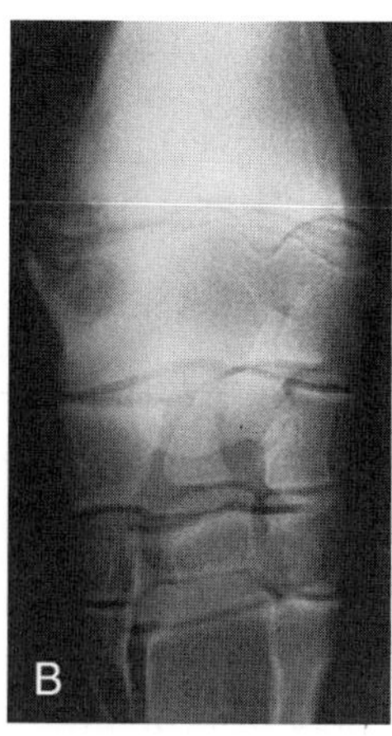

Figure 88-1. A, Lateral radiograph of the stifle joint of a foal with septic arthritis and osteomyelitis of the lateral trochlear ridge of the distal femur with radiolucent defects deep in the subchondral bone. The irregular margins of the proximal articular surface of the trochlear ridge are the normal ossification pattern observed in this location in growing foals. This foal was treated successfully with arthroscopic débridement, joint lavage, and intra-articular and systemic antibiotics. **B,** Craniocaudal radiograph of the carpus of a weanling foal with osteomyelitis in the distal radial physis. Note the large area of radiolucency because of severe lysis of bone around the medial physis. This foal was treated successfully with long-term (8 weeks) systemic antibiotic therapy.

In addition to efficacy against the most common bacterial isolates, expense of the drugs is a factor in selecting antibiotics. Cefazolin and amikacin may not be affordable at systemic doses in every patient, despite their broad spectrum and efficacy against isolates from horses with infected joints.[17] Penicillin and gentamicin are less expensive and still effective against many bacteria. Ceftiofur and cefazolin are antibiotics with a broad spectrum of efficacy and could be considered for initial intravenous antibiotic treatment.

Joint Lavage

Joint lavage is indicated in horses and foals with a septic joint. The decision to perform the lavage through needles or under arthroscopic guidance is usually based on the duration of the infection and the severity of the clinical signs. Acute cases may respond well to a through-and-through lavage accomplished with 14- or 16-gauge needles placed on opposite sides of the joint. This is a valuable technique in foals with multiple affected joints. Chronic septic joints frequently have a coagulum of fibrin and thickened synovium that makes adequate lavage via needles difficult. Fibrin and chronically thickened synovium can be removed from the joint when the lavage is accomplished under arthroscopic guidance. In addition, the health of the articular cartilage can be evaluated, and localized areas of osteitis or osteomyelitis can be débrided. The longer the infection has been present and the more inflamed the joint, the more likely it is that arthroscopic surgery will be necessary to achieve effective lavage. In foals, osteomyelitis in the subchondral epiphyseal bone requires surgical débridement under arthroscopic guidance, even in very acute cases. The value of arthroscopic lavage in the management of synovial sepsis in horses has been clearly demonstrated.[18]

A sterile, balanced electrolyte solution is recommended for flushing septic joints. Antiseptic solutions cause inflammatory changes in normal joints. Chlorhexidine solutions are too irritating to the joint to be recommended for lavage.[19,20] Even the minimal inflammatory response caused by 0.1% and 0.01% povidone-iodine does not offer an advantage over a balanced electrolyte solution.[21] Antibiotics can be included in the lavage solution, but because of the transient contact time of the fluid with the synovium, antibiotics are usually injected after the lavage to achieve higher synovial fluid concentrations.[8] Dimethyl sulfoxide (DMSO) in the lavage solution causes neither irritation nor significant inflammation in synovial structures.[22] The benefits of the drug include its superoxide radical–scavenging activity and suppression of prostaglandins; both actions decrease inflammation. The drug theoretically helps antibiotics penetrate the synovium. Despite these benefits, the value of including DMSO in the lavage fluid is debatable.

Joint lavage through needles can be accomplished in the standing animal with sedation and local anesthesia, although it is usually easier to accomplish distention and irrigation with the horse under general anesthesia. Small foals can normally have their joints flushed using sedation (diazepam, xylazine, or butorphanol) and local anesthesia injected into the joint 5 to 10 minutes before lavage. The use of the arthroscope usually requires general anesthesia.

Intra-articular Antibiotics

The intra-articular administration of antibiotics is a routine treatment in horses with septic arthritis. Gentamicin achieves high synovial fluid concentrations with relatively low intra-articular doses (150 mg) and causes minimal inflammation.[8] Amikacin, because of its similarity to gentamicin and its efficacy against a wide range of bacteria,[17] has become a routinely used intra-articular antibiotic. Ceftiofur,[23] Timentin (ticarcillin-clavulanic acid), methicillin, and imipenem-cilastatin[24] can be injected into joints with few inflammatory side effects on equine synovium. Imipenem-cilastatin, which is a suspension when 500 mg is diluted in 10 mL of sterile saline, causes only mild inflammation when it is injected once daily for 3 days.[24] Cefazolin injected into equine patients with septic arthritis causes no observed ill effects. The number of antibiotics that can be safely used intra-articularly will continue to increase; however, it is important that antibiotics be evaluated for their inflammatory effects on joint tissues before they are used in clinical patients. Some antibiotics may cause damage to the synovium or articular cartilage, or both. Synovial fluid levels measured after intra-articular injection of gentamicin, ceftiofur, ticarcillin-clavulanic acid, or Primaxin (imipenem-cilastatin) are 10 to 100 times the synovial fluid levels that can be achieved with systemic administration.[8,23,24] Organisms identified as resistant with antimicrobial susceptibility techniques used in the laboratory may be susceptible to the high concentrations of antibiotic achieved with intra-articular injection. Care must be taken not to exceed systemic doses of antibiotics in horses with multiple septic joints or tendon sheaths. This is most likely to occur in young foals with a relatively small body mass and multiple affected joints, especially because these foals receive systemic antibiotic therapy as well. Intra-articular antibiotics are usually administered after a joint lavage, and then once a day until clinical signs are resolving. Amikacin is the most frequently used intra-articular antibiotic because of its efficacy.[17] The use of the correct intra-articular antibiotic makes a dramatic difference in the clinical response to treatment. However, drugs such as ticarcillin-clavulanic acid and Primaxin should not be used routinely, to decrease the chances that bacteria will develop resistance to these antibiotics.

After lavage and intra-articular antibiotic injections, the affected joints are usually bandaged to decrease swelling and protect surgical incisions. The horses are maintained on a low dose of nonsteroidal anti-inflammatory medication, most commonly phenylbutazone (4 mg/kg PO once a day). This decreases inflammation and improves the use of the limb. Foals may also be placed on antiulcer medication (e.g., ranitidine [Zantac] and sucralfate [Carafate]) to combat the stress of hospitalization and treatment.

Regional Limb Perfusion

Another method that is used to deliver high concentrations of antibiotics to the joint and surrounding bones and soft tissues is regional limb perfusion.[25] The technique uses the vascular space to maximize antibiotic penetration into the synovial fluid and also into the tissues around the joint. It is of particular value in foals when penetration of bone and surrounding soft tissues is needed in sites of bacterial colonization. In the author's experience, it has been particularly valuable for treating foals that have osteomyelitis in the physis or epiphysis of hematogenous origin. The technique does not achieve synovial fluid concentrations as high as can be obtained through direct injection into the joint space, but synovial fluid levels exceeding 55 times the minimal inhibitory concentration (MIC) reported for most organisms can be reached with gentamicin.[25] Gentamicin concentration remains at or above the MIC for most sensitive organisms 24 hours after perfusion.[26]

Regional limb perfusion is performed by placing a tourniquet on the limb proximal to the area to be perfused. For the carpus and tarsus, a tourniquet also is placed distal to these joints. One gram of amikacin is diluted in 120 mL of sterile saline and injected through an intravenous catheter placed into a peripheral vein distal to the tourniquet using sterile technique. The tourniquet is maintained on the limb for 20 minutes to allow time for the antibiotic to penetrate into the synovial fluid, bone, and soft tissues. Antibiotics that have been used for this procedure in our hospital in addition to amikacin are gentamicin (500 mg), imipenem-cilastatin (250 mg), and cefotaxime (500 mg). Original studies performed with 300 mg of gentamicin have shown that a relatively small dose of antibiotics achieves high concentrations of the drug in the synovial fluid.[25] The procedure is frequently performed under general anesthesia after lavage of the joint. However, it can be performed on the distal limb of adults and in foals under sedation with local anesthesia.

Regional limb perfusion can be considered in any horse with a septic joint. It is recommended in horses that have cellulitis and edema around the joint and especially in cases where there is osteomyelitis. Penetration into bone using this technique has been shown to be just as effective as an intraosseous injection of antibiotics.[27] Perhaps more important has been the observation that a higher synovial fluid concentration of gentamicin is obtained by intra-articular injection than by regional limb perfusion.[28] Therefore, intra-articular injection of antibiotics is still the most effective way to obtain high synovial fluid concentrations of antibiotics.

Open Drainage

In horses that do not respond to treatment or have a chronic infection, open drainage of the joint is indicated. Clinical signs are used to monitor the response to treatment. Swelling around the joint decreases, the joint effusion resolves, there is less sensitivity to palpation, and the horse's use of the limb improves when the infection is being effectively controlled. The body temperature returns to normal, and systemic spread of the infection to another synovial structure is unlikely. This is especially important to monitor in young foals. The clinical signs persist or recur in joints where the infection is not controlled.

Open drainage is usually accomplished with the horse under anesthesia and using large-volume (3 to 5 L) lavage of the joint. Two or more 3- to 5-cm arthrotomy incisions are made to allow fibrin and fluid to drain from the joint. The arthrotomy incisions are left open so that chronic and effective drainage of the joint can be achieved, and they are placed in the best location to allow drainage, which varies with the joint.[10] Each arthrotomy is made sufficiently large to allow drainage without becoming sealed by fibrin and local swelling around the incision. Open arthrotomy incisions are protected by a sterile bandage that is changed daily. For joints such as the stifle, which cannot be bandaged, stent bandages may be sutured over the arthrotomy sites, especially in foals. Adult horses are cross-tied or tied on an overhead cable to keep them from lying down. The tail is wrapped, and the incisions are cleaned several times a day.

Open drainage and systemic antibiotics may be sufficient to resolve some infections, but usually, intra-articular antibiotics and repeated lavage of the joint are necessary when treating chronically infected joints. Repeat joint lavage is usually performed with the horse standing and sedated. The decision to perform a repeat lavage is based on examination of the joint. If effective drainage does not occur, the joint becomes distended, the arthrotomy plugs with fibrin, and the bandage or limb is not soaked by draining fluid. If this occurs, joint lavage through a large-gauge needle placed on the side of the joint opposite the incision allows fibrin to be flushed through the arthrotomy, opening the incision and promoting future drainage. Aseptic preparation of the skin is necessary both at the arthrocentesis site and around the arthrotomy. Distention irrigation of the joint is best accomplished with a 60-mL syringe and an extension tube connected to the needle. The syringe generates considerable pressure that can be controlled and regulated by the volume injected. Fibrin can be removed from the arthrotomy site with a sterile Kelly forceps. Intra-articular antibiotics are injected into the joint after the lavage. Joint lavage is performed only if necessary to maintain effective drainage from the joint. Antibiotics are injected through a small (18- to 20-gauge) needle placed in a location removed from the arthrotomy site under aseptic conditions once a day. Alternatively, a small sterile catheter may be passed into the joint through the arthrotomy once the incision has been cleaned with an antiseptic. It is important to pass the catheter several centimeters into the joint to keep the antibiotics from running back out of the joint immediately after injection.

When infection is eliminated, swelling and effusion resolve, and the synovial fluid draining through the incision becomes clear and viscous. The horse is maintained on systemic antibiotics until the arthrotomy heals. Once the infection resolves, the arthrotomy incision can be closed; the arthrotomy wound is débrided while the joint is lavaged and the incision is sutured closed.[10] Infection resolved after open drainage and closure of the arthrotomy in 30 horses. However, recurrence of infection has occurred in one horse 2 weeks after the arthrotomy was sutured. Early closure of the incision decreases hospitalization and the time that the horse must be on antibiotics with the joint protected by a bandage. However, the risk of recurrence of infection has devastating consequences to the horse and the owner because of the cost of starting over in the treatment of an infected joint.

Penrose drains can be used to improve drainage through openings in joints or tendon sheaths, but Penrose drains are foreign material, do not always contribute to effective drainage, and may be a pathway along which bacteria can migrate into the synovial cavity. Suction drains achieve more effective decompression of a joint through constant suction. Suction drains have been used to successfully treat horses with septic arthritis of the tarsocrural joint.[29] However, closed suction drains are more difficult to maintain than an open arthrotomy incision; they must be protected by a bandage, and the suction device must be continually monitored. Disconnection of the tubing could lead to ingress flow of air into the joint.

Which treatments are the most effective in eliminating infection in horses with septic arthritis is difficult to determine.[30] Arthrotomy and open drainage decrease fibrin accumulation in the joint in both experimental[30] and clinical[10] cases of septic arthritis. Intra-articular injection of antibiotics has improved success in treating horses with infectious arthritis.[8,10] It is possible to eliminate joint infection in adult horses with a one-time lavage of the joint followed by daily intra-articular injections of antibiotics, without administration of systemic antibiotics (because of economics). It is not recommended that systemic antibiotics be eliminated from the treatment regimen for horses with septic arthritis. However, in the future, early administration of intra-articular antibiotic treatments may be all that is necessary to eliminate infections in adult horses with a septic joint. Systemic antibiotics would appear to be necessary for all foals with infectious arthritis to avoid hematogenous dissemination of the infection to another synovial structure.

Adjunctive Treatment

Infection in a joint causes the release of most known mediators of inflammation and many catabolic enzymes from degenerating neutrophils that are part of the immune response. After the elimination of the infecting organism, anti-inflammatory medication returns the joint to normal and minimizes damage to the articular cartilage. Hyaluronan, polysulfated glycosaminoglycan (Adequan), and corticosteroids have beneficial effects in inflamed joints. The immunosuppressive properties of both glycosaminoglycan and cortisone increase the risk of recurrence of the infection if even a small number of bacteria have persisted in the joint.[31] Use of these drugs is controversial. The author uses hyaluronan IV (Legend) intra-articularly if all signs of the infection have resolved. This appears to help resolve the synovitis and joint capsule thickening that occur in infected joints.

Septic Physitis in Foals

Infection of a physis can occur simultaneously or secondary to infection of the synovial space in foals with hematogenous septic arthritis. Septic physitis may also occur as a primary disease, secondary to septicemia in foals, and must be considered a primary differential diagnosis for septic arthritis or tenosynovitis in young foals.[32] Foals with septic physitis have significant lameness, local heat and swelling around the growth plates, and intermittent fever. Because the physes are located near joints, careful palpation of the limb is necessary to distinguish physeal infection from septic arthritis.

Treatment of foals with septic physitis is different from treatment of foals with septic arthritis, because high concentrations of effective antibiotics must be achieved in the physis to successfully resolve infection at this site. The first and most important step in treating foals with septic physitis is to obtain a culture. A relatively easy method of obtaining a culture from an infected physis is to place a large-gauge needle (14 or 16 gauge) into the area of osteomyelitis that is identified on radiographs. In horses with large areas of lysis, purulent exudate may be obtained. Even in foals with a relatively small area of infection, an aspirate of blood can be obtained using suction from a 6-mL syringe; even small aspirates of blood can result in a positive culture.

Once a sample is obtained for culture, regional limb perfusion is performed. This is an effective method of achieving high concentrations of antibiotics in the physis. Although long-term systemic antibiotics also can be effective, a better response has been observed in foals treated with regional limb perfusion. The perfusion procedure is usually repeated at least two more times at weekly intervals; it can be repeated more frequently if necessary based on the clinical and radiographic evaluation of the foal. Although surgical drainage of purulent exudate is recommended, surgical curettage of the physis should be avoided to minimize irreversible damage to the growth plate. The use of regional limb perfusion has decreased the need to débride the area of bone infection and has proven to be an effective method of treatment for foals with septic physitis.

Prognosis

The survival rate and return to athletic use of horses with septic arthritis when treated aggressively have greatly improved. In a retrospective study of 192 treated horses, 85% of adults survived and more than 50% of the racehorses (Thoroughbred and Standardbred) returned to racing.[2] This is a significant improvement over prognoses that were given as recently as the early 1980s.[1] With improved techniques and early treatment, the prognosis may be even better.[10,18] The prognosis is not significantly affected by the joint involved,[2] although one study pointed out the difficulty in treatment of septic arthritis of the distal interphalangeal joint.[33] Tendon sheaths have a better prognosis for survival than joints,[2] perhaps because cartilage damage is not an issue in tendon sheaths. Although the chances for survival are better for a horse with an infected tendon sheath, these horses frequently develop fibrosis within the sheath that limits a return to soundness. The prognosis for foals is less than that of adults (62% survival) because of complications associated with septicemia and multiple-organ involvement. Therefore, treatment of foals is frequently more involved than treatment of a septic joint alone.

Despite improvements in management, not every horse with a joint infection can be successfully treated. Some joint infections are difficult to eliminate, and with time, either the bone is penetrated and osteomyelitis develops or irreversible damage to articular cartilage is caused, resulting in osteoarthritis. Laminitis in the opposite foot also complicates treatment. Some horses with refractory joint sepsis are candidates for arthrodesis, depending on the joint involved and the intended purpose of the horse. For horses with refractory joint infection, euthanasia may be the best option for the owner because of the costs and risks involved with further treatment.

ORTHOPEDIC INFECTIONS

Nothing complicates the treatment of a horse after surgical repair of a fracture or arthrodesis of a joint more than infection. Infection after these procedures increases the costs of care, decreases the use of the limb (which increases the chance for laminitis in the opposite limb), and delays healing of the fracture or arthrodesis.[11] The combination of infection and instability of an internal fixation is a reliable recipe for failure.[34] Therefore, every precaution should be taken to decrease the incidence of infection. Once it occurs, early recognition and aggressive treatment are necessary. In the 1970s, when internal fixation techniques were first applied to fractures in horses, infection of a major fracture repair almost always resulted in the death of the horse. Now, some horses with infected fractures can be saved, although treatment is expensive.

Etiology

Infection of a fracture site that has been surgically repaired occurs through an open wound in the skin before surgery, contamination of the surgery site during the open repair, or contamination through the surgical incision. The surgical incision is a source of contamination; excess swelling or motion leads to sutures cutting into the skin, allowing bacteria to invade and colonize the superficial tissues and facilitating the progress of infection deeper into the incision to colonize the implants, fracture site, or joint space. This is an important pathway for infection to invade the fracture site in horses, because there is relatively little soft tissue overlying the bones and joints in the distal limbs. Therefore, surgical incisions should always be protected by sterile bandages and dressings. The limb should be immobilized if the incision is located over a high motion area that will create tension on the sutured skin. Maintenance of a clean, dry seal of the surgical incision is important to avoid complications from infection.

Open fractures or the presence of even a small skin wound over the surgery site is a concern because contamination of the fracture site is difficult to avoid. These cases present difficult treatment decisions requiring experience and judgment regarding the initial treatment and the timing of any attempt at surgical repair. Despite the best decisions made or treatments implemented, treatment failure and loss of the horse may eventually occur.

Clinical Signs

Infection of a fracture site is not always recognized, especially when the incision is under a cast. The earliest and most consistent sign is a low-grade persistent fever observed even if the horse is receiving phenylbutazone. The development of a high fever of 39° to 40° C within the first 14 days after surgery is also a sign that infection may be present. In a review of 38 horses that developed infection after fracture repair or arthrodesis, the first clinical sign was a temperature elevation above 39° C that occurred an average of 10 days after surgery.[11] Therefore, an increased temperature is an indication to change the cast to allow examination of the incision and the surgical site.

Frequently, horses that develop infection decrease their use of the limb. This is variable and difficult to assess in horses that have a fracture or joint stabilized with internal fixation, because these horses already have reduced use of the limb. Pointing of the cast or injured limb, increased time lying down, increased pawing with the cast, an increase in hyperextension of the opposite fetlock joint, or an increase in ease of displacement of the limb from under the horse when the limb is in a weight-bearing position are all signs of the horse's decreased comfort on the operated limb. However, some horses that develop infection do not decrease their use of the repaired limb, making accurate recognition of the presence of infection even more difficult.

Evaluation of surgical incisions that are not covered by a cast is important. Horses that develop infection have increased swelling and heat at the surgery site. The skin frequently appears reddened or pink and may start to thin out as the infection progresses (Fig. 88-2). The sutures typically cut into the skin, and there may be drainage through the incision or along the sutures. Depending on the location of the incision, partial dehiscence may occur, with drainage of exudate. Early problems, such as drainage of serum through the incision, increase the risk of infection extending to the implants. An incision may drain a small amount of clear serous or serosanguineous fluid without developing infection; however, there is a higher incidence of infection in these horses than in horses in which the incision remains dry and sealed. An early sign of infection at the surgery site is an accumulation of fluid that can be detected through palpation. The surgical incision should be examined at every bandage change, especially in horses that develop an increased temperature, with the examiner wearing sterile gloves.

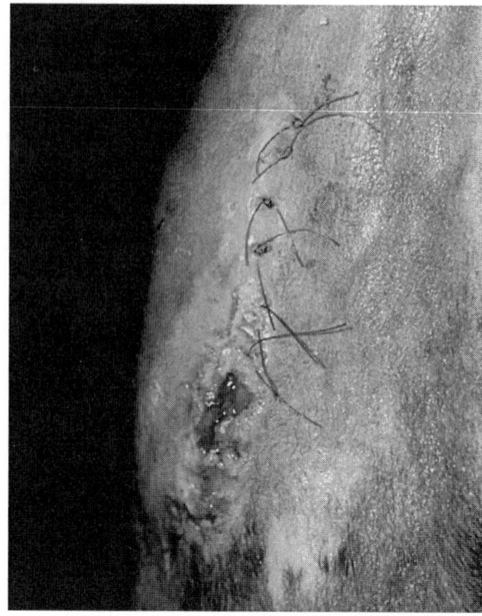

Figure 88-2. This surgical incision is infected; there is swelling and partial dehiscence, and the remaining sutures are cutting into the skin, which is pink.

Diagnosis

The most important step in recognizing that infection has occurred is to avoid denial. Because of the severe consequences of infection, it is easier and more optimistic to blame the elevation in temperature on a respiratory infection or other causes. However, early recognition is mandatory for successful management.

A complete blood count (CBC) demonstrating a leukocytosis with a neutrophilia confirms that infection is present, but a normal CBC does not rule out infection. A sample of fluid discharged from the wound or aseptically aspirated from deeper accumulations should be analyzed for cytology. A large number of neutrophils (more than 90%), bacteria, or both on a stained smear of the fluid confirms that infection is present. The continued production of excess fluid within or through the surgical wound is evidence that infection is present, especially if it is associated with a body temperature elevation.

Samples should be obtained for culture to identify the infecting organism or organisms and to perform antimicrobial sensitivity testing. If there is fluid accumulation, a needle aspirate can be obtained for culture using aseptic technique. If there is a draining tract or the incision has opened, a sterile swab (Culturette) can be advanced into the tract or into the incision (frequently down to the implant). Surgical preparation of the skin should be performed before passing the sterile swab into the wound to minimize the chance of inoculating the site with bacteria from the skin. In horses under anesthesia, it is possible to obtain tissue, bone, or a metal implant from the fracture site for culture. However, in a review of cultures from 38 horses, the culture results from swabs and fluid were very similar to results obtained from submitting bone or tissues from deep within the wound.[11] Samples should be submitted for both aerobic and anaerobic culture. It is difficult to accurately identify all of the infecting organisms because of bacterial adherence to the foreign material implant (plates and screws) and their production of a glycocalix that protects them from the wound environment.[30,31]

Treatment

Although systemic antibiotics help control infection, they cannot eliminate infection from surgical sites where infection exists around metal implants. Bacteria secrete a glycocalix (slime) that covers and protects them from antibiotics, antiseptics, antibodies, phagocytes, and mechanical removal by lavage solutions.[35,36] This is one reason why lavage with antiseptic (povidone-iodine) or antibiotic solutions has not been successful in eliminating infection in horses with infected orthopedic implants. Removal of the implant is usually necessary to resolve the infection.[3] Because of delayed healing, infection frequently causes lysis of bone and loosening of the implants or failure of the fixation from cyclic loading before healing occurs or laminitis develops in the opposite foot. This has made the treatment of infected fractures in horses a difficult and frequently unrewarding experience.

The new approach to horses that develop infection after the repair of a fracture or fusion of a joint is to achieve effective drainage and to maximize the concentrations of antibiotics at the surgery site[5] and in the surrounding tissues.[37] Once infection is confirmed, drainage is usually established by removing a few of the sutures from the bottom of the incision and creating an opening to the joint or fracture site. When the incision has healed or when preservation of the integrity of the suture line is desired, a 3- to 5-cm skin incision is made away from the incision to provide drainage from the surgery site. The incision is continued through any overlying soft tissues until drainage from the implants, fracture site, or joint has been established. Once there is an opening, antibiotic-impregnated polymethylmethacrylate (PMMA) implants are placed into the surgical wound, most frequently along the implants. If the infection is in an arthrodesed joint, antibiotic-impregnated PMMA implants may also be placed into the joint space or pouch. The wound is subsequently covered with a sterile bandage or a cast, depending on the location and orthopedic problem being treated. An antiseptic or antibiotic ointment is usually applied over the wound.

Antibiotic-impregnated PMMA has been used to treat infection in human orthopedic patients for years, and there has been considerable research evaluating the technique.[6,38] The antibiotic is released from the PMMA over time and achieves high concentrations of antibiotics locally at the fracture site and in surrounding tissues. Depending on the antibiotic, effective concentrations are maintained for many weeks (with gentamicin, concentrations are maintained for many months).[38] The use of antibiotic-impregnated PMMA has improved the treatment success of orthopedic infection in horses.[5] Before the use of this technique, successful treatment of infected fractures was rarely possible. Because of the persistence of infection deep within the fracture, removal of the implants was necessary to eliminate it. Several horses that developed infection after surgery have had the infection resolved without removal of the implants after treatment with antibiotic-impregnated PMMA.[5] This type of management has not eliminated infection in every case, and treatment failures still occur, but it has successfully eliminated infection in some horses. If signs of infection are not resolving, PMMA implants with different antibiotics should be considered. PMMA implants can be removed and replaced in most locations without too much difficulty. The use of other biomaterials (some absorbable) impregnated with antibiotics is described in Chapter 82.

Opening an incision or creating an opening through the skin to achieve drainage can be accomplished with sedation in many standing horses. The skin is desensitized with local anesthetic and prepared for aseptic surgery before making the incision. The more proximal the surgery site is on the limb, the easier it seems to be to establish drainage and insert the PMMA implants without general anesthesia.

Antibiotic-impregnated PMMA can be prepared at the surgery table or before surgery and sterilized with ethylene oxide. If the implants are gas sterilized, it is important to adequately aerate the implants before placing them in a wound. It is best to use a powdered form of the antibiotic to ensure equal mixing and distribution within the PMMA. The antibiotic (powder or liquid) is thoroughly mixed with the powdered polymer before acrylic resin is added (reagent-grade gentamicin in powdered form is available). Usually, 1 to 2 g of antibiotic is combined with 10 g of PMMA powder (1:10 or 1:5 ratio). Addition of antibiotic to PMMA weakens the biomechanical strength of PMMA.[39] This is not an concern where it is being used as a carrier for the sustained release of antibiotic, but it may be a consideration if PMMA is being used to lute plates,[40] where the biomechanical behavior of the material is important. After mixing, liquid resin is added to the powder and stirred. Within a few minutes, the material forms a thick liquid to claylike consistency. When it becomes like clay, the PMMA is rolled into beads and cylinders (Fig. 88-3). The PMMA is allowed to harden (3 to 5 minutes) before the cylinders or beads are implanted into the surgery site. The disadvantages of beads are that they are difficult to remove if the infection resolves and they become incorporated in the fibrous scar tissue. Cylinders of varying lengths (0.5 cm to several centimeters) are easier to remove (if necessary). PMMA implants can be saved and gas sterilized (by ethylene oxide) for future use.

Antibiotics selected for use in PMMA must be heat stable and released from the acrylic into surrounding tissues and fluids. Gentamicin, amikacin, cefazolin, tobramycin, and enrofloxacin have been used by the author in horses with orthopedic infection. With the exception of enrofloxacin, release of these antibiotics from PMMA has been demonstrated in the medical literature.[38]

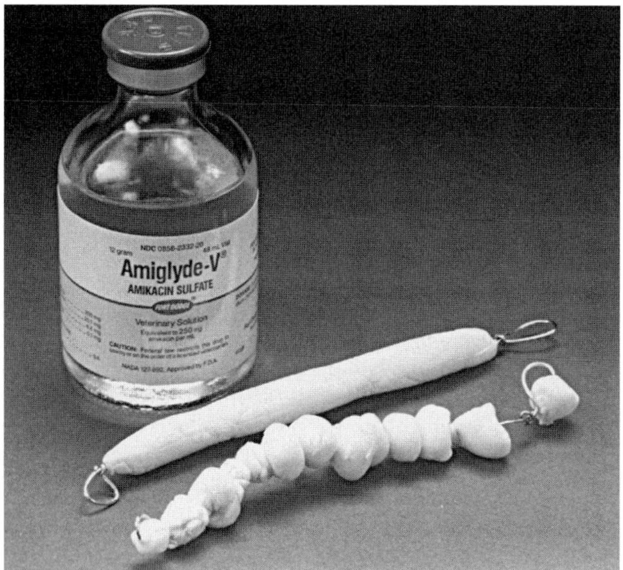

Figure 88-3. Polymethylmethacrylate, which is impregnated with antibiotics, can be rolled into beads or cylinders at the surgery table before implantation. Beads were originally strung on suture or wire for ease of removal. However, in most locations, the implants become incorporated into surrounding soft tissue, which makes it difficult to remove them. Sutures and wire frequently break or pull out. Many implants are left in place; however, for ease of removal, cylinders of varying lengths are currently recommended.

Antibiotic-impregnated PMMA has been left in horses for many years.[5] In two horses, infection and drainage recurred 5 months and 3 years, respectively, after all clinical signs of infection had resolved. In both cases, draining tracts were followed to the PMMA implants, and removal resolved the infection and drainage.

Regional limb perfusion should be considered in horses that develop postoperative orthopedic infections.[37] This technique has the advantage of delivering high concentrations of antibiotics not only to the surgery site but also to the surrounding soft tissues and bones. This treatment has been used to successfully treat three horses with postoperative infection after fracture repair or joint arthrodesis.[37] Regional perfusion is being performed with increasing frequency because of its success in treating horses with postoperative infection after fracture repair or surgical arthrodesis. The antibiotics and the procedure used are the same as previously described for septic joints.

Both antibiotic-impregnated PMMA implants and regional limb perfusion can be used in the same horse. Regional limb perfusion gets antibiotics into the bone and vascularized tissues around the site of the infection, and antibiotic PMMA implants provide sustained release of antibiotics over several days or, in the case of some antibiotics, several months. Because infection of a fracture repair or joint arthrodesis has severe consequences, every effective treatment should be considered. Treatment decisions regarding selection of the method for delivering local antibiotics or whether both treatments are used are based on the clinical signs, the anatomic location of the infection, and the preference of the surgeon.

Traditional treatments of aggressive débridement and daily lavage of the surgery site have not been effective in eliminating orthopedic infection in horses. These techniques have been replaced with an approach of establishing effective drainage and increasing the concentration of antibiotics at the site of infection. Exposure of the implants should be avoided. More aggressive débridement, autogenous cancellous bone grafts, and large-volume lavage still may be indicated as part of the treatment in chronic cases. However, even when this approach is used, the soft tissues should be closed to provide coverage for PMMA implants that are placed after débridement. Procedures that expose implants should be avoided. Antibiotic-impregnated PMMA is an effective method of maximizing antibiotic concentrations locally at the site of infection. Regional limb perfusion is another effective treatment for maximizing antibiotic concentrations in the vascularized tissues around an orthopedic infection. Finding new and better carriers or techniques to maintain antibiotics at the site of infection will be important in the future treatment of orthopedic infection.[41-43]

The treatment of orthopedic infection is expensive. The average days of hospitalization in 38 horses with an infected fracture or arthrodesis was 142 days (range, 16 to 804 days).[11] These horses were receiving systemic antibiotics, daily bandaging, wound care, periodic cast changes, or a combination. All of these treatments contribute to the expense.

Prognosis

The prognosis for horses with orthopedic infections has been unfavorable; only 52.9% of 38 horses with an infected fracture or arthrodesis site survived to be released from the hospital.[11] Horses were humanely destroyed as a result of long-term complications related to their fracture or joint fusion. The use of antibiotic-impregnated PMMA has resulted in successful fracture healing or joint fusion in 15 of 19 horses, but only 12 of 19 survived long term.[5] At this time, infection still causes complications and delayed healing that all too frequently result in the loss of the horse.

PREVENTION OF INFECTION

Because of the dire consequences of infection, everything possible should be done to prevent infection or decrease the risk of infection during major orthopedic surgery in horses. The importance of aseptic technique cannot be overemphasized. Despite efforts to avoid infection, there is a risk after any invasive surgery. The infection rate at The Ohio State University Veterinary Hospital for elective equine joint surgery during a 10-year period was 1.3% (out of 1352 horses).[44] Data included both arthroscopy and arthrotomy procedures and spanned the time when osteochondral fragment removal changed from an arthrotomy to an arthroscopic procedure. Four horses developed infection after surgery during a 7-day period, the cause of which was traced to a malfunctioning gas sterilization unit. During this same 10-year period, the infection rate in horses with major fracture repairs or arthrodesis procedures was 6.9% (452 horses),[44] including horses with open fractures. Ideally, the infection rate in both groups of horses should be lower; however, invasive surgery carries the risk of infection in all species. Estimates of the chance for infection in equine orthopedic surgery should be considered in preoperative discussions with horse owners regarding surgical risk. Principles of asepsis and prophylactic procedures discussed elsewhere in this book must be followed.

In the author's experience, the incision can be an important source of postoperative infection. Protection of the incision from the environment (in the horse's case, a stall with manure) is important. Some incisions are located over highly mobile areas, and a cast is necessary to allow the soft tissues to heal without excess tension. This is particularly true for incisions over the pastern. When these incisions are not immobilized, the skin sutures cut into the skin and cause local infection, or the incision dehisces. Horses develop infection when the skin sutures have been either left in too long or incompletely removed (the knot is cut off, leaving a loop of suture material deep in the skin incision).[44] Sutures removed between 10 and 14 days are almost never a problem. Skin sutures left in for longer than 14 days may be the cause of infection and drainage along the suture. This superficial infection beneath the skin can easily penetrate deeper tissues, especially if the skin incision is superimposed over an incision that penetrates deeper tissues. Even small arthroscopy incisions can develop infection that penetrates down the arthroscope or instrumental portal to the joint. When part or all of the suture is left in these sites, the horse may, in some cases 6 or 7 weeks after surgery, develop a septic joint.

Preventative antibiotic treatment in the horse has progressed beyond preoperative administration of systemic antibiotics. In horses with open fractures or contaminated joints undergoing internal fixation procedures, antibiotic-impregnated PMMA can be placed along the plates at the time of surgery to decrease the chance of infection. Similarly, regional limb perfusion can be performed at the time of surgical fixation, with the same rationale. When to use these procedures or choosing between the two is based on the judgment and the clinical experience of the surgeon.

REFERENCES

1. McIlwraith CW: Treatment of infectious arthritis, Vet Clin North Am Large Anim Pract 1983;5:353.
2. Schneider RK, Bramlage LR, Moore RM, et al: A retrospective study of 192 horses affected with septic arthritis/tenosynovitis, Equine Vet J 1992;24:435.
3. Bramlage LR: Long bone fractures, Vet Clin North Am Large Anim Pract 1983;5:285.
4. Snyder JR, Pascoe JR, Hirsh DC: Antimicrobial susceptibility of microorganisms isolated from equine orthopedic patients, Vet Surg 1987;16:197.
5. Holcombe SJ, Schneider RK, Bramlage LR, et al: Use of antibiotic-impregnated polymethyl methacrylate in horses with open or infected fractures or joints: 19 cases (1987-1995), J Am Vet Med Assoc 1997;211:889.
6. Tobias KMS, Schneider RK, Besser TE: Use of antimicrobial-impregnated polymethyl methacrylate, J Am Vet Med Assoc 1998;208:841.
7. Buchholz HW, Elson RA, Heinert K: Antibiotic loaded acrylic cement: Current concepts, Clin Orthop Rel Res 1984;190:96.
8. Lloyd KCK, Stover SM, Pascoe JR, et al: Plasma and synovial fluid concentrations of gentamicin in horses after intra-articular administration of buffered and unbuffered gentamicin, Am J Vet Res 1988;49:644.
9. Lloyd KCK, Stover SM, Pascoe JR, et al: Synovial fluid pH, cytologic characteristics, and gentamicin concentration after intra-articular administration of the drug in an experimental model of infectious arthritis in horses, Am J Vet Res 1990;51:1353.
10. Schneider RK, Bramlage LR, Moore RM, et al: Open drainage, intra-articular and systemic antibiotics in the treatment of septic arthritis/tenosynovitis in horses, Equine Vet J 1992;24:443.
11. Schneider RK, Bramlage LR: Unpublished data, 1989.
12. Curtis PH: The pathophysiology of joint infections, Clin Orthop Rel Res 1973;95:129.
13. Tulamo RM, Bramlage LR, Gabel AA: Sequential clinical and synovial fluid changes associated with acute infectious arthritis in the horse, Equine Vet J 1989;21:325.
14. Trotter GW, McIlwraith CW: Clinical features and diagnosis of equine joint disease. In McIlwraith CW, Trotter GW, editors: Joint Disease in the Horse, Philadelphia, 1996, WB Saunders.
15. Montgomery RD, Long IR Jr, Milton JL, et al: Comparison of aerobic culturette, synovial membrane biopsy, and blood culture medium in detection of canine bacterial arthritis, Vet Surg 1989;18:300.
16. Madison JB, Sommer M, Spencer PA: Relations among synovial membrane histopathologic findings, synovial fluid cytologic findings, and bacterial culture results in horses with suspected infectious arthritis: 64 cases (1979-1987), J Am Vet Med Assoc 1991;198:1655,
17. Moore RM, Schneider RK, Kowalski J, et al: Antimicrobial susceptibility of bacterial isolates from 223 horses with musculoskeletal infection during 1979-1989, Equine Vet J 1992;24:450.
18. Wright IM, Smith MRW, Humphrey TCJ, et al: Endoscopic surgery in the treatment of contaminated and infected synovial cavities, Equine Vet J 2003;35:613-619.
19. Bertone AL, McIlwraith CW, Powers BE, et al: Effect of four antimicrobial lavage solutions on the tarsocrural joint of horses, Vet Surg 1986;15:305.
20. Anderson MA, Payne JT, Kreeger J, et al: Effects of intra-articular chlorhexidine diacetate lavage on the stifle joint in healthy dogs, Vet Surg 1993;22:372.
21. Bertone AL, McIlwraith CW, Jones RL, et al: Povidone-iodine lavage treatment of experimentally induced equine infectious arthritis, Am J Vet Res 1987;48:712.
22. Welch RD, DeBowes RM, Liepold HW: Evaluation of the effects of intra-articular injection of dimethylsulfoxide on normal equine articular tissues, Am J Vet Res 1989;50:1180.
23. Mills ML, Moore BR, St Jean G, et al: Synovial fluid concentrations, cytologic characteristics, and effect on synovium of ceftiofur sodium after intra-articular injection in horses, Vet Orthop Soc Scientific Meeting, Big Sky, Mont, 1997.
24. Wooten TL, Schneider RK, Besser T, et al: The effect of intra-articular Timentin and Primaxin on normal equine synovium and articular cartilage, Unpublished data, 1998.
25. Whitehair KJ, Blevins WE, Fesler JF, et al: Regional perfusion of the equine carpus for antibiotic delivery, Vet Surg 1992;21:279.
26. Mattson S, Bouré L, Pearce S, et al: Intraosseous gentamicin perfusion of the distal metacarpus in standing horses, Vet Surg 2004;33:180.
27. Scheuch BC, Van Hoogmoed LM, Wilson WD: Comparison of intraosseous of intravenous infusion for delivery of amikacin sulfate to the tibiotarsal joint of horses, Am J Vet Res 2002;63:374.
28. Werner LA, Hardy J, Vertone AL: Bone gentamicin concentration after Intra-articular injection or regional intravenous perfusion in the horse, Vet Surg 2003;32:559.
29. Ross MW, Orsini JA, Richardson DW, et al: Closed suction drainage in the treatment of infectious arthritis of the equine tarsocrural joint, Vet Surg 1991;20:21.
30. Bertone AL, McIlwraith CW, Jones RL, et al: Comparison of various treatments for experimentally induced equine infectious arthritis, Am J Vet Res 1987;48:519.
31. Gustafson SB, McIlwraith CW, Jones RL: Comparison of the effect of polysulfated glycosaminoglycan, corticosteroids, and sodium

hyaluronate in the potentiation of a subinfective dose of *Staphylococcus aureus* in the midcarpal joint of horses, Am J Vet Res 1989;50:2014.
32. Firth C: Current concepts of infectious polyarthritis in foals, Equine Vet J 1983;15:5.
33. Honnas CM, Welch RD, Ford TS, et al: Septic arthritis of the distal interphalangeal joint in 12 horses, Vet Surg 1992;21:261.
34. Richarson DW: Long bone fractures: Evolving solutions (Rett), Equine J Vet 1992;24:333.
35. Mayberry-Carson KJ, Tober-Meyer B, Smith JK, et al: Bacterial adherence and glycocalix formation in osteomyelitis experimentally induced *Staphylococcus aureus*, Infect Immun 1984;43:825.
36. Gristina AG, Costerton JW: Bacterial adherence and the glycocalix and their role in musculoskeletal infection, Orthop Clin North Am 1984;15:517.
37. Whitehair KJ, Adams SB, Parker JE, et al: Regional limb perfusion with antibiotic in three horses, Vet Surg 1992;21:286.
38. Calhoun JH, Mader JT: Antibiotic beads in the management of surgical infections, Am J Surg 1989;157:443.
39. Nelson RC, Hoffman RO, Burton TA: The effect of an antibiotic addition on the mechanical properties of acrylic cement, J Biomed Mater Res 1978;12:473.
40. Nunamaker DM, Richardson DW, Butterweck DM: Mechanical and biological effects of plate luting, J Orthop Trauma 1991;5:138.
41. Gerhardt TN, Roux RD, Hanff RA, et al: Antibiotic-loaded biodegradable bone cement for prophylaxis and treatment of experimental osteomyelitis in rats, J Orthop Res 1993;11:250.
42. Jacob E, Cierney G, Gallon MT, et al: Evaluation of biodegradable cefazolin sodium microspheres for the prevention of infection in rabbits with experimental open tibia fractures stabilized with internal fixation, J Orthop Res 1993;11:404.
43. Sondhof AF, Booth LC, Rosenbusch RF, et al: In vitro biocompatibility of a novel biodegradable local drug delivery system intended for the treatment of orthopedic infections in the horse, Veterinary Orthopedic Society, Scientific Meeting, Snowmass, Colo, 1998.
44. Schneider RK, Bramlage LR, Gabel AA: Unpublished data, 1990.

CHAPTER 89

Angular Limb Deformities

Jörg A. Auer

The surgical techniques used for the management of angular limb deformities (ALD) in foals are well established.[1-11] However, when to use these techniques remains controversial. At one time, most foals showing some degree of angular deviation were surgically corrected, but a more conservative approach has been advocated recently. The following quote best represents the current thinking on managing ALD: "Foals should be expected to be born crooked and to correct with time. It is equally as wrong to disturb this process, as it is not to correct a variation from it."[12] Looking at ALD from this point of view allows objective criteria to be developed to manage them.

DEFINITION

Animals with ALD present with either a valgus deformity (lateral deviation of the limb distal to the location of the deformity) or a varus deformity (medial deviation of the limb distal to the location of the problem) (Fig. 89-1). Either type of deviation is usually associated with a certain degree of axial rotation. In foals with valgus deformity, this is displayed as an outward rotation (splay foot), and in cases of varus deformity, as a medial rotation of the feet (pigeon toes). In most cases, these deformities are initially merely postural, through a rotation of the limb axis toward either the outside or the inside, respectively. With time, however, the bone adapts to abnormal loading, according to Wolff's law,[13] and differential metaphyseal growth results in the development of a permanent rotational deformity.[9]

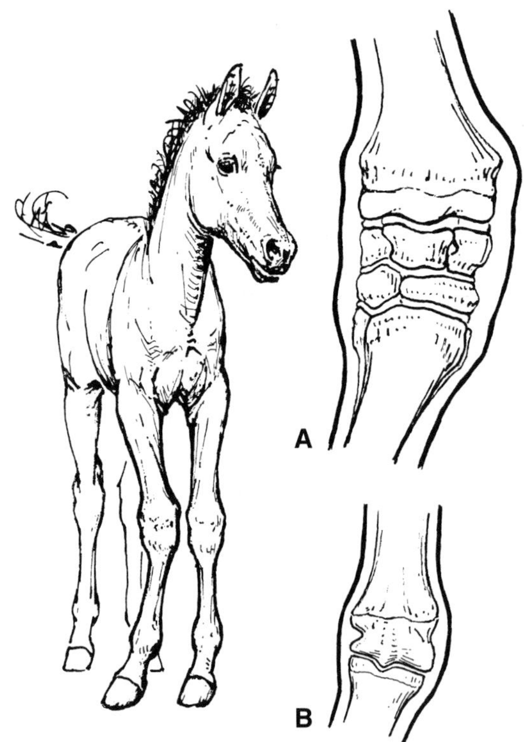

Figure 89-1. Drawing of a foal with a valgus deformity in the right carpal region (**A**) and a varus deformity in the left metacarpophalangeal region (**B**).

ANATOMY

Maturation of the skeleton from the primordial or precursor cartilage to bone is a very complicated process and occurs mainly during the later stages of gestation. Radiographs taken of the carpal and tarsal regions of aborted fetuses at 230 days of gestation reveal only partial ossification of the diaphyses and metaphyses of the long bones as well as of the calcaneus.[11] Other bones are not ossified at all at that time. For instance, intra-articular injections of contrast medium provide outlines of the bone templates in their normal shapes, although they consist of precursor cartilage only. Ossification of these structures begins in the center and expands spherically in all directions to the periphery.[11,14] At about 260 days of gestation, ossification centers are noticed in the distal radial epiphysis, distal tibial epiphysis, talus, and accessory carpal bone. Later, ossification centers in the intermediate, radial, and third carpal bones, and the central, third, and fourth tarsal bones develop. At around 290 days, the proximal epiphyses of the third metacarpus/third metatarsus (MCIII/MTIII) appear, and they unite shortly thereafter with the metaphyses of these bones (Fig. 89-2). At about 300 days of gestation, all bones of the carpus and tarsus are visible radiographically. The ulnar styloid process, which is the last ossification center to appear, is still not seen at this time. During the remaining days of gestation, ossification progresses toward the periphery, and the bones acquire their final shape. At birth, the edges of these bones are still somewhat rounded, but the "radiographic joint spaces" are within normal limits (Fig. 89-3). These spaces consist of two layers of cartilage in addition to the actual joint space.[6,15,16]

The vast majority of longitudinal growth in the long bones occurs at the level of the physis. Some growth is attributed to the epiphysis, growing both toward the articular cartilage and the physis. However, the vast majority of growth occurs in the metaphyseal region of the physis. The exact mechanisms responsible for this bone growth are not completely understood, but strides toward solving this mystery are being made with the help of molecular biology techniques. In mice, it was found that a feedback loop exists in the growth plate centered on the following molecules: parathyroid hormone–related protein (PTHrP), PTH/PTHrP receptors (PTHrPR) and Indian hedgehog (Ihh).[17] The feedback loop is regulated via the periosteum/perichondrium

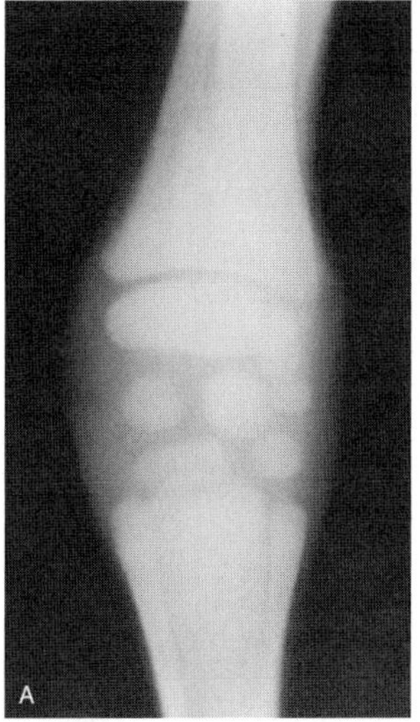

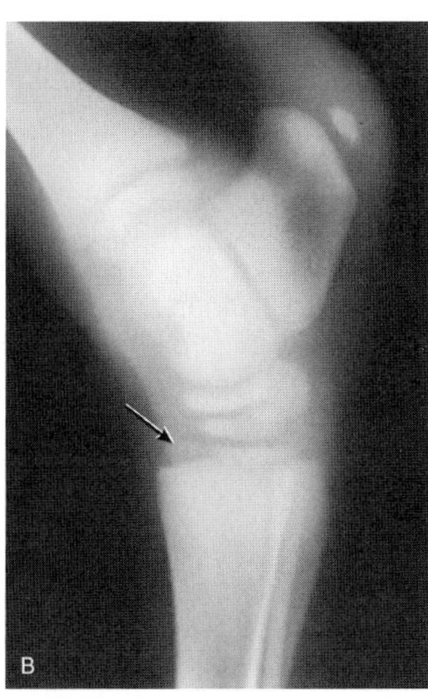

Figure 89-2. Dorsopalmar (DP) radiograph of a carpal region and lateromedial (LM) radiograph of a tarsal region of a premature foal. **A,** The DP view of the carpal region at 2 days of age shows incomplete ossification of the carpal bones. **B,** The LM view of the tarsal region shows inadequate ossification of the tarsal bones, especially the third and the central tarsal bones. Note the ununited proximal epiphysis of MTIII *(arrow)*.

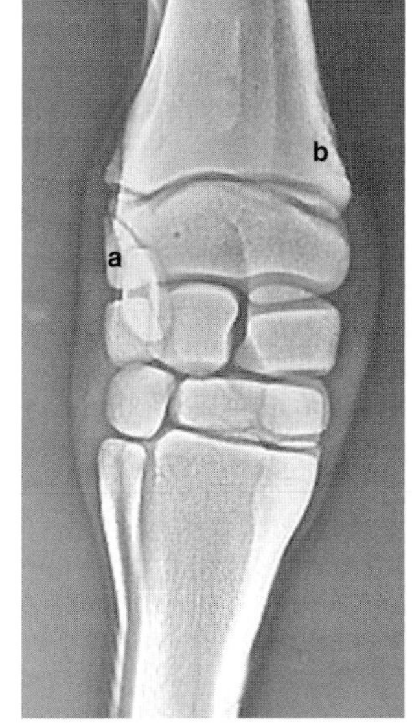

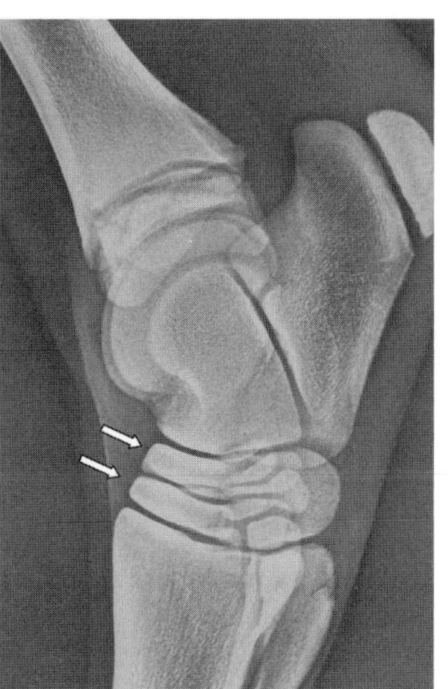

Figure 89-3. Normal ossification of the carpal and tarsal regions at the time of birth. **A,** Dorsopalmar radiograph of the carpal region. All the bones are ossified adequately, and the ulnar styloid process (a) is visible. The rough surface at the medial distal metaphysis of the radius (b) represents active endochondral ossification and is normal at that age. **B,** Lateromedial radiograph of the tarsal region showing adequate ossification of the central and third tarsal bones *(arrows)*. It is important that the ossification process proceed to the level of the proximal aspect of MTIII. These two radiographic views are the most relevant to evaluate ossification at the time of birth.

through the signaling molecules Patched1 (Ptc1), Gli, and Smoothend (Smo). If Ihh secretion is increased, PTHrP molecules are upregulated and inhibit differentiation of proliferating chondrocytes into hypertrophic chondrocytes, thus promoting longitudinal growth. Since Ihh and PTHrP are not expressed in the same vicinity and molecule diffusion through the extracellular matrix is limited, intermediates, such as Ptc1, transforming growth factor (TGF)-β_2, bone morphogenic proteins (BMPs), and fibroblast growth factor (FGF) that are located in the perichondrium participate in this regulatory process.[17] Once these mechanisms are understood in the horse, an explanation for the disproportionate long bone growth across a physis may become clear and specific molecular therapy may be developed.

The following *is* clear. Ideally, bone growth should occur evenly across the entire physis; immediately after birth, growth is most active; and each physeal region has an approximate time span during which new bone occurs. Closure of the physes of the different long bones occurs at predictable time points. Therefore, if manipulations to correct growth are to be effective, the closure time of the physes have to be considered.

ETIOLOGY

A variety of etiologies are responsible for the development of ALD, and can be grouped into two main categories (Fig. 89-4): perinatal factors, which include conditions that are present either during the later phases of gestation or in the immediate perinatal period, and developmental factors, which influence limb axes at a later stage.

ALD may originate at different locations of the appendicular skeleton: within the cuboidal bones of the carpus or tarsus, in the epiphyseal region of the long bones (epiphyses, physes, and metaphyses), and occasionally in diaphyses of the long bones. Most frequently, the deviation develops through disproportionate growth at the level of the metaphyseal growth plates. Physeal trauma, such as Salter-Harris type V or VI fractures,[18,19] can cause local retardation of growth at the medial or lateral aspect of the bone and result in the development of ALD. Compensatory ALD can occur in remote sites in the affected limb because of disproportionate loading of a growth plate distally. Such compensatory deviations may straighten the limb axis, but when the foal ambulates, the joint involved rotates, because the joint is not oriented at a right angle to the long axis of the limb.

Perinatal Factors

Incomplete Ossification

After a normal gestation period, a foal should be born with adequate ossification of the carpal and tarsal bones (see Fig. 89-3). A variety of events affecting the mare, including placentitis during pregnancy, severe metabolic disease over a prolonged period, heavy parasite infestation, and colic, may jeopardize the intrauterine environment of the foal and result in incomplete ossification at the time of birth.[11] Premature birth is usually associated with the same problem. Because the placenta of a mare does not provide as

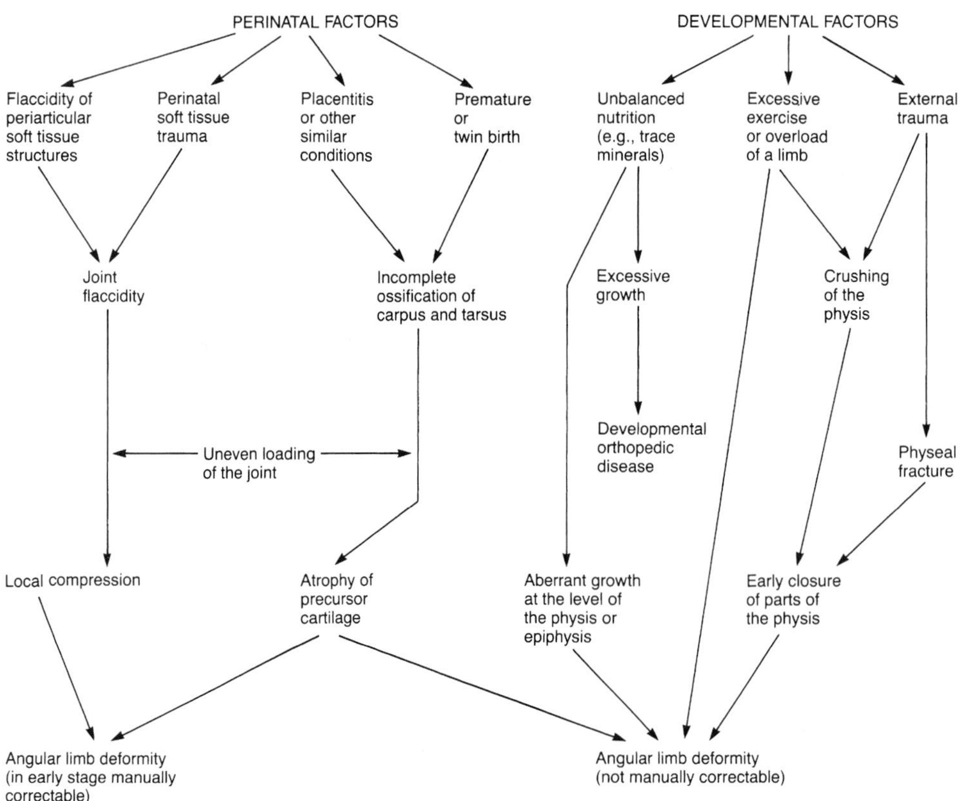

Figure 89-4. Interrelationship of perinatal and developmental factors and pathways and how they may contribute to the development of an angular limb deformity.

intricate a blood exchange between the fetus and the mare as it does in humans and dogs, normal intrauterine development of more than one fetus at the same time is not possible. Twin foals always exhibit incomplete ossification at birth. These immature foals do not mature properly and have a poor prognosis as athletes. Therefore, abortion of one of the twins during the early embryonic stages is standard.

Because most foals are born with a certain degree of angular limb deformity, they initially load their joints unevenly. The uneven pressure on the relatively thick layer of articular and precursor cartilage may deform that soft structure, especially in a dysmature foal. Incomplete ossification per se does *not* represent an ALD, but the uneven loading of the dysmature skeleton leads to it. Once ossification reaches the periphery, the abnormal shape of the bone results in a permanent ALD. Additionally, the force of digital extension is applied laterally in the carpal and tarsal regions and may impede longitudinal growth in these areas to a certain extent. In severely dysmature foals, osteochondral fractures may occur, which render the foal permanently lame because of osteoarthritis[9] (Fig. 89-5). This is especially true in the rear limb, where weight-bearing forces must change direction in the tarsal region from a cranioproximal-caudodistal direction to a vertical one. The most affected region is the dorsal aspect of the small tarsal bones. If these bones are incompletely ossified, loading causes thinning of the soft precursor cartilage. This may be followed by pathologic fracture and dislocation of a dorsal fragment.[6,9] This problem results in a partial collapse of the dorsal aspect of the tarsus and tilting of the proximal limb in a cranial direction (Fig. 89-6). Affected foals do not trot but rather "bunny hop" with their rear limbs. In chronic cases, a secondary flexural deformity of the forelimbs may result because of chronic overload.

If collapse of the cartilage template of cuboidal bones in dysmature foals is left untreated, the deformations worsen and eventually become impossible to correct. Therefore, early intervention and aggressive treatment are necessary to ensure normal development.

Laxity of Periarticular Structures

Some foals are born with severe ALDs in several regions, allowing oscillation between valgus and varus deviations depending on limb position during weightbearing. Rotational deformities of various degrees also are encountered during the first few days of birth (Fig. 89-7). These foals probably suffer from laxity of the periarticular supporting structures or from soft tissue trauma, both of which result in unstable joints. In most cases, several joints are involved at the same time. These deformities lead to abnormal loading of the articular surfaces and may, in the presence of incompletely ossified cuboidal bones, induce a severe ALD. It is unknown exactly how these problems develop. In some cases, the aberrant development of the long bones relative to the soft tissue structures may be caused by a hormonal imbalance or by intrauterine positioning.[20]

Developmental Factors

Unbalanced Nutrition

The common practice of "crib feeding" often leads to excessive grain intake. It is important that the nutrition be balanced, especially with regard to trace minerals.[21] If the

A

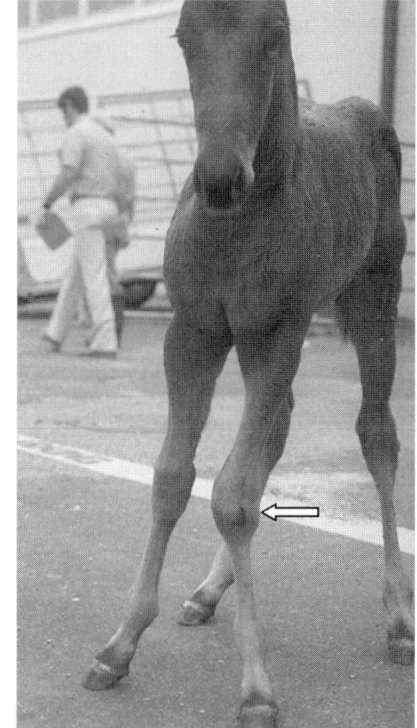

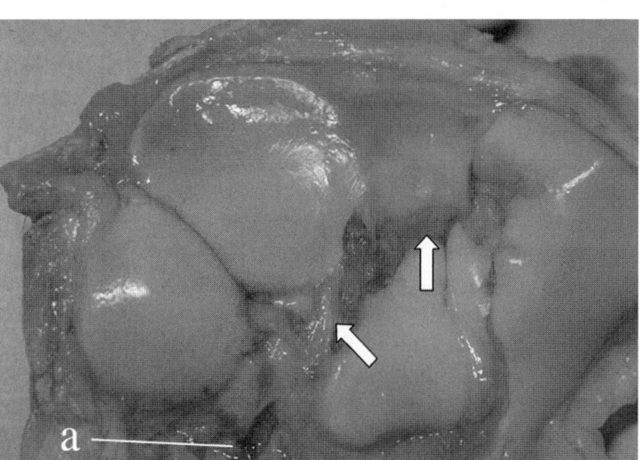

B

Figure 89-5. A, A 6-week-old foal with a marked carpal valgus deformity in the left limb. There is swelling *(arrow)* and the animal is lame. **B,** Postmortem picture of the articular surface of the third carpal bone, showing an osteochondral fracture *(arrows)*. There is also marked discoloration of the synovial membrane caused by intra-articular hemorrhage.

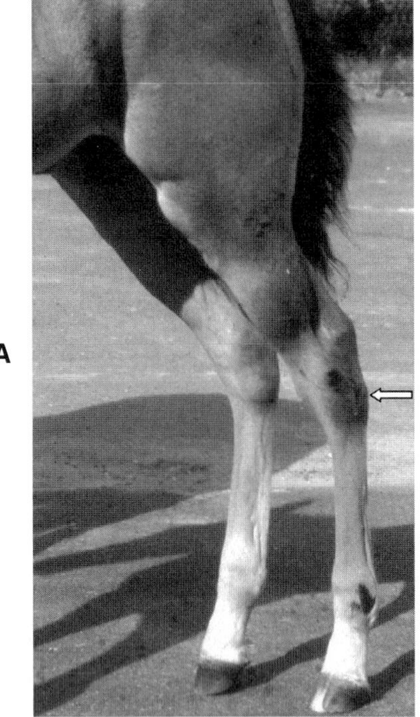

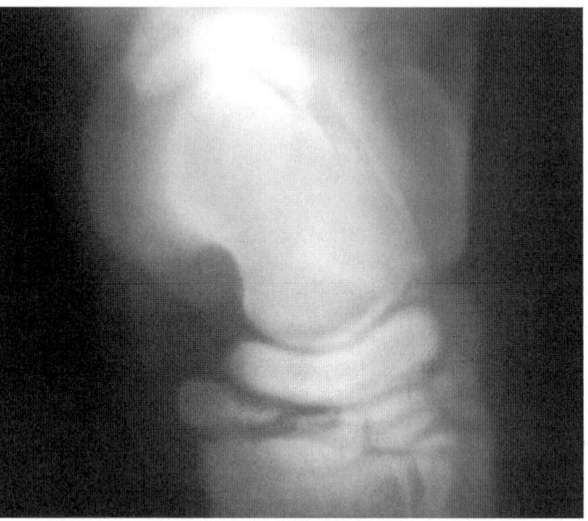

Figure 89-6. A, The hind limbs of a 1-month-old foal with a marked dorsal angulation at the level of the tarsus *(arrow)*. The foal showed the typical gait of a foal with collapsed third tarsal bones: it trotted with the forelimbs and "bunny-hopped" with the hindlimbs. **B,** Lateromedial radiograph showing the collapsed third tarsal bone, which is displaced dorsally.

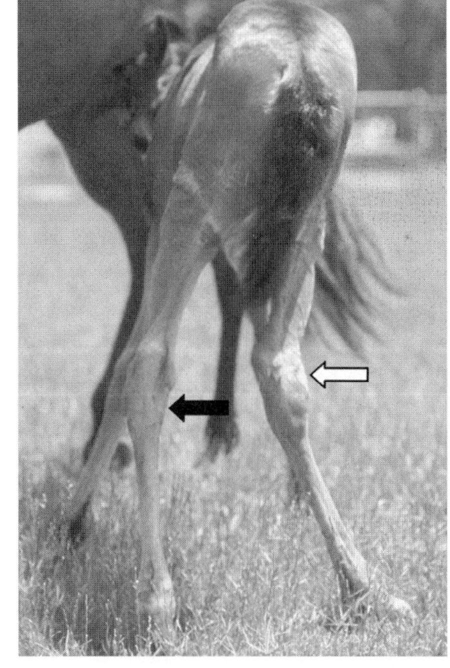

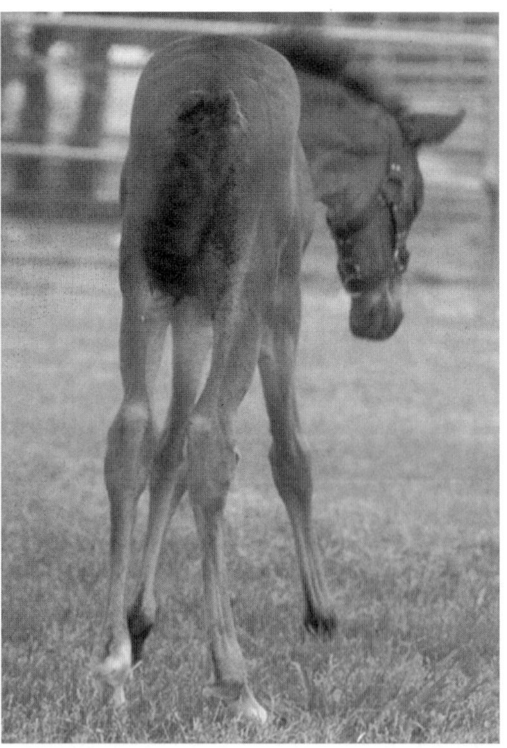

Figure 89-7. A, Photograph of a 1-week-old foal with a marked valgus deformity of the right tarsus *(white arrow)* and a varus deformity of the left tarsal region *(black arrow)*. The degree of ossification was normal. **B,** After 2 weeks of light hand-walking and no treatment, the deviations had corrected.

diet is not balanced, developmental orthopedic disease[22,23] may occur and jeopardize future athletic potential. Intake of trace minerals is further compromised by the exhaustion of grasslands and a lack of appropriate fertilization. A soil analysis of the local pasture may not be relevant, because forage (hay) is usually brought in from a distant source. Problems associated with unbalanced nutrition include flexural deformities, osteochondrosis,[22,23] and ALD, the latter being represented mainly by disproportionate growth at the level of the physes. Severe generalized osteochondrosis because of zinc toxicity or copper deficiency may cause ALD. On farms with a high occurrence of ALD, feeding practices should be evaluated through a complete feed and water analysis. If abnormalities are encountered, they should be corrected at once.[21]

Excessive Exercise and Trauma

Excessive exercise and trauma cause ALD. This trauma induces microfractures in and actual crushing of the proliferative zone at the base of the physis, altering cell proliferation and maturation. In severe cases, it leads early local closure. This type of injury has been classified as a Salter-Harris type V fracture.[18] Additionally, epiphyseal fractures caused by external trauma such as kicks from another mare may cause ALD.[18] Most physeal fractures heal with residual ALD because it is almost impossible to maintain viability of the entire physeal plate.[19]

DIAGNOSIS

Diagnosis is based on inspection, manipulation, and diagnostic imaging techniques. The foal is observed from several angles, most importantly from the front and back. To evaluate the limb, the clinician should be positioned perpendicular to a frontal plane through the examined limb. Splay-footed foals, with or without ALD, are therefore evaluated from a craniolateral position, allowing observation for proper alignment of the toe and carpus or tarsus, respectively (Fig. 89-8, *A*). It is very important that the toe point in the same direction as the carpus. Most newly born foals are weak, thin-chested, and, in relation to their size, long-legged. To provide some support to the forelimbs, which are connected to the chest only by seven muscles, the proximal ulna is positioned on the side of the chest. This results in an outward rotation of the entire limb and a toed-out posture. With increasing strength and age, the chest fills out and the connecting muscles become stronger, leading to an inward rotation of the limb and correction of the toed-out posture. Should, however, the carpus or tarsus point outward but the

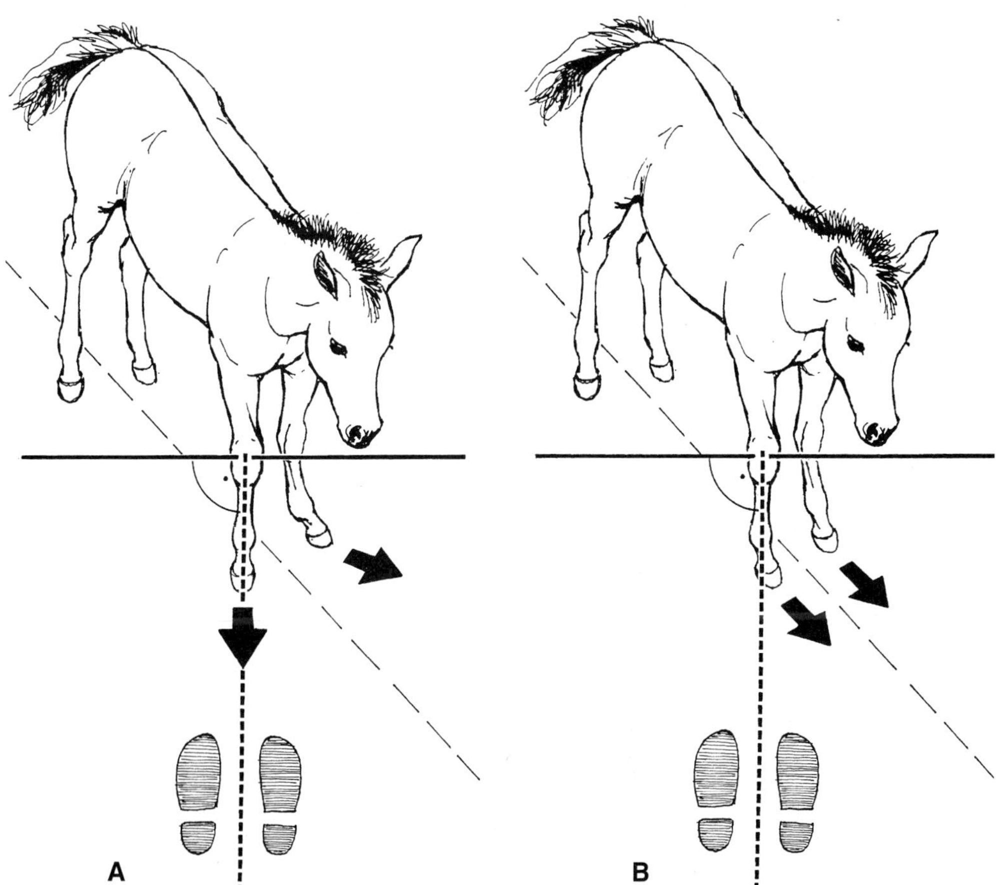

Figure 89-8. A, A valgus deformity of the carpal region is evaluated perpendicular to the frontal plane of the outward-rotated carpus. If the toe points in the same direction, the entire limb is rotated out and surgery can possibly be postponed. **B,** If the toes point forward and the carpus outward, surgical intervention is indicated to prevent the development of a varus deformity in the fetlock region.

toes point straight forward (see Fig. 89-8, *B*), a varus deformity of the distal limb is present, which may go unnoticed for a few months. Once the limb rotates into a normal position, the feet attain a toed-in posture. Unfortunately, the distal MCIII/MTIII experiences longitudinal growth only for 3 to 4 months, after which the physis closes. Frequently, this is when the problem is noticed.

Palpation and manipulation of the limb help differentiate between perinatal and developmental deformities. If application of manual pressure to the medial aspect of the carpal region straightens out a valgus deformity (Fig. 89-9), the cause of the deformity is either incomplete ossification or flaccidity of the periarticular supporting structures. If the limb cannot be straightened with manipulation, changes of the osseous structures of the region are involved.

Observation of the foal as it walks toward and away from the clinician also provides valuable clues. If the joints are aligned parallel to the ground, all the joint movements occur in the same planes and no outward or inward rotation of a joint is noticed. However pigeon-toed foals frequently rotate their metacarpophalangeal/metatarsophalangeal (MCP/MTP) joints outward while advancing the limb. This is caused by the joints not being oriented parallel to the ground.

The only diagnostic aid that allows exact determination of the location and degree of the deformity is radiography. It is important to use long, narrow cassettes for the radiographs and to include as much of the bones proximal and distal to the deformity as possible. The dorsopalmar/dorsoplantar views are most important, except in the tarsus, where the lateromedial view is preferred. The radiographs should be taken at a right angle to the frontal plane of the limb (the sagittal plane of the tarsus). The bones constituting the distal MCIII/MTIII and phalangeal region should be aligned in one plane for the radiographs, allowing interpretation of the articular orientation and differentiation of deformities.

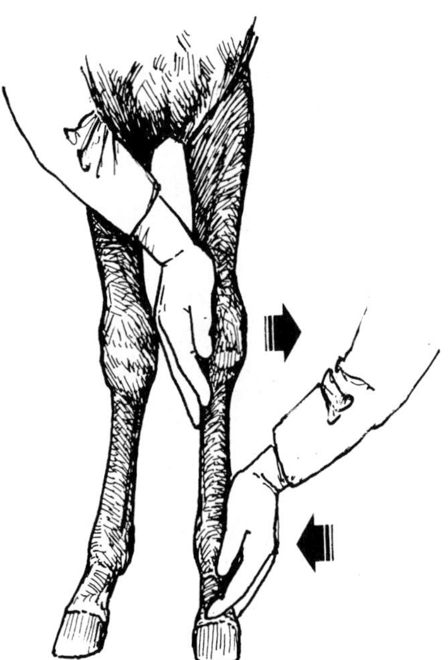

Figure 89-9. Manual pressure to the medial aspect of the carpal region of a foal suffering from bilateral valgus deformity corrects the deformity temporarily, indicating that conservative treatment is possible. Counterpressure is applied to the fetlock region of the same limb.

The need for early diagnosis cannot be overemphasized, especially in foals with incomplete ossification. The soft precursor cartilage is deformed through the uneven axial loads and, combined with the rapid progression of endochondral ossification, may result in a permanent deformity within 2 weeks after birth.

Compound and noncorrectable deformities present an added challenge. It is sometimes important to accept a compensatory deformity, if it aids the overall athletic soundness of the animal. A foal with a varus deformity in the metacarpophalangeal region would profit from a slight valgus deformity in the carpal region to balance the horse's weight-bearing axis over the foot. This necessitates the visual evaluation of the entire limb at the time of the diagnosis, and caution in using radiographs as the sole diagnostic aid.

TREATMENT

Two recent studies conducted in Thoroughbred horses have significantly changed the philosophy of the management of ALDs.[24,25] One study documented conformational changes with age.[24] The changes occurring from weanling age to 3 years in a population of racing Thoroughbreds were determined by recording specific body measurements. There was a strong relationship between long bone lengths and wither height in all age groups, supporting the theory that horses grow proportionally. Longitudinal bone growth in the distal limb increased only 5% to 7% from weanling age to 3 years and was presumably completed prior to the yearling year. This study provided objective information regarding conformation and skeletal growth in the Thoroughbred, which can be utilized for selection and recognition of significant conformational abnormalities.[24]

The other study investigated the relationship of conformation to injury.[25] It found that offset carpi (offset ratio) contributed to MCP joint problems. Long pasterns increased the odds of a fracture in the front limb. A certain degree of carpal valgus deformity exhibited a protective mechanism, since the odds for a carpal fracture and carpal effusion decreased with an increase in the carpal angle.[25]

Based on these studies, the goals of effective management of ALD have changed. Severe deformities that do not correct on their own (see Fig. 89-5) need to be distinguished from deviations that are a variation of the normal.[12,26] The art of management of ALD involves deciding which conditions require immediate aggressive management and which can tolerate a wait-and-see approach.

The following treatment methods are divided into nonsurgical and surgical procedures, according to the appearance and severity of the problem.

Nonsurgical Techniques

Stall Rest

Stall rest is an effective treatment in newborn foals with certain types of ALD. The following problems can be treated with stall rest:

Foals with incomplete ossification and straight limbs at the time of birth. Under no circumstances should these animals be turned out in a field.[6,9,10] Exercise on the weakened, partially ossified carpal and tarsal bones may result in abnormal ossification of the bones with subsequent development of osteoarthritis.[6,9,10] Stall rest should be maintained for a maximum of 1 month. While the animal is on stall rest, radiographs should be repeated at 2-week intervals to evaluate the progress of ossification.

Foals with adequate ossification and ALD because of disproportionate growth at the level of the physis (greater than 10 degrees) and foals with diaphyseal deformities. Stall rest may be continued for 4 to 6 weeks. If correction is not achieved during that time, surgical treatment should be attempted.

Foals with laxity of the periarticular supporting structures and a normal degree of ossification. Such animals should be exercised daily for 10 to 20 minutes through walking the mare, to stimulate muscle work and strengthening of the involved soft tissue structures. Three to 5 minutes of swimming daily is the best exercise if facilities are available (see Chapter 90). Growth of the foal usually resolves the deformity.

Predicting whether the problem will resolve with stall rest alone is not possible, and valuable time can be lost by waiting too long. This is the main reason for not prolonging stall rest treatment beyond 4 to 6 weeks. It is important to critically observe the foal continually during the stall rest period.

Splints and Casts

Foals with incomplete ossification of the carpal and tarsal bones may be treated effectively with splints or casts[6,9] (Fig. 89-10, *A*). The purpose of these devices is to maintain the limb in proper alignment and to allow the inadequately ossified cartilage template to ossify sufficiently and facilitate weightbearing without detrimental consequences.[10] It is of paramount importance that the cast or splint end at the fetlock. If the foot is incorporated in the splint, the musculotendinous flexor and extensor units weaken, resulting in a dropped fetlock and osteopenia. In most cases, this problem is of a temporary nature, but it should be prevented because it may lead to additional orthopedic problems. The limb

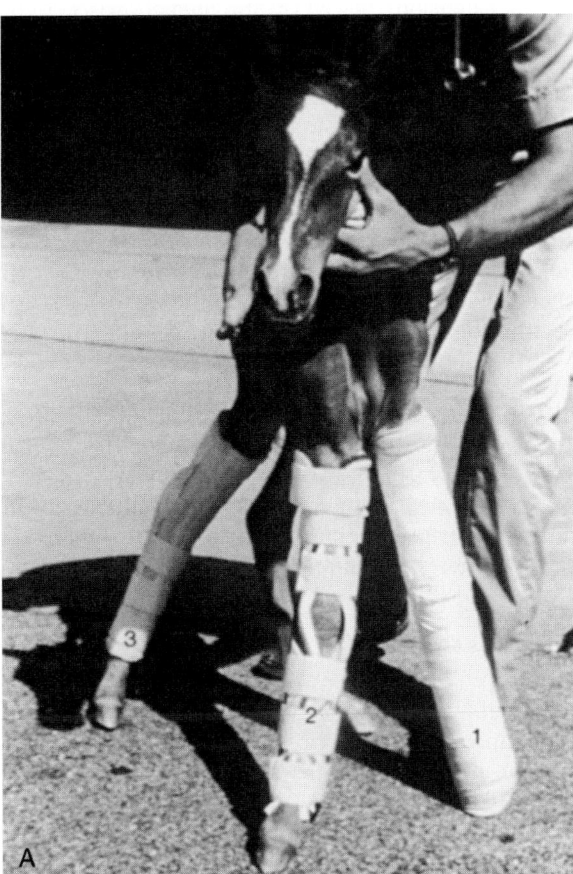

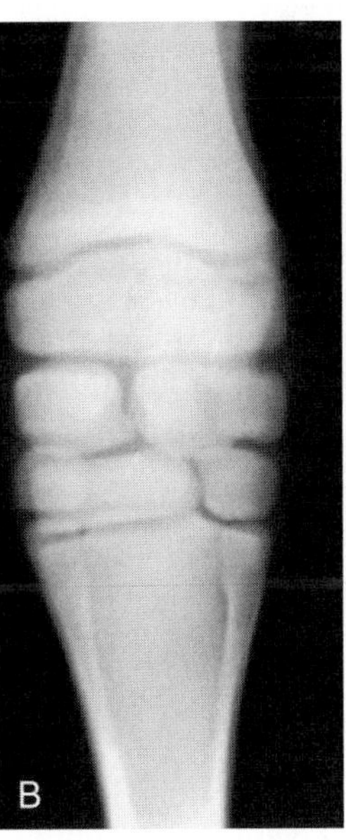

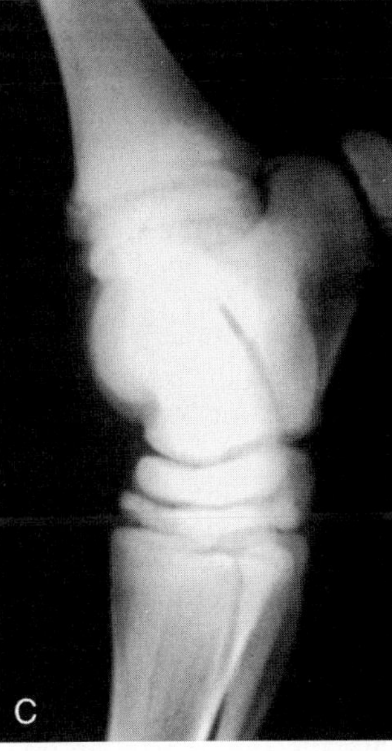

Figure 89-10. The foal mentioned in Figure 89-2 at 2 days of age. **A,** Splints are applied to three limbs. A polyvinylchloride (PVC) pipe splint is applied to the left forelimb (1). The PVC pipe is centered over the carpal region and reaches distally to the hoof because the animal also suffered from a ruptured common digital extensor tendon in that limb. The total limb is incorporated in the bandage. A commercial splint (2) (DePuy, Warsaw, Ind) is applied to the right forelimb. The splint is fastened with Velcro straps and contains medial and lateral metal strips for support. The right tarsal region is also splinted with a commercial splint (3) (DePuy, Warsaw, Ind). This splint is of the same material as the forelimb splint (2). Note that the commercial splints do not incorporate the phalanges. **B** and **C,** Radiographs carried out 30 days after the original radiographs: The dorsopalmar view of the carpal (**B**) and lateromedial view of the tarsal (**C**) regions show increased ossification compared with the previous radiographs. Ossification was sufficient to allow the foal to go without splints. The foal was maintained in bandages, kept in a stall for an additional week, and then turned out.

should be well padded before splint or cast application. The splint is changed every 3 to 4 days, and dry padding is placed next to the limb. Casts should be changed between 10 and 14 days after application. Leaving the cast on for too long results in skin damage because of the rapid growth of young foals. The radiographic evaluation is repeated at 2-week intervals and the change in degree of ossification is determined.

Casts and splints should be maintained as long as incomplete ossification is present. Depending on the degree of ossification at the time of birth, this may take 2 to 4 weeks (see Fig. 89-10, *B* and *C*). In twin foals, it may be continued for up to 2 months of age.

While the limb is under a cast or splint, the flexor carpi ulnaris and the ulnaris lateralis muscles are immobilized and become flaccid. This results in a temporary calf-kneed conformation immediately after the cast is removed (see Chapter 90). Additionally, pressure necrosis of the skin over the accessory carpal bone may develop. However, with time, these defects correct as strength returns to the muscles. Daily swim therapy is beneficial and helps in rapidly overcoming this condition. It is important to keep the limb bandaged for an additional 4 to 5 days after the cast or splints are removed.

If radiographs demonstrate that the deformity is located within the distal radius or tibia and is not caused by laxity of the periarticular supporting structures or incomplete ossification, splints and casts are ineffective and, in fact, contraindicated. Application of such devices almost invariably results in pressure sores without correction of the deformity.

Aside from somewhat labor-intensive management with the help of polyvinylchloride (PVC) half-shell splints, custom-fitted snap-on splints made of padded fiberglass (Endurasplint 2, Carapace Inc., New Tazewell, Tenn) can be used.[27] These splints have enough strength for foals younger than 6 weeks of age. The foal is sedated and placed in lateral recumbency, and a rectal sleeve is placed over the limb to protect it from contact with water and polyurethane resin. The splint material is immersed in warm water (21° to 23° C [69.8° to 73.4° F]) until it is soft and pliable. Excess water is squeezed out and the splint is swiftly applied to the limb with the felt positioned against the skin and covering half of the circumference of the limb. It is secured to the limb with gauze and allowed to dry, with care taken not to flex the limb during the setting time. The splint is removed and allowed to set for 5 to 7 minutes before reapplying it to the limb. Because the splint is padded and molded to the contour of the limb, it is easy to place, and only a single roll of self-adhesive elastic is needed to secure it, making it convenient for daily use. In a hospital setting, it is recommended that the splint be left on for 12 hours at a time to prevent pressure sores; it should be applied at night while the foal is less active.[27]

Special custom-fitted hinged braces, which allow the foal to move the carpal and tarsal regions while maintaining correct axial alignment, have been introduced to the market (Farley brace [Indialantic, Fla], Redden brace [International Equine Podiatry Center, Versailles, Ky]). Foals with incomplete ossification or laxity of the periarticular supporting structures can be successfully treated with these devices. Because these braces allow movement of the joints, this type of treatment is theoretically preferred over stiff splints or casts. However, this is the only application of such braces in foals with ALD.

Hoof Manipulation

Corrective hoof trimming is a frequent conservative treatment of ALD. In valgus deformities, the outside half of the hoof wall is slightly shortened. This causes the inside half of the foot to contact the ground first, and during the process of placing weight on the entire foot, it rotates medially. This type of hoof trimming is carried out with a rasp in young foals. In contrast, for varus deformities and pigeon-toed conformation, the inside wall is slightly lowered. In young foals, this type of treatment may be beneficial as an *adjunct* therapy to a surgical technique and should be maintained for only a few weeks to months because of the danger of the development of an abnormal hoof shape and of interphalangeal joint osteoarthritis.

The application of foot plates or shoes with an extension to the inside or outside may assist in correcting the deformity. Additionally, these devices prevent excessive wear-down at certain areas of the foot. For valgus deformities, extensions are placed on the medial side of the foot, and for varus deformities, on the lateral side. It is important to fill the extensions placed on the medial aspect of the hoof with acrylic to prevent stepping onto the plate with the other foot.

Corrective hoof trimming should *not* be used as the sole treatment for significant ALD in older foals. By forcing the foot into an uncomfortable, abnormal position, torsional and stress forces are created that cause early degenerative changes of cartilage and periarticular structures. Therefore, it is better to opt for surgical procedures at the location of the deformity than to try to bring about correction through altering the loading conditions of the entire limb up to the location of the deformity.

Surgical Techniques

The surgical techniques for correction of ALD are reviewed for the carpal region, because this is the area where ALD is diagnosed most frequently.[9] As the various techniques are discussed, consideration is given to the other anatomic regions where these surgical procedures may be used.

Growth Acceleration

Since its introduction into equine surgery, periosteal transection and elevation (stripping) has gained universal acceptance.[5,7,9,10,28-30] Periosteal transection is performed on the concave aspect of the limb (e.g., in an animal with a valgus deformity in the carpal region, on the lateral side). A 3-cm vertical skin incision is made between the common and lateral digital extensor tendons, starting from a point 4 to 5 cm proximal to the distal physis of the radius and continuing in a proximal direction (Fig. 89-11, *A*). The incision is carried down to the periosteum. With a curved hemostatic forceps, the subcutaneous tissues and tendons are separated from the periosteum parallel to the physis and perpendicular to the skin incision at its distal border. The forceps is abducted, with its slightly spread tips pressing onto the bone. Under this protection, a curved scalpel blade

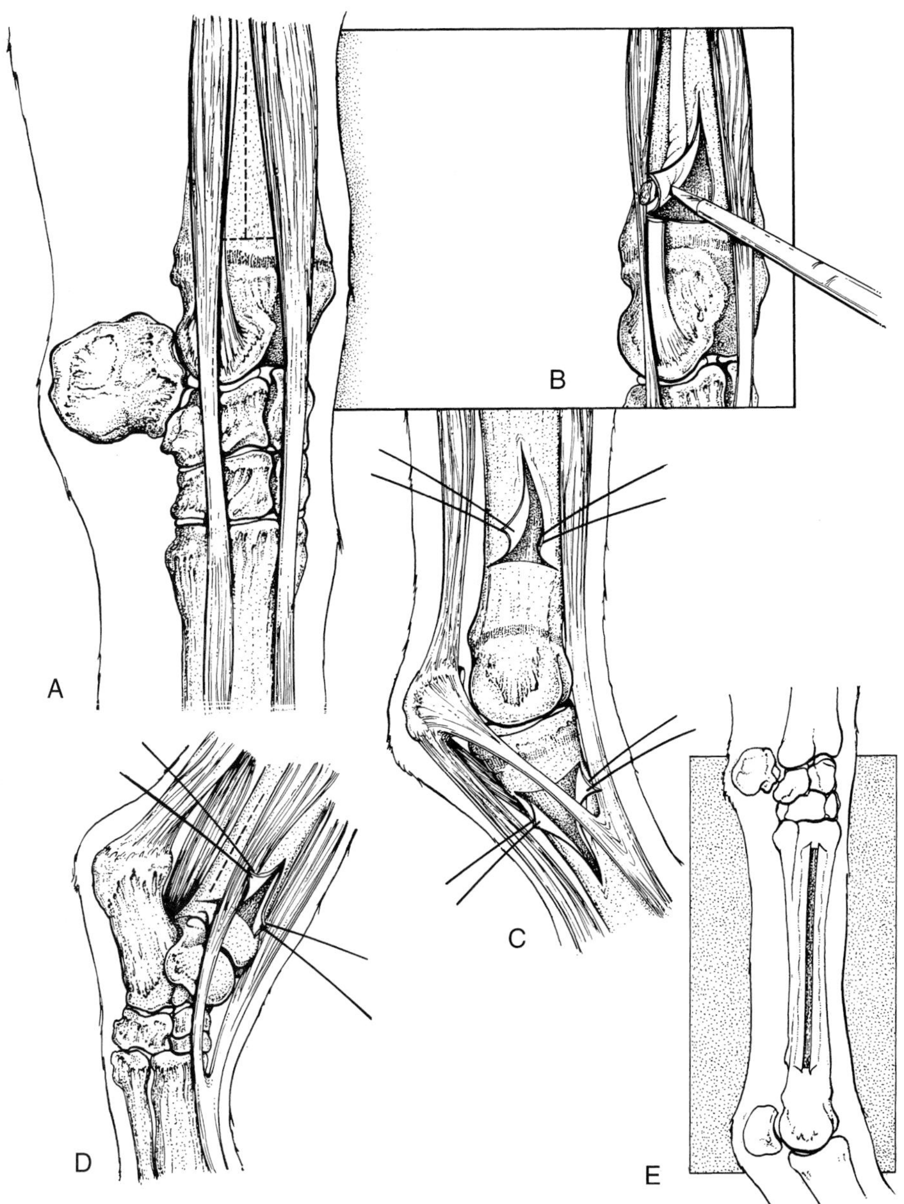

Figure 89-11. Locations at which growth acceleration may be carried out. **A,** Anatomic relationship of the landmarks for the surgical approach at the distal carpus (common digital extensor tendon cranially, lateral digital extensor tendon and rudimentary ulna caudally, and the distal radial physis distally). **B,** The periosteal transection is completed on the caudal aspect. The rudimentary ulna is transected, and the caudal periosteal flap is being elevated. **C,** Location of growth acceleration at the distal MCIII/MTIII and proximal phalanx. The procedures are performed, and the flaps are elevated. **D,** Anatomic relationship of the landmarks for the surgical approach at the distal tibia. The periosteal transection procedure was carried out through an approach cranial to the lateral digital extensor tendon. The vertical periosteal incision caudal to the lateral digital extensor tendon is an alternate site *(dotted line).* **E,** Location of the procedure carried out over the total length of the MCIII/MTIII. The procedure was performed and the two periosteal (barn-door) flaps were elevated.

(no. 12) is inserted cranially between the tips of the hemostatic forceps. Using moderate pressure, the scalpel blade is pulled back toward the level of the skin incision, transecting periosteum. Once the blade has reached the lateral aspect of the bone, the incision is stopped. The same procedures are repeated on the caudal aspect of the distal radius. The hemostat is first advanced to separate the lateral digital extensor tendon from the rudimentary ulna and then is redirected to a frontal plane to reach the caudal aspect of the distal radius. The scalpel blade is inserted under the protection of the forceps, and the periosteum, including the rudimentary ulna, is transected as described earlier. The cranial and caudal incisions are connected. Because this transection severs the rete carpi volaris, marked bleeding occurs. The periosteum is then incised parallel to the skin incision in a proximal direction over a length of 2 cm, starting at the horizontal periosteal incision, to create an inverted T. The periosteal elevator is advanced at a 45-degree angle to the periosteal incisions underneath the periosteum to elevate two triangular flaps (see Fig. 89-11, *B*). Once elevated, the periosteum is gently laid back onto the bone to prevent the ends from curling, which could result in new bone formation. The subcutaneous tissues are closed in a simple-continuous suture pattern, using 2-0 absorbable suture material, followed by a simple-continuous intradermal suture line. This results in an acceptable cosmetic appearance of the surgical site.

In about 20% of all cases, the rudimentary ulna is ossified and therefore has to be removed with rongeurs. It is important that the rudimentary ulna be transected, because it can act as a tethering mechanism and slow down growth at the concave aspect of the radius.

Postoperatively, a bandage, consisting of a nonadherent dressing (Telfa, Kendall Company, Boston, Mass) and unfolded 4×4 gauze sponges, covered by an adhesive elastic bandage (Elasticon, Johnson & Johnson Products Inc, New Brunswick, NJ), is applied. The elastic tape is attached directly to the skin for a width of 2 cm proximal and distal to the gauze sponges. The bandage is replaced 3 days postoperatively. The second bandage may stay in place for an additional week before it is removed. No skin sutures need to be removed because the sutures are below the skin surface (intradermally). It is advisable to keep the animal in a stall for 2 to 3 weeks and to allow minimal exercise during that time.

Postoperatively, the outside of the feet (in a valgus deformity) are rasped slightly every 2 weeks to assist in correction of the outward rotation of the feet and straightening of the limbs.

The surgery can be carried out in a foal as young as 2 weeks of age. The earlier the surgery is performed, the faster the correction occurs (Fig. 89-12). However, opting for surgical intervention at such an early age may include foals in which the deformity would have corrected spontaneously if the animal was allowed stall rest. Therefore, foals should be selected for this surgery after 4 weeks of age, unless the ALD is severe (greater than 10 degrees).

The landmarks for periosteal transection at the distal MCIII/MTIII are the distal-most aspect of the metaphysis of MCIII/MTIII or MCIV/MTIV and, depending on the location of the concavity of the deformed bone, the medial or lateral aspect of the bone (see Fig. 89-11, *C*). Care should be taken not to enter the palmar or plantar outpouching of the MCP/MTP joint. These surgical interventions must be performed prior to 3 months of age, because after that there is only limited growth at the distal physis of MCIII/MTIII.[31] The periosteum at the surgical site of MCIII/MTIII is markedly thinner than that of the distal radius or tibia.[9]

Surgery at the proximal phalanx should be carried out at the level where the extensor branch of the suspensory ligament curves over the lateral or medial aspect of the bone[32] (see Fig. 89-11, *C*). On this bone, the periosteal incisions are performed in a T-shaped configuration, with the horizontal incision about 1 cm distal to the physis and the vertical incision in a distal direction. At the palmar or plantar aspect of the horizontal incision, some attachments of the oblique

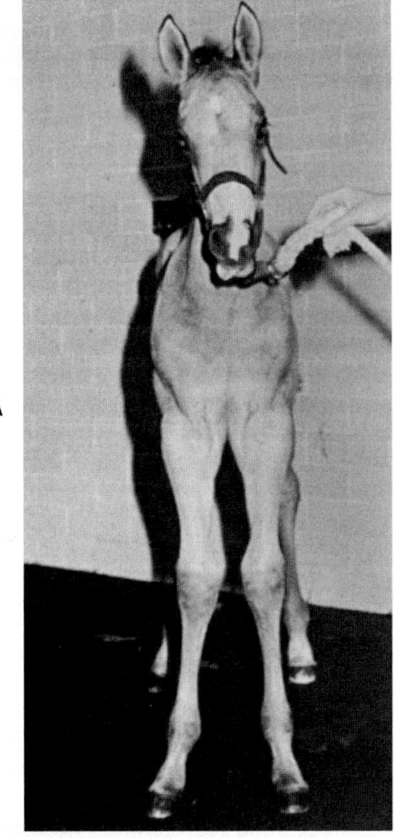

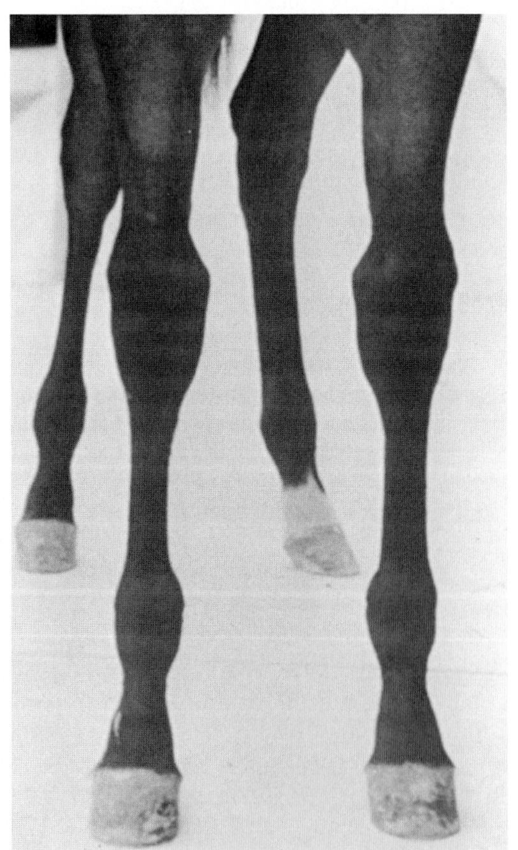

Figure 89-12. A 2-month-old Quarter Horse colt with a marked bilateral carpal valgus deformity (**A**) and the same foal 4 months after periosteal transection and elevation (stripping) at the lateral aspect of both forelimbs (**B**). Note the good correction and excellent cosmetic result. (From Auer JA, Martens RJ, Williams EH: J Am Vet Med Assoc 1982;181:459.)

distal sesamoidean ligaments will be transected. This appears to present no serious consequences but can result in minor new bone formation that resolves with time.

The surgical approach for the distal tibia is either cranial or caudal to the lateral digital extensor tendon (see Fig. 89-11, *D*). The rest of the procedure is carried out in a fashion analogous to that described for the distal radius. It is interesting to note that the periosteum in that area is thicker than that at any other surgical site discussed earlier.

"Bench knees" are a frequently encountered conformational defect that may continue to develop after 1 year of age.[24,25] These conformational defects are the result of two opposing ALDs—a valgus deformity at the distal radius and a varus deformity of the proximal third of MCIII[9,33] (Fig. 89-13). The limb has a straight appearance in the presence of bench-kneed (off-set) conformation. If this conformational defect is diagnosed within the first 2 months of life, periosteal stripping can be carried out at the lateral aspect of the distal radius and over the entire medial aspect of MCIII, starting 2 cm proximal to the distal physis and up to 3 cm below the carpometacarpal joint[33] (Fig. 89-14). A horizontal incision is carried out at each end of the longitudinal incision, producing an I-shaped incision in the periosteum (see Fig. 89-11, *E*). The two flaps are elevated, and the subcutaneous tissue and skin are closed as previously described.[10,29] Periosteal stripping over the total length of MCIII/MTIII is also effective in correcting diaphyseal or metaphyseal deformities of that bone in foals younger than 2 months[34] (Fig. 89-15).

Periosteal transection has its effect for approximately 2 months, which corresponds to the time needed to fill in the defect between the transected ends of the periosteum.[32,35] A prolonged effect is achieved through surgical excision of the elevated triangular flaps. Periosteal transection can be repeated if complete correction is not achieved. Overcorrection of the deformity does not occur.

It has been shown that periosteal transection carried out when the ALD is located within the carpus also corrects malformation of these bones to some degree.[31,32] Nevertheless, such problems should be recognized earlier and the incomplete ossification treated during the immediate postnatal period, as described previously. However, surgery accelerates correction even in these cases, allowing the foals pasture exercise at an earlier age while preventing the development of additional deformities further distally (e.g., digit, hoof).

Periosteal transection and elevation are routinely carried out on an outpatient basis, with the mare and foal returning home immediately after recovery from surgery. The most critical location for early diagnosis and surgery is the distal MCIII/MTIII, because longitudinal growth of MCIII/MTIII occurs mainly during the first 3 months after birth.[31] Later on, growth occurs at a very slow pace, and delaying surgery leads to incomplete correction. Additionally, the prolonged

A

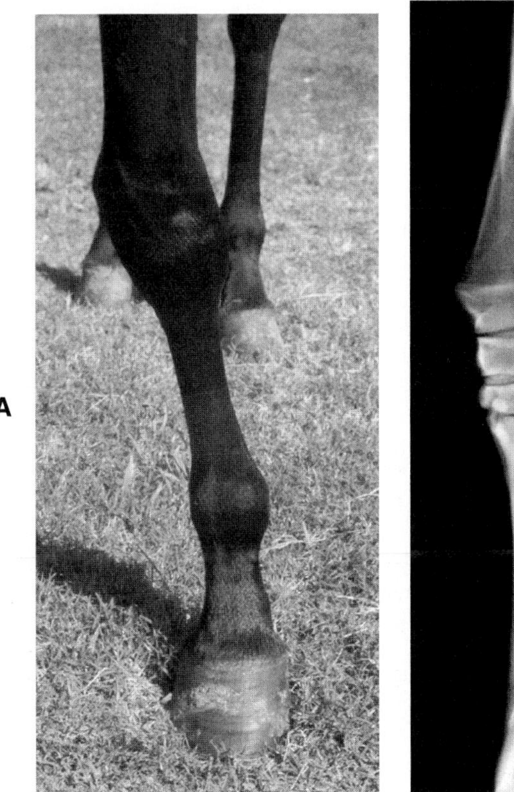

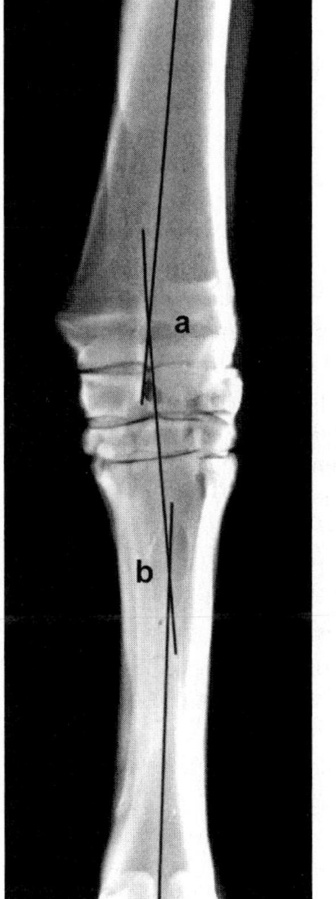

B

Figure 89-13. A, The frontal view of the left forelimb of the mare of the foal in Figure 14 showing marked "bench-knee" (off-set) conformation. **B,** The composite dorsopalmar radiograph of the radius, carpus, and MCII showing the combination of the distal radial valgus deformity and the proximal MCIII varus deformity, which results in an oblique orientation of the carpal region.

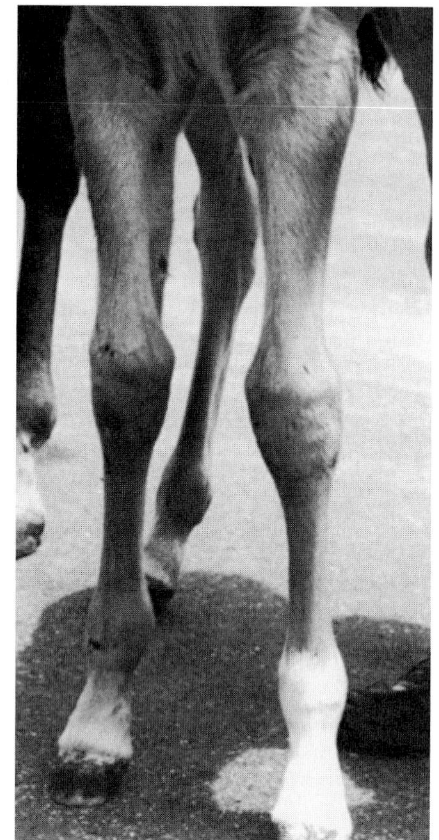

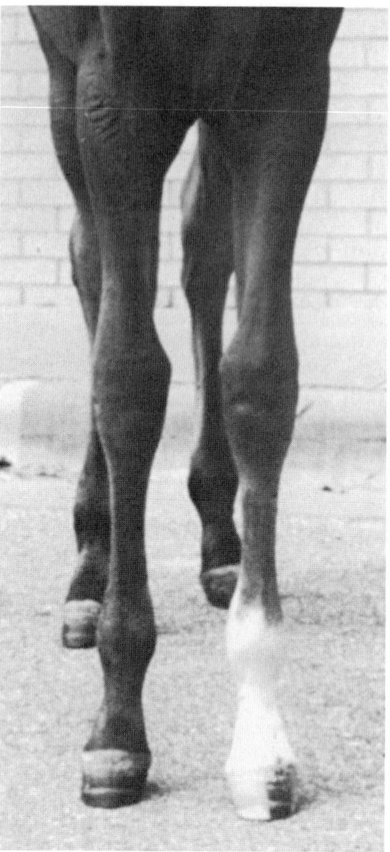

Figure 89-14. A 2-month-old foal with bench knees (**A**) and 2 months after growth acceleration at the lateral aspect of the distal radius and the medial aspect of MCIII (**B**). Note the good correction and excellent cosmetic result. (From Auer JA: Pferdeheilkunde 1989:5:201.)

abnormal loading of the metacarpophalangeal joints leads to the development of compensatory deformities in the proximal phalanx.[28,36] Thus, the limb may appear to be straight, but when the foal walks, an outward rotation is noted. This is caused by the orientation of the articular surfaces, which are not parallel to the ground (Fig. 89-16).

During the first weeks of life, affected foals show an outward rotation of the carpal region while their feet point straightforward (see Fig. 89-8, *B*). At that point, an actual varus deformity is hard to detect, especially for an inexperienced clinician. With time, the deformity is aggravated, making diagnosis easy but surgery difficult.

Recently, the effectiveness of hemi-circumferential periosteal transection and elevation in treating ALD was questioned.[37] In a controlled study, temporary transphyseal bridging was performed on the lateral aspect of the distal radius to induce a carpal valgus ALD of 15 degrees in normal young foals.[37] At the time of implant removal, the foals were divided into two groups. One group was subjected to an immediate hemi-circumferential periosteal transection and elevation on the same lateral aspect of the distal radius, whereas the other group underwent a sham surgical procedure at the same site to mimic the hemi-circumferential periosteal transection and elevation procedure. In both groups, the deformity corrected, leading to the erroneous conclusion that periosteal transection and elevation was ineffective. Three facts might explain the results: (1) the deformity was induced artificially through manipulation of the physis, (2) a clinical case with a carpal valgus deformity of 15 degrees does not correct without surgery, and (3) physeal growth is influenced by mechanical load, which in turn triggers signal molecules in a feedback loop between the cells of the different cartilage zones and the perichondrium or periosteum of the limb involved.[38] This regulatory mechanism of signaling molecules was triggered at the time of initial surgery, when the periosteum was disturbed, and it was accentuated by the second surgery, performed to remove the implants. Periosteal transection could not be expected to further trigger this cascade. Therefore, no difference between groups could be expected.

Preliminary data of ongoing research to elucidate the effects of hemi-circumferential transection of the periosteum and local periosteal stripping revealed that local signaling processes occurring at the physeal level involve the feedback loop of PTHrP, PTHrPR, and Ihh and determine the normal growth mechanism and its acceleration.[39] Additional work is needed, but there is a good chance that the phenomenon of growth acceleration through hemi-circumferential transection of the periosteum and local periosteal stripping can be explained through these processes and thus lay to rest the discussion on effectiveness once and for all.

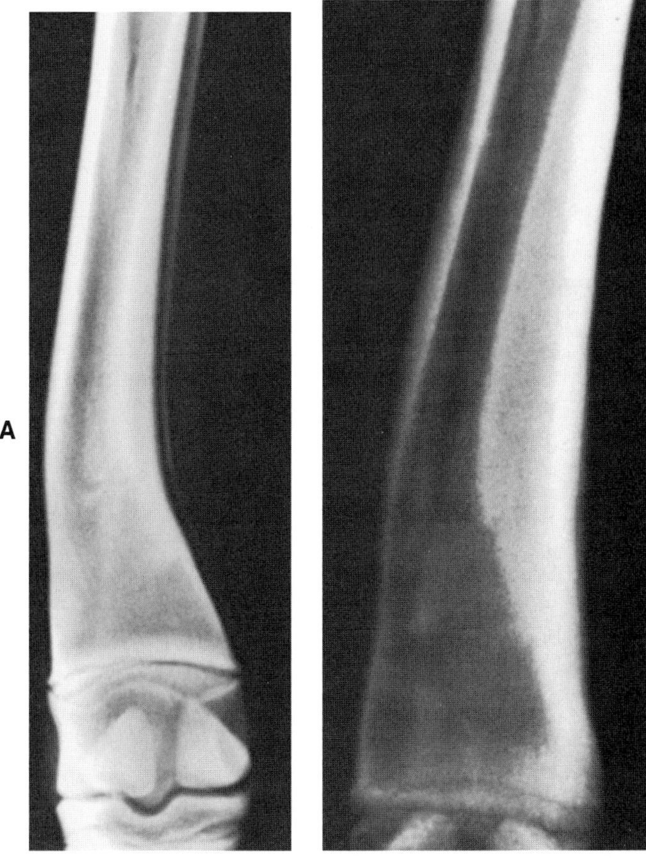

Figure 89-15. Dorsopalmar radiographs of the left MTIII region of a 2-month-old foal with a severe metaphyseal valgus deformity before periosteal transection and stripping of the entire lateral aspect of this bone (**A**). The 4-month follow-up radiograph (**B**) shows significant improvement of the deformity. For practical purposes, the foal had straight limbs at that time.

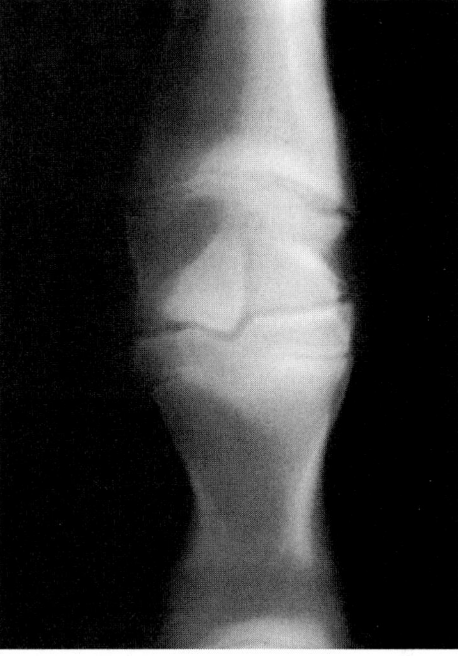

Figure 89-16. Dorsopalmar radiograph of the metatarsophalangeal region of a foal with a relatively straight limb. The proximal phalanx and distal MTIII have opposing deformities, resulting in an oblique orientation of the joint surface relative to the ground. (From Auer JA: J Am Vet Med Assoc 1985;187:496.)

Growth Retardation

Growth retardation is performed either in young foals (less than 3 months of age) with severe ALD or in foals with significant ALD in a bone after the rapid growth phase is over (MCIII/MTIII and proximal phalanx after 2 months, tibia after 4 months, radius after 6 months).[9,31] The techniques described for growth retardation use the same principle. Implants, applied on the convex aspect of the bone, bridge the physis temporarily, allowing the shorter aspect of the bone to continue to grow, eventually correcting the deformity.

Stapling was the first technique of growth retardation described in the foal.[40] The surgery is performed in some clinics with favorable results but is not discussed here because it has fallen into disfavor. Complications include implant and correction failures.

Screws and cerclage wires are the most frequently applied implants.[1-3,5,8,9,14] Implants are inserted through two stab incisions, one in the center of the epiphysis and the other proximal to the physis (Fig. 89-17, *A*). The soft tissues between these incisions are elevated with a hemostat (see Fig. 89-17, *B*). A 4.5-mm cortex screw is inserted through each incision but not completely tightened (see Fig. 89-17, *C*). A wire loop is inserted through the proximal incision and hooked over the distal screw head (see Fig. 89-17, *D*). The two wire ends are twisted together and tightened over the proximal screw head (see Fig. 89-17, *E*). Twisting the wire ends over the proximal screw rather than the distal screw results in less irritation of the surrounding soft tissues and produces a better cosmetic result.

The screws are tightened completely, which increases wire tension as the wires ride up on the shoulder of the screw heads. The stab incisions are then closed with two simple-interrupted skin sutures, and the area is protected with a light bandage for approximately 10 days. Sutures can be removed by the referring veterinarian. In foals with minor ALDs and laterally rotated forelimbs, surgery may be delayed for some time. However, foals with carpal valgus deformity and feet pointing straight forward should be treated immediately to prevent a toed-in conformation from developing. A second wire applied over the two screw heads strengthens the configuration and reduces the risk of wire failure and subsequent loss of growth retardation. The two stab incisions improve the overall cosmetic result considerably, compared with the large incision initially used.

Very recently, implantation of a transphyseal screw has been described as a method of retarding growth[41] (Fig. 89-18). The screws are inserted fully threaded and between the physes to arrest growth. They can be used in the physes of the distal MCIII/MTIII, distal radius, or distal tibia. The screws are removed when the desired conformation is reached. The advantages are ease of insertion and the improved cosmesis when a single screw is used. In the normal physis, the screw hole heals without affecting the foal's growth at the physis.

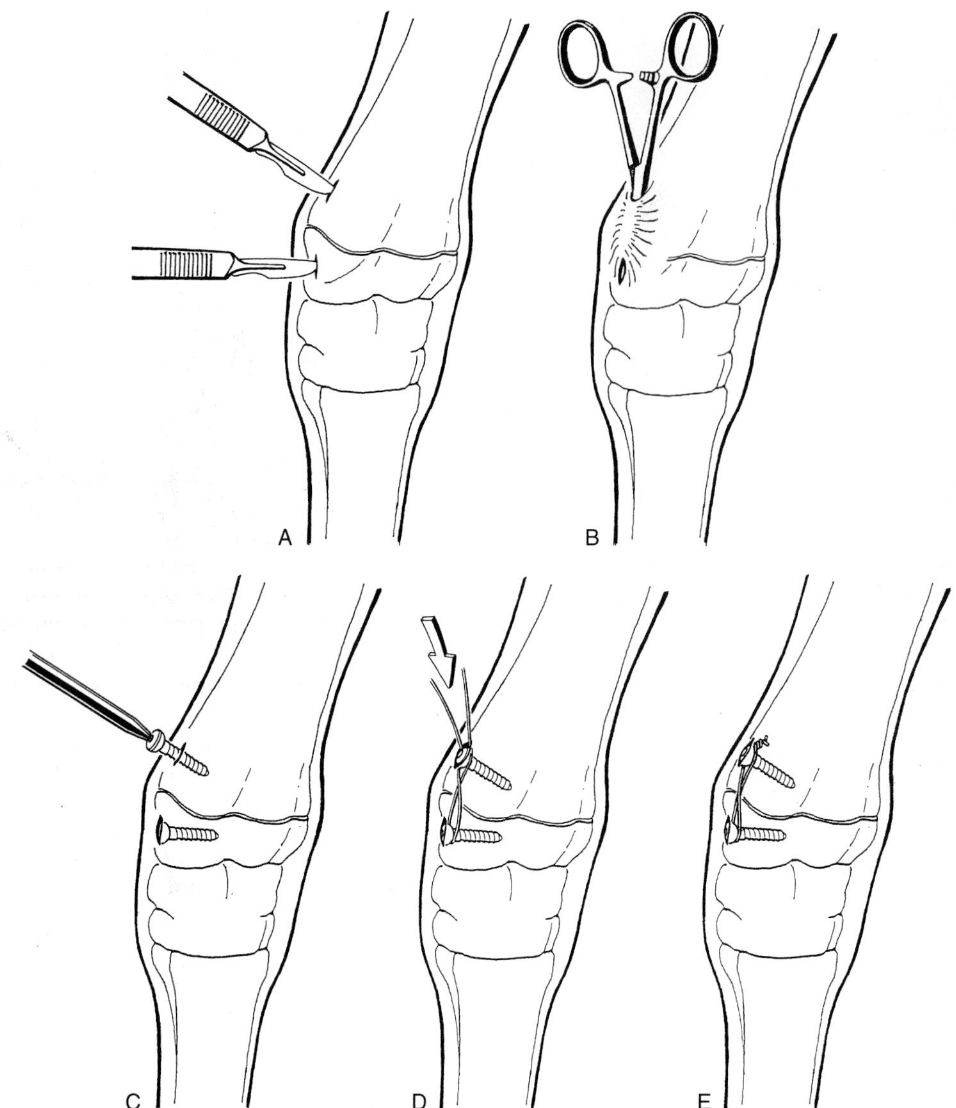

Figure 89-17. Growth retardation. **A,** A stab incision to the bone is carried out at the convex aspect of the epiphysis and the distal metaphysis. **B,** The soft tissue between the two incisions is elevated. **C,** A 4.5-mm screw is implanted through each incision but not tightened. **D,** A cerclage wire loop is introduced through the proximal incision, hooked over the distal screw head, and tightened in figure-eight fashion over the proximal screw (**E**). The screws are subsequently completely inserted, tightening the wire further.

A small, 2.7-mm bone plate can be used to correct ALD in older foals. The last hole on each side of the plate is enlarged to accept a 3.5-mm cortex screw. The plate can be implanted through stab incisions[9,10] (Fig. 89-19). This technique provides an excellent cosmetic appearance of the limb. The surgical approach consists of either a slightly curved incision centered over the physis or a stab incision on either side of the physis. The distal stab incision is carried out parallel to the fibers of the collateral ligament. A 2.5-mm hole is drilled and tapped into the physis parallel to the joint surface, which is readily palpable. A 2.7-mm bone plate of adequate length is manually contoured to the shape of the bone and slid through the proximal stab incision distally, where the 3.5-mm screw of about 26 mm in length is inserted through the distal hole of the plate.

An additional hole of the same diameter is drilled about 1 mm proximal to the last hole of the plate into the radial metaphysis. The hole is tapped, and the second screw is inserted into the hole. Both screws are tightened alternately until they are completely inserted into the bone (see Fig. 89-19). It is important that the distal screw be tightened completely to prevent it from protruding into the collateral ligament. The skin incisions are closed with simple-interrupted sutures. Radiographic evaluations should be carried out at monthly intervals to determine the correct time of implant removal and to prevent overcorrection of the deformity.

Growth retardation procedures also may be performed in the distal MCIII/MTIII, the proximal phalanx, and the distal tibia.[5,9,10] It is important to evaluate the anatomic

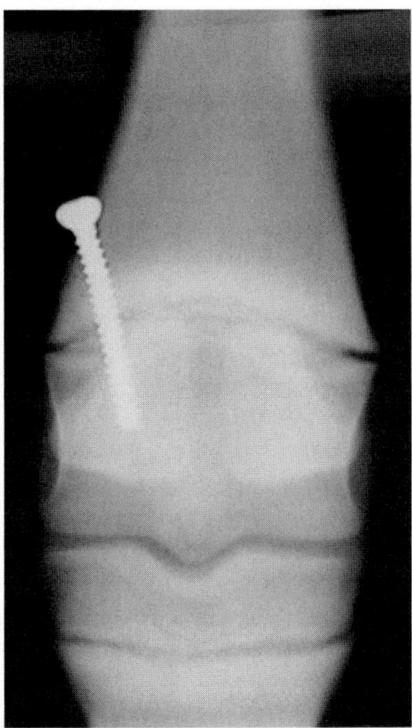

Figure 89-18. Dorsopalmar radiographic view of the distal MCIII. A single screw is inserted in an oblique proximodistal direction across the physis at the medial aspect of the bone. (Courtesy L. Bramlage, Lexington, Ky.)

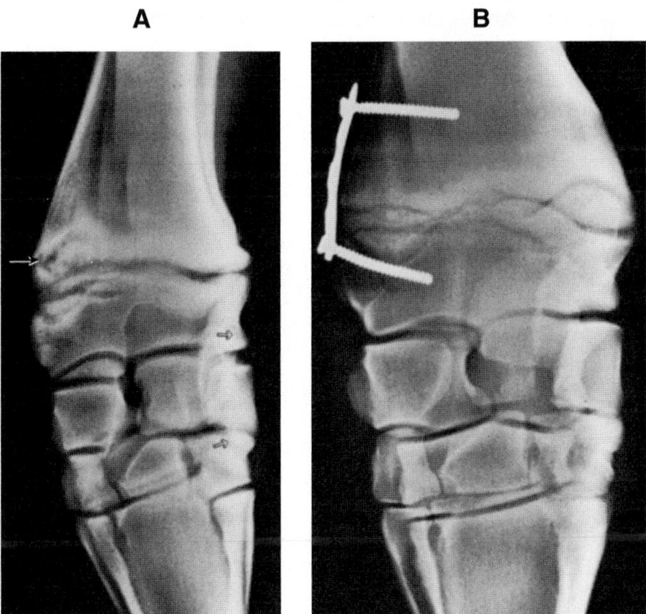

Figure 89-19. Dorsopalmar radiographic views of the left carpal region of a foal with severe bilateral valgus deformity. **A,** Preoperative radiograph at 3 months of age. Note the physeal ectasia located at the medial aspect of the distal radial metaphysis *(closed arrow).* The ulnar styloid process and the ulnar and fourth carpal bone have abnormal shapes because of increased weight-bearing and stress concentration in that region *(open arrows).* **B,** Three-month follow-up radiograph showing correction of the deformity. Note bending of the screws. The implants were removed, and the animal was discharged. The lateral aspect of the distal radius still shows some degenerative changes.

situation at each location. This is especially important for the distal tibia, where the epiphysis has an undulating configuration and the distal screw has to be inserted in a mediodistal to lateroproximal direction to avoid penetration of the joint.[5,9,10] A short screw is used to prevent penetration of the physis. However, the screw is at such a favorable angle, relative to the direction of the tension, that a short screw (22 mm) has adequate holding power. The proximal screw is easily inserted as previously described.

Once the correction is complete and verified radiographically, the implants must be removed through stab incisions over the screw heads, with the horse under short-term anesthesia.[9] The exact location of the screw heads is easily determined radiographically. It is important to be sure that the screwdriver is correctly seated in the hexagonal indentation in the screw head. Otherwise, stripping of the screw head may occur, making removal with a screwdriver difficult or impossible.[9] In that case, a screw removal device (see Fig. 81-13) should be used to remove the screws. The plate or wire is then removed through the proximal stab incision by introducing a curved hemostatic forceps into the hole and walking it off the edge of the hole in the bone, engaging the implant and pulling it through the incision. The stab incisions are closed using 2-0 absorbable suture material in a simple-interrupted pattern.

If implants are inserted in both forelimbs, it is important to remove the implants when each limb is straight. Waiting until both limbs are straight invariably results in overcorrection of one or undercorrection of the other limb. Implant removal can be carried out on an outpatient basis. Antibiotics are not routinely used.

As with growth acceleration, signal molecules from the proliferating and pre-hypertrophic zone in combination with the perichondrium are involved in retardation of the growth plate. It could be shown in rats that compressing the growth plate using surgical staples changed the feedback loop of PTHrP and Ihh, so that the pre-hypertrophic chondrocytes were pushed toward the osteogenic lineage, enhancing osteochondral ossification.[42] After stapling, the Ihh and Ptc molecules were modestly upregulated at 3 days, whereas BMP-2 and BMP-6 were inhibited.

Combination of Growth Acceleration and Retardation

In severe ALD, growth acceleration and growth retardation procedures are combined for a faster and more complete correction.[9,10] By combining the two techniques, there is a possibility that the deformity can be completely corrected. The advantage of using implants is that they can stay in place as long as they are needed, in contrast to periosteal transection, which has a time-limited effect.

In miniature horses, ALD is frequently diagnosed (Fig. 89-20, *A*). The presence of complete ulnas and fibulas is the predominant cause of ALD in this species and can be judged as an atavism (see Fig. 89-20, *B* and *C*). Early recognition of the problem is important in these animals. Miniature horses have less growth potential than regular horses; therefore, a 5-month-old foal with a moderate ALD will not achieve correction, even if growth acceleration and retardation procedures are combined. It is important to remove a portion of both the ulna and the fibula at the time of periosteal tran-

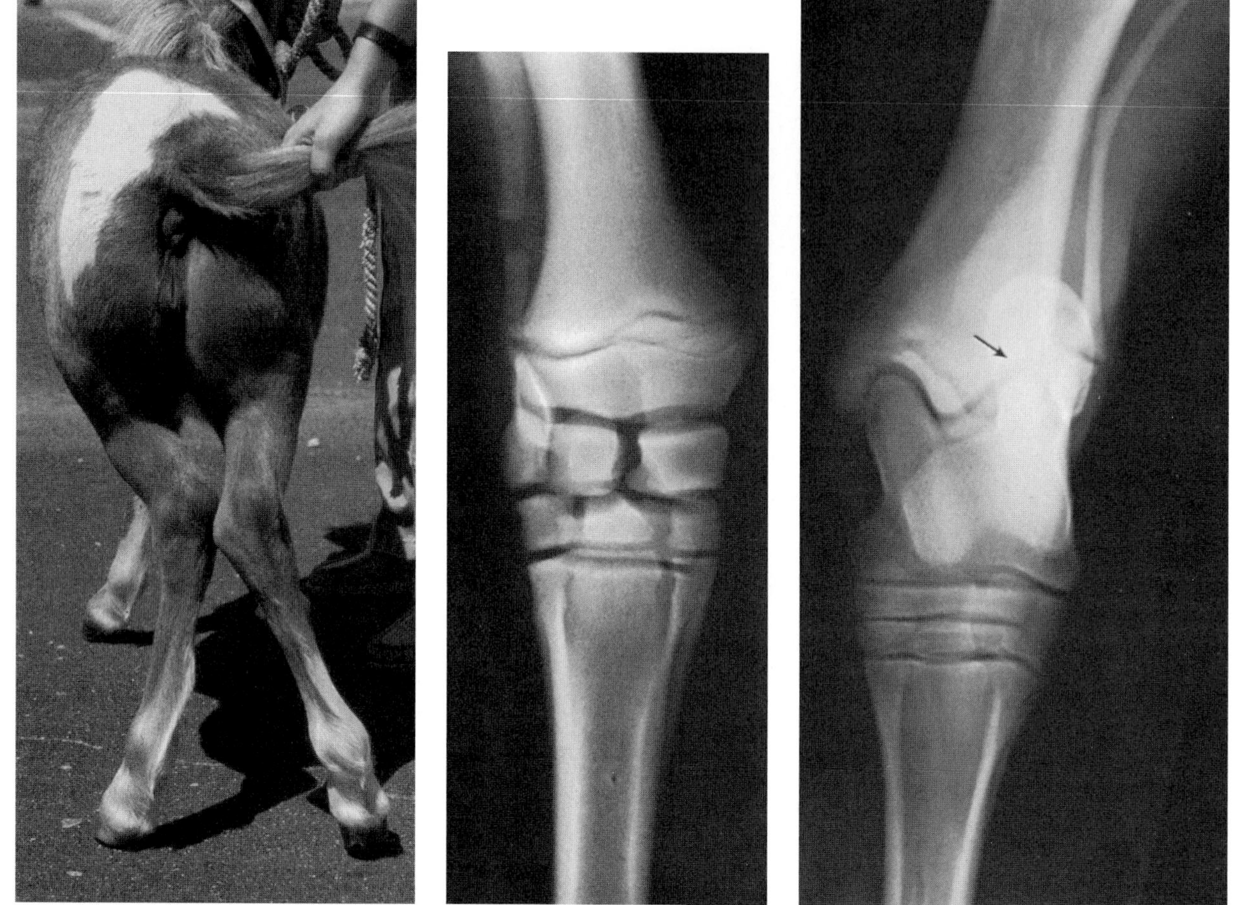

Figure 89-20. A, A 5-month-old miniature horse with severe tarsal valgus deformities in both rear limbs. Dorsoplantar radiographic views of the left carpal region showing a completely developed ulna (**B**) and of the left tibia showing a completely developed fibula (**C**). Note the acute angle of the lateral trochlear ridge of talus, representing early degenerative changes *(arrow)*.

section. However, the distal epiphyses of the complete fibula and the tibia are not united, and the continuous movement at their junction may result in abnormal development of the lateral trochlear ridge of the talus and associated osteoarthritis[43] (see Fig. 89-20). This problem is not as severe in the carpal region because of the architecture of the distal radius. In selected cases, transfixation of the distal fibular styloid process to the distal tibial epiphysis or metaphysis, or both, is needed to stop movement at the level of the joint. To insert the screws through the distal fibular metaphysis into the tibia, position screw technique (not lag technique) (see Chapter 81) should be applied to prevent alteration of the articular geometry.

Corrective Osteotomy/Ostectomy

Two types of ostectomy have been described in the literature: the closing wedge and the step. Closing wedge ostectomies (Fig. 89-21, *A*) have been used for correction of diaphyseal and metaphyseal/epiphyseal ALD in foals with closed growth plates.[44,45] However, the step ostectomy carried out in the sagittal plane and the step osteotomy carried out in the frontal plane are presently the preferred techniques and are discussed here.[46]

The skin incision is carried out over the lateral digital extensor tendon from the top of the MCIII/MTIII to the distal physis. At that point, the incision is continued medially (in a varus deformity) or laterally (in a valgus deformity) toward the MCP joint. The lateral digital extensor tendon together with the periosteum is split longitudinally. Subperiosteal dissection is carried out to gain access to the dorsal aspect of MCIII/MTIII. At the level of the proposed Z-shaped osteotomy, the periosteum is elevated circumferentially around the bone.

The step ostectomy in the sagittal plane removes a vertical wedge from the center of the bone (see Fig. 89-21, *B*).

The pivot point, which was previously established on radiographs (Fig. 89-22, *A*) by drawing the longitudinal bisecting lines through MCIII/MTIII and the phalanges, respectively, is identified relative to proper landmarks, and a 3.2-mm hole is drilled across the bone. A second hole is drilled parallel to the first one, approximately 4 cm further proximally. The oscillating saw is used to cut between the two drill holes across the bone. The previously prepared and sterilized aluminum template with the appropriate angle of the wedge to be removed is laid with one limb parallel to the saw cut and compared with the bisecting lines on the radiograph. A second saw cut is then made along the second

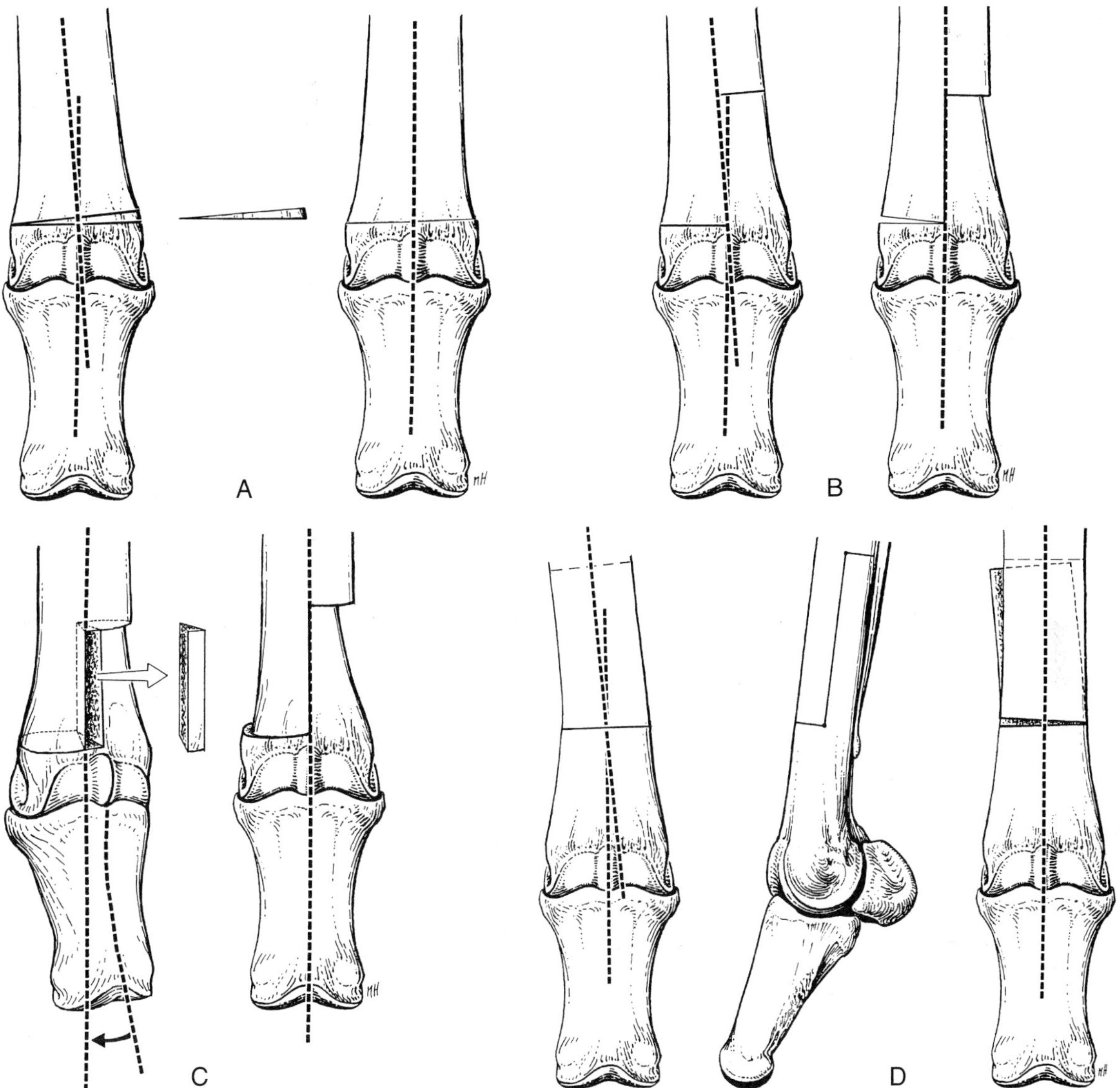

Figure 89-21. A, Closing wedge ostectomy. The bone wedge is removed from the horizontal plane near the physeal region. **B,** Step ostectomy. The wedge is removed from the center of MCIII in the sagittal plane. **C,** Derotational step ostectomy. By removing a vertical wedge with its wide aspect located either dorsally or in a palmar direction, a rotational deformity can be corrected. **D,** Step osteotomy. The Z-plasty is performed in the frontal plane, and the fragments are rotated into alignment.

limb of the template and parallel to the first one in the sagittal plane. The Z-shaped osteotomy is completed with the proximal cut through the thinner portion of MCIII/MTIII (lateral in a varus deformity) and the distal cut across the opposite side of the bone in a horizontal plane, parallel to the physis. The wedge is removed, and the two bone fragments are rotated into alignment. Final adjustments are made to ensure complete correction of the deformity and bone-on-bone contact at the palmar/plantar aspect of the bone. If an additional rotational deformity is present, it can be corrected at that point by removing an additional bone wedge from the palmar or dorsal aspect of the bone (see Fig. 89-21, *C*). Cortex screws are applied in lag fashion across the vertical section of the cut to reunite the two fragments of the bone. A bone plate is subsequently applied medially (in a varus deformity) or laterally (in a valgus deformity) to the bone and, along the vertical cut, the screws are inserted in lag fashion (see Fig. 89-22, *B* and *C*). The gap at the distal aspect of the osteotomy may be filled with some bone from the removed wedge as a cortical bone graft. The first row of sutures is placed into the split lateral digital extensor tendon using 2-0 absorbable suture material in a simple-continuous pattern. The subcutaneous tissues are closed, followed by intradermal closure of the skin, as previously described. In selected cases, skin sutures are applied.

Postoperatively, the limb is bandaged and supported by a splint or a cast for a few weeks. A cast would be applied in an adult horse, an excitable horse, or a foal whose step osteotomy was carried out near the physis, allowing only a limited number of screws in the distal fragment.

The holes drilled at the proximal and distal ends of the vertical saw cut reduce the concentration of stress at these locations and prevent postoperative fracture development.

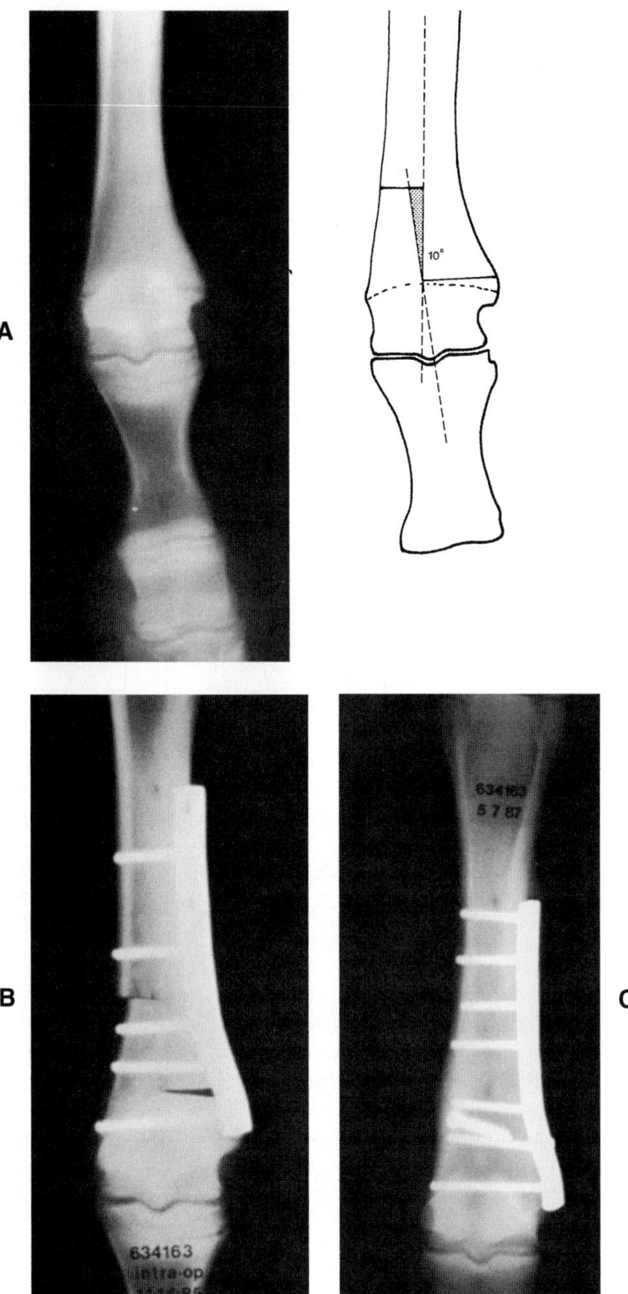

Figure 89-22. A, Dorsopalmar radiograph and diagram of the distal MCIII region with a varus deformity in an Arabian foal. The preoperative drawing shows the 10-degree wedge to be removed from the center of MCIII. **B,** Intraoperative radiograph of the corrected deviation showing a seven-hole DCP applied to MCIII with five screws inserted. The second and third screws from the bottom were inserted in lag fashion across the vertical aspect of the step osteotomy. The gap underneath the plate was filled with bone obtained from the wedge that was removed. The remaining screws were inserted through the plate, and an additional lag screw was placed across the vertical saw cut. **C,** Six-month follow-up radiograph of the corrected deformity. Note the excellent cosmetic result. The implants were subsequently removed. (From Auer JA: In White NA II, Moore JN, editors: Current Practice of Equine Surgery, Oxford, 1990, Blackwell.)

The step osteotomy in the frontal plane is carried out similarly (see Fig. 89-21, *D*). Again, a Z-shaped osteotomy is performed across the bone, but this time the vertical cut is placed in the frontal plane. In this type of osteotomy, no bone wedge is actually removed. Once the Z-shaped osteotomy is completed, the two fragments are rotated in alignment. At that point, lag screws are inserted and a plate is applied to the bone's dorsal surface. Performing the saw cuts is somewhat more difficult with this technique; nevertheless, careful handling of the periosteum ensures no inadvertent damage to other structures.

Step osteotomies are most frequently carried out in MCIII and MTIII. However, in selected cases, they can be performed in the proximal phalanx or the radius. The major advantages of a step ostectomy over a closing wedge ostectomy are maintenance of the bone length and the ability to create a lag effect across the vertical aspect of the saw cut and achieve good interfragmentary compression.[46] This cannot be accomplished in a closing wedge ostectomy. Also, the easy correction of rotational deformities is an advantage.

Step ostectomies are gaining in popularity, and a good prognosis can be given in many cases. The use of 5.5-mm bone screws is encouraged for these procedures.[45]

Prognosis

Several studies have reported the response to both nonsurgical and surgical treatment of foals with angular limb deformities. One study reported that in 81.5% of foals treated with hemi-circumferential periosteal transection and elevation (HCPTE) to correct angular deformities, total limb straightening was achieved and 60% of foals went on to be used at their intended performance level.[35,36] In a study that reported the results of transphyseal bridging, 80% of foals with carpal deformities and 27.3% of foals with metacarpo- or metatarsophalangeal deformities went on to a form of athletic use.[31] The poor results obtained in the foals treated for metacarpophalangeal or metatarsophalangeal deformities were attributed to the fact that several of these foals were operated on near or after the end of the rapid growth phase of the distal third metacarpal or metatarsal growth plate. Racing performance after HCPTE in Thoroughbreds has been reported; treated foals had fewer starts at 2 years of age and lower start percentile ranks.[32] However, it is difficult to rely heavily on these comparison numbers, because many foals that have undergone surgery for ALDs are not declared as such in yearling sales. A study reporting the results of treatment in foals with tarsal valgus demonstrated that only 52.4% met the expectations of their intended use, and these authors concluded that foals with tarsal valgus have a poorer prognosis for future athletic use than do foals with carpal deformities.[30] Another study showed that foals with incomplete ossification of the tarsal bones and greater than 30% collapse of the third and central tarsal bones had a poorer outcome than did similar foals with less than 30% collapse,[34] thereby stressing the importance of early recognition and treatment.

Conflicting results regarding the significance of the location of the pivot point and the presence of radiographic abnormalities in cases of carpal deformities have been published. According to one study, the more radiographic abnormalities that are seen distal to the distal radial physis and the more distal the location of the pivot point is, the poorer is the prognosis.[35] In another study, no such correlation could be made.[36] Also, it has been demonstrated that surgical manipulation of distal radial physeal growth can cause changes in the angles of all the carpal joints.[37] Thus surgical manipulation of physeal growth may be successful in correcting ALDs originating distal to the growth plate (e.g., epiphyseal deformities).

REFERENCES

1. Fackelman GE, Reid CF, Leitch MD, Cimprich R: Angular limb deformities in foals, Proc Am Assoc Equine Pract 1975;21:161.
2. Turner SA, Fretz PB: A comparison of surgical techniques and associated complications of transphyseal bridging in foals, Proc Am Assoc Equine Pract 1977;23:275.
3. Fretz PB, Donecker JM: Surgical correction of angular limb deformity in foals: A retrospective study, J Am Vet Med Assoc 1983;183:529.
4. McLaughlin BG, Doige CE, Fretz PB, Pharr JW: Carpal bone lesions associated with angular limb deformities in foals, J Am Vet Med Assoc 1981;178:224.
5. Auer JA, Martens RJ: Angular limb deformities in young foals, Proc Am Assoc Equine Pract 1980;26:81.
6. Auer JA, Martens RJ, Morris EL: Angular limb deformities in foals: Part 1. Perinatal factors, Comp Cont Educ Pract Vet 1982;4:330.
7. Auer JA, Martens RJ, Morris EL: Angular limb deformities in foals: Part 2. Developmental factors, Comp Cont Educ Pract Vet 1983;5:27.
8. Fackelman GE: Deformities of the appendicular skeleton. In Jennings BP, editor: The Practice of Large Animal Surgery, Philadelphia, 1984, WB Saunders.
9. Auer JA: Angular limb deformities. In Colahan PT, Mayhew IG, Merritt AM, Moore JN, editors: Equine Medicine and Surgery, ed 4, Santa Barbara, Calif, 1991, American Veterinary Publications.
10. Auer JA: Current treatment methods for angular limb deformity problems in foals, Proc Am Assoc Equine Pract 1988;34:263.
11. Auer JA: Zur intrauterinen Ossifikation der Karpal- und Tarsalknochen beim Fohlen und Behandlung von Ossifikationsstörungen, Pferdeheilkunde 1986;2:35.
12. Bramlage LR: Evaluation and management of foal limb deformities, Proc Am Assoc Equine Pract Resort Symp 2005:Jan.
13. Wolff J: The law of bone remodeling, New York, 1986, Springer Verlag.
14. Fretz PB: Angular limb deformities in foals, Vet Clin North Am Large Anim Pract 1980;21:125.
15. Auer JA, Smallwood JE, Morris EL, et al: The developing equine carpus from birth to six months of age, Equine Pract 1982;4:35.
16. Smallwood JE, Auer JA, Martens RJ, et al: The developing equine tarsus from birth to 6 months of age, Equine Pract 1984;6:7.
17. Vortkamp A, Lee K, Lanske B, et al: Regulation of rate of cartilage differentiation by Indian hedgehog and PTH-related protein, Science 1996;273:613.
18. Salter RB, Harris WR: Injuries involving the epiphyseal plate, J Bone Joint Surg 1963;45A:587.
19. Watkins JP, Auer JA: Physeal injuries, Comp Cont Educ Pract Vet 1984;6:226.
20. Shaver JR, Fretz PB, Doige CE, Williams DM: Skeletal manifestations of suspected hyperthyroidism in foals, Equine Vet Med 1979;3:269.
21. Knight DA, Gabel AA, Reed SM, et al: Correlation of dietary mineral to incidence and severity of metabolic bone disease in Ohio and Kentucky, Proc Am Assoc Equine Pract 1985;31:445.
22. Bridges CH, Womack JE, Harris ED, Scrutchfield WL: Consideration of copper metabolism in osteochondrosis of sucking foals, J Am Vet Med Assoc 1984;185:173.
23. Bridges CH, Harris ED: Experimentally induced cartilaginous fractures (osteochondritis dissecans) in foals fed low-copper diet, J Am Vet Med Assoc 1988;193:215.
24. Anderson TM, McIlwraith CW, Douay P: The role of conformation in musculoskeletal problems in the racing Thoroughbred, Equine Vet J 2004;36:571.
25. Anderson TM, McIlwraith CW: Longitudinal development of equine conformation from weanling to age 3 years in the Thoroughbred, Equine Vet J 2004;36:563.
26. Hintz HF, Schryver HF, Lowe JE: Delayed growth response and limb conformation in young horses, Proc Cornell Conference Feed Manufacturers 1976:94.
27. Jansson N, Ducharme NG: Angular limb deformities in foals: Treatment and prognosis, Comp Cont Educ Pract Vet, 2005;27:134.
28. Auer JA: Periosteal transection for correction of angular limb deformities, Proc Am Assoc Equine Pract 1982;28:223.
29. Mase CA: Observations on radial maturation in foals as they relate to skeletal pathology, Proc Am Assoc Equine Pract 1987;33:439.
30. Mase CA: The anatomy and response to surgical manipulation of the distal radial growth plate in foals, Master's thesis, University of Saskatchewan, 1986.
31. Fretz PB, Cyubaluk NF, Pharr JW: Quantitative analysis of longbone growth in the horse, Am J Vet Res 1984;45:1609.
32. Auer JA: Periosteal transection of the proximal phalanx in foals with angular limb deformities of the metacarpo/metatarsophalangeal area, J Am Vet Med Assoc 1985;187:496.
33. Auer JA: Beitrag zur Frühdiagnose und Behandlung einer speziellen Stellungsanomalie beim Pferd, Pferdeheilkunde 1989;5:201.
34. Honnas CM: Personal communication, 1987.
35. Bertone AL, Turner AS, Park RD: Periosteal transection and stripping for treatment of angular limb deformities in foals: Clinical observations, J Am Vet Med Assoc 1985;187:145.
36. Bertone AL, Park RD, Turner AS: Periosteal transection and stripping for treatment of angular limb deformities in foals: Radiographic observations, J Am Vet Med Assoc 1985;187:153.
37. Read EK, Read MR, Clark CW, et al: An evaluation of hemi-circumferential periosteal transection and evaluation in an angular limb deformity model, Proc Am Assoc Equine Pract 2001;47:478.
38. Wu Q, Zhang Y, Chen Q: Indian Hedgehog is an essential component of the mechanotransduction complex to stimulate chondrocyte proliferation, J Biol Chem 2001;276:35290.
39. von Rechenberg B: Personal communication, 2005.
40. Heinze CD: Epiphyseal stapling: A surgical technique for correction of angular limb deformities, Proc Am Assoc Equine Pract 1969;15:59.
41. Witte S, Thorpe PE, Hunt RJ, et al: Growth retardation at the distal tibial physis through single screw placement, Proc Am Assoc Equine Pract 2004;50:482.
42. Shao YY, Wang L, Ballock RT: The molecular basis of the Heuter-Volkman principle of physeal growth. In Proc Trans ORS, 51th annual meeting, poster 1054, 2005.
43. Shamis LD, Auer JA: Complete ulnas and fibulas in a pony foal, J Am Vet Med Assoc 1985;186:802.
44. Fretz PB, McIlwraith CW: Wedge osteotomy as a treatment for angular deformities of the fetlock in horses, J Am Vet Med Assoc 1983;182:245.
45. White KK: Diaphyseal angular limb deformities in three foals, J Am Vet Med Assoc 1983;182:272.
46. Auer JA: Corrective osteotomies. In Colahan PT, Mayhew IG, Merritt AM, Moore JN, editors: Equine Medicine and Surgery, ed 4, Santa Barbara, Calif, 1991, American Veterinary Publications.

CHAPTER 90

Flexural Limb Deformities

Jörg A. Auer

The complex problem of flexural limb deformities appears often in the equine veterinary literature,[1-5] and its treatment was documented as early as the 5th century AD in the *Mulomedicina* by Vegetius.[6] A flexural deformity represents a deviation of a limb in the sagittal plane and is expressed either as a persistent hyperflexion or hyperextension of a joint region. Persistent hyperflexion has been termed *contracted tendons,* even though in most cases the tendon units are not actually contracted, they are just functionally too short relative to the associated osseous structures.[7] By convention, the type of deformity is named according to the joint involved and not the tendon and is classified as a contractural deformity. Although hyperextension deformities are not part of the flexural deformity complex per se according to the definition for flexural deformities, these problems also are included and discussed in this chapter.

Flexural deformities are encountered in the distal interphalangeal joint, the metacarpophalangeal or metatarsophalangeal joint, the carpus, and, rarely, the tarsal region. Most often an animal suffers from one type of deformity only, but several areas can be affected in severe congenital contractural deformities. The forelimbs are more commonly affected, and the problem can be encountered in more than one limb at the same time. Flexural deformities present at birth are referred to as *congenital deformities. Acquired flexural deformities* develop during the remainder of the animal's life.

PATHOGENESIS

Congenital Deformities

Factors responsible for the development of congenital contractural deformities are shown in Figure 90-1. Some causes mentioned are speculative and lack scientific evidence of their existence. Work is needed to understand the intricate details that lead to the development of such deformities.

Intrauterine malpositioning is a commonly mentioned cause of the problem.[8-10] This could actually be the case in an abnormally large foal relative to the size of the mare, where intrauterine crowding leads to development of the problem. This, however, is the exception to the rule. More likely, congenital flexural deformities are multifactorial in their origin and hence are difficult to explain.

Diseases acquired by the mare during pregnancy can lead to the development of flexural deformities in the foal.[1] A multitude of agents and causes have been associated with the problem, including ingestion of locoweed[11] and hybrid Sudan grass[12] during pregnancy, a dominant gene mutation in a sire,[13] equine goiter,[14,15] an influenza outbreak,[1] neuromuscular disorders,[16] and defects in cross-linking of elastin and collagen caused by lathyrism.[17] The evidence in these cases may be only circumstantial, underscoring the need for further investigations into the development of congenital deformities.

An early report stated that 20% of 608 fetuses and newborn foals submitted for necropsy suffered from miscellaneous limb contractures,[18] which underscores the trend noted by clinicians that the incidence of flexural limb deformities is increasing.[19,20]

Acquired Deformities

There are several pathways for the development of acquired deformities (see Fig. 90-1). It has been suggested that acquired contractural deformities are part of the developmental orthopedic disease (DOD) complex, which also includes angular limb deformities, osteochondrosis, physitis, and cervical vertebral malarticulations or malformations.[20]

It has been postulated that in rapidly growing foals, the longitudinal growth of the bone is greater than the potential of the tendon unit to elongate passively at a corresponding rate.[4] Most acquired contractural deformities are encountered between 4 weeks and 4 months of age and again at the yearling age, an observation that supports the theory.[3-5,7] Rapid bone growth occurring between 4 weeks and 4 months can induce a contractural deformity in the distal interphalangeal joint. Passive elongation of the tendon might be limited because of the relatively unyielding accessory ligament of the deep digital flexor tendon, which originates at the proximal and palmar aspects of the third metacarpal bone (MCIII) and joins the tendon in the midmetacarpal region. Passive elongation proximal to that region, therefore, has little influence on prevention of the problem. Because of the functional shortening of the deep digital flexor tendon unit, excessive tension is exerted on the distal phalanx, which results in palmar rotation of the entire foot and the development of the typical club-footed stance.

The rate of bone growth is determined by genetics and nutrition. Foals can be overfed either by heavily lactating mares or by excessive supplementation with concentrates.[21] An abrupt change from inadequate—both in quality and quantity—nutrition to abundant nutrition also can induce the problem in yearlings.[22]

At 3 months of age, growth at the distal MCIII has ceased but continues to occur at the distal radius. The accessory ligament of the superficial digital flexor tendon originates just proximal to the distal radial growth plate from the caudal aspect of that bone. Rapid growth of the radius around 1 year of age can result in a functional shortening of the superficial flexor tendon unit and development of a contractural metacarpophalangeal deformity.[23] This theory was validated experimentally when foals previously kept on a poor ration were fed free-choice high-quality feed at the yearling age and subsequently developed flexural deformity.[24] However, the development of the problem might be more related to nutritional imbalances than excessive high-energy intake.[22,25]

Kidd and Barr have theorized that longitudinal bone growth is insufficient at any age to create a relative shortening of the flexor tendons.[26] They postulated that rapid

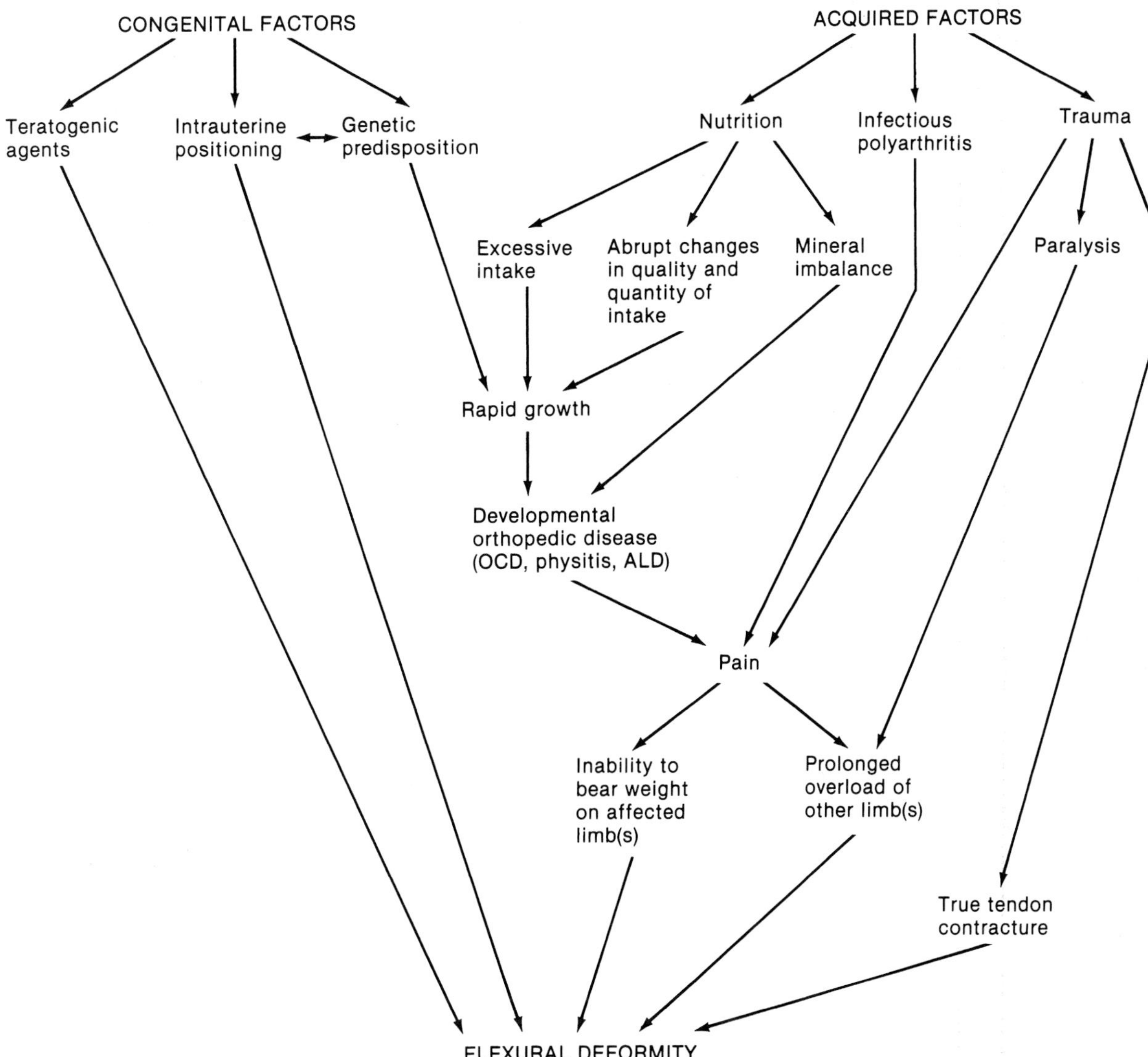
CONGENITAL FACTORS
ACQUIRED FACTORS
Teratogenic agents
Intrauterine positioning
Genetic predisposition
Nutrition
Infectious polyarthritis
Trauma
Excessive intake
Abrupt changes in quality and quantity of intake
Mineral imbalance
Paralysis
Rapid growth
Developmental orthopedic disease (OCD, physitis, ALD)
Pain
Inability to bear weight on affected limb(s)
Prolonged overload of other limb(s)
True tendon contracture
FLEXURAL DEFORMITY

Figure 90-1. Interrelationship between the various congenital and acquired factors and involvement in the development of flexural deformities. ALD, angular limb deformities; OCD, osteochondrosis.

growth increased tension within the flexor tendons and that this could induce pain, ultimately leading to the development of contractural deformities. Contractural deformities often have an acute onset of 24 to 48 hours, which also supports this theory. Whereas muscle contractions can develop in such a short period, bone lengthening would take longer.

A study of skeletally normal foals revealed that most of the cells in the deep digital flexor tendon and its accessory ligament are myofibroblasts.[27] These cells have contractile ability and therefore might play a role in the development of contractural deformities.

This leads to pain as the primary inciting factor associated with acquired contractural deformities.[9] Any painful condition could be responsible for the flexion withdrawal reflex and the resultant muscle contraction, leading to an altered stance. Osteochondrosis,[5,28] arthrosis,[28,29] infectious joint disease, acute severe trauma to osseous and soft-tissue structures, bruised feet as a result of prolonged exercise on hard ground,[30] and hoof problems[5] are just a few conditions associated with a non–weight-bearing lameness or continuous overload of limbs for prolonged periods. Such painful processes can induce muscle contractions, leading to the development of contractural deformities. Although pain can be the inciting factor in acute-onset contractural deformities, more permanent states of flexion of the musculotendinous unit can occur with contracture of the flexor aspect of the joint capsule and maintain the deformity, underscoring the need for early diagnosis and effective management.[28,29]

DIAGNOSIS

Congenital Deformities

A flexural limb deformity, whether a contractural or digital hyperextension deformity, is considered congenital when it is present at birth. The problem is easily recognized in most cases and should be evaluated by a veterinarian at that time.

Digital Hyperextension Deformities

Newborn foals might be presented with a mild degree of digital hyperextension (Fig. 90-2). Such foals might be unable to maintain their toes on the ground; while standing, their metacarpophalangeal or metatarsophalangeal joints are angled more acutely than normal, and the animals are reluctant to ambulate. The problem is caused by flaccidity of the flexor muscles[4] and usually corrects itself within a few weeks because of negative allometric growth of the tendons relative to the bones and increased muscle tone. In severe cases, the foals walk on the palmar or plantar aspect of the phalangeal region, where skin lesions rapidly develop as a result of abnormal loading. These severe hyperextension deformities have to be distinguished from the milder forms[4] and the skin must be protected accordingly.

A radiographic and ultrasonographic evaluation can be helpful in diagnosing the deformity; however, in most cases, no abnormal findings can be detected.

Contractural Deformities

The characteristic stance of foals with contractural deformities makes a diagnosis possible in most instances. The problem may be displayed in various degrees of severity and in several locations. Newborn foals with the deformity located in the distal interphalangeal joint walk on their toes (Fig. 90-3, *A*). The deformity can also be present in the metacarpophalangeal region. Newborn foals afflicted with this problem are not able to stand on their feet (see Fig. 90-3, *B*). The carpal region is another location where a deformity may be encountered. Some foals are able to stand but buckle forward in that region; others with severe deformities are not able to stand at all (see Fig. 90-3, *C*).

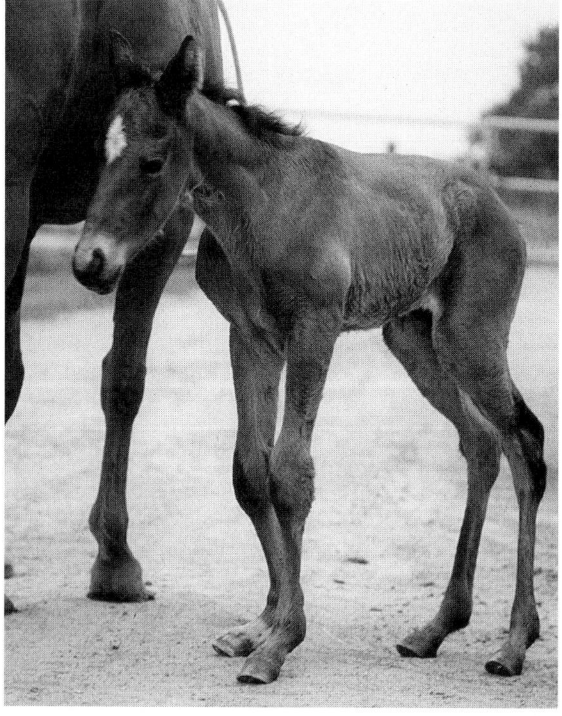

Figure 90-2. A newborn foal with digital hyperextension in all four feet. Additionally there is a mild flexural deformity present in both carpi.

The affected area should be palpated and manipulated with the animal in both weight-bearing and non–weight-bearing positions. In most cases the only abnormality noted is the lack of mobility in the affected joint or joint region. An attempt should be made to correct the deformity manually. The resistance toward such an effort is a good indicator of the prognosis and can help in deciding whether to treat a foal. Palpation of the flexor tendons during manipulation is helpful in determining which structures are involved. Both the deep and superficial digital flexor tendons and even the suspensory ligament are often involved.[31,32]

If manual correction is easily obtained, the animal should certainly be treated and has a good prognosis to respond positively to splint or cast management. In foals whose deformities are not manually correctable, the decision to treat depends on the severity of the deformity and prevailing economics. As examples, treatment should be initiated in a foal with a mild contractural deformity of the distal interphalangeal joint that is unresponsive to manual correction, whereas treatment might not be indicated in a foal with a severe deformity in the carpal region[33,34] (see Fig. 90-3, *C*).

Congenital contractural deformities of the proximal interphalangeal joint are rarely diagnosed and often involve osseous and soft tissue abnormalities.[34] Depending upon the severity of the problem, subluxations and ankyloses of this joint could be diagnosed.

A radiographic evaluation can be helpful in diagnosing congenital contractural deformities to determine whether bony abnormalities are associated (Fig. 90-4).

Ruptured Common Digital Extensor Tendon

This relatively common congenital disorder has some pathognomonic features that simplify the diagnosis.[4,5,35] Afflicted foals display a characteristic swelling in the tendon sheath at the dorsolateral aspect of the carpus (Fig. 90-5). The foal often has a slightly bowlegged and over-in-the-knees stance. This stance is caused by the lack of support at the dorsolateral aspect of the carpus, which is normally conferred by the intact common digital extensor tendon. Therefore, it is not truly a contractural deformity, but it clinically appears as one. The two ends of the partially or completely ruptured tendon can easily be palpated in the tendon sheath. With time, these ends proliferate, making their detection during palpation even easier.

During walking, afflicted animals throw their forelimbs forward, extend them completely, and retract them slightly before contacting the ground. A foal with a ruptured common digital extensor tendon often knuckles at the metacarpophalangeal joint during walking and might buckle in the carpal region while standing. In severe cases the foal may not be able to stand straight without knuckling forward (see Fig. 90-3, *B*).

Incomplete ossification of the cuboidal carpal and tarsal bones is usually diagnosed concomitantly in foals afflicted with ruptured common digital extensor tendons.

Acquired Deformities

Acquired contractural deformities are seen more often than acquired hyperextension deformities. Continuous overload

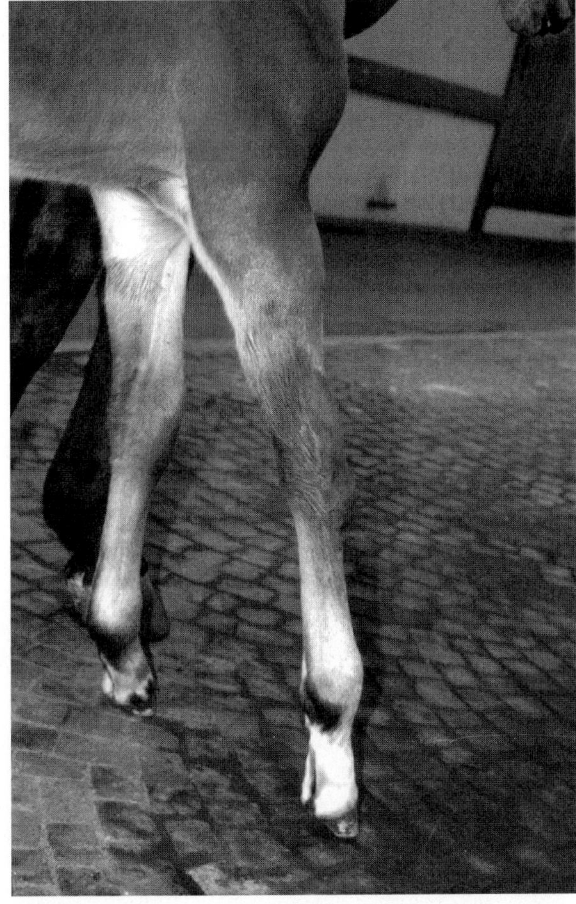

A

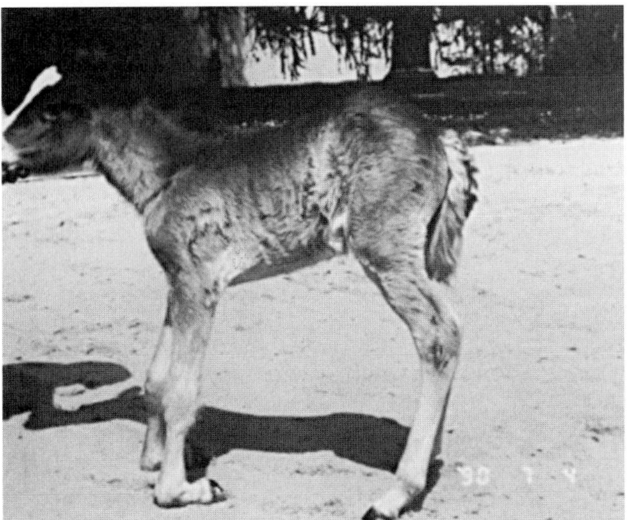

B

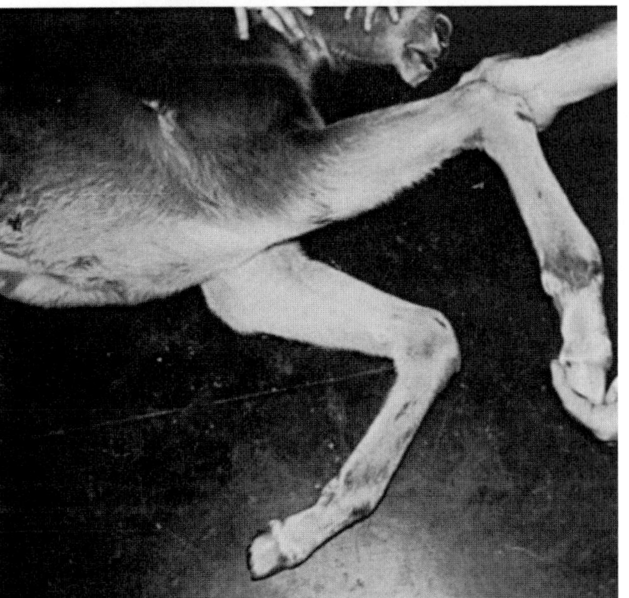

C

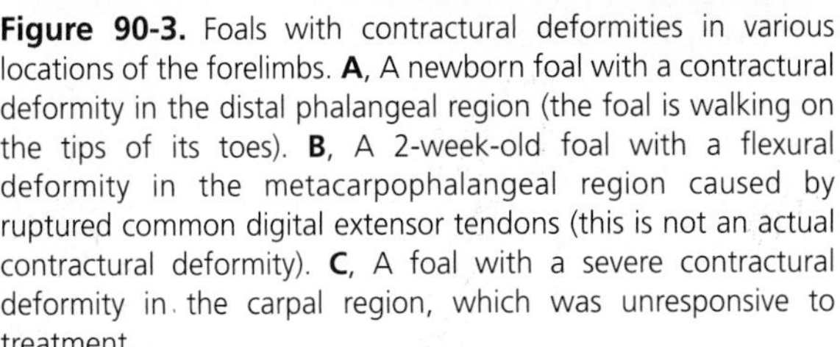

Figure 90-3. Foals with contractural deformities in various locations of the forelimbs. **A**, A newborn foal with a contractural deformity in the distal phalangeal region (the foal is walking on the tips of its toes). **B**, A 2-week-old foal with a flexural deformity in the metacarpophalangeal region caused by ruptured common digital extensor tendons (this is not an actual contractural deformity). **C**, A foal with a severe contractural deformity in the carpal region, which was unresponsive to treatment.

of certain limbs can, in selected cases, induce hyperextension deformities. Such problems can also be encountered after ruptures of flexor tendons (see Chapter 86). Flexural deformities develop over time, and careful examination of the animal can allow early diagnosis of the problem, when treatment is less complex.

Contractural Deformities

DISTAL INTERPHALANGEAL JOINT

Early signs of impending contractural deformity of the distal interphalangeal joint are a steeper dorsal hoof wall angle and a relatively short toe. With time, the typically boxy foot develops, in which the dorsal hoof wall and the heel are practically of the same length. As the heel grows, flexion of the distal interphalangeal joint and hyperextension of the metacarpophalangeal joint increase.

For diagnostic, therapeutic, and prognostic purposes, a classification of deformities has been proposed.[36] A stage I deformity is present when the angle described by the dorsal hoof wall and the sole is less than 90 degrees; in stage II contracture, the dorsal hoof axis passes beyond the vertical. The longer the condition is neglected, the worse the deformity becomes. Permanent changes of the associated soft-tissue structures occur, and the abnormally loaded bones remodel according to Wolff's law.[5]

METACARPOPHALANGEAL JOINT

Acquired contractural deformities of the metacarpophalangeal joint are initially characterized by a straight metacarpophalangeal angle. Palpation of the flexor tendons allows determination of which structure is tightest: the deep flexor tendon unit, the superficial flexor tendon unit, or the suspensory ligament. Application of pressure to the dorsal joint region in a palmar direction tenses the tendons. This diagnostic test is important to help select treatment. Palpation and passive manipulation of the involved region should be carried out with the limb in a non–weight-

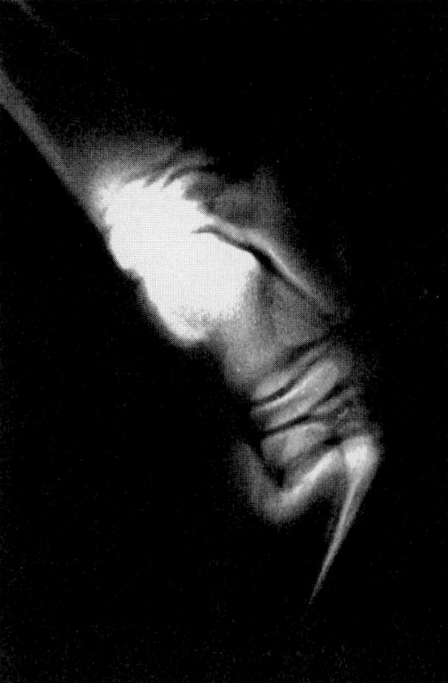

Figure 90-4. A lateromedial radiographic view of a newborn foal with an anomaly of the tarsometatarsal joint. The small tarsal bones have collapsed through the subchondral bone plate of the proximal third metatarsal bone. Surgical correction in such a case is not possible or at least not feasible.

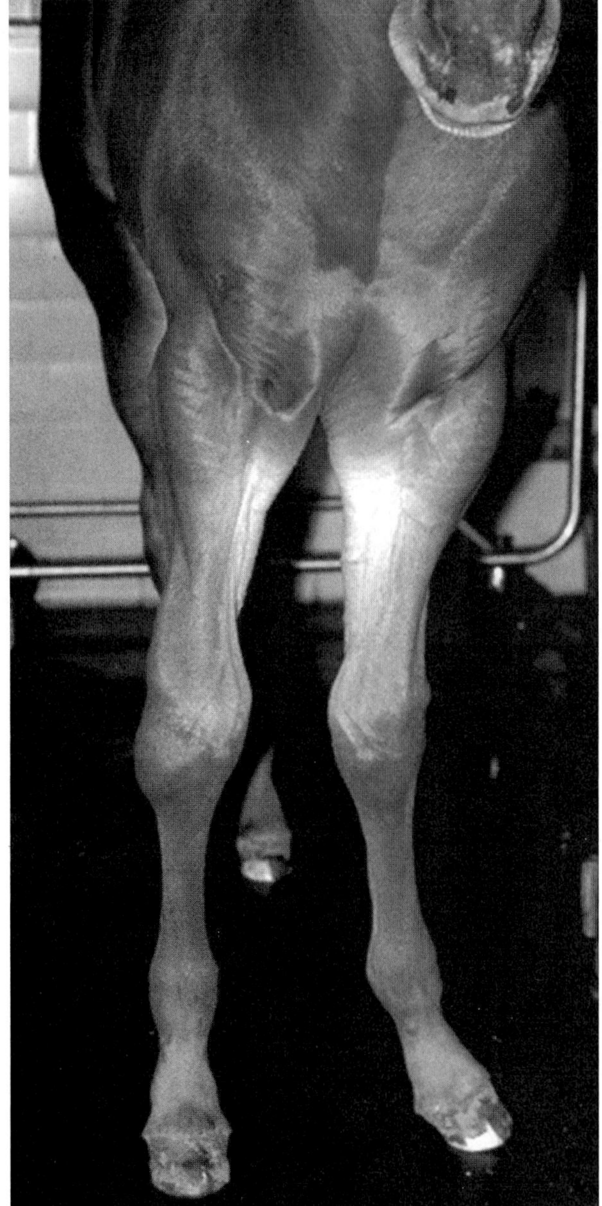

Figure 90-5. A 2-month-old foal with ruptured common digital extensor tendon in the right forelimb, a carpal varus deformity in the same limb, and a marked valgus deformity in the left forelimb. At the dorsolateral aspect of the right carpus a marked swelling is seen, which is caused by proliferation of the distal stump of the ruptured tendon within the tendon sheath.

bearing position to recognize potential adhesions between the tendinous structures.

Knuckling over in the metacarpophalangeal region is seen in more-severe cases in which treatment has been neglected for a long time. The speed at which such a deformity develops greatly depends on the degree of pain present, the pain threshold of the patient, the growth rate, the amount of exercise allowed, and possibly the foot-trimming techniques employed. It is important to diagnose a contractural deformity as early as possible, and promoting client awareness can be helpful in this regard.

Both front and back limbs can be affected, but acquired metatarsophalangeal joint contractural deformities are much less common than those affecting the metacarpophalangeal joint.[37] Acquired flexural deformities of the metacarpophalangeal joint have also been reported in mature horses secondary to desmitis of the accessory ligament of the deep digital flexor tendon.[38]

PROXIMAL INTERPHALANGEAL JOINT

Acquired contractural deformity of the proximal interphalangeal joint has been primarily diagnosed bilaterally in rapidly growing weanlings.[38] It occurs in foals with straight hindlimb conformation in the same time period as acquired contractural deformities of the metacarpophalangeal joint. The biomechanical basis of the condition has been postulated as shortening of the deep digital flexor musculotendinous unit and a concurrent laxity in the superficial digital flexor tendon, which inserts adjacent to the proximal interphalangeal joint.[39] Usually a dorsal subluxation is diagnosed and is accompanied by an audible click as the foal walks. Radiographs might show osteoarthritis in chronic cases.

Contractural deformities also develop after prolonged periods of not bearing weight, such as that occasioned by radial paralysis or often by conservative fracture treatment (Fig. 90-6). Depending on their management, deformities can become permanent and debilitating despite healing of the original ailment. The joint region involved with the contractural deformity can be fixed by the contracture, without osseous ankylosis present (fibrodesis).

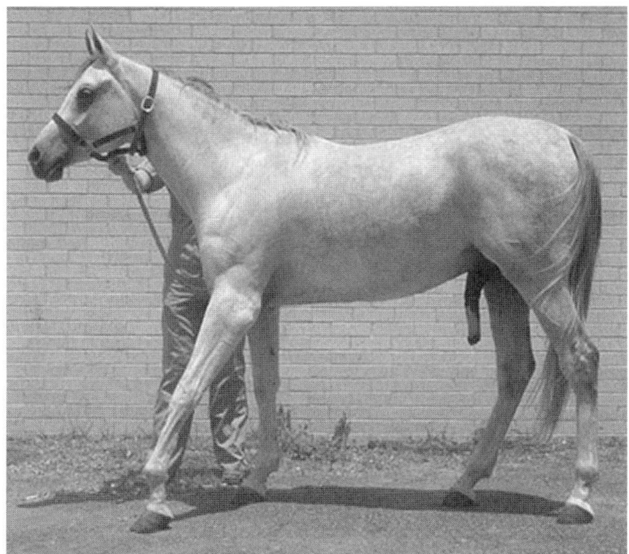

Figure 90-6. A three-year-old Arabian gelding showing a flexural deformity of the metacarpophalangeal region. The animal suffered an olecranon fracture, which was treated conservatively. Now the fracture has healed but the horse can't be ridden because of the flexural deformity.

TREATMENT

Congenital Deformities

Digital Hyperextension Deformities

Most foals with mild digital hyperextension do not need treatment other than minimal attention and trimming of the feet.[40] The animals should be carefully observed, and if the problem worsens, treatment should be promptly initiated. Moderate exercise is indicated; therefore, access to pasture is allowed. Excessive exercise is contraindicated because fatigue often aggravates the problem.

SWIMMING

Swimming has been advocated as excellent controlled physiotherapy.[4] The animal is supported in a swimming pool or pond by one or two helpers or a rescue net (Fig. 90-7). The paddling action of the foal in the water is carried out against the resistance of the water and without placing weight on the limbs. The resultant increase in muscle tone brings about rapid amelioration of symptoms.

Severe digital hyperextension problems must be treated immediately, because neglect soon leads to necrosis and traumatization of the skin in the palmar or plantar phalangeal region and jeopardizes treatment.

SHOEING

Application of glue-on shoes or similar devices with palmar or plantar extensions helps maintain the hoof sole on the ground[41] (Fig. 90-8). These devices constrict the foot and can cause problems if left in place too long. Application of a splint in combination with extension of the heel can help in treatment. However, care has to be taken not to overprotect the flexor tendons and their associated muscles.

BANDAGING

Light bandaging of the phalangeal region is indicated to minimize skin trauma. Splint bandages and casts incorporating the foot are contraindicated because they totally support the distal limb, leading to a further loss of tone of the already hypotonic flexor tendon units. Additionally, development of pressure sores on the delicate skin is a common untoward sequela.

Application of some padding between the elongated braces attached to the foot and the palmar or plantar aspect of the phalangeal region can supply support and decrease the excessive hyperextension angle. Daily swimming and carefully dosed anti-inflammatory drugs are indicated and should always be part of therapy.

SURGICAL MANAGEMENT

Tenoplasty has been described as a possible surgical management technique for severe digital hyperextension problems in small or miniature foal patients, but it is currently not recommended.[42]

Contractural Deformities

NONSURGICAL MANAGEMENT

Analgesics

Animals suffering from a contractural deformity, which is a painful condition, benefit from the administration of nonsteroidal anti-inflammatory drugs (NSAIDs). However, these drugs should be given judiciously because of the potentially detrimental side effects, including gastric ulcers and nephrotoxicity. Administration of phenylbutazone at 1.1 mg/kg body weight IV once a day and concurrent treatment with ranitidine (6.6 mg/kg orally three times a day, or 1.5 mg/kg IV three times a day) as a gastric protectant has been proposed.[26] Phenylbutazone plus cimetidine is another potentially useful combination of drugs to reduce pain in the treatment period.

Intravenous oxytetracycline

Administration of oxytetracycline has recently become popular as an initial treatment for congenital contractural deformities.[43] A single dose of 3 g oxytetracycline in 250 to 500 mL of physiologic saline is administered slowly by the intravenous route. An in vitro study showed that oxytetracycline induced a dose-dependent inhibition of collagen gel contraction by equine myofibroblasts. Oxytetracycline also induced a dose-dependent decrease in matrix metalloproteinase 1 (MMP-1) mRNA expression by equine myofibroblasts.[44] Results of this study indicate that oxytetracycline inhibits tractional structuring of collagen fibrils by equine myofibroblasts through an MMP-1–mediated mechanism.[44]

In young foals, oxytetracycline administration can make the developing ligaments and tendons more susceptible to elongation during normal weightbearing, resulting in correction of the deformity within 24 to 48 hours. The treatment may be repeated once or twice within the first weeks of life if necessary. No side effects have been mentioned, other than vital staining of the active osteons in the bone.

Mild cases of contractural deformities respond to this treatment with complete correction. In more severe cases or, more likely, those with a different cause, the response is

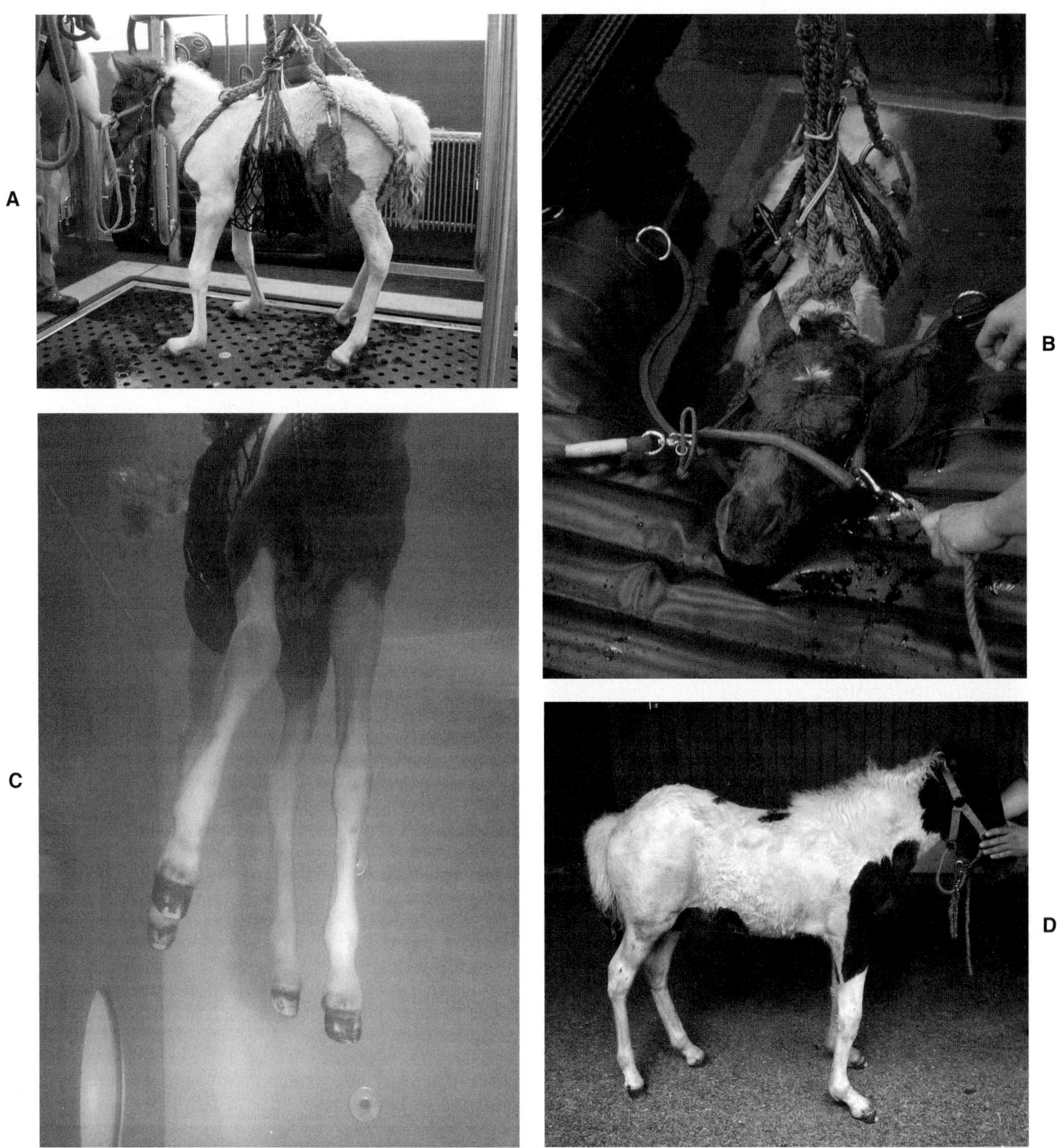

Figure 90-7. **A**, A 2-week-old Islandic pony is shown with marked digital hyperextension in both forelimbs. The foal wears a rescue net and stands on a scissor table. **B**, The table was lowered into warm water so that the foal was immmersed in it, protected by the rescue net, which was attached to a hoist. **C**, The foal is shown swimming and in doing so, effectively exercises its weak limb muscles. **D**, The same foal 4 weeks later. There is some improvement, but the fetlock angle is still hyperextended.

minimal and care must be taken to ensure that the foals are kept in a well-padded area with soft ground to prevent excessive wearing of hoof horn at the tip of the foot. If that is not possible, protection of the toes may be indicated. Addition of a splint bandage (see later) can support correction.

In a comparative study, a single dose of 44 mg/kg oxytetracycline was administered intravenously to normal newborn foals and newborn foals suffering from flexural deformities.[45] This treatment resulted in a significant decrease of the metacarpophalangeal joint angle in both groups. Within 4 days after the injection the foals regained

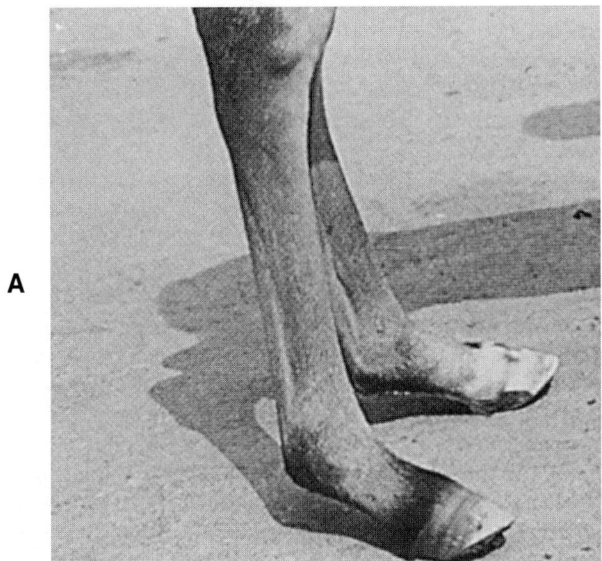

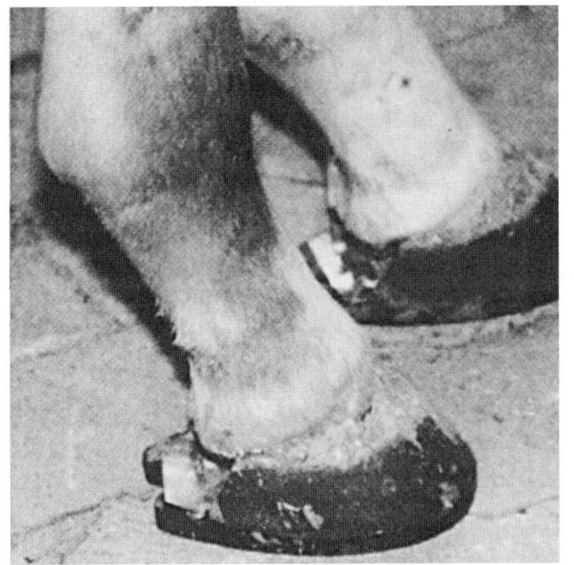

Figure 90-8. A, A newborn foal with marked digital hyperextension in the rear limbs. **B**, The same foal after application of a pair of Dalric glue-on shoes. Note the ability of the foal to bear weight on the soles after shoe application. (Photos courtesy H. Dallmer, Salzhausen-Putensen, Germany.)

their pretreatment angle. Based on this observation, one report accorded no clinical value to the oxytetracycline treatment of flexural deformities.[26]

Toe extensions

Application of a dorsal hoof extension using acrylic alone or in combination with a lightweight foot plate protects the toe from excessive wear and increases the tensile forces in the deep digital flexor tendons during ambulation. This probably helps in correcting the problem.

To maintain these devices on the feet, numerous holes of approximately 2 mm in diameter and depth are drilled into the dorsal hoof wall. The hoof acrylic used to achieve the dorsal extension is spread over the dorsal hoof wall and worked into the holes to add stability to the device. The acrylic, interdigitating with the dorsal hoof wall, serves as an anchoring device and prolongs the life of the extensions. Filling in the space between the extension and the dorsal hoof wall decreases the risk of the foal's stepping on the extensions or stumbling over them.

These devices may be successfully applied in newborn foals with mild contractural deformities of the metacarpophalangeal joints, when the foal cannot bear weight without knuckling over. Extending the dorsal hoof wall adds the necessary elongation to compensate for the lack of extension in the phalangeal region and allows the foal to stand without knuckling. Once the foal is able to ambulate, correction of the deformity is usually achieved within 2 weeks, at which time the extensions typically become detached.

The toes must be protected from excessive wear as foals are allowed free exercise. A special half-round glue-on shoe has been developed for this purpose, with a toe extension built into its design[46] (Fig. 90-9).

Splints and casts

Splints and casts are effective for treating contractural deformities. Foals suffering from contractural deformities of the distal interphalangeal joint that are unresponsive to hoof extensions can be treated with half-limb casts, incorporating the feet. This treatment causes relaxation of the muscle–tendon units within a few (10 to 14) days, correcting the problem.[3,4,47]

Some authors prefer splints applied over casts because they can be worn for several hours followed by a period without splints.[26] When the tone has returned into the muscle–tendon units, the animal may exercise, possibly with some concomitant anti-inflammatory drug therapy, and maintain the correction. Casts have to be changed at least every 2 weeks to keep pace with the growth of the foal.

Splints are more difficult to apply in the distal phalangeal region and are not as effective as casts; however, there are fewer complications associated with these devices. Splints are preferably used in contractural deformities of the metacarpophalangeal and carpal region, especially in mild carpal contractural deformities. In these cases care is taken to avoid incorporation of the phalangeal region into the splint.[47] Splints have to be well padded and changed every 3 to 5 days. It is important to use new, dry padding at each bandage change to minimize development of pressure sores (Fig. 90-10; see Fig. 90-3, C).

Splints may be used in combination with intravenous oxytetracycline, especially in treatment of severe carpal contractural deformities. These foals are unable to rise and nurse and have to be assisted many times daily.

Stretching of tendons and associated contracted soft-tissue structures (e.g., joint capsules) is painful; therefore, administration of low doses of anti-inflammatory drugs might be necessary. It is advisable to prolong the application intervals to prevent overdosing the patient. The doses should be reduced from the calculated dose per kilogram body weight regimen.

SURGICAL MANAGEMENT

Surgical intervention is seldom necessary with congenital contractural deformities. Surgical transection of the flexor carpi ulnaris and the ulnaris lateralis tendons resulted in the

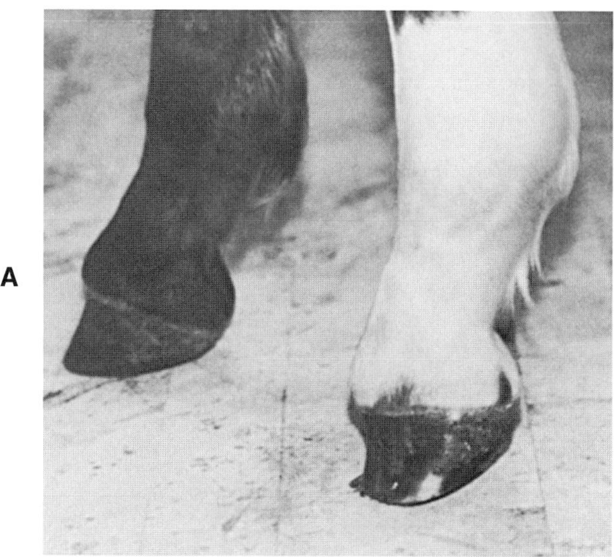

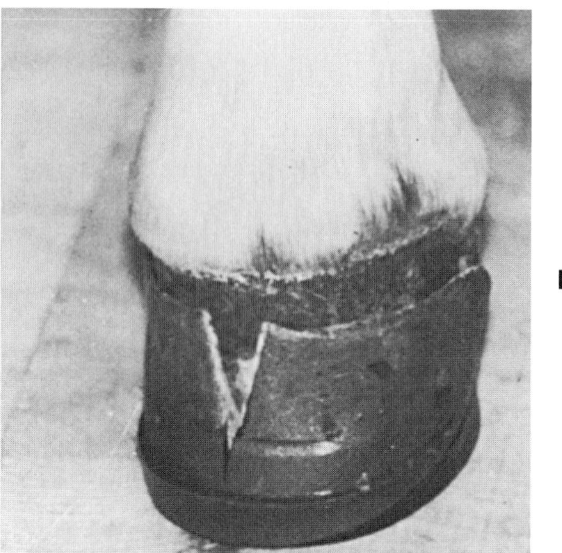

Figure 90-9. **A**, A 4-month-old foal with a stage I contractural deformity in the distal interphalangeal joint of the left forelimb. Note the dished appearance of the dorsal hoof wall. Allowing the foal to walk around like this would result in excessive wear at the toe and possible development of a painful condition or infection. **B**, A Dalric glue-on shoe was applied to protect the toe and to extend the footing surface dorsally, facilitating delayed breakover during walking. Note the spread cut in the region of the dorsal hoof wall. This allows better fit of the shoe to the foot because of the limited sizes available. (Photos courtesy H. Dallmer, Salzhausen-Putensen, Germany.)

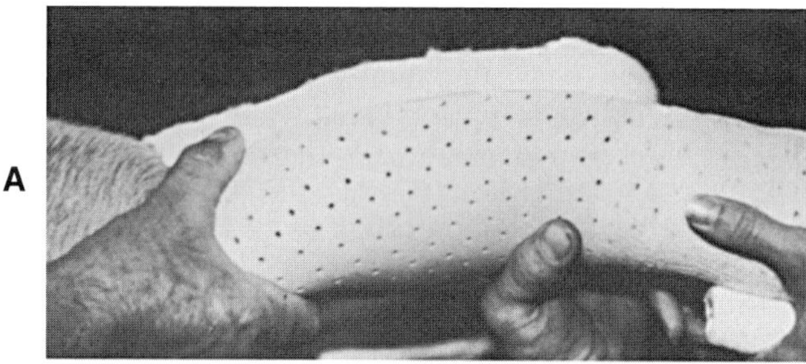

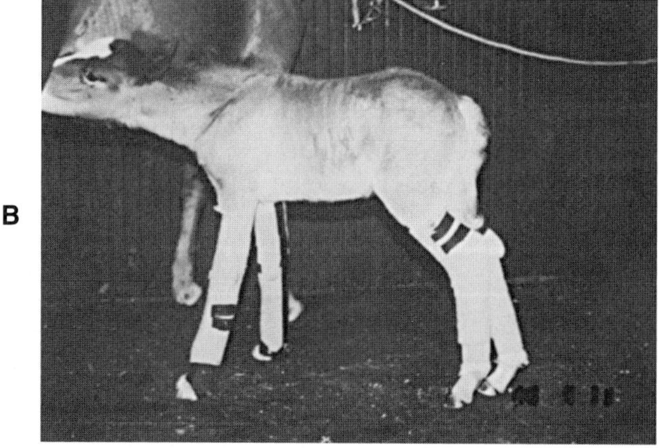

Figure 90-10. Splint application to the foal in Figure 90-3, *B*. **A**, A piece of Plastazote is applied to the dorsal and cranial aspect of MTIII and distal tibia, respectively, to manage incomplete ossification. This padding material is suited to application to the tarsal region. **B**, The foal with all four splints applied. Note that the splints were applied without incorporating the feet. In the forelimbs the splints are located palmarly and caudally, and in the hindlimbs they are located dorsally and cranially.

correction of mild carpal deformities.[48,49] The surgery is performed under general anesthesia with the foal in lateral recumbency. It is advisable to manipulate the limb immediately prior to surgery, while the foal is under anesthesia, to see if these tendons tighten when forceful carpal extension is applied. The tendons are easily identified and can be transected, if transection is deemed useful, through a small incision between the tendons. Routine aftercare is given to these patients.

Some success has been reported with surgical transection of the palmar ligament and capsule of the middle carpal and antebrachiocarpal joint[50] (see Fig. 90-3, *C*). The carpal canal is opened through a medial approach; the joints are identified and subsequently opened through a horizontal incision. This author has had little success with this technique on two foals with severe carpal contractural deformity. Release following transection was not adequate.

Ruptured Common Digital Extensor Tendon

NONSURGICAL MANAGEMENT

Foals with ruptured common digital extensor tendons are best confined to a box stall, because they tend to stumble frequently. Within a few weeks, locomotion normalizes and more exercise can be allowed.

Application of a well-padded splint bandage is the treatment of choice[35] (see Figs. 90-3, *B*, and 90-10). The use of a thermoplastic splinting material (Plastazote, Smith & Nephew, Hull, England) in combination with a polyvinylchloride pipe splint has had excellent results. These devices maintain a normal limb axis, which allows ossification of the often dysmature carpal bones to proceed under orthogonal loading conditions (see Chapter 89). Additionally, pressure exerted over the distended tendon sheath of the common digital extensor tendon in the carpal region decreases swelling.

The splint bandage is changed every 3 to 5 days over a period of 2 to 4 weeks. During this time, stall rest is indicated. Once the splint is removed, the bandage is maintained for an additional 3 to 4 weeks. Subsequently, the bandage is removed for a day. Should the swelling return, the bandage is reapplied immediately. Should the swelling not return, the bandage is left off another day, and so on, until the limb can be left unbandaged. Treatment is adapted to the response of the patient. In some cases, shorter intervals are successful.

In selected cases, full limb or tube casts are applied; however, the advantages of the polyvinylchloride splints are such that cast application for this purpose has decreased in popularity.

Aspiration of the synovial fluid from the tendon sheath is discouraged because of the risk of infection. Continuous external pressure quickly induces absorption of the excess fluid.

SURGICAL MANAGEMENT

It is generally accepted that ruptured common digital extensor tendons should not be treated surgically because of the good prognosis and success of splint application.[35] The risk of complications secondary to surgery outweighs any improvement of the prognosis. However, thorough removal of all fibrin clots from the tendon sheath through a surgical incision, followed by installation of a suction drain and cast immobilization, has resulted in excellent cosmetic appearance of the limbs.[48]

Acquired Contractural Deformities

Distal Interphalangeal (Coronopedal) Joint

NONSURGICAL MANAGEMENT

Nonsurgical management includes proper nutrition, physiotherapy, analgesics, application of a toe extension, and application of a cast.

Nutrition

Determination of the nutritional intake, especially the calcium-to-phosphorus ratio, is important because an aberrant ratio has been incriminated in the development of contractural deformities.[19] Balanced nutrition is important for normal development of the skeleton and enchondral ossification. Additionally, it is advisable to evaluate soil and drinking water samples for their mineral and trace mineral composition; adjustments should be implemented immediately after identifying inadequate levels. Foals still suckling should be weaned early, especially if they develop an angular limb deformity.[26]

Physiotherapy

It is important that afflicted foals exercise frequently. Extensive exercise can stretch the tendons and correct the problem; however, it is important that the toe region is protected to prevent excessive wear and possible development of a septic process.

Analgesics

Passive stretching of shortened or relatively shortened tendons is a painful process. To aid the foal in standing and moving around, nonsteroidal anti-inflammatory drugs are given at low doses. Foals with painful limbs tend to lie down a lot, which can aggravate the contractural problem.

Toe extensions

Application of a toe extension or a glue-on rubber shoe is effective for flexural deformities of the distal interphalangeal joint.[46] The purpose of this treatment is protection of the toe and prevention of excessive wear in that region. Additionally, the toe extension moves the weight-bearing surface of the foot farther forward, allowing a later breakover and greater tensile stress on the palmar soft-tissue structures of the phalangeal region.

Simple application of a shoe with a toe extension, without filling or bracing the extension against the dorsal hoof wall with hoof acrylic, can cause frequent stumbling and abnormal flaring of the dorsal hoof wall. Simple trimming of the excess heel of a club-footed foal is contraindicated as the only treatment, because it reduces the weight-bearing surface area and causes more rapid wearing of the tip of the toe. In most cases, a club foot develops initially because of the greater wear at the toe and lack of wear at the heel, not more rapid growth of the heel. Trimming of the heel combined with application of a toe extension and protection, however, can be an effective treatment (see Fig. 90-9).

Cast application

Cast application in foals causes temporary weakening of the tendons. The distal limbs of afflicted foals may be covered with a fiberglass cast that incorporates the feet for 10 days to a maximum of 14 days. After cast removal, the weakened tendons allow correction of the problem. Despite the fact that the weakening persists for only a few days, the author has achieved permanent correction of the problem with this technique. However, because of the potential complications associated with this type of treatment, cast application is rarely used.

SURGICAL MANAGEMENT

Surgical intervention is indicated in foals unresponsive to conservative treatment and in severely affected foals.

Desmotomy of the accessory (check) ligament of the deep digital flexor tendon

The treatment of choice for stage I contractural deformities is desmotomy of the accessory ligament of the deep digital flexor tendon (inferior or subcarpal check ligament)[4,5,36,51-53] (Fig. 90-11). The ligament may be approached from the lateral or medial aspect of the limb; with bilateral contractural deformity, this allows both surgical procedures to be performed without turning the foal on the table. However, because soft tissue proliferation is often encountered postoperatively, it is generally preferred to perform the procedure from the lateral side. A medial soft-tissue proliferation can be mistaken for a proliferation of the medial vestigial metacarpal bone and considered a blemish. Additionally, the check ligament is more easily identified from the lateral approach.

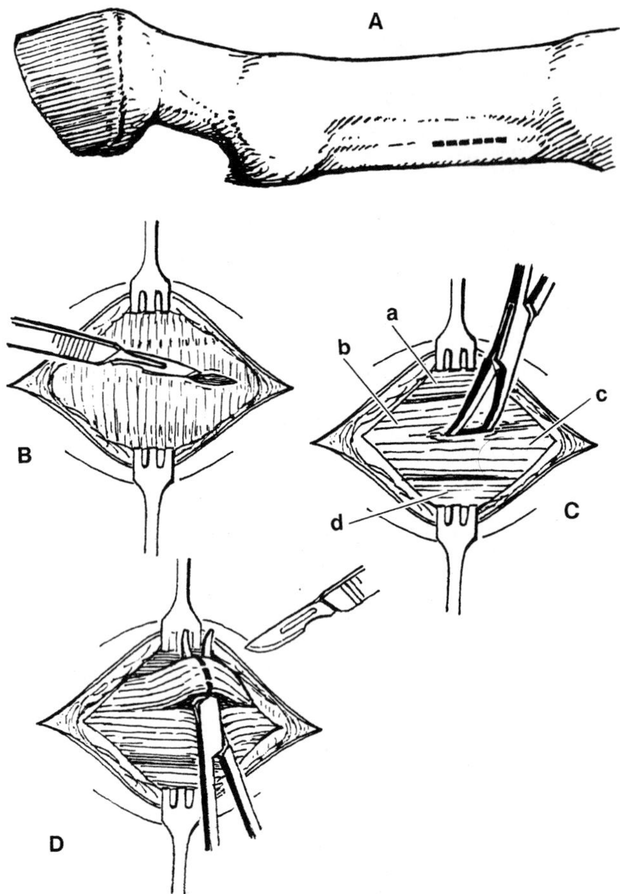

Figure 90-11. Surgical technique of desmotomy of the accessory ligament of the deep digital flexor tendon (inferior check ligament desmotomy). **A**, Location of the surgical site on the medial, or in most cases the lateral, side of the limb. **B**, The paratenon enclosing the deep flexor tendon and the accessory ligament is incised. **C**, The accessory ligament is isolated along its division plane with the deep digital flexor tendon. (*a*, Superficial digital flexor tendon; *b*, Deep digital flexor tendon; *c*, Accessory ligament of the deep digital flexor tendon; *d*, Suspensory ligament). **D**, The isolated and elevated accessory ligament is transected along the *dotted line*. (From Turner AS, McIlwraith CW: Techniques in Large Animal Surgery, ed 2, Oxford, 1989, Blackwell.)

A 5-cm skin incision, centered at the junction between the proximal and middle third of the MCIII, is made over the deep digital flexor tendon. The subcutaneous tissues are bluntly separated and the tendinous structures identified. With the medial approach, the neurovascular bundle overlying the deep digital flexor tendon and its accessory ligament are identified and reflected away from deeper structures. Palpation of the paratenon surrounding the deep digital flexor tendon and its accessory ligament allows separation between the two structures.

A curved hemostatic forceps is introduced and advanced following the slightly curved surface of the tendon to the opposite side, where the forceps is spread and turned. The accessory ligament of the deep digital flexor tendon lying palmar to the tendon is elevated to the level of the skin incision. Manipulation of the foot in a dorsal direction tightens the ligament and ensures the isolation of the correct structure. Once the ligament is positively identified, it is sharply transected with a scalpel blade. Dorsal rotation of the distal interphalangeal joint produces a 1-cm gap between the transected ends of the ligament. The gap is inspected and palpated, and any remaining fiber strands of the accessory ligament are transected.

The paratenon, subcutaneous tissues, and skin are closed using 2-0 or 3-0 absorbable suture materials in a continuous pattern. Intradermal placement of the skin suture is advised for a better cosmetic result. Postoperatively, a pressure bandage is applied and maintained for 2 to 3 weeks and changed at 3- to 4-day intervals.

Correction of the deformity is usually observed immediately. In some cases, however, it takes a few days until correction is complete. Occasionally, application of a toe protection or extension is needed. Young foals and those without long-standing contracture are allowed controlled exercise within 3 to 6 days after the surgery. Free pasture exercise is encouraged after 2 weeks. In older foals and those with chronic or severe contracture, limiting exercise for a period of months might prevent excessive fibroplasia at the surgery site. To relieve potential pain, nonsteroidal anti-inflammatory agents may be administered at low doses.

A minimally invasive ultrasonographically guided technique was developed some time ago. This technique can be performed in standing horses.[54]

Postoperative fibroplasia occurring at the surgery site reunites the transected ends of the ligament with time. In selected cases, fibroplasia in that region is excessive and results in a cosmetically undesirable appearance. Cosmetically unacceptable results can occur from tendinitis that can be induced from exercise when the tendon has been protected by the contracted accessory ligament for a long time. Tendinitis can be avoided with longer periods of controlled exercise. Daily massage of the swelling can reduce the size.

Long-term follow-up of Standardbred foals treated with a desmotomy of the accessory ligament of the deep digital flexor tendon revealed that young foals (younger than 8 months at the time of surgery) could reach their athletic potential.[55] No foals treated after 8 months of age had a favorable outcome.

Tenotomy of the deep digital flexor tendon

Stage II contractural deformities might not correct after desmotomy of the accessory ligament of the deep digital flexor tendon. Tenotomy of the deep digital flexor tendon can be used successfully for correction[56,57] (Fig. 90-12). Initially, such a tenotomy had been looked at as a salvage procedure; however, several animals have developed into sound riding horses.

Two main sites for the surgical procedure have been proposed. The distal approach centers at the palmar and median aspect of the pastern joint region and enters through the tendon sheath just distal to the bifurcation of the superficial digital flexor tendon.[57] The deep digital flexor tendon is identified, exteriorized, and transected with a scalpel blade. Immediate retraction of the proximal stump into the tendon sheath is noted. The tendon sheath may[53] or may not[57] be sutured using routine technique in addition to the subcutaneous tissue and the skin.

While the animal is under anesthesia, the feet are trimmed to a shape as normal as possible. Postoperative correction is often immediate and can be associated with substantial pain. Administration of nonsteroidal anti-inflammatory agents is therefore routine.

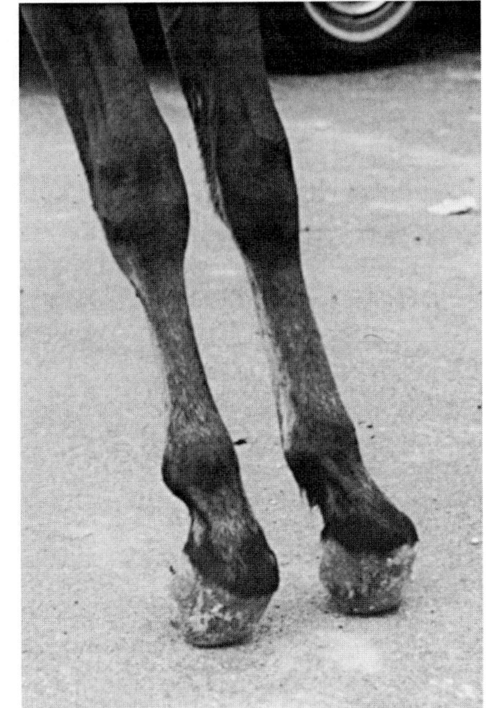

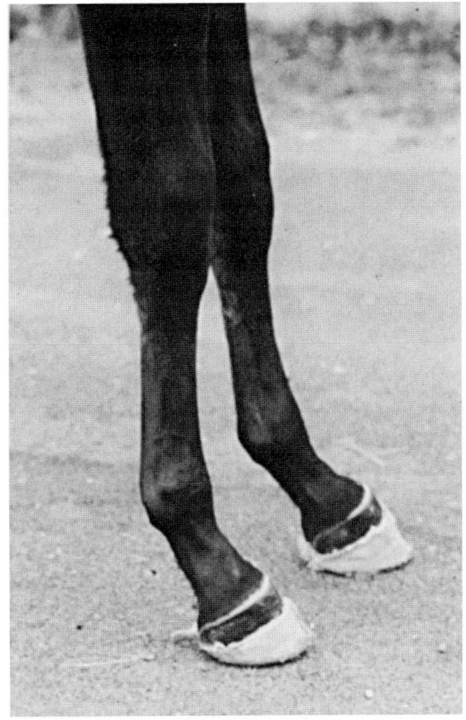

Figure 90-12. **A**, The forefeet of a 7-month-old foal with stage II contractural deformity of the coronopedal joint. Note the abnormal configuration and wear at the feet. **B**, The same foal 1 day after surgery. The deep digital flexor tendon was transected at the pastern level in both feet. Hoof acrylic was applied to the feet for protection. The animal has an almost normal stance.

Because of the long time it takes for a stage II contractural deformity to develop, the soft-tissue structures, such as joint capsule, ligaments, and periarticular tissues at the palmar aspect of the phalanges, are significantly contracted. Transection of the deep digital flexor tendon at the level of the proximal interphalangeal joint does not result in a marked elevation of the toe during weightbearing, as it does after rupture of this tendon in the region of the navicular bone. Nevertheless, in selected cases, application of a shoe with a heel extension is necessary.

Transection of the deep digital flexor tendon at the midmetacarpal level is advocated.[58] The procedure is carried out through a medial or lateral approach. The advantage of this approach is the greater distance from the feet and the fact that a tendon sheath is not invaded. Additionally, the procedure is easier to perform at the midmetacarpal level. However, scarring associated with marked disfigurement of the tenotomy site can be an undesirable sequela. Postoperative management is identical to that used with the other technique.

Metacarpophalangeal Joint

NONSURGICAL MANAGEMENT

Nonsurgical management includes proper nutrition, physiotherapy, analgesics, corrective shoeing, application of a vertical bar shoe, and application of splints.

Nutrition

The nutrition intake of the patient should be corrected first (see earlier discussion). Foals being conditioned for yearling sales should be checked carefully for early signs of contractural deformities of the metacarpophalangeal joint.

Physiotherapy

Hopping an animal is a further attempt to bring about correction of the deformity without surgery.[4] One limb of a foal is elevated and held in that position while a helper leads the animal at a walk. During the support phase of the elevated limb, most of the weight is transmitted to the person holding the limb. The opposite limb is quickly advanced and all the weight brought to bear on it. By repeating this type of physiotherapy several times daily, a potential stretching of the tendons can be achieved. Exercise is an important type of therapy, but it should be carried out in a controlled manner.[59] Excessive exercise leads to fatigue, which should be avoided.

Analgesics

Passive stretching of shortened or relatively shortened tendons as well as the physiotherapy manipulations are painful processes. Nonsteroidal anti-inflammatory agents are applied frequently to manage the pain involved in trying to stretch the tendons and their associated accessory ligaments. As mentioned earlier, foals with painful limbs tend to lie down a lot, which can aggravate the contractural problem.

Corrective shoeing

Corrective shoeing can eliminate contractural deformities of the metacarpophalangeal joint. Raising the heel with wedge pads results in a more acute angle of the metacarpophalangeal joint as a result of partial relaxation of the deep digital flexor tendon.[4,23,58] Some authors have questioned the effectiveness of such treatment, but clinically, an improvement is possible.[5] Toe extensions have been advocated and have proved very effective, especially when the problem was diagnosed early.[3-5,59] As the animal walks, breakover occurs later, and through this, greater tensile stress is exerted on the flexor tendons.

Vertical bar shoe

Application of a vertical bar shoe[4] in conjunction with the use of a piece of auto tire inner tube just proximal to the metacarpophalangeal joint can be an effective treatment (Fig. 90-13). The soft, stretchable inner tube prevents development of skin sores. Care must be taken to prevent the animal from interfering with the inner bars while moving about if the devices were applied to both forefeet.

Splints

Splint application can bring about some correction, especially in early-recognized cases. Care must be taken to prevent development of pressure sores.

SURGICAL MANAGEMENT

Horses that are unresponsive to conservative management are candidates for surgical correction. Depending on the result of palpation of the flexor tendons during the diagnostic work-up, the accessory ligament of either the deep or the superficial flexor tendon is transected.

Desmotomy of the accessory (check) ligament of the deep digital flexor tendon

If the deep digital flexor tendon was tighter during palpation and manipulation, its accessory ligament should be transected using the technique described earlier[60] (see Fig. 90-11). Application of a preshaped polyvinylchloride half-pipe splint is necessary for 2 to 3 weeks to maintain the metacarpophalangeal angle in the normal range.

Desmotomy of the accessory (check) ligament of the superficial digital flexor tendon

Transection of the accessory ligament of the superficial digital flexor tendon should be performed when this tendon was tighter during manipulation.[4,61] Two surgical approaches have been developed. The surgical landmarks for both approaches are the same and consist of the medial distal physis of the radius, the chestnut, and the cephalic vein. An approximately 10-cm skin incision is centered along the chestnut and made craniad to the cephalic vein. The subcutaneous tissue is bluntly separated, and communicating branches to the cephalic vein are isolated, double ligated, and transected between ligatures.

One surgical technique approaches the accessory ligament craniad to the flexor carpi radialis muscle.[4,23,62,63] The oval foramen in the carpal fascia can serve as the distal border of the desmotomy incision.[51] The carpal fascia is transected carefully, and the ensheathed flexor carpi radialis muscle is identified. Both the cephalic vein and the flexor carpi radialis muscle are displaced using a self-retaining

A

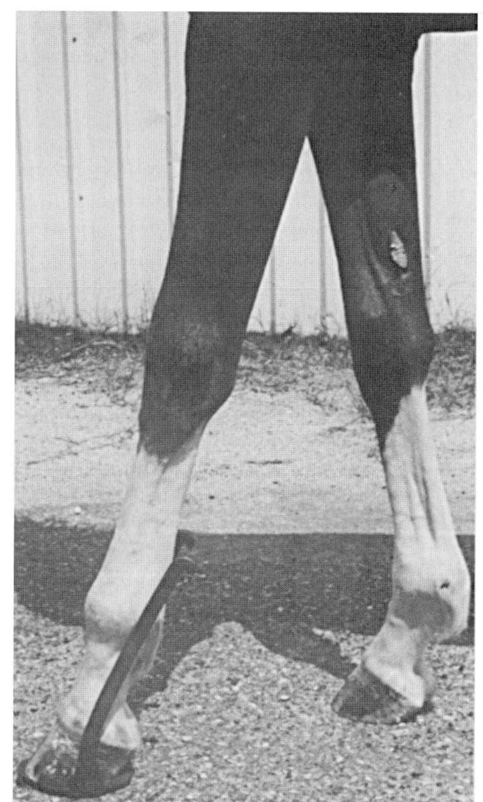

B

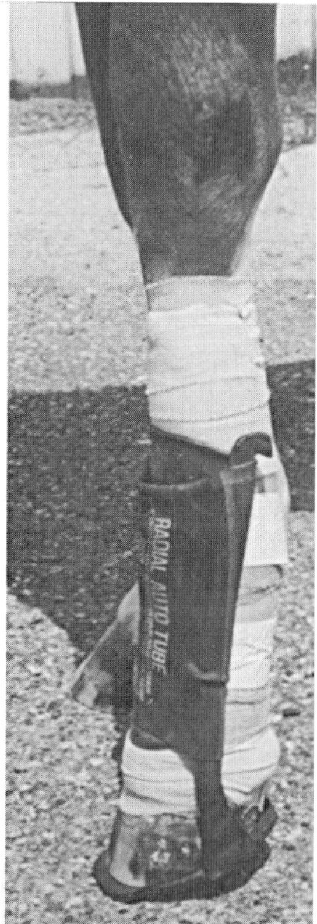

Figure 90-13. A, A yearling filly with a contractural deformity of the metacarpophalangeal joint. **B**, This animal was treated with a vertical bar shoe with a toe extension. A piece of tube from a radial auto tire was placed over the two bars to maintain the metacarpophalangeal region in a normal position.

retractor. The desmotomy of the fan-shaped accessory ligament is performed, and care is taken to avoid inadvertent injury to the palmar carpal rete. After transection of the ligament, the radial head of the deep digital flexor muscle appears and the carpal sheath becomes visible. Hemostasis is established, and routine closure of the carpal fascia, subcutaneous tissues, and skin is carried out.

An alternative approach is through the sheath of the flexor carpi radialis tendon[64,65] (Fig. 90-14). After reflecting the flexor carpi radialis tendon in the sheath with a self-retaining retractor, the craniolateral wall and accessory ligament are identified. A curved Kelly forceps is placed under the distal border and spread. Transection of the ligament is then performed in a proximal direction. Care is taken to avoid injury to the nutrient artery of the superficial flexor tendon, which enters along the proximal border of the accessory ligament. After transection, the same anatomic structures are visible as mentioned with the first technique. Inadvertent incision of the carpal sheath is of no consequence. Closure of the tendon sheath is carried out using

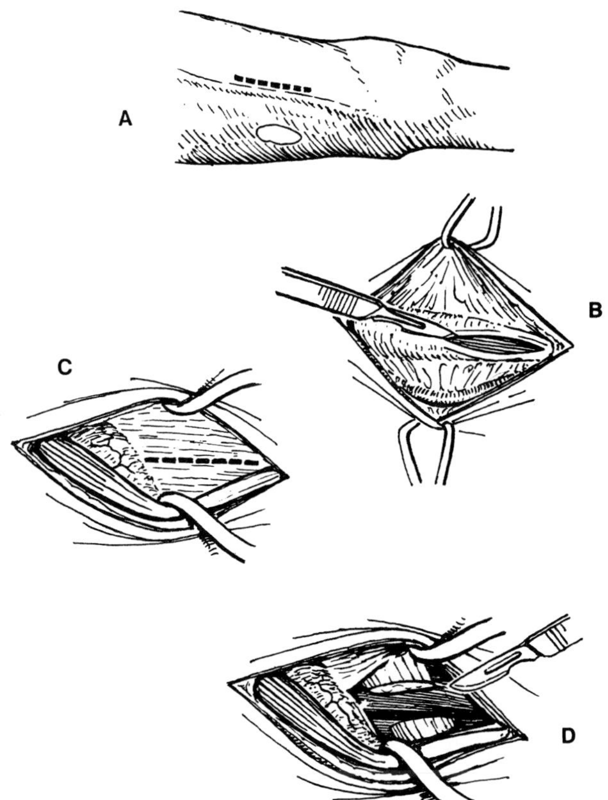

Figure 90-14. Surgical technique of accessory ligament desmotomy of the superficial digital flexor tendon (superior check ligament desmotomy). **A**, Location of the surgical site relative to the anatomic landmarks: cephalic vein, distal radial physis, and chestnut. **B**, The tendon sheath of the flexor carpi radialis muscle is incised. **C**, The flexor carpi radialis tendon is retracted, allowing visualization of the craniolateral tendon sheath wall. The site of the desmotomy incision is marked with a *dotted line* over the accessory ligament, which is at that location part of the craniolateral tendon sheath wall. **D**, The accessory ligament desmotomy is completed, allowing digital access to the radial head of the deep digital flexor muscle. **E**, The surgical incision is closed using routine technique. (From Turner AS, McIlwraith CW: Techniques in Large Animal Surgery, ed 2, Oxford, 1989, Blackwell.)

a continuous suture pattern with 2-0 or 3-0 synthetic absorbable material. The rest of the closure is routine.

A recent in vitro study revealed that desmotomy of the accessory ligament of the superficial digital flexor tendon was associated with significantly increased strains on the superficial digital flexor tendon and the suspensory ligament and significant alterations in the angles of the metacarpophalangeal and carpal joints.[65] Lengthening of the superficial digital flexor musculotendinous unit after desmotomy of the accessory ligament of the superficial digital flexor tendon can be associated with increased strain on the suspensory ligament.[65]

Postoperatively, a sterile pressure bandage is applied and maintained for 2 to 3 weeks. The bandage is changed at 3- to 4-day intervals.

In severe cases, the accessory ligaments of both the deep and the superficial digital flexor tendons are transected.[52] As an additional alternative procedure, desmotomy of the medial and lateral branch of the suspensory ligament may be performed for salvage purposes in persistent cases.[23] However, subluxation of the proximal interphalangeal joint is to be expected. A stab incision is performed directly over the suspensory branch, the subcutaneous tissues are separated with a Kelly forceps, and a curved tenotome is introduced. By applying pressure with a sawing motion, the previously undermined suspensory branch is transected. Care should be taken to avoid inadvertent injury to the palmar artery and vein and the metacarpophalangeal joint capsule. The skin is closed using a few simple interrupted sutures. The same procedure is performed on the other side of the limb.

Severe contractural deformities following prolonged non–weight-bearing lameness do not respond to desmotomy of either of the two accessory ligaments. Such cases should be treated either with a tenoplasty as the lengthening procedure in both flexor tendons, followed by long-term cast application, or with an osteotomy in conjunction with a fetlock arthrodesis (see Chapter 85).

Carpal Region

NONSURGICAL MANAGEMENT

Foals with long-term debilitating injuries that prevent weightbearing on the limb should be treated with splints early in the convalescent period to prevent development of a contractural deformity. Passive stretching exercises are indicated. These two therapies are combined with controlled exercise if the original injury allows it. A contracture typically occurs suddenly over a few days, after several weeks of not weightbearing on the limb. Therefore, physiotherapy should not be delayed. Care should be taken to prevent development of pressure sores under the splint.

SURGICAL MANAGEMENT

In cases resistant to conservative treatment, tenotomy of the ulnaris lateralis and flexor carpi ulnaris tendons can be performed with good results.[39] The same surgical procedure is performed as described earlier. Passive manipulation of the carpal region at that time demonstrates the greater mobility gained through this procedure.

Postoperatively, a well-padded pressure bandage is applied and a splint centered over the carpal region is incorporated. While the horse is under anesthesia, the limb is forced into a straight position. The splint bandage is changed at 4-day intervals and maintained for about 2 weeks. Hand-walking exercises are important for the first 3 to 4 weeks. As soon as the animal places good weight on the limb, the splint is removed.

Proximal Interphalangeal Joint

NONSURGICAL MANAGEMENT

Rest is not an effective management tool in these cases. The periarticular tissues may fibrose in, and eventually the clicking noise is not heard anymore. However, a marked bend at the joint level will be visible. Osteoarthritis could develop, necessitating a pastern arthrodesis to render the animal pain free again.

The clicking sound associated with dorsal snapping of the proximal interphalangeal and metacarpophalangeal area could also be observed in foals with persistent foal hoof at the tip of the hooves, resulting in an elongated hoof configuration. Trimming of the hoof was successful in eliminating the clicking sound and the snapping of the proximal interphalangeal and metacarpophalangeal area. This approach should be tried before a surgical intervention is performed.

SURGICAL MANAGEMENT

Surgical transection of the accessory ligament of the deep digital flexor tendon or transection of the tendon of the medial head of the deep digital flexor muscle at the level of the chestnut, or both, resulted in correction of the problem in three horses.[39]

COMPLICATIONS

Nonsurgical Management

Splint-associated pressure sores are the most often encountered complication. To avoid such complications, padding is placed around sites of predilection. Once necrosis is present, the local pressure has to be released in that area. Application of a donut-shaped pad around the periphery of the lesion can assist in that effort. Alternate application or temporary removal of the splint may be attempted. Daily topical wound care is necessary, especially in the initial period.

Surgical Management

Persistent hematoma formation, especially at the site of transection of the accessory ligament of the superficial flexor tendon, wound dehiscence, and infections are the most common complications encountered after surgical treatment. Whenever fever, leukocytosis, warmth at the surgery site, or increased pain are noted, an evaluation of the incision should be made and the necessary steps taken immediately. For additional information on wound dehiscence, please review Chapter 26.

REFERENCES

1. Fessler JF: Tendon disorders of the young horse, Arch ACVS 1977;6:19.
2. Rooney JR: Forelimb contracture in the young horse, J Equine Med Surg 1977;1:350.
3. Wagner PC, Reed SM, Hergeberg GA: Contracted tendons (flexural deformities) in the young horse, Comp Cont Educ Pract Vet 1982;4:S101.
4. Fackelman GE: Deformities of the appendicular skeleton. In Jennings PB, editor: The Practice of Large Animal Surgery, Philadelphia, 1984, WB Saunders.
5. McIlwraith CW: Diseases and problems of tendons, ligaments and tendon sheaths. In Stashak TS, editor: Adams' Lameness in Horses, 4th ed, Philadelphia, 1987, Lea & Febiger.
6. Von den Driesch A: Geschichte der Tiermedizin, Munich, 1989, Callwey Verlag.
7. Schneider RK: Contracted tendons: Pathophysiology, Proc Surg Forum ACVS 1989;17:310.
8. Badame EF: A corrective appliance for contracted tendons in foals, Proc Am Assoc Equine Pract 1963;9:91.
9. Rooney JR: Contracted foals, Cornell Vet 1966;56:173.
10. Johnson JH: Contracted tendons, Mod Vet Pract 1973;54:67.
11. McIlwraith CW, James LF: Limb deformities in foals associated with ingestion of locoweed by mares, J Am Vet Med Assoc 1982;181:255.
12. Prichard JT, Voss JL: Fetal ankylosis in horses associated with hybrid Sudan grass pasture, J Am Vet Med Assoc 1967;150:871.
13. Hutt FB: Genetic defects of bones and joints in domestic animals, Cornell Vet (Suppl) 1968;58:104.
14. Keeler RF, James LT: Failure of dietary supplementation to prevent abortions and congenital malformation of lathyrism and locoism in sheep, Can J Comp Med 1971;35:342.
15. McLaughlin BG, Doige CE: Congenital musculoskeletal lesions in hyperplastic goiter in foals, Can Vet J 1981;22:130.
16. Mayhew IG: Neuromuscular arthrogryposis multiplex congenita in a Thoroughbred foal, Vet Pathol 1984;2:187.
17. Baker JR, Lindsay JR: Equine goiter due to excess iodine, J Am Vet Med Assoc 1968;153:1618.
18. Crowe MW, Swerczek TW: Equine congenital defects, Am J Vet Res 1985;46:353.
19. Knight DA, Gabel AA, Reed SM, et al: Correlation of dietary mineral to incidence of metabolic bone disease in Ohio and Kentucky, Proc Am Assoc Equine Pract 1985;31:445.
20. Bramlage LR: Clinical manifestations of disturbed bone formation, Proc Am Assoc Equine Pract 1987;33:155.
21. Owen JM: Abnormal flexion of the coronopedal joint or "contracted tendons" in unweaned foals, Equine Vet J 1975;7:40.
22. Lewis LD: The role of nutrition in musculoskeletal development and disease. In Stashak TS, editor: Adams' Lameness in Horses, 4th ed, Philadelphia, 1987, Lea & Febiger.
23. Fackelman GE: Flexure deformity of the metacarpophalangeal joints in growing foals, Comp Cont Educ Pract Vet 1971;1:S1.
24. Hintz HF, Schryver HF, Lowe JE: Delayed growth responses and limb conformation in young horses, Proc Cornell Conference, 1976, p 94.
25. Potter G: Feeding young horses for sound development. In Pope SL, editor: Stud Manager's Handbook, vol 20, Sacramento, Calif, 1987, Spillmann Press.
26. Kidd JA, Barr ARS: Flexural deformities in foals, Equine Vet Educ 2002;14:311-321.
27. Hartzel DK, Arnoczky SP, Kilfoyle SJ, et al: Myofibroblasts in the accessory ligament (distal check ligament) and the deep digital flexor tendon of foals, Am J Vet Res 2001;62:823.
28. Shamis LD, Auer JA: Complete ulnas and fibulas in a pony foal, J Am Vet Med Assoc 1985;186:802.
29. Bridges CH, Harris ED: Experimentally induced cartilaginous fractures (osteochondritis dissecans) in foals fed low-copper diet, J Am Vet Med Assoc 1988;193:215.
30. McGladdery AJ: Three cases of acquired flexural deformity of the distal interphalangeal joint in growing foals on a stud farm, Equine Vet Educ 1992;4:173.

31. Cosgrove JSM: The veterinary surgeon and the newborn foal, Vet Rec 1955;67:961.
32. Collins SM: Discussion of Dr. Cosgrove's paper, Vet Rec 1955;67:961.
33. Wagner PC, Reed SM, Hegreburg GA: Contracted tendons (flexural deformities) in the young horse, Comp Cont Educ Pract Vet 1982;4:101.
34. Wagner von Matthiessen PC,: Case selection and management of flexural deformities in horses: Congenital flexural limb deformities, Part 2, Equine Pract 1994;16:7.
35. Yovich JV, Stashak TS, McIlwraith CW: Rupture of the common digital extensor tendon in foals, Comp Cont Educ Pract Vet 1984;6:S373.
36. McIlwraith CW, Fessler JF: Evaluation of inferior check ligament desmotomy for treatment of acquired flexor tendon contracture in the horse, J Am Vet Med Assoc 1978;172:293.
37. Wagner von Matthiessen PC: Case selection and management of flexural deformities in horses: Acquired flexural limb deformities, Part 1, Equine Pract 1993;15:51.
38. McDiarmid A: Acquired flexural deformities of the metacarpophalangeal joint in five horses associated with tendonous damage in the palmar metacarpus, Vet Rec 1999;144:475.
39. Shiorma JT, Engel HN, Wagner PC, et al: Dorsal subluxation of the proximal interphalangeal joint in the pelvic limb of three horses, J Am Vet Med Assoc 1989;195:777.
40. Myers VS, Lundvall RL: Corrective trimming for weak flexor tendons in a colt, J Am Vet Med Assoc 1966;148:1523.
41. Hertsch B: Durchtrittigkeit. In Dallmer H, editor: Müssen es immer Nägel sein? Arnsberg, Germany, 1986, Neheimer Druckerei.
42. Fackelman GE, Clodius L: Surgical correction of the digital hyperextension deformity in foals, Vet Med Small Anim Clin 1972;67:1116.
43. Lokai MD, Meyer RJ: Preliminary observation on oxytetracycline treatment of congenital flexural deformities in foals, Mod Vet Pract 1985;66:237.
44. Arnoczky SP, Lavagnino M, Gardner KL, et al: In vitro effects of oxytetracycline on matrix metalloproteinase-1 mRNA expression and on collagen gel contraction by cultured myofibroblasts obtained from the accessory ligament of foals, Am J Vet Res 2004;65:491.
45. Madison JB, Garber JL, Rice B, et al: Oxytetracycline decreases fetlock joint angle in new born foals, Proc Am Assoc Equine Pract 1992;38:745.
46. Hertsch B: Bockhuf. In Dallmer H, editor: Müssen es immer Nägel sein? Arnsberg, Germany, 1986, Neheimer Druckerei.
47. Kelly NJ, Watrous BJ, Wagner PC: Comparison of splinting and casting on the degree of laxity induced in thoracic limbs in young horses, Equine Pract 1987;9:10.
48. Wagner PC: Flexural deformity of the carpus. In White NA II, Moore JN, editors: Current Practice of Equine Surgery, Philadelphia, 1990, JB Lippincott.
49. Gerring EL: Flexural deformities of the limb in foals, Equine Vet Educ 1989;1:39.
50. Fackelman GE: Personal communication, 1990.
51. Soennichsen HV, Christiansen FR: Desmotomia capitis tendinei, Proc Eur Soc Vet Surg, 1975, p 1.
52. Wagner PC, Grant BD, Kaneps AJ, et al: Longterm results of desmotomy of the accessory ligament of the deep digital flexor tendon (distal check ligament) in horses, J Am Vet Med Assoc 1985;187:1351.
53. Nixon AJ: Deep digital flexor contracture deformity, Proc Surg Forum ACVS 1989;17:313.
54. White NA III: Ultrasound-guided transection of the accessory ligament of the deep digital flexor muscle (distal check ligament desmotomy) in horses, Vet Surg 1995;24:373.
55. Stick JA, Nickels FA, Williams MA: Long-term effects of desmotomy of the accessory ligament of the deep digital flexor muscle in Standardbreds: 23 cases (1979-1989), J Am Vet Med Assoc 1992;200:1131.
56. McGeady PA: General discussion following Dr. Cosgrove's paper, Vet Rec 1955;67:967.
57. Fackelman GE, Auer JA, Orsini J, von Salis B: Surgical treatment of severe flexural deformities of the distal interphalangeal joint in young horses, J Am Vet Med Assoc 1983;182:949.
58. Turner AS, McIlwraith CW: Techniques in Large Animal Surgery, 2nd ed, Philadelphia, 1989, Lea & Febiger.
59. Schneider RK: Treatment of horses with contraction of the superficial digital flexor tendon, Proc Surg Forum ACVS 1989;17:316.
60. Blackwell RB: Response of acquired flexural deformity of the metacarpophalangeal joint to desmotomy of the inferior check ligament, Proc Am Assoc Equine Pract 1982;28:107.
61. Soennichsen HV: Subcarpal check ligament desmotomy for the treatment of contracted deep flexor tendon in foals, Equine Vet J 1982;14:256.
62. Wagner PC, Shires MH, Watrous BJ, et al: Management of acquired flexural deformity of the metacarpophalangeal joint in *Equidae*, J Am Vet Med Assoc 1985;187:915.
63. Jann HW, Beroza GA, Fackelmann GE: Surgical anatomy for desmotomy of the accessory ligament of the superficial digital flexor tendon (proximal check ligament) in horses, Vet Surg 1986;15:378.
64. Bramlage LR: Superior check ligament desmotomy as a treatment for superficial digital flexor tendonitis: Initial report, Proc Am Assoc Equine Pract 1987;32:365.
65. Alexander GR, Gibson KT, Day RE, et al: Effects of superior check desmotomy on flexor tendon and suspensory ligament strain in equine cadaver limbs, Vet Surg 2001;30:522.

CHAPTER 91

Osteochondrosis

P. René van Weeren

The term *osteochondritis dissecans* was coined by König in 1887 and used to describe loose or semiloose bodies in joints of young persons that could have three causes: very severe trauma, lesser trauma and necrosis, or minimal trauma inducing an underlying lesion.[1] Although the name and concept have led to substantial confusion from the outset, this categorization is still valid today.[2]

It is the last, and most difficult to understand, of König's categories that is termed osteochondrosis (OC) in the equine veterinary literature. Osteochondrosis represents a disturbance of the process of endochondral ossification without a clearly understood etiology. This disturbance can eventually lead to the formation of semiloose or even completely loose fragments within a joint.

THE PROCESS OF ENDOCHONDRAL OSSIFICATION

In all mammals, the primordial skeleton is laid down first as a cartilaginous structure that, during the entire period of early development of the animal, is coupled in a process of simultaneous growth and transformation into bone. It is important to note that unlike mature articular cartilage, these fetal cartilaginous structures are well vascularized by vessels running through cartilage canals. Ossification of the primary centers of ossification in the diaphyses of the long bones starts early in fetal life, and at the time of birth, all the diaphyses are bony structures. This does not occur in many secondary centers of ossification located in the epiphyses of the long bones and in other sites such as apophyses and cuboidal bones in complex joints, which remain partly cartilaginous at the time of birth.

After birth, *longitudinal* growth of long bones results from the growth plates or physes where, from a germinal layer of cells (resting cells), chondrocytes proliferate and lay down a scaffold of extracellular matrix. These cells initially hypertrophy and later undergo apoptosis. The scaffold is used for the apposition of primary bone by osteoblasts originating from the metaphysis (Fig. 91-1). This primary spongiosa then undergoes continuous remodeling under the influence of biomechanical loading according to Wolff's law during the entire growth period of the foal. This remodeling con-

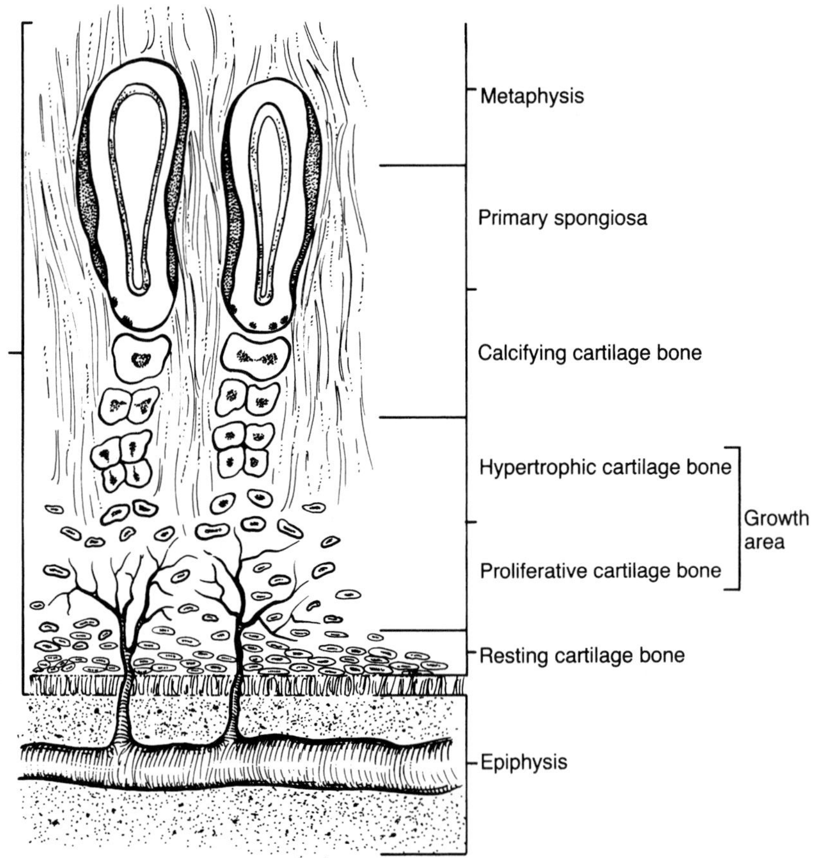

Figure 91-1. The relationship of the cartilage zones of the growth cartilage of a physis. (Redrawn from Watkins JW, Auer JA: Learning Systems 1984;6:S227.)

tinues in the adult with biomechanical loading changes; for instance, when the skeleton is exposed to athletic challenges.[3] The entire process of cartilage remodeling, followed by calcification of cartilage, deposition of primary bone, and successive remodeling into bony trabeculae, is known as endochondral ossification.[4]

The increase in *diameter* of the long bone during growth is the product of a different, but simultaneous and co-coordinated process, which is by appositional growth from the periosteum. This process results in the formation of compact cortical bone, characterized by the Haversian canals.

In the epiphyses of the long bones a growth process similar to that of the physis takes place, but it is not as completely developed as in the diaphyses at birth. This leads to large differences between joints in the times when ossification occurs. In some joints at birth, there is a complete ring of cartilage around the ossification center, connecting articular cartilage with the growth plate. Ossification of this cartilage ring takes place first at the border of the physis and at the perimeter of the epiphysis. The thick cartilage mass at the articular side of the epiphysis functions as a type of growth plate where the simultaneous processes of growth, remodeling, and ossification take place that finally result in a considerably thinner layer of articular cartilage in the mature animal. It is at this level that the characteristic lesions of equine osteochondrosis develop.

PATHOPHYSIOLOGY

There is little controversy about the gross pathogenetic mechanism of OC. Disturbances of the process of endochondral ossification result in irregularities in thickness of the epiphyseal cartilage. These create areas of focal weakness, which are exacerbated because the cartilage canals regress with increasing age and have disappeared in the horse by the age of 7 months.[5] This affects the nutrition of the deeper layers of the retained cartilage plugs, which cannot be sufficiently nourished by diffusion from the articular surface and can lead to necrosis. Biomechanical influences, mainly shearing forces, then lead to the formation of fissures and produce cartilage flaps, or detachment of cartilage or fragments of cartilage and subchondral bone. In some locations where biomechanical forces are mainly compressive, infolding of cartilage in these weakened areas can lead to the formation of subchondral bone cysts as another manifestation of OC.[6]

Many caveats concerning this seemingly straightforward mechanism have been made. In an extensive review of pathogenesis and possible etiologic factors of OC, some authors strongly question the view that defective ossification lies at the base of all lesions commonly qualified as osteochondrosis in the horse, based on clinical and pathologic observations.[4] One of their major arguments is the observation that after injury, bone and cartilage can manifest only a very limited reparative response. This makes it very difficult, if not impossible, to judge the stage of the process (recently originated or already in some phase of repair) and more so the origin of the lesion (delayed ossification or trauma, for example).[7] Things become even more difficult if one realizes that OC is generally assumed to be a multifactorial disease in which the problem is not to single out a specific causative factor but to determine to what extent, and in which order, a variety of factors play a role. These considerations are discussed in more detail in the section on etiology.

Along similar lines, comparisons between species should be dealt with cautiously. In the late 1970s, in-depth studies on the phenomenon of osteochondrosis in a multitude of species (including horses, poultry, dogs, and cattle, but with the emphasis on swine) concluded that because of the striking similarities in manifestation across the species, including humans, OC should have a common pathogenesis and etiology, the latter being principally growth rate that itself was determined by nutrition and hereditary factors.[8] Ever since, this paradigm of a "seemingly unified hypothesis"[4] has hovered over OC research, and the ease with which conclusions for the horse have been drawn based on research in entirely different species has been remarkable in some instances. It is questionable whether this simple explanation of the pathophysiology of osteochondrosis is justifiable, given many findings from more recent research that are discussed later.

CLINICAL AND RADIOGRAPHIC SIGNS

The typical OC patient is a yearling that is presented with effusion of the tibiotarsal or femoropatellar joint, which has been noted recently by the owner. The horse usually is not lame, and radiographic examination shows a fragment at the cranial end of the distal intermediate ridge of the tibia (Fig. 91-2) or irregularities at the lateral trochlear ridge of the femur (Fig. 91-3). However, as with any typical presentation of a disease, many variations on this theme are possible.

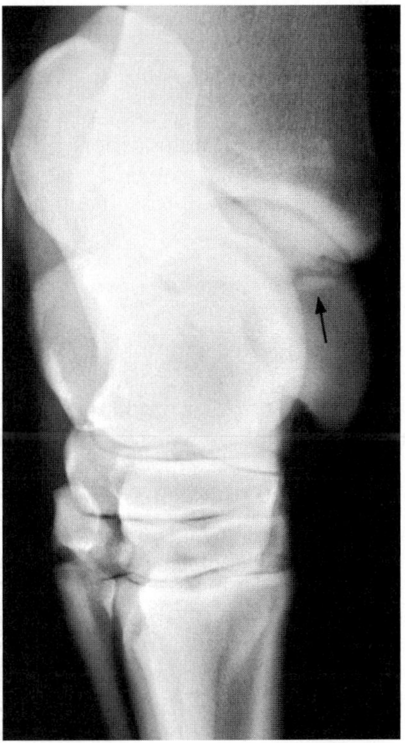

Figure 91-2. Radiograph showing a typical osteochondritic lesion of the dorsal aspect of the distal intermediate ridge of the tibia *(arrow)*. (Courtesy AJM van den Belt, University of Utrecht.)

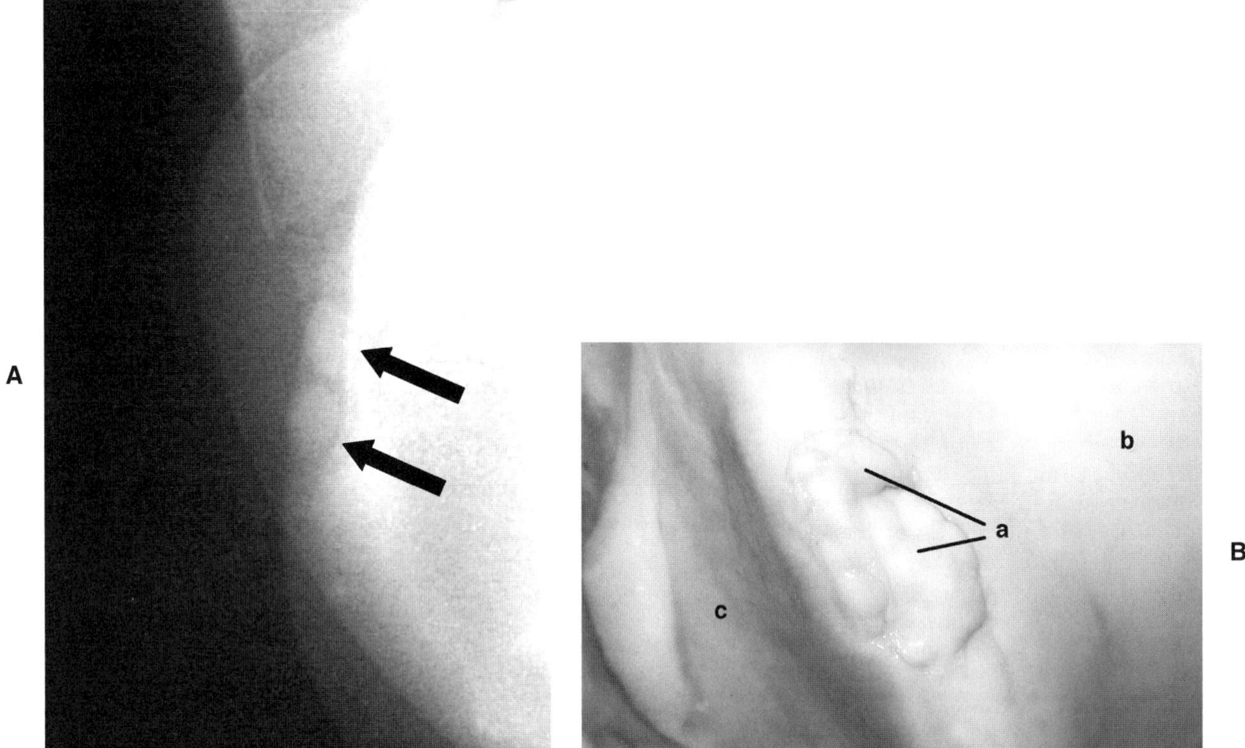

Figure 91-3. **A,** Radiograph view showing osteochondritic lesions on the lateral trochlear ridge of the distal femur *(arrows)*. **B,** Postmortem view of an osteochondritic lesion of the lateral trochlear ridge of the distal femur. *a,* OCD fragments at the lateral trochlear ridge; *b,* normal articular cartilage on the lateral aspect of the trochlea; *c,* patellar groove of the distal femur.

The age at which OC appears varies, although in the great majority of cases OC patients are juvenile animals. In severe cases of OC, which are more common in the stifle than in the hock, signs can be seen in foals as young as 6 months. OC can also manifest itself at the age the animals are put into training and the joints become challenged by athletic activity. The age at which this occurs varies with the branch of equestrian industry. Warmblood horses commonly are presented at about 3 years of age or older, and racing Thoroughbreds and Standardbreds manifest signs much earlier.

Distribution of Lesions

Osteochondrosis is most commonly diagnosed in tarsus, stifle, and metacarpophalangeal joints, but it has been described in almost every diarthrodial joint. In an experimental study, 43 Warmblood foals were used out of pairing OC-positive sires and partially OC-positive mares to produce offspring with a high prevalence of OC. Twenty-four foals were sacrificed at 5 months, all joints were inspected at necropsy, and macroscopic lesions were confirmed by microscopy.[9] Lesions were most numerous in the tarsocrural joint (average of two lesions per animal), followed by the femoropatellar and the cervical intervertebral (facet) joints (one lesion per animal), the metatarsophalangeal joint (0.6), the metacarpophalangeal and carpal joints (0.4), humeroradial joint (0.2), and scapulohumeral joint (0.04).[10]

Although the prevalence of OC in this study was artificially high, the relative distribution is in agreement with clinical experience in the Warmblood. Breed differences occur to a certain extent with regard to lesion distribution and relative clinical importance. Osteochondrosis in the femoropatellar joint is common in the racing Thoroughbred,[11] but in Warmbloods and Standardbreds, tarsocrural OC is seen more often.[12-16]

A hallmark of OC is that lesions almost always occur at certain predilection sites within a joint. In the tarsocrural joint, the most common site is the cranial end of the distal intermediate ridge of the tibia (see Fig. 91-2), followed by the distal end of the lateral trochlea of the talus and the medial malleolus of the tibia.[17] In the femoropatellar joint, the most common predilection site is the lateral trochlear ridge of the femur. Less common sites are the medial trochlear ridge of the femur, the trochlear groove, and the distal end of the patella.[6] Subchondral cysts that occur in the medial femoral condyle are a manifestation of osteochondrosis as well and are discussed in Chapter 92. The predilection site in the metacarpophalangeal joints is the dorsal end of the sagittal ridge of the metacarpus and metatarsus. Opinions on the nature of the fragments seen at the dorsal margin of the proximal phalanx differ, and the palmar or plantar osteochondral fragments (POFs) that were originally reported as being part of the osteochondrosis complex[18] are now considered traumatic in origin.[19,20] In the shoulder joint, osteochondrosis is commonly located on the glenoid and the humeral head.[21]

Lesions are often encountered bilaterally in the tarsocrural and femoropatellar joints and quadrilaterally in the metacarpophalangeal joints.[22] Bilateral presence, often with unilateral clinical manifestation only, can occur in the tarsocrural and femoropatellar joints in more than 50% of clinical cases.[6] Therefore, in horses with unilateral clinical signs, it is advisable to radiograph the contralateral joint. In contrast, concomitant occurrence in other joints or joint pairs is much less common. In a study of 225 horses with tarsocrural OC, lesions were found in other joints in only eight cases.[22] Therefore, joints other than the contralateral one do not need to be radiographed except when clinical signs exist.

Joint effusion is by far the most common clinical sign, but lameness can occur, especially when large radiographic lesions exist. Lameness is seen more in femoropatellar OC than in tarsocrural OC and is most likely when a loose or semiloose fragment is observed radiographically, thus when the osteochondritis dissecans form is present. Other, less-severe radiographic signs include irregularities in the articular contour of the subchondral bone and sometimes only a flattening of this contour.

Minor radiographic aberrations can be reliably classified as OC when judgments are made by an experienced radiologist. In one study, there was a correlation of 0.87 ($P < 0.001$) between radiographic classification of OC of the distal intermediate ridge of the tibia on a 0 to 4 scale[23] and histology.[10]

Nevertheless, the lesion severity as determined radiographically does not always correspond with arthroscopic or necropsy findings. In many cases, cartilage lesions are more severe than radiographic appearance suggests, or cartilaginous lesions are present without changes in the subchondral bone and hence do not show up on radiographs (Figs. 91-4 and 91-5). Severity of lesions can be assessed more accurately with more sophisticated imaging modalities such as magnetic resonance imaging (MRI). However, economic and physical constraints severely limit the wide clinical use of this kind of equipment, especially in the femoropatellar joint.

Breed Predilection

Osteochondrosis is common in many breeds of horses. In Swedish Standardbreds, Sandgren and colleagues found an incidence of 10.5% in the hock joints,[15] which was comparable to the 12% found by Schougaard and coworkers[13] but less than the 26% found earlier by Hoppe and Philipsson,[24] also in Standardbreds. Alvarado's group found an incidence of 35% in the femoropatellar and metacarpophalangeal joints of Standardbreds in a US population.[25] There are fewer studies in Thoroughbreds, but the incidence in that breed is reportedly high as well.[21,26,27]

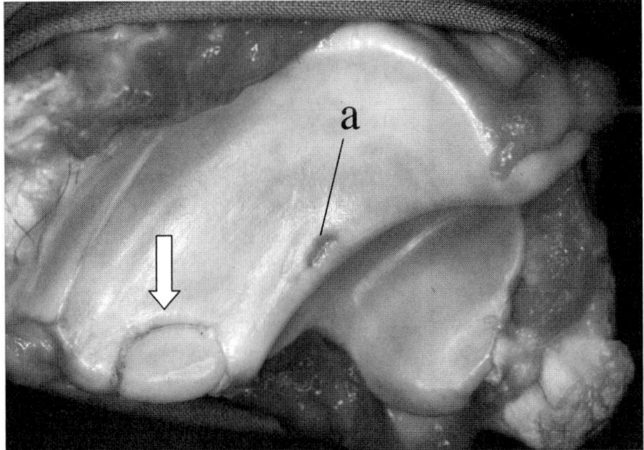

Figure 91-4. Typical osteochondrotic lesion of the distal intermediate ridge of the tibia in a cadaver specimen *(arrow)*. a, synovial groove.

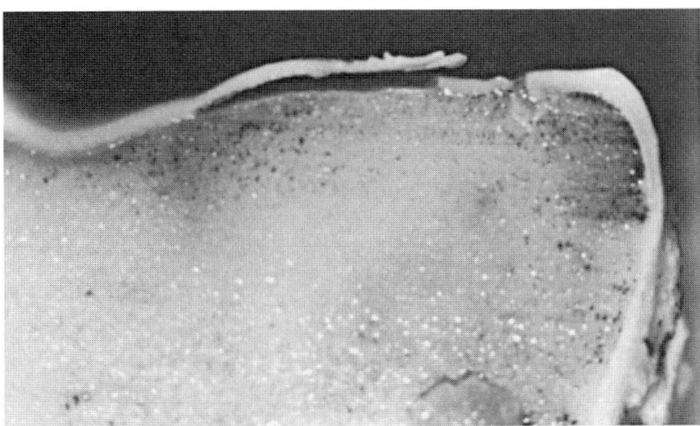
Figure 91-5. Example of an osteochondrotic lesion of the humeral condyle showing the formation of a large cartilage flap but relatively little damage to the subchondral bone.

In the Warmblood horse, early Swedish data mentioned an incidence of 15%[24]; more recent figures in the Dutch Warmblood population are higher (25% in the tarsocrural joint and 15% in the femoropatellar joint).[23] In a large study of 1180 horses in France (mainly Selle Français and Anglo-Arabs, a minority of Thoroughbreds), an incidence of 13.3% was reported in the tarsocrural joint.[16] A recent large-scale field study in Germany in several Warmblood breeds yielded figures of 19.5% for the metacarpophalangeal joints, 11.1% for the tarsocrural joint, and 7.2% for the femoropatellar joint.[28]

Overall, it has been estimated that in northwestern Europe alone annually 20,000 to 25,000 foals are born that will develop some degree of OC.[9] Osteochondrotic lesions are only rarely encountered in ponies.[29] Further, in a survey of 80 feral horses, extremely low incidences of 2.5% were found in the tarsocrural joint and 0% in the femoropatellar joint.[30] Because osteochondrosis is a relatively new disease (see next section), these observations strongly implicate breeding policies and possibly management aspects as key factors in this disease.

Osteochondrosis is a debilitating disease only in exceptional cases, where lesions are so extensive that no repair is possible. Nevertheless, the ailment has a strong impact on the economics of the equine industry, and to a certain extent on animal welfare, because tens of thousands of animals are operated upon each year. Apart from the direct economic loss, there is an even larger indirect cost of the disease, because many studbooks will not approve horses with (major or minor, depending on studbook policy) evidence of OC. It has been estimated that the strict breeding policy of the Royal Dutch Warmblood Studbook (KWPN) precludes 30% of all potential male breeding stock from participating in the selection procedures for becoming an approved sire. Apart from direct financial loss for the breeders, this also eliminates a large part of the gene pool. A last, but not insignificant, economic impact of OC is the loss in value of animals showing radiographic evidence of OC, regardless of their athletic capacities.

CHANGING CONCEPTS

In 1947 Nilsson, who described fragments in the stifle joints of Ardenner horses, gave the first description of what is retrospectively judged to have been OC.[31] Although in the following decades some reports describe intra-articular fragments that might have been osteochondrotic,[32] the real history of OC does not start before the publication of Birkeland and Haakenstad's paper in 1968.[33] These authors described a series of seven cases of OC of the distal ridge of the tibia, but they did not use the term *osteochondrosis*. In the early 1970s gradually more publications appeared,[34,35] and in the mid-1970s Olsson and Reiland with other Scandinavian coworkers published their comprehensive study on osteochondrosis in a multitude of species.[8,36-39]

Osteochondrosis was originally seen as a largely static condition, but this concept gradually changed. Strömberg reported changes in the radiographic appearance of femoropatellar OC after repeated radiographic examinations.[40] Dabareiner and colleagues recognized, after sequentially radiographing a number of foals, that osteochondrotic lesions of the distal femur could progress until the age of 9 months.[41] In the same year, Carlsten's group published a study in which they followed a cohort of 77 horses radiographically and found that no major osteochondrotic lesions in the tarsocrural joint were identified after 8 months of age. Interestingly, they noted a regression of a number of minor lesions before the age of 8 months, which had been detected between ages 1 and 3 months.[14]

Dik and colleagues radiographed the tarsocrural and femoropatellar joints of 43 foals on a monthly basis from the age of 1 month until age 5 months and of 19 of them until age 11 months. The study showed that not only minor lesions but also radiographically visible larger fragments ceased to exist. The ages at which lesions originated and the ages at which they became undetectable varied for each joint. In the tibiotarsal joint, lesions at the distal intermediate ridge of the tibia and at the distal aspect of the lateral trochlear ridge of the talus that were seen within the first few months of life had become undetectable before the age of 5 months. Thereafter no major changes occurred and existing lesions remained visible. In the femoropatellar joint, lesions originated later and peaked at approximately 6 months before declining in number until about 8 months, after which the lesions remained stable[23] (Fig. 91-6).

In a study in another group of Warmblood foals that was followed for 24 months, this general joint-specific pattern was confirmed.[42] In that study, very little change in radiographic appearance was noted from 12 to 24 months. Further confirmation of these patterns resulted from two studies. In one study, groups of horses were used to evaluate the relationship between liver copper content and OC,[43] and in the other study the influence of nutrition on OC was examined in the French Saddlebred.[44] The latter study also featured sequential radiographic examinations.

All these observations have led to the conclusion that OC is by no means a static condition, but in contrast is an extremely dynamic one in which lesions appear and apparently heal during the first months of life.[45] The acknowledgement of the dynamic character of OC has led to a profound change in the concept of this disease.

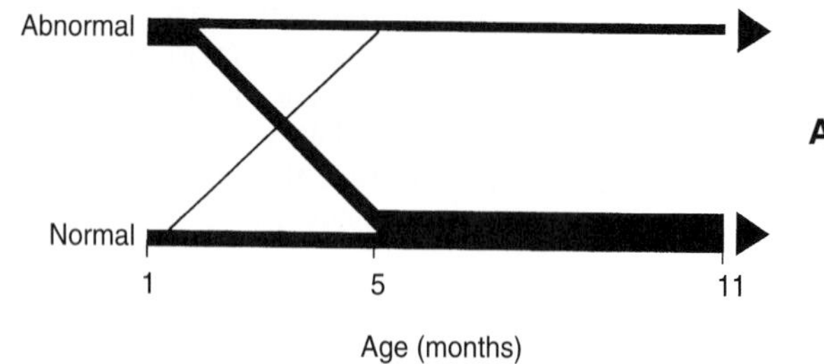

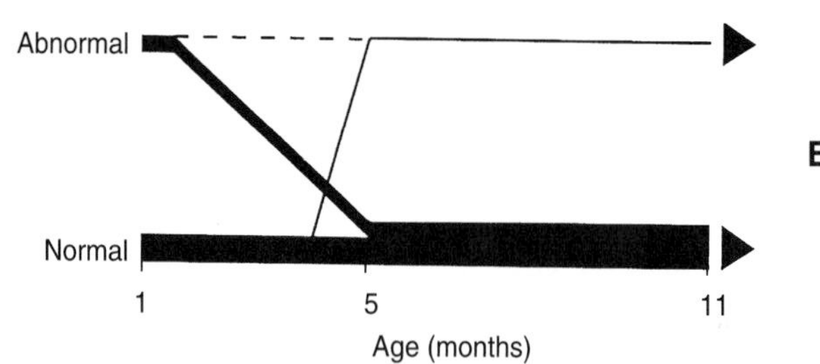

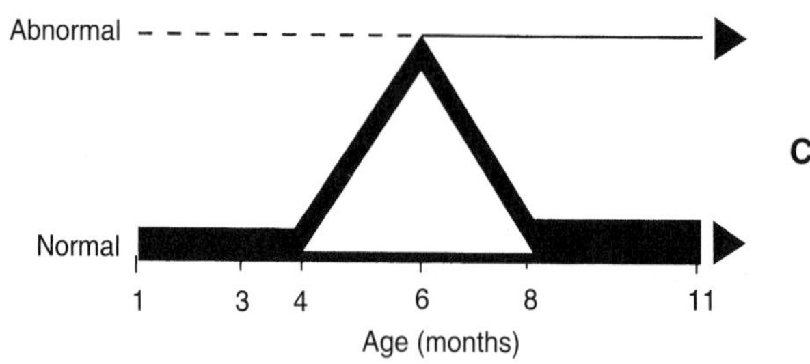

Figure 91-6. A, Schematic diagram of the early development of osteochondral lesions at the distal intermediate ridge of the tibia. At 1 month of age, there are several lesions that will heal. Only a few lesions originate after the age of 1 month, and at the age of 5 months, the situation remains stable. **B,** Schematic diagram of the early development of osteochondral lesions at the distal aspect of the lateral trochlear ridge of the talus. The same general pattern as in **A** is seen, but healing potential is better. **C,** Schematic diagram of the early development of osteochondral lesions of the lateral ridge of the femoral trochlea. The pattern is distinct from that of the hock. Lesions develop only after the age of 3 months, peak at about 6 months, and have resolved at the age of 8 months, although some lesions will remain. (From Dik KJ, Enzerink EE, van Weeren PR: Equine Vet J Suppl 1999;31:9, with permission from Equine Veterinary Journal Ltd.)

It is well known that the extracellular matrix of the articular cartilage goes through a phase of rapid remodeling in the neonatal animal. It is in this period that the topographic heterogeneity in biochemical composition that is necessary to withstand the locally different biomechanical challenges develops through the process of functional adaptation.[46,47] In this process, the collagen network of the articular cartilage is molded under biomechanical influences in a process not unlike that in bone.[3] However, whereas bone retains its capacity to remodel throughout the life of the horse, cartilage metabolism decreases quickly in the early juvenile period, and turnover times are very long in mature horses.[48,49]

The latter fact precludes any substantial remodeling or repair and makes the formation of the collagen network in the early juvenile phase a once-in-a-lifetime process that can have very important consequences for disease prevention in future life.[50] The sharp drop in collagen metabolism in the early juvenile period determines when the window for repair of lesions closes. Some lesions, either because they originate too late or are too large, do not have enough time for repair. These are the lesions that might eventually become clinically manifest. This means that in OC, a clear distinction should be made between the pathogenesis triggered by a number of etiologic factors on the one hand and the repair process on the other.[51,52] A flow chart for the putative mechanism of OC based on this concept is given in Figure 91-7.

ETIOLOGIC FACTORS

Osteochondrosis is a complex disease and multifactorial in origin. Biomechanical influences, exercise, failure of vascularization, nutrition imbalances, and genetic influences have all been incriminated and are probably interrelated.

Biomechanical Influences

Biomechanical loading plays a role in the pathogenesis of osteochondrosis. This assertion is supported by the consistency of predilection sites within specific joints. It is probable that the dramatic changes in biomechanical loading that take place after birth are an important trigger factor for initiating lesions. In a pathologic study of the stifles and hocks of nine fetuses and 10 foals aged 0 to 35 days, Rejnö and Strömberg found an osteochondrotic lesion in only one 3-day-old foal and none in any of the fetuses.[38] Other attempts to find osteochondrotic lesions in fetuses have failed.[53,54] Therefore, biomechanical loading most likely plays a role in all proposed mechanisms for OC.

Biomechanical loading can exert an influence late in the process, where it determines the formation and loosening of cartilage flaps after a faulty endochondral ossification, or early where it prematurely disrupts the vascular supply to neonatal cartilage (see next section). Biomechanical influences are strongly correlated with other etiologic factors such as exercise and genetics (through the determination of conformation of the animal). However, apart from direct blunt trauma that will cause an osteochondral fracture, biomechanical forces are considered a necessary additive factor rather than a sole cause of OC.

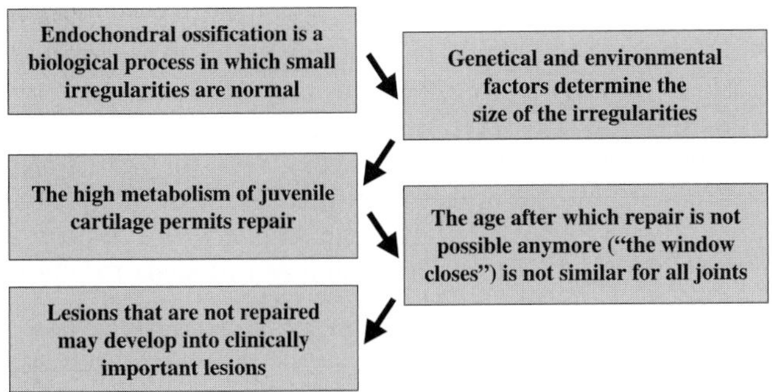

Figure 91-7. Flow chart outlining the supposed pathway along which clinical lesions eventually become manifest in equine osteochondrosis.

Failures of Vascularization

Wheeler Haines[55] described the existence of cartilage canals in the epiphyseal cartilage long ago. He stated that "the primary function of cartilage canals is . . . the nutrition of cartilage too large to be supplied by diffusion of nutriments through their substance. . . . Their presence retards rather than hastens the end of ossification." He also described the process of obliteration of these canals, called *chondrification*, that precedes ossification.

In the pig, extensive studies have been performed on the vascularization of cartilage, the physiologic process of regression of cartilage canals, and disturbances thereof as possible causes for OC. In this species, areas of chondronecrosis related to obliterated cartilage canals can be found, and they are much larger in commercial pig breeds than in miniature pigs from wild hog ancestry.[56] Artificial devascularization creates islands of cartilage without vascular supply, and these could create OC-like lesions.[57] These observations led to the hypothesis that premature interruption of the vascular supply of the growth cartilage of the articular–epiphyseal complex would lead to necrotic areas in the cartilage layer. These would later become engulfed in the ossification front and result in the typical irregularities and cartilage islands seen in OC.[58]

Later in-depth studies in this same area employed a more subtle and natural way of interrupting vascularization, in which only a limited number of cartilage canals was sectioned, which produced OC-like lesions.[59] No relationship between the overall regression pattern of cartilage canals and OC was shown. This led to the conclusion that OC is not the result of a general failure in endochondral ossification, and hence cannot be caused by a systemic factor such as growth rate, but is incited by local biomechanical factors.[60] This finding led, together with additional observations, to the hypothesis that OC was caused by local biomechanical damage to cartilage canals, especially to the anastomosing branches that run through the ossification front from the bone marrow.[61]

In the horse, cartilage canals are present in the juvenile period as well, and it is tempting to extrapolate the pathogenetic mechanism that now seems firmly established in the pig to the horse. However, there are several distinct interspecies differences. Focal islands of chondronecrosis seen in the pig are not frequent findings in the horse and are not a feature of the histologic description of OC as given by Henson and colleagues.[62] Although Carlson's group[5] showed a few necrotic areas near the ossification front, most of the irregularities and cartilage cores contain viable cartilage, not necrotic cartilage. This was supported by Shingleton and coworkers[63] in their study on equine cartilage canals, where they found patent canals in retained areas of viable cartilage. This led them to conclude that retention of cartilage canals, rather than disruption of them, might be necessary for the development of OC. Necrosis of cartilage would be the sequela, rather than the initiating factor.

Exercise

Exercise is known to be the steering factor in the process of functional adaptation during which the biochemical composition of the extracellular matrix of articular cartilage takes on a topographically heterogeneous character.[47,64,65] This process takes place principally in the first year of life, with emphasis on the first few months. Given the important role of exercise in the juvenile period for cartilage development, it may be hypothesized that this factor would be of importance in the development of osteochondrotic lesions too, because these originate in the same period that articular cartilage composition is molded.

Preliminary research in which controlled exercise was given to foals from 3 to 24 months of age using a high-speed horse walker yielded promising results. Osteochondrosis incidence was 6% in the high-exercise group and 20% in the low-exercise group, but results were flawed because of a concurrently running nutritional study employing different energy levels that were not consistently implemented.[66,67] A study focusing on the effect of exercise alone, given from 10 days until 5 months of age, did not yield conclusive results, although there was a tendency toward a decrease in severity of OC lesions in the exercised groups.[10]

In a large field study, Wilke found fewer OC lesions on the distal sagittal ridge of the metacarpus and metatarsus in the metacarpophalangeal and metatarsophalangeal joints of foals that got more exercise during the first months of life. There was, however, no effect on the incidence of OC in the tarsocrural joint.[68] Exercise might be a factor codetermining the final appearance of osteochondrotic lesions, but does not seem to be of primary pathogenetic importance.

Nutrition, Hormonal Factors, and Growth Rate

From the start of research into equine osteochondrosis, much effort has been dedicated to nutritional factors. The studies can be roughly divided into research on minerals and trace elements, mainly copper and zinc, to a lesser extent calcium and phosphorus, and on dietary energy level. The latter factor is closely related to growth rate, a factor heavily incriminated in OC pathogenesis in a large number of species. However, growth rate is determined not only by energy intake but also by genetic predisposition.

Interest in trace elements was raised by a report on the relationship between low copper levels in serum and ceruloplasmin and OC.[69] Studies followed on the effect of deliberately feeding low-copper diets[70] and the possible role of zinc in inducing a relative copper deficiency.[71] The mechanism was thought to act via the enzyme lysyl oxidase, a copper-dependent enzyme that is essential for the formation of collagen cross-links. Zinc, as well as cadmium, can antagonize copper by displacing it from the sulfhydryl binding sites on metallothionein.[72]

The epidemiologic studies on dietary mineral and trace element levels and the occurrence of developmental orthopedic disease in Ohio and Kentucky seemed to give further evidence for a key role of copper.[73] The original National Research Council (NRC) recommendation[74] of 10 ppm copper in dry matter, which was based on a study with a limited number of horses,[75] was challenged, and supplementation studies were started. These yielded positive results to some extent,[76-78] but they certainly were not conclusive enough to pinpoint copper deficiency as a sole cause of OC.[79] Higher dietary copper levels of 20 to 25ppm[78] or 50 ppm[80] were recommended, but they were later questioned following studies by Pearce and colleagues, who found that copper levels of 4.3 to 8.6 ppm in pasture were sufficient for a healthy development of bone and cartilage. Supplementation of copper to pregnant mares raised liver copper levels in both mares and foals at 150 days of age, but they did not abolish the occurrence of developmental orthopedic diseases.[81-83]

The proposed mechanism via lysyl oxidase was challenged[84] as in vitro research yielded additional information on the role of copper that appeared to have a chondroprotective effect through reduction of the activity of the proteinases cathepsin B and cathepsin D.[85] Another study showed that there was a relationship between neonatal liver copper concentration and the resolution of lesions, but there was no correlation with the initial occurrence. It was concluded from that study that copper had a positive effect on the repair of osteochondrotic lesions but not on their pathogenesis. This concept could explain many of the somewhat contradictory and inconclusive earlier findings. Copper retains a clinically important role because it is the outcome of both the pathogenetic process and the ensuing repair process that determines the eventual and clinically important lesions.[43]

High calcium levels did not influence the incidence of OC in foals, but high levels (four times the NRC recommendation) of phosphorus resulted in significantly more lesions.[86] The mechanism was supposed to be the induction of secondary hyperparathyroidism, which would lead to increased osteoporosis and subsequent weakening of the subchondral bone. The study is interesting because foals were studied in the period from 2.5 to 6.5 months of age, which is now known to be a period in which the dynamic process of OC is very active.

Dietary energy levels have been implicated in the pathogenesis of OC for decades.[87] This was mostly, but not solely, in relation to a high growth rate. In the early Scandinavian studies, it was stated that OC primarily occurred in large-framed, fast-growing animals, be they broilers, bulls, dogs, swine, or horses.[8,40] Later, the literature is more ambivalent on the subject of growth rate. Several authors found no relation to growth rate,[12,87,89] but others reported a larger prevalence in horses taller at the withers[15] or in horses having a higher average daily weight gain.[90] Sometimes this was true only for a limited period of development.[91]

Although the data about the effect of growth rate is conflicting and the concept of a high growth rate putting pressure on the process of endochondral ossification and thus leading to irregularities might be too simplistic, there is substantial evidence for other mechanisms. Excessive levels of energy, especially when fed in the form of easily digestible carbohydrates,[92,93] result in a strong postprandial hyperinsulinemia. Insulin and its derivatives insulin-like growth factor (IGF) I and IGF-II have a direct effect on the process of endochondral ossification, acting as mitogens for chondrocytes and stimulating chondrocyte survival or suppressing apoptosis.[94]

Insulin also stimulates a rapid removal from the circulation of the thyroid hormones T_3 and T_4,[95] which are involved in the final stages of chondrocyte differentiation and in the metaphyseal invasion of growth cartilage by blood vessels.[96] In fact, OC-positive foals have a significantly lower IGF-I activity than OC-negative foals.[97] In this way, high carbohydrate levels would induce a transient relative hypothyroidism and hence a retardation of the maturation of growth cartilage. Hypothyroidism in horses has been known to produce skeletal lesions, although they are not equivalent to those seen in OC.[98]

Interestingly, the effect of carbohydrates on thyroid hormone levels can be demonstrated in weanlings, but is not present in yearlings.[99] It has been possible to induce cartilaginous lesions by administering diets with high levels of digestible energy.[86,100] Further, horses with OC have been shown to have higher postprandial glucose and insulin responses to feeding high-grain ratios than did normal horses.[101]

Another indication of the importance of carbohydrate levels in the feed comes from a study in Kentucky on the influence of the season on the occurrence of OC. Early foals appeared to have a significantly higher incidence of OC in the tarsocrural joints, but late foals had a higher incidence in the femoropatellar joints. This seemingly contradictory effect of the season could be explained by the different windows of vulnerability of these joints, which appeared to coincide with the spring and autumn peaks in the high-energy value of the grass.[27]

There is hardly any doubt that the pathogenetic mechanism outlined here plays a certain role in the development of equine osteochondrosis. However, it is unlikely that it is the sole mechanism, because many lesions provoked by the administration of high-carbohydrate diets were similar, but they were not always identical to those seen in clinical OC. Besides, many lesions were seen in the growth plate,[89] and in contrast to other species, clinical OC is rarely, if ever, seen in the growth plate in the horse.

Genetics

In many species, the incidence of OC varies considerably with breed. In wild boars, the disease seems to be nonexistent, whereas it is common in many commercial pig breeds.[58] In horses, lesions are rarely found in ponies and have a much lower incidence in feral horses.[29,30] This suggests a considerable genetic influence. Further evidence comes from studies showing large differences in incidence of OC between progeny groups of different stallions.[13,39,102]

There is no doubt that OC is a polygenic trait and that the method of inheritance is complex.[103] Some estimates on heritability have been made, but they differed widely. For the tarsocrural joint, heritabilities of 0.24,[104] 0.26,[13] and 0.52[105] have been reported. A large progeny study in the Netherlands succeeded in establishing reliable heritabilities for navicular disease and bone spavin, but it did not give unequivocal results with respect to tarsocrural OC, which finally was estimated to be approximately 0.25.[106]

Heritabilities of 0.25 and higher are high enough to warrant selection programs, which indeed have been implemented by many studbooks. However, progress has been disappointing. The Royal Dutch Warmblood Studbook (KWPN) has rejected any candidate sire with even the slightest radiographic sign of tarsocrural OC since 1984 and any sign of femoropatellar OC since 1992, but no substantial decrease in incidence has been realized thus far. This is in contrast to the conditions of navicular disease and bone spavin, where a similar selection policy has been followed and resulted in a drastic reduction of the incidence of these orthopedic diseases.

There are various explanations for this. Osteochondrosis is classically seen as an all-or-none trait with an underlying continuous scale.[103] The genetic background may, however be much more complicated than originally supposed. First, there is mounting evidence that different genes are involved in different joints.[89,107] Second, the dynamic nature of OC allows many animals to be radiographically free of lesions at age 3 or 4 years when they enter the stallion selection procedures, yet they will have had evidence of the disease as a foal. Hence, they are genetically predisposed to OC and will pass on this trait.

Recently, studies have been undertaken to identify OC-related genes through modern molecular genetic techniques. These studies are difficult because they try to link the final phenotype, and thus the end product of various processes that most probably have different genetic backgrounds, to certain genes. It is highly unlikely that in the near future OC can be selected against using a simple genetic test that detects one or two culprit genes. Early results confirm the complexity of the disease because various candidate genes have been identified that differed per affected joint.[108]

THE MOLECULAR MECHANISM OF OSTEOCHONDROSIS

The need for a more fundamental approach to understanding and preventing osteochondrosis is obvious,[109] and in recent years most research on equine OC has focused on the molecular mechanisms involved. Both chondrocyte behavior and composition of the extracellular matrix have been targets of study. Lillich and colleagues found changes in proteoglycan composition of osteochondrotic fragments, but they could not tell whether this was primary or secondary.[110] This is a constant problem, because data from clinical cases and fragments collected at surgery are not representative of the initial phase of the disease.[7] Studies have focused on normal and abnormal (dyschondroplastic) cartilage, on the expression of various collagen types that are represented in the extracellular cartilage matrix (collagen types II, VI, and X), and on the expression of growth factors (transforming growth factor-β, IGF-I, IGF-II) that are known to play a role in the development and maturation of cartilage.[62,94,111-114]

There appeared to be distinct differences in expression patterns between normal and abnormal tissues, with notably high levels of activity around the chondrocyte clusters or chondrones in early cases of OC. This increase in activity is in line with the higher level of chondrocyte metabolism demonstrated by van den Hoogen and colleagues[115] and could be the primary cause, but is more likely a secondary event representing an attempt at repair.[116] Little work has been done on the subchondral bone underlying the cartilage defects. Van de Lest and coworkers showed changes in bone morphogenic enzymes and in membrane lipid composition of the cellular components of the subchondral bone.[117]

Levels of matrix metalloproteinases (MMPs) were found to be elevated in copper-deficient horses with clinical OC lesions,[78] and there is increasing evidence that changes in collagen metabolism play an important role in the molecular mechanism of OC. The Cambridge group performed in-depth studies on the distribution of cathepsins B, D, and L in normal and abnormal cartilage. They found physiologic differences in distribution[118-120] as well as a strong increase in cathepsin B activity in chondrocyte clonal clusters in OC.[121]

Al-Hizab and colleagues showed an increase in activity of gelatinases (MMP-2 and MMP-9) in osteochondrotic cartilage.[122] The increased collagen turnover in osteochondrotic cartilage is reflected by an increase in collagen split products that can be detected in the synovial fluid. Laverty's group showed an increase in the C-propeptide of collagen type II in synovial fluid from OC horses but a decrease in the epitope 846 of aggrecan, demonstrating different alterations in aggrecan and collagen turnover in OC.[123] This finding was confirmed in a later ex vivo study where no evidence was found for an increase in proteoglycan metabolism, but an increase in the levels of the $col_{2\text{-}3/4\ short}$ epitope was indicative of increased collagen breakdown.[124]

Billinghurst and colleagues were able to predict the presence of OC based on the detection of collagen markers in serum.[125] Additional evidence for the crucial role of collagen was provided by studies demonstrating a significant increase in the levels of MMP-1 (but not general MMP activity or specific activity of MMP-3) and the collagen degradation product hydroxyproline in synovial fluid from horses with OC compared to OC-free animals[126-128] and by the demonstration of differences in posttranslational modifications of collagen type II in samples from early lesions.[129] Overall, there now seems to be conclusive evidence that changes in collagen metabolism play a crucial role in the molecular mechanism of osteochondrosis. The question of whether this is a secondary or a primary event remains unanswered.

Parathyroid hormone related peptide (PTH-rp) and Indian hedgehog (Ihh) have a role in controlling cartilage differentiation and hypertrophy in the growth plate.[130] This influence is mediated by bone morphogenic proteins as signaling peptides. This led to the hypothesis that these molecules would have a similar role in cartilage differentiation in the equine articular–epiphyseal complex and could be implicated in the pathogenesis of OC. There was indeed a significant increase of PTH-rp protein and mRNA expression in chondrocytes from OC-affected cartilage, but not in Ihh.[131] Expression of bone morphogenic peptides 6 and 2 was not changed.[132]

TREATMENT OF OSTEOCHONDROSIS

Nonsurgical Management

Treatment of small osteochondrotic lesions might not always be necessary. Single small, radiographically obvious OC lesions in the tarsocrural joint without effusion did not influence performance in racing Standardbreds, in contrast to joints where there was significant effusion.[104] There was a negative effect on performance, however, if the lesions were more severe. Trotters with OC lesions in the tarsocrural joint had a significantly lower number of starts and somewhat lower earnings compared to controls.[133]

Treatment may be either conservative or surgical. Conservative treatment consists principally of rest and controlled exercise. Systemic NSAIDs and intra-articular medication (corticosteroids to enhance resolution of joint effusion and certain disease-modifying osteoarthritic drugs such as hyaluronic acid, chondroitin sulfate, or pentosan sulfate) may or may not be given, but they have not been reported to be of great value in OC. Given the nature of the disease described earlier, conservative management can only be expected to be successful in either very young animals, where there is still good capacity for regeneration, or in very mild cases.

A large study on the natural history of femoropatellar OC in three crops of Thoroughbred foals showed improvement and repair of several lesions, which was compatible with the age of the animals studied.[11] Laws and coworkers described a favorable outcome of conservative treatment of tarsocrural OC in a group of Standardbreds, half of which were treated conservatively and half surgically. The authors mentioned, however, that these results were biased, because the more severe cases tended to be treated surgically.[134]

Peremans and Verschooten concluded that conservative treatment of tarsocrural OC (consisting of simple box rest or a less-intense training program with a low-energy diet) was a good option in Warmbloods (80% success rate), but not in Standardbreds (25%). It should be noted that in Warmblood horses, especially those destined for dressage, resolution of joint effusion is often a therapeutic goal in itself. This aspect was not classified as such in this study.[135]

Surgical Management

Surgical treatment is the treatment of choice in most cases.[136,137] Clinical experience has taught that arthroscopic surgery presents definite advantages over arthrotomy.[136] Soft-tissue trauma is less, the convalescent period is considerably shorter, and functional and cosmetic recovery are better. An additional advantage is that a more comprehensive examination of the joint is possible.[6] In a direct comparison of arthroscopic treatment and treatment by conventional arthrotomy, Vatistas and colleagues demonstrated that hospitalization time was almost five times shorter after arthroscopy than after arthrotomy. Even more important, horses returned significantly more often to their intended use.[138]

Arthroscopic surgery is widely used at present in the femoropatellar, tarsocrural, and metacarpophalangeal and metatarsophalangeal joints to treat OC. In some other joints where OC is encountered less often but can present a serious clinical problem, such as the scapulohumeral joint, an arthroscopic approach is feasible too, but the technique is considerably more difficult.[21,139] The surgical techniques applied are discussed in more detail in Chapter 14 and in the relevant chapters discussing the respective joints.

PROGNOSIS

The prognosis after surgical intervention varies between joints and depends on the amount and extent of the lesion. It further depends on the definition of "favorable outcome." In most racing Thoroughbreds and Standardbreds, a favorable outcome means a sound horse that can compete at its maximal athletic capacity. In many show horses, the cosmetic appearance is important as well. In general, prognosis for a return to athletic activity is fair to good for the majority of joints involved.

For the femoropatellar joint, Foland's group reported a 64% success rate,[140] but this figure might be too pessimistic because the study included many horses operated on at a young age before their first performance. Therefore, it included a number of horses that would never have raced despite the OC lesions because attrition rates in Thoroughbred training are high and many young horses will never race. Jockey club records indicate that only about 60% of all Thoroughbreds intended for racing ever reach the starting gate in the United States.

In another study, 19 of 25 arthroscopically treated horses (76%) were able to perform their intended use.[138] Racing performance in Thoroughbreds treated for femoropatellar OC was not different from that in unaffected siblings, but fewer horses raced as 2-year-olds and earnings were less, both at 2 and 3 years of age.[141] Also, 2-year-old Thoroughbreds and Standardbreds that were operated on for OC in the tarsocrural joint were less likely to race, compared to unaffected siblings at 2 years of age, but findings were not different between groups at 3 years of age.[142] The differences might be mainly the result of the delay in training caused by the surgery.

McIlwraith and colleagues reported success rates of 73% and 83% for the tarsocrural joint in racehorses and nonracehorses, respectively. Synovial effusion resolved in 89% of racehorses and 74% of nonracehorses.[17] Of the other joints, prognosis is least favorable in the shoulder joint, with 46% success reported.[21] However, conservative treatment is not an option in this joint because the outcome is considerably worse.[6]

In the metacarpophalangeal and metatarsophalangeal joints there is some confusion about the extent to which radiographically detectable lesions are part of the OC complex. Fragments of the dorsal aspect of the distal metacarpus and metatarsus are commonly accepted to be osteochondrotic, and in these, 57% success has been reported after surgery. This figure is negatively biased because 18% of the cases were classified as unsuccessful for other reasons that made the horse unsuitable for use.[143] A more recent source mentions 90% return to athletic activity if the lesion is located in the more proximal part of the sagittal ridge but an unspecified lower rate for lesions in weight-bearing areas.[144]

Prognosis for arthroscopic removal of osteochondral fragments of the dorsal articular margin of the proximal phalanx, of which the osteochondrotic nature is still contentious, is given as nearly 100%.[144]

REFERENCES

1. König F: Über freie Körper in den Gelenken, Dtsch Z Klin Chir 1887;27:90.
2. Barrie HJ: Osteochondritis dissecans 1887-1987. A centennial look at König's memorable phrase, J Bone Joint Surg 1987;69-B:693.
3. Wolff, J: Das Gesetz der Transformation der Knochen, Berlin, 1892, Hirschwald.
4. Hurtig MB, Pool RR: Pathogenesis of equine osteochondrosis. In McIlwraith CW, Trotter GW, editors: Joint Disease in the Horse, Philadelphia, 1996, WB Saunders.
5. Carlson CS, Cullins LD, Meuten JD: Osteochondrosis of the articular-epiphyseal cartilage complex in young horses: Evidence for a defect in cartilage canal blood supply, Vet Pathol 1995;32:641.
6. Watkins, JP: Osteochondrosis. In Auer JA, Stick JA, editors: Equine Surgery, ed 2, Philadelphia, 1999, WB Saunders.
7. Pool RR: Difficulties in definition of equine osteochondrosis: Differentiation of developmental and acquired lesions, Eq Vet J Suppl 1993;16:5.
8. Olsson SE, Reiland S: The nature of osteochondrosis in animals, Acta Radiol Suppl 1978;358:299.
9. Van Weeren PR, Barneveld A: Study design to evaluate the influence of exercise on the development of the musculoskeletal system of foals up to age 11 months, Equine Vet J Suppl 1999;31:4.
10. Van Weeren PR, Barneveld A: The effect of exercise on the distribution and manifestation of osteochondrotic lesions in the Warmblood foal, Equine Vet J Suppl 1999;31:16.
11. McIntosh SC, McIlwraith CW: Natural history of femoropatellar osteochondrosis in three crops of Thoroughbreds, Equine Vet J Suppl 1993;16:54.
12. Hoppe F: Radiological investigations of osteochondrosis dissecans in Standardbred trotters and Swedish Warmblood horses, Equine Vet J 1984;16:425.
13. Schougaard H, Falk Rønne J, Philipsson J: A radiographic survey of tibiotarsal osteochondrosis in a selected population of trotting horses in Denmark and its possible genetic significance, Equine Vet J 1990;22:288.
14. Carlsten J, Sandgren B, Dalín G: Development of osteochondrosis in the tarsocrural joint and osteochondral fragments in the fetlock joints of Standardbred trotters. I. A radiological survey, Equine Vet J Suppl 1993;16:42.
15. Sandgren B, Dalin G, Carlsten J: Osteochondrosis in the tarsocrural joint and osteochondral fragments in the fetlock joints in Standardbred trotters. I. Epidemiology, Equine Vet J Suppl 1993;16:31.
16. Denoix, JM, Valette JP: Pathologie ostéo-articulaire chez le jeune cheval (incidence, évaluation clinique, facteurs de risque et conséquences), Proc Journée d'étude des Haras Nationaux 2001;27:101.
17. McIlwraith CW, Foerner JJ, Davis DM: Osteochondritis dissecans of the tarsocrural joint: Results of treatment with arthroscopic surgery, Equine Vet J 1991;23:155.
18. Sønnichsen HV, Kristoffersen J, Falk-Rønne J: Joint mice in the fetlock joint—osteochondritis dissecans, Nord Vet Med 1982;34:399.
19. Dalin G, Sandgren B, Carlsten J: Plantar osteochondral fragments in the metatarsophalangeal joints in Standardbred trotters: Results of osteochondrosis or trauma? Equine Vet J Suppl 1993;16:62.
20. Nixon AJ, Pool RR: Histologic appearance of axial osteochondral fragments from the proximoplantar/proximopalmar aspect of the proximal phalanx in horses, J Am Vet Med Assoc 1995;207:1076.
21. McIlwraith CW: Clinical aspects of osteochondrosis dissecans. In McIlwraith CW, Trotter GW, editors: Joint Disease in the Horse, Philadelphia, 1996, WB Saunders.
22. McIlwraith CW: Inferences from referred clinical cases of osteochondritis dissecans. Equine Vet J Suppl 1993;16:27.
23. Dik KJ, Enzerink EE, van Weeren PR: Radiographic development of osteochondral abnormalities, in the hock and stifle of Dutch Warmblood foals, from age 1 to 11 months, Equine Vet J Suppl 1999;31:9.
24. Hoppe F, Philipsson J: A genetic study of osteochondrosis dissecans in Swedish horses, Equine Pract 198;57:7.
25. Alvarado AF, Marcoux M, Breton L: The incidence of osteochondrosis in a Standardbred breeding farm in Quebec, Proc Am Assoc Equine Pract 1989;35:295.
26. O'Donohue DD, Smith FH, Strickland KL: The incidence of abnormal limb development in the Irish Thoroughbred from birth to 18 months, Equine Vet J 1992;24:305.

27. Paasch KM, Bramlage LR: Influence of birth month on location of osteochondrosis dissecans, Proc Am Assoc Equine Pract Focus on Joints Meeting, Louisville, Ky, July 22-24, 2004, p 17.
28. Arnan P, Hertsch B-W: Röntgenologische Untersuchung zur Erfassung der Osteochondrosis dissecans im Fessel-, Sprung- und Kniegelenk im Vergleich vom Fohlen zum Zweijährigen. In Bruns E, editor: Göttinger Pferdetage 2004, Warendorf, Germany, 2004, FN-Verlag.
29. Voûte LC, Henson FMD, Platt D, et al: Lesions of the lateral trochlear ridge of the distal femur in ponies with histological features of equine dyschondroplasia, Proc Brit Equine Vet Assoc 1997;36:153.
30. Valentino LW, Lillich JD, Gaughan EM, et al: Radiographic prevalence of osteochondrosis in yearling feral horses, Vet Comp Orthop Traumatol 1999;12:151.
31. Nilsson F: Hästens goniter, Svensk Vetidn 1947;52:1.
32. Numans SR, Wintzer HJ: Einige neue Indikationen zur Knochen- und Gelenkchirurgie des Pferdes, Berl Münchn Tierärztl Wschr 1961;74:205.
33. Birkeland R, Haakenstad LH: Intracapsular bony fragments of the distal tibia of the horse, J Am Vet Med Assoc 1968;152:1526.
34. Birkeland R: Chip fractures of the first phalanx in the metatarsophalangeal joint of the horse, Acta Radiol Suppl 1972;319:73.
35. De Moor A, Verschooten F, Desmet P, et al: Osteochondritis dissecans of the tibiotarsal joint of the horse, Equine Vet J 1972;4:139.
36. Reiland S: Morphology of osteochondrosis and sequelae in pigs, Acta Radiol Suppl 1978;358:45.
37. Reiland S, Strömberg B, Olsson SE, et al: Osteochondrosis in growing bulls. Pathology, frequency and severity on different feedings, Acta Radiol Suppl 1978;358:179.
38. Rejnö S, Strömberg B: Osteochondrosis in the horse: II. Pathology, Acta Radiol Suppl 1978;358:153.
39. Strömberg B, Rejnö S: Osteochondrosis in the horse I. A clinical and radiologic investigation of osteochondritis dissecans of the knee and hock joint, Acta Radiol Suppl 1978;358:139.
40. Strömberg B: A review of the salient features of osteochondrosis in the horse, Equine Vet J 1979;11:211.
41. Dabareiner RM, Sullins KE, White NA II: Progression of femoropatellar osteochondrosis in nine young horses. Clinical, radiographic and arthroscopic findings, Vet Surg 1993;22:515.
42. Enzerink E, Dik KJ, Knaap J, et al: Radiographic development of lesions in hock and stifle in a group of Dutch Warmblood horses from 1-24 months of age, Proc Brit Equine Vet Assoc 2000;39:195.
43. Van Weeren PR, Knaap J, Firth EC: Influence of liver copper status of mare and newborn foal on the development of osteochondrotic lesions, Equine Vet J 2003;35:67.
44. Martin-Rosset W: Personal communication, 2004.
45. Barneveld A, van Weeren PR: Conclusions regarding the influence of exercise on the development of the equine musculoskeletal system with special reference to osteochondrosis. Equine Vet J Suppl 1999;31:112.
46. Brama PAJ, TeKoppele JM, Bank RA, et al: Development of biochemical heterogeneity of articular cartilage: influences of age and exercise. Equine Vet J 2002;34:265.
47. Brama PAJ: Functional adaptation of equine articular cartilage, Proc Am Assoc Equine Pract Focus on Joints Meet Louisville, Ky, July 22-24, 2004, p 145.
48. Maroudas A: Metabolism of cartilaginous tissues: A quantitative approach. In Maroudas A, Holborrow EJ, editors: Studies in Joint Disease, vol 1, Tunbridge Wells, England, 1980, Pitman Medical.
49. Verzijl N, DeGroot J. Thorpe SR, et al: Effect of collagen turnover on the accumulation of advanced glycation end products, J Biol Chem 2000;275:39027.
50. Helminen HJ, Hyttinen MM, Lammi MJ, et al: Regular joint loading in the youth assists in the establishment and strengthening of the collagen network of articular cartilage and contributes to the prevention of osteoarthrosis later in life: A hypothesis, J Bone Min Metab 2000;18:245.
51. Van Weeren PR, Brama PAJ: Equine joint disease in the light of new developments in articular cartilage research, Pferdeheilkunde 2003;19:336.
52. Van Weeren PR: Osteochondrosis: Developmental disorder or disorderly development? (OC seen in the general framework of articular development in young animals), Proc Ann Sci Meet Eur Coll Vet Surg 13:164, 2004.
53. Hertsch B: Personal communication, 2004.
54. Van Weeren PR: Unpublished results, 2003.
55. Wheeler Haines R: Cartilage canals, J Anat 1933;68:45.
56. Ekman S, Rodriguez Martinez H, Plöen L: Morphology of normal and osteochondritic porcine articular-epiphyseal cartilage, Acta Anat 1990;139:239.
57. Carlson CS, Meuten DJ, Richardson DC: Ischemia of cartilage in spontaneous and experimental lesions of osteochondrosis, J Orthop Res 1991;9:317.
58. Ekman S, Carlson CS: The pathophysiology of osteochondrosis, Vet Clin North Am Small Anim Pract 1998;28:17.
59. Ytrehus B, Andreas Haga H, Mellum CN, et al: Experimental ischemia of porcine growth cartilage produces lesions of osteochondrosis, J Orthop Res 2004;22:1201.
60. Ytrehus B, Carlson CS, Lundeheim N, et al: Vascularization and osteochondrosis of the epiphyseal growth cartilage of the distal femur in pigs—development with age, growth rate, weight and joint shape, Bone 2004;34:454.
61. Ytrehus B: Osteochondrosis. A morphological study of aetiology and pathogenesis. Thesis. Oslo, 2004, Norwegian School of Veterinary Science.
62. Henson FMD, Davies ME, Jeffcott LB: Equine dyschondroplasia (osteochondrosis)—histological findings and type VI collagen localization, Vet J 1997;154:53.
63. Shingleton WD, Mackie EJ, Cawston TE, et al: Cartilage canals in equine articular/epiphyseal growth cartilage and a possible association with dyschondroplasia, Equine Vet J 1997;29:360.
64. Brama PAJ, TeKoppele JM, Bank RA, et al: Influence of different exercise levels and age on the biochemical characteristics of immature equine articular cartilage. Equine Vet J Suppl 1999;31:55.
65. Brama PAJ, teKoppele JM, Bank RA, et al: Functional adaptation of articular cartilage: The formation of regional biochemical characteristics during the first year of life in the horse, Equine Vet J 2000;32:217.
66. Bruin G, Creemers J: Het voorkómen van osteochondrose. In Bruin G, editor: Praktijkonderzoek paarden, Lelystad, Netherlands, 1994, Proefstation voor de Rundveehouderij, Schapenhouderij en Paardenhouderij.
67. Jeffcott LB: Osteochondrosis in the horse—searching for the key to pathogenesis, Equine Vet J 1991;23:33.
68. Wilke A: Der Einfluss von Aufzucht und Haltung auf Osteochondrose. Thesis. Hanover, 2003, Tierärztliche Hochshule.
69. Bridges CH, Womack JE, Harris ED, et al: Considerations of copper metabolism in osteochondrosis in suckling foals, J Am Vet Med Assoc 1984;185:173.
70. Bridges CH, Harris ED: Experimentally induced cartilaginous fractures (osteochondritis dissecans) in foals fed low-copper diets, J Am Vet Med Assoc 1988;193:215.
71. Bridges CH, Moffitt, PG: Influence of variable content of dietary zinc on copper metabolism of weanling foals, Am J Vet Res 1990;51:275.
72. Gunson DE, Kowalczyk DF, Shoop CR, et al: Environmental zinc and cadmium pollution associated with generalized osteochondrosis, osteoporosis, and nephrocalcinosis in horses, J Am Vet Med Assoc 1982;180:295.
73. Knight DA, Gabel AA, Reed SM, et al: Correlation of dietary mineral to incidence and severity of metabolic bone disease in Ohio and Kentucky. Proc Am Assoc Equine Pract 1985;31:445.
74. Committee on Animal Nutrition, National Research Council: The Nutrient Requirements of Horses, ed 5, Washington, DC 1989, National Academies Press.

75. Cupps PJ, Howell CE: The effects of feeding supplemental copper to growing foals. J Anim Sci 1949;8:286.
76. Knight DA, Weisbrode SE, Schmall LM, et al: The effects of copper supplementation on the prevalence of cartilage lesions in foals, Equine Vet J 1990;22:426.
77. Hurtig MB, Green SL, Dobson H, et al: Defective bone and cartilage in foals fed a low-copper diet, Proc Am Assoc Equine Pract 1990;36,637.
78. Hurtig M, Green SL, Dobson H, et al: Correlative study of defective cartilage and bone growth in foals fed a low-copper diet, Equine Vet J Suppl 1993;16:66.
79. Cymbaluk NF, Smart ME: A review of possible metabolic relationships of copper to equine bone disease, Equine Vet J Suppl 1993;16:19.
80. Lewis LD: Minerals for horses. In Lewis LD: Equine Clinical Nutrition: Feeding and Care, Baltimore, 1995, Williams & Wilkins.
81. Pearce SG, Grace ND, Wichtel JJ, et al: Effect of copper supplementation on copper status of pregnant mares and foals, Equine Vet J 1998;30:200.
82. Pearce SG, Grace ND, Firth EC, et al: Effect of copper supplementation on the copper status of pasture-fed young Thoroughbreds, Equine Vet J 1998;30:204.
83. Pearce SG, Firth EC, Grace ND, et al: Effect of copper supplementation on the evidence of developmental orthopaedic disease in pasture-fed New Zealand Thoroughbreds, Equine Vet J 1998;30:211.
84. Jeffcott LB, Davies ME: Copper status and skeletal development in horses: Still a long way to go. Equine Vet J 1998;30:183.
85. Davies ME, Pasqualicchio M, Henson F, et al: Effects of copper and zinc on chondrocyte behaviour and matrix turnover, Pferdeheilkunde 1996;12:367.
86. Savage CJ, McCarthy RN, Jeffcott LB: Effects of dietary phosphorus and calcium on induction of dyschondroplasia in foals, Equine Vet J Suppl 1993;16:80.
87. Savage CJ, McCarthy RN, Jeffcott LB: Effects of dietary energy and protein on induction of dyschondroplasia in foals, Equine Vet J Suppl 1993;16:74.
88. Glade MJ, Krook L, Schryver HF, et al: Growth inhibition by chronic dexamethasone treatment of foals, J Equine Vet Sci 1981;1:198.
89. Glade MJ, Belling TH: Growth plate cartilage metabolism, morphology and biochemical composition in over- and underfed horses, Growth 1984;48:473.
90. Sandgren B, Dalin G, Carlsten J, et al: Development of osteochondrosis in the tarsocrural joint and osteochondral fragments in the fetlock joints of Standardbred trotters. II. Body measurements and clinical findings, Equine Vet J Suppl 1993;16:48.
91. Van Weeren PR, Sloet van Oldruitenborgh-Oosterbaan MM, Barneveld A: The influence of birth weight, rate of weight gain and final achieved height and sex on the development of osteochondrotic lesions in a population of genetically predisposed Warmblood foals, Equine Vet J Suppl 1999;31:26.
92. Glade MJ: The control of cartilage growth in osteochondrosis: A review, J Equine Vet Sci 1986;6:175.
93. Glade MJ: The role of endocrine factors in equine developmental orthopedic disease, Proc Am Assoc Equine Pract 1987;33:171.
94. Henson FMD, Davenport C, Butler L, et al: Effects of insulin and insulin-like growth factors I and II on the growth of equine fetal and neonatal chondrocytes, Equine Vet J 1997;29:441.
95. Glade MJ, Gupta S, Reimers TJ: Hormonal responses to high and low planes of nutrition in weanling Thoroughbreds, J Anim Sci 1984;59:658.
96. Jeffcott LB, Henson FMD: Studies on growth cartilage in the horse and their application to aetiopathogenesis of dyschondroplasia (osteochondrosis), Vet J 1998;126:117.
97. Sloet van Oldruitenborgh-Oosterbaan MM, Mol JA, Barneveld A: Hormones, growth factors and other plasma variables in relation to osteochondrosis. Equine Vet J Suppl 1999;31:45.
98. Shavers JR, Fretz PB, Doige CE, et al: Skeletal manifestations of suspected hypothyroidism in two foals, J Equine Med Surg 1979;3:269.
99. Glade MJ, Reimers TJ: Effects of dietary energy supply on serum thyroxine, tri-iodothyronine and insulin concentrations in young horses, J Endocr 1985;104:93.
100. Glade MJ, Belling TH: A dietary etiology for osteochondrotic cartilage, J Equine Vet Sci 1986;6:151.
101. Ralston SL: Hyperglycaemia/hyperinsulinaemia after feeding a meal of grain to young horses with osteochondrosis dissecans (OCD) lesions, Pferdeheilkunde 1996;12:320.
102. Philipsson J, Andréasson E, Sandgren B, et al: Osteochondrosis in the tarsocrural joint and osteochondral fragments in the fetlock joints in Standardbred trotters. II. Heritability, Equine Vet J Suppl 1993;16:38.
103. Philipsson J: Pathogenesis of osteochondrosis: Genetic implications. In McIlwraith CW, Trotter GW, editors: Joint Disease in the Horse, Philadelphia, 1996, WB Saunders.
104. Brendov E: Osteochondrosis in Standardbred Trotters: Heritability and Effects on Racing Performance. Thesis. Uppsala, 1997, Swedish University of Agricultural Sciences.
105. Grøndahl AM, Dolvik NI: Heritability estimation of osteochondrosis in the tibiotarsal joint and of bony fragments in the palmar/plantar portion of the metacarpophalangeal and metatarsophalangeal joints of horses, J Am Vet Med Assoc 1993;203:101.
106. Van der Veen G, Kingmans J, van Veldhuizen AE, et al: The frequency and heredity of navicular disease, sesamoidosis, fetlock joint arthrosis, bone spavin, osteochondrosis of the hock: A radiographic progeny study. Zeist, Netherlands, 1994, Koninklijk Warmbloed Paardenstamboek Nederland.
107. Löhring K, Distl O: Entwicklung eines genomweiten Markersets für die Aufdeckung von QTL beim Pferd. In Bruns E, editor: Göttinger Pferdetage 2004, Warendorf, Germany, 2004, FN-Verlag.
108. Distl O: Personal communication, 2004.
109. Jeffcott LB: Problems and pointers in equine osteochondrosis. Equine Vet J Suppl 1993;16: 1.
110. Lillich JD, Bertone AL, Malemud CJ, et al: Biochemical, histochemical and immunohistochemical characterisation of distal tibial osteochondrosis in horses, Am J Vet Res 1997;58:89.
111. Henson FMD, Davies ME, Skepper JN, et al: Localisation of alkaline phosphatase in equine growth cartilage, J Anat 1995;187:151.
112. Henson FMD, Davies ME, Schofield PN, et al: Expression of types II, VI and X collagen in equine growth cartilage during development, Equine Vet J 1996;28:189.
113. Henson FMD, Schofield PN, Jeffcott LB: Expression of transforming growth factor-β1 in normal and dyschondroplastic articular growth cartilage of the young horse, Equine Vet J 1997;29:434.
114. Semovolos SA, Nixon AJ, Brower-Toland MA: Changes in molecular expression of aggrecan and collagen types I, II, and X, insulin-like growth factor-I, and transforming growth factor-β1 in articular cartilage obtained from horses with naturally acquired osteochondrosis, Am J Vet Res 2001;62:1088.
115. Van den Hoogen BM, van de Lest CHA, van Weeren PR: Changes in proteoglycan metabolism in osteochondrotic articular cartilage of growing foals, Equine Vet J Suppl 1999;31:38.
116. Muir H: The chondrocyte, architect of cartilage, Bio Essays 1995;17:1039.
117. Van de Lest CHA, van den Hoogen BM, van Weeren PR, et al: Changes in bone morphogenic enzymes and lipid composition of equine osteochondrotic subchondral bone, Equine Vet J Suppl 1999;31:31.
118. Hernandez-Vidal G, Davies ME, Jeffcott LB: Localization of cathepsins B and D in equine articular cartilage, Pferdeheilkunde 1996;12:371.
119. Hernandez Vidal G, Jeffcott LB, Davies ME: Cellular heterogeneity in cathepsin D distribution in equine articular cartilage, Equine Vet J 1997;29:267.

120. Gläser KE, Davies ME, Jeffcott LB: Differential distribution of cathepsins B and L in articular cartilage during skeletal development in the horse, Equine Vet J 2003;35:42.
121. Hernandez-Vidal G, Jeffcott LB, Davies ME: Immunolocalization of cathepsin B in equine dyschondroplastic cartilage, Vet J 1998;156:193.
122. Al-Hizab F, Clegg PD, Thompson CC, et al: Microscopic localization of active gelatinases in equine osteochondritis dissecans (OCD) cartilage, Osteoarthr Cart 2002;10:653.
123. Laverty S, Ionescu M, Marcoux M, et al: Alterations in cartilage type-III procollagen and aggrecan contents in synovial fluid in equine osteochondrosis, J Orthop Res 2000;18:399.
124. Laverty S, O'Kouneff S, Ionescu M, et al: Excessive degradation of type II collagen in articular cartilage in equine osteochondrosis, J Orthop Res 2002;20:1282.
125. Billinghurst RC, Brama PAJ, van Weeren PR, et al: Evaluation of serum concentrations of biomarkers of skeletal metabolism and results of radiography as indicators of severity of osteochondrosis in foals. Am J Vet Res 2004;65:143.
126. Brama PAJ, teKoppele JM, Beekman B, et al: Matrix metalloproteinase (MMP) activity in equine synovial fluid: Influence of age, osteoarthritis and osteochondrosis. Ann Rheum Dis 1998;57:697.
127. Brama PAJ, teKoppele JM, Beekman B, et al: Influence of development and joint pathology on stromelysin enzyme activity in equine synovial fluid, Ann Rheum Dis 2000;59:155.
128. Brama PAJ, van den Boom R, van Weeren PR: Collagenase (MMP-1) activity in synovial fluid as a marker for joint pathology in the horse. Proc Br Equine Vet Assoc 2002;41:192.
129. van de Lest CHA, Brama PAJ, van El B, et al: Extracellular matrix changes in early osteochondrotic defects in foals: A key role for collagen? Biochim Biophys Acta 2004;1690:54.
130. Kronenberg HM, Lee K, Lanke B, et al: Parathyroid hormone-related protein and Indian hedgehog control the pace of cartilage differentiation, J Endocrinol 1997;154:S39.
131. Semovolos SA, Brower-Toland BD, Bent SJ, et al: Parathyroid hormone–related peptide and Indian hedgehog expression patterns in naturally acquired equine osteochondrosis, J Orthop Res 2002;20:1290.
132. Semovolos SA, Nixon AJ, Strassheim ML: Expression of bone morphogenic protein-6 and -2 and a bone morphogenic protein antagonist in horses with naturally acquired osteochondrosis, Am J Vet Res 2004;65:110.
133. Grøndahl AM, Engeland A: Influence of radiographically detectable orthopedic changes on racing performance in Standardbred trotters, J Am Vet Med Assoc 1995;206:1013.
134. Laws EG, Richardson DW, Ross MW, et al: Racing performance of Standardbreds after conservative treatment and surgical treatment for tarsocrural osteochondrosis, Equine Vet J 1993;25:199.
135. Peremans K, Verschooten F: Results of conservative treatment of osteochondrosis of the tibiotarsal joint in the horse, J Equine Vet Sci 1997;17:322.
136. McIlwraith CW: Osteochondritis dissecans of the tibiotarsal (tarsocrural) joint, Proc Am Assoc Equine Pract 1993;39:69.
137. McIlwraith CW: Osteochondritis dissecans of the femoropatellar joint. Proc Am Assoc Equine Pract 1993;39:73.
138. Vatistas NJ, Wright IM, Dyson SJ: Comparison of arthroscopy and arthrotomy for the treatment of osteochondrotic lesions in the femoropatellar joint of horses, Vet Rec 1995;137:629.
139. McIlwraith CW: Diagnostic and Surgical Arthroscopy in the Horse, Philadelphia, 1990, Lea & Febiger.
140. Foland JW, McIlwraith CW, Trotter GW: Arthroscopic surgery for osteochondritis dissecans of the femoropatellar joint of the horse, Equine Vet J 1992;24:419.
141. Hopper SA, Bramlage LR: Postoperative racing performance of Thoroughbred weanlings and yearlings surgically treated for femoropatellar joint osteochondrosis, Proc Am Assoc Equine Pract 1996;42:168.
142. Beard WL, Bramlage LR, Schneider RK, et al: Postoperative racing performance in Standardbreds and Thoroughbreds with osteochondrosis of the tarsocrural joint: 109 cases (1984-1990), J Am Vet Med Assoc 1994;204:1655.
143. McIlwraith CW, Vorhees M: Management of osteochondritis disseccans of the dorsal aspect of the distal metacarpus and metatarsus, Proc Am Assoc Equine Pract 1990;36:547.
144. Richardson DW: Diagnosis and management of osteochondrosis and osseus cyst-like lesions. In Ross MW, Dyson SJ, editors: Diagnosis and Management of Lameness in the Horse, Philadelphia, 2003, WB Saunders.

CHAPTER 92

Subchondral Cystic Lesions

Brigitte von Rechenberg
Jörg A. Auer

DEFINITION

Subchondral cystic lesions (SCLs) are commonly referred to as *subchondral bone cysts* and are considered by some to be part of the developmental joint disease complex. SCLs in bone were once considered a coincidental finding in horses and not necessarily related to lameness or disease.[1,2] Currently they are recognized as a serious cause of lameness that can be difficult to treat.[3] They are characterized by radiolucent areas of bone (from several millimeters up to and even larger than 3 cm) often accompanied by a thin, but well-demarcated, sclerotic rim (Fig. 92-1). The center of the SCL is usually filled with a myxomatous tissue with or without fluid that resembles normal or slightly blood-tinged synovial fluid.[4] The SCL cavity was thought to be lined with a synovial-like membrane that was responsible for fluid production[5]; however, this membrane cannot be verified in all instances.[4]

SCLs can be uniloculated or multiloculated and occur usually in the subchondral bone underlying the articular cartilage in a weight-bearing area of the joint.[3-6] Occasionally they are also found in the metaphysis or close to the growth plate.[4,7]

SCLs occurring in the medial femoral condyle of the horse have been classified into three types according to Howard and colleagues.[1] Type 1 lesions are 10 mm or less in depth and have a shallow saucer or dome-shaped, concave appearance. Type 2 lesions exceed 10 mm in depth and typically are domed, conical, or spherical. Type 3 lesions

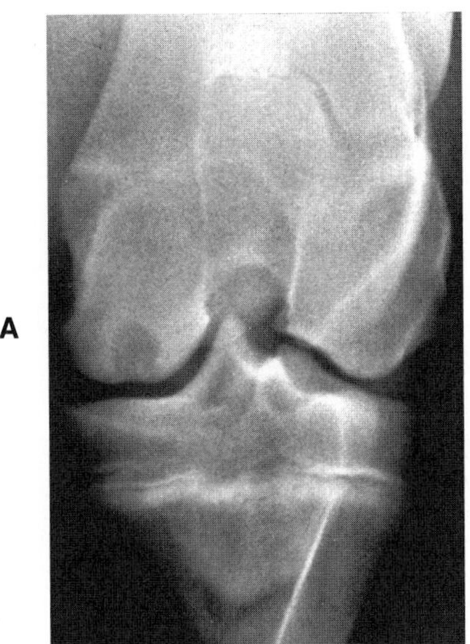

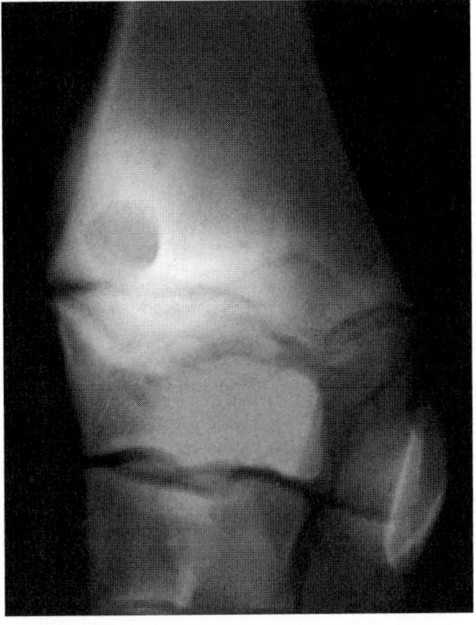

Figure 92-1. **A,** Radiographic view of a subchondral cystic lesion (SCL) in the medial femoral condyle of the stifle joint of a 3-year-old mare. The lesion is in the center of the weight-bearing area of the condyle and shows as a radiolucency, well demarcated from the surrounding normal bone by a thin sclerotic rim. **B,** Radiographic view of a SCL in the distal radius of a young foal. Note the periosteal new bone formation at the dorsomedial metaphysis.

have a flattened or irregular contour, or both. A similar classification system was proposed by Jeffcott and Kold, but lesions were divided into two types[6,8]: group A corresponds to the type 1 and 2 lesions of Howard and colleagues,[1] and group B includes type 3 lesions as well as those in the proximal part of the tibia.

In the past, SCLs were considered part of the osteochondrosis (OC) complex.[9-11] However, recently they were shown to be inflammatory in origin.[7] In addition, the location of OC lesions is different from that of SCLs. Normally, OC lesions occur at the transition from the weight-bearing to the non–weight-bearing articular surface,[11] whereas SCLs are found underneath the cartilage in a weight-bearing area of the joint.[4]

ETIOLOGY AND PATHOGENESIS

Many pathologic mechanisms leading to the development of SCL have been proposed. However, only two hypotheses have been supported experimentally in horses.

The first hypothesis is based on a hydraulic theory and was supported by an experiment in which a slit-like lesion created in the articular cartilage led to the development of SCLs over a period of several months.[12] Other coincidental findings of SCLs in experiments using osteochondral grafting procedures support this theory, because SCLs developed at the host–graft interface between the osteochondral transplants and the host bone.[13-15] These experiments had a common denominator: there was primary cartilage damage followed by secondary intrusion of synovial fluid. The fluid was thought to be responsible for mechanical pressure on the subchondral bone through its hydraulic action during weightbearing.

The second hypothesis evolved around cellular and molecular mechanisms, where inflammation could be demonstrated in tissues and cystic fluid harvested from SCLs in horses. The fibrous tissue harvested from the center of the lesion contained elevated concentrations of the local pro-inflammatory mediator prostaglandin E_2 (PGE_2), which also was found in high concentration in the cystic fluid.[16] In addition, an up-regulation of mRNA of interleukin 1 (IL-1) and IL-6 was documented in the SCL. Using quantitative real-time polymerase chain reaction (qRT-PCR), an up-regulation of IL-1 could be demonstrated at the periphery and IL-6 at the center of the lesion.[17] Lastly, increased recruitment and activation of osteoclasts could be elicited in vitro when media of cultured fibrous, cystic tissue, and cystic fluid was incubated with osteoclasts isolated from 1-day-old rats (the pit resorption assay).[16] This was attributed to the combined effect of the cytokines IL-1 and IL-6 and the mediator PGE_2, which are normally elevated in clinical cases of pathologic bone resorption and inflammation.[18-20]

Other mechanisms have been suggested in the development of SCL in horses. These include primary subchondral bone damage and secondary collapse of overlying cartilage, disturbances of endochondral ossification, primary intraosseous fibroplasias or metaplasia, herniation or protrusion of synovial membrane through a small fissure in the articular surface, and vascular disturbances.[1,4,6,21] In contrast to the two theories presented earlier, none of these have been supported experimentally.

EPIDEMIOLOGY OF SUBCHONDRAL CYSTIC LESIONS

An extensive literature review[4] involving 703 lesions in 619 horses (84 bilateral) revealed that SCLs occur mainly in the medial femoral condyle (45.8%), followed by the phalanges (26.2%) including the navicular bone (18.5% of all phalanges), carpal bones (7.1%), metacarpal and metatarsal bones (6%), tibia, radius, talus, proximal sesamoid bones, humerus, patella, scapula, distal tarsal bones, and hemimandible (all less than 5%). Sex distribution revealed that 62% of SCLs occur in males (including 41% stallions and 21% geldings). Thoroughbreds represented the majority of affected animals (39.5%), followed by Quarter Horses (14.1%), Crossbreds (12.2%), Standardbreds (9.9%), Arabian horses (8.5%), and Warmbloods (7.3%), with less than 5% in various other breeds. It seems that Warmbloods were overrepresented with cysts occurring in the phalanges,[22] often in combination with osteoarthritis, mostly in the phalangeal joints.[3,23]

CLINICAL SYMPTOMS

Horses are often presented with lameness in the affected limb with or without joint effusion.[1] Lameness is attributed to increased intracystic or intraosseous pressure, or both.[12] SCLs occur mostly in young horses between the ages of 1 and 3 years, when lameness commonly appears at the onset of training.[4] If SCLs are seen in older horses (Warmbloods), they often are accompanied by osteoarthritis (Fig. 92-2) and associated with a poor prognosis.[1] Although the onset of lameness can be acute, the lesions are usually longstanding, having been formed over time.

SCLs usually can be localized using routine lameness examinations followed by standard radiographic views of the affected joints. In rare cases, SCLs cannot be visualized using routine radiographic techniques,[1,5] and computed tomography has been of great value (Fig. 92-3). In a recent report, a variety of occult lesions in various bones of the tarsus, which were not radiographically visible, were localized using scintigraphy and confirmed with computed tomography.[24] SCLs can also be found unexpectedly during exploratory arthroscopic examination.

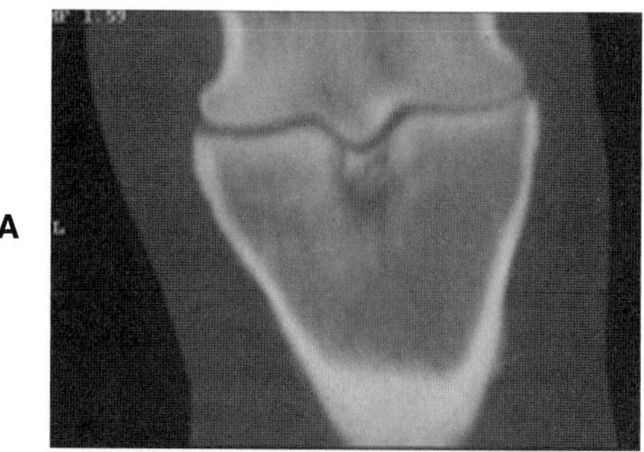

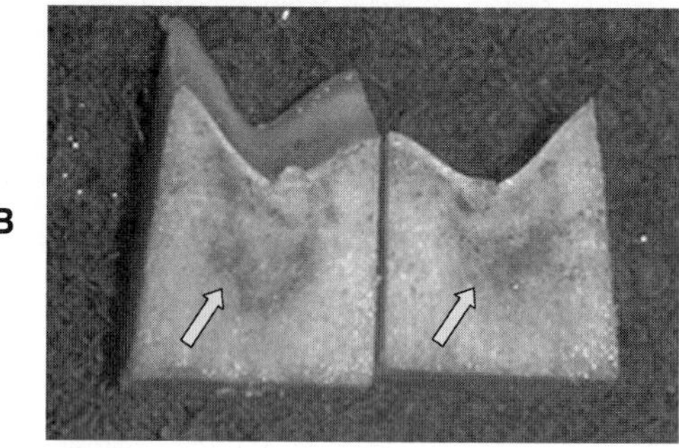

Figure 92-3. A, Computed tomographic image of a subchondral cystic lesion (SCL) in the metacarpophalangeal joint of a 4-year-old Warmblood mare, which was not clearly apparent on radiographs. **B,** The postmortem specimens demonstrate that the SCL is not completely formed and that bone was still present within the SCL cavity.

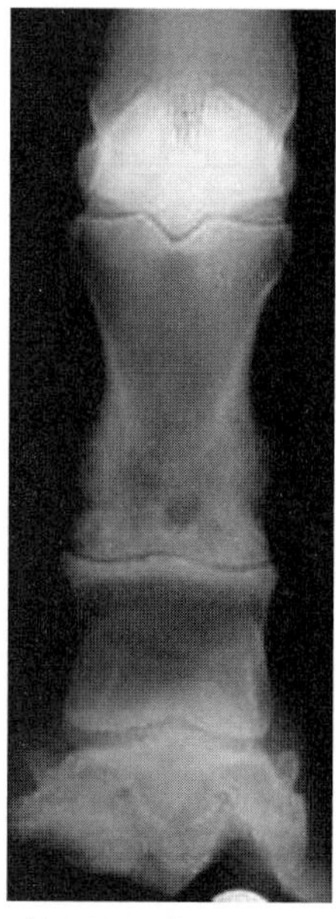

Figure 92-2. Radiographic view of a subchondral cystic lesion in the distal aspect of the proximal phalanx of a 9-year-old Warmblood gelding. The lesion is accompanied by osteoarthritis of the proximal interphalangeal joint.

Joint communication between the SCL and the overlying joint occurs only in a third of affected animals[4] and often can only be visualized during arthroscopic surgery (Fig. 92-4) if the overlying cartilage collapses into the SCL. The cartilage overlying an SCL might be normal except close to the canal, where signs of matrix degradation can be detected (Fig. 92-5). In cases where SCLs are associated with osteoarthritis, signs pertinent to osteoarthritic cartilage lesions are present (see Chapter 83).

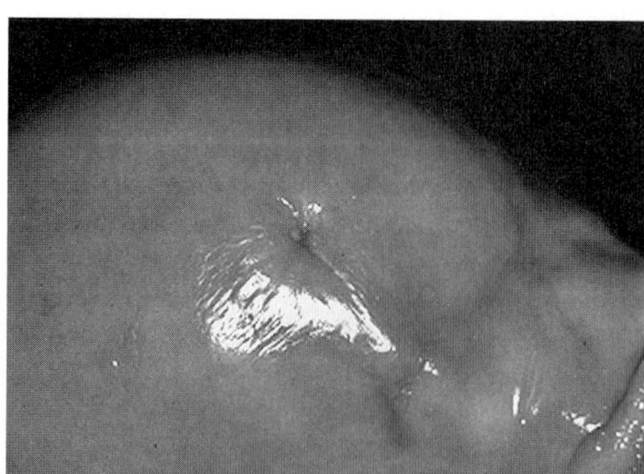

Figure 92-4. Postmortem specimen of a femoral condyle demonstrating a communication of a subchondral cystic lesion with the joint, which occurs in only 30% of the cases.

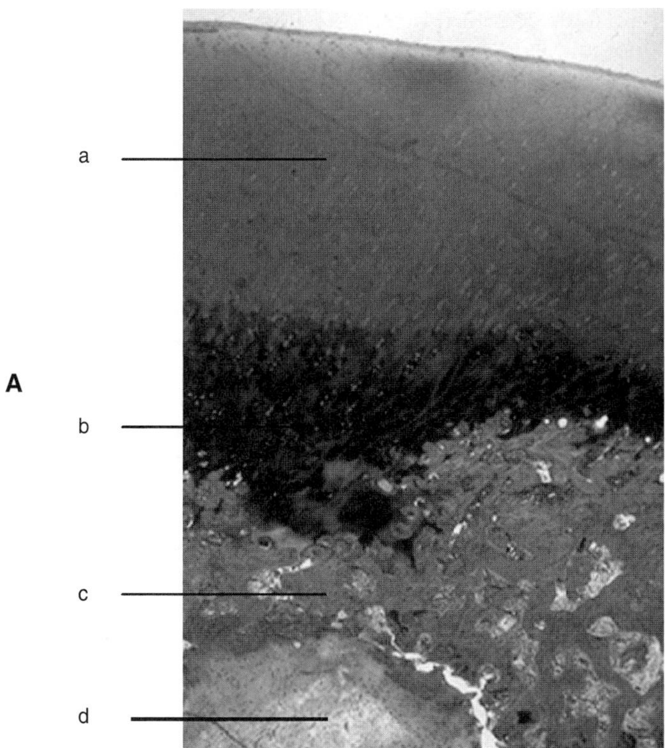

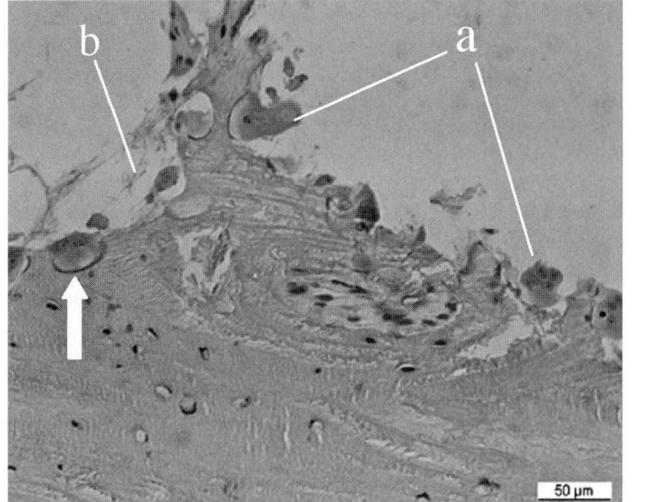

Figure 92-5. Histology specimen of a typical subchondral cystic lesion (SCL) of a horse. **A,** The cartilage overlying the SCL is normal except where it communicates with the joint. a, normal articular cartilage; b, calcified cartilage layer; c, subchondral bone, d, cyst cavity. (Undecalcified 5-μm section, embedded in acrylic resin, stained with toluidine blue.) **B,** Osteoclasts (a) are lining the calcified bone (b) at the periphery of the SCL. The lacunae are easily recognizable. (Undecalcified 5-μm section, embedded in acrylic resin, Pentachrom Movat stain.)

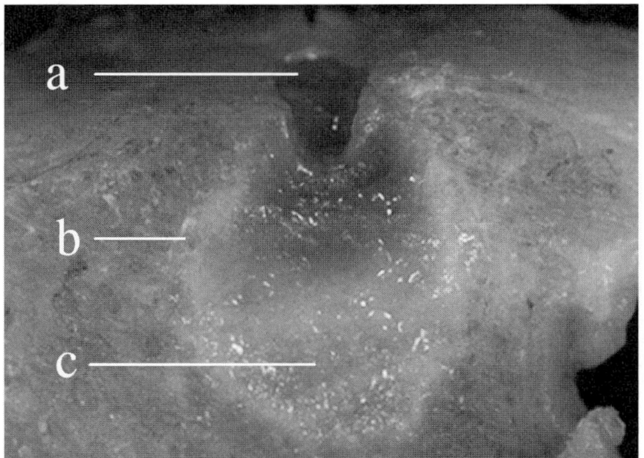

Figure 92-6. Postmortem specimen of a distal sesamoid bone showing a subchondral cystic lesion (SCL) in cross-section. a, communication into the joint; b, sclerotic border of the SCL; c, the contents of the SCL consist of a mixture of fibrous tissue, fibrocartilage, and necrotic bone and can be filled with synovial-like fluid.

Tissues harvested from SCLs at the time of surgery or necropsy (Fig. 92-6) reveal dense fibrous or myxomatous tissue containing necrotic bone, calcified or mineralized areas, or fibrocartilage in some instances.[4,8,21] The cystic wall consists of elongated fibroblasts aligned parallel to collagen bundles, scattered macrophages, and polymorphonuclear cells. Hypervascularity and thickened bone trabeculae can be noticed in the adjacent bone.[4]

MANAGEMENT OF SUBCHONDRAL CYSTIC LESIONS

Conservative treatment of SCLs using nonsteroidal anti-inflammatory drugs (NSAIDs), vitamin supplements, and anabolic drugs is not recommended because it is successful in only 33% of cases.[4] Surgical débridement of the lesion with a thorough curettage of the cystic tissue and lining is considered the treatment of choice, because a postoperative soundness up to 74% can be expected.[1,4]

The animal is anesthetized and, depending upon the location of the SCL, the preference of the surgeon, and the approach selected, the patient is positioned in lateral or dorsal recumbency on the surgery table. The surgical site is prepared for aseptic surgery and draped. Surgical débridement is performed either using an intra-articular approach[5] by arthroscopy or a trans-cortical approach.[25-27]

The arthroscope is introduced into the affected joint using routine technique. The lesion is identified either through the presence of a canal when the SCL has a communication with the joint or by a slight indentation or a "Mercedes star" irregularity. With the help of a hypodermic needle, the location for the instrument portal is identified. A no. 11 scalpel is used to make a small incision through the skin and into the joint along the needle path. The blunt obturator is used to identify the cyst either by advancing it through the small articular cartilage opening or by pushing it through the soft, slightly movable cartilage into the cyst.

A rongeur can be used to remove the articular cartilage overlying the SCL. A motorized cartilage resector also may be used to remove the cartilage, but it is often cumbersome and time consuming, because the cartilage is often too thick and pliable to be easily removed this way. Once all the cartilage not supported by underlying bone is removed, the contents of the cyst are evacuated with the help of a curet. Osteostixis of the adjacent bone is not recommended because it can lead to expansion of the cyst.[1,28]

The addition of intralesional corticosteroids at the time of surgery has been reported to improve the outcome considerably.[29] Packing the lesion with autogenous grafts also has been recommended.[30,31] However, a study comparing healing of surgically created subchondral defects filled with compacted cancellous bone grafts compared to unfilled defects revealed no difference in the healing patterns after 6 months.[32] This type of management is not used anymore. Closure of the arthroscopy portals is routine.

Some SCLs are not accessible through an articular approach and have to be débrided transosseously. Careful preplanning of the surgery is necessary.

The skin incision over the selected location is advanced down to the bone. Under fluoroscopic control, a 2.5-mm pilot hole is drilled across the bone into the cyst. If no fluoroscope is available, frequent radiographic images are needed to verify the correct drill direction. If the SCL communicates with the joint, distending it with saline solution may allow backflow through the drill hole once the drill penetrates the SCL. Once placement of the drill tip into the SCL has been verified, the drill hole is enlarged with a 5.5-mm drill bit so that it will accept a curet.

The contents of the cyst are evacuated, taking care to not traumatize the articular cartilage. This can be verified through fluoroscopy or radiography. The cystic lesion and drill hole can be filled with a cancellous bone graft. Other materials that have been used to successfully treat SCL include tricalcium phosphate granules (Fig. 92-7), hydraulic injectable biodegradable cements (Fig. 92-8), and composites of hydrogels and growth factors[25,26] (Fig. 92-9). Closure of the incision is routine.

Postoperative management of both treatment techniques is the same as for any arthroscopic surgical intervention. The healing of treated SCL normally is slow and can take several months to years if just surgical débridement is used, but the approach using bone replacements seems to enhance bone healing of the curetted lesion and thus to shorten healing time considerably. Younger horses have a better prognosis for complete recovery compared to older horses. This is especially true if SCLs are associated with osteoarthritis in older patients, and a cautious prognosis should be given.

A

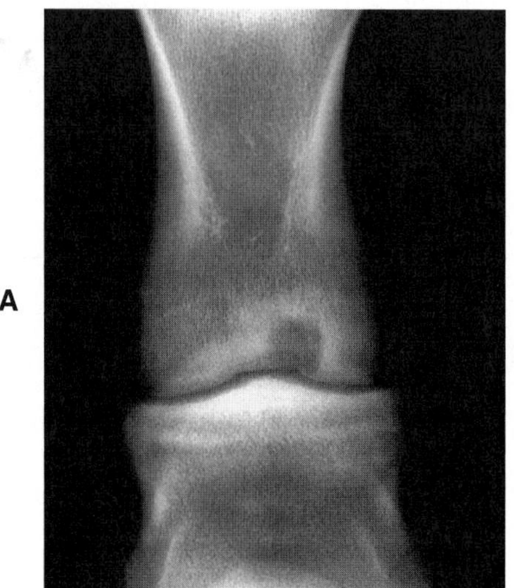

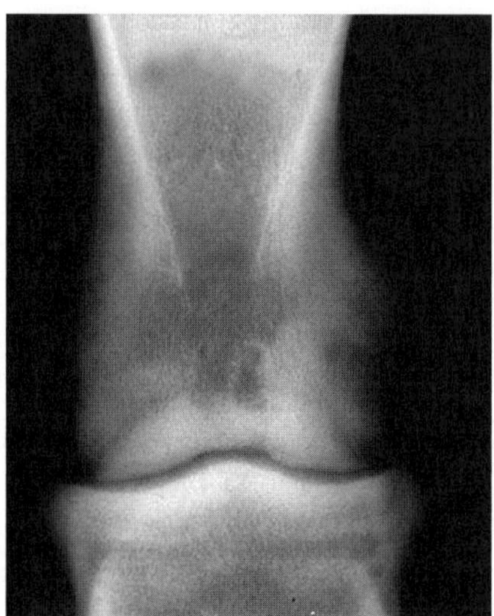

B

Figure 92-7. A, Preoperative dorsopalmar radiographic view of an SCL in the distal aspect of the proximal phalanx. The cyst was curetted and filled with tricalcium phosphate granules through a transcortical approach. **B,** Dorsopalmar radiographic view 2 years later. Complete healing has occurred.

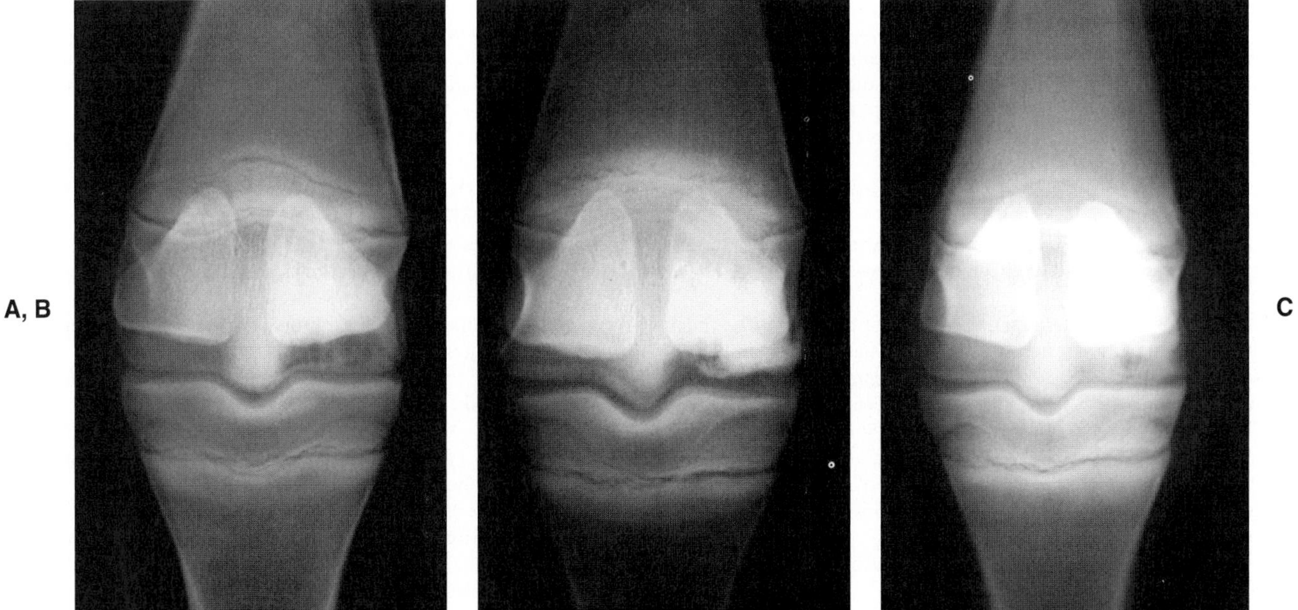

Figure 92-8. A, Dorsopalmar radiographic view of the distal MCIII depicting a cystic lesion, which involved the entire medial condyle. **B,** The defect was approached using an 8-mm diameter drill bit and filled with injectable biodegradable bone cement (chronOsInject: Synthes Inc, Solothurn, Switzerland). **C,** The 12-month follow-up radiograph shows satisfactory healing of the defect. The animal was pain free at a walk and trot.

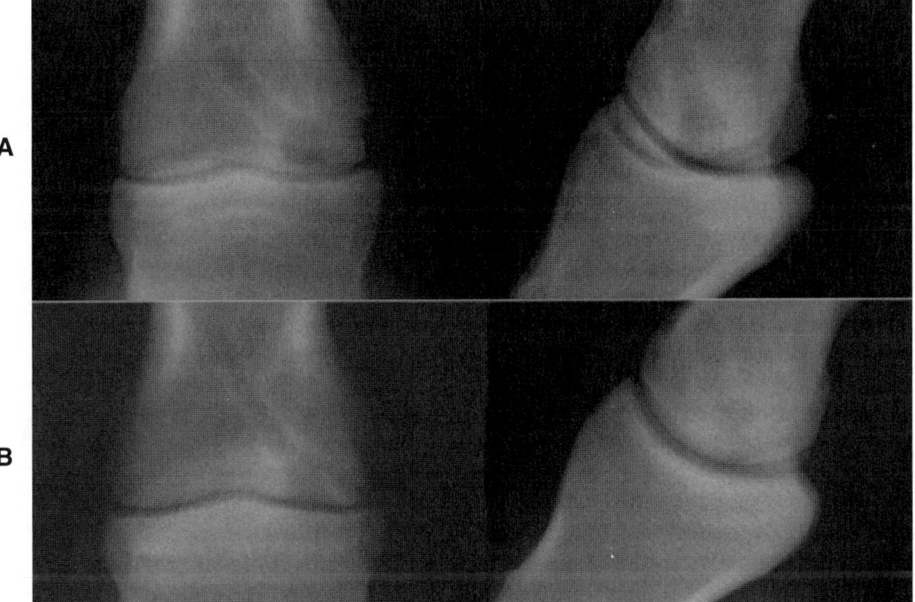

Figure 92-9. A, Immediate postoperative dorsopalmar (left) and lateromedial (right) radiographic views of a young horse with a subchondral cystic lesion (SCL) in the distal proximal phalanx. The cyst was enucleated through a transcortical approach and was treated with fibrin-based hydrogel and $PTH_{1\text{-}34}$. **B,** Four-month follow-up radiographs of the horse seen in **A**. Note that bone density has increased considerably and the SCL is hardly visible on radiographs.

REFERENCES

1. Howard RD, McIlwraith CW, Trotter GW: Arthroscopic surgery for subchondral cystic lesions of the medial femoral condyle in horses: 41 cases (1988-1991), J Am Vet Med Assoc 1995;206:842.
2. Petterson H, Sevelius F: Subchondral bone cysts in the horse: A clinical study, Equine Vet J 1966;1:75.
3. McIlwraith CW: Subchondral cystic lesions (osteochondrosis) in the horse, Comp Cont Ed 1982;4:394.
4. Rechenberg BV, McIlwraith CW, Auer JA: Cystic bone lesions in horses and humans: A comparative review, Vet Comp Orthop Traumatol 1998;11:8.
5. McIlwraith CW: Subchondral cystic lesions in the horse: The indications, methods and results of surgery, Equine Vet Educ 1990;2:75.
6. Kold SE: Clinical, Radiological and Therapeutical Aspects of Subchondral Bone Cysts in the Equine Femoro-Tibial Joint: A Clinical Investigation and Experimental Study. Thesis, Equine Clinical Unit, Animal Health Trust, Newmarket, England, Aarhus, Denmark, 1899, University Institute of Pathology.
7. Rechenberg BV: Subchondral Cystic Lesions in Horses. Thesis, Zurich 1999, University of Zurich.
8. Jeffcott LB, Kold SE: Clinical and radiological aspects of stifle bone cysts in the horse, Equine Vet J 1982;14:40.
9. Jeffcott L, Savage C: Nutrition and the development of osteochondrosis (dyschondroplasia), Pferdeheilkunde 1996;12:338.
10. Jeffcott LB: Osteochondrosis: An international problem for the horse industry, J Equine Vet Sci 1996;16:32.
11. McIlwraith CW: Inferences from referred clinical cases of osteochondrosis, Equine Vet J Suppl 1993;16:27.
12. Kold SE, Hickman J: An experimental study of the healing process of equine chondral and osteochondral defects, Equine Vet J 1986;18:18.
13. Ray CS, Baxter GS, McIlwraith CW, et al: Development of subchondral cystic lesions following subchondral bone trauma in horses, Vet Surg 1994;23:414.
14. Rechenberg Bv, Akens MK, Nadler D, et al: Changes in subchondral bone in cartilage resurfacing: An experimental study in sheep using different types of osteochondral grafts, Osteoarthritis Cartilage 2003;11:265.
15. Rechenberg Bv, Akens MK, Nadler D, et al: The use of photooxidized, mushroom structured osteochondral grafts for cartilage resurfacing: A comparison to photooxidized cylindrical grafts in an experimental study in sheep, Osteoarthritis Cartilage 2004;12:201.
16. Rechenberg Bv, McIlwraith CW, Guenther H, et al: Fibrous tissue of subchondral cystic lesions (SCL) in horses produce inflammatory mediators and matrix metalloproteinases and cause bone resorption in vitro, Vet Surg 2000;29:420.
17. Rechenberg Bv, Leutenegger CM, Zlinszky K, et al: Upregulation of mRNA of interleukin-1 and 6 in subchondral cystic lesions of four horses, Equine Vet J 2000;33:143.
18. Manolagas SC, Jilka RL, Girasole G, et al: Estrogen, cytokines, and the control of osteoclast formation and bone resorption in vitro and in vivo, Osteoporosis Int Suppl 1993;1:114.
19. Mundy GR: Inflammatory mediators and the destruction of bone, J Periodont Res 1991;26:213.
20. Lorenzo JA: The role of cytokines in the regulation of local bone resorption, Crit Rev Immunol 1991;11:195.
21. Jeffcott LB, Kold SE: Aspects of the pathology of stifle bone cysts in the horse, Equine Vet J 1983;15:304.
22. Haack D, Hertsch B, Baez C: Zystoide Defekte im Hufbein des Pferdes, Pferdeheilkunde 1988;4:143.
23. Trotter GW, McIlwraith CW: Osteochondritis dissecans and subchondral cystic lesions and their relationship to osteochondrosis in the horse, Equine Vet Sci 1981;1:156.
24. Garcia-Lopez JM, Kirker-Head CA: Occult subchondral osseous cyst-like lesions of the equine tarsocrural joint, Vet Surg 2004;33:557.
25. Deiss E, Fuerst A, Haas C, et al: Symptomatik, Diagnostik und Therapie von 5 Pferden mit traumatischen subchondralen Knochenzysten, Wien Tierarztl Mschr 2001;88:1.
26. Fürst A, Kaegi B, Rechenberg Bv, et al: Die Behandlung von 5 Pferden mit subchondralen zystoiden Defekten im Fesselbein, Pferdeheilkunde 1997;13:147.
27. Kold S, Hickman J: Three cases of subchondral bone cysts in the distal limb of the horse treated by bone grafting via an extra-articular approach, Equine Vet Educ 1990;2:70.
28. Bertone AL, McIlwraith CW, Powers BE, et al: Subchondral osseous cystic lesions of the elbow of horses: Conservative versus surgical treatment, J Am Vet Med Assoc 1986;189:540.
29. McIlwraith CW: Personal communication, 2003.
30. Kold SE, Hickman J: Results of treatment of subchondral bone cysts in the medial condyle of the equine femur with an autogenous cancellous bone graft, Equine Vet J 1984;16:414.
31. Kold SE, Hickman J: Use of an autogenous cancellous bone graft in the treatment of subchondral bone cysts in the medial femoral condyle of the horse, Equine Vet J 1983;15:312.
32. Jackson WA, Stick JA, Arnoczky SP, et al: The effect of compacted cancellous bone grafting on the healing of subchondral bone defects of the medial femoral condyle in horses, Vet Surg 2000;29:8.

CHAPTER 93

Foot

Anton E. Fürst
Christophorus J. Lischer

A multitude of disorders affect the equine foot. Once the problem is diagnosed, a decision has to be made whether to treat it conservatively or surgically. In some conditions, surgery serves as an option after conservative management has failed to bring about an improvement. For other problems, surgical intervention is the best or even the only treatment option. In this chapter, frequently encountered disorders of the foot managed by surgery are discussed.

DISORDERS OF THE HOOF CAPSULE

Often, changes in the hoof horn quality are noticed that jeopardize the use of the horse for competition or pleasure riding.[1,2] The old saying "no hoof, no horse" still holds true even nowadays with all the sophisticated treatment possibilities available in veterinary medicine, which clearly affirms the importance healthy hooves have for the everyday use of horses. Therefore, special attention should be given to the feet not only during lameness evaluations but also during prepurchase examinations, where the clinician is asked to provide the potential new owner of the horse with a statement regarding the future usefulness of the horse for its intended purpose.

Many hoof problems have a number of predisposing causes, such as faulty feeding regimens, including vitamin and mineral deficiencies, as well as excessive and uncontrolled work load, especially on hard and dry ground. Poor hygiene and inadequate hoof care propagate hoof problems because urine and manure weaken or in some cases destroy horn integrity. Trimming and shoeing practices can exacerbate problems with hooves that initially had minimal changes in horn quality. The hoof capsule can be damaged by different external insults. Last but not least, some horses are born with hooves of decreased quality, possibly triggered by genetic factors. These animals may be predisposed to hoof problems despite good stall hygiene, excellent feeding practices, and adequate exercise. Supplementation with biotin improves horn quality over time in some horses.[1,2]

Thrush

Etiology and Diagnosis

Thrush refers to infection that leads to necrotic processes in the frog area, especially in the central and lateral sulci.[3] The sulci become soft and slimy and emit a characteristic foul-smelling odor commonly recognized with this disorder. Horn damage can progress to involve the sensitive lamina; then it is referred to as pododermatitis. As a result of the soft nature of the altered horn, foreign body penetration is more likely.

Manure and urine accumulation in the foot dissolve horn in the frog area in association with bacteria and fungi. Therefore, this condition is seen in conjunction with poor stall hygiene and neglected hoof care. However, a contracted hoof and lack of exercise can also predispose a hoof to thrush. Different bacteria and fungi have been shown to colonize the horn of the frog and eventually destroy it.[4-6]

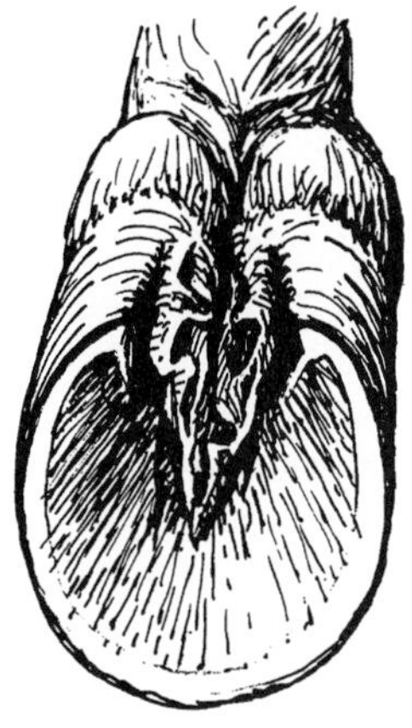

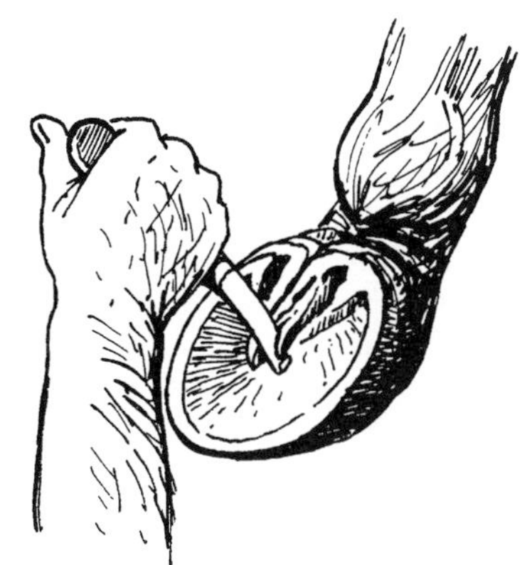

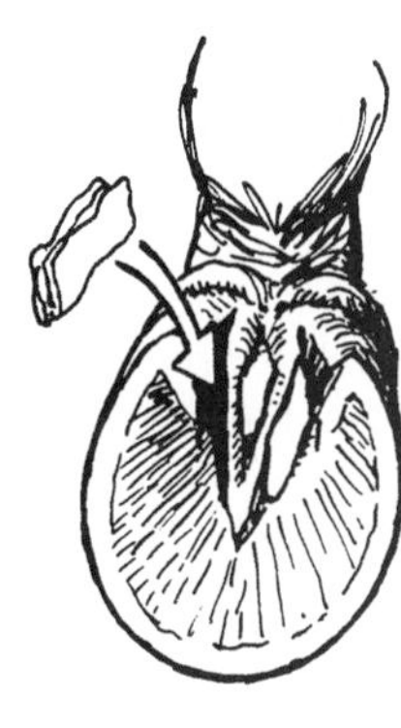

Figure 93-1. Hoof affected with thrush *(above)*. Initially the collateral sulci of the frog are thoroughly cleaned and subsequently medicated *(below)*.

Treatment and Aftercare

Meticulous hoof care and good stall hygiene are an important part of resolving this condition along with local treatment of the altered horn in the frog area. Box stalls should be thoroughly cleaned at regular intervals, and all urine-soaked straw or wood shavings should be removed. The sulci of the frog need to be cleaned twice daily to remove any manure packed into the hoof sole.

All damaged horn is removed, which effectively reduces bacteria and fungi colonization and provides better contact of locally applied medications to the affected tissues (Fig. 93-1). After removing the diseased horn, the sulci are cleaned with a disinfecting solution.[7] In cases where the sensitive lamina is involved, a protective bandage containing sponges soaked in povidone-iodine (Betadine) should be applied for a few days. Subsequently, the sulci are treated with solutions possessing disinfectant, drying, and hardening properties.[7] In most cases, solutions containing formalin in one form or another are used. These solutions are applied to gauze sponges or small cotton balls and pushed into the affected sulci.

The majority of thrush medication is toxic to epithelium, and therefore must be applied with utmost care, especially in the presence of severe horn damage and sensitive lamina. It is better to initiate treatment with povidone-iodine–soaked sponges and proceed to stronger medications once a thin horn layer has grown over the defect.

Prognosis

Horses suffering from thrush are predisposed to acquiring the problem again, mainly when the inciting causes of inadequate stall hygiene and neglect in hoof care and exercise have not been resolved. Therefore, complete resolution of the problem is possible only if good hygiene is maintained for the rest of the horse's life.

White Line Disease

Etiology and Diagnosis

White line disease refers to deterioration of the white line of the hoof capsule, resulting in the loss of the bond between the hoof wall and the sole. White line disease is incited through the presence of poor-quality horn, which allows the colonization of different bacteria and fungi.[8] These microorganisms are not able to grow in normal horn of the white line. They are more commonly encountered in geographic regions with a warm and humid climate.

Once the hoof wall begins to separate from the sole, the hoof wall is exposed to increased tensional forces, which leads to the development of inflammatory processes in the sensitive lamina; lameness is the result. Additionally, the selective placement of hoof nails into the white line is jeopardized, preventing solid attachment of horseshoes to the foot. If the necrotic processes extend farther proximally, entire parts of the hoof wall may be undermined and eventually form a hollow wall.

Treatment and Aftercare

Treatment consists of meticulous stall hygiene and local management of the affected hooves. All the altered and necrotic horn must be removed and the defects treated with solutions to destroy the remaining bacteria and fungi. The solutions used are the same ones used to manage thrush (see earlier). The débridement might need to include hoof wall resection (see later).

Hollow or Loose Hoof Wall

Etiology and Diagnosis

A hollow or loose hoof wall develops when there is a disruption of the most axial layers of the hoof wall, near the sensitive lamina[9] (Fig. 93-2). A loose, hollow wall can develop from an extension of white line disease. In other cases, bleeding into the hoof wall seems to be the inciting cause. Chronic tearing as a result of continuous excessive use can lead to a separation within the hoof wall. As an example, 50 years ago, hollow walls were commonly diagnosed in pulling horses. Soil, bacteria, and fungi can get access to the dead space between the hoof wall layers and induce a local infection.

As long as no infection is present and the sensitive lamina is not involved, it is possible to apply horseshoes to the foot. However, there is always a risk that the hollow wall will continue to extend proximally, which makes treatment more difficult. Therefore, effective treatment of a hollow wall should be initiated early in the course of events, especially in the presence of an infection.

Treatment and Aftercare

Successful therapy can be achieved only if all diseased, necrotic horn is removed. The remaining hoof defect must be treated with solutions effective against bacteria and fungi, using moist hoof bandages. Depending on the extent of the hollow wall, a considerable amount of horn may have to be removed (Fig. 93-3, *A*), which can result in a prolonged convalescent period. Treatment can last several months and the problem must be completely resolved before the horse can be ridden again.

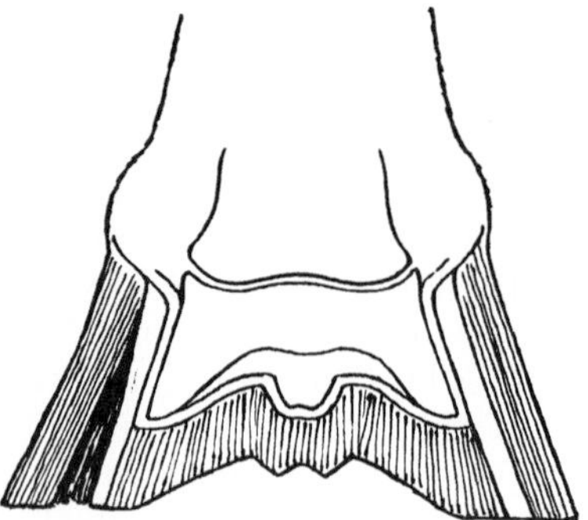

Figure 93-2. Hoof with a hollow wall shown on the left *(dark area)*.

Several artificial hoof products are on the market that allow the lost hoof wall to be replaced effectively. Products such as Keralit (Scheule GmbH, Kirchheim, Germany) or Sigafoos (Horsetec AG, Zeihen, Switzerland) have characteristics similar to normal hoof wall in respect to stability and flexibility, and they are ideally suited to replace horn defects.[10,11] The artificial horn products contain two components that are mixed together and develop into a sticky, easily moldable mass. Once molded into the clean and dry hoof wall defect, artificial horn is subsequently shaped to the contours of the hoof wall (see Fig. 93-3, *B*). Within a few minutes, the material hardens into hornlike material. The hoof replacement material can be reinforced with fiberglass webbing for additional strength.

The advantages of these products are that the susceptible laminae are covered with a durable protective layer, which increases the stability of the entire hoof wall. The artificial hoof wall also allows the placement of a horseshoe (see Fig. 93-3, *C*).

As a result of the continuous growth in the rest of the hoof wall, the artificial hoof wall has to be replaced repeatedly. There is a potential danger that an infection can

A, B

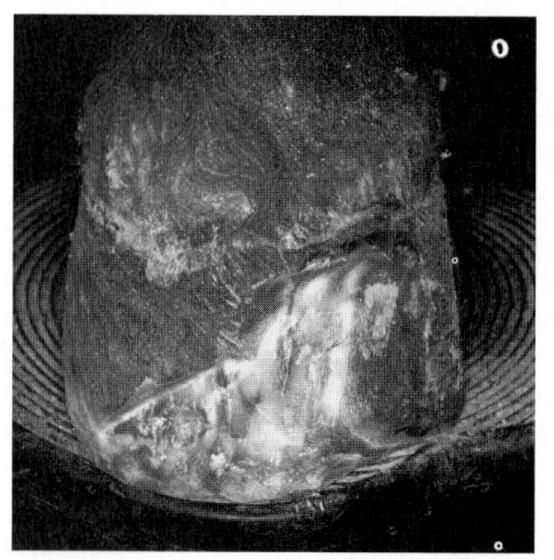

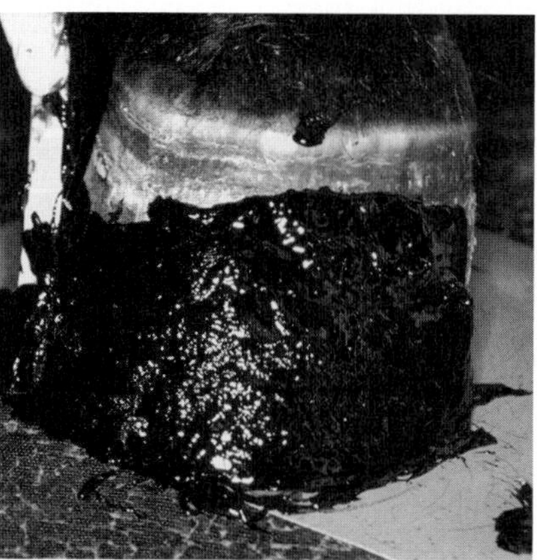

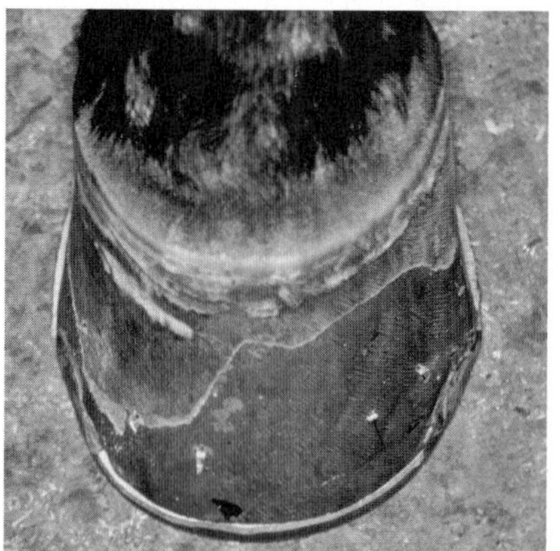

C

Figure 93-3. A hollow hoof wall is removed (**A**), the defect is filled with artificial horn (**B**), and a shoe is nailed to the foot (**C**), with nails placed into the artificial horn.

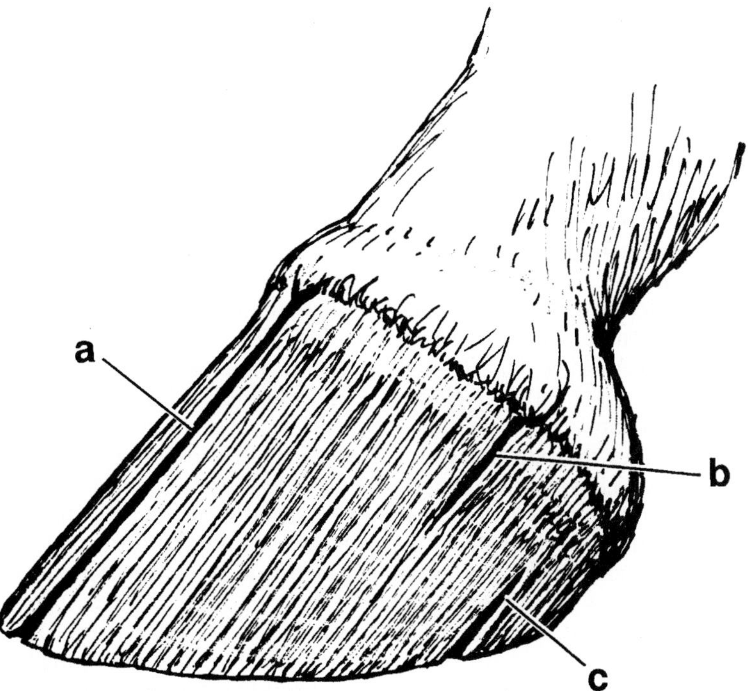

Figure 93-4. Different locations of hoof wall cracks. *a,* Dorsal crack extending over the entire length of the hoof wall. *b,* Proximal lateral hoof wall crack. *c,* distal lateral hoof wall crack.

develop under the artificial horn, necessitating its immediate removal. Therefore, careful monitoring of the healing process is required until the defect is completely replaced by new hoof wall, which will grow down from the coronary band.

Hoof Wall Cracks

Etiology

A hoof wall crack represents a longitudinal disruption of the hoof wall parallel to the horn tubules and lamellae. It can involve the entire length of the hoof wall, the proximal hoof wall near the coronary band only, or the distal hoof wall only (Fig. 93-4). The crack can penetrate the superficial layers only or can extend into the sensitive lamina. These cracks are called *deep* or *perforating hoof cracks;* the perforating hoof cracks result in inflammation and lameness (Fig. 93-5). Horizontally oriented hoof defects, at an angle parallel to the coronary band, are called *hoof crevices,* but they have the same etiology and treatment as hoof cracks.

The causes of the hoof cracks are diverse. Poor horn quality or a horn wall that is too thin are predisposing factors. Abnormal hoof angles can produce significant tension gradients within the hoof wall, which develop into cracks.[12]

DISTAL HOOF WALL CRACKS

Poor horn quality associated with excessive workload and poor hoof hygiene can lead to development of hoof cracks at the distal hoof wall (see Fig 93-5). Usually, these cracks are superficial initially and do not cause lameness unless they extend and develop into a perforating crack. A horizontal groove may be cut at the most proximal aspect of the crack, and the foot should be trimmed very short to prevent proximal and deep extension. If these management practices do not stop the progression of the crack, then more aggressive surgical techniques will be required (see later).

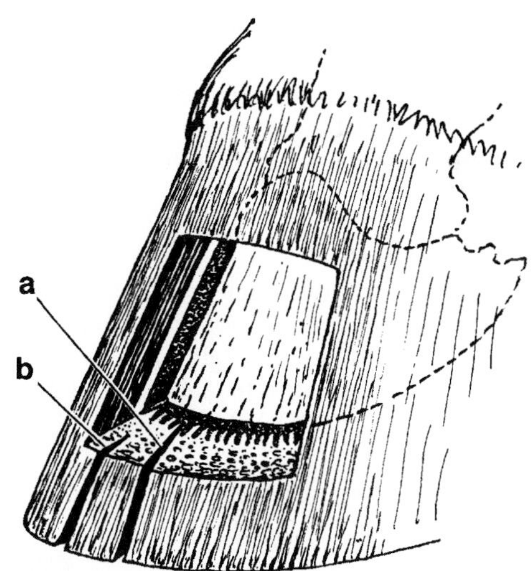

Figure 93-5. Hoof wall with a cut-away area, showing cracks penetrating to different depths. *a,* Superficial hoof wall crack. *b,* A deep or perforating hoof wall crack involving the sensitive lamina.

PROXIMAL HOOF WALL CRACKS

Proximal hoof wall cracks develop as a result of local trauma, inflammation, or scar tissue near the coronary band. Because of such damage, horn of poor quality is formed, facilitating the development of a hoof wall crack.

These cracks slowly extend distally with concomitant horn growth.

HOOF CRACKS INVOLVING THE ENTIRE LENGTH OF THE HOOF WALL

There are many etiologies of hoof cracks along the entire hoof wall, aside from local trauma to the coronary band. Most likely, tension gradients inside the hoof wall combined with extensive use and poor horn quality are major predisposing factors in their development. Often such hoof cracks are found in hooves with excessively long sidewalls (Fig. 93-6, *A* and *B*). Hoof cracks are more commonly seen on the medial hoof wall than on the lateral wall.

Uneven heels and displaced bulbs of the heel are predisposing factors. Hoof wall cracks can also be caused by faulty shoeing practices, such as shoes that are too short, branches that are too narrow or side clips applied too far back, uneven hoof soles, and hoof nails inserted too far caudally. When unphysiologic conditions such as these are present for several months, poor-quality horn can grow, predisposing the hoof wall to crack formation. The combination of long shoeing intervals and excessive work foster hoof crack development.[13]

Diagnosis

Most of the time the diagnosis is made on close visual inspection of the hoof. The deeper layers of the crack often are impacted with dirt and manure. Lameness is a prominent feature of deep or perforating hoof wall cracks. Conversely, superficial horn cracks are not associated with lameness and many do not require treatment. Nevertheless, there is always a risk that a superficial crack will extend into one that eventually initiates an inflammatory process.

Treatment and Aftercare

Because hoof cracks are encountered often and have been a common problem for hundreds of years, many treatment methods are described. However, although many methods and techniques exist, successful management of hoof cracks demands close cooperation among the clinician, the farrier, and the owner.

The type of treatment selected depends on the location and depth of the crack, and the duration of treatment can take from a few days to several weeks or even months. The first line of attack involves improvement of hoof care and shoeing.[14] The repair of the hoof crack without initial débridement can reduce the movement of the two sides relative to each other, effectively protecting the underlying sensitive laminae. In these instances, lameness will be attenuated. In rare cases, the crack can heal completely, allowing regrowth of normal horn from the coronary band distad. In most cases, however, more-involved techniques are necessary to bring about healing of the defect, especially if the crack is accompanied by infection and lameness.

First, the conditions of the shoes have to be assessed, correcting present abnormalities such as uneven heels and abnormal hoof angles. The old shoe is removed and the hoof is properly trimmed. By cutting the heels short, local pressure in the hoof wall can be partially reduced.

Subsequently, the horn adjacent to the crack is carefully removed with a Dremel tool[15] (Fig. 93-7). All altered horn down to the sensitive lamina is removed, taking special care to establish smooth transitions toward the sides. Once completely cleaned, the defect is covered with gauze sponges, and a hoof bandage is applied.

The foot is shod with a bar shoe, and the sole is filled with silicone and covered with a metal plate. This reduces pressure in the heel region, which is especially beneficial if the crack is located in this area. In some cases, the coronary band immediately proximal to the crack is displaced dorsally. Trimming the hoof wall short just below this crack reduces the continuous movement at the coronary band and leads to the production of better-quality horn.

Last, a fixation device should be applied to the crack. If the crack was débrided down to the sensitive lamina, fixation has to be delayed until a subtle layer of horn covers the defect.

An effective repair unites the two separated hoof parts and reduces individual movements at the transition to the normal horn proximally at the level of the coronary band.

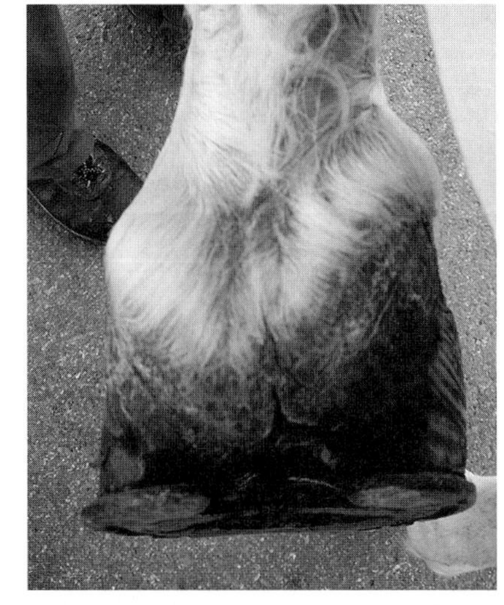

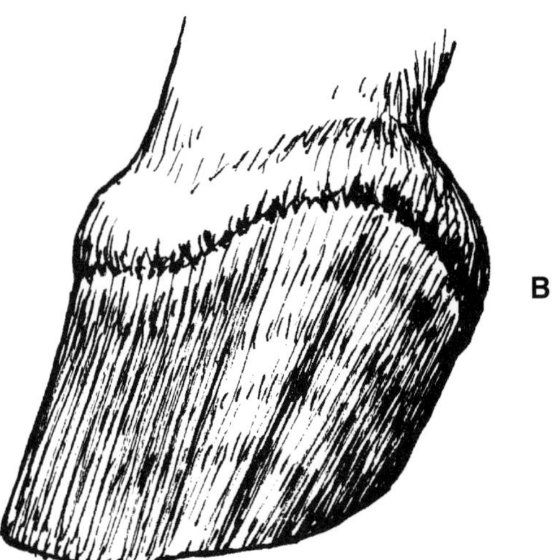

Figure 93-6. A, A hoof with a long and steep inside wall and uneven heels containing a hoof crack. **B,** Contracted hoof with a distorted coronary band and a hoof crack.

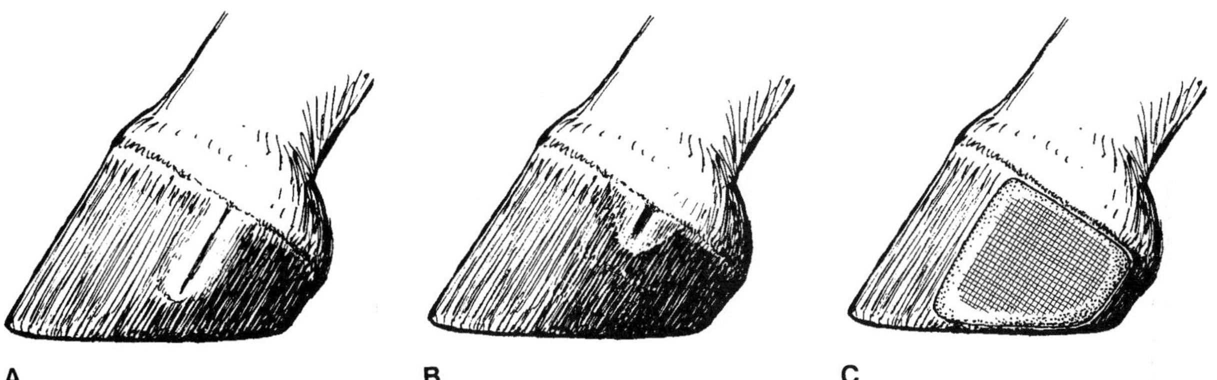

Figure 93-7. A and **B**, The hoof surrounding the crack is carefully removed, taking care to establish smooth transitions before it is covered with artificial horn (**C**).

There are a variety of methods that can be used to repair a hoof crack (Fig. 93-8). The introduction of the two-component hoof replacement materials mentioned earlier have significantly improved the effectiveness of hoof crack repair.[11] These materials provide a natural covering of the crack with a material having properties similar to the normal hoof wall. These materials cure with an exothermic reaction. Therefore, it is important that at least a thin layer of horn be present to protect the sensitive lamina. It is even possible to install a drainage system underneath the artificial horn.

The hoof wall must be covered over almost its entire length to prevent a recurrence of a crack (Fig. 93-9). Poor horn quality might dictate that a covering of artificial horn be maintained for several months. New horn growing from the coronary band eventually completely replaces the repaired hoof wall.

Immediately after the repair, the patient should be kept in a stall for a few days before gradually being returned to exercise. Depending on the quantity and quality of new horn production, the patient may be lightly used after 4 to 8 weeks.

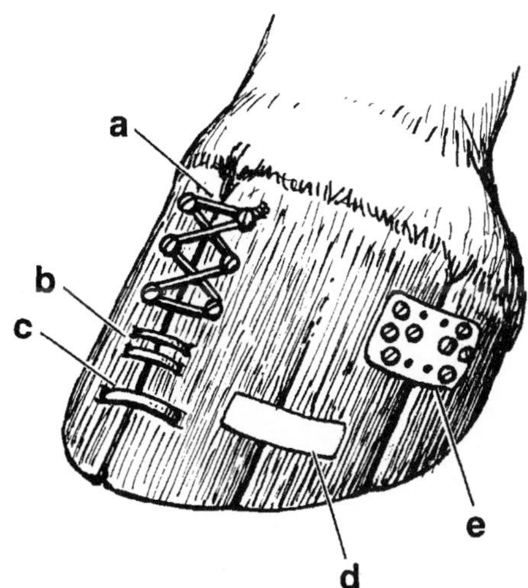

Figure 93-8. Various devices to repair hoof cracks. *a,* Umbilical tape laced around small protruding screws in the hoof wall. *b* and *c,* Different clamps whose sharp points were tapped into the hoof wall. *d,* A metal plate glued over the crack, *e,* A metal plate spanning the crack fixed to the hoof wall with small screws.

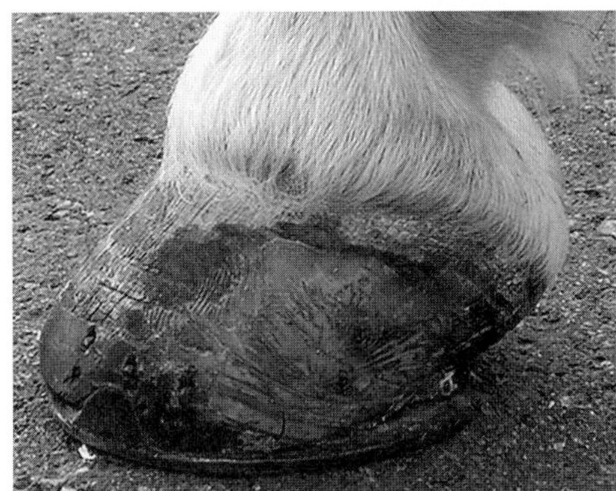

Figure 93- 9. A hoof crack covered with artificial horn.

Prognosis

The prognosis for a successful treatment of a hoof crack is good to guarded. Often, the crack recurs, especially if the predisposing factors are not abolished (Fig. 93-10). Because the properties of the horn vary with the location on the hoof,[16-18] the prognosis varies as well.

Keratoma

Etiology

A keratoma represents a columnar thickening of the hoof horn that extends toward the inside of the hoof (Fig. 93-11). Because it is rare, the disorder is often overlooked. In addition to the classic keratoma, with its cylindrical appearance and protrusion parallel to the horn tubules, a spherical form of keratoma has been described that can develop anywhere in the hoof capsule.[19]

Most keratomas are found in the dorsal aspect of the wall. A local inflammation reaction or trauma at the transition of the new horn produced at the coronary band and hoof wall is the most likely inciting cause. This results in the formation of scar tissue in that location, which gradually grows distad as new horn is produced.

A hoof abscess also can lead to the development of a keratoma. Because of the expansiveness of the keratoma, unphysiologic pressures are exerted on the sensitive laminae and the distal phalanx, leading to inflammation and lysis of

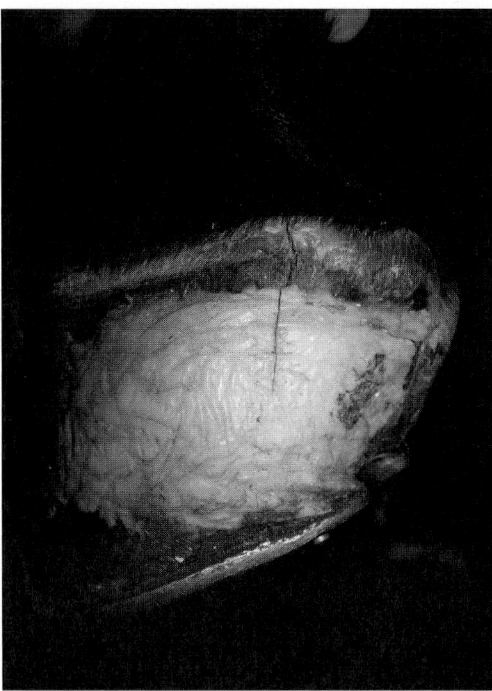

Figure 93-10. An inadequate repair with artificial horn led to recurrence, with the crack extending partially across the artificial horn.

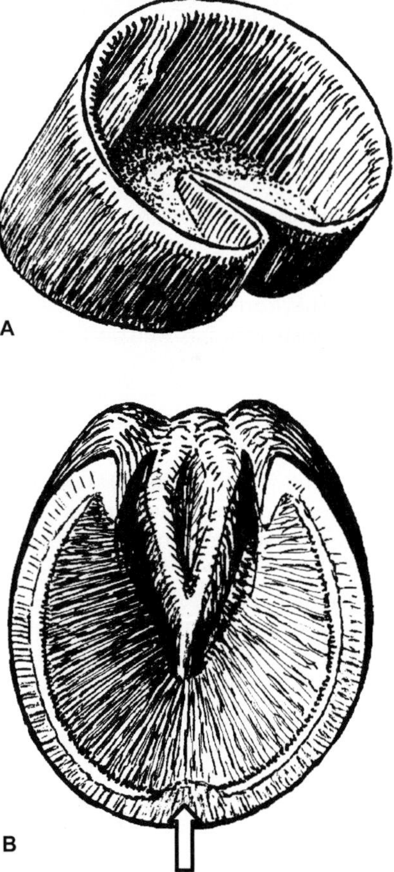

Figure 93-11. Keratoma in the hoof shell. **A,** Representation from the inside. **B,** First manifestation at the median of the white line *(arrow)*.

the underlying distal phalanx. The keratoma consists of poor quality horn, which decays early, allowing bacteria and fungi access to the inside of the hoof wall. Therefore, keratomas are often associated with local hoof wall infections and are the reason horses are presented to veterinarians. If a patient is presented with a chronic recurrent hoof abscess, it is prudent to assume a keratoma is the actual cause of the problem.

Diagnosis

Careful inspection of the sole is important for the diagnosis. Trimming and cleaning of the sole surface is necessary to recognize the abnormal configuration of the white line. Typically, the lamellar horn of the white line is replaced by tubular horn and scar tissue (Fig. 93-12 *A*). The pathologic tissue displaces the white line toward the sole. In advanced cases, a circular lytic area of the distal phalanx can be

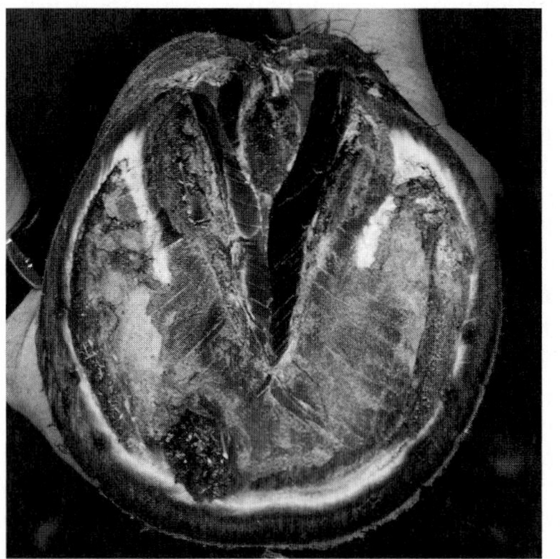

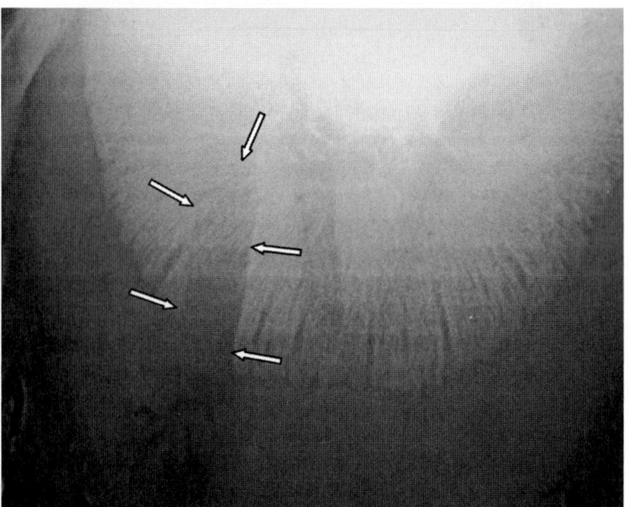

Figure 93-12. A, Clinical case with a local chronic infection in the sole. **B,** Radiograph of the same patient showing a lytic area in the distal phalanx extending up along the hoof wall (surrounding *white arrows*), which is typical of a keratoma.

recognized radiographically (see Fig. 93-12 *B*). This area should not be mistaken for the naturally occurring crena at the dorsal aspect of the distal margin of the distal phalanx. Often, a sclerotic border delineates the lytic area (see Fig. 93-12 *B*).

Treatment and Aftercare

In selected cases, it is possible to temporarily abolish the signs of a keratoma with the help of conservative management. However, even with meticulous hoof care and good hygiene it is not always possible to prevent the formation of a hoof abscess. Therefore, an early surgical approach toward solving the problem is advised. For successful resolution, two main principles must be observed[19,20]: the keratoma must be completely removed up to its origin, and support has to be given to the hoof wall.

The timing of the surgery depends to a certain extent on the condition of the patient and the intentions of the owner. The main dilemma is whether to first manage the inflammatory processes medically and remove the keratoma once it has resolved, or to immediately enucleate the structure. The choice should be based on the amount of pain shown by the patient; early intervention may be indicated in very lame patients to avoid laminitis in the contralateral foot. Aside from the altered horn, the altered sensitive laminae also must be removed. The hoof wall defect may be filled with artificial horn as soon as the sensitive lamina is healed. Additionally, a special shoe with large clips placed on either side of the defect should be applied to the foot.

The surgical intervention is performed in two steps, with a tourniquet applied above the foot. First, as much horn as possible is removed with the horse standing until the Dremel tool has to be exchanged for the scalpel and curets. The second stage of the procedure is carried out under aseptic conditions, and the altered lamina and the entire keratoma are removed in toto. This procedure also may be carried out on the standing horse if ring block at the level of the metacarpophalangeal joint is used. The advantages of performing the removal under general anesthesia are the more comfortable position for the surgeon and immobility of the patient. It is of utmost importance to remove *all* pathologically altered tissue in addition to the altered hoof horn. The keratoma usually has a characteristically round appearance at its origin.

At the end of the procedure, an aseptic pressure bandage is applied to the phalangeal region, and the tourniquet is removed. The bandage is changed at 3- to 4-day intervals under aseptic conditions. As soon as the bone is covered by granulation tissue, a medication plate shoe is applied. The hoof wall should be preserved to provide stability to the hoof capsule.

The horse remains confined to a box stall for 4 to 6 weeks, during which the wound is treated routinely with dressings. After this time, a new shoe is applied. Depending on the healing process, different avenues may be taken. If healing progresses normally, the defect may be filled with artificial horn and the patient subjected to light walking exercise and, after approximately 4 months, light riding work. If signs of infection recur, all affected tissues have to be removed and the process of postoperative management started again.

Prognosis

With surgical treatment, a significantly better prognosis can be given (83% success rate) compared to conservative management, where an approximate success rate of 43% has been published.[21]

SEPTIC AND ASEPTIC DISORDERS OF THE SOFT TISSUES

Acute Hoof Abscesses

Etiology

"Hoof abscesses have 1000 faces." Hoof abscesses are among the most frequently diagnosed causes of lameness seen in equine practice. It is interesting to realize how many symptoms a hoof abscess may generate. It is therefore not surprising that this problem is occasionally misdiagnosed.

Hoof abscesses develop in the unshod horse—often foals—as well as in shod horses. No breed or age predispositions are known. After penetration of bacteria across the hoof wall, infection develops in the region of the sensitive lamina, which includes the accumulation of purulent material within the hoof capsule (Fig. 93-13). Because the hoof capsule provides a solid external shield, increased pressure builds up inside, leading to severe, non–weight-bearing pain. Box 93-1 lists some possible etiologies for a hoof abscess. A sole bruise is the most likely to occur.

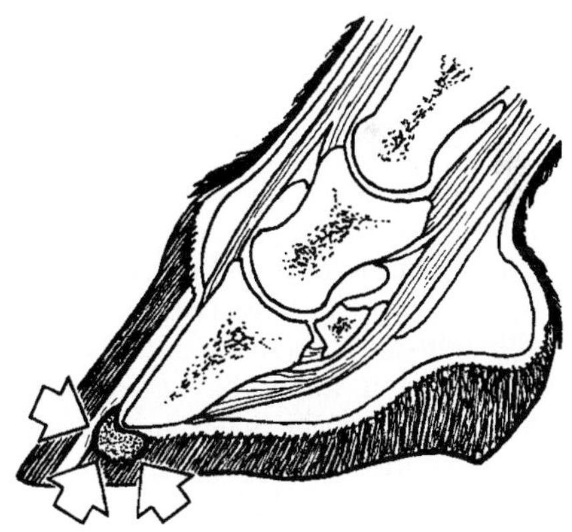

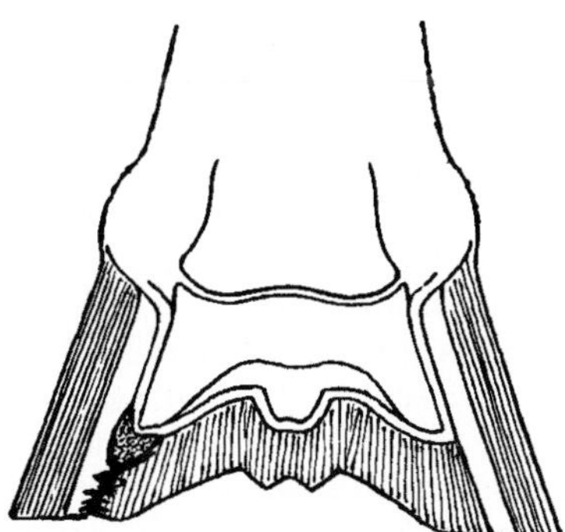

Figure 93-13. Location of a typical hoof abscess at the tip of the foot *(above)* and at the side *(below)*.

BOX 93-1. Possible Etiologies for a Hoof Abscess

- Placement of hoof nail too close to the sensitive lamina, allowing bacteria along the nail to induce an infection in close proximity to the sensitive lamina
- Insertion of a hoof nail into the sensitive lamina, resulting in an infection
- Small pointed rocks penetrating the solar horn
- Any penetrating foreign object, such as a street nail[22]
- Any sole bruise, which creates a blood culture medium for the growth of bacteria that enter the tubules in the horn normally

Diagnosis

The cardinal symptom is a sudden severe lameness, which might be described as "fracture lameness," resulting in the horse's being admitted to the clinic as a fracture patient. The horse might be febrile and have increased warmth of the foot, with strongly pulsating distal palmar and plantar arteries. A generalized swelling of the distal limb might be noticed, which can lead to the erroneous diagnosis of septic tenosynovitis or other similar conditions. Local application of pressure through the hoof tester generally elicits a marked positive response. Local perineural anesthetic blocks (deep palmar anesthesia, middle palmar/plantar anesthesia) aid in localizing the problem, allowing subsequent pain-free treatment. Complete blood count (CBC) and blood chemistry analyses are usually unrewarding, but in some cases radiography supports the tentative diagnosis of hoof abscess.

Treatment and Aftercare

If a hoof abscess is suspected, the shoe should be removed and each nail closely examined for wetness and odor. Subsequently, the exact location of the abscess is established with the help of the hoof testers. Location with the hoof tester can be difficult in the presence of thick and hard sole horn. In such a case, it might be necessary to apply a povidone-iodine or creosote bandage for overnight, which results in softening of the hoof horn, permitting localization of the abscess and subsequent drainage.

All the undermined and necrotic horn is carefully removed, piece by piece, until a smooth transition is achieved toward the surrounding normal sole (Fig. 93-14). Subsequently, the infected area is cleaned with iodine solution or H_2O_2 and covered with a povidone-iodine–soaked gauze sponge and a hoof bandage. The bandage is changed after 2 to 3 days under aseptic conditions. At that time, the defect is closely examined and any additional undermined sole is carefully removed. As soon as the site is dry, the horse can be reshod. It is prudent to cover the site with a leather or synthetic pad.

If the abscess is not managed properly or in a timely fashion, it can break through at the coronary band (Fig. 93-15) or extend deeper into the foot and involve the distal phalanx. In these cases, the draining tract has to be flushed daily with diluted povidone-iodine solution from the coronary band distad (Fig. 93-16). Distal exit of the flushing solution is important. The foot must be kept in a bandage until drainage has stopped.

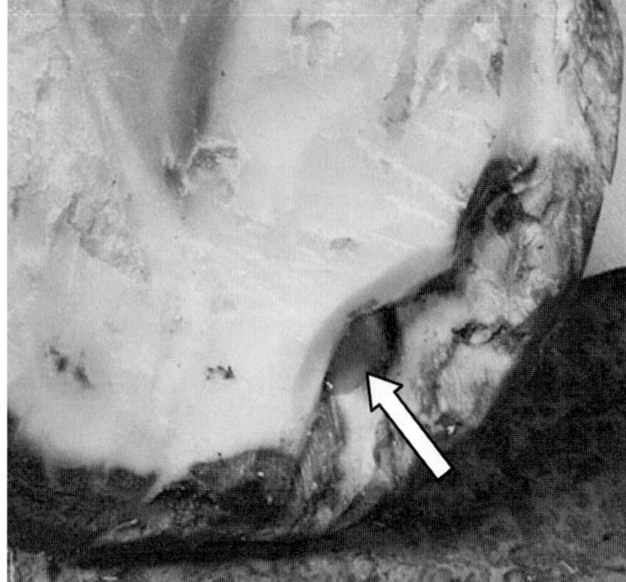

Figure 93-14. A subsolar abscess was opened; the purulent material is shown draining *(arrow)*.

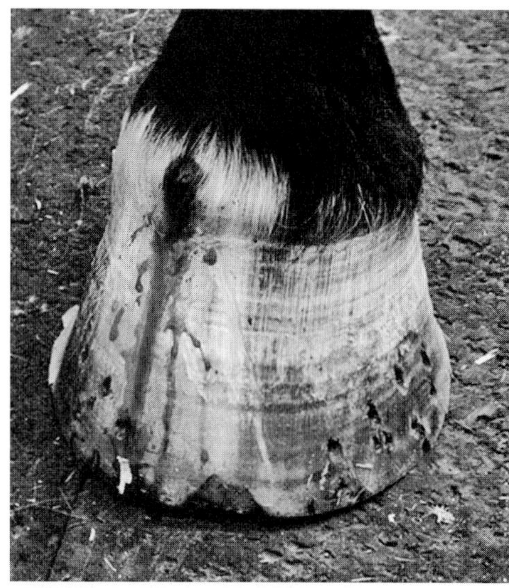

Figure 93-15. Delayed diagnosis or delayed treatment can lead to the abscess breaking out at the coronary band.

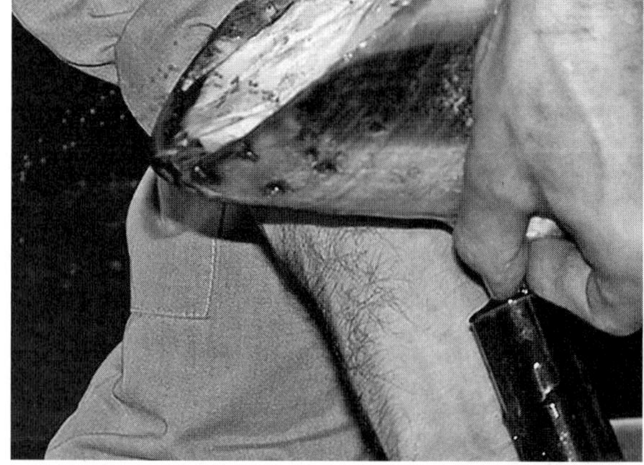

Figure 93-16. The abscess is flushed daily from the coronary band toward the sole with diluted povidone-iodine (Betadine) solution.

Administration of nonsteroidal anti-inflammatory drugs (NSAIDs; e.g., phenylbutazone) is indicated. Antimicrobials also are indicated, especially when bone involvement is suspected. Generally a good prognosis can be given, even though advanced abscesses can take weeks to heal completely.[22]

Chronic Hoof Abscesses

Etiology

On rare occasions, a hoof abscess might not be diagnosed right away, especially if the horse has been treated with pain-relieving medications for a period of time. The clinical symptoms are more or less effectively masked, preventing recognition of the problem and its treatment. Also, administration of NSAIDs prevents the abscess from maturing and can permit the microorganisms to invade other tissues within the foot. The abscess can extend into the foot along three avenues: along the dorsal and lateral hoof wall in a proximal direction, eventually breaking out at the coronary band (see Fig. 93-15); along the sole, potentially undermining it completely; or along the distal phalanx, resulting in septic pedal osteitis.[23,24]

Diagnosis

Physical examination of the foot might reveal a draining tract. A thorough radiographic evaluation, with or without a probe positioned in the draining tract, often helps make the diagnosis, because at this point radiographic changes usually are visible on the distal phalanx. Lytic changes can develop as a result of a chronic abscess as well as after aseptic local inflammation.

Treatment and Aftercare

The abscess needs to be opened and all the undermined sole removed until normal horn is encountered.[23,24] If the infection spreads out along the side wall, all the undermined wall must be carefully removed, again until normal wall is encountered. If the distal phalanx is involved, all the affected bone must be curetted. The treatment of a chronic abscess can take several weeks to months, especially if a substantial amount of hoof wall needs to be resected.

Aseptic Pododermatitis

Etiology

Aseptic pododermatitis is a severe bruising of the laminae and horn tissues of the foot and is a common cause of lameness in horses. Often this problem is not recognized immediately, and the concomitant lameness is attributed to navicular disease or osteoarthritis of the distal interphalangeal joint. There are many possible causes for this problem: poor shoeing technique, excessive use of the horse under difficult conditions such as hard, uneven ground, and frequent kicking against the stall wall.

Diagnosis

The symptoms are typical but not very specific, leading occasionally to a misdiagnosis (Fig. 93-17). The hoof is slightly warmer than normal and a positive pain reaction can be elicited with the hoof testers. Pulsation of the palmar arteries is usually increased. Palmar digital nerve anesthesia usually relieves the lameness. Radiography helps to differentiate the problem from a fracture in this region. Keratoma is part of the differential diagnosis in cases of chronic persistent pododermatitis.

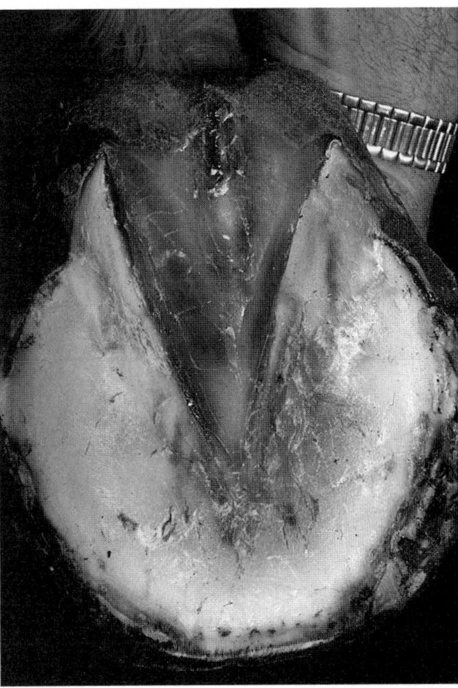

Figure 93-17. Marked reddening of the sole near the frog in a case of aseptic pododermatitis (severe bruising).

Treatment and Aftercare

Management of this disorder is directed at removing the actual cause. In most cases, the shoe must be removed. Application of creosote bandages for three or more days is very effective. These bandages are followed by dry bandages for a prolonged period. Some patients require NSAIDs because of persistent pain. Some hand-walking on soft ground is optional, and after 7 to 10 days the horse is reshod.

TRAUMATIC INJURIES

Puncture Wounds

Etiology

"Nail prick" refers to injury caused by inadvertently driving a nail through the sole and sensitive laminae during shoeing. "Street nail" refers to puncture of the solar surface of the hoof by nails or other sharp objects such as screws. A hoof is "nail bound" when a horseshoe nail is driven too deep into the horn, causing excessive pressure on the corium. All three types of injuries usually result in pain, inflammation, and infection.

Although puncture wounds of the sole can appear small (Fig. 93-18), they are often deep and can have disastrous

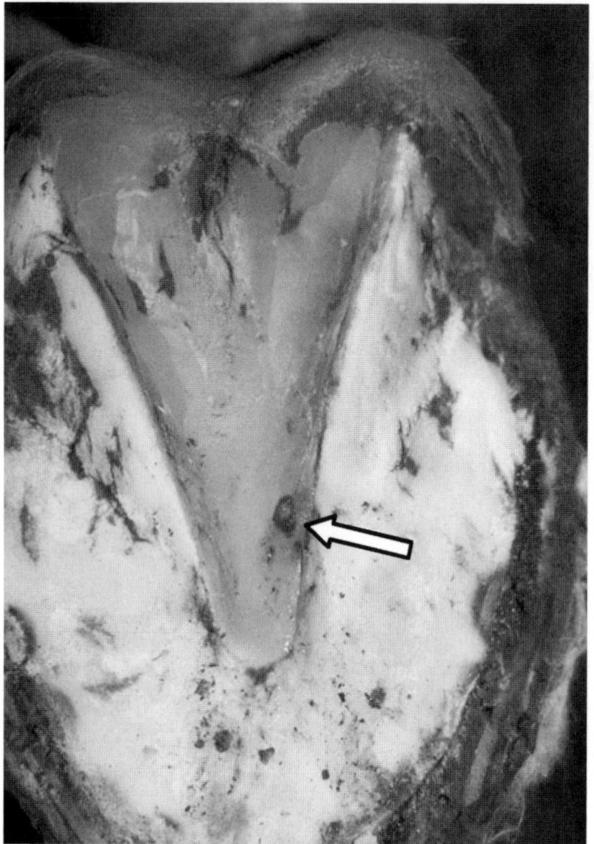

Figure 93-18. Typical appearance of a puncture wound near the apex of the frog *(arrow)*.

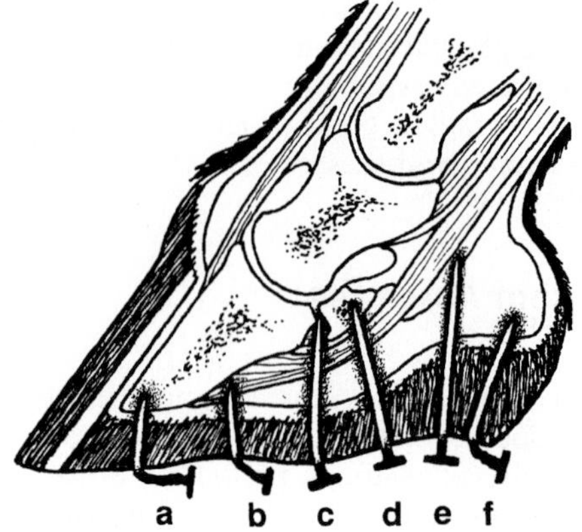

Figure 93-19. Potential puncture wound sites, resulting in the penetration of different anatomic structures. *a,* Tip of the sole, involving the distal phalanx. *b,* Dorsal third of the frog, involving the insertion of the deep digital flexor tendon. *c,* Middle of the frog, involving the deep digital flexor tendon, the impar ligament, and possibly the distal interphalangeal joint. *d,* Palmar third of the frog, involving the deep digital flexor tendon, distal phalanx, and navicular bursa. *e,* Palmar aspect of the frog, involving the hoof cushion, deep digital flexor tendon, and tendon sheath. *f,* Most palmar frog, involving the hoof cushion.

effects when structures such as the distal phalanx, distal sesamoid bone, distal interphalangeal joint, navicular bursa, deep digital flexor (DDF) tendon, or tendon sheath are penetrated (Fig. 93-19). The penetrating object is usually contaminated with soil, rust, or manure, which can lead to serious infection. The superficial wound in the sole usually seals quickly, leaving no area for drainage. The anaerobic environment created favors the growth of *Clostridium tetani,* the microorganism causing tetanus.

Depending on the location and depth of the puncture wound, various structures can be affected[25,26] (see Fig. 93-19). Deep puncture wounds are extremely serious and difficult to treat; affected horses are often referred to specialized clinics for surgical therapy. For these reasons, deep puncture wounds must be treated as an emergency to prevent the infection of bones, joints, and tendon sheaths.

Diagnosis

Horses usually have a moderate to severe supporting-leg lameness, often pointing the affected toe. The hoof is warmer than normal, and there is increased pulsation of the digital arteries. The horse might have a fever. Examination with hoof testers usually elicits severe pain. In horses with severe acute lameness, the hoof must be thoroughly cleaned and examined for a foreign body or puncture wound (see Fig. 93-18).

Treatment and Aftercare

The nail or foreign body should be promptly removed. However, it is imperative that the depth and direction of the tract be noted and the point of entry marked on the sole or recorded on paper, because it will rapidly become inapparent. The point of entry is cleaned, and the entire hoof is bandaged.

Based on the location, direction, and depth of the injury, the horse may be treated on site or referred to a clinic. When there is suspicion of injury to deeper structures, such as the navicular bursa, distal interphalangeal joint, or the DDF tendon sheath, the horse must be referred immediately for surgical treatment. Broad-spectrum antibiotics are started, and tetanus antitoxin and toxoid are administered.

TREATMENT IN A CLINIC

A thorough clinical examination is carried out, after which local anesthesia is administered. The shoe is removed and the entire hoof is trimmed (see Fig. 93-18). The decision to pursue further treatment is based on the results of clinical examination and radiography. The puncture tract is carefully cleaned and disinfected. A sterile metal probe is inserted into the puncture tract, and the hoof is radiographed in two planes (Fig. 93-20 *A*). Placing a needle into the navicular bursa using aseptic technique and injecting a contrast medium can enhance the diagnosis (see Fig. 93-20, *B*). A 20-gauge needle is placed in the distal interphalangeal joint and synovial fluid is collected into an EDTA tube. Approximately 10 mL of contrast medium is injected into the joint. After a few minutes, the hoof is radiographed again to determine whether the contrast medium is exiting through the puncture tract.[25] The same procedure is repeated for the DDF tendon sheath.

Surgical débridement and treatment of puncture wounds

Surgical débridement of puncture wounds is usually performed with the horse under general anesthesia. This

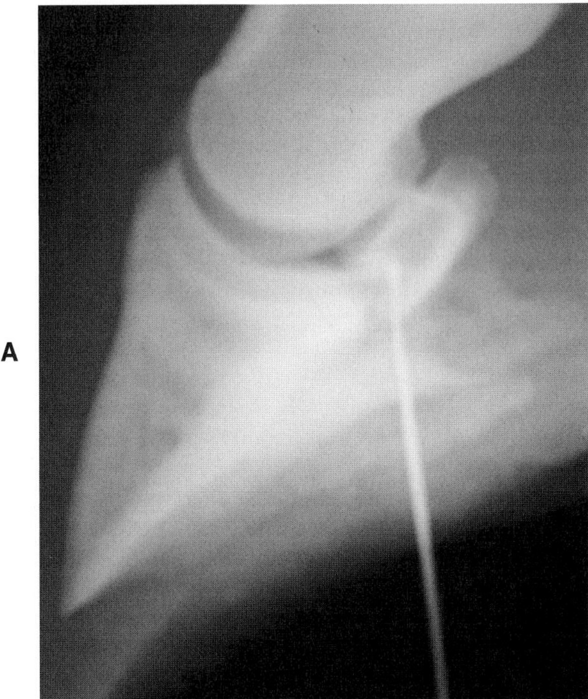

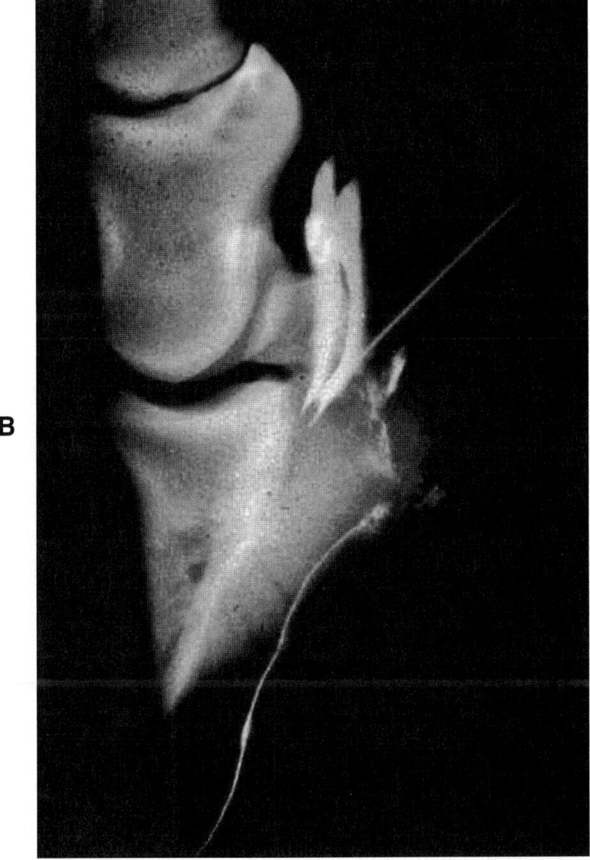

Figure 93-20. A, Lateral radiograph showing a probe inserted through a puncture wound, which penetrated the navicular bursa and distal sesamoid bone. **B,** Contrast study of the navicular bursa, showing contrast media exiting through the puncture wound.

procedure entails two parts: initial débridement of the sole followed by aseptic treatment of the hoof (Fig. 93-21).[27] With the horse sedated and standing, the hoof is cleaned and the horn around the puncture tract is carefully removed down to a thin layer of horn that can be cut with a scalpel blade. The hair from the hoof to the fetlock joint is clipped. The prepared area is cleaned with chlorhexidine scrub (Hibiscrub) and covered with a bandage.

The horse is positioned in lateral recumbency under general anesthesia and a tourniquet is applied. Occasionally, it is necessary to remove additional horn at this time. All affected structures around the puncture tract are excised. The horn around the tract is removed in an area measuring approximately 3 by 3 cm. The corium and subcutis are then removed and the underlying structures are exposed. When the foreign body has penetrated the DDF tendon, a 1.5 by 1.5 cm area of the tendon is resected (Fig. 93-22). Curettage is necessary if the foreign body penetrates the distal phalanx or the distal sesamoid bone (Fig. 93-23). With perforation of the impar ligament and penetration of the distal interphalangeal joint, the ligament must be resected and the joint lavaged. The flexor tendon sheath requires lavage when it is involved.

The affected synovial structures are lavaged with lactated Ringer's solution to which antibiotics have been added. A pressure bandage is applied, followed by a hoof bandage and a wedge under the heel. Regional intravenous perfusion with an antibiotic is recommended.[28]

An arthroscopic technique has been developed to lavage and treat a deep puncture wound that penetrates the navicular bursa or distal interphalangeal joint (Fig. 93-24). This technique has good results[29] and permits a less-invasive approach to the penetrated structures, because débridement is carried out under endoscopic guidance. Also, the area is under constant lavage during treatment, decreasing surgery time.

Depending on the severity of the injury, lavage may be repeated once or twice with the horse under general anesthesia. Afterward, with the horse standing and sedated, the bandage is changed under aseptic conditions. Systemic antibiotics and anti-inflammatory drugs are administered for at least 2 weeks. After a certain period of time, a medication-plate shoe can be applied (Fig. 93-25).

Prognosis

The prognosis for puncture wounds of the sole is generally guarded. Horses that receive prompt surgical treatment and have few deep structures affected have the best prognosis.[27] Injury to the distal sesamoid bone can eventually result in adhesions between the bone and the DDF tendon, necessitating neurectomy. Bursoscopic treatment can lessen the development of these types of morbidity.

Scalping Injuries

Etiology

Coronary band (Fig. 93-26) and heel injuries occur at the transition between the skin and hoof capsule. They are usually caused by overreaching, where one foot treads on the coronary band or heel of another foot. Heel calks on

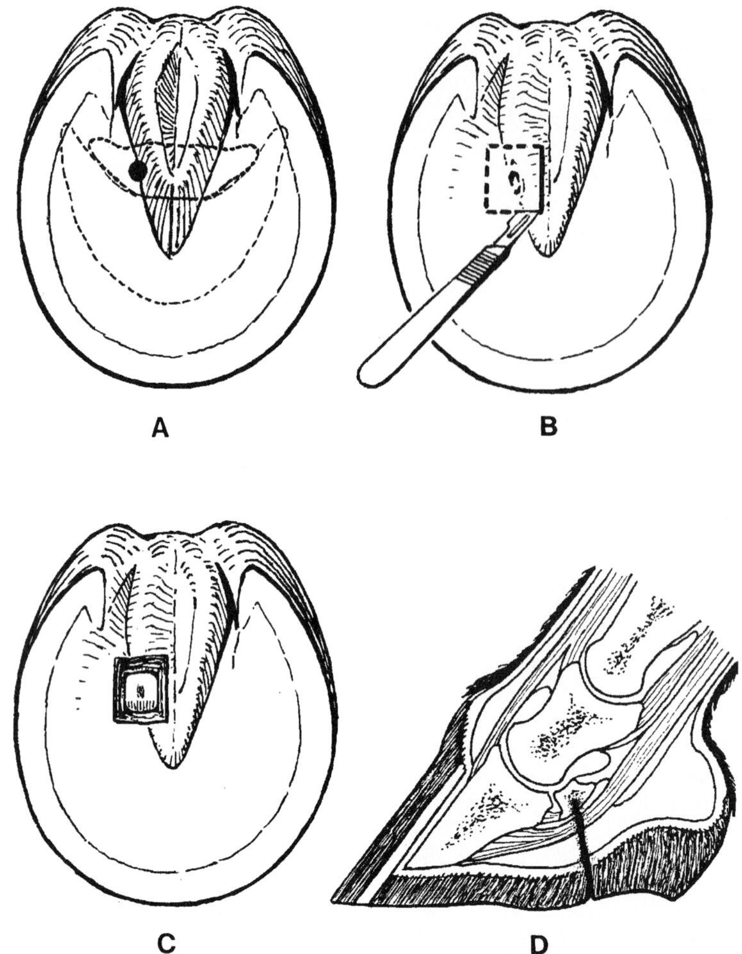

Figure 93-21. Street nail procedure. **A,** Localization of the entry point. **B,** Subcutis and sensitive lamina is removed. **C,** The deep digital flexor tendon is fenestrated. **D,** Representation of the puncture wound in a parasagittal plane.

shoes can result in very deep injuries and for this reason should always be removed before trailering.

Diagnosis

These injuries are usually quite painful in the acute stages and can cause severe lameness. Inadequate treatment can lead to infection within the hoof capsule. There is also a risk of permanent damage to the horn-producing cells, resulting in abnormalities of hoof growth such as cracks and ridges.

Treatment and Aftercare

The damaged horn should be removed to allow drainage of wound secretions. Heavy scissors or a hoof knife are ideal for this. The wound is then cleaned with a mild disinfectant solution and bandaged.

Other Hoof Lacerations

Injuries to the hoof capsule are relatively common. Trauma to the corium usually results in marked hemorrhage and severe pain. This type of injury is particularly problematic when the coronary corium is involved; damage to the horn-producing cells results in the production of poor-quality horn. A pressure bandage is applied to injuries that are bleeding severely. The bandage is changed daily until a stable and healthy layer of horn is formed.

DEGENERATIVE AND NEOPLASTIC DISEASES OF THE FOOT

Canker

Etiology

Canker used to be a common disease when draft horses were used for work. Therefore, detailed descriptions can be found in older textbooks. Canker of the frog represents abnormal horn proliferation in the frog region and is rarely seen in other areas of the hoof (Fig. 93-27). It is not a true neoplasm but rather a chronic inflammatory reaction characterized by massive parakeratosis.[30] There is hypertrophy of the sensitive lamina and degeneration of the superficial horn and corium. Canker can spread from the frog to the adjacent sole and even involve the hoof wall.

This disease is slowly progressive and spreads to adjacent structures over the course of months. In some horses, the skin adjacent to the hoof capsule is affected. The skin near

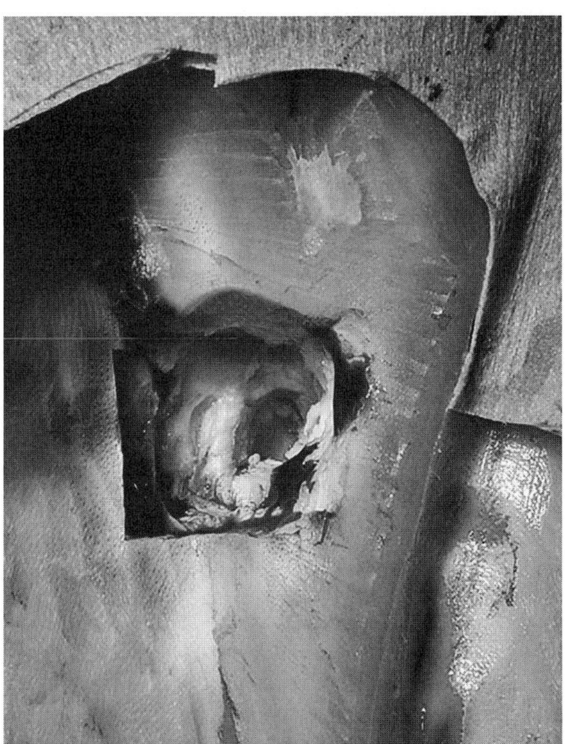

Figure 93-22. A window was cut through the frog and hoof cushion, the deep digital flexor tendon was fenestrated, and the navicular bursa was opened to allow flushing.

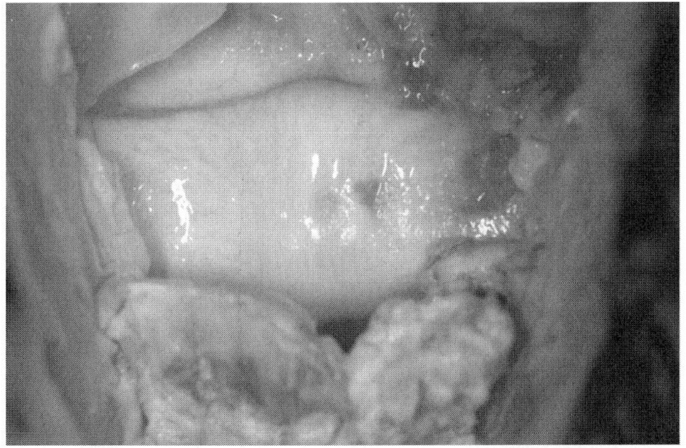

Figure 93-23. Ten-day post-operative appearance after a street nail procedure for a foreign body penetrating the distal sesamoid bone.

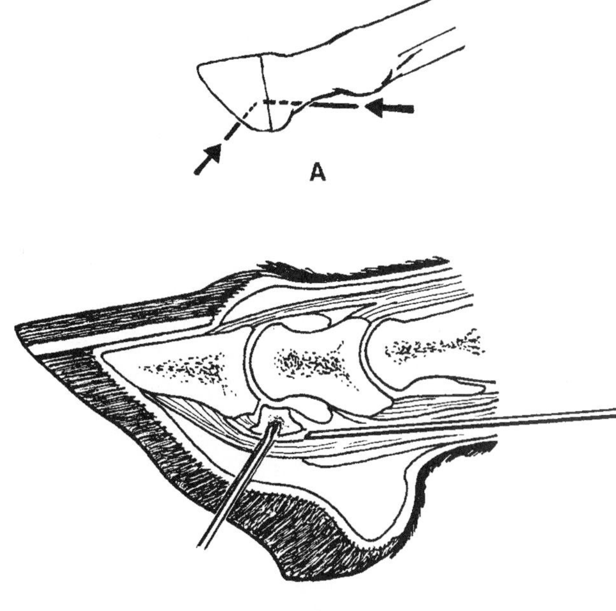

Figure 93-24. Bursoscopy in lateral recumbency. **A,** Overview of the surgical portals. **B,** Close-up view showing the anatomic structures involved.

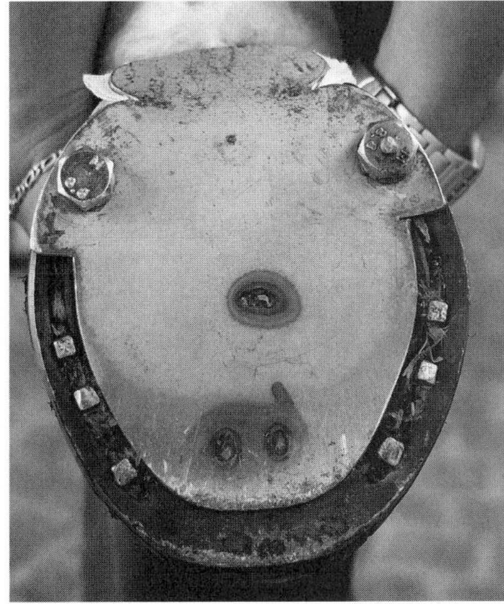

Figure 93-25. A medication-plate shoe used for postoperative protection of a foot after surgery. The wound may be dressed daily by removing the plate.

the coronary band is reddened, the hair grows in all directions, and the area is painful when palpated. In rare cases, the horn of the chestnuts is affected.

The cause of canker is not known, although unsanitary stall conditions appear to be a predisposing factor. Long-standing thrush is thought to result in canker formation, because it causes the original degeneration of the horn cells. Horses that are kept in moist and warm stalls with urine-soaked bedding often suffer from canker. Also, there seems to be a breed predilection; draft horses are most commonly affected, but the disease is also seen in Thoroughbreds, Standardbreds, ponies, and even donkeys. A genetic predisposition for this condition has been suggested. Young horses rarely have canker.

The hind hooves are more often affected than front hooves, and one or more hooves may be involved. Bacteriologic examination of affected tissue usually reveals gram-negative anaerobic bacteria. Although many micro-organisms can be isolated, anaerobic bacteria seem to be most important in this disease.

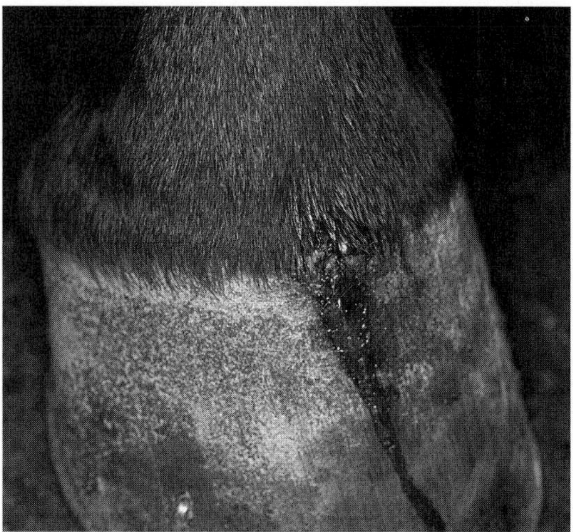

Figure 93-26. Fresh scalping injury at the coronary band.

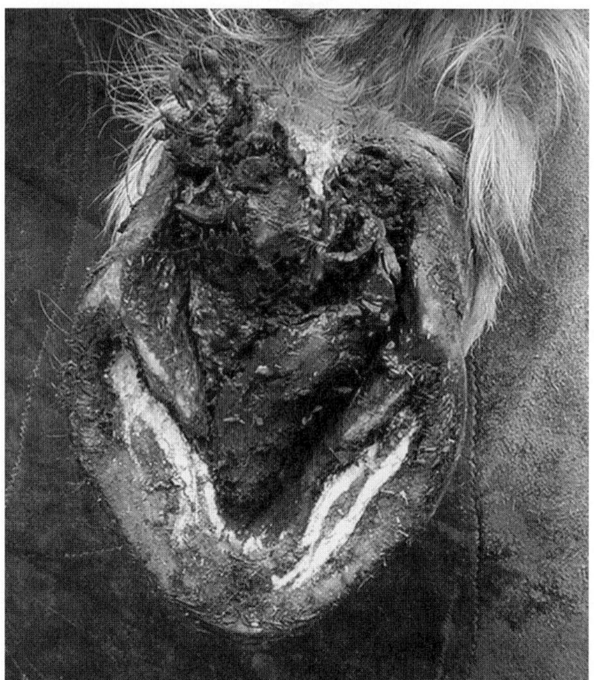

Figure 93-27. Canker in a horse showing a flaky, hypertrophic frog.

A differential diagnosis must include advanced thrush and fungal infection of the coronary band.

Diagnosis

Horn of rubber-like consistency that breaks easily on the surface is characteristic of canker. The horn produced by the epidermal cells affected by canker is soft, greasy, and friable. Cauliflower-like growths that are not cornified at the surface but covered with a greasy, grayish-white material are typical. These hypertrophic horn growths have a foul odor somewhat reminiscent of an abscessed tooth. Once traumatized, the area bleeds profusely. The poor horn quality can result in injury and infection of the underlying structures.

Treatment and Aftercare

Treatment of canker is very difficult and time-consuming, and it does not always result in a cure. All damaged cells must be removed to allow the growth of healthy horn tissue. Treatment must be as hygienic as possible and involves a number of steps.[31,32]

SURGERY

The first step is surgical débridement. All necrotic and abnormal horn is removed with the horse standing or, in severe cases, with the horse under general anesthesia. A tourniquet is applied to the limb in the middle metacarpal or metatarsal region. All abnormal horn is removed so that the area can be thoroughly cleaned and cut with a scalpel blade (Fig. 93-28).

The transition between abnormal and healthy horn is determined during paring with a hoof knife. A cut is made around the frog to define the surgical field. Then, beginning from the palmar or plantar surface, the entire frog is removed (Fig. 93-29). It is important not to cut too deeply

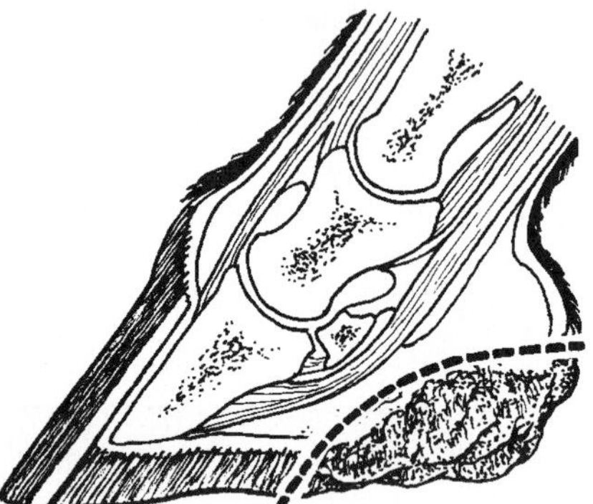

Figure 93-28. Sagittal view of a hoof with canker. The *dotted line* represents the level of the surgical cut needed for removing the frog.

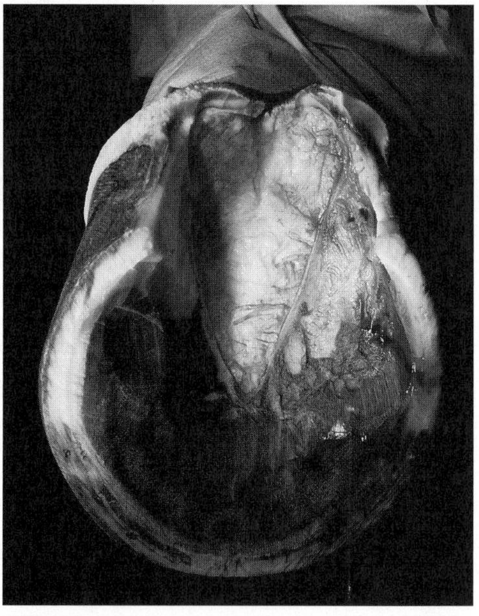

Figure 93-29. Postoperative picture of surgery for canker after removal of the entire frog.

in near the apex of the frog. Alternatively, cryotherapy can be used.[33] Normal epithelium is then able to grow from the remaining healthy tissue.

In most cases, removing the abnormal horn while sparing the stratum germinativum is adequate. A new frog grows within a few months (Fig. 93-30). The foot is bandaged during this time, so this treatment is labor intensive and time consuming for the owner.

LOCAL TREATMENT

The second step involves local treatment, which consists of disinfection, drying, and hardening of the horn. The hoof is cleaned and disinfected with povidone-iodine scrub and treated with povidone-iodine–soaked bandages for 2 to 3 days. Daily bandage changes are required thereafter.

When healing is observed, a shoe with a pad is applied. The pad must be removable so that the area can be cleaned with povidone-iodine scrub and rinsed with povidone-iodine solution daily. The defect is covered daily with a mixture of 20 g iodoform iodine, 20 g zinc oxide, 20 g tannic acid, and 40 g metronidazole; this mixture acts as a disinfectant, astringent, and drying agent. The wound is then bandaged or covered with gauze and protected with the pad.

Administration of local or systemic antibiotics might be necessary; chloramphenicol and metronidazole are particularly effective.[34] Systemic antibiotics should be administered when more than one hoof is affected. The horse should be given biotin and zinc supplements.

The horn defect becomes smaller as it heals (see Fig. 93-30). The persistence of soft greasy horn usually indicates recurrence of the disease. Repeated surgical débridement is required in some cases. Treatment entails many months and requires good owner compliance. Sanitary stall conditions also are important.

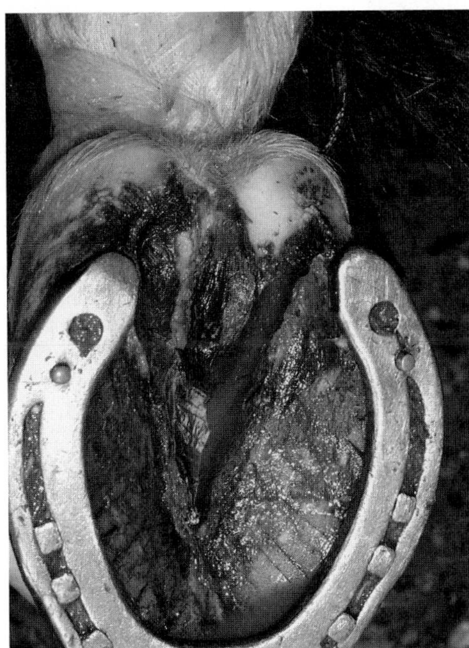

Figure 93-30. Progressive healing is shown 4 months after removal of the entire frog.

DISORDERS OF THE COLLATERAL CARTILAGES

Mineralization

Etiology

Mineralization of the collateral cartilages of the distal phalanx (side bone) is a common radiographic finding in the front feet of heavy horses.[35] Ossification of the collateral cartilages has been considered as a part of the normal aging process, and factors such as heavy bodyweight, working on hard surfaces, repetitive concussion, poor conformation, improper shoeing or trimming, and other foot problems are often mentioned as possible causes.

However, large side bones have also been found in young horses that have not yet started working; therefore an inherited tendency to develop side bones has been suspected. Side bones are more common in mares than in stallions and geldings.[36,37] Extensive ossification is more commonly found in the lateral than the medial cartilage.

Diagnosis

Ossification of the collateral cartilages is most often an incidental finding. Lameness associated with side bone is difficult to confirm. It is important to correlate radiographic findings with signs of pain. Radiographs reveal ectopic ossification emanating from the proximal aspects of the palmar or plantar eminences of the distal phalanx in the area of the collateral cartilages (Fig. 93-31). Because separate centers of ossification exist in these cartilages, these findings should not be confused with fractured side bones (Fig. 93-32), although in rare cases the side bone can fracture (Fig. 93-33).

Digital manipulation of the collateral cartilages can reveal loss of pliability and pain. Lameness is most marked when the horse is turned at a trot on a hard surface. A palmar digital nerve block on the suspected side of the hoof should improve the painful gait. Increased radiopharmaceutical uptake (scintigraphy) associated with a different radiographic appearance from that of other ossifications of the front feet was a conclusive sign of clinical significance in a recent report of 21 Finnish horses.[38] Ossification of the cartilages is commonly associated with obscure lameness problems, but most often ossification is not the cause.

Treatment

Once ossification of the collateral cartilage has started, it cannot be stopped, and specific treatment is not available. However, if the side bones are suspected as the cause of lameness, rest and administration of NSAIDs would be the logical initial treatment. Any foot imbalances should be corrected, and breakover should be moved caudally on the foot by rolling of the toe. The heels should have as much opportunity for expansion as possible, which is especially important for unbalanced or sheared heels.

A fracture of an ossified cartilage is treated conservatively with NSAIDs and an extended period of stall rest or small paddock turnout (8 to 12 weeks) followed by controlled exercise on level surfaces for 6 to 8 months. It is most likely that after this period of time, the fracture line will still be visible on radiographs but surrounded by proliferative

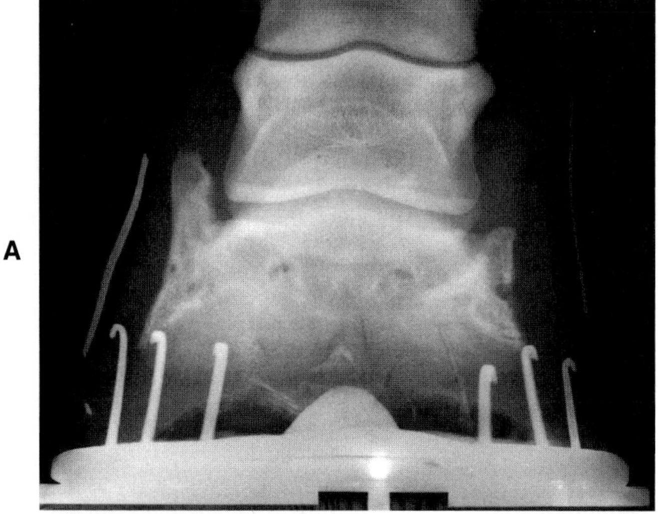

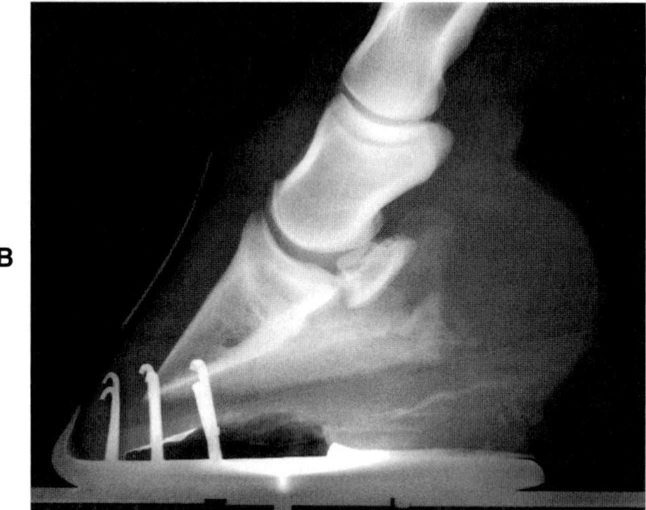

Figure 93-31. Dorsopalmar (**A**) and lateromedial (**B**) radiographs of a hoof with mild ossification of the lateral collateral cartilage at the palmar process of the distal phalanx.

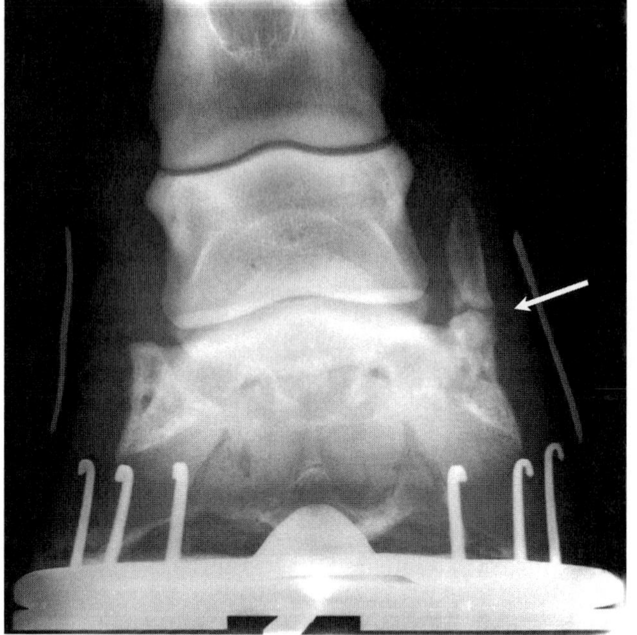

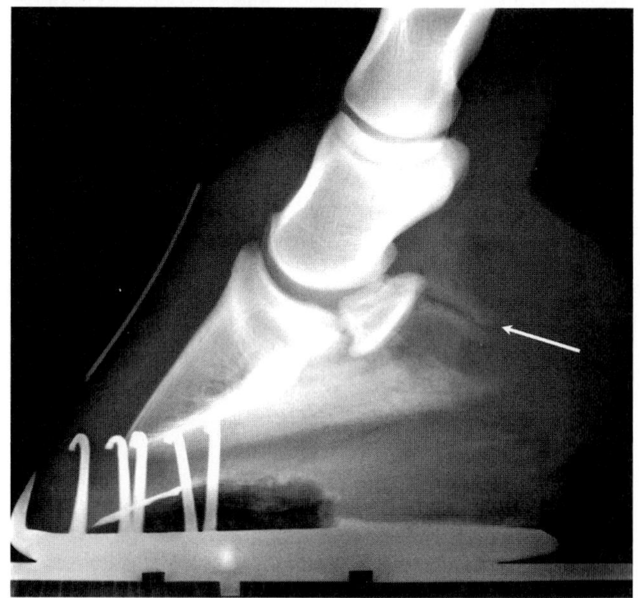

Figure 93-32. Ossification of the lateral collateral cartilage in a left forelimb. Note the radiolucent line *(arrows)* on the dorsopalmar (**A**) and the lateromedial (**B**) projection. This separate ossification center should not be confused with a fractured side bone. Dorsally and on each side of the foot, small wires were taped along the hoof wall to identify its surface.

exostosis (see Fig. 93-33). In refractory cases, unilateral palmar digital neurectomy can be performed.

Small fragments can be removed eventually if any signs of sequestrum formation are observed. An incision 1 to 2 cm parallel to the palmar or plantar coronary band gives access to the proximal part of the collateral cartilage. No attempts should be made to remove large proximal fragments.[39]

Necrosis

Necrosis of the collateral cartilage (quittor) is characterized by an intermittent purulent discharge and sinus tract formation at or proximal to the coronary band in proximity to the collateral cartilage. These lesions are chronic and do not heal. Lameness occurs in the acute stages but might show remission when the lesion appears to be healing. Usually a mixed bacterial infection is present, associated with subsequent necrosis of the cartilage, as the result of injury to the cartilage itself or to the adjacent soft tissue.[40] The quittor condition can develop secondary to a penetrating wound through the sole where infection has gained access to the collateral cartilage.

Diagnosis

Clinical signs of quittor include enlargement over the affected collateral cartilage with one or more chronic sinus tracts that continue to drain. The most important differential diagnosis is a chronic ascending infection of the white line that breaks and drains at or slightly proximal to the

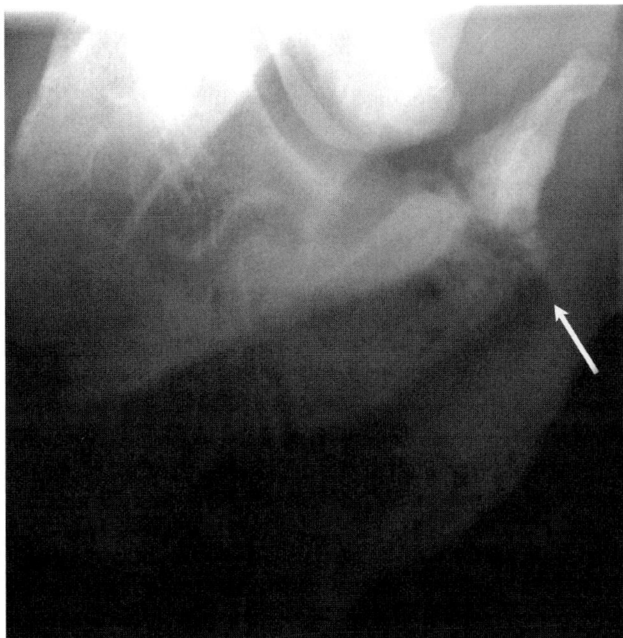

Figure 93-33. Oblique radiograph of the distal phalanx of an Arabian horse with a 6-month-old fracture of the medial side bone. Healing is in progress, but the fracture line *(arrow)* is still visible.

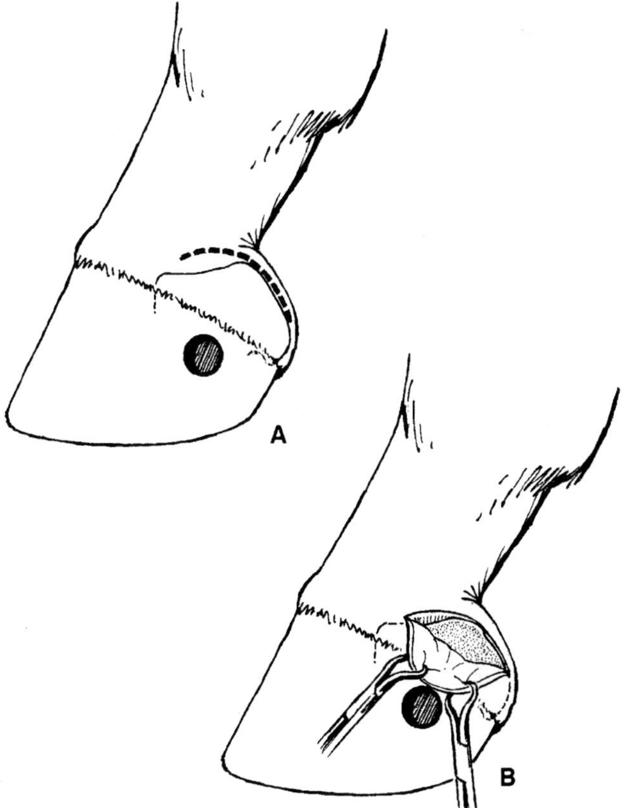

Figure 93-34. A and **B,** Surgical treatment for quittor, or necrosis of the collateral cartilage. A slightly curved incision beginning just dorsal to the coronary band over the diseased collateral cartilage produces a skin flap, which allows removal of the proximal part of the necrotic cartilage. A hole drilled in the hoof wall is required for adequate drainage if infection and necrosis extend distal to the coronary band.

coronary band. With quittor, the swelling is usually more diffuse and is located more proximally over the collateral cartilage.

Radiography can be helpful to detect foreign bodies or to rule out involvement of the middle or distal phalanx. The depth and direction of the draining tracts are determined radiographically after injection of a contrast medium or insertion of a flexible metal probe into the tract.[41]

Treatment

Prior to surgery the region is clipped and the hoof is trimmed and rasped, scrubbed, and placed in a povidone-iodine–soaked bandage for 24 hours. Once the horse is anesthetized, a tourniquet is applied. The foot is held in maximal extension during dissection to tighten the joint capsule and retract it from the area of dissection, minimizing the risk of accidental penetration into the distal interphalangeal joint.[40] A slightly curved incision beginning just dorsal to the coronary band over the diseased collateral cartilage is made (Fig. 93-34). The flap is dissected distad to expose the collateral cartilage, and a probe is used to identify the draining tract. Alternatively, diluted methylene blue can be injected into the tract to identify it during dissection.

Necrotic cartilage is recognized by its dark blue or reddish blue appearance. All of the necrotic tissue and cartilage is removed until healthy margins remain. Subsequently, arthrocentesis of the distal interphalangeal joint is performed and the joint is distended with polyionic fluid to assess the integrity of the joint capsule axial to the removed portions of the collateral cartilages. In case of accidental laceration of the joint capsule, the joint must be flushed with large amounts of fluid through a needle placed in the dorsal aspect of the joint capsule.

After débridement, the defect is closed with 2-0 monofilament absorbable suture material in a simple interrupted pattern. An injection of 2 mL gentamicin into the joint protects it from developing an infection. If necrotic cartilage extends distal to or below the coronary band, a hole is drilled in the hoof wall over the ventral-most limits of the excised cartilage to provide drainage (see Fig. 93-34). After extensive flushing, the proximal skin incision is closed with nonabsorbable tension sutures, and the wound is packed through the hole in the hoof wall using antiseptic-soaked gauze sponges. The surgical site is protected with a sterile bandage.

The following day the bandage is removed and the wound is flushed. Bandages are changed every other day until all evidence of infection has subsided and a healthy bed of granulation tissue is present. When this occurs, a short limb cast can be applied to the limb for 8 to 10 days to minimize movement at the suture line and to encourage primary healing. After removal of the sutures, bandaging is continued until granulation tissue fills the defect and epithelium begins to cornify.

FRACTURES OF THE DISTAL PHALANX

Fractures of the distal phalanx are diagnosed in horses of all ages, even very young foals.[42,43]

Etiology and Classification

Fractures of the distal phalanx are caused by acute trauma such as a kick toward a hard, nonmovable object. Most often fast or excessive work induces fractures of the distal phalanx.[44] Laceration of the hoof capsule results in fractures as well. The forelimb is more commonly involved than the hindlimb.[45]

Fractures of the distal phalanx are classified into the following types[45] (Fig. 93-35):

I. Abaxial fractures without joint involvement
II. Abaxial fractures with joint involvement
III. Axial fractures with joint involvement
IV. Fractures of the extensor process
V. Multifragment fractures with joint involvement
VI. Solar margin fractures

Some complicated fractures cannot be assigned to one of these classifications.[44,46]

Clinical Symptoms and Diagnosis

The patient usually shows an acute, moderate to severe lameness accentuated during turns. The hoof and distal phalangeal region are warm to the touch, and an increased pulse can be palpated over the palmar or plantar arteries.[42] Pressure exerted with the hoof testers might elicit a positive response. Arthrocentesis of the distal interphalangeal joint results in a blood-tinged synovial sample when there is articular involvement. Signs are relieved by regional anesthesia of the distal phalangeal region. In the differential diagnosis, a hoof abscess should be considered.

Radiography confirms the diagnosis in most cases. However, occasionally it is difficult to detect a fracture line because of minimal displacement. Additionally, the irregular border of the distal phalanx and debris on the hoof capsule can make recognition of the fracture difficult. It is important to take several radiographs from different angles.[45] Abaxial nonarticular fractures are usually difficult to recognize because they are normally only minimally displaced.

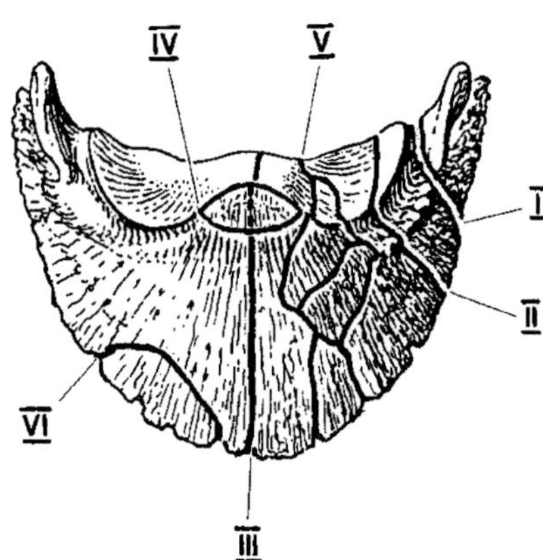

Figure 93-35. Classification of distal phalangeal fractures: I, Abaxial non-articular fracture; II, abaxial articular fracture; III, axial articular fracture; IV, extensor process fracture; V, multifragment articular fracture; VI, solar margin fracture.

It is important to distinguish vascular channels from potential fractures. The presence of thin lines crossing vascular channels at different angles indicates a fracture. If no fractures can be recognized, the animal should be placed in a box stall and the radiographs repeated after 7 to 10 days.[47] Because of the osteolysis occurring at the fracture margins, the radiographic fracture gap enlarges with time, aiding in recognition of the fracture. Scintigraphy, computed tomography (CT), and magnetic resonance (MR) imaging are often successful in delineating an obscure fracture[47,48] (see Chapters 75 and 76).

Treatment

Fractures of the distal fragment can be managed with fragment removal, cast application[49] and special shoeing[49], compression screw fixation[50], and neurectomy. Foals are best treated with stall rest.[43,50]

Abaxial Fractures (Types I and II)

These fractures are supported for 2 months by application of a fiberglass cast around the hoof capsule. Subsequently, a bar shoe with large side clips is applied to the hoof, providing support to the heels to limit hoof expansion during loading (Fig. 93-36). NSAIDs are administered to reduce the pain level and allow the horse to bear weight on the foot. Stall rest for 2 to 4 months is required. Follow-up radiographs are taken to evaluate fracture healing.

Usually after 4 months, the horses can be ridden at a walk on even terrain. Depending on the reaction, the workload is slowly increased.

A reasonable prognosis can be given for future use.[49,51] It usually takes 4 to 6 months for the fracture to heal. However, radiographically the fracture line is visible much longer. Initially a fibrous union develops, which ossifies at 6 to 12 months. In some cases, a nonunion develops.

Axial Fractures (Type III)

Axial fractures may be managed conservatively or surgically.

NONSURGICAL MANAGEMENT

The same type of treatment is used as that for abaxial fractures (see earlier). However, it is important to prolong the rest period: 4 months of stall rest followed by 4 months of hand-walking exercise. Additionally, the horses should be

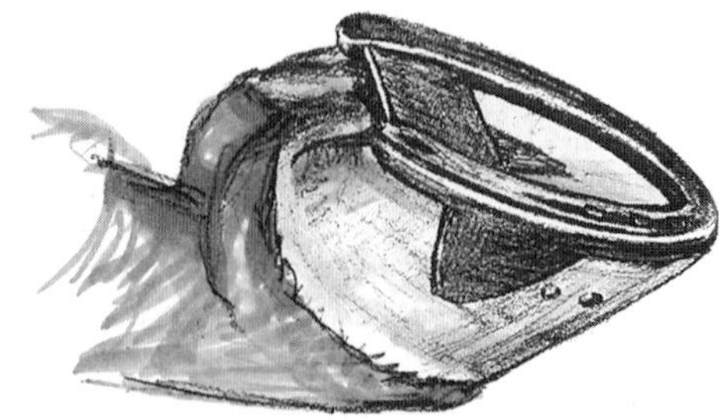

Figure 93-36. Bar shoe with large side clips to limit hoof expansion laterally during weightbearing. This shoe is often used after hoof wall resection is performed to access the interior of the hoof capsule.

shod for 6 to 8 months with a bar shoe. A guarded prognosis is given for horses older than 3 years that are to be used as future riding animals, whereas horses younger than 2 years have a good prognosis.[52]

SURGICAL MANAGEMENT

On the day prior to surgery,[52] the entire hoof is thoroughly cleaned and the sole trimmed and all crevices removed. The entire hoof wall surface is rasped and the foot placed overnight in a bandage soaked with an antiseptic (Betadine).

For surgery, the animal is anesthetized and positioned in lateral recumbency on the surgery table. The use of a fluoroscope during the surgery aids in achieving correct positioning of the screw. The entry point through the hoof capsule is determined by taping a radiodense object to the lateral hoof wall and taking a lateromedial radiograph. By comparing the radiographic image with the objects on the hoof wall, the entry point is determined and marked on the hoof wall with an awl. The final preparation of the hoof and phalangeal region for aseptic surgery is completed.

Using a 10-mm diameter drill bit, a hole is made through the hoof capsule parallel to the sole surface and aligned with the bulb of the heel. The hole is continued until the drill bit reaches the distal phalanx. A pilot hole is drilled into the third phalanx with a small drill bit until it crosses the fracture. This depth cannot usually be determined without the help of fluoroscopy or intraoperative radiographs. Once the desired location and direction of the drill bit is determined, the glide hole is prepared (Fig. 93-37). Frequent fluoroscopic views will help identify the moment when the fracture plane is crossed with the drill bit. At this point, the drill bit is removed and exchanged with the one used for drilling the thread hole, which is performed through an insert drill sleeve. Care is taken to identify the exit point through the opposite fragment to prevent inadvertent trauma to the sensitive lamina. After countersinking and tapping, a 5.5-mm cortex screw of predetermined length is inserted and solidly tightened.

Tangential radiographs are taken directed at the exit point of the screw tip to ensure correct length. Screws that are too long are exchanged for shorter ones. Conventionally, one screw is inserted without taking too big a risk of entering vital structures. With the help of computer-assisted navigation (see Chapter 14), two screws can safely be implanted.[53] The hole in the hoof capsule may be filled with an antibiotic-soaked sponge and placed under an aseptic pressure bandage or closed with antibiotic-impregnated polymethylmethacrylate (PMMA). Once the horn defect is dry (if it is not immediately filled with PMMA) it is filled with artificial horn.

Postoperatively the horse is kept in a box stall for 4 months followed by hand-walking exercise of an additional 4 months. Barring any complications, the screw may be left in place; otherwise it is removed when problems develop. The prognosis for a pleasure horse is guarded. Complications include postoperative infection and abscess formation.

Extensor Process Fragments (Type IV)

ETIOLOGY

These fragments have three known etiologies: hyperextension injury, avulsion by the extensor tendon, and a separate center of ossification (osteochondrosis, which may be bilateral).

CLINICAL SYMPTOMS AND DIAGNOSIS

Some horses show no clinical signs, and the presence of a fragment of the extensor process is found incidentally. Often the clinical signs are similar to those exhibited with other articular disorders of the distal interphalangeal joint. A routine lameness examination including perineural and

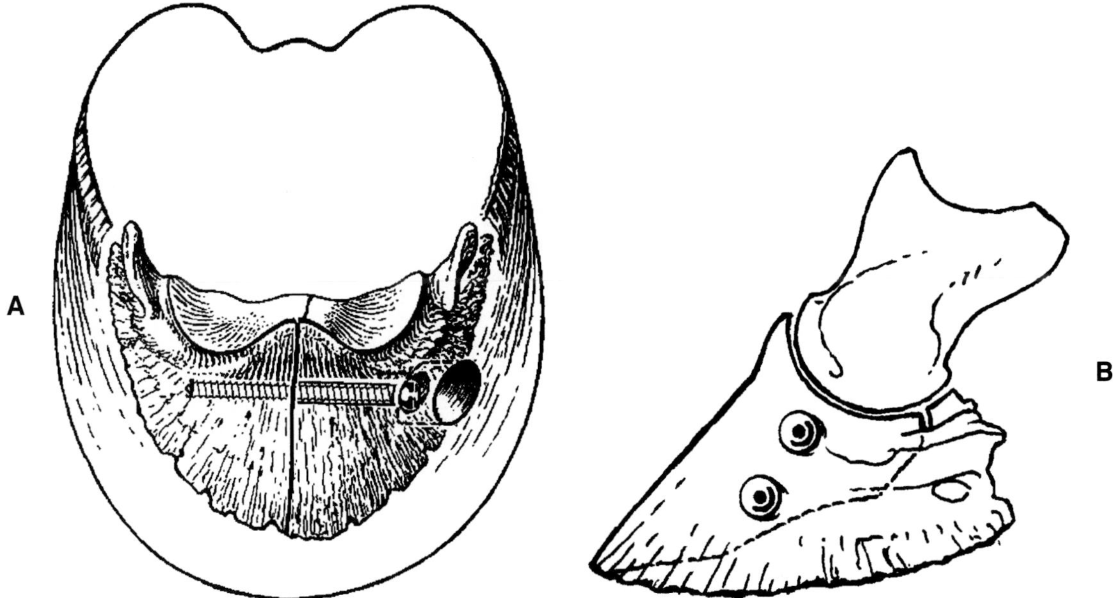

Figure 93-37. A, Dorsopalmar fixation of a type III fracture with one cortex screw inserted in lag fashion. **B,** Lateromedial fixation of a type III fracture with two cortex screws inserted in lag fashion.

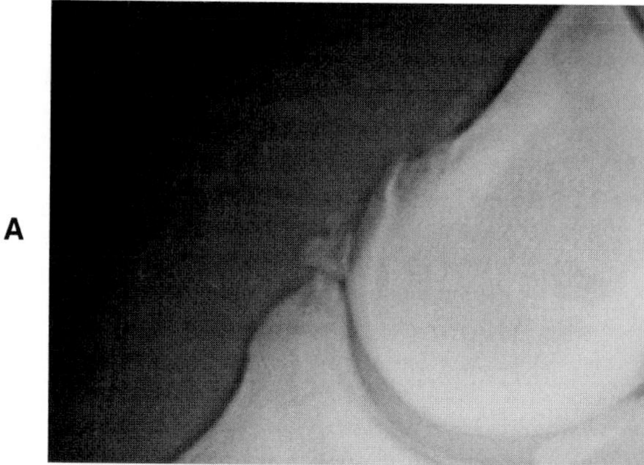

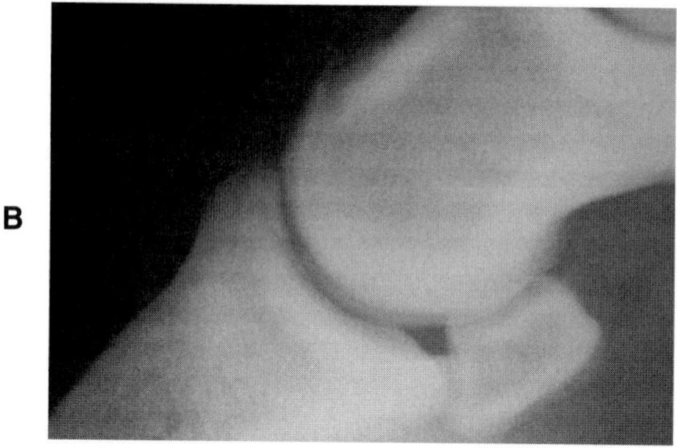

Figure 93-38. A, Preoperative lateromedial radiograph of an extensor process fracture. **B,** Postoperative lateromedial radiograph of the same horse after removing the fragment.

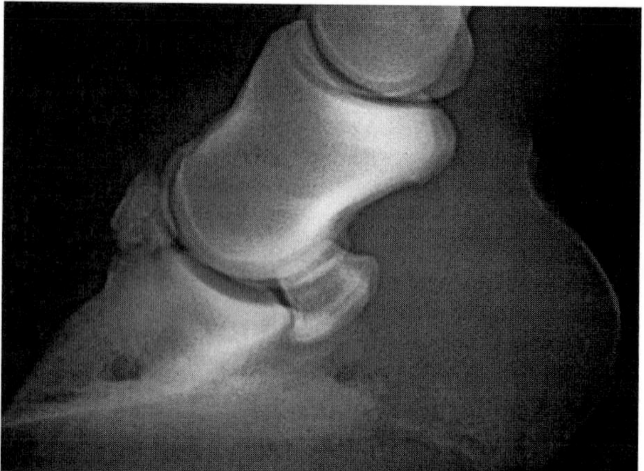

Figure 93-39. Lateromedial radiograph of a 3-year-old Friesian horse with a large fragment of the extensor process.

intra-articular anesthesia and a radiographic examination permit a definitive diagnosis (Fig. 93-38, *A*).

TREATMENT

Small fragments

Small fragments (see Fig. 93-38, *A*) should always be removed[54] because they are mobile and have contact with the articular surfaces. Fragment removal is accomplished by routine arthroscopy (see Fig. 93-38, *B*). Adjunctive therapy with intra-articular hyaluronan is encouraged. Postoperatively, the phalangeal region is kept under a bandage for 3 weeks and the horse rested for 6 to 8 weeks.

Large fragments

There is no ideal treatment for large fragments (Fig. 93-39). Therefore, conservative therapy is usually tried first. Insertion of one or two screws in lag fashion has been described,[55,56] but only rarely is a rigid fixation achieved. Therefore, if lameness persists after conservative management, surgical treatment is recommended. The fragment is divided into smaller pieces and these smaller pieces are removed under arthroscopic supervision. Generally, a good prognosis can be given.[57] Postoperatively a fiberglass cast or a compression bandage should be applied over the surgery site.

Multifragment Fractures (Type V)

Multifragment fractures are always associated with severe lameness. Radiographically, several fracture lines can be appreciated (Fig. 93-40). Application of a fiberglass cast may be tried; however, these fractures have a poor prognosis for future soundness. Therefore, euthanasia may be considered.

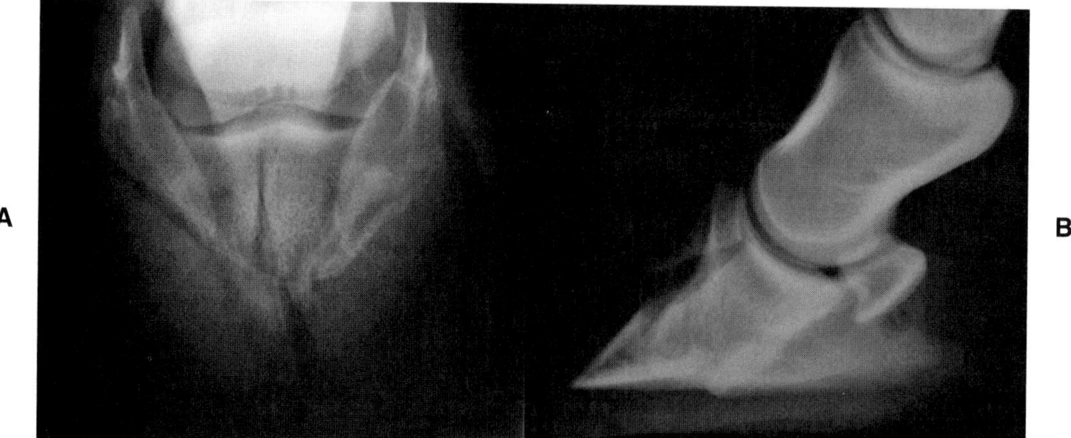

Figure 93-40. A, Dorsopalmar, and **B,** lateromedial radiographs of a Thoroughbred racehorse with a multifragment fracture of the distal phalanx.

Alternatively, a neurectomy can be performed if euthanasia is not an option for the owner.

Solar Margin Fractures (Type VI)

Solar margin fractures do occur often and are underdiagnosed.[45,58] Direct or blunt trauma, possibly caused when the horse kicks a hard, immobile object, are common causes of solar margin fractures. These fractures can also develop as a result of chronic laminitis.[45] Most solar margin fractures heal by bone union; rarely, resorption of small fragments can occur.[45] Surgical removal of fragments has been reported in individual cases.

Arthroscopy

Arthroscopy of the distal interphalangeal (DIP) joint (Fig. 93-41) has replaced arthrotomy, as it did in other joints. The advantages include the small approach portals, the small risk of postoperative infection, and the shortened convalescent period.[54] Indications for arthroscopic interventions include fragment removal from the extensor process, lavage in cases of infection, and curettage of subchondral cystic lesions.[59]

PREPARATION

The hoof should be thoroughly cleaned the day before surgery, and the coronary band and the phalangeal region should be clipped. The entire area is scrubbed and placed overnight in an antiseptic bandage. The shoe may be left in place.

For arthroscopic interventions in the forelimb, the animal is positioned in dorsal recumbency on the surgery table. Lateral recumbency is usually selected in the hind limb because the reciprocal apparatus makes manipulation easier in this position. An Esmarch bandage is applied to prevent intraoperative bleeding. Because of the location of the surgery site, meticulous attention is paid to the draping procedure. The use of a sterile incise drape (Ioban, Johnson & Johnson, Raritan, NJ) is advisable.

SURGICAL TECHNIQUE

Dorsal approach

With the DIP joint in an extended position, a needle is advanced in a dorsolateral to distomedial direction from 2 cm proximal to the coronary band. Withdrawal of synovial fluid ensures the correct placement of the needle. The joint is distended with gas or with 20 mL Ringer's lactate solution.

The arthroscope portal is prepared with a no. 11 scalpel blade introduced into the joint along the needle, and the needle is withdrawn. Immediately after the incision is prepared, the sleeve and the blunt obturator are carefully advanced together into the joint with a rotating movement. The obturator is replaced by the arthroscope.

Working with a dorsolateral arthroscope portal allows inspection of a medial fragment and its removal through an instrument portal positioned directly over the fragment (see Fig. 93-41). The joint is very small, providing little room for recognition of the anatomic landmarks. The middle phalanx is recognized by its articular cartilage surface and the proximal prominent ridge, which provides access to the dorsal outpouching of the joint. The synovial membrane, located at the dorsal aspect of the joint cavity, is covered with synovial villi, which partially obstructs the view. Often the osteochondral fragment of the extensor process is hidden behind the villi. The surface of the fragment is usually rough and irregular.

The first key to identifying the fragment is to recognize the separation between the fragment and the parent portion of the bone. The abaxial aspect of the joint should be inspected initially to provide an overview of the condition of the joint. It is possible that displaced small fragments can be found in these locations.

Most fragments are well attached. Insertion of an elevator between the fragment and the distal phalanx and careful manipulation loosens most fragments. It is important to remove a significant portion of the attachments of the extensor tendon and surrounding tissues from the fragment before attempting to remove the fragment with rongeurs. Once purchase is achieved on the fragment, rotating movements are performed to dislodge the remaining attachments.

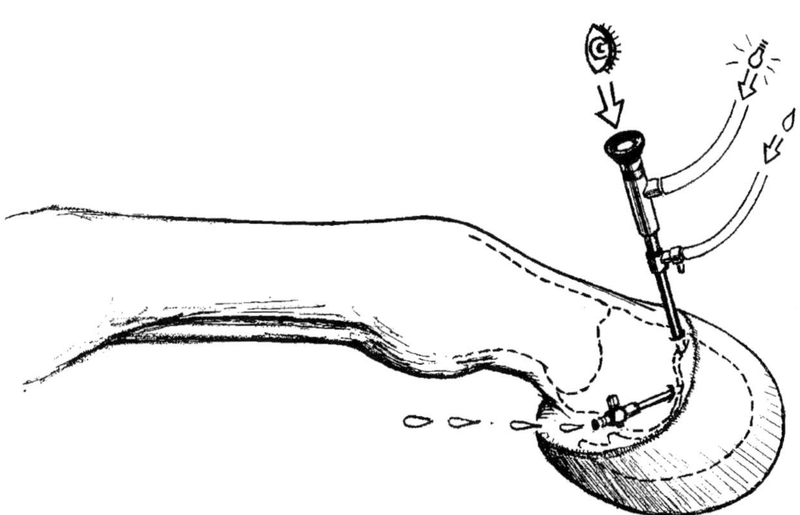

Figure 93-41. Typical positions of the arthroscope and instruments during arthroscopy of the distal interphalangeal joint.

Because of the softness of the fragment, it is usually removed in pieces.

The fracture bed is inspected and curetted. Introduction of the arthroscope through the instrument portal allows inspection of the fragment bed from a different view and occasionally the detection of other small fragments. The joint is then flushed and the portals closed with two simple interrupted sutures of an absorbable monofilament material.

A postoperative pressure bandage is maintained for 2 weeks.[60] The portals for the surgery heal slower than such portals in other joint regions. Therefore, there is an increased risk of infection. Additionally, intra-articular injections such as hyaluronan are delayed for about a week. The horse is kept in a box stall for 4 weeks and can then slowly return to work.

The prognosis depends on the nature of the problem, the age of the patient, and the arthroscopic findings during surgery. In young horses, a good prognosis usually can be given, whereas in older horses with concomitant osteoarthritis, the prognosis for successful return to work decreases.

Palmar approach

An arthroscopic approach to the palmar aspect of the distal interphalangeal joint has been described. The horse is positioned in lateral recumbency and the joint is distended through a dorsally placed needle. Observation of the process of joint distention allows identification of the best palmar location to access the joint. A needle is placed into the site to facilitate correct scope positioning.

Arthrotomy

Prior to the introduction of arthroscopy, fragments were removed through arthrotomy approaches. Arthrotomy[57] allows exploration of only a small part of the joint without a large skin incision. Therefore, this type of intervention is justified only under certain circumstances, such as for removing excessively large fragments.

The skin incision is made on the midline, starting 4 cm proximal to the coronary band and ending at the coronary band. The common digital extensor tendon is split, and a Gelpi retractor is inserted to allow inspection of the most proximal tip of the fragment. The fragment is grasped with Allis tissue forceps and an incision is made around it with a scalpel. The incision is closed using routine technique.

Occasionally, a trephine hole is made distal to the coronary band over the midline down to the distal phalanx. This can allow removal of a large fragment without causing extensive damage at the dorsal aspect of the joint and the coronary band. The defect in the hoof wall is managed as described earlier.

FRACTURES OF THE DISTAL SESAMOID BONE

Fractures of the distal sesamoid bone (DSB) occur rarely. They are diagnosed more often in the forelimbs. Four different types are distinguished: avulsion fractures, simple fractures of the body, comminuted fractures, and frontal fractures.

Avulsion fractures of the distal margin are often found in conjunction with navicular disease. Therefore, these fractures are considered part of an osteoarthritic syndrome (see later in this chapter).

Most of the simple fractures occur abaxially in a vertical or slightly oblique direction (Fig. 93-42). Some displacement is possible.

Multifragment fractures are rare and in most cases carry a poor prognosis.

Fractures in the frontal plane are highly unusual (Fig. 93-43).

Etiology

Most fractures of the DSB have a traumatic origin and are the result of excessive or repetitive loading through the middle and distal phalanx and the DDF tendon.[61] Occasionally, a pre-existing pathologic condition in the DSB predisposes it

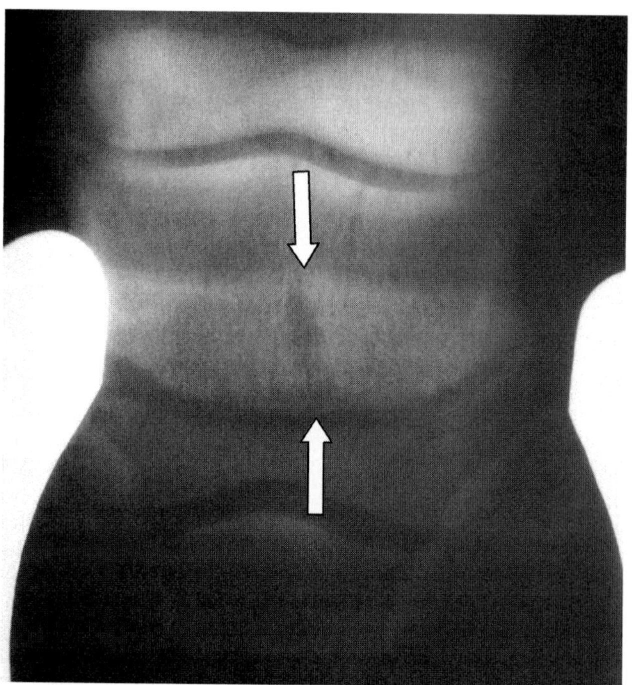

Figure 93-42. Dorsopalmar radiograph of an axial fracture of the distal sesamoid bone (between the *arrows*) with some displacement.

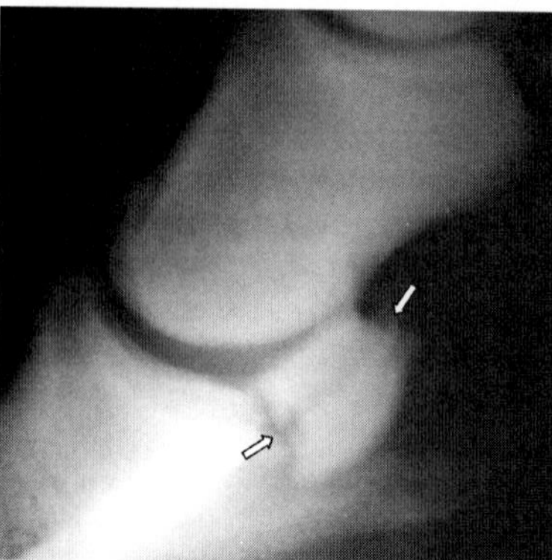

Figure 93-43. Lateromedial radiograph of a frontal plane fracture (between the *arrows*) of the distal sesamoid bone.

to fracture (Fig. 93-44). In these cases, chronic navicular disease is usually implicated.

Clinical Signs and Diagnosis

Clinical signs include an acute moderate to severe weight-bearing lameness associated with an intense pain reaction to turning, increased pulsation of the palmar or plantar arteries, and positive reaction to the application of hoof testers. The low palmar or plantar nerve block is usually diagnostic. All standard radiographic views of the DSB should be taken (lateromedial, tangential, and oblique) to rule out the potential presence of a bipartite DSB (two ossification centers) or other disorders. Air shadows of the sulci of the frog will project over the DSB and can be mistaken for fracture lines. Therefore, it is important to fill them with modeling compound (such as Play-Doh) before taking the radiographs.

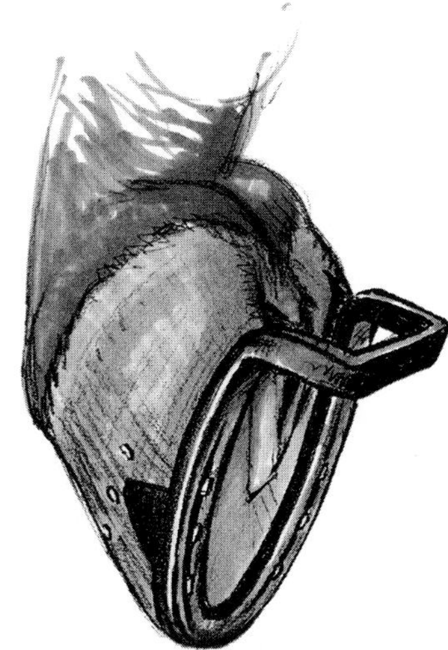

Figure 93-45. Elevated heel shoe.

Treatment

Management options for fractures of the DSB include conservative and surgical techniques. Callus formation is rare, and often syndesmoses are formed (fibrous tissue union).[61]

Nonsurgical Management

Corrective shoes are recommended to protect the DSB. Therefore, nonsurgical management involves stall rest and an elevated bar shoe (Fig. 93-45) for 4 months, followed by small paddock exercise and a shoe with thickened branches.[62] Even if the patient improves clinically during the first few months, an osseous union cannot be detected radiographically. Healing requires 10 to 12 months. The prognosis for future athletic activity is unfavorable.[63]

One option involves fixation of the distal limb in an extremely flexed position using a fiberglass cast, which relieves excessive stresses on the DSB. Acceptance of the cast takes a special patient, and healing requires about 6 months. Despite these measures, the prognosis for a future pleasure horse is guarded.

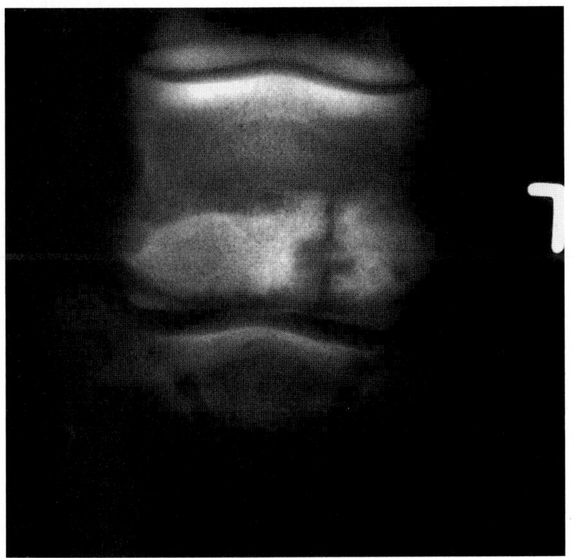

Figure 93-44. Dorsopalmar radiograph of pathologic fracture of the distal sesamoid bone. Note the large radiolucent area in the center of the fracture and the proliferative new bone formation on the proximal rim.

Surgical Management

The surgical options include screw fixation and neurectomy. Insertion of a cortex screw in lag fashion provides stability and promotes bone union.[64] The difficulty is in correct placement of the screw, avoiding penetration of the DIP joint and the palmar tendon sheath (Fig. 93-46). Close monitoring through fluoroscopy or multiple radiographic images is of utmost importance. The application of specially developed radiolucent aiming devices (Fig. 93-47) is mandatory for a correct screw placement. Computer-assisted navigation is an alternative technique (see Chapter 14).

Effective preoperative preparation of the hoof is initiated the day before surgery, as described earlier. The entry point through the hoof wall is determined and marked with the help of fluoroscopy. The horse is placed under general anesthesia and positioned in lateral recumbency on the surgery table. The surgical site is prepared for aseptic surgery.

The aiming device is applied to the hoof and adjusted with the help of fluoroscopy. The 3.5-mm glide hole is made, just crossing the fracture plane. The insert drill guide is inserted into the glide hole, and a 2.5-mm thread hole is drilled into the opposite fragment. After tapping, a 3.5-mm cortex screw of estimated length is inserted and tightened. With the help of a dorsopalmar radiograph, correct positioning and length are verified.

Healing of the fracture takes 6 to 8 months, during which stall rest and hand-walking exercise are implemented. Barring any complications,[65] the screw is left in place.

The prognosis for athletic competition is guarded, but for pleasure riding it is favorable.[64] Application of computer-assisted navigation greatly improves precision in screw placement and speeds up the surgery. To allow the horse to return to competitive work, it is often necessary to perform a neurectomy.[63]

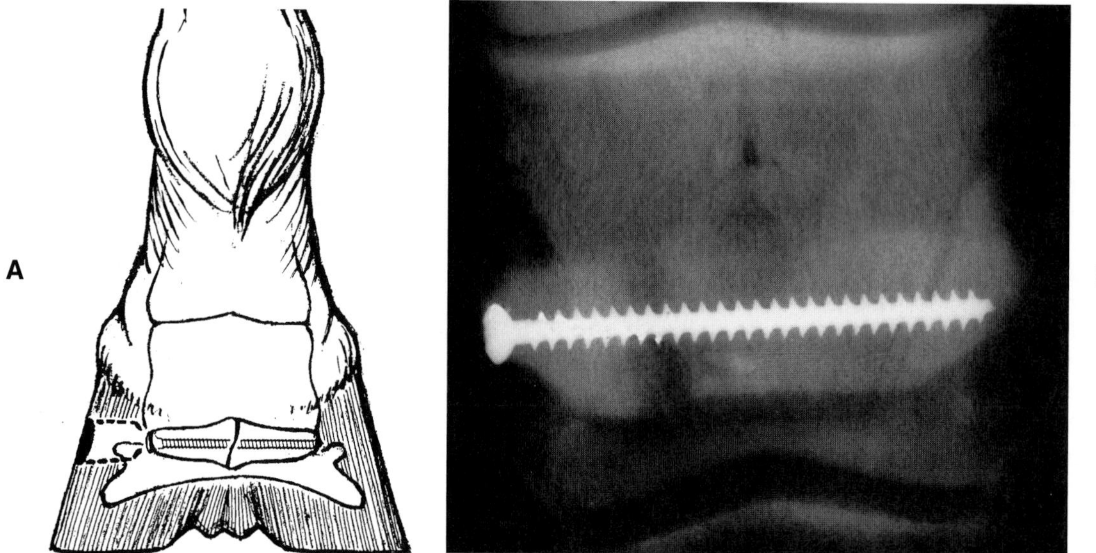

Figure 93-46. A, Illustration of screw inserted through the distal sesamoid bone, stabilizing the fracture. Note the larger hole drilled through the hoof wall to get access to the distal sesamoid bone. **B,** Dorsopalmar radiograph showing a 3.5-mm cancellous screw inserted across the fracture.

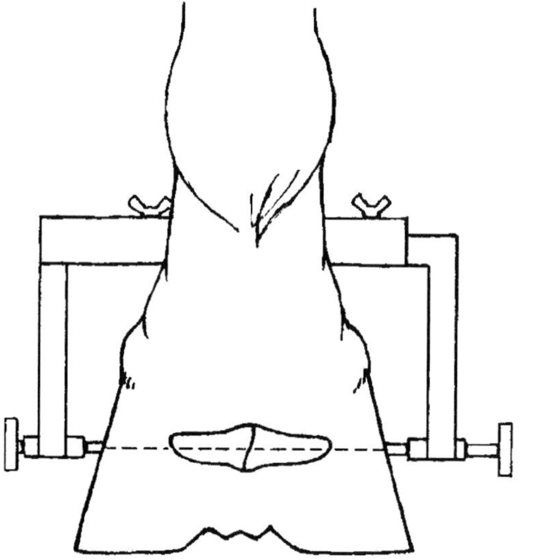

Figure 93-47. Illustration of the aiming device used to ensure intraosseous placement of a screw into the distal sesamoid bone.

PALMAR OR PLANTAR DIGITAL NEURECTOMY

General Considerations

Neurectomy is one of the oldest surgical procedures described in horses.[66] Palmar or plantar digital neurectomy is a viable option for alleviating pain in horses with certain kinds of chronic lameness, particularly navicular disease. A thorough clinical examination and proper case selection are critical. For example, digital neurectomy is contraindicated in horses with laminitis or infection of the distal interphalangeal joint.

Various techniques for digital neurectomy have been described. The operation may be performed with the horse standing[67] or in lateral or dorsal recumbency under general anesthesia.[68] There are various methods of denervation. With the horse standing, the procedure is carried out quickly and none of the risks of general anesthesia are encountered. With the horse in dorsal recumbency, repositioning the horse to access both sides of the limb is not required,[68] and a tourniquet is not necessary because minimal bleeding occurs. A nonsteroidal anti-inflammatory drug should be administered postoperatively and the horse kept in a box stall for 4 weeks. The horse is then slowly reconditioned by walking during another 4 weeks.

Re-innervation can occur when the severed nerve endings re-establish contact with each other. This can happen as early as 6 months postoperatively, depending on the technique used. However, ideally this does not happen for many years.[65,69] Neuritis and neuroma formation are common complications, particularly in the proximal nerve stump; depending on the study, up to 20% of patients are affected. These lesions are very painful, and in selected cases they must be treated with local injections of triamcinolone acetate (5 to 10 mg for each neuroma), sarrapin, or alcohol blocks. Rupture of the DDF tendon can occur after neurectomy, especially if it was compromised before surgery. Another sequela is laminitis, which can develop after a second operation or with injury of the blood vessels.

Special techniques are used in an attempt to prevent or at least delay regrowth of the severed nerve ends as well as to reduce the risk of neuroma formation. Various methods have been described for cutting the nerve and treating the severed nerve ends. The guillotine technique is the most commonly used.[65,69] This technique can be applied through one large or two small incisions, as described later.

Electrocoagulation is a less commonly used method. Other methods include epineural capping, inserting the nerve in a hole drilled into the proximal phalanx[70,71] or ligating the nerve. A valid alternative to digital neurectomy is cryoneurectomy, in which the nerve is frozen to as low as

−30° C.[72] Other alternatives include topical application of chemicals[73] and injection of neurotoxins such as cobra venom. Carbon dioxide laser treatment of the proximal nerve stump has reduced the development of neuromas.[74]

In certain countries, animal welfare legislation and equine sports associations (for instance, the International Equestrian Federation [FEI]) prohibit horses that have had a digital neurectomy from competing in official events. As a consequence, various methods of detecting a neurectomy have been developed.[75,76]

Palmar Digital Neurectomy in the Pastern Region Using One Skin Incision

The horse is positioned in dorsal recumbency,[68] and the limbs are extended and tied to restraints attached to the ceiling. The surgical field is clipped, prepared for aseptic surgery, and draped. The nerve is palpated, and an approximately 6- to 8-cm incision is made in the pastern skin directly over the nerve[65] (Fig. 93-48, *A* and *B*). Usually the skin incision is made along the dorsal edge of the DDF tendon, which directly exposes the nerve.

The ligament of the ergot is identified and split longitudinally (see Fig. 93-48, *C* and *D*), allowing access to the neurovascular bundle located beneath it. Splitting the ligament provides an extra layer to be closed over the severed nerve and potentially reduces postoperative irritation and subsequent neuroma formation. Additionally, mistakenly transecting the ligament instead of the nerve can be prevented with this technique. The nerve is isolated within the neurovascular bundle and well separated from the artery (see Fig. 93-48, *E* and *F*). The neurotomy is initially performed proximally and then distally, followed by removal of the loose piece of nerve (see Fig. 93-48, *G*).

The ligament of the ergot is closed in a continuous pattern, and the skin is closed with simple interrupted sutures. Aftercare is the same as that for the method using a small incision, described under "General Considerations."

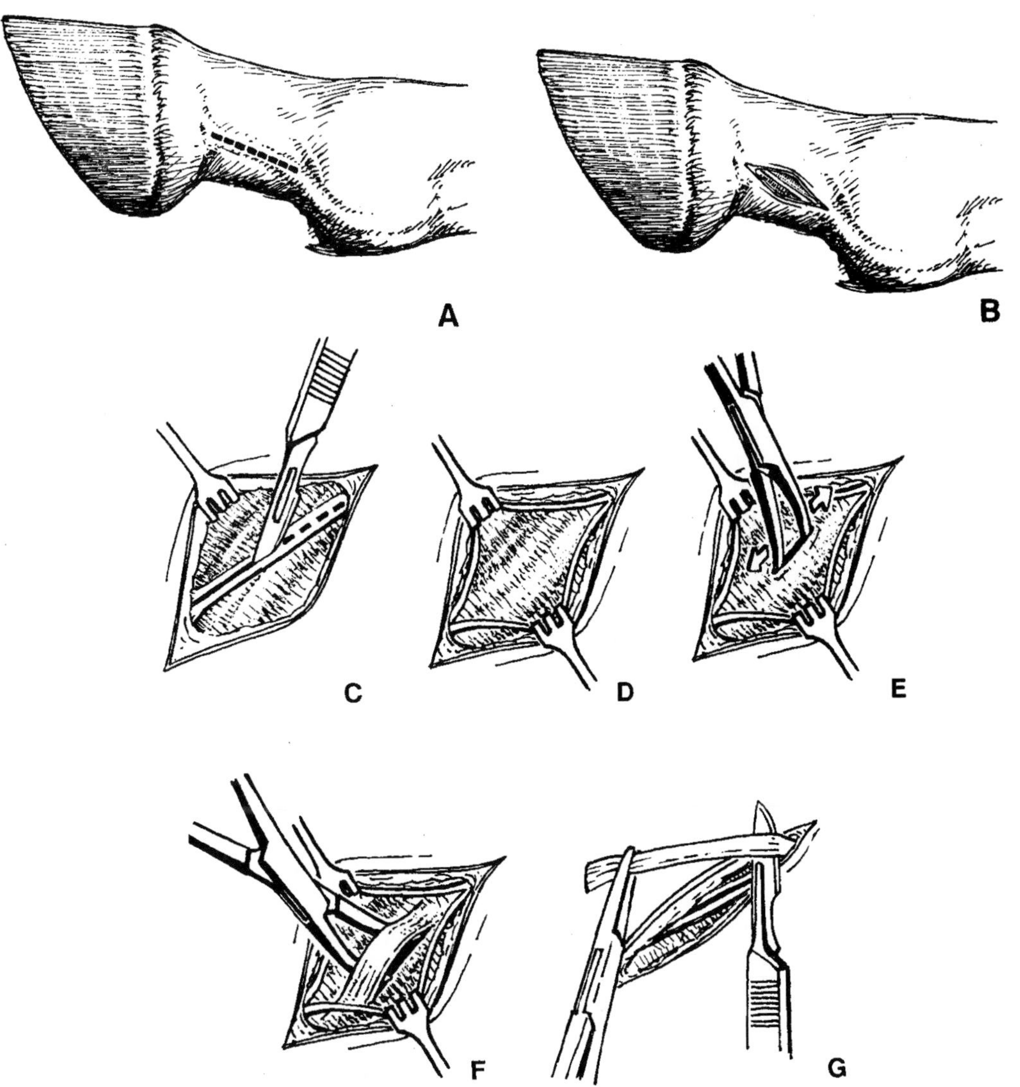

Figure 93-48. Illustration of the neurectomy procedure for the phalangeal region through one incision. **A,** Location of the skin incision. **B,** The skin incision has been made. **C,** The ligament of the ergot is split longitudinally and separated (**D**), giving access to the underlying tissues and the neurovascular bundle. **E,** The structures of the neurovascular bundle are separated, and **F,** the nerve is isolated. **G,** A 2-cm piece of nerve is excised.

Palmar Digital Neurectomy in the Pastern Region Using Two Small Incisions

The location of the nerve is palpated and two approximately 1.5-cm skin incisions are made directly over the nerve (Fig. 93-49, *A* and *B*). The distal skin incision is located at the distal end of the pastern region at the transition to the bulb of the heel. The proximal skin incision is selected at the proximal end of the pastern region at the transition to the metacarpophalangeal joint.

The tissue is bluntly dissected longitudinally with a mosquito forceps so that the dorsal and palmar aspects of the nerve are freed (see Fig. 93-49, *C*). It is important that the nerve and artery be well separated. Proximally the nerve might be obscured by the ligament of the ergot, which runs superficial to the nerve at a slightly different angle. The nerve is always covered by fascia, and it can be surprising how deep a dissection is required for its isolation.

Once the nerve has been freed proximally and distally, it is alternately pulled at either end to ensure that the correct structure has been exposed. The nerve is pulled up with a mosquito forceps, held with tissue forceps, and cut sharply as far distally and proximally as possible with a no. 15 scalpel blade (see Fig. 93-49, *D* and *E*). One clamp is applied to the proximal end and another one to the distal end of the severed nerve segment, and tension is applied to ensure that all attachments are eliminated and the nerve segment can be completely removed (see Fig. 93-49, *F* and *G*). The skin incisions are closed with 2-0 nonabsorbable suture material.

The advantages of this technique are the small size of the skin incisions, short time of surgery, and low incidence of neuroma formation.

Repeated Palmar Digital Neurectomy

A second neurectomy might be necessary when re-innervation occurs and the horse becomes lame again. For this procedure, a long incision is usually made so that the nerve can be adequately freed. This procedure is often more difficult than the initial operation because the nerve is generally very closely associated with the artery.

Small neuromas are always seen in the proximal aspect of the previous surgical field. These nodules can be easily palpated in horses that have had a neurectomy. Sometimes the regrown nerve is surrounded by a large amount of scar tissue, which makes the operation more difficult. Only the neuroma and part of the distal nerve should be removed. Skin closure and aftercare are the same as for the other neurectomy procedures.

High Lateral and Medial Palmar Neurectomy

The goal of high lateral and medial palmar neurectomy is to disrupt afferent and efferent nerve tracts proximal to the division into palmar and dorsal branches to prevent pain sensation from chronic disease processes innervated by the dorsal branches of the lateral and medial palmar nerve. This is usually performed proximal to the flexor tendon sheath, because locating and removing the nerve is easy in this location (Fig. 93-50). Also, there is little relative movement in this area, so that the nerve endings are less traumatized. The operation is carried out with the horse in dorsal recumbency. The skin is incised immediately proximal to the flexor tendon sheath on the lateral and medial aspects of the metacarpus. The nerve is located, isolated, and removed. Aftercare is the same as for the other techniques.

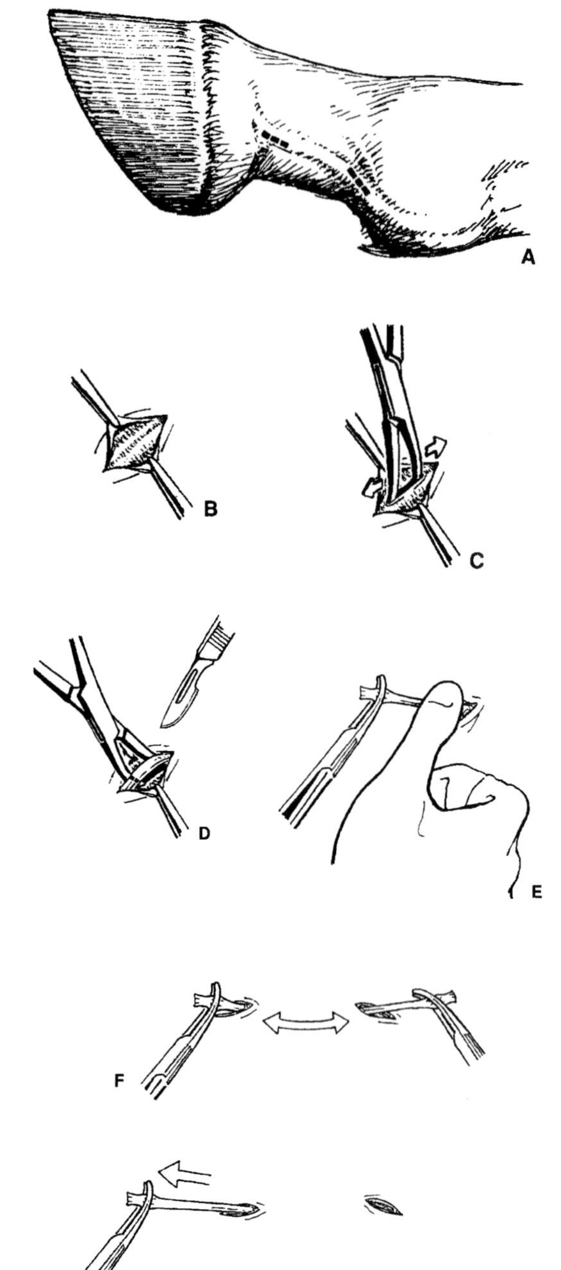

Figure 93-49. Digital neurectomy performed through two small incisions. **A,** Location of the two incisions. **B,** The neurovascular bundle is visible through an incision. **C,** The nerve is isolated, and **D,** elevated above the incision. **E,** The proximal end is transected, followed by the distal end (**F**) and the piece of nerve pulled out of the distal incision (**G**). The incisions are subsequently sutured.

SURGICAL MANAGEMENT OF NAVICULAR SYNDROME

Navicular disease is a degenerative disorder that involves the DSB and its surrounding structures. The etiopathogenesis of the condition is multifactorial, and many theories have been

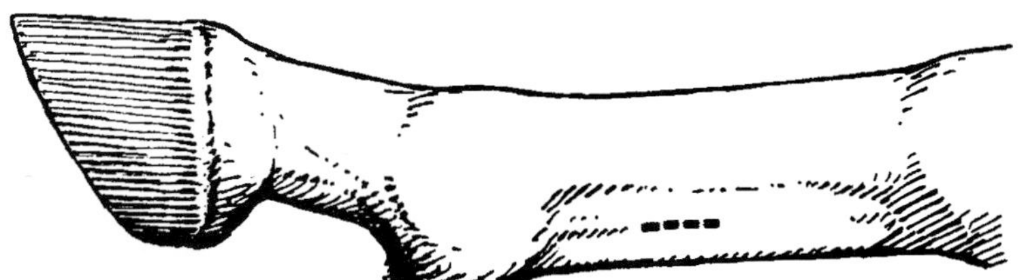

Figure 93-50. Location of the surgical site for the high palmar neurectomy.

proposed; these theories are discussed in detail in the literature.[77-79] Vascular and mechanical theories continue to be debated as the primary cause of the disease.

Treatment

There is no cure per se for navicular disease. Its management concentrates on abolishing the symptoms and clinical signs.

Nonsurgical Management

Management strategies include corrective shoeing, nonsteroidal anti-inflammatory drugs (NSAIDs), and vasodilators such as isoxsuprine or metrenperone.[80] Intra-articular administration of hyaluronan with or without corticosteroids into the distal interphalangeal joint or in the navicular bursa[81] can provide transient relief of clinical signs. The biphosphonate tiludronate (Sanofi-Aventis, Paris) has demonstrated positive effects in the treatment of recent cases (less than 6 months of lameness) of navicular disease.[82]

Another novel medical treatment is based on the pathophysiologic mechanism that podotrochlosis is associated with an increase of the intraosseous pressure in the navicular bone. The increase of pressure might be caused by an accumulation of osmotically active substances in the interstitium, as has been described in case of compartment syndrome. Therapy with coumarin is proposed.[83] This drug is successfully used in humans to reduce high-protein edemas.[84]

Surgical Management

Surgery is usually reserved for cases of navicular syndrome that have not responded to conservative treatments such as corrective shoeing and medical management. Three surgical procedures are currently available: navicular suspensory desmotomy, palmar digital neurectomy, and periarterial sympathectomy. These surgical procedures should be combined with balancing the feet and applying corrective shoes.

DESMOTOMY OF THE SUSPENSORY LIGAMENTS

Desmotomy of the suspensory ligaments (DSL) of the DSB has been proposed on the assumption that the syndrome has a mechanical basis. The proposed mechanism of action of the surgery reduces the forces on the navicular bone and perinavicular structures associated with the caudal weight-bearing phase of the stride (the portion of the stride where the suspensory ligaments are loaded).[85-87]

The DSB has its own supporting ligaments: proximally, the collateral sesamoidean ligaments (CSLs) and distally the impar ligament (IL) and the chondrosesamoidean ligaments (Fig. 93-51). The suspensory ligaments of the DSB are broad, elastic structures containing an abundance of nerve fibers. They originate at the dorsodistal aspect of the proximal phalanx and insert primarily on the proximal border of the DSB (Fig. 93-52, *A*). A branch of each ligament, the chondrosesamoidean ligament, also inserts on the axial surface of the adjacent collateral cartilage and the palmar process of the distal phalanx.

The biomechanics of the DSB and its suspensory apparatus are not completely understood and are explained mainly with the help of theoretical models. It is generally accepted that the CSLs anchor the DSB and prevent its descent during weight bearing.[86] However, the exact biomechanical implications of the CSL during loading are difficult to explain because the ligament passes over two joints, and time and maximum amount of tension depend on the foot or pastern axis and hoof conformation, as well as on the phase of the stride. Nevertheless, it is argued that

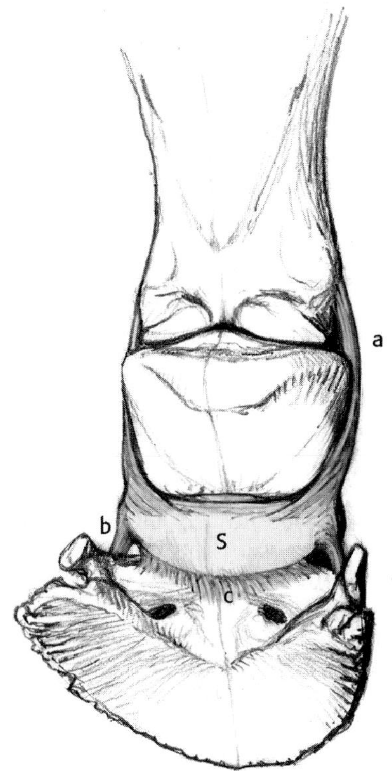

Figure 93-51. Supporting ligaments of the distal sesamoid bone (palmaromedial view). a, Collateral distal sesamoidean ligament; b, chondrosesamoidean ligament, c, impar ligament; S, distal sesamoid bone.

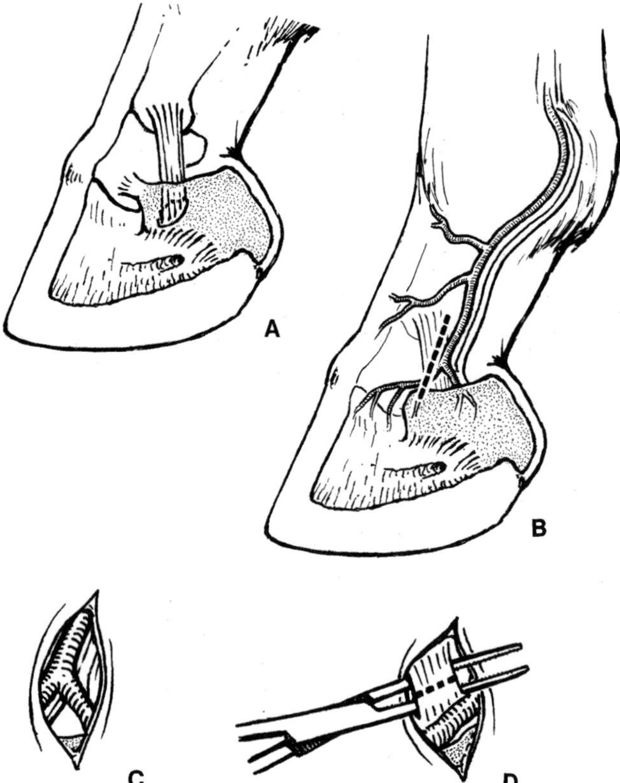

Figure 93-52. Desmotomy of the collateral distal sesamoidean ligament. **A,** Overview of the anatomic structures. **B,** Location of the skin incision over the ligament. **C,** After the skin is incised, the ligament can be seen underneath the superficial vessel. **D,** The ligament is isolated, elevated above the skin incision, and transected.

under maximal extension of the CSL, third-order acceleration (vibratory) forces between the DSB and the deep flexor tendon can develop.[88] Desmotomy of the CSL would remove these vibratory forces, which could potentially damage the DSB and IL with all the associated vasculature.

Surgical transection of the CSL is performed as described by Wright.[78,85] The horse is anesthetized and positioned in dorsal recumbency. An Esmarch bandage is applied as a tourniquet proximal to the metacarpophalangeal joint. A 4-cm vertical incision is made midway between the common digital extensor tendon and the distal eminence of the proximal phalanx, from the level of this eminence to the coronary band (see Fig. 93-52, *B*). The incision continues deeper through the subcutaneous fascia to permit identification and isolation of the coronary plexus (see Fig. 93-52, *C*) on the proximal margin of the collateral cartilage. Dissection axial to the cartilage allows identification of the dorsal margin of the CSL. A mosquito forceps is passed in the dorsopalmar direction under the CSL to elevate the ligament, and a no. 11 scalpel blade is used to transect it (see Fig. 93-52, *D*). The subcutaneous tissues are closed with a simple continuous suture pattern using 2-0 absorbable suture material. Skin closure is routine. The opposite CSL in the same limb and the ligaments of the opposite limb are transected with identical technique.

Postoperative care includes protective bandages for 10 days until the sutures or staples are removed. Hand-walking exercise should be initiated soon after surgery and is continued for 3 weeks. Thereafter, a gradually increasing exercise program is implemented with the goal of achieving full work levels by 3 months after surgery.[78] Postoperative complications are rare but include wound dehiscence, infection, local swelling, and postoperative scarring.

Preliminary results from the United Kingdom were encouraging: 13 of 16 horses treated with CSL desmotomy were able to work without lameness.[85] In the same year, another author reported clinical improvement in 50 % of 57 horses.[89] Two additional studies reported success rates of 15 of 21 horses and 12 of 17 horses,[90] respectively, with the latter horses being sound at least 6 months after surgery.[91] In a review of 118 horses suffering from navicular syndrome that were treated with navicular suspensory desmotomy, 76% were sound at 6 months, and 43% were sound after 36 months.[87]

All of the following conditions were associated with a diminished response: the presence of flexor cortex defects, the presence of proximal border enthesiophytes, mineralization of the DDF tendon, and medullary sclerosis of the DSB. Horses with more than 1 year's duration of clinical signs had a poor prognosis. The procedure is not recommended in horses with inflammatory disease of the distal interphalangeal joint and the navicular bursa, but horses with new bone growth at the site of insertion of the suspensory ligaments (enthesiophytes) are considered excellent candidates for this surgery. The procedure should be attempted early in the course of the syndrome.[92]

It was originally stated that desmotomy of the CSL should modify the biomechanical forces acting on the DSB, but clinical improvement could also be the result of transection of the sensory fibers that course within the suspensory ligaments. It seems that the procedure is more effective in improving clinical signs on a short-term basis (6 to 12 months), and the lameness can recur later on because of re-innervation of the sensory fibers in the CSL.

PALMAR DIGITAL NEURECTOMY

The most commonly performed surgical technique to abolish lameness associated with the navicular syndrome is palmar digital neurectomy (see earlier).

PERIVASCULAR SYMPATHECTOMY AND FASCIOLYSIS

Perivascular sympathectomy and fasciolysis around the lateral and medial digital artery and vein have been described for the treatment of navicular syndrome.[93] A 10-cm skin incision is centered over the lateral and medial proximal sesamoid bones. The subcutaneous tissues and fascia are carefully transected as well and the neurovascular bundle is identified. The artery and vein are isolated from their perivascular tissues and adventitia over the entire length of the surgical site. The nerve is isolated from its surroundings as well. Inadvertent traumatization of the vessels and the nerve should be avoided at all costs. Through this dissection the sympathetic nerve supply of the vessels is stripped, which results in a prolonged vasodilation. The subcutaneous tissues and the skin are closed in routine fashion.[94]

A significant increase in skin temperature caused by increased blood circulation in the region could be demonstrated at 8 and 20 weeks postoperatively with the help of thermography in 30 horses.[93] In each horse, one forelimb was operated on, whereas the other served as a control. A significant increase in hoof horn growth could be seen in the experimental limb compared to the control limb. In a review of 79 horses suffering from navicular syndrome that were treated with perivascular sympathectomy and fasciolysis, 73% were sound and returned to the intended use. The mean duration of follow-up was 23.6 months (range, 3 to 72 months).[93]

SURGICAL MANAGEMENT OF LAMINITIS

Laminitis is characterized by a breakdown of the connective tissue suspensory apparatus of the distal phalanx inside the hoof wall. As a result of lamellar pathology, the distal phalanx is no longer supported by the laminar attachment and starts to displace. As soon as the first signs of displacement are recognized, the disease becomes chronic.

There is a direct relationship between the degree and speed of movement of the distal phalanx away from the hoof capsule and the severity of damage to the laminae at the initial insult. Therefore, the most useful diagnostic and monitoring aids in the course of the disease are high-quality radiographs in both lateromedial and dorsopalmar (horizontal) projections.

Clinical Signs

Clinical signs, severity of damage, and response to therapy vary among individual horses, but it is widely accepted that the single most important factor influencing the final outcome of equine laminitis is the severity and extent of the initial damage to the internal anatomy of the foot.

Diagnosis

Clinical signs are very typical, and the radiographic examination further helps to diagnose this condition.

Treatment

Treatment of laminitis consists of dietary management, medical treatment, soft bedding, and hoof care. In all phases of the hoof care, corrective shoeing and trimming should aim to reduce stress to the damaged lamellae by minimizing the distracting forces affecting the displacement of the distal phalanx (rotation or sinking). DDF tenotomy is a salvage procedure for horses with chronic refractory laminitis accompanied by rotation of the distal phalanx and persistent pain. However, it is reported that even foundered horses with persistent draining tracts caused by osteomyelitis and excessive heel growth respond favorably to the procedure.[95]

Tenotomy of the Deep Digital Flexor Tendon

The rationale for tenotomy of the DDF tendon is based on the biomechanical forces in the foot. The procedure is performed to reduce the palmarly directed pulling forces of the DDF tendon on the distal phalanx and subsequently decrease the shearing stresses on the lamellae of the dorsal aspect of the hoof capsule. It also serves to reduce the pressure of the apex of the distal phalanx on the corium of the sole. Tenotomy of the DDF tendon permits lowering the heels to allow a more normal alignment (derotation) of the distal phalanx using orthopedic shoeing.[95]

DDF tenotomy can be performed at the midmetacarpal or the pastern area of the limb. Both procedures are equally effective, but tenotomy at the level of the midmetacarpus is preferred for various reasons. It is easier to perform and can be performed in a standing horse, the digital tendon sheath is not invaded, it bears less risk of postsurgical infection, and it leaves some support to the distal interphalangeal joint through fascial attachments. Pastern region DDF tenotomy must be performed under general anesthesia and should be reserved for cases that require a second tenotomy.

Before both surgeries, horses should be shod with a heel extension to stabilize the foot and help prevent postoperative hyperextension or subluxation of the distal interphalangeal joint.

MIDMETACARPAL APPROACH

The hair is clipped from the limb circumferentially from the level of the metacarpophalangeal joint to the carpus. The horse is sedated, and local anesthesia is achieved through a high palmar ring block.

After aseptic preparation of the limb, a vertical incision through the skin, subcutaneous tissue, and paratenon is made directly over the lateral aspect of the DDF tendon, centered at the junction of the proximal and middle third of the MCIII (Fig. 93-53, *A*). With the help of curved Kelly forceps, the DDF tendon is separated from the neurovascular bundle (Fig- 93-53B), the accessory ligament, and the superficial digital flexor (SDF) tendon. The DDF tendon is elevated out of the incision (see Fig. 93-53, *B*). During this part of the procedure, an assistant should lift the limb off the table to relieve the tension on the DDF tendon. Care must be taken to avoid elevating the neurovascular bundle located medially to prevent its inadvertent transection together with the tendon. The elevated tendon is subsequently transected with the scalpel blade. An immediate separation of the ends of 1 to 3 cm is usually noted after complete transection of the tendon.

An alternative tenotomy technique involves the blind transection of the DDF tendon with the help of a blunt bistoury while the animal is weightbearing.[96] Concomitant transection of the medially located neurovascular bundle can occur with this technique.

The subcutaneous tissue is closed with an absorbable monofilament suture material in a simple continuous pattern. The skin is closed with stainless steel staples.

DISTAL APPROACH

DDF tenotomy is performed with the horse in lateral recumbency under general anesthesia.[97] A 3-cm vertical skin incision is made along the palmar midline of the pastern region, 1 cm proximal to the bulb of the heel (Fig. 93-54, *A*). The skin, subcutaneous tissue, and sheath of the DDF tendon are incised, and the DDF tendon is exposed, elevated, and transected (see Fig. 93-54, *B* and *C*). The amount of separation of the tendon ends is greater after tenotomy at this level (6 to 10 cm) because there are no attachments to the distal tendon other than the insertion site to the distal

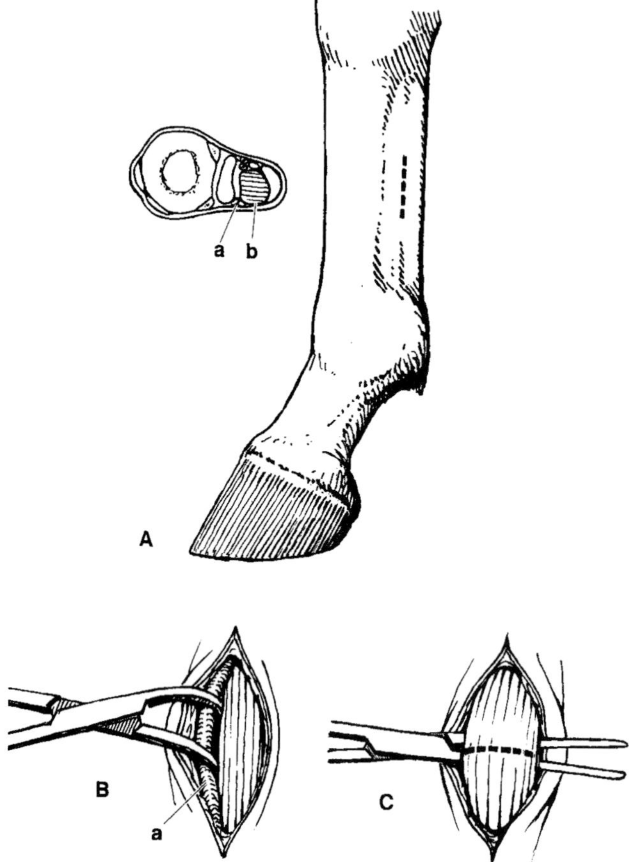

Figure 93-53. Deep digital flexor tenotomy in the mid-metacarpal region. **A,** Location of the surgical site on the lateral aspect of the limb. **B,** The deep digital flexor tendon is separated from the neurovascular bundle. **C,** The isolated deep digital flexor tendon is elevated above the incision and transected. a, Neurovascular bundle; b, deep digital flexor tendon.

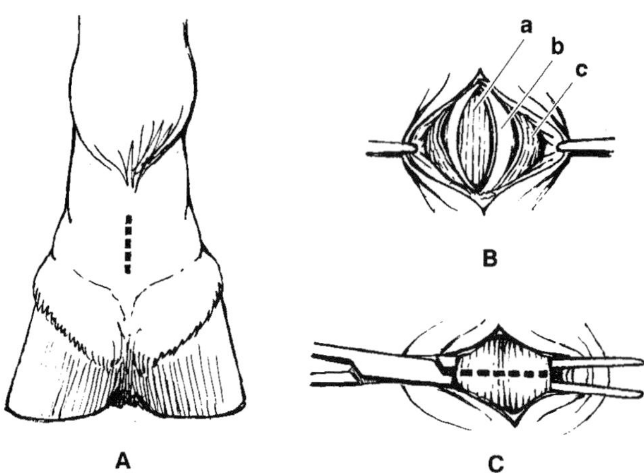

Figure 93-54. Deep digital flexor tenotomy in the mid-pastern region. **A,** Location of the surgical site. **B,** The skin, subcutaneous tissues (c), and tendon sheath (b) are sharply transected. **C,** The deep digital flexor tendon (a) is elevated above the incision and sharply transected.

phalanx.[96] Closure of the tendon sheath, subcutaneous tissue, and skin is routine.

Postoperative Management

Bandages should be maintained for a minimum of 6 weeks to minimize swelling and prevent contamination of the surgery site. The horse is administered phenylbutazone for pain as needed and confined to the stall, wearing a heel extension shoes for 6 to 8 weeks. For midmetacarpal tenotomy, this type of shoe seems to be less necessary.[95]

A mild degree of hyperextension of the distal interphalangeal joint occurs, but it is usually self-limiting.[92] Most horses show an initial improvement within 2 to 3 days of surgery. After tenotomy in either location, flexor support for the distal phalanx should develop through attachments of the distal tendon end by 6 to 8 weeks after surgery, and maintenance of a normal hoof–pastern axis without extended heels should be possible.[97] Tension relief after tenotomy appears to last for several months.[96]

Complications directly related to the surgery are rare but can include incision infection and postoperative pain. Chronic pain can result from overloading the SDF tendon before healing, osteoarthritis of the distal interphalangeal joint, or chronic infection of the digit.[96] A flexural deformity of the metacarpophalangeal joint (dorsiflexion) can develop from chronic pain, resulting in an inability to bear weight on the limb and contracture of scar tissue at the tenotomy site.

Prognosis

In a study of 13 horses with chronic laminitis and 12 to 36 degrees of rotation of the distal phalanx from the dorsal hoof wall, the first clinical improvement was noted by the third or fourth day after midpastern tenotomy of the DDF tendon. At the end of 2 weeks after surgery, the horses continued to improve and were willing to walk without the benefit of nerve blocks. Eventually, five horses could be lightly ridden, seven horses were pasture sound, and one horse was euthanized.[97] In another report of DDF tendon transection at the midmetacarpal level in 20 horses with severe acute or chronic laminitis unresponsive to conventional treatment, 11 patients survived less than 1 month after surgery and six horses survived longer than 6 months. Three horses remained lame, and no horse returned to athletic performance.[98]

One study evaluating the effect of DDF tenotomy as a treatment for chronic laminitis in 35 horses (midmetacarpal, 30 horses; midpastern, 5 horses) found that 27 horses (77%) were alive 6 months after surgery and 19 of 32 (59%) horses were alive for at least 2 years.[99] Bodyweight at the time of surgery and the degree of distal phalangeal rotation had no effect on the 2-year survival. Of the horses in this study, 10 became sound enough for light riding, and there was no correlation between the Obel grade of lameness, the degree of rotation, and the ability to be ridden.

Another study evaluating the effect of DDF tenotomy in the midcarpal region of nine horses with severe laminitis associated with complications such as intense pain, rotation more than 15 degrees, perforation of the sole, or evidence of infection of the sole or distal phalanx found an initial survival rate of 100%.[100] Six of the nine horses survived more than 21 months, and the other three were convalescing at the time the report was published. Four of the nine horses could be used for pleasure riding.

Although the recent studies report surprisingly good results, it should not be forgotten that these horses require prolonged and expensive supportive care and often additional surgical interventions. They suffer months of crippling foot pain and recumbency, and everyone involved must be dedicated to the patient.

REFERENCES

1. Josseck H, Zenker W, Geyer H: Hoof horn abnormalities in Lipizzaner horses and the effect of dietary biotin on macroscopic aspects of hoof horn quality, Equine Vet J 1995;27:175.
2. Geyer H, Schulze J: The long-term influence of biotin supplementation on hoof horn quality in horses, Schweiz Arch Tierheilkd 1994;136:137.
3. Roth F: Untersuchungen zur Strahlfäule und losen Wand beim Pferd, in Klinik für Pferde. Hannover, 1985, Tierärztliche Hochschule Hannover.
4. Kempson SA: Ultrastructural observation on the response of equine hoof defects to dietary supplementation with Farrier's Formula, Vet Rec 1990;127:494.
5. Kempson SA: Scanning electron microscope observations of hoof horn from horses with brittle feet, Vet Rec 1987;120:568.
6. Keller M, Krehon S, Stanek C, et al: Keratinopathogenic mould fungi and dermatophytes in healthy and diseased hooves of horses, Vet Rec 2000;147:619.
7. Kempson SA, Robb R: Use of a topical disinfectant as part of a hoof care programme for horses with diseases of the hoof capsule, Vet Rec 2004;154:647.
8. Tjalsma EJ, van Maurik JM: [The abnormal white line and hollow wall in horses, a comparative mycological study], Tijdschr Diergeneeskd 1995;120:526.
9. Hertsch B, Höppner S, Dallmer H: Lose Wand—Getrennte Wand. In Hertsch B, Höppner S, Dallmer H, editors: Der Huf und Sein Nagelloser Hufschutz, Warendorf, Germany, 2005, FN-Verlag.
10. Pollitt CC, Daradka M: Hoof wall wound repair, Equine Vet J 2004;36:210.
11. Moyer W, Sigafoos RD: Preliminary experience and uses of composite hoof wall repair, Proc Am Assoc Equine Pract 1991;37:681.
12. Hinterhofer C, Stanek C, Haider H: Finite element analysis (FEA) as a model to predict effects of farriery on the equine hoof, Equine Vet J Suppl 2001;Apr:58.
13. Pollitt CC: The Horse Foot, ed 1, London, 1995, Mosby-Wolfe.
14. O'Grady S: Quarter crack repair: An overview, Equine Vet Educ 2001;13:216.
15. Pardoe CH, Wilson AM: In vitro mechanical properties of different equine hoof wall crack fixation techniques, Equine Vet J 1999;31:506.
16. Kasapi MA, Gosline JM: Micromechanics of the equine hoof wall: Optimizing crack control and material stiffness through modulation of the properties of keratin, J Exp Biol 1999;202:377.
17. Kasapi MA, Gosline JM: Design complexity and fracture control in the equine hoof wall, J Exp Biol 1997;200:1639.
18. Kasapi MA, Gosline JM: Strain-rate-dependent mechanical properties of the equine hoof wall, J Exp Biol 1996;199:1133.
19. Greet TR: Keratoma of the hoof capsule. In Curtis S, editor: Corrective Farriery: A Textbook of Remedial Horseshoeing, Newmarket, England, 2002, R & W Publications.
20. Lloyd KC, Peterson PR, Wheat JD, et al: Keratomas in horses: 7 cases (1975-1986), J Am Vet Med Assoc 1988;193:967.
21. Bosch G, van Schie MJ, Back W: [Retrospective evaluation of surgical versus conservative treatment of keratomas in 41 lame horses (1995-2001)], Tijdschr Diergeneeskd 2004;129:700.
22. Stanek C: Management of foot abscesses, Presented at the 11th Annual Scientific Meeting, European College of Veterinary Surgeons, Vienna, Austria, July 5-7, 2002.
23. Cauvin ER, Munroe GA: Septic osteitis of the distal phalanx: Findings and surgical treatment in 18 cases, Equine Vet J 1998;30:512.
24. Pabst B, Kaegi B: Septic osteitis of the pedal bone in horses, Pferdeheilkunde 1990;6:197.
25. Richardson GL, O'Brien TR: Puncture wounds into the navicular bursa of the horse, Vet Radiol Ultrasound 1985;26:203.
26. Gibson KT, McIlwright CW, Park RP: A radiographic study of the distal interphalangeal joint and navicular bursa of the horse, Vet Radiol 1990;31:22.
27. Fürst A: Penetration wounds of the hoof, Presented at the 11th Annual Scientific Meeting, European College of Veterinary Surgeons, Vienna, Austria, July 5-7, 2002.
28. Murphy ED, Santschi EM, Papich MG: Regional intravenous perfusion of the distal limb of horses with amikacin sulfate, J Vet Pharmacol Ther 1999;22:68.
29. Wright IM, Phillips TJ, Walmsley JP: Endoscopy of the navicular bursa: A new technique for the treatment of contaminated and septic bursae, Equine Vet J 1999;31:5.
30. Marks G, Budras KD: Ultrastructure of the hoof epidermis in horses with canker, Vlaams-Diergeneeskundig-Tijdschrift 1985;54:287.
31. Reeves MJ, Yovich JV, Turner AS: Miscellaneous conditions of the equine foot, Vet Clin North Am Equine Pract 1989;5:221.
32. Prescott CW: Canker in the hoof of a horse, Aust Vet J 1970;46:449.
33. Mishra PN, Bose VS, Rao AT, et al: Cryotherapy for canker in a horse, Vet Rec 1998;142:284.
34. Wilson DG, Mays MB, Colahan PT: Treatment of canker in horses, J Am Vet Med Assoc 1989;194:1721.
35. Verschooten F, Van Waerebeek B: The ossification of cartilages of the distal phalanx in the horse: An anatomical, experimental, radiographic and clinical study, J Equine Vet Sci 1996;16:291.
36. Ruohoniemi M, Karkkainen M, Tervahartiala P: Evaluation of the variably ossified collateral cartilages of the distal phalanx and adjacent anatomic structures in the Finnhorse with computed tomography and magnetic resonance imaging, Vet Radiol Ultrasound 1997;38:344.
37. Ruohoniemi M, Laukkanen H, Ojala M, et al: Effects of sex and age on the ossification of the collateral cartilages of the distal phalanx of the Finnhorse and the relationships between ossification and body size and type of horse, Res Vet Sci 1997;62:34.
38. Ruohoniemi M, Makela O, Eskonen T: Clinical significance of ossification of the cartilages of the front feet based on nuclear bone scintigraphy, radiography and lameness examinations in 21 Finnhorses, Equine Vet J 2004;36:143.
39. Lundvall RL: Surgical removal of fractured sidebones, Proc Am Assoc Equine Pract.
40. Honnas CM, Ragle CA, Meagher DM: Necrosis of the collateral cartilage of the distal phalanx in horses: 16 cases (1970-1985), J Am Vet Med Assoc 1988;193:1303.
41. Honnas CM, Dabareiner RM, McCauley BH: Hoof wall surgery in the horse: Approaches to and underlying disorders, Vet Clin North Am Equine Pract 2003;19:479.
42. Hertsch B: Zur Diagnose und Behandlung der Hufbeinfraktur, Dtsch Tierärztl Wochenschr 1972;79:517.
43. Yovich JV, Stashak TS, DeBowes RM, et al: Fractures of the distal phalanx of the forelimb in eight foals, J Am Vet Med Assoc 1986;189:550.
44. Scott EA, McDole M, Shires MH: A review of third phalanx fractures in the horse: 65 cases, J Am Vet Med Assoc 1979;174:1337.
45. Honnas CM, O'Brien TR, Linford RL: Distal phalanx fractures in horses: A survey of 274 horses with radiographic assessment of healing in 36 horses, Vet Radiol 1988;29:98.
46. McDiarmid AM: An unusual case of distal phalanx fracture in a horse, Vet Rec 1995;137:613.

47. Keegan KG, Twardock AR, Losonsky JM, et al: Scintigraphic evaluation of fractures of the distal phalanx in horses: 27 cases (1979-1988), J Am Vet Med Assoc 1993;202:1993.
48. Martens P, Ihler CF, Rennesund J: Detection of a radiographically occult fracture of the lateral palmar process of the distal phalanx in a horse using computed tomography, Vet Radiol Ultrasound 1999;40:346.
49. Hertsch B, Haak D: Zur konservativen Behandlung der Sagittal- und Abrissfraktur des Hufbeins des Pferdes, Wien Tierärztl Monatsschr 74, 1987
50. Honnas CM, Vacek JR, Schumacher J: Diagnosis and treatment of articular fractures of the equine distal phalanx, Vet Med 1992;87:1208
51. O'Sullivan CB, Dart AJ, Malikides N, et al: Nonsurgical management of type II fractures of the distal phalanx in 48 Standardbred horses, Aust Vet J 1999;77:501.
52. Petterson H: Conservative and surgical treatment of fractures of the third phalanx, Proc Am Assoc Equine Pract 1972;18:183-191.
53. Andritzky J, Rossol M, Lischer C, et al: Comparison of computer assisted surgery with conventional technique for the treatment of axial distal phalanx fractures in horses: An in-vitro study, Vet Surg 2005;34:120.
54. Boening KJ, von Saldern FC, Leendertse I, et al: Diagnostische und operative Arthroskopie am Hufgelenk des Pferdes, Pferdeheilkunde 1988;4:155.
55. Haynes PF, Adams OR: Internal fixation of fractured extensor process of third phalanx in a horse, J Am Vet Med Assoc 1974;164:61.
56. MacLellan KN, MacDonald DG, Crawford WH: Lag screw fixation of an extensor process fracture in a foal with flexural deformity, Can Vet J 1997;38:226.
57. Dechant JE, Trotter GW, Stashak TS, et al: Removal of large fragments of the extensor process of the distal phalanx via arthrotomy in horses: 14 cases (1992-1998), J Am Vet Med Assoc 2000;217:1351.
58. Honnas CM, O'Brien TR, Linford RL: Solar margin fractures of the equine distal phalanx, Proc Am Assoc Equine Pract 1987;33:399.
59. Story MR, Bramlage L: Arthroscopic debridement of subchondral bone cysts in the distal phalanx of 11 horses (1994-2000), Equine Vet J 2004;36:356.
60. Kopp K, Bramlage L: Winning the battle of bowed tendons, Equus 116:47.
61. Wintzer HJ, Dämmrich K: Über Strahlbeinfrakturen beim Pferd, Schweiz Arch Tierheilk 1997;109:487.
62. Hertsch B, Königsmann D: Die Sagittalfrakturen des Strahlbeines beim Pferd—ein Beitrag zur Diagnose und Therapie, Pferdeheilkunde 1993;9:3.
63. Lillich JD, Ruggles AJ, Gabel AA, et al: Fracture of the distal sesamoid bone in horses: 17 cases (1982-1992), J Am Vet Med Assoc 1995;207:924.
64. Nemeth F, Dik KJ: Lag screw fixation of sagittal navicular bone fractures in five horses, Equine Vet J 1985;17:137.
65. Matthews S, Dart AJ, Dowling BA: Palmar digital neurectomy in 24 horses using the guillotine technique, Aust Vet J 2003;81:402.
66. Meier HP: [The history of neurectomy in horses with navicular disease], Schweiz Arch Tierheilkd 1996;138:15.
67. High JT, Miller SM, Swanson TD, Beeman GM: Standing guillotine neurectomy for the treatment of navicular pain in horses: 116 cases, Vet Comp Orthop Traumatol 2000;A5:13.
68. Black JB: Palmar digital neurectomy: An alternative surgical approach, Proc Am Assoc Equine Pract 1992;38:429.
69. Jackman BR, Baxter GM, Doran RE, et al: Palmar digital neurectomy in horses: 57 cases (1984-1990), Vet Surg 1993;22:285.
70. Lose MP, Hopkins EJ: Preliminary report of a modified surgical approach to posterior digital neurectomy in the horse, Vet Med Small Anim Clin 1976;71:317.
71. Harris JM, Kennedy MA: Modified posterior digital neurectomy for management of chronic heel pain in horses, Presented at the 40th Annual Convention of the American Association of Equine Practitioners, Vancouver, BC, December 4-7, 1994.
72. Tate LP, Jr., Evans LH: Cryoneurectomy in the horse, J Am Vet Med Assoc 1980;177:423.
73. Seino KK, Foreman JH, Greene SA, et al: Effects of topical perineural capsaicin in a reversible model of equine foot lameness, J Vet Intern Med 2003;17:563.
74. Haugland LM, Collier MA, Panciera RJ, et al: The effect of CO_2 laser neurectomy on neuroma formation and axonal regeneration, Vet Surg 1992;21:351.
75. Moorman GH, van Noort JH, Nemeth F, et al: Detection of neurectomy by testing skin sensitivity using an electrical stimulus, Equine Vet J 1988;20:194.
76. van Hoogmoed LM, Snyder JR: Use of infrared thermography to detect injections and palmar digital neurectomy in horses, Vet J 2002;164:129.
77. Dyson SJ: Navicular disease and other soft tissue causes of palmar foot pain. In Ross MW, Dyson SJ, editors: Diagnosis and Management of Lameness in the Horse, Philadelphia, 2003, WB Saunders.
78. Wright IM: A study of 118 cases of navicular disease: Clinical features, Equine Vet J 1999;25:488.
79. Wright IM, Kidd L, Thorp BH: Gross, histological and histomorphometric features of the navicular bone and related structures in the horse, Equine Vet J 1998;30:220.
80. Madison JB, Dyson SJ: Treatment and prognosis of horses with navicular disease. In Ross MW, Dyson SJ, editors: Diagnosis and Management of Lameness in the Horse, Philadelphia, 2003, WB Saunders.
81. Dabareiner RM, Carter GK, Honnas CM: Injection of corticosteroids, hyaluronate, and amikacin into the navicular bursa in horses with signs of navicular area pain unresponsive to other treatments: 25 cases (1999-2002), J Am Vet Med Assoc 2003;223:1469.
82. Denoix JM, Thibaud D, Riccio B: Tiludronate as a new therapeutic agent in the treatment of navicular disease: A double-blind placebo-controlled clinical trial, Equine Vet J 2003;35:407.
83. Fricker C, Bucher K, Stuker G: [Are degenerative joint diseases chronic compartment syndromes?], Schweiz Arch Tierheilkd 1995;137:137.
84. Casley-Smith JR, Casley-Smith JR: High-Protein Oedemas and the Benzo-Pyrones, Sydney, 1986, JB Lippincott.
85. Wright IM: Navicular suspensory desmotomy in the treatment of navicular disease: Technique and preliminary results, Equine Vet J 1986;18:443.
86. Wright IM, Douglas J: Biomechanical considerations in the treatment of navicular disease, Vet Rec 1993;133:109.
87. Wright IM: A study of 118 cases of navicular disease: Treatment by navicular suspensory desmotomy, Equine Vet J 1993;25:501.
88. Rooney JR: Biomechanics of Lameness in Horses, ed 1, Baltimore, 1969, Williams & Wilkins.
89. Diehl M: Desmotomy of the navicular collateral ligaments in horses with navicular disease, Eur Soc Vet Surg, 1986.
90. Watkins JP, McMullan WM, Morris EL: Navicular suspensory desmotomy in the management of navicular syndrome: A retrospective analysis, Proc Am Assoc Equine Pract 1993;39:261.
91. Bell B, Bridge I, Sullivan S: Surgical treatment of navicular syndrome in the horse using navicular suspensory desmotomy, N Z Vet J 1996;44:26.
92. Honnas CM: The foot. In Auer JA, Stick JA, editors: Equine Surgery, Philadelphia, 1999, WB Saunders.
93. Jaugstetter HP: Der Einfluss der perivaskulären Sympathektomie und Fasziolyse auf die Durchblutung der distalen Pferdeextremität: Thermographische Untersuchungen sowie Messungen des Hornwachstums nach perivaskulärer Sympathektomie und Fasziolyse beim Pferd. In Pferdechirurgie, Giessen, 2002, Justus-Liebig-Universität.
94. Jaugstetter H, Jacobi R, Litzke LF, et al: Perivaskuläre Sympathektomie: Eine Therapiemöglichkeit beim Podotrochlose-/Sesamoidose-Syndrom, Tierärztl Praxis 2003;31:46.
95. Redden RR: Complicated laminitis. Proc Am Assoc Equine Pract 1988;34:311.

96. Hunt RJ: Deep digital flexor tenotomy for managing laminitis. In Ross MW, Dyson SJ, editors: Diagnosis and Management of Lameness in the Horse, Philadelphia, 2003, WB Saunders.
97. Allen D Jr, White NA 2nd, Foerner JF, et al: Surgical management of chronic laminitis in horses: 13 cases (1983-1985), J Am Vet Med Assoc 1986;189:1604.
98. Hunt RJ, Allen D, Baxter GM, et al: Mid-metacarpal deep digital flexor tenotomy in the management of refractory laminitis in horses, Vet Surg 1991;20:15.
99. Eastman TG, Honnas CM, Hague BA, et al: Deep digital flexor tenotomy as a treatment for chronic laminitis in horses: 35 cases (1988-1997). J Am Vet Med Assoc 1999;214:517.
100. Nickels A: Deep digital flexor tenotomy: A personal perspective, Presented at the Thirteenth Annual Bluegrass Laminitis Symposium, Louisville, Ky, February 28–March 2, 1999.

CHAPTER 94

Phalanges and the Metacarpophalangeal and Metatarsophalangeal Joints

Alan J. Nixon

MIDDLE PHALANX

The middle phalanx is a relatively compact bone that is loaded predominantly in axial and torsional planes during athletic activity. It articulates with the distal phalanx through a high-motion joint and proximally with the proximal phalanx through a relatively low-motion joint. The middle phalanx is enclosed distally within the confines of the hoof and coronary band, but it is more exposed proximally, particularly over the palmar and plantar eminences.

The middle phalanx is bounded by multiple ligaments and tendons. The common (or long) digital extensor tendons dorsally and the digital flexor tendons palmarly (or plantarly) contribute to motion of the proximal and distal interphalangeal joints and provide resistance to overextension of the distal limb. In addition, the middle phalanx is stabilized by strong lateral and medial collateral ligaments of the proximal interphalangeal joint and the suspensory ligament of the navicular bone.

Fractures of the middle phalanx are most common in Quarter Horses but occur in all breeds.[1,2] Horses that turn predominantly on their hindlimbs, such as cutting and reining horses, incur comminuted fractures of the middle phalanx almost exclusively in the hindlimbs. More than 70% of middle phalanx fractures in one report involved the hindlimb.[2] Similarly, distraction fractures of the plantar eminences occur primarily in the hindlimbs because of the forces incurred during sudden stops and turns, most likely as an avulsion of the bony insertion of the superficial digital flexor (SDF) tendons.

Fracture Configurations

Middle phalangeal fractures are classified as simple or comminuted and fall into one of four categories: dorsal or palmar or plantar intra-articular osteochondral fractures, palmar or plantar eminence fractures, axial fractures, or comminuted fractures.[2]

Osteochondral Fractures

Dorsal or palmar or plantar osteochondral fractures are not common.[3-6] Most osteochondral fractures occur on the palmar or plantar aspect of the middle phalanx, either lateral or medial to the axial midline (Fig. 94-1). These fractures do not involve the insertion of SDF tendon or distal sesamoidean ligaments and therefore do not distract. Despite the size and intra-articular location of these fragments, development of osteoarthritis is relatively slow. Nevertheless, they have been reported as a cause of lameness, and surgical removal is recommended if a lameness examination confirms the mid-phalangeal region as the site of pain. They can be incidental findings.

Surgical removal of palmar or plantar fragments using arthroscopy is recommended, although open approaches through the digital sheath are described. The arthroscopic portal is made into the voluminous palmar pouch of the proximal interphalangeal (PIP) joint (Fig. 94-2). Access for instruments is provided by a second portal 2 cm distal to the arthroscope, and often an additional portal on the contralateral side of the palmar region of the pastern, especially when removing large palmar fragments. Fragment dissection and removal can be difficult.

Dorsal fragments also can be removed arthroscopically with an approach over the dorsal joint pouch.[6] Limited maneuverability results from the attachment of the extensor tendon immediately distal to the joint. Arthroscope entry is usually abaxial to the extensor tendon. The prognosis after surgical removal of dorsal and palmar fragments is favorable, unless the fragmentation is associated with early joint degeneration.

Palmar or Plantar Eminence Fractures

Fractures of the palmar or plantar eminence of the middle phalanx can be uniaxial or biaxial.[4] The treatment and

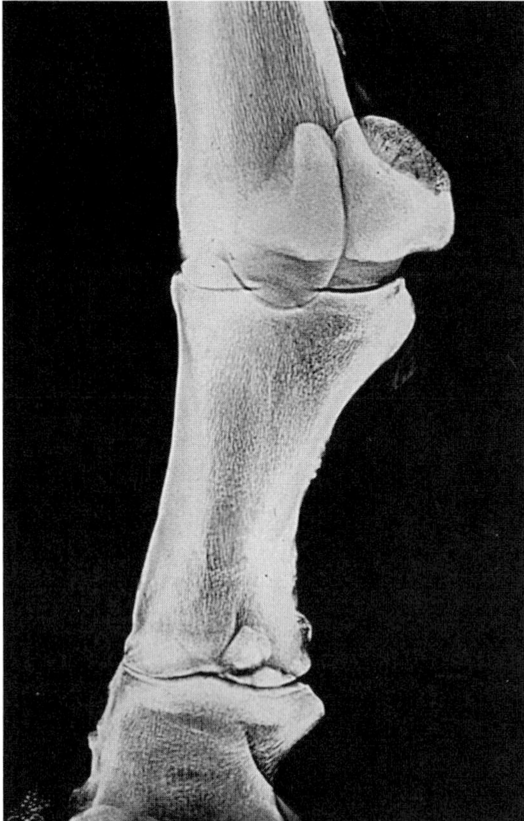

Figure 94-1. Plantar osteochondral fracture of the proximal margin of the middle phalanx. Arthroscopic access can be used to remove the fragments that cause lameness.

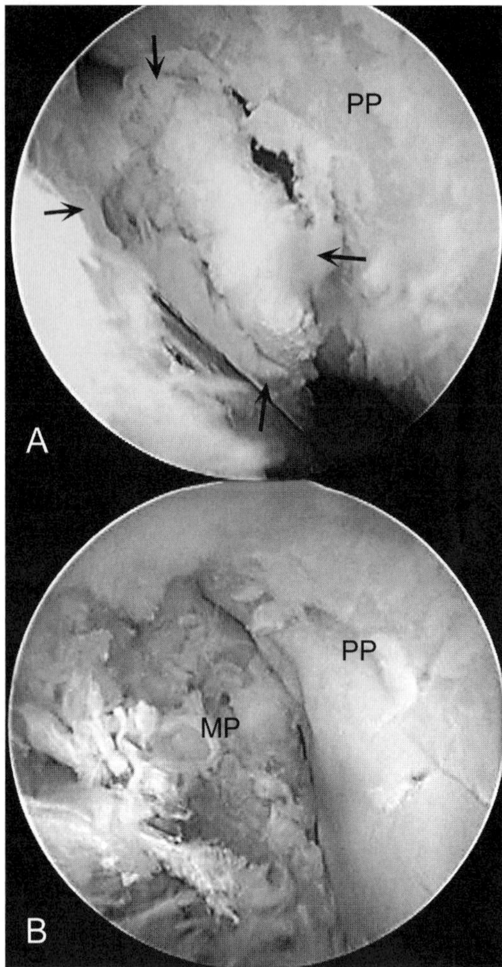

Figure 94-2. A, Arthroscopic appearance of a middle phalangeal palmar fragment *(arrows)*. Rongeurs have been introduced through an ipsilateral portal adjacent to the palmar condylar surface of the proximal phalanx (PP). **B,** After removal of the fracture fragment, the fracture bed on the proximal aspect of the middle phalanx (MP) is evident.

prognosis vary considerably depending on this configuration. These fractures result from hyperextension of the pastern joint, with tension on the palmar or plantar attachments of the SDF tendon or the distal sesamoidean ligaments. Uniaxial fracture does not result in pastern subluxation or the considerable lameness associated with biaxial fracture. Occasionally, fracture fragments do not involve the entire eminence. Rarely, the palmar soft-tissue structures are disrupted without fracture of the bony insertion. Radiographs verify the type and extent of the fracture.

Uniaxial palmar or plantar eminence fractures can be treated with screw fixation or pastern arthrodesis, depending on the duration and configuration of the fracture.[7] Screw fixation in lag fashion can be performed through stab incisions over the proximal extremity of the fractured eminence, with the screws inserted under radiographic control.

Fracture reduction can be difficult depending on the duration of the fracture. The interfragmentary screw is inserted in a distal axial direction, with the primary access to the eminence gained by splitting the insertion of the SDF tendon longitudinally. A delay in presentation or the presence of biaxial palmar eminence fractures necessitates pastern arthrodesis. Even with stable articulations and uniaxial eminence fracture, arthrodesis can be preferable and is best performed using two parallel 5.5-mm cortex screws inserted in lag fashion in addition to a three-hole narrow dynamic compression plate (DCP) dorsally[8,9] (see Chapter 85). The 5.5-mm cortex screws provide more rigid fixation than 4.5-mm screws. A bone graft is not usually necessary, although forage of the subchondral bone of the proximal and middle phalanx is used to improve access to bone-forming cells.

A postoperative cast is usually maintained for 10 days to 2 weeks. The prognosis after arthrodesis for uniaxial fractures is fair to favorable.[2,8,10] The outlook for return to active work is improved with fractures of hindlimb versus forelimb eminences. Recuperative periods of up to 12 months are required, which can be shortened by the use of plate fixation for pastern arthrodesis.

Biaxial fractures of the palmar or plantar eminences result in considerable lameness and instability of the PIP joint (Fig. 94-3). Pastern arthrodesis by dorsal plate application is preferred.[11,12] Plate configurations include a single broad DCP or two narrow DCPs placed on the dorsal aspect of the proximal and middle phalanges.[1,10] The palmar or plantar eminence fractures are stabilized by screw fixation placed in lag fashion through the distal plate screw holes (Fig. 94-4). Individual interfragmentary screws unassociated with the

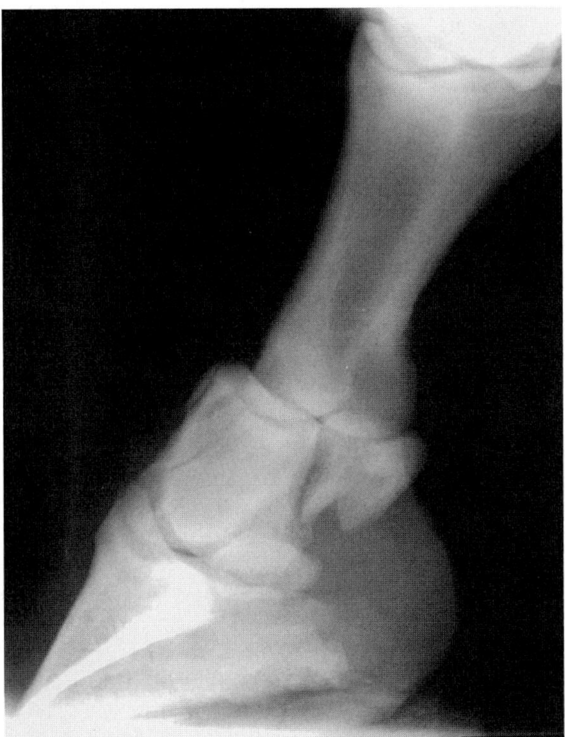

Figure 94-3. Biaxial fracture of the plantar eminences of the middle phalanx, with additional dorsal fractures. Stability is lost, and the most effective therapy is arthrodesis of the proximal interphalangeal joint.

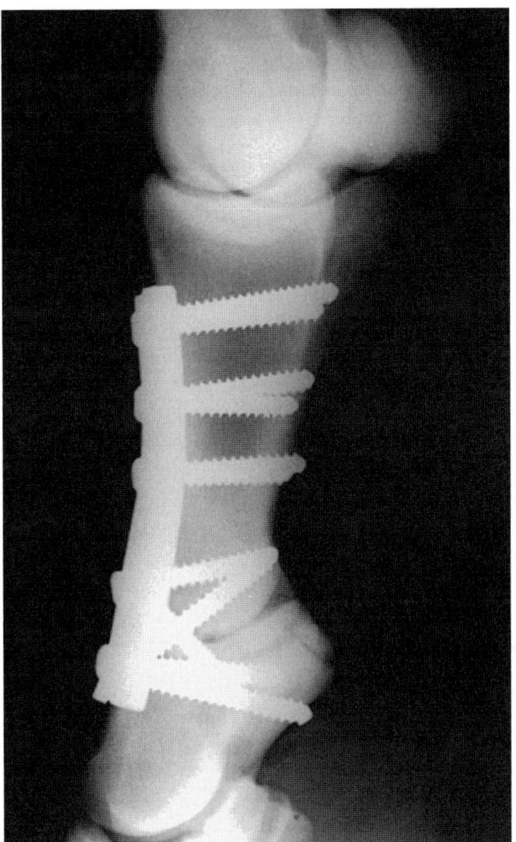

Figure 94-4. Repair of biaxial plantar eminence fractures using two narrow dynamic compression plates (DCPs) applied to the dorsal surface of the middle and proximal phalanges. The distal-most screw in both plates engages and lags the plantar eminence on either side.

plate can occasionally be added to strengthen the repair. Pastern arthrodesis by plate fixation without attempted perfect reduction of the individual eminence fractures is satisfactory; however, callus production and induced secondary lameness are minimized if the eminence fragments can be incorporated into the repair.

Prognosis after biaxial eminence fracture repair by arthrodesis is fair, particularly for fractures involving the hindlimbs.[2,8] For additional information on pastern arthrodesis, see Chapter 85.

Axial Fractures

Simple axial fractures of the middle phalanx occur rarely (Fig. 94-5). These fractures can be repaired with cortex or shaft screws applied in lag fashion. The fracture configuration dictates the approach. Adequate reduction is confirmed radiographically before placement of the first screw. Cast fixation during the initial 4 postoperative weeks is important. The prognosis is guarded for ambulation free of lameness because some proliferative new bone formation, especially at the articular margins, is expected as a result of the initial trauma.

Comminuted Middle Phalanx Fractures

Comminuted fractures are the most common configuration of middle phalangeal fracture.[2,4] Clinical appearance includes severe non–weight-bearing lameness with palpable instability and, occasionally, crepitus of the distal limb. The configuration of the fracture is confirmed with radiography, and the treatment is selected based on the extent of the fracture and possibility of adequate repair. Treatment options include screw fixation in lag fashion of minimally comminuted fractures, application of a single broad DCP or two narrow DCPs for fracture fixation and pastern arthrodesis, or application of a transfixation cast; another option is euthanasia.

An extensive series of preoperative radiographs is required to establish the extent of comminution. Most comminuted fractures involve proximal portions of the phalanx, and many extend into the distal interphalangeal (DIP) joint, reducing the prognosis (Fig. 94-6). A computed tomographic (CT) scan is particularly helpful in defining multiple fracture planes entering the DIP. Most are more complex than suggested by plain radiographs.

The aim of surgical repair is reconstruction of the distal and, to some extent, the proximal articular surfaces of the middle phalanx. If reconstruction of the DIP joint is inadequate or the bone is severely comminuted and unlikely to be adequately repaired with a plate and screws, humane destruction should be considered.

The most frequent configuration of comminuted fractures involves fractures in both a sagittal and frontal (transverse) plane, often with added comminution on the palmar or plantar proximal aspect. Marked instability because of

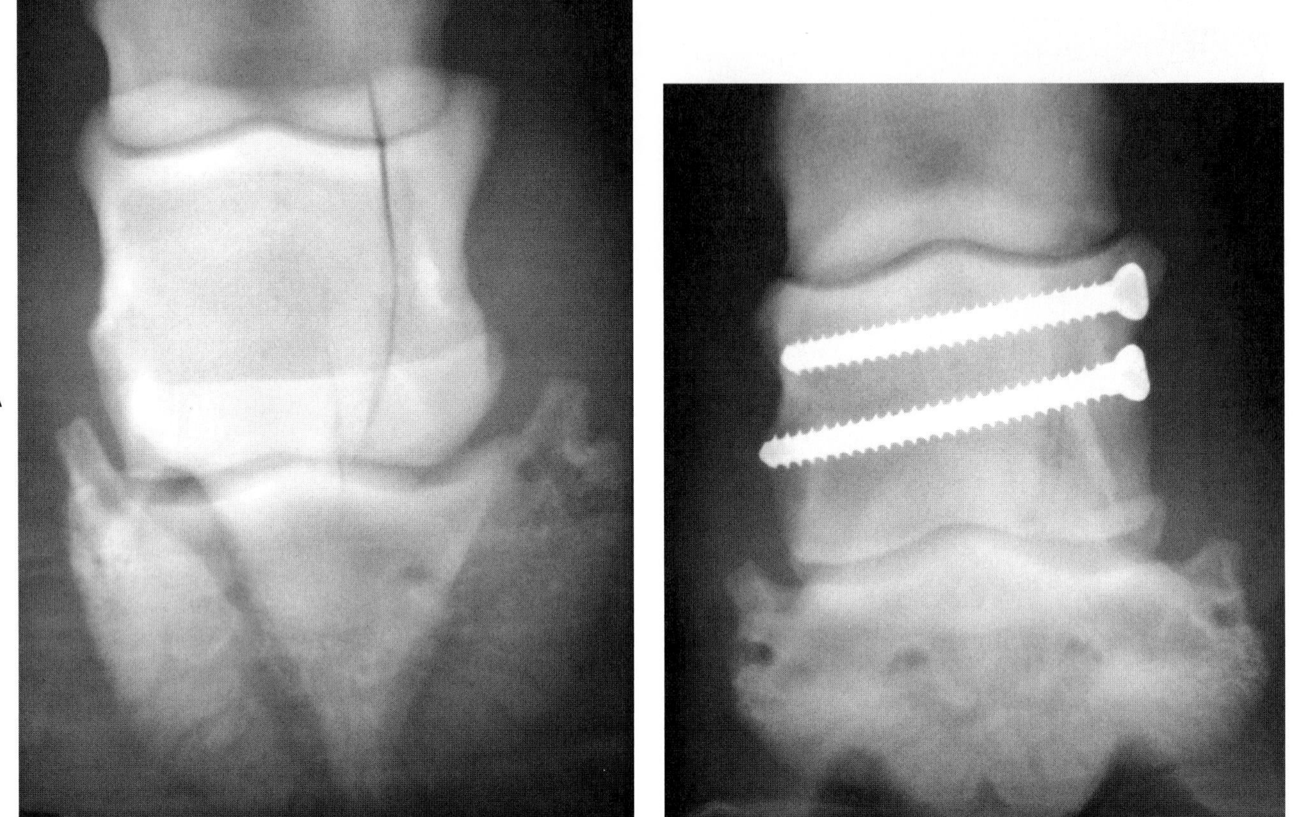

Figure 94-5. **A**, Dorsopalmar projection of a rarely occurring axial middle phalanx fracture. **B**, Dorsopalmar postoperative radiographic projection after implantation of two 5.5-mm cortex screws using lag technique. (Courtesy C. Lischer, University of Zurich.)

involvement of the attachments of the palmar or plantar ligaments and tendinous structures is common. Rarely, the distal sesamoid bone is also fractured. Treatment for most comminuted middle phalanx fractures involves application of two narrow DCPs,[4] although use of a single broad DCP and a T-plate has been described.[2,11,12]

Plate fixation in combination with pastern arthrodesis optimizes the chances for adequate reconstruction of the distal articular surface. An extensive dorsal approach to the proximal and middle phalanx is used. The application of two narrow DCPs allows greater versatility in screw placement than a single plate.

The proximal articular surface of the middle phalanx is exposed to allow initial reduction and stabilization of the palmar or plantar portions of the fracture to the dorsal struts of bone.[4] The sagittal fractures are reduced later with individual screws inserted in lag fashion. Intraoperative radiographs ensure reconstruction of the articular surface within the DIP joint.

The cartilage of the PIP joint is removed, and the plate screws in the proximal phalanx are implanted. If possible, one or two plate screws should be placed transarticularly (Fig. 94-7). Postoperative cast fixation for 4 to 8 weeks is used, particularly where fracture stability is tenuous. Follow-up radiographs at the time of cast removal dictate the period of stall confinement, which is an additional 6 to 12 weeks. Postfixation callus development can be extensive, depending on the extent of fracture line reduction and rigidity of the stabilization. The union of the proximal and middle phalanges usually progresses quickly. The most common cause of persisting lameness is osteoarthritis of the DIP joint.

Repair of severely comminuted fractures with cast or transfixation cast techniques is reserved for fractures that cannot be adequately reduced and stabilized by implants and when humane destruction is not an option for the owner. Fractures entering the DIP joint usually result in some osteoarthritis, and the degree of residual lameness varies accordingly. The prognosis is partly determined by the development of weight-bearing laminitis on the opposite limb. The selection of fixation should provide the earliest return of comfortable weightbearing on the fracture to minimize this complication.

Complete resolution of lameness with implant fixation can occur[1,2,4,11,12]; however, residual lameness is anticipated if there is inadequate reduction of the fracture fragments entering the DIP joint. Concurrent fractures of the distal sesamoid bone reduce the prognosis further. The vascular supply to the distal limb and the soft tissue integrity can occasionally be compromised through the initial fracture or during attempts at repair. Preoperative immobilization in a supporting splint is important for the long-term outcome of these cases (see Chapter 78). Infection can also be a serious complication, and local and systemic antibiotics are used to minimize bacterial growth. The prognosis is improved by the use of a pair of narrow DCPs, and this technique is recommended over others.[1,4]

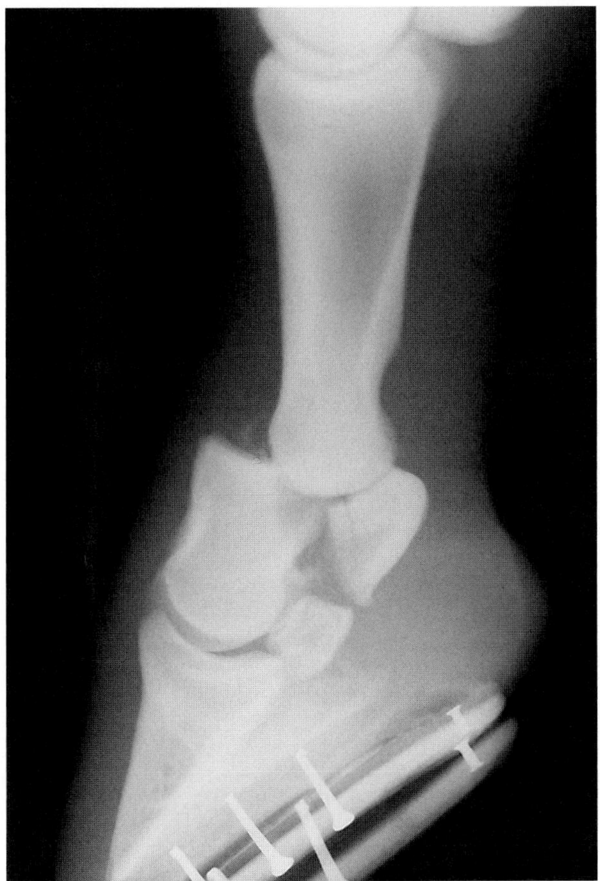

Figure 94-6. Lateromedial radiographic projection of comminuted middle phalanx fracture with pastern subluxation.

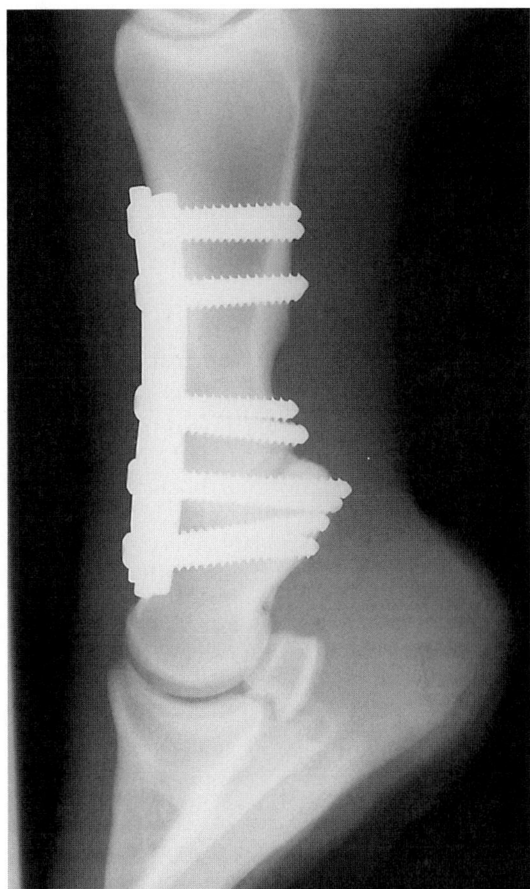

Figure 94-7. Double plate fixation of a comminuted middle phalanx fracture. Two distal screws in each plate and one independent lag screw secure the fracture planes. Same case as Figure 81-5.

PROXIMAL INTERPHALANGEAL JOINT

Osteoarthritis

Osteoarthritis of the PIP joint (high ringbone) is a relatively common condition affecting multiple breeds, particularly those with a tendency for short upright pastern conformation. In addition, horses that make quick stops and hard turns with rapid twisting, such as Western performance horses and show jumpers, have a high incidence of pastern osteoarthritis. In young horses, there is also the possibility of arthritic change induced by osteochondrosis (OC).[13]

Osteoarthritis can occur in the PIP joints of the forelimbs and hindlimbs and often results in grade II to III/IV lameness. Palpable enlargements of the PIP joints are a feature after the development of periarticular new bone. Confirmation of the PIP joint as a site of lameness usually requires perineural anesthesia and radiographs to confirm the involvement of the joint. Nonarticular new bone production can be misdiagnosed clinically as true intra-articular osteoarthritic change and should be assessed with radiography before any discussion of surgical therapy. Pain on manipulation of the PIP region is occasionally elicited, and the horse can have a positive response to flexion tests of the distal limb. Heat and swelling over the PIP joint are indicators of pastern arthritis. The lameness is usually chronic and exacerbated by increased work. Radiographic evidence of osteoarthritis can be confined to one limb but occasionally occurs in both, if the problem is conformational in origin.

Treatment of true intra-articular PIP osteoarthritis is usually surgical fusion of the involved joint.[8,10] The response to intra-articular medication with corticosteroid preparations is usually short term. Horses improve considerably with phenylbutazone therapy. Recalcitrant lameness is treated with surgical fusion of the PIP joint. For simple arthritic conditions, this can be accomplished by dorsal exposure of the affected joint, removal of articular cartilage, and application of two 5.5-mm cortex screws to provide lag screw compression across the articulation, as previously described. Additionally, a three-hole plate is applied to the dorsal aspect of the two phalanges involved. Postoperative cast fixation is needed for up to 2 weeks after arthrodesis. Cast bandage combinations may be substituted for the cast in the second week of the 2-week coaptation period.

The rate at which bone union is achieved depends on the degree of stability afforded by internal stabilization. Most horses continue to form periarticular callus for 6 months after surgical repair. Unstable repairs result in exuberant callus, which can interfere with the action of the flexor tendons on the palmar or plantar surface of the pastern and occasionally with the extensor tendons over the dorsal middle phalanx region. Digital extensor tendons can adhere to exostoses on the dorsal aspect of the distal phalanx and result in residual lameness.[8,14] Excessively long screws that penetrate the palmar or plantar surface of the middle phalanx and interfere with the action of the distal sesamoid bone are causes of residual lameness.

The prognosis for riding soundness is fair to favorable, particularly for conditions involving the hind limb. The outcome in one report indicated 16 of 22 horses returned to full function.[9] A second study indicated 16 of 21 clinical cases became sound after arthrodesis, with a better response in the hind limbs.[8]

Osteochondrosis and Subchondral Cystic Lesions

OC can occasionally develop in the PIP joint. Subchondral cystic lesions (SCLs) are diagnosed more often than dissecting cartilage flap lesions and involve the distal articular surface of the proximal phalanx (Fig. 94-8) or rarely the proximal articular surface of the middle phalanx. Late stages of OC with secondary osteoarthritis have been diagnosed in young horses unilaterally and bilaterally. Solitary SCLs are readily apparent on radiographs, whereas multiple SCLs are associated with a persistent lameness leading eventually to osteoarthritis.

Intra-articular hyaluronan injections provide temporary pain relief in solitary SCLs. Surgical curettage of solitary SCLs of the proximal phalanx has been performed in five horses (three foals and two adults).[15] Because the lesion is often not approachable arthroscopically, transosseous drilling is used. Initially, a small drill bit is advanced under fluoroscopic control into the cyst, confirmed by draining of saline previously injected into the PIP joint. Proper seating of the drill is verified radiographically, and the drill hole is enlarged with a 5.5-mm drill bit, allowing access with a curet to evacuate the cyst. After copious flushing from the joint, the cyst and drill hole are filled with tricalcium phosphate granules.[15] Long-term follow-up revealed that four of the five horses treated were serviceable and could engage in the intended athletic function. Additional information about this treatment is found in Chapter 92.

Multiple cystic lesions show a poor response to medical treatment, leaving elective arthrodesis of the joint as the only treatment (see Chapter 85). Simultaneous bilateral arthrodesis can be performed in foals, whereas staged fusion is elected in adult horses.

Luxation and Subluxation

Luxation and subluxation of the PIP joint are usually treated with arthrodesis. Subluxation is more common and occurs in either a dorsal or palmar direction. Dorsal subluxation is the result of damage to the suspensory ligament and its terminal extensor branches; it can occasionally be caused by contracture of the distal sesamoidean ligaments (Fig. 94-9). Palmar subluxation results from failure of the palmar

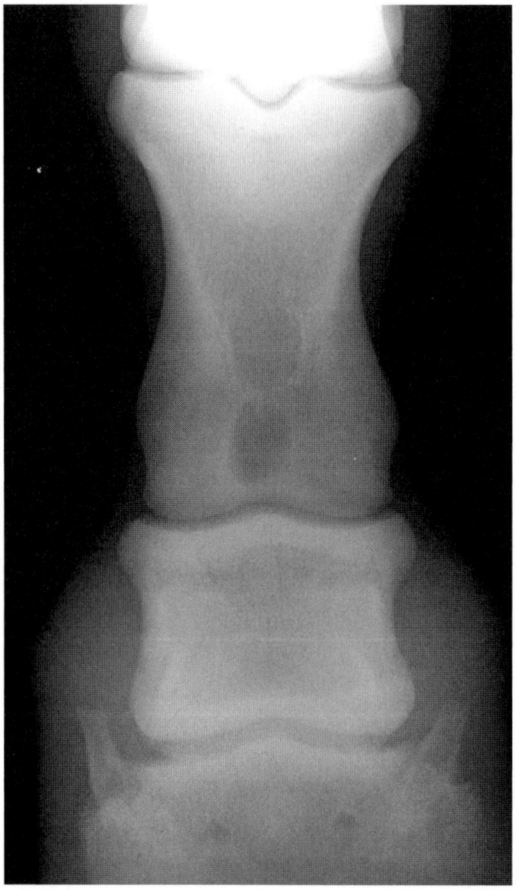

Figure 94-8. Subchondral cystic lesion of the distal aspect of the proximal phalanx. If conservative therapy fails, transcortical approaches either laterally or through the palmar cortex allow access to the cyst.

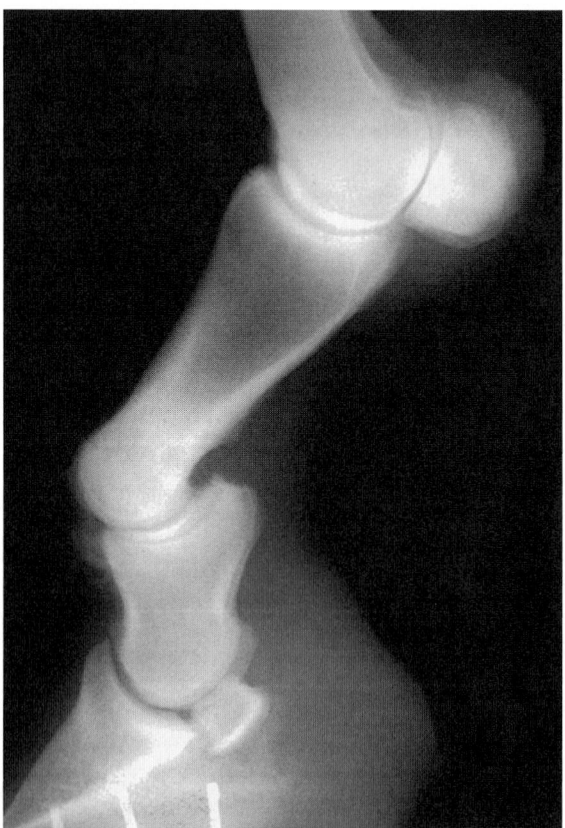

Figure 94-9. Dorsal subluxation of the proximal interphalangeal joint caused by loss of support from the extensor branches of the suspensory ligament. Note the distal location of the proximal sesamoid bones as a result of failure of the suspensory ligament.

supporting connective tissues such as the distal sesamoidean ligaments and SDF tendon insertions.

This condition is manifest by marked hyperextension of the PIP joint and considerable swelling associated with the soft tissue disruption. The clinical signs associated with dorsal and palmar subluxation include acute lameness initially, with the dorsal subluxations resulting in an obvious dorsal swelling over the PIP joint. Palmar subluxation, because of disruption of the support structures, usually results in hyperextension of the pastern and sinking of the metacarpophalangeal (MCP) joint. Radiographic examination is used to confirm the diagnosis of subluxation and to differentiate lesions associated with osteoarthritis or bony disruption of the middle phalanx. The lameness associated with PIP subluxation is less severe than that associated with fracture disruption.

Dorsal subluxation occurs bilaterally in the hind limbs of some horses with upright conformation. When this occurs, it can be managed with anti-inflammatory medication and a controlled exercise program. As the horse gains condition, the subluxations resolve.

Pastern arthrodesis is used to treat recalcitrant dorsal and palmar subluxations. Surgical arthrodesis is performed using either the slightly diverging lag screw technique or, preferably, the application of a single bone plate or a pair of bone plates as previously described. Some acquired dorsal subluxations are caused by excessive tension in the deep digital flexor (DDF) tendon, and successful resolution in three hindlimb cases resulted from release of the medial head of the DDF tendon.[16]

The prognosis after repair of subluxation is fair to favorable. With adequate reduction of the subluxation and stabilization, the pastern can be fused without excessive callus formation. Few cases are described in the equine literature that provide information on long-term follow-up, but horses can return to athletic activity, particularly if a hindlimb is involved. Rarely, bilateral subluxations develop, and a staged pastern arthrodesis can provide a return to soundness.

PROXIMAL PHALANX

Fractures of the proximal phalanx can be divided into two categories: proximal intra-articular osteochondral fractures and fractures involving the shaft or diaphyseal region of the proximal phalanx. The cause of most of these fractures is trauma, with hyperextension being particularly important for osteochondral fractures, and torsion with axial weight-bearing being more important for fractures of the shaft of the proximal phalanx.

Proximal Osteochondral Fractures

Proximodorsal Osteochondral Fractures

Osteochondral fractures of the proximal dorsal margin of the proximal phalanx within the MCP joint are common in racehorses.[17] They arise from hyperextension of the MCP joint with impact of the phalanx onto the dorsal region of the third metacarpus (MCIII). Proximodorsal fragments in immature horses have been described as OC, but it is uncommon to find histologic evidence to support these claims. Initial clinical symptoms include several days of moderate lameness associated with obvious synovial effusion and pain on flexion of the affected joint. Depending on the size of the fragment, lameness dissipates quickly. Radiography with four views, including horizontal beam oblique views, demonstrates the lesion adequately. The most prevalent site is the proximal medial eminence of the proximal phalanx. Occasionally, both lateral and medial eminences of the phalanx are involved.

The treatment of choice is surgical removal using arthroscopy.[17] However, small chip fractures (less than 2 mm in diameter) can be rapidly covered by synovial tissues, and many heal without causing clinical symptoms. Moderate to large dorsal fragments should be removed to prevent synovitis, cartilage degeneration, and villonodular synovitis mass development. Large chip fractures result in erosion of the opposing metacarpal condyle and often result in persistent lameness.

The arthroscope is placed into the joint just proximal to the middle of the dorsal joint pouch, next to the extensor tendon, because this facilitates examination of both lateral and medial portions of the joint without damage to the dorsal aspect of the sagittal ridge. A second entry portal is then made for instrument entry and fragment retrieval.

Postoperative convalescence includes 6 to 12 weeks' rest from race training, depending on the damage to the metacarpal cartilage. Results of arthroscopic surgery for the treatment of osteochondral fractures of the proximal phalanx in 336 horses revealed a return-to-use rate of 86% for racehorses.[18] Additionally, 68% of horses returned at the same or higher level of race performance. Removal of osteochondral fractures also may be useful even when moderate levels of osteoarthritis are present. Seventy-five percent of horses with other MCP lesions, including arthritis, were able to return to previous use.

Proximopalmar and Proximoplantar Osteochondral Fractures

Bone fragments associated with the plantar or palmar portions of the proximal phalanx within the metatarsophalangeal (MTP) or MCP joint have been recognized for many years.[19,20] The cause of fragmentation is controversial; one suggestion is that they are OC lesions. Recent data support a fracture etiology.[21]

The osteochondral fragments have been categorized as type I fractures when they are avulsed from the axial, proximal palmar, or plantar rim of the proximal phalanx and are mostly articular. Larger, abaxially located, partly articular osteochondral fragments have been categorized as type II fractures. Type II fractures extend distally 2 to 3 cm and contain minimal articular cartilage. Lameness associated with type I fractures is minimal and usually evident at higher speeds.[22,23] Type II fractures do not appear to produce lameness.

Affected MCP or MTP joints often exhibit synovial effusion, moderate pain on flexion, and a mild to moderate response to flexion tests. Intra-articular anesthesia is often required to confirm the diagnosis. The fragments are uncommon in the forelimb, possibly as a result of a more angled shape to the equine palmar aspect of the proximal phalanx compared with the plantar counterpart. Fragments have occurred in weanlings and yearlings, presumably as part of a form of OC.[22,24] Because most occur in younger animals, they are often covered by synovial tissue at the time of surgical removal. They are most prevalent in Standardbreds; 11.8% of all Standardbred yearlings in Norway[25] and 28.8% of yearlings in Sweden are affected.[26] In Warmblood horses, these lesions are diagnosed in 3- to 6-year-olds, when the training level for show jumping is increased.

Radiography is used to confirm the diagnosis. Routine oblique views are not particularly satisfactory for delineating type I fractures. A better projection results from raising the radiographic beam 20 degrees above horizontal and taking the oblique projections only 15 to 20 degrees dorsal to a standard lateromedial projection (Fig. 94-10).[27] These projections allow differentiation of type I axial fractures of the plantar aspect from the type II abaxial fractures (nonunited proximal plantar tuberosity of the proximal phalanx).[28,29] Type II fractures are quite evident on standard oblique radiographs. Both types of fragments are common in the MTP joints.

Type I plantar fractures are often removed in yearlings to prevent the development of lameness during training and racing. Lameness in yearlings is uncommon, and the prediction of later lameness induced by these plantar fragments is difficult. An arthroscopic approach through the plantar pouch of the MTP joint provides access to the intra-articular type I fractures.[30] The instrument portal is made at the base of the proximal sesamoid; the exact location of the portal is identified with a hypodermic needle. The fragments are dissected from the covering of synovial membrane and remnants of the attached short sesamoidean ligaments and removed with sturdy rongeurs. The use of motorized resectors, radio-frequency cutting loupes, or laser for removing excessive soft tissue proliferations and resection of the fragment reduces intraoperative bleeding and improves visualization.

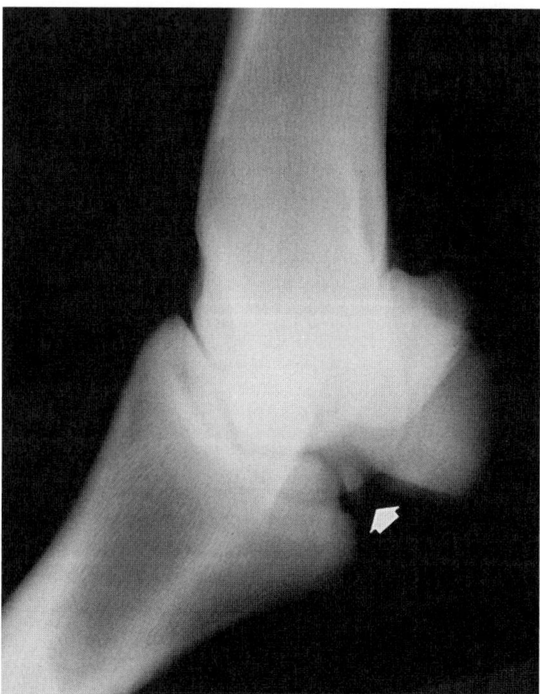

Figure 94-10. Elevated oblique radiograph (D15Pr20L-PlDiMO) of the rear fetlock of a Standardbred pacer with a type I (axial) osteochondral fracture *(arrow)* in the plantar pouch. These fragments need to be differentiated from type II fractures on the abaxial corner of the proximal phalanx, many of which do not need surgery.

Surgery is rarely indicated for type II abaxial osteochondral fractures. Additionally the incidence of these fragments is lower (2.4% of 753 Standardbred yearlings),[29] and they might not be fractures but rather might constitute a form of delayed ossification. Lesions in 11 of 18 horses had radiographically united to the parent proximal phalanx after 12 months. Occasionally nonhealing abaxial "fractures" and true traumatic fractures with fresh margins and associated lameness require screw fixation in lag fashion to achieve radiographic union. This type of fixation is only warranted when lameness is present, and simple absence of progressive bony fusion is not a cause for surgical fixation.

Convalescent care for type I fracture patients includes 6 to 12 weeks' rest from race training, depending on the damage to the distal sesamoidean ligaments at the time of surgery. In a review of 119 surgery cases, follow-up race performance information was available on 87.[23] Fifty-five horses (63%) returned to racing at or above their preoperative level. Abnormal arthroscopic findings with a negative impact on successful outcome included horses with articular cartilage loss over the palmar condyles and those with synovial proliferation.

Dorsal Frontal Fractures of the Proximal Phalanx

Dorsal frontal fractures entering the MCP joint are relatively rare; in a case series, they represented only 9 of 123 (7%) fractures involving the shaft of the proximal phalanx.[31] These fractures occur predominantly in Thoroughbreds and are prevalent in the hindlimbs. Dorsal frontal fractures tend to be short, extending from the articular surface 2 to 5 cm distally in the dorsolateral cortex of the proximal phalanx. Fractures are generally complete and minimally displaced. Fracture configuration and degree of displacement dictate the need for surgical repair.

Complete fractures are better repaired using screw fixation in lag fashion, although nondisplaced fractures heal with conservative therapy.[31] Complete and displaced fractures should be repaired with interfragmentary screws. The surgical repair can be supplemented by arthroscopic examination of the dorsal intra-articular region of the affected joint and débridement of associated cartilage damage. Insertion of one or two 3.5-mm cortex screws using the lag screw technique is recommended (Fig. 94-11).

Most horses recover in a soft bandage. Two weeks of complete stall rest is followed by 6 weeks of limited daily hand-walking. The implants are removed only where lysis or reaction has developed, associated with the screw heads. If conservative therapy is selected, adequate radiographic healing of the fracture occurs in 4 to 6 months.[31] The prognosis for a return to racing is favorable, with 6 to 9 horses reported to have returned to satisfactory performance with nonsurgical therapy.

Diaphyseal Fractures

Most axial fractures of the proximal phalanx occur in the sagittal plane and propagate distally from the articular surface of the MCP joint. The mid-sagittal groove is mechan-

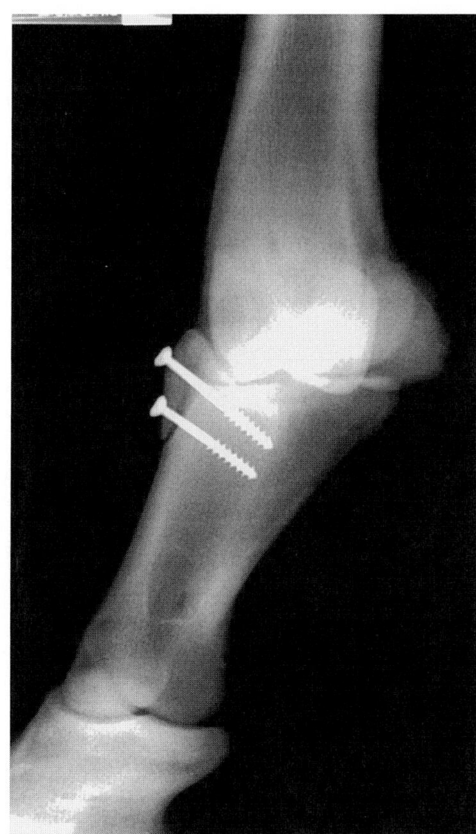

Figure 94-11. Dorsal frontal fracture of the dorsolateral cortex of the proximal phalanx in the rear limb. Repair using two 4-mm cancellous screws has resulted in improved joint congruity.

ically predisposed to the initiation of the fracture, possibly as a result of torsion applied to the sagittal groove from the opposing articular surface of the sagittal ridge of MCIII or MTIII. Fractures of the proximal phalanx are more common in the forelimbs and are particularly prevalent in racehorses, although proximal phalanx fractures are recorded in most breeds of horses.

The clinical signs associated with an axial fracture of the proximal phalanx depend on the extent of fracture propagation. Affected horses show moderate pain of relatively short duration with incomplete sagittal fractures. Fractures extending the full length of the proximal phalanx and those that tend to comminute result in non–weight-bearing lameness and moderate swelling of the pastern. Short, incomplete proximal fractures of the phalanx are sometimes difficult to isolate through a routine lameness examination, and perineural anesthesia is necessary to localize the site of lameness. The use of desensitizing nerve blocks in this situation increases the risk of propagation of the fracture lines during the lameness examination.

Radiographs define the extent of the fracture; most fractures commence in the sagittal groove and extend distally. Complete fractures exit on either the lateral or, rarely, medial cortex of the proximal phalanx or enter the proximal interphalangeal joint (Fig. 94-12, *A*). Short sagittal fractures can be difficult to localize on routine dorsopalmar radiographs. Several different dorsopalmar projections, using proximodistal and distoproximal dorsopalmar projections, better demonstrate the fracture. Short sagittal fractures are detected using nuclear scintigraphy or computed tomography, with radiographs performed to verify the extent of the fracture.

Most short sagittal fractures are treated conservatively because the fracture is incomplete and stable. Lag screw fixation is reserved for fractures that do not heal after 3 months of conservative therapy. Screw stabilization in lag fashion reduces the chance for further propagation of the fracture in the convalescent period.[32,33] Because of this, interfragmentary screw fixation may be considered as the initial treatment.

Complete nondisplaced and displaced fractures require surgical repair.[33-36] The extent of comminution varies considerably, and as a result, the inherent stability of the fracture configuration varies accordingly. Use of CT imaging can increase the success of surgical reconstruction by improved definition of the fracture planes for screw insertion. The prerequisite for selecting lag screw reconstruction of proximal phalanx fractures over transfixation casts or external fixator devices is the presence of an intact strut of bone spanning from the MCP to the PIP joint. Disruption of weight-bearing support without an intact bony column is generally a contraindication to screw repair alone. The articular surface of the MCP and PIP joints can be reconstructed with interfragmentary screws, but axial stabilization must be provided with a transfixation device.

Surgical Techniques

NONDISPLACED FRACTURES

For routine *nondisplaced* fractures, the proximal phalanx can be stabilized by insertion of screws in lag fashion through stab incisions (see Fig. 94-12, *B*). The most proximal screw in the series preferably should be a 5.5-mm cortex or shaft screw for additional compression of the articular surface, although 4.5-mm screws are adequate. Intraoperative radiographic monitoring is recommended to ensure that the proximal screw does not penetrate the MCP joint and the fracture planes are being adequately compressed.

Ideally, the proximal screw should pass within 5 mm of the most distal point of the sagittal groove of the proximal phalanx to provide maximum compression to the articular surface. This screw should penetrate the transcortex, and the screw head should be adequately countersunk to avoid torque on the screw shaft from the oblique angle of the cortex beneath the head. Additional screws are placed at intervals of 20 to 22 mm until the entire fracture line has been stabilized.

A less common configuration involves fractures in a frontal plane. These fractures can be repaired similarly, placing screws in a dorsal-to-palmar direction. However, in this configuration, potential trauma to the distal sesamoidean ligaments by sharp fragments can result in subluxation of the proximal interphalangeal joint after fracture healing. Therefore, pastern arthrodesis should be considered or at least discussed with the owner of the horse.

Postoperative support is provided using fiberglass casts if the fracture is extensive. Simple fractures that are repaired with several screws can be safely recovered in a firm bandage or a splint. Follow-up radiography is used to assess bone union, and most horses can return to light training 4 months after repair. Proximal phalanx fractures of the hindlimb are

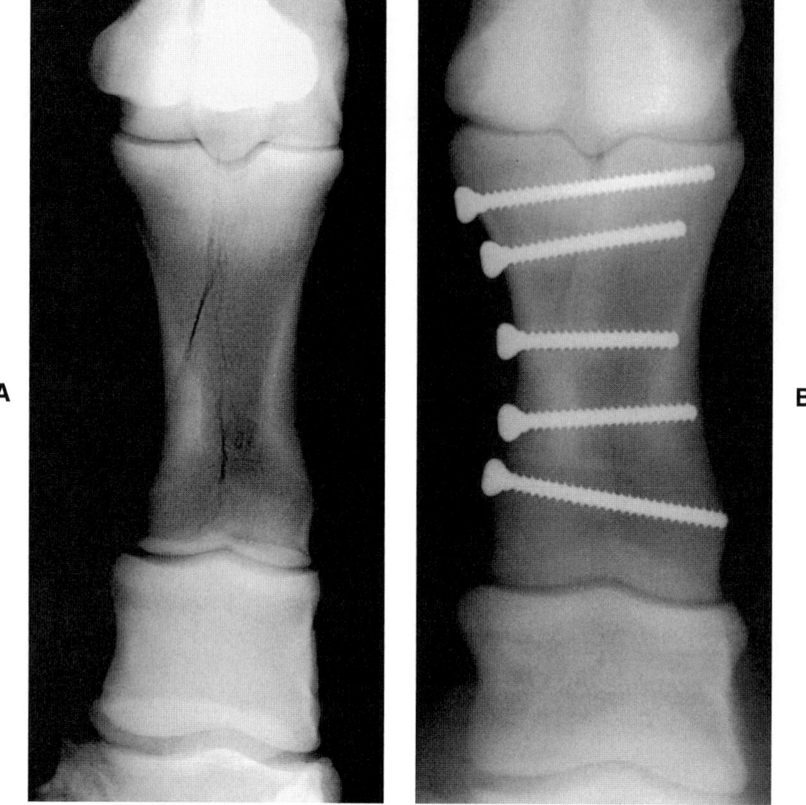

Figure 94-12. A, Complete nondisplaced fracture of the proximal phalanx commencing at the sagittal groove within the fetlock and spiraling distally to enter the pastern joint. **B**, Repair using 4.5-mm cortex screws placed in lag fashion through stab incisions.

more likely to require cast support for the recovery phase because of increased torsional loads on the hindlimbs during recovery.[34] Implant removal is unnecessary for fractures of the proximal phalanx. Lysis beneath the screw head, drainage from the wound, or excessively long screws are indications for screw removal.

MILDLY TO MODERATELY DISPLACED FRACTURES

Complete fractures that involve sagittal and oblique fracture planes with *mild to moderate displacement* can generally be better reduced with open approaches to the proximal phalanx followed by screw stabilization using lag technique.[34,35] Access for fracture débridement and reduction is provided by an incision over the dorsal aspect of the sagittal fracture. The incision usually enters the MCP joint for direct inspection of the articular surface, particularly to ensure accurate realignment of the subchondral bone plate and overlying cartilage. More extensive fractures require a more extensive longitudinal incision. Separate stab incisions are used for placing the screws in lag fashion in a lateral plane to stabilize the sagittal fracture.

Extensive fractures that have multiple sagittal and frontal plane fractures require an extensive open approach either using an I-shaped incision that exposes the entire dorsal and abaxial cortices of the proximal phalanx or an S-shaped incision.[35] The latter approach involves severing a collateral ligament of the MCP joint to expose the proximal articular surface of the proximal phalanx. The exposure of the fracture planes and the proximal articular surface allows placement of interfragmentary screws in lag fashion in multiple directions to anatomically reconstruct the bone around the residual intact strut. Most screws are placed in a lateromedial or dorsopalmar direction to provide stabilization of sagittal and frontal fracture planes, respectively. Alternatively, using the dorsal I-shaped incision, the dorsal articular margin of the proximal phalanx can be evaluated during screw insertion, and intraoperative radiographic control is used to ensure the remaining fracture planes are adequately aligned during reduction and stabilization (Fig. 94-13). This preserves the collateral ligaments and the metacarposesamoidean ligaments.

The limb is cast to the proximal aspect of MCIII or MTIII for recovery from anesthesia and for the next 6 weeks. Radiographic evaluation is then used to determine whether additional cast time is required. Preoperative antibiotics are continued for 3 to 5 days after surgery to minimize the risk of sepsis. Intraoperative culture during extensive and prolonged procedures might also be useful before closing the soft-tissue structures.

SEVERELY COMMINUTED FRACTURES

Fractures without an intact strut of bone are poor candidates for internal fixation. These fractures are generally high-energy fractures and the bone is extensively fragmented

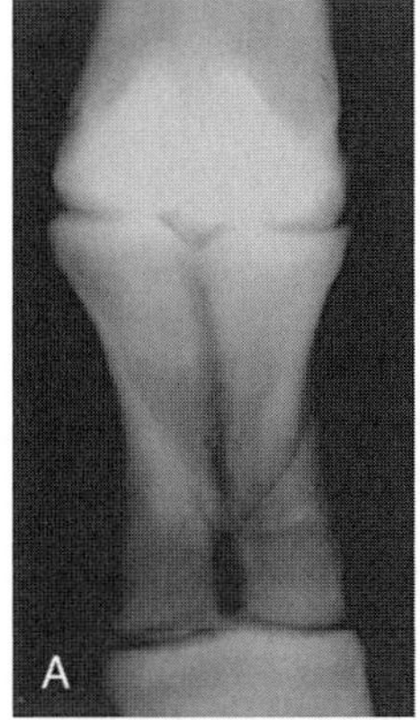

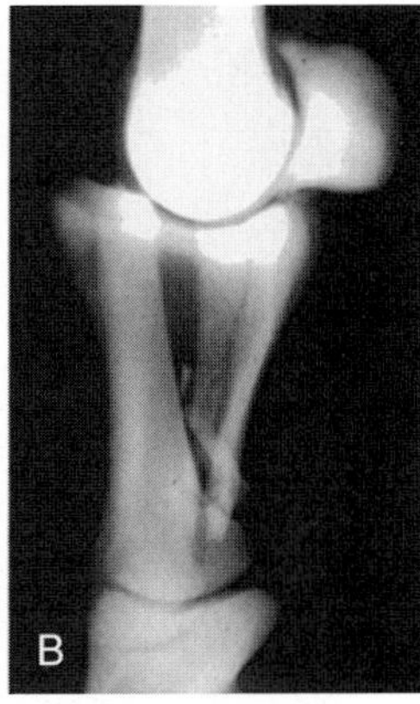

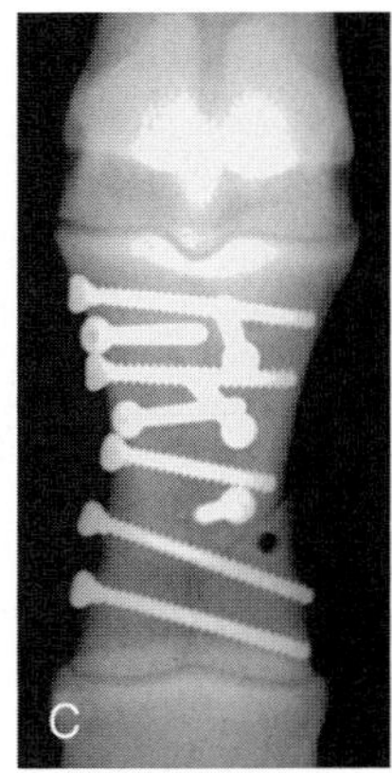

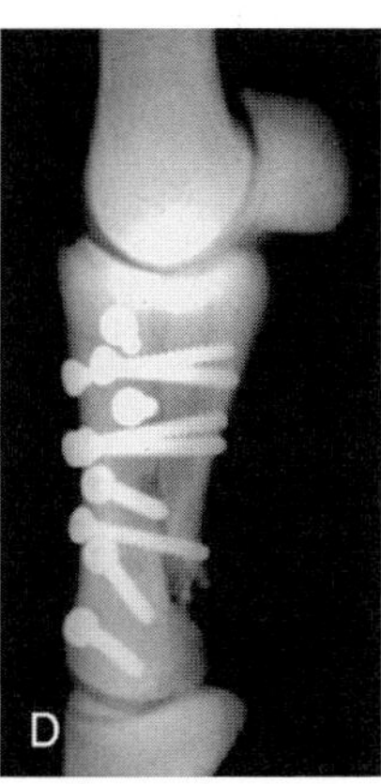

Figure 94-13. Comminuted displaced fracture of the proximal phalanx (**A** and **B**) with sagittal and frontal components, showing an intact medial strut of bone used in reconstructing the fragmented portions (**C** and **D**). Cortex screws are used in lag fashion to stabilize fractures in both planes and reconstruct the articular surfaces of the fetlock and pastern.

(Fig. 94-14). Lameness is marked, and considerable swelling can develop if the limb is left unbandaged for any length of time. Extensively comminuted fractures need to be stabilized within a cast before transfer of the horse for evaluation and surgery. Radiographs can often be taken through the cast to define the fracture configuration and the possibility for surgical repair or humane destruction. For cases where repair is desired, transfixation casts usually provide a reasonable possibility of salvaging the horse. Return to athletic activities is not an option.

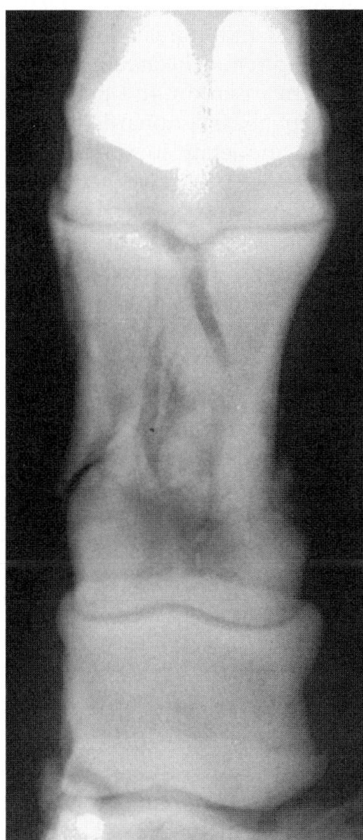

Figure 94-14. Extensively comminuted fracture of the proximal phalanx, without an intact strut and lacking inherent stability. Screw repair is generally inadequate, and transfixation casting or external fixators are required for salvage.

Simple cast fixation does not provide resistance to axial collapse of the fracture within the cast. The complications of collapse include continued lameness, a high risk for development of pressure necrosis of the skin leading to an open fracture, and laminitis of the unaffected weight-bearing limb. Transfixation techniques reduce the collapse of the fracture within the cast by using transcortical pins in the distal portion and mid portion of the MCIII or MTIII.[37] Pins with positive threads located in the center are preferable, and preparing the threads in the hole with a suitably sized tap is generally required before the pin is inserted (see Chapter 81).

An alternative to transfixation cast is the Nunamaker external skeletal fixator, which uses a series of transfixation pins through the MCIII or MTIII joined to side-connecting bars attached to a foot plate[38] (see Chapter 81). The most significant complications of transfixation casts and the external skeletal fixator is ring sequestrum formation around the pin tracts, especially in heavy horses, and subsequent fracture through a pin hole[39] (see Fig. 81-6). However, this fixator is a good choice for salvaging horses with massively comminuted fractures.

THE METACARPOPHALANGEAL JOINT

Palmar Metacarpal Fragmentation

Palmar fragmentation of the metacarpal condyles is a trauma-induced disorder, which results from the accumulated stress and sclerosis that develops during racing. Previously, this disease was thought to be OC of the palmar or plantar surface of the MCIII condyles.[40,41] However, there are no histologic data to verify this etiology, and classification as an OC lesion has been abandoned. Most patients are Thoroughbred racehorses that are 3 years old or older and have moderate to severe MCP lameness.

The palmar lesions are identified on standard lateromedial and flexed lateromedial projections (Fig. 94-15). Additional information can occasionally be derived from 125-degree dorsopalmar projections.[42] The radiographic lesions appear as different shapes including crescent, flat-

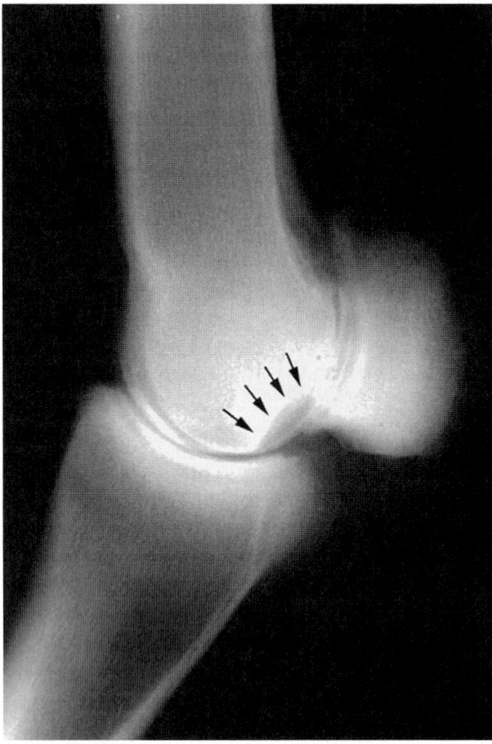

Figure 94-15. Radiograph of a 5-year-old Thoroughbred with marked palmar fragmentation, bone loss, and extensive subchondral sclerosis of the metacarpal condyles *(arrows)*. Enthesiophyte formation is noted at the proximal and distal ends of the proximal sesamoid bones, indicating chronic arthritis.

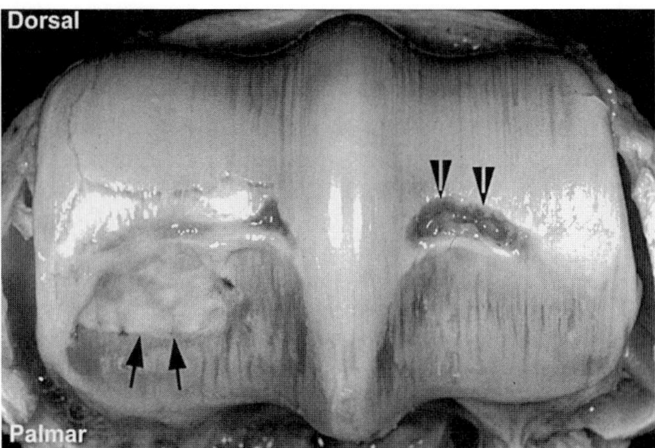

Figure 94-16. Palmar metacarpal fragmentation of the condyles in a 4-year-old Thoroughbred racehorse. Extensive score lines have developed over the entire cartilage surface, with fragmentation and granulation laterally *(arrowheads)* and fibrous healing tissue in the defect medially *(arrows)*.

tened, concave, oval, or circular. Secondary arthritic changes are common, with periarticular osteophytes or enthesiophytes, narrowing of the joint space, and supracondylar lysis. A prominent secondary feature is intense sclerosis of the palmar region of the condyle, deep to the lytic region. Morphologic assessment of these degenerate metacarpal condyles indicates an area of acellular and apparently necrotic bone over the entire distal palmar region of the affected metacarpus.[43] Deep to the necrotic area is a zone of new bone formation producing a sclerotic barrier that compensates for the biomechanical dysfunction of the palmar fracture. These remodeling and fracture changes are the result of accumulated stress fractures in the palmar region of the condyle, largely as a result of hyperextension of the MCP joint. Early lesions may have little overlying cartilage damage; however, eventual fracture and displacement of the subchondral bone result in complete bone and cartilage loss (Fig. 94-16). Lameness, although initially mild or moderate, then becomes severe.

Scintigraphy is sensitive in detecting the early stress fracture and bony deposition forming the sclerotic zone within the palmar region of the condyle. This is particularly helpful because the sclerosis can be reduced or allowed to remodel rather than progress to palmar fracture with prominent symptoms. This condition is difficult to treat, and efforts at prevention are important. Access to the palmar region of the distal metacarpus is very limited and is made more difficult because most of these lesions are close to the transverse ridge.

Proximal Sesamoid Bone Fractures

Fractures of the proximal sesamoid bones are relatively common, particularly those involving the apical portion.[44-55] Other configurations include basal, midbody, abaxial, sagittal, and comminuted fractures (Fig. 94-17). Most proximal sesamoid fractures occur because of excessive tension on the suspensory apparatus. Apical fractures are particularly common in the hindlimbs of Standardbreds, and the resultant prognosis often is dictated by the extent of loss of suspensory ligament insertion and pre-existing suspensory desmitis.[44] All except abaxial, nonarticular fractures result in MCP effusion and moderate to severe lameness of short duration.

Apical fractures involving the proximal one fourth to one third of the proximal sesamoid bone are always articular; however, they do not result in extensive suspensory derangement, and lameness diminishes rapidly. Removal of apical fragments up to one third of the proximodistal dimension

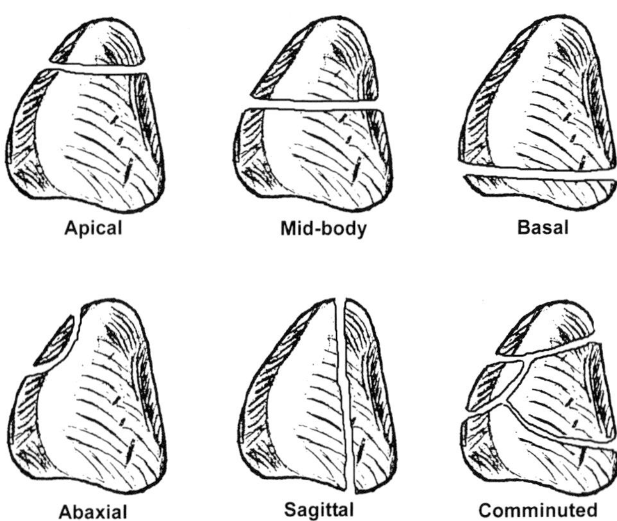

Figure 94-17. Proximal sesamoid fracture configurations.

of the proximal sesamoid bone is recommended,[44] although better results are evident with smaller apical fractures, where there is less disruption of suspensory ligament insertion.[46] Removal of the proximal third of the proximal sesamoid bone results in delay of return to racing and a considerably reduced likelihood of a successful postinjury career.

Arthroscopic removal of apical fractures results in less-extensive dissection and secondary fibrosis, but large apical fragments are best removed through arthrotomies. The arthroscope is inserted in the proximal aspect of the palmar or plantar pouch, and the instrument portal is made at the level of the fracture, allowing dissection of the fragment from the suspensory attachment.

Midbody and basal fractures present special problems for surgical fixation. Both of these injuries are slightly more prevalent in Thoroughbreds, and internal fixation is required for adequate fracture union. Midbody proximal sesamoid fractures should be repaired with either circumferential cerclage wire or lag screw fixation.[49,50] Previous therapy, including bone graft and extended periods of cast fixation, is unreliable in returning horses to work.

When *circumferential wiring* is used, either two separate approaches are made to access the lateral and medial aspect of the sesamoid bone or a combined, laterally based C-shaped incision is made that is centered over the sesamoid bone. The tendon sheath is opened palmarly, and a 2.5-mm drill hole is prepared across the apex. The drill bit is oriented parallel to the base of the bone in a slightly dorsopalmar direction. Exiting of the drill bit is observed through the open tendon sheath. A 14-gauge, 5-cm-long needle is placed into the hole. The beveled edge must be visible in the tendon sheath. Another 14-gauge hypodermic needle is placed laterally along the base of the fractured bone. A 1.2-mm-diameter wire is passed through the first needle, directed distally within the tendon sheath, and introduced into the pointed end of the second needle. By advancing the wire and retracting the second needle, the wire is exited at the lateral aspect of the bone. The proximal end of the wire is tunneled along the lateral aspect of the bone to the exiting point of the distal end of the wire, where the two ends are tightened solidly through even twisting using the Fastight (Synthes, Paoli, Penn) wire tightener. Excess wire is cut with a pair of cutters, and the end is turned toward the bone to reduce irritation of the surrounding soft tissues. The tendon sheath and soft-tissue incisions are closed using routine technique.

Screw fixation in lag fashion is performed from the base or the apex of the bone, depending on the configuration of the fracture. An oblique fracture with the fracture plane declining from medial to lateral is best treated with an interfragmentary screw placed from the apex, whereas a fracture declining from lateral to medial is best approached from the base. Interfragmentary compression and reduction during screw insertion is maintained with large pointed reduction forceps. Frequent intraoperative radiographs are essential for a high-quality repair. The screw head should come to lie between the oblique and straight distal sesamoidean ligaments in a natural fossa of the proximal sesamoid bone in the base approach, or proximolaterally at the apex of the bone, embedded in the insertion of the lateral suspensory branch. Insertion technique for the screws is routine once the correct screw position has been verified radiographically. Circumferential wiring and interfragmentary screw fixation in lag fashion return up to 60% of horses to active racing.[49,50]

Basal slab fractures involve the origin of all the distal sesamoidean ligaments, and the prognosis is certainly unfavorable. Lag screw fixation is rarely suitable because of the thin fragment profile, and the only recommended treatment has been circumferential wiring. There is an inverse relationship between fragment length and height and the likelihood of return to racing.[54] Basal osteochondral fragments that do not extend to the palmar surface have a much better prognosis, with 59% returning to racing in a recent study of 57 horses.[48] Many of these fractures can be removed arthroscopically. Similarly, in a second study, 57% of horses with fragments involving less than 25% of the base successfully returned to racing after fragment removal, compared to 40% with fragments involving more than 25% but not the entire base.[54]

Abaxial fractures must be assessed by a 60-degree skyline projection of the abaxial surface of the proximal sesamoid, which demonstrates whether the abaxial fracture is intra-articular or palmar and not involving the joint[51] (Fig. 94-18). Intra-articular fractures can be removed arthroscopically, whereas the nonarticular fractures are best treated conservatively.[52,53] Return to function is fair to good (61%), depending on the length of the intra-articular fracture.[53]

Sagittal fractures are rare and tend to occur on the axial margin of the sesamoid bone in conjunction with other MCP injuries such as condylar fractures[55] (see Fig. 95-5). Very rarely, they can develop as isolated fractures, but they

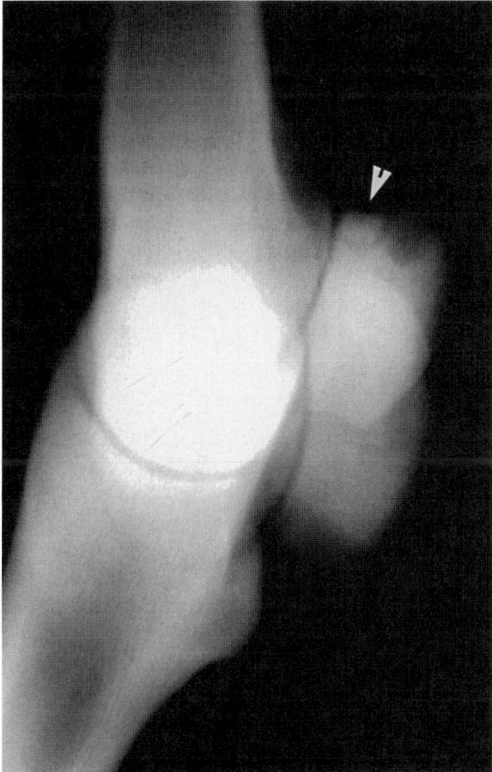

Figure 94-18. Elevated 60-degree lateromedial projection (Pr60L-DiMO) of the proximal sesamoid bones to evaluate the intra-articular component of an abaxial sesamoid fracture *(arrow).*

can be repaired using several lag screws placed in a lateral-to-medial orientation. Postoperatively, application of a cast is recommended for the initial 2 to 3 weeks. At that time, if everything looks satisfactory, the cast is exchanged for a heavy support bandage. The remainder of the postoperative management is routine.

Comminuted and biaxial fractures are severe breakdown injuries involving the MCP joint. In most cases, these horses require fetlock arthrodesis for a return to comfortable weightbearing[56] (see Chapter 85) (Fig. 94-19).

Follow-up on 109 horses with apical sesamoid fractures indicated that 64% of the horses treated surgically raced later,[44] whereas only 37% of those treated conservatively raced again. For midbody fractures repaired with lag screws, 9 of 12 horses were able to race after surgery.[49] Similarly, in horses with midbody fractures repaired by wiring, 11 of 15 were able to resume an athletic career, with half of these performing at the same level or better than before the injury.[50]

Chronic Proliferative (Villonodular) Synovitis

Development of soft-tissue masses in the dorsal aspect of the MCP joint is common secondary to chronic synovitis.[57-61] The most frequent cause is dorsal proximal phalangeal osteochondral fractures that are not immediately treated by fragment removal. In addition, villonodular masses commonly develop with advancing osteoarthritic changes within the joint. Horses with long pasterns are predisposed to this problem. A visible and palpable mass is evident in the proximal dorsal region of the affected fetlock. Lameness is usually moderate to moderately severe depending on the underlying disease. Radiographs occasionally show cortical lysis on the dorsal region of MCIII, under the enlarging mass. Definitive diagnosis requires either arthrography or ultrasonographic examination.[17] Ultrasonography is more convenient.

Most masses are 7 to 10 mm in diameter. The minimum width that warrants surgery is 4 mm; smaller masses can be treated with intra-articular atropine and steroids. The enlarged medial portion of the villonodular plica is usually thicker than the lateral portion.

A critical factor in the decision for surgery is the extent of osteoarthritis present in the joint. Osteochondral fragments and other fracture diseases in the MCP joint result in secondary fibrous mass development, and these fibrous masses can be removed without difficulty and with reasonably favorable prognoses.[17,60] Masses secondary to osteoarthritis are generally larger and more chronic, and the associated arthritis dictates the likelihood of successful return to work after the mass is removed. A critical evaluation of the joint space on preoperative radiographs and the use of ultrasonography to measure the dorsal articular cartilage thickness prevent inadvertent operation in these cases.

Primary villonodular masses can develop without an obvious initiating factor, and these most likely result from hyperextension of the MCP joint and impact trauma on the normal synovial plica, which forms a pad or cushion to lessen the impact of the dorsal margin of the proximal phalanx onto the metacarpal cortex.[57,60] Hemorrhage and

A
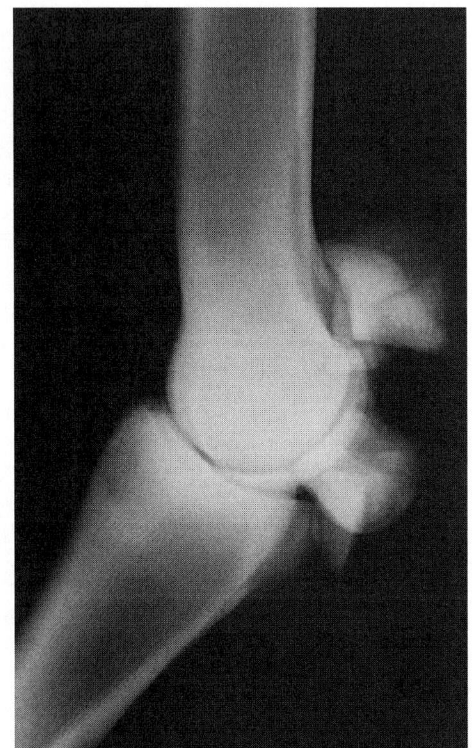
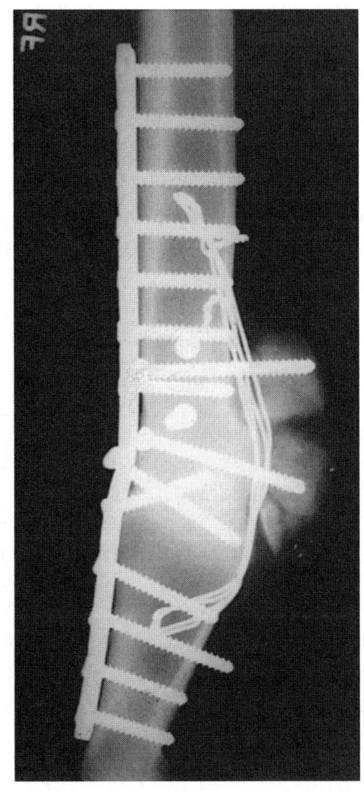
B

Figure 94-19. A, Suspensory breakdown injury with comminuted fracture and distraction of both sesamoid bones. **B,** Repair was achieved through a fetlock arthrodesis using a dynamic compression plate (DCP) applied to the dorsal surface of the limb and a tension band wire for palmar support.

fibrosis in this plica eventually result in significant enlargement, which is then more easily and repeatably injured during exercise. This is quite painful, but the horses do very well after surgery to remove the mass.

Arthroscopic approaches are suitable for removal of villonodular masses (Fig. 94-20), although some masses are so large that they require arthrotomy for excision.[17,60] Arthroscopic visualization allows mass removal using synovectomy instrumentation, guarded scalpels, or the biopsy suction punch for smaller masses (Dyonics, Smith & Nephew, Memphis, Tenn). Large masses can also be efficiently removed using CO_2 or holmium:yttrium-aluminum-garnet (holmium-YAG) laser where access to this equipment is available.[61]

Postoperative therapy includes intra-articular injections of 20 to 40 mg of hyaluronan. Repeat doses in 3 to 4 weeks are recommended. The use of polysulfated glycosaminoglycan (Adequan) is another option depending on the state of the articular cartilage. Return to race training depends on concurrent arthritis.

Osteoarthritis

Deterioration of articular cartilage is common in mature racehorses and can lead to moderate to severe unrelenting lameness, with the development of periarticular osteophytes, enthesiophytes, and joint space collapse, particularly medially. These horses respond poorly to intra-articular medication and require frequent injections to remain comfortable. Collapse of the medial compartment of the MCP joint is more prevalent than the lateral and often indicates the likelihood of a career-ending lameness.

Therapeutic options are limited. Pain relief can be effected by intra-articular steroid administration, but continued cartilage degradation is inevitable. In the final stages of joint deterioration, some improvement in the level of lameness has resulted from the administration of silicone oils to the joint and from desensitization of the synovial capsule with intra-articular cobra venom. The author has no first-hand experience with cobra venom as a form of therapy. Ultimately, some horses need MCP arthrodesis to become comfortable (see Chapter 85).

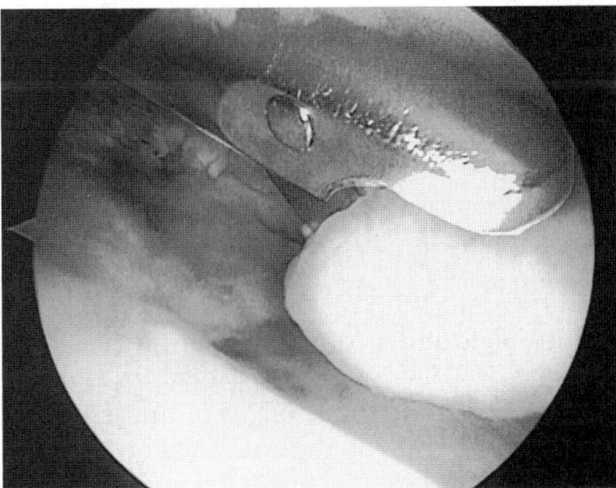

Figure 94-20. Arthroscopic removal of an 8-mm villonodular pad from the fetlock using a biopsy punch rongeur.

Osteochondrosis and Subchondral Cystic Lesions

Several manifestations of OC can occur in the MCP joint, and the incidence is relatively high. Two different types of MCP OC lesions are described.[62]

The first are dissecting cartilage flaps (osteochondritis dissecans [OCD]). They appear as mineralizing lesions on the dorsal sagittal ridge of the MCIII or MTIII and are common in young horses 8 to 24 months old.[63] These OCD lesions can affect all four MCP joints. They also appear as palmar metacarpal OCD lesions, which result in a debilitating lameness, often progressing to osteoarthritis and representing the most serious form of MCP OCD. These lesions occur in horses as young as 10 months but are more common in young race-age horses. (Distopalmar metacarpal fragmentation in 3- to 4-year-old racehorses was originally described as OCD but is a different disease from that described here as OCD.)

The second type of OC lesions in the MCP joint are subchondral cystic lesions (SCL) of the distal MCIII or MTIII condyle. They occur most commonly in weanlings and yearlings but can be first diagnosed in 2-year-olds in training. The resulting lameness is variable, and occasionally severe, but osteoarthritis is a rare sequela. Most subchondral cysts open to the joint just cranial to the transverse ridge by a narrow communicating channel. Occasionally, multiple cysts are present in the same bone, and the cysts can be bilateral. Cysts of the proximal articular surface of the proximal phalanx also can be seen, often opening near the sagittal groove.

The degree of lameness largely depends on the type of MCP OC. Dorsal sagittal ridge lesions result in mild to minimal lameness, although flexion tests of the involved joints are often positive. The other form of OC and SCL results in more significant lameness. Lameness and pain on flexion are most pronounced with palmar OCD lesions in yearlings. Regardless of the site, MCP effusion is a prominent feature. Most horses have sufficient lameness, synovial effusion, and exacerbation of the lameness with flexion tests that a tentative diagnosis can be reached without regional or intra-articular anesthesia. Radiographs are necessary to determine the exact cause of MCP disease and to provide prognostic guidelines. Dorsal sagittal ridge lesions often manifest as mineralized densities adjacent to the sagittal ridge (Fig. 94-21, *A*). They often arise from the proximal condylar cartilage and are more correctly termed *dorsal parasagittal* or *dorsal condylar* OCD lesions.

Treatment options vary according to the site of involvement. Palmar MCIII and plantar MTIII lesions are relatively inaccessible, and surgical therapy is not possible unless the lesion is located unusually far caudad on the condyles or sagittal ridge. Occasionally, part of these lesions can be débrided under arthroscopic guidance with a palmar or plantar pouch approach. On most occasions, however, the lesions are inaccessible, and osteoarthritis with permanent lameness is the usual sequela. These young horses rarely enter and sustain an athletic career.

Dorsal sagittal ridge and parasagittal condylar lesions should be surgically removed under arthroscopic guidance (see Fig. 94-21, *B*). The technique as described previously should be applied.[17] These lesions can achieve considerable size, and removal can leave a substantial subchondral defect. However, in this location, joint stability is unaffected, and

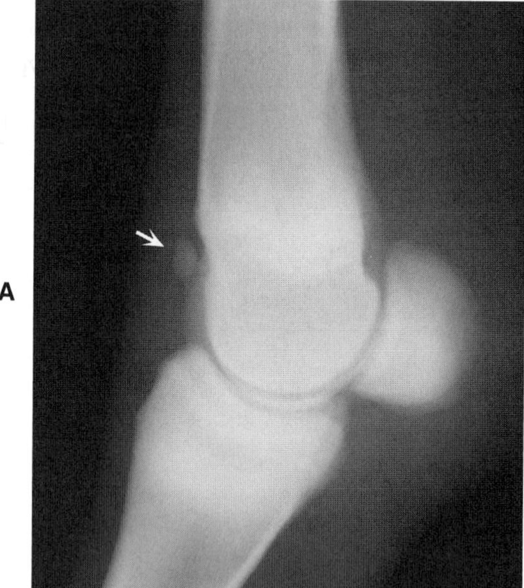

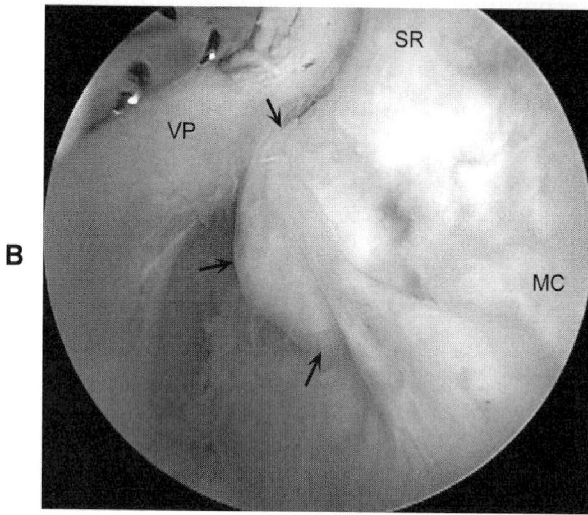

Figure 94-21. A, Lateromedial radiograph showing dorsal sagittal ridge OCD *(arrow)* that involved the adjacent condyle. **B,** Arthroscopic examination shows the sagittal ridge (SR) distal to the fragment *(arrows)*, the metacarpal condyle (MC), and villonodular pad (VP).

the outlook remains favorable. Subchondral cystic lesions of MCIII or MTIII that have narrow openings to the joint can be treated successfully with several injections of hyaluronan (Fig. 94-22, *A*). Most yearlings do well, and the lameness quickly resolves. The cystic cavity generally fills in but may take 1 to 2 years. Occasionally, lameness persists despite intra-articular medication and limited exercise, and surgery should then be considered.

Cystic lesions with wide channels to the articular surface do not respond to conservative therapy nearly as well as cysts with narrow openings, and débridement is often recommended at the initial diagnosis (see Fig. 94-22, *B*). Surgical débridement of the cysts can be accomplished via dorsal arthroscopy with the MCP joint flexed. Most cysts can be curetted; bone grafts are not usually necessary.

Arthroscopic techniques can be used only with cysts opening on or dorsal to the transverse ridge of MCIII. More palmar cysts are best approached transosseously through drilling. Cysts of the proximal phalanx can be débrided with difficulty from the articular surface, particularly in MTP joints where the joint separates with flexion.

The outlook for a sustained athletic career is favorable for subchondral cystic lesions of the distal MCIII or MTIII, reasonably favorable for dorsal sagittal ridge and parasagittal OCD, and poor for palmar metacarpal OCD flaps.[64]

Luxation

Lateral or medial complete luxation of the MCP and MTP joints occurs after rupture of either the medial or lateral collateral ligament.[65] Occasionally, there is an avulsion of the origin or insertion of one of these ligaments, resulting in marked instability. The condition is relatively rare and results primarily from entrapment of the distal limb in holes in the ground or cattle grates. The diagnosis is obvious when an angular deviation can be easily induced on manipulation (Fig. 94-23). Radiography with a dorsopalmar projection with the limb under lateral or medial bending stress usually provides clear evidence of the extent of the luxation. Some injuries associated with trailer accidents result in an open luxation with disruption of the collateral ligament and some loss of bone structure because of pavement injury.

The treatment of closed luxations is simple and involves cast fixation for 6 weeks.[65] Imbrication or repair of the collateral ligament is not usually necessary. The cast is applied with the horse anesthetized, maintaining the lateral–medial stability as the cast cures. Surgery for open luxations is necessary for adequate wound débridement and soft-tissue closure. Extensive antibiotic lavage and removal of all foreign matter are essential. Treatment of the luxation initially in a splint is an option for the acute inflammatory phase, until the infection has been controlled. Later, elective cast application for increased stabilization can be used, or arthrodesis by application of a DCP and screws can be used if the joint surface is extensively damaged (see Chapter 85).

A single case series involving 10 horses is reported in the literature; five horses had open luxation and five had closed luxation.[65] The open luxations were treated with joint lavage and cast immobilization, and the majority were sound at follow-up, including one horse that was being actively ridden.

The development of obvious sepsis within the MCP joint can be minimized by aggressive early therapy and the placement of lavage drains and ingress antibiotic portals. Later application of antibiotic-laden bone cement assists in bringing the infection under control. Overall, the prognosis after the development of infection is guarded, and chronic lameness can be expected. Some of these cases can be salvaged with aggressive débridement and elective arthrodesis later.

ANGULAR LIMB DEFORMITY OF THE DISTAL JOINT

Angular limb deformities originating at the distal physis of the MCIII or MTIII develop relatively often in foals; most are varus deformities. Concurrent valgus of the carpus or tarsus and a varus deformity of the MCP region are common. Many varus deformities are congenital and improve during the early postnatal period. A detailed discussion of angular limb deformity is found in Chapter 89.

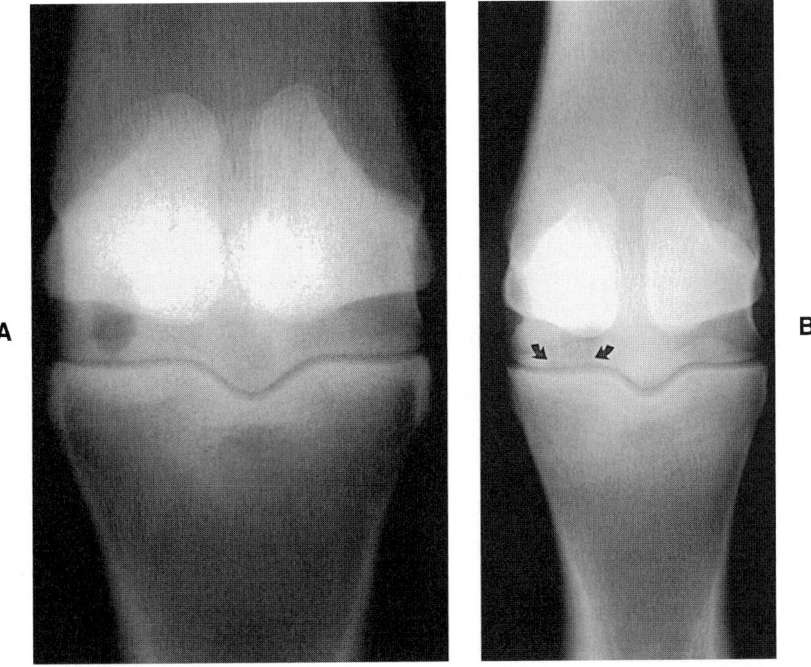

Figure 94-22. Subchondral cystic lesions of the distal metacarpus. Cysts with small communications into the joint **(A)** generally respond well to conservative therapy, whereas cysts with wide canals **(B)** *(arrows)* often need surgical débridement.

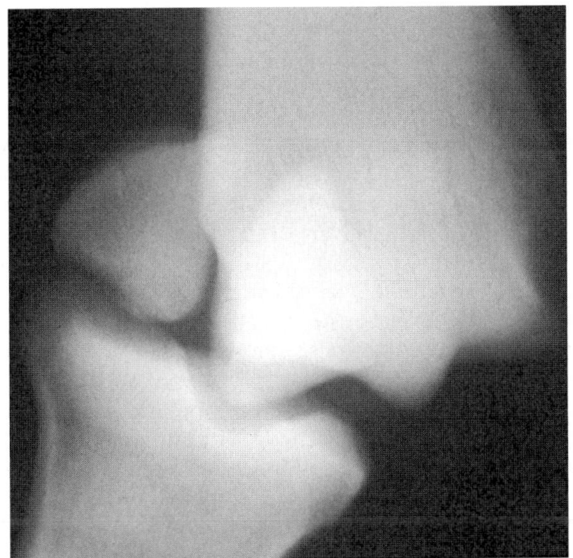

Figure 94-23. Luxation of the metacarpophalangeal joint. The lateral condyle interdigitates with the sagittal groove of the proximal phalanx, providing some stability to the limb. (Courtesy J. Auer, University of Zurich.)

FLEXURAL DEFORMITY OF THE METACARPOPHALANGEAL JOINT

Flexural deformities of the MCP joint can be classified as congenital or acquired.

Congenital Deformities

Congenital deformities are often relatively severe. If they are bilateral, the foal can have difficulty rising or, if it does stand, it tends to knuckle over at the MCP joint (Fig. 94-24). In some congenital cases, tension is apparent in both the deep and SDF tendons; in others, the common digital extensor tendon is ruptured. Occasionally, even the suspensory ligament is taut on palpation.

Acquired Deformities

Acquired flexural deformities can be unilateral or bilateral. Both forelimbs are commonly affected, one generally more severely than the other. The pathogenesis of the acquired form of flexural deformity is thought to involve pain-induced reflex loops in the ipsilateral limb, often precipitated by other skeletal disease. The diagnosis and management of these deformities are discussed in detail in Chapter 90.

ANNULAR LIGAMENT CONSTRICTION

Chronic tenosynovitis is a relatively common affliction in the digital sheaths of horses, developing mostly in the hindlimbs as an insidious reaction to increased workloads. Most cases of tenosynovitis are successfully treated by changing exercise intensity with or without intrasynovial medication. Untreated tenosynovitis or tenosynovitis associated with more serious disruption of the tendon sheath, the various mesotenons, the annular ligament, or the flexor tendons themselves can result in lameness and a self-

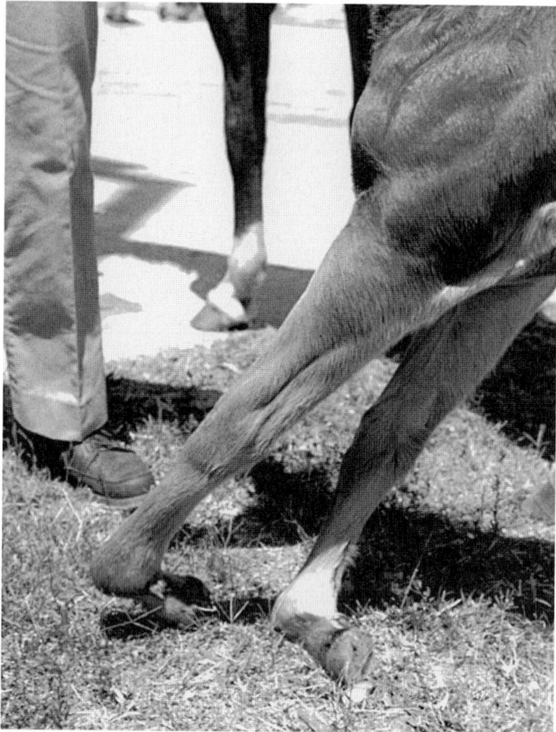

Figure 94-24. Congenital flexural deformity of the metacarpophalangeal joint, resulting in knuckling and collapse. This foal responded completely to combination proximal and distal check desmotomy.

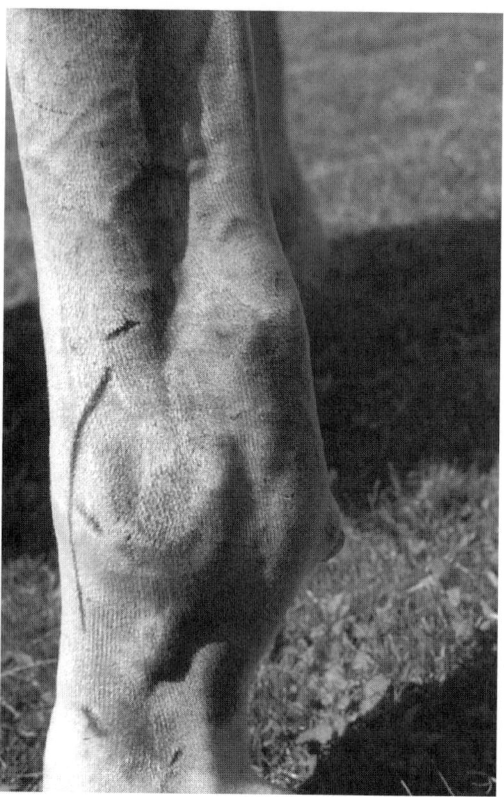

Figure 94-25. Lateral view of a horse suffering from constriction of the annular ligament, demonstrated by the synovial effusion in the tendon sheath and the characteristic notching of the tendons proximal to the annular ligament.

perpetuating cycle of tendon sheath fibrosis, repeat tearing, and annular ligament thickening.[66] Tenosynovial masses and adhesions can develop as a consequence of this chronic inflammatory action. These latter types of cases do not respond particularly well to medical therapy and not only require surgical intervention but also generally have a reduced prognosis for a cosmetic outcome and a return to complete soundness.

In animals in which the annular ligament causes constriction, chronic lameness (exacerbated by flexion of the fetlock), and tendon sheath effusion and thickening with a notching of the sheath over the width of the plantar annular ligament are common (Fig. 94-25). Ultrasonographic evaluation of the tendons within the canal is useful to determine the extent of tendon lesions and the thickness of the synovial tendon sheath and annular ligament and to define the number and attachments of tenosynovial masses. One report suggests that annular ligament desmitis can be the sole initiator of annular ligament constriction, and ultrasonographic evaluation is critical in making the diagnosis.[67] Tears within the DDF tendon also are recognized as a cause of chronic severe tenosynovitis.[68,69]

Treatment is commenced in chronic cases when a noticeable lameness has developed in conjunction with persistent swelling. Where tendon sheath masses and adhesions are evident on ultrasonographic examination or the annular ligament is thickened, surgical therapy is preferred for expeditious resolution of symptoms.

Mass Removal

Open tendon sheath approaches to mass and adhesion removal or resection have been successful. The disadvantage to extensive open approaches is the delay in the initiation of exercise postoperatively and adhesion formation or reformation. However, early postoperative walking increases the risk of wound dehiscence with the attendant risk of sepsis. For these reasons, endoscopic examination of the sheath (tenoscopy), using a standard rigid arthroscope, is preferred.[66,70]

The entry portal for routine tenoscopy of the digital sheath is on the palmarolateral or plantarolateral surface immediately distal to the annular ligament. This entrance allows examination of most regions of the sheath, and instrument portals can be made proximal to the annular ligament under tenoscopic guidance. Tenosynovial masses can be resected either with motorized synovial resectors or by division at their attachments with biopsy cutting forceps or retractable blades and subsequent removal with grasping forceps (Fig. 94-26). For extensive synovial resection, hemorrhage control is required, and a tourniquet is applied proximal to the digital sheath. If annular ligament transection also is needed, it can be accomplished initially to open further access for manipulation within the sheath, or at the end of the procedure, using the slotted cannula (Dyonics, Smith & Nephew, Memphis, Tenn) available for carpal tunnel release in humans.

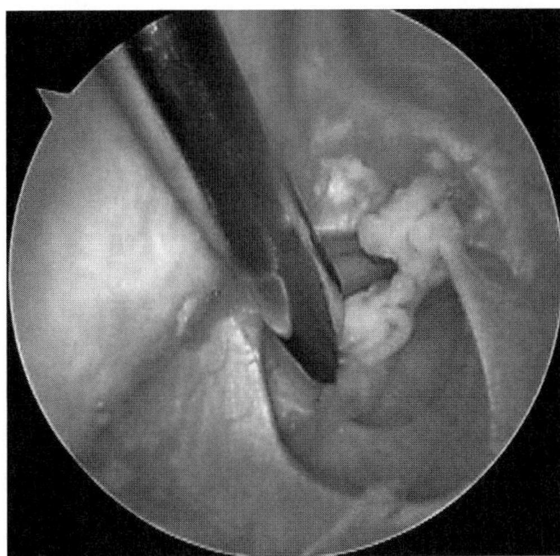

Figure 94-26. Tenoscopic removal of digital sheath masses from the dorsolateral recess of the sheath cavity using motorized equipment.

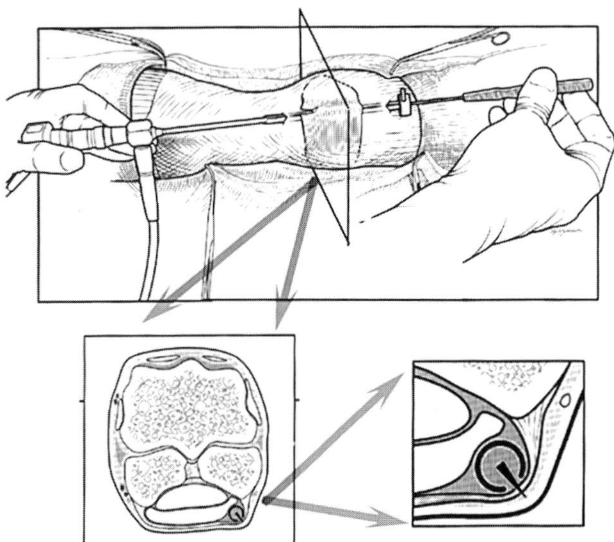

Figure 94-27. Tenoscopic annular ligament release, using a slotted cannula and arthroscopic visualization of an angled blade to sever the fibers of the annular ligament.

Annular Ligament Transection

The only effective treatment for the annular ligament constriction syndrome is division of the ligament. Depending on the presence of tendon core lesions or peripheral adhesions, other surgical procedures such as tendon injection, mass removal, or adhesiolysis are performed as indicated. Preoperative planning is important for determining the degree of exposure of the tendons required to optimize treatment. Where only the annular ligament is involved, the ligament can be severed in the standing animal with a curved bistoury introduced through a 1-cm incision proximal to the ligament. However, in the majority of cases, other structures are involved, and general anesthesia and a larger incision provide access to evaluate and surgically treat these components.

In original descriptions of surgical division of the annular ligament, the skin was incised over the entire proximodistal length of the annular ligament. This incision provided access to allow sectioning of the annular ligament and subsequent division of adhesions under direct view. Where the annular ligament is the only involved structure, the exposure required for division of the ligament can be reduced to a 2-cm skin incision over the proximal border of the annular ligament. Another surgical approach involved a paramedian skin incision over the entire length of the annular ligament, followed by palmar or plantar transection of the ligament over the tenaculum (mesotenon). This technique, if performed correctly, prevented opening of the tendon sheath. It can be applied if only the annular ligament is involved.

Tenoscopic examination of the digital sheath with an arthroscope entering distal to the annular ligament allows visual inspection of the entire sheath cavity and division of the annular ligament (Fig. 94-27). Second entry portals allow adhesion resection and mass removal, as previously described, and with a slotted cannula (Dyonics, Smith & Nephew, Memphis, Tenn), endoscopic release of the annular ligament can be accomplished.[71] The obvious advantages of tenoscopic annular ligament release include the extensive dissection that can be performed through limited entry wounds, allowing better wound healing with less risk of dehiscence and earlier postoperative exercise.

The entry and angle of the slotted cannula are critical to facilitate insertion of the arthroscope and 90-degree angled blade. The proximal entry portal should be dorsal in the digital sheath and the distal exit point should be plantar or palmar to allow the arthroscope or blades to clear the heel. The cannula with obturator in place is inserted under direct visualization from proximal to distal. The insertion path must be external to the manica flexoria, or this ring of the SDF will be divided along with the annular ligament. As the obturator nears the distal portal, the arthroscope is removed, and the obturator and cannula are exteriorized through the vacant portal.

The obturator is removed, and the unsheathed arthroscope is inserted to view and verify the flexor tendons, sesamoid surface, and annular ligament. The slot is oriented to open directly toward the annular ligament, and the 90-degree-angle sharp blade is drawn across the fibers of the annular ligament to sever the full thickness of this structure. Arthroscopic guided free-hand division of the annular ligament using right-angled blades, radio-frequency probes, or bistoury can also be used. Hemorrhage is flushed from the cannula, which is then removed, and the tendon sheath is flushed before the skin incision is closed.

Tendon Débridement

Linear tears or clefts within the DDF tendon, and occasionally the SDF tendon, present special problems in repair, with most requiring débridement and some requiring suture.[68] Ultrasonographic examination is not sensitive in detecting linear clefts in the tendon structure. Any ultrasonographic suggestion of echolucencies within the palmar or plantar third of the surface of the flexor tendons is highly suspicious, and this region should be carefully assessed

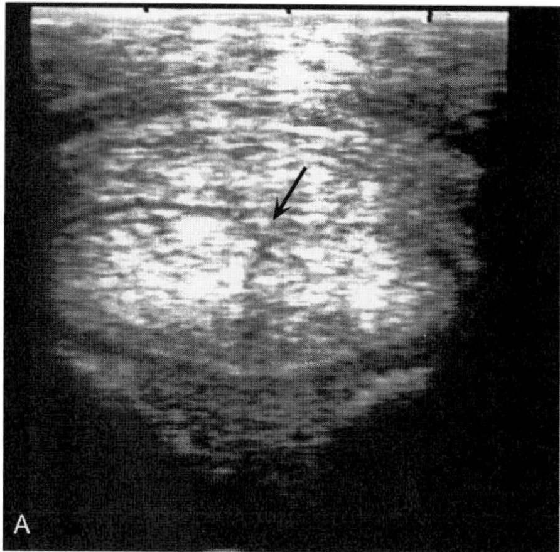

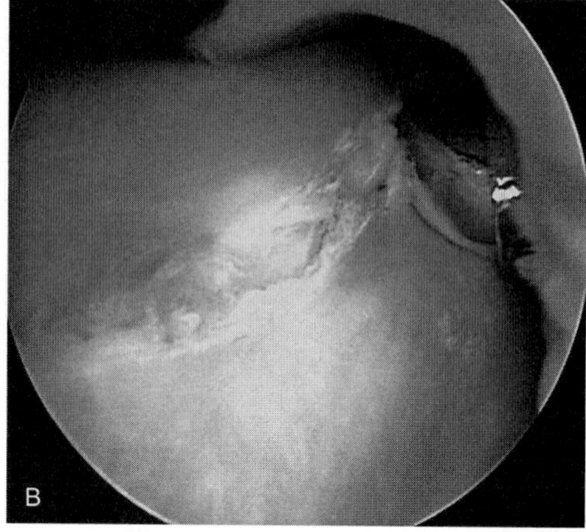

Figure 94-28. Deep digital flexor (DDF) tendon linear tears. **A**, Ultrasound image of DDF tendon with suspicious echolucency on the palmar surface of the tendon. **B**, Tenoscopic trimming of the linear cleft in the deep digital flexor.

during tenoscopic exploration. The linear clefts can penetrate a variable distance into the substance of the tendon.

The treatment of choice is tenoscopic débridement (Fig. 94-28). Débridement has proved superior to suture repair following open surgical approaches.[72] Tears in the DDF tendon can extend 4 to 10 cm. They often involve the DDF tendon from the level of the mid-proximal phalanx and extend beyond the level of the apex of the proximal sesamoid bones. The depth of the linear cleft varies from penetration to the center of the DDF tendon to more superficial fiber erosion. Trimming of exposed tendon fibers can be accomplished using a combination of biopsy punch rongeurs and motorized resectors with both side and forward aperture, which are also effective in trimming epitenal and tendon fiber damage. The aim should be a relatively smooth tendon surface.

Hyaluronan (20 to 40 mg) is injected into the tendon sheath at the time of wound closure. Research in horses and experimental animals indicates hyaluronan reduces the formation and re-formation of tendon adhesions in the sheath area and enhances intrinsic tendon healing.[73] The incidence of synovial fistulae associated with the extensive skin incision in the original description of annular ligament transection makes the smaller exposure and the use of tenoscopy attractive alternatives. Nevertheless, the maintenance of a firm bandage with careful changes and sterile nonadhesive padding is important. The limb is usually bandaged for 3 to 4 weeks after surgery. Although extensive tendon synovial mass and adhesion resection can be painful postoperatively, the majority of horses with simple annular ligament section do not require extensive analgesia.

Stall confinement without exercise is recommended initially, but hand-walking should be instituted after 5 days and the time period should be increased rapidly. Long periods of walking exercise are particularly helpful if tendon adhesions were present at surgery. If adhesiolysis was performed at surgery, a follow-up injection of hyaluronan is recommended 2 weeks postoperatively.

Tenoscopic mass removal and annular ligament division in 25 horses followed for 6 to 68 months revealed cosmetically acceptable results in 22 of the horses. Lameness resolved in 18 of the 25 horses (72%). The poorest response was evident in two horses with concurrent tendinitis in the region of the digital sheath. The cosmetic outcome was inversely related to the preoperative duration of signs and the thickness of the annular ligament. In addition, a longer history of symptoms led to a thicker annular ligament on preoperative ultrasonography.

Simple constrictive syndromes as a result of a wound, desmitis of the annular ligament, or chronic fibrosing synovitis of the tendon sheath have a good prognosis for return to work after sectioning of the annular ligament. The outlook is guarded where extensive tendon adhesions are resected, because these cases often have residual obliteration of the tendon sheath cavity with tendon tie-down in the proximal and distal limits of the sheath.

Constriction caused by tendinitis of the flexors in the MCP canal is readily relieved by annular ligament division; however, return to work is governed by the poorly healing bowed tendon. A guarded prognosis is common, and extended periods of measured increases in activity are recommended. Follow-up ultrasonograms are useful to evaluate the repair of tendon lesions, particularly where core lesions were injected at the time of annular ligament transection.

REFERENCES

1. Crabill MR, Watkins JP, Schneider RK, et al: Double-plate fixation of comminuted fractures of the second phalanx in horses: 10 cases (1985-1993), J Am Vet Med Assoc 1995;207:1459.
2. Colahan PT, Wheat JD, Meagher DM: Treatment of middle phalangeal fractures in horses, J Am Vet Med Assoc 1981;178:1182.
3. Welch RD, Watkins JP: Osteochondral fracture of the proximal palmar middle phalanx in a Thoroughbred, Equine Vet J 1991;23:67.
4. Watkins JP: Fractures of the middle phalanx. In Nixon AJ (ed): Equine Fracture Repair, Philadelphia, 1996, WB Saunders.
5. Modransky PD, Grant BD, Rantanen NW, et al: Surgical treatment of a palmar midsagittal fracture of the proximal second phalanx in a horse, Vet Surg 1982;11:129.
6. Schneider RK, Ragle CA, Carter BG, et al: Arthroscopic removal of osteochondral fragments from the proximal interphalangeal joint

of the pelvic limbs in three horses, J Am Vet Med Assoc 1994;205:79.

7. Turner AS, Gabel AA: Lag screw fixation of avulsion fractures of the second phalanx in the horse, J Am Vet Med Assoc 1975;167:306.
8. Martin GS, McIlwraith CW, Turner AS, et al: Long-term results and complications of proximal interphalangeal arthrodesis in horses, J Am Vet Med Assoc 1984;184:1136.
9. Schneider JE, Carnine BL, Guffy MM: Arthrodesis of the proximal interphalangeal joint in the horse: A surgical treatment for high ringbone, J Am Vet Med Assoc 1978;173:1364.
10. Steenhaut M, Verschooten F, De Moor A: Arthrodesis of the pastern joint in the horse, Equine Vet J 1985;17:35.
11. Doran RE, White NA, Allen D: Use of a bone plate for treatment of middle phalangeal fractures in horses: Seven cases (1978-1984), J Am Vet Med Assoc 1987;191:575.
12. Bukowiecki CF, Bramlage LR: Treatment of a comminuted middle phalangeal fracture in a horse by use of a broad dynamic compression plate, J Am Vet Med Assoc 1989;194:1731.
13. Trotter GW, McIlwraith CW, Nordin RW, et al: Degenerative joint disease with osteochondrosis of the proximal interphalangeal joint in young horses, J Am Vet Med Assoc 1982;180:1312.
14. Genetzky RM, Schneider EJ, Butler HC, et al: Comparison of two surgical procedures for arthrodesis of the proximal interphalangeal joint in horses, J Am Vet Med Assoc 1981;179:464.
15. Fürst A, Kaegi B, von Rechenberg B, et al: Die Behandlung von 5 Pferden mit subchondralen zystoiden Defekten im Fesselbein, Pferdeheilkunde 1997;13:147.
16. Shiroma JT, Engel HN, Wagner PC, et al: Dorsal subluxation of the proximal interphalangeal joint in the pelvic limb of three horses, J Am Vet Med Assoc 1989;195:777.
17. McIlwraith CW: Fetlock fractures and luxations. In Nixon AJ, editor: Equine Fracture Repair, Philadelphia, 1996, WB Saunders.
18. Kawcak CE, McIlwraith CW: Proximodorsal first phalanx osteochondral chip fragmentation in 336 horses, Equine Vet J 1994;26:392.
19. Birkeland R: Chip fractures of the first phalanx in the metatarsophalangeal joint of the horse, Acta Radiol Suppl 1970;319:73.
20. Petterson H, Ryden G: Avulsion fragments of the caudoproximal extremity of the first phalanx, Equine Vet J 1982;14:333.
21. Nixon AJ, Pool RR: Histologic appearance of axial osteochondral fragments from the proximoplantar/proximopalmar aspect of the proximal phalanx in horses, J Am Vet Med Assoc 1995;207:1076.
22. Barclay WP, Foerner JJ, Phillips TN: Lameness attributable to osteochondral fragmentation of the plantar aspect of the proximal phalanx in horses: 19 cases (1981-1985), J Am Vet Med Assoc 1987;7:855.
23. Fortier LA, Foerner JJ, Nixon AJ: Arthroscopic removal of axial osteochondral fragments of the plantar/palmar proximal aspect of the proximal phalanx in horses: 119 cases (1988-1992), J Am Vet Med Assoc 1995;206:71.
24. Sonnichsen HV, Kristoffersen J, Falk-Ronne J: Joint mice in the fetlock joint: Osteochondrosis dissecans, Nord Vet Med 1982;34:399.
25. Grondahl AM: The incidence of bony fragments and osteochondrosis in the metacarpo- and metatarsophalangeal joints of Standardbred trotters, J Equine Vet Sci 1992;12:81.
26. Sandgren B: Bony fragments in the tarsocrural and metacarpo- or metatarsophalangeal joints in the Standardbred horse: A radiographic survey, Equine Vet J Suppl 1988;6:66.
27. Dik KJ: Special radiographic projections for the equine proximal sesamoid bones and the caudoproximal extremity of the first phalanx, Equine Vet J 1985;17:244.
28. Bukowiecki CF, Bramlage LR, Gabel AA: Palmar/plantar process fractures of the proximal phalanx in 15 horses, Vet Surg 1986;15:383.
29. Grondahl AM: Incidence and development of ununited proximoplantar tuberosity of the proximal phalanx in Standardbred trotters, Vet Radiol 1992;33:18.
30. McIlwraith CW, Nixon AJ, Wright IM, et al: Diagnostic and Surgical Arthroscopy in the Horse, ed 3, London, 2005, Mosby-Elsevier.
31. Markel MD, Martin BB, Richardson DW: Dorsal frontal fractures of the first phalanx in the horse, Vet Surg 1984;514:36.
32. Holcombe SJ, Schneider RK, Bramlage LR, et al: Lag screw fixation of noncomminuted sagittal fractures of the proximal phalanx in racehorses: 59 cases (1973-1991), J Am Vet Med Assoc 1995;206:1195.
33. Markel MD, Richardson DW: Noncomminuted fractures of the proximal phalanx in 69 horses, J Am Vet Med Assoc 1985;186:573.
34. Markel MD, Richardson DW, Nunamaker DM: Comminuted first phalanx fractures in 30 horses: Surgical vs. nonsurgical treatments, Vet Surg 1985;14:135.
35. Richardson DW: Fractures of the proximal phalanx. In Nixon AJ, editor: Equine Fracture Repair, Philadelphia, 1996, WB Saunders.
36. Ellis DR, Simpson DJ, Greenwood RES, et al: Observations and management of fractures of the proximal phalanx in young Thoroughbreds, Equine Vet J 1987;19:43.
37. McClure SR, Watkins JP, Bronson DG, et al: In vitro comparison of the standard short limb cast and three configurations of short limb transfixation casts in equine forelimbs, Am J Vet Res 1994;55:1331.
38. Nunamaker D, Richardson D, Butterweck D, et al: A new external skeletal fixation device that allows immediate full weight-bearing application in the horse, Vet Surg 1986;15:345.
39. McClure SR, Watkins JP, Ashman RB: In vitro comparison of the effect of parallel and divergent transfixation pins on breaking strength of equine third metacarpal bones, Am J Vet Res 1994;55:1327.
40. Hornof WJ, O'Brien TR, Pool RR: Osteochondritis dissecans of the distal metacarpus in the adult racing Thoroughbred horse, Vet Radiol 1981;22:98.
41. Norrdin RW, Kawcak CE, Capwell BE, et al: Subchondral bone failure in an equine model of overload arthrosis, Bone 1998;22:133.
42. Hornof WJ, O'Brien TR: Radiographic evaluation of the palmar aspect of the equine metacarpal condyles: A new projection, Vet Radiol 1980;21:161.
43. Pool RR, Meagher DM: Pathologic findings and pathogenesis of racetrack injuries, Vet Clin North Am Equine Pract 1990;2:1.
44. Spurlock GH, Gabel AA: Apical fractures of the proximal sesamoid bones in 109 Standardbred horses, J Am Vet Med Assoc 1983;183:76.
45. Bukowiecki CF, Bramlage LR, Gabel AA: Proximal sesamoid bone fractures in horses: Current treatments and prognoses, Comp Cont Educ Pract Vet 1985;7:S683.
46. Petterson H, Ryden G: Prognosis in surgical treatment of sesamoid bone fractures in the horse, Pferdeheikunde 1986;2:253.
47. Woodie JB, Ruggles AJ, Bertone AL, et al: Apical fracture of the proximal sesamoid bone in Standardbred horses: 43 cases (1990-1996), J Am Vet Med Assoc 1999;214:1653.
48. Parente EJ, Richardson DW, Spencer P: Basal sesamoidean fractures in horses: 57 cases (1980-1991), J Am Vet Med Assoc 1993;202:1293.
49. Henninger RW, Bramlage LR, Schneider RK, et al: Lag screw and cancellous bone graft fixation of transverse proximal sesamoid bone fractures in horses: 25 cases (1983-1989), J Am Vet Med Assoc 1991;199:606.
50. Martin BB, Nunamaker DM, Evans LH, et al: Circumferential wiring of mid-body and large basilar fractures of the proximal sesamoid bone in 15 horses, Vet Surg 1991;20:9.
51. Palmer SE: Radiography of the abaxial surface of the proximal sesamoid bones of the horse, J Am Vet Med Assoc 1982;181:264.
52. Palmer SE: Arthroscopic removal of apical and abaxial sesamoid fracture fragments in five horses, Vet Surg 1989;18:347.
53. Southwood LL, Trotter GW, McIlwraith CW: Arthroscopic removal of abaxial fracture fragments of the proximal sesamoid bones in horses: 47 cases (1989-1997), J Am Vet Med Assoc 1998;213:1016.
54. Southwood LL, McIlwraith CW: Arthroscopic removal of fracture fragments involving a portion of the base of the proximal sesamoid bone in horses: 26 cases (1984-1997), J Am Vet Med Assoc 2000;217:236.

55. Barclay WP, Foerner JJ, Phillips TN: Axial sesamoid injuries associated with lateral condylar fractures in horses, J Am Vet Med Assoc 1985;186:278.
56. Bramlage LR: Fetlock arthrodesis. In Nixon AJ, editor: Equine Fracture Repair, Philadelphia, 1996, WB Saunders.
57. Nickels FA, Grant BD, Lincoln SD: Villonodular synovitis of the equine metacarpophalangeal joint, J Am Vet Med Assoc 1976;168:1043.
58. Rose PL: Villonodular synovitis in horses, Comp Cont Educ Pract Vet 1988;10:649.
59. Haynes PF: Disease of the metacarpophalangeal joint and metacarpus, Vet Clin North Am Large Anim Pract 1980;2:33.
60. Dabareiner RM, White NA, Sullins KE: Metacarpophalangeal joint synovial pad fibrotic proliferation in 63 horses, Vet Surg 1996;25:199.
61. Murphy DJ, Nixon AJ: Arthroscopic laser extirpation of metacarpophalangeal synovial pad proliferation in eleven horses, Equine Vet J 2001;33:296.
62. Nixon AJ: Osteochondrosis and osteochondritis dissecans of the equine fetlock, Comp Cont Educ Pract Vet 1990;12:1463.
63. Yovich JV, McIlwraith CW, Stashak TS: Osteochondrosis dissecans of the sagittal ridge of the third metacarpal and metatarsal bones in horses, J Am Vet Med Assoc 186:1985;1186.
64. Hogan PM, McIlwraith CW, Honnas CM, et al: Surgical treatment of subchondral cystic lesions of the third metacarpal bone: Results in 15 horses (1986-1994), Equine Vet J 1997;29:477.
65. Yovich JV, Turner AS, Stashak TS, et al: Luxation of the metacarpophalangeal and metatarsophalangeal joints in horses, Equine Vet J 1987;19:295.
66. Fortier LA, Nixon AJ, Ducharme NG, et al: Tenoscopic examination and proximal annular ligament desmotomy for treatment of equine "complex" digital sheath tenosynovitis, Vet Surg 1999;28:429.
67. McGhee JD, White NA, Goodrich LR: Primary desmitis of the palmar and plantar annular ligaments in horses: 25 cases (1990-2003), J Am Vet Med Assoc 2005;226:83.
68. Wright IM, McMahon PJ: Tenosynovitis associated with longitudinal tears of the digital flexor tendons in horses: A report of 20 cases, Equine Vet J 1999;31:12.
69. Wilderjans H, Boussauw B, Madder K, et al: Tenosynovitis of the digital flexor tendon sheath and annular ligament constriction syndrome caused by longitudinal tears in the deep digital flexor tendon: A clinical and surgical report of 17 cases in Warmblood horses, Equine Vet J 2003;35:270.
70. Nixon AJ: Endoscopy of the digital flexor tendon sheath in horses, Vet Surg 1990;19:266.
71. Nixon AJ, Sams AE, Ducharme NG: Endoscopically assisted annular ligament release in horses, Vet Surg 1993;22:501.
72. Nixon AJ: Arthroscopic surgery of the carpal and digital tendon sheaths, Clin Tech Equine Pract 2002;1:245.
73. Gaughan EM, Nixon AJ, Krook LP, et al: Effects of sodium hyaluronate on tendon healing and adhesion formation in horses, Am J Vet Res 1991;52:764.

CHAPTER 95

Metacarpal and Metatarsal Bones

Dean W. Richardson

ANATOMY

The third metacarpal bone (MCIII) and third metatarsal (MTIII) bones are important and vulnerable elements of the forelimbs and hindlimbs, respectively. The small metacarpal and metatarsal bones (splint bones, MC or MT II and IV) are often termed vestigial, but both MCII and MTII have major weight-bearing functions, and MCIV and MTIV serve as sites for important carpal and tarsal ligamentous insertions. MTIII is slightly longer and typically more round in cross-section than MCIII. The cross-section of MCIII changes dramatically in response to increased loading as the horse ages and trains.

There is little soft tissue coverage of MCIII or MTIII except for their palmar or plantar aspects where the superficial and deep digital flexor tendons, accessory (check) ligament of the deep digital flexor, and the suspensory (interosseous) ligament are located. The suspensory ligament originates in a broad attachment on the proximal palmar or plantar aspect of the bones. The soft tissues in the proximal palmar or plantar metacarpal and metatarsal regions also are invested in a retinacular sheath.

In the forelimb, the major neurovascular structures course along the length of the metacarpus both medially and laterally just dorsal to the flexor tendons. In the hindlimb, the great metatarsal (dorsal III) artery's location between MTIII and MTIV make it particularly vulnerable to accidental or surgical injury.

FRACTURES OF THE METACARPUS III AND METATARSUS III

Fractures of the metacarpus or metatarsus (MCIII or MTIII) are common long bone injuries of athletic horses. These are the most intensely loaded bones of the appendicular skeleton and are therefore vulnerable to single-event catastrophic failures as well as repetitive cyclic fatigue injuries. The most common site of major fracture of MCIII or MTIII is in the distal articulation. These bones are also common locations of kicking injuries in foals and adults, resulting in complete or incomplete fractures.

Condylar Fractures

Lateral Condylar Fractures

Vertical fractures in the sagittal plane occur in the distal condyle of MCIII or MTIII, predominantly in young racehorses, either during fast work or a race (Fig. 95-1). In Thoroughbreds, MCIII fractures are at least twice as common as MTIII fractures, but in Standardbreds, the ratio of forelimb to hindlimb fractures is more nearly equal.[1-3] Fractures in the right MCIII are significantly more likely to be displaced than those in the left.

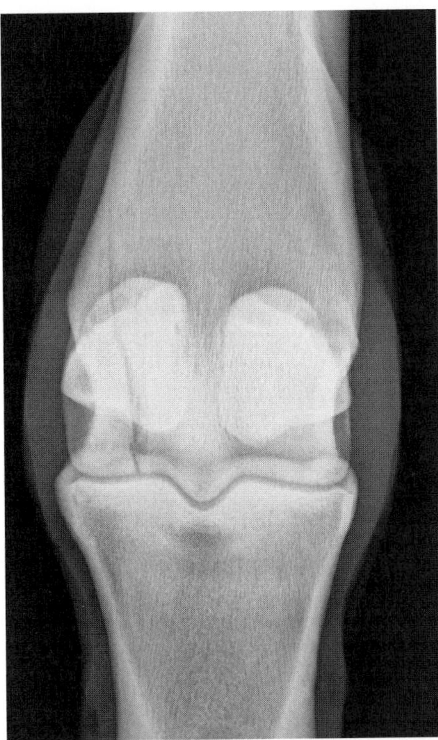

Figure 95-1. Dorsopalmar radiographic view of the distal third metacarpus (MCIII) depicting a nondisplaced lateral condylar fracture.

Clinical signs of lateral condylar fractures are typically straightforward, but incomplete fractures involving only the distal few centimeters of the condyle can present a diagnostic challenge. Horses might have a history of previous fetlock lameness preceding the onset of a more severe lameness; however, the most typical presentation is an acute onset of severe lameness after intense exercise or a race. The fetlock almost always develops effusion, and there is overt pain on manipulation of this joint. The degree of lameness is not well correlated with the amount of fracture displacement; many horses with nondisplaced fractures are extremely lame, whereas some horses with large displaced fractures walk fairly well on the fractured limb.

Approximately 85% of all condylar fractures involve the lateral condyle.[1-3] In the forelimbs, lateral fractures are seven times more common than medial fractures, and in the hindlimbs, lateral fractures are about three to four times more common.

Nearly all lateral condylar fractures propagate from the mid to mid-axial portion of the lateral condyle for a few centimeters in a sagittal plane and proximolaterally toward the lateral cortex. Their height varies, but the typical fracture exits 1 to 3 cm above the remnant of the physeal scar. Unlike medial condylar fractures, lateral condylar fractures rarely propagate in a spiral plane or course centrally through the diaphysis.

Radiographic diagnosis is not difficult when good-quality radiographs are obtained. An underexposed dorsopalmar or dorsoplantar (DP) projection or a radiograph in which the distal margins of the proximal sesamoid bones are superimposed over the metacarpophalangeal joint surface might not be diagnostic. This is avoided by taking the routine DP view in a slightly proximal-to-distal direction. Many horses have pre-existing degenerative disease involving the distal palmar or plantar condyle adjacent to the base of the ipsilateral proximal sesamoid bone, so an additional radiographic projection silhouetting this region is obtained by holding the fetlock in slight palmar flexion and taking a horizontal beam radiograph. This radiographic projection is used in all displaced condylar fractures because comminution along the fracture line is commonly identified in this location (Fig. 95-2). As imaging modalities such as computed tomography and magnetic resonance are used more, the repetitive stress injury in this location that predisposes to condylar fractures should be easier to recognize.

First aid for a lateral condylar fracture includes compression bandaging, nonsteroidal anti-inflammatory drugs, and absolute rest until definitive therapy is undertaken. The expense of cast coaptation is not justified because very few lateral condylar fractures will propagate if the horse is kept quiet in a heavy bandage. Manufactured splints and boots also are not indicated.

TREATMENT

Surgical management of lateral condylar fractures involves compression of the fracture with cortex or shaft screws applied in lag fashion. The screws prevent proximal propagation of the fracture and enhance articular healing, thus minimizing the potential for developing osteoarthritis. Surgical treatment is essential for displaced fractures because it provides anatomic reduction of the articular surface. Internal fixation renders the horse immediately more comfortable on the limb, thereby avoiding laminitis in the contralateral limb.

The disadvantages of surgery are those attendant on all general anesthetic procedures as well as the risk of infection and surgical error. However, condylar fractures can heal successfully without internal fixation, and a conservative approach is a reasonable consideration in nondisplaced fractures when there are economic limitations.

Nondisplaced fractures

Nondisplaced fractures are repaired with screws applied in lag fashion using minimum soft tissue dissection. The site of screw insertion is determined by topographic landmarks and intraoperative radiography or fluoroscopy. Radiopaque skin markers such as sterile skin staples can be used preoperatively to select the sites for screw insertion. Alternatively, needles or other markers can be used intraoperatively.

The distal screw is placed as centrally as possible in the lateral condylar fossa. This site can be accurately estimated by taking the midpoint of an imaginary line drawn between the proximal palmar prominence of the proximal phalanx and the most dorsal aspect of the lateral condyle, both readily palpable landmarks. A stab incision is made to the surface of the bone in this location and parallel with the collateral ligament fibers to minimize injury to them. The surgeon can feel the scalpel slide into the fossa, confirming accurate placement of the incision.

Standard lag technique is used (see Chapter 81). The author prefers to drill the thread hole completely through the bone to avoid creating a blind hole. A blind hole can

A

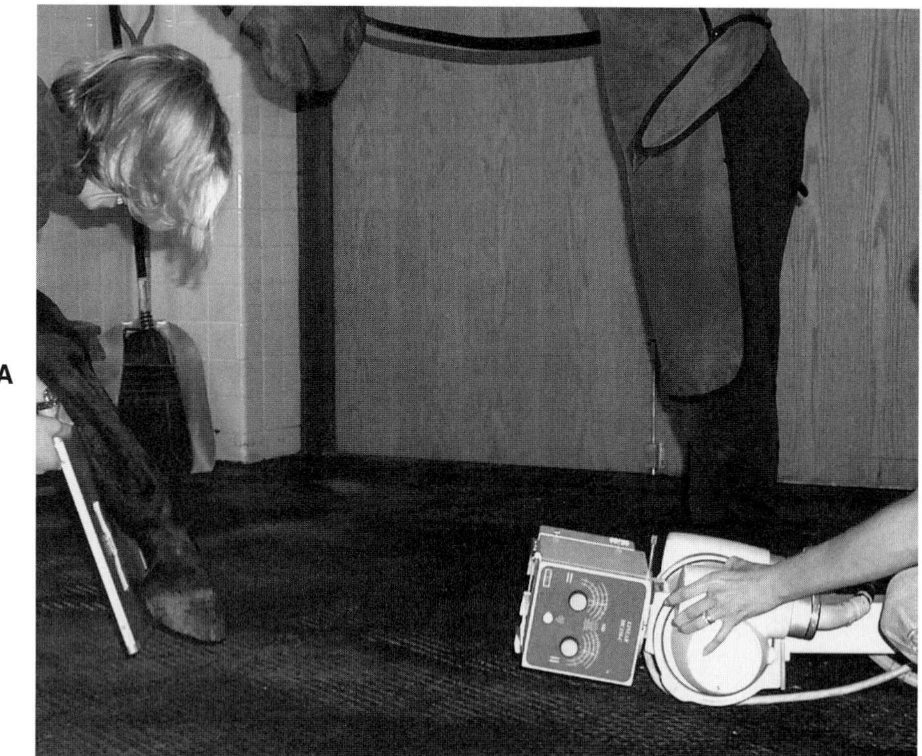

B

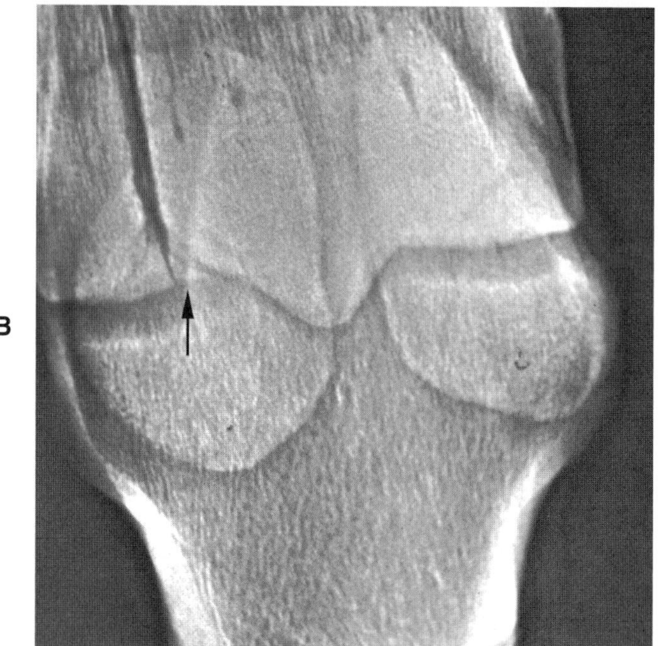

Figure 95-2. A, Positioning of the x-ray machine and corresponding x-ray plate to depict the distal articular surface of the third metacarpus (MCIII). **B**, Corresponding radiographic view that projects the distal palmar condyle. This view is essential in the preoperative evaluation of displaced condylar fractures because significant comminution may be present. Damage to this highly loaded portion of the condyle bears an unfavorable prognosis.

cause the tap to break inadvertently or a too-long screw to be inserted, preventing solid compression of the fracture. As many additional screws as needed are placed at 15- to 20-mm intervals more proximally. Blindly placing a screw too close (less than 20 mm) to the proximal end of the fracture increases of the risk of splitting the narrow end or entering a fracture line; a large majority of lateral condylar fractures can be treated with only two screws.

Correct positioning of the drill during the procedure is ensured through intraoperative radiographs (Fig. 95-3). Fluoroscopic image intensification is ideal, but plain films taken with small-diameter (2-mm) marker bits in place are

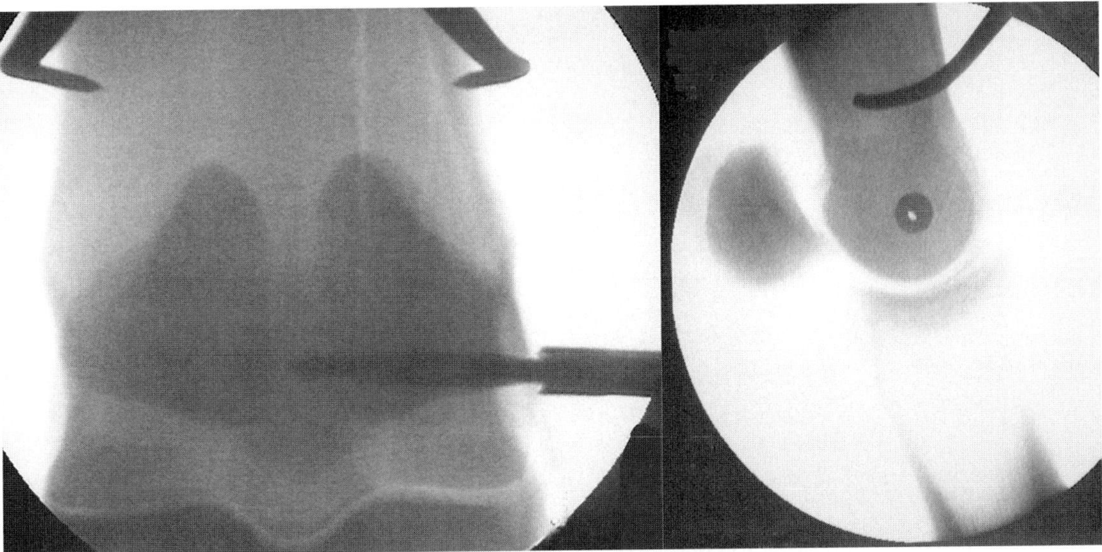

Figure 95-3. Correct positioning of the screws is checked intraoperatively and postoperatively with at least two perpendicular radiographic projections. The distal screw is usually positioned in the condylar fossa to maximize compression at the articular surface. The direction of drilling must be assessed with a lateromedial projection *(left picture)* to be certain of correct positioning. This image was taken with the insert drill guide in the glide hole. Because most horses' limbs are slightly externally rotated when they are in lateral recumbency, the implant will be positioned too far palmar or plantar if the surgeon drills perpendicularly to the floor. It is similarly easy to make an error in the proximal-to-distal direction if the limb is not positioned parallel to the floor.

acceptable. With either, two perpendicular views should be taken to check positioning in the dorsopalmar and lateromedial planes.

Either 4.5- or 5.5-mm cortex screws can be used. It remains unclear whether the larger screws yield improved results, because screw failure is rarely a problem. The 4.5-mm screws have the advantage of being replaceable with a larger cortex screw if the bone threads are inadvertently stripped. In vitro, greater resistance of shaft screws to shear stress occurred compared with cortex screws, indicating that shaft screws are an option for repair of clinical cases.[4]

The majority of lateral condylar fractures can be treated with two screws. A few will propagate proximally enough to justify more screws, but usually the more proximal portion of the fragment is quite narrow in its dorsopalmar thickness, and accurate positioning of the screw in the center of that part of the fragment is difficult.

The most common technical errors in lag screw fixation of nondisplaced condylar fractures include inadequate compression and incorrect drill or screw placement. The former can be avoided by drilling the thread hole fully through the transcortex and being certain to completely tap that cortex. To minimize the chances of incorrect proximal to distal aiming of the drill, the MCIII or MTIII should be positioned parallel to the ground before draping. Most horses have some degree of external rotation of the limb (especially hindlimbs) when they are in lateral recumbency. The surgeon must account for this or the drill will be directed toward the palmar or plantar articular surfaces. Palpation of the medial and lateral wings of the proximal phalanx provides a good topographical key for the surgeon to direct the drill in a true lateral to medial direction.

Unless there is a strong economic reason not to do so, the dorsal and palmar or plantar joint should be examined arthroscopically to confirm fracture reduction and characterize pre-existing or fracture-associated cartilage damage.

Displaced fractures

Similar lag technique and positioning of the screws are used to treat a displaced fracture. Unlike nondisplaced fractures, displaced fractures demand accurate anatomic reduction and often exhibit more severe injury to the joint surfaces. There is little room for error in reducing a displaced fracture in an athletic horse.

Complete radiographic obliteration of the entire fracture line does not always occur, even with accurate reduction and screw placement and correct technique, because of fibrin lodged within the fracture plane or bone loss along its margins. However, if the articular surfaces are aligned, the horse has a good chance to heal with minimal arthritic change. If there is a step on the major weight-bearing surface of the condyle, osteoarthritis is likely to develop. A significant malalignment of the condyle also will produce very high bending and shear loads that can lead to bending or breaking of the screws.

The best technique for reduction of displaced lateral condylar fractures in most cases is by arthroscopic guidance (Fig. 95-4). To tentatively hold the reduction, the metacarpophalangeal (MCP) or metatarsophalangeal (MTP) joint is dorsiflexed, and a large pointed bone-reduction forceps is used through the intact skin at about the level of the physeal scar. After preparing a stab incision through the skin and collateral ligament, as previously described, the 4.5-mm glide hole is drilled through the fracture fragment using radiographic or fluoroscopic guidance. The glide hole should be drilled exactly to the fracture plane; this can be facilitated by temporarily removing the clamp so that it is possible to feel the drill enter the fracture plane. The insert

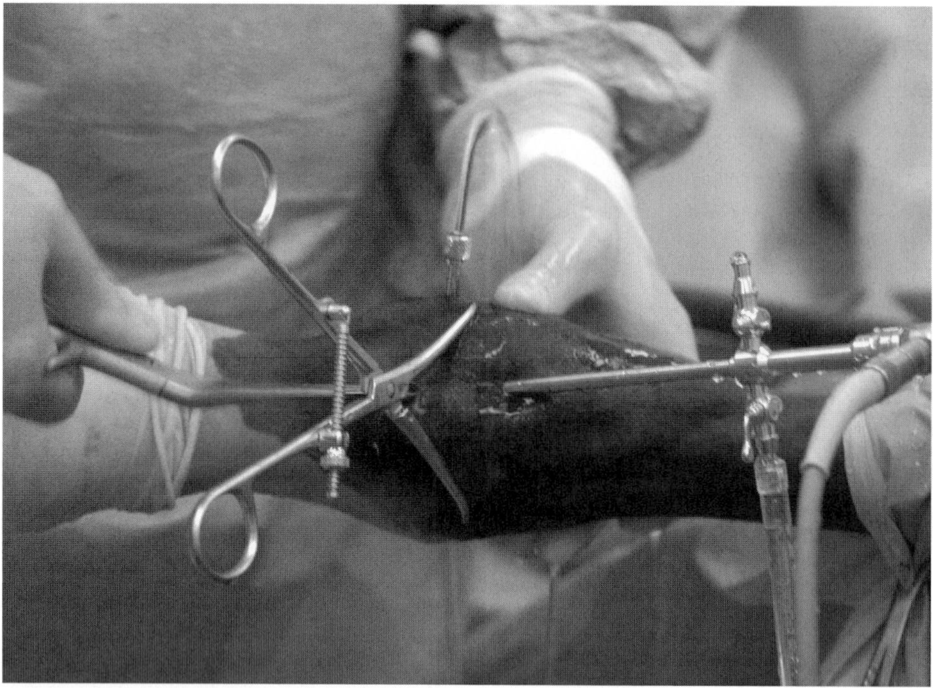

Figure 95-4. Arthroscopically assisted repair of lateral condylar fractures allows accurate fracture reduction and removal of loose fragments. In this image, the glide hole is complete and the insert drill sleeve is in place. The arthroscope is positioned proximodorsolateral. Pointed reduction clamps are in place to hold the fracture in reduction. A grasping forceps is used to remove a loose fragment from the fracture plane.

sleeve and a 3-mm pin are placed in the fragment to use as a handle.

The arthroscope is introduced into the proximal dorsolateral joint pouch. The MCP joint can be flexed, extended, or rotated and valgus or varus stresses can be applied until articular alignment is perfect. The pin inside the centering drill sleeve can be used for additional manipulation. When reduction is perfect, the reduction forceps are firmly reset and the remainder of the lag screw procedure performed.

The screw is inserted but not tightened. The arthroscope is repositioned and the articular compression and alignment are checked as the screw is firmly tightened. Subsequently, the palmar or plantar aspect of the joint is examined. Many comminuted fragments at the distal margin of MCIII or MTIII are immobilized by compression of the major fragment. If there are loose fragments, they can be removed under arthroscopic guidance. This is a difficult arthroscopic maneuver in some horses with chronic arthritis and capsular fibrosis. The instrument portal must be carefully positioned at the base of the lateral sesamoid, and instruments (curets, picks, and probes) with angled ends are invaluable.

Occasionally the fragment cannot be aligned properly because of interposed comminuted fragments. The pin and insert sleeve can be used to separate the dorsal aspect of the fracture plane to facilitate placement of the arthroscope and cannula into the fracture plane. A dorsal instrument portal exactly positioned over the fracture is made and the palmar fragments are retrieved.

If arthroscopic reduction is not feasible for some reason, enough of the fracture line should be exposed in displaced fractures to allow the surgeon to verify that reduction is accurate. In some cases this means a 2- to 3-cm incision over the proximal tip of the condylar fragment. In others, it means a longitudinal arthrotomy extending nearly to the proximal phalanx. In many horses, accurate reduction actually seems to get more difficult as the exposure is increased. It is always worthwhile to try to achieve accurate reduction using minimal exposure. It is imperative that postoperative radiographs are taken immediately to document correct surgical fixation of the fracture and create a comparative basis for follow-up radiographs.

Since arthroscopic examination of the entire joint has become a standard procedure, it has been recognized that sesamoid injury is often associated with condylar fractures. Most sesamoid damage involves varying degrees of erosion of articular cartilage, but more serious injuries also occur. Axial sesamoid fractures are often complications of displaced condylar fractures that should be identified preoperatively because they are associated with a very unfavorable prognosis. If an axial sesamoid fracture is present, repair of the condylar fracture should be done with the understanding that the horse has virtually no chance of returning to athletic competition. Axial sesamoid fractures are crescent shaped and represent an avulsion of the axial margin of the lateral proximal sesamoid bone by the intersesamoidean ligament (Fig. 95-5).

With large displaced fractures, the fragment can be fixed with one or two 3.5-mm cortex screws, but primary fetlock arthrodesis is probably a better option (see Chapter 85). In most axial fractures, a slender rim of articular surface is involved, but some fractures occur behind the articular surface and can be localized only with intraoperative radiographs or advanced imaging techniques such as computed tomography or magnetic resonance imaging.

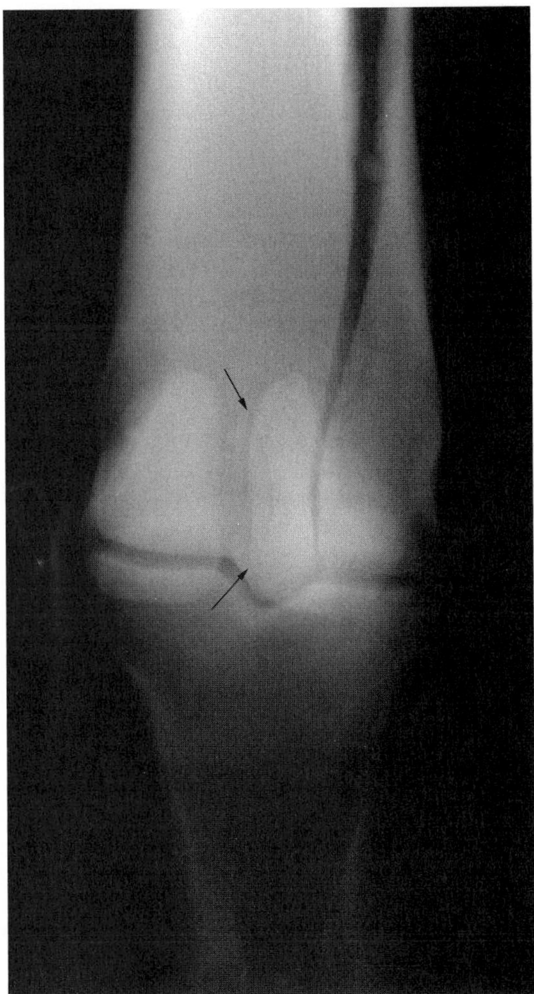

Figure 95-5. Axial sesamoid fractures are crescent shaped and always involve the lateral sesamoid. They represent an avulsion injury of the intersesamoidean ligament and bear an unfavorable prognosis for return to racing.

Nearly all lateral condylar fractures can be successfully treated with screws alone. On occasion, however, lateral condylar fractures of the MCIII also have diaphyseal spiral or oblique components that demand they be treated with more extensive fixation as described for medial condylar fractures.

Medial Condylar Fractures

Medial condylar fractures are seen in both the forelimb and hindlimb of racehorses. Horses typically develop severe lameness immediately after exercise or become lame a few hours afterward. There is rarely significant soft-tissue swelling unless there is displacement of the fracture.

In most cases, the site of the lameness is readily identified by manipulation of the MCP joint, and dorsopalmar or plantar radiographs clearly reveal the medial condylar fracture. Preoperative radiographs of any medial condylar fracture should include a full series of projections over the entire length of the MCIII or MTIII.

Medial fractures are quite different in terms of configuration, treatment, and complications. They are *not* the mirror image of a lateral fracture. Medial fractures nearly always propagate toward the axial aspect of the MCIII or MTIII, either spiraling up the diaphysis or remaining nearly sagittal to the mid-diaphysis, where oblique fractures can later develop. Medial condylar fractures of MTIII are particularly prone to catastrophic failure when the horse stands following general anesthesia or even for several weeks after repair.[5]

TREATMENT

Although internal fixation with multiple screws applied in lag fashion has been used successfully to treat many medial condylar fractures, plating techniques are preferable in most cases. Screws alone are not optimal for any fracture with a known oblique diaphyseal component; if an oblique or transverse diaphyseal fracture is identified in the preoperative radiographs, a plating technique should be used.

Approach

The plate and screws can be placed either medially or laterally. The fragments are equal enough in size and the bone is so dense that adequate fixation can be obtained with screws used in lag fashion, even if the threads are in the smaller fragment. The advantages of a dorsolateral approach are that the operated-on limb is uppermost and a lateral plate is easier to remove later under local anesthesia.

The incision is made in one layer down to the level of the bone surface. The periosteum is elevated, and the skin and underlying subcutaneous tissues are retracted together. When the surface of the cannon bone is exposed, the fracture line or lines are clearly defined (Fig. 95-6). The incision is continued distally to the level of the joint capsule, but the joint capsule is not incised.

The distal two screws are placed through stab incisions using radiographic control similar to that for nondisplaced lateral condylar fractures. If the limb is positioned uppermost, the glide hole must completely traverse the lateral fragment and the thread holes must engage the medial condylar fragment. This is ensured with intraoperative radiography or fluoroscopy.

A broad dynamic compression plate (DCP) is positioned extending from just above the second screw to the most

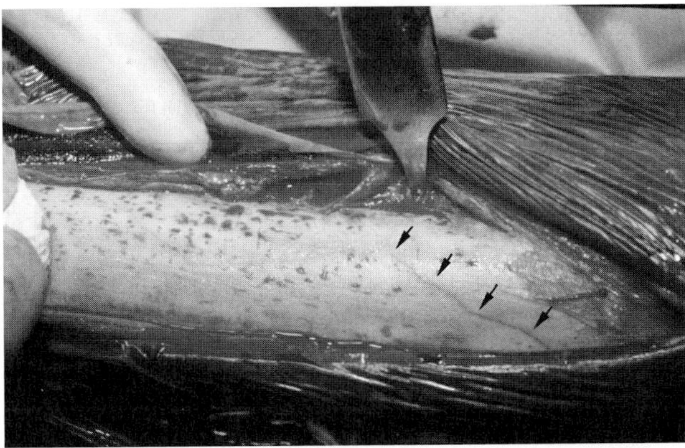

Figure 95-6. The simplest method of defining the configuration of a medial condylar fracture in the diaphyseal region is to make an open approach with periosteal elevation. The fracture line can easily be seen *(arrows)*, and screws can be placed accurately in a direction perpendicular to the fracture plane.

proximal aspect of the bone. Typically, 10-hole or 12-hole plates are used for the MCIII and 12-hole or 14-hole plates are used for the MTIII. It is possible to spirally conform the plate if the specific configuration of the fracture is evident, but a straight plate can usually be safely applied in these nondisplaced fractures. Exposure of the diaphyseal bone surface allows accurate placement of additional screws across the fracture plane and centrally within the fracture fragment. Either 4.5-mm or 5.5-mm cortex or shaft screws are used (Fig. 95-7). Although anatomic placement of screws through the plate is straightforward, the suspensory ligament or splint bones, or both, can be inadvertently injured. Obliquely directed screws or dorsopalmarly directed screws are drilled with care to avoid penetrating these structures, especially if using the 4-mm drill bit needed for the thread hole with 5.5-mm screws.

Closure of the incision is routine if initially it was made in one plane. A simple interrupted cruciate pattern or simple continuous pattern of synthetic absorbable suture in the subcutis followed by routine skin closure is adequate. If special recovery systems are not available, a full-length hindlimb cast should be considered for metatarsal fractures. Half-limb casts should not be used for metatarsal fractures. Forelimb medial condylar fractures are usually re-covered in a full limb Robert Jones bandage.

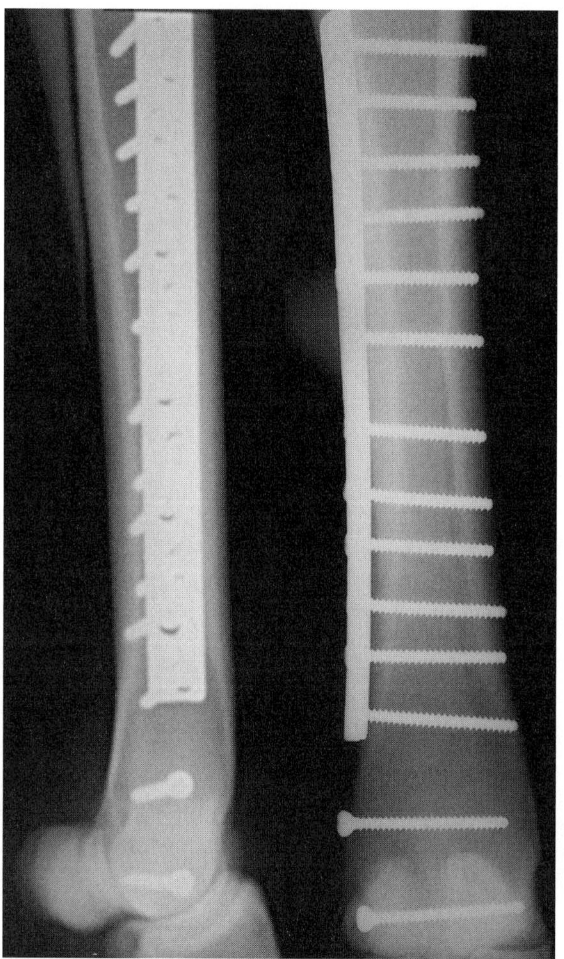

Figure 95–7. Medial condylar fractures that do not spiral and appear to either disappear in the middiaphysis or turn sharply in an oblique path across the bone can be repaired with a bone plate.

An alternative technique is to place the bone plate using a minimally invasive technique. This is particularly applicable if there is no obvious proximal spiraling of the fracture. A 2-cm incision is made adjacent to the extensor tendon in the proximal MCIII or MTIII. A (previously used) broad DCP that has a sharpened end and is attached to a handle can be used to prepare a subcutaneous tunnel for the plate.

After the tunnel is prepared, a roughly contoured 10-hole or 12-hole broad 5.5-mm limited-contact dynamic compression plate (LC-DCP) (see Fig. 81-17) with tapered ends is slid into it. The fit of the plate is assessed by palpation and with fluoroscopy. The plate is recontoured as needed and replaced. The holes in the plate can be easily palpated. Stab incisions are made over the holes in either end of the plate and screws are inserted routinely.

After inserting a screw through one proximal and one distal plate hole, a plate of the same length is placed on the surface of the skin and incisions are made through that plate's holes. The remaining screws are inserted using routine technique. The distal few screws in the plate may be placed in lag fashion if the fracture plane is radiographically visible at that level. Fluoroscopy or intraoperative radiography is used to check implant positioning. One or two skin sutures are used for each stab incision.

Caution should be used with this technique to avoid piercing the contralateral splint bone with drill bits and screws. It is important to carefully check that each screw is fully inserted into the plate. It is particularly difficult to accurately measure the depth of holes, and therefore, intraoperative radiographic control is needed. Although it is possible to inadvertently place a screw in a fracture line, the overall stability the plate appears to be adequate to prevent catastrophic failure of the bone. All possible precautions should be taken during recovery from anesthesia, especially in metatarsal fractures.

Another option for the treatment of high-risk condylar fractures is to place screws (typically two) to repair the distal portion of the fracture with the horse under sedation and local anesthesia. Although this still carries a risk of catastrophic post-fixation failure, the highest risk of fracture is during recovery from general anesthesia.

Aftercare

Convalescence of horses with condylar fractures involves stall rest with strictly controlled exercise for at least 2 months. Some turnout in a small paddock is allowed in the third month, and the patients usually are returned to regular exercise in the fourth or fifth month. Displaced fractures or those with articular comminution are rested longer. The average time from surgery to first racing start is approximately 11 months.

Although there is no uniform agreement on the need to remove screws from condylar fractures, many horses have returned to racing with screws in place, and most horses do not have screws removed after repair of typical fractures. When fractures extend into the mid-diaphyseal region, the screws are more likely to cause pain when horses return to intensive exercise. Therefore, diaphyseal screws are removed 3 to 4 months after surgery, usually with the horse under sedation and local anesthesia. The limb is clipped and scrubbed for routine aseptic surgery, and sterile skin staples are placed over the heads of the screws to be removed. Radiographs are taken to facilitate exact placement of the stab incisions over the screws if they cannot be clearly palpated. After the screws are removed, the horse is continued in a walking and jogging program for 60 to 90 days before returning to galloping exercise.

Plates used to treat medial condylar fractures are removed with the horse standing and under detomidine sedation and local anesthesia (see Chapters 20 and 74, respectively). These plates are typically removed about 70 to 80 days following surgery. Local anesthesia with direct infiltration over the implant or by means of a regional nerve block is performed, and a short incision is made over the proximal 2 cm of the plate (Fig. 95-8).

The most proximal screw is partially removed. A matching bone plate is placed on the skin, and stab incisions are made through its holes. Each screw is backed out above the skin edge but is not removed (Fig. 95-9). After the screws are all counted, they are removed. This helps prevent looking for a screw that has already been removed as well as preventing trying to remove a plate that still is secured with a screw. A battery-powered drill with the screwdriver attachment is quieter and easier to use in a standing horse.

A 12-mm osteotome is used to pry the plate up at its proximal end. The osteotome is left under the end of the plate, and the plate is grasped with sterile vise grips and extracted proximally. A single skin suture per screw is placed, and the larger proximal incision is closed in two layers.

The horse should be hand-walked for 60 days. It can be turned out into the paddock for another month and then gradually return to training.

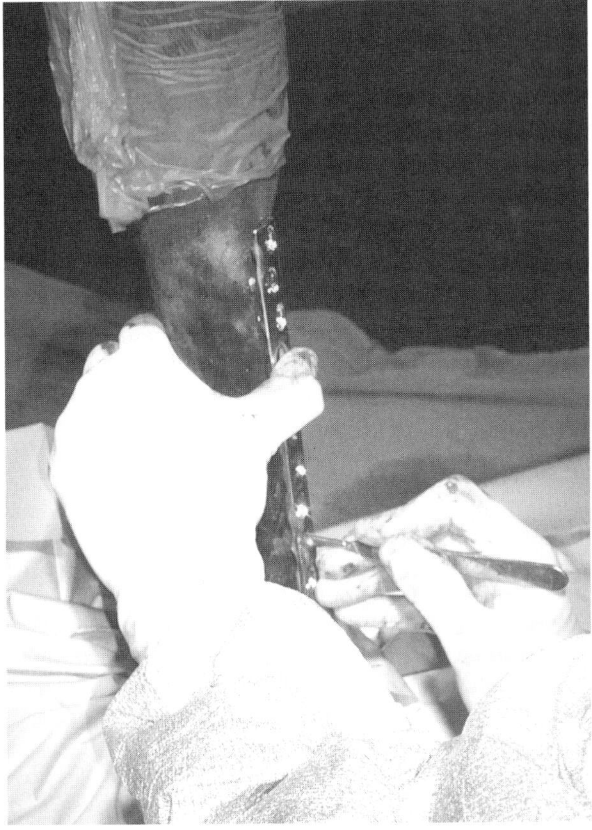

Figure 95-8. Bone plates are removed under sedation and local anesthesia. After identifying and partially removing one or two screws in the plate, a matching plate is used as a template to make stab incisions over each screw head.

Prognosis

Prognosis for condylar fractures is favorable (70% to 80% return to full function) if there is minimal pre-existing osteoarthritis and the fracture is not displaced.[1,2,6] Displacement requiring open reduction of the fracture lessens the prognosis considerably, both because of the surgical trauma and because there typically is more injury to the joint surfaces (comminution, degenerative changes, sesamoid injury).

The prognosis for displaced lateral condylar fractures of MCIII is about 50% for return to racing, less if there is serious comminution or sesamoid injury. Lateral condylar fractures of MTIII have a better prognosis than those of MCIII.

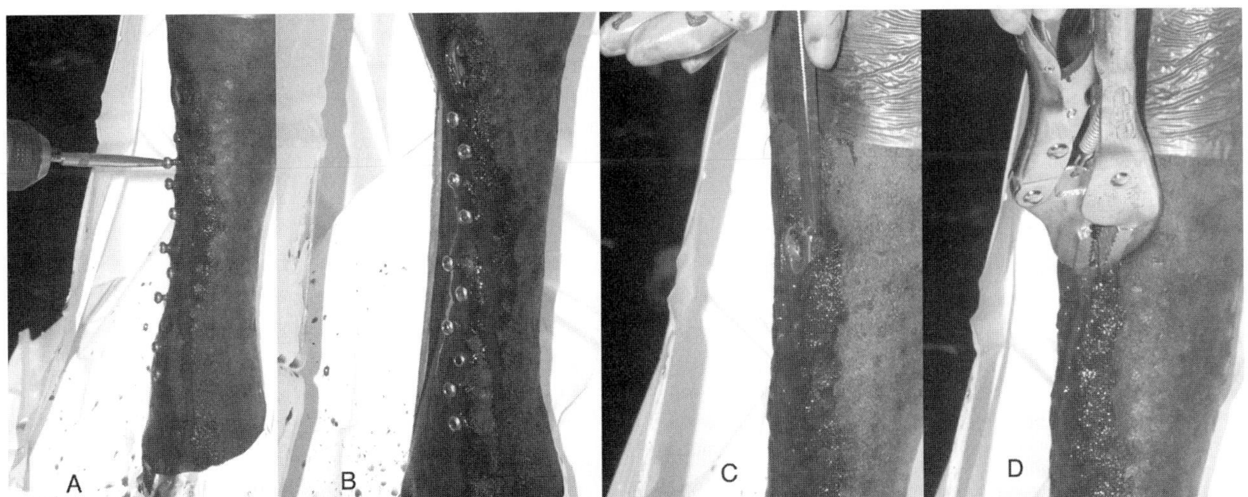

Figure 95-9. A and **B**, Each screw is removed partially until all are exposed. The screws are then removed and the proximal edge of the plate is elevated with an osteotome (**C**), grasped with a pair of pliers, and removed (**D**).

The prognosis for medial fractures is more variable and depends on the development of catastrophic complications. Complications of medial condylar fractures can occur before surgery, during recovery, or even weeks afterward. Therefore, by far the most important aspect of managing medial condylar fractures is to appropriately advise the owner of complications that can occur.

Diaphyseal Fractures

The most common major long bone fracture in horses is MCIII or MTIII, and diaphyseal fractures are the most often encountered. They occur in any age animal and during any type of activity. Many occur as pasture accidents.

There are favorable and unfavorable aspects to repairing fractures of MCIII or MTIII. Factors favoring successful repair are access and exposure of the entire diaphysis, making reduction and internal fixation feasible; strong bone to which screws and plates can be affixed; and the possibility of immobilization by external coaptation. Factors that do not favor repair are quite significant and include minimal soft-tissue coverage, which often leads to open fractures; no muscles adjacent to the fracture, resulting in poor extraosseous blood supply to the fracture site; sparse vascularity of the distal limb; and comminution, especially in older horses.

The diagnosis of diaphyseal MCIII or MTIII fractures is straightforward. In a frantic horse, radiography should be delayed until first aid has been administered and a preliminary decision has been made concerning treatment. It is particularly important not to risk opening a closed fracture by extended attempts to obtain radiographs. First aid for MCIII or MTIII fractures must include appropriate external coaptation (see Chapter 78).

Nonsurgical Management

Cast or splint coaptation as the sole treatment of displaced diaphyseal MCIII or MTIII fractures is rarely an acceptable approach. These fractures are unstable. Horses almost never become comfortable with simple external coaptation, and problems in the contralateral limb develop quickly. Furthermore, the lack of soft-tissue coverage over unstable MCIII or MTIII fractures can allow the fractures to open, even in a well-fitted cast.

In young animals, even though fracture healing occurs more quickly, cast coaptation is not the treatment of choice because permanent deformities develop rapidly in the contralateral limb and serious flexor or suspensory weakness occurs in the cast limb. Even if the fracture heals when treated in this manner, the problems associated with cast immobilization usually result in a less-than-optimal outcome.

Surgical Management

Internal fixation is the treatment of choice for diaphyseal cannon bone fractures. Although external skeletal fixation and intramedullary interlocking nails have been used, the optimal treatment remains double-plate fixation. Double-plating is usually necessary in foals and is always indicated in larger horses.

A dorsolateral surgical approach is used, splitting the digital extensor tendons. The skin incision is carried directly to the underlying bone through the periosteum (Fig. 95-10, *A*). The periosteum is elevated to allow reduction and reconstruction. Unlike in heavily muscled parts of the limb, reduction of MCIII or MTIII fractures is not usually difficult.

Reduction of simple fractures is maintained with large pointed reduction forceps or by inserting strategically placed compression screws. The sites for screw insertion are selected after planning plate application. If the only practical sites for the screws will be under a plate, 3.5-mm screws that are deeply countersunk are placed to hold the reduction while the plates are applied.

After reduction is secure with clamps, lag screws, or both, an aluminum template is used to help shape the two plates. The plates are placed dorsolaterally and dorsomedially at 90 degrees relative to each other unless fracture configuration dictates otherwise. In a large adult horse, two broad plates with 5.5-mm screws are used, but in a foal, one broad and one narrow plate are adequate. The plates are staggered so that screws placed perpendicularly through one plate will

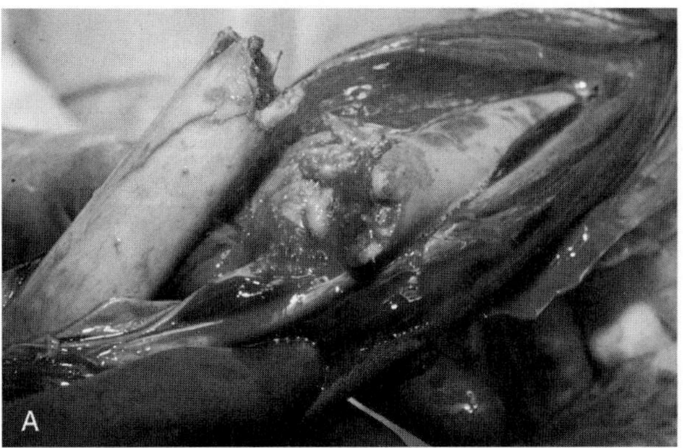

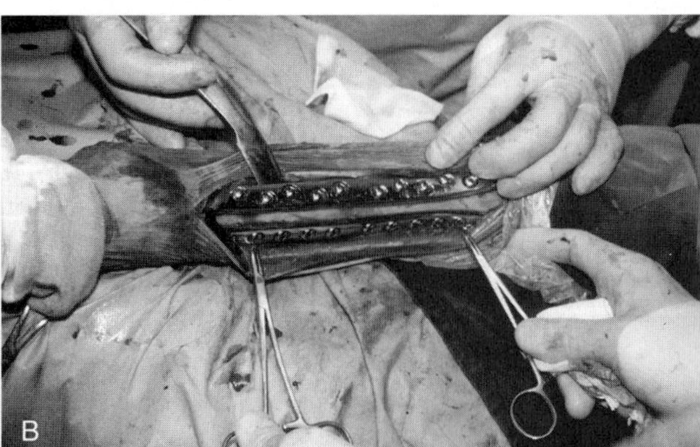

Figure 95-10. A, A fractured third metacarpus (MCIII) or third metatarsus (MTIII) is easily exposed and reduced through a straight incision along the margin of the extensor tendon. Minimal dissection of the underlying tissues will facilitate wound closure and lessen serum and blood accumulation at the surgical site. **B**, Most MCIII and MTIII diaphyseal fractures are repaired with two bone plates on the dorsolateral and dorsomedial aspects of the bone. Hohmann retractors provide necessary exposure at the bone ends.

not interfere with those from the other. All screw holes in the plates should be used; even if a hole is directly over a fracture line, a screw can nearly always be inserted that will engage at least one cortex. Both plates should be as long as possible without involving the joints or physis (see Fig. 95-10, *B*). Plate luting is recommended in larger horses with unstable fractures. The newer technology of locking compression plates (LCPs; see Chapter 81) should also be strongly considered if the additional expense of these implants can be justified.

An autologous cancellous bone graft should always be used if there are any cortical defects (see Chapter 82). It is best to perform the surgery as soon as possible after the injury because eburnation of the fragment ends makes reduction difficult and the repaired fracture less stable.

The incision is closed by initially apposing the tendon edges with interrupted synthetic absorbable sutures. Subcuticular and skin closure are routine.

The decision to use a cast versus a bandage on the limb depends on the horse's age, size, postoperative care, apparent stability of the repair, and available special recovery systems. A cast is used to protect the repair during recovery from anesthesia, but long-term protection of the repair with a cast is often undesirable because of the inevitable flexor weakness that develops. In general, foals younger than 1 year of age are not cast except for recovery. Casts are used in adult horses when the fixation is considered less than secure.

The major complication of MCIII or MTIII fractures is infection because of the relatively poor vascularity of the region, poor soft-tissue coverage, a large metal-to-bone ratio, and the commonness of open injury. Implant failure (loosening or breakage) is possible but less of a concern if correctly sized and positioned implants are used.

Distal Physeal Fractures

Distal physeal fractures of MCIII or MTIII are common injuries in suckling and weanling foals. Nearly all are Salter-Harris type II fractures with a variable length of metaphyseal involvement (Fig. 95-11, *A*). Such injuries usually heal relatively quickly with minimal surgical management. Young foals (younger than 6 weeks old) with these fractures can be treated with cast coaptation alone for 2 to 3 weeks followed by 2 to 3 additional weeks in a splinted bandage. If the fracture appears reasonably stable and the foal is comfortable, even less coaptation could be adequate.

In older, heavier foals or those with marked instability, the fracture can be repaired with compression screws through the metaphyseal component in addition to external coaptation (see Fig. 95-11, *B*). Although such minimal internal fixation is not inherently stable, it is adequate if combined with external coaptation in young foals because physeal injuries heal quite rapidly. It is preferable not to span this growth plate with any implants in animals intended for athletic function.

Regardless of the technique used to treat the fracture, the foal's return to exercise is carefully graduated over several weeks while the ligamentous and musculotendinous tissues regain strength.

Proximal Articular Fractures

Proximal articular fractures of MCIII or MTIII occur sporadically in racehorses and can be confusing because the lameness associated with them is typically eliminated by local anesthetic injected into the middle carpal or tarsometatarsal joint.

Sagittal fractures can be seen in any breed; most occur medial to the midline and are best diagnosed by nuclear scintigraphy and excellent-quality dorsopalmar or plantar radiographs. Occasionally, the fracture can be identified ultrasonographically as linear discontinuity in the proximal palmar or plantar cortex. *Frontal* plane fractures occur in MCIII or MTIII (Fig. 95-12, *A*). In Standardbreds, the fracture is most common in young pacers on the dorsomedial aspect of MCIII.[7]

All proximal articular fractures have been treated conservatively with good success, but displaced frontal plane fractures are best repaired with internal fixation using compression screws (see Fig. 95-12, *B*). The sagittal plane

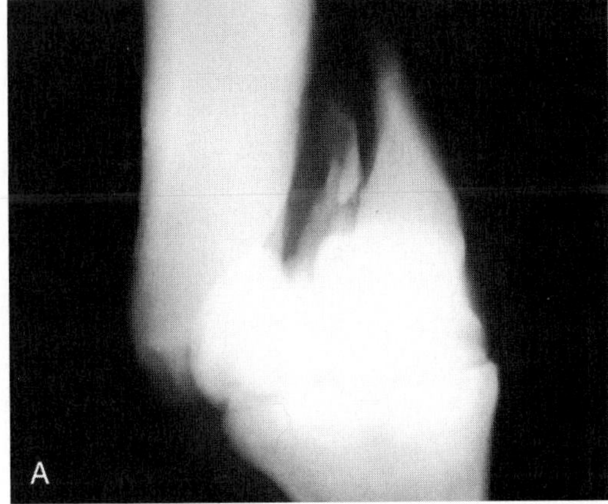

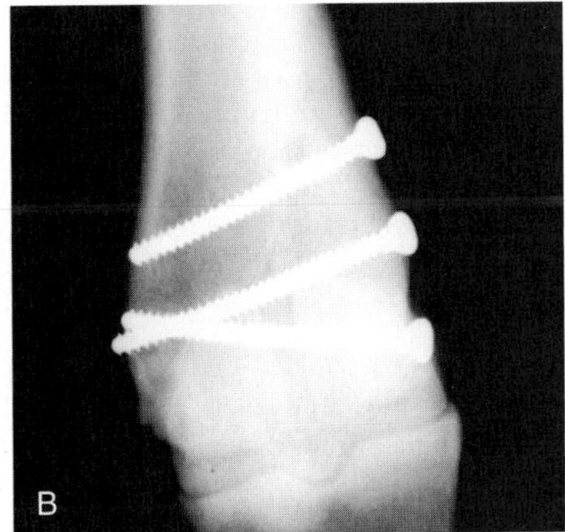

Figure 95-11. Most distal third metacarpal (MCIII) or third metatarsal (MTIII) fractures in foals are Salter-Harris type II injuries. Most can be treated with external coaptation, but older, larger foals are best repaired with bone screws placed in lag fashion coupled with a short period (4 weeks) of supporting external coaptation.

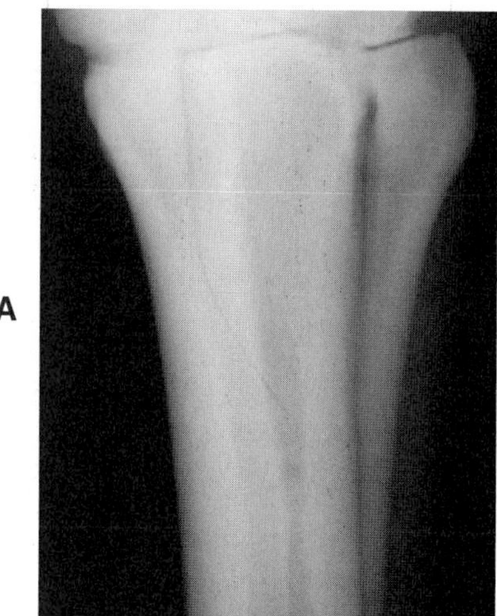

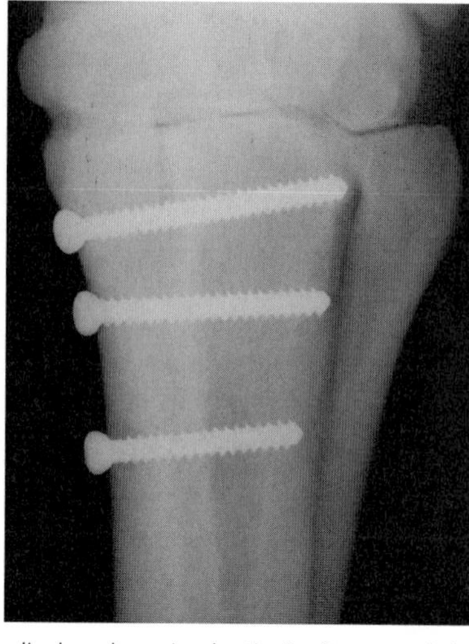

Figure 95-12. **A**, Radiographic view of a nondisplaced proximal articular fracture of the third metacarpus (MCIII). **B**, The fracture was repaired with three 5.5-mm cortex screws placed in lag fashion. Note the distal-most screw was not completely inserted, even though the hole was drilled completely across the bone. The fracture went on to heal because solid interfragmentary compression was achieved with the proximal two screws. (Courtesy J. Auer, University of Zurich.)

fractures are rarely displaced and will heal with stall rest alone.

Dorsal Cortical Fractures

A large percentage of young Thoroughbred horses in race training develop pain and lameness associated with the dorsal cortex of MCIII; this is called *bucked shins*. In the majority of horses, no specific fracture line is identified, but some develop one or more oblique radiolucent lines in the dorsal cortex accompanied by focal pain and swelling. These so-called stress fractures occur most commonly in 3-year-old Thoroughbreds after they experience bucked shin problems in their 2-year-old season.

The most common configuration of such fractures is a line coursing proximally at a 30- to 40-degree angle from the surface of the mid-distal dorsolateral cortex of the left MCIII (Fig. 95-13). Typically, the fissure extends approximately 60% to 70% through the dorsal cortex and disappears, but in some cases, the crack curves proximally and courses back to the dorsal cortex, forming a true saucer fracture. Fractures can occur in the opposite configuration (proximodorsal to distopalmar) as well as anywhere along the length of MCIII.

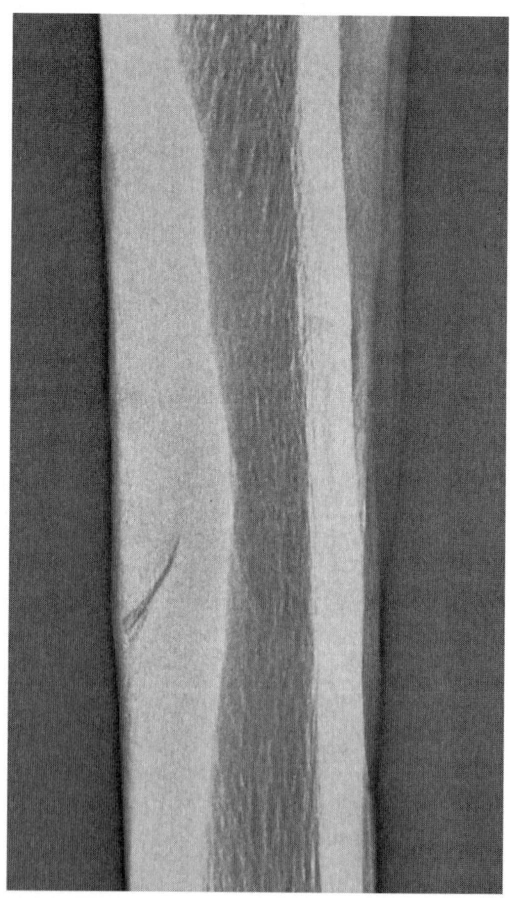

Figure 95-13. Xeroradiograph of a typical dorsal cortical stress fracture of the third metacarpus (MCIII) in a 3-year-old Thoroughbred racehorse. Optimal-quality films are always desirable to diagnose such injuries.

Nonsurgical Management

Treatment of dorsal cortical fractures can be conservative, with anti-inflammatory agents and rest (stall and paddock) until the fracture is radiographically healed. Some trainers return the horse to a diminished exercise program as soon as the overt lameness abates and then simply follow the progress of healing with sequential radiographs.

Many horses heal without surgical intervention, but a significant percentage have no signs of radiographic healing even after several months. The best candidates for conservative treatment are fractures in the distal or proximal metaphyseal regions of MCIII because they develop periosteal bridging callus much more rapidly than the typical intracortical fracture in the diaphysis.

Extracorporeal shock wave therapy has also been extensively used in the management of bucked shins and dorsal cortical fractures. There is controversy about its efficacy and whether or not a major effect of the shock wave treatment is primary analgesia.

Surgical Management

Surgical treatment of dorsal cortical fractures of MCIII is osteostixis alone or in combination with an intracortically placed 3.5-mm cortex screw.[8,9] The advantage of osteostixis alone is that it avoids a second operation to remove the screw. More-consistent results have been achieved with the combination treatment followed by routine screw removal at 60 days.

The surgery can be carried out under either general anesthesia or sedation and local anesthesia. Local anesthesia has the obvious advantage of avoiding the risks of general anesthesia and recovery, but it has the possible disadvantage of unexpected movement during drilling, leading to broken drill bits and taps.

It is important to accurately locate the exact site of the fracture preoperatively because it can often be very difficult to visually identify it at surgery. A useful technique is to take a radiograph of the limb after surgically preparing the skin and place multiple skin staples in a grid over the affected region, varying the orientation of the staples so that they can be easily identified (Fig. 95-14). This allows precise positioning of the incision over the fracture.

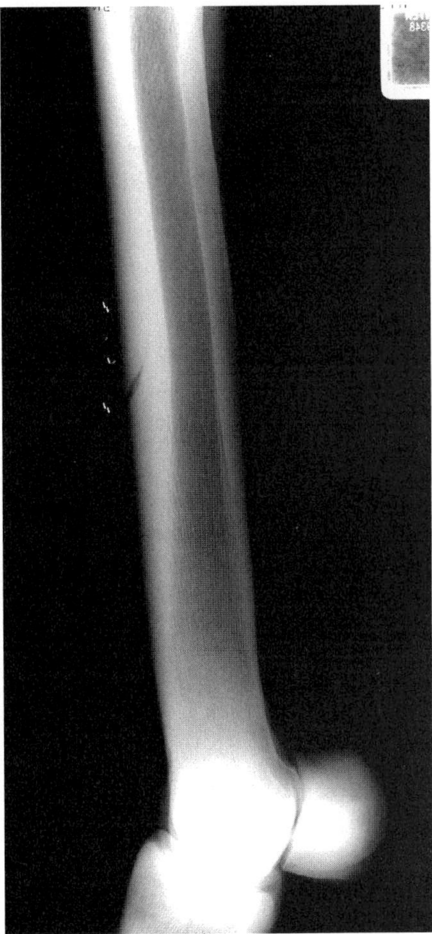

Figure 95-14. Perioperatively, sterile skin staples can be placed to help confirm the correct position for the incision and drilling of third metacarpal (MCIII) dorsal cortical fractures.

A 4- to 6-cm incision is made over the fracture site. In the typical dorsolateral fracture, the incision is between the common digital and lateral digital extensor tendons. The incision is made boldly directly to the level of the periosteum to minimize dissection. The periosteum is elevated, and self-retaining retractors are placed to expose the bone surface.

If a lag technique is used, the 3.5-mm glide hole is placed as perpendicular as possible to the middle of the radiographically identifiable fracture line. The depth of the glide hole is determined by measuring the actual depth of the hole and comparing it with the distance read off the radiograph. It is impossible to feel the drill cross the fracture line. Measuring the glide hole as it is drilled can result in error because the distance to the fracture line varies considerably with minor changes in the expected entrance point and obliquity of the drill path. Alternatively, because compression of the fracture is not necessary for successful treatment,[9] a position screw (without a glide hole) within the dorsal cortex is often placed.

A small bit is used to drill across the dorsal MCIII, with irrigation and frequent cleaning of the bit to avoid breaking the bit or causing thermal injury. Because the screw is inserted at an acute angle, countersinking is necessary to prevent the screw from bending at the head as it is tightened. The amount of countersinking should be minimal, however, because excessive depth of the head makes screw removal much more difficult. Most dorsal cortices accommodate a 22-mm screw. Because of the bending that occurs in the mid-diaphysis of the MCIII, a screw across both cortices is not recommended.

After the screw is implanted, six or seven osteostixis holes are drilled with a 3.2-mm or 2-mm drill bit across the dorsal cortex. The holes are drilled at a distance of approximately 20 mm between them all around the fracture (Fig. 95-15). Closure and bandaging of the area are routine.

Postoperative care includes stall rest and hand-walking for 2 to 4 weeks followed by 4 to 6 weeks of stall rest and paddock exercise. At 60 days postoperatively, the horse is returned for screw removal, which is easily performed in the standing animal under sedation and local anesthesia.

If the screw head cannot be palpated, a grid of sterile skin staples can be placed over the area and a radiograph taken to locate the ideal site for a small incision. Local infiltration at the site of the screw head is adequate. Because the hexagonal recess of the 3.5-mm screw head is quite shallow, it is easily stripped; therefore, the screw head recess should be completely cleaned with a needle, sharp hook, or small pin before inserting the screwdriver tip to prevent this complication. If it does strip, the head is grasped with locking pliers and removed.

Figure 95-15. If a screw is used, it is placed only in the dorsal cortex as close as possible to perpendicular to the fracture line. Multiple small (2- to 3.2-mm) drill holes are distributed around the fracture, each separated by at least 10 to 12 mm.

After the screw is removed, the horse is hand-walked for another month. The horse can begin a jogging program for about 6 to 8 weeks before returning to regular race training.

FRACTURES OF THE SMALL METACARPAL OR METATARSAL BONES

Fractures of the small metacarpal or metatarsal bones occur during exercise or as a result of direct trauma, such as kicks. The former are closed injuries, and the latter are often open. Clinical diagnosis is straightforward because pain and swelling are palpable and radiographs are simple to obtain and interpret. Ultrasonography is performed to assess concurrent injury to the suspensory ligament.

Distal Fractures

Distal splint bone fractures (those involving the distal half of the bone) are treated by surgical excision of the distal fragment (Fig. 95-16, *A*). The surgery is technically simple and can be successfully performed under general anesthesia or with the horse standing under local anesthesia.

Although this surgery can be carried out with an Esmarch bandage or tourniquet, bleeding is usually modest and rarely slows the procedure. In cases with extensive contamination, an Esmarch bandage can allow much more accurate débridement because foreign material is more easily recognized.

An incision is made directly over the bone, cutting down to the bone surface over the length of the fragment. The distal tip of the fragment is grasped with towel clamps or tissue forceps and elevated. The attachments between the distal fragment and MCIII are severed with heavy curved scissors or a 6-mm osteotome. As upward traction is applied on the fragment's extremity, sharp dissection is continued proximally to approximately 8 to 16 mm proximal to the fracture site.

After the distal fragment and the fracture callus are separated from MCIII or MTIII, the splint bone with its periosteum is transected obliquely in a proximal abaxial to distal axial direction with an osteotome and mallet. The distal stump and the bed of the removed fragment are checked for loose fragments or jagged edges (see Fig. 95-16, *B*). If found, these are removed with rongeurs or a curet. The wound is checked for bleeding vessels, which are cauterized or ligated.

The incision is closed in routine fashion in two layers, and an adhesive elastic pressure bandage is applied over a light sterile dressing. This is in turn covered with a padded bandage to further minimize bleeding into the dead space.

Prognosis depends to a great extent on the coexistence and degree of suspensory desmitis, sesamoiditis, or MCP joint disease. Thus it is essential to preoperatively evaluate adjacent tissues with physical examination, radiographs, and ultrasonography.

Prognosis after larger distal fragments of splint bones are removed depends on the size of the fragment removed as well as the specific bone involved. The entire MTIV can be

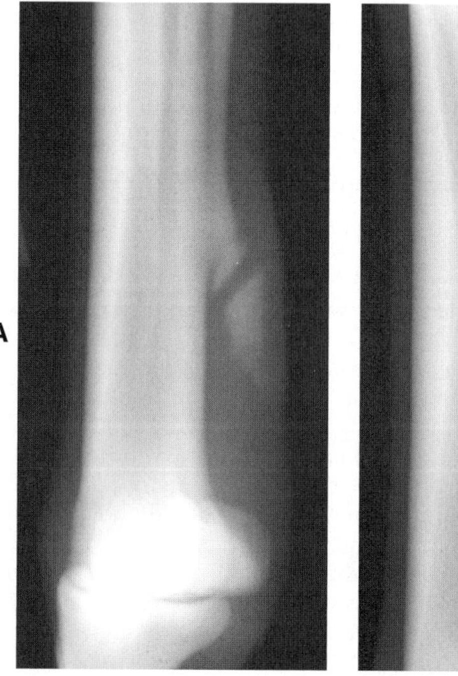

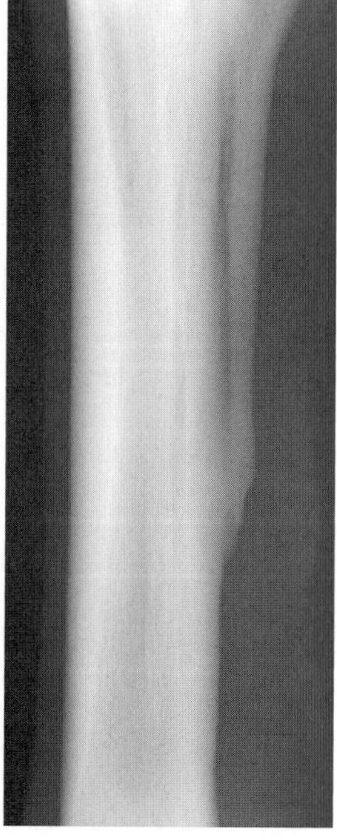

Figure 95-16. Fractures of the distal portion of splint bones are treated by removal. **A**, Preoperative radiographic view. **B**, Postoperative radiographic view.

removed with good results,[10] but removal of more than 50% of MCII can lead to carpometacarpal instability and lameness because MCII bears a substantial axial load. Therefore, an effort should be made to repair rather than remove fractures of the proximal half of MCII.

Proximal Fractures

Internal fixation of splint fractures is indicated for fractures involving the proximal half of MCII and the proximal third of MCIV, MTII, or MTIV. Although large fragments have been removed and the remaining portion successfully fixed to MCIII or MTIII, motion between the bones commonly leads to lameness.[11] Plate fixation in which the screws engage only the splint bone is the preferred technique for simple displaced fractures of the proximal splint bone. Comminuted fractures are treated conservatively because many heal adequately with bandaging and stall rest.

A slightly curved incision is made long enough so the plate is not positioned directly under it. A 3.5-mm narrow dynamic compression plate, a 3.5-mm semitubular plate, or a 3.5-mm reconstruction plate is used, even in a large horse. Principles of plate application do not differ from those of other fractures (see Chapter 81).

The ligamentous attachments on the abaxial surfaces of the proximal splints make the palmar or plantar abaxial aspect a tension surface, and the plate is best positioned there. Most fractures are oblique; thus the best technique is neutralization plating with screws applied in lag fashion across the fracture line (through the plate) (Fig. 95-17). A cancellous graft is placed in large defects, although the surgeon should be careful not to place it axially so that the suspensory ligament becomes entrapped in new bone. In open fractures, antibiotic-impregnated polymethylmethacrylate (PMMA) beads may also be placed at the fracture site.

Cast coaptation is not necessary postoperatively. If the fracture cannot be successfully plated without engaging the cannon bone, the plate will need to be removed about 3 to 4 months after surgery, before the horse goes back into strenuous work.

The plate can be removed through stab incisions. One screw in the plate is identified and removed. A matching plate is placed over the site, allowing accurate estimation of the other screw positions. Small stab incisions are made to remove the screws. A skin stab at the end of the plate is enlarged slightly, allowing the plate to be grasped with vise grips or a similar instrument and slid out of the incision.

The prognosis for most splint fractures repaired with plate fixation is excellent. The major complication is sepsis, particularly if the original injury was caused by external trauma. Fortunately, the limited weightbearing of the splint bone allows successful management when there is contamination and sepsis.

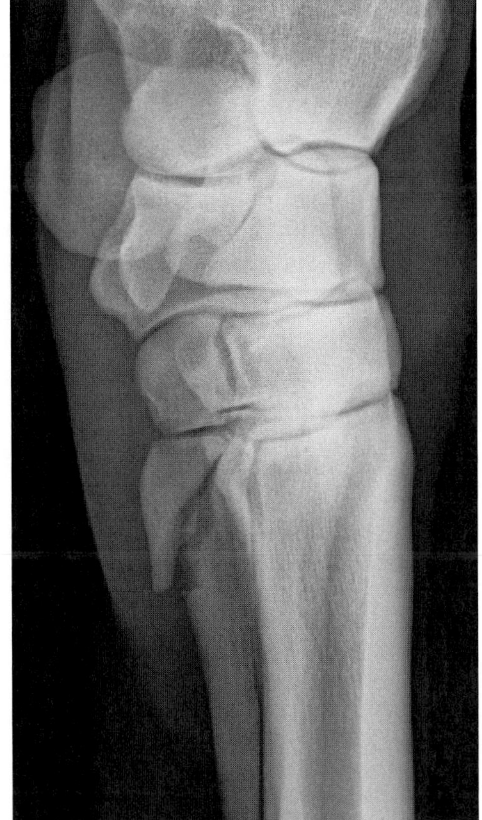

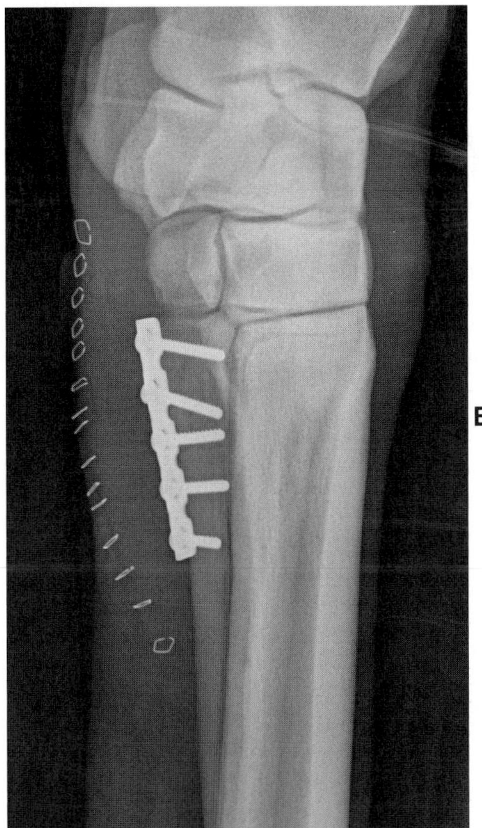

Figure 95-17. A, Most proximal fractures of MCII are oblique and involve the articular surface. **B,** A 3.5-mm reconstruction plate was applied. Screws alone are vulnerable to pull-out because of the collateral ligament attachment.

A, B

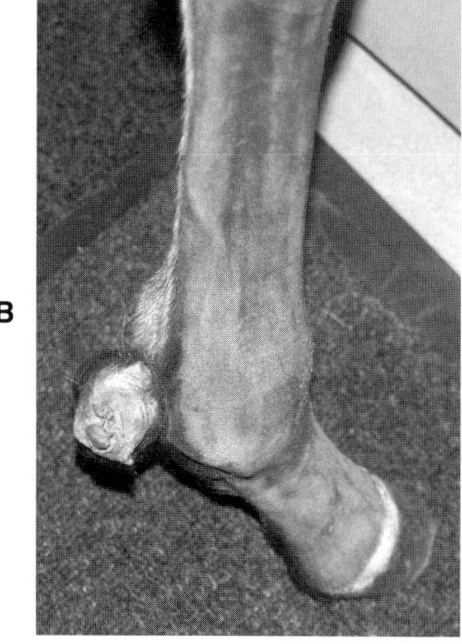

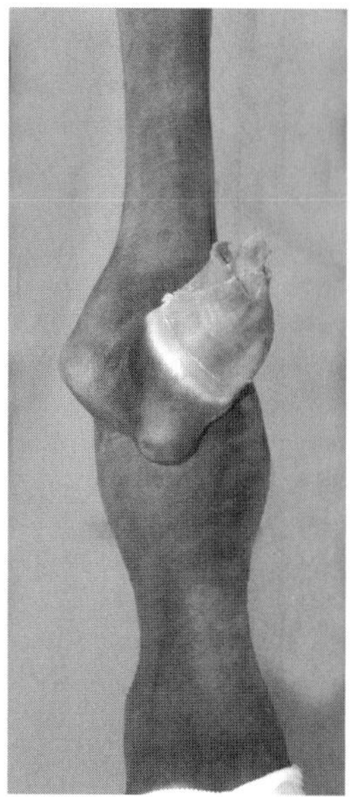

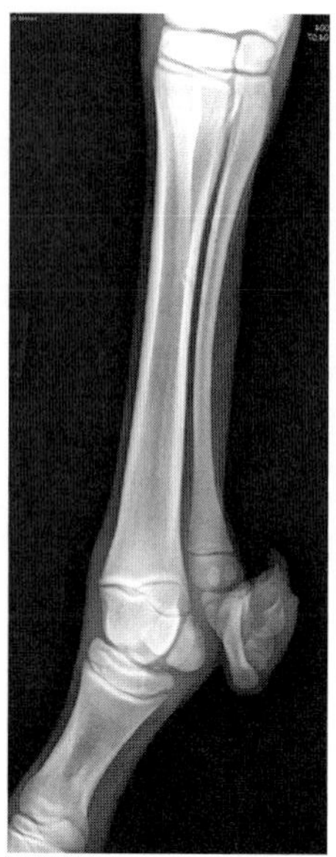

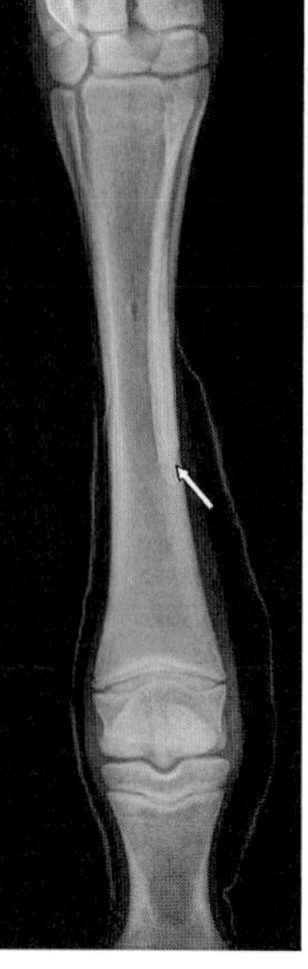

C, D

Figure 95-18. Polydactyly is a rare congenital anomaly. Most foals can be salvaged by removal of the extra digit. **A**, The rudimentary medial (second) digit shown on the limb from the side and **B**, from behind. **C**, Lateromedial radiographic view depicting the rudimentary digit. **D**, Postoperative dorsopalmar radiographic view.

Splint Exostoses

Most horses with exostoses involving the splint bone are not candidates for surgery except for cosmetic purposes. If cosmetic removal of a splint is undertaken, it is essential to inform the owner that the site might not have a blemish-free appearance. This is particularly true of splint exostoses that develop because of overt conformational abnormalities such as bench knees or carpus varus deformities.

Although there is no surgical technique that consistently produces elimination of a blemish, the best technique is a simple linear incision over the exostosis and en bloc excision of the entire bone mass. This excision should include the overlying periosteum. An oscillating saw or a sharp-bladed osteotome is used to cut the excessive bone and return it to a normal contour. Often, separation of the proliferative bone from normal bone occurs without effort once the level is identified. Transection of the metacarpal nerve coursing axially to the affected portion of the splint has been proposed to eliminate lameness.

Axial exostoses are the cause of lameness because of impingement on the suspensory ligament. The presence of such an exostosis (hidden splint) is diagnosed with dorsopalmar radiographs.[1] The problem is verified with computed tomography. In diagnosed cases, surgical removal of the splint can be attempted with the same restrictions discussed above. The lesion is approached through a skin incision over the palmar or plantar aspect of the splint bone involved. The axial fascia is transected, and the suspensory ligament is carefully displaced. Removal of the exostosis is routine. Care is taken to avoid damage to the suspensory ligament.

Good hemostasis is verified, the loose subcutaneous tissues are closed over the exposed bone surface, and the skin edges are apposed routinely. In very large exostoses, a portion of the skin margin is excised to reduce the tendency for hematoma or seroma to develop.

The most critical aspect of managing cosmetic splint removals is postoperative bandaging. A tight internal bandage applying direct pressure over the surgery site followed by an outer padded compression bandage should be kept in place for several weeks to minimize the accumulation of blood or serum at the surgical site.

POLYDACTYLY

Polydactyly of the metacarpal or metatarsal region occurs occasionally as a congenital defect (Fig. 95-18). The milder forms that do not compromise the carpus or tarsus too extensively can be successfully managed by surgical excision of the extra metacarpus and digit.

REFERENCES

1. Rick MC, O'Brien TR, Pool RR: Condylar fractures of the third metacarpal and third metatarsal bone in 75 horses: Radiographic features, treatments, and outcome, J Am Vet Med Assoc 1983;183:287.
2. Bassage LH, Richardson DW: Longitudinal fractures of the third metacarpal and metatarsal condyles in racehorses: 233 cases (1986–1995), J Am Vet Med Assoc 1998;212:1757.
3. Zekas LJ, Bramlage LR, Embertson RM, Hance SR: Characterisation of the type and location of fractures of the third metacarpal/metatarsal condyles in 135 horses in central Kentucky (1986-1994), Equine Vet J 1999;31:304.
4. Rahm C, Ito K, Auer JA: Lag screw fixation of equine cannon bone fractures: A biomechanical comparative study of shaft and shaftless cortex screws, Vet Surg 2000;29:564.
5. Richardson DW: Medial condylar fractures of the third metatarsal bone in horses, J Am Vet Med Assoc 1984;185:761.
6. Zekas LJ, Bramlage LR, Embertson RM, Hance SR: Results of treatment of 145 fractures of the third metacarpal/metatarsal condyles in 135 horses (1986-1994), Equine Vet J 1999;31:309.

7. Ross MW, Martin BB: Dorsomedial articular fracture of the proximal aspect of the third metacarpal bone in Standardbred racehorses: Seven cases, J Am Vet Med Assoc 1992;201:332.
8. Cervantes C, Madison JB, Ackerman N, et al: Surgical treatment of dorsal cortical fractures of the third metacarpal bone in Thoroughbred racehorses: 53 cases (1985–1989), J Am Vet Med Assoc 1992;200:1997.
9. Dallap B, Bramlage LR, Embertson RM: Results of screw fixation combined with cortical drilling for treatment of dorsal cortical stress fractures of the third metacarpal bone in 56 Thoroughbred racehorses, Equine Vet J 1999;31:252.
10. Baxter GM, Doran RE, Allen D: Complete excision of a fractured fourth metatarsal bone in eight horses, Vet Surg 1992;21:273.
11. Peterson PR, Pascoe JR, Wheat JD: Surgical management of proximal splint bone fractures in the horse, Vet Surg 1987;16:367.

CHAPTER 96

Carpus

Alan J. Ruggles

Carpal injuries in the horse occur most often in racing breeds. The expected outcome after injury and treatment is based on return to racing soundness.

ANATOMY

The carpus consists of three joints: antebrachiocarpal, middle carpal, and carpometacarpal. The middle carpal and carpometacarpal joints always communicate with each other. This fact is important when considering intra-articular and regional anesthesia of the proximal palmar metacarpus.

Injury of the carpometacarpal joint is mostly desensitized by intra-articular anesthesia of the middle carpal joint. Likewise, middle carpal joint injury can be desensitized if an anesthetic agent is inadvertently placed in the palmar aspect of the carpometacarpal joint during regional anesthesia of the proximal palmar metacarpus.[1] Studies have indicated that analgesia of the antebrachiocarpal and middle joints is not specific either. In one study, diffusion of mepivacaine between the antebrachiocarpal and middle carpal joints occurred in 84% of the tested limbs, and diffusion between the middle and antebrachiocarpal joints occurred in 96% of tested limbs.[2] Therefore, a positive response to intrasynovial anesthesia of one portion of the carpus might not specifically implicate that joint as the source of lameness. This information confirms clinical experiences in horses that block out variably in the carpal and proximal metacarpal region.

The bones that compose the carpus include the radius; the proximal row of carpal bones (radial carpal, intermediate carpal, and ulnar carpal); the distal row of carpal bones (second, third, and fourth carpal); the metacarpal (MC) bones II, III, and IV; the accessory carpal bone; and occasionally a first carpal bone (but rarely a fifth). The orientation of the carpal bones relative to themselves is maintained by their soft-tissue attachments, including the intercarpal ligaments, collateral ligaments, fibrous joint capsule, and palmar carpal ligament. The extensor carpi radialis and common digital extensor tendons as well as their sheaths span the carpus dorsally and dorsolaterally, respectively. They are maintained in their position over the dorsal surface of the carpus by the extensor retinaculum located at the distal radius approximately at the level of the physeal scar. The lateral digital extensor tendon courses over the lateral side of the carpus, as does the tendon of the ulnaris lateralis. Palmar and medial to the palmar carpal ligament is the carpal canal, a synovial structure in which the superficial and deep digital flexor tendons, median artery, and nerve are located. Immediately medial to the carpal canal is the tendon and tendon sheath of the flexor carpi radialis, which is an important surgical landmark for desmotomy of the proximal check ligament.

The function of the bony and ligamentous structures of the carpus is to dissipate axial loading during weight-bearing. The anatomic position of the carpal bones and the resultant transmission of forces to the intercarpal ligaments protect the weight-bearing surfaces of the carpal bones during exercise to prevent injury.[3] Loss of interosseous fibrous connections promotes instability, lameness, and osteoarthritis. The support of the cuboidal bones and the compressive stiffness of the hyaline cartilage are key to carpal function.

PATHOPHYSIOLOGY

Injury to the carpus most commonly occurs within the antebrachiocarpal and middle carpal joints. Injury of the proximal metacarpus, which can involve the carpometacarpal joint, is discussed in Chapter 95. Osteochondral fragments occur in both the dorsolateral and dorsomedial aspect of the antebrachiocarpal joint. Injury of the middle carpal joint nearly always involves the medial aspect of the joint—that is, the radial facet of the third carpal bone, the distal aspect of the radial carpal bone, and occasionally the medial aspect of the distal intermediate carpal bone.

High-energy injuries such as falls or kicks to the carpus cause acute single load failure. The resultant injury often causes open or comminuted fractures and carpal instability. (For additional details on stabilizing luxations of the carpus, see Chapter 85.) These injuries, however, are less common than those developing as a result of repetitive loading. During training, axial loading of the carpus occurs and stress-adaptive remodeling of the carpal bones is induced. Alterations in bone porosity and stiffness can predispose the bone to fracture.[4]

Exercise induces regional changes in bone density, which can be associated with the characteristic location of carpal injury. In one study, Thoroughbred horses exercised on a treadmill had increased trabecular thickening and increased bone mineral density in the third and radial carpal bones, in areas where cartilage degeneration and fractures occur commonly.[5] Previous work had identified increased areas of bone stiffness in the radial facet of the third carpal bone.[4] Loss of compressive stiffness of the subchondral bone plate subsequent to exercise, which is manifested by sclerosis on a radiograph, likely contributes to fractures of the carpus.

Likewise, cartilage injury has been correlated with underlying bone sclerosis.[6] Training has been shown to increase the thickness of the zone of calcified cartilage. The effect of this thickening is unknown, but it might be protective by maintaining the stiffness gradient between hyaline cartilage and subchondral bone of increased stiffness. Conversely, the relative increase in calcified to hyaline cartilage and resultant tidemark advancement could represent a pathologic process and predispose these areas of bone to failure.[7]

The result of repetitive loading of the carpal bones is stress-adaptive remodeling. In some horses, the loss of compressive stiffness of the subchondral bone plate and thickening of the calcified layer of cartilage can lead to cartilage injury and fracture.

Injury to the intercarpal ligaments can occur and usually involves the palmar medial intercarpal ligament within the middle carpal joint. Injury to the collateral ligaments is usually associated with avulsion fractures of the proximal aspect of the small metacarpal bones or distal radius. Injury to the extensor tendons usually develops in association with severe flexural deformities or lacerations. Injuries to the palmar aspect of the carpus occur, but they are less common than dorsal injury and have been associated with hyperextension of the carpus during recovery from anesthesia.

The role of conformation and carpal injury is complex and subject to personal opinion and anecdotal information. It is an area of intense concern in prepurchase examinations. One study found an association between offset carpi and lameness associated with the metacarpophalangeal joint and a protective effect of carpal valgus on carpal injury.[8] These observations are consistent with the author's clinical experience. Severe conformational abnormalities of foals can lead to malformation of the cuboidal bones and early osteoarthritis.

OSTEOCHONDRAL FRAGMENTS

Occurrence

Osteochondral fractures of the carpal bones, or carpal chips, are a common cause of lameness in horses. Racing breeds are particularly prone to carpal chip fractures, and the fractures are most likely to be a performance-limiting problem.

The occurrence of osteochondral fragmentation is a consequence of training and racing. In support of this, in Thoroughbred yearlings radiographed prior to sale, only 9 of 1121 horses (0.8%) had an osteochondral fragment in the carpus.[9] In racing Thoroughbreds and Quarter Horses, the distal aspect of the radial carpal bone is most often affected.[10] In another survey of osteochondral fragmentation in racing Thoroughbreds in Japan, 60% of the fractures occur in the antebrachiocarpal joint and 40% in the middle carpal joint.

Additional articular damage associated with osteochondral fragments tended to be greatest in the middle carpal joint.[11] If the injury involves the antebrachiocarpal joint, the distal lateral aspects of the radius and the proximal intermediate carpal bone are usually involved. If the middle carpal joint is involved, then the distal radial carpal and proximal third carpal bones are typically involved.[10]

Racing Standardbreds typically injure the carpal bones in the middle carpal joint. In a survey of 176 Standardbred horses undergoing carpal arthroscopy, only two antebrachial carpal joints had osteochondral fragments.[12]

Etiopathogenesis

Osteochondral fragments of the carpus are induced by trauma. The history usually includes a sudden onset of carpal swelling. Certainly, some carpal chips with sharp areas of demarcation and healthy subchondral bone represent acute single-event failure; however, degenerative bone and cartilage, compatible with chronic injury, most often are found both on radiographs and at surgery. The subchondral bone associated with the carpal chip undergoes stress-adaptive remodeling because of repetitive loading. The bone becomes sclerotic and acquires increased stiffness.

In the third carpal bone, reduction in vascular channels can lead to ischemic necrosis of the subchondral bone.[4] At surgery, degenerative bone appears discolored and brittle relative to the surrounding healthy bone. In racing Standardbreds, the prevalence of lameness was lower, 6.7% versus 45.4 %, in horses with mild versus severe sclerosis of the third carpal bone.[13] Resorption of the diseased bone predisposes development of a fracture at the junction of the compliant and noncompliant bone.[14]

Diagnosis

Diagnosis is based on clinical signs, including lameness, painful response to carpal flexion, joint effusion, and reduced performance. A complete set of well-exposed radiographs, including the tangential view of the distal row of carpal bones and flexed lateral projections, is needed. Occasionally, the tangential view of the proximal row of carpal bones is required for diagnosis. If a carpal chip is found, radiographs of the contralateral carpus are recommended, because it is common for fragments to be present bilaterally[10] (Fig. 96-1).

When a carpal chip is identified on a radiograph, it is important to document it as the cause of lameness, particularly in nonracing breeds, because it can represent an incidental finding. Intra-articular anesthesia in most cases confirms the associated joint as the source of lameness. Some horses become lame in the contralateral forelimb after anesthesia because of the presence of bilateral carpal chips.

When local anesthesia of the proximal suspensory region is induced, anesthetic may be injected into the palmar recesses of the carpometacarpal joint, anesthetizing both the carpometacarpal and middle carpal joints. Therefore, the relationship between the palmar recesses of the carpometacarpal joint and the proximal suspensory ligament

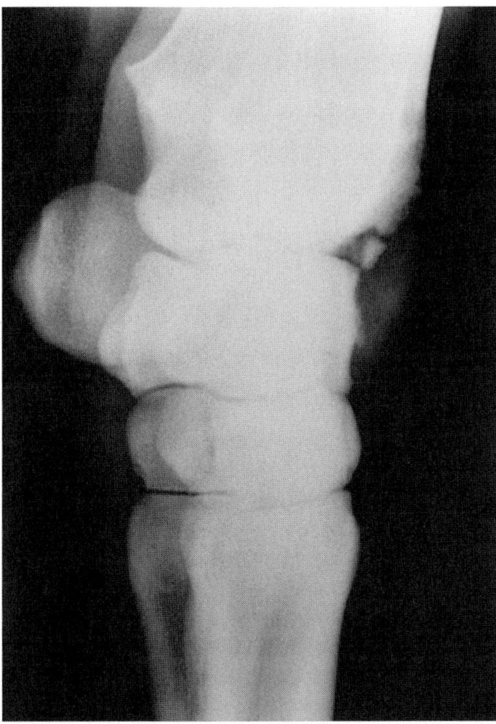

Figure 96-1. Dorsomedial to palmarolateral oblique radiograph of the carpus of a Thoroughbred with an osteochondral fragment of the distal lateral aspect of the radius. Note the enthesiophyte formation and subchondral lysis consistent with osteoarthritis.

should be considered when inducing local anesthesia in this area. Because of this, anesthesia of the middle carpal joint should be induced before the high palmar block if carpal lameness is suspected. Alternatively, the two-point high palmar block (see Chapter 74) is recommended for regional anesthesia of the proximal metacarpal region, because it prevents the anesthetic agent from entering the carpus.[1]

Case Selection

Most carpal chips are of clinical importance in racing breeds, and arthroscopic surgery to remove osteochondral fragments in the carpus is the treatment of choice. Factors that should be considered before chips are removed are the degree of lameness, the amount of degenerative change seen on the radiographs or lack thereof, previous intra-articular therapy, racing or training history, and economic concerns. Horses with carpal chip fractures are usually sound or mildly lame when jogged in hand, if examined a few days after the injury. If moderate or severe lameness is present, other conditions, such as slab fracture, moderate-to-severe cartilage damage, intercarpal ligament injury, or sepsis are suspected.

The radiographic findings of enthesiophytosis and subchondral bone lysis are associated with cartilage and subchondral bone damage at surgery (see Fig. 96-1). In one study, subchondral lysis of the radial carpal bone was associated with both osteochondral fragmentation and additional cartilage injury.[15] In another study, horses with cartilage degeneration involving more than 30% of the articular surface of the affected bone (Fig. 96-2) had reduced postoperative performance.[10]

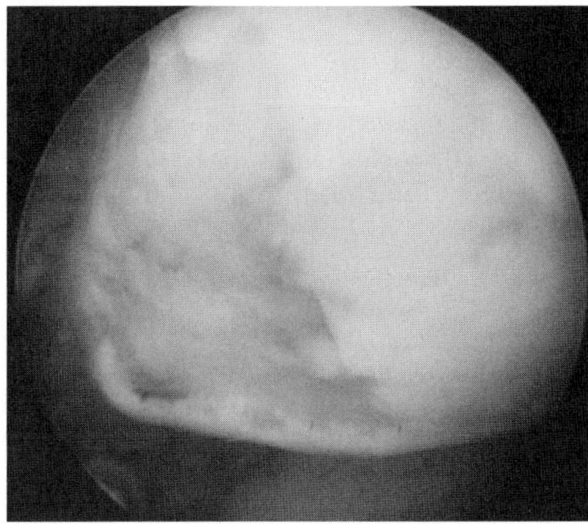

Figure 96-2. Arthroscopic view of the distal aspect of the radial carpal bone with moderate cartilage damage (grade II) and an osteochondral fragment. A greater than 30% loss of cartilage is associated with reduced postoperative performance.

Factors associated with reduced racing prognosis postoperatively include repeated joint injection, reduced response to joint injection, injury early in training, and a poor preoperative racing record. These factors, coupled with economic considerations, are important in the surgeon's case selection and the owner's willingness to have surgery performed.

Treatment

The horse is positioned in dorsal or lateral recumbency based on the site of the lesion and the surgeon's preference. If bilateral carpal arthroscopy is planned, or if both sides of a joint are to be examined, the author prefers to place the horse in dorsal recumbency with the limbs suspended from a rack or the ceiling. Antebrachiocarpal joint injury often occurs on both the lateral and medial sides simultaneously, and thus dorsal recumbency is usually selected.

The standard arthroscopy portals for the antebrachiocarpal and middle carpal joints are between the common digital and extensor carpi radialis tendons (lateral portal) and medial to the extensor carpi radialis tendon (medial portal). Portal locations for instruments and the arthroscope are determined by the lesion location, with the arthroscope portal placed farthest from the lesion.[16] The portals are made large enough to allow egress of fluid without the accumulation of fluid in the subcutaneous space (approximately 6 to 8 mm). Large portals should be avoided or adequate joint distention will be difficult to maintain. If gas is used as the arthroscopic medium, the portals should be very small and only allow access of the arthroscope and instruments.

Once the osteochondral fragment is identified, it is partially loosened with an elevator if needed, grasped with Ferris-Smith rongeurs, and removed through the instrument portal. Diseased cartilage and subchondral bone are removed with a curet. The lesion is débrided, minimizing the amount of cartilage removed, especially in weight-bearing areas of the joint. Débridement of partial-thickness cartilage lesions adjacent to the fragment is avoided unless the cartilage is detached from the underlying subchondral bone. An exception to this is partial-thickness cartilage injury overlying diseased subchondral bone (e.g., radial facet of the third carpal bone), which is typically débrided.

Aftercare

The postoperative use of intra-articular or intravenous hyaluronan and intramuscular or intra-articular polysulfated glycosaminoglycan (Adequan) varies among surgeons. The author's standard postoperative instructions for routine osteochondral carpal arthroscopy consists of 2 weeks of stall rest, 2 weeks of stall rest with hand-walking, and 2 weeks of pasture exercise, continued hand-walking, swimming physiotherapy, or a combination thereof. On occasion, a longer period of rest is given if substantial lameness or marked cartilage injury was present at the time of surgery. Bandaging is carried out until sutures are removed at approximately 12 days after the surgery.

Prognosis

A scale has been developed to grade cartilage injury observed at surgery. Grade I is minimal articular cartilage fibrillation or fragmentation extending no more than 5 mm from the fracture site. Grade II represents articular degeneration, including up to 30% of the articular surface of the bone. Grade III indicates loss of 30% to 50% of the articular surface. Grade IV represents severe loss of bone and cartilage associated with the fracture.[10]

Postoperative results of carpal arthroscopy for osteochondral fragments depend on the degree of cartilage injury and the horse's previous racing success. Horses with minimal to no cartilage injury (grades I or II) have a 72.8% chance of returning to racing at a level equal to or better than that before injury. If cartilage damage is greater than 30% of the visible surface of the affected bone (grades III or IV), then there is only a 53.5% chance of return to racing at a level equal to or better than that before injury.[10] In a survey of carpal arthroscopy in racing Standardbreds, 74% returned to racing after surgery and 61% raced at or above their previous level.[12] In another survey from Japan, 82.6% of racing Thoroughbreds returned to racing after carpal surgery, which is better than results in North America. A likely reason for the discrepancy is the higher percentage of antebrachiocarpal joint injuries with little additional cartilage injury in the Japanese study.[11] It is the author's experience that cartilage injury is greater and the prognosis worse with chip fractures of the middle carpal versus the antebrachiocarpal joint.

SUBCHONDRAL LUCENCY OF THE THIRD CARPAL BONE

Etiopathogenesis

Subchondral lucency or crush fracture of the third carpal bone is a common injury in racing breeds. It might be a prelude to slab fracture of the third carpal bone. Repetitive loading of the third carpal bone during training and racing leads to increased sclerosis of the radial facet, degeneration of the articular cartilage, and in some cases, loss of support from the subchondral bone. Subchondral lucency significantly influences the degree of carpal lameness in Standardbreds.[17]

Diagnosis

Clinical signs include lameness, reduced performance, and mild-to-moderate effusion of the middle carpal joint. Affected horses improve with intra-articular anesthesia of the middle carpal joint. A well-exposed tangential (skyline) projection of the third carpal bone is required for diagnosis. Radiographic signs include both sclerosis and lysis of the radial facet of the third carpal bone. In one study of racing Standardbreds and Thoroughbreds that improved after intra-articular anesthesia of the middle carpal joint and showed minimal to no degenerative changes on radiographs, 80% had cartilage damage, an incomplete fracture, or a crush fracture of the radial facet of the third carpal bone.[18] Radiographs of the contralateral carpus should be taken because disease affecting both carpi is not uncommon.

Treatment

Some horses respond to intra-articular therapy but many do not; therefore, arthroscopic débridement is the treatment of choice.[19] The articular cartilage often acquires partial- to full-thickness injury (Fig. 96-3). Removal of the abnormal cartilage reveals brittle, yellow-discolored, diseased subchondral bone and occasional fractures. In some cases, the mechanical strength of the cartilage and bone is very poor, and the arthroscopic probe sinks into the subchondral plate. The abnormal cartilage and bone are completely removed. If a dorsal rim remains on the third carpal bone, it is typically removed (Fig. 96-4). Prognosis for return to racing for horses with arthroscopic débridement of such lesions is 89%.[19]

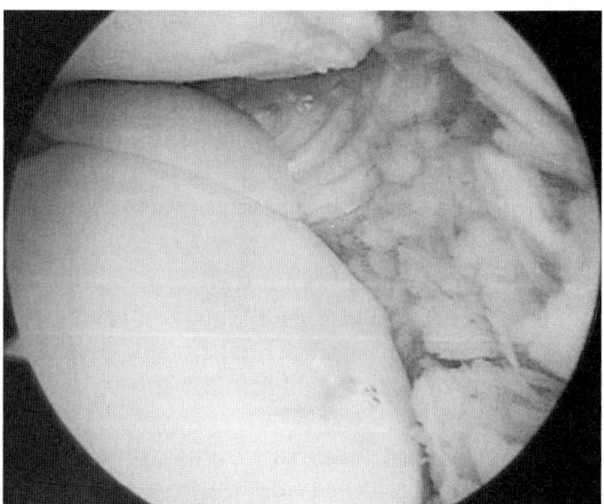

Figure 96-3. Arthroscopic view of the middle carpal joint of a 3-year-old racing Standardbred with a focal defect in the weight-bearing surface of the radial facet of the third carpal bone. On a tangential radiographic projection, subchondral lucency of the radial facet was seen.

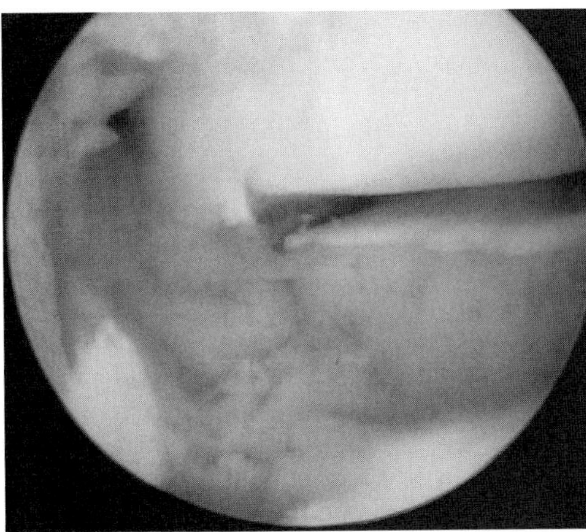

Figure 96-4. Postoperative appearance of the third carpal bone after débridement of degenerative cartilage and subchondral bone in a racing Standardbred. The diseased portion of the third carpal bone was resected until it was no longer in a weight-bearing position.

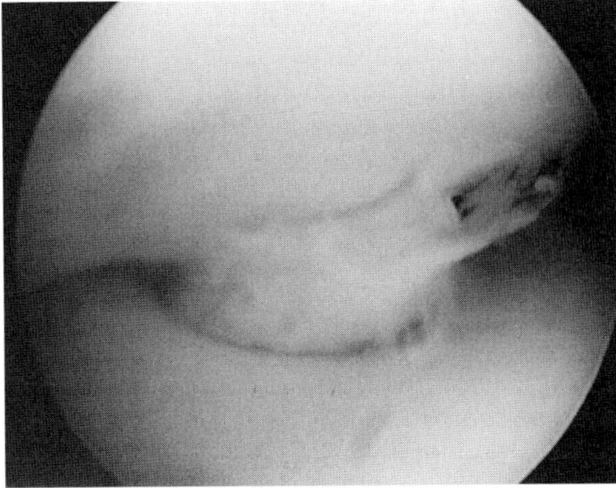

Figure 96-5. Arthroscopic view of the middle carpal joint of a racing Standardbred with a complete tear of the medial palmar intercarpal ligament. The lameness in this horse was isolated by intra-articular anesthesia of the middle carpal joint. The radiographs were normal.

MEDIAL PALMAR INTERCARPAL LIGAMENT INJURY

Etiopathogenesis

Diagnosis of partial or complete disruption of the medial palmar intercarpal ligament (MPICL) has become possible because of the use of arthroscopy in equine surgery. The medial and lateral palmar intercarpal ligaments prevent dorsal displacement of the middle carpal joint.[20] The frequency of injury to this ligament ranges between 8.7% and 70%.[21,22] Medial palmar intercarpal ligament injury can occur alone or with other types of carpal injury, including osteochondral fragments and cartilage damage.[21] One report found no association between intercarpal ligament injury (ICL) and cartilage injury.[23]

Diagnosis

Clinical signs of MPICL injury include moderate lameness and joint effusion. In acute cases, no radiographic signs specific to this injury are seen. In chronic cases, new bone formation on the distal dorsal aspect of the proximal row of carpal bones can be seen, which is related to a degree of joint instability. Intercarpal ligament injury is suspected by evaluation of clinical signs, absence of radiographic abnormalities, and response to middle carpal joint anesthesia. Ultrasonographic evaluation of the MPICL has been described in the standing horse.[24]

Confirmation of diagnosis is achieved through arthroscopic evaluation. Ligament disruption can be partial or complete (Fig. 96-5). A grading scale of injury from I to IV has been suggested. Grade I indicates rupture or fraying of a small number of fibers; grade II, rupture of up to one third of the ligament fibers; grade III, rupture of two thirds; and grade IV, complete rupture of the ligament. Mild (grade I) tears can be incidental findings at surgery and might not be associated with lameness.[23]

Treatment

No method of ligament repair is available, and the surgical procedure is limited to diagnosis, débridement of free strands of the ligament, and débridement of other lesions within the joint. Three months of stall confinement followed by 3 months of pasture turnout is recommended.

The prognosis is considered fair for partial tears (grades II and III) and guarded for complete tears (grade IV). In one study, injury to the MPICL combined with subchondral bone damage was the best indicator of postoperative performance. The presence of a complete MPICL tear or a mild tear with large subchondral bone defects was associated with a poor outcome.[25]

CARPAL SLAB FRACTURES

Etiopathogenesis

The third carpal bone is a common site for injury. Fracture types include osteochondral fragments, corner fractures, small and large frontal plane slab fractures, and sagittal slab fractures. Carpal slab fractures occur most often in the frontal plane of the radial facet of the third carpal bone.[26] Frontal slab fractures also can occur in the radial, fourth, and intermediate carpal bones.[27] Because the radial facet of the third carpal bone undergoes stress-adaptive remodeling during race training, repetitive loading of this area consistently leads to fracture in this location.[26] Additionally, subchondral lucency, cartilage injury, and incomplete fractures often occur in this area.[10,14,16,18,19]

Diagnosis

Horses with complete slab fractures of the third carpal bone have moderate to severe lameness, are reluctant to flex the carpus, and exhibit joint effusion. The right forelimb is more often affected in Thoroughbreds, but both forelimbs are equally affected in Standardbreds.[28,29] Horses with incomplete slab fractures have variable lameness and usually little joint effusion.

Radiographs, including the skyline projection, confirm the diagnosis and aid in the choice of treatment. Fragmentation at the articular margin of the middle carpal joint, third carpal bone sclerosis, and lysis can be present; these usually indicate advanced disease. Diagnosis of incomplete fractures is more difficult because localizing signs can be absent. Careful lameness examination, diagnostic anesthesia, well-positioned and well-exposed radiographs, and sometimes nuclear scintigraphy are necessary for diagnosis. Once a diagnosis is established, radiographs of the other carpus are obtained because bilateral slab fractures or other carpal disease can be present. Bilateral slab fractures occur most commonly in Standardbreds.

Treatment

Treatment options for complete slab fractures include removal of the slab or surgical repair of the fracture with interfragmentary bone screws placed in lag fashion. Surgery is recommended for all horses, even those to be retired from racing. Conservative management of complete slab fractures often results in moderate to severe osteoarthritis. Removal of slab fractures is recommended when thin fragments (less than 10 mm thick) are present or if there is significant loss of articular cartilage associated with the fracture.

In many complete slab fractures, there is a wedge-shaped piece of bone and cartilage present where the fracture enters the middle carpal joint (Fig. 96-6). This fragment might not be obvious on the preoperative radiographs. The consequence of this fragment is the potential loss of a large area of cartilage at the fracture site; in such cases, removal of the slab fracture may be elected. If cartilage loss is minimal or if the fracture is more than 10 mm thick or incomplete, compression of the fracture fragments with one or more bone screws is preferred.

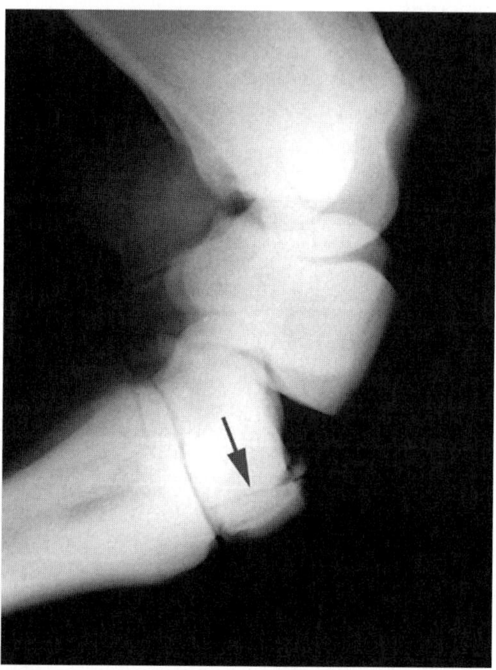

Figure 96-6. Lateral radiograph of the carpus of a Thoroughbred with a minimally displaced, complete frontal plane slab fracture of the third carpal bone *(arrow)*. Notice the osteochondral fragment (trough lesion) at the proximal articular surface.

Successful management of incomplete fractures is possible with rest alone; however, some horses refracture when they return to racing and eventually require surgery.

Surgical Technique

Internal fixation of frontal or sagittal slab fractures can be accomplished using arthroscopic or arthrotomy techniques. Arthroscopy has considerable advantages over arthrotomy in the management of third carpal slab fractures and is considered the treatment of choice. Arthroscopy provides a more complete examination of the joint and facilitates débridement of the fracture gap, but it is technically more difficult to properly orient the implant, and experience is necessary with the arthroscopic technique.[30]

In *arthroscopic* repair, the horse is positioned in lateral recumbency with the affected limb uppermost or in dorsal recumbency. The lateral portal is used to position the arthroscope for examination of the medial aspect of the middle carpal joint. The medial portal is used to débride the fracture. The joint is held in extension because this position opens the fracture gap.

Fracture hematoma and fragments of bone are removed. Subsequent flexion of the joint reduces the fracture. Hypodermic needles are placed at the lateral and medial extent of the fracture in the middle carpal joint and into the carpometacarpal joint to identify the borders of the fracture. The locations of the hypodermic needles and the reduction of the fracture are confirmed arthroscopically (Fig. 96-7). A 2.5-mm drill bit, oriented perpendicular to the dorsal surface of MCIII, is placed through a separate incision in the center of the fracture fragment. Its location is confirmed with radiography or image intensification (Fig. 96-8). Standard AO/ASIF (Association for the Study of Internal Fixation) technique is used to place a 3.5- or 4.5-mm cortex screw in lag fashion. During the placement of the marker bit and screw, it is important to maintain the carpus in flexion to provide adequate reduction.[31]

If *arthrotomy* is elected, an incision is made into the middle carpal joint over the radial facet of the third carpal bone just medial to the extensor carpi radialis tendon.[30] The fracture line is identified and débrided. Orientation of the drill bit is easier with an arthrotomy compared with the arthroscopic technique. The bit should be positioned perpendicular to MCIII and in the center of the fracture fragment (if only one screw is required).

The 3.5-mm AO ASIF system is used for most fractures and provides ample compression (Fig. 96-9). The 3.5-mm system has the advantage of easier placement of single or multiple screws because of its smaller size (Fig. 96-10). There is reduced risk of splitting the fracture fragment compared with the 4.5-mm system. The 3.5-mm screw also has a smaller head, which interferes less with the soft tissues over the carpus. Because of these features, 3.5-mm screws are used in thinner slabs. The 4.5-mm system is used for fractures that are large, typically involving both the radial and intermediate facet of the third carpal bone or other carpal bones (Fig. 96-11).

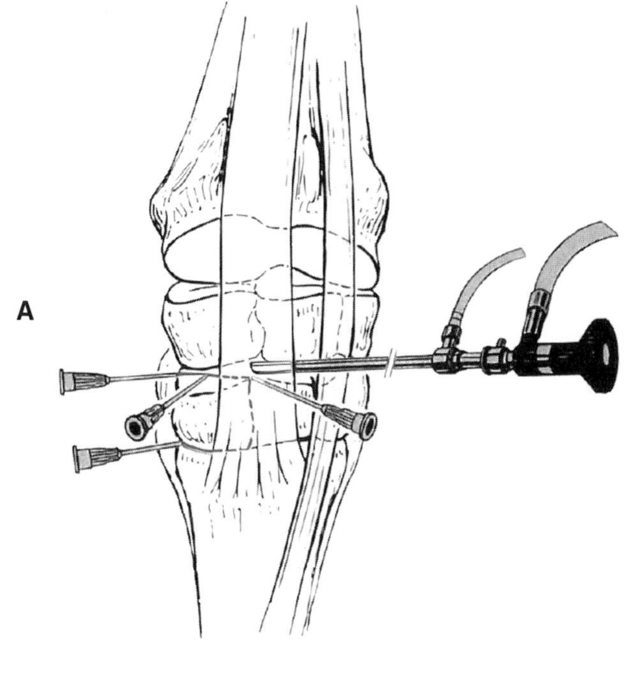

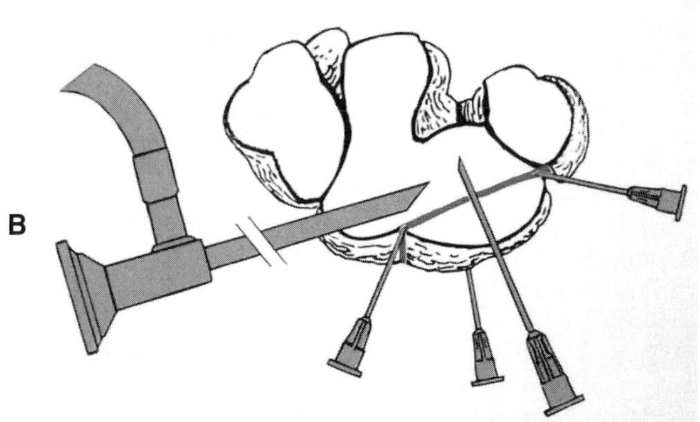

Figure 96-7. Schematic drawing of arthroscope and needle placement for the surgical repair for a third carpal bone slab fracture under arthroscopic guidance. **A** and **B**, One needle each is placed on each end of the fracture, one in the carpometacarpal joint and one centered over the middle of the slab fracture in the middle carpal joint to serve as guides for the location and direction of screw placement.

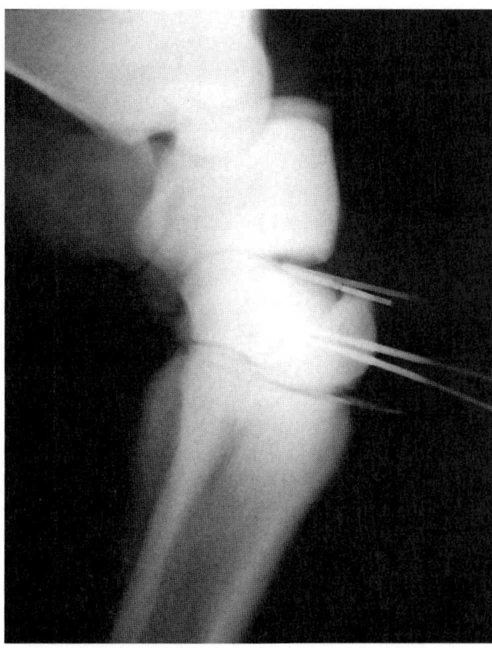

Figure 96-8. Intraoperative radiograph of the carpus of a Thoroughbred during surgery for repair of a third carpal bone slab fracture. Notice the placement of the needles to identify the borders of the fracture and the marker drill bits to confirm proper placement and orientation of the implants.

Careful intraoperative monitoring with radiographs or image intensification is required regardless of whether arthroscopy or arthrotomy is chosen.

Displaced sagittal slab fractures should be repaired with 3.5-mm screws. These fractures are usually located on the medial aspect of the third carpal bone. Both arthroscopy and arthrotomy techniques can be applied with intraoperative monitoring to guide placement of the implant. The surgical approach depends on location of the fracture. Screw placement should avoid contact of the screw head with the second carpal bone, which can cause lameness.

The presence of additional carpal pathology is typical in cases of third carpal slab fracture. A trough of cartilage and bone is usually present at the site where the fracture breaks

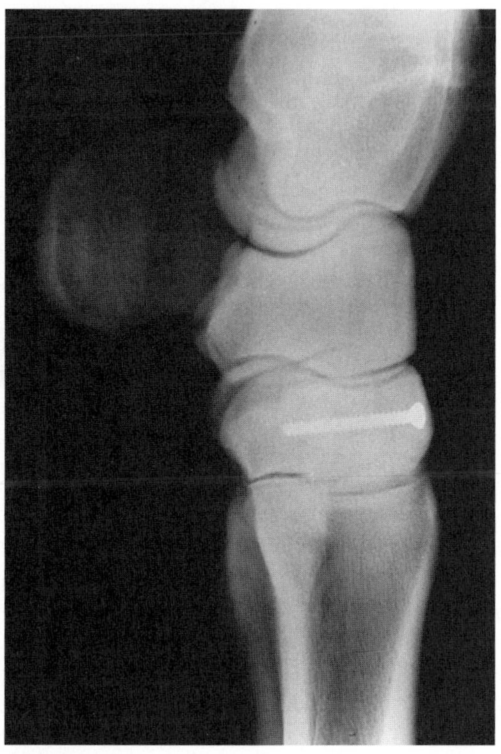

Figure 96-9. Lateral radiograph after repair of a third carpal bone frontal plane slab fracture with a single 3.5-mm cortex screw placed in lag fashion.

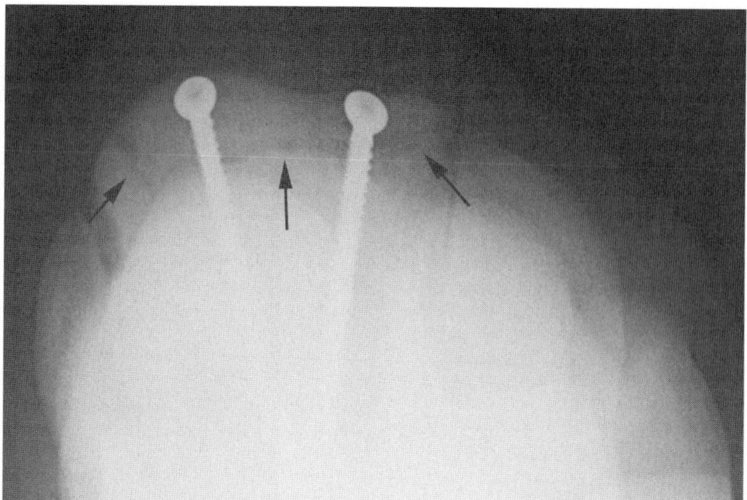

Figure 96-10. Tangential view of a third carpal bone of a Thoroughbred after repair of a frontal plane fracture *(arrows)* with two 3.5-mm cortex screws placed in lag fashion.

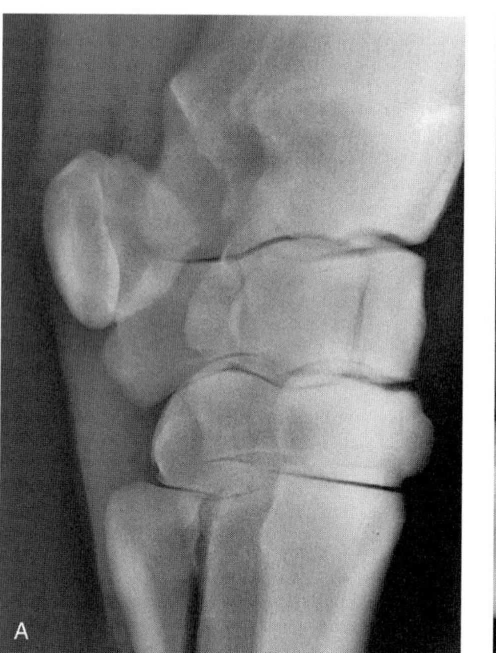

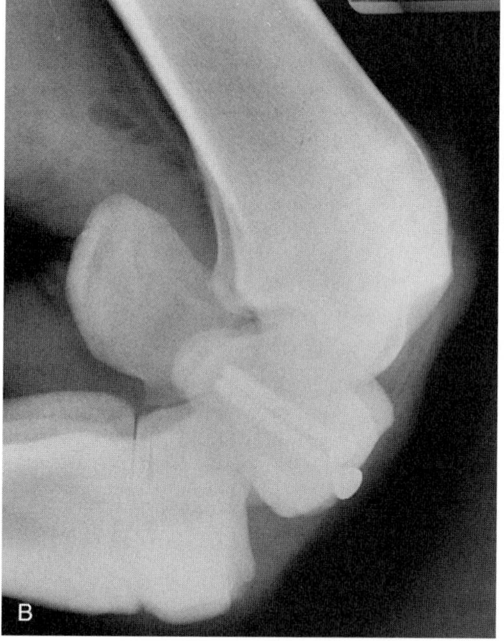

Figure 96-11. A, Dorsolateral to palmaromedial oblique radiograph of a frontal plane slab fracture of the radial carpal bone of a Thoroughbred. **B**, Flexed lateral radiograph after repair of the radial carpal slab fracture using two 4.5-mm cortex screws placed in lag fashion.

into the middle carpal joint. When a trough is left on the parent portion of the bone behind the slab, lag screw fixation is still an option. The slab is fixed to the parent portion of the bone with one or two screws, and the proximal 4 mm of the slab is removed with a chisel; depending on the size of the trough and the surgeon's preference, the proximal 4 mm could be left in place. By removing the articular surface, contact with the opposing bone is prevented, allowing undisturbed healing of the fracture. Additional pathology seen in the joint includes distal radial carpal bone chips, cartilage damage, and medial palmar intercarpal ligament injury.

Aftercare

Aftercare is routine, with bandaging for several weeks and a slow, gradual return to work. Most horses require approximately 4 months of recovery before returning to race training. Prognosis differs among breeds, with 77% of Standardbreds and 65% of Thoroughbreds returning to racing after surgery. Many horses return to racing at a lower level of performance.[28,29]

MULTIFRAGMENT FRACTURES

Etiopathogenesis

Multifragment fractures typically occur after kicks, falls, or collisions. Such injuries can also occur during racing. Non–weight-bearing lameness and carpal swelling are typical. The horse exhibits angular limb deformity and carpal hyperextension because of carpal collapse.

Diagnosis

Radiographs confirm the presence of multiple fracture lines involving several bones. Most of these fractures involve the medial aspect of the carpus and can include the radial, intermediate, second, or third carpal bones or a combination thereof. The loss of support of the bone column on the medial aspect of the carpus typically causes a carpal varus deformity.

Treatment

First aid is aimed at reconstructing the bone column by placing palmar and lateral splints over a bandage. The inherent instability and articular nature of the fractures usually makes external coaptation with casts or splints inadequate for treatment, however. Most horses remain severely lame, develop pressure necrosis of the skin, and are at high risk for developing laminitis in the supporting limb with coaptation alone.

Realignment of the bone column by reconstruction of the carpal bones with screws is recommended. If the bone column cannot be re-established, carpal arthrodesis with bone plates should be considered (see Chapter 85). Any attempt to treat such an injury is a salvage procedure. For carpal reconstruction, an arthrotomy over the appropriate joint space is performed, and the carpal bones are reconstructed using 5.5-mm, 4.5-mm, and 3.5-mm screws. In some cases arthroscopic reconstruction is possible.

Proper reduction of the fracture fragments is paramount during the reconstruction of the bone column for weight-bearing and load sharing with the implants. Additionally, a reduction in the development of osteoarthritis is achieved. At surgery, additional fracture lines and fragments are often found, which complicate the procedure. Coaptation in a sleeve cast for 4 to 6 weeks is recommended postoperatively.

Carpal arthrodesis is performed when the bone column cannot be reconstructed or in the presence of severe osteoarthritis, angular limb deformity, or instability caused by the fracture or luxation. Partial or pancarpal arthrodesis can be performed, and a variety of implants have been used.[32,33] For a more in-depth description of different arthrodesis procedures, please review Chapter 85.

CARPAL HYGROMA

Etiopathogenesis

Carpal hygroma is a subcutaneous swelling over the dorsum of the carpus. It is usually associated with a history of trauma to the region. Although the swelling is usually not infected, the potential for sepsis exists after drainage or injection, or both.

Diagnosis

Horses with sterile hygromas are not usually lame, but those with infected hygromas exhibit variable lameness depending on whether the area is draining. The skin is usually thickened. Purulent drainage is typical in infected hygromas, but joint involvement is rare.

Radiographs should be obtained to rule out bone involvement. Contrast radiography is helpful in determining joint or tendon sheath involvement and to outline the extent of the hygroma (Fig. 96-12). Filling of the joint by contrast medium from the hygroma in most cases is not expected because of the valve-like action of the tissues involved; therefore, communication between the joint and the hygroma is confirmed or ruled out through fluid injection into the middle carpal or antebrachiocarpal joint. An indirect filling of the hygroma confirms the communication. Ultrasonography helps to rule out the presence of a foreign body.

Treatment

Nonseptic carpal hygroma can be treated with rest, systemic and local anti-inflammatory agents, and bandaging. Hygromas that are refractory to treatment or that recur are treated with drainage and injection of corticosteroids or sclerosing agents as well as resection. Once sepsis is

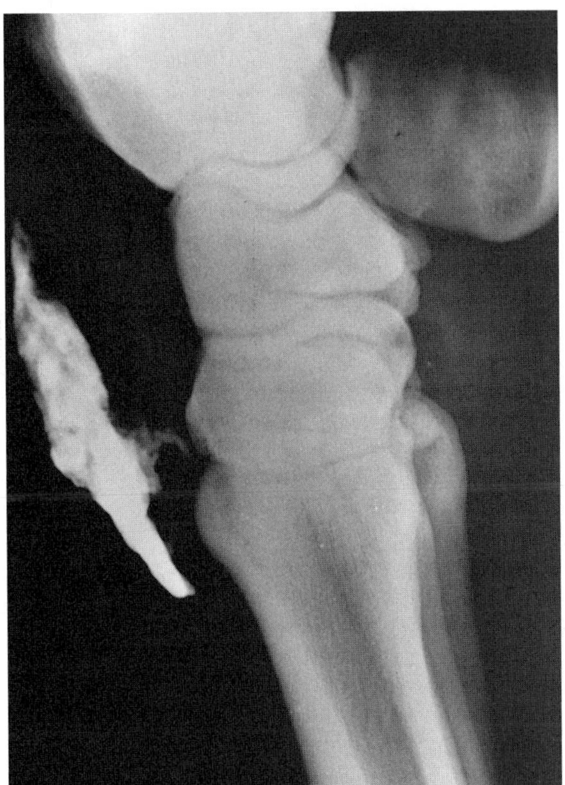

Figure 96-12. Lateral radiograph of a contrast study of a carpal hygroma in a Thoroughbred. The hygroma is isolated to the subcutaneous tissue.

established in the subcutaneous space, resolution is often difficult despite the use of lavage, drainage, and antimicrobial agents. When infection is present, resection of infected tissue is the treatment of choice.

Surgical Technique

The horse is placed under general anesthesia with the affected limb uppermost and the limb prepared for aseptic surgery. An elliptical incision is made over the hygroma and over a fistula, if one is present. The skin is reflected off the lining of the hygroma, retaining the subcutaneous tissue with the skin. Care is taken to avoid puncturing the hygroma. The dissection is continued to the fibrous layer of the carpal joint capsule and tendon sheaths of the extensor carpi radialis and common digital extensor tendons, and the hygroma is removed en bloc. Care is taken to avoid penetrating the carpal joints or tendon sheaths.

Once the hygroma is removed, excess skin is resected from the skin edges to reduce dead space. Two 6-mm Penrose drains are placed and secured to the top of the dead space and exited distally on the medial and lateral aspects of the incision. The subcutaneous tissue is secured to the joint capsule with multiple mattress sutures of absorbable material to decrease dead space. The subcutaneous tissue and the skin are closed routinely.

Elastic bandaging tape (such as Elastikon) is placed on the carpus directly over a sterile dressing as a pressure wrap. The limb is placed in a stack bandage followed by four layers of casting tape in which a polyvinylchloride splint is incorporated to the palmar surface. The casting tape and splint extend from below the elbow to the distal metacarpus. The cast bandage with splint effectively immobilizes the carpus and protects the skin incision during recovery from anesthesia and in the postoperative period.

Three days after surgery, or earlier if needed, the cast bandage is bivalved, and the dorsal portion is discarded. The wound dressing is changed, the stack bandage is replaced, and the palmar portion of the cast and splint is reapplied. The drains are removed 3 to 5 days postoperatively, and the splint is maintained for a total of 10 days. A bandage is maintained for 4 weeks after surgery. Antimicrobial and anti-inflammatory agents are used as needed. Hand-walking is initiated 1 month after surgery, and the horse is turned out to pasture or returned to exercise at 2 months.

DISTAL RADIAL EXOSTOSIS

Clinical Signs

Exostosis of the distal radius is a rare cause of lameness in horses. The development of exostosis on the caudal border of the distal radial physis causes a tenosynovitis of the carpal canal and irritation of the deep digital flexor tendon. Exostosis is differentiated from osteochondroma by its location and by histologic examination. Osteochondromas are present on the caudal border of the distal radial metaphysis typically 2 to 4 cm proximal to the distal radial physis. Exostoses are devoid of hyaline cartilage remnants, which are present in osteochondromas.[34]

Regardless of the origin of the mass, the resultant tenosynovitis caused by both conditions results in both a weight-bearing and swinging-limb lameness. The horse often carries the affected limb slightly abducted at the trot, and the lameness generally worsens with carpal flexion. Effusion of the carpal canal can be difficult to detect without careful inspection of the lateral aspect of the limb in the distal third of the forearm. Lameness is improved after intrasynovial anesthesia of the carpal canal.

Radiography confirms the presence of the exostoses on the caudal aspect of the distal radial physis (Fig. 96-13). Exostoses are occasionally seen as an incidental finding on survey radiography. Clinical exostoses generally measure at least 10 mm off the caudal aspect of the radius. It is important to confirm the exostosis as the cause of lameness by intrasynovial anesthesia.

Nonsurgical Management

Management of carpal canal tenosynovitis is by intrasynovial injection of hyaluronan and corticosteroids. In the author's experience, if the response to therapy is incomplete or short-lived, then surgical removal of the exostosis is the treatment of choice to remove the underlying cause of the tenosynovitis.

Surgical Management

Distal radial exostoses can be removed via carpal canal endoscopy, which represents the method of choice.[35] The horse is positioned with the affected limb positioned uppermost and the forelimb and carpus prepared for aseptic surgery. The carpal canal is distended with lactated Ringer's solution and the arthroscopic cannula is placed between the lateral digital extensor and the ulnaris lateralis tendons through a stab incision at a level of the proximal to the distal radial physis.

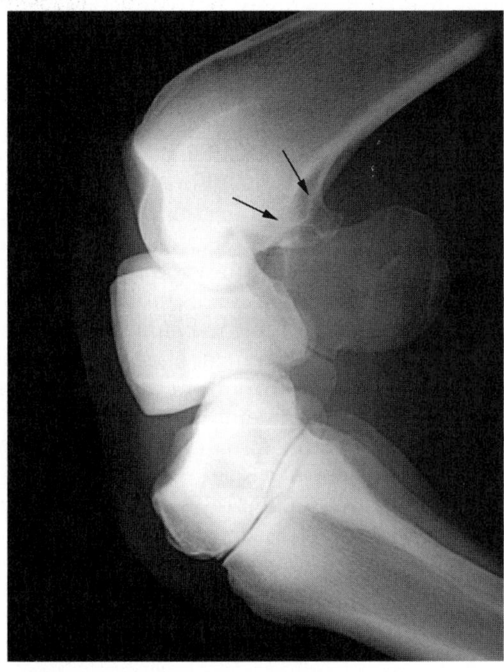

Figure 96-13. Flexed lateral radiograph of the carpus of a 7-year-old Thoroughbred with an exostosis of the caudal aspect of the distal radial physis.

The carpal canal is entered and a standard 4.0-mm 25-degree arthroscope is used for the examination. There is ample room within the carpal canal, and the arthroscope is usually positioned to examine the exostosis and any associated deep digital flexor tendon injury without difficulty. A needle is used to ascertain the proper location for the instrument portal distal to the arthroscopic portal. A 5-mm osteotome is used to loosen the exostosis from its bed. Care should be taken to remove the exostosis as close to its base as possible and not to completely dislodge it. The mass is grasped with a Ferris-Smith rongeur and removed. The associated bed can be further débrided with a rongeur or osteotome. Release of the carpal flexor retinaculum can also be accomplished via endoscopic guidance if constriction of the carpal canal is suspected.[36]

The canal is lavaged and the is skin closed with non-absorbable monofilament suture. Intraoperative radiographs are recommended to confirm that the entire exostosis was removed. A full limb bandage is used for recovery from general anesthesia. Postoperative recommendations include box stall confinement for 4 weeks and pasture turnout for 4 to 8 weeks thereafter.

Prognosis

Prognosis after removal of distal radial exostoses is good. In a clinical report, 9 of 10 horses returned to full athletic function after endoscopic removal of the exostosis. The remaining horse became sound after further intrasynovial medication with hyaluronan.[34]

ANGULAR LIMB DEFORMITIES

Angular limb deformities of the carpus occur commonly in foals. Valgus deformity is more common than varus deformity. Angular limb deformities of the carpal region can be caused by physeal dysplasia, joint laxity, and cuboidal bone hypoplasia or malformation.

Methods of treating angular limb deformities of the carpal region include splints, bandages, casts, growth retardation, and, most commonly, periosteal elevation and transection. Treatment varies depending on the age of the horse and the cause of the deformity. Treatment options are discussed in detail in Chapter 89.

ACCESSORY CARPAL BONE FRACTURES

Etiopathogenesis

Fracture of the accessory carpal bone occurs in Thoroughbred horses that race over fences, but it can be seen after collisions or falls in any breed. Relative to other carpal injuries, accessory carpal bone fractures are rare, representing 2% of all carpal fractures.[37] In a survey of Thoroughbred yearlings radiographed prior to sale, accessory carpal bone fractures were found in 0.4% of the horses.[9] Because of its location on the palmar aspect of the carpus and its multiple ligamentous attachments, the accessory carpal bone undergoes intense loading during extension of the carpus.

The preponderance of frontal plane fractures is likely caused by avulsion of the bone by its palmar attachments during carpal loading. Other suspected causes of accessory carpal bone fractures include compression between the radius and MCIII and direct trauma. It is typical for a small degree of comminution to be present at the fracture site in frontal plane fractures.[37] Nonarticular chip fractures and comminuted fractures are occasionally diagnosed.[38,39]

Diagnosis

Acute, severe lameness is typical. The carpus can be held in a somewhat flexed position to reduce loading. Carpal canal effusion might be present, but carpal joint effusion might be absent unless there is an articular component to the fracture.

Diagnosis is confirmed through radiographic examination. In acute fractures, displacement is usually present, although nondisplaced fractures occur. In nondisplaced fractures, another set of radiographs should be taken 10 to 14 days after injury. Nuclear scintigraphy and, if available, computed tomography are helpful in defining the fracture in detail. In chronic fractures, fragment edges are indistinct.

Treatment

Treatment options include conservative management or surgical reconstruction and compression with bone screws or plates. Conservative management has varying success. Stall rest for 3 months followed by turnout at pasture for 3 to 9 months is recommended. Of 19 horses with accessory carpal bone fractures, 17 were treated conservatively with rest for 3 to 6 months and two had internal fixation. All 11 horses available for follow-up were sound, and seven had returned to racing.[37]

Surgical repair with bone screws has been most often attempted in simple vertical fractures. Because of the location, the concave shape of the accessory carpal bone, and the narrow space for error in screw placement, attempts at surgical repair are infrequent. These difficulties, coupled with the low incidence of the injury, make the decision between conservative and surgical management difficult. In one study, vertical fractures were created experimentally, followed by treatment with immediate or delayed repair with bone screws or conservative management.[40] Three horses treated conservatively were still lame 6 months later, whereas all horses that had been surgically treated were sound at 6 months. Wound infection and screw breakage were reported complications. Another clinical study reports success with surgical management of vertical fractures with bone screws.[39]

The application of two four-hole 2.7-mm dynamic compression plates (DCPs) perpendicular to the vertical fracture plane resulted in solid bone union within 3 months and return of the horse to full athletic use.[41] The plate counteracts the tensile forces that displace the fracture, and the compression exerted across the fracture plane aids healing. The same result was achieved with a cervical fusion plate (Synthes, Paoli, Pa) applied to the lateral surface of the fractured accessory carpal bone[41] (Fig. 96-14).

Although conservative management of accessory carpal bone fractures can result in complete return to athletic soundness in fractures of many months' to years' duration, complete bone union is not usually present. In chronic fractures, the potential for carpal canal syndrome exists and should be evaluated during the examination.[42] Therefore, because surgical management of simple vertical fractures has

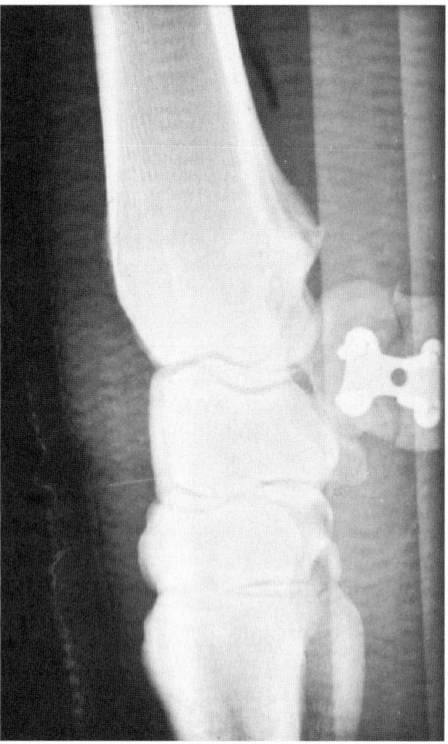

Figure 96-14. Lateral radiograph of a 5-year-old Thoroughbred with a vertical fracture of the accessory carpal bone that was repaired with a cervical fusion plate. (Courtesy J. Auer, Zurich.)

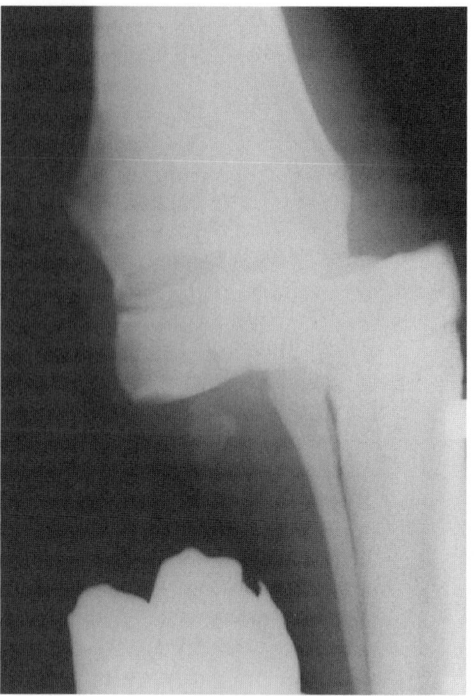

Figure 96-15. Craniocaudal radiographic view of the distal radius of a horse with complete luxation of the middle carpal joint. Note that the proximal and distal rows of carpal bones overlap and are rotated, resulting in a lateral view of the distal limb. A bone fragment is recognized below the intermediate carpal bone, indicating that an avulsion fracture of the palmar aspect of the intermediate carpal bone has occurred. (Courtesy J. Auer, Zurich.)

the potential to return the horse to athletic soundness with minimal callus formation and good bone union, it is the recommended treatment.

LUXATION (SUBLUXATION)

Etiopathogenesis

Carpal luxations are traumatic events caused by falling with one limb wedged in a fixed position, as a result of a car accident, or through a precise kick at a collateral ligament. Other causes are speculative because often the animal is found in the pasture with an obvious luxation whose origin was not observed.

Diagnosis

The animal might be presented with an obvious deformity in the carpus resulting in an abnormal position of the limb distal to the carpal region. In this instance, the diagnosis is obvious from radiographs (Fig. 96-15). Alternatively, the animal might bear weight on the limb but show a marked lameness. Standard radiographs might show some small bone chips in the periarticular region as the only abnormality. If the luxation is in association with skin trauma, crepitus is recognized in the periarticular soft tissues. A definitive diagnosis of joint involvement with the wound is made through arthrocentesis and stress radiographs under general anesthesia.

Treatment

Management of luxations may be carried out conservatively or through surgical intervention. Conservative treatment involves cast application for 3 months with two or three cast changes. During this time, the ruptured periarticular soft tissues heal by fibrosis. Depending on which joint is involved, decreased carpal flexion is the result. Careful management of the convalescent period helps in restoring a useful animal. Coaptation should only be considered if the bone column is intact and the bone column does not collapse during weightbearing.

Surgical management through partial or pancarpal arthrodesis is an option and is discussed in Chapter 85. Proximal fractures of the second or fourth metacarpal bone cause subluxation of the carpometacarpal joint. Small plates to repair these fractures are recommended to overcome the tension forces of the collateral ligaments, even in small foals. The author's experiences with coaptation or screw fixation alone have been disappointing. Plate fixation of proximal fractures of the small metacarpal bones is discussed in detail in Chapter 95.

CORONATION (COURONNEMENT)

Etiopathogenesis

Coronation refers to a severe soft-tissue injury of the dorsum of the carpus that occurs after a fall. It is characterized by the loss of skin over the carpus, and in more-severe cases, the wound involves the synovial sheaths of the extensor carpi radialis, common digital extensor tendons, or one of the carpal joints.

Diagnosis

Physical signs of injury are obvious, with a flap or degloving wound present over the dorsum of the carpus (Fig. 96-16). Entry into the tendon sheaths or joints might be obvious, but puncture wounds might go unnoticed.

If synovial involvement is suspected, a needle should be placed into the carpal joint or tendon sheath at a site distant from the wound after aseptic preparation and the structure distended with sterile saline to detect any defects. Care must be taken to avoid entry through traumatized or infected tissue to prevent inoculation of the synovial structure with bacteria. For the tendon sheath, a proximal location is chosen, and for the carpal joints, the palmar outpocketings may be used. Any draining fluid obtained is collected and submitted for cytologic examination and culture and susceptibility testing. Occasionally, the extensor carpi radialis or common digital extensor tendon is ruptured as well.

Radiographs should be obtained after cleaning the wound to assess bone injury and identify additional debris, especially gravel. Contrast radiography can be used to identify communications between the synovial structures and the wound. The use of ultrasonography is limited because of subcutaneous emphysema from the wound.

Treatment

Treatment consists of management of the wounds and any involved synovial structure. Wound management and management of synovial infections are discussed in Chapters 26 and 88, respectively. Some specific issues of management of these wounds deserve mention here (Fig. 96-17, *A*).

The author prefers to close acute wounds into synovial structures after lavage and intra-synovial antimicrobial therapy unless severe contamination exists. A 1- to 2-mm rim of skin is sharply dissected along the skin defect,

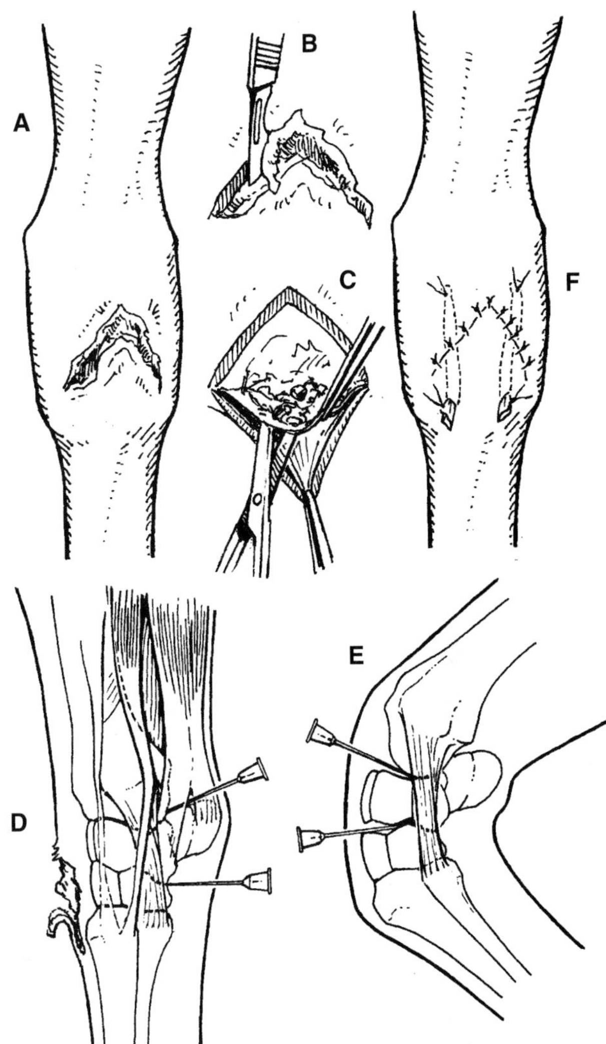

Figure 96-17. Treatment of a coronation injury. **A**, Appearance of the injury. **B**, A 1- to 2-mm rim is sharply removed around the skin defect. **C**, Careful débridement of the subcutaneous tissues aids in determining if the joint is involved as well. **D**, Needles placed from the palmar aspect of the carpus into the joints for joint lavage allows verification of any potential joint involvement. **E**, The needles may also be inserted from the dorsolateral or dorsomedial aspect of the carpus. **F**, After installing one or two drains, the skin is closed in routine fashion.

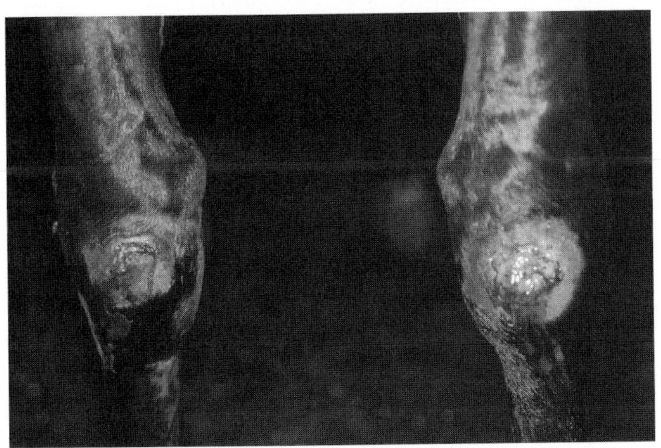

Figure 96-16. A Warmblood horse admitted for treatment of coronation, which occurred during a riding accident. (Courtesy J. Auer, Zurich.)

followed by careful sharp surgical débridement of the deeper tissues (Fig. 96-17, *B* and *C*). In cases where the joint capsule is opened as well, intra-articular lavage is mandatory. This can be accomplished through needles placed from the palmar aspect of the carpus (Fig. 96-17, *D*) or from the dorsolateral or dorsomedial aspect of the carpus (Fig. 96-17, *E*). The joint capsule is subsequently closed using simple interrupted sutures of a 2-0 monofilament absorbable suture material.

After implantation of one or two drains the skin is closed in routine fashion (Fig. 96-17, *F*). Delayed wound closure is sometimes necessary to identify the extent of injury and allow débridement. The use of splints, cast bandages, and casts is usually necessary to provide immobilization for wound healing. Supportive therapy such as repeated joint lavage, anti-inflammatory agents, and antimicrobial agents varies with the type and severity of the wound.

Horses can return to full athletic activity after injuries that involve superficial structures. Wounds that involve the tendon sheaths, joint, or carpal bones have a reduced prognosis, which is determined by the extent of the wound and use of the horse. Even wounds that have had significant loss of tissue over the dorsum of the carpus can heal and provide a satisfactory outcome if the synovial structures respond appropriately

REFERENCES

1. Ford TS, Ross MW, Orsini PG: Communications and boundaries of the middle carpal and carpometacarpal joints in horses, Am J Vet Res 1988;49:2161.
2. Gough MR, Mayhew IG, Munroe GA: Diffusion of mepivicaine between adjacent synovial structures in the horse. Part 1: Forelimb, foot and carpus, Equine Vet J 2002;34:80.
3. Bramlage LR: A clinical perspective on lameness originating in the carpus, Equine Vet J Suppl 1988;6:12.
4. Young DR, Richardson DW, Markel MD, et al: Mechanical and morphometric analysis of the third carpal bone in Thoroughbreds, Am J Vet Res 1991;52:402.
5. Firth EC, Delahunt J, Witchel JW, et al: Galloping exercise induces regional changes in bone density within the third and radial carpal bones of Thoroughbred horses, Equine Vet J 1999;31:111.
6. Anastasiou A, Skioldebrand E, Ekman S, et al: Ex vivo magnetic resonance imaging of the distal row of equine carpal bones: Assessment of bone sclerosis and cartilage damage, Vet Radiol Ultrasound 2003;44:501.
7. Murray RC, Whitton RC, Vedi, S, et al: The effect of training on the calcified zone of equine middle carpal articular cartilage, Equine Vet J Suppl 1999;30:274.
8. Anderson TM, McIlwraith CW, Douay P: The role of conformation in musculoskeletal problems in the racing Thoroughbred, Equine Vet J 2004;36:571.
9. Kane AJ, Park RD, McIlwraith CW, et al: Radiographic changes in Thoroughbred yearlings: Part 1. Prevalence at the time of yearling sales, Equine Vet J 2003;35:354.
10. McIlwraith CW, Yovich JV, Martin GS: Arthroscopic surgery for the treatment of osteochondral chip fractures in the equine carpus, J Am Vet Med Assoc 1987;191:531.
11. Shimozawa K, Ueno Y, Ushiya S, et al: Survey of arthroscopic surgery for carpal chip fractures in Thoroughbred racehorses in Japan, J Vet Med Sci 2001;63:329.
12. Lucas JM, Ross MW, Richardson DW: Arthroscopic surgery for the treatment of carpal chip fractures in racing Standardbreds: 176 cases (1986-1993), Proc Am Assoc Equine Pract 1995;41:198.
13. Hopper BJ, Steel C, Richardson JL, et al: Radiographic evaluation of sclerosis of the third carpal bone associated with exercise and the development of lameness in Standardbred racehorses, Equine Vet J 2004;36:441.
14. Pool RR, Meagher DM: Pathologic findings and pathogenesis of racetrack injuries, Vet Clin North Am Equine Pract 1990;6:1.
15. Dabrareiner RM, White NA, Sullins KE: Radiographic and arthroscopic findings associated with subchondral lucency of the distal radial carpal bone in 71 horses, Equine Vet J 1996;28:93.
16. McIlwraith CW: Diagnostic and surgical arthroscopy of the carpal joints. In McIlwraith CW: Diagnostic and Surgical Arthroscopy of the Horse, ed 2, Philadelphia, 1990, Lea & Febiger.
17. Ulhorn H, Carlstern J: Retrospective study of subchondral sclerosis and lucency in the third carpal bone of Standardbred trotters, Equine Vet J 1999;31:500.
18. Moore RM, Schneider RK: Arthroscopic findings in the carpal joints of lame horses without radiographically visible abnormalities: 41 cases (1986-1991), J Am Vet Med Assoc 1995;206:1741.
19. Ross MW, Richardson DW, Beroza GA: Subchondral lucency of the third carpal bone in Standardbred racehorses: 13 cases (1982-1988), J Am Vet Med Assoc 1989;195:789.
20. Whitton RC, Rose RJ: The intercarpal ligaments of the equine midcarpal joint: Part 2. The role of the palmar intercarpal ligaments in the restraint of the dorsal displacement of the proximal row of carpal bones, Vet Surg 1997;26:367.
21. McIlwraith CW: Tearing of the medial palmar intercarpal ligament in the equine midcarpal joint, Equine Vet J 1992;24:365.
22. Phillips TJ, Wright IM: Observations on the anatomy and pathology of the palmar intercarpal ligaments in the midcarpal joints of Thoroughbred racehorses, Equine Vet J 1994;26:486.
23. Whitton RC, Kannegieter NJ, Rose RJ: The intercarpal ligaments of the equine midcarpal joint: Part 3. Clinical observations in 32 racing horses with midcarpal joint disease, Vet Surg 1997;26:374.
24. Driver AJ, Barr FJ, Fuller CJ, et al: Ultrasonography of the medial palmar intercarpal ligament in the Thoroughbred: Technique and normal appearance, Equine Vet J 2004;36:402.
25. Whitton RC, Kannegieter NJ, Rose RJ: Postoperative performance of racing horses with tearing of the medial palmar intercarpal ligament, Aust Vet J 1999;77:713.
26. Schneider RK, Bramlage LR, Gabel AA, et al: Incidence, location and classification of 371 third carpal bone fractures in 313 horses, Equine Vet J Suppl 1988;6:33.
27. Auer JA, Watkins JP, White NA, et al: Slab fractures of the fourth and intermediate carpal bone in five horses, J Am Vet Med Assoc 1986;188:595.
28. Martin GS, Haynes PF, McClure JR: Effect of third carpal slab fracture and repair on racing performance in Thoroughbred horses: 31 cases (1977-1984), J Am Vet Med Assoc 1988;193:107.
29. Stephens PR, Richardson DW, Spencer PA: Slab fractures of the third carpal bone in Standardbreds and Thoroughbreds: 155 cases (1977-1984), J Am Vet Med Assoc 1988;193:353.
30. Richardson DW: Technique for arthroscopic repair of third carpal bone slab fractures in horses, J Am Vet Med Assoc 1986;188:288.
31. McIlwraith CW, Turner AS: Repair of the third carpal bone. In McIlwraith CW, Turner AS, editors: Equine Surgery Advanced Techniques, Philadelphia, 1987, Lea & Febiger.
32. Bertone AL, Scheiter HL, Turner AS, et al: Pancarpal arthrodesis for treatment of carpal collapse in the horse: A report of two cases, Vet Surg 1989;18:353.
33. Auer JA, Taylor JR, Watkins JP, et al: Partial carpal arthrodesis in the horse, Vet Comp Orthop Traumatol 1990;3:51.
34. Nixon AJ, Schachter BL, Pool RR: Exostoses of the caudal perimeter of the radial physis as a cause of synovial sheath tenosynovitis and lameness in horses: 10 cases (1999-2003), J Am Vet Med Assoc 2004;224:264.
35. Southwood LL, Stashak TS, Fehr JE, et al: Lateral approach for endoscopic removal of solitary osteochondromas from the distal radial metaphysis in three horses, J Am Vet Med Assoc 1997;210:1166.
36. Textor, JA Nixon AJ, Fortier LA: Tenoscopic release of the equine carpal canal, Vet Surgery 2003;32:378.
37. Barr ARS, Sinnott MJA, Denny HR: Fractures of the accessory carpal bone in the horse, Vet Rec 1990;126:342.
38. Dyson SJ: Fractures of the accessory carpal bone, Equine Vet Educ 1990;2:188.
39. Rijkenhuizen ABM, Nemeth J: Accessory carpal bone fractures in the horse, Vet Q 1994;16(Suppl 2):S101.
40. Easley KJ, Schneider JE: Evaluation of a surgical technique for repair of equine accessory carpal bone fractures, J Am Vet Med Assoc 1981;178:219.
41. Auer JA: Personal communication, 1998.
42. Radue P: Carpal tunnel syndrome due to fractures of the accessory carpal bone, Equine Pract 1981;3:8.

CHAPTER 97

Radius and Ulna

Jeffrey P. Watkins

The equine antebrachium consists of the radius and ulna in conjunction with the muscles that flex and extend the carpus and digit. The radius is the major weight-supporting bone in the antebrachium. The olecranon, by serving as the insertion site of the triceps muscle, acts as the lever arm during elbow extension. The primary indications for surgical intervention in this area are caused by traumatic events that result in fracture of either the ulna or the radius.

FRACTURES OF THE ULNA

Fractures of the ulna are relatively common in foals and adult horses. A wide variety of fracture configurations occur, and most are amenable to open reduction and internal fixation. The treatment of choice is fracture fixation using a bone plate applied as a tension band. Provided complications are not encountered, the prognosis is favorable for a return to full function.

Anatomy

The ulna has two components, the body and the olecranon. The body of the ulna extends distad from the level of the proximal radial physis. It is triangular in cross section and tapers distally, essentially ending in the mid-diaphyseal region of the radius. It is closely adherent to the radius, and distal to the interosseous space it is fused to the caudal cortex of the radius. Functionally, it serves as the distal attachment of the lever arm through which the triceps muscle functions.

Proximal to the body of the ulna is the olecranon. The olecranon is concave medially and has a proximal tuberosity for muscle attachment. Tendinous insertions on the olecranon tuberosity, principally by the triceps brachii muscle, provide elbow extension during locomotion. Equally important, by extending the elbow during standing, the triceps apparatus allows extension of the carpus through engagement of the stay apparatus of the forelimb. The olecranon is also an important component of the cubital joint, with articular cartilage present in the proximal aspect of the trochlear notch. In the distal aspect of the trochlear notch there is a synovial fossa, which is devoid of articular cartilage.

Foals have a physis in the proximal olecranon. Because the separate center of ossification of the physis is not involved in formation of a joint, it is termed an *apophysis*. Although growth at the olecranon physis is responsible for the ultimate size of the olecranon tuberosity, disturbances of physeal growth following injury or fracture repair are well tolerated and do not result in disability. However, because growth occurs at the proximal radial physis, the ulna must be able to displace proximad relative to the radius to maintain congruency between the humeral condyle and the trochlear notch of the olecranon.

Pathogenesis

A direct blow from a kick or a fall causes most fractures of the ulna. A common history includes injury during halter training of weanling foals. Often the fracture occurs when the foal rears up and falls onto its side. The body of the ulna or, more commonly, the olecranon fractures, and fragments are displaced during contraction of the triceps muscle when the foal jumps to its feet.

Ulnar fractures have been classified.[1] The most common configuration is for the fracture to traverse the caudal one third to one half of the physis, enter the metaphysis, and break into the proximal aspect of the trochlear notch near the anconeal process (type 1b) (Fig. 97-1). Less commonly, the fracture breaks out the cranial cortex of the olecranon proximal to the anconeal process and remains nonarticular (also type 1b). Occasionally, comminution occurs at the anconeal process.

Other configurations include physeal separations (type 1a), most common in neonates; transverse fractures entering the trochlear notch near its midpoint (type 2); distal olecranon–proximal ulnar body fractures, which usually have an oblique configuration traversing the bone in a proximal and cranial direction to enter the distal aspect of the trochlear notch (type 5); and comminuted fractures (type 4). Type 3 fractures—nonarticular, nonphyseal fractures of the olecranon extending from the caudal cortex to the cranial cortex proximal to the anconeal process—are rare.

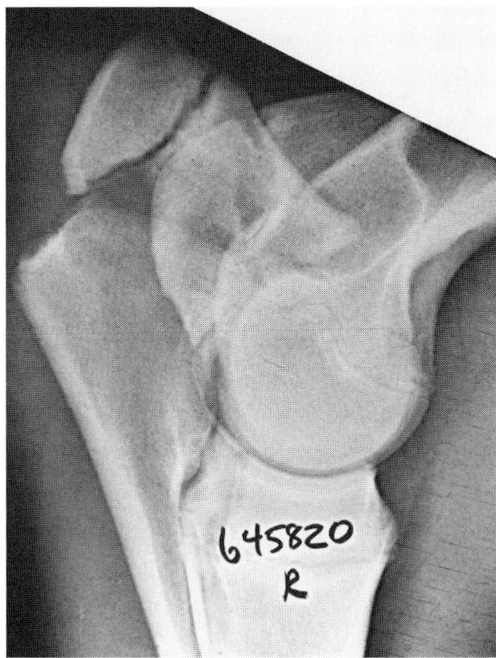

Figure 97-1. Mediolateral radiograph of type 1b, articular olecranon fracture.

The degree of soft tissue injury varies greatly. Contusions resulting from a kick are often accompanied by a skin wound at the site of impact. These wounds might communicate directly with the fracture, and if the fracture is articular, joint sepsis can develop secondary to bacterial colonization of the fracture. Displacement of the fracture is another indicator of the degree of soft tissue damage. Marked displacement indicates disruption of the aponeurosis of the ulnar head of the deep digital flexor muscle laterally and the ulnar head of the flexor carpi ulnaris muscle medially.

Diagnosis

The affected limb has a dropped-elbow appearance, because the carpus cannot be fixed in extension. Depending on the amount of displacement, the elbow might appear only slightly dropped, with the carpus held in flexion, the limb placed slightly craniad, and the toe touching the ground. With severe displacement, marked dropping of the elbow along with carpal flexion is evident (Fig. 97-2). The differential diagnosis for a dropped elbow stance includes ulnar fracture, humeral fracture, and radial neuropathy.

Soft tissue swelling is usually not severe in most ulnar fractures and is localized to the caudolateral aspect of the proximal antebrachium. This is distinct from humeral fractures, in which the swelling is typically much greater and best visualized by standing in front of the horse and comparing the relative thickness of the humeral regions on affected and unaffected sides. Pain on deep palpation and manipulation of the olecranon aids in localizing the fracture.

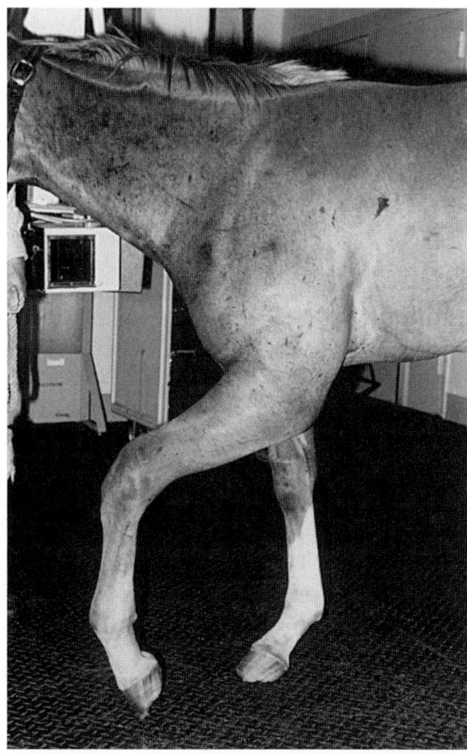

Figure 97-2. Photograph demonstrating the typical dropped elbow stance in a foal with a displaced olecranon fracture.

Definitive diagnosis is based on radiographic documentation of the fracture. Best detail of the area is obtained with a medial to lateral projection and the beam obliqued slightly cranial to caudal. When the affected limb is extended cranially, complete visualization of the cubital joint and olecranon is possible, and the fracture configuration and location can be determined. With type 1b fractures, it is important to visualize the anconeal process to delineate comminuted fragments. A cranial to caudal radiograph is necessary to detect concurrent injury to the proximal radius (Fig. 97-3). A contrast arthrogram determines the extent of communication between a soft tissue wound and an articular fracture.

Treatment

First Aid

Initial care for horses with fracture of the ulna accompanied by a wound should include appropriate wound therapy, removal of hair at the wound margins, and careful cleansing and débridement, followed by application of a sterile bandage to prevent further contamination before surgery. Systemic broad-spectrum bactericidal therapy should be initiated immediately.

It is important to ascertain the extent of soft tissue trauma. Fortunately, many wounds encountered with olecranon fractures are superficial and do not markedly affect therapy or prognosis. However, deep wounds that communicate with the fracture, particularly articular fractures, dictate aggressive therapy. Therapy for open articular fractures includes administration of intra-articular antimicrobial drugs. In addition, antimicrobial-impregnated polymethylmethacrylate (PMMA) beads placed into the depths of extensive soft tissue wounds help to reduce bacterial contamination before open reduction and internal fixation of the fracture.

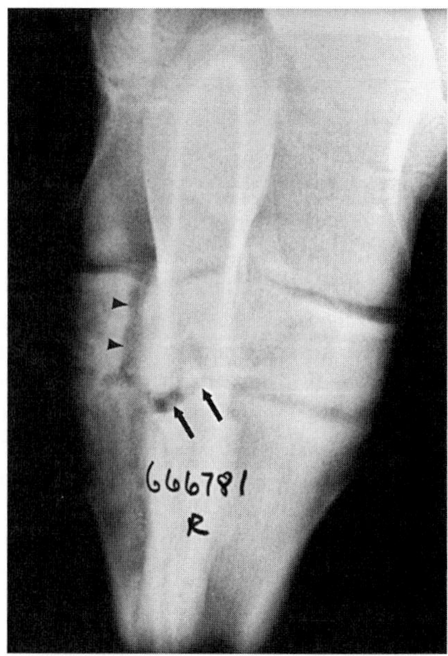

Figure 97-3. Craniocaudal radiograph demonstrating a Salter-Harris type III fracture of the proximal radius *(arrowheads)*, which occurred in conjunction with a fracture of the ulna *(arrows)*.

Many horses with displaced fractures cannot engage their stay apparatus and therefore are unable to support weight on the affected limb. If so, a splint is applied once wound therapy is complete. Although it is not possible to splint the fracture per se, splinting the carpus in extension allows weight to be supported on the affected limb. This markedly reduces the horse's anxiety and minimizes fatigue of the contralateral limb before internal fixation.

The splint should consist of rigid material applied over a well-padded full-limb bandage. Splints are fashioned from schedule 40 polyvinylchloride (PVC) pipe; an appropriate length is cut from a 15-cm (6-in.) diameter pipe and split longitudinally, using one third of the pipe's circumference. The splint should extend from the ground to the proximal antebrachium and is affixed to the bandage with nonelastic adhesive tape. Additional padding at the proximal aspect of the splint prevents soft tissue damage near the fracture site.

Nonsurgical Management

Conservative therapy has been advocated for nondisplaced, nonarticular fractures of the ulna (nondisplaced types 3 and 4). Conservative therapy includes strict stall confinement. If the patient does not bear full weight on the limb, a full-limb splint is applied. Functional soundness was reported in 7 of 10 horses with type 5 fractures managed conservatively.[2] Poor results are achieved following conservative therapy for other fracture configurations.

Horses with nondisplaced, nonarticular fractures that are managed conservatively have a prolonged convalescent period because of the instability of the fracture. Healing is slow, and lameness is protracted. Although type 5 fractures do not violate the articular surface of the cubital joint, they communicate with the synovial cavity. Therefore, inflammatory mediators released into the joint from the fracture have detrimental effects on the articular cartilage and lead to degenerative articular changes. Despite the inherent risk of surgery and anesthesia, surgical treatment is preferable, and the primary determinant for choosing conservative therapy over surgical therapy is economics.

Surgical Management

Open reduction and internal fixation is the treatment of choice for articular or displaced fractures of the ulna. By using the tension-band principle, stable fixation of nearly all fracture configurations can be achieved with minimal complications and a favorable prognosis. Tension-band fixation can be accomplished using a plate applied to the caudal aspect of the ulna or by using tension-band wire fixation.

The surgical approach to ulnar fractures has been described.[3] It is advisable to curve the skin incision proximally to avoid the point of the elbow. When possible, wounds should also be avoided when approaching the fracture. Once the skin and subcutaneous fascia have been incised, deep dissection between the ulnaris lateralis and ulnar head of the deep digital flexor tendon exposes the caudal and lateral aspects of the ulna.

Distally, the ulna is exposed for plate application by subperiosteal dissection. Proximally, the caudal and lateral aspects of the olecranon are closely invested in the dense fibrous connective tissue aponeuroses of the ulnar head of the deep digital flexor and flexor carpi ulnaris muscles. Sharp dissection of the fibrous connective tissue attachments from the olecranon is necessary for plate application. Additional dissection exposes the proximal aspect of the olecranon tuberosity for fixation of type 1 and 3 fractures. In these cases, the insertion of the triceps is sharply divided in the sagittal plane of the cranial olecranon and dissected abaxially for the approximate width of the fixation appliance.

Once the bone is exposed, the fracture hematoma is evacuated and the fracture line débrided of all fibrin or, in chronic cases, fibrous tissue. Assessment of the bone at this time might reveal hairline cracks in the ulna that might not have been evident radiographically. If the anconeal process is comminuted, the fracture is opened and the fragment is removed through the fracture gap. In displaced fractures, reduction is accomplished by grasping the olecranon process medially and laterally with a large pointed reduction forceps (Synthes, Paoli, Pa) and applying caudal and distal traction with the limb held in extension.

A soft aluminum template is used to provide a model for plate contouring. The plate is positioned to allow screw engagement of a minimum of five cortices on either side of the fracture. Usually a combination of 4.5- and 5.5-mm cortex screws in conjunction with a narrow limited-contact dynamic compression plate (LC-DCP) or dynamic compression plate (DCP) is used for fixation. In large patients or more comminuted fractures, a higher proportion of 5.5-mm cortex screws are used, and a broad LC-DCP or DCP may be chosen. In adult horses with comminuted fractures, double plate fixation with a broad LC-DCP or DCP applied caudally and a narrow LC-DCP or DCP applied laterally may be necessary.

The appropriately contoured plate is applied with the fracture held in reduction by positioning one screw proximal and another screw distal to the fracture. The initial screw is placed in the proximal fragment using the neutral drill guide. This screw is not tightened completely, and the plate is displaced distally before placing the screw in the distal fragment using the load drill guide. Tightening of these two screws compresses the fracture. Over-compression of minimally displaced fractures with comminution at the articular surface can result in fragment displacement. Therefore, screws should be applied in the neutral position with comminuted fractures.

At this point in the repair, an intraoperative lateromedial radiograph should be taken to assess the fixation (Fig. 97-4). The intraoperative radiograph can be used to evaluate the adequacy of reduction and screw position and as a guide for directing and gauging the approximate length of the remaining screws.

If further compression is needed, an additional screw on either side of the fracture can be placed in the load configuration. Before tightening these additional load screws, the previously placed screw in the same fragment should be loosened slightly. The remainder of the screws are placed in the neutral position.

Screw placement in the proximal fragment must avoid penetrating the concave medial cortex. Screws at the level of the trochlear notch should not penetrate into the joint.

Distally, screws should not engage the caudal cortex of the radius in foals. If the body of the ulna is transfixed to the

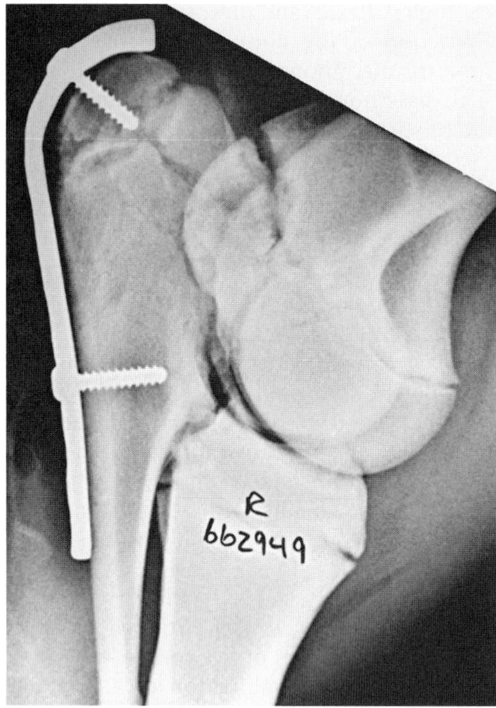

Figure 97-4. Intraoperative lateromedial radiograph documenting plate position and fracture reduction before cortex screws are placed in lag fashion through the plate into the cranial cortex of the olecranon in a type 1b fracture.

radius, growth of the proximal radial epiphysis forces the anconeal process into the humeral condylar notch, and subluxation of the cubital joint occurs, resulting in elbow dysplasia. The age at which it is safe to engage the caudal cortex is not well defined. In one study, there was growth at the proximal radial physis with relative displacement of the ulna until 18 months of age.[4] However, in another study in which the radius and ulna were transfixed, it appeared that subluxation was not a clinical problem in foals that were 7 months old or older at the time of surgery, even though subluxation was evident radiographically and at necropsy.[5]

Therefore, engagement of the caudal cortex of the radius should be avoided in foals younger than 1 year of age. If not, careful monitoring is necessary, and either the implants or the screws engaging the radius should be removed as soon as the fracture has healed (although subluxation can occur even after the implants are removed).[5] If subluxation occurs, it can be managed with an osteotomy of the body of the ulna at a level distal to the joint (Fig. 97-5). By not fixing the osteotomy, the ulna can adjust into a normal position during the postoperative period. Another alternative is active proximal displacement of the proximal fragment through flexion and extension of the joint and subsequent bridging of the osteotomy gap with a narrow plate.

The proximal location of types 1 and 3 fractures challenges the fixation, because the small size of the proximal fragment limits the number of screws available for purchase. With a type 1b fracture, the plate is contoured over the dorsal aspect of the apophysis to allow purchase with three short screws. The fourth and usually the fifth screw in the plate are placed in lag fashion across the metaphyseal portion of the fracture to engage the cranial cortex of the olecranon (Fig. 97-6). Purchase in the cranial cortex of the olecranon adds substantial stability to the fixation.

Compression at the fracture line improves fracture reduction; this is particularly important for type 1b fractures that enter the articulation. Care is taken with type 1b fractures to avoid overcompressing the caudal aspect of the fracture using a DCP, because the cranial aspect of the fracture can become displaced. In these fractures, the initial screw is placed in the apophysis through the second plate hole, and another screw is placed in the sixth or seventh hole of the plate. These screws are not completely tightened, allowing the fracture to be held in reduction while the lag screws are placed across the metaphyseal fracture. Once the lag screws are tight, the remainder of the fixation is routine.

Prognosis

The prognosis following plate fixation of ulnar fractures is favorable. Success, defined as fracture union, occurred in 13 of 19 patients (68%), with a return to full function in 11 of the 13 cases.[1] Another study reported return to full function in 16 of 21 patients (76%).[6] Type 2 was the most common fracture configuration in both studies. When both patient populations were combined, full function returned in 27 of 34 patients (79%). Type 4 fractures were the second most common configuration, but only two of seven patients returned to full function. In 17 adult horses with comminuted articular fractures (type 4), long-term follow-up was available for eight, and five were sound enough for riding or training.[7]

In a more recent retrospective study of 77 olecranon fractures, type 1b fractures were the most common configuration in young horses.[8] Twenty horses underwent plate fixation as previously described (see Fig. 97-6). Fracture healing occurred in 19 of the 20 repaired fractures. Sixteen horses were available for long-term follow-up, and 13 (81%) were reported to be sound. Twelve horses were older than 2 years of age at the time of follow-up, and nine of these were performing their intended purpose. The remaining four horses, which were not yet 2 years of age, were all reported to be in training for their intended use without evidence of complications related to their fracture. In this case series there were no catastrophic fixation failures, and other complications were minimal. Furthermore, four horses with comminution at the anconeal process did not appear to be negatively affected by removal of the anconeal process fragment.

Tension-band wire fixation has been used to manage olecranon fractures in horses. In 22 horses managed with tension-band wiring, fracture union was achieved in 18 cases,[9] and 13 of 17 horses returned to athletic function. Patients are candidates for tension-band wiring if they weigh 250 kg or less. When fractures are in close proximity to the physis, either pins or screws are positioned cranial to the apophysis and directed distally into the ulnar body. Distal fractures are repaired with wires alone or in conjunction with lag screws. Fractures in foals and weanlings are repaired with at least two or three 1.2-mm diameter wires, whereas four to six 1.5-mm diameter wires are used in older horses.

The advantages of tension-band wiring compared to plate fixation are less-expensive equipment, less risk of screws entering the joint space or engaging the caudal cortex of the

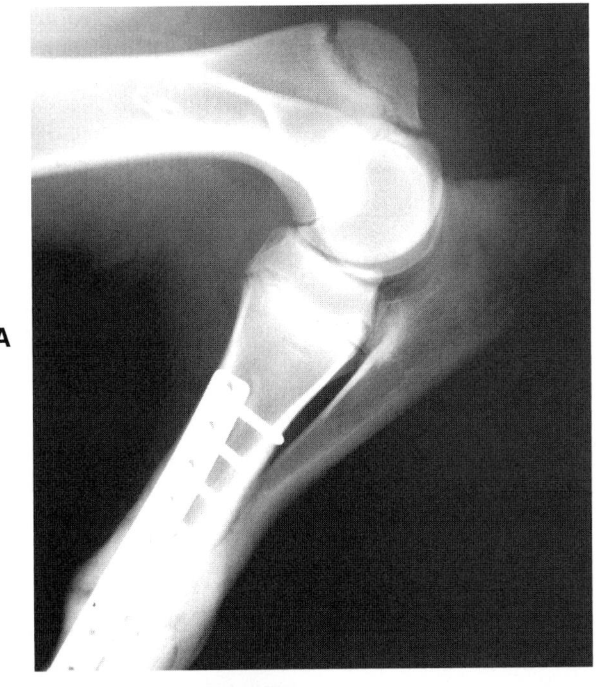

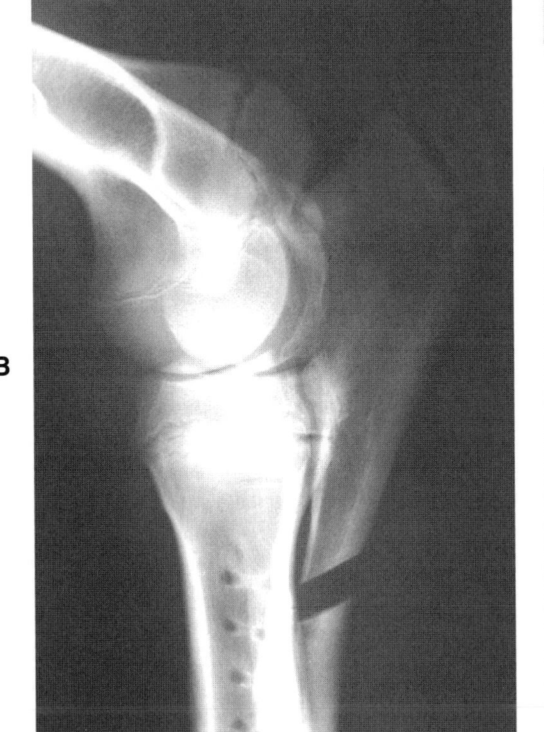

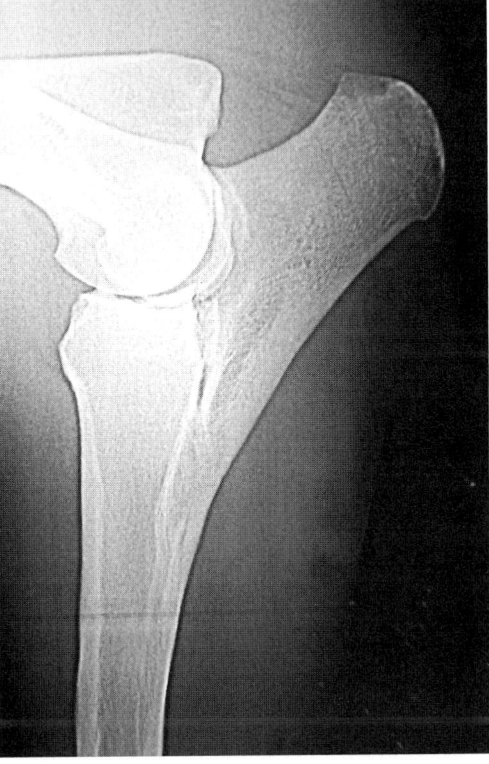

Figure 97-5. A, Follow-up radiograph of a mid-diaphyseal radius fracture in a foal treated with bone plates. The fracture shows progressive healing; however, there is a subluxation of the elbow joint. **B**, An ulnar osteotomy was performed 10 days prior to taking this radiograph, which resulted in correction of the subluxation and restoration of the normal joint anatomy. An osteotomy gap of 10 mm developed. **C**, The 6-year follow-up of the same animal shows a normal configuration of the joint without arthrosis and a sound animal. (Courtesy G. Bodo, Budapest.)

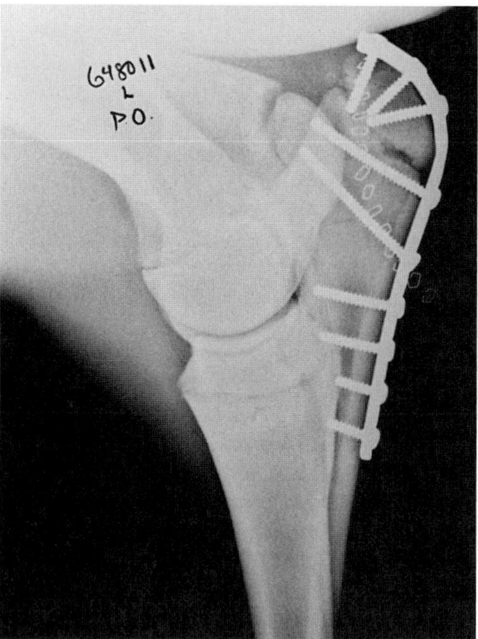

Figure 97-6. Postoperative mediolateral oblique radiograph of a repaired type 1b articular ulnar fracture.

radius, less risk of fracture of the apophysis because screw holes in the proximal fragment are not necessary for fixation, and, with more distal fractures, less tissue dissection required.

Complications

Complications of repair of ulnar fractures are infection, fixation failure, tendon contracture, support limb varus deformity, suspensory apparatus fatigue, and support limb laminitis.

Infection is most likely following repair of open, contaminated fractures. However, fractures with substantial soft tissue trauma also have an increased risk. Methods of reducing the infection potential include the use of perioperative systemic antimicrobial agents and, in high-risk patients, local application of antimicrobial-impregnated PMMA, usually as beads or in some cases as plate-luting material. If the fracture becomes infected, but the fixation is stable, a successful outcome is likely. However, the convalescent period is substantially prolonged, and lameness often persists until the infection is resolved. Resolution of infection requires implant removal once the fracture has healed. Infection in the presence of instability at the fracture invariably results in failure. Articular fractures that become infected have the additional risk of joint sepsis, which substantially worsens the prognosis.

Fixation failure can occur secondary to fracture of the apophysis in proximal olecranon fractures, especially with type 1a fractures in neonates, in which the apophysis is primarily cartilaginous. Following plate fixation of proximal fractures in older foals and adults, failure can result from fracture of the proximal fragment through the screw holes.[9] However, this complication did not occur following plate fixation of 20 patients with type 1b fractures.[8] Implant failure also can occur from using wire techniques, especially in large foals and adults.[9] Therefore, fractures in large foals and especially in adults deemed at risk for implant failure are candidates for fixation using a broad DCP.

Prolonged lameness for any reason results in a number of compensatory complications. Persistent lameness or increasing lameness in the postoperative period indicates fracture instability, infection, or both. With articular fractures, osteoarthritis secondary to incongruent joint surfaces or prolonged, severe synovitis causes persistent lameness. In foals, persistent lameness often results in varus deformities of both the carpus and the fetlock, as well as fatigue of the suspensory apparatus with hyperextension of the fetlock in the contralateral limb. The ipsilateral limb can develop flexural deformity of the carpus or fetlock, or both. In adults, ipsilateral flexor contracture may develop, but support limb laminitis is the most likely and potentially devastating complication.

FRACTURES OF THE RADIUS

In horses, radial fractures are not as common as ulnar fractures. When they occur, a wide variety of fracture configurations is possible. With most configurations, open reduction and internal fixation can be expected to produce a good to excellent outcome in horses weighing less than 250 kg. Fixation of radial fractures in adult horses, however, poses a substantial challenge. Although success has been reported, the prognosis for an adult horse with a completely displaced radial fracture is unfavorable.[10]

Anatomy

The radius is the major weight-supporting bone of the antebrachium. Proximally, it articulates with the humerus, and with the ulna it forms the cubital joint. Distally, along with the proximal row of carpal bones, it forms the antebrachiocarpal joint. Proximally, the biceps brachii inserts on its cranial surface, and distally, the tendons of the digital extensor muscles pass through their respective tendon sheaths as they traverse the carpus en route to the digit. Medially, the radius lacks overlying muscle and is covered only by skin and subcutaneous fascia. The bone is strongly curved in the sagittal plane and has a distinct cranial bow. Biomechanically, this places the caudal cortex under substantial compression. The cranial and craniolateral aspects of the radius are loaded in tension.

In foals, a proximal and a distal physis are present. These physes, along with their respective epiphyses, are subjected to compressive forces. Therefore, fractures involving these physes are classified according to the Salter-Harris scheme. Growth at these physes is responsible for the ultimate length of the bone and thereby affects limb length and conformation. Disproportionate growth at the distal radial physis is a common cause of carpus valgus limb deformity.

Pathogenesis

Most radial fractures result from external trauma. In foals, entrapment of the limb proximal to the carpus can result in proximal radial physeal fractures. However, direct blows to the antebrachium are the most common cause of fracture in both foals and adults. Often, the cause of the fracture is a kick from another horse.

Commonly, the fracture is comminuted, regardless of the patient's age. In adults, comminution almost always accompanies either a spiral or an oblique fracture of the diaphysis. The degree of comminution varies from single or multiple large butterfly fragments to multiple small fragments. Incomplete or complete nondisplaced fractures of the radius often occur in adult horses that have been kicked. Often these injuries are witnessed as a solid blow to the distal medial aspect of the antebrachium. A skin wound may be evident.

Because the fracture is not displaced and instability is not readily apparent, radiographs are occasionally omitted from the evaluation. Because the horse remains noticeably lame, the fracture is detected later, when it becomes unstable or radiographs are taken because the lameness fails to resolve. Therefore, radiographic examination is recommended in all cases in which there is evidence of a kick injury to the antebrachium.

Occasionally, if the initial radiographs are taken immediately after the incident, the fracture cannot be detected. Follow-up radiographs taken 5 to 7 days after the injury allows identification of the fracture lines.

The degree of fragmentation accompanying comminuted fractures in foals is less than that of comminuted fractures in adults. Fracture configurations in foals vary. Mid-diaphyseal transverse fractures result from a cranial blow to the antebrachium. A lateral blow results in an oblique fracture of the proximal metaphysis. Physeal fractures occur at both the proximal and the distal radial physes. Displacement with Salter-Harris type I and type II fractures of the proximal physis is accompanied by fracture of the ulna. If the radial metaphysis displaces cranially, injury to the radial nerve is possible. Salter-Harris type III fractures are encountered most commonly in the proximal epiphysis.

Diaphyseal fractures of the radius are at high risk of becoming open secondary to skin penetration by the sharp fracture fragments on the medial aspect of the antebrachium. Abduction of the distal limb displaces the fracture into the relatively thin soft tissues medially, and the fracture often becomes open. In addition, there is often substantial injury to the musculature covering the dorsal and lateral aspects of the antebrachium, accompanied by severe soft tissue swelling and hematoma. The degree of soft tissue injury accompanying radial fractures makes them highly susceptible to infection at the fracture site.

Diagnosis

Complete displaced radial fractures are easily identified on physical examination. Non–weight-bearing lameness accompanied by instability and crepitation in the antebrachial region is pathognomonic for these injuries. The patient usually holds the limb with the carpus and fetlock flexed and drags the toe. Attempts at weightbearing result in valgus angulation at the fracture. Soft tissue swelling is usually evident. Wounds or secondary penetration of the medial soft tissues are often present. Horses with incomplete fractures or with nondisplaced complete fractures do not demonstrate instability or crepitation. However, they are usually lame, and in many cases a wound is evident at the site of traumatic impact.

Radiographic evaluation confirms the presence of a fracture. Multiple views, including oblique projections, are advisable to delineate the severity of the fracture and to assist in determining a course of action and rendering a prognosis. It is important to delineate the extent and location of fragmentation in comminuted, completely displaced fractures. Nondisplaced fracture lines usually emanate proximal and distal from the displaced fracture. Occasionally, these are evident only after the fracture is surgically exposed, but complete radiographic evaluation before attempting internal fixation determines the feasibility of repair and the best method for managing the fracture.

Fractures with multiple small fragments that are likely to preclude anatomic reconstruction should be identified. This is especially important when these fragments are located along the caudal cortex, which must be reconstructed for repair to be successful.

Treatment

First Aid

As with ulnar fractures, wounds associated with a displaced fracture of the radius require immediate attention. There is a high probability that wounds at the medial aspect of the antebrachium communicate directly with the fracture. Initial management should include appropriate hair removal, cleansing, and topical and systemic antimicrobial therapy.

Immediate immobilization of a displaced fracture is paramount. With closed fractures, appropriate external coaptation can prevent fragments from displacing and the fracture from opening. Sedation is necessary for applying a bandage and splint with an unstable radius fracture. Once the patient is controlled, and after appropriate wound therapy in open fractures, a Robert Jones bandage is applied extending from the hoof to as far proximal on the antebrachium as possible.

The bandage should be applied in layers to increase rigidity. A *caudal* splint is applied that extends from the ground to the level of the olecranon process. A second *lateral* splint extends from the ground to the level of the midscapula. The portion of the splint extending proximal to the bandage should contact the brachium when the limb is directly beneath the body (Fig. 97-7). This provides counterpressure to prevent the limb from abducting with weightbearing. Nonelastic adhesive tape or fiberglass casting tape is used to affix the splints to the bandage. More information on bandaging and first aid for fracture patients can be found in Chapters 18 and 78.

Nonsurgical Management

Incomplete and nondisplaced complete fractures are candidates for conservative therapy[11-13] (Fig. 97-8). In one report, in only three of 10 horses, incomplete radial fractures became complete, displaced fractures with conservative management.[13] Predicting success based on the radiographic appearance of the fracture was not possible. An important aspect of therapy was preventing recumbency to reduce the

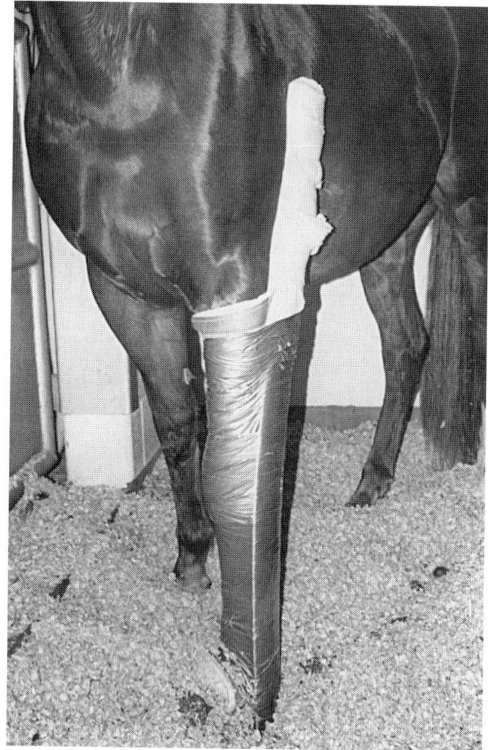

Figure 97-7. Photograph of appropriate external coaptation of a radial fracture in an adult horse before surgical repair.

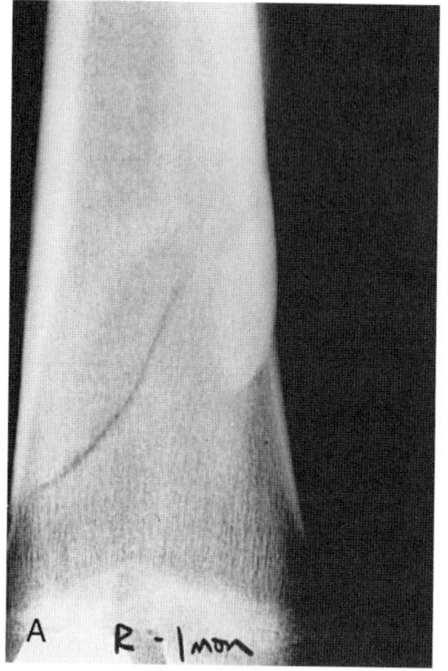

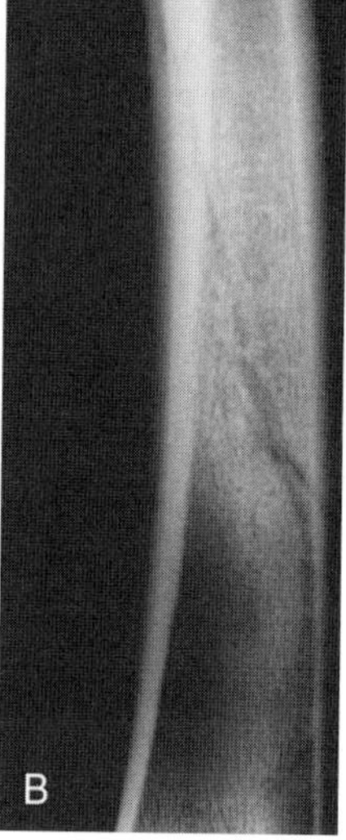

Figure 97-8. Craniocaudal (**A**) and lateromedial (**B**) radiographs of a nondisplaced fracture of the radius in an adult horse secondary to a kick injury.

likelihood of displacement secondary to forces experienced during standing up (see Fig. 81-1).

Phenylbutazone should be used judiciously to reduce inflammation and encourage limited weightbearing on the fractured limb. Care should be taken to avoid providing substantial pain relief, which could result in overuse of the fractured limb.

The horse is confined until there is evidence of advanced fracture healing. This usually requires a minimum of 3 to 4 months. During the last 30 days of confinement, a program of gradually increasing hand-walking is recommended. Access to free paddock exercise is allowed thereafter. An additional 30 days of paddock exercise is recommended before the horse is gradually returned to its intended function.

Surgical Management

ADULT HORSES

Open reduction and internal fixation of displaced radial fractures in adult horses is a monumental task that provides only a limited chance of survival.[10] In many cases, the fracture configuration and degree of soft tissue trauma preclude any reasonable likelihood of success. Even with fractures amenable to fixation, the biomechanical forces acting on the bone–implant construct place the fixation at risk for failure. Even the strongest, most stable construct has a high potential either to fail catastrophically during recovery or to fatigue and fail before fracture union.

Fixation with two plates is necessary; one plate is positioned cranially and the second plate is applied to either the medial or the lateral cortex. One of the plates should be a dynamic condylar plate, with the condylar screw placed in the smaller fracture segment. The second plate should be a broad 5.5-mm LC-DCP or DCP. As many 5.5-mm cortex screws as possible are implanted, and every opportunity to provide compression across fracture lines is used (Fig. 97-9). The entire length of the radius is spanned by the plates, and the plates should be offset to avoid ending at the same level in the transverse plane. Plate luting with antimicrobial-impregnated PMMA is recommended even though the PMMA loses some strength from the solvent that is added for the antibiotic. Cancellous bone grafts should be incorporated into the fixation to promote healing.

FOALS

Diaphyseal fractures in foals, other than simple transverse mid-diaphyseal fractures, are double plated as well. Implant selection depends upon the size of the foal, the fracture configuration, and the location. A broad LC-DCP or DCP is usually applied to the cranial cortex, and in most cases, 5.5-mm cortex screws are used throughout its length. The second plate may be either a broad or narrow LC-DCP or DCP fixed with a majority of 4.5-mm cortex screws. However, nearest the fracture and at the ends of the plate, 5.5-mm cortex screws should be inserted. With proximal oblique fractures, the second plate is placed lateral distally and twisted proximally to end on the craniolateral aspect of the proximal metaphysis, lateral to the insertion of the biceps brachii tendon on the radial tuberosity (Fig. 97-10).

Comminuted fractures

In foals with comminuted fractures, the repair is as described for adults, with the exception of implant selection. A second broad LC-DCP or DCP is used in place of the dynamic condylar screw plate. The author prefers to place the second plate laterally, unless the configuration of the fracture dictates medial placement. Lateral placement, although technically more demanding, avoids positioning

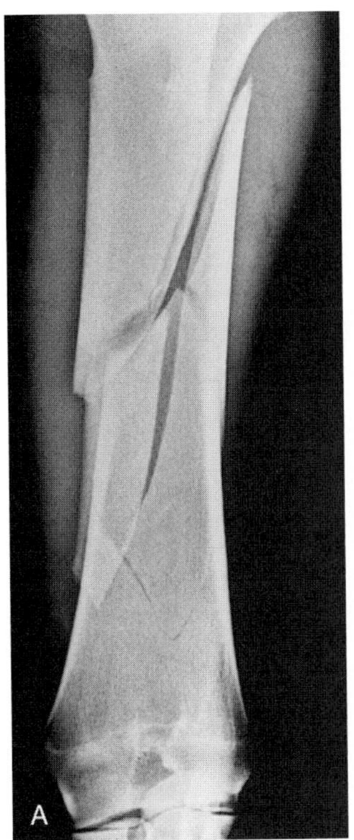

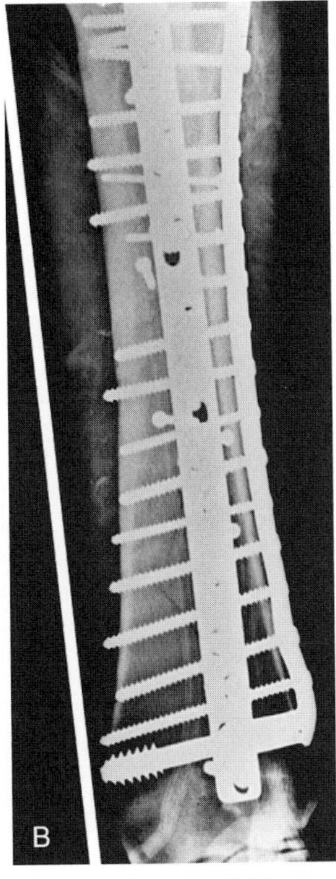

Figure 97-9. Craniocaudal radiograph of a comminuted radial fracture in an adult horse before internal fixation (**A**) and after application of a dynamic condylar screw plate applied to the lateral cortex and a broad dynamic compression plate applied to the cranial cortex (**B**). Most screws are 5.5-mm cortex screws, and the plates span the length of the radius.

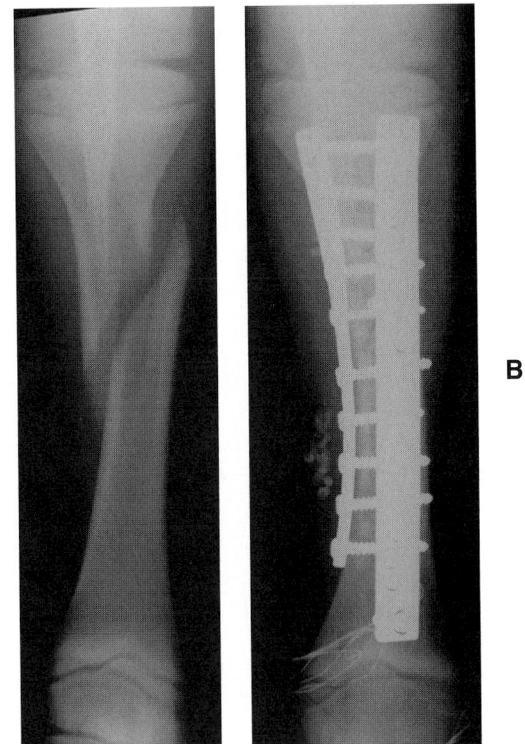

Figure 97-10. Craniocaudal radiograph of a proximal metaphyseal radial fracture in a foal, before internal fixation (**A**) and after application of a broad dynamic compression plate (DCP) to the cranial cortex and a narrow DCP applied to the lateral cortex distally and spiraled cranially at its proximal aspect (**B**).

the implant subcutaneously and, particularly in fractures that are open medially, avoids direct communication with the wound. In most cases, both implants can be placed using a lateral approach between the extensor carpi radialis and common digital extensor muscles. If the lateral plate is extended to the distal end of the radius, placement of the distal screws might require separate stab incisions lateral to the common digital extensor tendon.

Mid-diaphyseal fractures

Mid-diaphyseal transverse fractures are repaired with a single broad LC-DCP or DCP applied to the cranial cortex, provided the caudal cortex can be anatomically reconstructed. The strong cranial-to-caudal bending moment of the radius makes this a stable fixation in foals weighing less than 250 kg. With single-plate fixation, it is advisable to use 5.5-mm cortex screws throughout the entire length of the plate.

Proximal physeal fractures

Fractures at the proximal physis are less common than diaphyseal or metaphyseal fractures. They are candidates for internal fixation, with special considerations.

Type III fractures are uncommon, and conservative therapy is successful in nondisplaced fractures. However, anatomic reconstruction of the articular surface and compression across the fracture is the treatment of choice for displaced fractures. This is accomplished with lag screw fixation alone or in combination with tension band wire fixation.

Salter-Harris types I and II fractures of the proximal physis are accompanied by fracture of the ulna (Fig. 97-11, *A*). Plate fixation of the ulnar fracture, with screws engaging both cortices of the radius where possible, combined with a laterally applied narrow DCP with the most proximal screw in the radial epiphysis, is recommended (see Fig. 97-11, *B*). With small foals, transphyseal screw and wire fixation in place of the plate on the lateral aspect of the radius can be used.

Transfixion of the ulna and radius can result in elbow subluxation, but growth at the physis is minimal because of injury of the germinal layers of the growth plate and because the implants bridging the physis restrain growth. Because physeal growth is minimal, the ulna does not displace relative to the radius as the foal matures. The apparent disparity in bone length between limbs does not have an adverse effect on gait.

If the metaphyseal portion of the fracture displaces cranially (Fig. 97-12), the radial nerve can be traumatized, resulting in low radial nerve paresis. Difficulty in active extension of the digit occurs. Most foals learn to place the foot on the ground appropriately, and the paresis usually resolves.

Distal physeal fractures

Fractures of the distal physis are less common than fractures of the proximal physis. Salter-Harris type I physeal fractures result in displacement at the medial aspect of the physis (Fig. 97-13, *A*). The fractures occur in neonates and are

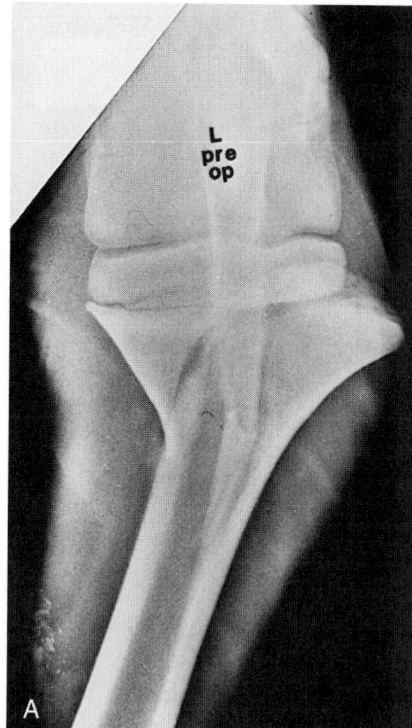

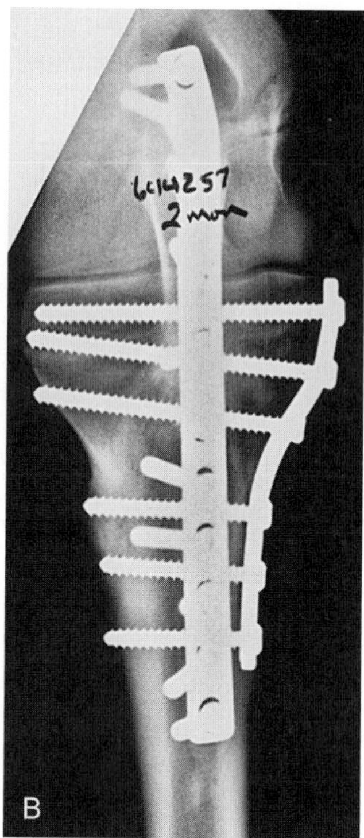

Figure 97-11. Craniocaudal radiograph of a Salter-Harris type II fracture of the proximal radius prior to repair (**A**) and after the application of a narrow dynamic compression plate (DCP) to the lateral aspect of the proximal radius and a second narrow DCP applied to the ulna with screws transfixing the ulna to the radius (**B**).

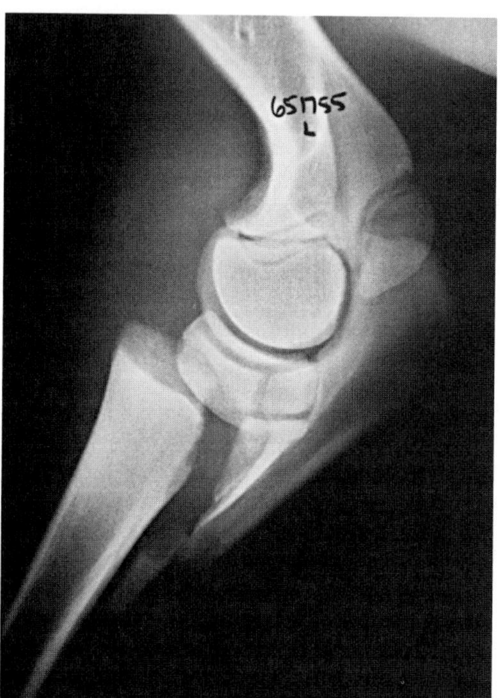

Figure 97-12. Lateromedial radiograph of Salter-Harris type II fracture of the proximal radius and ulnar fracture with cranial displacement of the distal fragment, resulting in temporary radial nerve paresis.

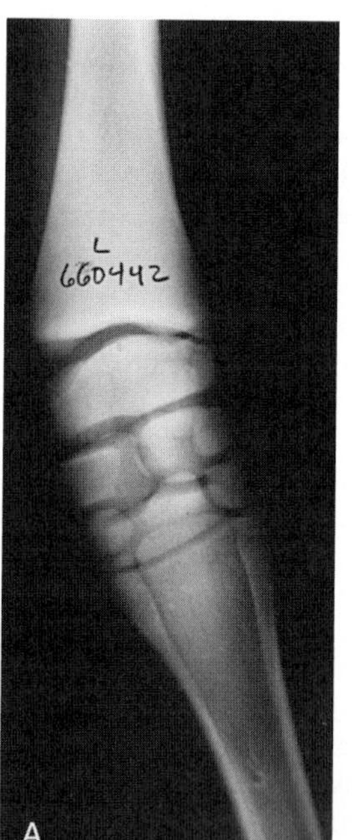

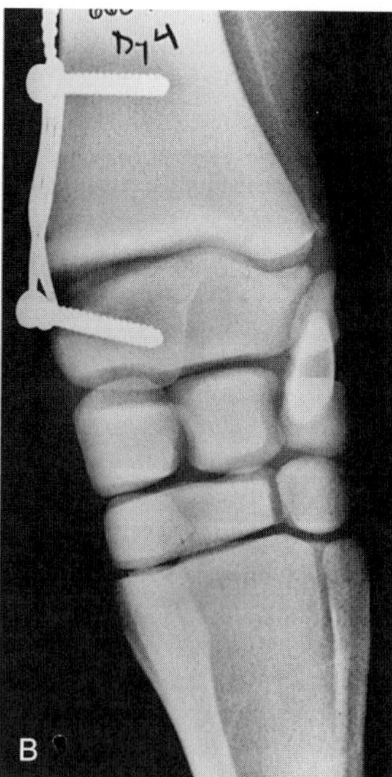

Figure 97-13. Craniocaudal radiograph of a foal with a Salter-Harris type I fracture of the distal radius before repair (**A**) and after repair with a transphyseal bridge using screws and wires (**B**).

treated by transphyseal bridging across the medial aspect of the physis. A T-plate or screws and wires can be used (Fig. 97-13, *B*). When the fractures are healed, the implants are removed.

Prognosis

Adults with displaced radial fractures have an unfavorable prognosis. In rare instances, successful internal fixation can be achieved.[10,12,14,15] In one report, internal fixation was attempted in six adult horses, none of which survived.[16] In another case series, nine of 15 horses that were presented for radial fracture had attempted internal fixation, and only two were discharged from the hospital.[10] However, with careful case selection and improved methods of increasing the strength and stability of the bone–implant construct, the success rate can be improved. The substantial expense associated with fixation, combined with the high risk of failure, often dissuades owners from pursuing repair.

Displaced radial fractures in foals, however, particularly if there is no comminution and when the fracture is closed, have a favorable prognosis. Physeal fractures and transverse fractures of the mid-diaphysis have an excellent prognosis.[16] In six of seven foals with mid-diaphyseal transverse fractures, and in two foals, one with Salter-Harris type I and another with a type II proximal physeal fracture, the fractures healed. Similarly, fixation of proximal oblique fractures in three of four foals had an excellent outcome.

Complications

Complications following repair of radial fractures are the same as for any equine long bone fracture repair. Infection, instability, failure of fixation, and support limb complications are the most common. The propensity for radial fractures to be open medially substantially increases the risk of infection. Even in closed fractures, the degree of soft tissue trauma and the lack of muscle covering of the medial aspect of the radius increase the potential for infection. The technical difficulty of the repair often prolongs surgery time. The quantity of implants used for repair significantly contributes to postoperative infection.

Fixation failure is the most common fatal complication. Catastrophic failure is a major risk during recovery from anesthesia, particularly in adult horses. Long surgery time and the condition of the patient at the time of anesthesia play major roles. Attention to the patient's physiologic status before and during anesthesia, along with a controlled recovery, can reduce the incidence of failure. The technical difficulty of the fixation dictates that an experienced surgical team be assembled. Every effort is made to minimize surgery time.

Fatigue failure of the implants is not uncommon. This is especially a problem in adults, where the high loads experienced by the bone–implant construct cause micromotion and cycle the implants. The greater the instability, the greater the probability of fatigue failure. Bone-to-bone contact is imperative at the caudal cortex. If that is not achieved, cyclic loading fatigue failure is inevitable (Fig. 97-14). Methods to reduce the likelihood of fatigue failure include using the strongest implants available and plate luting. Anatomic reconstruction of the fracture, especially at the caudal cortex, is an absolute necessity.

To prevent support limb complications, an early return to weightbearing on the fractured limb is best accomplished by restoring stability to the fracture site and preventing infection. In foals, the primary concern is for varus limb deformity and fatigue of the suspensory apparatus resulting in fetlock hyperextension. To reduce these complications, a foot plate with an extended heel and lateral bearing surface is applied. Support bandages are not advocated in foals because they tend to promote fetlock hyperextension rather than prevent it. In adults, to preclude support limb laminitis, appropriate footing is helpful. In addition, heart bar shoes are used, which reduce the frequency of support limb laminitis. Support wraps and judicious use of phenylbutazone are recommended in adults during the postoperative period.

OSTEOCHONDROMA

Osteochondromas originate from the dysplastic growth of aberrant growth cartilage. They are located adjacent to a physis and occur most commonly in adult horses at the caudal aspect of the distal radius.[17-19] Solitary osteochondromas have been reported in two foals; in one the calcaneus was affected, and in the other the distal palmar aspect of the middle phalanx was affected.[20,21]

Osteochondromas are exostoses composed of trabecular bone contiguous with cancellous bone of the adjacent medullary cavity. There is a characteristic cartilage cap composed of hyaline cartilage undergoing endochondral ossification. The histologic characteristics are identical to those of multiple cartilaginous exostoses of horses. However, the genesis of the lesion in the latter condition is hereditary. To date, a hereditary basis for solitary osteochondroma has not been identified.[22]

Pathogenesis

Causes of solitary osteochondroma include displacement of a growth cartilage fragment that rotates and grows transverse to the longitudinal axis of the bone, aberrant nest of subperiosteal growth cartilage, and herniation of growth cartilage through a perichondral defect. With continued growth, the expansile nature of the lesion impinges on adjacent structures and results in lameness. Osteochondromas of the caudal distal radial physis are located in the carpal canal and cause tenosynovitis. They also impinge on the deep digital flexor tendon as it passes through the area.[17-19] Bony projections that are not true osteochondromas, referred to as physeal remnant spikes, have been noted to cause the same clinical syndrome (see Chapter 96).[22,23]

Diagnosis

Horses with distal radial osteochondromas or physeal spikes are presented with effusion in the carpal canal. Lameness is mild and intermittent. Pain is evident on direct palpation and is induced by carpal flexion. In some cases, the bony projection can be identified by deep palpation. Radiography reveals the characteristic bone growth on the palmar aspect

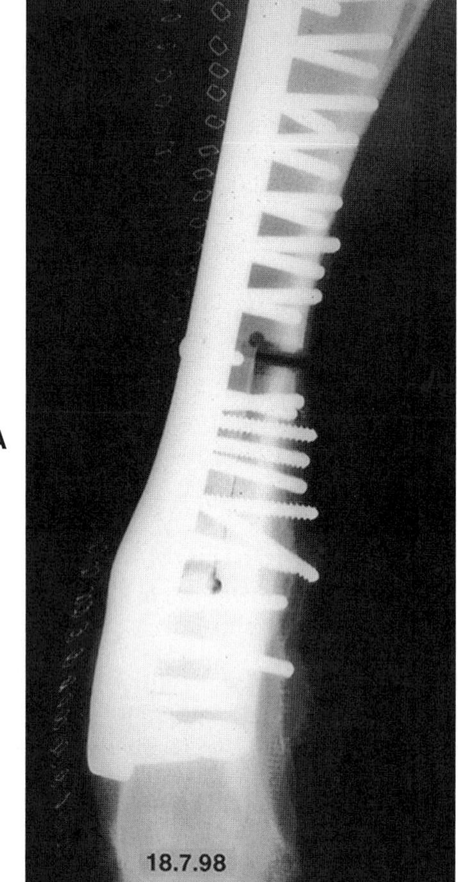

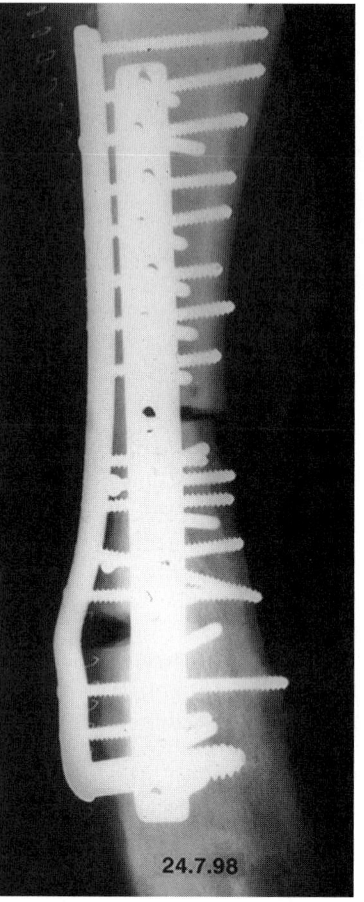

Figure 97-14. A, Lateromedial radiograph of corrective step osteotomy performed in the frontal plane of an adult Warmblood suffering from a severe varus deformity of the radius following abnormal healing of a radial fracture. Note the gap at the caudal osteotomy site. **B**, A 1-week follow-up radiograph showing narrowing of the gap at the caudal cortex and widening of the gap cranially. Screw loosening can be seen at the level of the proximal osteotomy in the lateral plate. Two days later, the dynamic condylar screw (DCS) plate broke at the level of the osteotomy, resulting in humane destruction of the animal. (Courtesy J. Auer, University of Zurich.)

of the radius adjacent to the physis (Fig. 97-15). There is a wide variation in the size and degree of ossification of the lesion. Ultrasonography can aid in determining the presence of deep digital flexor tendinitis. However, the absence of ultrasonographic changes does not preclude the presence of superficial injury to the tendon due to impingement by the osteochondroma or physeal spike.

Treatment

Instillation of corticosteroids into the tendon sheath temporarily resolves tenosynovitis in most instances. However, clinical signs usually recur. Surgical excision of the bony projection is curative and is the treatment of choice. Although excision via an open approach to the lateral aspect of the carpal canal was originally reported,[15] removal under arthroscopic guidance is currently advocated.[18,19]

With the affected limb positioned uppermost, the arthroscope is placed into the proximal aspect of the carpal canal through a stab incision located 3.5 cm proximal to the level of the physeal scar between the lateral digital extensor and ulnaris lateralis muscles.[19] Although a medial approach has been described, the surgeon is less likely to injure the median artery and vein from a lateral approach. Furthermore, the lateral approach makes it technically easier to manipulate the scope and instruments without interference from the opposite limb.

Once the arthroscope is in the carpal canal, the sheath is distended and the osteochondroma or physeal spike is readily identified (Fig. 97-16). The bony projection's attachment to the underlying bone is severed with a small osteotome positioned through a separate stab incision distal to the scope portal, and the bony projection is removed. Release of the carpal flexor retinaculum can also be accomplished via endoscopic guidance if chronic distention of the carpal canal is diagnosed as a complicating problem. The bone bed is curetted and the sheath is lavaged before closure of the skin incisions. Postoperative care is routine.

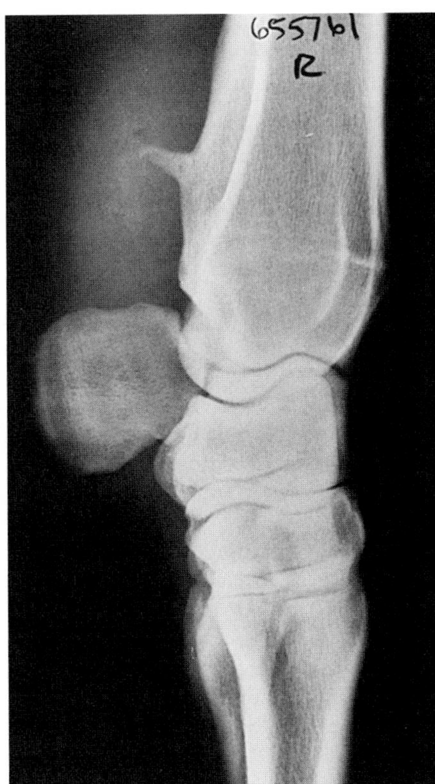

Figure 97-15. Lateromedial radiograph demonstrating a solitary osteochondroma of the caudal aspect of the radius adjacent to the physeal scar.

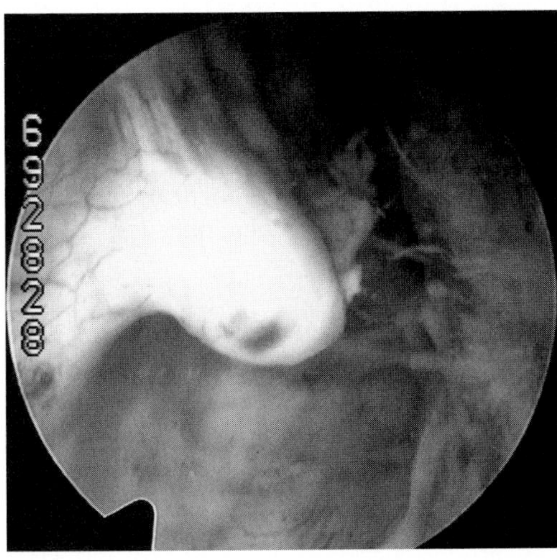

Figure 97-16. Endoscopic view of caudal radial osteochondroma before removal.

Prognosis

Horses are reported by their owners to be sound for their intended purpose following removal of the osteochondroma or physeal spike.[17-19,22,23] Distention of the carpal canal resolves. With chronic carpal canal distention, resolution of the effusion following osteochondroma removal can require additional medical therapy, including local corticosteroid injection.

REFERENCES

1. Donecker JM, Bramlage LR, Gabel AA: Retrospective analysis of 29 fractures of the olecranon process of the equine ulna, J Am Vet Med Assoc 1984;185:183.
2. Wilson DG, Riedesel E: Nonsurgical management of ulnar fractures in the horse: A retrospective study of 43 cases, Vet Surg 1985;14:283.
3. Milne DW, Turner AS: An Atlas of Surgical Approaches to the Bones of the Horse, Philadelphia, 1979, WB Saunders.
4. Smith BL, Auer JA, Taylor TS, et al: Use of orthopedic markers for quantitative determination of proximal radial and ulnar growth in foals, Am J Vet Res 1991;52:1456.
5. Clem MF, DeBowes RM, Douglass JP, et al: The effects of fixation of the ulna to the radius in young foals, Vet Surg 1988;17:338.
6. Denny HR, Barr ARS, Waterman A: Surgical treatment of fractures of the olecranon in the horse: A comparative review of 25 cases, Equine Vet J 1987;19:319.
7. Anderson DE, Allen D, DeBowes RM: Comminuted, articular fractures of the olecranon process in horses: 17 cases, Vet Comp Orthop Traumatol 1995;8:141.
8. Swor TM, Watkins JP, Bahr A, et al: Results of plate fixation of type 1b olecranon fractures in 24 horses, Equine Vet J 2003;35:670.
9. Martin F, Richardson DW, Nunamaker DM, et al: Use of tension band wires in horses with fractures of the ulna: 22 cases (1980-1992), J Am Vet Med Assoc 1995;207:1085.
10. Auer JA, Watkins JP: Treatment of radial fractures in adult horses: An analysis of 15 clinical cases, Equine Vet J 1987;19:103.
11. Martin BB, Reef VB: Conservative treatment of a minimally displaced fracture of the radius of a horse, J Am Vet Med Assoc 1987;191:847.
12. Barr ARS, Denny HR: Three cases of non-displaced radial fracture in horses, Vet Rec 1989;125:35.
13. Derungs S, Fuerst A, Haas C, et al. Fissure fractures of the radius and tibia in 23 horses: A retrospective study, Equine Vet Educ 2001;13:313.
14. Baxter GM, Moore JN, Budsberg SC: Repair of an open radial fracture in an adult horse, J Am Vet Med Assoc 1991;199:364.
15. Schneider RK, Andrea R, Barnes HG: Use of antibiotic-impregnated polymethyl methacrylate for treatment of an open radial fracture in a horse, J Am Vet Med Assoc 1995;207:1454.
16. Sanders-Shamis M, Bramlage LR, Gable AA: Radius fractures in the horse: A retrospective study of 47 cases, Equine Vet J 1986;18:432.
17. Held JP, Patton CS, Shires M: Solitary osteochondroma of the radius in three horses, J Am Vet Med Assoc 1988;193:563.
18. Squire KRE, Adams SB, Widmer WR, et al: Arthroscopic removal of a palmar radial osteochondroma causing carpal canal syndrome in a horse, J Am Vet Med Assoc 1992;201:1216.
19. Southwood LL, Stashak TS, Fehr JE, et al: Lateral approach for endoscopic removal of solitary osteochondromas from the distal radial metaphysis in three horses, J Am Vet Med Assoc 1997;210:1166.
20. Chan CC-H, Munroe GA, Callanan JJ: Congenital solitary osteochondroma affecting the tarsus in a filly foal, Equine Vet Educ 1996;8:153.
21. Easter JL, Watkins JP, Berridge B, et al: A digital osteochondroma as the cause of lameness in a foal, Vet Comp Orthop Traumatol 1998;11:44.
22. McIlwraith CW: Osteochondromas and physeal remnant spikes in the carpal canal, Equine Proc Am Coll Vet Surg 2002;12:168.
23. Nixon AJ, Schachter BL, Pool RR: Exostoses of the caudal perimeter of the radial physis as a cause of carpal synovial sheath tenosynovitis and lameness in horses: 10 horses, J Am Vet Med Assoc 2004;224:264.

CHAPTER 98

Shoulder

Lisa A. Fortier

Orthopedic abnormalities of the scapulohumeral (shoulder) joint are rare. Because shoulder pathologies are uncommon and relatively difficult to diagnose, treatment can be delayed, leading to an increase in secondary osteoarthritis. Further, there are very few large studies documenting treatment and outcome following specific injuries or treatments to guide the surgeon.

DIAGNOSIS OF SHOULDER LAMENESS

Localization of lameness to the shoulder region can be straightforward in cases when there is associated swelling or pain on palpation, but in many cases intra-articular or bursal anesthesia is necessary to confirm clinical examination findings. Horses with fractures of the shoulder region or luxation of the scapulohumeral joint are acutely, and initially, severely lame and have localized swelling. When the scapulohumeral joint is less severely affected, joint effusion cannot be palpated because of the overlying musculature, but a painful response can often be elicited following deep palpation of the notch between the cranial and caudal prominences of the greater tubercle of the humerus. Horses with biceps tendinitis or intertubercular bursitis (bicipital bursitis) often exhibit moderate pain when the biceps tendon or muscle is grasped and palpated. Less-specific signs of shoulder lameness include shoulder muscle atrophy, pain on extension or flexion of the shoulder joint, a narrow ipsilateral hoof with a long heel, and, typical of forelimb lameness, signs of a shortened anterior phase of the stride. Nuclear scintigraphy can help localize the cause of a subtle lameness to the shoulder joint.

When the lameness is localized to the shoulder region, radiographs should be obtained. If bicipital bursitis or biceps tendinitis is suspected, an ultrasonographic examination should be performed.[1] Although not currently available for imaging equine shoulders, magnetic resonance imaging (MRI) is considered the method of choice for evaluation of shoulder pain in people because it provides detailed information on all bone and soft-tissue components of the shoulder.[2]

Radiographs of the shoulder joint usually can be obtained in the standing horse, although higher-quality images are achieved when the horse is under general anesthesia because of the absence of motion artifact. The horse's leg is extended forward to center the shoulder joint over the trachea for a mediolateral projection. Normal survey radiographs do not exclude the shoulder as a cause of lameness, particularly in cases of osteochondrosis (OC) or other cartilaginous pathologies of the humeral head or glenoid cavity.[3,4] In cases where survey radiographs are normal and OC is suspected, positive-contrast radiography using 7 to 10 mL of a sterile water-soluble iodinated contrast medium should be performed.[5] Double-contrast radiography more clearly delineates the glenoid notch than positive-contrast radiography. To obtain a double-contrast image, 30 mL of air is injected following positive-contrast radiography.

INTRASYNOVIAL ANESTHESIA OR SYNOVIAL CENTESIS

When clinical examination findings do not definitively localize the lameness to the shoulder joint or bicipital bursa, diagnostic intrasynovial anesthesia can be useful. Local anesthetic (20 mL) is delivered into the shoulder joint using an 18-gauge, 8.9-cm spinal needle inserted in the notch between the cranial and caudal prominences of the greater tubercle of the humerus. The needle is directed toward the elbow of the opposite limb, parallel to the ground, and is advanced until bone or cartilage is contacted. Extrasynovial deposition or leakage of local anesthetic solution out of the shoulder joint can block the suprascapular nerve, resulting in lateral subluxation of the scapulohumeral joint, thereby producing the clinical appearance of sweeney. If the suprascapular nerve is inadvertently blocked, the horse should be placed in a box stall until the anesthetic wears off to prevent injury. In horses with intact cartilage that covers subchondral bone abnormalities, there might be minimal or no improvement in lameness following intra-articular anesthesia.

The bicipital bursa is entered approximately 4 cm proximal to the distal aspect of the deltoid tuberosity. An 18-gauge, 8.9-cm spinal needle is inserted between the biceps brachii muscle and the humerus and directed proximomedial to approximately 4 cm in depth, where 5 to 10 mL of local anesthetic is injected. Synovial fluid can usually be aspirated from both the shoulder joint and bicipital bursa to confirm intrasynovial needle placement and therefore deposition of local anesthetic or for synovial fluid analysis and culture in cases where infection is suspected.

OSTEOCHONDROSIS

Osteochondrosis (OC) occurs in the shoulder joint less often than in other sites such as the tarsocrural or femoropatellar joint. Clinical signs usually appear in horses 6 to 12 months old, and the lesions can be bilateral. Clinical examination in combination with conventional or contrast radiography reveals that the majority of shoulder OC lesions in horses are osteochondritis dissecans (OCD) lesions (cartilage flaps). Typical radiographic signs include irregular areas of subchondral bone with radiolucent areas surrounded by sclerosis. Contrast radiography more clearly delineates the presence and extent of undermined cartilage flaps and aids in determining a more accurate preoperative prognosis than one based on plain radiographs alone (Fig. 98-1). Subtle cartilage lesions might not be detected using current imaging modalities, and diagnostic arthroscopy should be used if clinical examination, intra-articular anesthesia, or nuclear scintigraphy implicates the shoulder joint as the source of lameness.[4]

Secondary osteoarthritis (OA) develops rapidly in cases of shoulder OCD, and radiographs should be carefully scruti-

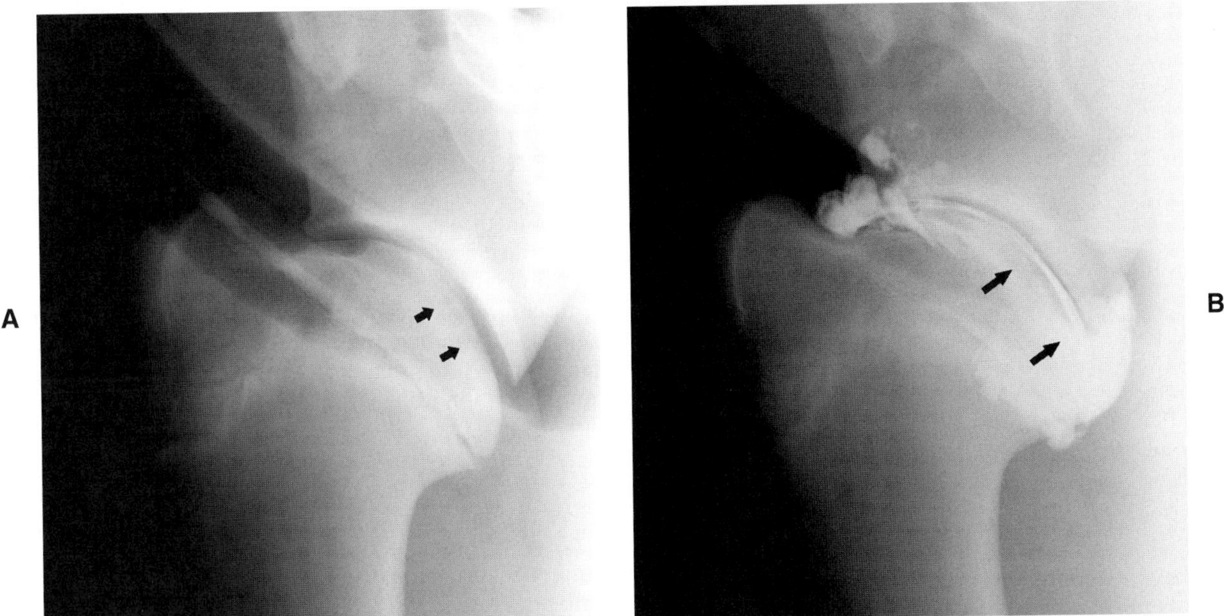

Figure 98-1. **A**, Mediolateral radiograph of the shoulder joint. A subchondral lucent region is present in the caudal humeral head *(arrows)*. The humeral head in this region also appears flattened. **B**, A positive contrast arthrogram of the same shoulder joint depicted in **A**. Contrast material outlines the shoulder joint and further delineates the extent of subchondral bone lysis *(arrows)*.

nized preoperatively for signs of OA, because the prognosis for future athletic function is poor in affected horses. Radiographic signs of shoulder OA include flattening of the humeral head and glenoid cavity, remodeling of the caudal rim of the glenoid, and subchondral bone sclerosis of the humeral head or glenoid cavity.[3]

Treatment

Arthroscopic surgery with débridement of loose cartilage flaps and curettage of abnormal underlying subchondral bone is the treatment of choice for shoulder OCD lesions. Repair of cartilage flaps using polydioxanone pins has been successful in select cases of OCD involving the femoropatellar and metacarpophalangeal joints and should be considered for cases of shoulder OCD.[6] Only cases with smooth, partially attached, unmineralized cartilage flaps should be considered for repair with polydioxanone pins.

Arthroscopy of the shoulder joint is technically more challenging than other joints. Lateral and craniolateral approaches have been reported.[7-9] The lateral approach is described here because it provides maximal visualization of the medial aspect of the humeral head and leaves the cranial portal (cranial to the infraspinatus tendon and proximal to the notch between the cranial and caudal prominences of the greater tubercle of the humerus) open for insertion of an egress cannula. The open cranial portal can also be used to introduce a large curved forceps, which can be engaged in the glenoid notch to distract the humeral head and gain access with the arthroscope to the medial side of the joint.

To perform shoulder arthroscopy, the horse is placed in lateral recumbency with the affected limb uppermost. The leg should be draped to allow adduction and traction during surgery in order to increase surgical exposure. The joint is distended with 60 mL lactated Ringer's solution using an 18-gauge, 8.9-cm spinal needle inserted in the notch between the cranial and caudal prominences of the greater tubercle of the humerus (this site becomes the cranial portal). The arthroscope is inserted 1 to 2 cm caudal to the infraspinatus tendon and cranial to the teres minor muscles. A third site 2 to 4 cm caudal to the arthroscope portal can be used as an instrument portal. The optimal site for instrument portal entry is determined using an 18-gauge, 8.9-cm spinal needle. If the lesions are extensive, or if they occur on the humeral head and glenoid cavity, more than one instrument portal might be required to complete the surgical débridement.

Cartilage flaps are removed and subchondral bone is débrided using several instruments including Ferris-Smith rongeurs, motorized resectors, periosteal elevators, and curets (Fig. 98-2). Lesions on the most medial aspect of the humeral head might be inaccessible. When débridement is complete, the joint is lavaged to remove cartilage and bone debris and the skin incisions are closed routinely.

Antibiotics and phenylbutazone are administered perioperatively, and phenylbutazone is continued for the next 5 to 10 days. Horses are restricted to stall rest for 14 days, at which time hand-walking begins for 5 minutes per day. After 30 days of stall rest with hand-walking, horses are turned out for 4 to 6 months before exercise is resumed.

Prognosis

The prognosis for return to soundness depends on the severity of the lesion and the presence of concomitant OA. The prognosis is poor when OA is detected on preoperative radiographs or when lesions are present on both the humeral head and opposing glenoid cavity. Typically, lesions identified during arthroscopy are more extensive than suggested by radiography.[4,7] The prognosis is fair to poor in horses with bilateral lesions, regardless of lesion size. However, in

A

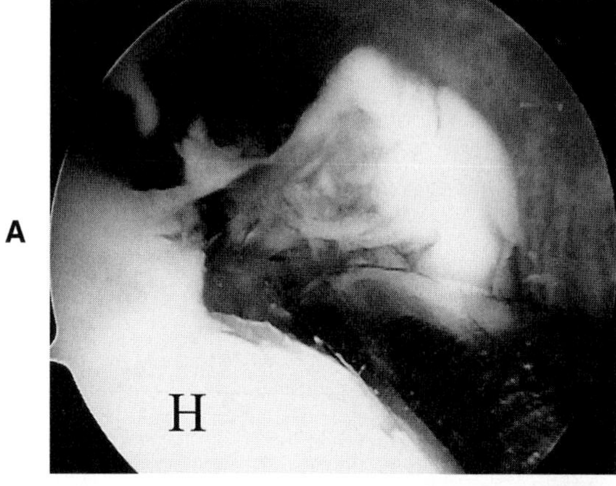

B

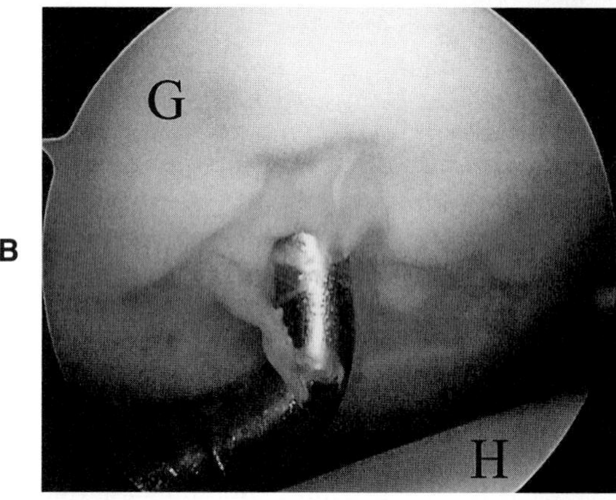

C

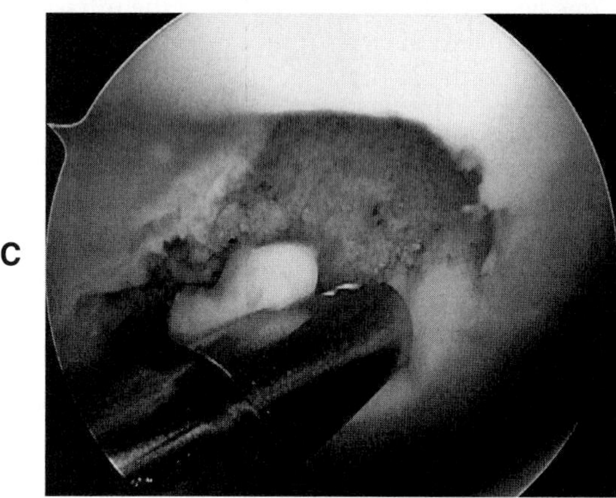

Figure 98-2. **A**, An arthroscopic image demonstrating elevation of an osteochondritis dissecans lesion of the humeral head (H). **B**, A probe inserted into a cystic defect in the glenoid cavity (G); humeral head (H). **C**, Use of a motorized burr to débride a lesion in the glenoid cavity.

cases where more subtle lesions are present, the prognosis for return to athletic function is good, even for middle-aged horses.[4]

FRACTURE OF THE SUPRAGLENOID TUBERCLE

Supraglenoid tubercle fractures are usually simple, intra-articular epiphyseal fractures. These fractures occur most commonly in horses younger than 2 years of age and are either the result of direct trauma or are avulsion fractures caused by tension from the biceps tendon, which originates on the supraglenoid tubercle. Horses with supraglenoid tubercle fractures are able to bear weight, but they are variably lame and reluctant to fully extend the affected limb.

Careful visual inspection and palpation of the cranial aspect of the shoulder will be suggestive of a supraglenoid tubercle fracture. In chronic cases, shoulder muscle atrophy will be present. Radiography of the shoulder is diagnostic. On a mediolateral projection, the fracture fragment is typically displaced in a cranioventral direction as a result of tension from the biceps brachii and coracobrachialis muscles, which originate on the supraglenoid tubercle (Fig. 98-3). The radiographs should be carefully evaluated for signs of OA (described previously), which will decrease the prognosis for athletic function.

Treatment

Several treatment options are available, and the therapy chosen will depend on the duration of the fracture and the intended use of the horse. Conservative management for all but the smallest fractures typically results in residual lameness and OA of the shoulder joint. Surgical options include repair of the fracture or removal of the fracture fragment. The goal of surgical repair should focus on restoring articular congruity of the glenoid cavity to prevent the development of OA. Therefore, if the fracture is chronic (longer than 1 week), enough bone remodeling will have occurred to preclude accurate reduction of the fracture, and the fragment should be removed. In acute fractures, if a substantial (one third or greater) portion of the glenoid cavity is involved, internal fixation should be considered to reconstruct the glenoid articular surface and provide maximal opportunity for future athletic performance. Acute

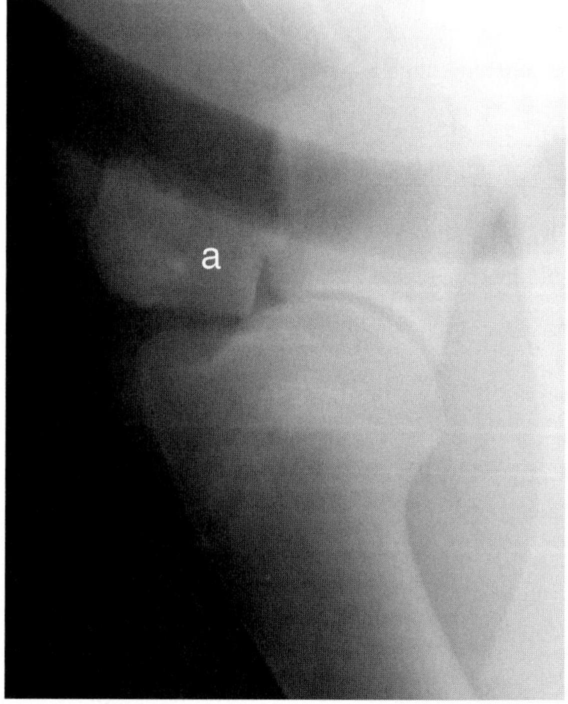

Figure 98-3. Mediolateral radiograph of the shoulder joint. A displaced fracture of the supraglenoid tubercle *(a)* is seen. The fracture fragment is displaced cranially and ventrally.

fracture fragments that involve only a small portion of the glenoid cavity can be removed with no apparent impact on future athletic performance.

Fracture Fragment Removal

The horse is placed in lateral recumbency with the affected limb uppermost. A 20-cm skin incision is made, beginning at the distal extent of the scapular spine, centering over the cranial aspect of the point of the shoulder, and extending distally over the deltoid tuberosity. The brachiocephalicus and supraspinatus muscles are separated and retracted; the brachiocephalicus is retracted caudally and the supraspinatus cranially.[10,11]

At this point, repeated palpation will guide the surgeon to the shoulder joint and fracture fragment. Care should be taken to identify and preserve the suprascapular nerve, artery, and vein as they course across the neck of the scapula. The articular surface of the humeral head and glenoid cavity should be inspected for signs of cartilage damage, which will diminish the prognosis for athletic function. The fracture fragment is grasped with a large bone-holding forceps and excised using a combination of blunt and sharp dissection to detach the muscular and tendinous attachments. The dissection can be challenging, particularly on the medial aspect of the fragment because of lack of visualization.

Following removal of the fragment, the area is lavaged and closed in several layers to diminish dead space. If substantial dead space remains, a closed suction device should be used to prevent development of a postoperative seroma. Assisted recovery from anesthesia is recommended. Antibiotics and phenylbutazone are administered perioperatively and continued until the there are no clinical signs of seroma formation.

Horses are restricted to stall rest for 60 days to allow time for the dead space to fill with fibrous tissue and the biceps to reattach. A carefully controlled rehabilitation program is important for these horses to regain strength and coordination in their shoulder joints. Percutaneous stimulation of the shoulder muscles during rehabilitation to minimize muscle atrophy should be considered. In humans, percutaneous muscle stimulation has been shown to minimize muscle atrophy after stroke or spinal cord injury.[12] Typically, physical therapy begins with range-of-motion exercises and hand-walking for 5 minutes per day, followed by walking over ground poles and gradual increases in duration of exercise each day. Horses are not usually ready to return to training or to be turned out into a paddock for 6 to 12 months after surgery.

Fracture Fixation

A variety of techniques have been described for internal fixation of supraglenoid tubercle fractures.[10,11,13,14] Tension from the biceps tendon is the primary force that needs to be neutralized when performing internal fixation. Partial or full transection of the biceps tendon to prevent tension on the fracture repair and facilitate internal fixation has been described,[11] but it is not routinely recommended.

The fracture site is approached as described previously for fragment removal. The fractured bone ends are débrided and the fracture is reduced using large bone-reduction forceps.

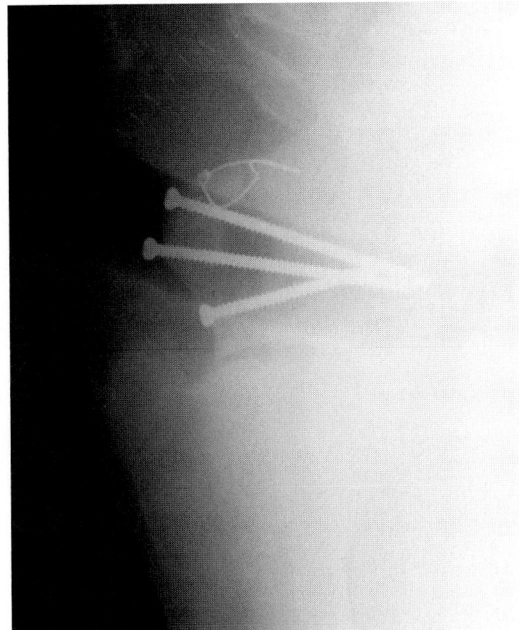

Figure 98-4. Internal fixation of a supraglenoid tubercle fracture using three 5.5-mm cancellous bone screws and a tension band wire. (Courtesy Alan J. Nixon, Cornell University.)

The fracture is repaired using two or three 5.5-mm cortical bone screws placed in lag fashion. Care is taken to implant the screws in a somewhat diverging pattern to increase resistance to the axial tension on the implants. Additional support is provided by tension band wiring between the supraglenoid tubercle and the cranial edge of the scapula using large-diameter (1.5-mm) wire[13,14] (Fig. 98-4). Wound closure and immediate postoperative care are similar to that described for fracture fragment removal.

Following internal fixation, horses are confined to a box stall for at least 8 weeks, until postoperative radiographs indicate sufficient fracture healing. An intense rehabilitation program involving physical therapy and a controlled exercise protocol should be prescribed until shoulder musculature returns to normal, at which time training may be resumed.

Prognosis

Return to athletic function depends on the amount of cartilage damage present at the time of surgery and, in cases where the fracture fragment is removed, the amount of glenoid cavity removed with the fracture fragment. Both of these factors are assumed to be directly related to development of shoulder OA. The few reports that are available regarding supraglenoid tubercle fractures in the horse suggest that the prognosis for athletic function is fair following either fracture removal or internal fixation but poor with conservative treatment.[10,11]

MISCELLANEOUS OTHER FRACTURES

Fractures of the neck or body of the scapula or proximal humerus are rare but have been described.[15,16] These fractures are usually the result of trauma, and horses are variably lame.

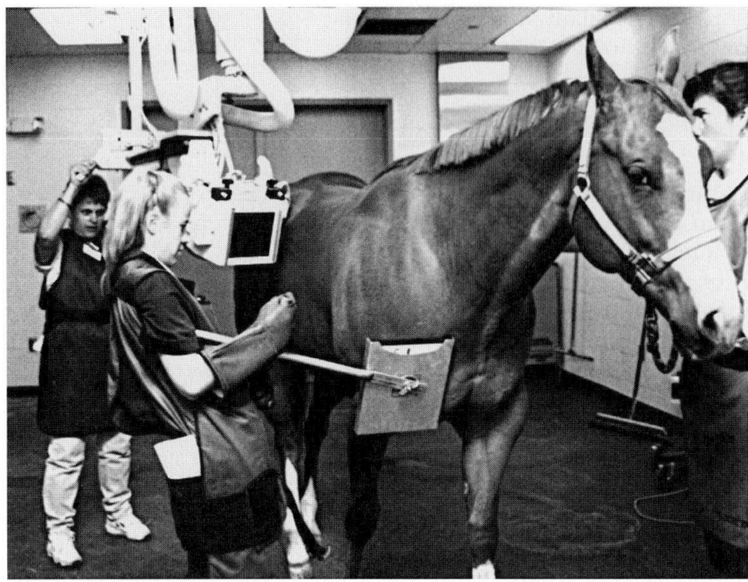

Figure 98-5. The position for obtaining a skyline view of the lateral tuberosity of the proximal humerus is shown. The x-ray beam is directed from a caudal to a cranial direction.

The cranial and caudal aspects of the greater tubercle of the proximal humerus can fracture in different configurations. If the entire greater tubercle fractures transversely, the scapulohumeral joint can luxate. When clinical examination or nuclear scintigraphy suggests involvement of the greater tubercle, a skyline radiograph of the proximal humerus should be obtained to diagnose the fracture (Fig. 98-5). Depending on the size of the fracture fragment and the muscular attachments involved, the fragment may be treated conservatively, removed, or repaired using cortex or shaft screws placed in lag fashion.

Horses with complete fractures of the body of the scapula or scapular neck will be unable to bear weight. A standing mediolateral radiograph with the affected limb pulled forward will reveal the fracture site. If the neck of the scapula is involved, function of the suprascapular nerve should be evaluated (described later in "Suprascapular Nerve Injury"). Internal fixation of complete fractures of the scapula has been described using two plates, one on each side of the scapular spine.[16,17] Incomplete fractures can be managed conservatively.[18]

SCAPULOHUMERAL JOINT LUXATION

Scapulohumeral joint luxations are rare in horses and are traumatic in origin. Because of their traumatic nature, concurrent fractures of the scapula or proximal humerus can occur.[19] The horses are non-weight-bearing and might have shoulder atrophy if the luxation is chronic. The humeral head can be palpated lateral, or less commonly cranial, to the scapula. Standing craniocaudal to mediolateral oblique-view radiographs best demonstrate the luxation (Fig. 98-6). The radiographs should be carefully evaluated for fractures

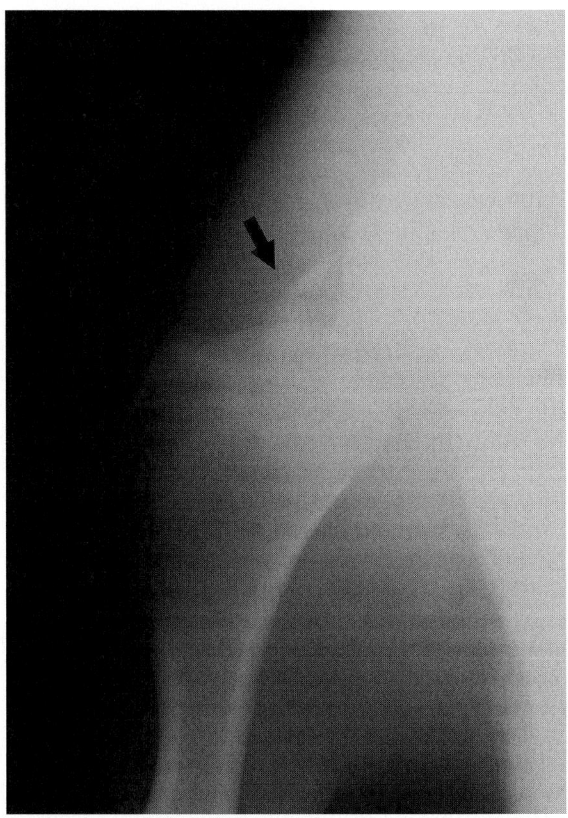

Figure 98-6. A craniocaudal to mediolateral oblique view of the shoulder joint. A scapulohumeral luxation is present, with the humeral head located lateral to the glenoid cavity. A concurrent fracture, presumably originating from the glenoid, is present *(arrow)*.

of the humeral head or scapula, particularly involving the lateral rim of the glenoid.

Treatment

Closed reduction followed by scapulohumeral joint arthroscopy to evaluate the articular surfaces and remove cartilage debris resulted in return to sound performance in one case.[20] Closed reduction should be attempted before an open approach is performed to preserve intact lateral musculature of the shoulder joint and minimize the potential for re-luxation of the shoulder joint postoperatively. Open reduction should be combined with some form of internal fixation such as scapulohumeral tension wires, although most types of internal fixation eventually fail.[19]

The ultimate outcome for most horses with scapulohumeral luxation is shoulder OA and severe lameness, resulting in euthanasia. Arthrodesis of the scapulohumeral joint has been successful in one small (250 kg) horse[21] and in miniature horses.[22,23] Arthrodesis is accomplished using a narrow dynamic compression plate contoured to the cranial surface of the scapula and cranial aspect of the humerus.[23] For more information, review Chapter 85.

Prognosis

There are very few reports detailing repair of scapulohumeral joint luxation, but the prognosis for soundness following repair appears to be poor because of resultant crippling shoulder OA.

PATHOLOGIES OF THE INTERTUBERCULAR BURSA AND BICEPS BRACHII

The biceps brachii muscle originates on the supraglenoid tubercle as a bilobed, tendinous structure, and it inserts, again as a tendon, on the medial radial tuberosity. It passes over the proximal, cranial aspect of the humerus, where it is bound to the intertubercular groove by a tendinous part of the superficial pectoral muscle. The intertubercular (bicipital) bursa lies between the proximal biceps tendon and the humerus.[24]

Horses with bicipital bursitis or biceps tendinitis exhibit pain when the biceps is grasped and pulled laterally. Nuclear scintigraphy can be helpful in any of the vascular, soft tissue, or bone phases, but a definitive diagnosis requires intrasynovial anesthesia. After localizing the lameness to the biceps region, an ultrasonographic and radiographic examination of the biceps region should be obtained. Normal ultrasonographic morphology of the biceps tendon and bicipital bursa have been reported.[25] Skyline radiographs of the proximal humerus are required to identify concurrent lesions involving the humeral tubercles (Fig. 98-7).

Various pathologies have been reported in association with the biceps tendon or bicipital bursa including bursitis,[26-28] tendinitis,[26] ossifying tendinitis,[29] medial displacement of the biceps tendon,[30] and infectious bursitis.[31,32] Simple biceps tendinitis is managed conservatively, but surgical intervention should be considered for horses with idiopathic or infectious bursitis or with chronic bicipital bursitis.

Treatment

Endoscopy

Infection of the bicipital bursa should be addressed using endoscopy and systemic antimicrobials. Endoscopy permits a thorough exploration of the infected bursa as well as a means of copious lavage and removal of adhesions. Synovial resection should be considered; however, it is controversial in cases of septic arthritis.

Endoscopy of the bicipital bursa in normal and infected bursae has been described.[31,33] The horse is positioned in lateral recumbency, with the affected limb uppermost. The bursa is distended with 100 mL lactated Ringer's solution as described under "Intrasynovial Anesthesia."

The arthroscope is inserted into the distal aspect of the bursa through a skin incision placed 2 to 3 cm proximal to the deltoid tuberosity on the dorsolateral aspect of the humerus. The arthroscope is advanced proximomedially through the brachiocephalicus muscle, beneath the biceps brachii muscle, and along the cranial surface of the humerus. When the distended bursa is entered, and fluid escapes from the cannula, the obturator is removed and replaced with the arthroscope. The instrument portal site is predetermined by placement of a spinal needle in the proximal aspect of the bursa, lateral to the biceps tendon. The bursa is explored and any foreign debris and adhesions are removed.

The type and duration of antibiotic and anti-inflammatory medications administered will depend on the presence or absence of sepsis. Similarly, postoperative rehabilitation and return to training or performance will be related to the degree of tendinitis or bursitis.

Biceps Tendon Transection

A combination of bicipital bursitis, biceps tendinitis, and humeral osteitis has been reported in horses.[27,28] This disease complex is thought to be a manifestation of chronic bursitis or tendinitis and can be infectious or traumatic in origin. Affected horses are severely lame and unresponsive to conservative therapy. Ultrasonography of the biceps bursa is consistent with bursitis, and skyline radiographs of the proximal humerus reveal osteolytic changes associated with the lateral tuberosity.

Complete transection of the biceps tendon results in a fair prognosis for return to soundness.[27] If purulent material is found within the biceps brachii tendon, then a tenectomy should be considered. The approach to the biceps tendon is the same as that described for removal of supraglenoid tubercle fractures. Postoperative management is also similar to that for removal of supraglenoid tubercle fractures because biceps tendon support is lost in both instances. There is, however, less dead space to be filled in by fibrous tissue.

Prognosis

There are too few reports of the various biceps tendon or bursa problems to provide an accurate prognosis. As with most synovial structures, the prognosis for return to sound function ranges from guarded to good depending on the structures involved and the duration of clinical signs.

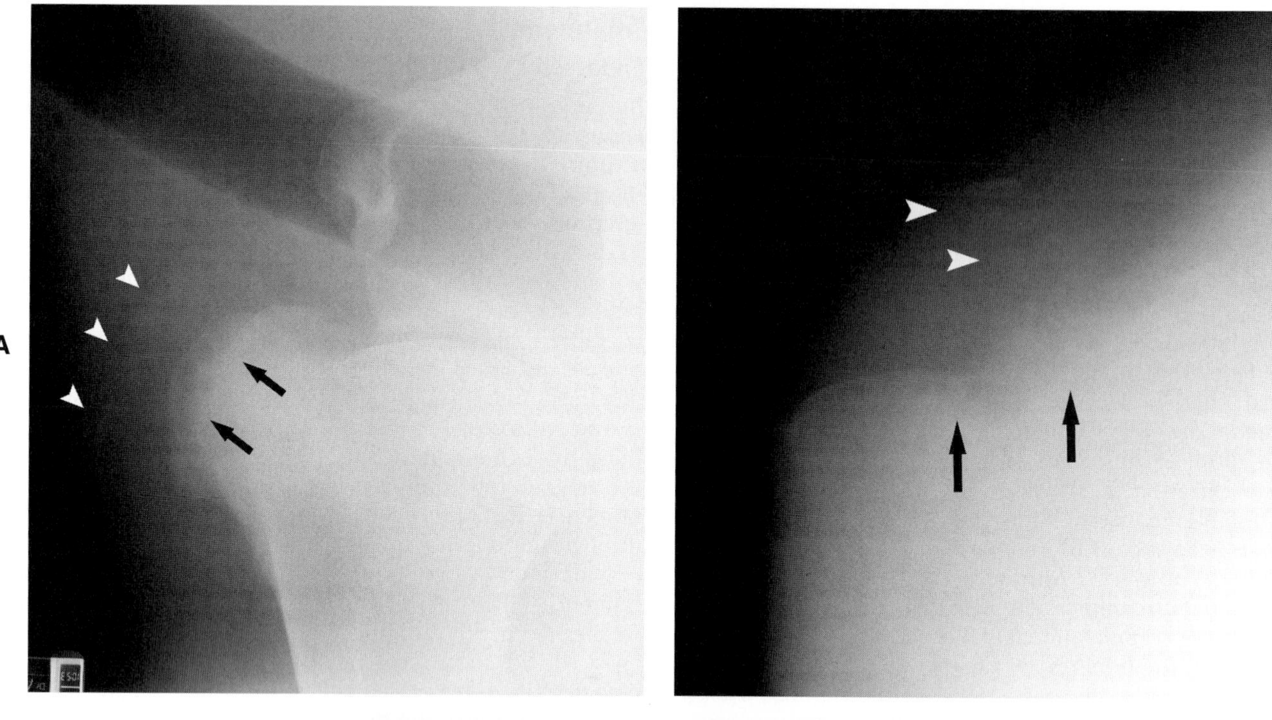

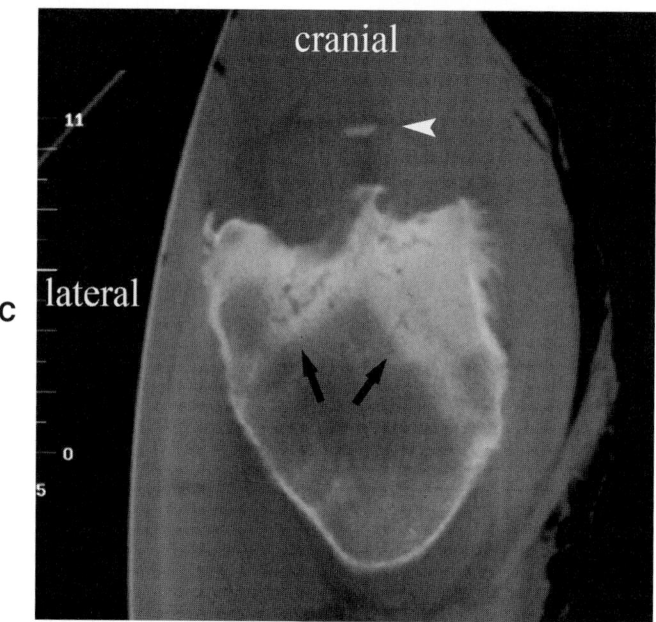

Figure 98-7. **A**, Mediolateral radiographs of the shoulder region. In the intermediate tubercle of the humerus, there are multifocal areas of irregular bone lysis *(black arrows)*. Cranial to the tubercles, there are linear foci of mineralization in the tendon of the biceps brachii *(white arrowheads)*. **B**, Skyline radiographic projection of the cranial proximal humerus. The lysis of the intermediate tubercle and mineralization of the bicipital tendon are confirmed and further defined in this radiographic projection. **C**, Postmortem transverse computed tomography evaluation of the affected shoulder region. The tubercles and medullary cavity of the cranial humerus are sclerotic *(black arrows)*. There is a focal mineral density in the tendon of the biceps *(white arrowhead)*.

SUPRASCAPULAR NERVE INJURY (SWEENEY)

The suprascapular nerve is typically damaged as the result of trauma to the cranial shoulder where the nerve courses across the neck of the scapula. The suprascapular nerve innervates the infraspinatus muscle, which provides the majority of lateral support to the shoulder. As a result, horses with suprascapular nerve injury have a lateral motion or shoulder slip during weightbearing on the affected limb.

If damage to the nerve is severe, the characteristic gait can be apparent immediately following injury, but more typically, a shoulder slip is not apparent for a few days to weeks after injury. Clinical signs do not indicate the degree of nerve damage, and there is no diagnostic method to determine the degree of recovery each horse will achieve.

Electromyography should be used to confirm that the suprascapular nerve, and not the brachial plexus, is the site of injury. Electromyography is only useful to evaluate nerve function from 7 days after injury on.

Treatment

Conservative Management

Conservative management consisting of box stall rest alone results in a good return to function.[34] However, shoulder stability takes an average of 7 months to return. Surgical decompression of the suprascapular nerve can hasten the return of shoulder stability, diminish the amount of shoulder muscle atrophy, and return the horse to function sooner than that accomplished with conservative therapy alone.[34,35]

The potential for a modestly decreased time to function needs to be weighed against the costs and risks associated with surgery, especially given the potential for postoperative supraglenoid tubercle or scapular neck fractures in horses following surgery.[36] A balance between the cost and benefit of each treatment is present in a staged approach consisting of conservative management for 3 months, and if little improvement is noted, then surgical nerve decompression.

Scapular Nerve Decompression

The horse is positioned in lateral recumbency with the affected limb uppermost. A 25-cm skin incision is made over the spine of the scapula and through the cutaneus trunci muscle. Fascia covering the spine of the scapula is incised, and the brachiocephalicus muscle is elevated from the spine of the scapula while preserving the fascia deep to the supraspinatus muscle to protect the suprascapular neurovascular bundle. The nerve is elevated from the scapula, and a small amount of bone is rasped off the cranial margin of the scapula. Care is taken to maintain smooth edges of the bone to decrease potential postoperative nerve injury. A tendinous band that limits the movement of the suprascapular nerve can be palpated on the medial side of the scapula and covering the nerve. This band should be incised to maximize nerve decompression from scar tissue. Incisional closure is routine, with attention to obliteration of dead space.

Assisted recovery from anesthesia is recommended given the shoulder instability and potential for fracture of the supraglenoid tubercle. The potential for postoperative fracture through the notch created in the scapula exists for 6 weeks postoperatively. Antibiotics and phenylbutazone are administered perioperatively, and low-dose phenylbutazone is continued for 3 to 5 days. Horses are confined to a box stall until shoulder stability is returned, typically 2 to 3 months. During stall confinement, muscle stimulation should be considered to minimize muscle atrophy. An intensive rehabilitation program then ensues to build shoulder strength prior to return to riding.

Prognosis

The prognosis for return to sound riding following conservative management or scapular nerve decompression is good.[34,36] Atrophy of the supraspinatus and infraspinatus muscles might not completely resolve in all cases.

REFERENCES

1. Tnibar MA, Auer JA, Bakkali S: Ultrasonography of the equine shoulder: Technique and normal appearance, Vet Radiol Ultrasound 1999;40:44.
2. Tirman PF, Smith ED, Stoller DW, et al: Shoulder imaging in athletes, Semin Musculoskelet Radiol 2004;8:29.
3. Dyson S: Interpreting radiographs 7: Radiology of the equine shoulder and elbow, Equine Vet J 1986;18:352.
4. Doyle PS, White NA: Diagnostic findings and prognosis following arthroscopic treatment of subtle osteochondral lesions in the shoulder joint of horses: 15 cases (1996-1999), J Am Vet Med Assoc 2000;217:1878.
5. Nixon AJ, Spencer CP: Arthrography of the equine shoulder joint, Equine Vet J 1997;22:107.
6. Nixon AJ, Fortier LA, Goodrich LR, et al: Arthroscopic reattachment of osteochondritis dissecans lesions using resorbable polydioxanone pins, Equine Vet J 2004;36:376.
7. McIlwraith CW, Nixon AJ, Wright IM, et al: Diagnostic and surgical arthroscopy of the scapulohumeral (shoulder) joint. In McIlwraith CW, Nixon AJ, Wright IM, Boening KJ, editors: Diagnostic and Surgical Arthroscopy in the Horse, Oxford, 2005, Elsevier Mosby.
8. Bertone AL, McIlwraith CW: Arthroscopic surgery for the treatment of osteochondrosis in the equine shoulder joint, Vet Surg 1987;16:303.
9. Nixon AJ: Diagnostic and operative arthroscopy of the equine shoulder joint, Vet Surg 1986;15:129.
10. Pankowski RL, Grant BD, Sande R, et al: Fracture of the supraglenoid tubercle: Treatment and results in five horses, Vet Surg 1986;15:33.
11. Bleyaert HF, Madison JB: Complete biceps brachii tenotomy to facilitate internal fixation of supraglenoid tubercle fractures in three horses, Vet Surg 1999;28:48.
12. Newsam CJ, Baker LL: Effect of an electric stimulation facilitation program on quadriceps motor unit recruitment after stroke, Arch Phys Med Rehabil 2004;85:2040.
13. Dart AJ, Snyder JR: Repair of a supraglenoid tuberosity fracture in a horse, J Am Vet Med Assoc 1992;201:95.
14. Adams SB: Surgical repair of a supraglenoid tubercle fracture in a horse, J Am Vet Med Assoc 1987;191:332.
15. Dyson S: Sixteen fractures of the shoulder region in the horse, Equine Vet J 1985;17:104.
16. Bukowiecki CF, van Ee RT, Schneiter HL: Internal fixation of comminuted transverse scapular fracture in a foal, J Am Vet Med Assoc 1989;195:781.
17. Shamis LD, Sanders-Shamis M, Bramlage LR: Internal fixation of a transverse scapular neck fracture in a filly, J Am Vet Med Assoc 1989;195:1391.
18. Davidson EJ, Martin BB Jr: Stress fracture of the scapula in two horses, Vet Radiol Ultrasound 2004;45:407.
19. Semevolos SA, Nixon AJ, Goodrich LR, et al: Shoulder joint luxation in large animals: 14 cases (1976-1997), J Am Vet Med Assoc 1998;213:1608.
20. Madison JB, Young D, Richardson D: Repair of shoulder luxation in a horse, J Am Vet Med Assoc 1991;198:455.
21. MacDonald DG, Bailey JV, Fowler JD: Arthrodesis of the scapulohumeral joint in a horse, Can Vet J 1995;36:312.
22. Arighi M, Miller CR, Pennock PW: Arthrodesis of the scapulohumeral joint in a miniature horse, J Am Vet Med Assoc 1987;191:713.
23. Semevolos SA, Watkins JP, Auer JA: Scapulohumeral arthrodesis in miniature horses, Vet Surg 2003;32:416.
24. Gyuru F, Zajer J: An anatomical study of the tendon of the equine biceps brachii muscle, Acta Vet Acad Sci Hung 1982;30:147.
25. Crabill MR, Chaffin MK, Schmitz DG: Ultrasonographic morphology of the bicipital tendon and bursa in clinically normal Quarter Horses, Am J Vet Res 1995;56:5.

26. Dyson SJ, Dik KJ: Miscellaneous conditions of tendons, tendon sheaths, and ligaments, Vet Clin North Am Equine Pract 1995;11:315.
27. Fugaro MN, Adams SB: Biceps brachii tenotomy or tenectomy for the treatment of bicipital bursitis, tendonitis, and humeral osteitis in 3 horses, J Am Vet Med Assoc 2002;220:1508.
28. Bohn A, Papageorges M, Grant BD: Ultrasonographic evaluation and surgical treatment of humeral osteitis and bicipital tenosynovitis in a horse, J Am Vet Med Assoc 1992;201:305.
29. Meagher DM, Pool RR, Brown MP: Bilateral ossification of the tendon of the biceps brachii muscle in the horse, J Am Vet Med Assoc 174:282, 1979.
30. McDiarmid A: Medial displacement of the biceps brachii in a foal: Clinical, pathological and comparative aspects, Equine Vet J 1997;29:156.
31. Tudor RA, Bowman KF, Redding WR, et al: Endoscopic treatment of suspected infectious intertubercular bursitis in a horse, J Am Vet Med Assoc 1998;213:1584, 1570.
32. Vatistas NJ, Pascoe JR, Wright IM, et al: Infection of the intertubercular bursa in horses: Four cases (1978-1991), J Am Vet Med Assoc 1996;208:1434.
33. Adams MN, Turner TA: Endoscopy of the intertubercular bursa in horses, J Am Vet Med Assoc 1999;214:221, 205.
34. Dutton DM, Honnas CM, Watkins JP: Nonsurgical treatment of suprascapular nerve injury in horses: 8 cases (1988-1998), J Am Vet Med Assoc 1999;214:1657.
35. Schneider JE, Adams OR, Easley KJ, et al: Scapular notch resection for suprascapular nerve decompression in 12 horses, J Am Vet Med Assoc 1985;187:1019.
36. Adams OR, Schneider RK, Bramlage LR, et al: A surgical approach to treatment of suprascapular nerve injury in the horse, J Am Vet Med Assoc 1985;187:1016.

CHAPTER 99

Tarsus

Jörg A. Auer

ANATOMY

The bones that make up the tarsus include the tibia, the talus and calcaneus, the central tarsal bone, the fused first and second tarsal bone, the third and fourth tarsal bones, and the metatarsal bones (MT II, III, and IV) (Fig. 99-1). The tarsal bones are maintained in intimate contact through their soft-tissue attachments, including the intertarsal ligaments, collateral ligaments, fibrous joint capsule, and plantar tarsal ligament. The medial collateral ligament connects the tibia and the proximal aspects of MTII and MTIII, whereas the lateral collateral ligament consists of a long part connecting MTIII and MTIV and a short part connecting the tibia to the calcaneus.[1]

The tarsus is composed of five joints: the tarsocrural (TC), proximal intertarsal (PIT), distal intertarsal (DIT), tarsometatarsal (TMT), and talocalcaneal (TCa) joints. Four of these five joints are almost immobile, and most of the movement of the tarsus is achieved in the tarsocrural joint. Micromovements occur during ambulation and weight-bearing in the three distal joints.

The three distal joints are often injected for diagnostic and therapeutic purposes. In one study, therapeutic con-

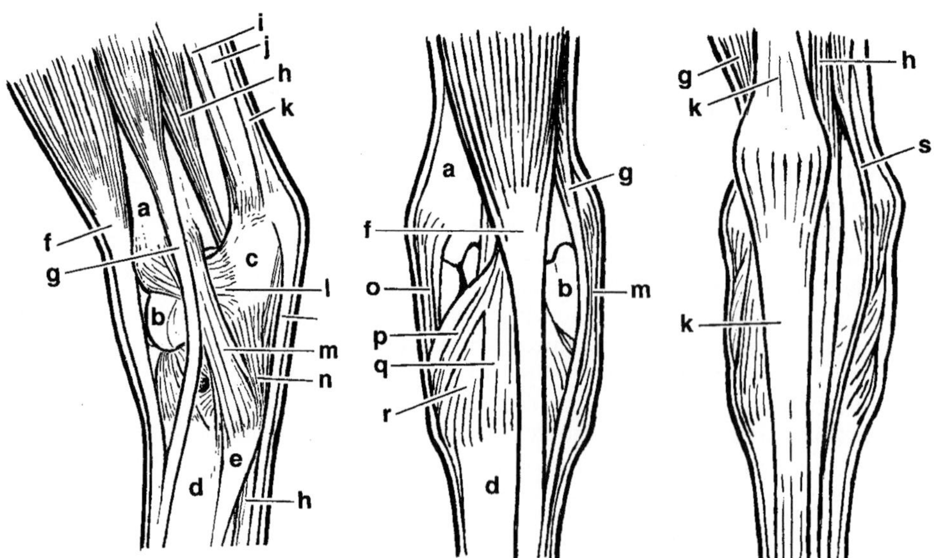

Figure 99-1. Anatomic structures associated with the tarsal region. a, distal tibia; b, talus; c, calcaneus; d, third metatarsus (MTIII); e, MTIV; f, long digital extensor muscle and tendon; g, lateral digital extensor tendon; h, flexor hallucis longus muscle and deep digital flexor tendon; i, soleus tendon; j, Achilles tendon; k, superficial digital flexor tendon; l, short lateral collateral ligament; m, long lateral collateral ligament; n, plantar ligament; o, medial collateral ligament; p, medial part of the tibialis anterior tendon (cunean tendon); q, middle part of the tibialis anterior tendon; r, fibularis tertius tendon; s, long digital flexor tendon.

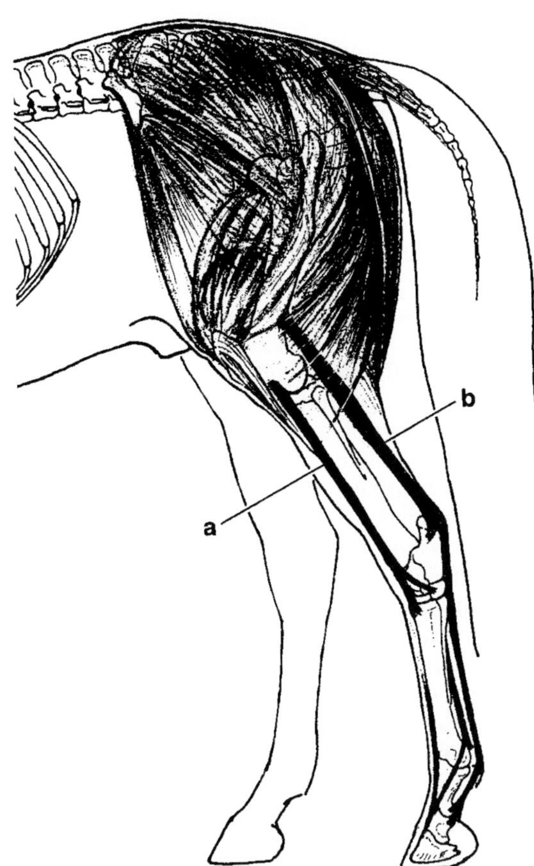

Figure 99-2. Correlation of the anatomic structures composing the reciprocal apparatus of the horse. *a,* Fibularis tertius tendon originating on the muscular fossa of the distal femur and inserting with the medial part on the central and third tarsal bones as well as at the third metatarsus (MTIII), whereas the lateral part courses towards the fourth tarsal bone. *b,* Gastrocnemius muscle, originating from the plantar fossa located at the distal aspect of the femur and the Achilles tendon, which unites with the soleus and accessory tendons before it inserts at the tuber calcanei.

centrations of methylprednisolone were measured in the DIT joint 6 hours after injection of methylprednisolone acetate into the TMT joint, confirming that communication between the TMT and DIT joints existed in 10 of 10 sampled joints (100%).[2] In an earlier study[3] communication was found between the TMT and DIT joints in four of 57 tarsi (7%); in one horse (2%), communication between the DIT and PIT could be established. In seven horses (14%), communication between the DIT joint and the tarsal canal existed, pointing out the potentially inconsistent results that can be found after intra-articular anethesia.[3] Other studies in the literature cite the communication between the TMT and DIT joints at 7%[4] and 38%.[5] Despite these conflicting reports, the most recent report is convincing to this author.

The TCa joint in horses is a multifaceted structure consisting of three facets between the two bones involved: the facet at the medial aspect of the calcaneus and talus, the angulated coracoid facet of the lateral aspect of the calcaneus and talus, and the facet at the lateral aspect of the calcaneus facing medially and talus facing laterally, respectively.[6] A strong interosseus ligament in the central tarsal sinus maintains the two bones in close proximity. The special relationship of the three facets relative to each other prevents motion in the joint.[6]

Dorsally, the long digital extensor tendon spans the entire tarsal region and is maintained in position by the retinaculi. Just distal to the tarsal region, the lateral digital extensor tendon unites with the long digital extensor tendon. The strong fibularis tertius (peroneus tertius) courses parallel to the long digital extensor tendon (Fig. 99-2). At the level of the tarsus, it divides into medial, middle, and lateral branches before inserting on the central, third, and fourth tarsal bones as well as in the proximal metatarsal region. The medial part is better known as the cunean tendon, which at one time was thought to be responsible for the development of spavin. The fibularis tertius forms the cranial part of the reciprocal apparatus (Fig. 99-3). The gastrocnemius muscle and tendon form the caudal part. Interspersed between these two parts, the tibia and tarsus function as weight-supporting structures. The intact reciprocal apparatus ensures that when one of the major joints of the rear limb is flexed, all others flex.

Plantarly, the superficial digital flexor tendon passes under the tarsal retinaculum at the proximal aspect of the calcaneus and from there distally to the digit. The deep digital flexor tendon passes medial to the calcaneus over the sustentaculum tali. The tendon of the long digital flexor muscle traverses the tarsal region medially and joins the deep digital flexor tendon in the proximal metatarsal region.

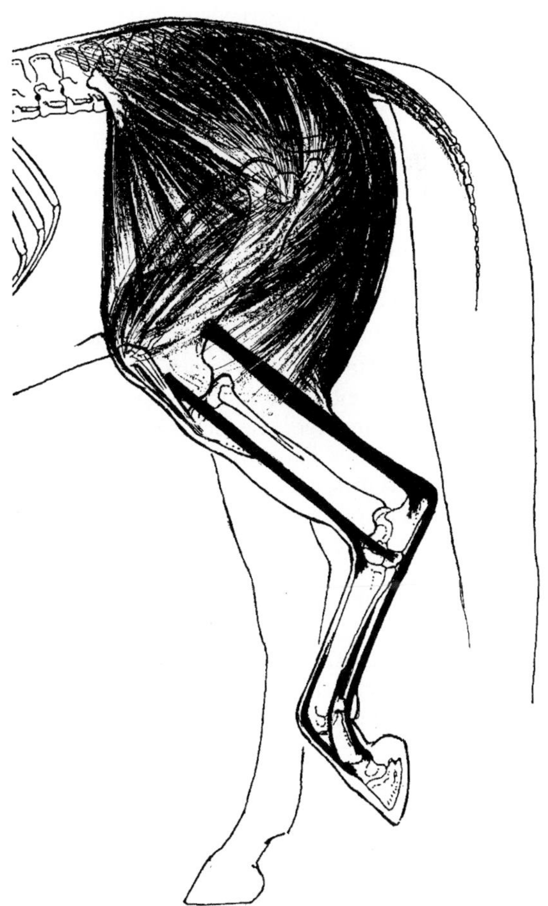

Figure 99-3. Flexion of the tarsus or stifle results in flexion of all remaining joints in the hind limb.

All tendons pass over the tarsal region embedded in a tendon sheath. The tarsal canal is the largest tendon sheath and surrounds the deep digital flexor tendon.

The function of the tarsus is to transform axial loading during weightbearing from the cranioproximal to caudodistal oblique forces exerted along the tibia into vertically and distally oriented forces through the metatarsal area.

ACQUIRED DISORDERS OF THE TARSAL REGION

Osteoarthritis is the most diagnosed acquired tarsal disorder causing lameness.[5] It is seen in three forms: one involves the distal tarsal joints (referred to as *bone spavin*), one is located at the talocalcaneal joint, and the other involves the tarsocrural joint (referred to as *bog spavin* when joint distention is present; see Chapter 91). Other acquired disorders include fractures, luxations, and tendon and ligament injuries.

Etiology

OA of the distal tarsal joints is the most common cause of hindlimb lameness in the horse.[7] The DIT and TMT joints are most often involved, but occasionally the PIT joint also is affected. A study in foals showed that bone density of the compact bone of the subchondral bone plate in the third tarsal bone reacts to variations in exercise at a very young age.[8] Low bone density caused by lack of exercise was reversed when exercise was increased later. Osteoarthritic radiographic signs (enthesiophytes) in the distal intertarsal joints were common at 5 months of age and increased in severity until 11 months of age. Although the clinical relevance of these abnormalities in foals is uncertain, they might be related to the development of osteoarthritis in this region later in life.[7]

Although the exact pathogenesis of distal tarsal OA is still unknown, compression and rotation of the distal tarsal bones, which occurs most forcefully at the gallop, can contribute to its development.[9] Dressage horses, western horses, pulling horses, and Standardbreds are prone to the disorder, which is associated with their type of athletic activity. Islandic horses are often affected, which is possibly related to the mismatch of the horse and the rider and the gaits at which these animals are used. The rack is a fast four-beat gait during which the horses place their hind limbs extremely far forward, and this extreme type of gait can be responsible for the development of bone spavin in these horses. Poor conformation also is a contributing factor to this disorder: bowlegged and sickle-hocked conformation results in abnormal loading of the small tarsal bones and leads to the development of OA.

Inciting causes of distal tarsal OA are septic arthritis, tarsal bone fractures, osteochondrosis, crushing of the central or third tarsal bones following incomplete ossification at birth, and excessive exercise.[6,10-12] OA also has been associated with increased intramedullary pressure within the cuboidal bones of the tarsal region.[13] Inciting causes for the less-often-encountered tarsocrural and to some extent talocalcaneal joint OA include intra-articular fracture, osteochondrosis, septic arthritis, and collateral ligament damage.[14]

For most other tarsal disorders, external trauma, such as a kick from another horse or being hit by or running into an object, is the inciting cause. Repetitive trauma as it occurs during racing or competitive events in general can lead to the development of lameness.

Clinical Signs

The cardinal sign of a tarsal problem is lameness, which can vary depending on the severity, location, and acuteness of the disorder. Toe dragging is a common early sign that occurs because of a reluctance to flex the tarsus. Horses with OA often have a reduced foot flight arc, shortened cranial phase of the stride, gradual axial deviation in the flight path of the foot during the cranial phase of the stride, and a rapid abaxial deviation at ground contact.[15] Affected horses often show pain to back palpation, and many horses are presented for a primary complaint of back pain. However, in most cases, a weight-bearing lameness is noted.

Joint distention is not a typical sign of OA of the distal tarsal joints, because the tarsal retinaculum over these small joints prevents its detection. However, new bone proliferation at the dorsomedial aspect of the limb might be noticeable in chronic cases (Fig. 99-4). A typical sign of a tarsocrural disorder is joint distention (bog spavin). However, as often noted in OCD, the swelling does not have to be painful.

An acute onset of a marked to severe weight-bearing lameness is a clear sign of trauma and is often associated

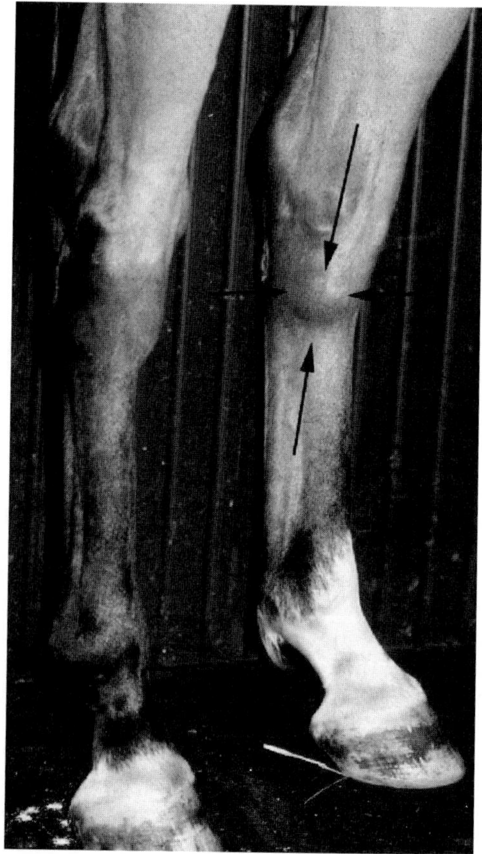

Figure 99-4. Marked enlargement at the dorsomedial aspect of the tarsal region in a horse suffering from osteoarthritis of the distal tarsal joints (bone spavin). Excessive new bone formation is responsible for this appearance.

with joint distention or swelling of the neighboring tissues, or both. Penetrating articular wounds lead in most cases to septic arthritis with all the accompanying signs including heat, swelling, and pain.

Diagnosis

The diagnosis of tarsal disorders involves a routine lameness examination, provided the animal is able to ambulate. In the presence of fractures and joint infections, the origin of which is often easy to localize, immediate attention should be given to the inciting cause, sidestepping the lameness examination. (This is not routine but an exception to the rule.)

Leading the horse in tight circles in both directions can exacerbate the lameness on the inside limb. Some horses initially show a marked lameness but with time warm out of it. Often the horse exhibits a barely detectable unevenness at the time of presentation or no evidence of lameness at all. A history that includes deterioration in the horse's attitude suggests subtle hock pain, which does not produce overt lameness. Evaluation of the shoes and looking for uneven wear can lead the clinician toward the diagnosis. Palpation of the tarsal region can allow detection of enlargement over the dorsomedial aspect of the tarsus; however, most lesions do not cause pain upon digital pressure. Cunean bursitis and effusion of the cunean bursa are rare, but they can be detected by palpation. Flexion tests often exacerbate the lameness.

Intra-articular anesthesia is a valuable aid in localizing the problem. Because there is controversy in the literature regarding communication between the TMT and DIT joints,[3,4,16-18] each joint should be anesthetized individually. Significant improvement in lameness 10 minutes after intra-articular injection of 2 to 4 mL mepivacaine hydrochloride is diagnostic, but complete resolution of lameness might not occur because of intraosseous pain in the tarsal bones.[13] Larger volumes of anesthetic should not be used because of the potential for periarticular extravasation and contact with nonarticular tissues, including the sensory nerve supply from the distal limb as it passes through the tarsus.[16] In young racing Standardbreds, it might be advantageous to anesthetize the cunean bursa, because cunean bursitis is diagnosed in the these animals.

The joint region to be injected is clipped and prepared as for aseptic surgery. Meticulous cleansing of the area without clipping of the hair (application of the antiseptic of choice, scrubbing for 5 minutes followed by removal of the antiseptic soap, repeated twice) has no higher risk of iatrogenic joint infection following arthrocentesis than clipping the hair prior to preparation and needle placement (see Chapter 74).

The TMT joint is the easiest of the distal tarsal joints to inject (Fig. 99-5). The needle is inserted laterally, 0.5 cm proximal to the head of MTIV, in a dorsomediodistal direction at a 45-degree angle to both the sagittal plane and the ground until it makes contact with bone, usually at a depth of approximately 2 cm.[13] This technique results in the needle tip's passing deep, medial, and slightly distal to the palpable lateral aspect of the head of MTIV, positioning it near the articulation between MTIV and the fourth tarsal bone. The steep angle is necessary to position the needle tip sufficiently distal to avoid penetrating the PIT joint, which is located only slightly proximal to the head of the MTIV.

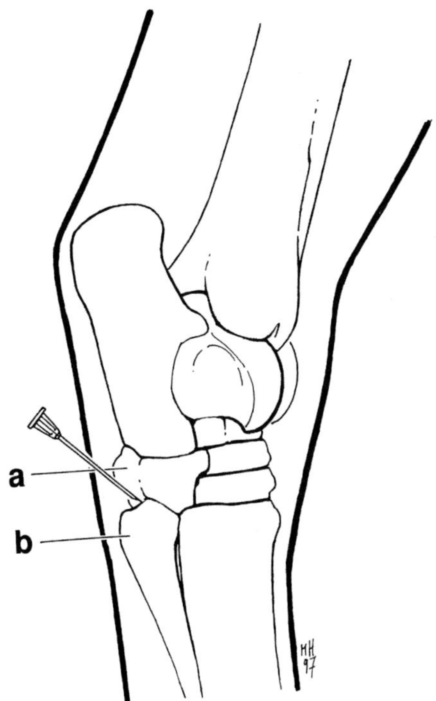

Figure 99-5. Graphic illustration of injection site for the tarsometatarsal joint. A 22-gauge 2.5-cm needle is inserted 0.5 cm proximal to the head of the fourth metatarsal bone (b) and directed in a dorsomediodistal direction at a 45-degree angle to both the sagittal plane and the ground until it contacts bone, usually at a depth of approximately 2 cm. The steep angle is critical to position the needle tip sufficiently distal to avoid penetration of the proximal intertarsal joint, which is located only slightly proximal to the head of the fourth metatarsal bone. a, fourth tarsal bone.

The DIT joint is injected medially in the space between the central tarsal bone, the third tarsal bone, and the fused first and second tarsal bones (Fig. 99-6). The location for needle placement is found by palpation of the distal border of the cunean tendon, approximately 2 cm caudal to a vertical line extended distally from the medial malleolus.[11] Ideally, the needle is inserted to the hub at a 45-degree angle in a plantarolateral direction and parallel to the ground.

Full penetration of a 2.5-cm needle in small horses can result in the needle's passing completely through the DIT joint and into connective tissue deep to the joint capsule.[7] Also, the TMT joint can be entered inadvertently on the medial aspect of the tarsus while attempting to enter the DIT joint, because the TMT joint capsule is located just slightly distal to the DIT joint capsule.[6] The PIT joint is rarely injected alone, because it communicates with the tarsocrural joint, and this injection is not discussed here.

The tarsocrural joint, of all joints composing the tarsus, is the easiest to inject, especially when it is distended. The dorsomedial pouch of the joint can be easily palpated. Taking care to avoid the saphenous vein, the needle is then inserted in a dorsocaudolateral direction, and depending on the degree of joint distention, 10 to 20 mL of synovial fluid is withdrawn prior to injection of 8 mL of mepivacaine hydrochloride.

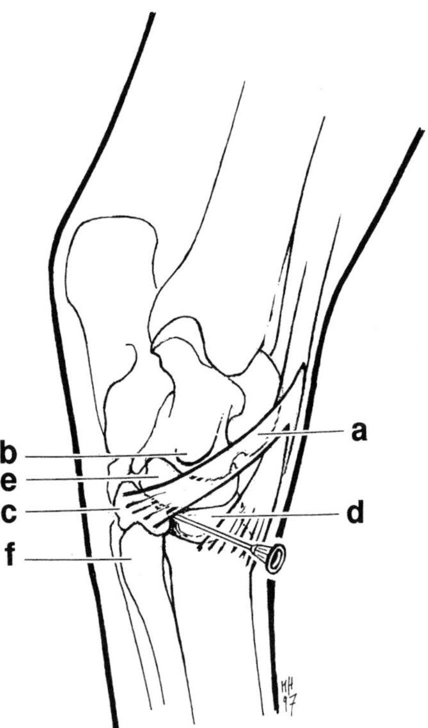

Figure 99-6. Graphic illustration of the injection site for the distal intertarsal (DIT) joint. The DIT joint is injected medially in the proximal aspect of the space that exists between the central tarsal bone (e), third tarsal bone (d), and fused first and second tarsal bone (c). The entrance to this space can often be felt with firm palpation and is found at the distal border of the cunean tendon (a), approximately 2 cm caudal to a vertical line extending distally from the medial malleolus. The location for needle entry can also be located along a line between the distal tubercle of the talus (b) and the palpable space between the second metatarsus (MTII) (f) and MTIII, where it intersects the cunean tendon.

Diagnosis is confirmed using standard radiographic views, including oblique projections. OA is commonly a bilateral condition; therefore, radiographs of both tarsal regions are recommended. Because some changes might be subtle, it is important to take good-quality radiographs. Lameness associated with the distal tarsal joints can exist with little or no radiographic abnormalities. Conversely, extensive radiographic changes might be present that are not associated with pain or lameness. Therefore, it is important to locate the site of lameness before obtaining radiographs. Fractures are best confirmed with good-quality radiographs. In rare cases, such as fractures of the central or third tarsal bones, this imaging technique does not provide evidence for an exact diagnosis.

Ultrasonography also can be used to arrive at a diagnosis as long as the lesions are peripheral. In-depth knowledge of the tarsal anatomy is a prerequisite if this imaging technique is applied. Scintigraphy has been used to localize lesions not visible on radiographs, especially in early cases where radiographic changes are not yet apparent.[19,20] Rarely is computed tomography necessary to localize a lesion. Computed tomography can be applied in the tarsus and provides valuable details for an exact diagnosis, especially in cases of hidden new bone formations and fractures. This technique is gaining in popularity.

Treatment of Fractures

Fractures of the tarsus, while rare because of the dense supporting structures that cover the bones in this area, occur when a significant external impact, such as a kick from another horse, is sustained in the tarsal region. Twisting and shearing of the tarsus while the lower limb is fixed can result in disruption of collateral and periarticular ligaments and subsequently lead to fractures.

Distal Tibia

Fractures of the distal tibia often involve the medial malleolus and can arise from external trauma, which results in avulsion of the medial malleolus from the tibia that is rarely accompanied by rupture of the medial short collateral ligament.[21,22] Fractures of the lateral malleolus can occur as avulsions and involve the short and long lateral collateral ligamants.[20,21] Avulsion fractures of the lateral malleolus are often comminuted. Arthroscopy can be used to remove fragments involving the medial malleolus; however, because of the soft-tissue coverage and intimate association with the joint capsule or lateral collateral ligaments, or both, lateral malleolar fragments can be removed more easily through an arthrotomy into the dorsolateral pouch of the TC joint or through a direct approach over the fracture through the lateral short collateral ligament, or a combination of these techniques and arthroscopy. If arthroscopy is attempted alone, the fragment might have to be divided into smaller pieces for removal using an osteotome and mallet.

Fragments larger than 3 cm are best reattached to the parent bone using 3.5-mm cortex screws placed in lag fashion.[10,23] Large avulsion fractures of the medial malleolus can be repaired with one or two 4.5- or 5.5-mm cortex or cancellous screws placed in lag fashion (Fig. 99-7). A full-limb cast is applied for recovery from anesthesia and the initial postoperative period, if fixation rather than removal has been used.

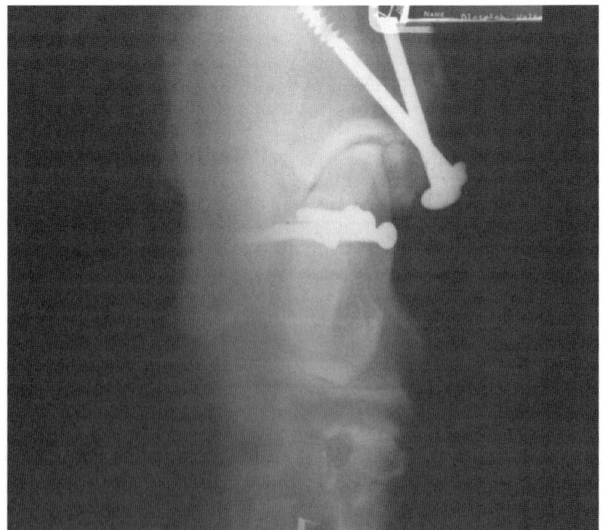

Figure 99-7. Dorsoplantar radiographic view of fixation of a medial malleolar fracture with two long cancellous screws and washers. Additionally, large fragments off the lateral trochlear ridge of the talus were reattached through three cortex screws, which were deeply countersunk into the articular surface.

Conservative management of nondisplaced distal tibial malleolar fractures is possible. Surgical management, either by removal of the fragment or by repair of the fracture, offers a favorable prognosis for return to previous performance levels in one report.[23] However, an unfavorable to guarded prognosis was given in another report.[9] A total of 4 to 6 months of rest is needed after surgery, particularly if fracture fixation was used as the surgical treatment.

Trochlear Ridges of the Talus

Fractures of the talus are acute injuries and are almost exclusively the result of external trauma such as a kick from another horse. The clinical signs vary considerably, depending on comminution, size, and displacement of the fracture. Significant effusion of the TC joint is seen with most fractures of the talus, and response to tarsal flexion is moderate to severe. Standard radiographic projections should be supplemented with flexed lateromedial and flexed lateromedial oblique projections and skyline views of the trochlear ridges.[11] The distal aspect of the lateral trochlear ridge and the proximal aspect of the medial trochlear ridge (see Fig. 99-7) are most often affected.[22,24,25]

Arthroscopic removal of small trochlear ridge fractures is generally the preferred treatment. The arthroscope portal for removing trochlear ridge lesions can be either dorsomedial or dorsolateral. The dorsolateral portal offers better visualization of the distal aspect of the lateral trochlear ridge, but the standard dorsomedial portal is preferred because triangulation is better and the surgeon can carry out a more thorough exploratory examination of the joint from a medial approach. The instrument portal is always dorsolateral and is usually slightly distal to that used for distal tibial lesions. Osteochondral defects or cartilage flaps might extend proximally along the lateral trochlear ridge, necessitating extension of the limb during surgery. Some surgeons prefer an arthrotomy approach directly over the lesion.[10,26]

Large trochlear ridge fractures can be repaired with interfragmentary compression using several screws[23] (Fig. 99-8). The fracture can be approached either through arthroscopy or an arthrotomy performed lateral to the ridge. After the fragment is identified and reduced, a glide hole is drilled perpendicular to the fracture plane from the dorsal aspect of the ridge. After preparing the thread hole, a deep countersink depression is prepared in the articular surface to accept the entire screw head. Therefore, it is better to use multiple 3.5-mm cortex screws, which have smaller heads, than to use 4.5- or 5.5-mm cortex screws. In large fragments, there is adequate solid bone to permit such a fixation. Anatomic reconstruction is a must if fixation is attempted. If this cannot be achieved, it is best to remove the fragment immediately to prevent the development of OA. Alternate fixation techniques include absorbable polydioxanone pins and cannulated screws.[23]

Spurs or fragments associated with the distal end of the medial trochlear ridge of the talus (dewdrop lesions) are usually incidental findings and are not an indication for surgery, because they are usually extra-articular[11,21] (Fig. 99-9). Arthroscopic removal has been described in the literature, although the technique is difficult because of extensive soft-tissue covering.[27] For removal of these fragments, both the arthroscope and instrument portals are made in the dorsomedial pouch of the tarsocrural joint, with the instrument portal placed distal and slightly medial to the arthroscope.

Fragments off the proximal medial trochlear ridge are best removed arthroscopically (Fig. 99-10). With the horse in dorsal recumbency, the limb is positioned in flexion. With the joint distended, the arthroscope portal is made in the center of the caudolateral pouch of the TC joint. This approach provides good visualization of the talocalcaneal

A, B

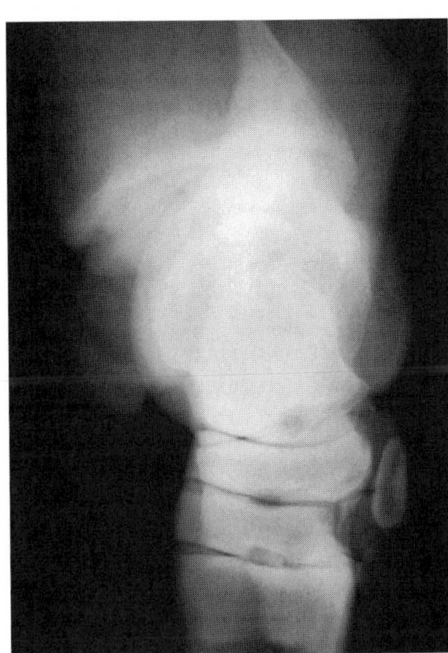

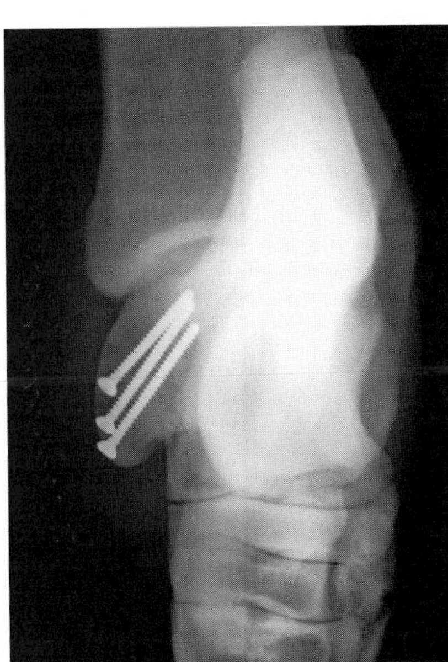

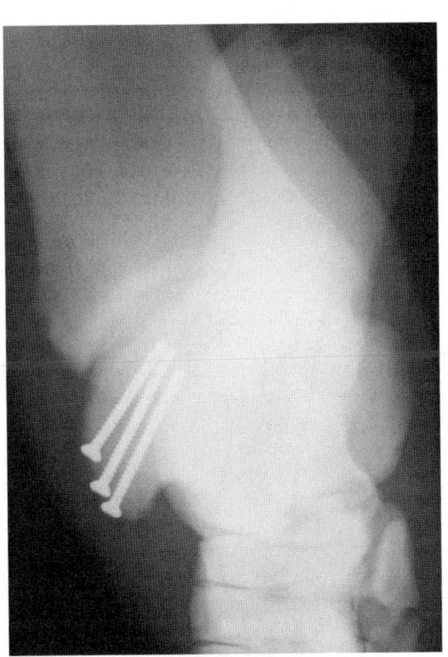

C

Figure 99-8. A, A large, slightly displaced slab fracture of the lateral trochlear ridge. **B,** The fracture was repaired with three 3.5-mm cortex screws inserted perpendicular to the fracture plane. The screws were inserted from the articular surface, and the screw heads were completely countersunk. **C,** A two-year follow-up revealed no osteoarthritis in the joint. The horse was successfully competing in show jumping events. (Courtesy C. Lischer, University of Zurich.)

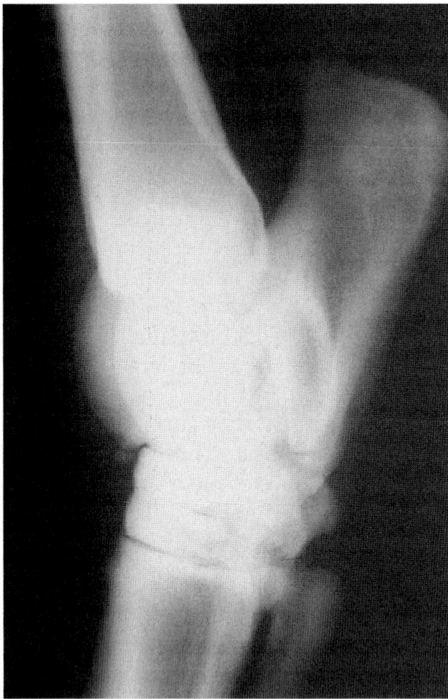

Figure 99-9. Dorsolateral–plantaromedial oblique radiographic view showing a teardrop lesion or fragmentation off of the distal aspect of the distal medial trochlear ridge of the talus. This finding is usually incidental and rarely has any clinical significance. (Courtesy C. W. McIlwraith, Colorado State University.)

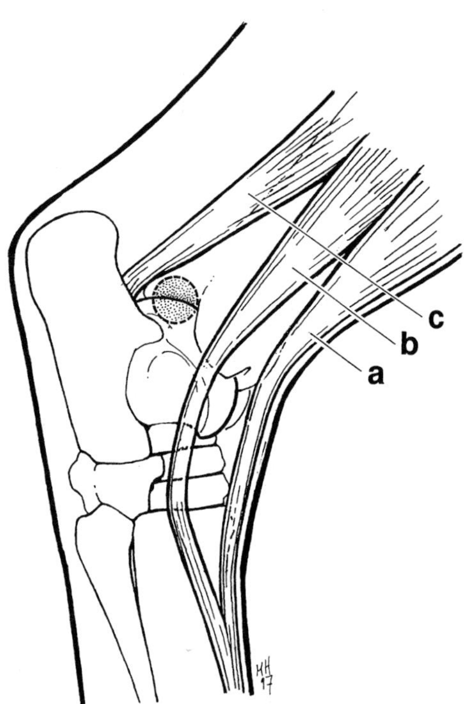

Figure 99-10. Graphic illustration of the arthroscope portal site for examining the plantar pouch and visualizing the plantar aspect of the trochlear ridges of the distal tibia. The arthroscope is placed contralateral, and the instrument is placed ipsilateral to the lesion. a, long digital extensor tendon; b, lateral digital extensor tendon; c, deep digital flexor tendon.

articulation, the proximocaudal aspect of the lateral trochlear ridge, the caudal aspect of the intermediate ridge of the tibia, and the medial trochlear ridge. Access to affected portions of the trochlear ridge can be accomplished as the degree of flexion is modified. The instrument portal is made in the caudomedial joint pouch using needle and visual guidance through the arthroscope.

Fractures of the distal lateral or medial aspect of the body of the talus occur rarely. Extreme angular forces need to be involved to cause such a fracture (Fig. 99-11, *A*). The animals are almost always non–weight-bearing lame and the tarsus is diffusely swollen. Radiography confirms the diagnosis. Conservative therapy in most cases is unrewarding. The horse shown in Figure 99-11 was readmitted for treatment after a year of limited pasture exercise because of continued lameness and pronounced joint distention of the tarsocrural and proximal intertarsal joint (see Fig. 99-11, *B*). The fracture subsequently was repaired with 3.5-mm cortex screws in lag fashion through an approach directly over the fragment. The lameness and joint distention resolved within 4 months postoperatively and the horse was returned to show jumping.

Recovery after surgery takes 8 to 10 weeks after arthroscopic removal of small fragments and 6 to 8 months or more if fracture repair is undertaken. Prognosis after fracture removal is favorable if soft-tissue damage at the time of injury is mild, secondary changes in the joint are minimal, and the fragment is shorter than 3 cm.[23]

Sagittal Fractures of the Talus

Sagittal fractures of the talus are rare.[23,28] The medial fragment is usually smaller, and fractures can be repaired with two or three 4.5- or 5.5-mm cortex screws placed in lag fashion. The fracture can be approached from either the medial or lateral side.[23,28] Arthroscopic visualization during the procedure is useful in assisting anatomic reduction of the fracture. Prognosis appears to be favorable if anatomic reduction can be achieved.[23] Severely comminuted fractures of the talus are associated with severe soft-tissue trauma and destabilization of the TC joint and are inoperable in most cases.[23]

Calcaneus

Calcaneal fractures are often open and can be complicated by osteomyelitis, septic calcaneal bursitis, sequestration, and chronic drainage. Major fractures of the calcaneus can result in displacement of the superficial flexor tendon or can involve the sustentaculum tali. An open wound and local infection can eventually extend into the tarsal sheath. Lameness is usually severe with calcaneus fractures, and diagnosis is straightforward. In addition to standard projections, stressed radiographs can provide additional important information for diagnosis and management. Skyline views are useful for evaluating the tuber calcis and sustentaculum tali.

Small fragments distant from the calcaneal bursa can be removed through a direct approach or left to heal conservatively if they are not infected, but larger fragments should be repaired by lag screw fixation. Transverse fractures of the shaft of the calcaneus require application of one or two

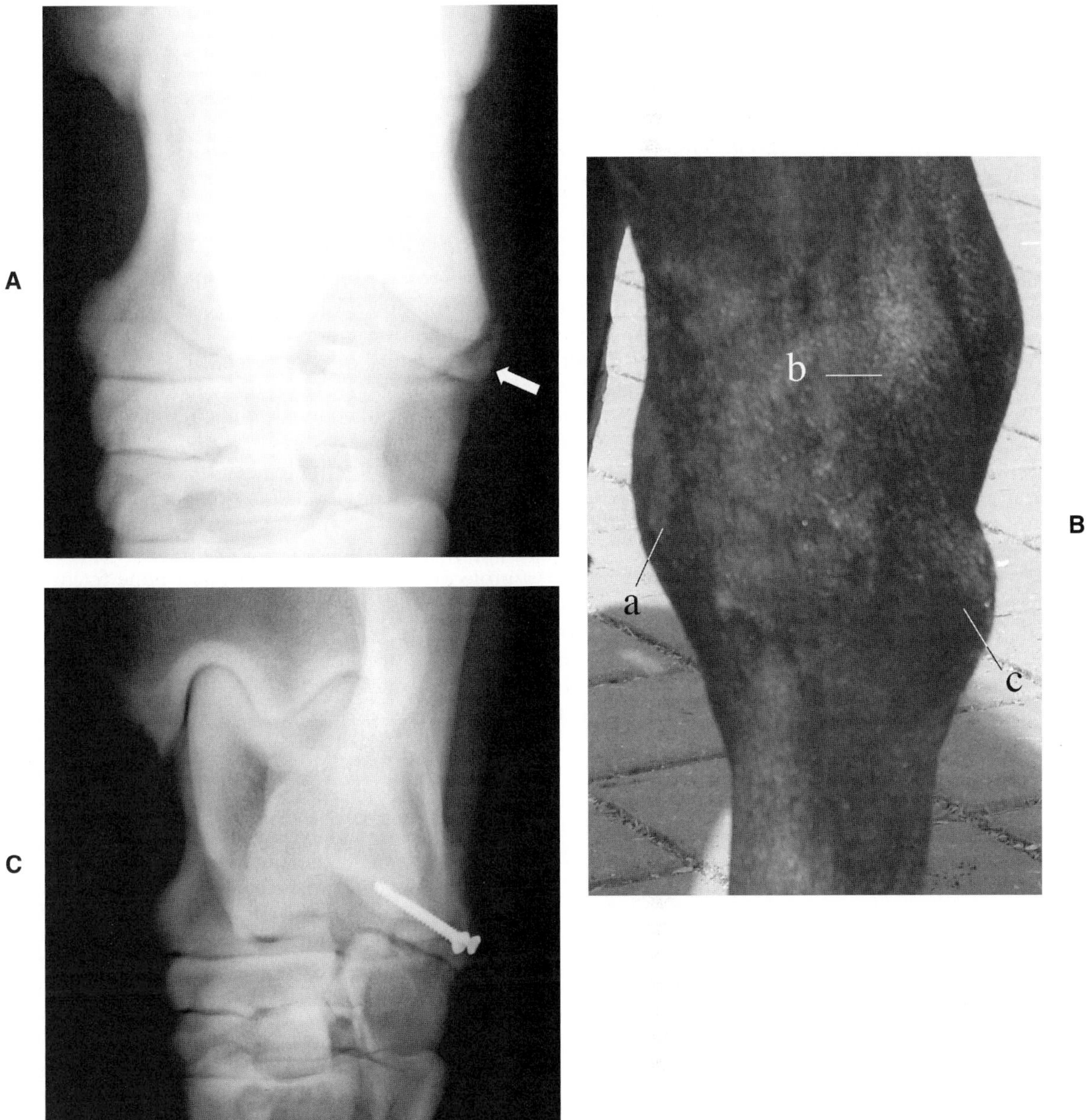

Figure 99-11. A, Avulsion fracture of the lateral aspect of the distal talus with proximal intertarsal (PIT) articular involvement. The horse was managed conservatively with rest for one year. **B,** Marked joint distention visible in the tarsocrural and proximal intertarsal joints. a, dorsomedial pouch; b, plantarolateral pouch; c, lateral aspect of the proximal intertarsal joint. **C,** Postoperative radiographic view showing the fixation of the fracture with two 3.5-mm cortex screws. Six months later, the horse competed successfully in show jumping events.

narrow 4.5-mm limited-contact dynamic compression plates (LC-DCPs) or one broad 4.5-mm LC-DCP to the plantarolateral aspect of the bone.[18] The superficial digital flexor tendon is reflected medially to allow placement of the plate, and the horse is recovered and maintained for 2 to 4 weeks in a full-limb cast that is removed with the horse standing. Removal of the implants after fracture healing can be helpful, but the overall prognosis to return to full performance for this type of fracture is guarded.[23,29,30]

Fractures involving the calcaneal bursa in the presence of an open wound from a kick usually have a poor prognosis for future soundness. Invariably the bursa gets infected, and eventually the patient has to be destroyed for humane reasons. Aggressive treatment should be implemented as soon as possible after the injury has occurred and includes meticulous débridement of the wound, removal of the fragment, curettage of the fracture bed, lavage of the bursa, broad-spectrum antibiotics for 3 weeks, and placement of the limb in a cast for 3 weeks. Subsequently, a half-shell cast should be applied for an additional 3 weeks, followed by a Robert Jones dressing, provided the horse doesn't show signs of infection at an earlier time. If signs of infection are present, the wound needs to be evaluated immediately and the owner should be informed of the complication and the potentially grave prognosis. If a decision is made at that time to euthanize the patient, massive costs can be avoided.

Chip Fractures of the Sustentaculum Tali

Fractures of the sustentaculum tali occur rarely. These injuries are caused by acute trauma, mainly in the form of kicking injuries. The skin can be perforated, resulting in communication with the tarsal sheath of the deep digital flexor tendon. The animals are acutely lame and, depending on the duration of the injury and possibly associated tendon sheath infection, a grade IV lameness may be present.

Diagnosis is by a radiographic examination using multiple views. The proximodistal flexed view best delineates the sustentaculum tali (Fig. 99-12). Analysis and culture of the tendon sheath fluid is indicated. Treatment should be initiated immediately, especially when the tendon sheath is penetrated. Chip fracture removal can be achieved with arthroscopic technique, although one study suggests that many of the bony lesions might be outside of the tendon sheath and are best approached directly.[31] Flushing of the tendon sheath with copious amounts of fluids is indicated after chip removal and careful curettage of the fracture bed. Tendovaginotomy and fragment removal represent another surgical approach.

Conservative management is contraindicated, especially in open injuries. Involvement of the sustentaculum is a key parameter in the decision for surgery. If the fracture involves a significant amount of the flexor surface, reattachment with cortex screws may be considered, especially if the tendon sheath was not penetrated at the time of injury. If treatment is delayed, proliferative changes can develop, leading to chronic lameness with a poor prognosis for future usefulness of the horse.

With immediate, effective treatment, a guarded prognosis for usefulness can be given. Neglected cases have a grave prognosis. Chip fracture removal can result in postoperative displacement of the deep digital flexor tendon, but this is rare.

Fractures of the Small Tarsal Bones

Slab fractures of the central or third tarsal bones occur after racing or other high-speed events. Fractures of the third tarsal bone are more common. Lameness is severe initially, but it diminishes over several weeks. Marked response to hock flexion persists over time, and persistent effusion of the TC joint is noted if the central tarsal bone is involved. When the central tarsal bone is fractured, intra-articular anesthesia of the TC joint partially alleviates lameness, but it can take 30 to 45 minutes for the maximal effect. Diagnosis of central and third tarsal bone fractures is confirmed with standard radiographic views but can require multiple oblique projections, because central tarsal bone fractures are often complex and comminuted.[32] Radiographic confirmation of these fractures can be difficult. Nuclear scintigraphy and computed tomography are helpful when available.[28,33]

Screw fixation of slab fractures of the central and third tarsal bones is the treatment of choice (Fig. 99-13). The horse is placed in dorsal or lateral recumbency, and the fracture is compressed using one or two 3.5- or 4.5-mm cortex screws placed in lag fashion through stab incisions

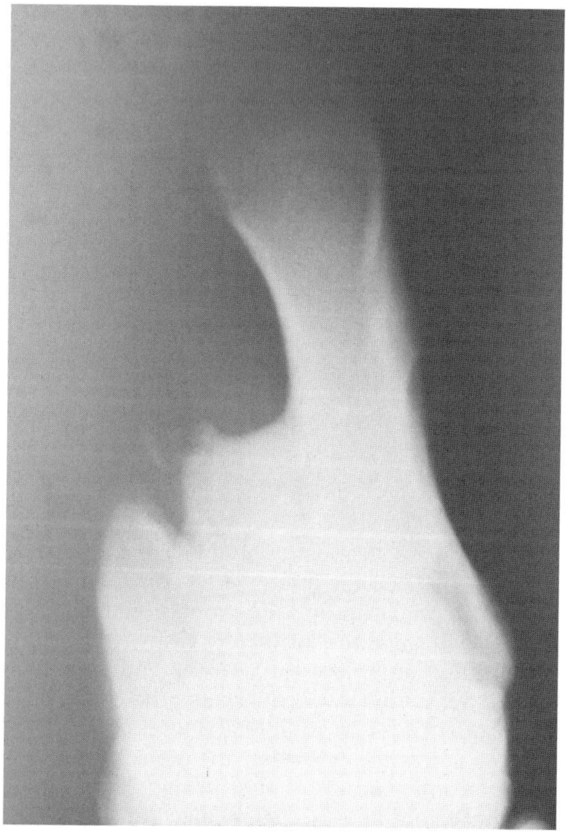

Figure 99-12. Flexed proximodistal radiographic view of the sustentaculum tali showing a chip fracture. The fracture was the result of a kicking injury to the medial aspect of the tarsus.

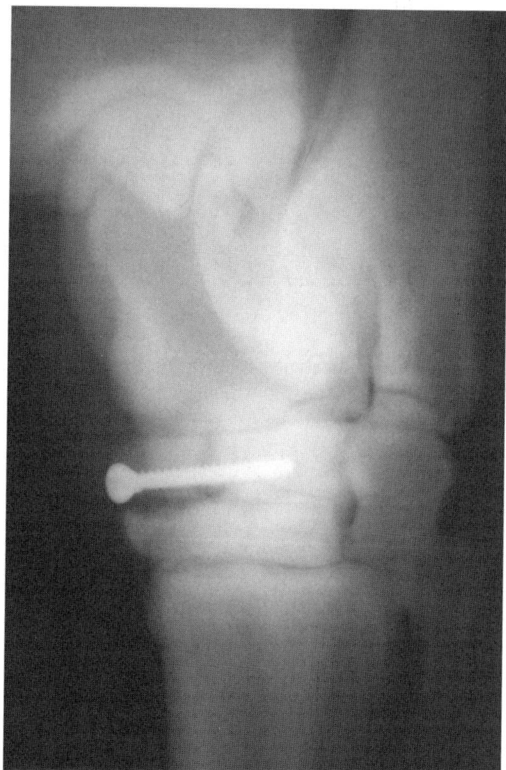

Figure 99-13. Radiographic view of a compression fixation of a slab fracture of the central tarsal bone. Lytic arthritis of the distal intertarsal joint is visible.

using intraoperative radiographic control. Conservative treatment (prolonged stall rest) has been successful, and some horses return to athletic use. However, treatment by screw fixation offers the best prognosis, because conservative management usually results in OA.[32,34-36] Horses are rested for 4 to 6 months after surgery.

Residual lameness can persist after either surgical or conservative management and eventually requires intra-articular medication, chemical or surgical arthrodesis (see Chapter 85), or screw removal after fracture healing.

Treatment of Osteoarthritis

Osteoarthritis of the Distal Intertarsal Joints (Bone Spavin)

Management of OA includes corrective shoeing, systemic and intra-articular anti-inflammatory medications, shock wave therapy, chemical and surgical arthrodesis, and cunean tenectomy.

CORRECTIVE SHOEING

Horses with bowlegged conformation profit from corrective shoeing in which the medial hoof wall is shortened and a special horseshoe with a wider, thicker outside branch is applied. The application of lateral wedges between shoes and hoof wall decreases tension on the medial patellar ligament and pressure on the medial side of the tarsal joint. However, the fetlock joint experiences considerably more stress.[37] A recent study revealed that proper conditioning also can have a protective effect against bone spavin and lateral luxation of the patella.[37]

EXTRACORPORAL SHOCK WAVE THERAPY

The systems used to apply extracorporal shock wave therapy in equine medicine are of the middle-energetic (0.2 mJ/mm^2) to high-energetic (0.4 mJ/mm^2) form. Therapy is generally applied in two or three sessions at approximately 3-week intervals. For treatment of soft-tissue calcifications, intervals between 3 and 6 weeks are used.

The skin overlying the target tissue is clipped or shaved. During application of the shock waves, horses are sedated. Depending upon the system used, a session takes 10 to 25 minutes. Some promising results have been achieved in the management of OA of the distal intertarsal joints, but insufficient clinical data are available to prove that there is a definite treatment benefit.[38]

MEDICAL MANAGEMENT

Nonsteroidal Anti-inflammatory Drugs

Nonsteroidal anti-inflammatory drugs (NSAIDs) can be used as adjunctive medication during the convalescent period after surgery, but as a sole treatment for distal tarsal OA they are only palliative. As long the medication is administered, the lameness might be reduced or even absent, but as soon as administration is stopped, the lameness returns.

Corticosteroids

Steroid treatment of OA involves intra-articular injection of long-acting corticosteroids into the involved joints (indicated only after diagnostic intra-articular anesthesia renders the animal free of pain or convincingly reduces the lameness). The TMT and DIT joints of both limbs can be treated simultaneously. With simultaneous treatment, the dose per joint should be reduced, because the total dose per horse should not exceed toxic levels (see Chapter 84 for specific drug dosages).

After injection, horses are rested for 2 or 3 days, after which work can be resumed. Most horses respond favorably to injection and are free of pain for several months. Aseptic technique is very important, because of the potential for inducing a postinjection flare or septic arthritis. A sudden onset of lameness within a few days of the injections should be managed immediately with joint lavage under general anesthesia. Oral anti-inflammatory therapy is indicated to maintain a reasonably comfortable patient during management of this complication.

Lameness usually recurs after a few weeks to months and can be managed by additional corticosteroid injections. The pain-free interval shortens with repeated injections. In such patients, surgical or chemical fusion should be considered to maintain a useful horse.

Hyaluronan and Polysulfated Glycosaminoglycan

Hyaluronan and polysulfated glycosaminoglycan (PSGAG; Adequan) are used to improve the joint environment and reduce inflammation in high-motion joints (see Chapter 84). It is the author's opinion that these drugs can provide temporary relief for distal tarsal OA. However, if the patient is to be used in athletic competition, return of lameness is inevitable. Therefore these drugs do not have a place in the management of OA of the distal tarsal joints, especially if costs are considered.

Chemical Fusion

Chemical fusion of the DIT and TMT joints by intra-articular injection of sodium monoiodoacetate (MIA) was introduced as an alternative to surgical arthrodesis for horses clinically affected with bone spavin. MIA blocks a specific enzyme pathway in chondrocyte metabolism, resulting in chondrocyte death, cartilage necrosis, joint collapse, and fusion of the distal tarsal joints.[39-42]

Horses receiving MIA should be premedicated with phenylbutazone (4.4 mg/kg IV q 12 hours) for 24 hours, beginning 12 hours before treatment. Injection with MIA should be preceded by contrast arthrography of each joint, because communication between the DIT and PIT joints and communication between the TMT and PIT joints has been documented[19] (Fig. 99-14). Using a 22-gauge 2.5-cm needle, joints are injected individually with 2 mL of diatrizoate meglumine, the needle is sealed with an injection cap, and dorsoplantar and lateral radiographs are taken immediately.[15] After radiographs are taken, the needle is uncapped to allow the contrast medium to drain out of the joint. If contrast arthrography reveals no evidence of communication between the distal tarsal joints and the PIT joint, 100 mg of MIA in 2 mL of 0.9% saline solution and sterilized with a 0.2-μm syringe filter is aseptically injected into each joint.[10] The DIT and TMT joints of both hindlimbs are routinely treated at the same time. Because of the danger of inadvertent periarticular injection, the procedure is performed best on the anesthetized horse (see Chapter 85).

Horses treated with MIA are likely to experience dramatic pain beginning 4 hours after treatment and lasting until

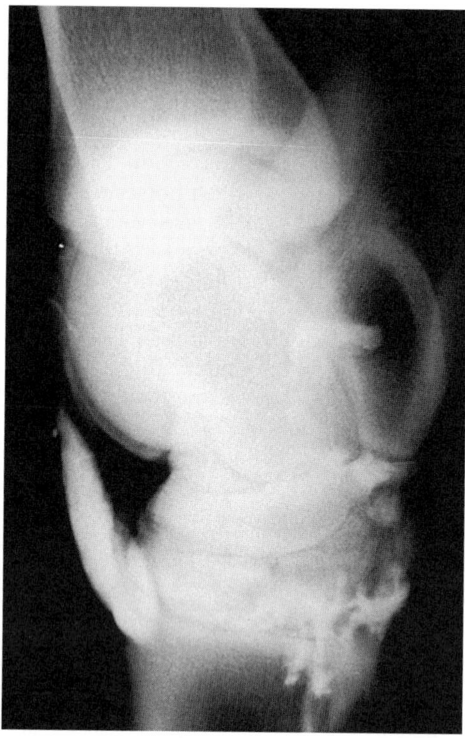

Figure 99-14. Positive contrast arthrogram showing communication of the tarsometatarsal joint with the proximal intertarsal and tarsocrural joints.

18 hours after treatment.[14] Because of this, horses should be hospitalized after treatment and medicated for pain with butorphanol tartrate and detomidine hydrochloride as needed. Anesthesia of the tibial and peroneal nerves with bupivacaine hydrochloride is also an effective technique for managing transient pain after injection of MIA.[15] Phenylbutazone is typically administered for 3 to 5 days after treatment, after which anti-inflammatory medications are usually unnecessary. Treated horses are exercised lightly the day following the injection, and these horses return to full work 2 days after the injection. Exercise sessions should consist of 45 to 60 minutes of full work in the horse's discipline 5 to 6 days per week for 60 days after treatment to provide physical disruption of the articular surface.

SURGICAL MANAGEMENT

Cunean Tenectomy

Cunean tenectomy is a relatively simple procedure performed with sedation and local anesthesia. Cunean tenectomy can improve lameness by decreasing rotational forces on the tarsus that occur when the obliquely oriented cunean tendon tightens. This surgical treatment for acute OA is controversial. In instances when distal tarsal OA is chronic and bone proliferation under the tendon is excessive, this technique can provide some pain relief. The procedure can be performed bilaterally.

The surgical site is anesthetized by an inverted V-shaped line block spanning from the chestnut to the dorsal aspect of the saphenous vein. A 4-cm vertical skin incision is made over the cunean tendon approximately 5 cm dorsal to the chestnut, where the tendon is easily palpable (see Fig. 85-14). A 4-cm section of tendon is removed with a no. 15 scalpel blade, and the skin is sutured. A compression bandage is applied and changed as needed until the sutures are removed.

Aftercare consists of stall rest for 12 days with limited daily hand-walking. After the sutures are removed, the amount of hand-walking is increased gradually through the 21st postoperative day and includes walking over poles. Three weeks after surgery, riding starts over poles, and full work resumes at 6 weeks. This exercise regimen is important for preventing formation of restrictive scar tissue between the severed tendon ends and the cunean bursa.

Arthrodesis

Various surgical procedures are used to arthrodese the distal tarsal joints.[15,43-48] Most procedures involve radiographically guided removal of cartilage by local drilling across part of the joint space. Bone plates, intra-articular stainless steel cylinders, transarticular screws placed in lag fashion, and cancellous bone grafts have been used to improve stability and hasten fusion after drill removal of cartilage and subchondral bone, but none of these treatments appears to offer substantial advantage to drilling alone.

Joint stability and pain relief can be obtained after bony bridging across only a small portion of the involved articular surface, which act as spot welds. Techniques have to be developed to provide better stabilization over a larger articular area, similar to the technique used for proximal interphalangeal arthrodesis, where a dorsal plate is supplemented by two screws that provide transarticular compression in the palmar region. However, in most of the currently used techniques, there is only a plate bridging the joints that are to be arthrodesed, and transarticular screws are avoided. Wyn-Jones and May also propose arthrodesis of the talocalcaneal joint with the help of four transarticular 5.5-mm cortex screws applied in lag fashion.[48] The lameness associated with this fixation can be attributed to osteoarthrosis of the proximal intertarsal joint and occasionally with the tarsocrural joint. For more information please review Chapter 85.

Articular drilling is another method of surgical arthrodesis. Articular drilling is performed bilaterally on both the DIT and TMT joints as a single procedure. The technique is described in detail in Chapter 85. Drilling too deeply can cause penetration of the tarsal canal, resulting in unnecessary periosteal reactions or profuse hemorrhage if the perforating branch of the cranial tibial artery is inadvertently traumatized. Avoiding these complications is preferable, but they appear to have no effect on the success of the procedure.[39-42]

Application of a four- or five-hole narrow dynamic compression plate (DCP) is described in detail in Chapter 85.

Aftercare

Horses can be lightly ridden 3 to 4 weeks after surgery. Administration of anti-inflammatory drugs maintains a reasonable level of comfort during the process of fusion. Most animals are free of lameness within 4 or 5 months of the procedure, but others show persistent lameness. Judgment on the outcome of the procedure is reserved until 12 months after surgery.

Prognosis

The prognosis for horses with distal tarsal OA treated with surgical arthrodesis is favorable, because most horses return to full function when the affected tarsal joints fuse.[15] Return to soundness over a 3- to 12-month period is reported in 66.7% to 85% of horses undergoing arthrodesis of the DIT and TMT joints.[44,46] Involvement of the PIT joint carries a less favorable prognosis because of its consistent communication with and concurrent involvement of the TC joint.[46]

The prognosis following chemical fusion of the distal tarsal joints with MIA is favorable. Most horses show dramatic improvement in the original level of lameness within 1 week after treatment, even though fusion might not be apparent radiographically for 3 to 6 months (Fig. 99-15).

Thirty-nine horses with OA that was treated with intra-articular MIA were evaluated.[40] Treatment was considered a short-term success when there was simultaneous documentation of radiographic fusion and soundness. At 1, 3, 6, and 12 months, success was achieved in 4 of 26 (8%), 15 of 27 (56%), 21 of 26 (81%), and 27 of 29 (93%) horses, respectively. Long-term evaluation showed that 16 of 16 (100%) horses had radiographic fusion of the treated distal tarsal joints, and 12 of 16 (75%) were free of lameness and the treatment was considered successful. OA of the PIT and TC joints was encountered in 4 of 39 horses (10%) and was diagnosed between 1 and 4 years after MIA treatment as acute severe lameness and swelling of the TC joint.[48] Each horse was treated with MIA before the potential for communication between the DIT and PIT joints was recognized, and none received contrast arthrograms. It is presumed that such a communication existed, resulting in contact of MIA with cartilage of the PIT and TC joints.

The efficacy of cunean tenectomy is debated, and there are no controlled clinical studies or experimental evidence in the literature to either support or refute the validity of the procedure. An owner survey of 285 cases of bone spavin treated by cunean tenectomy showed that most owners (83%) believed that lameness and performance improved after cunean tenectomy and that they would have the procedure performed again.[49]

Osteoarthritis of the Talocalcaneal Joint

The TCa joint has a curved contour, which is best recognized on lateromedial radiographs. The medial, lateral, proximal, and interosseous talocalcaneal ligaments support it.[1]

Osteoarthritis of the TCa is rarely described[14,50] (Fig. 99-16). However, two reports have renewed the interest in this disorder.[6,51] The clinical signs are not specific and resemble those of distal tarsal OA. Radiography and scintigraphy has been very beneficial in diagnosing the problem.[6,50]

Conservative therapy is usually unrewarding.[51] Stall rest, pasture exercise, and intra-articular corticosteroids with or without hyaluronan or PSGAG did not bring about consistent improvement of the lameness.

Surgical treatment involving partial tibial and fibular neurectomy cannot be recommended because of the poor results.[51] Forage also did not result in improvement of the lameness.[51] The best results were achieved with arthrodesis of the TCa joint.

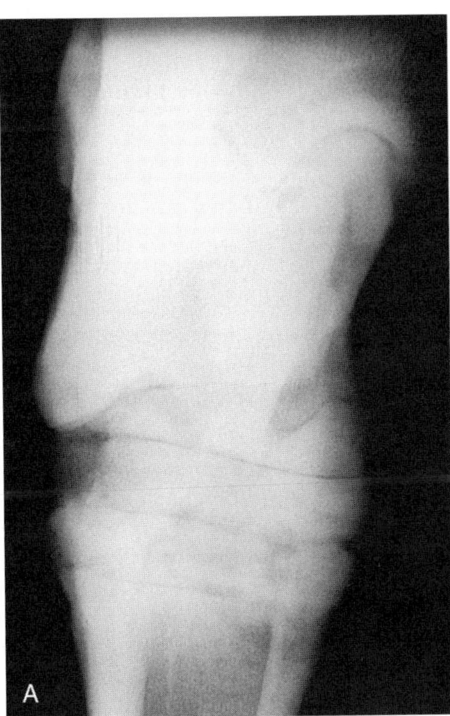

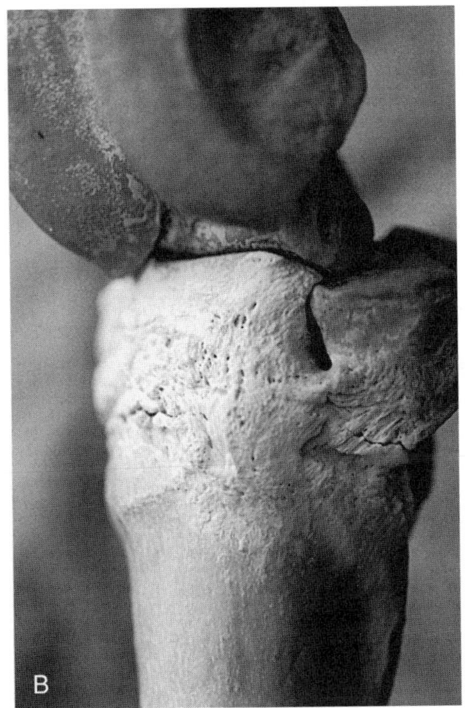

Figure 99-15. A, Dorsoplantar radiographic view demonstrating fusion of the tarsometatarsal and distal intertarsal joints 6 months after injection with sodium monoiodoacetate. **B,** Gross anatomic specimen of the same horse after it was euthanized 1 month later for an unrelated reason. Solid bone bridging is obvious in certain areas.

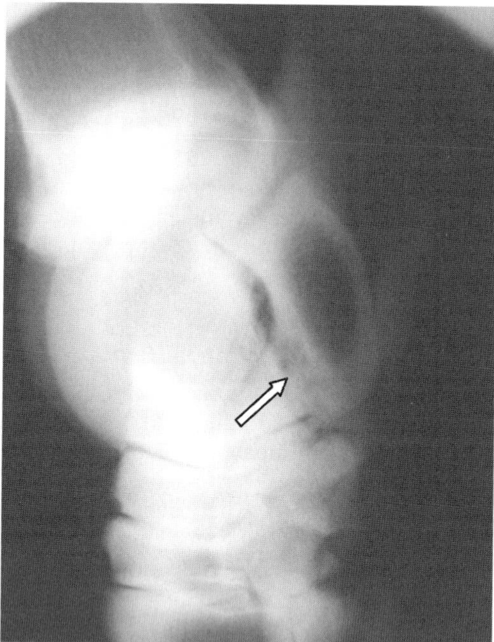

Figure 99-16. Lateromedial radiographic view of osteoarthritic changes located in the talocalcaneal joint *(arrow)*. (Courtesy R. Smith, Royal Veterinary College, London.)

Three techniques are described, all applying cortex screws across the joint.[6,51] One technique involves implanting three 5.5-mm cortex screws across the joint from the palmarolateral aspect of the calcaneus into the talus.[51] Lameness improved in all six horses subjected to this treatment. The other report described two techniques.[6] In a pony, three parallel 5.5-mm cortex screws were implanted in lag fashion from a dorsomedial arthrotomy approach to the talus across the medial talocalcaneal articular facet into the calcaneus. Successful fusion was achieved. In the other horse, two 5.5-mm cortex screws were implanted as described and two additional identical screws were inserted from the palmarolateral aspect of the calcaneus into the talus.[6] Successful fusion was achieved, allowing the horse to return to full daily work 1 year later. Additional information is found in Chapter 85.

Treatment of Luxations

Luxations usually occur at either the TMT joint or the PIT joint, but they occasionally involve the TC joint. Lameness is severe, with significant soft-tissue swelling, palpable instability, and crepitus. Luxations and subluxations of the tarsus might reduce spontaneously, but they can still be demonstrated with stressed dorsoplantar radiographs.

Luxations of the tarsus can be associated with fractures. The presence of fractures generally decreases the chances for a successful treatment. Open reduction and internal fixation is mandatory if fractures are present.

Luxations of the distal tarsal joints are best treated primarily with surgical arthrodesis, including débridement of the articular cartilage through an incision (if open, then on the open side of the joint), cancellous bone grafting, and joint stabilization with either trans-articular compression screws or bone plates (see Chapter 85).[17] Horses with good temperaments and subluxations can recover for breeding purposes with only stall rest if they are kept tied on an overhead wire or in a rescue net to prevent them from lying down. Horses with luxations of the distal tarsal joints might return to soundness after joint fusion or arthrodesis, but luxation of the TC joint has a poor prognosis for athletic soundness because of joint and ligament damage.[9,52]

Tarsal luxation is diagnosed as an acute traumatic event and can occur in any of the three distal tarsal joints or rarely in the tarsocrural joint. The animal is grade IV lame and might show an angular limb deformity in the tarsal region. However, lack of angular limb deformity does not rule out a luxation, because some luxations spontaneously reduce. Diagnosis is derived from palpation and a radiographic examination depicting the exact location of the injury (Fig. 99-17). In cases of reduced luxation, stress views should be taken under general anesthesia.

Tarsal luxation in the absence of major fractures can be treated with a full-limb cast for 3 months, with several cast changes during that time. This treatment is associated with the usual complications of prolonged cast applications, including pressure sores and cast disease.

Surgical arthrodesis of the TMT, DIT, and PIT joints has achieved superior results. The skin incision extends from the top of the calcaneus to the mid-MTIII on the plantarolateral aspect. The subcutaneous tissues are separated to expose the bone. The head of MTIV is trimmed with a chisel. An alternate approach involves removing the entire MTIV (see Chapter 85). A 12-hole 5.5-mm LC-DCP is contoured to the bones and applied with 5.5-mm cortex screws (see Fig. 99-17). Solid purchase of each screw in healthy bone is of great importance with this fixation. Therefore, the direction of each screw through the corresponding plate hole has to be carefully selected using radiographic control. It is important to insert several oblique transarticular screws across the luxated joint to provide additional stability.

After the subcutaneous tissues and skin are closed, a full-limb cast is applied for the initial 2-week period, after which a Robert Jones bandage is applied for 2 to 3 additional weeks. Hand-walking can be started after 2 months, and light riding can be resumed after 3 months. Full recovery is expected, barring no postoperative complications, such as infection or implant breakdown.

Treatment of Tendon Disorders

Luxation of the Superficial Digital Flexor Tendon

Superficial digital flexor (SDR) tendon luxations are seen in three forms in decreasing frequency: lateral displacement with disruption of the medial retinaculum, medial displacement with disruption of the lateral attachment, or splitting of the SDF tendon with a portion lying on either side of the tuber calcis.[5,26,53,54] The etiology can be direct trauma or excessive strain during partial flexion.[52]

Diagnosis of acute SDF tendon luxation can be difficult because of swelling, but palpation and observation during flexion and extension usually allow a diagnosis. Ultrasonography is the diagnostic aid of choice. Sometimes dislocation occurs only during motion, and the tendons maintain appropriate alignment when the limb is at rest. In more chronic cases of permanent luxation, the metacarpophalangeal joint can be hyperextended during weightbearing

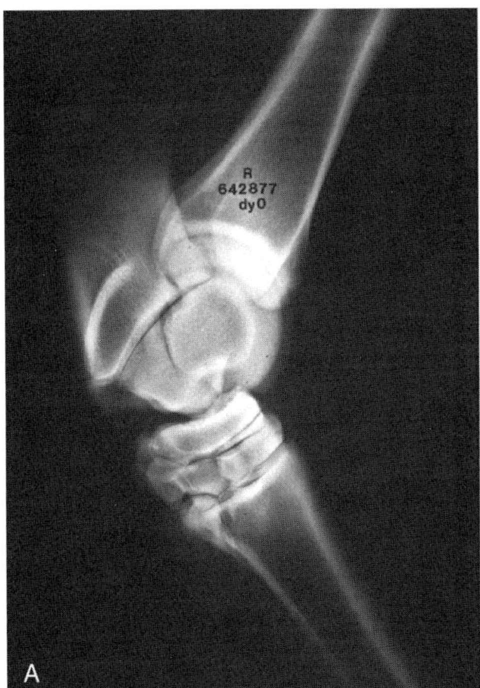

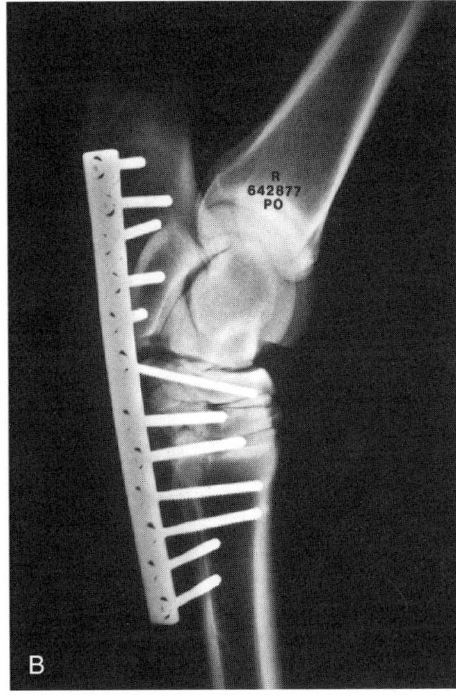

Figure 99-17. A, Cranial luxation of the proximal intertarsal joint after traumatic disruption of the plantar ligament. **B,** Repair of the luxation with 12-hole broad dynamic compression plate (DCP) applied with 5.5-mm cortex screws to the plantarolateral aspect of calcaneus, tarsal bones, and proximal third metatarsus (MTIII). (Courtesy J. P. Watkins.)

compared to the other limb. This occurs when the SDF tendon bypasses the tuber calcis in a course that is in a straighter line, which makes it functionally too long.

Partial or intermittent dislocations can heal with stall rest, with or without the benefit of a bandage or full-limb cast. Rest for 4 to 6 months is necessary.[54] Despite a clinical report claiming that conservative management allows a successful return to athletic competition,[55] the general thought is that surgical repair is mandatory for return to athletic function.[28,44,56,57]

The horse is placed in dorsal or lateral recumbency to allow exposure of the damaged side of the tarsal retinaculum. After débridement of the edges, horizontal mattress sutures are pre-placed on both sides of the defect well back from the defect margin. The ruptured ends are subsequently apposed and closed with interrupted horizontal mattress sutures of no. 0 monofilament absorbable material. A synthetic mesh graft is sutured over the defect using the pre-placed sutures.

After the incision is closed, the limb is placed in a full-length cast for recovery. Support of the repair can be provided by placement of bone screws into the calcaneus opposite the tear to provide a buttress against repeated dislocation.[48] Confinement for 4 to 6 months is necessary to allow for sufficient fibrosis.

Prognosis with surgical management diminishes as the anticipated level of performance increases. Prognosis for athletic soundness with conservative management is guarded for complete displacement, but it is favorable for cases involving partial rupture of the retinaculum. Medial dislocations have a better prognosis than do lateral displacements.[56]

Displacement of the Deep Digital Flexor Tendon

Luxation or displacement of the deep digital flexor (DDF) tendon is a rare congenital anomaly.[9] In this condition, the DDF tendon is located axial to its normal position and not within the groove formed by the sustentaculum tali. The malpositioned DDF tendon exerts a medial pull on the distal limb, and the first recognizable clinical sign is a varus deviation of the tarsus noted at 2 to 4 weeks after birth. Diagnosis is based on palpation, ultrasonography, and skyline radiography of the tarsus that demonstrates hypoplasia of the sustentaculum tali. Surgery to replace the DDFT in its normal position and augment the sustentaculum tali has been recommended.[9]

The foal is placed in lateral recumbency with the affected limb down. The DDF tendon and its tendon sheath are exposed from 10 cm proximal to 10 cm distal to the tarsus and freed from all soft-tissue attachments. The tendon sheath and tendon are placed back in the groove of the sustentaculum tali and sutured to underlying tissue. A cortical bone graft obtained from a rib is subsequently fixed onto the sustentaculum tali with bone screws to resist further medial displacement, and the incision is closed routinely. A cast is not necessary for recovery. Confinement is recommended for 4 weeks, and the prognosis for eventual soundness is good.[9]

Tenosynovitis of the Deep Digital Flexor Tendon

Chronic irritation and tenosynovitis of the DDF tendon can be a sequela to sustentaculum tali injury. Radiographically, new bone proliferations (Fig. 99-18, *A*) can be seen in the

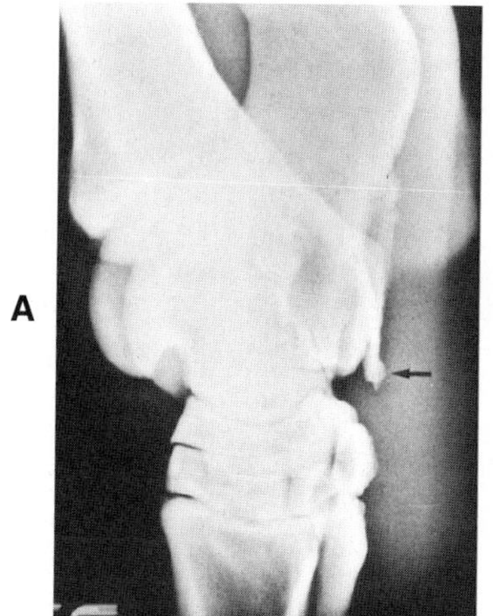

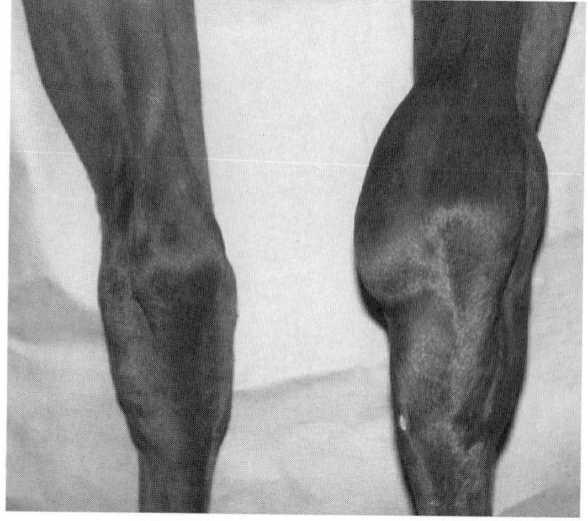

Figure 99-18. **A,** Lateral radiographic view showing osseous proliferation of the distal aspect of the sustentaculum tali. These lesions are associated with chronic irritation and inflammation of the sheath of the deep digital flexor tendon. **B,** Massive distention of the sheath of the deep digital flexor tendon medially in the tarsal region of a 6-year-old gelding. (**A,** Courtesy R. Welch.)

region, leading to tendon sheath distention (Fig. 99-18, *B*) and possible ossification. Contrast tenography can provide valuable information on the pathology present within the sheath.

Treatment of these problems involves tenoscopic exploration of the pathology and removal of any proliferative changes. Tendovaginotomy represents an alternate approach. However, chronic degenerative changes of the sustentaculum tali and overlying DDF tendon have a guarded prognosis for resuming normal work. After closing the skin incision in routine fashion, a pressure bandage is applied and maintained for 3 weeks. Intratendovaginal hyaluronan 1 week postoperatively is indicated.

Avulsion of the Gastrocnemius

Rupture of the gastrocnemius muscle occurs occasionally in foals and young horses. The disorder can be caused by external trauma or excessive running in the field, possibly associated with slipping or sudden unexpected turns. The diagnosis is straightforward, because the reciprocal apparatus is not functional. As the animal places weight on the limb, the tarsus collapses distally, and the stifle joint becomes extremely extended (Fig. 99-19, *A*).

Ultrasonography usually finds the gastrocnemius tendon intact but the origin of the muscle avulsed from the distal and caudal aspect of the femur. The avulsion can be complete or partial. Partial avulsion causes only slight dropping of the tarsus during weightbearing.

Management involves maintenance of a full-limb Robert Jones bandage with an incorporated splint for several weeks. An alternate treatment is application of a tube cast over the tarsal region (Fig. 99-19, *B*) for 3 weeks, followed by a Robert Jones bandage for an additional 3 to 5 weeks.

Both partial and complete avulsions have a favorable prognosis for a competitive future. Complications include all problems encountered with long-term casting and bandaging of the tarsal region.

DEVELOPMENTAL DISORDERS OF THE TARSAL REGION

Osteochondrosis

Etiology

Osteochondrosis (OC) in the equine tarsus occurs most commonly in the distal intermediate ridge of the tibia (Fig. 99-20, *A*), followed by the lateral trochlear ridge of the talus (see Fig. 99-20, *B*), the medial malleolus of the distal tibia, the medial trochlear ridge of the talus, and the lateral malleolus of the distal tibia.[58-60] Subchondral cystic lesions (see Chapter 92) have been identified in the distal tibia and talus, but they are considered unusual.[61] These lesions also have been identified in the cuboidal bones of the distal tarsus and are associated with an inflammatory reaction.[10,62]

Osteochondrosis results from failure of endochondral ossification or loss of blood supply to immature cartilage and subchondral bone[59,63-68] and can be influenced by various factors, including exercise, hormone imbalances, nutrition, heredity, and conformation (see Chapter 91). Heritability estimates suggest that 25% to 52% of the variation in occurrence of OC in the hock can be attributed to genetic factors.[69-73] Others conclude that distal tibial lesions arise from biomechanical trauma early in life[59] or represent supernumerary ossification centers that are not part of the OC complex.[74] One study documented 11 of 77 foals with obvious distal tibial fragments that were radiographically normal by 8 months of age.[75]

Diagnosis

Signs of tarsocrural OC are usually associated with the onset of training.[72,76] Synovial distention is the most common manifestation of the condition, sometimes followed by mild lameness (identified in only 66 of 144 affected limbs).[70] Pain on flexion of the tarsus is usually mild, and synovial fluid analysis is rarely indicated. Four standard radiographic views of the tarsus should be taken, but flexed views may

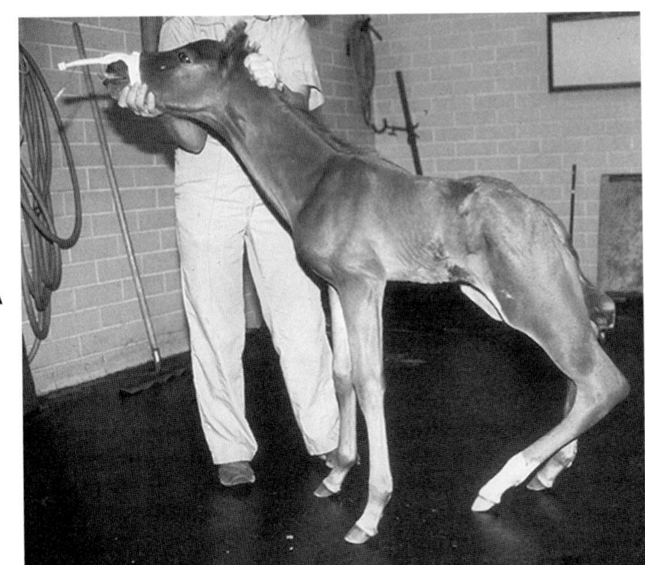

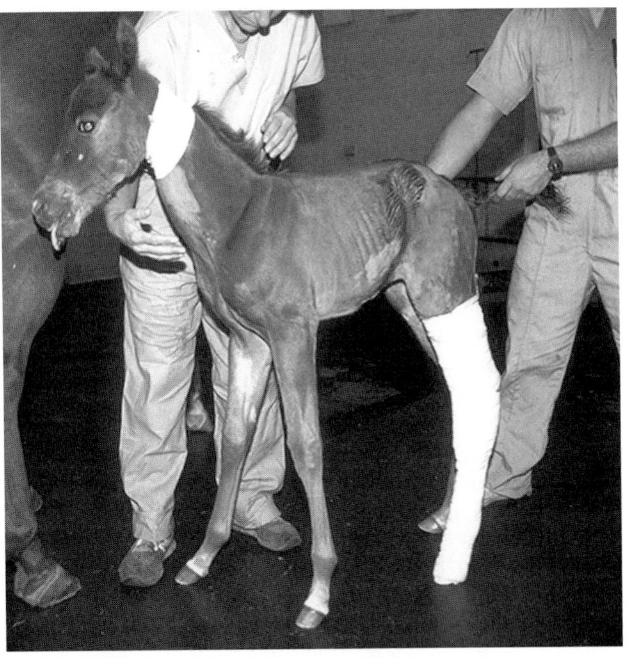

Figure 99-19. Three-week-old Quarter Horse foal with an avulsion of the gastrocnemius muscle. **A,** Weightbearing results in marked dropping of the tarsus and extension of the stifle. **B,** Application of a tube cast over the tarsal region allows the foal to bear weight.

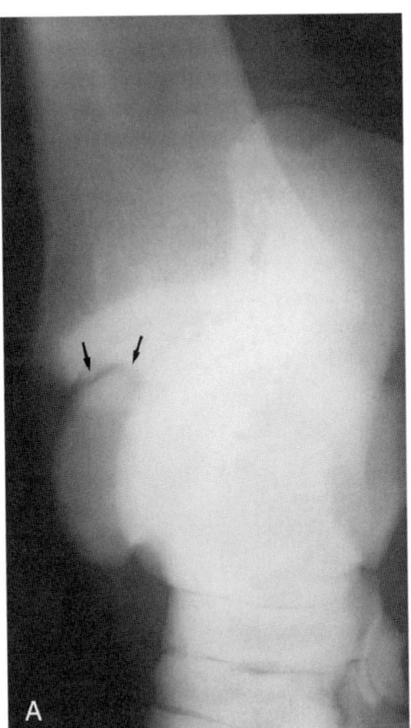

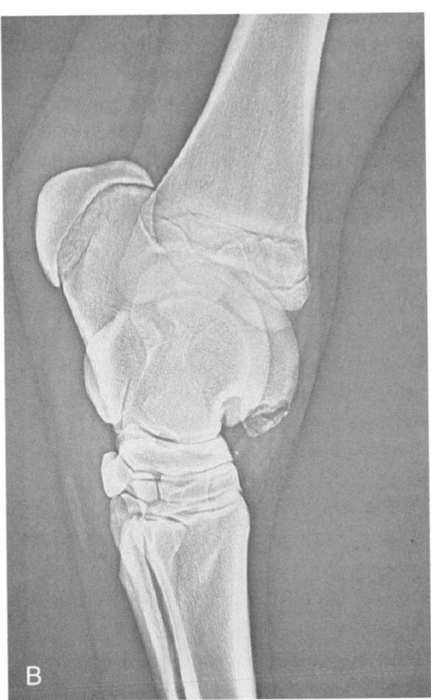

Figure 99-20. A, Dorsomedioplantarolateral oblique (DMPLO) radiographic view of the tarsus showing a distal intermediate ridge of the tibia OC lesion *(arrows)*. **B,** DMPLO xeroradiographic view of the tarsus showing a lateral trochlear ridge OC lesion. (Courtesy C. W. McIlwraith, Colorado State University.)

also be useful to demonstrate loose fragments or osteochondral defects in the caudal aspect of the joint. Bilateral lesions involve the distal tibia 20% to 45% of the time.[67,77] Distal lesions of the tibia vary dramatically in size, ranging from small fragments less than 5 mm in diameter to involvement of the entire intermediate ridge. OC lesions can be identified arthroscopically without radiographic evidence of their presence. These horses might or might not be presented with synovial effusion.[58]

Treatment

Arthroscopic removal of tarsocrural OC fragments is the treatment of choice, particularly if clinical signs of effusion or lameness are noted. Horses without clinical signs associated with radiographic evidence of OC can develop osteoarthritis of the TC and PIT joints and linear erosions along the side walls of the trochlear groove of the talus later in life.[3] Arthroscopic examination of the TC joint in mature horses with OC often reveals fibrillation of articular cartilage. These findings suggest that early surgical intervention is warranted to minimize secondary joint changes.[10]

DISTAL INTERMEDIATE RIDGE OF THE TIBIA

The horse is placed in dorsal recumbency with the limb in slight flexion. The arthroscope portal is made on the dorsal aspect of the dorsomedial pouch of the tarsocrural joint, centered over the pouch (Fig. 99-21). Placement of the arthroscopic portal too far medial makes it difficult to pass over the medial trochlear ridge, and placement too proximal or too distal also will jeopardize visualization. It is best to identify the saphenous vein before synovial distention and avoid it.

After the joint is distended, a stab incision is made through the synovial membrane, and the arthroscopic sleeve is inserted into the joint with a conical obturator. The limb is placed in 90 degrees of flexion, the arthroscope is inserted, and the joint is explored (Fig. 99-22, *A*).

The location of the instrument portal can be identified by passing the arthroscope laterally over the proximal aspect of the exposed lateral trochlear ridge into the dorsolateral pouch and palpating the tip through the skin. This procedure is also useful to demonstrate a vessel in the area by back-lighting it with the arthroscope when the surgery room lights are dimmed. Alternatively, a needle can be inserted through the dorsolateral pouch and advanced until it makes contact with the lesion.[14] Insertion of a hypodermic needle at the intended site allows the exploration of the range of motion possible with the instrument.

Once the ideal location is determined, a skin incision is made along the needle. A no. 11 scalpel blade is advanced into the joint along the needle, and a small incision is made into the synovial membrane. The needle and scalpel are removed and immediately exchanged with the arthroscopic probe. Intermediate ridge fragments may be loosely attached and elevated with the probe or may be firmly attached to the distal tibia, requiring partial separation with a periosteal elevator (Fig. 99-22, *B*) or an osteotome and mallet. Care should be taken not to damage the articular cartilage on the lateral trochlear ridge with the elevator or osteotome. After elevation, fragments are grasped with rongeurs, rotated to divide any remaining attachments, and removed. The sur-

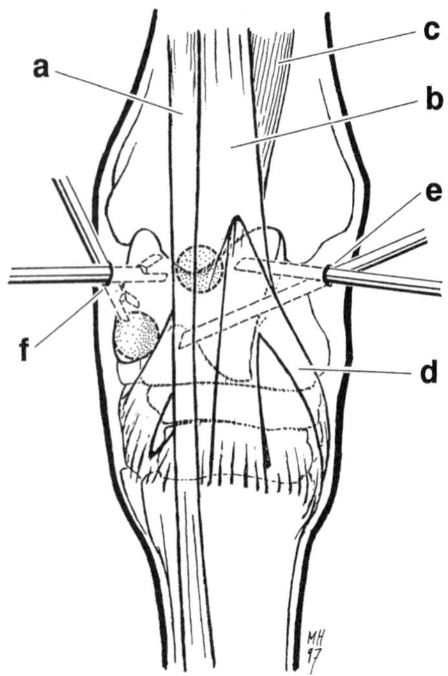

Figure 99-21. Graphic illustration of arthroscope and instrument portals for removing distal intermediate ridge OC lesions and lateral trochlear ridge OC lesions. These portals are also useful for diagnostic arthroscopy of the dorsal aspect of the tarsocrural joint and for removal of fragments from the proximal intertarsal joint. a, long digital extensor tendon; b, fibularis tertius; c, tibialis cranialis; d, medial branch of the fibularis tertius or cunean tendon; e, dorsomedial arthroscopic portal; f, dorsolateral instrument portal.

A

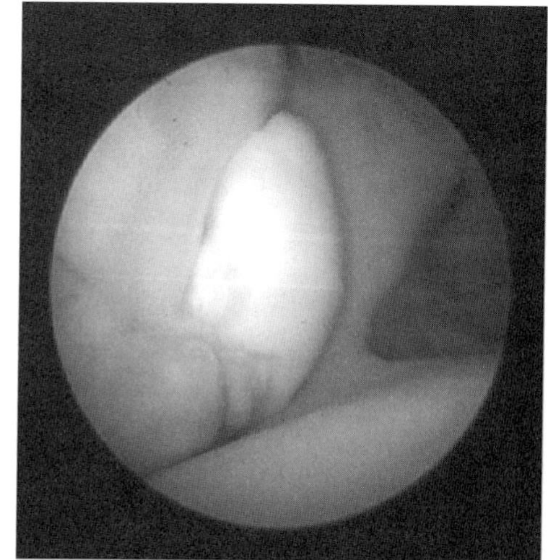

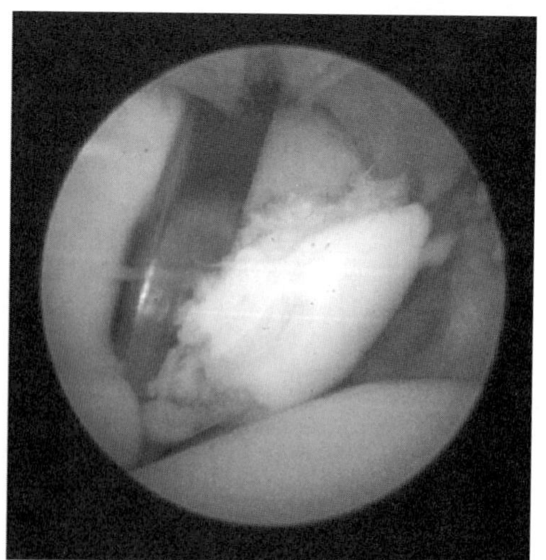

B

Figure 99-22. A, Arthroscopic view of a distal intermediate ridge (OC) lesion. **B,** Partial separation of the OC fragment from the distal tibia with the help of a periosteal elevator. These lesions are attached in most cases to the tibia by fibrous connective tissue.

geon should grasp fragments so that the minimum diameter is presented at the instrument portal. Increasing the size of the instrument portal is often necessary for removal. After the fragments are removed, the OC bed is examined for remaining tissue and curetted until firm subchondral bone remains in the site.

Occasionally, fragments of the intermediate ridge detach from the parent portion of the bone and are located in the distal end of the joint on preoperative radiographs (Fig. 99-23). Because these fragments can be free within the joint cavity or can pass into the PIT, removal can be problematic. If the fragments are free, they fall to the most distal aspect of the joint (which is into the dorsal aspect of the pouch [proximal] when the horse is in dorsal recumbency), especially if fluids are used to distend the joint. If fragments are located in the PIT, they can be left alone with minimal consequences or removed using a probe (see later). (The arthroscope can be passed into this joint through the normal communication just axial to the medial trochlear ridge.) Gas distention of the joint can aid in locating the fragment; however, if it cannot be localized intraoperatively, radiographs or fluoroscopy should be used to localize it. The instrument portal is selected in a place where the fragment can be accessed, and the fragment is removed.

MEDIAL MALLEOLUS

The arthroscope portal for medial malleolus lesions is made more ventral (more distal on the limb) than for intermediate ridge lesions to minimize the risk of accidentally pulling the arthroscope out of the joint during visualization.[14] The instrument portal (also ventromedial) is identified by prior insertion of a needle. Techniques for removing fragments are similar to those used for other lesions in the TC joint.

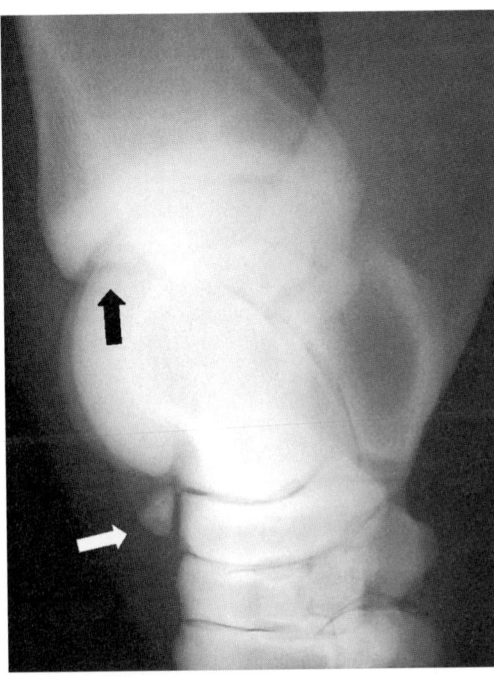

Figure 99-23. Lateromedial radiographic view of a tarsal region showing a loose fragment at the distal aspect of the joint cavity *(white arrow)*. The origin of the fragment is the distal intermediate ridge of the tibia *(black arrow)*.

LATERAL TROCHLEAR RIDGE

The arthroscope portal for removing lateral trochlear ridge lesions can be either medial or lateral. The lateral portal offers better visualization of the distal aspect of the lateral trochlear ridge, but the standard medial portal is preferred because triangulation is better and the surgeon can carry out a more thorough exploration of the joint from a medial approach.[14] The instrument portal is always lateral and is usually slightly distal to that used for distal tibial lesions. Both distal intermediate ridge and lateral trochlear ridge lesions can be treated with a single instrument portal when found concurrently within a single joint (see Fig. 99-21). Osteochondral defects or cartilage flaps can extend proximally along the lateral trochlear ridge, necessitating extension of the limb during surgery. Some surgeons prefer an arthrotomy approach directly over the lesion, but it is not the recommended approach.[9,25]

PROXIMAL INTERTARSAL JOINT

Loose fragments, usually shed from the intermediate ridge of the distal tibia, can lodge in the dorsal pouch or dorsal joint capsule of the PIT joint.[26] Although rarely of clinical significance, these fragments can be removed, if they are loose, by arthroscopically inserting an instrument into the pouch to blindly grasp the fragment or manipulate it into the TC joint for removal. Because of their limited clinical significance and the relative difficulty of finding and removing the fragments, it has been recommended that they be removed only if this can be easily accomplished during surgery for the primary lesion of the TC joint.[78]

Aftercare

Stab incisions are closed with skin sutures only. Bandages are applied and maintained for 21 days after surgery and are changed as necessary. Sutures are removed 14 days after surgery. Exercise is restricted to hand-walking for 4 to 8 weeks, and training can be resumed in 8 to 16 weeks, depending on the severity of the lesion and the amount of synovial distention before and after surgery. Postsurgical administration of phenylbutazone, hyaluronan, or PSGAG is useful to help resolve effusion, particularly in horses with prolonged synovial distention before surgery.

Prognosis

It is generally accepted that the prognosis for athletic soundness is improved with surgery compared to conservative management.[58,59,66,79,80] Seventy-seven percent of horses with OC of the tarsus raced successfully or performed their intended function following arthroscopy.[58] However, the prognosis decreases when articular cartilage degeneration or erosion is noted at the time of surgery, In one study,[58] resolution of synovial effusion after arthroscopy was higher in racehorses (83%) compared to non-racehorses (74%), and it was more likely with lesions of the distal tibia compared with other locations. There was no significant relationship between resolution of the effusion and successful performance outcome.[58]

Reports on the effects of OC on racing performance are contradictory. Although one study found no difference in the racing performance of Standardbreds demonstrating OC lesions compared with a radiographically normal control population,[81] another study reported that horses with OC of the TC joint had significantly fewer starts and lower earnings compared with horses without radiographic changes.[82] A third study found that the number of racing starts and race earnings for horses with surgically treated tarsocrural OC was reported to be lower than for age-matched siblings,[83] but a fourth study found that horses treated arthroscopically for OC of the distal tibia performed no worse than did their matched controls.[84] Despite these reports, the author recommends surgical treatment of this condition in all types of horses to prevent the development of OA in the TC joint.

Angular Limb Deformities

Angular limb deformities of the tarsus are seen less often than in the carpus or forelimb fetlocks, but they are diagnosed and treated in a similar fashion. Tarsus valgus is by far the most common presentation and can be caused by ligamentous laxity, malformation or incomplete ossification of the cuboidal bones of the tarsus, physeal dysplasia, or uneven growth of the distal tibial physis. A complete discussion of the etiology, diagnosis, and treatment of angular limb deformities can be found in Chapter 89.

REFERENCES

1. Wissdorf H, Gerhards H, Huskamp B: Praxisorientierte Anatomie des Pferdes, Hannover, 1988, Verlag M&H Alfred Schaper.
2. Serena A, Schumacher J, Schramme MC, et al: Concentration of methylprednisolone in the centrodistal joint after administration of methylprednisolone acetate in the tarsometatarsal joint, Equine Vet J 2005;37:172.
3. Bohanon TC: Contrast arthrography of the distal intertarsal and tarsometatarsal joints in horses clinically affected with osteoarthrosis, Proc Am Assoc Equine Pract 1994;40:192.
4. Kraus-Hansen AE, Jann HE, Kerr DV: Arthrographic analysis of communication between the tarsometatarsal and distal intertarsal joints of the horse, Vet Surg 1992;21:139.
5. Bell BTL, Baker GJ, Foreman JH, et al: In vivo investigation of communication between the distal intertarsal and tarsometatarsal joints in horses and ponies, Vet Surg 1993;22:289.
6. Pauwels FE, Adams SB, Blevins WB: Arthrodesis of the talocalcaneal joint for the treatment of two horses with talocalcaneal osteoarthritis, Vet Comp Orthop Traumatol 2005;18:7.
7. Stashak TS: The tarsus. In Stashak TS: Adams' Lameness in Horses, 4th ed, Philadelphia, 1987, Lea & Febiger.
8. Barneveld A, van Weeren PR: Early changes in the distal intertarsal joint of Dutch Warmblood foals and the influence of exercise on bone density in the third tarsal bone, Equine Vet J 1999;31:67.
9. Rooney JR: Biomechanics of Lameness in Horses, Huntington, NY, 1969, Krieger.
10. Foerner JJ: Surgical treatment of selected conditions of the rear limb. In Auer JA, editor: Equine Surgery, Philadelphia, 1992, WB Saunders.
11. Watrous BJ, Hultgren BD, Wagner PC: Osteochondrosis and juvenile spavin in equids, Am J Vet Res 1991;52:607.
12. Laverty S, Stover SM, Belanger D, et al: Radiographic, high detail radiographic, microangiographic and histological findings of the distal portion of the tarsus in weanlings, young and adult horses, Equine Vet J 1991;23:413.
13. Sonnichsen HV, Svalastoga E: Surgical treatment of bone spavin in the horse, Equine Pract 1985;7:6.
14. Dabareiner RM, Carter K, Dyson SJ: The tarsus. In Ross M, Dyson SJ, editors: Diagnosis and Management of Lameness in the Horse, Philadelphia, 2003, WB Saunders.
15. Bohanon TC: The tarsus. In Auer JA, Stick JA, editors: Equine Surgery, ed 2, Philadelphia, 1999, WB Saunders.
16. Sack WO, Orsini PG: Distal intertarsal and tarsometatarsal joints in the horse: Communication and injection sites, J Am Vet Med Assoc 1981;179:355.
17. Dyson SJ, Romero JM: An investigation of injection techniques for local analgesia of the equine distal tarsus and proximal metatarsus, Equine Vet J 1993;25:30.
18. Bohanon TC: Contrast arthrography of the distal intertarsal and tarsometatarsal joints in horses clinically affected with bone spavin, Vet Surg 1994;23:396.
19. Simpson CM, Lumsden JM: Unusual osteochondral lesions of the talus in a horse, Aust Vet J 2001;79:752.
20. Garcia-Lopez JM, Kirker-Head CA: Occult subchondral osseous cyst-like lesions of the equine tarsocrural joint, Vet Surg 2004;33:557.
21. Wright IM: Fractures of the lateral malleolus of the tibia in 16 horses, Equine Vet J 1992;24:424.
22. Jakovljevic S, Gibbs C, Yeats JJ: Traumatic fractures of the equine hock: A report of 13 cases, Equine Vet J 1982;14:62.
23. Nixon AJ: Fractures and luxations of the hock. In Nixon AJ, editor: Equine Fracture Repair, Philadelphia, 1996, WB Saunders.
24. McIlwraith CW: Surgery of the hock, stifle, and shoulder, Vet Clin North Am Equine Pract 1983;5:350.
25. Shelley J, Dyson S: Interpreting radiographs: 5. Radiology of the equine hock, Equine Vet J 1984;16:488.
26. McIlwraith CW, Foerner JJ: Diagnostic and surgical arthroscopy of the tarsocrural (tibiotarsal) joint. In McIlwraith CW, editor: Diagnostic and Surgical Arthroscopy in the Horse, ed 2, Philadelphia, 1990, Lea & Febiger.
27. Stephens PR, Richardson DW, Ross MW, et al: Osteochondral fragments within the dorsal pouch or dorsal joint capsule of the proximal intertarsal joint of the horse, Vet Surg 1989;18:151.
28. Meagher DM, Mackey VS: Lag screw fixation of a sagittal fracture of the talus in the horse, J Equine Vet Sci 1990;10:108.
29. Scott EA: Surgical repair of a dislocated superficial digital flexor tendon and fracture fibular tarsal bone in a horse, J Am Vet Med Assoc 1983;183:332.
30. Ferguson JG, Presnell KR: Tension band plating of a fractured equine fibular tarsal bone, Can Vet J 1976;17:314.
31. Hand DR, Watkins JP, Honnas DM, et al: Osteomyelitis of the sustentaculum tali in horses: 10 cases (1992-1998), J Am Vet Med Assoc 2001;219:431.
32. Tulamo RM, Bramlage LR, Gabel AA: Fractures of the central and third tarsal bone in horses, J Am Vet Med Assoc 1983;182:1234.
33. Stover SM, Hornof WJ, Richardson GL, et al: Bone scintigraphy as an aid in the diagnosis of occult distal tarsal bone trauma in three horses, J Am Vet Med Assoc 1986;188:624.
34. Lindsay WA, McMartin RB, McClure JR: Management of slab fractures of the third tarsal bone in five horses, Equine Vet J 1982;14:55.
35. Winberg FG, Pettersson H: Internal fixation of third and central tarsal bone fractures in the horse: A review, Proc Eur Coll Vet Surg 1993;2:252.
36. Murphy ED, Schneider RK, Adams SB, et al: Long-term outcome on conservative management of tarsal slab fractures in 25 horses (1976-1999), J Am Vet Med Assoc 2000;216:1949.
37. Back W, Remmen JL, Knaap J, et al: Effect of lateral heel wedges on sagittal and transverse plane kinematics of trotting Shetland ponies and the influence of feeding and training regimes, Equine Vet J 2003;35:606.
38. Schnewlin M, Lischer C: [Extracorporal shock wave therapy in veterinary medicine], Schweiz Arch Tierheilkd 2001;143:227.
39. Bohanon TC, Schneider RK, Weisbrode SE: Fusion of the distal intertarsal and tarsometatarsal joints in the horse using intra-articular sodium monoiodoacetate, Equine Vet J 1991;23:289.
40. Bohanon TC: Chemical fusion of the distal tarsal joints with sodium monoiodoacetate in 38 horses clinically affected with bone spavin, Vet Surg 1995;24:421.

41. Williams JM, Brandt KD: Immobilization ameliorates chemically-induced articular cartilage damage, Arthritis Rheum 1984;27:208.
42. Yovich JV, Trotter GW, McIlwraith CW, et al: Effects of polysulfated glycosaminoglycan on chemical and physical defects in equine articular cartilage, Am J Vet Res 1987;48:1407
43. Adams OR: Surgical arthrodesis for treatment of bone spavin, J Am Vet Med Assoc 1970;157:1480.
44. Archer RM, Schneider RK, Lindsay WA, et al: Arthrodesis of the equine distal tarsal joints by perforated stainless steel cylinders, Equine Vet J Suppl 1989;6:125.
45. Barber SM: Arthrodesis of the distal intertarsal and tarsometatarsal joints in the horse, Vet Surg 1984;4:227.
46. Edwards GB: Surgical arthrodesis for the treatment of bone spavin in 20 horses, Equine Vet J 1982;14:117.
47. McIlwraith CW, Turner AS: Arthrodesis of the distal tarsal joints. In McIlwraith CW, Turner AS: Equine Surgery: Advanced Techniques, Philadelphia, 1987, Lea & Febiger.
48. Wyn-Jones G, May SA: Surgical arthrodesis for the treatment of osteoarthrosis of the proximal intertarsal, distal intertarsal, and tarsometatarsal joints in 30 horses: A comparison of 4 different techniques, Equine Vet J 1986;18:59.
49. Eastman TG, Bohanon TC, Beeman GM, et al: Owner survey on cunean tenectomy as a treatment for bone spavin in performance horses, Proc Am Assoc Equine Pract 1997;43:121.
50. Butler JA, Colles CM, Dyson SJ, et al: The tarsus. In Butler JA, Colles CM, Dyson SJ, et al, editors: Clinical Radiology of the Horse, ed 2, Oxford, 2000, Blackwell Scientific.
51. Smith RKW, Dyson SJ, Schramme MC, et al: Osteoarthritis of the talocalcaneal joint in 18 horses, Equine Vet J 2005;37:166.
52. Reeves MJ, Trotter GW: Tarsocrural joint luxation in a horse, J Am Vet Med Assoc 1991;199:1051.
53. Meagher DM, Aldrete AV: Lateral luxation of the superficial digital flexor tendon from the calcaneal tuber in two horses, J Am Vet Med Assoc 1989;195:495.
54. Scott EA, Breuhaus B: Surgical repair of a dislocated superficial digital flexor tendon in a horse, J Am Vet Med Assoc 1982;181:171.
55. Bramlage LR: Personal communication, 2004.
56. Dik KJ, Leitch M: Soft tissue injuries of the tarsus, Vet Clin North Am Equine Pract 1995;11:235.
57. Hardy J: Diseases of soft tissue. In Kobluk CN, Ames TR, Geor RJ, editors: The Horse: Diseases and Clinical Management, Philadelphia, 1995, WB Saunders.
58. McIlwraith CW, Foerner JJ, Davis DM: Osteochondritis dissecans of the tarsocrural joint: Results of treatment with arthroscopic surgery, Equine Vet J 1991;23:155.
59. Hurtig MB, Pool RP: Pathogenesis of equine osteochondrosis. In McIlwraith C, Trotter G, editors: Joint Disease in the Horse, Philadelphia, 1966, WB Saunders.
60. Hoppe F: Radiological investigations of osteochondrosis dissecans in Standardbred trotters and Swedish Warmblood horses, Equine Vet J 1984;16:425.
61. McIlwraith CW: Current concepts in equine degenerative joint disease, J Am Vet Med Assoc 1982;180:239.
62. von Rechenberg Bv, McIlwraith CW, Guenther H, et al: Fibrous tissue of subchondral cystic lesions (SCL) in horses produce inflammatory mediators and matrix metalloproteinases and cause bone resorption in vitro, Vet Surg 2000;29:420.
63. Rooney JR: Osteochondrosis in the horse, Part 2, Mod Vet Pract 1975;56:112.
64. Rooney JR: Osteochondrosis in the horse, Part 1, Mod Vet Pract 1975;56:41.
65. Poole RR: Difficulties in definition of equine osteochondrosis: Differentiation of developmental and acquired lesions, Equine Vet J 1993;16(suppl):5.
66. McIlwraith CW: Clinical aspects of osteochondritis dissecans. In McIlwraith C, Trotter G, editors: Joint Disease in the Horse, Philadelphia, 1966, WB Saunders.
67. Gabel AA: Metabolic bone disease: Problems of terminology, Equine Vet J 1988;20:4.
68. Carsten J, Sandgren B, Dalin G: Development of osteochondrosis in the tarsocrural joint and osteochondral fragments in the fetlock joints of Standardbred trotters: I. A radiological study, Equine Vet J Suppl 1993;16:42.
69. Hoppe F, Philipsson J: A genetic study of osteochondrosis dissecans in Swedish horses, Equine Pract 1985;7:7.
70. Philipsson J: Pathogenesis of osteochondrosis: Genetic implications. In McIlwraith C, Trotter G, editors: Joint Disease in the Horse, Philadelphia, 1966, WB Saunders.
71. Schougaard H, Ronne JF, Phillipson J: A radiographic survey of tibiotarsal osteochondrosis in a selected population of trotting horses in Denmark and its possible genetic significance, Equine Vet J 1990;22:288.
72. Jeffcott LB: Osteochondrosis in the horse: Searching for the key to pathogenesis, Equine Vet J 1991;23:331.
73. Grondahl AM, Dolvik NI: Heritability estimations of osteochondrosis in the tibiotarsal joint and of bony fragments in the palmar/plantar portion of the metacarpo- and metatarsophalangeal joints of horses, J Am Vet Med Assoc 1993;203:101.
74. Grondahl AM, Jansen JH, Teige J: Accessory ossification centres associated with osteochondral fragments in the extremities of horses, J Comp Pathol 1996;114:385.
75. Sandgren B: Bony fragments in the tarsocrural and metacarpo- and metatarsophalangeal joints in the Standardbred horse: A radiographic study, Equine Vet J Suppl 1989;6:66.
76. Jeffcott LB, Kold SE: Clinical and radiological aspects of stifle bone cysts in the horse, Equine Vet J 1982;14:40.
77. McIlwraith CW: Osteochondrosis of the tibiotarsal (tarsocrural) joint, Proc Am Assoc Equine Pract 1993;39:69.
78. Little CB: Diseases of joints. In Kobluk CN, Ames TR, Geor RJ, editors: The Horse: Diseases and Clinical Management, Philadelphia, 1995, WB Saunders.
79. McIlwraith CW: Proceedings: Panel on developmental orthopedic disease, In Amarillo, Tex, 1986, American Quarter Horse Association.
80. Wagner PC, Watrous BJ: Equine pediatric orthopedics: Part 3. Tendon laxity and rupture, Equine Pract 1990;12:19.
81. Alvarado AF, Marcoux M, Breton L: The incidence of osteochondrosis in a Standardbred breeding farm in Quebec, Proc Am Assoc Equine Pract 1989;35:293.
82. Grondahl AM, Engeland A: Influence of radiographically detectable orthopedic changes on racing performance in Standardbred trotters, J Am Vet Med Assoc 1995;206:1013.
83. Beard WL, Bramlage LR, Schneider RK, et al: Postoperative racing performance in Standardbreds and Thoroughbreds with osteochondrosis of the tarsocrural joint: 109 cases (1984-1990), J Am Vet Med Assoc 1994;204:1655.
84. Laws EG, Richardson DW, Ross MW, et al: Racing performance of Standardbreds after conservative and surgical treatment for tarsocrural osteochondrosis, Equine Vet J 1993;25:199.

CHAPTER 100

Tibia

Larry R. Bramlage

The osseous structures of the tibial region include the tibia and fibula. The fibula is a rudimentary bone of variable shape and completeness. In most cases the fibula is incomplete and consists of several centers of ossification that are often mistaken for fibular fractures. Rarely, an atavistic complete fibula is identified radiographically in a pony or miniature horse foal.

The pathology associated with this condition creates limb deformities and tarsal arthritis (see Chapter 89). Other than traumatic injury, this is the only condition in which lameness is associated with the fibula.

By far the most common injuries of the tibial region are fractures. There are two common types of fractures of the tibia in the horse: the proximal physeal fracture and the diaphyseal fracture. The latter can be complete with displacement and instability, or it can be incomplete and stable.

PROXIMAL PHYSEAL FRACTURES

The most common tibial fracture in foals is the Salter-Harris type II proximal physeal fracture of the tibia (Fig. 100-1). It most often occurs when the foal is kicked from the lateral aspect on a weight-bearing rear limb. The soft tissue of the medial proximal tibial physis ruptures because of the tension created on the medial side of the limb when the traumatic bending force is applied. The fracture propagates across the tibial physis from medial to lateral approximately two thirds the width of the bone, at which point the medial bending force on the distal limb distracts the physis, changing the fracture plane orientation to vertical, leaving the lateral physis intact and a triangular metaphyseal fragment attached to the epiphysis.

With this fracture, the periosteal soft tissue is normally intact laterally but disrupted on the medial aspect. Occasionally, complete disruption of the soft tissue surrounding the physis occurs, rendering the fracture more unstable and creating more displacement.

Preoperative Considerations

The biomechanical force that creates the fracture is a tension force medially; therefore, fracture instability is best neutralized by re-establishing support on the medial aspect of the limb. This requires an implant that maintains the proximal tibial physis in a stable position on the metaphysis. Because normal bone formation, as part of bone growth, is already active in the growing physis, development of the vascular support system for fracture healing is unnecessary. Therefore, the fracture heals rapidly if it is stable, normally in 3 to 4 weeks (see Fig. 100-1).

Screw fixation,[1] pinning,[2] and external fixation[3] have been described for treating this fracture, and plate fixation has been used on the lateral aspect of the tibia.[4] A biomechanically stable fixation re-establishes the tension support on the medial aspect of the limb, a function that was previously provided by the soft tissue of the physis. If the lateral soft tissue is intact, stability is relatively easy to obtain. If the epiphysis is completely disrupted from the metaphysis, more elaborate fixation with more implants is required.

Although this fracture is usually closed, soft tissue damage occurs medially at the site where implants must be inserted. The close implant-to-skin location makes sepsis more difficult to avoid. Broad-spectrum antimicrobial agents and anti-inflammatory medications are administered preoperatively.

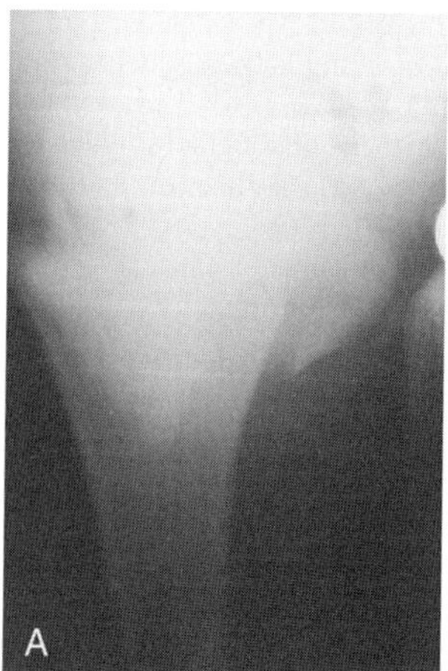

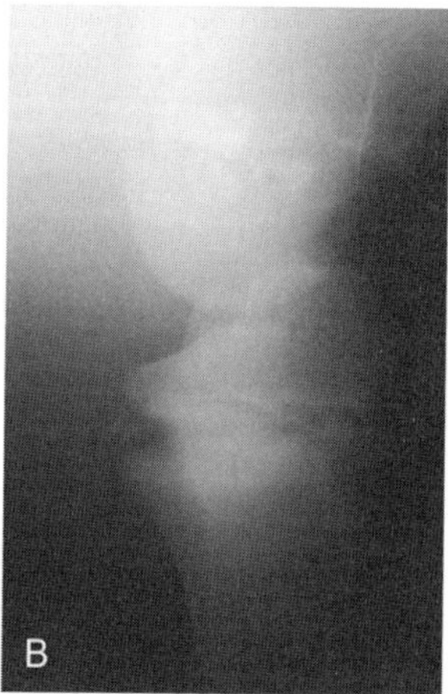

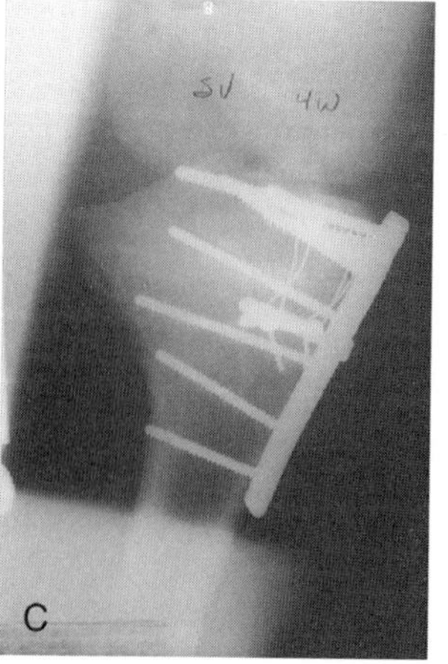

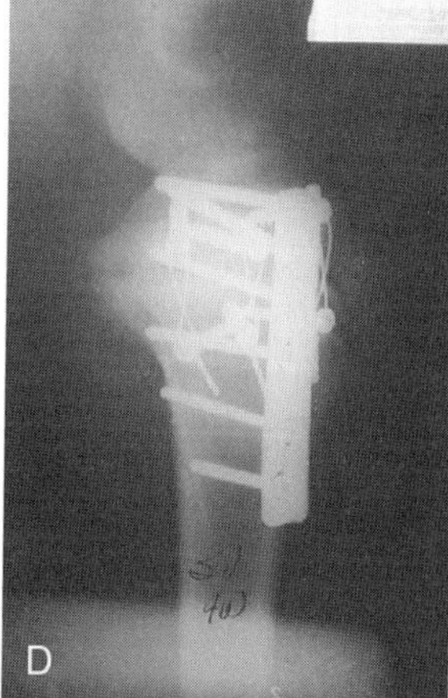

Figure 100-1. A and **B,** Craniocaudal and lateromedial radiographs of a Salter-Harris type II fracture of the proximal tibial physis, which was reduced and repaired with a 5-hole broad dynamic compression plate and two additional cortex screws placed in lag fashion. Two pairs of cortex screws also were inserted proximal and distal to the physes, respectively, and were each united with figure-eight cerclage for additional stability. **C** and **D,** Craniocaudal and lateromedial radiographs of the repaired fracture 4 weeks postoperatively, at the time of discharge from the clinic and resumption of normal exercise.

Treatment

The treatment of choice for proximal physeal fractures of the tibia in foals is medial plate fixation. The foal is positioned in either dorsal or lateral recumbency. When it is placed in lateral recumbency with the injured limb down, pressure on the proximal tibial physis facilitates reduction. The opposite rear limb is flexed, abducted, and tied vertically to prevent it from interfering with surgery on the medial aspect of the injured limb.

The approach to the proximal aspect of the tibia for medial plate application is along the caudal margin of the tibia. The soft tissue is elevated cranially, and the plate is placed on the medial aspect of the tibia. The close apposition of the tibia to the surface of the skin with no interposed muscle on the medial aspect of the limb complicates wound healing if the skin incision lies directly over the implant. Therefore, a slightly curved incision is initiated distally on the caudomedial aspect of the limb and extended cranioproximally across the proximal medial tibia. The proximal tibial physis is thin, and screws must be inserted sufficiently proximal to the growth plate to allow purchase in the bone but without endangering the articular surface. Placement of long needles along the plane of the proximal tibial physis permits orientation of the plane of the physis during drilling for screw placement.

Gentle traction on the physis separates the fracture plane and allows careful débridement. Removal of small fragments and blood clots permits accurate reduction of the physis. Damage to the growth cartilage of the physis is normally induced by the metaphysis near where the fracture plane changes from transverse to vertical. Evaluation of the physeal cartilage provides information on the likelihood of survival of proximal tibial growth plate function. The amount of damage depends on the time from injury to surgery and the adequacy of preoperative immobilization.

After the debris is removed from the fracture, the soft tissue must be elevated along the medial aspect of the proximal tibial physis. If this soft tissue is not elevated, it becomes trapped between the metaphyseal fragment and the physis, preventing complete reduction. Manual downward pressure on the medial aspect of the proximal tibial metaphysis places the intact soft tissue on the lateral aspect of the limb under tension and reduces the fracture. Reduction is maintained by the cranial placement of one 4.5-mm cortex screw in the epiphysis and one in the metaphysis. A figure-eight tension band wire is tightened between the two screws, maintaining reduction during placement of the primary implants.

Soft tissue dissection is carried to the bone surface on the metaphysis, but the soft tissue on the epiphysis should not be disturbed. A four-hole T-plate, right angle plate, or five-hole broad limited-contact dynamic compression plate (LC-DCP) or dynamic compression plate (DCP; see Fig. 100-1) is used for fixation. (T-plates and right-angle plates are named according to the number of vertical holes in the shaft; for example, a four-hole T-plate contains two horizontal holes and four additional holes in the vertical shaft.) The two transverse holes are positioned in the epiphysis closer to the posterior aspect of the proximal tibia, halfway between the stifle joint surface and the physis. The two proximal screws are inserted across the entire width of the epiphysis using needles in the physis for orientation. The use of 5.5-mm screws is ideal in the epiphysis. The four distal screws in the T-plate are inserted into the metaphysis after using the tension device or are placed in the load position to achieve compression. A second screw and wire insertion can be used to increase stability if needed (see Fig. 100-1).

Once fixation is complete, the soft tissue is closed. Closed suction drainage is optional. A stent bandage is sutured over the incision to reduce tension on and protect the incision. The area is difficult to bandage, but some compression of the soft tissue to reduce the hematoma can be obtained if elastic tape is used.

Aftercare

External coaptation is not used. The foal is assisted to its feet during recovery from anesthesia. Broad-spectrum antibiotic therapy along with anti-inflammatory treatment is continued until the swelling has subsided. The condition of the soft tissues postoperatively determines the length of antibiotic treatment. Foals are confined to the stall for 4 weeks, after which time radiographs are taken. If there is any indication of postoperative complications, radiographs are taken earlier. The foal should be bearing weight on the limb within 1 or 2 days and should begin walking soundly within 7 to 10 days. Absence of soundness indicates developing complications.

Complications

Three major complications are commonly encountered with this fracture: failure of the fixation, sepsis, and wound dehiscence. *Failure of the fixation* most commonly occurs by loss of purchase within the epiphysis. Failure seldom occurs from implant loosening in the metaphysis (Fig. 100-2) or by disruption of the implants themselves. Postoperative *sepsis* is possible, as with any equine fracture. A third complication that indirectly results in sepsis is *dehiscence* of the wound. The skin and subcutaneous tissue on the medial aspect of the limb are often traumatized by the sharp edge of the proximal tibial metaphysis if the duration from fracture to treatment was prolonged or if postinjury first aid was not adequate. Sepsis does not necessarily mean failure as long as it is appropriately treated with drainage and antibiotics sufficient to allow healing to occur and as long as stability is maintained.

Prognosis

The prognosis after repair of proximal physeal fractures is favorable, but the smaller the foal, the better the prognosis.[1-3] The preoperative condition of the soft tissues, the amount of soft tissue stability on the lateral aspect of the limb, the ability to reduce the fracture, and the security of the proximal epiphyseal implants all determine the outcome. Sufficient healing of the fracture and resolution of the injury to allow athletic activity are anticipated in 50% of cases. Closure of the proximal tibial physis occasionally occurs, but it is not a major complication. The proximal tibial physis of the horse does not close as readily as the physes of other animals or other sites, and the horse compensates for decreased limb length in spite of considerable damage if closure does occur.

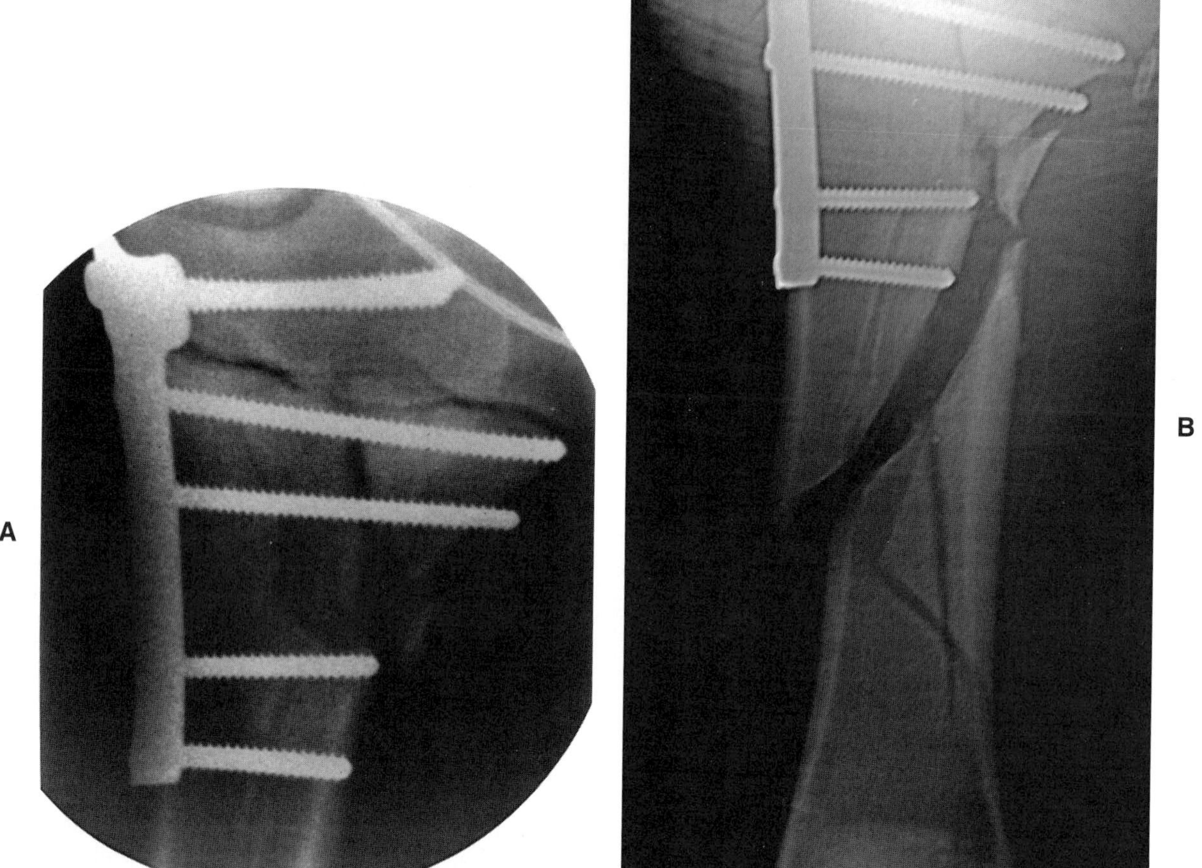

Figure 100-2. A, Craniocaudal intraoperative fluoroscopic view of a proximal tibial physeal fracture repaired with a four-hole T-plate. This fracture was more severe than a routine proximal tibial physeal fracture and required a more involved fixation. The metaphyseal component is comminuted and extends more than half the width of the bone. In addition, there is only one screw that is anchored in healthy bone distal to the comminuted fracture. This fracture probably required two implants and more distal fixation to resist the biomechanical instability the comminution created. **B,** The craniocaudal follow-up radiograph taken the next day, because the foal did not bear weight on the limb. A catastrophic bone failure occurred during the night. The fracture initiated at the distal end of the original fracture and spiraled distally, leading to a complete disruption of the bone. The owner did not want proceed with treatment and the foal was humanely destroyed. (Courtesy J. Auer, University of Zurich.)

DIAPHYSEAL FRACTURES

Diaphyseal fractures are the second common type of fracture of the tibia. Most diaphyseal fractures have a spiral configuration and are comminuted (Figs. 100-3 and 100-4). The fracture is created when the forces of loading, which in the tibia create considerable torque, are combined with an excessive external force. Diaphyseal fractures can occur in animals of any age. Appropriate first-aid therapy is necessary to minimize secondary soft tissue damage, as with any fracture (see Chapter 78). The trauma required to fracture a tibia often creates an open fracture.

Incomplete Fractures

Horses with incomplete fissure or stress fractures of the tibia have marked lameness that often resolves quickly. Pain can be elicited with palpation, but the diagnosis is made radiographically or with nuclear scintigraphy. It is important to include several oblique projections at different angles to identify the faint fracture planes. Occasionally, no fissure is seen at the initial examination. This is an indication for nuclear scintigraphy.

A stress fracture is suspected and the animal is placed in a stall. The radiographic examination is repeated 8 to 14 days later, at which time the fracture is usually identified. Stall rest is continued until the horse is sound. Initially, in tractable horses, it is prudent to prevent the horse from lying down either by tying it in front of a hay net or by applying a rescue net (see Fig. 81-1) This judgment must take into consideration the demeanor of the horse, because the risk of displacement might be increased in some horses because of restriction of movement.

Healing is monitored through monthly radiographs. Once healing has progressed adequately (usually in 3 to 4 months), a slowly increasing exercise program is begun. The prognosis for nondisplaced tibial fractures is favorable if they do not displace. The horse can resume work 30 days after the fracture is healed.

Complete Fractures

Preoperative Considerations

Usually, diaphyseal fractures of the adult tibia are high-energy, catastrophic injuries accompanied by extensive comminution and are quite often open. For these reasons, attempts at repair are seldom made. However, this fracture in foals usually has less comminution and repair has a greater chance of success.

Traction on the distal limb does not reduce a tibial fracture; in fact, it causes overriding because of the reciprocal apparatus. Placing the injured tibia down with the horse in lateral recumbency impedes surgical manipulation of the diaphyseal fracture and necessitates a medial surgical approach, where little soft tissue covers the bone and implant. Therefore, the horse is best positioned in dorsal recumbency or in lateral recumbency with the injured tibia uppermost.

Approaches to the tibia for diaphyseal fracture repair must take the following anatomy into consideration. The cranial tibial artery is located on the cranial lateral aspect of the tibia. The lateral outpouching (sulcus muscularis) of the lateral femorotibial joint compartment extends distally, surrounding the long digital extensor tendon on the proximal lateral aspect of the tibia. The tenuous soft tissue on the medial aspect of the tibia and the closely attached digital extensor tendons distally must be avoided near the tarsocrural joint.

Three surgical approaches are available: the medial approach directly over the tibia without muscle cover; the lateral approach between the long digital extensor and the cranial tibial muscles; and the cranial approach, in which the incision is made over the cranial tibial muscle.[5] The cranial approach over the muscle is the most versatile.

Deep dissection is extended slightly medially and the periosteum is incised, allowing the muscle and periosteum to be retracted as one unit laterally, permitting a cranial approach to the proximal tibial shaft. The cranial approach eliminates the necessity of dealing with any blood vessels, because all the vasculature is elevated with the periosteum and the cranial tibial muscle. Implants can be placed on the medial and lateral aspects of the bone through this incision, eliminating the need for two incisions, as with the medial and lateral approaches. The biomechanics of weightbearing of the tibia dictate that two plates be used, that one plate be placed craniolaterally[6] to neutralize torque loading, and that the major implant be placed on this tension surface of the bone (see Figs. 100-3 and 100-4).

Broad-spectrum antimicrobial agents and anti-inflammatory medications are administered preoperatively.

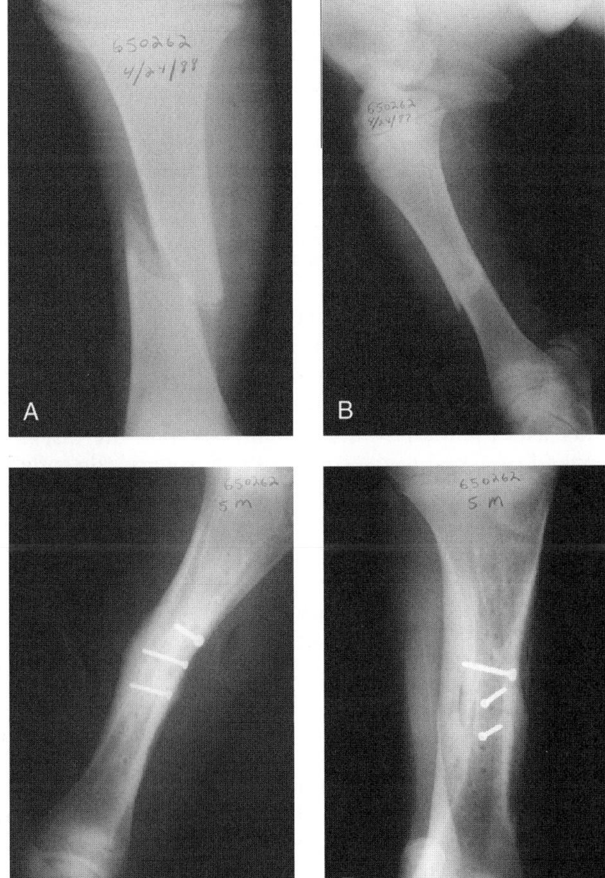

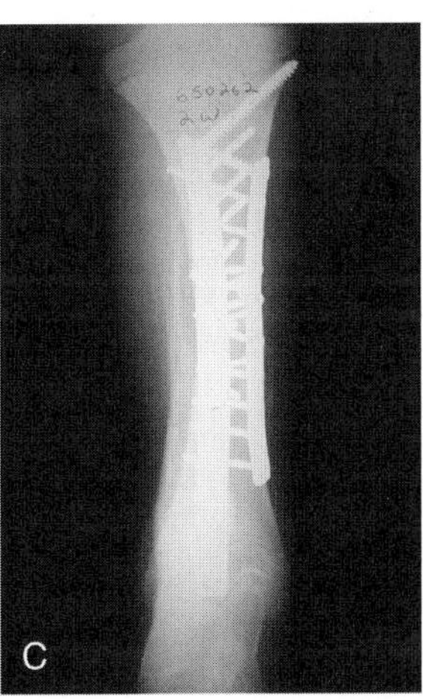

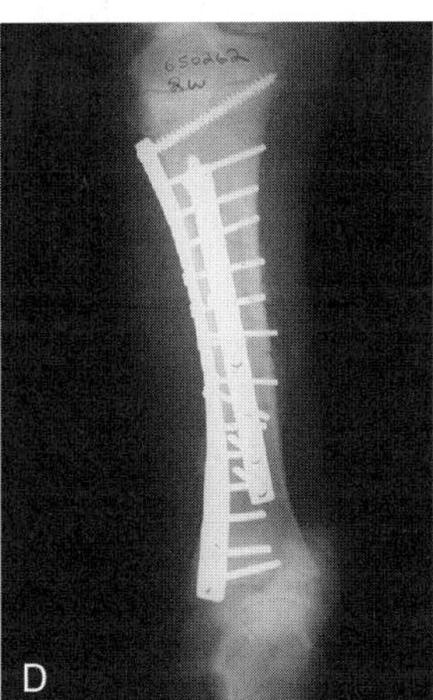

Figure 100-3. A and **B,** Craniocaudal and lateromedial radiographs of a mid-shaft tibial fracture in a foal. The fracture was repaired with three cortex screws applied across the fracture in lag fashion. Additionally, a long plate, spanning the tibia from one metaphysis to the other, and a shorter second plate at 90 degrees to the first was implanted. **C** and **D,** Craniocaudal and lateromedial radiographs of the repaired fracture when the foal was discharged from the hospital. **E** and **F,** Craniocaudal and lateromedial radiographs of the healed fracture –after the plates were removed 5 months after the fracture. The three initial screws were covered by bone and, therefore, were left in place.

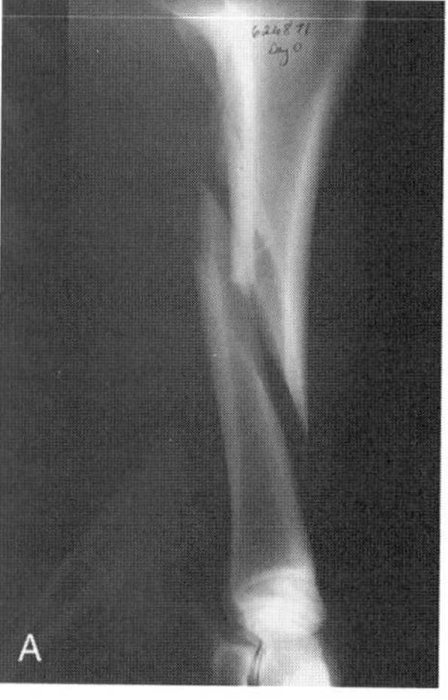
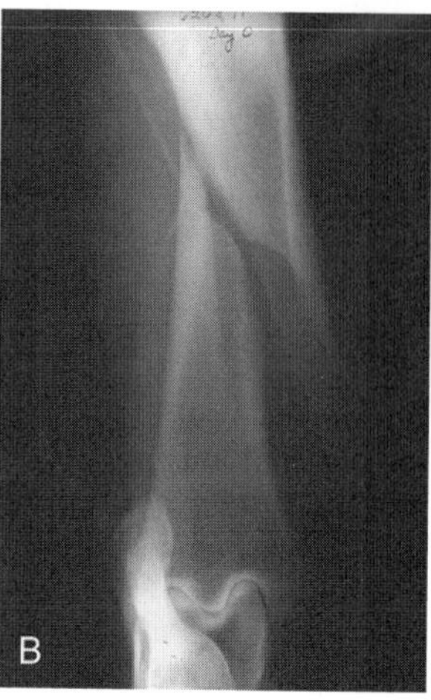
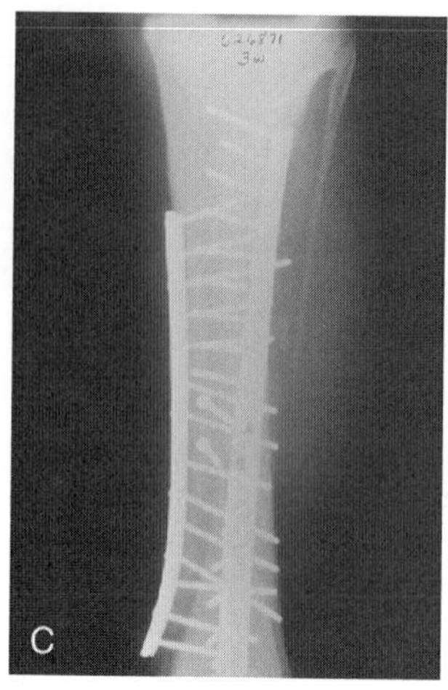
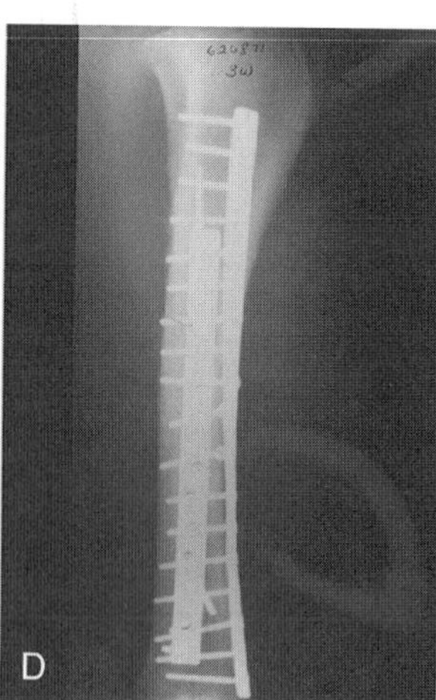

Figure 100-4. **A** and **B,** Craniocaudal and lateromedial radiographs of a fracture of the tibia in an adult horse. The fracture was repaired with two plates after initial compression screw fixation. **C** and **D,** Craniocaudal and lateromedial radiographic views of the same fracture at the time of the patient's discharge from the clinic, 3 weeks after surgery.

Treatment

The incision is initiated craniolaterally along the lateral patellar ligament, extended to the tibial crest, directed craniad over the cranial tibial muscle to the distal aspect of the limb, and curved slightly medially as the tarsocrural joint is approached. The incision is carried through the skin and subcutaneous fascia until the cranial tibial muscle is encountered. The cranial tibial muscle is elevated laterally, the periosteum is incised, and a subperiosteal dissection plane is established from cranial to lateral, exposing the lateral surface of the bone.

Positioning of the implant at the most proximal aspect of the tibia in proximal metaphyseal and mid-diaphyseal fractures necessitates entering the stifle joint through the sulcus muscularis, which surrounds the long digital extensor muscle. Normally, the long digital extensor and cranial tibial attachments are avoided by separating them, which allows placement of the implant near the proximal physis or physeal scar. Working on both sides of the cranial tibial muscle allows placement of the plate without damaging the muscle.

Fracture reduction is accomplished by traction on the distal tibia and appropriate reconstruction of the bone. The repair begins by reattaching comminuted fragments to the parent bone with lag screws to create a two-fragment fracture. The fracture is reduced to a proximal and distal fragment, and the plate is contoured to mimic the curve of the tibia from craniolateral proximally to cranial distally (see Figs. 100-3 and 100-4). The use of dynamic condylar screw (DCS) plates or 5.5-mm LC-DCPs is strongly encouraged, especially in older foals and the rare adult horse subjected to treatment. The screws are inserted in the order dictated by the individual fracture, which differs from case to case. Care must be taken to cross any fracture plane with screws placed in lag fashion and to create interfragmentary as well as axial compression during application of the plate for the most stable fixation.

Once the craniolateral plate is in place, the craniomedial plate is applied. It is contoured from craniomedial to medial and positioned in an envelope under the skin and subcutaneous tissue created by elevation of the periosteum medially. It is occasionally necessary to flex and abduct the limb to gain access to the medial aspect of the tibia. The medial plate is positioned to avoid the screws of the lateral plate. Interfragmentary and axial compression is created as needed. Both plates can be loaded to distribute the axial compression circumferentially around the bone. Plate luting has been advocated for repair of this fracture to increase stability and fatigue life of the implant construct. After placement of the plates, a suction drain is inserted, exiting proximolaterally, and attached to a suction reservoir.

Closure involves the fascia of the cranial tibial muscle, subcutaneous tissue, and skin. Release incisions can be made in the skin over the cranial tibial muscle to relieve tension on the closure if perioperative swelling and operative manipulation have increased the diameter of the limb.

Postoperatively, no cast is used. Cast immobilization increases the load on the implants because the cast cannot extend proximal to the stifle in the horse and the stifle joint cannot be immobilized. Stent bandages are sewn over the incision. The horse is allowed to recover from anesthesia unimpeded by bandages; bandages are placed once the horse is standing. The horse is always assisted in recovery; it should be helped to regain the standing position in one attempt, if possible. Bandaging is used as indicated during the postoperative period.

Aftercare

Antibiotics and anti-inflammatory drugs are continued for a prolonged period because tibial fractures are accompanied by considerable soft tissue damage. The health of the soft tissue and the postoperative use of the limb by the patient dictate the length of antibiotic and anti-inflammatory therapy.

Stall rest is maintained, with no exercise allowed for 6 to 8 weeks, depending on the age of the horse. Foals are often radiographed at 6 weeks, whereas follow-up radiographs are taken at 8 weeks in adults to ascertain whether bridging of the fracture has occurred. Postoperative use of the limb is the most accurate assessment of stability of the fracture. If use of the limb is not attained or diminishes, radiographs are taken.

Complications

The most common complication with tibial fractures is breakdown of the fixation because of bone or implant failure. Tibial fractures are most often comminuted in configuration, and the torsional force applied to a fractured bone that contains multiple drill holes often causes propagation of the fracture into additional sites. A single acute overload generally causes the bone to fail. Complications also include postoperative sepsis because of primary infection or breakdown of the incision. With any major long bone fracture, failure of the implants can occur with repeated cyclic loading.

Prognosis

Simple fractures in adult horses can be repaired successfully with internal fixation (see Fig. 100-4); however, this fracture configuration is the exception rather than the rule. Most diaphyseal tibial fractures are comminuted and accompanied by massive soft tissue damage. Therefore, the prognosis for tibial fractures is unfavorable in adults. In foals, however, internal fixation of tibial fractures can be successful when the fracture is immobilized and the implants protect the bone enough to allow healing[7] (see Fig. 100-3). The prognosis is guarded even in foals, but 60% success in healing of the fracture and dismissal of the horse postoperatively is attainable in selected fractures. Athletic activity is undertaken if the surgical procedure and stabilization proceed without complications.

DISTAL PHYSEAL FRACTURES

Fractures of the distal epiphysis occur rarely. Diagnosis is routine, and treatment involves external coaptation with a fiberglass cast alone or in conjunction with selective screw placement. The architecture of the undulating articular surface of the distal tibia and the corresponding physis makes implant placement into the epiphysis especially difficult, because neither should be endangered.

TIBIAL CREST FRACTURES

Tibial crest fractures are generally the result of direct trauma, often during attempts to jump a fence or from contact with other solid objects. By far the most common type of tibial crest fracture is the nondisplaced nonarticular fracture (Fig. 100-5). These fractures require no fixation because the patellar ligaments provide adequate stability for healing. Stall confinement for 60 days with follow-up radiographs at that time usually show adequate healing for gradual reintroduction to exercise.

If the tibial crest fracture is displaced or is articular (Fig. 100-6), the fracture is stabilized in much the same fashion as a proximal tibial physeal fracture with fixation and stabilization employing a tension band cranially and implants sufficient to stabilize the fracture and reconstruct the joint surface.

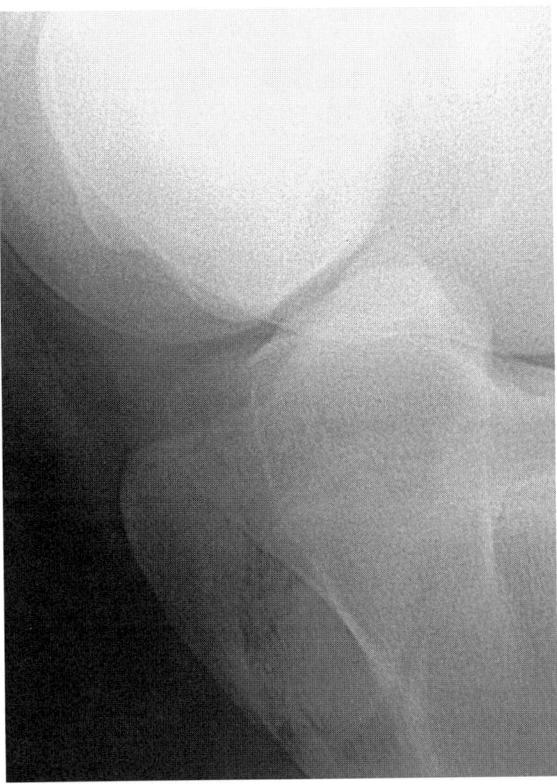

Figure 100-5. Lateromedial radiograph of the most commonly encountered tibial crest fracture. It usually results from impact of the hindlimb on a solid object such as a fence post or rail. If it is not displaced, it requires no fixation.

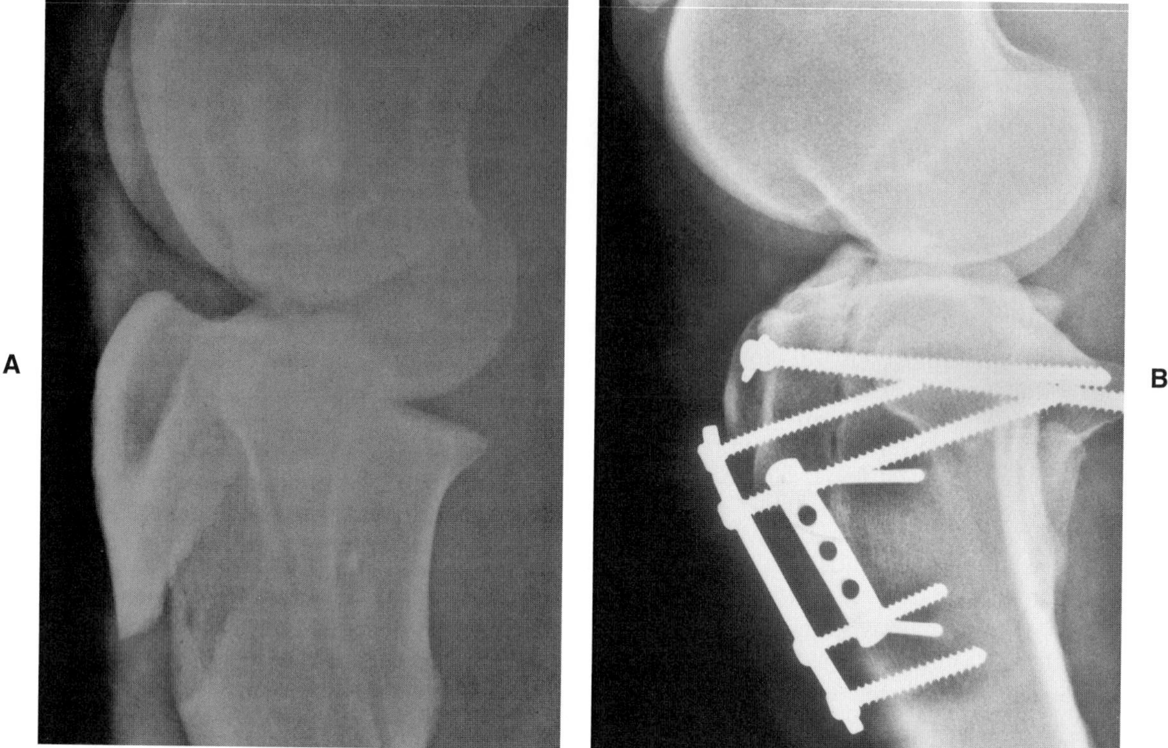

Figure 100-6. A, Lateromedial radiograph of a displaced tibial crest fracture, **B,** The fracture was repaired proximally with two 5.5-mm cortex screws applied in lag fashion perpendicularly across the fracture plane. In one screw, a washer was applied to avoid countersinking and concomitant weakening of the bone. Additionally a five-hole narrow dynamic compression plate (DCP) was applied over the medial ridge as a tension band and a five-hole 2.7-mm cuttable small animal plate with two 3.5-mm cortex screws over the lateral aspect of the fracture to provide a greater area of fixation and reduce stress concentration. The fracture healed without complications.

REFERENCES

1. Wagner PC, DeBowes RM, Grant BD, et al: Cancellous bone screws for repair of proximal growth plate fractures of the tibia in foals, J Am Vet Med Assoc 1984;184:688.
2. Watkins JP, Auer JA, Taylor TS: Crosspin fixation of fractures of the proximal tibia in three foals, Vet Surg 1985;14:153.
3. White NA, Wheat JD: An expansion and compression technique for reducing and stabilizing proximal epiphyseal fractures of the tibia in foals, J Am Vet Med Assoc 1975;167:733.
4. White NA, Blackwell RB, Hoffman PE: Use of a bone plate for repair of proximal physeal fractures of the tibia in two foals, J Am Vet Med Assoc 1982;181:252.
5. Bramlage LR, Hanes GE: Internal fixation of a tibial fracture in an adult horse, J Am Vet Med Assoc 1982;180:1090.
6. Schneider RK, Milne DW, Groom J: Multidirectional in vivo strain analysis of the equine radius and tibia during dynamic loading with and without a cast, Am J Vet Res 1982;43:1541.
7. Young DR, Richardson DW, Nunamaker DM, et al: Use of dynamic compression plates for treatment of tibial diaphyseal fractures in foals: Nine cases (1980-1987), J Am Vet Med Assoc 1989;194:1755.

CHAPTER 101

Stifle

John A. Stick

Because the stifle is the most complex and largest joint in the horse, it represents an important cause of hindlimb lameness.[1] Although it is cited as a common location of hindlimb lameness in the horse, the incidence is reported to be between 2% and 8% of all musculoskeletal problems that occur in lameness surveys.[2,3]

Stifle lameness clinically appears as swelling in the stifle region and is referred to as *gonitis*. The injury can be to soft tissue, bone, or cartilage, and it can range from simple sprains with a favorable prognosis to severely debilitating lameness necessitating humane destruction. With long-standing stifle involvement, atrophy of the gluteal muscles on the affected side may be apparent, and wearing of the toe of the affected hindlimb is common. The degree of lameness varies from almost occult to nonweightbearing, and when viewed from the rear, asymmetry of the gait is similar to hindlimb lameness seen from other causes.

Although minor injuries are generally accepted to originate in the soft tissue, bone involvement has been cited to have a higher incidence than soft tissue injury in one case study.[4] Uncertainty surrounding the diagnosis of conditions affecting the stifle joint in the horse 10 years ago have given way to accurate definitive descriptions of numerous disorders. With the advent of digital capture radiography techniques, fluoroscopy, scintigraphy, new applications of ultrasonography, and computed tomography, the definitive diagnoses of stifle lameness because of soft tissue injury have become more common. Likewise, surgical diagnosis and treatment by way of arthroscopy has become routine in most referral centers.

This chapter includes functional anatomy and diagnostic techniques pertaining to this complex joint in the horse, followed by disorders of the stifle joint, which have been divided into traumatic and developmental categories.

FUNCTIONAL ANATOMY

The stifle consists of two joints—the femoropatellar and the femorotibial[5] (Fig. 101-1). The femoropatellar joint has a large suprapatellar pouch, and the joint capsule inserts abaxially on the trochlear ridges, forming a lateral and a large medial cul-de-sac on each side. The femorotibial joint consists of two separate synovial sacs that do not communicate.[5-8] Each synovial sac is divided into a cranial pouch and a caudal pouch by the condyles (Fig. 101-2). The volume in the medial and lateral sacs of the femorotibial joints are reported to take, respectively, 41.67 ± 5.77 mL and 61.67 ± 2.89 mL of fluid injection. The cruciate ligaments are situated between the two synovial sacs of the femorotibial joint.

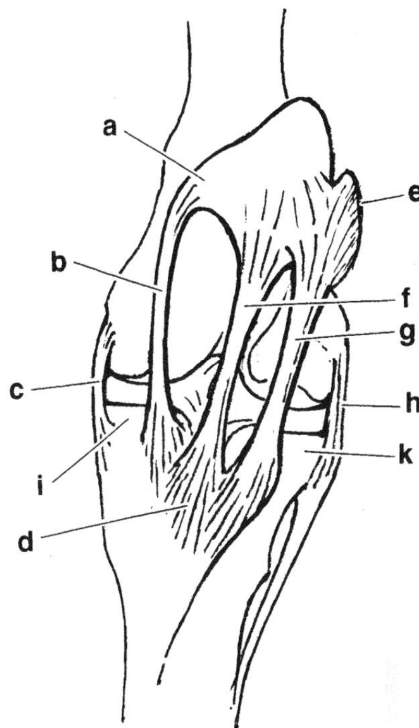

Figure 101-1. Anatomy of the equine stifle, cranial view, showing a, parapatellar ligament; b, medial patellar ligament; c, medial collateral ligament; d, tibial tuberosity; e, cut stump of the biceps femoris muscle; f, middle patellar ligament; g, lateral patellar ligament; h, lateral collateral ligament; i and k, medial and lateral condyles of tibia.

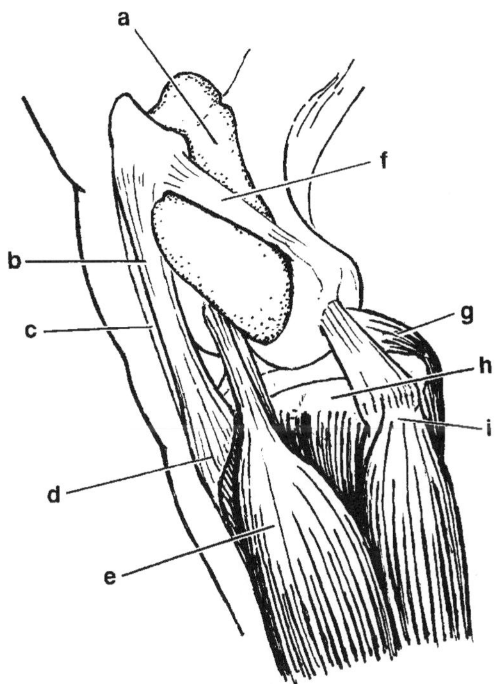

Figure 101-2. Anatomy of the equine stifle, lateral view, showing a, femoropatellar joint sac; b, middle patellar ligament; c, medial patellar ligament; d, cut stump of the lateral patellar ligament; e, extensor digitorum longus muscle; f, lateral femoropatellar ligament; g, popliteus muscle; h, lateral tibial condyle; i, extensor digitorum lateralis muscle.

There is communication between the femoropatellar joint and the medial femorotibial sac that is rarely absent, but the communication between the femoropatellar joint and the lateral sac of the femorotibial joint occurs in only 18% to 25% of horses.[5,9] In experimental studies, the communication between the femoropatellar joint and the medial sac of the femorotibial joint was found to be 60% to 65% and 1% to 17.5% between the femoropatellar joint and the lateral sac of the femorotibial joint.

DIAGNOSTIC TECHNIQUES

Inspection

Lameness evaluation of the stifle includes observation of the horse both at rest and during movement, palpation of the synovial structures of the joint and the patellar ligaments, and diagnostic aids such as manipulative tests and intra-articular anesthesia. Clinical signs depend on the severity and chronicity of the injury. Injuries causing pain such as fractures, sepsis, or instability of the joint (cruciate or collateral ligament damage) produce the most severe lameness. Chronic lameness of a rear limb results in atrophy of the gluteal muscles, causing an asymmetric appearance of the croup when viewed from the rear. The asymmetry is also exacerbated because the lame horse bears the weight on the affected limb for a shorter amount of time during movement. This results in a shortened anterior phase of the stride when viewed from the side. When viewed from the rear at the trot, there is a greater excursion (vertical displacement) of the tuber coxae on the affected than on the opposite side.[10]

Synovial distention of the femoropatellar joint may be visually obvious (Fig. 101-3) or quite subtle. Subtle changes can be detected by careful palpation between the patellar ligaments and over the patella and by comparing the two stifle joints. Synovial distention of the femorotibial joint sacs can be difficult to detect but can be palpated immediately cranial or caudal to the collateral ligaments. Palpation of swelling or crepitation of the patella indicates patellar fractures. Patellar ligament laxity is difficult to detect by palpation, but if manipulation of the patella proximad and laterad causes pain or the inability to flex the stifle, upward fixation of the patella should be suspected.

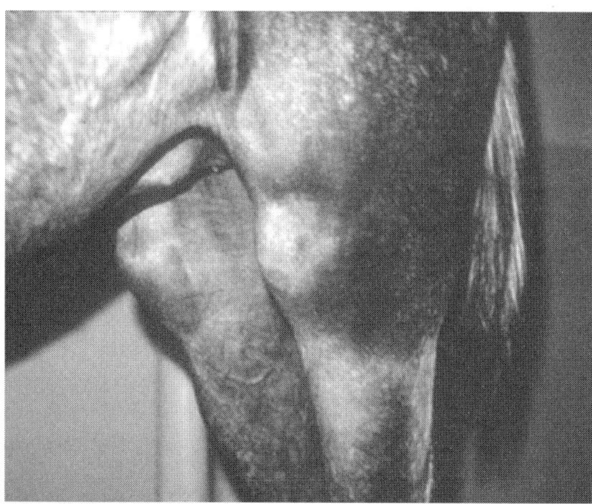

Figure 101-3. Appearance of bilateral femoropatellar effusion. Note the enlargement over both patellar regions.

Manipulation

Manipulative tests of the joint can exacerbate the lameness. These tests include the hock/stifle flexion test, the patellar test, the cruciate test, and an evaluation of the collateral ligaments.

Hock flexion also causes flexion of the stifle and is performed by grasping the distal metatarsus and holding the hindlimb in flexion for 1 to 2 minutes. The fetlock and phalangeal joints are only passively flexed by this method. A positive response to this test causes increased lameness but is not specific for either joint; therefore, one must differentiate by other diagnostic aids.

Two tests have been described for evaluation of the cruciate ligaments. These tests are supposed to elicit pain and lameness because of the abnormal movement created between the femur and the tibia if there is damage to the cruciate ligaments. The first test is for only the most cooperative horses. To perform this test, the examiner stands behind the affected limb and firmly grasps the proximal tibia with both hands (Fig. 101-4). If any movement or crepitation is detected when the examiner gives a quick pull backward, the test is said to be positive.[11] The second test is carried out with the examiner standing directly in front of the affected limb, placing the inside hand on the proximal tibia, and grasping and pulling the tail to load the limb while rapidly pushing and releasing the force on the tibia repeatedly 20 to 25 times. The horse is then trotted away to evaluate for increased lameness.

The medial collateral ligaments can be evaluated by elevating the limb off the ground and placing pressure on the lateral aspect of the stifle joint while abducting the distal limb. The lateral collateral ligament can be evaluated by elevating the limb off the ground and pulling the stifle joint laterally while adducting the distal limb.

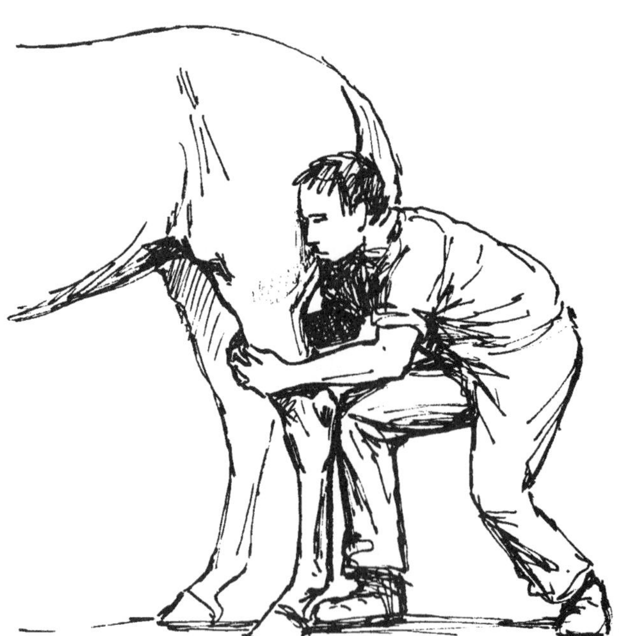

Figure 101-4. Cruciate ligament test used to detect rupture. The shoulder is placed against the back of the limb and the tibia is pulled caudad and released.

Anesthesia

Intra-articular anesthesia is an important diagnostic aid in determining articular involvement. Although local anesthesia diffuses between all stifle compartments about 75% of the time, when performing intra-articular anesthesia of the stifle, three synovial sites should be injected separately to ensure anesthesia of the intended synovial sac.[6,7,12]

Arthrocentesis of the *femoropatellar joint* can be performed through either a cranial or a lateral approach. The cranial approach is performed by inserting a 7.5-cm (3-in.) spinal needle between the medial and middle patellar ligaments or between the middle and lateral patellar ligaments and directing it proximally in the trochlear groove under the patella. The lateral approach is performed by inserting a 3.75-cm (1.5-in.) 18-gauge needle into the lateral cul-de-sac of the femoropatellar joint just caudal to the lateral patellar ligament and approximately 6 cm (2.5 in.) proximal to the lateral tibial condyle.[13]

The approach for the *lateral sac of the femorotibial joint* is performed by inserting a 3.75-cm 18-gauge needle between the lateral patellar ligament and the tendon of the long digital extensor muscle or between the previous tendon and the lateral collateral ligament above the proximal edge of the meniscus into the joint. The approach for the *medial sac of the femorotibial joint* is performed by inserting the 18-gauge needle between the medial patellar ligament and the medial collateral ligament above the proximal edge of the meniscus into the joint. The use of an 18-gauge needle and a bleb of local anesthetic in the skin at the insertion point to reduce limb flexion during the procedure reduces the chance of needle bending and breakage.

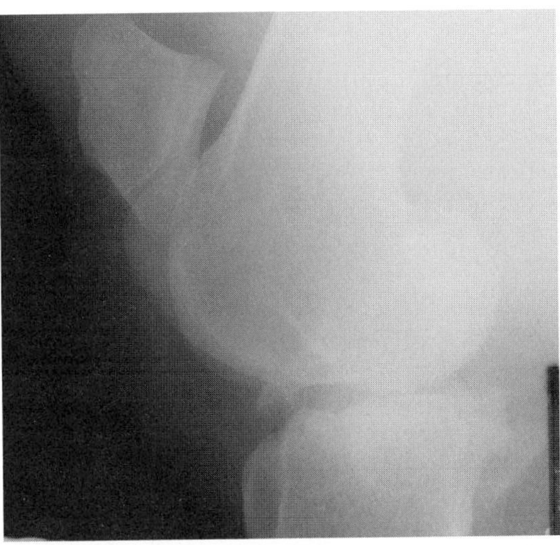

Figure 101-5. A lateromedial radiographic view of the stifle demonstrating an osseous fragment near the distal insertion of the cranial cruciate ligament, which represents an avulsion of the tibial eminence.

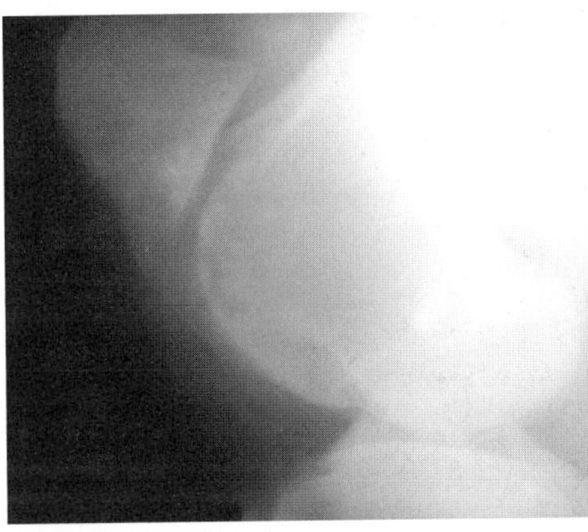

Figure 101-6. A caudal 30-degree lateral craniomedial oblique radiographic view of the stifle of a horse with osteochondrosis lesions of the lateral trochlear ridge of the femur.

DIAGNOSTIC IMAGING

Radiography

Four radiographic views are necessary for complete evaluation of the stifle: lateromedial, flexed lateromedial, caudocranial, and caudal 30-degree lateral craniomedial oblique. With the exception of the caudocranial view, these views can be taken with low-output portable equipment. However, for a complete examination, a caudocranial view of the stifle should be included. In mature horses, the x-ray machine will need a minimum output of 90 kV and 20 mA. Rare-earth screens and films are recommended, and a cassette holder should be used because of the amount of radiation necessary to obtain quality films of this large joint.

The lateromedial view highlights osseous irregularities near the insertion of the cranial cruciate ligament (Fig. 101-5). A flexed lateromedial view of the stifle, with the limb lifted and retracted caudally, permits patellar and condylar lesions to be seen more easily. The caudal 30-degree lateral craniomedial oblique view prevents superimposition of the images of the trochlear ridges and condyles of the femur (Fig. 101-6). The x-ray beam should be aligned 10 to 15 degrees proximodistally and 30 degrees caudolateral to craniomedial. Lateral trochlear ridge lesions are most easily seen with this view.

The caudocranial view is best obtained by angling the x-ray beam 10 to 20 degrees proximodistally and centered on a line bisecting the limb between the semimembranosus and semitendinosus muscles at a level of the distal third of these muscles. This view is best for demonstrating medial condylar cysts and osteoarthritis of the stifle (Fig. 101-7).

One special view that can be taken is a cranioproximal craniodistal oblique view (skyline) (Fig. 101-8). This view is used primarily to evaluate the patella, the intertrochanteric groove of the distal femur, and the trochlear ridges. It is most useful in demonstrating patellar fractures. In standing horses, the limb should be held semiflexed and drawn caudal to the horse. The cassette is held horizontally with its caudal edge against the cranial aspect of the tibia. The x-ray beam should be directed perpendicularly to the cassette as much as possible.

The stifle of the horse has six centers of ossification at birth. This makes radiographic assessment of the foal somewhat challenging. A summary of closure of growth plates and ossification sites is as follows: The patella is fully ossified by 4 months of age. The proximal portions of the trochlear ridges show irregular contours and granular subchondral bone opacity, which slowly becomes a smooth, regular subchondral bone outline between 3 and 5 months

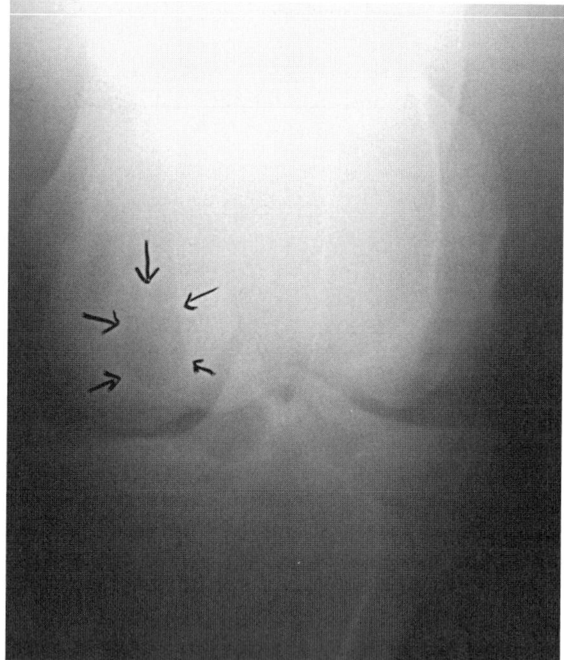

Figure 101-7. A caudocranial view of the stifle demonstrating a large bone cyst *(arrows)* in the medial femoral condyle.

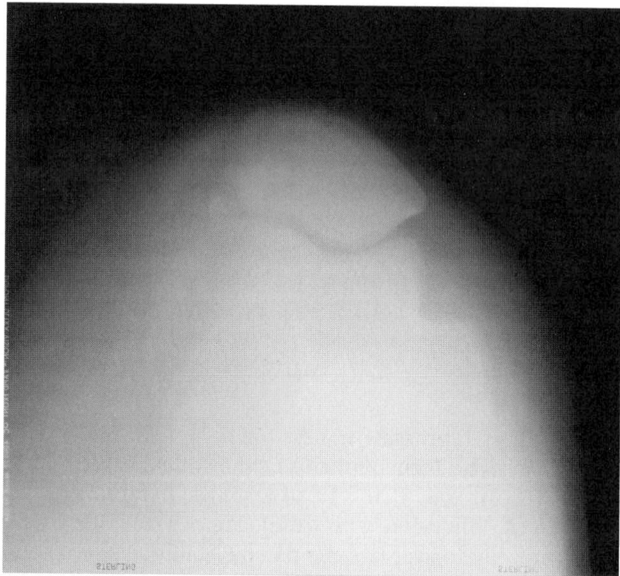

Figure 101-8. Cranioproximal craniodistal oblique radiographic view (skyline) of the equine stifle, which is used to evaluate the patella, intertrochanteric groove of the femur, and trochlear ridges. Note the sagittal fracture of the medial aspect of the patella.

of age. The distal femoral physis closes at 24 to 30 months of age. The femoral condyles are smoothly outlined, and any irregularity except in young foals should be interpreted as pathologic. At birth, the center of ossification of the tibial tuberosity (apophysis) is separated from the proximal tibial epiphysis as well as from the proximal tibial metaphysis. The apophyseal epiphyseal physis closes between 9 and 12 months of age, and the apophyseal metaphyseal physis closes at 30 to 36 months. The proximal tibial physis closes at 24 to 30 months of age. The fibula has multiple ossification centers that can remain incomplete throughout the life of the horse.

In adult horses, the trochlear ridges are smoothly curved in outline, but the medial trochlear ridge has a small, flattened area at its junction with the metaphysis of the femur. The medial trochlear ridge appears more prominent proximally and is flatter than the lateral ridge. On a caudocranial view in the adult horse, the patella is seen superimposed on the lateral cortex of the diaphysis of the femur. The medial femoral condyle is rounder than the lateral condyle, and the lateral joint space of the femoral tibial joint is narrower than the medial joint space. On the cranioproximal to craniodistal oblique view, the medial trochlear ridge is larger than the lateral ridge and is separated from it by a trochlear groove. The patella is approximately triangular, and its medial angle is blunter than the lateral angle.

Other Imaging Studies

Scintigraphy, computed tomography, fluoroscopy, and ultrasonography are additional imaging modalities that can be used to diagnose stifle pathology. The techniques used for scintigraphic examination are similar to those for other joint areas, and although its application for diagnosis of equine stifle lameness has been described, it is limited because of expense[14] (see Chapter 75). Computed tomography has been limited to research related to anatomic studies of the stifle (Fig. 101-9). Likewise, contrast techniques under fluoroscopic guidance have also been used for anatomic studies but are not of practical value in clinical cases (Fig. 101-10). Ultrasonographic examination of the

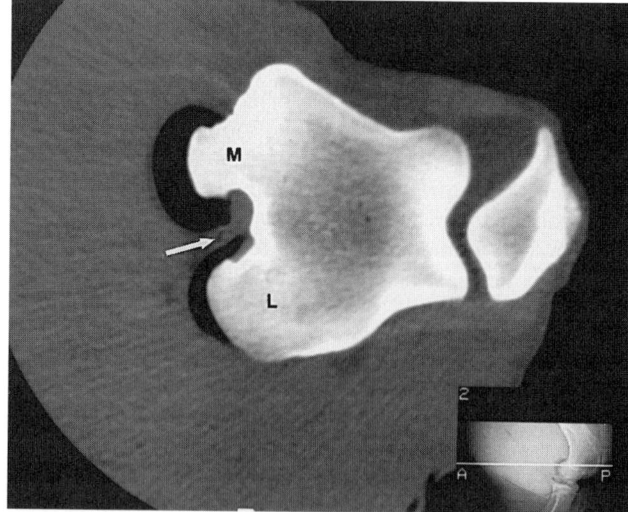

Figure 101-9. Computed tomographic (CT) image of a transverse cross-section of the right stifle of an equine cadaver limb after injection of the caudal pouches of the femorotibial joints with shaving cream, demonstrating the extent of distention of the caudal pouch of the medial femorotibial joint and caudal pouch of the lateral femorotibial joint at the level of the proximal aspect of the medial and lateral femoral condyles. The popliteal artery and vein *(arrow)* line the septum separating the caudal pouches. M, medial femoral condyle; L, lateral femoral condyle. (From Trumble TN, Stick JA, Arnoczky SP, Rosenstein D: Am J Vet Res 1994;55:1682.)

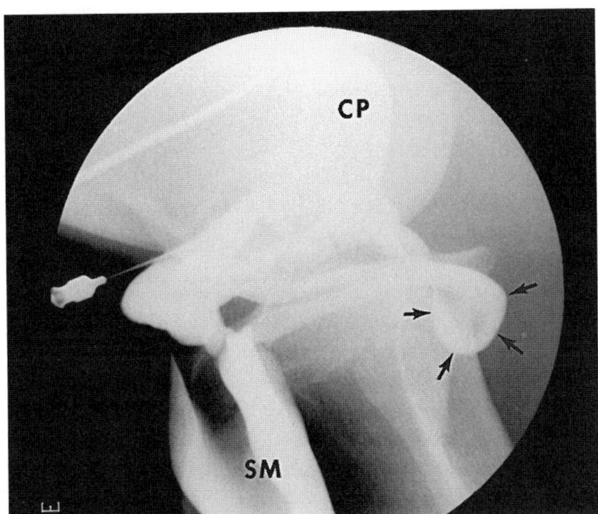

Figure 101-10. Fluoroscopic image of the lateral femorotibial joint of the stifle of an equine cadaver limb after injection of positive contrast medium into the caudal pouch of the lateral femorotibial joint, showing distention of the proximal compartment of the caudal pouch of the lateral femorotibial joint (CP), the sulcus muscularis (SM), and the area of the distal compartment of the caudal pouch of the lateral femorotibial joint *(arrows)*.

stifle, however, has been used to delineate injury in superficial structures, such as patellar and collateral ligaments.

Sonographic examination of the human knee is a widely established technique.[15-20] Although ultrasonography is widely used to diagnose specific equine orthopedic conditions, especially tendon injuries, and the ultrasonic anatomy of the metacarpophalangeal, metatarsophalangeal, shoulder, and tarsal joints have been established, ultrasonographic anatomy and pathology of the equine stifle were limited until recently.[21-23] Anatomic structures that can be identified include the cranial and medial third of both menisci, femoral and tibial articular cartilage, and tendons and ligaments surrounding the stifle.[23,24] However, only a small portion of the cruciate ligaments can be imaged. Pathologic conditions that can be identified include intra-articular bone fragments, thickening of the synovial membrane, joint effusion, and meniscal tears. This modality will continue to assume a more prominent role in the diagnosis of stifle problems in the horse in the future. Currently, the definitive method for determining the extent of intraarticular stifle injuries is arthroscopy.

ARTHROSCOPY

Diagnostic and surgical arthroscopy of the equine stifle is well established. Arthroscopy is most commonly performed to treat osteochondrosis of this joint, and most of the approaches have been developed based on the multiple locations of this disorder. Arthroscopy is also used routinely to establish a prognosis after traumatic injury that could involve damage to the menisci, cruciate ligaments, meniscal ligaments, and articular cartilage.

Complete arthroscopic examination of the stifle necessitates exploration of six separate synovial compartments. This, however, is rarely done because compartments are usually explored based on clinical and radiographic findings that often localize lesions to one aspect of the stifle. Because the stifle of the horse consists of two joints, the femoropatellar and the femorotibial, they are explored separately.

The femorotibial joint has two synovial sacs (medial and lateral) that do not communicate normally, and each of these synovial sacs can be divided into cranial and caudal pouches. Furthermore, the caudal pouch of the lateral femorotibial joint sac is divided into two separate pouches, proximal and distal, by the popliteal tendon. The following compartments can be explored:

- The cranial pouch of the medial femorotibial joint
- The caudal pouch of the medial femorotibial joint
- The cranial pouch of the lateral femorotibial joint
- The proximal pouch of the caudal pouch of the lateral femorotibial joint
- The distal pouch of the caudal pouch of the lateral femorotibial joint
- The femoropatellar joint.

Medial Femorotibial Synovial Sac

All compartments of the femorotibial joints are best approached with the horse in dorsal recumbency and the limb in flexion with the stifle joint at 70 to 90 degrees. Three arthroscopic approaches for diagnosis and surgical treatment of the cranial pouch of the medial femorotibial joint sac have been described.[25-27] The lateral approach, where the arthroscope portal is located caudal to the lateral patellar ligament, cranial to the long digital extensor tendon, and 2 cm proximal to the tibial spine, is most commonly used.

With a no. 11 blade, the portal is made through the skin and the deep fascia. Using a blunt trocar, the arthroscopic cannula is directed medially to penetrate the synovial membrane in the lateral aspect of the medial femorotibial joint (Fig. 101-11). Using this approach, the instrument portal is placed halfway between the tibial crest and the patella and midway between the medial and middle patellar ligaments. This allows examination of cranial portions of the medial meniscus, the tibial condyle, and the weight-bearing area of the femoral condyle as well as the medial meniscotibial ligament (Fig. 101-12). The caudal cruciate ligament can be seen under the synovial membrane (Fig. 101-13). Occasionally, the tibial attachment of the cranial cruciate ligament is found if the medial septum is disrupted.

Examination of the caudal pouch of the medial femorotibial synovial sac is best accomplished by locating the arthroscope portal 1 cm proximal and parallel to a line drawn from the tibial tuberosity to the medial condyle of the tibia and 3 cm caudal to the medial collateral ligament[8] (Fig. 101-14). The entire caudal aspect of the medial femoral condyle and the proximal aspect of the medial meniscus can be examined (Fig. 101-15). The caudal cruciate ligament is located extrasynovially and can be located with the probe through the synovial lining.

Lateral Femorotibial Synovial Sac

The arthroscopic portal for examination of the cranial pouch of the lateral femorotibial joint sac is best located midway between the patella and the tibial crest and halfway

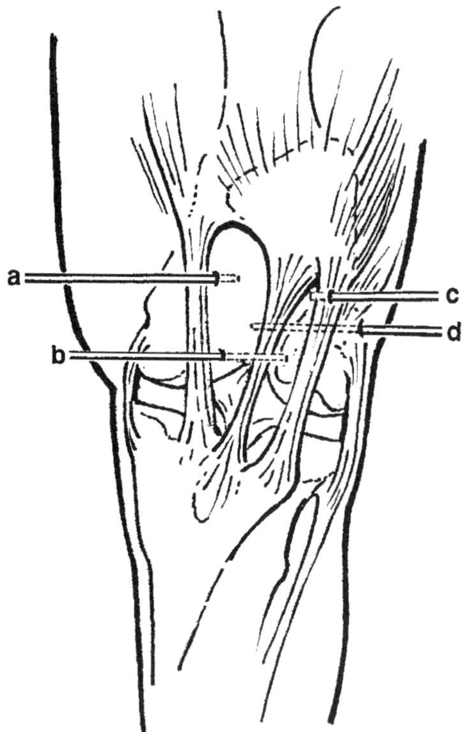

Figure 101-11. A schematic representation of the arthroscope portals used to explore the cranial pouches of the medial and lateral femorotibial joints and the femoropatellar joint. Portal a is used to position the arthroscope in the femoropatellar joint. Portal b is used to position the arthroscope in the lateral femorotibial joint (medial approach). Portal c either is used to position the arthroscope in the femoropatellar joint for closer examination of the lateral trochlear ridge or is used as an instrument portal to débride the lateral trochlear ridge. Portal d is used to position the arthroscope in the medial femorotibial joint (lateral approach).

between the medial and middle patellar ligaments. The arthroscope portal is directed laterally and caudad to enter the lateral joint pouch. The cranial cruciate ligament is seen from this approach lying in the medium septum. The lateral femoral condyle, the lateral meniscus, the lateral meniscotibial ligament, and the lateral tibial condyle can be visualized, but this joint compartment is much smaller than the cranial pouch of the medial femorotibial joint sac, and manipulation of the arthroscope is more limited. The opening into the synovial diverticulum of the long digital extensor tendon within the sulcus muscularis of the tibia can be seen; however, exploration of this compartment distally along the tendon is only accomplished through a cranial approach (see later).

The arthroscope portal that permits best examination of the proximal compartment of the caudal pouch of the lateral femorotibial joint sac is located 2.5 cm proximal and parallel to a line drawn from the tibial tuberosity to the lateral condyle of the tibia and 3 cm caudal to the lateral collateral ligament[8] (see Fig. 101-14). Most of the caudal aspect of the lateral femoral condyle and tendon of the popliteus muscle can be examined intrasynovially. Rotation of the hock laterally (clockwise rotation of the right hindlimb) loosens the popliteal tendon and creates a tunnel. Insertion

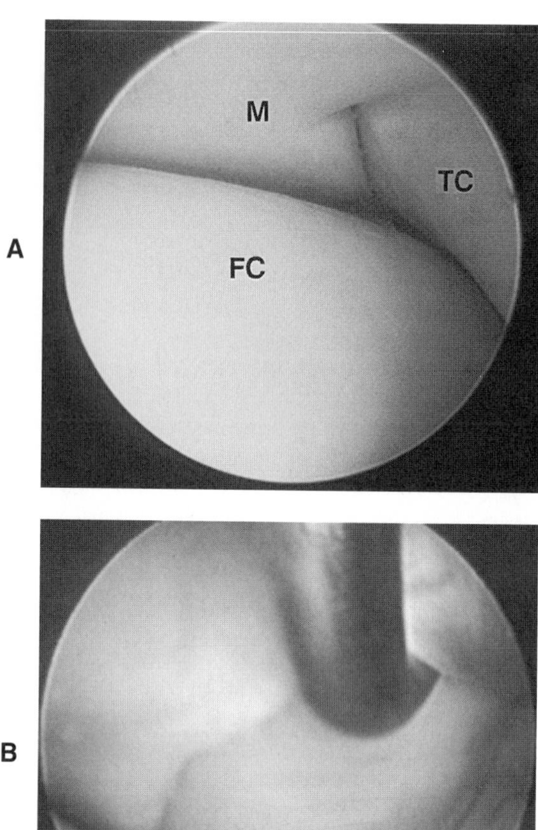

Figure 101-12. A, Arthroscopic view of the cranial pouch of the medial femorotibial joint as viewed from the lateral approach. The medial femoral condyle (FC) is seen ventrally, the medial meniscus (M) dorsally *(left)*, and tibial condyle (TC) dorsally *(right)*. **B,** A probe can be used to elevate the cranial pole of the meniscus and meniscotibial ligament exposing the medial tibial condyle.

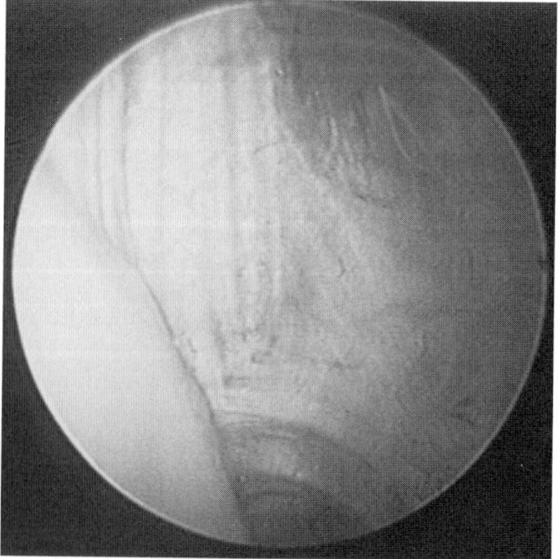

Figure 101-13. Arthroscopic view of the tibial attachment of the caudal cruciate ligament observed through the synovial membrane *(center)*.

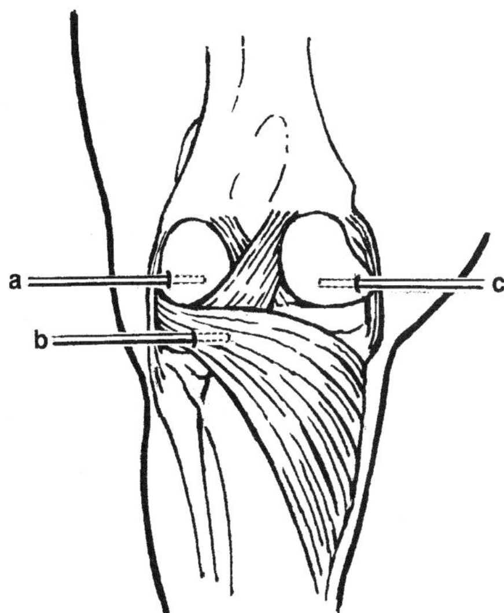

Figure 101-14. Schematic representation of the arthroscopic portals used to explore the caudal pouches of the medial and lateral femorotibial joints. a, The portal to the proximal compartment of the lateral caudal pouch is located at the level of the lateral femoral condyle, 2.5 cm proximal to the distal level of the lateral meniscus and 3 cm caudal to the lateral collateral ligaments. b, The portal to the distal compartment of the lateral caudal pouch is located at the level of the lateral meniscus, through popliteal tendon, 1.5 cm caudal to the lateral collateral ligament. c, The medial portal is located at the level of the medial femoral condyle, 1 cm proximal to the distal level of the medial meniscus and 3 cm caudal to the medial collateral ligament.

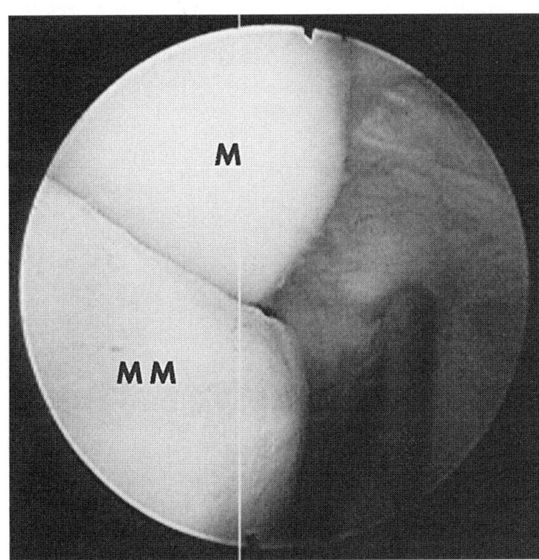

Figure 101-15. Arthroscopic view of the caudal pouch of the medial femorotibial joint of the stifle showing the medial femoral condyle (M), the medial meniscus (MM), and a probe placed on the caudal cruciate ligament located behind the synovial membrane.

of the arthroscope into the tunnel does not permit visualization of the lateral meniscus or of the tibial condyle. This is the most common portal used to approach this compartment.

The arthroscope portal that permits examination of the distal compartment of the caudal pouch of the lateral femorotibial joint sac is located on a line drawn from the tibial tuberosity to the lateral condyle of the tibia and 1.5 cm caudal to the lateral collateral ligament (see Fig. 101-14). Entrance to this level is directly through the popliteal tendon, permitting examination of the caudal lateral meniscus, part of the caudal aspect of the lateral femoral condyle, and the intra-articular portion of the popliteal tendon and the lateral tibial condyle (Fig. 101-16). Care should be taken when approaching the caudal pouch of the lateral femorotibial joint sac to avoid damage to the common peroneal nerve, which is located less than 7 cm caudal to the lateral collateral ligament. Additionally, the popliteal artery and vein are situated directly between the medial and lateral femoral condyles on the caudal aspect of this joint (see Fig. 101-9). Therefore the surgeon cannot pass safely from one pouch to the other across the caudal aspect of the joint without risk of injury to this vasculature, which is the major deep blood supply to the stifle.[28]

Femoropatellar Joint

Exploration and surgery on the femoropatellar joint are best accomplished with the horse placed in dorsal recumbency and the limb in extension. The portal for the arthroscope is located between the middle and lateral patellar ligaments and halfway between the tibial crest and the patella[29] (see Fig. 101-11).

The arthroscope sleeve, containing a blunt obturator, is inserted through the small skin incision and directed at an angle of 45 degrees up underneath the patella. The object is to place the sheath and obturator into the trochlear groove. Prior distention of the femoropatellar joint is usually not necessary to accomplish positioning of the arthroscope. The joint is then distended through the arthroscope sleeve, which allows sequential examination of the femoropatellar joint, along the entire lengths of both medial and lateral trochlear ridges, the articulating surface of the patella, and the attachments of both the medial and lateral patellar ligaments onto the patella.

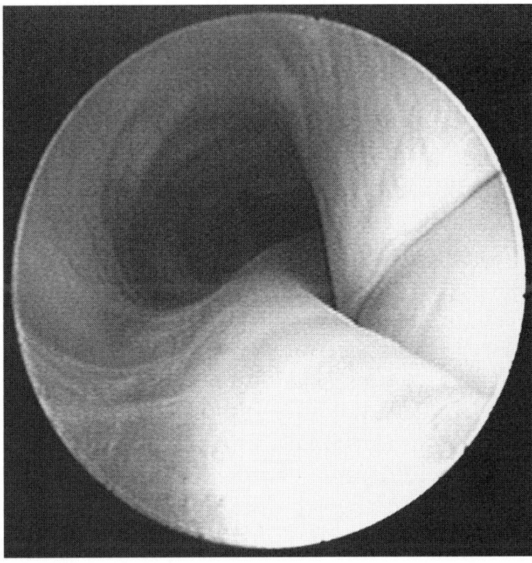

Figure 101-16. Arthroscopic appearance of the distal compartment of the caudal pouch of the lateral femorotibial joint sac, which permits examination of the caudolateral meniscus *(right dorsal)*, part of the caudal aspect of the lateral femoral condyle *(right middle)*, and the interarticular portion of the popliteal tendon *(center)*.

Instrument portals can be created between the middle and medial patellar ligaments for medial trochlear ridge lesions; portals can be created medial, lateral, or through the lateral patellar ligament for lateral trochlear ridge lesions. The instrument portal is located proximal and lateral to the arthroscope portal when it is passed through the lateral patellar ligament. If the portal is made lateral to the lateral patellar ligament, it is sometimes difficult to manipulate the instrument to operate effectively on lesions in this area.[30]

Cranial Arthroscopic Approach to the Cranial Stifle

An alternative arthroscopic approach for a complete examination of the cranial aspect of the stifle has been described,[31] wherein the endoscope portal is made through the middle patellar tendon into the femoropatellar joint. Thereafter, each femorotibial joint sac is entered via a cranial incision using arthroscopic hook scissors under arthroscopic guidance. This incision is made through the slit-like openings into the femorotibial joints at the distal end of the medial and lateral trochlear ridges. These are easily identified during routine examination of the femoropatellar joint pouches. Good visualization of the femoral and tibial condyles and the meniscus are obtained. An excellent image of the caudal cruciate ligament enhances evaluation and débridement of this structure.

Modification of this technique by entering the femoropatellar joint on either side of the middle patellar tendon avoids damage to this structure while permitting more mobility of the endoscope.[32] This technique has the advantage of easier scope placement through one portal, which allows access to the entire cranial aspect of the stifle joints. Single portal entry can decrease morbidity and permits better access to soft tissues of the femorotibial joints. This approach to the cranial stifle is used preferentially by the author and was evaluated in the treatment of 23 horses with various stifle disorders.[33]

The technique is as follows (Fig. 101-17 and 101-18). The horse is anesthetized and placed into dorsal recumbency, and the stifle joint is maintained in 60 degrees of flexion. An 8 mm long skin incision is made 2 cm medial to the middle patellar ligament and 1 cm distal to the distal end of the patella. The incision is extended through the superficial and deep fascia.

An arthroscopic cannula containing a blunt trocar is advanced through the incision distally and caudally within the femoropatellar joint without prior joint distention. The trocar is replaced by the arthroscope, and placement of the cannula in the joints is verified by observing the articular surface. Sterile polyionic fluids are delivered to distend the joint, and the femoropatellar joint is examined systematically.

The slit-like synovial membrane separating the cranial aspects of the femorotibial joint compartments from the femoropatellar joint are identified medially and laterally overlying the cranial and distal aspects of the femoral trochlea. The instrument entry portal is made into the femoropatellar joint lateral to the middle patellar ligament opposite the arthroscopic portal and at the same level. The instrument portal is placed at the same distance from the distal patellar margin and is of the same size and orientation described for the arthroscopic portal.

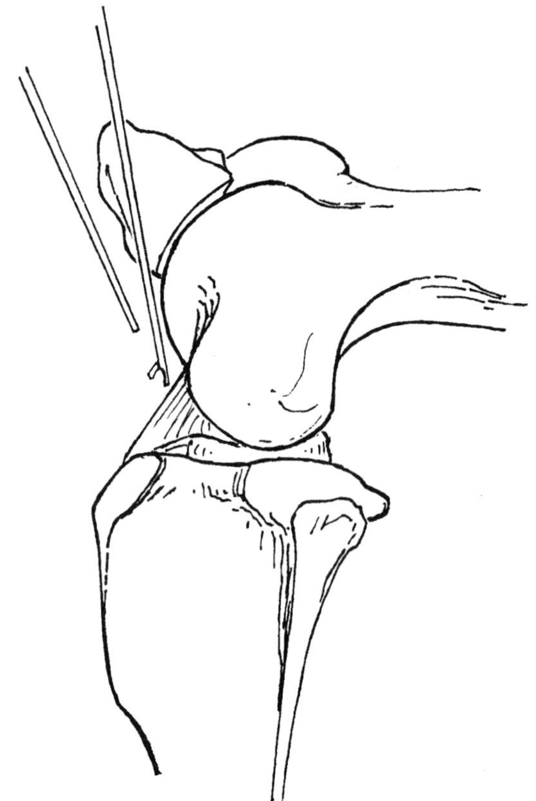

Figure 101-17. The cranial arthroscopic approach to the stifle joint in horses, lateral aspect. Arthroscope and hook scissors are drawn in the appropriate intraoperative positions close to the distal border of the patella.

Arthroscopic hook scissors (Fig. 101-19) are placed in the femoropatellar joint through this accessory portal. Synovial membrane overlying the medial femoral trochlea is transected with hook scissors (Fig. 101-20), allowing the arthroscope to advance into the medial femorotibial joint compartment (Fig. 101-21).

If indicated, the procedure is repeated using an identical approach to the lateral femorotibial joint compartment. The arthroscope does not need to be removed from its medial position and can be driven into the lateral femorotibial joint compartment after the incision is made with the hook scissors. This allows very good visualization of the cranial aspect of this compartment and also allows exploration of the sulcus muscularis containing the long digital extensor tendon.

The cranial pouches in both femorotibial joint compartments can be successfully evaluated through this single portal cranial arthroscopic approach, which uses the femoropatellar joint as a point of access. Arthroscope placement is critical to obtain optimal entry into the femorotibial joint. The arthroscope is positioned 1 cm distal to the palpable distal end of the patella. The view of the synovial membranes present over the trochlear ridges will be distorted or inaccessible if the arthroscope portal is located farther distally, as occurs with a traditional approach to the femoropatellar joint previously described.

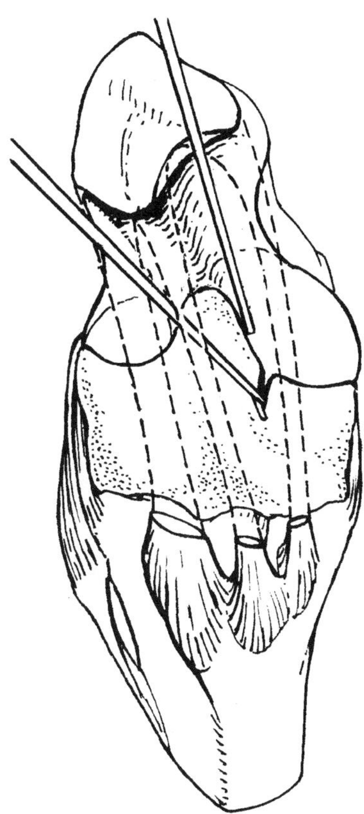

Figure 101-18. The cranial arthroscopic approach to the stifle joint in horses, lateral aspect. Arthroscope and hook scissors bisecting the synovium are drawn in the appropriate intraoperative positions. The *dotted lines* represent the medial, middle, and lateral patellar ligaments.

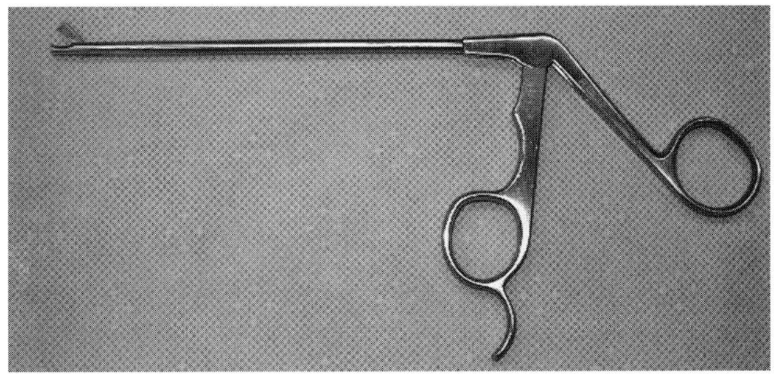

Figure 101-19. Hook scissors used in the cranial arthroscopic approach to the stifle joint in horses.

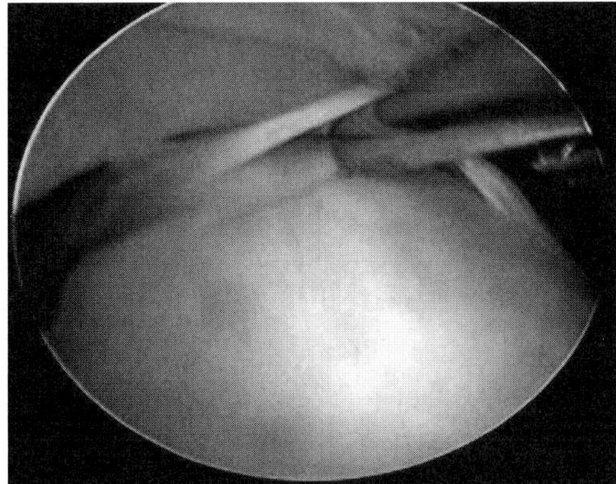

Figure 101-20. Arthroscopic view of the hook scissors engaging the synovium located over the cranial and distal aspect of the medial femoral trochlea in a horse.

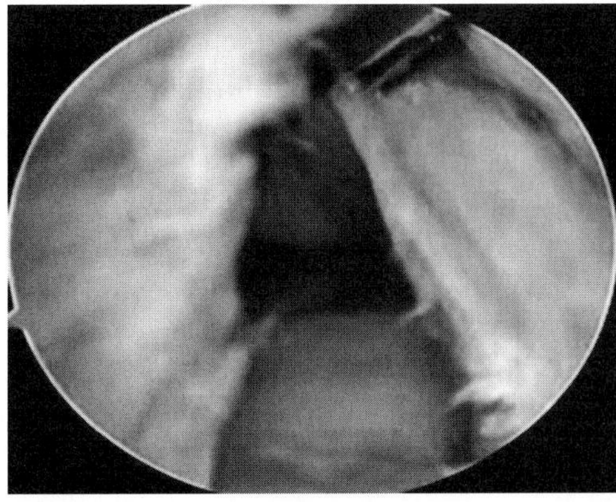

Figure 101-21. Arthroscopic view of the transected synovium located over the cranial and distal aspect of the medial femoral trochlea and the medial femoral condyle in a horse. Simultaneous telescope advancement and limb flexion were used to enhance the view of the condyle.

Using the hook scissors through a portal placed too far distal is awkward because of the acute angle formed between the synovial membrane and the instrument. Hook scissors are not effective despite correct instrument portal placement when the synovial membrane is thickened. This is particularly obvious in horses with chronic joint disease in which fibrous synovial membranes have to be transected with a scalpel blade inserted through the instrument portal. After incision, however, access to this joint is excellent. Directional movements of the arthroscope and examination of synovial structures within the femorotibial joint compartments will be facilitated once the synovial membrane located between the joints is transected.

Arthroscopic assistance of the cranial approach permits a controlled and atraumatic injury into the femorotibial joint compartments, thereby decreasing the reported risk of inadvertent meniscal damage from blind trocar insertion penetrating articular structures. This is particularly true when entering the lateral femorotibial joint compartment because a blind direct approach is complicated by the presence of the lateral collateral ligament, the lateral patellar ligament, and the origin of the long digital extensor tendon. Additionally, the controlled insertion eliminates the risk of extravasation of fluid in the periarticular tissues, which causes edema and renders the surgical approach difficult.

A unique feature of the single portal cranial arthroscopic approach to the stifle in horses is that a communication is created between the femoropatellar and femorotibial joints. Synovial fluid of all joint pouches freely communicates, and when joint lavage is performed at the completion of surgery it involves all compartments. When curetting medial femoral condylar cysts (see later) using this technique, it is important to remember that the suprapatellar pouch is explored before exiting the joint with the arthroscope. Some care should be taken not to allow a lot of debris to fall into the femorotibial joint because it can be difficult to extirpate from the cul-de-sacs of the suprapatellar pouch.

There are a few disadvantages to the cranial approach. These include the need for an additional instrument (hook scissors) and the learning period associated with mastering a new technique. Furthermore, the cranial approach might not lend itself to the evaluation of septic arthritis of the stifle joint. In horses that have only a single infected compartment, care should be taken not to contaminate other healthy synovial structures. However, because 70% of the time the medial femorotibial joint and the femoropatellar joint communicate, this might not be an issue, and the cranial arthroscopic approach can be used.

Because the cranial arthroscope approach eliminates the natural synovial barriers between both compartments, joint sepsis can be advantageously treated by vigorous joint lavage through a large opening created within the cranial arthroscopic approach. This is particularly important if the sepsis is in the lateral femorotibial joint compartment and involves the sulcus muscularis.

In summary, the cranial arthroscopic single portal approach is easy to perform, allows controlled access to the femorotibial joint, avoids accidental damage to articular structures, and requires fewer access portals to explore the entire cranial aspect of the stifle.

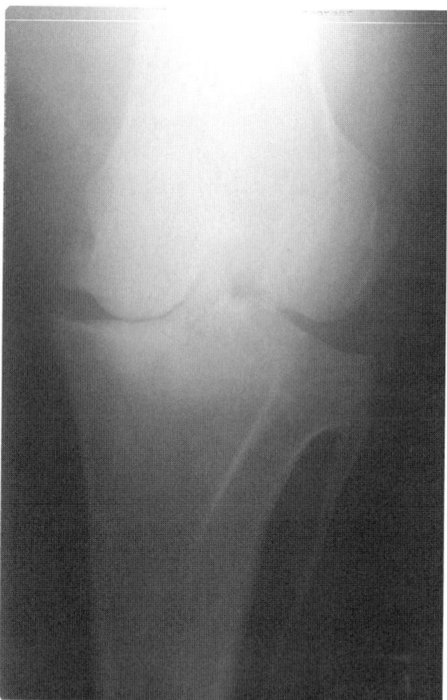

Figure 101-22. A caudocranial view of the stifle showing narrowing of the medial femorotibial joint space that occurs with advanced osteoarthritis.

DISORDERS OF THE STIFLE

Traumatic Disorders

Acute or chronic traumatic conditions of the stifle include osteoarthritis, synovitis, chondromalacia of the patella, meniscal tears, ligamentous disorders (e.g., sprains, avulsions, tears), and fractures. All of these disorders can exhibit the signs of gonitis, with joint distention and lameness.

Osteoarthritis

The earliest form of osteoarthritis in the equine stifle is recognized as cartilage damage on the medial femoral condyle, which results secondary to joint injury. These lesions produce lameness in the horse, and diagnostic arthroscopy is necessary to make an accurate diagnosis.[34] Therefore, horses with lameness localized to the stifle through diagnostic anesthesia or scintigraphy and in which radiography and ultrasonography did not yield a diagnosis are good candidates for arthroscopic exploration of the joint. Débridement of focal cartilage lesions allows some horses to successfully resume performance activities.

Osteoarthritis of the stifle in later stages is best detected on a craniocaudal radiographic view when the femorotibial joint is involved and manifests as articular osteophyte formation, flattening of the articular surfaces, sclerosis of the subchondral bone, or lucent zones in the subchondral bone. Narrowing of the femorotibial joint space is seen in advanced cases (Fig. 101-22). Positioning is important when making this determination; the horse should be bearing weight, with the limb centered under the body during this view. The lateromedial view demonstrates femoropatellar joint osteoarthritis, which is seen as periarticular osteophyte formation and changes along the distal aspect of the patella. Treatment for this condition is usually palliative, as with all other arthritic conditions, and includes intra-articular medications. Because of the size of these synovial compartments (with a volume of between 40 and 62 mL), intra-articular medications must be of sufficient quantity to be effective.

Osteoarthritis is usually established in the femorotibial joints as a result of some meniscal or ligamentous injury; however, advanced cases of osteoarthritis with complete denuding of articular cartilage from the medial femoral condyle can be seen in aged racing Standardbreds without evidence of other soft tissue injury (Fig. 101-23). Treatment of this condition by way of arthroscopy can include articular cartilage débridement and micropick techniques (Fig. 101-24).

Pannus formation of the femorotibial and femoropatellar joint compartments can be treated with anti-inflammatory medication but may best respond to arthroscopic débridement of synovial proliferation. If the surgeon is exploring a joint in which this is the only finding, mechanical débridement by way of mechanical synovial resectors or a holmium:yttrium-aluminum-garnet (holmium-YAG) laser is indicated.

Articular cartilage lesions on the surface of the patella are called chondromalacia (Fig. 101-25). The pathogenesis and significance of this condition in the horse are uncertain, but arthroscopic débridement of cartilage fragmentation using minimally traumatizing motorized cartilaginous débriders has resulted in clinical improvement.

Ligamentous Disorders

In addition to collateral ligaments common to most joints, the stifle of the horse includes ligaments associated with the menisci, cranial and caudal cruciate ligaments, and three

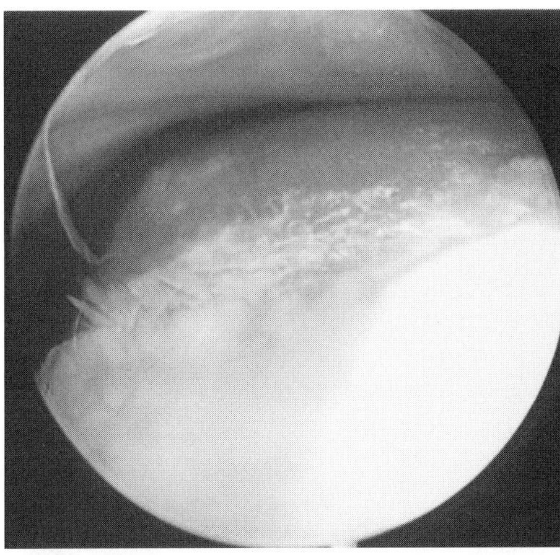

Figure 101-23. Arthroscopic appearance of advanced osteoarthritis of the medial femoral condyle. Articular cartilage débridement was accomplished using a motorized resector.

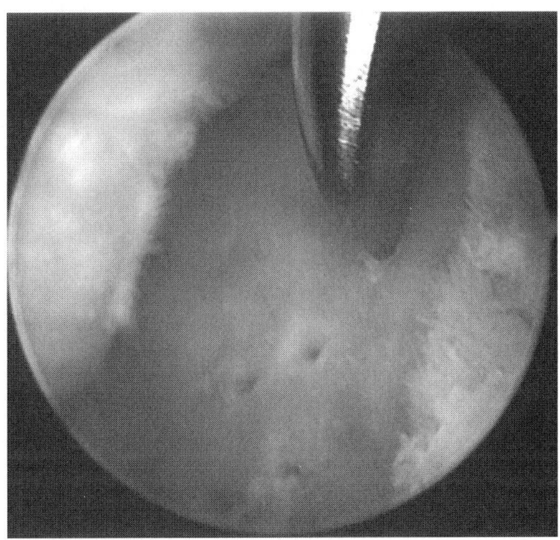

Figure 101-24. Arthroscopic appearance of the medial femoral condyle showing micropick technique.

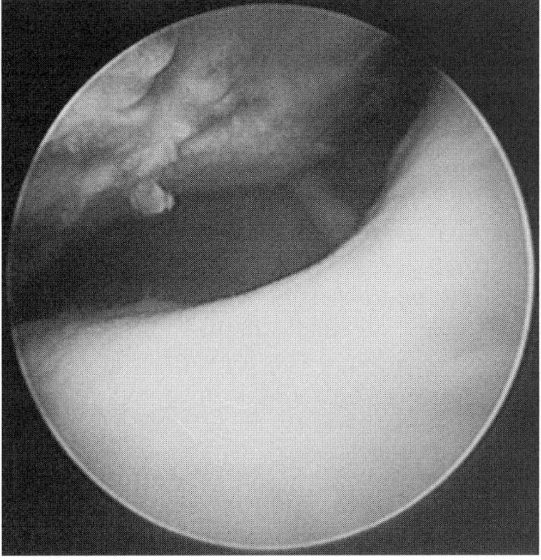

Figure 101-25. Arthroscopic appearance of chondromalacia of the patella (dorsal). The intertrochanteric fossa of the femur is seen ventrally.

patellar ligaments. All ligaments are subject to sprains, strains, and tears.

UPWARD FIXATION OF THE PATELLA

Upward fixation of the patella is a condition that is unique to the horse. It is believed that this condition occurs secondary to the beginning of training in young horses and is related to a straight hindlimb conformation.

Training

The treatment for this condition involves alterations in training rather than surgical treatment. As a treatment for this condition, medial patellar desmotomy has been associated with induction of chondromalacia of the patella and patellar fragmentation.[35,36] If this occurs, these fragments should be removed arthroscopically because they will lead to osteoarthritis. Except in Shetland ponies and miniature horses (horses that would not be expected to carry a rider), the treatment for this condition involves developing quadriceps muscle tone.

Quadriceps development is accomplished by riding at an extended trot up and down hills in deep, sandy, or loamy soil. Working the horse in a circle in an arena (and especially at a canter) should be avoided. This merely contributes to the trauma to the patella and the horse's continued lack of quadriceps development because of lameness. Rather than box stall confinement, anti-inflammatory medication and turnout for the horse are recommended.

Medial patellar desmotomy

If the appropriate conditioning and development of the quadriceps muscle tone with training does not resolve the condition, medial patellar desmotomy can be considered as a last resort in riding horses.

The surgical procedure is performed with the animal standing and the tail wrapped to avoid contamination of the surgical site. After preparation of the skin, local anesthetic is injected subcutaneously over the medial border of the middle patellar ligament. A 20-gauge 2.5-cm (1-inch) needle is inserted through this site, and the subcutaneous area around the distal part of the medial patellar ligament is infiltrated with local anesthetic.

A 1-cm incision is made over the medial border of the middle patellar ligament close to the attachment of the ligament to the tibial tuberosity. This is done because a fat pad is located in this area and the operator is less likely to enter the femoropatellar joint capsule at this site. Curved Kelly forceps are forced through the fascia and passed beneath the medial patellar ligament. A curved bistoury knife is inserted into this channel, the cutting edge is turned outward, and the ligament is cut. The blade should be placed completely on the other side of the medial patellar ligament before the ligament is severed. Once the ligament has been severed, the tendon of the sartorius muscle feels like a tense band and might lead the inexperienced operator to believe that the medial patellar ligament has not been completely severed. The skin is closed.

To avoid the complications discussed above, a prolonged period of rest is important before the animal is turned out to allow some scarring to occur at the surgery site, realigning the patella in the intertrochanteric groove.

Medial patellar ligament splitting

Medial patellar ligament splitting has been advocated for treating upward fixation of the patella when conservative methods have failed.[37] The authors claim numerous advantages over medial patellar desmotomy. The procedure is carried out under general anesthesia.

Using ultrasonographic guidance, multiple longitudinal splitting incisions are made in the distal aspects of the medial patellar ligament. This form of splitting results in a significant progressive increase in ligament size during the first 4 weeks after surgery. The final result is that the medial patellar ligament becomes thickened two to three times its initial diameter.

TEARING OF COLLATERAL LIGAMENTS

Collateral ligaments of the femorotibial joint can undergo partial tearing.[38,39] A diagnosis is made in acute cases with ultrasonography. Radiographs can be obtained with the joint under lateral or medial stress to confirm unilateral widening of the femorotibial joint space when complete rupture is suspected. Sprain of these ligaments can result in increased irregular new bone formation, which manifests as enthesiophyte formation at the insertions on the proximal tibia.

Treatment for this condition involves anti-inflammatory medication and rest. Healing should be monitored by periodic ultrasonographic examinations. The prognosis for horses undergoing partial tearing is guarded to favorable, depending on the degree of tearing and instability of the joint.[40]

Concurrent injury of the menisci or cruciate ligaments commonly occurs in horses with severe injuries or complete rupture of a collateral ligament. The medial collateral ligament and medial menisci are more commonly involved than the lateral aspect of the stifle. When concurrent structures such as the cruciate ligaments or menisci are involved, the prognosis is unfavorable for full return to athletic use.

RUPTURE OF THE CRUCIATE LIGAMENT

Complete rupture of the cranial cruciate ligament, or less commonly the caudal cruciate ligament, has been reported and carries an unfavorable prognosis for the horse's return to athletic function.[41-44] Weightbearing might return over time, but often extensive osteoarthritis prohibits even salvage of the horse as a breeding animal.

Much more commonly, sprain of the cruciate ligaments, with or without partial detachment of their distal insertions, occurs. Occasionally, avulsion of the tibial crest occurs or enthesiophytes develop in the ligament and can be seen on radiographs (see Fig. 101-5). Chronic cases can have proliferative bone changes, which can be seen in the flexed lateromedial view. Subchondral cystic lesions can develop at the sites of origin and insertion of the cruciate ligaments over time.

A definitive diagnosis is made after an arthroscopic examination of the femorotibial joint (Fig. 101-26). A lateral approach to the medial compartment has been used, and the septum between the two cranial compartments will have been ruptured with the traumatic injury, allowing examination of both cruciate ligaments through this approach. However, the cranial approach to both femorotibial joints permits more complete assessment. Treatment involves partial débridement. The prognosis is related to the amount of damage to the cruciate ligament.

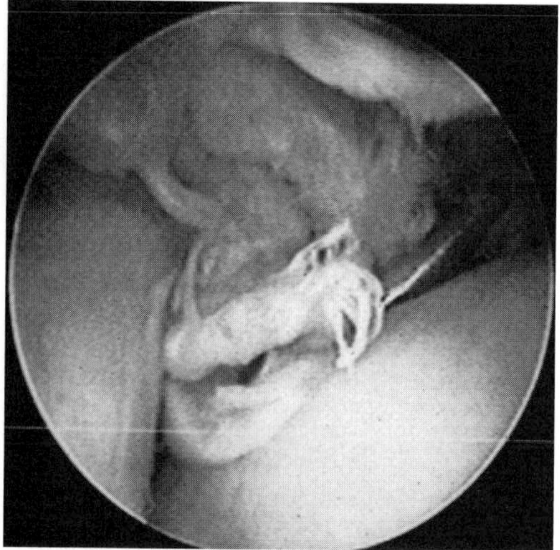

Figure 101-26. Endoscopic view of a torn cranial cruciate ligament as viewed from the cranial approach to the medial femorotibial joint sac. A probe easily separates the fibers of this ligament.

The majority of horses with minor superficial cranial cruciate tearing (Fig. 101-27) return to previous degrees of activity and can be used without further lameness. When the damage becomes moderate and approaches disruption of more than 50% of the ligament, the prognosis is unfavorable. Concurrent meniscal injury worsens the prognosis.

Meniscal Injury

Meniscal tears in the equine femorotibial joint have been recognized for more than a decade. Continued improvements in arthroscopic and ultrasonographic techniques have

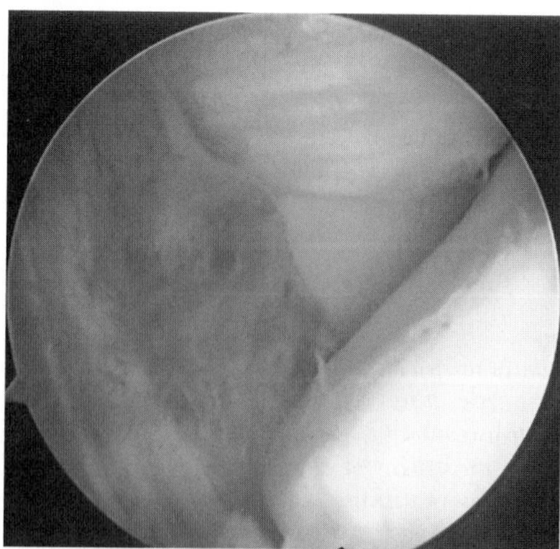

Figure 101-27. Arthroscopic appearance of a minor tear in the cranial cruciate ligament *(left)* as seen in the lateral femorotibial joint pouch. The lateral femoral condyle is ventral and the meniscotibial ligament and tibial condyle are dorsal.

led to an increase in this diagnosis. Although lameness is often acute and severe in onset after a traumatic incident in which the meniscal injury occurs, it usually becomes low grade and persistent after a period of time. The medial meniscus is involved 75% of the time and the cranial meniscotibial ligament of the menisci is almost always involved.

Distention of the joints can be expected in some horses; however, the most diagnostic clinical sign is severe lameness following the hindlimb flexion test. Traumatic injuries severe enough to cause damage to the menisci are usually the result of damage to other major structures such as the collateral ligaments, the meniscal ligaments, or the cruciate ligaments.[44,45] The diagnosis is made on arthroscopic assessment of the femorotibial joint compartments (Fig. 101-28). The medial meniscus is seen with a lateral or cranial approach to the cranial pouch of the medial femorotibial joint sac. However, lateral meniscal tears are less common and can be seen best through an approach to the caudal pouch. Treatment is by way of resection of the torn portion of the menisci using motorized meniscal resectors.

Because only the cranial and caudal poles of the menisci can be seen, arthroscopic assessment of meniscal injury is incomplete. A grading system has been established to determine prognosis as a meniscal tear is examined in the cranial pouch of the femorotibial joint[46]:

Grade 1: Tears extending longitudinally from the cranial ligament into the meniscus with minimal separation (Fig. 101-29)
Grade 2: Tears involving the cranial pole in which the extent of the injury is visible
Grade 3: Severe tears that extend beneath the femoral condyle and that cannot be completely assessed or débrided (see Fig. 101-28)

It has been reported that return to full athletic use can be expected in about 50% of horses overall. However, the best prognosis is in horses with lower grades of meniscal tears because only 25% of horses with grade 3 tears can be returned to athletic use. Concurrent damage to the cruciate ligament worsens the prognosis.

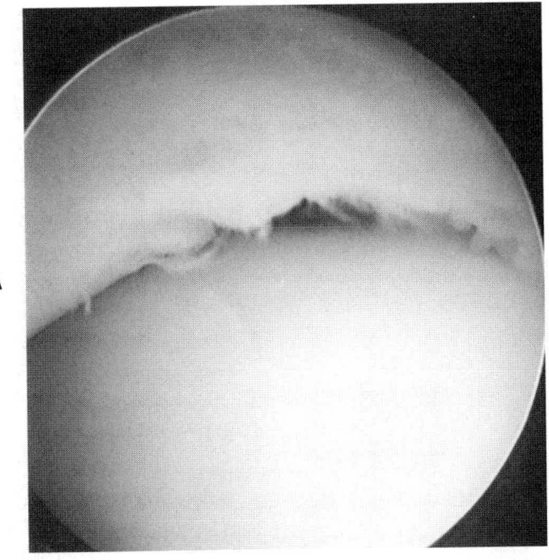

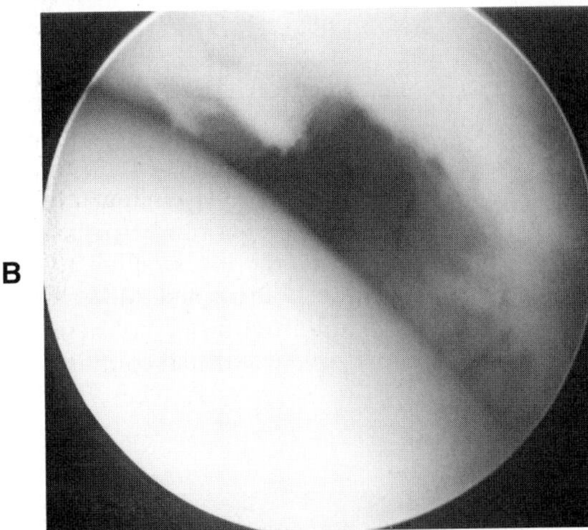

Figure 101-28. The arthroscopic appearance of a chronic medial meniscal tear before (**A**) and after (**B**) meniscal débridement.

Fractures

PATELLA

The patella is the largest sesamoid bone in the body and an integral portion of the quadriceps apparatus. Fractures of the patella are occasionally diagnosed and usually result from some direct trauma. These fractures cause variable lameness, soft tissue swelling, and effusion depending on the amount and configuration of the fracture. Radiographic evaluation should include not only the craniocaudal, lateromedial, flexed lateromedial, and caudal 30-degree lateral craniomedial oblique views but also the cranioproximal craniodistal (skyline) view of the patella to make a complete assessment of the fracture. Patellar fracture morphology is highly variable; however, sagittal fractures are most common and usually involve the medial aspect of the patella (see Fig. 101-8).

Techniques for partial patellectomy and internal fixation have been described; however, fractures located at the base

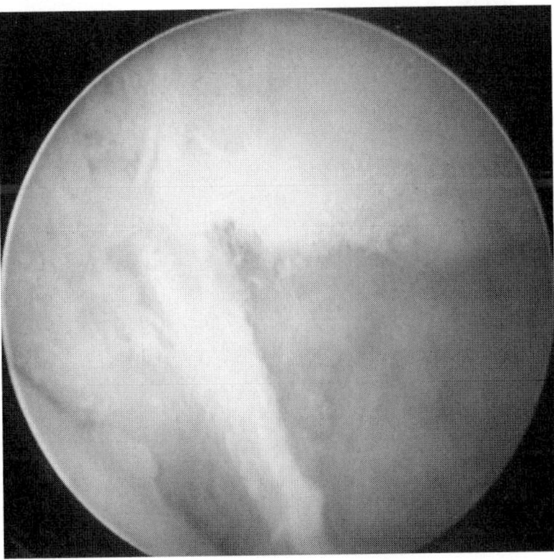

Figure 101-29. Example of a grade 1 meniscal tear that can be resected.

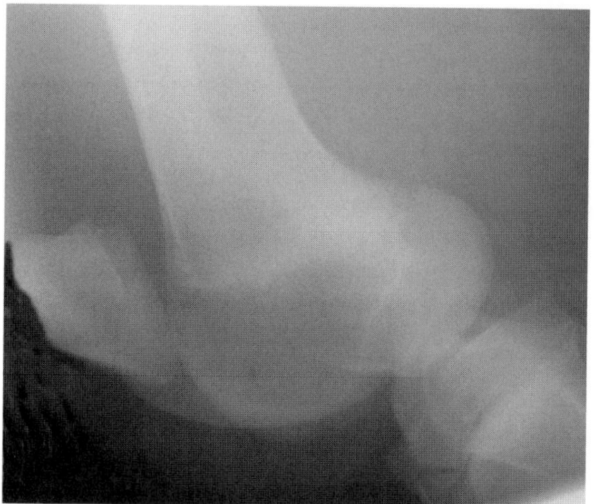

Figure 101-30. Lateromedial radiographic view of the stifle showing a fracture at the base of the patella.

of the patella are rarely emergencies and do not normally require surgical intervention[35,47,48] (Fig. 101-30). Surgery should be attempted only if the fracture gap is greater than 5 mm on radiographs, there is obvious malalignment of an articular fragment, or fragments can be palpated under the skin. One should allow for the swelling to decrease before surgical intervention is attempted. Medical management should include administration of nonsteroidal anti-inflammatory drugs for 2 weeks and stall confinement for 2 to 3 months.

Only when there is disruption of the quadriceps apparatus or a very large displaced articular fragment is internal fixation indicated (Fig. 101-31). Repairs have been performed through arthrotomy into the femoropatellar joint, and lag screw fixation using two or three 5.5-mm cortex screws placed from the apex to the base has been described. Partial patellectomy is indicated in sagittal medial articular fractures.[49,50] This can be carried out by removing up to one third of the patella through arthroscopy. A mechanical resector is used on the fragment to create a separation between the fragment and the parent portion of the bone. With an osteotome, the fragment is divided into smaller fragments, which subsequently are removed with Ferris-Smith rongeurs. However, it is often necessary to perform an arthrotomy, because dissection of the fragment from its extensive patellar ligament attachment can be difficult using only arthroscopic techniques. The prognosis after partial patellectomy for sagittal transverse fractures is favorable. When the quadriceps apparatus has been disrupted, the prognosis is guarded to unfavorable, depending on the success of the repair.

FEMORAL TROCHLEAR RIDGES

Fractures of the femoral trochlear ridges usually result from external trauma or wounds to the stifle. Either trochlear ridge can suffer fragmentation.[51] Clinical signs include sudden onset of moderate to severe lameness and effusion of the femoropatellar joint. Crepitus may be present on flexion of the joint. The fracture site might not be obvious unless a wound is present; however, the risk of sepsis is present when a skin wound is observed.

A

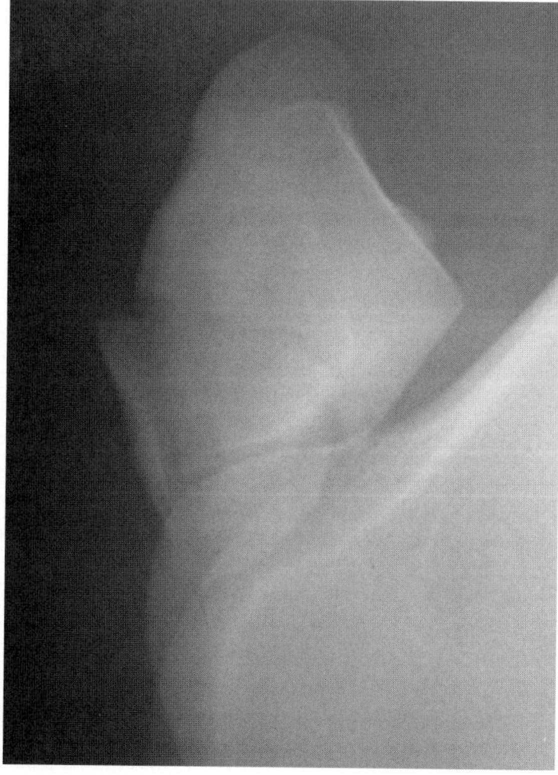

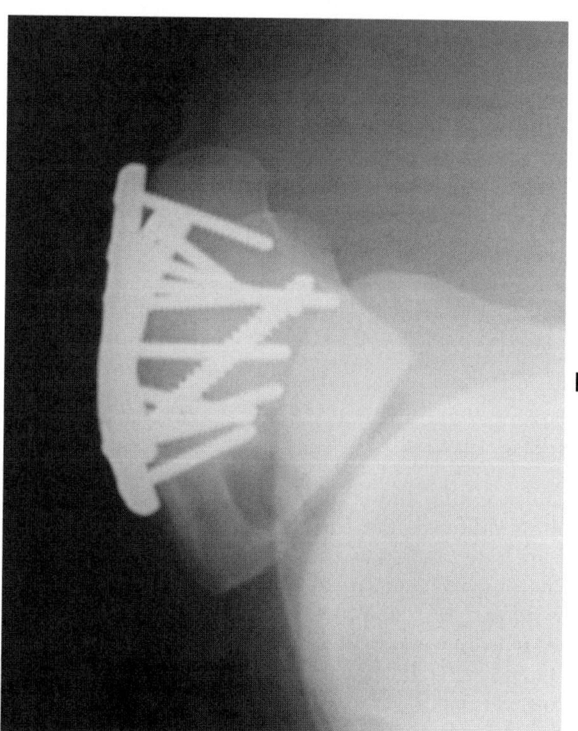

B

Figure 101-31. A, A lateromedial radiographic view of a patella fracture that resulted in complete disruption of the quadriceps apparatus. **B,** One 5.5-mm cortex screw used in lag fashion and two dynamic compression plates (DCPs) were used in the repair.

Fracture fragments should be removed. This is usually possible arthroscopically. Trochlear ridge fractures have a good prognosis after fracture removal, if no significant deeper structures are involved in the injury. Because of the non–weight-bearing articular surface where this usually occurs, horses can usually return to complete athletic activity.

Avulsion of the Origin of the Peroneus Tertius and Long Digital Extensor Tendon

This unusual condition in horses is commonly caused by a sudden forceful hyperextension of the hindlimb. Although mid-body tears of these structures are more common, usually from the horse lodging its foot in a gate and then forcibly extracting it, avulsions of the origin of the peroneus tertius and long digital extensor muscle do not have to occur with entrapment of the distal limb. Foals are most likely to suffer these avulsions, whereas the body of the structure tears in adult horses.[52]

Clinical signs are similar to those found with rupture of the peroneus tertius (see Chapters 86 and 99). However, distention of the femorotibial and femoropatellar joints is a cardinal sign that more might be involved than simply rupture. The condition can be recognized radiographically (Fig. 101-32).

Treatment is usually initiated by arthroscopic evaluation, which offers the opportunity to check the stifle for concurrent injury. Arthroscopy of the lateral femorotibial joint sac via a cranial approach can be used. The subchondral bone in the area of the extensor fossa and origin of the long digital extensor tendon can be débrided and bone fragments removed. Prognosis following this injury is guarded because many horses continue with some lameness following this injury.[52,53]

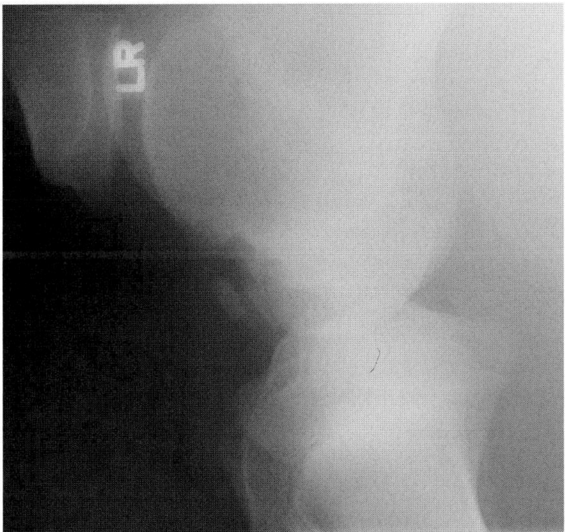

Figure 101-32. Lateromedial view of the stifle in a foal showing avulsion of the femoral insertion of the peroneus tertius and long digital extensor tendon.

Developmental Disorders

Osteochondrosis

Osteochondrosis (OC) is a term used to describe the developmental cartilaginous disease where failure of endochondral ossification results in thickening of the metaphyseal growth plate or the articular cartilage.[54,55] The etiopathogenesis of osteochondrosis and subchondral cystic lesions are discussed in detail in Chapters 91 and 92. For the purpose of discussion in this chapter, OC lesions have been divided into two categories: osteochondritis dissecans, which occurs as osteochondral fragments, and subchondral cystic lesions, seen as bone cysts.

OSTEOCHONDRITIS DISSECANS

Osteochondritis dissecans (OCD) is the most common cause of lameness in the stifle, and the femoropatellar joint is one of the principal sites in the horse.[56] The primary area involved is the lateral trochlear ridge of the femur (Fig. 101-33). The medial trochlear ridge, the patella, and the trochlear groove are involved less often.[56] Bilateral involvement is common. OCD has been reported in many breeds, but the Thoroughbreds, Quarter Horses, Arabians, and Warmbloods are over-represented. Most of the horses affected with OCD are between 1 and 2 years of age, but OCD has also been reported in very young horses.

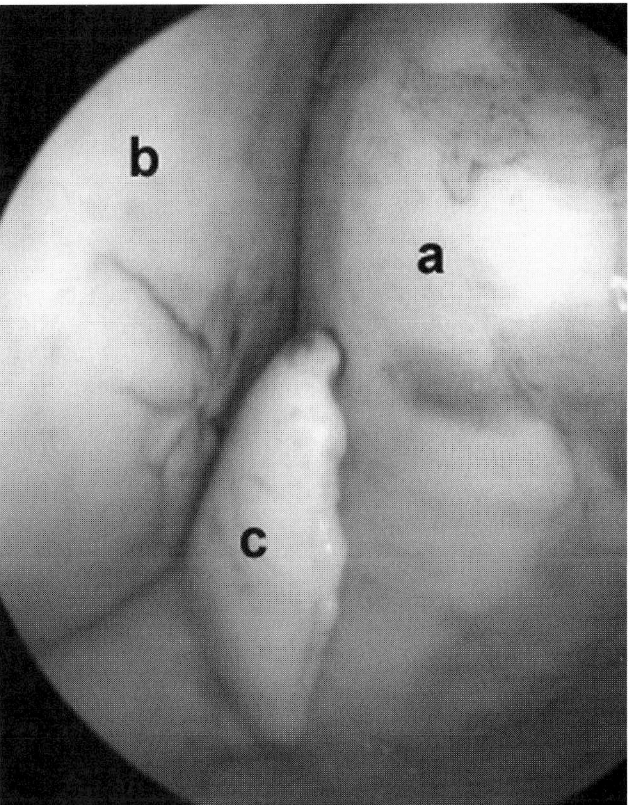

Figure 101-33. Arthroscopic appearance of osteochondritis dissecans of the lateral trochlear ridge demonstrating an osteochondral flap and an adjacent kissing lesion at the lateral aspect of the patella. *a,* lateral trochlear ridge of the distal femur; *b,* patella; *c,* OCD flap.

Radiographic examination of Thoroughbreds at the time of the yearling sales has become a common part of the selection process. This has allowed the prevalence of osteochondrosis of the stifle to be determined in a large group of Thoroughbred yearlings presented for sale.[57] The most common osteochondrosis lesion observed is flattening or fragmentation of the lateral trochlear ridge of the femur (6% of 660 horses).[58] This has a significant effect on future racing performance, and therefore stifle OCD is a detrimental finding in this breed.

Affected horses can be presented with acute, severe lameness or with a subtle lameness that becomes more obvious with increasing exercise.[54,59] Varying degrees of synovial effusion and lameness depend on the severity of the lesions. Young horses and horses that show clinical signs before training usually have more severe lesions from OCD than do those that do not show clinical signs until after training is initiated. In very young horses, the disease can be so severe as to cause difficulty in rising. Flexion test of the stifle usually increases the lameness.

A radiographic examination confirms the diagnosis, and the most common lesions are seen as flattening and irregularity of the trochlear ridge. This should not be confused with the irregularity of subchondral ossification of the trochlear ridges in foals younger than 5 months of age.[60] Smooth subchondral bone concavities, subchondral bone lysis, and osteochondral flaps and fragments are other lesions that are seen less often.[61] Radiographs usually underestimate the severity and the extent of the lesions, especially in foals younger than 9 months of age.[62] Therefore, if signs of stifle OCD are present (femoropatellar distention and lameness), arthroscopic treatment might need to be delayed until radiographic signs are obvious. During this time, these lesions have been observed to heal, with resolution of signs reported in young foals (see Chapter 91).

The treatment of choice for OCD is arthroscopic removal of osteochondral fragments and loose and undermined cartilage and débridement of the subchondral bone lesion.[56,59,63] Surgical success rates of approximately 64% without regard to sex, use, location of lesions, or bilateral or unilateral involvement have been reported. Conservative management of OCD has yielded poor results but might be appropriate under certain circumstances.[64] In one study, early detection and rest allowed lesions to heal and approximately 50% of horses were able to race; however, these animals tended to have less-severe lesions and no joint fragmentation.

MEDIAL FEMORAL CONDYLAR CYSTS

Subchondral bone cysts (SBCs) of the medial femoral condyle are an important and common cause of hindlimb lameness in the horse. There are two commonly proposed causes: articular damage with mechanical trauma of the subchondral bone and developmental orthopedic disease in the form of osteochondrosis. In support of the former theory, SBCs can be induced experimentally by creating a defect in the subchondral bone of the medial femoral condyle (see Chapter 92).[65]

Medial condylar cysts develop unilaterally in most cases but can be bilateral on presentation. Usually the medial femoral condyle is affected, but cysts have been described in the lateral condyle and proximal tibia.[66] The age of horses affected with cysts range from a few months up to 15 years of age, but most of the horses are between 1 and 3 years of age.

Lameness is the primary clinical sign and is usually obvious at the trot in one or both limbs. Flexion tests of the stifle can increase the lameness, but the change is usually not dramatic. The condition is usually observed as a stiffness in the limb or a reluctance to flex the limb at a walk or trot, and circling the horse in a trot toward the affected limb can increase the lameness.

Synovial distention is usually difficult to detect, especially in the medial femorotibial joint sac, but it is noticed occasionally in the femoropatellar joint. The condition responds to intra-articular anesthesia,[67] but radiographic examination provides a definitive diagnosis (see Fig. 101-7). Caudal to cranial and lateral to medial projections are important, but the former gives the best detail to the nature of the SBC. Radiographs of both limbs should be taken to detect bilateral lesions. The size of the lesions on the radiographs can vary from a slight indentation in the subchondral joint surface to a very round or oval lesion a few centimeters in height and width. There is usually a communication of the cyst with the joint that can range from being very narrow to quite broad. The size of the lesion and the amount of articular cartilage involvement has been suggested to correlate with clinical signs and prognosis, but this finding has not been confirmed in all studies.[68]

Recommendations for treatment involve arthroscopic surgery for débridement of the lesion followed by injection of betamethasone into the cyst. Débridement of the cyst lining and removal of all debris from the joint is the goal (Fig. 101-34). Compacted cancellous bone grafting and press-fit corticocancellous grafts or artificial cartilage implants have not produced an improved outcome.[69] However, novel bone replacement constructs are currently under evaluation, and early results are promising (see Chapter 92).

Postoperative intra-lesional corticosteroid therapy has been advocated to depress the anti-inflammatory mediators that are secreted from the lining in the cyst. Subchondral bone osteostixis is contraindicated because it can worsen the lesion. Additionally, débridement of small condylar defects that are asymptomatic is probably contraindicated because it can provoke an enlargement of the cyst. Therefore, these are quite often treated by intralesional injection of a corticosteroid using arthroscopic guidance.

The success rate for the horse's return to previous function after surgery ranges from 56% to 72%. Reports on conservative management of this condition, with or without the use of nonsteroidal anti-inflammatory medication, have been reported to be 64%.[70]

Lateral Luxation of the Patella

Lateral luxation of the patella in foals is uncommon, is usually congenital,[71,72] and can be inherited.[73,74] Luxations of the patella do occur in mature horses but are the result of trauma.

The condition can be unilateral or bilateral, and clinical signs depend on the severity of the displacement of the patella. Foals with complete luxation of the patellas are

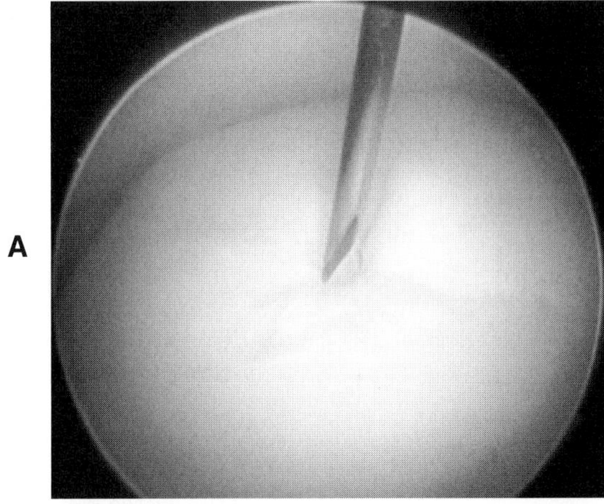

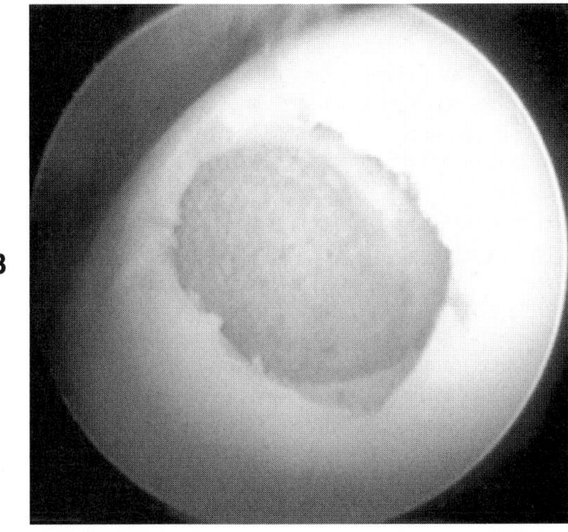

Figure 101-34. A, Arthroscopic appearance of a subchondral bone cyst showing the typical narrow opening. **B,** Appearance of the medial femoral condyle after débridement.

unable to stand (because the quadriceps acts as a flexor instead of an extensor of the joint) and assume a classic crouched position (Fig. 101-35, *A*). When patellas are not completely luxated, clinical signs include limb stiffness or lameness at the walk and trot. The patellas can usually be reduced manually. The femoropatellar joint is usually distended, and there may be crepitation on palpation of the patella.

Radiographic assessment of the stifle should include the degree of degeneration of the joint, the depth of the trochlear groove, the shape of the patella and trochlear ridges, and the amount of ossification of the trochlear ridges. (Pathology should not be confused with the irregularity of subchondral ossification of the trochlear ridges of foals up to 5 months.) On craniocaudal radiographic views, the patella is located lateral to the femur (Fig. 101-35, *B*); on the lateromedial view, it is projected over the femur or visible just caudal to it.

Surgical correction of patellar luxations includes lateral release incisions of the patellas combined with reinforcement of the medial patellar structures. In dorsal recumbency, under general anesthesia, surgical exposure is achieved with one large medially based curved incision extending from 6 cm above the patella distally to the tibial crest. Alternatively, two curved incisions can be used.

Lateral release of the patella is accomplished by incising the insertion of the biceps femoris, the lateral femoropatellar ligament, and the origin of the lateral patellar ligament without invading the joint.[75] The lateral release can sometimes be accomplished by partially transecting the tensor fascia and fibrous joint capsule while preserving the lateral femoropatellar ligament. The *medial joint capsule* from the base to the apex of the patella is imbricated with no. 5 braided polyester suture. Alternatively, suturing the tendon of the sartorius muscle and the parapatellar fascia to the joint capsule and the medial patellar ligament will be necessary. (The author has used a mesh implant to reinforce this imbrication in a 370-pound yearling.)

A sulcoplasty has been advocated for lateral ridge hypoplasia or instability of the patella in the trochlear groove.[76] In small animals, two different techniques are proposed.[77] These techniques are performed on young animals that have a thick hyaline cartilage layer covering the ossifying center of the epiphysis. One technique involves elevation of a U-shaped cartilage flap within the trochlear groove and removal of the subchondral bone (Fig. 101-36). The cartilage is incised at an angle, followed by careful elevation with the help of a periosteal elevator. The soft

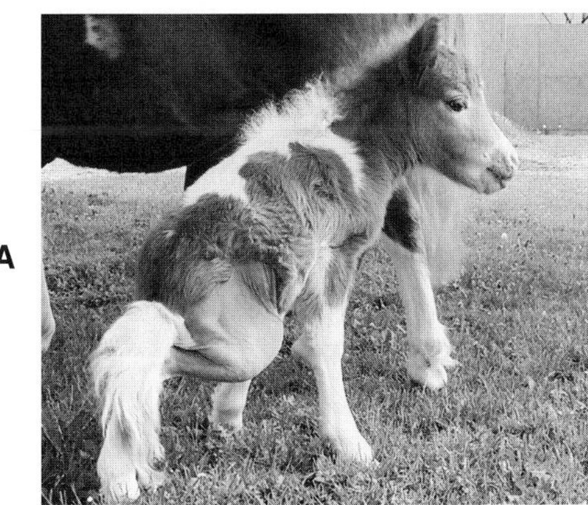

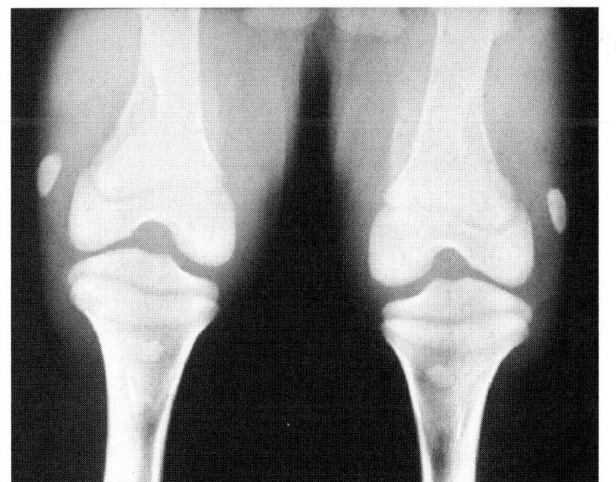

Figure 101-35. A, This 3-month-old pony foal shows the typical stance of an animal with complete lateral luxation of the patella. **B,** The craniocaudal radiographic views of both stifles show the patella located lateral to the distal femur. (Courtesy J. A. Auer, University of Zurich.)

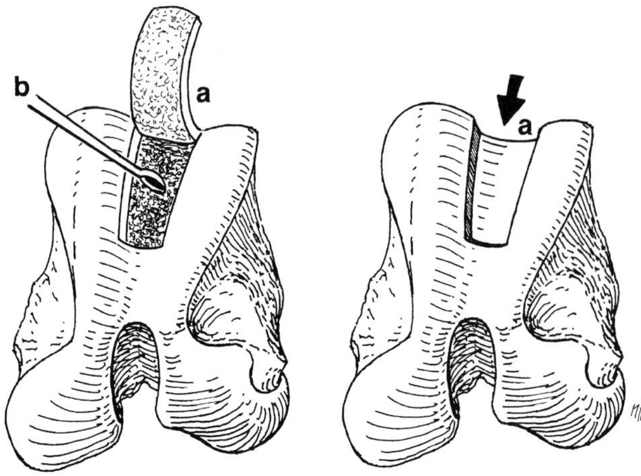

Figure 101-36. Sulcoplasty involving elevation of a U-shaped cartilage flap (a) and removal of the subchondral bone with rongeurs and a curet (b). The flap is repositioned *(arrow)* and, if necessary, the edges are smoothed out. The flap can be secured with suture.

bone is removed with rongeurs, and the surface is evened out with a curet. The cartilage flap is then repositioned and stabilized with sutures. If an abrupt change in trough angle on each side is noticed, additional cartilage can be removed with a scalpel to provide a smooth surface.

The other technique involves the removal of a wedge from the trochlear groove (Fig. 101-37) with a hand-held saw. Each saw cut removes some bone. By reapplying the wedge, some deepening of the groove is achieved. If additional deepening is desired, a parallel saw cut is carried out on one side, followed by replacement of the wedge. The edges are smoothed out. If the wedge is properly seated, no fixation is required. The soft tissue release and imbrication techniques discussed earlier are also performed.

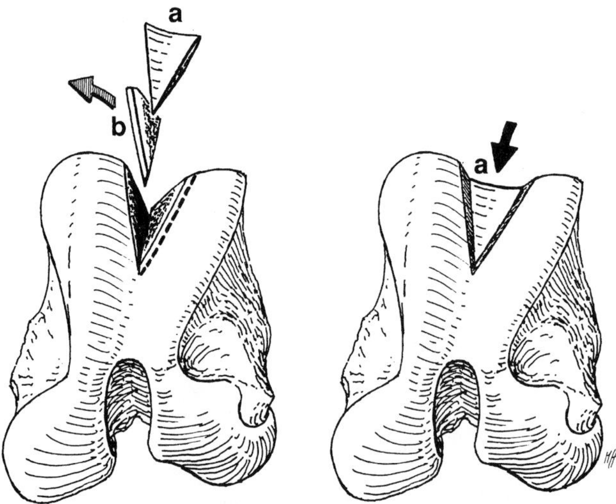

Figure 101-37. Sulcoplasty involving wedge (a) osteotomy of the intertrochlear groove. If necessary, an additional piece of bone (b) is removed with an additional saw cut parallel to a previous one. The wedge (a) is replaced in the trough and pressed into position, resulting in a functional intertrochlear groove.

Both procedures have been used successfully on foals. Postoperative care includes the use of systemic antibiotics, nonsteroidal anti-inflammatory medication, and good nursing care. Seromas do occur but resolve without treatment. Postoperative radiographs reveal correct positioning of the patella.

REFERENCES

1. Stashak TS: Lameness. In Stashak TS, editor: Adams' Lameness in Horses, ed 4, Philadelphia, 1987, Lea & Febiger.
2. Vaughan JT: Analysis of lameness in the pelvic limb and selected cases, Proc Am Assoc Equine Pract 1965;11:223.
3. Cook WR: British Equine Veterinary Association survey of equine diseases, 1962-1963. Vet Rec 1965;77:528.
4. Jeffcott LB, Kold SE: Stifle lameness in the horse: A survey of 86 referred cases, Equine Vet J 1982;14:31.
5. Sisson S: Equine syndesmology. In Getty R, editor: Sisson and Grossman's The Anatomy of the Domestic Animals, ed 5, vol 1, Philadelphia, 1975, WB Saunders.
6. Reeves MJ, Trotter GW, Kainer RA: Anatomical and functional communications between the synovial sacs of the equine stifle joint, Equine Vet J 1991;23:15.
7. Vacek JR, Ford TS, Honnas CM: Communication between the femoropatellar and medial and lateral femorotibial joints in horses, Am J Vet Res 1992;53:1431.
8. Trumble TN, Stick JA, Arnoczky SP, et al: Consideration of anatomic and radiographic features of the caudal pouches of the femorotibial joints of horses for the purpose of arthroscopy, Am J Vet Res 1994;55:1682.
9. deLahunta A, Habel RH: Applied Veterinary Anatomy, Philadelphia, 1986, WB Saunders.
10. May SA, Wyn-Jones G: Identification of hind leg lameness, Equine Vet J 1987;19:185.
11. Adams OR: Lameness in the Horse, ed 3, Philadelphia, 1974, Lea & Febiger.
12. Gough MR, Munroe GA, Mayhew G: Diffusion of mepivacaine between adjacent synovial structures in the horse. Part 2: Tarsus and stifle, Equine Vet J 2002;34:85.
13. Hendrickson DA, Nixon AJ: A lateral approach for synovial aspiration and joint injection of the femoropatellar joint of the horse, Equine Vet J 1992;24:397.
14. Devous MD, Twardock AR: Techniques and applications of nuclear medicine in the diagnosis of equine lameness, J Am Vet Med Assoc 1984;184:318.
15. Aisen AM, McCune WJ, MacGuine A, et al: Sonographic evaluation of the cartilage of the knee, Radiology 1984;153:781.
16. Friedl W, Glaser F: Dynamic sonography in the diagnosis of ligament and meniscal injuries of the knee, Arch Orthop Trauma Surg 1991;110:132.
17. Heikki RL, Harjula A, Peltokallio P: Ultrasound in the evaluation of the knee and patellar regions, J Ultrasound Med 1987;6:33.
18. Richardson ML, Selby B, Montana MA, et al: Ultrasonography of the knee, Radiol Clin North Am 1988;26:63.
19. Selby B, Richardson ML, Montana MA, et al: High resolution sonography of the menisci of the knee, Invest Radiol 1986;21:332.
20. Suzuki S, Kasahara K, Futami T, et al: Ultrasound diagnosis of pathology of the anterior and posterior cruciate ligaments of the knee joint, Arch Orthop Trauma Surg 1991;110:200.
21. Kalebo PL, Sward J, Karlsson J, Peterson L: Ultrasonography in the detection of partial patellar ligament ruptures (jumper's knee), Skeletal Radiol 1991;20:285.
22. Penninck DG, Nyland TG, Obrien TR, et al: Ultrasonography of the equine stifle, Vet Radiol 1990;31:293.
23. Denoix JM, Audigie F: Ultrasonographic examination of joints in

horses. Presented at the 47th AAEP Annual Convention, San Diego, Calif, November 24-28, 200.
24. Aschenbrenner M: Die sonographische Darstellung der Knieregion des Pferdes mit einem 7.5 MHz-Sektorscanner. Doctoral Thesis, 1996, University of Munich.
25. Nickels FA, Sande R: Radiographic and arthroscopic findings in the equine stifle, J Am Vet Med Assoc 1982;181:918.
26. Moustafa MAJ, Boero MJ, Baker GH: Arthroscopic examination of the femorotibial joints of horses, Vet Surg 1987;16:352.
27. Lewis RD: A retrospective study of diagnostic and surgical arthroscopy of the equine femorotibial joints of horses, Proc Am Assoc Equine Pract 1987;33:887.
28. Updike SJ, Diesem CD: Vascular supply of the equine stifle joint, Am J Vet Res 1980;41:1621.
29. Martin GS, McIlwraith CW: Arthroscopic anatomy of the equine femoropatellar joint and approaches for treatment of osteochondritis dissecans, Vet Surg 1985;14:99.
30. McIlwraith CW, Turner AS: Arthroscopic surgery of the femoropatellar joint. In McIlwraith CW, Turner AS, editors: Equine Surgery: Advanced Techniques, Philadelphia, 1987, Lea & Febiger.
31. Böhning KJ: Die Arthroskopie des Kniegelenkes beim Pferd über einen "zentralen" Zugang Teil 1: Methodik, Pferdeheilkunde 1995;11:247.
32. Brems R: Personal communication, 1998.
33. Peroni JF, Stick JA: Evaluation of a cranial arthroscopic approach to the stifle joint for the treatment of femorotibial joint disease in horses: 23 cases (1998-1999), J Am Vet Med Assoc 2002;220:1046.
34. Schneider RK, Jenson P, Moore RM: Evaluation of cartilage lesions on the medial femoral condyle as a cause of lameness in horses: 11 cases (1988-1994), J Am Vet Med Assoc 1997;210:1649.
35. McIlwraith CW: Osteochondral fragmentation of the distal aspect of the patella in horses, Equine Vet J 1990;22:157.
36. Riley CB, Yovich JV: Fracture of the apex of the patella after medial patellar desmotomy in a horse, Aust Vet J 1991;68:37.
37. Tnibar A: Treatment of upward fixation of the patella in the horse: An update, Equine Vet Educ 2003;5:306.
38. Bukowiecki CV, Sanders-Shamis MS, Bramlage LR: Treatment of a ruptured medial collateral ligament of the stifle in a horse, J Am Vet Med Assoc 1988;193:687.
39. Sanders-Shamis M, Bukowiecki CF, Biller DS: Cruciate and collateral ligament failure in the equine stifle: Seven cases (1975-1985), J Am Vet Med Assoc 1988;193:573.
40. Walmsley JP: The Stifle. In Ross MW, Dyson SJ, editors: Diagnosis and Management of Lameness in the Horse, Philadelphia, 2003, WB Saunders.
41. Edwards RB III, Nixon AJ: Avulsion of the cranial cruciate ligament insertion in a horse, Equine Vet J 1996;28:334.
42. Baker GJ, Moustafa MAI, Boero MJ, et al: Caudal cruciate ligament function and injury in the horse, Vet Rec 1987;121:319.
43. Mueller POE, Allen D, Watson E, et al: Arthroscopic removal of a fragment from an intercondylar eminence fracture of the tibia in a two-year-old horse, J Am Vet Med Assoc 1994;204:1793.
44. Prades M, Grant BD, Turner TA, et al: Injuries to the cranial cruciate ligament and associated structures: Summary of clinical, radiographic, arthroscopic and pathological findings from 10 horses, Equine Vet J 1989;21:354.
45. Walmsley JP: Vertical tears of the cranial horn of the meniscus and its cranial ligament in the equine femorotibial joint: 7 cases and their treatment by arthroscopic surgery, Equine Vet J 1995;27:20.
46. Walmsley JP, Phillips TJ, Townsend HGG: Meniscal tears in horses: an evaluation of clinical signs and arthroscopic treatment of 80 cases, Equine Vet J 2003;35:402.
47. Colbern GT, Moore JN: Surgical management of proximal articular fracture of the patella in a horse, J Am Vet Med Assoc 1984;185:543.
48. Hunt RJ, Baxter GM, Zamos DT: Tension-band wiring and lag screw fixation of a transverse, comminuted fracture of a patella in a horse, J Am Vet Med Assoc 1992;200:819.
49. Dyson S: Patellar injuries. In White NA II, Moore JN, editors: Current Techniques in Equine Surgery and Lameness, ed 2, Philadelphia, 1998, WB Saunders.
50. Marble GP, Sullins KE: Arthroscopic removal of patellar fracture fragments in horses: Five cases (1989-1998), J Am Vet Med Assoc 2000;216:1799.
51. Montesso F, Wright IM: Removal of chip fractures of the femoral trochlear ridges of three horses by arthroscopy, Vet Rec 1995; 137:94.
52. Blikslager AT, Beristol DG: Avulsion of the origin of the peroneus tertius tendon in a foal, J Am Vet Med Assoc 1994;204:1483.
53. Holcombe SJ, Bertone AL: Avulsion fracture of the origin of the extensor digitorum longus muscle in a foal, J Am Vet Med Assoc 1994;204:1652.
54. Stromberg B, Renjö S: Osteochondrosis in the horse. I: A clinical and radiologic investigation of osteochondritis dissecans of the knee and hock, Acta Radiol Suppl 1978;358:139.
55. Renjö S, Stromberg B: Osteochondrosis in the horse. II. Pathology, Acta Radiol Suppl 1978;358:153.
56. McIlwraith CW, Martin GS: Arthroscopic surgery for the treatment of osteochondritis dissecans in the equine femoropatellar joint, Vet Surg 1985;14:105.
57. Kane AJ, Park RD, McIlwraith CW, et al: Radiographic changes in Thoroughbred yearlings. Part 1: Prevalence at the time of the yearling sales, Equine Vet J 2003;35:354.
58. Kane AJ, McIlwraith CW, Park RD, et al: Radiographic changes in Thoroughbred yearlings. Part 2: Associations with racing performance, Equine Vet J 2003;35:366.
59. Foland JW, McIlwraith CW, Trotter GW: Osteochondritis of the femoropatellar joint: Results of treatment with arthroscopic surgery, Equine Vet J 1992;26:419.
60. Adams WM, Thilsted JP: Radiographic appearance of the equine stifle from birth to 6 months, Vet Radiol 1985;26:126.
61. Steinheimer DN, McIlwraith CW, Parks RD, et al: Comparison of radiographic subchondral bone changes with arthroscopic findings in the equine femoropatellar and femorotibial joints: A retrospective study of 72 joints (50 horses), Vet Radiol 1995;36:478.
62. Dabareiner RM, Sullins KE, White NA: Progression of femoropatellar osteochondrosis in nine young horses. Clinical radiographic and arthroscopic findings, Vet Surg 1993;22:515.
63. Wright IM, Deo MB, Vatistas NJ, et al: Osteochondrosis of the lateral trochlear ridge of the equine femoropatellar joint: A comparison between arthroscopy and arthrotomy, Proc Am Assoc Equine Pract 1992;38:151.
64. McIntosh SC, McIlwraith CW: Natural history of femoropatellar osteochondritis in three crops of Thoroughbreds, Equine Vet J Suppl 1993;16:54.
65. Ray CS, Baxter GM, McIlwraith CW, et al: Development of subchondral cystic lesions following subchondral bone trauma in horses, Vet Surg 1994;23:414.
66. Jeffcott LB, Kold SE: Clinical and radiological aspects of the stifle bone cysts in the horse, Equine Vet J 1982;14:40.
67. Lewis RD: A retrospective study of diagnostic and surgical arthroscopy of the femorotibial joint, Proc Am Assoc Equine Pract 1987;33:887.
68. Howard RD, McIlwraith CW, Trotter GW: Arthroscopic surgery for subchondral cystic lesions of the medial femoral condyle in the horse: 41 cases (1988-1991), J Am Vet Med Assoc 1995;206:842.
69. Jackson WA, Stick JA, Arnoczky SP, et al: The effect of compacted cancellous bone grafting on the healing of subchondral bone defects of the medial femoral condyle in horses, Vet Surg 2000;29:8.
70. Steward B, Reid CV: Osseous cyst-like lesions of the medial femoral condyle in the horse, J Am Vet Med Assoc 1982;180:254.
71. Rooney JR, Raker CW, Harmany KJ: Congenital lateral luxation of the patella in the horse, Cornell Vet 1971;61:670.

72. Van Pelt RW, Keahey KK, Dalley JB: Congenital bilateral patellar ectopia in a foal, Vet Med Small Animal Clin 1971;66:445.
73. Hermans WA, Kerjes AW, van der Mey GJW, et al: Investigation into the heredity of congenital lateral patellar (sub)luxation in the Shetland pony, Vet Q 1987;9:1.
74. Engelbert TA, Tate LP, Richardson DC, et al: Lateral patellar luxation in miniature horses, Vet Surg 1993;22:293.
75. Leitch M, Kotlikoff M: Surgical repair of congenital lateral luxation of the patella in the foal and a calf, Vet Surg 1980;9:1.
76. Kobluk CN: Correction of patellar luxation by recession sulcoplasty in three foals, Vet Surg 1993;22:298.
77. Vasseur PB: Stifle joint. In Slatter D, editor: Textbook of Small Animal Surgery, ed 2, Philadelphia, 1993, WB Saunders.

CHAPTER 102

Femur and Pelvis

Dean W. Richardson

FRACTURES OF THE FEMUR

Fractures of the femur occur primarily in foals and weanlings, although they can be found in a horse at any age. Most fractures follow a severe traumatic event, such as a fall or a kick.

The diagnosis is not difficult to make in most cases because of the acute onset as well as the marked lameness and swelling that localize the problem. Although crepitus is usually palpable with manipulation of the limb, hemorrhage and muscle swelling can be severe enough to separate the bone ends and minimize this sign. More severely comminuted fractures might not have crepitus, because motion between the individual fragments is limited. Less common presentations include shock caused by blood loss into the thigh musculature and dragging of the limb because of upward fixation of the patella.

Radiographs in any horse larger than a foal require general anesthesia unless the fracture is located distally. Alternatively, ultrasonography can be used to confirm a diagnosis of a displaced fracture.

Surgical treatment of mid-diaphyseal or proximal femoral fractures has generally been successful only in foals and small ponies. Distal metaphyseal fractures can also be successfully repaired in yearlings with plates and screws. Locking intramedullary nails are an option for mid-diaphyseal fractures in foals and even larger yearlings.[1]

Proximal (Head and Neck) Fractures

Proximal (head and neck) fractures are seen almost exclusively in foals and are the most difficult femoral fractures to diagnose without good-quality radiographs. Conservative treatment of such fractures is unlikely to result in a comfortable horse. Surgical repair is difficult to achieve, and the prognosis is guarded.

The favored surgical approach is craniodorsal, with a curved incision just cranial to the greater trochanter and that parallels the proximal shaft of the femur. Exposure is enhanced by either a tenotomy of the gluteal insertion or a trochanteric osteotomy. If an osteotomy is selected, the drill holes for later tension-band repair should be prepared before transecting the bone.

The bone can be cut with an oscillating saw or Gigli wire. The approach and arthrotomy are extended to allow palpation of the head and neck of the femur. Additional fractures that are not evident radiographically are detected in this manner. It is usually impossible to see the fracture site, but having fingers in the joint allows more accurate reduction of the fracture and alignment of the drill bit.

Although use of multiple pins has been described,[2] techniques involving screws provide more stability. These techniques include screws applied in lag fashion, cannulated screws, or a dynamic hip screw plate.[3,4] Regardless of the specific implant selected, alignment is critical to prevent damage to the articular surface. Cannulated screws have a major technical advantage for this particular fracture, because reduction is maintained by the guide wire during the entire procedure and the direction and depth of the drill or screw can be monitored constantly (see Chapter 81). Cannulated screws are significantly weaker in bending than solid screws, so there is a risk of screw failure in larger foals.

If a *cortex screw* and *lag technique* are used, the glide hole is drilled before reduction. This makes it possible to check for central positioning of the bit before entering the epiphysis with the thread hole. This central location maximizes the number of threads engaged in the small fragment. If the screw is not centered in the epiphysis or the epiphyseal fragment is penetrated off center with the large bit used for the glide hole, stability of the repair will be compromised.

Ease of reduction is variable and depends mainly on the degree of eburnation of the fracture surfaces. Smooth, eburnated fracture margins make reduction difficult. If the femoral shaft is held with forceps, leverage is provided when attempting reduction. However, reduction is maintained digitally because clamps cannot be applied. Predrilling the glide hole across the femoral shaft also minimizes the length of time that the fracture must be digitally maintained in reduction.

It is difficult to accurately estimate the ideal length of screw from preoperative radiographs; thus, intraoperative palpation and measurements are essential. To assess the depth and direction of drilling, a pin or drill bit of the same length is placed on the exterior of the bone in a parallel position as drilling is performed. This provides additional visual and tactile help for alignment as holes are drilled into the head of the femur. If at all possible, two screws should be used to ensure rotational stability.

Closure of the wound should be in layers with synthetic absorbable suture. Pre-placing several sutures in the joint capsule before tying is recommended. If a trochanteric osteotomy was performed, it must be repaired with a tension-band technique. Either two screws or two smooth pins can be used to replace the trochanter, but both must be supported distally with 1.25- or 1.5-mm-diameter wire. The wire is passed through a drill hole across the femoral shaft made 5 to 7 mm distal to the osteotomy. In larger foals, two wires are usually used. If screws are used to replace the trochanter, it might help to feed the screws through washers so that the tension-band wire comes to lie between the washer and the bone, which secures the fixation.

Other types of proximal femur fractures involve the greater trochanter or, more commonly, the third trochanter. These fractures can be diagnosed with physical examination or scintigraphy. Ultrasonography can then be used to more specifically define the injury without general anesthesia. Unless fractures are associated with a wound or become sequestrated, they should be treated conservatively with stall rest for several months.

Mid-Diaphyseal Fractures

Mid-diaphyseal fractures are the most common type and are the fractures most amenable to surgical repair.[5,6] Most have a spiral or long oblique shape or are comminuted.

The skin incision is made laterally over the length of the bone between the greater trochanter and the lateral condyle. After the fascia lata is incised, it is easy to separate the vastus lateralis and biceps femoris and identify the fracture hematoma. When the fracture hematoma is identified, the separation of the musculature is easier to define from the inside of the hematoma. The attachments to the third trochanter may need to be severed to provide exposure at the proximal end of the bone.

Comminuted fragments should be independently reduced with screws inserted in positions outside of the planned locations of the plates until the fracture is reconstructed into two main pieces. Comminution in some cases is severe and requires extensive reconstruction. It is useful to place 3.5-mm cortex screws in lag fashion to reduce small fragments, countersinking their relatively small heads deep enough that the plates can be placed over them (Fig. 102-1).

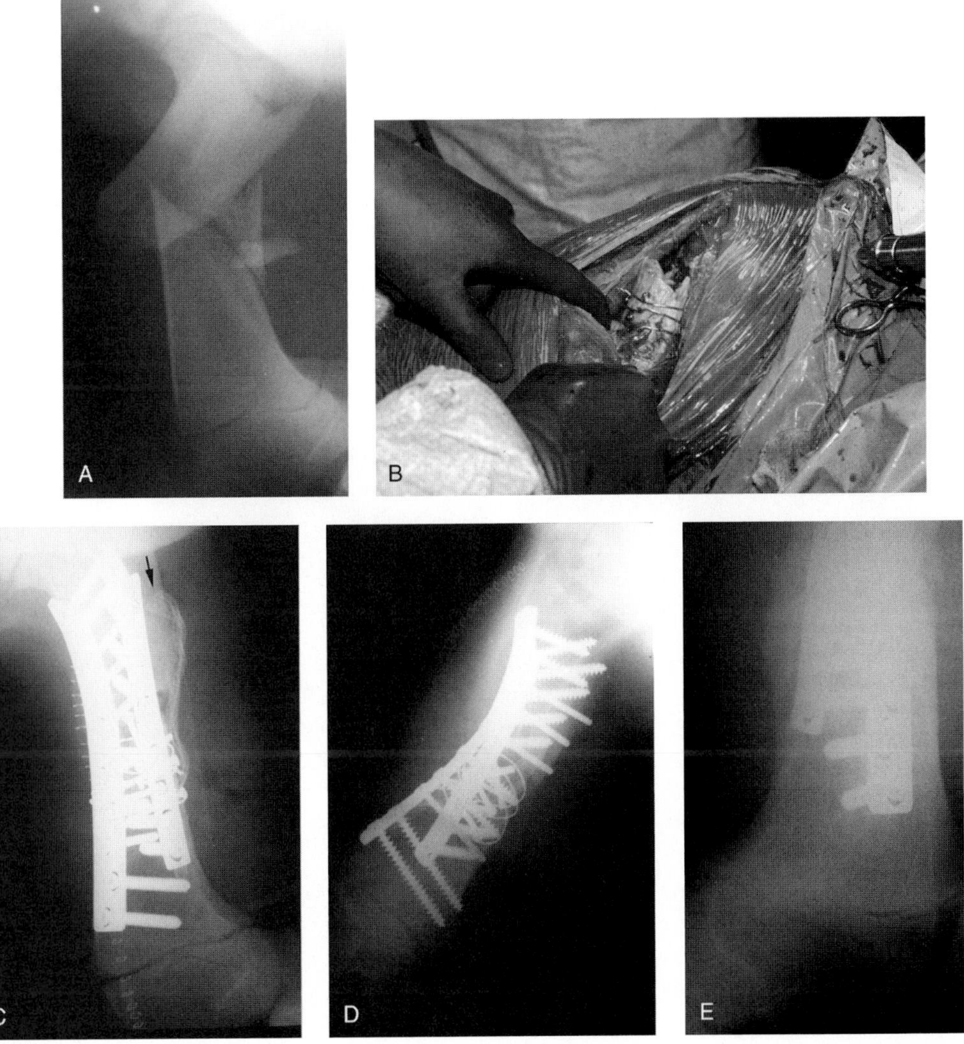

Figure 102-1. A and **B,** Femur fractures in foals often have incomplete cracks propagating along the longitudinal axis of the bone as well as complex comminution. Cerclage wires to stabilize the longitudinal splits and 3.5-mm screws placed in lag fashion help to maintain the reconstructed bone. **C-E,** Two plates, one laterally and one cranially, should be used to repair the femur fractures in foals. If wound complications can be avoided, healing is usually rapid because of the excellent blood supply.

If there is a barrel stave configuration to the fracture extending down the diaphysis, cerclage wires or cables can be used to prevent splitting the bone.

When the fracture is reconstructed to two pieces, reduction is usually possible by simply elevating the fragment ends out of the incision, aligning them properly, and folding the bone ends back into position. For long oblique fractures, it might be necessary to clamp the bone in an overriding position before sliding it incrementally by direct traction into reduction. Nylon cable ties or heavy cerclage wires can be pre-placed to help hold the reduction as it progresses. Vigorous traction might be necessary; therefore, it is essential that the foal's tail and body be tied securely with ropes and girths to the surgery table.

After reduction is obtained, bone clamps are applied. If possible, one or two screws are placed with lag technique across the oblique fracture in locations where they will not interfere with the lateral plate. The bone reduction forceps are removed, allowing application of a long, 5.5-mm limited-contact dynamic compression plate (LC-DCP), broad dynamic compression plate (DCP), or locking compression plate (LCP) with 5.5-mm cortex screws laterally. Alternatively, the plate can be placed with a bone clamp maintaining the reduction, but this is more difficult to achieve.

After applying the lateral plate, a shorter (usually also broad) LC-DCP, DCP, or LCP is placed cranially. Hohmann retractors provide adequate exposure to position the plates and insert the screws (see Fig. 102-1, *C* to *E*). Considerable effort at retraction is sometimes necessary to obtain exposure of the cranial plate for drilling and screw insertion. If necessary, it is possible to make stab incisions through the quadriceps muscle to drill, tap, and insert screws into the cranial plate. Lag technique is applied in plate screws crossing any fracture plane for additional compression and stability. Interfragmentary compression greatly increases the overall stability of the repair. The two plates must be staggered a half-hole apart, and the screws must be inserted perpendicular to the long axis of the plates to prevent interference of screws. The lateral plate should be luted. All cortex defects are filled with autologous cancellous bone.

The incision is closed in at least three layers: the fascial margins of the vastus lateralis and the biceps femoris, subcutaneous tissues, and skin. Interrupted sutures are recommended because wound problems are common and local drainage is sometimes necessary. Because of the considerable muscle trauma and compression, bandaging is impossible; closed suction drainage is essential to minimize accumulation of serum.

Although there is limited clinical experience to date with LCPs (see Chapter 81), they offer significant advantages in terms of stability, mainly because the locking screws prevent movement of the cortex screw heads within the combi hole[7] (Fig. 102-2).

An alternative technique for simple diaphyseal fractures of the femur is insertion of an interlocking intramedullary nail[8] (see Fig. 81-34). The axial position of the nail affords excellent bending stability, and the transfixing screws provide rotational stability. If possible, supplemental fixation in the form of lag screws, cerclage wires, or a plate with unicortical screws can be used in oblique or spiral fractures.

A 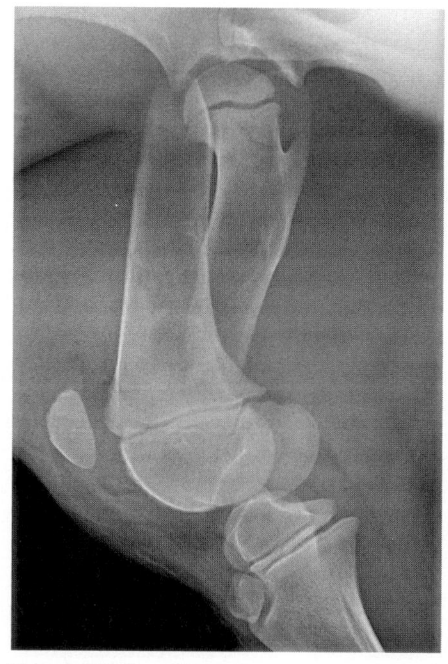

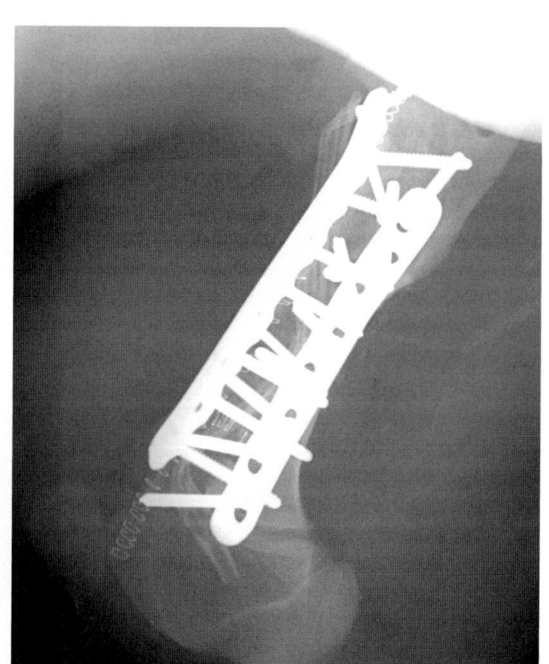 B

Figure 102-2. Locking compression plates with 5.5-mm locking screws can afford additional stability to the repair of femoral fractures in foals with thin cortices and relatively soft bone. **A,** Preoperative radiograph. **B,** Postoperative radiograph showing two 5.5 locking compression plates (LCPs) in place.

A routine incision is made as described earlier to reduce the fracture. A small incision is subsequently made over the medial aspect of the greater trochanter, and a 5.5-mm drill bit is used to prepare a hole across the bone into the medullary cavity. This hole and the medullary cavity are subsequently enlarged with reamers until a uniform-diameter path for the nail is created. The nail length is preselected based on measurements taken on radiographs of the contralateral intact bone. The nail is driven into the distal fragment, seating it securely but being careful not to penetrate the distal end of the bone. After the nail is fully inserted, an aiming device is attached to the proximal end of the nail, and 5.5-mm cortex screws are placed through the bone and the nail. At least two screws are applied at either end of the nail, in most cases more.

One major complication of interlocking intramedullary nails is the development of a fracture through the screw holes. The nails are more applicable in mid-diaphyseal fractures than in more distal or proximal injuries where it is difficult to adequately seat the nail in the distal fragment.

Distal Femoral Fractures

Distal femoral fractures are most commonly encountered in older weanlings and yearlings and are usually Salter-Harris type II, with the metaphyseal fragment positioned caudally. Salter-Harris types III and IV fractures have also been reported but are less common.[9,10] Any distal femoral fracture can be initially misdiagnosed as a stifle lesion because of the location of the swelling (Fig. 102-3). Fractures of the distal femur tend to be quite unstable and therefore require surgical repair.

The fracture is approached through a craniolateral incision between the vastus lateralis and biceps femoris muscles. The incision is extended distally to the level of the tibial crest. The lateral femoropatellar ligament must be transected to allow a parapatellar arthrotomy and patellar luxation. Reduction may be quite difficult to achieve. Like many physeal fractures, exact anatomic alignment is difficult to assess. The metaphyseal part of the fracture is not readily visible and is covered by the extensive soft tissues on the distal caudal femur.

After reduction is achieved, a long screw can be placed through the exposed intercondylar notch and into the metaphysis to maintain alignment while the lateral plate is applied. Because the epiphyseal fragment is small, a specialized plate is usually preferred. The strongest plate, which is best suited for larger yearlings, is a dynamic condylar screw (DCS) plate. The DCS plate is difficult to contour because of its large cross section.

Special care must be taken to fit the plate accurately on the horse's curved distal femur, because the plate was designed for the straight human femur. However, this plate provides superior stability in the distal fragment (Fig. 102-4). In horses weighing less than 175 kg, the condylar buttress plate with a flared end accommodating several screws is easier to apply and is strong enough despite its smaller cross section.[11] A cobra head plate may be used, although it is difficult to conform to the bone.[12] The broad LCPs with 5.0-mm locking screws also have potential for use in this location (see Fig. 102-2).

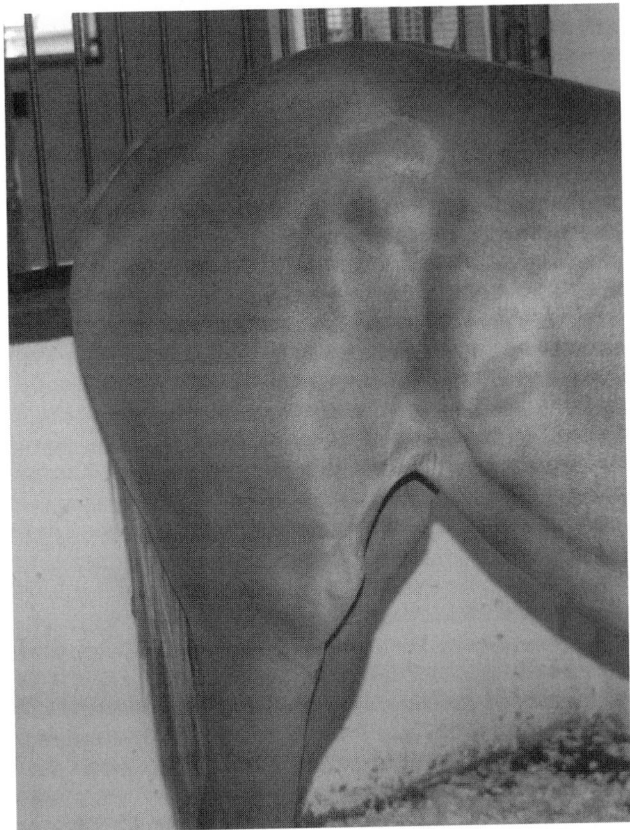

Figure 102-3. The swelling associated with a distal femoral fracture can be misinterpreted as a primary stifle joint problem. Typically, however, crepitus and instability are palpable.

Regardless of the plate selected, 5.5-mm cortex or 6.5-mm cancellous screws should be used. The para-patellar incision is closed with large tension-holding sutures (cruciate, overlap, or mattress), and a meticulously managed suction drain is used in the subcutaneous tissues.

Prognosis

The prognosis for fractures of the femur is guarded because of the high risk of complications.[6] As a result of muscle trauma and because a pressure bandage cannot be used on the area, surgical incisions are susceptible to extensive serum accumulations. Wound dehiscence and sepsis are common problems. If complications are avoided, however, healing of fractures of the femur is remarkably rapid in young animals because of excellent vascularity and muscle coverage. Callus is radiographically visible in foals within a few weeks.

Failure of plates and screws is rare, except when there is a bone defect in the caudal cortex. Such a defect leads to excessive cyclic loading of the implants and fatigue failure. If fracture healing is uncomplicated, it is not advisable to remove the implants because of the potential for healing problems. In distal physeal fractures, the plate might have to be removed if it is interfering with joint function or if there is significant remaining growth potential. Unfortunately, many physeal fractures of the distal femur result in

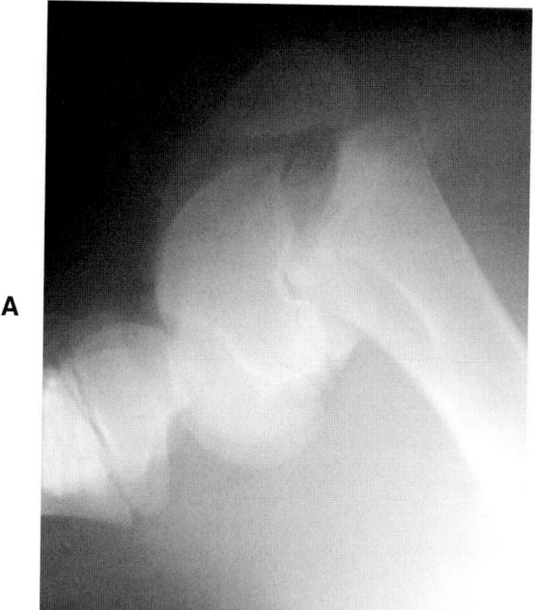

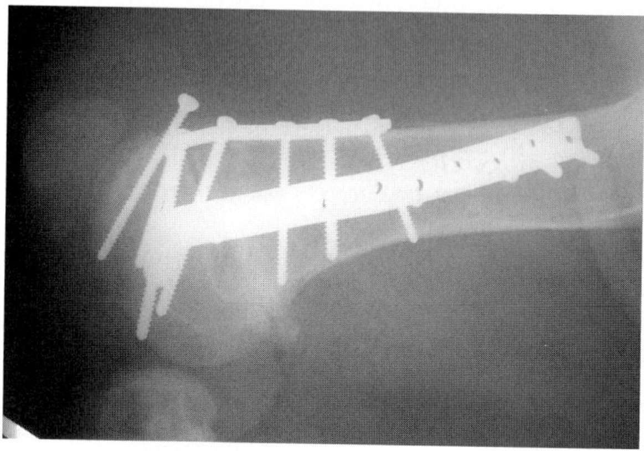

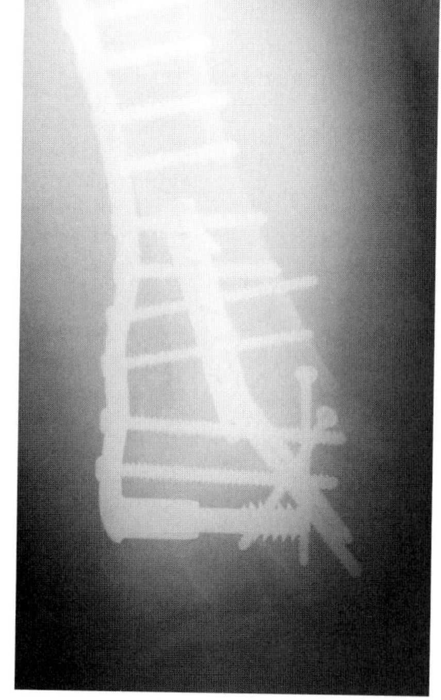

Figure 102-4. A, Salter-Harris type II fracture of the distal femur. **B** and **C,** The fracture was repaired with a dynamic compression screw (DCS) plate applied laterally and augmented with a five-hole narrow dynamic compression plate (DCP) containing long screws penetrating the medial condyle. One single screw was buried in the articular surface to provide additional stability to the cranial aspect of the reconstruction. Longitudinally placed screws should augment the plate fixation. (Courtesy C. Lischer, University of Zurich.)

permanent closure of the growth plate and consequently a shortened femur. This is acceptable for breeding soundness, because the animal can compensate somewhat by increasing its joint angles in the stifle and hock.

Although some fractures of the femur have been successfully managed conservatively, younger animals often rapidly develop a serious varus deformity in the contralateral limb (Fig. 102-5). Because these fractures can be repaired successfully in foals, the conservative approach should be reserved for older animals in which the surgical approach is too daunting or for cases where comminution is severe enough that reconstruction is not feasible.

FRACTURES OF THE PELVIS

Fractures of the pelvis occur in all animals of all ages but are disproportionately common in foals and yearlings.[13,14] Most follow a distinct traumatic event, such as a fall. In adult

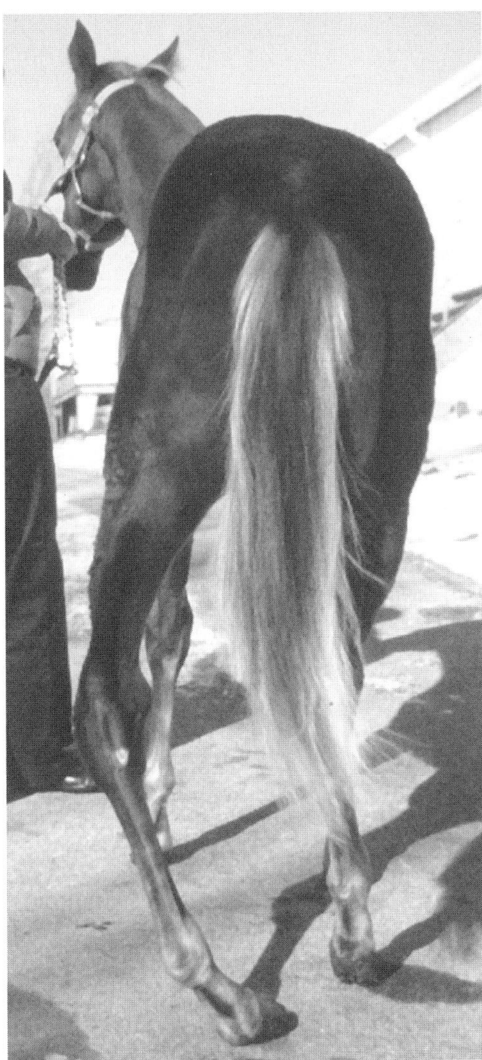

Figure 102-5. A 6-month old weanling suffering from a femoral shaft fracture of 1 month's duration in the right hindlimb, which was treated conservatively. Note the marked varus deformity in the left hindlimb.

horses, pelvic fractures can occur during intense exercise without obvious trauma.

The most obvious clinical sign is overt lameness either of the swinging or supporting limb type. External swelling or asymmetry of palpable pelvic landmarks (e.g., the tuber coxae, tuber ischii, tuber sacrale, and greater trochanters) can be present. It is helpful to measure the distances between these landmarks and to compare the two sides. Pain can be elicited by manipulation of the limb or by direct pressure over the trochanter or other prominences. Examination per rectum can reveal obvious asymmetry, especially with acetabular fractures in which there is often a rounded, firm swelling over the fractured region.

Crepitus can be difficult to appreciate externally in horses with pelvic fractures, but it is often more obvious if the horse's weight is shifted or if the horse is walked a few steps during a rectal examination. Vigorous manipulation of the limb by an assistant can also be helpful in some cases, although care should be taken to test the horse's pain response to such manipulation before the rectal examination is undertaken. Crepitus is usually appreciated more easily in the first day or two after the injury.

In chronic cases, pelvic musculature is usually atrophied, although this is obviously not specific for a pelvic injury. The medial thigh region should always be checked for asymmetry, because dependent swelling often develops in this area, especially with displaced acetabular and ileal fractures. The most dramatic presenting signs are seen with a laceration of a major artery (usually the internal iliac artery). This results in bleeding into the abdomen or thigh that is severe enough to cause shock or death.[14,15]

A definitive diagnosis of pelvic fractures is made with radiographs. This usually requires general anesthesia, although a technique for standing pelvic radiography has been described.[16] Even under general anesthesia, there are significant limitations in the sensitivity of radiographs of the pelvis in adult horses. Consequently, nuclear scintigraphy, either with an imaging or point-counting technique, is often used for screening.[17-19] Scintigraphy is the only technique that can identify subtle injuries such as ileal stress fractures. If a displaced fracture is suspected, a simpler and less expensive alternative is ultrasonography; it is possible to clearly identify discontinuities of a cortical surface in accessible locations.[20,21] Ultrasonography is particularly useful for diagnosing tuber coxae fractures.

Treatment

Treatment of pelvic fractures is almost always conservative, although displaced *iliac shaft fractures* in foals can be repaired successfully with internal fixation (Fig. 102-6). The ilium is approached by elevating the gluteal musculature sharply along its ventral attachments and forcefully retracting the musculature dorsally with Hohmann elevators. The fragments are reduced and secured with bone plates. In nonarticular fractures, anatomic reduction is not mandatory for a good result. Surgical repair of pelvic fractures in foals is restricted to those with marked displacement and a need for athletic function.

There are no reported cases of the successful repair of *acetabular fractures* in horses of any age, although it is feasible to approach the dorsal rim in younger foals or miniature horses. Displaced *tuber coxae fractures* (knocked-down hips) are usually not treated surgically either, although removal should be considered if they are open and draining.

In adult horses, stall rest for at least 3 to 4 months is combined with adequate analgesia, support bandaging, and frog support on the contralateral limb. Epidural analgesia can be used with caution, especially to manage the more intense pain in the initial period after the injury. Younger horses heal more quickly but also develop limb deformities more readily in the contralateral limb (see Fig. 102-5).

Prognosis

The prognosis for pelvic fractures depends primarily on the degree of displacement. Nondisplaced fractures of any portion of the pelvis, even those involving the acetabulum, heal without serious consequences, whereas displaced injuries that cause persistent pain lead to muscle wasting, contralateral limb and foot problems, and coxofemoral arthritis. In mares, markedly displaced fractures can

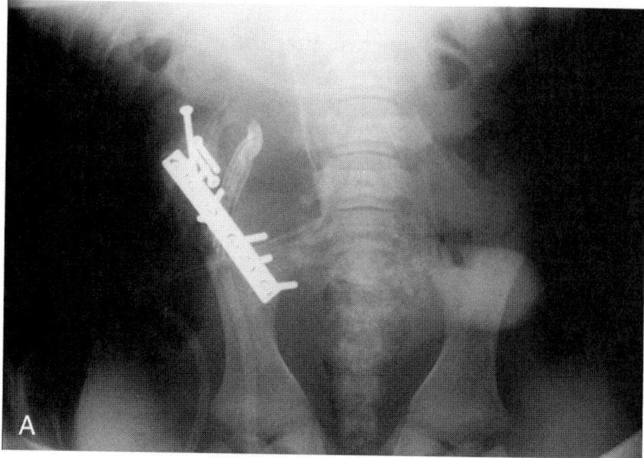

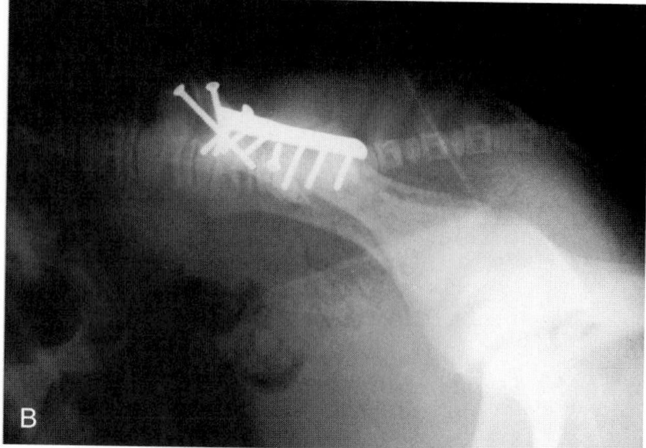

Figure 102-6. In selected cases (**A** and **B**) iliac shaft fractures can be repaired in young foals using internal fixation.

compromise the birth canal and lead to dystocia. In one study, a successful outcome occurred in 77% of horses that were not euthanized immediately after the pelvic fracture was diagnosed.[14] Because surprisingly rapid improvement and healing can occur, precipitous decisions to euthanize horses with pelvic fractures should be avoided, unless it is absolutely clear that recovery is impossible or the economic pressures dictate against continued treatment.

COXOFEMORAL LUXATIONS

Coxofemoral luxations are rare in equids but are more common in ponies and miniature horses than in larger animals.[22] Most occur after falls, after attacks by larger horses, or while the animal is struggling to extract an entrapped limb or straighten an upwardly fixed patella.[23] Coxofemoral luxations and femoral head fractures can occur in horses and foals wearing full hindlimb casts.[24]

Clinical diagnosis of coxofemoral luxation is not difficult except to distinguish it from a femoral head fracture, which can be achieved through radiography or ultrasonography. The affected horse is very lame and holds the distal limb externally rotated. Because most luxations occur craniodorsally, the point of the tarsus is higher than the normal side when the horse is viewed from behind. Manipulation of the limb might or might not yield a soft, clicking crepitus.

Treatment

Treatment of coxofemoral luxation in miniature horses and ponies has been accomplished by reduction and primary repair[25] or by excision arthroplasty.[26,27]

Surgical repair involves a craniodorsal approach to the hip[28] with or without greater trochanteric osteotomy. If a trochanteric osteotomy is elected, it is advisable to pre-drill one or two holes to facilitate tension-band repair during closure. Before the femoral head is reduced, the joint is cleaned of fibrin and any debris.

Reduction often requires mechanical assistance either with a calf jack or a pulley system rigged up in the operating room. A hip skid, which is a long lever with a curved spoon-like end, can be helpful in reducing the luxation. In most cases, replacement alone is not successful because of continued instability. Therefore, toggle pinning or augmentation of the lateral joint capsule with synthetic sutures attached to screws might be necessary. The latter technique involves placing screws above the cranial acetabular margin and lateral femoral shaft just distal to the neck. A large braided suture is tied around the screw heads to help prevent the head from moving proximolaterally. Washers can help to minimize slippage of the suture material from under the screw heads.

Femoral head and neck excision is unlikely to be successful, except in small ponies and miniature horses. The surgical exposure is achieved through a craniolateral approach, and an oscillating saw, Gigli wire, or wide osteotome is used to transect the femoral neck as close to the shaft as possible. Postoperatively, the horse should be kept on optimal footing to prevent the animal from slipping. Use of soft rope hobbles may be helpful to prevent abduction if the horse can tolerate them.

REFERENCES

1. Watkins JP: Personal communication, 2004.
2. Turner AS, Milne DW, Hohn RB, et al: Surgical repair of fractured capital femoral epiphysis in three foals, J Am Vet Med Assoc 1979;175:1198-1202.
3. Hunt DA, Snyder JR, Morgan JP, et al: Evaluation of an interfragmentary compression system for the repair of equine femoral capital physeal fractures, Vet Surg 1990;19:107-116.
4. Hunt DA, Snyder JR, Morgan JP, et al: Femoral capital physeal fractures in 25 foals, Vet Surg 1990;19:41-49.
5. Turner AS: Surgical repair of a fractured femur in a foal: A case report, J Equine Med Surg 1977;1:180-185.
6. Hance SR, Bramlage LR, Schneider RK, et al: Retrospective study of 38 cases of femur fractures in horses less than one year of age [see comments], Equine Vet J 1992;24:357-363.
7. Florin M, Arzdorf M, Linke B, et al: Assessment of stiffness and strength of four different implants available for equine fracture treatment: A study on a 20 degree oblique long bone fracture model using a bone substitute, Vet Surg 2005;34:231.
8 McClure SR, Watkins JP, Ashman RB: In vivo evaluation of intramedullary interlocking nail fixation of transverse femoral osteotomies in foals, Vet Surg 1998;27:29-36.
9. Byron CR, Stick JA, Brown JA, et al: Use of a condylar screw plate

for repair of a Salter-Harris type-III fracture of the femur in a 2-year-old horse, J Am Vet Med Assoc 2002;221:1292-1295.

10. Walmsley JP, Summerhays GES: Repair of a Salter-Harris type IV fracture of the distal femur of a yearling Thoroughbred by internal fixation, Equine Vet Educ 1990;2:177-179.
11. Orsini JA, Buonanno AM, Richardson DW, et al: Condylar buttress plate fixation of femoral fracture in a colt, J Am Vet Med Assoc 1990;197:1184-1186.
12. Kirker-Head CA, Fackelman GE: Use of the cobra head bone plate for distal long bone fractures in large animals. A report of four cases, Vet Surg 1989;18:227-234.
13. Little C, Hilbert B: Pelvic fractures in horses: 19 cases (1974-1984), J Am Vet Med Assoc 1987;190:1203-1206.
14. Rutkowski JA, Richardson DW: A retrospective study of 100 pelvic fractures in horses, Equine Vet J 1989;21:256-259.
15. Sweeney CR, Hodge TG: Sudden death in a horse following fracture of the acetabulum and iliac artery laceration, J Am Vet Med Assoc 1983;182:712-713.
16. May SA, Patterson LJ, Peacock PJ, et al: Radiographic technique for the pelvis in the standing horse, Equine Vet J 1991;23:312-314.
17. Pilsworth RC, Sheperd MC: The diagnosis and management of injuries to the equine pelvis, Ippologia 1997;8:35-59.
18. Davenport-Goodall CL, Ross MW: Scintigraphic abnormalities of the pelvic region in horses examined because of lameness or poor performance: 128 cases (1993-2000), J Am Vet Med Assoc 2004;224:88-95.
19. Dyson S, Murray R, Branch M, et al: The sacroiliac joints: Evaluation using nuclear scintigraphy. Part 2: Lame horses, Equine Vet J 2003;35:233-239.
20. Tomlinson JE, Sage AM, Turner TA, et al: Detailed ultrasonographic mapping of the pelvis in clinically normal horses and ponies. Am J Vet Res 2001;62:1768-1775.
21. Reef VB: Musculoskeletal ultrasonography. In Reef VB, editor: Equine Diagnostic Ultrasound, Philadelphia, 1998, WB Saunders.
22. Malark JA, Nixon AJ, Haughland MA, et al: Equine coxofemoral luxations: 17 cases (1975-1990), Cornell Vet 1992;82:79-90.
23. Clegg PD, Butson RJ: Treatment of a coxofemoral luxation secondary to upward fixation of the patella in a Shetland pony, Vet Rec 1996;138:134-137.
24. Trotter GW, Auer JA, Arden W, et al: Coxofemoral luxation in two foals wearing hindlimb casts, J Am Vet Med Assoc 1986;189:560-561.
25. Garcia-Lopez JM, Boudrieau RJ, Provost PJ: Surgical repair of coxofemoral luxation in a horse, J Am Vet Med Assoc 2001;219:1254-1258.
26. Field JR, McLaughlin R, Davies M: Surgical repair of coxofemoral luxation in a miniature horse, Can Vet J 1992;33:404-405.
27. Platt D, Wright IM, Houlton JEF: Treatment of chronic coxofemoral luxation in a Shetland pony by excision arthroplasty of the femoral head: A case report, Br Vet J 1990;146:374-379.
28. Milne D, Turner A: An Atlas of Surgical Approaches to the Bones of the Horse, Philadelphia, 1979, WB Saunders.

CHAPTER 103

Craniomaxillofacial Disorders

Jörg A. Auer

FRACTURES OF THE INCISORS, MANDIBLE, AND PREMAXILLA

Trauma to the head often results in fractures of the teeth, incisive bone, mandible, premaxilla, or maxilla. These injuries occur as blunt trauma from kicks, falls, and collisions or from being startled in the stall while cribbing on stall slats or mesh wire. Sudden jerking of the head while chewing on stationary objects results in avulsion fractures of the incisors.

Whatever the cause, these fractures can be repaired with good cosmetic and functional results. Several factors make this possible. There is good soft tissue covering with an abundant vascular supply. Because the bones of the head are not subjected to the same loading forces as the bones of the extremities, the requisites for fracture fixation are less demanding. The teeth serve as welcome stabilizing aids. Implants of adequate strength are available, and the instrumentation required is in most cases inexpensive and readily available.

Diagnosis

A thorough physical examination is the basis for a correct diagnosis. One of the first signs of a fracture of the jaws is excessive drooling and lack of appetite. Soft tissue swelling, hemorrhage, instability, and malalignment of the teeth and bones are usually noticed on closer inspection. A fetid odor is usually present with open fractures that are several days old.

Malocclusion of the incisors can be induced manually even in normal horses because of the normal side-to-side mobility of the temporomandibular joint. However, both mandibles will move in the same direction with manipulation unless a fracture is present, in which case, one side of the mandible can be manipulated independently of the other. Often, soft tissue swelling obscures the detection of a malalignment, especially if the fracture is located under the masseter muscles. Horses might object to manipulation and examination of the oral cavity because of pain. A protruding tongue should alert the clinician to suspect a bilateral fracture. Drooling occurs as a result of an inability to close the mouth.

The diagnosis is in most cases not difficult, but other structures might be injured concurrently; therefore, the nasal passages and cranial nerves should be examined. Horses can become significantly dehydrated after hemorrhage and salivary loss, which can be compounded by the patient's reluctance to drink. This is especially true if the fractures are not detected in a timely manner. The physical examination also should include cardiovascular parameters that would identify potential anesthetic risks. In by far the majority of the cases, repair is not an emergency procedure, allowing adequate time to arrive at a comprehensive surgical plan.

In most cases, radiographs are difficult to interpret because of the complexity of the bones in the head and the presence of the teeth, which often are superimposed over fracture lines.[1] Nevertheless, radiographs often demonstrate fractures even with minor malalignment and instability. Also, radiographs provide information about the precise location of the tooth roots in relation to the fracture, which helps in devising a surgery plan that avoids damage to the permanent teeth. Radiographs often aid in detecting potential sequestrum formation. Computed tomography greatly improves preoperative appreciation of the fracture configuration, especially when three-dimensional reconstruction of the fractured bone is obtained (Fig. 103-1).

Not all fractures require repair. Unilateral fractures of the mandible, maxilla, premaxilla, or incisive bone that are minimally displaced and do not result in significant malocclusion may be treated conservatively. Indications for repair include fractures that are unstable, result in malocclusion of the teeth, or are bilateral.[2] Other considerations that might favor surgical repair include improved cosmesis because of decreased callus formation, more rapid healing in the face of increased stability, and horses that are either unable or reluctant to eat because of pain.[2]

Preoperative Management

Simple dental fractures that do not require fixation devices that extend caudal to the canine teeth can be managed in the standing, sedated horse with regional anesthesia. Local anesthesia is easily accomplished by infiltrating 5 mL of lidocaine or mepivacaine around either the mental or infraorbital nerves at their exit point from their respective foramina.[3] Bilateral infiltration of the nerves is required in most cases.

The standing position facilitates observation of symmetry during surgical repair. However, general anesthesia is preferred because of the potential for injury to the surgeon by the patient in response to painful stimuli. Intravenous anesthetic regimens (see Chapter 20) are appropriate in most of the simple fractures, because patient and surgeon preparation and positioning requirements are minimal, so that repair may begin immediately after induction. To allow

A

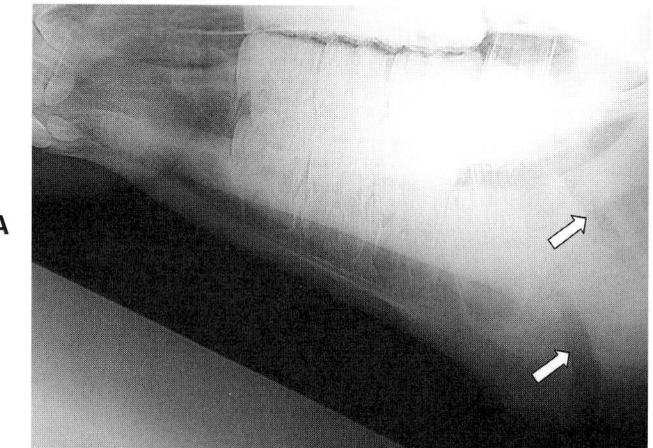

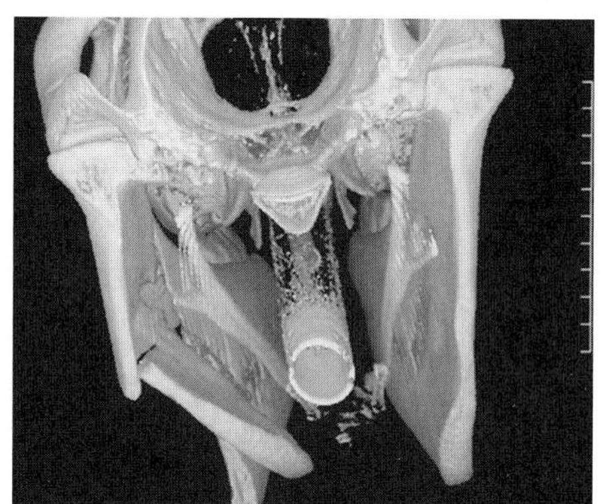

B

C

Figure 103-1. A, Lateromedial radiograph of a complicated mandible fracture in a foal. Two fracture lines are visible *(arrows)*; **B,** Lateral view, and **C,** caudal cross-sectional view of the three-dimensional reconstruction of the computed tomography study of this foal. The complexity of the fracture is easily visible.

unimpeded access to the fracture, nasotracheal intubation is preferred in most cases where inhalation anesthesia is desired or indicated.

The location of the fracture, its complexity, and the personal preferences of the surgeon dictate patient positioning on the surgery table. Most uncomplicated unilateral fractures are repaired in lateral recumbency. Access to both sides of the mouth is required for bilateral fractures and is most easily accomplished with the horse in dorsal recumbency, with the poll flexed so that the surgeon can look down into the horse's mouth.[2]

Preoperative planning should include the likelihood of fracture reduction and which implants will provide the best stability. All necessary equipment must be ready and sterilized. Additionally, any splint that might be required must be pre-shaped, ideally on a cadaveric specimen of approximately the same size to reduce anesthesia time.

Before repair, the mouth is rinsed with water to remove feed material; a dental pick is used to remove any feed material from fracture lines. The oral cavity is contaminated, and surgical scrubs are of dubious value if intraoral wiring alone is to be used.[2] Repair methods that use internal fixation devices deserve all of the precautions and considerations that internal fixation in other areas require because the implants are usually left in place. Prophylaxis against tetanus is indicated in all cases. Perioperative broad-spectrum antibiotics are strongly encouraged, because the surgery is usually performed in a contaminated field.

Surgical Considerations

The tension side of the jaw is the oral surface of both the mandible and the maxilla, and surgical repair should be directed accordingly when possible. Unilateral fractures of the mandible are partially supported by the intact contralateral side. This aids in the stability of the final repair. Avulsion fractures of the incisors, mandible, and premaxilla are usually simple fractures. The ends of the fractured bone usually interdigitate well and can be repaired using intraoral wiring.

Fractures of the incisors that result from kicks or collisions push the teeth caudally. These fractures are usually associated with a considerable amount of instability and some comminution of the bone caudal to the incisors. The extent of comminution can be assessed during physical examination by the stability of the fracture once it is reduced and by the resistance to collapse with manual manipulation.

Intraoral wiring alone tends to collapse comminuted fractures and results in malocclusion when the wires are tightened. In these cases, it is necessary to provide a buttress to maintain length and prevent collapse. This can be accomplished by intraoral splinting, external fixators, or bone plates applied in buttress fashion.[4]

Closed reduction is desirable to preserve blood supply and to leave soft tissues intact for support. Every effort should be made to prevent contamination of healthy tissues by exposure to the oral cavity.[2] Because accuracy of reduction is in most cases readily determined by visual inspection of the teeth, open reduction is often not necessary to ensure alignment of the fractures. The soft tissue attachments of the gingiva should not be disrupted. Small bone fragments devoid of their soft tissue attachments should be removed when the fracture is open. However, any bone fragment attached to the gingiva or periosteum should be left in place.

Loose teeth should never be removed until the fracture has healed and clear evidence is present that they are devitalized. Viability is not always easy to determine at the time of surgery, and many teeth will survive even if they are loose at the time of repair. More importantly, the teeth often serve a vital function as anchor sites in the thin flat bones of the jaws and quite often support the neighboring teeth when wires are used in the repair.

Intraoral wiring and external fixation methods have some advantages over internal fixation using plates and screws in fractures of the mandible and maxilla for several reasons. Intraoral wiring configurations are inexpensive and almost infinitely variable and adaptable to almost any fracture configuration. Bone in this area is soft, and screws can be easily stripped. The roots of both permanent and deciduous teeth occupy a large part of the mandible and maxilla and make placement of screws for plate fixation difficult without damaging the teeth.[2] Radiographic control is usually necessary if internal fixation methods are used. Accuracy of screw placement, screw length, and proper bone engagement of the screws are not easily determined without intraoperative radiographs.

The oral cavity contains a large population of resident microflora. Fractures are usually open and contaminated so that internal fixation often results in infection, thus necessitating eventual removal of the implant. Instrumentation for internal fixation requires more expertise, and the procedures are more time consuming. It is difficult to place bone plates on the tension surface. This does not preclude their use, and bone plates can result in satisfactory repair when placed on the lateral aspects of the mandible or maxilla because in this location the plates are loaded parallel to their width and not their thickness, which provides greater resistance against cyclic loading.

When repairing fractures of the teeth, mandible, and premaxilla, the goals are anatomic alignment and stable fixation to restore the ability to masticate. Involved incisors are best ground down to prevent contact with the opposing tooth arcade during mastication, which can cause decreased disturbance of fracture healing. Many successful methods have been reported, and the simplest method of repair that achieves these goals should be applied to any situation. Techniques are often combined as necessary.

Surgical Techniques

Intraoral Wires

WIRING OF THE INCISORS

Fractures involving the incisors, incisive bone, symphysis of the mandible, and premaxilla are amenable to intraoral wiring. The wound is properly cleaned and the potential damage to tooth roots or deciduous tooth buds is assessed. Fracture reduction is accomplished by manual manipulation.

A 14-gauge needle is inserted between the teeth at the gum line, and 1.25-mm diameter stainless steel wire is threaded through the needle (Fig. 103-2, *A*). Care is taken to prevent sharp bends in the wire from developing while weaving it around the teeth, because these bends prevent effective tightening of the wire. Additionally, cyclic loading of the wire during eating will straighten the wire and in

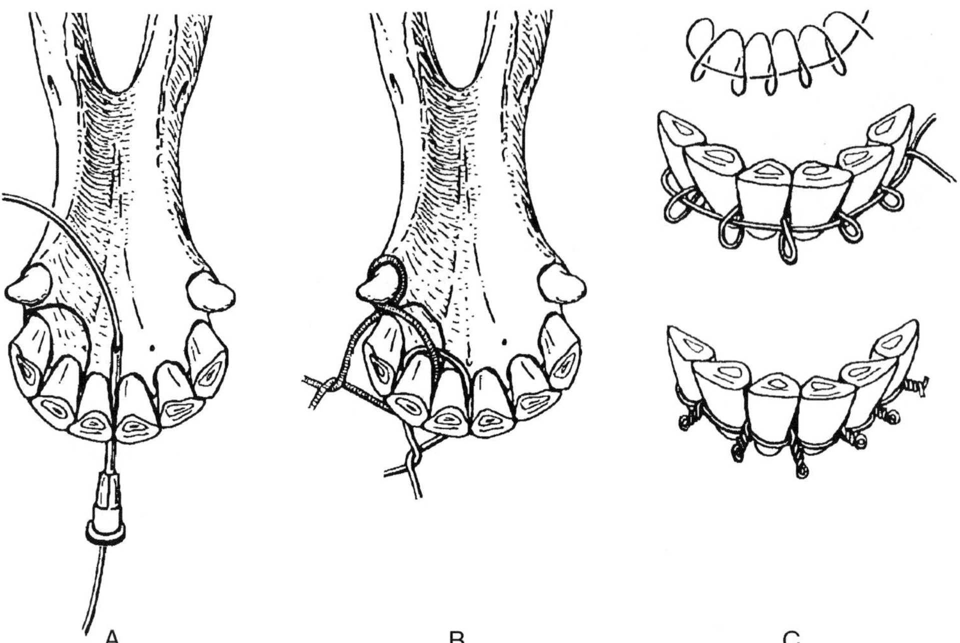

Figure 103-2. Cerclage wiring of a fracture involving 402 and 403. **A,** A 14-gauge needle is inserted between the teeth, and a 1.25-mm stainless steel wire is threaded into the needle as it is withdrawn. **B,** The fracture is treated with two cerclage wire loops, one around 401 and 402 and the other in figure-eight fashion around I_2 and the adjacent healthy canine tooth. **C,** An alternate method involves exiting wire loops from the lingual side and the labial side, followed by feeding one end of the wire through each loop. After tightening the two wire ends, each wire loop is tightened as well, resulting in the most stable of all wire fixations. The twisted ends are directed toward the gingiva.

doing so loosen the fixation. Sharp bends also predispose the wire to failure because of local weakening through prestressing. The wires are kept tight during application, and any slack in the wire is removed after each tooth is encircled. Fractured teeth are united to adjacent healthy ones with a figure-eight wire passed around all selected teeth and tightened at one end (Fig. 103-2, *B*). Another technique involves multiple overlapping cerclage wires placed around the selected teeth. Each wire fastens the unstable teeth and associated bone to the normal teeth until alignment and stability are achieved. The selection of the technique to be applied is at the discretion of the surgeon.

Wire fixation is most easily accomplished by simple interrupted wires encircling the teeth. One or two wires are usually sufficient to stabilize most simple fractures of the incisors. After each wire is tightened, the fracture is manipulated to ascertain the alignment and stability. Wire repair applying the figure-eight technique unites all teeth in one fixation, but because of the relatively long wire arranged in several circles around the involved teeth, tightening the wire is more difficult.[5] Repair is adequate if the incisors cannot be displaced by manual pressure.

A standard wiring technique applied in humans has been proposed.[6] Wire loops are inserted between each tooth from the oral to the labial side (Fig. 103-2, *C*). One end of the wire is fed through each loop and is tightened with the other end. Each wire loop is subsequently tightened, resulting in a constricting wire loop around each tooth and therefore increased stability. This technique provides a rigid fixation that allows the patient to eat for months while the fracture heals (Fig. 103-3).

Fractures that involve the corner incisors need some sort of anchoring farther caudally. In male horses the canine tooth may serve as such an anchor (Fig. 103-4). It is usually necessary to make a notch in the canine tooth at the gum line with a small triangular file to prevent the wire from slipping off of the tooth. An alternate approach to a caudal anchor is to insert a 4.5-mm cortex screw into the interdental space and wrap the wire around the screw head. Another technique is to drill a 2.5-mm hole across the lateral edge of the interdental space and feed the wire through it (see later). Tension band wiring can also be achieved by feeding the wire around the second premolar and tightening the wire.

In rare cases, cerclage wires may be applied in a circular manner around oblique unilateral fractures of the interdental space (Fig. 103-5). The intact opposite side of the mandible ensures maintenance of mandible length and some stability of the fracture ends, and the cerclage wires maintain the fragment ends in approximation and provide some compression across the fracture.

Hemicerclage wires are very useful in fractures of the mandible. Initially a K-wire of 2 to 2.5 mm is introduced across the fracture. The two ends of the pin are united across the surface of the bone in figure-eight fashion and solidly tightened, providing axial compression across the fracture (Fig. 103-6). This technique is also very effective in fractures of the symphysis of the mandible in very young foals, where the bone has inadequate strength for lag screw fixation (see later).

Interdental wiring becomes progressively more difficult as fractures occur more caudally on the mandible.[2] It is very

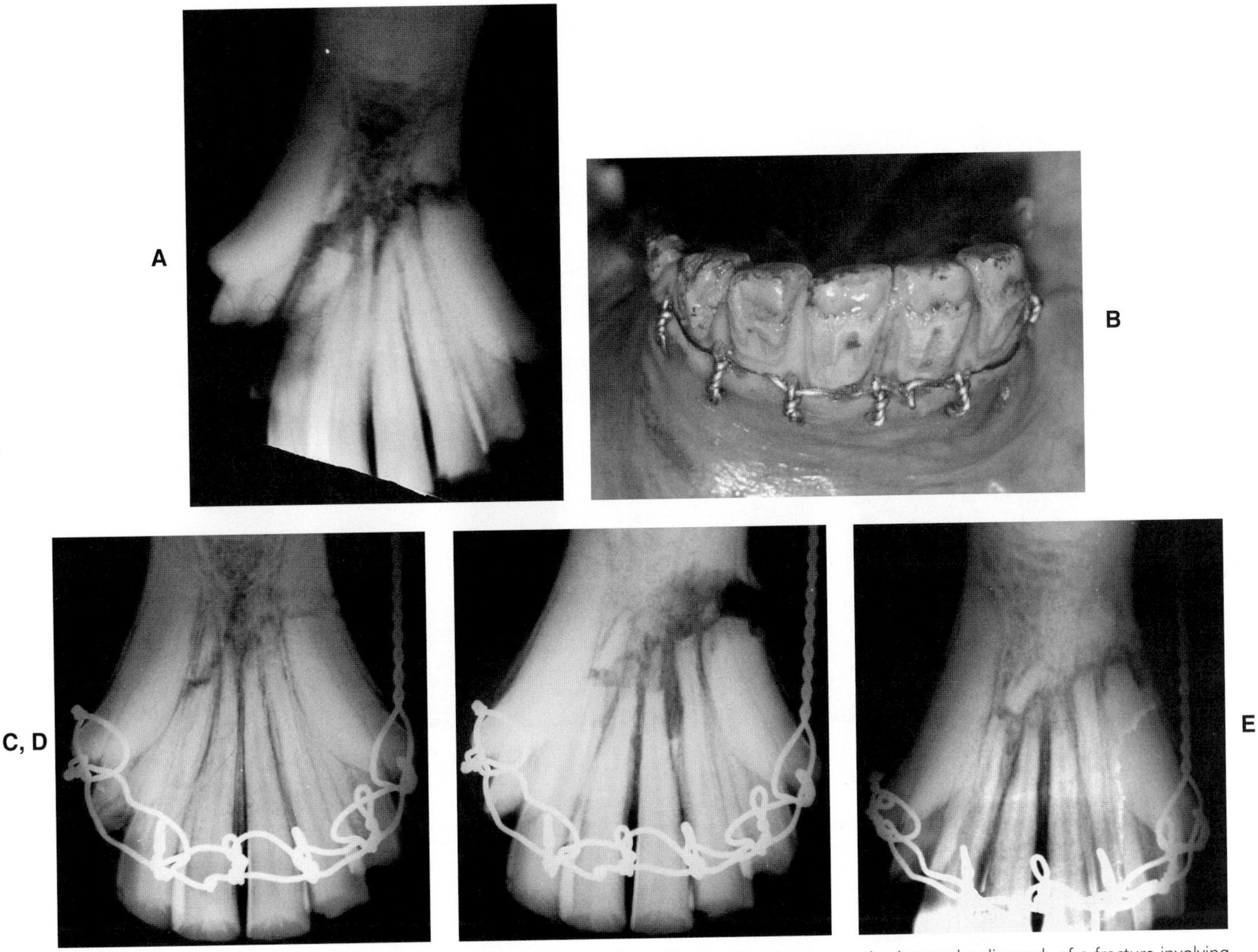

Figure 103-3. Intraoral wiring of a mandible fracture in an 11-year-old Arabian stallion. **A**, Preoperative intraoral radiograph of a fracture involving the base of the incisor teeth. **B**, The technique shown in Fig. 103-2, *C* was applied. Note the worn-down incisor teeth because of continuous crib biting. **C,** Postoperative intraoral radiograph of the fixation. Because the corner incisors were involved in the fracture as well, tension-band wiring was used. **D,** Four-month follow up intraoral radiograph after curetting of an abscess near the tooth roots. **E,** Seven-month follow-up at the time of wire removal. The fracture has healed and the infection has resolved.

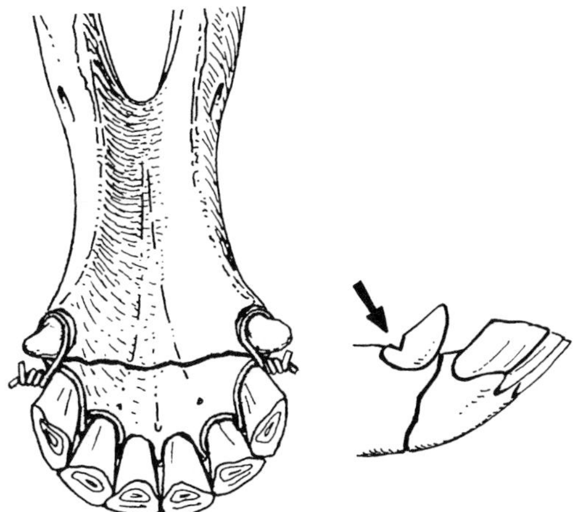

Figure 103-4. Tension-band wiring of incisors to the canine teeth used to repair a fracture involving the incisors. Note that an indentation *(arrow)* was created into the nuchal aspect of the canine teeth with a rasp to anchor the wire.

difficult to wire one cheek tooth to another one with the limited room to work in via an oral approach.

An alternative method of figure-eight wiring that does not use bone screws can be performed by anchoring the wire in the bone through holes drilled through the mandible on each side of the fracture (Fig. 103-7). The surgical approach is the same. A 2-mm drill bit is used to make a hole from a lateral to a medial direction through the mandible near the ventral border approximately 2 cm from the fracture. Figure-eight wiring is performed using the drill hole as an anchor site. This technique is adequate for young foals but not for adult horses with fractures of the interdental space.

TENSION-BAND WIRING TO THE CHEEK TEETH

Fractures of the diastema of the mandible are good candidates for repair with intraoral wiring. Unilateral fractures can be realigned and stabilized with a wire placed around the second premolar and secured to the incisors.

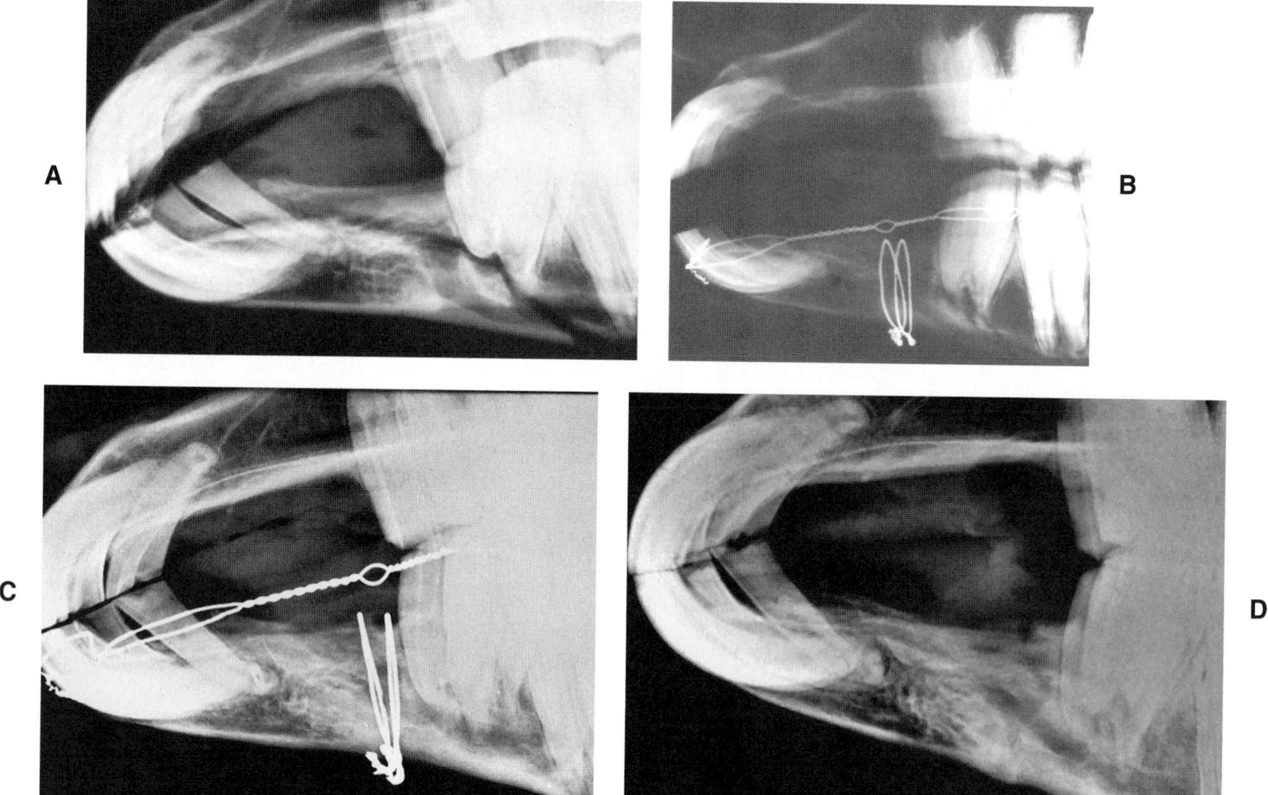

Figure 103-5. A, Preoperative radiograph of a long oblique fracture through the interdental space in a Shetland pony. **B,** Immediate postoperative radiograph showing the two circular wire loops in place, protected by a tension-band wire. **C,** Three-month follow-up radiograph showing the healed fracture. **D,** Radiograph after implant removal.

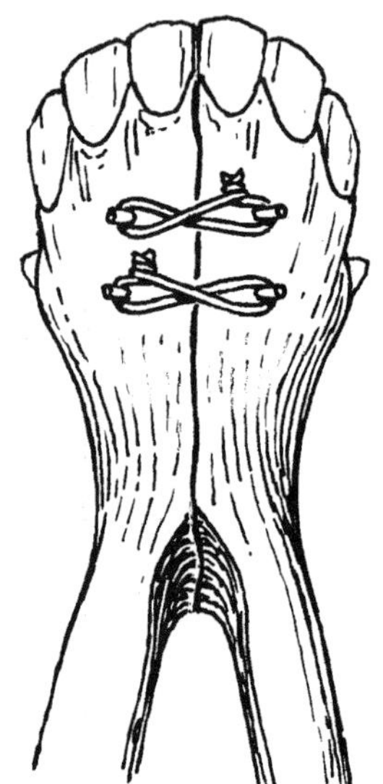

Figure 103-6. Hemicerclage fixation of a symphysis fracture. Two pins are placed across the symphysis. Figure-eight wires are placed around the protruding ends and solidly tightened to effectively stabilize the fracture. This type of fixation may also be applied to other locations.

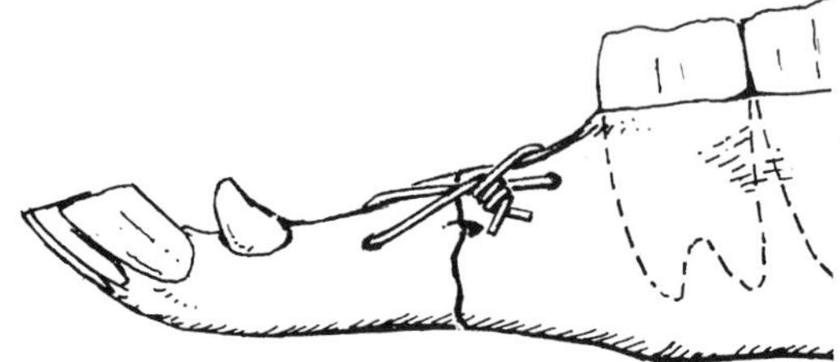

Figure 103-7. Figure-eight wiring of a vertical fracture of the mandible through the interdental space. The holes are created with a 2.5-mm drill bit or a Steinmann pin.

Under general anesthesia, the horse is placed in lateral recumbency on the surgery table with the fractured side toward the surgeon. With the help of hypodermic needles, the interdental space at the gingival level between 306 and 307 or 406 and 407 (see Chapter 30) is identified. Occasionally, the interdental space farther back is also used. Digital palpation facilitates identification as well.

Once the space is identified, a stab incision is made through the cheek. A 2.5-mm-diameter drill sleeve is introduced through the stab incision and placed over the interdental space, and a 2.5-mm hole is created between the teeth at the level of the gingiva (Fig. 103-8). A 1.25-mm diameter stainless steel wire is threaded through the cheek and the hole that was drilled between the teeth. Both ends of the wire are pulled into the mouth and drawn rostrally out of the mouth. The wire is crossed and looped around the intermediate and corner incisors by threading the wire between the teeth through a 14-gauge needle. The wire is twisted in the interdental space (Fig. 103-9). This results in a satisfactory repair because the wires compress the fractured

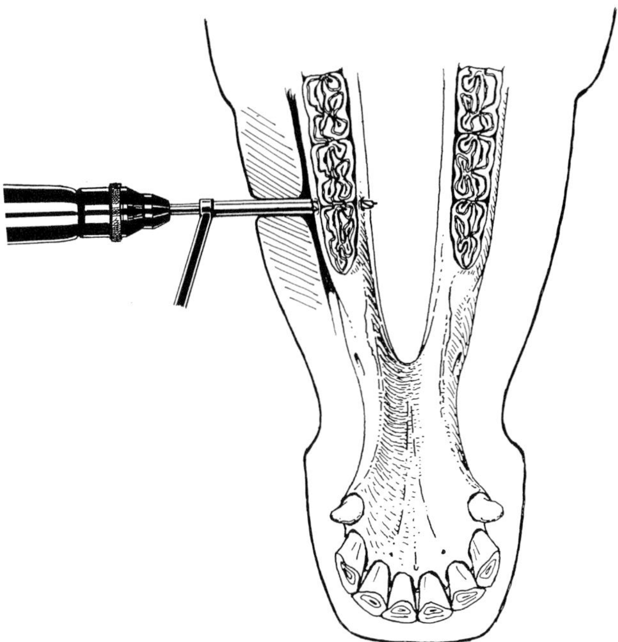

Figure 103-8. The drill guide is used to protect the cheek and gingiva as a drill bit creates a hole for passing the wire between the cheek teeth at the gum line. The wire is used to form a tension band across the interdental space.

bone ends, resulting in stability. Additional stability is provided by the contralateral intact hemi-mandible. Tension band wiring to the premolars may be performed bilaterally, if indicated.

Bilateral fractures are often comminuted. With comminution of the bone, tension-band wiring can collapse the fracture fragments and result in imperfect reduction. In these cases, additional support is required and can be provided by the methods described next.

ACRYLIC REINFORCEMENT OF INTRAORAL WIRING

In comminuted fractures, where wiring causes collapse of the mandible, some method of buttressing the bone is required to maintain its length. The simplest method uses acrylic reinforcement of the wires.

After the wires are placed, an intraoral splint is made by molding acrylic around the interdental wires and contouring it to fit the mouth (Fig. 103-10). The acrylic conforms to either the roof or floor of the mouth from the caudal surface of the incisors to 306 or 406. The acrylic serves as a buttress to maintain length and alignment. Additional wires are placed across the soft acrylic through drill holes in the bone and are tightened when the acrylic has set.

The surgeon should ensure that the acrylic splint is as form-fitting as possible and uses the least amount of material to serve the desired purpose. Excessive acrylic material in

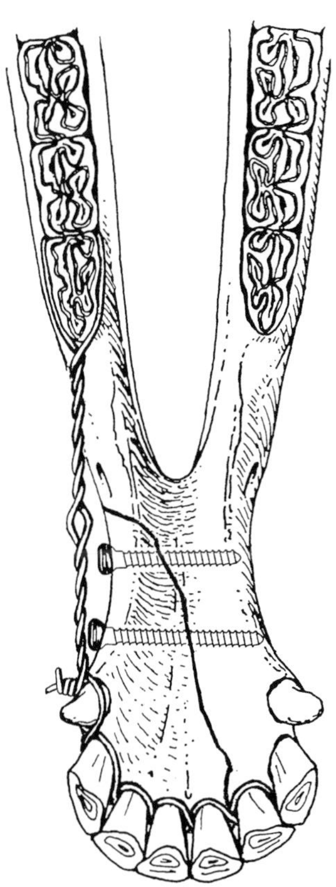

Figure 103-9. Lag screw repair of a unilateral fracture of the mandible containing a large osseous fragment. The fixation is protected with tension-band wiring of the incisors to the first cheek tooth.

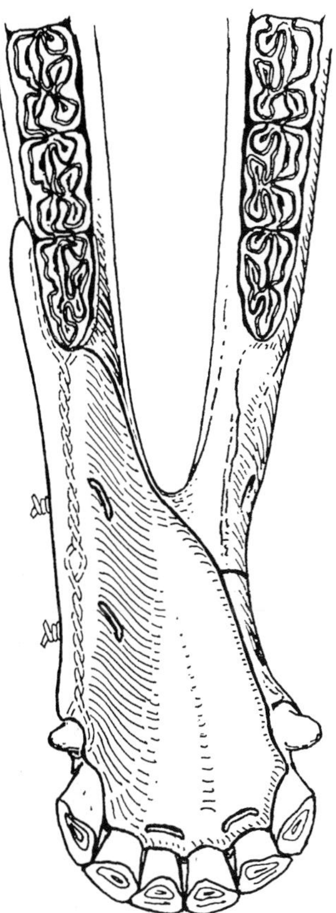

Figure 103-10. Intraoral splinting with dental acrylic (cold-curing type) formed around a tension-band wire between incisors and the first cheek tooth. Several additional wires are used to unite the splint with the mandible.

the mouth impedes eating by interfering with the horse's tongue. Ideally, dental acrylic should be used, because it sets with no appreciable exothermic reaction.

A more precise fit of methyl methacrylate to the oral surface can be obtained by molding methyl methacrylate to the mouth as well as possible and allowing it to harden. The methyl methacrylate is removed after it has cured, and the shaping is finished with a rasp or dermal tool to remove excess material and round any sharp edges. After smoothing, holes are drilled in the splint for wiring to the mandible, premolars, and incisors as necessary. Wiring configurations vary with the individual fractures.[7,8]

U-Bar Brace

Bilateral fractures almost always require support in the form of an intraoral brace or external fixator in addition to tension band wiring to maintain axial alignment, limit side-to-side mobility, and prevent collapse[2] (Fig. 103-11).

An intraoral splint is made from malleable brass or aluminum rods.[9,10] The pre-bent U-shaped brace is placed on the buccal surface of the incisors and spans the interdental space and the entire length of the dental arcade bilaterally. The brace is adaptable to fixation of fractures of the mandible, incisive bone, and premaxilla. The brace bar is fixed to the incisors and cheek teeth in multiple sites by cerclage wires encircling the teeth and bar. Wiring to the incisors is accomplished using individual cerclage wires, each encircling an incisor and the brace. Wiring to the cheek teeth is accomplished via stab incisions through the cheek and drilling between the teeth at the gum line.

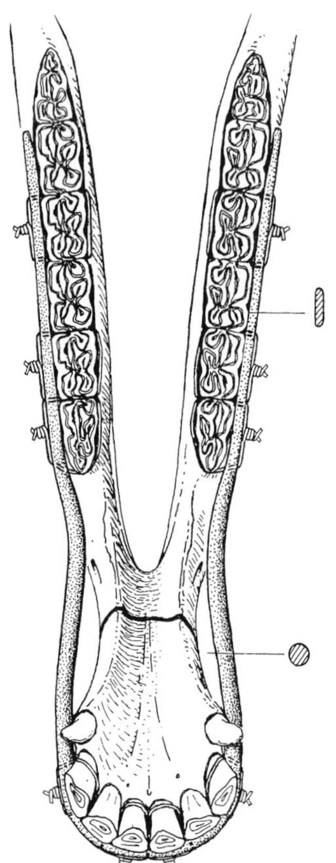

Figure 103-11. Intraoral splint made from an aluminum bar and molded around the contours of the mandible. The bar has a round cross-section in front and a flattened cross-section on each side. The aluminum bar is attached to selected teeth with cerclage wires.

This splint is very stable but is quite time consuming to apply (Fig. 103-12). The splint can be aided by application of tension-band wiring as previously described.

Intramedullary Pins

Intramedullary pins can, in selected cases, be a useful adjunct in the repair of mandibular fractures.[11] Indications for intramedullary pinning are rare, because pin placement options are limited by the tooth roots. Intramedullary pins provide axial alignment, and protruding pin ends can serve as fixation points for wires. When used alone, intramedullary pins are likely to migrate.

Screws

Lag screw fixation is used to repair selected fractures of the mandible in the region of the diastema and symphysis.[5,12] Lag screw fixation is useful in this area, especially in adult horses, because the bone is strong enough for purchase of the screw threads, and the screws can be used under biomechanically favorable circumstances (see Fig. 103-9). Symphyseal fractures are, however, rare.

The fractures are reduced manually and held in reduction by pointed reduction forceps. A stab incision is made through the gingiva, and 3.5-mm, 4.5-mm, or 5.5-mm cortex screws are inserted in lag fashion across the fracture plane. At least two screws should be placed to provide rotational stability. Lag screw fixation is appropriate if the fracture configuration allows screw placement without damaging the teeth and there is adequate bone for purchase of the screws. Screws are not removed unless they become infected and are the source of persistent drainage.

A cortex screw may also be placed unicortically on each side of the fracture line such that the screw heads are used as an anchor for figure-eight wiring. This provides a simple, minimally invasive method for tension wiring of the body of the mandible. This method also poses little risk to the tooth roots when the screws are placed on the ventral cortex.

A 5- to 7-cm longitudinal incision is made directly over the fracture on the ventral surface of the mandible. The fracture is reduced, and a 4.5- or 5.5-mm cortex screw is placed approximately 2 cm from the fracture line. Figure-eight wiring is completed with 1.25-mm stainless steel wire looped under each screw head and twisted until tight. Cortex screws can be inserted on the lateral surface of the mandible if preoperative or intraoperative radiographs are used to plan screw placement.

External Fixators

External fixators are good options for repairing fractures of the ramus or body of the mandible, premaxilla, and maxilla.[13,14] Advantages of external fixators include closed repair, reduced risk of sepsis to the fracture plane, easy removal of implants, and good stability. Disadvantages are additional technical expertise and the expense of additional equipment, potential of traumatizing tooth roots, and

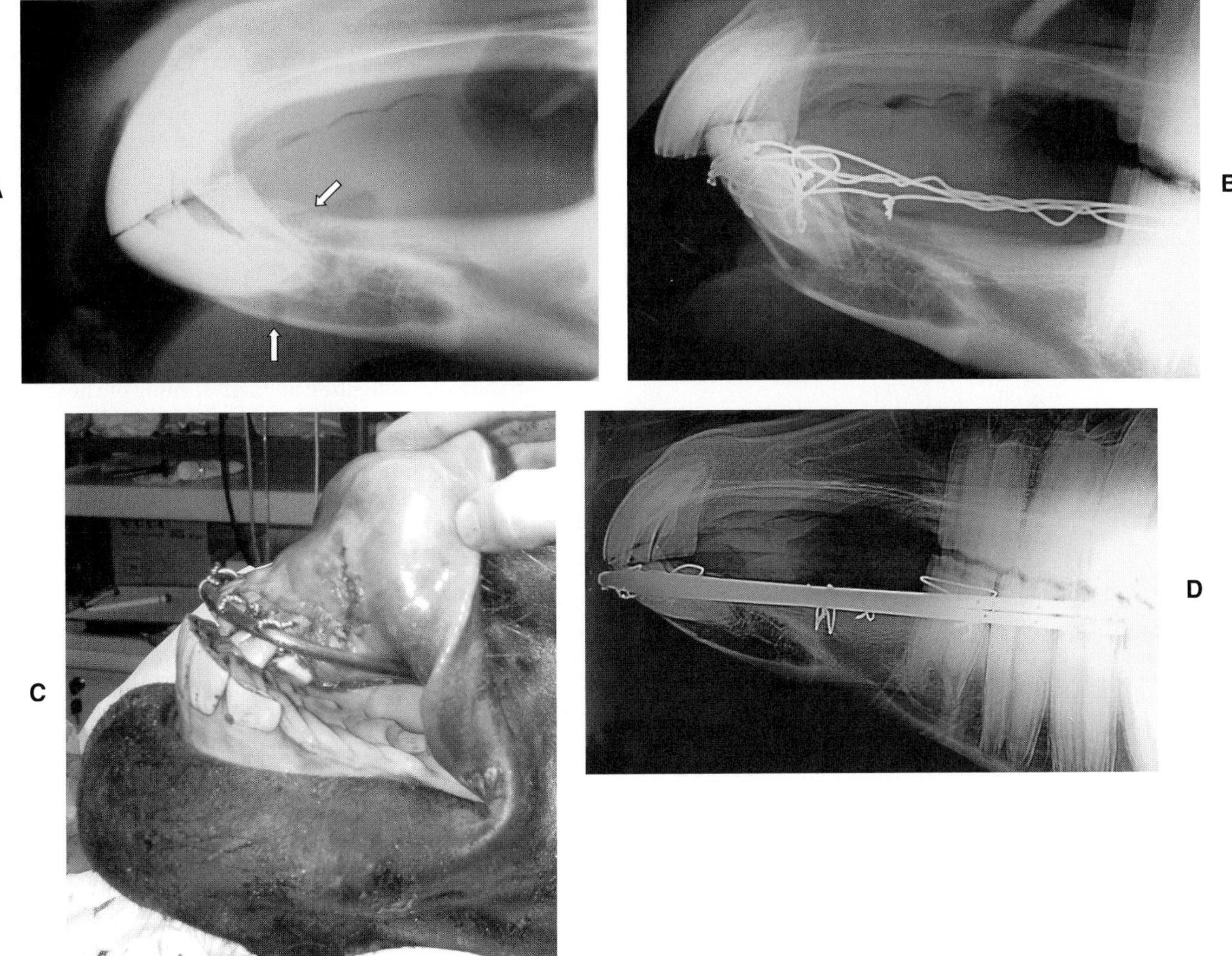

Figure 103-12. **A,** Preoperative lateromedial radiograph of a mandibular fracture. Good alignment is present and only slight disruptions at the cortex identify the fracture *(arrows)*. **B,** Postoperative lateromedial radiograph after intraoral and tension-band wiring. Note the marked caudal displacement and upward rotation of the fragment caused by tightening the wires. **C,** The wires were removed and an intraoral brace was applied to fix the fracture and maintain the length of the mandible. **D,** Lateromedial radiograph showing the brace in place.

frequent infection of pins associated with loosening. Intraoperative radiographic control is needed as well.

If a *type II* fixator is selected, each pin penetrates the medial and lateral cortex of both mandibles, and a connecting bar is placed on each side. Indications for a type II external fixator include bilateral fractures of the mandible or premaxilla or a highly unstable unilateral fracture (Fig. 103-13). Type II fixators are best applied with the horse in dorsal recumbency.

With *type I* external fixators, the pins engage both cortices of one side of the mandible. Indications would be a unilateral fracture of the horizontal ramus of the mandible. A type I fixator may be applied with the horse positioned in either lateral or dorsal recumbency. Ideally, at least two pins should be placed rostral and caudal to the fracture.

The usual pin size is 4 mm ($\frac{1}{8}$ inch) in diameter, and a 6-mm ($\frac{3}{16}$-inch) diameter connecting bar is used. In *type I* fixators, positive profile end-threaded pins are preferred to standard smooth pins because of their increased holding power in bone and decreased risk of pin loosening. In *type II* fixators, positive profile center-threaded pins are preferred. The pin holes should be predrilled before inserting the pins. Holes are drilled starting with a 2.5-mm hole and sequentially enlarging it ideally to a size 0.1 mm smaller than the pin size, which provides perfect axial preload to ensure solid fixation within the bone.[15] This type of drilling should be accompanied by continuous flushing of the drill bit to reduce heat production, which will prevent premature pin loosening caused by thermal necrosis of bone. High-torque, low-speed drills or hand drills are preferred to minimize thermal damage.

Steinmann pins are inserted through both cortices of both mandibles via stab incisions in the skin. Radiographic assistance is used to place the pins either ventral to, or between, tooth roots. Pin placement perpendicular to the sagittal plane prevents the pin from angling in either a rostral or caudal direction and damaging a tooth on the opposite mandible. All pins should be inserted in the same

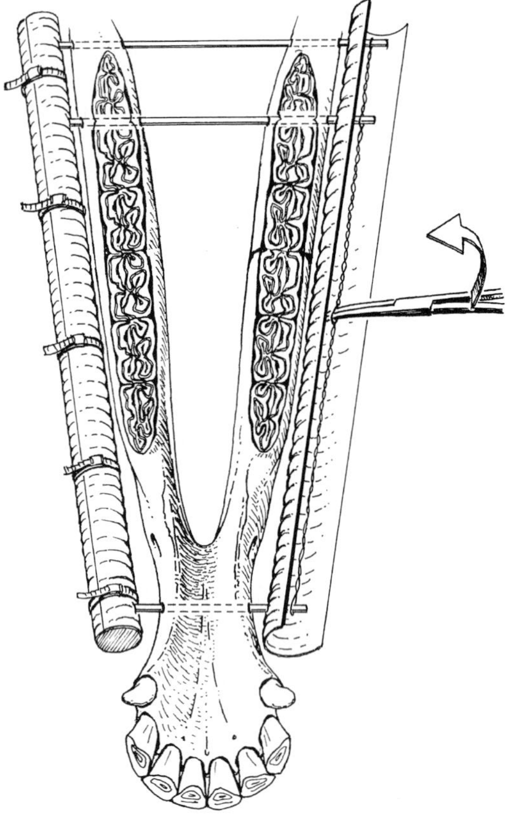

Figure 103-13. Type II external fixator is placed across both rami of the mandible. A tension-band wire is applied around the pins and tightened to achieve interfragmentary compression of the fracture. The previously open soft tubes are closed with parm bands, and the lumen is filled with epoxy material (e.g., polymethylmethacrylate, hoof acrylic).

horizontal plane to facilitate placement of the connecting clamps and rod.

An alternative technique that allows more variation in pin placement and is more forgiving of imperfect pin placement is to use an *acrylic side bar.* This obviates the need for all pins to be in the same plane. An acrylic side bar can be constructed with a piece of flexible rubber hose (25 mm inside diameter). The hose is skewered by the pins. The ends of the hose are occluded, and the lumen is filled with liquid polymethylmethacrylate, which is allowed to harden. An acrylic side bar can be molded to fit closer to the horse's head, which decreases the likelihood of inadvertently catching the fixator on objects in the stall. However, an acrylic side bar cannot be adjusted should the need arise.

A variation of this method involves opening the hose over the whole length (see Fig. 103-13). Wire is subsequently looped around the pins and tightened the same way as described for tension wiring of the teeth. This compresses the fracture, resulting in greater stability. The hose is then closed with parm bands, and the hose is filled with acrylic, as described earlier.

PINLESS EXTERNAL FIXATOR

A pinless external fixator attaches to the mandible via clamps instead of conventional transcortical pins (Fig. 103-14). This technique offers the advantage of a type I external fixator without the risk of damaging the tooth roots with pin placement. Clamps are made in a symmetric configuration with trocar-type points for attaching to the mandibular symphysis and an asymmetric clamp configuration with one trocar point and another bifurcated tip for fastening to the body of the mandible. Stab incisions are made in the soft tissues, and the tips of the bone clamp are embedded in

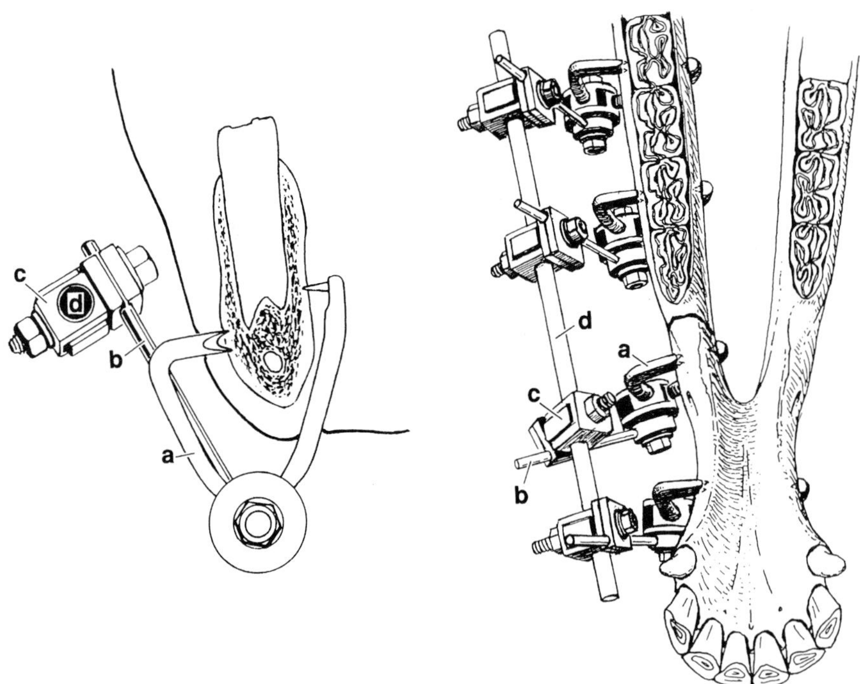

Figure 103-14. Pinless external fixator applied to a mandibular fracture. a, asymmetric clamp attached to the ramus; b, small adjustable connecting rod; c, single external fixator clamp; d, tubular connecting bar, which fits into the clamp [c].)

the mandibular cortex by an applicator instrument. Clamp placement avoids soft tissue structures and tooth roots because the clamps attach only to the cortex. Connector rods, clamps, and a rigid side bar complete the type I external fixator configuration.

Use of the pinless external fixator has been described in the horse and in adult cattle.[5,16] It may be applied to add stability to a fracture treated with wires and/or a bone plate during the initial postoperative period (Fig. 103-15). The benefits of this device include lack of pin tract infections, avoidance of traumatizing tooth roots, and flexibility for selecting the application point. One disadvantage is the increased cost; however, these clamps can be reused several times, partially offsetting the purchase costs.

With either method of external fixation, daily pin tract care is required to prevent soft tissue infection. The pin–skin interface should be cleaned as necessary and antibiotic ointment and a bandage should be applied.

External fixators can inadvertently catch on objects in the horse's environment. This problem is minimized by fitting the fixator as close to the horse as possible, wrapping the fixator to cover areas prone to snagging, and stabling the horse in an area free of projections.

Plates

Bone plates are used for repair of fractures of the ramus and body of the mandible.[3,5,17] Plating has several disadvantages that limit its usefulness for repair of fractures of the horizontal ramus of the mandible. Plates must be placed on the ventrolateral or lateral surface of the mandible. Exposure of the ventrolateral mandible is complicated by the presence of the parotid salivary duct. Screw placement is difficult because of the tooth roots. There is little soft tissue to cover the plates on the ventrolateral aspect of the mandible. Also, most fractures of the mandible are open, communicate with

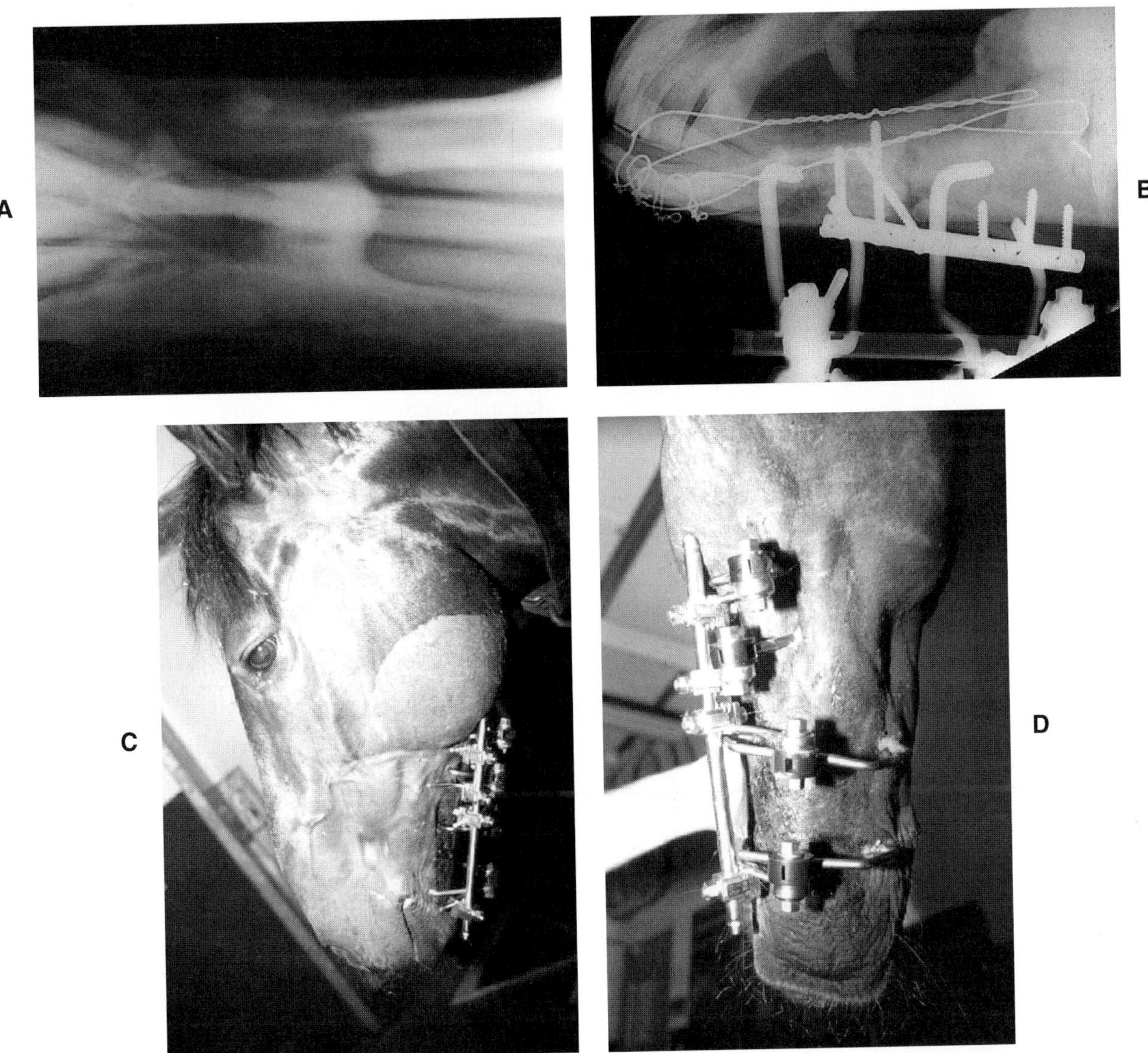

Figure 103-15. A, Ventrodorsal radiograph of a unilateral fracture of the horizontal ramus of the mandible with displacement. **B,** Postoperative oblique radiograph showing the plate implanted across the fracture supported by a tension-band wire. Additionally, a pinless external fixator was used to provide additional support during the initial postoperative period. **C,** Lateral, and **D,** ventrodorsal views of the head with the pinless external fixator applied.

the oral cavity, and result in contamination of the implants, which necessitates their eventual removal.

Nevertheless, there are indications for bone plates. Fractures of the horizontal ramus of the mandible involving the caudal cheek teeth and body of the mandible are difficult to repair with intraoral wiring procedures because of limited exposure. Severely comminuted fractures might benefit from bone plates used in buttress fashion. Broad or narrow 3.5-mm limited-contact dynamic compression plates (LC-DCPs) or reconstruction plates or 4.5-mm LC-DCPs with at least three screws on each side of the fracture are desirable. In selected cases, long plates are used and screws are inserted in selected holes along the plate.

Compression plating is an option for fractures of the *horizontal* ramus of the mandible in the interdental space (Fig. 103-16). Locking compression plates (LCPs) can improve stability of the fixation when used farther caudad (Fig. 103-17). However, the most appropriate indication for the use of bone plates is closed fractures of the body and *vertical* ramus of the mandible. Horses demonstrate less pain and return to feed quicker when these fractures are stabilized. These fractures are usually closed and have adequate soft tissue covering. The tooth roots do not pose an obstacle to screw placement in this area

A skin incision is made along the caudal edge of the mandible that parallels the caudal border of the mandible. In that location, the masseter muscle can be avoided and there is abundant bone to allow solid insertion of the screws. The lateral aspect of the vertical ramus is extremely thin and does not accept 4.5-mm screws. Smaller screws may be used, but the implants are not strong enough to withstand the cyclic loading occurring during chewing food. Additionally, the facial nerve and the transverse facial artery and vein are located superficially on the lateral aspect of the ramus.

A large periosteal elevator is used to expose the caudal rim of the vertical ramus.[18] A plate spanning the fracture and providing three to five screw holes on either side is selected (Fig. 103-18). Selecting a longer plate allows the surgeon to choose which plate holes to use. In selected cases, wire sutures may be used to appose fracture lines on the lateral surface of the ramus through small incisions (see Fig. 103-18). The plate is contoured to the surface of the bone and applied using routine technique. The subcutaneous tissues and skin are reapposed over the plate, with sutures in two separate layers.

A study has compared dynamic compression plate (DCP) fixation of an osteotomy in the diastema of the mandible with a fixation using an external fixator and interdental wiring and an intraoral splint and interdental wiring. This study revealed that DCP fixation had the greatest stiffness under monotonic bending to failure; however, the relatively low yield value might predispose it to earlier failure in fatigue testing without supplemental fixation.[19] The techniques using tension-band wiring in conjunction with an external fixator or an intraoral splint were similar to DCP constructs in yield, failure, and osteotomy displacement, whereas the external fixator constructs alone were biomechanically inferior to all others.

DCP fixation is therefore most likely the most stable form of fixation for comminuted fractures of interdental spaces.[19] However, for simple interdental space fractures, intraoral splinting together with interdental wire fixation should provide adequate stability with minimal invasiveness and decreased expense. Tension-band wiring significantly enhances the strength of type II external skeletal fixators and should be used to augment mandibular fracture repairs.[19]

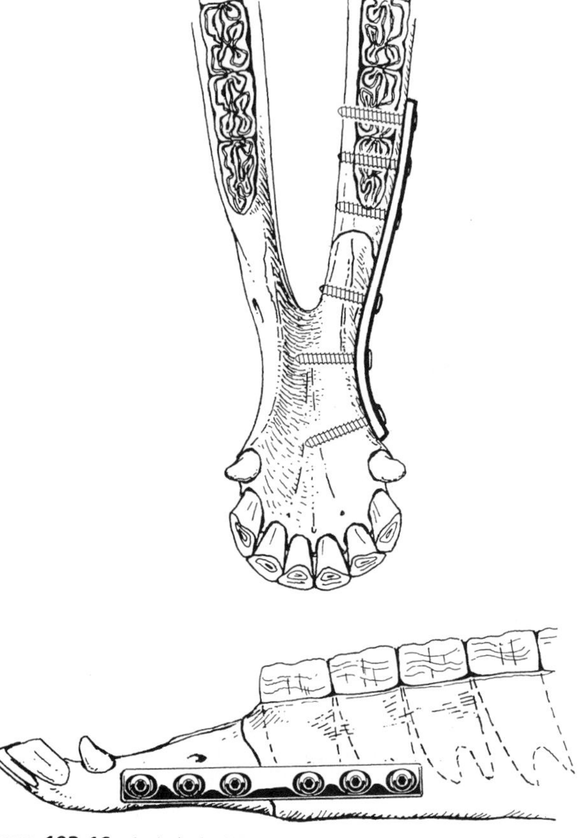

Figure 103-16. A six-hole 4.5-mm narrow dynamic compression plate is applied to the horizontal ramus of the mandible. The screws are inserted between the tooth roots.

Aftercare

Horses seldom demonstrate a reluctance to eat after fractures are stabilized, and they are quickly returned to routine feeding. The incisors are used only in prehension of food materials, and mastication is performed by the cheek teeth.[2] No attempt to modify the diet is made following repair of incisor fractures. Fractures involving the cheek teeth could give the horse more difficulty during mastication.

Horses should be provided a palatable diet that can be easily chewed. They usually prefer customary foodstuffs to the gruels and mashes sometimes recommended during convalescence. Therefore, there is little need to modify the diet unless there is a clear indication that the horse is having difficulty in masticating.

All foodstuffs tend to accumulate around the intraoral wires, rods, and acrylic. Frequent garden hose lavage of the mouth to remove accumulated debris is beneficial if the horse will tolerate it.

Phenylbutazone is routinely administered at 4.4 mg/kg by mouth for 7 days. The decision to administer antibiotics

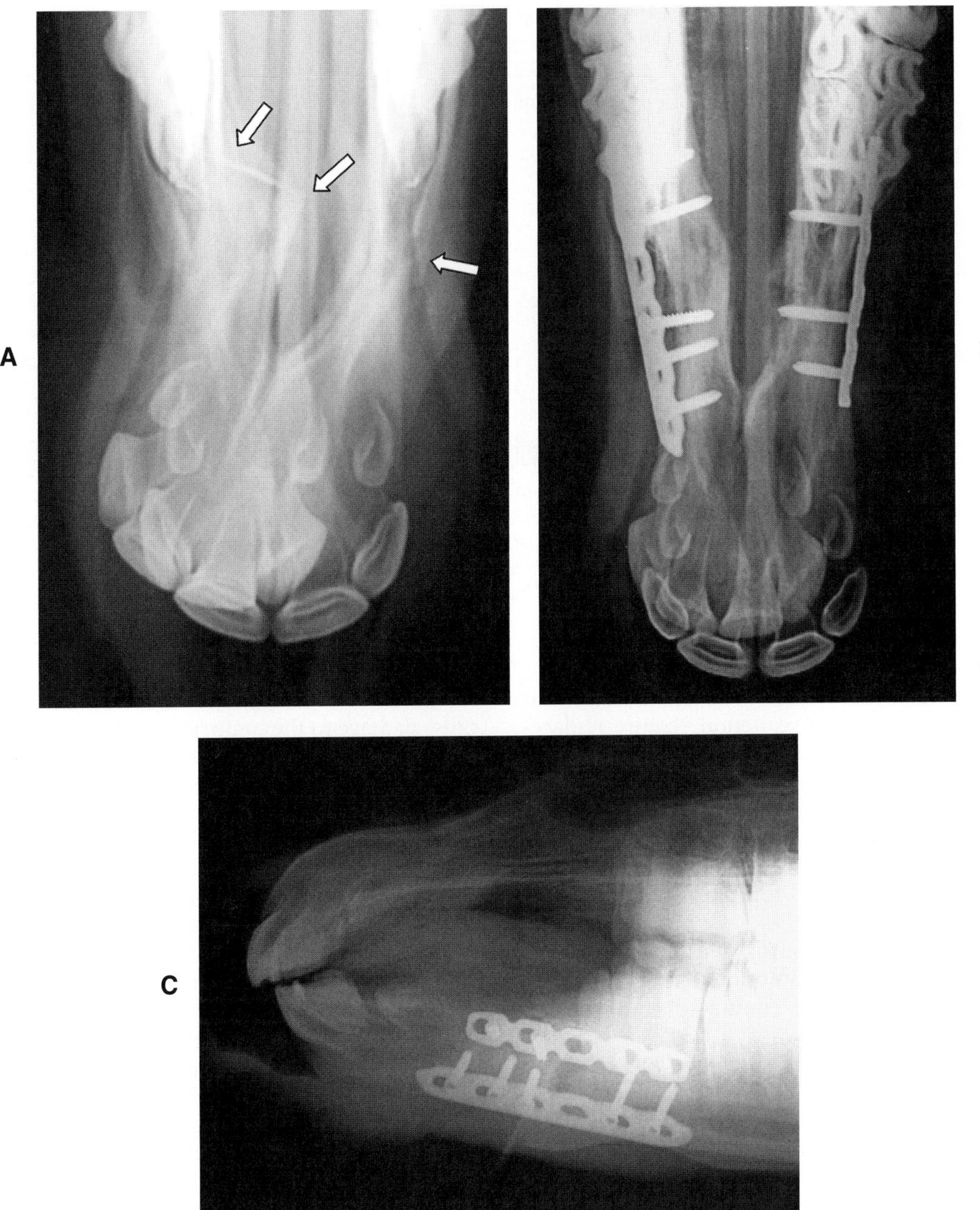

Figure 103-17. A, Ventrodorsal radiograph showing the mandible in a foal after it was kicked in the jaw 3 weeks earlier. Two fractures with marked medial displacement *(two arrows)* are shown in the left hemimandible with an additional fracture in the right *(one arrow)*. The fracture caused the rostral mandible to deviate to the left. **B,** Ventrodorsal, and **C,** lateromedial postoperative radiographs. The bone had partially healed and was refractured and repaired with a four-hole 3.5 locking compression plate (LCP) and a five-hole 3.5-mm reconstruction LCP. Note the slight caudal displacement of the mandible. The fixation healed without complications, and the implants were removed 5 weeks later.

is made on an individual basis. Most fractures are open and contaminated and benefit from administration of broad-spectrum antimicrobial agents.

Removal of the implant is usually carried out on the standing patient after healing has occurred, usually in 6 to 8 weeks. Bone plates and buried cerclage wires are not customarily removed unless the implants become infected.

Complications

Implants should be inspected regularly because wires loosen and break. Loose wires may be tightened by additional twisting. Undetected loosening of implants can result in malocclusion and delayed healing because of instability. The decision to replace broken implants should be based on the timing of implant failure. The wires can be removed if

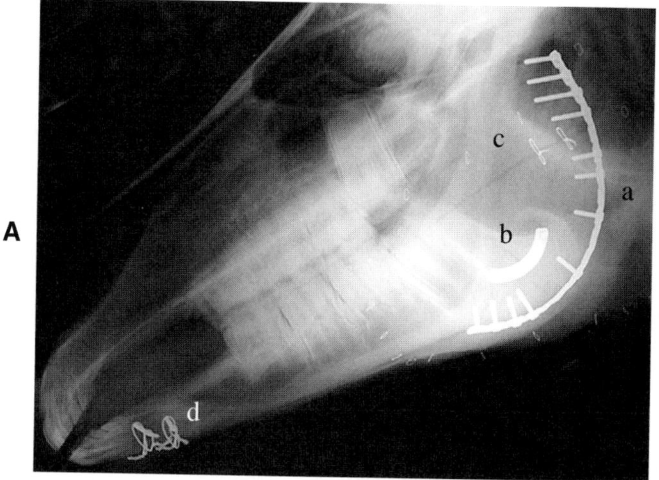

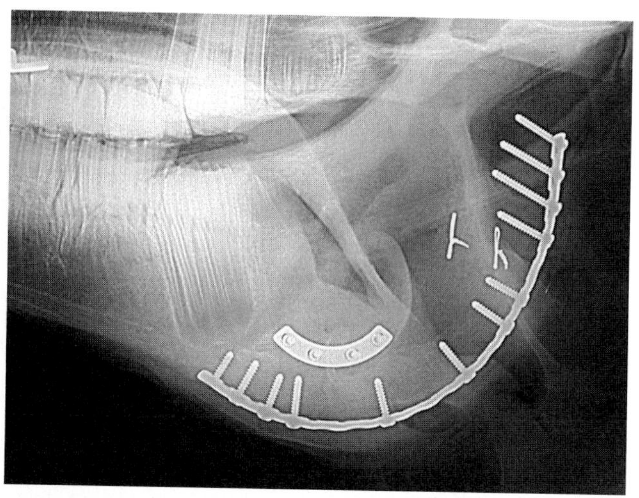

Figure 103-18. A, Immediate postoperative lateromedial radiograph of the same foal as in Figure 103-1. The fractures were repaired with different implants. a, A narrow 3.5-mm reconstruction plate was applied to the caudal edge of the ramus with 12 3.5-mm cortex screws placed in selected holes. At each end, four screws were placed. b, To provide additional stability to the triangular fragment, a four-hole small-animal 3.5-mm acetabular plate was implanted. c, The horizontal fracture was supported with two wire sutures. d, the fracture of the symphysis was repaired with two hemicerclage constructs. **B,** Four-month follow-up radiographs before implant removal. All fractures have healed.

the fracture is stable at the time of breakage. Failures that occur earlier in the postoperative period require replacement to maintain alignment and stability.

Drainage from the fracture is common following repair of open fractures, because infection is always present after exposure to the oral cavity. In most cases, the infection resolves with systemic antimicrobial agents and effective drainage. Drainage that persists for more than 4 weeks should be investigated.

With closed repair of comminuted fractures, small fragments of avascular bone commonly become sequestra. Radiographs should be taken to confirm the presence of sequestra if drainage persists. In many cases, the sequestra can be removed by curettage in the standing patient if the fragments are superficial.

Callus formation is to be expected with secondary bone healing of infected fractures and is more prominent with fractures that occur in the horizontal ramus of the mandible, because there is less soft tissue coverage. Factors that increase callus formation are comminution, infection, and instability in the repair. Efforts to attenuate these factors are rewarded with a more cosmetic outcome.

Prognosis

The prognosis for a serviceable outcome is favorable in most cases. Imperfect reduction of fractures leads to malocclusion. Fractures of the teeth themselves and fractures involving the alveolus sometimes result in tooth loss. Tooth loss (when it occurs) and irregular tooth wear because of malocclusion are managed effectively by regular dental care.

FRACTURES OF THE SKULL AND SINUSES

Fractures of the skull and sinuses are the result of blunt trauma from being kicked or from collisions. The most commonly injured bones include the nasal, frontal, and maxillary bones and the zygomatic process of the frontal bone. The trauma that causes fractures to these bones can cause damage to the brain, eye, and nasal passages, resulting in severe hemorrhage.[2] Depression fractures are often found.

Diagnosis

Initially, a minimally displaced depression fracture can be difficult to detect on physical examination because of the soft tissue swelling that obscures the depression. Other signs include obvious bone displacement, epistaxis, and skin lacerations. Emphysema can be palpated in the soft tissues as crepitus when fractures communicate with the nasal passages or sinuses. Radiographs with multiple oblique views are necessary to demonstrate the fracture. Computed tomography aids greatly with the final diagnosis and preoperative planning of the repair. Physical examination should include endoscopic examination of the upper airways as well as neurologic and ocular examinations to assess for additional undetected trauma.

Treatment

Initial therapy should be directed toward stabilizing the patient (see Chapter 8), because in most cases there is no urgency in the repair.[2] In fact, fracture repair is often difficult if significant soft tissue swelling has developed, and therefore repair is best delayed until swelling resolves. Skin lacerations should be repaired immediately to prevent infection to the soft tissues, even if fracture repair is delayed. Hyperosmotic wound dressings applied under pressure wraps will dissipate the edema.[2] Phenylbutazone is administered to decrease inflammation, and antimicrobial therapy is indicated for any open fractures or fractures that communicate with the sinuses. Tetanus prophylaxis is indicated in all cases.

Trauma to the facial bones often results in hemorrhage into the sinuses, which shows up on a lateral radiograph as a fluid line within the sinus. Consideration should be given to standing sinus lavage for removal of accumulated blood, when present, to prevent empyema of the sinus. Lavage is performed via an ingress portal made with a 6-mm (3/16-inch) Steinmann pin inserted into the frontal sinus and polyionic fluid lavage with a pressurized fluid delivery system.

Repair should be performed as soon as the soft tissue swelling is resolved. Delay in repair beyond a few days can result in difficulty in achieving reduction. The goals of repair are to maintain a patent airway and nasolacrimal duct, prevent ocular damage, and obtain a cosmetic appearance. Cosmetic considerations are the main purpose of repairing fractures that do not impair other body systems.

The typical configuration is a segmental depression fracture. Often, the skin and periosteal attachments are intact. Even so, the fractures usually communicate with the nasal passages or sinuses and will be contaminated, so that infection of soft tissues and of implants could be a problem.[20] Therefore, the surgical approaches should be performed as minimally invasively as possible to visualize the fracture, achieve reduction, and apply the implants. Many fractures can be reduced through stab incisions with no stabilization beyond that provided by the soft tissue attachments.[2]

Adequate reduction can often be achieved by elevating the fragments and wedging them back into place.[21] Whenever possible, closed reduction should be performed. The soft tissue attachments provide vascularity and the means for stabilizing the fractures once they are reduced. Adequacy of fracture reduction can be ascertained by direct inspection or evaluation of the facial contour; this is the reason for allowing the soft tissue swelling to resolve before attempting any repair.[2] The depressed fragments can be elevated by drilling holes in the bone and inserting an elevator to pry the fragment back into place.[22] A disadvantage of this approach is that commercially made elevators typically have a broad, flattened shaft that requires large drill holes to insert into the bone.

A better way to elevate the fracture fragment involves drilling a hole into the depressed segment with either a 3.5-mm drill bit or a Steinmann pin on a Jacob chuck. A 4-mm (1/8-inch) diameter Steinmann pin can be bent and inserted into the hole to elevate and wedge the fragment back into place. The end of the pin is bent at a right angle so that when the pin is inserted into the hole drilled in the fracture segment it has a broad area of contact and added leverage for elevating the fragment (Fig. 103-19). The length of the bent end should approximately match the width of the depressed bone segment. Another right angle bend is made in the opposite end of the pin to make a handle.[2] Axial traction is applied to pull the fragment back into place.

The skin over the drill holes is closed with a single suture. If necessary, multiple drill holes can be made with little or no disruption of the soft tissue attachments. In most cases the fragments can be wedged into place with no additional stabilization required because the fractures are not load bearing. If the fractures do require stabilization to maintain reduction, wire sutures can be applied in selected locations around the fragment. A small skin incision is made to expose the fracture line. A Steinmann pin (1.6 mm) and hand chuck or 2-mm drill bit is used to pre-drill holes for 0.8- to 1.0-mm cerclage wire sutures (see Fig. 103-19). Skin closure is routine.

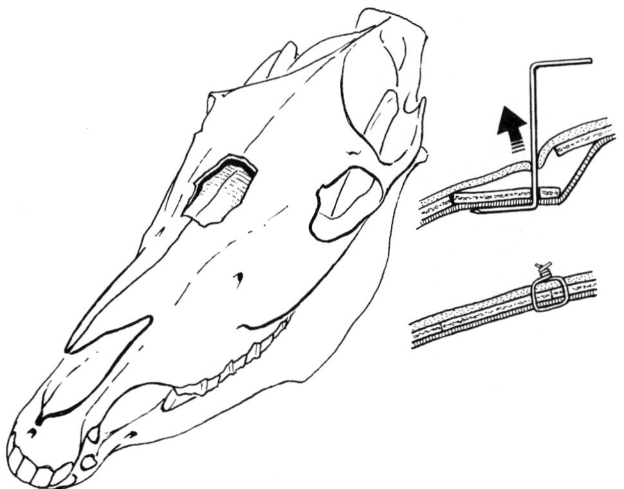

Figure 103-19. Insertion of a Steinmann pin through a small drill hole for elevation of a depressed bone fragment. If necessary, the fragment can be fixed with cerclage wire.

Occasional indications for the use of reconstruction plates arise with severely comminuted or unstable fractures. These plates are made in a variety of shapes and sizes and are easily contoured to fit specific fracture configurations.

Aftercare

Postoperatively, a pressure bandage is applied, and phenylbutazone is administered to decrease postoperative swelling and discomfort. Broad-spectrum antimicrobial agents are administered as necessary to treat soft tissue and sinus infections and prevent implant infections.

Complications

Inadequate reduction results in an inferior cosmetic outcome. Secondary bone healing results in callus formation, which causes an obvious blemish when it occurs over areas with no muscle. This is, however, only of temporary duration, because once the fracture is healed remodeling of the callus occurs, normalizing the contours of the skull. Hemorrhage into the paranasal sinuses can develop into a sinus empyema if untreated. Stenosis of the nasal passages can occur with severe injuries; however, this is rare. If the fragment is denuded of its blood supply through a loss of the periosteum, sequestration can occur, but it is less frequent than with mandible fractures.

When a sunken appearance is evident after healing because of inadequate reduction of depressed fragments or in cases that were left untreated (Fig. 103-20), refracture and proper alignment is not easily accomplished. The facial contour can be restored by implantation of prostheses of either a silicone or a fluorocarbon polymer and carbon fiber combination.[23,24] General anesthesia and strict asepsis are required.

With either technique, a slightly curved incision is made over the defect to expose the sunken bone. The implant material is sculpted to fill the defect and restore the normal facial contour. The silicone prosthetic material is sutured in place between the periosteum and the skin. A subperiosteal

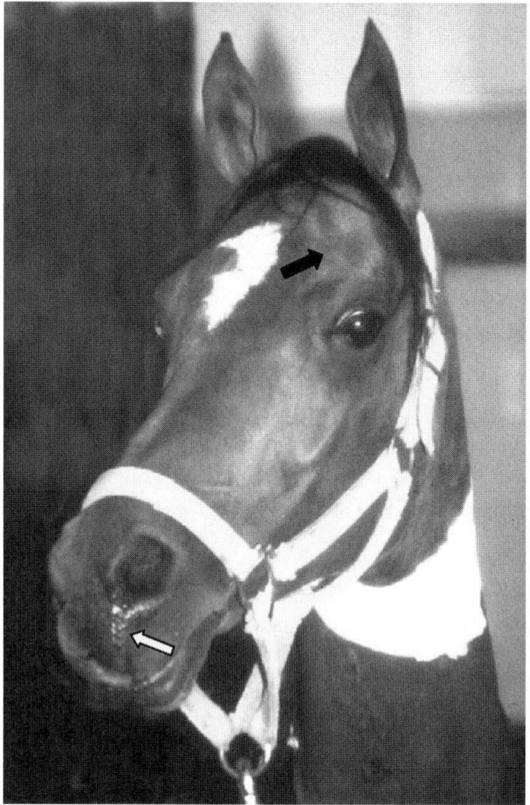

Figure 103-20. An Arabian horse with a depression fracture *(black arrow)*. There is some blood at the left nostril *(white arrow)*.

dissection is performed for insertion of the fluorocarbon polymer–carbon fiber prosthesis between the bone and periosteum. Skin closure is routine.

Prognosis

The prognosis for return to previous level of performance is usually good. The cosmetic outcome depends on the reduction achieved at surgery and is usually acceptable and often excellent depending on the severity of the injury.

PERIORBITAL FRACTURES

Fractures of the orbit are common in horses. The orbit serves as a protective housing for the eye and associated adnexa.[2] The orbit consists of the lacrimal, frontal, and zygomatic processes of the frontal and temporal bones. Fractures are the result of direct trauma and are usually of the depression type. Concurrent injury can be sustained to the central nervous system, eye, lacrimal duct, other skull bones, and the paranasal sinuses. These structures warrant examination as part of the physical examination prior to repair.

Diagnosis

Diagnosis is made by physical examination. Abnormal facial contour, soft tissue swelling, crepitus, and hemorrhage are usually present.[2] Acute soft tissue swelling can obscure the fracture and make detection difficult by physical examination alone. Pain can preclude a thorough physical examination in the unsedated patient.

Radiographs are indicated to identify trauma to the orbit but are also useful to identify concurrent injury and problems such as fluid in the maxillary sinuses. Fractures of the zygomatic arch are visible on the appropriate views; however, trauma to other parts of the orbit are difficult to image on radiographs.[2] Oblique views at different, sometimes acute, angles are often necessary to highlight the fractures. Ultrasonography might allow diagnosis of fractures and of tissue injuries lying deeper in the orbit.

The extent of ocular trauma is variable and ranges from chemosis to rupture of the eye. A thorough ocular examination should be performed, including an assessment of the patency of the lacrimal duct when fractures of the lacrimal bone are present.

Treatment

Fractures will heal without surgery, but in most cases they are associated with a facial deformity. Surgical repair is indicated to relieve impingement to the eye. Injury to the eye is treated as circumstances warrant (see Chapter 63). Repair is best attempted as soon as the patient is stabilized. The goal of reconstruction is to relieve impingement on the globe and adnexa and restore the normal anatomic contours to achieve a cosmetic outcome.[2] There are no muscle attachments to the orbit, except the small palpebral muscles that are inconsequential to any repair undertaken. Fractures often need only to be realigned to heal properly.[20] It is important to palpate the inner surface of the orbit to identify and remove any bone fragments that can damage the eye. These fragments are very difficult to identify with radiographs.

Fractures of the orbit that involve the zygomatic, lacrimal, or frontal bones are usually depression fractures and may be treated by elevation of the fragments via drill holes in the depressed segment as described in the previous section.

Zygomatic process fractures may be reduced noninvasively by use of a bone hook.[21] The horse is prepared for surgery with the affected side up. A finger is inserted into the orbit in the conjunctival space to palpate the fracture and guide the placement of a bone hook onto the ventral surface of the displaced fragment. Dorsal traction is used to elevate and wedge the fragment back into anatomic alignment[21] (Fig. 103-21). Fractures of more than 48 hours' duration are more difficult to reduce.

Most fractures are sufficiently stable that no other form of fixation is required. Fractures that do not maintain alignment after reduction require some form of stabilization in addition to that provided by the soft tissue attachments. These fractures are usually comminuted or involve portions of the orbital rim other than the zygomatic arch. Open reduction and interfragmentary wiring is the easiest but not the strongest method to provide additional stability when needed.

An incision is made directly over the fragments to be wired. Holes are drilled into the bone with a 2-mm drill bit. Cerclage wire of 0.8-mm to 1.0-mm diameter is pre-placed and twisted to tighten.[25]

Reconstruction plates can be used to repair severely comminuted fractures of the zygomatic arch (see Fig. 63-11).

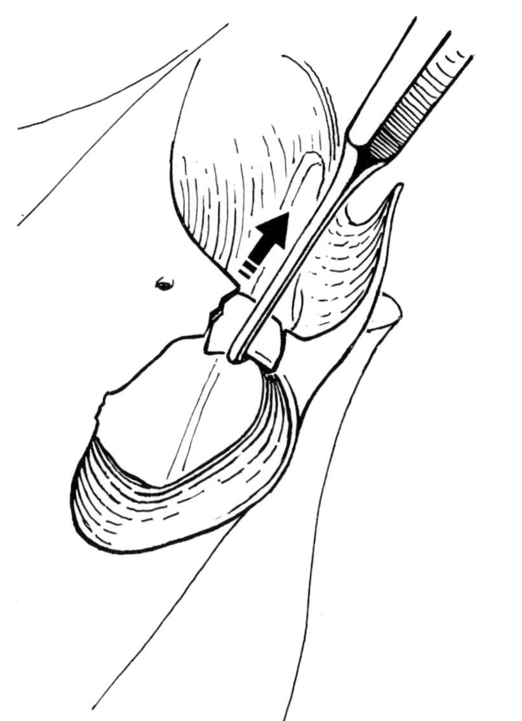

Figure 103-21. Use of a bone hook to reduce a depressed zygomatic arch fracture.

These plates have the advantage of being easily contoured. Bone plates should be reserved for cases in which easier methods will not achieve a satisfactory result.

Aftercare

Phenylbutazone is administered postoperatively to decrease discomfort and soft tissue swelling. Antimicrobial agents are not required if the fracture is reduced noninvasively. Systemic antibiotic agents should be administered if the fracture is open or communicates with the maxillary sinus, or if implants are used. Pressure bandages are not used because of the eye. Selection of any topical medication, if needed, should be based on safety of the substance for use in the eye.

Complications

Periorbital fractures are often associated with trauma to the eye. Rupture of the eye, proptosis, corneal ulceration and laceration, chemosis, and damage to the nasolacrimal duct are reported complications.[20,24] Empyema of the maxillary sinus can occur secondary to hemorrhage into the sinus.

Prognosis

Healing of the fractures usually proceeds uneventfully. The cosmetic appearance depends on the accuracy of surgical reduction and the amount of callus but is usually good. A prognosis for associated ocular trauma depends on the nature and severity of the injury.[2]

CRANIOFACIAL DEFECTS

Craniofacial defects can develop as a result of external trauma to the facial bones over the sinuses. If the fragments over a sinus are denuded of their blood supply, they can undergo necrosis, leading to the formation of sinus fistulas of various sizes[25] (Fig. 103-22). Rarely, congenital anomalies are also associated with bone defects in the skull.

Suturing skin over a bone defect in the skull usually results in failure of the repair. Underneath the skin flap is an air-filled cavity, which dehydrates the skin and results in necrosis. Periosteal[25] and occasionally muscle flaps[26] have been used to correct the problem. Periosteal flaps are dissected free from the area adjacent to the bone defect with a base at the edge of the bone defect. The vascularized periosteal flap is flipped over the bone defect and sutured to a similar flap taken from the opposite side (see Fig. 103-22, *B*). A cancellous bone graft or biodegradable bone cement is applied over the periosteum. To facilitate closure of the skin over the repaired defect, relief incisions or transportation flaps, or both, might have to be performed.

The surgery site should be protected from trauma during the recovery phase and the immediate postoperative period. Also, the animal should be kept from rubbing the area to prevent destroying the surgical repair. Drainage of the flaps should be aided through insertion of drains, with early removal once drainage has ceased. Anti-inflammatory drugs and antibiotics are indicated to control inflammation and prevent postoperative infection. Sutures should be removed 2 to 3 weeks postoperatively.

Complications include complete or partial breakdown of the repair, usually because of trauma, which can lead to disfigurement. Postoperative infection is always a risk because of the contaminated nature of the surgical site. Complications can require another surgical revision.

RESECTION OF THE ROSTRAL MANDIBLE, PREMAXILLA, AND MAXILLA

Ossifying fibromas of the rostral mandible are the most common indications for a rostral mandibulectomy[27] (Fig. 103-23, *A*). Other neoplasms, such as adamantinomas, and fungal and parasitic diseases can also be indications for the procedure. Inadequate local excision of these lesions results in a recurrence; therefore, block excision with wide non-affected margins is required. This procedure was developed in an attempt to completely excise the lesions in one surgical intervention.

Surgical Procedure

The animal is anesthetized and placed in dorsal recumbency on the surgery table. The endotracheal tube is placed either through the nasal passages or via a temporary tracheotomy, facilitating unimpeded access to the mouth. The oral cavity is washed, making sure that the cuff of the endotracheal tube is tight and prevents fluids from entering the lungs. The jaws are spread and maintained in that position by carefully placing a speculum between the cheek teeth. The dorsal aspect of the oral cavity and the upper lip is draped.

A transverse incision is made in the oral mucosa on the lingual side of the incisors. The gingiva is incised on the labial surface of the incisors ventral to the lesion, and this

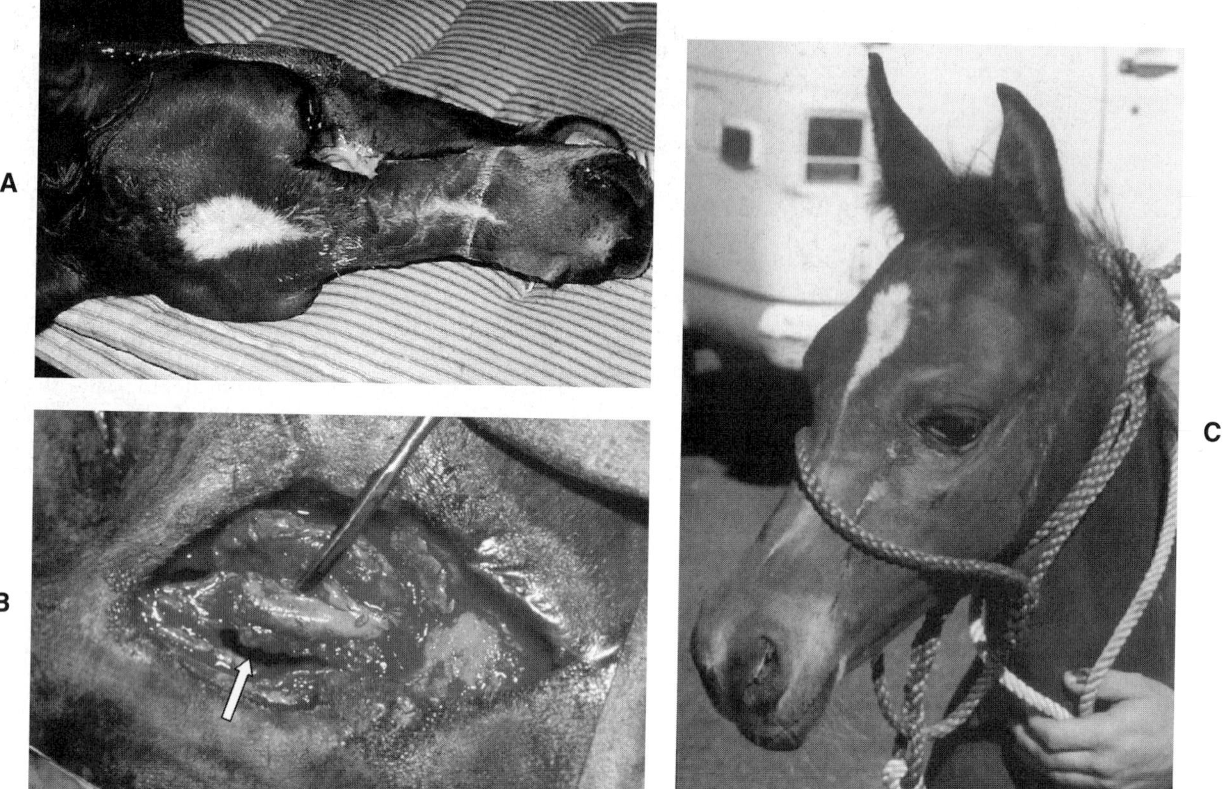

Figure 103-22. A, A 2-month-old foal with a sinus fistula just below the eye. The foal was kicked by a mare and subsequently sloughed a large bone sequestrum, which led to this fistula. **B,** Intraoperative picture showing the fistula *(arrow)* and the periosteal flap *(under the elevator)* that was sutured over the defect. A cancellous bone graft was placed over the flap (see Fig. 82-1). The skin was closed and healed without complication. **C,** Two-month follow-up of the foal with a cosmetically acceptable result.

incision is continued laterally and dorsally on both sides to connect with the initial incision. Both incisions are thus connected and continued down to the bone on the mandibular symphysis.

The soft tissues are elevated and reflected caudally with a periosteal elevator on the mandibular symphysis to expose normal bone. The soft tissues are preserved to allow coverage of the exposed mandibular stump.

The mandibulectomy procedure involves removing the incisive bone and as much of the symphysis of the mandible as needed, taking into account that part of the symphysis should be saved to ensure rostral continuity of the mandible. An oscillating bone saw or Gigli wire is used to transect the mandible at the selected level. After the bone edges are rounded off, the soft tissue on the lingual surface of the mandible is folded rostrally over the exposed mandible and trimmed to fit the mucosal flap from the labial surface (see Fig. 103-23, *B*). A Penrose drain is placed between the bone and the soft tissues.

Closure is performed to prevent the sutures from being subjected to trauma during mastication. An acceptable cosmetic appearance is retained as well as the ability to prehend feed despite significant shortening of the mandible (Fig. 103-24).

A similar procedure for excision of the premaxilla and maxilla caudal to the canine teeth has been described.[28]

Complications and Prognosis

For both procedures, a recurrence of the lesions can only be prevented by completely resecting them. The cosmetic outcome is acceptable to many owners.

Flaccidity of the lower lip may occur with rostral mandibular resection. Horses have no difficulty with prehension of hay and grain; however, they may have difficulty with prehension of short grass. Protrusion of the tongue may occur.[29]

WRY NOSE (CAMPYLORRHINUS LATERALIS)

This condition is present at birth and is assumed to be a congenital disorder. In Arabian horses it is possibly genetically linked, because of its frequency in this breed.[30] Intrauterine positioning as an etiology of this deformity is only a theory.

The foal is presented within the first few days to weeks after birth because of the cosmetic appearance. Clinically, a varying degree of premaxillar deviation is noticeable upon inspection of the foal's head; the deviation often results in malocclusion, with no contact between the incisors of the mandible and maxilla (Fig. 103-25). One side of maxilla or premaxilla is dysplastic, resulting in the lateral deviation toward this side. Often there is also a certain rotational component in the deviation. Close observation also reveals

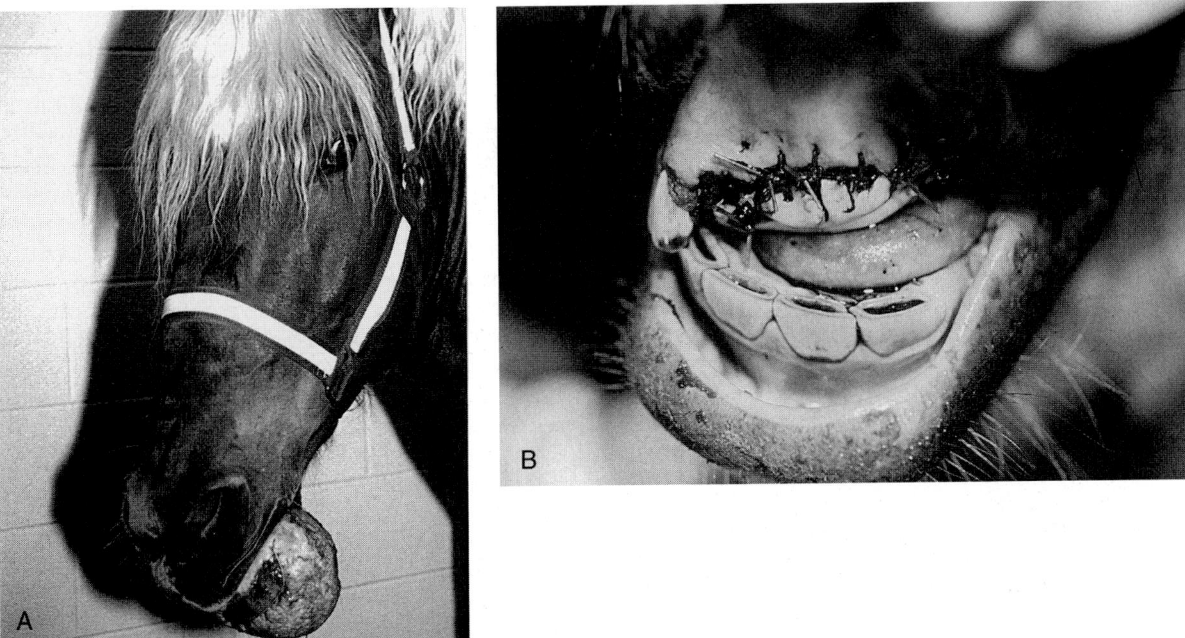

Figure 103-23. A, Preoperative picture of a 9-year-old Belgian horse with an ossifying fibroma of the mandible. **B,** Postoperative appearance after a partial rostral mandibulectomy. Note that the mucosa was sutured over the cut surfaces of the mandible.

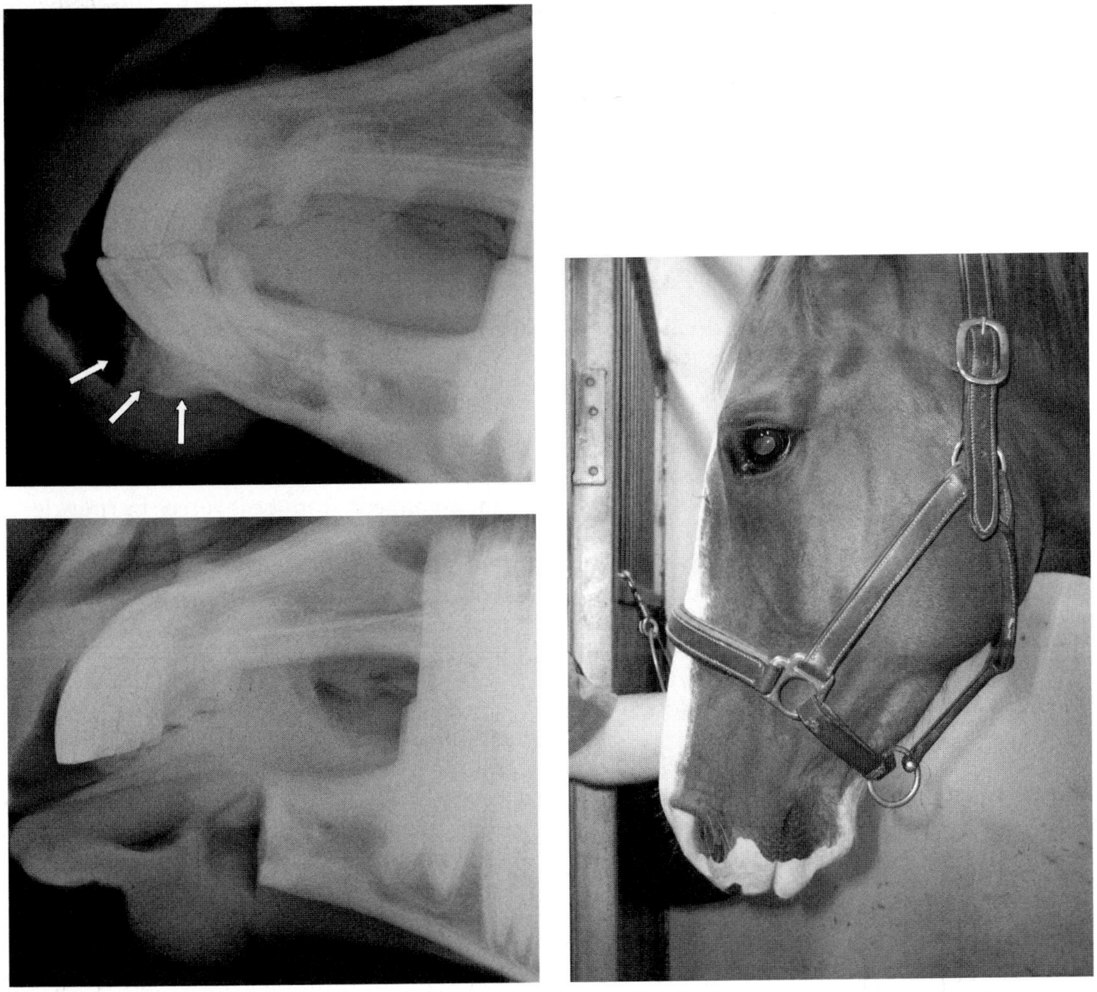

A

B

C

Figure 103-24. A, Lateromedial radiograph of an adamantinoma at the rostral end of the mandible *(arrows)*. **B,** Postoperative radiograph showing the missing rostral aspect of the mandible. **C,** Despite the mandibulectomy, the horse maintained an acceptable cosmetic appearance.

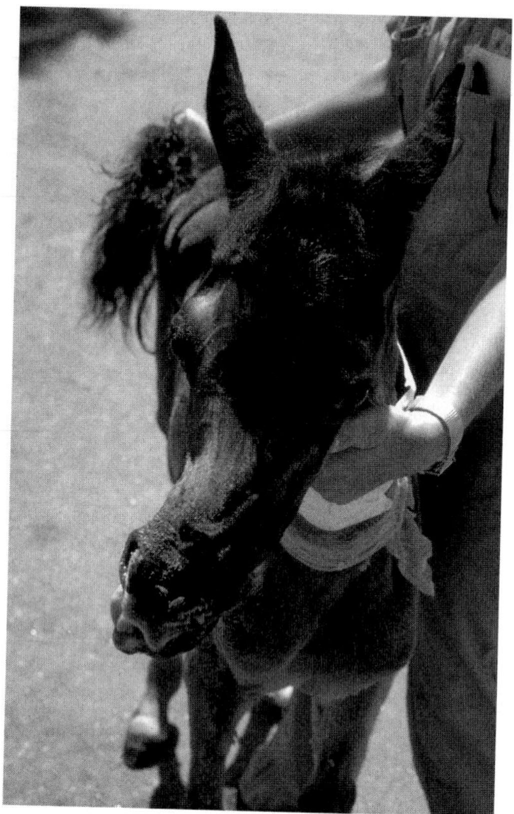

Figure 103-25. A 2-week-old Arabian foal with a wry nose.

an enhanced concavity of the hard palate in the interdental space region.

An incongruity of the nostrils and nasal septum are an additional anomaly. Some foals experience breathing difficulties or have increased respiratory sounds.

This condition will not self-correct, and a decision should be made to treat the foal using reconstructive techniques or to euthanize it to prevent it from suffering.

Surgical Procedure

Surgical correction should be delayed until the foal is 2 months old to allow the maxilla to gain enough strength to accept implants. The foal is anesthetized and positioned in dorsal recumbency on the surgery table. The endotracheal tube is inserted, the cuff is inflated, and the mouth is thoroughly washed.

Because the nasal septum is involved in the deviation, it is best to perform a resection of 8 cm of the rostral nasal septum at the onset of the surgery. This eliminates resistance against correction after the bilateral osteotomy of the maxilla. The nasal passages are packed with gauze sponges soaked in antiseptic solution. A surgical approach to the interdental space is made and the maxillary periosteum is elevated.

With an oscillating saw or a Gigli wire, both rami of the maxilla are transected. To achieve symmetry of the upper and lower jaws and normal interdental contact, the incisors of the maxilla and mandible should be temporarily wired shut. An individual wire brace is applied to the incisors of the mandible and maxilla respectively (see Figs. 103-2 and 103-3). Prior to tightening of the wire loops around each tooth, a double strand of wires is alternately pulled in a simple continuous fashion between the mandible and maxilla. The individual wires in the mandible are now tightened, followed by the wire loops in the maxilla. Lastly, the ends of the double-stranded wire suture between the incisors of the mandible and maxilla are connected and solidly tightened, effectively preventing opening of the mouth.

In the next step, 3.2-mm Steinmann pins are inserted from the rostral aspect of the mandible in a caudal fashion crossing the osteotomy sites, providing stability to the maxilla.[30-32] The application of an autogenous cortical bone graft in the form of a rib has been described in the literature.[32] An alternate approach is to apply locking compression plates (see Fig. 103-17).

The wiring of the tooth arcades ensures anatomic reconstruction and is maintained until the osteotomies have partially healed and can provide some stability. Enteral nutrition is provided for the foal (see Chapter 6), often by milking the mare and administering the milk through a stomach tube. Half of the packing of the nasal passages is removed one day postoperatively and the second half one day later. Some asymmetry of the rostral part of the nose will persist.

This correction can be performed without wiring the teeth; however, there might be inadequate stability across the osteotomy sites. In that case, the foal should be prevented from eating hay and grain.

Complications

Postoperative infection of the surgery sites and breakdown of the fixation are the most serious complications. Depending on the severity and duration of the problem, euthanasia of the patient has to be considered.

TEMPOROMANDIBULAR JOINT DISORDERS

Temporomandibular disease is diagnosed more often now than in the past. Different signs are being recognized, including reluctance to eat, attitude changes, and asymmetry of the head. Care must be taken to look at the entire head. An asymmetry can be caused by muscle atrophy or a swelling on the affected side. Sometimes it is difficult to recognize which side is involved without diagnostic imaging techniques. Most information can be gained from computed tomography (CT) (Fig. 103-26) or magnetic resonance (MR) imaging.

As expertise in the diagnosis and management of temporomandibular joint (TMJ) disorders increases, more techniques are being developed to treat them. In the future, arthroscopic techniques might be used to salvage the joint before radical surgical procedures are used. A recent cadaveric study demonstrated that a good portion of the TMJ can be evaluated arthroscopically.[33]

Infection

TMJ sepsis is rare in horses. However, standard diagnostic aids used to diagnose joint infections can be applied to the TMJ (see Chapter 88 for details).

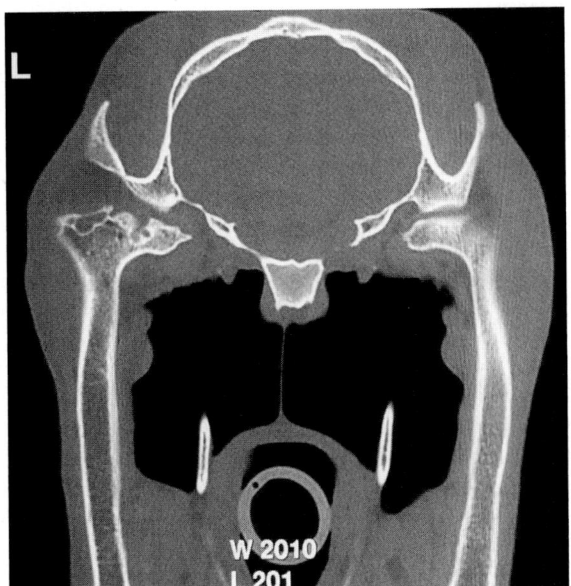

Figure 103-26. Severe osteoarthritic changes in the left temporomandibular joint shown on a computed tomographic image.

Arthroscopic investigation of the dorsal joint pouch of the TMJ can be performed through a stab incision into the dorsocaudal compartment. One report has described successful management of a septic TMJ with mechanized resection of synovium and fibrinous debris, copious lavage, and intra-articular and systemic antibiotics.[34] Eight months postoperatively, there was no clinical evidence of osteoarthritis or ankylosis of the TMJ.[34]

Condylectomy of the Mandible

Mandibular condylectomy is an option for treatment of fractures through the TMJ that are not amenable to repair. An alternate indication is management of osteoarthritis of the TMJ that causes chronic pain.[35] However, additional work is needed to find a practical solution to salvage the TMJ with osteoarthritis.

Surgical Procedure

A condylectomy is performed in lateral recumbency under general anesthesia.[2] A 6-cm horizontal skin incision is made, centered on the TMJ, extending rostrally and curving medially, caudal to the mandibular condyle. The soft tissues are reflected ventrally to expose the joint capsule.

The TMJ is opened by a horizontal incision of the joint capsule. The periosteum on the condyle is incised vertically, and a periosteal elevator is used to reflect the periosteum both rostrally and caudally. An oscillating bone saw or Gigli wire is used to make a 2-cm deep cut in the mandibular condyle 2.5 cm ventral to the articular surface (Fig. 103-27).

A chisel is inserted into the osteotomy and pried dorsally to fracture off the lateral portion of the mandibular condyle. It is necessary to remove the lateral portion of the condyle before continuing the cut through the condyle to provide room to introduce scissors to cut the capsular attachments. The oscillating saw is used to continue the osteotomy

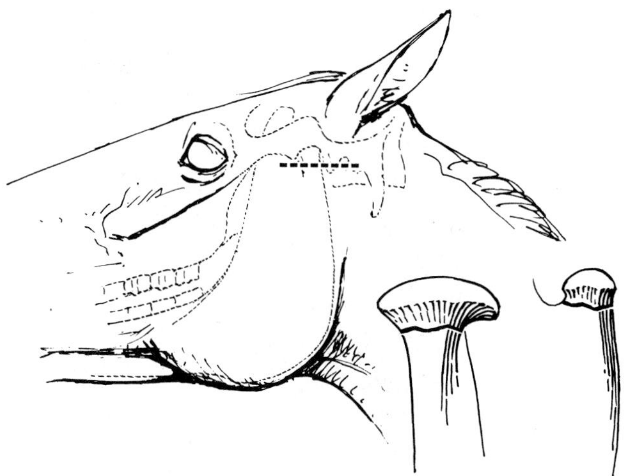

Figure 103-27. Mandibular condylectomy showing the line of incision and the level of resection of the mandibular condyle from two sides.

through the remaining portion of the mandibular condyle. The condyle is grasped with forceps for removal, and any joint capsule attachments are cut with scissors. The meniscus is removed by incising its attachments with scissors.[2] The bone edges are rounded.

Closure is performed in three layers: the periosteum and joint capsule, the subcutaneous tissue, and the skin. Additional information on temporomandibular joint disorders are found in Chapter 30.

Complications and Prognosis

The results of mandibular condylectomy have been summarized for normal horses. Remodeling of the condyle resulted in the formation of a pseudo-condyle with satisfactory function.[24] There are no reports of its use in clinically affected horses. Short-term complications in normal horses included masseter atrophy, malocclusion, weight loss, and difficulty in prehension and mastication.

RADICAL MANDIBULAR EXCISION

Neoplasia of the mandible is the indication for a radical mandibular resection. Tumors of the body of the mandible are rare and difficult to treat surgically.[2] One report describes en bloc resection of the horizontal ramus of the mandible for excision of a malignant tumor.[3] The mandibular defect is bridged using a bone plate of appropriate length as a buttress placed on the ventral surface of the mandible. A type II external fixator is used for additional support. The few occasions in which this type of treatment has been attempted makes formulation of a prognosis difficult.[2]

REFERENCES

1. Park RD: Radiographic examination of the equine head, Vet Clin North Am Equine Pract 1993;9:49.
2. Beard W: The skull, maxilla, and mandible. In Auer JA, Stick JA, editors: Equine Surgery, ed 2, Philadelphia, 1999, WB Saunders.
3. LeBlanc PH: Regional anesthesia, Vet Clin North Am Equine Pract 1990;6:693.

4. French DA, Fretz PB, Davis GD, et al: Mandibular adamantinoma in a horse: Radical surgical treatment, Vet Surg 1984;13:165.
5. Auer JA: Internal fixation of long bone fractures in cattle/ mandibular fractures in the horse, Proc Symp Am Assoc Vet Surg 1996;6:72.
6. Obwegeeser H: Über eine einfache Behandlung der freihändigen Drahtschienung von Kieferbrüchen, Österr Zeitschr Stomatol 1952;49:652.
7. Colahan PT, Pascoe JR: Stabilization of equine and bovine mandibular and maxillary fractures, using an acrylic splint, J Am Vet Med Assoc 1983;182:1117.
8. Dart AJ, Pascoe RR: Treatment of a bilateral mandibular fracture in a mare using an intraoral acrylic splint, Aust Vet J 1987;64:382.
9. Gabel AA: A method of surgical repair of the fractured mandible in the horse, J Am Vet Med Assoc 1969;155:1831.
10. Krahwinkel DJ, Hefferman HJ, Ewbank KL: Surgical repair of fractured maxillae and premaxillae in the horse, J Am Vet Med Assoc 1969;154:53.
11. Wallace CE: Repair by open reduction of fractured mandible in a stallion, Aust Vet J 1971;47:57.
12. DeBowes RM, Cannon JH, Grant BD, et al: Lag screw fixation of rostral mandibular fractures in the horse, Vet Surg 1981;10:153.
13. Meagher DM, Trout DR: Fractures of the mandible and premaxilla in the horse, Proc Am Assoc Equine Pract 1980;26:181.
14. Garner HE: Repair of bilateral fractures of the maxilla, premaxilla, and mandible in a horse, J Am Vet Med Assoc 1968;152:1402.
15. Müller ME, Allgöwer M, Schneider R, Willenegger H: Manual of Internal Fixation, ed 3, Berlin, 1990, Springer-Verlag.
16. Lischer CJ, Fluri E, Kaser-Hotlz B, et al: Pinless external fixation of mandible fractures in cattle, Vet Surg 1997;26:14.
17. Murch KM: Repair of bovine and equine mandibular fractures, Can Vet J 1980;21:69.
18. Wilson DG, Trent AM, Crawford WH: A surgical approach to the ramus of the mandible in cattle and horses: Case reports of a bull and a horse, Vet Surg 1990;19:191.
19. Peavey CL, Edward III RB, Escarcega AJ, et al: Fixation technique influences the monotonic properties of equine mandibular fracture constructs, Vet Surg 2003;32:350.
20. Burba DJ, Collier MA: T-plate repair of fracture of the nasal bones in a horse, J Am Vet Med Assoc 1991;199:909.
21. Blackford JT, Hanselka DV, Heitman JM, Boyd CL: Noninvasive technique for reduction of zygomatic process fractures in the horse, Vet Surg 1985;14:21.
22. Turner AS: Surgical management of depression fractures of the equine skull, Vet Surg 1979;8:29.
23. Bohanon TC, Gabel AA: Cosmetic repair of a facial deformity by use of a silicone implant in a horse, J Am Vet Med Assoc 1991;198:1957.
24. Valdez H, Rook JS: Use of fluorocarbon polymer and carbon fiber for restoration of facial contour in a horse, J Am Vet Med Assoc 1981;178:249.
25. Schumacher J, Auer JA, Shamis L: The use of periosteal flaps to repair facial defects in two horses, Vet Surg 1985;14:235.
26. Campbell ML, Peyton LC: Muscle flap closure of frontocutaneous fistula in a horse, Vet Surg 1984;13:185.
27. Caron JP, Barber SM, Bailey JV, et al: Periorbital skull fractures in five horses, J Am Vet Med Assoc 1986;188:280.
28. Richardson DW, Evans LH, Tulleners EP: Rostral mandibulectomy in five horses, J Am Vet Med Assoc 1991;199:1179.
29. Schumacher J, Kemper DL, Helman G, Edwards JL: Removal of the premaxilla and rostral portions of the maxillae of a horse, J Am Vet Med Assoc 1996;209:118.
30. Baker GJ: Abnormalities of development and eruption. In Baker GJ, Easley J, editors: Equine Dentistry, Philadelphia, 1999, WB Saunders.
31. Easley J: Basic orthodontics. In Baker GJ, Easley J, editors: Equine Dentistry, Philadelphia, 1999, WB Saunders.
32. Valdez H, McMullan W, Hobson P, et al: Surgical correction of a deviated nasal septum and premaxilla in a colt, J Am Vet Med Assoc 173:1001, 1978.
33. May KA, Moll HD, Howard RD, et al: Arthroscopic anatomy of the equine temporomandibular joint, Vet Surg 2001;30:564.
34. Carmalt JL, Wilson DG: Arthroscopic treatment of temporomandibular joint sepsis in a horse, Vet Surg 2005;34:55.
35. Barber SM, Doige CE, Humphreys SG: Mandibular condylectomy: Technique and results in normal horses, Vet Surg 1985;14:79.

INDEX

Page numbers followed by b indicate boxes; f, figures; t, tables.